Baillière's
ENCYCLOPAEDIC DICTIONARY OF

NURSING AND HEALTH CARE

BARBARA F. WELLER
EDITOR-IN-CHIEF

Baillière Tindall — 24–28 Oval Road
London NW1 7DX

W. B. Saunders — The Curtis Center
Independence Square West
Philadelphia, PA 19106–3399, USA

1 Goldthorne Avenue
Toronto, Ontario M8Z 5T9, Canada

ABP Australia Ltd, 32–52 Smidmore Street
Marrickville
NSW 2204, Australia

Harcourt Brace Jovanovich Japan Inc.
Ichibancho Central Building, 22-1 Ichibancho
Chiyoda-ku, Tokyo 102, Japan

First Published 1989

Editorial manager, book production, Christopher A. Gibson
Associate Nursing Editor, Sarah V. Smith

Lexicographical data system by Compulexis Ltd, Oxford

Typeset by Data-Sats Informatik A/S, Copenhagen, Denmark

Printed and bound in Great Britain by Mackays of Chatham PLC, Chatham, Kent

1. Medicine, Nursing. Encyclopaedias
I. Weller, Barbara F. (Barbara Fiona), **1933–**
610.73′03′21

ISBN 0–7020–1196–7

Acknowledgements

The permission to use the third edition of the *Encyclopedia and Dictionary of Medicine, Nursing, and Allied Health* by Benjamin F Miller and Claire Brackman Keane (W B Saunders, 1983, USA) for the basis of the dictionary database used in the preparation of this dictionary is acknowledged.

Contents

Publisher's Foreword

While planning this book it became apparent that the specialist dictionaries available to the United Kingdom's nursing and health care professionals did not adequately meet their needs. The many concise dictionaries were often too superficial, whilst most of the more comprehensive dictionaries were American and therefore largely inappropriate for the UK-trained and practising nurse. As a leading publisher of nursing books in the United Kingdom, it is appropriate that Baillière Tindall should fulfil this need with the present volume.

Under the expert supervision of Barbara Weller as Editor-in-Chief, a team of specialists in the nursing and medical professions, all experts in their own particular fields, were asked to review, originate and adapt the dictionary's entries. The intention was to create a dictionary that included all the terms encountered by the nurse as well as the majority of terms encountered by specialist health care personnel, such as physiotherapists, midwives and health visitors, and to define these in an up-to-date and relevant way. As a result, this dictionary will continue to serve as a comprehensive resource for nursing and allied health care professionals, for many years to come.

As the title indicates, this book is more than just a dictionary. In addition to defining the terms included, for all of the more important nursing topics articles include encyclopaedic information. For example, in the article on **diabetes**, as well as the definition there is further information including aetiology, progress, complications and nursing care. Consequently, this book can be used not only for checking the spelling, pronunciation and meanings of terms, but also as a study guide at the level of a concise textbook.

A unique feature of this specialist dictionary is the pronunciation guide. The words and terms are transcribed with a clear and easy-to-understand system based on a method of re-spelling the word or term. Ordinary letters are combined together in precise ways, thereby largely avoiding the use of unfamiliar symbols.

The preparation of this dictionary has been achieved with the help of the latest in sophisticated electronic publishing systems. This has ensured, among other things, consistency of style and accurate cross-referencing. Moreover, the dictionary exists as an electronic database, and can be continuously updated for future editions.

Baillière Tindall

Acknowledgements

The publishers wish to acknowledge their sincere gratitude and thanks to all those involved in this project, especially to Robert CJ Carling, formerly of Baillière Tindall, for his invaluable contribution to its earlier stages. We are also indebted to Jessica Andersen, Mairi Baker, Marie Carling, Rich Cutler, Paula Duggan, Sarah Dunstall, Peter Gill, Laila Grieg-Gran, Elizabeth Stockman, Dave Swinden, Lesley Ward and Di White.

Editor-in-Chief's Preface

"A common language is indispensable to a co-operative effort" — *Claire B Keane.*

The problem is, of course, that the common language, whatever it may be, must be a living entity. Otherwise it can never provide those who use it with a sufficiently adaptable tool with which to handle new concepts and ideas. If it is to survive, a language can never be static, rigid and inflexible like a stone carving — what Edward Gibbon once called 'the decent obscurity of a learned language' — but must be likened to a living organism forever evolving to meet new circumstances and challenges. Gibbonian obscurity is inappropriate when dealing with nursing and medical terms; clarity, simplicity and currency must be the aims.

The Healing Arts also have a language that is particularly their own, traditionally based upon Latin or Greek derivation. But increasingly over recent decades, science and technology call for a new and wider vocabulary. Never was this more relevant than today in the realm of health care, where all workers in this field need constantly to update their knowledge, learn new skills, as well as adapt or modify old ones. In order to do this, resources must be available, foremost of which must be a lexicon that is both informed and appropriate; I would also add attractive and readable for the user.

Adapting Miller and Keane's *Encyclopaedia and Dictionary of Medicine, Nursing, and Allied Health* for readers in the United Kingdom has been a challenge, and I hope that the original authors will approve of the result. Simply translating Americanisms into English — e.g. changing diaper into nappy, or substituting the appropriate UK statistics — is not enough. If one is not careful, one can ignore the many profound differences in the philosophies underlying the two nations' approach to health care. The situation can become even more confused by the very fact that we share what on the surface appears to be the same language, an illusion that many travellers on both sides of the Atlantic have come to realise.

Reviewers may question the wisdom of adapting an American text rather than starting from scratch. The answer relates to time and production costs. By using the database from the Miller and Keane dictionary, the time required by the specialist contributor to consider and review articles has been reduced so that costs have been kept to the minimum for the benefit of the purchaser.

In the book great efforts have been made by all the contributors to adapt and embrace the traditional approach to care and health education in the United Kingdom, whilst recognising developments relating to a conceptual approach of health care delivery for the patient and their family.

Acknowledgements

The delivery of health care is essentially about team work, and our team of contributors reflects that composition. I must record my debt and grateful thanks to all the contributors, who worked so diligently in ensuring that deadlines were met. I should like especially to thank Sarah V. Smith and Chris Gibson of Baillière Tindall for their support and understanding during the final stages of the collation of the dictionary.

Finally, very special gratitude to my husband David R. Fisher who eased all household burdens thus enabling me to concentrate on the work in hand.

Barbara F. Weller

Contributors

Editor-in-Chief

Barbara Weller RGN RSCN RNT, Professional Nursing Officer, Neonatal Nurses' Association; *Formerly*, Nursing Officer, DHSS, Alexander Fleming House, Elephant and Castle, London SE1 6BY

Editorial Advisors

Robin P Bolton BM BCh MRCP, Consultant Physician, Doncaster Royal Infirmary, Doncaster DN2 5LT
A Stuart Mason MB FRCP, Honorary Consulting Physician, The London Hospital, Whitechapel, London EC1
Bryan N Brooke MD MChir FRCS HonFRACS, Emeritus Professor of Surgery, University of London, St George's Hospital, London SW17

Specialist Contributors

Douglas Allan RGN RMN RCT Neuro Cert, Clinical Nurse Teacher, Glasgow South College of Nursing and Midwifery, Southern General Hospital, Govan Road, Glasgow G51 4TF
Rosamond Andrew SRN ONC RCN Certificate in Clinical Teaching, Clinical Teacher, Wolfson School of Nursing of Westminster, 30 Vincent Square, London SW1 2NW
J S A Ashley MB FFCM, Office of Population Censuses and Surveys, Medical Statistics Division, St Catherine's House, 10 Kingsway, London WC2B 6JP
Clive Andrews SRN RMN DN(Lond), Charge Nurse, The London Hospital, Whitechapel, London EC1
Graham E Ball BDS (Wales) FDS RCS (Eng), Community Dental Officer, Orkney Health Board, Kirkwall, Orkney KW17 2LH
Thomas Barrie MB FRCS, Consultant Ophthalmologist, Glasgow Eye Infirmary and Gartnavel General Hospital, 1053 Great Western Road, Glasgow G12 0YN
N Benjamin BM BS BMedSci MRCP (UK), Honorary Registrar, Department of Medicine, St George's Hospital Medical School, Blackshaw Road, Tooting, London SW17
Penelope J Bennett RGN OND RNT, Project Officer, Education and Training Management Development, North West Thames Regional Health Authority; formerly Acting Director of Nurse Education, North Hertfordshire School of Nursing, Stevenage
John R H Berrie MB ChB FFCM DPH DIH, Former Senior Medical Officer, DHSS, Alexander Fleming House, Elephant and Castle, London SE1 6BY
Carol M Black MD FRCP, Consultant Rheumatologist, West Middlesex University Hospital, Twickenham Road, Isleworth, Middlesex TW7 6AF
Alan Boylan Director of Nurse Education, Brighton School of Nursing, 157 Kingsway, Hove, Sussex BN3 4GR
Christine Chapman OBE BSc (Hons Soc) MPhil SRN SCM RNT FRCN, Professor of Nursing Education and Dean of Nursing Studies, University of Wales College of Medicine, Heath Park, Cardiff CF4 4XN
Stephen Chapman MB BS MRCS MRCP FRCR, Consultant Radiologist, The Children's Hospital, Ladywood Middleway, Birmingham B16 8ET

Contributors

Charmaine Childs BN MPhil, Research Fellow, University of Manchester NW Injury Research Centre and Regional Paediatric Burns Unit, Booth Hall Childrens Hospital, Charlestown Road, Blackley, Manchester M92AA

Morag Chisholm MB ChB MD FRCPath, Senior Lecturer, University of Southampton Medical School, Consultant Haematologist, Department of Haematology, Southampton General Hospital, Tremona Road, Southampton SO94 4XY

Robert C Chivers MA PhD CPhys FInstP FIOA, Senior Lecturer in Physics, Physics Department, University of Surrey, Guildford, Surrey GU2 5XH; Honorary Principal Grade Physicist, South West Surrey District Health Authority, Royal Surrey County Hospital, Guildford, Surrey

Vivien Coates BA SRN MPhil, Lecturer, Department of Nursing and Health Visiting, University of Ulster at Coleraine, Cromore Road, Coleraine, Co Londonderry, N Ireland BT52 1SA

David M Greenan MD PhD FRCP, Consultant and Senior Lecturer in Rheumatology, University of Manchester Rheumatic Diseases Centre, Hope Hospital, Eccles Old Road, Salford M6 8HD

Henry L Halliday MD FRCP (Ed) FRCP DCH D(Obst) RCOG, Consultant Neonatologist, Royal Maternity Hospital, Belfast, N Ireland BT12 6BB

Denise Victoria Hoare BSc MPS, Staff Pharmacist, Drug Information, Westminster Hospital, Dean Ryle Street, London SW1 2AP

Jeremy Hyde BPharm PhD, Formerly Assistant General Manager, Charing Cross Hospital, Fulham Palace Road, London W6 BRF

Joanna Ibarra BSc MRSH, Department of Biology, North East London Polytechnic, Romford Road, London E15 4LZ

Jack R Lyttle RMN RGN DipN(Lond) RNT, Senior Tutor, Inverclyde and Bute College of Nursing and Midwifery, Inverclyde Royal Infirmary, Larkfield Road, Greenock, Renfrewshire PA16 0XL

Penelope J Mawson SRN, Ward Sister, Renal Unit, Guy's Hospital, St Thomas' Street, London SE1 9RT

Rosemary C Methven SRN SCM MTD DN(Part A) DANS MSc RCNT, Senior Midwifery Tutor Post Basic Studies, The Clarendon Wing, General Infirmary of Leeds, St George Street, Leeds, LS1 3EX

G H Millward-Sadler BSc MB ChB FRCPath, Honorary Senior Lecturer, University of Southampton Medical School; Consultant Pathologist, Southampton General Hospital, Tremona Road, Southampton SO9 4XY

Rosemary Morris SRN SCM RSCN DN(Lond) RNT, Publisher, Scutari Press, The Royal College of Nursing, 20 Cavendish Square, London W1M 0AB

James F Mowbray BA MB BCh FRCP, Professor of Immunopathology, Department of Experimental Pathology, St Mary's Hospital Medical School, Norfolk Place, London W2 1PG

Rebecca Newbould SRN JBCNS, 134 Urology and Renal Nursing, Sister Nephrology/General Medical Ward, St Thomas' Hospital, London SE1 7EH

Doreen Norton OBE MSc RGN FRCN, Formerly Nursing Research Officer, SW Thames Regional Health Authority, London; Latterly Professor (1983/4) Florence Cellar Chair of Gerontological Nursing, Case Western Reserve University, Cleveland, Ohio, USA

Brian Perriss BSc MB BS FFARCS, Consultant Anaesthetist, Royal Devon and Exeter Hospital, Barrack Road, Exter, Devon EX2 5DW

Joan Ramsay SRN DipN(Lond) CertEd RNT, Senior Tutor, Charles West School of Nursing, Great Ormond Street, London WC1N 3JH

Jacqueline S Rogers SRN CMB(Part I) FETCert FPCert, Research Nurse, Academic Department of Genitourinary Medicine, James Pringle House, The Middlesex Hospital, London W1

Judy Skinner Grad Dip Phys MCSP, Senior Physiotherapist in Neurology, The National Hospital for Nervous Diseases, Queen Square, London WC1
Agnes Elizabeth Stalker BA DipNEd RGN RCNT ONC, Senior Tutor, Continuing and Post-Basic Education, Western College of Nursing and Midwifery, Glasgow; Chairman of the SNB Panels on Critical Care Nursing and Orthopaedic Nursing; Member of the Preview Panel for Professional Studies of the Scottish National Board
Elizabeth Ann Stevens RGN HV Diploma Health Services Management, Director of Nursing, Acute Unit, St Thomas' Hospital London SE1 7EH; Formerly Senior Nurse, Nephrology/General Unit, St Thomas' Hospital, London.
David R Thompson BSc PhD SRN RMN ONC, Senior Nurse, Coronary Care Unit, Leicester General Hospital, Gwendolen Road, Leicester LE5 4PW
Verena Tschudin BSc(Hon) SRN SCM Diploma in Counselling Skills, Counsellor and Writer
F. Mary Wellington RGN RNT, Senior Tutor, Wolfson School of Nursing of Westminster, 30 Vincent Square, London SW1 2NW
Richard Wells BA SRN RMN ONC FETC FRSH FRCN, Head of Rehabilitation Services, Marie Curie Rehabilitation Centre, Royal Marsden Hospital, Fulham Road, London SW3 6JJ; formerly Adviser in Oncology Nursing, The Royal College of Nursing, 20 Cavendish Square, London W1M 0AB
Margaret Ann Worsley SRN FETC, Senior Nurse, Infection Control, North Manchester Health Authority, Central Drive, Crumpsall, Manchester M8 6RL
Pat Young, Freelance Medical Journalist, Author and Editor, 8 Church Lane, Seaford, East Sussex BN25 1HJ

Pronunciation guide

Nigel D Turton MA, Lecturer in English and Applied Linguistics, English Department, Universiti Brunei Darussalam, Bandar Seri Begawan, Brunei

Notes on the Use of this Dictionary

This book is a compilation of words, terms, names, abbreviations and acronyms together with their pronunciation and definition. Many of the entries also have further 'encyclopaedic' information as well as their definition, e.g. in an article about a specific disease there is information about its aetiology, clinical features, nursing management and so on.

Terms within this Dictionary are located either as main or sub-entries. Main entries are printed in **bold type** (see Section 1 below) and stand out in the left hand margins from the main column of definitional material; these are followed by the pronunciation in parentheses (see Section 2 below). Sub-entries, also printed in **bold type**, occur after the main entry and its definition (see Section 3 below).

1. MAIN ENTRIES

The main entries of this Dictionary occur as single words, hyphenated words or two or more words separated by spaces. They are alphabetized as follows:

1.1 Single words: single words, acronyms and abbreviations are alphabetized letter by letter, with capital letters coming *before* lower-case letters. For example:

psyllium
Pt
pt
PTA
ptarmic

releasing factor
REM
rem
remedy

1.2 Multiple words: Main entries of more than one word that are separated by spaces, hyphens or dashes are alphabetized according to the first word and then (if needed) according to the second word (or other subsequent words). This means that all entries about a particular word (such as **heart** or **blood**) are collected together, followed by those words that use those letters for a different word or a word using that word element. For example:

heart
heart block
heart failure
heart–lung machine
heart murmur
heart rate
heart sounds
heartbeat

blood
blood bank
blood–brain barrier
blood clotting
"
"
blood vessel
blood volume
bloodstream
Blount's disease

(See also Compound terms, Section 1.3 below.)

However, where the hyphen simply separates two identical vowels, the word is treated as though it were a single word without a hyphen. For example:

intra-
intra vitam
intra-abdominal
intra-aortic balloon pump

gastromyxorrhoea
gastro-oesophageal
gastro-oesophagitis
gastro-oesophagostomy

intra-arterial
intra-articular
intra-atrial
intracanalicular
gastroparalysis

1.3 Compound terms: when a term is composed of two or more words, it will usually be found under more than one of the words, although discretion has been used to avoid unnecessary repetition of the definition. For example, although there is a brief description under **Fallot's tetralogy** in the **F**s, the article **tetralogy** has a more detailed subdefinition **t. of Fallot**. (See also Cross-referencing, Section 4 below.)

1.4 Combining forms (word elements): prefixes and suffixes are listed alphabetically, ignoring any characters in parentheses. Prefixes therefore usually appear immediately preceding those words that use them. For example:

lip
lip (o)-
lip reading
lipacidaemia
lipaciduria

macies
Mackenrodt's ligaments
macr (o)-
macrencephalia
macroamylasaemia

1.5 Terms with unusual characters: certain characters of the main entry are ignored in the alphabetization, i.e. Greek letters, numbers, small capital characters, and subscript/superscript characters. For example:

aminoaciduria
***p*-aminobenzoic acid**
γ-aminobutyric acid
ε-aminocaproic acid
aminoglutethimide
aminoglycoside
aminohippuric acid
δ-aminolaevulinic acid

Rh
Rh_{null}
Rh factor
Rh-null syndrome
RHA

1.6 Eponyms/possessive terms: where the suffix *'s* occurs, it is ignored in the alphabetization. For example:

Cushing's disease
Cushing's syndrome
cushingoid

1.7 Mc/Mac and St./Saint terms: entries beginning with Mc- are listed as if they were spelled Mac-. Similarly, those beginning St. (for Saint) are listed as if they were spelled Saint.

1.8 Variant forms and synonyms: common acceptable alternative spellings for particular entries are also included. These appear immediately after the first word, separated by comma. For example:

dilation, dilatation
desert fever, desert rheumatism
hypercapnia, hypercarbia
neuron, neurone

In many cases the more commonly used (or preferred) variant is placed first, but the order of variants should not be taken to imply that the first is the preferred since they may simply be truly equivalent variants.

In some entries, alternative spellings or terms are given within the definition. They are indicated by 'called also . . .'. For example:

hernia ('hərni·ə) the abnormal protrusion of part of an organ or tissue through the structures normally containing it. Called also a *rupture*. adj. **hernial**.

If the reader is likely to refer commonly to the secondary variant or synonym, this has often been included as a main entry in its own alphabetical location, but rather than defining the term in both places, there is a cross-reference to where the main definition occurs (see Cross-referencing, Section 3).

1.9 Homographs, i.e. words that have the same spelling but have different derivations etymologically, are designated as separate main entries with superscript **bold** numbers. For example:

lead[1] (led) a chemical element, atomic number 82, . . .
lead[2] (leed) a specific array (pair) of electrodes . . .

These must not be confused with alternative definitions of the same word — see Section 1.10 below.

1.10 Alternative definitions: Where two different usages of the same word exist, each definition is numbered, as in the example below (see Section 1.9 above homographs):

film (film) 1. a thin layer or coating. 2. a thin sheet of material (e.g., gelatin, cellulose acetate) specially treated for use in photography or radiography; . . .

2. PRONUNCIATION GUIDE

2.1. Introduction: the pronunciation of words, and medical words in particular, is often contentious and some unfamilar words can be daunting even for the highly literate native speaker. It is to a specialist dictionary that one turns to try to find the pronunciation of technical or specialist words, only to be disappointed if the dictionary in question does not contain a pronunciation guide. Moreover, most of the larger medical dictionaries available are published in the USA and therefore have American pronunciations. Added to this is the fact that many dictionaries have unfamiliar phonetic symbols. Many readers are therefore intimidated by the prospect of deciphering the symbols, even if there is a clear explanation of the use of such hieroglyphics in the preface.

After expert consultation, it was decided to develop a modern method of indicating how to pronounce words that is more transparent in its usage while not compromising accuracy and consistency. In this dictionary, therefore, instead of the reader trying to learn what sounds are represented by which phonetic symbol, the pronunciations are transcribed using ordinary English-spelling letters. So that the guide is consistent and unambiguous, these characters have been combined together in precise ways (see below). The avoidance of the use of phonetic symbols (with the exception of the upside-down 'e' or 'schwa' (ə) ensures that the guide is more-or-less immediately, and to some extent intuitively, understandable.

2.2 Style of transcription: all pronunciations are found in parentheses immediately following the bold main entry word (or variant, if one exists). The pronunciations reflect what could be called 'unaccented' or 'neutral' British English, i.e. regional variants have, as far as possible, been avoided, as have versions of pronunciations that have become old fashioned or obsolete.

Transcriptions given reflect *current, spoken usage* of the terms rather than how the term 'should' be pronounced, i.e. the guide does not atempt to be didactic or prescriptive.

2.3 Variant pronunciations: where alternative pronunciations for a word or term are given, they are separated by commas. Alternatives are often given in a truncated form with the use of hyphens. For example:

aminoacetic acid (əˌmeenoh·ə'seetik, əˌmienoh-, əˌminoh-)
encephalic (ˌenkə'falik, -ˌensə-)

Where alternative spellings and/or alternative words with the same meaning (synonyms) are given, the pronunciations for the first word or term and the second word or term are separated by semi-colons (again with the use of hyphens to abbreviate the first transcription if necessary). For example:

neuron, neurone ('nyooə·ron; 'nyooə·rohn)
motoneuron, motoneurone (ˌmohtoh'nyooə·ron; -rohn)

2.4 Entries with repeated words: note that once a transcription for a particular word has been given, subsequent entries that use the same word do not have a repeated transcription of that word again. For example **Duchenne's disease** is followed by **Duchenne's muscular dystrophy** and **Duchenne's paralysis** but only the first is transcribed. Immediately preceding **Duchenne's disease** is **Duchenne–Aran disease** which is also transcribed since the lack of the '*s* makes the word pronounce differently.
2.5 Homographs: since these are treated as separate entries (see Section 1.9 above) the pronunciations for each homograph (which are often distinct) are given after the appropriate homograph number. (See example in 1.9 above.)
2.6 Acronyms: these have been transcribed where appropriate. For example:

AIDS (aydz)
COHSE ('kohzee)

2.7 Characters and combinations used to represent sounds: in the pronunciation guide, single letters represent single sounds and where two or more characters are combined, as in the accompanying tables, these also represent precise sounds.

Pronunciation Style guide

Vowel sounds		*Nearest International Phonetic Alphabet Character*
a	as in **bad** (bad) **fat** (fat)	æ
ah	as in **father** ('fahdhə) **artery** ('ahtə·ree)	a:
air	as in **hair** (hair) **bare** (bair)	ɛə or eə
aw	as in **water** ('wawtə) **short** (shawt) **audio** ('awdioh) **aorta** (ay'awtə)	ɔ: (cf. **or**)
ay	as in **fatal** ('fayt'l) **vein** (vayn)	eɪ
e	as in **bed** (bed) **geriatric** (ˌjeri'atrik)	ɛ or e
ee	as in **fetus** ('feetəs) **key** (kee)	i:
i	as in **film** (film) **lick** (lik)	ɪ
ie	as in **bite** (biet) **light** (liet)	aɪ
i·ə	as in **chloropsia** (klor'ropsi·ə) **arterial** (ah'tiə·ri·əl)	ɪə
iə	as in **fear** (fiə) **hear** (hiə)	ɪə
ieə	as in **diet** ('dieət) **fire** ('fieə) **diabetic** (dieə'betik)	aɪə
o	as in **body** ('bodee) **cough** (kof)	
oh	as in **choke** (chohk) **bone** (bohn)	əʊ
oo	as in **boot** (boot)	u:
ooə	as in **cure** (kyooə)	ʊə
or	as in **claw** (klor) **sore** (sor)	ɔ: (cf. **aw**)
ow	as in **now** (now) **bough** (bow)	aʊ
owə	as in **hour** (owə) **power** ('powə)	aʊə
oy	as in **boy** (boy) **goitre** ('goytə)	ɔɪ
oyə	as in **soya** ('soyə)	ɔɪə
u	as in **cut** (kut) **tongue** (tung)	ʌ
uh	as in **put** (puht) **cook** (kuhk)	ʊ
ə	as in **mother** ('mudhə) **about** (ə'bowt)	ə
ər	as in **bird** (bərd) **murmur** ('mərmə)	ɜ:
y	as in **yet** (yet) **acute** (ə'kyoot)	j (semi vowel)

Consonant sounds

b	as in **baby** ('baybee)	b
ch	as in **chat** (chaht)	tʃ
d	as in **digit** ('dijit)	d
dh	as in **they** (dhay) **this** (dhis) **rhythm** ('ridhəm)	σ
f	as in **fever** ('feevə) **haemophilus** (hee'mofiləs)	f
g	as in **gag** (gag)	g
h	as in **heal** (heel) **hot** (hot)	h
j	as in **jump** (jump)	dʒ
k	as in **king** (king) **code** (kohd)	k
kh	as in **loch** (lokh)	χ or x
l	as in **light** (liet)	l
m	as in **man** (man) **medicine** ('medisin, 'medsin)	m
n	as in **need** (need) **sun** (sun)	n
ng	as in **sung** (sung)	η
nh	as in **restaurant** ('restəronh) **accouchement** (ə'kooshmonh) **brisement** (breez'monh)	ση or ƃ
ny	as in **nutrition** (nyoo'trishən)	nj
p	as in **pelvis** ('pelvis) **put** (puht)	p
r	as in **rod** (rod) **reactor** (ri'aktə)	r
s	as in **sack** (sak)	s
sh	as in **fish** (fish) **omission** (oh'mishən, ə'mishən) **shock** (shok)	ʃ
t	as in **test** (test)	t
th	as in **thirst** (thərst) **therapy** ('therəpee)	θ
v	as in **vein** (vayn)	v
w	as in **weight** (wayt) **water** ('wawtə)	w
z	as in **zero** ('ziə·roh) **zoonosis** (zoh·ə'nohsis, zooə'nohsis)	z
zh	as in **pleasure** ('plezhə) **vision** ('vizhən)	ʒ

2.8 Stress marks: these are used where the word or term has more than one syllable, with the stress mark placed *before* the syllable to be stressed. The primary stressed syllable is indicated by superior stress mark (') and secondary stress by a subscript stress mark (ˌ). For example:

Parkinson's disease ('pahkinsənz)
parkinsonian(ˌpahkin'sohni·ən)
parkinsonism('pahkinsəˌnizəm)

2.9 Syllabic apostrophe: where a consonant is preceded by an apostrophe, this indicates that the consonant should be pronounced. For example:

digital vascular imaging ('dijit'l)
hospital('hospit'l)

2.10 The use of the centred dot: where two letters occur together that may be mistaken for a different sound from that intended, a centred full point is added to separate the characters. For example:

myopia(mie'ohpi·ə)
chloropsia(klor'ropsi·ə)
arterial(ah'tiə·ri·əl)

3. SUB-ENTRIES

The term being sought may be a main entry or a sub-entry under the main entry.

Sub-entries are listed alphabetically under the main entry, with the initial letter(s) of the main entry repeated. For example:

enterocolitis . . .
antibiotic-associated e. . . .
haemorrhagic e. . . .
pseudomembranous e. . . .

The alphabetization of sub-entries ignores the repeated main entry abbreviation and such words as *a, and, in, of, on, the, to,* etc. For example:

organ . . .
o. of Corti . . .
effector o. . . .
enamel o. . . .
Golgi tendon o. . . .
reproductive o's . . .
sense o's, sensory o's . . .
spiral o. . . .
target o. . . .
vestigial o. . . .
o's of Zuckerkandl . . .

Occasionally, the repeated main entry is spelt out in full when needed. For example, when the irregular plural form is referred to:

linea . . .
l. alba . . .
lineae albicantes . . .

macula . . .
maculae acusticae . . .
m. atrophica . . .

4. CROSS-REFERENCING

Throughout the dictionary, cross-references are given with the text as SMALL CAPITALS. For example:

corticosteroid (ˌkawtikoh'stiə·royd) any of the hormones produced by the ADRENAL CORTEX; also, their synthetic equivalents. Called also *adrenocortical hormone* and *adrenocorticosteroid*.

When two or several entries have the same meaning (synonyms), the definition is placed under the most commonly used and best understood term. At the alternative entry(ies), a cross-reference is given. (See also Variant forms and synonyms, Section 1.8.) They appear as 'see'. For example:

adrenocortical . . .
a. hormone one of the steroids produced by the adrenal cortex (see also CORTICOSTEROID).

There are also situations where it is simply more convenient to define the word in a different location, to which the reader is then referred.

Cross-references are either to main entries (see the examples above) or to sub-entries. In the latter case, only the main entry appears as small capitals. For example:

Greenfield's disease ('greenfeeldz) the infantile form of metachromic LEUKODYSTROPHY.

leukodystrophy . . .
metachromic l. a hereditary . . . .

5. ADJECTIVAL FORMS

Adjectives are indicated in **bold type** immediately following the abbreviation adj. For example:

fetus ('feetəs) [L.] the developing young in the uterus, . . . adj. **fetal**.

6. IRREGULAR PLURALS

Where a noun takes an irregular plural, this is indicated in *italic type* immediately following the abbreviation pl.

fenestra (fə'nestrə) pl. *fenestrae* . . .

If both a regular plural and an irregular plural are in acceptable usage, both are given in italics.

7. TRANSLATIONS

Where a translation of a foreign term occurs, it is indicated in *italic type* immediately following the abbreviation for the language (which is in square brackets). For example:

aberratio (ˌabə'rayshioh) [L.] *aberration.*
-cele word element. [Gr.] *tumour, hernia.*

8. ABBREVIATIONS USED IN THIS DICTIONARY

adj.	adjective
Fr.	French
Ger.	German
Gr.	Greek
It.	Italian
L.	Latin
pl.	plural
Scand.	Scandinavian

9. DRUG NAMES

Where possible, only generic names are used. However, some proprietary drug names and names for preparations are included with information (and sometimes cross-references) concerning the generic drug(s) involved. Inclusion of a drug in the dictionary does not imply endorsement.

Combining Forms In Medical Terminology

The following is a list of combining forms encountered frequently in the vocabulary of medicine. A dash or dashes are appended to indicate whether the form usually precedes (as *ante-*) or follows (as *-agra*) the other elements of the compound or usually appears between the other elements (as *-em-*). Following each combining form, the first item of information is the Greek or Latin word, or both a Greek and a Latin word, from which it is derived. Greek words have been transliterated into Roman characters. Latin words are identified by [L.], Greek words by [Gr.]. Information necessary to an understanding of the form appears next in parentheses. Then the meaning or meanings of the words are given, followed where appropriate by reference to a synonymous combining form. Finally, an example is given to illustrate the use of the combining form in a compound English derivative.

a- *a-*[L.] (*n* is added before words beginning with a vowel) negative prefix. Cf. in-[3]. *a*metria

ab- *ab* [L.] away from. Cf. apo-. *ab*ducent

abdomin- *abdomen, abdominis* [L.] abdomen. *abdomin*oscopy

ac- See ad-. *ac*cretion

acet- *acetum* [L.] vinegar. *acet*ometer

acid- *acidus* [L.] sour. *acid*uric

acou- *akouō* [Gr.] hear. *acou*ethesia. (Also spelled acu-)

acr- *akron* [Gr.] extremity, peak. *acr*omegaly

act- *ago, actus* [L.] do, drive, act. reaction

actin- *aktis, aktinos* [Gr.] ray, radius. Cf. radi-. *actin*ogenesis

acu- See acou-. osteo*acu*sis

ad- *ad* [L.] (*d* changes to *c, f, g, p, s,* or *t* before words beginning with those consonants) to. *ad*renal

aden- *adēn* [Gr.] gland. Cf. gland-. *aden*oma

adip- *adeps, adipis* [L.] fat. Cf. lip- and stear-. *adip*ocellular

aer- *aēr* [Gr.] air. an*aer*obiosis

aem- *haima* [Gr.] blood. an*aem*ia. (See also haem(at)-)

aesthe- *aisthanomai, aisthē-* [Gr.] perceive, feel. Cf. sens-. an*aesthe*sia

af- See ad-. *af*ferent

ag- See ad-. *ag*glutinant

-agogue *agōgos* [Gr.] leading, inducing. galact*agogue*

-agra *agra* [Gr.] catching, seizure. pod*agra*

alb- *albus* [L.] white. Cf. leuk-. *alb*ocinereous

alg- *algos* [Gr.] pain. neur*alg*ia

all- *allos* [Gr.] other, different. *all*ergy

alve- *alveus* [L.] trough, channel, cavity. *alve*olar

amph- See amphi-. *amph*eclexis

amphi- *amphi* [Gr.] (*i* is dropped before words beginning with a vowel) both, doubly, *amphi*coelous

amyl- *amylon* [Gr.] starch. *amyl*osynthesis

an-[1] See ana-. *an*agogical

an-[2] See a-. *an*omalous

ana- *ana* [Gr.] (final *a* is dropped before words beginning with a vowel) up, positive. *ana*phoresis

ancyl- See ankyl-. *ancyl*ostomiasis

andr- *anēr, andros* [Gr.] man. gyn*andr*oid

angi- *angeion* [Gr.] vessel. Cf. vas*angi*emphraxis

ankyl- *ankylos* [Gr.] crooked, looped. *ankyl*odactylia. (Also spelled ancyl-)

ant- See anti-. *ant*ophthalmic

ante- *ante* [L.] before. *ante*flexion

anti- *anti* [Gr.] (*i* is dropped before words beginning with a vowel) against, counter. Cf. contra*anti*pyogenic

antr- *antron* [Gr.] cavern. *antr*odynia

ap-[1] See apo-. *ap*heter

ap-[2] See ad-. *ap*pend

-aph- *haptō, haph-* [Gr.] touch. dys*aph*ia. (See also hapt-)

apo- *apo* [Gr.] (*o* is dropped before words beginning with a vowel) away from, detached. Cf. ab-. *apo*physis

arachn- *arachnē* [Gr.] spider. *arachn*odactyly

arch- *archē* [Gr.] beginning, origin. *arch*enteron

arter(i)- *arteria* [Gr.] windpipe, artery. *arteri*osclerosis, peri*arter*itis

arthr- *arthron* [Gr.] joint. Cf. articulsyn*arthr*osis

articul- *articulus* [L.] joint. Cf. arthr-dis*articul*ation

as- See ad-. *as*similation

at- See ad-. *at*trition

aur- *auris* [L.] ear. Cf. ot-. *aur*inasal

aux- *auxō* [Gr.] increase. enter*aux*e

ax- *axōn* [Gr.] or *axis* [L.] axis. *ax*ofugal

axon- *axōn* [Gr.] axis. *axon*ometer

ba- *bainō, ba-* [Gr.] go, walk, stand. hypno*ba*tia

bacill- *bacillus* [L.] small staff, rod. Cf. bacter-.

actino*bacill*osis

bacter- *bacterion* [Gr.] small staff, rod. Cf. bacill-. *bacter*iophage

ball- *ballō, bol-* [Gr.] throw. *ball*istics. (See also bol-)

bar- *baros* [Gr.] weight. *bar*ometer

bi-[1] *bios* [Gr.] life. Cf. vit-. aero*bic*

bi-[2] *bi-* [L.] two (see also di-[1]). *bi*lobate

bil- *bilis* [L.] bile. Cf. chol-.; *bil*iary

blast- *blastos* [Gr.] bud, child, a growing thing in its early stages. Cf. germ-. *blast*oma, zygoto*blast*

blep- *blepō* [Gr.] look, see. haemia*blep*sia

blephar- *blepharon* [Gr.] (from *blepō;* see blep-) eyelid. Cf. cili*blephar*oncus

bol- See ball-. em*bol*ism

brachi- *brachiōn* [Gr.] arm. *brachi*ocephalic

brachy- *brachys* [Gr.] short. *brachy*cephalic

brady- *bradys* [Gr.] slow. *brady*cardia

brom- *brōmos* [Gr.] stench. podo*brom*idrosis

bronch- *bronch*os [Gr.] windpipe. *bronch*oscopy

bry- *bryō* [Gr.] be full of life. em*bry*onic

bucc- *bucca* [L.] cheek. disto*bucc*al

cac- *kakos* [Gr.] bad, abnormal. Cf. mal*cac*odontia, arthro*cace*. (See also dys-)

caec- *caecus* [L.] blind. Cf. typhl-. *caec*opexy

calc-[1] *calx, calcis* [L.] stone (cf. lith), limestone, lime. *calc*ipexy

calc-[2] *calx, calcis* [L.] heel. *calc*aneotibial

calor- *calor* [L.] heat. Cf. therm-. *calor*imeter

cancr- *cancer, cancri* [L.] crab, cancer. Cf. carcin-. *cancr*ology. (Also spelled chancr-)

capit- *caput, capitis* [L.] head. Cf. cephal-. de*capit*ator

caps- *capsa* [L.] (from *capio*; see cept-) container. en*caps*ulation

carbo(n)- *carbo, carbonis* [L.] coal, charcoal, *carbo*hydrate, *carbon*uria

carcin- *karkinos* [Gr.] crab, cancer. Cf. cancr-. *carcin*oma

cardi- *kardia* [Gr.] heart. lipo*cardi*ac

cary- See kary-. *cary*okinesis

cat- See cata-. *cat*hode

cata- *kata* [Gr.] (final *a* is dropped before words beginning with a vowel) down, negative. *cata*batic

caud- *cauda* [L.] tail. *caud*ad

cav- *cavus* [L.] hollow. Cf. coel-.con*cav*e

cel- See -cele. *cel*ectome

-cele *kēlē* [Gr.] tumour, hernia. gastro*cele*

cell- *cella* [L.] room, cell. Cf. cyt.*cell*iferous

cen- *koinos* [Gr.] common. *cen*aesthesia

cent- *centum* [L.] hundred. Cf. hect-. Indicates fraction in metric system. [This exemplifies the custom in the metric system of identifying fractions of units by stems from the Latin, as centimetre, decimetre, millimetre, and multiples of units by the similar stems from the Greek, as hectometre, decametre, and kilometre.] *cent*imetre, *cent*ipede

cente- *kenteō* [Gr.] to puncture. Cf. punct-. entero*cente*sis

centr- *kentron* [Gr.] or *centrum* [L.] point, centre. neuro*centr*al

cephal- *kephalē* [Gr.] head. Cf. capit-. en*cephal*itis

cept- *capio, -cipientis, -ceptus* [L.] take, receive. re*cept*or

cer- *kēros* [Gr.] or *cera* [L.] wax. *cer*oplasty, *cer*omel

cerat- See kerat-. a*cerat*osis

cerebr- *cerebrum* [L.] brain. *cerebr*ospinal

cervic- *cervix, cervicis* [L.] neck. Cf. trachel-. *cervic*itis

chancr- See cancr-. *chancr*iform

cheil- *cheilos* [Gr.] lip. Cf. labi-. *cheil*oschisis

cheir- *cheir* [Gr.] hand. Cf. man-. macro*cheir*ia. (Also spelled chir-)

chir- See cheir-. *chir*omegaly

chlor- *chlōros* [Gr.] green. a*chlor*opsia

chol- *cholē* [Gr.] bile. Cf. bil-. hepato*chol*angeitis

chondr- *chondros* [Gr.] cartilage. *chondr*omalacia

chord- *chordē* [Gr.] string, cord. peri*chord*al

chori- *chorion* [Gr.] protective fetal membrane. endo*chori*on

chro- *chrōs* [Gr.] colour. poly*chro*matic

chron- *chronos* [Gr.] time. syn*chron*ous

chy- *cheō, chy-* [Gr.] pour. ec*chy*mosis

-cid(e) *caedo, -cisus* [L.] cut, kill. infanti*cide*, germi*cid*al

cili- *cilium* [L.] eyelid. Cf. blephar-. super*cili*ary

cine- See kine-. auto*cine*sis

-cipient See cept-. in*cipient*

circum- *circum* [L.] around. Cf. peri*circum*ferential

-cis- *caedo, -cisus* [L.] cut, kill. ex*cis*ion

clas- *klaō* [Gr.] break. cranio*clast*

clin- *klinō* [Gr.] bend, incline, make lie down. *clin*ometer

clus- *claudo, -clusus* [L.] shut. Maloc*clus*ion

co- See con-. *co*hesion

cocc- *kokkos* [G.] seed, pill. gono*cocc*us

coel- *koilos* [Gr.] hollow. Cf. cav*coel*enteron

col-[1] See colon-. *col*ic

col-[2] See con-. *col*lapse

colon- *kolon* [Gr.] lower intestine. *colon*ic

colp- *kolpos* [Gr.] hollow, vagina. Cf. sin-. endo*colp*itis

com- See con-. *com*masculation

con- *con-* [L.] (becomes co- before vowels or *h*; col- before *l*; com- before *b*, *m*, or *p*; cor- before *r*) with, together. Cf. syn-. *con*traction

contra- *contra* [L.] against, counter. Cf. anti-. *contra*indication

copr- *kopros* [Gr.] dung. Cf. sterco-. *copr*oma

cor-[1] *korē* [Gr.] doll, little image, pupil. iso*cor*ia

cor-[2] See con-. *cor*rugator

corpor- *corpus, corporis* [L.] body. Cf. somat-. intra*corpor*al

cortic- *cortex, corticis* [L.] bark, rind. *cortic*osterone

cost- *costa* [L.] rib. Cf. pleur-. inter*cost*al

crani- *kranion* [Gr.] or *cranium* [L.] skull. peri*crani*um

creat- *kreas, kreato-* [Gr.] meat, flesh. *creat*orrhoea

-crescent *cresco, crescentis, cretus* [L.] grow. ex*crescent*

cret-[1] *cerno, cretus* [L.] distinguish, separate off. Cf. crin-. dis*crete*

cret-[2] See -crescent. ac*cret*ion

crin- *krinō* [Gr.] distinguish, separate off. Cf. cret-[1]. endo*crin*ology

crur- *crus, cruris* [L.] shin, leg. brachio*crur*al

cry- *kryos* [Gr.] cold. *cry*aesthesia

crypt- *kryptō* [Gr.] hide, conceal. *crypt*orchism

cult- *colo, cultus* [L.] tend, cultivate. *cult*ure

cune- *cuneus* [L.] wedge. Cf. sphen-. *cune*iform

cut- *cutis* [L.] skin. Cf. derm(at)-. sub*cut*aneous

cyan- *kyanos* [Gr.] blue. antho*cyan*in

cycl- *kyklos* [Gr.] circle, cycle. *cycl*ophoria

cyst- *kystis* [Gr.] bladder. Cf. vesic-. nephro*cyst*itis

cyt- *kytos* [Gr.] cell. Cf. cell-. plasmo*cyt*oma

dacry- *dakry* [Gr.] tear. *dacry*ocyst

dactyl- *daktylos* [Gr.] finger, toe. Cf. digit-. hexa*dactyl*ism

de- *de* [L.] down from. *de*composition

dec-[1] *deka* [Gr.] ten. Indicates multiple in metric system. Cf. dec-[2]. *dec*agram

dec-[2] *decem* [L.] ten. Indicates fraction in metric system. Cf. dec-[1]. *dec*ipara, *dec*imetre

dendr- *dendron* [Gr.] tree. neuro*dendr*ite

dent- *dens, dentis* [L.] tooth. Cf. odont-. inter*dent*al

derm(at)- *derma, dermatos* [Gr.] skin. Cf. cut-. endo*derm*, *dermat*itis

desm- *desmos* [Gr.] band, ligament. syn*desm*opexy

dextr- *dexter, dextr-* [L.] right-hand. ambi*dextr*ous

di-[1] *di-* [Gr.] two. *di*morphic. (See also bi-[2])

di-[2] See dia-. *di*uresis

di-[3] See dis-. *di*vergent

dia- *dia* [Gr.] (*a* is dropped before words beginning with a vowel) through, apart. Cf. per-. *dia*gnosis

didym- *didymos* [Gr.] twin. Cf. gemin-. epi*didym*al

digit- *digitus* [L.] finger, toe. Cf. dactyl-. *digit*igrade

diplo- *diploos* [Gr.] double, *diplo*myelia

dis- *dis-* [L.] (*s* may be dropped before a word beginning with a consonant) apart, away from. *dis*location

disc- *diskos* [Gr.] or *discus* [L.] disc. *disc*oplacenta

dors- *dorsum* [L.] back. ventro*dorsal*

drom- *dromos* [Gr.] course. haemo*drom*ometer

-ducent See duct-. ad*ducent*

-duct *duco, ducentis, ductus* [L.] lead, conduct. ovi*duct*

dur- *durus* [L.] hard. Cf. scler-. in*dur*ation

dynam(i)- *dynamis* [Gr.] power. *dynam*oneure, neuro*dynamic*

dys- *dys-* [Gr.] bad, improper. Cf. mal-. *dys*trophic. (See also cac-)

e- *e* [L.] out from. Cf. ec- and ex-. *e*mission

ec- *ek* [Gr.] out of. Cf. e- *ec*centric

-ech- *echō* [Gr.] have, hold, be. syn*ech*otomy

ect- *ektos* [Gr.] outside. Cf. extra-. *ect*oplasm

ede- See oede-

ef- See ex-. *ef*florescent

-elc- *helkos* [Gr.] sore, ulcer. enter*elc*osis. (See also *helc-*)

electr- *ēlectron* [Gr.] amber. *electr*otherapy

em- See en-. *em*bolism, *em*pathy, *em*phlysis

en- *en* [Gr.] (*n* changes to *m* before *b*, *p* or *ph*) in, on. Cf. in-[2]. *en*celitis

end- *endon* [Gr.] inside. Cf. intra-. *end*angium

enter- *enteron* [Gr.] intestine. dys*entery*

ep- See epi-. *ep*axial

epi- *epi* [Gr.] (*i* is dropped before words beginning with a vowel) upon, after, in addition. *epi*glottis

erg- *ergon* [Gr.] work, deed. en*ergy*

erythr- *erythros* [Gr.] red. Cf. rub(r)-. *erythr*ochromia

eso- *esō* [Gr.] inside. Cf. intra-. *eso*phylactic

esthe- See aesthe-

eu- *eu* [Gr.] good, normal. *eu*pepsia

ex- *ex* [Gr.] or *ex* [L.] out of. Cf. e-. *ex*cretion

exo- *exō* [Gr.] outside. Cf. extra-. *exo*pathic

extra- *extra* [L.] outside of, beyond. Cf. ect- and exo-. *extra*cellular

faci- *facies* [L.] face. Cf. prosop-. brachio*faci*olingual

-facient *facio, facientis, factus, -fectus* [L.] make. Cf. poie-. cale*facient*

-fact- See facient-. arte*fact*

fasci- *fascia* [L.] band. *fasci*orrhaphy

febr- *febris* [L.] fever. Cf. pyr-. *febr*icide

-fect- See -facient. de*fect*ive

-ferent *fero, ferentis, latus* [L.] bear, carry. Cf. phor-. ef*ferent*

ferr- *ferrum* [L.] iron. *ferr*oprotein

fibr- *fibra* [L.] fiber. Cf. in-[1]. chondro*fibr*oma

fil- *filum* [L.] thread. *fil*iform

fiss- *findo, fissus* [L.] split. Cf. schis-. *fiss*ion

flagell- *flagellum* [L.] whip. *flagell*ation

flav- *flavus* [L.] yellow. Cf. xanth-. ribo*flav*in

-flect- *flecto, flexus* [L.] bend, divert. de*flect*ion

-flex- See -flect-. re*flex*ometer

flu- *fluo, fluxus* [L.] flow. Cf. rhe-. *flu*id

flux- See flu-. af*flux*ion

for- *foris* [L.] door, opening. per*for*ated

-form *forma* [L.] shape. Cf. oid. ossi*form*

fract- *frango, fractus* [L.] break. re*fract*ive

front- *frons, frontis* [L.] forehead, front. naso*front*al

-fug(e) *fugio* [L.] flee, avoid. vermi*fuge*, centri*fug*al

funct- *fungor, functus* [L.] perform, serve, function. mal*funct*ion

fund- *fundo, fusus* [L.] pour. in*fund*ibulum

fus- See fund-. dif*fus*ible

galact- *gala, galactos* [Gr.] milk. Cf. lact-. dys*galact*ia

gam- *gamos* [Gr.] marriage, reproductive union. a*gam*ont

gangli- *ganglion* [Gr.] swelling, plexus. neuro*gangli*itis

gastr- *gastēr, gastros* [Gr.] stomach. cholangio*gastr*ostomy

gelat- *gelo, gelatus* [L.] freeze, congeal. *gelat*in

gemin- *geminus* [L.] twin, double. Cf. didym-. quadri*gemin*al

gen- *gignomai, gen-, gon-* [Gr.] become, be produced, originate, or *gennaō* [Gr.] produce, originate. cyto*gen*ic

germ- *germen, germinis* [L.] bud, a growing thing in its early stages. Cf. blast-. *germ*inal, ovi*germ*

gest- *gero, gerentis, gestus* [L.] bear, carry. con*gest*ion

gland- *glans, glandis* [L.] acorn. Cf. aden-. intra*gland*ular

-glia *glia* [Gr.] glue. neuro*glia*

gloss- *glōssa* [Gr.] tongue. Cf. lingu-. tricho*gloss*ia

glott- *glōtta* [Gr.] tongue, language. *glott*ic

gluc- See glyc(y)-. *gluc*ophenetidin

glutin- *gluten, glutinis* [L.] glue. ag*glutin*ation

glyc(y)- *glykys* [Gr.] sweet. *glyc*aemia, *glycy*rrhizin. (Also spelled gluc-)

gnath- *gnathos* [Gr.] jaw. ortho*gnath*ous

gno- *gignōsiō, gnō-* [Gr.] know, discern, dia*gno*sis

gon- See gen-. anphi*gon*y

grad- *gradior* [L.] walk, take steps. retro*grade*

-gram *gramma* [Gr.] letter, drawing. cardio*gram*

gran- *granum* [L.] grain, particle. lipo*gran*uloma

graph- *graphō* [Gr.] scratch, write, record.

histo*graphy*

grav- *gravis* [L.] heavy. multi*grav*ida

gyn(aec)- *gynē, gynaikos* [Gr.] woman, wife. andro*gyn*y, *gynae*cological

gyr- *gyros* [Gr.] ring, circle. *gyr*ospasm

haem(at)- *haima, haimatos* [Gr.] blood. Cf. sanguin-. *haem*angioma, *haemat*ocyturia. (See also -aem-)

hapt- *haptō* [Gr.] touch. *hapt*ometer

hect- *hekt-* [Gr.] hundred. Cf. cent-. Indicates multiple in metric system. *hect*ometre

helc- *helkos* [Gr.] sore, ulcer. *helc*osis

hem(at)- See haem(at)-

hemi- *hemi-* [Gr.] half. Cf. semi-. *hemi*ageusia

hen- *heis, henos* [Gr.] one. Cf. un-. *hen*ogenesis

hepat- *hēpar, hēpatos* [Gr.] liver. gastro*hepat*ic

hept(a)- *hepta* [Gr.] seven. Cf. sept-[2]. *hept*atomic, *hepta*valent

hered- *heres, heredis* [L.] heir. *hered*oimmunity

hex-[1] *hex* [Gr.] six. Cf. sex-. *hexyl-*. An *a* is added in some combinations

hex-[2] *echō, hex-* [Gr.] (added to *s* becomes *hex-*) have, hold, be. ca*chex*ia

hexa- See hex-[1]. *hexa*chromic

hidr- *hidros* [Gr.] sweat. hyper*hidr*osis

hist- *histos* [Gr.] web, tissue. *hist*odialysis

hod- *hodos* [Gr.] road, path. *hod*oneuromere. (See also od- and -ode[1])

hom- *homos* [Gr.] common, same. *hom*omorphic

horm- *ormē* [Gr.] impetus, impulse. *horm*one

hydat- *hydōr, hydatos* [Gr.] water, *hydat*ism

hydr- *hydōr, hydr-* [Gr.] water. Cf. lymph-. anclor*hydr*ia

hyp- See hypo-. *hyp*axial

hyper- *hyper* [Gr.] above, beyond, extreme. Cf. super-. *hyper*trophy

hypn- *hypnos* [Gr.] sleep. *hypn*otic

hypo- *hypo* [Gr.] (*o* is dropped before words beginning with a vowel) under, below. Cf. sub-. *hypo*metabolism

hyster- *hystera* [Gr.] womb. colpo*hyster*opexy

iatr- *iatros* [Gr.] physician. paed*iatr*ics

idi- *idios* [Gr.] peculiar, separate, distinct, *idi*osyncrasy

il- See in-[2,3]. *il*linition (in on), *il*legible (negative prefix)

ile- See ili- [ile- is commonly used to refer to the portion of the intestines known as the ileum]. *ile*ostomy

ili- *ilium (ileum)* [L.] lower abdomen, intestines [ili- is commonly used to refer to the flaring part of the hip bone known as the ilium]. *ili*osacral

im- See in-[2,3]. *im*mersion (in, on), *im*perforation (negative prefix)

in-[1] *is, inos* [Gr.] fibre. Cf. fibr-. *in*osteatoma

in-[2] *in* [L.] (*n* changes to *l*, *m*, or *r* before words beginning with those consonants) in, on. Cf. en-. *in*sertion

in-[3] *in-* [L.] (*n* changes to *l*, *m*, or *r* before words beginning with those consonants) negative prefix. Cf. a-. *in*valid

infra- *infra* [L.] beneath. *infra*orbital

insul- *insula* [L.] island. *insul*in

inter- *inter* [L.] among, between, *inter*carpal

intra- *intra* [L.] inside. Cf. end- and eso-. *intra*venous

ir- See in-[2,3]. *ir*radiation (in, on), *ir*reducible (negative prefix)

irid- *iris, iridos* [Gr.] rainbow, coloured circle. kerato*irid*ocyclitis

is- *isos* [Gr.] equal. *is*otope

ischi- *ischion* [Gr.] hip, haunch, *ischi*opubic

jact- *iacio, iactus* [L.] throw. *jact*itation

-ject *iacio, iectus* [L.] throw. in*ject*ion

jejun- *ieiunus* [L.] hungry, not partaking of food. gastro*jejun*osetomy

jug- *iugum* [L.] yoke. con*jug*ation

junct- *iungo, iunctus* [L.] yoke, join. con*junct*iva

kary- *karyon* [Gr.] nut, kernel, nucleus. Cf. nucle-. mega*kary*ocyte. (Also spelled cary-)

kerat- *keras, keratos* [Gr.] horn. *kerat*olysis. (Also spelled cerat-)

kil- *chilioi* [Gr.] one thousand. Cf. mill-. Indicates multiple in metric system. *kil*ogram

kine- *kineō* [Gr.] move. *kine*matograph. (Also spelled cine-)

labi- *labium* [L.] lip. Cf. cheil-. gingivo*labi*al

lact- *lac, lactis* [L.] milk. Cf. galact-. gluco*lact*one

lal- *laleō* [Gr.] talk, babble. glosso*lal*ia

lapar- *lapara* [Gr.] flank. *lapar*otomy

laryng- *larynx, laryngos* [Gr.] windpipe. *laryng*endoscope

lat- *fero, latus* [L.] bear, carry. See -ferent. trans*lat*ion

later- *latus, lateris* [L.] side. ventro*later*al

lent- *lens, lentis* [L.] lentil. Cf. phac-. *lent*iconus

lep- *lambanō, lēp-* [Gr.] take, seize. cata*lep*tic

leuc- See leuk-. *leuc*inuria

leuk- *leukos* [Gr.] white. Cf. alb-. *leuk*orrhoea. (Also spelled leuc-)

lien- *lien* [L.] spleen. Cf. splen-. *lien*ocele

lig- *ligo* [L.] tie, bind. *lig*ate

lingu- *lingua* [L.] tongue. Cf. gloss-. sub*lingu*al

lip- *lipos* [Gr.] fat. Cf. adip-. glyco*lip*in

lith- *lithos* [Gr.] stone. Cf. calc-[1]. nephro*lith*otomy

loc- *locus* [L.] place. Cf. top-. *loc*omotion

log- *legō, log-* [Gr.] speak, give an account. *log*orrhoea, embryo*log*y

lumb- *lumbus* [L.] loin. dorso*lumb*ar

lute- *luteus* [L.] yellow. Cf. xanth-. *lute*oma

ly- *lyō* [Gr.] loose, dissolve. Cf. solut-. kerato*ly*sis

lymph- *lympha* [Gr.] water. Cf. hydr-. *lymph*adenosis

macr- *makros* [Gr.] long, large. *macr*omyeloblast

mal- *malus* [L.] bad, abnormal. Cf. cac- and dys. *mal*function

malac- *malakos* [Gr.] soft. osteo*malac*ia

mamm- *mamma* [L.] breast. Cf. mast-. sub*mamm*ary

man- *manus* [L.] hand. Cf. cheir-. *man*iphalanx

mani- *mani* [Gr.] mental aberration. *mani*graphy, klepto*mani*a

mast- *mastos* [Gr.] breast. Cf. mamm-. hyper*mast*ia

medi- *medius* [L.] middle. Cf. mes-. *medi*frontal

mega- *megas* [Gr.] great, large. Also indicates multiple (1,000,000) in metric system. *mega*colon, *mega*dyne. (See also megal-)

megal- *megas, megalou* [Gr.] great, large. acro*megal*y

mel- *melos* [Gr.] limb, member. sym*mel*ia

melan- *melas, melanos* [Gr.] black. hippo*melan*in

men- *mēn* [Gr.] month. dys*men*orrhoea

mening- *mēninx, mēningos* [Gr.] membrane. encephalo*mening*itis

ment- *mens, mentis* [L.] mind. Cf. phren-, psych- and thym-. de*menti*a
mer- *meros* [Gr.] part. poly*mer*ic
mes- *mesos* [Gr.] middle. Cf. medi-. *mes*oderm
met- See meta-. *met*allergy
meta- *meta* [Gr.] (*a* is dropped before words beginning with a vowel) after, beyond, accompanying. *meta*carpal
metr-[1] *metron* [Gr.] measure. stereo*metry*
metr-[2] *metra* [Gr.] womb. endo*metr*itis
micr- *mikros* [Gr.] small. photo*micro*graph
mill- *mille* [L.] one thousand. Cf. kil-. Indicates fraction in metric system. *milli*gram, *milli*pede
miss- See -mittent. intro*miss*ion
-mittent *mitto, mittentis, missus* [L.] send. inter*mittent*
mne- *mimnērcō, mnē-* [Gr.] remember. pseudo*mne*sia
mon- *monos* [Gr.] only, sole. *mono*plegia
morph- *morphē* [Gr.] form, shape. poly*morph*onuclear
mot- *moveo, motus* [L.] move. vaso*mot*or
my- *mys, myos* [Gr.] muscle. inoleio*my*oma
-myces *mykēs, mykētos* [Gr.] fungus. myelo*myces*
myc(et)- See -myces. asco*mycet*es, strepto*myc*in
myel- *myelos* [Gr.] narrow. polio*myel*itis
myx- *myxa* [Gr.] mucus. *myx*oedema
narc- *narkē* [Gr.] numbness. topo*narc*osis
nas- *nasus* [L.] nose. Cf. rhin-. palato*nas*al
ne- *neos* [Gr.] new, young. *ne*ocyte
necr- *nekros* [Gr.] corpse. *necr*ocytosis
nephr- *nephros* [Gr.] kidney. Cf. ren-. para*nephr*ic
neur- *neuron* [Gr.] nerve. aesthesio*neur*e
nod- *nodus* [L.] knot. *nod*osity
nom- *nomos* [Gr.] (from *nemō* deal out, distribute) law, custom. taxo*nomy*
non- *nona* [L.] nine. *non*acosane
nos- *nosos* [Gr.] disease. *nos*ology
nucle- *nucleus* [L.] (from *nux, nucis* nut) kernel. Cf. kary-. *nucle*us
nutri *nutrio* [L.] nourish. mal*nutri*tion
ob- *ob* [L.] (*b* changes to *c* before words beginning with that consonant) against, toward, etc. *ob*tuse
oc- See ob-. *oc*clude
ocul- *oculus* [L.] eye. Cf. ophthalm-. *ocul*omotor
-od- See -ode[1]. peri*od*ic
-ode[1] *hodos* [Gr.] road, path. cath*ode*. (See also hod-)
-ode[2] See -oid. nemat*ode*
odont- *odous, odontos* [Gr.] tooth. Cf. dent-. orth*odont*ia
-odyn- *odynē* [Gr.] pain, distress. gastr*odynia*
oede- *oideō* [Gr.] swell. *oede*matous
oid- *eidos* [Gr.] form. Cf. -form. hy*oid*
-ol See ole-. cholester*ol*
ole- *oleum* [L.] oil. *ole*oresin
olig- *oligos* [Gr.] few, small. *olig*ospermia
omphal- *omphalos* [Gr.] navel. peri*omphal*ic
onc- *onkos* [Gr.] bulk, mass. haemat*onc*ometry
onych- *onyx, onychos* [Gr.] claw, nail. an*onych*ia
oo- *ōon* [Gr.] egg. Cf. ov-. peri*oo*thecitis
op- *horaō, op-* [Gr.] see. erythr*op*sia
ophthalm- *ophthalmos* [Gr.] eye. Cf. ocul-. ex*ophthalm*ic
or- *os, oris* [L.] mouth. Cf. stom(at)-. intra*or*al
orb- *orbis* [L.] circle. sub*orb*ital
orchi *orchis* [Gr.] testicle. Cf. test-. *orchi*opathy
organ- *organon* [Gr.] implement, instrument. *organ*oleptic
orth- *orthos* [Gr.] straight, right, normal. *orth*opedics
oss- *os, ossis* [L.] bone. Cf. ost(e)-. *oss*iphone
ost(e)- *osteon* [Gr.] bone. Cf. oss-. en*ost*osis, *oste*anaphysis
ot- *ous, ōtos* [Gr.] ear. Cf. aur-. par*ot*id
ov- *ovum* [L.] egg. Cf. oo-. syn*ov*ia
oxy- *oxys* [Gr.] sharp. *oxy*cephalic
pachy(n)- *pachynō* [Gr.] thicken. *pachy*derma, myo*pachyn*sis
paed- *pais, paidos* [Gr.] child. ortho*paed*ic, *paed*iatric
pag- *pēgnymi, pag-* [Gr.] fix, make fast. thoraco*pag*us
par-[1] *pario* [L.] bear, give birth to. primi*par*ous
par-[2] See para-. *par*epigastric
para- *para* [Gr.] (final *a* is dropped before words beginning with a vowel) beside, beyond. *para*mastoid
part- *pario, partus* [L.] bear, give birth to. *part*urition
path- *pathos* [Gr.] that which one undergoes, sickness, psycho*path*ic
pec- *pēgnymi, pēg-* [Gr.] (*pēk-* before *t*) fix, make fast. sym*pec*tothiene. (See also pex-)
pell- *pellis* [L.] skin, hide. *pell*agra
-pellent *pello, pellentis, pulsus* [L.] drive. re*pellent*
pen- *penomai* [Gr.] need, lack. erythrocyto*pen*ia
pend- *pendeo* [L]. hang down. ap*pend*ix
pent(a)- *pente* [Gr.] five. Cf. quinque-. *pent*ose, *penta*ploid
peps- *peptō, peps-* [Gr.] digest. brady*peps*ia
pept- *peptō* [Gr.] digest. dys*pept*ic
per- *per* [L.] through. Cf. dia-. *per*nasal
peri- *peri* [Gr.] around. Cf. circum-. *peri*phery
pet- *peto* [L.] seek, tend toward. centri*pet*al
pex- *pēgnumi, pēg-* [Gr.] (added to *s* becomes *pēx*) fix, make fast. hepato*pexy*
pha- *phēmi, pha-* [Gr.] say, speak. dys*pha*sia
phac- *phakos* [Gr.] lentil, lens. Cf. lent-. *phac*osclerosis. (Also spelled phak-)
phag- *phagein* [Gr.] eat. lipo*phag*ic
phak- See phac-. *phak*itis
phan- See phen-. dia*phan*oscopy
pharmac- *pharmakon* [Gr.] drug. *pharmac*ognosy
pharyng- *pharynx, pharyng-* [Gr.] throat. glosso*pharyng*eal
phen- *phainō, phan-* [Gr.] show, be seen. phos*phen*e
pher- *pherō, phor-* [Gr.] bear, support. peri*pher*y
phil- *phileō* [Gr.] like, have affinity for. eosino*phil*ia
phleb- *phleps, phlebos* [Gr.] vein. peri*phleb*itis
phleg- *phlogō, phlog-* [Gr.] burn, inflame. adeno*phleg*mon
phlog- See phleg-. anti*phlog*istic
phob- *phobos* [Gr.] fear, dread. claustro*phob*ia
phon- *phōne* [Gr.] sound. echo*phon*y
phor- See pher-. Cf. -ferent. exo*phor*ia
phos- See phot-. *phos*phorus
phot- *phōs, phōtos* [Gr.] light. *phot*erythrous
phrag- *phrassō, phrag-* [Gr.] fence, wall off, stop up. Cf. sept-[1]. dia*phrag*m
phrax- *phrassō, phrag-* [Gr.] (added to *s* becomes *phrax-*) fence, wall off, stop up. em*phrax*is
phren- *phrēn* [Gr.] mind, midriff. Cf. ment-. meta*phren*ia, meta*phren*on
phthi- *phthinō* [Gr.] decay, waste away. *phthsis*
phy- *phyō* [Gr.] beget, bring forth, produce,

be by nature. noso*phyte*

phyl- *phylon* [Gr.] tride, kind. *phyl*ogeny

-phyll *phyllon* [Gr.] leaf. xantho*phyll*

phylac- *phylax* [Gr.] guard. pro*phylac*tic

phys(a)- *physaō* [Gr.] blow, inflate. *phys*ocele, *physa*lis

physe- *physaō, physē-* [Gr.] blow, inflate, em*physe*ma

pil- *pilus* [L.] hair. e*pil*ation

pituit- *pituita* [L.] phlegm, rheum. *pituit*ous

placent- *placenta* [L.] (from *plakous* [Gr.]) cake. extra*placent*al

plas- *plassō* [Gr.] mould, shape. cine*plasty*

platy- *platys* [Gr.] broad, flat. *platy*rrhine

pleg- *plēssō* [Gr.] strike. di*pleg*ia

plet- *pleo, -pletus* [L.] fill. de*plet*ion

pleur- *pleura* [Gr.] rib, side. Cf. cost-. peri*pleur*al

plex- *plēssō, plēg-* (added to *s* becomes *plēx-*) strike. apo*plex*y

plic- *plico* [L.] fold. com*plic*ation

pnoe- *pneuma, pneumatos* [Gr.] breathing. traumato*pnoea*

pneum(at)- *pneuma, pneumatos* [Gr.] breath, air. *pneum*odynamics, *pneumat*othorax

pneumo(n)- *pneumōn* [Gr.] lung. Cf. pulmo(n)-. *pneumo*centesis, *pneumono*tomy

pod- *pous, podos* [Gr.] foot. *pod*iatry

poie- *poieō* [Gr.] make, produce. Cf. -facient. sarco*poie*tic

pol- *polos* [Gr.] axis of a sphere. peri*pol*ar

poly- *polys* [Gr.] much, many *poly*spermia

pont- *pons, pontis* [L.] bridge. *pont*ocerebellar

por-[1] *poros* [Gr.] passage. myelo*pore*

por-[2] *pōros* [Gr.] callus. *por*ocele

posit- *pono, positus* [L.] put, place. re*posit*or

post- *post* [L.] after, behind in time or place. *post*natal, *post*oral

pre- *prae* [L.] before in time or place, *pre*natal, *pre*vesical

press- *premo, pressus* [L.] press. *press*oreceptive

pro- *pro* [Gr.] or *pro* [L.] before in time or place. *pro*gamous, *pro*cheilon, *pro*lapse

proct- *prōktos* [Gr.] anus. entero*proct*ia

prosop- *prosōpon* [Gr.] face. Cf. faci-. di*prosop*us

pseud- *pseudēs* [Gr.] false. *pseudo*paraplegia

psych- *psychē* [Gr.] soul, mind. Cf. ment-. *psych*osomatic

pto- *piptō, ptō-* [Gr.] fall. nephro*pto*sis

pub- *pubes* and *puber, puberis* [L.] adult. ischio*pub*ic. (See also puber-)

puber- *puber* [L.] adult. *puber*ty

pulmo(n)- *pulmo, pulmonis* [L.] lung. Cf. pneumo(n)-. *pulmo*lith, cardio*pulmon*ary

puls- *pello, pellentis, pulsus* [L.] drive. pro*puls*ion

punct- *pungo, punctus* [L.] prick, pierce. Cf. cente-. *punct*iform

pur- *pus, puris* [L.] pus. Cf. py-. sup*pur*ation

py- *pyon* [Gr.] pus. Cf. pur-. nephro*py*osis

pyel- *pyelos* [Gr.] trough, basin, pelvis. nephro*pyel*itis

pyl- *pylē* [Gr.] door, orifice, *pyl*ephlebitis

pyr- *pyr* [Gr.] fire. Cf. febr-. galacto*pyr*a

quadr- *quadr-* [L.] four. Cf. tetra-. *quadr*igeminal

quinque- *quinque* [L.] five. Cf. pent(a)-. *quinque*cuspid

rachi- *rachis* [Gr.] spine. Cf. spin-. encephalo*rachi*dian

radi- *radius* [L.] ray. Cf. actin-. ir*radi*ation

re- *re-* [L.] back, again. *re*traction

ren- *renes* [L.] kidneys. Cf. nephr-. ad*ren*al

ret- *rete* [L.] net. *ret*othelium

retro- *retro* [L.] backwards. *retro*deviation

rhin- *rhis, rhinos* [Gr.] nose. Cf. nas-. basi*rhin*al

rot- *rota* [L.] wheel. *rot*ator

rrhag- *rhēgnymi, rhag-* [Gr.] break, burst, haemor*rhag*ic

rrhaph- *rhaphē* [Gr.] suture, gastror*rhaphy*

rrhoe- *rhaphē* [Gr.] flow. Cf. flu-. diar*rhoe*al

rrhex- *rhēgnymi, rhēg-* [Gr.] (added to *s* becomes *rhēx*) break, burst. metror*rhex*is

rub(r)- *ruber, rubri* [L.] red. Cf. erythr-. bili*rub*in, *rub*rospinal

salping- *salpinx, salpingos* [Gr.] tube, trumpet, *salping*itis

sanguin- *sanguis, sanguinis* [L.] blood. Cf. haem(at)-. *sanguin*eous

sarc- *sarx, sarkos* [Gr.] flesh. *sarc*oma

schis- *schizō, schid-* [Gr.] (before *t* or added to *s* becomes *schis-*) split. Cf. fiss-. *schis*torachis, rachi*schis*is

scler- *sklēros* [Gr.] hard. Cf. dur-. *scler*osis

scop- *skopeō* [Gr.] look at, observe. endo*scop*e

sect- *seco, sectus* [L.] cut. Cf. tom-. *sect*ile

semi- *semi* [L.] half. Cf. hemi-. *semi*flexion

sens- *sentio, sensus* [L.] perceive, feel. Cf. aesthe-. *sens*ory

sep- *sepō* [Gr.] rot, decay. *sep*sis

sept-[1] *saepio, saeptus* [L.] fence, wall off, stop up. Cf. phrag-. naso*sept*al

sept-[2] *septem* [L.] seven. Cf. hept(a)-. *sept*an

ser- *serum* [L.] whey, watery substance, *ser*osynovitis

sex- *sex* [L.] six. Cf. hex-[1]. *sex*digitate

sial- *sialon* [Gr.] saliva. poly*sial*ia

sin- *sinus* [L.] hollow, fold. Cf. colp-. *sin*obronchitis

sit- *sitos* [Gr.] food. para*sit*ic

solut- *solvo, solventis, solutus* [L.] loose, dissolve, set free. Cf. ly-. dis*solut*ion

-solvent See solut-. dis*solvent*

somat- *sōma, somatos* [Gr.] body. Cf. corpor-. psycho*somat*ic

-some See somat-. dictyo*some*

spas- *spaō, spas-* [Gr.] draw, pull. *spas*m, *spas*tic

spectr- *spectrum* [L.] appearance, what is seen. micro*spectr*oscope

sperm(at)- *sperma, spermatos* [Gr.] seed. *sperm*acrasia, *spermat*ozoon

spers- *spargo, -spersus* [L.] scatter. di*spers*ion

sphen- *sphēn* [Gr.] wedge. Cf. cune-. *sphen*oid

spher- *sphaira* [Gr.] ball. hemi*spher*e

sphygm- *sphygmos* [Gr.] pulsation. *sphygm*omanometer

spin- *spina* [L.] spine. Cf. rachi-. cerebro*spin*al

spirat- *spiro, spiratus* [L.] breathe. in*spirat*ory

splanchn- *splanchna* [Gr.] entrails, viscera, neuro*splanchn*ic

splen- *splēn* [Gr.] spleen. Cf. lien-. *splen*omegaly

spor- *sporos* [Gr.] seed. *spor*ophyte, zygo*spor*e

squam- *squama* [L.] scale. de*squam*ation

sta- *histēmi, sta-* [Gr.] make stand, stop. genesi*sta*sis

stal- *stellō, stal-* [Gr.] send. peri*stal*sis. (See also stol-)

staphyl- *staphylē* [Gr.] bunch of grapes, uvula. *staphyl*ococcus, *staphyl*ectomy

stear- *stear, steatos* [Gr.] fat. Cf. adip-. *stear*odermia

steat- See *stear-*. *steat*opygous

sten- *stenos* [Gr.] narrow, compressed. *sten*ocardia

ster- *stereos* [Gr.] solid. chole*ster*ol
sterc- *stercus* [L.] dung. Cf. copr-. *sterc*oporphyrin
sthen- *sthenos* [Gr.] strength, a*sthen*ia
stol- *stellō, stol-* [Gr.] send. dia*stol*e
stom(at)- *stoma, stomatos* [Gr.] mouth, orifice. Cf. or-. ana*stom*osis, *stomat*ogastric
strep(h)- *strephō, strep-* (before *t*) [Gr.] twist. Cf. tors-. *streph*osymbolia, *strep*tomycin. (See also stroph-)
strict- *stringo, stringentis, strictus* [L.] draw tight, compress, cause pain. con*strict*ion
-stringent See strict-. a*stringent*
stroph- *strephō, stroph-* [Gr.] twist. ana*stroph*ic. (See also strep(h)-)
struct- *struo, structus* [L.] pile up (against). ob*struct*ion
sub- *sub* [L.] (*b* changes to *f* or *p* before words beginning with those consonants) under, below. Cf. hypo-. *sub*lumbar
suf- See sub-. *suf*fusion
sup- See sub-. *sup*pository
super- *super* [L.] above, beyond, extreme. Cf. hyper-. *super*motility
sy- See syn-. *sy*stole
syl- See syn-. *syl*lepsiology
sym- See syn-. *sym*biosis, *sym*metry, *sym*pathetic, *sym*physis
syn- *syn* [Gr.] (*n* disappears before *s*, changes to *l* before *l*, and changes to *m* before *b*, *m*, *p*, and *ph*) with, together. Cf. con-. myo*syn*izesis
ta- See ton-. ec*ta*sis
tac- *tassō, tag-* [Gr.] (*tak-* before *t*) order, arrange, a*tac*tic
tact- *tango, tactus* [L.] touch. con*tact*
tax- *tassō, tag-* [Gr.] (added to *s* becomes *tax-*) order, arrange. a*tax*ia
tect- See teg-. pro*tect*ive
teg- *tego, tectus* [L.] cover, in*teg*ument
tel- *telos* [Gr.] end. *tel*osynapsis
tele- *tēle* [Gr.] at a distance, *tele*ceptor
tempor- *tempus, temporis* [L.] time, timely or fatal spot, temple. *tempor*omalar
ten(ont)- *tenōn, tenontos* [Gr.] (from *teinō* stretch) tight stretched band. *ten*odynia, *ten*onitis, *tenont*agra
tens- *tendo, tensus* [L.] stretch. Cf. ton-. ex*tens*or
test- *testis* [L.] testicle. Cf. orchi-. *test*itis
tetra- *tetra-* [Gr.] four. Cf. quadr-. *tetra*genous
the- *tithēmi, thē-* [Gr.] put, place. syn*the*sis
thec- *thēkē* [Gr.] repository, case. *thec*ostegnosis
thel- *thēlē* [Gr.] teat, nipple. *thel*erethism
therap- *therapeia* [Gr.] treatment. hydro*therapy*
therm- *thermē* [Gr.] heat. Cf. calor-. dia*therm*y
thi- *theion* [Gr.] sulphur. *thi*ogenic
thorac- *thōrax, thōrakos* [Gr.] chest. *thorac*oplasty
thromb- *thrombos* [Gr.] lump, clot. *thromb*openia
thym- *thymos* [Gr.] spirit. Cf. ment-. dys*thym*ia
thyr- *thyreos* [Gr.] shield (shaped like a door *thyra*). *thyr*oid
tme- *temnō, tmē-* [Gr.] cut. axono*tme*sis
toc- *tokos* [Gr.] childbirth. dys*toc*ia
tom- *temnō, tom-* [Gr.] cut. Cf. sect-. appendec*tom*y
ton- *teino, ton-* [Gr.] stretch, put under tension. Cf. tens-. peri*ton*eum
top- *topos* [Gr.] place. Cf. loc-. *top*aesthesia
tors- *torqueo, torsus* [L.] twist. Cf. strep-. ec*tors*ion
tox- *toxicon* [Gr.] (from *toxon* bow) arrow poison, poison. *tox*aemia
trache- *tracheia* [Gr.] windpipe, *trache*otomy
trachel- *trachēlos* [Gr.] neck. Cf. cervic-. *trachel*opexy
tract- *traho, tractus* [L.] draw, drag. pro*tract*ion
traumat- *trauma, traumatos* [Gr.] wound. *traumat*ic
tri- *treis, tria* [Gr.] or *tri-* [L.] three. *tri*gonid
trich- *thrix, trichos* [Gr.] hair. *trich*oid
trip- *tribō* [Gr.] rub. en*trip*sis
trop- *trepō, trop-* [Gr.] turn, react. sito*trop*ism
troph- *trepō, troph-* [Gr.] nurture. a*troph*y
tuber- *tuber* [L.] swelling, node. *tuber*cle
typ- *typos* [Gr.] (from *typto* strike) type. a*typ*ical
typh- *typhos* [Gr.] fog, stupor, adeno*typh*us
typhl- *typhlos* [Gr.] blind. Cf. cec-. *typhl*ectasis
un- *unus* [L.] one. Cf. hen-. *un*ioval
ur- *ouron* [Gr.] urine. poly*ur*ia
vacc- *vacca* [L.] cow. *vacc*ine
vagin- *vagina* [L.] sheath. in*vagin*ated
vas- *vas* [L.] vessel. Cf. angi-. *vas*cular
vers- See vert-. in*vers*ion
vert- *verto, versus* [L.] turn. di*vert*iculum
vesic- *vesica* [L.] bladder. Cf. cyst-. *vesic*ovaginal
vit- *vita* [L.] life. Cf. bi-[1]. de*vit*alize
vuls- *vello, vulsus* [L.] pull, twitch. con*vuls*ion
xanth- *xanthos* [Gr.] yellow, blond. Cf. flav- and lute-. *xanth*ophyll
-yl- *hyte* [Gr.] substance. cacod*yl*
zo- *zoē* [Gr.] life, *zōon* [Gr.] animal. micro*zo*aria
zyg- *zygon* [Gr.] yoke, union. *zyg*odactyly
zym- *zymē* [Gr.] ferment. en*zym*e

Compiled by Lloyd W. Daly, AM, PhD, LittD, Allen Memorial Professor of Greek, University of Pennsylvania, for *Encyclopedia and Dictionary of Medicine, Nursing and Allied Health*, 4th edn. Miller and Keane, W.B. Saunders.

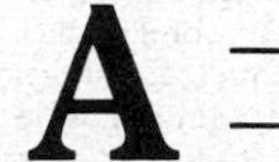

A accommodation; ampere; anode (anodal); anterior; axial; mass number.
A_2 aortic second sound (see HEART SOUNDS).
Å ångström.
a [L.] *arteria* (artery); symbol *atto-*.
a- word element. [L.] *without, not.*
AA achievement age; Alcoholics Anonymous; Association of Anaesthetists.
aa. pl. *arteriae* [L.] arteries.
Ab antibody.
ab preposition. [L.] *away from.*
ab- word element. [L.] *from, off, away from.*
abacterial (ˌaybak'tiə·ri·əl) indicating a condition not caused by bacteria.
abarognosis (ˌaybarog'nohsis) loss of sense of weight.
abasia (ə'bayzi·ə, -si·ə) inability to walk. adj. **abasic, abatic.**
a.-astasia astasia-abasia.
a. atactica abasia with uncertain movements, due to a defect of coordination.
choreic a. abasia due to chorea of the limbs.
paralytic a. abasia due to paralysis.
paroxysmal trepidant a., spastic a. abasia due to spastic stiffening of the legs on attempting to stand.
trembling a., a. trepidans abasia due to trembling of the legs.
abatement (ə'baytmənt) decrease in severity of a pain or symptom.
ABC aspiration biopsy cytology.
abdomen ('abdəmən, ab'doh-) the belly. The portion of the body between the thorax and the pelvis. adj. **abdominal.** The abdominal cavity, which is separated from the chest area by the diaphragm, is lined with a serous membrane known as the peritoneum. Contained within the peritoneum are the stomach, large and small intestines, appendix, liver, gallbladder, spleen, pancreas, major vessels, and other structures. Outside the peritoneum, but still within the abdominal cavity, are the kidneys, suprarenal glands, ureters and bladder.
For descriptive purposes, its area can be divided into ten regions: (1) right hypochondriac; (2) epigastric; (3) left hypochondriac; (4) right lumbar; (5) umbilical; (6) left lumbar; (7) right iliac; (8) hypogastric; (9) left iliac; (10) pubic.
acute a., surgical a. an acute intra-abdominal condition of sudden onset, usually associated with pain due to inflammation, perforation, obstruction, infarction or rupture of abdominal organs, and usually requiring emergency surgical intervention.
pendulous a. a condition in which the anterior part of the abdominal wall hangs down over the pubis.
scaphoid (navicular) a. a hollowing of the anterior wall, commonly seen in grossly emaciated people.
abdomin(o)- word element. [L.] *abdomen.*
abdominal (ab'domin'l) pertaining to the abdomen.
a. aneurysm a dilation of the abdominal aorta.
a. aorta that part of the aorta below the diaphragm.
a. breathing deep breathing—hyperpnoea using abdominal muscles; respiration involving excursion of the abdominal wall.
a. reflex reflex contraction of abdominal wall muscles observed when skin is lightly stroked.
a. section incision through the abdominal wall.
abdominocentesis (abˌdominohsen'teesis) paracentesis of the abdomen (see also abdominal PARACENTESIS).
abdominocystic (abˌdominoh'sistik) pertaining to the abdomen and gallbladder.
abdominohysterectomy (abˌdominohˌhistə'rektəmee) hysterectomy through an abdominal incision.
abdominohysterotomy (abˌdominohˌhistə'rotəmee) hysterotomy through an abdominal incision.
abdominopelvic (abˌdominoh'pelvik) concerning the abdomen and the pelvic cavity.
abdominoperineal (abˌdominohˌperi'neeəl) pertaining to the abdomen and the perineum.
a. excision an operation performed via the abdomen and the perineum for the excision of the rectum or other pelvic organs.
abdominoposterior (abˌdominohpo'stiə·ri·ə) indicating a position of the fetus with its abdomen turned towards the maternal back.
abdominoscopy (abˌdomi'noskəpee) examination of the abdomen.
abdominovaginal (abˌdominohvə'jien'l, -'vajin'l) pertaining to the abdomen and vagina.
abduce (ab'dyoos) to abduct, or draw away.
abducens (ab'dyoosənz) [L.] *drawing away.* **a. nerve** the sixth cranial nerve; it arises from the pons and supplies the lateral rectus muscle of the eyeball, allowing for motion. Paralysis of the nerve causes diplopia (double vision).
abducent (ab'dyoosənt) drawing away; causing separation.
a. nerve the sixth cranial nerve, which supplies the lateral rectus muscle.
abduct (ab'dukt) to draw away from an axis or the median plane.
abduction (ab'dukshən) the act of drawing away from the centre; the state of being away from the centre.
abductor (ab'duktə) that which draws away.
Aberdeen formula ('abədeen) a method developed in Aberdeen in 1974 of estimating the number of nurses needed on a ward, based on the number and dependency of the patients. The formula is $W = N(B + T) + A + D + E$ where:
W = average weekly nursing workload in hours.
N = average number of patients in ward.
B = time in hours per week required to maintain the standard of basic nursing care for a totally helpless bedfast patient.
T = time required for technical nursing of the ward speciality expressed as a percentage of the time spent on basic nursing.
A = time per patient per week for administrative duties.
D = time per patient per week for domestic work.
E = patient dependency factor for ward speciality.
Throughout the exercise of calculating nurse staffing establishments, it is important to remember that the purpose is to measure the amount of *time* required to give patients an acceptable standard of basic nursing care.
Abernethy's sarcoma (ˌabə'nethiz) a malignant fatty tumour occurring mainly on the trunk.
aberrant (a'berənt) taking an unusual course. Used of blood vessels and nerves.
aberratio (ˌabə'rayshioh) [L.] *aberration.*
aberration (ˌabə'rayshən) 1. deviation from the normal or usual. 2. imperfect refraction or focusing of a lens.
chromatic a. unequal refraction by a lens of light rays of different wavelengths passing through it, producing a blurred image and a display of colours.

dioptric a., spherical a. inability of a spherical lens to bring all rays of light to a point focus.

abetalipoproteinaemia (ay,beetə,lipoh,prohti'neemi·ə) a hereditary syndrome marked by a lack of β-lipoproteins in the blood and by acanthocytosis, hypocholesterolaemia, progressive ataxic neuropathy, atypical retinitis pigmentosa involving the macula, and malabsorption.

ability (ə'bilitee) the power to perform an act, either mental or physical, with or without training.

innate a. the ability with which a person is born.

abiosis (,aybie'ohsis) absence or deficiency of life. adj. **abiotic.**

abiotrophy (,aybie'otrəfee) progressive loss of vitality of certain tissues or organs leading to disorders or loss of function; applied especially to degenerative hereditary diseases of late onset, e.g., Huntington's chorea. adj. **abiotrophic.**

abirritant (ab'iritənt) 1. diminishing irritation; soothing. 2. an agent that relieves irritation.

abirritation (,abiri'tayshən) diminished irritability; atony.

ablactation (,ablak'tayshən) weaning.

ablate (ab'layt) to destroy or remove.

ablation (ab'layshən) 1. separation or detachment; extirpation; eradication. 2. removal by cutting or other means.

ablepharon (ay'blefə·ron) congenital reduction or absence of the eyelids. adj. **ablepharous.**

ablutomania (ə,blootoh'mayni·ə) compulsion to wash oneself frequently.

abnormality (,abnaw'malitee) 1. the state of being unlike the usual condition. 2. a malformation.

ABO a blood group system (see BLOOD GROUP).

aborad (ab'or·rad) away from the mouth.

aboral (ab'or·rəl) opposite to, or remote from, the mouth.

abort (ə'bawt) to arrest prematurely a disease or developmental process; to expel the products of conception before the fetus is viable.

abortifacient (ə,bawti'fayshənt) 1. causing abortion. 2. an agent that induces abortion.

abortion (ə'bawshən) the threatened, inevitable or induced termination of pregnancy before 28 weeks' gestation, i.e. before the fetus is considered viable and given legal status in British law. Abortion may be *spontaneous* (when the lay term *miscarriage* is often used) or *induced* for therapeutic reasons, when it is usually referred to as *termination of pregnancy*.

TYPES OF ABORTION

Spontaneous Abortion. Threatened abortion is a form of spontaneous miscarriage when the disturbance to pregnancy is so slight that it is possible for the pregnancy to continue to term if symptoms do not increase. The initial indication is slight, painless bleeding per vaginam. Intermittent pain felt low in the abdomen or as backache may follow. The cervical os remains closed and fetal membranes remain intact. There are three possible outcomes:

(1) Signs and symptoms subside and the pregnancy continues to term. Fetal growth and well-being should be monitored closely because of reduced placental function from the area of separation which caused the bleeding.

(2) Symptoms increase and bleeding occurs freely, accompanied by painful uterine contractions. The fetal membranes may rupture, and the uterine os begins to dilate so that abortion becomes *inevitable.* If the gestational sac is expelled complete containing the embryo/fetus and placenta, the abortion is said to be *complete*; if part, or all, of the products of conception are retained within the uterus, the abortion is said to be *incomplete.* The latter is a serious condition which may result in haemorrhage or infection. Dilation and curettage is required to remove all the retained products of conception. *Habitual or recurrent abortion* occurs when a woman has had three, or more, consecutive spontaneous abortions.

(3) Pain and bleeding subside because the degree of placental separation has resulted in death of the embryo/fetus. However, the products of conception are not expelled spontaneously and remain within the uterus. This is called *missed abortion.* Frequently symptoms also disappear. Diagnosis is confirmed by ultrasound. The products of conception are usually expelled with the use of prostaglandins. Occasionally a *blood mole* forms, when the decidua capsularis remains intact, permitting the ovum within to be surrounded by layers of blood. A reddish-brown clot is formed, measuring about 10 cm in diameter. If this is retained within the uterus for several months, fluid is extracted from the clot and becomes organized into a hard fleshy mass, called a *carneous mole.* When cut, this has the appearance of a small placenta, but what seem to be cotyledons are blebs of amnion with blood underneath. A tiny embryo, measuring less than half a centimetre, may be found attached to a short cord. Blood and carneous moles may lead to hypofibrinogenaemia.

Induced Abortion. May be legally or criminally performed.

Legal (therapeutic) abortion must be undertaken within the terms of the 1967 Abortion Act by a qualified medical practitioner. In the UK, excluding Northern Ireland where the 1967 Abortion Act does not apply, only an NHS hospital or a nursing home approved for this purpose may be used. Written consent must be given by the woman. Two registered medical practitioners must agree and sign on an approved form, HSA1, that 'in their opinion formed in good faith the continuance of the pregnancy would involve risk to the life of the pregnant woman, or of injury to the physical or mental health of the pregnant woman or any existing children of her family, greater than if the pregnancy were terminated or that there is a substantial risk that if the child were born it would suffer from such physical or mental abnormalities as to be seriously handicapped'.

It is important that the woman receives adequate, impartial counselling concerning all the options available to her and the state benefits that she could claim should she decide to continue with her pregnancy. She should also be made aware of the possible side-effects of termination of pregnancy: haemorrhage, infection, incompetent cervix and quite marked depression (sometimes due to feelings of suppressed guilt).

The nurse who strongly objects to abortion is legally and morally free to choose not to participate in the procedure itself.

All legal abortions have to be notified to the Chief Medical Officers of England, Wales and Scotland by the medical practitioner who performs the abortion.

Criminal abortion, i.e. termination of pregnancy outside the terms of the 1967 Abortion Act, may be undertaken in unregistered premises or by unqualified personnel. The hazards are greatly increased because of the methods that may be used. The 1967 legislation has greatly reduced both the incidence of and the complications associated with this procedure.

TECHNIQUES OF INDUCED ABORTION. The technique chosen to terminate pregnancy depends on the stage of pregnancy at the time the abortion is done and the policies of the doctor and institution.

Menstrual Extraction. This method can be used when

the expected menstrual period is less than 14 days overdue. It is a form of suctioning in which a flexible cannula is inserted through an undilated cervix for the purpose of removing the fertilized ovum and endometrium. The cannula is attached to a syringe, which is used to aspirate the uterine contents and induce the onset of the 'missed period'. There is some objection to the use of this technique; it is not always effective and a second procedure may be required.

Suction Curettage. This is the procedure of choice in pregnancies of up to 12 weeks gestation, the optimum time being 8 to 10 weeks, by which time pregnancy has been definitely established and the cervix has softened and is more easily dilated. The procedure involves dilation of the cervix followed by vacuum suctioning of the uterus. Some doctors follow the dilation and suctioning with gentle scraping of the uterine wall to assure removal of all fragments of the fetal body, placenta, and amniotic sac. A common though not frequent complication is infection related to pre-existing vaginitis and pelvic inflammatory disease.

Intra-amniotic method. The injection of a hypertonic saline solution of prostaglandin, usually combined with urea, via a needle and catheter inserted directly into the amniotic sac, is one of the most frequently used procedures for the termination of pregnancy in the second trimester. Such later abortions may be necessary when the diagnosis of fetal abnormality has been made by amniocentesis performed at 14 to 16 weeks. The patient is hospitalized for this procedure, because she goes into labour and therefore requires continuous care during labour, delivery, and the postpartum period.

After insertion of the needle through the abdominal and uterine wall, approximately 200 ml of amniotic fluid is withdrawn and replaced with the prostaglandin and urea solution. Contractions usually begin about 6–8 hours after injection of the solution, and abortion commonly occurs within 12–14 hours. A continuous oxytocin IV infusion drip may be given to hasten delivery. Subsequent curettage may be required to assure complete removal of residual tissue. When the saline procedure is done, there is considerable risk of accidental intravenous injection of the saline, which may cause renal and cardiac difficulties, hypernatraemia, and cerebral convulsions.

Extra-amniotic method. Sometimes used as an alternative for termination of pregnancy during the second trimester. In the extra-amniotic method a Foley catheter is passed through into the cervix. The balloon attached to the catheter is then filled with water to ensure that it remains in place. A slow infusion of prostaglandin is commenced and abortion normally takes place between 18–30 hours following commencement of the infusion.

Hysterotomy. This procedure is similar to a caesarean section and carries a higher morbidity than does intra-amniotic injection. It is recommended only for rare cases in which an injection procedure is contraindicated.

complete a. complete spontaneous expulsion of all the products of conception from the uterus.

criminal a. termination of pregnancy outside the terms of the 1967 Abortion Act. The mortality from criminal abortions is tragically high because most of these patients wait until too late to seek medical attention and the measures used are drastic and often dangerous. The most frequent complications are severe haemorrhage, sepsis, renal failure, and septic shock.

early a. abortion within the first 12 weeks of pregnancy.

habitual a. spontaneous abortion occurring in three or more successive pregnancies.

idiopathic a. spontaneous abortion for which no recognized organic cause can be found.

incomplete a. abortion in which parts of the products of conception are retained in the uterus.

induced a. abortion brought on intentionally by medication or instrumentation. This term usually refers to legal rather than criminal abortion.

inevitable a. a condition in which vaginal bleeding has been profuse and the cervix has become dilated or the fetal membranes ruptured so that abortion will invariably occur.

infected a. abortion associated with infection of the genital tract, usually due to retained products from an incomplete abortion.

legal a. abortion induced legally by a registered medical practitioner for medical or other reasons under the terms of the 1967 Abortion Act.

missed a. retention of a dead embryo for more than 8 weeks. See also CARNEOUS MOLE.

septic a. abortion associated with serious infection of the uterus leading to generalized infection.

spontaneous a. abortion occurring naturally. It has been estimated that 10 to 12 per cent of all pregnancies end in spontaneous abortion. Habitual aborters are uncommon, but they account for the high percentage of abortions of this type. The woman who has repeated abortions should have a comprehensive examination to determine the cause of this disorder. Early antenatal care, under the supervision of an obstetrician, may prevent a recurrence of spontaneous termination of pregnancy.

When spontaneous abortion does occur, the patient should notify her doctor at once in order to prevent serious complications that may develop. Any material such as clots or bits of tissue should be saved for laboratory examination, in order to assess whether the abortion is complete or incomplete. Haemorrhage, shock, and infection are the most frequent hazards of spontaneous abortion. Treatment usually consists of dilation and curettage (see above) to remove tissues that may be retained in the uterus. If the abortion is complete, the attending doctor may consider a surgical procedure unnecessary. In any event the patient should consult her doctor at the first sign of bleeding or cramping during pregnancy.

threatened a. a condition in which vaginal bleeding and pain is less than in inevitable abortion and the cervix is not dilated; abortion may or may not occur.

tubal a. expulsion of the gestational sac, via the open, fimbriated end of the uterine tube into the abdominal cavity following ectopic pregnancy.

abortionist (ə'bawshənist) one who performs criminal abortions.

abortive (ə'bawtiv) 1. incompletely developed. 2. abortifacient.

abortus (ə'bawtəs) a dead or nonviable fetus (weighing less than 17 ounces, or 500 g, at birth).

ABPN Association of British Paediatric Nurses.

abrachia (ə'brayki·ə) congenital absence of the arms.

abrachiocephalia (əˌbraykiohke'fayli·ə, -se'fayli·ə) a developmental anomaly with absence of the head and arms.

abrasion (ə'brayzhən) a wound caused by rubbing or scraping the skin or mucous membrane. A 'skinned knee' and a 'rope burn' are common examples. To treat the injury, the wound should be cleansed and covered with sterile gauze.

abrasive (ə'braysiv) 1. causing abrasion. 2. an agent that produces abrasion.

abreaction (ˌabri'akshən) the reliving of an experience

in such a way that previously repressed emotions associated with it are released.

abruptio (ə'brupshioh) [L.] *separation*.

a. placentae premature separation of a normally situated placenta (see also PLACENTA).

abscess ('abses) a localized collection of pus in a cavity formed by the liquefactive disintegration of tissue and a large accumulation of polymorphonuclear leukocytes. Abscesses are usually caused by specific microorganisms that invade the tissues, often by way of small wounds or breaks in the skin. An abscess results from a natural defence mechanism in which the body attempts to localize and 'wall off' an area of tissue damage. When such tissue damage is created by specific microorganisms invading tissue, e.g. through a break in the skin, this limits and prevents their spread throughout the body. As the tissue is destroyed, an increased supply of blood is created by opening of arterioles and capillaries in the area. The cells, bacteria, and dead neutrophil polymorphs leave these dilated postcapillary venules and actively migrate into the tissue. They phagocytose particulate matter including bacteria and liberate enzymes which digest and liquefy the dead tissue. The abscess sometimes 'comes to a head' (localizes) by itself and breaks through the skin or other tissues, allowing the pus to drain. Local applications of heat may be used to facilitate localization and drainage.

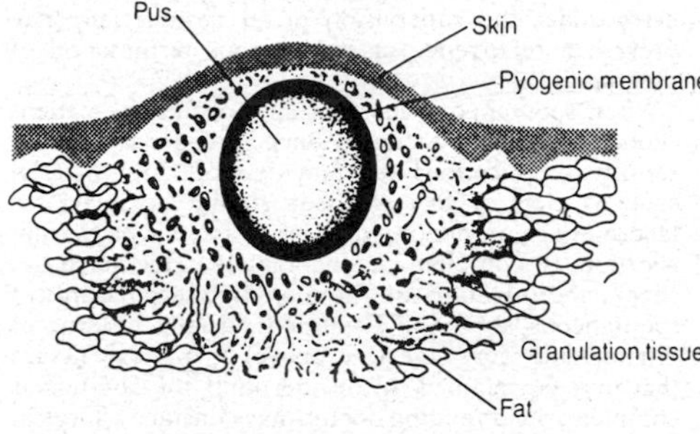

Abscess, cross-section

A skin abscess, no matter how small, should never be squeezed since pressure against the inflamed tissues is likely to spread the infection. Small abscesses frequently drain and heal themselves; larger abscesses and internal abscesses should always be treated by a surgeon, who may find it necessary to incise the abscess to allow for drainage of the exudate. Antibiotics often help combat the infection.

alveolar a. a localized suppurative inflammation of tissues about the apex of the root of a tooth.

amoebic a. an abscess cavity usually of the liver resulting from liquefaction necrosis due to entrance of *Entamoeba histolytica* into the portal circulation following amoebic infection of the colon (amoebic colitis); amoebic abscesses may also affect the lungs, brain, and spleen.

Bezold's a. one deep in the neck resulting from a complication of acute mastoiditis.

brain a. one in the brain as a result of extension of an infection (e.g., OTITIS MEDIA) from an adjacent area, or through bloodborne infection.

Brodie's a. a circumscribed abscess in bone, caused by haematogenous infection, that becomes a chronic nidus of infection.

cold a. one of slow development and with little acute inflammation, usually tuberculous.

diffuse a. a collection of pus not enclosed by a capsule.

gas a. one containing gas, caused by gas-forming bacteria such as *Clostridium welchii.* Called also Welch's abscess.

miliary a. one composed of numerous small collections of pus.

milk a. abscess of the breast occurring during lactation.

pancreatic a. one that occurs as a complication of acute pancreatitis or postoperative pancreatitis caused by secondary bacterial contamination.

perianal a. one beneath the skin of the anus and the anal canal.

peritonsillar a. a localized accumulation of pus in the peritonsillar tissue subsequent to suppurative inflammation of the tonsil; called also quinsy.

phlegmonous a. one associated with acute inflammation of the subcutaneous connective tissue.

primary a. one formed at the seat of the infection.

stitch a. one developed about a stitch or suture.

thecal a. one in the sheath of a tendon. **wandering a.** one that burrows into tissues and finally points at a distance from the site of origin.

Welch's a. gas abscess.

abscise (ab'siez) to cut off or remove.

abscissa (ab'sisə) the horizontal axis in a graph along which are plotted the units of one of the factors considered in the study, as time in a temperature–time study. The other (vertical) axis is called the ordinate. It is usual to plot the factor that can be independently varied on the abscissa and the other (dependent) variable on the ordinate.

abscission (ab'sizhən, -'sish-) removal of a part or growth by cutting.

abscopal (ab'skohp'l) pertaining to the effect on nonirradiated tissue resulting from irradiation of other tissues of the body.

absent-mindedness (absənt'miendidnəs) preoccupation to the extent of being unaware of one's immediate surroundings.

absorb (əb'sawb, -'zawb) 1. to take in or assimilate, as to take up substances into or across tissues, e.g., the skin or intestine. 2. to stop particles of radiation so that their energy is totally transferred to the absorbing material. 3. to stop the vibrating particles in an ultrasound beam so that their energy is converted into heat by the absorber.

absorbance (əb'sawbəns, -'zaw-) in radiology, a measure of the ability of a medium to absorb radiation, expressed as the logarithm of the quotient of the intensity of the radiation entering the medium divided by that leaving it.

absorbefacient (əb,sawbi'fayshənt, -,zaw-) 1. causing absorption. 2. an agent that promotes absorption.

absorbent (əb'sawbənt, -'zaw-) 1. able to take in, or suck up and incorporate. 2. a tissue structure involved in absorption. 3. a substance that absorbs or promotes absorption.

absorption (əb'sawpshən, -'zaw-) 1. the act of taking up or in by specific chemical or molecular action; especially the passage of liquids or other substances through a surface of the body into body fluids and tissues, as in the absorption of the end products of DIGESTION into the villi that line the intestine. 2. in psychology, devotion of thought to one object or activity only. 3. in radiology, uptake of energy by matter with which radiation or ultrasound interacts.

chemical a. any process by which one substance in liquid or solid form penetrates the surface of another substance.

a. coefficient the fraction of a beam of radiation that is absorbed in passing through a unit length of absorbing material.

digestive a. the passage of the end products of DIGESTION from the gastrointestinal tract into the blood and lymphatic vessels and the cells of tissues. Absorption of this kind can take place either by diffusion or by active transport.

radiation a. the dissipation of radiant energy as it passes through matter. This phenomenon is of particular importance in diagnostic and therapeutic radiology, which depends on the interaction between ionizing radiation and matter. As radiation passes through matter, it is absorbed by an amount dependent on the atomic and molecular structure and thickness of the substance, and the energy of the primary photons. If it passes through a medium of living or nonliving material without absorption (loss of energy), no biological or photographic effects can occur. In true absorption the photons of radiation waves give up or transfer all of their energy to electrons within the atoms of the matter through which they are passing. See also RADIATION.

ultrasound a. the absorption of sound of frequency greater than 20 kHz. Sound may be considered as vibrating particles. As a beam of sound passes through tissue, it is reduced in intensity by a combination of absorption, reflection, refraction and diffusion. In absorption, sound energy is converted into heat, the amount of heat generated depending on the frequency of the sound and the properties of the absorbing tissue.

absorptive (əb'sawptiv, -'zaw-) having the power of absorption; involving absorption.

abstinence ('abstinəns) a refraining from the use or indulgence in food, stimulants, or coitus.

a. syndrome withdrawal symptoms.

abstraction (ab'strakshən) 1. the mental process of forming abstract ideas. 2. the withdrawal of any ingredient from a compound.

abulia (ə'byooli·ə) loss or deficiency of will power, initiative, or drive. adj. **abulic.**

abuse (ə'byoos) misuse, maltreatment, or excessive use.

child a. see CHILD abuse.

drug a. use of illegal drugs or misuse of prescribed drugs.

solvent a. see SOLVENT ABUSE.

abutment (ə'butmənt) the anchorage tooth for a bridge.

Ac chemical symbol, *actinium.*

a.c. [L.] *ante cibum* (before meals).

acalculia (,aykal'kyooli·ə) inability to do mathematical calculations.

acampsia (ay'kampsi·ə) rigidity of a part or limb.

acanth(o)- word element. [Gr.] *sharp spine, thorn.*

acantha (ə'kanthə) 1. the spine. 2. a spinous process of a vertebra.

acanthaesthesia (ə,kanthis'theezi·ə) a sensation of a sharp point pricking the body.

acanthion (ə'kanthi·ən) a point at the base of the anterior nasal spine.

Acanthocephala (ə,kanthoh'kefələ, -sef-) a phylum of elongate, mostly cylindrical organisms (thorny-headed worms) parasitic in the intestines of all classes of vertebrates.

acanthocephaliasis (ə,kanthoh,kefə'lieəsis, -sef-) infection with worms of the phylum Acanthocephala.

acanthocyte (ə'kanthoh,siet) an erythrocyte with protoplasmic projections giving it a thorny appearance; seen in abetalipoproteinaemia.

acanthocytosis (ə,kanthohsie'tohsis) the presence in the blood of acanthocytes, characteristically seen in abetalipoproteinaemia.

acantholysis (,akən'tholisis) loss of cohesion between the cells of the prickle cell layer of the skin and between it and the layer above. adj. **acantholytic.**

a. bullosa epidermolysis bullosa.

acanthoma (,akən'thohmə) a tumour in the prickle cell layer of the skin.

acanthosis (,akən'thohsis) diffuse hypertrophy or thickening of the prickle cell layer of the skin. adj. **acanthotic.**

a. nigricans diffuse acanthosis with grey, brown, or black pigmentation, chiefly in the axillae and other body folds, occurring in an adult form, often associated with an internal carcinoma (called *malignant acanthosis nigricans*) and in a benign, naevoid form, more or less generalized. A benign form associated with obesity, which is sometimes due to endocrine disturbance, is called *pseudoacanthosis nigricans.*

acapnia (ay'kapni·ə) decrease of carbon dioxide in the blood. adj. **acapnic.**

acarbia (ay'kahbi·ə) decrease of bicarbonate in the blood.

acardia (ay'kahdi·ə) a developmental anomaly with absence of the heart.

acardiacus (,aykahdi'aykəs) [L.] *having no heart.*

acardius (ay'kahdiəs) an imperfectly formed twin fetus without a heart and invariably lacking other body parts.

acariasis (,akə'rieəsis) infestation with mites.

acaricide (a'karisied) an agent that destroys mites.

acarid ('akə·rid) a tick or a mite of the order Acarina.

Acarina (,akə'rienə) an order of arthropods (class Arachnoidea), comprising the mites and ticks.

acarinosis (,akə·ri'nohsis) any disease caused by mites; acariasis.

acarodermatitis (,akə·roh,dərmə'tietis) skin inflammation due to bites of parasitic mites (acarids).

acarophobia (,akə·roh'fohbi·ə) morbid dread or delusion of infestation by mites.

acatalasaemia (,aykatələ'seemi·ə) acatalasia.

acatalasia (,aykatə'layzi·ə) a rare hereditary disease seen mostly in the Japanese, marked by congenital absence of catalase; it may be associated with recurrent infections of oral structures.

acatalepsy (,ay'katə,lepsee) lack of understanding.

acatamathesia (,aykatəmə'theezi·ə) 1. loss or impairment of the power to understand speech. 2. impairment of any one of the perceptive faculties, due to a central lesion.

acataphasia (,aykatə'fayzi·ə) a speech disorder, with inability to express one's thoughts in a connected manner, due to a central lesion.

acathexia (,aykə'theksi·ə) inability to retain bodily secretions. adj. **acathectic.**

accelerator (ak'selə,raytə) [L.] an agent or apparatus that increases the rate at which something occurs or progresses.

a. globulin clotting factor V.

serum prothrombin conversion a. (SPCA) clotting factor VII.

acceptable risk (ak'septəb'l) see under RISK.

acceptor (ak'septə, ək-) a substance that unites with another substance.

hydrogen a. the molecule accepting hydrogen in an oxidation–reduction reaction.

accessory (ak'sesə·ri, ək-) supplementary or affording aid to another similar and generally more important thing.

a. nerve the eleventh cranial nerve; it originates in the medulla oblongata and provides motion for the sternocleidomastoid and trapezius muscles of the neck. Called also spinal accessory nerve.

accident prone ('aksidənt ,prohn) especially susceptible to accidents due to psychological factors.

accipiter (ak'sipitə) a facial bandage with tails like the claws of a hawk.

acclimation (ˌakli'mayshən) the process of becoming accustomed to a new environment.

accommodation (əˌkomə'dayshən) adjustment, especially adjustment of the eye for focusing on objects at various distances. This is accomplished by the ciliary muscle, which controls the shape of the LENS of the eye, allowing it to flatten or thicken as is needed for distant or near vision.

absolute a. the accommodation of either eye separately.

amplitude of a. the total amount of accommodative power of the eye; the difference in refractive power of the eye when adjusted for near and for far vision. The amplitude diminishes as age increases because elasticity of the lens is decreased. Called also *range of accommodation*.

histological a. changes in morphology and function of cells following changed conditions.

negative a. adjustment of the eye for long distances by relaxation of the ciliary muscle.

positive a. adjustment of the eye for short distances by contraction of the ciliary muscle.

a. reflex the coördinated changes that occur when the eye adapts itself for near vision; they are constriction of the pupil, convergence of the eyes, and ciliary muscle contraction, causing increased convexity of the lens.

accouchement (ə'kooshmonh) [Fr.] *childbirth*, *delivery*, *labour*.

a. forcé rapid forcible vaginal delivery by one of several methods; originally, rapid dilation of the cervix with the hands, followed by version and extraction of the fetus. Now considered unsafe practice.

accountable (ə'kowntəb'l) liable to be held responsible for a course of action. In nursing this refers to the responsibility the trained nurse takes for prescribing and initiating nursing care. The nurse is accountable to his/her patient, his/her peers, his/her employing authority.

accretion (ə'kreeshən) 1. growth by addition of material. 2. accumulation. 3. adherence of parts normally separated.

accumulator (ə'kyoomyuhˌlaytə) an apparatus for the collection and storage of electricity. A battery consisting of metal plates in an ionic solution that can be recharged.

ACE inhibitors (ays in'hibitəz) a new group of drugs used in the treatment of hypertension. Their name, angiotensin converting enzyme inhibitors, explains part of their mode of action, though it is thought that some of their other actions may also be important in reducing blood pressure.

acebutolol (ˌasi'byootəlol) a cardioselective beta-blocker having a greater effect on β_1-adrenergic receptors than β_2-adrenergic receptors.

acellular (ay'selyuhlə) not cellular in structure.

acentric (ay'sentrik) 1. not central; not located in the centre. 2. lacking a centromere, so that the chromosome will not survive cell divisions.

acephalic (ˌaykə'falik, -sə-) without a head.

acephalobrachia (ayˌkefəloh'brayki·ə, -ˌsef-) congenital absence of the head and arms.

acephalocardia (ayˌkefəloh'kahdi·ə, -ˌsef-) congenital absence of the head and heart.

acephalocardius (ayˌkefəloh'kahdi·əs, -ˌsef-) a fetus or infant without a head or heart.

acephalochiria (ayˌkefəloh'kieri·ə, -ˌsef-) congenital absence of the head and hands.

acephalogaster (ayˌkefəloh'gastə, -ˌsef-) a fetus without a head or stomach.

acephalogastria (ayˌkefəloh'gastri·ə, -ˌsef-) congenital absence of the head, chest, and stomach.

acephalopodia (ayˌkefəloh'pohdi·ə, -ˌsef-) congenital absence of the head and feet.

acephalopodius (ayˌkefəloh'pohdi·əs, -ˌsef-) a fetus without a head or feet.

acephalorachia (ayˌkefəloh'rayki·ə, -ˌsef-) congenital absence of the head and vertebral column.

acephalostomia (ayˌkefəloh'stohmi·ə, -ˌsef-) congenital absence of the head, with the mouth aperture on the upper aspect of the body.

acephalothoracia (ayˌkefəlohthor'rayki·ə, -ˌsef-) congenital absence of the head and thorax.

acephalous (ay'kefələs, -'sef-) headless.

acephalus (ay'kefələs, -'sef-) a headless fetus.

acervuline (ə'sərvyuhˌleen) aggregated; heaped up; said of certain glands.

acervulus (ə'sərvyuhˌləs) pl. *acervuli* [L.] sandy matter in or about the pineal body and other parts of the brain.

acetabular (ˌasi'tabyuhlə) pertaining to the acetabulum.

acetabulectomy (ˌasiˌtabyuh'lektəmee) excision of the acetabulum.

acetabuloplasty (ˌasi'tabyuhlohˌplastee) plastic repair of the acetabulum.

acetabulum (ˌasi'tabyuhləm) the cup-shaped cavity on the lateral surface of the hip bone, receiving the head of the femur.

acetal ('asiˌtal) an organic compound formed by a combination of an aldehyde with an alcohol.

acetaldehyde (ˌasi'taldiˌhied) a colourless volatile liquid, CH_3CHO, that is irritating to mucous membranes and has a general narcotic action. It is also an intermediate in the metabolism of alcohol.

acetanilide (ˌasi'tanilied) a white powder, slightly soluble in water, used previously as an analgesic and antipyretic. It has now been replaced by safer analgesics.

acetate ('asiˌtayt) a salt of acetic acid.

acetazolamide (əˌsetə'zoləmied) a diuretic of the carbonic anhydrase inhibitor type, useful in the treatment of cardiac oedema. It is used primarily to reduce intraocular pressure in the treatment of glaucoma. Side-effects may include paraesthesia of the limbs and gastrointestinal disturbances.

Acetest ('asiˌtest) trademark for reagent tablets containing sodium nitroprusside, aminoacetic acid, disodium phosphate, and lactose. A drop of urine is placed on a tablet on a sheet of white paper; if significant quantities of acetone are present the tablet changes from a purple tint (1+), to lavender (2+), to moderate purple (3+), or to deep purple (4+).

acetic (ə'seetik) pertaining to vinegar or its acid; sour.

a. acid a short-chain, saturated fatty acid, the characteristic component of vinegar. It has the odour of vinegar and a sharp acid taste. A 36.5 per cent solution of acetic acid is used topically as a caustic and rubefacient. A dilute acetic acid solution (6 per cent) may be used as an antidote to alkali. Glacial acetic acid is a 99.4 per cent solution.

acetoacetic acid (ˌasitoh·ə'seetik, əˌsee-) one of the KETONE BODIES formed in the body in metabolism of certain substances, particularly in the liver in the combustion of fats. It is present in the body in increased amounts in abnormal conditions such as uncontrolled DIABETES MELLITUS and starvation.

acetohexamide (ˌasitoh'heksəmied, əˌsee-) an oral hypoglycaemic.

acetonaemia (ˌasitə'neemi·ə, əˌsee-) ketonaemia.

acetone ('asiˌtohn) a compound, CH_3COCH_3, with solvent properties and characteristic odour, obtained by fermentation or produced synthetically; it is a by-product of acetoacetic acid. Acetone is one of the KETONE BODIES produced in abnormal amounts in uncontrolled DIABETES MELLITUS and metabolic ACIDOSIS. See also KETOSIS.

a. bodies acetone, acetoacetic acid, and beta-oxybutyric acid, being intermediates in fat metabolism. Also called KETONE BODIES.

acetonuria (,asitə'nyooə·ri·ə, ə,see-) ketonuria.

acetrizoate sodium (,asitrie'zoh·ayt 'sohdiəm) the sodium salt of acetrizoic acid, formerly used as a contrast medium but now largely superseded by safer compounds.

acetyl ('asitil, -,tiel, ə'seetiel) the monovalent radical, CH_3CO, a combining form of acetic acid.

acetylator (ə'seti,laytə) an organism capable of metabolic acetylation. Individuals that differ in their inherited ability to metabolize certain drugs, e.g., isoniazid, are termed fast or slow acetylators.

acetylcholine (,asitiel'kohleen, ,asitil-) the acetic acid ester of choline, normally present in many parts of the body and having important physiological functions. It is a neurotransmitter at cholinergic synapses in the central, sympathetic, and parasympathetic nervous systems. Used in medicine as a miotic. Abbreviated ACh.

acetylcholinesterase (,asitiel,kohlin'estə·rayz, ,asitil-) an enzyme present in nervous tissue, muscle, and red cells that catalyses the hydrolysis of acetylcholine to choline and acetic acid; called also CHOLINESTERASE. Abbreviated AChE.

acetylcoenzyme A (,asitielkoh'enziem, ,asitil-) acetyl-CoA, an important biochemical intermediate in the tricarboxylic acid (Krebs) cycle and the chief precursor of lipids; it is formed by the attachment to coenzyme A of an acetyl group during the oxidation of pyruvate, fatty acids, or amino acids.

acetylcysteine (,asitiel'sisti·een, -'sistayn, ,asitil-) a mucolytic agent used to reduce the viscosity of secretions of the respiratory tract and in paracetamol overdosage.

acetylene (ə'seti,leen) a colourless, combustible, explosive gas, the simplest triple-bonded hydrocarbon.

acetylsalicylic acid ('asitiel,salisilik, ,asitil) aspirin, a commonly used analgesic, antipyretic, and antirheumatic drug. It is available in pure form or in combination with a variety of drugs.

AcG accelerator globulin (clotting factor V).

ACh acetylcholine.

achalasia (akə'layzi·ə) failure to relax of the smooth muscle fibres of the gastrointestinal tract at any junction of one part with another; especially failure of the lower oesophagus to relax with swallowing, due to degeneration of ganglion cells in the wall of the organ.

The cause of achalasia is unknown, but anxiety and emotional tension seem to aggravate the condition and precipitate attacks. As the condition progresses there is dilation of the oesophagus (megaoesophagus) above the constriction and loss of peristalsis in the lower two-thirds of the organ.

SYMPTOMS. The patient complains of progressive dysphagia and a feeling of fullness in the sternal region; vomiting frequently occurs, and there may be aspiration of the oesophageal contents into the respiratory passages. As a result of this aspiration the patient may develop pneumonia or atelectasis.

Diagnosis is confirmed by x-ray studies using barium and by visual examination of the area by oesophagoscope.

TREATMENT. Conservative treatment of mild cases consists of advising the patient to eat a bland diet that is low in bulk. Very large meals should be avoided and all foods should be eaten slowly with frequent drinking of fluids during the meal. To reduce the possibility of aspiration of oesophageal contents during sleep, the patient is instructed to sleep with his head and shoulders elevated.

For severe constriction surgical relief may be necessary. The incision, which includes the lower oesophagus and upper stomach wall, is made down to but not through the intestinal mucosa. This allows for stretching of the mucosa to accommodate food passing through. Approach is made through an incision into the chest; thus, preoperative care and postoperative care are the same as for elective chest surgery (see also THORACIC SURGERY).

AChE acetylcholinesterase.

ache (ayk) 1. continuous pain, as opposed to sharp pangs or twinges. An ache can be either dull and constant, as in some types of backache, or throbbing, as in some types of headache and toothache. 2. to suffer such pain.

acheilia (ay'kieli·ə) a developmental anomaly with absence of the lips. adj. **acheilous**.

acheiria (ay'kieri·ə) 1. a developmental anomaly with absence of the hands. 2. a sensation of loss of the hands, seen in hysteria.

acheiropodia (ay,kieroh'pohdi·ə) a developmental anomaly characterized by absence of both hands and feet.

Achilles tendon (ə'kileez ,tendən) the strong tendon at the back of the heel that connects the calf muscles (triceps surae muscle) to the heel bone. The name is derived from the legend of the Greek hero Achilles, who was vulnerable only in one heel. Tapping the Achilles tendon normally produces the Achilles REFLEX, or ankle jerk. Failure or exaggeration of this reflex indicates disease or injury to the nerves of the leg muscles or of a part of the spinal cord.

achillobursitis (ə,kilohbər'sietis) inflammation of the bursae about the Achilles tendon.

achillodynia (ə,kiloh'dini·ə) pain in the Achilles tendon or its bursa.

achillorrhaphy (,aki'lo·rəfee) suturing of the Achilles tendon.

achillotenotomy, achillotomy (ə,kilohte'notəmee; ,aki'lotəmee) surgical division of the Achilles tendon.

plastic a. a plastic operation undertaken to lengthen the Achilles tendon.

achlorhydria (,ayklor'hiedri·ə) absence of hydrochloric acid in gastric juice; associated with PERNICIOUS ANAEMIA, stomach cancer, and pellagra. adj. **achlorhydric**.

achloropsia (,ayklor'ropsi·ə) inability to distinguish green colours.

acholia (ay'kohli·ə) lack or absence of bile secretion. adj. **acholic**.

acholuria (,aykə'lyooə·ri·ə) absence of bile pigments from the urine.

acholuric (,aykə'lyooə·rik) pertaining to acholuria.

a. jaundice jaundice without bile in the urine.

achondroplasia (ay,kondroh'playzi·ə) a hereditary disorder of cartilage formation in the fetus, leading to a type of DWARFISM. adj. **achondroplastic**.

achromasia (,aykroh'mayzi·ə) 1. lack of normal skin pigmentation. 2. the inability of tissues or cells to be stained.

achromat ('akrə,mat) 1. an achromatic objective. 2. monochromat.

achromatic (,akrə'matik, ,aykroh-) 1. producing no discoloration, or staining with difficulty. 2. refracting light without decomposing it into its component colours. Called also *apochromatic*. 3. pertaining to complete lack of colour discrimination. 4. monochromatic (2).

achromatin (ay'krohmətin) that part of the cell nucleus

not readily coloured by basic dyes (see CHROMATIN).

achromatism (ay'krohmə,tizəm, ə'krohmə-) 1. the quality or the condition of being achromatic. 2. monochromatism.

achromatophil (,aykroh'matəfil) 1. not easily stainable. 2. an organism or tissue that does not stain easily.

achromatopia (,aykrohmə'tohpi·ə) monochromatism. adj. **achromatopic.**

achromatopsia (,aykrohmə'topsi·ə) complete inability to distinguish colours.

achromatosis (,aykrohmə'tohsis) 1. deficiency of pigmentation in the tissues. 2. lack of staining power in a cell or tissue.

achromatous (ay'krohmətəs, ə-) colourless.

achromaturia (,aykrohmə'tyooə·ri·ə) colourless state of the urine.

achromia (ay'krohmi·ə) the lack or absence of normal colour or pigmentation, as of the skin. adj. **achromic.**

a. parasitica a term applied to the nonpigmented or whitish variety of macular patches occurring in tinea versicolor.

achromophil (ay'krohmə,fil) achromatophil.

Achromycin (,akroh'miesin) trademark for preparations of tetracycline hydrochloride, a broad-spectrum antibiotic.

achylia (ay'kieli·ə) absence of hydrochloric acid and enzymes in the gastric secretions.

achylous (ay'kieləs) deficient in chyle.

achymia (ay'kiemi·ə) deficiency of chyme.

acicular (ə'sikyuhlə) needle-shaped.

acid ('asid) 1. sour. 2. a substance that yields hydrogen ions in solution and from which hydrogen may be displaced by a metal to form a salt. All acids react with bases to form salts and water (neutralization). Other properties of acids include a sour taste and the ability to cause certain dyes to undergo a colour change. A common example of this is the ability of acids to change litmus paper from blue to red.

Inorganic acids are distinguished as *binary* or *hydracids*, and *ternary* or *oxacids*; the former contain no oxygen; in the latter, the hydrogen is united to an electronegative element by oxygen. The hydracids are distinguished by the prefix *hydro-*. The names of acids end in *-ic*, except in the case in which there are two degrees of oxygenation. The acid containing the greater amount of oxygen has the termination *-ic*, the one having the lesser amount has the termination *-ous*. Acids with the termination *-ic* form the salts ending in *-ate*; those ending in *-ous* form the salts ending in *-ite*. The salts of hydracids end in *-ide*. These rules are demonstrated by the acids and salts: hydrochloric acid (HCl), sodium chloride (NaCl), sulphuric acid (H_2SO_4), sodium sulphate (Na_2SO_4), sulphurous acid (H_2SO_3), sodium sulphite (Na_2SO_3). Acids are called *monobasic*, *dibasic*, *tribasic*, or *tetrabasic*, depending on whether they contain one, two, three or four replaceable hydrogen atoms, respectively.

The most common organic acids are carboxylic acids, containing the carboxyl group (—COOH); examples are acetic acid, citric acid, amino acids, and fatty acids. Their salts and esters end in *-ate*, e.g., ethyl acetate. Other organic acids are phenols and sulphonic acids.

Acids play a vital role in the chemical processes that are a normal part of the functions of the cells and tissues of the body. A stable balance between acids and bases in the body is essential to life. (See also ACID–BASE BALANCE.) For the various acids, see under the specific name, such as acetic acid.

amino a. any one of a class of organic compounds containing the amino and the carboxyl groups, occurring naturally in plant and animal tissues and forming the chief constituents of protein. See also AMINO ACID.

bile a's steroid acids derived from cholesterol. See also BILE ACIDS.

a. burn injury to tissues caused by an acid, such as sulphuric acid or nitric acid. Emergency first aid for an acid burn of the skin includes (1) immediate and thorough washing of the burn with water; (2) calling a doctor; and (3) continued bathing of the burn in water until the doctor arrives. See also BURN.

fatty a. any monobasic aliphatic acid containing only carbon, hydrogen, and oxygen. See also FATTY ACID.

inorganic a. an acid containing no carbon atoms.

keto a's compounds containing the groups CO (carbonyl) and COOH (carboxyl).

nucleic a's substances that constitute the prosthetic groups of the nucleoproteins and contain phosphoric acid, sugars, and purine and pyrimidine bases. See also NUCLEIC ACIDS.

a. perfusion test Bernstein test.

a. phosphatase a lysosomal enzyme that hydrolyses phosphate esters liberating inorganic phosphate and has an optimal pH of about 5.0. Serum activity of the prostatic isoenzyme is greatly increased in metastatic cancer of the prostate and is used to monitor the course of the disease.

acid–base balance ('asid,bays) a state of equilibrium between acidity and alkalinity of the body fluids; also called hydrogen ion (H^+) balance because, by definition, an acid is a substance capable of giving up a hydrogen ion during a chemical exchange, and a base is a substance that can accept it. The positively charged hydrogen ion (H^+) is the active constituent of all acids.

Most of the body's metabolic processes produce acids as their end products, but a somewhat alkaline body fluid is required as a medium for vital cellular activities. Therefore chemical exchanges of hydrogen ions must take place continuously in order to maintain a state of equilibrium. An optimal pH (hydrogen ion concentration) between 7.35 and 7.45 must be maintained; otherwise, the enzyme systems and other biochemical and metabolic activities will not function normally.

Although the body can tolerate and compensate for slight deviations in acidity and alkalinity, if the pH drops below 7.30, the potentially serious condition of ACIDOSIS exists. If the pH increases to more than 7.50, the patient is in a state of ALKALOSIS. In either case the disturbance of the acid–base balance is considered serious, even though there are control mechanisms by which the body can compensate for an upward or downward change in the pH. Shifts in the pH of body fluids are controlled by three major regulatory systems which may be classified as *chemical* (the buffer systems), *biological* (blood and cellular activity), and *physiological* (the lungs and kidneys).

CHEMICAL CONTROLS. The chemical buffer systems are dependent on the capability of certain substances to either combine with or release hydrogen ions. In the plasma and the intracellular and interstitial fluids there are three major buffer systems that regulate hydrogen ion activity: the carbonic acid-bicarbonate system, the protein buffer system, and the phosphate buffer system.

Of these three, the *carbonic acid–bicarbonate system* is the most important in fluids outside the cell. It is the most extensive and is the first to react to an acid-base imbalance. Carbonic acid and bicarbonate are both derived from water and carbon dioxide and therefore exist in large quantities in the body. Carbonic acid is, however, weakly ionized and needs to coexist with its salt in order to effectively remove excess hydrogen or hydroxyl ions from the extracellular fluids. Hence it is actually the *carbonic acid and sodium bicarbonate* buffer system that works to maintain normal levels of hydrogen ion concentrations in the extracellular fluids. It is important to remember that these two chemical components must be in the ratio of 1:20; that is, for every one part of carbonic acid (H_2CO_3) there must be twenty parts of sodium bicarbonate ($NaHCO_3$). It is not the absolute amount of each component that is crucial in the control of acid–base balance, but the ratio of the one substance to the other. The carbonic acid–bicarbonate buffer system is capable of either accepting or releasing hydrogen ions without forcing the pH to dangerous levels.

The *protein buffer system* is especially remarkable because proteins are powerful buffers that can function as either acid or base, depending on the state of the body fluids. This system is active in the plasma and in intracellular and extracellular fluids.

The *phosphate buffer system* operates in much the same way as the carbonic acid–bicarbonate system but is more active within the cell than in extracellular fluids. It is important in the regulation of pH in the red blood cells and kidney tubular fluids.

Although the chemical buffer systems react almost instantaneously to a change in the pH of the body fluids, they cannot provide sustained regulation of the pH because they are absorbed rapidly and cannot be replaced immediately. The hydrogen ions that are not handled by the chemical buffer systems become the responsibility of other regulatory controls which respond less rapidly but are not less important.

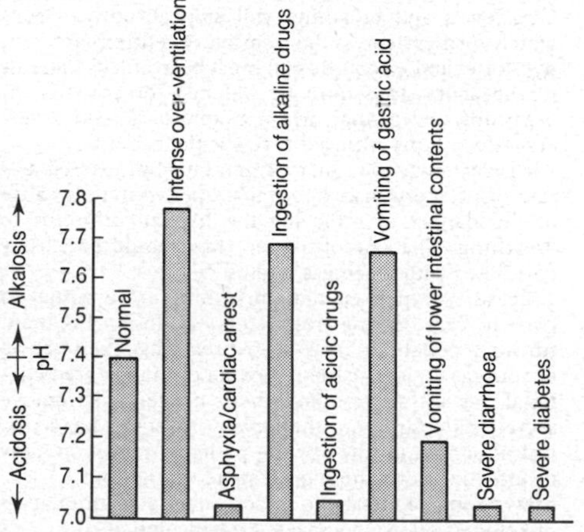

pH of the extracellular fluid in various acid-base disorders.

Biological Regulators. This type of control is concerned with the shifting of excess acid or alkali in and out of the cell. As excess ions cross over the cell membrane they must do so in combination with ions of the opposite charge, or in exchange for ions of the same charge. Sodium and potassium are the two cations most often exchanged for the positively charged hydrogen ion.

The haemoglobin–oxyhaemoglobin system is another regulatory control. As chloride leaves the oxygenated blood cells and enters the plasma, the bicarbonate moves from the plasma and crosses over into the cellular fluid. This reciprocal exchange between bicarbonate and chloride is a continuous process.

Physiological Regulators. The lungs begin to compensate for an acid–base imbalance within minutes of its onset. They do this by regulating the retention or the excretion of carbon dioxide. If acidosis is present, respiratory activity is increased so that CO_2 is blown off before it unites with the water in the blood to form carbonic acid. If alkalosis is present, respiratory activity is automatically decreased, CO_2 is retained, and carbonic acid is produced to neutralize the excess alkali.

The kidneys act as regulators by reabsorbing bicarbonate when it is needed to control excess acidity and by excreting it when there is a deficit of acid in the body. The kidneys also facilitate the excretion of excess hydrogen ions in combination with phosphate ions (in the form of phosphoric acid), or in combination with ammonia (excreted in the form of ammonium).

Imbalances of the acid–base ratio are discussed under acidosis and alkalosis. Diagnosis and monitoring of either of these conditions are greatly enhanced by periodic determination of the pH and by blood gas analysis.

acid-fast ('asid,fahst) not readily decolorized by acids after staining; said of bacteria, especially *Mycobacterium tuberculosis.*

acid-proof ('asid,proof) acid-fast.

acidaemia (,asi'deemi·ə) abnormal acidity of the blood.

acidic (ə'sidik) of or pertaining to an acid; acid-forming.

acidifier (ə'sidi,fie·ə) an agent that causes acidity; a substance used to increase gastric acidity.

acidity (ə'siditee) 1. the quality of being acid; the power to unite with positively charged ions or with basic substances. 2. excess acid quality, as of the gastric juice.

acidophil ('asidoh,fil, ə'sidə-) 1. a histological structure, cell, or other element staining readily with acid dyes. 2. an alpha cell of the anterior lobe of the pituitary gland or the pancreatic islets. 3. an organism that grows well in highly acid media. 4. acidophilic.

acidophilic (,asidoh'filik, ə,sidə-) 1. easily stained with acid dyes. 2. growing best on acid media.

acidosis (,asi'dohsis) a pathological condition resulting from accumulation of acid or depletion of the alkaline reserve (bicarbonate content) in the blood and body tissues, and characterized by increase in hydrogen ion concentration (decrease in pH). adj. **acidotic.** The optimal acid–base balance is maintained by chemical buffers, biological activities of the cells, and effective functioning of the lungs and kidneys. The opposite of acidosis is alkalosis.

It is rare that acidosis occurs in the absence of some underlying disease process but in cases of mild acidosis the symptoms may be overlooked. The more obvious signs of severe acidosis are muscle twitching, involuntary movement, cardiac arrhythmias, disorientation and coma.

In general, treatment consists of intravenous or oral administration of sodium bicarbonate or sodium lactate solutions and correction of the underlying cause of the imbalance. Many cases of severe acidosis can be prevented by careful monitoring of the patient whose primary illness predisposes him to respiratory problems or metabolic derangements that can cause increased levels of acidity or decreased bicarbonate levels. Such care includes effective teaching of self-care to the diabetic so that the disease remains under control. Patients receiving intravenous therapy, especially those having a fluid deficit, and those with biliary or intestinal intubation should be watched closely for early signs of acidosis. Others predisposed to acidosis are patients with shock, cardiac arrest, advanced circulatory failure, renal failure, respiratory disorders or liver disease.

compensated a. a condition in which the compensatory mechanisms have returned the pH toward normal.

diabetic a. a metabolic ACIDOSIS produced by accumulation of ketones in uncontrolled DIABETES MELLITUS.

hypercapnic a. respiratory acidosis.

hyperchloraemic a. renal tubular acidosis.

metabolic a. acidosis resulting from accumulation in the blood of keto acids (derived from fat metabolism) at the expense of bicarbonate, thus diminishing the body's ability to neutralize acids. This type of acidosis can occur when there is an acid gain, as in diabetic ketoacidosis, lactic acidosis, poisoning, and failure of the renal tubules to reabsorb bicarbonate. It can also result from bicarbonate loss due to diarrhoea or a gastrointestinal fistula.

The symptoms of metabolic acidosis include weakness, malaise, and headache. As the acid level goes up these symptoms progress to stupor, unconsciousness, coma, and death. The breath of the patient may have a fruity odour owing to the presence of acetone, and he may experience vomiting and diarrhoea. Loss of fluids can deplete his fluid content and aggravate the acidosis. Hyperventilation may occur as a result of stimulation of the hypothalamus. BLOOD GAS ANALYSIS will reveal a lowered pH and an elevated $P_{a}CO_2$.

TREATMENT AND PATIENT CARE. Treatment of metabolic acidosis is primarily concerned with control of the underlying causes. Diabetic ketoacidosis may be corrected by the administration of insulin and fluids. In acute renal failure the patient requires DIALYSIS, and in chronic uraemic acidosis the condition is controlled by restricting sodium intake and buffering with bicarbonate.

The patient's condition must be regularly assessed to monitor the effect of treatment. Alkalosis may ensue if the body's compensatory mechanisms combine with drugs and fluids to overcorrect the acidosis. A rising pulse rate may indicate respiratory compensation, a drop in blood pressure may indicate hypervolaemia or fluid overload. A rapid respiratory rate may indicate the body's attempt to blow off acid as carbon dioxide.

A careful recording of intake and output provides a means of determining the kidneys' ability to regulate the ACID–BASE BALANCE. Safety measures to avoid injury during involuntary muscular contractions should be carried out. (See also CONVULSIONS.) Mouth care using an alkaline mouthwash reduces the discomfort from mouth acids. Nursing measures to relieve discomfort from vomiting and to avoid the hazards of aspiration of vomitus are required. Education of the patient and his family in the prevention of acute episodes of metabolic acidosis is of primary importance.

renal tubular a. a metabolic acidosis resulting from impairment of the reabsorption of bicarbonate by the renal tubules, the urine being alkaline.

respiratory a. acidosis resulting from ventilatory impairment and subsequent retention of carbon dioxide. The respiratory system has an important role in maintaining acid-base equilibrium. In response to an increase in the hydrogen ion concentration in body fluids, the respiratory rate increases, causing more carbon dioxide to be released from the lung. When either an acute obstruction of the airways or a chronic condition involving the organs of respiration causes interference with the exhalation of the carbon dioxide produced by metabolic activity, carbon dioxide accumulates in the blood and unites with water to form carbonic acid.

Acute respiratory acidosis occurs when there is a relatively sudden malfunction of respiratory activities, as in upper airway obstruction, acute infections and inflammation of the lung and bronchial tissues, and pulmonary oedema. In acute respiratory acidosis the compensatory chemical buffer systems are of limited benefit in restoring the ACID–BASE BALANCE because they depend on normal blood circulation and tissue perfusion for optimal effect. The physiological regulators, the lungs and kidneys, are of little help because the lungs are malfunctioning and the kidneys require more time to compensate than the acute condition permits.

Chronic respiratory acidosis results from gradual and irreversible loss of ventilatory function, as in CHRONIC OBSTRUCTIVE AIRWAYS DISEASE (COAD). Although the patient in this condition does have an increased retention of CO_2, there is time for the kidneys to compensate by retaining bicarbonate and thereby maintaining a pH within tolerable limits. If, however, the patient develops even a minor respiratory infection, he is subject to a rapidly developing state of acute acidosis because his lungs cannot be depended upon to remove more than a minimal amount of CO_2.

TREATMENT AND PATIENT CARE. The initial treatment for acute respiratory acidosis is to establish an airway immediately and maintain adequate ventilation and hydration. Acute cases may require the use of an ENDOTRACHEAL TUBE or TRACHEOSTOMY tube. INTERMITTENT POSITIVE PRESSURE VENTILATION (IPPV) is used to avoid CO_2 narcosis. Beyond a certain point the respiratory centre may cease responding to the higher CO_2 levels and breathing will stop abruptly. Drugs which further depress the respiratory centre (narcotics, hypnotics and tranquillizers) must be avoided. Patients in the acute stage must be watched for cessation of breathing and cardiac arrest. CARDIOPULMONARY RESUSCITATION may be required to revive the patient.

It is recommended that oxygen be administered at a rate of no more than 1 to 2 litres per minute because of the danger of removing the hypoxic stimulus to breathing. The rate of oxygen flow should be closely correlated with blood gas studies.

Measures which facilitate breathing are essential to patient care during respiratory acidosis. Frequent turning, coughing, and deep breathing exercises to encourage oxygen–carbon dioxide exchange are beneficial, as is SUCTIONING when needed to remove secretions obstructing the airway. POSTURAL DRAINAGE, unless contraindicated by the patient's condition, may be effective in promoting adequate ventilation.

starvation a. a metabolic acidosis due to accumulation of ketones following a severe calorific deficit.

acidulous (ə'sidyuhləs) moderately sour.

acidum ('asiduhm) [L.] *acid.*

aciduria (ˌasi'dyooə·ri·ə) the excretion of acid in the urine. See also specific forms, such as aminoaciduria, orotic aciduria, etc.

acinar ('asiˌnah) pertaining to or affecting an acinus or acini.

acinetic (ˌaysi'netik) akinetic.

aciniform (ə'siniˌfawm) grapelike.

acinitis (ˌasi'nietis) inflammation of the acini of a gland.

acinose, acinous ('asiˌnohz; 'asinəs) made up of acini.

acinus ('asinəs) pl. *acini* [L.] any of the smallest lobules of a compound gland.

liver a. the smallest functional unit of the liver, a mass of liver parenchyma that is supplied by terminal branches of the portal vein and hepatic artery and drained by a terminal branch of the bile duct.

aclasia, aclasis (ay'klaysi·ə; ay'klaysis) pathological continuity of structure, as in chondrodystrophy.

diaphyseal a. a condition in which there is abnormal bone structure in the cartilage between the epiphysis and diaphysis; a form of dyschondroplasia in which bone development is impaired in fetal cartilage.

acleistocardia (ay,kliestoh'kahdi·ə) an open state of the foramen ovale of the fetal heart.

acme ('akmee) the critical stage or crisis of a disease.

acne ('aknee) a disorder of the skin affecting the pilosebaceous unit with eruption of papules or pustules, the primary cause of which appears to be excess keratin production; more particularly, ACNE VULGARIS.

conglobate a., a. conglobata severe acne with many comedones, marked by suppuration, cysts, sinuses, and scarring.

cystic a. acne with the formation of cysts enclosing a mixture of keratin and sebum in varying proportions.

a. indurata a progression of papular acne, with deep-seated and destructive lesions that may produce severe scarring.

keloid a. keloid folliculitis.

a. fulminans a rare form affecting teenage males, marked by sudden onset of fever and eruption of highly inflammatory, tender, ulcerative, and crusted lesions on the back, chest, and face.

a. necrotica acne varioliformis.

a. necrotica miliaris a rare and chronic form of folliculitis of the scalp, occurring principally in adults, with formation of tiny superficial pustules which are destroyed by scratching (see also ACNE VARIOLIFORMIS).

a. neonatorum a condition found in newborn infants with oily skins, characterized by comedones, papules, and pustules on nose, cheeks, and forehead.

a. papulosa acne vulgaris with the formation of papules.

a. rosacea a form of acne that most often occurs in persons over 25 years of age. Typically, the skin around each pustule is a rosy red; hence the name *rosacea.* This form of acne usually is resistant to treatment and often is associated with deep-seated emotional problems.

tropical a. a severe and extensive form of acne occurring in hot, humid climates, with nodular, cystic, and pustular lesions chiefly on the back, buttocks, and thighs; conglobate abscesses frequently form, especially on the back.

a. varioliformis a rare condition with reddish-brown, papulopustular umbilicated lesions, usually on the brow and scalp; probably a deep variant of acne necrotica miliaris.

a. vulgaris a chronic skin disorder usually occurring in adolescents and young adults, in which there is increased production of sebum (oil) from the sebaceous glands and the formation of comedones (blackheads and whiteheads) that plug the pores. Noninflammatory acne produces plugged follicles and a few pimples. Inflammatory acne is characterized by many pimples, pustules, nodules, and abscesses. The lesions are found on the face, neck, chest, and shoulders.

PREVENTION AND TREATMENT. The noninflammatory lesions usually respond to most nonprescription or over-the-counter soaps, scrubs and cleansers, masks, and foams. Inflammatory lesions require intensive and individualized medical treatment under the direction of a dermatologist. There is no evidence to support the belief that cleanliness will prevent or cure acne. Although frequent washing of the face and hands will remove accumulated secretions of oil and help prevent secondary bacterial infection, excessive scrubbing and drying of the skin can damage it, leaving it more susceptible to increased inflammation and the appearance of even more lesions.

For many years it was thought that certain foods contributed to the development of acne but current therapy emphasizes a well-balanced diet of a variety of foods. Sufficient rest and reduction of emotional stress are thought to be more important than the restriction of specific foods.

Acne is treated by both topical and systemic drugs. Salicylic acid and sulphur are helpful, but the drug most frequently recommended is benzoyl peroxide in a 5 or 10 per cent solution. The medication is applied to the skin daily or as frequently as necessary to produce mild dryness of the skin. A mainstay for treatment of acne continues to be oral tetracycline, which is known to be effective for most cases and safe even when taken for years. Other antibiotics that have been useful include co-trimoxazole, erythromycin and clindamycin. A relatively new systemic drug for severe, treatment-resistant acne is isotretinoin (13-*cis*-retinoic acid, 13-*cis*-RA). It inhibits the secretion of sebum and alters the lipid composition of the skin surface. Side-effects of the drug include dry mouth and dry eyes. Tretinoin (all-*trans*-retinoic acid, Retin-A) is applied topically to reduce the formation of inflammatory lesions. Oestrogens are effective in suppressing acne in female patients.

Acne therapy can continue for months and even years. Patients who conscientiously follow the prescribed regimen greatly increase their chances for improvement and the prevention of permanent scarring and pitting of the skin.

When acne has left permanent, disfiguring scars, there are medical techniques that can remove or improve the blemishes. One method is planing with a rotary, high-speed brush. This removes the outer layer of pitted skin, leaving the growing layer and the layers containing the glands and hair follicles. New epithelium grows from the layers underneath; it is rosy at first and gradually becomes normal in colour. The technique has also been used successfully in removing some types of disfigurations resulting from accidents. This so-called 'sand-paper surgery' or dermabrasion is recommended only for selected cases of acne. It must be performed by a qualified specialist.

acnegenic (,akni'jenik) producing acne.

acneiform (ak'nee·i,fawm) resembling acne.

acoelomate (ay'seeloh,mayt) 1. without a coelom or body cavity. 2. an acoelomate animal.

aconite ('akə,niet) dried tuberous root of *Aconitum napellus;* a counterirritant and local anaesthetic.

acorea (akə'reeə) absence of the pupil.

acoria (ay'kor·ri·ə, a'kor-) insatiable appetite.

acouaesthesia (ə,koois'theezi·ə) acoustic sensibility.

acousma (ə'koosmə) the hearing of imaginary sounds.

acoustic (ə'koostik) relating to sound or hearing.

acoustics (ə'koostiks) the science of sound and hearing..

ACP Association of Clinical Pathologists.

acquired (ə'kwieəd) incurred as a result of factors acting from or originating outside the organism; not inherited.

acquired immune deficiency syndrome (əkwie·əd) see AIDS.

acral ('akrəl) pertaining to an extremity.

acrania (ay'krayni·ə) partial or complete absence of the cranium. adj. **acranial.**

acranius (ay'krayni·əs) a fetus or infant in which the cranium is absent or rudimentary.

acrid ('akrid) bitter; pungent; irritating.

acridine ('akri,deen) a crystalline alkaloid from anthracene, the basis of certain dyes.

acriflavine (,akri'flayvin, -veen) an antiseptic dye used for topical application; average strength is 1:1000 to 1:8000 solution.

acritical (ay'kritik'l) having no crisis.

acro- word element. [Gr.] *extreme, top, extremity.*

acroaesthesia (,akrohes'theezi·ə) 1. exaggerated sensitiveness. 2. pain in the extremities.

acroagnosis (,akroh·ag'nohsis) lack of sensory recognition of a limb.

acroanaesthesia (,akroh,anəs'theezi·ə) anaesthesia of the extremities.

acroarthritis (,akroh·ah'thrietis) arthritis in the joints of the hands or feet.

acrobrachycephaly (,akroh,braki'kefəlee, -'sef-) abnormal height of the skull, with shortness of its anteroposterior dimension.

acrocentric (,akroh'sentrik) having the centromere toward one end of the replicating chromosome.

acrocephalia (,akrohke'fayli·ə, -se-) oxycephaly.

acrocephalic (,akrohkə'falik, -sə-) oxycephalic.

acrocephalosyndactyly (,akroh,kefəlohsin'daktilee, -,sef-) oxycephaly associated with webbing of the fingers or toes.

acrocephaly (,akroh'kefəlee, -'sef-) oxycephaly.

acrochordon (,akroh'kawdən) a pedunculated skin tag occurring principally on the neck, upper chest, and axillae in women of middle age or older.

acrocinesis (,akrohsi'neesis) acrokinesia.

acrocyanosis (,akroh,sieə'nohsis) persistent cyanosis of the fingers and hands or the toes and feet, with mottled blue or red discoloration, coldness, and profuse sweating of the digits.

acrodermatitis (,akroh,dərmə'tietis) inflammation of the skin of the hands or feet.

chronic atropic a., a. chronica atrophicans chronic inflammation of the skin of the extremities, leading to atrophy of the cutis.

continuous a., a. continua chronic inflammation of the skin of the extremities, in some cases becoming generalized.

enteropathic a., a. enteropathica a hereditary disorder of infancy associated with a defect of zinc uptake, with a vesiculopustulous dermatitis preferentially located periorificially and on the head, elbows, knees, hands, and feet, associated with gastrointestinal disturbances, chiefly manifested by diarrhoea, and total alopecia.

a. perstans acrodermatitis continua.

acrodermatosis (,akroh,dərmə'tohsis) any disease of the skin of the hands and feet.

acrodynia (,akroh'dini·ə) a disease of infancy and early childhood marked by pain and swelling in, and pink coloration of, the fingers and toes and by listlessness, irritability, failure to thrive, profuse perspiration, and sometimes scarlet coloration of the cheeks and tip of the nose. It is due to absorption of mercury. Called also *erythroedema polyneuropathy* and *pink disease.*

acrognosis (,akrog'nohsis) sensory recognition of the limbs.

acrohypothermy (,akroh'hiepoh,thərmee) abnormal coldness of the hands and feet.

acrokeratosis verruciformis (,akroh,kerə'tohsis və,roosi'fawmis) a hereditary dermatosis characterized by the presence of numerous flat wartlike papules on the dorsal aspect of the hand, foot, elbow, and knee.

acrokinesia (,akrohki'neezi·ə) abnormal motility or movement of the extremities.

acromegaly (,akroh'megəlee) abnormal enlargement of the extremities of the skeleton—nose, jaws, hands, and feet—resulting from hypersecretion of growth hormone (GH) from the PITUITARY GLAND. The condition is relatively rare and occurs in adults. In children overproduction of growth hormone stimulates growth of long bones and results in GIGANTISM, in which the child grows to an exaggerated height. With adults, however, growth of the long bones has already stopped, so that the bones most affected are those of the face, the jaw, and the hands and feet. Other signs and symptoms include amenorrhoea, diabetes mellitus, profuse sweating from loose thickened skin and hypertension.

Overproduction of GH is most often due to a tumour of the pituitary gland. Treatment usually requires either hypophysectomy or cobalt radiotherapy or a combination of the two.

Some acromegalic patients respond favourably to bromocriptine, a dopamine receptor agonist that lowers the secretion of growth hormone and also may diminish the size of the pituitary tumour.

acromelalgia (,akrohme'lalji·ə) erythromelalgia.

acromicria (,akroh'mikri·ə) abnormal smallness of the extremities of the skeleton—nose, jaws, hands, and feet.

acromio- word element. [Gr.] *acromion.*

acromioclavicular joint (ə,krohmioh,klə'vikyuhlə) the point at which the clavicle joins with the acromion.

acromiohumeral (ə,krohmioh'hyoomə·rəl) pertaining to the acromion and humerus.

acromion (ə'krohmi·ən) the lateral extension of the spine of the scapula, forming the highest point of the shoulder. adj. **acromial.**

acromionectomy (ə,krohmi·ə'nektəmee) resection of the acromion.

acromiothoracic (ə,krohmiohthor'rasik) pertaining to the acromion and thorax.

acromphalus (ə'kromfələs) 1. bulging of the navel; sometimes a sign of umbilical hernia. 2. the centre of the navel.

acroneurosis (,akrohnyuh'rohsis) any neuropathy of the extremities.

acronyx ('akrəniks) a toe- or finger-nail which becomes ingrown.

acropachy ('akroh,pakee) clubbing of the fingers.

acropachyderma (,akroh,paki'dərmə) thickening of the skin over the face, scalp, and extremities, clubbing of the extremities, and deformities of the long bones.

acroparaesthesia (,akroh,paris'theezi·ə) an abnormal sensation, such as tingling, numbness, pins and needles, in the digits.

acroparalysis (,akrohpə'ralisis) paralysis of the extremities.

acropathy (ə'kropəthee) any disease of the extremities.

acrophobia (,akroh'fohbi·ə) morbid fear of heights.

acroposthitis (,akrohpos'thietis) inflammation of the prepuce.

acroscleroderma (,akroh,skleroh'dərmə) acrosclerosis.

acrosclerosis (,akrohsklə'rohsis) a combination of Raynaud's disease and scleroderma of the distal parts of the extremities, especially of the digits, and of the neck and face, particularly the nose.

acrosome ('akrə,sohm) the caplike, membrane-bounded structure covering the anterior portion of the head of a spermatozoon; it contains enzymes involved in penetration of the ovum.

acrotism ('akrə,tizəm) absence or imperceptibility of the pulse. adj. **acrotic.**

acrylics (ə'kriliks) synthetic plastic materials derived from acrylic acid, from which dental and medical prostheses may be made. Used in ophthalmology in the manufacture of artificial eyes, intraocular lenses and hard contact lenses.

ACTH adrenocorticotrophic hormone, a hormone produced by the anterior lobe of the PITUITARY GLAND that stimulates the cortex of the ADRENAL GLAND to secrete its hormones, excluding aldosterone. If production of ACTH falls below normal, the adrenal cortex decreases in size, and production of the cortical hormones declines. Called also adrenocorticotrophin and corticotrophin. ACTH is prescribed to stimulate the adrenal glands in the treatment of some allergies, including asthma, and it has anti-inflammatory properties that sometimes help in the treatment of rheumatoid arthritis. It is also used in diagnostic tests of adrenocortical function and has been used experimentally in a large number of disorders.

Actifed ('akti,fed) trademark for a fixed combination preparation of triprolidine hydrochloride and pseudoephedrine hydrochloride.

actin ('aktin) a muscle protein localized in the I band of myofibrils; acting along with myosin particles, it is responsible for the contraction and relaxation of muscle.

acting out ('akting ,owt) the behavioural expression of hidden emotional conflicts, such as hostile feelings, in various kinds of neurotic behaviour, as a defence pattern analogous to somatic conversion.

actinic (ak'tinik) producing chemical action; said of rays of light beyond the violet end of the spectrum.

actinism ('akti,nizəm) the ability of rays of light to produce chemical changes.

actinium (ak'tini·əm) a chemical element, atomic number 89, atomic weight 227, symbol Ac. See table of elements in Appendix 2.

actino- word element. [Gr.] *ray, radiation.*

actinobacillosis (,aktinoh,basi'lohsis) an actinomycosis-like disease of domestic animals caused by *Actinobacillus lignieresii*, in which the bacilli form radiating structures in the tissues; sometimes seen in man.

Actinobacillus (,aktinohbə'siləs) a genus of gram-negative bacteria capable of infecting cattle and other domestic animals, but rarely man.

A. lignieresii the causative agent of actinobacillosis.

actinodermatitis (,aktinoh,dərmə'tietis) dermatitis from exposure to x-rays.

actinolyte (ak'tinə,liet) an apparatus for concentrating the rays of electric light in phototherapy.

Actinomadura (,aktinohmə'dyooə·rə) a genus of actinomycetes including *A. madurae*, the cause of madurомycosis in which the granules in the discharged pus are white, and *A. pelletierii*, the cause of maduromycosis in which the granules are red.

Actinomyces (,aktinoh'mieseez) a genus of actinomycetes.

A. bovis a gram-positive microorganism causing actinomycosis in cattle.

A. israelii a species causing actinomycosis in humans.

actinomyces (,aktinoh'mieseez) an organism of the genus *Actinomyces.* adj. **actinomycetic.**

actinomycete (,aktinoh'mieseet) a mouldlike bacterium (order Actinomycetales) occurring as elongated, frequently filamentous cells, with a branching tendency. adj. **actinomycetic.**

actinomycin (,aktinoh'miesin) a family of antibiotics from various species of *Streptomyces*, which are active against bacteria and fungi; it includes the antineoplastic agents cactinomycin (actinomycin C) and dactinomycin (actinomycin D).

actinomycoma (,aktinohmie'kohmə) a tumour-like reactive lesion due to *Actinomyces.*

actinomycosis (,aktinohmie'kohsis) an infection involving the deeper tissues of the skin and mucous membranes and caused by bacteria of the genus *Actinomyces.* The head and neck are most often involved, the lesions beginning as painless, tumour-like masses around the jaw and neck. Later these masses break down and begin to suppurate with discharge of the exudate through a network of sinuses extending through the skin. Intraperitoneal abscesses and lung abscesses may also occur. The source of infection is unknown, although the mouth is thought to be the portal of entry because the organisms are often found in decayed teeth and in the tonsillar crypts of persons who are otherwise normal.

The infection progresses slowly, without remission, and without at first seeming to affect the general health of the patient. If it is not treated successfully the condition may eventually be fatal.

Diagnosis is established by identifying the causative microorganisms in anaerobic culture from a lesion. The usual treatment is with penicillin, the drug of choice. In cases of allergy to this drug, tetracycline, clindamycin, or chloramphenicol can be used. Surgical measures include resection, incision, and drainage of chronic abscesses and sinuses.

actinotherapy (,aktinoh'therəpee) treatment of disease by rays of light, e.g. artificial sunlight.

action ('akshən) the accomplishment of an effect, whether mechanical or chemical, or the effect so produced.

cumulative a. the sudden and markedly increased action of a drug after administration of several doses.

reflex a. an involuntary response to a stimulus conveyed to the nervous system and reflected to the periphery, passing below the level of consciousness (see also REFLEX).

Action on Smoking and Health (ASH) a charity formed to mobilize, encourage and coordinate action in the UK to combat the illness and death caused by smoking. Further information can be obtained from ASH, 5–11 Mortimer Street, London W1N 7RH.

activator (,akti'vaytə) a substance that makes another substance active or that renders an inactive enzyme capable of exerting its proper effect.

plasminogen a. a substance that activates plasminogen and converts it into plasmin.

active ('aktiv) causing change; energetic.

a. immunity an immunity in which the individual has been stimulated with antigen to produce his or her own antibodies.

a. movements movements made by the patient as distinct from passive movements.

a. principle the ingredient in a drug which is primarily responsible for its therapeutic action.

active transport (,aktiv 'transpawt, -'trahn-) the movement of ions or molecules across the cell membranes and epithelial layers, usually against a concentration gradient, resulting directly from the expenditure of metabolic energy. For example, under normal circumstances more potassium ions are present within the cell and more sodium ions extracellularly. The process of maintaining these normal differences in electrolytic composition between the intracellular fluids is active transport. The process differs from simple diffusion or osmosis in that it requires the expenditure of metabolic energy.

activity (ak'tivitee) the quality or process of exerting energy or of accomplishing an effect.

displacement a. irrelevant activity produced by an excess of one of two conflicting drives in a person.

enzyme a. the catalytic effect exerted by an enzyme, expressed as units per milligram of enzyme (*specific* activity) or molecules of substrate transformed per minute per molecule of enzyme (*molecular* activity).

optical a. the ability of a chemical compound to rotate

the plane of polarization of plane-polarized light.

actomyosin (ˌaktoh'mieəsin) the complex of actin and myosin constituting muscle fibres and responsible for the contraction and relaxation of muscle.

acuity (ə'kyooitee) acuteness or clearness, especially of the vision.

acuminate (ə'kyoomiˌnayt) sharp-pointed.

acupressure ('akyuhˌpreshə) compression of a blood vessel by inserted needles.

acupuncture ('akyuhˌpungchə) the Chinese practice of inserting needles into specific points along the 'meridians' of the body to relieve the discomfort associated with painful disorders, to induce surgical anaesthesia, and for preventive and therapeutic purposes.

In general, acupuncture is employed to treat functional disorders rather than organic diseases that bring about severe tissue changes. It may be employed in combination with other therapies in the treatment of degenerative diseases. Acupuncture as a form of anaesthesia is considered by traditional Chinese practitioners to be a minor part of acupuncture practice.

Advocates of acupuncture base the practice on the concept of a vital energy flow or life force (*chi*) which circulates through the body along meridians similar to the blood, lymphatic, and neural circuits. It is believed that there are two energy flows and that these forces are in everything in the universe. *Yang*, the positive principle, tends to stimulate and to contract; *yin*, the negative principle, tends to sedate and to expand. Health depends upon the equilibrium of yang and yin, first in the body and secondly in the universe.

The therapeutic objective of acupuncture is to rectify an imbalance in the energy flow. This is accomplished by the insertion of needles, which are either of silver or gold, at specific points along the meridians. The needles are inserted in the skin to varying depths according to the point of insertion and the condition being treated. They may be left in place for varying lengths of time and are vibrated manually or electrically.

Traditionally an Oriental practice, acupuncture is becoming accepted in Western countries as a valid form of therapy. There is some experimental evidence that the procedure produces an analgesic effect because it causes the release of ENDORPHINS, the body's natural pain-suppressing substances.

acus ('akəs) a needle or needle-like process.

acute (ə'kyoot) 1. sharp. 2. having severe symptoms and a short course.

a. care the level of care in the HEALTH CARE SYSTEM that consists of emergency treatment and intensive care. Called also *secondary care*.

acyanotic (ayˌsieə'notik) not characterized or accompanied by cyanosis.

acyclic (ay'sieklik) occurring independently of a natural cycle of events (such as the menstrual cycle).

acyclovir (ay'sieklohviə) an antiviral agent used to treat herpes simplex. It is available as a cream, ophthalmic ointment, suspension, tablets and an intravenous infusion. The infusion is also used for patients with varicella zoster.

acyl ('asil, -siel) an organic radical derived from an organic acid by removal of the hydroxyl group.

acylation (ˌasi'layshən) introduction of an acyl radical into the molecules of a compound.

acystia (ay'sisti·ə) congenital absence of the bladder.

acystinervia (ayˌsisti'nərvi·ə) defective nervous tone of the bladder.

AD [L.] *auris dextra* (right ear).

ad (ad) preposition. [L.] *to*.

adactylia, adactyly (ˌaydak'tili·ə; ay'daktilee) congenital absence of the fingers or toes.

Adalat ('adəlat) trademark for a preparation of nifedipine, a coronary vasodilator.

Adam's apple ('adəmz) a subcutaneous prominence at the front of the throat produced by the thyroid cartilage of the LARYNX.

adamantine (ˌadə'manteen, -tien) pertaining to the enamel of the teeth.

Adams–Stokes disease (ˌadəmz'stohks) a condition characterized by sudden attacks of unconsciousness, with or without convulsions, which frequently accompanies heart block; called also *Stokes–Adams disease*.

adaptation (ˌadap'tayshən) adjustment, for example of an organism to environmental conditions. Used in ophthalmology to mean the adjustment of visual function according to the ambient illumination.

colour a. 1. changes in visual perception of colour with prolonged stimulation. 2. adjustment of vision to degree of brightness or colour tone of illumination.

dark a. adaptation of the eye to vision in reduced illumination.

light a. adaptation of the eye to vision in bright illumination (photopia), with reduction in the concentration of the photosensitive pigments of the eye.

adaptometer (ˌadap'tomitə) an instrument for measuring the time required for retinal adaptation, i.e., for regeneration of the visual purple (rhodopsin); used in detecting night blindness, vitamin A deficiency, and retinitis pigmentosa.

addict ('adikt) a person exhibiting addiction.

addiction (ə'dikshən) physiological or psychological dependence on some agent (e.g., alcohol, drug), with a tendency to increase its use (see also DRUG ADDICTION).

Addis count ('adis) the determination of the number of red blood cells, white blood cells, epithelial cells, casts, and the protein content in an aliquot of a 12-hour urine specimen, used in the diagnosis and management of kidney disease.

Addison's anaemia ('adis'nz) pernicious anaemia.

Addison's disease a syndrome resulting from destruction of both adrenal glands, with consequent insufficient production of adrenocortical hormones (glucocorticoids and mineralocorticoids). If gonadal function remains normal, the decreased secretion of adrenal sex hormones has no significant physiological effect.

Bilateral atrophy of the adrenal cortex caused by autoimmune disease is the most common form of Addison's disease; in this the adrenal medulla is preserved. Destruction of the whole adrenal gland by tuberculosis is no longer the most common pathology. Rare causes of Addison's disease include fungal infections, amyloidosis and metastatic carcinoma. Addison's disease must be distinguished from adrenocortical failure secondary to destructive lesions of the anterior pituitary causing loss of ACTH secretion (in Addison's disease ACTH secretion is excessive) and hence diminished cortisol secretion but continued secretion of mineralocorticoids whose production is not controlled by ACTH.

Serious and potentially life-threatening problems associated with Addison's disease are failure of the body to resist stress, fluid and electrolyte imbalance, and hypoglycaemia. Deficiency of mineralocorticoids leads to depletion of sodium (hyponatraemia), resulting in depletion of extracellular fluid and potassium retention (hyperkalaemia). The patient experiences generalized malaise and muscular weakness, muscle pain, and orthostatic hypotension, and may collapse when exposed to minor infection.

Deficiency of cortisol adversely affects the body's resistance to stress or trauma, so that collapse and shock prove fatal; hypoglycaemia also occurs. Gastrointestinal symptoms are anorexia, nausea, vomiting, flatulence, and diarrhoea. These symptoms, as well as anxiety, mental depression, and loss of mental acuity, are related to the low cortisol output.

Hyperpigmentation of certain areas of the skin and mucous membranes occurs, due to the direct pigmentary effect of excess ACTH. An insufficient supply of cortisol signals the pituitary gland to secrete more ACTH, which increases the brown pigmentation of fresh scars, skin folds, pressure areas, palmar tissues and the areolae of the nipples. Blue patches of pigmentation occur in the buccal mucosa.

PATIENT CARE. The medical treatment of Addison's disease is centred on replacement of the deficient hormones; that is, on administration of glucocorticoids and mineralocorticoids. Replacement therapy usually brings about a rapid recovery.

Nursing care is concerned with intensive support of the patient during *addisonian crisis*, prevention of problems related to hypoglycaemia and orthostatic hypotension, alleviation of gastrointestinal problems, and instruction of the patient in self-care. It includes providing regular feeds throughout the day and providing for adequate rest. When fasting is required for diagnostic studies or surgery, the patient will probably need intravenous glucose to avoid profound hypoglycaemia. Maintenance doses of glucocorticoids are especially important during fasting.

Gastrointestinal problems will disappear when glucocorticoid replacement is adequate.

The patient's intake and output are measured regularly, and postural blood pressure is checked periodically. The apical-radial pulse is taken along with other vital signs to identify early symptoms of hyperkalaemia. Cardiac monitoring may be indicated if cardiac arrhythmias develop. Safety measures must be taken to prevent falls during the spells of weakness and fainting that may occur.

Stress, even relatively mild physical and emotional stress, can quickly bring on an addisonian crisis. When this occurs, the physiological defence provided by cortisol no longer operates, and the patient suffers from hypotension and eventual circulatory collapse. Absence of mineralocorticoids compounds the problem by depletion of extracellular fluids and impairment of cardiac function.

A person with Addison's disease can usually lead a fairly normal life with optimal exogenous hormone therapy. Patient education is vital and includes instruction in the signs and symptoms of inadequate or excess steroid replacement, which indicate a need to return to the doctor, and in the importance of avoiding stressful situations or countering stress by increasing glucocorticoid dosage. If vomiting occurs, glucocorticoids must immediately be given by injection. The patient should wear a medical identification tag stating that he or she has the disease and is receiving steroid therapy.

addisonian crisis (ˌadi'sohniən) symptoms of fatigue, nausea and vomiting, weight loss, hypotension, and collapse accompanying an acute attack of ADDISON'S DISEASE.

addisonism ('adisəˌnizəm) symptoms seen in pulmonary tuberculosis, consisting of debility and pigmentation, resembling ADDISON'S DISEASE.

additive ('aditiv) 1. characterized by addition. 2. a substance added to another to improve its appearance, increase its nutritive value, etc.

adducent (ə'dyoos'nt) leading toward the midline.

adduct (ə'dukt) to draw toward a centre or median line.

adduction (ə'dukshən) the act of adducting; the state of being adducted.

adductor (ə'duktə) that which adducts.

adenalgia (adə'nalji·ə) pain in a gland.

adenasthenia (ˌadənas'theeni·ə) deficient glandular activity.

adendritic (ˌayden'dritik) without dendrites.

adenectomy (ˌadə'nektəmee) excision of a gland.

adenectopia (ˌadənek'tohpi·ə) displacement of a gland.

adeniform (ə'deeniˌfawm) gland-shaped.

adenine ('adəˌneen) a purine present in nucleoproteins of cells of plants and animals. Adenine and guanine are essential components of NUCLEIC ACIDS. The end product of the metabolism of adenine in man is uric acid.

a. arabinoside (ara-A) vidarabine.

adenitis (ˌadə'nietis) inflammation of a gland.

adenization (ˌadənie'zayshən) assumption by other tissue of an abnormal glandlike appearance.

adeno- word element. [Gr.] *gland*.

adenoacanthoma (ˌadənohˌakan'thohmə) adenocarcinoma in which some of the cells exhibit squamous differentiation.

adenoameloblastoma (ˌadənoh·əˌmeelohbla'stohmə) an odontogenic tumour with formation of ductlike structures in place of or in addition to a typical ameloblastic pattern.

adenoblast ('adənohˌblast) an embryonic forerunner of gland tissue.

adenocarcinoma (ˌadənohˌkahsi'nohmə) carcinoma derived from glandular tissue or in which the tumour cells form recognizable glandular structures.

adenocele ('adənohˌseel) a cystic adenomatous tumour.

adenocellulitis (ˌadənohˌselyuh'lietis) inflammation of a gland and the cellular tissue around it.

adenochondroma (ˌadənohkon'drohmə) a tumour containing both glandular and cartilaginous elements.

adenocystoma (ˌadənohsi'stohmə) adenoma in which there is cyst formation.

adenodynia (ˌadənoh'dini·ə) pain in a gland.

adenofibroma (ˌadənohfie'brohmə) a benign tumour of connective tissue which contains glandular structures.

adenogenous (ˌadə'nojənəs) orginating from glandular tissue.

adenohypophysis (ˌadənoh·hie'pofisis) the anterior or glandular portion of the hypophysis cerebri (see also PITUITARY GLAND). adj. **adenohypophyseal**.

adenoid ('adəˌnoyd) 1. resembling a gland. 2. in the plural, hypertrophy of the glandular tissue that normally exists in the nasopharynx of children and is known as the pharyngeal tonsil. Enlargement of this tissue may cause obstruction of the outlet from the nose so that the child breathes chiefly through the mouth, or the pharyngotympanic tube may be blocked, with pain in the ear or a sense of pressure resulting. It also may prepare the way for infections of the middle ear and occasionally interferes with hearing. Prolonged obstruction by enlarged adenoids produces a typical 'adenoid facies'. The child appears to be dull and apathetic, and has some degree of nutritional deficiency and hearing loss, and some delay in growth and development.

Surgical excision of the enlarged tissue is called adenoidectomy.

adenoidectomy (ˌadənoy'dektəmee) surgical excision of the adenoids. The operation is usually performed in conjunction with tonsillectomy since both the adenoids and palatine tonsils tend to become enlarged after repeated infections of the throat. The preoperative and postoperative care in adenoidectomy is similar to that in TONSILLECTOMY.

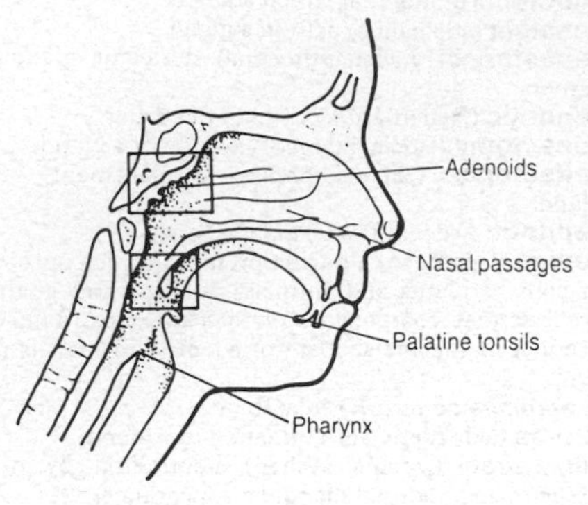

Adenoids

adenoiditis (,adənoy'dietis) inflammation of the adenoids.

adenolipoma (,adənohli'pohmə) a tumour composed of both glandular and fatty tissue elements.

adenolipomatosis (,adənoh,lipohmə'tohsis) the formation of numerous adenolipomas in the neck, axilla, and groin.

adenology (,adə'noləjee) the sum of knowledge regarding glands.

adenolymphitis (,adənohlim'fietis) lymphadenitis; inflammation of lymph nodes.

adenolymphoma (,adənohlim'fohmə) a cystic salivary-gland tumour containing epithelial and lymphoid tissue, affecting almost exclusively the parotid gland.

adenoma (,adə'nohmə) a benign epithelial tumour in which the cells form recognizable glandular structures or in which the cells are derived from glandular epithelium.

acidophilic a. a tumour of the alpha cells of the anterior lobe of the pituitary gland; called also eosinophilic adenoma. Such tumours produce ACROMEGALY and GIGANTISM.

basophilic a. a tumour of the beta cells of the anterior lobe of the pituitary gland, which may secrete an excess of corticotropin (ACTH) resulting in CUSHING'S SYNDROME.

chromophobe a. a tumour arising from the chromophobe cells of the anterior lobe of the pituitary gland.

eosinophilic a. acidophilic adenoma.

Hürthle cell a. see under HÜRTHLE CELL TUMOUR.

pituitary a. a benign neoplasm of the pituitary gland, such as acidophilic adenoma, basophilic adenoma, or chromophobe adenoma.

sebaceous a. hypertrophy or benign hyperplasia of a sebaceous gland.

a. sebaceum naevoid hyperplasia of sebaceous glands, forming multiple yellow papules or nodules on the face.

villous a. a large soft papillary polyp on the mucosa of the large intestine.

adenomalacia (,adənohmə'layshi·ə) undue softness of a gland.

adenomatome (,adə'nohmə,tohm) an instrument for the removal of adenoids.

adenomatosis (,adənohmə'tohsis) the formation of numerous adenomatous growths.

adenomatous (,adə'nohmətəs) pertaining to adenoma or to nodular hyperplasia of a gland.

adenomere ('adənoh,miə) the blind terminal portion of the glandular cavity of a developing gland, being the functional portion of the organ.

adenomyoma (,adənohmie'ohmə) a benign tumour made up of endometrium and muscle tissue, found in the uterus, or more frequently in the uterine ligaments.

adenomyometritis (,adənoh,mieohmi'trietis) adenomyosis of the uterus.

adenomyosarcoma (,adənoh,mieohsah'kohmə) adenosarcoma containing striated muscle.

adenomyosis (,adənohmie'ohsis) invasion of the muscular wall of an organ (e.g., uterus) by glandular tissue.

adenopathy (,adə'nopəthee) enlargement of glands, especially of the lymph nodes.

adenopharyngitis (,adənoh,farin'jietis) inflammation of the adenoids and pharynx, usually involving the tonsils.

adenosarcoma (,adənohsah'kohmə) a malignant tumour of mesenchyme with an admixed epithelial glandular component which may be benign or malignant.

adenosclerosis (,adənohsklə'rohsis) hardening of a gland.

adenosine (a'denoh,seen) a nucleoside composed of the pentose sugar D-ribose and adenine. It is a structural subunit of ribonucleic acid (RNA). Adenosine nucleotides are involved in the energy metabolism of all cells. Adenosine can be linked to a chain of one, two, or three phosphate groups to form *adenosine monophosphate* (AMP), *adenosine diphosphate* (ADP), or *adenosine triphosphate* (ATP). The bond between the phosphate groups in ADP or the two bonds between phosphate groups in ATP are called *high-energy bonds*, because hydrolysis of a high-energy bond provides a large amount of free energy that can be used to drive other processes that would not otherwise occur. The energy that is derived from the breakdown of carbohydrates, fats, or proteins is used to synthesize ATP. The energy stored in ATP is then used directly or indirectly to drive all other cellular processes that require energy, of which there are four major types: (1) the transport of molecules and ions across cell membranes against concentration gradients, which maintains the internal environment of the cell and produces the membrane potential for the conduction of nerve impulses; (2) the contraction of muscle fibres and other fibres producing the motion of cells; (3) the synthesis of chemical compounds; (4) the synthesis of other high-energy compounds.

cyclic a. monophosphate (cyclic AMP, cAMP, 3′,5′-AMP) a cyclic nucleotide, adenosine 3′,5′-cyclic monophosphate, involved in the action of many hormones, including catecholamines, ACTH, and vasopressin. The hormone binds to a specific receptor on the cell membrane of target cells. This activates an enzyme, adenylate cyclase, which produces cyclic AMP from ATP. Cyclic AMP acts as a second messenger activating other enzymes within the cell. **a. diphosphate (ADP)** a nucleotide, adenosine 5′-pyrophosphate, produced by the hydrolysis of adenosine triphosphate (ATP). It is then converted back to ATP by the metabolic processes oxidative phosphorylation, glycolysis, and the tricarboxylic acid cycle.

a. monophosphate (AMP) a nucleotide, adenosine 5′-phosphate, involved in energy metabolism and nucleotide synthesis. Called also adenylic acid.

a. triphosphatase (ATPase) a term used to refer to the enzymatic activity of certain intercellular processes that split ATP to form ADP and inorganic phosphate, when the energy released is not used for the synthesis

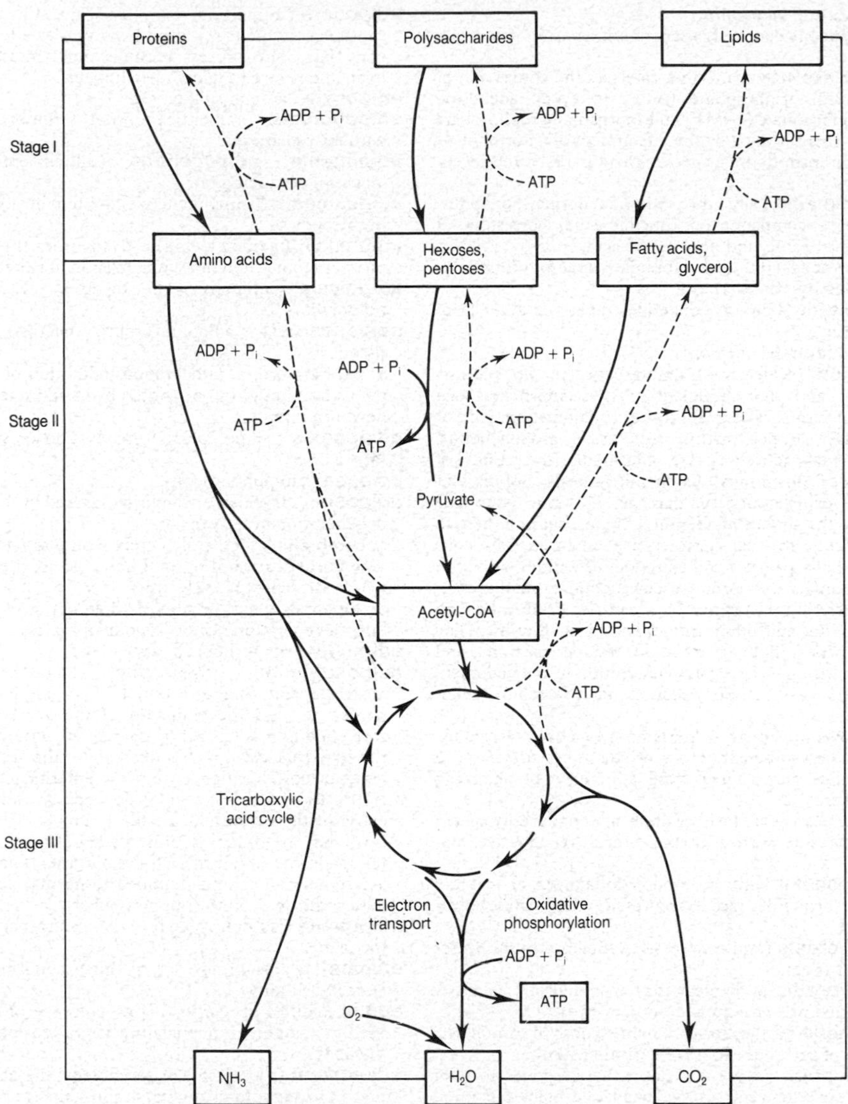

Adenosine triphosphate (ATP) in metabolism. Catabolic pathways (arrows pointing downward) converge to common end products and lead to ATP synthesis in Stage III. Anabolic (biosynthetic) pathways (arrows pointing upward) start from a few precursors in Stage III and utilize ATP energy to yield many different cell components

of chemical compounds. Examples are the splitting of ATP in muscle contraction and the transport of ions across cell membranes. **a. triphosphate (ATP)** a nucleotide, adenosine 5′-triphosphate, occurring in all cells, where it stores energy in the form of high-energy phosphate bonds. Free energy is supplied to drive metabolic reactions or to transport molecules against concentration gradients, when ATP is hydrolysed to ADP and inorganic phosphate or to AMP and inorganic pyrophosphate. ATP is also used to produce high-energy phosphorylated intermediary metabolites, such as glucose 6-phosphate.

adenosis (ˌadəˈnohsis) 1. any disease of a gland. 2. abnormal development of a gland.

adenotomy (ˌadəˈnotəmee) 1. anatomy, incision, or dissection of glands. 2. incision of adenoids.

adenotonsillectomy (ˌadənohˌtonsiˈlektəmee) removal of the tonsils and adenoids.

adenovirus (ˌadənohˈvierəs) any of a large group of viruses causing disease of the upper respiratory tract and conjunctiva, and also present in latent infections in normal persons; many induce malignancy in certain species. adj. **adenoviral**.

adenylate (ə'deni,layt) a salt, anion, or ester of adenylic acid.

a. cyclase an enzyme that catalyses the conversion of adenosine triphosphate (ATP) to cyclic adenosine monophosphate (cAMP) and inorganic pyrophosphate (PP_i). It is activated by the attachment of a hormone or neurotransmitter to a specific membrane-bound receptor.

adenylic acid (,adə'nilik, -'nie-) adenosine monophosphate; a component of nucleic acid, consisting of adenine, ribose, and phosphoric acid.

adeps ('adeps) [L.] *lard*, a foundation fat for ointments.

a. lanae hydrosus lanolin.

adermia (ay'dərmi·ə) congenital defect or absence of the skin.

ADH antidiuretic hormone.

adhesion (ad'heezhən) union between two surfaces which can be normal (anatomical) or abnormal as seen within serous cavities following inflammation, etc., or as may develop within soft tissue around joints. Abnormal adhesions are commonly the result of previous laparotomy. As an injury heals, fibrous scar tissue forms around the damage. This scar tissue may join to the surface of adjoining organs, causing them to kink when the scar contracts as it matures. Adhesions are usually painless and cause no difficulties, although occasionally they produce obstruction or malfunction by distorting the organ. They can also occur following peritonitis and other inflammatory conditions. They may occur in the pleura, in the pericardium, and around the pelvic organs, in addition to the abdomen. Surgery is sometimes recommended to relieve adhesions.

adhesive (əd'heesiv) 1. pertaining to, characterized by, or causing close adherence of adjoining surfaces. 2. a substance that causes close adherence of adjoining surfaces.

a. tape a strip of fabric or other material evenly coated on one side with a pressure-sensitive adhesive material.

adiadochokinesia (ə,deeədoh,kohki'neezi·ə) inability to perform fine, rapidly repeated, coordinated movements.

adiaphoresis (ay,dieəfə'reesis) deficiency in the secretion of sweat.

adiaphoretic (ay,dieəfor'retik) an anhidrotic agent. A drug that prevents the secretion of sweat.

adiaphoria (,aydieə'for·ri·ə) nonresponse to stimuli as a result of previous exposure to similar stimuli.

Adie's pupil ('aydeez) a pupil that responds to light and convergence in a slow, delayed fashion. The pupil is always dilated compared with the other eye. Called also *tonic pupil*.

Adie's syndrome a syndrome consisting of a pathological pupil reaction (pupillotonia), the most important element of which is a myotonic condition on accommodation; the pupil on the affected side contracts to near vision more slowly than does the pupil on the opposite side, and it also dilates more slowly. The affected pupil does not usually react to light (direct or indirect), but it may do so in an abnormal fashion. Certain tendon reflexes are absent or diminished, but there are no motor or sensory disturbances, nor are there demonstrable changes indicative of disease of the nervous system.

adip(o)- word element. [L.] *fat*.

adipectomy (,adi'pektəmee) excision of adipose tissue.

adipic (ə'dipik) pertaining to fat.

adipocele ('adipoh,seel) a hernia containing fat.

adipocellular (,adipoh'selyuhlə) composed of fat and connective tissue.

adipocere ('adipoh,siə) a swollen white stiffened waxy substance formed in a dead body due to alteration of body fats. The process requires time, moisture and heat, and is rare in temperate climates.

adipocyte ('adipoh,siet) fat cell.

adipofibroma (,adipohfie'brohmə) a fibrous tumour with fatty elements.

adipogenic, adipogenous (,adipoh'jenik; ,adi'pojənəs) producing fat.

adipokinesis (,adipohki'neesis) the mobilization of fat in the body.

adipokinin (,adipoh'kienin) a factor from the anterior pituitary that accelerates mobilization of stored fat.

adipolysis (,adi'polisis) the digestion of fats. adj. **adipolytic**.

adiponecrosis (,adipohnə'krohsis) necrosis of fatty tissue.

a. neonatorum, a. subcutanea induration of subcutaneous fat, thought to be caused by obstetric trauma, in newborn infants.

adipopexis (,adipoh'peksis) the fixation or storing of fat.

adipose ('adi,pohs, -z) fatty.

adiposis (,adi'pohsis) a condition marked by deposits or degeneration of fatty tissue.

a. cerebralis fatness from cerebral pituitary disease.

a. dolorosa a painful condition due to pressure on nerves caused by fatty deposits.

a. tuberosa simplex adiposis dolorosa in which the fatty degeneration occurs in nodular masses.

adiposity (,adi'positee) obesity.

adiposogenital dystrophy (,adipohsoh,jenit'l 'distrəfee) abnormal distribution of fat (obesity) accompanied by underdevelopment of the genitalia. This rare condition is caused by damage to certain parts of the HYPOTHALAMUS, with a decrease in the secretion of gonadotropic hormones from the anterior lobe of the PITUITARY GLAND. Treatment depends on the primary cause of the condition, usually a tumour or infection involving the hypothalamus. Called also adiposogenital syndrome and Fröhlich's syndrome. These terms are sometimes wrongly applied to normal obese boys with some delay in the onset of puberty.

adiposuria (,adipoh'syooə·ri·ə) the occurrence of fat in the urine.

adipsia (ay'dipsi·ə) absence of thirst; abnormal avoidance of drinking.

aditus ('aditəs) pl. *aditus* [L.] an entrance or opening; used in anatomic nomenclature for various passages in the body.

adjustment (ə'justmənt) in psychology, the ability of a person to adapt to changing circumstances or environment.

adjuvant ('ajəvənt) 1. assisting or aiding. 2. a substance that aids another, such as an auxiliary remedy.

Adler ('adlə) Alfred (1870–1937). Austrian psychiatrist who dissented from Freud's emphasis on the role of infantile sexuality in personality development. He started a psychological movement called *individual psychology* to indicate that the individual is viewed as a unified personality and indivisible unit of society. Adler introduced the terms *inferiority feelings* and *overcompensation*. He taught that the child has inferiority feelings in relation to both his parents and to society as a whole. This sense of inadequacy stems from the child's physical immaturity, uncertainty, dependence upon his parents and society, and a painful feeling of subordination to others. This leads to compensatory reactions and a drive to prestige, superiority, and achievement. In cases in which the feelings of inferiority are overpowering and a child fears that he will never be able to compensate for his weakness and inadequacy, he may develop an exaggerated striving for power and dominance (overcompensation), characterized by great haste and impatience, violent impulses, a lack of consideration for others, and grandiose goals. Many of Adler's views have been adopted by other schools of psychiatry.

ADM Advanced Diploma in Midwifery.

adnerval, adneural (ad'nərv'l; ad'nyooə-r'l) toward a nerve.

adnexa (ad'neksə) pl. *appendages* [L.] accessory organs, as of the eye (*adenxa oculi*) or uterus (*adnexa uteri*). adj. **adnexal.**

adolescence (ˌadə'lesəns) the period between the onset of puberty and the cessation of physical growth; it extends from about 12 to 21 years of age in females, and from about 14 to 25 years in males. adj. **adolescent.**

Adolescents vacillate between being children and being adults. They are adjusting to the physiological changes their bodies are undergoing and are working to establish a sexual identification and to use these changes for their personal benefit and for the benefit of society. Stress and illness can cause temporary setbacks in this progress toward maturation.

Adolescents are searching for personal identity and want freedom and independence of thought and action, but they continue to have a strong dependence on their parents and suffer feelings of loss in separating from them. In reaction to this they identify with their peers and tend to yield to peer pressure and conform to peer group values, behaviour, and tastes in such things as clothing, food, and entertainment.

Because of their sensitivity about questions of identity, it is especially important that an adolescent be treated as an individual having unique behaviour, attitudes, personal qualities, and traits. Prejudicial labelling of persons as 'adolescent' should be avoided.

Adolescents usually are narcissistic about their bodies and greatly concerned with personal appearance. An illness or injury that alters physical appearance or interferes with normal bodily function can be very distressing, perhaps more so than to an adult. They yearn to be their own persons, independent of their parents and other authority figures. Adolescents resent the isolation from friends that hospitalization brings about, probably because they view it as a return to dependence on their parents and other adults.

The health care of adolescents must take into account the particular needs of each patient. They should be provided with the information and support they need to adjust to the changes that are taking place in and around them. It is especially important that young people in this age group understand the relationships between their life style and their health. They should be informed of the kinds of illness and injury for which they are most at risk. Perhaps most importantly, they need to learn self-acceptance and to develop confidence in their ability to cope with the vagaries of life.

adoral (ad'or·rəl) 1. situated near the mouth. 2. directed toward the mouth.

ADP adenosine diphosphate.

adren(o)- word element. [L.] *adrenal glands.*

adrenal (ə'dreen'l) 1. near the kidney. 2. of or produced by the adrenal glands. 3. an adrenal gland.

a. gland a small endocrine gland situated in the retroperitoneal tissues at the upper pole of either kidney; called also suprarenal gland.

In man, the adrenal gland is the result of fusion of two organs, one forming the inner core or *medulla*, and the other forming an outer shell, or *cortex*. These two structures are quite different in their anatomy, and in the kinds of hormone they synthesize and secrete. Although both are endocrine in nature, the medulla is more akin to the autonomic nervous system than to other endocrine glands.

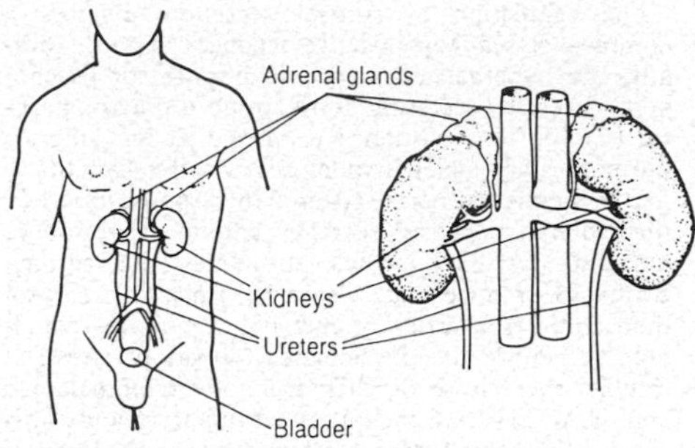

Adrenal glands

MEDULLA. The inner core of the adrenal gland is a glandular extension of sympathetic effector fibres or postganglionic neurons. The adrenal medullae release the hormones *adrenaline* and *noradrenaline* in response to stimulation of the sympathetic nervous system. These hormones enter the blood stream and are carried throughout the body, where they stimulate the organs sensitive to the sympathetic system. Their production and distribution by the blood usually occur at the same time that the organs are being stimulated by the sympathetic nerves. In this way, the adrenal medullae and the sympathetic nerves support one another and can act as substitutes for each other. Adrenaline and noradrenaline differ only in that adrenaline has a more prolonged effect because it is removed from the blood at a slower rate.

The effects of adrenaline and noradrenaline include elevation of cardiac output, increased metabolic rate, vasoconstriction, and increased peristaltic activity of the gastrointestinal tract.

CORTEX. The adrenal cortex synthesizes and secretes many related steroids. These are divided into three major groups: the GLUCOCORTICOIDS, the MINERALOCORTICOIDS, and the steriod sex hormones (ANDROGENS and OESTROGENS). The glucocorticoids derive their name from the fact that they cause an increase in blood glucose levels (*gluco-)*, are produced by the adrenal cortex (*corti-)*, and are synthesized from cholesterol, which is a steroid *(-oid)*. The mineralocorticoids, as their name implies, are chiefly concerned with the concentration of electrolytes (minerals) in the extracellular fluid. The adrenal cortex also secretes small amounts of androgens, which have the same masculinizing effect as *testosterone*, a hormone secreted by the testes.

Glucocorticoids. The principal glucocorticoid is *cortisol* (also known as hydrocortisone and compound F), which is responsible for more than 95 per cent of all glucocorticoid activity, the remainder being provided by *corticosterone* and *cortisone*. Glucocorticoids play a vital part in the body's reaction to stress and trauma. The degree of stress has to be matched by a sufficient secretion of cortisol.

The metabolic action of glucocorticoids is to promote the metabolic breakdown or anabolism of carbohydrates, proteins, and fats. Cortisol increases the rate of gluconeogenesis by the liver, decreases the utilization of glucose by the cells, reduces cellular protein and enhances utilization of amino acids by the liver, and promotes mobilization of fatty acids from adipose tissue into the plasma. The net effect of these actions is to make these noncarbohydrate nutritive elements readily available for energy.

The regulation of cortisol secretion involves a complex closed-loop negative feedback system. Initially, the hypothalamus reacts to physical or psychogenic stress by secreting corticotrophin-releasing factor (CRF). This substance is carried to the anterior pituitary gland (adenohypophysis) via the hypothalamic–hypophyseal portal system. In response to CRF, the adenohypophysis secretes adrenocorticotrophic hormone (ACTH), which stimulates the adrenal cortex to produce and release cortisol. The cortisol then initiates a series of metabolic activities which help to relieve the physiological effects of stress. It inhibits the release of CRF from the hypothalamus and of ACTH from the anterior pituitary gland. This exerts a negative feedback effect; high serum cortisol levels inhibit further production of cortisol. Thus, during times of relative calm when the body is not experiencing abnormal stress, the cortisol level returns to normal.

Another factor that influences the secretory rates of CRF, ACTH, and cortisol is a biological clock mechanism that establishes a cyclic pattern of signals from the hypothalamus. This is a 24-hour cycle that has its peak immediately after completion of the major portion of a night's sleep, usually about 4 or 5 a.m. About 18 hours later, the blood level of cortisol is at its lowest, being about one-third that of its early morning peak. This cycle is dependent on sleeping patterns; therefore, if a person changes his pattern and sleeps in the daytime, the cycle of hormonal levels changes accordingly. This information is significant in testing for cortisol levels as a means of diagnosing a disorder of the endocrine system. When blood is drawn for testing, the specimen should be clearly labelled as to the precise time it was taken.

Mineralocorticoids. The principal mineralocorticoid is *aldosterone*. This hormone and other mineralocorticoids prevent excessive loss of sodium and chloride in the urine by enhancing their reabsorption from the renal tubules. They have the same effect to a lesser degree on the sweat and salivary glands and on the intestines. Additionally, aldosterone promotes excretion of potassium in the urine. The net result of these activities is the maintenance of fluid and electrolyte balance in the blood and extracellular fluid, which, in turn, affects cardiac output and blood pressure.

A deficit of aldosterone secretion brings about a decrease in extracellular fluid and blood volumes, interference with the venous return to the heart, and a fall in cardiac output. If not corrected, the patient rapidly goes into profound shock.

DYSFUNCTION OF THE ADRENAL GLANDS. Either excessive or deficient secretion of adrenal hormones can produce various disorders. Primary aldosteronism (CONN'S SYNDROME) is caused by excess aldosterone secretion from an adrenocortical tumour or from bilateral hyperplasia of the aldosterone-producing cells. See also ALDOSTERONE, ALDOSTERONISM. Excess cortisol production (CUSHING'S SYNDROME) may arise from an adrenocortical tumour or from bilateral adrenocortical hyperplasia owing to excess stimulation by ACTH. Excess androgen secretion from an adrenal tumour or with congenital adrenal hyperplasia causes the adrenogenital syndrome. Tumours of the adrenal medulla produce excess noradrenaline.

a. insufficiency hypofunction of the adrenal gland; may be due to destructive disease of both adrenals (ADDISON'S DISEASE) or to failure of ACTH secretion by the anterior pituitary.

adrenalectomy (ə,dreenə'lektəmee) surgical excision of an adrenal gland. This procedure is indicated when a disorder of the adrenal gland, such as CUSHING'S SYNDROME or PHAEOCHROMOCYTOMA, causes an overproduction of adrenal hormone. Bilateral adrenalectomy is performed in some instances of severe Cushing's syndrome, and is sometimes undertaken in the treatment of metastatic breast cancer.

adrenaline (ə'drenəlin) a hormone produced by the medulla of the ADRENAL GLANDS; called also epinephrine (USA). Its function is to aid in the regulation of the sympathetic branch of the autonomic NERVOUS SYSTEM. At times when a person is highly stimulated, as by fear, anger, or some challenging situation, extra amounts of adrenaline are released into the bloodstream, preparing the body for energetic action. Adrenaline is a powerful vasopressor which increases blood pressure, heart rate and cardiac output. It also increases glycogenolysis and the release of glucose from the liver.

A pathological increase in adrenaline secretion is very rare and due to a tumour of the adrenal medulla (phaeochromocytoma). Such a tumour has bursts of adrenaline secretion. Acute hypertension is the result. Removal of the tumour cures the condition.

Adrenaline is also produced synthetically. It can be administered parenterally, topically, or by inhalation, and acts as a vasoconstrictor, antispasmodic, and sympathomimetic. It is used as an emergency heart stimulant and to relieve symptoms in allergic conditions such as urticaria and asthma. It is the first drug in the treatment of anaphylactic shock.

adrenergic (,adrə'nərjik) 1. activated by, characteristic of, or secreting adrenaline or substances with activities similar to those of adrenaline. The term is applied to those nerve fibres of the sympathetic nervous system that release noradrenaline (and possibly small amounts of adrenaline) at a synapse when a nerve impulse passes. 2. an agent that acts like adrenaline. Called also sympathomimetic.

a.-blocking agent a drug that blocks the secretion of adrenaline and noradrenaline at the post-ganglionic nerve endings of the sympathetic nervous system. By blocking these adrenergic substances, which cause constriction of blood vessels and increased cardiac output, adrenergic-blocking agents produce a dilation of the blood vessels and a decrease in cardiac output. They are classified as antihypertensive drugs. Guanethidine sulphate and bethanidine are examples of adrenergic-blocking agents. During therapy with these drugs, patients should avoid strenuous exercise, which is likely to produce a sudden drop in the blood pressure. Another difficulty to be expected with these drugs is postural hypotension.

a. receptors receptors for adrenaline or noradrenaline, such as those on effector organs innervated by postganglionic adrenergic fibres of the sympathetic nervous system. They are classified as α-adrenergic receptors, which are stimulated by noradrenaline and blocked by agents such as phenoxybenzamine, and β-adrenergic receptors, which are stimulated by adrenaline and blocked by agents such as propranolol. Each has two subtypes: α_1-receptors (which produce vasoconstriction) and α_2-receptors (which are thought to modulate the neural release of transmitter during presynaptic sympathetic nerve stimulation); and β_1-receptors (which produce lipolysis and cardiostimulation) and β_2-receptors (which produce bronchodilation and vasodilation).

adrenocortical (ə,dreenoh'kawtik'l) pertaining to or arising from the cortex of the adrenal gland.
a. hormone one of the steroids produced by the adrenal cortex (see also CORTICOSTEROID).
adrenocorticomimetic (ə,dreenoh,kawtikohmi'metik) having effects similar to those of hormones of the adrenal cortex.
adrenocorticotrophic (ə,dreenoh,kawtikoh'trohfik) having a stimulating effect on the adrenal cortex; corticotrophic.
a. hormone ACTH, a hormone secreted by the anterior PITUITARY GLAND that has a stimulating effect on the ADRENAL CORTEX. Called also *corticotrophin*.
adrenocorticotrophin (ə,dreenoh,kawtikoh'trohfin) adrenocorticotrophic hormone (ACTH), or corticotrophin.
adrenocorticotropic (ə,dreenoh,kawtikoh'trohpik) adrenocorticotrophic; corticotrophic.
adrenocorticotropin (ə,dreenoh,kawtikoh'trohpin) adrenocorticotrophic hormone; corticotrophin (see also ACTH).
adrenogenital syndrome (ə,dreenoh'jenit'l) a group of symptoms due to the excessive production of androgens by the adrenal cortex. The common form, seen in infants and children, is caused by a congenital defect in the enzyme systems that control the production of adrenal hormones. In consequence too little glucocorticoid and mineralocorticoid hormones are produced and too much androgen is secreted. In the male infant, the penis enlarges prematurely, with a precocious pseudopuberty (the testes do no develop as in true puberty). In the female infant, the genitalia at birth appear masculine, with gross hypertrophy of the clitoris. Masculinization proceeds during childhood. Both sexes are liable to addisonian crises, which may be fatal. Treatment with glucocorticoids and mineralocorticoids is successful in suppressing androgen production and correcting the deficiency in the production of these hormones.
In the adult woman, excess adrenal androgen production may be associated with the polycystic ovary syndrome. Rarely androgen-producing tumours of the adrenal cortex will cause severe virilization.
adrenoleukodystrophy (ə,dreenoh,lookoh'distrəfee) a hereditary disease transmitted as an X-linked recessive trait, characterized by diffuse abnormality of the cerebral white matter and adrenal atrophy.
adrenolytic (ə,dreenoh'litik) antagonizing the action of adrenaline or of the adrenal gland.
adrenomegaly (ə,dreenoh'megəlee) abnormal enlargement of the adrenal gland.
adrenomimetic (ə,dreenohmi'metik) having actions similar to those of adrenergic compounds; sympathomimetic.
adrenopathy (,adri'nopəthee) any disease of the adrenal glands.
Adriamycin (,aydri·ə'miesin) trademark for a preparation of doxorubicin, an antineoplastic antibiotic.
Adson's test ('adsənz) one for thoracic outlet syndrome; with the patient in a sitting position, his hands resting on thighs, the examiner palpates both radial pulses as the patient rapidly fills his lungs by deep inspiration and, holding his breath, hyperextends his neck and turns his head toward the affected side. If the radial pulse on that side is decidedly or completely obliterated, the result is positive.
adsorb (əd'sawb, -'zawb) to attract and retain other material on the surface.
adsorbent (əd'sawbənt, -'zawb-) 1. pertaining to or characterized by adsorption. 2. a substance that attracts other materials or particles to its surface.
gastrointestinal a. a substance, usually a powder, taken to adsorb gases, toxins, and bacteria in the stomach and intestines. Examples include activated charcoal and kaolin.
adsorption (əd'sawpshən, -'zawp-) the action of a substance in attracting and holding other materials or particles on its surface.
adtorsion (ad'tawshən) intorsion.
adult (ə'dult, 'adult) having attained full growth or maturity, or an organism that has done so.
a. respiratory distress syndrome (ARDS) a group of signs and symptoms that result in acute respiratory failure; characterized clinically by tachypnoea, dyspnoea, tachycardia, cyanosis, and low P_ao_2 that persists even with oxygen therapy (see also adult RESPIRATORY DISTRESS SYNDROME).
adulteration (ə,dultə'rayshən) addition of an impure, cheap, or unnecessary ingredient to cheat, cheapen, or falsify a preparation.
advancement (əd'vahnsmənt) detachment of a portion of tissue, especially muscle, and reattachment at an advanced point, thus increasing the distance between the origin and insertion of the muscle, as is done with an eye muscle for correction of strabismus.
adventitia (,adven'tishi·ə, -'tishə) the outer coat of an organ or structure, especially the outer coat of an artery.
adventitious (,adven'tishəs) not normal to a part.
adynamia (,adi'naymi·ə) lack of normal or vital powers. adj. **adynamic**.
Aedes (ay'eedeez) a genus of mosquitoes, comprising approximately 600 species.
A. aegypti the mosquito that most commonly transmits the causative organisms of yellow fever and dengue.
-aemia word element. [Gr.] *condition of the blood*.
aeration (air'rayshən) 1. the exchange of carbon dioxide for oxygen by the blood in the lungs. 2. the charging of a liquid with air or gas.
aeriform ('air·ri,fawm) resembling air; gaseous.
aero- word element. [Gr.] *air, gas*.
aerobe ('air·rohb) a microorganism that lives and grows in the presence of free oxygen. adj. **aerobic**.
facultative a. one that can live in the presence of oxygen, but does not require it.
obligate a. one that cannot live without oxygen.
aerocele ('air·roh,seel) a tumour formed by air filling an adventitious pouch, such as laryngocele and tracheocele.
aerodontalgia (,air·rohdon'talji·ə) pain in the teeth due to lowered atmospheric pressure at high altitudes.
aerodynamics (,air·rohdie'namiks) the science of air or gases in motion.
aeroembolism (,air·roh'embə,lizəm) obstruction of a blood vessel by air or gas.
aerogen ('air·roh,jen) a gas-producing bacillus.
aerogenesis (,air·roh'jenəsis) formation or production of gas.
aerogenous (air'rojənəs) gas-producing. Applied to microorganisms that give rise to the formation of gas, usually by the fermentation of lactose or other carbohydrate.
aerohydrotherapy (,air·roh,hiedrə'therəpee) therapeutic use of air and water. This is occasionally used in health spas.
aeropathy (air'ropəthee) bends (decompression sickness).
aerophagia (,air·roh'fayji·ə) habitual swallowing of air.
aerophagy (air'rofəjee) the excessive swallowing of air.
aerophilic, aerophilous (,air·roh'filik; ,air'rofiləs) requiring air for proper growth.
aeroplethysmograph (,air·rohple'thizmə,grahf, -graf) an apparatus for graphically recording respiratory

volumes.

aerosinusitis (ˌair·rohˌsienə'sietis) barosinusitis.

aerosol ('air·rəˌsol) a colloid system in which solid or liquid particles are suspended in a gas, especially a suspension of a drug or other substance to be dispensed in a cloud or mist.

Aerosol therapy is a major component of RESPIRATORY THERAPY in the treatment of bronchopulmonary disease. The major purpose of aerosol therapy is the delivery of medications or humidity or both to the mucosa of the respiratory tract and pulmonary alveoli.

Agents delivered by aerosol therapy may act in a number of ways: (1) to relieve spasm of the bronchial muscles and reduce oedema of the mucous membranes, (2) to render bronchial secretions more liquid so that they are more easily removed, (3) to humidify the respiratory tract, and (4) to administer antibiotics locally by depositing them in the respiratory tract.

Physical and chemical substances used as medical aerosols include drugs that act as BRONCHODILATORS and DECONGESTANTS, e.g., adrenaline, ephedrine, isoprenaline, atropine, and the steroids. Wetting agents administered as aerosols to render the bronchial secretions more liquid include tyloxapol and acetylcysteine. The selection of one or more antibiotics to be given as aerosol therapy is determined by the patient's specific condition and the preference of the doctor. Most standard antibiotic drugs are available in aerosol form.

In general, the doctor is concerned with factors that affect how deeply aerosol particles can penetrate into the bronchial tract and the locations at which these particles are deposited on the bronchial mucosa and alveolar tissues. Depth of penetration is affected by particle size. Particles as large as 100 μm and as small as 5 μm are trapped in the nose. Those which are 2–5 μm in size are deposited somewhere in the respiratory tract proximal to the alveoli. Deposition in the alveoli is 90% to 100% for particles 1–2 μm in size.

Because aerosol particles are so small, they present the phenomenon of brownian movement as they are bombarded by the molecules of the gas in which they are carried. The velocity with which these particles move about directly affects their diffusion and deposition onto nearby surfaces. Thus the type of aerosol generator used in aerosol therapy is of primary importance.

Another factor affecting penetration and deposition of aerosol particles that should be of concern to members of the health care team who are teaching patients the techniques of effective aerosol therapy is that of ventilatory pattern. The ideal pattern of breathing for optimum delivery of aerosol particles is that of slow, moderate deep breathing with breath holding at the end of each inspiration.

a. clearance removal of particles that have been deposited in the respiratory tissues. Clearance may occur by ciliary transport, by phagocytosis, by encapsulation and immobilization in a deposit of fibrous tissue (in which case the particles remain in the body), and by dissolving in tissue fluid and subsequently diffusing into the general circulation where the particles are metabolized.

a. deposition the depositing of aerosol particles onto a nearby surface, especially deposition or retention of the particles within the respiratory system. Closely related to aerosol penetration and affected by the same factors.

a. penetration the maximum distance aerosol particles can be carried into the respiratory tract by inhaled air. Depth of penetration increases as particle size decreases. Factors affecting where aerosol particles will be deposited and how deeply they can penetrate are: gravity, kinetic activity of gas molecules, inertial impaction, physical nature of the particle, and the ventilatory pattern.

Aerosporin (ˌair·roh'spor·rin) trademark for a preparation of polymyxin B sulphate, an antibiotic.

aerotitis (ˌair·roh'tietis) barotitis.

aerotolerant (ˌair·roh'tolə·rənt) surviving and growing in small amounts of air; said of anaerobic microorganisms.

Aerrane ('air·rayn) trademark for a preparation of isoflurane, a noninflammable anaesthetic agent.

Æsculapius ('eeskyuh'laypi·əs, 'es-) the god of healing in Roman mythology. The staff of Æsculapius, a rod or staff with a snake entwined around it, is a symbol of medicine.

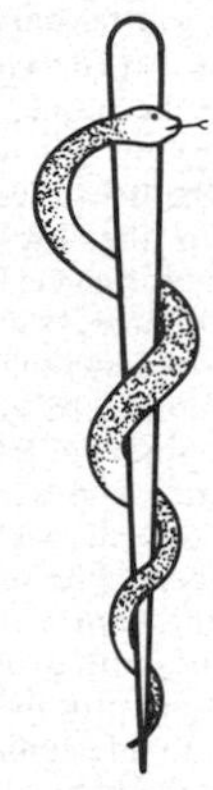

Staff of Aesculapius

aesthematology (esˌtheemə'toləjee) aesthesiology.

aesthesiogenic (esˌtheezioh'jenik) producing sensation.

aesthesiology (esˌtheezi'oləjee) the scientific study or description of the sense organs and sensations.

aesthesiometer (esˌtheezi'omitə) an instrument for measuring tactile sensibility; tactometer.

aesthesioneurosis (esˌtheeziohnyuh'rohsis) any disorder of the sensory nerves.

aesthesiophysiology (esˌtheeziohˌfizi'oləjee) the physiology of sensation and sense organs.

aesthesodic (ˌesthee'zodik) conducting or pertaining to conduction of sensory impulses.

aesthetics (ees'thetiks) the branch of philosophy dealing with beauty; in dentistry, a philosophy concerned especially with the appearance of a dental restoration, as achieved through its colour or form.

aestival (ee'stiev'l, 'esti-) pertaining to or occurring in summer.

aestivation (ˌeesti'vayshən, ˌes-) the dormant state in which certain animals pass the summer.

aestivoautumnal (ˌestivoh·aw'tumnəl) occurring in summer and autumn.

aetas ('eetas) [L.] *age;* abbreviated *aet.*

aetiology (ˌeeti'oləjee) the science dealing with causes of disease. adj. **aetiologic, aetiological**.

AFASIC (ay'fayzik) Association for all Speech Impaired Children.

afebrile (ay'feebriel, -'feb-) without fever.

affect (ə'fekt) emotional tone or feeling.

affection (ə'fekshən) a morbid condition or diseased state.

affective (ə'fektiv) pertaining to emotional tone or

feeling.

a. disorder any mental disorder characterized by a disturbance of mood accompanied by either manic or depressive symptoms or both. Major affective disorders are those in which the full syndrome of a manic or depressive episode is present: bipolar disorder (manic-depressive illness) and major depression. Other affective disorders include cyclothymic disorder and dysthymic disorder (depressive neurosis), which have less severe mood fluctuations.

afferent ('afə·rənt) conducting toward a centre or specific site of reference.

a. loop syndrome chronic partial obstruction of the proximal loop (duodenum and jejunum) after gastrectomy, resulting in duodenal distention, pain, and nausea following ingestion of food.

a. nerve any nerve that transmits impulses from the periphery toward the central nervous system (see also NEURON). Often used as a synonym for sensory pathways.

affiliation (ə,fili'ayshən) the judicial decision of paternity of a child with a view to a maintenance order.

affinity (ə'finitee) 1. attraction; a tendency to seek out or unite with another object or substance. 2. in chemistry, the tendency of two substances to form strong or weak chemical bonds forming molecules or complexes. 3. in immunology, the thermodynamic bond strength of an antigen–antibody complex.

afibrinogenaemia (,ayfiebrinəjə'neemi·ə) absence or deficiency of fibrinogen in the circulating blood. Congenital afibrinogenaemia—complete absence of fibrinogen—is a rare anomaly that is inherited. Acquired afibrinogenaemia is a deficiency of fibrinogen (*hypofibrinogenaemia*) and is usually secondary to disseminated intravascular coagulation (DIC). A common underlying cause of DIC is a complication of pregnancy such as septic abortion or ante partum haemorrhage. Other precipitating causes include severe infection, malignant disease (e.g. metastatic bone lesions, carcinoma of the prostate, leukaemia), transfusion of incompatible blood and the condition may sometimes complicate thoracic and abdominal surgery.

CLINICAL PICTURE. As fibrinogen plays an important role in the blood clotting mechanism, the chief symptom of fibrinogen deficiency is generalized bleeding, external or internal. The diagnosis is confirmed by the appropriate coagulation tests in the laboratory.

TREATMENT. Fibrinogen is present in fresh frozen plasma and this is usually administered intravenously to supply the body with this essential substance; transfusions of whole blood may also be indicated. Treatment of the underlying cause if possible, is necessary; for example in obstetric patients the fibrinogen level returns to normal after delivery has been accomplished and infection controlled.

AFP alpha-fetoprotein.

African sleeping sickness ('afrikən) African trypanosomiasis.

African tick fever disease caused by a spirochaete, *Borrelia duttoni.* Transmitted by ticks. See RELAPSING FEVER.

afterbirth ('ahftə,bərth) a lay expression to describe the special tissues associated with the development of a fetus in the uterus that are expelled after the birth of a baby. These are the PLACENTA, or the structure attached to the wall of the uterus through which nourishment passes from the mother of the fetus, the fetal membranes, which enclose the fetus and amniotic fluid *in utero*, and the UMBILICAL CORD, which attaches the fetus to the placenta.

afterbrain ('ahftə,brayn) metencephalon.

aftercare ('ahftə,kair) social, medical or nursing care following a period of hospital treatment.

afterhearing (,ahftə'hiə·ring) hearing of sounds after the stimulus has ceased.

afterimage ('ahftə,imij) a retinal impression remaining after cessation of the stimulus causing it.

afterpain ('ahftə,payn) pain that follows expulsion of the placenta, due to contraction of the uterus.

afterperception (,ahftəpə'sepshən) perception of after-sensations.

aftersensation (,ahftəsen'sayshən) sensation persisting after cessation of the stimulus that caused it.

aftersound ('ahftə,sownd) sensation of a sound after cessation of the stimulus causing it.

aftertaste ('ahftə,tayst) sensation of taste continuing after the stimulus has ceased.

afunctional (ay'fungkshənəl) lacking function.

Ag chemical symbol, *silver* (L. *argentum*); antigen.

A–G ratio ('aygee 'rayshioh) the ratio of albumin to globulin in blood serum, plasma, or urine.

agalactia (,aygə'lakshi·ə) absence or failure of secretion of milk.

agammaglobulinaemia (ay,gamə,globyuhli'neemi·ə) absence or severe deficiency of the plasma protein gamma globulin. There are three main types: transient, congenital, and acquired. The transient type occurs in early infancy, because gamma globulins are not produced in the fetus and the gamma globulins derived from the maternal blood are soon depleted. This temporary deficiency of gamma globulin lasts for the first 6 to 8 weeks, until the infant begins to synthesize the protein. Congenital agammaglobulinaemia is a rare condition, occurring in males, and resulting in decreased production of antibodies. Acquired agammaglobulinaemia is secondary to other disorders and is usually a hypogammaglobulinaemia, that is, a deficiency rather than total absence of this plasma protein. It is often secondary to malignant diseases such as leukaemia, myeloma, and lymphoma, and to diseases associated with hypoproteinaemia such as nephrotic syndrome and liver disease. Some patients have a family history of rheumatoid arthritis or allergies. This seems to indicate the presence of genetic factors in the development of agammaglobulinaemia.

Because gamma globulin is so important in the production of antibodies and thus in the body's ability to defend itself against infection, it follows that a deficiency or absence of gamma globulin would result in severe and recurrent infections.

aganglionic (ay,gangli'onik) lacking ganglion cells.

aganglionosis (ay,gangli·ə'nohsis) congenital absence of parasympathetic ganglion cells.

agar ('aygah) a dried hydrophilic, colloidal substance extracted from various species of red algae. It is used in culture media for bacteria and other microorganisms, in making emulsions, and as a supporting medium for immunodiffusion and immunoelectrophoresis. Because of its bulk it is also used in medicines to promote peristalsis and relieve constipation.

agastric (ay'gastrik) having no stomach.

age (ayj) 1. the duration, or the measure of time of the existence of a person or object. 2. to undergo change as a result of the passage of time.

achievement a. 1. see DEVELOPMENTAL MILESTONES. 2. proficiency in study expressed in terms of the chronological age of a normal child showing the same degree of attainment. 3. acquirement of a new interest or skill in old age or a praiseworthy accomplishment by an aged person, such as overcoming physical

handicaps.
chronological a. the actual measure of time elapsed since a person's birth.
gestational a. an expression of the age of a developing fetus, usually given in weeks. It is measured from the date of the mother's last menstrual period, and so is approximately two weeks greater than the length of time from conception. See PREGNANCY.
mental a. the age level of mental ability of a person as gauged by standard intelligence tests.
a.–sex register a list of patients in general practice or in other medical services classified by date of birth and sex.
a.-specific rate the number of deaths or cases of a disease in a specific age group in a specified time related to the number of persons in that age group and expressed per 1000 or other multiplier.

For example:

$$\text{Age-specific incidence of measles 0–5 years} = \frac{\text{number of cases in children aged 0–5 years in one year}}{\text{number of children aged 0–5 years at the mid point of the year}}$$

aged ('ayjid) persons of advanced age. It is convenient for statisticians to define everyone 65 years of age or older as 'aged', though 70 years is generally regarded as the commencement of old age. However, there is no definite age at which an individual become 'old'. Improvements in public health, nutrition, surgery, drugs and medical care since 1900 have added years to life expectancy, resulting in an ever larger 'ageing' population.

THE AGEING PROCESS. The reasons why we age are complex and only partially understood. It is probable that the ageing process is a combination of many factors, but researchers continue to look for one fundamental cause which can explain all its diverse effects.

The body continuously replaces worn-out cells, by the million, every day of our lives. With increasing age, the capacity to repair and replace damaged cells is reduced, this reduction proceeding throughout adult life. This is a very gradual change and may not result in any diminution of function. Most physiological functions have a reserve of capacity so that minor impairment will have no noticeable effect on function and a greater degree of impairment may only become apparent when the individual is under physiological stress, e.g. during exercise or when unwell. Some functions remain effectively unimpaired into old age, whilst others, e.g. strength of muscle contraction, deteriorate more evidently.

Genetic (hereditary) factors may play a part in determining how long a person lives and the functional quality of his life. Experiments with animals have shown that different groups of inbred animals (each inbred group having the same inherited characteristics) have different life-spans. Length of life may, therefore, be in part hereditary.

EFFECTS OF AGEING. Old age brings certain physical changes as a normal consequence of ageing. They may be discomforting, even limiting, but they are not necessarily incapacitating. Individuals vary in their rate of ageing and general fitness plays a part in some of this variation. The body has less strength and responds less well to stress as it ages. The speed of reaction and general agility are slowed. The basal metabolism or rate of energy production in the body cells is gradually lowered so that an old person tires more easily and is more sensitive to temperature changes. Sexual desire and ability decline, although they need never entirely end for either sex (though, of course, the reproductive capacity of the woman ceases at the MENOPAUSE). Those who have never used spectacles usually need them in later years, or their usual glasses need changing to bifocals (see also PRESBYOPIA). Hearing changes also occur. The elderly hear low tones fairly well, but their ability to perceive high tones declines. The capacity of soft tissue and bone to repair itself is slowed, as is cellular growth and division. Bones are more brittle. Skin becomes drier and loses some of its elasticity. Artificial teeth are often required. Taste and smell are blunted owing to a reduction in the number of receptors for these sensations. The mobility of the intestines is reduced, predisposing to constipation.

Much of the discomfort and disability that used to be considered a normal part of ageing can now be prevented with proper health care, including education in healthy living.

DISEASES OF OLD AGE. No disease is caused by old age, but age-related changes and the development of identifiable diseases are blurred and often interwoven, and certain diseases are more likely to occur in old age. ARTHRITIS, HERNIA, CATARACT, ATHEROSCLEROSIS, heart disease, MYOCARDIAL INFARCTION (heart attack), STROKE, DIABETES MELLITUS, CANCER, enlargement of the prostate in men, prolapse of the rectum or uterus, and other conditions tend to develop after decades of living. Worry, poor habits such as overeating, malnutrition, and lack of proper preventive attention to early signs probably accelerate the onset of these diseases in old age.

In the majority of cases, the disease originates during the middle years. This is why periodic health examinations are so important and become increasingly important after middle age.

AGE AND MENTAL POWERS. In most people ageing has little effect upon mental powers. It is one of the joys of old age that long after the body slows down and begins to limit physical activity, the mind can continue to seek and explore.

In older persons memory of recent events declines while important memories from long ago remain intact. This has been found to be largely a matter of interest and attention rather than an inability to remember. Older people do not learn new things as quickly as younger people, but once something has been learned, they remember it better and more accurately. The elderly have the further benefit of long experience and seasoned judgement to apply to the solution of new problems.

SOME RULES OF HEALTH AND HYGIENE FOR THE ELDERLY.
Periodic Health Examinations. The diseases that make invalids of the elderly, such as diabetes mellitus and heart disease, begin unnoticed in middle age; with regular checkups they can be detected in their early stages when they are easier to treat. Increasingly nurses, for example health vistors, clinic and domiciliary nurses, give advice on health care.
Proper Nutrition. Poor eating habits may stem from childhood but they begin to have their effects as people grow older. Poor nutrition has been demonstrated to have a definite adverse effect upon mental and physical vigour. Proper food can prolong life as well as preserve the strength and ability to fight off disease. Good nutrition is a vital aspect of successful ageing.

Many older people subsist on poor diets because they live alone and the preparation of proper meals requires too much effort. Some suffer from poor teeth or wear dentures that interfere with chewing. Others are victims of poor dietary habits, lack of interest, or, in some cases, misinformation.

The elderly need the same nutrients as those that must be supplied at any age. They must have all basic food elements every day, and this means not overloading the menu with any single type of food. The only kind of food that can be safely reduced in the diet is fat. Because of a gradual decrease in the amount of fat-digesting enzymes in the digestive tract of an older person, the ageing body manages fat less well. In general, the older person's diet tends to include too little of the foods that supply vitamin C, iron, vitamin A, vitamin B (thiamine), and vitamin B_2 (riboflavin).

Some older people believe that acid-containing foods such as citrus fruits and tomatoes, which are prime sources of vitamin C, cause acidity in the body. Actually, these acid-containing fruits are excellent alkalizers and rich sources of necessary vitamins and minerals as well, and should be included in the diet. Another common mistake is the belief that milk is only for children. It is an excellent food for adults too. Milk (full-cream or preferably skimmed or semi-skimmed) contains protein, calcium and riboflavin, and is readily digested and tolerated by most people of all ages.

If an older person has difficulty chewing, some foods will have to be chopped, strained, or cooked soft for his special requirements, but foods with important nutrient values must not be eliminated from the diet. As for persons of all ages, calorific intake should be adjusted according to the level of physical activity. See also NUTRITION.

Exercise. Proper exercise promotes good circulation and appetite, and helps to maintain good mental and physical functioning. Older people should be as active as possible, although never to the point of strain or exhaustion.

Rest. Rest becomes increasingly important in the later years. It is of great value to rest for half an hour after meals, and at intervals during the day. Older people whose work does not permit them to lie down should take advantage of 'breaks' or rest periods to relax as completely as possible, with their feet elevated, if at all feasible.

Avoidance of Inactivity. Following an illness, when the doctor says it is time to get out of bed, his instructions should be followed. A prolonged unnecessary stay in bed is harmful at all ages but especially in later years.

RETIREMENT PROBLEMS. Although many people look forward to retirement, it is not uncommon to hear of someone who, having worked hard all his life with that goal in mind, begins to fail mentally and physically when he actually reaches it. Successful retirement depends on far more than money in the bank. There must be a reserve of interests that make life worth living. Hobbies and recreational activities are important because they can be continued in later years. As Dr. George Lawton, an authority on gerontology, puts it: 'To grow old successfully, a man must learn to push around, not his body, but his mind. If his speed, strength, and endurance decline with the years, then he must train in advance skills which will hold up with age and even improve'.

MISCONCEPTIONS ABOUT THE ELDERLY. Concern about the health and welfare of elderly persons is praiseworthy but must not lead to stereotyping them as sick, poor, isolated, and pitiful. Surveys of older Americans show that fewer than one in five considers himself or herself to be in poor health. The number of the elderly officially counted as 'poor' has decreased in the past 20 years from 33 per cent in 1959 to 6 per cent in the 1980s. The reason for this is the additional noncash benefits and greatly increased retirement benefits for which they are now eligible. A large majority (over 80 per cent) of older Americans have children or other relatives living nearby with whom they are in almost daily contact. About the same percentage have their own home and live a life of relative independence.

The care of the elderly who are sick, infirm and financially unable to provide for themselves is a responsibility of those members of society who are younger and in their prime of health and productivity. But thinking of *all* elderly citizens as useless, burdensome, and unable to think and care for themselves is fallacious and does them a great injustice. An older person does have special needs, but then so do all of us.

ageing ('ayjing) the structural changes that take place in time that are not caused by accident or disease.

agenesis (ay'jenəsis) absence of an organ due to nonappearance of its primordium in the embryo.

agenitalism (ay'jenit'lizəm) a condition due to lack of secretion of the testes or ovaries.

agenosomia (ay,jenə'sohmi·ə) imperfect development of reproductive organs.

agent ('ayjənt) a person or substance by which something is accomplished.

adrenergic neuron blocking a. one that inhibits the release of noradrenaline from postganglionic adrenergic nerve endings.

alkylating a. a cytotoxic agent, e.g., a nitrogen mustard, which is highly reactive and can donate an alkyl group to another compound. Alkylating agents inhibit cell division by reacting with DNA and are used as ANTINEOPLASTIC agents.

anticholinergic a. cholinergic blocking agent.

chelating a. a compound that combines with metals to form weakly dissociated complexes in which the metal is part of a ring, and used to extract certain elements from a system.

cholinergic blocking a. one that blocks the action of acetylcholine at nicotinic or muscarinic receptors of nerves or effector organs.

ganglionic blocking a. one that blocks cholinergic transmission at autonomic ganglionic synapses.

A. Orange a herbicide containing 2,4,5-T, 2,4-D, and the contaminant dioxin and which is suspected of being carcinogenic and teratogenic.

oxidizing a. a substance that acts as an electron acceptor in a chemical oxidation–reduction reaction.

reducing a. a substance that acts as an electron donor in a chemical oxidation–reduction reaction.

surface-active a. a substance that exerts a change on the surface properties of a liquid, especially one, such as a detergent, that reduces its surface tension. Called also surfactant.

ageusia (ay'gyoozi·ə) absence or impairment of the sense of taste.

agger ('ajə) pl. *aggeres* [L.] an elevation.

a. nasi an elevation at the anterior free margin of the middle nasal concha.

agglutinable (ə'glootinəb'l) capable of agglutination.

agglutinant (ə'glootinənt) 1. acting like glue. 2. a substance that promotes union of parts.

agglutination (ə,glooti'nayshən) aggregation of separate particles into clumps or masses; especially the clumping together of bacteria by the action of a specific antibody directed against a surface antigen. See also AGGLUTININ. adj. **agglutinative.**

cross a. the agglutination of particulate antigen by an antibody raised against a different but related antigen; see also group agglutination.

group a. agglutination - usually to a lower titre - of various members of a group of biologically related organisms by an agglutinin specific for one of that group. For instance, the specific agglutinin of typhoid bacilli may agglutinate other members of the colon-typhoid group, such as *Escherichia coli* and *Salmonella enteritidis*.

intravascular a. clumping of particulate elements within the blood vessels; used conventionally to denote red blood cell agglutination.

platelet a. the clumping together of platelets owing to the action of platelet agglutinins. Such agglutinins are important in platelet typing.

agglutinin (ə'glootinin) any substance causing agglutination (clumping together) of cells, particularly a specific antibody formed in the blood in response to the presence of an invading agent. Agglutinins are proteins (IMMUNOGLOBULINS) and function as part of the immune mechanism of the body. When the invading agents that bring about the production of agglutinins are bacteria, the agglutinins produced bring about agglutination of the bacterial cells.

Erythrocytes also may agglutinate when agglutinins are formed in response to the entrance of noncompatible blood cells into the bloodstream. A transfusion reaction is an example of the result of agglutination of blood cells brought about by agglutinins produced in the recipient's blood in response to incompatible or foreign cells (the donor's blood). Anti-Rh agglutinins are produced in cases of Rh incompatibility and can result in a condition known as HAEMOLYTIC disease of the newborn when the maternal blood is Rh negative and the fetal blood is Rh positive (see also RH FACTOR).

cold a. one that acts only at low temperature.

group a. one that has a specific action on certain organisms, but will agglutinate other species as well.

H a. one that is specific for flagellar antigens of the motile strain of an organism.

immune a. a specific agglutinin found in the blood after recovery from the disease or injection of the microorganism.

incomplete a. one that at appropriate concentrations fails to agglutinate the homologous antigen.

normal a. a specific agglutinin found in the blood of an animal or of man that has neither had the associated disease nor been injected with the causative organism.

O a. one specific for somatic antigens of a microorganism.

partial a. one present in agglutinative serum which acts on organisms closely related to the specific antigen, but in a lower dilution.

warm a. an incomplete antibody that sensitizes and reacts optimally with erythrocytes at 37 °C.

agglutinogen (,agluh'tinəjən) a substance (antigen) that stimulates the animal body to form agglutinin (antibody).

aggregation (,agri'gayshən) 1. massing or clumping of materials together. 2. a clumped mass of material.

familial a. the occurrence of more cases of a given disorder in close relatives of a person with the disorder than in control families.

platelet a. platelet agglutination.

aggressin (ə'gresin) a substance said to be produced by some bacteria which increases their effect upon the host.

aggression (ə'greshən) ideas or behaviours that are angry and destructive and intended to be injurious, physically or emotionally, and aimed at domination of one person by another. It may be manifested by overt attacking and destructive behaviour or by covert attitudes of hostility and obstructionism.

agitation (,aji'tayshən) 1. shaking. 2. mental distress causing extreme restlessness.

aglaucopsia (,ayglaw'kopsi·ə) inability to distinguish green tints.

aglossia (ay'glosi·ə) congenital absence of the tongue.

aglossostomia (,ayglosoh'stohmi·ə) congenital absence of the tongue and the mouth opening.

aglutition (,aygloo'tishən) inability to swallow.

aglycaemia (,ayglie'seemi·ə) absence of sugar from the blood (see also HYPOGLYCAEMIA).

aglycone (ay'gliekohn) the noncarbohydrate portion of a glycoside molecule.

aglycosuric (ay,gliekoh'syooə·rik) free from glycosuria.

agnathia (ag'naythi·ə) congenital absence of the lower jaw.

agnogenic (,agnoh'jenik) of unknown origin.

agnosia (ag'nohzi·ə) inability to recognize the import of sensory impressions; the varieties correspond with several senses and are distinguished as auditory (acoustic), gustatory, olfactory, tactile, and visual.

finger a. loss of ability to indicate one's own or another's fingers.

time a. loss of comprehension of the succession and duration of events.

-agogue word element. [Gr.] *something that leads or induces.*

agonad (ay'gonad) an individual having no sex glands (gonads).

agonadal (ay'gonəd'l) having no sex glands; due to absence of sex glands.

agonal ('agənəl) pertaining to death or extreme suffering.

agonist ('agənist) a muscle which in contracting to move a part is opposed by another muscle (the antagonist). In pharmacology, a drug that has affinity for the cellular receptors of another drug or natural substance and which produces a physiological effect.

agony ('agənee) 1. death struggle. 2. extreme suffering.

agoraphobia (,agə·rə'fohbi·ə) fear of open or public spaces (literally 'fear of the market place')—the most commonly cited phobic disorder of persons seeking treatment.

-agra word element. [Gr.] *attack, seizure.*

agranular reticulum (ay'granyuhlə) smooth-surfaced endoplasmic reticulum.

agranulocyte (ay'granyuhloh,siet) a nongranular leukocyte.

agranulocytosis (ay,granyuhlohsie'tohsis) an acute disease in which there is a sudden drop in the production of leukocytes, leaving the body defenceless against bacterial invasion. A great majority of the cases of agranulocytosis are caused by sensitization to drugs or chemicals that affect the bone marrow and thereby depress the formation of granulocytes.

SYMPTOMS. The first manifestations of this disorder are usually produced by a severe infection and include high fever, chills, prostration, and ulcerations of mucous membrane such as in the mouth, rectum, or vagina. Laboratory tests reveal a profound leukopenia (low leukocyte count).

TREATMENT. Treatment is aimed at immediate withdrawal of the drug or chemical causing the disorder, and control of infection. In most cases control can be achieved by the administration of antibiotics, usually penicillin, streptomycin, or oxytetracycline. If the bone marrow is not irreparably damaged, the prognosis is good, with proper treatment, and the patient will recover as the production of granulocytes resumes. Rarely, the leukocyte-producing tissues are damaged beyond repair, and death ensues, unless a bone marrow transplant is successful.

agranuloplastic (ay,granyuhloh'plastik) forming nongranular cells only.

agranulosis (ay,granyuh'lohsis) agranulocytosis.

agraphia (ay'grafi·ə) loss of ability to express thoughts in writing.
ague (ˌaygyoo) 1. malaria. 2. a chill.
agyria (ay'jieri·ə) a malformation in which the gyri of the cerebral cortex are not normally developed; called also lissencephaly.
AHF antihaemophilic factor (clotting factor VIII).
AHG antihaemophilic globulin (clotting factor VIII).
AI aortic incompetence; aortic insufficiency; apical impulse; artificial insemination.
AID (ˌayie'dee) artificial insemination of a woman with donor semen. The woman must be menstruating regularly and be physically fit. The donor should be of the same race as the mother/husband and remains anonymous. He has no responsibility or legal right to the child, who is legally illegitimate (though changes in the law are expected). The husband may legally adopt the child.
AIDS (aydz) acquired immune deficiency syndrome. It is part of the spectrum of disease caused by human immunodeficiency virus (HIV) infection. This virus, previously known as human T-cell lymphotrophic virus III (HTLV-III) and lymphadenopathy associated virus (LAV), causes an impairment of the body's cellular immune system whiich may result in infection by organisms of normally no or low pathogenicity (opportunistic infections) principally *Pneumocystis carinii* pneumonia (PCP), or the development of unusual tumours, principally KAPOSI'S SARCOMA (KS).

Infection occurs after virus in the blood, semen, vaginal secretions or breast milk of a carrier gains entry to a particular form of lymphocyte—the helper T-lymphocyte—of the host. After a variable period, antibodies to the virus appear in the blood. This seroconversion may coincide with a transient glandular fever-like illness. These antibodies do not seem to be protective as the virus continues to be found in the helper T-lymphocytes where its continued replication destroys these cells and hence causes disordered immune function. The current experience of HIV-infected individuals is that many remain as asymptomatic infectious carriers. Some of the remainder may be asymptomatic but develop a persistent generalized lymphadenopathy. Others, in addition to the enlarged lymph nodes, develop symptoms such as night sweats, diarrhoea, weight loss and malaise; this latter condition is called AIDS-related complex. Examination of the blood may show abnormally low platelet and neutrophil counts as well as low lymphocyte counts.

Only individuals with an opportunistic infection or unusual tumour can be diagnosed as having AIDS. This has occurred in approximately 2.5% of infected British haemophiliacs and in about 30% of infected Manhattan homosexuals. This shows the error in calling the HIV antibody test the 'AIDS test'. Of the first 168 British AIDS cases, 41% had PCP (mean survival 12.5 months), 26% Kaposi's sarcoma (mean survival 21.2 months), 26% opportunistic infections other than PCP (mean survival 13.3 months) and 7% PCP and KS (mean survival 6.6 months).

A recently recognized development is the recognition of HIV nervous system involvement with late manifestations such as fits, presenile dementia and painful peripheral neuropathy. Early manifestations include personality changes and memory disturbance. As control measures depend on altering infected individual's behaviour the dementia may carry serious implications.

The causative organisms of Acquired Immune Deficiency Syndrome (HIV 1 and HIV 2) were both discovered concurrently by Professor Luc Montagnier of the Institute Pasteur in Paris, and Dr. Robert C. Gallo of the National Cancer Institute, Bethseda, USA. This development in finding a causative organism of this problem changed greatly the path of the disease and society's ability to monitor its spread. From this original work, tests were developed which could detect antibodies to the virus in an infected person's blood.

It is important to remember that not everyone who is infected with HIV goes on to develop AIDS, but for those who do, the incubation period may vary from between a few weeks to sixty months, and it is because of this extraordinary long incubation period that people who are desirous to be tested should first undergo very careful counselling about the implications of being discovered to be antibody positive. Society's reaction to this new illness has, on many occasions, been alarming, and those known to be infected have very often been shunned by society and indeed have difficulty in obtaining employment, housing and insurance.

The onset of AIDS and the potential for transmission from body fluids to body fluids highlights a potential risk to health care providers who are not skilled practitioners, and nurses should, without taking outrageous precautions against patients with AIDS, ensure that their practice is of a high enough standard to prevent them becoming accidentally comtaminated.

There are many laboratories around the world currently working to discover a vaccine against this virus, and indeed to develop new drugs to combat the opportunistic infections which result for patients with AIDS. Many of these are extremely new and not yet in the first trial stages. Others are currently undergoing clinical trials, and some of them offer a glimmer of hope for patients in the future.
AIH artificial insemination of a woman by her husband's semen.
ailment ('ailmənt) any minor disorder of the body.
ailurophobia (ˌiclyuhrə'fohbi·ə) morbid fear of cats.
AIMS Association for the Improvement of the Maternity Services.
AIMSW Associate of the Institute of Medical Social Workers.
ainhum ('ien·həm) a condition of unknown origin, occurring chiefly in dark-skinned races, leading to spontaneous amputation of the fourth of fifth toe.
air (air) the gaseous mixture that makes up the atmosphere.

a. hunger a distressing dyspnoea occurring in paroxysms, characteristic of diabetic acidosis and coma; called also Kussmaul's respiration.
airport malaria ('airpawt) see airport MALARIA.
airway ('airˌway) 1. the passage by which air enters and leaves the lungs. 2. a mechanical device used for securing unobstructed respiration during general anaesthesia or other occasions when the patient is not ventilating or exchanging gases properly.

In order to provide and maintain an open airway when there is cessation of breathing, the head is tilted back and the chin lifted up. This is accomplished by placing one hand on the forehead, pressing back, while the fingers of the other hand are placed under the chin and the lower jaw is lifted forward. This simple technique frequently is all that is needed to provide an open airway for spontaneous resumption of breathing.

OROPHARYNGEAL AIRWAY. This device is a hollow, flattened tube which is inserted into the mouth and back of the throat to prevent the tongue from slipping back into the throat and closing off the passage of air. It should not be used on alert or semiconscious patients as it may stimulate the gag reflex and cause vomiting unless the patient is deeply unconscious.

Selection of proper size is essential because an airway that is too short cannot lift the tongue away from the oropharynx, and one that is too long may damage the posterior pharynx or stimulate the larynx, causing laryngospasm. The airway should be gently inserted so as to avoid trauma to the mucous membranes. It must be inserted so that the tongue is not displaced back into the pharynx, where it will obstruct the air passage.

Endotracheal Tube. A tube with or without an inflatable cuff which is inserted into the mouth or nose and passed down into the trachea. It is used for the administration of anaesthetics and may be left in place after the completion of surgery until the patient is no longer in danger of asphyxiation. The endotracheal tube can be connected to a mechanical ventilator when necessary.

S-Tube Airway. This tube may be used to maintain a patent airway and to keep the mouth open during emergency resuscitation efforts. It does not, however, provide an adequate seal around the mouth, and may induce vomiting if not used properly.

Tracheostomy. This involves a surgical incision into the trachea to relieve obstruction of the respiratory tract above the level of the incision. A metal or plastic tracheostomy tube is inserted into the incision. See also tracheostomy.

Mini-tracheostomy. A method of managing excessive secretions in a patient unable to cough because of weakness or depressed consciousness, without the need for formal tracheostomy. A bougie is inserted through the cricothyroid membrane and a small plastic tube passed over it and into the trachea.

Cricothyrotomy. Passage of a cannula through the cricothyroid membrane and into the trachea as a last ditch method of securing the airway.

akaryocyte (ay'karioh,siet) a non-nucleated cell, e.g., an erythrocyte.

akaryote (ay'karioht) 1. non-nucleated. 2. a non-nucleated cell.

akathisia (,akə'thizi·ə) a condition marked by motor restlessness and anxiety.

akinaesthesia (,aykinəs'theezi·ə) absence of movement sense.

akinesia (,ayki'neezi·ə) 1. abnormal absence or poverty of movements. 2. the temporary paralysis of a muscle by the injection of procaine.

a. algera paralysis due to the intense pain of muscular movement.

akinetic (,ayki'netik) affected with akinesia.

Akineton (,aykie'neeton) trademark for preparations of biperiden, an anticholinergic used in the treatment of Parkinson's disease and certain forms of spasticity.

Al chemical symbol, *aluminium.*

ala ('aylə) pl. *alae* [L.] a winglike process. adj. **alate**.

a. nasi the cartilaginous flap on the outer side of either nostril.

alacrima (ay'lakrimə) a deficiency or absence of secretion of tears.

alalia (ə'layli·ə) impairment of the ability to speak.

alanine ('alə,neen, -nien) a naturally occurring, nonessential amino acid.

alanine aminotransferase ('alə,neen ə,meenoh'transfə,rayz, -'trahns-) an enzyme that catalyses the transfer of an amino group from an alpha amino acid to an alpha keto acid. Abbreviated ALT. It is present in many tissues and body fluids. The serum concentration is elevated especially when there is acute damage to liver cells, as in viral or toxic hepatitis, infectious mononucleosis, and obstructive jaundice. Called also *(serum) glutamic-pyruvic transaminase (GPT or SGPT).*

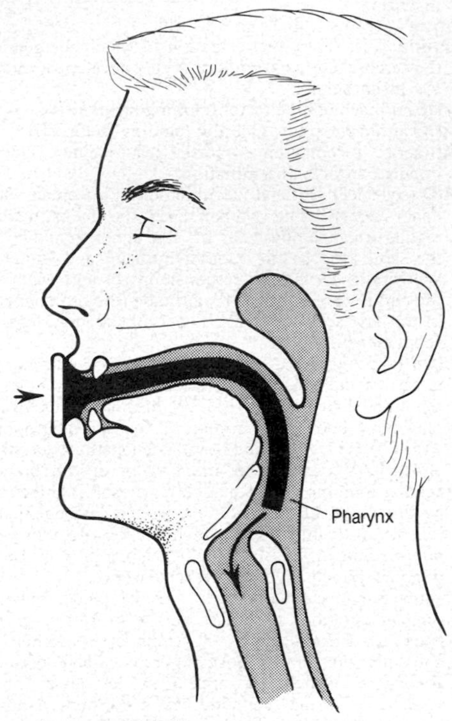

Oropharyngeal airway

alar ('aylə) pertaining to or like a wing.

alarm reaction (ə'lahm) the response of the sympathetic nervous system to either physical stress or to a strong emotional state; called also stress reaction and fight or flight reaction. It is an automatic and instantaneous response that increases the body's capability to cope with a sudden emergency.

The physiological changes occurring during this reaction increase physical strength and mental activity. The blood pressure is elevated, the blood glucose level is raised for additional energy, the blood coagulates more readily, and the flow of blood to muscles needed for activity is increased, while those organs not needed for 'fight' or 'flight' receive a diminished blood supply. One of the most striking manifestations of this reaction is the involution of lymphoid tissues due to the action of adrenal hormones.

alba ('albə) [L.] *white.*

Albers-Schönberg disease (,albairz'shərnbərg) a rare hereditary, congenital condition in which there are bandlike areas of condensed bone at the epiphyseal lines of long bones and condensation of the edges of smaller bones. Fractures occur frequently and deformities of the head, chest, or spine develop. There is no treatment and the prognosis is unfavourable. Called also *osteopetrosis* and *marble bones.*

albicans ('albi,kanz) [L.] *white.*

albiduria (,albi'dyooə·ri·ə) the discharge of white or pale urine.

Albini's nodules (al'beeneez) grey nodules of the size of small grains, sometimes seen on the free edges of the atrioventricular valves of infants; they are remains of fetal structures.

albinism ('albi,nizəm) congenital absence of normal pigmentation in the body (hair, skin, eyes).

albino (al'beenoh) a person affected with albinism.

albinuria (,albi'nyooə·ri·ə) albiduria.

Albl's ring ('alb'lz) a ring-shaped shadow in radiographs of the skull, caused by aneurysm of a cerebral artery.

Albright's syndrome ('awlbriets) a group of symptoms, including distortion of bone with fibrous changes in the bone marrow spaces, brownish pigmentation of the skin and precocious puberty in females, of unknown cause. Called also polyostotic fibrous dysplasia. The bone lesions may cause the bones to become bowed or shortened, resulting in difficulty in walking, and may make them more susceptible to fractures. Treatment is concerned with the complications of the disorder–fractures and deformities. Corrective orthopaedic surgery is often indicated.

albuginea (,albyoo'jini·ə) 1. a tough, whitish layer of fibrous tissue investing a part or organ. 2. the tunica albuginea.

albumin ('albyuhmin) 1. any protein that is soluble in water and moderately concentrated salt solutions and is coagulable by heat. 2. serum albumin; a plasma protein, formed principally in the liver and constituting about four-sevenths of the 6 to 8 per cent protein concentration in the plasma. Albumin is responsible for much of the colloidal osmotic pressure of the blood, and thus is a very important factor in regulating the exchange of water between the plasma and the interstitial compartment (space between the cells). Because of hydrostatic pressure, water is forced through the walls of the capillaries into the tissue spaces. This flow of water continues until the osmotic pull of protein (albumin) molecules causes it to stop. A drop in the amount of albumin in the plasma leads to an increase in the flow of water from the capillaries into the interstitial compartment. This results in an increase in tissue fluid which, if severe, becomes apparent as oedema. Albumin serves also as a transport protein carrying large organic anions, such as fatty acids, bilirubin, and many drugs, and also hormones, such as cortisol and thyroxine, when their specific binding globulins are saturated.

The presence of albumin in the urine (albuminuria) indicates malfunction of the kidney, and may accompany kidney disease or heart failure. A person with severe renal disease may lose as much as 20 to 30 g of plasma proteins in the urine in one day.

A decrease in the serum albumin level may occur with severe disease of the kidney. Other conditions such as liver disease, malnutrition, and extensive burns may result in serious decrease of plasma proteins.

aggregated a. heat-denatured human albumin, which is labelled with radioisotopes for pulmonary perfusion scanning. Called also macroaggregated albumin.

a.-globulin ratio the ratio of albumin to globulin in blood serum, plasma, or urine.

a. human a sterile, nonpyrogenic preparation of human serum albumin tested for absence of hepatitis B surface antigen, used in the treatment of shock and hypoproteinaemia.

iodinated I 131 a. a radiopharmaceutical used in blood pool imaging and plasma volume determinations, consisting of albumin human labelled with iodine-131.

macroaggregated a. (MAA) aggregated albumin.

normal human serum a. albumin human.

serum a. albumin of the blood.

albuminoid (al'byoomi,noyd) 1. resembling albumin. 2. an albumin-like substance; the term is sometimes applied to scleroproteins.

albuminoptysis (al,byoomi'noptisis) albumin in the sputum.

albuminuria (al,byoomi'nyooə·ri·ə) the presence in the urine of serum albumin. adj. **albuminuric**.

albumose ('albyuh,mohs, -,mohz) a substance formed during gastric digestion, intermediate between albumin and peptone.

Alcaligenes (,alkə'lijəneez) a genus of bacteria found in the intestines of vertebrates or in dairy products.

Alcock's canal ('awlkoks) a tunnel formed by a splitting of the obturator fascia, which encloses the pudendal vessels and nerve.

alcohol ('alkə,hol) 1. any organic compound containing the hydroxy (-OH) functional group except those in which the -OH group is attached to an aromatic ring, which are called *phenols*. Alcohols are classified as *primary*, *secondary*, or *tertiary* according to whether the carbon atom to which the -OH group is attached is bonded to one, two, or three other carbon atoms and as *monohydric*, *dihydric*, or *trihydric* according to whether they contain one, two, or three -OH groups; the latter two are called *diols* and *triols*, respectively. 2. common name for ethyl alcohol (ethanol).

absolute a. ethyl alcohol free from water and impurities.

denatured a. ethyl alcohol made unfit for consumption by the addition of substances known as denaturants. Although it should never be taken internally, denatured alcohol is widely used on the skin as a cooling agent and skin disinfectant.

ethyl a. the major ingredient of alcoholic beverages; called also ethanol and grain alcohol. It is sometimes used medically to stimulate the appetite of convalescent, weak, or elderly patients. **isopropyl a.** a transparent, volatile colourless liquid used as a rubbing compound; called also isopropanol.

methyl a. a mobile, colourless liquid used as a solvent; called also wood alcohol or methanol. It is a useful fuel, but is poisonous if taken internally. Consumption may lead to blindness or death.

wood a. methyl alcohol.

alcoholic (,alkə'holik) 1. containing or pertaining to alcohol. 2. a person suffering from alcoholism.

alcoholism ('alkə,holizəm) alcohol dependence; the term is used to denote a variety of conditions involving abuse of alcohol. Alcoholism in its many forms is considered to be a major drug problem in almost all Western societies. Problems related to intemperate consumption of alcohol are both immediate and long-term; it adversely affects the physical and mental health of the individual and the integrity of the society in which he or she lives.

The signs and symptoms associated with alcoholism include a wide range of behaviours, which vary among persons having alcohol-related health problems. These include drinking to the point of drunkenness in social situations, drinking alone or in secret, using alcohol to relieve insomnia in the evening or to help get started in the morning, using alcohol to modify stress, anger, and anxiety, and experiencing blackouts (palimpsests) in which the person has no memory of what happened during an episode of heavy drinking. Although any heavy social drinker has a risk of becoming physically dependent on alcohol, it is the compulsive nature of his drinking that sets the addicted alcoholic apart from the occasionally excessive drinker. Aside from the well-known signs of drunkenness, which include staggering, emotional lability, and incoherence of speech, the person suffering from chronic alcoholism also exhibits tremulousness, particularly of the hands, tachycardia, and sweating. The vast majority of alcoholics are ordinary people who constitute a cross-section of society.

AETIOLOGY. There is no universally accepted explanation of why one person becomes an alcoholic while another does not. In general, a person is more likely to become an alcoholic if his environment emphasizes drinking, presenting it as a fashionable, or indeed indispensable, social pastime. Although many alcoholics have no family history of alcohol abuse or addiction, a person who grew up in a family in which both parents had alcohol-related problems is at very high risk of becoming an alcoholic.

Psychological factors play an important role in the development of alcoholism in an individual. Unresolved conflicts, loneliness, financial difficulties, social rejection, and marital problems may contribute to the development of alcoholism in susceptible persons.

Studies performed in Denmark have shown that adopted children are more likely to become alcoholics if their biological parents abused alcohol. This gives support to the hypothesis that inheritance also plays a role in the development of alcoholism.

ASSOCIATED PATHOLOGIES. Alcohol is a toxic drug that is harmful to all of the body tissues. Protracted use can lead to a host of pathological changes in the central nervous system, the liver (which detoxifies the drug), and the heart, kidney, and gastrointestinal tract. Although cirrhosis of the liver is the most recognized complication of alcoholism, recent research indicates that intellectual impairment can arise in the early stages of the disease, and permanent and disabling brain damage can eventually occur. Prolonged and abusive intake of alcohol coupled with nutritional depletion and thiamine deficiency can produce WERNICKE-KORSAKOFF SYNDROME. Newborn infants of mothers who drink heavily during pregnancy are susceptible to FETAL ALCOHOL SYNDROME.

The interrelationships between alcohol and hepatic disease are not completely understood. There is still dispute about whether cirrhosis associated with alcohol abuse (Laennec's cirrhosis) results from the direct hepatotoxic effects of alcohol or from malnutrition associated with chronic alcohol abuse. Gastrointestinal disturbances are fairly common and include gastritis, excessive bowel activity, and oesophageal varices.

Coronary artery disease and hypertension are believed to be related to a high intake of alcohol, because it results in elevation of the level of triglycerides in the blood. Alcohol abusers have an increased risk of cancer of the mouth and oesophagus. Habitual drinking may lower resistance to infection by producing immunosuppression. Alcohol has been associated with sexual impotence, probably because of suppression of the production of testosterone.

'Hangovers'. The commonly experienced symptoms of headache, nausea, gastritis, emotional irritability, and mild tremors of the hands are most likely the result of the same physiological mechanisms as those associated with the withdrawal syndrome. Over-the-counter medicines and home remedies are of questionable value except as placebos. Quiet, rest, and sleep are usually sufficient for recovery from an occasional drinking bout and its resultant discomfort.

ALCOHOL ADDICTION. The hallmarks of addiction to alcohol, as to other central nervous system depressants, are tolerance and physical dependence. There is no firmly established limit to the amount of alcohol a person can consume before exhibiting signs of intoxication. Some can drink a large amount of liquor and maintain acceptable social behaviour and perform psychomotor feats without great difficulty, while others can become intoxicated by ingesting a very small quantity. However, a blood alcohol level of 80 mg per 100 ml makes a driver legally intoxicated. Blood levels above 200 mg per 100 ml can produce signs of severe intoxication.

Pharmacological tolerance to alcohol does not increase with use, as with barbiturates or heroin. Over a period of time the heroin addict can increase his tolerance gradually to the point that he is able to withstand 50 times the dose he began with. A person who consumes enough alcohol to raise his blood alcohol level to 400 mg per 100 ml will probably lapse into a coma no matter how many years he has been drinking to excess. If the level of blood alcohol reaches 600 mg per 100 ml, respiration is severely and sometimes fatally depressed. Tolerance for alcohol may, in fact, *decrease* as the various organs of the body are repeatedly insulted and the disease becomes more severe and chronic in nature.

Physical dependence is manifested most strikingly when the alcoholic is deprived of the drug and withdrawal symptoms appear. These symptoms are all manifestations of neurological impairment and range from mild tremors of the hands, to seizures or delirium tremens.

Tremulousness usually begins from 6 to 12 hours after drinking has diminished or ceased and may persist for 72 hours or more. Hallucinations can occur in an alcohol addict when the blood alcohol is very high as well as after drinking has ceased altogether and the level is relatively low. Hallucinations are also frequently a part of delirium tremens.

Grand mal seizures resulting from withdrawal of alcohol can occur 12 to 24 hours after cessation of drinking. There is usually no forewarning or aura as often occurs in epilepsy. Residual twitching in specific areas of the body or a stuporous condition sometimes follows the seizure. About one-third of those having seizures associated with alcohol withdrawal eventually develop delirium tremens.

DELIRIUM TREMENS is the rarest of all withdrawal syndromes and the one that is most severe. It is potentially fatal without proper treatment. A person who is suffering from this form of withdrawal needs hospitalization and intensive care.

MEDICAL TREATMENT AND PATIENT CARE DURING WITHDRAWAL. A patient experiencing detoxification and withdrawal from alcohol requires coordinated medical and nursing care. In the past decade, changing attitudes toward alcoholic patients and recognition of their physiological and psychosocial needs have led to improved care and to a decrease in the mortality rate during withdrawal. Symptoms of the withdrawal syndrome can last from days to weeks. During this time, the patient will probably exhibit problems related to: (1) fluid and electrolyte imbalance, (2) acid–base imbalance, (3) anxiety and psychomotor agitation, (4) nausea, vomiting, and possibly GI bleeding, and (5) a potentially severe nutritional deficit.

Fluid and electrolyte status should be assessed and any imbalance corrected, preferably by oral rather than intravenous therapy. Some alcoholic patients are dehydrated, while others are over hydrated and therefore need a diuretic to restore fluid balance. Transient hyperventilation associated with anxiety may produce respiratory ALKALOSIS, an increase in blood pH, and a decrease in magnesium levels.

Extreme irritability, restlessness, and insomnia can be relieved by the administration of a mild tranquillizer, and by sedatives that help the patient achieve adequate sleep and rest without interfering with normal daily activities. The agitated patient will benefit from a quiet, non-stimulating environment and calm assurance that he is safe and will be cared for. If hallucinating, he may or may not be frightened, but he will be confused and disoriented at times. Safety measures are necessary to prevent unintentional or intentional self-injury. There is always the possibility that an alcoholic patient will be suicidal; therefore expressions of depression and feelings of remorse should be taken seriously.

Anticonvulsant drugs, such as phenytoin (Epanutin), are sometimes prescribed to prevent and control seizures. Care for and protection of the patient before, during, and after a convulsive seizure is discussed under CONVULSION.

Nausea and vomiting should be controlled with medication and nursing measures in order to prevent upper GI tract trauma and haemorrhaging. If the patient has oesophageal varices, which are fairly common in conjunction with cirrhosis of the liver, they can rupture during an episode of strenuous vomiting and create an emergency situation.

The nutritional status of the alcoholic patient should be evaluated before therapy is begun. Many alcoholics have a vitamin deficiency, especially a deficiency of thiamine. Vitamin therapy of some kind is usually a valuable adjunct to other measures intended to improve the overall health status and produce a sense of well-being in the alcoholic patient. Some alcoholics may develop signs of BERIBERI during periods of drinking, when food intake may be drastically reduced.

Finally, it should be remembered that withdrawal symptoms may also be seen in an accident victim, surgical patient, or other patient with a medical problem unrelated to alcohol but who also has a hidden drinking problem. When early symptoms of withdrawal first appear in a hospitalized patient, his assessment should include a history of drinking patterns as well as an appraisal of his status with respect to physiological changes attributable to alcoholism. A care plan should be developed to help meet his specific needs.

Because of the social stigma of alcoholism, the patient and his family may not readily acknowledge and confront the problem. And, because it is such a difficult disorder to deal with, health professionals may ignore it and join them in denying the problem. This combination of attitudes all too often denies the patient any chance of receiving adequate treatment and control of his alcoholism. The delay in treatment of the early signs of withdrawal sets the stage for more serious and sometimes fatal progression of the syndrome.

TREATMENT OF CHRONIC ALCOHOLISM. Alcohol abuse and addiction are complex behaviour disorders for which there is no simple remedy. This is not to say that it is a hopeless condition. Many people are able to control their destructive drinking patterns when given the support and care they need.

There are several approaches to the treatment of alcoholism in addition to those which focus on correction of the patient's medical problems. Behavioural techniques, which include teaching the patient to recognize and cope with high-risk situations, are relatively new and are aimed at helping the individual find more acceptable and healthier ways to cope with the stresses of everyday living. Group therapy has been found to be particularly helpful when conducted under the direction of clinical psychologists, psychiatrists, and psychiatric nurse specialists who plan a programme of activities in conjunction with their clients and assist them in implementing it. Controlled drinking is an approach which aims to help the patient return to pre-alcoholic patterns of controlled drinking, well short of intoxication. The individual sets a limit and stops drinking once that limit has been reached. This approach is not suitable for patients who have alcohol-related organ damage or who lack social support, but the concept of controlled drinking is an interesting alternative to the traditional belief that complete abstinence is the only route to recovery.

Self-help groups such as Alcoholics Anonymous (AA) have a good record of success in helping alcoholics conquer their habitual drinking. From their own experiences, AA members have learned how to motivate and encourage others in their desire to stop drinking. Meetings and discussions give the alcoholic an opportunity to air his or her problems and to learn from the experiences of others who have similar problems. Hundreds of thousands of alcoholics and their families have been helped by AA since the organization was founded in 1935. Help in locating local groups and information about AA and alcoholism can be obtained from Alcoholics Anonymous (Great Britain), General Service Office, PO Box 1, Stonebow House, York YO1 2NJ.

Another resource for materials helpful to the patient and his family is The Medical Council on Alcoholism, 1 St. Andrew's Place, London NW1 4LB.

It is important to bear in mind that a person who is addicted to alcohol or is regularly drinking too much cannot change his drinking habits without continued support and encouragement. First, he must be confronted with the problem and helped to recognize it as one that he will have to overcome if he is to recover. The alcoholic will need to change his life style and break a firmly established pattern of habits. He must stop drinking completely, for there is little chance that he will ever be able to stop at just one or two drinks. Successful treatment is possible only if the alcoholic wants to stop drinking, and this happens only when he gains a full realization of the seriousness of his condition and the availability of continued help and support. Condemnation, sermonizing, and castigating the alcoholic usually reinforce his conviction that life is not worth the trouble. He needs hope of recovery and trust in those who have given him that hope. While the alcoholic does indeed need to admit his problem and often to commit himself to abstinence, he usually cannot do it alone.

alcoholuria (ˌalkəho'lyooə·ri·ə) the presence of alcohol in the urine. This may be estimated when excess blood levels of alcohol are suspected.

Aldactide (al'daktied) trademark for a fixed-combination preparation of spironolactone and hydrochlorothiazide, a diuretic.

Aldactone (al'daktohn) trademark for a preparation of spironolactone, an aldosterone antagonist used as a diuretic.

aldehyde ('aldiˌhied) an organic compound containing the aldehyde functional group (-CHO); that is, one with a carbonyl group (C=O) located at one end of the carbon chain.

Aldomet ('aldohˌmet) trademark for a preparation of methyldopa, an antihypertensive.

aldopentose (ˌaldoh'pentohz) any one of a class of sugars that contain five carbon atoms and an aldehyde group (-CHO).

aldose ('aldohs, -dohz) a sugar containing an aldehyde group (-CHO).

aldosterone (ˌaldoh'stiə·rohn, al'dostəˌrohn) the main MINERALOCORTICOID hormone secreted by the adrenal cortex, the principal biological activity of which is the regulation of electrolyte and water balance by promoting the retention of sodium (and, therefore, of water) and the excretion of potassium; the retention of water induces an increase in plasma volume and an increase in blood pressure. Its secretion is stimulated by angiotensin II.

aldosteronism (al'dostə·rə,nizəm) an abnormality of electrolyte balance caused by excessive secretion of aldosterone; hyperaldosteronism.

primary a. that arising from oversecretion of aldosterone by an adrenal adenoma, characterized typically by hypokalaemia, alkalosis, muscular weakness, polyuria, polydipsia, and hypertension. Called also Conn's syndrome.

pseudoprimary a. that caused by bilateral adrenal hyperplasia and having the same signs and symptoms as primary aldosteronism.

secondary a. that due to extra-adrenal stimulation of aldosterone secretion; it is commonly associated with oedematous states, as in nephrotic syndrome, hepatic cirrhosis, heart failure, and accelerated phase hypertension.

Aldrich syndrome ('awldrich) Wiskott–Aldrich syndrome.

alecithal (ay'lesithəl) having no distinct yolk.

aleukaemia (,ayloo'keemi·ə) 1. absence or deficiency of leukocytes in the blood. 2. aleukaemic leukaemia.

aleukia (ay'looki·ə) leukopenia; absence of leukocytes from the blood.

aleukocytosis (ay,lookohsie'tohsis) diminished proportion of leukocytes in the blood.

alexia (ə'leksi·ə, ay-) visual aphasia.

alexic (ə'leksik) 1. pertaining to alexia. 2. having the properties of an alexin.

alexin (ə'leksin) an obsolete name for complement.

aleydigism (ə'liedigizəm) absence of the interstitial cells of the testis (Leydig cells).

alfentanil (al'fentənil) an intravenously injected narcotic drug used to provide very rapid onset of analgesia of short duration during surgery. For longer operations it is often used as an infusion.

ALG antilymphocyte globulin.

algae ('aljee, -gee) a group of plants living in water, including all seaweeds, and ranging in size from microscopic cells to fronds hundreds of feet long.

algaesthesis (,aljis'theesis) a painful sensation.

algefacient (,aljee'fayshənt) cooling or refrigerant.

algesia (al'jeezi·ə) sensitiveness to pain; hyperaesthesia. adj. **algesic, algetic.**

algesimetry (,alji'simətree) measurement of sensitivity of pain.

-algia word element. [Gr.] *pain.*

algicide ('alji,sied) 1. destructive to algae. 2. an agent that destroys algae.

algid ('aljid) [L.] *chilly, cold.*

alginate ('alji,nayt) a salt of alginic acid, a colloidal substance from brown seaweed. The acid or sodium compound is used in pharmaceutical preparations to relieve heartburn and other symptoms of gastro-oesophageal reflux. Calcium, sodium, or ammonium alginate can be used as foam, clot, or gauze for absorbable surgical dressings.

algo- word element. [Gr.] *pain, cold.*

algodystrophy (,algoh'distrəfee) a combination of pain and dystrophic changes in bone.

algogenic (,algoh'jenik) 1. causing pain. 2. lowering temperature.

algology (al'goləjee) 1. the scientific study of pain. 2. phycology.

algometer (al'gomitə) a device used in testing the sensitiveness of a part.

algometry (al'gomətree) estimation of the sensitivity to painful stimuli.

algophobia (,algoh'fohbi·ə) morbid dread of pain.

algor ('algor) chill or rigor; coldness.

a. mortis the cooling of the body after death, which proceeds at a definite rate, influenced by the environmental temperature and protection of the body.

alienation (,ayli·ə'nayshən) a feeling of estrangement or separation from others or from self.

alienia (,aylie'eeni·ə) absence of the spleen.

aliform ('ali,fawm, 'ayli-) shaped like a wing.

alignment (ə'lienmənt) the state of being arranged in a line, i.e. in correct anatomical position.

aliment ('alimənt) food; nutritive material.

alimentary (,ali'mentə·ree, -tree) pertaining to or caused by food, or nutritive material.

a. canal all the organs making up the route taken by food as it passes through the body from mouth to anus; it comprises the oesophagus, stomach, and small and large intestines. Called also *digestive tract.* See also DIGESTIVE SYSTEM.

a. tract alimentary canal.

alimentation (,alimen'tayshən) giving or receiving of nourishment.

total parenteral a. (TPA) total parenteral nutrition. See under NUTRITION.

alinasal (,ali'nayz'l) pertaining to either of the cartilaginous flaps of the nose.

aliphatic (,ali'fatik) 1. fatty or oily. 2. pertaining to a hydrocarbon that does not contain an aromatic ring.

aliquot ('ali,kwot) 1. a sample that is representative of the whole. 2. a number that will divide another without a remainder; e.g., 2 is an aliquot of 6.

alkalaemia (,alkə'leemi·ə) abnormal alkalinity, or increased pH, of the blood.

alkali ('alkə,lie) any one of a class of compounds such as sodium hydroxide that form salts with acids and soaps with fats; a base, or substance capable of neutralizing acids. Other properties include a bitter taste and the ability to turn litmus paper from red to blue. Alkalis play a vital role in maintaining the normal functioning of the body chemistry. See also ACID–BASE BALANCE and BASE.

a. reserve the ability of the combined buffer systems of the blood to neutralize acid. The pH of the blood normally is slightly on the alkaline side, between 7.35 and 7.45. Since the principal buffer in the blood is bicarbonate, the alkali reserve essentially is represented by the plasma bicarbonate concentration. However, haemoglobin, phosphates, and other bases also act as buffers. A lowered alkali reserve means a state of acidosis; an increased reserve indicates alkalosis. Alkali reserve is measured by the combining power of carbon dioxide, which is the amount of carbon dioxide that can be bound as bicarbonate by the blood.

alkaline ('alkə,lien) having the reactions of an alkali.

a. phosphatase an enzyme localized on cell membranes that hydrolyses phosphate esters, liberating inorganic phosphate, and has an optimal pH of about 10.0. Serum alkaline phosphatase activity is elevated in hepatobiliary disease, especially in obstructive jaundice, and in bone diseases with increased osteoblastic activity such as HYPERPARATHYROIDISM, OSTEITIS DEFORMANS, and bone cancer. The liver and bone tissue each produce a distinct isoenzyme.

alkalinity (,alkə'linitee) 1. the quality of being alkaline. 2. the combining power of a base, expressed as the maximum number of equivalents of acid with which it reacts to form a salt.

alkalinuria (,alkəli'nyooə·ri·ə) an alkaline condition of the urine.

alkalization (,alkəlie'zayshən) the act of making alkaline.

alkalizer (,alkə'liezə) an agent that causes alkalization.

alkaloid ('alkə,loyd) one of a large group of organic,

basic substances found in plants. They are usually bitter in taste and are characterized by powerful physiological activity. Examples are morphine, cocaine, atropine, quinine, nicotine, and caffeine. The term is also applied to synthetic substances that have structures similar to plant alkaloids, such as procaine.

alkalosis (ˌalkə'lohsis) a pathological condition resulting from accumulation of base or from loss of acid without comparable loss of base in the body fluids, and characterized by decrease in hydrogen ion concentration (increase in pH). Alkalosis is the opposite of ACIDOSIS; see also ACID–BASE BALANCE.

compensated a. a condition in which compensatory mechanisms have returned the pH toward normal.

hypochloraemic a. a metabolic alkalosis in which gastric losses of chloride are disproportionately greater than sodium loss because of corresponding increase in potassium loss.

hypokalaemic a. a metabolic alkalosis associated with a low serum potassium level; retention of alkali or loss of acid occurs in the extracellular (but not intracellular) fluid compartment; although the pH of the intracellular fluid may be below normal.

metabolic a. a disturbance in which the acid–base status shifts toward the alkaline because of uncompensated loss of acids, ingestion or retention of excess base, or potassium depletion. The condition can occur in any patient who is vomiting frequently or has gastric suction, is taking a diuretic, or has hyperadrenocortical disease.

Metabolic alkalosis is characterized by a blood serum pH above 7.45, an increase of serum CO_2 above 32 mEq/l, and an unchanged $P\text{CO}_2$ when the lungs are compensating for the alkalosis. These values are determined by BLOOD GAS ANALYSIS. The symptoms may be mild at first, with muscle weakness, irritability, confusion, and muscle twitching. Respirations are shallow and slow as the lungs attempt to compensate by building up carbonic acid stores. If the condition progresses unchecked, the symptoms increase in severity and the patient lapses into coma. Convulsive seizures may occur. Respiratory paralysis can develop if potassium loss is great.

TREATMENT AND PATIENT CARE. The best control of metabolic alkalosis is careful monitoring of the patient because the condition is most often brought on by medication, especially diuretics, and by postoperative loss of acids through vomiting or gastric suctioning. One of the most frequent sources of increased alkali intake is the overzealous self-administration of antacids, particularly bicarbonate of soda, which is a systemic alkalizer. Education of the public in the hazards of such practices can do much to prevent metabolic alkalosis. Patients on diuretic therapy also must be taught to be alert for, and to report to their doctor the signs of potassium depletion and alkalosis.

The primary aim in the treatment of metabolic alkalosis is to re-establish fluid and electrolyte balance. Administration of potassium chloride and isotonic saline usually will correct the problem.

Vital signs should be checked frequently; hypotension and tachycardia may indicate potassium deficit, a decreased respiratory rate suggests compensation by the lungs. A record of fluid intake and output is helpful in planning fluid and electrolyte replacement. Blood gases and pH should be monitored. Signs of neural irritability, such as Trousseau's sign, are helpful in detecting early stages of tetany due to calcium deficiency. Muscle weakness and energy loss should be reported, as they may be symptomatic of hypokalaemia. Precautions are taken to prevent injury should disorientation or CONVULSIONS develop.

respiratory a. reduced carbon dioxide tension in the extracellular fluid caused by excessive excretion of carbon dioxide through the lungs (HYPERVENTILATION). Conditions commonly associated with respiratory alkalosis include anxiety, hysteria, pain, hypoxia, fever, high environmental temperature, poisoning, early pulmonary oedema, pulmonary embolism, stroke, central nervous system disease, and overuse of a mechanical VENTILATOR.

The condition is characterized by dizziness or light-headedness, inability to concentrate, tingling and numbness of the extremities and around the mouth, blurred vision, diaphoresis, dry mouth, muscle cramps, carpopedal spasms, and, in uncontrolled alkalosis, convulsions and syncope. Arterial blood gas values typically show a pH greater than 7.4 and a $P_a\text{CO}_2$ below 35 mmHg. The $P_a\text{O}_2$ may be normal except in cases in which hyperventilation is caused by anoxia. See also BLOOD GAS ANALYSIS.

Acute respiratory alkalosis is typified by the hyperventilation syndrome. The chronic form usually is manifested by few symptoms except those associated with CHRONIC OBSTRUCTIVE AIRWAYS DISEASE (COAD).

TREATMENT AND PATIENT CARE. Treatment is primarily aimed at removal of the underlying cause, particularly in cases of hyperventilation due to hysteria. Rebreathing carbon dioxide in a paper bag is helpful, as is encouraging the patient to hold his breath. The patient who has anoxia caused by pulmonary infection or congestive heart failure should be given oxygen to reduce respiratory effort and the resultant blowing off of carbon dioxide. If there is CNS involvement, sedation which suppresses activity of the respiratory centre may be indicated.

alkalotic (ˌalkə'lotik) pertaining to or characterized by alkalosis.

alkane ('alkayn) a saturated hydrocarbon, i.e., one that has no carbon–carbon multiple bonds.

alkapton (al'kapton) a class of substances with an affinity for alkali, found in the urine and causing the condition known as alkaptonuria. The compound commonly found, and most commonly referred to by the term, is homogentisic acid.

alkaptonuria (alˌkaptə'nyooə·ri·ə) excretion in the urine of homogentisic acid and its oxidation products as a result of a genetic disorder of phenylalanine-tyrosine metabolism.

alkavervir (ˌalkə'vərviə) a mixture of alkaloids extracted from *Veratrum viride*, used to lower blood pressure.

alkene ('alkeen) an aliphatic hydrocarbon containing a double bond.

alkyl ('alkil) the radical that results when an aliphatic hydrocarbon loses one hydrogen atom.

alkylate ('alkiˌlayt) to treat with an alkylating agent.

alkylating agent ('alkiˌlayting) a synthetic compound containing alkyl groups that combine readily with other molecules. Their action seems to be chiefly on the deoxyribonucleic acid (DNA) in the nucleus of the cell. They are used in chemotherapy of cancer although they do not damage malignant cells selectively, but also have a toxic action on normal cells. Locally they cause blistering of the skin and damage to the eyes and respiratory tract. Systemic toxic effects are nausea and vomiting, reduction in both leukocytes and erythrocytes, and haemorrhagic tendencies. Among the agents of this group used in therapy are the NITROGEN MUSTARDS, including mustine, chlorambucil and triethylenemelamine, and busulphan and cyclophosphamide.

alkyne ('alkien) an aliphatic hydrocarbon containing a triple bond.

ALL acute lymphoblastic (lymphoid) LEUKAEMIA.

all-or-none law (ˌawlor'nun) principle that states that in individual cardiac and skeletal muscle fibres there are only two possible reactions to a stimulus: either there is no reaction at all or there is a full reaction with no gradation of response according to the strength of the stimulus. Whole muscles can grade their response by increasing or decreasing the *number* of fibres involved.

all(o)- word element. [Gr.] *other, deviating from normal.*

allachaesthesia (ˌaləkis'theezi·ə) allaesthesia.

optical a. visual allaesthesia.

allaesthesia (ˌalis'theezi·ə) the experiencing of a sensation, e.g., pain or touch, as occurring at a point remote from where the stimulus is actually applied.

visual a. the transposition of visual images from one-half of the visual field to the other. Called also *optical allachaesthesia.*

allantochorion (əˌlantoh'kor·ri·ən) the allantois and chorion as one structure.

allantoid ('aləntoyd, ə'lantoyd) 1. sausage-shaped. 2. pertaining to the allantois.

allantoin (ˌalən'toh·in) a crystalline substance from allantoic fluid and fetal urine; used topically in ointments or lotions for certain skin conditions such as psoriasis or acne.

allantoinuria (əˌlantoh·i'nyooə·ri·ə) allantoin in the urine.

allantois (ə'lantoh·is) a ventral outgrowth of the hindgut of the early embryo, which becomes a small vestigial structure in the developing fetus. It stretches from the urachus at the apex of the bladder to the umbilicus and its blood vessels develop into those of the umbilical cord. adj. **allantoic.**

allele ('aleel, ə'leel) one of two or more alternative forms of a gene at the same site in a chromosome, which determine alternative characters in inheritance. adj. **allelic.**

silent a. one that produces no detectable effect.

allelomorph (ə'leeloh,mawf) allele.

allelotaxis (əˌleeloh'taksis) development of an organ from several embryonic structures.

Allen's law ('alənz) the more carbohydrates a diabetic takes, the less he utilizes.

allergen ('aləˌjen) 1. a substance, protein or nonprotein, capable of inducing allergy or specific hypersensitivity. 2. a purified protein of a food (such as milk, eggs, or wheat), bacterium, or pollen. adj. **allergenic.** Allergens are used to test a patient for hypersensitivity to specific substances (see SKIN TEST). They are also used to densensitize or hyposensitize allergic individuals (see IMMUNOTHERAPY).

Almost any substance in the environment can be an allergen. The list of known allergens includes plant pollens, spores of mould, animal dander, house dust, foods, feathers, dyes, soaps, detergents, cosmetics, plastics, and drugs. Allergens can enter the body by being inhaled, swallowed, touched, or injected. Once the allergen comes in contact with body cells it sets off a series of immune responses that can range from localized inflammation to a fatal systemic ANAPHYLAXIS.

allergid ('aləjid) a papular or nodular allergic skin reaction.

allergist ('aləjist) a doctor specializing in the diagnosis and treatment of allergic conditions.

allergization (ˌaləjie'zayshən) active sensitization by introduction of allergens into the body.

allergy ('aləjee) a state of abnormal and individual hypersensitivity acquired through exposure to a particular ALLERGEN, reexposure revealing an altered capacity to react.

Allergies can be divided into three major types: (1) delayed-reaction allergies caused by sensitized lymphocytes; (2) antigen–antibody allergies caused by a reaction between immunoglobulin G (IgG) antibodies (immunoglobulins) and antigens; and (3) atopic or inherited allergies, which are characterized by the presence of large amounts of sensitizing antibodies called *IgE antibodies.*

Examples of *delayed-reaction* allergies (also called cell-mediated hypersensitivity) include CONTACT DERMATITIS or skin eruptions resulting from exposure to certain drugs, to chemicals, such as those in cosmetics and household cleansers, or to certain plant toxins. On first contact with the allergen there is no response, but with repeated exposure some lymphocytes become sensitized. Once these lymphocytes are activated they remain in the body until a subsequent contact with the allergen to which they are sensitized. Then they diffuse into the skin and bring about a cell-mediated immune response. During this reaction toxins are released from the sensitized lymphocytes, and macrophages invade the tissues. If this process continues unchecked, there can be extensive destruction of the affected tissues.

Antigen–antibody allergies occur when an individual has built up a high titre of antibodies, usually of the IgG type, following exposure to a specific antigen. Subsequent exposure to a high level of that antigen results in the formation of an antigen–antibody complex that deposits small granules on the walls of blood vessels. Eventually, through the action of proteolytic enzymes released during the reaction, small blood vessels become inflamed and are severely damaged or destroyed. This kind of reaction is sometimes called *cytotoxic hypersensitivity.*

Examples of antigen–antibody reactions include TRANSFUSION reactions, haemolytic disease of the newborn secondary to incompatibility of Rh factor in the maternal and fetal blood, rejection of transplanted tissues and organs, AUTOIMMUNE DISEASE, and drug reactions.

Atopic allergies affect roughly 10 per cent of the population. The hypersensitivity is genetically transmitted and involves the production of excessive amounts of IgE antibodies. Allergens that react specifically with a type of IgE antibody include pollen, house dust, foods, and bee, wasp, and hornet venom. Reactions of this kind include hay fever, ASTHMA, urticaria, and potentially fatal ANAPHYLAXIS.

The injection, inhalation, ingestion of, or contact with an allergen by a person with an atopic allergy triggers a local inflammatory reaction with accompanying tissue damage. An anaphylactic reaction occurs throughout the body as a result of rupture of eosinophils and basophils followed by the release of histamine, eosinophil chemotactic factor of anaphylaxis (ECF-A), lysosomal enzymes, and other materials toxic to cells and tissues. The histamine causes dilation of blood vessels and decreased arterial pressure, increased capillary permeability and leakage of plasma from the blood into the interstitial spaces, and sometimes spasms of the bronchioles. These pathological changes produce circulatory shock that can be fatal in a matter of minutes. If the bronchioles are affected, the individual becomes dyspnoeic and has a wheezing-type respiration.

PREVENTION AND TREATMENT. The most successful means of preventing the symptoms of allergy is, of course, identification and avoidance of the offending allergen. In some instances, a cause-and-effect relationship can be clearly established, as in drug reactions, insect stings, and food allergies. In other cases, good detective work is needed to identify the allergen.

One diagnostic method that is fairly successful is testing. A minute quantity of various suspected allergens is applied to the skin of the person's inner forearm, either by means of a saturated adhesive patch (patch test) applied to the skin's surface, by intradermal injection, or by applying the substance to a small scratch (scratch test). (See also SKIN TEST.) When the substance so applied is the allergen, a mild allergic reaction takes place at the test site. Although the tests are not painful, they are tedious and cause some inconvenience to the patient.

Prevention of antigen–antibody reactions related to drug allergies and transfusion reactions is the responsibility of those delivering health care. Before any treatment is begun there should be a thorough assessment of the patient's current health status, and a history of his or her past illnesses and allergies and of family diseases should be obtained. Known allergies must be documented on the patient's record, and brought to the attention of everyone participating in the care of the patient or client. See TRANSFUSION for special precautions and the prevention and treatment of serious adverse reactions to blood components. Rejection of transplanted tissues and organs is discussed under TRANSPLANTATION.

Medications used for control of allergic reactions include ANTIHISTAMINES, ADRENALINE, ephedrine, aminophylline, and corticosteroids. A disadvantage of some antihistamines is that they produce drowsiness and other adverse effects that can interfere with a patient's activities.

An alternative to drug therapy is IMMUNOTHERAPY (desensitization or hyposensitization). This involves a series of injections that gradually increase the exposure to an allergen and stimulate the immune system to develop a resistance to the foreign substance. Although this process requires weekly injections over a period of 3 to 5 years without interruption, some patients are cured of their allergies by this method. Others, while not completely cured, do notice a marked reduction in the severity of their symptoms. Immunotherapy has been effectively used for rhinitis and asthma. There is no evidence that it is of value in the treatment of allergies to food and animal dander.

atopic a. an allergy with a hereditary predisposition. The tendency to develop some form of allergy is inherited, but the specific clinical form, e.g. hay fever, asthma, or eczema, is not. Reaginic antibodies of the IgE immunoglobulin class are involved.

bacterial a. a specific hypersensitivity to a particular bacterial antigen, e.g., *Mycobacterium tuberculosis*; it is dependent on previous infection with the specific organism and shows no circulating antibodies.

bronchial a. asthma.

cold a. a condition manifested by local and systemic reactions, mediated by histamine, which is released from mast cells and basophils as a result of exposure to cold.

delayed a. an allergic response which appears hours or days after application or absorption of an allergen. It includes CONTACT DERMATITIS and bacterial allergy.

food a., gastrointestinal a. allergy produced by ingested antigens, such as food or drugs; strawberries, milk, and eggs are the most common offenders. The organ affected usually is the skin.

hereditary a. atopic allergy. Called also *atopy*.

induced a. allergy resulting from the injection of an antigen, contact with an antigen, or infection with a microorganism, as contrasted with hereditary allergy; called also normal allergy, and physiological allergy.

physical a. a condition in which the patient is sensitive to the effects of physical agents, such as heat, cold, or light.

alloantibody (ˌaloh'antiˌbodee) see ISOANTIBODY.

alloantigen (ˌaloh'antijen, -jən) see ISOANTIGEN.

allocheiria (ˌaloh'kieri·ə) allaesthesia.

allochromasia (ˌalohkroh'mayzi·ə) change in colour of hair or skin.

allodiploidy (ˌaloh'diploydee) the state of having two sets of chromosomes derived from different ancestral species.

allodynia (ˌaloh'dini·ə) pain produced by a non-noxious stimulus.

alloeroticism (ˌaloh·i'rotiˌsizəm) direction of libido toward others. The opposite of autoeroticism.

allogeneic (ˌalohje'nee·ik, -'nayik) denoting individuals of the same species but of different genetic constitution (antigenically distinct).

allograft ('alohˌgrahft) a graft between allogeneic individuals.

alloimmunization (ˌalohˌimyuhnie'zayshən) see ISOIMMUNIZATION.

allokeratoplasty (ˌaloh'kerətohˌplastee) repair of the cornea, using a material foreign to the human body, e.g. a plastic substance.

allolalia (ˌaloh'layli·ə) any defect of speech of central origin.

alloploidy (ˌaloh'ploydee) the state of having any number of chromosome sets derived from different ancestral species.

allopolyploidy (ˌaloh'poliˌploydee) the state of having more than two sets of chromosomes derived from different ancestral species.

allopurinol (ˌaloh'pyooə·riˌnol) a drug that inhibits uric acid production and reduces serum and urinary uric acid levels; used in patients with hyperuricaemia and gout.

allorhythmia (ˌaloh'ridhmi·ə) irregularity of the pulse.

allosensitization (ˌalohˌsensitie'zayshən) sensitization to alloantigens (isoantigens), usually non-red blood cell antigens such as HLA antigens.

allosteric (ˌaloh'sterik) pertaining to an effect on the biological function of a protein, produced by a compound not directly involved in that function (an allosteric effector) or to regulation of an enzyme involving cooperativity between multiple binding sites (allosteric sites).

a. site that subunit of an enzyme molecule which binds with a nonsubstrate molecule, inducing a conformational change that results in inactivation of the enzyme for its substrate.

allotherm ('alohˌthərm) an organism whose body temperature changes with its environment.

allotriogeustia (əˌlotrioh'gyoosti·ə) perverted sense of taste.

allotropic (ˌaloh'tropik) 1. exhibiting allotropism. 2. concerned with others: said of a type of personality that is more preoccupied with others than with self.

allotropism (ə'lotrəˌpizəm) existence of an element in two or more distinct forms.

allotropy (ə'lotrəpee) 1. allotropism. 2. direction of one's interest more toward others than toward one's self.

alloxan (ə'loksan) an oxidized product of uric acid which tends to destroy the islet cells of the pancreas, thus producing diabetes. It has been obtained from intestinal mucus in diarrhoea and has been used in nutrition experiments.

alloxuraemia (əˌloksyuh'reemi·ə) the presence of purine bases in the blood.

alloxuria (ˌalok'syooə·ri·ə) the presence of purine bases in the urine.

alloy ('aloy) a solid mixture of two or more metals or metalloids that are mutually soluble in the molten condition.

aloes ('alohz) a drug made from the leaves of the aloe. An irritant purgative likely to cause griping. It is contraindicated in pregnancy, and its use is discouraged.

alogia (ə'lohji·ə) inability to speak, due to a central lesion.

alopecia (ˌalə'peeshi·ə) loss of hair; baldness. The cause of simple baldness is not yet fully understood, although it is known that the tendency to become bald is limited almost entirely to males, runs in certain families and is more common in certain racial groups than in others. Baldness is often associated with ageing.

a. areata hair loss in sharply defined areas, usually the scalp or beard.

a. capitis totalis loss of all the hair from the scalp.

cicatricial a., a. cicatrisata irreversible loss of hair associated with scarring, usually on the scalp.

a. congenitalis complete or partial absence of the hair at birth.

a. liminaris hair loss at the hairline along the front and back edges of the scalp.

male-pattern a. loss of scalp hair genetically determined and androgen-dependent, beginning with frontal recession and progressing symmetrically to leave ultimately only a sparse peripheral rim of hair.

a. medicamentosa hair loss due to ingestion of a drug.

symptomatic a., a. symptomatica loss of hair due to systemic or psychogenic causes, such as general ill health, infections of the scalp or skin, nervousness, or a specific disease such as typhoid fever, or to stress. The hair may fall out in patches, or there may be diffuse loss of hair instead of complete baldness in one area.

a. totalis loss of hair from the entire scalp.

a. universalis loss of hair from the entire body.

Alper's disease ('alpərz) poliodystrophia cerebri.

alpha ('alfə) the first letter of the Greek alphabet, α; used to denote the first position in a classification system; as, in names of chemical compounds, to distinguish the first in a series of isomers, or to indicate the position of substituent atoms or groups; also used to distinguish types of radioactive decay, brain waves or rhythms, adrenergic receptors, and secretory cells that stain with acid dyes, such as the alpha cells of the pancreas.

a.-blocking agents a group of drugs that selectively inhibit the activities of alpha receptors in the sympathetic nervous system. As with beta-blocking agents, alpha-adrenergic blocking agents compete with the catecholamines at peripheral autonomic receptor sites. This group includes ergot and its derivatives, and phentolamine.

a. brain waves brain-wave currents having a frequency of approximately 8 to 13 hertz (pulsations per second), best seen when patient's eyes are closed and he is physically relaxed. See also ELECTROENCEPHALOGRAPHY.

a. particles a type of emission produced by the disintegration of a radioactive substance. The atoms of radioactive elements such as uranium and radium are very unstable; they are continuously breaking apart with explosive violence and emitting particulate and nonparticulate types of radiation. The alpha particles, consisting of two protons and two neutrons, have an electrical charge and form streams of tremendous energy when they are released from the disintegrating atoms. These streams of energy (alpha rays) are used to advantage in the treatment of various malignancies. See also RADIATION and RADIATION THERAPY.

alpha$_1$-antitrypsin (ˌalfəwunˌanti'tripsin) a plasma protein (α_1-globulin) produced in the liver, which inhibits the activity of trypsin and other proteolytic enzymes. Deficiency of this protein is associated with development of emphysema. Written also α_1-antitrypsin.

alpha-fetoprotein (ˌalfəˌfeetoh'prohteen) a plasma protein produced by the fetal liver, yolk sac, and gastrointestinal tract and also by hepatocellular carcinoma, germ cell neoplasms, and other cancers in adults. Abbreviated AFP. The serum AFP level is used to monitor the effectiveness of cancer treatment, and the amniotic fluid AFP level is used in the prenatal diagnosis of neural tube defects.

Alport's syndrome ('awlpawts) a hereditary disorder marked by progressive nerve deafness, progressive pyelonephritis or glomerulonephritis, and occasionally ocular defects.

alprazolam (al'prayzəlam) a benzodiazepine tranquillizer used as an anxiolytic.

ALS antilymphocyte serum.

alseroxylon (ˌalsə'roksilon) a purified extract of *Rauwolfia serpentina*, used as a tranquillizer and sedative.

Alström's syndrome ('alstrohmz) a hereditary syndrome of retinitis pigmentosa with nystagmus and early loss of central vision, deafness, obesity, and diabetes mellitus.

ALT alanine aminotransferase.

alter ego ('altə 'eegoh, 'awl-) a non-technical term for a person so close to oneself that he or she seems to be a 'second self'.

altitude sickness ('altiˌtyood) a syndrome caused by exposure to altitude high enough to cause significant hypoxia, or lack of oxygen. At high altitudes the atmospheric pressure is decreased and consequently arterial oxygen content is also lowered.

Acute altitude sickness may occur after a few hours' exposure to a high altitude. Mental functions may be affected, and there may be lightheadedness and breathlessness. Eventually headache and prostration may occur. Older persons and those with pulmonary or cardiovascular disease are most likely to be affected. After a few hours or days of acclimatization the symptoms will subside.

Chronic altitude sickness (sometimes called Monge's disease or Andes disease) occurs in those living in the high Andes above 15,000 feet. It resembles POLYCYTHAEMIA, but is completely relieved if the patient is moved to sea level.

Aludrox ('alyoodroks) trademark for preparations of aluminium hydroxide gel, used as an antacid.

alum ('aləm) a substance formerly used, in the form of colourless crystals or white powder, as a styptic or haemostatic because of its astringent action.

aluminium (ˌalyə'mini·əm, ˌalə-) a chemical element, atomic number 13, atomic weight 26.982, symbol Al. See table of elements in Appendix 2.

a. acetate solution a preparation of aluminium subacetate and glacial acetic acid, used for its antiseptic and astringent action on the skin; called also Burow's solution.

a. chloride a deliquescent, crystalline powder used topically as an astringent solution and antiperspirant.

a. hydroxide gel an aluminium preparation, available in suspension or in dried form; used as an antacid in the treatment of peptic ulcer and gastric hyperacidity.

a. phosphate gel a water suspension of aluminium phosphate and some flavouring agents; used as a gastric antacid, astringent, and demulcent.

alveolectomy (ˌalvioh'lektəmee) surgical excision of part of the alveolar process.

alveolitis (ˌalvioh'lietis) inflammation of the alveoli.

extrinsic allergic a. inflammation of the alveoli of the lung caused by inhalation of an antigen such as pollen.

alveolodental (al,viohlə'dent'l) pertaining to teeth and the alveolar process.

alveolotomy (,alvioh'lotəmee) incision of the alveolar process.

alveolus (al'vi·ələs) pl. *alveoli* [L.] a little hollow, as the socket of a tooth, a follicle of an acinous gland, or one of the thin-walled chambers of the lungs (pulmonary alveoli), surrounded by networks of capillaries through whose walls exchange of carbon dioxide and oxygen takes place. adj. **alveolar.**

dental alveoli the cavities or sockets of either jaw, in which the roots of the teeth are embedded.

alveus ('alvi·əs) pl. *alvei* [L.] a canal or trough.

alymphia (ay'limfi·ə) absence or lack of lymph.

alymphocytosis (ay,limfohsie'tohsis) absence of lymphocytes in the blood.

alymphoplasia (ay,limfoh'playzi·ə) failure of development of lymphoid tissue.

thymic a. congenital agammaglobulinaemia in which there is thymic hypoplasia, sparsity of lymphocytes in the thymus, spleen, lymph nodes, and intestines, absence of plasma cells, and absence of Hassall's corpuscles.

Alzheimer's cells ('alts·hiemərz) 1. giant astrocytes with large prominent nuclei found in the brain in hepatolenticular degeneration and hepatic comas. 2. degenerated astrocytes.

Alzheimer's disease a progressive form of neuronal degeneration in the brain and the commonest cause of dementia in people of all ages. It is commoner in older than younger people and is not just a form of presenile dementia as was originally thought. The degeneration of neurons is accompanied by changes in the brain's biochemistry. At the moment this condition is irreversible and there is no effective treatment.

Am chemical symbol, *americium.*

amacrine ('aməkrin, -krien) without long processes.

a. cells modified nerve cells present in the retina and involved in the processing of visual information prior to its transmission along the optic nerve.

amalgam (ə'malgəm) an alloy of mercury with another metal.

amantadine (ə'mantə,deen) an antiviral agent used against the influenza A virus, and also used as an antidyskinetic in the treatment of Parkinson's disease.

amastia (ay'masti·ə) congenital absence of one or both mammary glands.

amaurosis (,amaw'rohsis) loss of sight without apparent lesion of the eye, as from disease of the optic nerve, spine, or brain.

a. fugax sudden temporary or fleeting blindness.

a. congenita of Leber, Leber's congenital a. hereditary blindness occurring at or shortly after birth, associated with an atypical form of diffuse pigmentation and commonly with optic atrophy and attenuation of the retinal vessels.

amaurotic (,amaw'rotik) pertaining to, or of the nature of, amaurosis.

a. familial idiocy a group of hereditary disorders characterized by cerebromacular degeneration, blindness, progressive dementia, and progressive and unremitting paralysis, usually of the spastic type. There is no cure and the prognosis is extremely poor. The disorders in this group are classified according to age of onset: TAY–SACHS DISEASE is the infantile form; BIELSCHOWSKY–JANSKY DISEASE is the late infantile form; SPIELMEYER–VOGT DISEASE is the juvenile form; and KUFS' DISEASE is the late juvenile, or adult form.

Amazon ('aməzon) a tall muscular woman (from the Greek myth of a race of female warriors). The term is still occasionally used, inaccurately, with the implication that such women are lesbian; there is no relationship between a woman's physical stature and her sexual preferences.

ambacksin (am'baksin) trademark for a preparation of bacampicillin, an antibacterial.

ambenonium (,ambə'nohni·əm) a cholinesterase inhibitor used to increase muscular strength in myasthenic patients.

ambidextrous (,ambi'dekstrəs) able to use either hand with equal dexterity.

ambilateral (,ambi'latə·rəl) pertaining to or affecting both sides.

ambilevous (,ambi'leevəs) unable to use both hands with equal dexterity.

ambisexual (,ambi'seksyooəl) denoting sexual characteristics common to both sexes, e.g., pubic hair.

ambivalence (am'bivələns) simultaneous existence of conflicting emotional attitudes toward a goal, object, or person. adj. **ambivalent.**

amblyacousia (,ambliə'koosi·ə) dullness of hearing.

amblyaphia (,ambli'afi·ə) bluntness of the sense of touch.

amblygeustia (,ambli'gyoosti·ə) dullness of the sense of taste.

Amblyomma (,ambli'omə) a genus of ticks, which comprises approximately 100 species, several of which are vectors of rickettsiae and probably other disease-producing organisms.

amblyopia (,ambli'ohpi·ə) reduced vision not due to organic defect or refractive errors. adj. **amblyopic.**

colour a. impairment of colour vision due to toxic or other influences.

amblyoscope ('amblioh,skohp) an instrument used in the assessment of binocular vision and in the measurement of strabismus.

ambo ('amboh) ambon.

amboceptor (,amboh'septə) haemolysin, particularly its double receptors, the one combining with the blood cell, the other with complement.

ambon ('ambon) the edge of the socket in which the head of a long bone is lodged.

ambulant, ambulatory ('ambyuhlənt; ,ambyuh'laytə·ree) walking or able to walk; not confined to bed.

amcinonide (am'sinə,nied) a glucocorticoid used for topical application in the treatment of corticosteroid-responsive dermatoses.

amelia (ay'meeli·ə) a developmental anomaly with absence of the limbs.

amelioration (ə,meelyə'rayshən) improvement of symptoms; a lessening of the severity of a disease.

ameloblast (ə'meloh,blast) a cell that takes part in forming dental enamel.

ameloblastoma (ə,melohbla'stohmə) a locally invasive, highly destructive tumour of the jaw.

pituitary a. craniopharyngioma.

amelodentinal (,aməloh'dentinəl) pertaining to dental enamel and dentine.

a. junction the joint between enamel and dentine. The plane of the joint is scalloped.

amelogenesis (,aməloh'jenəsis) formation of dental enamel.

a. imperfecta imperfect formation of enamel, resulting in brownish coloration and friability of the teeth.

amelogenic (,aməloh'jenik) forming enamel.

amelus (ay'meeləs) an individual exhibiting amelia.

amenorrhoea (a,menə'reeə, ay,men-) absence of the menses. adj. **amenorrhoeal.** *Primary* amenorrhoea refers to absence of the onset of menstruation at puberty. It may be caused by underdevelopment or malformation of the reproductive organs or by glandular disturbances. When menstruation has begun and then ceases, the term *secondary* amenorrhoea is used.

The most common cause is usually a disturbance of the endocrine glands concerned with the menstrual process. General ill health, a change in climate or living conditions, emotional shock or, frequently, either the hope or fear of becoming pregnant can sometimes stop the menstrual flow.

dietary a., nutritional a. cessation of menstruation accompanying loss of weight due to dietary restriction, the loss of weight and of appetite being less extreme than in ANOREXIA NERVOSA and unassociated with psychological problems.

amensalism (ay'mensalizəm) interaction between co-existing populations of different species, one of which is adversely affected and the other unaffected.

amentia (ay'menshi·ə) a term now rarely used indicating: 1. congenital mental handicap of varying extent. 2. a mental disorder characterized by marked mental confusion.

naevoid a. Sturge–Weber syndrome.

American Nurses' Association (ə'merikən) ANA, the US national organization and official spokesman for registered nurses. The ANA was founded in 1896 and exists for the purposes of improving the standards of nursing and promoting the general welfare of professional nurses. The association is a federation of 54 local organizations in the 50 US states, District of Columbia, Panama Canal Zone, Puerto Rico, and the Virgin Islands. The local organizations serve to implement the goals and carry out the functions of the national organization. The official publication of the ANA is the *American Journal of Nursing*. Offices of the organization are located at 2420 Pershing Road, Kansas City, MO 64108, USA.

americium (ˌamə'risi·əm) a chemical element, atomic number 95, atomic weight 243, symbol Am. See table of elements in Appendix 2.

amethocaine ('amethohˌkayn) A local anaesthetic of the ester group used to anaesthetize mucous membranes or injected as a spinal anaesthetic.

ametria (ay'meetri·ə) congenital absence of the uterus.

ametropia (ˌayme'trohpi·ə) a condition of the eye in which parallel rays fail to come to a focus on the retina. adj. **ametropic.**

amicrobic (ˌaymie'krohbik) not produced by microorganisms.

amiculum (ə'mikyuhləm) a dense surrounding coat of white fibres, as the sheath of the inferior olive and of the dentate nucleus.

amide ('amied, 'aymied) any compound derived from ammonia by substitution of an acid radical for hydrogen, or from an acid by replacing the -OH group by $-NH_2$.

amido ('amidoh) the monovalent radical $-NH_2$ united with an acid radical.

amikacin (ˌami'kaysin) a semisynthetic aminoglycoside antibiotic derived from kanamycin, used in the treatment of a wide range of infections due to susceptible organisms.

amiloride (ə'milor·ried) a potassium-sparing diuretic used concurrently with other diuretics for treatment of hypertension.

amimia (ay'mimi·ə) loss of the power of expression by the use of signs or gestures.

aminacrine (ə'minəˌkreen) an anti-infective agent used externally as the hydrochloride salt.

amine ('ameen, ə'meen, 'aymeen) an organic compound containing nitrogen.

biogenic a's amine neurotransmitters, e.g., noradrenaline, serotonin, and dopamine.

vasoactive a's amines that cause vasodilation and increase small vessel permeability, e.g., histamine and serotonin.

amino (ə'meenoh, ə'mienoh) monovalent radical NH_2, when not united with an acid radical.

a. acid any one of a class of organic compounds containing both amino ($-NH_2$) and carboxyl (-COOH) groups, occurring naturally in plant and animal tissues and forming the chief constituents of protein. They are the end products of protein digestion.

Twenty amino acids are necessary for protein synthesis. Eleven can be synthesized by the human body. Nine (the essential amino acids), histidine, isoleucine, leucine, lysine, methionine, phenylalanine, threonine, tryptophan, and valine, must be obtained from the diet.

Protein foods that provide the balance of essential amino acids required by the human body are known as *complete proteins*; these include proteins from animal sources, such as meat, eggs, fish, and milk. Proteins that cannot supply the body with all the essential amino acids are known as *incomplete proteins*; these are the vegetable proteins most abundantly found in peas, beans, and certain forms of wheat. Because different incomplete proteins lack different amino acids, specific combinations can provide all of the essential amino acids.

In certain inherited or acquired disorders of metabolism, specific amino acids accumulate in the blood (*aminoacidaemia*) or are excreted in excess in the urine (*aminoaciduria*). Urinary amino acid levels are increased in liver disease, muscular dystrophies, phenylketonuria (PKU), lead poisoning, and folic acid deficiency.

aminoacetic acid (əˌmeenoh·ə'seetik, əˌmienoh-, əˌminoh-) glycine.

aminoacidaemia (ˌaminohˌasi'deemi·ə, əˌmienoh-, əˌmeenoh-) an excess of amino acids in the blood.

aminoacidopathy (əˌmeenohˌasi'dopəthee, əˌmienoh-, əˌminoh-) any inborn error of amino acid metabolism producing a metabolic block that results in accumulation of one or more amino acids in the blood (aminoacidaemia) or excess excretion in the urine (aminoaciduria) or both.

aminoaciduria (ˌaminohˌasi'dyooə·ri·ə, əˌmienoh-, əˌmeenoh-) an excess in the urine of amino acids.

***p*-aminobenzoic acid** (ˌparəˌaminohben'zoh·ik, -əˌmienoh-, -əˌmeenoh-) a member of the B group of vitamins, a growth factor for certain organisms, and used in the treatment of certain rickettsial infections, including scrub typhus; called also PABA. See also PARA-AMINOBENZOIC ACID.

γ-aminobutyric acid ('gamə·əˌmeenohbyoo'tirik, -əˌmienoh-, -əˌminoh-) an amino acid that is one of the principal inhibitory neurotransmitters in the central nervous system. Abbreviated GABA.

ε-aminocaproic acid ('epsilonəˌmeenohkə'proh·ik, -əˌmienoh-, -əˌminoh-) an inhibitor of plasminogen and plasmin and so of fibrinolysis; used as a haemostatic.

aminoglutethimide (ˌaminohgloo'tethəˌmied, əˌmienoh-, əˌmeenoh-) formerly used as an anticonvulsant, this drug inhibits adrenal hormone synthesis. Its use is sometimes referred to as 'medical adrenalectomy'. The effects are reversible when the drug is discontinued. Used to treat metastatic breast and prostate cancers.

aminoglycoside (əˌmeenoh'gliekəˌsied, əˌmienoh-, əˌminoh-) any of a group of bacterial antibiotics derived from various species of *Streptomyces* that interfere with the function of bacterial ribosomes. These compounds contain an inositol moiety substituted with two amino or guanidino groups and with one or more sugars or aminosugars.

The aminoglycosides include gentamicin, netilmicin, streptomycin, tobramycin, amikacin, kanamycin, and neomycin. They are used to treat infections caused by gram-negative organisms and are classified as bactericidal agents because of their interference with bacterial replication. All of the aminoglycoside antibiotics are highly toxic, requiring monitoring of blood serum levels and careful observation of the patient for early signs of toxicity, particularly ototoxicity and nephrotoxicity.

aminohippuric acid (ˌaminoh·hi'pyooə·rik, əˌmienoh-, əˌmeenoh-) an acid used in renal function tests (see also PARA-AMINOHIPPURIC ACID).

δ-aminolaevulinic acid (ˌdeltə·əˌmeenohˌlevyuh'linik, -əˌmienoh-, -əˌminoh-) a precursor of porphyrins and haemoglobin. Serum levels of the acid are elevated in lead intoxication.

aminophylline (ˌami'nofəˌlin) a xanthine derivative used in the treatment of bronchospasm and left ventricular failure. Administration of the drug may be by mouth, intramuscularly, intravenously, or rectally. If given too rapidly by vein it may produce circulatory collapse. Intramuscular administration should be performed with caution because aminophylline is very irritating to the tissues. It also may cause gastric or urinary irritation when taken by mouth. Dose depends on the route of administration and the effect desired.

***p*-aminosalicylic acid** (ˌparəˌaminohˌsali'silik, -ə-ˌmienoh-, -əˌmeenoh-) an acid with antibacterial properties used in the treatment of tuberculosis (see also PARA-AMINOSALICYLIC ACID).

Aminosol (ə'meenəˌsol, ə'minə-, ə'mienə-) trademark for an amino acid preparation for intravenous injection.

aminotransferase (əˌmeenoh-, əˌmienoh-, əˌminoh-'transfəˌrayz, -'trahn-) an enzyme that catalyses the reversible transfer of an amino group from an α-amino acid to an α-keto acid using the coenzyme pyridoxal phosphate. Called also transaminase.

alanine a. (ALT) an enzyme that has high serum levels after acute damage to liver cells. See also ALANINE AMINOTRANSFERASE.

aspartate a. (AST) an enzyme that has high serum levels after a myocardial infarction or acute damage to liver cells. See also ASPARTATE AMINOTRANSFERASE.

aminuria (ˌami'nyooə·ri·ə) an excess of amines in the urine.

amiodarone (ˌamee'ohdərohn) an antiarrhythmic agent used to treat the Wolff–Parkinson–White syndrome and other arrhythmias where other agents are inappropriate.

amitosis (ˌami'tohsis) direct cell division; simple cleavage of the nucleus without the formation of a spireme spindle figure or chromosomes. adj. **amitotic.**

amitriptyline (ˌami'triptəˌleen) a compound used as an antidepressant.

AML acute myeloid LEUKAEMIA.

ammeter ('ameetə) an instrument for measuring in amperes the strength of a current flowing in a circuit.

ammonia (ə'mohni·ə, -nyə) a colourless alkaline gas, NH_3, with a pungent odour and acrid taste, and soluble in water.

ammoniaemia (əˌmohni'eemi·ə) hyperammonaemia.

ammoniate (ə'mohniˌayt) to combine with ammonia.

ammonium (ə'mohni·əm, -nyəm) a hypothetical radical, NH_4, forming salts analogous to those of the alkaline metals.

a. carbonate a mixture of ammonium compounds used as a liquefying expectorant in the treatment of chronic bronchitis and similar lung disorders. It is sometimes used as a reflex stimulant in 'smelling salts' because of the strong ammonia odour it gives off.

a. chloride colourless or white crystals, with a cool, salty taste, used as an expectorant because it liquefies bronchial secretions. In the body it is changed to urea and hydrochloric acid, and thus is useful in acidifying the urine and increasing the rate of urine flow. Excessive dosage may produce ACIDOSIS.

ammoniuria (əˌmohni'yooə·ri·ə) excess of ammonia in the urine.

amnalgesia (ˌamn'l'jeezi·ə) abolition of pain and memory of a painful procedure by the use of drugs or hypnosis.

amnesia (am'neezi·ə) pathological impairment of memory. adj. **amnestic.** Amnesia is usually the result of physical damage to areas of the brain from injury, disease, or alcoholism. It may also be caused by a decreased supply of blood to the brain, a condition that may accompany senility. Another cause is psychological. A shocking or unacceptable situation may be too painful to remember, and the situation is then retained only in the subconscious mind. The technical term for this is repression.

Rarely is the memory completely obliterated. When amnesia results from a single physical or psychological incident, such as a concussion suffered in an accident or a severe emotional shock, the victim may forget only the incident itself; he may be unable to recall events occurring before or after the incident or the order of events is confused, with recent events imputed to the past and past events to recent times. In another form, only certain isolated events are lost to memory.

Amnesia victims usually have a good chance of recovery if there is no irreparable brain damage. The recovery is often gradual, the memory slowly reclaiming isolated events while others are still missing. Psychotherapy may be necessary when the amnesia is due to a psychological reaction.

Amnesia takes different forms depending upon the area of the brain affected and how extensive the damage is. In auditory amnesia, or word deafness, the patient is unable to interpret spoken language. Words come to him as a jumble of sounds which he is unable to associate meaningfully with ideas. Similarly, in visual amnesia, or word blindness, the written language is forgotten. Tactile amnesia is the inability to recognize once familiar objects by the sense of touch.

anterograde a. amnesia for events subsequent to the episode precipitating the disorder.

retrograde a. amnesia for events prior to the episode precipitating the disorder. **transient global a.** a temporary episode of short-term memory loss without other neurological impairment.

amniocentesis (ˌamniohsen'teesis) transabdominal perforation of the amniotic sac. A sterile procedure for the purpose of obtaining a sample of amniotic fluid, which contains cells shed from the skin of the fetus as well as biochemical substances. Analyses of changes in chemical and cellular composition of the fluid are helpful in assessing the maturation and well-being of the fetus. Amniocentesis also provides for prenatal diagnosis of certain genetically transmitted errors of metabolism, congenital abnormalities, and chromosomal disorders. In all, it is currently feasible to detect the presence of over 40 different types of inherited disorders in fetuses of at least 15–16 weeks gestation.

Amniocentesis is useful when a mother with rhesus negative blood has a raised antibody titre in pregnancy. Examination of the liquor through light (spectrophotometric scanning) will indicate the concentration of bilirubin present and the management of pregnancy needed to prevent hydrops fetalis.

Another biochemical study involves measuring the level of alpha-fetoprotein (AFP) in the amniotic fluid.

Abnormally high levels may indicate an open defect of the spine; e.g., spina bifida or anencephaly.

Because of the ability to determine fetal maturation by amniotic fluid studies, it is possible to predict whether an infant will suffer from HYALINE MEMBRANE DISEASE at birth. A favourable ratio of lecithin to sphingomyelin indicates sufficient lung maturity.

PATIENT CARE DURING AND AFTER AMNIOCENTESIS. While the procedure for removal of amniotic fluid has minimal risk for the fetus and mother, there are slight risks of bleeding, leakage of fluid, or infection. There also is a small chance of miscarriage, or premature labour and possible damage to the fetus. Amniocentesis is usually recommended when the mother is older than 35 because of the risk of Down's syndrome or when there is a family history of a genetically transmitted disorder that can be detected by tests on the amniotic fluid, particularly, when both father and mother are known carriers of such a disorder. Parents who agree to amniocentesis must prepare to make a decision whether to abort the fetus if the laboratory tests indicate the presence of a birth defect.

During the procedure the obstetrician inserts a long pudendal needle into the mother's abdomen and into the amniotic cavity, avoiding the fetus and placenta by using ultrasound. Local anaesthesia is used to minimize discomfort. The woman is cautioned not to move during the procedure lest the needle become displaced. A syringe is attached and fluid is withdrawn.

Following amniocentesis the patient is observed for changes in blood pressure, excessive leakage of fluid, and signs of infection or contractions of the uterus. Haemorrhage from the placenta must be considered a possibility if the blood pressure begins to drop. Increased fetal activity or other signs of fetal distress such as changes in the fetal heart rate must be reported to the obstetrician at once as they may warrant immediate measures such as delivery of the infant if it is considered to be viable. Following amniocentesis, anti-D immunoglobulin should be given to Rh-negative women if antibodies are not already present.

Amniocentesis may also be used for the removal of excess fluid in cases of polyhydramnios.

See also CHORION BIOPSY.

amniochorial (ˌamnioh'kor·ri·əl) pertaining to amnion and chorion.

amniogenesis (ˌamnioh'jenəsis) the development of the amnion.

amniography (ˌamni'ogrəfee) radiography of the gravid uterus.

amnion ('amni·ən) the innermost membrane enclosing the developing fetus and the fluid in which the fetus is bathed.

a. nodosum a nodular condition of the fetal surface of the amnion, observed in oligohydramnios which may be associated with absence of the kidneys in the fetus.

amnionitis (ˌamnio'nietis) inflammation of the amnion.

amniorrhoea (ˌamni·ə'reeə) escape of the amniotic fluid.

amniorrhoexis (ˌamni·ə'reksis) rupture of the amnion.

amnioscope ('amni·əˌskohp) an endoscope that, by passage through the abdominal wall into the amniotic cavity, permits direct visualization of the fetus and amniotic fluid.

amnioscopy (ˌamni'oskəpee) 1. inspection of the amniotic sac, amniotic fluid and fetus by direct visualization using an endoscope passed through the abdominal wall. 2. visualization of the intact amniotic membranes and fluid per vaginam during labour by means of an amnioscope.

amniote ('amnioht) any animal with amnion.

amniotic (ˌamni'otik) pertaining to the amnion.

a. fluid the albuminous fluid contained in the amniotic sac; called also liquor amnii and 'waters'. The fetus floats in the amniotic fluid, which serves as a cushion against injury from sudden blows or movements and helps maintain a constant body temperature for the fetus. Normally the amniotic fluid is clear and slightly alkaline. Discoloration or excessive cloudiness of the fluid may indicate fetal distress or disease. The amount varies from 500 to 1500 ml.

A condition in which there is an excessive amount of amniotic fluid is called *polyhydramnios*; the amount may be as much as several litres. The cause of this condition is unknown but it frequently accompanies multiple pregnancy or some congenital defect of the fetus, especially hydrocephalus and meningocele.

A condition in which there is an abnormally small amount of amniotic fluid is referred to as *oligohydramnios*. In this condition there may be less than 100 ml of fluid present. The cause is unknown. A most important association is with interuterine growth retardation syndrome of the fetus. The condition may produce pressure deformities of the fetus, such as clubfoot or torticollis (wryneck). Adhesions may result from direct contact of the fetus with the amnion.

The technique for removal of a sample of amniotic fluid from the pregnant uterus is called AMNIOCENTESIS.

a. sac the amnion; the membranous sac enclosing the fetus suspended in the amniotic fluid.

amniotomy (ˌamni'otəmee) surgical rupture of the fetal membranes in order to induce labour.

amodiaquine (ˌamoh'dieəkween) a drug used as the hydrochloride salt in treatment of malaria, especially falciparum malaria.

Amoeba (ə'meebə) a genus of amoebae.

amoeba (ə'meebə) pl. *amoebaeamoebas* [L.] a minute, one-celled protozoan. The common laboratory example is *Amoeba proteus*. The usual cause of human amoebic infection is *Entamoeba histolytica*.

amoebiasis (ˌami'bieəsis) infection with amoebas, especially with *Entamoeba histolytica* (see also AMOEBIC DYSENTERY).

amoebic (ə'meebik) pertaining to, caused by, or of the nature of an amoeba.

a. abscess an abscess cavity of the liver resulting from liquefaction necrosis due to entrance of *Entamoeba histolytica* into the portal circulation in amoebiasis; amoebic abscesses may affect the lung, brain, and spleen.

a. dysentery a form of dysentery caused by *Entamoeba histolytica* and spread by contaminated food, water, and flies; called also amoebiasis. Amoebic dysentery is mainly a tropical disease, but many cases occur in temperate countries. Symptoms are diarrhoea, fatigue, and intestinal bleeding. Complications include involvement of the liver, liver abscess, and pulmonary abscess. For treatment several drugs are available, for example, emetine hydrochloride and chloroquine, which may be used singly or in combination.

amoebicide (ə'meebiˌsied) destructive to amoebas.

amoebocyte (ə'meebəˌsiet) a cell showing amoeboid movement.

amoeboid (ə'meeboyd) resembling an amoeba.

amoeboma (ˌami'bohmə) a tumour-like mass caused by granulomatous reaction in the intestines in amoebiasis.

amorph (ə'mawf) an inactive mutant gene, i.e., one that produces no detectable product.

amorphia, amorphism (ay'mawfi·ə; ay'mawfizəm) state of being amorphous.

amorphous (ə'mawfəs) having no definite form; shapeless and usually featureless.

Amoxil (ə'moksil) trademark for a preparation of amoxycillin, an antibiotic.

amoxycillin (ə,moksi'silin) a penicillin analogue similar in action to ampicillin but more efficiently absorbed from the gastrointestinal tract and therefore requiring less frequent dosage and not as likely to cause diarrhoea. It also penetrates sputum more readily than ampicillin.

AMP adenosine monophosphate.

cyclic AMP, 3',5'-AMP cyclic adenosine monophosphate.

amp. ampere, ampoule.

ampere ('ampair) a unit of electric current strength, the current yielded by one volt of electromotive force against one ohm of resistance.

amphetamine (am'fetə,meen, -min) 1. a white crystalline powder used as a central nervous system stimulant. It is odourless and has a slightly bitter taste. 2. any drug closely related to amphetamine and having similar actions, such as methamphetamine.

Amphetamine has the temporary effect of increasing energy and apparent mental alertness. It is used in some cases of mental depression and alcoholism, in the chronic rigidity following encephalitis, in attacks of narcolepsy, and to control the appetite in the overweight. It is also used to overcome the depressant effects of barbiturates.

Caution must be exercised in using amphetamine in persons hypersensitive to stimulants, those suffering from coronary or cardiovascular disease or hypertension, or women in the early stages of pregnancy. The drug should be used only under a doctor's supervision. The use of amphetamines as 'pep pills' or 'uppers' can lead to physical dependence.

amphi- word element. [Gr.] *both, on both sides.*

amphiarthrosis (,amfiah'throhsis) a joint in which the surfaces are connected by discs of fibrocartilage, as between vertebrae.

Amphibia (am'fibi·ə) a class of animals living both on land and in water.

amphicelous (,amfi'seeləs) concave on either side or end.

amphicentric (,amfi'sentrik) beginning and ending in the same vessel.

amphidiarthrosis (,amfi,die·ah'throhsis) a joint having the nature of both ginglymus and arthrodia, as that of the lower jaw.

amphitrichous (am'fitrikəs) having flagella at each end.

amphophil ('amfə,fil) an amphophilic cell or element.

amphophilic (,amfə'filik) staining with either acid or basic dyes.

amphoric (am'for·rik) pertaining to a bottle; resembling the sound made by blowing across the neck of a bottle.

amphoteric (,amfə'terik) capable of acting as both an acid and a base; capable of neutralizing either bases or acids.

amphotericin B (,amfə'terisin bee) an antifungal antibiotic used to treat deep-seated mycotic infections, especially histoplasmosis, and also to treat cutaneous and mucocutaneous candidiasis. It may be applied topically or administered intravenously. Toxic effects from the drug include anorexia, chills, fever, and headache may occur. Renal damage with evidence of renal tubular acidosis occurs, but usually clears when the drug is discontinued.

amphotony (am'fohtənee) hypertonia of the entire autonomic nervous system.

ampicillin (,ampi'silin) a broad-spectrum penicillin of synthetic origin, used in treatment of a number of infections, and available in oral preparations as well as ampoules for intramuscular injections. It is active against many of the gram-negative pathogens, in addition to the usual gram-positive ones that are affected by penicillin.

amplification (,amplifi'kayshən) the process of making larger, as the increase of an auditory or visual stimulus, as a means of improving its perception.

amplitude ('ampli,tyood) largeness, fullness; wideness or breadth of range or extent.

a. of accommodation the total amount of accommodative power of the eye.

ampoule ('ampyool) a small, hermetically sealed glass flask, e.g., one containing medication for parenteral administration.

ampulla (am'puhlə) pl. *ampullae* [L.] a flasklike dilation of a tubular structure, especially of the expanded ends of the semicircular canals of the ear.

a. chyli receptaculum chyli.

a. ductus deferentis the enlarged and tortuous distal end of the ductus deferens.

Henle's a. ampulla ductus deferentis.

hepatopancreatic a. ampulla of Vater; a flasklike cavity in the major duodenal papilla into which the common bile duct and pancreatic duct open.

Lieberkühn's a. the blind termination of the lacteals in the villi of the intestines.

ampullae membranaceae the dilations at one end of each of the three semicircular ducts.

ampullae osseae the dilations at one of the ends of the semicircular canals.

phrenic a. the dilation at the lower end of the oesophagus.

a. of rectum the dilated portion of the rectum just proximal to the anal canal.

a. of Thoma one of the small terminal expansions of an interlobar artery in the pulp of the spleen.

a. of uterine tube the longest and widest portion of the uterine tube, between the infundibulum and the isthmus of the tube.

a. of Vater hepatopancreatic ampulla; the term 'ampulla of Vater' is often mistakenly used instead of 'papilla of Vater', or major duodenal papilla.

amputation (,ampyuh'tayshən) the removal of a limb, in part or in whole, or other appendage such as the breast. The most common indication for amputation of an upper limb is trauma. Blood vessel disorders such as ATHEROSCLEROSIS, often associated with DIABETES MELLITUS, commonly account for lower leg amputations. Other indications may include malignancy, infection, and gangrene.

There are two general types of surgical procedure for amputation: (1) the closed or 'flap' amputation; and (2) the open procedure, which is often required when infection is present and there is a need for free drainage from the operative site. This is done only after the infection has been eliminated.

PATIENT CARE. The goal of patient care for the amputee is total rehabilitation with attainment of full function and normal active life. Such total rehabilitation is not always possible because of the physical and mental limitations of the patient. It requires that the patient be physically and psychologically able to accept and adapt to a PROSTHESIS and that each member of the health care team fulfil his responsibilities in preventing complications and in preparing the patient for optimum use of an artificial limb. Some patients, because of age or disease, do not have the necessary energy, muscular coordination, or mental capacity to undertake prosthetic training.

Preoperative Care. Unless time is a factor, as in emergency cases demanding immediate surgery, the preoperative care of the potential amputee should

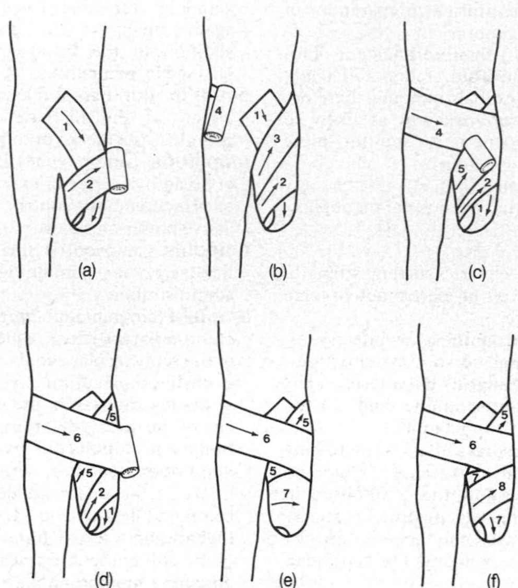

Bandaging an above-knee amputation stump. (a) Use 6″ ellastic bandage. Enclose medial, distal end of stump. Apply pressure via bandage to end of stump. Use diagonal, not circular, turns. (b) Turn 3 must be high in groin and then turn made around waist to hold 3 in place. Do not pull hip into flexion. (A second 6″ roll may be needed.) (c) Turn 5 must be high in groin and a loop made around waist again. (d) See diagram. (e) Enclose lateral, distal end of stump. (A 4″ roll may be needed.) Continue diagonal and figure-of-8 turns around stump. (f) Continue turns to shape end of stump

include emotional and vocational aspects as well as the physical. If the patient is fully involved in plans for his rehabilitation, understands what is expected of him, and knows the regimen of exercise and skills he will need to develop, his chances of full recovery and achievement of independence will be greatly enhanced. Much emotional support and encouragement can be offered by other amputees who are successfully mastering their prostheses and making progress toward their goal of total rehabilitation.

The patient will need help in dealing with the changes in his body image as he adjusts to the loss of a limb. He should be encouraged and given the opportunity to express feelings of anxiety, grief, anger, and depression, and given guidance in working toward a healthy acceptance of his handicap.

In general, physical preparation of the patient undergoing surgical amputation includes measures to promote optimum health and well-being, to establish nutritional and fluid balances, and to increase muscular strength and endurance levels. A programme of exercises may be started to help the patient develop skill in using a monkey pole, walking stick or walking frame and transferring himself between wheelchair and bed.

Immediately prior to surgery the affected limb may be shaved and thoroughly cleansed with an antiseptic. Special wrapping of the limb with sterile towels is sometimes requested by the surgeon.

Postoperative Care. Patient care during the immediate postoperative period is primarily centred on care of the stump and prevention of such complications as haemorrhage and infection. The stump dressing is checked at very frequent intervals, usually every 30 to 60 minutes for the first 12 hours. The area of bright red drainage on the dressing should be clearly marked with an indelible pencil and the time noted for each check for enlargement of the area. Dressings may be reinforced as necessary. Adequate analgesia must be given to the patient post-operatively. As PHANTOM PAIN may also be experienced, reassurance is necessary to dispel fear and anxiety.

Wound drainage is usually by a suction drain. Assessment of the amount of drainage is undertaken and the drain is generally removed about 72 hours after surgery.

Exercises are started as soon as possible to strengthen the muscles and prevent contractures. Early ambulation is encouraged to promote wound healing and facilitate fitting of a prosthesis. If all goes well and no complications develop, the patient may be fitted for a temporary prosthesis during the second or third postoperative week. He is allowed gradually to increase weight-bearing on the stump until he can tolerate his full weight on it. By the tenth or twelfth week a permanent prosthesis can be fitted to the stump of the lower extremity. Walking with the aid of a walking stick or walking frame is begun as soon as the patient's condition allows.

The patient with amputation of an upper extremity requires stump care similar to that of the lower extremity except that an upper extremity stump is bandaged more loosely, especially when trauma has necessitated removal of the limb. Exercises are begun the day after surgery and within ten to fourteen days the patient is fitted with a temporary prosthesis.

closed a. one in which skin flaps with subcutaneous tissue are sutured over the stump.

congenital a. absence of a limb at birth, attributed to constriction of the part by an encircling band during intrauterine development.

a. in contiguity amputation at a joint.

a. in continuity amputation of a limb elsewhere than at a joint.

diaclastic a. amputation in which the bone is broken by osteoclast and the soft tissues divided by an écraseur.

Dupuytren's a. amputation of the arm at the shoulder joint.

flap a. amputation in which the flaps, which are made of soft tissue, cover the stump.

forequarter (interscapulothoracic) a. removal of the arm with excision of the lateral portion of the shoulder girdle.

Gritti–Stokes a. amputation of the leg at the knee through condyles of the femur. The patella is retained and applied to the end of the stump.

guillotine a. open amputation; one in which the entire cross-section is left open (flapless) for dressing.

Hey's a. amputation of the foot between the tarsus and metatarsus.

hindquarter (interpelviabdominal) a. removal of the thigh with excision of the lateral portion of the pelvic girdle.

Lisfranc's a. amputation of the foot between the metatarsus and tarsus.

midtarsal a., Chopart's a. amputation of the foot, with the calcaneus, talus, and other parts of the tarsus being retained.

spontaneous a. loss of a part without surgical intervention, as in gangrene, etc.

Syme's a. disarticulation of the foot with removal of both malleoli.

Tripier's a. amputation of the foot through the calcaneus.

amputee (ˌampyuh'tee) an individual who has had a limb amputated.

a.m.u. atomic mass unit.

amusia (ay'myoozi·ə) loss of ability to produce (motor amusia) or to recognize (sensory amusia) musical sounds.

amyasthenia (ayˌmieəs'theeni·ə) failure of muscular strength.

amyasthenic (ayˌmieəs'theenik) 1. characterized by amyasthenia. 2. an agent that diminishes muscular power.

amyelia (ˌaymie'eeli·ə) congenital absence of the spinal cord.

amyelinic (ayˌmieə'linik) without myelin.

amyelonic (ayˌmieə'lonik) 1. having no spinal cord. 2. having no marrow.

amyelus (ay'mieələs) a fetus with no spinal cord.

amygdala (ə'migdələ) an almond-shaped structure; often used to refer to the corpus amygdaloideum.

amygdalin (ə'migdəlin) a glycoside from bitter almonds.

amygdaline (ə'migdəleen, -lin) 1. like an almond. 2. pertaining to tonsils.

amygdalolith (ə'migdələˌlith) a calculus in a tonsil.

amyl nitrite ('amil 'nietriet) a volatile, inflammable liquid with a pungent ethereal odour. It was administered by inhalation for the treatment of ANGINA PECTORIS (acting as a coronary vasodilator) and can be used by repeated inhalation in cyanide poisoning (producing methaemoglobin, which binds cyanide).

amyl(o)- word element. [Gr.] *starch.*

amylaceous (ˌami'layshəs) composed of or resembling starch.

amylase ('amiˌlayz) an enzyme that catalyses the hydrolysis of starch into simpler compounds. The α-amylases occur in animals and include pancreatic and salivary amylase; the β-amylases occur in higher plants. Measurement of serum α-amylase activity is an important diagnostic test for acute and chronic pancreatitis.

amylobarbitone (əˌmieloh'bahbitohn) one of the barbiturates, used as a short-acting hypnotic and sedative. Effects develop rapidly and the drug is eliminated more quickly than other barbiturates. Regular use may lead to habituation, and overdosage can produce narcosis and death. Classified as a controlled drug.

amylogenesis (ˌamiloh'jenəsis) the formation of starch. adj. **amylogenic.**

amyloid ('amiˌloyd) 1. starchlike; amylaceous. 2. an optically homogeneous, waxy, translucent, abnormal fibrillary protein that is deposited extracellularly in a variety of conditions.

amyloidosis (ˌamiloy'dohsis) the deposition in various tissues of amyloid. This protein is almost insoluble and once it infiltrates the tissues they become waxy and nonfunctioning. Primary amyloidosis is thought to be due to some obscure metabolic disturbance in which there is an abnormal protein in the plasma; the tissues most often affected are cardiac and smooth and skeletal muscle tissue. Secondary amyloidosis is related to chronic suppuration, especially those types associated with tuberculosis, lung abscess, osteomyelitis, or bronchiectasis; the most common sites of deposition are the spleen, kidney, liver, and adrenal cortex.

The symptoms of amyloidosis appear insidiously and progress slowly. They depend on the specific organ affected, and frequently in secondary amyloidosis they are overshadowed by symptoms of the disease causing the disorder. Primary systemic amyloidosis is treated symptomatically; there is no cure, and death usually occurs within 3 years of the onset. Heart failure is the most common cause of death. Secondary amyloidosis is best treated by eliminating the underlying cause. This includes control of suppuration by effective use of antibiotic drugs. There has been a reduction in incidence of secondary amyloidosis in recent years because of the development of drugs that are successful in controlling infection and suppuration.

amylopectin (ˌamiloh'pektin) the insoluble constituent of starch. The soluble constituent is amylose.

amylopectinosis (ˌamilohˌpekti'nohsis) glycogenosis (type IV) in which deficiency of the brancher enzyme amylo-1:4,1:6-transglucoside results in cirrhosis of the liver, hepatosplenomegaly, and progressive hepatic failure and death. Called also Andersen's disease.

amylopsin (ˌami'lopsin) an enzyme found in the pancreas. Amylase.

amylorrhoea (ˌamilə'reeə) the presence of an abnormal amount of starch in the stools.

amylose ('amiˌlohz, -lohs) 1. any carbohydrate other than a glucose or saccharose. 2. the soluble constituent of starch, as opposed to amylopectin.

amylum ('amiləm) [L.] *starch.*

amyocardia (ayˌmieoh'kahdi·ə) weakness of the heart muscle.

amyoplasia (ayˌmieoh'playzi·ə) lack of muscle formation or development.

a. congenita generalized lack in the newborn of muscular development and growth, with contracture and deformity at most joints.

amyostasia (ayˌmieoh'stayzi·ə) a tremor of the muscles.

amyotonia (ayˌmieoh'tohni·ə) atonic condition of the

muscles.

a. congenita any of several rare congenital diseases marked by general hypotonia of the muscles; called also Oppenheim's disease.

amyotrophia (ay,mieoh'trohfi·ə) amyotrophy.

amyotrophic lateral sclerosis (ay,mieoh'trofik) a type of motor disorder of the nervous system in which there is destruction of the anterior horn cells and pyramidal tract. The cause is unknown. Early symptoms include weakness of the hands and arms, difficulty in swallowing and talking, and weakness and spasticity of the legs. As the disorder progresses there is increased spasticity and atrophy of the muscles, with loss of motor control and overactivity of the reflexes. There is no known specific or effective treatment. Although there may be periods of remission, the disease usually progresses rapidly, death ensuing in 2 to 5 years in most cases.

amyotrophy (,aymie'otrəfee) a painful condition with wasting and weakness of muscle, commonly involving the deltoid muscle.

Amytal ('ami,tal) trademark for amylobarbitone, a short-acting hypnotic and sedative. Classified as a controlled drug.

amyxia (ay'miksi·ə) absence of mucus.

amyxorrhoea (ay,miksə'reeə) absence of mucous secretion.

An chemical symbol, *actinon*; anode.

ANA antinuclear antibody; American Nurses' Association.

ana- word element. [Gr.] *upward, again, backward, excessively*.

anabasis (ə'nabəsis) the stage of increase in a disease.

anabiosis (,anəbie'ohsis) restoration of life processes after their apparent cessation.

anabolic (,anə'bolik) relating to anabolism.

a. compound a substance that aids in the repair of body tissue, particularly protein. Androgens may be used in this way.

anabolism (ə'nabə,lizəm) the constructive phase of metabolism, in which the body cells synthesize protoplasm for growth and repair. adj. **anabolic.** The manner in which this synthesis takes place is directed by the genetic code carried by the molecules of deoxyribonucleic acid (DNA). The 'building blocks' for this synthesis of protoplasm are obtained from amino acids and other nutritive elements in the diet.

anachoresis (,anəkə'reesis) preferential collection or deposit of particles at a site, as of bacteria or metals that have localized out of the bloodstream in areas of inflammation.

anacidity (,anə'siditee) abnormal lack or deficiency of acid.

gastric a. achlorhydria.

anaclisis (,anə'klisis) generally reclining or leaning; typically an emotional dependence on others.

anaclitic (,anə'klitik) denoting the dependence of the infant on the mother or mother substitute for his sense of well-being.

a. choice a psychoanalytic term for the adult selection of a loved one who closely resembles one's mother (or another adult on whom one depended as a child).

a. depression severe and progressive depression found in children who have lost their mothers and have not found a suitable substitute.

anacrotism (ə'nakrə,tizəm) a pulse anomaly evidenced by the presence of a prominent notch on the ascending limb of the pulse tracing. adj. **anacrotic.**

anadipsia (,anə'dipsi·ə) intense thirst.

anadrenalism (,anə'dreenəlizəm) absence or failure of adrenal function.

anaemia (ə'neemi·ə) a reduction below normal in the packed red cell (erythrocyte) volume (see HAEMATOCRIT) or in the haemoglobin concentration in the blood. adj. **anaemic.**

Anaemia is not a disease but a symptom of many different disorders. Anaemia is caused by factors leading to failure of red cell production or to their increased destruction or loss. Aetiological factors include poor diet, blood loss, and primary diseases of the bone marrow.

Anaemias can be classified on the basis of their aetiology, but with the advent of electronic cell counters are more easily classified according to the morphological characteristics of the erythrocytes; that is, by their size and colour (haemoglobin concentration). Data defining the different types of red cells are known as red cell indices. These are: (1) mean corpuscular volume (MCV), the average erythrocyte volume; (2) mean corpuscular haemoglobin (MCH), the average amount of haemoglobin per erythrocyte; and (3) mean corpuscular haemoglobin concentration (MCHC), the average concentration of haemoglobin in erythrocytes. Based on the MCV and the MCH, three types of anaemia are described: (1) microcytic hypochromic; (2) normocytic normochromic; and (3) macrocytic. For example, microcytic hypochromic anaemia is characterized by very small erythrocytes that have a low haemoglobin concentration and hence poor coloration.

SYMPTOMS. Mild degrees of anaemia often cause only slight or no symptoms, perhaps little more than a lack of energy and easy tiring. In more severe anaemia, exertion causes shortness of breath. This may be accompanied by pounding of the heart and a rapid pulse and heart action. These symptoms are caused by the inability of anaemic blood to supply the body tissues with sufficient oxygen.

Pallor, particularly in the palms of the hands, the fingernails, and the conjunctiva (the lining of the eyelids), may also indicate anaemia. In severe anaemia, swelling of the ankles and other evidence of heart failure may appear.

COMMON CAUSES OF ANAEMIA

Loss of Blood. If there is massive bleeding from a wound or other lesion, the body may lose enough blood to cause severe anaemia. This acute anaemia is often accompanied by shock. Immediate transfusion is generally required to replace the lost blood. Chronic blood loss, such as excessive menstrual flow, or loss of blood from an ulcer or cancer of the stomach, may also lead to anaemia.

These anaemias disappear when the cause has been found and corrected. To help the blood rebuild itself, the doctor may prescribe iron, which is necessary to build haemoglobin, and foods with high iron content, such as kidney beans, liver, spinach, and wholewheat bread.

Diet Deficiency. Anaemia may develop if the diet does not provide enough iron, protein, folate, and other vitamins and minerals needed in the production of haemoglobin and the formation of erythrocytes. The combination of poor diet and chronic loss of blood makes for particular susceptibility to severe anaemia. For example, a child suffering from hookworm disease, living on an inadequate diet, is doubly likely to suffer from anaemia.

A good basic diet is the best way to combat diet-deficiency anaemia (see also NUTRITION). So-called 'blood tonics' containing iron or other vitamins or minerals are not necessary unless they are prescribed.

PATIENT CARE. Determining and treating the underlying cause is the first consideration in the management of the patient with anaemia. Observation for signs of blood loss through the intestinal tract or genitourinary tract may assist in diagnosis of the cause of anaemia. Tarry stools or hazy brown urine should be recognized as evidence of internal bleeding and should be reported.

Rest and limitation of physical activity may be necessary if the patient is very anaemic with reduced effort tolerance. Combating a lack of appetite and disinterest in food may be a problem in patients with anaemia. Fatigue, weakness, or soreness of the mouth must be considered as contributing factors. The patient may need to overcome poor eating habits developed through ignorance or indifference to the nutritional values of food.

Special mouth care is required when mouth and gums are tender and bleed easily. Brushing of the teeth may be traumatic and frequent cleansing of the mouth with gauze or sponge applicators dipped in a mild mouthwash can be substituted. The lips are kept lubricated with mineral oil or some other emollient to prevent dryness and cracking.

Extra warmth in the form of blankets and warm clothing should be available because many anaemic patients suffer from poor circulation and are easily chilled. The poor circulation also brings about decreased sensitivity to heat and these patients may be burned if care is not taken with hot water bottles and heating pads.

Decreased numbers of circulating erythrocytes result in inadequate supplies of oxygen to the tissues. Since hypoxic tissues are less easily healed, every effort should be made to avoid trauma to the skin and underlying tissues and to the mucous membranes.

Some anaemias are accompanied by a corresponding reduction in normally functioning leukocytes. This produces an increased susceptibility to infection and some loss of the ability to overcome an infection once it has occurred. Care must be taken to avoid introducing infectious agents into the patient's environment, and measures must be taken to promote healing and repair of injured tissues.

aplastic a. a form of anaemia, unresponsive to specific antianaemia therapy, often accompanied by granulocytopenia and thrombocytopenia; the bone marrow is usually acellular or hypoplastic and fails to produce adequate numbers of blood elements. Precipitating causes include drugs and viral infections. The cause is often not determined.

Cooley's a. the homozygous form of beta-THALASSAEMIA.

deficiency a. nutritional anaemia.

erythroblastic a. the homozygous form of beta-THALASSAEMIA.

haemolytic a. that due to shortened survival of mature erythrocytes and inability of the bone marrow to compensate for their decreased life span; it may be hereditary or acquired, as that resulting from infection, or as part of an autoimmune process (see also HAEMOLYTIC anaemia).

hypochromic a. anaemia in which the decrease in haemoglobin is proportionately much greater than the decrease in number of erythrocytes.

hypoplastic a. anaemia due to incapacity of blood-forming organs.

hypoplastic a., congenital 1. idiopathic progressive anaemia occurring in the first year of life, without leukopenia and thrombocytopenia; it is unresponsive to haematinics and requires multiple blood transfusions to sustain life. Called also erythrogenesis imperfecta. 2. Fanconi's syndrome.

iron-deficiency a. a form characterized by low or absent iron stores, low serum iron and ferritin concentration, low transferrin saturation, elevated transferrin, low haemoglobin concentration or haematocrit, and hypochromic, microcytic red blood corpuscles. See also IRON.

Lederer's a. an acute haemolytic anaemia of short duration and unknown aetiology.

macrocytic a. anaemia in which the erythrocytes are much larger than normal.

Mediterranean a. the homozygous form of beta-THALASSAEMIA.

megaloblastic a. anaemia characterized by the presence of megaloblasts in the bone marrow.

microcytic a. anaemia characterized by decrease in size of the erythrocytes.

myelopathic a., myelophthisic a. anaemia due to destruction or crowding out of haematopoietic tissues by space-occupying lesions.

normochromic a. that in which the haemoglobin content of the red cells as measured by the MCHC is in the normal range.

normocytic a. anaemia characterized by proportionate decrease in haemoglobin, packed red cell volume, and number of erythrocytes per cubic millimetre of blood.

nutritional a. anaemia due to a deficiency of an essential substance in the diet, which may be caused by poor dietary intake or by malabsorption; called also deficiency anaemia.

pernicious a. a megaloblastic anaemia due to vitamin B_{12} deficiency secondary to lack of secretion by the gastric mucous membrane of a factor (intrinsic factor) necessary for the absorption of vitamin B_{12}. Treatment consists of regular parenteral administration of vitamin B_{12}, which must be continued for life. See also PERNICIOUS ANAEMIA.

refractory a. a chronic acquired anaemia unresponsive to treatment with haematinics (iron, folate, vitamin B_{12}, etc.). A disease of older adults and often associated with blood and bone marrow abnormalities indicating myelodysplasia. One of the subgroups in the myelodysplastic syndrome when refractory anaemia is associated with an excess of blasts.

sickle cell a. a genetically determined defect of haemoglobin synthesis associated with poor physical development and skeletal anomalies, occurring usually in Afro-Caribbeans. See also SICKLE CELL DISEASE.

sideroblastic a. anaemia associated with disordered accumulation of iron in the red cells. The iron granules encircle the red cell nucleus forming 'ring' sideroblasts. It is usually secondary to causes such as multiple blood transfusions, alcoholism, drugs (e.g. some antituberculous agents) and lead. It can be classified as congenital or acquired (see table). Abnormalities of haem synthesis are usually present. The diagnosis is suggested by a mixed hypochromic and normochromic blood picture and confirmed on demonstrating excess iron granules in the nucleated red cells (i.e. sideroblasts) in the bone marrow.

spur-cell a. anaemia in which the red cells have a bizarre spiculated shape and are destroyed prematurely, primarily in the spleen; it is a rare acquired disorder in severe liver disease, and represents an abnormality in the cholesterol content of the red cell membrane.

anaemic (ə'neemik) pertaining to anaemia.

anaerobe (an'air·rohb, 'anə,rohb) an organism that lives and grows in the absence of molecular oxygen. adj. **anaerobic**.

facultative a. a microorganism that can live and grow with or without molecular oxygen.

obligate a. an organism that can grow only in the complete absence of molecular oxygen.

anaerosis (,anair'rohsis) interruption of the respiratory function.

anaesthecinesia (ˌanəsˌtheesi'neezi·ə) combined sensory and motor paralysis.

anaesthesia (ˌanəs'theezi·ə) loss of feeling or sensation. Anaesthesia may be produced by a number of agents capable of bringing about partial or complete loss of sensation. It is induced to permit the performance of surgery or other painful procedures. See also ANAESTHETIC.

PATIENT CARE. The patient recovering from general anaesthesia must be watched constantly until he has reacted. The vital signs (blood pressure, pulse and respiration) are checked regularly; any sudden or unacceptable change is reported immediately. The patient must be observed to ensure that the airway is patent at all times. If vomiting occurs, the patient is turned on his side in the slightly head-down position to prevent aspiration of vomitus into the respiratory tract. Suction is used when necessary to clear secretions.

In addition to the physical effects of general anaesthesia, the emotional and psychological aspects must also be considered. Fear of being rendered unconscious is common among patients. During recovery from anaesthesia noise should be kept at a minimum, as all sounds may be exaggerated to the patient. It is important to remember that conversations held within hearing of the patient may be misunderstood by him since he is not capable of interpreting words and phrases clearly as long as he is under the effects of the anaesthetic. When the patient is awakening from general anaesthesia he may be extremely restless, attempting to get out of bed or even striking out at those around him because he is afraid and disorientated.

Patients who have had local anaesthesia of the throat for diagnostic procedures or minor surgery should receive nothing by mouth for at least 4 hours to ensure that the anaesthetic has worn off and the cough reflex has returned. Otherwise any food or drink taken may be aspirated into the respiratory tract.

Local anaesthetic techniques should not be undertaken unless resuscitative equipment and drugs are available. This is to enable the rare case of local anaesthetic toxicity due to overdose or inadvertent intravascular injection to be treated. Allergic reactions to local anaesthetics are extremely rare and almost always only occur with ester-type drugs such as procaine.

block a. regional anaesthesia. See also BLOCK.

caudal a. injection of an anaesthetic into the sacral canal, usually done to relieve the pain of childbirth (see also CAUDAL ANAESTHESIA).

central a. lack of sensation caused by disease of the nerve centres.

closed a. that produced by partial or total rebreathing of expired gas in a circle or to-and-fro system. Sufficient oxygen is added to supply the body's needs and the carbon dioxide in the expired air is removed by passing it through soda-lime. Originally devised to effect economy in anaesthetic agents.

crossed a. loss of sensation on one side of the face and loss of pain and temperature sense on the opposite side of the body.

dissociated a., dissociation a. loss of perception of certain stimuli while that of others remains intact.

a. dolorosa pain felt in an area or region that is anaesthetic.

electric a. anaesthesia induced by passage of an electric current.

endotracheal a. anaesthesia produced by introduction of a gaseous mixture through a tube inserted into the trachea.

epidural a. anaesthesia produced by injection of the anaesthetic agent between the vertebral spines and beneath the ligamentum flavum in the extradural space; called also peridural anaesthesia.

general a. a state of unconsciousness produced by anaesthetic agents, with absence of pain sensation over the entire body and a greater or lesser degree of muscular relaxation; the drugs producing this state can be administered by inhalation, intravenously, intramuscularly, or rectally, or via the gastrointestinal tract.

gustatory a. loss of the sense of taste. **hysterical a.** loss of sensation or feeling occurring as part of a hysterical reaction and which has no physical cause but is an expression of repressed mental tensions. Like hysterical paralysis, with which it is often associated, it tends to have a neurologically improbable distribution. See also HYSTERIA.

infiltration a. local anaesthesia produced by injection of the anaesthetic solution directly into the area of terminal nerve endings.

inhalation a. anaesthesia produced by the breathing of a vapour from a volatile liquid or gaseous anaesthetic agent.

insufflation a. anaesthesia produced by introduction of a gaseous mixture into the trachea or the pharynx through a slender tube.

local a. that produced in a limited area, as by injection of a local anaesthetic or by freezing with ethyl chloride.

open a. general inhalation anaesthesia brought about by dropping the anaesthetic agent onto a Schimmelbusch mask.

paravertebral a. regional anaesthesia produced by the injection of a local anaesthetic around the spinal nerves at their exit from the spinal column, and outside the spinal dura.

peripheral a. lack of sensation due to changes in the peripheral nerves.

rectal a. anaesthesia produced by introduction of the anaesthetic agent into the rectum.

refrigeration a. local anaesthesia produced by applying a tourniquet and chilling the part to near freezing temperature; called also cryoanaesthesia.

regional a. insensibility caused by interrupting the sensory nerve conductivity of any region of the body; produced by: (1) field block, encircling the operative field by means of injections of a local anaesthetic; or (2) nerve block, making injections in close proximity to the nerves supplying the area.

saddle block a. the production of anaesthesia in the region of the body that impinges on the saddle when riding, corresponding roughly with the areas of the buttocks, perineum, and inner aspects of the thighs, by introducing a hyperbaric (i.e with a specific gravity greater than that of cerebrospinal fluid) local anaesthetic into the subarachnoid space with the patient in the sitting position.

segmental a. loss of sensation in a segment of the body due to a lesion of a nerve root.

spinal a. 1. anaesthesia due to a spinal lesion. 2. anaesthesia produced by injection of the agent into the subarachnoid space surrounding the spinal cord.

splanchnic a. block anaesthesia for visceral operation by injection of the anaesthetic agent into the region of the coeliac ganglia.

surgical a. that degree of anaesthesia at which operation may safely be performed.

tactile a. loss of the sense of touch.

topical a. that produced by application of a local anaesthetic directly to the area involved, for instance to the eye, nose or trachea.

twilight a. twilight sleep.

anaesthesiologist (ˌanəsˌtheeziˈoləjist) anaesthetist.

anaesthesiology (ˌanəsˌtheeziˈoləjee) that branch of medicine concerned with administration of anaesthetics and the condition of the patient while under anaesthesia.

anaesthetic (ˌanəsˈthetik) 1. pertaining to, characterized by, or producing anaesthesia. 2. a drug or agent used to abolish the sensation of pain, to achieve adequate muscle relaxation during surgery, to calm fear and allay anxiety, and to produce amnesia for the event.

Inhalational anaesthetics are gases or volatile liquids that produce general anaesthesia when inhaled. The commonly used inhalational agents are halothane (Fluothane), enflurane (Ethrane), isoflurane (Forane), and nitrous oxide. Older agents, such as ether and cyclopropane, are now used infrequently. The mechanism of action of all inhalational anaesthetics is thought to involve the uptake of the gas in the lipid bilayer of cell membranes and some interaction with the membrane proteins, resulting in an inhibition of the synaptic transmission of nerve impulses. For surgical anaesthesia, these agents are usually used with preanaesthetic medication, which includes sedatives or opiates to relieve preoperative and postoperative pain and tranquillizers to reduce anxiety. Neuromuscular blocking agents, such as tubocurarine, alcuronium and suxamethonium, are used to produce complete muscular relaxation during surgery.

Intravenous anaesthetics are sedative–hypnotic drugs that produce anaesthesia in large doses. The most commonly used intravenous anaesthetics are ultrashort acting barbiturates, such as thiopentone (Intraval) and methohexitone (Brietal), which can be used alone for brief surgical procedures or for rapid induction of anaesthesia maintained by inhalational anaesthetics.

Other types of intravenous methods of anaesthesia are *neuroleptanalgesia*, which uses a combination of the butyrophenone tranquillizer droperidol and an opioid such as fentanyl or phenoperidine; *neurolept-anaesthesia*, which uses neuroleptanalgesia plus nitrous oxide; and *dissociative anaesthesia*, which uses ketamine, a drug related to the hallucinogens that produces profound analgesia.

Local anaesthetics are drugs that block nerve conduction in the region where they are applied. They act by altering the permeability of the nerve cell to sodium ions and thus blocking the conduction of nerve impulses. They may be applied topically or injected into the tissues. The first local anaesthetic was cocaine. Synthetic local anaesthetics are all given names ending in *-caine*; examples are procaine (Novocain) and lidocaine (Xylocaine).

anaesthetist (əˈneesthətist) a doctor who specializes in anaesthetics.

anakatadidymus (ˌanəˌkatəˈdidiməs) a twin fetus or infant, separate above and below, but united in the trunk.

anakusis (ˌanəˈkyoosis) total deafness.

anal (ˈaynˈl) relating to the anus.

analbuminaemia (ˌanalˌbyoomiˈneemi·ə) absence or deficiency of serum albumins.

analeptic (ˌanəˈleptik) 1. a drug that acts as a stimulant to the central nervous system, such as caffeine and amphetamine. 2. a restorative medicine.

analgesia (ˌanˈlˈjeezi·ə) absence of sensibility to pain, particularly the relief of pain without loss of consciousness; absence of pain or noxious stimulation.

continuous caudal a. involves the passage of a catheter into the sacral canal, allowing local anaesthetics or other agents to be injected when required. Not often used because of risk of infection. Previously almost exclusively used during childbirth (see also CAUDAL ANAESTHESIA).

epidural a. analgesia induced by introduction of the analgesic agent into the epidural space of the vertebral canal.

infiltration a. paralysis of the nerve endings at the site of operation by subcutaneous injection of an anaesthetic.

surface a. local analgesia produced by an anaesthetic applied to the surface of mucous membranes, e.g., those of the eye, nose, throat, and urethra; called also *topical anaesthesia*.

analgesic (ˌanˈlˈjeezik, -sik) 1. relieving pain. 2. pertaining to analgesia. 3. a drug that relieves pain.

analgesiometer (ˌanˈlˌgeeziˈomitə) an instrument which indicates the degree of sensitiveness to pain.

analogous (əˈnaləgəs) resembling or similar in some respects, as in function or appearance, but not in origin or development.

analogue (ˈanəˌlog) 1. a part or organ having the same function as another, but of different evolutionary origin. 2. a chemical compound having a structure similar to that of another but differing from it in respect of a certain component; it may have similar or opposite action metabolically.

analogy (əˈnaləjee) the quality of being analogous; resemblance or similarity in function or appearance, but not in origin or development.

analysand (əˈnaliˌsand) a person undergoing psychoanalysis.

analysis (əˈnalisis) 1. separation into component parts. 2. psychoanalysis. adj. **analytic.**

qualitative a. determination of the nature of the constituents of a compound or mixture.

quantitative a. determination of the proportionate quantities of the constituents of a compound or mixture.

transactional a. a type of psychotherapy involving an understanding of the interpersonal interchanges between the components of the personalities of the participants (individuals or members of a group).

vector a. analysis of a moving force to determine both its magnitude and its direction, e.g., analysis of the scalar electrocardiogram to determine the magnitude and direction of the electromotive force for one complete cycle of the heart.

analyst (ˈanəlist) a person who performs analyses.

analyte (ˈanəˌliet) a substance or material determined by a chemical analysis.

analytical study (anəˈlitikˈl) an epidemiological study to determine the association between a disease and suspected causal factors. There are three types of study: (1) an incidence or cohort study; (2) a retrospective or case control study; and (3) a cross-sectional or prevalence study.

anamnesis (ˌanamˈneesis) 1. the faculty of memory. 2. the past history of a patient and his family.

anamnestic (ˌanamˈnestik) 1. pertaining to anamnesis. 2. aiding the memory.

anamniotic (ˌanamniˈotik) having no amnion.

anankastic (anənˈkastik) denoting a personality characterized by compulsive behaviour and inflexibility—also excessive frugality, obstinacy and cleanliness. Thought to be associated with fixation at the anal stage of psychosexual development. Called also *anal personality*.

anaphase (ˈanəˌfayz) the third stage of division of the nucleus of a cell in either meiosis or mitosis.

anaphia (əˈnafi·ə) lack or loss of the sense of touch.

anaphoresis (ˌanəfə'reesis) diminished activity of the sweat glands.

anaphoria (ˌanə'for·ri·ə) the tendency to tilt the head downward, with visual axes deviating upward, on looking straight ahead.

anaphrodisia (ˌanafrə'dizi·ə) absence or loss of sexual desire.

anaphrodisiac (ˌanafrə'diziˌak) 1. repressing sexual desire. 2. a drug that represses sexual desire.

anaphylactic shock (ˌanəfi'laktik) a serious and profound state of shock brought about by hypersensitivity (ANAPHYLAXIS) to an ALLERGEN, such as a drug, foreign protein, or toxin.

anaphylactogen (ˌanəfi'laktohjen) a substance that produces anaphylaxis.

anaphylactogenesis (ˌanəfiˌlaktoh'jenəsis) the production of anaphylaxis. adj. **anaphylactogenic.**

anaphylatoxin (ˌanəˌfilə'toksin) a substance produced in blood serum during complement fixation which serves as a mediator of inflammation by inducing mast cell degranulation and histamine release; on injection into animals, it causes anaphylactic shock.

anaphylaxis (ˌanəfi'laksis) an unusual or exaggerated allergic reaction of an organism to foreign protein or other substances. adj. **anaphylactic.**

Substances most likely to produce anaphylaxis include drugs, particularly antibiotics, local anaesthetics, and codeine; drugs prepared from animals, such as insulin, adrenocorticotrophic hormone, and enzymes; diagnostic agents, such as iodinated x-ray contrast media; biologicals used to provide immunity, such as vaccines, antitoxins, and gamma globulin; protein foods; the venom of bees, wasps, and hornets; and pollens, moulds, and animal dander.

PHYSIOLOGICAL BASIS. Anaphylaxis is the immediate reaction to allergens (often within a few seconds), causing the release of vasoactive substances as a result of antigen combining with IgE antibodies. Individuals who have an anaphylactic immune response may have a familial predisposition to produce an overabundance of IgE antibodies. When an allergen enters the body, IgE antibodies, which become bound to mast cells and basophils in the body, bind with the allergens.

During the interaction mast cells and eosinophils release histamine, slow-reacting substance of anaphylaxis (SRS-A), bradykinin, and enzymes. Histamine brings about bronchospasm, widespread peripheral vasodilation, and increased permeability of the capillaries. SRS-A causes increased constriction of the bronchioles and bronchi. Bradykinin has effects similar to those of histamine. Together they promote collapse of the vascular network by permitting the loss of fluid from the blood vessels into the interstitial fluid compartment.

CLINICAL MANIFESTATIONS. If the allergen comes into contact with cell-bound IgE in the respiratory tract, the released mediators produce the symptoms of ASTHMA and HAY FEVER. An insect bite or sting can produce localized swelling, redness, and itching, or a more severe systemic reaction.

Local anaphylactic reactions usually produce mildly irritating symptoms, which should not be ignored because the reaction can rapidly escalate into a general systemic response. The patient may then experience generalized itching, swelling, and urticaria. As the process continues respiration is impaired because of bronchospasm and laryngeal oedema. If an airway is not maintained and supplementary oxygen provided, the person will die of respiratory failure.

Another life-threatening series of events is related to vascular collapse resulting from a shift in body fluid. The symptoms are hypotension, decreasing levels of consciousness, tachycardia, and diminished production of urine. Without effective treatment these symptoms progress to profound shock and death.

PATIENT CARE. Mild anaphylaxis can be treated with antihistamines, local applications of cold to minimize swelling, and topical applications of medications to relieve itching and soothe the skin. *All* anaphylactic reactions require close monitoring, and the patient should be instructed to seek additional help if he or she experiences dizziness, palpitations, or prolonged or spreading oedema anywhere in the body. The drug of choice in the initial treatment of severe anaphylaxis is adrenaline, administered intravenously, subcutaneously, sublingually, or by intermittent positive pressure ventilation. The mode of administration is governed by the urgency of the situation and the presenting symptoms. Adrenaline causes bronchodilation, reduces laryngeal spasm, and elevates the blood pressure.

Steroid therapy is initiated to counteract the effects of histamine by decreasing capillary permeability. Acting as anti-inflammatory agents, steroids also stabilize mast cells and prevent further release of chemical mediators.

Supportive measures include administration of intravenous fluids and plasma to restore intravascular fluid volume. Pressor agents, such as dopamine, noradrenaline, and isoprenaline, are given to increase and maintain blood pressure.

The best way to control anaphylaxis is by preventing it from happening in the first place, but this is not always possible. A person engaging in normal activities outside the clinical setting can accidentally come in contact with an allergen. An allergic individual should be prepared for such an event by understanding his allergy and knowing what actions to take. Those with known atopic allergies should wear a medical identification necklace or bracelet, and those who undergo systemic reactions should carry with them at all times a kit containing diphenhydramine, a syringe and needle, and vials of adrenaline.

In the clinical setting, all health care personnel should be alert to the need for identifying patients with known allergies and communicating this information to their co-workers. Emergency equipment should be readily available in all places where drugs or diagnostic agents with a risk of provoking anaphylaxis are administered.

acquired a. that in which sensitization is known to have been produced by exposure to a foreign immunogen.

active a. that produced by injection of a foreign protein.

antiserum a. passive anaphylaxis.

cytotropic a. that induced by antigen reacting with antibody that has become fixed to mediator cells (e.g., mast cells, basophils) which release mediators of anaphylaxis when reacting with allergens.

heterologous a. passive anaphylaxis induced by transfer of serum from an animal of a different species.

homologous a. passive anaphylaxis induced by transfer of serum from an animal of the same species.

indirect a. that induced by an animal's own protein modified in some way.

passive a. that resulting in a normal person from injection of serum of a sensitized person.

passive cutaneous a. (PCA) localized anaphylaxis passively transferred by intradermal injection of an antibody and, after a latent period (about 24 to 72 hours), intravenous injection of the homologous antigen and Evans blue dye. Blueing of the skin at the site of the intradermal injection is evidence of a permeability reaction. A positive reaction demonstrates the presence of cytotropic antibody. Used in studies of antibodies causing immediate hypersensitivity reactions.

reverse a. that following injection of antigen, succeeded by injection of antiserum.

anaplasia (ˌanəˈplayzi·ə) loss of differentiation of cells, an irreversible alteration in adult cells toward more primitive (embryonic) cell types; a characteristic of tumour cells.

anaplastic (ˌanəˈplastik) 1. restoring a lost or absent part. 2. characterized by anaplasia.

anapophysis (ˌanəˈpofisis) an accessory vertebral process.

anaptic (əˈnaptik) pertaining to or characterized by loss of the sense of touch.

anarithmia (ˌanəˈridhmi·ə) inability to count, due to a lesion of the brain.

anarthria (anˈahthri·ə) severe dysarthria resulting in speechlessness.

a. literalis stuttering.

anasarca (ˌanəˈsahkə) generalized massive oedema.

anastalsis (ˌanəˈstalsis) 1. an upward-moving wave of contraction without a preceding wave of inhibition, occurring in the alimentary canal in addition to the peristaltic wave. 2. styptic action.

anastaltic (ˌanəˈstaltik) styptic; highly astringent.

anastole (əˈnastəlee) retraction, as of the lips of a wound.

anastomosis (əˌnastəˈmohsis) 1. communication between blood vessels by collateral channels. 2. surgical, traumatic, or pathological formation of a connection between two normally distinct structures. Also the restoration of the continuity of a hollow organ after resection of a part. adj. **anastomotic.**

arteriovenous a. anastomosis between an artery and a vein.

cruciate a. an arterial anastomosis in the upper part of the thigh.

intestinal a. establishment of continuity between two formerly distant portions of the intestine.

anatomical (ˌanəˈtomikˈl) pertaining to anatomy, or to the structure of the body.

anatomist (əˈnatəmist) one skilled in anatomy.

anatomy (əˈnatəmee) the science dealing with the form and structure of living organisms.

comparative a. description and comparison of the form and structure of different animals.

developmental a. structural embryology.

gross a., macroscopic a. that dealing with structures visible with the unaided eye.

microscopic a. histology.

morbid a., pathological a. anatomy of diseased tissues.

radiological a. x-ray anatomy.

special a. anatomy devoted to study of particular organs or parts.

topographic a. that devoted to determination of relative positions of various body parts.

x-ray a. study of organs and tissues based on their visualization by x-rays in both living and dead bodies.

anatriptic (ˌanəˈtriptik) a medicine applied by rubbing.

anatropia (ˌanəˈtrohpi·ə) upward deviation of the visual axis of one eye when the other eye is fixing. adj. **anatropic.**

anchorage (ˈangkəˌrij) fixation, e.g., surgical fixation of a displaced viscus or, in operative dentistry, fixation of fillings, or of artificial crowns or bridges. In orthodontics, the support used for a regulating apparatus.

anchylo- for words beginning thus, see those beginning *ankylo-*.

ancipital (anˈsipitˈl) two-edged.

Ancoloxin (ˌangkəˈloksin) trademark for preparations of meclozine, an antinauseant.

anconad (angˈkohnad) toward the elbow or olecranon.

anconal, anconeal (ˈangkohnˈl, angˈkohni·əl) pertaining to the elbow.

anconeus (angˈkohni·əs) an extensor muscle of the forearm.

ancrod (ˈankrod) a proteinase obtained from the venom of the Malayan pit viper *Agkistrodon rhodostoma*, acting specifically on fibrinogen; used as an anticoagulant in the treatment of retinal vein occlusion and deep vein thrombosis and to prevent postoperative rethrombosis.

ancylo- for words beginning thus, see also those beginning *ankylo-*.

Ancylostoma (ˌansiˈlostəmə) a genus of nematode parasites (HOOKWORMS).

A. americanum *Necator americanus*.

A. braziliense a species parasitic in dogs and cats in tropical and subtropical regions; its larvae may cause a creeping eruption in man.

A. caninum the common hookworm of dogs and cats.

a. duodenale a common hookworm of man, parasitic in the small intestine, which is widespread in the tropics and subtropics and also in temperate regions where sanitation is very poor.

ancylostomiasis (ˌansiˌlostəˈmieəsis) infection by worms of the genus *Ancylostoma* or by other hookworms (*Necator americanus*). See HOOKWORM.

Ancylostomidae (ˌansilosˈtohmidee) a family of nematode parasites having two ventrolateral cutting plates at the entrance to a large buccal capsule, and small teeth at its base; the hookworms.

Andersen's disease (ˈandəsənz) glycogenosis (type IV); see also AMYLOPECTINOSIS.

andr(o)- word element. [Gr.] *male, masculine.*

androblastoma (ˌandrohblaˈstohma) 1. a rare benign tumour of the testis histologically resembling the fetal testis. There are three varieties: diffuse stromal, mixed (stromal and epithelial), and tubular (epithelial). The epithelial elements contain Sertoli cells, which may produce oestrogen and thus cause feminization. 2. arrhenoblastoma.

androgen (ˈandrəˌjen) any steroid hormone that promotes male characteristics. The two main androgens are androsterone and testosterone. adj. **androgenic.**

The androgenic hormones are manufactured mainly by the testes under stimulation from the PITUITARY GLAND. To a lesser extent, androgens are produced by the adrenal glands in both sexes, as well as by the ovaries in women. Thus women normally have a small percentage of male hormones, in the same way that men's bodies contain some female sex hormones, the oestrogens.

The androgens are responsible for the growth of the penis and scrotum and for the secondary sexual characteristics, such as the beard and the deepening of the voice at puberty. They also stimulate the growth of muscle and bones throughout the body and thus account in part for the greater strength and size of men as compared to women.

Androgens stimulate erythropoiesis and have been used in the treatment of aplastic anaemia with moderate success.

android (ˈandroyd) resembling a man.

androphobia (ˌandrohˈfohbi·ə) morbid dread of the male sex.

androstane (ˈandrohˌstayn) the hydrocarbon nucleus, $C_{19}H_{32}$, from which androgens are derived.

androstanediol (ˌandrohˈstayndieol) an androgen, $C_{19}H_{32}O_2$, prepared by reducing androsterone.

androstanedione (ˌandrohˈstayndieohn) an androgen

formed in the testes.

androstene ('androh,steen) an unsaturated cyclic hydrocarbon, $C_{19}H_{30}$, forming the nucleus of testosterone and certain other androgens.

androstenediol (,androh'steendieol) a crystalline androgenic steroid, $C_{19}H_{30}O_2$.

androstenedione (,androh'steendieohn) an androgen, $C_{19}H_{26}O_2$, less potent than testosterone, secreted by the testis, ovary, and adrenal cortex.

androsterone (an'drostə,rohn, ,androh'stiə·rohn) an androgenic hormone, $C_{19}H_{30}O_2$, excreted in the urine of both men and women. When injected intramuscularly, it counteracts the effects of castration.

anectasis (ə'nektəsis) congenital atelectasis due to developmental immaturity.

anencephaly (,anən'kefəlee, -'sef-) congenital absence of the cranial vault, with the cerebral hemispheres completely missing or reduced to small masses. adj. **anencephalic, anencephalous.**

anephric (ay'nefrik) being without kidneys.

anergasia (,anə'gayzi·ə) generally, loss of function, psychosis due to organic lesions of the central nervous system.

anergy ('anəjee) diminished reactivity to specific antigen(s). adj. **anergic.**

anerythropsia (,aneri'thropsi·ə) inability to distinguish red colours.

anetoderma (,anetoh'dərmə) looseness and atrophy of the skin.

aneuploidy (,anyuh'ploydee) the state of having chromosomes in a number that is not an exact multiple of the haploid number. adj. **aneuploid.**

aneurine ('anyuh,reen) thiamine. An essential vitamin involved in carbohydrate metabolism. The main sources are unrefined cereals and pork. Vitamin B_1.

aneurysm ('anyə,rizəm) a sac formed by the dilation of the wall of an artery, vein, or the heart. adj. **aneurysmal.**

A *true* aneurysm results from dilation of the vascular wall. A *false* aneurysm develops in perivascular tissue following the rupture and slow leakage from a vessel (or a true aneurysm), its wall being formed of clot. Partial rupture of the wall of a large artery, commonly the aorta, may lead to a *dissecting* aneurysm, when the tissue planes of the vessel wall are stripped apart by blood being forced between them.

Although atherosclerosis is responsible for most arterial aneurysms, any injury to the arterial wall can predispose to the formation of a sac. Other diseases that can lead to an aneurysm include syphilis, cystic medionecrosis, certain nonspecific inflammations, and congenital defect in the artery.

It is possible to be unaware of a small aneurysm. About 80 per cent of all abdominal aneurysms are palpable and may be noticed on a routine physical examination. One should be particularly alert to the possibility of an aneurysm in persons with a history of cardiovascular disease, hypertension, or peripheral vascular disease.

Aneurysms tend to increase in size, presenting a problem of increasing pressure against adjacent tissues and organs and a danger of rupture. When an aneurysm ruptures a critical situation ensues. The patient with a ruptured aortic aneurysm exhibits severe pain and blood loss, leading to shock. A ruptured cerebral aneurysm produces neurological symptoms and can resemble the clinical picture of a STROKE.

Recent advances in surgical techniques have reduced the mortality rate for aneurysm repair. If an aneurysm occurs in a small blood vessel, the vessel can be tied off, relying on collateral flow in other vessels. There is also a more complex and serious operation which involves removing the segment of widened blood vessel and replacing it with a plastic graft or an artery or vein from a vascular bank.

arteriovenous a. an abnormal communication between an artery and a vein in which the blood flows directly into a neighbouring vein or is carried into the vein by a connecting sac.

atherosclerotic a. one arising as a result of weakening of the arterial wall due to atherosclerosis.

berry a. a small saccular aneurysm of a cerebral artery, usually at the junction of vessels in the circle of Willis.

cardiac a. thinning and dilation of a portion of the wall of the left ventricle, usually a consequence of myocardial infarction.

cirsoid a. a developmental abnormality, usually involving arterioles and capillaries, in which the vessels enlarge, extend and infold to form a sinuous vascular mass.

compound a. one in which some of the layers of the wall of the vessel are ruptured and some merely dilated; called also *mixed aneurysm.*

dissecting a. one resulting from haemorrhage that causes lengthwise splitting of the arterial wall, producing a tear in the inner wall (intima) and establishing communication with the lumen of the vessel; it usually affects the aorta.

Dissecting aortic aneurysms involve the ascending and descending aorta. Acute aortic dissection is fatal within one month of onset in approximately 83 per cent of the cases. Surgical treatment may be delayed in aneurysms involving the descending aorta until the blood pressure has been controlled and oedema and friability of the aorta are diminished. The usual course of treatment for an aneurysm of the ascending aorta is immediate surgery. The surgical procedure for either type is aimed at either repairing the intimal tear or removing the affected portion of the aorta. This may be done by suturing the separated aortic layers back together or by removing the damaged section of the aorta and replacing it with a synthetic graft.

fusiform a. a spindle-shaped aneurysm. **infected a.** one produced by growth of microorganisms (bacteria or fungi) in the vessel wall, or infection arising within a preexisting arteriosclerotic aneurysm.

mixed a. compound aneurysm.

mycotic a. an infected aneurysm caused by an infected embolus.

racemose a. cirsoid aneurysm.

sacculated a. a saclike aneurysm connected to the side of the main vessel by a narrow mouth.

varicose a. an aneurysm lying between an artery and its adjacent vein, forming a sac between the two.

aneurysmectomy (,anyə·riz'mektəmee) excision of an aneurysm.

aneurysmoplasty (,anyə'rizmə,plastee) plastic repair of an aneurysm from within the sac. See also ENDOANEURYSMORRHAPHY.

aneurysmorrhaphy (,anyə·riz'mo·rəfee) repair of an aneurysm by obliteration, reconstruction or removal.

anfractuous (an'frakchooəs) convoluted; sinuous.

angi(o)- word element. [Gr.] *vessel (channel).*

angiectasis (,anji'ektəsis) dilation of a vessel. adj. **angiectatic.**

angiectomy (,anji'ektəmee) excision of part of a blood or lymph vessel.

angiitis (,anji'ietis) inflammation of the coats of a vessel, chiefly blood or lymph vessels.

angina (an'jienə, 'anjienə) a sense of restrictive discomfort which can amount to severe pain, usually of ischaemic origin, brought on by effort and eased by rest. (See also intermittent CLAUDICATION). adj. **anginal.**

agranulocytic a. agranulocytosis.
intestinal a. generalized cramping abdominal pain occurring shortly after a meal and persisting for one to three hours.
a. ludovici, Ludwig's a., a. ludwigi cellulitis affecting neck and throat, causing obstruction of the airway.
a. parotidea mumps.
a. pectoris acute pain in the chest resulting from decreased blood supply to the heart muscle. The attacks occur during periods of physical activity, raised blood pressure or emotional stress.

Angina pectoris occurs more frequently in men than in women. It is not a disease entity but a symptom of underlying disease involving the arteries to the heart muscle. About 90 per cent of all cases can be attributed to coronary ATHEROSCLEROSIS. At least one of the three major coronary arteries is usually stenosed before angina develops; in most cases, all of the major coronary arteries are involved.

Angina pectoris also can result from stenosis of the aorta, pulmonary stenosis and ventricular hypertrophy, or connective tissue disorders such as systemic lupus erythematosus and periarteritis nodosa that affect the smaller coronary arteries.

SYMPTOMS. The chief symptom of angina pectoris is chest pain, usually of an unmistakable nature and readily distinguished by the patient as different from other types of pain. It is generally described as a feeling of tightness, strangling, heaviness, or suffocation. The pain is usually concentrated on the left side, beginning just under the sternum and radiating to the neck, throat and lower jaw, down the left arm and, more rarely, to the stomach, back or across to the right side of the chest. It seldom lasts more than 15 minutes and is usually relieved by rest and relaxation or by sublingual administration of nitrates. If the pain is not relieved in 10 to 15 minutes, the doctor should be notified and the patient ideally taken to a coronary care unit. The decreased blood supply to the heart makes it especially vulnerable to arrhythmias and MYOCARDIAL INFARCTION, which can be fatal. About one-half of all those who suffer from angina pectoris die suddenly, while about one-third succumb to a myocardial infarction.

Coronary arteriography and ventriculography are valuable in determining the prognosis for angina pectoris. The mortality rate for patients having a narrowing of all three main coronary arteries is higher than for those who have only one vessel involved. Severity of pain is not a good prognostic indicator; some patients with severe discomfort live for many years, while others with mild symptoms die suddenly. An enlarged heart, a third heart sound, ECG abnormalities at rest, and hypertension are all indicative of a poor prognosis.

TREATMENT AND PATIENT CARE. Relief from pain by rest and prevention of attacks by avoiding situations which precipitate them are the first steps in treatment. In most cases the patients are eager to learn about the process causing the pain and need to know how they can control their attacks. Compliance with the prescribed regimen usually requires a change in life style and the breaking of some lifelong habits. The known risk factors for coronary heart disease (see HEART) should be explained to the patient, and a regimen designed to avoid further damage to the arteries prescribed.

Organic nitrates may be administered orally or sublingually for relief from anginal pain. They act by dilating the arteries and may be used to treat acute attacks, for long-term prophylaxis and management, or for prophylaxis in situations likely to provoke an attack. Commonly used nitrates are isosorbide dinitrate and glyceryl trinitrate.

Beta-adrenergic receptor blockers, such as propranolol are used to treat patients who do not respond to weight control and treatment with vasodilators and whose angina significantly limits their activities. These agents decrease the heart rate, blood pressure, and myocardial oxygen consumption and increase the patient's exercise tolerance.

A group of drugs called CALCIUM CHANNEL BLOCKERS are particularly beneficial in relieving pain in those patients whose angina is the result of coronary artery spasm or constriction. These drugs act by selectively inhibiting the transport of calcium across the cell membrane of myocardial cells and also by reducing myocardial oxygen utilization. Patients most likely to obtain dramatic relief from drugs of this kind are those who experience chest pain while resting or sleeping, upon exposure to cold, or during emotional stress. Calcium channel blockers include drugs such as nifedipine, verapamil, and dilitiazem.

Surgical procedures to bypass the diseased portion of the coronary artery by suturing a vein graft from the aorta to one or more coronary arteries beyond the area of obstruction are now common practice. In most instances the graft is obtained from the patient's saphenous vein.

An attitude of calmness and efficiency is most important when caring for a person suffering from an attack of angina pectoris. His pain produces emotional reactions and the strongest of these is fear. Most of these patients know that their pain is resulting from an insufficient supply of oxygen to the heart and they frequently have a feeling of impending death. Much anxiety and pain can be eliminated if the patient is assured that someone will stay with him and is reminded that the pain will eventually subside. It usually helps to raise the patient to a sitting position so that he may breathe without difficulty. The prompt administration of glyceryl trinitrate or the specific drug ordered by the doctor usually shortens the attack and relieves pain. Above all, the calm presence of someone who knows how to care for him can do much to reassure the patient and help him relax, thus lessening the severity of the attack.

Prinzmetal's a. a variant of angina pectoris in which the attacks occur during rest, exercise capacity is well preserved, and attacks are associated electrocardiographically with elevation of the ST-segment.
variant a. Prinzmetal's angina.
Vincent's a. acute ulcerative gingivostomatitis associated with poor oral hygiene and malnutrition. Spirochaetes and fusiform bacilli predominate in the ulcers. Treatment is with metronidazole or penicillin. Called also *necrotizing ulcerative gingivostomatitis*.

anginoid ('anji,noyd) resembling angina.

anginophobia (,anjienə'fohbi·ə) morbid dread of angina pectoris.

anginose ('anji,nohz) characterized by angina.

angioblast ('anjioh,blast) 1. the earliest formative tissue from which blood vessels arise. 2. an individual vessel-forming cell. adj. **angioblastic.**

angioblastoma (,anjiohbla'stohmə) a term applied to certain blood-vessel tumours of the brain: those arising in the cerebellum (cerebellar angioblastomas) may be cystic and associated with von Hippel–Lindau disease; also, a blood-vessel tumour arising from the meninges of the brain or spinal cord (angioblastic meningioma).

angiocardiogram (,anjioh'kahdioh,gram) the film produced by angiocardiography.

angiocardiography (,anjioh,kahdi'ogrəfee) radiography of the heart and great vessels after introduction of an opaque contrast medium into a blood vessel or one of the cardiac chambers.

angiocardiokinetic (ˌanjiohˌkardiohki'netik) pertaining to movements of the heart and blood vessels.

angiocardiopathy (ˌanjiohˌkahdi'opəthee) disease of the heart and blood vessels.

angiocarditis (ˌanjiohkah'dietis) inflammation of the heart and blood vessels.

angiodysplasia (ˌanjiohdis'playzi·ə) small vascular abnormalities, especially of the intestinal tract.

angioectasis (ˌanjioh'ektəsis) abnormal enlargement of capillaries.

angiofibroma (ˌanjiohfie'brohmə) angioma containing fibrous tissue.

nasopharyngeal a. a relatively benign tumour of the nasopharynx composed of fibrous connective tissue with abundant endothelium-lined vascular spaces, usually occurring during puberty, most commonly in boys. It is marked by nasal obstruction which may become total, adenoid speech, discomfort in swallowing, and auditory tube obstruction.

angiofollicular (ˌanjiohfo'likyuhlə) pertaining to a lymphoid follicle and its blood vessels.

angiogenesis (ˌanjioh'jenəsis) the development of blood vessels in the embryo.

tumour a. the induction of the growth of blood vessels from surrounding tissue into a solid tumour by a diffusible chemical factor released by the tumour cells.

angioglioma (ˌanjiohglie'ohmə) a form of vascular glioma.

angiogram ('anjiohˌgram) a radiograph of a blood vessel.

angiography (ˌanji'ogrəfee) radiography of vessels of the body (arteriography, lymphangiography, or phlebography), after introduction into them of a suitable contrast medium.

angiohyalinosis (ˌanjiohˌhieəli'nohsis) hyaline degeneration of the muscular coat of blood vessels.

angioid ('anjioyd) resembling blood vessels.

angiokeratoma (ˌanjiohˌkerə'tohmə) a dermatosis marked by telangiectasia with secondary epithelial changes, including acanthosis and hyperkeratosis. **a. corporis diffusum** an inborn error of glycolipid metabolism characterized by purpuric skin lesions (angiokeratomas). See also FABRY'S DISEASE.

angiokinetic (ˌanjiohki'netik) vasomotor.

angioleiomyoma (ˌanjiohˌlieohmie'ohmə) a small tumour, most common in subcutaneous tissues, of blood vessels and smooth muscle.

angiolipoma (ˌanjiohli'pohmə) angioma containing fatty tissue.

angiolith ('anjiohˌlith) a calcareous deposit in the wall of a blood vessel. adj. **angiolithic**.

angiology (ˌanji'oləjee) scientific study or description of the blood and lymph vessels.

angiolupoid (ˌanjioh'loopoyd) a tuberculous skin lesion consisting of small, oval red plaques, chiefly on the side of the nose.

angiolysis (ˌanji'olisis) retrogression or obliteration of blood vessels, as in embryological development.

angioma (ˌanji'ohmə) a benign tumour made up of blood (haemangioma) or lymph vessels (lymphangioma). adj. **angiomatous**.

a. cavernosum, cavernous a. cavernous HAEMANGIOMA.

a. serpiginosum a skin disease marked by minute vascular points arranged in rings on the skin.

telangiectatic a. an angioma made up of dilated blood vessels.

angiomatosis (ˌanjiohmə'tohsis) the presence of multiple angiomas.

a. of retina a condition in which focal areas of dilated retinal blood vessels (i.e. angiomas) occur. May be associated with angiomas in the central nervous system (von Hippel's disease).

angiomegaly (ˌanjioh'megəlee) enlargement of blood vessels: especially a condition of the eyelid marked by great increase in its volume.

angiomyolipoma (ˌanjiohˌmieohli'pohmə) a benign tumour containing vascular, adipose, and smooth muscle elements, occurring most often in the kidney.

angiomyoneuroma (ˌanjiohˌmieohnyuh'rohmə) glomangioma.

angiomyosarcoma (ˌanjiohˌmieohsah'kohmə) angioma blended with myoma and sarcoma.

angioneurectomy (ˌanjiohnyuh'rektəmee) excision of vessels and nerves.

angioneurosis (ˌanjiohnyuh'rohsis) any neurosis affecting primarily the blood vessels; a disorder of the vasomotor system, as angioparalysis or angiospasm.

angioneurotic (ˌanjiohnyuh'rotik) caused by or of the nature of an angioneurosis.

a. oedema a condition characterized by the sudden and temporary appearance of large areas of painless swelling in the subcutaneous tissue or submucosa, usually around the face. It occurs in two types, sporadic and hereditary. The sporadic type, related to giant urticaria, is usually due to a food allergy but may also be caused by other allergens or by emotional factors. The hereditary type, transmitted as an autosomal dominant trait, is due to a deficiency of C'1 esterase inhibitor, a protein which also inhibits kallikrein and plasmin. The deficiency causes an increase in the levels of several vasoactive mediators of anaphylaxis. Respiratory and gastrointestinal symptoms can also occur in this type. Called also angiooedema and Quincke's disease.

angiooedema (ˌanjioh·i'deemə) angioneurotic oedema.

angioparalysis (ˌanjiohpə'ralisis) vasomotor paralysis of blood vessels.

angiopathy (ˌanji'opəthee) any disease of the vessels.

angioplasty ('anjiohˌplastee) plastic repair of blood vessels or lymphatic channels.

percutaneous transluminal a. (PCTA) dilation of a blood vessel by means of a balloon catheter inserted through the skin and into the chosen vessel and then passed through the lumen of the vessel to the site of the lesion, where the balloon is inflated to flatten plaque against the artery wall.

angiopoiesis (ˌanjiohpoy'eesis) the formation of blood vessels. adj. **angiopoietic**.

angiorrhaphy (ˌanji'o·rəfee) suture of a blood vessel.

angiosarcoma (ˌanjiohsah'kohmə) a malignant tumour of vascular tissue; called also *haemangiosarcoma*.

angiosclerosis (ˌanjiohsklə'rohsis) hardening of the walls of blood vessels.

angioscotoma (ˌanjiohskoh'tohmə) a defect in the visual field caused by the shadow of the retinal blood vessels.

angiospasm ('anjiohˌspazəm) spasmodic contraction of the walls of a blood vessel. adj. **angiospastic**.

angiostrongyliasis (ˌanjiohˌstronji'lieəsis) infection by nematodes of the genus *Angiostrongylus*.

Angiostrongylus (ˌanjioh'stronjiləs) a genus of nematode parasites.

A. cantonensis the rat lung worm, a species reported in cases of human meningoencephalitis in Hawaii and in other areas in the Pacific and in Asia. Human beings become infected through eating raw or undercooked slugs or snails, which are the intermediate hosts.

angiotelectasis (ˌanjiohtə'lektəsis) dilation of blood vessels.

angiotensin (ˌanjioh'tensin) a vasoconstrictive principle formed in the blood when RENIN is released from the juxtaglomerular apparatus in the kidney. The enzymatic action of renin cleaves a serum alpha$_2$-globulin, angiotensinogen, forming the decapeptide angiotensin I, which is relatively inactive. It in turn is acted upon by peptidases (converting enzymes), chiefly in the lungs, to form the octapeptide angiotensin II, a powerful vasopressor and a stimulator of aldosterone secretion by the adrenal cortex. By its vasopressor action, it raises blood pressure and diminishes fluid loss in the kidney by restricting blood flow. Angiotensin II is hydrolysed in various tissues to form heptapeptide angiotensin III, which has less vasopressor activity but more effect on the adrenal cortex.

a. amide an amide derivative of angiotensin II which is a powerful vasoconstrictor and vasopressor, and is used in the treatment of certain hypotensive states; usually administered by slow intravenous infusion, and sometimes intramuscularly or subcutaneously.

a.-converting enzyme inhibitors see ACE INHIBITORS.

angiotensinase (ˌanjioh'tensinayz) any of a group of peptidases in plasma and tissues that inactivate angiotensin.

angiotensinogen (ˌanjiohten'sinəjən) a serum α_2-globulin secreted in the liver which, on hydrolysis by renin, gives rise to angiotensin.

angiotomy (ˌanji'otəmee) incision of a blood vessel or lymphatic channel.

angiotonic (ˌanjioh'tonik) increasing vascular tension.

angiotribe ('anjiohˌtrieb) a strong forceps for crushing tissue containing an artery, for the purpose of checking haemorrhage.

angiotripsy (ˌanjioh'tripsee) haemostasis by means of an angiotribe.

angiotrophic (ˌanjioh'trofik) pertaining to the nutrition of vessels.

angle ('ang·g'l) the space or figure formed by two diverging lines, measured as the number of degrees one would have to be moved to coincide with the other.

acromial a. that between the head of the humerus and the clavicle.

alpha a. that formed by intersection of the visual axis with the optic axis.

cardiodiaphragmatic a. that formed by the junction of the shadows of the heart and diaphragm in posteroanterior x-rays of the heart.

costovertebral a. the angle formed on either side of the vertebral column between the last rib and the lumbar vertebrae.

filtration a., a. of the iris the angle between the iris and cornea at the periphery of the anterior chamber of the eye, through which the aqueous humour readily permeates.

a. of jaw the junction of the lower edge with the posterior edge of the lower jaw. **metre a.** the angle formed by intersection of the visual axis and the perpendicular bisector of the line joining the centres of rotation of the two eyes when viewing a point one metre distant (small metre angle) or the angle formed by intersection of the visual axes of the two eyes in the midline at a distance of one metre (large metre angle).

optic a. visual angle.

a. of pubis that between the pubic bones at the symphysis.

sternoclavicular a. that between the sternum and the clavicle.

visual a. the angle between two lines passing from the extremities of an object seen, through the nodal point of the eye, to the corresponding extremities of the image of the object seen.

Angle's classification ('ang·g'lz) a classification of dental malocclusion based on mesiodistal (anteroposterior) position of the mandibular dental arch and teeth relative to the maxillary dental arch and teeth.

ångström ('angstrom) a non-SI unit of length equal to 10^{-10} metre or 0.1 nanometre; symbol Å.

angulation (ˌang·gyuh'layshən) the formation of a sharp obstructive angle as in the intestine, the ureter, or similar tubes.

angulus ('ang·gyuhləs) pl. *anguli* [L.] angle; used in names of anatomical structures or landmarks.

anhedonia (ˌanhi'dohni·ə) inability to experience pleasure, or a general lack of interest in living. May occur in depression or schizophrenia.

anhidrosis (ˌanhi'drohsis) absence of sweating.

anhidrotic (ˌanhi'drotik) 1. checking the flow of sweat. 2. an agent that suppresses perspiration.

anhydraemia (ˌanhie'dreemi·ə) diminution of the fluid content of the blood.

anhydrase (an'hiedrayz) an enzyme that catalyses the removal of water from a compound.

carbonic a. an enzyme that catalyses the decomposition of carbonic acid into carbon dioxide and water, facilitating transfer of carbon dioxide from tissues to blood and from blood to alveolar air.

anhydration (ˌanhie'drayshən) the condition of not being hydrated.

anhydride (an'hiedried) a compound derived from an acid by removal of a molecule of water.

anhydrous (an'hiedrəs) containing no water.

anideus (ə'nidi·əs) a parasitic fetus consisting of a shapeless mass of flesh.

anidrosis (ˌani'drohsis) anhidrosis.

aniline ('aniˌleen, -lin) an oily liquid from coal tar and indigo or prepared by reducing nitrobenzene; the parent substance of colours or dyes derived from coal tar. It is an important cause of serious industrial poisoning associated with bone marrow depression as well as methaemoglobinaemia.

anilism ('aniˌlizəm) aniline poisoning.

anility (ə'nilitee) the state of being like an old woman.

anima ('animə) 1. the soul. 2. Jung's term for the unconscious, or inner being, of the individual, as opposed to the personality he presents to the world (persona). In jungian psychoanalysis, the more feminine soul or feminine component of a man's personality (see also ANIMUS).

animal ('animəl) 1. a living organism having sensation and the power of voluntary movement and requiring for its existence oxygen and organic food. 2. of or pertaining to such an organism.

a. bite a wound caused by the bite of an animal (see also BITE).

control a. an untreated animal otherwise identical in all respects to one that is used for purposes of experiment; used for checking results of treatment.

animation (ˌani'mayshən) the quality of being full of life.

suspended a. temporary suspension or cessation of the vital functions.

animus ('animəs) in jungian psychoanalysis, the more male soul or masculine component of a woman's personality (see also ANIMA).

anion ('anˌieən) an ion carrying a negative charge. In an electrolytic cell anions are attracted to the positive electrode (anode).

anion-exchange resin (ˌanieənˌiks'chaynj) ion-exchange resin.

aniridia (ˌani'ridi·ə) congenital absence of the iris.

anis(o)- word element. [Gr.] *unequal.*

anisakiasis (ˌanisə'kieəsis) infection with the third-stage larvae of the roundworm *Anisakis marina*, which burrow into the stomach wall, producing an eosinophilic granulomatous mass. Abdominal pain and vomiting result. Infection is acquired by eating undercooked marine fish.

Anisakis (ˌani'saykis) a genus of nematodes that parasitize the stomachs of marine mammals and birds.

aniseikonia (ˌanisie'kohni·ə) inequality of the size of the retinal images of the two eyes.

anisochromatic (anˌiesohkroh'matik) not of the same colour.

anisocoria (anˌiesoh'kor·ri·ə) inequality in size of the pupils of the eyes.

anisocytosis (anˌiesohsie'tohsis) the presence in the blood of erythrocytes showing abnormal variations in size.

anisokaryosis (anˌiesohkari'ohsis) inequality in the size of the nuclei of cells.

anisomastia (anˌiesoh'masti·ə) inequality in size of the breasts.

anisomelia (anˌiesoh'meeli·ə) a congenital condition in which one of a pair of limbs is longer than the other.

anisometropia (anˌiesohme'trohpi·ə) a considerable degree of inequality in the refractive power of the two eyes. adj. **anisometropic**.

anisopiesis (anˌiesohpie'eesis) difference in blood pressure recorded in corresponding arteries on the right and left sides of the body.

anisosthenic (anˌiesos'thenik) not having equal power; said of muscles.

anisotonic (anˌiesoh'tonik) 1. varying in tonicity or tension. 2. having different osmotic pressure; not isotonic.

anisotropic (anˌiesoh'tropik) 1. having unlike properties in different directions. 2. doubly refracting, or having a double polarizing power.

anisotropy (ˌanie'sotrəpee) the quality of being anisotropic.

anisuria (ˌanie'syooə·ri·ə) alternating oliguria and polyuria.

ankle ('angk'l) the part of the leg just above the foot; the joint between the leg and the foot. The ankle joint is a hinge joint and is formed by the junction of the tibia and fibula with the talus, or ankle bone. The bones are cushioned by cartilage and connected by a number of ligaments, tendons, and muscles that strengthen the joint and enable it to be moved.

Because it is in almost constant use, the ankle is particularly susceptible to injuries, such as SPRAIN and FRACTURE. It is also often one of the first joints to be affected by ARTHRITIS or GOUT.

Oedema or swelling of the tissues around the ankles is a fairly common occurrence in overweight people and pregnant women and is usually relieved by elevating the feet. It may, however, be a symptom of serious heart or renal disease.

a. jerk plantar extension of the foot elicited by a tap on the Achilles tendon, preferably while the patient kneels on a bed or chair, the feet hanging free over the edge; called also Achilles reflex and triceps surae reflex..

ankyl(o)- word element. [Gr.] *bent, crooked, in the form of a loop, adhesion.*

ankyloblepharon (ˌangkiloh'blefə·ron) adhesion of the eyelids to each other.

ankylocheilia (ˌangkiloh'kieli·ə) adhesion of the lips to each other.

ankyloglossia (ˌangkiloh'glosi·ə) tongue-tie; abnormal shortness of the frenulum of the tongue, resulting in limitation of its motion.

a. superior extensive adhesion of the tongue to the palate.

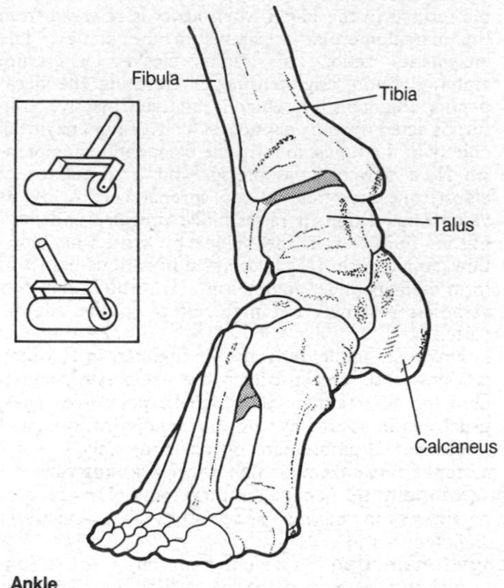

Ankle

ankylopoietic (ˌangkilohpoy'etik) producing ankylosis.

ankylosed ('angkiˌlohzd) affected with ankylosis.

ankylosing spondylitis ('angkiˌlohzing ˌspondi'lietis) a chronic inflammatory disease affecting sacroiliac joints (sacroiliitis) and spine (spondylitis) in particular but which may also cause a peripheral arthritis that is often asymmetrical and of medium or large joints. Associated features include iritis, apical lung fibrosis and rarely aortic incompetence. Disease onset is typically in young men and the disorder tends to be milder in women.

A characteristic pathological feature is invasion of bone–ligament entheses in both spine and peripheral regions by a chronic granulation tissue. In severe forms of the disease there is complete fusion of the sacroiliac joints and ossification of longitudinal ligaments in the spine, with production of a rigid 'bamboo spine'. Milder forms of spondylitis are more frequent and there is clinical overlap between ankylosing spondylitis and other forms of 'seronegative' arthritis (i.e. arthritis in which serological tests are persistently negative for rheumatoid factor), including psoriatic arthritis, Reiter's syndrome and the enteropathic arthritides found with Crohn's disease and ulcerative colitis.

The pathogenesis of ankylosing spondylitis remains undefined, but both genetic and environmental components are important.

The basis of management of the spondylitis and sacroiliitis is to maintain maximum spinal mobility with non-steroidal antiinflammatory drugs and an active exercise programme. The main principles of treatment of the peripheral joint disease are similar to those used in the management of rheumatoid arthritis except that gold and D-penicillamine tend to be less useful.

ankylosis (ˌangki'lohsis) immobility and consolidation of a joint. adj. **ankylotic**. Ankylosis may be caused by destruction of the membranes that line the joint or by faulty bone structure. It is most often a result of chronic rheumatoid arthritis, in which the affected joint tends to assume the least painful position and may become more or less permanently fixed in it.

Artificial ankylosis (arthrodesis), locking of a joint by surgical operation, is sometimes done in treatment of a severe joint condition.

bony a. union of the bones of a joint by proliferation of bone cells, resulting in complete immobility.

extracapsular a. that caused by rigidity of surrounding parts.

false a., fibrous a. reduced joint mobility due to proliferation of fibrous tissue.

intracapsular a. that caused by rigidity of structures within the joint.

spurious a. extracapsular ankylosis.

stapedial a. fixation of the footplate of the stapes in otosclerosis, causing a conductive hearing loss.

true a. bony ankylosis.

ankylotia (ˌangki'lohshi·ə) closure of the external meatus of the ear.

ankyroid ('angkiˌroyd) hooklike.

anlage ('anˌlahgə) pl. *anlagen* [Ger.] primordium.

anneal (ə'neel) to soften a material, such as a metal, by controlled heating and cooling, to make its manipulation easier.

annectent (ə'nektənt) connecting; joining together.

Annelida (ə'nelidə) a phylum of metazoan invertebrates, the segmented worms, including leeches.

annular ('anyuhlə) ring-shaped.

annuloplasty ('anyuhlohˌplastee) plastic repair of a cardiac valve.

annulorrhaphy (ˌanyuh'lo·rəfee) suture of a hernial ring or sac.

annulus ('anyuhləs) pl. *annuli* [L.] a small ring or encircling structure; also spelled anulus.

anococcygeal (ˌaynohkok'siji·əl) pertaining to the anus and coccyx.

anode ('anohd) the positive electrode or pole to which negative ions are attracted. adj. **anodal.**

anodontia (ˌanoh'donshi·ə) congenital absence of some or all of the teeth.

anodyne ('anəˌdien) 1. relieving pain. 2. a medicine that eases pain.

anodynia (ˌanə'dini·ə) freedom from pain.

anomalad (ə'nohməlad) a term proposed to designate a single, localized anomaly occurring during morphogenesis, together with the pattern of subsequent morphological defects that stem from it.

anomalopia (əˌnomə'lohpi·ə) a slight anomaly of colour vision.

anomaloscope (ə'noməlәˌskohp) an apparatus used to detect anomalies of colour vision.

anomaly (ə'noməlee) marked deviation from normal. adj. **anomalous.**

developmental a. absence, deformity, or excess of body parts as the result of faulty development of the embryo.

anomer ('anəmə, 'anohˌmər) one of two stereoisomers (designated α or β) of the furanose or pyranose form of a sugar, e.g., α-D-glucose. adj. **anomeric.**

anomia (ay'nohmi·ə) loss of power of naming objects or of recognizing names.

anomie, anomy ('anohmee) [Gr.] *without law,* used to describe states of disorganization, insecurity and loss of structure, whether affecting the equilibrium of a society, group or individual. Anomie may arise following catastrophes like war, famine or earthquake and may also be engendered when large numbers of persons undergo a period of abrupt social transition rendering previous values and norms irrelevant (e.g. immigrants and migrants from rural to urban settings). The feelings of alienation arising from the dissolution or loss of supportive social forces have been identified as a major cause of suicide.

anonychia (ˌanə'niki·ə) absence of the nails.

Anopheles (ə'nofiˌleez) a widely distributed genus of mosquitoes, comprising over 300 species, many of which are important vectors of MALARIA.

anophthalmia, anophthalmos (ˌanof'thalmi·ə; ˌanof'thalməs) a developmental anomaly marked by complete absence of one or both eyes or the presence of rudimentary eyes.

anoplasty ('aynohˌplastee) plastic repair of the anus.

anopsia (a'nopsi·ə) 1. nonuse or suppression of vision in one eye. 2. hypertropia.

anorchid (an'awkid) a person with no testes or with cryptorchidism (undescended testes).

anorchidism, anorchism (an'awkidizəm; an'awkizəm) congenital absence of one or both testes.

anorectic (ˌanə'rektik) 1. pertaining to anorexia. 2. an agent that diminishes the appetite for food. Most of the drugs used for this purpose are central nervous system stimulants (the amphetamines and similar sympathomimetic amines). Use of these drugs can lead to a short-term weight loss. However, the loss is rarely more than 10 per cent. These drugs have no role in a lifelong weight-control programme. Moreover, they are frequently abused and can lead to tolerance and psychological dependence.

anorectum (ˌaynoh'rektəm) the distal portion of the digestive tract, including the entire anal canal and the distal 2 cm. of the rectum. adj. **anorectal.**

anorexia (ˌanə'reksi·ə) lack or loss of appetite for food. Appetite is psychological, dependent on memory and associations, as compared with hunger, which is physiologically aroused by the body's need for food. Anorexia can be brought about by unattractive food, surroundings, or company.

a. nervosa loss of appetite due to emotional states, such as anxiety, irritation, anger, and fear. In true anorexia nervosa there is no real loss of appetite, but rather a refusal to eat or an aberration in eating patterns; hence, the term anorexia is probably a misnomer. The condition should be differentiated from restricted food intake such as that occurring in various psychiatric disorders.

The syndrome was first described more than 300 years ago and was once thought to be exceedingly rare. It is rapidly increasing throughout the world in developed countries as diverse as Russia, Japan, Australia, and the United States. The condition occurs mainly in girls after the age of puberty, and the prevalence may be as high as one in a hundred.

CAUSE. The cause of anorexia nervosa is unknown, but it is generally thought to be a disorder of psychological origins. These patients often have symptoms of depression and a faulty perception of body image; that is, they tend to overestimate the size of their own bodies, seeing themselves as wider and fatter than they really are. Starvation is self-imposed to reduce body size, and although the patient is skeleton-like in appearance, she vigorously defends her condition as not too thin.

There is some inconclusive evidence that anorexia nervosa may be a hypothalamic disorder owing to the fact that during the course of the disease gonadotrophins are not released from the anterior pituitary, there is a drop in the ovarian production of oestrogens, and ovulation fails to occur. These conditions often persist long after the nutritional status has been improved. In some cases menstruation ceases *before* the weight loss occurs. These factors indicate that the endocrine disturbance is not simply a sequel to malnutrition. In males there is a corresponding endocrine disorder with a drop in the level of gonadotropins and testosterone in the blood.

SYMPTOMS. Manifestations of anorexia nervosa, other than those previously mentioned, include signs of psychological maladjustment. There may be a history of difficulty in making friends, fear of meeting strangers, and changes in temperament consisting of irritability and depression.

The refusal to eat leads to malnutrition that may last for months or years. The diet often is limited to small amounts of fruits and vegetables and on some days only black coffee is taken. On occasion the fasting period may be alternated with eating sprees, usually at night, after which the patient forces herself to vomit.

Most patients resist their parents' suggestions that they see a doctor, insisting that they are not ill, in spite of progressive malnutrition and emaciation.

TREATMENT. The treatment of anorexia nervosa is difficult and lengthy. The primary goals are restitution of normal nutrition and resolution of the underlying psychological problems. Antidepressant drugs are helpful in some cases. Hospital admission may be necessary to avoid serious complications from malnutrition and electrolyte imbalance, but it should not be compulsory except as a last resort because, ultimately, success of treatment depends on the patient's cooperation.

Weight gain alone cannot be considered a sign of true progress. Relapses requiring readmission to the hospital occur in about half the cases. Psychotherapy utilizing techniques of behaviour modification is employed to correct the emotional problems underlying the condition. Family counselling and therapy are sometimes helpful in resolving familial conflicts that may have contributed to the development of the disorder.

anorexia–cachexia (ˌanə'reksi·əkə'keksi·ə) a systemic response to cancer occurring as a result of a poorly understood relationship between anorexia and cachexia, manifested by malnutrition, weight loss, muscular weakness, acidosis, and toxaemia. The basis of the anorexia may be a multifactorial severe metabolic disturbance that contributes to the development of cachectic wasting, which in turn reinforces the anorexia by the release from the tumour of an anorexigenic humoural product that stimulates the satiety centre in the hypothalamus, producing appetite loss.

anorexic (ˌanə'reksik) anorectic.

anorexigenic (ˌanəˌreksi'jenik) 1. producing anorexia. 2. an agent that diminishes or controls the appetite.

anorthography (ˌanaw'thogrəfee) loss of the ability to write.

anorthopia (ˌanaw'thohpi·ə) asymmetrical or distorted vision.

anorthosis (ˌanaw'thohsis) absence of penile erectility.

anoscope ('aynəˌskohp) a speculum or endoscope used in direct visual examination of the anal canal.

anoscopy (ay'noskəpee) examination of the anal canal with an anoscope.

anosigmoidoscopy (ˌaynohˌsigmoy'doskəpee) endoscopic examination of the anus and sigmoid.

anosmia (an'ozmi·ə) absence of the sense of smell. adj. **anosmatic, anosmic.**

anosognosia (əˌnohsog'nohzi·ə) failure to recognize one's own disease or defect.

anospinal (ˌaynoh'spien'l) pertaining to the anus and spinal cord.

anostosis (ˌano'stohsis) defective formation of bone.

anotia (an'ohshi·ə) congenital absence of the external ears.

anovaginal (ˌaynohvə'jien'l) pertaining to or communicating with the anus and vagina.

anovarism (an'ohvə·rizəm) absence of the ovaries.

anovesical (ˌaynoh'vesik'l) pertaining to the anus and bladder.

anovular, anovulatory (an'ohvyuhlə; anˌovyuh'laytə·ree, -tree) not associated with ovulation.

anoxaemia (ˌanok'seemi·ə) lack of sufficient oxygen in the blood. adj. **anoxaemic.**

anoxia (an'oksi·ə) absence of oxygen in the tissues; often used interchangeably with *hypoxia* to mean a reduction of oxygen in body tissues below physiological levels. The condition is accompanied by deep respirations, cyanosis, increased pulse rate, and impairment of coordination. adj. **anoxic.**

anaemic a. reduction of oxygen in body tissues because of diminished oxygen-carrying capacity of the blood.

anoxic a. reduction of oxygen in body tissues due to interference with the oxygen supply.

histotoxic a. condition resulting from diminished ability of cells to utilize available oxygen.

stagnant a. condition due to interference with the flow of blood and its transport of oxygen.

ansa ('ansə) pl. *ansae* [L.] a looplike structure.

a. cervicalis a nerve loop in the neck attached in front and above to the hypoglossal nerve and behind to the upper cervical spinal nerves. Its hypoglossal attachment is misleading since this part of the loop ultimately rejoins the upper spinal nerves.

a. of Henle Henle's loop or loop of Henle.

a. hypoglossi ansa cervicalis.

a. lenticularis a small nerve fibre tract arising in the globus pallidus and joining the anterior part of the ventral thalamic nucleus.

ansae nervorum spinalium loops of spinal nerves joining the anterior spinal nerves.

a. peduncularis a complex grouping of nerve fibres connecting the amygdaloid nucleus, piriform area, and anterior hypothalamus, and various thalamic nuclei.

Antabuse ('antəˌbyooz) trademark for a preparation of disulfiram, used in the treatment of alcoholism.

antacid (ant'asid) 1. counteracting acidity. 2. an agent that counteracts acidity. Substances that act as antacids include sodium bicarbonate, aluminium hydroxide gel, magnesium hydroxide, magnesium trisilicate, magnesium oxide, and calcium carbonate. They are often used in the treatment of peptic ULCER.

Since many substances used as medications are themselves weak acids or weak bases, there is a high potential for drug–drug interaction involving antacids. Antacids can form insoluble complexes, interfere with drug absorption, and affect renal excretion of drugs by changing the pH of urine.

In the most commonly used antacids the main active agents are magnesium hydroxide and aluminium hydroxide. Magnesium hydroxide, 'milk of magnesia', can produce diarrhoea. Aluminium hydroxide and calcium carbonate are constipating. It may be necessary to alternate types of antacids when they are taken on a long-term basis. The sodium content also varies; some antacids contain as much as ten times more sodium than others.

The sugar content of antacids must also be taken into account, particularly in the case of patients with diabetes mellitus or those who are on a low-calorie diet. It can range from none, as in Gelusil liquid, to 2.4 grams in a Gaviscon tablet.

antagonist (an'tagənist) 1. a muscle that counteracts the action of another muscle, its agonist. 2. a drug that binds to a cellular receptor for a hormone, neurotransmitter, or another drug blocking the action of that substance without producing any physiological effect itself. 3. a tooth in one jaw that articulates with one in the other jaw.

narcotic a. a drug that antagonizes the effects of narcotic analgesics. Some have analgesic properties when used alone (agonist–antagonists, e.g. pentazocine), while others are pure antagonists (e.g. naloxone). Usually used to reverse respiratory depression but does so at the expense of reducing analgesia.

ante ('antee) preposition. [L.] *before.*

ante- word element. [L.] *before* (in time or space).

ante mortem ('anti 'mawtəm) [L.] *before death.*

ante partum ('anti 'pahtəm) [L.] *before parturition.*

antebrachium (ˌanti'braykiəm) the forearm. adj. **antebrachial.**

antecedent (ˌanti'seedənt) a precursor.

plasma thromboplastic a. PTA; clotting factor XI.

antecurvature (ˌanti'kərvəchə) a slight anteflexion.

antefebrile (ˌanti'feebriel, -'feb-) preceding fever.

anteflexion (ˌanti'flekshən) the bending of an organ so that its top is thrust forward.

antemortem (ˌanti'mawtəm) performed or occurring before death.

antenatal (ˌanti'nayt'l) before birth.

antenna (an'tenə) one of the appendages on the head of arthropods.

Antepar ('antiˌpah) trademark for preparations of piperazine citrate and piperazine phosphate, anthelmintics.

Antepsin (an'tepsin) trademark for preparations of sucralfate.

antepyretic (ˌantipie'retik) occurring before the stage of fever.

anterior (an'tiə·ri·ə) situated at or directed toward the front; opposite of posterior.

a. chamber the part of the aqueous humour-containing space of the eyeball between the cornea and the iris.

anterior cord syndrome (an'tiə·ri·ə kawd) localized injury to the anterior portion of the spinal cord, characterized by complete paralysis and hypalgesia and hypaesthesia to the level of the lesion, but with relative preservation of posterior column sensations of touch, position, and vibration.

antero- word element. [L.] *anterior, in front of.*

anterograde ('antə·rohˌgrayd) extending or moving forward.

anteroinferior (ˌantə·roh·in'fiə·ri·ə) situated in front and below.

anterolateral (ˌantə·roh'latə·rəl) situated in front and to one side.

anteromedian (ˌantə·roh'meedi·ən) situated in front and on the midline.

anteroposterior (ˌantə·rohpos'tiə·ri·ə) directed from the front toward the back.

anterosuperior (ˌantə·rohsoo'piə·ri·ə) situated in front and above.

anteversion (ˌanti'vərzhən) the tipping forward of an entire organ.

anteverted (ˌanti'vərtid) tipped or bent forward.

anthelix (ant'heeliks, an'thee-) the semicircular ridge on the ear anterior and parallel to the helix.

anthelmintic (ˌant·hel'mintik, ˌanthel-) 1. destructive to worms. 2. an agent destructive to worms. Examples of anthelmintic drugs include: pyrantel for the treatment of the roundworm *Ascaris lumbricoides*; niclosamide for the treatment of tapeworms; and metronidazole for protozoan infection such as amoebic dysentery. Mebendazole is effective against a variety of intestinal worms.

Some anthelmintic drugs are toxic and should be given with care. The toxic effects of a specific drug should be known prior to administration and the patient observed carefully for these effects after the drug is given.

anthracene ('anthrəˌseen) a crystalline hydrocarbon, $C_{14}H_{10}$, from coal tar.

anthracoid ('anthrəˌkoyd) resembling anthrax.

anthracosilicosis (ˌanthrəkohˌsili'kohsis) a lung disease due to inhalation of coal dust (anthracosis) and fine particles of silica (silicosis).

anthracosis (ˌanthrə'kohsis) a lung disease due to inhalation of coal dust not containing silica (see also PNEUMOCONIOSIS).

anthracycline (ˌanthrə'siekleen) a class of antibiotics isolated from cultures of *Streptomyces peucetius*; it includes the antineoplastic agents epirubicin, daunorubicin, doxorubicin and mitozantrone.

anthraquinone (ˌanthrə'kwinohn) a yellow substance derived from anthracene, used in the manufacture of certain dyes.

anthrax ('anthraks) an acute,notifiable, infectious disease due to *Bacillus anthracis*, acquired through contact with infected animals or their byproducts, such as carcasses, bones or skins, usually by occupational exposure. The incubation period is 2–5 days.

A worldwide zoonosis, anthrax is now very uncommon in the UK, only five cases being notified in 1980–85.

cutaneous a. a malignant pustule due to lodgment of the causative organisms in wounds or abrasions of the skin, producing a black crusted elevation on a broad zone of oedema. Specific treatment: penicillin.

pulmonary a. (woolsorter's disease) a fulminating pneumonia due to inhalation of dust or animal hair containing the causative organism. Usually fatal.

A vaccine is available for persons likely to be exposed to infection in their occupation. Obtainable from the Public Health Laboratory Service in England and Wales.

anthropo- word element. [Gr.] *man (human being).*

anthropocentric (ˌanthrəpoh'sentrik) with a human bias; considering man the centre of the universe.

anthropoid ('anthrəˌpoyd) resembling man; the anthropoid apes, which include the chimpanzee, gibbon, gorilla, and orang-utan, are tailless.

Anthropoidea (ˌanthrə'poydi·ə) a suborder of Primates, including monkeys, apes, and man, characterized by a larger and more complicated brain than the other suborders.

anthropology (ˌanthrə'poləjee) the science that concerns man, his origins, historical and cultural development, and races.

cultural a. that branch of anthropology that concerns man in relation to his fellows and to his environment.

physical a. that branch of anthropology which concerns the physical characteristics of man.

anthropometric (ˌanthrəpə'metrik) pertaining to anthropometry.

anthropometry (ˌanthrə'pomətree) the science that deals with the measurement of the size, weight, and proportions of the human body. adj. **anthropometric.**

anthropomorphism (ˌanthrəpə'mawfizəm) the attribution of human characteristics to nonhuman objects.

anthropophilic (ˌanthrəpə'filik) preferring human beings to animals; said of certain mosquitoes.

anthropophobia (ˌanthrəpə'fohbi·ə) morbid dread of society.

anthropozoonosis (ˌanthrəpəˌzoh·ə'nohsis) a disease of either animals or man that may be transmitted from one species to the other.

anti- word element. [Gr.] *counteracting, effective against.*

anti-D (ˌanti'dee) a sterile solution of globulins derived from human blood plasma containing antibody to the erythrocyte factor Rh(D); used to suppress formation of active Rh antibodies in Rh-negative mothers after delivery or miscarriage of a Rh-positive baby or fetus, and thus to prevent HAEMOLYTIC DISEASE OF NEWBORN in the next pregnancy if the child is Rh-positive.

anti-Rh$_0$ anti-D.

antiadrenergic (,anti,adrə'nərjik) 1. sympatholytic: opposing the effects of impulses conveyed by adrenergic postganglionic fibres of the sympathetic nervous system. 2. an antiadrenergic agent.

antiagglutinin (,anti·əglootinin) a substance that opposes the action of an agglutinin.

anti-amoebic (,antiə'meebik) 1. destroying or suppressing the growth of amoebas. 2. an agent that destroys or suppresses the growth of amoebas.

antianaemic (,anti·əneemik) counteracting anaemia.

antianaphylaxis (,anti,anəfi'laksis) a condition in which the anaphylaxis reaction does not occur because of free antigens in the blood; the state of desensitization to antigens.

antiandrogen (,anti'andrəjən) any substance capable of inhibiting the biological effects of androgenic hormones.

antiantibody (,anti'antibodee) a substance that counteracts the effect of an antibody.

antianxiety (,antiang'zieətee) dispelling anxiety. The term *antianxiety agent* (called also an anxiolytic or minor tranquillizer) refers to a mild sedative, such as diazepam (Valium).

antiarrhythmic (,antiay'ridhmik) 1. preventing or alleviating cardiac arrhythmias. 2. an agent that prevents or alleviates cardiac arrhythmias.

antiarthritic (,antiah'thritik) 1. effective in treatment of arthritis. 2. an agent used in treatment of arthritis.

antibacterial (,antibak'tiə·ri·əl) 1. destroying or suppressing the growth or reproduction of bacteria. 2. an agent having such properties.

antibechic (,anti'bekik) 1. relieving cough. 2. an agent that relieves cough.

antibiosis (,antibie'ohsis) an association between two populations of organisms that is detrimental to one of them, or between one organism and an antibiotic produced by another.

antibiotic (,antibie'otik) 1. destructive of life. 2. killing microorganisms, or suppressing their multiplication or growth. 3. a chemical substance that has the capacity, in dilute solutions, to kill (biocidal capacity) or inhibit the growth (biostatic activity) of microorganisms. Called also *antimicrobial*.

Antibiotic agents are classified functionally according to the manner in which they adversely affect a microorganism. Some interfere with the synthesis of the bacterial cell wall. This results in cell lysis because the contents of the bacterial cell are hypertonic and therefore under high osmotic pressure. A weakening of the cell wall causes the cell to rupture, spill its contents, and be destroyed. The penicillins, cephalosporins, and bacitracin are examples of this group of antibiotics.

A second group interferes with the synthesis of nucleic acids. Without DNA and RNA synthesis a microorganism cannot replicate or translate genetic information. This interference with reproduction of the cell produces a bacteriostatic effect. Examples that exert this kind of bacteriostatic action are erythromycin and tetracycline.

A third group changes the permeability of the cell membrane, causing a leakage of metabolic substrates essential to the life of the microorganism. Their action can be either bacteriostatic or bactericidal. Examples include amphotericin B and polymyxin B.

A fourth group interferes with metabolic processes within the microorganism. They are structurally similar to natural metabolic substrates, but since they do not function normally, they interrupt metabolic processes. Most of these agents are bacteriostatic. Examples include the sulphonamides, aminosalicylic acid (PAS), and isoniazid (INH).

The side-effects of antibiotics can be widespread and dangerous to the patient. Damage to the central nervous system, blood components, liver, kidney, and lung are possible. (See accompanying table.) Additionally, debilitated and immunosuppressed patients are susceptible to a superinfection by a second microorganism that is resistant to the antibiotic that is being administered to them.

Local effects of antibiotic therapy involving the gastrointestinal tract are the result of destruction of large numbers of microorganisms that normally inhabit the intestines. This produces alterations in the balance of microbial flora in the body. Broad-spectrum antibiotics are likely to inhibit the growth of some normal flora and allow yeasts and moulds to flourish. An example of this is the occurrence of *candidiasis* when tetracycline is being taken. Other kinds of microorganisms that can replace normal gastrointestinal flora suppressed by antibiotic therapy are salmonellae and *Clostridium difficile*. Large numbers of salmonellae in the stools of patients on antibiotics greatly increase the possibility of cross-infection; hence, there is a need for enteric precautions in the care of these patients. *Clostridium difficile* produces a toxin that can cause severe pseudomembranous colitis (see antibiotic-associated COLITIS).

SPECIAL CONSIDERATIONS. Effective antibiotic therapy depends on maintaining an optimum and stable level of the drug in the serum and body tissues. This demands meticulous care in the administration of the drug by the correct route and at the correct time. Patients who take antibiotics at home need instruction in when and how to take the prescribed medication in order to obtain the desired effects. This includes knowledge of which foods to avoid because of food-drug interaction, whether to take the drug before or after meals, and the quantity of water or other liquid to take with the medication. Patients should be aware of the side-effects of their specific medication, and which ones should be reported immediately. Lay persons may not be aware of the hazards of ignoring directions and discontinuing the drug when their symptoms subside, or of taking an antibiotic prescribed for someone else. Failure to take only what is prescribed and in the full amount can contribute to the development of drug-resistant strains of microorganisms.

antiblennorrhagic (,anti,blenə'rayjik) 1. preventing or relieving gonorrhoea. 2. an agent that so acts.

antibody ('anti,bodee) an immunoglobulin molecule having a specific amino acid sequence, which property gives each antibody the ability to adhere to and interact only with the ANTIGEN that induced its synthesis. This antigen-specific property of the antibody is the basis of the antigen–antibody reaction that is essential to a humoral immune response. The antigen–antibody reaction begins as soon as substances interpreted as foreign invaders gain entrance into the body. Abbreviated Ab. See also IMMUNITY.

Antibodies, also called immune bodies, are synthesized by the plasma cells formed when antigen-specific groups *(clones)* of B-lymphocytes respond to the presence of antigen. The developmental process of antibody production begins when stem cells are transformed into B-lymphocytes, so called because they resemble the bursa-derived lymphocytes of birds. This transformation usually is completed a few

Major side effects of antibiotic agents

Organ system or condition	Antibiotic agent	Nursing observations
Central Nervous System		
Optic neuritis	Streptomycin, chloramphenicol	Blurred vision and amblyopia
Otoxicity	Aminoglycosides, vancomycin, streptomycin	Tinnitus, vertigo, roaring in the ears, hearing loss
Neuropathy	Nitrofurantoin, colistin, chloramphenicol, amphotericin B	Headache, dizziness, irritability, drowsiness, ataxia, slurring of speech paraesthesias (circumoral, lingual and extremities), confusion coma
Neuromuscular blockade	Aminoglycosides, colistin	Sense of uneasiness, dyspnoea hypoxia, hypercarbia, respiratory arrest
Gastrointestinal		
Pseudomembranous colitis	Clindomycin, lincomycin in particular but also penicillins, tetracyclines, co-trimoxazole, cephalosporins and gentamicin	Watery stools without blood, abdominal pain, cramps, fever and high leukocyte count
Haematoxicity		
Aplastic anaemia	Chloramphenicol	Weakness, pallor, breathlessness on exertion (*note*: this may happen long-after drug has been discontinued), ↓WBC
Leukopenia	Sulphonamides, penicillin	No clinical manifestations are expected as a result of leukopenia per se
Platelet defect	Carbenicillin, latamoxef	Multiple, spontaneous small vessel haemorrhages in the skin and mucous membranes
Hepatotoxicity	Erythromycin (base and salts), tetracycline, fusidic acid, sulphonamides	Nausea, vomiting, diarrhoea, fever, jaundice; ensure monitoring of liver functions
Hypersensitivity	Penicillins, cephalosporins, sulphonamides	Varies from stinging sensation at site of infection to anaphylactic shock. Symptoms of anaphylactic shock are itching, swelling, bronchospasm and signs of vascular collapse, i.e. hypotension, loss of consciousness and tachycardia
Nephrotoxicity	Aminoglycosides, amphotericin B, colistin, tetracycline, some cephalosporins	Casts or protein in the urine, oliguria, increased blood urea nitrogen, increased serum creatinine levels, decreased creatinine clearance
Pulmonary complications	Nitrofurantoin	Sudden onset of cough, fever and dyspnoea
Skin and appendages		
Grey baby syndrome	Chloramphenicol	Ashen grey cyanotic colour in skin, fall in body temperature, vomiting, irregular and rapid respiration mainly in new born infants

Adapted from Arking, L. and Saravolatz, L. (1980) Antimicrobial agents. *Nursing Clinincs of North America*, Vol. 15, p. 689.

months after birth, at which time the lymphocytes migrate to lymphoid tissue primarily located in the lymph nodes, but also found in the spleen, gastrointestinal tract, and bone marrow. Hence it is the lymphocyte that functions as the prime mover in antibody formation.

Antibody production, its interaction with a specific antigen, and the activation of complement (C), an interrelated group of eleven proteins, are the major components of the *humoral* system of IMMUNITY. Antibodies, the effectors of the immune response, can be transferred passively from one individual to another, as, for example, the transfer of maternal antibody across the placental barrier to the fetus, who has not yet developed a mature immune system.

Antibodies can be classified according to their mode of action as they react to and set about defending the body against foreign invaders. Some cause clumping together of bacterial cells (agglutination) and are called *agglutinins*. Agglutination also takes place when blood cells of one type are mixed with those of a different type. Those antibodies which cause bacterial cells to dissolve or liquefy are called *bacteriolysins*. This activity is assisted by COMPLEMENT, which interacts with the antigen–antibody complex in such a way that the cell ruptures and there is dissolution *(lysis)* of the cell body. *Opsonins* coat the outside of bacteria, making them more attractive to phagocytes. Other types of antibodies include those which neutralize the toxins of antigens *(antitoxins)*, and those which cause precipitation of antigens from a fluid medium *(precipitins)*. See also IMMUNOGLOBULIN.

anaphylactic a. a substance formed as a result of the first injection of a foreign anaphylactogen and responsible for the anaphylactic symptoms following the second injection of the same anaphylactogen.
antinuclear a's (ANAs) autoantibodies directed against components of the cell nucleus, e.g., DNA, RNA, and histones; they may be detected by immunofluorescence. A positive ANA test is characteristic of systemic lupus erythematosus. Antinuclear antibodies also occur in patients with rheumatoid arthritis, Sjögren's syndrome, and scleroderma.
blocking a. 1. one (usually IgG) that reacts preferentially with an antigen, preventing it from reacting with a cytotropic antibody (IgE), and producing a hypersensitivity reaction. 2. antibodies which bind to antigens sparsely distributed on a cell surface so that complement activation does not occur.
complete a. one that reacts with the antigen, producing an agglutination or precipitation reaction and may activate complement.
cross-reacting a. one that combines with an antigen other than the one that induced its production.
cytophilic a. cytotropic antibody.
cytotoxic a. any specific antibody directed against cellular antigens, which when bound to the antigen activates the complement pathway or activates killer cells, resulting in cell lysis.
cytotropic a. any of a class of antibodies that attach to tissue cells (such as mast cells and basophils) through their Fc segments to induce the release of histamine and other vasoconstrictive amines important in immediate hypersensitivity reactions. In man, this antibody, also known as *reagin*, is of the immunoglobulin class known as IgE. Called also cytophilic antigen.
immune a. one induced by immunization or by transfusion incompatibility, in contrast to natural antibodies.
incomplete a. 1. an antibody which combines with antigen without producing an observable reaction (i.e., without precipitation). 2. an antibody combining univalently specifically with heterozygous Rh-positive erythrocytes without causing visible agglutination, but which, in the presence of antihuman globulin (Coombs') serum or high molecular weight media, e.g., albumin, will cause red cell clumping. Homozygous Rh-positive cells will react in saline. Other red cell antibodies may demonstrate similar properties.
monoclonal a. antibodies produced by fusion of an immunoglobulin-producing cell with a lymphocyte making a specific antibody. The cell and its progeny continue to make a single antibody. Widely used to produce highly specific antibodies for diagnostic and, recently, therapeutic uses. Human lymphocytes may be fused with mouse tumour cells to make human-/mouse monoclonal antibodies.
natural a's ones that react with antigens to which the individual has had no known exposure; they play a major role in resistance to infection.
neutralizing a. one that reduces or destroys infectivity of a homologous infectious agent by partial or complete destruction of the agent.
protective a. one responsible for immunity to an infectious agent, observed in passive immunity.
Rh a's those directed against Rh antigen(s) of human erythrocytes. Not normally present, they may be produced when Rh-negative persons receive Rh-positive blood by transfusion or during separation of an Rh-positive placenta. Leakage of Rh-positive fetal cells into the maternal circulation occurs in the Rh-negative pregnant woman. This immunizes the woman to produce anti-Rh antibodies.
saline a. complete antibody.

antibrachium (ˌanti'brayki·əm) antebrachium, or forearm.
anticariogenic (ˌantiˌkair·rioh'jenik) effective in suppressing caries production.
anticholagogue (ˌanti'kohləgog) an agent that inhibits secretion of bile. adj. **anticholagogic**.
anticholinergic (ˌantiˌkohlin'ərjik) 1. blocking the action of acetylcholine, or of cholinergic agents; parasympatholytic. 2. an agent that blocks the action of acetylcholine in cholinergic areas, i.e., areas supplied by parasympathetic nerves, and voluntary muscles.
anticholinesterase (ˌantiˌkohli'nestəˌrayz) a drug that inhibits the enzyme acetylcholinesterase, thereby potentiating the action of acetylcholine at postsynaptic membrane receptors in the parasympathetic nervous system.
anticoagulant (ˌantikoh'agyuhlənt) 1. serving to prevent the coagulation of blood. 2. any substance that, *in vivo* or *in vitro*, suppresses, delays, or nullifies coagulation of the blood.

Anticoagulant therapy is indicated when there is danger of clot formation within a blood vessel. Its main purpose is preventive; once a clot has formed, the anticoagulant drug has no effect on it nor will the drug have a therapeutic effect on ischaemic tissue formerly supplied by the blood vessel in which the clot resides.

Conditions in which anticoagulant therapy is employed include occlusive vascular disease, such as coronary artery occlusion, cerebrovascular and venous thrombosis, and pulmonary embolism. It is administered prophylactically when major surgery is planned for a patient with a history of arterial stasis, and for patients who must be immobilized for a prolonged period of time.

Anticoagulant agents include those drugs that interfere with the formation of clots (*antithrombotics)*, for example: (1) the parenteral preparation heparin and the oral anticoagulants (coumarins); (2) those capable of disintegrating thrombi that have already formed (*thrombolytics)*, for example, streptokinase and urokinase; (3) a third group of anticoagulant agents, the anti-platelet-aggregating agents, are currently under investigation.

Oral anticoagulants are used mainly in the treatment of deep vein thrombosis and pulmonary embolism, and to prevent thrombosis in patients with heart valve protheses. Warfarin and other coumarins are the drugs of choice. They act by antagonizing vitamin K, reducing the synthesis of the vitamin K dependent factors II, VII, IX and X. They take up to 72 hours to be fully effective. Laboratory control (prothrombin time, thrombotest, etc.) is essential. Many drugs interact with warfarin and bleeding is not an uncommon complication of therapy. Major interactive drugs which potentiate the effect of oral anticoagulants are aspirin and other nonsteroidal anti-inflammatory drugs such as phenylbutazone, and broad-spectrum antibiotics. Phenobarbitone decreases the response to warfarin.

Patient Care. The major difficulties that may arise during the course of anticoagulant therapy are haemorrhage and drug interaction. Observation of the patient for early signs of internal as well as external spontaneous bleeding is of primary importance. Health care personnel responsible for the care of these patients must be knowledgeable about the various laboratory tests and interpretation of their results in the administration of anticoagulant drugs and assessment of the patient.

Since anticoagulants can be enhanced or inhibited by

many drugs, especially the salicylates, barbiturates, and antibiotics, ambulatory patients must not take any other drugs in combination with an anticoagulant agent without first consulting the doctor who prescribed the drug. This includes nonprescription or 'over-the-counter' drugs as well as prescription drugs. Dietary restrictions such as fasting diets or those that limit the intake or utilization of the fat-soluble vitamin K can result in increased pharmacological action of an anticoagulant.

The patient and his family should be given adequate instruction in the purposes of anticoagulant therapy, the effects and side-effects of other drugs, dietary intake and alcohol on anticoagulant agents. Regular contact with members of the health care team is necessary so that adequate laboratory and clinical monitoring of the patient's status can be continued as long as he is receiving an anticoagulant.

Instruction of the patient and associates should include prevention of accidental injury, basic first aid measures to control bleeding should an accident occur, education about the danger signs that warrant immediate medical attention, and assurance that bleeding can be controlled.

Women of childbearing age need counselling about the effects of anticoagulants on contraceptive methods and reproduction. Those who are taking an anticoagulant for prevention of emboli cannot use oral contraceptives or an intrauterine device, which could cause endometrial bleeding. Should a patient think she is or desires to be pregnant, the specialist should be notified at once. Warfarin crosses the placental barrier and can cause fetal abnormalities if taken early in pregnancy and fatal haemorrhage in the fetus at a later stage. It does not appear to enter the mother's milk and breast feeding is not contraindicated. Heparin does not have these properties and should be substituted for warfarin at critical stages during pregnancy.

anticodon (ˌanti'kohdon) a triplet of nucleotides in transfer RNA that is complementary to the codon in messenger RNA which specifies the amino acid.

anticomplement (ˌanti'komplimənt) a substance that counteracts a complement component (usually an inhibitor, e.g. C1s inhibitor).

anticonvulsant (ˌantikən'vulsant) 1. inhibiting convulsions. 2. an agent that suppresses convulsions. Drugs that act as anticonvulsants include phenytoin (Epanutin) and sodium valproate (Epilim). They are used in the treatment of EPILEPSY and in psychomotor and myoclonic seizures.

anticus ('antikəs) anterior.

antidepressant (ˌantidi'pres'nt) 1. effective against depressive illness. 2. a drug used for relief of symptoms of depression. The most commonly used are the *tricyclic antidepressants*, so called because of their chemical structure, which have three fused rings. These drugs block the reuptake of the neurotransmitters noradrenaline and serotonin at nerve endings. This group includes imipramine, amitriptyline, desipramine, doxepin, nortriptyline, and trimipramine. Two drugs with different chemical structures but similar effects are mianserin and maprotiline. These drugs vary in the degree to which they affect reuptake of the two neurotransmitters. Also, some are sedating while others are alerting. The patient must take the drug for about 2 to 3 weeks before the full therapeutic effect is established.

An older group of antidepressants are the *monoamine oxidase (MAO) inhibitors* isocarboxazid, phenelzine, and tranylcypromine. These drugs inhibit MAO, the enzyme that breaks down noradrenaline and serotonin released at nerve synapses. They are not as widely used as the tricyclic antidepressants because serious cardiovascular side-effects (hypertension, headache, stroke) can occur when tyramine is ingested, and foods containing tyramine, such as cheese, certain beans, beer, and wine, must be avoided by patients taking MAO inhibitors.

antidiarrhoeal (ˌantiˌdieə'reeəl) 1. counteracting diarrhoea. 2. an agent that counteracts diarrhoea.

antidinic (ˌanti'dinik) relieving giddiness or vertigo.

antidiuresis (ˌantiˌdieyuh'reesis) the suppression of secretion of urine by the kidneys.

antidiuretic (ˌantiˌdieyuh'retik) 1. pertaining to or causing suppression of rate of urine formation. 2. an agent that causes suppression of urine formation.

a. hormone vasopressin; a hormone that suppresses the excretion of urine; it has a specific effect on the epithelial cells of the renal tubules, stimulating the reabsorption of water independently of solids, and resulting in concentration of urine. Secreted by the hypothalmus, but stored and released by the posterior lobe of the PITUITARY GLAND, it also has vasopressor activity. Abbreviated ADH.

syndrome of inappropriate secretion of a. hormone (SIADH) one in which there is ectopic production of ADH by a tumour leading to hyponatraemia (see also SYNDROME OF INAPPROPRIATE SECRETION OF ANTIDIURETIC HORMONE).

antidote ('antiˌdoht) an agent that counteracts a poison. adj. **antidotal.**

chemical a. one that neutralizes the poison by changing its chemical nature.

mechanical a. one that prevents absorption of the poison.

physiological a. one that counteracts the effects of the poison by producing opposing effects.

universal a. a mixture formerly recommended as an antidote when the exact poison is not known. There is, in fact, no known universal antidote. Activated charcoal is now being used for many poisons.

antidromic (ˌanti'dromik) conducting impulses in a direction opposite to the normal.

antidysenteric (ˌantiˌdis'n'terik) counteracting dysentery.

antiemetic (ˌanti·i'metik) 1. useful in the treatment of vomiting. 2. an agent that relieves vomiting.

antiepileptic (ˌantiˌepi'leptik) 1. combating epilepsy. 2. a remedy for epilepsy.

antifebrile (ˌanti'feebriel, -'feb-) counteracting fever.

antifibrinolysin (ˌantiˌfiebri'nolisin) antiplasmin.

antifibrinolytic (ˌantiˌfiebrinoh'litik) inhibiting fibrinolysis.

antifungal (ˌanti'fung·g'l) 1. destructive to or checking the growth of fungi. 2. an agent that destroys or checks the growth of fungi, such as amphotericin, which is used for systemic fungal or yeast infections, or flucytosine (5-FC), which is used in systemic yeast infections only.

antigalactic (ˌantigə'laktik) 1. diminishing the secretion of milk. 2. an agent that so acts.

antigen ('antiˌjen, -jən) any substance which is capable, under appropriate conditions, of inducing a specific immune response and of reacting with the products of that response; that is, with specific ANTIBODY or specifically sensitized T-lymphocytes, or both. Antigens may be soluble substances, such as toxins and foreign proteins, or particulate, such as bacteria and tissue cells; however, only the portion of the protein or polysaccharide molecule known as the *antigenic determinant* or *epitope* combines with antibody or a specific receptor on a lymphocyte. Abbreviated Ag. adj. **antigenic.** See also IMMUNITY.

acetone-insoluble a. an antigen for the Wasserman

reaction consisting of the acetone-insoluble constitutents of an alcoholiç extract of beef heart.
allogeneic a. an antigen, occurring in some but not all individuals of the same species, which is capable of eliciting an immune response in genetically different individuals of the same species but not in an individual bearing it, e.g., histocompatibility antigens and human blood group antigens; called also isoantigen.
Au a., Australia a. hepatitis B surface antigen. Originally thought to be a plasma protein in Australian aborigines.
carcinoembryonic a. (CEA) an oncofetal glycoprotein antigen originally thought to be specific for adenocarcinoma of the colon, but now known to be found in many other cancers and some nonmalignant conditions. Its primary use is in monitoring the response of patients to cancer treatment.
common a. an antigenic determinant group (epitope) that is present in two or more different antigen molecules and leads to cross-reactions among them.
complete a. an antigen which both stimulates the immune response and reacts with the products (e.g., antibody) of that response.
conjugated a. antigen produced by coupling a hapten to a protein carrier molecule through covalent bonds; when it induces immunization, the resultant immune response is directed against both the hapten and the carrier.
cross-reacting a. 1. one that combines with antibody produced in response to a different but related antigen, owing to similarity of antigenic determinants. 2. identical antigens in two bacterial strains, so that antibody produced against one strain will react with the other.
D a. a red cell antigen of the Rh blood group system, important in the development of isoimmunization in Rh-negative persons exposed to the blood of Rh-positive persons.
E a. a red cell antigen of the Rh blood group system.
F a. a fast-migrating tumour-associated antigen first found in association with Hodgkin's disease and identified as a ferritin compound.
flagellar a. H antigen.
Forssman a. a heterogenetic antigen inducing the production of antisheep haemolysin, occurring in various unrelated species, mainly in the organs but not in the erythrocytes (guinea pig, horse), but sometimes only in the erythrocytes (sheep), and occasionally in both (chicken).
H a. [Ger.] *Hauch* (film) the antigen that occurs in the flagella of motile bacteria.
hepatitis a., hepatitis-associated a. (HAA) hepatitis B surface antigen.
hepatitis B core a. (HBcAg) the antigen of the DNA core of the hepatitis B virus, produced in the nucleus of hepatocytes in hepatitis B.
hepatitis B e a. (HBeAg) a virus coded antigen whose presence is usually associated with infectivity. It is generally agreed that the development of antibody to HB$_e$Ag is likely to be associated with loss of infectivity.
hepatitis B surface a. (HBsAg) one present in the serum of those infected with hepatitis B, consisting of the surface coat lipoprotein of the hepatitis B virus. Tests for serum Hb$_s$Ag are used in the diagnosis of hepatitis B and in screening blood and blood products for hepatitis B contamination. Many people carrying HB$_s$Ag in their blood are not making whole virus, and their blood and secretions may not be infectious. See HB$_e$Ag above. It was originally called Australia (Au) antigen because it was discovered in the blood of an Australian aborigine and was also called hepatitis-associated antigen (HAA) and serum-hepatitis (SH) antigen.
heterogenetic a., heterophil a. one capable of stimulating the production of antibodies that react with tissues from other animals or even plants.
histocompatibility a's genetically determined antigens present on the cell membranes of nucleated cells of most tissues, which incite an immune response when grafted onto a genetically disparate individual and thus determine the compatibility of tissues in transplantation.
HLA a's (*h*uman *l*eukocyte *a*ntigen), histocompatibility antigens on the surface of nucleated cells that are important in cross-matching procedures, and are partially responsible for the rejection of transplanted tissue when donor and recipient HLA antigens do not match. See also HLA.
H-Y a. a histocompatibility antigen determined by a locus on the Y chromosome. These antigens can cause rejection of a skin graft of male skin on females even in inbred strains of animals.
Ia a's class II histocompatibility antigens governed by the I region of the major histocompatibility complex (MHC), located principally on B cells, T cells, Langerhans skin cells and certain macrophages. First described in mice, the human analogues are the class II D+, DQ and D2 loci.
isogeneic a. allogeneic antigen.
Ly a's antigenic cell-surface markers of subpopulations of T lymphocytes, classified as Ly 1, 2, and 3.
lymphogranuloma venereum a. a sterile suspension of *Chlamydia lymphogranulomatis*; used as a dermal reactivity indicator.
M a. a type-specific antigen that appears to be located primarily in the cell wall and is associated with virulence of *Streptococcus pyogenes*.
mumps skin test a. a sterile suspension of mumps virus; used as a dermal reactivity indicator.
Nègre a. an antigen prepared from dead, dried, and triturated tubercle bacilli by means of acetone and methyl alcohol; used in serum tests for tuberculosis.
nuclear a's the components of cell nuclei with which antinuclear antibodies react.
O a. [Ger.] *ohne Hauch* (without film) the antigen that occurs in the bodies of bacteria.
oncofetal a. a gene product that is expressed during fetal development, but repressed in specialized tissues of the adult and that is also produced by certain cancers. In the neoplastic transformation, the cells dedifferentiate and these genes can be derepressed so that the embryonic antigens reappear. Examples are alpha-fetoprotein and carcinoembryonic antigen.
organ-specific a. any antigen that occurs exclusively in a particular organ and serves to distinguish it from other organs. Two types of organ specificity have been proposed: (1) first-order or tissue specificity, which is attributed to the presence of an antigen characteristic of a particular organ in a single species; (2) second-order organ specificity, which is attributed to an antigen characteristic of the same organ in many, even unrelated species.
partial a. an antigen that does not produce antibody formation, but gives specific precipitation when mixed with the antibacterial immune serum.
pollen a. the essential polypeptides of the pollen of plants extracted with a suitable menstruum, used in diagnosis, prophylaxis, and desensitization in hay fever.
a. presentation the presentation of ingested antigens on the surface of macrophages in close proximity to histocompatibility antigens. Some populations of T-lymphocytes can only be triggered by antigens that are presented in this way. Thus macrophages play a

role in inducing cell-mediated immunity.

private a's antigens that are restricted to an individual or a strain of inbred animals.

public a's antigens that are found in many individuals but are not universal and alternative antigens may replace them in some species.

recall a. an antigen to which an individual has previously been sensitized and which is subsequently administered as a challenging dose to elicit a hypersensitivity reaction.

self a. an autoantigen, a normal constituent of the body against which antibodies are formed in autoimmune disease.

sequestered a's the cellular constituents of tissue (e.g., the lens of the eye and the thyroid) sequestered anatomically from the lymphoreticular system during embryonic development and thus thought not to be recognized as 'self'. Should such tissue be exposed to the lymphoreticular system during adult life, an autoimmune response may be elicited.

tumour-specific a's cell-surface antigens of tumours tht elicit a specific immune response in the host; abbreviated TSA.

V a., Vi a. an antigen contained in the sheath of a bacterium, as *Salmonella typhosa* (the typhoid bacillus), and thought to contribute to its virulence.

xenogeneic a. an antigen common to members of one species but not to members of other species; called also heterogeneic antigen.

antigenaemia (ˌantijə'neemi·ə) the presence of antigen, such as hepatitis B surface antigen, in the blood.

antigenicity (ˌantijə'nisitee) the capacity to react with an antibody.

antiglobulin (ˌanti'globyuhlin) an antibody directed against gamma globulin, as used in the antiglobulin Coombs' test.

antihaemophilic (ˌantiˌheemoh'filik) 1. effective against the bleeding tendency in haemophilia. 2. an agent that counteracts the bleeding tendency in haemophilia.

a. factor AHF, one of the clotting factors, deficiency of which causes classic, sex-linked haemophilia; called also factor VIII and antihaemophilic globulin. It is available in a preparation for preventive and therapeutic use.

antihaemorrhagic (ˌantiˌhemə'rajik) 1. exerting a haemostatic effect and counteracting haemorrhage. 2. an agent that prevents or checks haemorrhage.

antihelix (ˌanti'heeliks) anthelix.

antihelmintic (ˌantihel'mintik) anthelmintic.

antihistamine (ˌanti'histəˌmeen, -min) a drug that counteracts the effects of histamine, a normal body chemical that is believed to cause the symptoms of persons who are hypersensitive to various allergens. Antihistamines are used to relieve the symptoms of allergic reactions, especially hay fever and other allergic disorders of the nasal passages. Some antihistamines have an antinauseant action that is useful in the relief of motion sickness. Others have a sedative and hypnotic action and may be used as tranquillizers.

Patients for whom an antihistamine has been prescribed should be warned of the side-effects of these drugs, including drowsiness, dizziness, and muscular weakness. These side-effects present a special hazard in driving a car or operating heavy machinery. Other side-effects include dryness of the mouth and throat, and insomnia.

antihistaminic (ˌantiˌhistə'minik) 1. counteracting the pharmacological effects of histamine. 2. an antihistamine.

antihormone (ˌanti'hormohn) a substance that counteracts a hormone.

antihypercholesterolaemic (ˌantiˌhiepəkohˌlestə·ro'leemik) 1. effective against hypercholesterolaemia. 2. an agent that prevents or relieves hypercholesterolaemia.

antihyperlipoproteinaemic (ˌantiˌhiepəˌlipohˌprohti'neemik) 1. promoting a reduction of lipoprotein levels in the blood. 2. an agent that so acts.

antihypertensive (ˌantiˌhiepə'tensiv) 1. effective against hypertension. 2. an agent that reduces high blood pressure.

Many different types of drugs are used in the treatment of hypertension. Diuretics inhibit the reabsorption of sodium in the renal tubules. This causes an increase in the urinary excretion of sodium and a decrease in the plasma volume and extracellular fluid volume. Other drugs act on adrenergic control of blood pressure. Beta-blockers, such as propranolol (Inderal), act at beta-adrenergic receptors in the heart and kidneys to reduce cardiac output and renin secretion. Other drugs, such as methyldopa (Aldomet), act on alpha-adrenergic mechanisms in the central or sympathetic nervous system to reduce peripheral vascular resistance. Vasodilators act directly on the arterioles to produce the same effect. Almost every case of hypertension can be controlled by one of these drugs or a combination of them. The proper combination is determined by the response of the individual patient. In some cases several drugs must be tried before the right combination is found.

PATIENT EDUCATION. Instruction of the patient and significant others is an essential part of antihypertensive therapy. Learning objectives are based on the patient's particular regimen of drug therapy, allowance of sodium intake, and other dietary restrictions, such as low-calorie diet to combat obesity.

Some antihypertensive drugs can produce acute hypotensive reactions. The patient will need to know how to prevent a hypotensive reaction and what measures to take should such a reaction occur.

Prevention of a hypotensive reaction includes avoiding hot baths and sudden immobility after exercise, both of which promote vasodilation and a lowering of arterial pressure. The patient also should be aware of the effect of sudden changes in position that can precipitate an attack of *orthostatic hypotension*. Pooling of blood in the lower extremities can divert the blood from the brain and other vital organs. This can sometimes be avoided by moving about frequently instead of standing motionless for long periods of time. Elastic stockings also help promote venous return from the legs and help prevent fainting from decreased cerebral blood supply.

Acute hypotension can be serious, but milder hypotensive reactions with faintness and weakness can be relieved at home if the patient lies down and elevates his lower extremities above the level of his head and flexes the thigh muscles to encourage the flow of blood from his feet and legs to his brain.

The patient on a diuretic that is not potassium-sparing will need instruction on the symptoms of potassium deficit, how to avoid potassium depletion, and when to notify the doctor should hypokalaemia occur.

Limitation of SODIUM intake can be very confusing and emotionally stressful to the uninstructed patient. In order to comply with his prescribed restriction of sodium he will need to know about satisfying substitutes and alternative seasonings for food, to be aware of the necessity of reading labels carefully when buying prepared food and over-the-counter medications, and to recognize the relationship between sodium and high blood pressure and the reasons why high sodium intake is harmful to his health and well-being.

antihypotensive (ˌantiˌhiepohˈtensiv) 1. counteracting low blood pressure. 2. an agent that so acts.

anti-immune (ˌanti·iˈmyoon) preventing immunity.

anti-infective (ˌanti·inˈfektiv) 1. counteracting infection. 2. a substance that counteracts infection. See also ANTIBIOTIC.

anti-inflammatory (ˌanti·inˈflamətə·ree, -tree) 1. counteracting or suppressing inflammation. 2. an agent that so acts.

antiketogenesis (ˌantiˌkeetohˈjenəsis) inhibition of the formation of ketone bodies.

antiketogenic (ˌantiˌkeetohˈjenik) preventing or suppressing the development of ketones (ketone bodies) and thus preventing development of ketosis.

antilewisite (ˌantiˈlooisiet) dimercaprol, a chelating agent used in poisoning with arsenic, gold, and mercury.

antilithic (ˌantiˈlithik) 1. preventing calculus formation. 2. an agent that prevents calculus formation.

antimalarial (ˌantiməˈlair·ri·əl) 1. therapeutically effective against malaria. 2. an agent that is therapeutically effective against malaria.

antimere (ˈantiˌmiə) one of the segments of the body bounded by planes at right angles to the long axis of the body.

antimetabolite (ˌantimeˈtabəˌliet) a substance bearing a close structural resemblance to one required for normal physiological functioning, and exerting its effect by interfering with the utilization of the essential metabolite.

antimethaemoglobinaemic (ˌantiˌmet·heeməˌglohbiˈneemik) 1. promoting reduction of methaemoglobin levels in the blood. 2. an agent that so acts.

antimetropia (ˌantimeˈtrohpi·ə) hypermetropia of one eye, with myopia in the other.

antimicrobial (ˌantimieˈkrohbi·əl) see ANTIBIOTIC.

antimony (ˈantimənee) a chemical element, atomic number 51, atomic weight 121.75, symbol Sb. (See table of elements in Appendix 2.) Antimony compounds are used in medicine as anti-infective agents in the treatment of tropical diseases, especially those of protozoan origin. All antimony compounds are potentially poisonous and must be used with caution. adj. **antimonial.**

a. potassium tartrate a compound used in treatment of parasitic infections, e.g., schistosomiasis or leishmaniasis.

a. sodium tartrate a compound used in the treatment of schistosomiasis.

antimorphic (ˌantiˈmawfik) in genetics, antagonizing or inhibiting normal activity (antimorphic mutant gene).

antimycotic (ˌantimieˈkotik) destructive to fungi.

antinauseant (ˌantiˈnawsi·ənt, -nawz-) 1. counteracting nausea. 2. an agent that counteracts nausea.

antineoplastic (ˌantiˌneeohˈplastik) 1. inhibiting the maturation and proliferation of malignant cells. 2. an agent having such properties.

a. therapy a regimen of treatment aimed at destruction of malignant cells and utilizing a variety of chemical agents that directly affect cellular growth and development. Called also *chemotherapy*. Antineoplastic therapy is but one of a variety of methods available in the treatment of CANCER. Chemotherapy is especially successful in curing choriocarcinoma, a highly malignant form of cancer that originates in the placenta, and Burkitt's lymphoma, a malignancy common among African children. Combinations of drugs have successfully controlled acute LEUKAEMIA in children and in persons with advanced stages of Hodgkin's disease.

TYPES OF ANTINEOPLASTIC AGENTS. The chemicals and drugs used in the treatment of cancer may be divided into three groups. The first group, the *alkylating* agents, are capable of damaging the DNA of cells, thereby interfering with the process of replication. Among these drugs are chlorambucil, cyclophosphamide, mustine hydrochloride, and triethylene thiophosphamide. Cytotoxic antibiotics affect DNA, RNA and protein synthesis. The antibiotic actinomycin D is included in this group, as is cisplatin and carboplatin.

The second type of drugs used in cancer chemotherapy is comprised of the *antimetabolites.* As the name suggests, these drugs interfere with the cancer cell's metabolism. Some replace essential metabolites without performing their function, while others compete with essential components by mimicking their functions and thereby inhibiting the manufacture of protein in the cell. Included in this group are cytosine arabinoside, fluorouracil, mercaptopurine, methotrexate and thioguanine.

The third group of chemicals employed in the treatment of cancer are *natural products* that directly affect the mechanism of cell division. The plant alkaloids, for example, vincristine and vinblastine, stop cell division at metaphase (a subphase in cell mitosis). The enzymes, for example, L-asparaginase, starve tumour cells by catabolizing substances (e.g., asparagine) which they need for survival. Hormones change cell metabolism by making the cellular environment unfavourable for growth of certain tumours.

PATIENT CARE. The drugs used in antineoplastic therapy are highly toxic and likely to produce troublesome and sometimes extremely dangerous reactions. They may be given singly or in combination, depending on the type of malignancy and the stage of its development. The complexity of this type of therapy, particularly when used in conjunction with surgery or radiation therapy, demands a team of specialists, including oncologists, radiotherapists, nurses and clinical pharmacologists, working cooperatively to accomplish the goals of the prescribed regimen.

It is especially important that members of the team be aware of and capable of dealing with the toxicity inherent in antineoplastic therapy. The management of drug toxicities requires a delicate balance between effective dosage to destroy malignant cells and the individual patient's tolerance of drug and dosage. Anorexia, alopecia, nausea, and vomiting are among the milder but more troublesome effects of antibiotics, alkylating agents and antimetabolites. It is necessary to work with each patient and help him establish a routine that will incorporate administration of the drug, taking an antiemetic, and spacing meals so that adequate nutrition is provided and excessive weight loss is avoided. STOMATITIS and DIARRHOEA are also likely to appear as early signs of toxicity from antimetabolic and antibiotic drug therapy.

Drugs that suppress bone marrow function produce leukopenia, which in turn increases susceptibility to infection. If the patient is also receiving an immunosuppressant such as prednisone, his resistance to infection is further compromised. He will need adequate rest, good nutrition, good habits of personal cleanliness, and avoidance of contact with persons who have infectious diseases. If an infection does develop, it should receive prompt attention to minimize its effects and inhibit its progress. It may be necessary to alter the dosage of the antineoplastic drug until the infection subsides.

Bone marrow-suppressing drugs can also affect the platelet count, reducing it to a level at which bleeding can readily occur. Normal clotting is impaired by some cancer therapeutic agents and there is therefore the danger of internal bleeding anywhere in the body. Should the situation become severe, the drug dosage may need to be reduced or stopped altogether and platelet transfusions may be given.

Hormonal therapy is frequently accompanied by fluid retention. Measurement of fluid intake and output, daily weight measurement, and observation for signs of surface oedema or congestive heart failure are essential parts of patient care. Care of the patient with OEDEMA must include meticulous skin care. If DIURETICS are given, the patient must be observed for signs of potassium depletion. Another side-effect of hormonal therapy may be changes in secondary sexual characteristics. These can be particularly embarrassing and emotionally disturbing to the patient.

Neurological disorders may result from treatment with the plant alkaloids. These conditions may manifest themselves as impaired sensation, loss of coordination, and severe constipation. Although these neurological effects are usually reversible, especially if caught in the early stages, it may take months for the nerve cells to recover and resume normal function.

antineoplaston (ˌantiˌneeoh'plaston) any of a number of peptides isolated from human urine that inhibit cell division in certain cancer cells but not in normal cells.

antinephritic (ˌantinə'fritik) effective against nephritis.

antineuralgic (ˌantinyuh'raljik) relieving neuralgia.

antineuritic (ˌantinyuh'ritik) relieving neuritis.

antinion (an'tini·ən) the frontal pole of the head.

antioestrogen (ˌanti'eestrəjən) 1. blocking the action of oestrogens. 2. an agent that so acts.

antiovulatory (ˌantiˌovyuh'laytə·ree) suppressing ovulation, as used with some forms of oral contraception.

antioxidant (ˌanti'oksidənt) a substance that in small amount will inhibit the oxidation of other compounds.

antiparasitic (ˌantiˌparə'sitik) 1. destroying parasites. 2. an agent that destroys parasites.

antiparkinsonian (ˌantiˌpahkin'sohni·ən) 1. effective in the treatment of parkinsonism. 2. an agent effective in the treatment of parkinsonism.

antiparticle (ˌanti'pahtik'l) either of a pair of elementary particles that have electric charges and magnetic moments of opposite sign and are the same in all other properties, such as mass, lifetime, and spin, e.g., the electron and positron. Every particle has an antiparticle. When antiparticles collide, they are annihilated, and their mass is converted to energy in the form of gamma rays.

antipediculotic (ˌantipeˌdikyuh'lotik) 1. effective against lice and in treatment of pediculosis. 2. an agent that is effective against lice.

antipepsin (ˌanti'pepsin) an antienzyme that counteracts pepsin.

antiperistalsis (ˌantiˌperi'stalsis) upward waves of contraction sometimes occurring normally in the lower ileum, competing with the normal downward peristalsis and retarding passage of intestinal contents into the caecum. adj. **antiperistaltic**.

antiplasmin (ˌanti'plazmin) a principle in the blood that inhibits plasmin.

antiplastic (ˌanti'plastik) unfavourable to healing.

antipolycythemic (ˌantiˌpolisie'theemik) 1. effective against polycythaemia. 2. an agent effective against polycythaemia.

antiport ('antiˌpawt) a cell membrane structure that transports two molecules at once through the membrane in opposite directions.

antiprothrombin (ˌantiproh'thrombin) a substance that retards the conversion of prothrombin into thrombin.

antipruritic (ˌantiˌprooə'ritik) 1. preventing or relieving itching. 2. an agent that counteracts itching.

antipsychotic (ˌantisie'kotik) effective in the management of manifestations of psychotic disorders; also, an agent that so acts. There are several classes of antipsychotic drugs (phenothiazines, thioxanthines, dibenzazepines, and butyrophenones), all of which may act by the same mechanism, i.e., blockade of dopaminergic receptors in the central nervous system. Called also NEUROLEPTIC and major tranquillizer.

antipyretic (ˌantipie'retik) 1. effective against fever. 2. an agent that relieves fever. Cold packs, aspirin and quinine are all antipyretics. Antipyretic drugs dilate the blood vessels near the surface of the skin, thereby allowing more blood to flow through the skin, where it can be cooled by the air. Also, an antipyretic can increase perspiration, the evaporation of which cools the body.

antipyrotic (ˌantipie'rotik) 1. effective in the treatment of burns. 2. an agent used in the treatment of burns.

antirachitic (ˌantirə'kitik) therapeutically effective against rickets.

anti-rhesus serum (ˌanti'reesəs) a substance containing rhesus agglutinins produced in the blood of those who are rhesus-negative if the rhesus-positive antigen obtains access to it, e.g. by blood transfusion. Haemolysis and jaundice are the result. See RHESUS FACTOR.

antirheumatic (ˌantiroo'matik) an agent that suppresses a rheumatic disease process.

antirickettsial (ˌantiri'ketsi·əl) 1. effective against rickettsiae. 2. an agent effective against rickettsiae.

antiscorbutic (ˌantiskor'byootik) 1. preventing or relieving scurvy. 2. an agent that prevents or cures scurvy.

antisecretory (ˌantisi'kreetə·ree) 1. inhibiting or diminishing secretion; secretoinhibitory. 2. an agent that so acts, such as certain drugs that inhibit or diminish gastric secretions.

antisepsis (ˌanti'sepsis) prevention of sepsis by destruction of microorganisms and infective matter.

antiseptic (ˌanti'septik) 1. preventing sepsis. 2. any substance that inhibits the growth of bacteria, in contrast to a germicide, which kills bacteria outright. Antiseptics are not considered to include antibiotics, which are usually taken internally. The term antiseptic includes disinfectants, although most disinfectants are too strong to be applied to body tissue and are generally used to clean inanimate objects such as floors and bathroom fixtures.

Antiseptics are divided into two types: physical and chemical. The most important physical antiseptic is heat, applied by boiling, autoclaving, flaming, or burning. These are among the oldest and most effective methods of disinfecting contaminated objects, water, and food.

Antiseptics have many applications. They are used in treating wounds and infections, in sterilizing, as before an operation, and in general hygiene. Antiseptics also have an application in the preservation of food and in the purification of sewage. The wide variety of antiseptics, their strength and the speed at which they work are all factors that influence the choice of which one to use for a specific job. See also STERILIZATION.

urinary a. a drug that is excreted mainly by way of the urine and performs its antiseptic action in the bladder. These drugs may be given before examination of or operation on the urinary tract, and they are sometimes used to treat urinary tract infections.

antiserum (ˌanti'siə·rəm) a serum containing antibodies. It may be obtained from an animal or human that has been subjected to the action of antigen either by injection into the tissues or blood or by infection. See also IMMUNITY and IMMUNIZATION.

antisialagogue (ˌantisie'aləgog) an agent that inhibits the flow of saliva.
antisialic (ˌantisie'alik) checking the flow of saliva.
antisocial (ˌanti'sohshəl) denoting a personality disorder marked by a basic lack of socialization and repeated conflict with society.
antispasmodic (ˌantispaz'modik) 1. preventing or relieving spasms. 2. an agent that prevents or relieves spasms.
antistatic (ˌanti'statik) relating to measures taken to prevent the build-up of static electricity.
antistreptococcal (ˌantiˌstreptə'kok'l) counteracting streptococcal infection.
antisudorific (ˌantiˌsyoodə'rifik) 1. inhibiting perspiration. 2. an agent that inhibits perspiration.
antisyphilitic (ˌantisifi'litik) 1. counteracting syphilis. 2. a remedy for syphilis.
antithenar (ˌanti'theenah) placed opposite to the palm or sole.
antithrombin (ˌanti'thrombin) any naturally occurring or therapeutically administered substance that neutralizes the action of thrombin and thus limits or restricts blood coagulation.
a. I a term referring to the capacity of fibrin to adsorb thrombin and thus neutralize it.
a. III a plasma protein (alpha$_2$-globulin) that inactivates thrombin; it is also a heparin cofactor and an inhibitor of certain coagulation factors.
antithrombocytic (ˌantiˌthrombə'sitik) 1. preventing the aggregation of blood platelets (thrombocytes). 2. an antithrombocytic agent.
antithromboplastin (ˌantiˌthromboh'plastin) any agent or substance that prevents or interferes with the interaction of blood clotting factors as they generate prothrombinase (thromboplastin).
antithrombotic (ˌantithrom'botik) 1. preventing or interfering with the formation of thrombi. 2. an agent that interferes with thrombus formation.
antithyroid (ˌanti'thieroyd) suppressing thyroid activity.
antitoxin (ˌanti'toksin) a particular kind of ANTIBODY produced in the body in response to the presence of a toxin (see also IMMUNITY). adj. **antitoxic.**
botulinum a. preparation from the serum of healthy horses immunized against botulinum toxins A, B and E. The polyvalent serum is used in the treatment of botulism. Stocks are maintained at selected hospital centres in the UK.
diphtheria a. preparation from the serum of healthy animals, usually the horse, immunized against diphtheria toxin. Used in the treatment of diphtheria and for the protection of previously unimmunized persons exposed to infection.
gas gangrene a. preparation from the serum of healthy animals, usually the horse, immunized against the toxins of gas-producing organisms of the genus *Clostridium*. Formerly used in the treatment of gas gangrene, but now replaced by penicillin treatment and high-pressure oxygen therapy.
tetanus a. preparation from the serum of healthy animals, usually the horse, immunized against tetanus toxin. Used in the treatment of tetanus and in the prevention of tetanus in the wounded. Now largely superseded by human tetanus immunoglobulin (HTIG).
antitragus (ˌanti'traygəs) a projection on the ear opposite the tragus.
antitrope ('antiˌtrohp) one of two structures that are similar but oppositely oriented, like a right and a left glove.
α_1-antitrypsin (ˌalfəwunˌanti'tripsin) alpha$_1$-antitrypsin.
antituberculotic (ˌantityuhˌbərkyuh'lotik) counteracting tuberculosis.
antitussive (ˌanti'tusiv) 1. effective against cough. 2. an agent that suppresses coughing.
antiulcerative (ˌanti'ulsəˌraytiv) 1. preventing the formation or promoting the healing of ulcers. 2. an agent that so acts.
antivenereal (ˌantivə'niə·ri·əl) counteracting venereal disease.
antivenin (ˌanti'venin) a material used to neutralize the venom of a poisonous animal.
antiviral (ˌanti'vierəl) 1. effective against viruses. 2. an agent effective against viruses.
antivitamin (ˌanti'vitəmin) a substance that inactivates a vitamin.
antixerotic (ˌantizə'rotik) preventing dryness.
antr(o)- word element. [L.] *chamber, cavity;* often used with specific reference to the maxillary antrum or sinus.
antrectomy (an'trektəmee) excision of an antrum.
antritis (an'trietis) inflammation of an antrum, especially of the antrum of Highmore (maxillary sinus).
antrocele ('antrohˌseel) accumulation of fluid in the maxillary antrum (sinus).
antronasal (ˌantroh'nayz'l) pertaining to the maxillary antrum (sinus) and nasal fossa.
antroscope ('antrəˌskohp) an instrument for inspecting the maxillary antrum (sinus).
antrostomy (an'trostəmee) incision of an antrum with drainage.
antrotomy (an'trotəmee) incision of an antrum.
antrotympanic (ˌantrohtim'panik) pertaining to the tympanic (mastoid) antrum and tympanum.
antrum ('antrəm) pl. *antra* [L.] a cavity or chamber. adj. **antral.**
a. of Highmore maxillary sinus.
mastoid a. an air space in the mastoid portion of the temporal bone communicating with the middle ear and the mastoid cells.
a. maxillare, maxillary a. maxillary sinus.
pyloric a., a. pyloricum the proximal, expanded portion of the pyloric part of the stomach.
tympanic a., a. tympanicum mastoid antrum.
Anturan ('antyuhˌran) trademark for a preparation of sulphinpyrazone, a uricosuric agent used in the longterm management of hyperuricaemia and gout.
anuclear (ay'nyookli·ə) having no nucleus.
anulus ('anyuhləs) pl. *anuli* [L.] alternative spelling of *annulus*; used in names of certain ringlike or encircling structures of the body.
anuresis (ˌanyuh'reesis) 1. retention of urine in the bladder. 2. anuria. adj. **anuretic.**
anuria (ə'nyooə·ri·ə) complete suppression of urine formation by the kidney. adj. **anuric.**
anus ('aynəs) the opening of the rectum on the body surface.
imperforate a. congenital absence of the normal opening of the rectum.
Anusol ('anyuhˌsol) trademark for a fixed combination preparation of bismuth subgallate, bismuth resorcin compound, benzyl benzoate, Peruvian balsam, zinc oxide, and either pramoxine hydrochloride or (in Anusol-HC) hydrocortisone acetate; used for relief of anorectal pain and itching.
anvil ('anvil) incus; the middle of the three bones of the ear.
anxiety (ang'zieətee) a feeling of uneasiness, apprehension, or dread. This may be rational, such as the anxiety about making good in a new job, about one's own or someone else's illness, about passing an examination or about moving to a new community. People also feel realistic anxiety about world dangers, such as the possiblity of nuclear war, and about social

and economic changes that may affect their livelihood or way of living. Modern mass communications tend to intensify normal anxieties about large issues by dramatizing minor incidents as though they were major crises.

A certain amount of unrealistic and irrational anxiety also is part of most people's experience. Some degree of generalized anxiety seems to be an unavoidable part of the human personality, since life is full of uncertainties and human beings have an awareness of past and future. Certain periods of life also generate increased anxiety; adolescence and middle age are especially anxious times for many. Persons who spend much of their time alone are likely to suffer more anxiety than those who live and work with others.

Most persons find healthy ways to deal with their normal quota of anxiety. They seek out friends and interesting activities; they take their minds off their own anxious feelings by listening to and doing things for other people. The enjoyment of art, music and literature, especially when it is shared, is an antidote to anxiety. The physical activity of games and sports, preferably with companions and out of doors, is one of the best antidotes. A good walk often dissipates an anxious mood.

Overindulgence in alcohol does not alleviate anxiety but only makes it worse. When a cause of anxiety is real, then the healthy step is to take realistic measures against it; for example, a real anxiety about money should be dealt with by improving money management or income or both.

When anxiety is chronic and not traceable to any specific cause, or when it interferes with normal activity, then it is neurotic, and the sufferer is in need of some wholesome self-examination and possible expert help.

Anxiety that needs attention can often be readily recognized by family or friends or by the general practitioner. Parents should be alert to symptoms of anxiety in their children. For instance, a child may develop compulsive habits, like overeating, or he may lose his appetite for no apparent reason. He may seem to want to spend an abnormal amount of time on his own, he may have difficulty with his schoolwork, or he may develop frequent headaches or stomach aches as a result of anxiety about school or friends. In a younger child, excessive thumbsucking or an unusual attachment to a particular plaything can sometimes be a sign of the kind of anxiety that needs professional help. Any important change in a young child's life, such as moving to a new home or the illness or absence of a parent, can give rise to behavioural problems stemming from anxiety. Similarly in adults, insomnia, recurrent headaches or the development of compulsive habits may be signs of chronic anxiety.

Whether it is purely psychological or arises from a real situation, severe anxiety can often be controlled by the proper use of medications, such as tranquillizers, under a doctor's care, though such drugs are only short-term solutions as there is a risk of dependence. PSYCHOTHERAPY is frequently the most effective method to relieve cases of chronic anxiety.

a.-equivalent a psychoanalytic term for the physical symptoms that substitute for conscious awareness of anxiety, such as a racing heart, trembling, light-headedness, sweating, rapid breathing, etc. It is not used for these sympathetic reactions when the individual is conscious of being anxious. **free-floating a.** fear in the absence of known cause for anxiety.

a. neurosis a neurosis characterized by anxiety or extreme fear without apparent cause. Anxiety is regarded as pathological when the individual cannot control his emotions and the anxiety interferes with effectiveness in living and the achievement of desired goals or satisfactions. The neurosis may be manifest as organic pain or physical illness.

separation a. apprehension due to removal of significant persons or familiar surroundings, common in infants 6 to 10 months old.

anxiolytic (ˌangzieoh'litik) a mild sedative, such as diazepam (Valium), used for relief of anxiety. Anxiolytics may, however, quickly cause dependence and are not suitable for long-term administration. Called also antianxiety agent and minor tranquillizer.

aorta (ay'awtə) pl. *aortae,aortas* [Gr.] the great artery arising from the left ventricle, being the main trunk from which the systemic arterial system proceeds. See CIRCULATORY SYSTEM.

overriding a. a congenital anomaly occurring in Fallot's tetralogy, in which the aorta is displaced to the right so that it appears to arise from both ventricles and straddles the ventricular septal defect.

aortalgia (ˌay·aw'talji·ə) pain in the region of the aorta.

aortic (ay'awtik) pertaining to the aorta.

a. arch syndrome any of a group of disorders leading to occlusion of the arteries arising from the aortic arch; such occlusion may be caused by atherosclerosis, arterial embolism, etc. See also PULSELESS DISEASE.

a. bodies small neurovascular structures on either side of the aorta in the region of the aortic arch, containing chemoreceptors that play a role in reflex regulation of respiration.

a. septal defect a congenital anomaly in which there is abnormal communication between the ascending aorta and the pulmonary artery just above the semilunar valves.

a. valve a semilunar valve that guards the orifice between the left ventricle and the aorta.

aortitis (ˌay·aw'tietis) inflammation of the aorta.

aortocoronary (ay·awtoh'korənə·ree) pertaining to or communicating with the aorta and coronary arteries.

aortogram (ay'awtohˌgram) the film produced by aortography.

aortography (ay·aw'tografee) radiography of the aorta after introduction into it of a water-soluble contrast medium.

catheter a. aortography via a catheter which has been introduced into the aorta via a peripheral artery, usually a femoral artery.

translumbar a. aortography following direct needle puncture of the aorta.

aortopathy (ˌay·aw'topəthee) any disease of the aorta.

aortorrhaphy (ˌay·aw'to·rəfee) suture of the aorta.

aortosclerosis (ayˌawtohsklə'rohsis) sclerosis of the aorta.

aortostenosis (ayˌawtohstə'nohsis) narrowing of the aorta.

aortotomy (ˌay·aw'totəmee) incision of the aorta.

AP angina pectoris; anteroposterior; arterial pressure.

apancreatic (ˌaypangkri'atik) due to absence of the pancreas.

aparalytic (ay'parə'litik) characterized by absence of paralysis.

apathic (ə'pathik) without sensation or feeling.

apathism ('apəˌthizəm) slowness of response to stimuli.

apathy ('apəthee) reactive absence of emotions. adj. **apathetic.**

aperient (ə'piəri·ənt) 1. mildly cathartic. 2. a gentle purgative.

aperistalsis (ˌayperi'stalsis) absence of peristaltic action.

Apert's syndrome (a'pairz) a congenital abnormality in which there is fusion at birth of all the cranial sutures in addition to syndactyly (webbed fingers).

apertura (ˌapə'tyoo·rə) pl. *aperturae* [L.] aperture.
aperture ('apəchə) an opening.
numerical a. an expression of the measure of efficiency of a microscope objective.
apex ('aypeks) pl. *apices* [L.] the pointed end of a cone-shaped part. adj. **apical.**
root a. the terminal end of the root of the tooth.
Apgar score ('apgah) a method for determining an infant's condition at birth by scoring the heart rate, respiratory effort, muscle tone, reflex irritability, and colour (see accompanying table). The infant is rated from 0 to 2 on each of the five items, the highest possible score being 10. Each of the factors is rated 60 seconds after birth and again five minutes later. The Apgar score is useful as a predictive measure of neonatal difficulties.

Apgar score

Signs	0	1	2
Colour	White	Blue	Pink
Respiratory effort	Absent	Weak irregular gasping	Good regular crying
Heart beat	Absent	Less than 100 beats/min	More than 100 beats/min, regular
Muscle tone	Limp and flaccid	Some flexion of extremities	Vigorous movement, limbs well flexed
Response to stimuli	Absent	Facial grimace only	Cough, sneeze, gasp or limb flexion

At one minute:

A score of 8–10 = No birth asphyxia
5–7 = Mild birth asphyxia
3–4 = Moderate birth asphyxia
0–2 = Severe birth asphyxia

At five minutes:

The score gives a more accurate prediction of the quality of life and survival. A low score at five minutes is more serious than a low score at one minute.

aphagia (ə'fayji·ə, ay-) loss of the power of swallowing.
aphakia (ay-, ə'fayki·ə, -'fak-) absence of the lens of an eye, occurring congenitally or as a result of trauma or surgery. adj. **aphakic.**
aphalangia (ˌayfə'lanji·ə) absence of fingers or toes.
aphasia (ə'fayzi·ə, ay-) defect or loss of the power of expression by speech, writing, or signs, or of comprehension of spoken or written language, due to disease or injury of the brain centres. Partial loss is called also DYSPHASIA.

PATIENT CARE. The recovery period typically is very long, sometimes extending to months and years. Because communication is such a vital part of everyday living, loss of the capacity for verbal expression, whether in speaking or writing, can profoundly affect the personality and behaviour of an aphasic patient. As a result he often becomes egocentric and frequently has an intense need for acceptance of his views and for immediate gratification of his desires.

Although aphasics usually require extensive treatment by specially trained speech therapists, all persons concerned with the care of the patient should practise simple techniques that will help minimize frustration and improve communication with the aphasic patient.

It is important to realize that inability to speak or write coherently does not necessarily mean that there is a loss of mental competence. The goal of care for an aphasic patient is to stimulate communication and gradually guide him to appropriate responses. Techniques that can help achieve this goal can be used by all members of the health care team and by family members and friends. For example, *self-talk* helps the aphasic associate activities with specific words. In essence, the nurse or other person who is engaged in the performance of a task in the presence of the patient talks about what he or she is doing while performing the activity. *Parallel-talk* describes what the *patient* is doing as he performs some activity. In *expansion*, the person communicating with the patient completes the patient's verbalization when he is unable to do so, but without adding new information. In *modelling*, the patient's sentences are completed and new information is added. All of these techniques must be used without being condescending to the patient or treating him as if he were a child.

Other helpful approaches include providing a quiet and orderly environment that does not overstimulate the patient. The patient should be spoken to slowly, distinctly, and in a normal tone; it certainly is not helpful to shout at a noncommunicative aphasic, because his problem is not with hearing but with responding. Aphasics often have difficulty reacting to a normal pace of speaking, and may complain when bombarded with too many words and messages at one time. In the process of communication the sender encodes or composes a message and transmits it. The receiver must decode or interpret the message and then respond to it. If there is too much information for the receiver to process, he becomes confused, frustrated, and unable to respond as he should.

The techniques and guidelines mentioned are but a few of the approaches one might take to help the aphasic patient cope with his problems and recover from his loss of communicating skills. In planning the care of an aphasic it is essential that specific problems are identified through assessment, that techniques and methods are planned and evaluated for their effectiveness, and that those which are most appropriate are conveyed to all persons who are responsible for the

patient's care.
amnestic a. anomic aphasia.
anomic a. amnestic or nominal aphasia; inability to name objects, qualities, or conditions.
ataxic a. expressive aphasia.
auditory a. loss of ability to comprehend spoken language; word deafness.
Broca's a. expressive aphasia.
conduction a. aphasia due to a lesion of the pathway between the sensory and motor speech centres.
expressive a. that in which the patient understands written and spoken words and knows what he wants to say, but cannot utter the words. Called also apraxia of speech, ataxic aphasia, Broca's aphasia, motor aphasia, and nonfluent aphasia.
fluent a. that in which speech is well articulated and grammatically correct but is lacking in content and meaning.
global a. total aphasia involving all the functions that go to make up speech and communication.
jargon a. paraphasia; aphasia characterized by utterance of meaningless phrases.
mixed a. combined expressive and receptive aphasia.
motor a. expressive aphasia.
nominal a. anomic aphasia.
nonfluent a. that in which little speech is produced and is uttered slowly, with great effort and poor articulation; due to a lesion in Broca's area.
receptive a. inability to understand written, spoken, or tactile speech symbols.
sensory a. receptive aphasia.
visual a. alexia.

aphasic (ə'fayzik, ay-) 1. pertaining to or affected with aphasia. 2. a person affected with aphasia.

aphasiologist (ə,fayzi'oləjist, ay-) a specialist in aphasiology.

aphasiology (ə,fayzi'oləjee, ay-) scientific study of aphasia and specific neurological lesions producing it.

aphemia (ə'feemi·ə, ay-) loss of the power of speech due to a central lesion.

apheresis (,afə'reesis) any procedure in which blood is withdrawn from a donor, a portion (plasma, leukocytes, platelets, etc.) is separated and retained, and the remainder is retransfused into the donor. It includes leukapheresis, thrombocytapheresis, etc. Called also pheresis.

aphonia (ə'fohni·ə, ay-) loss of the voice; inability to produce vocal sounds.
a. clericorum loss of the voice from overuse, as by clergymen.

aphonic (ay'fonik) 1. pertaining to aphonia. 2. without audible sound.

aphose ('ayfohz) any subjective visual sensation due to absence or interruption of light sensation.

aphrasia (ay'frayzi·ə) inability to speak.

aphrenia (ay'freeni·ə) dementia.

aphrodisiac (,afrə'diziak) 1. arousing sexual desire. 2. a drug that arouses sexual desire.

aphtha ('afthə) pl. *aphthae* [L.] (usually plural) small ulcers, especially the whitish or reddish spots in the mouth characteristic of aphthous stomatitis. adj. **aphthous.**

aphthosis (af'thohsis) a condition marked by presence of aphthae.

apical ('aypik'l) pertaining to an apex.

apicectomy (,aypi'sektəmee) 1. excision of the apex of the petrous portion of the temporal bone. 2. excision of the apical portion of the root of a tooth through an opening in overlying tissues of the jaw.

apicitis (,aypi'sietis) inflammation of the apex of the lung.

apicolysis (,aypi'kolisis) surgical collapse of the apex of the lung to obliterate the apical cavity.

aplasia (ə'playzi·ə, ay-) defective development or complete absence of an organ due to failure of development of the embryonic primordium.

aplastic (ay'plastik) pertaining to or characterized by aplasia; having no tendency to develop into new tissue.
a. anaemia a form of anaemia unresponsive to specific antianaemia therapy, often accompanied by granulocytopenia and thrombocytopenia, in which the bone marrow is usually acellular or hypoplastic and fails to produce adequate numbers of blood elements. Precipitating factors include drugs and viral infection, but the cause is often not determined.

apneumia (ap'nyoomi·ə) congenital absence of the lungs.

apneusis (ap'nyoosis) sustained, gasping inspiration followed by short, inefficient expiration, which can continue to the point of asphyxia. Often associated with lesions in the respiratory centre in the brain. adj. **apneustic.**

apnoea ('apni·ə, ap'neeə) 1. temporary cessation of breathing. 2. asphyxia. adj. **apnoeic.**
sleep a. transient attacks of failure of autonomic control of respiration, becoming more pronounced during sleep and resulting in acidosis and pulmonary arteriolar vasoconstriction and hypertension.

apo- word element. [Gr.] *away from, separated.*

apochromatic (,apəkroh'matik) free from chromatic aberration. Called also *achromatic.*

apocrine ('apəkrien, -krin) denoting that type of glandular secretion in which the secretory products become concentrated at the free end of the secreting cell and are thrown off, along with the portion of the cell where they have accumulated, as in the mammary gland; cf. holocrine and merocrine.

apodia (ay'pohdi·ə) congenital absence of the feet.

apoenzyme (,apoh'enziem) the protein component of an enzyme that requires the presence of the prosthetic group (coenzyme) to form the functioning enzyme.

apoferritin (,apoh'feritin) an apoprotein that can bind many atoms of iron per molecule to form ferritin, the form in which iron is stored in the liver and other tissues.

apogee ('apəjee) the state of greatest severity of a disease.

apolar (ay'pohlə) having neither poles nor processes; without polarity.

apolipoprotein (,apoh,lipoh'prohteen) a protein moiety occurring in plasma lipoproteins; there are five families of apolipoproteins, designated A–E.

apomorphine (,apoh'mawfeen) an alkaloid from morphine.

aponeurectomy (,apohnyuh'rektəmee) excision of an aponeurosis.

aponeurorrhaphy (,apohnyuh'ro·rəfee) repair of an aponeurosis.

aponeurosis (a,ponyuh'rohsis) pl. *aponeuroses* [Gr.] a sheetlike tendinous expansion, mainly serving to connect a muscle with the parts it moves. adj. **aponeurotic.**

aponeurositis (a,ponyuhroh'sietis) inflammation of an aponeurosis.

aponeurotomy (a,ponyuh'rotəmee) incision of an aponeurosis.

apophyseal (,apə'fizi·əl) pertaining to an apophysis.

apophysis (ə'pofisis) pl. *apophyses* [Gr.] any outgrowth or swelling, especially a bony outgrowth that has never been entirely separated from the bone of which it forms a part, such as a process, tubercle, or tuberosity.

apophysitis (ə,pofi'sietis) inflammation of an apophysis.

apoplectiform, apoplectoid (,apə'plekti,fawm, ,apə-

'plektoyd) resembling apoplexy.

apoplexy ('apə,pleksee) copious extravasation of blood into an organ; often used alone to designate such extravasations into the brain (cerebral apoplexy) after rupture of an intracranial blood vessel; stroke. The term is extended by some to include occlusive cerebrovascular lesions. See also STROKE. adj. **apoplectic.**

apoprotein (,apoh'prohteen) the protein moiety of a molecule or complex, as of a lipoprotein.

aporepressor (,apohri'presə) a repressor that is inactive until it combines with a corepressor.

apostasis (ə'postəsis) 1. an abscess. 2. the end or crisis of an attack or disease.

aposthia (ə'posthi·ə) congenital absence of the prepuce.

apothecaries' weights and measures (ə'pothi,kə·reez) a system used for measuring and weighing drugs and solutions. Now replaced by the metric system.

In the apothecaries' system fractions are used to designate portions of a unit of measure: e.g., one-fourth grain is written gr. 1/4. The fraction 1/2 is written ss.

There are two symbols in this system which are sometimes confused and always must be written clearly. These are the symbols for drams and ounces. Small Roman numerals are used after the symbols. For example, ʒiss reads drams one and one-half; ℥iii reads ounces three.

apothecary (ə'pothə,kə·ree) a pharmacist; a person who compounds and dispenses drugs.

apotripsis (,apoh'tripsis) removal of a corneal opacity.

apparatus (,apə'raytəs) an arrangement of a number of parts acting together to perform a special function.

Golgi a. a complex cellular organelle composed of a series of closely stacked, flattened, elongated vesicles that are involved in the synthesis of secretory proteins, particularly glycoproteins and lipoproteins; called also Golgi complex (see also GOLGI APPARATUS).

appendage (ə'pendij) a less important portion of an organ, or an outgrowth, such as a tail. Also, a limb or limblike structure.

appendectomy (,apən'dektəmee) excision of the vermiform appendix.

appendicectomy (ə,pendi'sektəmee) appendectomy.

appendicitis (ə,pendi'sietis) inflammation of the vermiform appendix. When performed early, appendectomy is comparatively simple and safe. When the appendix becomes inflamed and infected, rupture may occur within a matter of hours. Rupture of the appendix leads to PERITONITIS.

SYMPTOMS. The symptoms of appendicitis are pain, nausea, vomiting, and fever; children tend to have a high fever. The pain typically begins in the umbilical region and eventually localizes in the right lower quadrant of the abdomen over the site of the appendix, though this is not always so. It tends to be persistent and is aggravated by movement. Rebound tenderness occurs when the abdomen is deeply palpated on the right side and the hand is quickly removed from the abdomen. Rectal examination may elicit tenderness.

Other conditions which may be mistaken for appendicitis are cholecystitis, kidney infection on the right side, and salpingitis in women.

PATIENT CARE. When appendicitis is suspected because of symptoms exhibited by the patient, a doctor should be notified immediately. The patient should lie down and remain as quiet as possible. It is best to give him nothing by mouth, and because of the danger of aggravating the condition and possibly causing rupture of the appendix, cathartics and laxatives are contraindicated. After the patient has been seen by the doctor and a diagnosis of appendicitis has been established, surgical removal of the appendix (appendectomy) will probably be performed as soon as possible.

During the preoperative phase it may be necessary to hydrate the patient with intravenous fluids, especially when there has been prolonged nausea and vomiting. Removal of the gastric contents by aspiration at regular intervals using a nasogastric (NG) tube is necessary in some cases.

It should be remembered that the patient needing emergency surgery will have had little time to prepare for hospitalization or adjust to the idea of an operation and his stress levels will be high. Careful explanations of the need for such procedures should be given (and repeated as necessary) and the patient's questions answered.

Postoperative care is routine unless the appendix was ruptured. This warrants diligent nursing care to overcome the effects of peritonitis with the resultant shifting of body fluids, hypovolaemia, and septic shock. Antibacterial drugs are administered to combat the infection. Gastric and intestinal decompression via a NG tube is maintained, and some surgeons advocate intraperitoneal draining.

The most common complications of appendectomy and peritonitis are: (1) infection of the surgical wound, (2) paralytic ileus due to irritation of the small bowel, (3) intra-abdominal abscesses, and (4) obstruction and adhesions.

Ongoing assessment of the patient includes fluid balance charts, which are maintained until the passing of flatus and faecal material.

appendicolithiasis (ə,pendi,kohli'thieəsis) formation of calculi in the vermiform appendix.

appendicolysis (ə,pendi'kolisis) a method of removing an appendix fixed by adhesions.

appendicostomy (ə,pendi'kostəmee) surgical creation of an opening into the caecum via the appendix.

appendicular (,apen'dikyuhlə) 1. pertaining to an appendix or appendage. 2. pertaining to the limbs.

appendix (ə'pendiks) pl. *appendices* [L.] 1. a slender outgrowth or appendage. 2. the vermiform appendix, a small appendage near the juncture of the small intestine and the large intestine (ileocaecal valve). An apparently useless structure, it can be the source of a serious illness, APPENDICITIS. adj. **appendiceal.**

apperception (,apə'sepshən) conscious perception of a sensory stimulus.

appestat ('apistat) a brain centre (probably in the hypothalamus) concerned in controlling the appetite.

appetite ('api,tiet) the desire for food. It is stimulated by the sight, smell, or thought of food and accompanied by the flow of saliva in the mouth and gastric juice in the stomach. The stomach wall also receives an extra blood supply in preparation for its digestive activity.

Appetite is psychological, dependent on memory and associations, as compared with hunger, which is physiologically aroused by the body's need for food. Appetite can be discouraged by unattractive food, surroundings, or company, and by emotional states such as anxiety, irritation, anger, and fear.

Chronic loss of appetite is known as anorexia. It may be a symptom of physical disorders, or it may be related to emotional disturbances, in which case it is known as ANOREXIA NERVOSA. Excessive appetite may be an indication of metabolic disorders or may be caused by emotional disturbances. This latter condition is especially common among children, particularly girls, who may develop a habit of compulsive eating to compensate for a feeling of insecurity.

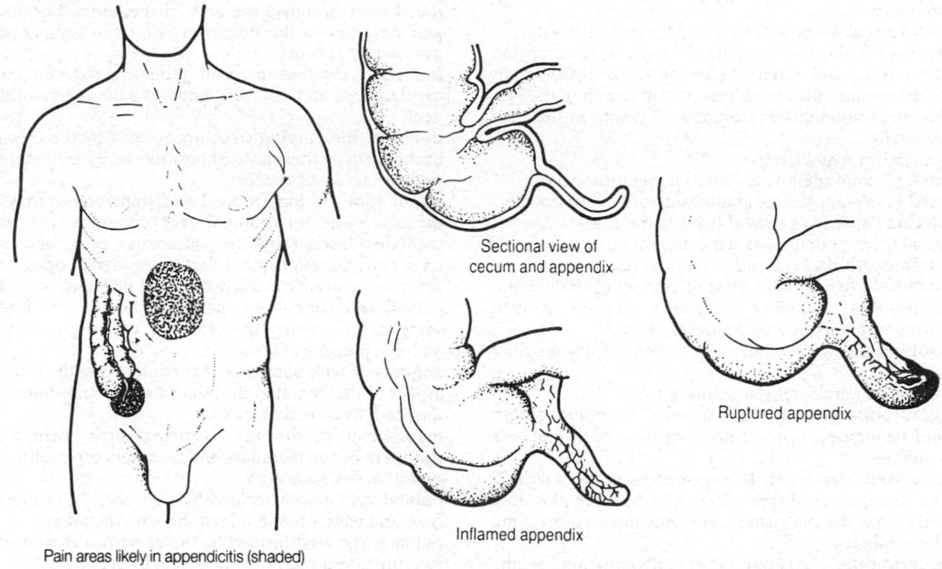

Appendix

applanation tonometer (aplə'nayshən) an instrument for determining intraocular pressure. Used clinically in the detection of glaucoma.

appliance (ə'plieəns) a device used for performing a particular function.

applicator ('aplı,kaytə) any device used to apply medication or treatment to a particular part of the body. See also PROBANG.

apposition (,apə'zishən) the placement or position of adjacent structures or parts so that they can come into contact.

apprehension (,apri'henshən) 1. perception and understanding. 2. anticipatory fear or anxiety.

approximal (ə'proksiməl) close together.

approximation (ə'proksi'mayshən) 1. the act or process of bringing into proximity or apposition. 2. a numerical value of limited accuracy.

successive a. a technique in behaviour therapy in which new behaviour is produced by providing reinforcement for progressively closer approximations of the final desired behaviour. Called also shaping.

apraxia (ə'praksi·ə) loss of ability to carry out familiar purposeful movements in the absence of sensory or motor impairment, especially impairment of the ability to use objects correctly.

amnestic a. loss of ability to carry out a movement on command due to inability to remember the command.

a. of gait a common disorder of the elderly in which the patient walks with a broad-based gait, taking short steps and placing the feet flat on the ground.

motor a. loss of ability to make proper use of an object, although its proper nature is recognized.

sensory a. loss of ability to make proper use of an object due to lack of perception of its purpose.

Apresoline (ə'presə,leen) trademark for preparations of hydralazine hydrochloride, an antihypertensive drug.

aproctia (ay'prokshi·ə) imperforate anus.

aprosopia (,ayproh'sohpi·ə) a developmental anomaly with partial or complete absence of the face.

aptitude ('apti,tyood) the natural ability or capacity to acquire mental and physical skills.

aptyalism (ap'tieə,lizəm) deficiency or absence of saliva.

APUD cells ('apəd) (*amine precursor uptake and decarboxylation*) a group of cells of common embryonic origin that secrete most of the body's hormones, with the exception of steroids. APUD cells comprise both specialized neurons and other endocrine cells. These cells synthesize structurally related polypeptides and biogenic amines. The acronym APUD derives from the fact that polypeptide production is linked to the uptake of a precursor amino acid and its decarboxylation in the cell to produce an amine. Examples of the peptide hormones are insulin, ACTH, glucagon, and antidiuretic hormone. Examples of the amine hormones are dopamine, noradrenaline, serotonin, and histamine.

apudoma (,apə'dohmə) a tumour derived from APUD cells, many of which secrete ectopic HORMONES.

apus ('aypəs) an individual without feet.

apyogenous (,aypie'ojənəs) not caused by pus.

apyretic (,aypie'retik) without fever.

apyrexia (,aypie'reksi·ə) absence of fever.

apyrogenic (ay,pierə'jenik) not producing fever.

aq. [L.] *aqua* (water).

aq. dest. *aqua destillata* (distilled water).

aqua ('akwə) [L] 1. water, H_2O. 2. a saturated solution of a volatile oil or other aromatic or volatile substance in purified water.

aquaphobia (,akwə'fohbi·ə) morbid fear of water.

aqueduct ('akwə,dukt) any canal or passage.

cerebral a. a narrow channel in the midbrain connecting the third and fourth ventricles and containing cerebrospinal fluid.

a. of cochlea a foramen in the temporal bone for a vein from the cochlea.

a. of Fallopius the canal for the facial nerve in pars petrosa of the temporal bone.

sylvian a., a. of Sylvius, ventricular a. cerebral aqueduct.

aqueous ('akwi·əs, 'ay-) watery; prepared with water.

a. humour the fluid produced in the eye, occupying the anterior and posterior chambers, and diffusing out of the eye into the blood; regarded as lymph of the eye, its composition differs from that of lymph in the body generally.

Ar chemical symbol, *argon.*

ara-A (a·rə'ay) adenine arabinoside; see VIDARABINE.

ara-C (a·rə'see) cytosine arabinoside; see CYTARABINE.

Arachis ('arəkis) a genus of leguminous plants.

A. oil peanut oil; used as substitute for olive oil.

arachnephobia (ə,rakni'fohbi·ə) arachnophobia.

Arachnida (ə'raknidə) a class of animals of the phylum Arthropoda, including 12 orders, comprising such forms as spiders, scorpions, ticks, and mites.

arachnidism (ə'rakni,dizəm) poisoning from a spider bite.

arachnitis (,arək'nietis) arachnoiditis.

arachnodactyly (ə,raknoh'daktilee) extreme length and slenderness of the fingers or toes, as in Marfan's syndrome.

arachnoid (ə'raknoyd) 1. resembling a spider's web. 2. the delicate membrane interposed between the dura mater and the pia mater, and with them constituting the meninges.

arachnoiditis (ə,raknoy'dietis) inflammation of the arachnoid membrane.

arachnophobia (ə,raknoh'fohbi·ə) morbid fear of spiders.

Aran–Duchenne disease (a'randoo'shen) spinal muscular atrophy.

araphia (ə'rayfi·ə) failure of closure of the embryonic neural tube, the spinal cord developing as a flat plate. adj. **araphic.**

arbor ('ahbə) pl. *arbores* [L.] a tree.

a. vitae 1. treelike outlines seen on median section of the cerebellum. 2. a series of branching ridges within cervix uteri, which are thought by some to assist passage of spermatozoa and allow dilation during delivery.

arborescent (,ahbə'res'nt) branching like a tree.

arborization (,ahbə·rie'zayshən) a collection of branches, as the branching terminus of a nerve-cell process.

arbovirus (,ahboh'vierəs) a group of viruses that are transmitted to man by mosquitoes and ticks. See also VIRUS. adj. **arboviral.**

ARC Arthritis and Rheumatism Council.

arc (ahk) a part of the circumference of a circle, or a regularly curved line.

binauricular a. the arc across the top of the head from one auricular point to the other.

reflex a. the circuit travelled by impulses producing a reflex action: receptor organ, afferent nerve, nerve centre, efferent nerve, effector organ in a muscle. See also REFLEX.

arcate ('ahkayt) curved; bow-shaped.

arch (ahch) a structure of bowlike or curved outline.

abdominothoracic a. the lower boundary of the front of the thorax.

a. of aorta the curving portion between the ascending aorta and the descending aorta, giving rise to the brachiocephalic trunk, the left common carotid and the left subclavian artery.

aortic a's six paired vessels arching from the ventral to the dorsal aorta through the branchial clefts of fishes and amniote embryos. The development of these vessels varies from species to species. In mammalian fetal development, the first two and the fifth pairs of vessels disappear. The third pair develops to connect the internal carotid and common carotid arteries. The fourth pair becomes the arch of the aorta. The sixth pair develops as the ductus arteriosus to become the pulmonary arteries.

branchial a's four pairs of mesenchymal and later cartilaginous arches of the embryo in the region of the neck.

dental a. the curving structure formed by the crowns of the teeth in their normal position, or by the residual ridge after loss of the teeth.

a's of foot the longitudinal and transverse arches of the foot. The longitudinal arch comprises the pars medialis, formed by the calcaneus, talus, and the navicular, cuneiform and first three tarsal bones; and the pars lateralis, formed by the calcaneus, and the cuboid and lateral two metatarsal bones. The transverse arch comprises the navicular, cuneiform, cuboid and five metatarsal bones.

lingual a. a wire appliance that conforms to the lingual aspect of the dental arch, used to secure movement of the teeth in orthodontic work.

mandibular a. the first branchial arch, being the rudiment of the maxillary and mandibular regions.

neural a. vertebral arch.

palatal a. the arch formed by the roof of the mouth from the teeth on one side to those on the other.

pubic a. the arch formed by the conjoined rami of the ischium and pubis of the two sides of the body.

pulmonary a's the most caudal of the aortic arches, which become the pulmonary arteries.

tendinous a. a linear thickening of fascia over some part of a muscle.

vertebral a. the dorsal bony arch of a vertebra, composed of the laminae and pedicles of a vertebra.

zygomatic a. the arch formed by the processes of the zygomatic and temporal bones.

arch(i)- word element. [Gr.] *ancient, beginning, first, original.*

archencephalon (,ahken'kefəlon, -'sef-) the primitive brain from which the midbrain and forebrain develop.

archenteron (ah'kentə,ron) the central cavity that is the provisional gut in the gastrula; the primitive digestive cavity of the embryo.

archeokinetic (,ahkiohki'netik) relating to the primitive type of motor nerve mechanism as seen in the peripheral and ganglionic nervous systems.

archetype ('ahki,tiep) in jungian psychology, a structural component of the collective unconscious, which is an inherited idea derived from the life experience of all of the members of the race and contained in the individual unconscious. The archetypes are the ideas, modes of thought, and patterns of reaction that are typical of all humanity and represent the wisdom of the ages. They appear in personified or symbolized form in dreams and visions and in mythology, legends, religion, fairy tales, and art. See also JUNG.

archinephron (,ahki'nefron) the pronephros.

archipallium (,ahki'pali·əm) that portion of the pallium, or cerebral cortex, which phylogenetically is the first to show the characteristic layering of the cellular elements.

arciform ('ahsi,fawm) arcuate.

arctation (ahk'tayshən) narrowing of an opening or canal.

arcuate ('ahkyoo·ət, -ayt) bent like a bow.

arcuation (,ahkyoo'ayshən) a bending or curvature.

arcus ('ahkəs) pl. *arcus* [L.] arch, bow.

a. adiposus arcus senilis.

a. juvenilis a condition identical to arcus senilis but occurring in young persons.

a. senilis an opaque line partially surrounding the margin of the cornea, usually occurring bilaterally in persons of 50 years or older as a result of lipoid degeneration. In younger subjects it can be associated with lipid abnormalities.

area ('air·ri·ə) pl. *areae,areas* [L.] a limited space or plane surface.

association a's areas of the cerebral cortex (excluding primary areas) connected with each other and with the neothalamus; they are responsible for higher mental and emotional processes, including memory, learning, etc.

Broca's motor speech a. an area comprising parts of the opercular and triangular portions of the inferior frontal gyrus; injury to this area may result in expressive APHASIA.

Broca's parolfactory a. see under BROCA.

Brodmann's a's specific occipital and preoccipital areas of the cerebral cortex, distinguished by differences in the arrangement of their six cellular layers, and identified by numbering each area. They are considered to be the seat of specific functions of the brain.

germinal a., a. germinativa embryonic disc.

Kiesselbach's a. an area on the anterior part of the nasal septum, richly supplied with capillaries, and a common site of epistaxis (nosebleed).

motor a. that area of the cerebral cortex which, on brief electrical stimulation, shows the lowest threshold and shortest latency for the production of muscle movement.

primary a. areas of the cerebral cortex comprising the motor and sensory regions.

psychomotor a. motor a.

silent a. an area of the brain in which pathological conditions may occur without producing symptoms.

a. subcallosa, subcallosal a. Broca's parolfactory area.

vocal a. the part of the glottis between the vocal cords.

areflexia (ˌayri'fleksi·ə) absence of the reflexes.

Arenaviridae (ˌarenə'viridee) a family of viruses comprising the arenaviruses.

arenavirus (ˌarenə'vierəs) any of a group of spherical or pleomorphic RNA viruses containing host cell-derived ribonucleoproteins, including the Lassa virus, lymphocytic choriomeningitis (LCM) virus, and Tacaribe viruses. The natural hosts are rodents.

areola (ə'reeələ) pl. *areolae* [L.] 1. a narrow zone surrounding a central area, e.g., the darkened area surrounding the NIPPLE of the mammary gland. 2. any minute space or interstice in a tissue.

Chaussier's a. the indurated area encircling a malignant pustule.

areolar (ə'reeələ) 1. containing minute spaces. 2. pertaining to an areola.

Argas ('ahgas) a genus of ticks parasitic in poultry and other birds and sometimes man.

Argasidae (ah'gasidee) a family of arthropods made up of the soft-bodied ticks.

argentaffin (ah'jentəfin) staining readily with silver salts without the prior use of a reducing agent; see also argentaffin CELL.

argentaffinoma (ahˌjentəfi'nohmə) a tumour arising from argentaffin cells, most frequently in the terminal ileum or the appendix; called also *carcinoid*. Such tumours produce CARCINOID SYNDROME.

argentum (ah'jentəm) [L.] *silver* (symbol Ag).

argillaceous (ˌahji'layshəs) composed of clay.

arginase ('ahjiˌnayz) an enzyme of the liver that splits arginine into urea and ornithine.

arginine ('ahjiˌneen, -ˌnin) a basic amino acid occurring in proteins.

argininosuccinic acid (ˌahji'neenohsukˌsinik) a compound normally formed in urea formation in the liver, but not normally present in urine.

argininosuccinicaciduria (ˌahjiˌneenohsukˌsinikˌasi'dyooə·ri·ə) excretion in the urine of argininosuccinic acid, a feature of an inborn error of metabolism marked also by mental handicap.

argon ('ahgon) a chemical element, atomic number 18, atomic weight 39.948, symbol Ar. See table of elements in Appendix 2.

Argyll Robertson pupil (ah'giel 'robətsən) a pupil that is miotic and responds to accommodative effort, but not to light.

argyria (ah'jieri·ə) poisoning by silver or its salts; chronic argyria is marked by a permanent ashen-gray discoloration of the skin, conjunctiva, and internal organs.

argyric (ah'jierik) pertaining to silver.

argyrism (ah'jierizəm) argyria.

argyrophil (ah'jierohfil) easily impregnated with silver once there has been pretreatment with a reducing agent.

argyrosis (ˌahjie'rohsis) argyria.

arhinia (ay'rieni·ə) congenital absence of the nose.

Arias-Stella reaction (ˌareeəs'stelə) nuclear and cellular hypertrophy of the endometrial epithelium, associated with the presence of chorionic tissue and seen in some cases of ectopic pregnancy.

ariboflavinosis (ayˌriebohˌflayvi'nohsis) deficiency of RIBOFLAVIN (vitamin B_2) in the diet, a condition marked by lesions in the corners of the mouth, on the lips, and around the nose and eyes, malaise, weakness, weight loss and, in severe cases, corneal or other eye changes and seborrhoeic dermatitis.

arm (ahm) 1. the upper extremity, from shoulder to elbow; often used to denote the entire extremity, from shoulder to wrist. 2. an armlike part.

brawny a. a hard, swollen condition of the arm due to lymphatic obstruction following mastectomy.

armamentarium (ˌahməmen'tair·ri·əm) the entire equipment of a practitioner, such as medicines, instruments, and books.

Arnold–Chiari malformation (deformity, syndrome) (ˌahn'ldki'ahree) a congenital anomaly in which the cerebellum and medulla oblongata protrude down into the cervical spinal canal through the foramen magnum; it is almost always associated with meningomyelocele and hydrocephalus.

Arnold's ganglion ('ahn'ldz) a parasympathetic ganglion immediately below the foramen ovale; its postganglionic fibres supply the parotid gland. Called also otic ganglion.

aromatic (ˌarə'matik) 1. having a spicy fragrance. 2. a stimulant, spicy medicine. 3. denoting a compound containing a resonance-stabilized ring, e.g., benzene or naphthalene.

arousal (ə'rowz'l) a state of alertness and increased response to stimuli.

arrachment (ˌarash'monh) the extraction of a membranous cataract via a corneal incision.

ARRC Associate, Royal Red Cross.

arrector (ə'rektə) pl. *arrectores* [L.] raising, or that which raises; an erector muscle.

a. pili pl. *arrectores pilorum* [L.] small muscle attached to the hair follicle of the skin; when contracted causes the hair to become more erect and produces the appearance known as goose flesh.

arrest (ə'rest) sudden cessation or stoppage.

cardiac a. sudden cessation of beating of the heart (see also CARDIAC ARREST).

epiphyseal a. premature arrest of the longitudinal growth of bone due to fusion of the epiphysis and diaphysis.

maturation a. interruption of the process of development, as of blood cells, before the final stage is reached.

ARRG Association for Research into Restricted Growth.

arrheno- (ə'reenoh) word element. [Gr.] *male, masculine.*

arrhenoblastoma (ə,reenohbla'stohmə) a rare ovarian tumour that causes virilization.

arrhinia (ay'rieni·ə) arhinia.

arrhythmia (ə'ridhmi·ə, ay-) variation from the normal rhythm, especially of the heartbeat. adj. **arrhythmic**.

sinus a. the physiological cyclic variation in heart rate related to vagal impulses to the sinoatrial node; it occurs commonly in children and in the aged.

arrhythmogenic (ə,ridhmə'jenik, ay-) producing or promoting arrhythmia.

arseniasis (,ahsə'nieəsis) arsenical poisoning.

arsenic ('ahsnik) a chemical element, atomic number 33, atomic weight 74.92, symbol As. (See table of elements in Appendix 2.) Arsenic compounds have been widely used in medicine; however, they have been replaced for the most part by antibiotics, which are less toxic and equally effective. Some of the arsenicals are used for infectious diseases, especially those caused by protozoa, and some skin disorders and blood dyscrasias also are treated with arsenic compounds. Since arsenic is highly toxic it must be administered with caution. The antidote for arsenic poisoning is DIMERCAPROL.

arsenical (ah'senik'l) 1. pertaining to arsenic. 2. a compound containing arsenic.

arsenoblast (ah'senohblast) the male element of a zygote; a male pronucleus.

Artane ('ahtayn) trademark for preparations of benzhexol hydrochloride, used as an anticholinergic in treatment of Parkinson's disease.

artefact ('ahti,fakt) a structure or appearance that is not natural, but is due to manipulation (man-made).

arteria (ah'tiə·ri·ə) pl. *arteriae* [L.] artery.

a. lusoria an abnormally situated vessel in the region of the aortic arch.

arterial (ah'tiə·ri·əl) pertaining to an artery or to the arteries.

a. thrombosis the presence of a thrombus in an artery. See also arterial THROMBOSIS.

arterialization (ah,tiə·ri·əlie'zayshən) the conversion of venous into arterial blood by the absorption of oxygen.

arteriectasis (ah,tiə·ri'ektəsis) dilation of an artery.

arteriectomy (ah,tiə·ri'ektəmee) excision of an artery.

arterio- word element. [L., Gr.] *artery.*

arteriogram (ah'tiə·rioh,gram) a radiograph of an artery.

arteriography (ah,tiə·ri'ografee) radiography of an artery or arterial system after injection of a contrast medium into the bloodstream.

catheter a. radiography of vessels after introduction of a contrast medium through a catheter inserted into an artery.

selective a. radiography of a specific vessel that is opacified by a contrast medium introduced directly into it, usually via a catheter.

translumbar a. see translumbar AORTOGRAPHY.

arteriol(o)- word element. [L.] *arteriole.*

arteriola (ah'tiə·ri'ohlə) pl. *arteriolae* [L.] arteriole.

arteriolae rectae renis branches of the arcuate arteries of the kidney that supply the renal pyramids.

arteriole (ah'tiə·ri,ohl) a minute arterial branch. adj. **arteriolar**.

arteriolith (ah'tiə·rioh,lith) a chalky concretion in an artery.

arteriolitis (ah,tiə·rioh'lietis) inflammation of arterioles.

arteriology (ah,tiə·ri'oləjee) sum of knowledge regarding the arteries.

arteriolonecrosis (ah,tiə·ri,ohlohna'krohsis) necrosis or destruction of arterioles.

arteriolosclerosis (ah,tiə·ri,ohlohsklə'rohsis) sclerosis and thickening of the walls of arterioles. The hyaline form may be associated with nephrosclerosis, the hyperplastic with malignant hypertension, nephrosclerosis, and scleroderma. adj. **arteriolosclerotic**.

arteriomotor (ah,tiə·rioh'mohtə) involving or causing dilation or constriction of arteries.

arteriomyomatosis (ah,tiə·rioh,mieohmə'tohsis) growth of muscular fibres in the walls of an artery, causing thickening.

arterionecrosis (ah,tiə·riohnə'krohsis) necrosis of arteries.

arteriopathy (ah,tiə·ri'opəthee) any disease of an artery.

hypertensive a. widespread involvement of the smaller arteries and arterioles, associated with hypertension and characterized primarily by hypertrophy of the tunica media.

arterioplasty (ah'tiə·rioh,plastee) plastic repair of an artery.

arteriopressor (ah,tiə·rioh'presə) increasing arterial blood pressure.

arteriorrhaphy (ah,tiə·ri'o·rəfee) suture of an artery.

arteriorrhoexis (ah,tiə·rioh'reksis) rupture of an artery.

arteriosclerosis (ah,tiə·riohsklə'rohsis) a group of diseases characterized by thickening and loss of elasticity of the arterial walls; popularly called 'hardening of the arteries'. adj. **arteriosclerotic**.

There are three main forms of arteriosclerosis: (1) ATHEROSCLEROSIS, in which plaques of fatty deposits form in the inner layer (*intima*) of the arteries; (2) Mönckeberg's arteriosclerosis, called also medial calcific sclerosis because of involvement of the middle layer (medial coat) of the arteries, where there is destruction of muscle and elastic fibres and formation of calcium deposits; and (3) arteriolar sclerosis (*arteriolosclerosis*), which is marked by thickening of the walls of small arteries (arterioles).

All three forms of arteriosclerosis may be present in the same patient, but in different blood vessels. Of the three types, atherosclerosis is the most common. When reference is made to hardening of the arteries, in most instances it is atherosclerosis that is meant. Frequently, the terms arteriosclerosis and atherosclerosis are used interchangeably.

a. obliterans arteriosclerosis in which proliferation of the intima has caused complete obliteration of the lumen of the artery.

arteriospasm (ah'tiə·rioh,spazəm) spasm of an artery.

arteriostenosis (ah,tiə·riohstə'nohsis) constriction of an artery.

arteriosympathectomy (ah,tiə·rioh,simpə'thektəmee) periarterial sympathectomy.

arteriotomy (ah,tiə·ri'otəmee) an incision into an artery.

arteriotony (ahtiə·ri'otənee) blood pressure.

arteriovenous (ah,tiə·rioh'veenəs) both arterial and venous; pertaining to both artery and vein.

arteritis (,ahtə'rietis) inflammation of an artery.

cranial a. temporal arteritis.

giant cell a. temporal arteritis.

a. obliterans endarteritis obliterans.

rheumatic a. generalized inflammation of arterioles and arterial capillaries occurring in rheumatic fever.

temporal a. a chronic vascular disease of unknown origin, occurring in the elderly, characterized by severe headache, fever, and accumulation of giant cells in the walls of medium-sized arteries, especially the temporal arteries. Ocular involvement may cause visual impairment or blindness.

Takayasu's a. pulseless disease.

artery ('ahtə-ree) a vessel through which the blood passes away from the heart to various parts of the body. The wall of an artery consists typically of an outer coat (tunica adventitia), a middle coat (tunica media), and an inner coat (tunica intima).

end a. one that undergoes progressive branching without development of channels connecting with other arteries.

arthr(o)- word element. [Gr.] *joint, articulation.*

arthralgia (ah'thralji·ə) pain in a joint.

arthrectomy (ah'threktəmee) excision of a joint.

arthritide ('ahthri,teed) a skin eruption of gouty origin.

arthritis (ah'thrietis) inflammation of a joint. adj. **arthritic.** The term is frequently used by the public to indicate any disease involving pain or stiffness of the musculoskeletal system and is incorrectly considered by many to be synonymous with rheumatism. In medical terminology arthritis is restricted to those types of rheumatic disease in which there is an inflammatory condition involving the joints. The term rheumatic diseases is a broader term, referring to conditions in which there are changes in connective tissues, including muscle, tendons, bursae, joints, and fibrous tissue.

Arthritis and the rheumatic diseases in general constitute the major cause of chronic disability in the United Kingdom, where it is estimated that 20 million persons have a rheumatic disease, of whom between 6 and 8 million are severely affected.

The two main types of arthritis are OSTEOARTHRITIS and rheumatoid arthritis. The treatment and care of patients suffering from these or other rheumatic diseases are included here under rheumatoid arthritis (see below), the most common, the most virulent, and one of the most disabling of these conditions.

acute a. arthritis marked by pain, heat, redness, and swelling.

acute rheumatic a. swelling, tenderness, and redness of many joints of the body, accompanying rheumatic fever.

colitic a. arthritis associated with ulcerative colitis which may affect both sacroiliac joints and spine as well as peripheral joints and which shares many of the features of ankylosing spondylitis. Treatment is directed at the underlying colitis as well as the arthritis.

hypertrophic a. term formerly used for rheumatoid arthritis marked by hypertrophy of the cartilage at the edge of the joints; OSTEOARTHRITIS.

infective a. arthritis caused by viral, fungal or bacterial infection of the joints. Viral forms of arthritis are quite common and usually self-limiting, while bacterial (septic) arthritis requires prompt antibiotic therapy if permanent joint change is not to occur. Fungal infections of joints are uncommon.

juvenile chronic a. (JCA) a chronic arthritis of children, with swelling, tenderness, and pain involving one or more joints, which in severe cases may lead to impaired growth and development, limitation of movement, and ankylosis and flexion contractures of the joints. It is subdivided by type of onset into pauciarticular (four or less joints affected), systemic and polyarticular forms. The systemic manifestations may include spiking fever, transient rash on the trunk and extremities, hepatosplenomegaly, generalized lymphadenopathy, and anaemia. Called also Still's disease.

Lyme a. a recurrent, tickborne form of arthritis affecting a few large joints, especially the knees, shoulders, and elbows, and associated with erythema chronicum migrans, malaise, and myalgia.

psoriatic a. that associated with psoriasis, which may affect the peripheral joints as well as the sacroiliac joints and spine. Various patterns of peripheral joint disease occur, including one classically affecting the terminal interphalangeal joints.

rheumatoid a. a chronic systemic disease with inflammatory changes occurring throughout the body's connective tissues. As such, it is classified as a COLLAGEN DISEASE.

This form of arthritis strikes during the most productive years of adulthood, with the majority of cases beginning between the ages of 20 and 40. No age is spared, however, and the disease may affect infants as well as the very old. For some reason the disease affects men and women about equally in number, but three times as many women as men develop symptoms severe enough to require medical attention.

AETIOLOGY. The cause of rheumatoid arthritis is unknown and it is doubtful that there is one specific cause. It is regarded by some researchers as an AUTOIMMUNE DISEASE, in which the body produces abnormal antibodies against its own cells and tissues. Evidence to support this theory is found in the fact that there is an abnormally high level of certain types of IMMUNOGLOBULINS in the blood of patients suffering from rheumatoid arthritis. Other researchers contend that the disease may be due to infection, perhaps from an undefined virus or some other microorganism (e.g., *Mycoplasma).* There also is a genetic element to rheumatoid arthritis, in which one inherits a predisposition to the disease.

Physical and emotional STRESS also plays some part in the onset of acute attacks; however, psychological stress is implicated as a causative factor in the onset of many illnesses.

SYMPTOMS AND PATHOLOGY. In about 75 per cent of patients the onset of rheumatoid arthritis is gradual with only mild symptoms at the beginning. Early symptoms include malaise, fever, weight loss, and morning stiffness of the joints. One or more joints may become swollen, painful, and inflamed. Some patients may experience only mild espisodes of acute symptoms with lengthy remissions. The more typical patient, however, experiences increasingly severe and frequent attacks with subsequent joint damage and deformity. The pattern of remissions and exacerbations continues throughout the course of the disease.

In severe untreated forms of the disease and sometimes in spite of treatment, the joint pathology goes through four stages: (1) proliferative inflammation of the synovium with increased exudate, which eventually leads to thickening of the synovium; (2) formation of a layer of granulation tissue (pannus), which erodes and destroys the cartilage and eventually spreads to contiguous areas, causing destruction of the bone capsule and parts of the muscles that control the joint; (3) fibrous ankylosis resulting from the invasion of the pannus by tough fibrous tissue; and (4) bony ankylosis as the fibrous tissue becomes calcified.

In addition to the joint changes there is atrophy of muscles, bones, and skin adjacent to the affected joint. The most characteristic lesions are subcutaneous nodules, which may be present for weeks or months and are most commonly found over bony prominences, especially near the elbow.

Because rheumatoid arthritis is a systemic disease, there is involvement of connective tissues other than those in the musculoskeletal system. Degenerative lesions may be found in the collagen in the lungs, heart, blood vessels, and pleura.

Patients with rheumatoid arthritis appear undernourished and chronically ill. Most are anaemic because of the effect of the disease on blood-forming organs. The erythrocyte sedimentation rate is elevated and the WBC may be slightly elevated.

TREATMENT AND PATIENT CARE. Management of rheumatoid arthritis is aimed at providing rest and freedom from pain, minimizing emotional stress, preventing or correcting deformities, and maintaining or restoring function so that the patient can enjoy as much independence and mobility as possible.

Rest and Exercise. It is recommended that the patient with rheumatoid arthritis allow himself from 10 to 12 hours sleep out of each 24. During the time the patient is lying in bed he should be careful to maintain good posture and avoid pillows or other devices that support the joints in a flexed position. A firm mattress is recommended, with only one pillow under the head. During periods of severe attacks, the patient may require continuous bed rest.

The purpose of rest is to allow the body's natural defences against inflammation to work at their optimal level. It is necessary, however, even in the acute phase to balance rest with prescribed exercises which take into account the severity of the case, the joints affected, and the patient's individual needs and tolerance.

Physiotherapy. The goals of physiotherapy for the patient with rheumatoid arthritis are to prevent and correct deformities, control pain, strengthen weakened muscles, and improve function.

Therapeutic EXERCISE is of major importance in the physiotherapy programme established for the patient. It is necessary to enlist his cooperation, and this can be done most effectively by explaining the purposes of the exercises and teaching him ways to exercise which will not increase pain. In many instances proper exercise can actually diminish pain. The patient's tolerance for exercises must be carefully monitored. While it is expected that some discomfort may be present during exercise, there should not be persistent pain that continues for hours after the exercises have been done. If such pain and fatigue do occur, the exercise programme should be reviewed and revised so that a good balance of rest and exercise is obtained. It should be remembered that overactivity can contribute to the inflammatory process.

Applications of HEAT or COLD may be used in the management of rheumatoid arthritis. Heat applications improve circulation, promote relaxation, and relieve pain. When used in conjunction with exercise, heat can allow more freedom of joint movement. Various forms of heat therapy may be used, including dry heat, moist heat, DIATHERMY, and ultrasound. For dry heat a therapeutic infrared heat lamp may be most convenient during home care. Hot-water bottles or electric heating pads also may be used. For treatment of the hands, paraffin baths are effective. Wet heat can be applied by hot baths with the water temperature not exceeding 39 °C (102 °F) or by means of a towel dipped in hot water, wrung out, and applied to the joint. Whirlpool baths are effective, especially when prolonged treatment is indicated.

Relief from pain and stiffness can be provided for some patients by applications of cold packs to the affected joints. This can be done by placing ice packs directly over the joint. When either heat or cold is used, care must be taken to protect the patient's skin. It should be remembered that rheumatoid arthritis affects the skin as well as other tissues.

Whenever it is necessary to handle the joints and limbs of a patient with rheumatoid arthritis, it is extremely important to move slowly and gently, avoiding sudden, jarring movements which stimulate muscle contraction and produce pain. The affected joints should be supported so that there is no excessive motion.

Medication. There is no drug that will cure arthritis. There are a variety of medications that may be prescribed, depending on the individual patient, his needs and tolerance. It is important that the patient be advised of the expected results and possible undesirable side-effects that may accompany the ingestion of certain drugs. He should also be advised that therapeutic trials of several different drugs may be necessary. With this information at hand, he can work cooperatively with the doctor in determining which drug or drugs can be most beneficial for treatment of his condition.

The nonsteroidal antiinflammatory drugs (NSAIDs) are the drugs of first choice in the treatment of inflammation of active rheumatoid arthritis. They include soluble aspirin and enteric-coated aspirin; propionic acid derivatives such as ibuprofen and naproxen; the phenulacetic acid derivative diclofenac; indomethacin; azapropazone, and piroxicam. The main side-effects of all NSAIDs are gastrointestinal ulceration and bleeding and they provide only symptomatic relief of pain and stiffness.

Gold compounds, D-penicillamine and the antimalarial drugs chloroquine or hydroxychloroquine, may be prescribed for selected patients who cannot tolerate or are not responding well to more conservative methods of treatment. Careful monitoring for haemotological and renal toxicity is mandatory in all patients receiving gold and penicillamine, while the antimalarials, although generally better tolerated, may cause retinal toxicity.

Oral corticosteroids are usually reserved for patients with severe forms of rheumatoid arthritis that have not responded to the above or for patients with severe systemic features of the disease such as vasculitis. Drugs included in this group are cortisone, hydrocortisone, prednisone, prednisolone, and dexamethasone.

Surgical Intervention and Orthopaedic Devices. In the past, surgical intervention was reserved for patients who had already suffered severe joint deformity. There is presently a trend toward the use of surgery in the early stages of the disease so that deformities and serious mechanical abnormalities can be prevented or at least modified.

One surgical procedure employed is *synovectomy* (excision of the synovial membrane of a joint). The goal of this treatment is to interrupt the destructive inflammatory processes which eventually lead to ankylosis and invasion of surrounding cartilage and bone tissues.

Surgical repair of a hip joint (*arthroplasty*) may be performed when there is extensive damage. The purpose of this procedure is to restore, improve, or maintain joint function or to relieve persistent pain not responding to conservative measures. Operations to replace destroyed hips and knees are now commonplace and replacements of other joints such as shoulders, elbows and small joints of the fingers are available in special centres.

Braces, casts, or splints are sometimes used to immobilize the affected part so that it can rest during an active stage of the disease. Devices which immobilize the affected joint may also allow for motion of adjacent muscle, thereby improving muscle strength and permitting more independence on the part of the patient. Braces may also be used to prevent deformities by maintaining good position of the joints.

Patient Education. The arthritic patient and his family should be encouraged to work closely with the health care team in order to devise the most effective programme of care for the individual.

Unfortunately, arthritis is so widespread and such a crippling disease that its victims are easy prey for charlatans and promoters of miraculous 'cures'. The nature of the disease, with its unexplained remissions and relief of symptoms, makes it easy for unscrupulous individuals to convince the arthritic patient that some bizarre treatment they have used has indeed 'cured' the arthritis.

Home care is an essential part of the management of arthritis. To help in the education of the public the Arthritis and Rheumatism Council (ARC) provides a number of pamphlets and other educational materials. The Council also supports a broad programme of research, education and training. The address of the Council is The Arthritis and Rheumatism Council, 41 Eagle Street, London WC1R 4AR.

Arthritis Care, at 6 Grosvenor Crescent, London SW1 7ER, is a self-help organization open to people with rheumatism and arthritis, and to anyone interested in the welfare of people with a rheumatic disease.

seronegative a. arthritis associated with negative serological tests for the IgM antiglobulin, rheumatoid factor. The classical seronegative joint diseases, where serological tests for rheumatoid factor are persistently negative, are ankylosing spondylitis, Reiter's syndrome, psoratic arthritis and Crohn's and colitic arthritis.

seropositive a. arthritis associated with positive serological tests for the IgM antiglobulin, rheumatoid factor. Seventy-five per cent of rheumatoid arthritis patients are seropositive at some time in their course.

suppurative a. inflammation of a joint with a purulent effusion into the joint, due chiefly to bacterial infection.

arthrocentesis (,ahthrohsen'teesis) surgical puncture of a joint cavity for aspiration of fluid.

arthroclasia (,ahthrə'klayzi·ə) surgical breaking down of an ankylosis to permit a joint to move freely.

arthrodesis (,ahthrə'deesis) surgical fusion of a joint.

arthrodia (ah'throhdi·ə) a type of synovial joint that allows only a gliding motion; called also gliding joint. adj. **arthrodial.**

arthrodynia (,ahthrə'dini·ə) arthralgia.

arthrodysplasia (,ahthrohdis'playzi·ə) any abnormality of joint development.

arthrogram ('ahthrə,gram) the film produced by arthrography.

arthrography (ah'throgrəfee) radiography of a joint, following injection of a suitable contrast medium into the joint space.

air a. pneumoarthrography.

arthrogryposis (,ahthrohgrie'pohsis) 1. persistent flexion of a joint. 2. tetanoid spasm.

arthrolith ('ahthrə,lith) a calculous deposit within a joint.

arthrology (ah'throləjee) scientific study or description of the joints.

arthrolysis (ah'throlisis) operative loosening of adhesions in an ankylosed joint.

arthrometer (ah'thromitə) an instrument for measuring the angles of movements of joints.

arthropathy (ah'thropəthee) any joint disease.

Charcot's a., neuropathic a. chronic progressive degeneration of the stress-bearing portion of a joint, with hypertrophic changes at the periphery; it is associated with neurological disorders involving loss of sensation in the joint.

chondrocalcific a. progressive polyarthritis with joint swelling and bony enlargement, most commonly in the small joints of the hand but also affecting other joints, characterized radiologically by narrowing of the joint space with subchondral erosions and sclerosis and frequently chondrocalcinosis.

osteopulmonary a. clubbing of fingers and toes, and enlargement of ends of the long bones, in cardiac or pulmonary disease.

arthroplasty ('ahthrə,plastee) surgical reconstruction of a joint.

total hip a. replacement of the femoral head and acetabulum with prostheses that are cemented into the bone.

arthropod ('ahthrə,pod) an individual of the phylum Arthropoda.

a.-borne viral diseases viral diseases transmitted by insects, of which there are two principal types: ENCEPHALITIS or HAEMORRHAGIC fever.

Arthropoda (ah'thropədə) a phylum of the animal kingdom including bilaterally symmetrical animals with hard, segmented bodies bearing jointed appendages; embracing the largest number of known animals, with at least 740,000 species, divided into 12 classes. It includes the arachnids, crustaceans, and insects.

arthroscintigram (,ahthroh'sinti,gram) a radionuclide scan of a joint.

arthroscintigraphy (,ahthrohsin'tigrəfee) scintigraphy of a joint.

arthrosclerosis (,ahthrohskle'rohsis) stiffening or hardening of the joints.

arthroscope ('ahthrə,skohp) an endoscope for examining the interior of a joint.

arthroscopy (ah'throskəpee) examination of the interior of a joint with an arthroscope.

arthrosis (ah'throhsis) 1. a joint or articulation. 2. disease of a joint.

arthrostomy (ah'throstəmee) surgical creation of an opening into a joint, as for drainage.

arthrosynovitis (,ahthroh,sienoh'vietis) inflammation of the synovial membrane of a joint.

arthrotomy (ah'throtəmee) incision of a joint.

arthroxesis (,ahthrok'sesis) scraping of an articular surface.

Arthus reaction (phenomenon) (ah'toos) an inflammatory reaction due to repeated exposure to antigen, causing oedema, haemorrhage and necrosis. Classically an ulcer develops within hours after injection of an antigen into a subject with antibodies to that antigen. Caused by immune complexes that, in the presence of COMPLEMENT, adhere to the vessel walls and are surrounded by fibrin, platelets and neutrophils.

articular (ah'tikyuhlə) pertaining to a joint.

articulare (ah,tikyuh'lahree) the point of intersection of the dorsal contours of the articular process of the mandible and the temporal bone.

articulate (ah'tikyuh,layt) 1. to unite by joints; to join. 2. united by joints. 3. capable of expressing oneself orally.

articulatio (ah,tikyuh'layshioh) pl. *articulationes* [L.] an articulation or joint.

articulation (ah'tikyuh'layshən) 1. a joint; the place of union or junction between two or more bones of the skeleton. 2. enunciation of words and sentences.

articulator (ah'tikyuh,laytə) a device for effecting a jointlike union.

dental a. a device that simulates movements of the temporomandibular joints or mandible, used in dentistry.

articulo mortis (ah,tikyuhloh 'mawtis) at the point or moment of death.

artificial (,ahti'fishəl) made by art; not natural or

pathological.

a. eye see under EYE.

a. kidney a popular name for an extracorporeal haemodialyser. See also artificial KIDNEY and HAEMODIALYSIS.

a. limb a replacement for a natural limb (see also PROSTHESIS).

a. organ a mechanical device that can substitute temporarily or permanently for a body organ. The development of artificial organs represents one of the outstanding achievements of contemporary medicine. The field of organ substitution has progressed rapidly over a brief span of years. Most of the artificial organs in use today are hospital devices that are connected temporarily to patients in order to do the work of an organ that is either disabled or undergoing surgery. Recent advances in electronics (principally the development of the transistor and the low-drain battery), together with advances in surgical techniques, have made possible the development of miniature artificial organs that can be surgically implanted in a patient and function independently for long periods.

The development of artificial organs has paved the way for other medical advances in the field of organ TRANSPLANTATION, the replacement of a disabled organ with a healthy living organ from a 'donor'. The surgical techniques of artificial organ implantation and living organ transplantation have much in common. Also, it is often necessary to use an artificial organ to temporarily take over the functions of an organ undergoing transplantation surgery.

The HEART-LUNG MACHINE is a surgery aid that permits previously impossible operations on the heart, lungs, and great vessels, and also allows other kinds of surgery to be performed on seriously weakened patients without fear of heart failure.

Cardiac patients suffering from HEART BLOCK (a defect in the transmission of nerve impulses between the separate pumping chambers of the heart) are kept alive with an electronic heart stimulator called the artificial PACEMAKER. The device is also used in certain cardiac operations in which heart block is a possible complication. A compact version of the hospital pacemaker can be surgically implanted in the chest of a patient. Miniature pacemakers of this kind are keeping thousands of heart block victims alive today.

Researchers in cardiac disease are experimenting with several types of artificial hearts. It is hoped that a mechanical pump implanted permanently in a patient can match the output of a normal heart. Another experimental device along similar lines is called a 'booster heart', designed to reduce the workload of the left ventricle.

Artificial heart valves are used to replace those damaged by disease. The mitral valve, which controls the passage of blood between the left atrium and left ventricle, is often impaired by rheumatic fever. Some cardiac disorders impair the aortic valve, which controls blood flow from the heart to the body. Artificial aortic and mitral valves have been successfully implanted in human hearts and are now routinely performed on many patients. Damaged blood vessels (which in the past could be replaced only by the difficult procedure of transplantation from donors who had died suddenly) are now replaced with tubes made of Teflon or Dacron.

Normal kidneys filter waste products from the blood, expelling these substances in the urine. When the kidneys fail, waste products can build up in the blood to poisonous levels, causing uraemia. Treatments for this condition include dialysis and transplantation. Dialysis (the essential features of which are similar for haemodialysis or peritoneal dialysis) is the process whereby crystalloid and colloid substances are separated from a solution by placing a semipermeable membrane, e.g. cellophane or the peritoneum, between the solution and pure water. Renal transplantation is the alternative unless patients are unsuitable for medical reasons. Patients are followed up with long-term immunosuppressive drugs to prevent graft rejection.

a. respiration any method of forcing air into and out of the lungs to start breathing in a person whose breathing has stopped. Artificial respiration can be given with no equipment whatsoever, so that it is an ideal emergency first-aid procedure.

INDICATIONS. Artificial respiration can save a life whenever breathing has stopped but heartbeat has not, as in near-drowning, electric shock, choking, gas poisoning, drug poisoning, injury to the chest, or suffocation from other causes. Usually one can tell that breathing has stopped by noting the lack of up-and-down movement of the chest. Often the cause of the stoppage of breathing is obvious, as when a drowning person is pulled out of the water. But sometimes it is impossible to tell what stopped the breathing—accident or disease—and therefore whether artificial respiration would or would not be helpful. In such cases, the rule to follow is: when in doubt, give artificial respiration and continue until additional medical help is available.

WHAT TO DO. To be effective, artificial respiration must be begun immediately. A person dies in minutes after his breathing stops. A delay of seconds may be the difference between life and death. That is why it is so important to learn how to apply artificial respiration before an accident happens.

At the same time that artificial respiration is begun someone should call a doctor or the ambulance service, but if there is no one to send to summon help, artificial respiration should be given in preference.

Any obstruction in the victim's mouth that would interfere with the passage of air—mud, sand, chewing gum, or displaced false teeth, for example—is removed immediately. Clothing that is tight around the neck is loosened.

Once begun, artificial respiration should be continued until the victim begins to breathe regularly by himself, until a doctor takes charge, or until it is obvious that the victim will not revive. Do not give up easily. Victims have recovered as long as 4 hours after artificial respiration was started. If cardiac arrest or weakness occurs, a second person who knows how should give CARDIAC MASSAGE. If only one person is present, he should provide both alternately. See also CARDIOPULMONARY RESUSCITATION.

When the victim has revived, he is kept quiet, covered to prevent chills, and given other first aid for SHOCK.

METHODS. There are three methods of artificial respiration: the mouth-to-mouth method, the chest pressure–arm lift (Silvester) method, and the back pressure–arm lift (Holger–Nielsen) method.

The mouth-to-mouth technique, called also transanimation, is recognized by authorities as the most effective method that can be given by an individual. Some persons feel squeamish at the thought of using it, but in an emergency such doubts usually vanish. Anyone who hesitates about putting his mouth on another person's, even in an emergency, can place a handkerchief over the victim's mouth. Air will pass readily through the cloth. The rescuer should close the patient's nose by pinching the nostrils, or if the latter is a child, by placing his mouth over the child's mouth and nose to make a seal.

If the patient has had a laryngectomy and has a stoma at the trachea, the lips of the rescuer are placed around the stoma so as to make a seal. The procedure is followed in the same manner as in mouth-to-mouth resuscitation.

The other two methods are recommended only (1) if a person cannot bring himself to use the mouth-to-mouth technique, (2) if circumstances (such as a severe mouth injury in the victim) prevent him from using it, or (3) if he feels more familiar with another method at the time of the emergency.

aryl- in organic chemistry, a prefix denoting any radical having the free valency on a carbon atom in an aromatic ring.

arytenoid (ˌari'teenoyd) shaped like a jug or pitcher, as the arytenoid cartilage or arytenoid muscle of the larynx.

arytenoidectomy (ˌariˌteenoy'dektəmee) excision of an arytenoid cartilage.

arytenoiditis (ˌariˌteenoy'dietis) inflammation of the arytenoid muscle or cartilage.

arytenoidopexy (ˌaritee'noydəˌpeksee) surgical fixation of arytenoid cartilage or muscle.

AS [L.] *auris sinistra* (left ear).

As chemical symbol, *arsenic*.

Asacol ('asəkol) trademark for a preparation of mesalazine.

ASBAH Association for Spina Bifida and Hydrocephalus.

asbestiform (as'bestˌfawm) resembling asbestos.

asbestos (as'bestos, -təs) fibrous magnesium and calcium silicate, a nonburning compound used in roofing and insulating materials. See ASBESTOSIS.

a. bodies golden-yellow, long, slender bodies of various shapes in the sputum, lung secretions, and faeces of patients with ASBESTOSIS, formed by deposition of calcium and iron salts and proteins on spicules of asbestos.

asbestosis (ˌasbes'tohsis) increasing fibrosis of lung parenchyma and of pleura associated with the regular inhalation of ASBESTOS as a powder or dust. Associated with mesothelioma and bronchogenic carcinoma (see also PNEUMOCONIOSIS).

ascariasis (ˌaskə'rieəsis) infection with *Ascaris*.

ascaricide (as'kariˌsied) an agent destructive to ascarids. adj. **ascaricidal**.

ascarid ('askə·rid) any of the phasmid nematodes (roundworms) of the Ascaridoidea, which includes the genera *Ascaridia*, *Ascaris*, *Toxocara*, and *Toxascaris*.

Ascaris ('askə·ris) a genus of nematode (roundworm) parasites found in the intestines of man and other vertebrates.

A. lumbricoides a species parasitic in man, which may cause colicky pains and diarrhoea, especially in children. See also WORMS.

Aschheim–Zondek test ('ash·hiem'tsondek) AZ test; a biological test formerly used to determine pregnancy, in which urine from a woman suspected of being pregnant was injected into immature female mice; if the woman was pregnant, marked changes in the appearance of the mice ovaries occurred within 100 hours. See also PREGNANCY TESTS.

Aschoff's bodies (nodules) ('ashofs) submiliary collections of cells and leukocytes in the interstitial tissues of the heart in rheumatic myocarditis.

ascites (ə'sieteez) abnormal accumulation of serous (oedematous) fluid within the peritoneal cavity. adj. **ascitic.** Sometimes called *hydroperitoneum*. The condition may be associated with numerous disorders, including neoplastic and inflammatory disorders of the peritoneum which produce increased permeability of the peritoneal capillaries; severe hypoalbuminaemia of any cause; portal and hepatic venous hypertension associated with cirrhosis of the liver and advanced congestive heart failure and constrictive pericarditis; and hyperaldosteronism with increased retention of sodium and water. In portal and venous hepatic hypertension there is increased pressure within the sinusoids and hepatic veins. As the pressure increases there is movement of protein-rich plasma filtrate into the hepatic lymphatics. Some of the fluid enters the thoracic duct, but if the pressure is high enough, the excess fluid will ooze from the surface of the liver into the peritoneal cavity. Because the fluid has a high colloidal osmotic pressure owing to its high protein content, it is not readily reabsorbed from the peritoneal cavity.

TREATMENT. Because ascites is symptomatic of an underlying disorder that can range from liver failure to endocrine disease, treatment of the primary disorder is a major goal. The problems of fluid and electrolyte imbalance that are associated with ascites, and the potential for mechanical trauma due to pressure against internal organs adjacent to the abdominal cavity necessitate some kind of symptomatic relief.

Medical treatment of ascites includes restriction of fluid and sodium intake and administration of diuretics. Supplementation of potassium and chloride may be necessary during diuretic therapy to avoid an imbalance of these electrolytes. Careful measurement of fluid intake and output is essential, and laboratory values for the electrolytes must be monitored frequently.

Surgical control of ascites was at one time almost entirely limited to abdominal PARACENTESIS for removal of large accumulations of ascitic fluid. It is, however, only a temporary measure that poses problems of rapid fluid shift, loss of protein, and the potential for introducing infectious agents into the peritoneum.

A more effective procedure is the insertion of a peritoneal-venous SHUNT (LeVeen shunt), which provides a means for continuous reinfusion of ascitic fluid into the venous system. A perforated peritoneal tube is inserted into the peritoneal cavity and connected to a one-way valve that prevents a backflow of blood from the vein. The other end of the shunt is a tube that empties into either the jugular vein or the superior vena cava. The shunt is triggered into action by the patient's breathing, which increases pressure within the peritoneal cavity each time air is inhaled and the diaphragm descends toward the abdomen.

PATIENT CARE. Assessment of the degree of fluid accumulation and the problems it presents to the patient can be done by measuring abdominal girth, recording daily weight gain and loss, and determining the extent to which pressure from the fluid is interfering with respiration, circulation, and digestion.

Most patients with ascites are more comfortable when sitting well supported by pillows. When a change of position is necessary to maintain integrity of the skin and promote circulation, small pillows can be used to support the rib cage while the patient is lying on his side. Ascites is usually a chronic condition that is difficult to control. Management must include an explanation to the patient so he can better understand his condition and the need for compliance with the prescribed treatment. He and significant others will need instruction in self-care and management of his problems at home and continued support as they cope with a difficult and uncomfortable situation.

ascorbate (əs'korbayt) a compound or derivative of ascorbic acid.

ascorbic acid (əs'kawbik) vitamin C, called also

cevitamic acid; a substance found in many fruits and vegetables, especially citrus fruits, such as oranges and lemons, and tomatoes. Ascorbic acid is an essential element of the diet; lack of vitamin C can lead to SCURVY or to less severe conditions, such as delayed healing of wounds. Solutions of ascorbic acid deteriorate very rapidly and the vitamin is not stored in the body to any extent. Large doses of commercial preparations of ascorbic acid may cause gastrointestinal irritation. There is no general agreement as to the normal and therapeutic daily requirements of vitamin C. It is believed that ascorbic acid requirements in stress are abnormally high. Under moderate stress circumstances authorities recommend about 300 mg daily.

ascospore ('askə,spor) a spore contained or produced in an ascus.

ascus ('askəs) the spore case of certain fungi.

-ase suffix used in forming the names of enzymes, affixed to a stem indicating the substrate (luciferase), the general nature of the substrate (proteinase), or the type of reaction effected (hydrolase).

asemasia (,ayse'mayzi·ə) inability to make or comprehend signs or tokens of communication.

asemia (ay'seemi·ə) inability to understand or to use speech or signs, due to a cerebral lesion. Aphasia.

ASEP trademark for a solution of gluteraldehyde.

asepsis (ay'sepsis) absence of septic matter; freedom from infection or infectious material. adj. **aseptic**. Surgical asepsis refers to the achievement of a bacteria-free environment in the operating theatre by controlling the air-flow, the use of sterile instruments and drapes, and the wearing of appropriate clothing, such as sterile gowns, caps, masks, and gloves, by the theatre staff.

ASEPTIC TECHNIQUE. A method of carrying out sterile procedures so that there is the minimum risk of introducing infection. Achieved by the sterility of equipment and a non-touch method.

asexual (ay'seksyooəl, a'sek-) without sex; not pertaining to or involving sex.

ASH Action on Smoking and Health.

asialia (,aysie'ayliə) aptyalism.

asiderosis (,aysidə'rohsis) deficiency of iron reserve of the body.

Asilone ('asilohn) trademark for a proprietary compound antacid mixture.

asparaginase (ə'sparəji,nayz) an enzyme that catalyses the deamination of asparagine; used as an antineoplastic agent against cancers, e.g., acute lymphocytic leukaemia, in which the malignant cells require exogenous asparagine for protein synthesis.

asparagine (a'sparə,jeen, -jin) the β-amide of aspartic acid, a nonessential amino acid occurring in proteins.

aspartame (ə,spahtaym) a synthetic compound of two amino acids (L-aspartyl-L-phenylalanine methyl ester) used as a low-calorie sweetener. It is 180 times as sweet as sucrose (table sugar); the amount equal in sweetness to a teaspoon of sugar contains 0.1 calorie. Aspartame does not promote the formation of dental caries. The amount of phenylalanine in aspartame must be taken into account in the low-phenylalanine diet for patients with phenylketonuria.

aspartate (ə,spahtayt) any salt of aspartic acid; aspartic acid in dissociated form.

aspartate aminotransferase (ə,spahtayt) an enzyme that catalyses the transfer of an amino group from an alpha amino acid to an alpha keto acid. Abbreviated AST. It is present in many tissues and body fluids. The serum concentration is elevated when damage to tissue cells, especially of the heart and liver, causes a release of the enzyme. Elevated values are observed after a myocardial infarction. Very high values occur in viral or toxic hepatitis, and high values in infectious mononucleosis and obstructive jaundice. AST values are also increased in some muscle diseases, such as progressive muscular dystrophy. Called also *(serum) glutamic-oxaloacetic transaminase* (*GOT* or *SGOT*).

aspartic acid (ə'spahtik) a nonessential dibasic amino acid, widely distributed in proteins.

aspecific (,ayspə'sifik) not specific; not caused by a specific organism.

aspect ('aspekt) 1. that part of a surface viewed from a particular direction. 2. the look or appearance.

dorsal a. that surface of a body viewed from the back or, in veterinary anatomy, from above.

ventral a. that surface of a body viewed from the front or, in veterinary anatomy, from below.

aspergilloma (,aspəji'lohmə) a tumour-like granulomatous mass formed by colonization of *Aspergillus* in a bronchus or pulmonary cavity; the organism may disseminate through the blood stream to the brain, heart, and kidneys.

aspergillosis (,aspəji'lohsis) a disease caused by species of *Aspergillus*, marked by inflammatory granulomatous lesions in the skin, ear, orbit, nasal sinuses, lungs, and sometimes bones and meninges.

Aspergillus (,aspə'jiləs) a genus of fungi (molds), several species of which are endoparasitic and opportunistic pathogens.

aspermia (ay'spərmi·ə) failure of formation or emission of semen.

aspheric (ay'sferik) correcting or not affected by spherical aberration.

asphyxia (as'fiksi·ə) a condition in which there is a deficiency of oxygen in the blood and an increase in carbon dioxide in the blood and tissues. adj. **asphyxial.** The symptoms include irregular and disturbed respirations, or a complete absence of breathing, and pallor or cyanosis. Asphyxia may occur whenever there is an interruption in the normal exchange of oxygen and carbon dioxide between the lungs and the outside air. Some common causes are drowning, electric shock, lodging of a foreign body in the air passages, inhalation of smoke and poisonous gases, and trauma to or disease of the lungs or air passages. Treatment includes immediate remedy of the situation by ARTIFICIAL RESPIRATION and removal of the underlying cause whenever possible.

asphyxiant (as'fiksi·ənt) any substance capable of producing asphyxia.

asphyxiate (as'fiksi,ayt) to suffocate; to deprive of oxygen for utilization by the tissues.

aspidium (a'spidi·əm) the dried products of a genus of plants known as male fern.

aspirate ('aspi,rayt) 1. to withdraw fluid by negative pressure, or suction. 2. the fluid obtained by aspiration.

aspiration (,aspi'rayshən) 1. the act of inhaling. Pathological aspiration of vomitus or mucus into the respiratory tract may occur when a person is unconscious or under the effects of general anaesthesia. This can be avoided by keeping the head turned to the side and removing foreign material such as vomitus, mucus, or blood from the air passages. 2. withdrawal of liquid or gas by physical or mechanical suction.

a. biopsy, fine needle the removal of a minute amount of tissue by aspiration through a fine needle for rapid cytological diagnosis.

meconium a. fetal inhalation of MECONIUM-stained liquor. The hypoxic fetus passes meconium into the liquor. Premature inhalation prior to, or immediately following, delivery draws the meconium-stained liquor into the lungs, where it causes chemical pneumonitis and plugging of the airways. The ball-valve obstructions produce areas of consolidation and under-aeration, as well as hyperinflation, contributing to the potentially pathological condition *meconium aspiration syndrome*.

vacuum a. removal of the uterine contents by application of a vacuum through a hollow curet or a cannula introduced into the uterus. See under ABORTION, *Suction Curettage*.

aspirator ('aspi,raytə) an instrument for evacuating liquid or gas by suction.

aspirin ('asprin) acetylsalicylic acid, a common drug generally used to relieve pain and reduce fever, and specifically prescribed for rheumatic and arthritic disorders. See SALICYLATE for adverse reactions and poisoning. Aspirin should not be given to children under 12 years of age except under medical supervision, because this has been associated with the subsequent development of REYE'S SYNDROME.

asplenia (ay'spleeni·ə) absence of the spleen.

asporogenic (,ay·spor·roh'jenik) not producing spores; not reproduced by spores.

asporous (ay'spor·rəs) having no true spores.

assay ('asay, ə'say) determination of the purity of a substance or the amount of any particular constituent of a mixture.

biological a. bioassay; determination of the potency of a drug or other substance by comparing the effects it has on animals with those of a reference standard.

assertiveness (ə'sərtivnəs) a form of behaviour characterized by a confident declaration or affirmation of a statement without need of proof. To assert oneself is to compel recognition of one's rights or position without either aggressively transgressing the rights of another and assuming a position of dominance or submissively permitting another to deny one's rights or rightful position.

a. training instruction and practice in techniques for dealing with interpersonal conflicts and threatening situations in an assertive manner, avoiding the extremes of aggressive and submissive behaviour. Such training has as its goals enabling the learner to express personal feelings freely, speak up for his or her rights, communicate disagreement effectively, accept compliments comfortably, persist in expressing a legitimate complaint, and negotiate mutually satisfying solutions to interpersonal situations in which there is some type of conflict.

assessment (ə'sesmənt) the critical analysis and valuation or judgement of the status or quality of a particular condition, situation, or other subject of appraisal.

In the NURSING PROCESS, assessment involves the gathering of information about the health status of the patient/client, analysis and synthesis of that data, and the making of a clinical nursing judgement. The outcome of the nursing assessment is the establishment of a nursing DIAGNOSIS, that is, the identification of the nursing problems.

assimilation (ə,simi'layshən) 1. conversion of nutritive material into living tissue; anabolism. 2. psychologically, absorption of new experiences into the existing psychological makeup.

assistant (ə'sistənt) one who aids or helps another; an auxiliary.

association (ə,sohsi'ayshən, -,sohshi-) close relation in time or space. In neurology, correlation involving a high degree of modifiability and also consciousness. In genetics, the occurrence together of two characteristics (e.g., blood group O and peptic ulcers) at a frequency greater than would be predicted on the basis of chance.

a. areas areas of the cerebral cortex (excluding primary areas) connected with each other and with the neothalamus; they are responsible for higher mental and emotional processes, including memory, learning, etc.

free a. oral expression of one's ideas as they arrive spontaneously; a method used in psychoanalysis.

AST aspartate aminotransferase.

astasia (a'stayzi·ə) motor incoordination with inability to stand. adj. **astatic.**

a.-abasia inability or refusal to stand or walk, although the legs are otherwise under control.

astatine ('astə,teen, -tin) a chemical element, atomic number 85, atomic weight 210, symbol At. See table of elements in Appendix 2.

asteatosis (,aystiə'tohsis) any disease in which persistent dry scaling of the skin suggests scantiness or absence of sebum.

astemizole (as'temizohl) an antihistamine.

aster ('astə) a structure occurring in dividing cells, composed of microtubules radiating from a centrosome. The two asters are the poles of the spindle apparatus.

astereognosis (ay,stiə·ri·əg'nohsis) inability to recognize familiar objects by feeling their shape.

asterixis (,aystə'riksis) a motor disturbance marked by intermittent lapses of an assumed posture as a result of intermittency of sustained contraction of groups of muscles; called liver flap because of its occurrence in coma associated with liver disease, but also observed in other conditions.

asternal (ay'stərnəl) 1. not joined to the sternum. 2. pertaining to asternia.

asternia (ay'stərni·ə) congenital absence of the sternum.

asteroid ('astə,royd) star-shaped.

asthen(o)- word element. [Gr.] *weak, weakness.*

asthenia (as'theeni·ə) debility; loss of strength and energy; weakness. adj. **asthenic.**

neurocirculatory a. a symptom complex characterized by breathlessness, giddiness, a sense of fatigue, pain in the region of the precordium, and palpitation. It occurs chiefly in soldiers in active war service, though it is also seen in civilians, and is a form of NEUROSIS.

tropical anhidrotic a. a condition due to generalized absence of sweating in conditions of high temperature, characterized by a tendency to overfatigability, irritability, anorexia, inability to concentrate, and drowsiness, with headache and vertigo.

asthenocoria (as,thenoh'kor·ri·ə) sluggishness of the pupillary light reflex.

asthenometer (,asthe'nomitə) a device used in measuring the degree of muscular asthenia or of asthenopia.

asthenopia (,asthe'nohpi·ə) weakness or easy fatigue of the eye, with pain in the eyes, headache, dimness of vision, etc. Called also *eyestrain*. adj. **asthenopic.**

accommodative a. asthenopia due to strain of the ciliary muscle, usually due to uncorrected refractive errors.

muscular a. asthenopia due to weakness of the external ocular muscles.

asthenospermia (,asthenoh'spərmi·ə) reduced motility of spermatozoa in the semen.

asthma ('asmə) adj. **asthmatic.** It is also known as *bronchial asthma.* Attacks vary greatly from occasional periods of wheezing and slight dyspnoea to severe attacks that almost cause suffocation. An acute attack that lasts for days or weeks is called *status asthmaticus.* This is a medical emergency condition that can be fatal.

CAUSES. Asthma can be classified into three types

according to causative factors. *Extrinsic asthma* is due to an allergy to antigens; usually the offending allergens are suspended in the air in the form of pollen, dust, smoke, fumes from exhausts, and animal dander. More than half of the cases of asthma in children and young adults are of this type. It is responsive to disodium cromoglycate (see below). This type is called also atopic or allergic asthma. *Intrinsic or nonallergic asthma* is usually secondary to chronic or recurrent infections of the bronchi, sinuses, or tonsils and adenoids and is not due to allergic reactions. It is not responsive to disodium cromoglycate. The condition is made worse by respiratory infections, especially with *Haemophilus influenzae*. There is evidence that this type of asthma develops from a hypersensitivity to the bacteria causing the infection. Attacks can be precipitated by infections, emotional factors, and exposure to nonspecific irritants. The third type of asthma, *mixed*, is due to a combination of extrinsic and intrinsic factors.

There is an inherited tendency toward the development of extrinsic asthma. It is related to a hypersensitivity reaction of the IMMUNE RESPONSE. The patient often gives a family medical history that includes allergies of one kind or another and a personal history of allergic disorders.

Secondary factors affecting the severity of an attack or triggering of its onset include events that produce emotional stress, environmental changes in humidity and temperature, and exposure to noxious fumes or other airborne allergens.

SYMPTOMS. Typically, an attack of asthma is characterized by dyspnoea and a wheezing type of respiration. The patient usually assumes a classical sitting position, leaning forward so as to use all the muscles of respiration. The skin is usually pale and moist with perspiration, but in a severe attack there may be cyanosis of the lips and nailbeds. In the early stages of the attack coughing may be dry; but as the attack progresses the cough becomes more productive of a thick, tenacious, mucoid sputum.

TREATMENT. The treatment of extrinsic asthma begins with attempts to determine the allergens causing the attacks. The cooperation of the patient is needed to relate onset of attacks with specific environmental substances and emotional factors which trigger or intensify his symptoms. The patient with nonallergic asthma should avoid infections, nonspecific irritants, such as cigarette smoke, and other factors that provoke attacks.

Drugs given for the treatment of asthma are primarily used for the relief of symptoms. There is no cure for asthma but the disease can be controlled with an individualized regimen of rest, relaxation, and avoidance of causative factors. Bronchodilators such as adrenaline and aminophylline may be used to dilate the bronchioles, thus relieving respiratory embarrassment. Other drugs that thin the secretions and help in their ejection (expectorants) may also be prescribed.

The treatment of extrinsic asthma has been revolutionized by the use of inhaled particulate disodium cromoglycate (DSG). The life of children with asthma has been completely altered by prophylactic inhalation of DSG two or more times daily. Special schools for asthmatics are no longer needed for children with extrinsic asthma. Adults also respond well but DSG is quite ineffective in intrinsic asthma. Treatment for intrinsic asthma should be directed to treating infection and the use of bronchodilators.

The patient with status asthmaticus is very seriously ill and must receive special attention and medication to avoid excessive strain on the heart and severe respiratory difficulties that can be fatal.

PATIENT CARE. Because asthma is a chronic condition with an irregular pattern of remissions and exacerbations, education of the patient is essential to successful treatment. The care plan must be individualized to meet the needs of the patient and designed so that he can participate actively in his own care. He may need to adjust his life style so that he works and plays at a more leisurely pace. Most patients welcome the opportunity to learn more about their disorder and ways in which they can exert some control over the environmental and emotional events which are likely to precipitate an attack. Exercises that improve posture are helpful in maintaining good air exchange. Special deep-breathing exercises can be taught to the patient so that he maintains elasticity and full expansion of lung and bronchial tissues. (See also LUNG and CHRONIC OBSTRUCTIVE AIRWAYS DISEASE.) Some asthmatic patients develop a protective breathing pattern that is shallow and ineffective because of a fear that deep breathing will bring on an attack of coughing and wheezing. They will need help in breaking this pattern and learning to breathe deeply and fully expand the bronchi and lungs.

The patient should be encouraged to drink large quantities of fluids during an attack unless otherwise contraindicated. The extra fluids are needed to replace those lost during respiratory distress and seizures of coughing. The increased intake of fluids also can help thin the bronchial secretions so that they are more easily removed by coughing and deep breathing.

The patient should be warned of the hazards of extremes in eating, exercise, and emotional events such as prolonged laughing or crying. The key words are modification and moderation to avoid overtaxing and overstimulating the body systems. Relaxation techniques can be very helpful, especially if the patient can find a method that works well for him in reducing tension.

Asthmatic patients fare better if they feel that they do have some control over their disease and are not necessarily helpless victims of a debilitating incurable illness. There is no cure for asthma but there are ways in which one can adjust to the illness and minimize its effects.

allergic a., atopic a. extrinsic asthma; bronchial asthma due to allergy.

bronchial a. asthma.

cardiac a. a term applied to breathing difficulties due to pulmonary oedema in heart disease, such as left ventricular failure.

extrinsic a. asthma due to allergy to antigens (see above).

intrinsic or infectious a. asthma not due to allergic reactions (see above).

astigmatism (əˈstigməˌtizəm) an error of refraction in which a ray of light is not sharply focused on the retina, but is spread over a more or less diffuse area, and where the refractive power of the eye varies in different meridians; it is due to differences in curvature in various meridians of the refractive surfaces (cornea and lens) of the eye. adj. **astigmatic.** The exact cause of astigmatism is not known. Common types of astigmatism seem to run in families and are believed to be inherited. Everyone has a degree of astigmatism, since it is rare to find perfectly shaped curves in the cornea and lens. The defect may not be sufficient to make treatment necessary; however, corrective lenses may be needed when the refractive error is troublesome.

compound a. that in which both principal meridians are hypermetropic (compound hypermetropic astigmatism) or myopic (compound myopic astigmatism).

corneal a. that due to the presence of abnormal curvatures on the anterior or posterior surface of the cornea.

hypermetropic a. that in which the light rays are brought to a focus behind the retina.

irregular a. that in which the curvature varies in different parts of the same meridian or in which refraction in successive meridians differs irregularly.

lenticular a. astigmatism due to a defect of the crystalline lens.

mixed a. that in which one principal meridian is hypermetropic and the other myopic.

myopic a. that in which the light rays are brought to a focus in front of the retina.

regular a. that in which the refraction changes gradually in power from one principal meridian of the eye to the other, the two meridians always being at right angles; this condition is further classified as being *against the rule* when the meridian of greatest refractive power tends toward the horizontal, *with the rule* when it tends toward the vertical, and *oblique* when it lies 45 degrees from the horizontal and vertical.

ASTMS ('aztəmz) Association of Scientific, Technical and Managerial Staffs.

astomia (ay'stohmi·ə) congenital atresia of the mouth. adj. **astomatous.**

astragalectomy (ə,stragə'lektəmee) excision of the astragalus.

astragalus (ə'stragələs) talus. adj. **astragalar**.

astringent (ə'strinjənt) 1. causing contraction or arresting discharges. 2. an agent that causes contraction or arrests discharges. Astringents act as protein precipitants; they arrest discharge by causing shrinkage of tissue.

Some astringents, such as tannic acid, have been used in treating diarrhoea. Skin preparations such as shaving lotions often contain astringents such as aluminium acetate that help to reduce oiliness and excessive perspiration. Witch hazel is a common household astringent used to reduce swelling. Styptic pencils, used to stop bleeding from small cuts, contain astringents. Zinc oxide and calamine are astringents used in lotions, powders, and ointments to relieve itching and chafing in various forms of dermatitis. Astringents have some bacteriostatic properties, though they are not generally used as antiseptics.

astroblast ('astroh,blast) a cell that develops into an astrocyte.

astroblastoma (a,strohblas'tohmə) an astrocytoma of Grade II, composed of cells with abundant cytoplasm and two or three nuclei.

astrocyte ('astroh,siet) a neuroglial cell of ectodermal origin, characterized by fibrous or protoplasmic processes; collectively called astroglia, or macroglia.

astrocytin (,astroh'sietin) an antigen present on the cell membrane of astrocytes, found in the serum of patients with malignant glial tumours.

astrocytoma (,astrohsie'tohmə) a tumour composed of astrocytes; classified in order of malignancy as: *Grade I*, consisting of fibrillary or protoplasmic astrocytes; *Grade II* (astroblastoma); *Grades III* and *IV* (glioblastoma multiforme).

astroglia (ə'strogli·ə) neuroglia tissue made up of astrocytes.

astrosphere ('astrə,sfiə) 1. the central mass of an aster, excluding the rays. 2. aster.

asymbolia (,aysim'bohli·ə) loss of ability to understand symbols, such as words, figures, gestures, signs.

asymmetry (ay'simitree, a-) lack or absence of symmetry; dissimilarity in corresponding parts or organs on opposite sides of the body which are normally alike. In chemistry, lack of symmetry in the special arrangements of the atoms and radicals within the molecule or crystal. adj. **asymmetrical.**

asymphytous (ay'simfitəs) separate or distinct; not grown together.

asymptomatic (,aysimptə'matik, a-) showing no symptoms.

asynchronism (ay'sinkrə,nizəm, a-) occurrence at different times; disturbance of coordination.

asynclitism (ay'sinkli,tizəm) 1. oblique presentation of the fetal head in labour, called anterior asynclitism when the anterior parietal bone is designated the point of presentation, and posterior asynclitism when the posterior parietal bone is so designated. It is diagnosed by palpating the sagittal suture in the transverse diameter of the pelvis well above the ischial spines on vaginal examination. 2. maturation at different times of the nucleus and of the cytoplasm of blood cells.

asyndesis (ay'sindəsis) a language disorder in which related elements of a sentence cannot be welded together in a whole.

asynechia (aysi'neki·ə) absence of continuity of structure.

asynergia (aysi'nərji·ə) lack of coordination among parts or organs normally acting in unison. adj. **asynergic.**

asynovia (aysi'nohvi·ə, -sie-) absence or insufficiency of synovial secretion.

asyntaxia (aysin'taksi·ə) lack of proper and orderly embryonic development.

asystole (ay'sistəlee) cardiac standstill or arrest; absence of heartbeat. adj. **asystolic.**

At chemical symbol, *astatine.*

at. atomic.

at.no. atomic number.

at.wt atomic weight.

atactic (ə'taktik) pertaining to or characterized by ataxia; marked by incoordination or irregularity.

ataractic (aytə'raktik) 1. pertaining to or characterized by ataraxia. 2. an agent that induces antaraxia; a tranquillizer.

ataralgesia (,aytarəl'jeezi·ə) combined sedation and analgesia intended to abolish mental distress and pain attendant on surgical procedures, with the patient remaining conscious and alert.

Atarax ('atə,raks) trademark for preparations of hydroxyzine hydrochloride, an anxiolytic.

ataraxia (,atə'raksi·ə) a state of detached serenity with depression of mental faculties or impairment of consciousness.

atavism ('atə,vizəm) apparent inheritance of characters from remote ancestors. adj. **atavistic.**

ataxia (ə'taksi·ə) failure of muscular coordination; irregularity of muscular action. adj. **atactic, ataxic.**

cerebellar a. ataxia due to disease of the cerebellum.

Friedreich's a. the spinal form of hereditary sclerosis (see also FRIEDREICH'S ATAXIA).

frontal a. disturbance of equilibrium occurring in tumour of the frontal lobe.

hereditary a. Friedreich's ataxia.

locomotor a. tabes dorsalis.

sensory a. ataxia due to loss of proprioception (joint position sense), resulting in poorly judged movements and becoming aggravated when the eyes are closed.

a.-telangiectasia a severe hereditary progressive ataxia, transmitted as an autosomal recessive trait, associated with oculocutaneous telangiectasia, sinopulmonary disease with frequent respiratory infections, immunodeficiency, and abnormal eye movements. Called also Louis-Bar syndrome.

ataxiaphasia (ə,taksi·ə'fayzi·ə) inability to arrange

words into sentences.

ataxophaemia (ə,taksoh'feemi·ə) lack of coordination of speech muscles.

atel(o)- word element. [Gr.] *incomplete*, *imperfectly developed.*

atelectasis (,atə'lektəsis) a collapsed or airless state of the lung, which may be acute or chronic, and may involve all or part of the lung. adj. **atelectatic.** The primary cause of atelectasis is obstruction of the bronchus serving the affected area. In fetal atelectasis the lungs fail to expand normally at birth. This condition may be due to a variety of causes, including prematurity (and may accompany HYALINE MEMBRANE DISEASE), diminished nervous stimulus to breathing and crying, fetal hypoxia from any cause, including oversedation of the mother during labour and delivery and obstruction of the bronchus by a mucous plug.

SYMPTOMS. In acute atelectasis in which there is sudden obstruction of the bronchus, there may be pain in the affected side, dyspnoea and cyanosis, elevation of temperature, a drop in blood pressure or shock. In the chronic form, the patient may experience no symptoms other than gradually developing dyspnoea and weakness.

Radiological examination may show a shadow in the area of collapse. If an entire lobe is collapsed, the radiograph will show the trachea, heart, and mediastinum deviated toward the collapsed area, with the diaphragm elevated on that side.

TREATMENT. Atelectasis in the newborn is treated by suctioning the trachea to establish an open airway, positive-pressure breathing, and administration of oxygen (40 per cent concentration). High concentrations of oxygen given over a prolonged period tend to promote atelectasis and may lead to the development of retrolental fibroplasia in preterm infants.

Acute atelectasis is treated by removing the cause whenever possible. To accomplish this, coughing (sometimes using a cough-inducing machine), suctioning, and BRONCHOSCOPY may be employed. A detergent AEROSOL, used with a mist-producing apparatus, may be administered at regular intervals. Chronic atelectasis usually requires surgical removal of the affected segment or lobe of lung. Antibiotics are given to combat the infection that almost always accompanies secondary atelectasis.

congenital a. that present at (primary atelectasis) or immediately after (secondary atelectasis) birth.

lobar a. that affecting only a lobe of the lung.

lobular a. that affecting only a lobule of the lung.

primary a. congenital atelectasis in which the alveoli have never been expanded with air.

secondary a. congenital atelectasis in which resorption of the contained air has led to collapse of the aveoli.

atelia (ə'teeli·ə) imperfect or incomplete development.

ateliosis (ə,teeli'ohsis) 1. a condition characterized by failure to develop completely. 2. hypophyseal infantalism.

atelocardia (,atəloh'kahdi·ə) imperfect development of the heart.

atelocephaly (,atəloh'kefəlee, -sef-) imperfect development of the skull. adj. **atelocephalic, atelocephalous.**

atelomyelia (,atəlohmie'eeli·ə) imperfect development of the spinal cord.

atenolol (ə'tenə,lol) a cardioselective BETA-BLOCKER having a greater effect on β_1-adrenergic receptors of the heart than on the β_2-adrenergic receptors of the bronchi and blood vessels; used for treatment of hypertension.

athelia (ay'theeli·ə) congenital absence of the nipples.

athermic (ay'thərmik) without rise of temperature.

athermosystaltic (ay,thərmohsi'staltik) not contracting under the action of cold or heat.

atheroembolism (,athə·roh'embə,lizəm) embolism due to blockage of a blood vessel by an atheroembolus.

atheroembolus (,athə·roh'embələs) pl. *atheroemboli;* an embolus composed of cholesterol or its esters (typically lodging in small arteries) or of fragments of atheromatous plaques.

atherogenesis (,athə·roh'jenəsis) formation of atheromas in arterial walls. adj. **atherogenic.**

atheroma (,athə'rohmə) an abnormal mass of fatty or lipid material with a fibrous covering, existing as a discrete, raised plaque within the intima of an artery. adj. **atheromatous.**

atheromatosis (,athə·rohmə'tohsis) the presence of multiple atheromas.

atherosclerosis (,athə·rohsklə'rohsis) an extremely common form of ARTERIOSCLEROSIS in which deposits of yellowing plaques (atheromas) containing cholesterol, other lipoid material, and lipophages are formed within the intima of large and medium-sized arteries. adj. **atherosclerotic.** The word *atherosclerosis* comes from the Greek, *athere*, meaning 'soft, fatty, gruel-like', and *scler-* meaning 'hard'. These terms are descriptive of the material deposited on the inner lining (*intima*) of an artery and of the state of the arterial muscle walls once they have been affected by the disease.

In a normal artery the endothelial lining is tightly packed with cells that allow for the smooth passage of blood and act as a protective covering against harmful substances circulating in the bloodstream. The endothelial lining is surrounded by a sheath of muscle cells. In the earliest stage of atherosclerosis fatty streaks form along the intima. The lesions are widely scattered at first, but as the disease progresses they become more numerous and can eventually cover the entire intimal surface of an artery. Later, *atheromas* or plaques of newly formed muscle cells filled with cholesterol build up and protrude into the lumen of the vessel. These deposits cause the inner wall to become roughened and also cause the muscle wall to be rigid and inelastic. Narrowing of the lumen and hardening of the muscle wall decrease the rate at which blood can flow through the vessel and may lead to ischaemia of the tissues served by the vessel and the development of clots within the vessel itself. The process also damages and deforms the muscle wall to the extent that it becomes weakened and may develop an ANEURYSM.

The eventual outcome of the atherosclerotic process in large arteries can be a STROKE or occlusion of one or more of the coronary arteries and MYOCARDIAL INFARCTION.

AETIOLOGY. The exact cause of atherosclerosis is not yet known and is most likely a combination of factors rather than a single aetiologic agent. Heredity seems to play some role; men in certain families have been found to be more susceptible than the average. The fact that women seldom are affected by the disease before menopause suggests that the female sex hormones are associated with the disease. Atherosclerosis is accelerated by HYPERTENSION, probably because of the added stress on the linings of the large blood vessels. Persons suffering from disorders of metabolism, particularly DIABETES MELLITUS, are especially susceptible and tend to develop atherosclerosis earlier in life than persons who do not have these disorders.

Another major factor is *hyperlipaemia*, particularly high serum cholesterol, which is closely associated with the development of coronary heart disease. Studies of well-defined population groups, notably the

USA Framingham, Massachusetts Study, have shown that in male and female subjects between 35 and 44 years of age high total serum cholesterol levels (265 mg/100 ml or over) present a five times higher risk of coronary artery disease than levels below 220 mg/100 ml. When the LIPOPROTEINS were analysed more definitively, it was found that low-density lipoprotein (LDL), which is rich in cholesterol, was positively related to risk for both men and women up to 70 years of age. In contrast, high-density lipoprotein (HDL) was *inversely* related to risk for ischaemic heart disease. It is thought that HDL facilitates the transport of cholesterol from smooth muscle cells, including those in the arterial walls, to the liver where it is excreted and therefore unavailable for recycling in the synthesis of LDL.

Although heart disease, stroke, and other diseases related to atherosclerosis remain a major cause of death in the United Kingdom, the death rate for these diseases has been declining in the past decade. It is thought that the decline is at least in part due to changes in diet with emphasis on reduced intake of cholesterol and animal fats, the popularity of regular exercise programmes and jogging, success in efforts to control HYPERTENSION, reduction in smoking, weight reduction, and careful monitoring of persons known to be at high risk for diseases associated with atherosclerosis.

athetoid ('athitoyd) 1. resembling athetosis. 2. affected with athetosis.

athetosis (ˌathi'tohsis) repetitive involuntary, slow, sinuous, writhing movements.

athlete's foot ('athleets) a fungal infection of the skin of the foot; called also *tinea pedis*. Athlete's foot causes itching and often blisters and cracks, usually between the toes. Causative agents are *Candida albicans*, *Epidermophyton floccosum*, and species of *Trichophyton*, which thrive on warmth and dampness.

If not arrested, athlete's foot can cause a rash and itching in other parts of the body as well. It is likely to be recurrent, since the fungus survives under the toenails and reappears when conditions are favourable. Although athlete's foot is usually little more than an uncomfortable nuisance, its open sores provide excellent sites for more serious infections. Early treatment and medical advice insure correct diagnosis and prevention of complications. Specific diagnosis is made by microscopic examination or culture of skin scrapings for the fungus.

Prevention of athlete's foot includes keeping the feet dry and open to the air as much as possible, especially the areas between the toes. Small cotton pads may be used between the toes if this area is difficult to keep dry. A dusting powder may be used on the feet and sprinkled in the shoes to reduce the accumulation of moisture.

For treatment, there are a number of compounds that can be applied locally for both the acute and chronic stages. Benzoic acid together with salicylic acid (Whitfield's ointment) is the most effective treatment.

athrepsia (ay'threpsi·ə) marasmus. adj. **athreptic.**

athymia (ay'thiemi·ə) 1. dementia. 2. absence of functioning thymus tissue.

athymism (ay'thiemizəm) absence of the thymus or the condition induced by absence or removal of the thymus.

athyreosis (ˌaythieri'ohsis) absence of the thyroid. adj. **athyreotic.**

athyria (ay'thieri·ə) 1. absence of functioning thyroid tissue. 2. hypothyroidism.

Ativan ('atiˌvan) trademark for a preparation of lorazepam, an anxiolytic.

atlantal (at'lant'l) pertaining to the atlas.

atlas ('atləs) the first cervical vertebra, the uppermost segment of the backbone which supports the skull.

atloaxoid (ˌatloh'aksoyd) pertaining to the atlas and axis.

atmosphere ('atməsˌfiə) 1. the entire gaseous envelope surrounding the earth, extending to an altitude of 10 miles. 2. a unit of pressure, equivalent to that on a surface at sea level, being about 14.7 lb per square inch (= 100 kPa), or equivalent to that of a column of mercury 760 mm high.

atmospheric (ˌatməs'ferik) of or pertaining to the atmosphere.

a. pressure the pressure exerted by the atmosphere, about 14.7 lb per square inch (= 100 kPa) at sea level.

atom ('atəm) the smallest particle of an element that has all the properties of the element. adj. **atomic.** There are two main parts of an atom: the nucleus and the electron cloud. The nucleus is made up of protons, which have one unit of mass and carry a positive electrical charge, and (except in hydrogen) neutrons, which have an identical unit of mass but carry no electrical charge. The electron cloud is made up of particles called electrons, which carry a negative electrical charge and move in orbits or 'shells' around the nucleus. Different atoms have different numbers of protons, neutrons, and electrons in their makeup.

In a chemical change, atoms do not break up but act as individual units. The chemical behaviour of an atom is controlled by the number and spatial arrangement of electrons in orbit around the nucleus. The atoms of radioactive elements are very unstable and are capable of emitting nuclear particles and electromagnetic radiation in a stream or 'ray'. These are called radiations. See also ELEMENT and RADIATION.

atomic mass unit (ə'tomik) dalton; unit for specifying the masses of different elements. The isotope ^{12}C represents the standard of 12 atomic mass units. One a.m.u. is approximately 1.67×10^{-27} kg.

atomic number the number of protons in the nucleus of an atom; it is equal to the net positive charge of the nucleus.

atomic weight the average weight of the atoms of an element in ATOMIC MASS UNITS.

atomization (ˌatəmie'zayshən) the act or process of breaking up a liquid into a fine spray.

atomizer ('atəˌmiezə) an instrument for dispensing liquid in a fine spray.

atonia, atony (ay'tohni·ə; 'atənee) absence or lack of normal tone. adj. **atonic.**

atopen ('atəˌpen) the antigen responsible for atopy.

atopic (ay'topik) 1. displaced; ectopic. 2. pertaining to atopy.

atopy ('atəpee) a clinical hypersensitivity state or ALLERGY with a hereditary predisposition; i.e., the tendency to develop an allergy is inherited, but the specific clinical form (hay fever, asthma, etc.) is not. IgE antibodies are involved.

atoxic (ay'toksik) not poisonous; not due to a poison.

ATP (ˌaytee'pee) adenosine triphosphate.

ATPase (ˌaytee'peeayz) adenosine triphosphatase.

ATPS ambient temperature and pressure, saturated; denoting a volume of gas saturated with water vapour at ambient temperature and barometric pressure.

atracurium (ˌatrə'kyooə·ri·əm) a new neuromuscular blocking agent of the non-depolarizing type remarkable for spontaneously breaking down in the blood. It has a relatively short duration of action and is particularly useful for providing muscle relaxation in patients with kidney or liver disease undergoing surgery.

atraumatic (ˌaytraw'matik) not producing injury or damage.

atresia (ə'treezi·ə) congenital absence or closure of a normal body opening or tubular structure. adj. **atretic**.
anal a., a. ani imperforate anus.
aortic a. absence of the opening from the left ventricle of the heart into the aorta.
aural a. absence of closure of the auditory canal.
biliary a. congenital obliteration or hypoplasia of one or more components of the bile ducts, resulting in persistent jaundice and liver damage.
oesophageal a. congenital lack of continuity of the oesophagus, commonly accompanied by tracheo–oesophageal fistula, and characterized by accumulations of mucus in the nasopharynx, gagging, vomiting when fed, cyanosis, and dyspnoea. Treatment is by surgical repair by oesophageal anastomosis and division of the fistula.
follicular a., a. folliculi degeneration and resorption of an ovarian follicle before it reaches maturity and ruptures.
tricuspid a. absence of the opening between the right atrium and right ventricle, circulation being made possible by an atrial septal defect.

atria ('aytri·ə) plural of *atrium*.

atrial ('aytri·əl) pertaining to an atrium.
a. fibrillation see atrial FIBRILLATION.
a. septal defect a CONGENITAL HEART DEFECT in which there is persistent patency of the atrial septum, owing to failure of closure of the ostium primum or ostium secundum.

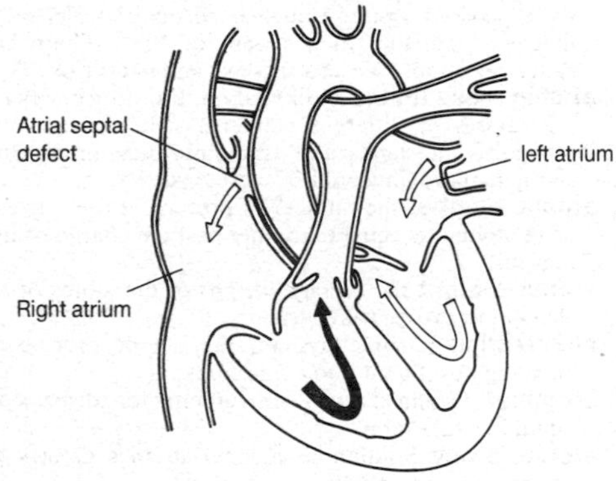

Atrial septal defect.

atrichia (ay'triki·ə) absence of hair or of flagella or cilia.

atrichous (ay'trikəs) 1. having no hair. 2. having no flagella.

atriomegaly (ˌaytrioh'megəlee) abnormal enlargement of an atrium of the heart.

atrioseptopexy (ˌaytrioh'septohˌpeksee) surgical correction of a defect in the interatrial septum.

atrioseptoplasty (ˌaytrioh'septohˌplastee) plastic repair of the interatrial septum.

atrioventricular (ˌaytriohven'trikyuhlə) pertaining to an atrium and ventricle of the heart.
a. bundle bundle of His.
a. canal the common canal connecting the primitive atrium and ventricle; it sometimes persists as a congenital anomaly.
a. node a mass of cardiac muscle fibres (Purkinje fibres) lying on the right lower part of the interatrial septum of the heart. Its function is the transmission of the cardiac impulse from the sinoatrial node to the muscular walls of the ventricles. The conductive system is organized so that transmission is slightly delayed at the atrioventricular node, thus allowing time for the atria to empty their contents into the ventricles before the ventricles begin to contract.

atrioventricularis communis (ˌatriohvenˌtrikyuhˌlahris ko'myoonis) a congenital cardiac anomaly in which the endocardial cushions fail to fuse, the ostium primum persists, the atrioventricular canal is undivided, a single atrioventricular valve has anterior and posterior cusps, and there is a defect of the membranous interventricular septum.

atrium ('aytri·əm) pl. *atria* [L.] a chamber affording entrance, especially the upper chamber (atrium cordis) on either side of the heart, transmitting to the ventricle of the same side blood received (left atrium) from the pulmonary veins and (right atrium) from the venae cavae.

Atromid-S ('atrəmid·əs) trademark for a preparation of clofibrate, an antihyperlipoproteinaemic.

atrophia (a'trohfi·ə) [L.] *atrophy*.

atrophoderma (ˌatrohfoh'dərmə) atrophy of the skin.

atrophy ('atrəfee) 1. gradual decrease in size of a normally developed organ or tissue with a reduction in size and number of its functional parenchymal components; wasting. 2. to undergo or cause atrophy. adj. **atrophic**.
acute yellow a. the shrunken, yellow liver which is a complication, usually fatal, of fulminant hepatitis with massive hepatic necrosis. Not a true atrophy.
disuse a. atrophy of a tissue or organ as a result of inactivity or diminished function.
gyrate a. of choroid and retina a rare hereditary, slowly progressive atrophy of the choroid and pigment epithelium of the retina; inherited as an autosomal recessive trait.
Leber's optic a. hereditary bilateral atrophy of the optic nerve affecting postpubertal males; there is rapid loss of vision resulting in permanent central scotoma.
myelopathic muscular a. muscular atrophy due to lesion of the spinal cord, as in spinal muscular atrophy.
progressive neuromuscular a., progressive neuropathic (peroneal) muscular a. hereditary muscular atrophy beginning in the muscles supplied by the peroneal nerves, progressing slowly to involve the muscles of the hands and arms. Called also *Charcot–Marie–Tooth disease*.
spinal muscular a. progressive degeneration of the motor cells of the spinal cord, beginning usually in the small muscles of the hands, but in some cases (scapulohumeral type) in the upper arm and shoulder muscles, and progressing slowly to the leg muscles. Called also *Aran–Duchenne disease*, *Cruveilhier's disease*, and *Duchenne's disease*.
subacute yellow a. submassive necrosis of liver associated with broad zones of necrosis, due to viral, toxic, or drug-induced hepatitis; it may have an acute course with death from liver failure occurring after several weeks, or there may be clinical recovery associated with regeneration of the parenchymal cells.

atropine ('atrəˌpeen, -pin) an anticholinergic alkaloid occurring in belladonna, hyoscyamus, and strammonium. It acts as a competetive antagonist of acetylcholine at muscarinic receptors, blocking stimulation of muscles and glands by parasympathetic and cholinergic sympathetic nerves; used as a smooth muscle relaxant, as a preanaesthetic to reduce secretions, and as an antidote to organophosphate poisoning.
a. poisoning severe toxic reaction due to overdosage of

atropine. Symptoms include dryness of mouth, thirst, difficulty in swallowing, dilated pupils, tachycardia, fever, delirium, stupor, and a rash on the face, neck, and upper trunk. Treatment consists of gastric suction or the inducement of vomiting to remove the poison from the stomach; the stomach is then washed with 2 to 4 litres of water containing activated charcoal. The lavage is followed with a solution of 30 gm of sodium sulphate in 200 ml of water, which is left in the stomach. Barbiturates may be used to control excitability. There may be a need for treatment of respiratory difficulty. Measures also are taken to reduce the high body temperature.

atropinic (,atrə'pinik) muscarinic.

ATS anti-tetanus serum.

attack (ə'tak) an episode or onset of illness.

a. rate number of cases of a disease in a particular group, e.g. a school, over a given period related to the population of that group.

transient ischaemic a's brief attacks (a few hours or less) of cerebral dysfunction of vascular origin, without lasting neurological deficit. See also TRANSIENT ISCHAEMIC ATTACK.

attention deficit syndrome (ə'tenshən) a disorder of childhood characterized by marked failure of attention, impulsiveness and increased motor activity. The syndrome tends to decline somewhat after puberty, although attentional difficulties often persist.

attenuation (ə,tenyoo'ayshən) 1. the act of thinning or weakening. 2. the change in the virulence of a pathogenic microorganism induced by passage through another host species, decreasing its virulence for the native host and increasing it for the new host. This is the basis for the development of live vaccines. 3. the change in a beam of radiation as it passes through matter. The intensity of the electromagnetic radiation decreases as its depth of penetration increases.

attic ('atik) a small upper space of the middle ear, containing the head of the malleus and the body of the incus.

atticoantrotomy (,atikoh·an'trotəmee) surgical exposure of the attic and mastoid antrum.

atticotomy (,ati'kotəmee) incision into the attic.

attitude ('ati,tyood) 1. a posture or position of the body; in obstetrics, the relation of the various parts of the fetal body to one another. 2. a pattern of mental views established by cumulative prior experience.

atto- word element. [Scand.] *eighteen;* used in naming units of measurement to indicate a quantity 10^{-18} (one-million-million-millionth) of the unit with which it is joined; symbol a.

attraction (ə'trakshən) the force or influence by which one object is drawn toward another.

capillary a. the force that causes a liquid to rise in a fine-calibre tube.

attributable risk (ə'tribyuhytəb'l) see under RISK.

atypia (ay'tipi·ə) deviation from the normal or typical state.

atypical (ay'tipik'l) irregular; not conformable to the type.

Au chemical symbol, *gold* (L. *aurum*).

audi(o)- word element. [L.] *hearing.*

audioanalgesia (,awdioh,anəl'jeezi·ə, -,an'l'jeezi·ə) reduction or abolition of pain by listening to recorded music to which has been added a background of so-called white sound.

audiogenic (,awdioh'jenik) produced by sound.

audiogram ('awdioh,gram) a graphic record of the findings by audiometry.

audiologist (,awdi'oləjist) an allied health professional specializing in audiology, who provides services that include: (1) evaluation of hearing function to detect hearing impairment and, if there is a hearing disorder, to determine the anatomical site involved and the cause of the disorder, (2) selection of appropriate hearing aids, and (3) training in lip reading, hearing aid use, and maintenance of normal speech.

audiology (,awdi'oləjee) the science concerned with the sense of hearing, especially the evaluation and measurement of impaired hearing and the rehabilitation of those with impaired hearing. See also AUDIOLOGIST.

audiometer (,awdi'omitə) an apparatus used in audiometry.

audiometry (,awdi'omətree) measurement of the acuity of hearing for the various frequencies of sound waves. adj. **audiometric.**

electrocochleographic a. measurement of electrical potentials from the middle ear or external auditory canal (cochlear microphonics and eighth nerve action potentials) in response to acoustic stimuli.

pure tone a. audiometry utilizing pure tones that are relatively free of noise and overtones.

speech a. that in which the speech reception threshold in decibels and the ability to understand speech (speech discrimination) are measured.

audit ('awdit) systematic review and evaluation of records and other data to determine the quality of the services or products provided in a given situation.

a. Monitor an adaptation for the UK of the USA Rush Medicus system of assessing quality of nursing care. It consists of 'checklists' for quality leading to a scoring system. The closer the score to 100 per cent the better the care being given. The master list has over 200 criteria which are divided into four categories based on patient dependency levels.

nursing a. an evaluation of structure, process, and outcome as a measurement of the quality of nursing care. *Concurrent audits* are conducted at the time the care is being provided to clients/patients. They may be conducted by means of observation and interview of clients/patients, review of open charts, or conferences with groups of consumers and providers of nursing care.

Retrospective audits are conducted after the patient's discharge. Methods include the study of closed patients' charts and nursing care plans, questionnaires, interviews, and surveys of patients and families.

Evaluations are based on criteria and standards developed by leaders in the field of nursing. Among these are the Standards of Nursing Practice Scale developed by Doris Slater Stewart, and a revision of the Slater Scale that is called Qualpacs, the Quality Patient Care Scale. See also EVALUATION, MONITOR, NURSING AUDIT, and NURSING PROCESS.

audition (aw'dishən) perception of sound; hearing.

chromatic a. chromaesthesia.

auditory ('awditə·ree, -tree) pertaining to the ear or the sense of hearing.

a. bulb the membranous labyrinth and cochlea.

a. nerve the eighth cranial nerve; called also VESTIBULOCOCHLEAR NERVE and *acoustic nerve.*

a. tube the narrow channel connecting the middle ear and the nasopharynx (see also PHARYNGOTYMPANIC TUBE).

Auerbach's plexus ('owə,bahkhs) the ganglionic neurones of the vagus nerve that supply the muscle fibres of the intestine.

Augmentin (awg'mentin) trademark for a combination of amoxycillin and clavulanic acid.

augnathus (awg'naythəs) a fetus with a double lower jaw.

aura ('or·rə) a peculiar sensation preceding the appearance of more definite symptoms. An epileptic aura precedes the convulsive seizure and may involve visual disturbances, dizziness, numbness, or any of a number of sensations which the patient may find difficult to describe exactly. In epilepsy the aura serves a useful purpose in that it warns the patient of an impending attack and gives him time to seek privacy and a safe place to lie down before the seizure actually begins.

A migraine aura sometimes precedes migraine headache, warning the patient that an attack is imminent. When it occurs the patient should lie down in a quiet, darkened room. A warm bath before lying down sometimes increases relaxation and helps to prevent a severe attack.

aural ('or·rəl) 1. pertaining to the ear. 2. pertaining to an aura.

aurantiasis (ˌor·ran'tieəsis) yellowness of skin caused by intake of large amounts of food containing carotene.

auric ('or·rik) pertaining to gold.

auricle ('or·rik'l) 1. the flap of the ear. 2. the ear-shaped appendage of either atrium of the heart; formerly used to designate the entire atrium.

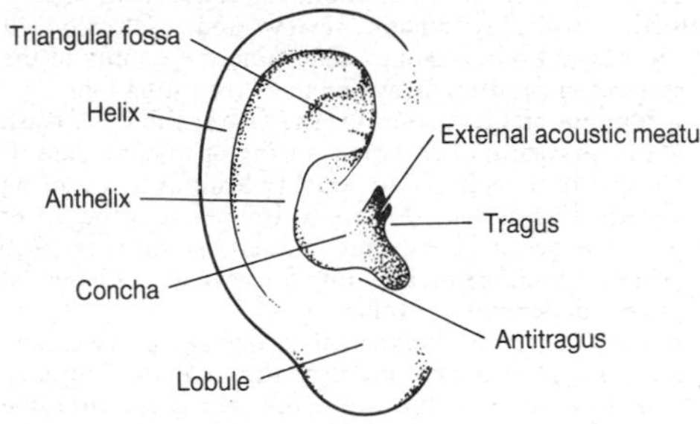

Auricle

auricula (or'rikyuhlə) pl. *auriculae* [L.] auricle.

auricular (or'rikyuhlə) pertaining to an auricle or ear.

auricularis (orˌrikyuh'lahris) [L.] pertaining to the ear.

auriculotemporal (orˌrikyuhloh'tempə·rəl, -'temprəl) pertaining to the ear and the temporal region.

auripuncture ('or·riˌpungkchə) myringotomy; surgical puncture of the tympanic membrane.

auris ('or·ris) pl. *aures* [L.] ear.

auriscope ('or·riˌskohp) otoscope; an instrument for examining the ear.

aurum ('or·rəm) [L.] *gold* (symbol Au).

auscultate ('awskəlˌtayt) to examine by auscultation.

auscultation (ˌawskəl'tayshən) listening for sounds produced within the body, chiefly to ascertain the condition of the thoracic or abdominal viscera and to detect pregnancy; it may be performed with the unaided ear (direct or immediate auscultation) or with a stethoscope (mediate auscultation).

auscultatory (aw'skultətə·ree) pertaining to auscultation.

Australia antigen (o'strayli·ə) antigen found in the blood of patients with serum hepatitis. Originally discovered in Australian aborigines.

aut(o)- word element. [Gr.] *self.*

autacoid ('awtəˌkoyd) a term once proposed to replace the term *hormone* and recently suggested as a general term for various physiologically active, endogenous substances (histamine, serotonin, angiotensin, prostaglandins, etc.) that do not yet fit into existing functional classifications.

autism ('awtizəm) a form of thinking in which the content is either entirely subjective or has a subjective meaning and emphasis including fantasies, delusions, and hallucinations; a fundamental symptom of schizophrenia.

akinetic a. coma vigil.

early infantile a. a syndrome beginning in infancy, characterized by extreme withdrawal and an obsessive desire to maintain the status quo. It becomes apparent in the first or second year of life. The child is self-absorbed, inaccessible, and unable to relate to others. He may play happily alone for hours but has temper tantrums if interrupted. Language disturbances include repetition of previously heard speech and reversal of the pronouns 'I' and 'you'. The cause of the syndrome is unknown and the prognosis is poor; affected children rarely recover completely. Called also kannerian psychosis.

infantile a. early infantile autism.

autistic (aw'tistik) pertaining to or exhibiting autism.

a. child a child suffering from infantile autism.

autoagglutination (ˌawtoh·əˌglooti'nayshən) 1. clumping or agglutination of an individual's cells by his own serum, as in autohaemagglutination. Autoagglutination occurring at low temperatures is called *cold agglutination.* 2. agglutination of particulate antigens, e.g., bacteria, in the absence of specific antigens.

autoagglutinin (ˌawtoh·ə'glootinin) a factor in serum capable of causing clumping together of the subject's own cellular elements.

autoamputation (ˌawtohˌampyuh'tayshən) spontaneous detachment from the body and elimination of an appendage or an abnormal growth, such as a polyp.

autoantibody (ˌawtoh'antiˌbodee) an antibody formed in response to, and reacting against, an antigenic constituent of the individual's own tissues.

autoantigen (ˌawtoh'antijən) a tissue constituent that stimulates production of autoantibodies in the organism in which it occurs.

autocatalysis (ˌawtohkə'talisis) catalysis in which a product of the reaction hastens or intensifies the catalysis.

autochthonous (aw'tokthənəs) 1. originating in the same area in which it is found. 2. denoting a tissue graft to a new site on the same individual.

autoclasis (ˌawtoh'klaysis) destruction of a part by influences within itself.

autoclave ('awtəˌklayv) an automatically regulated apparatus for the sterilization of materials by steam under pressure. The autoclave allows steam to flow around each article placed in the chamber. The vapour penetrates cloth or paper used to package the articles being sterilized. Autoclaving is an effective method for destruction of spore-bearing microorganisms. The amount of time and degree of temperature necessary for sterilization depend on the articles to be sterilized and whether they are wrapped or left directly exposed to the steam.

autocytolysin (ˌawtohsie'tolisin) autolysin.

autocytolysis (ˌawtohsie'tolisis) autolysis.

autodigestion (ˌawtohdie'jeschən, -di-) dissolution of tissue by its own secretions.

autoecholalia (ˌawtohˌekoh'layli·ə) repetition of one's own words.

autoeczematization (ˌawtohˌeksimətie'zayshən, -ˌeksmə-) the spread, at first locally and later more generally, of lesions from an originally circumscribed focus of eczema.

autoeroticism, autoerotism (ˌawtoh·i'rotiˌsizəm; ˌawtoh'erəˌtizəm) erotic behaviour directed toward one's self. adj. **autoerotic.**

autoerythrocyte sensitization syndrome (ˌawtoh·i'rithrohsiet) a reaction occurring chiefly in young women, in which spontaneous, painful, recurrent single or multiple ecchymoses occur on any part of the body without trauma or after insufficient trauma. Sensitivity to a component of the erythrocytes' structural framework is responsible in many cases, but in some cases the leukocytes seem to be responsible. Emotional upsets are believed to be a precipitating factor. Called also painful bruising syndrome.

autogeneic (,awtohjə'nee·ik, -'nay-) arising from self; pertaining to an autograft.

autogenesis (,awtoh'jenəsis) self-generation; origination within the organism. adj. **autogenetic, autogenous.**

autograft ('awtə,grahft) a graft transferred from one part of the patient's body to another part.

autohaemagglutination (,awtoh,heemə,glooti'nayshən) agglutination of erythrocytes by a factor produced in the subject's own body.

autohaemagglutinin (,awtoh,heemə'glootinin) a substance produced in a person's body that causes agglutination of his own erythrocytes.

autohaemolysin (,awtoh·hee'molisin) a haemolysin produced in the body of an animal which causes destruction of its own erythrocytes.

autohaemolysis (,awtoh·hee'molisis) haemolysis of the blood cells of an individual by his own serum. adj. **autohaemolytic.**

autohaemotherapy (,awtoh,heemə'therəpee) treatment by reinjection of the patient's own blood.

autohypnosis (,awtoh·hip'nohsis) self-induced hypnosis; the act or process of hypnotizing oneself.

autoimmune disease (,awtoh·i'myoon) disease due to immunological action of an individual's own cells or antibodies on components of the body.

The immunological mechanism of the body is dependent on two major factors: (1) the inactivation and rejection of foreign substances; and (2) the ability to differentiate between the body's own material ('self') and that which is foreign ('nonself'). Prevention of self reaction that is damaging is largely by the development of controlling feedback processes. Of these, two are most important: T suppressor lymphocytes and anti-idiotypic antibodies. Both of these can inhibit responses to foreign antigens and usually prevent self responses. Several possibilities have been identified as pertinent to the development of autoimmunity.

(1) There may be a leakage of normally *inaccessible* tissue antigen from its isolated location into an area where it comes into contact with the immunocompetent cells of the reticuloendothelial system (RES). These RES cells do not recognize the formerly inaccessible antigen as 'self' and react accordingly.

(2) The antigens that are normally accessible to the RES cells may suddenly stimulate the production of autoantibodies. It is thought that this occurs as a result of the emergence of 'forbidden clones' (colonies) of cells. Normally these cells are inactivated by suppressor T cells and anti-idiotypic antibodies. For reasons not yet fully explained, these 'forbidden clones' survive and emerge to produce an autoimmune reaction. It is believed that they may be activated by injury, disease, or a metabolic change in the body, or there may be a mutation of the forbidden clone cells and immunologically competent cells. It appears that there may be a genetic tendency to fail to inhibit some autoimmune reactions.

(3) Certain body proteins may be so altered by viral infection, by combination with a drug or chemical, or by extensive trauma (as in a severe burn and myocardial infarction) that they are not recognized by the body as 'self' and are therefore rejected as foreign.

Many B cells secrete autoreactive antibodies of IgM class that do not cause damage and may be important in normal homeostasis. On the other hand, it is believed that healthy autoreactive T lymphocytes are usually deleted during their development. If this does not happen, they may be aggressive and cytotoxic and also help B cells in the production of tissue damaging autoantibodies of IgG class.

Autoimmune disease can be viewed as a spectrum of disorders. At one end are *organ-specific* diseases, in which there is localized tissue damage resulting from the presence of specific antibodies. An example is *Hashimoto's disease* of the thyroid, characterized by a specific lesion in the thyroid gland with infiltration by mononuclear cells, destruction of follicular cells, and production of antibodies with absolute specificity for certain thyroid constituents.

In the middle of the spectrum are disorders in which the lesion tends to be localized in one organ, but the antibodies are non-organ specific. An example is *primary biliary cirrhosis*, in which there is inflammatory cell infiltration of the small bile ductule, but the serum antibodies are not specific to liver cells.

At the other end of the spectrum are *non-organ specific* diseases, in which lesions and antibodies are widespread throughout the body and not limited to one target organ. Systemic LUPUS ERYTHEMATOSUS (SLE) is an example of this type of autoimmune disease. In the early 1970's researchers using fluorescent-labelling techniques were able to identify antinuclear antibody (ANA) in the diseased tissue of the kidneys of patients with SLE. The antinuclear antibodies attack the nucleic acids DNA and RNA and other components of the body's own cells. Identification of ANA in SLE victims established once and for all the existence of autoimmune disease. Recently, antibodies specific to *hormone receptors* on the surface of cells have been found. These autoantibodies are partially responsible for such conditions as MYASTHENIA GRAVIS, in which anti-acetylcholine-receptor antibodies are involved, GRAVES' DISEASE, in which antibodies against components of thyroid cell membranes including the receptors for thyroid stimulating hormone (TSH) are responsible, and certain cases of insulin-resistant DIABETES MELLITUS, in which the antibodies affect insulin receptors on cells.

Other diseases involving autoimmune mechanisms include rheumatic fever, rheumatoid arthritis, autoimmune haemolytic anaemia, idiopathic thrombocytopenic purpura, and postviral encephalomyelitis.

Treatment of autoimmune diseases varies with each specific disease, but in all cases the doctor must strive to achieve a delicate balance between adequate suppression of the autoimmune reaction to avoid continued damage to the body tissues, and maintenance of sufficient functioning of the immune mechanism to protect the patient against foreign invaders.

In general, autoimmune diseases are treated by immunosuppression with corticosteroids, azathioprine or cyclophosphamide. Plasmapheresis is also used in some conditions to remove damaging antibodies. High dose intravenous IgG is used to provide anti-idiotypic antibodies which can neutralize autoantibodies.

autoimmunity (,awtoh·i'myoonitee) a condition characterized by a specific humoural or cell-mediated immune response against the constituents of the body's own tissues (autoantigens); it may result in hypersensitivity reactions or, if severe, in AUTOIMMUNE DISEASE.

autoimmunization (,awtoh,imyuhnie'zayshən) induction in an organism of an immense response to its own tissue constituents.

autoinfection (,awtoh·in'fekshən) self-infection, transferred from one part of the body to another by fingers, towels, etc.

autoinoculation (,awtoh·i,nokyuh'layshən) inoculation with microorganisms from one's own body.

autointoxication (,awtoh·in,toksi'kayshən) poisoning by uneliminated material (toxins) formed within the body.

autoisolysin (,awtoh·ie'solisin) a substance that lyses cells (e.g., blood cells) of the individual in which it is formed and also those of other individuals of the same species.

autokeratoplasty (,awtoh'kerətoh,plastee) grafting of corneal tissue from one eye to the other.

autokinesis (,awtohki'neesis) voluntary motion. adj. **autokinetic.**

autolesion (,awtoh'leezhən) a self-inflicted injury.

autologous (aw'toləgəs) related to self; belonging to the same organism.

autolysate (aw'toli,sayt) a substance produced by autolysis.

autolysin (aw'tolisin, ,awtə'liesin) a lysin originating in an organism and capable of destroying its own cells and tissues.

autolysis (aw'tolisis) the disintegration of cells or tissues by endogenous enzymes. adj. **autolytic.**

automatic (,awtə'matik) spontaneous; done involuntarily; self-regulating.

automatism (aw'tomə,tizəm) mechanical, often repetitive motor behaviour performed without conscious control.

command a. uncritical response to commands, as in hypnosis and certain mental states.

autonomic (,awtə'nomik) not subject to voluntary control.

a. nervous system the branch of the nervous system that works without conscious control. The voluntary nervous system governs the striated or skeletal muscles, whereas the autonomic nervous system governs the glands, the cardiac muscle, and the smooth muscles, such as those of the digestive system, the respiratory system, and the skin. The autonomic nervous system is divided into two subsidiary systems, the sympathetic system and the parasympathetic system.

autonomotropic (,awtə,nohmoh'trohpik, -'trop-) having an affinity for the autonomic nervous system.

autopathy (aw'topəthee) idiopathic disease; one without apparent external causation.

autophagia (,awtoh'fayji·ə) 1. eating or biting of one's own flesh. 2. nutrition of the body by consumption of its own tissues. 3. autophagy.

autophagosome (,awtoh'fagə,sohm) a secondary lysosome in which elements of a cell's own cytoplasm are digested.

autophagy (aw'tofəjee) 1. lysosomal digestion of a cell's own cytoplasmic material. 2. autophagia.

autopharmacological (,awtoh,fahməkə'lojik'l) pertaining to substances (e.g., hormones) produced in the body that have pharmacological activities.

autophilia (,awtoh'fili·ə) pathological self-esteem; narcissism.

autoplasmotherapy (,awtoh,plazmə'therəpee) therapeutic reinjection of one's own plasma.

autoplasty ('awtoh,plastee) 1. replacement or reconstruction of diseased or injured parts with tissues taken from another region of the patient's own body. 2. in psychoanalysis, instinctive modification within the psychic systems in adaptation to reality. adj. **autoplastic.**

autopolyploidy (,awtoh'poli,ploy) the state of having more than two chromosome sets as a result of redoubling of the chromosomes of a haploid individual or cell. adj. **autopolyploid.**

autopsy (aw'topsee, 'awtəp-) examination of a body after death to identify the distribution and extent of any disease present; called also postmortem examination and necropsy. An autopsy is ordered by a coroner or medical examiner whenever the cause of death is unknown or the death takes place under suspicious circumstances. Unless an autopsy is demanded by public authorities, it cannot be performed without the permission of the next of kin of the deceased.

autoradiograph (,awtoh'raydiə,grahf, -,graf) the film produced by autoradiography. Called also *radioautograph.*

autoradiography (,awtoh,raydi'ogrəfee) the making of a radiograph of an object or tissue by recording on a photographic plate the radiation emitted by radioactive material within the object. Called also *radioautography.*

autoreactive (,awtohri'aktiv) pertaining to an immune response directed against the body's own tissues.

autoregulation (,awtoh,regyuh'layshən) control of certain phenomena by factors inherent in a situation; specifically, (1) maintenance by an organ or tissue of a constant blood flow despite changes in arterial pressure, and (2) adjustment of blood flow through an organ in accordance with its metabolic needs.

heterometric a. those intrinsic mechanisms controlling the strength of ventricular contractions that depend on the length of myocardial fibres at the end of diastole.

homeometric a. those intrinsic mechanisms controlling the strength of ventricular contractions that are independent of the length of myocardial fibres at the end of diastole.

autosensitization (,awtoh,sensitie'zayshən) development of sensitivity to one's own serum or tissues.

autosepticaemia (,awtoh,septi'seemi·ə) septicaemia from poisons developed within the body.

autoserum (,awtoh'siə·rəm) serum administered to the patient from whom it was derived.

autosite ('awtoh,siet) the larger, more normal member of asymmetrical conjoined twin fetuses, to which the other twin (the parasite) is attached.

autosome ('awtoh,sohm) any of the 22 pairs of chromosomes in man not concerned with determination of sex.

autosplenectomy (,awtohspli'nektəmee) almost complete disappearance of the spleen due to progressive fibrosis and shrinkage.

autosuggestion (,awtohsə'jeschən) suggestion arising in one's self.

autotomography (,awtohtə'mogrəfee) a method of body-section radiography involving movement of the patient instead of the x-ray tube.

autotopagnosia (,awtoh,topəg'nohzi·ə) inability to orient correctly different parts of the body.

autotoxin (,awtoh'toksin) a toxin developed within the body.

autotransfusion (,awtohtrans'fyoozhən, -trahns-) reinfusion of a patient's own blood.

autotransplantation (,awtoh,transplahn'tayshən) transfer of tissue from one part of the body to another part.

autotroph ('awtoh,trohf) an autotrophic organism.

autotrophic (,awtoh'trofik) capable of synthesizing necessary nutrients if water, carbon dioxide, inorganic salts, and a source of energy are available.

autoxidation (,awtoksi'dayshən, aw,toksi-) the spontaneous reaction of a compound with molecular oxygen at room temperature.

auxesis (awg'zeesis, awk'see-) increase in size of an organism, especially that due to growth of its individual cells rather than increase in their number. adj. **auxetic.**

auxodrome ('awksə,drohm) the course of growth of a child as plotted on a specially devised graph (Wetzel grid).

auxotroph ('awksə,trohf) an auxotrophic organism.

auxotrophic (,awksə'trofik) 1. requiring a growth factor not required by the parental or prototype strain; said of microbial mutants. 2. requiring specific organic growth factors in addition to the carbon source present in a minimal medium.

AV, A-V arteriovenous; atrioventricular.

av. avoirdupois.

avascular (ay'vaskyuhlə) not vascular; bloodless.

avascularization (ay,vaskyuhlə·rie'zayshən) diversion of blood from tissues, as by bandaging.

Avellis' syndrome (a'veleez) ipsilateral paralysis of the vocal cord and soft palate, loss of pain and temperature sensibility in the contralateral leg, trunk, arm, neck, and in the skin over the scalp.

aversion therapy (ə'vərshən) see THERAPY.

aversive control (ə'vərsiv) in BEHAVIOUR THERAPY, the use of unpleasant stimuli to change undesirable behaviour, as the undesirable behaviour becomes associated with the unpleasant stimuli.

avidity (ə'viditee) in immunology, an imprecise measure of the strength of antigen–antibody binding based on the rate at which the complex is formed.

avirulence (ay'viryuhləns) lack of virulence; lack of competence of an infectious agent to produce pathological effects. adj. **avirulent.**

avitaminosis (ay,vitəmi'nohsis) disease due to deficiency of vitamins in the diet. adj. **avitaminotic.**

Avloclor ('avlohklor) trademark for a preparation of chloroquine, an antimalarial used also in treatment of amoebic abscess and lupus erythematosus.

Avogadro's law (,avoh'gadrohz) equal volumes of perfect gases at the same temperature and pressure contain the same number of molecules.

Avogadro's number the number of particles of the type specified by the chemical formula of a certain substance in 1 gram-molecule of the substance. Called also Avogadro's constant.

avoidance (ə'voydəns) a conscious or unconscious defensive reaction intended to escape anxiety, conflict, danger, fear, or pain.

avoir. avoirdupois.

avoirdupois (,avwahdyoo'pwah, ,avədə'poyz) a system of weight used in English-speaking countries for all commodities except drugs, precious stones, and precious metals.

avulsion (ə'vulshən) forcible separation of a structure from its natural attachment.

a. fracture see under FRACTURE.

phrenic a. extraction of a portion of the phrenic nerve, producing one-sided paralysis of the diaphragm and partial collapse, usually of the lower lobe of the corresponding lung.

axenic (ay'zeenik) not contaminated by or associated with any foreign organisms; used in reference to pure cultures of microorganisms or to germ-free animals.

axilla (ak'silə) pl. *axillae* [L.] the armpit.

axillary (ak'silə·ree) of or pertaining to the armpit.

axio- word element. [L., Gr.] denoting relation to an axis; in dentistry, used in special reference to the long axis of a tooth.

axis ('aksis) pl. *axes* [L., Gr.] 1. a line through the centre of a body, or about which a structure revolves. 2. the second cervical vertebra. adj. **axial.**

coeliac a. coeliac trunk.

a. cylinder axon.

dorsoventral a. one passing from the back to the belly surface of the body.

electrical a. of heart the resultant of the electromotive forces within the heart at any instant.

frontal a. an imaginary line running from right to left through the centre of the eyeball.

a. of heart. a line passing through the centre of the base of the heart and the apex.

optic a. 1. visual axis. 2. the hypothetical straight line passing through the centres of curvature of the front and back surfaces of a simple lens. **sagittal a.** an imaginary line extending through the anterior and posterior poles of the eye.

visual a. an imaginary line passing from the midpoint of the visual field to the fovea centralis.

axoaxonic (,aksoh·ak'sonik) referring to a synapse between the axon of one neuron and the axon of another.

axodentritic (,aksohden'dritik) referring to a synapse between the axon of one neuron and dentrites of another.

axolemma (,aksoh'lemə) the surface membrane of an axon.

axolysis (ak'solisis) degeneration of an axon.

axon ('akson) the process of a nerve cell along which impulses travel away from the cell body. It branches at its termination, forming synapses at other nerve cells or effector organs. Many axons are covered by a myelin sheath formed from the cell membrane of a glial cell. adj. **axonal.**

axonapraxia (,aksonə'praksi·ə) neurapraxia.

axoneme ('aksə,neem) the central core of a cilium or flagellum, consisting of two central fibrils surrounded by nine peripheral fibrils.

axonotmesis (,aksonət'meesis) nerve injury characterized by disruption of the axon and myelin sheath but with preservation of the connective tissue fragments, resulting in degeneration of the axon distal to the injury site; regeneration of the axon is spontaneous and of good quality.

axoplasm ('aksoh,plazəm) the cytoplasm of an axon; called also hyaloplasm. adj. **axoplasmic.**

axosomatic (,aksohsə'matik) referring to a synapse between the axon of one neuron and the cell body of another.

Ayerza's disease (ə'yəirsəz) a form of polycythaemia vera marked by chronic cyanosis, chronic dyspnoea, chronic bronchitis, bronchiectasis, hepatosplenomegaly, and hyperplasia of bone marrow, and associated with sclerosis of the pulmonary artery.

AZ test ('ayzed) Aschheim–Zondek test (for pregnancy).

azapropazone (,ayzə'prohpəzohn) a nonsteroidal anti-inflammatory drug.

azatadine (ə'zatə,deen, -din) an antihistamine used in the treatment of allergic rhinitis and chronic urticaria.

azathioprine (,azə'thieə,preen) a mercaptopurine derivative used as a cytotoxic and immunosuppressive agent in the treatment of leukaemia and autoimmune diseases and in transplantation therapy.

azeotrope (ə'zeeə,trohp) a mixture of two substances that has a constant boiling point and cannot be separated by fractional distillation.

azlocillin (azloh'silin) a systemic antibiotic, particularly active against *Pseudomonas aeruginosa.*

azoospermia (,ayzoh·oh'spərmi·ə) absence of spermatozoa in the semen, or failure of formation of spermatozoa.

azotaemia (,azə'teemi·ə) the presence of nitrogen-containing compounds in the blood. adj. **azotaemic.** See URAEMIA.

azote (ə'zoht, 'azoht) nitrogen.

azotenesis (,azohtə'neesis) any disease due to excess

nitrogen in system.

azotorrhoea (ˌazohtə'reeə) discharge of excessive quantities of nitrogenous matter in the stools.

azoturia (ˌazoh'tyooə·ri·ə) excess of urea in the urine.

azovan blue (ˌayzohvan 'bloo) an odourless green, bluish-green, or brown powder dye, used in the estimation of blood volume. The dye is injected into the bloodstream and after a sufficient period of time samples of the blood are taken to determine the degree of dilution of the dye.

azure ('azhə, 'ay-, -zhuh·ə) one of three metachromatic basic dyes (azures A, B, and C).

azuresin (ˌazyuh'rezin) a complex combination of azure A dye and carbacrylic cation-exchange resin used as a diagnostic aid in detection of gastric secretion.

azurophil (a'zyooə·rohfil) a tissue constituent staining with azure or a similar metachromatic thiazin dye.

azurophilia (ˌazyuhroh'fili·ə) a condition in which the blood contains cells having azurophilic granules.

azurophilic (ˌazyuhroh'filik) staining with azure or similar metachromatic thiazin dyes; pertaining to azurophilia.

azygogram ('azigohˌgram) the film obtained by azygography.

azygography (ˌazi'gogrəfee, ˌazie-) radiography of the azygous venous system.

azygos ('aziˌgos, a'zie-) 1. any unpaired part, as the azygos vein. 2. unpaired.

a. vein a vein beginning in the abdomen as a continuation of the ascending lumbar vein which is a tributary of the inferior vena cava. The azygos vein and its tributaries serve as vessels for the return of blood from the thorax to the superior vena cava. The azygos vein also serves as a connecting link, through the ascending lumbar vein, between the venae cavae, returning blood from above and below the heart.

azygous ('azigəs, a'zie-) having no fellow; unpaired.

azymic (ay'ziemik) not giving rise to fermentation.

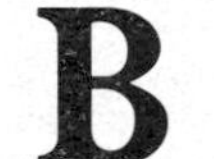

B

B chemical symbol, *boron*; Baumé scale; boils at.

BA Bachelor of Arts.

Ba chemical symbol, *barium*.

Babcock's test ('babkoks) one for determination of the fat content of milk.

Babès–Ernst granules (ˌbabayz'ərnst) metachromatic granules, present in many bacterial cells.

Babinski reflex (bə'binskee) a reflex action of the toes, indicative of abnormalities in the motor control pathways leading from the cerebral cortex and widely used as a diagnostic aid in disorders of the central nervous system. It is elicited by a firm stimulus (usually scraping) on the sole of the foot, which results in dorsiflexion of the great toe and fanning of the smaller toes. Normally such a stimulus causes all the toes to bend downward. Called also Babinski's sign.

Babkin reflex ('babkin) pressure by the examiner's thumbs on the palms of both hands of the infant results in opening of the infant's mouth; it is elicited in many newborn infants, normal and abnormal, except when lethargic or comatose.

baby ('baybee) an infant; a child not yet able to walk.

blue b. an infant born with cyanosis due to a congenital heart lesion or to congenital atelectasis (see also BLUE BABY).

collodion b. an infant affected with lamellar EXFOLIATION OF THE NEWBORN.

bacampicillin (bəˌkampi'silin) an ester of ampicillin that in vivo becomes ampicillin and has the actions and uses of the parent drug.

bacillaemia (ˌbasi'leemi·ə) the presence of bacilli in the blood.

bacillary (bə'silə·ree) pertaining to bacilli or to rodlike structures.

bacilli (bə'silie) plural of *bacillus*.

bacilliform (bə'siliˌfawm) having the appearance of a bacillus.

bacillosis (ˌbasi'lohsis) infection with bacilli.

bacilluria (ˌbasi'lyooə·ri·ə) bacilli in the urine.

Bacillus (bə'siləs) a genus of bacteria that are gram-positive, aerobic, spore-forming rods.

B. anthracis the causative agent of anthrax.

B. cereus a genus causing food poisoning.

B. subtilis a common saprophytic soil and water form, often occurring as a laboratory contaminant, and rarely, in apparently causal relation to pathological processes, such as conjunctivitis.

bacillus (bə'siləs) pl. *bacilli* [L.] 1. an organism of the genus *Bacillus*. 2. any rod-shaped bacterium.

Calmette–Guérin b. *Mycobacterium bovis*, rendered completely avirulent by cultivation over a long period on bile-glycerol-potato medium (see BCG VACCINE).

colon b. *Escherichia coli*.

Döderlein's b. a non-pathogenic lactobacillus occurring naturally within a healthy vagina from the menarche to the menopause. The production of lactic acid creates a pH of 4.5, which effectively inhibits ascending infection.

Friedländer's b. *Klebsiella pneumoniae*. **glanders b.** *Pseudomonas mallei*.

Hansen's b. *Mycobacterium leprae*.

tubercle b. *Mycobacterium tuberculosis*.

typhoid b. *Salmonella typhosa*.

bacitracin (ˌbasi'traysin) an antibacterial substance elaborated by the licheniformis group of *Bacillus subtilis*, found in a contaminated wound, and named after the patient, Margaret Tracy; useful in a wide range of infections, applied topically or given intramuscularly.

back (bak) dorsum; posterior trunk from neck to pelvis.

hunch b. kyphosis.

b. bone the vertebral column.

b. slab plaster or plastic splint in which a limb is supported.

back-cross ('bakˌkros) a mating between a heterozygote and a homozygote.

double b. the mating between a double heterozygote and a homozygote.

backache ('bakˌayk) any pain in the back, usually the lower part. The pain is often dull and continuous, but sometimes sharp and throbbing.

Backache, or lumbago, is one of the commonest ailments and can be caused by a wide variety of disorders, some serious and some not. Occasionally backache is a symptom of spinal arthritis, peptic ulcer, pancreatic lesions, SCIATICA, diseases of the kidney or other serious disorders, but usually it is caused simply by strain of the back in such a way that the bones, ligaments, nerves or muscles of the spine are compressed or stretched. A sudden action, using muscles that are already fatigued or out of condition, is particularly likely to cause acute strain. In such cases, rest and time usually bring recovery, although a doctor should always be consulted. A very sharp and persistent pain, following the use of unusual force against something—for example, when trying to open a jammed window—could indicate a prolapsed intervertebral DISC or sacroiliac strain.

TREATMENT. The initial treatment for backache is usually conservative. It includes bedrest, a bed board under the mattress, muscle relaxant medication, analgesics, and pelvic or cervical traction. Epidural and subarachnoid injections of steroids also are helpful in some cases. Surgical treatment is usually a last resort, and involves excision of a herniated disc, laminectomy, or some other type of orthopaedic surgery, depending on the cause of the back pain.

Chronic back pain that does not respond to other modes of treatment sometimes is relieved by transcutaneous neural stimulation (TNS). Electrodes are applied to the skin over the painful area and attached to a hand-held, battery-operated pulse generator. Mild electrical stimulation transmitted by the electrodes interferes with the transmission of pain messages and helps suppress the sensation of pain in the area.

backbone ('bak,bohn) the vertebral column.

backflow ('bak,floh) abnormal backward flow of fluids; regurgitation.

pyelovenous b. drainage from the renal pelvis into the venous system occurring under certain conditions of back pressure.

backscatter ('bak,skatə) in radiology, radiation deflected by scattering processes at angles greater than 90 degrees to the original direction of the beam of radiation.

baclofen ('bakloh,fen) an analogue of gamma-aminobutyric acid which acts on the central venous system to relieve muscle spasm or spasticity.

bacter(io)- word element. [Gr.] *bacteria.*

bacteraemia (,baktə'reemi·ə) the presence of bacteria in the blood.

bacteria (bak'tiə·ri·ə) plural of *bacterium.* adj. **bacterial.**

bacteriaemia (bak,tiə·ri'eemi·ə) bacteraemia.

bactericidal (bak,tiə·ri'sied'l) destructive to bacteria.

bactericide (bak'tiə·ri,sied) an agent that destroys bacteria.

bactericidin (,baktiə·ri'siedin) bacteriocidin.

bacterid ('baktiə·rid) a skin eruption due to bacterial infection elsewhere in the body.

bacterin ('baktə·rin) bacterial vaccine; suspension of bacteria used either prophylactically or therapeutically to stimulate the production of antibodies or antisera.

bacteriocidin (bak,tiə·rioh'siedin) a bactericidal antibody.

bacteriologist (bak,tiə·ri'oləjist) an expert in the study of bacteria.

bacteriology (bak,tiə·ri'oləjee) the scientific study of bacteria. adj. **bacteriological.**

bacteriolysin (bak,tiə·ri'olisin, -rioh'liesin) an antibody that lyses bacterial cells.

bacteriolysis (bak,tiə·ri'olisis) destruction or dissolution of bacteria. adj. **bacteriolytic.**

bacteriophage (bak'tiə·ri·ə,fayj, -fahzh) a virus that destroys bacteria by lysis; several varieties exist, and usually each attacks only one kind of bacteria. Certain types of bacteriophages attach themselves to the cell membrane of the bacterium and instill a charge of DNA into the cytoplasm. DNA carries the genetic code of the virus, so that rapid multiplication of the virus can and does take place inside the bacterium. The growing viruses act as parasites, using the metabolism of the bacterial cell for growth and development. Eventually the bacterial cell bursts, releasing many more viruses capable of destroying similar bacteria. Called also bacterial virus. adj. **bacteriophagic.**

temperate b. one whose genetic material (prophage) becomes an intimate part of the bacterial genome, persisting and being reproduced through many cell division cycles; the affected bacterial cell is known as a lysogenic BACTERIUM.

bacteriopsonin (bak,tiə·ri'opsənin) an opsonin that acts on bacteria.

bacteriospermia (bak,tiə·rioh'spərmi·ə) the presence of bacteria in the semen.

bacteriostatic (bak,tiə·rioh'statik) arresting the growth or multiplication of bacteria; also, an agent that so acts.

bacteriotherapy (bak,tiə·rioh'therəpee) treatment of a disease by the injection of bacteria into the blood.

bacterium (bak'tiə·ri·əm) pl. *bacteria* [L., Gr.] any prokaryotic organism. Bacteria are single-celled microorganisms that differ from all other organisms (the eukaryotes) in lacking a true nucleus and organelles such as mitochondria, chloroplasts, and lysosomes. Their genetic material consists of a single loop of double-stranded DNA, whereas the genetic material of eukaryotes consists of multiple chromosomes, which are complex structures of DNA and protein.

Bacteria reproduce by cell division about every 20 minutes, giving them a very high rate of population growth and evolution. Genetic material can be transferred between bacteria by three processes: *transformation* (absorption of naked DNA), *transduction* (transfer by a virus), and *conjugation* (transfer by independently replicating DNA molecules, called *plasmids*, which can be inserted into the bacterial DNA). Some bacteria can also form *spores*, dehydrated forms that are relatively resistant to heat, cold, lack of water, toxic chemicals, and radiation.

Most bacteria have a rigid cell wall outside the cell membrane primarily composed of a dense layer of peptidoglycan, a network of polysaccharide chains with polypeptide crosslinks. Some antibiotics, the penicillins and cephalosporins, act by interfering with peptidoglycan synthesis. Bacteria can have any of three types of external structures: *flagella*, which are whiplike locomotor organelles; *pili* or fimbriae, which are minute filamentous appendages; and a *capsule*, which is a layer of gelatinous material around the cell. Various types of pili are involved in conjugation and in the adherence of bacteria to mucosal surfaces. The capsule protects the bacterium from phagocytosis.

CLASSIFICATION OF BACTERIA. Bacteria are classified into two major groups (gram-positive and gram-negative) based on their reaction to the Gram stain, a four step procedure: staining with crystal violet, mordanting in iodine, decolorization in alcohol, and counterstaining with safranin. Gram-positive bacteria have a thick peptidoglycan cell wall, which resists decolorization, and are stained violet. Gram-negative bacteria have a thin peptidoglycan layer covered by an outer membrane; they are decolorized and counterstained pink.

Other important characteristics used in the classification of bacteria are morphology and metabolic reactions. Spherical bacteria are called *cocci.* Some species do not always completely separate when the cells divide and characteristically occur in pairs *(diplococci)*, clusters *(staphylococci)*, or chains *(streptococci).* Rod-shaped bacteria are called *bacilli.* Some species have tapered ends *(fusiform bacilli)* or are shaped like long threads *(filamentous bacilli)* or spirals *(spirochetes, spirilla).*

On the basis of their requirements for atmospheric oxygen, bacteria can be divided into *obligate aerobes*, which require oxygen; *obligate anaerobes*, which grow only in the absence of oxygen; and *facultative anaerobes*, which adapt to either environment. On the basis of their growth on a specific medium under aerobic and anaerobic conditions, certain groups are divided into *oxidizers*, those that use oxygen to metabolize sugars; *fermenters*, those that metabolize sugars in the absence of oxygen; and *nonutilizers*, which do not grow on the medium.

Two groups of prokaryotic organisms are sometimes not classified as bacteria. These are the cyanobacteria (blue-green algae), which have aerobic photosynthesis like plants; and the mycoplasmas, which lack cell walls.

BACTERIAL INFECTION. The skin, respiratory tract, and gastrointestinal tract are inhabited by a variety of bacteria. These normal flora are harmless or even helpful, protecting their host by interference with the growth of harmful bacteria. An opportunistic infection occurs when an organism indigenous to one part of the body invades another part where it is pathogenic. A commonly occurring example is infection of the urinary tract with *Escherichia coli* or other enteric bacilli.

There are many mechanisms by which pathogenic bacteria can be transmitted from person to person, including airborne infection, direct contact, contact with animals, transmission by insect vectors, or indirect transmission in drinking water, milk, or food, or on inanimate objects. Although some diseases, such as CHOLERA and BOTULISM, are caused by toxins absorbed in the intestine, most diseases occur from bacteria that can attach to a mucosal surface, multiply, and invade tissue. To be pathogenic, bacteria must also be able to resist the host defences: bactericidins, such as complement and lysozyme in the blood, and phagocytosis and subsequent intracellular destruction by leukocytes.

Bacteria can cause disease by producing *toxins*, by causing inflammation or the formation of granulomas, or by inducing a hypersensitivity reaction. *Exotoxins* are extremely potent poisons produced by some gram-positive bacteria. These include neurotoxins, such as tetanus toxin and botulinum toxin; enterotoxins, such as cholera toxin; and diphtheria toxin, which blocks protein synthesis, thereby causing tissue necrosis. *Endotoxins* are lipopolysaccharides that are components of the outer membrane of gram-negative cell walls and are released on cell lysis. They can cause hypotension, fever, disseminated intravascular coagulation, and shock. Other toxins include haemolysins and leukocidins, which destroy red and white blood cells; kinases, which lyse blood clots; and enzymes that attack tissue.

Host resistance to infection is lowered in weak and debilitated patients and in those with a decreased ability to mount an effective immune response because of disease or the effects of drugs (such as corticosteroids, immunosuppressive agents, or cytotoxic agents).

A major problem in antibiotic therapy is the evolution of antibiotic-resistant strains of bacteria, which are an important cause of serious nosocomial (hospital-acquired) infections. Unnecessary overuse of ANTIBIOTIC agents speeds up the evolution of resistant strains. This problem is exacerbated by the transfer of resistance between different species by plasmids, producing multiple drug-resistant strains.

DISEASES CAUSED BY BACTERIA. The different kinds of bacteria tend to affect different organs and systems of the body, producing infectious diseases, each with its own group of symptoms.

Staphylococci are generally found on the surface of the skin. When they invade the body tissue, for instance through a cut, they usually produce a local infection with inflammation and pus. Occasionally a strain of staphylococcus develops that can cause an infection affecting more than a local area of the body, but this is relatively rare.

The diseases produced by streptococci are often more serious. Streptococci tend to resist localization and may spread through the bloodstream. Among the diseases caused by streptococci are streptococcal sore THROAT, RHEUMATIC FEVER, and SCARLET FEVER.

PNEUMONIA, MENINGITIS, and GONORRHOEA are produced by different types of diplococci. The pneumococcus, which produces pneumonia, has its special effect on the lungs; the meningococcus has an affinity for the coverings, or meninges, of the brain and spinal cord. Both types of bacteria enter the body via the respiratory tract. The gonorrhoea bacteria (gonococci) are usually spread by coitus.

CHOLERA, caused by a spirillum and spread by unsanitary water supplies, was formerly a dread epidemic disease. SYPHILIS, like gonorrhoea, is spread most often by coitus. It also is caused by a spirochaete.

Bacilli are responsible for many serious diseses, including PLAGUE, DIPHTHERIA, LEPROSY, TUBERCULOSIS, and TYPHOID FEVER. Prevention and control of the spread of many infectious diseases can be accomplished through IMMUNIZATION and proper sanitary conditions.

acid-fast b. one that is not readily decolorized by acids after staining, especially *Mycobacterium tuberculosis*.

coliform bacteria a general term for those members of the Enterobacteriaceae that usually ferment lactose.

haemophilic bacteria microorganisms of the genera *Haemophilus* and *Bordetella*, which have a nutritional affinity for constituents of fresh blood or whose growth is significantly stimulated on blood-containing media.

lactic acid bacteria bacteria that, in suitable media, produce fermentation of carbohydrate materials to form lactic acid.

lysogenic b. any bacterial cell harbouring in its genome the genetic material (prophage) of a temperate BACTERIOPHAGE and thus reproducing the bacteriophage in cell division; occasionally the prophage develops into the mature form, replicates, lyses the bacterial cell, and is free to infect other cells.

bacteriuria (bak,tiə·ri'yooə·ri·ə) bacteria in the urine. adj. **bacteriuric.**

bacteroid ('baktə,royd) 1. resembling a bacterium. 2. a structurally modified bacterium.

Bacteroides (,baktə'roydeez) a genus of anaerobic bacteria occurring as normal flora in the mouth and large bowel, and often in necrotic tissue, where it is frequently pathogenic.

bacteroides (,baktə'roydeez) 1. any highly pleomorphic rod-shaped bacteria. 2. an organism of the genus *Bacteroides*.

bacteruria (,baktiə'yooə·ri·ə) bacteriuria.

Bactrim ('baktrim) trademark for preparations of trimethoprim and sulphamethoxazole, an antibiotic.

Bactroban ('baktroh,ban) trademark for mupirocin.

BAD British Association of Dermatologists.

bag (bag) a sac or pouch.

colostomy b. a receptacle worn over the stoma by a COLOSTOMY patient, to receive the faecal discharge.

Douglas b. a receptacle for the collection of expired air, permitting measurement of respiratory gases.

ice b. a rubber or plastic bag half-filled with pieces of ice and applied near or to a part of the body.

ileostomy b. any of various plastic or latex pouches attached to the stoma for the collection of faecal material following ILEOSTOMY.

Politzer b. a soft bag of rubber for inflating the pharyngotympanic tube.

urine b. a receptacle used for urine by ambulatory patients with urinary incontinence.

b. of waters the membranes enclosing the AMNIOTIC

FLUID and the developing fetus in utero.

bagassosis (ˌbagə'sohsis) a lung disease due to inhalation of dust from the residue of cane after extraction of sugar (bagasse).

Bainbridge reflex ('baynbrij) an increase in the heart rate caused by an increase in right atrial pressure.

Baker's cyst ('baykəz) a knee bursa found in the popliteal fossa behind the knee, which may communicate with the knee joint itself and which occasionally extends into the calf.

BAL dimercaprol (British antilewisite), a chelating agent used in poisoning with arsenic, gold, mercury, and certain other metals.

balance ('baləns) 1. an instrument for weighing. 2. harmonious adjustment of different elements or parts; harmonious performance of functions.

acid–base b. the proportion of acid and base required to keep the blood and body fluids within narrowly defined limits (see also ACID–BASE BALANCE).

analytical b. a laboratory balance sensitive to variations of the order of 0.05 to 0.1 mg.

fluid b. the state of the body in relation to ingestion and excretion of water and electrolytes (see also FLUID BALANCE).

nitrogen b. the state of the body in regard to ingestion and excretion of nitrogen. In negative nitrogen balance the amount of nitrogen excreted is greater than the quantity ingested. In positive nitrogen balance the amount excreted is smaller than the amount ingested. See also NITROGEN BALANCE.

water b. fluid balance.

balanic (bə'lanik) pertaining to the glans penis or glans clitoridis.

balanitis (ˌbalə'nietis) inflammation of the glans penis.

gangrenous b. erosion of the glans penis leading to rapid destruction, believed to be due to continually unhygienic conditions together with secondary spirochetal infection.

balanoposthitis (ˌbalənohpos'thietis) inflammation of glans penis and prepuce.

balanopreputial (ˌbalənohpri'pyooshəla) pertaining to the glans penis and prepuce.

balanorrhagia (ˌbalənoh'rayji·ə) balanitis with free discharge of pus.

balantidiasis (ˌbalanti'dieəsis) infection by protozoa of the genus *Balantidium*; in man, *B. coli* may cause diarrhoea and dysentery, with ulceration of the colon mucosa.

Balantidium (ˌbalan'tidi·əm) a genus of ciliated protozoa, including many species found in the intestine in vertebrates and invertebrates. See CILIATA.

B. coli a common parasite of swine, rarely in man, in whom it may cause dysentery.

baldness ('bawldnəs) total or partial loss or absence of hair, especially absence of the hair from the scalp; called also ALOPECIA. Baldness is a common condition that occurs much more often in men than in women. Ordinary baldness is usually a permanent and incurable condition; symptomatic baldness occurs as a result of some other condition or disorder and is usually temporary.

Balkan beam ('bawlkən) an apparatus consisting of overhead bars fixed to a bed, to which pulleys are attached for the suspension of a splint or slings to give support to a leg and extension to the limb in treatment of fractures of the femur.

ball (bawl) a more or less spherical mass.

fungus b. aspergilloma.

ballismus (bə'lizməs) violent flinging movements of the limbs, sometimes affecting only one side of the body (hemiballismus).

ballottement (bə'lotmənt) [Fr.] *tossing;* a palpatory manoeuvre to test for a floating object, especially a manoeuvre for detecting pregnancy by inserting two fingers into the vagina and pushing the fetal head or breech, causing the fetus to leave and quickly return to the fingers. It can be diagnostic for polyhydramnios. It is also used later in pregnancy to identify the fetal head in a breech presentation on abdominal examination.

balm (bahm) 1. a balsam. 2. a soothing or healing medicine.

balsam ('bawlsəm) a semifluid, fragrant, resinous, vegetable juice. Balsams are resins combined with oils, used in various preparations to treat irritated or denuded areas of the skin and mucous membranes. Stains from these preparations are extremely difficult to remove. Friar's balsam, called also compound benzoin tincture, is used as a topical protectant. Balsam of Peru, or Peruvian balsam, is used as a local protectant and rubefacient. Tolu balsam is used as an ingredient in compound benzoin and as an expectorant.

Balser's fatty necrosis ('bahlzəz) gangrenous pancreatitis with omental bursitis and disseminated patches of necrosis of fatty tissues.

Bamberger–Marie disease (ˌbambərgəmə'ree) hypertrophic pulmonary osteoarthropathy.

BAN British Approved Name; British Association of Neurologists.

bancroftosis (ˌbankrof'tohsis) infection with *Wuchereria bancrofti*.

band (band) 1. a part, structure, or appliance that binds. 2. in dentistry, a thin metal strip fitted around a tooth or its roots. 3. in histology, a zone of a myofibril of striated muscle. 4. in cytogenetics, a segment of a chromosome stained brighter or darker than the adjacent bands; used in identifying the chromosomes and in determining the exact extent of chromosomal abnormalities. Called *Q-bands*, *G-bands*, *C-bands*, *T-bands*, etc., according to the staining method used.

bandage ('bandij) 1. a strip or roll of gauze or other material for wrapping or binding any part of the body. 2. to cover by wrapping with such material. Bandages may be used to stop the flow of blood, to provide a safeguard against contamination, or to hold a dressing in place. They may also be used to hold a splint in position or otherwise immobilize an injured part of the body to prevent further injury and to facilitate healing.

APPLICATION OF BANDAGES. In applying a bandage: (1) If the skin is broken a dressing should be placed over the wound before adhesive tape or a bandage is applied. Adhesive tape is only applied directly to an incised wound. (2) The bandage should not be so tight that it interferes with circulation; a pressure bandage should be applied only for the purpose of arresting haemorrhage.

Esmarch's b. a flat rubber bandage applied to a limb from the distal to the proximal end in order to expel blood from it and provide a bloodless field for subsequent surgery. It must be released after 20 minutes. It can also be used as a tourniquet.

figure-of-8 b. one in which the turns cross each other like the figure 8.

many-tailed b. a rectangular piece of cloth with overlapping strips attached at the sides. When the bandage is applied, usually to the abdomen, the strips from each side are tied, from below upwards on the abdomen and above downwards on the chest.

plaster b. a bandage containing plaster of Paris in an unhydrated state. It is applied wet to set in the form of the part to which it is applied, usually to immobilize it.

pressure b. a firmly applied bandage, for the purpose of arresting haemorrhage or to limit swelling.

roller b. a tightly rolled, circular bandage of varying widths and materials, often prepared commercially. In an emergency, strips may be torn from a sheet or piece of cotton or linen cloth and rolled. When more than a few inches of length is needed, rolling is essential for quick and clean bandaging.

triangular b. one made by folding or cutting a large square of cloth diagonally to form a sling.

banding ('banding) 1. the act of encircling and binding with a thin strip of material. 2. in genetics, any of several techniques of staining chromosomes so that a characteristic pattern of transverse dark and light bands becomes visible, permitting identification of individual chromosome pairs.

Bandl's ring ('band'lz) a complication of prolonged, obstructed labour marked by excessive stretching and thinning of the circular fibres at the junction of the lower and upper uterine segment and the excessive stretching and thinning of longitudinal fibres. When present, a transverse ridge appears on the maternal abdomen. Called also pathological retraction ring.

bank (bank) a stored supply of human material or tissues for future use by other individuals, as blood bank, bone bank, skin bank, eye bank, etc.

Bankart's operation ('bangkhahts) an operation carried out for recurrent anterior dislocation of the shoulder. The anterior capsule and glenoid limbus are reattached to the anterior rim of the glenoid fossa of the scapula.

Banti's disease ('banteez) a disease originally described as a primary disease of the spleen with splenomegaly and pancytopenia, now considered secondary to portal hypertension.

Banting ('banting) Sir Frederick Grant (1891–1941). Canadian scientist. Born in Allison, Ontario, and educated at the University of Toronto, Banting undertook research on the internal secretion of the pancreas, and in 1921, with Charles Herbert Best, he discovered insulin. Banting and J. J. R. Macleod shared the Nobel prize for medicine in 1923. The Banting Research Foundation was established in 1924, and the Banting Institute was opened at Toronto in 1930. Banting was knighted in 1934.

Banting treatment treatment of obesity by a low carbohydrate diet rich in nitrogenous matter.

BAO Bachelor of the Art of Obstetrics; British Association of Otolaryngologists.

BAPhysMed British Association of Physical Medicine.

BAPS British Association of Paediatric Surgeons; British Association of Plastic Surgeons.

bar (bah) 1. a unit of pressure, equivalent to 10^5 Pa (or 10^5 N/m^2). 2. a heavy wire or a wrought or cast metal segment, longer than its width, used to connect parts of a removable partial denture.

median b. a fibrotic formation across the neck of the prostate, producing obstruction of the urethra.

bar diagram (bah 'di·əgram) a chart showing the number or rate of particular observations in the form of bars, the length of each bar representing the frequency of each observation.

baraesthesia (,baris'theezi·ə) sensibility for weight or pressure.

baraesthesiometer (,baris,theezi'omitə) an instrument for estimating the acuteness of the sense of weight or pressure.

baragnosis (,barag'nohsis) impairment of the ability to perceive differences in weight or pressure.

barber's itch ('bahbəz) an infection of the hair follicles on the face and neck, caused by staphylococci; called also SYCOSIS BARBAE.

barbitone ('bahbitohn) the first of the barbiturates, being a long-acting hypnotic and sedative.

barbiturate (bah'bityuh·rət, -'rayt) any of a group of organic compounds derived from barbituric acid. Available by prescription only, barbiturates may be used to reduce anxiety, induce sedation or promote sleep. The many types of barbiturates differ in their strength and in the rapidity and duration of their effect. To varying degrees, all serve to depress the central nervous system, depress respiration, affect the heart rate, and decrease blood pressure and temperature.

The use of barbiturates has declined sharply in recent years, their being replaced as sedatives, anxiolytics and hypnotics by the benzodiazepine group of drugs. Oral barbiturates should be avoided as far as possible because of the risks of dependence and cumulation. Abrupt withdrawal can cause severe withdrawal symptoms.

Barbiturates are still used under certain circumstances: (1) phenobarbitone as an anticonvulsant, (2) intermediate-acting drugs, e.g. for severe intractable insomnia—though never in the elderly—and (3) ultra-short-acting drugs, such as thiopentone and methohexitone, which are given intravenously either as the sole anaesthetic, for short procedures, or as an induction agent, for longer procedures.

Since barbiturates can become habit-forming, they should be used only by the person for whom they have been prescribed and only according to specific directions. Barbiturate abuse is particularly hazardous and is not uncommon.

Barbiturate overdose can be fatal and should be treated with utmost promptness. It produces drowsiness, coma, respiratory depression, hypotension and hypothermia. A doctor should be called immediately. Until he arrives, the victim should be made to vomit by sticking a finger down his throat, but *only if he is awake* and only if it is likely that the drugs have been ingested within the past four hours; he should be kept warm and his breathing should be facilitated by removing constricting clothing and proper positioning. See also POISONING.

barbituric acid (,bahbi'tyooə·rik) a compound, $C_4H_4N_2O_3$, the parent substance of BARBITURATES.

barbotage (,bahbə'tahzh) [Fr.] repeated alternate injection and withdrawal of fluid with a syringe, as in gastric lavage or administration of an anaesthetic agent into the subarachnoid space by alternate injection of part of the anaesthetic and withdrawal of cerebrospinal fluid into the syringe.

bariatrics (,bari'atriks) a field of medicine encompassing the study of overweight, its causes, prevention, and treatment.

baritosis (,bari'tohsis) inhalation of barite or barium dust resulting in pneumoconiosis.

barium ('bair·ri·əm) a chemical element, atomic number 56, atomic weight 137.34, symbol Ba. See table of elements in Appendix 2.

b. examination radiological examination using a barium sulphate preparation to help locate disorders in the oesophagus, stomach, duodenum, and the small and large intestines. Such conditions as peptic ulcer, benign or malignant tumours, colitis, or enlargement of organs that might be causing pressure on the stomach may be readily identified with the use of barium tests.

Barium sulphate is a harmless chalky, water-insoluble compound that does not permit x-rays to pass through it. Taken before or during an examination, it causes the intestinal tract to stand out in silhouette when viewed through a fluoroscope or seen on a radiograph.

The principal examinations using barium are the

barium enema, barium follow through, barium meal, barium swallow and small bowel enema.

Barium Enema. The barium enema may be performed for diagnosis or therapy. The diagnostic enema is usually double contrast, i.e. barium sulphate is used to coat the mucosa and air is inflated to distend the lumen, but is frequently single contrast in children where anatomical rather than mucosal abnormalities predominate. The diagnostic enema is undertaken to define suspected colonic pathology.

For the double contrast method it is essential that the colon is clean. A combination of low residue diet, oral laxative and colonic washout is usual. The patient lies on the fluoroscopy table and an enema tube is inserted. Barium sulphate solution is infused as far as the splenic flexure. Air is then gently puffed into the rectum which forces the column of barium round towards the caecum. Under fluoroscopic guidance the radiologist positions the patient to demonstrate each segment of colon and radiographs are taken.

The barium enema may be used therapeutically to reduce hydrostatically the head of an intussusception. Barium is infused via a rectal catheter from a bag which is held 1 metre above the patient.

Barium Follow Through. This is the simplest technique of examining the small bowel with barium. The patient is given a laxative on the evening prior to the examination and arrives following a 6-hour fast. A low density (100% w/v) barium sulphate suspension is drunk and the patient lies on his right side so that a single column of barium is delivered into the small bowel. Radiographs are exposed at 20–30 minute intervals until barium reaches the colon.

Barium Meal. This is indicated when there is suspected upper gastrointestinal tract pathology, e.g. in those patients with dyspepsia, gastrointestinal bleeding, obstruction or weight loss. The technique may involve either a single contrast method, i.e. barium sulphate suspension only, or double contrast, in which carbon dioxide gas is used in addition. The single contrast method is used in children and very ill adults in which only gross anatomical abnormalities need to be excluded. The double contrast method is used to demonstrate mucosal abnormalities.

The examination is undertaken following a 6-hour fast. In the double contrast method the patient swallows a gas-producing agent followed by a high density (250% w/v) barium sulphate solution. The patient is turned so that the barium coats the mucosa and the gas distends the stomach. A smooth muscle relaxant (Buscopan 20 mg or glucagon 0.3 mg i.v.) is given. The radiologist observes the stomach and duodenum by fluoroscopy and numerous radiographs are taken.

The patient is warned that his stools will be white for the next few days and laxatives may be necessary to keep the bowels open. Called also gastrointestinal *series*.

Barium Swallow. This examination is undertaken for pharyngeal and oesophageal symptoms. It may be performed on its own or as part of a barium meal. There is no patient preparation unless the stomach is also to be examined. Using fluoroscopy the radiologist watches the patient swallow a low density (150% w/v) barium sulphate solution and radiographs are exposed as required. If there is a suspected perforation a water-soluble contrast medium should be used instead of barium as the latter is harmful in the mediastinum.

Small Bowel Enema. This technique provides better visualization of the small bowel than that achieved by a conventional barium follow through examination because rapid infusion of a large continuous column of contrast medium into the jejunum avoids segmentation of the barium column and does not allow time for flocculation to occur. It does however have the disadvantages of being unpleasant for the patient and more time consuming for the radiologist.

The patient is prepared with laxatives and a low residue diet and arrives following a 6-hour fast. A special tube is passed through the mouth or nose and advanced until its tip has passed beyond the duodenal–jejunal flexure. Very dilute barium sulphate suspension or barium sulphate followed by a non-opaque agent (e.g. methyl cellulose) is infused until the colon is reached. The leading edge of the barium column is observed by fluoroscopy and radiographs exposed by the radiologist as required.

Because of the large volume of fluid infused the patient is warned that diarrhoea is likely.

b. sulphate a water-insoluble salt used as an opaque contrast medium for radiological examination of the digestive tract.

Barlow's syndrome ('bahlohz) mitral valve prolapse, heard on auscultation during ventricular contraction as a high-pitched clicking sound followed by a murmur; called also *click–murmur syndrome*.

barognosis (,barog'nohsis) conscious perception of weight; the faculty by which weight is recognized.

baro-otitis (,baroh·oh'tietis) barotitis.

barophilic (,barə'filik) growing best under high atmospheric pressure; said of bacteria.

baroreceptor (,barohri'septə) a sensory nerve terminal that is stimulated by changes in pressure, as those in blood vessel walls.

barosinusitis (,baroh,sienə'sietis) a symptom complex due to differences in environmental atmospheric pressure and the air pressure in the paranasal sinuses.

barotaxis (,baroh'taksis) stimulation of living matter by change of atmospheric pressure.

barotitis (,barə'tietis) a morbid condition of the ear due to exposure to differing atmospheric pressures.

b. media a symptom complex due to a difference between the atmospheric pressure of the environment and air pressure in the middle ear.

barotrauma (,baroh'trawmə) injury due to pressure, such as to structures of the ear owing to differences between atmospheric and intratympanic pressures. See also barotitis and barosinusitis.

Barr body (bah) sex chromatin; the optically visible mass of chromatin attached to the nuclear membrane and representing the inactivated X chromosome in cells of normal females.

Barrett's syndrome ('barəts) peptic ulcer of the lower oesophagus, often with stricture, due to the presence of columnar-lined epithelium, which may contain functional mucous cells, parietal cells, or chief cells, in the oesophagus instead of normal squamous cell epithelium.

barrier ('bari·ə) an obstruction; a partition between two fluid compartments in the body.

blood–air b. alveolocapillary membrane. **blood–aqueous b.** the physiological mechanism that prevents exchange of materials between the chambers of the eye and the blood.

blood–brain b. (BBB) the barrier separating the blood from the brain parenchyma everywhere except the hypothalamus (see also blood–brain barrier).

blood–gas b. alveolocapillary membrane.

blood–testis b. a barrier separating the blood from the seminiferous tubules, consisting of special junctional complexes between adjacent Sertoli cells near the base of the seminiferous epithelium.

b. contraceptive a mechanical barrier preventing the sperm entering the cervical canal, e.g. diaphragm, condom.

b. nursing precautions taken by nurses to prevent infection from a patient spreading to other patients and/or staff. This normally involves nursing the patient in a separate room or cubicle. The nurses wear gowns, and frequently gloves, masks and overshoes, when carrying out nursing care. All items used by the patient, such as crockery, toilet requisites, etc., are sterilized after use. Excreta are disinfected prior to disposal; laundry is collected separately and either washed in a special container or disinfected prior to joining the main wash. Articles that cannot be disinfected or sterilized are burnt after use.

In some cases, a patient who is highly susceptible to infection may be barrier nursed. This is to prevent infection from outside reaching the patient, and such care is often called 'reverse barrier nursing'. In this case, the patient is nursed inside an air-conditioned room or tent. All items intended for the patient are sterilized prior to use, and some, such as food, may be irradiated to destroy organisms.

placental b. the tissue layers of the placenta which regulate the exchange of substances between the maternal and fetal blood.

Barron's ligator ('barənz 'liegay,tə) instrument for surgical treatment of haemorrhoids by binding them with rubber ligatures so that the ligated portion sloughs away after several days. Called also *rubber band ligator*.

Bartholin's cyst ('bahtəlin) a retention cyst affecting a Bartholin's gland, and usually developing as a consequence of an earlier infection of the gland.

Bartholin's duct ('bahtəlinz) the larger of the sublingual glands, which opens into the submandibular duct.

Bartholin's glands two small glands, one on each side of the vaginal orifice, that secrete mucus; their ducts open on the vulva. Called also the vulvovaginal glands. Their exact function is not clear but they are believed to secrete large amounts of mucus during sexual excitement, thereby providing lubrication for the vagina during coitus. The Bartholin glands are homologues of the bulbourethral glands in the male.

bartholinitis (,bahtəlin'ietis) inflammation of the Bartholin glands.

Barton's fracture ('bahtənz) fracture of the distal end of the radius into the wrist joint.

Bartonella (,bahtə'nelə) a genus of the family Bartonellaceae.

B. bacilliformis the aetiological agent of Carrión's disease (Oroya fever).

Bartonellaceae (,bahtəne'laysi·ee) a family of the order Rickettsiales, occurring as pathogenic parasites in the erythrocytes of man and other animals.

bartonellaemia (,bahtəne'leemi·ə) the presence in the blood of organisms of the genus *Bartonella*.

bartonellosis (,bahtəne'lohsis) an infectious disease of South America due to *Bartonella bacilliformis*, and transmitted by the sandfly *Phlebotomus verrucarum*; an acute febrile anaemic stage (Oroya fever) is followed by the appearance of a nodular cutaneous eruption (verruga peruana). Called also *Carrión's disease*.

Bartter's syndrome ('bahtərz) hypertrophy and hyperplasia of the juxtaglomerular cells, producing hypokalemic alkalosis and hyperaldosteronism, characterized by absence of hypertension in the presence of markedly increased plasma renin concentration and by insensitivity to the pressor effects of angiotensin. It usually affects children and is perhaps hereditary.

baryaesthesia (,bari·is'theezi·ə) baraesthesia.

barylalia (,bari'layli·ə) indistinct, thick speech, resulting from a lesion of the central nervous system.

baryphonia (,bari'fohni·ə) deepness and hoarseness of the voice.

basal ('bays'l) pertaining to or situated near a base; in physiology, pertaining to the lowest possible level.

b. metabolism test a method of measuring the body's expenditure of energy by recording its rate of oxygen intake and consumption. Once a major test of THYROID GLAND function, it is being replaced by diagnostic tests requiring less extensive preparation and capable of producing more accurate test results, e.g., the determination of the levels of thyroid hormones in the blood and the RADIOACTIVE IODINE UPTAKE test.

base (bays) 1. the lowest part or foundation of anything (see also BASIS). 2. the main ingredient of a compound. 3. the nonacid part of a salt; a substance that combines with acids to form salts. In the chemical processes of the body, bases are essential to the maintenance of a normal ACID–BASE BALANCE. Excessive concentration of bases in the body fluids leads to ALKALOSIS.

nitrogenous b. an aromatic, nitrogen-containing molecule that serves as a proton acceptor, e.g., purine or pyrimidine.

purine b's a group of compounds of which purine is the base, including uric acid, adenine, guanine, xanthine, and theobromine.

pyrimidine b's a group of chemical compounds of which pyrimidine is the base, including uracil, thymine, and cytosine, which are common constituents of nucleic acids.

Basedow's disease ('basidohz) exophthalmic goitre.

Basedow's goitre a colloid goitre which has become hyperfunctioning after administration of iodine.

baseline ('bays,lien) a known value or quantity used to measure or assess an unknown.

basement membrane ('baysmənt) the delicate layer of extracellular condensation of mucopolysaccharides and Type IV collagen underlying the epithelium of mucous membranes and secreting glands.

basic ('baysik) 1. pertaining to or having properties of a base. 2. capable of neutralizing acids.

basicity (bay'sisitee) 1. the quality of being a base, or basic. 2. the combining power of an acid.

Basidiobolus (ba,sidioh'bohləs) a genus of fungi of the group Phycomycetes, including *B. haptosporus*, the cause of subcutaneous phycomycosis.

basidiospore (ba'sidioh,spor) a spore of certain higher fungi formed on a basidium following karyogamy and meiosis.

basidium (ba'sidi·əm) pl. *basidia* [L.] the clublike organ bearing basidiospores.

basihyoid (,baysi'hieoyd) the body of the hyoid bone.

basilad ('basi,lad) toward the base.

basilar ('basilə) pertaining to a base or basal part.

basilateral (,baysi'latə·rəl) both basilar and lateral.

basilemma (,baysi'lemə) basement membrane.

basilic (bə'silik) prominent.

b. vein a large vein on the inner side of the arm.

basiloma (,baysi'lohmə, ,basi'lohmə) a basal cell carcinoma.

basion ('baysi·ən) the midpoint of the anterior border of the foramen magnum.

basipetal (bay'sipit'l) descending toward the base; developing in the direction of the base.

basis ('baysis) the lower, basic, or fundamental part of an object, organ, or substance. In anatomical nomenclature, used as a general term to designate the base of a structure or organ, or the part opposite to or distinguished from the apex.

basisphenoid (,baysi'sfeenoyd) an embryonic bone that becomes the back part of the body of the sphenoid.

basophil ('baysə,fil) adj. **basophilic**. 1. any structure, cell, or histological element staining readily with basic dyes. 2. a granular leukocyte with an irregularly shaped, relatively pale-staining nucleus that is partially constricted into two lobes, and with cytoplasm containing coarse bluish-black granules of variable size. 3. a beta cell of the adenohypophysis.

basophilia (ˌbaysə'fili·ə) 1. an affinity of cells or tissues for basic dyes. 2. the reaction of relatively immature erythrocytes to basic dyes whereby the stained cells appear blue, grey, or greyish-blue, or bluish granules appear. 3. abnormal increase of basophilic leukocytes in the blood. 4. basophilic leukocytosis.

basophilic (ˌbaysə'filik) staining readily with basic dyes.

basophilism (bay'sofilizəm) abnormal increase of basophilic cells.

basoplasm ('baysəˌplazəm) cytoplasm that stains with basic dyes.

BASW British Association of Social Workers.

Batchelor plaster ('bachələ) a plaster of Paris splint used in the correction of congenital dislocation of the hip.

bath (bahth) 1. a medium, e.g., water, vapour, sand, or mud, with which the body is washed or in which the body is wholly or partially immersed for therapeutic or cleansing purposes; application of such a medium to the body. 2. the equipment or apparatus in which a body or object may be immersed.

contrast b. alternate immersion of a part in hot water and cold water.

cool b. one in water from 15 to 24 °C.

emollient b. a bath in a soothing and softening liquid, used in various skin disorders. It is prepared by adding soothing agents, such as gelatin, starch, bran, or similar substances to the bath water, for the purpose of relieving skin irritation and pruritus. The patient is dried by patting rather than rubbing the skin. Care must be taken to avoid chilling.

hot b. one in water from 36 to 44 °C. Care must be taken to avoid faintness.

sitz b. see SALT bath.

sponge b. one in which the patient's body is not immersed but is wiped with a wet cloth or sponge. Sponge baths are most often employed for reduction of body temperature in the presence of a fever, in which case the water used is tepid and may contain alcohol to increase evaporation of moisture from the skin.

tepid b. one in water 30 to 33 °C.

warm b. one in water 32 to 40 °C.

whirlpool b. one in which the water is kept in constant motion by mechanical means. It has a gentle massaging action that promotes relaxation.

bathrocephaly (ˌbathroh'kefəlee, -'sef-) a developmental anomaly marked by a steplike posterior projection of the skull, caused by excessive growth of the lambdoid suture.

bathy- word element. [Gr.] *deep*.

bathyaesthesia (ˌbathi·is'theezi·ə) deep sensibility.

bathyanaesthesia (ˌbathiˌanəs'theezi·ə) loss of deep sensibility.

bathyhypaesthesia (ˌbathiˌhiepəs'theezi·ə) abnormally diminished deep sensibility.

bathyhyperaesthesia (ˌbathiˌhiepə·ris'theezi·ə) abnormally increased sensitiveness of deep body structures.

bathypnoea (ˌbathi'neeə) deep breathing.

battered-baby syndrome (ˌbatəd'baybee) a clinical presentation of CHILD ABUSE, multiple traumatic lesions, wilfully inflicted by an adult, of the bones and soft tissues of young children, often accompanied by subdural haematomas. See also NON-ACCIDENTAL INJURY. First described by John Caffey (1895–1966), paediatrician, USA.

BAUS British Association of Urological Surgeons.

Bayle's disease (baylz) progressive general paralysis of the insane.

Bazin's disease (ba'zanhz) erythema induratum; a chronic necrotizing vasculitis, usually occurring on the calves of young women; it was thought to be a form of tuberculosis of the skin complicated by vasculitis, but now the role of tuberculosis is in dispute.

BCG vaccine (ˌbeecee'gee) bacille Calmette–Guérin vaccine, a tuberculosis vaccine, containing live, attenuated bovine tubercle bacilli (*Mycobacterium bovis*). In the UK, BCG vaccine (intradermal) is supplied as a freeze-dried vaccine with diluent provided in a separate ampoule. It is given by intradermal injection in a dose of 0.1 ml. A special concentrated vaccine is available and used in other countries, administered by the multiple puncture technique. In the UK, vaccination is recommended for contacts of cases of tuberculosis, for health service staff, for particularly susceptible immigrant populations, and for all schoolchildren between their 10th and 14th birthdays. The vaccine is given only to persons who are tuberculin-test negative or weakly positive (Heaf test grades 0 and 1), although in other countries, direct vaccination of all persons irrespective of tuberculin sensitivity is practised. In British schoolchildren, vaccination is over 70 per cent effective in protecting against primary infection with tuberculosis and this protection persists for at least 15 years. Vaccination is contraindicated in persons on steroid therapy or who are immunosuppressed, including those with HIV infection, and in persons with skin disease at the vaccination site. About 6 weeks after vaccination with BCG, the subject will usually have a positive response to the tuberculin test, usually Heaf grade 1 or 2.

BCNU carmustine.

BDA British Dental Association.

Bdellovibrio (ˌdeloh'vibrioh) a genus of small, rod-shaped or curved, actively motile bacteria that are obligate parasites of certain gram-negative bacteria, including *Pseudomonas*, *Salmonella*, and coliform bacteria.

bdellovibrio (ˌdeloh'vibrioh) any microorganism of the genus *Bdellovibrio*.

BDS Batchelor in Dental Surgery.

Be chemical symbol, *beryllium*.

beaker ('beekə) a laboratory vessel of various materials, sometimes conical but usually with parallel sides, open at the top and often with a pouring spout.

beat (beet) a throb or pulsation, as of the heart or of an artery.

apex b. the beat felt over the apex of the heart, normally in the fifth left intercostal space.

capture b's occasional ventricular responses to a sinus impulse that reaches the atrioventricular node in a nonrefractory phase.

ectopic b. a heartbeat originating at some point other than the sinus node.

escaped b's heart beats that follow an abnormally long pause.

forced b. an extrasystole produced by artificial stimulation of the heart.

fusion b. in electrocardiography, the complex resulting when an ectopic ventricular beat coincides with normal conduction to the ventricle.

premature b. an extrasystole.

Beau's lines (bohz) transverse furrows on the fingernails, usually a sign of a systemic disease but also due to other causes.

bechic ('bekik) pertaining to cough.

Bechterew's disease ('bekhtə·rets) ankylosing spondylitis.

Beck's triad (beks) rising venous pressure, falling arterial pressure, and small, quiet heart; characteristic of cardiac compression.

Becker's dystrophy, Becker's muscular dystrophy ('bekəz) a form closely resembling Duchenne's muscular dystrophy, but having a later onset and milder course; transmitted as an X-linked recessive trait.

beclomethasone dipropionate (ˌbekloh'methəzohn) a glucocorticoid administered by aerosol inhalation to patients who require chronic treatment with corticosteroids for control of bronchial asthma symptoms. A nasal spray is available for treating allergic rhinitis, and creams and ointments are available to treat severe inflammatory skin conditions.

Becotide ('bekətied) trademark for a beclomethasone dipropionate metered-dose inhaler, a glucocorticoid used for bronchial asthma.

becquerel (be'krel) the SI unit of radioactivity, defined as the quantity of a radionuclide that undergoes one decay per second (s^{-1}). The non-SI unit CURIE is equivalent to 3.7×10^{10} becquerels. Abbreviated Bq.

bed (bed) 1. a supporting structure or tissue. 2. a couch or support for the body during sleep.

capillary b. the capillaries of a tissue, area, or organ considered collectively, and their volume capacity.

b. cradle a frame placed over the body of a bed patient for application of heat or cold or for protecting injured parts from coming into contact with the bed clothes. Cradles vary in size according to their intended purpose and can be used over the entire body or over one or more extremities.

fracture b. a bed for the use of patients with broken bones.

King's Fund b. a bed fitted with jointed springs, which may be adjusted to various positions. See also KING'S FUND.

nail b. the area of modified epidermis beneath the nail over which the nail plate slides as it grows.

bed-wetting ('bed,weting) enuresis; involuntary voiding of urine. See also ENURESIS.

bedbug ('bed,bug) a bug of the genus *Cimex*, a flattened, oval, reddish insect that inhabits houses, furniture and neglected beds, and feeds on man, usually at night.

bedpan ('bed,pan) a shallow vessel used for defaecation or urination by patients confined to bed.

bedsore ('bed,sor) an ulcerlike sore caused by prolonged pressure of the patient's body against the bed.

bee sting (bee sting) injury caused by the venom of a bee. The pain from a bee sting can be relieved by sodium bicarbonate, a few drops of ammonia, or calamine lotion. Cold compresses help prevent swelling. The skin should not be scratched as this may lead to infection. The insect's 'stinger' should be scraped out with a fingernail or removed with tweezers held flat against the skin. If the pain or swelling persists, or if the sting is on the tongue or in the mouth, a doctor should be consulted at once. Symptoms of a severe allergic reaction, such as collapse or swelling of the body, indicate ANAPHYLAXIS and require that medical help be sought immediately.

Beer's knife (biəz) one with a triangular blade used in cataract operations for incising the cornea preparatory to the removal of the lens.

beeswax ('beez,waks) yellow wax secreted by bees, and used in the manufacture of ointments.

behaviour (bi'hayvyə) those activities of an organism that can be observed—the visible, 'public' realm of activities, as opposed to the invisible 'private' realm of thoughts and feelings. adj. **behavioural.**

b. modification an approach to correction of undesirable behaviour that focuses on changing observable actions. Modification of the behaviour is accomplished through systematic manipulation of the environmental and behavioural variables related to the specific behaviour to be changed. The principles and techniques of behaviour modification have been utilized in the treatment of both physical and mental disorders; for example, in control of alcoholism, smoking, obesity, and stress. See also CONDITIONING.

b. therapy a therapeutic approach in which the focus is on the patient's observable behaviour, rather than on conflicts and unconscious processes presumed to underlie his maladaptive behaviour. This is accomplished through systematic manipulation of the environmental and behavioural variables related to the specific behaviour to be modified; operant conditioning, systematic desensitization, token economy, aversive control, flooding, and implosion are examples of techniques that may be used in behaviour therapy.

behavioural sink (bi'hayvyooə·rəl sink) disorganized and aberrant environment thought by some theorists to be the result of overcrowding.

behaviourism (bi'hayvyə,rizəm) a theory of psychology based upon objectively observable, tangible, and measurable data, rather than subjective phenomena, such as ideas and emotions.

Behçet's syndrome ('baysets) severe uveitis and retinal vasculitis, optic atrophy, and aphtha-like lesions of the mouth and genitalia, often with other signs and symptoms suggestive of a diffuse vasculitis; it most often affects young males. Called also Behçet's disease.

bejel ('bayjəl) a non-venereal form of syphilis caused by a treponema indistinguishable from that which causes syphilis. It is spread by direct or indirect contact with lesions of skin or mucous membrane of an infected person, usually in conditions of poor hygiene, and is limited to Africa, Asia and the Eastern Mediterranean.

bel (bel) a unit used to express the ratio of two powers, usually electric or acoustic powers; an increase of 1 bel in intensity approximately doubles the loudness of most sounds (see also DECIBEL).

belching ('belching) eructation.

belemnoid (bə'lemnoyd) 1. dart-shaped. 2. the styloid process.

Bell's palsy (belz) neuropathy of the facial nerve, resulting in paralysis of the muscles of the face, usually on one side. The victim usually is unable to close his mouth, so that he drools and cannot whistle. If he is unable to close the eye on the affected side, it may become tearful and inflamed.

Bell's palsy is often no more than a temporary condition lasting a few days or weeks. Occasionally facial paralysis results from a tumour pressing on the nerve, or from physical trauma to the nerve. In this event, recovery will depend on the success in treating the tumour or injury. More often, however, the cause is unknown. In many cases the deformity can be reduced by plastic surgery.

belladonna (ˌbelə'donə) 1. *Atropa belladonna* (deadly nightshade), a plant that is the source of various alkaloids, e.g., atropine, hyoscyamine, etc. 2. belladonna leaf; the dried leaves and fruiting tops of *Atropa belladonna*, used previously as an anticholinergic in the management of peptic ulcer and other gastrointestinal disorders.

b. poisoning a severe toxic condition due to overdosage of belladonna or accidental ingestion of large amounts of the drug. Symptoms include dryness of the mouth, thirst, dilated pupils, flushed skin or rash on the face, neck, and upper trunk, tachycardia, fever, delirium, and stupor. Treatment consists of removal of the poison from the stomach by inducing vomiting or gastric suction. This is followed by gastric lavage with water containing activated charcoal and an instillation of a solution of 200 ml of water and 30 g of sodium sulphate. Tranquillizers are administered to reduce excitability. Respiratory difficulties may require administration of oxygen or in extreme cases tracheostomy. Measures are also taken to reduce high body temperature and maintain an adequate blood pressure.

belle indifference (,bel in'difə·ronhs) a bland indifference to distressing symptoms or disabilities in mental disorder. Most commonly displayed in hysterical conversion disorders.

belly ('belee) 1. the abdomen. 2. the fleshy, contractile part of a muscle.

Benadryl ('benə,dril) trademark for diphenhydramine, an antihistamine.

Bence Jones protein (,bens 'johnz) a low molecular weight, heat-sensitive urinary protein found in patients with multiple myeloma, which coagulates on heating to 45–55 °C and redissolves partially or wholly on boiling.

bendrofluazide (,bendroh'flooə,zied) an oral diuretic of the thiazide group. Used primarily to treat mild hypertension and cardiac failure.

bends (bendz) decompression sickness; a condition resulting from a too-rapid decrease in atmospheric pressure, as when a deep-sea diver is brought too hastily to the surface. The term 'bends' is derived from the bodily contortions its victims undergo when atmospheric pressure is abruptly changed from a high pressure to a relatively lower one. Decompression sickness in underwater construction workers is referred to as *caisson disease*. Bends may also be a complication in a type of oxygen therapy called HYPERBARIC OXYGENATION, in which the patient is placed in a high-pressure chamber to increase the oxygen content of his blood. Nurses, doctors, and the patient within the chamber must be protected from bends when they emerge from the high-pressure chamber.

CAUSE. The phenomenon of bends is explained in terms of a law of physics: the greater the atmospheric pressure, the greater the amount of gas that can be dissolved in a liquid. The gas involved in bends is the air we breathe, composed chiefly of nitrogen and oxygen. Under normal atmospheric pressure, nitrogen is present in the blood in dissolved form. If the atmospheric pressure is substantially increased, a proportionately greater amount of nitrogen will be dissolved in the blood. The same is true of oxygen, and this is the basis for hyperbaric oxygenation in the treatment of oxygen deficiency.

The increase in pressure causes no ill effects. Nor will there be any ill effects if the pressure is gradually brought back to normal. When the decrease in pressure is slow, the nitrogen escapes safely from the blood as it passes through the lungs to be exhaled. If the pressure drops abruptly back to normal, the nitrogen is suddenly released from its state of solution in the blood and forms bubbles. Although the body is now under normal air pressure, expanding bubbles of nitrogen are present in the circulation and force their way into the capillaries, blocking the normal passage of the blood. This blockage (or embolism) starves cells dependent on a constant supply of oxygen and other blood nutrients. Some of these cells may be nerve cells located in the limbs or in the spinal cord. When they are deprived of blood, an attack of bends occurs.

The oxygen in the blood reacts similarly when abnormal pressure is abruptly relieved. But because oxygen is dissolved more easily than nitrogen, and because some of the oxygen combines chemically with haemoglobin, the oxygen released in decompression forms fewer bubbles, and is therefore less troublesome.

SYMPTOMS AND TREATMENT. The symptoms of bends include joint pain, dizziness, staggering, visual disturbances, dyspnoea, and itching of the skin. Partial paralysis occurs in severe cases; collapse and insensibility are also possible. Only rarely is the condition itself fatal, although a diver while in this condition may suffer a fatal accident unless he is rescued.

Bends is treated by placing the victim in a decompression chamber where the air pressure is at the level to which he was originally exposed. If the victim is a diver, this is the pressure at the depth where he was working. Pressure in the chamber is then reduced to normal at a safe rate.

Benedict's solution ('beni,dikts) a chemical solution used to determine the presence of glucose and other reducing substances in the urine; called also Benedict's reagent.

Benedikt's syndrome ('beni,dikts) ipsilateral oculomotor paralysis, contralateral hyperkinesia, contralateral tremor and paralysis of the arm and leg, and ipsilateral ataxia; due to damage to the third cranial nerve with involvement of the nucleus ruber and corticospinal tract.

Benemid ('benəmid) trademark for probenecid, a uricosuric agent used mainly in the treatment of chronic gout and also for some forms of arthritis. It is also used to increase blood levels of penicillin by reducing the excretion of penicillin.

benign (bi'nien) not malignant; not recurrent; favourable for recovery.

Bennett's fracture ('benits) fracture of the base of the first metacarpal bone running into the carpometacarpal joint, complicated by subluxation.

benorylate (be'nor·rilayt) an ester of paracetamol and aspirin used as an anti-inflammatory and analgesic.

Benson's disease ('bensənz) a unilateral condition of unknown origin, sometimes occurring with age, characterized by spherical and stellate opacities in the vitreous body, which appear to sparkle when illuminated by an examining light. Called also *asteroid hyalosis*.

Benylin Expectorant ('beni,lin) trademark for a preparation of ammonium chloride, diphenhydramine hydrochloride, methol and sodium citrate, a compound cough mixture.

benzalkonium chloride (,benzal'kohni·əm) a quaternary ammonium compound used as a surface disinfectant and detergent and as a topical antiseptic and antibiotic preservative.

benzathine penicillin (,benzətheen,peni'silin) a long-acting antibiotic. Used in treatment of infections and also in rheumatic fever prophylaxis.

benzene ('benzeen) a liquid hydrocarbon, C_6H_6, from coal tar; used as a solvent.

b. hexachloride a chloronated hydrocarbon, one isomer, gamma benzene hexachloride (LINDANE) was used as an insecticide, to kill lice. Its use is not currently recommended because of the emergence of resistant strains. Abbreviated BHC.

b. ring the closed hexagon of carbon atoms in benzene, from which the different benzene compounds are derived by replacement of the hydrogen atoms.

benzhexol (benz'heksol) an anticholinergic drug which helps to overcome the tremors and rigidity of Parkinson's disease.

benzidine ('benzi,deen) a compound used as a test for traces of blood (benzidine test).

benzoate ('benzoh,ayt) a salt of benzoic acid.

benzocaine ('benzoh,kayn) a local anaesthetic used

topically for the relief of pain or to anaesthetize the oropharynx or anus. Available as lozenges or ointment.

benzodiazepine (,benzohdie'azi,peen) any of a group of drugs having similar molecular structure. The group includes the sedative-hypnotics chlordiazepoxide, diazepam, oxazepam, flurazepam, and clorazepate, which are used as antianxiety agents; and the anticonvulsant clonazepam. Prolonged use of these drugs often causes dependence.

benzoic acid (ben'zoh·ik) an acid from benzoin and other resins and from coal tar, used as an antifungal agent in pharmaceutical preparations and as a germicide. The sodium salt of benzoic acid, sodium benzoate, is used as an antifungal agent in pharmaceutical preparations, and may be used as a test for liver function.

benzol ('benzol) benzene.

benzoyl ('benzoh·il, -zoh·iel) the acyl radical formed from benzoic acid, C_6H_5CO–.

b. peroxide dibenzoyl peroxide, used as a topical keratolytic in the treatment of acne vulgaris.

benztropine (benz'trohpeen) a parasympatholytic agent, used as the mesylate salt in Parkinson's disease.

benzydamine (ben'zidəmeen) an analgesic used as a mouthwash.

benzyl ('benzil, -ziel) the hydrocarbon radical, C_7H_7.

b. alcohol a colourless liquid used as a bacteriostatic in solutions for injection, and also topically as a local anaesthetic.

b. benzoate a clear, oily liquid used as a scabicide and with dimercaprol as an antidote in metal poisoning.

benzylpenicillin (,benzil,peni'silin, ,benziel-) penicillin G.

Berger's disease ('bərgəz) a chronic glomerulonephritis marked by recurring episodes of haematuria and by deposits of IgA immunoglobulin in the mesangial areas of the renal glomeruli. Called also IgA glomerulonephritis and IgA nephropathy.

Berger rhythm ('bərgə) alpha rhythm.

beriberi (,beri'beri) an endemic form of polyneuritis due to an unbalanced diet, chiefly a lack of vitamin B_1, or thiamine. The disease is more common in areas in which refined rice is the main staple in the diet; however, improved refining processes and dietary habits have decreased the incidence of this disease.

Mild forms of the disease occasionally occur in persons who are on extremely restricted diets. Alcoholics, who tend to decrease food intake drastically during periods of drinking, may show signs of beriberi. (See also ALCOHOLISM.) The disease also occurs in persons whose diet consists of highly refined and overcooked food.

Berkefeld's filter ('bərkə,felts) a filter composed of diatomaceous earth, impermeable to ordinary bacteria.

berkelium (bər'keeli·əm, 'bərkli·əm) a chemical element, atomic number 97, atomic weight 247, symbol Bk. See table of elements in Appendix 2.

Berkow formula ('bərkof) a method for estimating the extensiveness of a burn or scald. The seriousness of a burn is generally considered to indicate morbidity and mortality. The importance of estimating the extent of a burn had been recognized for a long time and many methods of classification relating to the depth of burned tissue have been proposed. In 1924 Samuel Berkow recognized that the *extent* as well as the depth of a burn was important, but difficult to measure in practice. Berkow proposed a method for estimating the extensiveness of a burn by considering the area of the burn as a percentage of the region it affected (e.g. the arm, leg, or trunk) and then calculating what percentage this is of the total body surface. In adults the proportions of the body surface do not vary very much. The head represents 6%, the trunk 38%, the upper extremities 18% and the lower extremities 38%, making a total of 100%. A burn or scald affecting half the trunk (which is 38%) would therefore represent 19% of the total body surface area.

The 'rule of nines', a method by which the body regions are represented as multiples of nine, is a simple and quick way to estimate the size of a burn. It is based on the Berkow formula but is less accurate.

In the child the body surface area proportions are quite different from the adult; the head and lower extremities vary considerably with age. Consideration of the areas of the body affected by growth is important if accurate assessment of the extent of a burn in a child is to be made (see LUND AND BROWDER CHART).

Bernstein test ('bərnstien, -steen) an acid perfusion test useful in differentiating oesophageal pain from ANGINA PECTORIS. Very rarely used, the test requires passage of a nasogastric tube and instillation of an acid solution into the oesophageal area. A lack of discomfort from the presence of the acid rules out oesophagitis.

berylliosis (bə,rili'ohsis) a morbid condition caused by exposure to fumes or finely divided dust of beryllium salts, marked by formation of granulomas, usually involving the lungs and, rarely, the skin, subcutaneous tissues, lymph nodes, liver, and other organs.

beryllium (bə'rili·əm) a chemical element, atomic number 4, atomic weight 9.012, symbol Be. See table of elements in Appendix 2.

Besnier–Boeck disease (,baynyay'bərk) sarcoidosis.

Besnier's prurigo (,bezni·əz prooə'riegoh) diathetic prurigo, seen in young children.

Best's disease (bestz) congenital macular degeneration; mainly presents in infants and very young children.

bestiality (,besti'alitee) sexual connection with an animal. See also BUGGERY.

beta ('beetə) second letter of the Greek alphabet, β; used to denote the second position in a classification system. Often used in names of chemical compounds to distinguish one of two or more isomers or to indicate the position of substituent atoms or groups in certain compounds. Also used to distinguish types of radioactive decay; brain rhythms or waves; adrenergic receptors; secretory cells of the various organs of the body that stain with basic dyes, such as the beta cells of the pancreas; and the type of haemolytic streptococci that produce a zone of decolorization when grown on blood media.

b.-adrenergic receptors specific sites on effector cells that respond to adrenaline. There are two types: β_1-receptors, found in the heart and small intestine, and β_2-receptors, found in the bronchi, blood vessels, and uterus.

b.-blocker a drug that blocks the action of adrenaline at beta-adrenergic receptors on cells of effector organs. There are two types of these receptors: β_1-receptors in the myocardium and β_2-receptors in the bronchial and vascular smooth muscles. The principal effects of beta-adrenergic stimulation are increased heart rate and contractility, vasodilation of the arterioles that supply the skeletal muscles, and relaxation of bronchial muscles.

Because of their effects on the heart, beta-blockers are used to treat angina pectoris, hypertension, and cardiac arrhythmias. And, because they decrease the workload of the heart, they are effective in reducing the long-term risk of mortality and reinfarction after recovery from the acute phase of a myocardial infarction. They are also used for the prophylaxis of migraine.

Nonselective beta-blockers affect both types of receptors and can produce bronchospasm in patients with asthma or chronic obstructive airways disease. If such patients need a beta-blocker, they should be given a cardioselective beta-blocker that preferentially blocks the β_1-receptors in the heart.

Nonselective beta-blockers include propranolol, used for treatment of angina, hypertension, arrhythmias, and migraine and for prophylaxis after the acute phase of a myocardial infarction; and timolol, used as an ophthalmic preparation for treatment of glaucoma and as an oral preparation for treatment of hypertension and for prophylaxis after the acute phase of a myocardial infarction. Cardioselective beta-blockers are used for treatment of hypertension, angina, arrhythmias and for prophylaxis against future infarction and include atenolol and metoprolol.

b. brain waves those having a frequency of more than 10 hertz (pulsations per second); seen during wakefulness. See also ELECTROENCEPHALOGRAPHY.

b. particles negatively charged particles emitted by radioactive elements. These particles are the result of the disintegration of neutrons, their source being the unstable atoms of radioactive metals such as radium and uranium. There are three general types of emissions from radioactive substances: alpha and beta particles and gamma rays. Beta particles are less penetrating than gamma rays and may be used to treat certain conditions on or near the surface of the body. See also RADIATION and RADIATION THERAPY.

beta-hydroxybutyric acid (ˌbeetəhieˌdroksibyoo'tirik) see β-HYDROXYBUTYRIC ACID.

beta-ketobutyric acid (ˌbeetəˌketohbyoo'tirik) acetoacetic acid.

betacism ('beetəˌsizəm) excessive use of the *b* sound in speaking.

Betadine ('betəˌdeen, -din) trademark for preparations of providone-iodine, which have a longer antiseptic action than most iodine solutions.

betaine ('beetəˌeen) the carboxylic acid derived by oxidation of choline; it acts as a transmethylating metabolic intermediate. The hydrochloride salt is used as a gastric acidifier.

betamethasone (ˌbeetə'methəˌzohn) a synthetic glucocorticoid, the most active of the anti-inflammatory steroids; available as a cream or tablet for topical or oral use.

betatron ('beetəˌtron) an apparatus for accelerating electrons to millions of electron volts by magnetic induction.

bethanechol (bə'thaniˌkol) a derivative of a choline-like substance, the chloride salt is used as a cholinergic in the treatment of abdominal distention and urinary retention. Hypotension and dyspnoea may occur as side-effects. If they do, atropine is usually administered.

bethanidine (bə'thaniˌdeen) an adrenergic blocking agent used in the treatment of essential hypertension, especially the malignant phase.

Betnovate ('betnəvayt) trademark for preparations containing betamethasone.

Betz cells (bets) large pyramidal neurons within a specific layer of the grey matter of the brain.

bezoar ('beezor) a mass formed in the stomach by compaction of repeatedly ingested material that does not pass into the intestine.

BGS British Geriatrics Society.

Bi chemical symbol, *bismuth.*

bi- word element. [L.] *two.*

biarticular (ˌbieah'tikyuhlə) affecting two joints.

biarticulate (ˌbieah'tikyuhˌlət) having two joints.

bias ('bie·əs) a term used in epidemiological investigations to mean any effects on the investigations which may cause the results to differ from their true values.

bibliotherapy (ˌbiblioh'therəpee) use of books and the reading of them in treatment of psychiatric disorders.

bicameral (bie'kamə·rəl) having two chambers or cavities.

bicapsular (bie'kapsyuhlə) having two capsules.

bicarbonate (bie'kahbəˌnayt, -nət) any salt containing the HCO_3^- anion.

blood b., plasma b. the bicarbonate of the blood plasma, an important parameter of ACID–BASE BALANCE measured in BLOOD GAS ANALYSIS.

b. of soda sodium bicarbonate.

bicaudal, bicaudate (bie'kawd'l; bie'kawdayt) having two tails.

bicellular (bie'selyuhlə) made up of two cells.

bicephalus (bie'kefələs, -'sef-) a two-headed fetus or infant.

biceps ('bieseps) a muscle having two heads. The biceps muscle of the arm flexes and supinates the forearm; the biceps muscle of the thigh flexes and rotates the leg laterally and extends the thigh.

Bichat's fissure (bi'shahz) transverse fissure.

Bichat's tunic (bi'shahz) tunica intima.

bichloride (bie'klor·ried) a chloride containing two equivalents of chlorine.

Bicillin ('biesilin) trademark for a mixture of procaine penicillin and benzylpenicillin sodium.

bicipital (bie'sipit'l) having two heads; pertaining to a biceps muscle.

biconcave (bie'konkayv) having two concave surfaces.

biconvex (bie'konvex) having two convex surfaces.

bicornate, bicornuate (bie'kawnayt; bie'kawnyooayt) having two horns, or cornua.

bicorporate (bie'kawpə·rət, -prət) having two bodies.

bicuspid (bie'kuspid) 1. having two cusps. 2. bicuspid (mitral) valve. 3. a premolar tooth.

b.i.d. [L.] *bis in die* (twice a day).

bidet ('beeday) a low narrow basin on a stand for washing the perineum and genitalia.

biduous ('bidyoo·əs) lasting two days.

Bielschowsky–Jansky disease (beelˌshovskeejanskee) the late infantile form of AMAUROTIC FAMILIAL IDIOCY, differing from the infantile form (TAY–SACHS DISEASE) in that it occurs between 3 and 4 years of age, progresses more slowly, and the cherry-red retinal spot is frequently absent, but there are pigmentary changes of the retina.

Bier's block (biəz 'blok) a form of regional analgesia in which the local anaesthetic solution is injected into a vein of a limb made ischaemic by a tourniquet. It is most useful for operations on the arm, but can also be used in the leg. The drug of choice is prilocaine (0.5% in 30–50 ml for an arm). Analgesia comes on in about 5–10 minutes and continues while the tourniquet remains inflated. Resuscitation equipment must be to hand to combat local anaesthetic toxicity should the cuff accidentally deflate in the first 20 minutes after injection. Called also *intravenous regional analgesia.*

bifid ('biefid) cleft into two parts or branches.

Bifidobacterium (ˌbiefidohbak'tiə·ri·əm) a genus of obligate anaerobic bacteria commonly occurring in the faeces, particularly in breast-fed infants.

bifocal spectacles (bie'fohk'l) spectacles in which each lens is made up of two segments of different refractive powers, or strength. Generally, the upper part of the lens is used for ordinary or distant vision, and the smaller, lower section for near vision, for close work such as reading or sewing. Bifocal spectacles are usually prescribed for PRESBYOPIA, which occurs as part of the ageing process. For advanced cases of presbyopia, and for special purposes such as watchmaking, trifocal glasses are available.

biforate (bie'for·rayt) having two perforations or foramina.

bifurcate (bie'fərkayt) divided into two branches.

bifurcation (ˌbiefə'kayshən) 1. a division into two branches. 2. the point at which division into two branches occurs.

bigeminal (bie'jemin'l) double.

b. pulse two pulse beats which occur together, regular in time and force. A regular irregularity.

biguanide (bie'gwahnied) an oral hypoglycaemic drug for treating diabetes, most commonly used in overweight diabetics.

bilateral (bie'latə·rəl) having two sides; pertaining to both sides.

bile (biel) a clear yellow or orange fluid produced by the liver. It is concentrated and stored in the gallbladder, and is poured into the small intestine via the bile ducts when needed for digestion. Bile helps in alkalinizing the intestinal contents and plays a roll in the emulsification, absorption, and digestion of fat; its chief constitutents are conjugated bile salts, cholesterol, phospholipid, bilirubin, and electrolytes. The bile salts emulsify fats by breaking up large fat globules into smaller ones so that they can be acted on by the fat-splitting enzymes of the intestine and pancreas. A healthy liver produces bile according to the body's needs and does not require stimulation by drugs. Infection or disease of the liver, inflammation of the gallbladder, or gallstones can interfere with the flow of bile.

b. acids steroid acids derived from cholesterol; classified as primary, those synthesized in the liver, e.g., cholic and chenodeoxycholic acid, or secondary, those produced from primary bile acids by intestinal bacteria and returned to the liver by enterohepatic circulation, e.g., deoxycholic and lithocholic acid.

b. ducts the canals or passageways that conduct bile. There are three bile ducts: the hepatic duct drains bile from the liver; the cystic duct is an extension of the gallbladder and conveys bile from the gallbladder; and the common bile duct passes through the wall of the small intestine at the duodenum and joins with the pancreatic duct to form the hepatopancreatic ampulla, or ampulla of Vater. The first two ducts may be thought of as branches which drain into the 'trunk'. At the opening into the small intestine there is a sphincter that automatically controls the flow of bile into the intestine.

The bile ducts may become obstructed by GALLSTONES, benign or malignant tumours, or a severe local infection. Various disorders of the GALLBLADDER or bile ducts are often diagnosed by CHOLECYSTOGRAPHY and CHOLANGIOGRAPHY, i.e., radiological examination of the gallbladder and bile ducts, using a special contrast medium so that these hollow structures can be clearly outlined on the radiographs.

b. pigment any one of the colouring matters of the bile; they are bilirubin, biliverdin, bilifuscin, biliprasin, choleprasin, bilihumin, and bilicyanin.

bilharziasis (ˌbilhah'tsieəsis) schistosomiasis.

bili- word element. [L.] *bile.*

biliary ('bilyə·ree) pertaining to the bile, to the bile ducts, or to the gallbladder.

b. drainage test an examination of the contents of the duodenum at the site where the common bile duct empties into it. The test is used when other, more conventional diagnostic tests for gallbladder disease reveal no pathology but the patient's symptoms persist. Specimens are collected and examined for leukocytes, cholesterol crystals, and parasites.

b. tract the organs, ducts, etc., participating in secretion (the liver), storage (the gallbladder), and delivery (hepatic and bile ducts) of bile into the duodenum.

biligenesis (ˌbili'jenəsis) production of bile.

biligenic (ˌbili'jenik) producing bile.

Biligrafin (ˌbili'grafin) trademark for a preparation of meglumine iodipamide, an i.v. cholangiographic agent.

Biligram ('biligram) trademark for a preparation of meglumine ioglycamate, an i.v cholangiographic agent.

biliousness ('biliəs,nəs) a symptom complex comprising nausea, abdominal discomfort, headache, and constipation, formerly attributed to excessive bile secretion.

bilirachia (ˌbili'raki·ə) the presence of bile pigments in the spinal fluid.

bilirubin (ˌbili'roobin) an orange bile pigment produced by the breakdown of haem and reduction of biliverdin; it normally circulates in plasma and is taken up by liver cells and conjugated to form bilirubin diglucuronide, the water-soluble pigment excreted in the bile. Failure of the liver cells to excrete bile, or obstruction of the BILE DUCTS, can cause an increased amount of bilirubin in the body fluids and thus lead to obstructive jaundice.

Another type of jaundice results from excessive destruction of erythrocytes (haemolytic jaundice). The more rapid the destruction of red blood cells and the degradation of haemoglobin, the greater the amount of bilirubin in the body fluids.

Laboratory tests for the determination of bilirubin content in the blood are of value in diagnosing liver dysfunction and in evaluating HAEMOLYTIC ANAEMIAS. Bilirubin may be classified as indirect ('free' or unconjugated) while en route to the liver from its site of formation by reticuloendothelial cells, and direct (bilirubin diglucuronide) after its conjugation in the liver with glucuronic acid. Elevated indirect bilirubin levels indicate prehepatic jaundice, such as haemolytic jaundice, or certain types of hepatic jaundice involving inability to conjugate bilirubin. Elevated direct bilirubin levels indicate other types of hepatic jaundice, such as in viral or alcoholic hepatitis, or posthepatic jaundice, as in biliary obstruction.

Normally the body produces a total of about 260 mg of bilirubin per day. Almost 99 per cent of this is excreted in the faeces; the remaining 1 per cent is excreted in the urine as UROBILINOGEN.

bilirubinaemia (ˌbiliˌroobi'neemi·ə) the presence of bilirubin in the blood.

bilirubinuria (ˌbiliˌroobi'nyooə·ri·ə) the presence of bilirubin in the urine.

Biliscopin (ˌbili'skopin) trademark for a preparation of meglumine iotroxate, an i.v. cholangiographic agent.

biliuria (ˌbili'yooə·ri·ə) the presence of bile acids in the urine.

biliverdin (ˌbili'vərdin) a green bile pigment formed by catabolism of haemoglobin and converted to bilirubin in the liver.

Billings method ('bilingz) ovulation method of CONTRACEPTION.

Billroth's operation ('bilrohts) gastrectomy.

bills of mortality (bilz əv maw'talitee) lists of deaths published principally in London, first in the plague years in the 16th century and later weekly or annually until the early 19th century.

bilobate (bie'lohbayt) having two lobes.

bilobular (bie'lobyuhlə) having two lobules.

bilocular (bie'lokyuhlə) having two compartments.

biloma ('bielohmə) an encapsulated collection of bile in the peritoneal cavity.

Biloptin (bie'loptin) trademark for a preparation of sodium ipodate, an oral cholecystographic contrast medium.

bimanual (bie'manyooəl) with both hands.

bimastoid (bie'mastoyd) pertaining to both mastoid processes.

binary ('bienə·ree) made up of two elements, or of two equal parts; denoting a number system with a base of two.

b. fission the halving of the nucleus and then of the cytoplasm of the cell, as in protozoa.

binaural (bie'nor·rəl) pertaining to both ears.

binauricular (,bienor'rikyuhlə) pertaining to both auricles of the ears.

binder ('biendə) a girdle or large bandage for support of the abdomen or breast.

abdominal b. one applied to the abdomen to hold an abdominal dressing.

breast b. one used to give support and hold the breasts firmly in proper position.

double T b. one used for male patients to hold perineal or rectal dressings in place.

many-tailed b. one applied with the tails overlapping each other and held in position by safety pins.

T b. one used to hold perineal or rectal dressings in place.

Binet's test, Binet–Simon test ('beenayz; ,beenay-'siemən) a method of ascertaining a child's or youth's mental age by asking a series of questions adapted to, and standardized on, the capacity of normal children at various ages.

Bing test (bing) a vibrating tuning fork is held to the mastoid process and the auditory meatus is alternately occluded and left open; an increase and decrease in loudness (positive Bing) is perceived by the normal ear and in sensorineural hearing impairment, but in conductive hearing impairment no difference in loudness is perceived (negative Bing).

binocular (bi'nokyuhlə, bie-) 1. pertaining to both eyes. 2. having two eyepieces, as in a microscope.

binomial (bie'nohmi·əl) composed of two terms, e.g., names of organisms formed by combination of genus and species names.

b. distribution probability distribution of two mutually exclusive variables.

binotic (bi'notik) binaural.

binovular (bi'novyuhlə) pertaining to or derived from two distinct ova. Binovular or dizygotic twins result from the fertilization of two separate ova by two distinct spermatozoa. They are three times more common than uniovular twins.

Binswanger's dementia ('binsvangəz) dementia due to demyelination of the subcortical white matter of the brain with sclerotic changes in the blood vessels supplying it.

binuclear (bie'nyookli·ə) having two nuclei.

binucleation (,bienyookli'ayshan) formation of two nuclei within a cell through division of the nucleus without division of the cytoplasm.

binucleolate (bie'nyookli·ə,layt) having two nucleoli.

bio- word element. [Gr.] *life, living.*

bioactive (,bieoh'aktiv) having an effect on or eliciting a response from living tissue.

bioamine (,bieoh'ameen) biogenic amine.

bioaminergic (,bieoh,amin'ərjik) of or pertaining to neurons that secrete biogenic amines.

bioassay (,bieoh'asay) determination of the active power of a drug sample by comparing its effects on a live animal or an isolated organ preparation with those of a reference standard.

bioavailability (,bieoh·ə,vaylə'bilitee) the degree to which a drug or other substance becomes available to the target tissue after administration.

biochemistry (,bieoh'kemistree) the chemistry of living organisms and of their chemical constituents and vital processes.

biocidal (,bieə'sied'l) destructive to living organisms.

biocompatibility (,bieohkəmpatə'bilitee) the quality of not having toxic or injurious effects on biological systems. adj. **biocompatible.**

biodegradable (,bieohdi'graydəb'l) susceptible of degradation by biological processes, as by bacterial or other enzymatic action.

biodegradation (,bieoh,degrə'dayshən) the series of processes by which living systems render chemicals less noxious to the environment.

bioequivalence (,bioh·i'kwivələns) the relationship between two preparations of the same drug in the same dosage form that have a similar bioavailability. adj. **bioequivalent.**

biofeedback (,bieoh'feed,bak) the provision of visual or auditory evidence to a person of the status of an autonomic body function as a method of teaching control of certain visceral responses previously thought to be exclusively dictated by the autonomic nervous system and therefore involuntary or unconscious.

Examples of the kinds of biological feedback that can be provided include information about changes in skin temperature, muscle tonicity, cardiovascular activities, blood pressure, and brain wave activities. With the aid of such sensitive electronic equipment as the electrocardiogram, electromyelogram, and electroencephalogram, it is possible for the person to become consciously aware of the response being measured and to learn to control it. The feedback may be presented in the form of musical tones, lights, or direct visualization of scales or meters which indicate variance in the response.

In clinical biofeedback, the patient must practise the particular desired response many times under the supervision of professional persons who are skilled in the techniques of psychophysiology and have a thorough understanding of sophisticated electronics. An example in which biofeedback may be used clinically is in the treatment of RAYNAUD'S DISEASE, in which the patient learns to consciously raise skin temperature in the extremities and thus reduce vasoconstriction.

While clinical biofeedback is still an emerging field, encouraging results have been reported in the treatment of a variety of diseases, particularly PSYCHOSOMATIC ILLNESS. Examples include modifying insomnia and phobias, the control of certain types of epileptic seizures, and cardiac arrhythmias. It has also been used in muscle retraining in cases of hemiplegia, paralysis, and spasticity.

alpha b. the visual presentation of his own brain-wave pattern to a subject who is instructed to try to produce alpha brain-wave activity to achieve the alpha state of relaxation and peaceful wakefulness. An acoustic tone is used to indicate nonproduction of alpha waves.

biogenesis (,bieoh'jenəsis) 1. origin of life, or of living organisms. 2. the theory that living organisms originate only from other living organisms.

biogenic (,bieoh'jenik) originating in a biological process.

b. amine an amine neurotransmitter, such as adrenaline, noradrenaline, serotonin, or dopamine.

bioimplant (,bieoh'implahnt) denoting a prosthesis made of biosynthetic material.

biokinetics (,bieohki'netiks) the science of the movements of tissue and related phenomena that occur during the development of organisms.

biological (ˌbieə'lojik'l) 1. pertaining to biology. 2. a medicinal preparation made from living organisms and their products; these include serums, vaccines, etc.

b. clock the physiological mechanism that governs the rhythmic occurrence of certain biochemical, physiological, and behavioural phenomena in living organisms. See also biological RHYTHM.

biologist (bie'oləjist) a specialist in biology.

biology (bie'oləjee) scientific study of living organisms. adj. **biological.**

molecular b. study of molecular structures and events underlying biological processes, including relation between genes and the functional characteristics they determine.

radiation b. scientific study of the effects of ionizing radiation on living organisms.

bioluminescence (ˌbieohˌloomi'nes'ns) chemoluminescence occurring in living cells.

biomass ('biohˌmas) the entire assemblage of living organisms of a particular region, considered collectively.

biomaterial (ˌbieohmə'tiə·ri·əl) a synthetic dressing with selective barrier properties, used in the treatment of burns; it consists of a liquid solvent (polyethylene glycol-400) and a powdered polymer.

biome ('bieˌohm) a large, distinct, easily differentiated community of organisms arising as a result of complex interactions of climatic factors, biota, and substrate; usually designated, according to kind of vegetation present, as tundra, coniferous or deciduous forest, grassland, etc.

biomechanics (ˌbieohmə'kaniks) the application of mechanical laws to living structures.

biomedicine (ˌbieoh'medisin, -'medsin) clinical medicine based on the principles of the natural sciences—biology, biochemistry, etc. adj. **biomedical.**

biomembrane (ˌbieoh'membrayn) any membrane, e.g., the cell membrane, of an organism. adj. **biomembranous.**

biometrics, biometry (ˌbieə'metriks; bie'omətree) the application of statistical methods to biological facts.

biomicroscope (ˌbieoh'miekrəˌskohp) a microscope for examining living tissue in the body.

biomicroscopy (ˌbieohmie'kroskəpee) microscopic examination of living tissue in the body.

biomolecule (ˌbieoh'moliˌkyool) a molecule produced by living cells, e.g., a protein, carbohydrate, lipid, or nucleic acid.

bionecrosis (ˌbieohnə'krohsis) necrobiosis.

bionics (bie'oniks) scientific study of functions, characteristics, and phenomena observed in the living world, and application of knowledge gained therefrom to nonliving systems.

biophysics (ˌbieoh'fiziks) the science dealing with the application of physical methods and theories to biological problems. adj. **biophysical.**

biophysiology (ˌbieohˌfizi'oləjee) that portion of biology including organogenesis, morphology, and physiology.

biopsy ('bieopsee) removal for examination, usually microscopic, of tissue from the living body. Biopsies are usually done to determine the diagnosis, e.g. whether a tumour is malignant or benign, but are also used to assess the stage to which a known disease has progressed and to analyse the effects of the treatment.

aspiration b. biopsy in which tissue is obtained by application of suction through a hollow needle attached to a syringe.

brush b. removal of cells and tissue fragments using a brush with stiff bristles to obtain samples from sites accessible only to endoscopy or intubation.

cone b. biopsy in which an inverted cone of tissue is excised, as from the uterine cervix.

endoscopic b. removal of tissue through an endoscope.

excisional b., incisional b. biopsy of tissue removed from the body by simple excision.

fine needle b. removal of very small amounts of tissue by aspiration through a very fine needle, usually for the purpose of a very rapid cytological diagnosis.

needle b. biopsy in which tissue is obtained within the lumen of a needle and is detached by rotation, the needle then being withdrawn.

punch b. biopsy in which tissue is obtained by a punch.

sternal b. biopsy of bone marrow of the sternum removed by puncture or trephining (see also STERNAL PUNCTURE).

bioptome ('bieopˌtohm) a cutting instrument for taking biopsy specimens.

bioreversible (ˌbieohri'vərsəb'l) capable of being changed back to the original biologically active chemical form by processes within the organism; said of drugs.

biorhythm ('bieohˌridhəm) biological RHYTHM.

bioscience (ˌbieoh'sieəns) the study of biology wherein all the applicable sciences (physics, chemistry, etc.) are applied.

biosphere ('bieəˌsfiə) 1. that part of the universe in which living organisms are known to exist, comprising the atmosphere, hydrosphere, and lithosphere. 2. the sphere of action between an organism and its environment.

biostatistics (ˌbieohstə'tistiks) the biomedical application of STATISTICS; that branch of biometry dealing with the data and laws of human mortality, morbidity, and natality.

biosynthesis (ˌbieoh'sinthəsis) creation of a compound by physiological processes in a living organism. adj. **biosynthetic.**

Biot's respirations ('beeohz) a type of respiration associated with spinal meningitis and other central nervous system disorders; respirations are faster and deeper than normal, interspersed with abrupt pauses in breathing.

biota (bie'ohtə) all the living organisms of a particular area; the combined flora and fauna of a region.

biotelemetry (ˌbieohtə'lemətree) the recording and measuring of certain vital phenomena occurring in living organisms that are at a distance from the measuring device.

biotic (bie'otik) 1. pertaining to life or living organisms. 2. pertaining to the biota.

biotin ('bieətin) a member of the vitamin B complex, required by or occurring in all forms of life tested.

biotoxicology (ˌbieohˌtoksi'koləjee) scientific study of poisons produced by living organisms, their cause, detection, and effects, and treatment of conditions produced by them.

biotoxin (ˌbieoh'toksin) a poisonous substance produced by a living organism.

biotransformation (ˌbieohˌtransfə'mayshən, -ˌtrahns-) the series of chemical alterations of a compound (e.g., a drug) occurring within the body, as by enzymatic activity.

biotype ('bieəˌtiep) 1. a group of individuals having the same genotype. 2. any of a number of strains of a species of microorganisms having differentiable physiological characteristics.

biovular (bie'ohvyuhlə) binovular.

biparental (ˌbiepə'rent'l) derived from two parents, male and female.

biparietal (biepə'rieət'l) pertaining to both parietal

eminences or bones.

b. diameter (BPD) the distance between the two parietal eminences measured through (not around) the fetal skull. It has a value of 9.5 cm in a normal baby at birth, and forms an important obstetric measurement. It may be determined by ultrasonic cephalometry from 9 weeks' gestation using an A scan. Serial measurement of the BPD in pregnancy is used to assess fetal maturity and well-being. The fetal head is said to be *engaged* when the BPD, which is the widest transverse diameter of the skull, has passed through the brim of the maternal pelvis; this indicates that delivery by the vaginal route should be possible. *Crowning* occurs when the BPD distends the vulva during delivery and the head no longer recedes during contractions.

bipenniform (bie'penifawm) doubly feather-shaped; said of muscles whose fibres are arranged on each side of a tendon like barbs on a feather shaft.

biperiden (bie'peridən) a synthetic anticholinergic used to reduce the tremors of parkinsonism and certain other forms of spasticity and for the treatment of drug-induced extrapyramidal reactions. Side-effects are minor and include dryness of the mouth, blurring of vision, drowsiness, and nausea. Biperiden is contraindicated in patients with epilepsy and should be given with great care to patients with glaucoma.

biphenyl (bie'feenil, -niel) diphenyl, $(C_6H_5)_2$.

polybrominated b's (PBBs) brominated derivatives of biphenyl; uses and toxic hazard are similar to polychlorinated biphenyls.

polychlorinated b's (PCBs) chlorinated derivatives of biphenyl, used as heat-transfer agents and as electrical insulators; they are toxic and not biodegradable.

bipolar (bie'pohlə) 1. having two poles. 2. pertaining to both poles.

bipotentiality (ˌbiepəˌtenshi'alitee) ability to develop or act in either of two different ways.

BIPP an antiseptic paste composed of bismuth, iodoform and paraffin.

BIR British Institute of Radiology.

biramous (bie'rayməs, 'birəməs) having two branches.

birefractive (ˌbieri'fraktiv) doubly refractive.

birefringence (ˌbieri'frinjəns) the bending of light, exhibited by anisotropic materials, such that the light is split into rays which are polarized in mutually perpendicular planes and travel at different speeds. Called also *double refraction*.

birth (bərth) a coming into being; the act or process of being born.

b. canal the canal through which the fetus passes in birth. Its contours and size are determined by the pelvic capacity. It comprises the cervix and vagina.

b. certificate a statement issued by the registrar for births, marriages and deaths for the district in which the child was born. It certifies details of parentage, name and sex of the child, and date and place of birth. This certificate must be obtained by the parents, or failing them, anyone present at the delivery, within 42 days of the birth in England (21 days in Scotland). It gives legal status to the child and is necessary before he can receive Child Benefit. A birth certificate is issued to any child born alive, irrespective of the period of gestation. A stillbirth certificate is issued for babies of 28 weeks maturity or longer who did not breathe or show other signs of life after complete expulsion from the mother.

b. control the concept of limiting the size of families by measures designed to prevent conception. The movement of that name began in modern times as a humanitarian reform to conserve the health of mothers and the welfare of children, especially among the poor. More recently it has been superseded by the term 'family planning', which means planning the arrival of children to correspond with the desire and resources of the married couple and to provide greater happiness for the children. (See also CONTRACEPTION.) Family planning is concerned not only with controlling fertility but also with overcoming apparent sterility in those couples who want a child but have been unsuccessful in having one.

b. interval the period of time which elapses between two or more successive pregnancies or births. A term used in family planning in connection with family spacing.

multiple b. the birth of two or more offspring produced in the same gestation period.

b. notification in the UK, notification of birth is required by the doctor, midwife or any other person in attendance at birth, within 36 hours of the birth, to the District Medical Officer or Chief Administrative Officer of the locality in which the birth takes place.

premature b. expulsion of the fetus from the uterus before termination of the normal gestation period, but after independent existence has become a possibility. See also PRETERM INFANT.

b. rate the number of births during one year per 1000 total estimated mid-year population (crude birth rate), per 1000 estimated mid-year female population (refined birth rate), or per 1000 estimated mid-year female population of childbearing age (true birth rate), that is, between the ages of 15 and 45.

b. registration in the UK, registration of birth is required by the parent or person having charge of the child to the local registrar of births, deaths and marriages within 42 days of birth.

b. weight the weight of a baby immediately following delivery. This should be checked by two people to ensure accuracy because it forms the baseline for assessing future development and acts as an important national statistic. The average birth weight for a healthy infant born at term is currently 3.5 kg.

birthmark ('bərthˌmahk) a congenital blemish or spot on the skin, usually visible at birth or shortly after. Those appearing later occur at the location of a skin defect present at birth. The cause is unknown. See also NAEVUS.

physiological b. one so common as to be considered normal; once applied to naevus flammeus in the suboccipital region.

vascular b. one caused by an unusual clustering of small blood vessels near the surface of the skin; called also HAEMANGIOMA. These birthmarks include 'strawberry' or 'raspberry' marks, 'port-wine stains', and an elevated type called cavernous haemangiomas.

bis in die (ˌbis in 'dee·ay) [L.] *twice a day;* abbreviated b.i.d.

bisacodyl (ˌbisə'kohdil) a stimulant laxative.

bisacromial (ˌbisə'krohmi·əl) pertaining to the two acromial processes.

bisalbuminaemia (ˌbisalˌbyoomi'neemi·ə) a congenital abnormality marked by the presence of two distinct serum albumins that differ in mobility on electrophoresis.

bisection (bie'sekshən) division into two parts by cutting.

bisexual (bie'seksyooəl) 1. having gonads of both sexes. 2. hermaphrodite. 3. having both active and passive sexual interests or characteristics. 4. capable of the function of both sexes. 5. both heterosexual and homosexual. 6. an individual who is both heterosexual and homosexual. 7. of, relating to, or involving both sexes, as bisexual reproduction.

bisexuality (bieˌseksyoo'alitee) 1. the condition of being bisexual or of being a bisexual. 2. hermaphroditism.

bisferious (bis'feri·əs) dicrotic; having two beats.

Bishop score ('bishəp) a gauge for estimating the likelihood of successful induction of labour, by assessing the state or 'ripeness' of the cervix (see accompanying table).

biteplate ('biet,playt) an appliance, usually plastic or wire, worn in the palate as a diagnostic or therapeutic adjunct in orthodontics or prosthodontics.

Bitot's spots ('beetohz) foamy grey, triangular spots of keratinized epithelium on the conjunctiva, associated with vitamin A deficiency.

Bishop score

Cervical features	Score			
	0	1	2	3
Degree of effacement (%)	0–30	40–50	60–70	80 +
Dilation of the external os (cm)	Closed (pinhole os)	1–2	3–4	5
Consistency	Firm	Medium	Soft	—
Position	Posterior	Midline	Anterior	—
Station of presenting part above or below the ischial spines	−3	−2	−1	+1 or +2

Favourable features for successful induction of labour result in a score of 6–13.
Unfavourable features for successful induction of labour result in a score of 0–5.

bisiliac (bis'ili,ak) pertaining to the two iliac bones or to any two corresponding points on them.

bismuth ('bizməth) a chemical element, atomic number 83, atomic weight 208.980, symbol Bi. (See table of elements in Appendix 2.) Its salts have been much used in inflammatory diseases of the stomach and intestines and in syphilis.

b. subgallate a bright yellow, amorphous powder, applied locally in skin diseases.

bismuthosis (,bizmə'thohsis) chronic bismuth poisoning, with anuria, stomatitis, dermatitis, and diarrhoea.

bistoury ('bistə·ree) a long, narrow, straight or curved surgical knife used in opening sinuses and fistulas, and incising abscesses.

bisulphate (bie'sulfayt) an acid sulphate.

bite (biet) 1. seizure with the teeth. 2. a wound or puncture made by a living organism. 3. an impression made by closure of the teeth upon some plastic material, e.g., wax. 4. occlusion (2).

ANIMAL BITE. Any animal bite that breaks the skin should be treated rapidly and with care. The wound should be washed at once with soap and water.

In countries where RABIES is present, a doctor should be consulted so that necessary steps may be taken to prevent the development of rabies.

HUMAN BITE. Any human bite that penetrates the skin should be considered dangerous. The wound should be washed immediately with soap and water and a doctor consulted. Antibiotic therapy may be needed as there is a serious danger of infection, a danger that is more serious with human bites than with animal bites, since many of the organisms carried by animals do not affect humans.

anterior open b. failure of the anterior teeth to establish an occlusal contact when the posterior teeth are closed.

over-b. overbite.

bite-wing ('biet,wing) a wing or fin attached along the centre of the tooth side of a dental x-ray film and bitten on by the patient, permitting production of images of the corona of the teeth in both dental arches and their contiguous peridontal tissues.

bitemporal (bie'tempə·rəl, -'temprəl) pertaining to both temples or temporal bones.

bitrochanteric (,bietrohkan'terik) pertaining to both trochanters on one femur or to both greater trochanters.

bitters ('bitəz) drugs characterized by bitter taste; used to stimulate the appetite.

bituminosis (,bityuhmi'nohsis) a form of PNEUMOCONIOSIS due to dust from soft coal.

biuret (bie'yooə·rət) a urea derivative; its presence is detected after addition of sodium hydroxide and copper sulphate solutions by a pinkish-violet colour (protein test) or a pink and finally a bluish colour (urea test).

bivalent (bie'vaylənt, 'bivə-) 1. having a valency of two. 2. denoting homologous chromosomes associated in pairs during the first meiotic prophase.

bivalve ('bie,valv) 1. having two valves, as the shells of molluscs such as oysters. 2. to cut a plaster cast into an anterior and a posterior section.

bivalved speculum ('bie,valv'd) a vaginal speculum, having two blades that can be adjusted for easy insertion.

biventral (bie'ventrəl) 1. having two bellies. 2. digastric muscle.

biventricular (,bieven'trikyuhlə) pertaining to or affecting both ventricles of the heart.

bizygomatic (,bieziegoh'matik) pertaining to the two most prominent points of the two zygomatic arches.

Bk chemical symbol, *berkelium*.

black eye ('blak,ie) a bruise of the tissue around the eye marked by discoloration, swelling, and pain.

blackhead ('blak,hed) comedo; a plug of keratin and sebum within the dilated orifice of a hair follicle. The colour of blackheads is caused not by dirt but by the discolouring effect of air on the sebum in the clogged pore. Infection may cause the comedo to develop into a pustule or boil. See also ACNE VULGARIS.

blackout ('blakowt) temporary loss of vision and momentary unconsciousness due to diminished circulation to the brain and retina. Blackout refers specifically to a condition which sometimes occurs in aviators resulting from increased acceleration, which causes a decrease in blood supply to the brain cells. The term can also refer to other forms of temporary loss of consciousness and to FAINTING, as well as to temporary loss of memory and to certain forms of vertigo.

blackwater fever ('blak,wawtə) a dangerous and poorly understood complication of falciparum malaria, characterized by the passage of dark red to black urine, severe toxicity, and high mortality, especially for Europeans.

bladder ('bladə) a musculo-membranous sac which acts as a receptacle for secretion, especially the urinary bladder. The urinary bladder is situated in the anterior part of the pelvis; the symphysis pubis lies anteriorly and the small intestine lies superiorly. In the female the uterus lies posteriorly and the urethra and pelvic floor muscles lie inferiorly. In the male the rectum and seminal vesicles lie posteriorly and the urethra and prostate gland lie inferiorly. The bladder is joined to the kidneys by the ureters, which open on to the posterior wall of the bladder. The urethra connects the bladder to the exterior and opens on to the inferior bladder wall. A thickening of smooth muscle around the urethral origin forms the internal sphincter and controls passage of urine from the bladder to the urethra. The external urethral sphincter is found at the distal end of the urethra and is controlled at will. The three orifices in the bladder wall form a triangular area called the trigone. The arterial blood supply is from the anterior internal iliac artery and venous drainage is into the internal iliac vein. The nerve supply is from the third and fourth sacral nerves and the pelvic plexus of the sympathetic nervous system.

The bladder is roughly pear-shaped, becoming more oval when distended with urine. The kidneys produce urine every few seconds which moves via the ureter to the bladder and collects. The bladder adapts to accommodate the increased volume, initially with little change in pressure. When 250–350 ml of urine have collected, the autonomic nerve endings within the bladder wall are stimulated. Nerve impulses are conveyed to consciousness and, when convenient, micturition occurs.

Micturition is the expulsion of urine to the exterior and occurs when the internal sphincter dilates, the muscular wall of the bladder contracts and the external sphincter is voluntarily relaxed. It may be assisted by voluntarily increasing the intra-abdominal pressure. In the adult the sphincters can prevent urination even when the bladder is uncomfortably full, but in children full bladder control is slow to develop. BED-WETTING may normally continue to the age 3 or 4 years.

DISORDERS OF THE BLADDER. Infections of the bladder are common, especially in females, as the female urethra is shorter than that of the male, allowing easier entry of pathogens, very commonly *Escherichia coli*. Most infections are successfully treated with antibiotics.

Inflammation of the bladder, or CYSTITIS, may be caused by many different agents, and can vary greatly in severity. Its most usual symptoms are a persistent desire to urinate, and a burning sensation at urination. Haematuria may occur due to small haemorrhages in the oedematous muscle.

Various deformations of the bladder are found. The most common and least serious is the formation of a diverticulum. This may be caused by pressure from inside the bladder, when for some reason the urine is obstructed, or it may have existed from birth.

An abnormal opening in the bladder causes a fistula, which conducts escaping urine to other parts of the body, or to the exterior through the skin. The most common varieties are fistulas which lead into the intestine or directly into the vagina (vesicovaginal fistula). They occur sometimes after childbirth or after diverticulitis of the colon. The condition may be repaired by surgery.

Stones (calculi) may form in the bladder and often lead to painful and difficult urination. They are usually caused by obstructions in the mouth of the bladder, brought about, for example, by an enlarged prostate. They may be removed by surgery, or more commonly by cystoscopy, or shattered by lithotripsy and passed through the urethra.

Urinary INCONTINENCE can occur as a result of *neurogenic bladder*, trauma to and weakening of the external urinary sphincter muscle, or inflammation, infection, or other transient disorders. In many instances, a bladder training programme can help overcome the problem of incontinence. Other techniques for management of inability to control urination are discussed under INCONTINENCE.

In *urinary retention* there is an inability to initiate and complete micturition, resulting in accumulation of urine in the bladder. The most common cause is obstruction to the flow of urine through the urethra, usually because of constriction by an enlarged prostate gland. Obstruction from outside the bladder or urethra may also be caused by invasive pelvic tumours, haemorrhage or collections of fluid, retroperitoneal fibrosis, or phimosis. Obstruction from inside may be caused by a stone or blood clot, fibrosis following infection, or precipitation of crystals due to treatment with sulphonamides. Other causes include anxiety, hysteria, and diminished neural function, either motor or sensory. Certain medications, vaginal and rectal surgery, haemorrhoids, and faecal impaction also can interfere with the ability to urinate normally, with resultant retention of urine in the bladder.

Benign tumours of the bladder are relatively rare. Small, superficial ones can be treated by fulguration, using a cystoscope and an electric cautery. Normally, after fulguration there is minimal bleeding and the patient can usually be treated as a day patient.

The bladder is the most common site of malignancy of the urinary system. It affects men more frequently than women, and it occurs most frequently in persons over the age of 50. Suspected contributing factors in the development of malignant tumours of the bladder include exposure to industrial substances, such as aniline dyes, and toxins in cigarette smoke. The artificial sweeteners saccharine and cyclamate have been shown to cause bladder tumours in animal studies; however, these substances have not been shown to cause bladder tumours in humans.

In the UK, the TNM classification of malignant tumours (UICC) is generally used for bladder tumours (see also CANCER).

The classification applies only to epithelial tumours. Papilloma is excluded but such cases may be listed under category T_0 (no evidence of anaplasia). The suffix m may be added to the appropriate T category to indicate multiple tumours.

T_{is} = preinvasive carcinoma (carcinoma in situ).

T_x = the minimum requirements to assess fully the extent of the tumour cannot be met.

T_0 = no evidence of primary tumour.

T_1 = on bimanual examination, a freely mobile mass may be felt: this should not be felt after complete transurethral resection of the lesion and/or microscopically the tumour does not extend beyond the lamina propria.

T_2 = on bimanual examination, there is induration of the bladder wall which is mobile. There is no residual induration after complete transurethral resection of the lesion and/or there is microscopic invasion of superficial muscle.

T_3 = on bimanual examination, induration or a nodular mobile mass is palpable in the bladder wall which persists after transurethral resection of the exophytic portion of the lesion and/or there is microscopic invasion of deep muscle or extension through the bladder wall.

T_{3a} = invasion of deep muscle.

T_{3b} = extension through the bladder wall.

T_4 = tumour fixed or invading neighbouring structures and/or there is microscopic evidence of such involvement.

T_{4a} = tumour invading prostate, uterus or vagina.

T_{4b} = tumour fixed to pelvic wall and/or infiltrating the abdominal wall.

The most common symptom of tumour of the bladder is painless haematuria. It may come and go during the early stages of the disease, which gives the patient a false sense of security or causes him or her to be indifferent about seeking treatment. Later, there can be urinary frequency and dysuria.

DIAGNOSTIC PROCEDURES. The most common diagnostic procedure for bladder disorders is CYSTOSCOPY, which allows direct visualization of the interior of the bladder. CYSTOGRAPHY is used to detect filling defects. A contrast medium or air is instilled into the bladder and radiographs are taken. *Cystometrography* is used to assess the motor and sensory function of the bladder when the patient is incontinent or has difficulty voiding or completely emptying the bladder.

TREATMENT. Treatment of bladder cancer depends on the type of tumour, its stage of development when first diagnosed, the patient's general state of health, and other factors. There are several chemotherapeutic agents that are applied locally by instillation and others that are given systemically. These ANTINEOPLASTIC agents have been shown to be of some use, particularly when they are used in combination. Radiotherapy is often used in cases in which the disease is more advanced.

Surgery of the Bladder. Surgical treatment of bladder cancer ranges from electric cauterization of the tumour mass to removal of the entire bladder (cystectomy) and diversion of the urinary flow through a surgically created opening to the skin. In some cases, only a portion of the bladder (*segmental resection*) is done. This is the procedure of choice when a tumour is located in the dome of the bladder or near the points at which the ureters empty into the bladder. *Cystostomy* is surgical incision into the bladder for removal of stones that cannot be passed through the urethra, for drainage, or for access to an enlarged prostate gland.

Patient Care. Following all types of surgery involving the bladder the major concerns are maintenance of the flow of urine and prevention of infection. The urinary system fulfils its primary function, the excretion of wastes, by continuously producing urine. If for any reason there is an obstruction to the flow of urine from the bladder, it will continue to fill, causing extreme discomfort and leading to possible rupture, or backflow of urine into the renal pelvis with resultant hydronephrosis. It is therefore essential that catheters and drainage tubes be monitored frequently and carefully.

The urine must be observed for signs of haemorrhage, the presence of clots or bits of tissue, unusual colour, odour, and concentration during both the preoperative and the postoperative periods. It is extremely important that intake and output be measured accurately. If an irrigation fluid is used either continuously or intermittently, the amount of fluid that is instilled into the bladder must be subtracted from the total amount of fluid collected in the drainage bag to calculate the urine output.

In order to prevent infection extreme care must be used in the handling of catheters, drainage tubes, and collecting devices. If dressings are applied, as in cystostomy, they should be changed frequently to reduce the hazard of infection and to avoid the unpleasant odour that accompanies the leakage of urine from the incision.

atonic b. a condition marked by a dilated, poorly contracting urinary bladder without evidence of a lesion of the central nervous system.

atonic neurogenic b. neurogenic urinary bladder caused by destruction of the sensory nerve fibres from the bladder to the spinal cord (lateral spinal tracts), marked by the absence of awareness of bladder filling and of the desire to void. This leads to overdistention of the bladder, and an abnormal amount of residual urine with a tendency toward overflow incontinence. It is most frequently associated with tabes dorsalis, diabetic neuropathy, and pernicious anaemia. Called also *paralytic bladder* and *sensory paralytic bladder*.

automatic b. neurogenic urinary bladder due to complete resection of the spinal cord above the sacral segments, marked by complete loss of micturition reflexes and bladder sensation, violent involuntary voiding, and an abnormal amount of residual urine. Called also *reflexneurogenic bladder*.

autonomous b. neurogenic urinary bladder due to a lesion in the sacral portion of the spinal cord that interrupts the reflex arc that controls the bladder. The lesion may be in the cauda equina, conus medullaris, sacral roots, or pelvic nerve. It is marked by loss of normal bladder sensation and reflex activity, inability to initiate urination normally, and stress incontinence.

gall b. see GALLBLADDER.

irritable b. a state of the urinary bladder marked by increased frequency of contraction with associated desire to urinate.

motor paralytic b. neurogenic urinary bladder due to impairment of the motor neurons or nerves controlling the bladder. The *acute* form is marked by painful distention and inability to initiate micturition; the *chronic* form is marked by difficulty in initiating micturition, straining, a decrease in the size and force of the stream, interrupted stream, and recurrent infection of the urinary tract.

nervous b. a colloquial term for a functional condition characterized by a constant desire to urinate without the power to do so completely.

neurogenic b. any condition of dysfunction of the urinary bladder caused by a lesion of the central or peripheral nervous system.

paralytic b. atonic neurogenic bladder.

reflex neurogenic b. automatic bladder. **sensory paralytic b.** atonic neurogenic bladder.

b. training a programme designed to assist the patient having difficulties controlling the flow of urine. The training programme and techniques used will depend on the optimal neural and muscular control that can be realistically expected, as in PARAPLEGIA and hemiplegia, and on the mental and emotional status of the patient. The cause of urinary incontinence must be known and the specific symptoms manifested by the patient clearly defined. This would include information about difficulty in initiating voiding, degree of awareness of the need to void, ability to empty the bladder completely and amount of residual urine, signs of distention and dribbling of overflow, night incontinence, stress incontinence, and usual times for voiding.

Spinal cord injuries and lesions produce what is

known as a cord bladder or neurogenic bladder. Patients with disorders of this type are not aware of the need to void and must be trained in techniques to initiate voiding and empty the bladder. If the lesion is above the 2nd, 3rd, and 4th sacral segment of the spinal cord, it is sometimes possible for the bladder to empty partially by reflex, and so training is centred on techniques to improve emptying of the bladder. This is done because pooling of residual urine in the bladder can lead to infection and the formation of bladder stones. If the lesion is located at the site of the 2nd, 3rd, and 4th sacral segment, the bladder is flaccid because of interference with the reflex arc. Bladder training in these cases is concerned with emptying the bladder to prevent distention and the dribbling of overflow.

Some urinary problems can be relieved by a simple scheduling of times to void at regular intervals. Many elderly patients wet the bed at night because they are not fully awake or are not aware of the need to void. Noting the time of bed–wetting and offering the bedpan or urinal about 30 minutes before that time each night can avoid this type of night incontinence. This same technique can be used to control incontinence during the day. It is especially important not to assume that an incontinent patient cannot be helped. With diligence and genuine interest, the problem can often be resolved.

Those patients with neural damage and paralysis require more intensive training for bladder control. An indwelling catheter may be inserted at the onset of incontinence and some patients may never become catheter free. This does not mean, however, that every effort should not be made to teach urinary control so that whenever possible the patient can achieve some degree of independence and avoid the hazards that an indwelling catheter presents.

When bladder training specific techniques planned for the individual patient are initiated. Aids to stimulate voiding may be used for those patients who have difficulty initiating it. The CREDÉ TECHNIQUE for manual expression of urine often is successful in removing urine from a flaccid bladder.

If training is not successful at first, encouragement and perseverance are essential.

uninhibited neurogenic b. neurogenic bladder due to a lesion in the region of the upper motor neurons with subtotal interruption of the corticospinal pathways, marked by urgency, frequent involuntary voiding, and a small-volume threshold of activity. It is associated with stroke, multiple sclerosis, and myelomeningocele.

Blakemore–Sengstaken tube (ˌblaykmor-ˈsengztaykən) Sengstaken–Blakemore tube.

Blalock–Taussig operation (ˌblaylokˈtawsig) anastomosis of the subclavian artery to the pulmonary artery to shunt some of the systemic circulation into the pulmonary circulation; undertaken to overcome congenital pulmonary stenosis.

blanch (blahnch) to become pale.

bland (bland) non-irritating, soothing.

b. fluids mild and non-irritating fluids such as barley water and milk.

blast (blahst) 1. an immature stage in cellular development before appearance of the definitive characteristics of the cell; used also as a suffix, as in ameloblast, etc. 2. the wave of air pressure produced by the detonation of high-explosive bombs or shells or by other explosions; it causes pulmonary damage and haemorrhage (lung blast, blast chest), laceration of other thoracic and abdominal viscera, ruptured eardrums, and effects in the central nervous system.

blastema (blaˈsteemə) 1. the primitive substance from which cells are formed. 2. a group of cells that will give rise to a new individual, in asexual reproduction, or to an organ or part, in either normal development or in regeneration.

blasto- word element. [Gr.] *a bud, budding.*

blastocoele (ˈblastohˌseel) the fluid-filled central segmentation cavity of the mass of the blastula.

blastocyst (ˈblastohˌsist) the mammalian conceptus in the post-morula stage, consisting of the trophoblast and an inner cell mass.

blastocyte (ˈblastohˌsiet) an undifferentiated embryonic cell.

blastocytoma (ˌblastohsieˈtohmə) blastoma.

blastoderm (ˈblastohˌdərm) the single layer of cells forming the wall of the blastula, or the cellular cap above the floor of segmented yolk in the discoblastula of telolecithal ova.

blastodisc (ˈblastohˌdisk) the convex structure formed by the blastomeres at the animal pole of an ovum undergoing incomplete cleavage.

blastogenesis (ˌblastohˈjenəsis) 1. development of an individual from a blastema, i.e., by asexual reproduction. 2. transmission of inherited characters by the germ plasm. 3. morphological transformation of mature small lymphocytes into larger cells resembling blast cells on exposure to stimuli such as phytohaemagglutin and/or antigens to which the donor is immunized.

blastoma (blaˈstohmə) a neoplasm composed of embryonic cells derived from the blastema of an organ or tissue. adj. **blastomatous.**

blastomatosis (ˌblastohməˈtohsis) the formation of blastomas; tumour formation.

blastomere (ˈblastohˌmiə) one of the cells produced by cleavage of a fertilized ovum.

Blastomyces (ˌblastohˈmieseez) a genus of pathogenic fungi growing as mycelial forms at room temperature and as yeastlike forms at body temperature; applied to the yeasts pathogenic for man and animals.

B. brasiliensis *Paracoccidioides brasiliensis.*

B. dermatitidis the species causing North American blastomycosis.

blastomycete (ˌblastohˈmieseet) any organism of the genus *Blastomyces*; also, any yeastlike organism.

blastomycosis (ˌblastohmieˈkohsis) 1. infection with *Blastomyces.* 2. infection with any yeastlike organism.

North American b. a chronic infection caused by *Blastomyces dermatitidis*, marked by suppurating tumours in the skin (cutaneous blastomycosis) or by lesions in the lungs, bones, subcutaneous tissues, liver, spleen, and kidneys (systemic blastomycosis).

South American b. paracoccidioidomycosis.

blastopore (ˈblastohˌpor) the opening of the archenteron to the exterior of the embryo at the gastrula stage.

blastospore (ˈblastohˌspor) a spore formed by budding, as in yeast.

blastula (ˈblastyuhlə) the usually spherical body produced by cleavage of a fertilized ovum, consisting of a single layer of cells (blastoderm) surrounding a fluid-filled cavity (blastocoele); it follows the morula stage.

blastulation (ˌblastyuhˈlayshən) conversion of the morula to the blastula by development of a blastocoele.

bleb (bleb) a large flaccid vesicle, usually at least 1 cm in diameter.

bleeder (ˈbleedə) 1. the popular term for a person who bleeds freely, especially one suffering from a condition in which the blood fails to clot properly; a haemophiliac (see also HAEMOPHILIA). 2. any large blood vessel cut during surgery.

bleeding (ˈbleeding) 1. the escape of blood, as from an injured vessel. See also HAEMORRHAGE. 2. the purposeful withdrawal of blood from a vessel of the body; venesection; phlebotomy.

decidual b. that occurring at 4, 8 or 12 weeks of pregnancy when the normal period could have been anticipated. The decidua vera, lining the uterine cavity, is shed. Decidual bleeding is sometimes mistaken for the last menstrual period.

functional b. bleeding from the uterus when no organic lesions are present (see MENSTRUATION).

implantation b. that occurring at the time of implantation of the fertilized ovum in the decidua.

occult b. escape of blood in such small quantity that it can be detected only by chemical tests or by microscopic or spectroscopic examination.

b. time the time required for a small inflicted wound to cease bleeding. If done properly, the test can be helpful in determining the functional capacity of platelets and of vasoconstriction. The test for bleeding time involves making a small cut with a lancet into a fingertip, earlobe (Duke method), or forearm (Ivy method). The Ivy method is the most accurate: a blood pressure cuff is placed on the arm and a pressure of 40 mmHg is maintained. A lancet or spring-loaded device which makes a standardized cut is used to make a small wound on the inner surface of the forearm and the blood is absorbed gently by filter paper at intervals until bleeding ceases. The normal range depends on the method used. The Ivy lancet time is less than 7 minutes. A prolonged bleeding time is found in patients with vascular abnormalities, with deficiencies in the platelet count and/or platelet function, and in other rare conditions.

vascular b. disorders a group of disorders in which bleeding occurs secondary to a vascular or perivascular connective tissue abnormality. The coagulation factors and platelets are normal. Examples include hereditary haemorrhage, telangiectasia, senile purpura and Henoch–Schönlein purpura.

blenn(o)- word element. [Gr.] *mucus.*

blennadenitis (ˌblenadəˈnietis) inflammation of mucous glands.

blennogenic (ˌblenohˈjenik) producing mucus.

blennoid (ˈblenoyd) resembling mucus.

blennorrhagia (ˌblenəˈrayji·ə) 1. any excessive discharge of mucus; blenorrhoea. 2. gonorrhoea.

blennorrhoea (ˌblenəˈreeə) any free discharge of mucus, especially a gonococcal discharge from the urethra or vagina; gonorrhoea.

inclusion b. inclusion conjunctivitis.

blennostasis (bleˈnostəˌsis) suppression of an abnormal mucous discharge, or correction of an excessive one. adj. **blennostatic.**

blennothorax (ˌblenohˈthor·raks) an accumulation of mucus in the chest.

blennuria (blenˈyooə·ri·ə) mucus in the urine.

bleomycin (ˌbliohˈmiesin) a polypeptide antibiotic mixture having ANTINEOPLASTIC properties, obtained from cultures of *Streptomyces verticellus.* Evidence indicates that bleomycin inhibits cell division, thymidine incorporation into DNA, and DNA synthesis.

blephar(o)- word element. [Gr.] *eyelid, eyelash.*

blepharadenitis (ˌblefəˌradəˈnietis) blepharoadenitis.

blepharal (ˈblefə·rəl) pertaining to the eyelids.

blepharectomy (ˌblefəˈrektəmee) partial or complete excision of an eyelid.

blepharism (ˈblefəˌrizəm) blepharospasm.

blepharitis (ˌblefəˈrietis) inflammation of the eyelids.

angular b. inflammation involving the outer angle of the eyelids.

squamous b. that in which the edge of the eyelid is covered with small white or grey scales.

ulcerative b. that marked by small ulcerated areas along the eyelid margin, multiple, suppurative lesions, and loss of lashes.

blepharoadenitis (ˌblefə·rohˌadəˈnietis) inflammation of the meibomian glands of the eyelids.

blepharoatheroma (ˌblefə·rohˌathəˈrohmə) an encysted tumour or sebaceous cyst of an eyelid.

blepharochalasis (ˌblefə·rohˈkaləsis) hypertrophy and loss of elasticity of the skin of the upper eyelid.

blepharoconjunctivitis (ˌblefə·rohkənˌjungktiˈvietis) inflammation of the eyelids and conjunctiva.

blepharoncus (ˌblefəˈrongkəs) a tumour on the eyelid.

blepharophimosis (ˌblefə·rohfieˈmohsis) abnormal narrowness of the palpebral fissures.

blepharoplasty (ˈblefə·rohˌplastee) plastic surgery of an eyelid.

blepharoplegia (ˌblefə·rohˈpleeji·ə) paralysis of an eyelid.

blepharoptosis (ˌblefə·ropˈtohsis) drooping of an upper eyelid; ptosis.

blepharospasm (ˈblefə·rohˌspazəm) spasm of the orbicularis muscles of the eyelid.

blepharostenosis (ˌblefə·rohstəˈnohsis) blepharophimosis.

blepharosynechia (ˌblefə·rohsiˈneeki·ə) growing together or adhesion of the eyelids.

blepharotomy (ˌblefəˈrotəmee) surgical incision of an eyelid; tarsotomy.

blind (bliend) not having the sense of sight.

b. spot the area marking the site of entrance of the optic nerve on the retina; it is not sensitive to light and therefore produces a round defect in the monocular visual fields.

blind loop syndrome (ˌbliend ˈloop) a condition of stasis in the small intestine which aids bacterial multiplication, leading to diarrhoea and salt deficiencies. The cause may be intestinal obstruction or surgical anastomosis.

blindness (ˈbliendnəs) lack or loss of ability to see; lack of perception of visual stimuli. Legally, blindness is defined as less than 6/60 vision with glasses (vision of 6/60 is the ability to see only at 6 metres what the normal eye can see at 60 metres).

CAUSES. A major cause of blindness is CATARACT, clouding of the lens of the eye. Removal of the clouded lens from the eye restores sight to most cataract patients.

A second major cause is chronic simple GLAUCOMA, an increase in the fluid pressure inside the eyeball. This disease, which can usually be controlled if discovered and treated early enough, often causes no pain and gives no warning. People over 45 are more susceptible to glaucoma than younger persons, and there is a familial tendency toward the disease.

DETACHMENT OF THE RETINA is a condition in which the retina becomes separated from the underlying tissues. It once led to incurable blindness, but now can often be repaired by surgery.

Scarring of the cornea may result from a local infection and can usually be checked by medical treatment. If it becomes so severe as to interfere seriously with vision, the condition may require a corneal graft.

TRACHOMA, a viral infection of the conjunctiva, was once a major cause of blindness in Europe and still is in many of the developing countries. Improvements in hygiene, sulphonamide drugs and antibiotics can halt the disease.

Blindness may occur as an effect of various infectious diseases, including scarlet fever, smallpox, and syphilis. Modern techniques of IMMUNIZATION and the development of antibiotics have brought most of these diseases under control. There is still grave danger to the sight of the child whose mother contracts rubella (German measles) during the early months of pregnancy. See also OPHTHALMIA NEONATORUM and RETROLENTAL FIBROPLASIA.

Some cases of blindness are caused by hereditary factors. Little is known about this aspect of heredity, but an increasing amount of research is being done.

EDUCATION AND TRAINING. Today a blind person is no longer thought of as helpless or dependent on others for everything. New methods of education and recreation have made it possible for more than half the blind children in school to attend schools with sighted children. Many colleges provide special funds to enable blind students to hire readers and tape recorders to help them in their studies. Closed circuit television may also be available.

Those of working age who are legally blind are entitled to special counselling, vocational training, and placement through local authorities and the Royal National Institute for the Blind. Other programmes provide work for blind people who are home-bound, visiting teachers for those who want to learn to read and write Braille, and recreation facilities.

The Royal National Institute for the Blind publishes many excellent pamphlets to help those who deal with the special problems involved in blindness.

PATIENT CARE. The patient who is blind often presents a special challenge to those assigned to his care. They must strive to know the patient well and quickly learn his degree of dependence and his attitude toward his loss of vision. Their handling of the situation will depend on whether the patient has been deprived of his sight recently or has been blind for several years. If he is to adjust to a recent loss of vision, they must delicately balance sympathy with a sincere desire to help him adjust to a new life in which he must learn again the simple activities of daily living. A patient who has been blind for years and has adjusted to his handicap most often wishes to be treated as any other patient.

Feeding the Blind Patient. A blind person should be told what different types of food he has on his tray. Before he is given hot foods or iced liquids he should be warned that they are hot or cold. Liquids are usually easier for the blind patient to handle if they are served in a cup, without a straw. The cup is placed in his hand so that he can drink from it himself. Solid foods are given to the patient in the same manner in which one would eat them oneself, with variety and combining of foods that go well together. The patient should be allowed to feed himself 'finger foods' and liquids.

The Ambulatory Patient. When walking with a blind patient it is best to walk beside him allowing him to hold your arm. Directions are given in advance so that he will know to turn to the left or right or go down steps, as well as how many steps. The prevention of accidents is an important part of the care of the blind patient who is up and about. Aside from the physical effects of bumping into objects or falling over them, the blind person also suffers from a loss of self-confidence and security if he cannot move about safely and independently. Doors should be kept closed or completely open. They must never be left ajar. If it is necessary to move a piece of furniture in the patient's room, he should be told of its new location.

Other rules that should be observed in caring for the blind include: (1) Remember that the person is blind, not deaf. There is no reason to shout at him or address him as if he were a child or mentally handicapped. Speak normally and naturally. (2) Speak to the blind person as you enter his room and do not touch him until after you have spoken to him. Otherwise he may be startled or frightened if he has not heard you enter his room. (3) When you leave the room tell the patient you are going. He will not then resume the conversation later and find that he is talking to someone who is not there. (4) Pity is neither expected nor appreciated by the blind. They want to be treated as normal people, and would rather ask for help than have someone do everything for them. It is important to remember that there are no such things as 'extra senses of blindness', which many people mistakenly believe blind people are given to compensate for their loss of sight. Whatever a blind person has learned about living with his blindness he has accomplished through hard work and determination.

blue b. tritanopia.

blue-yellow b. 1. tritanopia. 2. tetartanopia (2).

colour b. popular term for any deviation from normal perception of colour (see also COLOUR BLINDNESS).

day b. defective vision in bright light.

green b. deuteranopia.

night b. failure or imperfection of vision in conditions of diminished illumination (see also NIGHT BLINDNESS).

red b. protanopia.

snow b. dimness of vision, usually temporary, due to the glare of the sun upon snow.

BLISS baby life support systems.

blister ('blistə) a vesicle, especially a bulla.

blood b. a vesicle having bloody contents, as may be caused by a pinch or bruise.

fever b. a lesion on the skin or mucous membrane, due to infection with the virus of HERPES SIMPLEX, which often accompanies fever, and is most common about the lips or nose. Called also *herpes fibrilis*.

water b. one with clear watery contents.

Blocadren ('blokə,dren) trademark for a preparation of timolol maleate; a beta-blocker used as an antihypertensive.

block (blok) 1. an obstruction or stoppage. 2. regional anaesthesia.

bundle-branch b. a form of HEART BLOCK involving obstruction in one of the bundle branches of the cardiac conduction system.

epidural b. anaesthesia produced by injection of the anaesthetic between the vertebral spines and beneath the ligamentum flavum into the extradural space.

field b. regional anaesthesia obtained by blocking conduction in nerves with chemical or physical agents.

heart b. impairment of conduction in heart excitation; often applied specifically to atrioventricular heart block (see also HEART BLOCK).

mental b. obstruction to thought or memory, particularly that produced by emotional factors.

metabolic b. the blocking of a biosynthetic pathway due to a genetic enzyme defect or to inhibition of an enzyme by a drug or other substance.

nerve b. regional anaesthesia secured by injection of an anaesthetic in close proximity to the appropriate nerve.

paracervical b. anaesthesia of the inferior hypogastric plexus and ganglia produced by injection of the local anaesthetic into the lateral fornices of the vagina.

parasacral b. regional anaesthesia produced by injection of a local anaesthetic around the sacral nerves as they emerge from the sacral foramina.

paravertebral b. infiltration of the cervicothoracic ganglion with an anaesthetic agent.

perineural b. regional anaesthesia produced by injection of the anaesthetic agent close to the nerve.

presacral b. anaesthesia produced by injection of the local anaesthetic into the sacral nerves on the anterior aspect of the sacrum.

pudendal b. anaesthesia produced by blocking the pudendal nerves, accomplished by injection of the local anaesthetic into the tuberosity of the ischium.
sacral b. anaesthesia produced by injection of the local anaesthetic into the extradural space of the spinal canal.
saddle b. the production of anaesthesia in a region corresponding roughly with the areas of the buttocks, perineum, and inner aspects of the thighs, by introducing the anaesthetic agent low in the dural sac.
sinoatrial b. a disturbance in which the atrial response is delayed or omitted because of partial or complete interference with the propagation of impulses from the sinoatrial node to the atria.
sinus b. pain in the paranasal sinuses due to air being trapped in them in decompression sickness.
subarachnoid b. anaesthesia produced by the injection of a local anaesthetic into the subarachnoid space around the spinal cord.
vagal b., vagus nerve b. blocking of vagal impulses by injection of a solution of local anaesthetic into the vagus nerve at its exit from the skull.

blockade (blo'kayd) 1. in pharmacology, the blocking of the effect of a neurotransmitter or hormone by a drug. 2. in histochemistry, a chemical reaction that modifies certain chemical groups and blocks a specific staining method.
adrenergic b. selective inhibition of the response to sympathetic impulses transmitted by adrenaline or noradrenaline at alpha or beta receptor sites of an effector organ or postganglionic adrenergic neuron.
cholinergic b. selective inhibition of cholinergic nerve impulses at autonomic ganglionic synapses, postganglionic parasympathetic effectors, or neuromuscular junctions.

blocker ('blokə) something that blocks or obstructs passage, activity, etc.
α-b., alpha-b. a drug that induces adrenergic blockade at α-adrenergic receptors.
β-b., beta-b. a drug that induces adrenergic blockade at either β_1- or β_2-adrenergic receptors, or both (see also BETA-BLOCKER).
calcium channel b. a drug that selectively inhibits the influx of calcium ions through a specific ion channel of cardiac muscle and smooth muscle cells (see also CALCIUM CHANNEL BLOCKER).
H_2-receptor b. a drug, such as cimetidine or ranitidine, that inhibits the secretion of gastric acid stimulated by histamine, pentagastrin, food and insulin, and also basal secretion; used in the treatment of peptic ulcer.

blocking ('bloking) 1. interruption of an afferent nerve pathway (see BLOCK). 2. inhibition of an intracellular biosynthetic process; metabolic block. 3. difficulty in recollection, or interruption of a train of thought or speech, due to emotional factors, usually unconscious.

blood (blud) the fluid that circulates through the heart, arteries, capillaries, and veins. Blood is the chief means of transport within the body. It transports oxygen from the lungs to the body tissues, and carbon dioxide from the tissues to the lungs. It transports nutritive substances and metabolites to the tissues and removes waste products to the kidneys and other organs of excretion. It has an essential role in the maintenance of fluid balance.

When required, blood cells and antibodies carried in the blood are brought to a site of infection, or blood-clotting substances are carried to a break in a blood vessel. The blood distributes hormones from the endocrine glands to the organs they influence. It helps in the regulation of body temperature by carrying excess heat from the interior of the body to the surface layers of the skin, where the heat is dissipated to the surrounding air.

Blood varies in colour from a bright red in the arteries to a duller red in the veins. The total quantity of blood within an individual depends upon his weight and is of the order of 65 ml per kg body weight. An average (60 kg) person will have a blood volume of about 4 litres.

Blood is composed of two parts: (1) plasma, the fluid portion, and (2) formed elements, the blood cells and platelets suspended in the fluid.

PLASMA. The plasma accounts for about 55 per cent of the total volume of the blood. It consists of about 92 per cent water, 7 per cent proteins, and less than 1 per cent inorganic salts, organic substances other than proteins, dissolved gases, hormones, antibodies, and enzymes. Plasma from which the fibrinogen has been removed is called serum.

Plasma contains many specialized proteins such as serum albumin, the globulins, and fibrinogen. Serum albumin is important to the nutrition of body cells and helps prevent the escape of body water from the intravascular fluid compartment. It probably originates in the liver, as does fibrinogen, which is essential to the normal clotting of blood. The globulins are divided into three major groups. Many of the alpha and beta globulins aid in transporting nutritive elements and other substances in the blood; others are involved in physiological processes such as clotting. Almost all gamma globulins are immunoglobulins, the antibodies that play an important role in IMMUNITY.

Plasma volume is sometimes measured in order to calculate the total BLOOD VOLUME. One method for determining plasma volume is by injection of a dye (azovan blue) into the circulating blood and later calculating the total blood volume.

BLOOD CELLS AND PLATELETS. The suspended particles of the blood comprise the other 45 per cent of the total volume of blood. They include erythrocytes (red blood cells), leukocytes (white blood cells), and platelets (thrombocytes). The red and white blood cells are also known as corpuscles (Latin for 'little bodies').

Erythrocytes (*Red Blood Cells*). The great majority of the cells in the blood are red blood cells. There are about 5×10^6 red blood cells in a speck of blood the size of a pinhead, and about 35×10^{12} in the average adult. Although microscopic in size, these cells have a total surface area almost the size of a football pitch. This vast surface area is important in the blood's task of carrying oxygen from the lungs to the tissues, because the exchange of oxygen in both places takes place across the cell surfaces and must be accomplished quickly as the blood flows by.

The erythrocytes owe their oxygen-carrying ability to HAEMOGLOBIN, a combination of an iron-containing prosthetic group, *haem*, with a protein, *globin*. Haemoglobin has the special ability of attracting and forming a loose connection with free oxygen, and its presence enables blood to absorb some 60 times the amount of oxygen that the plasma by itself absorbs. Oxyhaemoglobin is red, which gives oxygenated blood its red colour. See also COLOUR INDEX.

Red blood cells are stored in the SPLEEN, which acts as a reservoir for the blood system and discharges the cells into the blood as required. The spleen also discharges extra red blood cells into the blood during emergencies such as haemorrhage or shock.

Red blood cells originate in the red bone marrow of the ribs, sternum, skull, pelvic bone, vertebrae, and the ends of the long bones of the limbs. The average red cell has a life of 110 to 120 days. Aged red cells are ingested by macrophages in the spleen and liver. The iron is transported by the plasma protein *transferrin* to the bone marrow, where it is incorporated into new red cells. The haem group is converted to bilirubin, a bile pigment secreted by the liver. About 180 million red blood cells are destroyed every minute. Since the number of cells in the blood remains more or less constant, this means that about 180 million red blood cells are manufactured every minute.

Determination of the red blood cell volume is usually done as a preliminary step in the determination of the total BLOOD VOLUME. A radioactive substance, usually chromium, is used to 'tag' cells of a sample of blood drawn from the patient. The sample is then reintroduced into the circulating blood and subsequent samples are taken to be evaluated for degree of radioactivity. The degree of dilution is used to calculate total blood volume.

Leukocytes (*White Blood Cells*). The leukocytes are the body's primary defence against infections. They have no haemoglobin and thus are colourless and, unlike red blood cells, they can move about under their own power. White blood cells are larger than red blood cells and fewer in number. Normally the blood has about 8×10^9 white blood cells per litre.

Leukocytes originate in the bone marrow and lymph tissue. There are six types of white blood cells. Three are polymorphonuclear cells or 'polymorphs': *neutrophils*, which make up about 63 per cent of all leukocytes; *eosinophils*, which make up about 2.5 per cent; and *basophils*, which make up 0.4 per cent. All have a granular cytoplasm and are often grouped together under the name *granulocytes*. The remaining three kinds of leukocytes are the monocytes, lymphocytes, and plasma cells.

Leukocytes are actively engaged in the destruction or neutralization of invading microorganisms and are quickly transported to sites of infection and inflammation. For this reason, their life span in the blood is usually very short. When infection is present their numbers are greatly increased and they also become more mobile and move back and forth between the blood, lymph, and tissues. The granulocytes and monocytes are phagocytic, i.e., they swallow or ingest the foreign particles with which they come in contact. During the process of phagocytosis the phagocytes themselves are destroyed. The two types of lymphocytes involved in immunity are: *B-cells* (B-lymphocytes), which play a role in humoral immunity, and *T-cells* (T-lymphocytes), which are important in cell-mediated immunity. Activated B-cells that secrete antibodies are called *plasma cells*. Monocytes are also involved in some immune processes.

Platelets. Platelets or *thrombocytes* are small, clear, disc-shaped bodies about one-third the size of red blood cells or even smaller, which initiate blood clotting and are concerned in contraction of a clot. When they encounter a leak in a blood vessel, they adhere to the edges of the injured tissue and create a matrix on which the clot forms. There are about 350 to 500×10^9 platelets per litre of blood.

Platelets are actually fragments of very large cells called *megakaryocytes*, formed in the bone marrow. The bone marrow produces from 30 to 50×10^9 platelets per litre of blood daily, which means that every 10 days all the platelets in the body have been completely replaced.

BIOCHEMICAL TESTS. Chemical analyses of various substances in the blood are invaluable aids in (1) the prevention of disease by alerting the patient and doctor to potentially dangerous levels of blood constituents that could lead to more serious conditions, (2) diagnosis of pathological conditions already present, (3) assessment of the patient's progress when a disturbance in blood chemistry exists, and (4) assessment of the patient's status by establishing a baseline or 'normal' levels for each individual patient.

In recent years, with the increasing attention to preventive medicine and rapid progress in technology and automation, the use of a battery of screening tests performed by automated instruments has become quite common. These instruments are capable of performing simultaneously a variety of blood chemistry tests on as many as 60 patients.

Some of the more common screening tests performed on samples of blood include evaluation of ELECTROLYTES, ALBUMIN, and BILIRUBIN levels, blood urea nitrogen (BUN), CHOLESTEROL, total protein, and such enzymes as lactate dehydrogenase (LDH) and aspartate aminotransferase (AST).

The plasma proteins are separated by ELECTROPHORESIS, according to the speed at which they migrate in an electric field. The speed of migration (electrophoretic mobility) depends on the electric charge, size, and shape of the protein. Routine serum protein electrophoresis separates the plasma proteins into five bands: prealbumin, albumin, and the alpha, beta, and gamma globulins. Studies of this type are valuable in diagnosing and treating many diseases in which the protein constituents of blood have been affected. The technique of electrophoresis also is used in separating and identifying types of human HAEMOGLOBIN.

Blood urea nitrogen (BUN) tests measure the blood's content of urea, one of the nitrogenous waste products of protein metabolism (see also UREA NITROGEN). Measurement of nonprotein NITROGEN (NPN) also may be used as a test of kidney function, after severe injury or extended infection or when the body is overloaded with fluid; a high level of NPN may indicate poisoning, hormonal disorders, or shock.

Analysis of blood gases is useful in the care of patients having difficulty with oxygen and carbon dioxide transport and maintenance of a normal ACID–BASE BALANCE. BLOOD GAS ANALYSIS determines oxygen and carbon dioxide levels and their partial pressure in arterial and venous blood. The pH or hydrogen ion concentration as determined by blood gas analysis is extremely important in evaluating a patient's status in regard to states of ACIDOSIS and ALKALOSIS.

Determinations of glucose as in a GLUCOSE TOLERANCE TEST are helpful in identifying disorders of carbohydrate metabolism.

Iron determinations may be used to identify and differentiate certain anaemias. In cases of iron deficiency, a test of the blood's iron-binding capacity can indicate the extent to which the patient will be helped by increasing his intake of iron, either by diet or by taking iron preparations.

central b. blood from the pulmonary venous system; sometimes applied to splanchnic blood, or blood obtained from chambers of the heart or from bone marrow.

citrated b. blood treated with sodium citrate to prevent its coagulation.

cord b. that contained in the umbilical vessels at the time of delivery of the infant.

defibrinated b. whole blood from which fibrin has been separated during the clotting process.

occult b. that present in such small amounts as to be detectable only by chemical tests or by spectroscopic or microscopic examination.

peripheral b. that obtained from acral areas, or from the circulation remote from the heart; the blood in the systemic circulation.

splanchnic b. that circulating in thoracic, abdominal, and pelvic viscera, further distinguished on the basis of specific organ, e.g., pulmonary, hepatic, splenic.

whole b. that from which none of the elements has been removed, especially that drawn from a selected donor under aseptic conditions; it contains added citrate ion or heparin, and is used as a blood replenisher.

blood bank 1. a place of storage for blood. 2. an organization that collects, processes, stores, and transfuses blood. In most hospitals the blood bank is located in the pathology laboratory.

blood–brain barrier ('bludbrayn) the barrier separating the blood from the brain parenchyma everywhere except in the hypothalamus. Abbreviated BBB. It is permeable to water, oxygen, carbon dioxide, and nonionic solutes, such as glucose, alcohol, and general anaesthetics, and is only slightly permeable to electrolytes and other ionic substances. Some small molecules, e.g., amino acids, are taken up across the barrier by specific transport mechanisms.

blood clotting, coagulation see CLOTTING.

blood count the number of blood cells in a given sample of blood, usually expressed as the number of cells per litre of blood (as red blood cell, white blood cell, or platelet count). A differential white cell count determines the number of various types of leukocytes in a sample of blood. The cell count is useful in the diagnosis of various blood dyscrasias, infections or other abnormal conditions of the body and is one of the most common tests done on the blood. For normal ranges in the blood count see the table of normal values in Appendix 2.

blood gas analysis laboratory studies of arterial and venous blood for the purpose of measuring oxygen and carbon dioxide levels and pressure or tension, and hydrogen ion concentration (pH). (See accompaning table.) Analyses of blood gases provide the following information:

P_ao_2—partial pressure (*P*) of oxygen (o_2) in the arterial blood ($_a$).

Sao_2—percentage of available haemoglobin that is saturated (Sa) with oxygen (o_2).

P_aco_2—partial pressure (*P*) of carbon dioxide (co_2) in the arterial blood ($_a$).

pH—an expression of the extent to which the blood is alkaline or acidic.

HCO_3^-—the level of plasma bicarbonate; an indicator of the metabolic acid–base status.

These parameters are important tools for assessment of a patient's ACID–BASE BALANCE. They reflect the ability of the lungs to exchange oxygen and carbon dioxide, the ability of the kidneys to control the retention or elimination of bicarbonate, and the effectiveness of the heart as a pump. Because the lungs and kidneys act as important regulators of the respiratory and metabolic acid-base balance, assessment of the status of a patient with any disorder of respiration and metabolism includes periodic blood gas measurements.

The partial pressure of a particular gas in a mixture of gases, as of oxygen in air, is the pressure exerted by that gas alone. It is proportional to the relative number of molecules of the gas; for example, the fraction of all the molecules in the air that are oxygen molecules. The partial pressure of a gas in a liquid is the partial pressure of a real or imaginary gas that is in equilibrium with the liquid.

P_ao_2 measures the oxygen content of the arterial blood, most of which is bound to haemoglobin, forming oxyhaemoglobin. The Sao_2 measures the oxygen in oxyhaemoglobin as a percentage of the total haemoglobin oxygen-carrying capacity.

A P_ao_2 of 8 kPa (60 mmHg) represents an Sao_2 of 90 per cent, which is sufficient to meet the needs of the body's cells. However, as the P_ao_2 falls, the Sao_2 decreases rapidly. A P_ao_2 below 7.3 kPa (55 mmHg) indicates a state of hypoxaemia that requires correction. Normal P_ao_2 values at sea level are 10.7 kPa (80 mmHg) for elderly adults and 13.3 kPa (100 mmHg) for young adults. However, some patients with CHRONIC OBSTRUCTIVE AIRWAYS DISEASE can tolerate a P_ao_2 as low as 9.3 kPa (70 mmHg) without becoming hypoxic. In caring for patients with this condition, it is important to know that attempts to elevate the P_ao_2 level to the normal level can be dangerous and even fatal. It is best to establish a baseline for each individual patient before supplementary oxygen is given, and then to assess his condition and the effectiveness of his therapy according to this baseline.

P_aco_2 gives information about the cellular production of carbon dioxide through metabolic processes, and the removal of it from the body via the lungs. The normal range is 4.3 to 6 kPa (32 to 45 mmHg). Values outside this range indicate a primary respiratory problem associated with pulmonary function, or a metabolic problem for which there is respiratory compensation. Blood pH gives information about the patient's metabolic state. A pH of 7.4 is considered normal: a value lower than 7.4 indicates acidaemia and one higher than 7.4 alkalaemia.

Because the amount of CO_2 in the blood affects its pH, abnormal P_aco_2 values are interpreted in relation to the pH. If the P_aco_2 value is elevated, and the pH is below normal, *respiratory acidosis* from either acute or chronic hypoventilation is suspected. Conversely, a P_aco_2 below normal and a pH above normal indicates *respiratory alkalosis*. When both the P_aco_2 and the pH are elevated, there is respiratory retention of CO_2 to compensate for *metabolic acidosis*. If both values are below normal, there is respiratory elimination of CO_2 (HYPERVENTILATION) to compensate for metabolic acidosis.

Abnormal levels of bicarbonate (HCO_3^-) in the plasma are also interpreted in relation to the pH in the diagnosis of disturbances in the *metabolic* component of the acid-base balance. The normal range for HCO_3^- is 22 to 26 mmol (22 to 26 mEq) per litre. Abnormally low levels of both HCO_3^- and pH indicate acidosis of metabolic origin. Conversely, elevations of both of these values indicate metabolic alkalosis. The kidneys maintain bicarbonate levels by filtering bicarbonate and returning it to the blood; they also produce new bicarbonate to replace that which is used in buffering. Therefore, a decreased HCO_3^- and an increased pH level indicate either retention of hydrogen ions by the kidneys or the elimination of HCO_3^- in an effort to compensate for respiratory alkalosis. Conversely, if the HCO_3^- level is increased and the pH is decreased, the kidneys have compensated for respiratory acidosis by retaining HCO_3^- or by eliminating hydrogen ions.

COLLECTION OF BLOOD SAMPLES FOR GAS ANALYSES. The manner in which specimens of blood for blood gas analysis are obtained is important to the accuracy of the test results. Arterial blood samples may be taken from an indwelling arterial catheter or by a femoral puncture performed by a doctor. Because peripheral venous blood does not usually present a true pH, electrolyte, or gaseous picture, it is recommended that a sample of venous blood collected for analysis of these factors be drawn from a CENTRAL VENOUS CATHETER or from a catheter in the pulmonary artery.

During the process of drawing blood for gas analyses

Clinical method of blood gas interpretation

Status	pH	P_{CO_2}	HCO_3^-	Base excess
Ventilatory failure (respiratory acidosis)				
Acute	↓ 7.30	↑ 50	Normal	Normal
Chronic	7.30–7.50	↑ 50	↑ 27	↑ +2
Alveolar hyperventilation (respiratory alkalosis)				
Acute	↑ 7.50	↓ 30	Normal	Normal
Chronic	7.40–7.50	↓ 30	↓ 22	↓ −2
Metabolic acidosis				
Uncompensated	↓ 7.30	Normal	↓ 22	↓ −2
Partially compensated	↓ 7.30	↓ 30	↓ 22	↓ −2
Compensated	7.30–7.40	↓ 30	↓ 22	↓ −2
Metabolic alkalosis				
Uncompensated	↑ 7.50	Normal	↑ 27	↑ +2
Partially compensated*	↑ 7.50	↑ 50	↑ 27	↑ +2
Compensated	7.40–7.50	↑ 50	↑ 27	↑ +2

* In general, partially compensated or compensated metabolic alkalosis is rarely seen clinically because of the body's mechanism to prevent hypoventilation.

From Kacmarek, R. M., Dimas, S. and Mack, C. W. (1979) *The Essentials of Respiratory Therapy*, Year Book Medical Publishers, Inc., Chicago.

care is taken to avoid getting any air bubbles into the sample. The amount drawn may vary from 0.5 to 2.5 ml, depending on the type of analyser used in the laboratory. The sample usually is collected in a heparinized vacuum tube or plastic syringe. Heparin is used because unclotted blood is needed for the analyses; care is exercised in the strength and amount of heparin used because heparin in excessive amounts will cause falsely low blood pH values.

It is extremely important that the container for the blood sample be labelled correctly. Values and norms for venous and arterial blood differ. Therefore, the container should indicate the source of the blood sample and this information also should be written on the report of the results.

blood group the phenotype of erythrocytes defined by one or more cellular antigenic structural groupings under the control of allelic genes. In clinical practice there are four main blood types: A, B, O, and AB. In addition to this major grouping there is a rhesus (Rh) system that is important in the prevention of HAEMOLYTIC DISEASE OF THE NEWBORN resulting from incompatibility of blood groups in mother and fetus.

The ABO blood group system was first introduced in 1900 by Karl Landsteiner; in 1920 group AB was discovered by van Descatello and Sturli. Identification of these four major blood groups represented a major step toward resolving the problem of blood transfusion reactions resulting from donor-recipient incompatibility. In 1938 Landsteiner and Weiner discovered another blood factor related to maternal-fetal incompatibility. The factor was named rhesus because the researchers were using rhesus monkeys in their studies. Further research has uncovered additional factors in the Rh group.

Although more than 90 factors have been identified, many of these are not highly antigenic and are not, therefore, a cause for concern in the typing of blood for clinical purposes.

The term *factor*, in reference to blood groups, is synonymous with antigen, and the reaction occurring between incompatible blood types is an antigen-antibody reaction. In cases of incompatibility, the antigen, located on the red blood cells, is an agglutinogen and the specific antibody, located in the serum, is an agglutinin. These are so named because whenever red blood cells with a certain factor come in contact with the agglutinin specific for it, there is agglutination or clumping of the erythrocytes.

In determining blood group, a sample of blood is taken and mixed with specially prepared sera. One serum, anti-A agglutinin, causes blood of group A to agglutinate; another serum, anti-B agglutinin, causes blood of group B to agglutinate. Thus, if anti-A serum alone causes clumping, the blood is group A; if anti-B serum alone causes clumping, it is group B. If both cause clumping, the blood group is AB, and if it is not clumped by either, it is identified as group O..

blood plasma see BLOOD.

blood poisoning the term used by laypersons to refer to the presence of infective agents (bacteria) or their toxins in the blood stream, i.e., septic shock or SEPTICAEMIA. The condition is characterized by elevated body temperature, chills, and weakness. Small abscesses may form on the surface of the body and red and blue streaks become apparent along the pathway of surface blood vessels leading to and from the site of the primary infection. A blood culture confirms the diagnosis and helps identify the most effective anti-infective drug for therapy.

Blood poisoning is a serious disease that must be treated promptly. Otherwise, the process of infection leads to circulatory collapse, profound shock, and death.

blood pressure the pressure of the blood against the walls of the blood vessels. The term usually refers to the pressure of the blood within the arteries, or arterial blood pressure. This pressure is determined by several interrelated factors, including the pumping action of the heart, the resistance to the flow of blood in the arterioles, the elasticity of the walls of the main arteries, the blood volume and extracellular fluid volume, and the blood's viscosity, or thickness.

The pumping action of the heart includes how hard the heart pumps the blood (force of heartbeat), how much blood it pumps (the cardiac output), and how efficiently it does the job. Contraction of the heart, which forces blood through the arteries, is the phase known as systole. Relaxation of the heart between contractions is called diastole.

Human blood group systems and erythrocytic antigenic determinants

Blood group system	Antigenic determinants
ABO	A, A_1, B
H	H
I	I, i, I^T, I^D, I^F
MN	M, N, S, s, U, Cl^a, Far, He, Hill, Hu, M^A, M^C, M^e, M^g, M_1, Mi^a, Mt^a, Mur, M^V, Ny^a, Ri^a, S^B, Sj , St^a, Sul, Tm, U^B, Vr, Vw, N^A, Z
P	P1, P2, (Tj^a), P3 (P^K)
Rh	Rh1 (D, Rh_0), Rh2 (C, rh′), Rh3 (E, rh″), Rh4 (c, hr′), Rh5 (e, hr″), Rh6 (f, ce, hr), Rh7 (Ce, rh), Rh8 (C^W, rh″), Rh9 (C^x, rh^x), Rh10 (V, ce^s, hr^v), Rh11 (E^w, rh^{w2}), Rh12 (G, rh^G), Rh13 (Rh^A), Rh14 (Rh^B), Rh15 (Rh^C), Rh16 (Rh^D), Rh17 (Hr_0), Rh18 (Hr), Rh19 (hr^s), Rh20 (VS, e^s), Rh21 (C^G), Rh22 (CE), Rh23 (D^W), Rh24 (E^T), Rh26, Rh27 (cE), Rh28 (hr^H), Rh29 (RH), Rh30 (Go^a), Rh31 (hr^B), Rh32, Rh33
Lutheran	Lu^a (Lu1), Lu^b (Lu2), Lu^{ab} (Lu3), Lu4, Lu5, Lu6, Lu7, Lu8, Lu9, Lu10, Lu11, Lu12, Lu13, Lu14 (Sw^a)
Kell	K1 (K), K2 (k), K3 (Kp^a), K4 (Kp^b), K5 (Ku), K6 (Js^a), K7 (Js^b), K8 (kw), K9 (KL), K10 ($U1^a$), K11, K12, K13, K14, K15, K16
Lewis	Le^a (Le1), Le^b (Le2), Le^x (Le^{ab}, Le3), Mag (Le4), Le^c (Le5), Le^d
Duffy	Fy^a (Fy1), Fy^b (Fy2), Fy^{ab} (Fy3), Fy4
Kidd	Jk^a (Jk1), Jk^b (Jk2), Jk^{ab} (Jk3)
Cartwright	Yt^a, Yt^b
Xg	Xg^a
Dombrock	Do^a, Do^b
Auberger	Au^a
Cost-Sterling	Cs^a, Yk^a
Wright	Wr^a, Wr^b
Diego	Di^a, Di^b
Vel	Vel 1, Vel 2
Sciana	Sm, Bu^a
Bg	Bg^a, Bg^b, Bg^c, Ho, Ho-like, Ot, Sto, DBG (similar to HL-A7 of lymphocytes)
Gerbich	Ge1, Ge2, Ge3 (anti-Ge1 = M.Y.; anti-Ge1,2 = Ge; anti-Ge1,2,3 = Yus)
Coltan	Co^a, Co^b
Stolzfus	Sf^a

Low-incidence antigenic determinants not thus far associated with a blood group system:

Be^a, Bec, Bi, Big Charles, Bp^a, Bx^a, By, Cad, Chr^a, Coates, Craig, Dahl, Donaviesky, Driver, Duch, Evans, Evelyn, Fin, Fuerhart, Gf^a, Gilbraith, Good, Green, Hands, Heibel, Hil, Ht^a, Je^a, Jn^a, Job, Kam, Ken, Kosis, Lev, Lw^a, McCall, Man, Mar, Mo^a, Nij, Orr, Pt^a, Rd^a, Reid, Rm, Skjelbred, Th^a, To^a, Tr^a, Ven, Wb, Weeks, Wu, Yh^a, Za, 754

High-incidence antigenic determinants not thus far associated with a blood group system:

An^a, At^a, Bou, Bra, Car, Chido (Gursha), Cip, Dp, El, En^a, Fuj, Gn^a, Go^b, Gy^a, Hen, Hy, Jo^a, Jr, Kelly, Knops, Lan, MZ443, Ola, Pea, Savior, Sch, Sd^a, Simon, Ters, Todd, Vennera, Wil, Winbourne

Antigenic determinants that depend on gene interactions:

ABO/I	IH, IA, IB, iH
P/I	IP1, IP2(ITj^a), I^TP1, iP1
Lewis/I	ILe^{bh}
Lewis/ABO	A_1Le^b
P/ABO	Luke
Xor/Duffy	Fy5
Rh/LW	Rh25 (LWO)

Systematized according to observed and assumed independent assortment of their responsible genes. Within many systems, alleles are responsible for differing combinations of antigenic determinants. Symbols within parentheses are those of alternative nomenclatures. (Compiled by Dr. Fred H. Allen, Jr.)

The main arteries leading from the heart have walls with strong elastic fibres capable of expanding and absorbing the pulsations generated by the heart. At each pulsation the arteries expand and absorb the momentary increase in blood pressure. As the heart relaxes in preparation for another beat, the aortic valves close to prevent blood from flowing back to the heart chambers, and the artery walls spring back, forcing the blood through the body between contractions. In this way the arteries act as dampers on the pulsations and thus provide a steady flow of blood through the blood vessels.

Because of this, there are actually two blood pressures within the blood vessels during one complete beat of the heart; a higher blood pressure during *systole* (contraction phase) and a lower blood pressure during *diastole* (relaxation phase). These two blood pressures are known as the systolic pressure and the diastolic pressure, respectively.

It is generally agreed that a reading of 120 mmHg systolic and 80 mmHg diastolic are the norms for a blood pressure reading; that is, these represent the *average* blood pressure obtained from a large sample of healthy adults. In general, a blood pressure of 95 mmHg systolic and 60 mmHg diastolic indicates HYPOTENSION. However, a reading equal to or below this level must be interpreted in the light of each patient's 'normal' reading as determined by baseline data.

Normal upper limits for blood pressure have been the subject of much debate and controversy, especially in determining degrees of HYPERTENSION. On the basis of validated research on the long-term effects of an elevated blood pressure, it is generally agreed that some degree of risk for major cardiovascular disease exists when the systolic pressure is greater than or equal to 140 mmHg, and the diastolic pressure is greater than or equal to 90 mmHg. Life expectancy is reduced at all ages and in both males and females when the diastolic pressure is above 90 mmHg.

MEASUREMENT OF THE BLOOD PRESSURE. The blood pressure is usually measured in the artery of the upper arm, with a sphygmomanometer. This consists of a rubber cuff connected to a glass tube containing a column of mercury. Alongside the glass tube are numbers that indicate the height of the column of mercury in millimetres. In some sphygmomanometers the mercury column is replaced by a gauge. The rubber cuff is wrapped about the patient's arm, and then air is pumped into the cuff by means of a rubber bulb. As the pressure inside the rubber cuff increases, the flow of blood through the artery is momentarily checked. The pressure within the cuff causes the mercury to rise or the gauge's needle to move.

A stethoscope is then placed over the artery at the elbow and the air pressure within the cuff is slowly released. The pressure begins to fall slowly. As soon as blood begins to flow through the artery again, KOROTKOFF'S SOUNDS are heard. The first sounds heard are tapping sounds that gradually increase in intensity. The initial tapping sound that is heard for at least two consecutive beats is recorded as the *systolic* blood pressure.

The first phase of the sounds may be followed by a momentary disappearance of sounds that can last from 30 to 40 mmHg as the mercury column or gauge needle descends. It is important that this auscultatory gap *not* be missed; otherwise, either an erroneously low systolic pressure or high diastolic pressure will be obtained.

During the second phase following the temporary absence of sound there are murmuring or swishing sounds. As deflation of the cuff continues, the sounds become sharper and louder. These sounds represent phase three. During phase four the sounds become muffled rather abruptly and then are followed by silence, which represents phase five.

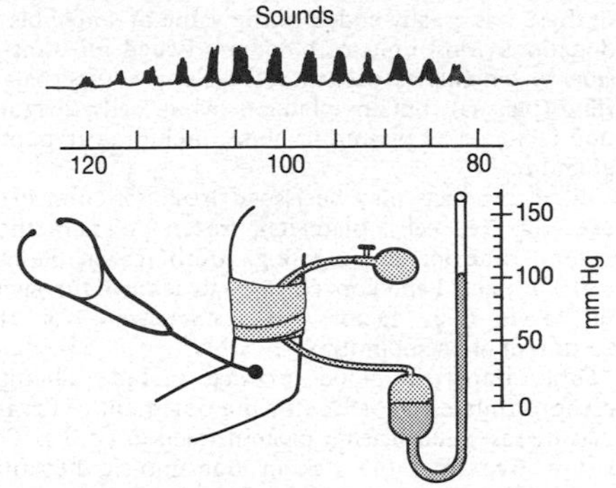

Blood pressure measurement

Although there is some disagreement as to which of the latter phases should represent the diastolic pressure, it is usually recommended that phase five, the point at which sounds disappear, be used as the diastolic pressure for adults, and phase four be used for children. The reason for this is that children, having a high cardiac output, often will continue to produce sounds when the gauge is at a very low reading or even at zero. In some adult patients whose arterioles have lost their elasticity, the fifth phase is also extremely low or nonexistent. In these cases, it is recommended that three readings be recorded: phase one and phases four and five. For example, the blood pressure would be written as 140/96/0. On most occasions, however, the blood pressure is written as a fraction. The systolic pressure is written as the top number, a line is drawn, and the diastolic pressure is written as the bottom number.

The blood pressure can vary considerably between the sexes, among different age groups, and even between two persons of the same age and sex. At birth, the systolic blood pressure is about 80 mmHg. In young people it usually varies from 100 to 140 mmHg, and in people over 60 it may range up to 170 mmHg.

Blood pressure also varies according to the time of day and the kind of activity a person is engaged in. It is usually lowest just before awakening in the morning. Strenuous physical activity can increase the systolic blood pressure 60 to 80 mmHg above normal. Excitement, nervous tension or fright also raises the systolic blood pressure. Increased weight tends to lead to increased blood pressure. See also HYPERTENSION and HYPOTENSION.

Errors in blood pressure measurement can result from failure of the cuff to reach and compress the artery. The cuff diameter should be 20 per cent greater than the diameter of the limb, the bladder of the cuff must be centred over the artery, and the cuff must be wrapped smoothly and snugly to assure proper inflation. When a mercury gauge is used the meniscus should be at eye level to avoid a false reading.

Critically ill patients who require continuous monitoring of the blood pressure may have a catheter inserted into an artery and attached to a catheter-monitor-transducer system. The blood pressure is displayed on an oscilloscope at the bedside so that the patient's pressure can be determined at a glance. This intra-arterial technique of blood pressure monitoring provides accurate, objective, and continuous data on the patient's status.

blood products a group of products derived from blood. The increased manufacture of a large number of these has greatly added to the value of whole blood donations. Most units of blood are issued for transfusion to patients as packed red cells; the supernatant fluid (plasma) contains platelets, white cells, coagulation factors, and plasma proteins, including immunoglobulin.

Blood products may be issued fresh for immediate use (e.g., red cells, platelets), frozen down in their natural state for late use (e.g., fresh frozen plasma, FFP) or pooled and concentrated to achieve therapeutic levels (e.g., factor VIII concentrate for the treatment of haemophilia).

Other important blood products include albumin, cryoprecipitate, factor IX (for the treatment of Christmas disease) and plasma protein fraction (PPF). The last is free from the risk of transmitting hepatitis, unlike FFP.

Blood products are submitted to rigorous quality control and infection screening and where possible are treated to prevent the transmission of infections such as the human immunodeficiency virus (HIV), the agent responsible for AIDS.

blood serum see BLOOD.

blood transfusion see TRANSFUSION.

blood type 1. blood group. 2. the phenotype of an individual with respect to a blood group system.

blood vessel any of the vessels conveying the blood; an artery, arteriole, vein, venule or capillary.

blood volume the total quantity of blood in the body. The regulation of blood volume in the circulatory system is affected by the intrinsic mechanism for fluid exchange at the capillary membranes and by hormonal influences and nervous reflexes that affect the excretion of fluids by the kidneys. A rapid decrease in the blood volume, as in haemorrhage, greatly reduces the cardiac output and creates a condition called SHOCK or circulatory shock. Conversely, an increase in blood volume, as when there is retention of water and salt in the body because of renal failure, results in an increase in cardiac output. The eventual outcome of this situation is increased arterial blood pressure.

The blood volume in the pulmonary circulation is approximately 12 per cent of the total blood volume. Conditions such as left-sided heart failure and mitral stenosis can greatly increase the pulmonary blood volume while decreasing the systemic volume. As would be expected, right-sided heart failure has the opposite effect. The latter condition has less serious effects because the volume of the systemic circulation is about seven times that of the pulmonary circulation and it is therefore better able to accommodate a change in fluid volume.

Clinical assessment of blood volume can be accomplished in a number of ways, for example, by measuring the patient's blood pressure while he is lying down, sitting, and standing. The quality and volume of peripheral pulses will give information about blood volume, as does determining the ease and speed with which a compressed vein will refill after pressure is released. Neck veins that are engorged indicate hypervolaemia; the collapse of these veins indicates hypovolaemia. A more accurate assessment can be done through the use of intravascular catheters such as the CENTRAL VENOUS PRESSURE catheter, which measures pressure in the right atrium, and the SWAN–GANZ CATHETER, which measures pressure on both sides of the heart.

Measurement of blood volume is accomplished by using substances that combine with red blood cells, for example, iron, chromium, and phosphate, or substances that combine with plasma proteins. In either case the measurement of the blood volume is based on the 'dilution' principle. That is, the volume of any fluid compartment can be measured if a given amount of a substance is dispersed evenly in the fluid within the compartment, and then the extent of dilution of the substance is measured.

For example, a small amount of radioactive chromium (^{51}Cr), which is widely used to determine blood volume, is mixed with a sample of blood drawn from the patient. After about 30 minutes the ^{51}Cr will have entered the red blood cells. The sample with the tagged red blood cells is then returned by injection into the patient's blood stream. About 10 minutes later a sample is removed from the patient's circulating blood and the level of radioactivity of the sample is measured. The total blood volume is calculated according to the following formula:

$$\text{volume in ml} = \frac{\text{quantity of test substance instilled}}{\text{concentration per ml of dispersed fluid}}$$

When *plasma volume* is used to arrive at the total blood volume, a dye (usually azovan blue) is injected into the circulating blood. The dye immediately combines with the blood proteins and within 10 minutes is dispersed throughout the circulatory system. A sample of blood is then drawn and the exact quantity of dye is measured. Using the information about plasma volume obtained by applying the above formula, the total blood volume can be calculated, provided the haematocrit is also known. The formula for this calculation is:

$$\begin{matrix}\text{Blood}\\ \text{volume}\end{matrix} = \begin{matrix}\text{plasma}\\ \text{volume}\end{matrix} \times \frac{100}{100 - 0.87\ \text{haematocrit}}$$

bloodstream ('blud,streem) the blood flowing through the CIRCULATORY SYSTEM in the living body.

Blount's disease (blunts) lateral bowing of the legs owing to impaired growth of the upper part of the medial tibial condyle.

blowpipe ('bloh,piep) a tube through which a current of air is forced upon a flame to concentrate and intensify the heat.

BLROA British Laryngological, Rhinological and Otological Association.

blue baby (bloo) an infant born with cyanosis, with a bluish colour that is due to an abnormally low concentration of oxygen in the circulating blood. The term is commonly used to designate an infant born with congenital atelectasis or with one or more defects of the heart and great vessels (see also CONGENITAL HEART DEFECT).

blue dome cyst (bloo dohm) a benign retention cyst of the breast that shows a brown to blue colour (see also CYSTIC DISEASE OF BREAST).

Blumberg's sign ('blumbərgz) pain on abrupt release of steady pressure (rebound tenderness) over the site of a suspected abdominal lesion, indicative of peritonitis.

blush (blush) sudden, brief erythema of the face and neck, resulting from vascular dilation due to emotion or heat.

BM Bachelor of Medicine.

BMA British Medical Association.

BMR basal metabolic rate.

BMUS British Medical Ultrasound Society.

BNA Basle Nomina Anatomica, a system of anatomical

nomenclature adopted at the annual meeting of the German Anatomic Society in 1895; superseded by NOMINA ANATOMICA.

BNF British National Formulary.

Bobath technique ('bohbahth, -bath) an approach to the treatment of neurological conditions developed by Dr. and Mrs Bobath. It aims to facilitate movement by inhibiting abnormal tone, abnormal patterns of movement and abnormal balance reactions. It is used mainly in the treatment of hemiplegia to facilitate active movement on the affected side of the body.

body ('bodee) 1. the trunk, or animal frame, with its organs. 2. the largest and most important part of any organ. 3. any mass or collection of material.

acetone b's ketone bodies.

acidophil b's individual cells that have undergone necrosis, become shrunken and show an increased affinity for acidophil dyes such as eosin. Also referred to as *apoptosis*.

alkapton b's a class of substances with an affinity for alkali, found in the urine and resulting from the condition known as alkaptonuria. The compound commonly found, and most commonly referred to by the term, is homogentisic acid.

amygdaloid b. a small mass of subcortical grey matter within the tip of the temporal lobe, anterior to the inferior horn of the lateral ventricle of the brain.

aortic b's small neurovascular structures on either side of the aorta in the region of the aortic arch, containing chemoreceptors that play a role in reflex regulation of respiration.

asbestos b's golden yellow bodies of various shapes in sputum, and lung secretions of patients with asbestosis (see also ASBESTOS BODIES).

Aschoff's b's submiliary collections of mononuclear cells around a microscopic focus of degenerate collagen in the interstitial tissues of the heart in rheumatic myocarditis; called also *Aschoff's nodules*.

asteroid b. an irregularly star-shaped inclusion body found in the multinucleate giant cells in sarcoidosis and other diseases.

Barr b. sex chromatin; the persistent mass of the material of the inactivated X-chromosome in cells of normal females.

basal b. a modified centriole that occurs at the base of a flagellum or cilium.

carotid b's small neurovascular structures lying in the bifurcation of the right and left carotid arteries, containing chemoreceptors that monitor the oxygen content of the blood and help to regulate respiration.

ciliary b. the thickened part of the vascular tunic of the eye, connecting the choroid and iris (see also CILIARY BODY).

Dohle b's small blue inclusions, occasionally seen in the cytoplasm of neutrophils and eosinophils, which may be a congenital or acquired abnormality. When congenital, they are a feature of the May-Hegglin anomaly. Acquired causes include various infections, burns and normal pregnancy.

Donovan b's encapsulated bacteria (*Calymmatobacterium granulomatis*) found in lesions of granuloma inguinale.

fimbriate b. corpus fimbriatum.

foreign b. a mass of material that is not normal to the place where it is found.

geniculate b's, lateral two metathalamus eminences, one on each side, just lateral to the medial geniculate bodies, marking the termination of the optic tract.

geniculate b's, medial two metathalamus eminences, one on each side, just lateral to the superior colliculi, concerned with hearing.

Heinz b's small inclusions of denatured haemoglobin in the cytoplasm of red cells, best seen in a wet-stained film. They indicate red cell instability, are often drug induced and may be found in a number of congenital haemolytic anaemias.

Howell's b's, Howell–Jolly b's smooth, round remnants of nuclear chromatin seen in erythrocytes in megaloblastic and haemolytic anaemia, in various leukemias and after splenectomy.

inclusion b's round, oval, or irregular-shaped bodies in the cytoplasm and nuclei of cells, as in disease caused by viral infection, such as rabies, smallpox, herpes, etc.

ketone b's acetone, acetoacetic acid, and β-hydroxybutyric acid; except for acetone (which may arise spontaneously from acetoacetic acid), they are normal products of lipid metabolism within the liver, and are oxidized by muscles (see also KETONE BODIES).

Lafora's b's intracytoplasmic inclusions consisting of a complex of glycoprotein and acid mucopolysaccharide; widespread deposits are found in myoclonus epilepsy.

Leishman–Donovan b's round or oval bodies found in the reticuloendothelial cells, especially those of the spleen and liver, in kala-azar; they are nonflagellate intracellular forms of *Leishmania donovani.* Also used to designate similar forms of *L. tropica* found in macrophages in lesions of cutaneous leishmaniasis.

mamillary b. either of the pair of small spherical masses in the interpeduncular fossa of the midbrain, forming part of the hypothalamus.

Masson b's cellular tissue that fills the pulmonary alveoli and alveolar ducts in rheumatic pneumonia.

molluscum b's peculiar round or oval, encapsulated bodies found in the lesions of molluscum contagiosum, a focal viral infection of skin.

multilamellar b. any of the osmiophilic, lipid-rich, layered bodies found in the great alveolar cells of the lung.

Negri b's oval or round inclusion bodies in the nerve cells of animals dead of rabies and composed of masses of rabies virions.

Nissl b's large granular bodies that stain with basic dyes, forming the reticular substance of the cytoplasm of neurons, composed of rough endoplasmic reticulum and free polyribosomes.

olivary b. a rounded elevation, lateral to the upper part of each pyramid of the medulla oblongata. Called also *olive*.

para-aortic b's enclaves of chromaffin cells near the sympathetic ganglia along the abdominal aorta, which secrete catecholamines during prenatal and early postnatal life, aiding the adrenal medulla. Tumours of these structures produce symptoms similar to those of PHAEOCHROMOCYTOMA Called also *organs of Zuckerkandl*.

pineal b. a small, conical structure attached by a stalk to the posterior wall of the third ventricle of the cerebrum. It secretes the hormone melatonin. See also PINEAL BODY.

pituitary b. pituitary gland.

polar b's 1. the small cells consisting of a tiny bit of cytoplasm and a nucleus that result from unequal division of the primary oocyte (*first polar body*) and, if fertilization occurs, of the secondary oocyte (*second polar body*). 2. metachromatic granules located at the ends of bacteria.

psammoma b's microscopic, discrete, rounded, laminated masses of calcareous material, occurring in both benign and malignant epithelial tumours, usually of a papillary character.

quadrigeminal b's corpora quadrigemina.

striate b. corpus striatum.

trachoma b's inclusion bodies found in clusters in the

cytoplasm of the epithelial cells of the conjunctiva in trachoma.

vitreous b. the transparent gel filling the inner portion of the eyeball between the lens and retina. Called also vitreous and vitreous humour.

wolffian b. mesonephros.

body image the total concept, including conscious and unconscious feelings, thoughts, and perceptions, that a person has of his or her own body as an object in space, which is independent and apart from other objects. The body image develops during infancy and childhood from exploration of the body surface and orifices, from development of physical abilities, and from play and comparison of the self with others. Changes in body image are particularly important in adolescence when attention is focused on appearance and attractiveness and relations with others. Body image is strongly influenced by parental attitudes, which give the child a perception of certain body parts as good, clean, and attractive, or bad, dirty, and repulsive. The evolution of body image continues throughout life and incorporates such factors as a person's style of dress, hair style, and use of makeup, which symbolize social and professional status and other feelings about the self.

ALTERATIONS IN BODY IMAGE. Many clinical syndromes involve disturbances of body image. Surgery or trauma involving disfigurement or loss of a body part can be very threatening to a patient. Diseases involving a loss of body function, such as stroke, paraplegia, quadriplegia, coronary heart disease, and bowel or bladder incontinence, and diseases involving disfiguring skin lesions or the feeling of 'rotting away' as in cancer or gangrene, can all cause changes in body image. Rape or violent physical assault can disturb the feeling of being secure in one's own body. Changes in body image involving sexual attractiveness or sexual identity, such as surgery or trauma involving the genitals or breasts and tubal ligation, hysterectomy, or vasectomy, can be especially difficult for the patient to deal with. Intrusive therapeutic or diagnostic procedures, such as insertion of a nasogastric tube, bladder catheterization, administration of intravenous fluids, endoscopy, and cardiac catheterization, can also threaten a patient's body image.

The reaction of a patient to an alteration in body image can include mourning the loss of the former body image, fear of rejection by significant others, hostility, and experiencing of 'phantom' sensations from missing body parts. Patients with less ability to cope with their loss may respond with denial or depression. This can lead to a rejection of the altered body image and feelings of depersonalization that can involve avoidance of interpersonal contact and an unwillingness to discuss the deformity or to accept corrective medical treatment or vocational rehabilitation.

PATIENT CARE. The patient who has undergone a traumatic change in body image may need help in acknowledging the loss and reconstructing his body image. It is important that the patient and his significant others be given an opportunity to prepare for the changes that will occur in an elective surgical procedure. Significant others should also be helped to adjust to changes in a patient's body due to trauma or emergency surgery and be allowed to express their feelings before they visit the patient. Passive or active movement of the affected body part provides kinaesthetic feedback that helps the patient rebuild his body image. It is also important to encourage the patient's attention to personal appearance and to involve the patient in his care.

body language the expression of thoughts or emotions by means of posture or gestures.

Boeck's sarcoid (beks) sarcoidosis.

Bohr effect (bor) displacement of the oxyhaemoglobin dissociation curve by a change in carbon dioxide tension.

boil (boyl) a painful nodule formed in the skin by circumscribed inflammation of the corium and subcutaneous tissue, enclosing a central slough or 'core'. Called also *furuncle.* Boils occur most frequently on the neck and buttocks, although they may develop wherever friction or irritation, or a scratch or break in the skin, allows the bacteria resident on the surface to penetrate the outer layer of the skin. A CARBUNCLE is a group of interconnected boils and is more serious than a simple boil.

CAUSE. When bacteria gain entrance into the skin, the infection settles in the hair follicles or the sebaceous glands. To combat the infection, large numbers of leukocytes travel to the site and attack the invading bacteria. Some bacteria and white cells are killed and they and their liquefied products form pus. The body's defences may succeed in overcoming the invaders so that the boil subsides by itself, or the pus may build up pressure against the skin surface so that it ruptures, drains and heals.

Boils may afflict healthy persons but often their appearance is a sign that the resistance is low, usually as a result of poor nutrition or illness. Persons suffering from dermatitis or untreated DIABETES MELLITUS are particularly susceptible to boils.

TREATMENT. In most cases, a single boil is not serious and will respond to careful treatment, but there are some important exceptions. Medical attention is necessary if the patient is an infant, a young child, or an elderly person. A boil on or above the upper lip, on the nose or scalp or in the outer ear can be very serious because in these areas infection has easy access to the brain. Other danger zones are the armpit, the groin, and the breast of a woman who is nursing. If bacteria from a boil enter the bloodstream, septicaemia may result. See also BLOOD POISONING and SEPTICAEMIA.

bolometer (boh'lomitə) 1. an instrument for measuring the force of the heart beat. 2. an instrument for measuring minute degrees of radiant heat.

bolus ('bohləs) 1. a rounded mass of food or pharmaceutical preparation ready to be swallowed, or such a mass passing through the gastrointestinal tract. 2. a concentrated mass of pharmaceutical preparation, e.g., an opaque contrast medium, given intravenously. 3. a mass of scattering material, such as wax or paraffin, placed between the radiation source and the skin to achieve a precalculated isodose pattern in the tissue irradiated.

alimentary b. the mass of food, made ready by mastication, that enters the oesophagus at one swallow.

Bolvidon ('bolvidon) trademark for mianserin.

bombesin ('bombi,sin) a tetradecapeptide neurotransmitter and hormone found in the brain and gut.

bond (bond) the linkage between atoms or radicals of a chemical compound, or the symbol representing this linkage and indicating the number and attachment of the valencies of an atom in constitutional formulas, represented by a line or a pair of dots between atoms, e.g., H–O–H, H–C≡C–H or H:O:H, H:C:::C:H.

coordinate covalent b. a covalent bond in which one of the bonded atoms furnishes both of the shared electrons.

covalent b. a chemical bond between two atoms or radicals formed by the sharing of a pair (single bond), two pairs (double bond), or three pairs of electrons (triple bond).

disulphide b. a strong covalent bond, -S-S-, important in linking polypeptide chains in proteins, the linkage arising as a result of the oxidation of the sulphhydryl (SH) groups of two molecules of cysteine.

high-energy phosphate b. an energy-rich phosphate linkage present in adenosine triphosphate (ATP), phosphocreatine, and certain other biological molecules. On hydrolysis at pH 7 it yields about 33.4 kJ per mole, in contrast to the 12.5 kJ per mole yielded by phosphate esters. The bond stores energy that is used to drive biochemical processes, such as the synthesis of macromolecules, contraction of muscles, and the production of the electrical potentials for nerve conduction.

high-energy sulphur b. an energy-rich sulphur linkage, the most important of which occurs in the acetyl-CoA molecule, the main source of energy in fatty acid biosynthesis.

hydrogen b. a weak, primarily electrostatic, bond between a hydrogen atom bound to a highly electronegative element (such as oxygen or nitrogen) in a given molecule, or part of a molecule, and a second highly electronegative atom in another molecule or in a different part of the same molecule.

ionic b. a chemical bond in which electrons are transferred from one atom to another so that one bears a positive and the other a negative charge, the attraction between these opposite charges forming the bond.

peptide b. the -CO-NH- linkage formed between the carboxyl group of one amino acid and the amino group of another; it is an amide linkage that joins amino acids to form peptides.

bonding ('bonding) the development of a close emotional tie to a mate or to a newborn infant. It is now thought that optimal bonding of the parents to a newborn infant requires a period of close contact with the infant in the first few hours after birth. The infant's responses to the mother, such as body and eye movements, are a necessary part of the process, and the presence of the father during the birth increases his bonding to the infant.

bone (bohn) 1. the hard, rigid form of connective tissue constituting most of the skeleton of vertebrates, composed chiefly of calcium salts. 2. any distinct piece of the skeleton of the body.

There are 206 separate bones in the human body. Collectively they form the SKELETAL SYSTEM, a structure bound together by ligaments at the joints and set in motion by stimulation of the muscles, which are secured to the bones by means of tendons. Bones, ligaments, muscles, and tendons are the tissues of the body responsible for supporting and moving the body.

Some bones have chiefly a protective function. An example is the skull, which encloses the brain, the back of the eyeball, and the inner ear. Some, such as the pelvis, are mainly supporting structures. Other bones, such as the jaw and the bones of the fingers, are concerned chiefly with movement. The MARROW contained in bones manufactures the blood cells. The bones themselves act as a storehouse of calcium, which must be maintained at a certain level in the blood for the body's normal chemical functioning.

STRUCTURE AND COMPOSITION. Bone is not uniform in structure but is composed of several layers of different materials. The outermost layer, the periosteum, is a thin, tough membrane of fibrous tissue. It gives support to the tendons that secure the muscle to the bone and also serves as a protective sheath. This membrane encloses all bones completely, except at the joints where there is a layer of cartilage. Beneath the periosteum lie the dense, hard layers of bone tissue called compact bone. Their composition is fibrous rather than solid and they give bone its resiliency. Encased within these layers is the tissue that makes up most of the volume of bone, called cancellous or spongy bone because it contains little hollows like those of a sponge. The innermost portion in long bones is a hollow cavity containing marrow. Blood vessels course through every layer of bone, carrying nutritive elements, oxygen, and other products. Bone tissue also contains a large number of nerves. The basic chemical in bone, which gives bone its hardness and strength, is calcium phosphate.

DEVELOPMENT. Cartilage forms the major part of bone in the very young; this accounts for the great flexibility and resiliency of the infant skeleton. Gradually, calcium phosphate collects in the cartilage, and it becomes harder and more brittle. Some of the cartilage cells break loose, so that channels develop in the bone shaft. Blood vessels enter the channels, bearing with them small cells of connective tissue, some of which become osteoblasts, cells that form true bone. The osteoblasts enter the hardened cartilage, forming layers of hard, firm bone. Other cells, called osteoclasts, work to tear down old or excess bone structure, allowing the osteoblasts to rebuild with new bone. This renewal continues throughout life, although it slows down with age.

Cartilage formation and the subsequent replacement of cartilage by hard material is the mechanism by which bones grow in size. During the period of bone growth, cartilage grows over the hardened portion of bone. In time, this layer of cartilage hardens as calcium phosphate is added, and a fresh layer grows over it, and it too hardens. The process continues until the body reaches full growth. Bone growth is influenced by many factors, including growth hormone (see also GROWTH and HORMONE). Long bones grow in length because of special cross-sectional layers of cartilage located near the flared ends of the bone. These harden and new cartilage is produced by the same process as previously described.

BONE DISORDERS. FRACTURE, a break in the bone, is the most common injury to the bone; it may be closed, with no break in the skin, or open, with penetration of the skin and exposure of portions of the broken bone.

OSTEOPOROSIS is rarefaction of bone, owing to lack of physical activity, lack of oestrogens or androgens, nutritional deficiency or long-term corticosteroid therapy; it is most commonly found in the elderly. OSTEOMYELITIS is a bone infection similar to a boil on the skin, but much more serious because the infection can destroy the bone and invade other body tissues. OSTEOMALACIA is the term used for RICKETS when it occurs in adults. In these diseases there is softening of the bones, due to inadequate concentration of calcium or phosphorus in the body. The usual cause is deficiency of vitamin D, which is required for utilization of calcium and phosphorus by the body.

In OSTEITIS FIBROSA CYSTICA, bone is replaced by fibrous tissue because of abnormal calcium metabolism. The condition is due to overactivity of the parathyroid glands and is associated with cyst formation.

OSTEOMA refers to abnormal benign new growth of the tissue of the bones. Although it is not common, it may occur in any of the bones of the body, and at any age.

ankle b. talus.

brittle b's osteogenesis imperfecta.

cancellated b., cancellous b. bone composed of thin intersecting lamellae, usually found internal to compact bone.

cartilage b. bone developing within cartilage, ossification taking place within a cartilage model.

cheek b. zygomatic bone.

collar b. clavicle.

compact b. bone substance that is dense and hard.

cortical b. the compact bone of the shaft of a bone that surrounds the marrow cavity.

flat b. one whose thickness is slight, sometimes consisting of only a thin layer of compact bone, or of two layers with intervening cancellated bone and marrow; usually curved rather than flat.

heel b. calcaneus.

incisive b. the portion of the maxilla bearing the incisors; developmentally, it is the premaxilla, which in humans later fuses with the maxilla, although in most other vertebrates it persists as a separate bone.

jaw b. the mandible or maxilla, especially the mandible.

jugal b. zygomatic bone.

lingual b. hyoid bone.

long b. one whose length far exceeds its breadth and thickness.

malar b. zygomatic bone.

marble b's osteopetrosis.

mastoid b. the mastoid process.

membrane b. bone that develops within a sheet of mesenchyma.

petrous b. the petrous portion of the temporal bone; pars petrosa.

pneumatic b. bone that contains air-filled spaces.

premaxillary b. premaxilla.

pterygoid b. pterygoid process.

rider's b. localized ossification sometimes seen on the inner aspect of the lower end of the tendon of the adductor muscle of the thigh in horseback riders.

shin b. tibia.

short b. one of approximately equal length, width, and thickness.

solid b. compact bone.

spongy b. cancellous bone.

squamous b. the upper forepart of the temporal bone, forming an upright plate.

sutural b's variable and irregularly shaped bones in the sutures between the bones of the skull.

thigh b. femur.

turbinated b. nasal conchae.

tympanic b. the part of the temporal bone surrounding the middle ear.

wormian b's sutural bones.

bone marrow (bohn 'maroh) the soft, organic, spongelike material in the cavities of bones, which has as its principal function the manufacture of erythrocytes, leukocytes, and platelets. See also MARROW.

b. m. transplantation a procedure used to treat aplastic anaemia, acute leukaemia and some rare congenital disorders with varying success. Healthy bone marrow is taken from the donor and infused into the blood stream of the recipient, where it 'homes' into the bone marrow where it will grow. Histocompatibility between the donor (usually a sibling) and recipient is essential, and even then there are many problems and the immediate mortality is high. Long-term success is achieved for about half the patients. The role of bone marrow transplantation in acute leukaemia is to restore bone marrow function following massive doses of chemotherapy or total body irradiation aimed at eradicating the leukaemia cells. A new approach is to use the patient's own bone marrow, taken during remission, to repopulate the marrow.

b. m. trephine biopsy a core of bone marrow 1 to 4 cm long, taken from sites such as the iliac crest, using a special biopsy needle (e.g., Jamshidi), is cut into thin sections and stained for microscopic examination. The advantage of the biopsy technique over the usual aspiration of a sample by a syringe is that it provides a much larger sample of tissue, maintains the structure of the bone marrow, enables cellularity to be assessed and is usually superior for the diagnosis of malignant infiltration of the marrow.

bonelet ('bohnlet) an ossicle, or small bone.

Bonner's position ('bonəz) flexion, abduction, and outward rotation of the thigh in coxitis.

Bonnevie–Ullrich syndrome (bon,vee'uhlrikh) pterygium colli, lymphangiectatic oedema of the hands and feet, ocular hypertelorism, short stature, and other developmental anomalies.

Bonney's blue (,boniz 'bloo) brilliant green and crystal violet paint.

booster dose ('boostə) see under DOSE.

boot (boot) an encasement for the foot; a protective casing or sheath.

Unna's paste b. a dressing for varicose ulcers, consisting of a paste made from gelatin, zinc oxide and glycerin, and spiral bandages. The entire leg is covered with paste and bandage, applied in alternate layers until they make a rigid boot.

borate ('bor·rayt) any salt of boric acid.

borax ('bor·raks) sodium borate.

borborygmus (,bawbə'rigməs) a rumbling noise caused by propulsion of gas through the intestines. See also BOWEL SOUNDS.

border ('bawdə) a bounding line, edge, or surface.

brush b. a specialization of the free surface of a cell, consisting of minute cylindrical processes (microvilli) that greatly increase the surface area.

vermilion b. the exposed red portion of the upper or lower lip.

borderline substances ('bawdə,lien) generally foods which in some cases can be considered as drugs and issued on a standard prescription. Guidance on these agents is obtained in the *British National Formulary* (BNF).

Bordetella (,bawdə'telə) a genus of bacteria.

B. parapertussis a species found occasionally in whooping cough (pertussis).

B. pertussis the causative agent of whooping cough (pertussis).

Bordet–Gengou bacillus (baw,day·zhanh'goo) *Bordetella pertussis.*

Bordet–Gengou phenomenon complement fixation.

boric acid ('bor·rik) a crystalline powder used as a buffer. It was formerly used as a household antiseptic for treating minor irritations of the skin and eyes. Because the powder is highly poisonous when taken internally, and since other antiseptics are more effective, boric acid is no longer recommended. Boric acid ointment (for external use only) occasionally helps in cases of mild skin irritations and keeps gauze dressing from sticking to a wound.

borism ('bohrizəm) poisoning by a boron compound.

Bornholm disease ('bawn,holm) epidemic pleurodynia, an epidemic disease due to coxsackievirus B, and marked by a sudden attack of violent pain in the chest or epigastrium, fever of brief duration, and a tendency to recrudescence on the third day; called also devil's grip, epidemic myalgia, and epidemic myositis.

boron ('bor·ron, 'boh-) a chemical element, atomic number 5, atomic weight 10.811, symbol B. See table of elements in Appendix 2.

Borrelia (bor'reeli·ə) a genus of bacteria.

B. recurrentis a causative agent of relapsing fever, transmitted by the human body louse.

B. vincentii a species parasitic in the human mouth, occurring in large numbers with a fusiform bacillus in necrotizing ulcerative gingivitis (trench mouth) and in necrotizing ulcerative gingivostomatitis.

borreliosis (bo,reli'ohsis) infection with *Borrelia.*

boss (bos) a rounded eminence.

bosselated ('bosi,laytid) marked or covered with bosses.

botryoid ('botri·oyd) shaped like a bunch of grapes.

botuliform (bo'tyooli,fawm) sausage-shaped.

botulin ('botyuhlin, 'bochə-) a neurotoxin produced by *Clostridium botulinum* sometimes found in imperfectly preserved or canned foods.

botulinal (,botyuh'lien'l, ,bochə-) pertaining to *Clostridium botulinum* or to its toxin (botulin).

botulism ('botyuh,lizəm, 'bochə-) an extremely severe form of food poisoning due to a neurotoxin (botulin) produced by *Clostridium botulinum*, sometimes found in improperly canned or preserved foods.

The symptoms include vomiting, abdominal pain, headache, weakness, constipation, and nerve paralysis, which causes difficulty in seeing, breathing, and swallowing. Death is usually due to paralysis of the respiratory organs.

This is a highly dangerous form of food poisoning, and to prevent it home canning and preserving of all nonacid foods–that is, all foods other than fruits and tomatoes–must be done according to proper specific directions.

Treatment consists of removing unabsorbed toxin from the intestinal tract through gastric lavage and induced emesis, administration of antitoxin to neutralize the circulating toxin (care should be taken in considering the risk of ANAPHYLAXIS), and providing required respiratory support.

infant b. that affecting infants, thought to result from toxin produced in the gut by ingested organisms, rather than from preformed toxins.

wound b. a form resulting from infection of a wound with *Clostridium botulinum.*

Bouchard's nodes (boo'shahz) cartilaginous and bony enlargements of the proximal interphalangeal joints of the fingers in degenerative joint disease.

bougie ('boozhee, boo'zhee) a slender, flexible, solid, cylindrical instrument for introduction into the urethra or other ducts, usually for calibrating or dilating constricted areas.

filiform b. a bougie of very slender calibre.

bougienage (,boozhi'nahzh) passage of a bougie.

Bouillaud's syndrome ('booiyohz) the coincidence of pericarditis and endocarditis in acute articular rheumatism.

bouquet (boo'kay) a structure resembling a cluster of flowers.

Bourneville's disease ('bawnvilz) tuberous sclerosis.

bouton ('bootonh) [Fr.] *button.*

boutonneuse fever (,booton'ərz) a tickborne disease endemic in the Mediterranean and Black Sea areas, Africa, and India, due to infection with *Rickettsia conorii*, with chills, fever, primary skin lesion (tache noire), and a generalized maculopapular rash appearing on about the fourth day.

bovine ('bohvien) pertaining to, characteristic of, or derived from the ox (cattle).

bowel ('bowəl) the intestine.

b. sounds relatively high-pitched abdominal sounds caused by the propulsion of the intestinal contents through the lower alimentary tract. Auscultation of bowel sounds is best accomplished by using a diaphragm-type stethoscope rather than a bell-shaped one. Normal bowel sounds are characterized by bubbling and gurgling noises that vary in frequency, intensity, and pitch. In the presence of distention from flatus, the sounds are hyperresonant and can be heard over the entire abdomen.

The *absence* of bowel sounds is symptomatic of greatly decreased or totally absent peristaltic movement. This can occur in such conditions as paralytic ileus, advanced intestinal obstruction, gangrene of the bowel, enterocolic ulceration, myxoedema, and spinal cord injury. In the early stages of bowel obstruction, high-pitched splashing sounds are heard in the intestine proximal to the obstruction. As the obstruction continues to constrict the lumen of the bowel, the sounds are of shorter duration and eventually cease altogether as the obstruction to the lumen of the bowel becomes complete.

Increased motility of the bowel usually results from some sort of irritating stimulus, such as gastroenteritis with diarrhoea, bleeding in the intestine, and emotional disorders. The propulsion of gas through the bowel produces a rush of sounds, with waves of loud, gurgling and tinkling sounds called *borborygmi* (see also BORBORYGMUS).

b. training a programme designed to assist the patient having difficulty with the regulation and control of defecation. A programme of this type may be indicated in a variety of cases ranging from chronic constipation to paralysis, as in PARAPLEGIA and HEMIPLEGIA. Patients who suffer from lesions or congenital anomalies of the intestinal tract also may benefit from a programme of training.

Before planning a programme of bowel control it is necessary to determine the cause of the difficulty, the patient's former bowel habits, and his specific symptoms. The plan devised will depend on the patient's needs and his physical, mental, and emotional capacities for cooperation in the planning and implementation of the programme. It is necessary to know whether he can realistically be expected to achieve complete control, or if neural damage or anatomical and structural changes in the intestine prevent his reaching this goal. For example, a COLOSTOMY patient cannot achieve complete control over his bowel movements, but regulation of his diet and fluid intake can affect the number and consistency of the stools, giving him some sense of security. Diet also is important in all other types of bowel training in which the goal is regularity of defecation and stools of normal consistency.

It is important that the patient participate as much as possible in planning the programme. He will need to give an accurate history of his bowel habits, his former use of laxatives and enemas, his usual time of day for bowel movements, and the frequency, and whether or not he is aware of the urge to defecate. As the programme is carried out, revisions may be necessary as the patient learns which techniques are most helpful to him.

The major components of a bowel training programme are choosing the location to ensure some degree of privacy, getting the patient into a sitting position, having him attempt defecation at a specific time that is most natural for him, regulating the food and fluid intake, and establishing some plan of regular exercise and physical activity.

In some cases of paralysis it may be necessary to stimulate bowel function through the use of suppositories and digital stimulation. Enemas, laxatives, and bulk-forming medications are used only if necessary, not on a regular basis if at all possible. These measures may be necessary, however, at the beginning of a bowel training programme to remove constipated stool and FAECAL IMPACTION.

Bowen's disease ('boh·ənz) intraepidermal squamous cell carcinoma, often occurring in multiple sites.

bowleg ('boh,leg) an outward curvature of one or both legs near the knee; genu varum.

Bowman's capsule ('bohmənz) a two-layered cellular envelope enclosing the tuft of capillaries constituting the glomerulus of the kidney; called also *glomerular capsule*.

Bowman's disc one of the flat, disclike plates making up a striated muscle fibre.

Bowman's glands small mucous glands in olfactory mucosa; called also *olfactory glands*.

Boyle's anaesthetic machine (boylz) a continuous-flow anaesthetic machine which supplies oxygen and nitrous oxide together with cyclopropane, halothane and other anaesthetic agents as required. Named after Henry Boyle, an anaesthetist at St. Bartholomew's Hospital, who described the original machine in 1917.

Strictly speaking, the term 'Boyle's machine' applies only to those pieces of equipment manufactured by the British Oxygen Company, but nowadays it is colloquially applied to all continuous-flow anaesthetic machines.

Boyle's law at a constant temperature and mass the volume of a perfect gas varies inversely with pressure; that is, as increasing pressure is applied, the volume decreases. Conversely, as pressure is reduced, volume is increased.

Bozeman's position ('bohzmənz) the knee-elbow position with straps used for support.

BP 1. blood pressure. 2. boiling point. 3. British Pharmacopoeia, a publication of the General Medical Council, describing and establishing standards for medicines, preparations, materials, and articles used in the practice of medicine, surgery, or midwifery.

b.p. boiling point.

BPA British Paediatric Association.

BPC British Pharmaceutical Codex.

BPD biparietal diameter, skull measurement during ultrasound scanning of the fetus in utero.

Bq becquerel.

Br chemical symbol, *bromine*.

brace (brays) an orthopaedic appliance or apparatus (orthosis), usually made of thermoplastic materials, metal or leather, applied to the body, particularly the trunk and lower extremities, to support the weight of the body, to correct deformities, to prevent deformities, or to control involuntary movements, such as occur in spastic conditions. In some cases bracing is needed after remedial surgery. Back braces are used to treat certain kinds of backache.

Dental braces are used to support the teeth or to change their position in treatment of malocclusion.

brachi(o)- word element. [L., Gr.] *arm*.

brachial ('brayki·əl, 'brak-) pertaining to the arm.

b. plexus a nerve plexus originating from the ventral branches of the last four cervical and the first thoracic spinal nerves. It gives off many of the principal nerves of the shoulder, chest, and arms.

brachialgia (,brayki'alji·ə) pain in the arm.

brachiocephalic (,braykiohkə'falik, -sə'falik) pertaining to the arm and head.

brachiocrural (,braykioh'kroo·ə·ral) pertaining to the arm and leg.

brachiocubital (,braykioh'kyoobit'l) pertaining to the arm and forearm.

brachiocyrtosis (,braykiohsər'tohsis) crookedness of the arm.

brachium ('brayki·əm) pl. *brachia* [L.] 1. the arm; specifically the arm from shoulder to elbow. 2. any armlike process or structure.

b. conjunctivum cerebelli the superior cerebellar peduncle, a fibrous band extending from each hemisphere of the cerebellum upward over the pons, the two joining to form the sides and part of the roof of the fourth ventricle.

b. pontis the brachium of the pons, the middle cerebellar peduncle.

brachy- word element. [Gr.] *short*.

brachybasia (,braki'baysi·ə) a slow, shuffling, short-stepped gait.

brachycardia (,braki'kahdi·ə) bradycardia.

brachycephalic (,brakikə'falik, -sə'falik) having a short, wide head.

brachycephaly (,braki'kefəlee, -'sef-) the state of being brachycephalic.

brachycheilia (,braki'kieli·ə) shortness of the lip.

brachydactyly (,braki'daktilee) abnormal shortness of the fingers and toes.

brachygnathia (,braki'nathi·ə) abnormal shortness of the mandible.

brachymetacarpia (,braki,metə'kahpi·ə) abnormal shortness of the metacarpal bones.

brachymetatarsia (,braki,metə'tahsi·ə) abnormal shortness of the metatarsal bones.

brachyphalangia (,brakifə'lanji·ə) abnormal shortness of one of the phalanges.

brachytherapy (,braki'therəpee) radiotherapy delivered into or adjacent to a tumour by means of an intracavitary or interstitial radioactive source.

brady- word element. [Gr.] *slow*.

bradyacusia (,bradiə'kyoosi·ə) dullness of hearing.

bradyaesthesia (,bradi·is'theezi·ə) slowness or dullness of perception.

bradyarrhythmia (,bradi·ə'ridhmi·ə) bradycardia associated with arrhythmia.

bradycardia (,bradi'kahdi·ə) slowness of the heart beat, as evidenced by slowing of the pulse rate to less than 60 per minute. adj. **bradycardiac.** A heart rate and pulse of less than 60 beats per minute can occur in normal persons, particularly during sleep. Trained athletes usually have a slow pulse and heart rate.

bradyglossia (,bradi'glosi·ə) abnormal slowness of utterance.

bradykinesia (,bradiki'neezi·ə) abnormal slowness of movement; sluggishness of physical and mental responses. adj. **bradykinetic.**

bradykinin (,bradi'kienin) a nonapeptide kinin formed from a plasma protein, high-molecular-weight (HMW) kininogen, by the action of kallikrein; it is a very powerful vasodilator that increases capillary permeability and, in addition, constricts smooth muscle and stimulates pain receptors.

bradylalia (,bradi'layli·ə) abnormally slow utterance due to a central nervous system lesion; bradyphasia.

bradylexia (,bradi'leksi·ə) abnormal slowness in reading, due neither to defect in intelligence or of vision, nor to ignorance of the alphabet.

bradylogia (,bradi'lohji·ə) abnormal slowness of speech, due to slowness of thinking, as in a mental disorder.

bradyphaemia (,bradi'feemi·ə) slowness of speech.

bradyphagia (,bradi'fayji·ə) abnormal slowness of eating.

bradyphasia (,bradi'fayzi·ə) slow utterance of speech.

bradyphrasia (,bradi'frayzi·ə) slowness of speech due to mental disorder.

bradypnoea (,bradi'neeə) respirations that are regular in rhythm but slower than normal in rate. This is normal during sleep; otherwise it is associated with disturbance in the brain's respiratory control centre, as when the centre is affected by opiate narcotics, alcohol, a tumour, a metabolic disorder, or a respiratory decompensation mechanism.

bradyspermatism (ˌbradiˈspərməˌtizəm) abnormally slow ejaculation of semen.
bradysphygmia (ˌbradiˈsfigmi·ə) abnormal slowness of the pulse.
bradystalsis (ˌbradiˈstalsis) abnormal slowness of peristalsis.
bradytachycardia (ˌbradiˌtakiˈkahdi·ə) alternating attacks of bradycardia and tachycardia.
bradyuria (ˌbradiˈyooə·ri·ə) slow discharge of urine.
braille (ˈbrayl) a method of printing developed by Louis Braille (1809–1852) for the blind. Letters of the alphabet are represented by patterns of raised dots. These dots are read by passing the finger tips over them.
brain (brayn) encephalon; that part of the central nervous system contained within the cranium, comprising the forebrain, midbrain, and hindbrain, and developed from the embryonic neural tube. It is connected at its base with the spinal cord. The brain is a mass of soft, spongy, pinkish grey nerve tissue which, in the human, weighs about 1.5 kg.

The brain is made up of millions of nerve cells, intricately connected with each other. It contains centres (groups of NEURONS and their connections) which control many involuntary functions, such as circulation, temperature regulation, and respiration, and interpret sensory impressions received from the eyes, ears, and other sense organs. Consciousness, emotion, thought, and reasoning are functions of the brain. It also contains centres or areas for associative memory which allow for recording, recalling, and making use of past experiences.

CEREBRUM. The largest and main portion of the brain, the cerebrum is made up of an outer coating, or cortex, of grey cells, several layers deep, which covers the cerebral hemispheres. The cortex is the thinking and reasoning brain, the intellect, as well as the part of the brain that receives information from the senses and directs the conscious movements of the body.

The cerebrum is made up of two cerebral hemispheres, divided incompletely by the longitudinal cerebral fissure. A bed of matted white fibres, the corpus callosum, joins the right and left hemispheres, at their base. The major folds (the sulci) divide each hemisphere into four sections or lobes, each of which is named according to the bones of the cranium under which it lies. The frontal lobe is separated from the parietal lobe by the central sulcus. The lateral sulcus separates the frontal and parietal lobe from the temporal lobe and the parieto-occipital sulcus divides the parietal and occipital lobes. Between the sulci there are many exposed ridges, termed the gyri; these give the cortex its convoluted appearance.

The Senses. The major senses of sight and hearing are well mapped in the cortex; the centre for vision is at the back, in the occipital lobe, and the centre for hearing is at the side, in the temporal lobe. Two other areas have been carefully explored; these are the sensory and motor areas for the body, which parallel each other along the central sulcus (or fissure).

In the sensory strip are located the brain cells that register all sensations. In the motor strip are the nerves that control the voluntary muscles. In both, the parts of the body are represented in an orderly way.

It is in the sensory areas of the brain that all perception takes place. Here sweet and sour, hot and cold, and the form of an object held in the hand are recognized. Here are sorted out the sizes, colours, depth, and space relationships of what the eye sees, and the timbre, pitch, intensity, and harmony of what the ear hears. The significance of these perceptions is interpreted in the cortex and other parts of the brain.

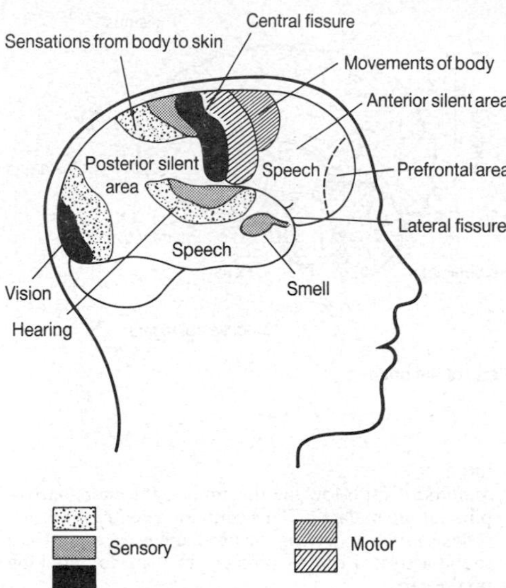

Projection areas of the brain

A face is not merely seen; it is recognized as familiar or interesting or attractive. Remembering takes place at the same time as perception, so that other faces seen in the past, or experiences linked to that face are called up. Emotions may also be stirred. For this type of association the cortex draws on other parts of the brain by way of the communicating network of nerves.

A large part of the cortex that remains unmapped is thought to be involved in associative response. Factual knowledge and technical skills depend upon a background of experience and relationships between one kind of thing and another. Whether the mind is daydreaming, thinking rationally, or experiencing a surge of emotion, it draws upon an intensely personal and private background of association. The richer a person's life is in experiences that have made their imprint on thought and feeling, the richer will be the patterns upon which the conscious mind can draw.

For a long time, the frontal lobe, which particularly distinguishes man's brain from that of the lower orders, was thought to be an associative area. It was called a 'silent' area because it seemed to have no specific function. This appears to be true for most of the frontal area, but it has been learned that in the frontal lobe, close to the small centre for the sense of smell, is the centre for speech.

Memory. In the temporal lobe, near the auditory area, is a centre for memory. This centre appears to be a storehouse where memories are filed. When this area alone is stimulated, a particular event, a piece of music, or an experience long forgotten or deeply buried is brought to the individual's mind, complete in every detail. This is a very mechanical type of memory; when the stimulation is removed the memory ends. When it is applied again, the memory begins again, not where it left off, but from the beginning. See also MEMORY.

BRAIN STEM. This is the stemlike portion of the brain connecting the cerebral hemispheres with the spinal cord, and comprising midbrain, pons, and medulla oblongata. Some consider it to include the diencepha-

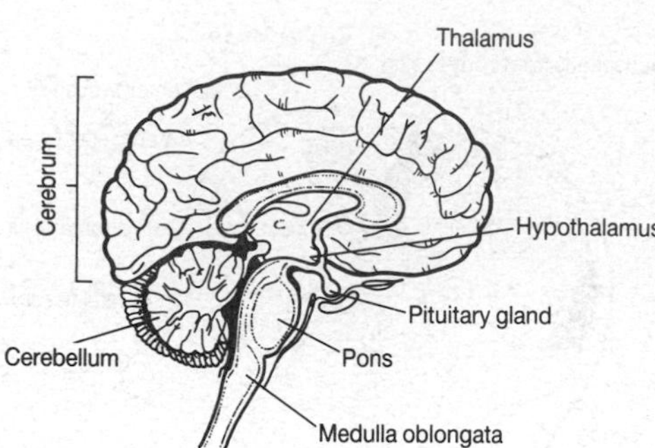

Parts of the brain

lon.

Midbrain. Just below the thalamus is the short narrow pillar of the midbrain. This contains a centre for visual reflexes, such as moving the head and eyes, as well as a sound-activated centre, obsolete in man, for pricking up the ears.

Pons Varolii. Located between the midbrain and the medulla. The fifth, sixth, seventh and eighth cranial nerves connect to the brain in the pons and it also exerts some control over respiratory function.

Medulla Oblongata. Below the midbrain is the medulla oblongata, the continuation upwards of the spinal cord. In the medulla, the great trunk nerves, both motor and sensory, cross over, left to right and right to left, producing the puzzling phenomenon by which the left hemisphere of the cerebrum controls the right half of the body, while the right hemisphere controls the left half of the body. This portion of the brain also contains the centres that activate the heart, blood vessels, and respiratory system.

Thalamus. Beneath the cortex, deep within the cerebral hemispheres, lies the THALAMUS. This organ is a relay station for body sensations; it also integrates these sensations on their way to the cortex. The thalamus is an organ of crude consciousness and of sensations of rough contact and extreme temperatures, either hot or cold. It is principally here that pain is felt. In the thalamus responses are of the all-or-nothing sort; even mild stimuli would be felt as acutely painful if they were not graded and modified by the cortex.

Hypothalamus. Below the thalamus, at the base of the cerebrum, is the HYPOTHALAMUS. This organ, no larger than a lump of sugar, takes part in such vital activities as the ebb and flow of the body's fluids and the regulation of metabolism, blood sugar levels, and body temperature. It directs the body's many rhythms, including those of activity and rest, appetite and digestion, sexual desire, and menstrual and reproductive cycles. The hypothalamus is also the body's emotional brain. It is the integrating centre of the autonomic NERVOUS SYSTEM, with its sympathetic and parasympathetic branches, and is situated close to the PITUITARY GLAND.

CEREBELLUM. The cerebellum, or 'little brain', is attached to the back of the brain stem, under the curve of the cerebrum. It is connected, by way of the midbrain, with the motor area of the cortex and with the spinal cord, as well as with the SEMICIRCULAR CANALS, the organs of balance.

The function of the cerebellum appears to be to blend and coordinate motion of the various muscles involved in voluntary movements. It does not direct these movements; that is the function of the cortex. The cortex, however, operates in terms of movements, not of muscles. As a conscious function the cortex may, for example, direct the arm to pick up a glass of water; the cerebellum, which operates entirely below the level of consciousness, then translates this instruction into detailed actions by the 32 different muscles in the hand, plus several more in the arm and shoulder. When the cerebellum is injured, the patient's movements are jerky and uncoordinated.

CRANIAL NERVES. From the brain stem there emerge on their separate pathways the CRANIAL NERVES. They arise within the skull and, with one important exception, the VAGUS NERVE, serve the head and neck.

PROTECTION OF THE BRAIN. The brain is protected by the bony skull and by three layers of membranes, the meninges. Between the middle and inner layer (the subarachnoid space), CEREBROSPINAL fluid can be found. The cerebrospinal fluid has several protective functions, including supporting and protecting the delicate nervous tissue, maintaining uniform pressure and acting as a shock absorber. The same system of membranes and fluid protects the spinal cord.

The brain is protected from harmful substances in the bloodstream by a barrier (the BLOOD–BRAIN BARRIER) that keeps some of the substances out of the brain entirely and delays the entry of others for hours or even days after they have penetrated the rest of the body.

DISORDERS OF THE BRAIN. In spite of protection of the brain by the skull and membranes and by the blood–brain barrier, a number of functional disorders and diseases may affect the brain.

Concussion or fracture of the skull may occur as a result of a severe shock or blow to the head. An interruption to the flow of blood to the brain may result from haemorrhage from one of the blood vessels serving the brain, or an obstruction caused by formation of a thrombus. A stroke occurs when brain cells are deprived of their supply of blood.

Several diseases affect the brain specifically, including epilepsy, meningitis, and encephalitis.

Hydrocephalus is caused by an abnormal accumulation of cerebrospinal fluid in the head.

Cerebral palsy is a name given to a motor disorder that results in inability to control muscle movement. It is usually the result of brain damage before, during, or immediately after birth.

Many diseases that originate in other parts of the body may affect the brain and nerves. Rabies and tetanus (lockjaw) are two examples of diseases that can cause brain damage. Others are syphilis, rheumatic fever, and alcoholism.

Brain Abscess. Brain abscess is a localized suppurative lesion within the intracranial cavity. The majority of cases are secondary to chronic middle ear infections. Other causes include compound fracture of the skull with contamination of the brain tissue, sinusitis, and infections of the face, lung or heart. Symptoms include fever, malaise, irritability, severe headache, convulsions, vomiting, and other signs of intracranial hypertension. Treatment consists of surgical removal and drainage of the infected area and administration of antibiotic drugs.

Brain Tumour. Any abnormal growth within the skull creates a special problem because it is in a confined space and will press on normal brain tissue and interfere with the functions of the body controlled by the affected parts. This is true whether the tumour itself is benign or malignant. Fortunately, the functions of certain areas of the brain are well known, and a disturbance of some specific function guides doctors readily to the affected area. If diagnosed early, a benign tumour often can be removed surgically with a good chance of recovery. Malignant tumours are more difficult to remove.

The causes of brain tumour are not known. It is not a common disease, but it can occur at any age, and it can appear in any part of the brain. It may originate in the brain or may metastasize from a tumour in another part of the body.

The symptoms of brain tumour vary. Headache together with nausea is sometimes the first sign. The headache can be generalized or localized in one part of the head, and the pain is usually intense. Vomiting can be significant if it is sudden and without nausea. Disturbances of vision, loss of coordination in movement, weakness, and stiffness on one side of the body are also possible symptoms. Loss of sight, hearing, taste, or smell may result from brain tumour. A tumour can also cause a distortion of any of these senses, such as seeing flashes at the sides of the field of vision, or smelling odours or hearing sounds that do not exist. It can affect the ability to speak clearly or to understand the speech of others. Varying degrees of weakness or paralysis in the arms or legs may appear. A tumour may cause convulsions.

Changes in personality or mental ability are rare in cases of brain tumour. When such changes occur they may take the form of lapses of memory or absent-mindedness, mental sluggishness, or loss of initiative.

Brain tumour is treated surgically. As a result of recent progress in the methods of diagnosis and brain surgery, many cases of brain tumour can now be operated on successfully.

BRAIN SURGERY. There are two types of brain surgery —that which corrects damage to the brain itself, and that which seeks to remedy a condition in another part of the body. The first type includes operations to relieve tumours, brain injuries, abscesses, and infections, hydrocephalus, and PARKINSON'S DISEASE. The second includes surgery for pain and movement disorders.

Brain's reflex (braynz) quadrupedal extensor reflex.

brain death irreversible coma; see DEATH.

brain failure a deterioration in brain function occurring predominantly in old age, characterized by mental impairment and behavioural disorder. Formerly inappropriately termed 'senility', brain failure is classified as organic (biological/pathological) and functional (psychogenic) and as acute and chronic.

ACUTE BRAIN FAILURE. Acute brain failure or 'confusional state' equates with delirium in younger persons in that most of its many causes are potentially reversible; these include infections and toxic states, the effect of drugs, trauma, metabolic imbalance, disorders of or affecting cerebral circulation, severe depression and stress from abrupt change of environment and loss.

Symptoms include tremulousness, agitation and restlessness or clouding of consciousness, fluctuating awareness of persons and environment, thought disturbance and impaired concentration; the confusion may include visual hallucinations and delusions.

The sudden onset of change in the mental and physical status of an old person requires prompt medical attention to identify and treat the cause.

CHRONIC BRAIN FAILURE. Chronic brain failure, organic brain syndrome or senile dementia is a condition of insidious onset, which is slowly progressive and irreversible. The commonest causes are Alzheimer's disease and atherosclerosis.

By the age of 70, many people normally have some degree of change in functioning ability, such as a slowing of reflexes, greater susceptibility to fatigue and mild forgetfulness, especially for names. In organic brain syndrome such changes are extreme in nature.

The characteristic features are progressive impairment of memory and judgement, loss of interest in wordly affairs, disorientation in time and place, and eventually dementia, commonly accompanied by loss of excetory control; sudden outbursts of joy, rage or despair may occur for no apparent reason and verbally disruptive behaviour and wandering may be constant.

The condition can also be psychogenic in origin (functional brain failure) and a secondary condition aggravating behaviour can occur (acute-on-chronic), but as the patient may not be able to communicate feeling unwell, this can go undetected without discerning observation.

Medication may be prescribed in some cases to reduce the severity of the dementia, but as anxiety and fear are often paramount in the behaviour, the best medicine is constant reassurance and comforting of the individual. Care includes kindly supervision, maintenance of nutrition, personal hygiene and adequate rest, engagement in activities (although attention span is often short)—including those of self-care, like washing and dressing—and applying techniques, use of signs and symbols, and any reminders which aid the individual to keep in touch with reality and location in time and place. In the home situation, the emphasis is on giving the carer support and relief from the constant stress and strain that is often involved in looking after an elderly relative with this condition.

brain scanning an imaging technique used to detect abnormalities of the brain. Several different methods of imaging currently exist. Computed TOMOGRAPHY is the best known and most frequently used. It uses computer processing to generate an image of the tissue density of the brain and will demonstrate tumours, haematomas, abscesses, areas of infarction and cerebral oedema, and other intracranial lesions. Isotope scanning involves injecting a radioisotope, such as technetium-99m, and then using a scintillation camera to make an image of the distribution of radioactivity, in which a lesion appears as a region of increased radioactivity. With the advent of computed tomography, this technique is now not nearly so often performed. A combination of computed tomography and scintillation scanning, termed positron emission tomography, has been developed for the brain. Magnetic resonance imaging is a new technique involving the use of a strong magnetic field and radiofrequency pulse waves, which has been developed to provide a safe, non-invasive method of producing tissue images without many of the usual radiological hazards. Images produced by magnetic resonance are based on hydrogen distribution within the body; by applying different scanning techniques, information on the chemistry and physiology of living tissues, as well as anatomical differences, can be obtained.

brain stem, brainstem ('braynstem) the stemlike portion of the brain connecting the cerebral hemispheres with the spinal cord, and comprising the pons, medulla oblongata, and midbrain; considered by some to include the diencephalon. Contains the vital centres which exert control over the visual reflexes, heart rate, blood pressure and respiration.

brainwashing ('brayn,woshing) systematic emotional and mental conditioning of an individual or a group of individuals designed to secure attitudes and beliefs conformable to the wishes of those administering the conditioning, accomplished by means of propaganda, torture, drugs, distorted psychiatric procedures, or other means.

bran (bran) the husk of grain. The coarse outer coat of cereals. High in roughage and vitamins of the B complex. Frequently recommended as a dietary component both for those with alimentary disorders and for those in normal health.

branch (brahnsh) ramus; a division or offshoot from a main stem, especially of blood vessels, nerves, or lymphatics.

bundle b. a branch of the bundle of His.

branched-chain ketoaciduria ('brahnchd,chayn) maple syrup urine disease.

branchial ('brangki·əl) pertaining to, or resembling, gills of a fish or derivatives of homologous parts in higher forms.

b. arches paired arched columns that bear the gills in lower aquatic vertebrates and which, in embryos of higher vertebrates, become modified into structures of the ear and neck.

b. clefts the clefts between the branchial arches of the embryo, formed by rupture of the membrane separating corresponding entodermal pouch and ectodermal groove.

b. cyst a cyst formed deep within the neck from an incompletely closed branchial cleft, usually located between the second and third branchial arches. The branchial arches develop during the first two months of embryonic life and are separated by four clefts, which correspond to the gills of a fish. As the fetus develops, these arches grow to form structures within the head and neck. Two of the arches grow together and enclose the cervical sinus, a cavity in the neck. A branchial cyst may develop within the cervical sinus. Called also *branchiogenic* or *branchiogenous cyst*.

b. groove an external furrow lined with ectoderm, occurring in the embryo between two branchial arches.

Branham's sign ('branhamz) bradycardia produced by digital closure of an artery proximal to an arteriovenous fistula.

Branhamella (,branhə'melə) a genus of aerobic, nonmotile, non-spore-forming cocci. The type species, *B. catarrhalis*, is a normal inhabitant of the nasopharynx, which occasionally causes opportunistic infections.

brash (brash) heartburn.

water b. heartburn with regurgitation of sour fluid or almost tasteless saliva into the mouth.

weaning b. diarrhoea in infants occurring as a result of weaning.

Braun frame ('brawn fraym) a metal frame, used to elevate the lower limb in fractures of the tibia and fibula.

Braxton Hicks contractions (,brakstən 'hiks) light, usually painless, irregular contractions of the uterus throughout pregnancy, gradually increasing in intensity and frequency and becoming more rhythmic during the third trimester; are often mistaken for true labour, and sometimes referred to as 'false labour' or *false pains* (see PAIN). The contractions do not effect change in the shape of the cervix or uterus. They may be stimulated by the descent of the head of the fetus into the pelvic inlet. Braxton Hicks contractions are not as regular and rhythmic as are true LABOUR contractions.

Brazelton behavioural scale ('brayzəltən) a method for assessing infant behaviour by responses to environmental stimuli.

BRCS British Red Cross Society.

breast (brest) the front of the chest, especially the modified cutaneous, glandular structure it bears, the mamma. In women the breasts are secondary sex organs with the function of producing milk after childbirth. The term breast is less commonly used to refer to the breasts of the human male, which neither function nor develop.

At the tip of each breast is an area called the areola, usually reddish in colour; at the centre of this area is the NIPPLE. About 20 separate lactiferous ducts empty into a depression at the top of the nipple. Each duct leads from alveoli within the breast called lobules, where the milk is secreted. Along their length, the ducts have widened areas that form reservoirs in which milk can be stored. The ducts and lobules form the glandular tissue of the breasts. Connective tissue covers the glandular tissue and is itself sheathed in a layer of fatty tissue. The fatty tissue gives the breast its smooth outline and contributes to its size and firmness.

ABNORMALITIES AND DISORDERS OF THE BREAST. *Amastia* is the absence of one or both breasts at birth. *Hypomastia* is abnormal smallness of the breasts. Hypertrophy of the breasts, abnormal enlargement of the breasts, may be idiopathic or due to an endocrine disorder. Enlargement of the breasts in the male is called gynaecomastia and is a not uncommon occurrence during adolescence. Polymastia is the presence of more than two breasts; it is more common in men than in women.

MASTITIS, inflammation of the breast, may occur in a variety of forms and in varying degrees of severity. Persistent cases may require MASTECTOMY, but usually medical treatment suffices.

Breast Tumour. Benign tumours are growths of breast tissue that are usually encapsulated, do not metastasize, and usually can be removed by surgery without difficulty. Once removed, they do not recur. The most common of these is fibroadenoma, which is found most frequently in women between 21 and 25, although it can develop during and after menopause. This tumour grows rapidly during pregnancy, is seldom painful, and can be removed surgically. Another benign breast tumour is intraductal papilloma. It occurs most frequently in women between 35 and 55. Its primary symptom is discharge of blood or fluid containing blood from the nipples when the breast is compressed.

The breast is the most common site of malignant tumours in women. In the United Kingdom 13,000 women a year die of this condition and although the survival rates for breast cancer continue to increase, albeit slowly, the incidence of the disease in the western world increases. Improvement in these survival rates has come from increased public awareness, breast self-examination, breast screening programmes, and improved methods of treatment.

Breast cancer first appears as a small, painless lump, most frequently in the outer, upper portion of the breast. If the lump is near the surface, there is often a visible dimpling of the skin. A biopsy of cells from the lump can establish a diagnosis of malignancy. However, most breast lumps are not malignant; eight out of ten are benign, and those that are malignant can usually be treated successfully if diagnosed and treated in the early stages of the disease.

The International Union Against Cancer (UICC) classification of staging breast cancer is used in the United Kingdom (see Table accompanying CANCER).

Improvements in x-ray techniques have made it possible to diagnose breast tumours in the early stages. Radiological examination of the breast is called *mammography*. Another imaging technique, called *thermography*, uses infrared rays and shows the variation in temperature over the skin surface.

Treatment of malignant tumours of the breast varies according to the patient's condition. The type of

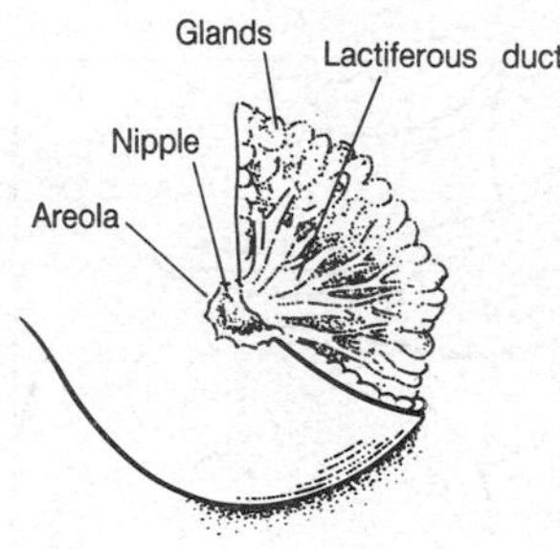

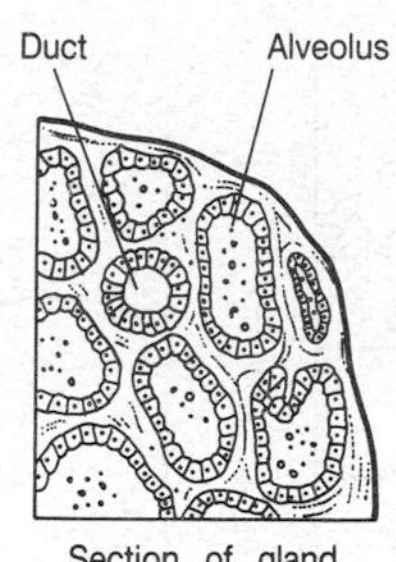

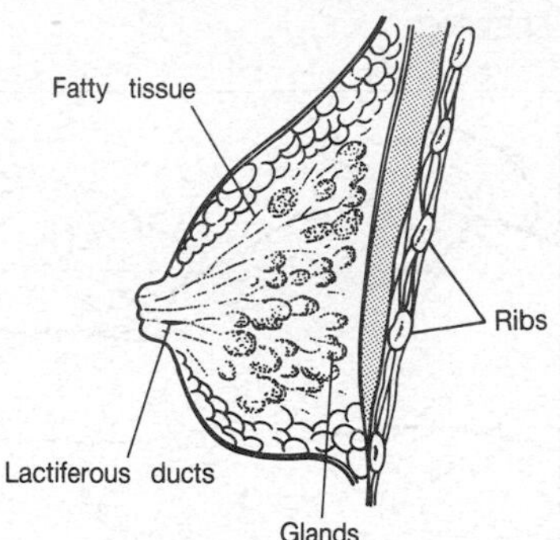

Breast, with detail and cross-section.

surgical procedure that will be recommended, and whether radiation therapy or chemotherapy will be used, depends on the type, size, location, and extent of the growth, as well as other factors.

SELF-EXAMINATION OF THE BREAST. Women should train themselves to perform a simple self-examination of the breasts, described in the accompanying diagrams. The best time for this is just after menstruation when the breasts are normally soft. If any lump in the breast can be felt, a doctor should be consulted immediately. More than 90 per cent of breast cancers are discovered by the patients themselves.

SURGERY OF THE BREAST. Surgical operations of the breast may be done for a variety of reasons.

Mammoplasty refers to reconstructive surgery of the breast and is usually done for the purpose of reducing the size of large, pendulous breasts or to augment the size of very small breasts.

MASTECTOMY is surgical removal of breast tissue; it is most often performed to treat cancer of the breast. Procedures vary from extended radical mastectomy to partial mastectomy to LUMPECTOMY.

Patient Care. The psychological aspects of surgery of the breast are paramount. The breast is a symbol of femininity, motherhood, and sexual attractiveness; thus, a surgical procedure involving its partial or complete removal will always bring about some degree of emotional upheaval for the patient. Many women, out of fear of mutilation or even death, resist surgical treatment of the breast even though the procedure may be necessary to save their lives. The patient should be reassured that modern prostheses and specially designed brassières, swimsuits and other clothes eliminate many of the outward signs of the loss of a breast.

There are two approaches to the diagnosis and surgical treatment of breast tumours. In the *one-step* approach, a biopsy of the tumour is taken in the operating theatre and the specimen is immediately sent to the pathologist. The patient remains under anaesthesia until the results are reported. If the tumour is diagnosed as malignant, the surgery continues, and a mastectomy is performed. This is the least desirable approach. In the *two-step* approach, there is a waiting period of several days or more between the biopsy and the surgery. It is the consensus of most surgeons that the two-step approach is best. However, there are advantages and disadvantages to each approach.

Some patients are disturbed that a decision to remove the breast could be made while they are under anaesthesia. These patients prefer the two-step approach because they are given time to discuss the test results with the surgeon and their family, and to obtain a second opinion if they wish. There is also time to deal with personal matters, and begin to adjust emotionally to the idea of having a breast removed. Others prefer to 'get it over with' as quickly as possible. Delay only adds to their anxiety and creates more emotional stress. It is at these times that the services of a Breast Care Nurse are invaluable in helping patients and families through psychologically trying times.

Oedema of the arm occurs commonly on the side from which axillary lymph tissue has been removed. Arm exercises, such as the ones described later, are helpful in preventing some oedema, as are elastic bandages and pressure gradient elastic sleeves, which are worn until collateral lymphatic pathways have been established. Excision of the lymph nodes also reduces the patient's ability to combat infection in the affected arm. She will need instruction in prevention of injury to the hand and arm from cuts, burns, and other breaks in the skin. In addition, she should be told to not allow any injections in the swollen arm. If the arm becomes red, warm, and unusually hard and swollen, these signs indicate cellulitis, which should be reported to the surgeon immediately.

Special exercises are essential to recovery from mastectomy. They are begun as soon as ordered by the surgeon/nurse and should be continued after the patient has returned home. Combing and brushing the hair, buttoning clothes at the back, 'wall climbing' with the fingers, and arm-swinging exercises are all useful in preserving muscle tone and preventing contracture of the joints. The Mastectomy Association of Great Britain, 26 Harrison Street, London WC1H 8JG, has useful leaflets which describe these exercises.The Association also offers help and support to women with breast cancer.

chicken b. pectus carinatum.

breast feeding, breastfeeding (brest'feeding) the method of feeding a baby with milk directly from the mother's breasts. Most paediatricians agree that breast feeding is usually better for baby and mother, both physically and emotionally.

ADVANTAGES AND DISADVANTAGES. Breast milk is easily digested by the baby, for whom nature especially made it. It is safe and clean and contains practically everything the baby needs during the first months of his life. Babies who are breast fed are less susceptible to certain respiratory and gastrointestinal infections

FEELING

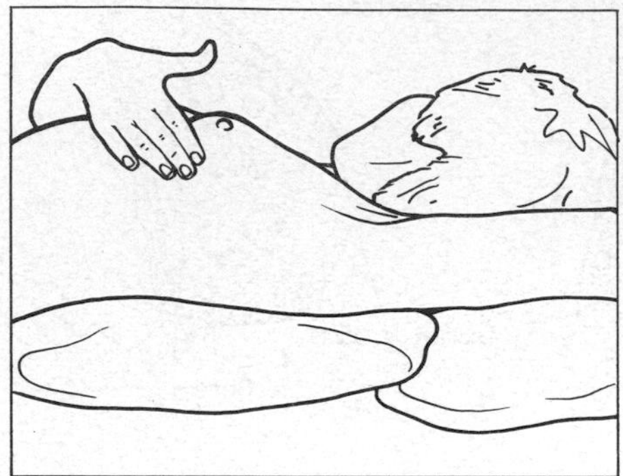

Lie down on your bed and make yourself comfortable with your head on a pillow.

Examine one breast at a time.

Put a folded towel under your shoulder-blade on the side you are examining. This helps to spread the breast tissue so that it is easier to examine.

Use your right hand to examine your left breast and vice versa. Put the hand you're not using under your head.

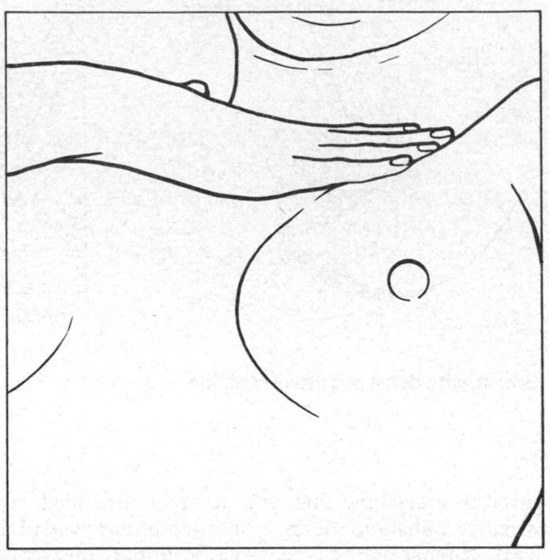

Keep your fingers together and use the flat of the fingers, not the tips.

Start from the collarbone above your breast.

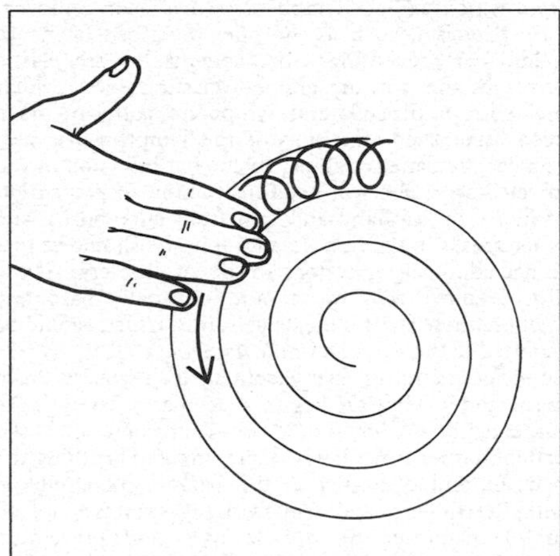

Trace a continuous spiral round your breast moving your fingers in small circles. Feel gently but firmly for any unusual lump or thickening.

Work right round the outside of your breast first. When you get back to your starting point, work round again in a slightly smaller circle, and so on. Keep on doing this until you have worked right up to the nipple. Make sure you cover every part of your breast.

You may find a ridge of firm tissue in a half-moon shape under your breast. This is quite normal. It is tissue that develops to help support your breast.

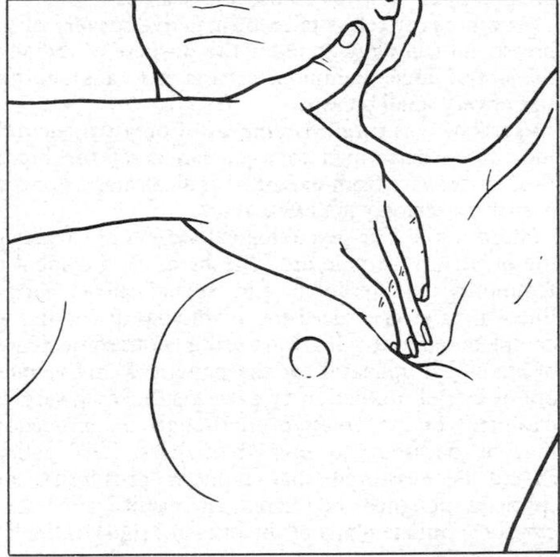

Finally, examine your armpit. Still use the flat of your fingers and the same small circular movements to feel for any lumps.

Start right up in the hollow of your armpit and gradually work your way down towards your breast.

It's important not to forget this last part of the examination.

LOOKING

When you examine your breasts you're looking for anything that's unusual. For this, looking is just as important as feeling.

Undress to the waist and sit or stand in front of a mirror in a good light. When you look at your breasts, remember that no two are the same – not even your own two. One will probably be slightly larger than the other, and one a little lower on the chest.

Here's what to look for:

- ☐ any change in the size of either breast
- ☐ any change in either nipple
- ☐ bleeding or discharge from either nipple
- ☐ any unusual dimple or puckering on the breast or nipple
- ☐ veins standing out more than is usual for you.

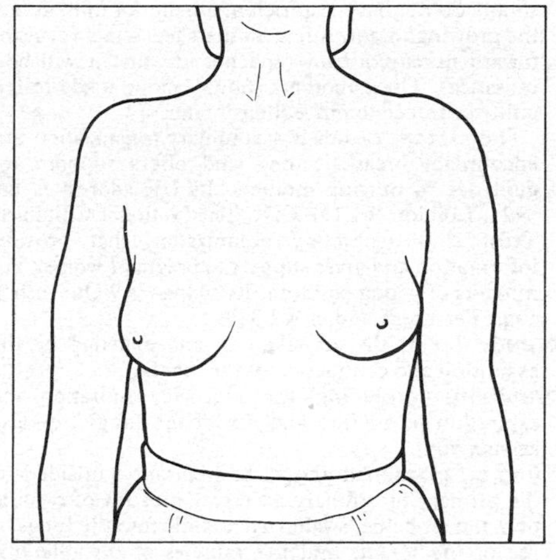

1. First let your arms hang loosely by your sides and look at your breasts in the mirror.

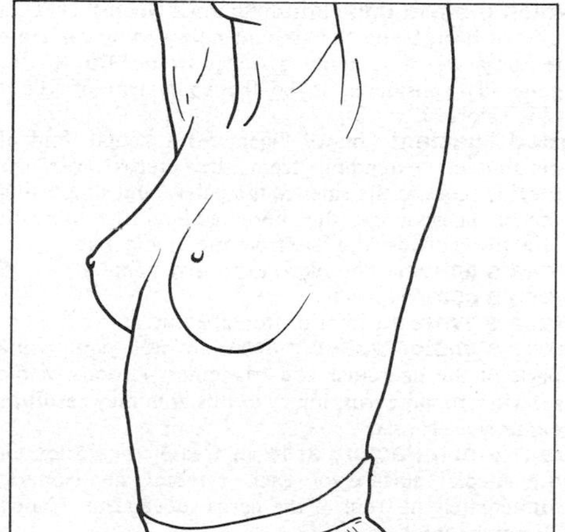

2. Next raise your arms above your head. Watch in the mirror as you turn from side to side to see your breasts from different angles.

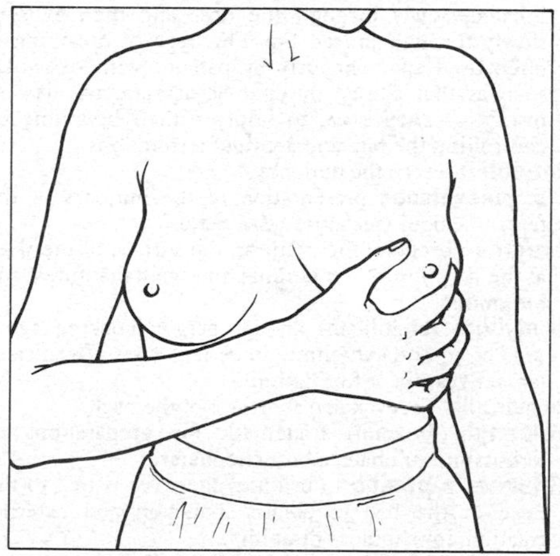

3. Now look down at your breasts and squeeze each nipple gently to check for any bleeding or discharge that's unusual for you.

than are babies given a formula containing cow's milk. Also, it is believed that breast feeding and the restriction of semisolid foods during the first 4–6 months of life help prevent the development of food allergies.

Most unbiased studies of the nutritional state of growing infants and children living in the developed countries show no significant differences between breast-fed and bottle-fed babies. However, in the underdeveloped countries, where sanitation is poor and community water, milk, and food supplies are likely to be contaminated, breast-fed babies have a significantly lower mortality rate.

For the mother, nursing causes contraction of the muscles of the uterus, bringing about its rapid return to normal size after birth. Suckling also strengthens the emotional bond between the mother and child. Breast feeding is also more economical than bottle feeding.

Another advantage of breast feeding is its contraceptive effect. When an infant suckles the breast, endocrinological effects result in lactation amenorrhoea, or failure to menstruate. This occurs *only* when breast milk is the sole source of food for the infant and breast feeding is done throughout the entire day on 'demand-feeding'.

Some women feel that breast feeding is more convenient than bottle feeding, while others are not willing or able to change their life styles to accommodate the schedule of breast feeding. Other mothers simply do not have a sufficient amount of milk to feed the growing infant. A few mothers feel a real revulsion toward nursing a baby (and not just that it will be a nuisance). These mothers should not be made to feel guilty or forced to nurse their infants.

The LALECHE LEAGUE is a voluntary organization that encourages breast feeding and offers support and guidance to nursing mothers. Its UK address is BM 3424, London WC1N 3XX. The National Childbirth Trust is as voluntary organization that provides information and gives support to pregnant women and mothers of young children. Its address is 9 Queensborough Terrace, London W2 3TB.

breath (breth) the air taken in and expelled by the expansion and contraction of the thorax.

breathing ('breedhing) the alternate inspiration and expiration of air into and out of the lungs (see also RESPIRATION).

frog b., glossopharyngeal b. respiration unaided by the primary or ordinary accessory muscles of respiration, the air being 'swallowed' rapidly into the lungs by use of the tongue and the muscles of the pharynx; used by patients with chronic muscle paralysis to augment their vital capacity.

intermittent positive pressure b. (IPPB) see INTERMITTENT positive pressure ventilation.

pursed-lip b. a breathing technique in which air is inhaled slowly through the nose and then exhaled slowly through pursed lip. This type of breathing is often used spontaneously by patients with DYSPNOEA, such as that caused by CHRONIC OBSTRUCTIVE AIRWAYS DISEASE or EMPHYSEMA, to improve their breathing by controlling the rate and depth of respirations.

breech (breech) the buttocks.

b. presentation presentation of the buttocks of the fetus in labour (see also PRESENTATION).

bregma ('bregmə) the point on the surface of the skull at the junction of the coronal and sagittal sutures. adj. **bregmatic.**

bretylium (bre'tili·əm) an adrenergic blocking agent used as an antiarrhythmic in certain cases of ventricular tachycardia or fibrillation.

brevicollis (,brevi'kolis) shortness of the neck.

Bricanyl ('brikənil) trademark for preparations of terbutaline sulphate, a bronchodilator.

Brickner's position ('briknəz) the wrist is tied to the head of the bed to obtain abduction and external rotation, for shoulder disability.

bridge (brij) 1. a dental prosthesis bearing one or more artificial teeth attached to adjacent natural teeth. 2. pons. 3. a protoplasmic structure uniting adjacent elements of a cell, similar in plants and animals.

disulphide b. disulphide bond.

fixed b. one retained with crowns or inlays cemented to the natural teeth.

removable b. one retained by attachments which permit its removal.

Brietal ('brie·ətal) trademark for a preparation of methohexitone sodium, an ultrashort-acting barbiturate.

Bright's disease (briets) a broad descriptive term once used for kidney disease with proteinuria, usually glomerulonephritis. The name Bright's disease is derived from a description of the diseases published in 1827 by Richard Bright, an English physician.

Brill's disease (brilz) recrudescent typhus.

Brill–Symmers disease (,bril'siməz) giant follicular lymphadenopathy.

Brill–Zinsser disease (,bril'zinsə) recrudescent typhus.

brilliant green and crystal violet paint ('brili·ənt) an antiseptic made from aniline dyes. It consists of 0.5% *brilliant green* and 0.5% *crystal violet* in alcohol. Both skin and linen are badly stained by it.

brim (brim) the edge of the superior strait of the pelvis.

Briquet's syndrome ('brikayz) chronic multiple complaint syndrome in which patients present repeatedly with numerous different bodily complaints and in whom there is little evidence of significant physical illness and a marked tendency to chronicity. The symptoms are essentially a form of hysterical conversion.

brisement (breez'monh) [Fr.] a crushing, especially the breaking up of an ankylosis.

British antilewisite ('british ,anti'looisiet) BAL; dimercaprol, a chelating agent used against poisoning with arsenic, gold, mercury, and certain other metals.

British National Formulary ('british 'nashən'l 'fawmuhlə·ree) a publication produced twice a year by the British Medical Association and The Pharmaceutical Society of Great Britain, containing details of nearly all the drugs currently available on prescription in the United Kingdom. Abbreviated BNF.

British Pharmacopoeia (,british ,fahməkə'peeə) list of 'official' drugs which is published by HM Stationery Office on behalf of the Health Minister. The drugs are listed on the recommendations of the Medicines Commission in accordance with the Medicines Act 1968. Abbreviated BP.

British thermal unit ('british 'thərməl 'yoonit) BTU, a unit of heat, being the amount necessary to raise the temperature of 1 pound of water from 39 to 40 °F, generally considered to be the equivalent of 1053J (252 calories).

broad ligament (,brawd 'ligəmənt) a double fold of peritoneum extending from the uterus over the uterine tubes to the sides of the pelvis, and supporting the blood vessels to the uterus and uterine tubes. It effectively divides the fore from the hind pelvis.

Broca's aphasia ('brohkəz) expressive aphasia.

Broca's centre speech centre.

Broca's gyrus the inferior frontal gyrus.

Broca's motor speech area an area comprising parts of the opercular and triangular portions of the inferior frontal gyrus; injury to this area may result in expressive APHASIA.

Broca's parolfactory area an area of the cortex on the medial surface of each cerebral hemisphere, immediately in front of the gyrus subcallosus. Called also *area subcallosa.*

Brock syndrome (brok) middle lobe syndrome.

Brodie's abscess (,brohdiz) a chronic abscess of bone, usually the head of the tibia, caused by prolonged staphylococcal infection.

Brodmann's areas ('brodmanz) specific occipital and preoccipital areas of the cerebral cortex, distinguished by differences in the arrangement of their six cellular layers, and identified by number. They are considered to be the seat of specific functions of the brain.

bromelain ('brohmə,layn) any of a group of proteolytic and milk-clotting enzymes derived from the pineapple plant, *Ananas sativus.* In the plural, a concentrate of these enzymes, used as an anti-inflammatory agent. Also used in tenderizing meat, preparing protein hydrolysates, and chill-proofing beer.

bromhexine (,brom'hekseen) a mucolytic available as an elixir, tablets and an injection.

bromhidrosis (,bromhi'drohsis) the secretion of foul-smelling perspiration.

bromide ('brohmied) any binary compound of bromine. Bromides produce depression of the central nervous system, and were once widely used for their sedative effect. Because overdosage causes serious mental disturbances they are now seldom used.

bromidrosis (,bromi'drohsis) bromhidrosis.

bromine ('brohmeen) a chemical element, atomic number 35, atomic weight 79.909, symbol Br. See table of elements in Appendix 2.

brominism ('brohminizəm) poisoning by excessive use of bromine or its compounds. This condition occurs when the bromine concentration in the body fluids is high enough to have a toxic and depressant action on the central nervous system. The toxic level varies with each individual and is also somewhat dependent on chloride intake because the bromide ion and the chloride ion are equally absorbed and distributed throughout the same fluid compartments. This means that in a person with a limited salt intake bromine accumulates more quickly and severe poisoning can occur after ingestion of an amount of bromine that would be relatively harmless for a person with a normal or high salt intake.

Many cases of brominism result from indiscriminate use of patent medicines advertised as 'nerve tonics' and 'headache remedies' containing bromide. The early symptoms may be similar to the symptoms for which the patient is taking the patent medicine, and correct diagnosis and treatment of the condition may be delayed. The symptoms of bromine poisoning include acne, coldness of arms and legs, fetid breath, sleeplessness, impotence, headache, irritability, emotional instability, malaise, and mental aberrations such as hallucinations, amnesia, and disorientation.

Treatment consists of immediate curtailment of bromine ingestion and efforts to eliminate the substance from the body. Mercurial diuretics aid in bromine removal. Enteric-coated tablets of ammonium and sodium chloride are prescribed if they are not contraindicated by cardiac or renal disease. The removal of bromine from the system may take as long as several months. In severe, acute poisoning the bromine may be removed by HAEMODIALYSIS.

When an emotional disturbance or mental illness is the primary cause of brominism, psychotherapy is indicated.

bromocriptine (,brohmoh'kripteen) a dopamine agonist, a derivative of ergot alkaloids used to inhibit prolactin secretion. It may be used to suppress lactation. It also raises serum growth hormone levels in normal persons, but lowers them in persons with acromegaly.

bromoderma (,brohmoh'dərmə) a skin eruption due to use of bromides.

bromomania (,brohmoh'mayni·ə) a mental disorder induced by misuse of bromides.

bromomenorrhoea (,brohmoh,menə'reeə) menstruation characterized by an offensive odour.

brompheniramine (,bromfe'nrə,meen) a pyridine derivative used as an antihistamine in the form of the maleate salt.

Brompton Cocktail ('bromptən 'koktayl) name given to mixtures containing various combinations of morphine, diamorphine and cocaine. These mixtures often also contained gin and/or chlorpromazine. They were used in the relief of pain in terminal care. They have now been replaced by a simple solution of morphine in chloroform water.

bronchadenitis (,brongkadə'nietis) inflammation of the bronchial glands.

bronchi ('brongkee) plural of *bronchus*.

bronchial ('brongki·əl) pertaining to or affecting one or more bronchi.

b. asthma asthma.

b. calculus a hard concretion formed in a bronchus by accretion about an inorganic nucleus or from calcified portions of lung tissue or adjacent lymph nodes.

b. spasm bronchospasm.

b. tree the bronchi and their branching structures.

bronchiarctia (,brongki'ahkshi·ə) bronchostenosis.

bronchiectasis (,brongki'ektəsis) chronic dilation of the bronchi and bronchioles with secondary infection, usually involving the lower lobes of the lung. The condition may occur as a congenital malformation of the alveoli with resultant dilation of the terminal bronchi. Most often it is an acquired disease secondary to partial obstruction of the bronchi with necrotizing infection. Primary diseases leading to bronchiectasis include chronic sinusitis, allergy, whooping cough, pneumonia, influenza, tuberculosis, and lung tumour. The presence of a foreign body in the respiratory tract can produce bronchiectasis.

SYMPTOMS. The most immediate symptom of bronchiectasis is persistent coughing. The coughing may be mild, often occurring when the patient first gets up in the morning. In severe cases, the coughing becomes more violent as the walls of the bronchial tubes thicken and secrete quantities of mucus. The muscles may become so weak that even violent coughing fails to expel the mucus. Pus may also be secreted, and the cilia destroyed. In advanced cases the sputum and breath may become foul-smelling, and the patient may suffer loss of appetite, anaemia, fever, intermittent attacks of pneumonia, and a general lowering of resistance to infection.

TREATMENT. To maintain the strength and general health of the patient, fresh air and sunshine, a good diet, and plenty of rest are essential. A move to a mild climate may be of great benefit. Cigarette smoking should be stopped. If the disease is fairly well localized, it may be relieved by surgery. Penicillin or other antibiotics are sometimes useful, particularly in controlling other infections, which may weaken the patient and further lower his resistance.

Long-term care is essentially the same as for any patient with CHRONIC OBSTRUCTIVE AIRWAYS DISEASE.

bronchiloquy (brong'kilə,kwee) high-pitched pectoriloquy due to lung consolidation.

bronchiocele ('brongkioh,seel) dilation or swelling of a bronchiole.

bronchiogenic (,brongkioh'jenik) bronchogenic.

bronchiole ('brongki,ohl) one of the successively smaller channels into which the segmental bronchi divide within the bronchopulmonary segments. adj. **bronchiolar.**

respiratory b. the final branch of a bronchiole, communicating directly with the alveolar ducts; a subdivision of a terminal bronchiole, it has alveolar outcroppings and itself divides into several alveolar ducts.

bronchiolectasis (,brongkioh'lektəsis) dilation of the bronchioles.

bronchiolitis (,brongkioh'lietis) inflammation of the bronchioles; bronchopneumonia.

acute obliterating b. cirrhosis of the lung due to hardening of the walls of the bronchioles.

b. exudativa, exudative b. inflammation of the bronchioles with exudation of Curschmann's spirals (coiled mucinous fibrils) and grey, tenacious sputum; often associated with asthma.

b. fibrosa obliterans bronchiolitis marked by ingrowth of connective tissue from the wall of the terminal bronchi, with occlusion of their lumina.

vesicular b. bronchopneumonia.

bronchiolus (,brongki'ohləs) pl. *bronchioli* [L.] bronchiole.

bronchiospasm ('brongkioh,spazəm) bronchospasm.

bronchiostenosis (ˌbrongkiohstəˈnohsis) bronchostenosis.

bronchitis (brongˈkietis) inflammation of one or more bronchi. adj. **bronchitic.** Bronchitis may be either an acute or chronic disorder and frequently involves the trachea as well as the bronchi (tracheobronchitis). The acute stage of the disease often is an extension of an upper respiratory infection which is usually viral in origin. Causes other than infectious agents are physical and chemical irritants that are inhaled in air polluted by dust, car exhaust fumes, industrial fumes, and tobacco smoke.

ACUTE BRONCHITIS. Acute bronchitis is most often encountered in small children and in the elderly or the debilitated. It is particularly serious in infants and small children because their bronchi are smaller and more easily obstructed. The elderly and debilitated are prime targets for complications of bronchitis because they are more susceptible to secondary infections.

Symptoms of acute bronchitis include the early symptoms of an upper respiratory infection or common cold, which progress to chest pain, fever, and a dry, irritating cough. Later the cough becomes more productive of mucopurulent to purulent sputum. There may be moderate fever with accompanying chills, muscle soreness, and headache.

The condition is treated conservatively, with antibiotics being administered only as indicated by a positive sputum culture. Symptoms may be relieved through the use of humidifying devices that produce either warm or cool moist air, cough mixtures and AEROSOLS to reduce coughing and soothe the irritated tracheal and bronchial mucosa, and bed rest to promote healing and minimize the effects of the inflammation. Fluids are forced and a well-balanced bland diet is recommended.

Acute bronchitis and tracheobronchitis require a period of convalescence to avoid development of a chronic condition. Although the disease in its acute form occurs most often in the winter months, repeated bouts indicate a chronic bronchitis.

CHRONIC BRONCHITIS. This condition is characterized by increased secretion from the bronchial mucosa and obstruction of the respiratory passages. It is a stubborn disease that interferes with the flow of air to and from the lungs, causes shortness of breath, induces persistent coughing and expectoration, breeds infection, and causes necrosis and fibrosis of the respiratory tract.

The symptoms and treatment of chronic bronchitis are the same as those of any CHRONIC OBSTRUCTIVE AIRWAYS DISEASE. There is no cure for the disorder and its management requires long-range planning involving patient education and cooperation in carrying out the prescribed regimen.

bronchoadenitis (ˌbrongkohˌadəˈnietis) inflammation of bronchial glands.

bronchocandidiasis (ˌbrongkohˌkandiˈdieəsis) candidiasis of the respiratory tree, occurring in a mild afebrile form manifested as chronic bronchitis, and in a usually fatal form resembling tuberculosis.

bronchocavernous (ˌbrongkohkavˈərnəs) both bronchial and cavitary.

bronchocele (ˈbrongkohˌseel) localized dilation of a bronchus.

bronchoconstriction (ˌbrongkohkənˈstrikshən) bronchostenosis.

bronchoconstrictor (ˌbrongkohkənˈstriktə) 1. narrowing the lumina of the air passages of the lungs. 2. an agent that causes such constriction.

bronchodilation (ˌbrongkohˌdielyshən) a dilated state of a bronchus, or the site at which a bronchus is dilated.

bronchodilator (ˌbrongkohdieˈlaytə) 1. expanding the lumina of the air passages of the lungs. 2. an agent that causes dilation of the bronchi.

The most commonly used class of drugs are the sympathomimetic amines, which are used in the management of ASTHMA and COAD where BRONCHOSPASM is prominent. Although adrenaline and isoprenaline are still used occasionally in the management of acute bronchospasm, they have both been largely superseded by the more safe and effective selective β_2-adrenoceptor stimulants, for example salbutamol or terbutaline. These agents are generally available in various forms for administration: in pressurized aerosols for inhalation, as solution which can be nebulized, in tablet form for oral medication, or for parenteral use in severe attacks.

Atropine-like agents, e.g. Atrovent, and the theophylline derivatives have different modes of action and are often used in combination with β-sympathomimetic agents.

bronchofibrescope (ˌbrongkohˈfieboˌskohp) a flexible bronchoscope utilizing fibreoptics.

bronchofibroscopy (ˌbrongkohfieˈbroskəpee) examination of the bronchi through a bronchofibrescope.

bronchogenic (ˌbrongkohˈjenik) originating in the bronchi.

bronchogram (ˈbrongkohˌgram) the film obtained by bronchography.

bronchography (brongˈkografee) radiography of the lungs after instillation of an opaque medium into the bronchi.

broncholith (ˈbrongkohlith) a bronchial calculus.

broncholithiasis (ˌbrongkohliˈthieəsis) a condition in which calculi are present within the lumen of the tracheobronchial tree.

bronchology (brongˈkoləjee) the study and treatment of diseases of the tracheobronchial tree. adj. **bronchological.**

bronchomalacia (ˌbrongkohməˈlayshi·ə) a deficiency in the cartilaginous wall of the trachea or a bronchus that may lead to atelectasis or obstructive emphysema.

bronchomoniliasis (ˌbrongkohˌmoniˈlieəsis) bronchocandidiasis.

bronchomotor (ˌbrongkohˈmohtə) affecting the calibre of the bronchi.

bronchomucotropic (ˌbrongkohˌmyookohˈtropik) augmenting secretion by the respiratory mucosa.

bronchomycosis (ˌbrongkohmieˈkohsis) an industrial disease chiefly affecting agricultural workers, stablemen, etc., and due to inhalation of microfungi which infect the air passages. Causes can be *Actinomyces* or *Aspergillus* species. Symptoms are similar to those of pulmonary tuberculosis.

broncho-oesophageal (ˌbrongkoh·iˌsofəˈjeeəl) pertaining to or communicating with a bronchus and the oesophagus.

broncho-oesophagology (ˌbrongkoh·iˌsofəˈgoləˌjee) the branch of medicine concerned with the air passages (bronchi) and oesophagus.

broncho-oesophagoscopy (ˌbrongkoh·iˌsofəˈgoskəpee) instrumental examination of the bronchi and oesophagus.

bronchopancreatic (ˌbrongkohˌpangkriˈatik) communicating with a bronchus and the pancreas, as in a bronchopancreatic fistula.

bronchopathy (brongˈkopəthee) any disease of the bronchi.

bronchophony (brongˈkofənee) the sound of the voice as heard through the stethoscope applied over a healthy bronchus. Heard elsewhere, it indicates solidification of the lung tissue.

pectoriloquous b. that which is accompanied by the

sound of the voice through the chest wall.

whispered b. that which is heard while the patient is whispering.

bronchoplasty ('brongkoh,plastee) plastic surgery of a bronchus; surgical closure of a bronchial fistula.

bronchoplegia (,brongkoh'pleeji·ə) paralysis of the muscles of the walls of the bronchial tubes.

bronchopleural (,brongkoh'plooə·rəl) pertaining to a bronchus and the pleura, or communicating with a bronchus and the pleural cavity.

bronchopneumonia (,brongkohnyoo'mohni·ə) inflammation of the bronchi and lungs, usually beginning in the terminal bronchioles (see also PNEUMONIA).

bronchopneumopathy (,brongkohnyoo'mopəthee) disease of the bronchi and lung tissue.

bronchopulmonary (,brongkoh'pulmənə·ree, -'puhl-) pertaining to the bronchi and lungs.

b. segment one of the smaller divisions of the lobe of a lung, separated from others by a connective tissue septum and supplied by its own branch of the bronchus leading to the particular lobe.

bronchorrhagia (,brongkoh'rayji·ə) haemorrhage from the bronchi.

bronchorrhaphy (brong'ko·rəfee) suture of a bronchus.

bronchorrhoea (,brongkə'reeə) excessive discharge of mucus from the bronchi.

bronchoscope ('brongkoh,skohp) an endoscope especially designed for passage through the trachea to permit inspection of the interior of the tracheobronchial tree and carrying out of endobronchial diagnostic and therapeutic manoeuvres, such as taking specimens for culture and biopsy and removing foreign bodies. adj. **bronchosopic.**

fibreoptic b. bronchofibrescope.

bronchoscopy (brong'koskə,pee) inspection of the interior of the tracheobronchial tree through a bronchoscope. Bronchoscopy is used as a diagnostic and therapeutic aid.

As an aid to diagnosis the bronchoscope allows visualization of the bronchial mucosa and removal of tissue for biopsy. Bronchial washings and collection of secretions are done at the time of bronchoscopy to obtain samples for culture and cytological examination. Therapeutically, the bronchoscope permits removal of foreign bodies that have been aspirated into the bronchial tree and also may be used to facilitate suctioning of the lower airway. The latter technique is done at the bedside and anaesthesia is not considered necessary.

If the fibreoptic bronchoscope is used at the bedside as an adjunct to bronchial hygiene and removal of secretions, it should be used only by personnel who have been trained in the technique. It has the advantage of allowing for precise suctioning with less trauma to the respiratory tract, because it is possible to visualize the areas needing suctioning and to reach lower segments not accessible to the larger suction catheter.

PATIENT CARE. Bronchoscopy requires preparation and instruction of the patient in regard to the purpose of the procedure, what he can expect to be done, and how he may cooperate during the procedure. A topical anaesthetic is used most often, but in some cases the patient may have general anaesthesia.

Food and fluids are withheld for 8 hours before bronchoscopy is performed. The patient should brush his teeth and wash out his mouth carefully before the procedure to lessen the danger of introducing bacteria from the mouth into the bronchi. Dentures are removed and any loose teeth are brought to the attention of the doctor. A mild sedative may be given prior to the bronchoscopy. This medication plus instructions to the patient and a full explanation of what is going to be done will help him relax and make the passing of the bronchoscope into the bronchi easier and less traumatic.

After bronchoscopy, fluids and food are withheld until the effects of the local anaesthetic have worn off and the gag reflex has returned completely. The patient must be observed for signs of bleeding from the throat and respiratory embarrassment. Since swelling of the larynx may necessitate a TRACHEOSTOMY, the equipment should be readily at hand. The patient should be kept quiet and discouraged from talking or coughing.

Potential problems following bronchoscopy include arterial hypoxaemia, bleeding, pneumothorax, bronchial and laryngeal spasm, and anaphylactic reaction to anaesthetic drugs.

Bronchospasm and laryngeal spasm necessitate the intravenous administration of medications such as prednisolone and aminophylline. If an intravenous line was not established before the procedure, the equipment should be at the bedside in case it is needed. Indications that bronchospasm is occurring include pallor, respiratory distress, and an elevation of the pulse rate and rate of respirations.

Supplementary oxygen is needed if arterial BLOOD GAS ANALYSIS indicates a drop in the $P_{a}O_2$. Blood gases should be monitored before and after the procedure, because hypoxaemia can occur at either time. The amount and character of the sputum should be observed in case bleeding occurs, especially when a biopsy has been done during bronchoscopy. A foul-smelling, purulent sputum in the postoperative period probably indicates an infection. A sputum culture for bacteria and an antibiotic sensitivity test are then commonly ordered.

Pneumothorax is not a common complication of bronchoscopy; should it occur, a thoracotomy tube must be inserted as soon as possible to allow for reexpansion of the lung. A trocar thoracic kit should be readily available.

fibreoptic b. bronchofibroscopy.

bronchospasm ('brongkoh,spazəm) bronchial spasm; spasmodic contraction of the muscular coat of the smaller divisions of the bronchi, such as occurs in asthma.

bronchospirography (,brongkohspie'rogrəfee) the recording of bronchospirometry results.

bronchospirometry (,brongkohspie'romətree) determination of vital capacity, oxygen intake, and carbon dioxide excretion of a single lung, or simultaneous measurements of the function of each lung separately.

differential b. measurement of the function of each lung separately.

bronchostaxis (,brongkoh'staksis) bleeding from the bronchial wall.

bronchostenosis (,brongkohstə'nohsis) stricture or cicatricial diminution of the calibre of a bronchial tube.

spasmodic b. a spasmodic contraction of the walls of the bronchi.

bronchostomy (brong'kostəmee) surgical creation of an opening through the chest wall into the bronchus.

bronchotomy (brong'kotəmee) incision of a bronchus.

bronchotracheal (,brongkoh'traki·əl, -trə'keeəl) pertaining to the bronchi and trachea.

bronchovesicular (,brongkohve'sikyuhlə) pertaining to the bronchi and alveoli.

bronchus ('brongkəs) pl. *bronchi* [L.] any of the larger passages conveying air to (right or left principal bronchus) and within the lungs (lobar and segmental bronchi). See also RESPIRATION.

bronze diabetes (bronz ˌdieə'beetis, -teez) a disorder of iron metabolism, with deposits of iron-containing pigments in the body tissues, bronze pigmentation of the skin, diabetes mellitus, and cirrhosis of the liver; called also *haemochromatosis* and *iron storage disease*.

brow (brow) the forehead, or either lateral half of it.

brown adipose tissue (brown 'adipohs) a special type of adipose tissue found in the newborn infant, and which is widely distributed throughout the body. The tissue is highly vascular and owes its colour to the large number of mitochondria found in the cytoplasm of its cells. It allows the infant to increase its metabolic rate and thus its heat production when subjected to cold. At the same time the fat itself is used up.

Brown-Séquard's syndrome (brown'saykahdz) paralysis and loss of discriminatory and joint sensation on one side of the body and of pain and temperature sensation on the other, due to a lesion involving one side of the spinal cord.

Brucella (broo'selə) a genus of bacteria.

B. abortus the causative agent of infectious abortion in cattle and the commonest cause of BRUCELLOSIS in man in the UK.

B. melitensis the causative agent of BRUCELLOSIS (UNDULANT FEVER), occurring primarily in goats and sheep as the reservoir of infection. Common in Mediterranean countries and some others.

B. suis a species found in swine that is capable of producing severe disease in man.

brucella (broo'selə) pl. *brucellae;* any member of the genus *Brucella.* adj. **brucellar**.

Brucellin (broo'selin) trademark for a solution of nucleoproteins derived from *Brucella*; used in a skin test for brucella infection.

brucellosis (ˌbroosi'lohsis) a generalized infection involving primarily the reticuloendothelial system, marked by remittent undulant fever, malaise, headache, and anaemia. It is caused by various species of *Brucella* and is transmitted to man from domestic animals such as pigs, goats, and cattle, especially through infected milk or contact with the carcass of an infected animal.

The disease is also called undulant fever because one of the major symptoms in man is a fever that fluctuates widely at regular intervals. The symptoms in the beginning stages are difficult to notice and include loss of weight and increased irritability. As the illness advances, headaches, chills, sweating, and muscle aches and pains appear. It is possible for these symptoms to persist for years, either intermittently or continuously, although most patients recover completely within 2 to 6 months. Diagnosis is confirmed by blood tests.

Treatment consists of bed rest, antibiotics, and a high intake of vitamins.

Prevention is best accomplished by the pasteurization of milk and a programme of testing, vaccination, and elimination of infected animals.

Brudzinski's sign (broo'jinskiz) 1. in meningitis, bending the patient's neck usually produces flexion of the knee and hip. 2. in meningitis, passive flexion of the lower limb on one side causes a similar movement in the opposite limb.

Brufen ('broofen) trademark for a preparation of ibuprofen; a nonsteroidal anti-inflammatory agent.

Brugia ('brooji·ə) a genus of filarial worms. **B. malayi** a species similar to, and often found in association with, *Wuchereria bancrofti*, which causes human filariasis and elephantiasis (usually below the knee only) throughout Southeast Asia, in countries bordering the China Sea, and in parts of India.

bruise (brooz) superficial discoloration due to haemorrhage into the tissues from ruptured blood vessels beneath the skin surface, without the skin itself being broken; called also CONTUSION.

bruit ('brooee) [Fr.] a sound or murmur heard in auscultation, especially an abnormal one (see SOUFFLE).

Brunner's glands ('bruhnəz) glands in the submucosa of the duodenum, opening into the glands of the small intestine; called also *duodenal glands*.

brush border (brush 'bawdə) a specialization of the free surface of a cell, consisting of minute cylindrical processes (microvilli) that greatly increase the surface area.

bruxism ('brooksizəm) gnashing, grinding, or clenching the teeth, usually during sleep. Repeated and continuous grinding of the teeth over a long period of time can wear down and loosen teeth and cause bone loss. Bruxism can also cause headache, muscle spasm, and chronic pain in the face and jaw.

Possible causes of bruxism include dental problems, such as malocclusion and high fillings, emotional problems associated with tension and anxiety, and intense concentration for a long period of time during which the person unknowingly tightens the jaw and grinds the teeth.

A dentist can diagnose bruxism and also correct the dental problem, if that is the cause, or prescribe and fit a night guard to protect the teeth during sleep. If stress is the underlying cause, methods to reduce tension and promote relaxation are sometimes helpful.

BS Bachelor of Surgery.

BSA body surface area.

BSc Bachelor of Science.

BSCC British Society of Clinical Cytology.

BSI British Standards Institute.

BSP sulphobromophthalein sodium, a dye formerly used in testing liver function.

BTA British Thoracic Association.

BTPS body temperature and pressure, saturated; denoting a volume of gas saturated with water vapour at 37 °C and ambient barometric pressure.

BTS Blood Transfusion Service.

BTU British thermal unit.

bubo ('byooboh) an enlarged and inflamed lymph node, particularly in the axilla or groin, resulting from absorption of infective material and occurring in various diseases, e.g., lymphogranuloma venereum, plague, syphilis, gonorrhoea, chancroid, and tuberculosis.

indolent b. a hard, nearly painless bubo that shows no tendency to break.

bubonalgia (ˌbyoobo'naji·ə) pain in the groin.

bubonic (byoo'bonik) characterized by or pertaining to buboes.

b. plague a severe infectious disease caused by the bacillus *Yersinia pestis* (previously classified as *Pasteurella pestis*) carried in infected rats and transmitted to man by the rat flea (see also PLAGUE).

bubonocele (byoo'bonəˌseel) inguinal or femoral hernia forming a swelling in the groin.

bucardia (byoo'kahdi·ə) extreme enlargement of the heart as in cor bovinum.

bucca ('bukə) [L.] *the cheek.*

buccal ('buk'l) pertaining to or directed toward the cheek.

buccinator ('buksiˌnaytə) a muscle of the cheek, between the mandible and the maxilla.

bucco- word element. [L.] *cheek*.

Buck's extension (buks) traction applied to a fractured leg by the use of weights, the foot of the bed being raised so that the body acts as countertraction.

buckling ('bukling) the process or an instance of

becoming crumpled or warped.

scleral b. a technique for repair of detachment of the retina, in which indentations or infoldings of the sclera are made over the tears in the retina so as to promote apposition and adherence of the retina to the overlying tissues.

buclizine ('byookli,zeen) an antihistamine, used mainly as an antinauseant in the management of motion sickness.

bucnaemia (buk'neemi·ə) diffuse, tense, inflammatory swelling of the leg.

bud (bud) a structure resembling the bud of a plant, especially a protuberance in the embryo from which an organ or part develops.

end b. the remnant of the embryonic primitive knot, from which arises the caudal part of the trunk.

limb b. one of the four lateral swellings appearing in vertebrate embryos, which develop into the two pairs of limbs.

tail b. 1. the primordium of the caudal appendage. 2. end bud.

taste b's end organs of the gustatory nerves containing the receptor surfaces for the sense of TASTE.

ureteric b. an outgrowth of the mesonephric duct giving rise to all but the nephrons of the permanent kidney.

b. of urethra bulb of urethra.

Budd–Chiari syndrome (,budki'ahri) a condition in which thrombosis of the hepatic vein(s) causes vomiting, jaundice, enlargement of the liver and ascites.

budding ('buding) gemmation; asexual reproduction in which a portion of the cell body is thrust out and then becomes separated, forming a new individual.

budesonide (,byoo'desənied) a corticosteroid used in a metered-dose inhaler for the treatment of bronchial asthma.

Buerger–Allen exercises (,bərgə'alən) specific exercises intended to improve circulation to the feet and legs. The lower extremities are elevated to a 45 to 90 degree angle and supported in this position until the skin blanches (appears dead white). The feet and legs are then lowered below the level of the rest of the body until redness appears (care should be taken that there is no pressure against the back of the knees); finally, the legs are placed flat on the bed for a few minutes. The length of time for each position varies with the patient's tolerance and the speed with which colour change occurs. Usually the exercises are prescribed so that the legs are elevated for 2 to 3 minutes, down for 5 to 10 minutes, and then flat on the bed for 10 minutes.

Buerger's disease ('bərgəz) a disease affecting the medium-sized blood vessels, particularly the arteries of the legs, which can cause severe pain and in serious cases lead to gangrene; called also *thromboangiitis obliterans*, a term that refers to the clotting, pain, and inflammation occurring in this disease and to the fact that it can obliterate, or destroy, blood vessels.

The cause of this violent reaction has been thought to be excessive use of tobacco over a long period of time. The number of cases has diminished strikingly in recent years.

The intense pain that is a symptom of the disease is caused by the formation of blood clots, or THROMBOSIS, in the lining of the arterial blood vessels.

When the clots grow larger, the blood flow slows and may stop entirely. Since every part of the body depends on the continuous flow of blood, affected areas such as fingers and toes, for example, soon begin to atrophy or develop ulcers. If the causes of the disease are not completely arrested, amputation may be necessary.

To treat the disease, the patient must stop smoking at once and entirely. This generally results in the partial healing of the affected membrane with a renewed flow of blood. However, more blood may have to be brought to damaged tissue by surgical methods of channelling detours or making canals in the clot itself.

Special exercises called BUERGER–ALLEN EXERCISES are sometimes used to empty the engorged blood vessels and stimulate collateral circulation. These exercises can be done at home by the patient and are usually prescribed to be done several times during the day. The patient is also instructed to avoid wearing any tight clothing, such as tight girdles, garters, constricting belts, and other items that may impair circulation. He should also avoid sitting or standing in one position for long periods of time. Care should be used in the selection of shoes and stockings so that they fit properly and do not cause pressure against the blood vessels. The patient should be told to avoid walking barefoot or otherwise subjecting himself to the hazards of trauma to the feet and legs. Should such an accident occur, no matter how minor it may seem, he must notify the doctor so that treatment may be begun and infection and ulceration can be prevented.

buffer ('bufə) 1. a physical or physiological system which tends to oppose change within that system, e.g. the reflexes involved in blood pressure homeostasis. 2. a chemical system that acts to prevent change in the concentration of another chemical substance. The most important chemical buffers in physiological systems are those which oppose changes in pH by means of accepting or donating protons.

bicarbonate b. this is the principal buffering system in the blood and involves the bicarbonate ion and carbon

$$HCO_3^- + H^+ \rightleftharpoons H_2CO_3 \rightleftharpoons CO_2 + H_2O$$

dioxide:

phosphate b. an important buffering system regulating pH in the renal tubules:

$$HPO^{2-} + H^+ \rightleftharpoons H_2PO_4^-$$

buffy coat ('bufee) reddish-grey layer observed above packed red cells in centrifuged blood.

buggery ('bugə·ree) anal intercourse, either heterosexual or homosexual. In law the term also includes sexual contact with an animal.

bulb (bulb) a rounded mass or enlargement. adj. **bulbar.**

b. of aorta the enlargement of the aorta at its point of origin from the heart.

auditory b. the membranous labyrinth and cochlea.

b. of eye the eyeball.

gustatory b's taste buds.

hair b. the bulbous expansion at the proximal end of a hair, in which the hair shaft is generated.

Krause's b's end-bulbs.

olfactory b. the bulblike expansion of the olfactory tract on the under surface of the frontal lobe of each cerebral hemisphere.

b. of penis bulb of urethra.

taste b's taste buds.

b. of urethra the enlarged proximal part of the corpus spongiosum.

b. of vestibule, vestibulovaginal b. a body consisting of paired masses of erectile tissue, situated one on either side of the vaginal orifice.

bulbar ('bulbə) pertaining to a bulb; pertaining to or involving the medulla oblongata, as bulbar paralysis.

bulbiform ('bulbi,fawm) bulb-shaped.

bulbitis (bul'bietis) inflammation of the bulb of the urethra.

bulbourethral (ˌbulbohyuh'reethrəl) pertaining to the bulb of the urethra.

b. glands two glands embedded in the substance of the sphincter of the male urethra, just posterior to the membranous part of the urethra. Their secretion, which is slippery and viscous, lubricates the urethra. Called also bulbocavernous glands and Cowper's glands.

bulbous ('bulbəs) having the form or nature of a bulb; bearing or arising from a bulb.

bulbus ('bulbəs) pl. *bulbi* [L.] bulb.

bulimia (byoo'limi·ə) abnormal increase in the sensation of hunger. adj. **bulimic**.

b. nervosa a pattern of 'binge eating', or episodes of uncontrolled and compulsive overeating occurring in response to stress. Bulimic 'binges' often occur in anorexia nervosa.

bulla ('buhlə) pl. *bullae* [L.] a blister; a circumscribed, fluid-containing, elevated lesion of the skin, usually more than 5 mm in diameter. adj. **bullate, bullous**.

Buller's shield ('buhləz) a type of protection placed over one eye when the other is infected. A watch glass is placed over the eye and fixed with adhesive strapping. Now rarely used.

bullosis (buh'lohsis) the production of, or a condition characterized by, bullous lesions.

bumetanide (byoo'metəˌnied) a diuretic drug which prevents the resorption of urine from Henle's loop in the renal tubule.

BUN blood urea nitrogen (see UREA NITROGEN).

bundle ('bund'l) a collection of fibres or strands, as of muscle fibres, or a fasciculus or band of nerve fibres.

atrioventricular b. bundle of His.

fundamental b., ground b. that part of the white matter of the spinal cord bordering the grey matter and containing fibres that travel for a distance of only a few segments of the cord.

b. of His a band of cardiac muscle connecting the atria with the ventricles of the heart; called also *atrioventricular bundle*.

Keith's b. a bundle of fibres in the wall of the atrium of the heart between the venae cavae.

medial forebrain b. a group of nerve fibres connecting the midbrain tegmentum and elements of the limbic system.

sinoatrial b. Keith's bundle.

b. of Vicq d'Azyr a band of fibres from the mamillary body to the anterior nucleus of the thalamus.

bundle branch ('bund'l ˌbrahnsh) a branch of the bundle of His.

bunion ('bunyən) an abnormal prominence on the inner aspect of the first metatarsal head, with bursal formation, and lateral or valgus displacement of the great toe. Bunions can be caused by congenital malformation of the bony structure of the foot or by joint disease such as rheumatoid arthritis, but they are most often caused by wearing shoes with pointed toes, especially ones that are high-heeled and too short. When the shoes do not fit properly they force the great toe toward the outer side of the foot. The result is continued pressure on the joint where the great toe articulates with the first metatarsal head. Chronic irritation causes a build-up of soft tissue and underlying bone in the area. Symptoms are swelling, redness, and pain.

Mild cases can be relieved by changing to properly fitting shoes. If there is severe pain making ambulation difficult or impossible, anti-inflammatory agents may be effective. Surgical correction (*bunionectomy*) is indicated when all other measures fail.

bunionectomy (ˌbunyə'nektəmee) excision of a bunion.

bunionette (ˌbunyə'net) enlargement of the lateral aspect of the fifth metatarsal head.

BUPA ('boopə, 'byoopə) British United Provident Association.

buphthalmos (buf'thalməs) abnormal enlargement of the eyes in congenital GLAUCOMA.

bupivacaine (byoo'pivəˌkayn) a local anaesthetic used for peripheral nerve block, infiltration, and sympathetic, caudal, or epidural block. It is a member of the amide group of local anaesthetics and has a long duration of action.

burette, buret (byuh'ret) a glass tube with a capacity of the order of 25 to 100 ml and graduation intervals of 0.05 to 0.1 ml, with stopcock attachment, used to deliver an accurately measured quantity of liquid.

Burinex K (ˌbyooə·rineks 'kay) trademark for a combination of a loop diuretic with potassium.

Burkitt's lymphoma (tumour) (bərkits) a form of undifferentiated malignant lymphoma, usually found in central Africa, but also reported from other areas, and manifested most often as a large osteolytic lesion in the jaw or as an abdominal mass; called also *African lymphoma*.

The Epstein–Barr virus (EB virus), a herpesvirus, has been isolated from Burkitt's lymphoma cells in culture, and has been implicated as a causative agent.

burn (bərn) injury to tissues caused by exposure of the body surface to temperatures greater than 45 °C. A variety of skin surface lesions can occur and in some instances deeper structures may be involved. Whilst irreversible cell damage occurs at higher temperatures (60–70 °C), different severities of injury occur in the temperature range 45–55 °C. Cell recovery in the lower range depends upon the duration of exposure to the heat source as well as the intensity of heat. For example, greater destruction to skin will occur in a patient who is in contact with a hot radiator for 1 hour compared with contact for 5 minutes. In addition the intense heat from flame burns causes greater cell destruction than burns caused by scalding with hot water.

Although damage or destruction to the skin from heat is usually called a burn, different terms are sometimes used. *Thermal injury* is usually used to describe injuries resulting from dry heat (flame burns, contact with hot objects) as well as injuries from steam or liquid (scalds). There are numerous causes of tissue destruction from burning (burns and scalds) in both adults and children, but many injuries are common to certain age groups. In infancy and early childhood, scalds are the most common injuries seen. These injuries occur in the home and are caused by spillage of hot beverages, pulling the flex of boiling kettles, and falls into boiling bathwater. Many of these accidents could be prevented if the public were made aware of dangers in and around the kitchen and bathroom. Shortening the kettle flex reduces the possibility of a toddler pulling over a boiling kettle, and more (rather than less) attention to the movements of infants placed in babywalkers would reduce some of the devastating injuries seen in the younger age groups.

Older children (particularly boys) and adults are more likely to receive injuries from flame burns and chemicals. Both are a hazard of many occupations. House fires are less common, largely because open fires have been replaced by central heating, but when house fires do occur mortality is high.

The depth of a burn has traditionally been classified as first, second or third degree, indicating the depth of tissue destroyed. This has now largely been replaced by a classification which takes into account the gross and microscopic changes which occur, and is clinically more useful, in which burn injuries are divided into partial thickness or full thickness skin loss.

Partial thickness skin loss includes burns to the epidermis and dermis, and may be superficial or deep. Erythema does not alter the classification, but its presence should be noted. A *superficial partial thickness burn* involves loss of some of the epidermis. Since epithelium is repaired from germinating cells within the epidermis, healing is rapid (7–10 days). Superficial burns are bright pink, usually blistered and painful. When pressed the burn blanches, indicating that there is good capillary return. A *deep partial thickness burn* involves loss of all the epidermis and some epidermal appendages within the dermis (see Figure) such as dermal papillae. The hair follicles and sweat glands are usually spared and it is from these structures that healing takes place, as well as from spread of epithelium from the wound margin. Healing may take place within 10–14 days, but a skin GRAFT may be necessary if the wound is large. Dermal burns are red, orange or white. They blister and are painful. Capillary return is sometimes rather slow.

By definition, the *full thickness burn* involves destruction of the epidermis and all the epidermal appendages, as well as the dermis. Spontaneous healing cannot occur from the wound but only from the edges. If the wound is large, migrating epithelial cells from the wound margin fail to provide a satisfactory cover and the wound must ultimately be grafted to ensure complete re-epithelialization. Full thickness burns may be white, brown, black or cherry-red. They have a tough, dry leathery ESCHAR within which thrombosed blood vessels are seen. The burn eschar is inelastic and causes compression upon deeper structures as oedema develops underneath it. When a circumferential eschar is formed around a limb the circulation to that area may be affected since the dry inelastic eschar acts as a tourniquet. If obstruction to the flow of blood to a limb is suspected then an incision into the burn wound (escharotomy) will alleviate the pressure and improve circulation. The full thickness burn has no sensation. When patients with full thickness burns experience pain at the burn site it is usually because there are areas of partial thickness injury which have intact nerve endings surrounding the full thickness burn.

FIRST AID. Unless extremely small, most burns in children should be referred to a doctor, health professional or Accident and Emergency Department. The ambulance should therefore be called to allow quick transport to hospital. Fluids should not be given since the patient frequently vomits.

In both adults and children the clothing should be removed and cold water applied. Exceptions are electrical injuries where the current has not been broken. In these injuries no attempt to perform first aid of any kind should be undertaken until the electrical source has been switched off. If the burn has been caused by chemicals, copious amounts of running (or stirred) water should be applied. The patient should then be wrapped in clean towels or sheets. Patients from house fires often have 'sooty' or carbonaceous substances in the mouth and nostrils and singed nasal hairs. These should not be wiped away, for they indicate to medical staff that there may be some degree of inhalation injury or respiratory damage.

Unless the first aider has access to a chart specifically designed for calculation of the extent of the burn (see BERKOW FORMULA and LUND AND BROWDER CHART) it is very difficult to assess the size of the burn and the next course of action. A simple method of assessing the size of the burn is to take the surface of the patient's palm as representing 1% of the body surface area. The number of 'palms' can then be totalled to give a rough approximation of the total burn size. Burns of the face, hands or genitalia should always be referred to a doctor, as should any burn covering 10% or more of the body surface in a child or 15% in an adult. Obviously there are no hard rules about referral and when there is an element of doubt regarding the severity of the injury, advice should always be sought.

CLINICAL MANAGEMENT OF MAJOR BURNS DURING THE FIRST 48 HOURS (THE SHOCK PHASE). Children with burns of 10% or more of the body surface and adults with burns of 15% require resuscitation with intravenous fluid because there is a rapid loss of fluid from the burn surface as well as from the intravascular space. This fluid 'leak' occurs because thermal injury causes the capillaries to become more permeable to water and solutes and thus fluid escapes from the intravascular compartment into the interstitial spaces. The amount of fluid lost is proprtional to the size of the burn and must be replaced. Oral replacement is successful if the burn is small, but in burns covering 10% of the body surface area in children and 15% in adults intravenous infusion with crystalloid (dextrose with saline) and colloid (plasma) is essential and oral intake should be avoided. After approximately 24–36 hours the capillaries recover and fluid ceases to escape from the blood vessels. At approximately 72 hours the fluid lost to the interstitial spaces early in the shock phase is reabsorbed and eliminated through the kidneys. The end of the shock phase is heralded by a diuresis. During the shock phase close observation and hourly monitoring is essential. Parameters which should be monitored include core and surface temperature, pulse and respiratory rate, sinus rhythm (particularly in electrical burns), and all fluid intake and urine output.

The relief of pain is vital. Morphine sulphate is frequently administered during the early period to ensure that the patient is made as comfortable and free from anxiety as possible. Inadequate analgesia allows the development of a vicious circle where pain leads to anxiety and the anxious and frightened patient has a low pain threshold.

During the early post-burn period many clinical problems arise due to disturbances in homeostatic mechanisms and the complex pathophysiological changes occurring at this time.

CARE OF THE BURN WOUND. Before any attempt is made to clean the wound, swabs should be taken and sent to the laboratory for culture. This procedure establishes a baseline for the types of microorganisms colonizing the surface of the burn. Although the wound is thought to be sterile initially, cross contamination (usually from other areas on the patient's skin) occurs within hours, usually with gram-positive organisms such as *Staphylococcus aureus*. It is important to prevent over-colonization and invasion of bacteria into underlying tissues because overwhelming sepsis is still the major cause of death in burn patients. Most Burn Centres have their own policies on wound cleansing and dressings and there are a wide selection of antibiotics on the market. They should be used selectively because resistant strains of bacteria are a hazard in a Burns Unit, and are difficult to eradicate once they emerge. One particular gram-positive organism which is a hazard in a Burns Unit is beta-haemolytic streptococcus group A. This organism creates unhealthy granulation tissue and is the cause of many failed skin grafts. Once the skin has been

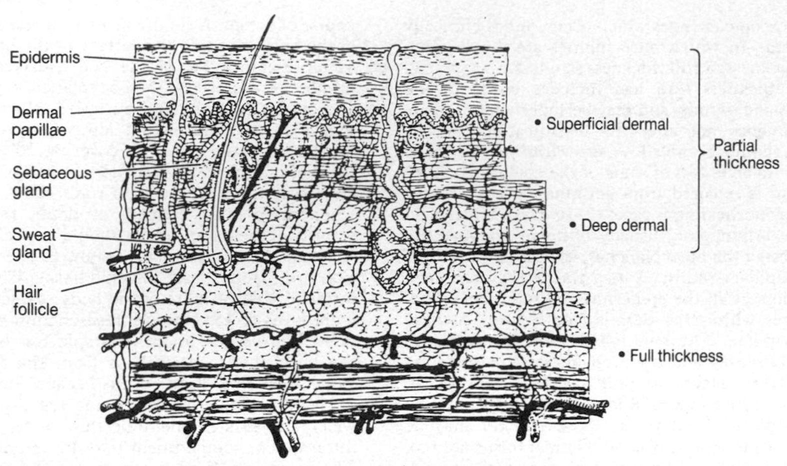

The relative depth of burn in superficial dermal, deep dermal, and full thickness injuries of the skin

cleaned and nonviable tissue removed, the burn is covered with wet soaks of an antiseptic preparation and wrapped in gauze and bandages. After approximately 48 hours the dressings are removed and an assessment of subsequent burn wound management made. Two options are currently practised in the UK. In some centres the burn will be dressed frequently for about 14 days. If the wound has large areas of deep partial thickness burn or is full thickness, skin grafts may be applied to close the wound. This is the conservative approach to burn wound management. An increasing number of centres have now adopted an approach to wound management which involves surgical removal of nonviable skin within 48–72 hours using tangential excision (shaving of dead skin in layers until healthy tissue is visible). Early application of a skin graft to an area which is not going to heal spontaneously prevents the patient from a lengthy stay in hospital and reduces the number of painful dressings which need to be frequently performed if surgery is delayed. Early surgery, early application of skin grafts and early discharge is obviously a great step forward in reducing the distress of hospitalization, particularly for the young child.

burn out a term used to describe the result of chronic stress on members of the helping professions. Burn out is characterized by chronic low energy, defensiveness and emergence of manoeuvres designed to create distance between helper and patient/client. Dissatisfaction and tension may be carried over from the work situation into the personal one and self-esteem and confidence may suffer badly.

Burow's solution ('boorovz) a preparation of aluminium subacetate, glacial acetic acid, and water; used topically on the skin as an astringent, and as a topical antiseptic and antipruritic in various skin disorders. Called also *aluminium acetate solution*.

burr, bur (bər) a bit for a surgical drill, used for cutting bone or teeth.

b. hole a circular hole drilled in the cranium to permit access to the brain or to release raised intercranial pressure.

bursa ('bərsə) pl. *bursae,bursas* [L.] a small fluid-filled sac or saclike cavity situated in places in tissues where friction would otherwise occur. adj. **bursal**. Bursae function to facilitate the gliding of muscles or tendons over bony or ligamentous surfaces. They are numerous and are found throughout the body; the most important are located at the shoulder, elbow, knee, and hip. Inflammation of a bursa is known as BURSITIS.

b. of Fabricius an epithelial outgrowth of the cloaca in chick embryos, which develops in a manner similar to that of the thymus in mammals, atrophying after 5 or 6 months and persisting as a fibrous remnant in sexually mature birds. It contains lymphoid follicles, and before involution is the site of formation of B-lymphocytes associated with humoural IMMUNITY.

b. mucosa, synovial b. a closed synovial sac interposed between surfaces that glide upon each other; it may be subcutaneous, submuscular, subfascial, or subtendinous in location.

bursectomy (bər'sektə,mee) excision of a bursa.

bursitis (bər'sietis) inflammation of a bursa. The bursa of the shoulder is most commonly affected, but inflammation may develop in almost any bursa in the body. Excessive use of the joint or chilling or a draft on the joint may be the cause.

Acute bursitis comes on suddenly; severe pain and limitation of motion of the affected joint are the principal symptoms. Resting the joint in a sling and applications of moist heat frequently are sufficient treatment. In some cases it may be necessary to aspirate fluid and calcium salts from the inflamed area. Steroids, such as cortisone, hydrocortisone, and ACTH, injected into the joint, may be effective in relieving acute attacks. X-ray therapy is also frequently effective.

Chronic bursitis may follow the acute attacks. There is continued pain and limitation of motion around the joint. Radiological examination will usually reveal the deposit of calcium salts. If rest, heat, and medications do not relieve the condition, x-ray therapy or surgery may be required to remove the calcium deposits or free the area of chronic inflammation.

bursolith ('bərsoh,lith) a calculus in a bursa.

bursopathy (bər'sopə,thee) any disease of a bursa.

bursotomy (bər'sotə,mee) incision of a bursa.

Buschke–Löwenstein tumour (,buhshkə'lərvən-,stien) a large cauliflower-like mass of warts occurring in the prepuce in the perianal region. Called also *giant condyloma acuminatum*.

Buscopan ('buskəpan) trademark for a preparation of

hyoscine butylbromide.

Busse–Buschke disease (ˌbuhse'buhshkə) cryptococcosis.

busulphan (byoo'sulfan) an alkylating agent that acts selectively on the bone marrow, depressing granulocyte formation, and is therefore used in the treatment of myelocytic (granulocytic) leukaemias. Side-effects include nausea and vomiting, and heavy doses may lead to excessive bone marrow depression. Complete blood counts (including platelet counts) must be done frequently while the drug is being administered and are used as a guide to dosage and effects on bone marrow production.

butane ('byootayn, byoo'tayn) an aliphatic hydrocarbon, C_4H_{10}, from petroleum.

Butazolidin (ˌbyootə'zolidin) trademark for a preparation of phenylbutazone, an analgesic, anti-inflammatory, and antipyretic. Only available in hospitals for the treatment of ankylosing spondylitis.

butobarbitone (ˌbyootoh'bahbiˌtohn) an intermediate-acting barbiturate, formerly much used as a sedative. Now used only in severe insomnia. It is classified as a controlled drug.

butorphanol (byoo'tawfənol) a synthetic opioid having analgesic and antitussive properties.

buttock ('butək) either of the two fleshy prominences formed by the gluteal muscles on the lower part of the back.

butyl ('byootil, -tiel) a hydrocarbon radical, C_4H_9.

butyraceous (ˌbyooti'rayshəs) of a buttery consistency.

butyrate ('byootiˌrayt) a salt of butyric acid.

butyric acid (byoo'tirik) a saturated fatty acid found in butter.

butyroid ('byootiˌroyd) resembling butter.

butyrophenone (ˌbyootiroh'feenohn) a chemical class of major tranquillizers especially useful in the treatment of manic and moderate to severe agitated states and in the control of the vocal utterances and tics of Gilles de la Tourette's syndrome.

butyrous ('byootirəs) resembling butter.

bypass ('bieˌpahs) an auxiliary flow; a shunt; a surgically created pathway achieved by anastomosis or graft circumventing the normal anatomical pathway, e.g., an aortoiliac or an intestinal bypass.

aortocoronary b. a section of saphenous vein or suitable substitute grafted between the aorta and a coronary artery distal to an obstructive lesion in the latter.

aortoiliac b. insertion of a vascular prosthesis from the abdominal aorta to the femoral artery to bypass intervening atherosclerotic segments.

cardiopulmonary b. diversion of the flow of blood from the entrance to the right atrium directly to the aorta, usually via a pump oxygenator, avoiding both the heart and the lungs; a form of extracorporeal circulation used in HEART surgery.

femoropopliteal b. insertion of a vascular prosthesis or vein graft from the femoral to the popliteal artery to bypass occluded segments.

intestinal b., jejunoileal b. a surgical procedure in which all but a few centimetres of the proximal jejunum and terminal ileum are bypassed in order to reduce obesity (see also INTESTINAL BYPASS).

left heart b. diversion of the flow of blood from the pulmonary veins directly to the aorta, avoiding the left atrium and the left ventricle.

right heart b. diversion of the flow of blood from the entrance of the right atrium directly to the pulmonary arteries, avoiding the right atrium and right ventricles.

byssinosis (ˌbisi'nohsis) pneumoconiosis due to inhalation of cotton dust. adj. **byssinotic**.

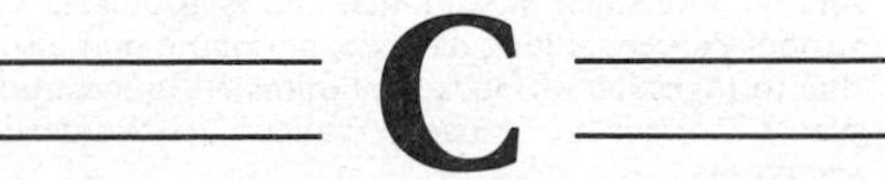

C chemical symbol, *carbon*; cathode (cathodal); Celsius or centigrade (scale); cervical; clearance; clonus; closure; contraction; cylinder; in the electrocardiogram; symbol for *complement*.

$\mathbf{C_L}$ lung compliance.

$\mathbf{C_{LT}}$ total lung–thorax compliance.

$\mathbf{C_T}$ thoracic compliance.

c symbol, *centi-*.

C-reactive protein (ˌsee·ri'aktiv) a globulin that forms a precipitate with the C-polysaccharide of the pneumococcus. Abbreviated CRP. For reasons not clearly understood, inflammation and tissue breakdown give rise to the C-reactive protein. Blood from patients with inflammatory conditions or disorders accompanied by necrosis gives a positive result with the test, and it is therefore of some use in diagnosing or determining the progress of such disorders as rheumatoid arthritis, acute rheumatic fever, widespread malignancy, and bacterial infections.

C-terminal ('seeˌtərmin'l) the end of the peptide chain carrying the free alpha carboxyl group of the last amino acid, conventionally written to the right.

Ca chemical symbol, *calcium*; cathode (cathodal).

cac(o)- word element. [Gr.] *bad, ill.*

cacaesthesia (ˌkakis'theezi·ə) disordered sensibility.

cachet (ka'shay, 'ka-) [Fr.] a dish-shaped wafer or capsule enclosing a dose of medicines.

cachexia (kə'keksi·ə) a profound and marked state of constitutional disorder; general ill health and malnutrition. adj. **cachectic**.

malarial c. the physical signs resulting from antecedent attacks of severe malaria, including anaemia, sallow skin, yellow sclera, splenomegaly, hepatomegaly, and, in children, retardation of growth and puberty.

pituitary c. that due to diminution or absence of pituitary function (see also PANHYPOPITUITARISM and SIMMONDS' DISEASE).

cachinnation (ˌkaki'nayshən) excessive, hysterical laughter.

cacogeusia (ˌkakoh'gyoozi·ə) a bad taste; a complaint of some patients with idiopathic epilepsy or those receiving antipsychotic agents or lithium, and a somatic delusion in psychoses.

cacomelia (ˌkakoh'meeli·ə) congenital deformity of a limb.

cacosmia (ka'kozmi·ə) 1. foul odour; stench. 2. a hallucination of unpleasant odour.

cacumen (kə'kyoomen) pl. *cacumina* [L.] 1. the top or apex of an organ. 2. the top of a plant. 3. the anterior and upper part of the monticulus cerebelli; called also *culmen*.

cadaver (kə'davə, -'day-) a dead body; generally applied to a human body preserved for anatomical study. adj. **cadaveric, cadaverous**.

cadaverine (kə'davəˌreen) a relatively nontoxic ptomaine, $C_5H_{14}N_2$, formed by decarboxylation of lysine; it is sometimes one of the products of *Vibrio proteus* and of *V. cholerae*, and is occasionally found in the urine in cystinuria.

cadmiosis (ˌkadmi'ohsis) pneumoconiosis due to inhalation of and tissue reaction to CADMIUM dust.

cadmium ('kadmi·əm) chemical element, atomic number 48, symbol Cd; its salts are poisonous. (See table of elements in Appendix 2.) Inhalation of cadmium fumes causes pulmonary oedema, followed by proliferative interstitial pneumonia, and is associated with various degrees of lung damage; poisoning may also be due to ingestion of foods contaminated by cadmium-plated containers, causing violent gastrointestinal symptoms.

c. sulphide a salt used, in a 1 per cent suspension, in treatment of seborrhoeic dermatitis of the scalp (dandruff).

caduceus (kə'dyoosi·əs) the wand of Hermes or Mercury; used as a symbol of the medical profession.

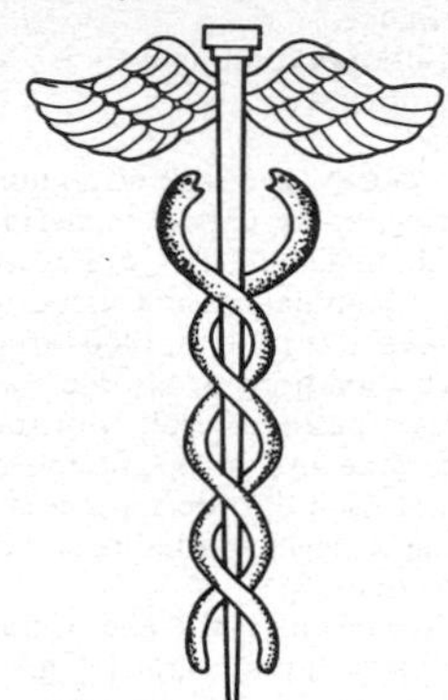

Caduceus

caecal ('seek'l) pertaining to the caecum.

caecectomy (see'kektəmee) excision of the caecum.

caecitis (see'kietis) inflammation of the caecum.

caeco- word element. [L.] *caecum*.

caecocele ('seekoh,seel) a hernia containing part of the caecum.

caecocolopexy (,seekoh'kohlə,peksee) an operation for fixation or suspension of the caecum and ascending colon.

caecocolostomy (,seekohkə'lostəmee) surgical anastomosis of the caecum and the colon.

caecopexy ('seekoh,peksee) fixation or suspension of the caecum to correct excessive mobility.

caecoplication (,seekohplie'kayshən) plication of the caecal wall to correct ptosis or dilation.

caecorrhaphy (see'ko·rəfee) suture or repair of the caecum.

caecosigmoidostomy (,seekoh,sigmoy'dostəmee) formation of an anastomosis between the caecum and sigmoid.

caecostomy (see'kostəmee) surgical creation of an artificial opening or fistula into the caecum.

caecotomy (see'kotəmee) incision of the caecum.

caecum ('seekəm) 1. the first or proximal part of the large intestine, forming a dilated pouch distal to the ileum and proximal to the colon, and giving off the vermiform appendix. 2. any blind pouch.

caelotherapy (,seeloh'therəpee) the therapeutic use of religion and religious symbols.

caesarean section (si'zairi·ən) delivery of a fetus by incision through the abdominal wall and uterus ater 28 weeks of pregnancy. The procedure takes its name from the Latin word *caedere*, to cut, and has no relation to the birth of Caesar as is sometimes believed. Indications for caesarean section include dystocia, pre-eclampsia, haemorrhage from abruptio placentae or placenta praevia, fetal distress, and breech presentation.

The incidence of caesarean section has increased, probably due to the development of safer anaesthetics and surgical procedures and improved monitoring of the fetus, which can warn the obstetrician that the fetus is in distress during labour. Prolonged labour is now recognized as a serious threat to the fetus as well as the mother. Brain damage and other serious injuries can be avoided by performance of a caesarean section in such cases.

Another factor contributing to the increase in caesarean deliveries is adherence to the old dictum 'once a caesarean, always a caesarean'. The possibility of rupture of the uterus during a subsequent labour is greatly reduced when a lower segment caesarean section is performed, i.e. the incision is made low in the abdomen and horizontally. Classical caesarean section involves a vertical incision in the body of the uterus, the scar of which is more likely to rupture in subsequent pregnancies.

Normal vaginal delivery is preferred to a caesarean delivery, but when the mother or the fetus is in jeopardy, the surgical procedure provides a relatively safe alternative to prolonged labour and the application of forceps. Subsequent labours and deliveries can be accomplished by the vaginal route after a caesarean section with minimal risk, provided the patients are carefully selected and closely monitored during labour in a fully equipped obstetric unit that is staffed for any emergency.

caesium ('seezi·əm) a chemical element, atomic number 55, atomic weight 132.905, symbol Cs. See table of elements in Appendix 2.

café au lait spot ('kafay oh 'lay) pigmented macules of a distinctive light brown colour, like coffee with milk, as in neurofibromatosis and Albright's syndrome.

Cafergot ('kafə,got) trademark for a preparation of ergotamine, an alkaloid of ergot used to treat migraine.

caffeine ('kafeen, 'kafi,een) a central nervous system stimulant from coffee, tea, guarana, and maté; it also acts as a mild diuretic.

caffeinism ('kaf,ee·inizəm) an agitated state induced by excessive ingestion of caffeine.

Caffey's disease ('kafeez) infantile cortical hyperostosis.

caisson disease ('kays'n) decompression sickness, a condition occurring in underwater workers, and caused by too-rapid decrease in atmospheric pressure. The condition is named after the pressurized, watertight compartments (caissons) in which underwater construction men work. The main symptoms are dizziness, staggering, muscle spasms, difficulty in breathing, abdominal pain, and partial paralysis. Caisson disease is a form of BENDS.

cal calorie.

calamine ('kalə,mien) a preparation of zinc and ferric oxides, used topically in lotion form as a protectant, antipruritic and astringent.

calcaemia (kal'seemi·ə) excessive calcium in the blood; hypercalcaemia.

calcaneoapophysitis (kal,kaynioh·ə,pofi'sietis) inflammation of the posterior part of the calcaneus, marked by pain and swelling.

calcaneoastragaloid (kal,kaynioh·ə'stragəloyd) pertaining to the calcaneus and astragalus.

calcaneodynia (kal,kaynioh'dini·ə) pain in the heel.

calcaneus, calcaneum (kal'kayni·əs; kal'kayni·əm) the irregular quadrangular bone at the back of the tarsus; called also heel bone and os calcis.

calcar ('kal,kah) a spur or spur-shaped structure.

c. avis the lower of two medial elevations in the lateral cerebral ventricle, produced by the lateral extension of the calcarine sulcus; called also *hippocampus minor*.

calcareous (kal'kair·ri·əs) pertaining to or containing lime; chalky.

calcarine ('kalkareen) 1. spur-shaped. 2. pertaining to the calcar avis.
c. sulcus a sulcus of the medial surface of the occipital lobe, separating the cuneus from the lingual gyrus.

calcariuria (,kalkari'yooə·ri·ə) the presence of lime (calcium) salts in the urine.

calcibilia (,kalsi'bili·ə) the presence of calcium in the bile.

calcic ('kalsik) of or pertaining to lime or calcium.

calcicosis (,kalsi'kohsis) a lung disease due to inhalation of marble dust.

calciferol (kal'sifə·rol) 1. see VITAMIN D. 2. ergocalciferol.

calcific (kal'sifik) forming lime.

calcification (,kalsifi'kayshən) the deposit of calcium salts in a tissue. The normal absorption of calcium is facilitated by parathyroid hormone and by vitamin D. When there are increased amounts of parathyroid hormone in the blood (as in HYPERPARATHYROIDISM), there is deposition of calcium in the alveoli of the lungs, the renal tubules, the thyroid gland, the gastric mucosa, and the arterial walls. Normally calcium is deposited in the bone matrix to insure stability and strength of the bone. In OSTEOMALACIA there is decalcification of bone because of a failure of calcium and phosphorus deposition in the bone matrix.
dystrophic c. the deposition of calcium in abnormal tissue, such as scar tissue or atherosclerotic plaques, without abnormalities of blood calcium.

calcinosis (,kalsi'nohsis) a condition characterized by abnormal deposition of calcium salts in the tissues.
c. circumscripta localized deposition of calcium in small nodules in subcutaneous tissues or muscle.
c. universalis widespread deposition of calcium in nodules or plaques in the dermis, panniculus, and muscles.

calcipenia (,kalsi'peeni·ə) deficiency of calcium in the system.

calcipexis, calcipexy (,kalsi'peksis; ,kalsi'peksee) fixation of calcium in the tissues. adj. **calcipectic, calcipexic.**

calciphilia (,kalsi'fili·ə) a tendency to calcification.

calciphylaxis (,kalsifi'laksis) the formation of calcified tissue in response to administration of a challenging agent after induction of a hypersensitive state. adj. **calciphylactic.**

calciprivia (,kalsi'privi·ə) deprivation or loss of calcium. adj. **calciprivic.**

calcitonin (,kalsi'tohnin) a polypeptide hormone secreted by the parafollicular or C cells of the thyroid gland, which is involved in plasma calcium homeostasis. Salmon calcitonin, which has a longer duration of action than human calcitonin, is administered in the treatment of severe hypercalcaemia and Paget's disease of bone. It acts to decrease the rate of bone resorption. Called also *thyrocalcitonin*.

calcitriol (,kalsi'trieol) a nonproprietary name for 1,25-dihydroxycholecalciferol; used as a calcium regulator in the management of hypocalcaemia in patients undergoing renal dialysis, and in hypoparathyroidism.

calcium ('kalsi·əm) a chemical element, atomic number 20, atomic weight 40.08, symbol Ca. (See table of elements in Appendix 2.) Calcium is the most abundant mineral in the body. In combination with phosphorus it forms calcium phosphate, the dense, hard material of the bones and teeth. It is an important cation in intra- and extracellular fluid and is essential to the normal clotting of blood, the maintenance of a normal heartbeat, and the initiation of neuromuscular and metabolic activities.

Within the body fluids calcium exists in three forms. Protein-bound calcium accounts for about 47 per cent of the calcium in plasma; most of it in this form is bound to albumin. Another 47 per cent of plasma calcium is ionized. About 6 per cent is complexed with phosphate, citrate, and other anions.

Ionized calcium is physiologically active. One of its most important physiological functions is control of the permeability of cell membranes. Parathyroid hormone, which causes transfer of exchangeable calcium from bone into the blood stream, maintains calcium homeostasis by preventing either calcium deficit or excess.

When the level of serum calcium rises above normal, neuromuscular activity begins to diminish. This condition, known as *hypercalcaemia*, is characterized by lethargy and muscle weakness, which, as the level of calcium increases, can progress to depressed reflexes, hypotonic muscles, nausea, thirst, constipation, mental confusion, and coma. Hypercalcaemia also slows the heartbeat, and therefore potentiates the effects of digitalis.

In contrast, *hypocalcaemia*, which is indicated by a serum level below normal, is manifested by increased neuromuscular irritability. When there is a deficit of ionized calcium, the nerve cells become more permeable, allowing leakage of sodium and potassium from the cells. This produces excitation of the nerve fibres and triggers uncontrollable activity of the skeletal muscles. Hence, as the calcium level continues to drop, the patient begins to experience muscle twitching and cramping, grimacing, and carpopedal spasm, which can quickly progress to tetany, laryngospasm, convulsions, cardiac arryhthmias, and eventually to respiratory and cardiac arrest. Relatively early signs of hypocalcaemia are a positive TROUSSEAU'S SIGN and a positive CHVOSTEK'S SIGN.

Dietary sources of calcium include dairy products such as milk and cheese, which are the best sources of the mineral. Other sources include dark green leafy vegetables, and sardines, clams, and oysters. The recommended daily dietary intake of calcium is 800 mg for children and adults, and 1200 mg for teenagers and for pregnant and lactating women. It is difficult to meet this requirement without including milk or milk products in the daily diet.
c. carbonate an insoluble salt occurring naturally in bone, shells, and chalk; used as an antacid.
c. chloride a salt used in solution to restore electrolyte balance and as an antidote to magnesium poisoning.
c. glubionate a calcium replenisher.
c. gluceptate a calcium replenisher.
c. gluconate a calcium replenisher and antidote to fluoride or oxalate poisoning.
c. hydroxide an astringent compound used topically in solution or lotions.
c. lactate a calcium supplement.
c. levulinate a calcium supplement.
c. mandelate a white, odourless powder used as a urinary antiseptic.
c. oxalate a compound occurring in the urine in crystals and in certain calculi.
c. pantothenate a calcium salt of the dextrorotatory isomer of pantothenic acid; used as a growth-promoting vitamin.
c. phosphate one of three salts containing calcium and the phosphate radical: dibasic and tribasic calcium phosphate are used as sources of calcium; monobasic calcium phosphate is used in fertilizer and as a calcium and phosphorus supplement.
c. polycarbophil a hydrophilic agent used as a bulk laxative in the treatment of constipation and diar-

rhoea.

c. propionate a salt used as an antifungal preservative in foods and as a topical antifungal agent.

c. resonium a polystyrene sulphonate ion-exchange resin used for removal of potassium ions in hyperkalaemia.

c. sulphate a compound of calcium and sulphate, occurring as gypsum or as plaster of Paris.

calcium channel blocker a drug, such as nifedipine, verapamil or diltiazem, that selectively blocks the influx of calcium ions through a specific ion channel (the slow channel or calcium channel) of cardiac muscle and smooth muscle cells; used in the treatment of Prinzmetal's angina, chronic stable angina, and cardiac arrhythmias. Calcium channel blockers act to control arrhythmias by slowing the rate of sinoatrial (SA) node discharge and the conduction velocity through the atrioventricular (AV) node. They act in Prinzmetal's angina to relax and prevent coronary artery spasm. The mechanism of action in classical angina is a lowering of myocardial oxygen utilization by dilating peripheral arteries and thereby reducing total peripheral resistance and the work of the heart. Nifedipine is also used in the treatment of hypertension. Called also *calcium blocker*.

calciuria (ˌkalsi'yooə·ri·ə) calcium in the urine.

calcospherite (ˌkalkoh'sferiet) one of the minute globular bodies formed during calcification by chemical union of calcium particles and albuminous matter of cells.

calculifragous (ˌkalkyuh'lifrəgəs) breaking up calculi.

calculogenesis (ˌkalkyuhloh'jenəsis) the formation of calculi.

calculosis (ˌkalkyuh'lohsis) a condition characterized by the presence of calculi; lithiasis.

calculus ('kalkyuhləs) pl. *calculi* [L.] an abnormal concretion, usually composed of mineral salts, occurring within the animal body, chiefly in the hollow organs or their passages. Called also stones, as in kidney stones (see also KIDNEY) and GALLSTONES. adj. **calculous.**

biliary c. a gallstone.

bronchial c. lung calculus.

dental c. calcium phosphate and carbonate, with organic matter, deposited on tooth surfaces.

lung c. a concretion formed in the bronchi (see also LUNG CALCULUS).

renal c. a calculus occurring in the kidney.

urinary c. a calculus in any part of the urinary tract.

vesical c. one in the urinary bladder.

Caldwell–Luc operation (ˌkawldwel'look) an antrostomy operation to drain the maxillary sinus through an incision above the upper canine tooth.

Caldwell–Moloy classification (ˌkawldwelmə'loy) the classification of female pelves as gynecoid, android, anthropoid, and platypelloid (see also PELVIC inlet and accompanying illustration).

calefacient (ˌkali'fayshənt) causing a sensation of warmth; an agent that so acts.

calf (kahf) SURA; the fleshy back part of the leg below the knee.

calibration (ˌkali'brayshən) determination of the accuracy of an instrument, usually by measurement of its variation from a standard, to ascertain necessary correction factors.

calibrator ('kaliˌbraytə) an instrument for dilating a tubular structure or for determining the calibre of such a structure.

calibre ('kalibə) the diameter of the lumen of a canal or tube.

calicectasis (ˌkali'sektəsis) dilation of a calix of the kidney.

calicectomy (ˌkali'sektəmee) excision of a calix of the kidney.

calices ('kaliˌseez) plural of *calix*.

caliculus (ke'likyuhləs) a small cup or cup-shaped structure.

californium (ˌkali'fawni·əm) a chemical element, atomic number 98, atomic weight 249, symbol Cf. See table of elements in Appendix 2.

calipers ('kalipəz) an instrument with two bent or curved legs used for measuring thickness or diameter of a solid.

calix ('kayliks) pl. *calices* [L.] a cuplike organ or cavity, e.g., one of the recesses of the kidney pelvis which enclose the pyramids. adj. **caliceal.**

Calliphora (ka'lifor·rə) a genus of flies, the blowflies or bluebottle flies, which deposit their eggs in decaying matter, on wounds, or in body openings; the maggots are a cause of myiasis.

callisthenics, calisthenics (ˌkalis'theniks) mild gymnastics for developing the muscles and producing a graceful carriage.

callosity (kə'lositee) a callus (1).

callosum (kə'lohsəm) corpus callosum.

callous ('kaləs) of the nature of a callus; hard.

callus ('kaləs) 1. localized hyperplasia of the horny layer of the epidermis due to pressure or friction. 2. an unorganized network of woven bone formed about the ends of a broken bone; it is absorbed as repair is completed (provisional callus), and ultimately replaced by true bone (definitive callus).

calmative ('kahmətiv) 1. sedative; allaying excitement. 2. an agent having such effects.

calor ('kalə) [L.] heat; one of the cardinal signs of inflammation.

calorie ('kalə·ree) any of several units of heat defined as the amount of heat required to raise the temperature of 1 gram of water by 1 degree Celsius (1 °C) at a specified temperature. The calorie used in chemistry and biochemistry is equal to 4.184 joules. Symbol cal.

In referring to the energy content of foods it is customary to use the 'large calorie' or Calorie, which is equal to 1 kilocalorie (kcal), 1000 cal. Every bodily process—the building up of cells, motion of the muscles, the maintenance of body temperature—requires energy, and the body derives this energy from the food it consumes. Digestive processes reduce food to usable 'fuel', which the body 'burns' in the complex chemical reactions that sustain life.

The amount of energy required for these chemical processes varies. Factors such as weight, age, activity, and metabolic rate determine a person's daily calorie requirement. Nutrition experts have computed daily calorie requirements in terms of age and other factors. These tabulations serve only as guides; they cannot, of course, embrace all individual variations.

From its daily intake of energy foods, the body uses only the amount it needs for energy purposes. The remainder is stored as fat; hence the utility of calorie counting in weight control. If the average adult male consumes more than his 2900-calorie daily requirement, he will gain weight. However, if he consumes less than 2900 calories, the body will supplement its energy sources by drawing upon fat which the body has stored away, and he will lose weight.

A person can usually gain or lose weight as he wishes by keeping to a daily diet with a calorie count above or below his daily requirement. See also NUTRITION.

calorific (ˌkalə'rifik) 1. heat-producing. 2. pertaining to heat or to calories.

calorimeter (ˌkalə'rimitə) an instrument for measuring the amount of heat produced in any system or organism.

calorimetry (ˌkaləˈrimətree) measurement of the heat eliminated or stored in any system.

Calpol (ˈkalpol) trademark for a paracetamol elixir for children.

Calthor (ˈkalthor) trademark for a preparation of ciclacillin, a semisynthetic penicillin.

calvaria, calvarium (kalˈvair·ri·ə; kalˈvair·ri·əm) the domelike superior portion of the cranium, comprising the superior portions of the frontal, parietal, and occipital bones.

Calvé–Perthes disease (ˌkalvayˈpərtayz) osteochondrosis of the epiphysis at the head of the femur.

calvities (kalˈvishiˌeez) baldness.

calx (kalks) 1. lime or chalk. 2. the hindmost part of the foot; the heel.

calyculus (kəˈlikyuhləs) caliculus.

Calymmatobacterium (kəˌlimətohbakˈtiə·ri·əm) a genus of bacteria made up of gram-negative rods.

C. granulomatis the species causing granuloma inguinale (granuloma venereum).

calyx (ˈkayliks, ˈkal-) calix.

camera (ˈkamə·rə, ˈkamrə) pl. *camerae* [L.] a cavity or chamber.

cAMP cyclic adenosine monophosphate.

Campbell de Morgan's spot (kambˈl de mawgənz) a small localized haemangioma common in later life localized mostly to the trunk.

camphor (ˈkamfə) a ketone derived from a cinnamon tree, *Cinnamomum camphora*, or produced synthetically; used as an antipruritic agent.

campimetry (kamˈpimətree) assessment of the central part of the visual field.

campotomy (kamˈpotəmee) the stereotaxic surgical technique of producing a lesion in Forel's fields, beneath the thalamus, for correction of tremor in Parkinson's disease.

camptocormia (ˌkamptohˈkawmi·ə) a static deformity consisting of forward flexion of the trunk.

camptodactyly (ˌkamptohˈdaktilee) permanent flexion of one or more fingers.

camptomelia (ˌkamptohˈmeeli·ə) bending of the limbs, producing permanent bowing or curving of the affected part. adj. **camptomelic**.

camptospasm (ˈkamptohˌspazəm) camptocormia.

Campylobacter (ˈkampilohˌbaktə) a genus of bacteria, family Spirillaceae, made up of gram-negative, non-spore-forming, motile, spirally curved rods, which are microaerophilic to anaerobic.

C. fetus a species, certain subspecies of which cause acute gastroenteritis in man.

Canada–Cronkhite syndrome (ˌkanədəˈkrongkiet) familial polyposis of the gastrointestinal tract associated with alopecia, nail dystrophy, and hyperpigmentation of the skin.

canal (kəˈnal) a relatively narrow tubular passage or channel.

adductor c. Hunter's canal.

Alcocks' c. a tunnel formed by a splitting of the obturator fascia, which encloses the pudendal vessels and nerve.

alimentary c. the digestive tube from mouth to anus (see also ALIMENTARY CANAL).

anal c. the terminal portion of the alimentary canal, from the rectum to the anus.

atrioventricular c. the common canal connecting the primitive atrium and ventricle; it sometimes persists as a congenital anomaly.

birth c. the canal through which the fetus passes in birth.

carotid c. one in the pars petrosa of the temporal bone, transmitting the internal carotid artery to the cranial cavity.

cervical c. the part of the uterine cavity lying within the cervix.

condylar c. an occasional opening in the condylar fossa for transmission of the transverse sinus; called also *posterior condyloid foramen*.

c. of Corti a space between the outer and inner rods of Corti.

femoral c. the cone-shaped medial part of the femoral sheath lateral to the base of Gimbernat's ligament.

haversian c. any of the anastomosing channels of the haversian system in compact bone, containing blood and lymph vessels, and nerves.

Hunter's c. a fascial tunnel in the middle third of the medial part of the thigh, containing the femoral vessels and saphenous nerve. Called also *adductor canal*.

hypoglossal c. an opening in the occipital bone, transmitting the hypoglossal nerve and a branch of the posterior meningeal artery; called also *anterior condyloid foramen*.

infraorbital c. a small canal running obliquely through the floor of the orbit, transmitting the infraorbital vessels and nerve.

inguinal c. the oblique passage in the lower anterior abdominal wall on either side, through which passes the round ligament of the uterus in the female, and the spermatic cord in the male.

medullary c. 1. spinal canal. 2. the cavity, containing marrow, in the diaphysis of a long bone; called also *marrow cavity* or *medullary cavity*.

optic c. a passage for the optic nerve and ophthalmic artery at the apex of the orbit; called also *optic foramen*.

pulp c. root canal.

root c. that part of the pulp cavity extending from the pulp chamber to the apical foramen. Called also *pulp canal*.

sacral c. the continuation of the spinal canal through the sacrum.

Schlemm's c. the venous sinus of the sclera, a circular canal at the junction of the sclera and cornea (see also venous SINUS of sclera).

semicircular c's the long canals (anterior, lateral, and posterior) of the bony labyrinth of the ear (see also SEMICIRCULAR CANALS).

spinal c., vertebral c. the canal formed by the series of vertebral foramina together, enclosing the spinal cord and meninges.

Volkmann's c's canals communicating with the haversian canals, for passage of blood vessels through bone.

canaliculus (ˌkanəˈlikyuhləs) pl. *canaliculi* [L.] an extremely narrow tubular passage or channel. adj. **canalicular**.

bile canaliculi fine tubular channels forming a three-dimensional network within the parenchyma of the liver. They join to form the bile ductules and eventually the hepatic duct.

bone canaliculi branching tubular passages radiating like wheel spokes from each bone lacuna to connect with the canaliculi of adjacent lacunae, and with the haversian canal.

lacrimal c. the short passage in an eyelid, beginning at the lacrimal point and draining tears from the lacrimal lake to the lacrimal sac; called also *lacrimal duct*. See also LACRIMAL APPARATUS.

mastoid c. a small channel in the temporal bone transmitting the tympanic branch of the vagus nerve.

canalis (kəˈnaylis) pl. *canales* [L.] a canal or channel.

canalization (ˌkanəlieˈzayshən) 1. the formation of canals, natural or pathological. 2. the surgical establishment of canals for drainage.

canaloplasty (kəˈnalohˌplastee) plastic reconstruction

of a passage, as of the external acoustic meatus.

Canavan's disease ('kanə,vanz) spongy degeneration of central nervous system.

cancellated ('kansi,laytid) having a lattice-like structure.

cancellous ('kansələs) of a reticular, spongy, or lattice-like structure; said mainly of bone tissue.

cancellus (kan'seləs) pl. *cancelli* [L.] the lattice-like structure in bone; any structure arranged like a lattice.

cancer ('kansə) any malignant, cellular tumour. adj. **cancerous.** The term *cancer* encompasses a group of neoplastic diseases in which there is a transformation of normal body cells into malignant ones. This probably involves some change in the genetic material of the cells, deoxyribonucleic acid (DNA), perhaps as a result of faulty repair of damage to the cell caused by carcinogenic agents or ionizing radiation. The altered cells pass on inappropriate genetic information to their offspring and begin to proliferate in an abnormal and destructive way. Normally, the cells of tissues are regularly replaced by new growth, which stops when the cells are replaced; new cells form to repair tissue damage and stop forming when healing is complete. Why they stop forming is unknown, but clearly the body in its normal processes regulates cell growth. In cancer, cell growth is unregulated.

As the cancer cells continue to proliferate, the mass of abnormal tissue that they form enlarges, penetrating neighbouring tissues, destroying normal cells and taking their place. Cells are spread from this primary site via lymphatics or blood vessels to distant sites. This migration is called *metastasis.* Another way of spread is by entering a body cavity and coming into contact with a healthy organ by diffusion.

CAUSES. It is doubtful that one process is involved in the aetiology of all cancers. The exact cause of the conversion of normal cells into cancerous ones is still not known. An important factor is permanent alteration in the DNA of the cell, which is passed on to subsequent generations, but we do not know what triggers the change in DNA structure and why some people succumb to a cancer and others do not. Cellular immunity undoubtedly plays some part in one's ability to stop the growth of cancer cells; it is believed by some that most persons develop many small cancers in their lifetime but do not develop clinical signs because their defence mechanisms destroy the malignant cells and prevent their replication.

Oncologists recognize that environmental, hereditary, and biological factors play an important role in the development of cancer. Environmental causes are believed to account for at least 50 per cent and perhaps, in some types, as much as 80 per cent of all cancers. For example, cigarette smoking is directly related to approximately 90 per cent of all cancers of the lung. Other environmental carcinogens include industrial pollutants and radiation. Among the chemical carcinogens are arsenic from mining and smelting industries; asbestos from insulation, at construction sites and power plants; benzene from oil refineries, solvents, and insecticides; and products from coal combustion in steel and petrochemical industries. Each year new products that in all probability are carcinogenic are being produced by industrial operations. A major concern is the occupational and environmental hazards these chemicals present to those who work in or live near these plants.

Radiation from prolonged exposure to the ultraviolet rays from the sun and from injudicious use of diagnostic and therapeutic procedures involving x-rays and radioactive substances is also a significant factor in the incidence of cancer, particularly in the development of cancer of the skin, bone marrow, and thyroid.

Hormones, especially the synthetic oestrogens given to forestall the effects of menopause and to prevent spontaneous abortion, are directly related to some cancers of the female reproductive organs.

Viruses as causal agents in the development of cancers have been subjected to intensive research efforts in recent years. A number of cancers can be produced in experimental laboratory animals, but irrefutable evidence that cancers in humans are caused by viruses is slender. Exceptions may be the Epstein-Barr virus, which may have a causal association with Burkitt's lymphoma and certain cases of nasopharyngeal cancer, the hepatitis B virus with hepatocellular carcinoma, and certain strains of papilloma virus with carcinoma of the uterine cervix. Viruses are capable of introducing new genetic material into a normal cell and transforming it into a malignant one, and cell reproduction may be altered when viruses interact with such carcinogens as chemicals and radiation. It is not known exactly how these properties enhance the ability of malignant cells to thrive under adverse conditions and to metastasize to other parts of the body and produce another cancerous tumour. Recent studies have implicated oncogenes in the pathogenesis. The oncogenes may be of viral origin and directly inserted into the host DNA at a point where it can magnify its replicative activity or where it can inhibit normal regulatory mechanisms. Alternatively, they may already exist in the cell (cellular oncogenes) with a normal function but insertion of non-oncogenic viral DNA may disrupt the cell's normal growth regulatory mechanisms and so 'free' them from its restraining and inhibiting control.

The incidence of cancer in certain populations suggests that other factors are important in its development. It is known, for example, that some families show a high incidence of malignancy among its members, but there is no definite hereditary pattern. There also is a high incidence of cancer in persons receiving drugs for immunosuppression, yet cancer itself is immunosuppressive. It is suggested that prolonged suppression of the body's immune response may eventually impair its ability to distinguigh between self and nonself and thus render it unable to destroy malignant cells. When cancer itself acts to suppress the immune response, it may be the result of an overwhelming demand on the body to destroy more foreign cells than it is prepared to cope with at any given time.

CLASSIFICATION. Cancers are classified on the basis of two factors: the type of tissue and the type of cell in which they arise. Using this classification system, it is possible to identify over 150 types of cancer in humans. In the classification of cancers according to the type of tissue from which they evolve, there are two main groups: *sarcomas* and *carcinomas.* Sarcomas are of mesenchymal origin and affect such tissues as the bones and muscles. They tend to grow rapidly and to be very destructive. The carcinomas are of epithelial origin and make up the great majority of the glandular cancers and cancers of the breast, stomach, uterus, skin, and tongue.

Cell type affects the appearance, rate of growth, and degree of malignancy. Thus, classification of tumours according to the type of cell from which they are derived is important in deciding the course of treatment for a specific malignancy.

Staging. An approach to describing and categorizing malignant tumours has been developed by the International Union Against Cancer (UICC). It is hoped that by standardizing the classification and staging of tumours, treatment protocols can be established and end-results reporting can be utilized to determine the effectiveness of the suggested treatment.

Whereas classification of tumours refers to the anatomical and histological descriptions of the tumour (see above), staging refers to the extent of the tumour. The three basic components of the staging system are the primary tumour (T), regional nodes (N), and metastasis (M). Subscripts may be used to describe the extent to which the malignancy has increased in size, its involvement of regional nodes, and its metastatic development (see Table). For example, a tumour may be described $T_1N_2M_0$.

At the present time, the UICC system is the most widely used.

TNM staging to breast cancer

Tis		In situ			
T1		≤ 2 cm			
	T1a	≤ 0.5 cm			
	T1b	> 0.5 to 1 cm			
	T1c	> 1 to 2 cm			
T2		> 2 to 5 cm			
T3		> 5 cm			
T4		Chest wall/skin			
	T4a	Chest wall			
	T4b	Skin oedema/ulceration, satellite skin nodules			
	T4c	Both 4a and 4b			
	T4d	Inflammatory carcinoma			
N1		Movable axillary	pN1		
				pN1a	Micrometastasis only ≤ 0.2 cm
				pN1b	Gross metastasis
					i 1–3 nodes/ > 0.2 to < 2 cm
					ii ≥ 4 nodes/ > 0.2 to < 2 cm
					iii through capsule/ < 2 cm
					iv ≥ 2 cm
N2		Fixed axillary	pN2		
N3		Internal mammary	pN3		

Precancers. Some potentially dangerous cancers appear first in the form of non-invasive changes in the body's tissues. Their danger lies in the fact that they have a tendency to become malignant. Hence they are known as precancers. Among these are lesions that appear as thickened white patches in the mouth, and on the vulva and uterine cervix. Polyps of the large intestine also are possible precancers.

Hodgkin's Disease. This disease is generally considered a form of cancer. It usually afflicts young people, causing a progressive enlargement of the lymph nodes, in most cases starting in the neck, groin, or armpit. Treatment may be by surgery, radiotherapy, use of certain chemicals, or a combination of these (see HODGKIN'S DISEASE).

Leukaemias. In these diseases, abnormal leukocytes are produced in enormous quantities. The leukaemias respond to much the same treatment as cancer and are commonly considered cancers (see LEUKAEMIA).

PREVENTION. Because man-made conditions play an important role in the aetiology of many cancers, prevention is aimed at identifying carcinogens, educating the general public about them, and encouraging their avoidance. Equally important, if not more so, is recognition of causative factors related to life style and personal habits. Perhaps the best example of this is the relationship between smoking and lung cancer. When heavy consumption of alcohol is combined with cigarette smoking, the risk for cancer of the larynx, oesophagus, and mouth is greatly increased.

Nutritional balance may also be important in the prevention of cancer. Foods and food additives could contain specific carcinogenic agents. Nutritional deficiency can lower resistance and increase the risk of certain types of cancers. The decrease in the incidence of stomach cancer in most Western countries is thought to be perhaps the result of an increase in the consumption of fruits and vegetables.

Studies have shown that a relationship, but not necessarily a causal one, exists between obesity and cancer, and between dietary excess, particularly the consumption of large amounts of fats, and certain types of cancers. In general, overweight women are at increased risk for cancer of the endometrium, the gallbladder, and the kidney. Cancers associated with a high dietary intake of fat, with or without the presence of obesity, are those affecting the breast, ovary, endometrium, prostate, colon, and pancreas. Neither saturated nor unsaturated fats are themselves carcinogenic. The relationship of fat consumption to colon cancer is thought to be due to the effect of bile acids and their metabolites, which have been shown to act as tumour promoters in laboratory animals. In humans, patients with cancer of the colon typically have elevated levels of bile acid metabolites.

The judicious use of hormones for therapeutic purposes also can reduce the incidence of some cancers. The widespread use of stilboestrol to prevent threatened or habitual abortion and premature labour, beginning in the 1940s, eventually resulted in the development of vaginal and cervical cancer in a significant number of the female offspring of women who were given the drug while pregnant. As was previously mentioned, oestrogens prescribed for the relief of menopausal symptoms have been implicated in cancer in women. These drugs are known to increase the risk of endometrial cancer by as much as four to eight times.

Cancer of the skin and malignant melanoma are related to prolonged exposure to the ultraviolet radiation in sunlight. The incidence of cancer of the skin is increasing in those persons who value a deep suntan and spend a significant amount of time engaged in outdoor leisure activities. Also at risk are those whose work requires that they be exposed to sunlight for prolonged periods of time, e.g., farmers.

Since most occupational cancers are preventable, increased awareness on the part of industry and the provision of a safe workplace environment can decrease the incidence of many kinds of cancer. It is also necessary for workers to cooperate in reducing exposure to carcinogens by complying with rules for preventive measures.

Ultimately, the prevention of cancer depends upon knowledge of each person's risk factors for development of cancer, and that person's decision to avoid whenever possible those habits and practices that predispose to the disease. There also should be frequent examination and monitoring of those who are known to be at greater risk because of hereditary or environmental conditions.

Detection. It is well known that early diagnosis of most cancers results in cure or greatly extended survival times. Screening is an excellent method of achieving this, and although health education about screening is sparse, and the facilities for screening are deficient, the following is intended as a guide for the education of patients/clients on the desirability of screening/self-examination in order to reduce the mortality from late-diagnosed cancers.

Early danger signs of cancer

1. Any lump or thickening, especially in the breast, lip, or tongue
2. Any irregular or unexplained bleeding. Blood in the urine or bowel movements. Blood or bloody discharge from the nipple or any body opening. Unexplained vaginal bleeding or discharge, or any bleeding after the menopause
3. A sore that does not heal, particularly around the mouth, tongue, or lips, or anywhere on the skin
4. Noticeable changes in the colour or size of a wart, mole, or birthmark
5. Loss of appetite or continual indigestion
6. Persistent hoarseness, cough, or difficulty in swallowing
7. Persistent change in normal elimination (bowel habits)

Special note: Pain is not usually an early warning sign of cancer

Colon and Rectum. Cancer of the colon and/or rectum is more common after 40 years of age. Patients should be made aware of the necessity to consult their doctor immediately if there is a change in or fluctuation of bowel habits. Digital or proctoscopic examination will reveal malignant involvement. In the USA it is common for men and women over 50 years of age to have their stools tested for occult blood, and research along similar lines is now being carried out in the UK.

Cervix. A Papanicolaou test (Pap test, smear) should be available for all women over the age of 21 (and for sexually active women under the age of 21). At present this test is available every five years for women over 21 (unless an abnormal smear has been seen), though many authorities believe that a three-year interval is desirable. The Government have asked all Health Authorities to operate efficient call/recall schemes for cervical cancer. At present over 2000 women die each year from cervical cancer in the UK.

Breast. All women should be taught how to examine their breasts for abnormalities. Ideally this should be taught to young girls in schools, at an appropriate age. Breast self-examination (BSE) should be carried out every month. Routine mammographic screening of women aged 50 years or more has been shown to reduce the mortality from breast cancer in this age group by one-third.

Lung. The number of deaths from lung cancer, especially in women, continues to increase. 'Stop smoking' and 'Don't start' campaigns are widely available, and health-care providers should seek to influence this habit by discouraging smoking on health-care premises, and by acting as role models.

High-risk Exceptions. More frequent and thorough examinations are advisable for: (1) women with personal family histories of breast cancer; (2) women who began having sexual intercourse at an early age or those with many partners; (3) women who have a history of obesity, infertility, failure of ovulation, abnormal uterine bleeding or oestrogen therapy; and (4) persons who have a personal or family history of cancer of the rectum, familial polyposis, Gardner's syndrome, ulcerative colitis or a history of polyps.

Symptoms of Cancer. There are seven early warning signs of cancer. *These signs do not necessarily signify cancer, but should they occur, a doctor should be consulted and an examination is advisable.* Other symptoms depend on location and type of malignancy present. *Stomach cancer:* continued lack of appetite; persistent indigestion; pain after eating; loss of weight; vomiting; anaemia.

Cancer of the rectum: changes in bowel habits, such as periods of constipation followed by episodes of diarrhoea; abdominal cramps and a sensation of incomplete elimination or a feeling that there is a mass in the rectum; rectal pain and bleeding.

Cancer of the uterus: increased or irregular vaginal discharges; return of vaginal bleeding after the menopause; bleeding between menstrual periods or after coitus.

Cancer of the breast: painless lumps in the breast; bleeding or discharging from the nipple. Many kinds of lumps in the breast are innocent, but since this form of cancer is now the leading cause of death from cancer among women, any breast nodule or tumour should be examined by a doctor.

Skin cancer: sores and ulcers that do not heal; sudden changes in colour, size, and texture in moles, warts, scars, and birthmarks.

Lung cancer: a persistent cough that lasts beyond 2 weeks; wheezing or other noises in the chest; coughing up of blood or bloody sputum; shortness of breath not caused by obvious exertion, such as climbing stairs or running; chest ache or pain.

Cancer of the mouth, tongue and lips: any sore that does not heal in 2 weeks; any white patch taking the place of the normal pink colour of the tongue or inside of the mouth; hoarseness lasting more than 2 weeks.

Cancer of the larynx: persistent hoarseness.

Kidney, bladder and prostate cancers: bloody urine or reddish or pink urine; difficulty in starting urination; increasing frequency of urination during the night.

Brain tumours and cancers: headaches; changes in vision; dizziness; nausea and vomiting; paralysis.

Diagnosis. The detection of cancer can be accomplished by a number of tests and examinations. By palpation, a tumour can be felt as a lump or nodule below the surface of the skin or mucous membrane. By visualization of the hollow organs with instruments such as the cystoscope, gastroscope, colonoscope, or bronchoscope, abnormal growths of cells can be seen. Laboratory examination of the tissue removed by biopsy can determine whether a tumour is malignant or benign. This test is considered the most accurate and dependable aid to diagnosis of cancer.

The papanicolaou test is used for diagnosing early cancers of the uterine cervix, mouth, bronchi, stomach, and other organs lined with mucous membrane. In this technique washings or scrapings from the mucous membrane are removed by the doctor, placed on a glass slide and sent to a laboratory for cytological examination. Radiological studies can reveal tumours which may not be detected by palpation or direct visualization. These include gastrointestinal studies, chest x-rays and pyelography, angiography and mammography. Radioisotopes and photoscanners may be introduced into the body orally or by injection to locate tumours of the brain, pancreas, thyroid, liver, and kidney. Special instruments are used to trace and 'photograph' the distribution of radioisotopes, thereby pinpointing the location of the tumour by identifying abnormal variations. Other diagnostic techniques include ultrasonography, xerography, thermography, and colposcopy.

A number of laboratory tests are useful in the diagnosis of specific types of cancers. For example, cancer of the prostate can secrete an acid phosphatase isoenzyme, increasing its level in the blood. Determination of the level of prostatic acid phosphatase can be used as an indication of the extent of the disease. There are several tumour-specific markers (oncofetal antigens), which are proteins synthesized only by fetal tissues and certain cancers. These include alpha-fetoprotein (AFP) and carcinoembryonic antigen (CEA). The measurement of these proteins in the patient's serum provides useful information about the extent of cancer involvment. Plasma gamma globulins are secreted in excessive amounts by the plasma cells of a myeloma. Microscopic analysis of the blood cells and bone marrow cells is necessary in diagnosing leukemias.

TREATMENT. The current treatment of cancer includes any one or a combination of the following: (1) surgical removal of the tumour and possibly adjacent tissue, (2) RADIATION THERAPY, (3) chemotherapy using ANTINEOPLASTIC agents, and (4) IMMUNOTHERAPY, which helps bolster the body's own defences against malignant cells. The selection of treatment modalities is based on the type of cancer, its location, and the extent of involvement.

Surgical removal of the tumour and the areas to which it has metastasized is aimed at removal of all cancerous and potentially cancerous tissue. This method of treatment is most successful when the growth is small and localized and is situated in areas where adjacent tissues, particularly lymphatic tissues, also can be excised.

Radiotherapy. Therapeutic radiation utilizes ionizing radiations to destroy cells by inhibiting their ability to multiply. Radiation damages tissue, particularly tissue that is growing rapidly, and because malignant tissue does grow more rapidly than normal tissue, it is more readily affected by radiation. Cells vary in their susceptibility to radiation and not all malignancies respond to this form of treatment.

Techniques vary in respect to the source of radiation and method of delivery. In teletherapy the source of radiation is either a radioactive element that is housed in a shielded unit located some distance from the patient or a megavoltage x-ray machine. Interstitial therapy requires placement or implantation of a radioactive substance directly into the tissues of the malignant growth.

Although normal tissue can be damaged by radiation, instruments that deliver precisely targeted beams of energy keep damage to normal tissue near the tumour to a minimum.

In teletherapy there is no danger that the patient will become a source of radiation or be hazardous to those with whom he comes in contact. However, when radioactive materials are implanted in the body tissues, those materials do emit radiations that could be harmful to others. See also RADIATION.

Chemotherapy is most frequently used against disseminated cancers that cannot be removed surgically or do not respond to radiotherapy and against neoplasias of the blood cells and their precursors. There are several classes of antineoplastic agents. Most of these act by interfering with cell division and are as likely to damage normal cells undergoing division as malignant cells. They are thus extremely toxic and generally nonselective. For example, the bone marrow is often greatly depressed by cancer chemotherapy. See also ANTINEOPLASTIC THERAPY.

Alkylating agents are drugs that react chemically with various cellular constituents. Their principal effects are produced by reacting with the genetic material, introducing cross-links between the DNA strands of the double helix; this prevents DNA replication and cell division. These drugs have also been called *radiomimetic agents* because ionizing radiation also acts by damaging DNA.

Antimetabolites are molecules that resemble natural metabolites in their chemical structure. There are three types: purine analogues, pyrimidine analogues, and folic acid antagonists. They can bind to enzymes like their analogous metabolites: the purine and pyrimidine bases and folic acid. The bases are building blocks of DNA, and folic acid is a coenzyme involved in the synthesis of these bases. The antimetabolite cannot perform the function of its analogous metabolite and thereby stops DNA synthesis and cell division.

Vinca alkaloids (vincristine and vinblastine) stop cell division by binding to the protein tubulin and disrupting the mitotic spindle. This prevents the even division of chromosomes between the two daughter cells and causes cell death.

Several *antibiotics* have specific antineoplastic effects. These act by damaging DNA and thereby preventing DNA replication or by binding to DNA and preventing transcription of the genetic code into messenger RNA. The first effect stops cell division; the second stops protein synthesis and cell growth.

Certain *hormones* control the growth of specific tissues. Corticosteroids are used for treatment of leukaemias, progestins for endometrial carcinoma, and oestrogens and androgens for cancers of the breast, ovaries and prostate.

An *enzyme, LA heavy-metal complex* (cisplatin, a central platinum atom surrounded by two chlorine atoms and two ammonia molecules) is used to treat metastatic tumours of the testes, ovaries, bladder, and head and neck. Its mechanism of action is similar to that of the alkylating agents.

Adjuncts to chemotherapy with highly toxic agents must include the use of other drugs and techniques to improve the patient's well-being by restoring normal tissue function, replacing blood elements destroyed or prevented from forming, encouraging ossification of bone lesions, and removing pressure and obstruction of blood vessels, lymphatic vessels, and neural pathways. *Immunotherapy*. This is another recent and still investigational addition to the arsenal of weapons against cancer. It is most effective in treating bronchogenic carcinoma, malignant melanoma, cancer of the bladder, head and neck tumours, osteogenic sarcoma, and carcinoma of the colon and ovaries. There are three basic approaches to immunotherapy: active (specific and nonspecific), passive, and adoptive.

As in other kinds of immunity, *active* immunity against cancer depends on the patient's ability to produce resistance to the tumour. In active, specific immunotherapy, the patient is vaccinated with allogenic tumour cells of the same histological type as his own tumour. These cells can stimulate an immune response to tumour-specific antigens, but they cannot grow in the patient because of histoincompatibility. In contrast, nonspecific immunotherapy involves the use of vaccine extracts to stimulate a general immune response, especially the cell-mediated immunity provided by the T-cells. The most frequently used nonspecific immunotherapeutic agent is BCG vaccine, an attenuated form of *Mycobacterium bovis* that has been used for many years to prevent tuberculosis.

Passive immunotherapy involves giving the patient an immune serum produced by another person who is immune to the cancer.

Adoptive immunotherapy provides a means by which live immune lymphocytes are transferred from a compatible donor to the cancer patient.

c. registry department or office, usually (though not always) attached to a cancer research institute, which maintains records of the incidence, types, age features, epidemiology and mortality associated with cancers in a given area or country.

canceraemia (ˌkansə'reemi·ə) the presence of cancer cells in the blood.

cancericidal (ˌkanseri'sied'l) destructive to cancer cells.

cancerophobia, cancerphobia (ˌkansə·roh'fohbi·ə; ˌkansə'fohbi·ə) carcinophobia; morbid dread of cancer.

cancriform ('kangkriˌfawm) resembling cancer.

cancroid ('kangkroyd) 1. cancer-like. 2. a skin cancer of a low grade of malignancy.

cancrum ('kangkrəm) [L.] *canker*.

c. oris see NOMA.

c. pudendi see NOMA.

candela (kan'deelə, -'daylə) the SI unit of luminous intensity. Abbreviated cd.

Candida ('kandidə) a genus of yeastlike fungi that are commonly part of the normal flora of the mouth, skin, intestinal tract, and vagina, but can cause a variety of infections (see also CANDIDIASIS).

C. albicans the usual pathogen in human infection.

candidaemia (ˌkandi'deemi·ə) the presence in the blood of fungi of the genus *Candida.*

candidiasis (ˌkandi'dieəsis) infection by fungi of the genus *Candida*, generally *C. albicans*, most commonly involving the skin, oral mucosa (thrush), respiratory tract, and vagina; rarely there is a systemic infection or endocarditis.

candidid ('kandidid) a secondary skin eruption that is an expression of hypersensitivity to infection with *Candida* elsewhere on the body.

candidin ('kandidin) a skin test antigen derived from *Candida albicans*, used in testing for the development of delayed-type hypersensitivity to the microorganism.

candidosis (ˌkandi'dohsis) candidiasis.

candiduria (ˌkandi'dyooə·ri·ə) the presence of *Candida* organisms in the urine.

Canesten ('kanestən) trademark for a preparation of clotrimazole, an antifungal.

canine ('kaynien) 1. pertaining to or characteristic of dogs. 2. pertaining to a canine tooth (cuspid).

canker ('kangkə) an ulceration, especially of the lip or oral mucosa.

cannabinoid (kə'nabiˌnoyd) any of the active principles of *Cannabis*, including tetrahydrocannabinol, cannabinol, and cannabidiol.

cannabinol (kə'nabiˌnol) a physiologically inactive principle from *Cannabis*; its tetrahydro derivatives are active.

cannabis ('kanəbis) a preparation of the hemp plant (*Cannabis sativa)* containing isomers of tetrahydrocannabinol (THC) and used for its psychoactive effect including a sense of euphoria and alterations in the sense of time. Its possession is illegal in many countries. Cannabis resin (exuded by the flowering tips of the female hemp plant and known as 'hash') is the most widely used preparation in the UK and is usually smoked, though it may be eaten. The dried plant material ('grass') is less potent and is smoked after mixing with tobacco. See also HASHISH, MARIJUANA. Hash oil is obtained by percolating a solvent through cannabis resin and is a very potent preparation of cannabis which is rarely used in the UK. The most potent preparation is synthetic THC and 'designer drug' analogues of THC are now circulating in the illicit drugs market in the USA.

Contradictory data exists regarding the chromosomal damaging effects of prolonged cannabis use and some researchers have suggested an amotivational syndrome associated with prolonged heavy use. In some parts of the world cannabis is an accepted recreational drug and plays a similar part to the Western use of recreational drugs like alcohol, tobacco and caffeine.

Slang terms for cannabis include marijuana, hashish, hash, grass, pot, the weed, ganga, kaya, kif, and bhang.

cannabism ('kanəbizəm) a state produced by misuse of cannabis.

Cannon's ring ('kanənz) a focal contraction seen radiographically at the mid-third of the transverse colon, marking an area of overlap between the superior and inferior nerve plexuses.

cannula ('kanyuhlə) a tube for insertion into a duct or cavity; during insertion its lumen is usually occupied by a trocar.

cannulate ('kanyuhˌlayt) to introduce a cannula, which may be left in place.

cannulation (ˌkanyuh'layshən) introduction of a cannula into a tubelike organ or body cavity.

cantharidin (kan'tharidin) the most active principle of cantharides, the dried Spanish fly, *Lytta vesicatoria*; preparations containing cantharidin are used topically as a vesicant to remove warts and lesions of molluscum contagiosum.

canthectomy (kan'thektəmee) excision of a canthus.

canthitis (kan'thietis) inflammation of a canthus.

cantholysis (kan'tholisis) surgical section of a canthus or a canthal ligament.

canthoplasty ('kanthohˌplastee) plastic surgery of a canthus.

canthotomy (kan'thotəmee) incision of a canthus.

canthus ('kanthəs) pl. *canthi* [L.] the angular junction of the eyelids at either corner of the eyes. adj. **canthal**.

capacitance (kə'pasitəns) 1. the property of being able to store an electric charge. 2. the ratio of charge to potential in a conductor.

capacitation (keˌpasi'tayshən) the process by which spermatozoa become capable of fertilizing an ovum after it reaches the ampullar portion of the uterine tube.

capacitor (kə'pasitə) a device for holding and storing charges of electricity.

capacity (kə'pasitee) the power to hold, retain, or contain, or the ability to absorb; usually expressed numerically as the measure of such ability.

closing c. (CC) the volume of gas in the lungs at the time of airway closure (see also CLOSING VOLUME).

forced vital c. the maximal volume of gas that can be exhaled from full inspiration, exhaling as forcefully and rapidly as possible (see also PULMONARY FUNCTION TESTS).

functional residual c. the amount of gas remaining at the end of normal quiet respiration.

heat c. thermal capacity.

inspiratory c. the volume of gas that can be taken into the lungs in a full inspiration, starting from the resting inspiratory position; equal to the tidal volume plus the inspiratory reserve volume.

maximal breathing c. maximal voluntary ventilation.

thermal c. the amount of heat absorbed by a body in being raised 1 °C.

total lung c. the amount of gas contained in the lung at the end of a maximal inspiration.

virus neutralizing c. the ability of a serum to inhibit

the infectivity of a virus. **vital c.** the volume of gas that can be expelled from the lungs from a position of full inspiration, with no limit to duration of expiration; equal to inspiratory capacity plus expiratory reserve volume.

CAPD continuous ambulatory PERITONEAL DIALYSIS.

capillarectasia (ka,pilə·rek'tayzi·ə) dilation of capillaries.

Capillaria (,kapi'lair·ri·ə) a genus of parasitic nematodes.

C. hepatica a species parasitic in the liver of rats and other mammals; rarely, man may be affected.

C. philippinensis a species found in the human intestine in the northern Philippines and also in Thailand, causing severe diarrhoea, malabsorption, and high mortality.

capillariasis (ka,pilə'rieəsis) infection with nematodes of the genus *Capillaria*, especially *C. philippinensis*.

capillariomotor (ka,pilə·rioh'mohtə) pertaining to the functional activity of the capillaries.

capillaritis (ka,pilə'rietis) inflammation of the capillaries.

capillarity (,kapi'laritee) the action by which the surface of a liquid where it is in contact with a solid, as in a capillary tube, is elevated or depressed.

capillary (kə'pilə·ree) 1. pertaining to or resembling a hair. 2. one of the minute vessels connecting arterioles and venules, the walls of which act as a semipermeable membrane for interchange of various substances between the blood and tissue fluid. (See CIRCULATORY SYSTEM.) The walls consist of thin endothelial cells through which dissolved substances and the body fluids can pass. At the arterial end, the blood pressure within the capillary is higher than the osmolality of the blood that opposes it. Thus the watery parts of the plasma and some dissolved solid substances pass through the capillary wall into the surrounding tissues. At the venous end of the capillary, the osmolality of the blood is higher than the blood pressure, which results in fluids from the tissues passing back into the capillary.

capillus (kə'piləs) pl. *capilli* [L.] a hair; used in the plural to designate the aggregate of hair on the scalp.

capitellum (,kapi'teləm) 1. capitulum. 2. the bulb of a hair.

capitular (kə'pityuhlə) pertaining to a capitulum or the head of a bone.

capitulum (kə'pityuhləm) pl. *capitula* [L.] a small eminence on a bone, as on the distal end of the humerus, by which it articulates with another bone.

Capnocytophaga (,kapnohsie'tofəgə) a genus of anaerobic, gram-negative, rod-shaped bacteria that have been implicated in the pathogenesis of periodontal disease.

capotement (kə'pohtmonh) [Fr.] a splashing sound heard in dilation of the stomach.

Capoten ('kapoh,ten) trademark for a preparation of captopril.

capping ('kaping) the provision of a protective or obstructive covering.

pulp c. the covering of an exposed dental pulp with some material to provide protection against external influences and to encourage healing.

capreomycin (,kaprioh'miesin) a polypeptide antibiotic produced by *Streptomyces capreolus*, which is active against human strains of *Mycobacterium tuberculosis* and has four microbiologically active components. It is used when other agents have failed.

caproate ('kaproh·ayt) any salt or ester of caproic acid (hexanoic acid).

capsid ('kapsid) the shell of protein that protects the nucleic acid of a virus; it is composed of structural units, or capsomers. According to the number of subunits possessed by capsomers, they are called dimers (2), trimers (3), pentamers (5), or hexamers (6).

capsomer, capsomere ('kapsəmə; 'kapsoh,miə) a morphological unit of the capsid of a virus.

capsula ('kapsyuhlə) pl. *capsulae* [L.] capsule.

capsulation (,kapsyuh'layshən) enclosure in a capsule.

capsule ('kapsyool) 1. an enclosing structure, as a soluble container enclosing a dose of medicine. 2. a cartilaginous, fatty, fibrous, or membranous structure enveloping another structure, organ, or part. adj. **capsular**.

articular c. the saclike envelope that encloses the cavity of a synovial joint by attaching to the circumference of the articular end of each involved bone.

bacterial c. a gelatinous envelope surrounding a bacterial cell, usually polysaccharide but sometimes polypeptide in nature; it is associated with the virulence of pathogenic bacteria.

Bowman's c. the globular dilation forming the beginning of a uriniferous tubule within the kidney, and surrounding the glomerulus. Called also *glomerular capsule* and *malpighian capsule*.

c's of the brain two layers of white matter in the substance of the brain; external capsule and internal capsule.

external c. the layer of white fibres between the putamen and claustrum.

Glisson's c. a sheath of connective tissue accompanying the hepatic ducts and vessels through the hepatic portal.

glomerular c. Bowman's capsule.

c. of heart pericardium.

internal c. the fanlike mass of white fibres separating the lentiform nucleus laterally from the head of the caudate nucleus, the dorsal thalamus, and the tail of the caudate nucleus medially.

joint c. articular capsule.

c. of lens the elastic sac enclosing the lens of the eye.

malpighian c. Bowman's capsule.

renal c., adipose the investment of fat surrounding the fibrous capsule of the kidney, continuous at the hilus with the fat in the renal sinus.

renal c., fibrous the connective tissue investment of the kidney, which continues through the hilus to line the renal sinus.

Tenon's c. the connective tissue enveloping the posterior eyeball.

capsulectomy (,kapsyuh'lektəmee) excision of a capsule, especially a joint capsule or lens capsule.

capsulitis (,kapsyuh'lietis) inflammation of a capsule, as that of the lens.

capsulolenticular (,kapsyuhlohlen'tikyuhlə) pertaining to the lens of the eye and its capsule.

capsuloma (,kapsyuh'lohmə) a capsular or subcapsular tumour of the kidney.

capsuloplasty ('kapsyuhloh,plastee) plastic repair of a joint capsule.

capsulorrhaphy (,kapsyuh'lo·rəfee) suturing of a joint capsule.

capsulotomy (,kapsyuh'lotəmee) incision of a capsule, as that of the lens or of a joint.

captopril ('kaptohpril) an angiotensin-converting enzyme (ACE) inhibitor used, usually with a diuretic, for treatment of hypertension in patients who have failed to respond to or developed unacceptable side-effects with multiple drug regimens that usually include an adrenergic blocking agent, diuretic, and vasodilator. Serious adverse reactions associated with its use include proteinuria, neutropenia, and agranulocytosis.

caput ('kapuht) pl. *capita* [L.] the head; a general term applied to the expanded or chief extremity of an organ or part.

c. medusae the dilated cutaneous veins around the umbilicus, seen mainly in the newborn and in patients suffering from cirrhosis of the liver.

c. succedaneum oedema occurring in and under the fetal scalp during labour.

carbachol ('kahbə,kol) a drug related to and acting like acetylcholine, but more stable. It causes contraction of plain muscle and relaxation of voluntary sphincters. It may be used to relieve postoperative retention of urine. Also rarely used in the treatment of glaucoma as an alternative to pilocarpine.

carbamazepine (,kahbə'mazi,peen) an anticonvulsant and analgesic used in the treatment of pain associated with trigeminal neuralgia and for control of complex partial seizures or generalized tonic–clonic seizures.

carbamide ('kahbə·mied) urea in anhydrous, lyophilized, sterile powder form; injected intravenously in dextrose or invert sugar solution to induce diuresis.

carbaminohaemoglobin (kah,baminoh,heemə'glohbin) a combination of carbon dioxide and haemoglobin, CO_2HHb, being one of the forms in which carbon dioxide exists in the blood.

carbamoyl ('kahbəmoyl) the radical NH_2–CO–.

carbamoyltransferase (,kahbəmoyl'transfə,rayz, -'trahns-) an enzyme that catalyses the transfer of carbamoyl, as from carbamoylphosphate to L-ornithine to form orthophosphate and citrulline in the synthesis of urea.

carbenicillin (,kahbeni'silin) a semisynthetic antibiotic of the penicillin group, prepared as the disodium salt and used in infections due to *Pseudomonas*.

carbenoxolone (,kahbe'noksə,lohn) an anti-inflammatory drug used in the treatment of gastric ulcers.

carbidopa (,kahbi'dohpə) an inhibitor of the decarboxylation of levodopa (L-dopa) in peripheral tissues, which does not cross the blood–brain barrier. It is used in combination with levodopa to control the symptoms of PARKINSON'S DISEASE. In the presence of carbidopa, levodopa enters the brain in larger quantities, thus avoiding the need for excessively high doses of it.

carbimazole (kah'bimə,zohl) an antithyroid drug used in the treatment of thyrotoxicosis.

carbinoxamine (,kahbi'noksə,meen) a potent antihistamine used in the treatment of allergic disorders.

carbo ('kahboh) charcoal.

c. ligni medical wood charcoal. Used for the relief of digestive disorders and diarrhoea.

carbohydrase (,kahboh'hiedrayz) any of a group of enzymes that catalyse the hydrolysis of higher carbohydrates to lower forms.

carbohydrate (,kahboh'hiedrayt) a compound of carbon, hydrogen, and oxygen, the latter two usually in the proportions of water, i.e., $(CH_2O)_n$. They are classified into mono-, di-, tri-, poly-, and heterosaccharides. Carbohydrates in food are an important and immediate source of energy for the body; 1 g of carbohydrate yields 17kJ (4 kcal). They are present, at least in small quantities, in most foods, but the chief sources are the sugars and starches. The sugars include granulated sugar, maple sugar, honey, and molasses. The simple sugars (monosaccharides) include glucose, called also dextrose or grape sugar, and fructose, called also laevulose or fruit sugar. Galactose is a simple sugar produced by the digestion or hydrolysis of lactose (milk sugar). The double sugars (disaccharides) include sucrose, which is found in sugar cane or sugar beet, maltose or malt sugar, and lactose or milk sugar. All ripe fruits and many vegetables contain some natural sugars. The starches are present in such foods as rice, wheat, and potatoes.

Carbohydrates may be stored in the body as glycogen for future use. If they are eaten in excessive amounts, however, the body changes them into fats and stores them in that form.

carbohydraturia (,kahboh,hiedrə'tyooə·ri·ə) excess of carbohydrates in the urine.

carbolfuchsin (,kahbol'fooksin) a mixture of carbolic acid and fuchsin used for staining purposes, especially in bacteriology.

carbolic acid (kah'bolik) called also PHENOL, a caustic poison obtained by distillation of coal tar or produced synthetically; used as an antiseptic and disinfectant.

carbolism ('kahbə,lizəm) PHENOL (carbolic acid) poisoning.

carbon ('kahbən) a chemical element, atomic number 6, atomic weight 12.011, symbol C. See table of elements in Appendix 2.

carbon dioxide ('kahbən die'oksied) an odourless, colourless gas, CO_2, resulting from oxidation of carbons, formed in the tissues and eliminated by the lungs; used with oxygen to stimulate respiration and in solid form (CARBON DIOXIDE SNOW) as an escharotic.

c. d. combining power the ability of blood plasma to combine with carbon dioxide; indicative of the alkali reserve and a measure of the acid–base balance of the blood.

c. d. content the amount of carbonic acid and bicarbonate in the blood; reported in millimoles per litre.

c. d. narcosis respiratory acidosis.

c. d. snow solid carbon dioxide, formed by rapid evaporation of liquid carbon dioxide; it gives a temperature of about −79 °C (−110 °F), and is used as an escharotic in various skin diseases. Called also *dry ice*.

c. d. tension the partial pressure of carbon dioxide in the blood; noted as P_{CO_2} in BLOOD GAS ANALYSIS. See also RESPIRATION.

carbon dioxide–oxygen therapy (,kahbən die-,oksied'oksi,jən) administration of a mixture of carbon dioxide and oxygen (commonly 5 per cent CO_2 and 95 per cent O_2 or 10 per cent CO_2 and 90 per cent O_2); used for improvement of cerebral blood flow, stimulation of deep breathing, or treatment of singultation (hiccupping). Carbon dioxide acts by stimulating the respiratory centre, it also increases heart rate and blood pressure. Therapy is given for 6 minutes or less with a 5 per cent mixture and 2 minutes or less with a 10 per cent mixture. Potential adverse effects include headache, dizziness, dyspnoea, nausea, tachycardia and high blood pressure, blurred vision, mental depression, coma, and convulsions.

carbon monoxide ('kahbən mon'oksied) a colourless, odourless, tasteless gas, CO, formed by burning carbon or organic fuels with a scanty supply of oxygen; inhalation causes central nervous system damage and asphyxiation. Carbon monoxide is present in the exhaust of petrol engines, in the smoke of wood and coal fires, in manufactured gas such as that used in the household, and wherever carbon burns without a sufficient supply of oxygen.

c. m. poisoning poisoning by carbon monoxide; one of the most common types of gas poisoning. When carbon monoxide is inhaled, it comes in contact with the blood and combines with haemoglobin. Since carbon monoxide combines more readily with haemoglobin than does oxygen, it takes the place of oxygen in the erythrocytes, and the tissues are thus deprived of their normal oxygen supply. Death from asphyxia results if a large enough quantity of carbon monoxide is inhaled.

SYMPTOMS AND TREATMENT. The symptoms of carbon monoxide poisoning are dizziness, headache, weakness, shortness of breath, possibly nausea, and then unconsciousness. The skin and mucous membranes become cherry red in colour.

Emergency treatment consists of opening doors and windows, and turning off the source of the gas, if possible. The victim should be dragged or carried out into the air. If breathing has stopped or is irregular, ARTIFICIAL RESPIRATION should be undertaken immediately. The police or the emergency ambulance services should be called and the nature of the accident described so that emergency equipment to administer oxygen may be rushed to the scene. The victim is kept lying down.

PREVENTION. Cases of carbon monoxide poisoning are usually accidental. It should be remembered that carbon monoxide has no odour and its presence may not be detected unless other gases, such as exhaust fumes from a vehicle motor, are also escaping. Care should be taken to ensure proper ventilation of working and sleeping areas. It is extremely dangerous to leave a vehicle motor running in a closed garage. Stoves and furnaces should be kept in good repair. Burners using gas, especially in a bedroom, should have a ventilator pipe to carry the exhaust to the outside.

carbon tetrachloride ('kahbən ˌtetrə'kloried) a clear, colourless, mobile liquid; the inhalation of its vapours can depress central nervous system activity and cause degeneration of the liver and kidneys.

carbonate ('kahbəˌnayt) a salt of carbonic acid.

carbonic acid (kah'bonik) aqueous solution of carbon dioxide, H_2CO_3.

c. a. anhydrase an enzyme that catalyses the decomposition of carbonic acid into carbon dioxide and water, facilitating transfer of carbon dioxide from tissues to blood and from blood to alveolar air.

carbonuria (ˌkahbə'nyooə·ri·ə) the presence in the urine of carbon dioxide or other carbon compounds.

carbonyl ('kahbənil, -ˌniel) the bivalent organic radical, =CO, characteristic of aldehydes, ketones, carboxylic acid, and esters.

carboplatin (ˌkahboh'playtin) a derivative of cisplatin associated with reduced toxicity.

carboxyhaemoglobin (kahˌboksiˌheemə'glohbin) haemoglobin combined with carbon monoxide, which occupies the sites on the haemoglobin molecule that normally bind with oxygen and which is not readily displaced from the molecule; exposure to carbon monoxide thus results in cellular anoxia.

carboxyl (kah'boksil, -siel) the monovalent radical, -COOH, found in those organic acids termed carboxylic acids.

carboxylase (kah'boksiˌlayz) an enzyme that catalyses the removal of carbon dioxide from the carboxyl group of alpha amino keto acids.

carboxylation (kahˌboksi'layshən) the addition of a carboxyl group, as to pyruvate to form oxaloacetate.

carboxylesterase (kahˌboksi'lestəˌrayz) an enzyme that catalyses the hydrolysis of the esters of carboxylic acids.

carboxylic acid (ˌkahbok'silik) an organic compound containing the carboxy group (-COOH), which is weakly ionized in solution, forming a carboxylate ion ($-COO^-$).

carboxyltransferase (kahˌboksil'transfəˌrayz, -'trahns-) an enzyme that catalyses carboxylation.

carboxylyase (kahˌboksi'lieayz) any of a group of lyases that catalyse the removal of a carboxyl group; it includes the carboxylases and decarboxylases.

carboxymyoglobin (kahˌboksiˌmieoh'glohbin) a compound formed from myoglobin on exposure to carbon monoxide.

carboxypeptidase (kahˌboksi'peptiˌdayz) an exopeptidase that acts only on the peptide linkage of a terminal amino acid containing a free carboxyl group.

carbuncle ('kahbungk'l) a necrotizing infection of skin and subcutaneous tissue composed of a cluster of BOILS (furuncles), usually due to *Staphylococcus aureus*, with multiple formed or incipient drainage sinuses. These organisms are often present on the skin but are unable to do any damage unless resistance is lowered by such conditions as irritating friction, cuts, poor health, nutritional deficiency, ordiabetes mellitus. adj. **carbuncular.**

Treatment includes administration of antibiotics and incision and drainage when necessary to remove exudate. Efforts are made to determine the cause of the carbuncles so that it can be eliminated.

malignant c. anthrax.

carbunculoid (kah'bungkyuhˌloyd) resembling a carbuncle.

carbunculosis (kahˌbungkyuh'lohsis) a condition marked by the formation of numerous carbuncles.

carcinoembryonic antigen (ˌkahsinohˌembri'onik) an oncofetal glycoprotein antigen found in colonic adenocarcinoma and other cancers and in certain nonmalignant conditions (see also carcinoembryonic ANTIGEN). Abbreviated CEA.

carcinogen ('kahsinəˌjen, kah'sinəjən) a substance that causes cancer. adj. **carcinogenic.**

carcinogenesis (ˌkahsinoh'jenəsis) production of cancer.

carcinogenicity (ˌkahsinohje'nisitee) the ability or tendency to produce cancer.

carcinoid ('kahsiˌnoyd) a tumour of the gastrointestinal tract formed from the enterochromaffin cells of the enteric canal. Although potentially malignant, the majority behave as benign tumours and occur as incidental findings at operation or autopsy. Rarely, they produce the carcinoid syndrome (see below).

c. syndrome a symptom complex associated with carcinoid tumours, marked by attacks of severe cyanotic flushing of the skin lasting from minutes to days and by diarrhoeal watery stools, bronchoconstrictive attacks, sudden drops in blood pressure, oedema, and ascites. Symptoms are caused by serotonin, prostaglandins, and other biologically active substances secreted by the tumour.

The specific symptoms associated with this disorder depend upon the site of the primary tumour, which is found most commonly in the terminal third of the ileum but can be located in the bronchi, ovaries, testes, and anywhere along the entire length of the alimentary tract. The full set of carcinoid symptoms are manifested only when the liver is involved.

Diagnosis of the condition is established by a 24-hour urine test for 5-hydroxyindole acetic acid (5-HIAA), which is the end-product of the breakdown of tryptophan to serotonin. Patients with carcinoid syndrome may have very high levels, 100 to 500 mg in 24 hours.

Treatment of the condition depends upon the patient's symptoms. Surgical resection of the primary tumour and partial hepatectomy to remove the bulk of tumour tissue may give prolonged survival but are rarely curative. Hepatic embolization offers an alternative nonoperative approach for reducing the bulk of tumour with alleviation of symptoms. Drugs are administered as indicated to manage the hypotension, diarrhoea, flushing, and other symptoms. Efforts are made to improve nutrition and at the same time avoid serotonin-containing foods, such as walnuts and bananas, which are known to precipitate an attack.

carcinolysis (ˌkahsi'nolisis) destruction of cancer cells.

adj. **carcinolytic.**

carcinoma (ˌkahsi'nohmə) a malignant new growth made up of epithelial cells tending to infiltrate surrounding tissues and to give rise to metastases. A form of CANCER, carcinoma is much more common than sarcoma and makes up the majority of the cases of malignancy of the lung, breast, uterus, bladder, intestinal tract, skin, and tongue.

adenocystic c., adenoid cystic c. carcinoma marked by cylinders or bands of hyaline or mucinous stroma separated or surrounded by nests or cords of small epithelial cells, occurring in the mammary and salivary glands, and mucous glands of the respiratory tract. Called also cylindroma.

alveolar c. alveolar adenocarcinoma.

basal cell c. an epithelial tumour of the skin that seldom metastasizes but has potential for local invasion and destruction.

basosquamous c. carcinoma that histologically exhibits both basal and squamous elements.

bronchogenic c. carcinoma of the lung, so called because it arises from the epithelium of the bronchial tree.

cholangiocellular c. primary carcinoma of the liver originating in bile duct cells.

chorionic c. choriocarcinoma.

colloid c. mucinous carcinoma.

cylindrical cell c. carcinoma in which the cells are cylindrical or nearly so.

embryonal c. a highly malignant primitive form of carcinoma, probably of germinal cell or teratomatous derivation, usually arising in a gonad.

epidermoid c. that in which the cells tend to differentiate in the same way as those of the epidermis; i.e., they tend to form prickle cells and undergo cornification.

giant cell c. carcinoma containing many giant cells.

hepatocellular c. primary carcinoma of the liver cells.

Hürthle cell c. Hürthle cell tumour.

c. in situ a neoplastic entity wherein the tumour cells have not invaded the basement membrane but are still confined to the epithelium of origin; popularly applied to such cells in the uterine cervix.

large-cell c. a bronchogenic tumour of undifferentiated (anaplastic) cells of large size.

medullary c. that composed mainly of epithelial elements with little or no stroma.

mucinous c. adenocarcinoma producing significant amounts of mucin.

nasopharyngeal c. a malignant tumour arising in the epithelial lining of the space behind the nose (nasopharynx), and occurring at high frequency in southern China. The Epstein–Barr virus has been implicated as a causative agent.

oat-cell c. small-cell carcinoma.

papillary c. carcinoma in which there are papillary excrescences; called also *papillocarcinoma.*

renal cell c. carcinoma of the renal parenchyma, composed of tubular cells in varying arrangements.

scirrhous c. carcinoma with a hard structure owing to the formation of dense connective tissue in the stroma.

c. simplex an undifferentiated carcinoma.

small-cell c. a radiosensitive tumour composed of small, oval, undifferentiated cells that are intensely haematoxyphilic and typically arise from bronchus. Called also *oat-cell carcinoma.*

spindle cell c. squamous cell carcinoma marked by fusiform development or rapidly proliferating cells.

squamous cell c. that arising from squamous epithelium and having cuboid cells, showing squamous differentiation.

carcinomatosis (ˌkahsiˌnohmə'tohsis) the condition of widespread dissemination of cancer throughout the body.

carcinomatous (ˌkahsi'nohmətəs) pertaining to or of the nature of cancer; malignant.

carcinophilia (ˌkahsinoh'fili·ə) special affinity for cancerous tissue. adj. **carcinophilic.**

carcinophobia (ˌkahsinoh'fohbi·ə) morbid dread of cancer.

carcinosarcoma (ˌkahsinohsah'kohmə) a malignant tumour composed of carcinomatous and sarcomatous tissues. **embryonal c.** a rapidly developing, malignant mixed tumour of the kidneys, made up of embryonal elements, and occurring chiefly in children before the fifth year; called also *Wilms' tumour.*

carcinosis (ˌkahsi'nohsis) carcinomatosis.

miliary c. that marked by development of numerous nodules resembling miliary tuberculosis.

Cardarelli's sign (kahdə'reliz) transverse pulsation of the laryngotracheal tube in aneurysms and in dilation of the arch of the aorta.

cardi(o)- word element. [Gr.] *heart.*

cardia ('kahdi·ə) 1. the cardiac opening. 2. the cardiac part of the stomach; that part of the stomach surrounding the oesophagogastric junction, distinguished by the presence of cardiac glands.

cardiac ('kahdiˌak) 1. pertaining to the heart. 2. pertaining to the cardia.

c. arrest sudden and often unexpected stoppage of effective heart action. Either the periodic impulses which trigger the coordinated heart muscle contractions cease or ventricular fibrillation or flutter occurs in which the individual muscle fibres have a rapid irregular twitching. The majority of victims of cardiac arrest suffer from ventricular fibrillation, and most of them have severe coronary artery disease (CAD). The only chance for survival for many of those who experience unexpected cardiac arrest is successful implementation of emergency cardiac care and CARDIOPULMONARY RESUSCITATION (CPR).

Programmes aimed at achieving the goal of reduced mortality from cardiac arrest include education of the general public in ways to avoid the development of CAD in the first place, and secondarily, training lay people and health care professionals in the techniques of CPR.

Although cardiac arrest usually is related to preexisting coronary artery disease, there are other events in which the prompt delivery of CPR alone could mean survival for the victim. These include the cessation of heart and lung action as a result of drowning, suffocation, electrocution, drug overdose, and severe accidental trauma.

c. catheterization the insertion of a catheter into a vein or artery under fluroscopic control and guiding it into the interior of the heart for purposes of measuring cardiac output, determining the oxygen content of blood in the heart chambers, and evaluating the structural components of the heart. It is indicated whenever it is necessary to establish a precise and definite diagnosis in order to determine whether heart surgery is necessary and to plan the surgical approach.

c. compression an emergency measure to empty the ventricles of the heart in an effort to circulate the blood, and also to stimulate the heart so that it will resume its pumping action. In both external cardiac compression and internal cardiac massage, mouth-to-mouth resuscitation must be carried out at the same time. If available, an automatic resuscitator with mask and rebreathing bag can be used. See also CARDIOPULMONARY RESUSCITATION.

CLOSED OR EXTERNAL CARDIAC COMPRESSION. This closed-chest method of cardiopulmonary resuscitation is a rhythmic compression of the heart between the lower sternum in the front and the vertebral column in the back. It is a drastic measure that should be undertaken only by trained personnel because of the risk of causing injuries such as rib fractures, damage to the heart and liver, and puncture of the lungs or blood vessels that can lead to internal bleeding, fat emboli, and other serious complications.

Open or Internal Cardiac Massage. This involves a surgical incision directly over the heart and manual massage of the heart or stimulation with an electric current.

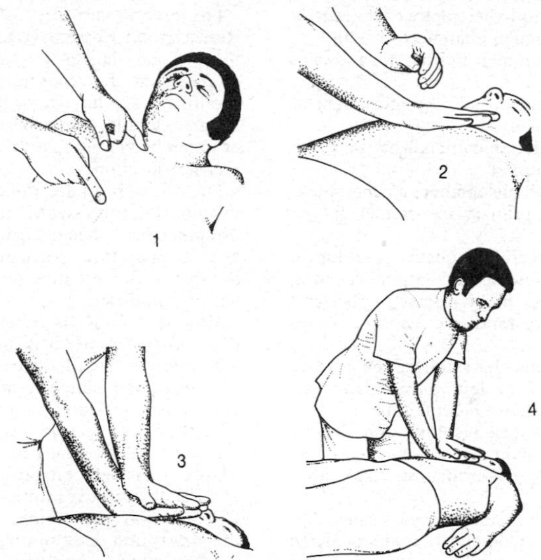

Closed cardiac massage. 1. Locate lower half of sternum. 2. Apply heel of one hand over lower half of sternum 1 to 1½ inches above the tip of the sternum. 3. Place second hand over first, bringing shoulders directly over victim's sternum. 4. Apply pressure so that sternum is depressed 1½ to 2 inches.

cardialgia (ˌkahdi'alji·ə) cardiodynia.

cardinal ('kahdin'l) of first importance; fundamental.

c. ligaments deep transverse cervical ligaments; Mackenrodt's ligaments.

Cardio Green ('kahdioh ˌgreen) trademark for a preparation of indocyanine green, a dye used intravenously as a diagnostic aid in the determination of blood volume, cardiac output, and hepatic function.

cardioaccelerator (ˌkahdioh·ak'seləˌraytə) quickening the heart action; an agent that so acts.

cardioactive (ˌkahdioh'aktiv) having an effect on the heart.

cardioangiology (ˌkahdiohˌanji'oləjee) the medical speciality dealing with the heart and blood vessels.

cardiocele ('kahdiohˌseel) hernial protrusion of the heart through a fissure of the diaphragm or through a wound.

cardiocentesis (ˌkahdiohsen'teesis) surgical puncture into the pericardial space and aspiration of fluid for therapeutic or diagnostic purposes. The procedure is used in an emergency to relieve cardiac tamponade, pericardial effusion, traumatic perforation or rupture of the myocardium, or effusion secondary to a tumour or chest injury.

cardiochalasia (ˌkahdiohkə'layzi·ə) relaxation or incompetence of the sphincter action of the cardiac opening of the stomach.

cardiocirculatory (ˌkahdioh'sərkyuhlətree, -ˌsərkyuh'laytə·ree) pertaining to blood flow through the heart and vascular system.

cardiocirrhosis (ˌkahdiohsi'rohsis) cirrhosis of the liver complicating heart disease, with recurrent intractable congestive heart failure.

cardiodiaphragmatic (ˌkahdiohˌdieəfrag'matik) pertaining to the heart and the diaphragm.

cardiodilator (ˌkahdiohdie'laytə) an instrument for dilating the cardia of the stomach.

cardiodiosis (ˌkahdiohdie'ohsis) dilation of the gastric cardia.

cardiodynamics (ˌkahdiohdie'namiks) study of the forces involved in the heart's action.

cardiodynia (ˌkahdioh'dini·ə) pain in the heart.

cardiogenesis (ˌkahdioh'jenəsis) development of the heart in the embryo.

cardiogenic (ˌkahdioh'jenik) originating in the heart.

cardiogram ('kahdiohˌgram) a tracing of a cardiac event produced by cardiography (see also ELECTROCARDIOGRAM).

cardiograph ('kahdiohˌgrahf, -ˌgraf) an instrument for recording some element of the heart beat.

cardiography (ˌkahdi'ografee) the graphic recording of a physical or functional aspect of the heart, e.g., electrocardiography, kinetocardiography, phonocardiography, vibrocardiography.

apex c. graphic recording of low-frequency pulsations at the anterior chest wall over the apex of the heart.

ultrasonic c. echocardiography.

vector c. vectorcardiography.

cardiohepatic (ˌkahdioh·hi'patik) pertaining to the heart and liver.

cardioinhibitor (ˌkahdioh·in'hibitə) an agent that restrains the heart's action.

cardioinhibitory (ˌkahdioh·in'hibitə·ree) restraining or inhibiting the heart movements.

cardiokinetic (ˌkahdiohki'netik) 1. exciting or stimulating the heart. 2. an agent that excites or stimulates the heart.

cardiokymography (ˌkahdiohkie'mogrəfee) the recording of the motion of the heart by means of the electrokymograph. adj. **cardiokymographic**.

cardiologist (ˌkahdi'oləjist) a doctor skilled in the diagnosis and treatment of heart disease.

cardiology (ˌkahdi'oləjee) study of the heart and its functions.

cardiolysis (ˌkahdi'olisis) the operation of freeing the heart from its adhesions to the sternal periosteum in adhesive mediastinopericarditis.

cardiomalacia (ˌkahdiohmə'layshi·ə) morbid softening of the muscular substance of the heart.

cardiomegaly (ˌkahdioh'megəlee) enlargement of the heart, which can be due to hypertrophy of its muscle fibres, dilation of its ventricular chambers, or both.

cardiomelanosis (ˌkahdiohˌmelə'nohsis) melanosis of the heart.

cardiomotility (ˌkahdiohmoh'tilitee) the movement of the heart; motility of the heart.

cardiomyoliposis (ˌkahdiohˌmieohli'pohsis) fatty degeneration of the heart muscle.

cardiomyopathy (ˌkahdiohmie'opəthee) a general diagnostic term designating primary myocardial disease with obvious cause.

alcoholic c. a congestive cardiomyopathy resulting in cardiac enlargement and low cardiac output occurring in chronic alcoholics; the heart disease in beriberi (thiamine deficiency) may rarely be associated with alcoholism.

congestive c. a syndrome characterized by cardiac enlargement, especially of the left ventricle, myocardial dysfunction, and congestive heart failure.

infiltrative c. myocardial disease resulting from deposition in the heart tissue of abnormal substances, as may occur in amyloidosis, haemochromatosis, and other disorders.

cardiomyopexy (ˌkahdioh'mieohˌpeksee) surgical removal of the epicardium and application of a pedicled flap of pectoralis major muscle to the denuded myocardium and pericardium, as a means of supplying collateral circulation to the heart.

cardionector (ˌkahdioh'nektə) the structures that regulate the heart beat, comprising the sinoatrial node, bundle of His, and atrioventricular node.

cardionephric (ˌkahdioh'nefrik) pertaining to the heart and kidney.

cardioneural (ˌkahdioh'nyooə·rəl) pertaining to the heart and nervous system.

cardioneurosis (ˌkahdiohnyuh'rohsis) neurocirculatory asthenia.

cardio-oesophageal (ˌkahdioh·iˌsofə'jeeəl) pertaining to the cardia of the stomach and the oesophagus, as the cardio-oesophageal junction or sphincter.

cardio-omentopexy (ˌkahdioh·oh'mentəˌpeksee) suture of a portion of the omentum to the heart, as a means of supplying collateral circulation to the heart.

cardiopaludism (ˌkahdioh'palyuhˌdizəm) heart disease due to falciparum malaria.

cardiopathy (ˌkahdi'opəthee) any disorder or disease of the heart.

cardiopericardiopexy (ˌkahdiohˌperi'kahdiohˌpeksee) surgical establishment of adhesive pericarditis, for relief of coronary disease.

cardiopericarditis (ˌkahdiohˌperikah'dietis) inflammation of the heart and pericardium.

cardiophobia (ˌkahdioh'fohbi·ə) morbid dread of heart disease.

cardioplasty ('kahdiohˌplastee) oesophagogastroplasty.

cardioplegia (ˌkahdioh'pleeji·ə) arrest of myocardial contraction, as by use of chemical compounds or cold in cardiac surgery. adj. **cardioplegic**.

cardiopneumatic (ˌkahdiohnyoo'matik) pertaining to the heart and respiration.

cardiopneumograph (ˌkahdioh'nyoomohˌgrahf, -ˌgraf) an apparatus for registering cardiopneumatic movements.

cardioptosis (ˌkahdiop'tohsis) downward displacement of the heart.

cardiopulmonary (ˌkahdioh'pulmənə·ree, -'puhl-) pertaining to the heart and lungs.

c. resuscitation (CPR) the reestablishment of heart and lung action as indicated for CARDIAC ARREST The CPR procedure is an essential component of basic life support (BLS), basic cardiac life support (BCLS), and advanced cardiac life support (ACLS).

The preliminary steps of CPR, as defined by the Resuscitation Council (UK) are: (1) establishing that there is no danger to yourself or the patient; (2) establishing the consciousness of the patient by shouting 'wake up' two or three times and shaking the shoulder gently, remembering the possibility of a neck or upper body injury; and (3) placing the patient in the recovery position.

These first steps are initiated as quickly as possible. Prompt action is essential to the successful outcome of the procedure. When cardiac arrest occurs at normal body temperature, permanent brain damage can be avoided with certainty only if CPR is commenced within 3 minutes.

Although CPR is strongly recommended as a life-saving measure, it is not without danger; specifically, there is risk of rib fracture, damage to the liver and heart, and puncture of the lungs and large blood vessels. Anyone interested in learning the techniques of CPR should receive instruction and practice under the direction of a qualified CPR instructor.

Once it has been established that a person is in need of CPR, the rescuer immediately begins the 'ABC's' of CPR—Airway, Breathing, and Circulation. Opening the airway and determining by look, sound, and feel is the first step for determining whether the person will be able to resume unassisted breathing. This is accomplished by lifting the chin and tilting the head back to lift the tongue away from the back of the throat. If there is no evidence of spontaneous breathing, the rescuer corrects obstruction of the airway by a foreign body, when this is indicated. This is done first by finger sweeps in the mouth if the jaw is relaxed. If this is not successful, firm blows to the back may dislodge a foreign body by compressing what air remains in the lungs, thereby causing an upward force behind the obstructing material. Once the airway is open, rescue breathing is started by means of mouth-to-mouth resuscitation (see ARTIFICIAL RESPIRATION).

The third element of CPR is circulation, which begins by establishing the presence or absence of a pulse in a major artery (preferably the carotid artery). If there is no pulse, compression of the chest is begun. External cardiac compression consists of rhythmic applications of pressure on the lower half of the sternum (NOT on the xiphoid process, which may injure the liver). For a normal-sized adult, sufficient force is used to depress the sternum about 4 to 5 cm (1½ to 2 inches). This raises intrathoracic pressure and produces the output of blood from the heart. When the pressure is released, blood is allowed to flow into the heart. Compressions should be maintained for one-half second; the same length of time is allowed for the relaxation period.

Cardiac compression is always accompanied by artificial respiration. The two must be coordinated so that there is regular and uninterrupted compression of the heart, circulation of blood, and aeration of the lungs.

The techniques of CPR provide basic life support

(BLS) in all cases of respiratory and cardiac arrest. Unfortunately, at present there is no recognized national training programme for basic or advanced life support in nursing or medical schools in the UK. However, the Resuscitation Council (UK) has issued guidelines which are now being used in many centres. Further information may be obtained from the Resuscitation Council (UK), Department of Anaesthetics, Hammersmith Hospital, Du Cane Road, London W12 0HS.

THE PRECORDIAL THUMP. Although the subject of debate, delivering a sharp blow to the sternum to revive heart action may be useful in specific types of cardiac arrest cases. The precordial thump is recommended in cases of witnessed cardiac arrest, with patients who are being monitored during advanced life support, and those with known atrioventricular block. In delivering the precordial thump one should strike a single, sharp and quick blow over the midportion of the sternum. The blow is delivered with the bottom, fleshy portion of the fist, striking from 8 to 12 inches over the chest. If there is no immediate response from the heart, CPR is begun at once.

cardiopuncture (ˌkahdioh'pungkchə) penetration of the heart by a needle or due to trauma.

cardiopyloric (ˌkahdiohpie'lorik) pertaining to the cardiac opening of the stomach and the pylorus.

cardiorenal (ˌkahdioh'reen'l) pertaining to the heart and kidneys.

cardiorrhaphy (ˌkahdi'o·rəfee) suture of the heart muscle.

cardiorrhexis (ˌkahdioh'reksis) rupture of the heart.

cardiosclerosis (ˌkahdiohsklə'rohsis) fibrous induration of the heart.

cardioselective (ˌkahdiohsi'lektiv) having greater activity on heart tissue than on other tissue.

cardiospasm ('kahdioh,spazəm) achalasia of the oesophagus.

cardiosphygmograph (ˌkahdioh'sfigmoh,grahf, -ˌgraf) a combination of the cardiograph and sphygmograph for recording the movements of the heart and an arterial pulse.

cardiosplenopexy (ˌkahdioh'splenoh,peksee) suture of the parenchyma of the spleen to the denuded surface of the heart for revascularization of the myocardium.

cardiotachometer (ˌkahdiohta'komitə) an instrument for continuously portraying or recording the heart rate.

cardiotachometry (ˌkahdiohta'komitree) continuous recording of the heart rate for long periods.

cardiotherapy (ˌkahdioh'therə,pee) the treatment of diseases of the heart.

cardiotocograph (ˌkahdioh'tohkoh,grahf, -ˌgraf) the recording demonstrating the interrelation between fetal heart rate and maternal uterine contractions in labour and indicating the presence of any fetal distress. Called also *tocograph*.

cardiotocography (ˌkahdiohtə'kogrəfee) the simultaneous monitoring of the fetal heart rate and maternal uterine contractions, as during delivery. Also a non-stress test for fetal well-being. Called also *tocography*. See also FETAL MONITORING.

cardiotocometer (ˌkahdiohtə'komitə) the instrument used in cardiotocography. Called also *tocometer, tokodynamometer*.

cardiotomy (ˌkahdi'otəmee) 1. surgical incision of the heart. 2. surgical incision into the cardia of the stomach.

cardiotonic (ˌkahdioh'tonik) having a tonic effect on the heart; an agent that so acts.

cardiotoxic (ˌkahdioh'toksik) having a poisonous or deleterious effect upon the heart.

cardiovalvular (ˌkahdioh'valvyuhlə) pertaining to the valves of the heart.

cardiovalvulotome (ˌkahdioh'valvyuhlə,tohm) an instrument for incising a heart valve.

cardiovascular (ˌkahdioh'vaskyuhlə) pertaining to the heart and blood vessels.

cardioversion (ˌkahdioh'vərshən) the delivery of a direct-current shock synchronized with the QRS complex to the myocardium as an elective treatment to end tachydysrhythmias; called also *countershock* and *precordial shock*. For *emergency* treatment by precordial shock using a nonsynchronized current to terminate arrhythmia, see DEFIBRILLATION.

The goal of cardioversion is to restore sinoatrial control of the heart rhythm by depolarizing the entire myocardium at the moment of shock. The depolarization interrupts re-entrant circuits, thus ending myocardial fibrillation and some other types of dysrhythmias. The electric shock can be delivered directly to the myocardium in an open chest procedure, or through externally applied paddles placed on the chest.

Cardioversion is most effective in terminating arrhythmias due to continuous reentry, including atrial flutter, atrial fibrillation, paroxysmal supraventricular tachycardia, ventricular tachycardia, and ventricular fibrillation. Patients who have had a recent myocardial infarction and resultant atrial, nodal, or ventricular tachycardia are the most frequent candidates for cardioversion. Patients with severe, long standing arrhythmias due to chronic extensive heart disease usually do not benefit from cardioversion.

The procedure should be done only by qualified doctors in a setting where resuscitation equipment and respiratory support are readily at hand. Serum potassium levels must be within normal limits at the time of procedure because hypokalaemia increases the patient's chance of developing deadly postconversion dysrhythmias. If necessary, potassium salts can be given prior to the procedure. Digitalis toxicity predisposes the patient to life-threatening dysrhythmias *during* cardioversion and the drug should be withheld several days prior to the anticipated procedure. Hypoxia and acidosis also preclude conversion because they can prevent conversion to a normal rhythm after cardioversion.

cardioverter ('kahdioh,vərtə) an energy-storage capacitor-discharge type of condenser that is discharged with an inductance; it delivers a direct-current shock which restores normal rhythm of the heart.

carditis (kah'dietis) inflammation of the heart; MYOCARDITIS.

cardivalvulitis (ˌkahdi,valvyuh'lietis) inflammation of the heart valves.

Carey Coombs murmur (ˌkair·ree 'koomz) a rumbling mid-diastolic murmur occurring in the early stages of rheumatic fever.

caries ('kair·reez, -ri·eez) decay, as of bone or teeth. adj. **carious**.

dental c. a disease which commences on the tooth surface and results in the gradual destruction of enamel and dentine.

Decayed and infected teeth may result in pain, loss of function and even be the source of other infections throughout the body.

CAUSES. Dental caries is a bacterial disease. The initial lesion occurs after the outer enamel layer has been breached by the action of acid-producing bacteria contained in dental plaque.

Refined carbohydrate taken in the diet is metabolized by the plaque bacteria, which in turn produce acid waste products. If the plaque remains on the tooth surface, the initial breach of the enamel will progress, forming a carious cavity.

Dental caries needs the following factors to be present: (1) a susceptible host; (2) suitable acid-producing bacteria within the dental plaque; and (3) a diet containing substances which the bacteria can readily metabolize.

TREATMENT. The only treatment for dental caries is regular dental care. Where caries is active, it must be removed by cavity preparation and a suitable restoration placed in the tooth.

The restoration may commonly be of silver amalgam or composite material or, less commonly, of gold.

If the decay has reached the pulp of the tooth, a pulp necrosis may result. This may mean that an extraction or, more commonly, endodontic treatment of the tooth is required. Endodontic or root treatment techniques now mean that many teeth which formerly would have been lost can now be saved.

PREVENTION. Dental caries is usually an entirely preventable disease. Methods of prevention include: (1) increasing the patient's resistance—for example, by fluoride taken in drinking water or as a mouthwash, as this strengthens the enamel, thereby producing a dramatic reduction in dental caries; (2) removal of plaque—by toothbrushing, dental flossing and other methods of oral hygiene, and also the use of certain substances such as chlorhexidine, which are known to be effective in reducing the activity of the plaque bacteria; (3) modifying the diet—avoiding highly cariogenic foods, such as biscuits, sweets and soft drinks, which are easily metabolized by the plaque bacteria.

dry c., c. sicca a form of tuberculous caries of the joints and ends of bones.

carina (kə'rienə, -'reena) pl. *carinae* [L.] a ridgelike structure.

c. tracheae a downward and backward projection of the lowest tracheal cartilage, forming a ridge between the openings of the right and left principal bronchi.

c. urethralis vaginae the column of rugae in the lower anterior wall of the vagina, immediately below the urethra.

cariogenesis (ˌkair·rioh'jenəsis) the development of caries.

cariogenic (ˌkair·rioh'jenik) conducive to caries.

carisoprodol (kəˌriesoh'prohdol) an analgesic and skeletal muscle relaxant.

carminative (kah'minətiv) 1. relieving flatulence. 2. an agent that relieves flatulence.

carmustine (kah'musteen) BCNU; a nitrosourea, used as an ANTINEOPLASTIC agent.

carneous ('kahni·əs) fleshy.

c. mole a mass of clotted blood surrounding a dead embryo and retained by the uterus. See ABORTION.

carnitine ('kahniˌteen) a vitamin of the B complex present in meat extracts.

carnivore ('kahniˌvor) any animal that eats primarily flesh, particularly mammals of the order Carnivora, which includes cats, dogs, bears, etc. adj. **carnivorus**.

carnosinaemia (ˌkahnohsi'neemi·ə) excessive amounts of carnosine in the blood; it has been associated with a progressive neurological disease characterized by severe mental defect and myoclonic seizures, and is probably due to a genetic deficiency of carnosinase in the serum.

carnosinase ('kahnohˌsienayz) an enzyme that hydrolyses carnosine (amino-acyl-L-histidine) and other dipeptides containing L-histidine into their constituent amino acids.

carnosine ('kahnohˌseen) a dipeptide composed of beta-alanine and histidine, found in skeletal muscle of vertebrates.

carnosinuria (ˌkahnohsi'nyooə·ri·ə) an aminoacidurea characterized by excess of carnosine in the urine; it occurs in carnosinaemia or may be dietary in origin, especially in young children.

carotenaemia (ˌkarotə'neemi·ə) the presence of carotene in the blood; sometimes occurring in sufficient amounts to cause yellowing of the skin.

carotenase (kə'rotəˌnayz) an enzyme that converts carotene into vitamin A.

carotene ('karəˌteen) a yellow or red pigment from carrots, sweet potatoes, milk and body fat, egg yolk, etc.; it is a chromolipoid hydrocarbon existing in several forms (α-, β-, and γ-carotene), which can be converted into vitamin A in the body.

carotenodermia (kəˌrotənoh'dərmi·ə) yellowness of the skin due to carotenaemia.

carotenoid (kə'rotəˌnoyd) 1. any member of a group of red, orange, or yellow pigmented polyisoprenoid lipids found in carrots, green leaves, and some animal tissues; examples are the carotenes, lycopene, and xanthophyll. 2. marked by yellow colour. 3. lipochrome.

carotenosis (ˌkarotə'nohsis) deposition of carotene in tissues, especially the skin.

caroticotympanic (kəˌrotikohtim'panik) pertaining to the carotid canal and tympanum.

carotid (kə'rotid) relating to the carotid artery, the principal artery of the neck.

c. body a small neurovascular structure lying in the bifurcation of the right and left carotid arteries, containing chemoreceptors that monitor oxygen content in blood and help to regulate respiration.

c. canal a canal in the pars petrosa of the temporal bone, transmitting the internal carotid artery to the cranial cavity.

c. endarterectomy the surgical removal of atherosclerotic plaques within an extracranial carotid artery, usually the common carotid, to prevent stroke in certain patients. This procedure may be performed in those who have experienced TRANSIENT ISCHAEMIC ATTACKS (TIAs), patients who have already had a stroke and have good neurological recovery but are known to have severe stenosis of a carotid artery, and those with severe stenosis of one internal carotid artery and total occlusion of the other but who have not yet had a stroke. **c. sinus** a dilation of the proximal portion of the internal carotid or distal portion of the common carotid artery, containing in its wall baroreceptors which monitor changes in blood pressure and initiate adjustments to maintain homeostasis.

c. sinus reflex slowing of the heart beat when pressure is exerted on the carotid artery at the level of the cricoid cartilage.

c. sinus syndrome syncope sometimes associated with convulsive seizures due to overactivity of the carotid sinus reflex. Transient attacks of numbness or weakness of the face, arm, or leg, headache, and in some cases aphasia may occur in susceptible persons due to sudden turning of the head or the wearing of a tight collar.

Diagnosis can be confirmed by a gentle massage of the carotid sinus area, which will cause profound slowing of the heart and may precipitate an attack. However, this must only be done when resuscitation and monitoring facilities are available. Drugs used to terminate attacks or to prevent their occurrence include atropine sulphate, but insertion of a pacemaker may be required in severe cases.

carotidynia (kəˌroti'dini·ə) tenderness along the course of the carotid artery.

carpal ('kahp'l) pertaining to the carpus, or wrist.
c. tunnel the osseofibrous passage for the median nerve and the flexor tendons, formed by the flexor retinaculum and the carpal bones.
c. tunnel syndrome a symptom complex resulting from compression of the median nerve in the carpal tunnel, with pain and burning or tingling paraesthesias in the fingers and hand, sometimes extending to the elbow. The disorder is found most often in middle-aged women. Excessive wrist movements, arthritis, hypertrophy of the bone and connective tissue in ACROMEGALY, and swelling of the wrist can produce the carpal tunnel syndrome. Treatment is usually conservative and consists of splinting the wrist to immobilize it for several weeks until the irritation of the median nerve has healed. In severe cases surgical resection of the carpal ligament is helpful.
carpectomy (kah'pektəmee) excision of a carpal bone.
Carpenter's syndrome ('kahpintəz) a hereditary disorder, transmitted as an autosomal recessive trait, characterized by acrocephalopolysyndactyly, brachydactyly, peculiar facies, obesity, mental handicap, hypogonadism, and other anomalies.
carphology (kah'foləjee) involuntary picking at the bedclothes, seen in states of great exhaustion and hyperpyrexia.
carpometacarpal (ˌkahpohˌmetə'kahp'l) pertaining to the carpus and metacarpus.
carpopedal (ˌkahpoh'ped'l, -'peed'l) affecting the wrist and foot.
carpophalangeal (ˌkahpohfə'lanji·əl) pertaining to the carpus and phalanges.
carpoptosis (ˌkahpoh'tohsis) wristdrop.
carpus ('kahpəs) the joint between the arm and hand, made up of eight bones; the WRIST.
carrier ('kari·ə) 1. one who harbours disease organisms in his body without manifest symptoms, thus acting as a carrier or distributor of infection. 2. a heterozygote, i.e., one who carries a recessive gene, autosomal or sex-linked, together with its normal allele.
carrier-free ('kari·əˌfree) a term denoting a radioisotope of an element in pure form, i.e., essentially undiluted with a stable isotope carrier.
Carrión's disease (kari'onz) bartonellosis.
Cartesian (kah'teezi·ən) pertaining to French philosopher René Descartes (1591–1650); see DUALISM.
cartilage ('kahtilij) a specialized, fibrous connective tissue present in adults, and forming most of the temporary skeleton in the embryo, providing a model in which most of the bones develop, and constituting an important part of the organism's growth mechanism; the three most important types are hyaline cartilage, elastic cartilage, and fibrocartilage. Also, a general term for a mass of such tissue in a particular site in the body.
alar c's the cartilages of the wings of the nose.
aortic c. the second costal cartilage on the right side.
arthrodial c., articular c. that lining the articular surfaces of synovial joints.
arytenoid c's two pyramid-shaped cartilages of the larynx.
connecting c. that connecting the surfaces of an immovable joint.
costal c. a bar of hyaline cartilage that attaches a rib to the sternum in the case of true ribs, or to the immediately above rib in the case of the upper false ribs.
cricoid c. a ringlike cartilage forming the lower and back part of the larynx.
diarthrodial c. articular cartilage.
elastic c. cartilage that is more opaque, flexible, and elastic than hyaline cartilage, and is further distinguished by its yellow colour. The ground substance is penetrated in all directions by frequently branching fibres that give all of the reactions for elastin.
ensiform c. xiphoid process.
fibrous c. fibrocartilage.
floating c. a detached portion of semilunar cartilage in the knee joint.
hyaline c. flexible, somewhat elastic, semitransparent cartilage with an opalescent bluish tint, composed of a basophilic fibril-containing substance with cavities in which the chondrocytes occur.
permanent c. cartilage that does not normally become ossified.
reticular c. elastic cartilage.
semilunar c. one of the two interarticular cartilages of the knee joint. **temporary c.** cartilage that is normally destined to be replaced by bone.
thyroid c. the shield-shaped cartilage of the larynx.
vomeronasal c. either of the two narrow strips of cartilage, one on each side, of the nasal septum supporting the vomeronasal organ.
yellow c. elastic cartilage.
cartilaginiform (ˌkahtilə'jinifawm) resembling cartilage.
cartilaginous (ˌkahti'lajinəs) consisting of or of the nature of cartilage.
cartilago (ˌkahti'laygo) pl. *cartilagines* [L.] cartilage.
caruncle ('karəngk'l, kə'rung-) a small fleshy eminence, often abnormal.
hymenal c's small elevations of mucous membrane around the vaginal opening, being relics of the ruptured hymen.
lacrimal c. the red eminence at the medial angle of the eye.
sublingual c. an eminence on either side of the frenulum of the tongue (frenulum linguae), on which the major duct of the sublingual gland and the duct of the submandibular gland open.
urethral c. a small, polypoid, red growth on the mucous membrane of the female urinary meatus, sometimes causing difficulty in voiding.
caruncula (kə'rungkyuhlə) pl. *carunculae* [L.] caruncle.
caryo- for words beginning thus, see those beginning *karyo-*.
cascade (kas'kayd) a series of steps or stages (as of a physiological process) which, once initiated, continues to the final step by virtue of each step being triggered by the preceding one, sometimes with cumulative effect.
cascara (kas'kahrə) bark.
c. sagrada dried bark of *Rhamnus purshiana*, used as a cathartic.
case (kays) a particular instance of disease; as a case of leukaemia; sometimes used incorrectly to designate the patient with the disease.
c. control study an epidemiological study in which the characteristics of cases of disease are compared with a matched control group of persons without the disease. Called also *retrospective study, case referent study*.
c. fatality rate the number of persons dying of a particular disease expressed as a proportion of the total contracting the disease and usually expressed as a percentage.
c. history the collected data concerning an individual, his family, and environment, including his medical history and any other information that may be useful in analysing and diagnosing his case or for instructional or research purposes.
c. referent study see case control study (above).
caseation (ˌkaysi'ayshən) 1. the precipitation of casein. 2. a form of necrosis typical of tuberculosis, in which tissue is changed into a dry, amorphous mass resem-

bling cheese.

casein ('kaysi·in, -seen) the chemical product of the action of rennin on caseinogen.

caseinogen (,kaysi'inəjən, kay'seenə-) a phosphoprotein, the principal protein of milk, the basis of curd and of cheese. NOTE: In American nomenclature caseinogen is called casein, and casein is called paracasein.

caseous ('kaysi·əs) resembling cheese or curd; cheesy.

Casoni's test (kə'sohneez) intradermal injection of hydatid fluid followed by production of wheal-flare reaction denoting hydatid infection.

cassette (ka'set) [Fr.] a light-proof housing for x-ray film, containing front and back intensifying screens, between which the film is placed; a magazine for film or magnetic tape.

cast (kahst) 1. a positive copy of an object, e.g., a mould of a hollow organ (a renal tubule, bronchiole, etc.), formed of effused plastic matter and extruded from the body, as a urinary cast; named according to constituents, as epithelial, fatty, waxy, etc. 2. a positive copy of the tissues of the jaws, made in an impression, over which denture bases or other restorations may be fabricated. 3. to form an object in a mould. 4. a stiff dressing or casing, usually made of plaster of Paris, used to immobilize body parts. 5. strabismus.

PATIENT CARE. If the patient is confined to bed after a plaster of Paris cast is applied, it is necessary to provide a firm mattress protected by a waterproof material until the cast is dry. Several small pillows should be available for placing under the curves of the cast to prevent remoulding or cracking of the plaster and to provide adequate support of the patient. When handling a wet cast only the palm or flat of the hand is used so that the fingertips will not make indentations that might produce pressure against the patient's skin.

While the cast is drying it is left uncovered to allow sufficient circulation of air around it. The parts of the body not included in the cast are covered with a sheet or light blanket to avoid chilling. Extreme heat should not be used to hasten drying as this may produce burns under the cast. The patient is turned frequently to ensure proper drying and to avoid prolonged pressure on any one area.

Parts of the cast that may become soiled by urine or faeces can be covered with a plastic material which can be changed as necessary. To minimize crumbling of the edges and irritation of the skin around and under the cast, a strip of stockinette or adhesive tape is applied so that the rim of the cast is thoroughly covered. Observation of the patient for signs of impaired circulation or pressure against a nerve is extremely important. Any numbness, recurrent pain, or tingling should be reported at once. If an extremity is enclosed in a cast, it should be elevated to reduce swelling. Cyanosis or blanching of the fingers or toes extending from a cast usually indicates impaired blood flow which may lead to serious complications if not corrected immediately.

The patient should be encouraged to move joints on either side of the cast to prevent stiffness. He should be warned not to drop anything inside the cast and to avoid wetting it.

castor oil ('kahstə) a fixed oil obtained from the seed of the castor bean plant *(Ricinus communis)*; it has an irritant effect on the intestines and acts as a powerful purgative. Castor oil is a powerful cathartic, and should not be used as a treatment for constipation or any digestive disorder. It is used primarily in the preparation of the bowel for diagnostic tests and surgery. Its unpleasant taste can be disguised if it is given in iced orange juice. Castor oil is also used externally as an emollient in seborrhoeic dermatitis and other skin diseases.

castrate (ka'strayt) 1. to remove the testes. 2. a castrated individual.

castration (ka'strayshən) removal of the testes, or their destruction, as by radiation or disease.

female c. removal of the ovaries, or bilateral OOPHORECTOMY; spaying.

casualty ('kazhooəltee, -zyooəl-) 1. an accident; an accidental wound; death or disablement from an accident; also the person so injured. 2. in the armed forces, one missing from his unit as a result of death, injury, illness, capture, because his whereabouts are unknown, or other reasons.

CAT computerized axial tomography (see computed TOMOGRAPHY).

cat-bite fever ('katbiet) an infectious disease of man transmitted by the bite of a cat, caused by *Pasteurella multocida* and marked by the formation of an abscess at the site of inoculation.

NOTE: Not to be confused with CAT-SCRATCH DISEASE.

cat-scratch disease (fever) ('katskratch) a benign, subacute, regional lymphadenitis resulting from a scratch or bite of a cat or a scratch from a surface contaminated by a cat.

No specific causative agent has been isolated, but a viral aetiology is suspected. Cats thought to be associated with human infection show no signs of illness, and probably act only as vectors of the disease, conveying the causative agent on claws or teeth.

In half the cases, after several days there is a persistent sore at the site of the scratch, and fever and other symptoms of infection may develop. There is also swelling of the lymph nodes draining the infected part.

In milder cases, the symptoms soon disappear, with no after-effects. Sometimes the attack is more serious and the glands may require surgical incision and drainage. Occasionally meningoencephalitis is a serious complication. The disease is generally mild and lasts for about 2 weeks. In rare cases, it may persist for a period of up to 2 years.

No specific remedy exists for cat-scratch disease, although certain antibiotics appear to shorten its course. The main treatment consists simply of keeping the patient as comfortable as possible. The disease can, however, usually be prevented by avoiding cat scratches or bites or by thoroughly washing and disinfecting any wound that does occur.

NOTE: Not to be confused with CAT-BITE FEVER.

cat(a)- word element. [Gr.] *down, lower, under, against, along with, very.*

catabasis (kə'tabəsis) the stage of decline of a disease. adj. **catabatic.**

catabiosis (,katəbie'ohsis) the natural senescence of cells. adj. **catabiotic.**

catabolism (kə'tabə,lizəm) any destructive process by which complex substances are converted by living cells into simpler compounds, with release of energy (see also METABOLISM). adj. **catabolic.**

catabolite (kə'tabə,liet) a compound produced in catabolism.

catacrotism (kə'takrə,tizəm) a pulse anomaly in which a small additional wave or notch appears in the descending limb of the pulse tracing. adj. **catacrotic.**

catadicrotism (katə'dikrə,tizəm) a pulse anomaly in which two small additional waves or notches appear in the descending limb of the pulse tracing. adj. **catadicrotic.**

catagenesis (,katə'jenəsis) involution or retrogression.

catalase ('katə,layz) a crystalline enzyme that specifically catalyses the decomposition of hydrogen peroxide

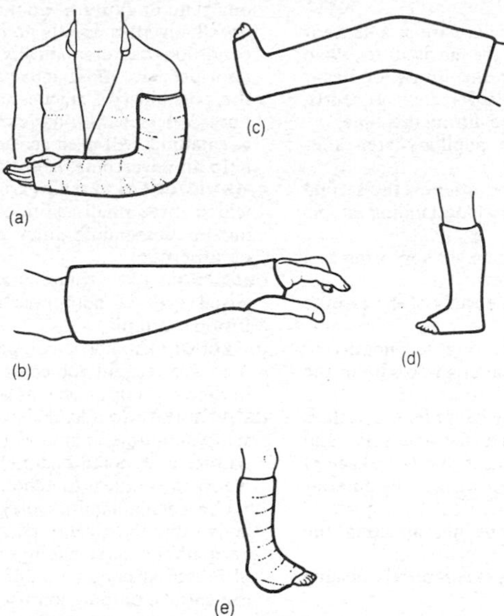

Casts. (a) Long arm cast. (b) Short arm cast. (c) Long leg cast. (d) Short leg cast. (e) Weight bearing cast.

and is found in almost all cells except certain anaerobic bacteria. adj. **catalatic.**

catalepsy ('katəlepsee) catatonia.

cataleptiform (ˌkatə'leptiˌfawm) resembling catatonia (catalepsy).

catalyse ('katəˌliez) to cause or produce catalysis.

catalysis (kə'talisis) increase in the velocity of a chemical reaction or process produced by the presence of a substance that is not consumed in the net chemical reaction or process; negative catalysis denotes the slowing down or inhibition of a reaction or process by the presence of such a substance. adj. **catalytic.**

catalyst ('katəˌlist) any substance that brings about catalysis.

catamenia (ˌkatə'meeni·ə) menstruation.

cataphasia (ˌkatə'fayzi·ə) speech disorder with constant repetition of a word or phrase.

cataphora (kə'tafə·rə) lethargy with intervals of imperfect waking.

cataphoria (ˌkatə'for·ri·ə) a downward turning of the visual axes of both eyes after visual functional stimuli have been removed. adj. **cataphoric.**

cataphylaxis (ˌkatəfi'laksis) movement of leukocytes and antibodies to the site of an infection. adj. **cataphylactic.**

cataplasia (ˌkatə'playzi·ə) atrophy with tissues reverting to earlier, or more embryonic conditions.

cataplasm ('katəˌplazəm) a poultice, which acts as a counter-irritant. It is generally made from kaolin and glycerin.

cataplexy ('katəˌpleksee) a condition, often associated with narcolepsy; marked by abrupt attacks of muscular weakness and hypotonia triggered by an emotional stimulus, such as mirth, anger, fear, etc. adj. **cataplectic.**

Catapres ('katəˌpres) trademark for preparations of clonidine used for moderate to severe hypertension.

cataract ('katəˌrakt) opacity of the lens of the eye. adj. **cataractous.**

Causes and Symptoms. Cataract may result from injuries to the eye, exposure to great heat or radiation, or inherited factors. The great majority of cases, however, are senile cataracts, which are apparently a part of the ageing process of the human body.

Blurred and dimmed vision are often the first symptoms of cataract. The patient may find that he needs a brighter reading light, or must hold objects closer to his eyes. The continued clouding of the lens may cause double vision. Finally a need for frequent changes of spectacles may be caused by the presence of cataract. However, these symptoms do not necessarily indicate cataract.

Treatment. The only known effective treatment for cataract is surgical removal of the lens (lens extraction or cataract extraction). This may be an intracapsular extraction, which involves total removal of the lens within its capsule, or extracapsular extraction, which involves removal of the lens nucleus and cortex with retention of the posterior lens capsule. See also cryoextraction.

The lens of the eye serves only to focus light rays upon the retina. After cataract extraction the loss of the natural lens is compensated for by either special spectacles or contact lenses. Implantation of a permanent intraocular lens, either during cataract surgery or later, is an alternative to use of cataract spectacles or a removable contact lens.

Patient Care. Special pre-operative care may include the trimming of eyelashes, the instillation of mydriatic drops to the appropriate eye, and rarely the taking of conjunctival cultures. Following surgery, nursing care should aim to minimize the risk of further damage to the eye from trauma or infection. Anti-emetics will reduce the possibility of trauma from vomiting and any signs of rising intra-ocular pressure require immediate treatment.

On discharge, following either day care or a 48 hour admission, the patient should be advised to avoid sudden movement, bending or the lifting of heavy loads for the next few weeks. Participation in sports, e.g. swimming, should be avoided during this time.

after-c. any membrane of the pupillary area after extraction or absorption of the lens.

atopic c. cataract occurring, most often in the second to third decade, in those with longstanding atopic dermatitis.

brown c., brunescent c. senile cataract appearing as a brown opacity.

capsular c. one consisting of an opacity of the capsule of the lens.

complicated c. a cataract occurring secondarily to other intraocular disease. **cortical c.** an opacity in the cortex of the lens.

hypermature c. one in which the entire lens capsule is wrinkled and the contents have become solid and shrunken, or soft and liquid. This is due to leakage of denatured lens protein from the lens into the anterior chamber.

lenticular c. opacity of the lens not affecting the capsule.

mature c. one in which the lens is completely opaque and usually white in colour.

secondary c. complicated cataract.

senile c. the cataract of old persons.

cataractogenic (ˌkatəˌraktoh'jenik) tending to induce the formation of cataracts.

catarrh (kə'tah) inflammation of a mucous membrane (particularly of the head and throat), with free discharge. adj. **catarrhal.**

catatonia (ˌkatə'tohni·ə) a condition of diminished responsiveness usually characterized by a trancelike state and constantly maintained immobility, often with flexibilitas cerea (WAXY FLEXIBILITY). The patient with catatonia may remain in one position for minutes, days, or even longer. adj. **catatonic.** Called also *catalepsy.*

Catatonia may occur in several mental illnesses. It is most common and indeed considered typical in cases of catatonic SCHIZOPHRENIA. The patient may sit with his hands flat on his knees and his head bowed, or may remain in an awkward and uncomfortable position. He is not necessarily unaware of what is going on, but he does not respond. This apathetic condition may end as suddenly as it begins.

PATIENT CARE. Regular skin care and exercise of the muscles and joints are necessary to prevent circulatory complications in the patient with catalepsy. Attention must also be given to his nutritional status and an adequate diet provided. Even though the patient may not be able to respond to spoken directions or conversation and is physically unable to move, he cannot be left in one position for long periods of time any more than can the patient who is physically paralysed. The patient's mental state is such that he cannot recognize numbness or pain, nor can he communicate his need for attention.

Care must be used in conversations held within the patient's hearing. His total apathy does not mean that he cannot hear or see what is going on around him. Sometimes it is of great help to this type of patient to have someone sit quietly beside him so that he is aware that someone cares and is genuinely interested in his welfare. Above all, he should not be ignored simply because he is quiet and undemanding of the staff's time and attention.

A sudden change in the patient's condition, with increased activity, may indicate his progression from one state of extreme emotion to another. Restlessness or talkativeness usually do not indicate that his mental condition has dramatically improved. When the patient becomes more active the staff should be alert to the possibility of SUICIDE and attempts at self-mutilation. A person who has exhibited symptoms as severe as catatonia will need continued and long-term care to help him overcome his serious emotional problems.

catatricrotism (ˌkatə'triekroˌtizəm) a pulse anomaly in which three small additional waves or notches appear in the descending limb of the pulse tracing. adj. **catatricrotic.**

catatropia (ˌkatə'trohpi·ə) a downward turning of the visual axes of both eyes in the presence of visual fusional stimuli.

catechol ('katiˌkol) a compound, *o*-dehydroxybenzene, used as a reagent and comprising the aromatic portion in the synthesis of catecholamines.

catecholamine (ˌkatikol'aymeen) any of a group of sympathomimetic amines (including dopamine, adrenaline, and noradrenaline), the aromatic portion of whose molecule is catechol.

The catecholamines play an important role in the body's physiological response to stress. Their release at sympathetic nerve endings increases the rate and force of muscular contraction of the heart, thereby increasing cardiac output; constricts peripheral blood vessels, resulting in elevated blood pressure; elevates blood glucose levels by hepatic and skeletal muscle glycogenolysis; and promotes an increase in blood lipids by increasing the catabolism of fats.

catecholaminergic (ˌkatikolˌami'nərjik) activated by or secreting catecholamines.

catgut ('katˌgut) an absorbable suture material obtained from the submucous layer of sheep's intestine.

catharsis (kə'thahsis) 1. a cleansing or purgation. 2. the bringing into consciousness and the emotional reliving of a forgotten (repressed) painful experience as a means of releasing anxiety and tension.

cathartic (kə'thahtik) 1. causing bowel evacuation; an agent that so acts. 2. producing catharsis.

bulk c. one stimulating bowel evacuation by increasing faecal volume.

lubricant c. one that acts by softening the faeces and reducing friction between them and the intestinal wall.

saline c. one that increases fluidity of intestinal contents by retention of water by osmotic forces, and indirectly increases motor activity.

stimulant c. one that directly increases motor activity of the intestinal tract.

cathectic (kə'thektik) pertaining to cathexis.

cathepsin (kə'thepsin) a proteinase found in most cells, which takes part in cell autolysis and self-digestion of tissues.

catheter ('kathitə) a tubular, flexible instrument, passed through body channels for withdrawal of fluids from (or introduction of fluids into) a body cavity.

angiographic c. one through which a contrast medium is injected for visualization of the vascular system of an organ. Such catheters usually have preformed ends to facilitate selective locating (as in a renal or coronary vessel) from a remote entry site. They may be named according to the site of entry and destination, e.g., *femoral-renal*, or shape of end, e.g., pigtail, or after their designer, e.g., Judkins.

arterial c. one inserted into an artery and utilized as part of a catheter-transducer-monitor system to continuously observe the BLOOD PRESSURE of critically ill patients. An arterial catheter also may be inserted for radiological studies of the arterial system and for delivery of chemotherapeutic agents directly into the

arterial supply of malignant tumours. **cardiac c.** a long, fine catheter especially designed for passage, usually through a peripheral blood vessel, into the chambers of the heart under fluoroscopic control. See also CARDIAC CATHETERIZATION.
central venous c. a long, fine catheter inserted into a vein for the purpose of administering through a large blood vessel parenteral fluids (as in parenteral NUTRITION), antibiotics, and other therapeutic agents. This type of catheter is also used in the measurement of CENTRAL VENOUS PRESSURE. See also CENTRAL VENOUS CATHETERIZATION.
de Pezzer's c. a self-retaining bladder catheter inserted suprapubically; called also *Pezzer's catheter*.
double-current c. one having two channels; one for injection and one for removal of fluid.
elbowed c. a catheter bent at an angle near the beak; used principally in cases of enlarged prostate. A one-elbow catheter is termed a coudé catheter; a two-elbow catheter is termed a bicoudé catheter.
faucial c. a pharyngotympanic catheter for passage through the fauces.
Foley's c. self-retaining catheter.
indwelling c. one especially designed so that it is held in place in the urethra using an inflatable balloon for the purpose of draining urine from the bladder.
nasal c., oropharyngeal c. one made of soft flexible rubber or plastic with several holes in the terminal 1 inch; used for the administration of oxygen.
pharyngotympanic c. one for inflating the pharyngotympanic tube.
prostatic c. one with a short, angular tip; called also *Tiemann's catheter*.
self-retaining c. one constructed to remain in the bladder, effecting constant drainage; called also *Foley's catheter*.
Tiemann's c. prostatic catheter.
tracheal c. one with small holes at the terminal 1 inch, especially designed for removal of secretions during tracheal SUCTIONING.
ureteral c. a long, extremely small gauge catheter designed for insertion directly into a ureter.
urethral c. any of various types of catheters designed for insertion via the urethra into the urinary bladder. See also CATHETERIZATION.

catheterization (ˌkathitə·rie'zayshən) passage of a catheter into a body channel or cavity. (See also CARDIAC CATHETERIZATION and CENTRAL VENOUS CATHETERIZATION.) The most common usage of the term is in reference to the introduction of a catheter via the urethra into the urinary bladder. This is often a nursing procedure, one that demands strict adherence to the principles of asepsis so that pathogenic microorganisms are not introduced into the urinary system. Since the urinary tract is normally sterile, any break in technique during the insertion of a catheter, or in the care of an indwelling catheter may result in a serious infection.

PATIENT CARE. About 40 per cent of all hospital-acquired infections are urinary tract infections (UTIs), and of these, about 75 per cent are related to indwelling bladder catheters. Prevention of these infections is a challenge to the nursing staff.

The smallest gauge catheter that will drain the bladder should always be chosen. It should be inserted gently to avoid trauma, especially to the vesical TRIGONE, and under aseptic conditions to avoid introducing microorganisms into the urinary system. Once an indwelling catheter has been inserted, an absolutely closed drainage system must be maintained. Special care must be taken to guard against tension on the catheter and kinking of the tubing, which can obstruct the flow of urine. Catheters should never be pinned to the bedclothing as this can result in accidental removal of the catheter or unnecessary pulling when the patient moves about in bed. The catheter is taped securely to the patient's body. Male, bedridden patients can have the catheter taped to the abdomen to avoid pressure at the junction of the penis and scrotum.

The tubing and collection bag should be arranged so that there is continuous gravity flow of urine. Modern drainage bags have a one-way valve, to prevent backflow of urine should the bag be inverted. The catheter should not be clamped nor should it be *routinely* irrigated and changed. Most authorities agree that catheters need changing only if they are obstructed, if contamination is suspected, or if there is a malfunction of the apparatus. When the collecting bag is being emptied, care must be taken to avoid contamination of the spout.

Patient care must also include attention to the area surrounding the urinary meatus. At least twice daily, or more often if necessary, the genital area should be washed gently with soap and water and dried thoroughly. Crusts and secretions around the catheter may be removed by gentle wiping with a gauze or cotton square saturated with a mild antiseptic. These measures will reduce the possibility of infection and ensure the comfort of the patient by eliminating unpleasant odours and irritation.

Because of the ever-present danger of UTI, routine catheterization to relieve bladder distention should be avoided and alternatives to an indwelling catheter should be considered. Catheterization following surgery may not be necessary if other measures to induce voiding are tried. Patients who require continuous care because of incontinence or an inability to void normally may respond favourably to measures other than indwelling catheterization, such as condom drainage, suprapubic catheter drainage, and, for some carefully selected patients, self-catheterization.
cardiac c. introduction of a catheter into the heart chambers in order to confirm a diagnosis or to evaluate the extent of the disease process (see also CARDIAC CATHETERIZATION).

catheterize ('kathitəˌriez) to introduce a catheter into a body cavity, usually into the urinary bladder for the withdrawal of urine.

cathexis (kə'theksis) the charge or attachment of mental or emotional energy upon an object or idea. adj. **cathectic.**

cathode ('kathohd) 1. the negative electrode, from which electrons are emitted and to which positive ions are attracted. 2. the electrode through which current leaves a nerve or other substance.

cathodic (kə'thodik, -'thoh-) pertaining to or emanating from a cathode.

cation ('katie·ənə) a positively charged ion.

cation-exchange resin (ˌkatie·ənˌiks'chayng) ion-exchange resin.

cauda ('kawdah) pl. *caudae* [L.] a tail or tail-like appendage.
c. equina the collection of spinal roots descending from the lower spinal cord and occupying the vertebral canal below the cord.

caudad ('kawdad) directed toward the tail or distal end; opposite of cephalad.

caudal ('kawd'l) 1. pertaining to a cauda. 2. situated more toward the cauda, or tail, than some specified reference point; toward the inferior (in humans) or posterior (in animals) end of the body.
c. anaesthesia a type of epidural anaesthesia whereby local anaesthetics or other agents are injected into the

caudal area of the spinal canal through the lower end of the sacrum. It affects the sacral nerves and can be used to cover operations on the anus, lower birth canal and perineum. It has occasionally been used during childbirth. In continuous caudal anaesthesia a catheter is inserted into the sacral canal and the patient is given either intermittent boluses or a continuous infusion of a local anaesthetic. Care must be taken to ensure that the solution does not extend too high or the injection be given inadvertently into the subarachnoid space. For this reason resuscitation equipment must be available and the procedure only be done by personnel trained in resuscitation.

caudate ('kawdayt) having a tail.

caudatum (kaw'daytəm) the caudate nucleus.

caul (kawl) a part of the amnion that sometimes envelops the head of the fetus at birth.

cauliflower ear ('koli,flowə) a thickened and deformed ear caused by the accumulation of fluid and blood clots in the tissue following repeated injury. It is most commonly seen in boxers.

caumaesthesia (,kawmis'theezi·ə) a sensation of burning heat even though the body temperature is not elevated.

causalgia (kaw'zalji·ə) a burning pain often associated with trophic skin changes in the hand or foot, caused by peripheral nerve injury. The syndrome may be aggravated by the slightest stimulus or it may be intensified by the emotions. Causalgia usually begins several weeks after the initial injury and the pain is described as intense, with the patient sometimes taking elaborate precautions to avoid any stimulus he knows to be capable of causing a flare-up of symptoms. He often will go to great extremes to protect the affected limb and becomes preoccupied with such protection.

Any one of a variety of injuries to the hand, foot, arm, or leg can lead to causalgia, but in most cases there has been some injury to the median or the sciatic nerve. Sympathectomy may be necessary to eliminate the severe pain, and in the majority of cases it is quite successful. Psychotherapy may be necessary when emotional instability is suspected. Emotional problems may have been present before the initial injury, or they may result from the intense suffering characteristic of severe causalgia.

causality (kaw'zalitee) the relationship between cause and effects.

principle of c. the postulate that every phenomenon has a cause or causes; i.e., that events do not occur at random but in accordance with physical laws so that in principle causes can be found for each effect.

caustic ('kostik, 'kaw-) 1. burning or corrosive; destructive to tissue. 2. having a burning taste. 3. a corrosive or escharotic agent.

cauterant ('kawtə·rənt) 1. any caustic material or application. 2. caustic.

cauterization (,kawtə·rie'zayshən) the application of heat sufficient to sear tissue; used to obtain haemostasis.

cautery ('kawtə·ree) 1. the application of searing heat by a hot instrument, an electric current, or other means such as a laser. 2. an agent so used.

cold c. cauterization by carbon dioxide, called also *cryocautery*.

cava ('kayvə) [L.] 1. plural of *cavum*. 2. a vena cava.

Cavell ('kəvel) Edith (1865–1915). Born in Norfolk, Miss Cavell commenced her nurse training at the age of 30 years at the London Hospital. After completion of her training she was appointed night superintendent at St. Pancras Infirmary, and then assistant matron at Shoreditch Infirmary.

Miss Cavell later moved to Brussels to establish the first Belgian School of Nursing. Despite the onset of the First World War, when Brussels was handed over to the Germans on August 20th, 1914, Miss Cavell remained at the Edith Cavell–Marie Depage Institute.

On August 15th, 1915, Edith Cavell and her assistant were arrested on the charge of aiding the escape of allied soldiers; the assistant was later released. At her trial on October 6th, 1915, Miss Cavell admitted helping 200 men to the frontier. For this she was condemned to death on October 8th, 1915, and was executed in Brussels on October 12th, 1915, wearing her blue nurse's uniform.

As she waited in her prison cell a few hours before her execution, she wrote: 'Now that I am face to face with God and eternity, I realize that patriotism is not enough. I must not feel hate or bitterness towards anyone'.

caveola (,kavi'ohlə) pl. *caveolae* [L.] one of the minute pits or incuppings of the cell membrane formed during pinocytosis.

caverna (ka'vərnə) pl. *cavernae* [L.] a cavity.

cavernitis (,kavə'nietis) inflammation of the corpora cavernosa or corpus spongiosum of the penis.

cavernoma (,kavə'nohmə) cavernous haemangioma (see also HAEMANGIOMA).

cavernositis (,kavənoh'sietis) cavernitis.

cavernous ('kavənəs, kə'vərnəs) pertaining to a hollow, or containing hollow spaces.

cavitary ('kavitə·ree) characterized by the presence of a cavity or cavities.

cavitas ('kavi,tas) pl. *cavitates* [L.] cavity.

cavitation (,kavi'tayshən) the formation of cavities; also, a cavity.

cavitis (kay'vietis) inflammation of a vena cava.

cavity ('kavitee) a hollow or space, or a potential space, within the body or one of its organs. In dentistry, the lesion produced by dental CARIES.

abdominal c. the cavity of the body between the diaphragm above and the pelvis below, containing the abdominal organs.

absorption c's cavities in developing compact bone due to osteoclastic erosion, usually occurring in the areas laid down first.

amniotic c. the closed sac betwen the embryo and the amnion, containing the amniotic fluid.

cranial c. the space enclosed by the bones of the cranium.

glenoid c. a depression in the lateral angle of the scapula for articulation with the humerus.

medullary (marrow) c. the cavity, containing marrow, in the diaphysis of a long bone; called also *medullary canal*.

nasal c. the proximal part of the respiratory tract, within the nose, separated by the nasal septum and extending from the nares to the pharynx. **oral c.** the cavity of the mouth, bounded by the jaw bones and associated structures (muscles and mucosa).

pelvic c. the space within the walls of the pelvis.

pericardial c. the potential space between the epicardium and the parietal layer of the serous pericardium.

peritoneal c. the potential space between the parietal and the visceral peritoneum.

pleural c. the potential space between the parietal and the visceral pulmonary pleura.

pulp c. the pulp-filled central chamber in the crown of a tooth.

serous c. a coelomic cavity, like that enclosed by the pericardium, peritoneum, or pleura, not communicating with the outside of the body and lined with a serous membrane, i.e., one which secretes a serous fluid.

tension c. cavities of the lung, in which the air pressure is greater than that of the atmosphere.
thoracic c. the portion of the ventral body cavity situated between the neck and the diaphragm.
tympanic c. the middle ear.
uterine c. the flattened space within the uterus communicating proximally on either side with the uterine tubes and below with the vagina.
cavography (kay'vogrəfee) radiography of the vena cava.
cavum ('kayvəm) pl. *cava* [L.] cavity.
cavus ('kayvəs) [L.] *hollow*.
CC closing capacity.
cc cubic centimetre.
CCD Central Council for the Disabled.
CCHE Central Council for Health Education.
c.cm. cubic centimetre.
CCNU lomustine.
CD controlled drug.
Cd chemical symbol, *cadmium*.
cd candela.
CDC CENTERS FOR DISEASE CONTROL.
CDSC Communicable Diseases Surveillance Centre (Public Health Laboratory Services, Colindale, England).
Ce chemical symbol, *cerium*.
ce- for words beginning thus, see also those beginning *cae-, coe-*.
CEA carcinoembryonic antigen.
cebocephaly (ˌseeboh'kefəlee, -'sef-) a monkey-like deformity of the head, with the eyes close together and the nose defective.
Cedocard ('seedohkahd) trademark for preparations of isosorbide dinitrate.
cefaclor ('kefəklor) a semisynthetic broad-spectrum cephalosporin antibiotic administered orally in the treatment of otitis media and infections of the respiratory tract, urinary tract, and the skin due to susceptible organisms.
cefadroxil (ˌkefə'droksil) a semisynthetic cephalosporin antibiotic.
cefotaxime (ˌkefoh'takseem) a third generation cephalosporin antibiotic having a broad spectrum of activity, used to treat intra-abdominal infections, bone and joint infections, gonorrhoea, and other infections due to susceptible organisms, including penicillinase-producing strains.
cefoxitin (ke'foksitin) a semisynthetic cephalosporin antibiotic, especially effective against gram—negative organisms, with strong resistance to degradation by β-lactamase.
cefsulodin (kef'soolohdin) a cephalosporin with activity against *Pseudomonas aeruginosa*.
ceftazidime (kef'tazideem) a third-generation cephalosporin with activity against a wide range of organisms.
ceftizoxime (kefti'zokseem) a third-generation cephalosporin with activity against a wide range of organisms.
cefuroxime (ˌkefyuh'rokseem) a second-generation cephalosporin commonly used for surgical prophylaxis.
-cele word element. [Gr.] *tumour, hernia*.
cell (sel) 1. the basic structural unit of living organisms. 2. a small more or less enclosed space.

All living cells arise from other cells, either by division of one cell to make two, as in MITOSIS and MEIOSIS, or by fusion of two cells to make one, as in the union of the sperm and ovum to make the zygote in sexual reproduction.

All cells are bounded by a structure called the *cell membrane* or *plasma membrane*, which is a *lipid bilayer* composed of two layers of phospholipids with various admixed proteins. Each layer is one molecule thick with the charged, hydrophilic end of the lipid molecules on the surface of the membrane and the uncharged hydrophobic fatty acid tails in the interior of the membrane.

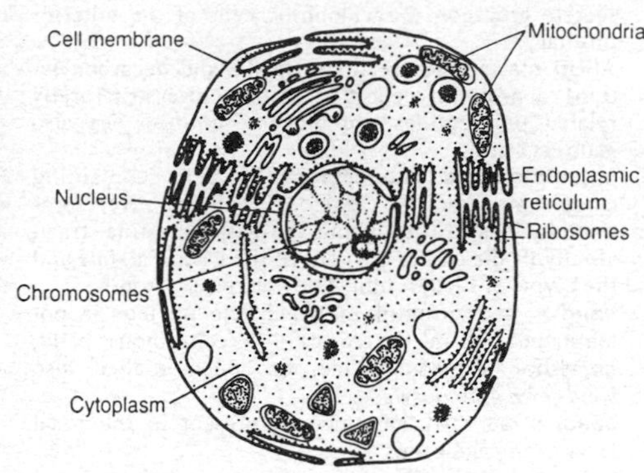

Major parts of a cell

Cells are divided into two classes, eukaryotic cells and prokaryotic cells. *Eukaryotic cells* have a true nucleus, which contains the genetic material, composed of the *chromosomes*, which are long linear structures composed of DEOXYRIBONUCLEIC ACID (DNA) and protein. The nucleus is bounded by a nuclear envelope, which is composed of two lipid bilayer membranes. *Prokaryotic cells*, the bacteria, have no nucleus, and their genetic material, consisting of a single loop of naked DNA, is not separated from the rest of the cell. Eukaryotic cells are larger and more complex than prokaryotic cells. They also have membrane-bounded structures, such as mitochondria, chloroplasts, the Golgi apparatus, the endoplasmic reticulum, and lysosomes, that prokaryotic cells lack.

The contents of a cell are referred to collectively as the *protoplasm*. In eukaryotic cells the contents of the nucleus are referred to as the *nucleoplasm* and the rest of the protoplasm as the *cytoplasm*.

The lipid bilayer of eukaryotic cells is impermeable to many substances, such as ions, sugars, and amino acids; however, membrane proteins move specific substances through the cell membrane by active or passive transport. Water, gases such as oxygen and carbon dioxide, and nonpolar compounds pass through the cell membrane by DIFFUSION. Materials can also be engulfed and taken into the cell enclosed in a portion of the cell membrane. This is called *phagocytosis* when solids are ingested and *pinocytosis* when liquids are ingested. The reverse process is called *exocytosis*. All of these processes permit the cell to maintain an internal environment different from its exterior. See also body FLUIDS.

The cells of the body differentiate during development into many specialized types with specific tasks to perform. Cells are organized into tissues and tissues into organs.
accessory c's macrophages involved in the processing and presentation of antigens, making them more immunogenic.
acinar c., acinous c. any of the cells lining an acinus, especially applied to the zymogen-secreting cells of the pancreatic acini.
alpha c's 1. cells in the islets of Langerhans that

secrete glucagon. 2. acidophilic cells of the anterior pituitary.
APUD c's (*a*mine *p*recursor *u*ptake and *d*ecarboxylation), a group of cells that manufacture structurally related polypeptides and biogenic amines. See also APUD CELLS.
argentaffin c's enterochromaffin cells containing cytoplasmic granules capable of reducing silver compounds, located throughout the gastrointestinal tract, chiefly in the basilar portions of the gastric glands and the crypts of Lieberkühn. They secrete serotonin.
band c. a neutrophil in which the nucleus is not lobulated but in the form of a continuous band, horseshoe shaped, twisted, or coiled. Called also *band-form granulocyte.*
basal c. an early keratinocyte, present in the basal layer of the epidermis.
beta c's 1. basophilic cells in the pancreas that secrete insulin and make up most of the bulk of the islands of Langerhans; they contain granules that are soluble in alcohol. 2. basophilic cells of the anterior pituitary.
Betz c's large pyramidal neurons forming a layer of the grey matter of the brain.
blood c. one of the formed elements of the blood (see also BLOOD).
bone c. a nucleated cell in the lacunae of bone. Called also *osteocyte.*
cartilage c. chondrocyte.
chromaffin c's cells whose cytoplasm shows fine brown granules when stained with potassium bichromate, occurring in the adrenal medulla and in scattered groups in various organs and throughout the body.
cleavage c. any of the cells derived from the fertilized ovum by mitosis; a blastomere.
daughter c. a cell formed by division of a mother cell.
foam c. a cell with a vacuolated appearance due to the presence of complex lipoids; seen in xanthoma.
ganglion c. a large nerve cell, especially one of those of the spinal ganglia.
Gaucher's c. a large cell characteristic of Gaucher's disease (see also GAUCHER'S CELLS).
germ c. an ovum or spermatozoon.
giant c. a very large, multinucleate cell; applied to megakaryocytes of bone marrow, to giant cells formed by coalescence and fusion of macrophages occurring in the lesions of tuberculosis and other infectious granulomas and about foreign bodies, and to certain cancer cells.
glial c's neuroglia cells.
goblet c. a mucus-secreting epithelial cell in which the mucin accumulates intracellularly in the apical portion of the cell and gives the cell its characteristic appearance, found extensively in the epithelium lining the respiratory tract, and large and small intestines.
Golgi's c's Golgi neurons.
granular c. one containing granules, such as a keratinocyte in the stratum granulosum of the epidermis, when it contains a dense collection of darkly staining granules.
heart failure c's, heart-lesion c's iron-containing macrophages found in the pulmonary alveoli and sputum in chronic congestive heart failure.
HeLa c's cells of the first continuously cultured carcinoma strain, descended from a human cervical carcinoma of the cervix.
helper c's a subtype of T-lymphocytes; they cooperate with B-lymphocytes for the synthesis of antibody to many antigens, and they play an integral role in immunoregulation.
Hürthle c's large eosinophilic cells sometimes found in the thyroid gland. See also HÜRTHLE CELL TUMOUR.
interstitial c's the cells of the connective tissue of the ovary or of the testis (Leydig's cells) which furnish the internal secretion of those structures.
islet c's cells composing the islets of Langerhans.
Ito c's perisinusoidal cells found only in the liver. Also known as fat-storing cells, their functions include the storage of vitamin A. They are believed to contribute to fibrogenesis, once stimulated.
juxtaglomerular c's specialized cells, containing secretory granules, located in the tunica media of the afferent glomerular arterioles. They cause aldosterone production by secreting the enzyme renin and play a role in the regulation of blood pressure and fluid balance.
K c's, killer c's T-lymphocytes or null lymphocytes that have cytotoxic activity against target cells coated with specific IgG antibody.
Kupffer's c's large, stellate or pyramidal, intensely phagocytic cells lining the walls of the hepatic sinusoids and forming part of the reticuloendothelial system.
Langhans' giant c's giant cells in which the multiple nuclei tend to lie at the periphery of the cells in a horseshoe pattern; seen in chronic granulomatous conditions such as tuberculosis.
LE c. a mature neutrophilic polymorphonuclear leukocyte characteristic of lupus erythematosus (see also LE CELL).
Leydig's c's interstitial cells of the testis, which secrete testosterone.
luteal c's, lutein c's the plump, pale-staining, polyhedral cells of the corpus luteum.
lymph c. lymphocyte.
lymphoid c's lymphocytes and plasma cells.
mast c. a connective tissue cell capable of elaborating basophilic, metachromatic, cytoplasmic granules that contain histamine, heparin, hyaluronic acid, slow-reacting substance of anaphylaxis (SRS-A), and, in some species, serotonin.
mastoid c's air spaces of various sizes and shapes in the mastoid process of the temporal bone.
mother c. a cell that divides to form new, or daughter, cells.
natural killer c's, NK c's cells capable of mediating cytotoxic reactions without themselves being specifically sensitized against the target.
nerve c. any cell of the nervous system; a NEURON.
neuroglia c's, neuroglial c's the branching non-neural cells of the supporting tissue (the neuroglia) of the central nervous system; they are of three types: astroglia (macroglia), oligodendroglia, and microglia.
null c's lymphocytes that lack the surface antigens characteristic of B- and T-lymphocytes; such cells are seen in active systemic lupus erythematosus and other disease states.
olfactory c's a set of specialized cells of the mucous membrane of the nose; the receptors for smell.
parafollicular c's ovoid epithelial cells located in the thyroid follicles, which secrete calcitonin.
Pick's c's round, oval, or polyhedral cells with foamy, lipid-containing cytoplasm found in the bone marrow and spleen in Niemann–Pick disease.
plasma c. a spherical or ellipsoidal cell with a single nucleus containing coarsely clumped chromatin, an area of perinuclear cytoplasmic clearing, and generally abundant, basophilic cytoplasm. Plasma cells are involved in the synthesis, storage, and release of antibody. Called also *plasmacyte* and *plasmocyte.*
prickle c. a dividing keratinocyte of the prickle-cell layer of the epidermis, with delicate radiating processes connecting with other similar cells.
Purkinje's c's large branching cells of the middle layer

of the cerebellar cortex.
red c., red blood c. erythrocyte.
Reed–Sternberg c's large, generally binucleate cells. They classically show a mirror-image arrangement of their nuclei; their precise histogenesis is uncertain. They are the common histological characteristic of Hodgkin's disease.
reticular c's the cells forming the reticular fibres of connective tissue; those forming the framework of lymph nodes, bone marrow, and spleen form part of the reticuloendothelial system and may differentiate into macrophages.
reticuloendothelial c. a cell of the RETICULOENDOTHELIAL SYSTEM.
Schwann c. any of the large nucleated cells whose cell membrane spirally enwraps the axons of myelinated peripheral neurons supplying the myelin sheath between two nodes of Ranvier.
Sertoli c's elongated cells in the tubules of the testes to which the spermatids become attached; they provide support, protection, and, apparently, nutrition until the spermatids are transformed into mature spermatozoa.
sickle c. a crescentic or sickle-shaped erythrocyte, the abnormal shape of which is caused by the presence of varying proportions of haemoglobin S when in its reduced form (see also SICKLE CELL DISEASE).
signet-ring c. a cell in which the nucleus has been pressed to one side by an accumulation of intracytoplasmic mucin.
somatic c's the cells of the somatoplasm; undifferentiated body cells.
squamous c's flat, scalelike epithelial cells.
stellate c. any star-shaped cell, as a Kupffer cell or astrocyte, having many filaments extending in all directions.
stem c. a primitive precursor cell which has the capacity to differentiate to form mature cells. *Pluripotent stem cells* have several differentiating pathways that they may follow, e.g., the haemopoietic stem cell may give rise to red cells, white cells or platelets. *Differentiated stem cells* have much less potential and are committed to become forms of a particular cell line.
Sternberg's giant c's, Sternberg–Reed c's See Reed–Sternberg cells (above).
stipple c. an erythrocyte containing granules that take a basic or bluish stain with Wright's stain.
suppressor c's lymphoid cells, especially T-lymphocytes, that inhibit humoural and cell-mediated immune responses. They play an integral role in immunoregulation, and are believed to be operative in various autoimmune and other immunological disease states.
target c. 1. an abnormally thin erythrocyte showing, when stained, a dark centre and a peripheral ring of haemoglobin, separated by a pale, unstained zone containing less haemoglobin; seen in various anaemias and other disorders. 2. any cell selectively affected by a particular agent, such as a hormone or drug.
taste c's cells in the taste buds associated with the nerves of taste.
totipotential c. an embryonic cell that is capable of developing into any variety of body cell.
visual c's the neuroepithelial elements of the retina.
white c., white blood c. leukocyte.

cell division (sel di'vizhən) the process by which cells reproduce; fission of a cell.

cell marker (sel 'mahkə) a technique used to identify the nature of a cell (e.g., lymphoid or myeloid, haemic or nonhaemic). Techniques that identify the lineage of cells include cytochemistry (to define staining characteristics), enzymatic reactions, immunological reactions and chromosomal studies. They are particularly helpful in diagnosing acute leukaemias and the malignant lymphomas.

cellobiase (ˌseloh'bieayz) β-glucosidase.

cellular ('selyuhlə) pertaining to, or made up of, cells.

cellularity (ˌselyuh'laritee) the state of a tissue or other mass as regards the number of its constituent cells.

cellulase ('selyuhˌlayz) a concentrate of cellulose-splitting enzymes derived from *Aspergillus niger* and other sources; used as a digestive aid.

cellulicidal (ˌselyuhli'sied'l) destroying cells.

cellulitis (ˌselyuh'lietis) a diffuse inflammatory process within solid tissues, characterized by oedema, redness, pain, and interference with function. It may be caused by infection with streptococci, staphylococci, or other organisms.

Cellulitis usually occurs in the loose tissues beneath the skin, but may also occur in tissues beneath mucous membranes or around muscle bundles or surrounding organs.

ERYSIPELAS, a surface cellulitis of the skin, is characterized by patches of skin that are red with sharply defined borders and that feel hot to the touch. Other types of skin cellulitis are also characterized by hot red patches, but the borders are less clearly defined. Red streaks extending from the patch indicate that the lymph vessels have been infected. Ludwig's angina is a cellulitis of the tissues of the floor of the mouth and neck, in the area around the submaxillary gland. Orbital cellulitis is an acute inflammation of the eye socket. Pelvic cellulitis involves the tissues surrounding the uterus and is called parametritis.

Cellulitis is potentially dangerous but usually can be treated successfully with antibiotics. Any cellulitis on the face must be given special attention because the infection may extend directly to the cavernous sinuses of the brain.

cellulofibrous (ˌselyuhloh'fiebrəs) partly cellular and partly fibrous.

celluloid ('selyuhˌloyd) a plastic compound of pyroxylin and camphor.

celluloneuritis (ˌselyuhlohnyuh'rietis) inflammation of neurons.

cellulose ('selyuhˌlohs, -ˌlohz) a carbohydrate forming the skeleton of most plant structures and plant cells.
absorbable c., oxidized c. an absorbable oxidation product of cellulose, applied locally to stop bleeding.

celoschisis (see'loskisis) congenital fissure of the abdominal wall.

celosomia (ˌseeloh'sohmi·ə) congenital fissure or absence of the sternum, with hernial protrusion of the viscera.

Celsius scale ('selsi·əs) a temperature scale with the ice point at 0 and the normal boiling point of water at 100 degrees (100 °C). For equivalents of Celsius and Fahrenheit temperatures, see Appendix 2.

Celsius thermometer a centigrade thermometer employing the Celsius scale. The abbreviation 100 °C should be read 'one hundred degrees Celsius'.

cement (si'ment) 1. a substance that produces a solid union between two surfaces. 2. in dentistry, a material used to insulate the tooth pulp and also to aid the retention of inlays, crowns and bridges.
dental c. cementum.

cementicle (si'mentik'l) a small, discrete globular mass of cementum in the region of a tooth root.

cementoblast (si'mentohˌblast) a large cuboidal cell, found between fibres on the surface of cementum, which is active in the formation of cementum.

cementoblastoma (siˌmentohbla'stohmə) periapical ossifying FIBROSIS.

cementoclasia (si,mentoh'klayzi·ə) resorption of the cementum of a tooth.

cementocyte (si'mentoh,siet) a cell found in lacunae of cellular cementum, frequently having long processes radiating from the cell body toward the periodontal surface of the cementum.

cementogenesis (si,mentoh'jenəsis) development of cementum on the root dentine of a tooth.

cementoma (,seemen'tohmə) a mass of cementum lying free at the apex of a tooth, probably a reaction to injury.

cementum (si'mentəm) the bonelike connective tissue covering the root of a tooth and assisting in tooth support.

cenaesthesia (,seenəs'theezi·ə) the general feeling or sense of conscious existence; the sense of normal functioning of body organs. adj. **cenaesthesic, cenaesthetic.**

ceno- word element. [Gr.] *new, empty;* or denoting relationship to a common feature.

cenosis (si'nohsis) a morbid discharge. adj. **cenotic.**

censor ('sensə) 1. a member of a committee on ethics or for critical examination of a medical or other society. 2. the psychic influence which prevents unconscious thoughts and wishes coming into consciousness.

censorship ('sensə,ship) in psychiatry, the process of selecting, accepting or rejecting conscious ideas, memories and impulses arising from the individual's subconscious.

census ('sensəs) enumeration of a population. The national census was first introduced in England and Wales in 1801 and has since been repeated every 10 years (except in 1941). It usually records name, address, age, sex, occupation, marital status and other social information.

Centers for Disease Control ('sentəz) an agency of the US Department of Health and Human Services, located in Atlanta, Georgia, which serves as a centre for the control, prevention, and investigation of diseases. Abbreviated CDC. A similar function is performed in England and Wales by the COMMUNICABLE DISEASES SURVEILLANCE CENTRE and in Scotland by the COMMUNICABLE DISEASES (SCOTLAND) UNIT.

-centesis word element. [Gr.] *puncture and aspiration of.*

centi- word element. [L.] *hundred;* used to indicate one-hundredth (10^{-2}) of the unit designated by the root with which it is combined, e.g., centimetre; symbol c.

centigrade ('senti,grayd) having 100 gradations (steps or degrees), as the Celsius scale; abbreviated C. For equivalents of Celsius and Fahrenheit temperatures, see Appendix 2.

centimetre ('senti,meetə) one-hundredth of a metre, or approximately 0.3937 inch; abbreviated cm.

cubic c. a unit of capacity, being that of a cube 1 cm on a side; abbreviated cm^3, cu.cm., c.cm. or cc.

centrad ('sentrad) toward a centre.

central ('sentrəl) pertaining to a centre; located at the midpoint.

c. cord syndrome injury to the central portion of the cervical spinal cord resulting in disproportionately more weakness or paralysis in the upper extremities than in the lower; pathological change is caused by haemorrhage or oedema.

c. fissure fissure of Rolando.

c. nervous system the portion of the NERVOUS SYSTEM consisting of the brain and spinal cord.

c. sulcus fissure of Rolando.

c. venous catheterization insertion of an indwelling catheter into a central vein for the purpose of administering fluid and medications and for the measurement of CENTRAL VENOUS PRESSURE. The most common sites of insertion are the jugular and subclavian veins; however, such large peripheral veins as the saphenous and femoral veins can be used in an emergency, even though they offer some disadvantages. The procedure is performed under sterile conditions and placement of the catheter is verified by radiographs before fluids are administered or central venous pressure measurements are made.

Selection of a large central vein in preference to a smaller peripheral vein for the administration of therapeutic agents is based on the nature and amount of fluid to be injected. Central veins are able to accommodate large amounts of fluid when shock or haemorrhage demand rapid replacement. The larger veins are less susceptible to irritation from caustic drugs and from hypertonic nutrient solutions administered during parenteral NUTRITION.

Long-term use of an indwelling venous catheter demands strict attention to technique to avoid contamination when fluids and medications are added. The site of insertion must be kept free from contamination; dressings must be sterile.

c. venous pressure (CVP) the pressure of blood in the right atrium. Measurement of central venous pressure is made possible by the insertion of a catheter through the median cubital vein to the superior vena cava. The distal end of the catheter is attached to a manometer on which can be read the amount of pressure being exerted by the blood inside the right atrium. The manometer is positioned at the bedside so that the zero point is at the level of the right atrium. Each time the patient's position is changed the zero point on the manometer must be reset.

The normal range for CVP is 0 to 5 mmH_2O. A CVP of 15 to 20 mmH_2O usually indicates inability of the right atrium to accommodate the current BLOOD VOLUME. However, the trend of response to rapid administration of fluid is more significant than the specific level of pressure. Normally the right heart can circulate additional fluids without an increase in CVP. If the CVP is elevated in response to the rapid administration of a small amount of fluid, there is indication that the patient is hypervolaemic in relation to the pumping action of the right heart. Thus, the CVP is used as a guide to the safe administration of replacement fluids intravenously, particularly in patients who are subject to pulmonary OEDEMA.

A high venous pressure may indicate congestive HEART FAILURE, hypervolaemia (increased blood volume), cardiac tamponade in which the heart is unable to fill, or vasoconstriction, which affects the heart's ability to empty its chambers. Conversely, a low venous pressure indicates hypovolaemia (low blood volume) and possibly a need to increase fluid intake.

centre ('sentə) a point from which a process starts, especially a plexus or ganglion giving off nerves that control a function.

accelerating c. one in the brain stem involved in acceleration of heart action.

apneustic c. a nerve centre in the brain stem controlling normal respiration.

auditory c. the centre for hearing, in the more anterior of the transverse temporal gyri.

Broca's c. speech centre.

cardioinhibitory c. one in the medulla oblongata that exerts an inhibitory influence on the heart.

deglutition c. a nerve centre in the medulla oblongata that controls swallowing.

germinal c. the area in the centre of a lymph node containing aggregations of actively proliferating lym-

phocytes.
gustatory c. the cerebral centre supposed to control taste.
health c. see HEALTH centre.
medullary respiratory c. the centre in the medulla oblongata that coordinates respiratory movements.
motor c. any centre that originates, controls, inhibits, or maintains motor impulses.
nerve c. a collection of nerve cells in the central nervous system that are associated together in the performance of some particular function.
c. of ossification any point in bones at which ossification begins.
pneumotaxic c. one in the upper pons that rhythmically inhibits inspiration.
reflex c. any nerve centre at which afferent sensory impressions are converted into efferent motor impulses.
respiratory c's a series of the centres (the apneustic, pneumotaxic, and medullary respiratory centres) in the medulla and pons that coordinate respiratory movements.
speech c. one in the left (or right) inferior frontal gyrus concerned with the motor aspects of speech.
swallowing c. deglutition centre.
thermoregulatory c's hypothalamic centres regulating the conservation and dissipation of heat.
Wernicke's c. the speech centre in the cortex of the left temporo-occipital convolution.
word c. one concerned with the recognition of words, different areas being involved for recognition of written and of spoken words.

centrencephalic (ˌsentrenkəˈfalik, -səˈfalik) pertaining to the centre of the encephalon.
centric (ˈsentrik) pertaining to a centre.
centriciput (senˈtrisipuht) the central part of the upper surface of the head, located between the occiput and sinciput.
centrifugal (sentriˈfyoog'l) moving away from a centre.
centrifugate (senˈtrifyuh,gayt) material subjected to centrifugation.
centrifugation (ˌsentrifyuhˈgayshən) the process of separating lighter portions of a solution, mixture, or suspension from the heavier portions by centrifugal force.
centrifuge (ˈsentri,fyooj) 1. to rotate, in a suitable container, at extremely high speed, to cause the deposition of solids in solution. 2. a laboratory device for subjecting substances in solution to relative centrifugal force up to 25,000 times gravity.
centrilobular (ˌsentriˈlobyuhlə) pertaining to the central portion of a lobule.
centriole (ˈsentri,ohl) either of the two cylindrical organelles located in the centrosome and containing nine triplets of microtubules arrayed around their edges; centrioles migrate to opposite poles of the cell during cell division and serve to organize the spindles. They are capable of independent replication and of migrating to form basal bodies.
centripetal (senˈtripit'l, ˈsentri,peet'l) moving toward a centre.
centro- word element. [L., Gr.] *centre, central location.*
centrokinesia (ˌsentrohkiˈneezi·ə) movement originating from central stimulation. adj. **centrokinetic.**
centromere (ˈsentroh,miə) the clear constricted portion of the chromosome at which the chromatids are joined and by which the chromosome is attached to the spindle during cell division. adj. **centromeric.**
centrosclerosis (ˌsentrohskləˈrohsis) osteosclerosis of the marrow cavity of a bone.
centrosome (ˈsentrə,sohm) a specialized area of condensed cytoplasm containing the centrioles and playing an important part in mitosis.
centrosphere (ˈsentrə,sfiə) centrosome.
centrostaltic (ˌsentrohˈstaltik) pertaining to a centre of motion.
centrum (ˈsentrəm) pl. *centra* [L.] 1. a centre. 2. the body of a vertebra.
c. commune the solar plexus.
cephal(o)- word element. [Gr.] *head.*
cephalad (ˈkefə,lad, ˈsef-) toward the head.
cephalalgia (ˌkefəˈlalji·ə, ˌsef-) pain in the head; headache.
cephalexin (ˌkefəˈleksin, ˌsef-) an oral cephalosporin used in the treatment of pneumococcal and Group-A streptococcal respiratory infections and infections of the urinary tract, skin, and soft tissue.
cephalhaematocele (ˌkefəlˈheemətoh,seel, ˌsef-) a haematocele under the pericranium, communicating with the sinuses of the dura mater.
cephalhaematoma (ˌkefəlˌheeməˈtohmə, ˌsef-) a localized effusion of blood beneath the periosteum of the skull of a newborn infant, due to disruption of the vessels during birth.
cephalic (kəˈfalik, sə-) pertaining to the head, or to the head end of the body.
c. index 100 times the maximal breadth of the skull divided by its maximal length.
cephalin (ˈkefəlin, ˈsef-) a group of phospholipids found particularly in the brain and other nerve tissue.
cephalitis (ˌkefəˈlietis, ˌsef-) encephalitis.
cephalocele (ˈkefəloh,seel, ˈsef-) protrusion of a part of the cranial contents.
cephalocentesis (ˌkefəlohsenˈteesis, ˌsef-) surgical puncture of the skull and brain for the purpose of drainage by aspiration.
cephalodactyly (ˌkefəlohˈdaktilee, ˌsef-) malformation of the head and digits.
cephalodynia (ˌkefəlohˈdini·ə, ˌsef-) pain in the head; headache.
cephaloedema (ˌkefəliˈdeemə, ˌsef-) oedema of the head.
cephalogram (ˈkefəloh,gram, ˈsef-) a radiograph of the structures of the head; cephalometric radiograph.
cephalography (ˌkefəˈlogrəfee, ˌsef-) radiographic examination of the contours of the head.
cephalogyric (ˌkefəlohˈjierik, ˌsef-) pertaining to turning motions of the head.
cephalohaematoma (ˌkefəloh,heeməˈtohmə, ˌsef-) cephalhaematoma.
cephalomelus (ˌkefəˈlohmeləs, ˌsef-) a fetus or infant with an accessory limb growing from the head.
cephalometer (ˌkefəˈlomitə, ˌsef-) an instrument for measuring the head; an orienting device for positioning the head for radiographic examination and measurement.
cephalometry (ˌkefəˈlomətree, ˌsef-) a branch of anthropometry, being the measurement of the dimensions of the head of a living person, taken either directly or by radiography. adj. **cephalometric.**
cephalomotor (ˌkefəlohˈmohtə, ˌsef-) moving the head; pertaining to motions of the head.
cephalonia (ˌkefəˈlohni·ə, ˌsef-) a condition in which the head is abnormally enlarged, with sclerotic hyperplasia of the brain.
cephalopathy (ˌkefəˈlopəthee, ˌsef-) any disease of the head.
cephalopelvic (ˌkefəlohˈpelvik, ˌsef-) pertaining to the relationship of the fetal head to the maternal pelvis.
c. disproportion a misfit between the fetal head and the maternal pelvis. This may be due to a small pelvis or, more often, the attitude of the fetal head causing larger diameters to present at the pelvic brim. It is diagnosed when the fetal head will not engage in the

pelvis after 36 weeks of pregnancy. See also BIPARIETAL DIAMETER.

cephaloridine (ˌkefə'lo·rideen, ˌsef-) a broad-spectrum cephalosporin antibiotic, administered parenterally for the treatment of infections of the respiratory and genitourinary tracts, bones and joints, soft tissue, skin and bloodstream due to sensitive organisms.

cephalosporin (ˌkefəloh'spor·rin, ˌsef-) any of a group of broad-spectrum, penicillinase-resistant antibiotics from *Cephalosporium*, a genus of soil-inhabiting fungi, including cephazolin, cefotaxime, cephalexin, cephaloridine, cephalothin, and cephradine, which share the nucleus 7-aminocephalosporanic acid.

cephalosporinase (ˌkefəloh'spor·riˌnayz, ˌsef-) an enzyme that hydrolyses the CO–NH bond in the lactam ring of cephalosporin, converting it to an inactive product.

cephalostat ('kefəlohˌstat, 'sef-) a head-positioning device which assures reproducibility of the relations between an x-ray beam, a patient's head, and an x-ray film.

cephalothin ('kefəlohˌthin, 'sef-) a broad-spectrum, semisynthetic cephalosporin antibiotic, administered parenterally for the treatment of infections of the respiratory, gastrointestinal and genitourinary tracts, bones and joints, skin and soft tissue, and bloodstream due to sensitive organisms, including many penicillin-resistant staphylococci.

cephalothoracic (ˌkefəlohthor'rasik, ˌsef-) pertaining to the head and thorax.

cephalothoracopagus (ˌkefəlohˌthor·rə'kopəgəs, ˌsef-) a twin fetus or infant united at the head, neck, and thorax.

cephamandole (ˌsefə'mandohl) a semisynthetic broad-spectrum cephalosporin antibiotic administered parenterally in the treatment of infections of the lower respiratory tract, urinary tract, bones and joints, and skin, and in peritonitis and septicaemia due to susceptible organisms.

cephazolin (se'fazohlin) a semisynthetic cephalosporin antibiotic effective against a wide range of gram-negative and gram-positive bacteria.

cephradine ('kefrədeen, 'sef-) a broad-spectrum, acid-stable, semisynthetic cephalosporin antibiotic administered orally or parenterally for the treatment of infections of the respiratory and urinary tracts, ear, skin and bloodstream due to susceptible pathogens.

cera ('seerə) [L.] *wax.*

ceramidase (se'ramiˌdayz) an enzyme occurring in most mammalian tissue that catalyses the reversible acylation–deacylation of ceramides.

ceramide ('serəˌmied) any of a group of naturally occurring sphingolipids in which the NH_2 group of sphingosine is acylated with a fatty acyl CoA derivative to form *N*-acylsphingosine.

c. glucoside the major sphingolipid accumulated in Gaucher's disease.

c. lactosidosis a sphingolipidosis in which ceramide lactoside accumulates in neural and visceral tissues owing to a deficiency of a β-galactosidase.

c. trihexoside the major sphingolipid accumulated in Fabry's disease.

cerate ('seeə·rayt) a medicinal preparation for external use, compounded of fat or wax, or both, intermediate in consistency between an ointment and a plaster.

cerato- for words beginning thus, see those beginning *kerato-*.

cercaria (sə'kair·ri·ə) pl. *cercariae* [Gr.] the final, free-swimming larval stage of a trematode parasite.

cerclage (sər'klahzh) [Fr.] encircling of a part with a ring or loop, as for correction of an incompetent cervix uteri or fixation of the adjacent ends of a fractured bone (see also SHIRODKAR'S SUTURE).

cercus ('sərkəs) a bristle-like structure.

cerebellar (ˌseri'belə) pertaining to the cerebellum.

c. cortex the superficial grey matter of the cerebellum.

cerebellitis (ˌseribe'lietis) inflammation of the cerebellum.

cerebellum (ˌseri'beləm) the part of the metencephalon situated on the back of the brain stem, to which it is attached by three cerebellar peduncles on each side; it consists of a median lobe (vermis) and two lateral lobes (the hemispheres). See also BRAIN.

cerebral ('seribrəl) pertaining to the cerebrum.

c. contusion contusion of the brain following a HEAD INJURY (see also cerebral CONTUSION).

c. cortex the convoluted layer of grey matter covering the cerebral hemispheres, which governs thought, reasoning, memory, sensation, and voluntary movement. See also BRAIN.

c. gigantism gigantism in the absence of increased levels of growth hormone, attributed to a cerebral defect (see also cerebral GIGANTISM).

c. palsy a nonspecific term used to describe a persistent qualitative motor disorder caused by non-progressive damage to the brain. Although manifested primarily by motor dysfunction, the disorder also may involve sensory deficits and impairment of the intellect. Prior to age eight or nine, function lost by damage to one part of the brain can be taken over by another part of the brain. Hence, many people consider that brain damage occurring any time prior to this age can lead to cerebral palsy. Most cases, however, are diagnosed before the age of three.

AETIOLOGY. The exact cause of a case of cerebral palsy cannot always be determined, but the condition usually develops before or during birth or in infancy. Damage to the fetal brain can occur as a result of maternal infections, drug and alcohol abuse, anaemia, and rubella. Other causes are related to faulty implantation of the fertilized ovum, maternal and fetal blood incompatibilities, and genetic factors.

The majority of cases are caused during labour and delivery or during the first month of extrauterine life. Prematurity is a factor, as are prolonged labour and traumatic delivery, which can cause intracranial haemorrhage. Any situation that interferes with fetal oxygen supply can produce brain damage and cerebral palsy. These include premature separation of the placenta, prolapsed cord, and excessive sedation during labour and delivery. Other causes during the perinatal period include *hypoglycaemia*, which leads to cerebral hypoxia; *hypernatraemia*, which results in cellular hyperosmolality, vascular lesions, and intracranial haemorrhage; and *hyperbilirubinaemia*.

Damage to the brain after birth and in the early years of life can result from infections of the meninges and of the brain cells, head injury, toxicosis, and stroke.

CLASSIFICATION. The system most commonly used for typing the various forms of cerebral palsy is based on the predominant clinical manifestations. There are three main types: (1) spastic type, in which there are exaggerated stretch relexes, muscle spasm, and increased deep tendon reflexes; (2) athetoid, with purposeless, uncontrollable movements and muscle tension; and (3) atactic, in which the child has poor balance, poor coordination, and a staggering gait. Visual, hearing, and speech defects may be present. Mental handicap may or may not be a manifestation of the brain damage.

TREATMENT. Treatment varies according to the nature and extent of brain damage. Muscle relaxants may help reduce spasms. Anticonvulsant drugs are necessary when seizures are among the symptoms of the disorder. Orthopaedic surgery, casts, braces, and traction can be used to correct some types of disability associated with cerebral palsy. Early muscle training and special exercises often help the child lead a useful, productive life. If muscle training is not begun early, extensive rehabilitation may be necessary to correct faulty habits and poor muscle patterns established by the child. However, it is never too late for a complete evaluation of the condition of a patient with cerebral palsy. A rehabilitation programme can produce good results later in life as well as in childhood.

cerebration (ˌseri'brayshən) functional activity of the brain.

cerebritis (ˌseri'brietis) inflammation of the cerebrum.

cerebrocerebellar (ˌseribrohˌseri'belə) pertaining to the cerebrum and the cerebellum.

cerebrohepatorenal syndrome (ˌseribrohˌhepətoh'reen'l) a hereditary disorder, transmitted as an autosomal recessive trait, characterized by craniofacial abnormalities, hypotonia, hepatomegaly, polycystic kidneys, jaundice, and death in early infancy.

cerebroid ('seribroyd) resembling brain substance.

cerebroma (ˌseri'brohmə) any abnormal mass of brain substance.

cerebromacular (ˌseribroh'makyuhlə) pertaining to or affecting the brain and the macula retinae.

cerebromalacia (ˌseribrohmə'layshi·ə) abnormal softening of the substance of the cerebrum.

cerebromeningitis (ˌseribrohˌmenin'jietis) meningoencephalitis.

cerebronic acid (ˌseri'bronik) a fatty acid derived from sphingomyelin, which is the principal hydroxy saturated acid from the brain.

cerebropathy (ˌseri'bropəthee) any brain disorder.

cerebrophysiology (ˌseribrohˌfizi'oləjee) the physiology of the brain.

cerebropontile (ˌseribroh'pontiel) pertaining to the cerebrum and pons.

cerebrosclerosis (ˌseribrohsklə'rohsis) morbid hardening of the substance of the cerebrum.

cerebroside ('seribrohˌsied) a general designation for sphingolipids in which sphingosine is combined with galactose or glucose; found chiefly in nervous tissue.

cerebrosis (ˌseri'brohsis) any disease of the cerebrum.

cerebrospinal (ˌseribroh'spien'l) pertaining to the brain and spinal cord.

c. fluid the fluid within the subarachnoid space, the central canal of the spinal cord, and the four ventricles of the brain. The fluid is formed continuously by the choroid plexus in the ventricles, and, so that there will not be an abnormal increase in amount and pressure, it is reabsorbed into the blood by the arachnoid villi at approximately the same rate as that at which it is produced.

The cerebrospinal fluid aids in the protection of the brain, spinal cord, and meninges by acting as a watery cushion surrounding them to absorb the shocks to which they are exposed. There is a blood–cerebrospinal fluid barrier that prevents harmful substances, such as metal poisons, some pathogenic organisms, and certain drugs from passing from the capillaries into the cerebrospinal fluid.

The normal cerebrospinal fluid pressure is 5 mmHg (100 mmH_2O) when the individual is lying in a horizontal position on his side. Fluid pressure may be increased by a brain tumour or by haemorrhage or infection in the cranium. HYDROCEPHALUS, or excess fluid in the cranial cavity, can result from either excessive formation or poor absorption of cerebrospinal fluid. Blockage of the flow of fluid in the spinal canal may result from a tumour, blood clot, or severance of the spinal cord. The pressure remains normal or decreases below the point of obstruction but increases above that point.

Cell counts, bacterial smears, and cultures of samples of cerebrospinal fluid are done when an inflammatory process or infection of the meninges is suspected. Since the cerebrospinal fluid contains nutrient substances such as glucose, proteins, and sodium chloride and also some waste products such as urea, it is believed to play a role in metabolism. The major constituents of cerebrospinal fluid are water, glucose, sodium chloride, and protein, and changes in their concentrations are helpful in diagnosis of brain diseases.

Samples of cerebrospinal fluid may be obtained by SPINAL PUNCTURE (lumbar puncture), in which a hollow needle is inserted between two lumbar vertebrae (below the lower end of the spinal cord), or into the cisterna cerebellomedullaris just below the occipital bone of the skull (cisternal puncture). Pressure of the cerebrospinal fluid is measured by a manometer attached to the end of the needle after it has been inserted.

cerebrotendinous (ˌseribroh'tendinəs) pertaining to the cerebrum and the tendons.

cerebrotomy (ˌseri'brotəmee) anatomy or dissection of the brain.

cerebrovascular (ˌseribroh'vaskyuhlə) pertaining to the blood vessels of the cerebrum, or brain.

c. accident an outdated term for STROKE.

cerebrum ('seribrəm) the main portion of the brain, occupying the upper part of the cranial cavity; its two cerebral hemispheres, united by the corpus callosum, form the largest part of the central nervous system in man. The term is sometimes applied to the postembryonic forebrain and midbrain together or to the entire brain. See also BRAIN.

cerium ('siə·ri·əm) a chemical element, atomic number 58, atomic weight 140.12, symbol Ce. See table of elements in Appendix 2.

ceruloplasmin (siˌrooloh'plazmin) an alpha$_2$-globulin of the plasma, being the form in which most of the plasma copper is transported.

cerumen (si'roomen) a waxy secretion of the glands of the external acoustic meatus; ear wax. adj. **ceruminal, ceruminous.**

ceruminolysis (siˌroomi'nolisis) dissolution or disintegration of cerumen in the external acoustic meatus. adj. **ceruminolytic.**

ceruminosis (siˌroomi'nohsis) excessive or disordered secretion of cerumen.

cervic(o)- word element. [L.] *neck, cervix.*

cervical ('sərvik'l, sə'vie-) pertaining to the neck or to the cervix.

c. canal the part of the uterine cavity lying within the cervix.

c. erosion see cervical EROSION.

c. os this term usually refers to the external outlet to the uterine cervix. The cervix, a 2.5 cm long tube forming the neck of the uterus or womb, is constricted at its ends by the internal and external os (see accompanying illustration).

In pregnancy the internal os gradually dilates before delivery occurs. In primigravidae this occurs during the last month of pregnancy to achieve effacement or taking up of the cervix into the lower uterine segment, so that the cervical canal becomes obliterated. The external os remains closed. In multigravidae this process occurs simultaneously with dilation of the external os during labour. See also EFFACEMENT.

The degree of effacement of the cervix achieved by dilation of the internal os is an important indicator of the suitability of the cervix for induction of labour. See also BISHOP SCORE.

Progress of labour is assessed by dilation of the external cervical os. This dilates slowly during the latent phase of labour, usually taking up to eight hours to achieve 2 cm dilation. Progress speeds up during the active phase of labour, which lasts for about four hours. Full dilation of the external cervical os (cervix) is about 10 cm and marks the end of the first stage of labour and completion of the birth canal. See also LABOUR.

c. plexus a network of nerve fibres formed by the first four cervical nerves and supplying the structures in the region of the neck. One important branch is the phrenic nerve, which supplies the diaphragm.

c. polyp a small, pedunculated, relatively innocuous tumour arising from the mucous membrane of the endocervical canal. It is composed of loose stroma containing mucus-secreting glands. It may cause irregular vaginal bleeding.

c. rib a supernumerary rib arising from a cervical vertebra.

c. rib syndrome pain over the shoulder, often extending down the arm or radiating up the back of the neck, due to compression of the nerves and vessels between a cervical rib and the anterior scalene muscle.

c. vertebrae the upper seven vertebrae, constituting the skeleton of the neck.

cervicoplasty ('sərvikoh,plastee) plastic surgery of the neck or the cervix uteri.

cervicovesical (,sərvikoh'vesik'l) relating to the cervix uteri and urinary bladder.

cervix ('sərviks) pl. *cervices* [L.] neck; the front portion of the neck (collum), or a constricted part of an organ (e.g., cervix uteri).

incompetent c. a cervix uteri that is abnormally prone to dilate before termination of the normal period of gestation, resulting in premature expulsion of the fetus.

c. uteri the narrow lower end of the uterus between the isthmus and the opening of the uterus into the vagina.

Cervical cancer is surpassed only by breast cancer as a cause of female cancer deaths in the UK. Its victims are usually women over 40. One of the first warning signs of cervical cancer is vaginal bleeding between menstrual periods, after coitus, or after menopause is established. There may also be increased vaginal discharge. The PAPANICOLAOU TEST (Pap test; smear) should be available for all women over 21 (and for sexually active women under 21). At present in the UK this test is available every five years for women over 21 (unless an abnormal smear has already been seen), though many authorities believe that a three-year interval is desirable. This test identifies cancer in its earliest stages while the malignancy is still capable of relatively easy eradication.

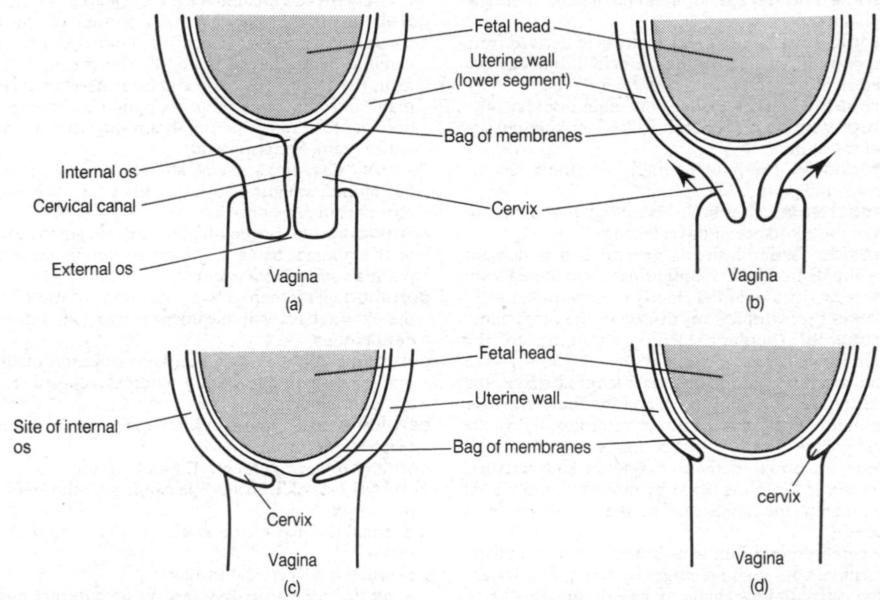

'Taking up' of the cervix (a, b) and dilatation of the os uteri (c, d). The cervix is fully effaced in (c)

Traditionally, a positive finding of abnormal cells from the cervix was an indication for cervical biopsy, which, if positive for malignancy, was an indication for total hysterectomy. Currently, this sequence is giving way to more selective methods of diagnosis and treatment. Special stains and colposcopy are used to define more clearly the nature and extent of abnormal changes in cervical cells. These techniques have permitted a greater use of localized excision of cervical

cervicectomy (,sərvi'sektəmee) excision of the cervix uteri.

cervicitis (,sərvi'sietis) inflammation of the cervix uteri. Called also *trachelitis*.

cervicobrachialgia (,sərvikoh,brayki·'alji·ə) pain in the neck radiating to the arm, due to compression of nerve roots of the cervical spinal cord.

cervicocolpitis (,sərvikohkol'pietis) inflammation of the cervix uteri and vagina.

cervicofacial (,sərvikoh'fayshəl) pertaining to the neck and face.

tissues (conization) and CRYOSURGERY of early cancer zones, thereby avoiding total removal of the uterus.

Cervical erosion refers to the destruction of the squamous epithelium covering the intravaginal portion of the cervix. An overgrowth of columnar epithelium from around the external os results in a ring of red, friable tissue. Treatment, if necessary, is by cautery. *Cervical lacerations* are likely to occur during childbirth. Most small lacerations heal by themselves; more extensive tears in the cervix may require surgical repair. *Cervical polyps* are fleshy growths that may form on the cervix, causing bleeding. They are removed surgically.

Cestan-Chenais syndrome (se'stanshen'ayz) an association of contralateral hemiplegia, contralateral hemianaesthesia, ipsilateral lateropulsion and hemiasynergia, Horner's syndrome, and ipsilateral laryngoplegia, due to scattered lesions of the pyramid, sensory tract, inferior cerebellar peduncle, nucleus ambiguus, and oculopupillary centre.

cesticidal (ˌsesti'sied'l) destructive to cestodes.

Cestoda (se'stohdə) a subclass of Cestoidea comprising the true tapeworms, which have a head (scolex) and segments (proglottides). The adults are endoparasitic in the alimentary tract and associated ducts of various vertebrate hosts; their larvae may be found in various organs and tissues.

cestode ('sestohd) 1. any individual of the class Cestoidea, especially any member of the subclass Cestoda. 2. cestoid.

cestoid ('sestoyd) resembling a tapeworm.

Cestoidea (se'stoydi·ə) a class of tapeworms (phylum Platyhelminthes), characterized by a noncellular cuticular layer covering their bodies and by the absence of a mouth and digestive tract. The true tapeworms are included in the subclass Cestoda.

cetrimide ('setrimied) a quaternary ammonium antiseptic and detergent, applied topically to disinfect the skin.

cetylpyridinium chloride (ˌseetil,piri'dini·əm) a cationic disinfectant used as a local anti-infective applied topically or sublingually to intact skin or mucous membrane.

cevitamic acid (ˌsevi'tamik) ascorbic acid; vitamin C.

Cf chemical symbol, *californium*.

cGMP cyclic guanosine monophosphate.

CGS, c.g.s. centimetre-gram-second (system), a system of measurements based on the centimetre as the unit of length, the gram as the unit of mass, and the second as the unit of time.

Chaddock's sign (reflex) ('chadoks) dorsiflexion of the big toe when the foot is stroked around the lateral malleolus and along the dorsum laterally. It occurs in lesions of the pyramidal tract.

chafe (chayf) to irritate the skin by friction, usually from clothing, or the rubbing together of body surfaces, such as the thighs, when they are damp with perspiration, or the rubbing together of opposing skin folds. The skin folds of the obese are particularly subject to chafing. Tight shoes, badly fitting brassieres, and other clothing that binds, all cause chafing. Babies are particularly susceptible.

The irritation can usually be cleared up by keeping the parts dry, using a plain talcum powder, and, if necessary, substituting clothing that does not bind or rub. The best prevention is to keep the skin clean and dry and to wear clothing that fits properly.

Chagas' disease ('shahgəs) trypanosomiasis due to *Trypanosoma cruzi* (see also South American TRYPANOSOMIASIS).

chagasic (shə'gasik) pertaining to or due to Chagas' disease.

chain (chayn) a collection of objects linked together in linear fashion, or end to end, as the assemblage of atoms or radicals in a chemical compound, or an assemblage of individual bacterial cells. **branched c.** an open chain of atoms, usually carbon, with one or more side chains attached to it.

heavy c. any of the large polypeptide chains of five classes that, paired with the light chains, make up the antibody molecule. Heavy chains bear the antigenic determinants that differentiate the immunoglobulin classes. See also HEAVY-CHAIN DISEASE.

J c. a polypeptide occurring in polymeric IgM and IgA molecules.

light c. either of the two small polypeptide chains (molecular weight 22,000) that, when linked to heavy chains by disulphide bonds, make up the antibody molecule; they are of two types, kappa and lambda, which are unrelated to immunoglobulin class differences as these are defined by the heavy chains.

side c. a chain of atoms attached to a larger chain or to a ring.

chalasia (kə'layzi·ə) relaxation of a bodily opening, such as the cardiac sphincter (a cause of vomiting in infants).

chalazion (kə'lazi·ən) a small eyelid mass resulting from chronic inflammation of a meibomian gland due to retained secretions. A chalazion can sometimes be treated at home with the application of hot compresses, but while this method is usually successful with a STY, a similar infection that has not yet formed a cyst, chalazion often requires incision and drainage.

chalcosis (kal'kohsis) copper deposits in tissue.

chalicosis (ˌkali'kohsis) pneumoconiosis due to inhalation of particles of stone.

chalone ('kalohn) a group of tissue-specific, water-soluble substances that are produced within a tissue and inhibit mitosis of the cells of that tissue, and whose action is reversible.

chalybeate (ka'libi,ayt) containing or charged with iron.

chamaecephaly (ˌkami'kefəlee, -'sef-) the condition of having a low, flat head, i.e., a cephalic index of 70 or less. adj. **chamaecephalic.**

chamber ('chaymbə) an enclosed space.

anterior c. the part of the aqueous humour-containing space of the eyeball between the cornea and iris.

hyperbaric c. an enclosed space in which gas (oxygen) can be raised to greater than atmospheric pressure (see also HYPERBARIC OXYGENATION).

ionization c. an enclosure containing two or more electrodes between which an electric current may be passed when the enclosed gas is ionized by radiation; used for determining the intensity of x-rays and other rays.

posterior c. that part of the aqueous humour-containing space of the eyeball between the iris and the lens.

vitreous c. the vitreous humour-containing space in the eyeball, bounded anteriorly by the lens and ciliary body and posteriorly by the posterior wall of the eyeball.

Chamberlen forceps ('chaymbərlen) the original form of obstetric forceps.

chancre ('shangkə) 1. the primary lesion of SYPHILIS, occurring at the site of entry of the infection. Called also *hard*, *hunterian*, or *true chancre*. 2. a papular lesion occurring at the site of entry of infection in tuberculosis of the skin or in sporotrichosis.

A true chancre begins as a papule which breaks down into a reddish ulcer. It is generally firm with little or no pain, and is accompanied by painless enlargement of regional lymph nodes (usually inguinal). Although most frequently located on the external genitalia, it may be on the lips or fingers. In women, a chancre is sometimes concealed in the internal genitalia where it may not be seen or felt. Two or three may develop simultaneously. A chancre heals of its own accord without treatment, thus leading many persons infected with syphilis to believe they are cured. They are not, and if adequate medical treatment is not begun at this early and curable stage of syphilis, the disease will progress, doing irreparable damage.

chancroid ('shangkroyd) a soft nonsyphilitic venereal sore caused by *Haemophilus ducreyi.* As in syphilis, the first symptom of the disease may be the appearance of a sore, but the sore is soft, as distinguished from the hard chancre of syphilis.

Chancroid is almost always spread by sexual contact, but in rare instances it may be transmitted indirectly from soiled dressings or towels. Three to five days after exposure one or more small soft sores appear on or near the external genitalia. These sores soon develop into ulcers with irregular edges and surrounding areas which become red and swollen. In many cases, the infection spreads to the lymph nodes of the groin, causing swelling and tenderness. These glandular masses usually require aspiration.

Chancroid is successfully treated with sulphafurazole or the antibiotics tetracycline and streptomycin.

chancrous ('shangkrəs) of the nature of chancre.

character ('kariktə) a quality or attribute indicative of the nature of an object or an organism; in genetics, the expression of a gene or group of genes as seen in a phenotype.

acquired c. a noninheritable modification produced in an animal as a result of its own activities or of environmental influences.

dominant c. a mendelian character that is expressed when it is transmitted by a single gene.

mendelian c's in genetics, the separate and distinct traits exhibited by an animal or plant and dependent on the genetic constitution of the organism.

recessive c. a mendelian character that is expressed only when transmitted by both genes (one from each parent) determining the trait.

sex-conditioned c., sex-influenced c. an autosomal trait whose full expression is conditioned by the sex of the individual, e.g., human baldness.

sex-linked c. one transmitted consistently to individuals of one sex only, being carried in the sex chromosome.

characteristic (ˌkariktə'ristik) 1. character. 2. typical of an individual or other entity.

demand c's behaviour exhibited by the subject of an experiment in an attempt to accomplish certain goals as a result of cues communicated by the experimenter (expectations or hypothesis).

primary sexual c's those characteristics of the male and female directly concerned in reproduction.

secondary sexual c's those characteristics specific to the male and female but not directly concerned in reproduction.

charcoal ('chahkohl) carbon prepared by charring wood or other organic material.

activated c. the residue of destructive distillation of various organic materials, treated to increase its adsorptive power; used as a general purpose antidote.

Charcot's arthropathy (disease) (shah'kohz) chronic progressive degeneration of the stress-bearing portion of a joint, with hypertrophic changes at the periphery; it is associated with neurological disorders involving loss of sensation in the joint. Called also *neuropathic arthropathy.*

Charcot–Marie–Tooth disease (shah'kohmə'reetooth) progressive neuropathic (peroneal) muscular atrophy.

Charcot's triad (shah'kohz) nystagmus, intention tremor and scanning speech. A trio of signs of disseminated sclerosis.

charlatan ('shahlətan) a pretender to knowledge or skills not possessed; in medicine, a quack.

Charles' law (shahlz) at a constant pressure the volume of a given mass of perfect gas varies directly with the absolute temperature.

Charnley's arthroplasty ('chahnliz) the replacement of the hip joint using a plastic acetabulum and a steel femoral head.

chart (chaht) a record of data in graphic or tabular form.

genealogical c. a graph showing various descendants of a common ancestor, used to indicate those affected by genetically determined disease.

reading c. a chart with material printed in gradually increasing type sizes, used in testing acuity of near vision.

Reuss' c's charts with coloured letters printed on coloured backgrounds, used in testing colour vision.

Snellen's c. a chart printed with block letters in gradually decreasing sizes, used in testing visual acuity.

charting ('chahting) the keeping of a clinical record of the important facts about a patient and the progress of his illness. The patient's chart usually contains a medical history, a nursing history, results of physical examinations, laboratory reports, results of special diagnostic tests, and the observations of the nursing staff. Medical treatments, medications, and nursing approaches to problems are recorded on the chart, as are the patient's response to treatment. See also PROBLEM-ORIENTED RECORD.

chauffage (shoh'fahzh) [Fr.] a form of therapy using heat transfer by convection and radiation from a source close to but not in contact with the skin.

ChB [L.] *Chirurgiae Baccalaureus* (Bachelor of Surgery).

CHC Community Health Council.

Chédiak–Higashi syndrome (ˌchaydeeakhie'gashee) a lethal, progressive, autosomal recessive, systemic disorder associated with oculocutaneous albinism, massive leukocyte inclusions (giant lysosomes), histiocytic infiltration of multiple body organs, development of pancytopenia, hepatosplenomegaly, recurrent or persistent bacterial infections, and a possible predisposition to development of malignant lymphoma.

cheek (cheek) a fleshy, rounded protuberance, especially the fleshy portion of either side of the face. Called also *bucca.*

cleft c. facial cleft caused by developmental failure of union between the maxillary and primitive frontonasal processes.

cheil(o)- word element. [Gr.] *lip.*

cheilectropion (ˌkielek'trohpi·ən) eversion of the lip.

cheilitis (kie'lietis) inflammation of the lips.

actinic c., c. actinica involvement of the lips after exposure to actinic rays, with pain and swelling, and development of a scaly crust on the vermilion border. See also solar CHEILITIS.

angular c. an infection of the fissures at the corners of the mouth. Commonly associated with *Candida albicans* but other organisms can sometimes be isolated from the fissure. In some patients there may be an associated vitamin deficiency, in others an overclosure of the jaws which requires the construction of new dentures.

solar c. involvement of the lips after exposure to solar radiation; it may be acute (actinic cheilitis), or chronic, with alteration of the epithelium and sometimes

fissuring or ulceration.
cheilognathopalatoschisis (ˌkielohˌnathohˌpalə'toskisis) cleft of the lip, upper jaw, and hard and soft palates.
cheiloplasty ('kielohˌplastee) plastic repair of a lip defect.
cheilorrhaphy (kie'lorəfee) suture of the lip; surgical repair of a cleft lip.
cheiloschisis (kie'loskisis) cleft lip.
cheiloscopy (kie'loskəpee) study of the surface configuration of the vermilion border of the lips to identify individual patterns (lip-print patterns).
cheilosis (kie'lohsis) fissuring and dry scaling of the vermilion surface of the lips and angles of the mouth, a characteristic of riboflavin deficiency.
cheilotomy (kie'lotəmee) incision of the lip.
cheir(o)- word element. [Gr.] *hand;* see also words beginning *chir(o)-*.
cheiralgia (kie'ralji·ə) pain in the hand.
cheiroarthropathy (ˌkieroah'thropəthee) flexion tendon contracture of fingers, contracture of large joints and sometimes dermal sclerosis found in association with insulin-dependent diabetes mellitus.
cheirognostic (ˌkierog'nostik) pertaining to or characterized by the ability to distinguish stimuli as originating on the right or left side of the body.
cheirokinaesthesia (ˌkierohˌkinis'theezi·ə) subjective perception of movements of the hand, especially in writing.
cheiroplasty ('kierohˌplastee) plastic surgery on the hand.
cheiropodalgia (ˌkierohpo'dalji·ə) pain in the hands and feet.
cheiropompholyx (ˌkieroh'pomfohliks) pompholyx.
cheiropractic (ˌkierə'praktik) see CHIROPRACTIC.
cheirospasm ('kierohˌspazəm) spasm of the muscles of the hand.
chelating agent (ki'layting) a substance which combines with a metal in complexes in which the metal is part of a ring; by extension, a chemical compound in which a metallic ion is sequestered and firmly bound into a ring within the chelating molecule. Chelates are used in chemotherapy of metal poisoning. See DIMERCAPROL and PENICILLAMINE.
cheloid ('keeloyd) keloid.
chem(o)- word element. [Gr.] *chemical, chemistry.*
chemabrasion (ˌkeemə'brayzhən) superficial destruction of the epidermis and the upper layer of the dermis by application of a cauterant to the skin; done to remove scars, tattoos, etc.
chemexfoliation (ˌkeemeksˌfohli'ayshən) chemabrasion.
chemical ('kemik'l) 1. pertaining to chemistry. 2. a substance composed of chemical elements, or obtained by chemical processes.
cheminosis (ˌkemi'nohsis) any disease due to chemical agents.
chemist ('kemist) 1. an expert in chemistry. 2. a PHARMACIST, especially one who dispenses prescribed medicines from a retail shop. Called also *dispensing chemist.* 3. a retail shop where medicines are dispensed.
chemistry ('kemistree) the science that treats of the elements and atomic relations of matter, and of the various compounds of the elements.
colloid c. chemistry dealing with the nature and composition of colloids.
inorganic c. the branch of chemistry dealing with inorganic compounds.
organic c. the branch of chemistry dealing with organic compounds, those characterized by carbon–carbon bonds, i.e., all compounds containing carbon except oxides of carbon, carbides, and carbonates.
chemoattractant (ˌkeemohə'traktənt, ˌkem-) a chemical (chemotactic) agent that induces an organism or a cell (e.g., a leukocyte) to migrate toward it.
chemoautotroph (ˌkeemoh'awtohˌtrohf, ˌkem-) a chemoautotrophic organism.
chemoautotrophic (ˌkeemohˌawtoh'trofik, ˌkem-) capable of synthesizing cell constituents from carbon dioxide by means of energy derived from inorganic reactions.
chemodectoma (ˌkeemohdek'tohmə, ˌkem-) any tumour of the chemoreceptor system, e.g., a carotid body tumour.
chemohormonal (ˌkeemoh·haw'mohnəl, ˌkem-) pertaining to drugs having hormonal activity.
chemolithotroph (ˌkeemoh'lithohˌtrohf, ˌkem-) an organism that derives its energy from oxidation of inorganic compounds and its carbon from carbon dioxide.
chemolithotrophic (ˌkeemohˌlithoh'trofik, ˌkem-) deriving energy from the oxidation of reduced inorganic compounds such as ferrous iron, ammonia, hydrogen sulphide, or hydrogen; said of bacteria.
chemoluminescence (ˌkeemohˌloomi'nes'ns, ˌkem-) luminescence produced by the direct transformation of chemical energy into light energy.
chemonucleolysis (ˌkeemohˌnyookli'olisis, ˌkem-) dissolution of a portion of the nucleus pulposus of an intervertebral disc by injection of a chemolytic agent for treatment of a herniated intervertebral disc.
chemoorganotroph (ˌkeemoh'awgənohˌtrohf, ˌkem-) an organism that derives its energy and carbon from organic compounds.
chemoorganotrophic (ˌkeemohˌawgənoh'trofik, ˌkem-) deriving energy from the oxidation of organic compounds; said of bacteria.
chemopallidectomy (ˌkeemohˌpali'dektəmee, ˌkem-) destruction of tissue of the globus pallidus by a chemical agent.
chemoprophylaxis (ˌkeemohˌprofi'laksis, ˌkem-) prevention of disease by chemical means.
chemopsychiatry (ˌkeemohsie'kieətree, ˌkem-) the treatment of mental and emotional disorders by the use of drugs.
chemoreceptor (ˌkeemohri'septə, ˌkem-) any of the special cells or organs adapted for excitation by chemical substances and located outside the central nervous system. There are chemoreceptors in the large arteries of the thorax and the neck; called carotid and aortic bodies. These receptors are responsive to changes in the oxygen, carbon dioxide, and hydrogen ion concentration in the blood. When oxygen concentration falls below normal in the arterial blood, the chemoreceptors send impulses to stimulate the respiratory centre so that there will be an increase in alveolar ventilation, and consequently, an increase in the intake of oxygen by the lungs.

Other chemoreceptors are the taste buds, which are sensitive to chemicals in the mouth, and the olfactory cells of the nose, which detect certain chemicals in the air.
chemosensitive (ˌkeemoh'sensitiv, ˌkem-) sensitive to changes in chemical composition.
chemosensory (ˌkeemoh'sensə·ree, ˌkem-) relating to the perception of chemical substances, as in odour detection.
chemosis (kee'mohsis) oedema of the conjunctiva of the eye.
chemosurgery (ˌkeemoh'sərjə·ree, ˌkem-) the destruction of tissue by chemical agents for therapeutic purposes; originally applied to chemical fixation of malignant, gangrenous, or infected tissue, with use of

frozen sections to facilitate systematic microscopic control of its excision.

chemosynthesis (ˌkeemoh'sinthəsis, ˌkem-) the building up of chemical compounds under the influence of chemical stimulation, specifically the formation of carbohydrates from carbon dioxide and water as a result of energy derived from chemical reactions. adj. **chemosynthetic.**

chemotaxin (ˌkeemoh'taksin, ˌkem-) a substance, e.g., an activated complement component, that induces chemotaxis.

chemotaxis (ˌkeemoh'taksis, ˌkem-) taxis in response to the influence of chemical stimulation. adj. **chemotactic.**

leukocyte c. the response of leukocytes to products formed in immunological reactions, wherein leukocytes are attracted to and accumulate at the site of the reaction; a part of the inflammatory response. See also INFLAMMATION.

chemotherapy (ˌkeemoh'therəpee, ˌkem-) the treatment of illness by chemical means; that is, by medication. adj. **chemotherapeutic.** The term was first applied to the treatment of infectious diseases, but it is now used to include the treatment of mental illness and CANCER with drugs. See also ANTINEOPLASTIC THERAPY.

chemotic (kee'motik) pertaining to or affected with chemosis.

chemotrophic (ˌkeemoh'trofik, ˌkem-) deriving energy from the oxidation of organic (chemoorganotrophic) or inorganic (chemolithotrophic) compounds; said of bacteria.

chemotropism (ˌkeemoh'trohpizəm, ˌkem-) tropism in response to the influence of chemical stimulation.

chenodeoxycholic acid (ˌkeenohdiˌoksi'kohlik) a primary bile acid, $C_{24}H_{40}O_4$, administered to dissolve gallstones.

Chenofalk ('keenohfalk) trademark for a preparation containing chenodeoxycholic acid. Used in the dissolution of cholesterol gallstones.

chenotherapy (ˌkeenoh'therəpee) treatment with chenodeoxycholic acid, as for dissolution of gallstones.

cherry-red spot ('chereeˌred) the normal red appearance of the foveal area of the retina contrasted with the grey-white colour of the rest of the retina occurring as a result of central retinal artery occlusion. Also occurs in the rare degenerative condition known as Tay–Sachs disease.

cherubism ('cherəbizəm) hereditary and progressive bilateral swelling at the angle of the mandible, sometimes involving the entire jaw, imparting a cherubic look to the face, in some cases enhanced by upturning of the eyes.

chest (chest) the thorax; the part of the body enclosed by the ribs and sternum, especially its anterior aspect.

c. drain a tube inserted into the thoracic cavity for the purpose of removing air or fluid, or both. In some cases more than one drain is inserted so that both fluid and air can be removed. Chest drains are attached to a closed drainage system or one-way valve system device so that normal pressures within the alveoli and the pleural cavity can be restored. These pressures are essential to adequate expansion and deflation of the lung.

Chest drains are indicated when the normally airtight pleural space has been penetrated through surgery or trauma, when a defect in the alveoli allows air to enter the intrapleural space, and when there is an accumulation of fluid, as from pleural EFFUSION. The effect of excessive amounts of air and fluid within the pleural space is collapse of the lung and the danger of MEDIASTINAL shift.

PATIENT CARE. It is important that those responsible for the personal care of a patient who has chest drains inserted understand the basic mechanics of lung inflation and deflation (see under LUNG), and the purpose of the drains and their location in each patient. In some cases one drain is inserted higher in the thorax (usually in the 2nd intercostal space) to remove air, and a second drain is placed lower (in the 8th or 9th intercostal space) to drain off fluids.

Chest drains may be connected to a variety of closed drainage systems: a water-seal drainage system with one, two, or three bottles; and a vacuumed self-contained system. Whatever the type, the purpose of the system is to allow for drainage from the pleural cavity and at the same time prevent the entry of atmospheric air into the pleural cavity.

Precautions that must be taken in the maintenance of the drainage system are:

(1) The bottles and collection apparatus of the system must be kept below the level of the chest to prevent backflow.

(2) The lumens of the drains must be kept open to allow for drainage. If they are obstructed there will be no fluctuation of the fluid level in the tube that is connected to the chest drain at one end and kept under water in the bottle at the other end. In the vacuumed self-contained system the liquid in the chamber should rise on the right side and fall on the left side. If there is evidence that the system is not working properly, this must be corrected immediately. Occlusion of the drains can lead to a buildup of air and fluids in the pleural cavity and create a tension PNEUMOTHORAX.

(3) The system must be a *closed* system. There can be no leaks around connections, and the lower end of the drain must remain under water in the bottle.

The amount, colour, and consistency of the fluid drainage should be checked at least once each hour for the first 24 hours after surgery. The chest drains may be milked and stripped at intervals to assure patency and adequate drainage. The removal of air is indicated by occasional bubbling in the water-seal chamber.

Following pneumonectomy, the patient with chest drains will normally be asked to lie on the operated side for the first 24 hours to allow consolidation of the lung space. In all other instances patients should be encouraged to be as active as possible within the limits of their condition. Chest physiotherapy, frequent changes of postition (avoiding kinking or putting tension on the drainage tube), coughing and deep breathing will all encourage drainage from the chest.

Clamps should be available at all times for use if the chest drains should become disconnected. Any signs of respiratory distress or malfunctioning of the system should be dealt with at once or death may quickly ensue.

On removal of the chest drains, the wound must be promptly sealed by tightening the purse-string suture around the wound and applying an occlusive dressing.

flail c. one whose wall moves paradoxically with respiration, owing to multiple fractures of the ribs (see also FLAIL CHEST).

funnel c. depression of the sternum and rib cartilage; PECTUS EXCAVATUM.

pigeon c. prominence of the sternum and rib cartilage; PECTUS CARINATUM.

c. tube see chest drain (above).

Cheyne–Stokes respiration ('chaynˌstohks) breathing characterized by rhythmic waxing and waning of the depth of respiration; the patient breathes deeply for a short time and then breathes very slightly or stops breathing altogether. The pattern occurs over and over again every 45 seconds to 3 minutes. Periodic breathing of this type is caused by disease affecting the respiratory centres, usually heart failure or brain damage.

chi-squared test ('kie,skwaird) a statistical test to determine whether two or more groups of observations differ significantly from one another, i.e., more than would be expected by chance.

chiasm ('kieazəm) a decussation or Y-shaped crossing.

optic c. a structure in the forebrain formed by the decussation of fibres of the optic nerve from each half of each retina.

chiasma (kie'azmə) pl. *chiasmata* [L., Gr.] chiasm; in genetics, the points at which members of a chromosome pair are in contact during the prophase of meiosis and because of which recombination, or crossing over, occurs on separation.

c. formation the process by which a chiasma is formed; it is the cytological basis of genetic recombination, or crossing over.

chickenpox ('chikin,poks) an acute, generalized viral infection, with mild constitutional symptoms and a maculopapular vesicular skin eruption, caused by the varicella-zoster (V-Z) virus, a *herpesvirus*. The same virus causes herpes zoster (shingles), which is due to reactivation of the infection in persons previously infected with the virus.

Chickenpox is a very common, usually mild childhood disease worldwide, but severe disease may occur in neonates, adults and in persons who are immunocompromised. It is a specifically human disease and the source of infection is a person with lesions in the mouth or respiratory tract and less commonly the skin; scabs are not infectious. There are no 'carriers'. Spread of the disease is via the airborne route by droplet infection, the early prodromal stage of the disease before the rash appears being highly infectious. The period of communicability lasts for about a week. The incubation period is usually 15 to 18 days, but may extend from one to three weeks. One attack usually gives lifelong immunity. Chickenpox is a notifiable disease in Scotland.

SYMPTOMS. Chickenpox may begin with a slight fever, headache, sore throat and malaise for 1 to 2 days, but often in children these prodromal symptoms are absent. The rash appears mainly on the trunk and evolves rapidly from macules to papules, vesicles and then pustules. All stages of the rash may be seen on a patient at any one time and it persists for about a week. Severe disseminated infection may occur in persons with leukaemia or who are immunosuppressed. The infection sometimes causes a primary viral pneumonia.

TREATMENT. Most cases of chickenpox are mild and require no special treatment. Antihistamines by mouth and calamine lotion to the skin may be useful if itching is severe, and antibiotics may be given if secondary infection of the rash occurs. In severe disease antiviral drugs such as acyclovir should be given.

PREVENTION. A chickenpox vaccine is not yet generally available. Leukaemics and other highly susceptible persons exposed to infection, for example when a case occurs in a hospital ward, should be given zoster immune globulin (ZIG) as soon as possible. Neonates of mothers with chickenpox within 5 days of delivery should also be protected with ZIG.

It is usual to exclude children with chickenpox from school until one week after the appearance of the rash, though it is doubtful whether this prevents the spread of infection, as they are most infectious before they become ill.

chigger ('chigə) the six-legged red larva of mites of the family Trombiculidae, which attach to their host's skin, and whose bite produces a wheal, usually with intense itching and severe dermatitis. Some species are vectors of the rickettsiae of scrub typhus. Called also *harvest mite* and *red bug*.

chigoe ('chigoh) the sand flea, *Tunga penetrans*, of tropical America and Africa. The pregnant female flea burrows into the skin of the feet, legs, or other part of the body, causing intense irritation and resulting in ulceration, and secondary infection.

chilblain ('chil,blayn) one of the mildest forms of cold injury, characterized by recurrent localized itching, swelling, painful erythema, and sometimes blistering and ulceration, caused by exposure to cold and dampness. It occurs chiefly on the fingers, toes, ears, and face, but may involve other areas of the body. Called also *pernio*. The basic cause of chilblain is sensitivity to cold, sometimes resulting from circulatory disturbances, which may be corrected in part by exercise and proper diet; severe cases require medical attention. This condition should not be confused with FROSTBITE, another type of skin damage caused by exposure to cold.

child (chield) the human young, from infancy to puberty.

c. abuse the nonaccidental use of physical force or the nonaccidental act of omission by a parent or other custodian responsible for the care of a child. Child abuse encompasses malnutrition and other kinds of neglect through ignorance as well as deliberate withholding from the child the necessary and basic physical care, including the medical and dental care necessary for the child to grow up without threat to his or her physical and emotional survival. Examples of physical abuse range from burns and exposure to extreme cold to beating, poisoning, strangulation, and withholding food and water.

Abusive parents come from all socioeconomic groups. Many have themselves been abused as children. They typically lack parenting skills and do not understand the normal developmental stages through which children progress and demand performance from their children that is clearly beyond a child's capability. Some engage in role reversal, looking to the child for protection and loving response, while at the same time denying the child satisfaction of his or her own needs.

Members of the health care team should be alert for signs of child abuse and aware of the proper procedure for reporting suspected cases to local authorities.

deprived c. a vague term usually implying that the child in question has been raised in a situation lacking in love, affection and consistent parenting responses from adults. Sometimes used to suggest that the child has experienced a generalised deficit of life opportunities, both interpersonal and social.

childbed ('chield,bed) the puerperal state or period.

c. fever puerperal fever.

childbirth ('chield,bərth) the act or process of giving birth to a child (see also LABOUR). Called also *parturition*.

natural c. a term used to describe an approach to labour and delivery in which the parents are prepared for the event so that the mother is awake and cooperative and the father is able to assume an active and supportive role during the birth of their child. Medical interference, drugs and other stimuli to labour are avoided. See also NATURAL CHILDBIRTH.

chill (chil) a sensation of cold, with convulsive shaking of the body. See RIGOR.

Chilomastix (,kieloh'mastiks) a genus of parasitic

protozoa found in the intestines of vertebrates.

C. mesnili a very common, widely distributed species found as a commensal in the human caecum and colon.

Chilopoda (kie'lopohdə) a class of the phylum Arthropoda embracing the centipedes.

chimera (kie'miə·rə, ki-) an organism whose body contains different cell populations derived from different zygotes of the same or different species, occurring spontaneously or produced artificially.

chimerism (ki'miərizəm, 'kiemə·rizəm) the state of being a chimera; the presence in an individual of cells of different origin.

chin (chin) the anterior prominence of the lower jaw; the mentum.

Chinese restaurant syndrome ('chieneez 'restəronh) transient arterial dilation due to ingestion of monosodium glutamate, which is used liberally in seasoning Chinese food, marked by throbbing head, lightheadedness, tightness of the jaw, neck, and shoulders, and backache.

chir(o)- word element. [Gr.] *hand;* see also words beginning *cheir(o)-*.

chiropodist (ki'ropədist, shi-) alternative name for podiatrist.

chiropody (ki'ropədee, shi-) the study and care of the feet and the treatment of foot diseases.

chiropractic (,kierə'praktik) a system of treating disorders by manipulation of the vertebral column. Chiropractic is based on the theory that most disorders are caused by problems in nerve transmission and therefore mode function because of faulty alignment of the vertebrae. Called also cheiropractic.

chiropractor (,kierə'praktə) a practitioner in chiropractic.

chirurgery (kie'rərjə·ree) surgery.

chitin ('kietin) a horny polysaccharide, the principal constituent of shells of arthropods and shards of beetles, and found in certain fungi.

chlamydaemia (,klami'deemi·ə) the presence of chlamydiae in the blood.

Chlamydia (klə'midi·ə) a genus of bacteria comprising two species: *C. trachomatis*, which causes lymphogranuloma venereum, trachoma and inclusion conjunctivitis, and some cases of nongonococcal urethritis; and *C. psittaci*, which causes psittacosis (parrot fever). They are obligate intracellular parasites that are totally dependent on the host cell for energy in the form of adenosine triphosphate (ATP), which they cannot synthesize. Outside of a host they exist as elementary bodies, which have a rigid cell wall and are unable to grow or divide. The elementary bodies attach to host cells and are taken in by phagocytosis. Inside the phagosome they become reticulate bodies, which have flexible cell walls and grow and divide. After about 40 hours elementary bodies are formed, the host cell dies, and the elementary bodies are released.

chlamydia (klə'midi·ə) pl. *chlamydiae;* any member of the genus *Chlamydia.*

Chlamydiaceae (kla,midi'aysi·ee) a family of bacteria containing a single genus, *Chlamydia.*

chlamydiosis (klə,midi'ohsis) any infection or disease caused by *Chlamydia.*

chlamydospore ('klamidoh,spor, kla'midə-) a thick-walled intercalary or terminal asexual spore formed by the rounding-up of a cell; it is not shed.

chloasma (kloh'azmə) hyperpigmentation in circumscribed areas of the skin; called also melasma.

c. gravidarum melasma gravidarum.

c. hepaticum generalized discoloration of the skin allegedly due to disorder of the liver.

c. uterinum melasma gravidarum.

chloracetone (,klor'asitohn) tear-gas.

chloracne (klor'raknee) an acneiform eruption, caused by exposure to chlorine compounds.

chloraemia (klor'reemi·ə) 1. chlorosis. 2. hyperchloraemia.

chloral ('klor·ral) 1. an oily liquid with a pungent, irritating odour, prepared by the mutual action of alcohol and chlorine; used in the manufacture of chloral hydrate and DDT. 2. chloral hydrate.

c. hydrate a hypnotic and sedative with mild action as a pain reliever but used most commonly to induce sleep.

Chloral hydrate is available in liquid and in capsule form. It may be habit-forming. It should not be given with alcohol. The drug is now rarely used.

chloralism ('klor·rəlizəm) a morbid condition due to excessive use of chloral.

chlorambucil (klor'rambyuhsil) a nitrogen mustard derivative used as an antineoplastic agent.

chloramphenicol (,klor·ram'fenikol) a broad-spectrum antibiotic with specific therapeutic activity against rickettsiae and many different bacteria. Side-effects include serious, even fatal, blood dyscrasias in certain patients. Frequent blood tests are recommended during therapy.

Chlorasol ('klorəsol) trademark for a sterile solution of sodium hypochlorite.

chlorcyclizine (klor'siekli,zeen) an antihistamine, used as the hydrochloride salt.

chlordane ('klordayn) a poisonous substance of the chlorinated hydrocarbon group, used as an insecticide.

chlordiazepoxide (,klordie,azi'poksied) a minor tranquillizer.

chlorhexidine (klor'heksi,deen) an antibacterial compound used in antibiotic skin cleansers for surgical scrub, preoperative skin preparation, and cleansing skin wounds.

chlorhydria (klor'hiedri·ə) an excess of hydrochloric acid in the stomach.

chloride ('klor·ried) a salt of hydrochloric acid; any binary compound of chlorine.

chloridorrhoea (,klor·ridə'reeə) diarrhoea with an excess of chlorides in the stool.

chloriduria (,klor·ri'dyooə·ri·ə) an excess of chlorides in the urine.

chlorinated ('klor·ri,naytid) charged with chlorine.

chlorination (,klor·ri'nayshən) the addition of chlorine to water or sewage to kill germs. Liquid or gaseous chlorine has been found to be the most effective water disinfectant, and is used for the purification of both public water supplies and swimming pools. This addition of chlorine is harmless, since enough chlorine to affect the health of those using the chlorinated water would also make the water too unpalatable to drink.

chlorine ('klor·reen, -rin) a gaseous chemical element, atomic number 17, atomic weight 35.453, symbol Cl. (See table of elements in Appendix 2.) It is a disinfectant, decolorizer, and irritant poison. It is used for disinfecting, fumigating, and bleaching, either in an aqueous solution or in the form of chlorinated lime.

chlormethiazole (,klormə'thieə,zohl) a hypnotic, sedative and anticonvulsant drug with a depressant action on the central nervous system. It is used to treat insomnia, agitation and confusion, chiefly in the elderly. It is also used to treat acute withdrawal symptoms in alcoholism and drug addiction, and for the control of sustained epileptic fits.

chlormezanone (klor'mezənohn) a muscle relaxant used to treat muscle spasms; also an anxiolytic.

chloroacetone (,klor·roh'asi,tohn) tear-gas.

Chlorocain ('klor·rohkayn) trademark for a preparation

of mepivacaine, a local anaesthetic.

chlorocresol (ˌklor·roh'kreesol) a coal tar product with a bactericidal action more powerful than phenol and with a lower toxicity. Used as an antiseptic and as a preservative in injection fluids.

chloroform ('klo·rəˌfawm) a colourless, mobile liquid with an ethereal odour and sweet taste, used as a solvent; once used widely as an inhalation anaesthetic and analgesic, and as an antitussive, carminative, and counterirritant.

chlorolabe ('klor·rohlayb) the pigment in retinal cones that is more sensitive to the green portion of the spectrum than are the other pigments (cyanolabe and erythrolabe).

chloroleukaemia (ˌklor·rohloo'keemi·ə) myelogenous leukaemia in which no specific tumour masses are observed at autopsy, but the body organs and fluids show a definite green colour.

chloroma (klor'rohmə) a malignant, green-coloured tumour arising from myeloid tissue, associated with myelogenous leukaemia, and occurring anywhere in the body.

Chloromycetin (ˌklor·rohmie'seetin) trademark for preparations of chloramphenicol, a broad-spectrum antibiotic.

chloropexia (ˌklor·roh'peksi·ə) the fixation of chlorine in body tissues.

chlorophyll ('klo·rəˌfil) any of a group of green pigments, containing a magnesium-porphyrin complex, that are involved in oxygen-producing photosynthesis. Preparations of water-soluble chlorophyll derivatives are applied topically for deodorization of skin lesions, and administered orally to deodorize ulcerative lesions and the urine and faeces in colostomy, ileostomy or incontinence.

chloroplast ('klor·rohˌplast) the photosynthetic unit of a plant cell, containing all the chlorophyll.

chloroprivic (ˌklor·roh'prievik) deprived of chlorides; due to loss of chlorides.

chloropsia (klor'ropsi·ə) a defect of vision in which objects appear to have a greenish tinge.

chloroquine ('klor·rohˌkween) an antimalarial and lupus erythematosus suppressant.

chlorosis (klor'rohsis) a disorder, generally of pubescent females, characterized by greenish yellow discoloration of the skin and hypochromic erythrocytes; believed to be related to iron deficiency. adj. **chlorotic**.

chlorothiazide (ˌklor·roh'thieəzied) a diuretic drug that also has an antihypertensive effect. It is used in treatment of the oedema of congestive heart failure, and in hypertension. Possible side-effects include potassium depletion and other electrolyte imbalances; bone marrow depression with a lowering of the platelet and leukocyte counts, agranulocytosis, and aplastic anaemia are rare adverse reactions.

chlorotrianisene (ˌklor·rohtrie'aniseen) a long-acting synthetic oestrogen, used for treatment of vasomotor symptoms or urogenital atrophy associated with menopause and for palliative treatment of prostatic carcinoma.

chloroxylenol (ˌklor·roh'zielənol) a broad-spectrum antibiotic used in the treatment of bacterial, fungal, and yeast infections of the skin and nails.

chlorpheniramine (ˌklorfe'nirəˌmeen) a pyridine derivative used as an antihistamine in the form of the maleate salt.

chlorpromazine (klor'prohməˌzeen) a phenothiazine used as an antipsychotic agent and antiemetic. Side-effects include drowsiness and slight hypotension. In prolonged therapy the patient should be observed for jaundice. Some patients on long-term therapy develop persistant tardive dyskinesia.

chlorpropamide (klor'prohpəˌmied) an oral hypoglycaemic drug useful in the treatment of diabetes mellitus in the adult whose condition is stabilized. The drug is contraindicated in patients with impairment of renal or hepatic function. Dosage is individually adjusted.

chlorprothixene (ˌklorproh'thikseen) a major tranquillizer.

chlortetracycline (ˌklortetrə'siekleen) a broad-spectrum antibiotic obtained from *Streptomyces aureofaciens*, used in the form of the hydrochloride salt as an antibacterial (effective against both gram-positive and gram-negative bacteria) and as an antiprotozoal. It is available in capsules, in ampoules for intravenous injection, and in ointment for topical use. Side-effects include gastrointestinal disturbances, especially diarrhoea.

chlorthalidone (klor'thaliˌdohn) a diuretic and antihypertensive.

chloruresis (ˌkloryuh'reesis) excretion of chlorides in the urine. adj. **chloruretic**.

chloruria (klor'yooə·ri·ə) an excess of chlorides in the urine.

ChM [L.] *Chirurgiae Magister* (Master of Surgery).

choana ('koh·anə, koh'ahnə) pl. *choanae* [L.] 1. any funnel-shaped cavity or infundibulum. 2. *choanae*, the paired openings between the nasal cavity and the nasopharynx.

choke (chohk) 1. to interrupt respiration by obstruction or compression, or the condition resulting from such interruption. 2. *chokes*, a burning sensation in the substernal region, with uncontrollable coughing, occurring during decompression.

chol(o)- word element. [Gr.] *bile*.

cholaemia (ko'leemi·ə) bile or bile pigment in the blood. adj. **cholaemic**.

cholagogue ('kohləgog) an agent that stimulates gallbladder contraction to promote bile flow. adj. **cholagogic**.

cholangiectasis (kəˌlanji'ektəsis) dilation of a bile duct.

cholangiocarcinoma (kəˌlanjiohˌkahsi'nohmə) adenocarcinoma of the bile ducts. Called also *cholangiocellular carcinoma*.

cholangioenterostomy (kəˌlanjiohˌentə'rostəmee) surgical anastomosis of a bile duct to the intestine.

cholangiogastrostomy (kəˌlanjiohga'strostəmee) surgical anastomosis of a bile duct to the stomach.

cholangiogram (kə'lanjiohˌgram) the film obtained by cholangiography.

cholangiography (kəˌlanji'ogrəfee) x-ray examination of the bile ducts, using a radiopaque contrast medium. adj. **cholangiographic**.

intravenous c. method in which the contrast medium is administered intravenously, usually as a slow infusion but occasionally as a bolus. It is unlikely to be successful if the serum bilirubin is greater that 50 μmol per litre. The patient should be well hydrated prior to the examination and a laxative may be given so that faecal material does not obscure the biliary tract. The contrast medium is excreted via the liver into the bile ducts. Radiographs are taken at the end of the infusion and at 15-minute intervals until contrast medium is seen in the duodenum. If the ducts or gallbladder are not seen after 2 hours, further films are taken every 30 minutes until 4 hours post-infusion. If no opacification has occurred by this time, the examination is terminated.

operative c. demonstration of the bile ducts during surgery prior to exploration or in order to avoid surgical exploration of the common bile duct. Radiographs are taken of the biliary tree following cannulation of the cystic duct and injection of contrast medium.

percutaneous transhepatic c. technique used to further evaluate the cause of obstructive jaundice, especially when this is believed to be due to an extrahepatic cause. The demonstration of dilated intrahepatic bile ducts by ultrasound usually precedes the investigation. (Intravenous cholangiography is unsuccessful in the jaundiced patient.) Under fluoroscopic control a skinny needle is inserted through the skin into the liver and a dilated duct is located. Contrast medium is injected into a bile duct to ascertain the nature and level of obstruction. If the patient is not intended for early surgical relief of the obstruction, it is possible to drain the obstructed ducts by inserting a catheter. Drainage may be either external, through the skin, or the catheter may be threaded past the obstruction so that bile drains normally into the duodenum.

post-operative c. see T-tube cholangiography (below).

T-tube c. technique performed after biliary tract surgery, usually to exclude residual biliary tract calculi. The contrast medium is injected directly into a T-shaped tube which has been left in the bile duct since surgery. Radiographs are exposed by the radiologist whilst examining the patient under fluoroscopy.

cholangiohepatoma (kə,lanjioh,hepə'tohmə) primary carcinoma of the liver of mixed liver cell and bile duct cell origin.

cholangiole (kə'lanji·ohl) one of the fine terminal elements of the bile duct system. adj. **cholangiolar**.

cholangiolitis (kə,lanjioh'lietis) inflammation of the cholangioles. adj. **cholangiolitic**.

cholangioma (kə,lanji'ohmə) cholangiocellular carcinoma.

cholangiostomy (kə,lanji'ostəmee) fistulization of a bile duct.

cholangiotomy (kə,lanji'otəmee) incision into a bile duct.

cholangitis (,kohlan'jietis) inflammation of a bile duct. adj. **cholangitic**.

cholanopoiesis (,kohlənohpoy'eesis) the synthesis of bile acids or of their conjugates and salts by the liver.

cholanopoietic (,kohlənohpoy'etik) 1. promoting cholanopoiesis. 2. an agent that promotes cholanopoiesis.

cholate ('kohlayt) a salt or ester of cholic acid.

chole- word element. [Gr.] *bile*.

Cholebrin ('kolebrin) trademark for iocetamic acid (an oral cholecystographic contrast medium).

cholecalciferol (,kohlikal'sifə·rol) vitamin D_3, an oil-soluble antirachitic vitamin (see also VITAMIN D).

cholecystagogue (,kohli'sistəgog) an agent that promotes evacuation of the gallbladder.

cholecystalgia (,kohlisi'stalji·ə) biliary colic.

cholecystectasia (,kohli,sistek'tayzi·ə) distention of the gallbladder.

cholecystectomy (,kohlisi'stektəmee) excision of the gallbladder (see also surgery of the GALLBLADDER and CHOLECYSTITIS).

cholecystenterostomy (,kohli,sistentə'rostəmee) formation of a new communication between the gallbladder and the intestine.

cholecystic (,kohli'sistik) pertaining to the gallbladder.

cholecystitis (,kohlisi'stietis) inflammation of the GALLBLADDER, acute or chronic.

ACUTE CHOLECYSTITIS. The most frequent cause of acute cholecystitis is GALLSTONES. Other causes include typhoid fever and a malignant tumour obstructing the biliary tract. The inflammation may be secondary to a systemic staphylococcal or streptococcal infection.

The symptoms of a mild inflammation may be very slight and include indigestion, moderate pain and tenderness in the upper right quadrant of the abdomen that is usually aggravated by deep breathing, malaise, and a low-grade fever. When gallstones or other disorders cause complete obstruction of the bile ducts, the symptoms are much more extreme. The pain becomes unbearable, the temperature may rise to 40 °C (104 °F), and there is nausea and vomiting.

Treatment of acute cholecystitis may entail either cholecystectomy or cholecystostomy. In some cases the surgery may be postponed until the attack subsides, the initial treatment consisting of administration of antibiotics and parenteral fluids and, after a period of no oral intake, administration of a special gallbladder diet.

CHRONIC CHOLECYSTITIS. Chronic cholecystitis progresses more slowly than acute cholecystitis, but it also is usually the result of gallstones or other conditions that lead to obstruction of the bile ducts and impaired gallbladder function. It is the most common disorder of the gallbladder.

The characteristic symptom of chronic cholecystitis is indigestion manifested by discomfort after eating, with flatulence and nausea. If the meal has been larger than usual, or high in fat content, the symptoms are more pronounced and there is eructation (belching) and regurgitation. There may also be vomiting and some pain in the upper right quadrant of the abdomen. It is not unusual for patients to suffer repeated episodes before seeking medical attention. Neglect of the situation may lead to permanent damage to the gallbladder and liver.

Diagnosis of cholecystitis is aided by the use of CHOLECYSTOGRAPHY, radiological examination after administration of a radiopaque contrast medium that is concentrated by the gallbladder.

The preferred treatment of chronic cholecystitis with gallstones is cholecystectomy. If surgery is contraindicated for some reason, then the symptoms may be controlled to some extent by low-fat diet, restriction of alcohol intake and spacing of meals so that large amounts of food are avoided and there is not a long interval between meals.

emphysematous c. that due to gas-producing organisms, marked by gas in the gallbladder lumen, often infiltrating into the gallbladder wall and surrounding tissues.

cholecystoduodenostomy (,kohli,sistoh,dyooədi'nostəmee) surgical anastomosis of the gallbladder and the duodenum.

cholecystogastrostomy (,kohli,sistohga'strostəmee) surgical anastomosis between the gallbladder and stomach.

cholecystogram (,kohli'sistə,gram) a radiograph of the gallbladder.

cholecystography (,kohlisi'stogrəfee) radiology of the gallbladder, using a radiopaque contrast medium taken orally. adj. **cholecystographic.**

The purpose of the examination is to determine the ability of the gallbladder to fill, concentrate bile and empty and to demonstrate radiolucent gallstones not demonstrated on the plain radiograph of the abdomen. The examination is unlikely to be successful when the serum bilirubin is greater than 34 μmol per litre.

Overlying bowel gas and faeces may obscure the gallbladder, so a laxative is prescribed for 2 days prior to the procedure. On the evening before the examination, the patient eats a fatty meal to empty the gallbladder and allow better filling with contrast medium. The cholecystographic agent is taken 14 hours prior to the patient's appointment. Food is forbidden until the examination is completed, though water is encouraged. On the morning of the examination, radiographs are taken of the gallbladder. The ability of the gallbladder to empty is studied by taking further films after a fatty meal.

cholecystojejunostomy (ˌkohliˌsistohjejuh'nostəmee) surgical anastomosis of the gallbladder and jejunum.

cholecystokinin (ˌkohliˌsistoh'kienin) a polypeptide hormone secreted in the small intestine, which stimulates gallbladder contraction and secretion of pancreatic enzymes.

cholecystolithiasis (ˌkohliˌsistohli'thieəsis) cholelithiasis.

cholecystopexy (ˌkohli'sistohˌpeksee) surgical suspension or fixation of the gallbladder.

cholecystorrhaphy (ˌkohlisi'sto·rəfee) suture or repair of the gallbladder.

cholecystostomy (ˌkohlisi'stostəmee) the creation of an opening into the gallbladder for drainage.

cholecystotomy (ˌkohlisi'stotəmee) incision of the gallbladder.

choledochal (ˌkohli'dohk'l) pertaining to the common bile duct.

choledochectomy (ˌkohlidoh'kektəmee) excision of part of the common bile duct.

choledochitis (ˌkohlidoh'kietis) inflammation of the common bile duct.

choledocho- word element. [Gr.] *common bile duct*.

choledochoduodenostomy (ˌkohliˌdohkohˌdyooədi'nostəmee) surgical anastomosis of the common bile duct to the duodenum.

choledochoenterostomy (ˌkohliˌdohkohˌentə'rostəmee) surgical anastomosis of the common bile duct to the intestine.

choledochogastrostomy (ˌkohliˌdohkohga'strostəmee) surgical anastomosis of the common bile duct to the stomach.

choledochogram (ˌkohli'dohkohgram) cholangiogram.

choledochojejunostomy (ˌkohliˌdohkohjejuh'nostəmee) surgical anastomosis of the common bile duct to the jejunum.

choledocholithiasis (ˌkohliˌdohkohli'thieəsis) calculi in the common bile duct.

choledocholithotomy (ˌkohliˌdohkohli'thotəmee) incision into the common bile duct for removal of stone.

choledochoplasty (ˌkohli'dohkohˌplastee) plastic surgery of the common bile duct.

choledochorrhaphy (ˌkohlidoh'ko·rəfee) suture or repair of an incision into the common bile duct.

choledochoscope (ˌkohlee'dohkohskohp) an endoscope used to examine the interior of the common bile duct.

choledochoscopy (ˌkohleedoh'koskəpee) the examination of the common bile duct using a choledochoscope.

choledochostomy (ˌkohlidoh'kostəmee) creation of an opening into the common bile duct for drainage.

choledochotomy (ˌkohlidoh'kotəmee) incision into the common bile duct.

choledochus (kohlee'dohkəs) the common bile duct.

Choledyl (koh'leedil) trademark for a preparation of choline theophyllinate, a bronchodilator.

choleic (koh'lee·ik) pertaining to the bile.

cholelith ('kohliˌlith) gallstone.

cholelithiasis (ˌkohlili'thieəsis) the presence or formation of GALLSTONES. adj. **cholelithic**.

cholelithotomy (ˌkohlili'thotəmee) incision of the biliary tract for the removal of gallstones.

cholelithotripsy, cholelithotrity (ˌkohli'lithohˌtripsee; ˌkohlili'thotritee) crushing of a gallstone.

cholemesis (koh'leməsis) vomiting of bile.

choleperitoneum (ˌkohliˌperitə'neeəm) the presence of bile in the peritoneum.

cholepoiesis (ˌkohlipoy'eesis) the formation of bile in the liver. adj. **cholepoietic**.

cholera ('kolə·rə) an acute,notifiable, infectious enteritis endemic and epidemic in Asia, and, within the past twenty years, also in Africa. It is caused by *Vibrio cholerae*, and is marked by frequent watery diarrhoea and occasional vomiting, with, in severe cases, extreme fluid and electrolyte depletion, and by muscle cramps and prostration.

INCIDENCE. Modern methods of sanitation have all but eliminated cholera epidemics in Europe and the United States, but they are still a danger in many other parts of the world, e.g., in the tropics, and particularly in India. Travellers to areas where cholera is endemic should protect themselves by vaccination, though this only provides partial immunity. The local drinking water should be boiled and uncooked foods avoided. Food should be protected from flies, and fruits and vegetables peeled and the rinds discarded.

TRANSMISSION. *Vibrio cholerae*, a spiral microorganism, is carried in the cholera patient's faeces, and vomitus, and transmitted to others in contaminated water or food.

SYMPTOMS. Symptoms begin to appear at any time from a few hours to 5 days after contact; the usual incubation period is 3 days. When a severe case of the disease is at its peak, diarrhoea, and sometimes vomiting, occur with such frequency and abundance that dehydration results very rapidly. The skin is cyanotic and shrivelled, the eyes are sunken and the voice is feeble. There may be painful muscular cramps throughout the body.

TREATMENT. Because alkaline substances are lost in the vomitus and faeces, ACIDOSIS and HYPOKALAEMIA, as well as dehydration, must be combated. The fluids and electrolytes are replaced where necessary by intravenous infusions.

PATIENT CARE. Measures must be taken to maintain normal body temperature because of the loss of body heat, which often causes the body temperature to drop dangerously low. Antiemetic drugs are seldom indicated.

Patients suffering from cholera (and proved carriers of the disease) should be isolated. The vomitus and faeces of the patient must be promptly and thoroughly disinfected. Eating utensils, dishes, and all other contaminated articles must be disinfected or burned. See also COMMUNICABLE DISEASE and ISOLATION TECHNIQUE.

pancreatic c. a condition marked by profuse watery diarrhoea, hypokalaemia, and usually achlorhydria, and due to an islet-cell tumour (other than beta cell) of the pancreas.

choleragen ('kolə·rəˌjen) the exotoxin produced by the cholera vibrio, which is thought to stimulate electrolyte and water secretion into the small intestine and to block the absorption of sodium.

choleraic (ˌkolə'rayik) of or pertaining to cholera, or of the nature of cholera.

choleresis (ˌkohlə'reesis) the secretion of bile by the liver.

choleretic (ˌkohlə'retik) 1. stimulating bile production by the liver. 2. an agent that stimulates bile production by the liver.

choleria (koh'leri·ə) an irritable or hostile temperament.

choleriform (ko'leriˌfawm) resembling cholera.

cholerine ('kolə·reen) 1. the earliest stage of cholera. 2. a relatively mild form of cholera.

choleroid ('koləˌroyd) resembling cholera.

cholestasis (ˌkohli'staysis) stoppage or suppression of bile flow, due to factors within the liver (intrahepatic cholestasis) or outside the liver (extrahepatic cholestasis). adj. **cholestatic.**

cholesteatoma (ˌkohliˌsteeə'tohmə) a cystlike mass with a lining of stratified squamous epithelium, filled with desquamating debris frequently including cholesterol, which occurs in the meninges, central nervous system, and bones of the skull, but most commonly in the middle ear and mastoid region.

cholesteatosis (ˌkohliˌsteeə'tohsis) fatty degeneration due to cholesterol esters.

cholesteraemia (kəˌlestə'reemi·ə) hypercholesterolaemia.

cholesterol (kə'lestəˌrol) a steroid alcohol found in animal fats and oils, bile, blood, brain tissue, milk, egg yolk, myelin sheaths of nerve fibres, liver, kidneys, and adrenal glands. It is a precursor of bile acids and steroid hormones, and it occurs in the most common type of gallstone, in atheroma of the arteries, in various cysts, and in carcinomatous tissue. Most of the body's cholesterol is synthesized, but some is obtained in the diet.

The role that cholesterol plays in the formation of atherosclerotic plaques in the coronary arteries has been the subject of dispute for several decades. High levels of *total* serum cholesterol have repeatedly been shown to be associated with a high risk for coronary artery disease and myocardial infarction. Further research has drawn a distinction between high-density lipoprotein (HDL) and low-density lipoprotein (LDL), two fractions of the serum lipoproteins, the form in which lipids are transported in the blood. It is now believed that the *balance* between HDL and LDL is more significant than the *total* concentration of cholesterol in the blood. The risk of coronary heart disease increases as LDL increases and HDL decreases.

Because HDL promotes the removal of excess cholesterol from the cells and its excretion from the body, it is thought to be beneficial rather than harmful. In contrast, LDL picks up cholesterol from ingested fats and from cells that synthesize it in the body and delivers it to blood vessels and muscles, where it is deposited in the cells. The concentration of cholesterol in cells within the linings of the arteries contributes to the build-up of atherosclerotic plaques. See also ATHEROSCLEROSIS and LIPOPROTEIN.

The question of whether or not the dietary intake of fats affects the pattern of HDL and LDL cholesterol levels has not yet been answered to everyone's satisfaction. All experts do agree, however, that those persons who are at high risk for heart disease, already have a heart condition or are obese would do well to limit the amount of fats and cholesterol in the foods they eat.

BLOOD CHOLESTEROL. Laboratory testing of cholesterol in the blood is often used as a preliminary test for a disorder of blood lipids. Although the normal values for total blood cholestrol vary according to age, diet and nationality, levels above 6.5 mmol/l indicate a need for further testing of the triglycerides.

Increased levels of cholesterol in the blood are found in cardiovascular disease and atherosclerosis, obstructive jaundice, hypothyroidism, nephrotic syndrome, and uncontrolled diabetes mellitus. Cholesterol exists in both a free and esterified form; the ratio of free to esterified cholesterol is significant in the diagnosis of certain diseases. For example, there is a markedly abnormal ratio of these two forms of cholesterol in hepatic biliary disease, infectious diseases, and extreme cholesterolaemia. Decreased levels of cholesterol in the blood are noted when there is malabsorption of cholestrol from the intestinal tract, as in pernicious anaemia, haemolytic jaundice, hyperthyroidism, and terminal cancer.

cholesterolaemia (kəˌlestə·ro'leemi·ə) hypercholesterolaemia.

cholesterolosis (kəˌlestə·ro'lohsis) focal collections of cholesterol-laden macrophages within the papillary fronds of the mucosa of the gallbladder.

cholesteroluria (kəˌlestə·ro'lyooə·ri·ə) the presence of cholesterol in the urine.

cholesterosis (kəˌlestə'rohsis) a condition in which cholesterol is deposited in tissues in abnormal amounts.

cholestyramine resin (ˌkohli'stierəmeen) a synthetic, strongly basic anion-exchange resin that chelates bile salts in the intestine, thus preventing their reabsorption; used in the symptomatic relief of pruritus associated with bile stasis.

choletherapy (ˌkohli'therəpee) treatment by administration of bile salts.

choleuria (ˌkohli'yooə·ri·ə) choluria.

cholic acid ('kohlik) an acid formed in the liver from cholesterol that plays, with other bile acids, an important role in digestion.

choline ('kohleen) a quaternary amine which occurs in the phospholipid phosphatidylcholine and the neurotransmitter acetylcholine, and is an important methyl donor in intermediary metabolism. Choline is a lipotrophic agent, a substance that decreases liver fat content by increasing phospholipid turnover. It was formerly considered to be a B vitamin and was used to treat fatty degeneration of the liver.

c. acetylase, c. acetyltransferase an enzyme that brings about the synthesis of acetylcholine.

c. magnesium trisalicylate a combination of choline salicylate and magnesium salicylate used as an antiarthritic.

c. salicylate the choline salt of salicylic acid, which has analgesic, antipyretic, and anti-inflammatory properties.

cholinergic (ˌkohli'nərjik) 1. parasympathomimetic; activated or transmitted by acetylcholine; said of nerve fibres that liberate acetylcholine at a synapse when a nerve impulse passes, i.e., the parasympathetic fibres. 2. an agent that resembles acetylcholine or simulates its action.

c. receptors receptor sites on effector organs or at nerve synapses that are stimulated by acetylcholine released by the nerve terminal. There are two types: muscarinic receptors, present primarily on autonomic effector cells, and nicotinic receptors, present primarily on autonomic ganglion cells and on the motor end-plates of skeletal muscle.

cholinesterase (ˌkohli'nestəˌrayz) an enzyme that splits acetylcholine into acetic acid and choline. Called also *acetylcholinesterase.*

This enzyme is present throughout the body, but is particularly important at the neuromuscular junction, where the nerve fibres terminate. Acetylcholine is released when a nerve impulse reaches a neuromuscular junction. It diffuses across the synaptic cleft and binds to cholinergic receptors on the muscle fibres, causing them to contract. Cholinesterase splits acetylcholine into its components, thus stopping stimulation of the muscle fibres. The end products of the metabolism of acetylcholine are taken up by nerve fibres and resynthesized into acetylcholine.

The drugs neostigmine, physostigmine, and pyridostigmine inhibit cholinesterase. These drugs are used to treat MYASTHENIA GRAVIS, a disease in which the cholinergic receptors are attacked by autoantibodies. The drug extends the effect of acetylcholine on the muscle fibre.

cholinoceptive (ˌkohlinoh'septiv) pertaining to the sites on effector organs that are acted upon by cholinergic transmitters.
cholinoceptor (ˌkohlinoh'septə) cholinergic receptor.
cholinomimetic (ˌkohlinohmi'metik) having an action similar to that of acetylcholine; parasympathomimetic.
cholohaemothorax (ˌkohlohˌheemə'thor·raks) the presence of bile and blood in the thorax.
chololithiasis (ˌkohlohli'thieəsis) cholelithiasis.
cholothorax (ˌkohloh'thor·raks) cholohaemothorax.
Choloxin (koh'loksin) trademark for a preparation of dextrothyroxine, an antihyperlipoproteinaemic agent reserved for patients unresponsive to other agents.
choluria (koh'lyooə·ri·ə) the presence of bile in the urine; discoloration of the urine with bile pigments. adj. **choluric.**
chondr(o)- word element. [Gr.] *cartilage.*
chondral ('kondrəl) pertaining to cartilage.
chondralgia (kon'dralji·ə) pain in a cartilage.
chondrectomy (kon'drektəmee) excision of a cartilage.
chondrification (ˌkondrifi'kayshən) conversion into cartilage.
chondrio- word element. [Gr.] *cartilage, granule.*
chondritis (kon'drietis) inflammation of a cartilage.
chondroadenoma (ˌkondrohˌadə'nohmə) adenochondroma.
chondroblast ('kondrohˌblast) an immature cartilage-producing cell.
chondroblastoma (ˌkondrohbla'stohmə) a benign tumour arising from young chondroblasts in the epiphysis of a bone.
chondrocalcinosis (ˌkondrohˌkalsi'nohsis) deposition of calcium salts in the cartilage of joints. When accompanied by attacks of goutlike symptoms, it is called pseudogout.
chondroclast ('kondrohˌklast) a giant cell believed to be concerned in absorption of cartilage.
chondrocostal (ˌkondroh'kost'l) pertaining to the ribs and costal cartilages.
chondrocranium (ˌkondroh'krayni·əm) the cartilaginous cranial structure of the embryo from the seventh week to the middle of the third month, when it is a unified cartilaginous mass without clear boundaries indicating the limits of future bones.
chondrocyte ('kondrohˌsiet) a mature cartilage cell embedded in a lacuna within the cartilage matrix. adj. **chondrocytic.**
chondrodermatitis (ˌkondrohˌdərmə'tietis) an inflammatory process involving cartilage and skin; used almost exclusively to mean chondrodermatitis nodularis chronica helicis, a condition marked by a painful nodule on the helix of the ear.
chondrodynia (ˌkondroh'dini·ə) pain in a cartilage.
chondrodysplasia (ˌkondrohdis'playzi·ə) enchondromatosis.
chondrodystrophia, chondrodystrophy (ˌkondrohdis'trohfi·a; ˌkondroh'distrəfee) a disorder of cartilage formation.
chondroepiphysitis (ˌkondrohˌepifi'zietis) inflammation of the epiphyseal cartilages.
chondrofibroma (ˌkondrohfie'brohmə) a fibroma with cartilaginous elements.
chondrogenesis (ˌkondroh'jenəsis) formation of cartilage.
chondrogenic (ˌkondroh'jenik) giving rise to or forming cartilage.
chondroid ('kondroyd) resembling cartilage.
chondroitin sulphate (kon'droh·itin) a glycosaminoglycan (mucopolysaccharide) which is widespread in connective tissue, particularly cartilage, and in the cornea.
chondrolipoma (ˌkondrohli'pohmə) a tumour containing cartilaginous and fatty tissue.
chondroma (kon'drohmə) a tumour or tumour-like growth of cartilage cells. It may remain in the interior or substance of a cartilage or bone (true chondroma, or enchondroma), or may develop on the surface of a cartilage and project under the periosteum of a bone (ecchondroma, or ecchondrosis).
chondromalacia (ˌkondrohmə'layshi·ə) literally softening of cartilage.
c. patellae chondromalacia affecting the patella, causing pain behind one or both knees.
chondromatosis (ˌkondrohmə'tohsis) formation of multiple chondromas.
synovial c. a rare condition in which cartilage is formed in the synovial membrane of joints, tendon sheaths, or bursae, sometimes becoming detached and producing a number of loose bodies.
chondromere ('kondrohˌmiə) a cartilaginous vertebra of the fetal vertebral column.
chondrometaplasia (ˌkondrohˌmetə'playzi·ə) a condition characterized by metaplastic activity of the chondroblasts.
chondromyoma (ˌkondrohmie'ohmə) a benign tumour with myomatous and cartilaginous elements.
chondromyxoma (ˌkondrohmik'sohmə) myxoma with cartilaginous elements.
chondromyxosarcoma (ˌkondrohˌmiksohsah'kohmə) a sarcoma containing cartilaginous and mucous tissue.
chondro-osseous (ˌkondroh'osi·əs) composed of cartilage and bone.
chondro-osteodystrophy (ˌkondrohˌostioh'distrəfee) Morquio's disease.
chondropathy (kon'dropəthee) any disease of cartilage.
chondroplasia (ˌkondroh'playzi·ə) the formation of cartilage by specialized cells (chondrocytes).
chondroplast ('kondrohˌplast) chondroblast.
chondroplasty ('kondrohˌplastee) plastic repair of cartilage.
chondroporosis (ˌkondrohpor'rohsis) the formation of sinuses or spaces in cartilage.
chondrosarcoma (ˌkondrohsah'kohmə) a malignant tumour derived from cartilage cells or their precursors.
chondrosis (kon'drohsis) the formation of cartilage.
chondrosteoma (ˌkondrosti'ohmə) osteochondroma.
chondrosternal (ˌkondroh'stərnəl) pertaining to the costal cartilages and sternum.
chondrosternoplasty (ˌkondroh'stərnohˌplastee) surgical correction of pectus excavatum (funnel chest).
chondrotomy (kon'drotəmee) the dissection or the surgical divison of cartilage.
chondroxiphoid (ˌkondroh'zifoyd) pertaining to the xiphoid process.
chord (kawd) cord.
chorda ('kawdə) pl. *chordae* [L.] a cord or sinew. adj. **chordal.**
c. magna Achilles tendon.
chordae tendineae tendinous cords connecting the two atrioventricular valves to the appropriate papillary muscles in the heart ventricles.
c. tympani a nerve originating from the facial nerve, distributed to the submandibular, sublingual, and lingual glands and the anterior two-thirds of the tongue; it is a parasympathetic and special senory nerve.
c. umbilicalis umbilical cord.
c. vocalis vocal cord.
Chordata (kaw'dahtə) a phylum of the animal kingdom comprising all animals having a notochord during some developmental stage.
chordate ('kawdayt) 1. an animal of the Chordata. 2.

having a notochord.

chordee (kaw'dee) downward deflection of the penis, due to a congenital anomaly (hypospadias) or to urethral infection.

chorditis (kaw'dietis) inflammation of vocal or spermatic cords.

chordoma (kaw'dohmə) a malignant tumour arising from embryonic remains of the notochord.

chordotomy (kaw'dotəmee) cordotomy (2).

chorea (ko'reeə) the ceaseless occurrence of rapid, jerky involuntary movements. adj. **choreic.**

acute c. Sydenham's chorea.

chronic c. Huntington's chorea.

c. gravidarum Sydenham's chorea occurring in early pregnancy, with or without a previous history of rheumatic fever.

hereditary c., Huntington's c. a hereditary disease marked by chronic progressive chorea and mental deterioration (see also HUNTINGTON'S DISEASE).

Sydenham's c. an acute, usually self-limiting disorder, chiefly occurring between the ages of 5 and 15, or during pregnancy, closely linked with rheumatic fever, and marked by involuntary movements that gradually become severe, affecting all motor activities (see also SYDENHAM'S CHOREA).

choreiform (ko'ree·ifawm) resembling chorea.

choreoathetosis (ˌko·rioh,athi'tohsis) a condition characterized by choreic and athetoid movements. adj. **choreoathetoid.**

chorioadenoma (ˌko·rioh,adə'nohmə) adenoma of the chorion.

c. destruens a form of hydatidiform mole in which molar chorionic villi penetrate into the myometrium and may invade the parametrium. Hydropic villi may be transported to distant sites, most often the lungs, but they do not grow as metastases.

chorioallantois (ˌko·rioh·ə'lantoh·is) an extraembryonic structure formed by union of the chorion and allantois, which by means of vessels in the associated mesoderm serves in gas exchange; in many mammals, it forms the placenta. adj. **chorioallantoic.**

chorioamnionitis (ˌko·rioh,amnioh'nietis) inflammation of the fetal membranes.

chorioangioma (ˌko·rioh,anji'ohmə) a collection of fetal blood cells in WHARTON'S JELLY, forming a tumour on the placenta. It is of little clinical significance, but is rarely associated with HYDRAMNIOS.

choriocapillaris (ˌko·rioh,kapi'lair·ris) the capillary layer of the choroid, the lamina choriocapillaris.

choriocarcinoma (ˌko·rioh,kahsi'nohmə) a malignant tumour of trophoblastic cells which develops in about 3 per cent of hydatiform moles and is detected by raised levels of chorionic gonadotrophin in serum or urine and by radioimmunoassay. It is treated by cytotoxic chemotherapy (hysterectomy is a last resort).

chorioepithelioma (ˌko·rioh,epi,theeli'ohmə) choriocarcinoma.

choriogenesis (ˌko·rioh'jenəsis) the development of the chorion.

chorioid ('ko·ri,oyd) choroid.

chorioma (ˌko·ri'ohmə) any trophoblastic proliferation, benign or malignant.

choriomeningitis (ˌko·rioh,menin'jietis) cerebral meningitis with lymphocytic infiltration of the choroid plexus.

lymphocytic c. a form of viral meningitis.

chorion ('ko·rion, 'kor·ri·ən) the outermost of the fetal membranes. It is opaque and friable in nature, and may sometimes be retained following delivery. Together with the placenta, it is formed from the trophoblast when the chorion frondosum sheds its villi to become the chorion laeve (bald).

c. biopsy tissue removed from the gestational sac early in pregnancy so that chromosome and other inherited disorders can be identified. Because this can be done as early as 8 weeks gestation, termination (where necessary) can be undertaken before 12 weeks, which is not possible with amniocentesis.

c. frondosum the part of the chorion covered by villi in the early weeks of embryonic development before the placenta is formed.

c. laeve the nonvillous, membranous part of the trophoblast which develops into the chorion.

chorionic (ˌko·ri'onik) pertaining to the chorion.

c. gonadotropin a substance produced from the blastocyst, which stimulates the corpus luteum to produce oestrogen and progesterone as the pituitary gonadotrophins are decreasing, so ensuring the continuation of the pregnancy. The presence of the human chorionic gonadotrophin (HCG) in a woman's urine is diagnostic of pregnancy. See also PREGNANCY TESTS.

chorioretinal (ˌko·rioh'retinəl) pertaining to the choroid and retina.

chorioretinitis (ˌko·rioh,reti'nietis) inflammation of the choroid and retina.

chorioretinopathy (ˌko·rioh,reti'nopəthee) a noninflammatory process involving both the choroid and retina.

chorista (ko'ristə) defective development due to, or marked by, displacement of the primordium.

choristoma (ˌko·ri'stohmə) a mass of histologically normal tissue in an abnormal location.

choroid ('ko·royd) the middle, vascular coat of the eye, between the sclera and the retina. adj. **choroidal.** It contains an abundant supply of blood vessels and a large amount of brown pigment which serves to reduce reflection or diffusion of light when it falls on the retina. Adequate nutrition of the eye is dependent upon blood vessels in the choroid.

c. plexus vascular fringelike folds in the pia mater in the third, fourth, and lateral ventricles of the brain; concerned with formation of cerebrospinal fluid.

choroidea (ko'roydi·ə) choroid.

choroideremia (ko,roydə'reemi·ə) hereditary (X-linked) primary choroidal degeneration which, in males, eventually leads to blindness as degeneration of the retinal pigment epithelium progresses to complete atrophy; in females, it is nonprogressive and vision is usually normal.

choroiditis (ˌko·roy'dietis) inflammation of the choroid.

choroidocyclitis (ko,roydohsie'klietis) inflammation of the choroid and ciliary processes.

choroidoiritis (ko,roydoh·ie'rietis) inflammation of the choroid and iris.

choroidoretinitis (ko,roydoh,reti'nietis) inflammation of the choroid and retina.

Chotzen's syndrome ('chotzenz) a hereditary disorder, transmitted as an autosomal dominant trait, characterized by acrocephalosyndactyly in which the syndactyly is mild and by hypertelorism, ptosis, and sometimes mental handicap.

Christian–Weber disease (ˌkrischən'webə) nodular nonsuppurative panniculitis.

Christmas disease ('krisməs) a hereditary haemorrhagic diathesis clinically similar to haemophilia A (classic haemophilia) but due to deficiency of clotting factor IX; called also *haemophilia B.*

chrom(o)- word element. [Gr.] *colour.*

chromaesthesia (ˌkrohmis'theezi·ə) association of imaginary colour sensations with actual sensations of taste, hearing, or smell.

chromaffin (kroh'mafin) taking up and staining strongly with chromium salts; said of certain cells occurring in the adrenal glands and the carotid bodies, along with the sympathetic nerves, and in various organs.

chromaffinoma (kroh,mafi'nohmə) 1. any tumour containing predominantly chromaffin cells. 2. phaeochromocytoma.

chromat(o)- word element. [Gr.] *colour, chromatin.*

chromate ('krohmayt) any salt of chromic acid.

chromatelopsia (,krohmatə'lopsi·ə) imperfect perception of colours.

chromatic (kroh'matik) 1. pertaining to colour; stainable with dyes. 2. pertaining to chromatin.

chromatid ('krohmətid) either of two parallel filaments joined at the centromere which make up a chromosome, and which divide in cell division, each going to a different pole of the dividing cell and each becoming a chromosome of one of the two daughter cells.

chromatin ('krohmətin) the substance of the chromosomes, composed of DNA and basic proteins (histones), the material in the nucleus that stains with basic dyes.

sex c. Barr body; the persistent mass of the material of the inactivated X chromosome in cells of normal females.

chromatin-negative (,krohmətin'negətiv) lacking sex chromatin; characteristic of the nuclei of cells in a normal male.

chromatin-positive (,krohmətin'pozətiv) containing sex chromatin; characteristic of the nuclei of cells in a normal female.

chromatism ('krohmə,tizəm) 1. hallucinatory perception of colour. 2. abnormal pigmentation.

chromatogenous (,krohmə'tojənəs) producing colour or colouring matter.

chromatogram (kroh'matoh,gram) the record produced by chromatography.

chromatograph (kroh'matoh,grahf, -,graf) 1. to analyse by chromatography. 2. the apparatus used in chromatography.

chromatography (,krohmə'togrəfee) a technique for analysis of chemical substances. The term *chromatography* literally means colour writing, and denotes a method by which the substance to be analysed is poured into a vertical glass tube containing an adsorbent, the various components of the substance moving through the adsorbent at different rates, according to their degree of attraction to it, and producing bands of colour at different levels of the adsorption column. The term has been extended to include other methods utilizing the same principle, although no colours are produced in the column. adj. **chromatographic.**

The mobile phase of chromatography refers to the fluid that carries the mixture of substances in the sample through the adsorptive material. The stationary phase (or adsorbent) refers to the solid material that takes up the particles of the substance passing through it. Kaolin, alumina, silica, and activated charcoal have been used as adsorbing substances or stationary phases.

Classification of chromatographic techniques tends to be confusing because it may be based on the type of stationary phase, the nature of the adsorptive force, the nature of the mobile phase, or the method by which the mobile phase is introduced.

The technique is a valuable tool for the research biochemist and is readily adaptable to investigations conducted in the clinical laboratory. For example, chromatography is used to detect and identify in body fluids certain sugars and amino acids associated with inborn errors of metabolism.

adsorption c. that in which the stationary phase is an adsorbent.

column c. the technique in which the various solutes of a solution are allowed to travel down a column, the individual components being adsorbed by the stationary phase. The most strongly adsorbed component will remain near the top of the column; the other components will pass to a position further and further down the column, according to their affinity for the adsorbent. If the individual components are naturally coloured, they will form a series of coloured bands or zones.

Column chromatography has been employed to separate vitamins, steroids, hormones, and alkaloids and to determine the amount of these substances in samples of body fluids.

exclusion c. that in which the stationary phase is a gel having a closely controlled pore size. Molecules are separated based on molecular size and shape, smaller molecules being temporarily retained in the pores.

gas c. a type of automated chromatography in which the mobile phase is an inert gas. Volatile components of the sample are separated in the column and measured by a detector. The method has been applied in the clinical laboratory to separate and quantify steroids, barbiturates, and lipids.

gas–liquid c. gas chromatography in which the substances to be separated are moved by an inert gas along a tube filled with a finely divided inert solid coated with a nonvolatile oil; each component migrates at a rate determined by its solubility in oil and its vapour pressure.

gel-filtration c., gel-permeation c. exclusion chromatography.

ion-exchange c. that utilizing resins to which are coupled either cations or anions that will exchange with other cations or anions in the material passed through their meshwork.

molecular sieve c. exclusion chromatography.

paper c. a form of chromatography in which a sheet of blotting paper, usually filter paper, is substituted for the adsorption column. After separation of the components as a consequence of their different migratory velocities, they are stained to make the chromatogram visible. In the clinical laboratory, paper chromatography is employed to detect and identify sugars and amino acids.

partition c. a form of separation of solutes utilizing the partition of the solutes between two liquid phases, namely the original solvent and the film of solvent on the adsorption column.

thin-layer c. that in which the stationary phase is a thin layer of an adsorbent such as silica gel coated on a flat plate. It is otherwise similar to paper chromatography.

chromatolysis (,krohmə'tolisis) 1. the solution and disintegration of the chromatin of cell nuclei. 2. disintegration of the Nissl bodies of a neuron as a result of injury, fatigue, or exhaustion.

chromatometry (,krohmə'tomətree) the measurement of colour perception.

chromatophil (kroh'matəfil) a cell or structure that stains easily. adj. **chromatophilic.**

chromatophore (kroh'matə,for) any pigmentary cell or colour-producing plastid.

chromatopsia (,krohmə'topsi·ə) perversion of colour vision, in which objects are seen as abnormally coloured.

chromatoptometer (,krohmətop'tomitə) a device for measuring colour perception.

chromatoptometry (,krohmətop'tomətree) measurement of colour perception.

chromaturia (,krohmə'tyooə·ri·ə) abnormal coloration

of the urine.

chromhidrosis (ˌkrohmi'drohsis) secretion of coloured sweat.

chromic acid ('krohmik) 1. a dibasic acid, H_2CrO_4; its salts are called chromates. 2. chromium trioxide.

chromidium (kroh'midi·əm) pl. *chromidia;* a granule of extranuclear chromatin in the cytoplasm of a cell.

chromidrosis (ˌkrohmi'drohsis) chromhidrosis.

chromium ('krohmi·əm) a chemical element, atomic number 24, atomic weight 51.996, symbol Cr. See table of elements in Appendix 2.

c.-51 a radioisotope of chromium having a half-life of 27.8 days; used to label red blood cells to determine red cell volume and red cell survival time. Symbol ^{51}Cr.

chromoblast ('krohmohˌblast) an embryonic cell that develops into a pigment cell.

chromoblastomycosis (ˌkrohmohˌblastohmie'kohsis) chromomycosis.

chromoclastogenic (ˌkrohmohˌklastoh'jenik) giving rise to or inducing chromosomal disruption or damage.

chromocystoscopy (ˌkrohmohsi'stoskəpee) cystoscopy of the ureteral orifices after oral administration of a dye which is excreted in the urine.

chromocyte ('krohmohˌsiet) any coloured cell or pigmented corpuscle.

chromodacryorrhoea (ˌkrohmohˌdakri·ə'reeə) the shedding of bloody tears.

chromogen ('krohməˌjen) any substance giving rise to a colouring matter.

chromogenesis (ˌkrohmoh'jenəsis) the formation of colour or pigment.

chromogenic (ˌkrohmoh'jenik) producing colour or pigment.

chromolysis (kroh'molisis) chromatolysis.

chromomere ('krohməˌmiə) 1. any of the beadlike granules occurring in series along a chromonema. 2. granulomere.

chromomycosis (ˌkrohmohmie'kohsis) a chronic fungal infection of the skin, producing wartlike nodules or papillomas that may ulcerate. Called also *chromoblastomycosis*.

chromonema (ˌkrohmoh'neemə) pl. *chromonemata* [Gr.] the coiled central thread of a chromatid along which lie the chromomeres. adj. **chromonemal.**

chromophil ('krohmohˌfil) any easily stainable structure. adj. **chromophilic.**

chromophobe ('krohmohˌfohb) any cell, structure, or tissue that does not stain readily; applied especially to the chromophobe cells of the anterior lobe of the pituitary gland.

chromophobia (ˌkrohmoh'fohbi·ə) the quality of staining poorly with dyes. adj. **chromophobic.**

chromophore ('krohməˌfor) any chemical group whose presence gives a decided colour to a compound and which unites with certain other groups (auxochromes) to form dyes; called also *colour radical*.

chromophoric (ˌkrohmoh'for·rik) 1. bearing colour. 2. pertaining to a chromophore.

chromophose ('krohmohˌfohz) a subjective sensation of colour.

chromopsia (kroh'mopsi·ə) chromatopsia.

chromoscopy (kroh'moskəpee) the diagnosis of renal function by the colour of urine following the administration of dyes.

gastric c. diagnosis of gastric function by the colour of the gastric contents: a test for achylia gastrica.

chromosome ('krohməˌsohm) in animal cells, a structure in the nucleus, containing a linear thread of DEOXYRIBONUCLEIC ACID (DNA), which transmits genetic information and is associated with RIBONUCLEIC ACID and histones. adj. **chromosomal.** During cell division the material composing the chromosome is compactly coiled, making it visible with appropriate staining and permitting its movement in the cell with minimal entanglement. Each organism of a species is normally characterized by the same number of chromosomes in its somatic cells, 46 being the number normally present in man—22 pairs of autosomes, and the two sex chromosomes (XX or XY), which determine the sex of the organism. (See also HEREDITY.) In bacterial genetics, a closed circle of double-stranded DNA which contains the genetic material of the cell and is attached to the cell membrane; the bulk of this material forms a compact bacterial nucleus.

CHROMOSOME ANALYSIS. Fetal cells obtained by AMNIOCENTESIS or lymphocytes from a blood sample can be cultured in the laboratory until they divide. Cell division is arrested in mid-metaphase by the drug colchicine. The chromosomes can be stained by one of several techniques that produce a distinct pattern of light and dark bands along the chromosomes, and each chromosome can be recognized by its size and banding pattern. The chromosomal characteristics of an individual are referred to as his *karyotype*. This also refers to a photomicrograph of a cell nucleus that is cut apart and rearranged so that the individual chromosomes are in order and labelled. The autosomes are numbered 1–22, roughly in order of decreasing length. The sex chromosomes are labelled X and Y. Karyotyping is useful in determining the presence of chromosome defects.

Before the chromosomes could be precisely identified they were placed in seven groups: A (chromosomes 1–3), B (4–5), C (6–12 and X), D (13–15), E (16–18), F (19–20), and G (21–22 and Y).

CHROMOSOMAL ABNORMALITIES. The prevalence of chromosomal disorders cannot be fully and accurately determined because many of these disorders do not permit full embryonic and fetal development and therefore end in spontaneous abortion. About one in every 100 newborn infants does, however, have a gross demonstrable chromosomal abnormality. A large majority of cytogenetic abnormalities can be identified by cytogenetic analysis either before birth, by means of AMNIOCENTESIS, or after birth.

Cytogenetic disorders with visible chromosomal abnormalities are evidenced by either an abnormal number of chromosomes or some alteration in the structure of one or more chromosomes. In the language of the geneticist, *trisomy* refers to the presence of an additional chromosome that is homologous with one of the existing pairs so that that particular chromosome is present in triplicate. An example of this type of disorder is a form of Down's syndrome (*trisomy 21*). Another example is Patau's syndrome (*trisomy 13*) which produces severe anatomical malformations and profound mental handicap.

The term *monosomy* refers to the absence of one of a pair of homologous chromosomes. Monosomy involving an autosome usually results in the loss of too much genetic information to permit sufficient fetal development for a live birth. Either trisomy or monosomy involving the sex chromosomes yields relatively mild abnormalities.

A condition known as *mosaicism* results from an error in the distribution of chromosomes between daughter cells during an early embryonic cell division, producing two and sometimes three populations of cells with different chromosome numbers in the same individual. Mosaicism involving the sex chromosomes is not uncommon.

Other abnormal structural changes in the chromosome are consequences of some kind of chromosomal breakage, with either the loss or rearrangement of genetic material. *Translocation* involves the transfer of a segment of one chromosome to another. *Inversion* refers to a change in the sequence of genes along the chromosome, which occurs when there are two breaks in a chromosome and the segment between the breaks is reversed and reattached to the wrong ends. *Deletion* occurs when a portion of a chromosome is lost. An example of this type of chromosomal abnormality is cri du chat syndrome, a deletion in the short arm of chromosome 5, (5p-), marked by mental handicap and, in about one-quarter of the cases, congenital heart defects. When deletion occurs at both ends of the chromosome, the two damaged ends can unite to form a circle and the rearrangement produces a *ring chromosome. Isochromosomes* form when the centromere divides along the transverse plane rather than the normal long axis of the chromosome so that both arms are identical. All of the previously described structural abnormalities can affect both autosomal and sex chromosomes.

The causes of chromosomal errors are not completely understood. In some conditions such as Down's syndrome, late maternal age seems to be a factor. Other factors may include the predisposition of chromosomes to nondisjunction (failure to separate during meiosis), exposure to radiation, and viruses.

homologous c's the chromosomes of a matching pair in the diploid complement that contain alleles of specific genes.

Ph[1] c., Philadelphia c. an abnormality of chromosome 22, characterized by shortening of its long arms, seen in the marrow cells of most patients with chronic myelogenous leukaemia.

ring c. a chromosome in which both ends have been lost (deletion) and the two broken ends have reunited to form a ring-shaped figure.

sex c's the chromosomes responsible for determination of the sex of the individual that develops from a zygote, in mammals constituting an unequal pair, the X and the Y chromosome.

somatic c. autosome.

X c. the female sex chromosome, being carried by half the male gametes and all female gametes; female diploid cells have two X chromosomes.

Y c. the male sex chromosome, being carried by half the male gametes and none of the female gametes; male diploid cells have an X and a Y chromosome.

chronaxie, chronaxy ('krohnaksee, kro'naksee) the minimum time for which an electric current must flow at a voltage twice the rheobase to cause a muscle to contract.

chronic ('kronik) persisting for a long time; applied to a morbid state, designating one showing little change or extremely slow progression over a long period.

c. obstructive airways disease (COAD) a functional category designating a chronic condition of persistent obstruction of bronchial air flow. Called also *chronic obstructive lung disease* (*COLD*), *chronic obstructive pulmonary disease* (*COPD*) and *diffuse obstructive lung disease* (*DOLD*). ASTHMA, chronic BRONCHITIS, and chronic pulmonary EMPHYSEMA are the diseases mainly associated with this condition; others are BRONCHIECTASIS, pulmonary TUBERCULOSIS, and SILICOSIS.

COAD is the most significant chronic pulmonary disorder in Britain in regard to morbidity rate. Chronic bronchitis and emphysema have traditionally been regarded as British diseases and together represent the largest single cause of loss of work (with about 30 million days lost each year). Exact figures for prevalence are difficult to determine because of problems of definition.

The incidence of COAD is increasing and, although the specific cause is not known, factors contributing to its development and affecting its degree of severity have been identified. Of these known factors heavy cigarette smoking appears to be most important. There is evidence that smoking increases the levels of certain body chemicals that destroy *elastin*, a protein that gives resilience to lung tissue. Other factors are related to industrial pollution and occupational exposure to irritating inhalants, allergy, autoimmunity, genetic predisposition, and chronic infections.

Prevention of COAD is best accomplished through education of the public about the hazards of cigarette smoking and air pollution and the need for early detection and prompt treatment of respiratory disorders that could become chronic in nature.

SYMPTOMS. COAD is an insidious disease that can develop into advanced lung damage almost before its victim is aware that his condition is serious. The early symptoms are shortness of breath upon exertion, a mild cough, sometimes called 'smoker's cough', which occurs most often in the morning, and excessive tiredness that follows even minimal physical effort. Prompt treatment of these symptoms can forestall the more serious effects of extensive lung damage; however, the destruction of lung tissue and bronchial mucosa damage that has already occurred by the time these symptoms appear is irreversible.

As COAD progresses, the symptoms of dyspnoea, weakness, and cough become more severe. The patient has difficulty expelling air from his lungs and his cough becomes more productive of thick, tenacious sputum. He looks anxious and drawn and may speak in short, hesitant sentences. Symptoms related to disturbances of the respiratory and circulatory systems and ACID–BASE BALANCE may appear as these complications develop.

COMPLICATIONS. Destructive involvement of respiratory structures and the resultant impairment of circulatory function can produce serious life-threatening complications in patients with COAD. Among these are acute respiratory failure, disturbance in the acid–base balance (which can occur either as uncompensated respiratory ACIDOSIS or metabolic ALKALOSIS), bronchopulmonary infections, COR PULMONALE (occurring as a result of increased resistance in the pulmonary circulation), and pulmonary EMBOLISM (especially if polycythaemia is severe). PATHOLOGY. In COAD there is an irreversible change in the structure and function of the bronchi and bronchioles, and in the lungs and the blood vessels that serve them. The bronchial mucosa becomes swollen, cilia are destroyed, and the mucus-producing glands hypertrophy. These changes bring about difficulty in removal of mucus and increased obstruction of the air passages.

The walls of the alveoli break down, resulting in large, nonfunctioning air spaces and enlargement of the surviving alveoli. The destruction of alveoli is accompanied by a loss of the capillaries serving them, thus diminishing the diffusion of gases and exchange of carbon dioxide and oxygen. Loss of the capillary bed also interferes with pulmonary circulation, which in turn increases the work load of the right side of the heart. The normal elasticity of the lungs, which allows for their expansion during inspiration and return to normal volume during expiration, is severely impaired.

DIAGNOSIS. A history of heavy cigarette smoking over a period of years or long-term exposure to air pollutants is almost invariably found in patients with COAD. In addition the patient may have suffered from a chronic allergy manifested by respiratory symptoms, a chronic respiratory infection, or a congenital lung defect.

The triad of dyspnoea, cough, and excessive tiredness is strongly indicative of COAD. A more definitive diagnosis is made through laboratory studies and pulmonary function tests.

Physical examination using palpation, percussion, and auscultation usually reveals symptoms of pathological changes that are confirmed by radiography films and fluoroscopy. COAD is demonstrated by an *obstructive pattern* seen in the results of PULMONARY FUNCTION TESTS. The residual volume (air remaining in the lungs at the end of maximal expiration) is likely to be increased, as is the $FEV_{1.0}$ (forced expiratory volume—one second) and the ratio of $FEV_{1.0}$ to FVC (forced vital capacity).

BLOOD GAS ANALYSIS is helpful in evaluating effectiveness of blood gas exchange across alveolar walls. In severe COAD, the P_aco_2 level is high while the P_ao_2 and the Sao_2 is low.

TREATMENT AND PATIENT CARE. In general, the treatment of COAD is concerned with restoring and maintaining existing lung function, relieving symptoms, and planning a programme of rehabilitation tailored to accommodate the individual patient's physiological needs, physical stamina, vocational needs, life style, and personality.

Specific measures of patient care are concerned with (1) initial and periodic assessment of patient status, (2) maintenance of general health in so far as possible, (3) prevention and control of infection, (4) improvement of ventilation, and (5) patient education.

COAD is a chronic disease for which there is no cure. The nature of the disease demands an on-going programme of assessment and long-term care that is planned and revised as the patient's needs dictate. Whatever the patient care setting, the elements of care presented below are essential to the effective management of COAD.

Assessment. Patient assessment begins with the taking of the patient's history and performing physical examination and lung function tests at the time the diagnosis is established. These measures, along with blood gas analysis at rest and after exercise, provide a baseline for periodic evaluation of the patient's status to determine the progress of the disease and the effectiveness of treatment.

When patients are informed about the purpose of the tests they are more likely to participate in the planned regimen of care and to become motivated to continue carrying out their responsibilities in the management of their illness. Those who work with the patient should clarify for him the goals to be achieved and offer encouragement when he makes progress toward those goals. All members of the health care team must have an understanding of the disease, the meaning of various test values, and the purpose of each aspect of care.

Maintenance of Health. It is important to communicate to the patient the concept of good health, particularly in regard to his position on the health-illness continuum. He cannot be completely healthy again or restored to his former state of health, before the development of COAD. He can, however, hold his own against the disease for periods of time and even make progress toward a better state of health.

Adequate nutrition can be assured by careful planning of well-balanced meals, spacing them so that the stomach is not overloaded at any one time, perhaps as five small meals a day. If POSTURAL DRAINAGE or deep breathing exercises are a part of his daily routine, they should be scheduled for a time when the stomach is not full. Each time these procedures are done they should be followed by good oral hygiene measures to remove the unpleasant taste of sputum and thereby reduce anorexia and nausea.

Physical activity may be severely limited by COAD because of inadequate ventilation and decreased circulation. As with all other aspects of patient care, plans to increase exercise tolerance and promote physical activity should be designed according to the patient's cardiopulmonary status. Techniques that promote muscular relaxation and breathing control are the first step, followed by gradual increase in activity as the patient's progress and general physical condition permit.

Adequate rest is essential, but the well-known hazards of immobility must be avoided, especially in patients who are fearful that any physical activity may precipitate an exhausting episode of coughing and dyspnoea.

Prevention and Control of Infection. Acute respiratory infection can be fatal in patients with COAD. Chronic infections inflict further damage to the respiratory structures, lead to increased debilitation, and increase the likelihood of severe complications. Both acute and chronic infections produce increased secretions in the air passages, which further restrict the flow of air.

Contact with others who have an upper respiratory infection should be avoided, as should being in large crowds during the season when such infections are common. A high level of resistance should be maintained through good personal hygiene and adequate nutrition. Vaccines to guard against influenza are recommended.

Because the lungs of the patient with COAD are never entirely free of bacteria, he is a prime candidate for severe bacterial infections. He should be taught to watch for changes in colour and amount of sputum. If a change in sputum or any other symptoms of infection appear, he should report to his doctor for medication and reassessment of his condition. A small maintenance dose of antibiotics may be prescribed during the winter season as a prophylactic measure. Should an infection develop, the doctor may increase the dosage or switch to another drug to avoid the development of drug-resistant organisms.

Improvement of Ventilation. Improvement of ventilation is of primary importance in the care of patients with COAD. Most difficulty will be experienced during the expiratory phase due to air trapped in the lungs, copious bronchial secretions and weakened bronchial walls. Most patients are anxious and apprehensive in addition.

The following methods may be employed to improve ventilation and the choice of method(s) will depend on the patient's physical condition and his ability to cooperate.

Hydration is considered especially valuable in improvement of ventilation. Inhaled air should be moist to facilitate removal of secretions and soothe the irritated mucous membranes. This can be accomplished through the use of vaporizers and humidifiers, either for environmental humidification in his room or in conjunction with oxygen therapy and the administration of AEROSOLS. Although many other agents can be used for humidification, water remains the most effective. The patient is encouraged to maintain a daily intake of fluids equal to 10–12 glasses daily.

BRONCHODILATORS in the form of aerosols, oral medications, injections, or rectal suppositories are usually prescribed.

Controlled breathing patterns are especially helpful in emptying the lungs and providing adequate ventilation. The patient with COAD is taught to expand his lower chest and to use his abdominal muscles and diaphragm to improve his breathing pattern. He is probably not in the habit of breathing in the most efficient manner, making optimum use of his remaining pulmonary function.

He is taught breathing control, gentle breathing using the lower chest while relaxing the upper chest and shoulder girdle. Inspiration is active and expiration relaxed. The patient breathes at his own rate, gradually slowing as he becomes more comfortable.

A correct breathing pattern should be coordinated with all of the patient's daily activities so that it becomes habitual and he does it without too much thought.

Effective coughing does not come easily to the patient with COAD. He may have experienced too many episodes which exhausted him. He must be convinced that coughing and huffing, when done correctly, can remove mucus plugs and relieve rather than produce dyspnoea.

A huff, a forced expiration, from mid lung volume to low lung volume, will aid the clearance of secretions from the smaller airways. A huff at a high lung volume will clear secretions from the upper airways. It is important to use breathing control after any huff or cough to prevent an increase in airflow obstruction and exhaustion. Paroxysmal coughing is ineffective and exhausting and should be discouraged by using breathing control.

When the patient is unable to cooperate with deep breathing, huffing and coughing, it may be necessary to use a mechanical ventilator. These patients may require SUCTIONING. This procedure is particularly effective when done correctly, but should be undertaken by persons trained in the technique and aware of its inherent dangers.

POSTURAL DRAINAGE is also valuable in facilitating the removal of mucus from the air passages. Chest percussion and vibration may be employed during postural drainage to loosen secretions.

OXYGEN THERAPY is used as a supportive measure when there is decreased oxygenation of arterial blood. Blood gas analysis is an excellent guide in determining the need for initiating oxygen therapy and for monitoring dosage.

Patient Education. As with all chronic diseases that require long-term planning and management, patient education is of primary importance in successful execution of the plan. Full and clear explanation of the need for all aspects of his treatment will mean that the patient is more likely to participate actively in his care. His opinions should be sought and respected whenever possible and he should be encouraged to accept his limitations as well as striving to control his disease pattern.

chron(o)- word element. [Gr.] *time.*

chronobiology (ˌkronəbie'oləjee, ˌkrohnə-) the scientific study of the effect of time on living systems and of biological rhythms. adj. **chronobiological.**

chronognosis (ˌkronog'nohsis) perception of the lapse of time.

chronograph ('kronəˌgrahf, -ˌgraf, 'krohnə-) an instrument for recording small intervals of time.

chronotropic (ˌkronə'tropik) affecting the time or rate.

chronotropism (kro'notrəpizəm) interference with regularity of a periodical movement, such as the heart's action.

chrys(o)- word element. [Gr.] *gold.*

chrysiasis (kri'sieəsis) deposition of gold in living tissue.

chrysoderma (ˌkrisə'dərmə) permanent pigmentation of the skin due to gold deposit.

Chrysops ('kriesops) a genus of bloodsucking tropical flies, the grove flies, including *C. silacea* (and other species), an intermediate host of *Loa loa*, and *C. discalis* (deer fly), a vector of tularaemia in the western USA.

chthonophagia (ˌthonə'fayji·ə) the habit of eating clay or earth; geophagia.

Chvostek's sign, Chvostek–Weiss sign (ˌvosteks; ˌvostek'vies) a spasm of the facial muscles elicited by tapping the facial nerve in the region of the parotid gland; seen in tetany.

chylaemia (kie'leemi·ə) the presence of chyle in the blood.

chylangioma (kieˌlanji'ohmə) a tumour of intestinal lymph vessels filled with chyle.

chyle (kiel) the milky fluid taken up by the lacteals from the intestine during digestion, consisting of lymph and triglyceride fat (chylomicrons) in a stable emulsion, and conveyed by the thoracic duct to empty into the venous system.

chylifaction, chylification (ˌkieli'fakshən; ˌkielifi'kayshən) the formation of chyle.

chyliform ('kieliˌfawm) resembling chyle.

chylocele ('kielohˌseel) distention of the tunica vaginalis testis with effused chyle.

chyloderma (ˌkieloh'dərmə) elephantiasis filariensis.

chylomediastinum (ˌkielohˌmeedi·ə'stienəm) the presence of effused chyle in the mediastinum.

chylomicron (ˌkieloh'miekron) a stable droplet containing principally triglyceride fat, but also cholesterol, phospholipids, and protein; found in intestinal lymphatics (lacteals) and blood during and after meals.

chylomicronaemia (ˌkielohˌmiekroh'neemi·ə) an excess of chylomicrons in the blood.

chylopericardium (ˌkielohˌperi'kahdi·əm) the presence of effused chyle in the pericardium.

chyloperitoneum (ˌkielohˌperitə'neeəm) the presence of effused chyle in the peritoneal cavity.

chylopneumothorax (ˌkielohˌnyoomoh'thor·raks) the presence of effused chyle and air in the pleural cavity.

chylopoiesis (ˌkielohpoy'eesis) chylification. adj. **chylopoietic.**

chylothorax (ˌkieloh'thor·raks) the presence of effused chyle in the pleural cavity.

chylous ('kieləs) pertaining, mingled with, or of the nature of chyle.

chyluria (kie'lyooə·ri·ə) the presence of chyle in the urine, giving it a milky appearance, due to obstruction of lymph flow, which causes rupture of lymph vessels into the renal pelves, ureters, bladder, or urethra.

chyme (kiem) the semifluid, homogeneous, creamy or gruel-like material produced by action of the gastric juice on ingested food and discharged through the pylorus into the duodenum.

chymification (ˌkiemifi'kayshən) conversion of food into chyme; gastric digestion.

chymodenin (ˌkiemoh'deenin) a polypeptide secreted by the duodenum that specifically stimulates pancreatic secretion of chymotrypsinogen.

chymopapain (ˌkiemohpə'pie·in, pə'payin) a proteolytic enzyme (a sulphhydryl proteinase) from the tropical tree *Carica papaya*, used in chemonucleolysis.

chymotrypsin (ˌkiemoh'tripsin) an endopeptidase with action similar to that of trypsin, produced in the intestine by activation of chymotrypsinogen; a product crystallized from an extract of the pancreas of the ox has been used clinically as an anti-inflammatory agent and for enzymatic zonulolysis and débridement.

chymotrypsinogen (ˌkiemohtrip'sinəjən) the inactive precursor of chymotrypsin, the form in which it is secreted by the pancreas.

Ci curie.
cib. [L.] *cibus* (food).
cicatrectomy (ˌsikə'trektəmee) excision of a cicatrix or scar.
cicatricial (ˌsikə'trishəl) pertaining to a cicatrix or scar.
cicatrix ('sikətriks) pl. *cicatrices* [L.] the fibrous tissue left after the healing of a wound; a scar.
cicatrization (ˌsikətrie'zayshən) the formation of a cicatrix or scar; scarring.
ciclacillin (ˌsieklə'silin) a semisynthetic penicillin of the ampicillin class used in the treatment of infections of the respiratory tract, urinary tract, and skin and skin structures due to susceptible organisms.
-cide word element. [L.] *destruction or killing, an agent that kills or destroys.* adj. **-cidal.**
CIF clone-inhibiting factor.
cili(o)- word element. [L.] *cilia, ciliary (body).*
cilia ('sili·ə) [L.] plural of *cilium.* 1. the eyelids or their outer edge. 2. the eyelashes. 3. minute hairlike processes that extend from a cell surface, composed of nine pairs of microtubules around a core of two microtubules. They beat rhythmically to move the cell or to move fluid or mucus over the surface.
ciliary ('sili·əˌree) pertaining to or resembling cilia; used particularly in reference to certain eye structures, as the ciliary body or muscle.
c. body the thickened part of the vascular tunic of the eye, connecting choroid and iris, made up of the ciliary muscle and the ciliary processes. These processes radiate from the ciliary muscle and give attachment to ligaments supporting the lens of the eye.
c. glands sweat glands that have become arrested in their development, situated at the edges of the eyelids.
c. muscle the muscle that forms the main part of the ciliary body and functions in accommodation of the eye.
c. reflex the movement of the pupil in accommodation.
Ciliata (ˌsili'aytə) a class of protozoa (subphylum Ciliophora) whose members possess cilia throughout the life cycle; a few species are parasitic. See BALANTIDIUM.
ciliate ('siliˌayt) 1. having cilia. 2. any individual of the Ciliata.
ciliated ('siliˌaytid) provided with cilia.
ciliectomy (ˌsili'ektəmee) 1. excision of a portion of the ciliary body. 2. excision of the portion of the eyelid containing the roots of the eyelashes.
Ciliophora (ˌsili'ofə·rə) a subphylum of Protozoa, distinguished from the other subphyla by the presence of cilia at some stage in the existence of the member organisms.
cilium ('sili·əm) [L.] singular of *cilia.*
cillosis (si'lohsis) spasmodic quivering of the eyelid.
cimbia ('simbi·ə) a white band running across the ventral surface of the crus cerebri.
cimetidine (si'metiˌdeen) a histamine H_2-receptor antagonist that inhibits the action of histamine at cell surface receptors of the gastric parietal cells and reduces basal gastric acid secretion and secretion stimulated by food, histamine, gastrin, caffeine, and insulin. It is used for short-term (two months) treatment of peptic ulcer and for treatment of pathological hypersecretory conditions, such as Zollinger–Ellison syndrome. Treatment of peptic ulcer with cimetidine brings prompt relief and speeds ulcer healing. Antacids are also taken as needed for relief of pain.
Cimex ('siemeks) a genus of flightless blood-sucking insects (order Hemiptera), the bedbugs.
C. lectularius the common bedbug of temperate regions; other species are limited to tropical and subtropical areas and feed on other animals as well as man.
cinchocaine ('sinchohkayn) a local anaesthetic of the amide group used mainly as a spinal anaesthetic.
cinchona (sing'kohnə) the dried bark of the stem or root of various South American trees of the genus *Cinchona*; it is a source of quinine, quinidine, cinchonine, and other alkaloids.
cinchonism ('singkəˌnizəm) toxicity due to cinchona alkaloid overdosage; symptoms are tinnitus and slight deafness, photophobia and other visual disturbances, mental dullness, depression, confusion, headache, and nausea.
cine- word element. [Gr.] *movement;* see also words beginning *kine-.*
cineangiocardiography (ˌsiniˌanjiohˌkardi'ografee) the photographic recording of fluoroscopic images of the heart and great vessels by motion picture techniques.
cineangiography (ˌsiniˌanji'ografee) the photographic recording of fluoroscopic images of the blood vessels by motion picture techniques.
cinefluorography (ˌsiniˌflooə'rografee) cineradiography.
cinemicrography (ˌsinimie'krografee) the making of motion pictures of a small object through the lens system of a microscope.
cinephlebography (ˌsinifli'bografee) cineradiography of the veins after administration of a contrast medium.
cineradiography (ˌsiniˌraydi'ografee) the making of a motion picture record of successive images appearing on a fluoroscopic screen.
cinerea (si'niə·ri·ə) the grey matter of the nervous system. adj. **cinereal.**
cineroentgenofluorography (ˌsinirontjənohˌflooə'rografee) cineradiography.
cinesi- for words beginning thus, see those beginning *kinesi-.*
cineto- for words beginning thus, see those beginning *kineto-.*
cingulectomy (ˌsing·gyuh'lektəmee) bilateral extirpation of the anterior half of the gyrus cinguli.
cingulotomy (ˌsing·gyuh'lotəmee) the creation of precisely placed lesions in the cingulum of the frontal lobe for relief of intractable pain.
cingulum ('sing·gyuhləm) pl. *cingula* [L.] 1. an encircling part or structure; a girdle. 2. a bundle of association fibres partly encircling the corpus callosum not far from the median plane, interrelating the cingulate and hippocampal gyri. 3. the lingual lobe of an anterior tooth. adj. **cingulate.**
cingulumotomy (ˌsing·gyuhlə'motəmee) cingulotomy.
cinnamon ('sinəmən) an extract from the bark of an East Indian laurel, sometimes used as a digestive and carminative.
cinnarizine (si'nariˌzeen) an antihistamine drug which may also be used to treat nausea, vertigo, labyrinthine disorders and motion sickness.
Cinobac ('sinohˌbak) trademark for a preparation of cinoxacin, an antibiotic agent used in the treatment of urinary tract infections.
cinoxacin (si'noksəˌsin) a synthetic antibiotic agent administered orally in the treatment of urinary tract infections due to *Escherichia coli*, *Proteus mirabilis*, *P. vulgaris*, *Klebsiella* species, including *K. pneumoniae*, and *Enterobacter* species.
circadian (sər'kaydi·ən) denoting a period of about 24 hours.
c. rhythm the regular recurrence of certain phenomena in cycles of approximately 24 hours, e.g., biological activities that occur at about the same time each day (or night) regardless of constant darkness or other

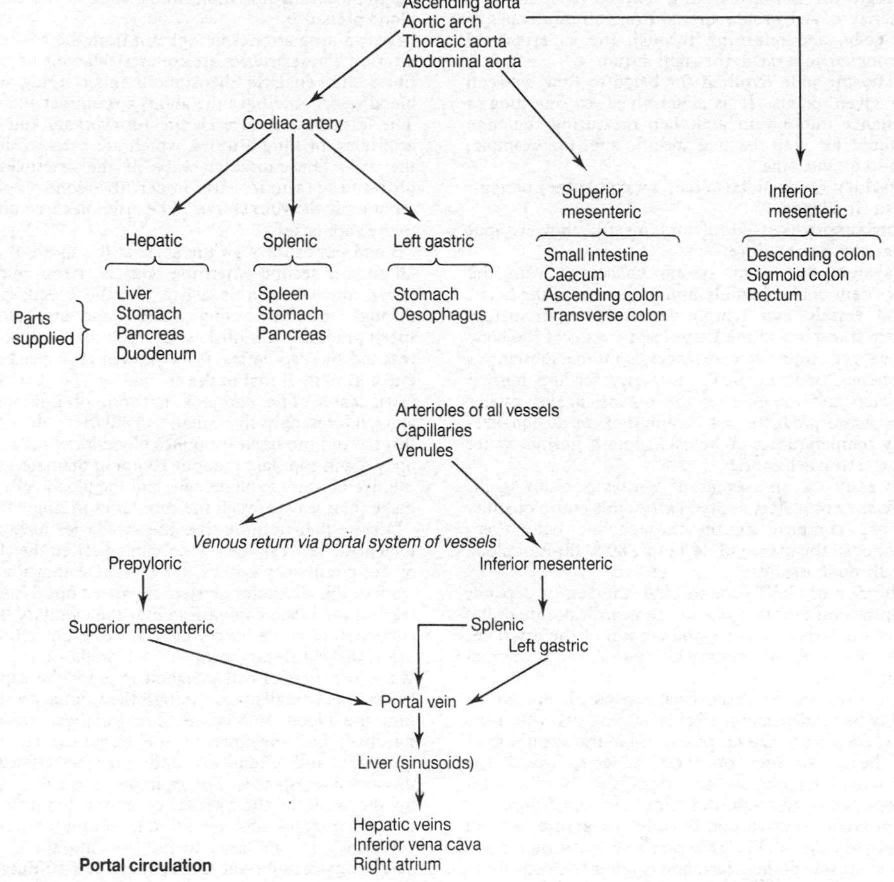

Portal circulation

conditions of illumination.

circinate ('sərsi,nayt) resembling a ring, or circle.

circle ('sərk'l) a round figure, structure, or part.
Berry's c's charts with circles on them for testing stereoscopic vision.
sensory c. a body area within which it is impossible to distinguish separately the impressions arising from two sites of stimulation.
c. of Willis the anastomatic loop of arteries at the base of the brain, formed by the branches of the internal carotids and the branches of the basilar artery.

CircOlectric bed (,sərkoh'lektrik) an electrically operated frame similar in principle to the STRYKER FRAME. The bed can be rotated so that the patient may be placed in a prone, supine, or sitting position, or an erect position. It may be utilized to facilitate turning of a patient with severe burns, a patient in traction, or a patient with various types of spinal injuries.

circulation (,sərkyuh'layshən) movement in a regular or circuitous course, returning to the point of origin, as the circulation of the blood through the heart and blood vessels (see also CIRCULATORY SYSTEM).
collateral c. that carried on through secondary channels after obstruction of the principal channel supplying the part.
coronary c. that within the coronary vessels; which supply the muscle of the heart.
enterohepatic c. the cycle in which bile salts and other substances excreted by the liver are absorbed by the intestinal mucosa and returned to the liver via the portal circulation.
extracorporeal c. circulation of blood outside the body, as through a HAEMODIALYSER or a HEART–LUNG MACHINE.
fetal c. circulation of blood through the body of the fetus and to and from the placenta through the umbilical cord (see also FETAL CIRCULATION).
portal c. a general term denoting the circulation of blood through larger vessels from the capillaries of one organ to those of another; applied especially to the passage of blood from the gastrointestinal tract and spleen through the portal vein to the liver. See accompanying illustration.
pulmonary c. the flow of blood from the right ventricle through the pulmonary artery to the lungs, where carbon dioxide is exchanged for oxygen, and back through the pulmonary vein to the left artrium (see also PULMONARY CIRCULATION) and to the hypothalamopituitary portal system which connects the hypothalamus with the anterior portion of the pituitary gland (see also PITUITARY).
systemic c. the flow of blood from the left ventricle

through the aorta, carrying oxygen and nutrient material to, and waste material from, all the tissues of the body, and returning through the superior and inferior venae cavae to the right atrium.

c. time the time required for blood to flow between two given points. It is determined by injecting a substance into a vein and then measuring the time required for it to reach a specific site, for example, arm-to-tongue time.

circulatory (ˌsərkyuhˈlaytə·ree, ˈsərkyuhlətree) pertaining to circulation.

c. collapse SHOCK; circulatory insufficiency without congestive heart failure.

c. system the major system concerned with the movement of blood and lymph; it consists of the heart, blood vessels, and lymph vessels. The circulatory system transports to the tissues and organs of the body the oxygen, nutritive substances, immune substances, hormones, and chemicals necessary for the normal function and activities of the organs; it also carries away waste products and carbon dioxide. It equalizes body temperature and helps maintain normal water and electrolyte balance.

An adult has an average of 5 litres of blood in his body; the circulatory system carries this entire quantity on one complete circuit through the body every minute. In the course of 24 hours, 8000 litres of blood pass through the heart.

The rate of blood flow through the vessels depends upon several factors: force of the heartbeat, rate of the heartbeat, venous return, and control of the arterioles and capillaries by chemical, neural, and thermal stimuli.

PULMONARY AND SYSTEMIC CIRCULATION. There are in reality two independent circulatory systems within the body, each with its own pump inside the sheathing of the heart. In one of these systems, called the pulmonary circulation, the right side of the heart pumps blood through the lungs. In the lungs, the blood gives up its carbon dioxide and absorbs a fresh supply of oxygen. The reoxygenated blood then flows to the left side of the heart, and is pumped out again to all the systems and organs of the body. This major circulatory system is called the systemic circulation.

The circulation of blood through the fetus bypasses the pulmonary circuit (see also FETAL CIRCULATION).

ARTERIAL SYSTEM. Blood pumped from the left side of the heart enters the aorta, the main arterial trunk of the systemic circulation. The aorta, which is about 2.5 cm in diameter, arches upward and toward the left side of the body. Just above the heart two coronary arteries branch off from the aorta. These arteries supply the muscles of the heart with blood.

Branching from the top of the aortic arch are three large arteries which supply the upper part of the body, the brachiocephalic trunk (which divides into the right carotid and right subclavian arteries) and the left carotid and left subclavian arteries. The carotid arteries supply the head and neck; the subclavian arteries supply the arms. The aorta then turns downward and passes through the trunk of the body, close to the vertebral column. Smaller arteries branch off from the aorta to supply the lungs, stomach, spleen, pancreas, kidneys, intestines, and other organs of the body. At about the level of the umbilicus, the aorta divides into two branches, the two iliac arteries, which supply the vessels of the pelvic organs and the legs.

The arteries so far named are the main conducting arteries. They consist of a smooth inner lining covered largely by elastic fibres that absorb the pulsations of the heart. As the heart beats, the elastic arterial walls damp the strong pulsations into a more nearly constant blood pressure.

Distributing arteries branch out from the conducting arteries. These arteries are composed largely of muscle fibres that encircle the smooth inner lining of the blood vessels and have the ability to contract and relax. The distributing arteries in turn branch out into arterioles, or little arteries, which are barely visible to the eye. The muscular walls of the arterioles and distributing arteries are under the control of the autonomic NERVOUS SYSTEM. The arterioles lead directly to the capillaries.

Blood passes through the aorta at the speed of about 40 cm per second when the body is at rest, and at a faster rate when it is active. As the blood spreads through the distributing arteries and arterioles, its speed gradually diminishes. By the time the blood has reached the capillaries, it has slowed to a speed about one-eightieth of that in the arteries.

CAPILLARIES. The complex network of innumerable and microscopically small capillaries distributed throughout the tissues supplies blood to all cells in the body. Each capillary is about 10 μm in diameter, about the size of a single blood cell, and the blood cells must make their way through the capillaries in single file.

Despite their minute size, the capillaries have a vast total area. The capillary 'lake' can be called the climax of the circulatory system, for it is here that the vital work of the circulatory system is carried out. Nutrients leaving the blood capillaries enter the capillary lake, a collection of tissue fluid which bathes each cell. From there the nutrients permeate the walls of the cells. Waste products of cell metabolism enter the capillary lake and eventually pass through the capillary wall and into the blood circulation. The capillary walls are selective; i.e., they permit the exchange of special nutrients and chemicals and bar the passage of unwanted substances. For example, the cells making up the walls of the capillaries in the brain bar the passage of many substances that might injure the brain cells, and the capillaries in the placenta also act as a barrier against substances that might be harmful to the developing fetus.

VENOUS SYSTEM. From the capillaries the blood returns to the heart via the veins, which together make up the venous system. The blood flows from the capillaries to minute venules, and then to the veins, in a network of blood vessels of ever increasing size that parallels in reverse the branching of the arterial system. The walls of the veins, however, are thinner, less elastic and less muscular than those of the arteries. And whereas the arteries are for the most part buried deep within the body for protection, the venous system has many superficial veins that run close to the surface of the skin. If an arterial blood vessel is cut, the blood flows from the cut in spurts, whereas blood from a cut vein flows steadily.

The blood returning to the heart collects into two main veins. Blood returning from the arms, head and upper chest flows into the superior vena cava; blood returning from the rest of the body flows into the inferior vena cava. Both these veins return the blood to the right side of the heart.

The blood from the lower part of the body must return to the heart against the force of gravity, since all the pressure built up by the heart has been dissipated in the capillaries. This is accomplished in several ways. The veins themselves contain one-way venous valves which work in pairs. When the blood is flowing in the correct direction, the venous valves are pressed against the walls of the veins, permitting unobstructed flow. If the blood should tend to flow backward, however, the venous valves fall inward and press against each other, effectively stopping the backward flow of blood. The blood is 'milked' upward toward the heart principally by the massaging action of the abdominal and leg muscles as they press against the veins. Inspirations of air also force the blood through the venous system, as do the movements of the intestines. If the leg muscles do not move for long periods of time, the blood collects in the lower part of the body and the amount available for the brain is decreased.

SYSTEMIC CIRCUITS. The circulatory system has been discussed so far as if the blood flowed through the body in a simple circular path. In fact, the blood can take one of several circuits through the body. Among these circuits are the coronary circuit through the arteries and veins of the heart; a circuit through the neck, head, and brain; a circuit through the digestive organs; and the renal circuit through the kidneys. The importance of the renal circulation lies in the fact that the kidneys act as the cleansing filter of the circulatory system, removing a variety of products that have been cast off from the cells and body tissues. At any given time, about one-quarter of all the blood pumped through the body is passing through the renal circuit.

The most complex circuit (portal circulation) is that which flows through the digestive system, picking up proteins, carbohydrates, fats, and chemicals from the intestines and delivering them to the tissues. Separate distributing arteries conduct the blood to the lower intestine, upper intestine, stomach, spleen, and pancreas. The veins leading from these organs combine to form the portal vein, which leads to the liver. Within the liver, the artery leading to the liver (the hepatic artery) and the portal vein subdivide into a complex network of capillary-like vessels called sinusoids which bring the blood into closer contact with the cells of the liver. The liver cells withdraw glucose from the blood for storage as glycogen or release it as needed, and remove from the blood many harmful substances that might be toxic to body tissues. The blood leaving the liver flows to the inferior vena cava.

LYMPHATIC SYSTEM. The cells, chemicals, and other components of the blood are suspended within the blood vessels in plasma. Similar fluid also fills the spaces between the tissue cells. Nutrients reaching the cells are carried there by this tissue fluid, and it also carries waste products from the cells to the capillaries. One function of the lymphatic system is to collect and return some of this fluid via the lymphatic vessels to the circulatory system. When this tissue fluid is within the lymphatic system, it is called lymph. In addition to draining off excess tissue fluid, the lymphatic capillaries also transport some waste products as well as dead blood cells, pathogenic organisms in case of infection, and malignant cells from cancerous growths. From the lymphatic capillaries the lymph is carried into larger lymphatic vessels which contain one-way valves similar to those in the veins. Lymph nodes are interspersed among the lymph vessels and filter their fluids. Eventually large lymph ducts (the thoracic duct and right lymphatic duct) empty into the right and left subclavian veins. The lymph is propelled by the same massaging action that causes the blood to circulate through the venous system. There are larger masses of lymphatic tissue called lymphatic organs, and among them are the SPLEEN, TONSILS, and THYMUS. These organs produce specialized leukocytes (lymphocytes) that help protect the body against infections (see also IMMUNITY).

CONTROL OF CIRCULATION. The organs and systems of the body vary greatly in the quantity of blood they require at different times. The needs of the brain are constant; the demands of the muscles are more varied. Heavy physical exertion may increase the rate of blood flow to the muscles eight times above the normal resting rate. In hot weather, a larger percentage of blood flows through the skin to cool the body. After every meal an extra supply of blood is required by the stomach to help digest and absorb the meal.

These changes in blood supply are accomplished automatically by the autonomic nervous system, which acts through the muscle fibres that surround the distributing arteries and arterioles. These muscle fibres either contract or relax, according to the specific nerve signal transmitted to them by the medulla oblongata in the deepest part of the brain. As these muscle fibres contract or relax, they alter the diameter of the blood vessels and, therefore, the rate of blood flow. Certain chemicals, such as adrenaline, ephedrine, histamine, and alcohol, as well as tobacco, can also affect the size of the blood vessels. These changes in the size of the blood vessels are entirely reflexive and the individual has no conscious control over them at all. Ordinarily, the autonomic nervous system maintains the muscles surrounding the arteries in a state of mild tension, which keeps the blood pressure at its normal level.

The brain requires a constant, unvarying supply of blood. Except for the presence of a special control system, this would be impossible to maintain, since every time a person moved or shifted position the quantity of blood flowing to the brain would change. The control system consists of the action of two nerves, one located in the aorta and the other in the carotid artery in the neck, which, acting together, register any changes in the blood pressure and cause the autonomic nervous system to change the rate of heartbeat and the size of the blood vessels to maintain the correct blood pressure.

circum- word element. [L.] *around*.

circumcise ('sərkəm,siez) to perform circumcision.

circumcision ('sərkəm,sizhən) surgical removal of the prepuce.The operation is done for hygienic and medical reasons, and also for religious reasons.

Circumcision is not without risk from complications, the most common of which are haemorrhage, infection, and amputation of the tip of the penis, resulting later in a urethral stricture. Although there is some evidence that there may be a relationship between lack of circumcision and penile cancer, which is relatively rare, lack of hygiene seems equally important as an aetiologic factor.There is some evidence of a relationship between cervical cancer in females and coitus with an uncircumcised spouse.

There would appear to be no valid medical reasons for routine circumcision of newborn infants. Continuous good personal hygiene is a viable alternative to routine circumcision with all its attendant surgical risks.

PATIENT CARE. Preoperative care for the child or adult undergoing circumcision includes laboratory tests to determine coagulation or clotting time.

The patient is watched closely after the operation for signs of bleeding; however, excessive bleeding is extremely rare. Other observations include watching for signs of infection and difficulty in urination.

A sterile lubricated dressing is usually placed over the penis when surgery is completed. The dressing is changed frequently, in young children and adults, after each urination. Healing usually takes place in five to seven days.

circumclusion (,sərkəm'kloozhən) compression of an artery by a wire and pin.

circumduction (ˌsərkəm'dukshən) circular movement of a limb or of the eye.

circumflex ('sərkəmˌfleks) curved like a bow.

circumoral (ˌsərkəm'or·rəl) around the mouth.

c. pallor a pale area around the mouth contrasting with the flushed cheeks, e.g. in scarlet fever.

circumscribed ('sərkəmˌskriebd) bounded or limited; confined to a limited space.

circumstantiality (ˌsərkəmˌstanshi'alitee) a disturbance in the flow of thought in which a patient's conversation is characterized by unnecessary elaboration of trivial details.

circumvallate (ˌsərkəm'valayt) surrounded by a ridge or trench, as the vallate (circumvallate) papillae.

cirrhosis (si'rohsis) a liver disease characterized pathologically by the loss of the normal microscopic lobular architecture and regenerative replacement of necrotic parenchymal tissue with fibrous bands of connective tissue which eventually constrict and partition the organ into irregular nodules. The term is sometimes used to refer to chronic interstitial inflammation of any organ. adj. **cirrhotic**.

Cirrhosis of the liver constitutes a group of chronic diseases. The disorder has a lengthy latent period, usually followed by the sudden appearance of abdominal pain and swelling, haematemesis, dependent oedema, with or without jaundice. In advanced stages, ASCITES, pronounced jaundice, portal hypertension, and central nervous system disturbances, which may end in hepatic coma, predominate.

CLINICAL MANIFESTATIONS. The signs and symptoms of hepatic cirrhosis are manifestations of interference with the major functions of the liver; that is: (1) the storage and release of blood to maintain adequate circulating volume, (2) the metabolism of nutrients and the detoxification of poisons absorbed from the intestines, (3) the regulation of fluid and electrolyte balance, and (4) production of clotting factors.

The patient with alcoholic cirrhosis (Laënnec's cirrhosis) may be admitted to the hospital with acute alcoholic hepatitis, marked by fever and dehydration. Prominent spider angiomata and redness of the palms of the hands (palmar erythema) are usually present. Delirium tremens may prove difficult to treat during the early phase. Liver function tests usually show elevated transaminase and bilirubin levels, and decreased values for albumin and clotting factors. See also ALCOHOLISM.

Continued fluid and electrolyte imbalance and inefficient metabolism of nutrients produce ascites, hypoglycaemia, and hypoproteinaemia. Obstruction to the return of blood from the portal system causes increased pressure within the veins of the oesophagus and stomach, which engorge to become *varices* and which may rupture with subsequent haemorrhage, exacerbated by clotting disorders. JAUNDICE develops as a result of biliary obstruction and as a result of hepatocellular damage.

Neurological symptoms (hepatic encephalopathy) begin with subtle changes in mental acuity, mild memory loss, poor reasoning ability, and irritability. Tremor of the outstretched hands (asterixis) is common. These symptoms become more severe and may eventually progress to delirium, suicidal tendencies, and coma.

TREATMENT AND PATIENT CARE. The major goals of care are: (1) to maintain liver function at its current level and prevent further deterioration of the organ, (2) to alleviate anxiety of the patient and his family, (3) to maintain electrolytes within normal limits, (4) to maintain sufficient respiratory function, (5) to prevent or resolve gastrointestinal bleeding, and (6) to provide adequate nutritional intake and a positive nitrogen balance.

To prevent further deterioration of the liver cells, any identifiable primary cause must be removed; for example, restriction of the intake of alcohol or other toxic agent, treatment of infection, and providing an adequate nutritional intake.

In the early stages of the disease, rest and adequate nutrition in the form of a normal to high-protein, high-calorific diet are essential for the repair of damaged liver cells; supplementary vitamins are administered.

Observations for signs of bleeding are necessary because the liver is no longer able to produce normal amounts of prothrombin, which plays an important role in the clotting of blood. The patient may have haematemesis, tarry stools, bleeding gums, frequent and severe nosebleeds, and bleeding under the skin. Care should be taken in brushing the teeth, and the patient is instructed to avoid blowing his nose with force.

Severe acute blood loss is compensated for by transfusions of whole blood and plasma fractions to provide extra clotting factors. Intravenous agents, such as pitressin, glypressin or nitroglycerine can be used to lower portal pressure. Excessive bleeding from oesophageal varices may necessitate the temporary insertion of a Sengstaken–Blakemore tube. This device has four channels: one for inflation of the oesophageal balloon, one for inflation of the gastric balloon, one for pharyngeal aspiration, and a fourth for aspiration of stomach contents.

Relief of portal hypertension is sometimes accomplished by a portacaval shunt. The portal vein is surgically connected to the inferior vena cava, thus allowing for drainage of excessive amounts of blood from the portal system to the general circulation. A similar procedure, the splenorenal shunt, involves connecting the splenic vein to the renal vein. Neither procedure alters the mortality. Both are giving way to endoscopic injection of oesophageal varices as a less traumatic procedure, though this has yet to be shown definitely to lower the mortality. Transection of the lower oesophagus using a stapling gun to divide and resuture the oesophagus, thereby interrupting the varices, is another means of treatment which is being increasingly used for bleeding varices. The varices tend to recur subsequently and obliteration by endoscopic sclerotherapy can then be performed.

Fluid and electrolyte status in patients with advanced cirrhosis is carefully monitored. A record of intake and output is kept and the patient is weighed daily. Sodium intake may be restricted and DIURETICS, especially spironolactone, are prescribed to assist in the control of oedema and ascites. Gross ascites, unresponsive to these measures, can be treated by repeated small volume paracentesis, with replacement of albumin intravenously. Reinfusion of ascites into the circulation can be performed externally using a surgically inserted peritoneal-venous shunt (LeVeen shunt). Progressive renal impairment is a major problem in patients with decompensated cirrhosis and may lead to hepatorenal syndrome when both the liver and kidneys fail. This carries a very high mortality.

Hepatic coma demands total restriction of protein intake, but a high-calorific diet utilizing fats and carbohydrates is recommended.

Drugs that may be used include the laxative lactulose and broad-spectrum antibiotics, such as neomycin, to alter the bowel flora and thereby decrease the production of ammonia by intestinal bacteria. Although an increased level of ammonia in the blood does not directly cause hepatic coma, a reduction of serum ammonia has a beneficial effect.

The semicomatose or completely comatose patient requires continued monitoring of the vital signs, and measures to avoid complications from immobility. See also COMA.

Hepatic transplantation offers a potential solution in some cases of liver failure in endstage cirrhosis and can be expected to play an increasingly important role.

acholangic c. a liver disorder affecting children up to 12 years of age, due to complete or partial agenesis of the intrahepatic, intralobular bile ducts, with manifestations similar to those seen in obstructive biliary cirrhosis; called also *biliary atresia.*

alcoholic c. Laënnec's cirrhosis.

atrophic c. cirrhosis in which the liver is decreased in size; it may be seen in the alcoholic, but is more common in posthepatic or postnecrotic cirrhosis.

biliary c. cirrhosis of the liver due to obstruction or infection of the major extra- or intrahepatic bile ducts (except in *primary biliary cirrhosis*). It is marked by jaundice, abdominal pain, steatorrhoea, and enlargement of the liver and spleen.

cardiac c. fibrosis of the liver, probably following central haemorrhagic necrosis, in association with congestive heart disease.

fatty c. cirrhosis in which liver cells are infiltrated with fat (triglyceride), the infiltration usually being due to alcohol ingestion; see Laënnec's cirrhosis (below).

Laënnec's c. cirrhosis of the liver closely associated with chronic excessive alcohol ingestion. In the early stages, liver enlargement may reflect fatty infiltration of liver cells (fatty cirrhosis) with necrosis and inflammation due to acute alcohol injury; progressive fibrosis extending from portal areas separates uniform small regenerating nodules. Some attribute the condition to a nutritional deficiency associated with alcoholism and others to chronic exposure to alcohol as a hepatotoxin. Called also *alcoholic cirrhosis.*

metabolic c. cirrhosis of the liver associated with metabolic diseases, such as haemochromatosis, Wilson's disease, glycogenosis, galactosaemia, and disorders of amino acid metabolism.

portal c. Laënnec's cirrhosis.

posthepatic c. cirrhosis (usually macronodular) resulting as a sequel to acute hepatitis.

postnecrotic c. cirrhosis which follows submassive necrosis of the liver (subacute yellow atrophy) due to toxic or viral hepatitis.

primary biliary c. a less common form of biliary cirrhosis of unknown aetiology, occurring without obstruction or infection of the major bile ducts, sometimes developing after the administration of such drugs as chlorpromazine and arsenicals. Affecting chiefly middle-aged women, it is characterized by chronic cholestasis with pruritus and jaundice, hypercholesterolaemia with xanthomas, and malabsorption.

secondary biliary c. cirrhosis of the liver resulting from chronic bile obstruction due to congenital atresia or stricture.

cirsectomy (sər'sektəmee) excision of a portion of a varicose vein.

cirsoid ('sərsoyd) resembling a varix.

cirsomphalos (sər'somfələs) caput medusae.

cis (sis) [L.] in organic chemistry, having certain atoms or radicals on the same side; in genetics, having the two mutant genes of a pseudoallele on the same chromosome. Compare *trans.*

cis-platinum (sis'platinəm) cisplatin.

cisplatin ('sisplə,tin) an antineoplastic agent whose main mode of action resembles that of alkylating agents—production of cross-links between the two strands of DNA in the double helix so that DNA cannot be replicated and the cells cannot divide. It was serendipitously discovered when Dr. Barnett Rosenberg noted that the platinum electrodes used in a laboratory study of *Escherichia coli* inhibited cell division in the organism under study. Called also *cis*-platinum. Its full chemical name is diamminedichloroplatinum, abbreviated to DDP.

Cisplatin is used in the treatment of metastatic tumours of the testis, ovary, bladder, and head and neck. Like other chemotherapeutic agents used in the treatment of cancer, cisplatin produces major toxicities. It can cause serious damage to the kidney, the eighth cranial nerve, gastrointestinal tract, and bone marrow. It also can upset metabolic processes and produce hypocalcaemia and hypomagnesaemia.

cistern ('sistən) a closed space serving as a reservoir for lymph or other body fluids, especially one of the enlarged subarachnoid spaces containing cerebrospinal fluid.

cisterna (si'stərnə) pl. *cisternae* [L.] cistern.

c. cerebellomedullaris the enlarged subarachnoid space between the undersurface of the cerebellum and the posterior surface of the medulla oblongata; called also cisterna magna.

c. chyli the dilated portion of the thoracic duct at its origin in the lumbar region; called also receptaculum chyli.

cisternal (si'stərnəl) pertaining to a cistern, especially the cisterna cerebellomedullaris.

c. puncture puncture of the cisterna magnum with a hollow needle inserted just between the occipital bone, to obtain a specimen of CEREBROSPINAL FLUID (see also SPINAL PUNCTURE).

Preparation of the patient for this procedure should include a detailed explanation, because insertion of a needle so close to the brain may cause apprehension. The neurologist may request that the back of the neck be shaved. Some patients may be given sedation prior to the procedure. Cisternal puncture is performed with the patient in the sitting position with his head tilted forward or in the face down position on the couch. A graduated needle is used so that the operator knows exactly to what depth it has been inserted. Following the procedure, assessment of vital signs and neurological status is performed along with observation for cyanosis, dyspnoea and haemorrhage from the puncture site.

cisternography (,sistər'nogrəfee) radiography of the basal cistern of the brain after subarachnoid injection of a contrast medium.

cistron ('sistron) the smallest unit of genetic material that must be intact to function as a transmitter of genetic information; as traditionally construed, approximately synonymous with gene.

citrate ('sitrayt, 'sietrayt) any salt of citric acid.

citric acid ('sitrik) a tricarboxylic acid occurring in citrus fruits and acting as an antiscorbutic and diuretic. It functions as an anticoagulant in the blood preservatives, acid citrate dextrose and citrate phosphate dextrose, and is a metabolic intermediate in the tricarboxylic acid cycle.

c. a. cycle tricarboxylic acid cycle.

citronella (,sitrə'nelə) a fragrant grass, the source of a volatile oil (citronella oil) used in perfumes and insect repellents.

citrovorum factor (,sitroh'vor·rəm) folinic acid.

citrulline ('sitrə,leen) an alpha amino acid involved in the urea cycle.

citrullinuria (sit,ruli'nyooə·ri·ə) the presence in the

urine of large amounts of citrulline, with increased levels also in both plasma and cerebrospinal fluid.

citta (si'tah) craving for unusual foods during pregnancy; cravings for starch, sweets, fruits, vegetables, pickles, or raw cereals are common and are sometimes associated with PICA, eating of non-nutritive substances, such as ice, clay, or chalk.

cittosis (si'tohsis) pica.

Cl chemical symbol, *chlorine.*

cladosporiosis (ˌkladohˌspor·ri'ohsis) any infection with *Cladosporium.*

Cladosporium (ˌkladoh'spor·ri·əm) a genus of fungi, including *C. herbarum*, which produces 'black spot' on meat in cold storage, growing at a temperature of −8 °C (18 °F); and *C. carrioni*, an agent of chromomycosis.

Claforan ('kləfəˌran) trademark for a preparation of cefotaxime sodium.

clairvoyance (klair'voyəns) [Fr.] a form of extrasensory perception in which knowledge of objective events is acquired without the use of the senses.

clamp (klamp) a surgical device for compressing a part or structure.

clap (klap) gonorrhoea.

clapotement (klə'pohtmonh) [Fr.] a splashing sound, as in succussion.

clapping ('klaping) in physiotherapy, a term used to denote rhythmic beating with cupped hands. Frequently used over the chest to aid expectoration.

clarificant (klə'rifikənt) a substance that clears a liquid of turbidity.

Clark's rule (klahks) the dose of a drug for a child is obtained by multiplying the adult dose by the child's weight in pounds and dividing the result by 150.

Clarke–Hadfield syndrome (klahk'hadfiəld) congenital pancreatic infantilism, with hepatomegaly, bulky stools, and extensive atrophy of the pancreas in an undersized and underweight child.

class (klahs) 1. a taxonomic category subordinate to a phylum and superior to an order. 2. a group of variables all of which show a value falling between certain limits.

clastic ('klastik) 1. undergoing or causing division. 2. separable into parts.

clastogenic (ˌklastoh'jenik) giving rise to or inducing disruption or breakages, as of chromosomes.

clastothrix ('klastohˌthriks) trichorrhoexis nodosa.

clathrate ('klathrayt) 1. having the shape or appearance of a lattice; pertaining to clathrate compounds. 2. clathrate compounds: inclusion complexes in which molecules of one type are trapped within cavities of the crystalline lattice of another substance.

Claude's syndrome (klawdz) paralysis of the third (oculomotor) nerve on one side and asynergia on the other side, together with dysarthria.

claudication (ˌklawdi'kayshən) limping or lameness.

intermittent c. a complex of symptoms characterized by absence of pain or discomfort in a limb when at rest, the commencement of pain, tension, and weakness after walking is begun, intensification of the condition until walking is impossible, and the disappearance of symptoms after the limb has been at rest. It is seen in occlusive arterial disease of the limbs.

venous c. intermittent claudication caused by venous stasis.

claustrophilia (ˌklostrə'fili·ə, ˌklaw-) an abnormal desire to be in a closed room or space.

claustrophobia (ˌklostrə'fohbi·ə, ˌklaw-) morbid fear of closed places.

claustrum ('klawstrəm) pl. *claustra* [L.] the thin layer of grey matter lateral to the external capsule of the brain, separating it from the white matter of the insula.

Claviceps ('klaviˌseps) a genus of parasitic fungi that infest various seed plants.

C. purpurea the source of ergot.

clavicle ('klavik'l) an elongated, slender, curved bone lying horizontally at the root of the neck, in the upper part of the thorax; called also *collar bone.* adj. **clavicular.**

clavicotomy (ˌklavi'kotəmee) surgical division of the clavicle.

clavicula (klə'vikyuhlə) pl. *claviculae* [L.] the clavicle.

clavulanic acid (ˌklavuh'lanik) an agent capable of enhancing the antibacterial activity of other agents by inhibiting the activity of beta-lactamase.

clavus ('klayvəs) a corn.

c. hystericus a sensation as if a nail were being driven into the head.

clawfoot (ˌklor'fuht) a high-arched foot with the toes hyperextended at the metatarsophalangeal joint and flexed at the distal joints.

clawhand (ˌklor'hand) flexion and atrophy of the hand and fingers.

clearance ('kliə·rəns) the act of clearing; specifically, complete removal by the kidneys of a solute or substance from a specific volume of blood per unit of time.

blood-urea c. the volume of the blood cleared of urea per minute by renal elimination.

creatinine c. the volume of plasma cleared of creatinine in a unit of time by the kidney system. See also CREATININE.

inulin c. an expression of the renal efficiency in eliminating inulin from the blood, a measure of glomerular function.

urea c. blood-urea clearance.

cleavage ('kleevij) 1. division into distinct parts. 2. the early successive splitting of a fertilized ovum into smaller cells (blastomers) by mitosis.

cleft (kleft) a fissure or longitudinal opening, especially one occurring during embryonic development.

branchial c's the slit-like openings in the gills of fish between the branchial arches; also, the homologous branchial grooves between the branchial arches of mammalian embryos.

c. lip, c. palate congenital fissure, or split, of the lip (cleft lip) or of the roof of the mouth (cleft palate).

Cleft palate and cleft lip occur in about one birth per thousand and are sometimes associated with clubfoot (talipes) or other anatomical defects. Parents who were born with cleft palate or cleft lip are more likely than other parents to have children with these defects.

Cleft palate and cleft lip result from failure of the two sides of the face to unite properly at an early stage of prenatal development. The defect may be limited to the outer flesh of the upper lip (the term harelip, suggesting the lip of a rabbit, is both inaccurate and unkind), or it may extend back through the midline of the upper jaw through the roof of the palate. Sometimes only the soft palate, located at the rear of the mouth, is involved.

The infant with a cleft palate is unable to suckle properly, because the opening between mouth and nose through the palate prevents suction. Feeding must be done by other means, with a dropper, a cup, a spoon, or an obturator, a device inserted in the mouth to close the cleft while the baby is sucking. Cleft palate allows food to get into the nose, and it causes difficulty in chewing and swallowing. Later it will hinder speech, because consonants such as *g*, *b*, *d*, and *f*, which are normally formed by pressure against the roof of the mouth, are distorted by resonance in the nasal cavity. The cleft may also prevent movements of the soft palate essential in clear speech.

Treatment of cleft palate and cleft lip is by surgery, followed by measures to improve speech.

c. tongue a tongue whose anterior portion is divided by a longitudinal fissure.

cleid(o)- word element. [Gr.] *clavicle.*

cleidocranial (ˌkliedoh'krayni·əl) pertaining to the clavicles and head.

c. dysostosis a rare hereditary condition in which there is defective ossification of the cranial bones; complete or partial absence of the clavicles, so that the shoulders may be brought together in front; and dental and vertebral anomalies.

cleidotomy (klie'dotəmee) surgical division of the clavicle of the fetus in difficult labour to facilitate delivery.

clemastine ('kleməsteen) an antihistamine used in the treatment of allergic rhinitis and allergic skin disorders.

click (klik) a brief, sharp sound, especially any of the short, dry clicking heart sounds during systole, indicative of various heart conditions.

click–murmur syndrome (klik'mərmə) mitral valve prolapse.

clidinium bromide (klie'dini·əm) an anticholinergic used in combination with chlordiazepoxide.

climacteric (klie'maktə·rik, ˌkliemək'terik) menopause.

climatotherapy (ˌkliemətoh'therəpee) treatment of disease by means of a favourable climate.

climax ('kliemaks) the period of greatest intensity, as in the course of a disease.

clindamycin (ˌklində'miesin) a semisynthetic antibiotic derivative of lincomycin, which it has largely replaced; used as an antibacterial agent, but causes potentially fatal pseudomembranous colitis.

clinic ('klinik) 1. a session held by medical practitioners for the diagnosis and treatment of outpatients, e.g., antenatal clinic. 2. a building where patients attend for medical care.

clinical ('klinik'l) pertaining to or founded on actual observation and treatment of patients, as distinguished from theoretical or experimental.

c. trial assessment of effectiveness of modes of treatment by carefully following response to therapy in defined patient groups. A controlled clinical trial is one where a comparison is made of one or more active treatments against each other and against placebo.

double-blind c. trial comparison of different treatments (active and placebo) in which neither patients nor observers know which patient is receiving which treatment until a trial code is decoded after completion of the study.

clinician (kli'nishən) a medical practitioner involved in clinical medicine.

nurse c. see clinical NURSE specialist.

clinicopathological (ˌklinikoh,pathə'lojik'l) pertaining to both symptoms of disease and its pathology.

clinicoradiological (ˌklinikoh,raydi·ə'lojik'l) relating the bedside observations to the results of radiological investigations.

Clinistix ('klini,stiks) trademark for glucose oxidase reagent strips used to test for glucose in urine. The strip is dipped into the urine and results of positive or negative are indicated by the colour of the strip.

Clinitest ('klini,test) trademark for alkaline copper sulphate reagent tablets used to test for reducing substances, such as sugars, in urine. Ten drops of water and 5 of urine are placed in a test tube. The tablet, which generates heat, is added and the solution is allowed to boil. Within a few moments the colour of the solution is compared to a colour chart.

clinocephaly (ˌklienoh'kefəlee, -'sef-) congenital flatness or concavity of the vertex of the head.

clinodactyly (ˌklienoh'daktilee) permanent deviation or deflection of one or more fingers.

Clinoril ('klinə,ril) trademark for a preparation of sulindac, an anti-inflammatory agent.

clinoscope ('klienoh,skohp) an instrument for measuring the paralysis of the ocular muscles as shown by torsion of the eyeballs.

clip (klip) a metallic device for approximating the edges of a wound or for the prevention of bleeding from small individual blood vessels.

clition ('klieti·ən) the midpoint of the anterior border of the clivus.

clitorectomy, clitoridectomy (ˌklitə'rektəmee; ˌklitə·ri'dektəmee) excision of the clitoris.

clitoriditis (ˌklitə·ri'dietis) clitoritis.

clitoridotomy (ˌklitə·ri'dotəmee) incision of the clitoris.

clitorimegaly (ˌklitə·ri'megəlee) enlargement of the clitoris.

clitoris ('klitə·ris, 'kliet-) the small, elongated, erectile body in the female, situated at the anterior angle of the rima pudendi, and homologous with the penis in the male.

clitorism ('klitə,rizəm) 1. hypertrophy of the clitoris. 2. persistent erection of the clitoris.

clitoritis (ˌklitə'rietis) inflammation of the clitoris.

clitoromegaly (ˌklitə·roh'megəlee) clitorimegaly.

clitoroplasty ('klitə·roh,plastee) plastic surgery of the clitoris.

clivography (klie'vogrəfee) radiographic visualization of the clivus, or posterior cranial fossa.

clivus ('klievəs) pl. *clivi* [L.] a bony surface in the posterior cranial fossa sloping upward from the foramen magnum to the dorsum sellae.

cloaca (kloh'aykə) pl. *cloacae* [L.] 1. a common passage for faecal, urinary, and reproductive discharge in most lower vertebrates. 2. the terminal end of the hindgut before division into rectum, bladder, and genital primordia in mammalian embryos. 3. an opening in the involucrum surrounding necrosed bone. adj. **cloacal.**

cloacogenic (ˌkloh·əkoh'jenik) originating from the cloaca or from persisting cloacal remnants; said of a group of rare transitional-cell nonkeratinizing epidermoid anal cancers.

clobetasol (ˌkloh'beetəzol) a very potent corticosteroid used topically when other, weaker agents have failed.

clofibrate (kloh'fiebrayt) an anticholesterolaemic.

Clomid ('klohmid) trademark for a preparation of clomiphene.

clomiphene ('klohmi,feen) a nonsteroid oestrogen analogue used as the citrate salt to stimulate ovulation. Unfortunately the dose is difficult to determine and multiple pregnancy may result in some cases.

clomipramine (kloh'miprə,meen) an antidepressant drug used to treat patients with obsessional fears.

clonality (kloh'nalitee) the ability to form clones.

clonazepam (kloh'nazi,pam) a benzodiazepine derivative used as an oral anticonvulsant.

clone (klohn) 1. the genetically identical progeny produced by the natural or artificial asexual reproduction of a single organism, cell, or gene, e.g., plant cuttings, a cell culture descended from a single cell, or genes reproduced by recombinant DNA technology. 2. to establish or produce such a line of progeny. adj. **clonal.**

clonic ('klonik) pertaining to or characterized by clonus.

clonicity (klo'nisitee) the condition of being clonic.

clonicotonic (ˌklonikoh'tonik) both clonic and tonic.

clonidine ('klohni,deen) a centrally acting antihypertensive agent, also used in smaller doses to treat migraine.

clonism ('klonizəm) a succession of clonic spasms.

clonogenic (ˌklonoh'jenik) giving rise to a clone of cells.

clonograph ('klonohˌgrahf, -ˌgraf) an instrument for recording spasmodic movements of parts and tendon reflexes.

clonorchiasis (ˌklonor'kieəsis) infection of the biliary passages with the liver fluke *Clonorchis sinensis*, which may lead to inflammation of the biliary tree, proliferation of the biliary epithelium, and progressive portal fibrosis; extension into the liver parenchyma may lead to fatty changes and cirrhosis.

Clonorchis (klo'nawkis) a genus of Asiatic liver flukes.

C. sinensis a species prevalent in the Far East, particularly Japan, Korea, China, and Vietnam. Infection is contracted by eating uncooked freshwater fish containing encysted larvae.

clonospasm ('klonohˌspazəm) clonic spasm.

clonus ('klohnəs) alternate involuntary muscular contraction and relaxation in rapid succession.

ankle c., foot c. a series of abnormal reflex movements of the foot, induced by sudden dorsiflexion, causing alternate contraction and relaxation of the triceps surae muscle.

toe c. abnormal rhythmic contraction of the great toe, induced by sudden passive extension of its first phalanx.

wrist c. spasmodic contraction of the hand muscles, induced by forcibly extending the hand at the wrist.

clorazepate (klor'raziˌpayt) a benzodiazepine compound used as an antianxiety agent.

closing volume ('klohsing) the volume of gas in the lungs in excess of the residual volume (RV) at the time when small airways in the dependent portions of the lungs close during maximal exhalation; abbreviated CV. CV normally increases with age and is also increased in obstructive airways disease. It can be used to detect the disease in high-risk patients before symptoms appear. CV is measured by the single-breath nitrogen test. From RV the patient inhales pure oxygen to total lung capacity (TLC), and then expires slowly and evenly while the nitrogen concentration of the exhaled gas is recorded. Because the lower portions of the lung expand more during inspiration, the nitrogen remaining in the alveoli is mixed with more oxygen in the lower portions than in the upper portions. Thus when the closing volume is reached there is a sharp rise in the nitrogen concentration, because most of the gas is coming from upper air spaces. The closing capacity (CC) is equal to CV plus RV.

Clostridium (klo'stridi·əm) a genus of anaerobic spore-forming bacteria (family Bacillaceae).

C. bifermentans a species common in faeces, sewage, and soil, and associated with gas gangrene.

C. botulinum the agent causing botulism in man.

C. difficile a species often occurring transiently in the gut of infants, it is the aetiological agent of antibiotic-associated COLITIS.

C. histolyticum a species found in faeces and soil.

C. novyi a species that is an important cause of gas gangrene.

C. perfringens see *C. welchii* below.

C. septicum a species commonly occurring in animal intestines and soil, strikingly pathogenic for various animals and sometimes associated with gaseous infections in man. Called also *vibrion septique*.

C. tetani a common inhabitant of soil and human and horse intestines, and the cause of TETANUS in man and domestic animals.

C. welchii the most common causative agent of gas gangrene. Called also *Clostridium perfringens*.

clostridium (klo'stridi·əm) pl. *clostridia* [Gr.] any individual of the genus *Clostridium*.

clot (klot) 1. a semisolidified mass, as of blood or lymph. 2. to form such a mass.

c. retraction the drawing away of a blood clot from a vessel wall, a function of blood platelets.

clotrimazole (kloh'triemaˌzohl) a synthetic broad-spectrum antifungal agent applied topically in the treatment of diseases caused by dermatophytes and yeasts.

clotting ('kloting) the formation of a jellylike substance over the ends or within the walls of a blood vessel, with resultant stoppage of the blood flow. Clotting is one of the natural defence mechanisms of the body when injury occurs. A clot will usually form within 5 minutes after a blood vessel wall has been damaged. The exact process of clotting is not known; however, it is believed that the mechanism is triggered by the platelets, which disintegrate as they pass over rough places in the injured surface. As they disintegrate they release serotonin and thromboplastin. Serotonin causes constriction of the blood vessels and reduction of local blood pressure. Thromboplastin unites with calcium ions and other substances which promote the formation of fibrin. When examined under a microscope, a clot consists of a mesh of fine threads of fibrin in which are embedded erythrocytes and leukocytes and small amounts of fluid (serum).

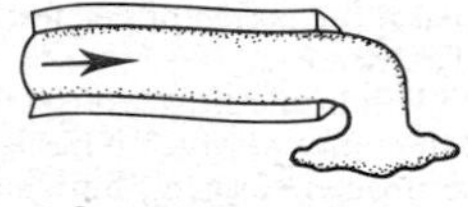

1. Severed vessel

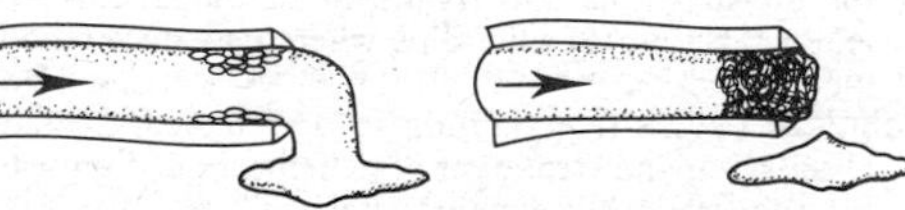

2. Platelets agglutinate

4. Fibrin clot forms

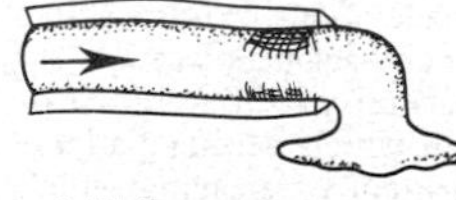

3. Fibrin appears

5. Clot retraction occurs

The clotting process in the traumatized blood vessel

At least twelve factors essential to normal blood clotting, whose absence, diminution, or excess may lead to abnormality of the clotting mechanism, have been described; they are designated by Roman numerals (I to V and VII to XIII; VI is no longer considered to have a clotting function).

Factor I. Usually called *fibrinogen*. A high-molecular-weight plasma protein that is converted to fibrin through the action of thrombin and that participates in stages 3 and 4 of blood clotting. Deficiency results in afibrinogenaemia or hypofibrinogenaemia.

Factor II. Usually called *prothrombin*. A glycoprotein present in the plasma that is converted into thrombin by extrinsic thromboplastin during the second stage of blood clotting. Deficiency leads to hypoprothrombinaemia.

Factor III. Usually referred to as *tissue factor* or *tissue thromboplastin*. A material that has a number of sources in the body and is important in the formation of extrinsic thromboplastin.

Factor IV. An appellation that is, in the scheme of haemostasis, assigned to calcium, because of its requirement in the first, second, and probably the third stages of blood clotting.

Factor V. A heat- and storage-labile material, present in plasma and not in serum, and functioning in the formation of intrinsic and extrinsic thromboplastins. Deficiency leads to parahaemophilia. Called also *accelerator globulin* and *proaccelerin*.

Factor VI. A factor previously called accelerin and thought to be an intermediate product of prothrombin conversion; it no longer is considered in the scheme of haemostasis, and hence it is assigned neither a name nor a function.

Factor VII. A heat- and storage-stable material, present in plasma and in serum and participating only in the formation of extrinsic thromboplastin. Deficiency, either hereditary or acquired (possibly owing to VITAMIN K deficiency), leads to haemorrhagic tendency. Called also *prothrombinogen* and *serum prothrombin conversion accelerator*, *SPCA*.

Factor VIII. A relatively storage-labile material present in plasma and not in serum, and involved in the formation of intrinsic thromboplastin. Deficiency, a sex-linked recessive trait, results in classical haemophilia. Called also *antihaemophilic factor* (*AHF*) and *antihaemophilic globulin* (*AHG*).

Factor IX. A relatively storage-stable substance, present in plasma and in serum, that is involved in the generation of intrinsic thromboplastin; a deficiency of this factor results in a haemorrhagic syndrome called haemophilia B or Christmas disease, which is similar to classical haemophilia A; called also *Christmas factor*, *plasma thromboplastin component*, *PTC*.

Factor X. A heat-labile material with limited storage stability at room temperature, present in plasma and in serum, that functions in the common pathway. Deficiency may result in a systemic coagulation disorder. Called also *Stuart factor*.

Factor XI. A stable factor, present in both serum and plasma, that together with factor XII forms a complex that activates factor IX in the formation of intrinsic thromboplastin. Deficiency results in haemophilia C. Called also *plasma thromboplastin antecedent*, *PTA*.

Factor XII. A stable factor, present in plasma and serum, that is activated by contact with glass or other foreign substances and initiates the process of blood coagulation in vitro; its precise role during in vivo haemostasis remains unclear; called also *Hageman factor*.

Factor XIII. A factor that polymerizes fibrin monomers. Deficiency causes a clinical haemorrhagic diathesis.

At least four platelet factors also exist that have a part in clotting.

It is possible for a clot to form within a blood vessel if the inner wall of the vessel has been roughened by injury or disease. Clots may form in conditions such as arteriosclerosis, varicose veins, and thrombophlebitis. An internal clot that remains at the place where it forms is called a thrombus; the general condition is called THROMBOSIS. If the clot (or pieces of it) breaks loose and flows through the blood vessels, it is called an embolus, and the condition is called EMBOLISM.

Clotting of the blood can be hastened by contact with injured tissue, by warming, by adding such coagulants as calcium, or by combination with thromboplastin and thrombin. The process can be retarded by cooling, by dilution, by adding oxalates and citrates, or by administration of substances such as heparin and dicoumarol, called ANTICOAGULANTS.

c. time the time required for blood to clot in a glass tube. Called also *coagulation time*.

cloxacillin (ˌkloksə'silin) a semisynthetic penicillin; its sodium salt is used in treating staphylococcal infections due to penicillinase-producing organisms.

clubbing ('klubing) proliferation of soft tissue about the terminal phalanges of fingers or toes, sometimes with osseous change.

clubfoot (ˌklub'fuht) a deformity in which the foot is twisted out of normal position. The medical term for this condition is talipes. The deformity is usually congenital but a few cases of clubfoot in older children may have been caused by injury or poliomyelitis. There are several types of clubfoot; the foot may be turned inward, outward, upward, or downward. Sometimes a combination of these defects may be present. See also illustration accompanying TALIPES.

There are several theories as to the cause of clubfoot. A familial tendency or arrested growth during fetal life may contribute to its development, or it may be caused by a defect in the ovum. It sometimes accompanies meningomyelocele as a result of paralysis. In mild clubfoot there are slight changes in the structure of the foot; more severe cases involve orthopaedic deformities of both the foot and leg.

Treatment varies according to the severity of the deformity. Milder cases may be corrected with casts that are changed periodically, the foot being manipulated into position each time the cast is changed so that it gradually assumes normal position. A specially designed splint also may be used. More severe deformities require surgery of the tendons and bones, followed by the application of a cast to maintain proper position of the joint.

clubhand (ˌklub'hand) deformity of the hand, resembling that of the foot in clubfoot; talipomanus.

clumping ('klumping) the aggregation of particles, such as bacteria or other cells, into irregular masses.

cluneal ('klooni·əl) pertaining to the buttocks.

clunis ('kloonis) pl. *clunes* [L.] buttock.

cluster sampling ('klustər) a method of sampling in which groups of persons rather than individuals are selected (for example, selecting whole family units or households).

clustering ('klustə·ring) a grouping of cases or other events in time or place (for example, a clustering of cases of legionnaires' disease in persons who visited a particular hotel at a particular time).

Clutton's joint ('klutənz) painless hydrarthrosis of the knee occurring in congenital syphilis.

clysis ('kliesis) the administration other than orally of any of several solutions to replace lost body fluid, supply nutriment, or raise blood pressure; also, the solution so administered.

CM [L.] *Chirurgiae Magister* (Master in Surgery).

Cm chemical symbol, *curium*.

cm centimetre.

cm² square centimetre.

cm³ cubic centimetre.

CMF Christian Medical Fellowship.

CMI cell-mediated immunity.

CMS Christian Medical Society.

cnemial ('neemi·əl) pertaining to the shin.

CNS central nervous system.

Co chemical symbol, *cobalt*.

co-codamol (koh'kohdəmol) preparations containing paracetamol and codeine used as an alalgesic.

co-codaprin (koh'kohdəprin) preparations containing codeine and aspirin used as an analgesic.

co-danthramer (koh'danthrəmə) preparations containing danthron and poloxamer used as a laxative.

Recently withdrawn from the UK market. See also DORBANEX.

co-dergocrine mesylate (koh'dərgohkrien 'mesilayt, -krin) a mixture of hydrogenated ergot alkaloids used for relief of signs and symptoms of idiopathic decline in mental capacity (including impairment of recent memory, confusion, and disorientation) in persons over 60.

co-dydramol (koh'didrəmol) preparations containing paracetamol and dihydrocodeine used as an analgesic.

co-proxamol (koh'proksəmol) preparations containing paracetamol and dextropropoxyphene.

co-trimoxazole (ˌkohtrie'moksəˌzohl) a mixture of trimethoprim and sulphamethoxazole; an antibiotic.

CoA coenzyme A.

COAD chronic obstructive airways disease.

coadaptation (ˌkoh·adap'tayshən) the mutual, correlated, adaptive changes in two interdependent organs.

coagglutination (ˌkoh·əˌglooti'nayshən) the aggregation of particulate antigens by agglutinins of more than one specificity.

coagulability (kohˌagyuhlə'bilitee) the state of being capable of forming or of being formed into clots.

coagulant (koh'agyuhlənt) promoting, accelerating, or making possible coagulation of blood; also, an agent that so acts.

coagulase (koh'agyuhˌlayz) an antigenic substance of bacterial origin, produced chiefly by staphylococci, which may be causally related to thrombus formation.

coagulate (koh'agyuhˌlayt) 1. to cause to clot. 2. to become clotted.

coagulation (kohˌagyuh'layshən) 1. formation of a clot. 2. in surgery, the disruption of tissue by physical means to form an amorphous residuum, as in electrocoagulation and photocoagulation.

disseminated intravascular c. (DIC) a disorder characterized by reduction in the elements involved in blood coagulation due to their utilization in widespread blood clotting within the vessels; the activation of the clotting mechanism may arise from any of a number of disorders. In the late stages, it is marked by profuse haemorrhage. See also DISSEMINATED INTRAVASCULAR COAGULATION.

c. factors factors essential to normal blood clotting, whose absence, diminution, or excess may lead to abnormality of the clotting; several factors, commonly designated by Roman numerals, have been described (see CLOTTING).

c. time clotting time.

coagulopathy (kohˌagyuh'lopəthee) any disorder of blood coagulation.

consumption c. disseminated intravascular coagulation.

coagulum (koh'agyuhləm) pl. *coagula* [L.] a clot.

coal tar (kohl tah) a by-product obtained in destructive distillation of bituminous coal; used in ointment or solution in treatment of eczema and psoriasis.

coalescence (ˌkoh·ə'lesəns) a fusion or blending of parts.

coapt (koh'apt) to approximate, as the edges of a wound.

coarctate (koh'ahktayt) 1. to press close together; contract. 2. pressed close together; restrained.

coarctation (ˌkoh·ahk'tayshən) stricture or narrowing.

c. of aorta a localized malformation characterized by deformity of the tunica media of the aorta, causing narrowing, usually severe, of the lumen of the vessel.

reversed c. pulseless disease.

coat (koht) a membrane or other tissue covering or lining an organ; in anatomical nomenclature called also *tunica*.

buffy c. the thin yellowish layer of leukocytes overlying the packed erythrocytes in centrifuged blood.

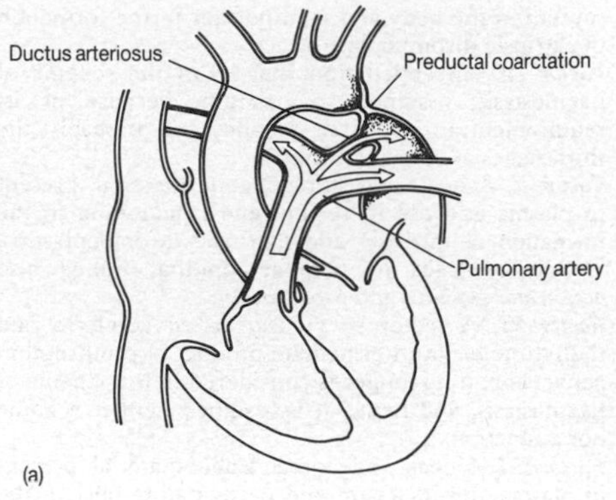

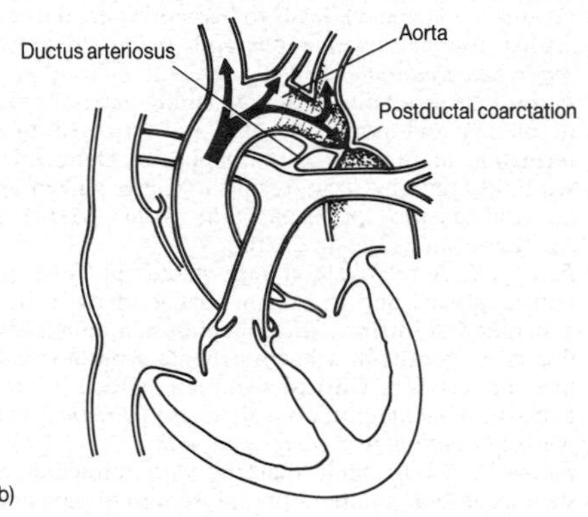

Coarctation of aorta. (a) Preductal. (b) Postductal

Coats' disease (kohts) chronic progressive retinopathy usually affecting male children, in which the fundus reveals an exudative retinal detachment associated with telangiectatic blood vessels and multiple haemorrhages; it may lead to total retinal detachment, iritis, glaucoma, and cataract.

cobalamin (koh'baləmin) a cobalt-containing complex common to all members of the vitamin B_{12} group.

cobalt ('kohbawlt) a chemical element, atomic number 27, atomic weight 58.933, symbol Co. See table of elements in Appendix 2.

c.-57 a radioisotope of cobalt having a half-life of 270 days; used as a label for cyanocobalamin. Symbol ^{57}Co.

c.-60 a radioisotope of cobalt having a half-life of 5.27 years and a principal gamma-ray energy of 1.33 MeV; used as a radiation therapy source. Symbol ^{60}Co.

Cobelli's glands (koh'beliz) mucous glands in the oesophageal mucosa just above the cardia.

cocaine (hydrochloride) (koh'kayn) an alkaloid derived from the leaf of the coca plant (*Erythroxylon coca*) which has a powerful but brief stimulant action. The drug is usually taken intranasally ('snorted'), though sometimes it is injected in combination with heroin. Long-term abuse is associated with a toxic psychosis similar to that caused by amphetamines. 'Crack' is a highly purified and extremely potent preparation of cocaine which is smoked and (in the USA) is rapidly replacing crystalline cocaine hydrochloride as a drug of abuse. Cocaine is also called coke, snow, 'C'.

cocainism (koh'kaynizəm) 1. addiction to cocaine. 2. the condition following continued use of cocaine, when the initial stimulation and feeling of well-being is followed by mental and physical deterioration.

cocarcinogen (ˌkohkah'sinəjən) an agent that increases the effect of a carcinogen by direct concurrent local effect on the tissue.

cocarcinogenesis (kohˌkahsinoh'jenəsis) the development, according to one theory, of cancer only in preconditioned cells as a result of conditions favourable to its growth.

cocci ('koksie) plural of *coccus*.

Coccidia (kok'sidi·ə) an order of sporozoa commonly parasitic in epithelial cells of the intestinal tract, but also found in the liver and other organs; it includes two genera, *Eimeria* and *Isospora*.

coccidia (kok'sidi·ə) plural of *coccidium*.

coccidial (kok'sidi·əl) of, pertaining to, or caused by Coccidia.

coccidian (kok'sidi·ən) 1. pertaining to Coccidia. 2. any member of the Coccidia; coccidium.

Coccidioides (kokˌsidi'oydeez) a genus of pathogenic fungi.

C. immitis the aetiological agent of coccidioidomycosis.

coccidioidin (kokˌsidi'oydin) a sterile preparation containing by-products of growth products of *Coccidioides immitis*, injected intracutaneously as a test for coccidioidomycosis.

coccidioidoma (kokˌsidioy'dohma) residual pulmonary granulomatous nodules seen radiographically as solid round foci in coccidioidomycosis.

coccidioidomycosis (kokˌsidi·oydohmie'kohsis) a fungal disease caused by infection with *Coccidioides immitis*. This fungus grows in hot, dry areas, especially in the southwestern United States, Mexico, and parts of Central and South America. The disease occurs in a primary and in a secondary form. The primary form, due to inhalation of windborne spores, varies in severity from that of the common cold to symptoms resembling those of influenza; called also *desert fever*, *desert rheumatism*, and *San Joaquin Valley fever*. The secondary form is a virulent and severe, chronic, progressive, granulomatous disease resulting in involvement of cutaneous and subcutaneous tissues, viscera, central nervous system, and lungs.

Treatment consists primarily of rest. Antibiotics may be given to prevent secondary bacterial infection. Amphotericin B or ketokonazole may be used to reduce the risk of extrapulmonary dissemination or to obtain remission after dissemination occurs.

coccidioidosis (kokˌsidioy'dohsis) coccidioidomycosis.

coccidiosis (kokˌsidi'ohsis) infection by coccidia. In man, applied to the presence of *Isospora belli* in stools; such infection is often asymptomatic, rarely causing a severe watery mucous diarrhoea.

coccidium (kok'sidi·əm) pl. *coccidia* [L.] any member of the Coccidia; coccidian.

coccobacillus (ˌkokohbə'siləs) an oval bacterial cell intermediate between the coccus and bacillus forms. adj. **coccobacillary**.

coccobacteria (ˌkokohbak'tiə·ri·ə) a common name for spheroid bacteria, or for various bacterial cocci.

coccoid ('kokoyd) resembling a coccus.

coccus ('kokəs) pl. *cocci* [L.] a spherical bacterium, usually slightly less than 1 μm in diameter, belonging to the Micrococcaceae family. It is one of the three basic forms of bacteria, the other two being bacillus (rod-shaped) and spirillum (spiral-shaped). Almost all of the pathogenic cocci are either staphylococci, which occur in clusters, or streptococci, which occur in short or long chains. Both staphylococci and streptococci are gram-positive and do not form spores.

The staphylococci are responsible for many serious infections, especially *Staphylococcus aureus*, which is the causative agent in boils, abscesses, osteomyelitis, and a large variety of other infections. The staphylococcus has received much attention in recent years because of the ability of most strains to develop a resistance to antibiotics.

The most dangerous streptococci are those of the beta-haemolytic type. Various species of streptococci cause sore throat, scarlet fever, mastoiditis, and septicaemia.

coccyalgia, coccydynia (ˌkoksi'alji·ə; ˌkoksi'dini·ə) coccygodynia.

coccygeal (kok'siji·əl) pertaining to or located in the region of the coccyx.

coccygectomy (ˌkoksi'jektəmee) excision of the coccyx.

coccygeus (kok'siji·əs) pertaining to the coccyx.

coccygodynia (ˌkoksigoh'dini·ə) pain in the coccyx and neighbouring region.

coccygotomy (ˌkoksi'gotəmee) incision of the coccyx.

coccyx ('koksiks) the small bone caudad to the sacrum in man, formed by the union of four (sometimes five or three) rudimentary vertebrae, and forming the caudal extremity of the vertebral column; called also os coccygis.

cochlea ('kokli·ə) a spiral tube forming part of the inner ear, shaped like a snail shell, which is the essential organ of hearing. adj. **cochlear**.

The cochlea is filled with fluid and is connected with the middle ear by two membrane-covered openings, the oval window (fenestra vestibuli) and the round window (fenestra cochleae). Inside the cochlea is the organ of Corti, a structure of highly specialized cells that translate sound vibrations into nerve impulses. The cells of this organ have tiny hairlike strands (cilia) that protrude into the fluid of the cochlea.

Sound vibrations are relayed from the tympanic membrane (eardrum) by the bones of hearing in the middle ear of the oval window of the cochlea, where they set up corresponding vibrations in the fluid of the cochlea. These vibrations move the cilia of the organ of Corti, which then sends nerve impulses to the brain. See also HEARING.

cochleariform (ˌkokli'ariˌfawm) spoon-shaped.

cochleitis (ˌkokli'ietis) inflammation of the cochlea.

cochleotopic (ˌkoklioh'topik) relating to the organization of the auditory pathways and auditory area of the brain.

cochleovestibular (ˌkokliohve'stibyuhlə) pertaining to the cochlea and vestibule of the ear.

coconsciousness (koh'konshəsnəs) consciousness secondary to the main stream of consciousness.

cod liver oil (kod livə) an oil pressed from the fresh liver of the cod and purified. It is one of the best-known natural sources of vitamin D, and a rich source of vitamin A. Because cod liver oil is more easily absorbed than other oils, it was formerly widely used as a nutrient and tonic, but it is rarely used today since more efficient sources are available. See also VITAMIN.

code (kohd) 1. a set of rules governing one's conduct. 2. a system by which information can be communicated.

genetic c. the arrangement of nucleotides in the polynucleotide chain of a chromosome that governs the transmission of genetic information to proteins, i.e., determines the sequence of amino acids in the polypeptide chain making up each protein synthesized by the cell (see also GENETIC CODE).

codeine ('kohdeen) an alkaloid obtained from opium or prepared from morphine by methylation; used as a narcotic analgesic and antitussive.

Codivilla's extension (ˌkohdi'viləz) extension of a limb by calipers or pins, transfixing or fixed into the bone.

Codman's triangle ('kodmənz 'trieˌang·g'l) a radiological sign in bone tumours.

codon ('kohdon) a series of three adjacent bases in one polynucleotide chain of a DNA or RNA molecule, which codes for a specific amino acid.

coefficient (ˌkoh·i'fishənt) 1. an expression of the change or effect produced by the variation in certain factors, or of the ratio between two different quantities. 2. in chemistry, a number or figure put before a chemical formula to indicate how many times the formula is to be multiplied.

absorption c. 1. the extent to which a beam of x-rays or other radiation is absorbed in a homogeneous material, equal to the fraction absorbed in a thin layer of material divided by the thickness of the layer. 2. a number indicating the volume of a gas absorbed by a unit volume of a liquid at 0 °C and at a pressure of 760 mmHg.

Bunsen c. absorption coefficient (2).

correlation c. a measure of the relationship between two statistical variables, most commonly expressed as their covariance divided by the standard deviation of each.

phenol c. a measure of the bactericidal activity of a compound in relation to phenol (see also PHENOL COEFFICIENT).

-coele word element. [Gr.] *cavity, space.*

Coelenterata (ˌseelentə'rahtə) a phylum of invertebrates including the hydras, jellyfish, sea anemones, and corals.

coelenterate (ˌsee'lentəˌrayt) 1. pertaining or belonging to Coelenterata. 2. an individual member of the phylum Coelenterata.

coeli(o)- word element. [Gr.] *abdomen, through the abdominal wall.*

coeliac ('seeliˌak) pertaining to the abdomen.

c. disease a malabsorption syndrome characterized by marked atrophy and loss of function of the villi of the jejunum (and rarely, the caecum). Called also *coeliac sprue, gluten-induced enteropathy, nontropical sprue,* and *adult, childhood,* or *infantile coeliac disease.*

The condition is related in some way to dietary gluten and is either a hypersensitive reaction to a protein in certain cereal grains or a local toxic inflammatory reaction to gluten. A hereditary factor has been implicated because the disease occurs in familial clusters. Diagnosis is usually made in young to middle-aged adults, but the onset of symptoms often is traced to early childhood. Until recently, it was thought that the infantile form (called also GEE'S DISEASE) and the adult form (called also GEE–THAYSEN DISEASE) were separate entities, but it is now believed that they are the same.

The symptoms of coeliac disease are fairly typical of all malabsorption syndromes. Manifestations include large, foul-smelling, bulky, frothy, and pale-coloured stools containing much fat. There are recurrent attacks of diarrhoea, with accompanying stomach cramps, alternating with constipation. There is some oedema and abdominal distention as in severe malnutrition, extreme weight loss, asthenia, deficiency of vitamins B, D, and K, and electrolyte depletion.

Diagnosis is based on intestinal biopsy and demonstrated pathological changes in the structure of the absorbing cells of the small intestine. In many cases, elimination of gluten from the diet produces a dramatic improvement in symptoms and restoration of normal function of the small intestine. Some patients experience remission within a few days, while others continue to have symptoms for months.

Treatment consists of placing the patient on a gluten-free diet that excludes all cereal grains except corn and rice. Since many prepared foods contain wheat, barley, rye and oats to provide bulk, the patient must be cautioned to read *all* labels on packaged foods, even ice cream, salad dressings, condiments, and many other foods one would not expect to contain cereal products. Further information can be obtained from the Coeliac Society of the UK, PO Box 181, London NW2 2QY.

The administration of corticosteroids may be necessary for some adults who do not respond to a gluten-free diet.

There is evidence that coeliac disease is associated with lymphoma and carcinoma of the small bowel. This is especially true of patients who have not been treated with a gluten-free diet.

c. crisis an attack of severe watery diarrhoea and vomiting producing dehydration and acidosis, which sometimes occurs in infants with COELIAC DISEASE.

coeliectomy (ˌseeli'ektəmee) 1. excision of the coeliac branches of the vagus nerve. 2. excision of an abdominal organ.

coeliocentesis (ˌseeliohsen'teesis) puncture into the abdominal cavity.

coeliocolpotomy (ˌseeliohkol'potəmee) incision into the abdomen through the vagina.

coelioenterotomy (ˌseeliohˌentə'rotəmee) incision through the abdominal wall into the intestine.

coeliogastrotomy (ˌseeliohga'strotəmee) incision through the abdominal wall into the stomach.

coelioma (ˌseeli'ohmə) a tumour of the abdomen.

coeliomyomectomy (ˌseeliohˌmieoh'mektəmee) myomectomy by abdominal incision.

coeliomyositis (ˌseeliohˌmieoh'sietis) inflammation of the abdominal muscles.

coelioparacentesis (ˌseeliohˌparəsen'teesis) paracentesis of the abdominal cavity.

coeliopathy (ˌseeli'opəthee) any abdominal disease.

coeliorrhaphy (ˌseeli'o·rəfee) suture of the abdominal wall.

coelioscope ('seeliohˌskohp) an endoscope for use in coelioscopy.

coelioscopy (ˌseeli'oskəpee) examination of a body cavity, especially the abdominal cavity, through a coelioscope.

coeloblastula (ˌseeloh'blastyuhlə) the common type of blastula, consisting of a hollow sphere composed of blastomeres.

coelom ('seelom, -lohm) body cavity, especially the cavity in the mammalian embryo between the somatopleure and splanchnopleure, which is both intra- and extraembryonic; the principal cavities of the trunk arise from the intraembryonic portion. adj. **coelomic.**

coeloscope ('seelohˌskohp) coelioscope.

coelosomy (ˌseeloh'sohmee) a developmental anomaly characterized by protrusion of the viscera from and their presence outside the body cavity.

coelothelioma (ˌseelohˌtheeli'ohmə) mesothelioma.

coelozoic (ˌseeloh'zoh·ik) inhabiting the intestinal canal of the body; said of parasites.

coenzyme (koh'enziem) an organic molecule, usually containing phosphorus and some vitamins, sometimes separable from the enzyme protein; a coenzyme and an apoenzyme must unite in order to function (as a holoenzyme).

c. A a coenzyme essential for carbohydrate and fat metabolism; among its constituents are pantothenic acid and a terminal SH group, which forms thioester linkages with various acids, e.g., acetic acid (acetyl CoA) and fatty acids (acyl CoA); abbreviated CoA.

c. Q any of a group of related quinones with isoprenoid units in the side chains (the ubiquinones), occurring in the lipid fraction of mitochondria and serving, along with the cytochromes, as an intermediate in electron transport; they are similar in structure and function to vitamin K_1.

coeur (kər) [Fr.] *heart*.

c. en sabot a heart whose shape on a radiograph vaguely resembles that of a wooden shoe; noted in tetralogy of Fallot.

cofactor ('kohfaktə) an element or principle, e.g., a coenzyme, with which another must unite in order to function.

cogener ('kohjinə) congener.

Cogentin (koh'jentin) trademark for preparations of benztropine mesylate.

cognition (kog'nishən) a broad term used to describe such mental activities as thinking, reasoning, etc. Often used loosely to describe any form of mental activity. adj. **cognitive**.

cohesion (koh'heezhən) the force causing various particles to unite. adj. **cohesive**.

Cohnheim's theory ('kohnhiemz) 1. the emigration of leukocytes is the essential feature of inflammation. 2. tumours develop from embryonic rests which do not participate in the formation of normal surrounding tissue.

cohort ('koh·hawt) in statistics, a group of individuals who share a characteristic acquired at the same time. The term usually refers to a birth cohort, which contains persons born in a specified time period.

c. study see INCIDENCE STUDY.

COHSE ('kohzee) Confederation of Health Service Employees.

coil (koyl) a winding structure or spiral; called also *helix*.

coition (koh'ishən) coitus.

coitophobia (ˌkoytoh'fohbi·ə) morbid fear of coitus.

coitus ('koytəs, 'koh·itəs) sexual union between human beings; usually called 'sexual intercourse'. adj. **coital**.

c. incompletus, c. interruptus coitus in which the penis is withdrawn from the vagina before ejaculation.

c. reservatus coitus in which ejaculation of semen is intentionally suppressed.

colation (koh'layshən) the process of straining or filtration, or the product of such a process.

colchicine ('kolchi,seen) a poisonous alkaloid from *Colchicum autumnale* (meadow saffron), used in treatment of gout and usually effective in terminating an attack of acute gout. Also used in CHROMOSOME analysis. Side-effects include gastrointestinal symptoms and hypotension.

cold (kohld) 1. coryza, an acute infection of the upper respiratory tract (see also COMMON COLD). 2. a relatively low temperature; the lack of heat. A total absence of heat is absolute zero, at which all molecular motion ceases.

A body temperature below 34.5 °C (94 °F) results in impairment of the heat-regulating centre in the hypothalamus. As the temperature drops, sleepiness and coma develop, and as a result the central nervous system heat-control mechanism is depressed and shivering (a means of heat production) is prevented. FROSTBITE is a local freezing of a surface area of the body and results from exposure to extremely low temperatures. Circulatory disturbances and gangrene can result from frostbite.

Induced HYPOTHERMIA, in which the body temperature is deliberately lowered and maintained below 32 °C (90 °F), is sometimes used during heart surgery and other types of surgery when it is necessary to slow or stop the heart action for several minutes. This type of prolonged cooling does not have any seriously harmful effects on the body provided that it is achieved slowly and that subsequent warming of the body is also carefully controlled.

USE OF COLD APPLICATIONS.

Effects. The primary effect of cold on the surface of the body is constriction of the blood vessels. Cold also causes contraction of the involuntary muscles of the skin. These actions result in a reduced blood supply to the skin and produce a marked pallor. If cold is prolonged there may be damage to the tissues because of the decreased blood supply.

Cold acts as a depressant to the activity of the cells and slows the heart action and pulse rate. By causing constriction of the blood vessels it may elevate the blood pressure. Intense cold numbs the sensory nerve endings so that impulses are not transmitted and sensations such as pain and taste are lost.

The secondary effects of cold are the opposite of its primary action. There is increased cell activity, dilation of the blood vessels, and increased sensitivity of the nerve endings. The outward appearance of the skin is a characteristic mottled blue or purple colour, and there is stiffness and numbness of the affected part.

Purposes. Cold applications may be used to control bleeding or to check an inflammatory process. Application of cold may inhibit the swelling and relieve pain and loss of motion in an inflamed area; however, it will not reduce oedema that is already present in the tissues. Because cold slows down activity of all living cells it may be used to check the growth of bacteria in a local infection.

Cold applications may be used in the emergency treatment of burns because the cold reduces the loss of fluids from the blood vessels into the tissue spaces and thus controls oedema.

Cool sponge baths, using cool water or occasionally alcohol, may be used to lower the body temperaure when FEVER is present.

Cold compresses are most often applied to the eyes for relief of swelling and inflammation. They also may be used to relieve the symptoms of haemorrhoids.

cold sore ('kohld ˌsaw) a lesion caused by the virus of HERPES SIMPLEX, usually on the border of the lips or nares.

colectomy (koh'lektəmee) excision of the colon or of a portion of it.

Colestid (koh'lestid) trademark for a preparation of colestipol, an antihyperlipoproteinaemic.

colestipol (koh'lesti,pol) an antihyperlipidaemic agent used as adjunctive therapy to diet for the reduction of elevated serum cholesterol in patients with primary hypercholesterolaemia.

colibacillaemia (ˌkohlie,basi'leemi·ə) the presence of *Escherichia coli* in the blood.

colibacillosis (ˌkohlie,basi'lohsis) infection with *Escherichia coli*.

colibacilluria (ˌkohlie,basi'lyooə·ri·ə) the presence of *Escherichia coli* in the urine.

colibacillus (ˌkohliebə'siləs) *Escherichia coli*.

colic ('kolik) 1. pertaining to the colon. 2. acute paroxysmal abdominal pain.

Colic usually refers to an attack of abdominal pain caused by spasmodic contractions of the intestine, most common during the first 3 months of life. The infant may pull up his arms and legs, cry loudly, turn red-faced, and expel gas from the anus or belch it up from the stomach.

The exact cause of infant colic is not known but several factors may contribute to its occurrence. These include excessive swallowing of air, too rapid feeding or overfeeding, overexcitement, and anxious parents. The infant can usually be relieved by being picked up, 'burped' gently, and given some warm water to drink. To relieve his tenseness he should be held and soothed with tender loving care. His condition is not serious and most infants gain weight and are healthy in spite of the colic.

biliary c. colic due to passage of gallstones along the bile duct.

lead c. colic due to lead poisoning.

menstrual c. dysmenorrhoea.

renal c. intermittent and acute pain usually resulting from the presence of one or more calculi in the kidney or ureter. The pain begins in the kidney region and radiates forward and downward to envelop the abdomen, genitalia, and legs. Other symptoms include nausea, vomiting, diaphoresis, and a desire to urinate frequently.

colicky ('kolikee) pertaining to or affected by colic.

colicoplegia (ˌkohlikoh'pleeji·ə) combined colic and paralysis produced by lead poisoning.

Colifoam ('kolifohm) trademark for an aerosol foam containing 10 per cent hydrocortisone acetate; used as an intrarectal anti-inflammatory.

coliform ('kohliˌfawm) pertaining to fermentative gram-negative enteric bacilli, sometimes restricted to those fermenting lactose, i.e., *Escherichia*, *Klebsiella*, *Enterobacter* and *Citrobacter*.

coliplication (ˌkohliplie'kayshən) COLOPLICATION.

colipuncture ('kohliˌpungkchə) colocentesis.

colisepsis (ˌkohli'sepsis) infection with *Escherichia coli*.

colistin (koh'listin) an antibiotic produced by *Bacillus polymyxa* var. *colistinus*, or the same substance produced by other means; it is related chemically to polymyxin, and is used in the treatment of urinary tract infections by bladder instillation. (It is not absorbed when given orally.) It is also used in bowel sterilization regimens in neutropenic patients.

c. sulphomethate a colistin derivative; the sodium salt is used in the treatment of infections, particularly those of the urinary tract.

colitides (kohli'tiedeez) plural of *colitis*; inflammatory disorders of the colon considered collectively.

colitis (kə'lietis, koh-) inflammation of the colon. There are many types of colitis, each having different aetiologies. The differential diagnosis involves the clinical history, stool examinations, sigmoidoscopy, and radiological studies such as a lower gastrointestinal series and fluoroscopy.

One of the most common forms of colitis is *idiopathic ulcerative colitis*, which is characterized by extensive ulcerations along the mucosa and submucosa of the bowel. Other types of colitis often can be traced to such aetiological factors as bacteria and viruses, drugs such as antibiotics, and radiation from x-rays or radioactive materials. Emotions can cause hypermotility of the gut and thereby produce symptoms typical of colitis.

There is a difference between true colitis and *irritable bowel syndrome* (formerly referred to by many names, including mucous colitis, irritable colon, and spastic colon), in which there is no actual inflammation of the gastrointestinal mucosa.

Almost all forms of colitis cause lower abdominal pain, bleeding from the bowel, and diarrhoea. The patient may have as many as 20 bowel movements a day, resulting in serious depletion of body fluids and electrolytes.

Treatment is aimed at eliminating or mitigating the underlying cause of the inflammatory process, resting and soothing the inflamed bowel, and restoring the nutritional status and fluid and electrolyte balance to normal.

antibiotic-associated c. colitis associated with antibiotic therapy, most commonly with lincomycin or clindamycin, but also with other broad-spectrum antibiotics, such as ampicillin and tetracycline. It can range from mild nonspecific colitis and diarrhoea to severe fulminant pseudomembranous colitis with profuse watery diarrhoea, abdominal cramps, and fever. The inflammation may be caused by a toxin produced by *Clostridium difficile*, a microorganism that is normally present in the resident bowel flora of infants, but is rarely found in adults. Presumably, the disruption of the normal flora allows the growth of *C. difficile*.

ischaemic c. acute vascular insufficiency of the colon, usually involving the portion supplied by the inferior mesenteric artery; symptoms include pain at the left iliac fossa, bloody diarrhoea, low-grade fever, abdominal distention, and abdominal tenderness. The classic radiological sign is thumbprinting, due to localized elevation of the mucosa by submucosal haemorrhage or oedema. Ulceration may follow.

pseudomembranous c. a severe acute inflammation of the bowel mucosa, with the formation of pseudomembranous plaques. It is most commonly associated with antibiotic therapy (see antibiotic-associated colitis above). The common symptoms are watery diarrhoea, abdominal cramps and fever. The pathological lesions are yellow-green pseudomembranous plaques of mucinous inflammatory exudate distributed in patches over the colonic mucosa and sometimes also in the small intestine. Called also pseudomembranous enterocolitis.

ulcerative c. chronic, recurrent ulceration of the colon, chiefly in the mucosa and submucosa, of unknown origin; it is manifested clinically by cramping abdominal pain, rectal bleeding, and loose discharges of blood, pus, and mucus with scanty faecal particles. Complications include haemorrhoids, abscesses, fistulas, perforation of the colon, pseudopolyps, and carcinoma. The patient with longstanding ulcerative colitis is at extremely high risk for the development of carcinoma of the colon (see also ULCERATIVE COLITIS).

colitoxicosis (ˌkohliˌtoksi'kohsis) toxaemia caused by *Escherichia coli*.

colitoxin (ˌkohli'toksin) a toxin from *Escherichia coli*.

coliuria (ˌkohli'yooə·ri·ə) the presence of *Escherichia coli* in the urine.

collagen ('koləjən) a fibrous structural protein that constitutes the protein of the white fibres (collagenous fibres) of skin, tendon, bone cartilage, and all other connective tissues. It also occurs dispersed in a gel to provide stiffening, as in the vitreous humour of the eye. It is made of monomers of tropocollagen. adj. **collagenous**.

c. diseases a group of diseases having in common certain clinical and histological features that are manifestations of involvement of CONNECTIVE TISSUE, i.e., those tissues that provide the supportive framework (musculoskeletal structures) and protective covering (skin and mucous membranes and vessel linings) for the body.

The basic components of connective tissue are cells and extracellular protein fibres embedded in a matrix or ground substance of large carbohydrate molecules and carbohydrate-protein complexes called mucopolysaccharides. For the sake of clarity and organization, collagen diseases may be divided into two major groups: (1) those that are genetically determined and are a result of structural and biochemical defects, and (2) those that are acquired and in which immmunological and inflammatory reactions are taking place within the tissues. Among the first group are those diseases caused by a lack of a specific enzyme necessary for proper storage and excretion of one or more mucopolysaccharides. Also included in this group are osteogenesis imperfecta, Ehlers–Danlos syndrome, and Marfan's syndrome. These disorders are distinguished by structural defects affecting the formation of the extracellular fibres called collagen.

Acquired connective tissue diseases are believed to develop as a result of at least two causative factors: a genetic factor and an abnormal immunological response. The exact role of these factors in the development of connective tissue diseases has not been firmly established, but there is strong evidence that immunological mechanisms are involved. Examples of collagen diseases that are most probably the result of an aberration of the immunological reactions that mitigate injury and inflammation of connective tissues are systemic lupus erythematosus, scleroderma, rheumatoid arthritis, rheumatic fever, polymyositis, and dermatomyositis.

collagenase (ko'laji,nayz) an enzyme that catalyses the degradation of collagen.

collagenation (ko,laji'nayshən) the appearance of collagen in developing cartilage.

collagenic (,kolə'jenik) 1. producing collagen. 2. pertaining to collagen.

collagenoblast (ko'lajinoh,blast) a cell arising from a fibroblast and which, as it matures, is associated with collagen production; it may also form cartilage and bone by metaplasia.

collagenocyte (ko'lajinoh,siet) a mature collagen-producing cell.

collagenogenic (ko,lajinoh'jenik) pertaining to or characterized by collagen production; forming collagen or collagen fibres.

collagenolysis (,kolaji'nolisis) dissolution or digestion of collagen. adj. **collagenolytic.**

collagenosis (,kolaji'nohsis) collagen disease.

collapse (kə'laps) 1. a state of extreme prostration and depression, with failure of circulation. 2. abnormal falling in of the walls of a part or organ.

circulatory c. shock; circulatory insufficiency without congestive heart failure.

c. therapy operative collapse and immobilization of the lung in treatment of pulmonary disease; artificial pneumothorax (see also surgery of the LUNG).

collar-bone ('kolə,bohn) the clavicle.

collateral (kə'latə·rəl) 1. secondary or accessory; not direct or immediate. 2. a small side branch, as of a blood vessel or nerve.

c. fissure, c. sulcus a longitudinal fissure on the inferior surface of the cerebral hemisphere between the fusiform and parahippocampal gyri.

Colles' fracture ('koliz) a break in the lower end of the radius, the distal fragment being displaced backward. If the lower fragment is displaced forward, it is a reversed Colles' fracture.

Colles' law an apparently healthy mother who gives birth to a child affected with congenital syphilis can breast feed her child without developing signs of syphilis.

colliculectomy (ko,likyuh'lektəmee) excision of the seminal colliculus.

colliculitis (ko,likyuh'lietis) inflammation about the seminal colliculus.

colliculus (ko'likyuhləs) pl. *colliculi* [L.] a small elevation.

seminal c. a prominent portion of the male urethral crest, on which are the opening of the prostatic utricle and, on either side of it, the orifices of the ejaculatory ducts; called also *verumontanum*.

collimation (,koli'mayshən) in microscopy, the process of making light rays parallel; the adjustment of two or more optical axes with respect to each other. In radiology, the elimination of the more divergent portion of an x-ray beam.

collimator ('koli,maytə) a device used in radiotherapy machines and also in diagnostic machines to help in determining the limits of the treatment field.

colliquative (ko'likwətiv) characterized by excessive liquid discharge, or by liquefaction of tissue.

collodiaphyseal (,koloh,dieə'fizi·əl) pertaining to the neck and shaft of a long bone, especially the femur.

collodion (kə'lohdi·ən) a highly flammable syrupy liquid compounded of pyroxylin dissolved in ether and alcohol, which dries to a clear tenacious film; used as a topical protectant applied to the skin to close small wounds, abrasions, and cuts, to hold surgical dressings in place, and to keep medications in contact with the skin.

flexible c. a mixture of collodion, camphor, and castor oil; used topically as a protectant.

salicylic acid c. flexible collodion containing salicylic acid, used topically as a keratolytic.

colloid ('koloyd) 1. gluelike. 2. the translucent, yellowish, gelatinous substance resulting from colloid degeneration. 3. a chemical system composed of a continuous medium (continuous phase) throughout which are distributed small particles, 1 to 1000 nm in size (disperse phase), which do not settle out under the influence of gravity. For example, if the disperse phase is a solid and the dispersing phase a liquid, the system is called a *sol*, such as glue. Milk is an example of an *emulsion*, in which both phases are liquid, one an oil and one water. Colloidal particles are not capable of passing through a semipermeable membrane, as in DIALYSIS. Solutes that can pass through a semipermeable membrane are sometimes called crystalloids.

c. degeneration the assumption by the tissues of a gumlike or gelatinous character.

sulphur c. a colloid formed by reacting sodium thiosulphate with hydrochloric acid, used with a radioactive label of technetium-99m for radioisotope imaging of liver and spleen.

colloidal (ko'loyd'l) of the nature of a colloid.

c. gold test a test of cerebrospinal fluid based on alterations in the albumin–globulin ratios that occur in certain disorders of the central nervous system. Normal spinal fluid, when diluted and added to a colloidal gold suspension, will not precipitate the colloidal gold. The extent of precipitation is indicative of various diseases such as multiple sclerosis, poliomyelitis, and encephalitis. A positive reaction also occurs in the presence of neurosyphilis. The sample of spinal fluid must not contain blood because this will cause a false-positive reaction.

colloidin (ko'loydin) a jelly-like principle produced in colloid degeneration.

collum ('koləm) pl. *colla* [L.] the neck, or a necklike part.

c. distortum torticollis.

c. valgum coxa valga.

collutory ('kolyuh,tə·ree) mouthwash or gargle.

colo- word element. [Gr.] *colon*.

coloboma (,koloh'bohmə) an apparent absence or defect of some ocular tissue, usually due to failure of a part of the fetal fissure to close; it may affect the choroid, ciliary body, eyelid (palpebral coloboma,

coloboma palpebrale), iris (coloboma iridis), lens (coloboma lentis), optic nerve, or retina (coloboma retinae).

colocaecostomy (ˌkohlohsee'kostəmee) caecocolostomy.

colocentesis (ˌkohlohsen'teesis) surgical puncture of the colon.

coloclysis (koh'loklisis) irrigation of the colon.

coloclyster (ˌkohloh'klistə) an enema introduced into the colon through the rectum.

colocolostomy (ˌkohlohkə'lostəmee) surgical formation of an anastomosis between two portions of the colon.

colocutaneous (ˌkohlohkyoo'tayni·əs) pertaining to the colon and skin, or communicating with the colon and the cutaneous surface of the body.

coloenteritis (ˌkohlohˌentə'rietis) enterocolitis.

colofixation (ˌkohlohfik'sayshən) the fixation of the colon in cases of ptosis.

Cologel ('kolohˌjel) trademark for a preparation of methylcellulose, which acts as a mild laxative by increasing intestinal bulk.

coloileal (ˌkohloh'ili·əl) ileocolic.

Colomycin (ˌkohloh'miesin) trademark for preparations of colistin sulphate or colistimethate sodium, antibiotics.

colon ('kohlon) the part of the large intestine extending from the caecum to the rectum. adj. **colonic.** The colon is divided into the *ascending colon*, which passes upward from the caecum to the lower edge of the liver, where it bends and becomes the transverse colon; the *transverse colon*, which lies across the abdominal cavity from right to left, below the stomach, and then bends downward to become the descending colon; the *descending colon*, which extends downward along the left side of the abdomen; and the *sigmoid colon*, which extends downward in an S-shaped curve from the brim of the pelvis to the sacrum, where it becomes the rectum. See also DIGESTIVE SYSTEM.

irritable c., nervous c., spastic c. terms formerly used for IRRITABLE BOWEL SYNDROME.

colonitis (ˌkohlə'nietis) inflammation of the colon; colitis.

colonize, colonization ('koləniez; ˌkoləniez'ayshən) the multiplication of pathogenic organisms in the body without causing disease.

colonopathy (ˌkohlə'nopəthee) any disease or disorder of the colon.

colonorrhagia (ˌkohlonə'rayji·ə) haemorrhage from the colon.

colonorrhoea (ˌkohlonə'reeə) mucous colitis.

colonoscope (koh'lonəˌskohp) an elongated flexible fibreoptic endoscope which permits visual examination of the entire colon.

colonoscopy (ˌkohlə'noskəpee) endoscopic examination of the colon, either transabdominally during laparotomy, or transanally by means of a colonoscope.

colony ('kolənee) a discrete group of organisms, as a collection of bacteria in a culture.

colopexy ('kohlohˌpeksee) surgical fixation or suspension of the colon.

coloplication (ˌkohlohplie'kayshən) the operation of taking in a dilated colon, a pleat or fold.

coloproctectomy (ˌkohlohprok'tektəmee) surgical removal of the colon and rectum.

coloproctitis (ˌkohlohprok'tietis) inflammation of the colon and rectum; colorectitis.

coloproctostomy (ˌkohlohprok'tostəmee) anastomosis of the colon to the rectum.

coloptosis (ˌkohlop'tohsis) downward displacement of the colon.

colopuncture ('kohlohˌpungkchə) colocentesis.

Colorado tick fever (ˌkulə'rahdoh) a nonexanthematous febrile disease occurring in the Rocky Mountain regions of the United States where the tick vector (*Dermacentor andersoni)* of the causative virus is prevalent.

colorectitis (ˌkohlohrek'tietis) inflammation of the colon and rectum; coloproctitis.

colorectostomy (ˌkohlohrek'tostəmee) coloproctostomy.

colorectum (ˌkohloh'rektəm) the distal 25 cm of the bowel, including the distal portion of the colon and the rectum, regarded as a unit. adj. **colorectal.**

colorimeter (ˌkulə'rimitə) an instrument for measuring colour differences; especially one for measuring the colour of the blood in order to determine the proportion of haemoglobin.

colorrhaphy (koh'lo·rəfee) suture of the colon.

coloscope ('kohlohˌskohp) colonoscope.

coloscopy (koh'loskəpee) colonoscopy.

colosigmoidostomy (ˌkohlohˌsigmoy'dostəmee) the surgical anastomosis of a formerly remote portion of the colon to the sigmoid.

colostomy (kə'lostəmee) an artificial opening (stoma) created in the large intestine and brought to the surface of the abdomen for the purpose of evacuating the bowels; also the opening (STOMA) so created. Conditions necessitating colostomy include INTESTINAL OBSTRUCTION, perforation of the bowel, CANCER, and birth defects. The operation may be required in occasional cases of ulcerative colitis.

The artificial anus may be permanent or temporary, depending on the primary condition being treated. A colostomy in the transverse or descending colon is unsuitable as a permanent stoma, sigmoid colostomy being the only acceptable permanent stoma.

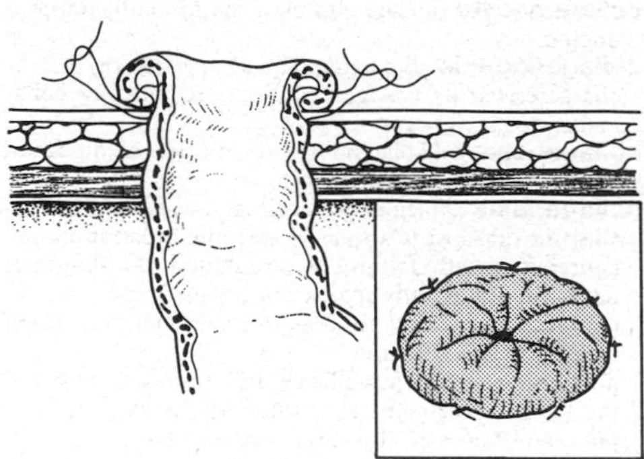

Single-barrelled end colostomy. The margins of the stoma are fixed to the skin with sutures

A double-barred, or a loop, colostomy is appropriate for temporary faecal deflection, ultimate closure being achieved by simple anastomosis of the proximal functioning opening to the distal end which is returned to the abdomen. End colostomy is *de rigueur* for a permanent opening, achieved by division of the sigmoid colon, the distal end being either closed and returned to the abdomen or brought on to the abdominal wall separately.

PATIENT CARE. Unless otherwise prohibited by physical weakness or mental incompetence, colostomy care is directed toward helping the patient become totally self-sufficient in the care of his colostomy. He is taught to care for the physical aspects of his colostomy and is assisted in adjusting psychologically to a new method of handling solid body waste. This is accomplished in stages, doing for the patient those things he cannot do, showing him the way they can be done, and encouraging him to accept responsibility for his own care. Once having overcome initial shock and revulsion at the prospect of colostomy care, most patients welcome the opportunity to care for themselves in privacy.

Before operation the procedure is explained to the patient and he is encouraged at this time to ask questions which concern him. The idea of an artificial anus in the abdominal wall may well be overwhelming to someone who has never heard of the operation. It is best to be open and matter-of-fact in discussing this with the patient, remembering that he cannot be expected to absorb too much information at one time. He should be assured that his questions will be answered as they occur to him, that there will be someone to listen to him when he wants to talk, and that there are many sources of information available to help him through his adjustment.

When the patient is ready to learn about caring for his own colostomy, information can be obtained from the Colostomy Welfare Group, 38–39 Eccleston Square, London SW1V 1PB, and from the Colostomy Advisory Service, Saltair House, Lord Street, Nechells, Birmingham B7 4DS (which has several branches in the UK). It is often helpful for the patient to talk to someone who has a colostomy and is living a normal active life. The certificated STOMA care nurse, is specially trained to work with colostomy patients and others who have permanent stomas.

Devices for collection of waste passing through the stoma vary in design according to the patient's progress. An open-ended bag is needed until bowel control is developed and then a closed pouch is used. Eventually the patient may need nothing more than a simple dressing over the stoma. Selection of a drainage pouch should be based on the size of the stoma. As the stoma shrinks following surgery, the pouch size is changed so that it fits correctly, not so small as to constrict the stoma, and not so large as to permit leakage around the stoma.

Skin care around the stoma is planned so the area is kept clean and protected from the enzymes and acid in the digestive fluid. The area is washed with soap and water, dried thoroughly, and then a medicated skin barrier such as karaya gum is applied.

Colostomy management is based upon obtaining a normal motion at a predictable time. To this end daily habits and meals are undertaken at routine intervals, as far as possible, and the patient learns in the postoperative period the items of food most likely to assist regularity of bowel function with passage of a formed stool. Recourse to colostomy irrigation is only had after the natural routine has proved to be inadequate; irrigation is by water enema at the beginning of the day. It is cumbersome and time-consuming.

The diet of a patient with a colostomy need not be severely restricted. He will need to notice which foods produce gas, diarrhoea and constipation, and then adjust his diet to reduce difficulties arising from his own individual problems with certain foods.

Odours may be a source of worry for the patient until he learns to control them with cleanliness, avoidance of gas-producing foods, and the use of deodorants within the pouch. Commercially produced deodorants are available, but if these cannot be found it is possible to eliminate much of the odour by placing four aspirin tablets in the pouch.

Patients with temporary colostomies may undergo barium studies of the intestines. Preparation of the bowel for these radiological studies should be carried out with care as the fluid and electrolyte balance of the patient can be easily upset. When the studies are completed, the barium must be removed in order to avoid intestinal obstruction.

Suppositories can be inserted into a colostomy stoma. If the patient has had a double-barred colostomy, the choice of stoma for insertion of the suppository will depend on the desired action of the drug. A glycerine suppository to facilitate passage of faecal material through the stoma would be inserted into the *proximal* limb to achieve the desired action. Conversely, a drug that is to be absorbed from the intestine, for example for the relief of pain, is inserted into the *distal* limb, from which it will not be expelled through the stoma.

Before inserting any kind of medication or a catheter for irrigation, the stoma should be digitally examined. The gloved finger is gently inserted into the stoma to determine the direction of the lumen of the intestine.

colostrum (kə'lostrəm) the thin, yellow, milky fluid secreted by the mammary gland from 16 weeks of pregnancy and for 3 to 4 days following birth until lactation is initiated. Colostrum is high in protein, and initially low in lactose; its fat content is equivalent to breast milk. It is an important source of passive antibody.

colotomy (kə'lotəmee) incision of the colon.

colour ('kulə) 1. a property of a surface or substance due to absorption of certain light rays and reflection of others within the range of wavelengths (roughly 370 to 760 nm) adequate to excite the retinal receptors. 2. radiant energy within the range of adequate chromatic stimuli of the retina, i.e., between the infrared and ultraviolet. 3. a sensory impression of one of the rainbow hues.

c. blindness inability to distinguish between certain colours. Genuine colour blindness, a complete inability to see colours, is quite rare, affecting only one person in 300,000. Generally the term describes some form of deficiency of colour vision. The most common form is red-green confusion, which affects approximately 8 per cent of males. There is no known cure for colour deficiency.

Colour vision is a function of the cones in the retina of the eye, which are stimulated by light and transmit impulses to the brain. It is now thought that there are three types of cones, each type stimulated by one of the primary colours in light (red, green, and violet). Most cases of colour deficiency affect either the red or green receptors, so that the two colours do not appear distinct from each other.

Colour vision is usually tested with cards called pseudoisochromatic colour plates. These have a letter, number, or symbol printed in dots of one colour in the midst of dots of grey or other colours. The normal person can see the symbol with no difficulty, but the person with colour deficiency cannot distinguish it from the background.

Although colour deficiency may occasionally result from injuries, diseases, or certain drugs, most cases are hereditary. The deficiency is most often inherited by males through the mother, who carries the trait from her father although she is not colour-deficient herself. In some cases, if the grandfather is colour-deficient and the mother carries the trait, a daughter may inherit the disability. The ratio of men to women affected with inherited colour deficiency is about 20 to 1.

colour index ('kulə,indeks) an index of the amount of haemoglobin in red blood cells. It is often estimated in examination of the blood, and is obtained by dividing the percentage of haemoglobin by the percentage of red cells of the norm. A normal colour index will give a value of 1. See BLOOD.

colovaginal (ˌkohlohvəˈjien'l) pertaining to or communicating with the colon and vagina.

colovesical (ˌkohlohˈvesik'l) pertaining to or communicating with the colon and urinary bladder.

colp(o)- word element. [Gr.] *vagina.*

colpalgia (kolˈpalji·ə) pain in the vagina.

colpatresia (ˌkolpəˈtreezi·ə) atresia, or occlusion of the vagina.

colpectasia (ˌkolpekˈtayzi·ə) distention or dilation of the vagina.

colpectomy (kolˈpektəmee) excision of the vagina.

colpeurysis (kolˈpyooə·risis) operative dilation of the vagina.

colpitis (kolˈpietis) inflammation of the vaginal mucosa; vaginitis.

colpocele (ˈkolpohˌseel) vaginal hernia.

colpocleisis (ˌkolpohˈkliesis) surgical closure of the vaginal canal.

colpocystitis (ˌkolpohsiˈstietis) inflammation of the vagina and bladder.

colpocystocele (ˌkolpohˈsistohˌseel) hernia of the bladder into the vagina.

colpocytogram (ˌkolpohˈsietohˌgram) a differential listing of the cells observed in smears from the vaginal mucosa.

colpocytology (ˌkolpohsieˈtoləgee) the quantitative and differential study of cells exfoliated from the epithelium of the vagina.

colpohysterectomy (ˌkolpohˌhistəˈrektəmee) removal of the uterus through the vagina, usually for prolapse of uterus.

colpomicroscope (ˌkolpohˈmiekrəˌskohp) an instrument for examining stained tissues of the cervix in situ.

colpomicroscopy (ˌkolpohmieˈkroskəpee) examination by means of a colpomicroscope.

colpoperineoplasty (ˌkolpohˌperiˈneeohˌplastee) plastic repair of the vagina and perineum.

colpopexy (ˈkolpohˌpeksee) suture of a relaxed vagina to the abdominal wall.

colpoplasty (ˈkolpohˌplastee) plastic surgery involving the vagina.

colpoptosis (ˌkolpopˈtohsis) prolapse of the vagina.

colporrhaphy (kolˈpo·rəfee) repair of the vagina.

anterior c. correction of a cystocele.

posterior c. correction of a retrocele.

colporrhoexis (ˌkolpəˈreksis) laceration of the vagina.

colposcope (ˈkolpəˌskohp) a speculum for examining the vagina and cervix by means of a magnifying lens; used for the early detection of malignant changes. adj. **colposcopic**.

colpospasm (ˈkolpohˌspazəm) vaginal spasm.

colpostenosis (ˌkolpohstəˈnohsis) contraction or narrowing of the vagina.

colpostenotomy (ˌkolpohstəˈnotəmee) a cutting operation for stricture of the vagina.

colpotomy (kolˈpotəmee) incision of the vagina with entry into the cul-de-sac.

colpoxerosis (ˌkolpohziˈrohsis) abnormal dryness of the vulva and vagina.

columella (ˌkolyuhˈmelə) pl. *columellae* [L.] a little column.

c. nasi the fleshy external termination of the septum of the nose.

column (ˈkoləm) an anatomical part in the form of a pillar-like structure; anything resembling a pillar.

anal c's vertical folds of mucous membrane at the upper half of the anal canal; called also rectal columns.

anterior c. the anterior portion of the grey substance of the spinal cord, in transverse section seen as a horn.

grey c. the longitudinally oriented parts of the spinal cord in which the nerve cell bodies are found, comprising the grey matter of the spinal cord.

lateral c. the lateral portion of the grey substance of the spinal cord, in transverse section seen as a horn; present only in the thoracic and upper lumbar regions.

posterior c. the posterior portion of the grey substance of the spinal cord, in transverse section seen as a horn.

rectal c's anal columns.

spinal c., vertebral c. the rigid structure in the midline of the back, composed of the vertebrae. See also SPINE.

columna (koˈlumnə) pl. *columnae* [L.] column.

coma (ˈkohmə) a state of unconsciousness from which the patient cannot be aroused, even by powerful stimuli.

PATIENT CARE. The patient in coma requires meticulous care and almost constant surveillance to maintain the integrity and function of all body organs. In the absence of gagging and swallowing reflexes, he must be fed intravenously or by TUBE FEEDING; SUCTIONING is necessary to remove secretions from the mouth and throat and maintain an open AIRWAY. In some cases TRACHEOSTOMY may be performed and a mechanical VENTILATOR used to maintain adequate respiration.

The comatose patient should be turned at least every two hours to relieve pressure on the skin and prevent pressure sores, to aerate the lungs and avoid hypostatic pneumonia, and to maintain good circulation in an effort to prevent formation of blood clots within the blood vessels. In order to minimize the danger of orthopaedic deformities he must be positioned so that the body is in good alignment, and his joints are kept functional by range of movement EXERCISES at least once daily.

Incontinence of urine is usually relieved at least once daily by an indwelling catheter and drainage apparatus. Loss of bowel control requires initiating a basic bowel programme to prevent faecal impaction. This involves regular digital removal of stool from the rectum or the insertion of a rectal suppository at the same time each day.

The patient's vital signs are taken and recorded at regular intervals throughout the day and night. Electronic monitoring equipment may be used. A very important part of assessment of the status of the comatose patient is determination of the level of CONSCIOUSNESS. This is done periodically by noting his response to various kinds of stimuli.

In carrying out the many details of the physical care and assessment of the comatose patient, health care personnel must not lose sight of the fact that the patient is a fellow human being and a member of a family. One cannot always be sure exactly how much the patient is aware of the quality of care he is receiving, the gentleness with which he is handled, or the courtesy and respect with which he is treated. Whether he is aware of or totally oblivious to what is being done to and for him, he deserves the same respect afforded an alert and aware patient. Members of his family can be greatly reassured and supported in their ordeal by the knowledge that he is receiving the best of care. Close relatives may wish to participate actively in the care of the comatose patient and this should be encouraged wherever possible since it may help to relieve their feeling of helplessness and may also aid the patient's recovery. With the life support devices now available it is possible for persons in deep coma to live for months and even years.

alcoholic c. stupor accompanying severe alcoholic intoxication.

alpha c. coma in which there are electroencephalographic findings of dominant alpha-wave activity.
diabetic c. the coma of severe diabetic ACIDOSIS (see also DIABETES MELLITUS).
hepatic c. coma accompanying cerebral damage resulting from degeneration of liver cells, especially that associated with CIRRHOSIS of the liver. **irreversible c.** brain DEATH.
Kussmaul's c. the coma and air hunger of diabetic acidosis (see also DIABETES MELLITUS).
c. vigil apparent wakefulness with absent or grossly diminished response to outside stimuli; called also akinetic autism.

comatose ('kohmə,tohs, -,tohz) pertaining to or affected with coma.

combustion (kəm'buschən) rapid oxidation with emission of heat.

comedo (ko'meedoh) pl. *comedones;* a blackhead; a plug of keratin and sebum within the dilated orifice of a hair follicle frequently containing the bacteria *Corynebacterium acnes*, *Staphylococcus albus*, and *Pityrosporon ovale* (see also ACNE VULGARIS).

comedogenic (ko,meedoh'jenik) producing comedones.

comedomastitis (ko,meedohma'stietis) mammary duct ectasia.

comes ('kohmeez) pl. *comites* [L.] an artery or vein accompanying a nerve trunk.

commensal (kə'mensəl) living on or within another organism, and deriving benefit without harming or benefiting the host individual.

commensalism (kə'mensəlizəm) symbiosis in which one population (or individual) is benefited and the host is neither benefited nor harmed.

comminuted ('komi,nyootid) broken or crushed into small pieces, as a comminuted fracture.

comminution (,komi'nyooshən) the act of breaking, or condition of being broken, into small fragments.

commissura (,komi'syooə·rə) pl. *commissurae* [L.] commissure.

commissure ('komis,yooə) a site of union of corresponding parts, as the angle of the lips or eyelids; used also with specific reference to the sites of junction between adjacent cusps of the heart valves.
anterior c. the band of fibres connecting the parts of the two cerebral hemispheres.
middle c. a band of grey matter joining the optic thalami; it develops as a secondary adhesion and may be absent.
posterior c. a large fibre bundle crossing from one side of the cerebrum to the other dorsal to where the aqueduct opens into the third ventricle.

commissurorrhaphy (,komisyooə'ro·rəfee) suture of the components of a commissure, to lessen the size of an orifice.

commissurotomy (,komisyooə'rotəmee) surgical incision or digital disruption of the components of a commissure to increase the size of an orifice.
mitral c., mitral valvotomy the breaking apart of the adherent leaves (commissure) of the mitral valve. This surgical procedure is indicated when the leaflets of the mitral valve have become scarred, usually as a complication of rheumatic fever, which prevents them opening and closing (mitral stenosis) with a resultant increase of pressure in the pulmonary artery and hypertrophy of the left ventricle.

Mitral valvotomy can be achieved either by rupture of the scar tissue by direct insertion of a finger into the heart and through the valve, or by open operation which necessitates maintenance of the circulation by a HEART-LUNG MACHINE.

If the valve is badly scarred or there are calcareous deposits, only partial relief can be obtained. Reoperation may become necessary when stenosis of the valve recurs.

Committee on Safety of Medicines (kə'mitee) an organization responsible for controlling the release of new drugs in the United Kingdom; abbreviated CSM. All manufacturers wishing to market a product require a licence from the CSM acting on behalf of the Department of Health (DH). The CSM will provide guidance on the data they require before issuing a licence. If they refuse to grant a licence, the manufacturer has the right to appeal to the Medicines Commission.

The CSM also collect data on adverse reactions to drugs via the yellow card system. This data enables the committee to issue warnings about serious adverse effects.

common cold ('komən) an acute infection of the upper respiratory tract, usually caused by one of a group of over 100 different rhinoviruses and sometimes by other respiratory and enteroviruses. Called also CORYZA. It occurs throughout the world, particularly in the winter and spring in temperate zones. Spread is from person to person by the airborne route by droplet infection or by direct contact with infected secretions. An individual is probably most infectious before the onset of symptoms and communicability lasts for up to five days. The incubation period is usually two days, but may range from 12 hours to three days.

SYMPTOMS. Usually the common cold starts with a runny nose, sneezing, a sore throat, slight headache, watering of the eyes, and malaise. Fever is uncommon. Symptoms usually persist for one to two weeks. Sinusitis, otitis media, laryngitis, and bronchitis may occur as complications. Antibiotics are of no value.

TREATMENT. There is no specific treatment. Asprin may be helpful in adults, but should not be used in children because of the possible association of this drug with Reye's syndrome.

common source outbreak an outbreak owing to exposure of individuals to the same infective or toxic source (for example, an outbreak of food poisoning as a result of eating the same contaminated food). Called also a *point source outbreak.*

communicability (kə'myoonikə,bilitee) transmissibility; ability to spread from infected to susceptible hosts.
period of c. the period of time during which an infection may be transmitted from an infected person to a susceptible individual.

communicable disease (kə'myoonikəb'l) a disease, the causative agents of which may pass or be carried from a person, animal or the environment to a susceptible person either directly or indirectly. Modes of transmission include: (1) airborne—directly by droplets or indirectly by droplet nuclei or dust; (2) contact—directly by physical contact with skin, mucous membrane or body secretions and excretions, or indirectly by contact with contaminated inanimate objects; (3) foodborne—by the consumption of contaminated food, milk or water; (4) percutaneous—by injection, abrasion or biting insects; and (5) transplacental—from mother to fetus.

PATIENT CARE. The goals of patient care include identification of the causative organism, control of the spread of the disease, protection of others from contamination, and specific measures to combat the disease and provide symptomatic relief. Specific techniques of disinfection of contaminated objects and isolation of the patient vary according to the type of causative organism and mode of transmission. See also ISOLATION TECHNIQUE.

Communicable Disease Surveillance Centre (CDSC) the national centre for the surveillance and control of communicable disease in England and Wales, for monitoring immunization and vaccination programmes, for epidemiological research in communicable diseases, and for training in this field. It is part of the Public Health Laboratory Service and has close links with the Department of Health and Social Security and the Welsh Office.

Communicable Diseases (Scotland) Unit the national centre for the surveillance and control of communicable disease in Scotland, with a function similar to that of the CDSC.

community (kə'myoonitee) a group of individuals living in an area, having a common interest, or belonging to the same organization.

c. health see community HEALTH.

c. medicine see community MEDICINE.

therapeutic c. any treatment setting (usually psychiatric) which provides a living-learning situation through group processes emphasizing social, environmental and personal interactions and which encourages the individual to learn socially from these processes. Self-determination, trust, respect and group consensus contrast with the usual hierarchical and authoritarian organization of therapeutic services. Feedback from the peer group increases self-awareness and group support increases the motivation to revise self-damaging or negative behaviours and attitudes.

commutator ('komyuh,taytə) a device by which the direction of an electrical current can be interrupted or reversed.

compaction (kom'pakshən) a complication of labour in twin births in which the pressure of one twin against the other causes the true pelvic cavity to be filled so that further descent is prevented. Called also *impacted* or *locked twins*.

compatibility (kəm,patə'bilitee) mutual suitability. Mixing together of two substances without chemical change or loss of power. See BLOOD GROUPING.

compensation (,kompən'sayshən) the counterbalancing of any defect of structure or function. In psychoanalysis, the mechanism by which an approved character trait is put forward to hide from the ego the existence of an opposite trait. In cardiology, the maintenance of an adequate blood flow without distressing symptoms. adj. **compensatory**.

complement ('kompliment) a complex series of enzymatic proteins occurring in normal serum that interact to combine with the antigen-antibody complex, producing lysis when the antigen is an intact cell. Complement comprises eleven discrete proteins, or nine functioning components symbolized as C1 through C9, with C1 being divided into subcomponents C1q, C1r, and C1s. Components C3 and C5 are involved in the generation of anaphylatoxin and in the promotion of leukocyte chemotaxis, the result of these two activities being the inflammatory response. The complement system is known to be activated by the IMMUNOGLOBULINS IgM and IgG, or by a variety of polysaccharide surfaces of low negative charge (low sialic acid content); the immunoglobulins activate via the 'classical pathway', and surfaces via the 'alternative' pathway. The latter are used in the classical pathway as an amplification step. Both cause activation of C3, leading to chemotaxis, phagocytosis and release of lysosomal enzymes.

c. fixation when antigen unites with its specific ANTIBODY, the first complement C1, if present, is bound. Its presence or absence as free, active complement can be shown by adding antibody-coated blood cells to the mixture. If free complement is present, haemolysis occurs; if not, no haemolysis is observed. This reaction is the basis of many serological tests for infection, including the Wassermann test for syphilis, and reactions for gonococcus infection, glanders, typhoid fever, tuberculosis, and amoebiasis. Called also *Bordet–Gengou phenomenon*. See also IMMUNITY.

complementary (,kompli'mentə·ree) pertaining to that which completes or makes perfect.

c. feed feed given to infants to supplement breast feeding when the mother has insufficient milk of her own.

complex ('kompleks) 1. the sum or combination of various things, like or unlike, as a complex of symptoms. 2. a group of associated, partially or wholly repressed ideas, usually outside of awareness, which can evoke emotional forces that influence an individual's behaviour. 3. that portion of an electrocardiographic tracing that represents the systole of an atrium or ventricle.

antigen–antibody c. a complex formed by the binding of antigen to antibody.

Electra c. libidinous fixation of a daughter toward her father. See also OEDIPUS COMPLEX.

factor IX c. a sterile, freeze-dried powder containing coagulation factors II, VII, IX, and X, extracted from plasma of healthy human donors.

Ghon c. primary complex (1).

Golgi c. a complex cellular organelle involved in the synthesis of glycoproteins, lipoproteins, membrane-bound proteins, and lysosomal enzymes; called also *Golgi apparatus* (see also GOLGI APPARATUS).

immune c. antigen–antibody complex.

inferiority c. unconscious feelings of inferiority, producing timidity or, as a compensation, exaggerated aggressiveness and expression of superiority (superiority complex).

major histocompatibility c. (MHC) the chromosomal region containing genes that control the histocompatibility antigens. In man, it controls the HLA antigens.

Oedipus c. libidinous fixation of a son toward his mother (see also OEDIPUS COMPLEX).

primary c. 1. the combination of a parenchymal pulmonary lesion (*Ghon focus*) and a corresponding lymph node focus, occurring in primary tuberculosis, usually in children. Similar lesions may also be associated with other mycobacterial infections and with fungal infections. 2. the primary cutaneous lesion at the site of infection in the skin, e.g., chancre in syphilis and tuberculous chancre.

superiority c. see inferiority COMPLEX.

complexion (kəm'plekshən) the colour and appearance of the skin of the face.

compliance (kəm'plieəns) the quality of yielding to pressure or force without disruption, or an expression of the measure of ability to do so, as an expression of the distensibility of an air- or fluid-filled organ, e.g., the lung or urinary bladder, in terms of unit of volume per unit of pressure.

The compliance of the lungs (C_L) and thorax (C_T) determine the elastic resistance to ventilation. The total compliance of the lungs and thorax (C_{LT}) is given by the formula $1/C_{LT} = 1/C_L + 1/C_T$. C_L is measured by determining the intrapleural pressure at different end-inspiratory volumes. A balloon-tipped catheter is used to determine the intrapleural pressure, which is transmitted through the soft wall of the oesophagus. C_L is usually divided by the functional residual capacity to give the specific compliance. Lung compliance is decreased in congestive heart failure and interstitial lung disease and increased in emphysema. C_{LT} can be measured by determining the change in lung volume for various amounts of pressure differ-

ence between the mouth and chest surface using a body plethysmograph.
complication (kompli'kayshən) 1. a disease(s) concurrent with another disease. 2. the occurrence of two or more disease in the same patient.
compos mentis ('kompəs 'mentis) [L.] *sound of mind, sane.*
compound ('kompownd) 1. made up of diverse elements or ingredients. 2. a substance made up of two or more materials. 3. in chemistry, a substance made up of two or more elements in union. The elements are united chemically, which means that each of the original elements loses its individual characteristics once it has combined with the other element(s). When elements combine in this way they do so in definite proportions by weight. Water, sugar, and salt are examples of compounds.

Organic compounds are those containing carbon atoms; inorganic compounds are those that do not contain carbon atoms.

quaternary ammonium c. an organic compound containing a quaternary ammonium group, i.e., a nitrogen atom carrying a single positive charge bonded to four carbon atoms. An example of a quarternary ammonium compound is choline.
compress ('kompres) a square of gauze or similar dressing, for application of pressure or medication to a restricted area, or for local applications of heat or cold.
compression (kəm'preshən) 1. the act of pressing upon or together; the state of being pressed together. 2. in embryology, the shortening or omission of certain developmental stages.
compromised ('komprə,miezd) lacking adequate resistance to infection, or lacking the ability to mount an adequate immune response, owing to a course of treatment (e.g., irradiation) or to an underlying disorder (e.g., leukaemia).
compulsion (kəm'pulshən) an overwhelming urge to perform an irrational act or ritual. adj. **compulsive.**

repetition c. in psychoanalytic theory, the impulse to reenact earlier emotional experiences.
computed tomography (kəm'pyootid tə'mogrəfee) a radiological imaging technique that produces images of 'slices' 1–10 mm thick through a patient's body; abbreviated CT (see also computed TOMOGRAPHY).
computerized axial tomography (kəm'pyootə·riezd 'aksiəl) computed tomography; abbreviated CAT.
conarium (koh'nair·ri·əm) the pineal body.
conation (koh'nayshən) in psychology, the power that impels effort of any kind; the conscious tendency to act.
conative ('konətiv, 'kohn-) pertaining to the basic strivings of a person, as expressed in his behaviour and actions.
concanavalin (,kongkə'navəlin) either of two phytohaemagglutinins isolated along with canavalin from the meal of the Jack bean (*Canavalia ensiformis* and other species of *Canavalia*), which agglutinate the blood of mammals as a result of reaction with polyglucosans. Concanavalin A has been shown to inhibit the growth of ascites tumours.
Concato's disease (kon'kahtohz) progressive malignant polyserositis with large effusions into the pericardium, pleura, and peritoneum.
concave ('konkayv, kon'kayv) rounded and somewhat depressed or hollowed out.
concavity (kon'kavitee) a depression or hollowed surface.
conceive (kon'seev) 1. to become pregnant. 2. take in, grasp, or form in the mind.
concentrate ('konsən,trayt) 1. to bring to a common centre; to gather at one point. 2. to increase the strength by diminishing the bulk of, as of a liquid; to condense. 3. a drug or other preparation that has been strengthened by evaporation of its nonactive parts.
concentration (,konsən'trayshən) 1. increase in strength by evaporation. 2. the ratio of the mass or volume of a solute to the mass or volume of the solution or solvent.

hydrogen ion c. an expression of the degree of acidity or alkalinity of a solution. See also ACID–BASE BALANCE and pH.

mass c. the mass of a constituent substance divided by the volume of the mixture, usually given as milligrams per litre (mg/l).

molar c., substance c. the amount of a constituent substance in moles divided by the volume of the mixture, usually given as millimoles per litre (mmol/l).

c. test a test of renal function based on the patient's ability to concentrate urine.
concept ('konsept) the image of a thing held in the mind.
conception (kən'sepshən) 1. the onset of pregnancy, marked by implantation of the blastocyst; the formation of a viable zygote. 2. concept.
conceptus (kon'septəs) the whole product of conception at any stage of development, from fertilization of the ovum to birth, including extraembryonic membranes as well as the embryo or fetus.
concha ('kongkə) pl. *conchae* [L.] a shell-shaped structure.

c. of auricle the hollow of the auricle of the external ear, bounded anteriorly by the tragus and posteriorly by the antihelix.

nasal c., inferior a bone forming the lower part of the lateral wall of the nasal cavity.

nasal c., middle the lower of two bony plates projecting from the inner wall of the ethmoidal labyrinth and separating the superior from the middle meatus of the nose.

nasal c., superior the upper of two bony plates projecting from the inner wall of the ethmoidal labyrinth and forming the upper boundary of the superior meatus of the nose.

nasal c., supreme a third thin bony plate occasionally found projecting from the inner wall of the ethmoidal labyrinth, above the two usually found.

sphenoidal c. a thin curved plate of bone at the anterior and lower part of the body of the sphenoid bone, on either side, forming part of the roof of the nasal cavity.
conchitis (kong'kietis) inflammation of a concha.
conchotomy (kong'kotəmee) incision of a nasal concha.
conclination (,konkli'nayshən) inward rotation of the upper pole of the vertical meridian of each eye.
concordance (kən'kawdəns) in genetics, the occurrence of a given trait in both members of a pair of twins. adj. **concordant.**
concrescence (kən'kresens) a growing together of parts originally separate.
concretio (kon'kreeshioh) [L.] *concretion.*

c. cordis adhesive pericarditis in which the pericardial cavity is obliterated.
concretion (kən'kreeshən) 1. a calculus or inorganic mass in a natural cavity or in tissue. 2. abnormal union of adjacent parts. 3. a process of becoming harder or more solid.
concussion (kən'kushən) a violent jar or shock, or the condition that results from such an injury.

c. of the brain loss of consciousness, transient or prolonged, due to a blow to the head; there may be transient amnesia, vertigo, nausea, and weak pulse.

Breathing often is unusually rapid or slow. Outward evidence of the injury may include bleeding and contusions (bruises). When the patient regains consciousness, he is likely to have severe headache, and may have blurred vision. If severely injured, he may lapse into a coma.

First Aid. The patient is kept lying down and quiet. He should be covered with a blanket or coat, and medical assistance should be obtained. Artificial respiration is given if breathing stops. Stimulants or drugs that may be depressants, e.g., pain relievers, should not be given; these drugs may mask the symptoms and make an accurate diagnosis difficult. See also HEAD INJURY.

condensation (ˌkonden'sayshən) 1. the act of rendering, or the process of becoming, more compact. 2. the fusion of events, thoughts, or concepts to produce a new and simpler concept. 3. the process of passing from a gaseous to a liquid or solid phase.

condenser (kən'densə) 1. a vessel or apparatus for condensing gases or vapors. 2. a device for illuminating microscopic objects.

condition (kən'dishən) to train; to subject to conditioning.

conditioned response (kən'dishənd) a response that does not occur naturally in the animal but that may be developed by regular association of some physiological function with an unrelated outside event, such as ringing of a bell or flashing of a light. Soon the physiological function starts whenever the outside event occurs. Called also conditioned reflex. See also CONDITIONING.

conditioning (kən'dishəning) a form of learning in which a response is elicited by a neutral stimulus which previously had been repeatedly presented in conjunction with the stimulus that originally elicited the response. Called also *classical* and *respondent conditioning*.

The concept had its beginnings in experimental techniques for the study of reflexes. The traditional procedure is based on the work of Ivan P. Pavlov, a Russian physiologist. In this technique the experimental subject is a dog that is harnessed in a sound-shielded room. The neutral stimulus is the sound of a metronome or bell which occurs each time the dog is presented with food, and the response is the production of saliva by the dog. Eventually the sound of the bell or metronome produces salivation, even though the stimulus that originally elicited the response (the food) is no longer presented.

In the technique just described, the conditioned stimulus is the sound of the bell or metronome, and the conditioned response is the salivation that occurs when the sound is heard. The food, which was the original stimulus to salivation, is the unconditioned stimulus and the salivation that occurred when food was presented is the unconditioned response.

Reinforcement is said to take place when the conditioned stimulus is appropriately followed by the unconditioned stimulus. If the unconditioned stimulus is withheld during a series of trials, the procedure is called extinction because the frequency of the conditioned response will gradually decrease when the stimulus producing the response is no longer present. The process of extinction eventually results in a return of the preconditioning level of behaviour.

classical c. see CONDITIONING.

instrumental c., operant c. learning in which a particular response is elicited by a stimulus because that response produces desirable consequences (reward).

Instrumental conditioning differs from classical conditioning in that the reinforcement takes place only after the subject performs a specific act that has been previously designated. If no unconditioned stimulus is used to bring about this act, the desired behaviour is known as an operant. Once the behaviour occurs with regularity the behaviour may be called a conditioned response. The classic example of instrumental or operant conditioning involves the use of the Skinner box, named after B.F. Skinner, an American behavioural psychologist. In this example the subject, a rat, is kept in the box and becomes conditioned to press a bar by being rewarded with food pellets each time its early random movements caused it to press against the bar.

The principles and techniques related to instrumental conditioning are used clinically in BEHAVIOUR THERAPY to help patients eliminate undesirable behaviour and substitute for it newly learned behaviour that is more appropriate and acceptable.

respondent c. see CONDITIONING.

condom ('kondəm) a sheath or cover worn over the penis in coitus, to prevent impregnation or infection.

conductance (kən'duktəns) ability to conduct or transmit, as electricity or other energy or material; in studies of respiration, an expression of the amount of air reaching the alveoli per unit of time per unit of pressure, the reciprocal of resistance.

conduction (kən'dukshən) conveyance of energy, as of heat, sound, or electricity.

aerial c., air c. conduction of sound waves to the organ of hearing through the air.

bone c. conduction of sound waves to the inner ear through the bones of the skull.

conductivity (ˌkonduk'tivitee) capacity for conduction.

conductor (kən'duktə) 1. a substance through which electricity, light, heat or sound may pass. 2. any part of the nervous system which conveys impulses.

conduit ('kondit, -dyuh·it) a channel for the passage of fluids.

ileal c. the surgical anastomosis of the ureters to one end of a detached segment of ileum, the other end being used to form a stoma on the abdominal wall.

condylarthrosis (ˌkondielah'throhsis) a modification of the spheroidal form of synovial joint, in which the articular surfaces are ellipsoidal rather than spheroidal.

condyle ('kondiel, -dil) a rounded projection on a bone, usually for articulation with another bone.

condylectomy (ˌkondi'lektəmee) excision of a condyle.

condylion (kon'dili·ən) the most lateral point on the surface of the head of the mandible.

condyloid ('kondiˌloyd) resembling a condyle.

condyloma (ˌkondi'lohmə) pl. *condylomata;* an elevated wartlike lesion of the skin. adj. **condylomatous.**

condylomata acuminata small, pointed papillomae of viral origin, usually occurring on the skin or mucous surfaces of the external genitalia or perianal region. See also genital WARTS.

flat condylomata condylomata lata.

giant c. acuminatum Buschke–Löwenstein tumour.

condylomata lata wide, flat, syphilitic condylomata occurring on moist skin, especially about the genitals and anus.

condylotomy (ˌkondi'lotəmee) transection of a condyle.

condylus ('kondiləs) pl. *condyli* [L.] condyle.

cone (kohn) 1. a solid figure or body having a circular base and tapering to a point, especially one of the conelike structures of the retina, which, with the retinal rods, form the light-sensitive elements of the retina. The cones make possible the perception of colour. 2. in radiology, a conical or open-ended cylindrical structure used as an aid in centring the radiation beam and as a guide to source-to-film distance. 3. surgical cone.

ether c. a cone-shaped device used over the face in administration of ether for anaesthesia.

c. of light the triangular reflection of light seen on the tympanic membrane.

pressure c. the area of compression exerted by a mass in the brain, as in transtentorial herniation.

retinal c's see cone (1) (above).

surgical c. a cone of tissue removed surgically, as in partial excision of the cervix uteri.

conexus (ko'neksəs) a connecting structure.

confabulation (kən,fabyuh'layshən) the recitation of imaginary experiences to fill gaps in memory.

confection (kən'fekshən) a preparation of sugar or honey containing drugs, e.g. senna.

configuration (kən,figyuh'rayshən) the general form of a body. In chemistry, the arrangement in space of the atoms of a molecule.

confinement (kən'fienmənt) restraint within a specific area; used especially to designate the natural termination of pregnancy with delivery of an infant.

conflict ('konflikt) a painful state of consciousness caused by presence of opposing emotional forces or desires and failure to resolve them, found to a certain extent in all persons.

extrapsychic c. that between the self and the external environment.

intrapsychic c. that between forces within the personality.

confluence ('konflooəns) a running together; a meeting of streams.

c. of sinuses the dilated point of confluence of the superior sagittal, straight, occipital, and two transverse sinuses of the dura mater.

confluent ('konflooənt) running together.

confounding variable (kən'fownding) see confounding VARIABLE.

confusion (kən'fyoozhən) disturbed orientation in regard to time, place, or person, sometimes accompanied by disordered consciousness.

congener (kən'jeenə, 'konjinə) something closely related to another thing, as a member of the same genus, a muscle having the same function as another, or a chemical compound closely related to another in composition and exerting similar or antagonistic effects, or something derived from the same source or stock. adj. **congeneric, congenerous.**

congenital (kən'jenit'l) present at and existing from the time of birth.

c. heart defect a structural defect of the heart or great vessels or both, present at birth. Any number of defects may occur, singly or in combination. They result from improper development of the heart and blood vessels during the prenatal period. Cardiac anomalies are found in 8 of every 1000 liveborn children in the UK.

A fairly common defect is TETRALOGY OF FALLOT, so-called because it involves four major defects and was first described by Fallot. It can, in some instances, be corrected by surgery. Another defect, PATENT DUCTUS ARTERIOSUS, involves the persistent presence of a passage, the ductus arteriosus, between the aorta and pulmonary artery. Normally this passage closes at birth.

VENTRICULAR SEPTAL DEFECT is an opening between the ventricles, often described by laymen as a 'hole in the heart'. This defect results in a flow of blood directly from one ventricle to the other, resulting in a bypassing of the pulmonary circulation and producing varying degrees of cyanosis because of oxygen deficiency. Defective valves affecting the flow of blood to and from the heart may be associated with this.

A rarer congenital condition is transposition of the great vessels. In this defect the position of the chief blood vessels of the heart is reversed. The aorta rises from the right ventricle instead of the left, and the pulmonary artery emerges from the left ventricle rather than from the right. The result of this circulatory confusion is that oxygen-poor blood returning from the systemic circulation to the right side of the heart is pumped back into the general circulation instead of being transported to the lungs. Meanwhile, oxygen-rich blood flows aimlessly to and from the lungs. Transposition of the great vessels can sometimes be corrected by surgery.

Another congenital defect results when the ostium primum or ostium secundum, openings in the septum primum of the embryonic heart, fails to close completely after birth. This condition is called atrial septal defect. When an opening remains between the atria, some of the oxygen-rich blood from the left atrium passes into the right atrium and travels back to the lungs without being first transported through the body. Coarctation of the aorta is a narrowing of a portion of the aorta.

In many cases—depending on the severity of the defect and the physical condition of the patient—these congenital conditions can be treated by surgery. Some congenital defects are so minor that they do not significantly affect the action of the heart; these kinds of defects do not require surgery.

The cause of most congenital abnormalities is unknown. In a small number of cases, rubella (German measles) when contracted by the mother during the first 2 or 3 months of pregnancy can cause congenital defects in the baby.

c. infection an infection which takes place in utero. The most important congenital infections are rubella, cytomegalovirus, herpes simplex, acquired immune deficiency syndrome (AIDS), syphilis, and toxoplasmosis. Some of these and many other infections may be acquired during or shortly after birth and are termed neonatal infections.

congestion (kən'jeschən) abnormal accumulation of blood in a part.

congestive (kən'jestiv) pertaining to or associated with congestion.

c. heart failure a broad term denoting conditions in which the heart's pumping capability is impaired (see also congestive HEART FAILURE).

conglobation (,kong·gloh'bayshən) the act of forming, or the state of being formed, into a rounded mass.

conglutinant (kən'glootinənt) promoting union, as of the lips of a wound.

conglutination (kən,glooti'nayshən) 1. the adherence of tissues to each other. 2. agglutination of erythrocytes that is dependent upon both complement and antibodies.

Congo red ('kong·goh) a synthetic dye, a derivative of benzidine and naphthionic acid. It is used for staining of amyloid in tissue sections, when a characteristic salmon-pink staining is produced, which when viewed through a polarizing filter show pathognomonic anomalous colours, particularly a bright apple green. Congo red undergoes a change in hue with acidity and thus can be used as an indicator of pH, turning red in the presence of alkalies (bases) and blue when exposed to acids.

C. r. test an obsolete laboratory test used in the diagnosis of AMYLOIDOSIS.

coniofibrosis (,kohniohfie'brohsis) pneumoconiosis with exuberant growth of connective tissue in the lungs.

coniosis (ˌkohniˈohsis) a diseased state due to inhalation of dust.

coniosporosis (ˌkohniohspoˈrohsis) a condition characterized by asthmatic symptoms and acute pneumonitis, caused by inhalation of spores of *Coniosporium corticale*, a fungus growing under the bark of certain trees; observed in workers engaged in peeling logs.

coniotoxicosis (ˌkohniohˌtoksiˈkohsis) pneumoconiosis in which the irritant affects the tissues directly.

conization (ˌkohnieˈzayshən) the removal of a cone of tissue, as in partial excision of the cervix uteri.

cold c. that done with a cold knife, as opposed to electrocautery, to better preserve the histological elements.

conjugate (ˈkonjuhˌgayt) 1. paired, or equally coupled; working in union. 2. a conjugate diameter of the pelvic inlet; used alone usually to denote the true conjugate diameter (see also PELVIC DIAMETER).

conjugation (ˌkonjuhˈgayshən) a joining. In unicellular organisms, a form of sexual reproduction in which two individuals join in temporary union to transfer genetic material. In biochemistry, the joining of a toxic substance with some natural substance of the body to form a detoxified product for elimination from the body.

conjunctiva (ˌkonjungkˈtievə) pl. *conjunctivae* [L.] the delicate membrane lining the eyelids and covering the anterior surface of the eyeball. adj. **conjunctival**. Its epithelium is continuous with that of the CORNEA.

conjunctivitis (kənˌjungktiˈvietis) inflammation of the conjunctiva. The disorder may be caused by bacteria or a virus, or by allergic, chemical, or physical factors. The bacterial and viral forms are infectious.

acute haemorrhagic c. a highly infectious form due to infection with enteroviruses.

gonorrhoeal c. a severe form due to infection with gonococci.

inclusion c. conjunctivitis primarily affecting newborn infants, caused by a strain of *Chlamydia trachomatis*, beginning as acute purulent conjunctivitis and leading to papillary hypertrophy of the palpebral conjunctiva.

conjunctivoma (kənˌjungktiˈvohmə) a tumour of the eyelid composed of conjunctival tissue.

conjunctivoplasty (ˌkənjungkˈtievohˌplastee) plastic repair of the conjunctiva.

Conn's syndrome (konz) primary hyperaldosteronism. The condition is characterized by an expanded extracellular fluid volume and marked potassium depletion, secondary to continuous elevation in aldosterone levels. If unchecked, the increased extracellular fluid volume can lead to cardiac decompensation and congestive heart failure. The hypokalaemia produces muscle weakness and fatigue and can affect the renal tubules, causing excessive loss of free water and a resultant hypernatraemia.

The most common aetiological factors in primary aldosteronism are adrenal adenoma, idiopathic hyperplasia of the adrenal cortex, and, rarely, carcinoma of the adrenal gland. Most adenomas affect only one of the pair of adrenal glands and therefore can be removed surgically without depriving the patient of a sufficient supply of adrenal cortical hormones. If total adrenalectomy is necessary, the removal of both glands creates a serious and potentially fatal insufficiency of the hormones these glands produce.

connective tissue (kəˈnektiv) a fibrous type of body tissue with varied functions. The connective tissue system supports and connects internal organs, forms bones and the walls of blood vessels, attaches muscles to bones, and replaces tissues of other types following injury.

Connective tissue consists mainly of long fibres embedded in noncellular matter, the ground substance. The density of these fibres and the presence or absence of certain chemicals make some connective tissues soft and rubbery and others hard and rigid. Compared with most other kinds of tissue, connective tissue has few cells. The fibres contain a protein called collagen.

Connective tissue can develop in any part of the body, and the body uses this ability to help repair or replace damaged areas. Scar tissue is the most common form of this substitute. See also COLLAGEN DISEASES.

Conray (ˈkonray) trademark for preparations of meglumine and/or sodium iothalamate used as a radiological contrast medium.

consanguinity (ˌkonsang·gwinitee) blood relationship; kinship. adj. **consanguineous**.

conscience (ˈkonshəns) an individual's set of moral values, the conscious part of the superego.

conscious (ˈkonshəs) capable of responding to sensory stimuli and having subjective experiences; awake; aware.

consciousness (ˈkonshəsnəs) the state of being conscious; responsiveness of the mind to impressions made by the senses. **clouding of c.** a moderate degree of lowering of consciousness, such as is found in mild confusional states, owing to disturbance of brain function.

levels of c. the somewhat loosely defined states of awareness of and response to stimuli, essential for the assessment of an individual's neurological status. The level of consciousness is an accurate indicator of the degree of brain (dys)function.

Consciousness depends upon close interaction between the intact cerebral hemispheres and the central grey matter of the upper brain stem. Although the hemispheres contribute most of the specific components of consciousness (memory, intellect, and learned responses to stimuli), there must be arousal or activation of the cerebral cells before they can function. For this reason, it is suggested that a detailed description of the patient's response to specific auditory, visual, and tactile stimuli will be more meaningful to those concerned with neurological assessment than would the use of such terms as 'alert', 'drowsy', 'stuporous', 'semiconscious', or other equally subjective labels.

An example of such a system is the Glasgow Coma Scale, now in wide use. It logically and independently evaluates three modes of behaviour, i.e. eye opening, verbal response and motor response. By the use of increasingly greater stimuli, ranging from verbal commands to painful stimuli, it arranges the responses in an order of increasing dysfunction, on a graph.

Reliability of the scale has been tested and proven and it greatly facilitates assessment of the patient with a compromised conscious level. A paediatric version has now also been developed.

consent (kənˈsent) in law, voluntary agreement with an action proposed by another. Consent is an act of reason; the person giving consent must be of sufficient mental capacity and be in possession of all essential information in order to give valid consent. A person who is an infant, is mentally incompetent, or is under the influence of drugs is incapable of giving consent. Consent must also be free of coercion or fraud.

In nonemergency situations, written informed consent is generally required before many clinical procedures, such as surgery, including biopsies, endoscopy, and radiographic procedures involving catheterization. The doctor must explain to the patient the diagnosis, the nature of the procedure, including the risks involved and the chances of success, and the alternative methods of treatment that are available. Nurses or other members of the health care team may be involved in filling out the consent form and witnessing the signature of the patient, or the parent or guardian if the patient is a minor. In medical research, the patient must be informed that the procedure is experimental and that consent can be withdrawn at any time. In addition, he must be informed of the risks and benefits of the experimental procedure and of alternative treatments.

conservative (kən'sərvətiv) the use of non-radical methods to restore health and preserve function.

consolidation (kən,soli'dayshən) solidification; the process of becoming solidified or the condition of being solid; said especially of the lung as it fills with exudate in pneumonia.

constipation (,konsti'payshən) ordinarily a condition in which the waste matter in the bowels is too hard to pass easily, or in which bowel movements are so infrequent that discomfort or uncomfortable symptoms result. Many people also use the term when referring to a sense of incomplete evacuation or when they feel they should have more frequent bowel movements. The frequency of bowel movements varies according to individual body make-up, type of intestine, eating habits, physical activity, and custom.

CAUSES. An organic cause of constipation may be a disease such as hypothyroidism. Or there may be a structure or obstruction that prevents wastes from being passed through the intestines, as in the case of hernia, tumour, or cancerous growth. Often constipation from such obstructions comes on suddenly.

SYMPTOMS. Prolonged constipation, called obstipation, can cause such uncomfortable symptoms as nausea, heartburn, headache, or distress in the rectum or intestines, which may last until the stool is passed. These symptoms are not due to the absorption of poisons from the waste material, as some people believe. Rather they are a reaction of the nerves when the rectum is distended by the matter it contains. This condition is uncomfortable rather than harmful.

PREVENTION AND TREATMENT. Elimination is largely a matter of habit. Therefore it is desirable to establish a regular routine for it. Sensible living can also help to prevent or combat constipation. Emotional tension and strain can cause constipation. Therefore, it is important to avoid unnecessary tensions and worry, including concern over constipation itself.

When constipation does not respond to addition of fibre to the diet and an effort to improve bowel habits, an enema may be advisable, or a mild laxative such as liquid paraffin, aromatic cascara sagrada, or milk of magnesia may be taken. Laxatives should be resorted to only after the bowels have been given a chance to function by themselves. The frequent and often unnecessary use of laxatives can be the cause of constipation, rather than its cure. Cathartics, such as castor oil, which are more powerful in their purgative action than laxatives, should never be used unless prescribed by a doctor. See also BOWEL TRAINING.

constitution (,konsti'tyooshən) 1. the make-up or functional habit of the body. 2. the order in which the atoms of a molecule are joined together.

constitutional (,konsti'tyooshənəl) 1. affecting the whole constitution of the body; not local. 2. pertaining to the constitution.

constriction (kən'strikshən) 1. a narrowing or compression of a part; a stricture. 2. a diminution in range of thinking or feeling, associated with diminished spontaneity.

constrictor (kən'striktə) that which causes constriction.

consultant (kən'sult'nt) a doctor or surgeon whose opinion on diagnosis or treatment is sought by the doctor originally attending a patient.

consultation (,kons'l'tayshən) a deliberation of two or more doctors about diagnosis or treatment in a particular case.

consumption (kən'sumpshən) 1. the act of consuming, or the process of being consumed. 2. a wasting away of the body; once applied especially to pulmonary tuberculosis.

contact ('kontakt) 1. a mutual touching of two bodies or persons. 2. an individual known to have been in association with an infected person or animal or a contaminated environment which might have exposed him to infection.

c. dermatitis a skin rash marked by itching, swelling, blistering, oozing, and scaling. It is caused by direct contact between the skin and a substance to which the person is allergic or sensitive. The rash usually occurs only on that area of the body that has come into contact with the irritating substance. Contact dermatitis may be caused by industrial oils, medicines, cosmetics, perfumes, mouthwashes, deodorants, rubber, plastics, metals, some plants, and clothing made of various materials and treated with certain preservatives and dyes. A nonallergic form, primary-irritant dermatitis, may be induced by a substance acting as an irritant rather than as a sensitizer or allergen. Some soaps, detergents, and other cleansing products can cause a condition of the hands often referred to as 'housewives' dermatitis' or 'housewife's eczema'. See also DERMATITIS.

direct c., immediate c. the contact of a healthy person with a person having a communicable disease or carrying a pathogenic organism (for example, direct skin contact or contact of mucous membranes, as in kissing or sexual intercourse).

indirect c. the contact of a healthy person with a pathogenic organism indirectly by means of inanimate objects (fomites) or vectors such as insects.

c. lenses corrective lenses that fit directly over the cornea of the eye, for correction of refractive errors. They do not actually touch the surface of the eye, but float on a thin layer of the fluid that naturally moistens the eyeball.

There are two main types of contact lenses: hard and soft. The hard lenses were the first to be developed and are still used because they are durable, easy to care for, and relatively inexpensive. They also provide good vision, especially in the correction of ASTIGMATISM. Their chief disadvantage is their inflexibility, which makes them difficult to fit to the shape of the eyeball.

The newer, soft lenses are more comfortable because of their flexibility. However, they do not provide such sharp vision as do conventional glasses and hard lenses. Moreover, the surface of soft lenses can harbour bacteria; therefore there is a higher risk of infection. For this reason, the lenses must be periodically disinfected; thus they require more care than do hard lenses. Another disadvantage is that soft lenses are more easily damaged and must be replaced more frequently than the hard ones.

A more recent development is gas-permeable lenses. They have the same advantages as hard lenses; that is, they are durable, easy to care for, and have a high optical quality. In addition, they allow the cornea to 'breathe' by permitting the passage of oxygen and carbon dioxide to and from the cornea, and tears flow more easily across the eye when these lenses are worn.

As newer materials are developed, there will be an even greater variety of contact lenses from which to choose. There is the possibility that inexpensive disposable contact lenses will soon become available.

Contact lenses are convenient to wear and cosmetically more appealing to most people than are conventional glasses. Moreover, because they correct vision problems through the entire visual field, contact lenses are more desirable for certain kinds of eye disorders. For example, they eliminate the difficulties associated with the thick lenses of the cataract glasses previously required for all patients following CATARACT extraction. Irregular scarring of the cornea cannot be helped by spectacles but contact lenses can improve vision when the cornea has been injured.

There are relatively few serious problems caused by wearing contact lenses. If the lenses are properly fitted and the patient regularly has his eyes checked, there should be no great difficulty. Signs of continued irritation and infection should be reported to the ophthalmologist promptly in order to avoid scarring and permanent loss of vision.

mediate c. indirect contact.

contactant (kon'taktənt) an allergen capable of inducing delayed contact-type hypersensitivity of the epidermis after one or more episodes of contact.

contagion (kən'tayjən) 1. the spread of disease from one person to another by contact/touch. 2. a contagious disease.

contagious (kən'tayjəs) capable of being transmitted by touch from person-to-person. See also contagious DISEASE.

containment (kən'taynmənt) a term used in communicable disease control, meaning prevention of spread of disease from a focus of infection. For example, if a case of diphtheria is imported into the UK, containment is achieved by searching for and isolating other cases and carriers, and by protecting all close contacts by immunization or chemotherapy.

contaminant (kən'taminənt) something that causes contamination.

contamination (kən,tami'nayshən) 1. presence of pathogenic organisms on the body surface or in wounds, in food or drink, and on inanimate objects. 2. the deposition of radioactive material in any place where it is not desired.

content ('kontent) that which is contained within a thing.

latent c. the part of a dream that is hidden in the unconsciousness.

manifest c. the part of a dream that is remembered after awakening.

continence ('kontinəns) the ability to exercise voluntary control over natural impulses, such as the urge to defecate or urinate. adj. **continent.**

c. adviser a nurse who specializes in the maintenance of continence and management of incontinence.

contingency table (kən'tinjənsee) a statistical term used to mean a cross-tabulation of two or more characteristics (for example, in a study of vaccine efficacy, the duration of time after vaccination of individuals might be recorded horizontally across the table and their antibody levels vertically). The tabulation permits statistical tests to detect any significant variation in antibody levels with time.

continuing care (kə'tinyooing) the level of care in the HEALTH CARE SYSTEM that consists of ongoing care of the physically, mentally and emotionally handicapped, and those suffering from chronic incapacitating illness.

continuing education further study after the attainment of basic qualifications. This is vital for all professional practitioners so that they may keep up to date within their field and is accomplished in the form of organized study days or courses, or by individual reading.

continuing source outbreak an outbreak in which new cases continue to occur over a long period of time, owing to persistence of the source of infection.

continuous positive airway pressure a method of medical gas administration in which gas is delivered to the patient at positive pressure in order to hold open alveoli that would normally close at the end of expiration and thereby increase oxygenation and reduce the work of breathing. Abbreviated CPAP. CPAP is used with patients who are breathing spontaneously. When the same principle is used in mechanical ventilation, it is called *positive end-expiratory pressure* (*PEEP*).

continuous variable see continuous DATA.

contra- word element. [L.] *against, opposed.*

contra-aperture (,kontrə'apəchə) a second opening made in an abscess to facilitate the discharge of its contents.

contraception (,kontrə'sepshən) prevention of conception or impregnation. Contraception may be achieved by several methods. See also BIRTH CONTROL.

RHYTHM METHOD. This is called the natural method since it uses no artificial means and is based on the natural cycle of ovulation in the female. The period of possible conception usually lasts from 2 days before ovulation until 1 day after it, or 3 days in all; during this time if conception is to be prevented, the woman must abstain from coitus. The other days of the cycle constitute the so-called 'safe period'. In practice, however, the safe period is considered to be shorter, since ovulation generally occurs between the twelfth and sixteenth days of the cycle, so that any of these days must be counted as days of possible conception. The first day of the cycle is the first day of menstruation.

To calculate the fertile period, it is necessary to keep an accurate record of menstrual cycles for 8 to 12 months. The length of the longest and shortest cycles must be carefully noted over this time.

It is also possible to determine when ovulation takes place by daily readings of body temperature since the temperature is elevated by 0.3 °C the day after ovulation takes place. These readings need to be continued over a period of several months. Even when such measurements are used, this method has a 20% failure rate.

OVULATION METHOD. Recent research into 'rhythm failures' has led to the development of a more reliable technique of natural contraception, the ovulation method (or Billings method). It is based on an awareness of days of 'dryness' and days of 'wetness' during the menstrual cycle, and recognition of the significance of a unique 'fertile mucus' which appears in the vaginal area at the time of ovulation. According to proponents of this method, appearance of the mucus signals the onset of the period during which impregnation can occur. See also LEUKORRHOEA.

Success of the ovulation method depends on the female's ability to observe and recognize the characteristics of a vaginal discharge which gives warning of the period of ovulation. The cycle begins with the onset of menstruation. Following menses there are 'early dry days' during which no mucus is seen or felt in the vaginal area. With the ripening of the ovum just prior to ovulation, there is production of some opaque and sticky mucus which is generally yellow or white, non-irritating and non-offensive. As the menstrual cycle proceeds and hormonal changes take place, the blood oestrogen level reaches a critical stage, at which point the cervical glands begin to produce the fertile mucus. This mucus usually appears three days prior to

(a)

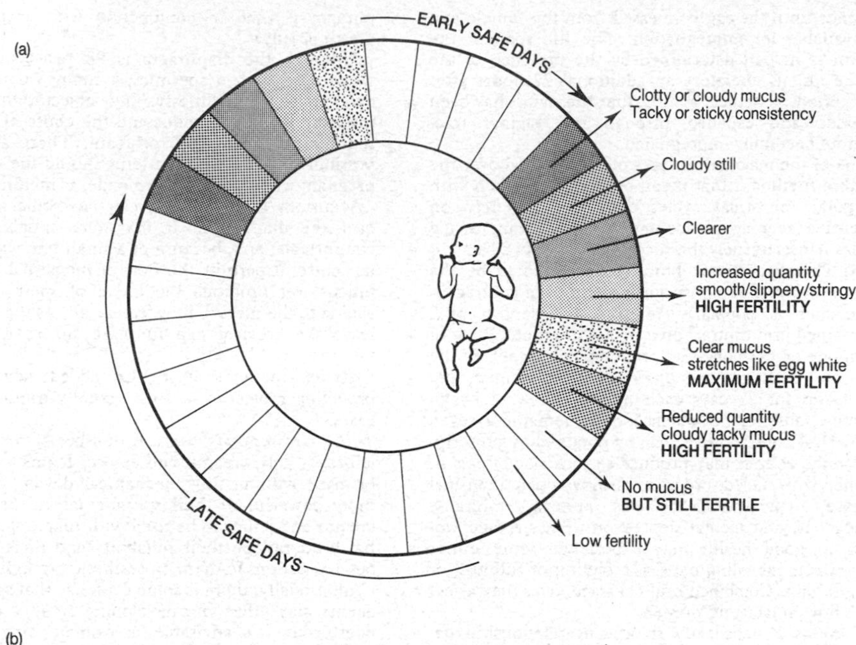

(b)

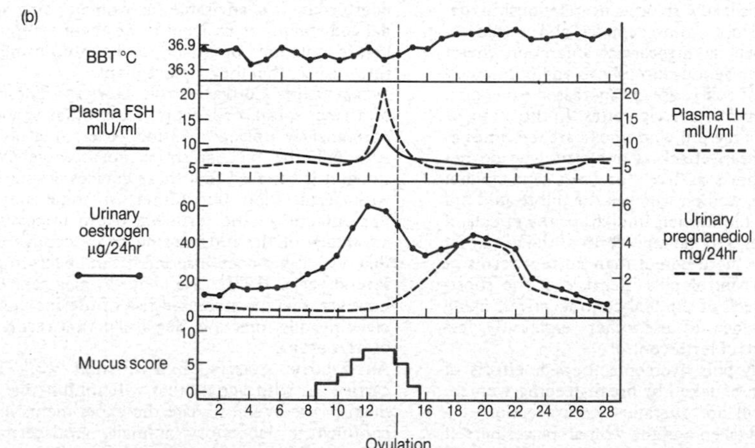

Billings Mucus Observation Chart and the Menstrual Cycle

(a) Billings mucus identification chart used to help patients identify the type of cervical mucus which is felt in the vagina each day. This illustration is merely a guide since the mucus consistency will not necessarily follow the exact pattern or length of days indicated here. Observation of change in mucus enables approximately 50% of women to have 6 days' warning of impending ovulation.

(b) Basal temperature, plasma follicle stimulating hormone and luteinizing hormone, urinary oestrogen and pregnanediol excretion, and cervical mucus score during the normal menstrual cycle. Time of ovulation is shown by the vertical dotted line. Cervical mucus is rated on volume and characteristics (dry sensation (1), yellow or white minimal (2), yellow or white sticky (3), cloudy becoming clear (4), thinner more stretchy (7), stretchy, lubricative clear (7), wet slippery (9)). The urinary oestrogen peak occurs 36 hours before ovulation which is triggered by the LH surge. Progesterone from the corpus luteum causes the temperature rise and also inhibits cervical mucus production and changes its characteristics. (Courtesy of Professor James Brown).

ovulation, though the time may vary with individuals. It is cloudy at first and then becomes clear, similar in appearance and consistency to the white of an uncooked egg. The vaginal area has a sensation of wetness or lubrication. The egg is released from the follicle within 24–48 hours of the peak of wetness.

It is recommended that those persons using the ovulation method of contraception refrain from sexual intercourse from the first appearance of the fertile mucus through the height of the sensation of wetness and then for an additional 72 hours. The reason for this precaution is that the fertile mucus produced by the glands at the time of ovulation helps keep the sperm alive and active and facilitates penetration of the ovum. Should there be sperm present before ovulation occurs, the mucus can help maintain their potency until the egg is released from the follicle and is available for impregnation. The life span of the sperm is in part determined by the presence of the fertile mucus, therefore an additional 72 hours after the period of wetness assures that the ovum has been released and expelled through the vaginal tract without becoming impregnated.

One of the major advantages of this method over the rhythm method is that it can be used by women with irregular menstrual cycles and does not rely on extensive keeping of accurate records of menstrual cycles. Unfortunately the success rate is only 80%.

ORAL CONTRACEPTIVES. This is considered to be the most reliable of all nonsurgical methods of contraception, and is popularly referred to as 'the pill'. Combined oral contraceptives contain an oral form of hormone or hormone-like products that duplicate the action of oestrogen and progesterone in women, and are taken for 21 days each month, followed by an inactive tablet or no tablets for the remaining seven days. Oral contraceptives can be obtained by prescription only, as they may produce serious side-effects in women with such disorders as cardiovascular and renal disease, hypertension, diabetes, epilepsy, migraine headaches, and mental depression. The average woman in good health may experience some minor side-effects including nausea, a feeling of fullness, or weight gain. Combined oral contraceptives may affect milk flow in lactating women.

There is a statistically significant relationship between the use of oral contraceptives and cardiovascular disease, such as myocardial infarction (heart attack), stroke, deep venous thrombosis and pulmonary embolism, and this risk is greatly increased in women who use the pill and smoke cigarettes. In the 30 to 39 age group, users of the pill who smoke are ten times as likely to have a heart attack as nonusers who do not smoke and five times as likely as users who do not smoke. Therefore, women who use the pill should not smoke. However, the women studied for the effects of oral contraceptives were taking a form of the drug that is about ten times more potent than current forms of oestrogenic birth-control pills. Because of the short- and long-term effects of the oral contraceptives, many women have decided to use other apparently less hazardous methods of birth control.

Progestogen-only pills overcome the side-effects of oestrogen and can be taken by breast-feeding women. However, they will not guarantee contraception if a single tablet is not taken and the woman places herself at risk. Low-dose oestrogen pills are also available and no pill may contain more than 50 micrograms of oestrogen.

Other hormonal contraceptives are currently being tested. These include the once-a-month pill, the morning-after pill, and the every-three-month injection. Research on hormonal contraceptives for the male is currently being conducted.

PERMANENT STERILIZATION. Irreversible contraceptive techniques involving surgical procedures include SALPINGECTOMY, tubal ligation, and VASECTOMY. Newer techniques utilizing endoscopy include hysteroscopic, culdoscopic, and laparoscopic STERILIZATION.

BARRIER METHODS.

Condom and Cervical Diaphragm. The condom is a thin flexible sheath worn over the penis to prevent entry of spermatozoa into the vagina during coitus. The diaphragm is a cup-shaped device of moulded rubber or other soft plastic material, with a flexible spring forming the circular outer edge. It is inserted in the vagina in such a position that it covers the cervix uteri and prevents entry of spermatozoa. The diaphragm is used in conjunction with a spermicidal cream or jelly.

Although the diaphragm is 98 per cent effective when used with a spermicide, many women find it awkward to use and messy. They object to the need for inserting it prior to coitus and the chore of using the spermicidal cream, gel, or foam. There also is the possibility of affecting the fetus should the woman be pregnant when using a spermicide, as mentioned later.

A custom fitted cervical cap has some advantages over the diaphragm. It fits more snugly, is more comfortable, and, because of a small one-way valve in its centre, it permits the flow of menstrual blood and mucus, yet prohibits the travel of sperm from the vagina to the uterus. This feature allows the woman to leave the cervical cap in place for as long as 12 months.

Barrier methods have the added advantage of providing protection against sexually transmitted diseases.

Jellies, Creams and Foams. A number of contraceptive jellies, or gels, creams, and aerosol foams are made to be used without any mechanical device. These are more powerful in their spermicidal effects than the creams and jellies to be used with diaphragms. Doubt has been cast on their reliability and there have also been objections to them on aesthetic grounds.

Additionally, there is some evidence that spermicidal agents may affect the developing fetus if pregnancy does occur. It is advisable for women using spermicidal contraceptives to avoid using them several months before a planned pregnancy and to stop using them if they suspect that they are pregnant.

INTRAUTERINE CONTRACEPTIVE DEVICES. These consist of a ring, spiral, coil, loop, T, or other shape that is permanently placed inside the uterine cavity. Although the mechanism is not completely understood, it is believed that these devices do not interfere with fertilization but rather in some way render implantation of the fertilized ovum impossible. The advantage of the intrauterine contraceptive device is that once it has been inserted it can be left in place for several years. IUCDs are about 97 per cent effective; however, there is increased risk of uterine perforation, bleeding, and infection. See also INTRAUTERINE CONTRACEPTIVE DEVICE.

ANTIZYGOTIC AGENTS. Experimental work is being carried on with agents that will inhibit the development of the ovum; to date the experiments have been confined to laboratory animals. Antispermatogenic agents, which would inhibit the development of sperm, are also being studied.

contraceptive (ˌkontrəˈseptiv) 1. diminishing the likelihood of or preventing conception. 2. an agent that diminishes the likelihood of or prevents conception. See also CONTRACEPTION.

contractile (kənˈtraktiel) having the power or tendency to contract in response to a suitable stimulus.

contractility (ˌkontrakˈtilitee) a capacity for becoming short in response to suitable stimulus.

contraction (kənˈtrakshən) a drawing together; a shortening or shrinkage.

Braxton Hicks c's light, usually painless, irregular uterine contractions during pregnancy, gradually increasing in intensity and frequency and becoming more rhythmic during the third trimester (see also BRAXTON HICKS CONTRACTIONS).

carpopedal c. the condition resulting from chronic shortening of the muscles of the fingers and toes. Transient spasm of carpopedal muscles is a feature of tetany.

Dupuytren's c. Dupuytren's contracture.

Hicks c's Braxton Hicks contractions.
isometric c. see ISOMETRIC CONTRACTION.
isotonic c. see ISOTONIC CONTRACTION.
postural c. the state of muscular tension and contraction that just suffices to maintain the posture of the body.
spurious c's abdominal pains occurring in pregnancy which are not the real pains of labour.
tetanic c., tonic c. sustained muscular contraction of all or part of the uterus, which causes extreme maternal distress and fetal anoxia, and may obstruct the second and third stages of labour. It may result from overdose of an oxytocic agent, or cephalopelvic disproportion, and is relieved only by a general anaesthetic or amyl nitrite. See also HOUR-GLASS CONTRACTION.
Volkmann's c. Volkmann's contracture.

contracture (kən'trakchə) abnormal shortening of muscle tissue, rendering the muscle highly resistant to stretching. A contracture can lead to permanent disability. It can be caused by fibrosis of the tissues supporting the muscle or the joint, or by disorders of the muscle fibres themselves.

Improper support and positioning of joints affected by arthritis or injury, and inadequate exercising of joints in patients with paralysis can result in contractures. For example, a patient with arthritis or severe burns may assume a position most comfortable for him and will resist changing position because motion is painful. If the joints are allowed to remain in this position, the muscle fibres that normally provide motion will stretch or shorten to accommodate the position and eventually they will lose their ability to contract and relax.

In many cases contractures can be prevented by proper exercise (active or passive), and by adequate support of the joints to eliminate constant shortening or stretching of the muscles and surrounding tissues.
Dupuytren's c. a flexion deformity of the fingers or toes, due to shortening, thickening, and fibrosis of the palmar or plantar fascia.
ischaemic c. muscular contracture and degeneration due to interference with the circulation due to pressure or to injury or cold.
Volkmann's c. contraction of the fingers and sometimes of the wrist, or of analogous parts of the foot, with loss of power, after severe injury or improper use of a tourniquet or cast in the region of the elbow.

contrafissure (ˌkontrə'fishə) a fracture in a part opposite the site of the blow.

contraindication (ˌkontrəˌindi'kayshən) any condition that renders a particular line of treatment improper or undesirable.

contralateral (ˌkontrə'latə·rəl) pertaining to, situated on, or affecting the opposite side.

contrast medium ('kontrahst) a substance employed to increase or create a density difference in diagnostic radiology. X-ray contrast media may be more dense than surrounding tissues (radiopaque) or less dense (radiolucent). A contrast medium may also be used in ultrasonography of the heart to demonstrate an intracardiac shunt; in this case it is a simple saline infusion, which is visible on the ultrasound scan because of the microbubbles within it. Gadolinium–DTPA is a contrast medium used in magnetic resonance imaging.

contrecoup (ˌkontrə'koo) [Fr.] denoting an injury, as to the brain, occurring at a site opposite to the point of impact.

control (kən'trohl) 1. the governing or limitation of certain objects or events. 2. a standard against which experimental observations may be evaluated, as a procedure identical to the experimental procedure except for the absence of the one factor being studied. Also, any individual of the group exhibiting the standard characteristics.
aversive c. in behaviour therapy, the use of unpleasant stimuli to change undesirable behaviour.
birth c. deliberate limitation of childbearing by measures designed to prevent conception (see also BIRTH CONTROL and CONTRACEPTION).
stimulus c. any influence exerted by the environment on behaviour.

controlled drugs (kən'trol'd) preparations subject to the Misuse of Drugs Act (1971), Misuse of Drugs (Notification of and Supply to Addicts) Regulations (1973), and the Misuse of Drugs Regulations (1985) which regulate the prescribing and dispensing of psychoactive drugs, including narcotics, hallucinogens, depressants, and stimulants.

contuse (kən'tyooz) to bruise; to injure without breaking the skin.

contusion (kən'tyoozhən) injury to tissues without breakage of skin; a bruise. In a contusion, blood from the broken vessels accumulates in surrounding tissues, producing pain, swelling, and tenderness. A discoloration appears as a result of blood seepage under the surface of the skin.

Most contusions heal without special treatment, but cold compresses may reduce bleeding, and thus reduce swelling and discoloration, and relieve pain. If a contusion is unusually severe, the injured part should be rested and slightly elevated. Later the application of heat may hasten the absorption of blood.

Serious complications may develop in some cases of contusion. Normally blood is drawn off from the bruised area in a few days, but there is a possibility that blood clotted in the area will form a cyst or calcify and require surgical treatment. The contusion may also be complicated by infection.
cerebral c. contusion of the brain following a HEAD INJURY. It may occur with extradural or subdural collections of blood, in which case the patient may be left with neurological defects or EPILEPSY. See also cranial HAEMATOMA.

Chronic subdural haematoma may occur after relatively mild head injuries especially in the elderly, alcoholics or those with impaired coagulation. Headache is the commonest presenting feature, associated with mood changes, drowsiness, irritability and vomiting. This condition should also be suspected in any patient who deteriorates after an initial period of improvement after head injury. Diagnosis is by CT scan or isotope scan and treatment is by evacuation of the haematoma through burr holes.

conus ('kohnəs) pl. *coni* [L.] 1. a cone or cone-shaped structure. 2. posterior staphyloma of the myopic eye.
c. arteriosus the anterosuperior portion of the right ventricle of the heart, at the entrance to the pulmonary trunk.
c. medullaris the cone-shaped lower end of the spinal cord, at the level of the upper lumbar vertebrae.

convalescence (ˌkonvə'les'ns) the stage of recovery from an illness, operation, or injury.

convalescent (ˌkonvə'les'nt) 1. pertaining to or characterized by convalescence. 2. a patient who is recovering from a disease, operation, or injury.

convection (kən'vekshən) the act of conveying or transmission; specifically, transmission of heat in a liquid or gas by circulation of heated particles.

convergence (kən'vərjəns) 1. a moving together, or inclination toward a common point; the coordinated movement of the two eyes toward fixation of the same near point. 2. the point of meeting of convergent lines.

adj. **convergent.**

conversion (kən'vərshən) 1. the act of changing into something of different form or properties. 2. the transformation of emotions into physical manifestations. 3. manipulative correction of malposition of a fetal part during labour.

c. reaction, c. hysteria a mental mechanism that is unconsciously employed by an individual to solve a strong emotional conflict. In conversion reaction the patient 'converts' his emotional distress into any of a wide variety of physical symptoms, none of which have any organic basis. Among the symptoms which may develop are deafness, blindness, and paralysis of a limb. The symptom chosen by the patient can be related to his particular emotional conflict, and his reaction to the symptom appears to be one of indifference. This is not surprising when one realizes that the patient is using the symptom to obtain relief from a distressing conflict in his mind, and that such a symptom often provokes sympathy and a solicitous attitude from the person or persons involved in the conflict. Treatment of conversion reaction is aimed at helping the patient find more realistic ways of solving his emotional conflict.

convertase (kən'vərtays) an enzyme that converts a substance to its active state.

convex ('konveks, kon'veks) having a rounded, somewhat elevated surface.

convolution (ˌkonvə'looshən) a tortuous irregularity or elevation caused by the infolding of a structure upon itself.

convulsion (kən'vulshən) a series of involuntary contractions of the voluntary muscles. Convulsive seizures are symptomatic of some neurological disorder; they are not in themselves a disease entity. Convulsions can be produced by any of a number of chemical disorders, such as HYPOGLYCAEMIA and hypocalcaemia; metabolic disturbances and hormonal imbalances; brain cell injury from head trauma, tumours, degenerative neural disease, and stroke; anoxia and haemorrhage which deprive brain cells of vital substances; acute cerebral oedema which interferes with normal brain cell function; and infection and high fever (*febrile convulsions*). Finally, EPILEPSY is one of the most common of all disorders associated with convulsions.

PATIENT CARE. The plan for patient care should take into account the potential for injury to the patient during a seizure; should include observing the patient before, during, and after each convulsion; and should, when possible, prevent or minimize environmental factors and events in the patient's daily life that are believed to precipitate a convulsion.

Protection of the patient from injury is of primary concern. If it is known that the patient has had seizures in the past, side rails padded with cotton blankets or some other soft material should be applied to the bed. The head of the bed also should be padded to prevent head injury during an attack. Once a seizure has begun, the nurse or other person with the patient should remain calm, summon help, and try to help the patient prevent injury to himself, using mild restraint in order to avoid allowing the extremities to strike nearby hard objects. Vigorous restraint can cause orthopaedic injuries, as the muscles contract strongly against resistance. If the patient has fallen to the floor, he should not be moved until after the seizure is over. If the patient has some warning and there is time before the seizure actually begins, a soft oral airway or folded towel can be placed between the teeth to prevent tongue biting. Hard objects should never be used to force open the mouth. It is not only useless to attempt this once the jaws are firmly fixed, but teeth can be broken and soft tissues severely injured by trying to force something into the mouth and between the teeth.

It is especially important to observe and report what happened before, during, and immediately after a seizure. This is a critical source of information in the diagnosis of epilepsy. Observations should include: (1) the time the convulsion began, whether the patient had any warning or specific symptoms just before the convulsion occurred, and the length of time the seizure lasted; (2) where the seizure began and what parts of the body were involved; (3) whether the eyes deviated, and a description of the patient's level of consciousness before and during the seizure; (4) whether there was incontinence of urine or stool, vomiting, bleeding, or foaming or frothing at the mouth; (5) the effects of the seizure on the patient's pulse and respirations, and any other objective signs, such as change in skin colour or profuse perspiration; and (6) the condition of the patient after the seizure was over (*postictal* symptoms and signs), such as lethargy, mental confusion, or speech impairment.

Careful attention to environmental factors such as noise or bright light, pain, exhaustion, and other seizure triggers can help identify conditions that might have precipitated seizure activity. Emotional events should also be considered as possible stimulants that can elicit uncontrollable activity.

If the seizures are recurring, as in epilepsy, the patient and his significant others will need instruction in the nature of his illness, an explanation of his prescribed regimen for medications, a list of potential seizure triggers that could precipitate an attack, how to prevent injury during a seizure, and when notification of his doctor is indicated.

central c. a convulsion not triggered by any external cause but due to a lesion of the central nervous system; called also *spontaneous convulsion* and *essential convulsion*.

clonic c. a convulsion marked by alternating contracting and relaxing of the muscles.

epileptiform c. any convulsion attended by loss of consciousness.

febrile c. a convulsion occurring almost exclusively in children aged 6 months to 5 years of age, and associated with a fever of 40 °C (104 °F) or higher. Treatment of children with febrile convulsions who have no evidence of neurological dysfunction is usually limited to measures to lower the temperature by tepid sponging, cooling blankets (hypothermia blankets), or antipyretics (although aspirin must be avoided, see REYE'S SYNDROME). Phenobarbitone and phenytoin are sometimes prescribed to decrease seizure activity. See also FEVER.

tetanic c. a tonic spasm without loss of consciousness and often associated with hypocalcaemia (see also TETANY).

tonic c. prolonged contraction of the muscles, as a result of an epileptic discharge.

uraemic c. one due to uraemia, or retention in the blood of material that should have been expelled by the kidneys.

convulsive (kən'vulsiv) pertaining to, characterized by, or of the nature of a convulsion.

Cooley's anaemia ('kooleez) the homozygous form of β-THALASSAEMIA.

Coolidge tube ('koolij) a vacuum tube formerly used for the generation of x-rays; the cathode consisted of a spiral filament of incandescent tungsten, and the anode (the target) of massive tungsten.

Coombs tests (koomz) laboratory tests that reveal certain antigen–antibody reactions; used in differentiating between various types of haemolytic anaemias, for determining minor blood types, including the RH FACTOR, and for testing for anticipated HAEMOLYTIC DISEASE OF THE NEWBORN.

direct C. t. the test used to detect the presence of cell-bound antibodies that may damage erythrocytes but will not cause visible agglutination. The red cells are washed free of serum and unbound antibody, and antiglobulin (antiserum directed against human antibodies and complement components) is added. Agglutination indicates the presence of antibody. Clinically its most important use is in early diagnosis of haemolytic disease of the newborn and autoimmune HAEMOLYTIC ANAEMIAS. It is used also in crossmatching blood for transfusions. Venous blood or blood from the umbilical cord may be used.

indirect C. t. a test for detecting incompatibility in transfusions when the recipient has a greater than normal risk of TRANSFUSION REACTION. The test also can reveal the presence of anti-Rh antibodies in maternal blood during pregnancy. Either clotted blood or blood with an anticoagulant may be used. The patient's serum is incubated with donor red cells, the cells are washed, and antiglobulin added. Agglutination indicates the presence of antibody.

coordination (koh,awdi'nayshən) the harmonious functioning of interrelated organs and parts. Applied especially to the process of the motor apparatus of the brain which provides for the coworking of particular groups of muscles for the performance of definite adaptive useful responses.

COPD chronic obstructive pulmonary disease (see CHRONIC OBSTRUCTIVE AIRWAYS DISEASE).

coping ('kohping) the process of contending with life difficulties in an effort to overcome or work through them.

c. mechanisms conscious or unconscious strategies or mechanisms that a person uses to cope with stress or anxiety, including turning to a comforting person for love and support, self-discipline, acting out or working off tension, talking and expressing feelings by crying or laughing, and also unconscious DEFENCE MECHANISMS, such as avoidance and rationalization.

copolymer (koh'polimə) a polymer containing monomers of more than one kind.

copper ('kopə) a chemical element, atomic number 29, atomic weight 63.54, symbol Cu. (See table of elements in Appendix 2.) It is necessary for bone formation and for the formation of blood because it occurs in several oxidative enzymes including one involved in the transformation of inorganic iron into haemoglobin. There is little danger of deficiency in ordinary diets because of relatively abundant supply and minute daily requirements.

copremesis (kop'remisis) the vomiting of faecal matter.

coproantibody (,koproh'anti,bodee) an antibody (chiefly IgA) present in the intestinal tract, associated with immunity to enteric infection.

coprolalia (,koproh'layli·ə) the utterance of obscene words, especially words relating to faeces.

coprolith ('koprohlith) a hard faecal concretion in the intestine.

coprology (kop'roləjee) the study of the faeces.

coprophagia (,koproh'fayji·ə) coprophagy.

coprophagy (kop'rofəjee) the ingestion of dung or faeces.

coprophilia (,koproh'fili·ə) a psychopathological interest in filth, especially in faeces and defecation.

coprophilic (,koproh'filik) 1. pertaining to or characterized by coprophilia. 2. inhabiting dung or faeces; said of bacteria.

coprophobia (,koproh'fohbi·ə) abnormal repugnance to defecation and to faeces.

coproporphyria (,koprohpaw'firi·ə) hereditary PORPHYRIA marked by excessive excretion of coproporphyrin, chiefly in the faeces.

coproporphyrin (,koproh'pawfirin) a porphyrin formed in the blood-forming organs and intestine and found in the urine and faeces in coproporphyrinuria.

coproporphyrinogen (,koproh,pawfi'rinəjən) the fully reduced, colourless compound giving rise to coproporphyrin by oxidation.

coproporphyrinuria (,koproh,pawfiri'nyooə·ri·ə) the presence of coproporphyrin in the urine.

coprostasis (kop'rostəsis) faecal impaction.

coprozoic (,koproh'zoh·ik) living in faecal matter.

copula ('kopyuhlə) any connecting part or structure.

copulation (,kopyuh'layshən) sexual union or coitus; usually applied to animals lower than man.

cor (kor) [L.] *heart*.

c. adiposum a heart that has undergone fatty degeneration or that has an accumulation of fat around it.

c. bovinum a greatly enlarged heart due to a hypertropied left ventricle.

c. pulmonale a serious cardiac condition in which there is right ventricular heart failure due to pulmonary hypertension secondary to disease of the blood vessels of the lungs. Acute cor pulmonale is an emergency situation arising from a sudden dilation of the right ventricle as a result of pulmonary embolism. Chronic cor pulmonale develops gradually and is associated with CHRONIC OBSTRUCTIVE AIRWAYS DISEASES, such as EMPHYSEMA, SILICOSIS, and fibrosis of the lung following, an infection. These conditions impair pulmonary circulation and thus create a 'damming' effect on the blood flowing through the pulmonary artery. This in turn slows down the flow of blood from the right ventricle, and the ventricle becomes hypertrophied and dilated.

SIGNS AND SYMPTOMS. Symptoms are similar to those of congestive heart failure from other causes: dyspnoea, oedema of the lower extremities, enlargement of the liver, and distention of the veins in the neck. The haematocrit is increased as the body attempts to compensate for impaired circulation by producing more erythrocytes.

TREATMENT. Treatment is ultimately aimed at relief of the lung disorder causing the condition and relieving the pulmonary insufficiency. This includes the administration of bronchodilators and the use of a mechanical VENTILATOR to reduce hypoxia and dyspnoea. Severe polycythaemia and hypervolaemia may require phlebotomy to lower the blood volume and red cell count. The heart failure is treated with digitalis, diuretics, adequate rest, and dietary measures. See also HEART FAILURE.

coracoid ('ko-rə,koyd) CORONOID.

cord (kawd) any long, cylindrical, flexible structure.

spermatic c. the strucutre extending from the abdominal inguinal ring to the testis, comprising the pampiniform plexus, nerves, ductus deferens, testicular artery, and other vessels.

spinal c. that part of the central nervous system lodged in the spinal canal, extending from the foramen magnum to upper part of the lumbar region.

umbilical c. the structure connecting the fetus and placenta, and containing the channels through which fetal blood passes to and from the placenta (see also UMBILICAL CORD).

vocal c's folds of mucous membrane in the larynx, the superior pair being called the false, and the inferior pair the true, vocal cords (see also VOCAL CORDS).

cordal ('kawdəl) pertaining to a cord; used specifically in referring to the vocal cords.

cordate ('kawdayt) heart-shaped.

cordectomy (kaw'dektəmee) excision of a cord, as of a vocal cord.

Cordilox ('kawdiloks) trademark for preparations of verapamil, a calcium channel blocker.

corditis (kaw'dietis) inflammation of the spermatic cord.

cordopexy ('kawdoh,peksee) surgical fixation of a vocal cord.

cordotomy (kaw'dotəmee) 1. section of a vocal cord. 2. surgical division of the anterolateral tracts of the spinal cord.

Cordylobia anthropophaga (kawdi'lohbiə ,anthropoh'fayjə) tumbu fly; a species of tropical African fly whose larvae burrow under the skin of man and animals, causing one form of myiasis.

core(o)- word element. [Gr.] *pupil of the eye.*

corectopia (,ko·rek'tohpi·ə) abnormal location of the pupil of the eye.

coredialysis (,kor·ridie'aləsis) surgical separation of the external margin of the iris from the ciliary body; now an obsolete procedure.

corediastasis (,kor·ridie'astəsis) dilation of the pupil.

corelysis (ko'relisis) operative destruction of the pupil; especially detachment of adhesions of the pupillary margin of the iris from the lens.

corepressor (,kohri'presə) a substance (e.g., the product of a metabolic pathway) that activates a repressor by combining with it.

Corgard ('korgəhd) trademark for a preparation of nadolol, an antihypertensive (beta-blocker).

Cori's disease ('kohreez) Forbes' disease.

corium ('kor·ri·əm) the true skin, or DERMIS.

corn (kawn) a circumscribed, conical, horny induration and thickening of the stratum corneum that causes severe pain by pressure on nerve endings in the corium. Corns are always caused by friction or pressure from poorly fitting shoes or hose. There are two kinds: the hard corn, usually located on the outside of the little toe or on the upper surfaces of the other toes; and the soft corn, found between the toes, usually the fourth and fifth toes, kept softened by moisture.

cornea ('kawni·ə) the clear, transparent anterior portion of the EYE. The cornea is subject to injury by foreign bodies in the eye, bacterial infection, and viral infection, especially by the herpesvirus that causes HERPES SIMPLEX. The herpesvirus that causes HERPES ZOSTER (shingles), can also infect the cornea. Prompt treatment of any corneal injury or infection is essential to avoid ulceration and loss of vision.

corneal ('kawni·əl) pertaining to the cornea.

c. reflex a reflex action of the eye resulting in automatic closing of the eyelid when the cornea is stimulated. The corneal reflex can be elicited in a normal person by gently touching the cornea with a wisp of cotton. Absence of the corneal reflex indicates deep coma or injury of one of the nerves carrying the reflex arc.

corneosclera (,kawnioh'skliə·rə) the cornea and sclera regarded as one organ.

corneous ('kawni·əs) hornlike or horny; consisting of keratin.

corneum ('kawni·əm) the horny layer of the skin.

cornification (,kawnifi'kayshən) 1. conversion into keratin, or horn. 2. conversion of epithelium to the stratified squamous type.

cornified ('kawni,fied) converted into horny tissue (keratin); keratinized.

cornu ('kawnyoo) pl. *cornua* [L.] horn; a hornlike excrescence or projection; an anatomical structure that appears horn-shaped, especially in section. adj. **cornual.**

c. ammonis hippocampus.

c. sacrale either of two hook-shaped processes extending downward from the arch of the last sacral vertebra.

cornua ('kawnyooa) plural of CORNU.

cornual, cornuate ('kawnyooəl; 'kawnyoo,ayt) pertaining to a horn, especially to the horns of the spinal cord.

corona (kə'rohnə) pl. *coronae* [L.] a crown; in anatomic nomenclature, a crownlike eminence or encircling structure. adj. **coronal.**

c. radiata 1. the radiating crown of projection fibres passing from the internal capsule to every part of the cerebral cortex. 2. an investing layer of radially elongated follicle cells surrounding the zona pellucida of the ovum. Called also *cumulus oophorus.*

coronary ('ko·rənə·ree) encircling in the manner of a crown; a term applied to vessels, ligaments, nerves, etc.

c. arteries two large arteries that branch from the ascending aorta and supply all of the heart muscle with blood.

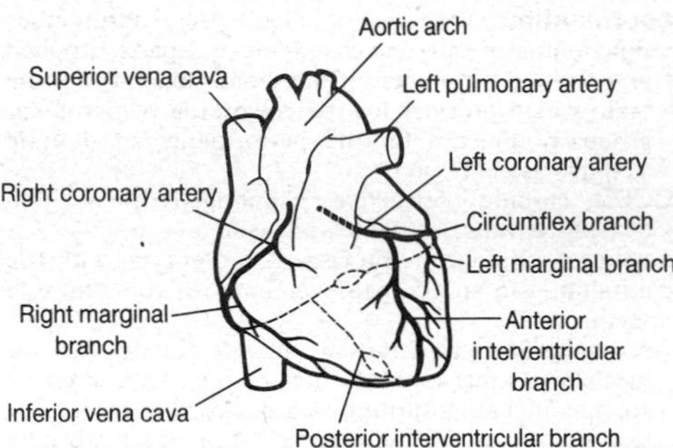

Coronary arteries

c. insufficiency decreased supply of blood to the myocardium resulting from constriction or obstruction of the coronary arteries, but not accompanied by necrosis of the myocardial cells. Called also *myocardial ischaemia.*

c. occlusion the occlusion, or closing off, of a coronary artery. The occlusion may result from formation of a clot (thrombosis), but it is most often caused by a narrowing of the lumen of the blood vessels by the plaques of ATHEROSCLEROSIS. If there is adequate collateral circulation to the heart muscle at the time of the occlusion, there may be little or no damage to the myocardial cells. When occlusion is complete, however, with no blood being supplied to an area of the myocardium, MYOCARDIAL INFARCTION results.

c. sinus the terminal portion of the great cardiac vein, which lies in the cardiac sulcus between the left atrium and ventricle, and empties into the right atrium.

c. thrombosis formation of a clot in a coronary artery. See also MYOCARDIAL INFARCTION.

coronavirus ('ko·rənə,vierəs) any of a group of morphologically similar, ether-sensitive viruses, probably RNA, causing infectious bronchitis of birds, hepatitis in mice, gastroenteritis in swine, and respiratory infections in humans.

coroner ('ko·rənə) a public official (e.g. a barrister,

solicitor or doctor) who holds inquests concerning sudden, violent, or suspicious deaths.

coronoid ('ko·rə,noyd) shaped like a crow's beak.

c. process a projection from the upper part of the neck of the scapula, overhanging the shoulder joint.

coronoidectomy (,ko·rənoy'dektəmee) surgical removal of the coronoid process of the mandible.

corpse (kawps) a dead body; cadaver.

corpulence, corpulency ('kawpyuh,ləns; 'kawpyuh-,lənsee) undue fatness; OBESITY.

corpulent ('kawpyuhlənt) obese.

corpus ('korpəs) pl. *corpora* [L.] body.

c. albicans white fibrous tissue that replaces the regressing corpus luteum in the human ovary in the latter half of pregnancy, or soon after ovulation when pregnancy does not supervene.

c. amygdaloideum a small mass of subcortical grey matter within the tip of the temporal lobe, anterior to the inferior horn of the lateral ventricle of the brain; it is part of the limbic system.

corpora amylacea small hyaline masses of degenerate cells found in the prostate, neuroglia, etc.

c. callosum an arched mass of white matter in the depths of the longitudinal fissure, and made up of transverse fibres connecting the cerebral hemispheres.

c. cavernosum either of the two columns of erectile tissue forming the body of the penis or clitoris.

c. fimbriatum a band of white matter bordering the lateral edge of the lower cornu of the lateral ventricle of the brain.

c. geniculatum geniculate body; see geniculate BODIES, LATERAL and geniculate BODIES, MEDIAL.

c. haemorrhagicum 1. an ovarian follicle containing blood. 2. a corpus luteum containing a blood clot.

c. luteum a yellow glandular mass in the ovary formed by an ovarian follicle that has matured and discharged its ovum. During pregnancy this is responsible for the production of oestrogen and progesterone from the granulosa cells until the placenta is able to take over this function at twelve weeks. See also OVULATION.

corpora quadrigemina four rounded eminences on the posterior surface of the mesencephalon.

c. spongiosum penis a column of erectile tissue forming the urethral surface of the penis, in which the urethra is found.

c. striatum a subcortical mass of grey and white substance in front of and lateral to the thalamus in each cerebral hemisphere.

corpuscle ('kawpəs'l) any small mass or body. adj. **corpuscular.**

blood c's formed elements in the BLOOD, i.e., erythrocytes and leukocytes.

colostrum c's large rounded bodies in colostrum, containing droplets of fat and sometimes a nucleus.

Krause's c's small, encapsulated nerve endings of sensory nerve fibres in skin, mucous membranes, muscles, and other areas. Called also *end-buds* and *Krause's bulbs.*

malpighian c. the funnel-like structure constituting the beginning of the structural unit of the kidney (nephron) and comprising Bowman's capsule and its partially enclosed glomerulus. Called also *renal corpuscle.*

Purkinje's c's large, branched nerve cells composing the middle layer of the cortex of the cerebellum.

red blood c. erythrocyte.

renal c. malpighian corpuscle.

tactile c's medium-sized nerve endings in the skin, chiefly in the palms and soles; called also *tactile papillae.*

white blood c. leukocyte.

corrective (kə'rektiv) a corrigent; a drug which modifies the action of other drugs.

correlation (,ko·ri'layshən) in neurology, the union of afferent impulses within a nerve centre to bring about an appropriate response. In statistics, the degree of association of variable phenomena.

correspondence (,ko·ri'spondəns) the condition of being in agreement or conformity.

retinal c. the state concerned with the impingement of image-producing stimuli on the retinas of the two eyes.

Corrigan's pulse ('ko·rigənz) a jerky pulse with full expansion and sudden collapse.

corrosive (kə'rohsiv, -ziv) having a caustic and locally destructive effect; an agent having such an effect.

cortex ('kawteks) pl. *cortices* [L.] an outer layer, as the bark of the trunk or root of a tree, or the outer layer of an organ or other structure, as distinguished from its inner substance. adj. **cortical.**

adrenal c. the outer, firm layer comprising the larger part of the ADRENAL GLAND; it secretes various hormones.

cerebellar c. the superficial grey matter of the cerebellum.

cerebral c., c. cerebri the convoluted layer of grey matter covering each cerebral hemisphere (see also cerebral cortex of BRAIN).

renal c. the smooth-textured outer layer of the kidney, composed mainly of glomeruli and convoluted tubules, extending in columns between the pyramids constituting the renal medulla.

Corti's canal ('kawteez) a space between the outer and inner rods of Corti.

Corti's ganglion the ganglion of the cochlear nerve, located within the modiolus, sending fibres peripherally to the organ of Corti and centrally to the cochlear nuclei of the brain stem. Called also spiral ganglion.

Corti's organ the terminal acoustic apparatus within the scala media of the inner ear, including the rods of Corti and the auditory cells, with their supporting elements.

Corti's rods (fibres) rodlike bodies in the inner ear, having their heads joined and their bases on the basilar membrane widely separated so as to form a spiral tunnel.

corticate ('kawti,kayt) having a cortex or bark.

corticectomy (,kawti'sektəmee) excision of an area of cerebral cortex, as of a scar or microgyrus in the treatment of focal epilepsy.

corticifugal (kaw,tisi'fyoog'l) proceeding, conducting, or moving away from the cortex.

corticipetal (kaw,tisi'pet'l) proceeding, conducting, or moving toward the cortex.

corticoadrenal (,kawtikoh·ə'dreen'l) pertaining to the adrenal cortex; adrenocortical.

corticobulbar (,kawtikoh'bulbə) pertaining to or connecting the cerebral cortex and the medulla oblongata or brain stem.

corticoid ('kawti,koyd) corticosteroid; a hormone of the adrenal cortex, or other natural or synthetic compound with similar activity.

corticopontine (,kawtikoh'pontien) pertaining to or connecting the cerebral cortex and the pons.

corticospinal (,kawtikoh'spien'l) pertaining to or connecting the cerebral cortex and spinal cord.

corticosteroid (,kawtikoh'stiə·royd) any of the hormones produced by the ADRENAL CORTEX; also, their synthetic equivalents. Called also *adrenocortical hormone* and *adrenocorticosteroid.* All the hormones are steroids having similar chemical structures, but quite different physiological effects. Generally they are divided into GLUCOCORTICOIDS (cortisol, or hydrocortisone, and cortisone and corticosterone), MINERALOCOR-

TICOIDS (aldosterone and desoxycorticosterone, and also corticosterone) and androgens. Patients who must take exogenous adrenal corticosteroids to supplement a deficit in endogenous cortisol or as a treatment for metastatic breast cancer should be thoroughly instructed in self-medication. Their needs are somewhat similar to those of the insulin-dependent diabetic patient. They should know the prescribed dosage and basic therapeutic action of the oral corticosteroid preparation they are taking and should be aware of the importance of taking the medication at the same time every day. The medication should never be discontinued abruptly for any reason. If the patient is to be away from home at the time the medication is due to be taken, or travelling for an extended period of time, he or she must be very careful not to misplace the medication or pack it in luggage that might be lost. It is advisable that the patient carry an extra prescription in case the supply is used up before returning home.

These patients also need to wear some form of medical identification so that all health care professionals with whom they may come in contact will know that they are receiving hormones of this kind. This includes dentists, oral surgeons, accident and emergency personnel, and others who might not be familiar with the patient's medical history.

corticosterone (,kawti'kostə·rohn) a steroid hormone of the adrenal cortex; it is usually classified as a GLUCOCORTICOID, but it also has slight MINERALOCORTICOID activity.

corticotrope ('kawtikoh,trohp) a cell of the anterior pituitary gland that secretes ACTH.

corticotrophic (,kawtikoh'trohfik) having a stimulating effect on the adrenal cortex; pertaining to corticotrophin; adrenocorticotrophic.

corticotrophin (,kawtikoh'trohfin) 1. adrenocorticotrophic hormone (see also ACTH). 2. a pharmaceutical preparation derived from the anterior pituitary of mammals used to stimulate adrenal cortical activity in various conditions, such as allergy, hypersensitivity, and rheumatoid arthritis. It has also been used experimentally in a large number of disorders.

corticotropic (,kawtikoh'trohpik) corticotrophic.

corticotropin (,kawtikoh'trohpin) corticotrophin.

cortilymph ('kawti,limf) the fluid filling the intercellular spaces of the organ of Corti.

cortisol ('kawti,sol) a hormone from the adrenal cortex; the principal GLUCOCORTICOID. Called also *17-hydroxycorticosterone* and, pharmaceutically, *hydrocortisone*. A synthetic preparation is used for its anti-inflammatory actions and in replacement therapy for adrenocortical insufficiency.

cortisone ('kawti,zohn, -,sohn) a GLUCOCORTICOID with significant MINERALOCORTICOID activity, isolated from the adrenal cortex, largely inactive in man until it is converted to hydrocortisone (cortisol). Cortisone is no longer used for adrenal replacement therapy.

coruscation (,ko·rəs'kayshən) the subjective sensation of a flash of light before the eyes.

corybantism (,ko·ri'bantizəm) wild, frenzied, and sleepless delirium.

corymbiform (ko'rimbi,fawm) clustered; said of lesions grouped around a single, usually larger, lesion.

Corynebacteriaceae (ko,rienibak,tiə·ri'aysi·ee) a family of bacteria, made up of usually nonmotile rods, sometimes showing marked variation in form and sometimes beaded or banded with metachromatic granules.

Corynebacterium (ko,rienibak'tiə·ri·əm) a genus of bacteria (family Corynebacteriaceae).

C. acnes a species usually present in acne lesions.

C. diphtheriae the causative agent of diphtheria.

C. minutissimum the causative agent of erythrasma.

C. pseudodiphtheriticum a nonpathogenic microorganism present in the upper respiratory tract.

C. vaginale *Gardnerella vaginale.*

coryneform (ko'rieni,fawm) denoting or resembling organisms of the family Corynebacteriaceae.

coryza (kə'riezə) acute infection of the upper respiratory tract, characterized by perfuse discharge from nasal mucous membranes, sneezing and watering of the eyes. See also COMMON COLD.

coryzavirus (kə,riezə'vierəs) rhinovirus.

cosmetic (koz'metik) 1. beautifying; tending to preserve, restore, or confer comeliness. 2. a beautifying substance or preparation.

cost(o)- word element. [L.] *rib.*

costa ('kostə) pl. *costae* [L.] a rib. adj. **costal**.

costalgia (kos'talji·ə) pain in the ribs.

costectomy, costatectomy (ko'stektəmee; ,kostə'tektəmee) excision of a rib.

costive ('kostiv) 1. pertaining to, characterized by, or producing constipation. 2. an agent that depresses intestinal motility.

costiveness ('kostivnəs) constipation.

costocervical (kostoh'sərvik'l, -sə'vie-) pertaining to the ribs and neck.

costochondral (,kostoh'kondrəl) pertaining to a rib and its cartilage.

costoclavicular (,kostohklə'vikyuhlə) pertaining to the ribs and clavicle.

costocoracoid (,kostoh'korə,koyd) pertaining to the ribs and coracoid process.

costosternal (,kostoh'stərnəl) pertaining to the ribs and sternum.

costosternoplasty (,kostoh'stərnoh,plastee) surgical repair of funnel chest, a segment of rib being used to support the sternum.

costotomy (ko'stotəmee) incision or division of a rib or costal cartilage.

costotransverse (,kostohtranz'vərs, -trahnz-) lying between the ribs and the transverse processes of the vertebrae.

costovertebral (,kostoh'vərtibrəl) pertaining to a rib and a vertebra.

costoxiphoid (,kostoh'zifoyd) connecting the ribs and xiphoid cartilage.

cot death (kot) sudden infant death syndrome.

Cotard's syndrome ('kohtahdz) a syndrome characterized by nihilistic delusions in which the patient denies his own existence and that of the outside world, Although some claim this as a distinct clinical entity, it is perhaps best regarded as a nihilistic delusion which may occur in some severe depressions of a psychotic nature or certain organic states.

cotton-wool spot ('kotən,wuhl) white or grey soft-edged opacities in the retina represent impaired axoplasmic transport; seen in hypertensive retinopathy, diabetic retinopathy, lupus erythematosus, and numerous other conditions.

cotyledon (,koti'leedən) any subdivision of the uterine surface of the placenta.

couching ('kowching) surgical displacement of the lens of the eye in cataract.

cough (kof) 1. a sudden noisy expulsion of air from the lungs. 2. to produce such an expulsion of air.

dry c. cough without expectoration.

productive c. cough attended with expectoration of material from the bronchi.

c. reflex the sequence of events initiated by the sensitivity of the lining of the passageways of the lung and mediated by the medulla as a consequence of impulses transmitted by the vagus nerve, resulting in coughing, i.e., the clearing of the passageways of foreign matter.

whooping c. pertussis, an infectious disease caused by *Bordetella pertussis*, characterized by coryza, bronchitis, and a typical cough (see also WHOOPING COUGH).

coulomb ('koolom) the unit of electrical charge, defined as the quantity of electrical charge transferred by 1 ampere in 1 second.

coumarin ('koomə·rin) 1. a principle extracted from the tonquin bean, from which several anticoagulants are derived that inhibit hepatic synthesis of vitamin K-dependent coagulation factors. 2. any of these derivatives.

counselling ('kownsəling) a generic term used to describe a process of consultation and discussion in which one individual (the counsellor) listens and offers guidance or advice to another who is experiencing difficulties (the client). The counsellor does not direct or make decisions for the client. The general aim is to solve problems, increase awareness and promote constructive exploration of difficulties so that the future may be approached more confidently and more constructively. The term is often used as a synonym for psychotherapy of the supportive type, and the approach is widely used by psychiatric nurses and social workers.

genetic c. a type of counselling in which the counsellor explains the possible effects of genetic inheritance to the client, so as to assist them in deciding whether or not to have a child.

count (kownt) a numerical computation or indication.

Addis c. the determination of the number of erythrocytes, leukocytes, epithelial cells, casts, and the protein content in an aliquot of a 12-hour urine specimen.

blood c. determination of the number of formed elements in a measured volume of blood, usually a cubic millimetre (as of red blood cells, white blood cells, or a platelet count).

differential c. a count on a stained blood smear, of the proportion of different types of leukocytes (or other cells), expressed in percentages.

platelet c. the count of the total number of platelets per cubic millimetre of blood.

counter ('kowntə) an instrument or apparatus by which numerical value is computed; in radiology, a device for enumerating ionizing events.

Geiger c., Geiger–Müller c. a radiation counter using a gas-filled tube that indicates the presence of ionizing particles.

scintillation c. a device for detecting beta and gamma rays, permitting determination of the concentration of radioisotopes in the body or other substance. The rays interact with the material in the device to produce short light flashes (scintillations), which are detected by a photomultiplier tube and counted.

countercurrent ('kowntə,kurənt) flowing in an opposite direction.

counterelectrophoresis (,kowntə·i,lektrohfə'reesis) counterimmunoelectrophoresis.

counterextension (,kowntə·rik'stenshən) traction in a proximal direction coincident with traction in opposition to it.

counterimmunoelectrophoresis (,kowntə-,imyuhnoh·ilektrohfə'reesis) abbreviated CIE; a laboratory technique in which an electric current is used to accelerate the migration of antibody and antigen through a buffered diffusion medium. Most antigens in a gel medium in which the pH is controlled are strongly negatively charged and will migrate rapidly across the electric field toward the anode. The majority of antibody molecules in such a medium are less negatively charged and will migrate in an opposite or 'counter' direction toward the cathode. If the antigen and antibody are specific for each other, they combine and form a distinct precipitin line.

The technique of CIE has been applied clinically to detect many antibodies to the antigens of infectious agents. The antigens themselves are sometimes identified by CIE. It can be especially valuable as an aid to accurate diagnosis of clinical bacterial infections and the selection of specific therapeutic agents for control of infections once the causative organisms have been identified.

counterincision (,kowntə·in'sizhən) a second incision made to promote drainage or to relieve tension on the edges of a wound.

counterirritant (,kowntə·iritənt) 1. producing counterirritation. 2. an agent that produces counterirritation.

counterirritation (,kowntə,iri'tayshən) superficial irritation intended to relieve some other irritation.

counteropening (,kowntə'ohpəning) a second incision made across an earlier one to promote drainage.

counterpulsation (,kowntəpul'sayshən) a technique for assisting the circulation and decreasing the work of the heart by synchronizing the force of an external pumping device with cardiac systole and diastole. *External* counterpulsation is a noninvasive procedure in which the legs are encased in rigid tubular bags filled with air or water and connected to a pumping unit. *Internal* counterpulsation requires insertion of an intra-aortic balloon-tipped catheter, the distal end of which is attached to a pump that inflates the balloon. See also INTRA-AORTIC BALLOON PUMP.

External counterpulsation is less effective than internal counterpulsation, but it is easier to use and less hazardous to the patient. It employs the same general principles as internal counterpulsation by applying pressure against the blood vessels of the legs during diastole and release of pressure during systole. This has the effect of increasing venous return and enhancing systolic unloading of the left ventricle. The end result of external counterpulsation is that of augmenting coronary circulation and improving blood flow to the myocardium, improving systemic circulation, and reducing the workload of the heart, thereby lessening myocardial demand for and consumption of oxygen. Indications for external counterpulsation include cardiogenic shock and severe heart failure in acute situations such as myocardial infarction and open-heart surgery. It is a temporary measure that does not benefit patients with chronic heart failure.

counterpuncture ('kowntə,pungkchə) a second opening made opposite another.

counterstain ('kowntə,stayn) a stain applied to render the effects of another stain more discernible.

countertraction ('kowntə,trakshən) traction opposed to traction; used in reduction of fractures.

countertransference (,kowntə'transfə·rəns, -'trahns-) in psychoanalysis, the emotional reaction aroused in the doctor by the patient.

counting chamber ('kownting ,chaymbə) a specially designed microscope slide which is divided into 0.05 × 0.05 mm squares. It allows for the accurate counting of blood cells.

coup (koo) [Fr.] *stroke*.

c. de sabre a linear, circumscribed lesion of scleroderma on the forehead or scalp, so called because of its resemblance to the scar of a sabre wound.

coupling ('kupling) in cardiology, the frequent occurrence of a normal heartbeat followed by an extraventricular one. May be found following digitalis overdose.

couvade (koo'vahd) the experiencing of the rigours of labour and childbirth by the father. This psychosomatic phenomenon is common in many societies and

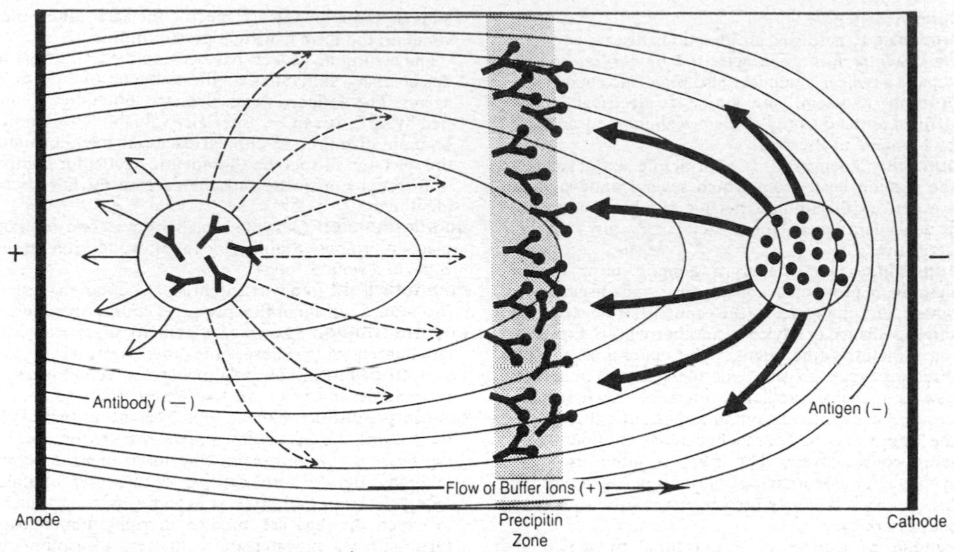

Counterimmunoelectrophoresis (CIE) test depends upon reactions to electric current of antibody and antigen molecules and buffer. At the pH used, antigen is strongly negative and migrates rapidly toward the anode. Although weakly negative antibody tends to migrate slowly toward the anode, it becomes swept along (dashed arrows) toward the cathode with positive buffer ions of the agar, in the 'counter' motion of CIE. Antibody and antigen meet between wells (space here is exaggerated), combine and precipitate if they are specific for each other, forming precipitin line characteristic of the test

occurs to some extent in all.

covalency (koh'vaylənsee) a chemical bond between two atoms in which electrons are shared between the two nuclei. adj. **covalent.**

coverglass ('kuvə,glahs) coverslip.

coverslip ('kuvə,slip) a very thin glass plate that covers a tissue, culture or object mounted on a glass slide for microscopic examination. Called also *coverglass.*

Cowper's glands ('koopəz) bulbourethral glands.

cowperitis (,koopə'rietis) inflammation of the bulbourethral (Cowper's) glands, located in the urethral sphincter.

cowpox ('kow,poks) an acute virus infection characterized by skin lesions which progress from papules to vesicles and then pustules, accompanied by fever and lymphadenopathy. It is a zoonosis usually acquired from bovines either by milking animals with infectious lesions on the udder or by handling meat. It is also sometimes acquired from domestic cats.

Edward Jenner, a general practitioner in Berkeley, Gloucestershire, in the 18th century, discovered that infection with cowpox protected against smallpox. From this discovery, vaccination against smallpox was developed using the vaccinia virus derived from the cowpox virus and enabled the eradication of smallpox from the world.

coxa ('koksə) pl. *coxae* [L.] the hip, loosely, the hip joint.

c. plana flattening of the head of the femur resulting from osteochondrosis of its epiphysis.

c. valga deformity of the hip joint with increase in the angle of inclination between the neck and shaft of the femur.

c. vara deformity of the hip joint with decrease in the angle of inclination between the neck and shaft of the femur.

coxalgia (kok'salji·ə) pain in the hip joint.

Coxiella (,koksi'elə) a genus of microorganisms of the order Rickettsiales.

C. burnetii the causative agent of Q fever.

coxitis (kok'sietis) inflammation of the hip joint.

coxodynia (,koksoh'dini·ə) pain in the hip.

coxofemoral (,koksoh'femə·rəl) pertaining to the hip and thigh.

coxotuberculosis (,koksohtyuh,bərkyuh'lohsis) tuberculosis of the hip joint; hip-joint disease.

coxsackievirus (kok'saki,vierəs) one of a heterogeneous group of enteroviruses producing, in man, a disease resembling poliomyelitis, but without paralysis. Called also *Coxsackie virus.*

c. A disease herpangina.

CPAP continuous positive airway pressure.

CPH Certificate of Public Health.

c.p.m. counts per minute.

CPR cardiopulmonary resuscitation.

c.p.s. cycles per second.

CR conditioned reflex (response).

Cr chemical symbol, *chromium.*

crab louse ('krab ,lows) *Phthirus pubis.* See LOUSE.

Crabtree effect ('krab,tree) the inhibition of oxygen consumption on the addition of glucose to tissues or microorganisms having a high rate of aerobic glycolysis; the converse of the Pasteur effect.

crack (krak) crystallized cocaine base obtained by 'cooking' cocaine powder with water and baking soda. The cooking process removes impurities and results in a highly potent cocaine preparation (70 to 90% pure). This illicit reprocessing results in a paste which is dried and then 'cracked' into small pieces (hence the name) before sale. Crack is smoked in a water pipe or may be inserted into a cannabis cigarette. Risk of overdose, cardiac arrest and uncontrolled or criminal behaviour after use is high. In the USA, crack seems to be replacing cocaine hydrochloride in the illicit drugs market and the substance is already beginning to appear on the European black market.

cradle ('krayd'l) a frame placed over the body of a bed patient for application of heat or cold or for protecting injured parts from coming in contact with the bed clothes. Cradles vary in size according to their intended purpose and can be used over the entire body or over one or more extremities.

c. cap an oily yellowish crust that sometimes appears on the scalp of nursing infants; also called milk crust (crusta lactea). The crust is caused by excessive secretion of the sebaceous glands in the scalp. Treatment consists of applications of oil or a bland ointment and frequent scalp shampoos until the crust is removed. It is usually a self-limiting disorder which clears after 3 to 6 months.

electric c., heat c. a tunnel- or hood-shaped cradle equipped with light bulbs, for applications of heat to the patient's body.

cramp (kramp) a painful spasmodic muscular contraction.

heat c. spasm accompanied by pain, weak pulse, and dilated pupils; seen in workers in intense heat.

recumbency c's cramping in the muscles of the legs and feet occurring while resting or during light sleep.

writers' c. an occupational neurosis marked by spasmodic contraction of the muscles of the fingers, hand, and forearm, with neuralgic pain.

crani(o)- word element. [L.] *skull.*

craniad ('krayniad) in a cranial direction; toward the anterior (in animals) or superior (in humans) end of the body.

cranial ('krayni·əl) pertaining to the cranium or to the anterior (in animals) or superior (in humans) end of the body.

c. nerves nerves that are attached to the brain and pass through the openings of the skull. There are 12 pairs of cranial nerves, symmetrically arranged so that they are distributed mainly to the structures of the head and neck. The one exception, the vagus nerve, extends beyond the head and carries among its fibres the motor fibres that go to the bronchi, stomach, gallbladder, small intestine, and part of the large intestine. It also carries the fibres that control the release of secretions of the gastric glands and the pancreas, and inhibitory fibres to the heart.

Some of the cranial nerves are both sensory and motor; i.e., they control motion as well as conduct sensory impulses. Others are sensory or motor only.

Cranial nerves

I	Olfactory	Sensory
II	Optic	Sensory
III	Oculomotor	Mixed
IV	Trochlear	Mixed
V	Trigeminal	
	Ophthalmic	Sensory
	Maxillary	Sensory
	Mandibular	Mixed
VI	Abducens	Motor
VII	Factal	Mixed
VIII	Vestibulocochlear	
	Cochlear	Sensory
	Vestibular	Sensory
IX	Glossopharyngeal	Mixed
X	Vagus	Mixed
XI	Accessory	Motor
XII	Hypoglossal	Motor

craniectomy (ˌkrayni'ektəmee) excision of a segment of the skull.

craniocele ('kraynioh,seel) protrusion of part of the brain through the skull.

craniocerebral (ˌkraynioh'seribrəl) pertaining to the skull and cerebrum.

cranioclasis (ˌkrayni'oklasis) craniotomy (2).

cranioclast ('kraynioh,klast) an instrument for performing craniotomy (2).

craniocleidodysostosis (ˌkraynioh,kliedoh,disos'tohsis) cleidocranial dysostosis.

craniodidymus ('kraynioh'didimus) a fetus or infant with two heads.

craniofacial (ˌkraynioh'fayshəl) of or pertaining to the cranium and face.

craniomalacia (ˌkrayniohmə'layshi·ə) abnormal softness of the bones of the skull.

craniometer (ˌkrayni'omitə) an instrument for measuring the skull in craniometry. adj. **craniometric.**

craniometry (ˌkrayni'omitree) a branch of anthropometry, being the measurement of the dimensions and angles of a bony skull.

craniopagus (ˌkrayni'opəgəs) a double fetus or infant joined at the head.

craniopharyngeal (ˌkrayniohfə'rinji·əl, -ˌfarin'jeeəl) pertaining to the cranium and pharynx.

craniopharyngioma (ˌkrayniohfaˌrinji'ohmə) a tumour arising from the cell rests derived from the infundibulum of the hypophysis or Rathke's pouch.

cranioplasty ('kraynioh,plastee) any plastic operation on the skull.

craniopuncture ('kraynioh,pungkchə) exploratory puncture of the brain.

craniorachischisis (ˌkrayniohrə'kiskisis) congenital fissure of the skull and vertebral column.

craniosacral (ˌkraynioh'saykrəl) pertaining to the skull and sacrum.

cranioschisis (ˌkrayni'oskisis) congenital fissure of the skull.

craniosclerosis (ˌkrayniohsklə'rohsis) abnormal calcification and thickening of the cranial bones.

cranioscopy (ˌkrayni'oskəpee) diagnostic examination of the head.

craniospinal (ˌkraynioh'spien'l) pertaining to the skull and spine.

craniostenosis (ˌkrayniohstə'nohsis) deformity of the skull due to premature closure of the cranial sutures.

craniostosis (ˌkrayni'ostəsis) congenital ossification of the cranial sutures.

craniosynostosis (ˌkrayniohsi'nostəsis) premature closure of the cranial sutures.

craniotabes (ˌkraynioh'taybeez) reduction in mineralization of the skull, with abnormal softness of the bone, usually affecting the occipital and parietal bones along the lambdoidal sutures.

craniotome ('kraynioh,tohm) a cutting instrument used in craniotomy.

craniotomy (ˌkrayni'otəmee) 1. any operation on the cranium. 2. puncture of the skull and removal of its contents to decrease the size of the head of a dead fetus and facilitate delivery.

craniotympanic (ˌkrayniohtim'panik) pertaining to the skull and tympanum.

cranium ('krayni·əm) pl. *crania* [L.] the skeleton of the head, variously construed as including all of the bones of the head, all except the mandible, or the eight bones forming the vault lodging the brain.

crater ('kraytə) an excavated area surrounded by an elevated margin, such as is caused by ulceration.

craterization (ˌkraytə·rie'zayshən) excision of bone tissue to create a crater-like depression.

creatinaemia (ˌkreeəti'neemi·ə) excessive creatine in the blood.

creatinase (kree'atiˌnayz) an enzyme that catalyses the decomposition of creatine into urea and ammonia.

creatine ('kreeəˌteen, -tin) a nonprotein substance synthesized in the body from three amino acids: arginine, glycine (aminoacetic acid), and methionine. Creatine readily combines with phosphate to form phosphocreatine, or creatine phosphate, which is present in muscle, where it serves as the storage form of high-energy phosphate necessary for muscle contraction.

c. kinase an enzyme catalysing the transfer of a phosphate group from phosphocreatine to ATP. It has three isoenzymes: CK_1, found primarily in the brain; CK_2, found in the myocardium; and CK_3, found in both skeletal muscle and the myocardium. The presence of CK_2 in the blood is strongly indicative of a recent myocardial infarction; it is present until about 72 hours after the attack.

creatinine (kree'atiˌneen) a nitrogenous compound formed as the end-product of creatine metabolism. It is formed in the muscle in relatively small amounts, passes into the blood and is excreted in the urine.

A laboratory test for the creatinine level in the blood may be used as a measurement of kidney function. Since creatinine is normally produced in fairly constant amounts as a result of the breakdown of phosphocreatine and is excreted in the urine, an elevation in the creatinine level in the blood indicates a disturbance in kidney function or an abnormal muscle-wasting process. To determine the creatinine clearance, urine is collected for 24 hours and the serum creatinine is measured by a venous blood sample. Thus the rate of creatinine excretion per minute can be calculated.

creatinuria (kreeˌati'nyooə·ri·ə) increased concentration of creatine in the urine.

creatorrhoea (ˌkreeətə'reeə) the presence of muscle fibres in the faeces. It occurs in certain diseases of the pancreas.

Credé's technique (manoeuvre, method) ('kredayz) a technique for manual expression of urine from the bladder used in BLADDER TRAINING for paralysed patients: the hands are held flat against the abdomen, just below the umbilicus. A firm downward stroke toward the bladder is repeated six or seven times, followed by pressure from both hands placed directly over the bladder to manually remove all urine.

cremaster muscle (kri'mastə) the muscle that elevates the testis.

cremasteric (ˌkrimə'sterik) pertaining to the cremaster muscle.

crenate, crenated ('kreenayt; 'kreenaytid) scalloped or notched.

crenation (kri'nayshən) the formation of abnormal notching around the edge of an erythrocyte; the notched appearance of an erythrocyte due to its shrinkage after suspension in a hypertonic solution.

crenocyte ('kreenohˌsiet) a crenated erythrocyte.

creosol ('kreeəˌsol) one of the active constituents of creosote.

creosote ('kreeəˌsoht) a mixture of phenols from wood tar; used externally as an antiseptic and internally in chronic bronchitis as an expectorant. A mixture of the carbonates of various constituents of creosote (creosote carbonate) is used.

crepitant ('krepitənt) having a dry, crackling sound.

crepitation (ˌkrepi'tayshən) a dry, crackling sound or sensation, such as that produced by the grating of the ends of a fractured bone.

crepitus ('krepitəs) 1. the discharge of flatus from the bowels. 2. crepitation. 3. a crepitant rale.

crescent ('kres'nt, -z'nt) 1. shaped like a new moon. 2. a crescent-shaped structure. adj. **crescentic.**

Giannuzzi's c's crescent-shaped patches of serous cells surrounding the mucous tubercles in mixed glands.

sublingual c. the crescent-shaped area on the floor of the mouth, bounded by the lingual wall of the mandible and the base of the tongue.

cresol ('kreesol) a phenol from coal or wood tar; a preparation consisting of a mixture of isomeric cresol from coal tar or petroleum is used as a disinfectant.

crest (krest) a projection, or projecting structure or ridge, especially one surmounting a bone or its border.

dental c. the maxillary ridge passing along the alveolar processes of the fetal maxillary bones.

iliac c. the thickened, expanded upper border of the ilium.

cretin ('kretin) a patient exhibiting cretinism.

cretinism ('kretiˌnizəm) arrested physical and mental development with dystrophy of bones and soft tissues, due to congenital lack of thyroid gland secretion from hypofunctioning or absence of the gland. The child has a large head, short limbs, puffy eyes, a thick and protruding tongue, excessively dry skin, lack of coordination, and mental handicap. The acquired or adult form of thyroid deficiency is MYXOEDEMA.

Administration of thyroid extract, which must be continued for life, can result in normal growth and mental developmment. If untreated, the child will become permanently dwarfed, probably mentally handicapped, and often sterile.

cretinoid ('kretiˌnoyd) resembling a cretin, or suggestive of cretinism.

cretinous ('kretinəs) affected with cretinism.

Creutzfeld–Jakob disease (ˌkroytsfelt'yakob) a rare, usually fatal encephalopathy due to a transmissible agent with a very long incubation period, termed a slow virus. It is manifested by confusion, dementia and ataxia, usually in persons over the age of 40 years.

The only known source of infection is man. The mode of transmission is unknown in most cases, but transmission by cortical electrodes, by corneal transplant and by human growth hormone has been reported. (Human growth hormone is no longer available and has been replaced by a synthetic preparation).

crevice ('krevis) a fissure.

gingival c. the space between the cervical enamel of a tooth and the overlying unattached gingiva.

CRF corticotrophin-releasing factor.

cri du chat syndrome (ˌkree doo 'shah) [Fr.] a hereditary congenital syndrome characterized by hypertelorism, microcephaly, severe mental deficiency, and a plaintive catlike cry, due to deletion of part of the short arm of chromosome 5.

cribriform ('kribriˌfawm) perforated like a sieve.

cricoarytenoid (ˌkriekohˌari'teenoyd) pertaining to the cricoid and arytenoid cartilages.

cricoid ('kriekoyd) 1. ring-shaped. 2. the cricoid cartilage.

c. cartilage a ringlike cartilage forming the lower and

back part of the larynx.

cricoidectomy (ˌkriekoy'dektəmee) excision of the cricoid cartilage.

cricopharyngeal (ˌkriekohfə'rinji·əl, -ˌfarin'jeeəl) pertaining to the cricoid cartilage and pharynx.

cricothyreotomy (ˌkriekohˌthieri'otəmee) incision through the cricoid and thyroid cartilages.

cricothyroid (ˌkriekoh'thieroyd) pertaining to the cricoid and thyroid cartilages.

cricothyrotomy (ˌkriekohthie'rotəmee) incision through the skin and cricothyroid membrane to secure a patent airway for emergency relief of upper airway obstruction.

cricotomy (krie'kotəmee) incision of the cricoid cartilage.

cricotracheotomy (ˌkriekohˌtraki'otəmee) incision of the trachea through the cricoid cartilage.

Crigler–Najjar disease (syndrome) (ˌkriglə'najə) a congenital hereditary non-haemolytic jaundice due to absence of the hepatic enzyme glucuronide transferase, marked by excessive amounts of unconjugated bilirubin in the blood, kernicterus, and severe central nervous system disorders.

Crimean–Congo haemorrhagic fever (krieˌmeeən-'kong·goh) an acute-onset fever with haemorrhagic rash caused by a virus of the Bungavirus group. The disease occurs in Asia, Eastern Europe, the Middle East and Africa; it has not been reported in the UK. It is a zoonosis, the source of infection probably being wild rodents, domestic cattle, sheep and goats, with transmission to man by tick bites. Person-to-person spread in hospitals by accidental inoculation of blood or tissue fluid has been described. The incubation period is 3 to 12 days. Treatment is in strict isolation; convalescent serum may be helpful.

crinogenic (ˌkrinoh'jenik, ˌkrienoh-) causing secretion in a gland.

crisis ('kriesis) pl. *crises* [L.] 1. the turning point of a disease for better or worse; especially a sudden change, usually for the better, in the course of an acute disease. 2. a sudden paroxysmal intensification of symptoms in the course of a disease. 3. life crisis; a period of disorganization that occurs when a person meets an obstacle to an important life goal, such as the sudden death of a family member, a difficult family conflict, an incident of domestic violence (spouse or child abuse), a serious accident, loss of a limb, loss of a job, or rape or attempted rape.

addisonian c., adrenal c. symptoms of fatigue, nausea and vomiting, and collapse accompanying an acute attack of adrenal failure (see ADDISON'S DISEASE).

blast c. a sudden, severe change in the course of chronic myelocytic leukaemia, in which the clinical picture resembles that seen in acute myelogenous leukaemia, with an increase in the proportion of myeloblasts.

coeliac c. an attack of severe watery diarrhoea and vomiting producing dehydration and acidosis, sometimes occurring in infants with COELIAC DISEASE.

identity c. a period in the psychosocial development of an individual, usually occurring during adolescence, manifested by a loss of the sense of the sameness and historical continuity of one's self, and inability to accept the role the individual perceives as being expected of him by society.

c. intervention counselling or psychotherapy for patients in a life crisis that is directed at supporting the patient through the crisis and helping the patient to cope with the stressful event that precipitated it.

salt-losing c. see SALT-LOSING CRISIS.

tabetic c. a painful paroxysm occurring in tabes dorsalis.

thyroid c., thyrotoxic c. a sudden and dangerous increase of the symptoms of thyrotoxicosis.

crista ('kristə) pl. *cristae* [L.] crest.

cristae cutis ridges of the skin produced by the projecting papillae of the corium on the palm of the hand and sole of the foot, producing a fingerprint and footprint characteristic of the individual; called also dermal ridges.

c. galli a thick, triangular process projecting upward from the cribriform plate of the ethmoid bone.

criterion (krie'tiə·ri·ən) pl. *criteria;* the basis on which a decision is made, e.g. for drug dosage, treatment plans, research trials, etc.

critical care unit ('kritikəl kair) see INTENSIVE CARE UNIT.

Crohn's disease (krohnz) an inflammatory disease which may affect the whole alimentary tract from mouth to anus. The term inflammatory bowel disease (IBD) is conveniently used to include both Crohn's disease and ULCERATIVE COLITIS, which are non-specific inflammatory diseases of the bowel, with a tendency to involvement of extra colonic tissue. There is, however, one fundamental difference, namely that ulcerative colitis involves only the colon, whereas Crohn's disease may affect the whole alimentary tract.

The cause of Crohn's disease is unknown. It is largely a disease of adults 20 to 40 years of age, although it may manifest itself in children or the elderly. In contrast to ulcerative colitis, which affects only the mucosa and submucosa, Crohn's disease involves the full thickness of the bowel wall. Other differences are that people with Crohn's disease may develop internal or external fistulas of the bowel, form abscesses, develop strictures, and their lesions may be single or they may have multiple affected areas separated by normal bowel. Aphthous ulcers of buccal mucosa commonly occur, and the oral mucous membrane may show hyperplasia, deep ulceration and fissure, chronic oedema and a cobblestone appearance.

CLINICAL MANIFESTATIONS. The disease may manifest itself as an acute illness or in a subacute form. Diarrhoea, abdominal pain, weight loss, anaemia and fever are common problems, but the patient can present with acute surgical abdominal problems. Some patients experience relatively few attacks during their lifetime, while others have frequent, prolonged and severe problems. Surgery for intestinal strictures is often necessary, and patients with Crohn's disease may have a series of operations over a number of years.

PATIENT CARE. The patient will most likely present problems related to intestinal obstruction, pain, electrolyte and fluid imbalance, alteration in nutrition, diarrhoea, infection, lethargy and anxiety. Treatment is symptomatic; the goals are maintenance of good nutrition and prevention of a secondary infection. Antibiotics may be prescribed to prevent secondary infection and anti-inflammatory agents, normally corticosteroids, are given to promote healing. It is becoming more common also to use immunosuppressive agents. Diet remains controversial. Some believe that dietary requirements are individual and that no specific diet helps, while others believe elemental diets or parenteral nutrition may have a role to play.

There is no cure for Crohn's disease. Long-term problems occur owing to some patients having regular 'attacks', with episodes of diarrhoea and pain, intestinal obstruction, and anaemia. It is a debilitating disease, particularly if a series of operations is required. The aim should be to provide physiological, psychological and social support.

Crookes' tube (kruhks) an early form of vacuum tube by use of which x-rays were discovered.

Crosby capsule ('krozbee) a capsule attached to the end of a flexible tube which is swallowed by the patient. When the capsule reaches the small intestine, as seen on radiological examination, a biopsy of the intestinal mucosa may be taken.

cross (kros) 1. a cross-shaped figure or structure. 2. any organism produced by crossbreeding; a method of crossbreeding.

cross dressing (kros 'dresing) dressing in clothes designed for those of the opposite sex, generally to arouse feelings of sexual pleasure. One who habitually does so is referred to as a TRANSVESTITE.

cross-eye ('krosie) STRABISMUS in which there is manifest deviation of the visual axis of one eye toward that of the other eye, resulting in diplopia. Called also *esotropia, squint* and *convergent strabismus*.

cross matching ('kros ,maching) a procedure vital in blood transfusions and organ transplantation. The donor's erythrocytes or leukocytes are placed in the recipient's serum and vice versa. Absence of agglutination, haemolysis, and cytotoxicity indicates that the donor and recipient are blood group compatible or histocompatible.

cross-reactivity (,krosriak'tivitee) the degree to which an antibody participates in cross-reactions.

cross-sectional study (kros'sekshən'l) an epidemiological study to compare disease or other health characteristics with possible causative factors at one point of time (point prevalence) or over a limited period of time (period prevalence).

crossbite ('kros,biet) malocclusion in which the normal tooth relationship is reversed—the mandibular teeth occluding bucally to the maxillary teeth.

crossbreeding ('kros,breeding) hybridization; the mating of organisms of different strains or species.

crossing over (,krosing'ovə) the exchanging of material between homologous chromosomes, during the first meiotic division, resulting in new combinations of genes.

crossover design ('krosohvə) a type of epidemiological study in which two treatments (*x* and *y*) are compared between two groups of patients, where one group of patients receives treatment *x* then *y*, while the other receives treatment *y* then *x*.

crotamiton (kroh'tamiton) an acaricide used in the treatment of scabies and as an antipruritic.

croup (kroop) a condition resulting from acute obstruction of the larynx caused by allergy, foreign body, infection, or new growth, occurring chiefly in infants and children. adj. **croupous**.

CHARACTERISTICS. Croup in itself is not a disease but a group of symptoms of varied origin with the following general characteristics: (1) obstruction of the upper respiratory tract, usually at the level of the larynx or just below it in the trachea; (2) hoarseness; (3) a resonant cough, usually described as 'barking'; and (4) a croaking sound, called stridor, during inspiration.

A typical attack of croup usually begins at night, often precipitated by exposure to cold air. The onset is sudden, with hoarse, 'croupy' voice or cough, and what seems like difficult breathing. Spasms of choking that seem close to strangulation follow.

Croup can be a frightening experience for the child and his or her parents. If the child becomes dyspnoeic at home, cool mist and hydration may be all that is needed to relieve the child's respiratory difficulties.

Although croup is very frightening, with a sudden onset and dramatic symptoms of asphyxia, it is rarely fatal and the prognosis is very good.

Crouzon's disease (kroo'zonz) craniofacial dysostosis.

crown (krown) 1. the topmost part of an organ or structure, e.g., the top of the head. 2. artificial crown.

anatomical c. the upper, enamel-covered part of a tooth.

artificial c. a metal, porcelain, or plastic reproduction of a crown affixed to the remaining natural structure of a tooth.

crowning ('krowning) the moment during birth when the suboccipitobregmatic and biparietal diameters of the fetal head are descending the vulval ring, and the head no longer recedes between contractions.

CRP C-reactive protein.

crucial ('krooshəl) 1. shaped like a cross, e.g., an incision. 2. decisive. 3. critical or severe.

cruciate ('krooshiayt) shaped like a cross.

crucible ('kroosib'l) a vessel for melting refractory substances.

cruciform ('kroosi,fawm) cross-shaped.

crural ('kroo ə·rəl) relating to the thigh.

crus (krus) pl. *crura* [L.] 1. the leg, from knee to foot. 2. a leglike part.

c. cerebri a structure comprising fibre tracts descending from the cerebral cortex to form the longitudinal fascicles of the pons.

c. of clitoris the continuation of the corpus cavernosum of the clitoris, diverging posteriorly to be attached to the pubic arch.

crura of diaphragm two fibroelastic bands that arise from the lumbar vertebrae and insert into the central tendon of the diaphragm.

crura of fornix two flattened bands of white matter that unite to form the body of the fornix of the cerebrum.

c. of penis the continuation of each corpus cavernosum of the penis, diverging posteriorly to be attached to the pubic arch.

crush syndrome (krush) the oedema, oliguria, and other symptoms of acute renal failure that follow crushing of a part, especially a large muscle mass, causing the release of myoglobin (see also lower nephron NEPHROTIC SYNDROME).

crust (krust) a formed outer layer, especially an outer layer of solid matter formed by drying of a bodily exudate or secretion.

crusta ('krustə) pl. *crustae* [L.] 1. a crust. 2. crus cerebri.

Crustacea (kru'stayshi·ə) a class of arthropods including the lobsters, crabs, shrimps, wood lice, water fleas, and barnacles.

crutches ('kruchiz) artificial supports, made of wood or metal, used by those who need aid in walking because of injury, disease, or a birth defect.

TYPES. Crutches are usually adjustable in handgrip-to-ground length, and are made in different sizes to suit people of various heights.

The standard type of crutch is the elbow crutch, which consists of an adjustable aluminium tube with a horizontal handgrip and a plastic foerarm grip (see accompanying illustration). The user can release his hold on the handgrip, as in grasping a handrail to climb stairs, without dropping the crutch. The end is covered with a rubber ferrule to prevent slipping.

Another type of crutch, less commonly used now, is the wooden axillary crutch. This is a tall crutch which fits under the armpit, with double uprights and a small horizontal handbar between them.

In walking with crutches, the means of locomotion is transferred from the legs to the arms. The muscles of the arms, shoulders, back, and chest work together to manipulate the crutches. The kind of crutches used depends largely on the nature of the disability. In some cases, the legs may be partially able to function and bear some of the body's weight, so that there is less dependence on the crutches. In other cases, leg braces

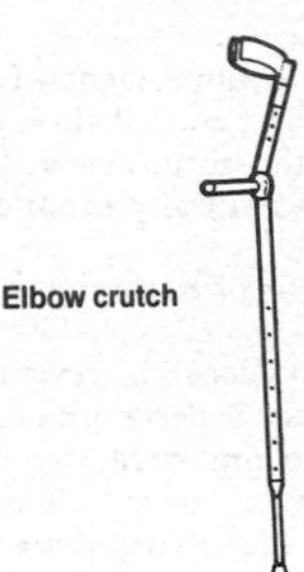
Elbow crutch

may be needed to supplement the crutches.

GAITS. The user is taught one of several standard methods or gaits, according to his condition.

In describing a gait each foot and crutch is called a point, so that a two-point gait, for example, means that two points of the total of four are in contact with the ground during the performance of one step. A three-point gait may be used when one leg is stronger than the other, meaning that two crutches and the weaker leg hit the ground simultaneously while the next step is made by the stronger leg alone. (See also GAIT).

Crutchfield tongs ('kruchfeeld) a metal appliance inserted into the parietal bones of the skull to allow the application of skeletal traction to the cervical spine.

Cruveilhier–Baumgarten murmur (kroovayl'yay-'bowmgahtən) a murmur heard at the abdominal wall over veins connecting the portal and caval systems.

Cruveilhier–Baumgarten syndrome cirrhosis of the liver with portal hypertension associated with congenital patency of the umbilical and paraumbilical veins.

Cruveilhier's disease (kroovayl'yayz) 1. simple ulcer of the stomach. 2. spinal muscular atrophy.

cry(o)- word element. [Gr.] *cold.*

cryaesthesia (ˌkrieis'theezi·ə) abnormal sensitiveness to cold.

cryalgesia (ˌkrieal'jeezi·ə) pain on application of cold.

cryanaesthesia (ˌkrieanəs'theezi·ə) loss of power of perceiving cold.

cryoanalgesia (ˌkrieohˌan'l'jeezi·ə, -si·ə) the relief of pain by application of cold by cryoprobe to peripheral nerves.

cryobank ('krieohˌbank) a facility for freezing and preserving semen at low temperatures (usually −196.5 °C) for future use.

cryobiology (ˌkrieohbie'oləjee) the science dealing with the effect of low temperatures on biological systems.

cryocautery (ˌkrieoh'kawtə·ree) cold cautery.

cryoextraction (ˌkrieoh·ik'strakshən) application of extremely low temperature probe for the removal of a cataractous lens (see also CATARACT).

cryoextractor (ˌkrieoh·ik'straktə) a cryoprobe used in cryoextraction.

cryofibrinogen (ˌkrieohfie'brinəjən) an abnormal fibrinogen that precipitates at low temperatures and redissolves at 37 °C.

cryofibrinogenaemia (ˌkrieohˌfiebrinohjə'neemi·ə) the presence of cryofibrinogen in the blood.

cryogenic (ˌkrieoh'jenik) producing low temperatures.

cryoglobulin (ˌkrieoh'globyuhlin) an abnormal globulin that precipitates at low temperatures and redissolves at 37 °C.

cryoglobulinaemia (ˌkrieohˌglobyuhli'neemi·ə) the presence of cryoglobulin in the blood, which is precipitated in the microvasculature upon exposure to cold.

cryohypophysectomy (ˌkrieohˌhiepohfi'zektəmee) destruction of the pituitary gland by the application of cold.

cryometer (krie'omitə) a thermometer for measuring very low temperature.

cryophilic (ˌkrieoh'filik) preferring or growing best at low temperatures; psychrophilic.

cryophylactic (ˌkrieohfi'laktik) resistant to very low temperatures; said of bacteria.

cryoprecipitate (ˌkrieohpri'sipiˌtayt) any precipitate that results from cooling. Of particular therapeutic value is the cryoprecipitate from fresh plasma. which is rich in factor VIII and is used to treat haemophilia.

cryopreservation (ˌkrieohˌprezə'vayshən) maintenance of the viability of excised tissue or organs by storing at very low temperatures.

cryoprobe ('krieohˌprohb) an instrument for applying extreme cold to tissue.

cryoprotective (ˌkrieohprə'tektiv) capable of protecting against injury due to freezing, as glycerol protects frozen red blood cells.

cryoprotein (ˌkrieoh'prohteen) a blood protein that precipitates on cooling.

cryoscopy (krie'oskəpee) examination of fluids based on the principle that the freezing point of a solution varies according to the amount and nature of the solute. adj. **cryoscopic**.

cryospray ('krieohˌspray) the use of a liquid nitrogen spray in cryosurgery.

cryostat ('krieohˌstat) 1. a device by which temperature can be maintained at a very low level. 2. in pathology and histology, a chamber containing a microtome for sectioning frozen tissue.

cryosurgery (ˌkrieoh'sərjə·ree) the ablation of tissue by application of extreme cold, as in the destruction of lesions in the thalamus for the treatment of Parkinson's disease, for the treatment of certain malignant lesions of the skin and mucous membranes, and for the early removal of malignant lesions of the uterine cervix. The method has also been used successfully in some types of surgery of the eye, for example, in the removal of cataracts and the repair of retinal detachment.

cryothalamectomy (ˌkrieohˌthalə'mektəmee) destruction of a portion of the thalamus by application of extreme cold.

cryotherapy (ˌkrieoh'therəpee) the therapeutic use of cold (see also HYPOTHERMIA).

cryotolerant (ˌkrieoh'tolə·rənt) able to withstand very low temperatures.

crypt (kript) a blind pit or tube on a free surface.

anal c's furrows, with pouchlike recesses at the lower end, separating the rectal columns; call also *anal sinuses*.

c's of Lieberkühn intestinal glands on the surface of the intestinal mucous membrane.

c's of tongue deep, irregular invaginations from the surface of the lingual tonsil.

tonsillar c's epithelium-lined clefts in the palatine tonsils.

crypt(o)- word element. [Gr.] *concealed, pertaining to a crypt.*

cryptaesthesia (ˌkriptis'theezi·ə) subconscious perception of occurrences not ordinarily perceptible to the senses.

cryptectomy (krip'tektəmee) excision or obliteration of a crypt.

cryptitis (krip'tietis) inflammation of the mucous membrane of the anal crypts.

cryptocephalus (ˌkriptoh'kefələs, -'sef-) a fetus or

infant with an inconspicuous head.

cryptococcosis (ˌkriptohkok'ohsis) infection caused by the fungus *Cryptococcus neoformans*, having a predilection for the brain and meninges but also invading the skin, lungs, and other parts. It particularly affects persons immunocompromized by disease or therapy. The source of infection is the environment. Transmission is probably airborne; person-to-person transmission does not occur. Treatment is by antifungal drugs, of which amphotericin B is the most effective.

Cryptococcus (ˌkriptoh'kokəs) a genus of yeastlike fungi.

C. neoformans a species of worldwide distribution, causing cryptococcosis in man.

cryptodeterminant (ˌkriptohdi'tərminənt) hidden determinant.

cryptodidymus (ˌkriptoh'didiməs) a twin fetus or infant, one twin being enclosed within the body of the other.

cryptogenic (ˌkriptoh'jenik) of obscure or doubtful origin.

cryptoglioma (ˌkriptohglie'ohmə) a stage of retinal glioma in which the eyeball shrinks, masking the presence of the growth.

cryptolith ('kriptohˌlith) a concretion in a crypt.

cryptomenorrhoea (ˌkriptohˌmenə'reeə) the occurrence of menstrual symptoms without external bleeding, as in imperforate hymen.

cryptomerorachischisis (ˌkriptohˌmerohrə'kiskisis) spina bifida occulta.

cryptomnesia ('kriptom'neezi·ə) subconscious memory. adj. **cryptomnesic**.

cryptophthalmia, cryptophthalmos, cryptophthalmus (ˌkriptof'thalmi·ə; -'thalmos; -'thalməs) congenital absence of the palpebral fissure, the skin extending from the forehead to the cheek, and the eye malformed or rudimentary.

cryptopodia (ˌkriptoh'pohdi·ə) swelling of the lower leg and foot, covering all but the sole of the foot.

cryptorchid (krip'tawkid) a person with undescended testes.

cryptorchidectomy (ˌkriptawki'dektəmee) excision of an undescended testis.

cryptorchidism, cryptorchism (krip'tawkiˌdizəm; krip'tawkizəm) failure of one or both of the testes to descend into the scrotum. In the embryo, the testes develop in the abdomen at about the level of the kidneys. At approximately the seventh month of fetal life they begin to descend to the groin and from there they move into the inguinal canal and so to the scrotum. The descent of a testis may be halted within the abdomen or the inguinal canal.

An improperly developed testis may never leave the abdomen, and so fail to produce the hormones necessary for secondary sexual characteristics. A testis lodged in the canal may well produce the hormones necessary for secondary sexual characteristics, but not spermatozoa.

Failure of both testes to descend is most uncommon. Usually only one testis is involved and the other produces sufficient numbers of spermatozoa.

cryptosporidosis (ˌkriptohspori'dohsis) a self-limiting parasitic infection of the intestine which causes mild diarrhoea in normal persons, and possibly severe and prolonged diarrhoea in the immunocompromised; a common manifestation of AIDS. It is probably a zoonosis, but person-to-person infection by the faecal-oral route may be common. Food-, milk- and water-borne outbreaks have been reported. The incubation period is over a week. Treatment consists of symptom management, no specific treatment being available.

cryptozygous (ˌkriptoh'ziegəs) having the calvaria wider than the face, so that the zygomatic arches are concealed when the head is viewed from above.

crystal ('kristəl) a naturally produced angular solid of definite form.

crystallin ('kristəˌlin) a globulin in the crystalline lens of the eye.

crystalline ('kristəˌlien) 1. resembling a crystal in nature or clearness. 2. pertaining to crystals.

c. lens the transparent organ behind the pupil of the eye (see also LENS).

crystallography (ˌkristə'logrəfee) the science dealing with the study of crystals.

x-ray c. the determination of the three-dimensional structure of molecules by means of diffraction patterns produced by x-rays.

crystalloid ('kristəˌloyd) 1. resembling a crystal. 2. a noncolloid substance. Crystalloids form true solutions and therefore are capable of passing through a semipermeable membrane, as in DIALYSIS. The physical opposite of a crystalloid is a COLLOID, which does not dissolve and does not form true solutions.

crystalluria (ˌkristə'lyooə·ri·ə) the excretion of crystals in the urine, causing irritation of the kidney.

Crystapen ('kristəpen) trademark for preparations of penicillin G potassium.

Cs chemical symbol, *caesium*.

CSF cerebrospinal fluid.

CSM Committee on Safety of Medicines.

CSP Chartered Society of Physiotherapy.

CSSD Central Sterile Supply Department.

CT computed tomography.

CT number the density assigned to a voxel in a CT (computed TOMOGRAPHY) scan on an arbitrary scale on which air has a density −1000; water, 0; and compact bone +1000. CT numbers are sometimes expressed in 'Hounsfield units'.

Cu chemical symbol, *copper* (L. *cuprum*).

cu. cubic.

cu.cm. cubic centimetre.

cu.mm. cubic millimetre.

cubitus ('kyoobitəs) 1. the elbow. 2. the upper limb distal to the humerus: the elbow, forearm, and hand. 3. ulna. adj. **cubital**.

c. valgus deformity of the elbow in which it deviates away from the midline of the body when extended.

c. varus deformity of the elbow in which it deviates toward the midline of the body when extended.

cuboid ('kyooboyd) resembling a cube; applied particularly to a bone of the foot.

cuffing ('kufing) formation of a cufflike surrounding border, as of leukocytes about a blood vessel observed in certain infections.

cuirass (kwi'ras) a covering for the chest.

cul-de-sac ('kuldaˌsak, -'kuhl-) [Fr.] *a blind pouch*.

Douglas' c. a sac or recess formed by a fold of the peritoneum dipping down between the rectum and the uterus. Called also *rectouterine excavation* or *pouch*.

culdocentesis (ˌkuldohsen'teesis) transvaginal puncture of Douglas' pouch for aspiration of fluid.

culdoscope ('kuldohˌskohp) an endoscope used in culdoscopy.

culdoscopy (kul'doskəpee) direct visual examination of the female viscera through an endoscope introduced into the pelvic cavity through the posterior vaginal fornix.

Culex ('kyooleks) a genus of mosquitoes found throughout the world; many species transmit various disease-producing agents, e.g. microfilariae, and viruses.

culicide ('kyooliˌsied) an agent that destroys mosquitoes.

culicifuge (kyoo'lisi,fyooj) an agent that repels mosquitoes.

culicine ('kyoolisin) 1. any member of the genus *Culex* or related genera. 2. pertaining to, involving, or affecting mosquitoes of the genus *Culex* or related species.

Cullen's sign ('kulənz) bluish discoloration around the umbilicus sometimes occurring in intraperitoneal haemorrhage, especially following rupture of the uterine tube in ectopic pregnancy. A similar discoloration is seen in acute haemorrhagic pancreatitis.

culmen ('kulmən) pl. *culmina* [L.] the anterior and upper part of the monticulus cerebelli; called also *cacumen*.

cultivation (,kulti'vayshən) the propagation of living organisms, applied especially to the growth of microorganisms or other cells in artificial media.

culture ('kulchə) 1. the propagation of microorganisms or of living tissue cells in special media conducive to their growth. 2. to induce such propagation. 3. the product of such propagation. 4. a collective noun for the symbolic and acquired aspects of human society, including convention, custom and language. 5. a singular noun for the customs and features of an ethnic (racial, religious or social) group. adj. **cultural**.

cell c. a growth of cells of a tissue in vitro; although the cells proliferate, they do not organize into tissue.

continuous flow c. the cultivation of bacteria in a continuous flow of fresh medium to maintain bacterial growth in logarithmic phase.

hanging-drop c. a culture in which the material to be cultivated is inoculated into a drop of fluid attached to a coverglass inverted over a hollow slide.

c. medium any substance or preparation used for the cultivation of living cells.

primary c. a cell or tissue culture started from material taken directly from an organism, as opposed to that from an explant from an organism.

slant c. one made on the surface of solidified medium in a tube which has been tilted to provide a greater surface area for growth.

stab c. a culture into which the organisms are introduced by thrusting a needle deep into the medium.

streak c. one in which the medium is inoculated by drawing an infected wire across it.

suspension c. a culture in which cells multiply while suspended in a suitable medium.

tissue c. the maintaining or growing of tissue, organ primordia, or the whole or part of an organ in vitro so as to preserve its architecture and function.

type c. a culture of a species of microorganism usually maintained in a central collection of type or standard culture.

cumulative ('kyoomyuhlətiv) adding to.

c. action the toxic effects produced by prolonged use of a drug given in comparatively small doses. Usually occurs due to slow excretion of the drug.

c. incidence rate the proportion of persons in a group becoming ill over a fixed period of time.

cumulus ('kyoomyuhləs) pl. *cumuli* [L.] a small elevation.

c. oophorus a mass of follicular cells surrounding the ovum in the vesicular ovarian follicle. Called also *corona radiata*.

cuneate ('kyooni,ayt) wedge-shaped.

cuneiform ('kyooni,fawm) wedge-shaped; applied particularly to three bones of the foot.

cuneus ('kyooni·əs) pl. *cunei* [L.] a wedge-shaped lobule on the medial aspect of the occipital lobe of the cerebrum.

cuniculus (kyoo'nikyuhləs) pl. *cuniculi* [L.] a burrow in the skin made by the itch mite, *Sarcoptes scabiei*.

cunnilingus (,kuni'lingəs) [L.] oral stimulation of the female genitals.

cup (kup) a depression or hollow.

glaucomatous c. a depression of the optic disc due to persistently increased intraocular pressure, broader and deeper than a physiological cup, and occurring first at the temporal side of the disc.

physiological c. a slight depression sometimes observed in the optic disc.

cupola ('kyoopələ) cupula.

cupping ('kuping) 1. the formation of a cup-shaped depression with the hand. Its effects are (a) to produce a skin erythema, thereby improving local circulation, and (b) to loosen excessive secretions from air passages, and perhaps induce coughing; it may also evoke a stretch reflex of the muscle, leading to a momentary increase in tone. 2. the use of a cupping glass to stimulate skin blood flow.

cupric ('kyooprik) pertaining to or containing divalent copper.

cuprous ('kyooprəs) pertaining to or containing monovalent copper.

cupruresis (,kyoopruh'reesis) the urinary excretion of copper.

cupula ('kyoopyuhlə) pl. *cupulae* [L.] a small, inverted cup or dome-shaped cap over a structure.

cupulogram ('kyoopuhloh,gram) the record, in the form of a tracing, made during cupulometry.

cupulolithiasis (,kyoopuhlohli'thieəsis) the presence of calculi in the cupula of the posterior semicircular duct.

cupulometry (,kyoopyuh'lomətree) a method of testing vestibular function, in which subjects are accelerated in a rotational chair and the duration of postrotational vertigo and nystagmus are plotted against rates of angular momentum.

curare (kyoo'rahree) any of a wide variety of highly toxic extracts from various botanical sources, including various species of *Strychnos*, a genus of tropical trees; used originally as arrow poisons in South America. A form extracted from the shrub, *Chondodendron tomentosum*, has been used as a skeletal muscle relaxant.

curarization (,kyuh,rahri'zayshən) administration of drugs that cause muscle relaxation by blocking transmission at the neuromuscular junction. The term is derived from curare, the first neuromuscular-blocking agent.

curative ('kyooə·rətiv) anything which promotes healing by overcoming disease.

cure (kyooə) 1. the course of treatment of any disease, or of a special case. 2. the successful treatment of a disease or wound. 3. a system of treating diseases. 4. a medicine effective in treating a disease.

curettage (,kyooə·ri'tahzh, kyuh'retij) [Fr.] the scraping of a surface with a curette for therapeutic purpose or to obtain biopsy material (see also DILATION AND CURETTAGE).

suction c., vacuum c. removal of the uterine contents, after dilation, by means of a hollow curette introduced into the uterus, through which suction is applied (see also ABORTION).

curette, curet (kyuh'ret, kyooə'ret) 1. a spoon-shaped instrument for cleansing a diseased surface. 2. to use a curette.

curie ('kyooə·ree) a non-SI unit of radioactivity, defined as the quantity of any radioactive nuclide in which the number of disintegrations per second is 3.700×10^{10}; abbreviated Ci. Superseded by the BECQUEREL.

curie-hour ('kyooə·ree,owə) a unit of dose equivalent to that obtained by exposure for one hour to radioactive material disintegrating at the rate of 3.7×10^{10} atoms per second.

curietron ('kyooə·ri,tron) an apparatus used for the treatment of cancer of the cervix and body of the uterus. The applicators are placed in the patient, and the radioisotope is then moved in and out of the applicators by remote control.

curium ('kyooə·ri·əm) a chemical element, atomic number 96, atomic weight 247, symbol Cm. See table of elements in Appendix 2.

Curling's ulcer ('kərlingz) an ulcer of the duodenum seen after severe burns of the body.

current ('kurənt) that which flows; electric transmission in a circuit.

alternating c. a current that periodically flows in opposite directions.

direct c. a current whose direction is always the same.

curvature ('kərvəchə) a nonangular deviation from a normally straight course.

greater c. of stomach the left or lateral and inferior border of the stomach, marking the inferior junction of the anterior and posterior surfaces.

lesser c. of stomach the right or medial border of the stomach, marking the superior junction of the anterior and posterior surfaces.

Pott's c. abnormal posterior curvature of the spine occurring as a result of Pott's disease.

spinal c. abnormal deviation of the vertebral column, as in KYPHOSIS, lordosis, and SCOLIOSIS.

curve (kərv) a line that is not straight, or that describes part of a circle, especially a line representing varying values in a graph.

frequency c. a curve representing graphically the probabilities of different numbers of recurrences of an event.

growth c. the curve obtained by plotting increase in size or numbers against the elapsed time.

Cushing's disease ('kuhshingz) Cushing's syndrome in which the hyperadrenocorticism is secondary to excessive pituitary excretion of adrenocorticotrophic hormone.

Cushing's syndrome a group of symptoms produced by an excess of free-circulating cortisol from the ADRENAL CORTEX. Circumstances that can bring about the manifestations typical of Cushing's syndrome are: (1) excessive secretion of adrenocorticotrophic hormone (ACTH) from the pituitary gland, which may actually result from faulty release of corticotrophin-releasing factor (CRF) from the hypothalamus; (2) tumour of the adrenal cortex, causing hypersecretion of the glucocorticoids; (3) ectopic production of ACTH by extrapituitary tumours, most commonly lung carcinoma, medullary thyroid carcinoma, and thymoma; and (4) *iatrogenic* Cushing's syndrome resulting from overzealous administration of exogenous glucocorticoids.

Diagnosis of Cushing's syndrome is established by laboratory findings indicating a continuous elevation of plasma cortisol. The symptoms and signs exhibited by the patient are a result of the action of this hormone. They include painful, fatty swellings in the interscapular area (buffalo hump) and in the facial area (moon face), distention of the abdomen, ecchymoses following even minor trauma, impotence, amenorrhoea, high blood pressure, and general weakness due to excessive protein catabolism and loss of muscle mass. There also can be an unusual growth of body hair (hirsutism) in females and broad streaked purple markings (atrophic striae) in the abdominal area as a result of collections of body fat. Patients who have a familial predisposition to diabetes mellitus frequently develop insulin-dependent diabetes mellitus as a result of the anti-insulin, diabetogenic properties of cortisol.

Treatment of Cushing's syndrome is becoming more effective as new modes of therapy become available. Pituitary Cushing's syndrome can be treated by surgical excision of the neoplasm using microsurgical techniques. Radiation with cobalt also is helpful in some cases. Drug therapy using adrenocorticolytic agents may be used as an adjunct to surgery and radiation or as an alternative when these modes of therapy are not feasible.

The syndrome is named for Dr. Harvey Cushing, the celebrated American brain surgeon and endocrinologist, who in 1932 was the first to describe it.

cushingoid ('kuhshing,oyd) resembling Cushing's syndrome, said of signs and symptoms.

cusp (kusp) a pointed or rounded projection, such as on the crown of a tooth, or a segment of a cardiac valve.

semilunar c. any of the semilunar segments of the aortic valve (having posterior, right, and left cusps) or the pulmonary valve (having anterior, right, and left cusps).

cuspid ('kuspid) 1. the third tooth on either side from the midline in each jaw; called also *canine tooth*. 2. having one cusp.

cuspis ('kuspis) pl. *cuspides* [L.] a cusp.

cutaneous (kyoo'tayni·əs) pertaining to the skin.

cutdown ('kut,down) creation of a small incised opening, especially in a vein (venous cutdown), to facilitate venipuncture and permit the passage of a needle or cannula for transfusion of blood or infusion of fluids.

cuticle ('kyootik'l) 1. a layer of more or less solid substance covering the free surface of an epithelial cell. 2. the narrow band of epidermis extending from the nail wall onto the nail surface; called also eponychium.

cutin ('kyootin) 1. a waxy constituent of the cuticle of plants. 2. a preparation of the gut of cattle used as suture material.

cutireaction (,kyootiri'akshən) an inflammatory or irritative reaction of the skin, occurring in certain infectious diseases, or on application or injection of a preparation of the organism causing the disease.

cutis ('kyootis) the outer protective covering of the body; the skin.

c. anserina transitory erection of the hair follicles due to contraction of the arrectores muscles, a reflection of sympathetic nerve discharge; goose flesh.

c. hyperelastica Ehlers–Danlos syndrome.

c. laxa a hereditary disorder in which the skin and subcutaneous tissues hypertrophy, so that the skin hangs in folds. Called also *dermatomegaly*.

cuvette (kyoo'vet) [Fr.] a glass container generally having well-defined characteristics (dimensions, optical properties), to contain solutions or suspensions for study.

CV closing volume.

CVA cerebrovascular accident (see STROKE).

CVP central venous pressure.

cyan(o)- word element. [Gr.] *blue*.

cyanhaemoglobin (,siean,heemə'glohbin) a bright cherry-red compound believed previously to be formed by the combination of hydrogen cyanide with haemoglobin. The colour of the blood characteristic of cyanide poisoning is due to the action of hydrocyanic acid, preventing the utilization of oxygen; the red coloration is thus thought to be due to oxyhaemoglobin.

cyanide ('siə,nied) a binary compound of cyanogen. Some inorganic compounds, such as cyanide salts, potassium cyanide, and sodium cyanide, are important in industry for extracting gold and silver from their ores and in electroplating. Other cyanide compounds are used in the manufacture of synthetic rubber and textiles. Cyanides are also used in pesticides.

Most cyanide compounds are deadly poisons. Treatment for cyanide poisoning varies according to the nature of the poison. In the case of a swallowed poison, such as hydrocyanic acid, the poison itself will cause vomiting. If the victim is able to swallow, milk or water may be given. A large dose of hydrocyanic acid will cause almost instant death.

If a gas, such as hydrogen cyanide, has been inhaled, the victim should be taken into open air and given artificial respiration.

cyanmethaemoglobin (ˌsieanˌmet·heemə'glohbin) a compound formed by combination of hydrocyanic acid with methaemoglobin. It is formed when methylene blue is administered as an antidote in cyanide poisoning. In laboratory methods, haemoglobin is converted to cyanmethaemoglobin and measured spectrophotometrically.

cyanmetmyoglobin (ˌsieanmetˌmieə'glohbin) a compound formed from metmyoglobin by addition of the cyanide ion.

cyanocobalamin (ˌsieənohkoh'baləmin) a substance having haematopoietic activity found in liver, fish meal, eggs, and other natural sources, or produced from cultures of *Streptomyces griseus*; it combines with intrinsic factor for absorption and is needed for erythrocyte maturation. Absence of intrinsic factor leads to malabsorption of cyanocobalamin and results in pernicious anaemia. Called also *antianaemia factor*, *extrinsic factor*, and VITAMIN B_{12}.

^{57}Co-labelled c. a radiopharmaceutical used in the Schilling test for the diagnosis of pernicious anaemia.

cyanolabe ('sieənohˌlayb) the pigment in retinal cones that is more sensitive to the blue range of the spectrum than are chlorolabe and erythrolabe.

cyanopia, cyanopsia (ˌsieə'nohpi·ə; siea'nopsi·ə) a defect of vision in which objects appear tinged with blue.

cyanosed ('sieəˌnohzd) cyanotic.

cyanosis (ˌsieə'nohsis) a bluish discoloration of the skin and mucous membranes due to excessive concentration of reduced haemoglobin in the blood. adj. **cyanotic.**

central c. that due to arterial unsaturation, the aortic blood carrying reduced haemoglobin.

enterogenous c. a syndrome due to absorption of nitrites and sulphides from the intestine, principally marked by methaemoglobinaemia and/or sulphhaemoglobinaemia associated with cyanosis, and accompanied by severe enteritis, abdominal pain, constipation or diarrhoea, headache, dyspnoea, dizziness, syncope, anaemia, and, occasionally, digital clubbing and indicanuria.

peripheral c. that due to an excessive amount of reduced haemoglobin in the venous blood as a result of extensive oxygen extraction at the capillary level.

cybernetics (ˌsiebə'netiks) the science of communication and control in the animal and in the machine.

cycl(o)- word element. [Gr.] *round, recurring, ciliary body of the eye.*

cyclamate ('sieklәˌmayt, 'sikləmayt) a non-nutritive sweetener.

cyclandelate (sie'klandəˌlayt) a vasodilator for peripheral vascular disease.

cyclarthrosis (ˌsieklah'throhsis) a pivot joint.

cyclase ('sieklayz) an enzyme that catalyses the formation of a cyclic phosphodiester.

cycle ('siek'l) a succession or recurring series of events.

cardiac c. a complete cardiac movement, or heart beat, including systole, diastole, and the intervening pause.

cell c. the cycle of biochemical and morphological events occurring in a reproducing cell population; it consists of the S phase, occurring toward the end of interphase, in which DNA is synthesized; the G_2 phase, a relatively quiescent period; the M phase, consisting of the four phases of mitosis; and the G_1 phase of interphase, which lasts until the S phase of the next cycle. **citric acid c.** tricarboxylic acid cycle.

oestrous c. the recurring periods of heat (estrus) in adult females of most mammals and the correlated changes in the reproductive tract from one period to another.

Krebs c. tricarboxylic acid cycle.

menstrual c. the period of the regularly recurring physiological changes in the endometrium which culminate in its shedding (MENSTRUATION) (see also MENSTRUAL CYCLE).

ovarian c. the sequence of physiological changes in the ovary involved in ovulation (see also OVULATION and REPRODUCTION).

reproductive c. the cycle of physiological changes in the reproductive organs, from the time of fertilization of the ovum through gestation and parturition (see also REPRODUCTION).

sex c., sexual c 1. the physiological changes recurring regularly in the reproductive organs of female mammals when pregnancy does not supervene. 2. the period of sexual reproduction in an organism that also reproduces asexually.

tricarboxylic acid c. the cyclic metabolic mechanism by which the complete oxidation of the acetyl moiety of acetyl-coenzyme A is effected; the process is the chief source of mammalian energy, during which carbon chains of sugars, fatty acids, and amino acid are metabolized to yield carbon dioxide, water, and high-energy phosphate bonds. Called also *citric acid cycle* and *Krebs cycle.*

urea c. a cyclic series of reactions that produce urea, a major route for removal of the ammonia produced in the metabolism of amino acids in the liver and kidney (see also UREA).

cyclectomy (sie'klektəmee) 1. excision of a piece of the ciliary body. 2. excision of a portion of the ciliary border of the eyelid.

cyclic ('sieklik) pertaining to or occurring in a cycle or cycles. The term is applied to chemical compounds that contain a ring of atoms in the nucleus.

cyclic AMP ('sieklik 'ayempee) cyclic adenosine monophosphate.

cyclic GMP ('sieklic 'gee·empee) cyclic guanosine monophosphate.

cyclitis (sie'klietis) inflammation of the ciliary body.

cyclizine ('siekliˌzeen) an antihistamine used in the form of the hydrochloride salt as an antinauseant to prevent motion sickness.

cyclobarbitone (ˌsiekloh'bahbiˌtohn) a short-acting barbiturate drug administered orally in cases of insomnia. Prolonged use may lead to dependence. Classified as a controlled drug.

cyclochoroiditis (ˌsiekloh,ko·roy'dietis) inflammation of the ciliary body and choroid.

cyclocryotherapy (ˌsiekloh,krieoh'therəpee) freezing of the ciliary body; done in the treatment of glaucoma.

cyclodialysis (ˌsieklohdie'aləsis) creation of a communication between the anterior chamber of the eye and the suprachoroidal space, in glaucoma surgery.

cyclodiathermy (ˌsiekloh,dieə'thərmee) destruction of a portion of the ciliary body by diathermy.

cyclogram ('sieklohˌgram) a tracing of the visual field made with a cycloscope.

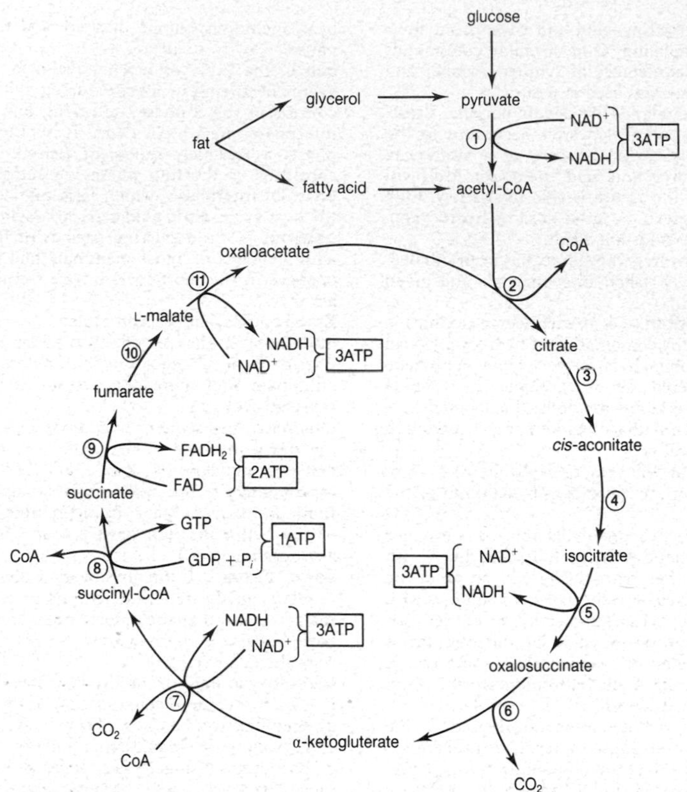

Tricarboxylic acid (Krebs) cycle. 1. pyruvate dehydrogenase; 2. citrate synthase; 3. aconitate dehydrogenase; 4. aconitate dehydrogenase; 5. isocitrate dehydrogenase; 6. isocitrate dehydrogenase; 7. α-ketogluterate dehydrogenase; 8. succinyl-CoA synthetase; 9. succinate dehydrogenase; 10. fumarase; 11. malate dehydrogenase. CoA = coenzyme A.

cycloid ('siekloyd) 1. containing a ring of atoms; said of organic chemical compounds. 2. cyclothymic (2). 3. cyclothyme.

cyclopenthiazide (ˌsieklohpen'thieəˌzied) an oral diuretic used in the treatment of oedema and hypertension.

cyclopentolate (ˌsiekloh'pentəˌlayt) used as 0.5% or 1% preparation as drops for dilating pupils. Short duration of action. Functions by blocking parasympathetic supply to ciliary muscle and sphincter of iris.

cyclophoria (ˌsiekloh'for·ri·ə) heterophoria in which there is torsional deviation of one eye from the anteroposterior axis in the absence of visual fusional stimuli, i.e. when the fellow eye is covered.

cyclophosphamide (ˌsiekloh'fosfəˌmied) a neoplastic suppressant used in the treatment of lymphomas and leukaemias.

cyclopia (sie'klohpi·ə) a developmental anomaly characterized by a single orbital fossa, with the globe absent or rudimentary, apparently normal, or duplicated, or the nose absent or present as a tubular appendix located above the orbit.

cycloplegia (ˌsiekloh'pleeji·ə) paralysis of the ciliary muscle; paralysis of accommodation.

cycloplegic (ˌsiekloh'pleejik) 1. pertaining to, characterized by, or causing cycloplegia. 2. an agent that produces cycloplegia.

cyclopropane (ˌsiekloh'prohpayn) a highly explosive gas, which is stored in orange cylinders and is used as an inhalational anaesthetic agent. It should only be used in areas where precautions against flames and sparks have been taken. Little used now, it retains a place as an induction agent in children because of its rapid onset of action. Once the child is asleep another inhalational agent is substituted and the cyclopropane is turned off.

Cyclops ('sieklops) a genus of minute crustaceans, species of which act as hosts of *Diphyllobothrium* and *Dracunculus*.

cyclops ('sieklops) a fetus or infant exhibiting cyclopia.

cycloscope ('siekloh,skohp) a form of perimeter for mapping the visual fields.

cycloserine (ˌsiekloh'siə·rien) a antibiotic substance elaborated by *Streptomyces orchidaceus* or produced synthetically, used as a tuberculostatic in patients resistant to first-line therapy and in the treatment of urinary tract infections.

cyclosis (sie'klohsis) movement of the cytoplasm within a cell, without external deformation of the cell wall.

Cyclospasmol (ˌsiekloh'spazmol) trademark for preparations of cyclandelate, a peripheral vasodilator.

cyclosporin (sieklohspo·rin, -spor·rin) an immunosuppressant commonly used to prevent rejection following transplantation.

cyclothyme ('siekloh,thiem) an individual with a cyclothymic personality or exhibiting cyclothymia.

cyclothymia (ˌsiekloh'thiemi·ə) 1. cyclothymic personality. 2. a condition characterized by alternating moods of elation and mild depression.

cyclothymic (ˌsiekloh'thiemik) 1. pertaining to or characterized by cyclothymia. 2. a cyclothymic personality. 3. cyclothyme. **c. personality** a personality marked by alternate moods of elation and dejection.

cyclotron ('siekloh,tron) an apparatus for accelerating protons or deuterons to high energies by means of a constant magnetic field and an oscillating electric field.

cyclotropia (ˌsiekloh'trohpi·ə) STRABISMUS in which there is permanent torsional deviation of the eye in the presence of visual fusional stimuli, resulting in diplopia.

cyesis (sie'eesis) pregnancy. adj. **cyetic.**

cylindroid ('silin,droyd) 1. shaped like a cylinder. 2. a urinary cast of various origins, which tapers to a slender tail that is often twisted or curled upon itself.

cylindroma (ˌsilin'drohmə) 1. adenocystic carcinoma. 2. a benign skin tumour, usually on the face and scalp, consisting of cylindrical masses of small, dark epithelial cells surrounded by a thick band of eosinophilic hyaline material. adj. **cylindromatous.**

cylindruria (ˌsilin'drooə·ri·ə) the presence of cylindroids in the urine.

cymbocephaly (ˌsimboh'kefəlee, -'sef-) scaphocephaly.

cynanthropy (sie'nanthrəpee) a delusion in which the patient believes himself a dog.

cynophobia (ˌsienoh'fohbi·ə) morbid fear of dogs.

cyotrophy (sie'otrəfee) nutrition of the fetus.

cyproheptadine (ˌsieproh'heptədeen) a histamine and serotonin antagonist used as an antipruritic and antihistaminic.

cyproterone (sie'prohtə·rohn) an anti-androgen used to treat male hypersexuality and prostatic carcinoma.

cyrtometer (sər'tomitə) a device for measuring the curved surfaces of the body.

cyst (sist) 1. a closed epithelium-lined sac or capsule containing a liquid or semisolid substance. Most cysts are harmless. Nevertheless they should be removed when possible because some types occasionally may change into malignant growths, become infected, or obstruct a gland. There are four main types of benign cysts: retention cysts, exudation cysts, embryonic cysts, and parasitic cysts. 2. a stage in the life cycle of certain parasites, during which they are enveloped in a protective wall.

alveolar c's dilations of pulmonary alveoli, which may fuse by breakdown of their septa to form large air cysts (pneumatoceles).

blue dome c. a benign retention cyst of the breast that shows a blue colour (see also CYSTIC DISEASE OF BREAST).

branchial c., branchiogenic c., branchiogenous c. one formed from an incompletely closed branchial cleft (see also BRANCHIAL CYST).

chocolate c. one filled with haemosiderin following local haemorrhage, such as may occur in the ovary in ovarian endometriosis.

daughter c. a small parasitic cyst developed from the walls of a larger cyst.

dentigerous c. see DENTIGEROUS cyst.

dermoid c. a tumour containing bone, hair, teeth, etc. May occur in the region of the eye (see also DERMOID CYST).

echinococcus c. hydatid cyst.

embryonic c. one developing from bits of embryonic tissue that have been overgrown by other tissues, or from developing organs that normally disappear before birth. An example is a BRANCHIAL CYST.

epidermal c., epidermoid c. an intradermal or subcutaneous cyst containing keratinizing squamous epithelium. It may arise from occluded hair follicles.

exudation c. a cyst formed by the slow seepage of an exudate into a closed cavity.

follicular c. one due to occlusion of the duct of a follicle or small gland, especially one formed by enlargement of a graafian follicle as a result of accumulated transudate.

hydatid c. the larval stage of the tapeworms *Echinococcus granulosis* and *E. multilocularis* (see also HYDATID DISEASE).

keratin c. one arising in the pilosebaceous apparatus, lined by stratified squamous epithelium and containing largely macerated keratin and often sufficient sebum to render the contents greasy and often rancid.

meibomian c. chalazion.

myxoid c. a nodular lesion usually overlying a distal interphalangeal finger joint in the dorsolateral or dorsomedial position, consisting of focal mucinous degeneration of the collagen of the dermis; not a true cyst, lacking an epithelial wall, it does not communicate with the underlying synovial space.

Naboth's c's, nabothian c's cystlike formations caused by occlusion of the necks of glands in the mucosa of the uterine endocervix, causing them to be distended with retained secretion. Called also *Naboth's*, or *nabothian, follicles.*

parasitic c. one forming around the larvae of parasites (tapeworms, amoebae, trichinae) that enter the body.

pilar c. a type of epidermal cyst, almost always found on the scalp, arising from the outer root sheath of the hair follicle.

pilonidal c. a hair-containing sacrococcygeal dermoid cyst or sinus, often opening at a postanal dimple (see also PILONIDAL CYST).

retention c. a tumour-like accumulation of a secretion formed when the outlet of a secreting gland is obstructed. These cysts may develop in any of the secretory glands—the breast, pancreas, kidney, salivary or sebaceous glands, and mucous membranes.

sarcosporidian c's cylindrical cysts containing parasitic spores, found in the muscles of mammals infected with *Sarcocystis*; rare in man.

sebaceous c. a retention cyst of a sebaceous gland (see also SEBACEOUS CYST).

vitelline c. a congenital cyst lined with ciliated epithelium occurring along the gastrointestinal canal; the remains of the omphalomesenteric duct or yolk sac.

cyst(o)- word element. [Gr.] *cyst, bladder.*

cystadenocarcinoma (siˌstadənohˌkahsi'nohmə) adenocarcinoma with extensive cyst formation.

cystadenoma (siˌstadə'nohmə) a benign glandular tumour forming a large cystic space or spaces, containing secretions.

mucinous c. a multilocular, usually benign, tumour produced by ovarian epithelial cells and having mucin-filled cavities.

papillary c. any benign tumour producing patterns that are both papillary and cystic.

serous c. a cystic tumour of the ovary containing thin, clear yellow serum and some solid tissue.

cystalgia (si'stalji·ə) pain in the bladder.

cystathioninuria (ˌsistəˌthieohni'nyooə·ri·ə) a hereditary disorder of cystathionine metabolism, marked by increased concentrations in the urine, and due to deficiency of γ-cystathionase; mental handicap may be associated.

cystectasia (ˌsistek'tayzi·ə) dilation of the bladder.

cystectomy (si'stektəmee) 1. excision of a cyst. 2. excision or resection of the urinary bladder.

cysteine ('sisti,een, sis'tayn) a sulphur-containing amino acid produced by enzymatic or acid hydrolysis of proteins, readily oxidized to cystine; sometimes found in urine.

cystencephalus (ˌsisten'kefələs, -'sef-) a fetus or infant with a membranous sac in place of a brain.

cystic ('sistik) 1. pertaining to or containing cysts. 2. pertaining to the urinary bladder or to the gallbladder.

c. disease of breast a form of mammary dysplasia with formation of cysts containing a semitransparent, turbid fluid that imparts a brown to blue colour to the unopened cysts (blue dome cysts). The condition is due to abnormal hyperplasia of the ductal epithelium and dilation of the ducts of the mammary gland. Called also *Schimmelbusch's disease* and *fibrocystic disease of breast*.

c. duct the excretory duct of the gallbladder (see also BILE DUCTS).

c. fibrosis a generalized hereditary disorder associated with widespread dysfunction of the exocrine glands, with accumulation of excessively thick and tenacious mucus and abnormal secretion of sweat and saliva; called also *cystic fibrosis of the pancreas*, and *mucoviscidosis*. The disease is inherited as a recessive trait; both parents must be carriers. The cause of the disease is presumably the absence, insufficiency, or abnormality of some essential hormone or enzyme.

Symptoms and severity of cystic fibrosis vary widely. Although it is congenital, it may not manifest itself to any appreciable degree during the early weeks or months of life, or it may cause intestinal obstruction and perforation in the newborn. The chief cause of complications in cystic fibrosis is the extremely thick mucus produced. Normal mucus bathes and protects internal surfaces and transports chemicals produced in one organ through intricate small ducts for use in another organ. Normal mucus flows easily, carrying with it bacteria, dirt, and wastes that will be eliminated from the body. The mucus of cystic fibrosis, in contrast, is highly adhesive. Bacteria and other matter stick to it, and it in turn clogs the lungs and usually interferes with the flow of digestive enzymes from the pancreas to the small intestine.

In the lungs, the mucus blocks the bronchioles, creating breathing difficulties. Infection develops, thereby increasing obstruction of the air passages. Air becomes trapped in the lungs (emphysema), and scattered small areas eventually collapse (patchy atelectasis). Repeated infections follow, inflaming and damaging lung tissue, leading to chronic lung disease. About 50 per cent of children with cystic fibrosis have symptoms related to lung involvement.

When mucus prevents the pancreatic enzymes from reaching the duodenum (which occurs in approximately 80 per cent of cystic fibrosis patients), digestion is hindered. Fats especially are poorly digested and absorbed. The child may have a voracious appetite, yet fail to grow normally or gain weight. There may be marked signs of malnutrition. The outstanding symptom associated with pancreatic enzyme deficiency is frequent bulky, fatty, and foul-smelling faeces.

Between 5 and 10 per cent of cystic fibrosis babies are born with intestines obstructed by putty-like intestinal secretions (meconium ileus) and die unless the condition is diagnosed promptly and relieved by surgery within the first few days of life. Such relief does not protect the child against the other manifestations of cystic fibrosis, although these may not appear until later.

Because cysts and scar tissue on the pancreas were observed during autopsy when the disease was first being differentiated from other conditions, it was given the name cystic fibrosis of the pancreas. Although this term describes a secondary rather than primary characteristic, it is still used in some places.

DIAGNOSIS. Sweat in cystic fibrosis is excessively salty. Collapse of cystic fibrosis patients in the USA from salt loss during a heat wave led, in 1953, to recognition of the sweat abnormality. The sweat chloride test, introduced the next year, remains the cornerstone of diagnosis of cystic fibrosis. In children, a sweat chloride level above 60 mEq/l indicates cystic fibrosis. Newborn infants do not produce sufficient sweat for the test, but nurses have noted that these babies 'taste salty' when kissed. Supporting evidence can confirm the sweat test finding.

Caucasians appear more susceptible to cystic fibrosis than Afro-Caribbeans, and among Orientals it seems to be rare.

cysticercosis (ˌsistisər'kohsis) an infection of the tissues with the larval forms (Cysticercus cellulosae) of the pork tapeworm *Taenia solium* which penetrate the intestinal wall and invade such tissues as the subcutaneous tissue, brain, eye, muscle, heart, liver, lung, and peritoneum. If the brain is penetrated, epilepsy and raised intracranial pressure may result. It occurs worldwide, but has been eliminated from the UK and is very rare in Europe and North America. The infection is transmitted by eating undercooked infected pork, and cysticercosis results when the tapeworm eggs produced in the intestine are ingested by spread through food or by the faecal–oral route.

cysticercus (ˌsisti'sərkəs) pl. *cysticerci;* a larval form of tapeworm.

cystiform ('sistiˌfawm) resembling a cyst.

cystigerous (si'stijə·rəs) containing cysts.

cystinaemia (ˌsisti'neemi·ə) the presence of cystine in the blood.

cystine ('sisteen, -tin) a naturally occurring amino acid, the chief sulphur-containing component of the protein molecule. It is sometimes found in the urine and in the kidneys in the form of minute hexagonal crystals, frequently forming cystine calculus in the bladder.

c. storage disease Fanconi's syndrome (2).

cystinosis (ˌsisti'nohsis) a hereditary disorder of childhood, usually appearing after 6 months of age, and marked by osteomalacia, aminoaciduria, phosphaturia, and deposition of cystine throughout the tissues of the body, including the liver, bone marrow, spleen, and cornea. It is the most common cause of FANCONI'S SYNDROME (2).

cystinuria (ˌsisti'nyooə·ri·ə) a hereditary condition of persistent excessive urinary excretion of cystine, lysine, ornithine, and arginine, due to impairment of renal tubular reabsorption of these amino acids. The predominant clinical manifestation is the formation of urinary cystine calculi.

cystistaxis (ˌsisti'staksis) oozing of blood from the mucous membrane into the bladder.

cystitis (si'stietis) acute or chronic inflammation of the urinary bladder, usually caused by ascending infection from the exterior via the urethra which may be associated with tissue trauma, urine stagnation or bladder distortion or compression by an enlarged neighbouring organ or mass. Cystitis is common in pregnant women, as the enlarged uterus compresses the bladder. It may also be caused by radiotherapy of the pelvis, administration of certain drugs (e.g. cyclophosphamide), bladder calculi, tumours or neurological diseases impairing normal function of the bladder.

Cystitis is more common in females, as the shorter, wider-calibre urethra is more likely to allow the entry of micro-organisms. In acute cystitis, inflammation is confined to the bladder mucosa which is hyperemic, and oedematous with haemorrhagic areas. In chronic cystitis the inflammation may extend into the detrusor muscle. Persistent inflammation may cause fibrosis of tissues and reduction of bladder capacity, increasing the problem of frequency.

Prevention of recurrent cystitis in females that is not attributable to abnormal structures or other factors mentioned previously may be simply a matter of good personal hygiene and some common sense measures: (1) always wipe the anal region from front to back after a bowel movement; (2) avoid wearing nylon tights, tight trousers, or any clothing that traps perineal moisture and prevents evaporation; (3) do not wash underclothing in strong soap, and rinse underclothing well; (4) do not use bubble bath, perfumed soap, feminine hygiene sprays, or products containing hexachlorophene; (5) try to drink at least 1500 ml of water a day; (6) do not ignore vaginal discharge or other signs of vaginal infection; and (7) empty the bladder promptly after sexual intercourse, and drink two glasses of water to help flush out microorganisms that might have entered the urethra during coitus.

SYMPTOMS AND TREATMENT. The presenting symptoms are dysuria, nocturia, frequency and urgency of urination, and sometimes haematuria. Shivers and fever indicate involvement of the entire urinary tract and are not symptomatic of uncomplicated cystitis.

Treatment of acute cystitis may consist of a copious fluid intake to flush out organisms in the bladder, or antibiotics and a fluid intake of about 2 litres, which is sufficient to allow antibiotics excreted into the urinary tract to be effective, while not diluting them to beyond a useful concentration. Hot baths give some relief of the discomfort, and spasms of the bladder wall may respond to an antispasmodic drug such as emepronium or propantheline. Chronic cystitis is more difficult to cure and may require surgical dilation of the urethra and antiseptic bladder instillations. In many cases removal of the underlying cause, such as chronic vaginal infection, relieves the cystitis.

cystitomy (si'stitəmee) surgical division of the capsule of the crystalline lens.

cystocarcinoma (ˌsistohˌkahsi'nohmə) carcinoma associated with cysts.

cystocele ('sistohˌseel) herniation of the urinary bladder into the vagina.

cystodiathermy (ˌsistoh'dieəˌthərmee) the application of a high-frequency electric current to the bladder mucosa, usually for fulguration of papilloma.

cystodynia (ˌsistoh'dini·ə) pain in the bladder; cystalgia.

cystoelytroplasty (ˌsistoh'elitrohˌplastee) surgical repair of a vesicovaginal fistula.

cystoepithelioma (ˌsistohˌepiˌtheeli'ohmə) a tumour with cystic and epitheliomatous elements.

cystofibroma (ˌsistohfie'brohmə) a fibroma containing cysts.

cystogastrostomy (ˌsistohga'strostəmee) surgical anastomosis of a pancreatic cyst to the stomach for drainage.

cystogram ('sistohˌgram) the film obtained by cystography.

micturating c. a radiogram of the urinary tract made while the patient is urinating.

cystography (si'stogrəfee) radiography of the urinary bladder using a contrast medium. Imaging of the urethra is frequently included in the technique (see CYSTOURETHROGRAPHY). The principal indications are abnormalities of the bladder, vesicoureteric reflux, abnormalities of the urethra during micturition, and stress incontinence. Conventional cystography is undertaken using a water-soluble, iodine-containing contrast medium.

double contrast c. a technique for demonstrating a bladder tumour within a diverticulum. The mucosa is outlined by coating it with contrast medium and the bladder is then distended with gas.

radionuclide c. a method of evaluating the severity of vesicoureteric reflux using radionuclides instead of a contrast medium. The method does not provide the anatomical information of conventional cystography but the radiation dose to the patient is considerably less. Two techniques are possible: direct, in which sodium pertechnetate followed by saline are instilled in the bladder following catheterization; and indirect, which is possible at the end of a renogram, when all the intravenously administered isotope has passed through the kidneys and is within the bladder. In both cases vesicoureteric reflux is assessed by observing the urinary tract with a gamma camera during micturition.

cystoid ('sistoyd) 1. resembling a cyst. 2. a cystlike, circumscribed collection of softened material, having no enclosing capsule.

cystojejunostomy (ˌsistohjejuh'nostəmee) surgical anastomosis of a pancreatic cyst to the jejunum.

cystolith (sistohˌlith) a vesical calculus.

cystolithectomy (ˌsistohli'thektəmee) surgical removal of a stone by cutting into the urinary bladder.

cystolithiasis (ˌsistohli'thieəsis) formation of vesical calculi.

cystolithic (ˌsistoh'lithik) pertaining to a vesical calculus.

cystolithotomy (ˌsistohli'thotəmee) cystolithectomy.

cystoma (si'stohmə) a tumour containing cysts of neoplastic origin; a cystic tumour.

cystometer (si'stomitə) an instrument for studying the neuromuscular mechanism of the bladder by means of measurements of pressure and capacity.

cystometrogram (ˌsistoh'metrohˌgram) the record obtained by cystometrography.

cystometrography (ˌsistohme'trogrəfee) the graphic recording of intravesical volumes and pressures.

cystometry (si'stomətree) the study of pressure changes within the bladder and of variations in its capacity.

cystomorphous (ˌsistoh'mawfəs) resembling a cyst or bladder.

cystopexy ('sistohˌpeksee) fixation of the bladder to the abdominal wall.

cystoplasty ('sistohˌplastee) plastic repair of the bladder.

cystoplegia (ˌsistoh'pleeji·ə) paralysis of the bladder.

cystoproctostomy (ˌsistohprok'tostəmee) surgical creation of a communication between the urinary bladder and the rectum.

cystoptosis (ˌsistop'tohsis) prolapse of part of the inner coat of the bladder into the urethra.

cystopyelitis (ˌsistohˌpieə'lietis) inflammation of the bladder and renal pelvis.

cystopyelonephritis (ˌsistohˌpieəlohnə'frietis) combined cystitis and pyelonephritis.

cystorrhaphy (si'sto·rəfee) suture of the bladder.

cystorrhoea (ˌsistə'reeə) mucous discharge from the bladder.

cystosarcoma (ˌsistohsah'kohmə) an unusually large tumour of the mammary gland, with a cellular, sarcoma-like stoma; it is locally aggressive and sometimes metastasizes.

cystoscope ('sistəˌskohp) an endoscope especially designed for passing through the urethra into the bladder to permit visual inspection of the interior of that organ.

cystoscopy (si'stoskəpee) visual examination of the

bladder by means of an endoscope, a narrow telescope introduced into the urethra and passed into the bladder.

Catheters can be passed through the endoscope into the bladder and beyond into the ureters and kidneys. Thus samples of urine can be obtained for diagnostic purposes and radiopaque fluids can be injected for radiographs of the urinary tract (see also PYELOGRAPHY).
PATIENT CARE. Prior to the procedure the patient should be given an adequate explanation of its purpose and expected outcome, and of the need for proper preparation. Because the full cooperation of the patient is of crucial importance to a successful test, it is essential that the patient be told what is expected of him when the procedure is done under local anaesthesia. During the procedure, if the patient is awake, the nurse or other attendant should be alert for indications of sudden pain, which could signify perforation of the urethra or other structures. Cardiac arrhythmia may occur in patients with a history of heart disease.

The plan of care following cystoscopy should include observation of the amount and character of the urine. Some slight coloration from blood should be expected, but any frank bleeding and passing of clots should be reported to the surgeon. Other problems likely to require nursing intervention are discomfort from bladder spasms, back pain, a feeling of fullness and burning in the bladder region, and possible urinary retention. Nursing measures would include warm baths, relaxation techniques to promote rest and provide relief from pain, and administration of prescribed medications.

If chilling and fever occur and do not respond to attempts to provide warmth and to increased fluid intake, there could be an infection in the urinary tract requiring antibacterial therapy.

cystostomy (si'stostəmee) surgical formation of an opening into the bladder.

cystotomy (si'stotəmee) incision into the urinary bladder for the purpose of removing calculi, tumours, etc.

cystoureteritis (ˌsistoh·yuhˌreetə'rietis) inflammation involving the urinary bladder and ureters.

cystoureterogram (ˌsistoh·yuh'reetə·rəˌgram) a radiograph of the bladder and ureter.

cystourethrography (ˌsistohˌyooə·ri'throgrəfee) radiology of the urinary bladder and urethra.

chain c. that in which a sterile beaded metal chain is introduced via a modified catheter into the bladder and urethra; used in evaluating anatomical relationships of the bladder and urethra.

micturating c. radiology of the bladder and urethra during micturition using a water-soluble, iodine-containing contrast medium. The principle indications are vesicoureteric reflux and abnormalities of micturition.

cystourethroscope (ˌsistoh·yuhreethrəˌskohp) an instrument for examining the posterior urethra and bladder.

cyt(o)- word element. [Gr.] *a cell.*

cytapheresis (sieˌtafə'reesis) a procedure in which cells of one or more kinds (leukocytes, platelets, etc.) are separated from whole blood and retained, the plasma and other formed elements being retransfused into the donor; it includes leukapheresis and thrombocytapheresis.

cytarabine (si'tarəˌbeen) an antimetabolite that inhibits DNA synthesis, and hence has antineoplastic and antiviral properties. Also called cytosine arabinoside.

-cyte (siet) word element. [Gr.] *a cell.*

cytoanalyser (ˌsietoh'anəliezə) an electronic optical apparatus for the detection of malignant cells in smears.

cytochalasin (ˌsietoh'kaləsin) any of a group of fungal metabolites that affect the motility of polymorphonuclear leukocytes.

cytochemistry (ˌsietoh'kemistree) the identification and localization of the different chemical compounds and their activities within the cell.

cytochrome ('sietohˌkrohm) any of a class of haemoproteins, widely distributed in animal and plant tissue, whose main function is electron transport; distinguished according to their prosthetic group as *a*, *b*, *c*, and *d*.

cytoclasis (sie'tokləsis) the destruction of cells. adj. **cytoclastic.**

cytodiagnosis (ˌsietohˌdieəg'nohsis) diagnosis based on examination of cells. adj. **cytodiagnostic.**

cytodifferentiation (ˌsietohˌdifəˌrenshi'ayshən) the development of specialized structures and functions in embryonic cells.

cytodistal (ˌsietoh'dist'l) denoting that part of an axon remote from the cell body.

cytogenesis (ˌsietoh'jenəsis) the origin and development of the cell.

cytogenetics (ˌsietohjə'netiks) that branch of genetics devoted to the cellular constituents concerned in heredity, i.e., the chromosomes.

clinical c. the branch of cytogenetics concerned with relations between chromosomal abnormalities and pathological conditions.

cytogenic (ˌsietoh'jenik) 1. pertaining to cytogenesis. 2. forming or producing cells.

cytoglucopenia, cytoglycopenia (ˌsietohˌglookoh'peeni·ə; ˌsietohˌgliekoh'peeni·ə) deficient glucose content of the body or blood cells.

cytohistogenesis (ˌsietohˌhistoh'jenəsis) development of the structure of cells.

cytohistology (ˌsietoh·hi'stoləjee) the combination of cytological and histological methods. adj. **cytohistological.**

cytokinesis (ˌsietohki'neesis) the division of the cytoplasm between daughter cells in MITOSIS or MEIOSIS.

cytologist (sie'toləjist) a specialist in cytology.

cytology (sie'toləjee) the study of cells, their origin, structure, function, and pathology. adj. **cytological.**

aspiration biopsy c. (ABC) the microscopic study of cells obtained from superficial or internal lesions by suction through a fine needle.

exfoliative c. microscopic examination of cells desquamated from a body surface or lesion as a means of detecting malignancy and microbiological changes, to measure hormonal levels, etc. Such cells may be obtained by such procedures as aspiration, washing, smear, and scraping, and the technique may be applied to vaginal secretions, sputum, urine, abdominal fluid, prostatic secretion, etc.

fine needle c. see ASPIRATION biopsy, fine needle.

cytolysin (sie'tolisin) a substance or antibody that produces cytolysis.

cytolysis (sie'tolisis) the dissolution of cells.

immune c. cell lysis produced by antibody with the participation of complement.

cytolysosome (ˌsietoh'liesohˌsohm) a lysosome fused with mitochondria and other cell organelles and associated with cell autolysis. Called also *autophagosome.*

cytomegalic inclusion disease (ˌsietoh'megəlik in'kloozhən) an infection due to cytomegalovirus and marked by nuclear inclusion bodies in enlarged infected cells. In the congenital form, there is hepatosplenomegaly with cirrhosis, and microcephaly with mental or motor handicap. Acquired disease may cause a clinical state similar to infectious mononucleosis. When acquired by blood transfusion, postperfusion syndrome results.

cytomegalovirus (ˌsietohˌmegəloh'vierəs) any of a group of highly host-specific herpesviruses infecting man, monkeys, or rodents, producing unique large cells with inclusion bodies; the virus specific for man causes cytomegalic inclusion disease, and it has been associated with a syndrome resembling infectious mononucleosis.

cytometaplasia (ˌsietohˌmetə'playzi·ə) change in function or form of cells.

cytometer (sie'tomitə) a device for counting cells.

cytometry (sie'tomətree) the counting of cells, especially blood cells.

cytomorphology (ˌsietohmaw'foləjee) the morphology of body cells.

cytomorphosis (ˌsietohmaw'fohsis) the changes through which cells pass in development.

cytopathic (ˌsietoh'pathik) pertaining to or characterized by pathological changes in cells.

cytopathogenesis (ˌsietohˌpathoh'jenəsis) the mechanism of production of pathological changes in cells. adj. **cytopathogenetic**.

cytopathological (ˌsietohˌpathə'lojik'l) relating to cytopathology; denoting the changes in cells in disease.

cytopathologist (ˌsietohpə'tholəjist) an expert in the study of cells in disease; a cellular pathologist.

cytopathology (ˌsietohpə'tholəjee) the study of cells in disease; cellular pathology.

cytopenia (ˌsietoh'peeni·ə) deficiency in the cells of the blood.

cytophagy (sie'tofəjee) the ingestion of cells by phagocytes.

cytophilic (ˌsietoh'filik) having an affinity for cells.

cytophylaxis (ˌsietohfi'laksis) 1. the protection of cells against cytolysis. 2. increase in cellular activity.

cytopipette (ˌsietohpi'pet) a pipette for taking cytological smears.

cytoplasm ('sietohˌplazəm) the protoplasm of a cell surrounding the nucleus (nucleoplasm). adj. **cytoplasmic**.

cytoscreener (ˌsietoh'skreenə) a person specializing in cytology who can process and stain specimens of exfoliated cells from the female genital tract and from other accessible organs, and then screen the resulting microscopic preparations. Abnormalities are positively identified and referred directly to a pathologist specializing in cytology.

cytosine ('sietohˌseen) a pyrimidine base found in NUCLEIC ACIDS.

cytoskeleton (ˌsietoh'skelitən) a conspicuous internal reinforcement in the cytoplasm of a cell, consisting of tonofibrils, filaments of the terminal web, and other microfilaments. adj. **cytoskeletal**.

cytosol ('sietohˌsol) the liquid medium of the cytoplasm, e.g., cytoplasm minus organelles and nonmembranous insoluble components. adj. **cytosolic**.

cytosome ('sietohˌsohm) the body of a cell apart from its nucleus.

cytostatic (ˌsietoh'statik) 1. suppressing the growth and multiplication of cells. 2. an agent that so acts.

cytotaxis (ˌsietoh'taksis) the movement and arrangement of cells with respect to a specific source of stimulation. adj. **cytotactic**.

cytothesis (sie'tothəsis) restitution of cells to their normal condition.

cytotoxic (ˌsietoh'toksik) 1. having a deleterious effect upon cells. 2. an agent that destroys cells.

cytotoxin (ˌsietoh'toksin) a toxin having a specific toxic action on cells of special organs.

cytotrophoblast (ˌsietoh'trofohˌblast) the cellular (inner) layer of the trophoblast.

cytotropism (ˌsietoh'trohpizəm) 1. cell movement in response to external stimulation. 2. the tendency of viruses, bacteria, drugs, etc., to exert their effect upon certain cells of the body.

Cytoxan (sie'toksan) trademark for preparations of cyclophosphamide, an antineoplastic agent.

cyturia (sie'tyooə·ri·ə) the presence of cells of any sort in the urine.

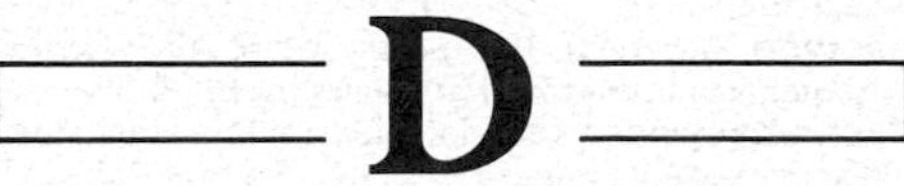

D

D chemical symbol, *deuterium*.

2,4-D a toxic chlorphenoxy herbicide (2,4-dichlorophenoxyacetic acid), a component of Agent Orange.

D- chemical prefix (small capital) specifying that the substance corresponds in chemical configuration to the standard substance D-glyceraldehyde. Opposed to L-. For carbohydrates, the configuration of the highest numbered asymmetric carbon atoms determines whether the substance is D- or L-; for amino acids the lowest numbered asymmetric carbon atom is the key.

d symbol, *deci-*.

***d*-** prefix, *dextro-*.

D & C, D. and C. dilation (of cervix) and curettage (of uterus).

DA Diploma of Anaesthetics.

dacarbazine (də'kahbəˌzeen) an antineoplastic used in the treatment of metastatic malignant melanoma.

dacry(o)- word element. [Gr.] *tears;* or *the lacrimal apparatus of the eye*.

dacryagogic (ˌdakri·ə'gojik) 1. inducing a flow of tears. 2. serving as a channel for discharge of secretion of the lacrimal glands.

dacryagogue ('dakri·əˌgog) 1. an agent that induces a flow of tears. 2. a lacrimal duct.

dacryoadenalgia (ˌdakriohˌadə'nalji·ə) pain in a lacrimal gland.

dacryoadenectomy (ˌdakriohˌadə'nektəmee) excision of a lacrimal gland.

dacryoadenitis (ˌdakriohˌadə'nietis) inflammation of a lacrimal gland.

dacryoblennorrhoea (ˌdakriohˌblenə'reeə) mucous flow from the lacrimal apparatus.

dacryocele ('dakriohˌseel) dacryocystocele.

dacryocystalgia (ˌdakriohsi'stalji·ə) pain in the lacrimal sac.

dacryocystectomy (ˌdakriohsi'stektəmee) excision of the wall of the lacrimal sac.

dacryocystitis (ˌdakriohsi'stietis) inflammation of the lacrimal sac.

dacryocystocele (ˌdakrioh'sistohˌseel) hernial protrusion of the lacrimal sac; dacryocele.

dacryocystography (ˌdakriohsi'stogrəfee) radiological examination of the lacrimal passages using a radiopaque contrast medium.

dacryocystoptosis (ˌdakriohˌsistop'tohsis) prolapse of the lacrimal sac.

dacryocystorhinostenosis (ˌdakriohˌsistohˌrienohstə'nohsis) narrowing of the duct leading from the lacrimal sac to the nasal cavity.

dacryocystorhinostomy (ˌdakriohˌsistohrie'nostəmee) surgical creation of an opening between the lacrimal sac and nasal cavity.

dacryocystorhinotomy (ˌdakriohˌsistohrie'notəmee) passage of a probe through the lacrimal sac into the nasal cavity.

dacryocystostenosis (ˌdakrioh ˌsistohstəˈnohsis) narrowing of the lacrimal sac.
dacryocystostomy (ˌdakriohsiˈstostəmee) surgical creation of a new opening into the lacrimal sac with drainage.
dacryocystotomy (ˌdakriohsiˈstotəmee) incision of the lacrimal sac and duct.
dacryohaemorrhoea (ˌdakrioh ˌheeməˈreeə) the discharge of tears mixed with blood.
dacryolith (ˈdakrioh ˌlith) a lacrimal calculus.
dacryolithiasis (ˌdakriohliˈthieəsis) the presence of dacryoliths.
dacryon (ˈdakrion) the point where the lacrimal, frontal, and upper maxillary bones meet.
dacryopyorrhoea (ˌdakrioh ˌpieəˈreeə) the discharge of tears mixed with pus.
dacryorrhoea (ˌdakriəˈreeə) excessive flow of tears.
dacryoscintigraphy (ˌdakriohsinˈtigrəfee) scintigraphy of the lacrimal ducts.
dacryosolenitis (ˌdakrioh ˌsohleˈnietis) inflammation of a lacrimal duct.
dacryostenosis (ˌdakriohstəˈnohsis) stricture or narrowing of a lacrimal duct.
dactinomycin (ˌdaktinohˈmiesin) an antibiotic of the actinomycin complex (actinomycin D), produced by several species of *Streptomyces;* used as an antineoplastic agent.
dactyl (ˈdaktil) a digit.
dactyl(o)- word element. [Gr.] *digit, finger* or *toe.*
dactylion (dakˈtili·ən) webbed fingers. See SYNDACTYLISM.
dactylitis (ˌdaktiˈlietis) inflammation of a finger or toe.
dactylography (ˌdaktiˈlogrəfee) the study of fingerprints.
dactylogryposis (ˌdaktilohgriˈpohsis) permanent flexion of the fingers.
dactylology (ˌdaktiˈloləjee) communication between individuals by signs made with the hands and fingers.
dactylolysis (ˌdaktiˈlolisis) loss of a digit, usually from disease such as leprosy.
dactylomegaly (ˌdaktilohˈmegəlee) abnormally large fingers or toes.
dactyloscopy (ˌdaktiˈloskəpee) examination of fingerprints for identification.
dactylus (ˈdaktiləs) pl. *dactyli* [L.] a digit.
Dakin's solution (ˈdaykinz) an aqueous solution containing sodium hypochlorite, boric acid and sodium carbonate; used as a local antibacterial and to irrigate wounds.
Daktarin (dakˈtahrin) trademark for preparations containing miconazole.
Dalacin-C (ˌdaləsinˈsee) trademark for preparations of clindamycin, an antibiotic.
Dalmane (ˈdalmayn) trademark for a preparation of flurazepam hydrochloride, a hypnotic.
dalton (ˈdawltən) an arbitrary unit of mass, being one-twelfth the mass of the nuclide of carbon-12, equivalent to 1.657×10^{-24}g. Called also *atomic mass unit.*
Dalton's law (ˈdawltənz) the pressure exerted by a mixture of nonreacting gases is equal to the sum of the partial pressures of the separate components.
daltonism (ˈdawltə ˌnizəm) red–green colour blindness.
dam (dam) a sheet of latex rubber used to isolate teeth from the fluids of the mouth during dental treatments; also used occasionally in surgical procedures to isolate certain tissues or structures. Called also *rubber-dam.*
damping (ˈdamping) steady diminution of the amplitude of successive vibrations of a specific form of energy, as of electricity.
danazol (ˈdanə ˌzol) a synthetic progestogen that suppresses the ovarian-pituitary axis by inhibiting the release of gonadotrophins from the pituitary gland, used for treatment of endometriosis and fibrocystic disease of the breast and for prevention of attacks of hereditary angiooedema.
dander (ˈdandə) small scales from the hair or feathers of animals, which may be a cause of allergy in sensitive persons.
dandruff (ˈdandruf) 1. a scaly material shed from the scalp; applied to that normally shed from the scalp epidermis as well as to the excessive scaly material asssociated with disease. The condition may spread unless checked and in rare cases may extend to the eyebrows, ears, nose, and neck, causing a reddening of the skin in those areas. 2. SEBORRHOEIC DERMATITIS of the scalp.
Dandy-Walker syndrome (ˌdandiˈwawkə) congenital hydrocephalus due to obstruction of the foramina of Magendie and Luschka.
Dane particle (dayn) an intact hepatitis B viron.
Danol (ˈdanol) trademark for a preparation of danazol, an anterior pituitary suppressant.
danthron (ˈdanthron) a cathartic.
Dantrium (ˈdantri·əm) trademark for preparations of dantrolene used as a skeletal muscle relaxant and in the treatment of malignant hyperthermia.
dantrolene (ˈdantrə ˌleen) muscle relaxant producing its primary action on muscle and only secondarily on the central nervous system. Drug of choice in the treatment of malignant hyperpyrexia.
dapsone (ˈdapsohn) an antibacterial used as a leprostatic and a dermatitis herpetiformis suppressant.
Daranide (ˈdarə ˌnied) trademark for a preparation of dichlorphenamide, a carbonic anhydrase inhibitor.
Darier's disease (ˈdari ˌayz) keratosis follicularis.
Darling's disease (ˈdahlingz) histoplasmosis.
dartoid (ˈdahtoyd) resembling the dartos.
dartos (ˈdahtos) the contractile tissue under the skin of the scrotum; called also tunica dartos.
darwinism (ˈdahwi ˌnizəm) the theory of evolution according to which higher organisms have been developed from lower ones through the influence of natural selection.
data (ˈdaytə, ˈdahtə) plural of *datum;* a collection of facts.
continuous d. data which have a continuous set of values, e.g. for variables such as height, weight, and antibody titres in response to vaccination.
discrete d. data with a single value or characteristic, e.g. colour of hair.
d. processing the storage and analysis of data to produce statistical tabulations, often by computer.
daughter (ˈdawtə) 1. decay product. 2. arising from cell division, as a daughter cell.
daunomycin (ˌdawnohˈmiesin) daunorubicin.
daunorubicin (ˌdawnohˈroobisin) an anthracycline antibiotic produced by a strain of *Streptomyces coeruleorubidus* that has antimitotic, cytotoxic, and immunosuppressive effects. It is used in the treatment of acute nonlymphocytic leukaemia in adults. Called also daunomycin.
dB, db decibel.
DCH Diploma of Child Health.
DCh Doctor of Surgery.
DChO Doctor of Ophthalmic Surgery.
DCMT Doctor of Clinical Medicine of the Tropics.
D_{L}co diffusing capacity of the lung for carbon monoxide.
DCP Diploma in Clinical Pathology.
DDA Dangerous Drugs Act.
DDAVP trademark for a preparation of desmopressin acetate, a synthetic analogue of vasopressin used to treat diabetes insipidus.

DDH Diploma in Dental Health.
DDP diamminedichloroplatinum, an alternative name for CISPLATIN.
DDPH Diploma in Dental Public Health.
DDRB Doctors and Dentists Review Body.
DDT dichloro-diphenyl-trichloroethane, a powerful insect poison; used in dilution as a powder or in an oily solution as a spray.
de- word element. [L.] *away from;* sometimes negative or privative, and often intensive.
de Musset's sign (də 'muhsayz) rhythmic jerky movements of the head; seen in cases of aortic aneurysm and aortic insufficiency. Called also *Musset's sign*.
de Pezzer's catheter (de'petsəz) see PEZZER'S CATHETER.
de Quervain's disease (dəkair'vanh) see QUERVAIN'S DISEASE.
deactivation (dee,akti'vayshən) the process of making or becoming inactive.
dead space (ded spays) 1. a space remaining in the tissues as a result of failure of proper closure of surgical or other wounds. 2. the portions of the respiratory tract that are ventilated but not perfused by pulmonary circulation. The *anatomical dead space* consists of the airways of the mouth, nose, pharynx, larynx, trachea, bronchi and bronchioles. The *alveolar dead space* consists of alveoli that are not perfused owing to disease, the influence of gravity on blood flow, or other reasons. The *physiological dead space* is the sum of the anatomic and alveolar dead spaces. The volume of the physiological dead space (V_D) is determined by measuring the partial pressure of carbon dioxide in a sample of exhaled gas (P_Eco_2) and in the arterial blood (P_aco_2) and the tidal volume (V_T) and using the formula:
$V_D/V_T = (P_aco_2 - P_Eco_2)/P_aco_2$.
deaf (def) lacking the sense of hearing or not having the full power of hearing; exhibiting DEAFNESS.
deaf-mute (,def'myoot) a person unable to hear or speak.
deafness ('defnəs) lack or loss, complete or partial, of the sense of HEARING. Total deafness is quite rare, but partial deafness is common. Partial or complete deafness is also referred to as *hearing loss*.
CAUSES. The two major types of deafness are conductive deafness and sensorineural (nerve) deafness. In some cases both types may be present; this is called mixed deafness.
In conductive deafness sound vibrations are interrupted in the outer or middle ear before they reach the nerve endings of the inner ear. In the outer ear, a foreign body or an accumulation of cerumen (earwax) may block the external acoustic meatus. These cases generally can be cured by removal of the obstruction. In the middle ear, infections, often entering through a perforated tympanic membrane (eardrum) or the pharyngotympanic tube, may fill the chamber with fluid, hampering the passage of vibrations. The small bones of the middle ear (ossicles) may be damaged by injury or fixed in place by otosclerosis.
In sensorineural deafness, the outer and middle ear function normally, but damage to the nerve endings of the inner ear, the cochlear portion of the vestibulocochlear (eighth cranial) nerve, or the hearing centre in the brain causes either interruption or confusion of the sound messages. This damage may be caused by disease, head injury, tumour, excessively loud and sudden noise, or continuous loud noise.
A great many cases of congenital deafness are caused by infectious diseases, especially viral infections, contracted by the mother during pregnancy. Of these, rubella (German measles) is the most common.
Impaired hearing or a predisposition to ear diseases may be inherited. The laws of heredity with respect to deafness, though not yet fully understood, are the subject of continuing research.
Two of the greatest contributing factors to deafness are pride and neglect. Many ear diseases that can be cured if treated early are allowed to lead to deafness because of these two factors. Symptoms such as ringing in the ears, a feeling of pressure in the ear, or increasing hearing difficulty call for prompt medical consultation, if necessary with an ear specialist.
DETECTION OF HEARING LOSS. Hearing loss in the young child is evidenced by a lack of response to the sounds of his environment. As the infant matures and begins to talk there is a noticeable defect in his speech development and he may rely more on gestures than on words to communicate with others.
Emotional and behavioural disorders frequently are signs of hearing loss in children and in adults. The frustration they feel in trying to cope with their disability may be manifested by irritability, hyperactivity, hostility, and withdrawal from contact with others.
Special tests to determine hearing loss include the use of the tuning fork and the audiometer. The vibrating tuning fork produces sound waves that can be heard in both ears by a person with normal hearing when the stem of the fork is placed on the top of the head. The sound is heard louder in the affected ear in conductive hearing loss and softer in the affected ear in sensorineural loss. The audiometer produces sounds at varying levels of intensity and frequency. It is useful in determining the degree and type of hearing ability.
TREATMENT. Medical science has made great progress in the treatment of conditions that are capable of causing deafness. Middle ear infections now yield to the antibiotics and sulphonamide drugs. The greatest progress, however, has been in the field of microsurgery. Special binocular microscopes and miniature surgical instruments have enabled the surgeon to operate freely in the small crowded chambers of the ear. Two examples of this type of microsurgery are TYMPANOPLASTY and STAPEDECTOMY.
There still remain many cases of deafness that cannot be improved by drugs or surgery. These patients require guidance to make the best use of what hearing remains. With proper training and the use of a suitable hearing aid where necessary, the deaf person can continue to lead a normal, useful life.
An important tool in rehabilitation is training in lip-reading. The patient is taught to use visual clues, such as the movements of the lips and tongue of the speaker, to supplement his hearing.
Another important tool is a correct HEARING AID. This should be selected with the help of an otologist, as different types of deafness require different instruments. Careful training in the use of the hearing aid also is necessary. After the silence of deafness, the patient may find it impossible at first to disregard the background noises that the instrument picks up. Also, some types of nerve deafness 'scramble' sounds; training in the use of the hearing aid may enable the patient to distinguish among these sounds.
A third important component of rehabilitation is speech therapy. Since the deaf person is no longer able to hear his own voice, his speech often deteriorates. Proper training can help the patient prevent this deterioration, as well as correcting any speech defect that may already have developed.
DEAFNESS IN CHILDREN. The problems of a child who is deaf from birth or shortly afterward are somewhat different from those of a person who loses his hearing

during adult life. Children learn to speak by imitating the sounds they hear; a child who cannot hear will be mute unless he is taught speech. This calls for special methods of teaching.

cortical d. that due to disease of the cortical centres of the cerebrum.

hysterical d. that which may appear or disappear in a hysterical patient without an organic cause being present.

word d. auditory aphasia; receptive aphasia in which sounds are heard but convey no meaning to the mind.

deamidase (dee'ami,dayz) an enzyme that splits amides to form a carboxylic acid and ammonia.

deamidization (dee,amidie'zayshən) liberation of the ammonia from an amide.

deaminase (dee'ami,nayz) an enzyme causing deamination, or removal of an amino group from organic compounds, named according to its substrate as adenosine deaminase, cytidine deaminase, guanine deaminase, etc.

deamination (dee,ami'nayshən) removal of the amino group, $-NH_2$, from a compound.

death (deth) the cessation of all physical and chemical processes that occurs in all living organisms or their cellular components.

black d. bubonic plague.

brain d. the diagnosis of clinical brain stem death is governed, in the UK, by a set of guidelines ratified by the Medical Royal Colleges and their Faculties.

Prior to the consideration of brain death, the examiner must satisfy himself that the patient has positively diagnosed structural brain damage and that at least six hours have elapsed since the onset of apnoeic coma.

A number of pre-conditions must be fulfilled prior to testing of brain stem function. These comprise potentially reversible phenomena including the ingestion of depressant drugs or administration of a neuromuscular blocking agent, hypothermia or severe metabolic disturbances such as uncontrolled diabetes.

The next stage involves testing the integrity of the brain stem reflexes. These include the pupillary reaction to light and corneal reflexes, the latter being tested by drawing a wisp of cotton wool across the exposed cornea and observing for a blink response. The oculovestibular (calorific) reflex is checked by syringing 20 ml of ice cold water into each ear in turn. A positive response comprises eye movement to the stimulated side. Deep painful stimuli are applied to several sites including the cranium to ascertain the presence of cranial nerve motor responses. Movement of the patient's endotracheal tube or vigorous suctioning and observing the throat muscles for movement will determine whether the pharyngeal and laryngeal reflexes have been affected.

The final part of the test schedule is to confirm apnoea. The patient is disconnected from the ventilator and is given oxygen via a tracheal catheter at 6 litres per minute to avoid hypoxaemia. The $P\text{CO}_2$ level must be allowed to build up to what is termed the 'threshold level', i.e. $P\text{CO}_2$ of 50 mmHg or above. This will determine the length of time that the patient is disconnected; in most cases this is no more than five minutes. The object of achieving a threshold level is to provide the maximum stimulus to the patient for breathing. Whilst disconnected, the respiratory chest wall is observed for movement.

It is not considered necessary, under the UK code, to perform an electroencephalogram or angiogram.

Special consideration must be given to those patients who may display features which affect the outcome of these tests. These include: (1) a third cranial nerve palsy or local injury preventing a pupillary reaction to light; (2) corneal oedema due to local injury preventing a normal blinking response; (3) wax or other debris blocking the passageway between the external ear and the tympanic membrane or the membrane itself may be torn; (4) a cervical cord injury preventing normal cranial nerve motor responses below the level of the lesion; (5) the patient's $P\text{CO}_2$ level which may not be within normal limits to start with, e.g. it may be lowered in the patient who has been hyperventilated or raised in the patient who has long-standing chronic obstructive airways disease.

The entire testing procedure is performed twice by two different doctors to eliminate any observer error. The time interval between testing is not specified. For medicolegal purposes, the time of death is that time when the second examination has been completed and the patient fulfils the criteria.

Performance of the brain death criteria under the appropriate circumstances allows the patient a dignified death, reduces the agony of the relatives and releases scarce resources for other seriously ill patients.

d. certificate certificate issued by the registrar for deaths after receipt of a preliminary certificate completed and signed by an attending doctor, indicating the date and probable cause of death. Only after issue of this certificate, indicating that the death has been registered, can the body be disposed of.

clinical d. the absence of heart beat (no pulse can be felt) and cessation of breathing.

cot d. sudden infant death syndrome (SIDS).

d. instinct a concept introduced by Freud, but not now widely accepted in psychoanalysis, proposing a self-destructive drive opposed by the sexual instinct which perpetually seeks a renewal of life. Still adopted by followers of the contemporary psychologist, Melanie Klein, who view life as a struggle against death, with the death instinct as the most powerful human instinct. May manifest itself as a repetition COMPULSION with the aim to annihilate oneself.

d. rate the number of deaths per stated number of persons (100 or 10,000 or 100,000) in a certain region in a certain time period.

debility (di'bilitee) lack or loss of strength; weakness.

débride (di'breed, day-) [Fr.] to remove by débridement.

débridement (di'breedmonh, day-) [Fr.] the surgical removal of all foreign material and contaminated and devitalized tissue from a wound until the surrounding healthy tissue is exposed.

debris ('debree, 'day-) devitalized tissue or foreign matter. In dentistry, soft foreign matter loosely attached to the surface of a tooth.

Debrisan ('debrizan) trademark for a preparation of dextranomer beads used to assist wound cleaning and the de-sloughing of ulcers.

debrisoquine (de'briesoh,kween) a powerful oral drug used in the treatment of resistant hypertension. It causes postural hypertension and this has accounted for its fall from more widespread use.

debt (det) something owed.

oxygen d. the extra oxygen that must be used in the oxidative energy processes after a period of strenuous exercise to reconvert lactic acid to glucose and decomposed ATP and creatine phosphate to their original states.

deca- word element. [Gr.] *ten;* also spelled *deka-;* used in naming units of measurement to indicate a quantity 10 times the unit designated by the root with which it is combined; symbol da.

Decadron ('dekə,dron) trademark for preparations of dexamethasone, an anti-inflammatory adrenocortical steroid.

decalcification (dee,kalsifi'kayshən) 1. the process of removing calcareous matter. 2. the loss of calcium salts from bone or teeth.

decalcify (dee'kalsi,fie) to deprive of calcium or its salts.

decannulation (dee,kanyuh'layshən) the removal of a cannula.

decantation (,deekan'tayshən) the pouring of a clear supernatant liquid from a sediment.

decapitation (di,kapi'tayshən) removal of the head, as of an animal, fetus, or bone.

decapsulation (dee,kapsyuh'layshən) removal of a capsule, especially the renal capsule.

decarboxylase (,deekah'boksi,layz) any of the lyase class of enzymes that catalyse the removal of a carbon dioxide molecule from a compound.

decarboxylation (,deekah,boksi'layshən) removal of the carboxyl group from a compound.

decay (di'kay) 1. the gradual decomposition of dead organic matter. 2. the process or stage of ageing of living matter.

radioactive d. the process by which an unstable atom loses energy by the emission of gamma rays, beta or alpha particles and is transformed to a more stable atom.

radioactive d. curve a graphic plot of the rate of radionuclide transformation against time.

radioactive d. rate also known as the activity of a radionuclide. The number of nuclear transformations which occur in a unit of time.

deceit (di'seet) misrepresentation; deception.

facial d. in psychology, misrepresentation, in terms of facial expressiveness, of one's true emotional state.

decerebrate (dee'seri,brayt) to eliminate cerebral function by transecting the brain stem or by ligating the common carotid arteries and basilar artery at the centre of the pons; an animal so prepared, or a brain-damaged person with similar neurological signs.

d. rigidity see under RIDIGITY.

decerebration (dee,seri'brayshən) the act of decerebrating.

decholesterolization (deekə,lestə·rolie'zayshən) reduction of cholesterol levels in the blood.

deci- word element. [L.] *one-tenth;* used to indicate one-tenth (10^{-1}) of the unit designated by the root with which it is combined; symbol d.

decibel ('desi,bel) a unit used to express the ratio, r, of two powers, usually electric or acoustic powers, equal to one-tenth of a bel. The powers are said to differ by s decibels if $s = 10 \log_{10} r$. One decibel equals approximately the smallest difference in acoustic power the human ear can detect. Abbreviated dB or db.

decidua (di'sidyooə) a name applied to the endometrium during pregnancy, all of which except for the deepest layer is shed after childbirth; called also the *decidual* or *deciduous membrane*. adj. **decidual**.

basal d., d. basalis that portion on which the implanted ovum rests.

capsular d., d. capsularis that portion directly overlying the implanted ovum and facing the uterine cavity.

menstrual d., d. menstrualis the hyperaemic uterine mucosa shed during menstruation.

parietal d., d. parietalis, true d., d. vera the decidua exclusive of the area occupied by the implanted ovum. This is sometimes shed at 4, 8 or 12 weeks (of pregnancy) when menstruation could have been expected if pregnancy had not occurred. See decidual BLEEDING.

deciduate (di'sidyoo,ayt) characterized by shedding.

deciduitis (di,sidyoo'ietis) a bacterial disease leading to changes in the decidua.

deciduoma (di,sidyoo'ohmə) an intrauterine mass containing decidual cells.

deciduosis (di,sidyoo'ohsis) the presence of decidual tissue or of tissue resembling the endometrium of pregnancy in an ectopic site.

deciduous (di'sidyooəs) falling off; subject to being shed, as deciduous teeth.

declination (,dekli'nayshən) cyclophoria.

declive (di'kliev) a slope or a slanting surface. In anatomy, the part of the vermis of the cerebellum just caudal to the primary fissure.

declivis (di'klievis) [L.] *declive.*

decoloration (dee,kulə'rayshən) 1. removal of colour; bleaching. 2. lack or loss of colour.

decolorizer (dee'kulə,riezə) an agent that removes colour, bleaches.

decompensation (,deekompən'sayshən) 1. inability of the heart to maintain adequate circulation; it is marked by dyspnoea, venous engorgement, cyanosis, and oedema. 2. in psychiatry, the failure of defence mechanisms as occurs in relapses of schizophrenics.

decomposition (dee,kompə'zishən) the separation of compound bodies into their constituent smaller components.

decompression (,deekəm'preshən) return to normal environmental pressure after exposure to greatly increased pressure.

cerebral d. removal of a flap of the skull and incision of the dura mater for the purpose of relieving intracranial pressure.

d. sickness a disorder characterized by joint pains, respiratory manifestations, skin lesions, and neurological signs, occurring as a result of rapid reduction in air pressure. Aviators flying at high altitudes and persons breathing compressed air in caissons and diving apparatus are particularly susceptible to this disorder (see also BENDS and CAISSON DISEASES).

decongestant (,deekən'jestənt) 1. tending to reduce congestion or swelling. 2. an agent that reduces congestion or swelling, usually of the nasal membranes. Decongestants may be inhaled, taken as spray or nose drops, or used orally in liquid or tablet form. The medication acts by reducing swelling of the nasal membranes and thus opening up the nasal passages. Among the leading medications used as decongestants are adrenaline, ephedrine, and phenylephrine. Antihistamines, alone or in combination with decongestants, may also be effective.

A decongestant must be used several times a day to be helpful; but excessive use may cause headaches, dizziness, or other disorders and sometimes the medicine itself may cause reactive nasal swelling.

decongestive (,deekən'jestiv) reducing congestion.

decontamination (,deekən,tami'nayshən) the freeing of a person or an object of some contaminating substance such as war gas, radioactive material, etc.

decortication (dee,kawti'kayshən) 1. removal of the outer covering from a plant, seed, or root. 2. an operation to strip the outer layer of an organ, e.g. the removal of the thickened pleura in the treatment of chronic empyema.

Decortisyl (de'kawtisil) trademark for a preparation of prednisone, a glucocorticoid.

decrudescence (,deekroo'desəns) diminution or abatement of the intensity of symptoms.

decubitus (di'kyoobitəs) pl. *decubitus;* 1. the act of lying down; the position assumed in lying down. 2. a decubitus ulcer. adj. **decubital**.

Andral's d. lying on the unaffected side in the early stages of pleurisy.

dorsal d. lying on the back.

lateral d. lying on one side, designated right lateral decubitus when the subject lies on the right side and left lateral decubitus when he lies on the left side.

d. ulcer an ulcer due to interference with the local circulation from prolonged or severe pressure on the surface body tissue resulting in tissue anoxia and cell death; called also *bedsore* and *pressure sore*. Although the term decubitus ulcer is derived from the Latin word meaning 'lying down', these lesions can develop in any position when local pressure is unrelieved, especially over bone prominences. See PRESSURE SORE.

ventral d. lying on the stomach.

decussate (di'kusayt) 1. to cross in the form of an Y. 2. crossed like the letter Y.

decussation (deekə'sayshən) a crossing over; the intercrossing of fellow parts or structures in the form of a Y.

d. of pyramids the anterior part of the lower medulla oblongata in which most of the fibres of each pyramid intersect as they cross the midline and descend as the lateral corticospinal tracts.

dedifferentiation (dee,difə,renshi'ayshən) regression from a more specialized or complex form to a simpler state.

deerfly fever ('diə,flie) tularaemia.

defatted (dee'fatid) deprived of fat.

defecation (,defi'kayshən) elimination of wastes and undigested food, as faeces, from the rectum.

defect ('deefekt) an imperfection, failure, or absence.

filling d. an interruption in the contour of the inner surface of stomach or intestine revealed by radiology, indicating excess tissue or substance on or in the wall of the organ.

septal d. a defect in the cardiac septum resulting in an abnormal communication between opposite chambers of the heart. See also AORTIC SEPTAL DEFECT, ATRIAL SEPTAL DEFECT, and VENTRICULAR SEPTAL DEFECT.

defective (di'fektiv) 1. imperfect. 2. a person lacking in some physical, mental, or moral quality.

defeminization (dee,feminie'zayshən) loss of female sexual characteristics.

defence (di'fens) behaviour directed to protection of the individual from injury.

character d. any character trait, e.g., a mannerism, attitude, or affectation, which serves as a DEFENCE MECHANISM.

insanity d. a legal concept that a person cannot be convicted of a crime if he lacked criminal responsibility by reason of insanity at the time of commission of the crime.

d. mechanism in psychology, an unconscious mental process or coping pattern that lessens the anxiety associated with a situation or internal conflict and protects the person from mental discomfort. In psychoanalytic theory, the EGO, following the reality principle, conforms to the demands of the outside world, but the ID (repressed unconscious), following the pleasure principle, pursues immediate gratification of desires and reduction of psychic tension. The SUPEREGO (conscience or morality) may take either side. Defence mechanisms develop in order to control impulses or feelings that lead to inner conflicts, to reach compromises between conflicting impulses, and to reduce inner tensions. They help to manage or avoid anxiety, aggression, hostility, resentment, and frustration. Defence mechanisms are not pathological in themselves; they can be a means of dealing with unbearable situations.

There are many common defence mechanisms. *Repression* is the exclusion of unacceptable ideas, fantasies, or feelings from the consciousness. The repressed material cannot be recalled but may emerge in disguised form in dreams or associations. *Rationalization* is the creation of plausible explanations for behaviour. The person believes that his behaviour is the result of thoughtful deliberation and unbiased judgement rather than of unacceptable unconscious motives. *Projection* is the unconscious attribution of traits, attitudes, motives, or desires, which a person cannot accept in himself, to other persons, whom he then criticizes for having the traits he disavows. *Identification* is the adoption of behaviour patterns of significant others. The identification of a child with his parents is important in his normal psychological growth and development. *Reaction-formation* is the adoption of feelings, ideas, attitudes, and behaviours that are the exact opposite of unconscious motives and impulses. *Sublimation* is the channelling of unacceptable impulses into socially acceptable forms of expression. *Displacement* is the transfer of unacceptable emotions or wishes from the original object to an acceptable substitute. *Denial* is the blocking from consciousness of painful or intolerable perceptions, the reality of the situation being ignored or disregarded.

deferens ('defə,renz) [L.] *deferent*.

deferent ('defə·rent) conducting or progressing away, as from a centre or specific site of reference.

deferentectomy (,defə·ren'tektəmee) excision of a ductus deferens. Called also *vasectomy*.

deferential (,defə'renshəl) pertaining to the ductus deferens.

deferentitis (,defə·ren'tietis) inflammation of the ductus deferens.

defervescence (,deefə'vesəns) the period of abatement of fever.

defibrillation (dee,fibri'layshən) 1. termination of atrial or ventricular fibrillation, usually by electric shock. 2. separation of tissue fibres by blunt dissection.

Defibrillation by precordial shock is accomplished by delivering a nonsynchronized direct current to the myocardium. It is an emergency procedure, used to terminate a life-threatening ventricular arrhythmia. The electric shock is delivered by means of metal paddles applied directly to the heart muscle, as in cardiac surgery, or by placing the paddles on the chest (closed defibrillation).

The high-voltage electrical current delivered during precordial shock causes complete depolarization of the heart muscle, disrupting all of the electrical circuits that are activating the heart muscle and causing ventricular fibrillation. This allows the heart's natural pacemaker to regain control and regulation of the heart rate and rhythm.

The procedure carries some risk and should be done only by specially trained doctors, nurses, and paramedical staff. Cardiopulmonary resuscitation and the administration of intravenous fluids and drugs are essential components of defibrillation. Sodium bicarbonate is given to combat acidosis; lignocaine is given to forestall arrhythmias that may develop during and after defibrillation.

Electrocardiographic readings and assessment of ECG patterns are done prior to the procedure to verify the presence of a lethal arrhythmia, and afterwards to evaluate the effectiveness of the treatment. Some ECG machines and cardiac monitors can continue to function during defibrillation because they have been designed to withstand the electrical shock when it is delivered to the patient.

Burns of the skin frequently occur under the paddles at the time of defibrillation; steroid or lanolin-based ointments or creams are usually prescribed as treatment. More serious complications of defibrillation include cardiac arrest, respiratory arrest, neurological impairment, pulmonary oedema, and pulmonary and systemic emboli. The patient must be monitored carefully after the procedure for return of ventricular fibrillation. He should be frequently and regularly observed for changes in blood pressure; pulse rate, rhythm, and character; state of consciousness; and adequacy of ventilation.

defibrillator (di'fibri,laytə) an apparatus used to produce defibrillation by application of brief electroshock to the heart, directly or through electrodes placed on the chest wall.

defibrination (dee,fibri'nayshən) the destruction or removal of fibrin, as from the blood.

deficiency (di'fishənsee) a lack or shortage; a condition characterized by the presence of less than the normal or necessary supply or competence.

d. disease a condition caused by dietary or metabolic deficiency, including all diseases due to an insufficient supply of essential nutrients.

deficit ('defisit) a lack or deficiency.

oxygen d. a lack of OXYGEN, as in hypoxia or anoxia.

deflection (di'flekshən) a turning aside. In psychoanalysis, an unconscious diversion of ideas from conscious attention. In the electrocardiogram, a deviation of the curve from the isoelectric baseline, that is, any wave or complex.

defluvium (dee'floovi·əm) [L.] a falling out, as of the hair.

defluxion (di'flukshən) 1. a sudden disappearance. 2. a copious discharge, as of catarrh. 3. a falling out, as of hair.

deformability (di,fawmə'bilitee) the ability of cells, such as erythrocytes, to change shape as they pass through narrow spaces, such as the microvasculature.

deformation (,deefaw'mayshan, ,defə-) 1. deformity, especially an alteration in shape or structure. 2. the process of adapting in shape or form.

deformity (di'fawmitee) distortion of any part or general disfigurement of the body; malformation.

defundation (,deefun'dayshən) excision of the fundus of the uterus and uterine (fallopian) tubes.

degenerate (dee'jenərayt, -'jenə·rət) 1. to change from a higher to a lower form. 2. characterized by degeneration. 3. a person whose moral or physical state is below the normal.

degeneration (di,jenə'rayshən) deterioration; change from a higher to a lower form, especially change of tissue to a lower or less functionally active form. When there is chemical change of the tissue itself it is true degeneration; when the change consists of the deposit of abnormal matter in the tissues, it is infiltration. adj. **degenerative.**

albuminoid d., albuminous d. cloudy swelling, an early stage of degenerative change characterized by swollen, parboiled-appearing tissues which revert to normal when the cause is removed.

amyloid d. degeneration with deposit of amyloid in the extracellular tissues.

caseous d. caseation (2).

cerebromacular d., cerebroretinal d. degeneration of brain cells and of the macula retinae, as occurs in TAY-SACHS DISEASE.

colloid d. degeneration with conversion of the tissues into a gelatinous or gumlike material.

congenital macular d. a congenital, hereditary form of macular degeneration, often marked by the presence of a cystlike lesion that in the early stages resembles egg yolk (vitelline dystrophy).

cystic d. degeneration with formation of cystic spaces filled with fluid but not lined by epithelium.

fatty d. deposit of fat globules in a tissue.

fibroid d. degeneration into fibrous tissue.

hepatolenticular d. a hereditary disorder of copper metabolism, marked by a pigmented ring at the outer margin of the cornea, degenerative changes in the brain, cirrhosis of the liver, splenomegaly, tremor, rigidity, contractures, psychic disturbances, dysphagia, and increasing weakness and emaciation. Called also *Wilson's disease.*

hyaline d. a regressive change in cells in which the cytoplasm takes on a homogeneous, glassy appearance; also used loosely to describe the histological appearance of tissues.

hydropic d. a form in which the epithelial cells are distended by absorbing much water.

lattice d. of retina a frequently bilateral, often asymptomatic condition, characterized by patches of fine grey or white lines that intersect at irregular intervals in the peripheral retina, usually associated with numerous, round, punched-out areas of retinal thinning or retinal holes. It predisposes to the development of retinal tears and detachment.

macular d. degenerative changes in the macula retinae.

mucoid d. degeneration with deposit of myelin and lecithin in the cells.

mucous d., myxomatous d. degeneration with accumulation of mucus in epithelial tissues.

spongy d. of central nervous system, spongy d. of white matter a rare hereditary form of leukodystrophy marked by early onset, widespread demyelination and vacuolation of the cerebral white matter giving rise to a spongy appearance, and by severe mental handicap, megalocephaly, atony of the neck muscles, spasticity of the arms and legs, and blindness; death usually occurs at about 18 months of age. Called also *Canavan's disease.*

subacute combined d. of spinal cord degeneration of both the posterior and lateral columns of the spinal cord, producing various motor and sensory disturbances; it is due to vitamin B_{12} deficiency and usually associated with pernicious anaemia. Called also *Lichtheim's syndrome* and *Putnam–Dana syndrome.*

wallerian d. fatty degeneration of a nerve fibre that has been severed from its nutritive source.

Zenker's d. Zenker's necrosis.

degloving (dee'gluving) 1. intra-oral surgical exposure of the bony mandibular chin; it can be performed in the posterior region if necessary. 2. the tearing off of the skin of the forearm, hand, leg or foot by an injury.

deglutition (,deegloo'tishən) the act of swallowing.

degradation (degrə'dayshən) conversion of a chemical compound to one less complex, as by splitting off one or more groups of atoms.

degree (di'gree) 1. a grade or rank awarded to scholars by a college or university. 2. a unit of measure of temperature. 3. a unit of measure of arcs and angles, one degree being 1/360 of a circle.

degrees of freedom (di'greez ov 'freedəm) a statistical term used in significance testing to mean the number of values independently contributing to a sample.

degustation (,deegu'stayshən) the act or function of tasting.

dehiscence (di'hisəns) a splitting open.

wound d. separation of the layers of a surgical wound.

dehumidifier (,deehyoo'midi,fie·ə) an apparatus for reducing the content of moisture in the atmosphere.

dehydratase (dee'hiedrə,tayz) any enzyme of the lyase class that catalyses the removal of H_2O, leaving double bonds (or adding groups to double bonds).

dehydration (,deehie'drayshən) removal of water from the body or a tissue; or the condition that results from undue loss of water. Severe dehydration is a serious condition that may lead to fatal SHOCK, ACIDOSIS, and the accumulation of waste products in the body, as in URAEMIA.

Water accounts for more than half the body weight. Under normal conditions, a certain amount of fluid is lost daily. About 1.5 litres is removed by urination, and another 90 ml is lost from the digestive tract in the faeces. Through vaporization another litre is given off through the skin and lungs. To make up for these losses, about 2.5 litres of fluid must be taken into the body in food and fluids, and the cells contribute another 250 ml through chemical activities.

When the fluid intake is insufficient or the output is excessive, FLUID VOLUME DEFICIT occurs. See also FLUID BALANCE.

dehydrocholesterol (dee,hiedrohkə'lestə,rol) a sterol found in the skin which, when properly irradiated by ultraviolet rays, forms vitamin D.

activated 7-d. cholecalciferol.

dehydrocholic acid (dee,hiedrə'kohlik) a white, fluffy, bitter, odourless powder used to increase output of bile by the liver and the filling of the gallbladder. Preparations of this acid are used to aid the digestion of fats and increase absorption of fat-soluble vitamins. Drugs containing dehydrocholic acid are contraindicated in cases of biliary obstruction. Because of its bitter taste on the tongue when injected into a vein, it is used to provide an end point for the measurement of arm-tongue circulation time. Not currently available in the UK.

11-dehydrocorticosterone (i'levəndee,hiedroh,kawti'kostə·rohn) one of the least active of the GLUCOCORTICOSTEROIDS produced by the adrenal cortex.

dehydroepiandrosterone (dee,hiedroh,epian'drostə,rohn) an androgen occurring in normal human urine.

dehydrogenase (,deehie'drojə,nayz, dee'hiedrəjə-) an enzyme that mobilizes the hydrogen of a substrate so that it can pass to a hydrogen acceptor.

glucose-6-phosphate d. an enzyme necessary for the oxidation of glucose-6-phosphate, an intermediate in carbohydrate metabolism. Hereditary deficiency of this enzyme in the erythrocytes is associated with a tendency toward haemolysis with certain antimalarial and sulphonamide drugs and fava beans (favism).

lactate d. (LDH) an enzyme that catalyses the interconversion of lactate and pyruvate. It is widespread in tissues and is particularly abundant in kidney, skeletal muscle, liver, and myocardium. It appears in elevated concentrations when these tissues are injured.

dehydrogenate (dee'hiedrəjə,nayt) to remove hydrogen from.

dehydroretinal (dee,hiedroh'retinəl) the aldehyde of dehydroretinol, derived from the visual pigment porphyropsin, found in fresh-water fishes and certain vertebrates and amphibians; its metabolic role is analogous to that of rhodopsin in other animals.

dehydroretinol (dee,hiedroh'reti,nol) vitamin A_2, the form of vitamin A found in the retina and liver of fresh-water fishes and certain invertebrates and amphibians; it differs from retinol (vitamin A_1) in having one more conjugated double bond and has approximately one-third the biological activity of retinol. Called also *retinol*$_2$.

deionization (dee,iənie'zayshən) the production of a mineral-free state by the removal of ions.

déjà vu (,dayzhah 'voo) [Fr.] an illusion that a new situation is a repetition of a previous experience.

dejecta (di'jektə) excrement.

dejection (di'jekshən) 1. a mental state marked by depression and melancholy. 2. discharge of faeces; defecation. 3. excrement; faeces.

Dejerine's disease (,dezhə'reenz) progressive hypertrophic interstitial neuropathy.

Dejerine–Sottas disease (,dayzhə·reen'sotəs) progressive hypertrophic interstitial neuropathy.

deka- see DECA-.

delacrimation (di,lakri'mayshən) excessive and abnormal flow of tears.

delactation (,deelak'tayshən) 1. weaning. 2. cessation of lactation.

delayed primary closure (di'layd) the suture of a wound several days after injury when contamination and infection have subsided. Abbreviated DPC. Called also *delayed primary suture*.

deleterious (,deli'tiə·ri·əs) injurious; harmful.

deletion (di'leeshən) in genetics, loss from a chromosome of genetic material.

delinquency (di'lingkwənsee) criminal or antisocial conduct, especially among juveniles.

delinquent (di'lingkwənt) 1. lacking in some respect; characterized by antisocial, illegal, or criminal behaviour. 2. a person exhibiting such behaviour, especially a minor (juvenile delinquent).

deliquescence (,deli'kwes'ns) the condition of becoming moist or liquified as a result of absorption of water from the air.

delirium (di'liri·əm) a mental disturbance of relatively short duration usually reflecting a toxic state, marked by illusions, hallucinations, delusions, excitement, restlessness, and incoherence. Almost any acute illness accompanied by very high fever can bring on delirium. Other causes are metabolic derangements, such as those resulting from liver failure, end stage renal disease, and hypoglycaemia; neurological trauma, as from a physical injury or from a stroke; congestive heart failure; thyrotoxicosis; physical and mental exhaustion; drug and alcohol intoxication and withdrawal; and senility. PATIENT CARE. A thorough assessment of the patient's mental status is needed in order to distinguish delirium from other altered states of consciousness and to identify specific behaviours that require attention. Delirious patients have special safety needs for the prevention of self-injury and avoidance of harm from medications and procedures that can exacerbate their condition. A patient who is hallucinating, severely confused, or paranoid may endanger others while trying to escape an imagined threat to his well-being. He thus requires constant attendance and possible restraint while receiving intravenous fluids or when dressings, catheters, and drains are necessary. Even though the patient might not fully understand, he should be given a brief explanation of the need for restraint. Restricting the movements of a patient brings with it all of the hazards of immobility and consequently a need to plan his care so that these problems can be avoided.

A confused patient needs help in orientation to reality. Clocks, radio, television, newspapers, and magazines should be available to the patient as normal aids to orientation. Any necessary sensory aids such as glasses or a hearing aid must be available to the patient. One should speak directly to the patient and face him when talking to him. Speak slowly and provide new information in small bits so as to avoid adding to his confusion. When the patient makes statements that are not factual, it is better to gently provide him with the truth than to reinforce his delusions by ignoring him or agreeing with him. If he has frightening hallucinations, express empathy for his feelings but do not concur with his misperceptions, allow him to dwell on them, or otherwise add to his fear and anxiety.

A calm and reassuring manner, consistent responses, and concise explanations of what is going on around him can give stability to his fragmented thoughts. It is helpful for the nursing staff to know that many delirious and confused patients can eventually recover and that for some the state of confusion is in part an attempt to adapt to and deal with profound physical and emotional shock.

d. tremens an acute alcohol withdrawal syndrome that can occur in any person who has been drinking heavily. It can be caused by any form of alcoholic beverage, including beer and wine, and is most commonly seen in chronic alcoholics. The severity of the symptoms usually depends on the length of time the patient has had a problem of alcohol abuse and the amount of alcohol he had drunk before the abstinence that precipitated the delirium. See also ALCOHOLISM.

CLINICAL COURSE. Delirium tremens can be heralded by a variety of signs and symptoms. Some patients exhibit only mild tremulousness, irritability, difficulty in sleeping, tachycardia and hypertension, and pyrexia. Others have generalized convulsions as the first sign of difficulty.

Hallucinations are likely to follow the early signs and usually, but not always, are unpleasant and threatening to the patient. These hallucinations can be of all three types: auditory, visual, or tactile. Delusions often follow or accompany the hallucinations. The patient is unable to think clearly and sometimes becomes paranoid and greatly agitated. At this point he can become dangerous to himself and others. Generalized, grand mal seizures can occur in delirium tremens. The hallucinations and delusions may continue, contributing to the state of agitation and precipitating seizures.

TREATMENT AND PATIENT CARE. The person with delirium tremens is very ill and has multiple short-term and long-term problems. He should be kept in a quiet, nonstimulating environment and approached in a calm, reassuring manner. He must be watched closely and protected from self-injury during the period of delirium and also when he is convalescing from his illness and is likely to feel great remorse and depression. He should be observed for signs of extreme fatigue, pneumonia, or heart failure. Respiratory infections are quite common in these patients because of their weakened condition and inattention to personal hygiene.

The diet should be of high fluid intake and high in protein and carbohydrate content and low in fats. Dietary supplements usually include vitamin preparations, especially the B complex vitamins. If the patient is unable to cooperate by taking fluids and food by mouth, tube feeding and intravenous fluids may be necessary. Tranquillizing agents and sedatives may be useful.

deliver (di'livə) 1. to aid in childbirth. 2. to remove, as a fetus, placenta, or lens of the eye.

delivery (di'livə·ree) natural expulsion or extraction of the child, placenta and fetal membranes at birth (see also LABOUR).

abdominal d. delivery of an infant through an incision made into the uterus through the abdominal wall (CAESAREAN SECTION).

instrumental d. delivery facilitated by the use of instruments, particularly forceps.

spontaneous d. delivery occurring without assistance of forceps or other mechanical aid.

vaginal d. complete expulsion of the baby, placenta and membranes via the birth canal. Normally the head comes first presenting by the vertex. Breech delivery is also possible.

dellen ('delən) saucer-shaped excavations at the periphery of the cornea, usually on the temporal side. These irregularities may affect the corneal tear film.

delomorphous (,deloh'mawfəs) having definitely formed and well-defined limits, as a cell or tissue.

delouse (dee'lows) to free from lice.

delta ('deltə) 1. the fourth letter of the Greek alphabet, Δ or δ; used in chemical names to denote the fourth of a series of isomeric compounds or the carbon atom fourth from the carboxyl group, or to denote the fourth of any series. 2. a triangular area.

deltoid ('deltoyd) 1. triangular. 2. the deltoid muscle.

d. muscle the muscular cap of the shoulder, an inverted triangle that abducts the arm. It is often used as a site for intramuscular injections.

delusion (di'loozhən) a false personal belief based on incorrect inference about external reality and firmly maintained in spite of incontrovertible and obvious proof or evidence to the contrary. adj. **delusional.**

demecarium (,demə'kair·ri·əm) a cholinesterase inhibitor used in the treatment of glaucoma and convergent strabismus.

demeclocycline (di,mekloh'siekleen) a broad-spectrum tetracyclic antibiotic produced by a mutant strain of *Streptomyces aureofaciens*, effective against certain gram-negative bacteria, rickettsias, chlamydias, and *Mycoplasma pneumonia*.

dementia (di'menshi·ə) a global and progressive deterioration of the mental faculties which is irreversible and affects memory, intellect, judgement, personality and emotional control. Dementia is the result of an organic brain syndrome. The term *brain failure* is gradually replacing the term dementia as it is less stigmatizing and conveys that brain failure is a process while the term dementia simply suggests a state, and one associated with nihilistic views on treatment and prognosis.

Binswanger's d. dementia due to demyelination of the subcortical white matter of the brain, with sclerotic changes in the blood vessels supplying it.

paralytic d., d. paralytica a chronic meningoencephalitis characterized by degeneration of the cortical neurons, progressive dementia, and generalized paralysis, which, if untreated, is ultimately fatal; it results from antecedent syphilitic infection; called also *general paresis*.

d. praecox a former name for schizophrenia.

senile d. mental deterioration in old age.

demilune ('demi,loon) a crescent-shaped structure or cell.

demineralization (dee,minə·rəlie'zayshən) excessive elimination of mineral or organic salts from the tissues of the body.

demodectic (,deemoh'dektik) pertaining to or caused by *Demodex*.

Demodex ('deemoh,deks) a genus of mites parasitic within the hair follicles of the host, including the species *D. folliculorum* in man, and several other species in domestic and other animals.

demography (di'mogrəfee) the statistical science dealing with populations, including matters of health, disease, births, and mortality.

demulcent (di'mulsənt) 1. soothing; bland. 2. a soothing mucilaginous or oily medicine or application.

demyelinate (di'mieəli,nayt) to destroy or remove the myelin sheath of a nerve or nerves.

demyelination (di'mieəli'nayshən) destruction, removal, or loss of the myelin sheath of a nerve or nerves.

demyelinization (di,mieəlinie'zayshən) demyelination.

denarcotize (dee'nahkətiez) to deprive of narcotics or of narcotic properties.

denasality (,deenay'zalitee) hyponasality.

denaturant (dee'naychə·rənt) a denaturing agent.

denaturation (dee,naychə'rayshən) a change in the usual nature of a substance, as by the addition of methanol or acetone to alcohol to render it unfit for drinking, or the change in molecular structure of proteins due to splitting of hydrogen bonds caused by heat or certain chemicals.

protein d. any nonproteolytic change in the chemistry, composition, or structure of a native protein which causes it to lose some or all of its unique or specific characteristics.

dendr(o)- word element. [Gr.] *tree, treelike.*

dendraxon (den'drakson) a nerve cell whose axon splits up into terminal filaments immediately after leaving the cell.

dendric ('dendrik) pertaining to a dendrite.

dendriform ('dendri,fawm) tree-shaped.

dendrite ('dendriet) any of the threadlike extensions of the cytoplasm of a neuron; dendrites, which typically branch into treelike processes, compose most of the receptive surface of a neuron.

dendritic (den'dritik) 1. branched like a tree. 2. pertaining to or possessing dendrites.

dendrodendritic (,dendrohden'dritik) referring to a synapse between dendrites of two neurons.

dendroid ('dendroyd) branched like a tree.

dendron ('dendron) dendrite.

denervation (,deenər'vayshən) interruption of the nerve supply to an organ or part.

dengue ('deng·gee) a painful viral disease that occurs in tropical countries throughout the world. The virus that causes the disease, one of four types of a group B arbovirus, is carried by *Aedes* mosquitoes. Because of the intense pain in the bones, dengue is also known as *breakbone fever*. People who have had dengue are generally immunized against the particular type of virus involved for 5 years, but only for a few months against the other types. Explosive epidemics may occur if a type new to, or long absent from, an area is introduced.

SYMPTOMS. The symptoms of dengue begin within a week after the bite of the infective mosquito. The onset is marked by a severe headache and pain behind the eyes. Within hours the characteristic pain in the back and joints begins. Movement is difficult, and the temperature may rise as high as 41 °C (106 °F). Congested eyeballs, a flushed face and sometimes general erythema are outward symptoms. The disease often has two stages of about 3 days and 2 days separated by a period of 24 hours in which the symptoms disappear, raising hopes of the end of the attack. An itchy red rash appears in many cases about the fifth day of illness, starting on the hands and feet then spreading rapidly to the arms and legs and sometimes to the trunk. The total course of the acute illness is rarely more than 6 or 7 days although the sufferer is exhausted and depressed and convalescence may be slow. Dengue by itself is rarely fatal, unless the infection produces dengue haemorrhagic fever.

TREATMENT AND PREVENTION. As there is no known remedy for dengue, the treatment is mainly palliative.

The best method of preventing dengue is by controlling the mosquito, and in some areas this has been successful. In areas lacking mosquito control, personal protection (repellants, protective clothing, bed nets) reduces the risk.

d. haemorrhagic fever a severe form of dengue which occurs in many parts of tropical Asia, mainly in children. Various haemorrhagic phenomena may develop. Some cases proceed into a state of shock with a high mortality. Fluid replacement therapy is indicated.

denial (di'nieəl) a defence mechanism in which the existence of intolerable actions, ideas, etc., are unconsciously denied.

denidation (,deni'dayshən) the degeneration and expulsion, during menstruation, of certain epthelial elements, potentially the nidus of an embryo. The term used to describe the intended shedding of the uterine lining when postcoital contraceptive pills are used.

Denis Browne splint (,denis 'brown) a splint for the correction of clubfoot, consisting of two metal footplates connected by a crossbar.

denominator (di'nominaytə) the lower part of a fraction of a rate or ratio.

dens (dens) pl. *dentes* [L.] a tooth or toothlike structure.

densimeter, densitometer (,den'simitə; ,densi'tomitə) an instrument for determining density or specific gravity of a liquid.

densitometry (,densi'tomitree) determination of variations in density by comparison with that of another material or with a certain standard.

density ('densitee) 1. the ratio of the mass of a substance to its volume. 2. the quality of being compact. 3. the quantity of matter in a given space.

charge d. the quantity of electrostatic charge per unit area of a surface or per unit volume.

current d. the quantity of electrical current flowing through unit area of a surface.

optical d. the degree of blackening in an area of a photograph or radiograph.

dent(o)- word element. [L.] *tooth, toothlike.*

dental ('dent'l) pertaining to the teeth.

d. caries tooth decay (see also CARIES).

d. hygienist a dental health specialist whose primary concern is maintenance of dental health and the prevention of oral disease. Patient education in the area of proper brushing and flossing also is a major responsibility for the dental hygienist.

The dental hygienist must undergo a training course which lasts 9 to 12 months and takes place at a number of dental hospitals. The course ends in an examination for the Certificate of Proficiency in Dental Hygiene. To practise the hygienist must register on the Roll of Dental Hygienists kept by the General Dental Council.

dentalgia (den'talji·ə) toothache.

dentate ('dentayt) notched; tooth-shaped.

dentia ('denshi·ə) a condition relating to development or eruption of the teeth.

d. praecox premature eruption of the teeth; presence of teeth in the mouth at birth.

d. tarda delayed eruption of the teeth, beyond the usual time for their appearance.

denticle ('dentik'l) 1. a small toothlike process. 2. a distinct calcified mass within the pulp chamber or in the dentine of a tooth.

dentifrice ('dentifris) see TOOTHPASTE.

dentigerous (den'tijə·rəs) bearing teeth.

d. cyst a common odontogenic cyst of developmental origin associated with an unerupted tooth. Multiple dentigerous cysts may be found adjacent to unerupted teeth in the jaws of cleidocranial dysostosis.

dentine ('denteen) the chief substance of the teeth, surrounding the tooth pulp and covered by the enamel on the crown and by cementum on the roots. adj. **dentinal.**

dentinoblastoma (,dentinohbla'stohmə) dentinoma.

dentinogenesis (,dentinoh'jenəsis) the formation of dentine.

d. imperfecta a hereditary condition marked by imperfect formation and calcification of dentine, giving the teeth a brown or blue opalescent appearance known as hereditary opalescent dentine.

dentinoma (ˌdenti'nohmə) tumour of odontogenic origin, consisting mainly of dentine; called also *dentinoblastoma.*

dentist ('dentist) a person who has received a degree in dentistry and who is authorized to practise dentistry.

dentistry ('dentistree) 1. that branch of the healing arts concerned with the teeth and associated structures of the oral cavity, including prevention, diagnosis, and treatment of disease and restoration of defective or missing teeth. 2. the work done by dentists, e.g., the creation of restoration, crowns, and bridges, and surgical procedures performed in and about the oral cavity. 3. the practice of the dental profession collectively.

operative d. dentistry concerned with restoration of parts of the teeth that are defective as a result of disease, trauma, or abnormal development to a state of normal function, health, and aesthetics.

preventive d. dentistry concerned with maintenance of a normal masticating mechanism by fortifying the structures of the oral cavity against damage and disease.

prosthetic d. prosthodontics.

dentition (den'tishən) the teeth in the dental arch; ordinarily used to designate the natural teeth in position in the alveoli.

deciduous d. the complement of teeth that erupt first and are later succeeded by the permanent teeth.

mixed d. the complement of teeth in the jaws after eruption of some of the permanent teeth, but before all the deciduous teeth are shed.

permanent d. the complement of teeth that erupt and take their places after the deciduous teeth have been shed.

denture ('denchə) a complement of teeth, either natural or artificial; ordinarily used to designate an artificial replacement for the natural teeth and adjacent tissues.

complete d. an appliance replacing all the teeth of one jaw, as well as associated structures of the jaw.

immediate d. a partial or complete denture constructed beforehand which is fitted immediately after the teeth have been extracted.

overlay d. a complete denture supported both by soft tissue (mucosa) and by a few remaining natural teeth that have been altered, as by insertion of a long or short coping, to permit the denture to fit over them.

partial d. a removable (removable partial denture) or permanently attached (fixed partial denture) appliance replacing one or more missing teeth in one jaw and receiving support and retention from underlying tissues and some or all of the remaining teeth.

denucleated (dee'nyookliˌaytid) deprived of the nucleus.

denudation (ˌdenyuh'dayshən, ˌdee-) stripping or laying bare.

Denver classification ('denvə) the classification of human CHROMOSOMES on the basis of size and centromere position; the 23 pairs of chromosomes are classified in seven groups (A to G), in order of decreasing length. Used before it was possible to distinguish among the chromosomes of the groups.

deodorant (di'ohdə·rənt) 1. destroying or masking odours. 2. an agent that masks offensive odours.

deodorize (di'ohdəˌriez) to neutralize or absorb odour.

deodorizer (di'ohdəˌriezə) a deodorizing agent.

deorsumversion (diˌorsəm'vərshən) the turning downward of a part, especially of the eyes.

deossification (diˌosifikayshən) loss or removal of the mineral elements of bone.

deoxidation (ˌdeeoksi'dayshən) the removal of oxygen from a chemical compound.

deoxy- a chemical prefix designating a compound containing one less atom of oxygen than the reference substance. For words beinning thus, see also those beginning *desoxy-.*

deoxycholic acid (deeˌoksi'kohlik) one of the bile acids, capable of forming soluble, diffusible complexes with fatty acids, and thereby allowing for their absorption in the small intestine.

deoxycorticosterone (deeˌoksiˌkawti'kostə·rohn) deoxycortone.

deoxycortone (deeˌoksi'kawtohn) a naturally occurring mineralocorticoid, $C_{21}H_{30}O_3$, with no glucocorticoid activity, secreted in small amounts by the human adrenal cortex.

d. acetate and d. pivalate synthetic preparations used in the treatment of adrenocortical insufficiency.

deoxygenation (deeˌoksijə'nayshən) the act of depriving of oxygen.

2-deoxy-D-glucose ('toodeeˌoksideeˌglookohs) an antimetabolite of glucose tried as an antiviral; it acts by inhibiting the glycosylation of glycoproteins and glycolipids; it has been investigated for treatment of herpesvirus infections.

deoxyhaemoglobin (diˌoksiˌheemə'glohbin) haemoglobin not combined with oxygen, formed when oxyhaemoglobin releases its oxygen to the tissues.

deoxyribonuclease (diˌoksiˌrieboh'nyookliˌayz) an enzyme that catalyses the hydrolysis (depolymerization) of deoxyribonucleic acid (DNA). Abbreviated DNase.

deoxyribonucleic acid (diˌoksiˌriebohnyoo'klee·ik, -'klay-) a NUCLEIC ACID of complex molecular structure occurring in cell nuclei as the basic structure of the GENES. Abbreviated DNA. DNA is present in all body cells of every species, including unicellular organisms and DNA viruses. The structure of DNA was first described in 1953 by J.D. Watson and F.H.C. Crick.

DNA molecules are linear polymers of small molecules called *nucleotides*, each of which consists of one molecule of the five-carbon sugar *deoxyribose* bonded to a *phosphate* group and to one of four heterocyclic nitrogenous compounds referred to as *bases.* A single strand of DNA is made by linking the nucleotides together in a chain with bonds between the sugar and phosphate groups of adjacent nucleotides. It thus consists of a backbone of alternating sugar and phosphate groups with a base attached to each sugar as a side chain. The four bases are two purines, *adenine* (A) and *guanine* (G), and two pyrimidines, *cytosine* (C) and *thymine* (T). Single-stranded DNA can be synthesized with any specified sequence of bases, but in living cells the base sequence has a meaning: it specifies the amino acid sequence of all of the polypeptides and proteins made by the cell. And since all of the enzymes that catalyse biochemical reactions are proteins, the DNA contains the specifications for all of the biochemistry and structure of the cell.

The chemical basis of the genetic code lies in the ability of the bases to form hydrogen bonds with each other. Unlike the covalent bonds holding together the atoms of a single strand of DNA, hydrogen bonds are weak and easily broken and reformed. Hydrogen bonding is governed by the base pairing rule: A always bonds with T, and C always bonds with G. A and T (or C and G) are called *complementary bases.* The genetic information is read and preserved by the matching up of complementary bases.

In cells, the DNA is double-stranded. The configuration of the DNA molecule resembles a ladder in which the sides are the sugar-phosphate backbones, which are antiparallel (they run in opposite directions), and the rungs are hydrogen-bonded complementary bases;

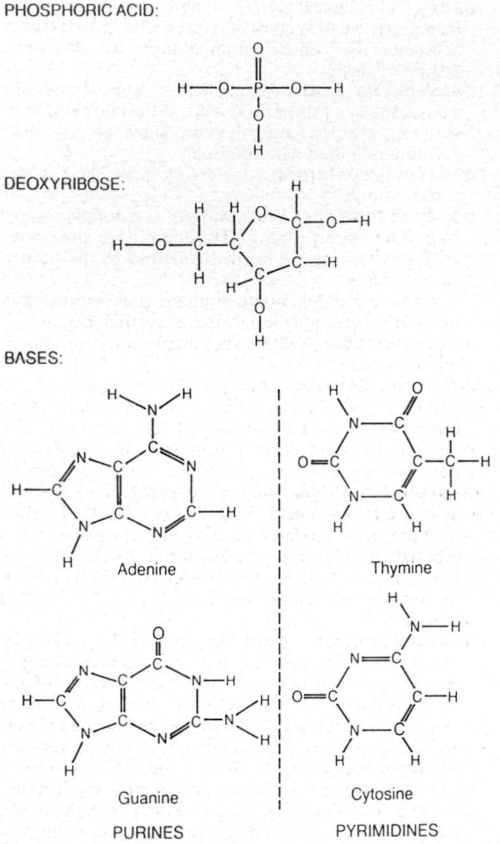

PHOSPHORIC ACID:

DEOXYRIBOSE:

BASES:

Adenine

Thymine

Guanine

Cytosine

PURINES

PYRIMIDINES

The basic building blocks of DNA

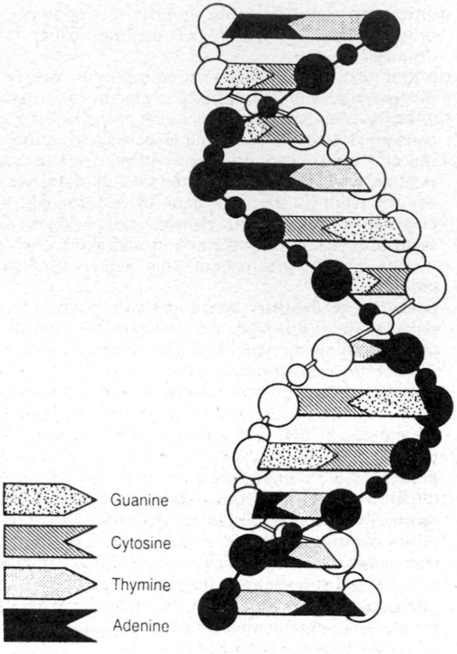

Diagrammatic representation of DNA helix

thus, the entire sequence along the two strands is complementary. This whole structure is twisted so that the two strands form a double helix. Once before each cell division, a group of proteins splits the two strands apart, and as complementary nucleotides bond to the bases of each strand they are joined to form a new strand. This process if called *replication.* It results in the exact duplication of the DNA molecule, because each strand serves as a *template* (pattern) for the synthesis of its complementary strand. When the cell divides, one copy goes to each daughter cell. Thus, the genetic information is passed on from generation to generation without change except for rare mutations, which result from copying errors or incorrectly repaired breaks in the DNA molecule that change the base sequence.

The reading of the genetic code involves two processes: *transcription* and *translation.* In transcription, a length of DNA is used as a template to make a complementary strand of *messenger RNA* (mRNA). RNA (ribonucleic acid) is a nucleic acid like DNA. The only differences are that the sugar, *ribose,* has an extra oxygen atom, and the pyrimidine base, *uracil* (U), which also pairs with adenine, replaces thymine.

In translation, the mRNA molecule is read by a structure called a *ribosome,* which produces the polypeptide specified by the mRNA message.

The genetic code is a triplet code. Every triplet of bases along the strand specifies a single amino acid. There are 64 possible triplets (codons) that can be formed from the four bases. Each one specifies that one of 20 different amino acids be inserted in a growing polypeptide chain or marks either the start or the end of a chain.

Two other types of RNA are involved in translation. *Ribosomal RNA* (rRNA) forms a large part of the ribosome. *Transfer RNA* (tRNA) is the means by which codons are matched with amino acids. tRNAs are small molecules with several self-complementary sections so that they fold up into a compact structure owing to bonding between complementary bases. One end of the molecule is a three-base anticodon, which bonds to its complementary codon on mRNA molecules. The other end is recognized by a specific enzyme which attaches the correct amino acid to it. During translation, the ribosome proceeds along the mRNA molecule and, as each codon is matched by a specific tRNA, the amino acid it carries is transferred to the growing polypeptide chain, and the process is repeated until the 'stop' codon is reached. Like the mRNA molecules, rRNA and tRNA molecules are formed on DNA templates; the genetic material contains not only the information for polypeptide sequences but also for rRNA and tRNA sequences.

There is an enormous amount of information stored in the DNA of a cell. The 48 chromosomes of a human cell contain a total length of about 6 billion base pairs of DNA. This is enough to code for the thousands of enzymes and structural proteins in the cell. DNA is the molecule that directs all of the activities of living cells, including its own reproduction and perpetuation in generation after generation.

deoxyribonucleoprotein (di,oksi,rieboh'nyooklioh-'prohteen) a nucleoprotein in which the sugar is D-2-deoxyribose.

deoxyribonucleoside (di,oksi,rieboh'nyooklioh,sied) a nucleoside having a purine or pyrimidine base bonded to deoxyribose.

deoxyribonucleotide (di,oksi,rieboh'nyooklioh,tied) a nucleotide having a purine or pyrimidine base bonded to deoxyribose, which in turn is bonded to a phosphate group.

deoxyribose (di,oksi'riebohs, -bohz) an aldopentose found in deoxyribonucleic acid, deoxyribonucleotides, and deoxyribonucleosides.

dependence (di'pendəns) the total psychophysical state of a drug user, in which the usual or increasing doses of the drug are required to prevent the onset of WITHDRAWAL SYMPTOMS.

dependency (di'pendənsee) a state of relying on another for love, affection, mothering, comfort, security, food, warmth, shelter, protection and the like.

d.studies the measurement of the need for care required by a patient based on his/her level of ability to carry out self-care. The main self-care activities measured are ability to feed, carry out toilet requirements and level of mobility, including dressing.

d. studies for staffing ratios studies undertaken to determine the number of staff required to provide the appropriate skills to care for specific types and numbers of patients (see ABERDEEN FORMULA).

depersonalization (dee,pərsənəlie'zayshən) alteration in the perception of self so that the usual sense of one's own reality is temporarily lost or changed; it may be a manifestation of a neurosis or another mental illness or can occur in mild form in normal persons.

dephosphorylation (,deefos,fo·ri'layshən) removal of a phosphate group from an organic molecule.

depilate ('depi,layt) to remove hair.

depilatory (di'pilətə·ree) 1. having the power to remove hair. 2. an agent that removes or destroys the hair.

depolarization (dee,pohlə·rie'zayshən) the process or act of neutralizing polarity.

depolymerization (dee,polimə·rie'zayshən) the conversion of a compound into one of smaller molecular weight and different physical properties without changing the percentage relations of the elements composing it.

Deponit ('depohnit) trademark for a preparation of glyceryl trinitrate transdermal infusion, a coronary vasodilator.

deposit (di'pozit) 1. sediment or dregs. 2. extraneous inorganic matter collected in the tissues or in an organ of the body.

depot ('depoh) a body area in which a substance, e.g., a drug, can be accumulated, deposited, or stored and from which it can be distributed.

fat d. a site in the body in which large quantities of fat are stored, as in adipose tissue.

depressant (di'pres'nt) 1. diminishing any function or activity. 2. an agent that retards any function, especially a drug that acts on the central nervous system to depress activity at all levels by stabilizing neuronal membranes. CNS depressants, e.g., barbiturates and inhalational anaesthetics, are used as sedatives, hypnotics, and anaesthetics. Alcohol is also a depressant, although its first effect is sometimes stimulating.

depressed (di'prest) carried below the normal level; associated with depression.

depression (di'preshən) 1. a hollow or depressed area. 2. a lowering or decrease of functional activity. 3. in psychiatry, a morbid sadness, dejection, or melancholy, distinguished from grief, which is realistic and proportionate to a personal loss. Profound depression may be symptomatic of a psychiatric disorder or it may constitute the principal manifestation of a neurosis or psychosis. adj. **depressive**.

Treatment of profound and chronic depression is often very difficult, requiring in most cases intensive psychotherapy to help the patient understand the underlying cause of his depression. Antidepressant drugs such as imipramine hydrochloride and amitriptyline are often used in the treatment of depression. They are not true stimulants of the central nervous system, but they do alter the function of the reticular system in the midbrain and of the nuclei of the thalamus. Monoamine oxidase (MAOI) inhibitors are also used. When antidepressants fail, some form of shock therapy such as electric shock or insulin shock treatments may be used in conjunction with the psychotherapy.

PATIENT CARE. Mild, sporadic depression is a relatively common phenomenon experienced by almost everyone at some time in his life, but hospitalized patients are particularly susceptible to feelings of depression and a sense of loss and despair. Early signs of depression of this kind include pessimistic statements about one's illness and its prognosis, refusal to eat, diminished concern about personal appearance, and reluctance to make decisions. When depression is noted in a patient, his care plan should list this problem and suggest some approaches to helping him deal with it.

Consistency of care is helpful to the depressed patient. He knows what to expect, and thus is not repeatedly disappointed when his expectations are not met. An example is consistency in scheduling and carrying out treatments and routine care at the same time each day. If the patient has a supportive family and interested friends, they should be involved in choosing and planning activities that can help overcome his depression.

When a patient is depressed, he is likely to isolate himself and avoid social contact even with those who are trying to help him. Since loss of contact with others contributes to his depression, members of the health care team should persist in attempts to talk with the patient, by asking him questions, and actively listening when he attempts to express his feelings. One should be especially careful to avoid being judgemental when the patient does express despair, anger, hostility, or some negative feeling. Above all, it is important not to be condescending and respond to his statements with some meaningless cliché, such as 'Don't worry', or 'I'm sure everything will turn out OK'. These convey a lack of empathy with the patient's suffering and are an unrealistic approach to a problem that is very real.

Physical contact and touching may be misunderstood by a depressed patient. Sometimes, it is better just to sit with the patient and calmly observe him without making him feel uncomfortable. Honest dialogue and expressions of support and concern can often improve his mood and sense of self-worth.

The severely depressed patient usually expresses three basic feelings associated with his mental state. These are physical inactivity and a lack of desire to socialize, feelings of worthlessness, and loss of self-esteem and thoughts of self-injury or destruction. In planning the care of the depressed patient, one must always consider these attitudes and strive for some understanding as to why the patient behaves as he does. Although an optimistic approach should be used when helping the patient overcome his depression, one must guard against excessive cheerfulness and attempts to 'jolly' the patient into a better mood. Only by gradually gaining his attention and pointing out to him encouraging signs of his progress can he be helped in his early attempts to return to reality and socialize with others. As he progresses out of his depression the patient may become overdependent on the therapist and then later show signs of hostility toward her. She must, however, remain consistent in her relationship with him, demonstrating warmth and a sincere interest in him no matter what type of behaviour he may exhibit.

The patient's physical inactivity will require attention to adequate nutrition, a normal balance of fluid intake and output, proper elimination, and good skin care. He will need help in maintaining a pleasing personal appearance and good personal hygiene. At first it may be necessary for the hospital staff to initiate all such activities as bathing, dressing, and even eating and drinking. As his condition improves the patient should take over responsibility for his personal care and grooming. If he is severely depressed he may be totally out of touch with reality and completely unresponsive to anyone else's presence. In such instances the therapist may be able to do little more than sit with the patient, letting him know by her presence that she is interested in his problem and that she cares enough to try to help him.

Constant vigilance must be maintained to prevent the profoundly depressed patient from injuring himself or committing SUICIDE. Self-destructive behaviour is a manifestation of the patient's feeling of worthlessness and loss of self-esteem. An awareness of the potential dangers in such a situation should help the therapist plan and provide a safe and congenial atmosphere. She should be alert to the early signs of a patient's intention to harm or destroy himself. In most cases suicide is most likely to occur when the patient is recovering from severe depression.

congenital chrondrosternal d. a congenital deformity with a deep, funnel-shaped depression in the anterior chest wall.

involutional d. a major depression occurring in late middle life. Called also *involutional melancholia.*

reactive d., situational d. depression due to some external situation, and often relieved when the situation is removed.

depressomotor (di,presoh'mohtə) 1. retarding or abating motor activity. 2. an agent that so acts.

depressor (di'presə) anything that depresses, as a muscle, agent, or instrument, or an afferent nerve, whose stimulation causes a fall in blood pressure.

tongue d. an instrument for pressing down the tongue.

deprivation (,depri'vayshən) loss or absence of parts, organs, powers, or things that are needed.

emotional d. deprivation of adequate and appropriate interpersonal or environmental experience, usually in the early developmental years.

maternal d. syndrome a group of symptoms, including stunted emotional and physical development, arising in infants who have been deprived of care and love provided by a mother or mothering figure. Deprivation of maternal care during the first three years of life is thought to be particularly critical as this is the optimal period for the forming of social attachments. Maternal deprivation, in children who have been abandoned or institutionalized, may lead to psychological problems in later life and the syndrome has also been described in several mammalian species.

sensory d. deprivation of usual external stimuli and the opportunity for perception.

deradelphus (,derə'delfəs) a twin fetus or infant fused at or near the navel, and having one head.

derangement (di'raynjmənt) 1. mental disorder. 2. disarrangement of a part or organ.

Derbyshire neck ('dahbishə) see GOITRE.

Dercum's disease ('dərkəmz) adiposis dolorosa.

dereism ('deeri,izəm) mental activity in which fantasy runs unhampered by logic and experience. adj. **dereistic.**

derencephalus (,deren'kefələs, -'sef-) a fetus or infant with a rudimentary skull and bifid cervical vertebrae, the brain resting in the bifurcation.

derepression (,deeri'preshən) 1. elevation of the level of an enzyme above the normal, either by lowering the corepressor concentration or by a mutation that decreases the formation of aporepressor or the response to the complete repressor. 2. the inhibition of the repressor substance produced by the regulator genes with the result that the operator gene is free to initiate the process of polypeptide formation.

derma ('dərmə) the corium, or true skin.

dermabrasion (,dərmə'brayzhən) PLANING of the skin done by mechanical means, e.g., sandpaper, wire brushes, etc.

Dermacentor (,dərmə'sentə) a genus of ticks parasitic on various animals, and vectors of disease-producing microorganisms.

D. andersoni a species of tick common in the western United States, parasitic on numerous wild mammals, most domestic animals, and man. It is an important vector of Rocky Mountain spotted fever, and also transmits, in the United States, tularaemia, Colorado tick fever, and Q fever. It is the commonest cause of tick paralysis.

D. variabilis the chief vector of Rocky Mountain spotted fever in the central and eastern United States, the dog being the principal host of the adult forms, but also parasitic on cattle, horses, rabbits, and man.

dermal ('dərməl) pertaining to the true skin, or corium.

dermat(o)- word element. [Gr.] *skin.*

dermatic (dər'matik) dermal.

dermatitides (,dərmə'titi,deez) plural of *dermatitis;* inflammatory conditions of the skin considered collectively.

dermatitis (,dərma'tietis) inflammation of the skin. Dermatitis can result from contact with various animal, vegetable, and chemical substances, from heat or cold, from mechanical irritation, from certain forms of malnutrition, or from infectious disease. In some cases, dermatitis may have a psychological rather than a physical cause. The symptoms may include itching, redness, crustiness, blisters, watery discharges, fissures, or other changes in the normal condition of the skin. The treatment of dermatitis varies greatly and is determined by the cause.

TYPES OF DERMATITIS. One of the most common forms of the disorder, CONTACT DERMATITIS, results from contact of the skin with various substances. There are two types: allergic contact dermatitis and primary-irritant dermatitis. Familiar examples of the allergic type include rubber and plastics, industrial chemicals, cosmetics, clothing dyes, costume jewellery, some animals and plants, detergents, insecticides, and paints.

The second type of contact dermatitis is due to a direct irritating effect on the skin of certain chemical, physical, or mechanical agents. In contrast to the allergic type, which affects only people who have a specific sensitivity, these agents cause dermatitis in everyone upon sufficient exposure. Acids, alkalis, petroleum products, and mineral dusts are some of the chemical causes. A mild form is the familiar 'housewife's eczema', resulting from contact with strong soaps and detergents.

Such physical agents as excessive cold or heat may cause inflammation of the skin. Prolonged exposure to extreme cold may result in chilblains or in frostbite, and exposure to a hot sun may cause sunburn. When heat causes unusual sweating, miliaria (commonly called prickly heat) may result. All these familiar complaints are forms of dermatitis. Exposure to x-rays is another factor which may cause skin inflammation. Mechanical agents, such as chafing, pressure, or scratching, are other common causes of dermatitis. Pressure and friction resulting from ill fitting shoes cause corns and calluses, and pressure on bony parts of the body incurred in extended bed rest may cause PRESSURE SORES.

PATIENT CARE. The patient with dermatitis is frequently uncomfortable, irritable, and emotionally upset because of itching and the unsightly appearance produced by his condition. Efforts should be made to provide a quiet atmosphere that is conducive to rest, and to give the patient individual attention to help him feel acceptable to others.

If large areas of the skin are involved there will be increased sensitivity to cold, making the patient more susceptible to chilling. Care must be used to protect the patient and the bed linen from dampness when wet compresses are prescribed.

Bathing with ordinary soap and water is usually contraindicated and special colloid or medicated baths may be ordered to cleanse and soothe irritated or pruritic skin. After the bath the skin is dried by patting with a soft towel, *never* by rubbing. Scales, crusts, and other exudates are *not* removed without specific medical instruction. The skin should be handled gently, and great care used in changing the bedclothes or the patient's clothing.

actinic d., d. actinica that produced by exposure to actinic radiation, such as that from the sun, ultraviolet waves, or x- or gamma radiation.

atopic d. a chronic pruritic eruption of unknown aetiology, although allergic, hereditary, and psychogenic factors appear to be involved.

contact d. acute dermatitis due to direct contact of the skin with various substances (see also CONTACT DERMATITIS). **d. exfoliativa neonatorum** exfoliative dermatitis supervening in bullous impetigo of the newborn; called also *Ritter's disease*.

exfoliative d. virtually universal erythema, desquamation, scaling, and itching of the skin and loss of hair; it may result from internal medication with such drugs as penicillin, quinine, sulphonamides, gold salts, and iodides.

d. herpetiformis chronic dermatitis marked by successive crops of grouped, symmetrical, erythematous, papular, vesicular, eczematous, or bullous lesions, accompanied by itching and burning; a granular deposition of IgA immunoglobulin around the lesion almost always occurs.

d. medicamentosa an eruption or solitary skin lesion caused by a drug taken internally.

photocontact d. allergic CONTACT DERMATITIS caused by the action of sunlight on skin sensitized by contact with a substance capable of causing this reaction, such as sandalwood oil, hexachlorophene and drugs such as phenothiazines, tetracyclines and sulphonamides.

primary-irritant d. CONTACT DERMATITIS induced by a substance acting as an irritant rather than as a sensitizer or allergen.

seborrhoeic d., d. seborrhoeica a chronic, usually pruritic, dermatitis with erythema, dry, moist, or greasy scaling, and yellow crusted patches on various areas, especially the scalp, with exfoliation of an excessive amount of dry scales (dandruff). In mild forms frequent shampooing may be all that is required. In more severe involvement a keratolytic preparation may be necessary (see also SEBORRHOEIC DERMATITIS).

stasis d. an eczematous eruption of the lower legs, usually due to impeded circulation, with oedema, pigmentation, and often chronic ulceration.

d. venenata severe allergic contact dermatitis.

x-ray d. radiodermatitis; inflammatory reaction of the skin to radiotherapy.

Dermatobia (ˌdərməˈtohbi·ə) a genus of botflies; the larvae of *D. hominis* are parasitic in the skin of man and domestic animals in Central and South America.

dermatocele (ˈdərmətohˌseel) cutis laxa.

dermatofibroma (ˌdərmətohfieˈbrohmə) a fibrous tumour-like nodule of the skin.

dermatofibrosarcoma (ˌdərmətohˌfiebrohsahˈkohmə) a fibrosarcoma of the skin.

dermatoglyphics (ˌdərmətohˈglifiks) the study of the patterns of ridges of the skin of the fingers, palms, toes, and soles; of interest in anthropology and law enforcement as a means of establishing identity and in medicine, both clinically and as a genetic indicator, particularly of chromosomal abnormalities.

dermatographia (ˌdərmətohˈgrafi·ə) dermatographism.

dermatographism (ˌdərmətohˈgrafizəm) urticaria due to physical allergy in which a pale, raised welt or wheal with a red flare on each side is elicited by stroking or scratching the skin with a dull instrument. adj. **dermatographic**.

dermatoheteroplasty (ˌdərmətohˈhetə·rohˌplastee) the grafting of skin derived from an individual of another species.

dermatological (ˌdərmətəˈlojikˈl) pertaining to dermatology; of or affecting the skin.

dermatologist (ˌdərməˈtoləjist) a doctor who specializes in dermatology.

dermatology (ˌdərməˈtoləjee) the medical speciality concerned with the diagnosis and treatment of skin diseases.

dermatome (ˈdərməˌtohm) 1. an instrument for cutting split skin grafts. 2. the area of skin supplied with afferent nerve fibres by a single posterior spinal root. 3. the lateral part of an embryonic somite.

dermatomegaly (ˌdərmətohˈmegəlee) cutis laxa.

dermatomere (ˈdərmətohˌmiə) any segment of the embryonic integument.

dermatomycosis (ˌdərmətohmieˈkohsis) a superficial fungal infection of the skin or of its appendages.

dermatomyoma (ˌdərmətohmieˈohmə) a dermal leiomyoma.

dermatomyositis (ˌdərmətohˌmiehohˈsietis) an acute, subacute, or chronic disease marked by nonsuppurative inflammation of the skin, subcutaneous tissue, and muscles, with necrosis of muscle fibres. It is included among the group of illnesses known as COLLAGEN DISEASES.

Among a variety of symptoms that point to the onset of the disease are fever, loss of weight, skin lesions, and aching muscles. As the disease progresses there may be loss of the use of the arms and legs. Overlap forms of the disease with systemic connective sclerosis may occur. Steroids are the main form of treatment.

dermatopathic (ˌdərmətohˈpathik) pertaining to or attributable to disease of the skin.

dermatopathology (ˌdərmətohpəˈtholəjee) pathology that is especially concerned with lesions of the skin.

dermatopathy (ˌdərmə'topəthee) any disease of the skin; dermopathy.
Dermatophagoides pteronyssinus (ˌdərmətohfa'goydeez ˌterohni'sienəs) the house dust mite, which can produce allergic asthma in susceptible persons.
dermatophilosis (ˌdərmətohfi'lohsis) an actinomycotic disease caused by *Dermatophilus congolensis*, affecting cattle, sheep, horses, goats, deer, and sometimes man. In man, it is marked by nonpainful pustules on the hands and arms; the lesions break down and form shallow red ulcers which regress spontaneously, leaving some scarring.
Dermatophilus (ˌdərmə'tofiləs) a genus of pathogenic actinomycetes.
D. congolensis the aetiological agent of dermatophilosis.
dermatophyte ('dərmətohˌfiet) a fungus parasitic upon the skin, including *Microsporum*, *Epidermophyton*, and *Trichophyton*.
dermatophytid (ˌdərmə'tofitid) a secondary skin eruption which is an expression of hypersensitivity to a dermatophyte infection, occurring on an area remote from the site of infection.
dermatophytosis (ˌdərmətohfie'tohsis) a fungal infection of the skin; often used to refer to ATHLETE'S FOOT (tinea pedis).
dermatoplasty ('dərmətohˌplastee) a plastic operation on the skin; operative replacement of lost skin. adj. **dermatoplastic.**
dermatosclerosis (ˌdərmətohsklə'rohsis) scleroderma.
dermatosis (ˌdərmə'tohsis) any skin disorder, especially one not characterized by inflammation.
precancerous d. any skin condition in which the lesions—warts, naevi, or other excrescences—are likely to undergo malignant degeneration.
stasis d. a chronic, usually eczematous dermatitis almost always of the anteromedial aspect of the lower leg, and often complicated by ulceration; probably due to deficient venous return. Called also *stasis dermatitis*.
dermatotherapy (ˌdərmətoh'therəpee) treatment of skin diseases.
dermatotropic (ˌdərmətoh'tropik, -'trohpik) having a specific affinity for the skin.
dermatozoon (ˌdərmətoh'zoh·on) any animal parasite on the skin; an ectoparasite.
dermis ('dərmis) the true skin; the fibrous inner layer of skin just beneath the epidermis, derived from the embryonic mesoderm and varying from 0.5 to 3 mm in thickness. It is well supplied with nerves and blood vessels and contains hair roots and sebaceous and sweat glands. On the palms and soles the dermis bears ridges whose arrangement in whorls and loops is peculiar to the individual. Called also *corium*. adj. **dermal, dermic.**
dermoblast ('dərmohˌblast) the part of the mesoderm that develops into the true skin.
dermographia (ˌdərmoh'grafi·ə) dermatographism.
dermoid ('dərmoyd) skinlike.
d. cyst a tumour consisting of a fibrous wall lined with stratified epithelium containing pulpy material in which epithelial elements such as hair may be found.
dermoidectomy (ˌdərmoy'dektəmee) excision of a dermoid cyst.
dermomycosis (ˌdərmohmie'kohsis) dermatomycosis.
dermopathy (dər'mopəthee) any skin disease; dermatopathy.
diabetic d. any of several cutaneous manifestations of diabetes.
dermophyte ('dərmohˌfiet) dermatophyte.
dermosynovitis (ˌdərmohˌsienoh'vietis) inflammation of the skin overlying an inflamed bursa or tendon sheath.
dermotropic (ˌdərmoh'tropik, -'trohpik) dermatotropic.
dermovascular (ˌdərmoh'vaskyuhlə) pertaining to the skin and blood vessels of the skin.
derodidymus (ˌdiroh'didiməs) a monster with two heads; dicephalus.
Descemet's membrane ('desiˌmayz) the posterior lining membrane of the cornea, a thin hyaline membrane between the substantia propria and the endothelial layer.
descemetocele (ˌdese'metohseel) hernial protrusion of Descemet's membrane.
descensus (di'sensəs) pl. *descensus* [L.] downward displacement or prolapse.
d. testis normal migration of the testis from its fetal position in the abdominal cavity to its location within the scrotum, usually during the last 3 months of gestation.
d. uteri prolapse of the uterus.
desensitization (deeˌsensitie'zayshən) 1. the prevention or reduction of immediate hypersensitivity reactions by the administration of graded doses of allergen; hyposensitization. See also IMMUNOTHERAPY. 2. in behaviour therapy, the treatment of phobias and related disorders by intentionally exposing the patient, in imagination or in real life, to emotionally distressing stimuli.
desensitize (dee'sensiˌtiez) 1. to deprive of sensation. 2. to subject to desensitization.
desert fever, desert rheumatism ('desərt) the primary form of COCCIDIOIDOMYCOSIS.
desferrioxamine (ˌdezferee'oksəmeen) an iron-chelating agent isolated from *Streptomyces pilosus*, used to treat iron poisoning either in the acute situation or as a result of an iron storage disease.
desiccant ('desikənt) 1. promoting dryness. 2. an agent that promotes dryness.
desiccate ('desiˌkayt) to render thoroughly dry.
desiccation (ˌdesi'kayshən) the act of drying.
designer drug (di'zienə) originally coined to describe drugs illicitly produced to suit the tastes of individual clients but now widely used to describe synthetic variants (drug analogues) of potent controlled drugs (including narcotics and stimulants) but which are not themselves controlled. These substances currently circumvent existing drug legislation and many are relatively easy to synthesize from common industrial chemicals. Many designer drugs are extremely potent (some synthetic analogues of heroin are 1000 times as potent as heroin) and are consequently extremely dangerous.

Designer drugs first appeared in the late 1960s (analogues of mescaline and amphetamine) and the range available began to increase steadily in the mid 1970s (analogues of methaqualone and phencyclidine). The 1980s have been characterized by an alarming increase in the domestic production of drug analogues and three main groups of analogues have begun to dominate the illicit market:

FENTANYL ANALOGUES. Modelled around the parent drug fentanyl (used as an anaesthetic and postoperative analgesic) which is approximately 100 times as potent as morphine. Some illicit fentanyl analogues are 6000 times as potent as morphine and are abused for their heroin-like effects. The alphamethyl analogue of fentanyl (known on the streets as 'China White') was the first narcotic designer drug to appear in substantial amounts on the US illicit market. Fentanyl analogues carry a major risk of death from overdose or respiratory depression as the margin between the euphoriant and the lethal dose may be very small and difficult to estimate accurately.

PETHIDINE ANALOGUES. Modelled around the perioperative analgesic and known as meperidine (Demerol) in most journal articles as they are more frequently mentioned in American journals. Some derivatives (MPP and PEPAP) are 30–70 times more potent than pethidine. These substances carry a high risk of inducing an irreversible state of drug-induced pseudoparkinsonism, characterized by muscular rigidity, tremors, slowness of movement and speech, and the expressionless 'Parkinsonian Mask'.

METHAMPHETAMINE ANALOGUES. Modelled on the stimulant methamphetamine or related substances. One substance (MDMA, XTD or ADAM) with the street name of 'Ecstasy' is an analogue of the hallucinogen MDA and the stimulant methamphetamine and induces states of altered consciousness with associated euphoria and hallucinations. Use of MDMA carries a risk of panic reactions, depression or paranoia.

Designer drugs are largely an American problem at present but have figured in British seizures of illicit drugs. Given the internationalism of the illicit drugs market (and of many aspects of the drug subculture) it would be complacent to assume that the problem will remain American.

desipramine (de'siprə,meen) a tricyclic antidepressant, which is a metabolite of imipramine; used for relief of symptoms of depression.

desm(o)- word element. [Gr.] *ligament*.

desmitis (dez'mietis) inflammation of a ligament.

desmocranium (dezmoh'krayni·əm) the mass of mesoderm at the cranial end of the notochord in the early embryo, forming the earliest stage of the skull.

desmography (dez'mografee) a description of ligaments.

desmoid ('dezmoyd) 1. an unencapsulated, locally invasive, and rarely metastasizing fibromatous tumour arising in the muscle sheath, usually of the abdominal wall, which closely resembles fibrosarcoma. An example of one of a group of similar fibrous tumours collectively designated as fibromatoses. 2. fibrous or fibroid.

desmology (dez'moləjee) the science of ligaments.

desmoma (dez'mohmə) desmoid tumour.

desmopathy (dez'mopəthee) any disease of the ligaments.

desmoplasia (,dezmoh'playzi·ə) the formation and development of fibrous tissue. adj. **desmoplastic**.

desmopressin (,desmoh'presin) a synthetic analogue of 8-argininevasopressin used for antidiuretic replacement therapy in the management of cranial diabetes insipidus and for the temporary polyuria and polydipsia associated with trauma to or surgery in the pituitary region. It is also used to treat mild haemophilia and von Willebrand's disease because of its ability to induce release of Factor VIII from vascular endothelial cells.

desonide ('dezo,nied) a synthetic corticosteroid used as a topical anti-inflammatory agent in the treatment of steroid-responsive dermatoses including psoriasis and eczema.

desorb (dee'sawb, -'zawb) to remove a substance from the state of absorption or adsorption.

desorption (dee'zawpshən) the process or state of being desorbed.

desoximetasone (dez,oksi'metə,sohn) an anti-inflammatory, antipruritic, and vasoconstrictive corticosteroid used topically to relieve inflammation in corticosteroid-responsive dermatoses when bacterial infection is present or suspected.

desoxy- for words beginning thus, see also those beginning *deoxy-*.

desquamation (,deskwə'mayshən) the shedding of epithelial elements, chiefly of the skin, in scales or sheets. adj. **desquamative**.

desulphhydrase (,deesulf'hiedrayz) an enzyme that splits cysteine into hydrogen sulphide, ammonia, and pyruvic acid.

detachment (di'tachmənt) the condition of being separated or disconnected.

d. of retina, retinal d. separation of the inner layers of the retina from the pigment epithelium, which remains attached to the choroid. Called also sublatio retinae. Retinal detachment occurs most often as a result of degenerative changes in the peripheral retina and vitreous body, which produce holes or tears in the retina that can range from minute breaks no larger than 0.1 mm to extensive breaks. About two-thirds of all patients with retinal detachment are myopic (nearsighted). Trauma to the eyeball, severe contusions, inflammatory lesions, and sometimes ocular surgery can lead to retinal detachment.

SYMPTOMS. The onset of symptoms may be gradual or sudden, depending on the cause, size, number, and location of retinal holes. The patient usually sees flashes of light and then days or weeks later notices cloudy vision or loss of central vision. Another common manifestation is the sensation of spots or moving particles in the field of vision. In severe retinal detachment there can be complete loss of vision.

TREATMENT. Retinal detachment is corrected surgically. Two outpatient modes of therapy for flat retinal breaks without retinal detachment are *photocoagulation*, using the light source of an argon laser or a xenon photocoagulator, and *cryosurgery*, in which a freezing probe is used to penetrate the tissues of the eye and cover the hole or tear in the retina. Scar tissue eventually forms and seals the opening.

Where the retina is detached a surgical procedure called *scleral buckling* is required. The buckle places the retinal breaks in contact with the pigment epithelium and choroid. Adhesions form and bind the sensory retinal layers to these structures. In some cases, where there is an associated vitreous haemorrhage, the surgeon performs a closed vitrectomy and internal retinal repair. The purpose of the surgery is to remove the vitreous body that is opaque because of accumulated blood, and to stabilize the retina in apposition to the choroid. Aqueous humour eventually fills the space.

Preoperative and postoperative care of the patient requires a thorough knowledge of the type of detachment afflicting the patient and the surgical procedure performed. Positioning of the patient and the level of physical activity allowed after surgery are determined by the surgeon.

detergent (di'tərjənt) 1. purifying, cleansing. 2. an agent that purifies or cleanses.

deterioration (di,tiə·ri·ə'rayshən) progressive impairment of function; worsening.

determinant (di'tərminənt) a factor that establishes the nature of an entity or event.

antigenic d. the structural component of an antigen molecule responsible for its specific interaction with antibody molecules elicited by the same or related antigen.

hidden d. an antigenic determinant located in an unexposed region of a molecule so that it is prevented from interacting with receptors on lymphocytes, or with antibody molecules, and is unable to induce an immune response; it may appear following stereochemical alterations of molecular structure.

determination (di,tərmi'nayshən) the establishment of the exact nature of an entity or event.

embryonic d. that precise stage of development of any embryonic tissue where it loses the potential to become any part and starts to develop to become a specific part.

sex d. the process by which the sex of an organism is fixed, associated, in man, with the presence or absence of the Y chromosome.

determinism (di'tərmi,nizəm) the theory that all phenomena are the result of antecedent conditions and that nothing occurs by chance.

detoxicate (dee'toksi,kayt) detoxify.

detoxication (dee,toksi'kayshən) detoxification.

detoxification (dee,toksifi'kayshən) 1. reduction of the toxic properties of a substance. 2. treatment designed to assist in recovery from the toxic effects of a drug.

metabolic d. reduction of the toxic properties of a substance by chemical changes induced in the body, producing a compound which is less poisonous or more readily eliminated.

detoxify (dee'toksi,fie) to subject to detoxification.

detrition (di'trishən) the wearing away, as of teeth, by friction.

detritus (di'trietəs) particulate matter produced by or remaining after the wearing away or disintegration of a substance or tissue.

detrusor (di'troozə) a general term for a body part, e.g., a muscle, that pushes down.

detumescence (,deetyuh'mesəns) the subsidence of congestion and swelling.

deutan ('dyootan) a person exhibiting deuteranomalopia or deuteranopia.

deuteranomalopia (,dyootə·rə,nomə'lohpi·ə) a variant of normal colour vision with imperfect perception of the green hues.

deuteranope ('dyootə·rə,nohp) a person exhibiting deuteranopia.

deuteranopia, deuteranopsia (,dyootə·rə'nopi·ə; ,dyootə·rə'nopsi·ə) defective colour vision, with confusion of greens and reds, and retention of the sensory mechanism for two hues only—blue and yellow. adj. **deuteranopic.**

deuterium (dyoo'tiə·ri·əm) the mass 2 isotope of hydrogen, symbol ^2H or D; it is available as a gas or heavy water and is used as a tracer or indicator in studying fat and amino acid metabolism.

deuteropathy (dyootə'ropəthee) a disease that is secondary to another disease.

devascularization (dee,vaskyuhlə·rie'zayshən) interruption of circulation of blood to a part due to obstruction or destruction of blood vessels supplying it.

development (di'veləpmənt) the process of growth and differentiation.

cognitive d. the development of intelligence, conscious thought, and problem-solving ability that begins in infancy.

psychosexual d. development of the psychological aspects of sexuality from birth to maturity. In psychoanalytic theory, the development of object relations has five stages: the *oral* stage from birth to 2 years, the *anal* stage from 2 to 4 years, the *phallic* stage from 4 to 6 years, the *latent* stage from 6 years until puberty, and the *genital* stage from puberty onward (see also SEXUAL DEVELOPMENT).

psychosocial d. the development of the personality, including the acquisition of social attitudes and skills, from infancy through maturity.

developmental (di,veləp'ment'l) pertaining to development.

d. anomaly absence, deformity, or excess of body parts as the result of faulty development of the embryo.

d. milestones significant behaviours which are used to mark the process of development (see AGE achievement). Walking is a developmental milestone in locomotor development, conversation in cognitive development, production of functional sex cells in sexual development, etc.

deviance ('deevi·əns) generally any pattern of behaviour which violates prevailing standards of morality or behaviour within a society. The term is usually qualified to indicate the specific form of deviance, e.g. sexual deviance.

deviant ('deevi·ənt) 1. varying from a determinable standard. 2. a person with characteristics varying from what is considered standard or normal.

colour d. a person whose colour perception varies from the norm.

sexual d. a person exhibiting sexual deviation.

deviation (,deevi'ayshən) variation from the regular standard or course. In ophthalmology, a tendency for the visual axes of the eye to fall out of alignment owing to muscular imbalance.

sexual d. sexual behaviour that varies from that normally considered biologically or socially acceptable.

standard d. a measure of statistical dispersion. See STANDARD DEVIATION.

devil's grip ('dev'lz) epidemic pleurodynia. An acute infection caused by the Coxsackie B group of viruses giving rise to stabbing pains in the chest and abdomen. First described in an outbreak on the island of Bornholm in Denmark. The Coxsackie viruses are human enteroviruses spread by the faecal–oral route or by droplets. The incubation period is 3 to 5 days. Treatment is symptomatic. Called also *Bornholm disease.*

devitalized (dee'vietə,liezd) devoid of vitality or life; dead.

dexamethasone (,deksə'methə,zohn) a synthetic glucocorticoid used primarily as an anti-inflammatory agent in various conditions, including collagen diseases and allergic states; it is also used in a screening test for the diagnosis of CUSHING'S SYNDROME.

dexter ('dekstə) [L.] *right, on the right side.*

dextr(o)- word element. [L.] *right.*

dextrality (dek'stralitee) the preferential use, in voluntary motor acts, of the right member of the major paired organs of the body, as the right eye, hand, or foot.

dextran ('dekstran) polyanhydroglucose, a water-soluble polysaccharide of glucose produced by the action of *Leuconostoc mesenteroides* on sucrose; used as a plasma volume expander. It is metabolically inert.

dextraural (dek'strawrəl) hearing better with the right ear.

dextrin ('dekstrin) any of a range of glucose polymers of varying sizes formed during the hydrolysis of starch.

dextrin-1,6-glucosidase (,dekstrin,wunsiksgloo'kohsi,dayz) dextrin 6-glucanohydrolase: an enzyme that catalyses the hydrolysis of α-1-6-glucan links in dextrins containing short 1,6-linked side chains.

dextrinosis (,dekstri'nohsis) a condition characterized by accumulation in the tissues of an abnormal polysaccharide.

limit d. glycogenosis, type III (see also FORBES' DISEASE).

dextrinuria (,dekstri'nyooə·ri·ə) presence of dextrin in the urine.

dextroamphetamine (,dekstroh·am'fetə,meen, -min) the dextrorotatory isomer of amphetamine, having a more conspicuous stimulant effect on the central nervous system than the laevorotatory (laevamphetamine) racemic forms of amphetamine in the same dosage. Abuse of this drug may lead to dependence. See also AMPHETAMINE.

dextrocardia (,dekstroh'kahdi·ə) location of the heart in the right side of the thorax, the apex pointing to the right.

mirror-image d. location of the heart in the right side of the chest, the atria being transposed and the right ventricle lying anteriorly and to the left of the left ventricle.

dextrocularity (ˌdekstrokyuh'laritee) having greater visual power in the right eye, therefore using it more than the left.

dextromanual (ˌdekstroh'manyooəl) right-handed.

dextromethorphan (ˌdekstrohme'thorfan) a synthetic morphine derivative used as an antitussive in the form of the hydrobromide salt.

dextromoramide (ˌdekstroh'mo·rəˌmied) a narcotic used in the treatment of chronic pain in terminal disease. A drug of addiction.

dextropedal (dek'stropid'l) right-footed.

dextroposition (ˌdekstrohpə'zishən) displacement to the right.

dextropropoxyphene (ˌdekstrohproh'poksiˌfeen) an analgesic.

dextrorotatory (ˌdekstrohroh'taytə·ree) turning the plane of polarization, or rays of light, to the right.

dextrose ('dekstrohz, -trohs) an old chemical name for D-glucose, an important energy source for all tissues and the sole energy source for the brain. The term dextrose continues to be used to refer to glucose solutions administered intravenously for fluid or nutrient replacement. See also GLUCOSE.

dextrosinistral (ˌdekstroh'sinistrəl) extending from right to left; also applied to a left-handed person trained to use the right hand in certain performances.

dextrosuria (ˌdekstroh'syooə·ri·ə) the presence of dextrose in the urine; called also *glucosuria*.

dextrothyroxine (ˌdekstrohthie'rokseen) the dextrorotatory isomer of thyroxine without the biological activity of laevothyroxine.

dextroversion (ˌdekstroh'vərshən, -zhən) 1. version to the right, especially movement of the eyes to the right. 2. location of the heart in the right chest, the left ventricle remaining in the normal position on the left, but lying anterior to the right ventricle.

DF 118 trademark for preparations of dihydrocodeine.

DH Department of Health.

DHSS Department of Health and Social Security, now divided into the Department of Health (DH), and the Department of Social Security (DSS).

DHyg Doctor of Hygiene.

di- word element. [Gr., L.] *two.*

dia- word element. [Gr.] *through, between, apart, across, completely.*

diabetes (ˌdieə'beetis, -teez) a general term referring to a variety of disorders characterized by excessive urination (polyuria), as in diabetes mellitus and diabetes insipidus.

bronze d. a primary disorder of iron metabolism, with deposits of iron-containing pigments in the body tissues, and often with bronze or grey-blue pigmentation of the skin, diabetes mellitus, and cirrhosis of the liver; called also *haemochromatosis* and *iron storage disease.*

gestational d. that in which onset or recognition of impaired glucose tolerance occurs during pregnancy.

d. insipidus a disorder characterized by an excessive urinary output of up to 10 litres per day. The urine is colourless and very dilute. It does not contain abnormal constituents. A raging thirst accompanies the polyuria.

d. insipidus (central), d. insipidus (pituitary) a metabolic disorder due to damage to the neurohypophyseal system, which results in a deficient quantity of antidiuretic hormone (ADH or vasopressin) being produced or released, so that the renal tubules do not reabsorb water. As a consequence, there is the passage of a large amount of urine having a low specific gravity, and great thirst; it is often attended by voracious appetite, loss of strength, and emaciation. It may be acquired through infection, neoplasm, trauma, or radiation injuries to the posterior lobe of the pituitary gland or it may be inherited or idiopathic.

Pituitary diabetes insipidus is treated by instilling into the nose drops containing lysine-vasopressin or the longer acting desmopressin (a synthetic form of antidiuretic hormone). The dosage and frequency of administration is controlled so that the patient no longer has excessive thirst and polyuria. The cumbersome injection of vasopressin tannate in oil is now outdated. Patients with this condition should wear some form of medical identification at all times.

d. insipidus (nephrogenic) a rare congenital and familial form of diabetes insipidus, resulting from failure of the renal tubules to reabsorb water; there is excessive production of antidiuretic hormone but the tubules fail to respond to it. Thiazide diuretics will alleviate the condition.

d. mellitus a broadly applied term used to denote a complex group of syndromes that have in common a disturbance in the oxidation and utilization of glucose, which is secondary to a malfunction of the beta cells of the pancreas, whose function is the production and release of INSULIN. Because insulin is involved in the metabolism of carbohydrates, proteins, and fats, diabetes is not limited to a disturbance of glucose homeostasis alone.

There are at least two major types and several subtypes of diabetes mellitus. The major types require very different forms of therapy.

Type I or *insulin-dependent diabetes mellitus* (IDDM) accounts for about 5 to 10 per cent of all cases. As the name implies, persons having this type of diabetes require injections of exogenous insulin. In general, persons with IDDM are more prone to ketoacidosis and are more likely to develop the disease early in life. In fact, this type was formerly called 'juvenile-onset' diabetes.

Type II or *non-insulin-dependent diabetes mellitus* (NIDDM) occurs in the remaining 90 to 95 per cent of the diabetic population. It is believed to be related to some *inappropriate* insulin secretion, such as an insufficient quantity or a delayed response to a glucose load. NIDDM has a tendency to develop later in life than Type I; however, the terms 'juvenile-onset' and 'maturity-onset', which were formerly used to distinguish between the two types of diabetes, are misleading because either Type I or Type II can occur in the very young or the very old.

AETIOLOGY. There are at least four sets of factors that influence the development of diabetes mellitus: genetic, metabolic, microbiological, and immunological. They are related to an inherited predisposition, to injury or insult to the beta cells and, in IDDM, a defective capacity for regeneration. However, the various types do not have the same basic causes.

Genetic Factors. Diabetes mellitus is a familial disease with a multifactorial mode of inheritance. Particular susceptibility to diabetes is shown by people with certain HLA tissue types. The risk of developing some form of diabetes increases in proportion to the number of relatives who are affected, the severity of their disease, and the closeness of an individual's family ties to diabetic relatives. Familial inheritance is far more common in NIDDM.

Metabolic Factors. The number and complexity of these factors contribute to the difficulty of research into the cause of diabetes. Pregnancy has a diabetogenic influence because of increased metabolic workload and insulin resistance. However, this occurs only in women who have a genetic predisposition to the disease.

Emotional or physical stress can unmask an inherited predisposition to the disease, probably as a result of gluconeogenesis induced by the adrenal GLUCOCORTICOIDS, and increased secretion of CATECHOLAMINES. Some pharmacological agents such as phenytoin and the thiazide diuretics suppress the release of insulin.

Perhaps most significant is the association between obesity and NIDDM. The majority of NIDDM patients (about 80%) are obese, and there is a higher incidence of diabetes among the obese that increases with the degree of over-weight, but only a minority of obese people develop diabetes. With weight reduction and increased physical activity their blood glucose can be restored to normal levels and maintained there. It is thought that repeated demands for the production of insulin to metabolize large quantities of ingested carbohydrates may 'exhaust' the beta cells and lead to the symptoms of NIDDM. Once these demands are diminished by a reduction in dietary intake, the beta cells recover and are able to supply sufficient quantities of insulin. In NIDDM, there also seems to be an age-related reduction in the function of the beta cells and the secretion of insulin.

Microbiological Factors. Studies have suggested that some forms of IDDM are due to viral destruction of the beta cells. The occurrence of diabetes in clusters associated with some common viral epidemics gives support to this theory. It is also thought that this might account for seasonal fluctations in the onset of diabetes. During the late autumn and winter months there is an increase in the onset of diabetes mellitus. This corresponds to the time of year when some common childhood viral diseases are most prevalent.

Immunological Factors. Research studies have presented some strong evidence that IDDM can be classified as an AUTOIMMUNE DISEASE. At the time IDDM is diagnosed, about three-quarters of the cases studied have shown the presence of islet cell antibodies. The number of antibodies gradually decreases and they can be found in only about 20 per cent of all cases three to four years after onset of the disease.

Postmortem studies of infants and children who died shortly after developing diabetes mellitus have shown that in some cases the islets of Langerhans had been infiltrated by lymphocytes, monocytes, and occasionally eosinophils. These data strongly suggest that in some cases of juvenile diabetes there is both cell-mediated and antibody-related autoimmunity.

INCIDENCE AND PREVALENCE. Diabetes mellitus is a common endocrine disorder affecting about 30 million people world-wide. The incidence has increased greatly during the last thirty years. Improved methods of case finding and reporting account for some of this increase. In Europe and the USA about 6 per cent of all adults have the disease, although many of those affected are unaware of the condition and may remain undetected. There is a clinical impression that the incidence of clinical diabetes is rising and this may be related to the increasing prevalence of obesity. Although death rates are crude indicators of prevalence, they do show very marked regional differences in the prevalence of diabetes. However, it is clear that the disease is one of the leading causes of death in about 30 countries. The older the population, the greater the number of diabetics. Rates of disability are about twice as great in diabetics as in non-diabetics and blindness is ten times more common (facts derived from WHO statistics).

The large number of diabetics is partly explained by more effective treatment, increasing the life span of diabetics. Successful management has saved the lives of diabetic infants who formerly did not survive more than a few months. Improved treatment has also allowed diabetics of child-bearing age to have children safely, and their offspring have an increased risk of developing the disease.

DIAGNOSIS. The most common diagnostic tests for diabetes mellitus are chemical analyses of the urine and the blood. A simple test useful in screening large segments of a population for diabetes is one that tests for glucose in the urine. Glucose is excreted in the normal person in minute amounts; diabetic persons 'spill' glucose into the urine when their blood glucose level is above normal. A positive result for glucose in the urine is an indication for further, more definitive testing.

The *fasting blood sugar* (glucose) level should be within the normal limits of 4.4 and 6.7 mmol/l. A reading above the upper limit suggests diabetes mellitus.

The GLUCOSE TOLERANCE TEST does not indicate the clinical severity of diabetes mellitus, nor can it be depended on to rule out the disease conclusively in every case. It is, however, reliable in establishing the presence of diabetes and is commonly used for that purpose.

Essentially, the test evaluates the subject's ability to dispose of a glucose load appropriately. In normal persons the blood glucose level rises to about 7.8 mmol/l one hour after ingesting a glucose load of 1 g/kg of body weight, then drops back down to a normal level within two to three hours. In contrast, the diabetic person's blood glucose level slowly rises for two to three hours after ingestion of the glucose and only then drops back to the original level after five or six hours.

CLINICAL MANIFESTATIONS. Diabetes mellitus can present a wide variety of symptoms, ranging from asymptomatic to profound ketosis and coma. If the disease manifests itself late in life, the patient may not know he has diabetes until it is discovered during a routine examination, or when the symptoms of chronic vascular disease, insidious renal failure, or impaired vision cause him to seek medical help.

The typical symptoms of diabetes mellitus are the three 'polys' —*polyuria*, *polydipsia*, and *polyphagia*. Because of insulin deficiency, the assimilation and storage of glucose in muscle, adipose tissues, and the liver is greatly diminished. This produces an accumulation of glucose in the blood and creates an increase in its osmolarity. In response to this increased osmotic pressure there is depletion of intracellular water and osmotic diuresis. The water loss creates intense thirst and increased urination.

The occasionally increased appetite (polyphagia) is not as clearly understood. With a severe insulin deficiency, protein and fat are catabolized, and amino acids and fatty acids are released into the blood. Certain of the amino acids are converted into glucose by the liver; others are metabolized for energy in muscle and the liver. The energy for gluconeogenesis comes primarily from the oxidation of fatty acids in the liver, which results in the release of ketone bodies (acetoacetic and β-hydroxybutyric acids) into the blood. This is the body's normal response to a lack of glucose from fasting. With insulin deficiency it occurs despite a high blood glucose level. Raised blood levels of ketone bodies cause *ketoacidotic diabetid coma*, a potentially fatal medical emergency that may be the presenting condition in IDDM. Diabetics already treated with insulin may develop this severe metabolic disturbance if the dose of insulin is not sufficient to meet the extra demands of infection. Coma itself is heralded by persistent vomiting, dehydration and collapse.

The destruction of muscle and adipose tissue to provide sufficient energy can produce weight loss and emaciation, especially in those patients who have IDDM. On the other hand, NIDDM patients are usually obese because of their high calorific intake and production of insulin to utilize the food that is eaten.

Another manifestation of diabetes mellitus is susceptibility to infections. This probably is due to decreased blood supply to the infected area and the fact that sugar provides a good medium for the growth of microorganisms. In addition, there is decreased leukocyte chemotaxis and diminished bactericidal activity when blood glucose levels are high.

In females, high blood glucose often results in susceptibility to fungal and bacterial infections of the external genitalia. Pruritus and inflamed tissues of the vulva sometimes signal the onset of diabetes.

SEQUELAE. Despite treatment the life expectancy of childhood-onset IDDM is about 50 per cent of normal. Older people who develop NIDDM have a life expectancy that is around 70 per cent of normal. Diabetic coma still causes some deaths but it is the sequalae of the disease that contribute most to its morbidity and mortality. The long-term consequences of diabetes mellitus can involve both large and small blood vessels throughout the body. *Macrovascular* disease of the coronary arteries, cerebral arteries, and arteries of the lower extremities can eventually lead to myocardial infarction, stroke, or gangrene of the feet and legs.

Atherosclerosis is far more likely to occur in diabetics than in normal persons. About half of all diabetics suffer a premature death from myocardial infarction, and for those who do have a nonfatal attack the survival time is about half that of nondiabetic persons. The predisposition of diabetics of all ages to develop an accelerating atherosclerosis is not clearly understood. The question of the effectiveness of strict biochemical control is still unanswered but there is no conclusive evidence to indicate that a rigid control of blood glucose levels slows down the process of atherosclerosis. Some believe that diabetics inherit the tendency to develop severe atherosclerosis as well as an aberration in glucose metabolism, and that the two are not necessarily related.

There is strong evidence, however, to substantiate the claim that optimal control will either prevent or mitigate the *microvascular* complications of diabetes, particularly in the young and middle-aged who are at greatest risk for developing complications involving the arterioles.

Pathological changes in the small blood vessels serving the kidney lead to nephrosclerosis, pyelonephritis, and other disorders that eventually result in renal failure. Many of the deaths of juvenile and adult diabetics are caused by renal failure.

Visual impairment and blindness are common sequelae of diabetes mellitus. The three most frequently occurring problems involving the eye are diabetic RETINOPATHY, cataracts, and glaucoma. Techniques involving photocoagulation of destructive lesions of the retina with laser beams can now be used to delay further progress of pathological changes and thereby preserve sight in the affected eye.

Another area of pathological changes associated with diabetes mellitus is the nervous system, particularly the peripheral nerves in the lower extremities. The patient typically experiences a 'stocking-type' anaesthesia begining about 10 years after the onset of the disease. There may eventually be almost total anaesthesia of the affected part with the potential for serious injury to the part without the patient being aware of it. In contrast, some patients experience debilitating pain and *hyper*aesthesia, with loss of deep tendon reflexes.

Other problems related to the destruction of nerve tissue are the result of autonomic nervous system involvement. These include orthostatic hypotension, delayed gastric emptying, diarrhoea or constipation, and asymptomatic retention of urine in the bladder.

Although age of onset and length of the disease process are related to the frequency with which vascular, renal, and neurological complications develop, there are some patients who remain relatively free of sequelae even into the later years of their lives. Because diabetes mellitus is not a single disease but rather a complex constellation of syndromes, each patient has a unique response to the disease process.

MANAGEMENT. There is no cure for diabetes; the goal of treatment is to maintain blood glucose and lipid levels within normal limits and to prevent complications. There is strong support for the concept that microvascular sequelae of the disease can be minimized by optimal control. However, it may prove very difficult to achieve such control, even in the cooperative patient. However, too rigid a regime increases the potential for a serious hypoglycaemic reaction should the patient taking insulin miss a meal or engage in unusual physical activity, and it also restricts the patient's life style and daily activities. The induced tendency to hypoglycaemia may make the patient eat more and become obese, with the various problems of obesity. These aspects must be balanced by the near certainty that good control of the blood sugar will allow most diabetic patients to avoid many of the serious and debilitating consequences of the disease.

In general, good control is achieved when the following occur: fasting blood glucose is within normal limits and blood glucose is not above 10 mmol/l two hours after breakfast or lunch, urine is negative for glucose and acetone before meals, the patient's weight is normal, blood lipids remain within normal limits, and the patient has a sense of health and well-being.

The protocol for therapy is determined by the type of diabetes mellitus. Both IDDM and NIDDM patients must pay attention to their diet and exercise regimens. Insulin therapy may occasionally be prescribed for NIDDM patients as well as those who are dependent on insulin for survival. In most cases, the NIDDM patient can be treated effectively by reducing calorific intake and body weight and promoting physical exercise. This regimen can be aided by the use of sulphonylurea HYPOGLYCAEMIC agents which promote insulin secretion in NIDDM patients and/or the use of metformin which enhances sugar metabolism.

Diet. A diet adjusted to individual needs is prescribed for each diabetic patient. For mild cases, there is no need to measure food intake precisely, but patients must avoid foods that have a high sugar content, and they must keep their weight within normal limits.

When the disease is more severe and stricter control is required, a quantitative diet is prescribed. Such a diet will be low in animal fats and high in fibre. Refined sugar will be avoided but carbohydrate is given in normal proportions provided it is contained in high fibre foods such as beans or coarse ground wheat flour. The total calorie intake will be set according to the patient's physical activity and the need to lose weight. It is important for the patient to have a list of

Differences between hyper- and hypoglycaemia in patients with diabetes mellitus

	Hyperglycaemia	**Hypoglycaemia**
Onset	Slow (2–3 days)	Rapid
History	Has not taken insulin/acute infection	Taken insulin ½–4 h previously, but has not eaten/has eaten but had unusual burst of energy
Patient reactions	Thirst Nausea Abdominal pain Constipation Vomiting	Irrational Bad tempered Disorientated (may be mistaken for drunk)
Leads to	Ketoacidosis Drowsiness BP ↓ Pulse weak and rapid Skin dry Tongue dry	Respirations normal No drowsiness BP normal Pulse normal Skin moist Tongue moist
Leads to	Coma	Coma
Needs	Insulin Restoration of fluid/balance	Glucose
Avoided by	Recognition of early symptoms and taking appropriate action	

From Faulkner, A. (1985) *Nursing: A Creative Approach*, 1st edn, Baillière Tindall, p. 232.

alternative foodstuffs and, preferably, a recipe book so that the meals are pleasant to taste and not boring. Most clinics provide dietary advice and the British Diabetic Association, like its American counterpart, will provide details of diets and recipes.Three meals a day are to be advised for all and the time of eating is especially important for the patient taking insulin. Since the insulin-dependent diabetic needs to match food consumption with exercise and available insulin it is wise for snacks to be taken between meals and at bedtime.

Insulin-dependent diabetics who are unable to eat the prescribed diet during short-term illnesses, such as gastrointestinal upset and influenza, need to substitute carbohydrate liquids and semiliquids and to ask their doctor for advice on adjustment of the insulin dosage. On no account must they stop taking insulin.

Exercise. A programme of regular exercise gives anyone a sense of good health and well-being; for the diabetic it gives added benefits by helping to control blood glucose and lipid levels. Exercise helps prevent obesity, increases the utilization of glucose in muscle tissue and thereby reduces blood glucose levels and promotes circulation to peripheral tissues. In addition, there is evidence that exercise increases the number of insulin receptor sites on the surface of cells and thus facilitates the metabolism of glucose.

Diabetics who take insulin must be careful about indulging in unplanned exercise. Strenuous physical activity can rapidly lower their blood sugar and precipitate a hypoglycaemic reaction.

Insulin Therapy. Insulin is prepared from beef or pork pancreas, or by biogenetic engineering as human insulin. Insulin was previously available in various types and strengths but has now been standardized at 100 units per ml. Soluble, or regular, insulin is short-acting but modifications of insulin with added zinc and protein allow slower absorption and hence more prolonged action. Combinations of soluble insulin with slower-acting preparations can be tailored to suit the individual patient in the 24-hour control of blood sugar. All insulin has to be given by injection, usually subcutaneously. Pump systems to deliver continuous insulin under the skin are available, Most diabetics requiring insulin will need twice daily injections for optimum control.

The emergency treatment of KETOACIDOTIC DIABETIC COMA demands a constant intravenous infusion of soluble insulin together with adequate volumes of tissue repair fluids. The problem is so grave that the best supervision requires an intensive care unit or the equivalent in facilities.

Oral hypoglycaemic agents are not a substitute for insulin. The sulphonylureas are drugs that prompt secretion of insulin. This is effective in NIDDM, but will not occur in IDDM where the islet cells are destroyed. The biguanides enhance the action of whatever endogenous insulin is available.

Biomedical engineers are working on an 'artificial pancreas' that will monitor the patient's blood glucose and automatically inject appropriate amounts of insulin directly into the patient's blood stream. Such a device may be of practical use in the future (see also INSULIN PUMP).

Patient Education. The diabetic patient and his family need instruction so that the patient can be as independent as possible and will have support from those close to him. The instructions should be tailored to the individual patient and should include information about diet, planned exercise, and the effect of these factors on the disease. Patients should learn to administer accurately their own insulin when prescribed, or if this is not possible, a member of the family or close friend must learn how to administer it. All concerned need to learn the symptoms and emergency treatment of hypoglycaemia (lower than normal blood glucose) and hyperglycaemia (diabetic ketoacidosis) (see accompanying table).

Monitoring glucose in the urine and the blood is an important part of achieving good control. The testing of urine is a relatively simple procedure requiring minimal skills. A paper or plastic strip coated with reagents is dipped in the urine specimen. After a specified time period, the strip is compared with a colour chart. The colour of the reagent area indicates the glucose concentration.

In addition to testing his urine at prescribed times each day, the diabetic patient must continue to have periodic laboratory testing of blood glucose. This is needed by those monitoring their own blood glucose as a check on the accuracy of home measurement. He usually is asked to have a fasting blood sugar, and one taken two hours after a meal, every two to three months. These tests only give information about blood glucose levels at the time of testing. An important test, based on the binding of glucose to haemoglobin, can determine the *average* level of blood glucose during the previous four to six weeks, indicating the adequacy of blood glucose control over this period of time. Therefore, this test is less subject to manipulation by a patient who might follow his regimen of diet, exercise, and insulin only on the few days prior to having routine blood sugar tests. A measurement of HbA_{ic} should be made every four to six months (see also HAEMOGLOBIN A_{ic}).

Home measurement of blood glucose is now available for diabetic patients who require close monitoring to control blood glucose levels. A small electronic meter that gives a digital readout of the glucose concentration in a drop of blood makes this procedure relatively easy, and provides more accurate information than urine testing for adjustments in insulin dosage.

Patient instruction must also include basic principles of good personal hygiene. The importance of cleanliness and the prompt treatment of minor skin irritations in the prevention of complications must be stressed. Gangrene and possible loss of a lower extremity can often be avoided by scrupulous foot care, which includes properly fitting shoes and stockings, correct trimming of the toenails, and protection of the feet and legs from injury.

There are many teaching aids available to help the diabetic patient understand his disease and comply with his prescribed therapy. Most will be supplied by the diabetic clinic. Information is always available from the British Diabetic Association or its equivalent in other countries, and it will even arrange holidays. The address of the British Diabetic Association is 10 Queen Anne Street, London W1M OBD.

unstable d. diabetes mellitus that is difficult to control; characterized by unexplained oscillation between hypoglycaemia and diabetic ketoacidosis.

diabetic (ˌdieə'betik) 1. pertaining to or characterized by diabetes. 2. a person affected with diabetes.

diabetogenic (ˌdieəˌbeetoh'jenik) producing diabetes.

diabetogenous (ˌdieəbee'tojənəs) caused by diabetes.

Diabinese (die'abiˌneez) trademark for chlorpropamide, an oral hypoglycaemic drug.

diabrotic (ˌdieə'brotik) 1. ulcerative; caustic. 2. a corrosive substance.

diacetic acid (ˌdieə'setik) acetoacetic acid.

diacetylmorphine (dieˌasitil'mawfeen) heroin; a highly addictive narcotic derived from opium.

diacrisis (die'akrisis) 1. diagnosis. 2. a disease characterized by a morbid state of the secretions. 3. a critical discharge or excretion.

diacritic (ˌdieə'kritik) diagnostic; distinguishing.

diadochokinesia (dieˌadəkohki'neezi·ə) the function of arresting one motor impulse and substituting one that is diametrically opposite.

diagnose ('dieəgˌnohz) to identify or recognize a disease.

diagnosis (ˌdieəg'nohsis) 1. determination of the nature of a case of a disease. 2. a concise technical description of the cause, nature, or manifestations of a condition, situation, or problem. adj. **diagnostic.**

clinical d. diagnosis based on signs, symptoms, and laboratory findings during life.

differential d. the determination of which one of several diseases may be producing the symptoms.

medical d. diagnosis performed by a doctor and based on information gleaned from a variety of sources, including (1) findings from a physical examination, (2) interview with the patient or his family or both, (3) a medical history of the patient and his family, and (4) findings reported by pertinent laboratory tests and radiological studies.

nursing d. see NURSING process.

physical d. diagnosis based on information obtained by inspection, palpation, percussion, and auscultation.

diagnostician (ˌdieagno'stishən) an expert in diagnosis.

diagnostics (ˌdieəg'nostiks) the science and practice of diagnosis of disease.

diakinesis (ˌdieəki'neesis) the stage of first meiotic prophase, in which the nucleolus and nuclear envelope disappear and the spindle fibres form.

dialysance (die'alisəns) the minute rate of net exchange of solute molecules passing through a membrane in dialysis.

dialysate (di'aliˌsayt) the material passing through the membrane in dialysis.

dialyser ('dieəˌliezə) an apparatus for performing dialysis; a haemodialyser.

dialysis (die'aləsis) the process of separating components of a solution using the ability of those of small molecular size to pass through a semipermeable membrane. Dialysis of the blood is used in acute and chronic renal failure to restore fluid balance, to correct electrolyte imbalance, and to lower blood levels of toxins and metabolic waste products such as urea and creatinine.

The blood is separated from a specially prepared solution known as dialysis fluid by a semipermeable membrane through which water and some solutes may pass. Molecules and ions of solutes which are small enough, e.g. crystalloids such as sodium, potassium, glucose, and urea, pass through the membrane by diffusion along a concentration gradient (from a higher concentration to a lower concentration) in an attempt to achieve equilibrium. The membrane pore size only allows the passage of small molecules and prevents the passage of large molecules such as proteins and blood cells. The osmolality of the solution on each side of the membrane determines the movement of water, which will pass from the side with a lower osmotic pressure to the side with a higher osmotic pressure. The semipermeable membrane used may be the patient's peritoneum (see PERITONEAL DIALYSIS) or a synthetic material such as cuprophane (see HAEMODIALYSIS).

diameter (die'amitə) the length of a straight line passing through the centre of a circle and connecting opposite points on its circumference; hence the distance between the two specified opposite points on the periphery of a structure such as the cranium or pelvis.

cranial d's, craniometric d's imaginary lines connecting points on opposite surfaces of the cranium; the most important are: biparietal, that joining the parietal eminences; bitemporal, that joining the extremities of the coronal suture; submentobregmatic, that joining the centre of the anterior fontanelle and the junction of the neck with the floor of the mouth; frontomental, that joining the forehead and chin; occipitofrontal, that joining the external occipital protuberance and the most prominent midpoint of the frontal bone; occipitomental, that joining the external occipital protuberance and most prominent midpoint of the chin; suboccipitobregmatic, that joining the lowest posterior point of the occiput and the centre of the anterior fontanelle; mentovertical, that joining the tip of the chin with the centre point of the vertex.

fetal d. this forms important obstetric landmarks (see BIPARIETAL DIAMETER). At term the diameters of an average size fetal skull are:

suboccipitobregmatic	9.5cm	biparietal	9.5cm
suboccipitofrontal	10.0cm	bitemporal	8.2cm
occipitofrontal	12.0cm	mentovertical	13.5cm
submentobregmatic	9.5cm		

See also MOULDING.

pelvic d. any of the diameters of the pelvis (see also PELVIC DIAMETER).

diamniotic (die,amni'otik) having or developing within separate amniotic cavities, as dizygotic twins (see TWINS).

diamorphine hydrochloride (dieə'mawfeen) a morphine derivative similar to heroin. A powerful analgesic and drug of addiction.

Diamox ('dieəmoks) trademark for preparations of acetazolamide, a diuretic.

diapedesis (,dieəpe'deesis) the outward passive passage of blood cells through apparently intact vessel walls.

diaphanoscope (,dieə'fanoh,skohp) an instrument for transilluminating a body cavity.

diaphemetric (,dieəfi'metrik) pertaining to measurement of tactile sensibility.

diaphoresis (,dieəfə'reesis) perspiration, especially profuse perspiration.

diaphoretic (,dieəfor'retik) 1. pertaining to, characterized by, or promoting diaphoresis. 2. an agent that promotes diaphoresis (sweating).

diaphragm ('dieə,fram) 1. the musculomembranous partition separating the thoracic and abdominal cavities. On its sides, it is attached to the six lower ribs; at the front, to the sternum; at the back, to the spine. The oesophagus, the aorta and vena cava, and nerves pass through the diaphragm. When relaxed, the diaphragm is convex but it flattens as it contracts during inhalation, thereby enlarging the chest cavity and allowing for expansion of the lungs. See also RESPIRATION. 2. any separating membrane or structure. 3. a disc with one or more openings or with an adjustable opening, mounted in relation to a lens or source of radiation, by which part of the light or radiation may be excluded from the area. 4. contraceptive diaphragm. adj. **diaphragmatic**.

Bucky d., Bucky-Potter d. a device used in radiography to prevent scattered radiation from reaching the film, thereby securing better contrast and definition.

contraceptive d. a device of moulded rubber or other soft plastic material, fitted over the cervix uteri to prevent entrance of spermatozoa. See also CONTRACEPTION.

pelvic d. the portion of the floor of the pelvis formed by the coccygeus muscles and the levator ani muscles, and their fascia.

urogenital d. the musculomembranous layer superficial to the pelvic diaphragm, extending between the ischiopubic rami and surrounding the urogenital ducts. Called also *deep pelvic fascia* or *urogenital trigone of the pelvic floor*.

vaginal d. contraceptive diaphragm.

diaphragmatocele (,dieəfrag'matoh,seel) diaphragmatic hernia.

diaphragmitis (,dieəfrag'mietis) inflammation of the diaphragm.

diaphyseal (,dieə'fizi·əl) pertaining to or affecting the shaft of a long bone (diaphysis).

diaphysectomy (,dieəfi'zektəmee) excision of part of a diaphysis.

diaphysial (,dieə'fizi·əl) diaphyseal.

diaphysis (di'afisis) pl. *diaphyses;* 1. the portion of a long bone between the ends or extremities, which are usually articular, and wider than the shaft; it consists of a tube of compact bone, enclosing the medullary cavity. Called also *shaft*. 2. the portion of a bone formed from a primary centre of ossification.

diaplasis (di'apləsis) the setting of a fracture or reduction of a dislocation.

diapophysis (,dieə'pofisis) an upper transverse process of a vertebra.

diapyesis (,dieəpie'eesis) suppuration. adj. **diapyetic**.

diarrhoea (,dieə'reeə) rapid movement of faecal matter through the intestine resulting in poor absorption of water, nutritive elements, and electrolytes and producing abnormally frequent evacuation of watery stools. adj. **diarrhoeic, diarrhoeal.**

The major causes are local irritation of the intestinal mucosa by infections with bacteria or viruses or by chemical agents (gastroenteritis), and emotional disorders which bring about increased peristalsis and increased secretion of mucus in the colon (psychogenic diarrhoea or irritable colon); chronic recurrent diarrhoea is a major symptom of CROHN'S DISEASE and of ULCERATIVE COLITIS. In all types of diarrhoea there is rapid evacuation of water and electrolytes resulting in a loss of these essential substances. Potassium supply especially is depleted by diarrhoea, thus producing ACIDOSIS as well as FLUID VOLUME DEFICIT.

SYMPTOMS. Diarrhoea is accompanied by frequent and liquid bowel movements, abdominal cramps, and general weakness. The stools often contain mucus and may be blood streaked. In chronic diarrhoea the patient is likely to be anaemic and suffering from malnutrition.

TREATMENT. Mild cases of diarrhoea of short duration can be treated conservatively with a bland diet, increased intake of liquids, and the administration of kaolin compounds to relieve the symptoms.

More severe and chronic cases of diarrhoea may be symptomatic of a wide variety of disorders including glandular disturbances, deficiency diseases, allergies, and tumours of the intestinal tract. Since diarrhoea is a symptom rather than a disease, extensive diagnostic procedures may be necessary to determine the underlying cause. In the meantime symptomatic treatment must be instituted to relieve the dehydration, nutritional deficiencies, and disturbances of acid–base balance produced by the loss of water, food elements, and electrolytes in the stools. Liquids and semisolids may be given orally at frequent intervals if they can be tolerated by the patient. In cases in which vomiting accompanies the diarrhoea or the stools occur with serious frequency, the fluids may be given intravenously.

When diarrhoea is psychogenic, psychotherapy may be used in conjunction with other methods of management.

PATIENT CARE. The patient should be provided with an atmosphere conducive to rest and relaxation. Emotional factors must always be considered in cases of diarrhoea, even though nervous tension may not always be the major cause of the disorder. The patient is likely to be embarrassed and inconvenienced by frequent trips to the bathroom or requests for the bedpan.

If the diarrhoea is chronic and recurrent, the patient may have problems related to altered self-concept and anxiety, anger, and a lack of understanding about the cause and prognosis of his condition.

During hospitalization, the care plan for the patient should include the following observations and techniques of assessment: measurement of daily intake, output, and weight, auscultation of bowel sounds, recording of the exact number and character of stools, and, when the condition is persistent, monitoring blood gases and electrolytes for abnormalities indicating acid–base imbalance or potassium depletion. Other tests include stool cultures and testing for occult blood.

The patient should have his physiological needs for comfort and rest attended to. If his diarrhoea is chronic, discharge planning will be necessary to help him cope with problems related to dietary restrictions, self-medication, and the need for understanding his illness and coping with any fear or anxiety he may be experiencing.

diarrhoeogenic (ˌdieəˌreeoh'jenik) giving rise to diarrhoea.

diarthric (die'ahthrik) pertaining to or affecting two different joints; biarticular; diarticular.

diarthrodial (dieah'throhdi·əl) of the nature of a diarthrosis.

diarthrosis (ˌdieah'throhsis) pl. *diarthroses* [Gr.] a specialized form of articulation in which there is more or less free movement, the union of the bony elements being surrounded by an articular capsule enclosing a cavity lined by synovial membrane; called also *synovial joint*.

d. rotatoria a joint characterized by mobility in a rotary direction.

diarticular (ˌdiah'tikyuhlə) pertaining to two joints; diarthric.

diaschisis (die'askisis) loss of function and electrical activity in an area of the brain due to a lesion in a remote area that is neuronally connected with it.

diascope ('dieəˌskohp) a glass plate pressed against the skin to permit observation of changes produced in the underlying areas after the blood vessels are emptied and the skin is blanched.

diascopy (die'askəpee) 1. examination by means of a diascope. 2. transillumination.

diastase ('dieəˌstays, -stayz) a combination of enzymes produced during germination of seeds, and contained in malt; it converts starch into maltose and then into dextrose.

diastasis (die'astəsis) 1. dislocation or separation of two normally attached bones between which there is no true joint. Also, an abnormally large separation between associated bones, as between the ribs. 2. diastasis cordis, the rest period of the cardiac cycle, occurring just before systole.

diastema (ˌdieə'steemə) a space or cleft, often between adjacent teeth.

central d. a space between the upper central incisors.

diastematocrania (ˌdieəˌsteemətoh'krayni·ə) congenital longitudinal fissure of the cranium.

diastematomyelia (ˌdieəˌsteemətohmie'eeli·ə) abnormal congenital division of the spinal cord by a bony spicule or fibrous band protruding from a vertebra or two, each of the halves being surrounded by a dural sac.

diastematopyelia (ˌdieəˌsteemətohpie'eeli·ə) congenital median fissure of the pelvis.

Diastix ('dieəˌstiks) trademark for a reagent strip used for the semiquantitative determination of glucose in urine.

diastole (die'astəlee) the phase of the cardiac cycle in which the heart relaxes between contractions; specifically, the period when the two ventricles are dilated by the blood flowing into them (see also BLOOD PRESSURE and HEART). adj. **diastolic.**

diastrophic (ˌdieə'strofik) bent or curved; said of structures, such as bones, deformed in such manner.

diataxia (ˌdieə'taksi·ə) ataxia affecting both sides of the body.

diathermal, diathermic (ˌdieə'thərməl; ˌdieə'thərmik) pertaining to diathermy; permeable by heat waves.

diathermy ('dieəˌthərmee) the use of high-frequency electrical currents as a form of physiotherapy and as a coagulative, cutting and haemostatic agent in surgical procedures. The term diathermy is derived from the Greek words *dia* and *therma*, and literally means 'heating through'.

Diathermy is used in physiotherapy to deliver moderate heat directly to pathological lesions in the deeper tissues of the body. Surgically, the extreme heat that can be produced by diathermy may be used to destroy neoplasms, warts, and infected tissues, and to cauterize blood vessels to prevent excessive bleeding. The technique is particularly valuable in neurosurgery and surgery of the eye.

The three forms of diathermy employed by physiotherapists are shortwave, ultrasound, and microwave. The application of moderate heat by diathermy increases blood flow and speeds up metabolism and the rate of ion diffusion across cellular membranes. The fibrous tissues in tendons, joint capsules, and scars are more easily stretched when subjected to heat, thus facilitating the relief of stiffness of joints and promoting relaxation of the muscles and decrease of muscle spasms.

Short wave diathermy machines utilize two condenser plates that are placed on either side of the body part to be treated. Another mode of application is by induction coils that are pliable and can be moulded to fit the part of the body under treatment. As the high-frequency waves travel through the body tissues between the condensers or the coils, they are converted into heat. The degree of heat and depth of penetration depend in part on the absorptive and resistance properties of the tissues that the waves encounter.

The frequencies assigned for short wave diathermy operations are 13.66, 27.33, and 40.98 megahertz. Most commercial machines operate at a frequency of 27.33 megahertz and a wavelength of 11 metres.

Short wave diathermy usually is prescribed for treatment of deep muscles and joints that are covered with a heavy soft-tissue mass, for example, the hip. In some instances short wave diathermy may be applied to localize deep inflammatory processes, as in pelvic inflammatory disease.

Ultrasound diathermy employs high-frequency acoustic vibrations which, when propelled through the tissues, are converted into heat. This type of diathermy is especially useful in the delivery of heat to selected musculatures and structures because there is a difference in the sensitivity of various fibres to the acoustic vibrations; some are more absorptive and some are more reflective. For example, in subcutaneous fat, relatively little energy is converted into heat, but in muscle tissues there is a much higher rate of conversion to heat.

The therapeutic ultrasound apparatus generates a high-frequency alternating current, which is then converted into acoustic vibrations. The apparatus is moved slowly across the surface of the part being treated. Ultrasound is a very effective agent for the application of heat, but it should be used only by a therapist who is fully aware of its potential hazards and the contraindications for its use.

Microwave diathermy uses radar waves, which are of higher frequency and shorter wavelength than radio waves. Most, if not all, of the therapeutic effects of microwave therapy are related to the conversion of energy into heat and its distribution throughout the body tissues. This mode of diathermy is considered to be the easiest to use, but the microwaves have a relatively poor depth of penetration.

Microwaves cannot be used in high dosage on oedematous tissue, over wet dressings, or near metallic implants in the body because of the danger of local burns. Microwaves and short waves cannot be used on or near persons with implanted electronic cardiac pacemakers.

As with all forms of heat applications, care must be taken to avoid burns during diathermy treatments, especially to patients with decreased sensitivity to heat and cold.

surgical d. electrosurgery.

diathesis (die'athəsis) an unusual constitutional susceptibility or predisposition to a particular disease. adj. **diathetic.**

diatomic (ˌdieə'tomik) 1. containing two atoms. 2. dibasic.

diatrizoate (ˌdieətrie'zoh·ayt) a water-soluble, iodine-containing, radiopaque x-ray contrast medium. Used as the sodium or meglumine salt. Trademarks Hypaque and Urografin.

Diazemuls (ˌdie'azeemuhlz) trademark for an emulsion of diazepam as an injection. It is reportedly less painful than the aqueous injection for the patient.

diazepam (die'aziˌpam) a benzodiazepine tranquillizer used primarily as an antianxiety agent, and also used as a skeletal muscle relaxant, as an anticonvulsant, as preoperative medication to relieve anxiety and tension, and in the management of alcohol withdrawal symptoms and delirium tremens. Diazepam (Valium) is one of the most widely prescribed drugs in the United Kingdom. Diazepam therapy creates the risk of dependence if treatment is prolonged.

diazo- the group $-N_2-$.

diazotize (die'azohˌtiez) to introduce the diazo group into a compound.

diazoxide (dieaz'oksied) a rapid-acting antihypertensive having no diuretic activity. Diazoxide has a longer duration of action than other rapid-acting antihypertensives, and is used intravenously in the treatment of malignant hypertension. It also inhibits insulin release and may be used to treat hypoglycaemia due to organic hyperinsulinism.

dibasic (die'baysik) containing two replaceable hydrogen atoms, or furnishing two hydrogen ions.

Dibothriocephalus (dieˌbothrioh'kefələs, -'sef-) *Diphyllobothrium.*

DIC disseminated intravascular coagulation.

dicephalous (die'kefələs, -'sef-) having two heads.

dicephalus (die'kefələs, -'sef-) a fetus or infant with two heads.

dichloralphenazone (dieˌklor·ral'fenəˌzohn) a complex of chloral and phenazone (antipyrine), a sedative and hypnotic.

dichlorophen (die'klor·rohfen) an anthelmintic, used specifically against tapeworms. No preliminary starvation is necessary and one dose can cause the worm to disintegrate.

dichlorphenamide (ˌdieklor'fenəˌmied) a diuretic used to reduce intraocular pressure in glaucoma. Acts by reducing the secretion of aqueous humour.

dichorial, dichorionic (die'kor·ri·əl, dieˌko·ri'onik) having two distinct chorions, said of dizygotic twins.

dichotomy (die'kotəmee) division into two parts.

dichroic (die'kroh·ik) characterized by dichroism.

dichroism ('diekrohˌizəm, die'kroh·izəm) the quality or condition of showing one colour in reflected and another in transmitted light. adj. **dichroic.**

dichromate (die'krohmayt) a salt containing the bivalent Cr_2O_7 radical.

dichromatic (ˌdiekroh'matik) pertaining to or characterized by dichromatism.

dichromatism (die'krohməˌtizəm) 1. the quality of existing in or exhibiting two different colours. 2. dichromatopsia.

dichromatopsia (dieˌkrohmə'topsi·ə) a condition in which only two of the retinal cone pigments (red, green, and blue) are present and only two colours can be perceived.

Dick test (dik) an intracutaneous test for determination of susceptibility to scarlet fever.

diclofenac (die'klohfənak) a nonsteroidal anti-inflammatory drug.

dicoelous (die'seeləs) 1. hollowed on each of two sides. 2. having two cavities.

Diconal ('diekənal) trademark for the combination of the controlled drug dipipanone hydrochloride and cyclizine.

dicoria (die'kor·ri·ə) double pupil.

dicoumarol (die'kyoomə·rol, -koo-) a coumarin anticoagulant that acts by inhibiting the synthesis of vitamin K-dependent clotting factors (prothrombin and factors VII, IX, and X) in the liver; used in the prevention and treatment of thromboembolic disorders. Formerly called bishydroxycoumarin. Not available in the UK.

Dicrocoelium (ˌdikroh'seeli·əm) a genus of flukes.

D. dentriticum a species of liver flukes that infest ruminants, especially sheep, and have been reported in man.

dicrotism ('diekroˌtizəm) the occurrence of two sphygmographic waves or elevations to one beat of the pulse. adj. **dicrotic.**

dictyoma (ˌdikti'ohmə) diktyoma.

dicyclomine (die'siekloh,meen) an anticholinergic used as a gastrointestinal antispasmodic.

didactylism (die'daktiˌlizəm) the presence of only two digits on a hand or foot.

didelphia (die'delfi·ə) the condition of having a double uterus.

Didronel (die'drohnel) trademark for a preparation of etidronate, a bone calcium regulator.

didymalgia (didi'malji·ə) pain in a testis.

didymitis (ˌdidi'mietis) inflammation of a testis.

didymous ('didiməs) occurring in pairs.

didymus ('didiməs) a testis; also used as a word termination designating a fetus with duplication of parts or one consisting of conjoined symmetrical twins.

dieldrin (die'eldrin) an insecticide.

diembryony (die'embriˌonee) the production of two embryos from a single egg.

diencephalon (ˌdie·en'kefəlon, -'sef-) 1. the posterior part of the forebrain, consisting of the hypothalamus, thalamus, metathalamus, and epithalamus; the subthalamus is often considered to be a distinct division. 2. the posterior of the two brain vesicles formed by specialization of the prosencephalon in the developing embryo (see also BRAIN STEM).

dienoestrol (ˌdie·en'eestrol) a synthetic oestrogen used in the treatment of atrophic vaginitis and kraurosis vulvae.

Dientamoeba (ˌdie·entə'meebə) a genus of amoebae

commonly found in the colon and appendix of man.

D. fragilis a species that has been associated with diarrhoea.

diet ('dieət) the customary amount and kind of food and drink taken by a person from day to day; more narrowly, a diet planned to meet specific requirements of the individual, including or excluding certain foods.

bland d. one that is free from any irritating or stimulating foods.

elemental d. one consisting of a well-balanced, residue-free mixture of all essential and nonessential amino acids combined with simple sugars, electrolytes, trace elements, and vitamins.

elimination d. one for diagnosis of food allergy, based on omission of foods that might cause symptoms in the patient.

high-calorie d. one that furnishes more calories than needed to maintain weight, often more than 3500–4000 kilocalories per day.

high-fat d. ketogenic diet.

high fibre d. one relatively high in dietary fibres, which decreases bowel transit time and relieves constipation.

high-protein d. one containing large amounts of protein, consisting largely of meats, fish, milk, legumes, and nuts.

hospital d. a routine diet plan provided in a hospital that includes general, soft, and liquid diets and modifications of them to suit the needs of specific patients.

ketogenic d. one containing large amounts of fat (see also KETOGENIC DIET).

liquid d. a diet limited to liquids or to foods that can be changed to a liquid state (see also LIQUID DIET).

low-calorie d. one containing fewer calories than needed to maintain weight, e.g. less than 1200 kilocalories per day for an adult.

low-fat d. one containing limited amounts of fat.

low-fibre d. low-residue diet.

low-purine d. one for mitigation of gout, omitting meat, fowl, and fish and substituting milk, eggs, cheese, and vegetable protein.

low-residue d. one with a minimum of cellulose and fibre and restriction of connective tissue found in certain cuts of meat. It is prescribed for irritations of the intestinal tract, after surgery of the large intestine, in partial intestinal obstruction, or when limited bowel movements are desirable, as in colostomy patients. Called also *low-fibre diet*.

protein-sparing d. one in which enough energy is eaten with the protein to ensure that the protein is not used as an energy source.

purine-free d. low-purine diet.

dietary ('dieətree) 1. pertaining to diet. 2. a course or system of diet.

dietetic (ˌdieə'tetik) pertaining to diet or proper food.

dietetics (ˌdieə'tetiks) the science of diet and nutrition.

diethylcarbamazine (dieˌethilkah'baməˌzeen) an antifilarial agent used as the citrate salt.

diethylenetriamine pentaacetic acid (dieˌethileentrie'ameen pentə·əˌseetik) a chelating agent; abbreviated DTPA. When combined with technetium-99m it is used as a radiopharmaceutical in nuclear medicine. Technetium-99m-DTPA given as an intravenous injection is excreted by the kidney, enabling the kidneys to be imaged using a gamma camera to show abnormalities of excretion such as obstruction. Relative renal functions may be determined and, because the radiopharmaceutical is eliminated by glomerular filtration only, quantitative studies will produce an estimation of glomerular filtration rate. This type of study of the kidneys is called a RENOGRAM.

Gadolinium-DTPA is a contrast agent used in magnetic resonance imaging.

diethylpropion (dieˌethil'prohpion) a sympathomimetic amine similar to amphetamine, used as an anorectic. It is a controlled drug.

diethyltoluamide (dieˌethil'tolyooəmied) an insect repellent.

dietitian (ˌdieə'tishən) one who is concerned with the promotion of good health through proper diet and with the therapeutic use of diet in the treatment of disease. The dietitian may work in a variety of settings, including hospitals and other health care agencies, schools, hotels, and other commercial institutions where her duties are primarily administrative, or she may choose to enter the fields of education and research. Some dietitians practice independently either as a consultant or private practitioner in the area of therapeutic dietetics.

Many dietitians belong to the British Dietetic Association, which acts as both a professional body and a trade union. However, membership is not mandatory. Further information may be obtained from the British Dietetic Association, Daimler House, Paradise Street, Birmingham B1 2BJ.

State Registered D. one who has undertaken one of the following forms of training: (1) a bachelor's degree in nutrition which incorporates state registration as a dietitian (4 years' duration); (2) a bachelor's degree in dietetics (4 years' duration); (3) a 2-year postgraduate course in dietetics after gaining a bachelor's degree in a relevant subject.

State registration can be obtained by application to the Council for Professions Supplementary to Medicine. Only State Registered Dietitians are permitted to work in the National Health Service. Once qualified dietitians can specialize in a particular aspect of dietetics, such as renal, paediatric or community dietetics.

differential (ˌdifə'renshəl) making a difference.

d. blood count see BLOOD COUNT.

d. diagnosis see DIAGNOSIS.

differentiation (ˌdifəˌrenshi'ayshən) 1. the distinguishing of one thing from another. 2. the act or process of acquiring completely individual characteristics, such as occurs in the progressive diversification of cells and tissues in the embryo. 3. increase in morphological or chemical heterogeneity.

Difflam ('diflam) trademark for benzydamine oral rinse.

diffraction (di'frakshən) the bending or breaking up of a ray of light into its component parts.

diffusate (di'fyooˌzayt) material that has diffused through a membrane.

diffuse (di'fyoos, -'fyooz) 1. not definitely limited or localized. 2. to pass through or to spread widely through a tissue or substance.

diffusing capacity (di'fyoozing kəˌpasitee) the rate at which a gas diffuses across the alveolar-capillary membrane per unit difference in the partial pressure of the gas across the membrane, expressed in ml/min/mmHg. Because of their high affinity for haemoglobin both oxygen and carbon monoxide are limited in their rate of diffusion by their diffusing capacity. The diffusing capacity of the lung for these gases is symbolized by D_LO_2 and D_LCO. The parameter usually measured is D_LCO. The normal value for the diffusing capacity of oxygen is 20 ml/min/mmHg. If, during quiet breathing, the pressure difference of oxygen averages 11 mmHg, a total of approximately 220 ml of oxygen diffuses through the respiratory membrane each minute. During strenuous exercise or other conditions that increase pulmonary activity, the diffusion capacity may increase to three times as much as that during rest. Pulmonary diseases that damage the respiratory membrane greatly interfere with the capacity of the oxygen to pass through the membrane and oxygenate the blood.

diffusion (di'fyoozhən) 1. the state or process of being widely spread. 2. the spontaneous mixing of the molecules or ions of two or more substances resulting from random thermal motion; its rate is proportional to the concentrations of the substances and it increases with the temperature.

In the body fluids the molecules of water, gases, and the ions of substances in solution are in constant motion. As each molecule moves about, it bounces off other molecules and loses some of its energy to each molecule it hits, but at the same time it gains energy from the molecules that collide with it.

The rate of diffusion is influenced by the size of the molecules; larger molecules move less rapidly, because they require more energy to move about. Molecules of a solution of higher concentration move more rapidly toward those of a solution of lesser concentration; in other words, *the rate of movement from higher to lower concentration is greater than the movement in the opposite direction.*

Other factors influencing the rate of diffusion from one substance to another are the size of the chamber in which the diffusion is taking place and the temperature within the chamber. *The rate of diffusion increases as the size of the chamber increases.* Molecular motion never ceases except at absolute zero; as the temperature increases so does the rate of motion of molecules. Thus, *the higher the temperature, the greater the molecular activity and, consequently, the greater the rate of diffusion.*

Many of the substances passing through the cell membrane are transported actively or passively by the process of diffusion. Without this constant motion of molecules there would be no exchange of nutrients and end products of cellular metabolism between the intracellular and extracellular fluid and the cell could not survive. The diffusion of water across cell membranes is called OSMOSIS.

The diffusion of gases through the respiratory membrane is essential to normal respiration. The rapidity and ease with which oxygen and carbon dioxide are diffused through the membrane are affected by the thickness of the membrane and its surface area, the diffusion coefficient of the gas in the water within the membrane, and the difference between the partial pressures of the gases in the alveoli and the blood. The respiratory membrane is at most only 1 micron in thickness, yet it is composed of three layers within the alveolus (surfactant and fluid layers and alveolar epithelium), an interstitial space between the alveolar epithelium and capillary membrane, and two layers in the capillary membrane. The thickness of the respiratory membrane can be affected by the presence of oedematous fluid and by fibrotic changes in the membrane resulting from certain pulmonary diseases. An increase of fluid within the respiratory membrane and alveoli reduces the rate of diffusion because the gases must pass through the additional fluid as well as the other layers of the membrane. Thickening of the epithelial layers of the membrane, as in fibrosis, imposes additional restriction on the passage of gases.

The difference in the partial pressure of a gas in the alveoli and that same gas in the blood is a measure of the net tendency of that gas to pass through the respiratory membrane. The term *partial pressure* refers to the amount of pressure being exerted by a particular gas in a mixture of gases, the word *partial* referring to the part that is a particular gas in relation to the whole mixture. The partial pressure of oxygen, for example, reflects the number of oxygen molecules striking the surface of the membrane at any given point. The difference in the partial pressure refers to the difference in the amount of pressure being exerted by the oxygen molecules on the alveolar side of the membrane and the amount of pressure being exerted by the oxygen striking the same point from the opposite side. When the partial pressure of oxygen in the alveoli is greater than that of the oxygen in the blood, the oxygen molecules move across the membrane in the direction of the blood. The same is true in regard to carbon dioxide, which moves in the opposite direction when its partial pressure in the blood is greater than that in the alveoli. Partial pressures of oxygen and carbon dioxide are discussed in more detail under BLOOD GAS ANALYSIS.

d. coefficient the number of millilitres of a gas that will diffuse at a distance of 0.001 mm over a square centimetre surface per minute, at 1 atm of pressure. The diffusion coefficient for any given gas is proportional to the solubility and molecular weight of the gas. The diffusion coefficient for oxygen is 1.0, for carbon dioxide it is 20.3, and for nitrogen it is 0.53. The diffusion capacity of a gas varies directly with the diffusion coefficient.

diflunisal (die'flooni,sal) a salicylic acid derivative that, like aspirin, has analgesic and anti-inflammatory properties, but it has fewer side-effects than aspirin, does not affect bleeding time or function, and has a long half-life that permits twice daily dosage.

digastric (di'gastrik) 1. having two bellies. 2. digastric muscle.

digenetic (diejə'netik) having two stages of multiplication, one sexual in the mature forms, the other asexual in the larval stages.

digestant (die'jestənt, di-) 1. assisting or stimulating digestion. 2. an agent capable of aiding digestion.

digestion (die'jeschən, di-) 1. the act or process of converting food into chemical substances that can be absorbed into the blood and utilized by the body tissues. 2. the subjection of a substance to prolonged heat and moisture, so as to disintegrate and soften it.

Digestion is accomplished by physically breaking down, churning, diluting, and dissolving the food substances, and also by splitting them chemically into simpler compounds. Carbohydrates are eventually broken down to monosaccharides (simple sugars); proteins are broken down into amino acids; and fats are absorbed as fatty acids and glycerol (glycerin).

The digestive process takes place in the alimentary canal or DIGESTIVE SYSTEM. The salivary glands, liver, gallbladder, and pancreas are located outside the alimentary canal, but they are considered accessory organs of digestion because their secretions provide essential enzymes.

gastric d. digestion by the action of gastric juice.

intestinal d. digestion by the action of intestinal juices.

pancreatic d. digestion by the action of pancreatic juice.

peptic d. gastric digestion.

primary d. digestion occurring in the gastrointestinal tract.

salivary d. the change of starch into maltose by the saliva.

digestive (die'jestiv) pertaining to digestion.

d. system the organs that have as their particular function the ingestion, digestion, and absorption of food or nutritive elements. They include the mouth, teeth, tongue, pharynx, oesophagus, stomach, and

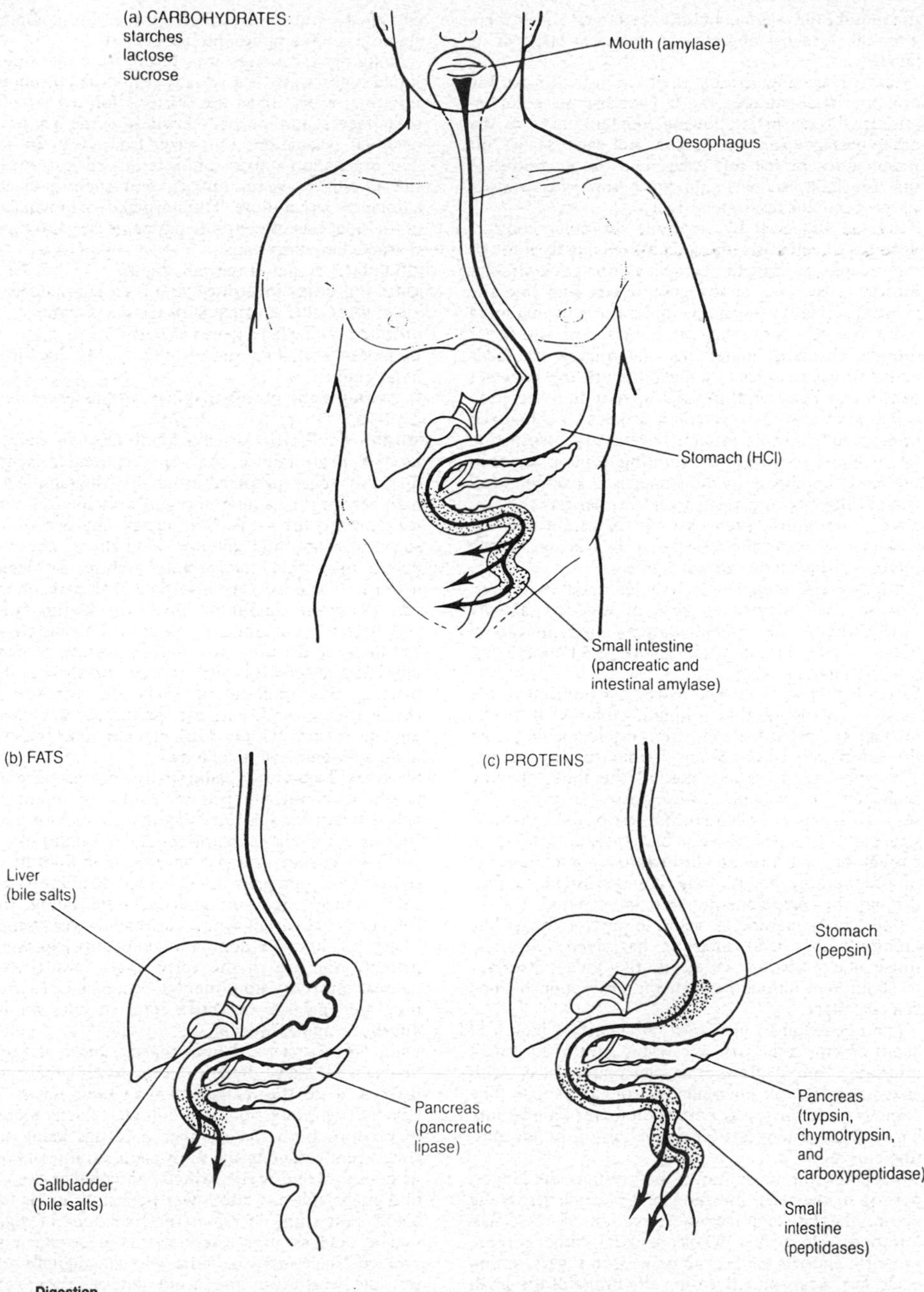

Digestion

intestines. The accessory organs of digestion, which contribute secretions important to digestion include the salivary glands, pancreas, liver, and gallbladder.

Mouth. The entrance to the alimentary canal is the **mouth**, where the teeth, tongue, and jaws begin the process of digestion by mastication. Saliva is secreted into the mouth by three separate pairs of salivary glands located under the tongue, inside the lower jaw, and in the cheek. Saliva softens and lubricates the food, dissolves some of it, and begins the conversion of the starches into sugar by the action of ptyalin, the enzyme of the saliva. The saliva moistens the inside of the mouth, the tongue, and the teeth, and rinses them after the food has departed on the next stage of its journey.

Four passageways meet at the back of the throat: the oral and nasal passages, the larynx, and the oesophagus. In the act of swallowing, the entrances to the nasal passages and the larynx are each sealed off momentarily by the soft palate and the epiglottis, so that the food can pass into the oesophagus without straying into the respiratory tract.

STOMACH. Propelled by rhythmic muscular contractions called peristalsis, the food moves rapidly through the oesophagus, past the cardiac sphincter—a circular muscle at the base of the oesophagus—and into the STOMACH. Here the peristaltic motions are stronger and more frequent, occurring at the rate of three per minute, churning, liquefying, and mixing the foods with the gastric juice. In the juice are the enzymes pepsin and lipase and, in infants, rennin; a secretion called mucin, which coats and protects the stomach lining; and hydrochloric acid. Together the pepsin and hydrochloric acid begin the splitting of the proteins in the food. The lipase in the stomach is a rather weak fat-splitting enzyme, able to act only on fats that are already emulsified, such as those in cream and the yolk of egg; more powerful lipase is available in the intestine, where most fats are digested.

The average adult stomach holds about 1.7 litres. The stomach reaches its peak of digestive activity nearly 2 hours after a meal and may empty in 3 to 4½ hours; a heavy meal may take as long as 6 hours to pass into the small intestine.

SMALL INTESTINE. The food leaves the stomach in the form of *chyme*, a thick, liquid mixture. It passes through the pylorus, a sphincter muscle opening from the lower part of the stomach into the duodenum. This sphincter is closed most of the time, opening each time a peristaltic wave passes over it. The stomach is much wider than the rest of the canal and also has a J-shaped curve at its bottom, so that the passage of food through the pylorus is automatically slowed until the food is of the right consistency to flow through the narrow opening into the intestine.

The small intestine is about 6 metres long. The lining of the small intestine has deep folds and finger-like projections called villi that give it a surface of about 9 m^2 through which the absorption of food can take place.

The duodenum, a C-shaped curve with a length of about 25 cm, is the first and widest part of the small intestine. Into it flows the pancreatic juice, with enzymes that break down starch, protein, and fats. The common bile duct also empties into the duodenum. The bile emulsifies fats for the action of the fat-splitting enzymes.

Just below the duodenum is the jejunum, the longest portion of the small intestine, and beyond that is the ileum, the last and narrowest section of the small intestine. Along this whole length, carbohydrates, proteins, and fats are broken down into sugars, amino acids, fatty acids, and glycerin. The lining of the small intestine absorbs these nutrient compounds as rapidly as they are produced. The bulky and unusable parts of the diet pass into the large intestine.

LARGE INTESTINE. At the junction of the small and large intestines is the ileocaecal valve, so called because it is at the end of the ileum and the beginning of the caecum. A small blind tube called the vermiform appendix is attached to the caecum. The longer part of the large intestine is called the colon and is divided into the ascending, transverse, and descending colon, and the sigmoid flexure, an S-shaped bend at the distal end of the colon. The sigmoid colon empties into the rectum.

Along the 1.7 metres or so of the large intestine, the liquid in the waste is gradually reabsorbed through the intestinal walls. Thus the waste is formed into fairly solid faeces and pushed down into the rectum for eventual evacuation. This takes from 10 to 20 hours. The evacuation consists of bacteria, cells cast off from the intestines, some mucus, and such indigestible substances as cellulose. The normal dark brown colour of the stool is caused by bile pigments (see also FAECES).

d. tract alimentary canal.

digit ('dijit) a finger or toe. adj. **digital.**

digital vascular imaging ('dijit'l) see SUBTRACTION.

digital vascular subtraction see SUBTRACTION.

Digitalis (ˌdiji'taylis) a genus of herbs.

D. lanata a Balkan species that yields digoxin and lanatoside.

D. purpurea the purple foxglove, whose leaves furnish digitalis.

digitalis (ˌdiji'taylis) dried leaf of *Digitalis purpurea;* used in heart failure and supraventricular tachycardias. All drugs prepared from this digitalis leaf are members of the same group and principles of administration are the same. The drugs vary according to speed of action and potency. Digitalis is, however, a potent drug that can produce severe problems of toxicity. It can be very effective in the treatment of various cardiac conditions, but its therapeutic range is very narrow; a therapeutic dose is only about one-third less than the dose that will induce toxicity. Moreover, physiological changes due to age, electrolyte disturbances, renal impairment, metabolic disorders, and certain heart conditions can predispose a patient to digitalis toxicity. Other drugs can also alter the effects of digitalis and lead to toxicity.

SIGNS OF TOXICITY. Traditionally, nurses have been taught to count the patient's pulse or monitor his apical heartbeat for rate and rhythm before administering a digitalis preparation. A decreased pulse rate of 60 per minute or less is an indication that the drug should be temporarily discontinued. While this is the most typical sign of digitalis intoxication, there frequently are earlier symptoms that deserve attention.

Some of the more common complaints expressed by patients who are in the early stages of toxicity are nausea, blurred vision, mental depression, disorientation, and malaise. Objective signs include vomiting, diarrhoea, and confusion.

DRUG INTERACTIONS. Unfortunately, most of the patients who take digitalis also have other drugs prescribed for the management of their illness. The risk of drug interactions and digitalis toxicity increases in proportion to the number of drugs being taken concurrently. One of the most common interactions is with a thiazide diuretic, which can enhance the effect of digitalis and can also lower potassium levels in the blood. Potassium decreases the likelihood of digitalis toxicity and so it is essential that hypokalaemia be avoided. Since many patients who take digitalis are on restricted calorific and fluid intake, they cannot adequately replace lost potassium by eating enough potassium-rich foods and need a potassium supplement.

PATIENT EDUCATION. There is a danger of complacency about this drug because it is so familiar and so frequently prescribed for self-medication. Without unduly alarming the patient, it is imperative that the action of the drug and its potential for harm if it is not taken as prescribed and with caution are explained to him.

The patient must be informed about the interactions

of digitalis with over-the-counter drugs such as antacids and cold remedies that contain ephedrine. He should know the signs and symptoms of digitalis toxicity and appreciate the importance of notifying his doctor should any of these signs appear. If he does not know how to check his pulse for rate and rhythm, he will need to learn how and to learn why it is important to stop taking the drug and notify the doctor should his pulse rate fall outside his normal range. There is so much that a patient needs to know in order to avoid the problems of toxicity inherent in the particular digitalis preparation he is taking that it is probably unrealistic to expect him to remember all that he is told about taking his medication safely. Therefore it is best to give him the information in written form and go over the instructions with him and a member of his family in order to be sure that the instructions are understood.

digitalization (ˌdijitəlie'zayshən) the administration of digitalis in a dosage schedule designed to produce and then maintain optimal therapeutic concentrations of its cardiotonic glycosides.

digitation (ˌdiji'tayshən) 1. a finger-like process. 2. surgical creation of a functioning digit by making a cleft between two adjacent metacarpal bones, after amputation of some or all of the fingers.

digitiform ('dijitiˌfawm) finger-like.

digitoxin (ˌdiji'toksin) a cardiotonic glycoside obtained from *Digitalis purpurea* and other species of the same genus; used in the treatment of congestive heart failure. It has a slowly developing action and slow elimination. Parenteral solutions should be diluted when given by vein.

diglossia (die'glosi·ə) bifid tongue.

diglyceride (die'glisəˌried) a glyceride containing two fatty acid molecules in ester linkage.

dignathus (die'naythəs) a fetus with two lower jaws.

digoxin (di'joksin) a cardiotonic glycoside obtained from the leaves of *Digitalis lanata*; used in the treatment of congestive heart failure. It has a relatively rapid action and rapid elimination and is used in preference to digitoxin.

DIH Diploma in Industrial Health.

dihydrocodeine (dieˌhiedroh'kohdeen) a synthetic narcotic analgesic and antitussive.

dihydroergotamine (dieˌhiedroh·ər'gotaˌmeen) hydrogenated ergotamine, an alpha adrenergic blocking agent and vasoconstrictor, used in the treatment of migraine.

dihydrotachysterol (dieˌhiedrohtaki'stiə·rol) a synthetic steroid derived from tachysterol; an antihypocalcaemic agent used in the treatment of hypocalcaemic tetany.

dihydroxycholecalciferol (ˌdie·hieˌdroksiˌkohlikal'sifə·rol) a group of active metabolites of cholecalciferol (vitamin D_3) numbered according to the carbon atom(s) on which a hydroxyl group is substituted. 1,25-Dihydroxycholecalciferol (calcitriol) is the most active derivative; it increases intestinal absorption of calcium and phosphate, enhances bone resorption, and prevents rickets, and, because of these activities at sites distant from the site of its synthesis, is considered to be a hormone.

diktyoma (ˌdikti'ohmə) a tumour of the ciliary epithelium resembling embryonic retinal tissue in structure.

dilaceration (dieˌlasə'rayshən) 1. a tearing apart. 2. in dentistry, an abnormal angulation or curve in the root or crown of a formed tooth.

dilation, dilatation (die'layshən; ˌdielə'tayshən) 1. the act of dilating or stretching. 2. the condition, as of an orifice or tubular structure, of being dilated or stretched beyond normal dimensions.

d. and curettage expanding of the ostium uteri to permit scraping of the walls of the uterus; called also *D & C* (see also ABORTION, *Suction Curettage*).

d. of the heart compensatory enlargement of the cavities of the heart, with thinning of the walls.

dilator (die'laytə) a structure (muscle) that dilates, or an instrument used to dilate.

diltiazem (diltee'ayzem) a calcium-channel blocking drug used in the treatment of angina.

diluent ('dilyooənt) 1. diluting. 2. an agent that dilutes or renders less potent or irritant.

dilution (die'looshən) 1. reduction of concentration of an active substance by admixture of a neutral agent. 2. a substance that has undergone dilution.

serial d. 1. the progressive dilution of a substance in a series of tubes in predetermined ratios. 2. a method of obtaining a pure bacterial culture by rapid transfer of an exceedingly small amount of material from one nutrient medium to a succeeding one of the same volume.

Dimelor ('diemilor) trademark for acetohexamide, an oral hypoglycaemic agent of the sulphonylurea group.

dimenhydrinate (ˌdiemen'hiedriˌnayt) an antihistamine used as an antinauseant and antiemetic.

dimercaprol (ˌdiemə'kaprol) a colourless, liquid chelating agent used in the treatment of heavy metal poisoning; called also *British antilewisite* (*BAL*). The drug forms a relatively stable compound with arsenic, mercury, gold, and certain other metals, thus protecting the vital enzyme systems of the cells against the effects of the metals. It is sometimes diluted with water and used to wash out the stomach, some of the solution being permitted to remain in the stomach.

Side-effects include tachycardia, hypertension, nausea and vomiting, severe headaches, and a sense of constriction of the chest. Barbiturates are usually ordered to relieve the symptoms, which should subside within an hour. The drug has a very disagreeable skunklike odour and should be handled carefully to avoid spilling.

dimercaptosuccinic acid (ˌdiemərkaptohˌsuk'sinik) when tagged to technetium-99m, a radiopharmaceutical used in nuclear medicine to demonstrate functioning renal tubules. Abbreviated DMSA.

dimethicone a silicone oil used as a skin protective; available as an ointment, spray, and cream.

dimethindene (ˌdieme'thindeen) an antihistaminic, used as the maleate salt.

dimethyl sulphoxide (die'methil sul'foksied, -'meethiel) a powerful solvent which has the ability to penetrate animal and plant tissues and to preserve living·cells during freezing; abbreviated DMSO. It has been proposed as a topical analgesic and anti-inflammatory agent and to increase penetrability of other substances. Herpid, used for severe herpetic skin infections, contains idoxuridine in DMSO.

dimethylphthalate (dieˌmethil'thalayt) an insect repellent in liquid or ointment form that is effective for several hours when applied to the skin. Abbreviated DIMP.

dimetria (die'metri·ə) a condition characterized by a double uterus.

dimorphism (die'mawfizəm) the quality of existing in two distinct forms. adj. **dimorphous.**

sexual d. 1. physical or behavioural differences associated with sex. 2. having some properties of both sexes, as in the early embryo and in some hermaphrodites.

Dimotane ('diemohtayn) trademark for preparations of brompheniramine, an antihistaminic.

Dimotapp ('diemohtap) trademark for a fixed combination preparation of brompheniramine maleate, phenylephrine hydrochloride, and phenylpropanolamine hydrochloride.

dinoprost trometamol ('dienoh,prost) a PROSTAGLANDIN ($PGF_2\alpha$) administered intra-amniotically and intravenously to induce abortion.

dioctyl sodium sulphosuccinate (die'oktil 'sohdi·əm) docusate sodium; a faecal softener, wetting agent, and cathartic.

dioecious (die'eeshəs) sexually distinct; denoting species in which male and female genitals do not occur in the same individual. In botany, having staminate and pistillate flowers on separate plants.

diopter (die'optə) a unit adopted for calibration of lenses, being the reciprocal of the focal length when expressed in metres; symbol D.

dioptometry (die·op'tomətree) the measurement of ocular accommodation and refraction.

dioptric (die'optrik) pertaining to refraction or to transmitted and refracted light; refracting.

dioptrics (die'optriks) the science of refracted light.

dioxin (die'oksin) a highly toxic and teratogenic chlorinated hydrocarbon that is a trace contaminant in the herbicide 2,4,5-T.

dioxybenzone (die,oksi'benzohn) a topical sun—screening agent.

Dipetalonema (die,petəloh'neemə) a genus of nematode parasites of the superfamily Filarioidea, including *D. perstans* and *D. streptocerca*, species primarily parasitic in man, other primates serving as reservoir hosts.

diphallus (die'faləs) a developmental anomaly characterized by duplication of the penis.

diphenhydramine (,diefen'hiedrə,meen) an antihistamine used in treatment of allergic disorders and also for its sedative, antiemetic, antitussive, local anaesthetic, and anticholinergic effects.

diphenoxylate (,diefe'noksi,layt) a synthetic narcotic related to meperidine used for the management of diarrhoea.

diphenylpyraline (die,feenil'piera,leen) an antihistaminic, used as the hydrochloride salt.

diphonia (die'fohni·ə) the production of two different voice tones in speaking.

diphtheria (dif'thiə·ri·ə, dip-) a severe,notifiable,infectious disease, usually of children, characterized by the formation of membranes in the throat and nose and rarely the skin, following an open wound, and toxic neurological and cardiac complications; caused by the bacillus *Corynebacterium diphtheriae*. adj. **diphtherial, diphtheric, diphtheritic.**

The disease occurs worldwide but has been virtually eliminated from most Western countries by routine immunization in childhood. Less than five cases per year are reported in the UK in unimmunized or inadequately immunized children and are often associated with imported infection. The source of infection is a human case or carrier and spread by close contact with infected nasal or pharyngeal secretions or exudate from skin lesions. The incubation period of the disease is usually between 1 and 3 days, sometimes longer, and the period of communicability lasts until virulent organisms have been eliminated from the nose and throat, which may be from 2 to 4 weeks after recovery.

SYMPTOMS. The first symptoms of diphtheria include insidious onset of sore throat, low grade fever, malaise and formation of a greyish coloured membrane in the throat. This membrane, combined with swelling of the throat, may interfere with swallowing or breathing, especially in young infants because of their narrow windpipe, and may require tracheostomy.

The diphtheria bacillus produces a toxin which may cause myocarditis about 8–10 days after onset and death through cardiac failure at about the 15th day. Toxic neurological manifestations occur later, the commonest being palatal paralysis between the 14th and 21st day causing regurgitation of fluid through the child's nose.

TREATMENT. Treatment consists of immediate administration of diphtheria antitoxin, isolation, strict bed rest and chemotherapy with penicillin or erythromycin to eradicate the infection.

PREVENTION. Primary prevention is provided by the routine immunization of the population in childhood. In the UK diphtheria toxoid is given in combination with tetanus toxoid and pertussis vaccine as 'triple-antigen' at 3 months, 4½–5 months and 8½–11 months of age. A reinforcing dose of diphtheria–tetanus toxoid is given at school entry at the age of about 5 years.

In the event of a case or outbreak of diphtheria, a search should be made for missed cases and carriers by taking nose and throat swabs of all close contacts of known cases and carriers so that they may be isolated and treated. At the same time as the swabs are collected, reinforcing doses of diphtheria toxoid should be given to those previously immunized (a special low dose preparation is available for contacts over 10 years of age), and chemotherapy, usually with erythromycin, to those unimmunized.

d. and tetanus vaccine, adsorbed (DT/Vac/Ads) a mixture of diphtheria and tetanus formol toxoids with a mineral carrier. Used for immunization of children in infancy in whom pertussis vaccine is contraindicated and for reinforcing immunity at school entry.

d., tetanus and pertussis vaccine, adsorbed (DTPer/Vac/Ads) a mixture of diphtheria and tetanus formol toxoids and pertussis vaccine with a mineral carrier. Used in the routine immunization schedule in the UK at 3 months, 4½–5 months and 8½–11 months. Called also *triple antigen*.

d. vaccine, adsorbed (Dip/Vac/Ads) prepared from diphtheria formol toxoid with a mineral carrier. Used for immunization of children. A special low dose preparation is available for adults.

diphtheroid ('difthə,royd) 1. resembling diphtheria or the diphtheria bacillus. 2. pseudodiphtheria.

diphthongia (dif'thonji·ə) the production of double vocal sounds.

diphyllobothriasis (,diefilohbo'thrieəsis) infection with *Diphyllobothrium*.

Diphyllobothrium (die,filoh'bothri·əm) a genus of large TAPEWORMS.

D. latum the broad or fish tapeworm, a species found in the intestines of man, dogs, cats, and other fish-eating mammals.

diphyodont ('difioh,dont) having two dentitions, a deciduous and a permanent.

dipipanone (die'pipə,nohn) a potent analgesic used for the relief of severe pain.

diplacusis (,diplə'kyoosis) the perception of a single auditory stimulus as two separate sounds.

diplegia (die'pleeji·ə) paralysis of like parts on either side of the body. adj. **diplegic.**

diplobacillus (,diplohbə'siləs) a short, rod-shaped organism occurring in pairs; diplobacterium.

diplobacterium (,diplohbak'tiə·ri·əm) diplobacillus.

diploblastic (,diploh'blastik) having two germ layers.

diplocardia (,diploh'kahdi·ə) separation of the two halves of the heart.

Diplococcus (,diploh'kokəs) former name for a genus of bacteria (tribe Streptococceae).

D. pneumoniae *Streptococcus pneumoniae.*

diplococcus (,diploh'kokəs) pl. *diplococci;* 1. any of the spherical, lanceolate, or coffee-bean-shaped bacteria occurring usually in pairs as a result of incomplete separation after cell division in a single plane. 2. any organism of the genus *Diplococcus*.

diplocoria (ˌdiploh'kor·ri·ə) double pupil.

diploë ('diploh·ee) the spongy layer between the inner and outer compact layers of the flat bones of the skull. adj. **diploetic, diploic.**

diplogenesis (ˌdiploh'jenəsis) the production of a double embryo or fetus.

diploid ('diployd) 1. having a pair of each chromosome characteristic of a species (2n or, in man, 46). 2. a diploid individual or cell.

diploidy (di'ploydee) the state of being diploid.

diplomyelia (ˌdiplohmie'eeli·ə) lengthwise fissure and seeming doubleness of the spinal cord.

diplonema (ˌdiploh'neemə) the double chromosomes in the diplotene stage.

diploneural (ˌdiploh'nyooə·rəl) having a double nerve supply.

diplopia (di'plohpi·ə) the perception of two images of a single object (double vision).

binocular d. perception of a separate image of a single object by each of the two eyes.

crossed d. horizontal diplopia in which the image belonging to the right eye is displaced to the left of the image belonging to the left eye (divergent strabismus).

direct d. horizontal diplopia in which the image belonging to the right eye appears to the right of the image belonging to the left eye (convergent strabismus).

horizontal d. diplopia in which the two images lie in the same horizontal plane, being either direct or crossed.

vertical d. diplopia in which one image appears above the other in the same vertical plane.

diplosomatia (ˌdiplohsoh'mayshi·ə) a condition in which complete twins are joined at some of their body parts.

diplosomia (ˌdiploh'sohmi·ə) diplosomatia.

diplotene ('diplohˌteen) the stage of the first meiotic prophase, following the pachytene, in which the two chromosomes in each bivalent begin to repel one another and a split occurs between the chromosomes.

dipole ('diepohl) 1. a pair of electric charges or magnetic poles separated by a finite distance. 2. a molecule having separated charges of equal and opposite sign.

diprophylline (die'prohfileen) a theophylline derivative used as a bronchodilator in the treatment of bronchial asthma or bronchospasm associated with chronic bronchitis or emphysema.

diprosopus (ˌdieproh'sohpəs) a fetus or infant with varying degrees of duplication of the face.

dipsomania (ˌdipsoh'mayni·ə) alcoholism.

dipsotherapy (ˌdipsoh'therəpee) the therapeutic limitation of the amounts of fluids ingested.

Diptera ('diptə·rə) an order of insects, including flies, gnats, and mosquitoes.

dipterous ('diptə·rəs) 1. having two wings. 2. pertaining to insects of the order Diptera.

Dip/Vac/Ads diphtheria vaccine, adsorbed.

dipygus (di'piegəs) a fetus with a double pelvis.

dipylidiasis (ˌdipili'dieəsis) infection with *Dipylidium caninum.*

Dipylidium (ˌdipi'lidi·əm) a genus of TAPEWORMS.

D. caninum the dog tapeworm, parasitic in dogs and cats and occasionally found in man.

dipyridamole (ˌdiepi'ridəˌmohl) a coronary vasodilator.

director (die'rektə, di-) a grooved instrument for guiding a knife or other surgical instrument.

Dirofilaria (ˌdierohfi'lair·ri·ə) a genus of nematode parasites of the superfamily Filarioidea which occur in dogs and cats and occasionally cause infection.

dirofilariasis (ˌdierohˌfilə'rieəsis) infection with organisms of the genus *Dirofilaria.*

dis- word element. [L.] *reversal* or *separation* [Gr.] *duplication.*

disability (ˌdisə'bilitee) any restriction or lack (resulting from an impairment) of ability to perform an activity in the manner or within the range considered normal for a human being.

developmental d. a substantial handicap of indefinite duration, with onset before the age of 18 years, and attributable to mental handicap, autism, cerebral palsy, epilepsy, or other neuropathy.

disaccharide (die'sakəˌried) any of a class of sugars each molecule of which yields two molecules of monosaccharide on hydrolysis.

disarticulation (ˌdisahˌtikyuh'layshən) amputation or separation at a joint.

disc (disk) a circular or rounded flat plate.

articular d. a pad of fibrocartilage or dense fibrous tissue present in some synovial joints.

Bowman's d. one of the flat, disclike plates making up a striated muscle fibre. **choked d.** papilloedema.

embryonic d. a flattish area in a cleaved ovum in which the first traces of the embryo are seen.

intervertebral d. the layer of fibrocartilage between the bodies of adjoining vertebrae (see also slipped DISC).

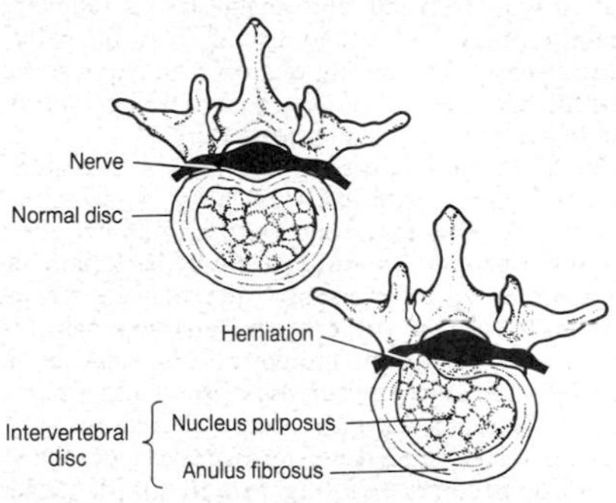

Vertebral disc. Transverse section showing normal intervertebral disc and ruptured intervertebral disc with herniation of the nucleus pulposus (slipped disc)

intra-articular d. articular disc.

optic d. the intraocular part of the optic nerve formed by fibres converging from the retina and appearing as a pink to white disc in the retina.

prolapsed intervertebral d. rupture of an intervertebral disc. The condition occurs most commonly in the lower back, occasionally in the neck, and rarely in the upper portion of the spine.

Pads of cartilage and fibre enclosing a rubbery tissue known as the nucleus pulposus lie between the vertebrae. They act as cushions between the vertebrae, absorbing ordinary shocks and strains and shifting position to accommodate the various movements of the spine. Excessive strain may weaken the cartilage to the extent that the nucleus pulposus protrudes through it and forms a bulge. This bulge may push against the nerve roots in the spinal canal, causing pain.

CAUSES AND SYMPTOMS. Rupture, or herniation, of the discs may be caused by injury or by sudden straining with the spine in an unnatural position. The condition may come on gradually as a result of a progressive deterioration of the discs.

Symptoms depend upon the location and the extent to which the disc material has been pushed out. Most cases involve the discs between the fourth and fifth lumbar vertebrae or between the fifth lumbar vertebra and the sacrum. There is severe pain in the lower back and difficulty in walking. The sciatic nerve, which originates in the lower part of the spinal cord, is affected, with resulting pain at the back of the thigh and lower leg. A cough, sneeze, or strain will send the pain along the course of the sciatic nerve to the calf or ankle.

When the discs of the cervical vertebrae are affected, severe pain in the back of the neck radiates down the arms to the fingers. Neck movements are restricted. Any neck motion, coughing, sneezing, or straining will accentuate the pain.

DIAGNOSIS AND TREATMENT. Careful examination, including laboratory tests and radiological examination, is necessary to distinguish the condition from other disturbances of the spine. The radiographs may reveal pathological changes in the spine and narrowing of the space between the vertebrae.

Treatment for prolapsed intervertebral disc varies according to the seriousness of the condition. Conservative treatment for a ruptured disc of the lower back consists of bed rest on a firm mattress over a bed board and local application of heat, which should not be prolonged because it may aggravate the congestion, and muscle relaxants and analgesics to relieve pain. Traction may be applied to the legs or pelvis. In chronic cases the wearing of a surgical support may be helpful. Care must be taken to avoid aggravating the condition by excessive physical effort.

Cases of ruptured disc of the neck are treated in a similar manner with bed rest, heat, analgesics, and traction. A collar may be worn to immobilize the neck when the patient is out of bed. Acute back pain caused by a prolapsed intervertebral disc may be treated by chemonucleolysis. An enzyme (chymopapain) is injected into the nucleus pulposus. The enzyme slowly dissolves the nucleus pulposus producing pain relief and resolution of nerve root compression.

If the response to these measures is poor or if the condition becomes disabling, surgery may be necessary to relieve the pressure on the injured disc (see LAMINECTOMY).

PATIENT CARE. The patient receiving conservative treatment for a prolapsed intervertebral disc must always have his spine in good alignment so as to avoid pressure on the adjacent nerves. In addition to the firm mattress and bed boards, he should be instructed in the proper method of turning himself by 'log-rolling'. To accomplish this the patient crosses his arms over his chest, flexes the knee opposite the side onto which he is to turn, and then rolls over in 'one piece', being sure that his spine is not bent forward or twisted.

A bed cradle should be used to eliminate the weight of the bed clothes and also to prevent footdrop. A small bedpan is recommended for the patient's use so that he can roll onto it without discomfort. A folded towel or small pillow is placed under his lower back for support of the lumbar region. Measures must be taken to avoid constipation which is quite common and likely to cause increased pain as the patient strains to defecate. A nonconstipating diet may be sufficient; however, a mild laxative, such as one of the bulk laxatives, may also be necessary.

HEAT, in the form of a heating pad or infrared lamp, often relieves the pain caused by muscle spasms. Care should be taken in the application of heat because of the danger of burning the patient who has a loss of sensory perception because of nerve damage caused by the prolapsed intervertebral disc.

Most orthopaedic surgeons prescribe a special corset to be worn by the patient whenever he is out of bed. The corset is designed to give proper support to the vertebral column and to relieve tension on the back muscles. Support devices of this kind are usually removed after symptoms are relieved, because they weaken the musculature of the back. Training in good posture and body mechanics, especially during lifting or stooping, are important in preventing recurrence of acute episodes. Special exercises may be prescribed to strengthen the back muscles.

slipped d. popular name for PROLAPSED INTERVERTEBRAL DISC.

discectomy (dis'kektəmee) excision of an intervertebral disc.

discharge ('dischahj) 1. a setting free, or liberation. 2. material or force set free. 3. an excretion or substance evacuated.

disciform ('disi,fawm) in the shape of a disc.

discission (di'sishən) incision, or cutting into, as of a soft cataract.

discitis (di'skietis) inflammation of a disc, especially of an intervertebral disc.

discogenic (,diskoh'jenik) caused by derangement of an intervertebral disc.

discography (dis'kogrəfee) radiology of the vertebral column after injection of radiopaque material into an intervertebral disc.

discoid ('diskoyd) 1. disc-shaped. 2. a disc-like medicated tablet.

discordance (dis'kawdəns) the occurrence of a given trait in only one member of a twin pair. adj. **discordant.**

discrete (di'skreet) made up of separated parts; characterized by lesions that do not become blended.

discus ('diskəs) pl. *disci* [L.] disc.

d. oophorus, d. ovigerus, d. proligerus cumulus oophorus.

disease (di'zeez) a definite pathological process having a characteristic set of signs and symptoms. It may affect the whole body or any of its parts, and its aetiology, pathology, and prognosis may be known or unknown. For specific diseases, see under the specific name, as ADDISON'S DISEASE.

autoimmune d. any of a group of disorders in which tissue injury is associated with humoral or cell-mediated immune responses to body constituents; they may be systemic or organ-specific (see also AUTOIMMUNE DISEASE).

chronic granulomatous d. genetically determined defect in the intracellular bactericidal function of leukocytes, associated with a chronic suppurative lymphadenitis, eczematoid dermatitis, hepatosplenomegaly, and chronic pulmonary disease.

chronic obstructive airways d. (COAD) a functional category designating a chronic condition of persistent obstruction of bronchial air flow (see also CHRONIC OBSTRUCTIVE AIRWAYS DISEASE).

collagen d's a group of poorly understood diseases that have in common widespread pathological changes in association with circulating immune complexes. These diseases include systemic lupus erythematosus, polyarteritis nodosa, scleroderma, dermatomyositis, and perhaps rheumatoid arthritis and rheumatic fever (see also COLLAGEN DISEASES).

communicable d. a disease the causative agents of which may pass or be carried from one person to another directly or indirectly (see also COMMUNICABLE DISEASE).

complicating d. one that occurs in the course of some other disease as a complication.

constitutional d. one involving a system of organs or one with widespread symptoms.
contagious d. disease conveyed by touch (used only when the disease is transmitted by direct contact or by infected secretions).
cystine storage d. cystinosis.
deficiency d. a condition due to dietary or metabolic deficiency, including all diseases caused by an insufficient supply of essential nutrients.
degenerative joint d. osteoarthritis.
demyelinating d. any condition characterized by destruction of myelin as seen in multiple sclerosis.
diverticular d. a general term including the prediverticular state, diverticulosis, and diverticulitis usually applied to the colon.
epizootic d. a disease that affects a large number of animals in some particular region within a short period of time.
extrapyramidal d. any of a group of clinical disorders marked by abnormal involuntary movements, alterations in muscle tone, and postural disturbances; it includes parkinsonism, chorea, athetosis, etc.
focal d. a localized disease.
functional d. any disease involving body functions but not associated with detectable organic lesion or change.
glycogen d., glycogen storage d. any of a group of genetically-determined disorders of glycogen metabolism, marked by abnormal storage of glycogen in the body tissues (see also GLYCOGEN STORAGE DISEASE).
haemolytic d. of newborn see HAEMOLYTIC disease of the newborn.
haemorrhagic d. of newborn see HAEMORRHAGIC DISEASE OF NEWBORN.
heavy-chain d. a rare monoclonal gammopathy characterized by neoplastic proliferation of plasma cells and precursors that secrete immunoglobulin heavy chains. It is often accompanied by hepatosplenomegaly, lymphadenopathy, and soft tissue tumours. There are three variants, characterized by a specific heavy chain: alpha-chain disease and gamma-chain disease resemble a malignant lymphoma; mu-chain disease is very rare and occurs most frequently in patients with chronic lymphocytic leukaemia.
hookworm d. see HOOKWORM.
idiopathic d. one that exists without any known cause.
immune-complex d. 1. disease induced by the deposition of or association with antigen–antibody–complement complexes in the microvasculature of tissues. Activation of complement by the complexes may occur and initiates inflammation. In other examples the complexes react with platelets without complement participation. The platelets then may release prostaglandins and other mediators producing proteinuria or oedema. 2. serum sickness.
infectious d. disease resulting from multiplication of microorganisms in the body. Most are communicable but not all. See also COMMUNICABLE DISEASE.
intercurrent d. a disease occurring during the course of another disease with which it has no connection.
iron storage d. haemochromatosis.
lysosomal storage d. any inborn error of metabolism in which the deficiency of a lysosomal enzyme results in the accumulation of the substance normally degraded by that enzyme in the lysosomes of certain cells. These diseases are further classified, depending on the nature of the stored substance, as glycogen storage diseases (glycogenoses), sphingolipidoses, mucopolysaccharidoses, and mucolipidoses.
Mediterranean d. the homozygous form of beta-THALASSAEMIA.
metabolic d. one caused by some defect in the chemical reactions of the cells of the body.
molecular d. any disease in which the pathogenesis can be traced to a single chemical substance, usually a protein, which is either abnormal in structure or present in reduced amounts.
motor neuron d. any disease of the motor neurons, including spinal muscular atrophy, progressive bulbar paralysis, amyotrophic lateral sclerosis, and lateral sclerosis.
notifiable d. a disease whose occurrence must by law be reported to the public health authorities. Some diseases are notifiable in certain circumstances, e.g., certain industrial diseases.
occupational d. a disease arising from various factors involved with the patient's occupation (see also OCCUPATIONAL DISEASES).
organic d. one due to or accompanied by structural changes in organs or tissues.
periodontal d. any disease or disorder of the periodontium (see also PERIODONTITIS and PERIODONTOSIS).
secondary d. 1. a morbid condition subsequent to or a consequence of another disease. 2. a condition due to introduction of incompatible, immunologically competent cells into a host rendered incapable of accepting them by heavy exposure to ionizing radiation.
self-limited d. one that by its very nature runs a limited and definite course.
sexually transmitted d. (STD) an infectious disease that is usually acquired by sexual intercourse or other genital contact (see also SEXUALLY TRANSMITTED DISEASE).
storage d. a metabolic disorder in which a specific substance (a lipid, a protein, etc.) accumulates in certain cells in unusually large amounts.
systemic d. a generalized disease affecting the whole body.
thyrocardiac d., thyrotoxic heart d. see THYROTOXIC HEART DISEASE.
venereal d. (VD) an infectious disease usually acquired in sexual intercourse or other genital contact and legally defined: in the UK SYPHYLIS, GONORRHOEA and CHANCROID are defined as venereal diseases. See also VENEREAL disease and SEXUALLY TRANSMITTED DISEASE.
wasting d. any disease marked especially by progressive emaciation and weakness.

disequilibrium (ˌdiseekwi'libri·əm) unstable equilibrium.

disimpaction (ˌdisim'pakshən) reduction of an impacted fracture.

disinfect (ˌdisin'fekt) to destroy microorganisms but not usually bacterial spores, reducing the number of mircoorganisms to a level which is not harmful to health.

disinfectant (ˌdisin'fektənt) an agent that destroys infection-producing organisms. Heat and certain other physical agents such as live steam can be disinfectants, but in common usage the term is reserved for chemical substances such as gluteraldehyde, sodium hypochlorite or phenol. Disinfectants are usually applied to inanimate objects since they are too strong to be used on living tissues. Chemical disinfectants are not always effective against spore-forming bacteria.

disinfection (ˌdisin'fekshən) the act of disinfecting.
terminal d. disinfection of a sick room and its contents at the termination of a disease.

disinfestation (ˌdisinfe'stayshən) destruction of insects, rodents, or other animal forms present on the person or his clothes or in his surroundings, and which may transmit disease.

disintegrant (di'sintiˌgrənt) an agent used in pharma-

Activity and uses of disinfectants

Group	Examples	Activity against:			Resistant to inactivation	Use	Remarks
		Bacteria	Spores	Viruses			
Phenols	Hycolin Stericol Izal	+	−	+/−	+/−	Environment	
Chlorine	Milton Sterite Presept	+	+/−	+	−	Environment Equipment	Corrosive to metals
Diguanide	Hibitane Hibiscrub	+	−	+/−	−	Skin	
Alcohols	Ethanol Isopropanol	+	−	+	+	Skin Surfaces	Inflammable
Iodine	Aqueous Tincture Betadine Disadine	+	+/−	+	−	Skin	Aqueous and tincture can irritate
Hexachlorophane	Ster-Zac	+	−	+/−	−	Skin	Avoid routine use in neonates
Triclosan	Manusept Cidal	+	−	+/−	−	Skin	—
Glutaraldehyde	Cidex Asep Totacide	+	+	+	+	Instrument	Irritating vapour
Quaternary ammonium compounds	Roccal Zephiran Cetavlon Dettox	+	−	+/−	−	Instrument Skin	Contamination problems use with caution

From Caddow, P.(ed.) (1989) *Applied Microbiology*, Scutari Press.

ceutical preparation of tablets, which causes them to disintegrate and release their medicinal substances on contact with moisture.

disintegration (di,sinti'grayshən) 1. the process of breaking up or decomposing; specifically the spontaneous fission of a nucleus to produce ionizing radiation. 2. radioactive decay (see DECAY).

disjunction (dis'jungkshən) the act or state of being disjoined. In genetics, the moving apart of bivalent chromosomes at the first anaphase of meiosis.

disk (disk) disc.

diskitis (di'skietis) discitis.

diskography (dis'kogrəfee) discography.

dislocation (,dislə'kayshən) displacement of a bone from a joint. The most common dislocations are those involving a finger, thumb, or shoulder. Less common are those of the mandible, elbow, knee, or hip. Symptoms include loss of motion, temporary paralysis of the involved joint, pain and swelling, and sometimes shock.

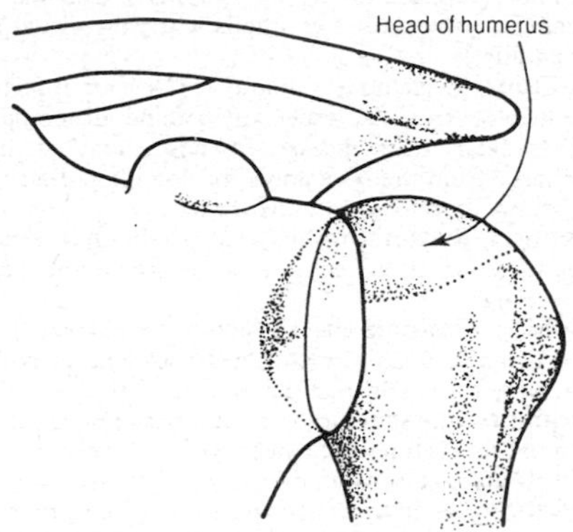

Posterior dislocation of the shoulder

A dislocation is usually caused by a blow or fall, although unusual physical effort may lead to this condition. Some dislocations, especially of the hip, are congenital, usually resulting from a faulty construction of the joint. Such a condition is best treated in infancy, with a cast and possibly surgery to correct the dislocation.

A dislocation should be treated as a fracture when first aid is administered. As soon as possible the dislocation is reduced by an orthopaedic surgeon. Traction, slight flexion, abduction, and rotation will often reduce a dislocation. The affected joint is then immobilized to allow for healing of the torn ligaments, tendons, and capsules. In some cases surgery may be necessary to stabilize the joint.

complete d. one in which the surfaces are entirely separated.

compound d. one in which the joint communicates with the outside air through a wound.

pathological d. one due to disease of the joint or to paralysis of the muscles.

simple d. one in which there is no communication with the air through a wound.

dismemberment (dis'membəmənt) amputation of a limb or a portion of it.

dismutase (dis'myootayz) any of a group of enzymes that have the ability to catalyse the reaction of two molecules of the same compound to yield two molecules in different oxidation states.

disodium etidronate (die'sohdi·əm e'tidrənayt) a bone calcium regulator used in the treatment of Paget's disease and for the prevention of heterotopic ossification due to spinal cord injury or following total hip replacement.

disomus (die'sohməs) a double-bodied fetus or infant.

disopyramide (,diesoh'pirə,mied) an antiarrhythmic agent used for suppression and prevention of recurrence of both unifocal premature ventricular contractions and those of multifocal origin, paired premature ventricular contractions, and episodes of ventricular tachycardia that are not persistent.

disorder (dis'awdə) a derangement or abnormality of function; a morbid physical or mental state.

affective d's the group of psychoses characterized chiefly by a predominant mood (extreme depression or elation) or by alternations between such moods, including involutional melancholia and manic-depressive psychosis.

attention deficit d. see ATTENTION DEFICIT SYNDROME.

bipolar affective d. a major disorder of mood in which both manic and depressive episodes occur. Also known as *manic-depressive disorder* or *manic-depressive psychosis*.

character d. a mental disorder characterized by maladaptive behaviour, emotional responses that are socially unacceptable, and minimal feelings of anxiety or other symptoms that usually accompany neuroses.

functional d. a disorder not associated with any clearly defined physical or structural change.

mental d. any psychiatric illness or disease, whether functional or of organic origin.

personality d. a mental disorder which stems from the personality of the individual and in which there is minimal feeling of subjective anxiety and little or no feeling of distress, coupled with poor social learning.

psychophysiological d., psychosomatic d. a mental disorder in which physical symptoms are presumed to be of psychogenic origin.

disorganization (dis,awgənie'zayshən) the process of destruction of any organic tissue; any profound change in the tissues of an organ or structure which causes the loss of most or all of its proper characters.

disorientation (dis,or·rien'tayshən) the loss of proper bearings, or a state of mental confusion as to time, place, or identity.

dispensary (di'spensə·ree) any place where drugs or medicines are actually dispensed.

disperse (di'spərs) to scatter the component parts, as of a tumour or the fine particles in a colloid system; also, the particles so dispersed.

dispersion (di'spərshən) 1. the act of scattering or separating; the condition of being scattered. 2. the incorporation of one substance into another. 3. a colloid solution.

displacement (dis'playsmənt) removal to an abnormal location or position; in psychology, unconscious transference of an emotion from its original object onto a more acceptable substitute.

disposition (,dispə'zishən) a tendency to suffer from certain diseases.

disproportion (,disprə'pawshən) a lack of the proper relationship between two elements or factors.

cephalopelvic d. abnormally large size of the fetal skull in relation to the maternal pelvis, leading to difficulties in delivery.

dissect (die'sekt, di-) to cut apart, separate or expose structures at operation or in a cadaver.

dissection (die'sekshən, di-) 1. the act of dissecting. 2. a part or whole of an organism prepared by dissecting to expose anatomical features.

blunt d. separation of tissues along natural lines of cleavage, by means of a blunt instrument or finger.
sharp d. separation of tissues by means of the sharp edge of a knife or scalpel, or with scissors.

disseminated (di'semi,naytid) scattered; distributed over a considerable area.
d. intravascular coagulation (DIC) widespread formation of thromboses in the microcirculation, mainly within the capillaries. It is a secondary complication of a diverse group of obstetrical, surgical, haemolytic, and neoplastic disorders, all of which activate the coagulation sequence in some way. Paradoxically, the intravascular clotting ultimately produces haemorrhage because of rapid consumption of fibrinogen, platelets, prothrombin, and clotting factors V, VIII, and X. Because of this pathology, DIC is sometimes called *defibrination syndrome* or *consumption coagulopathy*.
The condition may present signs and symptoms related to tissue hypoxia and infarction caused by the many microthrombi, but it is more often seen as an acute or chronic haemorrhagic disorder related to excessive and diffuse depletion of the elements needed for haemostasis.
DIC should be suspected in any patient who has an unexplained tendency toward bleeding, and is suffering from one of the following types of clinical conditions: (1) those that introduce coagulation-promoting factors into the circulation, as in abruptio placentae, retained dead fetus, amniotic fluid embolism, metastatic carcinoma of the pancreas, lung, stomach, or prostate, and acute promyelotic leukaemia; (2) those that lead to stagnant blood flow, as in hypotension and shock; (3) those accompanied by widespread endothelial injury, as in severe burns, trauma, heat stroke, and surgery, particularly surgery involving extracorporeal circulation; (4) various types of infections and bacteraemias; and (5) snake bite and fat embolism.
The tendency toward excessive bleeding can appear suddenly and, with little warning, rapidly progress to severe or even fatal haemorrhage. Signs of DIC include continued bleeding from a venipuncture site, occult and internal bleeding, and, in some cases, profuse bleeding from all orifices. Other less obvious and more easily missed signs are generalized sweating, cold and mottled fingers and toes (due to capillary thrombi and hypoxia), and petechiae.
The diagnosis of DIC is confirmed by laboratory tests which show prolonged thrombin time, prothrombin time, and partial thromboplastin time; depressed platelet count; elevated fibrin split products (FSP); and a strongly positive protamine sulphate test. Assays for coagulation factors and, in particular, fibrinogen may be done to diagnose DIC; if the condition is present, the levels of these factors are reduced.
Treatment of DIC consists of replacement of the inadequate blood products and correction, when possible, of the underlying cause. When the primary disease cannot be treated, intravenous injections of heparin may inhibit the clotting process and raise the level of the depleted clotting factors.

dissociation (di,sohsi'ayshən, -,sohshi-) 1. the act of separating or the state of being separated. 2. an intrapsychic defence process in which one or more groups of mental processes become separated off from normal consciousness and then function as a unitary whole.
atrial d. independent beating of the left and right atria, each with normal rhythm or with various combinations of normal rhythm, atrial flutter, or atrial fibrillation.
atrioventricular d. control of the atria by one pacemaker and of the ventricles by another, independent pacemaker.

dissolution (disə'looshən) 1. the process in which one substance is dissolved in another. 2. separation of a compound into its components by chemical action. 3. liquefaction. 4. death.

dissolve (di'zolv) 1. to cause a substance to pass into solution. 2. to pass into solution.

distad ('distad) in a distal direction.

distal ('dist'l) remote; further from any point of reference.

Distalgesic (,distal'jeezik) trademark for a combination of dextropropoxyphene and paracetamol not used as widely as in the past due to consequences of overdose.

distance ('distəns) the measure of space intervening between two objects or two points of reference.
interocclusal d. the distance between the occluding surfaces of the maxillary and mandibular teeth with the mandible in physiological rest position.
interocular d. the distance between the eyes, usually used in reference to the interpupillary distance (the distance between the two pupils when the visual axes are parallel).

distemper (di'stempə) a name for several infectious diseases of animals, especially canine distemper, a highly fatal viral disease of dogs, marked by a discharge from the nose and eyes, vomiting, diarrhoea, coughing, dyspnoea, and seizures.

distention, distension (dis'tenshən) the state of being distended, or stretched out or enlarged; the act of distending.

distichia, distichiasis (di'stiki·ə; ,disti'kieəsis) the presence of a double row of eyelashes, one or both of which are turned against the eyeball.

distigmine (die'stigmeen) a cholinesterase inhibitor used in the treatment of a neurogenic bladder.

distillate ('disti,layt) a product of distillation.

distillation (,disti'layshən) vaporization; the process of vaporizing and condensing a substance to purify the substance or to separate a volatile substance from less volatile substances.
fractional d. separation of volatilizable substances into a number of fractions, based on their different boiling points.

distobuccal (,distoh'buk'l) pertaining to or formed by the distal and buccal surfaces of a tooth, or by the distal and buccal walls of a tooth cavity.

distoclusion (,disto'kloozhən) malrelation of the dental arches, with the lower jaw in a distal or posterior position in relation to the upper.

distomiasis (,distoh'mieəsis) infection due to trematodes or flukes.

distortion (di'stawshən) the state of being twisted out of normal shape or position; in psychiatry, the conversion of material offensive to the superego into acceptable form.

distraction (di'strakshən) 1. diversion of attention. 2. separation of joint surfaces without rupture of their binding ligaments and without displacement. 3. surgical separation of the two parts of a bone after it is transected. 4. separation of bone fragments in a fracture of a long bone, usually resulting from excessive traction.

distress (di'stress) physical or mental anguish or suffering.

disturbance (di'stərbəns) a departure or divergence from that which is considered normal.

disulfiram (die'sulfi,ram) Antabuse; a compound that, when used in the presence of alcohol, produces distressing symptoms of severe nausea and vomiting. It is a dangerous drug, should always be given under the supervision of a doctor and is never given to a patient in a state of intoxication or without his full knowledge. Disulfiram inhibits the oxidation of acetaldehyde produced by the metabolism of alcohol, so that acetaldehyde accumulates in the body and produces nausea, vomiting, palpitation, dyspnoea, lowered blood pressure, and occasionally profound collapse.

dithranol ('dithrə,nol) a yellowish-brown crystalline powder used topically in eczema and psoriasis.

diurese (,dieyuh'rees) the act of effecting diuresis.

diuresis (,dieyuh'reesis) increased excretion of the urine.

diuretic (,dieyuh'retik) 1. increasing urine excretion or the amount of urine. 2. an agent that promotes urine secretion. Certain common substances such as tea, coffee, and water act as diuretics. The *thiazides* are the most frequently prescribed diuretics because they are moderately potent and have relatively few side-effects. Most act within 1 hour after being taken and are excreted in 3 to 6 hours. They decrease reabsorption of sodium by the kidney and thereby increase the loss of water and sodium. Thiazides also increase urinary secretion of chloride, potassium, and, to some extent, bicarbonate ions. Patients who are taking a thiazide diuretic should be monitored for electrolyte imbalances, metabolic acidosis, and, in the case of diabetic patients, hyperglycaemia, which may necessitate an increase in their insulin dosage. Because gastrointestinal irritation can occur, it is advisable to take these diuretics at mealtimes.

The *potassium-sparing diuretics* do not carry the threat of potassium loss, but they do present a potential problem of hyperkalaemia. Triamterene, one of the diuretics in this group, also can lead to hyperglycaemia in diabetic patients.

The *loop diuretics* block the active transport of chloride in the ascending limb of the loop of Henle, which stops the coupled passive reabsorption of sodium. Precautions when giving these drugs are generally the same as for other diuretics. In addition, some of them produce ototoxicity, which can result in reversible impaired hearing, and nephrotoxicity, which damages the kidney, and therefore are contraindicated in renal disease. Frusemide, which belongs to this group, is a sulphonamide; hence, hypersensitivity reaction can develop in persons with a specific allergy.

Osmotic diuretics produce a very rapid loss of sodium and water by inhibiting their reabsorption in the kidney tubules and the loop of Henle. Mannitol is clinically the most useful of these diuretics, but it has some serious side-effects, such as pulmonary oedema and congestive heart failure.

In addition to the observations mentioned previously, all hospitalized patients receiving diuretic therapy should have their fluid intake and urine output measured and be weighed daily. Those on diuretics that are not potassium sparing will need an increased potassium intake, either by means of high-potassium foods or potassium-containing medicines. Discharge planning should include information about food sources of potassium and a warning that enemas can further deplete blood potassium levels. As with all patients who continue drug therapy after discharge, they will need to understand the desired effect of the diuretic they are taking, ways to avoid its side-effects, the signs of toxicity, and other events that should be brought to the attention of the doctor or nurse.

Diuretic drugs are used chiefly in the treatment of oedema resulting from conditions other than kidney disease since the abnormal kidney rarely responds fully to them. They are most useful in relieving oedema accompanying congestive heart failure or diminished plasma proteins.

Many diuretics, especially the thiazides, are used in the management of hypertension, particularly when used in conjunction with other kinds of antihypertensive agents.

diurnal (die'ərnəl) pertaining to or occurring during the daytime, or period of light.

divagation (,dievə'gayshən) incoherent or wandering speech.

divalent (die'vaylənt) 1. bivalent. 2. carrying an electronic charge of two units.

divergence (die'vərjəns) a moving apart, or inclination away from a common point. adj. **divergent.**

diverticular (,dievə'tikyuhlə) pertaining to or resembling a diverticulum.

diverticulectomy (,dievə,tikyuh'lektəmee) excision of a diverticulum.

diverticulitis (,dievə,tikyuh'lietis) inflammation of a diverticulum, especially inflammation involving diverticula of the colon. Weakness of the muscles of the colon, sometimes produced by chronic constipation, leads to the formation of diverticula, small blind pouches that form in the lining and wall of the colon. Inflammation may occur as a result of collections of bacteria or other irritating agents trapped in the pouches.

Symptoms of diverticulitis include muscle spasms and cramplike pains in the abdomen, especially in the lower left quadrant. Diagnosis is confirmed by barium enema (see BARIUM TEST), in which the diverticula are clearly shown.

Treatment consists of bed rest, cleansing enemas, a bland or low-residue diet, and drugs to reduce infection. In severe cases portions of the affected bowel may require surgical removal and a temporary *colostomy*.

diverticulosis (,dievə,tikyuh'lohsis) the presence of diverticula in the absence of inflammation. See DIVERTICULITIS.

diverticulum (dievə'tikyuhləm) pl. *diverticula* [L.] a circumscribed pouch or sac occurring normally or created by herniation of the lining mucous membrane through a defect in the muscular coat of a tubular organ.

intestinal d. a pouch or sac formed by hernial protrusion of the mucous membrane through a defect in the muscular coat of the intestine.

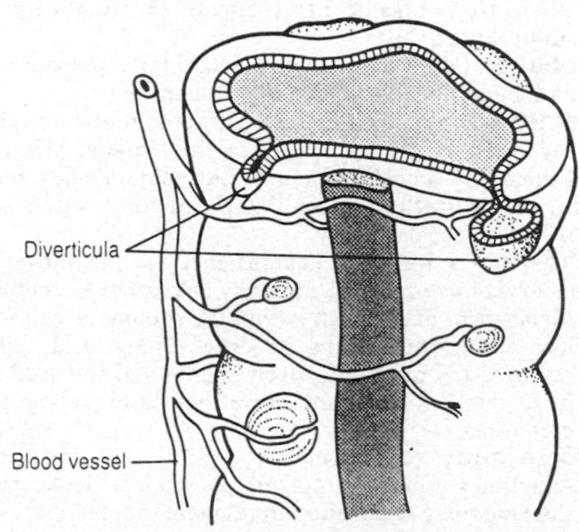

Diverticula of the large intestine

Meckel's d. an occasional sacculation or appendage of the ileum, derived from an unobliterated yolk stalk.

pressure d., pulsion d. a sac or pouch formed by hernial protrusion of the mucous membrane through the muscular coat of the oesophagus or colon as a result of pressure from within.

traction d. a localized distortion, angulation, or funnel-shaped bulging of the oesophageal wall, due to adhesions resulting from external lesion.

division (di'vizhən) the act of separating into parts.

cell d. fission of a cell, the process by which cells reproduce.

divulsion (die'vulshən) avulsion.

divulsor (die'vulsə) an instrument used for forcible dilation.

dizygotic, dizygous (ˌdiezie'gotik; die'ziegəs) pertaining to or derived from two separate zygotes (fertilized ova); said of twins.

dizziness ('dizinəs) a disturbed sense of relationship to space; a sensation of unsteadiness and a feeling of movement within the head; lightheadedness; disequilibrium; vertigo is sometimes used erroneously as a synonym.

dk symbol, *deka-*.

DL- chemical prefix (small capitals) denoting that the substance is an equimolecular mixture of two catamorphs, one of which corresponds in configuration to D-glyceraldehyde, the other to L-glyceraldehyde.

DLE discoid lupus erythematosus.

DM Doctor of Medicine (Oxford University).

DMF *d*ecayed, *m*issing, *f*illed (teeth): an index used in dental surveys.

DMSA dimercaptosuccinic acid.

DMSO dimethyl sulphoxide.

DN Diploma in Nursing; District Nurse; Doctor of Nursing.

DNA deoxyribonucleic acid; District Nursing Association.

DNase deoxyribonuclease.

DNE Diploma in Nursing Education; Director of Nurse Education.

DNS Director of Nursing Services.

DO Diploma in Ophthalmology.

D_{LO_2} diffusing capacity of the lung for oxygen.

DObstRCOG Diploma in Obstetrics, of the Royal College of Obstetricians and Gynaecologists.

dobutamine (doh'byootəˌmeen) a synthetic catecholamine administered parenterally for inotropic support in short-term treatment of adults with cardiac decompensation due to depressed contractility resulting either from organic heart disease or from cardiac surgical procedures.

Dobutrex ('dohbyuhˌtreks) trademark for a preparation of dobutamine, a synthetic catecholamine.

doctor (doktə) 1. registered medical practitioner (on the Medical Register maintained by the General Medical Council). 2. a holder of a university doctorate degree.

docusate sodium ('dokyuhˌsayt) an ionic surfactant used as a faecal softener.

Döderlein's bacillus ('dardəˌlienz) a nonpathogenic lactobacillus occurring normally in vaginal secretions. Metabolism of glycogen within the squamous epithelium lining the vagina produces lactic acid. The resulting pH of 4.5 effectively counteracts the alkalinity of cervical mucus and proves hostile to pathogenic organisms.

Döhle body (dərlə) small (1–2 μm) oval inclusion sometimes found in polymorphonuclear leukocytes showing toxic granulation in response to infection.

dol (dol) a unit of pain intensity.

DOLD diffuse obstructive lung disease (see CHRONIC OBSTRUCTIVE AIRWAYS DISEASE).

dolich(o)- word element. [Gr.] *long*.

dolichocephalic (ˌdolikohkə'falik, -sə'falik) having a narrow, long head.

dolichofacial (ˌdolikoh'fayshəl) having a long face.

dolicomorphic (ˌdolikoh'mawfik) having a long, thin, asthenic body type.

Dolobid ('dolohbid) trademark for a preparation of diflunisal, an anti-inflammatory and analgesic drug used in the treatment of osteoarthritis and rheumatoid arthritis.

dolor ('dolə, 'dohlə) [L.] *pain;* one of the cardinal signs of inflammation.

d. capitis headache.

dolorific (ˌdohlə'rifik) producing pain.

dolorimeter (ˌdohlə'rimitə) an instrument for measuring pain in dols.

dominance ('dominəns) 1. the supremacy, or superior manifestation, in a specific situation of one of two or more competitive or mutually antagonistic factors. 2. the appearance, in the phenotype of a heterozygote, of one of two mutually antagonistic parental characters.

dominant ('dominənt) 1. exerting a ruling or controlling influence; in genetics, capable of expression when carried by only one of a pair of homologous chromosomes. 2. a dominant allele or trait.

d. gene one that produces an effect (the phenotype) in the organism regardless of the state of the corresponding allele. An example of a trait determined by a dominant gene is brown eye colour (see also HEREDITY).

domperidone (dom'peridohn) used in the treatment of nausea and vomiting. Cardiac problems associated with the intravenous use of domperidone have meant that its use has now been restricted to named patients only.

Donath–Landsteiner test (ˌdohnath'landstienə) a test for paroxysmal cold haemoglobinuria based on the fact that the blood of patients with this disease contains isohaemolysin and autohaemolysin that unites with erythrocytes only at low temperatures (2 to 10 °C), haemolysis occurring only after warming with the complement to 37 °C.

donor ('dohnə) 1. an organism that supplies living tissue to be used in another body, as a person who furnishes blood for transfusion, or an organ for transplantation. 2. a substance or compound that contributes part of itself to another substance (acceptor).

universal d. a person with group O blood; such blood is sometimes used in emergency transfusion. Transfusion of blood cells rather than whole blood is preferred.

Donovan bodies ('donəvən) encapsulated bacteria (*Calymmatobacterium granulomatis)* found in lesions of granuloma inguinale.

Donovania granulomatis (ˌdonoh'vayni·ə ˌgranyuh'lohmətis) *Calymmatobacterium granulomatis.*

dopa ('dohpə) L-3,4-dihydroxyphenylalanine, produced by oxidation of tyrosine by tyrosinase; it is the precursor of dopamine and an intermediate product in the biosynthesis of noradrenaline and adrenaline. It is used in PARKINSON'S DISEASE and manganese poisoning. Called also *L-dopa* and *levodopa.*

dopa-oxidase (ˌdohpə'oksiˌdays) an enzyme that oxidizes dopa to melanin in the skin, producing pigmentation.

dopamine ('dohpəˌmeen) a compound, hydroxytyramine, produced by the decarboxylation of dopa; an intermediate product in the synthesis of noradrenaline. It is a neurotransmitter in the central nervous system. It is administered intravenously to correct haemodynamic imbalance in shock syndrome.

dopaminergic (ˌdohpəmiˈnərjik) activated or transmitted by dopamine; pertaining to tissues or organs affected by dopamine.

Doppler effect (ˈdoplə) the relationship of the apparent frequency of waves, as of sound, light, and radio waves, to the relative motion of the source of the waves and the observer, the frequency increasing as the two approach each other and decreasing as they move apart.

The Doppler effect can be experienced when a train whistle or car horn produces a continuous sound as it approaches and passes a listener. The pitch of the sound suddenly falls as the source passes the listener.

Doppler ultrasound flowmeter a device for measuring blood flow that transmits sound at a frequency of several megahertz along a blood vessel. Some of the sound waves are reflected by the moving red blood cells back toward the transducer. The difference in pitch between the transmitted and reflected sounds is produced as an audible tone and is proportional to the velocity of blood flow. The flowmeter can be incorporated into a real-time ultrasound machine so that quantitative measurements of the flow of blood through arteries and veins and across cardiac valves can be obtained. The Doppler flowmeter is capable of recording very rapid pulsatile changes in flow as well as steady flow; hence, it is helpful in assessing intermittent claudication, thrombus obstruction of deep veins, and other abnormalities of blood flow in the major arteries and veins. Changes in flow may be correlated with pressure gradients across stenosed vessels and valves. It is often incorporated with ultrasonic imaging scanners to make a 'duplex' diagnostic instrument.

Dorbanex (ˈdawbəneks) trademark for the combination of danthron with poloxamer, recently withdrawn from the UK market. See also CO-DANTHRAMER.

Dormia basket (ˈdawmi·ə) a cage-like instrument which is attached to a CHOLEDOCHOSCOPE and used to remove gallstones. The basket is positioned in the bile duct alongside the stone, and then opened, trapping the stone. The basket and stone are then removed along with the choledochoscope.

dornase (ˈdawnayz) a shortened term for *deo*xy*r*ibo*n*ucle*ase*; also a word termination, as in strepto*dornase*.

dors(o)- word element. [L.] *the back, dorsal aspect*.

dorsad (dawsad) toward the back.

dorsal (ˈdaws'l) directed toward or situated on the back surface; opposite the ventral.

dorsalgia (dawˈsalji·ə) pain in the back.

dorsalis (dawˈsaylis) [L.] *dorsal*.

dorsiflexion (ˌdawsiˈflekshən) backward flexion or bending, as of the hand or foot.

dorsocephalad (ˌdawsohˈkefəlad, -ˈsef-) toward the back of the head.

dorsolateral (ˌdawsohˈlatə·rəl) pertaining to the back and side.

dorsoventral (ˌdawsohˈventrəl) 1. pertaining to the back and belly surfaces of a body. 2. passing from the back to the belly surface.

dorsum (ˈdawsəm) pl. *dorsa* [L.] 1. the back; the posterior or superior surface of a body or body part, as of the foot or hand. 2. the aspect of an anatomical structure or part corresponding in position to the back; posterior in the human.

DOrth Diploma in Orthodontics.

dosage (ˈdohsij) the determination and regulation of the size, frequency, and number of doses.

dose (dohs) the quantity to be administered at one time, as a specified amount of medication or a given quantity of radiation.

absorbed d. that amount of energy from ionizing radiations absorbed per unit mass of matter, expressed in rads or Grays.

air d. the intensity of a roentgen-ray or gamma-ray beam in air, expressed in roentgens.

booster d. an amount of immunogen (vaccine, toxoid, or other antigen preparation), usually smaller than the original amount, injected at an appropriate interval after primary immunization to sustain the immune response to that immunogen.

curative d. (CD) a dose that is sufficient to restore normal health.

curative d. (median) (CD_{50}) a dose that abolishes symptoms in 50 per cent of test subjects.

divided d. a fraction of the total quantity of a drug prescribed to be given at intervals, usually during a 24-hour period.

erythema d. that amount of x-radiation which, when applied to the skin, causes temporary reddening.

fatal d. lethal dose.

genetically significant d. that aspect of radiation damage that is expressed in the descendants.

infective d. (ID) that amount of pathogenic microorganisms that will cause infection in susceptible subjects.

infective d. (median) (ID_{50}) that amount of pathogenic microorganisms that will produce infection in 50 per cent of the test subjects.

lethal d. (LD) that quantity of an agent that will or may be sufficient to cause death. See also LD_{50}.

lethal d. (median) see LD_{50}.

lethal d. (minimum) 1. the amount of toxin that will just kill an experimental animal. 2. the smallest quantity of diphtheria toxin that will kill a guinea pig of 250 g weight in 4 to 5 days when injected subcutaneously.

maximum permissible d. the largest amount of ionizing radiation that onc may safely receive according to recommended limits in radiation protection guides.

skin d. 1. the air dose of radiation at the skin surface, comprising the primary radiation plus backscatter. 2. the absorbed dose in the skin.

threshold erythema d. TED, the single skin dose that will produce in 80 per cent of those tested, a faint but definite erythema within 30 days, and in the other 20 per cent, no visible reaction.

tolerance d. the largest quantity of an agent that may be administered without harm.

dosimeter (dohˈsimitə) an instrument used to detect and measure exposure to radiation.

dosimetry (dohˈsimətree) scientific determination of amount, rate, and distribution of radiation emitted from a source of ionizing radiation.

dothiepin (dohˈthieəpin) a tricyclic antidepressant and sedative drug.

double bind (ˈdub'l biend) in psychiatry, a type of communication in which one individual directs contradictory verbal remarks to another who is unable to perceive the lack of congruence and cannot respond effectively or escape from the situation. Also, the situation produced by such interaction.

double-blind (ˌdub'lˈbliend) see double blind CLINICAL trial.

douche (doosh) [Fr.] a stream of water or air directed against a part of the body or into a cavity.

air d. a current of air blown into a cavity, particularly into the tympanum to open the pharyngotympanic tube.

vaginal d. irrigation of the vagina to cleanse the area, to apply medicated solutions to the vaginal mucosa and the cervix, or to apply heat in order to relieve pain, inflammation, and congestion. For the treatment to be effective the patient must be in the dorsal recumbent position with the hips level with the chest. Excessive pressure in administering the solution should be avoided so that the solution is not forced beyond the ostium uteri.

Douglas bag ('dugləs) a bag which is used to collect expired air when oxygen consumption has to be measured.

Douglas' fold a crescentic line marking the termination of the posterior layer of the sheath of the rectus abdominis muscle, just below the level of the iliac crest.

Douglas' pouch (cul-de-sac) a sac or recess formed by a fold of the peritoneum dipping down between the rectum and the uterus. Called also *rectouterine excavation* or *pouch*.

down (down) see LANUGO.

Down's syndrome (downz) a congenital condition characterized by physical malformations and some degree of mental handicap. The disorder was formerly known as mongolism because the patient's facial characteristics resemble those of persons of the Mongolian race. It is also called *trisomy 21 syndrome* because the disorder is concerned with a defect in CHROMOSOME 21.

The causes of Down's syndrome are not known. There is, however, a relatively high incidence in children of mothers who are in the older childbearing age. A particular type of Down's syndrome that occurs in children of younger mothers seems to have a tendency to occur in certain families.

The term trisomy refers to the presence of three representative chromosomes in a cell instead of the usual pair. In Down's syndrome the twenty-first chromosome pair fails to separate when the germ cell (usually the ovum) is being formed. Thus the ovum contains 24 chromosomes, and when it is fertilized by a normal sperm carrying 23 chromosomes, the child is born with an extra chromosome (or total of 47) per cell.

Although not all of the physical characteristics of Down's syndrome are always found in a child suffering from this disorder, there usually is a combination of several of them so that diagnosis can be made without difficulty at birth. These characteristics include a small, flattened skull, a short, flat-bridged nose, wide-set eyes, epicanthus, a protruding tongue that is furrowed and lacks a central fissure, short, broad hands and feet with a wide gap between the first and second toes, and a little finger that curves inward. The muscles are hypotonic and there is excessive mobility of the joints. The genitalia are often underdeveloped and congenital heart defects are not uncommon.

As the child grows older he remains below average in height and shows some degree of mental handicap.

There is no cure for Down's syndrome. Depending on the level of intelligence, the child can be helped to live productively. See also MENTAL HANDICAP.

doxapram ('doksə,pram) a respiratory stimulant, used as the hydrochloride salt.

doxepin ('doksipin) a tricyclic ANTIDEPRESSANT used for treatment of depression.

doxorubicin (,doksoh'roobisin) an antineoplastic antibiotic, which binds to DNA and inhibits synthesis of nucleic acids and cell division. It is used intravenously to produce regression in various neoplastic conditions. The side-effects include bone marrow depression, alopecia, and cardiac toxicity. Electroencephalogram monitoring is required during administration of the drug.

doxycycline (,doksi'siekleen) a broad-spectrum antibiotic, synthetically derived from oxytetracycline, active against a wide range of gram-positive and gram-negative organisms, which can be given once a day and whose absorption is not significantly affected by food or milk.

DPH Diploma in Public Health.

DPhil Doctor of Philosophy.

DPM Diploma in Psychological Medicine.

DR Diploma in Radiology.

Dr. Doctor.

dr. dram.

drachm (dram) dram.

dracontiasis (,drakon'tieəsis) a tropical disease caused by infestation with the guinea-worm; acquired by drinking contaminated water. Called also DRACUNCULIASIS.

dracunculiasis (dra,kungkyuh'lieəsis) infection by nematodes of the genus *Dracunculus*. Called also DRACONTIASIS.

Dracunculus (dra'kungkyuhləs) a genus of nematode parasites.

D. medinensis the guinea-worm, a threadlike worm widely distributed in Africa, the Middle East and India; found in the subcutaneous and intermuscular tissues of man and certain other animals; acquired by drinking contaminated water.

drain (drayn) 1. to withdraw liquid gradually. 2. any device by which a channel or open area may be established for exit of fluids or purulent material from a cavity, wound, or infected area. See also WOUND HEALING.

cigarette d., Penrose d. a drain made by drawing a small strip of gauze or surgical sponge into a tube of thin flexible plastic material.

drainage ('draynij) systematic withdrawal of fluids and discharges from a wound, sore, or cavity.

capillary d. that effected by material of solid core small calibre facilitating capillary attraction.

closed d. hermetically sealed drainage of a closed cavity.

open d. drainage through an opening not sealed against the entrance of outside air.

postural d. drainage by gravity, thus necessitating an appropriate posture such as recumbency in the head-down position in order to drain a lung. See also POSTURAL DRAINAGE.

tidal d. drainage of the urinary bladder by an apparatus that alternately fills the bladder with fluid to a predetermined pressure and empties it by a combination of siphonage and gravity flow.

dram (dram) a unit of weight in the avoirdupois (27.344 grains, 1/16 ounce) or apothecaries' (60 grains, 1/8 ounce) system; symbol ʒ. Sometimes also spelled *drachm*.

fluid d. a unit of liquid measure of the apothecaries' system, containing 60 minims, and equivalent to 3.697 ml. Abbreviated fl. dr.

Dramamine ('dramə,meen) trademark for preparation of dimenhydrinate, an antihistamine effective against nausea and vomiting, especially in motion sickness.

draught (drahft) a potion or dose.

drawsheet ('dror,sheet) a narrow sheet placed across the bed under a patient to prevent soiling of the main sheet. The sheet is twice the width of the bed to enable a clean piece to be drawn under the patient without the whole sheet being changed.

DRCPath Diploma of the Royal College of Pathologists.

dream (dreem) a series of images, emotions, or thoughts occurring during SLEEP.

drepanocyte ('drepənoh,siet) a sickle cell. adj. **drepanocytic.**

drepanocytosis (,drepənohsie'tohsis) occurrence of drepanocytes (sickle cells) in the blood.

dressing ('dresing) any of various materials used for covering and protecting a wound. A pressure dressing is used for maintaining pressure in order to control bleeding. A protective dressing is applied to shield a part from injury or from contamination.

APPLICATION AND REMOVAL. All dressings applied to wounds and open areas should be sterile and must be handled with antiseptic technique to avoid contamination of the wound. Before applying or changing a dressing, assemble all equipment and medications to be used. The hands are always washed with soap and running water immediately before changing dressings, even if sterile gloves are to be used.

A soiled dressing is removed by starting at the outer edges and releasing tape or other adhesive bandages, pulling *toward* the wound so as to avoid strain or damage to the healing tissues. This is done gently and slowly, and if there is dried exudate holding the dressing to the wound, sterile saline solution is applied until it loosens. All soiled dressings are placed in a paper bag, or wrapped in several thicknesses of newspaper. They are never left in the patient's room. They should be discarded in an incinerator or in a container provided for this purpose.

If sterile technique is required for the changing of a dressing, sterile gloves are worn during the procedure. The first step is to open a sterile towel or wrapper and establish a sterile field from which to work. All principles of an aseptic technique must be observed when handling equipment. Containers of drugs to be applied are opened and the wrappings from dressings to be used are removed. After the equipment is ready and the soiled dressings are removed, either gloves are put on or sterile forceps are used and the clean dressings applied. The wound is cleansed with a mild antiseptic each time a dressing is changed, unless otherwise directed by the doctor.

Dressings may be held in place by a variety of tapes, bandages, or binders. The type chosen will depend on the location of the wound and the tolerance of the patient's skin to different adhesives. If there is profuse drainage from the wound, absorbent pads may be applied and then covered with a moisture-proof dressing. After the procedure is completed all equipment is removed and the patient's unit is left in order. The hands should be washed immediately after leaving the patient's room or unit.

DRESSING MATERIALS. A wide variety of materials may be used as dressings for open wounds, both dry and wet. Dry materials include traditional cotton and synthetic gauze which absorb exudate but stick to the wound when dry. Other synthetic 'non-stick' gauze type pads stick less but may still adhere if allowed to dry out. There are a range of dressings which are non-adherent, such as foam dressings and biological dressings (the latter are made from seaweed and degraded by the body). Occlusive dressings, normally transparent, semi-permeable film, are left over a wound until the wound is healed and/or they drop off. Medicated dressings are pads of gauze or bandages which include another substance, e.g., tulle gras, zinc paste bandages. Materials to secure dressings include gauze, crepe and stretch mesh bandages, adhesive tapes, some of which may be waterproof and others of 'non-allergic' material. Cleansing dressing materials include swabs of cotton wool, gauze, some of which may be mounted on sticks for ease of use. Solutions used to cleanse wounds are sterile water, saline and a wide range of antiseptics. See also ASEPSIS.

drift (drift) 1. a chance variation, as in gene frequency from one generation to another; the smaller the population, the greater are the random variations. 2. a small but steady change in the calibration of an instrument due, for example, to heating effects.

Drinker respirator (drinkə) a type of VENTILATOR that provides controlled, automatic breathing for a patient whose respiratory muscles are paralysed (see also IRON LUNG).

drip (drip) the slow, drop-by-drop infusion of a liquid.

postnasal d. drainage of excessive mucous or mucopurulent discharge from the postnasal region into the pharynx.

drive (driev) the force that activates human impulses.

dromotropic (,drohmoh'tropik) affecting conductivity of a nerve fibre.

drop (drop) 1. a minute sphere of liquid as it hangs or falls. 2. a descent or falling below the usual position.

d. foot a condition in which the foot hangs in a plantar-flexed position, due to lesion of the peroneal nerve.

droperidol (droh'peri,dol) a tranquillizer of the butyrophenone series, used as a narcoleptic preanaesthetic and, in combination with fentanyl citrate, as a neuroleptanalgesic.

droplet infection ('droplət) infection due to inhalation of respiratory pathogens suspended on liquid particles exhaled from someone already infected.

dropper ('dropə) a pipette or tube for dispensing liquids in drops.

dropsical ('dropsik'l) affected with or pertaining to dropsy.

dropsy ('dropsee) an abnormal accumulation of serous fluid in a body cavity or in the cellular tissues; called also *hydrops*.

drostanolone propionate (dro'stanəlohn 'prohpeeonayt) an androgenic, anabolic steroid compound; used for palliative treatment of advanced metastatic breast cancer (second or third line) in post-menopausal women.

drowning ('drowning) death from suffocation resulting from aspiration of water or other substance or fluid. Drowning occurs because the liquid prevents breathing. The lungs of a drowned person contain very little water or other liquid.

First-aid measures are begun as soon as the individual is rescued from the water. He should not be allowed to walk or remain standing if he has undergone a prolonged struggle to stay afloat because of the strain on his heart. Shock should be prevented by keeping the victim in a prone position with the head lower than the rest of the body. Blankets and other coverings are used only to prevent loss of body heat; the victim should not be kept overwarm. *No time should be lost in administering* ARTIFICIAL RESPIRATION *to anyone who has stopped breathing.* If the victim is unconscious but still breathing, he should be placed in a reclining position, preferably on his side. If the victim is not breathing and there is no evidence of a heartbeat, CARDIOPULMONARY RESUSCITATION is begun immediately.

drug (drug) 1. any medicinal substance. 2. a narcotic. 3. to administer a drug.

d. abuse the use of one or more drugs for purposes other than those for which they are prescribed or recommended. The major groups of drugs and medicines generally considered to be most commonly misused are stimulants ('uppers'), depressants ('downers'), psychedelics, and narcotics.

The stimulants affect the central nervous system, producing increased physical and mental activity, excitability, and prevention of sleep. Among the more popular stimulants are the amphetamines, for example methamphetamine, or 'speed'. Prolonged use of these drugs can lead to acute toxic psychosis accompanied by hallucinations and delusions.

The depressant drugs favoured by drug abusers are the barbiturates, tranquillizers, and alcohol. Their effect is opposite to that of stimulants and they often are taken as a means of 'coming down' from a 'high' produced by a stimulant. Sudden withdrawal from depressants can cause convulsions and even death. Combinations of barbiturates and alcohol, which compound the effect of each other, frequently lead to death.

Probably the best known of the psychedelic drugs is LSD (lysergic acid diethylamide). Its use has declined in recent years because of public awareness of its long-term, if not permanent, effects on the psyche, producing 'flashbacks' of an acute psychotic state, and its implication in chromosomal damage. Another popular psychedelic drug is mescaline, which is derived from the peyote cactus.

The narcotic drugs of choice for the addict or drug abuser are heroin and cocaine. Both of these drugs are extremely potent, highly addictive, and frequently present the complication of overdose.

MARIJUANA is a controversial drug that is thought by many authorities to be the least dangerous of all drugs commonly used by drug abusers. Extensive research has not as yet led to valid conclusions about the physical or mental health hazards presented by marijuana.

There is little evidence to substantiate the frequently heard claim that experimentation with 'soft' drugs, such as marijuana, will lead to stronger drugs and narcotic addiction. There is no denying that many narcotic addicts do begin by abuse of milder drugs and experimentation with their effects on them. However, many factors enter into drug addiction, including individual personality, life style, social environment, and physical status.

'Designer drugs' are highly potent synthetic drugs, illicitly produced and may mimic the action of narcotics and psychedelic drugs, though they are often more potent than the substances they are designed to mimic. See also DESIGNER DRUG.

d. addiction a state of periodic or chronic intoxication produced by the repeated consumption of a drug, characterized by (1) an overwhelming desire or need (compulsion) to continue use of the drug and to obtain it by any means, (2) a tendency to increase the dosage, (3) a psychological and usually a physical dependence on its effects, and (4) a detrimental effect on the individual and on society.

REASONS FOR ADDICTION. Addiction can result from extensive exposure to drugs for the relief of pain, although this is rare. The majority of persons who become addicted do so because of psychological or emotional needs to avoid facing deep personal problems. The use of drugs can create a false sense of well-being that temporarily, if inadequately, helps the user to escape from his problems. The use of drugs for this purpose only adds to a person's difficulties, because he is faced with additional problems of obtaining a supply of drugs through illegal sources. The main purpose in an addict's life frequently centres on how to obtain the money necessary to purchase more drugs for his addiction. Because of this, many addicts resort to criminal acts in their effort to maintain their addiction.

WITHDRAWAL AND TREATMENT. There are differences of opinion on the treatment methods of withdrawal from narcotic addiction. The most extreme method, often known as 'cold turkey', is abrupt and uncomfortable. It is the natural process that occurs when no more drugs are taken. In the prison system, the method of withdrawal is a matter for the independent clinical judgement of the prison medical officer in charge of the case. Many consider that a quick, well supervised withdrawal with constant medical and nursing observation and care, is the best method. In these circumstances, tranquilizers will often be used to ease the process. It is arguable that methadone is as addictive, if not more so, as heroin, and in the security of the prison system, and in the hospital unit within a prison establishment, the possibility of resuming the drug habit is removed. Thus, the need to extend the withdrawal process by drug substitution is not necessary.

If the narcotic addict's dosage has been mild, his withdrawal is equally mild and may include yawning, sneezing, watering eyes, perspiring, and running nose. In the case of the heavy user, the symptoms become increasingly severe. These include severe cramps, vomiting, diarrhoea, and muscle spasms. Withdrawal in this manner lasts approximately 2 to 4 days. Since he cannot eat, an addict may lose 5 to 10 lb during this period.

In the controlled withdrawal method, under the supervision of a doctor, a synthetic drug, such as methadone, is substituted for the narcotic, and the dosage is gradually decreased over a period of about 10 days.

HELP FOR THE ADDICT. Help available to the addict who wants to be cured of his addiction varies throughout the UK. In most of the major cities treatment is available in the larger hospitals, in some of which beds are available for controlled withdrawal. The amount of help or treatment available varies greatly. Some hospitals maintain a staff of psychiatrists, psychologists, and social workers who offer the addict treatment for his psychological addiction and help him to look realistically at some of the problems that drove him to drugs. Many of these treatment programmes are known as 'aftercare' because the addict returns regularly for additional care following his release from the hospital. For those addicts who are sent to prison, similar programmes of individual and group treatment are offered to help him prepare for his return to the community.

The crucial period in the addict's adjustment following withdrawal is his attempt to find a place in community life. Job-hunting is difficult because he is often unable to explain his periods of unemployment and hospitalization. Many social service agencies offer treatment and support to these individuals during this period. It is often the difficulty in readjusting to community life that leads the addict to return to his previous habit of drug-taking.

d. interaction modification of the potency of one drug by another (or others) taken concurrently or sequentially. Some drug interactions are harmful and some may have therapeutic benefits. Present knowledge of drug interactions is limited and no single chart of drug interactions can be completely accurate in predicting the effects of a drug combination on an individual patient. For this reason any person responsible for administration of medications must be ever alert to the possibility of dangerous drug interaction any time drugs are given in combination. It is recommended that a clinical pharmacologist be consulted whenever the possibility of incompatibility is suspected in a multiple-drug regimen.

Additives, for example, in an intravenous infusion may produce an adverse chemical interaction. Factors influencing these interactions include pH and chemical composition, especially the various buffering, stabilizing, and preserving chemicals present in commercially prepared intravenous solutions. Due to the variety and volume of drugs and chemicals available and the high potential of incompatibility, it is recommended that admixtures be restricted to a single additive in each intravenous solution administered.

Drugs may also interact with various foods. In general, these interactions fall into three categories: (1) food malabsorption; (2) nutritional status; and (3) alteration of drug response by nutrients. In teaching patients self-care in the taking of prescribed medications, one should explain the need for meticulously following directions related to the intake of food and drink while the medication regimen is being followed.

druggist ('drugist) pharmacist.

drusen ('droozən) 1. hyaline excrescences in Bruch's membrane, the inner layer of the choroid of the eye, usually due to ageing. 2. rosettes of granules occurring in the lesions of actinomycosis.

dry ice (drie 'ies) carbon dioxide snow.

DSc Doctor of Science.

DSS Department of Social Security.

DTM&H Diploma in Tropical Medicine and Hygiene.

DTPA diethylenetriaminepentaacetic acid.

DTPer/Vac/Ads diphtheria, tetanus and pertussis vaccine, adsorbed.

DT/Vac/Ads diphtheria and tetanus vaccine, adsorbed.

dualism (dyooə·lizəm) pertaining to the theories of the French philosopher and mathematician Rene Descartes (1591–1650), and is hence often referred to as CARTESIAN dualism. He suggested a strong form of dualism with the mind being indivisible and to be understood by rational study. The body he identified as being divisible and mechanical and to be understood by physical and mathematical study.

Dubin–Johnson syndrome (ˌdoobin'jonsən) hereditary chronic nonhaemolytic jaundice thought to be due to defective excretion of conjugated bilirubin and certain other organic anions by the liver; a brown coarsely granular pigment in hepatic cells is pathognomonic.

Duchenne–Aran disease (dooˌshena'ran) spinal muscular atrophy.

Duchenne's disease (doo'shenz) 1. spinal muscular atrophy. 2. bulbar paralysis. 3. tabes dorsalis.

Duchenne's muscular dystrophy the childhood type of MUSCULAR DYSTROPHY.

Duchenne's paralysis 1. Erb-Duchenne paralysis. 2. progressive bulbar paralysis.

Ducrey's bacillus (doo'krayz) *Haemophilus ducreyi*, the organism causing soft chancre. See CHANCROID.

duct (dukt) a passage with well-defined walls, especially a tubular structure for the passage of excretions or secretions. adj. **ductal**.

alveolar d's small passages connecting the respiratory bronchioles and the alveolar sacs.

d. of Bartholin the larger and longer of the sublingual ducts.

bile d's, biliary d's the passages for the conveyance of bile in and from the liver (see also BILE DUCTS).

cochlear d. a spiral membranous tube in the bony canal of the cochlea divided into the scala tympani, scala vestibuli, and spiral lamina.

common bile d. a duct formed by the union of the cystic and hepatic ducts (see also BILE DUCTS).

cystic d. the passage connecting the gallbladder neck and the common bile duct.

efferent d. any duct that gives outlet to a glandular secretion.

ejaculatory d. the duct formed by union of the ductus deferens and the duct of the seminal vesicles, opening into the prostatic urethra on the colliculus seminalis.

endolymphatic d. a canal connecting the membranous labyrinth of the ear with the endolymphatic sac.

excretory d. one through which the secretion is conveyed from a gland.

hepatic d. the excretory duct of the liver, or one of its branches in the lobes of the liver (see also BILE DUCTS).

lacrimal d. the excretory duct of the lacrimal gland (see also LACRIMAL APPARATUS). Called also *lacrimal canaliculus*.

lacrimonasal d. nasal duct.

lactiferous d's ducts conveying the milk secreted by the lobes of the breast to and through the nipples.

lymphatic d., left thoracic duct.

lymphatic d., right a vessel draining lymph from the upper right side of the body, receiving lymph from the right subclavian, jugular, and mediastinal trunks when those vessels do not open independently into the right brachiocephalic vein.

mammary d. lactiferous ducts.

mesonephric d. an embryonic duct of the mesonephros, which in the male becomes the epididymis, ductus deferens and its ampulla, seminal vesicles, and ejaculatory duct, and in the female is largely obliterated.

müllerian d. either of the two paired embryonic ducts developing into the vagina, uterus, and uterine tubes, and becoming largely obliterated in the male. **nasal d., nasolacrimal d.** the downward continuation of the lacrimal sac, opening on the lateral wall of the inferior meatus of the nose (see also LACRIMAL APPARATUS).

pancreatic d. the main excretory duct of the pancreas, which usually unites with the common bile duct before entering the duodenum at the major duodenal papilla (see also BILE DUCTS).

papillary d's the straight excretory or collecting portions of the renal tubules, which descend through the renal medulla to a renal papilla.

paramesonephric d. müllerian duct.

paraurethral d's Skene's glands.

parotid d. the duct by which the parotid glands empty into the mouth (see also PAROTID GLANDS).

prostatic d's minute ducts from the prostate, opening into or near the prostatic sinuses on the posterior wall of the urethra.

salivary d's the ducts of the salivary glands.

semicircular d's the long ducts of the membranous labyrinth of the ear.

seminal d's the passages for conveyance of spermatozoa and semen.

sublingual d's the excretory ducts of the sublingual salivary glands.

submandibular d., submaxillary d. the duct that drains the submandibular gland and opens at the sublingual caruncle.

tear d. lacrimal duct.

thoracic d. a duct beginning in the cisterna chyli and emptying into the venous system at the junction of the left subclavian and left internal jugular veins. It acts as a channel for the collection of lymph from the portions of the body below the diaphragm and from the left side of the body above the diaphragm.

ductile ('duktiel) susceptible to being drawn out without breaking.

ductless ('duktləs) having no excretory duct.

d. glands endocrine glands. See ENDOCRINE.

ductule ('duktyool) a minute duct.

ductulus ('duktyuhləs) pl. *ductuli* [L.] ductule.

ductus ('duktəs) pl. *ductus* [L.] duct.

d. arteriosus a fetal blood vessel that joins the aorta and pulmonary artery.

d. arteriosus, patent abnormal persistence of an open lumen in the ductus arteriosus after birth (see also PATENT DUCTUS ARTERIOSUS).

d. deferens the excretory duct of the testis, which joins the excretory duct of the seminal vesicle to form the ejaculatory duct; called also *vas deferens*.

d. venosus a major blood channel that develops through the embryonic liver from the left umbilical vein to the inferior vena cava.

dullness ('dulnəs) a quality of sound elicited by percussion, being short and high-pitched with little resonance.

dumb (dum) unable to speak; mute.

dumping syndrome ('dumping) nausea, weakness, sweating, palpitation, syncope, often a sensation of warmth, and sometimes diarrhoea, occurring after ingestion of food in patients who have had partial gastrectomy (see also surgery of the STOMACH).

duodenal (ˌdyooə'deenəl) of or pertaining to the duodenum.

d. ulcer peptic ulcer of the duodenum (see also peptic ULCER).

duodenectomy (ˌdyooədi'nektəmee) total or partial excision of the duodenum.

duodenitis (ˌdyooədi'nietis) inflammation of the duodenum.

duodenocholedochotomy (ˌdyooəˌdeenohˌkohlidoh'kotəmee) incision of the duodenum and common bile duct.

duodenoenterostomy (ˌdyooəˌdeenohˌentə'rostəmee) anastomosis of the duodenum to some other part of the small intestine.

duodenography (ˌdyooədi'nogrəfee) radiography of the duodenum.

duodenohepatic (ˌdyooəˌdeenoh·hi'patik) pertaining to the duodenum and liver.

duodenojejunostomy (ˌdyooəˌdeenohˌjejuh'nostəmee) anastomosis of the duodenum to the jejunum.

duodenorrhaphy (ˌdyooədi'no·rəfee) suture of the duodenum.

duodenoscopy (ˌdyooədi'noskəpee) examination of the duodenum by an endoscope.

duodenostomy (ˌdyooədi'nostəmee) surgical formation of a permanent opening into the duodenum.

duodenotomy (ˌdyooədi'notəmee) incision of the duodenum.

duodenum (ˌdyooə'deenəm) the first or proximal portion of the small intestine, extending from the pylorus to the jejunum. It is about 25 cm long. It plays an important role in digestion of food because both the common bile duct and the pancreatic duct empty into it. (See also DIGESTIVE system.) It is subject to various disorders, the most common of which are peptic ULCER and obstruction due to dilation of the intestine and stasis of the duodenal contents. The duodenum also may be the site of diverticula, fistulas and, rarely, tumours.

Duphalac ('dyoofəlak) trademark for a preparation of lactulose used to decrease blood ammonia levels in portosystemic encephalopathy. It is also used as a laxative.

duplication (ˌdyoopli'kayshən) a doubling; in genetics, the presence of an extra segment of chromosome.

dupp (dup) a syllable used to represent, or mimic the second sound heard at the apex of the heart in auscultation (see also HEART SOUNDS).

Dupuytren's contracture (ˌduhpwi'trenz) a flexion deformity of the fingers or toes, due to shortening, thickening, and fibrosis of the palmar or plantar fascia.

Dupuytren's fracture Pott's fracture.

dura mater ('dyooə·rə mahtə, -maytə) [L.] the outermost, toughest and most fibrous of the three membranes (meninges) covering the brain and spinal cord.

dural ('dyooə·rəl) pertaining to the dura mater.

Durham rule ('durəm) a court decision which states that the McNaghten rule and irresistible impulse test are not compatible with modern psychiatric thought, and holds that 'an accused is not criminally responsible if his unlawful act was the product of mental disease or mental defect'.

Durham's tube ('durəmz) a jointed tracheotomy tube.

duroarachnitis (ˌdyooə·rohˌarək'nietis) inflammation of the dura mater and arachnoid.

Duromine ('dyuhrohmeen, -ien) trademark for a preparation of phentermine hydrochloride, an anorexic.

Duroziez's disease (duh'rohziˌayz) congenital mitral stenosis.

Duroziez's murmur (sign) in aortic insufficiency, a double murmur over the femoral artery or other large peripheral artery.

Duvadilan (dyoo'vadilan) trademark for preparations of isoxsuprine, a vasodilator.

Duverney's fracture (duh'vərnayz) fracture of the ilium just below the anterior inferior spine.

DVI digital vascular imaging, see SUBTRACTION.

DVS digital vascular subtraction, see SUBTRACTION.

dwarf (dwawf) an abnormally undersized person.

dwarfism ('dwawfizəm) the state of being a dwarf; retarded growth, underdevelopment of the body. Dwarfism may be the result of a developmental anomaly, of nutritional or hormone deficiencies, or of other diseases. The size of pygmies found in some parts of the world, such as the Philippines and equatorial Africa, is not the result of dwarfism; their small stature is a hereditary trait.

An adult short in stature may be as small as 0.75 m (2½ feet) tall. The proportions of body to head and limbs may be normal or abnormal. The dwarf may also be deformed, and may suffer from mental handicap, depending on the cause of his condition.

Achondroplasia is a developmental anomaly that affects the growth of the bones. The patient's trunk is usually normal, but his head is unusually large and his arms and legs unusually short. Most fetuses with achondroplasia are stillborn. Those who reach adulthood do not suffer any lessening of their mental or sexual abilities, and may have unusual muscular strength. Achondroplasia does not significantly shorten the patient's life span.

An infant who suffers from an insufficiency of thyroxine, a hormone secreted by the thyroid gland, may develop the symptoms of CRETINISM. These include an enlarged head, short limbs, puffy eyes, a thick and protruding tongue, very dry skin, and lack of coordination. Cretinism is treated by giving the child thyroxine; early treatment can result in normal growth and development. If the condition is not treated, however, the child will grow up mentally handicapped, sexually sterile, and short.

Growth hormone, a hormone that plays a major role in the process of growth is produced in the pituitary gland. If this hormone is not produced in sufficient quantity, the patient's growth will be abnormally slight, although his head and limbs will be in normal proportion to his small torso. Administration of growth hormone has been shown to induce skeletal growth in patients with pituitary dwarfism.

Dy chemical symbol, *dysprosium.*

Dyazide ('dieə,zied) trademark for a fixed combination preparation of triamterene and hydrochlorothiazide, a diuretic.

dydrogesterone (,diedroh'jestə·rohn) an orally effective, synthetic progestin used mainly in the diagnosis and treatment of primary amenorrhoea and severe dysmenorrhoea, and in combination with oestrogen in dysfunctional menorrhagia.

dye (die) any of various coloured substances containing auxochromes and thus capable of colouring substances to which they are applied; used for staining and colouring, as test reagents, and as therapeutic agents.

dynamic (die'namik) pertaining to or manifesting force.

dynamics (die'namiks) 1. the scientific study of forces in action; a phase of mechanics. 2. the motivating or driving forces, physical or moral, in any field.

group d. see GROUP DYNAMICS.

dynamograph (die'namoh,grahf, -graf) a self-registering dynamometer.

dynamometer (,dienə'momitə) an instrument for measuring the force of muscular contraction.

dyne (dien) a unit of force; one dyne will produce an acceleration of 1 cm per second of a particle of 1 gram mass. It is equal to 10^{-5} newtons.

dynein ('dieneen) a protein from the microtubules of cilia and flagella, which functions as an ATP-splitting enzyme and is essential to the motility of cilia and flagella.

dys- word element. [Gr.] *bad, difficult, disordered.*

dysacousia, dysacousis (,disə'koosi·ə, ,disə'koosis) dysacusis.

dysacusis (,disə'kyoosis) 1. a hearing impairment in which the loss is not measurable in decibels, as in disturbances in discrimination of speech or tone quality, pitch, loudness, etc. 2. a condition in which certain sounds produce discomfort.

dysadrenalism, dysadrenia (,disə'drenə,lizəm; ,disə'dreni·ə) any disorder of adrenal function, whether of decreased or heightened function.

dysaesthesia (,disis'theezi·ə) 1. impairment of any sense, especially of the sense of touch. 2. a painful, persistent sensation induced by a gentle touch of the skin.

dysaphia (dis'afi·ə) impairment of the sense of touch.

dysarthria (dis'ahthri·ə) imperfect articulation of speech due to disturbances of muscular control resulting from central or peripheral nervous system damage.

dysarthrosis (,disah'throhsis) 1. deformity or malformation of a joint. 2. dysarthria.

dysaudia (di'sawdi·ə) impaired hearing.

dysautonomia (,disawtoh'nohmi·ə) a hereditary condition marked by defective lacrimation, skin blotching, emotional instability, motor incoordination, total absence of pain sensation, and hyporeflexia.

dysbarism (dis'barizəm) any clinical syndrome caused by difference between the surrounding atmospheric pressure and the total gas pressure in the various tissues, fluids, and cavities of the body, including such conditions as barosinusitis, barotitis media, or expansion of gases in the hollow viscera.

dysbasia (dis'baysi·ə) difficulty in walking, especially that due to a nervous lesion.

dysbetalipoproteinaemia (dis,beetə,lipoh,prohti'neemi·ə) the accumulation of abnormal β-lipoproteins in the blood.

familial d. familial hyperlipoproteinaemia, type III.

dysbulia (disbyooli·ə) weakness or perversion of the will. adj. **dysbulic.**

dyscephaly (dis'kefəlee, -'sef-) malformation of the cranium and bones of the face. adj. **dyscephalic.**

dyschezia (dis'keezi·ə) difficult defecation. A form of constipation due to delay in the passage of faeces from the pelvic colon into the rectum for evacuation.

dyschiria (dis'kieri·ə) loss of power to tell which side of the body has been touched.

dyscholia (dis'kohli·ə) a disordered condition of the bile.

dyschondroplasia (,diskondroh'playzi·ə) enchondromatosis.

dyschromatopsia (,diskrohmə'topsi·ə) disorder of colour vision.

dyschromia (dis'krohmi·ə) any disorder of pigmentation of the skin or hair.

dyschronism (,diskrohnizəm) separate in time; disturbance of any time relation.

dyscoria (dis'kor·ri·ə) abnormality in shape or form of the pupil or in the reaction of the two pupils.

dyscorticism (dis'kawtisizəm) disordered functioning of the adrenal cortex.

dyscrasia (dis'krayzi·ə) a morbid condition, usually referring to an imbalance of component elements. adj. **dyscratic.**

blood d. any abnormal or pathological condition of the blood.

dysdiadochokinesis (,disdie,adəkohki'neesis) a sign of cerebellar disease in which the ability to perform rapid alternating movements, such as rotating the hands, is lost.

dysembryoma (,disembri'ohmə) teratoma.

dysencephalia splanchnocystica (dis,enke'fayli·ə ,splangknoh'sistikə, -se'fayli·ə) Meckel's syndrome.

dysentery ('dis'ntree) any of a number of disorders marked by inflammation of the intestine, especially of the colon, with abdominal pain, tenesmus, and frequent stools often containing blood and mucus. The causative agent may be chemical irritants, bacteria, protozoa, viruses, or parasitic worms. adj. **dysenteric.** Dysentery has declined in areas with improved hygiene and sanitation. Some forms of dysentery give rise to severe illness, especially in infants, the elderly and those with intercurrent disease.

In dysentery, there is an unusually fluid discharge of stool from the bowels, as well as fever, stomach cramps, and spasms of involuntary straining to evacuate, with the passage of little faeces. The stool is often mixed with pus and mucus and may be streaked with blood.

amoebic d. a form common in tropical countries but also found elsewhere; caused by the protozoon *Entamoeba hstolytica.* Spread is exceptional in places with high standards of hygiene and sanitation. It is a notifiable disease in the UK. It is usually less acute and violent than bacillary dysentery, but it frequently becomes chronic and causes unexplained attacks of diarrhoea over a long period of time. It rarely causes death, but complications may result, including involvement of the liver, liver abscess, and pulmonary abscess. Drugs used in treatment include metronidazole, emetine hydrochloride and chloroquine. Prevention is by maintaining high standards of hygiene and sanitation. Close contacts of cases should be screened and those found to be infected treated. Called also AMOEBIASIS.

bacillary d. the most common and acute form of the disease, caused by bacteria of the genus *Shigella*; *S. sonnei* is the most frequent cause in the UK. It is a notifiable disease. Called also *shigellosis*.

Bacillary dysentery is common worldwide, but especially in the tropics and subtropics. The source of the infection is the faeces of cases or carriers and spread is by the faecal-oral route or by the contamination of food or water.

Attacks of bacillary dysentery are usually acute after the incubation period of 2–3 days. Mild cases occur, particularly in infections with *Shigella sonnei*. Temperature may rise as high as 40 °C (104 °F), sometimes with symptoms of dehydration, shock, and delirium. Bowel movements of blood-stained mucus may be as many as 30 to 40 a day. Running its normal course, without special medicines, it is usually over within a few weeks from its outset, although an attack in a child may be more serious and last longer.

Treatment is by fluid replacement by oral or intravenous administration to correct the FLUID VOLUME DEFICIT and electrolyte imbalance, and appropriate chemotherapy. Antibiotics such as chlortetracycline and chloramphenicol are often effective in shortening the duration of illness but should be reserved for the more severe cases and preferably given only after drug sensitivity tests on the organisms isolated have indicated which antibiotic is the most appropriate.

Prevention is by maintaining high standards of hygiene and sanitation. Contacts of cases need only be screened if they are food handlers, health care workers or children under 5 years of age or where there are poor standards of personal hygiene. They should be excluded from work or school until three negative faeces specimens have been obtained.

dyserethesia (ˌdiseri'theezi·ə) 1. impairment of sensibility. 2. an unpleasant abnormal sensation produced by a stimulus.

dysergasia (ˌdisər'gayzi·ə) a behaviour disorder due to organic changes in the nervous system, with disorientation, hallucination, and delirious reactions.

dysergia (di'sərji·ə) motor incoordination due to defect of efferent nerve impulse.

dysfunction (dis'fungkshən) disturbance, impairment, or abnormality of functioning of an organ.

minimal brain d. a disturbance of children and adolescents of normal or above normal intelligence without signs of major neurological or psychiatric disorder who have central nervous system deficits that affect their behaviour and ability to learn.

dysgalactia (ˌdisgə'lakshi·ə) disordered milk secretion.

dysgammaglobulinaemia (disˌgaməˌglobyuhli'neemi·ə) an immunological deficiency state marked by selective deficiencies of one or more, but not all, classes of immunoglobulins, resulting in heightened susceptibility to those infectious diseases vulnerable to immunoglobulin-associated defence mechanisms. adj. **dysgammaglobulinaemic.**

dysgenesis (dis'jenəsis) defective development; malformation.

gonadal d. any of a variety of gonadal developmental anomalies, including gonadal dysplasia, Turner's syndrome, etc.

dysgerminoma (ˌdisjərmi'nohmə) a solid, often radiosensitive, malignant ovarian neoplasm derived from undifferentiated germinal cells; the counterpart of seminoma of the testis.

dysgeusia (dis'gyoozi·ə) impairment of the sense of taste.

dysglycaemia (ˌdisglie'seemi·ə) any disorder of blood sugar metabolism.

dysgnathia (dis'naythi·ə) any oral abnormality extending beyond the teeth to involve the maxilla or mandible, or both. adj. **dysgnathic.**

dysgnosia (dis'nohzi·ə) any abnormality of the intellect.

dysgonic (dis'gonik) seeding badly; said of bacterial cultures that grow poorly.

dysgraphia (dis'grafi·ə) inability to write properly; it may be part of a language disorder due to disturbance of the parietal lobe or of the motor system.

dyshaematopoiesis (disˌheemətohpoy'eesis) defective blood formation. adj. **dyshaematopoietic.**

dyshesion (dis'heezhən) 1. disordered cell adherence. 2. loss of intercellular cohesion; a characteristic of malignancy.

dyshidrosis (dis·hi'drohsis) 1. a skin eruption on the sides of the digits or on the palms and soles. Called also *pompholyx*. 2. any disorder of the eccrine sweat glands.

dyskaryosis (ˌdiskari'ohsis) abnormality of the nucleus of a cell. adj. **dyskaryotic.**

dyskeratoma (ˌdiskerə'tohmə) a dyskeratotic tumour.

warty d. a solitary brownish red nodule with a soft, yellowish, central keratotic plug, most commonly occurring on the face, neck, scalp, or axilla, or in the mouth; histologically it resembles an individual lesion of keratosis follicularis.

dyskeratosis (ˌdiskerə'tohsis) abnormal, premature, or imperfect keratinization of the keratinocytes. adj. **dyskeratotic.**

dyskinesia (ˌdiski'neezi·ə) impairment of the power of voluntary movement.

d. tarda, tardive d. involuntary repetitive movements of the facial, buccal, oral, and cervical musculature, affecting chiefly the elderly; induced by long-term use of antipsychotic agents, often persisting after withdrawal of the agent.

dyslalia (dis'layli·ə) impairment of ability to speak associated with abnormality of external speech organs.

dyslexia (dis'leksi·ə) impairment of ability to comprehend written language, due to a central lesion. adj. **dyslexic.**

dyslipoproteinaemia (disˌlipohˌprohti'neemi·ə) the presence of abnormal lipoproteins in the blood.

dyslogia (dis'lohji·ə) impairment of the power of reasoning; also, impairment of speech, due to mental disorders.

dysmaturity (ˌdismə'tyooə·ritee) the condition of being small or immature for gestational age; said of fetuses that are the product of a pregnancy involving placental insufficiency or dysfunction. Called also *small for dates* or *light for gestational age*.

pulmonary d. Wilson–Mikity syndrome.

dysmelia (dis'meeli·ə) malformation of a limb or limbs due to disturbance in embryonic development.

dysmenorrhoea (disˌmenə'reeə) painful menstruation. adj. **dysmenorrhoeal.** Dysmenorrhoea is characterized by cramplike pains in the lower abdomen, and sometimes accompanied by headache, irritability, mental depression, malaise, and fatigue. There are a variety of causes, but in many cases the factors involved may be extremely elusive. Relief can often be obtained by simple hygienic measures such as adequate rest, avoidance of constipation, moderate exercise, applications of moderate heat to the abdomen, and removal of restricting clothing.

Severe dysmenorrhoea requires more aggressive therapy with analgesics and, in some cases, hormonal contraceptives and other prescription drugs. Prostaglandins have been found to be a cause of some forms of dysmenorrhoea, which respond well to drugs that act as antiprostaglandins. Antiprostaglandins show promise in the relief of selected cases of dysmenorrhoea, but they have potentially serious side-effects and must be prescribed and taken with caution.

congestive d. that accompanied by great congestion of the uterus.

essential d. painful menstruation for which there is no demonstrable cause.

inflammatory d. that due to inflammation.

membranous d. that marked by membranous exfoliation derived from the uterus.

obstructive d. that due to mechanical obstruction to the discharge of menstrual fluid.

dysmetria (dis'metri·ə) inability to properly direct or limit motions.

dysmimia (dis'mimi·ə) impairment of the power to express thoughts by gestures.

dysmnesia (dis'neezi·ə) disordered memory.

dysmorphism (dis'mawfizəm) 1. appearing under different morphological forms. 2. an abnormality in morphological development. adj. **dysmorphic**.

dysmyelopoietic syndrome (dis,mieəlohpoy'eetik) myelodysplastic syndrome.

dysmyotonia (,dismieoh'tohni·ə) muscular dystonia; abnormal tonicity.

dysodontiasis (,disohdon'tieəsis) defective, delayed, or difficult eruption of the teeth.

dysontogenesis (,disontoh'jenəsis) defective embryonic development. adj. **dysontogenetic**.

dysopia (dis'ohpi·ə) defective vision.

dysorexia (,disə'reksi·ə) impaired or deranged appetite.

dysosmia (dis'ozmi·ə) impairment of the sense of smell.

dysostosis (,diso'stohsis) defective ossification; a defect in the normal ossification of fetal cartilages.

cleidocranial d. a rare hereditary condition in which there is defective ossification of the cranial bones, complete or partial absence of the clavicles, so that the shoulders may be brought together, or nearly together, in front, and dental and vertebral anomalies.

craniofacial d. a hereditary condition marked by acrocephaly, exophthalmos, hypertelorism, strabismus, parrot-beaked nose, and hypoplastic maxilla with relative mandibular prognathism. Called also *Crouzon's disease*.

mandibulofacial d. a hereditary disorder occurring in a complete form (Franceschetti's syndrome) with antimongoloid slant of the palpebral fissures, coloboma of the lower lid, micrognathia and hypoplasia of the zygomatic arches, and microtia, and in an incomplete form (Treacher Collins syndrome) with the same anomalies in lesser degree.

metaphyseal d. a skeletal abnormality in which the epiphyses are normal or nearly so, and the metaphyseal tissues are replaced by masses of cartilage, producing interference with endochondral bone formation and expansion and thinning of the metaphyseal cortices.

orodigitofacial d. orofaciodigital syndrome.

dyspancreatism (dis'pankri·ə,tizəm) disorder of function of the pancreas.

dyspareunia (,dispa'rooni·ə) difficult or painful coitus in women.

dyspepsia (dis'pepsi·ə) impairment of the power or function of digestion; usually applied to epigastric discomfort after meals. adj. **dyspeptic**.

acid d. dyspepsia associated with excessive acidity of the stomach.

dysphaemia (dis'feemi·ə) stuttering or other speech disorder due to psychoneurosis.

dysphagia (dis'fayji·ə) difficulty in swallowing.

There are numerous underlying causes of dysphagia, including stroke and other neurological conditions, local trauma and muscle damage, and a tumour or swelling that partially obstructs the passage of food. The condition can range from mild discomfort, such as a feeling that there is a lump in the throat, to a severe inability to control the muscles needed for chewing and swallowing.

Dysphagia can seriously compromise the nutritional status of a patient. Temporary measures such as tube feeding and parenteral nutrition can remedy the immediate problem, but long-term goals for rehabilitation must focus on helping the patient recover the ability to swallow sufficient amounts of food and drink to assure adequate nutrition.

Nursing measures intended to accomplish the goal of oral feeding are implemented only after determining the particular techniques that are most helpful for the individual patient. In general, placing the patient in an upright position, providing a pleasant and calm environment, being sure the lips are closed as the patient begins to swallow, and preparing and serving foods of the proper consistency are all helpful techniques.

dysphasia (dis'fayzi·ə) impairment of speech consisting of lack of coordination and failure to arrange words in their proper order; due to a central lesion. See also APHASIA.

dysphonia (dis'fohni·ə) any voice impairment; difficulty in speaking. adj. **dysphonic**.

d. clericorum loss of the voice from overuse, as by clergymen.

dysphoria (dis'for·ri·ə) disquiet; restlessness; malaise.

dysphrasia (dis'frayzi·ə) imperfection of speech due to a central or cerebral defect.

dyspigmentation (,dispigmen'tayshən) any abnormality of pigmentation of the skin or hair.

dysplasia (dis'playzi·ə) an abnormality of development; in pathology, alteration in size, shape, and organization of adult cells. adj. **dysplastic**.

bronchopulmonary d. a chronic lung disease of infants, possibly related to oxygen toxicity or barotrauma, characterized by bronchiolar metaplasia and interstitial fibrosis.

congenital alveolar d. respiratory distress of the newborn.

cretinoid d. a developmental abnormality characteristic of cretinism, consisting of retarded ossification and smallness of the internal and reproductive organs.

fibrous d. (of bone) thinning of the cortex of bone and replacement of bone marrow by gritty fibrous tissue containing bony spicules, causing pain, disability, and gradually increasing deformity; it may affect a single bone (monostotic fibrous dysplasia) or several or many bones (polyostotic fibrous dysplasia).

dyspnoea (disp'neeə) laboured or difficult breathing. adj. **dyspnoeic.** Dyspnoea is a symptom of a variety of disorders and is primarily an indication of inadequate ventilation, or of insufficient amounts of oxygen in the circulating blood.

Difficult or painful breathing can be symptomatic of a variety of disorders, both acute and chronic. Acute conditions causing dyspnoea include acute infections and inflammations of the respiratory tract, obstruction by an inhaled foreign object, anaphylactic swelling of the tracheal and bronchial mucosa, and traumatic injury to the chest. Chronic disorders manifested by dyspnoea usually fall into the category of CHRONIC OBSTRUCTIVE AIRWAYS DISEASE (COAD), or are associated with pulmonary OEDEMA and congestive HEART FAILURE. A fat embolism resulting from the release of fat particles from bone marrow at the time of a fracture of a long bone also can cause dyspnoea.

Patient Care. The dyspnoeic patient has some degree of difficulty in meeting the basic physiological need for adequate levels of oxygen in the blood and the transportation of that oxygen to all cells of the body. Whatever the cause of dyspnoea, the plan of care begins with a thorough assessment of the patient's condition in order to ascertain the extent of his problem and the urgency of his need. A current and past history are obtained and a physical examination completed as soon as possible. If the patient is acutely short of breath, corrective measures should be instituted promptly. In cases of acute airway obstruction, it may be necessary to intubate the patient, begin oxygen therapy, and obtain laboratory arterial blood gas data.

If the patient is suffering from an acute attack of dyspnoea and has a history of COAD, certain nursing measures can help relieve anxiety and improve ventilation. The patient should respond favourably to a calm, reassuring manner and an explanation of what is being done to relieve his shortness of breath. Placing him in high Fowler's position or in orthopnoeic position with his arms resting on pillows on an overbed table will help improve chest expansion. Helping the patient relax muscles not needed for breathing conserves oxygen and promotes rest. Once the dyspnoeic patient is more comfortable and less apprehensive, he may need instruction in prolonged, controlled exhalation. If he already knows how to do pursed-lips breathing (i.e., inhaling slowly through the nose and then exhaling slowly through pursed lips), he may need to be reminded of this technique and encouraged to use it to improve his breathing.

Special observations and methods of assessment of a patient who has dyspnoea include: auscultation of the chest for abnormal breath and voice sounds, lung aeration, rales, and ronchi; inspection of the chest for respiratory rate and rhythm and for symmetrical expansion; inspection of the skin, lips, and nail beds for cyanosis; and percussion of the chest for abnormal resonance. Results of arterial BLOOD GAS ANALYSES should be monitored and the patient observed for fatigability when engaged in various levels of activity.

functional d. respiratory distress not caused by organic disease and unrelated to exertion but associated with anxiety states.

paroxysmal nocturnal d. respiratory distress related to posture (especially reclining at night), usually attributed to congestive heart failure with pulmonary oedema.

dyspragia (dis'prayji·ə) painful performance of any function.

dyspraxia (dis'praksi·ə) partial loss of ability to perform coordinated movements.

dysprosium (dis'prohzi·əm, -si·əm) a chemical element, atomic number 66, atomic weight 162.50, symbol Dy. See table of elements in Appendix 2.

dysproteinaemia (dis,prohti'neemi·ə) disorder of the protein content of the blood.

dysrhythmia (dis'ridhmi·ə) disturbance of rhythm.

cerebral d., electroencephalographic d. disturbance or irregularity in the rhythm of the brain waves as recorded by electroencephalography.

dyssebacea (,disi'bayshi·ə) disorder of sebaceous follicles; specifically, a condition seen (but not exclusively) in riboflavin deficiency, marked by greasy seborrhoea on the midface, with erythema in the nasal folds, canthi, or other skin folds.

dyssocial (di'sohshəl) denoting a personality disorder that is not antisocial, but is characterized by disregard for social codes, predation, and more or less criminality.

dysspermia (di'spərmi·ə) impairment of the spermatozoa, or of the semen.

dysstasia (di'stayzi·ə) difficulty in standing. adj. **dysstatic.**

dyssynergia (,disi'nərji·ə) muscular incoordination.

d. cerebellaris myoclonica dyssynergia cerebellaris progressiva associated with myoclonus epilepsy.

d. cerebellaris progressiva a condition marked by generalized intention tremors associated with disturbance of muscle tone and of muscular coordination; due to disorder of cerebellar function.

dystaxia (dis'taksi·ə) difficulty in controlling voluntary movements.

dystectia (dis'tekshi·ə) defective closure of the neural tube.

dysthymia (dis'thiemi·ə) mental depression; also, any intellectual abnormality.

dysthyroid, dysthyroidal (dis'thieroyd; ,dis·thie'royd'l) denoting defective functioning of the thyroid gland.

dystocia (dis'tohsi·ə) abnormal labour or childbirth.

fetal d. that due to shape, size, or position of the fetus.

maternal d. that due to some condition inherent in the mother.

placental d. difficult delivery of the placenta.

shoulder d. difficulty in delivering the shoulders.

dystonia (dis'tohni·ə) impairment of muscular tonus. adj. **dystonic.**

dystopia (dis'tohpi·ə) malposition; displacement. adj. **dystopic.**

dystrophia (dis'trohfi·ə) [Gr.] dystrophy.

d. adiposogenitalis adiposogenital dystrophy.

d. epithelialis corneae dystrophy of the corneal epithelium, with erosions.

d. myotonica a rare, slowly progressive, hereditary disease, marked by myotonia followed by muscular atrophy (especially of the face and neck), cataracts, hypogonadism, frontal balding, and cardiac disorders. Called also *myotonia dystrophia.*

d. unguium changes in the texture, structure, and/or colour of the nails due to no demonstrable cause, but presumed by some to be attributable to some disturbance of nutrition.

dystrophoneurosis (dis,trohfohnyuh'rohsis) 1. any nervous disorder due to poor nutrition. 2. impairment of nutrition due to a nervous disorder.

dystrophy ('distrəfee) any disorder due to defective or faulty nutrition. adj. **dystrophic.**

adiposogenital d. a condition marked by adiposity of the feminine type, genital hypoplasia, changes in secondary sexual characteristics, and metabolic disturbances; seen with lesions of the hypothalamus.

muscular d., progressive muscular d. a group of genetically determined, painless, degenerative myopathies marked by muscular weakness and atrophy without nervous system involvement (see also MUSCULAR DYSTROPHY).

myotonic d. dystrophia myotonica.

pseudohypertrophic muscular d. muscular dystrophy affecting the shoulder and pelvic girdles, beginning in childhood and marked by increasing weakness, pseudohypertrophy of the muscles, followed by atrophy, and a peculiar swaying gait with the legs kept wide apart. Called also *pseudohypertrophic paralysis.*

dysuria (dis'yooə·ri·ə) painful or difficult urination. adj. **dysuric.**

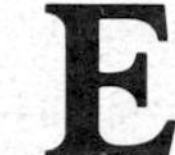

E symbol, *exa-*.

E45 a combination cream which hydrates and soothes the skin.

E-book a method of recording consultations by diagnostic category in general practice enabling epidemiological studies to be made.

ear (iə) the organ of hearing and of equilibrium. The ear is made up of the outer (external) ear, the middle ear, and the inner (internal) ear.

The outer ear consists of the auricle, or pinna, and the external acoustic meatus. The auricle collects sound waves and directs them to the external acoustic meatus which conducts them to the tympanum (the cavity of the middle ear).

The tympanic membrane (eardrum) separates the outer ear from the middle ear. In the middle ear are the three ossicles, the malleus (hammer), incus (anvil), and stapes (stirrup), so called because of their resemblance to these objects. These three small bones form a chain across the middle ear from the tympanum to the oval window in the membrane separating the middle ear from the inner ear. The middle ear is connected to the nasopharynx by the pharyngotympanic tube, through which the air pressure on the inner side of the eardrum is equalized with the air pressure on its outside surface. The middle ear is also connected with the cells in the mastoid bone just behind the outer ear. Two muscles attached to the ossicles contract when loud noises strike the tympanic membrane, limiting its vibration and thus protecting it and the inner ear from damage.

In the inner ear (or labyrinth) is the cochlea, containing the nerves that transmit sound to the brain. The inner ear also contains the SEMICIRCULAR CANALS, which are essential to the sense of balance.

When a sound strikes the ear it causes the tympanic membrane to vibrate. The ossicles function as levers, amplifying the motion of the tympanic membrane, and passing the vibrations on to the cochlea. From there the vestibulocochlear (eighth cranial) nerve transmits the vibrations, translated into nerve impulses, to the auditory centre in the brain. See also HEARING.

DISEASES OF THE EAR. Infections and inflammations of the ear include OTOMYCOSIS, a fungal infection of the outer ear; OTITIS MEDIA, an infection of the middle ear; and MASTOIDITIS, an infection of the mastoid cells. DEAFNESS may result from infection or from other causes such as old age, injury to the ear, or hereditary factors. Another cause of deafness is OTOSCLEROSIS. Disorders of equilibrium may be caused by imperfect functioning of the semicircular canals of the inner ear or from labyrinthitis, an inflammation of the inner ear. MENIÈRE'S DISEASE, believed to result from dilation of the lymphatic channels in the cochlea, may also cause disturbances in balance.

SURGERY OF THE EAR. Surgical procedures on the ear usually are indicated when chronic infection has resulted in some destruction of the bones of the middle ear or mastoid. An exception is myringotomy, incision of the tympanic membrane, which is sometimes necessary to relieve pressure behind the eardrum and allow for drainage from an inflammatory process in the middle ear. Surgical procedures involving plastic reconstruction of the small bones of the middle ear are extremely delicate and have been made possible by the development of special instruments and technical equipment. STAPEDECTOMY and TYMPANOPLASTY are examples of this type of surgery, which has done much to preserve hearing that would otherwise be lost as a result of infectious destruction or sclerosis of these bones.

Within the past decade techniques have been developed for treatment of sensorineural hearing loss. Techniques such as implantation of electronic receivers offer relief to patients who have profound sensory deafness but some remaining functional nerve cells.

PATIENT CARE. Care following surgery of the ear is aimed at prevention of infection and promoting the comfort of the patient. Since the ear is so close to the brain, it is extremely important to avoid introducing pathogenic organisms into the operative site. The external ear and surrounding skin must be kept scrupulously clean. If the patient's hair is long it should be plaited or arranged so that it does not come in contact with the patient's ear and side of the face. Aseptic technique must be used in all procedures carried out immediately before and after surgery.

The patient should be instructed to avoid nose blowing, especially after surgery, when there is a possibility that such an action can alter pressure within the ear. Observation of the patient after surgery of the ear includes watching for signs of injury to the facial nerve. The patient will not be able to wrinkle his forehead, close his eye, pucker his lips, or bare his teeth if the facial nerve has been damaged. This is often a temporary situation resulting from oedema, and will subside as the oedema is reduced. Some permanent damage may result, however, and signs of facial nerve damage should be reported to the surgeon. Vertigo is another common occurrence after surgery of the ear. It too is usually only temporary and will subside as the operative site heals. The situation does require special protective measures such as side rails, and support of the patient while he is up out of bed, so as to avoid falling and accidental injury.

Most surgeons prefer that the dressings around the ear not be changed during the immediate postoperative period. Should excessive drainage require more dressings, these can be applied over the basic dressing. Any drainage should be noted and recorded and excessive drainage reported immediately. See also care of the patient with impaired HEARING.

cauliflower e. a partially deformed auricle due to injury and subsequent perichondritis (see also CAULIFLOWER EAR).

earache ('iə-rayk) pain in the ear; otalgia.

eardrum ('iə,drum) tympanic membrane.

earwax ('iə,waks) cerumen.

Eaton agent ('eetən) *Mycoplasma pneumoniae.*

Eaton–Lambert syndrome ('eetən'lambət) a myasthenia-like syndrome in which the weakness usually affects the limbs but ocular and bulbar muscles are spared; often associated with oat-cell carcinoma of the lung.

EBM expressed breast milk.

Ebner's glands ('ebnəz) serous glands at the back of the tongue near the taste buds.

Ebola virus disease (ee'bohlə) a central African viral haemorrhagic fever with acute onset and characteristic morbilliform rash, identical clinically with Marburg disease but due to an antigenically different virus. The incubation period is 2–21 days. Outbreaks have been reported in Sudan and Zaire. It has no known source, although it is probably a zoonosis. Person-to-person spread in hospitals and laboratories by accidential inoculation of blood and tissue fluids has occurred. A single case has been reported in a laboratory worker in the UK.

EBS Emergency Bed Service.

Ebstein's anomaly ('ebstienz) a malformation of the tricuspid valve, usually associated with an atrial septal defect.

eburnation (ˌeebə'nayshən, ˌeb-) conversion of bone into a hard, ivory-like mass.

EBV Epstein–Barr virus.

ecaudate (ee'kawdayt) tail-less.

ecbolic (ek'bolik) oxytocic, i.e., makes uterine muscles contract.

ecchondroma, ecchondrosis (ˌekon'drohmə; ˌekon-'drohsis) a benign growth of cartilaginous tissue on the surface of a cartilage or projecting under the periosteum of a bone.

ecchymoma (ˌeki'mohmə) swelling due to blood extravasation.

ecchymosis (ˌeki'mohsis) pl. *ecchymoses* [Gr.] a haemorrhagic spot, larger than a petechia, in the skin or mucous membrane, forming a flat, rounded or irregular, blue or purplish patch. adj. **ecchymotic**.

eccrine ('ekrien, -rin) exocrine, with special reference to ordinary sweat glands.

eccritic (e'kritik) 1. promoting excretion. 2. an agent that promotes excretion.

ECF-A eosinophil chemotactic factor of anaphylaxis; a primary mediator of Type I anaphylactic hypersensitivity. It is an acidic peptide (molecular weight 500) released by mast cells, which attracts eosinophils to areas where it is present.

ECG electrocardiogram.

echinococcosis (eˌkienohko'kohsis) an infection, usually of the liver, caused by larval forms (hydatid cysts) of TAPEWORMS of the genus *Echinococcus*, marked by the development of expanding cysts (see also HYDATID DISEASE).

Echinococcus (eˌkienoh'kokəs) a genus of small TAPEWORMS.

E. granulosus a species parasitic in dogs, wolves and other canidae; its larvae may develop in nearly all mammals, including man, forming hydatid cysts in the liver, lungs, kidneys, and other organs.

E. multilocularis a species whose adult forms usually parasitize foxes, wolves, etc; the larvae develop in wild rodents, although man is sporadically infected. It resembles *E. granulosus*, but the larvae form alveolar or multilocular rather than unilocular cysts.

echo-ranging ('ekohˌraynjing) in ultrasonography, determination of the position or depth of a body structure on the basis of the time interval between the moment an ultrasonic pulse is transmitted and the moment its echo is received.

echoacousia (ˌekoh·ə'koosi·ə) the subjective experience of hearing echoes after normally heard sounds.

echocardiogram (ˌekoh'kahdiohˌgram) the record produced by echocardiography.

echocardiography (ˌekohˌkahdi'ogrəfee) recording of the position and motion of the heart walls or internal structures of the heart and neighbouring tissue by the echo obtained from beams of ultrasonic waves directed through the chest wall.

Echocardiography is based on the same principle as the oceanographic technique of depth-sounding; that is, it utilizes ultrasound to delineate anatomical structures by recording on a graph the echoes from the heart structures. The methods commonly used are the M-mode and the two-dimensional mode. The former records the motion of the intra-cardiac structures, and the latter records a cross-sectional view of cardiac structures. It is particularly useful in demonstrating, without danger to the patient, valvular and other structural deformities of the heart which formerly required CARDIAC CATHETERIZATION or some other elaborate procedure for accurate diagnosis. See also ULTRASONOGRAPHY.

echogenic (ˌekoh'jenik) in ultrasonography, giving rise to reflections (echoes) of ultrasound waves.

echogram ('ekohˌgram) the record made by echography.

echography (e'kogrəfee) ultrasonography; the use of ultrasound as a diagnostic aid.

echolalia (ˌekoh'layli·ə) automatic repetition by a patient of what is said to him.

echolucent (ˌekoh'loos'nt) permitting the passage of ultrasonic waves without giving rise to echoes, the representative areas appearing black on the sonogram.

echomimia (ˌekoh'mimi·ə) echopraxia.

echomotism (e'kohməˌtizəm) echopraxia.

echophonocardiography (ˌekohˌfohnohˌkahdi-'ogrəfee) the combined use of echocardiography and phonocardiography.

echophony (e'kofənee) the echo of the voice heard in the chest on auscultation.

echopraxia (ˌekoh'praksi·ə) the spasmodic and involuntary imitation of the movements of others.

echovirus ('ekohˌvierəs) a group of viruses (enteroviruses) isolated from man, the name of which was derived from the first letters of the description 'enteric cytopathogenic human orphan'. At the time of the isolation of the viruses the diseases they caused were not known, hence the term 'orphan', but it is now known that these viruses produce many different types of human disease, especially aseptic meningitis, and diarrhoea and various respiratory diseases.

Eck's fistula (eks) an artificial communication made between the portal vein and the vena cava.

eclabium (ek'laybi·əm) eversion of a lip.

eclampsia (i'klampsi·ə) a serious complication of pregnancy characterized by fits and accompanied by severe hypertension, pitting oedema and proteinuria. adj. **eclamptic.** The condition may be acute or fulminating when it develops quickly in mid-pregnancy; it is then usually necessary to terminate the pregnancy in order to save the life of the mother. More usually, eclampsia develops from pre-eclampsia. The prodromal symptoms of impending eclampsia are severe frontal headache, flashing before the eyes and other visual disturbances, epigastric or abdominal pain, nausea, and exacerbation of the three cardinal signs: hypertension, oedema and proteinuria. The aetiology of this condition is still not clear, so the only effective management is to remove the fetus and placenta. Where possible the condition should be prevented by early detection of pre-eclampsia in the antenatal period. Treatment with salt restriction, diuretics and hypertensive drugs is largely ineffective. The timing of delivery is determined by the maturity and well-being of the fetus and the condition of the mother. Labour may be induced using Syntocinon with care and monitoring the condition of the fetus closely. Alternatively caesarean section may be necessary.

An eclamptic fit is described in four phases. In the *premonitory phase* or *aura* the mother becomes restless, her face may twitch, and she may draw her arm over her face; this lasts 10–12 seconds. In the *tonic phase* the body goes into a state of muscular spasm, and adopts a hypertonic position (opisthotonos). Respiration ceases so cyanosis develops. The teeth are clenched so that passage of an airway is impossible. Fetal hypoxia develops and death may ensue. This phase lasts 10–20 seconds. The *clonic phase* is characterized by violent convulsive movements of the whole body, when physical injury is possible. Foaming occurs at the mouth, saliva may be blood-stained if the tongue is bitten, and inhalation may occur. The woman's face is congested and distorted, her breathing stertorous and her pulse full and bounding. She is unconscious. The convulsion gradually subsides within 60 to 90 seconds. The coma may last a few moments or several hours. Occasionally a further fit may occur before consciousness is regained.

The principles of management during a fit are to maintain a clear airway and prevent injury. The mother is sedated until her condition will allow delivery.

Complications of eclampsia are cerebral haemorrhage or thrombosis, liver damage, myocardial failure, acute renal failure, pulmonary oedema and bronchopneumonia, abruptio placenta and Sheehan's syndrome. Twenty per cent of fits occur antepartum, 45 per cent occur during labour, and 35 per cent occur immediately postpartum; the latter are thought to be the most serious. The current mortality rate from eclampsia is 2 per cent and the perinatal mortality rate in Britian is 6.2 per cent. With expert management, however, it is possible for the mother to make a good recovery, though some suffer residual hypertension. There is an increased risk of recurrence in subsequent pregnancies. Susceptible mothers are those with diabetes, multiple pregnancy, renal or hypertensive conditons, or hydatidiform mole, and those under 15 and over 35 years of age.

PRE-ECLAMPSIA. Pre-eclampsia is traditionally described with three cardinal signs: (1) a diastolic blood pressure 10 mmHg higher than that at booking or any blood pressure reaching 140/90 on two occasions during pregnancy; (2) excess weight gain (occult oedema) manifesting as clinical, pitting oedema in the last trimester; and (3) proteinuria—the most serious sign.

Recently a new classification of hypertensive conditions in pregnancy has been made: (1) *hypertension*, when the maternal blood pressure is 140/90 or more when first recorded in early pregnancy; pre-eclampsia may be superimposed upon this condition; (2) *gestational hypertension*, when a rise in the diastolic blood pressure to 90 mmHg or more is sustained or recurs within 24 hours at any time in the second half of pregnancy when the booking blood pressure was normal; and (3) *pre-eclampsia*, when gestational hypertension occurs as above together with proteinuria of 0.3 grams or more per litre in any 24-hour period; this condition usually manifests only the the second half of pregnancy.

Oedema is no longer considered part of the definition of pre-eclampsia because this is frequently found in normal pregnancies, when the fetal birth weight is not impaired unless proteinuria develops. Similarly excess weight gain does not affect the fetal birth weight in the absence of proteinuria. However, oedema and excess weight gain should be considered possible premonitory signs of potential pre-eclampsia.

Pre-eclampsia occurs most frequently in the first pregnancy and is more likely in mothers under 15 or over 35. The incidence falls with subsequent pregnancies. Management consists of prevention, early detection, and when diagnosed, rest and regular monitoring of the fetal condition. Placental blood flow is reduced and placental insufficiency results in a malnourished light-for-gestational-age fetus (see DYSMATURITY). Labour is induced when the fetus is thought capable of surviving better outside the uterus than within it.

puerperal e. that occurring after childbirth.

uraemic e. eclampsia due to uraemia.

eclamptogenic (i,klamptə'jenik) causing eclampsia.

ecmnesia (ek'neezi·ə) forgetfulness of recent events with remembrance of more remote ones.

ecologist (i'koləjist, ee-) a person skilled in ecology.

ecology (i'koləjee, ee-) the science of organisms as affected by environmental factors; the study of the environment and the life history of organisms. adj. **ecological.**

ecomania (,eekoh'mayni·ə) an attitude of mind that is dominating toward members of the family but humble toward those in authority.

econazole (i'konə,zohl) an antifungal similar to clotrimazole and miconazole.

Economo's encephalitis (i'konəmohz) see Economo's ENCEPHALITIS.

economy (i'konəmee) the management of money or domestic affairs.

token e. in behaviour therapy, a programme of treatment in which the patient earns tokens, exchangeable for tangible rewards, by engaging in appropriate personal and social behaviour and loses tokens for antisocial behaviour.

ecosystem (,eekoh'sistəm, ,ekoh-) the fundamental unit in ecology, comprising the living organisms and the nonliving elements interacting in a certain defined area.

ecotaxis (,eekoh'taksis) the movement or 'homing' of a circulating cell, e.g., a lymphocyte, to a specific anatomical compartment.

ecothiopate iodide (eekoh'thieohpayt) a cholinesterase inhibitor previously used to reduce intraocular pressure in glaucoma.

écraseur (,aykrə'zər) [Fr.] a snare of wire, cord or chain used to enclose a part and divide it.

ECT electroconvulsive therapy; electroplexy.

ect(o)- word element. [Gr.] *external, outside.*

ectasia (ek'tayzi·ə) expansion, dilation, or distention. adj. **ectatic.**

mammary duct e. a benign condition occurring in postmenopausal women, characterized by dilation of the ducts, inspissation of breast secretions, and periductal inflammation. Called also *comedomastitis.*

ectental (ek'tentəl) pertaining to the ectoderm and entoderm, and to their line of junction.

ecthyma (ek'thiemə) a shallowly eruptive form of impetigo, chiefly on the shins and forearms.

ectoantigen (,ektoh'anti,jən) 1. an antigen that seems to be loosely attached to the outside of bacteria. 2. an antigen formed in the ectoplasm (cell membrane) of a bacterium.

ectoblast ('ektoh,blast) the ectoderm.

ectocardia (,ektoh'kahdi·ə) congenital displacement of the heart; exocardia.

ectocervix (,ektoh'sərviks) portio vaginalis. adj. **ectocervical.**

ectoderm ('ektoh,dərm) the outermost of the three primitive germ layers of the embryo; from it are derived the epidermis and epidermic tissues, such as the nails, hair, and glands of the skin, the nervous system, external sense organs (eye, ear, etc.) and mucous membrane of the mouth and anus. adj. **ectodermal, ectodermic.**

ectodermosis (,ektohdər'mohsis) a disorder based on congenital maldevelopment of organs derived from the ectoderm.

ectoentad (,ektoh'entad) from without inward.

ectoenzyme (,ektoh'enziem) an extracellular enzyme.

ectogenous (ek'tojənəs) originating outside the organism.

ectoglobular (,ektoh'globyuhlə) formed outside the blood cells.

ectomere ('ektoh,miə) one of the blastomeres taking part in formation of the ectoderm.

ectomorph ('ektə,mawf) an individual exhibiting ectomorphy.

ectomorphy ('ektə,mawfee) a type of body build in which tissues derived from the ectoderm predominate; a somatotype in which both visceral and body structures are relatively slightly developed, the body being linear and delicate. adj. **ectomorphic**.

-ectomy word element. [Gr.] *excision, surgical removal.*

ectoparasite (,ektoh'parə,siet) a parasite living on the surface of the host's body. adj. **ectoparasitic**.

ectophyte ('ektə,fiet) a vegetable parasite living on the surface of the host's body.

ectopia (ek'tohpi·ə) [L.] *ectopy.*

e. cordis congenital displacement of the heart outside the thoracic cavity.

ectopic (ek'topik) 1. pertaining to or characterized by ectopy. 2. located away from normal position. 3. arising or produced at an abnormal site or in a tissue where it is not normally found.

e. pregnancy pregnancy in which the fertilized ovum becomes implanted outside the uterus instead of in the wall of the uterus. Called also *extrauterine pregnancy*. The ovum may rarely develop in the abdominal cavity, ovary, or uterine cervix, but ectopic pregnancy is almost always found in one of the uterine (fallopian) tubes (see PREGNANCY). A spontaneous abortion may then occur, but more often the fetus will grow to a size large enough to burst the tube. This is an emergency situation requiring immediate treatment. The symptoms of a uterine tube ruptured by ectopic pregnancy are vaginal bleeding and severe pain in one side of the abdomen. Prompt surgery is necessary to remove the damaged tube and the fetus, and to stop the bleeding. Fortunately, the removal of one tube usually leaves the other one intact, so that future pregnancy is possible. The differential diagnosis includes threatened abortion; however, in ectopic pregnancy the pain precedes the bleeding, but in abortion the bleeding precedes the pain.

ectopy ('ektə,pee) displacement or malposition, especially if congenital.

ectosteal (ek'tosti·əl) pertaining to or situated outside a bone.

ectostosis (,ekto'stohsis) ossification beneath the perichondrium of a cartilage or the periosteum of a bone.

ectothrix ('ektə,thriks) a fungus that grows inside the shaft of a hair, but produces a conspicuous external sheath of spores.

ectozoon (,ektoh'zoh·on) ectoparasite.

ectro- word element. [Gr.] *miscarriage, congenital absence.*

ectrodactyly (,ektroh'daktilee) congenital absence of all or part of a digit.

ectrogeny (ek'trojənee) congenital absence or defect of a part. adj. **ectrogenic**.

ectromelia (,ektroh'meeli·ə) gross hypoplasia or aplasia of one or more long bones of one or more limbs. adj. **ectromelic**.

ectromelus (ek'tromələs) an individual with rudimentary arms and legs.

ectropion (ek'trohpi·ən) eversion or turning outward, as of the margin of an eyelid.

ectrosyndactyly (,ektrəsin'daktilee) a condition in which some digits are absent and those that remain are webbed.

eczema ('eksimə, 'eksmə) 1. a general term for any superificial inflammatory process involving primarily the epidermis, marked early by redness, itching, minute papules and vesicles, weeping, oozing, and crusting, and later by scaling, lichenification, and often pigmentation. 2. atopic dermatitis.

Eczema is a common allergic reaction in children but it also occurs in adults, usually in a more severe form. Childhood eczema often begins in infancy, the rash appearing on the face, neck, and folds of elbows and knees. It may disappear by itself when the offending food is removed from the diet, or it may become more extensive and in some instances cover the entire surface of the body. Severe eczema can be complicated by skin infections.

Childhood eczema may persist for several years or return when the child is older. Persons suffering from childhood eczema may develop another allergic condition later, most often hay fever or asthma.

CAUSE AND CLASSIFICATION. The cause of eczema can either be *exogenous* (due to external or traumatic factors) or *endogenous* (due to internal or constitutional factors).

Exogenous eczema is usually subdivided into *allergic eczema* caused by an allergy to a certain substance and *irritant eczema* caused by direct damage to the skin by a known irritant substance (e.g. strong acids or alkalis).

Endogenous eczema is classified according to its appearance. There are four main varieties:

Atopic Eczema. The commonest form of eczema in childhood. Usually associated with a marked familial tendency to allergy.

Seborrhoeic Eczema. Eczema related to the areas where sebum production is greatest (scalp, back, chest).

Nummular or Discoid Eczema. This occurs as small circular lesions.

Pompholyx Eczema. A form of eczema in which the lesions are usually symmetrical and occur on the palms of the hands and soles of the feet.

Any type of exogenous or endogenous eczema can spread to cause generalized involvement of the skin. Complete involvement of the skin by autosensitization is termed *erythroderma* or *exfoliative dermatitis*.

TREATMENT. Exogenous eczema can be prevented by health screening of applicants in jobs where dermatitis is a known risk. Protective clothing, dust extractors and good ventilation should be available in such industries. In non-industrial cases the patient should endeavour to avoid the problem substance.

Curative treatment of the exogenous eczema must include removal of the source of the problem. In the acute phase, the skin can be treated as endogenous eczema.

The treatment of endogenous eczema depends upon the features present. The principles are as follows:

Dry Skin. Topical corticosteroid preparations can be used, with a polythene covering if extra protection is required. Emulsifying agents may be used for washing.

Weeping, Oozing Lesions. Drying lotions and wet compresses are used such as potassium permanganate and physiological saline. Such treatments can be followed by an application of a weak corticosteroid cream.

Irritation. Itching should be controlled to prevent further damage to the skin by scratching. Antihistamines such as promethazine hydrochloride and trimeprazine tartrate are useful, especially at night. Cool cotton clothing, cool baths and the avoidance of extremes of temperature also help to overcome irritation.

Infection. Any type of eczema can become secondarily infected. To avoid further trauma to the skin systemic antibiotics are usually given rather than antibiotic topical preparations.

Stress and Depression. Support should be available for the patient and his family to aid in the avoidance of physical and/or psychological stress which exacerbates the condition. A positive approach with an opportunity to discuss problems can be useful.

e. herpeticum disseminated herpes simplex (see KAPOSI'S VARICELLIFORM ERUPTION).

stasis e. stasis dermatitis.

e. vaccinatum disseminated vaccinia (see KAPOSI'S VARICELLIFORM ERUPTION).

eczematoid (ek'semə,toyd) resembling eczema.

eczematous (ek'semətəs) characterized by or of the nature of eczema.

EDC expected date of confinement (obstetrics).

EDD expected date of delivery (obstetrics).

edentia (ee'denshi·ə) absence of the teeth; called also *anodontia.*

edentulous (ee'dentyuhləs, -'dench-) without teeth.

edetate ('edi,tayt) any salt of ethylenediaminetetraacetic acid (EDTA), including *edetate disodium calcium*, used in the diagnosis and treatment of lead poisoning, and *edetate disodium*, used in the treatment of poisoning with lead and other heavy metals, and, because of its affinity for calcium, in the treatment of hypercalcaemia.

edetic acid (i'detik) ethylenediaminetetraacetic acid (EDTA).

edrophonium (,edrə'fohni·əm) a cholinergic used in the form of the chloride salt as a curare antagonist and diagnostic agent in myasthenia gravis.

EDTA ethylenediaminetetraacetic acid.

educable ('edyuhkəb'l) capable of being educated; used with special reference to persons with mild mental handicap (IQ approximately 52–67).

Edward's syndrome ('edwədz) trisomy 18 syndrome.

EEC European Economic Community.

EEG electroencephalogram.

Efcortelan (ef'kawtilan) trademark for preparations of hydrocortisone, an adrenocortical steroid.

effacement (i'faysmənt) obliteration; used especially of the 'taking-up' of the uterine cervix. This commences at 8 weeks of pregnancy when the isthmus is incorporated into the lower uterine segment. In primigravidae, obliteration of the cervical canal occurs after 36 weeks of pregnancy. In multigravidae effacement usually accompanies dilation of the external os. See also CERVICAL OS.

effect (i'fekt) a result produced by an action.

additive e. the combined effect produced by the action of two or more agents, being equal to the sum of their separate effects.

Bohr e. displacement of the oxyhaemoglobin dissociation curve by a change in carbon dioxide tension.

Crabtree e. the inhibition of oxygen consumption on the addition of glucose to tissues or microorganisms having a high rate of aerobic glycolysis; the converse of the Pasteur effect.

cumulative e. cumulation action.

Doppler e. the relationship of the apparent frequency of waves, as of sound, light, and radio waves, to the relative motion of the source of the waves and the observer, the frequency increasing as the two approach each other and decreasing as they move apart (see also DOPPLER EFFECT).

experimenter e's demand characteristics.

Pasteur e. the decrease in the rate of glycolysis and the suppression of lactate accumulation by tissues or microorganisms in the presence of oxygen.

position e. in genetics, the changed effect produced by alteration of the relative positions of various genes on the chromosomes.

pressure e. the sum of the changes that are due to obstruction of tissue drainage by pressure.

side-e. a consequence other than that for which an agent is used, especially an adverse effect on another organ system.

Somogyi e. a rebound phenomenon occurring in diabetes mellitus (see also SOMOGYI EFFECT).

effectiveness (i'fektivnəs) the ability to produce a specific result or to exert a specific measurable influence.

relative biological e. an expression of the effectiveness of other types of radiation in comparison with that of gamma or x-rays.

effector (i'fektor) 1. a muscle or gland that contracts or secretes, respectively, in direct response to nerve impulses. 2. a molecule that binds to an enzyme with an effect on its catalytic activity, i.e., either an activator or inhibitor.

allosteric e. one that binds to an enzyme at a site other than the active site.

effemination (i,femi'nayshən) feminization.

efferent ('efə·rənt) conducting or progressing away from a centre or specific site of reference, as an efferent nerve.

e. nerve any nerve that carries impulses from the central nervous system toward the periphery, as a motor nerve (see also NEURON).

effervescent (,efə'ves'nt) foaming or giving off gas bubbles.

effleurage (,eflə'rahzh) [Fr.] stroking movement in massage. In NATURAL CHILDBIRTH, a light circular stroke of the lower abdomen, done in rhythm to control breathing, to aid in relaxation of the abdominal muscles, and to increase concentration during a uterine contraction. The stroking is accomplished by moving the wrist only. Concentrating on the coordination of stroking and breathing is believed to block out some of the sensations created by the contracting uterus.

efflorescence (,eflor'res'ns) 1. the quality of being efflorescent. 2. a rash or eruption.

efflorescent (,eflor'res'nt) becoming powdery by losing the water of crystallization.

effluvium (i'floovi·əm) pl. *effluvia* [L.] 1. an outflowing or shedding, as of the hair. 2. an exhalation or emanation, especially one of noxious nature.

effusion (i'fyoozhən) 1. escape of a fluid into a part; exudation or transudation. 2. an exudate or transudate.

pleural e. accumulation of fluid in the space between the membrane encasing the lung and that lining the thoracic cavity. The normal pleural space contains only a small amount of fluid to prevent friction as the lung expands and deflates. If, however, there is a disturbance in either the production of this fluid or its removal, the fluid accumulates and threatens collapse of the lung. In extreme cases there is total collapse of the lung and MEDIASTINAL SHIFT.

Excess fluid in the pleural space may be removed by THORACENTESIS or by insertion of CHEST drains to allow for drainage of the fluid and, through a closed-drainage system, gradual re-expansion of the lung.

Conditions that may lead to pleural effusion include infections, inflammatory processes, and malignancies affecting the pulmonary structures, and renal and cardiac disease. See also PLEURISY.

egesta (ee'jestə) undigested material discharged from the body.

egestion (ee'jeschən) the casting out of undigested material.

egg (eg) 1. an ovum; a female gamete. 2. an oocyte. 3. a female reproductive cell at any stage before fertilization and its derivatives after fertilization and even after some development.

ego ('eegoh, 'eg-) in psychoanalytic theory, one of the three major parts of the personality, the others being the ID and the SUPEREGO. The word ego is Latin for 'I', that is, self or individual as distinguished from other persons. The ego is represented by certain mental mechanisms, such as perception and memory, and specific defence mechanisms that are used to adjust to the demands of primitive instinctual drives (the id) and the demands of the external world (superego). The ego may be considered the psychological aspect of one's personality, the id comprising the physiological aspects and the superego the social aspects. The ego controls and directs an individual's actions and seeks compromises between the id impulses, social and parental prohibitions and the pressures of reality.

The word ego also is commonly used to express conceit or self-centredness. This should not be confused with the psychiatric meaning described above.

e. ideal the standard of perfection unconsciously created by a person for himself.

e. strength according to psychoanalytic theory, the share of psychic energy available to the ego. Theoretically the 'stronger' the ego the greater the resoluteness of character and, according to some, the more likely the individual will be able to withstand stress.

ego-dystonic (ˌegohdis'tonik) denoting any impulse, idea, or the like, that is repugnant to and inconsistent with an individual's conception of himself.

ego-syntonic (ˌegohsin'tonik) denoting any impulse, idea, or the like, that is in harmony with an individual's conception of himself.

egobronchophony (ˌeegohbrong'kofənee) increased vocal resonance with a high-pitched bleating quality of the transmitted voice, detected by auscultation of the lungs, especially over lung tissue compressed by pleural effusion. Called also *egophony*.

egocentric (ˌeegoh'sentrik, ˌeg-) having all one's ideas centred on one's self.

egoism ('eegohˌizəm, ˌeg-) a self-seeking for advantage at the expense of others; overevaluation of the self.

egomania (ˌeegoh'mayni·ə, ˌeg-) morbid self-esteem.

egophony (ee'gofənee) egobronchophony.

egotism ('eegəˌtizəm, 'eg-) overevaluation of one's self.

egotropic (ˌegə'tropik) egocentric.

Ehlers–Danlos syndrome ('aylərz'danlos) a congenital hereditary syndrome of joint hyperextensibility, hyperelasticity and fragility of the skin, poor wound healing leaving parchment-like scars, capillary fragility, and subcutaneous nodules after trauma. Called also *cutis hyperelastica*.

Ehrlich's side-chain theory ('airliks) an explanation of the phenomena of immunity, in which protoplasmic cells are said to possess certain chemical attachments or side-chains. These side-chains are capable of uniting with bacterial toxins and in so doing render them harmless. Named after Paul Ehrlich (1854–1915), winner, with Metchnikoff, of the Nobel prize for medicine and physiology in 1908.

eidetic (ie'detik) denoting exact visualization of events or objects previously seen; a person having such an ability.

eidoptometry (ˌiedop'tomətree) measurement of the acuteness of visual perception.

einsteinium (ien'stieni·əm) a chemical element, atomic number 99, atomic weight 254, symbol Es. See table of elements in Appendix 2.

Eisenmenger's syndrome ('iez'nˌmengəz) ventricular septal defect with pulmonary hypertension and cyanosis due to right-to-left (reversed) shunt of blood. Sometimes defined as pulmonary hypertension (pulmonary vascular disease) and cyanosis with the shunt being at the atrial, ventricular, or great vessel area.

ejaculate (i'jakyuhlayt) 1. to expel semen. 2. the products of ejaculation.

ejaculatio (iˌjakyuh'layshioh) [L.] *ejaculation*.

e. praecox premature ejaculation in coitus.

ejaculation (iˌjakyuh'layshən) forcible, sudden expulsion; especially expulsion of semen from the male urethra, a reflex action that occurs as a result of sexual stimulation. adj. **ejaculatory.** The three components of semen are expelled in quick succession. First to emerge is a lubricating fluid produced by the bulbourethral glands in the penis. Next comes a fluid released into the urethral channel by the prostate; this fluid provides a neutral medium within which the sperm cells can swim. Lastly, the spermatic fluid, which has been stored in the seminal vesicles, is likewise injected into the urethral channel and ejaculated. See also REPRODUCTION.

ejecta (i'jektə) refuse cast off from the body.

Ekbom's syndrome called also RESTLESS *legs syndrome* (see LEG).

elaborate (i'labəˌrayt) to produce complex substances out of simpler materials.

elaboration (iˌlabə'rayshən) 1. the process of producing complex substances out of simpler materials. 2. in psychiatry, an unconscious mental process of expansion and embellishment of detail, especially of a symbol or representation in a dream.

elastance (i'lastəns) the quality of recoiling on removal of pressure without disruption, or an expression of the measure of the ability to do so in terms of unit of volume change per unit of pressure change; it is the reciprocal of compliance.

elastase (i'lastayz) an enzyme capable of catalysing the digestion of elastic tissue.

elastic (i'lastik) capable of resuming normal shape after distortion.

e. cartilage a substance that is more opaque, flexible, and elastic than hyaline cartilage, and is further distinguished by its yellow colour. The ground substance is penetrated in all directions by frequently branching fibres that give all of the reactions for elastin.

e. tissue connective tissue made up of yellow elastic fibres, frequently massed into sheets.

elasticity (iˌla'stisitee, ˌeela-, ˌela-) the quality of being elastic.

elastin (i'lastin) a yellow scleroprotein, the essential constituent of elastic connective tissue; it is brittle when dry, but flexible and elastic when moist.

elastofibroma (iˌlastohfie'brohmə) a tumour consisting of both elastin and fibrous elements.

elastoidosis (nodular) (iˌlastoy'dohsis) a condition characterized by comedones and yellowish, circumscribed, thickened plaques around the orbits or the nose, or the nape.

elastolysis (ˌeela'stolisis) the digestion of elastic substance or tissue.

elastoma (ˌeela'stohmə) a tumour or focal excess of elastic tissue fibres or abnormal collagen fibres of the skin.

elastometer (ˌeela'stomitə) an instrument for measuring the elasticity of tissues.

elastorrhexis (iˌlastə'reksis) a rupture of fibres composing elastic tissue.

elastosis (ˌeela'stohsis) 1. degeneration of elastic tissue. 2. degenerative changes in the dermal connective tissue with increased amounts of elastotic material. 3. any disturbance of the dermal connective tissue.

e. perforans serpiginosa, perforating e. an elastic tissue defect, occurring alone or in association with other disorders, including Down's syndrome and Ehlers–Danlos syndrome, in which elastomas are extruded through small keratotic papules in the epidermis; the lesions are usually arranged in arcuate serpiginous clusters on the sides of the nape, face, or arms.

elastotic (ˌeela'stotik) 1. pertaining to or characterized by elastosis. 2. resembling elastic tissue; having the staining properties of elastin.

elation (i'layshən) emotional excitement marked by acceleration of mental and bodily activity.

elbow ('elboh) 1. the bend of the arm; the joint connecting the arm and forearm. 2. any angular bend.

The elbow joint connects the large bone of the upper arm, or humerus, with the two smaller bones of the lower arm, the radius and ulna. It is one of the body's more versatile joints, with a combined hinge and rotating action allowing the arm to bend and the hand to make a half turn. The flexibility of the elbow and shoulder joints together permits a nearly infinite variety of hand movements.

The action of the elbow is controlled primarily by the biceps and the triceps muscles. When the biceps contracts, the arm bends at the elbow. When the triceps contracts the arm straightens. In each action, the opposite muscle exerts a degree of opposing tension, moderating the movement so that it is smooth and even instead of sudden and jerky.

As in other joints, the ends of the bones meeting at the elbow have a smooth covering of cartilage, a tough rubbery substance that minimizes friction when the joint is moved. The elbow joint is lubricated with synovia. The bursa, a small sac of connective tissue, eases its movement. The bones forming the joint are held together by tough, fibrous ligaments.

The 'funny bone' is not a bone but the ulnar nerve, a vulnerable and sensitive nerve that lies close to the surface near the point of the elbow. Hitting it causes a tingling pain or sensation that may be felt all the way to the fingers.

DISORDERS OF THE ELBOW. The elbows, like the knees, are continually exposed to bumps, twists, and wrenches. A common injury of the elbow is a fracture of a bone near the joint. Another injury of the elbow is dislocation, in which the hinge joint is pulled apart by a violent twist or pull. Tendons and ligaments may be torn. In some cases, dislocation and fracture may occur together.

ARTHRITIS may affect the elbow and make it stiff or impossible to move. Special exercises, manipulation and heat therapy may be prescribed to help restore flexibility. BURSITIS can also cause pain in the elbow. It often results from excessive use of the joint. 'Tennis elbow', which may affect people who have never held a tennis racket, is a term often used for bursitis of the elbow but is more accurately a tendinitis, or inflammation of the tendons. Rest and heat therapy are usually effective in relieving the condition.

ele(o)- word element. [Gr.] *oil.*

elective (i'lektiv) that which is chosen by the patient or doctor, as opposed to an emergency procedure.

Electra complex (i'lektrə) libidinous fixation of a daughter toward her father. See also OEDIPUS COMPLEX.

electric shock (i'lektrik) shock caused by electric current passing through the body. The longer the contact with electricity, the smaller the chance of survival. The victim's breathing may stop, and his body may appear stiff.

In giving first aid for electric shock, first the electric contact is broken as quickly as possible; this must be done with care to avoid exposure to the current. The rescuer, keeping in mind that water and metals are conductors of electricity, stands on a *dry* surface and does not touch the victim or electric wire with his bare hands.

The victim may have stopped breathing and have no

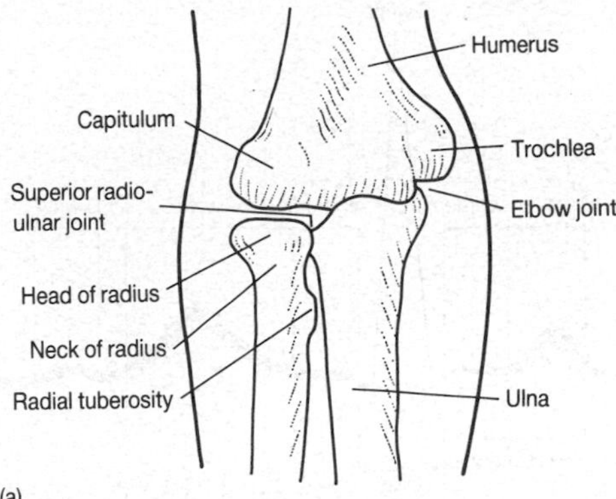

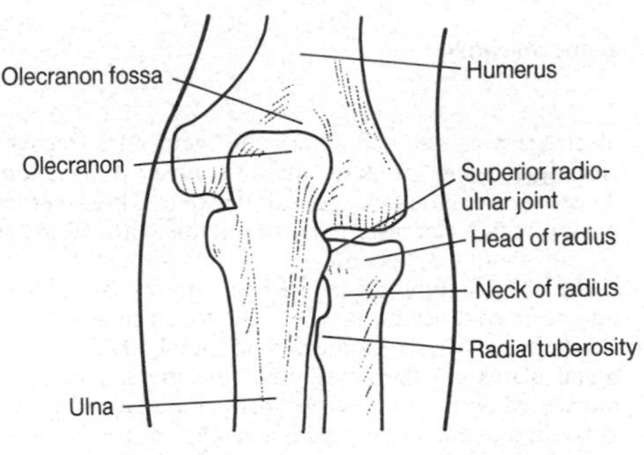

Elbow. (a) Anterior view, right arm. (b) Posterior view, right arm

pulse. In this case CARDIOPULMONARY RESUSCITATION is begun immediately.

electro- word element. [Gr.] *electricity.*

electroaffinity (iˌlektrohˌə'finitee) electronegativity.

electroanalgesia (iˌlektrohˌan'l'jeezi·ə) the reduction of pain by electrical stimulation of a peripheral nerve or the dorsal column of the spinal cord.

electrocardiogram (iˌlektroh'kahdiohˌgram) the record produced by ELECTROCARDIOGRAPHY; a tracing representing the heart's electrical action derived by amplification of the minutely small electrical impulses normally generated by the heart. Abbreviated ECG.

electrocardiograph (iˌlektroh'kahdiohˌgrahf, -ˌgraf) the apparatus used in electrocardiography.

electrocardiography (iˌlektrohˌkahdi'ogrəfee) the graphic recording from the body surface of the potential of electric currents generated by the heart, as a means of studying the action of the heart muscle. adj. **electrocardiographic.** With the modern electrocardiograph, the current that accompanies the action of the heart is amplified 3000 times or more, and it moves a small, sensitively balanced lever in contact with moving paper. The pattern of heart waves that is traced on the paper indicates the heart's rhythm and other actions.

The normal electrocardiogram is composed of a P wave, Q, R, and S waves known as the QRS COMPLEX, or QRS wave, and a T wave. The P wave occurs at the beginning of each contraction of the atria. The QRS wave occurs at the beginning of each contraction of the ventricles. The T wave seen in a normal

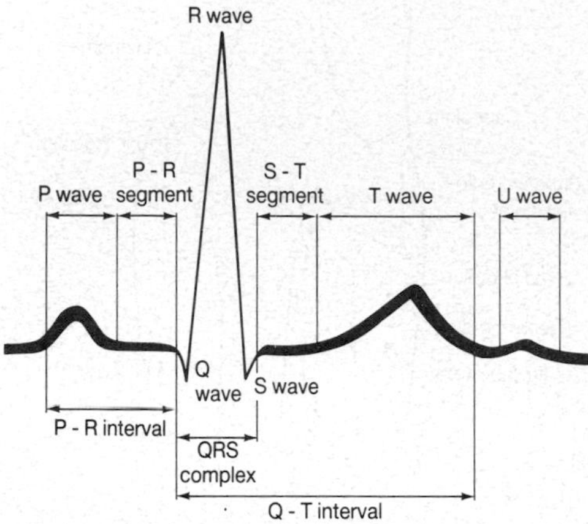

Electrocardiogram

electrocardiogram occurs as the ventricles recover electrically and prepare for the next contraction. There is a refractory period between these waves during which the muscle is inexcitable; this period is usually about 0.30 second.

The electric impulses in the heart muscle are picked up and conducted to the electrocardiograph by electrodes or leads connected to the body by small metal plates or other methods. The metal plates are moistened with a conductive paste and attached to the arms, legs, and chest (cardiac area) of the patient.

Electrocardiography is a valuable diagnostic tool, used in some routine physical examinations and when a heart disorder occurs or is suspected. It helps diagnose the damage that may have been inflicted on the heart muscle by a coronary occlusion, the progress of rheumatic fever, the presence of abnormal rhythms, or the effect of digitalis or other drugs. An electrocardiogram cannot always detect impending heart disease or all cardiovascular disorders. The readings are interpreted together with the results of other diagnostic tests.

electrocardiophonograph (i,lektroh,kahdioh'fohnə,grahf, -,graf) an electrical machine for recording graphically the heart sounds; a phonocardiograph.

electrocautery (i,lektroh'kawtə·ree) cauterization by means of an electrode of wire held in a holder and heated by either direct or alternating current. The term *electrocautery* is used to refer to both the procedure and to the instrument used in the procedure.

electrochemistry (i,lektroh'kemistree) the study of chemical changes produced by electric action.

electrocoagulation (i,lektrohkoh,agyuh'layshən) a surgical method of achieving haemostasis and dissection simultaneously which employs moderately damped or modulated undamped alternating current.

electrocochleogram (i,lektroh'kokli·ə,gram) the record obtained by electrocochleography.

electrocochleograph (i,lektroh'kokli·ə,grahf, -,graf) the instrument used in electrocochleography.

electrocochleography (i,lektroh,kokli'ogrəfee) measurement of electrical potentials of the eighth cranial nerve in response to acoustic stimuli applied by an electrode to the external acoustic canal, promontory, or tympanic membrane.

electrocontractility (i,lektrohkontrak'tilitee) contractility in response to electrical stimulation.

electroconvulsive therapy (i,lektrohkən'vulsiv) electroshock therapy; called also *electroplexy*; abbreviated ECT. A form of somatic therapy in which an electric current is used to produce convulsions. ECT is used primarily to treat depression or the depressive phase of manic-depressive psychosis; it has also been used to treat some forms of schizophrenia. It is most effective in treating depression precipitated by external events in patients with no previous history of mental illness. ECT does not provide insight to the patient and is of no value in the treatment of neuroses. Many cases formerly treated by ECT are now treated with antidepressants.

The convulsion is produced by a 60 hertz electric current applied to electrodes placed on the forehead. A voltage of 70 to 130 volts is applied for 0.1 to 0.5 seconds. The current produces a generalized tonic-clonic seizure, with a tonic phase lasting about 10 seconds and a clonic phase lasting about 40 seconds. This is followed by a coma lasting about 5 minutes and an acute confusional state lasting an hour or more. There is a loss of memory, particularly of recent events. Memory gradually improves until full memory returns after a few weeks or months.

In order to prevent injury during the seizure the patient is given a muscle relaxant, such as succinylcholine. An intravenous anaesthetic, such as thiopentone is also usually given to relieve anxiety about the treatment.

electrocorticography (i,lektroh,kawti'kogrəfee) electroencephalography with the electrodes applied directly to the cerebral cortex.

electrode (i'lektrohd) either of two terminals of an electrically conducting system or cell.

active e. therapeutic electrode.

calomel e. one capable of both collecting and giving up chloride ions in neutral or acidic aqueous media, consisting of mercury in contact with mercurous chloride; used as a reference electrode in pH measurements.

depolarizing e. an electrode that has a resistance greater than that of the portion of the body enclosed in the circuit.

hydrogen e. an electrode made by depositing platinum black on platinum and then allowing it to absorb hydrogen gas to saturation; used in determination of hydrogen ion concentration.

indifferent e. one larger than a therapeutic electrode, dispersing electrical stimulation over a larger area.

point e. an electrode having on one end a metallic point; used in applying current.

therapeutic e. one smaller than an indifferent electrode, producing electrical stimulation in a concentrated area; called also *active electrode*.

electrodermal (i,lektroh'dərməl) pertaining to the electrical properties of the skin, especially to changes in its resistance.

electrodesiccation (i,lektroh,desi'kayshən) a method of electrosurgery using high frequency, high voltage, low amperage current imparted to the tissue through a needle electrode to achieve fulguration with the minimum of coagulation (see also ELECTROSURGERY).

electrodialyser (i,lektroh'dieə,liezə) a blood dialyser utilizing an applied electric field and semipermeable membranes for separating the colloids from the solution.

electroencephalogram (i,lektroh·en'kefələ,gram, -'sef--) the record produced by ELECTROENCEPHALOGRAPHY; a tracing of the electric impulses of the brain. Abbreviated EEG.

electroencephalograph (i,lektroh·en'kefələ,grahf,

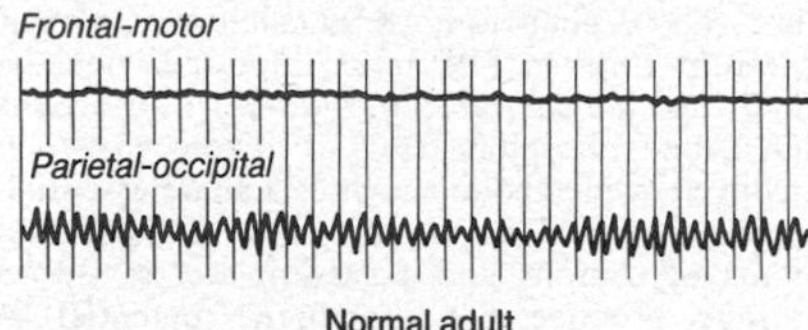

Normal adult
10/s activity in occipital area

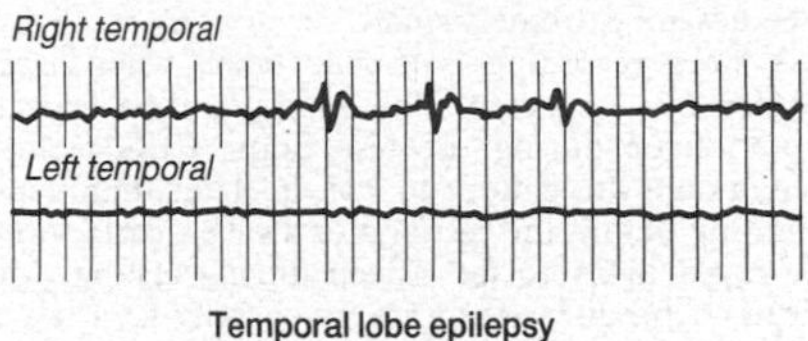

Temporal lobe epilepsy
Right temoral spike focus

Petit mal seizure
Synchronous 3/s spikes & waves

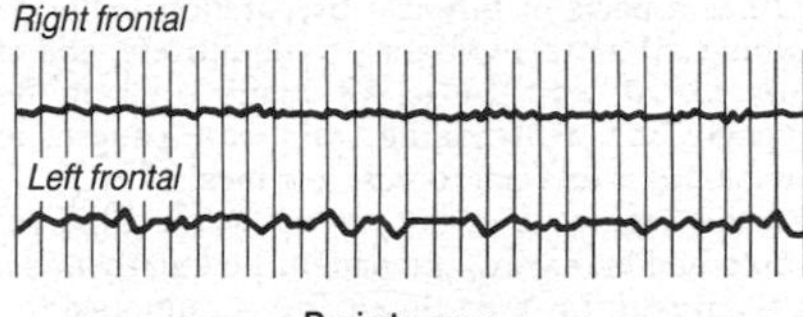

Brain tumour
Left frontal slow wave focus

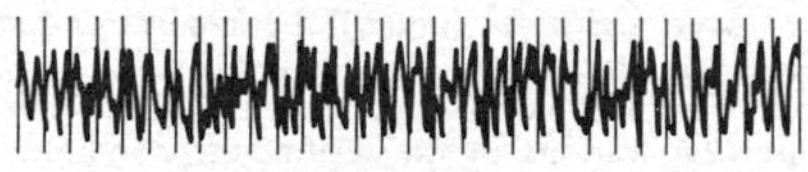
Grand mal seizure
High voltage spikes, generalized

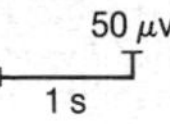

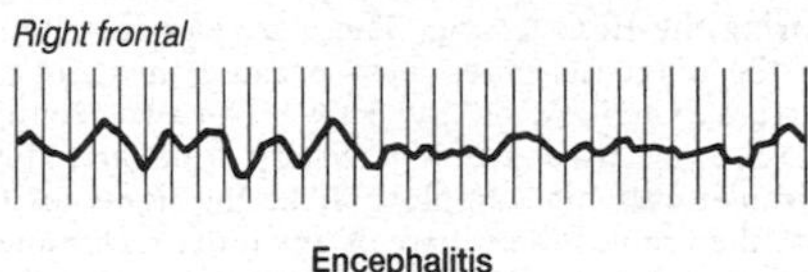

Encephalitis
Diffuse slowing

Examples of normal and abnormal EEGs

-ˌgraf, -'sef-) the instrument used in electroencephalography.

electroencephalography (iˌlektroh·enˌkefə'logrəfee, -ˌsefə-) the recording of changes in electric potentials in various areas of the brain by means of electrodes placed on the scalp or on or in the brain itself, and connected to a vacuum tube radio amplifier, which amplifies the impulses more than a million times. The impulses are of sufficient magnitude to move an electromagnetic pen that records the brain waves. adj. **electroencephalographic**.

The rate, height, and length of the waves vary in different parts of the brain, and each individual has a unique and characteristic EEG pattern. Age and degree of consciousness also cause the wave patterns to differ. Most of the recorded waves in a normal adult's EEG are the occipital alpha waves, which are best obtained from the back of the head (occipital region) when the subject is resting quietly, but not asleep, with his eyes closed (see ALPHA brain waves). These waves are blocked by excitement or by opening the eyes.

The beta waves, obtained from the central and front parts of the head are more closely related to the sensory-motor parts of the brain (see BETA brain waves). These waves are blocked in the same way as are alpha waves, by opening the eyes. In a normal EEG the frequencies are predominately within the range of alpha and beta rhythms at the rate of 8 to 30 hertz (cycles per second). During sleep the brain cells generate higher voltage electrical waves, but the rhythm is slowed down to 2 or 3 hertz, sometimes with short 'sleep' spindles of about 15 hertz. One should use the word 'normal' with caution when speaking of EEG readings. Some persons with mild deviations from normal may have no evidence of cerebral disease, while others with readings within normal ranges may be suffering from a serious disorder.

Irregular slow waves of 2 to 3 hertz, called delta waves or the delta pattern, are normally found in deep sleep and in infants and young children, but indicate an abnormality in the awake adult. Rhythmic slow waves of 4 to 7 hertz are called theta waves.

Electroencephalography is widely used in studying brain function and in tracing the connections between the parts of the central nervous system. It is particularly valuable in diagnosing EPILEPSY, brain tumour, and other diseases of and injury to the brain.

An electroencephalogram is of little use in the study of those mental disorders and diseases that do not cause gross brain damage.

PATIENT CARE. The electroencephalograph is an extremely sensitive instrument and readings can be greatly influenced by the actions of the subject and his physiological status. It is apparent, then, that the cooperation of the patient is needed, and that he is properly prepared physically and psychologically in order to obtain an accurate and useful record of brain activity. The patient is more likely to be cooperative if he has had adequate preparation in the purpose of the test, how the procedure will be carried out, and what will be expected of him during the testing. His fears about electricity and how it will be used must be allayed. He should know that the electrodes carry minute amounts of electrical charge *from* his body and that there is no danger of electric shock and no relationship of this procedure to electroconvulsive therapy. In most instances the test is painless because the electrodes are attached to the scalp with collodion. If needle electrodes are to be used, however, he should be told there will be mild discomfort because the needles are extremely small.

A sleep recording is usually taken when a seizure disorder is suspected. The patient will be expected to go to sleep during the test. Some EEG technicians encourage the patient to stay up later than usual the evening before the test and to awaken early so he will be more likely to fall asleep during testing. Medications to produce sleep are given only as a last resort because these drugs alter brain wave patterns. Infants and small children are not allowed to nap before the test.

Other aspects of physical preparation include withholding all anticonvulsants, tranquillizers, and stimulants for at least 24 to 48 hours prior to testing. Hypoglycaemia affects the brain wave patterns and so the patient is told not to miss any meals.

At the beginning of the test a baseline EEG reading is obtained by having the patient lie quietly in a dimly lit room with his eyes closed. He is cautioned to avoid movement of the eyelids, mouth, or tongue because these activities can be particularly disruptive. Provocative or 'stressing' techniques are sometimes used during the EEG testing. These are particularly useful in the diagnosis of epilepsy because they can evoke seizure potentials on the EEG. The two techniques most often used are HYPERVENTILATION and 'photic' stimulation which employs flickering lights to stimulate the brain. When these or any other techniques are anticipated, the patient should be informed so he can avoid becoming unduly apprehensive before and during the testing.

electrofulguration (i,lektroh,fulgyuh'rayshən) electrodesiccation.

electrogastrograph (i,lektroh'gastrə,grahf, -,graf) an instrument for recording the electrical activity of the stomach by means of swallowed gastric electrodes.

electrogastrography (i,lektrohga'strogrəfee) the recording of the electrical activity of the stomach as measured between its lumen and the body surface. adj. **electrogastrographic.**

electrogram (i'lektroh,gram) any record produced by changes in electrical potential.

His bundle e. an intracardiac electrocardiogram of potentials in the bundle of His (atrioventricular bundle), done through a cardiac catheter.

electrogustometry (i,lektrohgu'stomətree) the testing of the sense of taste by application of galvanic stimuli to the tongue.

electrohaemostasis (i,lektroh,hee'mostəsis, -,heemoh'staysis) arrest of haemorrhage by electrocautery.

electrohysterography (i,lektroh,histə'rogrəfee) the recording of changes in electric potential associated with contractions of the uterine muscle. Called also *topography.*

electrokymogram (i,lektroh'kiemoh,gram) the record produced by electrokymography.

electrokymograph (i,lektroh'kiemoh,grahf, -,graf) the instrument used in electrokymography.

electrokymography (i,lektrohkie'mogrəfee) the photography on x-ray film of the motion of the heart or of other moving structures which can be visualized radiographically.

electrolysis (,ilek'trolisis, ,elek-) destruction by passage of a galvanic current, as in disintegration of a chemical compound in solution or removal of excessive hair from the body.

electrolyte (i,lektrə,liet) a chemical substance which, when dissolved in water or melted, dissociates into electrically charged particles (*ions*), and thus is capable of conducting an electric current. The principal positively charged ions in the body fluids (*cations*) are sodium (Na^+), potassium (K^+), calcium (Ca^{2+}), and magnesium (Mg^{2+}). The most important negatively charged ions (*anions*) are chloride (Cl^-), bicarbonate (HCO_3^-), and phosphate (PO_4^{3-}). These electrolytes are involved in metabolic activities and are essential to the normal function of all cells. Concentration gradients of sodium and potassium across the cell membrane produce the membrane potential and provide the means by which electrochemical impulses are transmitted in nerve and muscle fibres.

The concentration of the various electrolytes in body fluids is maintained within a narrow range. However, the optimal concentrations differ in the extracellular fluid and intracellular fluid. For example, as shown in the accompanying table, the concentration of sodium in extracellular fluid (serum) is about 15 times higher than in the intracellular fluid. Conversely, the concentration of potassium is about 30 times higher within the cell than in the serum or extracellular fluid.

An electrolyte imbalance exists when the serum concentration of an electrolyte is either too high or too low. The terms for excessive and deficient blood levels of electrolytes are derived from the Greek prefixes *hyper-* (over) and *hypo-* (under), the English or Latin name of the electrolyte, and the Latin suffix *-aemia* (blood). For example, if there is an excess of sodium (L. *natrium*) cations in the serum, the condition is referred to as *hypernatraemia.* A deficit of these ions is called *hyponatraemia.*

Stability of the electrolyte balance depends on adequate intake of water and the electrolytes, and on homeostatic mechanisms within the body that regulate the absorption, distribution, and excretion of water

Average Electrolyte Concentrations of the Body Fluids (meq./l)

	Plasma	Interstitial fluid	Intra-cellular fluid
Cations			
Na^+ (Sodium)	142	147	15
K^+ (Potassium)	5	4	150
Ca^{2+} (Calcium)	5	2.5	2
Mg^{2+} (Magnesium)	2	1	27
	154	154.5	194
Anions			
Cl^- (Chloride)	103	114	1
HCO_3^- (Bicarbonate)	27	30	10
PO_4^{2-} (Phosphate)	2	2	100
SO_4^{2-} (Sulphate)	1	1	20
Organic acids	5	7.5	—
Proteinate	16	0	63
	154	154.5	194

and its dissolved particles. Many conditions can interfere with these processes and result in an imbalance. For example, renal disease, in which the kidney nephron is unable to function normally, causes a retention of water, sodium, chloride, bicarbonate, and calcium as the glomerular filtration rate falls. Even when the kidney structures are intact, electrolyte imbalances can result from an inadequate supply of blood to the nephrons or from imbalances of regulatory hormones, such as aldosterone and antidiuretic hormone (ADH).

The effects of an electrolyte imbalance are not isolated to a particular organ or system. In general, however, imbalances in CALCIUM concentrations affect the bones, kidney, and gastrointestinal tract. Calcium also influences the permeability of cell membranes and thereby regulates neuromuscular activity. SODIUM affects the osmolality of blood and therefore influences blood volume and pressure and the retention or loss of interstitial fluid. POTASSIUM affects muscular activities, notably those of the heart, intestines, and respiratory tract, and also affects neural stimulation of the skeletal muscles.

electrolytic (i,lektrə'litik) pertaining to electrolysis or to an electrolyte.

electromagnet (i,lektroh'magnit) a piece of metal rendered temporarily magnetic by passage of electricity through a coil surrounding it.

electromagnetism (i,lektroh'magnə,tizəm) magnetism developed by an electric current.

electromotive force (i,lektroh'mohtiv) the force that, by reason of differences in potential, causes a flow of electricity from one place to another, giving rise to an electric current.

electromyogram (i,lektroh'mieoh,gram) the record obtained by electromyography.

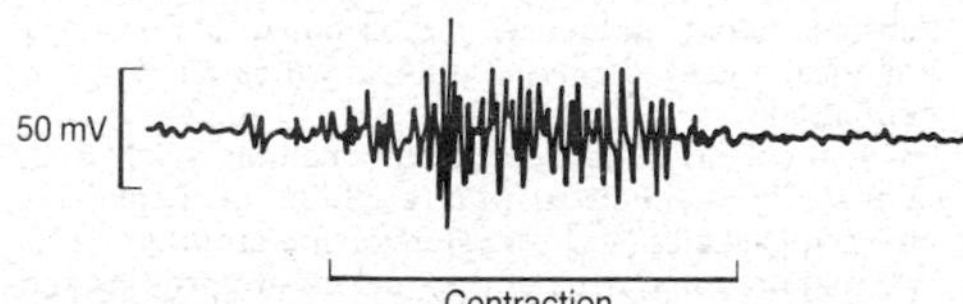

Electromyogram recorded during contraction of the gastrocnemius muscle

electromyograph (i,lektroh'mieoh,grahf, -,graf) the instrument used in electromyography.

electromyography (i,lektrohmie'ogrəfee) the recording and study of the intrinsic electrical properties of skeletal muscle. adj. **electromyographic.** When it is at rest, normal muscle is electrically silent, but when the muscle is active, an electrical current is generated. In electromyography the electrical impulses are picked up by needle electrodes inserted into the muscle and amplified on an oscilloscope screen in the form of wavelike tracings. The visual recording may be accompanied by auditory monitoring in which the sounds are amplified.

Electromyography is useful in diagnosing disorders of the nerves supplying the muscle (as in AMYOTROPHIC LATERAL SCLEROSIS and POLIOMYELITIS) and in disorders affecting the muscle tissues. Recordings usually are obtained while the muscle is relaxed, during voluntary contraction, and during muscle activity that is produced by nerve stimulation. In this way it is possible to determine the presence of a disorder, localize the site, and identify the specific disease producing muscle weakness.

electron (i'lektron) any of the negatively charged particles arranged in orbits around the nucleus of an atom and determining all of the atom's physical and chemical properties except mass and radioactivity. Electrons flowing in a conductor constitute an electric current; when ejected from a radioactive substance, they constitute beta particles.

The number of electrons revolving around the nucleus of an atom is equal to its atomic number. An atom of oxygen, for instance, which has an atomic number of 8, has eight electrons in orbit around the nucleus in a manner similar to the planets revolving around the sun in our solar system.

Electrons greatly influence the behaviour of an atom toward other atoms. The combination of various ELEMENTS to form compounds is brought about by losing or gaining electrons; the process is sometimes called 'sharing' of electrons. For example, the combination of the elements sodium and chlorine produce the compound sodium chloride (table salt). This is accomplished by the transfer of one electron from the outer orbit of the sodium atom to the outer orbit of the chlorine atom. This combining of elements by the loss or gain of electrons is called electrovalency. After the electron exchange, the atoms become charged particles called ions.

electron-dense (i'lektron,dens) in electron microscopy, having a density that prevents electrons from penetrating.

electronarcosis (i,lektrohnah'kohsis) anaesthesia produced by passage of an electric current through electrodes placed on the temples.

electronegative (i,lektroh'negətiv) bearing a negative electric charge or an excess of electrons.

electronegativity (i,lektroh,negə'tivətee) the relative power of an atom to attract electrons.

electroneurography (i,lektrohnyuh'rogrəfee) the measurement of the conduction velocity and latency of peripheral nerves.

electroneuromyography (i,lektroh,nyooə·rohmie'ogrəfee) electromyography in which the nerve of the muscle under study is stimulated by application of an electric current.

electronic (,ilek'tronik, ,eelek-, ,elek-) pertaining to or carrying electrons.

electronystagmogram (i,lektrohni'stagmə,gram) the record obtained by electronystagmography.

electronystagmograph (i,lektrohni'stagmə,grahf, -,graf) the instrument used in electronystagmography; abbreviated ENG.

electronystagmography (i,lektroh,nistag'mogrəfee) electroencephalographic recordings of eye movements that provide objective documentation of induced and spontaneous nystagmus.

electro-oculogram (i,lektroh'okyuhloh,gram) the electroencephalographic tracings made while moving the eyes a constant distance between two fixation points, inducing a deflection of fairly constant amplitude; abbreviated EOG.

electro-olfactogram (i,lektroh·ol'faktə,gram) a recording of electrical potential changes detected by an electrode placed on the surface of the olfactory mucosa as the mucosa is subjected to an odorous stimulus. Abbreviated EOG.

electropherogram (i,lektroh'feroh,gram) electrophoretogram.

electrophile (i'lektroh,fiel) a chemical compound that serves as an electron acceptor in a chemical reaction. adj. **electrophilic.**

electrophoresis (i,lektrohfə'reesis) the movement of

charged particles suspended in a liquid on various media (e.g., paper, gel, liquid) under the influence of an applied electric field. adj. **electrophoretic.** The various charged particles of a particular substance migrate in a definite and characteristic direction—toward either the anode or the cathode—and at a characteristic speed. This principle has been widely used in the separation of proteins and is therefore valuable in the study of diseases in which the serum and plasma proteins are altered. The principle also has been applied in the separation and identification of various types of human haemoglobin.

electrophoretogram (i,lektrohfə'retə,gram) the record produced on or in a supporting medium by bands of material which have been separated by the process of electrophoresis.

electroplexy (i'lektroh,pleksee) electroconvulsive therapy.

electropositive (i,lektroh'pozətiv) bearing a positive electric charge.

electroresection (i,lektrohri'sekshən) electrosection.

electroretinogram (i,lektroh'retinoh,gram) a recording of the electrical response of the retina to light stimulation; abbreviated ERG.

The ERG is obtained using a contact lens containing an electrode, which is placed on the surface of the eye. Electrical activity of the retina is magnified and recorded as waves similar to those seen on an electrocardiograph. Signals from a diseased retina are reduced in size and slower than normal. The ERG is useful in confirming the diagnosis of conditions such as RETINITIS PIGMENTOSA before visible signs can be detected with an ophthalmoscope.

electroscission (i,lektroh'sizhən, -shan) cutting of tissue by means of electric cautery.

electroscope (i'lektrə,skohp) an instrument for measuring radiation intensity.

electrosection (i,lektroh'sekshən) a method of electrosurgery used to incise or excise tissue, which employs a slightly damped, modulated undamped, or undamped alternating electrical current, and requires both an active concentrating electrode and an inactive dispersing electrode. Called also *electroresection*. See also ELECTROSURGERY.

electroshock therapy (i'lektroh,shok) electroconvulsive therapy.

electrosleep (i'lektroh,sleep) see cerebral ELECTROTHERAPY.

electrostimulation (i,lektroh,stimyuh'layshən) electric stimulation of tissues.

electrostriatogram (i,lektrohstrie'aytə,gram) an electroencephalogram showing differences in electric potential recorded at various levels of the corpus striatum.

electrosurgery (i,lektroh'sərjə·ree) the use of high-frequency alternating current to remove, incise, or destroy tissue. This is accomplished by converting the electrical energy into heat through tissue resistance to the passage of the electrical current. Called also *surgical diathermy*. adj. **electrosurgical.**

Two types of current are utilized in electrosurgery, damped and undamped; a damped current destroys and coagulates tissue and stops bleeding, and undamped current destroys minimal tissue and incises tissue. Basically, there are three types of electrosurgical techniques: ELECTRODESICCATION, ELECTROCOAGULATION, and ELECTROSECTION.

electrotaxis (i,lektroh'taksis) taxis in response to electric stimuli.

electrotherapeutics (i,lektroh,therə'pyootiks) electrotherapy.

electrotherapy (i,lektroh'therəpee) treatment of disease by means of electricity passed through tissues in order to stimulate muscles and nerves. See also DIATHERMY.

cerebral e. the use of low-intensity electricity, usually employing positive pulses or direct current in the treatment of insomnia, anxiety, and neurotic depression. Misleadingly called electrosleep—the treatment does not induce sleep.

electrotonic (i,lektroh'tonik) 1. pertaining to electrotonus. 2. denoting the direct spread of current in tissues by electrical conduction, without the generation of new current by action potentials.

electrotonus (i,lektroh'tohnəs) the altered electrical state of a nerve or muscle cell when a constant electric current is passed through it.

electroureterography (i,lektrohyuh,reetə'rogrəfee) electromyography in which the action potentials produced by peristalsis of the ureter are recorded.

electrovalency (i,lektroh'vaylənsee) the number of charges an atom acquires in a chemical reaction by gain or loss of electrons.

electroversion (i,lektroh'vərshən) the act of electrically terminating a cardiac dysrhythmia.

electrovert (i'lektroh,vərt) to apply electricity to the heart or precordium to depolarize the heart and terminate a cardiac dysrhythmia.

electuary (i'lektyooə·ree) a medicinal preparation consisting of a powdered drug made into a paste with honey or syrup.

eledoisin (,eli'doysin) a decapeptide from the posterior salivary gland of a species of snail (*Eledone*), which is a precursor of a large group of biologically active peptides; it has vasodilator, hypotensive, and extravascular smooth muscle stimulant properties.

eleidin (el'ee·idin) a substance, allied to keratin, found in the cells of the stratum lucidum of the skin.

element ('elimənt) 1. any of the primary parts or constituents of a thing. 2. in chemistry, a simple substance that cannot be decomposed by ordinary chemical means; the basic 'stuff' of which all matter is composed.

Chemical elements are made up of atoms. Each atom consists of a nucleus with a cloud of negatively charged particles (ELECTRONS) revolving around it. The two major components of the nucleus are protons and neutrons. The number of protons in the atoms of a particular element is always the same, and therefore the physical and chemical properties of the element are always the same. It is possible, however, for a chemical element to exist in several different forms, the difference depending on the number of neutrons in the nucleus of its atoms. Different forms of the same element are called isotopes.

There are at least 109 different chemical elements known. The table in Appendix 2 lists the elements and their symbols. The atomic number of an element is determined by the number of protons in the nucleus of an atom of the element. The mass number of an isotope is determined by the total number of neutrons and protons in the nucleus.

STABLE CHEMICAL ELEMENTS. A stable chemical element is one that contains an optimal ratio or range of ratios between the number of protons and neutrons in the nucleus. A stable element does not spontaneously transmute into another element and therefore does not give off radiations. The stable elements are those that have an atomic number below 84, except for a few, such as potassium and rubidium, which are weakly radioactive.

RADIOACTIVE CHEMICAL ELEMENTS. A radioactive chemical element does not contain an optimal proton-to-neutron ratio in its atomic nuclei and therefore readily gives off nuclear particles until all nuclei have attained the optimal combination of protons and neutrons. The spontaneous releasing of its nuclear particles changes the radioactive atom into a new atom (transmutation).

As radioactive elements disintegrate and form new chemical elements, a tremendous amount of energy is released. This emission of energy and nuclear particles is called RADIATION. The radiations may be electrically charged particles having size and mass, such as ALPHA PARTICLES and BETA PARTICLES, or they may be nonparticulate and contain no electrical charges, such as GAMMA RAYS. Most radioactive elements give off either alpha or beta particles and at the same time emit gamma radiation.

formed e's (of the blood) erythrocytes, leukocytes, and platelets.

trace e. a chemical element present or needed in extremely small amounts by plants and animals, such as manganese, copper, cobalt, zinc, iron.

eleoma (ˌeli'ohmə) a tumour or swelling caused by injection of oil into the tissues.

elephantiasis (ˌelifən'tieəsis) a chronic disease marked by inflammation and obstruction of the lymphatics and hypertrophy of the skin and subcutaneous tissues, chiefly affecting the legs and external genitalia. The disease derives its name from the symptoms, particularly swelling of the legs, which makes them look like those of an elephant. The term is often applied to hypertrophy and thickening of the tissues from any cause.

True elephantiasis, or elephantiasis filariensis, is most often caused by a slender, threadlike parasite, the filarial worm, *Wuchereria bancrofti*, which enters the lymphatic system, causing an obstruction to drainage. The disease, sometimes called FILARIASIS, is transmitted by mosquitoes which carry blood infected with filaria larvae. Elephantiasis is most often encountered in Central Africa, in some Pacific Islands, and in other tropical and subtropical areas. It is rare or nonexistent in the temperate zone.

The first visible signs are inflammation of the lymph nodes, with temporary swelling in the affected area, red streaks along the leg or arm, pain, and tenderness. Specific drugs are administered for destruction of the parasites; bandages and elevation of the affected area help relieve the swelling. Sanitary control to eliminate the carrier insects is the most effective approach to elimination of this disease.

e. scroti that in which the scrotum is the main site affected by the disease.

elephantoid fever (ˌeli'fantoyd) a recurrent acute febrile condition occurring with filariasis; it may be associated with elephantiasis or lymphangitis.

elevator ('eliˌvaytə) 1. an instrument used as a lever for raising a depressed portion of bone. 2. an instrument with a curved tip used for removing teeth or root fragments from their socket. There are many shapes and sizes. 3. a levator muscle.

periosteal e. instrument for stripping the periosteum in bone surgery.

zygomatic e. instrument used to elevate a fractured zygomatic arch via an incision in the temporal region.

elimination (iˌlimi'nayshən) discharge from the body of indigestible materials and of waste products of body metabolism.

e. diet one for diagnosing food allergy, based on the sequential omission of foods that might cause the symptoms in the patient.

ELISA assays (i'liezə) assays of antibodies or antigens in which one or the other is bound to the surface of a multi-well plastic plate. Antibodies labelled with an enzyme are bound in the test and the enzyme bound measured by chemical techniques. The amount of antigen or antibody present is related to the amount of enzyme bound. Widely used to measure hormones and drugs.

elixir (i'liksə) a clear, sweetened, usually hydroalcoholic liquid containing flavouring substances and sometimes active medicinal ingredients, for oral use.

elliptocyte (i'liptəˌsiet) an elliptical erythrocyte.

elliptocytosis (iˌliptohsie'tohsis) a hereditary disorder in which the erythrocytes are largely elliptical and which is characterized by increased red cell destruction; anaemia, if present, is usually mild.

Eltroxin (el'troksin) trademark for a preparation of levothyroxine sodium, used for replacement therapy in hypothyroidism.

eluate ('elyooˌayt) the substance separated out by, or the product of, elution or elutriation.

eluent ('elyooənt) the solution used in elution.

elution (i'looshən) in chemistry, separation of material by washing; the process of pulverizing substances and mixing them with water in order to separate the heavier constituents, which settle out in solution, from the lighter.

elutriation (iˌlootri'ayshən) purification of a substance by dissolving it in a solvent and pouring off the solution, thus separating it from the undissolved foreign material.

Em. emmetropia.

emaciation (iˌmaysi'ayshən) excessive leanness; a wasted condition of the body.

emanation (ˌemə'nayshən) that which is given off, such as a gaseous disintegration product given off from radioactive substances, or an effluvium.

emasculation (iˌmaskyuh'layshən) removal of the penis or testes.

embalming (em'bahming) treatment of a dead body to retard decomposition.

embarrass (em'barəs) to impede the function of; to obstruct.

Embden–Meyerhof pathway (ˌemdən'mieəhof) the series of enzymatic reactions in the anaerobic conversion of glucose to lactic acid, resulting in energy in the form of adenosine triphosphate (ATP).

embedding (em'beding) fixation of tissue in a firm medium, in order to keep it intact during cutting of thin sections.

embole ('embəlee) the reducing of a dislocated limb.

embolectomy (ˌembə'lektəmee) surgical removal of an embolus.

emboli ('embəlie) plural of *embolus*.

embolic (em'bolik) pertaining to embolism or an embolus.

embolism ('embəˌlizəm) the sudden blocking of an artery by a clot of foreign material (embolus) that has been brought to its site of lodgment by the blood current. The obstructing material is most often a blood clot, but may be a fat globule, air bubble, piece of tissue, or clump of bacteria.

SYMPTOMS. The symptoms of an embolism usually do not appear until the embolus lodges within a blood vessel and suddenly obstructs the blood flow. Emboli usually lodge at divisions of an artery, where the vessel narrows. The signs of obstruction appear almost immediately with severe pain at the site. If the embolus lodges in an extremity the area becomes pale, numb, and cold to the touch, and normal arterial pulse below the site is absent. Fainting, nausea and vomiting and eventually severe shock may occur if a large vessel is occluded. Unless the obstruction is relieved, gangrene of the adjacent tissues served by the affected vessel develops.

PREVENTION. Venous THROMBOSIS is the most common

predisposing cause of embolism. In order to prevent the development of emboli it is necessary to avoid venous stasis in patients who are confined to bed because of surgery, illness, or injury. In addition to physical inactivity, heart failure and pressure on the veins of the legs and pelvis can inhibit blood flow and thus set the stage for inflammation, clot formation, and the possibility of embolism.

Although frequent changing of position, exercise, and early ambulation are necessary to the prevention of thrombosis and embolism, sudden and extreme movements should be avoided. Under no circumstances should the legs be massaged to relieve 'muscle cramps', especially when the pain is located in the calf and the patient has not been up and about; pain in the calf may be symptomatic of thrombosis.

The occurrence of an air embolism can be avoided by careful handling of equipment used for intravenous therapy and correct technique in administering intramuscular injections.

Treatment and Patient Care. Immediate care of the patient with an embolism of an extremity must be prompt, especially if the affected blood vessel is large and gangrene is a real possibility. The purpose of initial treatment is facilitation of blood flow to the part. This is accomplished by lowering the limb to a dependent position and wrapping it to prevent loss of body warmth and combat constriction of the blood vessels. Direct heat is not applied to ischaemic tissue because it may further damage the tissues and accelerate the development of gangrene. Heparin may be given immediately to decrease the possibility of further clot formation. Spasms of the blood vessels may be relieved by an antispasmodic drug or by blocking the sympathetic nerves by local injection of procaine. If conservative measures are not effective, surgery may be necessary to remove the obstructing clot and restore circulation.

Postoperatively the patient's vital signs—pulse, blood pressure and respirations—are monitored and the extremity evaluated frequently to assess circulation. The affected limb should show signs of adequate circulation, that is, warmth, return of colour and feeling, and normal pulse. If these are not present or the limb shows signs of increasing ischaemia, the surgeon should be notified. Signs of bleeding at the operative site also should be reported, particularly if the patient has received anticoagulant medication. Exercise of the limb and ambulation are begun only after the surgeon has assessed the patient's status and given permission.

cerebral e. embolism of a cerebral artery, one of the three main causes of stroke.

pulmonary e. (PE) obstruction of the pulmonary artery or one of its branches by an embolus. The embolus is usually a blood clot swept into circulation from a large peripheral vein, particularly one in the leg or pelvis.

Factors that predispose a patient to PE include: (1) *stasis of blood flow*, as in a patient who is on prolonged bed rest, is immobilized for some reason, or is aged, obese, or suffering from a burn, or has recently delivered a child; (2) *venous injury*, as from surgical procedures or trauma and fractures of the legs or pelvis; (3) *predisposition to clot formation* because of malignancy or use of oral contraceptives; (4) *cardiovascular disease*; (5) *chronic lung disease*; and (6) *diabetes mellitus*.

The effects of PE will depend on the size of the embolus and the amount of lung tissue involved. When an embolus becomes lodged in a pulmonary blood vessel, it prevents adequate blood supply to the lung, interferes with ventilation, and results in arterial hypoxaemia. As pressure within the obstructed pulmonary artery increases there is strain on the right ventricle and it may eventually fail. Two other complications of PE are pulmonary infarct and pulmonary haemorrhage.

Signs and symptoms of PE vary greatly, depending on the extent to which the lung is involved, the size of the clot, and the general condition of the patient. Simple, uncomplicated embolism produces such cardiopulmonary symptoms as dyspnoea, tachypnoea, persistent cough, pleuritic pain, and haemoptysis. Apprehension is a common symptom. On rare occasions the cardiopulmonary symptoms may be acute, occurring suddenly and quickly producing cyanosis and shock.

The drug most often used in the treatment of PE is heparin, which prolongs clotting time and allows the body time to resolve the existing clot. Patients with massive embolism or an ascending thrombophlebitis are sometimes treated with fibrinolytic agents, such as streptokinase and urokinase, which dissolve the clot.

Prevention of PE includes measures to avoid venous stasis: that is, turning, coughing, deep breathing, and early ambulation following surgery. Signs of thrombophlebitis should be reported promptly; any evidence of redness, tenderness, or pain in the calf with dorsiflexion of the foot should alert one to the possibility of thrombophlebitis. Under no circumstances should the legs be massaged because of the danger of breaking loose any clots that might form in the legs of a patient predisposed to PE. Vital signs should be monitored frequently and the patient instructed not to use a pillow under the knees, which can slow down venous return and lead to the formation of a clot.

embolization (ˌembəlie'zayshən) 1. occlusion of a blood vessel by particulate matter impacting within it, such as fragments of clot, air or fat. 2. therapeutic introduction of a substance into a vessel in order to occlude it.

embololalia (ˌembəloh'layli·ə) the interpolation of meaningless words or phrases in a spoken sentence.

embolophrasia (ˌembəloh'frayzi·ə) embololalia.

embolus ('embələs) pl. *emboli* [Gr.] a clot or other plug, usually part or all of a thrombus, brought by the blood from another vessel and forced into a smaller one, thus obstructing circulation (embolism).

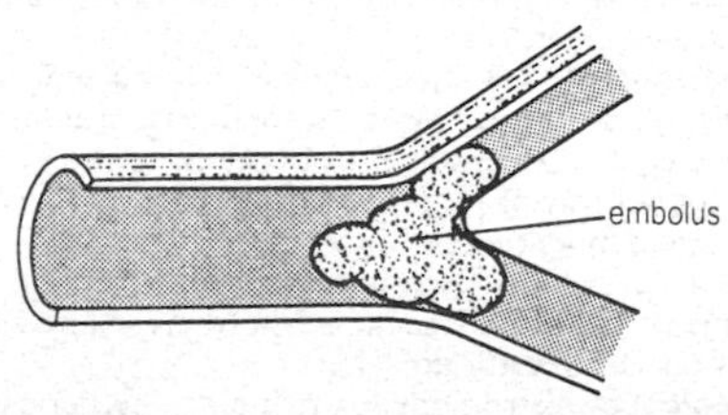

Embolus

saddle e. one situated at the bifurcation of a large artery, sometimes blocking both branches.

embrocation (ˌembroh'kayshən) a liquid applied to the body by rubbing to treat strains; a liniment.

embryectomy (ˌembri'ektəmee) excision of an extrauterine embryo or fetus.

embryo ('embriˌoh) a new organism in the earliest stage of development; the human young from the time of fertilization of the ovum until the beginning of the third month. After the second month the unborn baby is usually referred to as the fetus. adj. **embryonal, embryonic.**

Immediately after fertilization takes place, cell division begins and progresses at a rapid rate. At approximately 4 weeks the cell mass becomes a recognizable embryo from 7 to 10 mm long with rudimentary organs. The beginnings of the eyes, ears, and extremities can be seen. By the end of the second month the embryo has grown to a length of 2 to 2.5 cm, and the head is the most prominent part because of the rapid development of the brain; the sex can be distinguished at this stage.

At the time of fertilization the ovum contains the potential beginnings of a human being. As cell division takes place the cells of the blastoderm (embryonic disc) gradually form three layers from which all the body structures develop. The ectoderm (outer layer) gives rise to the epidermis of the skin and its appendages, and to the nervous system. The mesoderm (middle layer) develops into muscle, connective tissue, the circulatory organs, circulating lymph and blood cells, endothelial tissues within the closed vessels and cavities, and the epithelium portion of the urogenital system. From the entoderm (internal layer) are derived those portions not arising from the ectoderm, the liver, pancreas, and the lungs.

embryocardia (ˌembrioh'kahdi·ə) a symptom in which the heart sounds resemble those of the fetus, there being very little difference in the quality of the first and second sounds.

embryologist (ˌembri'oləjist) an expert in embryology.

embryology (ˌembri'oləjee) the science of the development of the individual during the embryonic stage and, by extension, in several or even all preceding and subsequent stages of the life cycle. adj. **embryological.**

embryoma (ˌembri'ohmə) a general term applied to neoplasms thought to be derived from embryonic cells or tissues, including dermoid cysts, teratomas, embryonal carcinomas, etc.

e. of kidney Wilms' tumour.

embryonization (ˌembri·ənie'zayshən) reversion of a tissue or cell to the embryonic form.

embryonoid ('embri·əˌnoyd) resembling an embryo.

embryopathy (ˌembri'opəthee) a morbid condition of the embryo or a disorder resulting from abnormal embryonic development, with consequent congenital anomalies.

rubella e. congenital deformities in an infant due to RUBELLA (German measles) in the mother during early pregnancy; called also *rubella syndrome*.

embryoplastic (ˌembrioh'plastik) pertaining to or concerned in formation of an embryo.

embryotoxon (ˌembrioh'tokson) a ringlike opacity at the margin of the cornea.

anterior e. embryotoxon.

posterior e. a developmental anomaly in which there is a ringlike opacity at Schwalbe's ring, with thickening and anterior displacement of the latter.

embryotroph ('embri·əˌtrohf) the total nutriment (histotroph and haemotroph) made available to the embryo.

embryotrophy (ˌembri'otrəfee) the nutrition of the early embryo.

emedullate (ee'medəˌlayt) to remove bone marrow.

emergent (i'mərjənt) 1. coming out from a cavity or other part. 2. coming on suddenly.

emesis ('eməsis) the act of vomiting. Also used as a word termination, as in *haematemesis*.

emetic (i'metik) 1. causing vomiting. 2. an agent that causes vomiting. A strong solution of salt (1 tablespoon to 1 cup of water), mustard water (1 tablespoon to 1 cup of water), and powdered ipecac or ipecac syrup are examples of emetics.

Emetics should not be used when strong alkalis or acids have been swallowed, since vomiting may rupture the already weakened walls of the oesophagus. Among the acids and alkalis for which emetics should not be used are sodium hydroxide (caustic soda), potassium hydroxide (caustic potash), and carbolic acid. Emetics should be avoided also when kerosene, gasoline, nail polish remover, or lacquer thinner has been swallowed, since vomiting of these substances may draw them into the lungs.

emetine ('eməˌteen) an alkaloid derived from ipecac or produced synthetically. Its hydrochloride salt is used as an amoebicide.

emetocathartic (ˌemətohkə'thahtik) 1. both emetic and cathartic. 2. an emetocathartic agent.

EMF electromotive force.

EMI elderly mentally infirm.

emigration (ˌemi'grayshən) the escape of leukocytes through the walls of small blood vessels; diapedesis.

eminence ('eminəns) a projection or boss.

eminentia (ˌemi'nenshi·ə) pl. *eminentiae* [L.] eminence.

emissary ('emisə·ree) affording an outlet, referring especially to the venous outlets from the dural sinuses through the skull.

emission (i'mishən) a discharge; specifically an involuntary discharge of semen.

nocturnal e. reflex emission of semen during sleep.

emmenagogue (i'menəˌgog, -'mee-) an agent or measure that promotes menstruation.

emmenia (e'meeni·ə) menstruation. adj. **emmenic.**

emmenology (ˌemə'noləjee) the sum of knowledge about menstruation and its disorders.

emmetrope ('emeˌtrohp) a person who has no refractive error of vision.

emmetropia (ˌeme'trohpi·ə) the ideal optical condition, parallel rays coming to a focus on the retina. adj. **emmetropic.**

emollient (i'moli·ənt, -'moh-) 1. soothing and softening, as an emollient bath given for various skin disorders. 2. an agent that softens or soothes the skin, or soothes an irritated internal surface.

emotion (i'mohshən) feeling or affect; a state of arousal characterized by alteration of feeling tone and by physiological behavioural changes. adj. **emotional.** The physical form of emotion may be outward and evident to others, as in crying, laughing, blushing, or a variety of facial expressions. However, emotion is not always reflected in one's appearance and actions even though psychic changes are taking place. Joy, grief, fear, and anger are examples of emotions.

empathize ('empəˌthiez) to experience or feel empathy; to enter into another's feelings.

empathy ('empəthee) the recognition of and entering into another's feelings. adj. **empathic.**

emperipolesis (ˌemperipo'leesis) lymphocytic penetration of and movement within another cell.

emphysema (ˌemfi'seemə, -fie-) a pathological accumulation of air in tissues or organs. The term is generally used to designate chronic pulmonary emphysema, a lung disorder in which the terminal bronchioles become plugged with mucus. Eventually there is a loss of elasticity in the lung tissue so that inspired air cannot be expelled, making breathing difficult.

bullous e. emphysema in which bullae form in areas of lung tissue so that these areas do not contribute to respiration.

chronic pulmonary e. emphysema of the lungs that develops slowly over a period of years and in some persons may gradually lead to serious disability. The disease becomes disabling between the ages of 50 and

80, but ventilatory deficits can be detected earlier.

In many cases, it occurs as a result of prolonged respiratory disorders, such as chronic bronchial ASTHMA, BRONCHITIS, or TUBERCULOSIS, that have caused partial obstruction of the smaller divisions of the bronchi. (See also CHRONIC OBSTRUCTIVE AIRWAYS DISEASE.) Chronic emphysema may also occur without serious preceding respiratory problems. It has been one of the major causes of death in industrialized countries. Sufferers have difficulty with breathing and a persistent cough that is moist and wheezing in nature. Cardiac complications, especially enlargement and dilation of the right ventricle with resultant right heart failure (COR PULMONALE), may ultimately develop.

TREATMENT AND PATIENT CARE. See CHRONIC OBSTRUCTIVE AIRWAYS DISEASE.

hypoplastic e. pulmonary emphysema due to a developmental abnormality, resulting in a reduced number of alveoli, which are abnormally large.

interlobular e. accumulation of air in the septa between lobules of the lungs.

interstitial e. presence of air in the peribronchial and interstitial tissues of the lungs.

lobar e. emphysema involving less than all the lobes of the affected lung.

lobar e., congenital, lobar e., infantile a condition characterized by overinflation, commonly affecting one of the upper lobes and causing respiratory distress in early life.

panacinar e., panlobular e. generalized obstructive emphysema affecting all lung segments, with atrophy and dilation of the alveoli and destruction of the vascular bed.

subcutaneous e. air or gas in the subcutaneous tissues.

surgical e. air or gas which has escaped along tissue planes following operation or trauma.

unilateral e. emphysema affecting only one lung, frequently due to congenital defects in circulation.

vesicular e. panacinar emphysema.

emphysematous (ˌemfi'seemətəs, -fie-) of the nature of or affected with emphysema.

empiricism (em'piriˌsizəm) skill or knowledge based entirely on experience. adj. **empirical.**

emprosthotonos (ˌempros'thotənəs) tetanic forward flexure of the body.

empty-sella syndrome (ˌemptee'selə) a clinical syndrome in which the diaphragm of the sella turcica is vestigial, the sella turcica forms an extension of the subarachnoid space and is filled with cerebrospinal fluid, and the pituitary fossa appears to be empty, although the pituitary gland is present in a flattened form.

empyema (ˌempie'eemə) accumulation of pus in a body cavity, particularly the presence of a purulent exudate within the pleural cavity (pyothorax). It occurs as an occasional complication of pleurisy or some other respiratory disease. Symptoms include dyspnoea, coughing, chest pain on one side, malaise, and fever. Thoracentesis may be done to confirm the diagnosis and determine the specific causative organism. The condition is treated with antibiotics, rest, and sedative cough mixtures.

empyesis (ˌempie'eesis) a pustular eruption.

emulgent (i'muljənt) 1. effecting a straining or purifying process. 2. a renal artery or vein. 3. an emulsifying agent.

emulsion (i'mulshən) a mixture of two immiscible liquids, one being dispersed throughout the other in small droplets; a colloid system in which both the dispersed phase and the dispersion medium are liquids. Margarine, cold cream, and various medicated ointments are emulsions. In some emulsions the suspended particles tend to join together and settle out; hence the container must be shaken each time the emulsion is used.

Emulsions are used in dermatology as lubricants and ointments. They are also used as an alternative to soap for washing eczematous skin.

emulsoid (i'mulsoyd) a colloid system in which the dispersion medium is liquid, usually water, and the disperse phase consists of highly complex organic substances, such as starch or glue, which absorb much water, swell, and become distributed throughout the dispersion medium.

emunctory (i'mungktə·ree) 1. excretory or cleansing. 2. an excretory organ or duct.

EN(G) Enrolled Nurse (General).

EN(M) Enrolled Nurse (Mental).

EN(MH) Enrolled Nurse (Mental Handicap).

enalapril (e'naləpril) an angiotensin converting enzyme inhibitor used in hypertension and heart failure.

enamel (i'naməl) the white, compact, and very hard substance covering and protecting the dentine of the crown of a tooth.

mottled e. dental fluorosis; defective enamel, with a chalky white appearance or brownish stain, caused by excessive amounts of fluorine in drinking water and food preparations during the period of enamel calcification.

e. organ a process of epithelium forming a cap over a dental papilla and developing into the enamel.

enanthema (en'anthəmə) an eruption upon a mucous surface. adj. **enanthematous.**

enantiomorph (e'nantiohˌmawf) one of a pair of isomeric substances, the molecular structures of which are mirror opposites of each other.

enarthrosis (ˌenah'throhsis) a joint in which the rounded head of one bone is received into a socket in another, permitting motion in any direction; called also *ball-and-socket joint.*

ENB English National Board.

encanthis (en'kanthis) a small fleshy growth at the inner canthus of the eye which may form an abscess.

encapsulation (enˌkapsyuh'layshən) enclosure within a capsule.

encephal(o)- word element. [Gr.] *brain.*

encephalalgia (enˌkefə'lalji·ə, -ˌsef-) cephalalgia; pain within the head; headache.

encephalatrophy (enˌkefə'latrəfee, -ˌsef-) atrophy of the brain.

encephalic (ˌenkə'falik, -ˌensə-) 1. pertaining to the brain. 2. within the skull.

encephalitis (enˌkefə'lietis, -ˌsef-) inflammation of the brain. adj. **encephalitic.**

There are many types of encephalitis, depending on the causative agent and the structures involved. Many cases are caused by viruses; some are transmitted from animals to man, as in equine encephalitis, and some from man to man, as in HERPES SIMPLEX encephalitis. The symptoms may be mild, with headache, general malaise and muscle ache similar to that associated with influenza. The more acute and serious symptoms may include fever, delirium, convulsions and coma, and in a significant number of patients result in death.

ACUTE VIRAL ENCEPHALITIS. This may be caused by mumps virus, herpes simplex virus, varicella zoster virus, cytomegalovirus, Epstein–Barr virus, enteroviruses, influenza virus, rabies virus, lymphocytic choriomeningitis virus or arboviruses.This condition is a statutorily notifiable disease.

Arbovirus encephalitis is transmitted by insects and can be classified into two types: (1) the *mosquito-borne type*, which includes *equine encephalitis* found in

North and South America (divided into Eastern, Western and Venezuelan equine encephalitis), *St. Louis encephalitis* found throughout most of the USA, *lacrosse encephalitis* found in forest areas of the USA and Canada, *Murray Valley encephalitis* found in Australia and New Guinea, and *Japanese B encephalitis* found in Japan and the Western Pacific, for which a vaccine is available in Japan, where it is made and may be obtained in the UK for travellers to endemic areas. The source of these viral encephalitides is not known; transmission is by mosquito bite with an incubation period of 5–15 days. Person-to-person spread does not occur. (2) *The tick-borne type*, which includes *Russian spring-summer encephalitis* found in Russia and the Far East, and *Central European tick-borne encephalitis* found in forest areas of Austria, Poland, Hungary and parts of Germany; a vaccine is available in the UK for travellers who are likely to be exposed to infection in these forest areas. It also includes *louping-ill*, which has been reported in Scotland but is very rare. The source of these tick-borne viral encephalitides appears to be wild mammals; rodents and deer have been implicated. Transmission to man is by the bite of a tick. The incubation period is 7–14 days. Person-to-person spread does not occur.

OTHER CAUSES OF ENCEPHALITIS. Encephalitis may occur in bacterial infections such as leptospirosis, tuberculosis and syphilis, in fungal infections such as histoplasmosis and cryptococcosis, and protozoal infections such as malaria, toxoplasmosis, trypanosomiasis (sleeping sickness) and primary amoebic meningoencephalitis.

Economo's e. a form of epidemic encephalitis, the original type described by von Economo, marked by increasing languor, apathy, and drowsiness, passing into lethargy; observed in various parts of the world between 1915 and 1926. In the UK epidemic of 1920 to 1929 there were over 18,000 notified cases. Then the disease disappeared although sporadic cases have been reported from time to time. Called also *lethargic encephalitis*.

post-infectious e. an allergic encephalitis following 2–12 days after infection with measles, rubella, mumps, influenza, varicella zoster or vaccinia virus (when it is termed post-vaccinial encephalitis).

slow virus e. viral encephalitis with a long incubation period, including subacute sclerosing panencephalitis after measles and Creutzfeldt–Jakob disease.

encephalocele (en'kefəloh,seel, -'sef-) hernial protrusion of brain substance through a congenital or traumatic opening of the skull.

encephalocystocele (en,kefəloh'sistə,seel, -,sef-) hernial protrusion of the brain distended by fluid.

encephalogram (en'kefələ,gram, -'sef-) the film obtained by encephalography.

encephalography (en,kefə'logrəfee, -,sef-) radiography demonstrating the intracranial fluid-containing spaces after the withdrawal of cerebrospinal fluid and introduction of air or other gas; it includes pneumoencephalography and ventriculography.

encephaloid (en'kefə,loyd, -'sef-) 1. resembling the brain or brain substance. 2. medullary carcinoma.

encephalolith (en'kefəloh,lith, -'sef-) a brain calculus.

encephalology (en,kefə'loləjee, -,sef-) the sum of knowledge regarding the brain, its functions, and its diseases.

encephaloma (en,kefə'lohmə, -,sef-) 1. any swelling or tumour of the brain. 2. medullary carcinoma.

encephalomalacia (en,kefəlohmə'layshi·ə, -,sef-) softening of the brain.

encephalomeningitis (en,kefəloh,menin'jietis, -,sef-) meningoencephalitis; inflammation of the brain and meninges.

encephalomeningocele (en,kefəlohmə'ning·gohseel, -,sef-) meningocephalocele; protrusion of the brain and meninges through a defect in the skull.

encephalomeningopathy (en,kefəloh,mening-'gopəthee, -,sef-) meningoencephalopathy; disease involving the brain and meninges.

encephalomere (en,kefəloh,miə, -,sef-) one of the segments making up the embryonic brain.

encephalometer (en,kefə'lomitə, -,sef-) an instrument used in locating certain of the brain regions.

encephalomyelitis (en,kefəloh,mieə'lietis, -,sef-) inflammation of the brain and spinal cord. Caused by agents which cause MENINGITIS and ENCEPHALITIS.

encephalomyeloneuropathy (en,kefəloh-,mieəlohnyooə'ropəthee, -,sef-) a disease involving the brain, spinal cord, and nerves.

encephalomyelopathy (en,kefəloh,mieə'lopəthee, -,sef-) a disease involving the brain and spinal cord.

encephalomyeloradiculitis (en,kefəloh,mieəlohra-,dikyuh'lietis, -,sef-) inflammation of the brain, spinal cord, and spinal nerve roots.

encephalomyeloradiculopathy (en,kefəloh-,mieəlohra,dikyuh'lopəthee, -,sef-) a disease involving the brain, spinal cord, and spinal nerve roots.

encephalomyocarditis (en,kefəloh,mieohkah'dietis, -,sef-) a viral disease characterized by degenerative and inflammatory changes in skeletal and cardiac muscle and by lesions of the central nervous system resembling those of poliomyelitis.

encephalon (en'kefəlon, -'sef-) the brain; with the spinal cord (medulla spinalis) constituting the central nervous system.

encephalopathy (en,kefə'lopəthee, -,sef-) a non-specific term meaning diffuse disease or damage of the brain.

biliary e., bilirubin e. kernicterus.

boxer's e. traumatic encephalopathy.

dialysis e. a degenerative disease of the brain associated with long-term use of haemodialysis, marked by speech disorders and constant myoclonic jerks, progressing to global dementia.

hepatic e. a condition, usually occurring secondarily to advanced liver disease, marked by disturbances of consciousness that may progress to deep coma (hepatic coma), psychiatric changes of varying degree, flapping tremor, and fetor hepaticus.

hypernatraemic e. a severe haemorrhagic encephalopathy induced by the hyperosmolarity accompanying hypernatraemia and dehydration.

lead e. brain disease caused by lead poisoning.

portal–systemic e. hepatic encephalopathy.

progressive subcortical e. Schilder's disease.

traumatic e. general slowing of mental functions, occasional confusion, and scattered memory loss, due to cumulative punishment absorbed in the boxing ring. Called also *boxer's encephalopathy*.

Wernicke's e. an inflammatory haemorrhagic form due to thiamine deficiency associated with alcoholism (see also WERNICKE'S ENCEPHALOPATHY).

encephalopuncture (en,kefəloh'pungkchə, -,sef-) surgical puncture of the brain.

encephalopyosis (en,kefəlohpie'ohsis, -,sef-) suppuration or abscess of the brain.

encephalorrhagia (en,kefələ'rayji·ə, -,sef-) haemorrhage within or from the brain.

encephalosclerosis (en,kefəlohsklə'rohsis, -,sef-) hardening of the brain.

encephalosis (en,kefə'lohsis, -,sef-) any organic brain disease.

encephalotomy (en,kefə'lotəmee, -,sef-) 1. craniotomy (2). 2. dissection or anatomy of the brain.

enchondroma (ˌenkon'drohmə) a benign tumour of cartilage arising within the marrow cavity of a bone. adj. **enchondromatous.**

enchondromatosis (enˌkondrohmə'tohsis) a condition characterized by hamartomatous proliferation of cartilage cells within the metaphysis of several bones, causing thinning of the overlying cortex and distortion of the growth in length. Called also *dyschondroplasia.*

enchondrosarcoma (enˌkondrohsah'kohmə) central chondrosarcoma.

enclave ('enklayv) tissue detached from its normal connection and enclosed within another organ.

encopresis (ˌenkə'preesis) incontinence of faeces not due to organic defect or illness.

encysted (en'sistid) enclosed in a sac, bladder, or cyst.

end-artery ('endˌahtə-ree) an artery that does not anastomose with other arteries.

end-bulb ('endˌbulb) one of the small encapsulated bodies at the end of sensory nerve fibres in skin, mucous membranes, muscles, and other areas. They are called also *Krause's bulbs* or *corpuscles.*

end-feet ('endˌfeet) button- or knoblike terminal enlargements of naked nerve fibres which end in a synapse with dendrites of another cell.

end-organ ('endˌawgən) one of the larger, encapsulated endings of sensory nerves.

end-plate ('endˌplayt) a flattened discoid expansion at the neuromuscular junction, where a myelinated motor nerve fibre joins a skeletal muscle fibre.

end(o)- word element. [Gr.] *within, inward.*

endadelphos (ˌendə'delfos) a fetus or infant in which a parasitic twin is enclosed within the body of the other twin (the autosite).

Endamoeba (ˌendə'meebə) a genus of amoebas parasitic in the intestines of invertebrates.

endangiitis (ˌendanji'ietis) inflammation of the endangium.

endangium (en'danji·əm) tunica intima (inner coat) of a blood vessel.

endaortitis (ˌenday·aw'tietis) inflammation of the membrane lining the aorta.

endarterectomy (ˌendahtə'rektəmee) removal of thickened atheromatous areas of the innermost coat of an artery.

carotid e. endarterectomy within an extracranial carotid artery, usually the common carotid (see also CAROTID ENDARTERECTOMY).

endarterial (ˌendah'tiə·ri·əl) within an artery.

endarteritis (ˌendahtə'rietis) inflammation of the innermost coat (tunica intima) of an artery.

e. obliterans a form in which the lumen of the smaller vessels becomes narrowed or obliterated as a result of proliferation of the tissue of the intimal layer.

endaural (end'awrəl) within the ear.

endbrain ('endˌbrayn) telencephalon.

endemic (en'demik) a disease or infection constantly present in a community.

endergonic (ˌendə'gonik) characterized or accompanied by the absorption of energy; requiring the input of free energy.

ending ('ending) a termination, especially the peripheral termination of a nerve or nerve fibre.

endoaneurysmorrhaphy (ˌendohˌanyə·riz'mo·rəfee) an operation to cure an aneurysm by evacuating its contents and closing all the vascular connections by suturing from within the sac.

endoangiitis (ˌendohˌanji'ietis) endangiitis.

endoappendicitis (ˌendoh·əˌpendi'sietis) inflammation of the mucous membrane of the vermiform appendix.

endoarteritis (ˌendohˌahtə'rietis) endarteritis.

Endobil ('endohbil) trademark for a preparation of meglumine iodoxamate (an intravenous cholangiographic agent).

endoblast ('endohˌblast) entoderm.

endobronchitis (ˌendohbrong'kietis) inflammation of the epithelial lining of the bronchi.

endocardial (ˌendoh'kahdi·əl) 1. situated or occurring within the heart. 2. pertaining to the endocardium.

e. cushions elevations on the atrioventricular canal of the embryonic heart which later help form the interatrial septum.

endocarditis (ˌendohkah'dietis) exudative and proliferative inflammatory alterations of the endocardium, characterized by the presence of vegetations on the surface of the endocardium or in the endocardium itself, and most commonly involving a heart valve, but also affecting the inner lining of the cardiac chambers or the endocardium elsewhere. adj. **endocarditic.**

atypical verrucous e. nonbacterial endocarditis found in association with systemic lupus erythematosus. Called also *Libman–Sacks encocarditis.*

bacterial e. infectious endocarditis, acute or subacute, caused by various bacteria, including streptococci, staphylococci, enterococci, gonococci, and gram-negative bacilli.

infectious e., infective e. that due to infection with microorganisms, especially bacteria and fungi: the *acute* form may be due to staphylococci, pneumococci, gonococci, streptococci, and other bacteria or to other microorganisms; the *subacute* form may be caused by viridans streptococci, fungi, or other microorganisms.

Libman–Sacks e. atypical verrucous endocarditis.

Löffler's e., Löffler's fibroplastic parietal e. endocarditis associated with eosinophilia, marked by fibroplastic thickening of the endocardium, resulting in congestive heart failure, persistent tachycardia, hepatomegaly, splenomegaly, serous effusions into the pleural cavity, and oedema of the limbs.

mural e. that affecting the lining of the walls of the heart chambers only.

mycotic e. infectious endocarditis, usually subacute, due to various fungi, most commonly species of *Candida, Aspergillus,* and *Histoplasma.*

nonbacterial thrombotic e. that in which the vegetations, single or multiple, consist of fibrin and other blood elements.

parietal e. mural endocarditis.

prosthetic valve e. infectious endocarditis as a complication of implantation of a prosthetic valve in the heart; the vegetations usually occur along the line of suture.

rheumatic e. that associated with rheumatic fever.

rickettsial e. endocarditis caused by invasion of the heart valves with *Coxiella burnetii*; it is a sequela of Q fever, usually occurring in persons who have had rheumatic fever.

syphilitic e. endocarditis resulting from extension of syphilitic infection from the aorta.

tuberculous e. that resulting from extension of a tuberculous infection from the pericardium and myocardium.

valvular e. that affecting the membrane over the heart valves only.

vegetative e., verrucous e. endocarditis, infectious or noninfectious, the characteristic lesions of which are vegetations or verrucae on the endocardium.

endocardium (ˌendoh'kahdi·əm) the endothelial lining membrane of the cavities of the heart and the connective tissue bed on which it lies.

endocervicitis (ˌendohˌsərvi'sietis) inflammation of the endocervix.

endocervix (ˌendoh'sərviks) 1. the mucous membrane lining the canal of the uterine cervix. 2. the region of the opening of the cervix into the uterine cavity. adj. **endocervical.**

endochondral (,endoh'kondrəl) situated, formed, or occurring within cartilage.

endocolitis (,endohkə'lietis) inflammation of the mucous membrane of the colon.

endocranial (,endoh'krayni·əl) within the cranium.

endocranitis (,endohkray'nietis) inflammation of endocranium.

endocranium (,endoh'krayni·əm) the endosteal layer of the dura mater of the brain.

endocrine ('endoh,krin, -,krien) 1. secreting internally. 2. pertaining to internal secretions; hormonal.

e. glands ductless organs or groups of cells that secrete regulatory substances that are released directly into the circulation (hormones). The endocrine or hormonal system and the nervous system are the two major control systems of the body, and their functions are interrelated. Hormonal activity is mostly concerned with regulating metabolic activities by controlling the rates at which chemical reactions take place within cells, the transport of substances across the cell membrane, and activities related to growth and reproduction. The word HORMONES is applied to substances released by the endocrine glands that have physiological effects on target organs (which can be other endocrine glands) and tissues distant from the gland. There are, however, local hormones (autacoids) secreted at the site of the tissue being affected, for example, acetylcholine and serotonin.

The interactions between hormones and metabolic activities throughout the body are controlled by negative feedback. The system is a closed loop in which either an excess or deficit of some hormone initiates a response that results in its return to a level within normal range. For example, the level of thyroxine in the serum is responsive to the level of thyroid-stimulating hormone (TSH) released by the anterior pituitary gland, which in turn responds to the level of TSH-releasing hormone (TRH), released by the hypothalamus; the release of these hormones responds to the level of thyroxine. Excessive amounts of thyroxine eventually result in reduction in the amount of thyroxine released from the thyroid gland. Similarly, a lower than normal concentration of thyroxine in the serum will initiate changes that eventually raise the level of thyroxine by stimulating its release from the thyroid gland.

The major endocrine glands are the HYPOTHALAMUS, the PITUITARY, THYROID, PARATHYROID, and ADRENAL GLANDS, the alpha and beta cells of the PANCREAS, and the gonads (OVARIES and TESTES).

Disorders of the endocrine glands are not simply a matter of overproduction or underproduction of a particular hormone. Hyperfunction and hypofunction of the endocrine glands can be classified according to the source of the dysfunction.

A *primary* disorder is one in which the gland responsible for synthesis and production of one or more specific hormones is not functioning normally and is releasing too much or too little of one or more hormones. An example is hypothyroidism resulting from surgical or radiotherapeutic destruction of the thyroid gland.

A *secondary* endocrine disorder is one in which dysfunction of one gland, usually the pituitary, causes dysfunction of another gland. An example is hyposecretion of adrenocorticotrophic hormone (ACTH) from the anterior lobe of the pituitary gland. This results in secondary adrenocortical insufficiency and a deficit of glucocorticoids and some mineralocorticoids.

In a *tertiary* endocrine disorder, two control steps are involved, as when a disorder of the hypothalamus causes improper inhibition or release of a releasing hormone that influences the pituitary. Dysfunction of the pituitary gland then affects some other endocrine gland that is normally stimulated by a pituitary hormone.

endocrinism (,endoh'krienizəm) endocrinopathy.

endocrinologist (,endohkri'noləjist) an individual skilled in endocrinology, and in the diagnosis and treatment of disorders of the glands of internal secretion, i.e., the endocrine glands.

endocrinology (,endohkri'noləjee) study of the endocrine system.

endocrinopathy (,endohkri'nopəthee) any disease due to disorder of the endocrine system. adj. **endocrinopathic.**

endocrinotherapy (,endoh,krinoh'therəpee) treatment of disease by the administration of endocrine preparations; hormonotherapy.

endocrinous (en'dokrinəs) of or pertaining to an internal secretion (hormone) or to a gland producing such a secretion, i.e., to an endocrine gland.

endocystitis (,endohsi'stietis) inflammation of the bladder mucosa.

endocytosis (,endohsie'tohsis) the uptake by a cell of material from the environment by invagination of the plasma membrane; it includes both phagocytosis and pinocytosis.

endoderm ('endoh,dərm) entoderm.

endodontia (,endoh'donshi·ə) endodontics.

endodontics (,endoh'dontiks) the branch of dentistry concerned with the aetiology, prevention, diagnosis, and treatment of conditions that affect the tooth pulp, root, and periapical tissues.

endodontist (,endoh'dontist) a dentist who specializes in endodontics.

endoenteritis (,endoh,entə'rietis) inflammation of the intestinal mucosa.

endogamy (en'dogəmee) 1. fertilization by union of separate cells having the same chromatin ancestry. 2. restriction of marriage to persons within the same community. adj. **endogamous.**

endogenous (en'dojənəs) produced within or caused by factors within the organism.

endointoxication (,endoh·in,toksi'kayshən) poisoning by an endogenous toxin.

endolaryngeal (,endoh,larin'jeeəl, -lə'rinji·əl) situated on or occurring within the larynx.

Endolimax (,endoh'liemaks) a genus of amoebas found as a commensal in the colon of man (*E. nana)*, and also in other mammals, birds, amphibians, and cockroaches.

endolymph ('endoh,limf) the fluid within the membranous labyrinth of the ear.

endolysin (,endoh'liesin, en'dolisin) a bactericidal substance in cells; acting directly on bacteria.

endometriosis (,endoh,meetri'ohsis) a condition in which tissue more or less perfectly resembling the uterine mucous membrane occurs aberrantly in various locations in the pelvic cavity. adj. **endometriotic.** The condition may be characterized by pelvic pain, abnormal uterine or rectal bleeding, dysmenorrhoea, and symptoms of pressure within the pelvic cavity. Sterility and dyspareunia also may be present.

Treatment is based on the age of the patient and the extent of the endometrial growth. In young women exogenous hormone therapy is employed, and, whenever feasible, the patient is encouraged to become pregnant since interruption of menstruation is thought to retard the progress of the disease. In older women and in cases of extensive growth, surgical treatment involving complete hysterectomy is indicated. X-ray

Principal endocrine hormones and their actions

Endocrine gland and hormone	Acts on (target)	Actions
Posterior pituitary		
Antidiuretic hormone (ADH)	Distal tubules of kidney	Stimulates conservation of water by reabsorption
Oxytocin	Uterus and mammary glands	Stimulates uterine contraction and ejection of milk into ducts
Anterior pituitary		
Adrenocorticotrophic hormone (ACTH)	Adrenal cortex	Formation and secretion of adrenal cortex hormones (see below)
Thyroid-stimulating hormone (TSH)	Thyroid gland	Formation and secretion of thyroid hormones (see below)
Gonadotrophic hormones (follicle-stimulating hormone and luteinising hormone)	Gonads	Stimulates gonad hormone production (see below)
Human growth hormone (HGH)	General	Stimulates growth — promotes protein synthesis, raises blood glucose level, mobilizes fat
Prolactin	Mammary glands	Stimulates milk secretion
Thyroid		
Thyroxine (T_4) and tri-iodothyronine (T_3)	General	Control metabolic rate, mobilize fat, affect metabolism of carbohydrates essential to normal development
Calcitonin	Bone	Lowers blood calcium level by inhibiting breakdown of bone
Adrenal cortex		
Aldosterone	Kidney tubules	Maintains sodium balance
Cortisol	General	Promotes synthesis of glucose in liver to raise blood glucose, mobilizes fat
Adrenal medulla		
Adrenaline and noradrenaline	General	Helps body to cope with stress, e.g. by increasing heart rate, metabolic rate, rerouting blood, increasing blood sugar
Parathyroids		
Parathyroid hormone	Bone, gut, kidneys	Increases blood calcium level
Pancreas		
Insulin	General	Lowers blood sugar by allowing glucose to enter the cells for use, stimulates fat storage and protein synthesis
Glucagon	Adipose tissue, liver	Increases blood glucose by stimulating fat breakdown and glucose production in the liver
Testes		
Testosterone	General	Maturation of reproductive organs of male, development of secondary sexual characteristics in male, bone growth and fusion of epiphyses
Ovaries		
Oestrogen	General	Preparation of endometrium for pregnancy and maintenance during pregnancy
Progesterone	Uterus, breasts	Maturation of female reproductive organs, development of secondary sexual characteristics in female, thickening of endometrium, development of breast lobules and areoli
Placenta		
Production of oestrogen and progesterone is taken over from ovaries at about the twelfth week of pregnancy		

From Faulkner, A. (1985) *Nursing: A Creative Approach*, 1st edn, Baillière Tindall, p. 28.

therapy in doses large enough to produce destruction of the reproductive organs is sometimes used when there is definite evidence of advanced endometriosis and surgery is contraindicated or refused.

endometritis (ˌendohmi'trietis) inflammation of the endometrium.

puerperal e. endometritis following childbirth.

syncytial e. a benign tumour-like lesion with infiltration of the uterine wall by large syncytial trophoblastic cells.

tuberculous e. inflammation of the endometrium, usually also involving the uterine tubes, due to infection by *Mycobacterium tuberculosis*, with the presence of tubercles.

endometrium (ˌendoh'meetri·əm) the mucous membrane lining the uterus. adj. **endometrial**.

endomitosis (ˌendohmie'tohsis) mitosis taking place without dissolution of the nuclear membrane, and not followed by cytoplasmic division, resulting in doubling of the number of chromosomes within the nucleus. adj. **endomitotic**.

endomorph ('endohˌmawf) an individual having the type of body build in which endodermal tissues predominate; there is relative preponderance of soft roundness throughout the body, with large digestive viscera and fat accumulations, and with large trunk and thighs and tapering extremities.

endomorphy ('endohˌmawfee) the condition of being an endomorph. adj. **endomorphic**.

endomyocarditis (ˌendohˌmieohkah'dietis) inflammation of the endocardium and myocardium.

endomysium (ˌendoh'misi·əm) the sheath of delicate reticular fibrils that surrounds each muscle fibre.

endoneuritis (ˌendohnyooə'rietis) inflammation of the endoneurium.

endoneurium (ˌendoh'nyooə·ri·əm) the interstitial connective tissue in a peripheral nerve, separating individual nerve fibres. adj. **endoneurial**.

endonuclease (ˌendoh'nyookliˌayz) a nuclease that cleaves internal bonds of polynucleotides.

restriction e's enzymes that cleave large DNA molecules at specific sequences of four to six nucleotides. See also RECOMBINANT DNA.

endoparasite (ˌendoh'parəˌsiet) a parasite that lives within the body of the host. adj. **endoparasitic**.

endopelvic (ˌendoh'pelvik) within the pelvis.

endopeptidase (ˌendoh'peptiˌdayz) a peptidase capable of acting on any peptide linkage in a peptide chain.

endopericarditis (ˌendohˌperikah'dietis) inflammation of the endocardium and pericardium.

endoperimyocarditis (ˌendohˌperiˌmieohkah'dietis) inflammation of the endocardium, pericardium, and myocardium.

endoperitonitis (ˌendohˌperitə'nietis) inflammation of the serous lining of the peritoneal cavity.

endophlebitis (ˌendohfli'bietis) inflammation of the intima of a vein.

endophthalmitis (ˌendofthal'mietis) inflammation of the ocular cavities and their adjacent structures.

endophyte ('endohˌfiet) a parasitic plant organism living within its host's body.

endophytic (ˌendoh'fitik) 1. pertaining to an endophyte. 2. growing inward; proliferating on the interior of an organ or structure.

endoreduplication (ˌendohreeˌdyoopli'kayshən) replication of chromosomes without subsequent cell division.

endorphin (en'dawfin) one of a group of opiate-like peptides produced naturally by the body at neural synapses at various points in the central nervous system pathways where they modulate the transmission of pain perceptions. The term *endorphin* was coined by combining the words *endogenous* and *morphine*. Like morphine, endorphins raise the pain threshold and produce sedation and euphoria; the effects are blocked by naloxone, a narcotic antagonist.

endorrhachis (ˌendoh'rakis) the spinal dura mater.

endosalpingitis (ˌendohˌsalpin'jietis) inflammation of the endosalpinx.

endosalpingoma (ˌendohˌsalping'gohmə) ADENOMYOMA of the uterine tube.

endosalpingosis (ˌendohˌsalping'gohsis) 1. endometriosis involving the uterine tube. 2. ovarian endometriosis in which the abnormal mucosa resembles tubal mucosa rather than endometrium.

endosalpinx (ˌendoh'salpingks) the mucous membrane lining the oviduct (uterine tube).

endoscope ('endəˌskohp) an instrument used for direct visual inspection of hollow organs or body cavities. Specially designed endoscopes are used for such examinations as BRONCHOSCOPY, URETHROSCOPY, CYSTOSCOPY, OESOPHAGOSCOPY, GASTROSCOPY, SIGMOIDOSCOPY and PROCTOSCOPY. Although the design of an endoscope may vary according to its specific use, all endoscopes have similar working elements. The viewing part (scope) may be a hollow metal or fibre tube fitted with a lens system that permits viewing in a variety of directions. The endoscope also has a light source, power cord, and power source. Accessories that might be used with an endoscope for diagnostic or therapeutic purposes include suction tip, tubes, and suction pump; forceps for removal of biopsy tissue or a foreign body; and an electrode for cauterization.

The diagnostic and therapeutic capacity of endoscopy has been immeasurably enhanced by the introduction of fibreoptic systems. These have replaced rigidity by flexibility of the instruments making them more manoeuvrable. Instruments can now be made longer and finer with the result, for example, that the flexures of the large bowel can be negotiated, the colon be examined throughout its length and the ileocaecal valve be seen and passed to reveal the terminal ileum beyond. Removal of stones from the common bile duct by endoscopy is becoming the method of choice rather than choledochotomy. Such is the improvement of vision and flexibility that fibreoptic gastroscopy takes precedence over contrast radiology for gastric and duodenal lesions and is mandatory in cases of haematemesis. Similar advantages have accrued in other systems; arthroscopy has been developed and is in common use for disorders of the knee; meniscectomy is now undertaken through an arthroscope.

endoscopy (en'doskəpee) visual examination of interior structures of the body with an endoscope. adj. **endoscopic**.

endosepsis (ˌendoh'sepsis) septicaemia originating from causes inside the body.

endoskeleton (ˌendoh'skelitən) the cartilaginous and bony skeleton of the body, exclusive of that part of the skeleton of dermal origin.

endosmosis (ˌendoz'mohsis) inward osmosis; inward passage of liquid through a membrane of a cell or cavity, by which one fluid passes through a septum into a cavity that contains fluid of a different density. adj. **endosmotic**.

endosteal (en'dosti·əl) 1. pertaining to the endosteum. 2. occurring or located within a bone.

endosteitis (ˌendosti'ietis) inflammation of the endosteum.

endosteoma (enˌdosti'ohmə) a tumour in the medullary cavity of a bone.

endosteum (en'dosti·əm) the tissue lining the medullary cavity of a bone.

endostoma (ˌendo'stohmə) endosteoma.

endotendineum (ˌendohten'dini·əm) the delicate connective tissue separating the secondary bundles (fascicles) of a tendon.

endothelia (ˌendoh'theeli·ə) [Gr.] plural of *endothelium*.

endothelial (ˌendoh'theeli·əl) pertaining to or made up of endothelium.

endotheliocyte (ˌendoh'theeliohˌsiet) a large mononuclear phagocytic wandering cell of the circulating blood and tissues. Called also *endothelial leukocyte*.

endothelioid (endoh'theeli,oyd) resembling endothelium.

endothelioma (,endoh,theeli'ohmə) a tumour arising from the endothelial lining of blood vessels.

endotheliosis (,endoh,theeli'ohsis) proliferation of endothelial elements.

endothelium (,endoh'theeli·əm) pl. *endothelia* [Gr.] the layer of epithelial cells that lines the cavities of the heart and of the blood and lymph vessels, and the serous cavities of the body.

endothermal, endothermic (,endoh'thərməl; ,endoh-'thərmik) 1. characterized by the absorption of heat. 2. pertaining to endothermy.

endothermy ('endoh,thərmee) diathermy.

endothrix ('endoh,thriks) a dermatophyte whose growth and spore production are confined chiefly within the shaft of a hair.

endotoxaemia (,endohtok'seemi·ə) the presence of endotoxins in the blood.

endotoxic (,endoh'toksik) pertaining to or possessing endotoxin.

endotoxin (,endoh'toksin) a heat-stable toxin present in the intact bacterial cell but not in cell-free filtrates of cultures of intact bacteria. They are found primarily in enteric bacilli, in which they are identical with the O antigen, but are also found in certain of the gram-negative cocci and in *Pasteurella* and *Brucella* species. The endotoxins are lipopolysaccharide complexes that occur in the cell wall. They are pyrogenic and increase capillary permeability, the activity being substantially the same regardless of the species of bacteria from which they are derived.

endotracheal (,endohtrə'keeəl) within the trachea.

e. tube an AIRWAY catheter inserted in the trachea during endotracheal INTUBATION to assure patency of the upper airway. It also allows for the removal of secretions. Endotracheal intubation may be accomplished through the mouth using an orotracheal tube, or through the nose using a nasotracheal tube. A variety of endotracheal tubes is available. The tubes are almost always 'cuffed' to allow for their use with a mechanical ventilator. The cuff is a balloon-like device that fits over the lower end of the tube. It is attached to a narrow tube that extends outside the body and allows for inflation of the cuff. Once the cuff is inflated there is no flow of air through the trachea other than that going through the endotracheal tube.

Passage of an endotracheal tube during surgery is a well established and long used technique. In recent years the procedure has become a part of medical management of ventilatory failure as an alternative to TRACHEOTOMY. Endotracheal intubation has the advantage of not requiring a surgical procedure as does tracheotomy, removal of the tube (extubation) is less involved, and the procedure can be repeated as necessary.

When endotracheal intubation is used for ventilatory failure, plastic inert tubes with high-volume, low-pressure cuffs are used to lessen damage to the trachea and larynx. These can be left in for weeks (how long exactly varies with local practice). Some conscious patients cannot tolerate the tube and may need to be sedated.

Complications of endotracheal intubation include damage to the vocal cords, ulceration, and eventual subglottic stricture of the larynx. Pulmonary infections may result from interference with the normal protective mechanisms of the glottis and from the introduction of pathogenic organisms into the respiratory tract and difficulty in their removal by coughing.

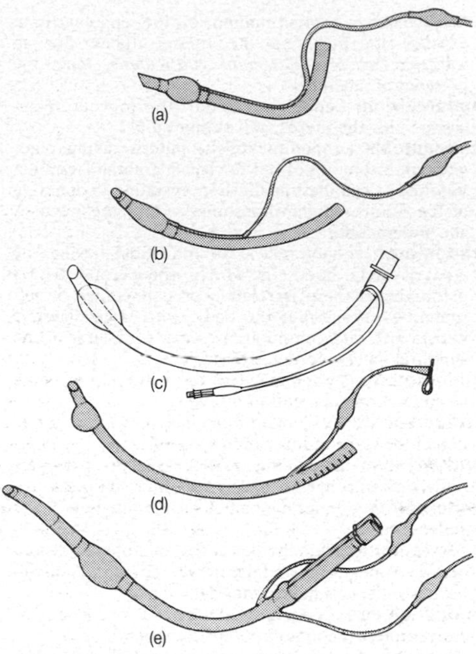

Endotracheal tubes. (a) Oxford non-kink orotracheal tube. Requires an introducer to pass it into the trachea. (b) Magill red-rubber orotracheal tube with inflatable cuff. (c) Nylon armoured non-kink tube. Note the two lines on the tube. If the vocal cords are placed between these lines then the tube will remain in the trachea and not pass into the right bronchus. (d) Nasotracheal tube. Thinner than an orotracheal tube, the tube to the inflatable cuff is attached further back and is buried in the main tube to prevent damage to the nasal mucosa. (e) Robertshaw double-lumen tube that allows one-lung ventilation during thoracic surgery. Note the individual inflatable cuffs for the trachea and left bronchus

PATIENT CARE. After the tube has been inserted by the doctor and the cuff inflated, the orotracheal tube is secured to the patient's face. Secure anchoring of the tube and apparatus is necessary to prevent tension on or misplacement of the endotracheal tube.

The inhaled air must be of adequate humidity and protected from contamination as much as possible. SUCTIONING of secretions via the tube is done with gentleness and according to the basic guidelines established for this procedure. Suctioning often causes a marked rise in blood pressure. Where these effects may be dangerous, e.g., in the patient with head injury, the procedure is only carried out after appropriate sedation of the patient. The patient will require mouth care and frequent observation for signs of pressure against the lips and nose. An emergency tracheotomy tray and an extra endotracheal tube are kept at the patient's bedside.

endovasculitis (,endoh,vaskyuh'lietis) endangiitis.

Enduron ('endyuhron) trademark for a preparation of methyclothiazide, a diuretic.

enema ('enimə) 1. introduction of fluid into the rectum. 2. a solution introduced into the rectum to promote evacuation of faeces or as a means of administering nutrient or medicinal substances. 3. introduction of a radiopaque material in a radiological examination of the colon (barium enema) or via a tube inserted into the jejunum in a radiological examination of the small bowel (small bowel enema).

energy ('enəjee) power that may be translated into motion, overcoming resistance, or effecting physical change; the ability to do work. Energy assumes several forms; it may be thermal (in the form of heat), electrical, mechanical, chemical, radiant, or kinetic. In doing work, the energy is changed from one form to another or to several forms. In these changes some of the energy is 'lost' in the sense that it cannot be recaptured and used again. Usually there is loss in the form of heat, which escapes or is dissipated unused. All energy changes give off a certain amount of the energy as heat.

All activities of the body require energy, and all needs are met by the consumption of food containing energy in chemical form. The human diet comprises three main sources of energy: carbohydrates, proteins, and fats. Of these three, carbohydrates most readily provide the kind of energy needed to activate muscles. Proteins work to build and restore body tissues. The body transforms chemical energy derived from food by the process of METABOLISM, an activity that takes place in the individual cell. Molecules of the food substances providing energy pass through the cell wall. Inside the cell, chemical reactions occur that produce the new forms of energy and yield by-products such as water and waste materials. See also ADENOSINE TRIPHOSPHATE.

free e. the energy equal to the maximum amount of work that can be obtained from a process occurring under conditions of fixed temperature and pressure.

nuclear e. energy that can be liberated by changes in the nucleus of an atom (as by fission of a heavy nucleus or by fusion of light nuclei into heavier ones with accompanying loss of mass).

enervation (ˌenə'vayshən) 1. lack of nervous energy. 2. removal of a nerve or a section of a nerve.

enflagellation (enˌflajə'layshən) the formation of flagella; flagellation.

enflurane (en'flooə·rayn) a general anaesthetic similar to halothane but with a more rapid onset of action and a faster recovery. It is more depressant on the cardiovascular and respiratory systems but is less likely to cause arrhythmias. It damages liver less when inhaled frequently, and hepatitis following its use is unlikely.

ENG electronystagmograph.

engagement (in'gayjmənt) the entry of the presenting part of the fetus, generally the head, into the true pelvis. A head is said to be engaged when its greatest presenting transverse diameter, the biparietal diameter, has passed the plane of the pelvic brim. In a primigravida the fetal head usually becomes engaged after the 36th week of pregnancy; in a multigravida it is usually later and may not occur until after the onset of labour.

engastrius (en'gastri·əs) a double fetus or infant in which one fetus is contained within the abdomen of the other.

engorgement (en'gorjmənt) local congestion; distention with fluids; hyperaemia.

engram ('engram) a lasting mark or trace. In psychology, it is the lasting trace left in the psyche by anything that has been experienced psychically; a latent memory picture.

enkatarrhaphy (ˌenkə'tarəfee) the operation of burying a structure by suturing together the sides of tissues adjacent to it.

enkephalin (en'kefəlin) either of two naturally occurring pentapeptides (methionine enkephalin and leucine enkephalin) isolated from the brain, which have potent opiate-like effects and probably serve as neurotransmitters. They are classified as ENDORPHINS.

enol ('eenol) one of two tautomeric forms of a substance, the other being the keto form; the enol is formed from the keto by migration of hydrogen from the adjacent carbon atom to the carbonyl group.

enolase ('eenəˌlayz) an enzyme in glycolytic systems that changes phosphoglyceric acid into phosphopyruvic acid.

enophthalmos (ˌenof'thalmos) a backward displacement of the eyeball into the orbit.

enostosis (ˌeno'stohsis) a bony growth within a bone cavity or on the internal surface of the bone cortex.

ensiform ('ensiˌfawm) sword-shaped; xiphoid.

e. cartilage the xiphoid process.

ensomphalus (en'somfələs) a double fetus or infant with blended bodies, two separate navels, and two umbilical cords.

enstrophe ('enstrəfee) inversion; especially of the margin of the eyelids.

ENT ear, nose, and throat.

entad ('entad) toward a centre; inwardly.

ental ('entəl) inner; central.

Entamoeba (ˌentə'meebə) a genus of amoebas parasitic in the intestines of vertebrates.

E. coli a nonpathogenic form found in the intestinal tract of man.

E. gingivalis a nonpathogenic species found in the human mouth.

E. histolytica a species causing AMOEBIC DYSENTERY and abscess of the liver.

entamoebiasis (ˌentəmi'bieəsis) infection by *Entamoeba.*

entasia (en'tayzi·ə) a constrictive spasm; tonic spasm.

enter(o)- word element. [Gr.] *intestine.*

enteral ('entə·ral) within, by way of, or pertaining to the small intestine.

e. nutrition the provision of nutrients in fluid form to the alimentary tract by mouth, nasogastric tube, or via an opening into the tract such as a gastrostomy.

enteralgia (ˌentə'ralji·ə) pain in the intestines; colic.

enterectomy (ˌentə'rektəmee) excision of a portion of the intestine.

enterelcosis (ˌentə·rel'kohsis) ulceration of the intestine.

enteric (en'terik) pertaining to the small intestine.

e.-coated designating a special coating applied to tablets or capsules which prevents release and absorption of their contents until they reach the intestine.

enteritis (ˌentə'rietis) inflammation of the intestine, especially the small intestine, a general condition that can be produced by a variety of causes. Bacteria and certain viruses may irritate the intestinal tract and produce symptoms of abdominal pain, nausea, vomiting, and diarrhoea. Similar effects may result from poisonous foods such as mushrooms and berries, or from a harmful chemical present in food or drink. Enteritis may also be the consequence of overeating, alcoholic excesses, or emotional tension.

Rest and a bland diet are generally prescribed. In cases of bacterial infection antibiotics may be helpful. Severe dehydration, which may accompany enteritis, is treated with replacement of lost fluids and electrolytes.

membranous e., mucomembranous e., mucous e. mucous colitis.

e. necroticans an inflammation of the intestines due to *Clostridium welchii* type F, characterized by necrosis.

phlegmonous e. a condition with symptoms resembling those of peritonitis, which may be secondary to other intestinal diseases, e.g., chronic obstruction, strangulated hernia, carcinoma.

e. polyposa enteritis marked by polypoid growths in the intestine, due to proliferation of the connective tissue.

regional e. a chronic inflammatory disorder of the intestinal tract that may involve any area of the intestine but is characteristically located in the terminal ileum (see CROHN'S DISEASE).

enteroanastomosis (ˌentə·roh·əˌnastə'mohsis) anastomosis between intestinal loops.

Enterobacter (ˌentə·roh'baktər) a genus of bacteria that includes two species, *E. aerogenes* and *E. cloacae.*

Enterobacteriaceae (ˌentə·rohbaktiə·ri'aysi·ee) a family of gram-negative, rod-shaped bacteria (order Eubacteriales) occurring as plant or animal parasites or as saprophytes.

enterobiasis (ˌentə·roh'bieəsis) infection with nematodes of the genus *Enterobius*, especially *E. vermicularis.*

Enterobius (ˌentə'rohbi·əs) a genus of nematode worms.

E. vermicularis the seatworm or pinworm, a small white worm parasitic in the upper part of the large intestine. Gravid females migrate to the anal region to deposit their eggs, sometimes causing severe itching. Infection is frequent in children. See also WORMS.

enterocele ('entə·rohˌseel) intestinal hernia.

enterocentesis (ˌentə·rohsen'teesis) surgical puncture of the intestine.

enteroclysis (ˌentə'roklisis) the injection of liquids into the intestine.

enterococcus (ˌentə·roh'kokəs) pl. *enterococci* [Gr.] any streptococcus of the human intestine.

enterocoele (ˌentə·roh'seel) the body cavity formed by outpouchings from the archenteron.

enterocolectomy (ˌentə·rohkə'lektəmee) resection of part of the intestine, including the ileum, caecum, and colon.

enterocolitis (ˌentə·rohkə'lietis, -koh-) inflammation of the small intestine and colon.

antibiotic-associated e. that in which treatment with antibiotics alters the bowel flora and results in diarrhoea or pseudomembranous enterocolitis. See antibiotic-associated COLITIS.

haemorrhagic e. enterocolitis characterized by haemorrhagic breakdown of the intestinal mucosa, with inflammatory cell infiltration.

pseudomembranous e. an acute inflammation of the bowel mucosa, with the formation of pseudomembranous plaques, usually associated with antibiotic therapy (see pseudomembranous COLITIS).

enterocolostomy (ˌentə·rohkə'lostəmee) surgical anastomosis of the small intestine to the colon.

enterocutaneous (ˌentə·rohkyoo'tayni·əs) pertaining to or communicating with the intestine and the skin, or surface of the body.

enterocyst ('entə·rohˌsist) a cyst proceeding from subperitoneal tissue.

enterocystocele (ˌentə·roh'sistohˌseel) hernia of the bladder and intestine.

enterocystoma (ˌentə·rohsi'stohmə) vitelline cyst.

enterodynia (ˌentə·roh'dini·ə) pain in the intestine.

enteroenterostomy (ˌentə·rohˌentə'rostəmee) surgical anastomosis between two segments of the intestine.

enteroepiplocele (ˌentə·roh·e'piplohˌseel) hernia of the intestine and omentum.

enterogastritis (ˌentə·rohga'strietis) inflammation of the small intestine and stomach.

enterogastrone (ˌentə·roh'gastrohn) a hormone of the duodenum that mediates the humoural inhibition of gastric secretion and motility produced by ingestion of fat. Called also *anthelone E.*

enterogenous (ˌentə'rojənəs) 1. arising from the primitive foregut. 2. originating within the small intestine.

enterogram ('entə·rohˌgram) an instrumental tracing of the movements of the intestine.

enterohepatitis (ˌentə·rohˌhepə'tietis) inflammation of the intestine and liver.

enterohepatocele (ˌentə·roh'hepətohˌseel) an umbilical hernia containing intestine and liver.

enterohydrocele (ˌentə·roh'hiedrohˌseel) hernia with hydrocele.

enterokinase (ˌentə·roh'kienayz) an intestinal enzyme that converts trypsinogen into trypsin; enteropeptidase.

enterokinesia (ˌentə·rohki'neezi·ə) peristalsis.

enterokinetic (ˌentə·rohki'netik) pertaining to or stimulating peristalsis.

enterolith ('entə·rohˌlith) a calculus in the intestine.

enterolysis (ˌentə'rolisis) surgical separation of intestinal adhesions.

enteromegaly (ˌentə·roh'megəlee) enlargement of the intestines.

enteromerocele (ˌentə·roh'miə·rohˌseel) femoral hernia containing an intestinal loop.

enteromycosis (ˌentə·rohmie'kohsis) fungal disease of the intestine.

enteron ('entə·ron) the gut or alimentary canal; usually used in medicine with specific reference to the small intestine.

enteroparesis (ˌentə·rohpə'reesis) relaxation of the intestine resulting in dilation.

enteropathogen (ˌentə·roh'pathəˌjen) a microorganism which causes disease of the intestine. adj. **enteropathogenic.**

enteropathogenesis (ˌentə·rohˌpathə'jenəsis) the production of disease or disorder of the intestine.

enteropathy (ˌentə'ropəthee) any disease of the intestine.

gluten e. coeliac disease.

protein-losing e. a nonspecific term referring to conditions, e.g., adult COELIAC DISEASE, associated with excessive loss of enteric plasma proteins.

enteropeptidase (ˌentə·roh'peptiˌdayz) an enzyme of the intestinal juice which activates the proteolytic enzyme of the pancreatic juice by converting trypsinogen into trypsin.

enteropexy ('entə·rohˌpeksee) surgical fixation of the intestine to the abdominal wall.

enteroplasty ('entə·rohˌplastee) plastic repair of the intestine.

enteroplegia (ˌentə·roh'pleeji·ə) adynamic ileus.

enteroptosis (ˌentə·rop'tohsis) abnormal downward displacement of the intestine. adj. **enteroptotic.**

enterorrhagia (ˌentə·roh'rayji·ə) intestinal haemorrhage.

enterorrhaphy (ˌentə'ro·rəfee) suture of the intestine.

enterorrhoexis (ˌentə·roh'reksis) rupture of the intestine.

enterosepsis (ˌentə·roh'sepsis) sepsis developed from the intestinal contents.

enterospasm ('entə·rohˌspazəm) intestinal colic.

enterostasis (ˌentə·roh'staysis) intestinal stasis.

enterostenosis (ˌentə·rohstə'nohsis) narrowing or stricture of the intestine.

enterostomal (ˌentə·roh'stohməl) relating to an enterostomy.

enterostomy (ˌentə'rostəmee) the artificial formation of a permanent opening into the intestine through the abdominal wall (see also COLOSTOMY and ILEOSTOMY).

enterotome ('entə·rətohm) a crushing clamp used to break down the spur of a colostomy, now obsolescent.

enterotomy (ˌentə'rotəmee) incision of the intestine.

enterotoxaemia (ˌentə·rohtok'seemi·ə) a condition characterized by the presence in the blood of toxins produced in the intestines.

enterotoxigenic (ˌentə·roh,toksi'jenik) producing, produced by, or pertaining to production of enterotoxin.
enterotoxin (ˌentə·roh'toksin) 1. a toxin specific for the cells of the intestinal mucosa. 2. a toxin arising in the intestine. 3. an exotoxin that is protein in nature and relatively heat-stable, produced by staphylococci.
enterotoxism (ˌentə·roh'toksizəm) autointoxication of enteric origin.
enterotribe ('entə·rohtrieb) enterotome.
enterotropic (ˌentə·roh'tropik) affecting the intestines.
enterovaginal (ˌentə·rohvə'jien'l) pertaining to or communicating with the intestine and the vagina, as an enterovaginal fistula.
enterovenous (ˌentə·roh'veenəs) communicating between the intestinal lumen and the lumen of a vein.
enterovesical (ˌentə·roh'vesik'l) pertaining to or communicating with the intestine and urinary bladder.
enterovirus (ˌentə·roh'vierəs) any of a subgroup of picornaviruses infecting the gastrointestinal tract and discharged in the excreta, including the poliovirus, coxsackievirus, and echovirus. adj. **enteroviral.**
enterozoon (ˌentə·roh'zoh·on) an animal parasite in the intestines. adj. **enterozoic.**
enthesis (en'theesis) 1. the use of artificial material in the repair of a defect or deformity of the body. 2. the site of attachment of a muscle or ligament to bone.
enthetobiosis (enˌthetohbie'ohsis) a term suggested to denote the dependency of an organism on a mechanical device implanted within the body, for example, dependency of a patient on an electronic cardiac pacemaker to regulate the heart beat. The relationship between the organism and the device is critical. Called also *epenthetobiosis*.
ento- word element. [Gr.] *within, inner.*
entoblast ('entohˌblast) the entoderm.
entocele ('entohˌseel) an internal hernia.
entoderm ('entohˌdərm) the innermost of the three primitive germ layers of the embryo; from it are derived the epithelium of the pharynx, respiratory tract (except the nose), digestive tract, bladder, and urethra. adj. **entodermal, entodermic.**
entoectad (ˌentoh'ektad) from within outward.
entomere ('entohˌmiə) a blastomere normally destined to become entoderm.
entomion (en'tohmi·ən) the tip of the posteroinferior, or mastoid, angle of the parietal bone.
entomology (ˌentə'moləjee) that branch of biology concerned with the study of insects.
medical e. that concerned with insects that cause disease or serve as vectors of pathogens.
entopic (en'topik) occurring in the proper place.
entoptic (en'toptik) originating within the eye.
entoretina (ˌentoh'retinə) the nervous or inner layer of the retina.
entotic (en'totik) situated in or originating within the ear.
entozoon (entoh'zoh·on) an internal animal parasite. adj. **entozoic.**
entropion (en'trohpi·ən) inversion, or the turning inward, as of the margin of an eyelid.
e. uveae inversion of the margin of the pupil.
entropy ('entrəpee) 1. in thermodynamics, a measure of the part of the internal energy of a system that is unavailable to do work. In any spontaneous process, such as the flow of heat from a hot region to a cold region, entropy always increases. 2. in information theory, the negative of information, a measure of the disorder or randomness in a physical system. The theory of statistical mechanics proves that this concept is equivalent to entropy as defined in thermodynamics. 3. in jungian psychology, the tendency of psychic energy to move from a stronger to a weaker value until a state of equilibrium is reached.
enucleate (i'nyookliˌayt) to remove whole and clean, as the eye from its socket.
enucleation (iˌnyookli'ayshən) removal of an organ or other mass intact from its supporting tissues, as of the eyeball from the orbit.
enuresis (ˌenyuh'reesis) involuntary discharge of urine, usually referring to involuntary discharge of urine during sleep at night; bed-wetting. adj. **enuretic.** It occurs most often in children who are very sound sleepers or who have small bladder capacity. In many cases enuresis is due to emotional rather than physical causes. If it persists after the age of 6, a physical or emotional disorder is likely to be present.
envelope ('envəˌlohp) an encompassing structure or membrane. In virology, a coat surrounding the capsid and usually furnished, at least partially, by the host cell. In bacteriology, the cell wall and the plasma membrane considered together.
nuclear e. the condensed double layer of lipids and proteins enclosing the cell nucleus and separating it from the cytoplasm; its two concentric membranes, inner and outer, are separated by a perinuclear space.
envenomation (inˌvenə'mayshən) the poisonous effects caused by the bites, stings, or effluvia of insects and other arthropods, or the bites of snakes.
environment (in'vierənmənt) the sum total of all the conditions and elements that make up the surroundings and influence the development of an individual.
enzygotic (ˌenzie'gotik) developed from one zygote.
enzymatic (ˌenzie'matik) of, relating to, caused by, or of the nature of an enzyme.
enzyme ('enziem) any protein that acts as a catalyst, increasing the rate at which a chemical reaction occurs. The human body probably contains about 10,000 different enzymes. At body temperature, very few biochemical reactions proceed at a significant rate without the presence of an enzyme. Like all catalysts, an enzyme does not control the direction of the reaction; it increases the rates of the forward and reverse reactions proportionally.

Enzymes work by binding molecules so that they are held in a particular geometric configuration that allows the reaction to occur. Enzymes are very specific; few molecules closely fit the binding site. Each enzyme catalyses a specific type of chemical reaction between a few closely related compounds, which are called *substrates* of the enzyme.

Enzymes are given names ending in *-ase.* In older names, the suffix is added to the name of the substrate, as in amylase, an enzyme that breaks down the polysaccharide amylose. In newer names, the suffix is added to the type of reaction, as in lactate dehydrogenase, an enzyme that converts lactate to pyruvate by transferring a hydrogen atom to nicotinamide-adenine dinucleotide (NAD).

REGULATION OF ENZYMES. The reaction rate of an enzyme-catalysed reaction varies with the pH, temperature, and substrate concentration. Under physiological conditions the rates of many reactions are controlled by substrate concentrations. Certain key reactions are controlled by one of three different mechanisms.

In *allosteric regulation*, the enzyme can bind molecules, which are referred to as *effectors*, at a site other than the active site, which is referred to as an *allosteric site.* In many biochemical pathways the enzyme that catalyses the first reaction in the pathway is inhibited by the final product of the last reaction, so that when sufficient product is present the whole pathway is shut down. This is an example of negative FEEDBACK.

Many enzymes are regulated by *phosphorylation.* A

phosphate group is attached to the enzyme by another enzyme, called a *protein kinase*. When the enzyme is phosphorylated it changes its shape and thus its activity. Phosphorylation activates some enzymes and inactivates others; by this means one protein kinase can control several enzymes.

All enzymes are controlled by their rate of synthesis. Like all proteins enzymes are synthesized by ribosomes, which translate the genetic information coded in the DEOXYRIBONUCLEIC ACID (DNA) of the CHROMOSOMES into the specific amino acid sequence of the enzyme. The expression of many genes is controlled by the processes of *genetic regulation*. Thus, although each cell contains the information to make all of the body's enzymes, it actually makes only those appropriate for its specific type of cell. The synthesis of some enzymes can be induced or repressed by the action of specific hormones, substrates, or products so that the enzyme is produced only when metabolic conditions require its presence.

INBORN ERRORS OF METABOLISM. Hundreds of genetic diseases that result from deficiency of a single enzyme are now known. Many of these diseases fall into two large classes. The *aminoacidopathies* result from deficiency of an enzyme in the major pathway for the metabolism of a specific amino acid. The amino acid accumulates in the blood, and it or its metabolites are excreted in the urine. The *lysosomal storage diseases* result from deficiency of a lysosomal enzyme and the accumulation of the substance degraded by that enzyme in lysosomes of cells throughout the body. The stored material is usually a complex substance, such as glycogen, a sphingolipid, or a mucopolysaccharide.

An example of an aminoacidopathy is PHENYLKETONURIA (PKU), which results from a deficiency of the enzyme phenylalanine hydroxylase, which converts the amino acid phenylalanine to tyrosine. Phenylalanine accumulates in the blood and phenylpyruvic acid is excreted in the urine. The phenylalaninaemia eventually results in mental handicap due to defective formulation of myelin. However, PKU can be detected at birth by a screening test for phenylalanine in the blood, and clinical symptoms can be avoided by strict adherence to a low-phenylalanine diet.

An example of a lysosomal storage disease is TAY–SACHS DISEASE, which results from a deficiency of the enzyme hexosaminidase A. The stored substance is a sphinogolipid, GM_2-ganglioside, which accumulates in nerve tissue, causing blindness and mental deterioration. No cure is possible, but antenatal diagnosis can be made by determining hexosaminidase A activity in fetal fibroblasts from an amniotic fluid specimen drawn by AMNIOCENTESIS. It is also possible to identify carriers (heterozygotes) who are at risk of having children with the disease.

ENZYME ASSAYS. Several enzymes are important in clinical pathology. Enzymes characteristic of a tissue are released into the blood when the tissue is damaged, and enzyme levels in the blood can aid in the diagnosis or monitoring of specific diseases. Lipase and amylase levels are useful in pancreatic diseases; alkaline phosphatase (ALP), lactate dehydrogenase (LD), aspartate aminotransferase (AST), and alanine aminotransferase (ALT) in liver diseases; and LD and creatine kinase (CK) in myocardial infarction. ALP is also released in bone diseases. Many enzymes have different forms (*isoenzymes)* in different organs. The isoenzymes can be separated by electrophoresis in order to determine the origin of the enzyme. Isoenzymes of LD, CK, and ALP have the most clinical use.

activating e. one that activates a given amino acid by attaching it to the corresponding transfer ribonucleic acid.

brancher e., branching e. α-glucan-branching glycosyltransferase: an enzyme involved in conversion of amylose to amylopectin; deficiency of this enzyme causes amylopectinosis.

constitutive e. one produced by a microorganism regardless of the presence or absence of the specific substrate acted upon.

debrancher e., debranching e. dextrin-1,6-glucosidase: an enzyme that acts on glucose residues of the glycogen molecule, and is important in glycogenolysis; deficiency of this enzyme causes Forbes' disease.

induced e., inducible e. one whose production requires or is stimulated by a specific small molecule, the inducer, which is the substrate of the enzyme or a compound structurally related to it.

proteolytic e. one that catalyses the hydrolysis of proteins and various split products of proteins, the final product being small peptides and amino acids.

repressible e. one whose rate of production is decreased as the concentration of certain metabolites is increased.

respiratory e's enzymes of the mitochondria, e.g., cytochrome oxidase, which serve as catalysts for cellular oxidations.

enzymic (en'ziemik) enzymatic.

enzymology (ˌenzie'moləjee) the study of enzymes and enzymatic action.

enzymopathy (ˌenzie'mopəthee) an inborn error of metabolism consisting of defective or absent enzymes, as in the glycogenoses or the mucopolysaccharidoses.

EOG electro-oculogram; electro-olfactogram.

eonism ('eeəˌnizəm) tranvestism in the male.

eosin ('eeohsin) any of a class of rose-coloured stains or dyes, all being bromine derivatives of fluorescein; eosin Y, the sodium salt of tetrabromfluorescein, is much used in histological and laboratory procedures.

eosinopenia (ˌeeəˌsinə'peeni·ə) abnormal deficiency of eosinophils in the blood.

eosinophil (eeə'sinəfil) an element readily stained by eosin; specifically, a granular leukocyte with a nucleus that usually has two lobes connected by a thread of chromatin, and cytoplasm containing coarse, round granules of uniform size.

eosinophilia (ˌeeəˌsinə'fili·ə) 1. the formation and accumulation of an abnormally large number of eosinophils in the blood. 2. the condition of being readily stained with eosin. adj. **eosinophilic.**

tropical e. a disease characterized by anorexia, malaise, cough, leukocytosis, and an increase in eosinophils.

eosinophilic (ˌeeəˌsinə'filik) staining readily with eosin; pertaining to eosinophils or to eosinophilia.

epallobiosis (eˌpalohbie'ohsis) dependency on an external life-support system, as on a HEART–LUNG MACHINE or haemodialyser (see HAEMODIALYSIS).

Epanutin (epə'nyootin) trademark for phenytoin, an anticonvulsant used in the treatment of all forms of epilepsy except petit mal.

epaxial (e'paksi·əl) situated above or upon an axis.

epencephalon (ˌepen'kefəlon, -'sef-) 1. cerebellum. 2. metencephalon.

ependyma (e'pendimə) the membrane lining the cerebral ventricles and the central canal of the spine. adj. **ependymal.**

ependymoma (eˌpendi'mohmə) a neoplasm arising from the lining cells of the ventricles or central canal of the spinal cord.

epenthetobiosis (ˌepenˌthetohbie'ohsis) enthetobiosis.

ephapse ('efaps) a point of lateral contact (other than a synapse) between nerve fibres across which impulses are conducted directly through the nerve membranes. adj. **ephaptic**.

ephebiatrics (i,feebi'atriks) the branch of medicine that deals especially with the diagnosis and treatment of diseases and problems peculiar to youth.

ephebic (i'feebik) pertaining to youth or the period of puberty and adolescence.

ephebogenesis (,efiboh'jenəsis) the bodily changes occurring at puberty. adj. **ephebogenetic**.

ephebology (,efi'boləjee) the study of puberty.

ephedrine ('efi,dreen, -drin) an adrenergic alkaloid obtained from several species of the shrub *Ephedra* or produced synthetically; used as a bronchodilator, antiallergic, central nervous system stimulant in narcolepsy, mydriatic, and pressor agent.

ephelis (e'feelis) pl. *ephelides* [Gr.] a freckle.

ephidrosis (,efi'drohsis) profuse sweating; hyperhidrosis.

epi- word element. [Gr.] *upon*.

epiandrosterone (,epian'drostə,rohn) an androgenic steroid less active than androsterone and excreted in small amounts in normal human urine.

epiblepharon (,epi'blefə·ron) a developmental anomaly in which a horizontal fold of skin stretches across the border of the eyelid, pressing the lashes against the eyeball.

epibulbar (,epi'bulbə) situated upon the eyeball.

epicanthus (,epi'kanthəs) a vertical fold of skin on either side of the nose, sometimes covering the inner canthus; a normal characteristic in persons of certain races, but anomalous in others. adj. **epicanthal**, **epicanthic**.

epicardia (,epi'kahdi·ə) the lower portion of the oesophagus, extending from the oesophageal hiatus to the cardia, the upper orifice of the stomach.

epicardial (,epi'kahdi·əl) pertaining to the visceral pericardium (epicardium) or to the epicardia.

epicardium (,epi'kahdi·əm) the inner layer of the serous pericardium, which is in contact with the heart.

epichorion (,epi'kor·ri·ən) the portion of the uterine mucosa enclosing the implanted conceptus.

epicondyle (,epi'kondiel) an eminence upon a bone, above its condyle.

epicondylitis (,epi,kondi'lietis) inflammation of an epicondyle or of tissues adjoining the humeral epicondyle.

epicranium (,epi'krayni·əm) the structures collectively that cover the skull.

epicritic (,epi'kritik) determining accurately; said of cutaneous nerve fibres sensitive to fine variations of touch or temperature.

epicystotomy (,episi'stotəmee) cystotomy by the suprapubic method.

epicyte ('epi,siet) cell membrane.

epidemic (,epi'demik) the presence in a population of disease or infection in excess of that usually expected.

epidemicity (,epidə'misitee) the quality of being widely diffused and rapidly spreading throughout a community.

epidemiologist (,epi,deemi'oləjist) an expert in epidemiology.

epidemiology (,epi,deemi'oləjee) the study of the distribution of factors determining health and disease in human populations, and the application of this study to the prevention and control of disease. adj. **epidemiological**.

epidermis (,epi'dərmis) the outermost and nonvascular layer of the skin, derived from the embryonic ectoderm, varying in thickness from 0.07 to 1.4 mm. On the palmar and plantar surfaces it comprises, from within outward, five layers: (1) *basal layer* (stratum basale), composed of columnar cells arranged perpendicularly; (2) *prickle-cell* or *spinous layer* (stratum spinosum), composed of flattened polyhedral cells with short processes or spines: (3) *granular layer* (stratum granulosum), composed of flattened granular cells; (4) *clear layer* (stratum lucidum), composed of several layers of clear, transparent cells in which the nuclei are indistinct or absent; and (5) *horny layer* (stratum corneum), composed of flattened, cornified, non-nucleated cells. In the epidermis of the general body surface, the clear layer is usually absent. adj. **epidermal, epidermic**.

epidermitis (,epidər'mietis) inflammation of the epidermis.

epidermodysplasia (,epi,dərmohdis'playzi·ə) faulty development of the epidermis.

e. verruciformis a skin condition due to a virus identical with or closely related to the virus of common warts, in which the lesions are red or red-violet and widespread and tend to become malignant.

epidermoid (,epi'dərmoyd) 1. resembling the epidermis. 2. any tumour occurring at a noncutaneous site and formed by inclusion of epidermal cells.

epidermoidoma (,epi,dərmoy'dohmə) a cerebral or meningeal tumour formed by inclusion of ectodermal elements at the time of closure of the neural groove.

epidermolysis (,epidər'molisis) a loosened state of the epidermis with formation of blebs and bullae either spontaneously or at the site of trauma.

e. bullosa a variety with development of bullae and vesicles, often at the site of trauma; in the hereditary forms, there may be severe scarring after healing, or extensive denuded areas after rupture of the lesions.

epidermomycosis (,epi,dərmohmie'kohsis) dermatophytosis.

epidermophytid (epi,dərmoh'fietid) dermatophytid.

epidermophytin (epi,dərmoh'fietin) a filtrate of Epidermophyton cultures that induces a hypersensitivity reaction of the tuberculin type; used in treatment of epidermophytosis.

Epidermophyton (epi,dərmoh'fieton) a genus of fungi. *E. floccosum* attacks both skin and nails but not hair, and is one of the causative organisms of tinea cruris, tinea pedis (athlete's foot), and onychomycosis.

epidermophytosis (,epi,dərmohfie'tohsis) a fungal skin infection, especially one due to *Epidermophyton*; dermatophytosis.

epididymectomy (,epi,didi'mektəmee) excision of all or part of the epididymis.

epididymis (,epi'didimis) pl. *epididymides* [Gr.] an elongated, cordlike structure along the posterior border of the testis, whose coiled duct provides for the storage, transport, and maturation of spermatozoa. adj. **epididymal**.

epididymitis (,epi,didi'mietis) inflammation of the epididymis. Nonspecific epididymitis may result from an infection in the urinary tract, especially in the prostate. Rarely it may be traced to an infection elsewhere in the body. Tuberculosis, mumps, and gonorrhoea may be complicated by epididymitis. Symptoms include sudden severe pain in the testes followed by scrotal swelling and tenderness. Treatment is usually with antibiotics, rest in bed, and avoidance of alcoholic beverages, spiced foods, sexual excitement, and physical exercise until all symptoms have disappeared.

epididymo-orchitis (,epi,didimoh·aw'kietis) inflammation of the epididymis and testis.

epididymotomy (,epi,didi'motəmee) incision of the epididymis.

epididymovasostomy (,epi,didimohva'sostəmee) surgical anastomosis of the epididymis to the vas (ductus) deferens.

epidural (ˌepi'dyooə·rəl) situated upon or outside the dura mater.

epidurography (ˌepidyooə'rogrəfee) radiographic visualization of the epidural space following the injection of air or contrast medium into it.

epigastralgia (ˌepiga'stralji·ə) pain in the epigastrium.

epigastrium (ˌepi'gastri·əm) the upper and middle region of the abdomen, located within the sternal angle. adj. **epigastric.**

epigenesis (ˌepi'jenəsis) the development of an organism from an undifferentiated cell, consisting in the successive formation and development of organs and parts that do not preexist in the fertilized egg. adj. **epigenetic.**

epiglottis (ˌepi'glotis) the lidlike cartilaginous structure overhanging the entrance to the larynx. adj. **epiglottic.** The muscular action of swallowing closes the opening to the trachea by placing the larynx against the epiglottis. This prevents food and drink from entering the larynx and trachea, directing it instead into the oesophagus.

epilation (ˌepi'layshən) the removal of hair by the roots.

epilemma (ˌepi'lemə) endoneurium.

epilepsy ('epiˌlepsee) paroxysmal transient disturbances of nervous system function resulting from abnormal electrical activity of the brain. It is not a specific disease, but rather a group of symptoms that are manifestations of any of a number of conditions that overstimulate nerve cells of the brain. The estimated incidence of epilepsy is 0.5 per cent of the population, making it a relatively common disease. Over 70 per cent of those having epilepsy experience their first attack during childhood or after age 50. The type of seizure varies with age of onset.

TYPES. There are several methods for classifying the various types of epilepsy. On the basis of origin, epilepsy is idiopathic (cryptogenic, essential, genetic) or symptomatic (acquired, organic). Symptomatic epilepsy has a physical cause, for example, brain tumour, injury to the brain at birth, a wound or blow to the head, or an endocrine disorder.

The taxonomy of epileptic seizures, called the Clinical and Electroencephalographical Classification of Epileptics of the International League Against Epilepsy, identifies four main types and subtypes. The *first* major group, Partial Seizures, includes those that begin locally. They are further divided into: (1) Partial Seizures with Elementary Symptomatology, (2) Partial Seizures with Complex Symptomatology, including those with impairment of consciousness only, psychomotor symptomatology, and psychosensory symptomatology, and (3) Partial Seizures That Are Secondarily Generalized. The *second* major group comprises generalized seizures that are bilaterally symmetrical and without local onset. The *third* major group includes unilateral seizures; that is, those involving only one hemisphere. The *fourth* major group includes all other unclassified epileptic seizures.

SYMPTOMS. The manifestations of epilepsy depend on the area of the brain where the abnormal discharge occurs. *Elementary partial seizures*, called also *simple* or *focal seizures*, result from a localized cortical discharge. The symptoms may be either motor, sensory, or autonomic, or any combination of the three. *Complex partial seizures*, called also *psychomotor* or *temporal lobe seizures*, usually, but not always, originate in the temporal lobe of the brain. There may be an aura before the seizure. As the name implies, there are many different cognitive, affective, and psychomotor symptoms. There is either loss or alteration of consciousness when the seizure begins; after the attack the patient may feel drowsy or confused.

Absence or *petit mal seizures* last only a few seconds. There is a sudden onset with no aura or warning and no postictal symptoms. Seizures of this type usually affect children between the ages of 5 and 12 years and disappear during puberty. There typically is a twitching about the eyes or mouth, the patient remains sitting or standing, and appears to have had no more than a lapse of attention or a moment of absentmindedness.

Grand mal or *tonic–clonic seizures* usually begin with bilateral jerks of the extremities or focal seizure activity. There is loss of consciousness and both tonic and clonic type convulsions. The patient may be incontinent during the attack and there is danger of tongue biting. In the postictal phase the patient is confused and drowsy.

Atonic or *akinetic seizures* are characterized by loss of body tone that can produce nodding of the head, weakness of the knees, or total collapse and falling. The patient usually remains conscious during the attack.

There are six commonly used antiepileptic drugs. Phenytoin, phenobarbitone, primidone, and carbamazepine are used for maintenance therapy for generalized tonic–clonic seizures and focal and complex partial seizures. Ethosuximide and sodium valproate are used for generalized absence seizures. Clonazepam is also used for absence seizures when ethosuximide or sodium valproate is ineffective.

A complete assessment of the patient's status is necessary, including a complete history, physical and neurological examination, and laboratory studies of the blood and spinal fluid. The latter are especially useful in determining whether an infection is the cause of the seizures. Radiographic examination of the skull is usually done. The diagnosis is confirmed by ELECTROENCEPHALOGRAM and ECHOENCEPHALOGRAM, which are helpful in locating the site and possibly the cause of the seizures.

TREATMENT AND PATIENT CARE. Surgical removal of the brain lesion, for example, tumour or scar tissue, is indicated in a limited number of patients. The large majority of cases are treated by medications that prevent disabling effects of the disease.

DIAGNOSIS. An important source of information for the diagnostician who is trying to determine the type of epilepsy that a patient has is an accurate and detailed description of the symptoms exhibited or felt before, during and after the seizure. The source of this information can be the patient himself, members of his family, a health care professional, or anyone else who has witnessed the attack. See also CONVULSIONS.

In the continued management of his illness, the patient and his family should be aware of seizure triggers that can precipitate an attack. These include HYPERVENTILATION, physical stress from trauma, lack of sleep, poor nutrition, fever, and illnesses; emotional stress; bright light; hormonal changes such as those occurring during menstruation and pregnancy; fluid and electrolyte imbalances; and alcohol and other drugs. Another common trigger is inadequate dosage of an antiepileptic drug or use of an ineffective drug. The patient should be encouraged to work cooperatively with his doctor to help identify the best medical regimen for treating his individual case. Members of his family should be taught the proper care of a person having a convulsive seizure. See also CONVULSION.

The British Epilepsy Association, New Wokingham Road, Wokingham, Berkshire, supplies information on all aspects of epilepsy and can refer patients and their families to specialists and clinics in their locality.

One of the major challenges to persons working in the health field and concerned with the care of patients with epilepsy is the dispelling of myths and superstitions about the disease and the propagation of accurate information. Most persons with epilepsy can lead normal lives with few restrictions, but many are subjected to unfair employment practices and social stigma because of prejudices resulting from the general public's ignorance of the effects of epilepsy.

myoclonus e. see MYOCLONUS EPILEPSY.

epileptic (ˌepi'leptik) 1. pertaining to or affected with epilepsy. 2. a person affected with epilepsy.

epileptiform (ˌepi'leptiˌfawm) 1. resembling epilepsy or its manifestations. 2. occurring in severe or sudden paroxysms.

epileptogenic (ˌepiˌleptoh'jenik) causing an epileptic seizure.

epileptoid (ˌepi'leptoyd) epileptiform.

Epilim ('epilim) trademark for preparations of sodium valproate.

epiloia (ˌepi'loyə) tuberous sclerosis; a congenital disorder with areas of hardening in the cerebral cortex and other organs, characterized clinically by mental deficiency and epilepsy.

epimer ('epimə) one of two or more isomers which differ only in the position of one carbon atom.

epimerase (i'piməˌrayz) an isomerase that catalyses the inversion of asymmetric groups in substrates (epimers) having more than one centre of asymmetry.

epimere ('epiˌmiə) the dorsal portion of a somite, from which is formed muscles innervated by the dorsal ramus of a spinal nerve.

epimerite (ˌepi'meriet) an organelle of certain protozoa by which they attach themselves to epithelial cells.

epimerization (iˌpimə·rie'zayshən) the changing of one epimeric form of a compound into another, as by enzymatic action.

epimorphosis (ˌepimaw'fohsis) the regeneration of a piece of an organism by proliferation at the cut surface. adj. **epimorphic.**

epimysium (ˌepi'misi·əm) the fibrous sheath around an entire skeletal muscle.

epinephrectomy (ˌepinə'frektəmee) adrenalectomy.

epinephrine (ˌepi'nefrin) see ADRENALINE.

epineural (ˌepi'nyooə·rəl) situated upon a neural arch.

epineurium (ˌepi'nyooə·ri·əm) the sheath of a peripheral nerve. adj. **epineurial.**

epinosis (ˌepi'nohsis) a psychic or imaginary state of illness secondary to an original illness.

epioestriol (ˌepi'eestriol) an oestrogenic steroid found in pregnant women.

epiphora (i'pifə·rə) persistent overflow of tears, often due to obstruction in the lacrimal passages or to ectropion.

epiphysiolysis (ˌepiˌfizi'olisis) separation of the epiphysis from the diaphysis of a bone.

epiphysis (i'pifisis) pl. *epiphyses* [Gr.] 1. the end of a long bone, usually wider than the shaft, and either entirely cartilaginous or separated from the shaft by a cartilaginous disc. 2. part of a bone formed from a secondary centre of ossification, commonly found at the ends of long bones, on the margins of flat bones, and at tubercles and processes; during the period of growth epiphyses are separated from the main portion of the bone by cartilage. adj. **epiphyseal.**

e. cerebri pineal body.

epiphysitis (ˌepifi'zietis) inflammation of an epiphysis or of the cartilage joining the epiphysis to a bone shaft.

epipial (ˌepi'pieəl) situated upon the pia mater.

epiplocele (i'piplohˌseel) omental hernia.

epiploenterocele (ˌepiploh'entə·rohˌseel) a hernia containing intestine and omentum.

epiplomerocele (ˌepiploh'miə·rohˌseel) a femoral hernia containing omentum.

epiplomphalocele (ˌepi'plomfəlohˌseel) an umbilical hernia containing omentum.

epiploon (epi'ploh·on) pl. *epiploa* [Gr.] the greater omentum. adj. **epiploic.**

epirubicin (ˌepiroo'bisin) an oncolytic similar to adriamycin but claimed to be less toxic.

episclera (ˌepi'skliə·rə) the loose connective tissue forming the sclera and the conjunctiva.

episcleral (ˌepi·skliə·rəl) 1. overlying the sclera. 2. pertaining to the episclera.

episcleritis (ˌepi·sklə'rietis) inflammation of the episclera and adjacent tissues.

episioperineoplasty (əˌpeeziohˌperi'neeohˌplastee) plastic repair of the vulva and perineum.

episioperineorrhaphy (əˌpeeziohˌperini'o·rəfee) suture of the vulva and perineum.

episioplasty (ə'peeziohˌplastee) plastic repair of the vulva.

episiostenosis (əˌpeeziohstə'nohsis) narrowing of the vulvar orifice.

episiotomy (əˌpeezi'otəmee) surgical incision of the perineum in order to enlarge the vaginal outlet and facilitate delivery of the fetus. Episiotomy should normally be preceded by infiltration of the perineum with 5 ml of 1 per cent or 10 ml or 0.5 per cent lignocaine. A single, sufficient cut of approximately 3–4 cm should be made at the height of a contraction. The ideal incision is the right mediolateral, which commences at the centre of the fourchette and is directed at a 45 degree angle away from the anus. This avoids Bartholin's ducts, is relatively avascular, is easy to repair, and if extension does occur the tear is usually away from the anus. This is the only episiotomy recommended for use by midwives. Doctors may use a median, J-shaped or occasionally a lateral incision. Episiotomies may be made for fetal distress, for delivery of a preterm infant to avoid pressure on the soft skull bones if forceps are not used, or for abnormal presentation of the fetus, especially occipitoposterior position. Episiotomy will also avoid uncontrolled tearing of an overstretched perineum or where there are varicosities, and prevent delay in the second stage of labour due to a rigid perineum or maternal exhaustion. Episiotomy is performed by doctors prior to instrumental delivery using forceps. Repair of episiotomy should be undertaken as soon as possible by a midwife or doctor. A sutured perineum is painful to the mother, and unnecessary episiotomy should be avoided.

episode ('epiˌsohd) a noteworthy happening occurring in the course of a continuous series of events.

episome ('epiˌsohm) in bacterial genetics, any accessory extrachromosomal replicating genetic element that can exist either autonomously or integrated with the chromosome.

epispadias (ˌepi'spaydi·əs) a congenital malformation with absence of the upper wall of the urethra, occurring in both sexes, but more commonly in the male, the urethral opening being located anywhere on the dorsum of the penis. adj. **epispadiac, epispadial.**

episplenitis (ˌepisplə'nietis) inflammation of the capsule of the spleen.

epistaxis (ˌepi'staksis) haemorrhage from the nose, usually due to rupture of small vessels overlying the anterior part of the cartilaginous nasal septum; nosebleed. A minor nosebleed may be caused by a blow on the nose, irritation from foreign bodies, or vigorous nose-blowing during a cold. Sometimes it occurs in connection with menstruation. If bleeding persists in spite of the following first-aid measures, medical attention is advisable.

The victim should sit up with the head tilted back. The soft portion of the nose is grasped firmly between the thumb and forefinger. If this does not stop the bleeding, small wads of cotton or gauze are gently inserted into the nose and then the nostrils are pressed firmly together again. This often helps a clot to form. If a clot fails to form, cold compresses are applied about the nose, the lips, and the back of the neck. If the bleeding still persists, cauterization of the blood vessel may be necessary.

Sometimes nosebleed has serious underlying causes. Arteriosclerosis is a possible cause in the elderly. Polyps and other fleshy growths in the nose, food allergy, hypertension, vitamin deficiencies, or any disease producing a bleeding tendency may produce nosebleed. If the nose bleeds often or profusely or if the bleeding is difficult to stop, a doctor should be consulted.

episternal (ˌepi'stərnəl) 1. situated on or over the sternum. 2. pertaining to the episternum.

episternum (ˌepi'stərnəm) the manubrium, or upper piece of the sternum.

epitendineum (ˌepiten'dini·əm) the fibrous sheath covering a tendon.

epithalamus (ˌepi'thaləməs) the part of the diencephalon just superior and posterior to the thalamus, comprising the pineal body and adjacent structures; considered by some to include the stria medullaris.

epithelial (ˌepi'theeli·əl) pertaining to or composed of epithelium.

epithelialization (ˌepiˌtheeli·əlie'zayshən) healing by the growth of epithelium over a denuded surface.

epithelialize (ˌepi'theeli·əˌliez) to cover with epithelium.

epitheliitis (ˌepiˌtheeli'ietis) inflammation of the epithelium.

epithelioid (ˌepi'theeliˌoyd) resembling epithelium.

epitheliolysis (ˌepiˌtheeli'olisis) destruction of epithelial tissue. adj. **epitheliolytic.**

epithelioma (ˌepiˌtheeli'ohmə) any tumour derived from epithelium. adj. **epitheliomatous.**

e. adenoides cysicum trichoepithelioma.

epitheliosis (ˌepiˌtheeli'ohsis) proliferation of conjunctival epithelium, forming trachoma-like granules.

epitheliotropic (ˌepiˌtheelioh'tropik, -'trohpik) having a special affinity for epithelial cells.

epithelium (ˌepi'theeli·əm) pl. *epithelia* [Gr.] the cellular covering of internal and external surfaces of the body, including the lining of vessels and other small cavities. It consists of cells joined by small amounts of cementing substances. Epithelium is classified into types on the basis of the number of layers deep and the shape of the superficial cells.

ciliated e. epithelium bearing vibratile, hairlike processes (cilia) on its free surface.

columnar e. epithelium whose cells are of much greater height than width.

cuboidal e. epithelium whose cells are of approximately the same height and width, and appear square in transverse section.

germinal e. thickened peritoneal epithelium covering the gonad from earliest development; formerly thought to give rise to germ cells.

glandular e. that composed of secreting cells.

pigmentary e., pigmented e. that made of cells containing granules of pigment.

sense e., sensory e. neuroepithelium (1).

simple e. that composed of a single layer of cells.

squamous e. that composed of layers of flattened platelike cells.

stratified e. epithelium made up of cells arranged in layers.

transitional e. a type characteristically found lining hollow organs, such as the urinary bladder, that are subject to great mechanical change due to contraction and distention, originally thought to represent a transition between stratified squamous and columnar epithelium.

epithelization (ˌepiˌtheelie'zayshən) epithelialization.

epitonic (ˌepi'tonik) abnormally tense or tonic.

epitope ('epitohp) a part of an antigen which fits into the binding site of an antibody. A single antigen molecule may have many epitopes which fit different antibodies.

epitrichium (ˌepi'triki·əm) periderm.

epitrochlea (ˌepi'trokli·ə) the inner condyle of the humerus.

epitympanum (ˌepi'timpənəm) the upper part of the tympanum. adj. **epitympanic.**

epizoic (ˌepi'zoh·ik) pertaining to or caused by an epizoon.

epizoon (ˌepi'zoh·on) pl. *epizoa* [Gr.] an external animal parasite.

epizootic (ˌepizoh'otik) 1. attacking many animals in any region at the same time; widely diffused and rapidly spreading. 2. a disease of high morbidity which is only occasionally present in an animal community.

eponychium (ˌepə'niki·əm) 1. the narrow band of epidermis extending from the nail wall onto the nail surface; commonly called cuticle. 2. the horny fetal epidermis at the site of the future nail.

eponym ('epohˌnim, 'epə-) a name or phrase formed from or including a person's name, e.g., Hodgkin's disease, Cowper's gland, Schick test. adj. **eponymic, eponymous.**

epoophoron (ˌepoh'ofə·ron) a vestigial structure associated with the ovary.

epoxy (i'poksee) 1. containing one atom of oxygen bound to two different carbon atoms. 2. a resin composed of epoxy polymers and characterized by adhesiveness, flexibility, and resistance to chemical actions.

epsilon-aminocaproic acid ('epsilonəˌmeenohkə'proh·ik, -ə'mienoh-) an amino acid that is a potent inhibitor of plasminogen and plasmin and indirectly of fibrinolysis; used as a haemostatic.

Epsom salt ('epsəm) magnesium sulphate, a cathartic.

Epstein–Barr virus (ˌepstien'bah) a herpesvirus that is the aetiological agent of infectious mononucleosis. It has been isolated from cells cultured from Burkitt's lymphoma, and has been found in certain cases of nasopharyngeal cancer. Called also *EB virus.*

epulis (e'pyoolis) pl. *epulides* [Gr.] a POLYP of the gingiva.

epulosis (ˌepyuh'lohsis) a scarring over; cicatrization. adj. **epulotic.**

Eq equivalent; see chemical EQUIVALENT.

Equagesic (ˌekwə'jeezik) trademark for a fixed combination preparation of meprobamate, ethoheptazine citrate, and aspirin.

Equanil ('ekwənil) trademark for preparations of meprobamate, a minor tranquillizer.

equation (i'kwayzhən) an expression of equality between two parts.

Henderson–Hasselbalch e. a formula for calculating the pH of a buffer solution such as blood plasma:

$$pH = pK' + \log \frac{[BA]}{[HA]}$$

where [HA] is the concentration of a weak acid, [BA] is the concentration of a weak salt of this acid, and pK' is the pK of the buffer system.

equilibration (ˌeekwilieˈbrayshən, iˌkwili-) the achievement of a balance between opposing elements or forces.

equilibrium (ˌeekwiˈlibri·əm, ˌekwi-) a state of balance between opposing forces or influences. In the body, equilibrium may be chemical or physical. A state of chemical equilibrium is reached when the body tissues contain the proper proportions of various salts and water. (See also ACID–BASE BALANCE and FLUID BALANCE.) Physical equilibrium, such as the state of balance required for walking, standing, or sitting, is achieved by a very complex interplay of opposing sets of muscles. The labyrinth of the inner ear contains the semicircular canals, or organs of balance, and relays to the brain information about the body's position and also the direction of body motions.

dynamic e. the condition of balance between varying, shifting, and opposing forces that is characteristic of living processes.

equine (ˈekwien) pertaining to, characteristic of, or derived from the horse.

equinovalgus (iˌkwienohˈvalgəs) talipes equinovalgus.

equinovarus (iˌkwienohˈvair·rəs) talipes equinovarus; a foot deformity in which the heel is turned inward and the foot is plantar flexed.

equipotential (ˌeekwipəˈtenshəl) having similar and equal power or capability.

equipotentiality (ˌeekwipəˌtenshiˈalitee) the quality or state of having similar and equal power; the capacity for developing in the same way and to the same extent.

equivalent (iˈkwivələnt) 1. of equal force, power, value, etc. 2. something that has equivalent properties. 3. chemical equivalent.

chemical e. that weight in grams of a substance that will produce or react with 1 mole of hydrogen ion or 1 mole of electrons. Symbol Eq.

The concentrations of electrolytes are sometimes specified in milliequivalents per litre (mEq/l).

epilepsy e. any disturbance, mental or physical, that may take the place of an epileptic seizure.

Er chemical symbol, *erbium*.

erasion (iˈrayzhən) removal by scraping or curettage.

Erb–Duchenne paralysis (ˌairpdooˈshen) paralysis of the upper roots of the brachial plexus due to destruction of the fifth and sixth cervical roots, without involvement of the small muscles of the hand. Called also *Duchenne's paralysis* and *Erb's palsy*.

Erb–Goldflam disease (ˌairpˈgoltflahm) myasthenia gravis.

Erb's palsy (airps) Erb–Duchenne paralysis.

erbium (ˈərbi·əm) a chemical element, atomic number 68, atomic weight 167.26, symbol Er. See table of elements in Appendix 2.

ERCP endoscopic retrograde cholangiopancreatography. See also GALLBLADDER.

erectile (iˈrektiel) capable of erection.

erection (iˈrekshən) the condition of becoming rigid and elevated, as erectile tissue when filled with blood; applied especially to the swelling and rigidity that occur in the penis as a result of sexual or other types of stimulation. Impulses received by the nervous system stimulate a flow of blood from the arteries leading to the penis, where the erectile tissue fills with blood, and the penis becomes firm and erect. Erection makes possible the transmission of semen into the body of the female (see REPRODUCTION). Erection can also occur in the clitoris and the nipples of the female.

erector (iˈrektə) [L.] a structure that erects, as a muscle that holds up or raises a part.

erepsin (iˈrepsin) the enzyme of succus entericus, secreted by the intestinal glands, which splits peptones into amino acids.

erethism (ˈeriˌthizəm) excessive irritability or sensitivity to stimulation. adj. **erethismic, erethistic**.

erethisophrenia (ˌeriˌthizohˈfreeni·ə) exaggerated mental excitability.

erg (ərg) a unit of work or energy, equivalent to 1.0×10^{-7} joules, to 2.4×10^{-8} calories, or to 0.624×10^{12} electron volts.

ergasia (ərˈgayzi·ə) any mentally integrated function, activity, reaction, or attitude of an individual. adj. **ergastic**.

ergocalciferol (ˌərgohkalˈsifə·rol) vitamin D_2; an oil-soluble antirachitic vitamin (see also VITAMIN D and table of the principal VITAMINS).

ergograph (ˈərgohˌgrahf, -graf) an instrument for measuring work done in muscular action.

ergography (ərˈgogrəfee) a method of measuring the amount of work done during muscular activity.

ergometrine (ˌərgohˈmetreen) an alkaloid of ergot which stimulates contraction of the uterine muscle and is used to control sustained bleeding after childbirth. The usual dose, 0.5 mg acts in 7 minutes if given intramuscularly, and in 45 seconds if given intravenously.

ergonomics (ˌərgəˈnomiks) the scientific study of man in relation to his work and the effective use of human energy.

ergosterol (ərˈgostə·rol) a sterol occurring in animal and plant tissues which on ultraviolet irradiation becomes a potent antirachitic substance, vitamin D_2 (ergocalciferol).

ergot (ˈərgot) the dried sclerotium of the fungus *Claviceps purpurea*, which attacks rye plants. Ergot alkaloids are used as oxytocics and in the treatment of migraine. See also ERGOTISM.

ergotamine (ərˈgotəˌmeen) an alkaloid derived from ergot, used as an oxytocic and in the treatment of migraine.

ergotherapy (ˌərgohˈtherəpee) treatment of disease by physical effort.

ergotism (ˈərgəˌtizəm) chronic poisoning produced by ingestion of ergot, marked by cerebrospinal symptoms, spasm, cramps, or by a kind of dry gangrene.

erogenous (iˈrojənəs) arousing erotic feelings.

e. zones areas of the body stimulation of which produces erotic desire, e.g., the oral, anal, and genital orifices and the nipples.

erosion (iˈrohzhən) an eating or gnawing away; a shallow or superficial ulceration; in dentistry, the loss of substance of a tooth by a chemical process that does not involve known bacterial action. adj. **erosive**.

cervical e. destruction of the squamous epithelium covering the intravaginal portion of the cervix. An overgrowth of columnar epithelium from around the external os results in a ring of red, friable tissue. Treatment, if necessary, is by cautery.

erotic (iˈrotik) pertaining to sexual love or to lust.

eroticism, erotism (iˈrotiˌsizəm; ˈerəˌtizəm) a sexual instinct or desire; the expression of one's instinctual energy or drive, especially the sex drive.

anal e. fixation of libido at (or regression to) the anal phase of infantile development, producing egotistic, dogmatic, stubborn, miserly character.

genital e. achievement and maintenance of libido at the genital phase of psychosexual development, permitting acceptance of normal adult relationships and responsibilities.

oral e. fixation of libido at (or regression to) the oral phase of infantile development, producing passive, insecure, sensitive character.

eroticize, erotize (iˈrotiˌsiez; ˈerəˌtiez) to endow with erotic meaning or significance.

erotogenic (i,rotoh'jenik) producing erotic feeling.
erotomania (i,rotoh'mayni·ə) morbidly exaggerated sexual behaviour or reaction; preoccupation with sexuality.
erotopathy (,erə'topəthee) any perversion of the sexual impulse.
erotophobia (i,rotoh'fohbi·ə) morbid dread of sexual love.
errhine ('erien) promoting a nasal discharge; an agent that so acts.
eructation (,iruk'tayshən) the oral ejection of gas or air from the stomach; belching.
eruption (i'rupshən) 1. the act of breaking out, appearing, or becoming visible, as eruption of the teeth. 2. visible efflorescent lesions of the skin due to disease, with redness, prominence, or both; a rash. adj. **eruptive.**
creeping e. a peculiar eruption that appears to migrate, due to burrowing beneath the skin of certain larvae (see also LARVA MIGRANS).
drug e. dermatitis medicamentosa.
Kaposi's varicelliform e. a generalized and serious vesiculopustular eruption of viral origin, superimposed on preexisting atopic dermatitis; it may be due to the herpes simplex virus (eczema herpeticum) or vaccinia (eczema vaccinatum).
ERV expiratory reserve volume.
erysipelas (,eri'sipələs) a febrile disease characterized by inflammation and redness of the skin and subcutaneous tissues, and due to Group A haemolytic streptococci.
The visible symptoms of erysipelas, a form of cellulitis, are round or oval patches on the skin that promptly enlarge and spread, becoming swollen, tender, and red. The affected skin is hot to the touch, and, occasionally, the adjacent skin blisters. Headache, vomiting, fever, and sometimes complete prostration can occur. Sulphonamide compounds or antibiotics are used in the treatment. Care must be taken to avoid spreading the disease to other areas of the body.
swine e. an infectious and highly fatal disease of pigs, caused by *Erysipelothrix insidiosa.*
erysipelatous (,erisi'pelətəs) pertaining to or of the nature of erysipelas.
erysipeloid (,eri'sipə,loyd) an infective dermatitis or cellulitis due to infection with *Erysipelothrix insidiosa*; it usually begins in a wound (often the result of a prick by a fish bone) and remains localized, rarely becoming generalized and septicaemic.
Erysipelothrix (,eri'sipiloh,thriks) a genus of bacteria containing a single species.
E. insidiosa (E. rhusiopathiae) the causative organism of swine erysipelas, which also infects sheep, turkeys, and rats. An erythematous, oedematous lesion, commonly on the hand, resulting from contact with infected meat, hides, or bones, represents the usual type of infection in man (see also ERYSIPELOID).
erythema (,eri'theemə) redness of the skin caused by congestion of the capillaries in the lower layers of the skin. It occurs with any skin injury, infection, or inflammation.
e. ab igne that due to exposure to radiant heat.
e. chronicum migrans an annular erythema due to the bite of a tick (*Ixodes*); it begins as an erythematous plaque several weeks after the bite and spreads peripherally with central clearing.
e. induratum a chronic necrotizing vasculitis, usually occurring on the calves of young women (see also BAZIN'S DISEASE).
e. marginatum a type of erythema multiforme in which the reddened areas are disc-shaped, with elevated edges.
e. migrans geographic tongue; called also ERISIPELOID tongue.
e. multiforme a symptom complex with highly polymorphic skin lesions, including macular papules, vesicles, and bullae, predominantly on the extensor surfaces of hands, forearms and feet; attacks of the disorder are usually self-limited but recurrences are the rule. It is commonly caused by sulphonamides and penicillin.
toxic e., e. toxicum a generalized erythematous or erythematomacular eruption due to administration of a drug or to bacterial toxins or other toxic substances.
erythematous (,eri'theemətəs) characterized by erythema.
erythr(o)- word element. [Gr.] *red, erythrocyte.*
erythraemia (,eri'threemi·ə) polycythaemia vera.
erythrasma (,eri'thrazmə) a chronic bacterial infection of the major skin folds due to *Corynebacterium minutissimum*, marked by red or brownish patches on the skin.
erythrism ('eri,thrizəm) redness of the hair and beard with a ruddy complexion. adj. **erythristic.**
erythroblast (i'rithroh,blast) originally, any nucleated erythrocyte, but now more generally used to designate the nucleated precursor from which an erythrocyte develops.
basophilic e. see under NORMOBLAST.
orthochromatic e. see under NORMOBLAST. **polychromatophilic e.** see under NORMOBLAST.
erythroblastaemia (i,rithrohbla'steemi·ə) the presence in the peripheral blood of abnormally large numbers of nucleated red cells; erythroblastosis.
erythroblastoma (i,rithrohbla'stohmə) a tumour-like mass composed of nucleated red cells.
erythroblastomatosis (i,rithroh,blastohmə'tohsis) a condition marked by the formation of erythroblastomas.
erythroblastopenia (i,rithroh,blastə'peeni·ə) abnormal deficiency of erythroblasts.
erythroblastosis (i,rithrohbla'stohsis) the presence of erythroblasts in the circulating blood. adj. **erythroblastotic.**
e. fetalis, e. neonatorum see HAEMOLYTIC DISEASE OF THE NEWBORN.
erythrochloropia (i,rithrohklor'rohpi·ə) ability to distinguish only red and green, not blue and yellow.
erythrochromia (i,rithroh'krohmi·ə) haemorrhagic, red pigmentation of the cerebrospinal fluid.
Erythrocin (i'rithrə,sin) trademark for preparations of erythromycin, an antibiotic.
erythrocyanosis (i,rithroh,sieə'nohsis) coarsely mottled bluish or red discoloration on the legs and thighs, especially of girls; thought to be a circulatory reaction to exposure to cold.
erythrocytapheresis (i,rithroh,sietəfe'reesis) the withdrawal of blood, separation and retention of red blood cells, and retransfusion of the remainder into the donor.
erythrocyte (i'rithrə,siet) a red BLOOD cell, or corpuscle; one of the formed elements in the peripheral blood. For immature forms see NORMOBLAST. Normally, in the human, mature erythrocytes are biconcave discs that have no nuclei and are about 7.7 micrometres in diameter, consisting mainly of haemoglobin and a supporting framework, called the stroma. Erythrocyte formation (erythropoiesis) takes place in the red bone marrow in the adult, and in the liver, spleen, and bone marrow of the fetus. Erythrocyte formation requires an ample supply of certain dietary elements such as iron, cobalt, and copper, amino acids, folic acid, and vitamin B_{12}.
The functions of erythrocytes include transportation

of oxygen and carbon dioxide. They are also important in the maintenance of a normal ACID–BASE BALANCE, and, since they help determine the viscosity of the blood, they also influence its specific gravity.

The average life span of a red blood cell is 120 days. They are subjected to much wear and tear in circulation and eventually are removed by cells of the RETICULOENDOTHELIAL SYSTEM, particularly in the liver, bone marrow, and spleen. In spite of this constant destruction and production of red cells, the body maintains a fairly constant number of erythrocytes: between 4 and 5×10^{12} per litre of blood in women and 5 to 6×10^{12} per litre in men. A decreased number of erythrocytes constitutes one form of ANAEMIA.

Red blood cells are destroyed whenever they are exposed to solutions that are not isotonic to blood plasma. If the erythrocyte is placed in a solution that is more dilute than plasma (distilled water for example) the cell will swell until osmotic pressure bursts the cell membrane. If the erythrocyte is placed in a solution more concentrated than plasma, the cell will lose water and shrivel or crenate. It is for this reason that solutions to be given intravenously must be isotonic to plasma.

e. sedimentation rate an expression of the extent of settling of erythrocytes in a column of fresh citrated or otherwise treated blood, per unit of time (see also SEDIMENTATION RATE).

erythrocythaemia (i,rithrohsie'theemi·ə) an increase in the number of erythrocytes in the blood, as in erythrocytosis.

erythrocytic (i·rithroh'sitik) 1. pertaining to, characterized by, or of the nature of erythrocytes. 2. pertaining to the erythrocytic series.

erythrocytolysin (i,rithrohsie'tolisin) a substance that produces erythrocytolysis.

erythrocytolysis (i,rithrohsie'tolisis) dissolution of erythrocytes and escape of haemoglobin.

erythrocytosis (i,rithrohsie'tohsis) increase in the total red cell mass secondary to any of a number of nonhaematogenic systemic disorders in response to a known stimulus (secondary polycythaemia), in contrast to primary polycythaemia (polycythaemia vera).

stress e. an apparent polycythaemia seen in active, anxiety-prone persons, often overweight and smokers, resulting from diminished plasma volume.

erythroderma (i,rithrə'dərmə) abnormal redness of the skin over widespread areas of the body.

congenital ichthyosiform e. a generalized hereditary dermatitis with scaling, occurring in bullous and nonbullous forms.

e. desquamativum a condition resembling and probably identical with severe seborrhoeic dermatitis, affecting newborn breast-fed infants, characterized by generalized exfoliative dermatitis and marked erythroderma. Called also *Leiner's disease*.

lymphomatous e. widespread redness of the skin associated with lymphoma.

maculopapular e. a reddish eruption composed of maculae and papules.

psoriatic e. a generalized psoriasis vulgaris, showing the chemical characteristics of exfoliative dermatitis.

erythrodontia (i,rithroh'donshi·ə) reddish-brown pigmentation of the teeth.

erythroedema polyneuropathy (i,rithri'deemə ,poli-,nyooə'ropəthee) a disease of infancy and early childhood marked by pain and swelling in, and pink coloration of, the fingers and toes, and by listlessness, irritability, failure to thrive, profuse perspiration, and sometimes scarlet coloration of the cheeks and tip of the nose. Called also *acrodynia, pink disease*.

erythrogenesis (i,rithroh'jenəsis) the production of erythrocytes.

e. imperfecta congenital hypoplastic anaemia.

erythrogenic (i,rithroh'jenik) 1. producing erythrocytes. 2. producing a sensation of red. 3. producing or causing erythema.

erythroid (i'rithroyd) 1. of a red colour; reddish. 2. pertaining to the developmental series of cells ending in erythrocytes.

erythrokeratodermia (i,rithroh,kerətoh'dərmi·ə) a reddening and hyperkeratosis of the skin.

e. figurata variabilis, e. variabilis a rare hereditary disorder marked by circumscribed erythematous and hyperkeratotic plaques on the skin which vary in size and shape within hours or days; they appear shortly after birth and persist into adolescence or adulthood.

erythrokinetics (i,rithrohki'netiks) the quantitative, dynamic study of in vivo production and destruction of erythrocytes.

erythrolabe (i'rithroh,layb) the pigment in retinal cones that is more sensitive to the red range of the spectrum than the other pigments (chlorolabe and cyanolabe).

erythroleukaemia (i,rithrohloo'keemi·ə) a malignant blood dyscrasia, one of the myeloproliferative disorders, with atypical erythroblasts and myeloblasts in the peripheral blood.

erythrolysin (,eri'throlisin) erythrocytolysin.

erythrolysis (,eri'throlisis) erythrocytolysis; dissolution of erythrocytes and escape of haemoglobin.

erythromania (i,rithroh'mayni·ə) uncontrollable blushing.

erythromelalgia (i,rithrohmə'lalji·ə) paroxysmal, bilateral vasodilation, particularly of the extremities, with burning pain and increased skin temperature and redness.

erythromycin (i,rithroh'miesin) a broad-spectrum antibiotic produced by a strain of *Streptomyces erythreus*. It is effective against a wide variety of organisms, including gram-negative and gram-positive bacteria. It may be administered orally or parenterally.

erythron ('eri,thron) the circulating erythrocytes in the blood, their precursors, and all the body elements concerned in their production.

Erythroped (i'rithrohped) trademark for a preparation of erythromycin, an antibiotic.

erythropenia (i,rithroh'peeni·ə) deficiency in the number of erythrocytes.

erythrophage (i'rithroh,fayj) a phagocyte that ingests erythrocytes.

erythrophagia, erythrophagocytosis (i,rithroh-'fayji·ə; i,rithroh,fagohsie'tohsis) phagocytosis of erythrocytes.

erythropheresis (i,rithrohfə'reesis) erythrocytapheresis.

erythrophil (i'rithroh,fil) 1. a cell or other element that stains easily with red dyes. 2. erythrophilous.

erythrophilous (,eri'throfiləs) easily staining red.

erythrophobia (i,rithroh'fohbi·ə) 1. a neurotic manifestation marked by blushing at the slightest provocation. 2. morbid aversion to red.

erythroplasia (i,rithroh'playzi·ə) a condition of the mucous membranes characterized by erythematous papular lesions.

e. of Queyrat squamous cell carcinoma in situ, manifested as a circumscribed, velvety, erythematous papular lesion on the glans penis, coronal sulcus, or prepuce, leading to scaling and superficial ulceration.

erythropoiesis (i,rithrohpoy'eesis) the formation of erythrocytes. adj. **erythropoietic**.

erythropoietin (i,rithroh'poyitin, -poy'ee-) a glycoprotein hormone secreted by the kidney in the adult and by the liver in the fetus, which acts on stem cells of the bone marrow to stimulate red blood cell production (erythropoiesis).

erythroprosopalgia (i,rithroh,prohsə'palji·ə) a nervous disorder marked by redness and pain in the face.

erythropsia (,eri'thropsi·ə) a defect of vision in which objects appear tinged with red.

erythrosine (i'rithroh,seen) a colouring agent used to disclose plaque on teeth.

erythrosis (,eri'throhsis) 1. reddish or purplish discoloration of the skin and mucous membranes, as in polycythaemia vera. 2. hyperplasia of the haematopoietic tissue.

erythrostasis (i,rithroh'staysis) the stoppage of erythrocytes in the capillaries, as in sickle cell anaemia.

erythruria (,eri'throoə·ri·ə) excretion of red urine.

Es chemical symbol, *einsteinium.*

es- for words beginning thus, see also those beginning *aes-*.

escape (i'skayp, e-) the act of becoming free.

vagal e. the exhaustion of or adaptation to neural chemical mediators in the regulation of systemic arterial pressure.

ventricular e. extrasystole in which a ventricular pacemaker becomes effective before the sinoatrial pacemaker; it usually occurs with slow sinus rates and often, but not necessarily, with increased vagal tone.

eschar ('eskah) 1. a slough produced by a thermal burn, a corrosive application, or by gangrene. 2. tache noire.

escharotic (,eskə'rotik) 1. capable of producing an eschar; corrosive. 2. a corrosive or caustic agent.

escharotomy (,eskə'rotəmee) surgical incision of the eschar and superficial fascia of a circumferentially burned limb in order to permit the cut edges to separate and restore blood flow to unburned tissue distal to the eschar. Oedema may form beneath the inelastic eschar of a full-thickness burn and compress arteries, thus impairing blood flow and necessitating an escharotomy. The incision is protected from infection with the same antibiotic being used on the burn wound.

Escherichia (,esh·ə'riki·ə) a genus of widely distributed gram-negative bacteria (family Enterobacteriaceae), occasionally pathogenic for man.

E. coli a species constituting a large part of the normal intestinal flora of man and other animals; called also *colon bacillus*. Pathogenic strains are the cause of many cases of urinary tract infections and of epidemic diarrhoeal diseases, especially in children.

Escherichieae (,esh·ə'riki·ee) a tribe of bacteria (family Enterobacteriaceae), comprising *Escherichia* and *Shigella.*

eschrolalia (,eskroh'layli·ə) coprolalia.

escutcheon (is'kuchən) the pattern of distribution of the pubic hair.

eserine ('esəreen, -in) physostigmine.

Esidrex ('ezidreks) trademark for a preparation of hydrochlorothiazide, a diuretic.

-esis word element. [Gr.] *state, condition.*

Esmarch's bandage ('ezmahks) see under BANDAGE.

ESMI elderly severe mentally ill.

ESN educationally subnormal; a relatively mild degree of mental handicap.

eso- word element. [Gr.] *within;* for words beginning *eso-*, see also *oeso-*.

esoethmoiditis (,eesoh,ethmoy'dietis) inflammation of the ethmoid sinuses.

esogastritis (,eesohga'strietis) inflammation of the gastric mucosa.

esophoria (,eesoh'for·ri·ə) heterophoria in which there is deviation of the visual axis of one eye toward that of the other eye in the absence of visual fusional stimuli.

esosphenoiditis (,eesoh,sfeenoy'dietis) osteomyelitis of the sphenoid bone.

esotropia (,eesoh'trohpi·ə) STRABISMUS in which there is deviation of the visual axis of one eye toward that of the other eye, resulting in diplopia. adj. **esotropic.**

ESP extrasensory perception.

ESPR European Society of Paediatric Radiology.

ESR erythrocyte sedimentation rate.

essence ('esəns) 1. the distinctive or individual principle of anything. 2. a mixture of alcohol with a volatile oil.

essential (i'senshəl) 1. constituting the necessary or inherent part of a thing; giving a substance its peculiar and necessary qualities. 2. indispensable; required in the diet, as essential fatty acids. 3. idiopathic; self-existing; having no obvious external exciting cause.

ester ('estə) a compound formed from an alcohol and an acid by removal of water.

esterase ('estə,rayz) any enzyme that catalyses the hydrolysis of esters into its alcohol and acid.

esterification (e,sterifi'kayshən) conversion of an acid into an ester by combination with an alcohol and removal of a molecule of water.

esterify (e'steri,fie) to combine with an alcohol with elimination of a molecule of water, forming an ester.

esterolysis (,estə'rolisis) the hydrolysis of an ester into its alcohol and acid. adj. **esterolytic.**

estramustine (,estrə'musteen, -in) a combination of mustine and an oestrogen used in prostatic carcinoma.

e.s.u. electrostatic unit.

et- for words beginning thus, see also those beginning *aet-*.

ethacrynic acid (,ethə'krinik) a powerful diuretic used orally or parenterally, and effective in promoting sodium and chloride excretion.

ethambutol (e'thambyuh,tol) a tuberculostatic agent.

ethanol ('ethə,nol, 'eethə-) the major ingredient of alcoholic beverages; called also *ethyl alcohol* and *grain alcohol.*

ethanolamine (,ethə'nolə,meen) a colourless, moderately viscous liquid with an ammoniacal odour contained in cephalins and phospholipids, and derived metabolically by decarboxylation of serine. The oleate is used as a sclerosing agent in the treatment of varicose veins.

ethene ('etheen) ethylene.

ether ('eethə) 1. diethyl ether: a colourless, transparent, mobile, very volatile, highly inflammable liquid with a characteristic odour; given by inhalation to produce general ANAESTHESIA. 2. any organic compound containing an oxygen atom bonded to two carbon atoms.

ethereal (i'thiə·ri·əl) 1. pertaining to, prepared with, containing, or resembling ether. 2. evanescent; delicate.

etherization (,eethə·rie'zayshən) induction of anaesthesia by means of ether.

ethics ('ethiks) rules or principles which govern right conduct, and personal and social values. Each practitioner, upon entering a profession, is also invested with the responsibility to adhere to the standards of ethical practice and conduct set by that profession.

medical e. the values and guidelines governing decisions in medical practice, expressed in various codes and declarations.

nursing e. the values and ethical principles governing nursing practice, conduct, and relationships, expressed in various codes and declarations.

The Code of Professional Conduct for the Nurse, Midwife and Health Visitor (see Appendix 1), adopted by the UNITED KINGDOM CENTRAL COUNCIL FOR NURSING, MIDWIFERY AND HEALTH VISITING (UKCC) in 1984, provides guidance and advice for standards of practice and conduct that are essential for the ethical discharge of the nurse's responsibility. The Code is subject to periodic review.

The Code for Nurses, issued by the International Council of Nurses (ICN) in 1973, and the Code of Professional Conduct – A Discussion Document, 1976, of the Royal College of Nursing provide similar guidelines for professional conduct. See also PATIENT'S RIGHTS.

ethionamide (ˌethie'onəmied) a tuberculostatic agent.

ethmocarditis (ˌethmohkah'dietis) inflammation of the connective tissue of the heart.

ethmoid ('ethmoyd) 1. sievelike; cribriform. 2. the ethmoid bone.

e. bone the sievelike bone that forms a roof for the nasal fossae and part of the floor of the anterior cranial fossa.

ethmoidal (eth'moyd'l) pertaining to the ethmoid bone.

ethmoidectomy (ˌethmoy'dektəmee) excision of the ethmoid cells or of a portion of the ethmoid bone.

ethmoiditis ('ethmoy'dietis) inflammation of the ethmoid bone or ethmoid sinuses.

ethmoidotomy (ˌethmoy'dotəmee) incision into the ethmoid sinus.

ethnic ('ethnik) pertaining to a social group who share cultural bonds or physical (racial) characteristics.

e. minority a social grouping of people who share cultural or racial factors but who constitute a minority within the greater culture or society.

ethnology (eth'noləjee) the science dealing with the races of man, their descent, relationship, etc.

ethoglucid (ˌethoh'gloosid) an antineoplastic agent which may be used to treat bladder cancers by intravesical instillations.

ethologist (ee'tholəjist) a person skilled in ethology.

ethology (ee'tholəjee) the scientific study of animal behaviour, particularly in the natural state. adj. **ethological.**

ethosuximide (ˌethoh'suksiˌmied) an anticonvulsant.

ethotoin (ˌethoh'toh·in) an anticonvulsant used in the treatment of generalized tonic–clonic seizures and psychomotor seizures, but less effective than phenytoin.

Ethrane ('eethrayn) trademark for the inhalation anaesthetic enflurane.

ethyl ('ethil, 'eethil, -thiel) the monovalent radical, C_2H_5.

e. alcohol ALCOHOL, the major ingredient of alcoholic beverages; called also *ethanol* and *grain alcohol.*

e. chloride a local anaesthetic applied topically to intact skin.

ethylene ('ethiˌleen) a colourless, highly flammable gas with a slightly sweet taste and odour that was used as an inhalation anaesthetic to induce general ANAESTHESIA.

e. oxide a gaseous, flammable alkylating agent with a broad spectrum of activity, being sporicidal and viricidal. It is used (mixed with CO_2 or fluorocarbons because it is explosive above 3 per cent) for disinfecting and sterilizing equipment and instruments that are used in the hospital, surgery, dentistry, and the pharmaceutical and other industries and that are thermolabile or will be adversely affected by immersion in water or other media.

Ethylene oxide is toxic because it alkylates tissue constituents. Inhalation may cause nausea, vomiting, and neurological disorders, and severe exposure may be fatal.

Before items exposed to ethylene oxide can be used they must be aired to remove any trace of the gas. This is also true for articles of clothing, such as gloves and shoes, that have been exposed because chemical burns can occur when the contaminated clothing comes in contact with the skin.

ethylenediaminetetraacetic acid (ˌethileenˌdieəmeenˌtetrə·ə'seetik) a chelating agent that binds calcium and other metals; abbreviated EDTA; used as an anticoagulant for preserving blood specimens. Also used medicinally; see EDETATE.

ethyloestrenol (ˌethil'eestrəˌnol) an anabolic steroid that may be used to treat severe weight loss, debility and osteoporosis.

ethynodiol diacetate (ˌethinoh'dieol) a progestin used in combination with an oestrogen as an oral contraceptive.

ethynyl (ˌethinil, -iel) the group -C≡CH, when it occurs in organic compounds.

etiolation (ˌeeti·ə'layshən) 1. blanching or paleness of a plant grown in the dark due to lack of chlorophyll. 2. the process by which the skin becomes pale when deprived of sunlight.

etomidate (i'tomidayt) intravenous anaesthetic induction agent associated with rapid recovery and little hangover. It does not release histamine and is notable for its lack of depressant effect on the cardiovascular system. It causes pain on injection and has recently been shown to depress the adrenal cortex leading to low levels of cortisol.

etoposide (i'topəsied) a cytotoxic drug acting in a similar way as the vinca alkaloids. It is available as capsules and as an injection.

Eu chemical symbol, *europium.*

eu- word element. [Gr.] *normal, good, well, easy.*

euaesthesia (yoois'theezi·ə) a normal state of the senses.

Eubacteriales (ˌyoobakˌtiə·ri'ayleez) an order of Schizomycetes comprising the true bacteria.

Eubacterium (ˌyoobak'tiə·ri·əm) a genus of bacteria found in the intestinal tract as parasites, and as saprophytes in soil and water.

eucalyptol (ˌyookə'liptol) a colourless liquid obtained from eucalyptus oil and other sources; used as an expectorant, flavouring agent, and local anaesthetic.

eucalyptus oil (ˌyookə'liptəs) a volatile oil from the fresh leaf of a species of *Eucalyptus*, the chief constituent of which is eucalyptol.

Eucaryotae (yooˌkaree'ohtee) a kingdom of organisms that includes higher plants and animals, fungi, protozoa, and most algae (except blue-green algae), all of which are made up of eukaryotic cells. See also EUKARYOTE.

euchlorhydria (yooklor'hiedri·ə) the presence of the normal amount of hydrochloric acid in the gastric juice.

eucholia (yoo'kohli·ə) normal condition of the bile.

euchromatin (yoo'krohmətin) that state of chromatin in which it stains lightly, is genetically active, and is considered to be partially or fully uncoiled.

euchromatopsy (yoo'krohməˌtopsee) normal colour vision.

eucrasia (yoo'krayzi·ə) 1. a state of health; proper balance of different factors constituting a healthy state. 2. a state in which the body reacts normally to ingested or injected drugs, proteins, etc.

eudiemorrhysis (ˌyoodie·i'mo·risis) the normal flow of blood through the capillaries.

eudipsia (yoo'dipsi·ə) ordinary, normal thirst.

euergasia (ˌyooə'gayzi·ə) normal psychobiological functioning.

eugenics (yoo'jeniks) the study and control of procreation as a means of improving hereditary characteristics of future generations.

negative e. that concerned with prevention of reproduction by individuals having inferior or undesirable traits.

positive e. that concerned with promotion of optimal mating and reproduction by individuals having desirable or superior traits.

eugenol ('yooji,nol) the chief constituent of clove oil, also obtained from other sources, used in dentistry as a constituent of some dental cements and for its antiseptic qualities.

euglobulin (yoo'globyuhlin) one of a class of globulins characterized by being insoluble in water but soluble in saline solutions.

euglycaemia (,yooglie'seemi·ə) a normal level of glucose in the blood. adj. **euglycaemic**.

eugonic (yoo'gonik) growing luxuriantly; said of bacterial cultures.

eukaryon (yoo'karion) 1. a highly organized nucleus bounded by a nuclear membrane, a characteristic of cells of higher organisms. 2. eukaryote.

eukaryosis (,yookari'ohsis) the state of having a true nucleus.

Eukaryotae (yoo,kari'ohtee) Eucaryotae.

eukaryote (yoo'kari,oht) an organism of the Eucaryotae, whose cells have a true nucleus bounded by a nuclear membrane and containing the CHROMOSOMES and which divide by MITOSIS. Eukaryotic cells also contain membrane-bound organelles, such as mitochondria, chloroplasts, lysosomes, and the Golgi apparatus. Plants and animals, protozoa, fungi, and algae (except blue-green algae) are eukaryotes. Other organisms (the bacteria) are prokaryotes.

eukaryotic (,yookari'otik) pertaining to a eukaryon or to a eukaryote.

eukinesia (yooki'neezi·ə) normal or proper motor function or activity. adj. **eukinetic**.

eulaminate (yoo'lami,nayt) having the normal number of laminae, as certain areas of the cerebral cortex.

Eulenburg's disease ('oylen,booəgz) myotonia congenita.

eumetria (yoo'meetri·ə) a normal condition of nerve impulse, so that a voluntary movement just reaches the intended goal; the proper range of movement.

eunuch ('yoonək) a male deprived of the testes or external genitalia, especially one castrated before puberty (so that male secondary sexual characteristics fail to develop).

eunuchoid ('yoonə,koyd) 1. resembling a eunuch. 2. a person who resembles a eunuch.

eunuchoidism ('yoonəkoy,dizəm) deficiency of the testes or of their secretion, with impaired sexual power and eunuchoid symptoms.

female e. hypogonadism in which the ovaries fail to function at puberty, resulting in infertility, absence of development of secondary sexual characteristics, infantile sexual organs, and excessive growth of the long bones.

hypergonadotrophic e. that associated with secretion of high levels of gonadotrophins, as in Klinefelter's syndrome.

hypogonadotrophic e. that due to lack of gonadotrophin secretion.

eupancreatism (yoo'pankri·ə,tizəm) normal functioning of the pancreas.

eupepsia (yoo'pepsi·ə) good digestion; the presence of a normal amount of pepsin in the gastric juice. adj. **eupeptic**.

euphoretic (,yoofə'retik) 1. pertaining to, characterized by, or producing euphoria. 2. an agent that produces euphoria.

euphoria (yoo'for·ri·ə) bodily comfort; well-being; absence of pain or distress. In psychiatry, abnormal or exaggerated sense of well-being. adj. **euphoric**.

euphoriant (yoo'for·ri·ənt) euphoretic.

euplastic (yoo'plastik) readily becoming organized; adapted to tissue formation.

euploid ('yooployd) 1. having a balanced set or sets of chromosomes, in any number. 2. a euploid individual or cell.

euploidy (yoo'ploydee) the state of being euploid.

eupnoea (yoop'ni·ə) normal respiration. adj. **eupnoeic**.

eupraxia (yoo'praksi·ə) intactness of reproduction of coordinated movements. adj. **eupractic**.

eurhythmia (yoo'ridhmi·ə) regularity of the pulse.

europium (yuh'rohpi·əm) a chemical element, atomic number 63, atomic weight 151.96, symbol Eu. See table of elements in Appendix 2.

eury- word element. [Gr.] *wide, broad.*

eurycephalic (,yoorikə'falik, -sə'falik) having a wide head.

euryon ('yoorion) a point on either parietal bone marking either end of the greatest transverse diameter of the skull.

eusol ('yoosol) the commonly used name for chlorinated lime and boric acid solution. The name is derived from the initials of Edinburgh University Solution of Lime.

e. equivalents solutions of sodium hypochlorite with the same quantity of available chlorine as eusol.

eustachian tube (yoo'stayshən) see PHARYNGOTYMPANIC TUBE.

euthanasia (,yoothə'nayzi·ə, -zhə) 1. an easy or good death. 2. the deliberate ending of life of a person suffering from an incurable disease; this can be voluntary or involuntary.

Voluntary euthanasia is requested by the sufferer, and can be described as assisted suicide. Involuntary euthanasia is an act by society or an individual, to end the life of a person who cannot exercise any will in this matter. This includes severely handicapped infants and the demented. In no country is either form of euthanasia legal. Any 'right to die' is fraught with possible abuse.

Good medical and nursing practice, including pain relief and a recognition of the process of dying, should lead to a good death whatever the circumstances.

euthermic (yoo'thərmik) characterized by the proper temperatures; promoting warmth.

euthyroid (yoo'thieroyd) having a normally functioning thyroid gland.

eutocia (yoo'tohsi·ə) normal labour, or childbirth.

Eutrombicula (,yootrom'bikyuhlə) a subgenus of *Trombicula* (see also CHIGGER).

eutrophia (yoo'trohfi·ə) a state of normal (good) nutrition.

eutrophication (yoo,trohfi'kayshən) the accidental or deliberate promotion of excessive growth (multiplication) of one kind of organism to the disadvantage of other organisms in the same ecosystem.

eV electron volt.

evacuant (i'vakyooənt) 1. promoting evacuation. 2. an agent that promotes evacuation.

evacuation (i,vakyoo'ayshən) 1. an emptying or removal, especially the removal of any material from the body by discharge through a natural or artificial passage. 2. material discharged from the body, especially the discharge from the bowels.

evacuator (i'vakyoo,aytə) an instrument used to evacuate a cavity such as the bladder or rectum; in particular, an instrument designed to wash out small particles of stone from the bladder after lithotrity.

evagination (i,vaji'nayshən) an outpouching of a layer or part.

evaluation (i,valyoo'ayshən) a critical appraisal or

assessment; a judgement of the value, worth, character, or effectiveness of that which is being assessed. In the health care field, this includes assessment of the patient's position on the health/illness continuum, and evaluation of the effectiveness of patient care activities in bringing about a change in his position. See also NURSING PROCESS and NURSING AUDIT.

The basic components of evaluation are (1) identifying the parameters of the subject of appraisal, (2) developing criteria specific to the topic within the parameters, (3) data gathering, (4) measuring the data against the criteria, and (5) employing the results of assessment for improvement of the process, status, behaviour, or activity evaluated.

Parameters are the exact dimensions or fixed limits that clearly define the area of evaluation. They establish the frame of reference within which the process will take place and are essential to accurate interpretation and meaningful use of the results of the evaluation. Parameters to be considered might include the framework of time within which the data gathering will take place, description of the kinds of data to be obtained, and specification of the patient population selected for evaluation of patient care. In a NURSING AUDIT, for example, the medical records chosen for audit might be those of patients whose admission and discharge dates were within a specific period of time, and whose age range and diagnoses were similar. Since it is a *nursing* audit, the kind of data collected should be limited to information related to the area of nursing activities and the resulting patient care outcomes recorded on the patient's chart.

In the assessment of a patient's position on the health/illness continuum, the parameters might limit the appraisal to respiratory function, neuromuscular function, emotional state, or any of a number of areas that are important to accomplishing the overall goals and objectives of health care for that specific patient.

Parameters may vary widely, then, depending on what is being appraised and the goals and purposes of the evaluation. They focus the attention of the evaluators on specifics rather than generalities and allow for a more analytic and logical approach to the task of evaluation.

A *criterion* is a standard on which a judgement is based; a set of criteria is useful only insofar as it provides a sound basis for decision-making and action. The criteria developed for the purpose of evaluation may be stated in a number of ways, but they must be pertinent to the previously established parameters and objectives. If, for example, the parameters limit an assessment to nursing activities related to adult patients with new colostomies, the objectives would be concerned with the ability of the patient to manage his colostomy and resume his daily life at home and at work. The criteria must be stated within the confines of these parameters and they must be compatible with the objectives. The criteria are written as positive outcomes; that is, they clearly state the specific things the patient has demonstrated an ability to do as a result of the nursing care he has received. It should be noted that, although objectives project future desired ends, and criteria state outcomes in terms of what has been accomplished, both are based on the same concept.

Criteria should be measurable, that is, stated in terms that denote logical and sequential steps in the progression toward a desirable goal. In some instances criteria may be relatively easy to define because they are based on previously and scientifically determined norms and values. In the area of assessment of a patient's physiological state one could use as criteria the normal range of values for laboratory tests, the acceptable limits of vital sign readings, the normal range of joint motion, or any of the established quantifiable values and standards.

Criteria related to patient care activities also should reflect a systematic and analytical approach. If they are related to patient education, they should be written in behavioural terms that describe the specific units of behaviour one would look for to determine whether a change is taking or has taken place. For example, is the patient able to change his colostomy drainage bags without assistance?

Criteria represent the 'ideal', but they should not be considered as inflexible and permanently fixed. They may, and often do, require revision after having been tested in the process of evaluation and found to be irrelevant, impractical, or unachievable because of factors that are difficult or impossible to control. They may prove to be invalid because they do not measure what they were intended to measure, or they may be of little use because they do not lead to the detection of deficiencies that need correction. When criteria do fail to serve the function for which they are intended, it may be that those developing the criteria are not sufficiently knowledgeable about the area of assessment and thus need the help of practitioners who are more experienced.

Data gathering involves the collection of information that gives factual and objective evidence about the subject being evaluated. The evidence may be obtained through observation, interview, the review of patient records, and, as in the case of assessment of a patient's health/illness status, through such procedures as laboratory analysis and testing, radiological studies, and other diagnostic techniques, as well as a physical assessment or examination and history taking.

The data collected become documented evidence, which is then measured against the established criteria. If the evidence indicates that all of the criteria are being met, there is no indication of a problem in the area of evaluation. If the evidence shows that certain criteria are not met, these deficiencies are identified as the ones needing attention so that there can be progress toward the stated goals.

eventration (ˌeeven'trayshən) 1. protrusion of the bowels through the abdomen. 2. removal of the abdominal viscera.

e. of the diaphragm, diaphragmatic e. elevation of the dome of the diaphragm into the thoracic cavity, usually due to phrenic nerve paralysis.

eversion (i'vərshən) a turning inside out; a turning outward.

evert (i'vərt) to turn inside out; to turn outward.

evisceration (iˌvisə'rayshən) 1. extrusion of the viscera, or internal organs; disembowelment; eventration (2). 2. removal of the contents of an organ, particularly the eyeball. Evisceration of the eyeball, leaving the sclera in place, is used only in very severe panophthalmitis, when removal of the intact eye is not possible. It was performed more often in the pre-antibiotic era, since infection was less likely to spread to the meninges if the optic nerve was left intact.

evolution (ˌeevə'looshən) the process of development in which an organ or organism becomes more and more complex by the differentiation of its parts; a continuous and progressive change according to certain laws and by means of resident forces.

convergent e. the development, in animals that are only distantly related, of similar structures or functions in adaptation to similar environment.

evulsion (i'vulshən) extraction by force.

Ewing's tumour (sarcoma) ('yooingz) a malignant tumour of bone that arises in medullary tissue, occurring more often in cylindrical bones, with pain, fever, and leukocytosis as prominent symptoms.

ex- word element. [L.] *away from*, *without*, *outside;* sometimes used to denote *completely.*

ex vivo (eks 'veevoh) outside the living body; denoting removal of an organ (e.g., the kidney) for reparative surgery, after which it is returned to the original site.

exa- ('eksə) word element; used in naming units of measurement to designate a quantity 10^{18} (a trillion) times the unit to which it is joined; symbol E.

exacerbation (ek,sasə'bayshən, ig,zasə-) increase in severity of a disease or any of its symptoms.

examination (eg,zami'nayshən) inspection or investigation, especially as a means of diagnosing disease, qualified according to the methods used, as physical, cystoscopic, etc.

exanthem (eg'zanthəm, ek's-) 1. any cutaneous eruptive disease or fever. 2. the eruption which characterizes an eruptive fever.

e. subitum an acute viral disease of infants and young children, with continuous or remittent fever, falling by crises, and followed by a rash on the trunk (see also ROSEOLA INFANTUM).

exanthema (,egzan'theemə, ,eks-) pl. *exanthemata* [Gr.] exanthem.

exanthematous (,egzan'themətəs, eks-) characterized by or of the nature of an eruption or rash.

exarticulation (,eksah,tikyuh'layshən) amputation at a joint; partial removal of a joint.

excavation (,ekskə'vayshən) 1. the act of hollowing out. 2. a hollowed-out space, or pouchlike cavity.

atrophic e. cupping of the optic disc, due to atrophy of the optic nerve fibres.

e. of optic disc, physiological e. a normally occurring depression in the centre of the optic disc.

excavator ('ekskə,vaytə) a scoop or gouge for surgical use.

excerebration (,ekseri'brayshən) removal of the brain.

excipient (ek'sipi·ənt) any more or less inert substance added to a drug to give suitable consistency or form to the drug; a vehicle.

excise (ek'siez) to remove by cutting.

excision (ek'sizhən) removal, as of an organ, by cutting.

excitability (ek,sietə'bilitee) readiness to respond to a stimulus; irritability.

excitant (ek'sietənt) an agent producing excitation of the vital functions, or of those of the brain.

excitation (,eksie'tayshən) an act of irritation or stimulation; a condition of being excited or of responding to a stimulus; the addition of energy, as the excitation of a molecule by absorption of photons.

indirect e. electrostimulation of a muscle by placing the electrode on its nerve.

excitement (ek'sietmənt) a physiological and emotional response to a stimulus.

excitomotor (ek,sietoh'mohtə) tending to produce motion or motor function; an agent that so acts.

excitosecretory (ek,sietohsi'kreetə·ree) producing increased secretion.

excitovascular (ek,sietoh'vaskyuhlə) causing vascular changes.

exclave ('eksklayv) a detached part of an organ.

exclusion (ek'skloozhən) a shutting out or elimination; surgical isolation of a part, as of a segment of intestine, without removal from the body.

excoriation (ek,skor·ri'ayshən) any superficial loss of substance, such as that produced on the skin by scratching.

excrement ('ekskrəmənt) faecal matter; matter cast out as waste from the body.

excrementitious (,ekskrimen'tishəs) pertaining to or of the nature of excrement.

excrescence (ek'skresəns) an abnormal outgrowth; a projection of morbid origin. adj. **excrescent**.

excreta (ek'skreetə) excretion products; waste material excreted or eliminated from the body, including FAECES, URINE, and PERSPIRATION. Mucus and carbon dioxide also can be considered to be excreta. The organs of excretion are the intestinal tract, kidneys, lungs, and skin.

excrete (ek'skreet) to throw off or eliminate, as waste matter, by a normal discharge.

excretion (ek'skreeshən) 1. the act, process, or function of excreting. 2. material that is excreted. adj. **excretory.** Ordinarily, what is meant by excretion is the evacuation of faeces. Technically, excretion can refer to the expulsion of any matter, whether from a single cell or from the entire body, or to the matter excreted.

excursion (ek'skərshən) a range of movement regularly repeated in performance of a function, e.g., excursion of the jaws in mastication. adj. **excursive**.

excystation (,eks·si'stayshən) escape from a cyst or envelope, as in that stage in the life cycle of parasites occurring after the cystic form has been swallowed by the host.

exenteration (eg,zentə'rayshən) evisceration.

exercise ('eksə,siez) performance of physical exertion for improvement of health or correction of physical deformity.

active e. motion imparted to a part by voluntary contraction and relaxation of its controlling muscles.

active assisted e. voluntary contraction of muscles controlling a part, assisted by a therapist or by some other means.

active resisted e. voluntary contraction of muscles with mechanical or manual resistance applied.

Buerger–Allen e's specific exercises intended to improve circulation to the feet and legs (see also BUERGER–ALLEN EXERCISES).

corrective e. therapeutic exercise.

isometric e. active exercise performed against stable resistance, without change in the length of the muscle. No movement occurs at any joints over which the muscle passes.

isotonic e. active exercise without appreciable change in the force of muscular contraction, with shortening of the muscle.

Kegel e's a programme of exercises designed to strengthen the pelvic–vaginal muscles in stress incontinence in women (see also KEGEL EXERCISES).

muscle-setting e. voluntary contraction and relaxation of skeletal muscles without movement of the associated part of the body; called also *static exercise.*

passive e. motion imparted to a segment of the body by another individual, machine, or other outside force, or produced by voluntary effort of another segment of the patient's own body.

range of movement (ROM) e's exercises that move each joint through its full range of movement, that is, to the highest degree of movement of which each joint normally is capable. See accompanying figure.

static e. muscle-setting exercise.

e. testing a technique for evaluating circulatory response to physical stress; called also stress testing. The procedure involves continuous electrocardiographic monitoring during physical exercise, the objective being to increase the intensity of physical exertion until a target heart rate is reached or signs and symptoms of cardiac ischaemia appear.

Clinical exercise testing has become an important tool in screening for and diagnosing early ischaemic heart disease that cannot be detected by a standard resting ECG, and in predicting the probability of the

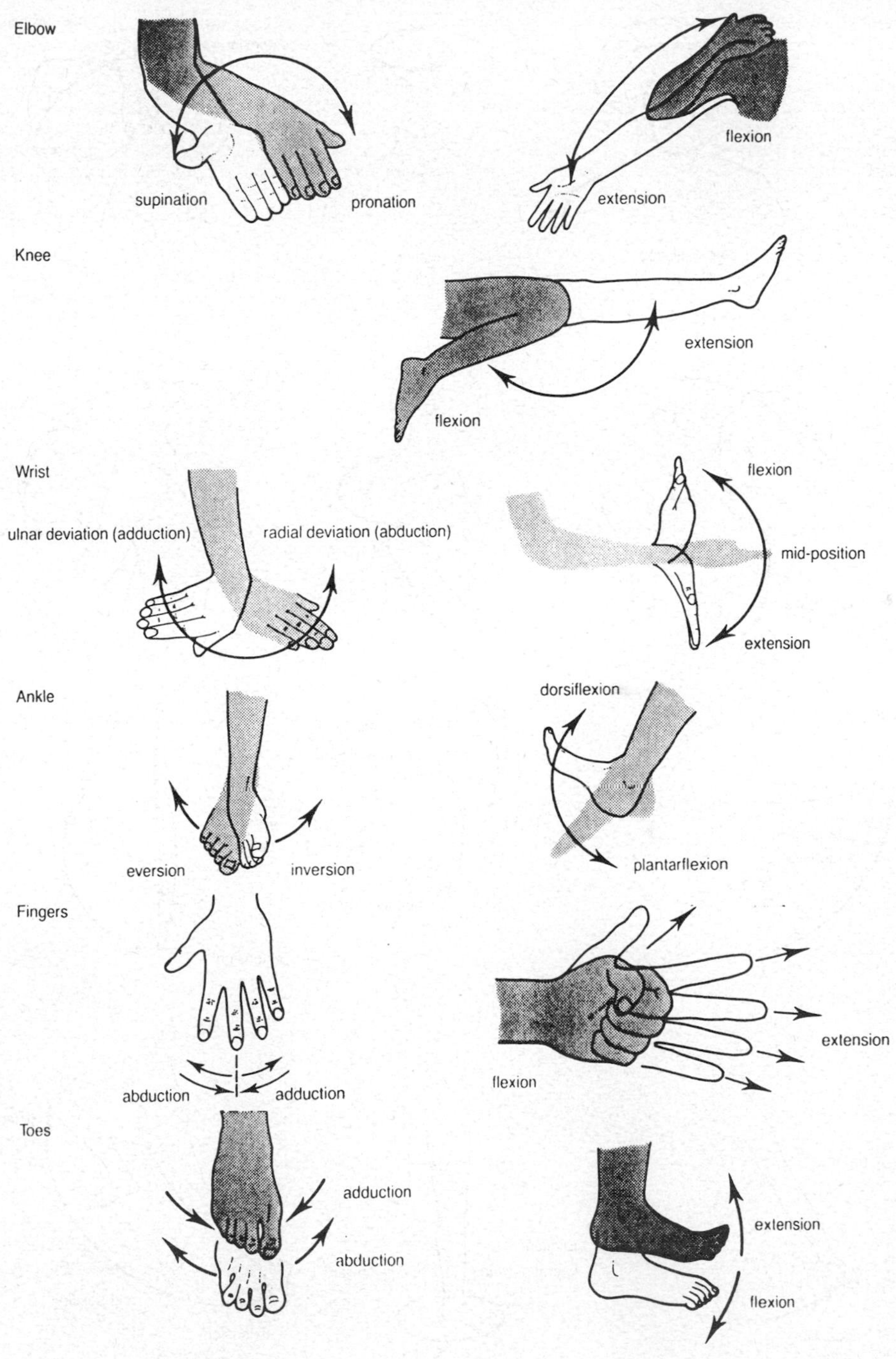

Ranges of motion. All **exercises** can be performed from the supine position in bed except extension of the spine, hips and shoulders and flexion of the knees, for which the person must lie prone or on his side

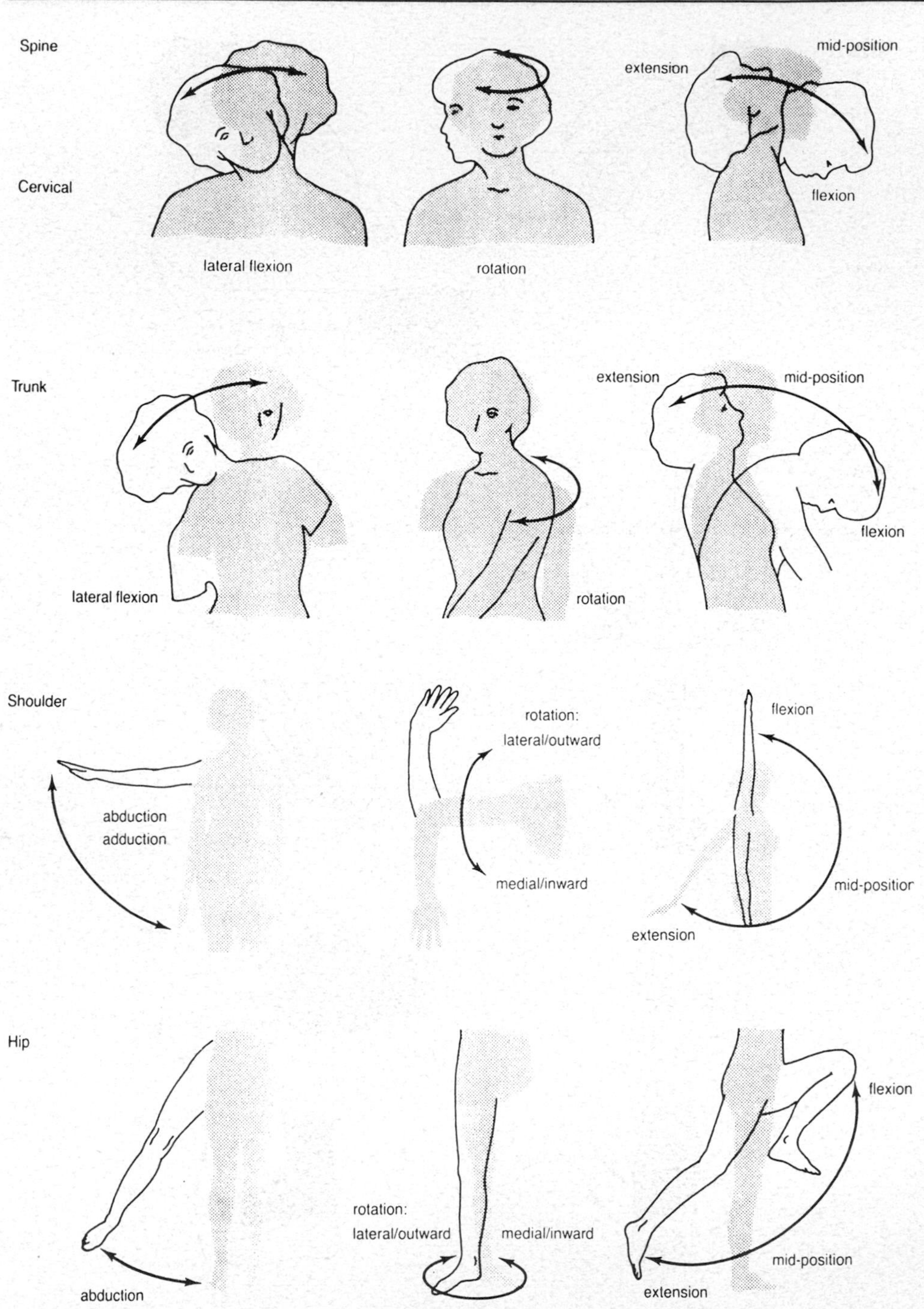

development of the condition in later years. The technique cannot determine the location of the lesion causing cardiac ischaemia and therefore must be supplemented with angiocardiography when coronary occlusion is detected.

Three basic forms of exercise are used: the treadmill, step climbing, and the bicycle ergometer. The procedure must be performed in a clinical setting where medical personnel are available in the event that symptoms of dyspnoea, vertigo, extreme fatigue, severe arrhythmias, and other abnormal ECG readings develop during the exercise.

Exercise testing also may be used to assess the pulmonary status of a patient with a respiratory disease. As the patient performs specific exercises, blood samples are drawn for BLOOD GAS ANALYSIS, and ventilatory function tests such as tidal volume, total lung capacity, and vital capacity are conducted. An example of the kind of exercise test that may be used is the *step test*, in which the patient steps up and down on a 20-cm-high platform 30 times a minute.

therapeutic e. the scientific use of bodily movement to restore normal function in diseased or injured tissues or to maintain a state of well-being. Called also *corrective exercise*. As with any type of therapy, a therapeutic exercise programme is designed to correct specific disabilities of the individual patient. The programme is evaluated periodically and modified as indicated by the progress of the patient and his response to the prescribed regimen. Exercises affect the body locally and systemically, and bring about changes in the nervous, circulatory, and endocrine systems as well as the musculoskeletal system.

Among the types of therapeutic exercise are those that (1) increase or maintain mobility of the joints and surrounding soft tissues, (2) develop coordination through control of individual muscles, (3) increase muscular strength and endurance, and (4) promote relaxation and relief of tension.

JOINT MOBILITY. In the absence of a disability that prohibits mobility, the regular day-to-day activities of living maintain the normal movements of the joints. If, however, motion is restricted for any reason, the soft tissues become dense and hard and adaptive shortening of the connective tissues takes place. These changes begin to develop within four days after a joint has been immobilized and are evident even in a normal joint that has been rendered immobile. It is for this reason that therapeutic exercises to prevent loss of joint motion are so important and should be begun as soon as possible after an injury has occurred or a disease process has begun.

Prevention of the loss of joint movement is much less costly and time-consuming than correction of tissue changes that seriously impair joint mobility. It is recommended that each joint should be put through its full range of movement three times at least twice daily. If the patient is not able to carry out these exercises, he is assisted by a physiotherapist or member of his family who has been instructed in the exercises. Inflammation of the joint, as in arthritis, may cause some pain on motion, and so passive exercises are done slowly and gently with the joint as relaxed as possible. Procedures that stretch tight muscles to increase joint motion should be done only by a skilled physiotherapist who understands the hazards of fracture and bleeding within the joint, which can occur if the exercises are done improperly or too strenuously.

MUSCLE TRAINING. Exercises of this type are taught to the patient who has lost some control over a major skeletal muscle. By learning precise and conscious control over a specific muscle, the patient is able to strengthen and coordinate its movement with normal motor patterns and thus enhance his mobility. Muscle training or neuromuscular re-education demands full cooperation of the patient. He must be capable of understanding the purpose of the exercises and able to follow directions and give his full attention to the muscle isolated for retraining. The training sessions are held in a quiet, comfortable atmosphere in which the patient is able to concentrate on the task of controlling the activity of the specific muscle.

The development of conscious control over individual muscles is useful in the rehabilitation of patients with a variety of disorders, including physical trauma, diseases such as poliomyelitis that affect the motor neurons, and congenital disorders such as cerebral palsy. It demands full concentration and mental awareness on the part of the patient and involves a systematic programme of sequential activities carried out under the direction of a physiotherapist who is knowledgeable in the technique. Although it requires much effort on the part of the patient and the therapist, the attainment of muscle control and coordination is a very satisfying reward.

MUSCLE STRENGTH AND ENDURANCE. Improvement of muscle strength and endurance is particularly important in the rehabilitation of patients whose goal is to return to an active and productive life after a debilitating illness or disabling injury. The exercises are prescribed according to the individual needs of the patient and usually involve more than one group of muscles. Endurance exercises, usually of the low-resistance type, demand repetition and persistence beyond the point of fatigue. When developing a programme of this type it is necessary to take into account the patient's need for motivation and the pitfalls of boredom from monotony. The various activities included in occupational therapy can be useful in maintaining the patient's interest and cooperation.

RELIEF OF TENSION. Exercises that promote relaxation of the muscles and provide relief from the effects of tension are useful in a wide variety of disorders ranging from mild tension headache to insomnia. Patients who are especially tense may require several sessions of instruction in relaxation before they can learn the technique.

exeresis (ek'serisis) surgical removal, or excision.

exergonic (ˌeksə'gonik) accompanied by the release of free energy.

exflagellation (eksˌflaji'layshən) the protrusion or formation of flagelliform microgametes from a microgametocyte in malarial parasites and some related sporozoa.

exfoliation (eksˌfohli'ayshən) a falling off in scales or layers. adj. **exfoliative.**

lamellar e. of newborn a congenital hereditary disorder in which the infant is born completely covered with a collodion- or parchment-like membrane that peels off within 24 hours, after which there may be complete healing, or the scales may re-form and the process repeated. In the more severe form, the infant (harlequin fetus) is completely covered with thick, horny, armour-like scales, and is usually stillborn or dies shortly after birth. Called also *ichthyosis congenita*, *ichthyosis fetalis*, and *lamellar ichthyosis of newborn*.

exhalation (ˌeks·hə'layshən) 1. the giving off of watery or other vapour, or of an effluvium. 2. a vapour or other substance exhaled or given off. 3. the act of breathing out.

exhaustion (ig'zawschən) 1. privation of energy with consequent inability to respond to stimuli; lassitude. 2. withdrawal. 3. a condition of emptiness caused by withdrawal. 4. emptying by a process of withdrawal.

heat e. an effect of excessive exposure to heat (see also HEAT EXHAUSTION).

exhibitionism (ˌeksi'bishəˌnizəm) a sexual deviation in which pleasure is gained by exposure of the genitals to persons of the opposite sex in socially unacceptable circumstances. It is more common in men than in women, and in adults it is difficult to correct. It may be resorted to by an individual who is unable for physical or psychological reasons to gain sexual gratification by normal means. A common cause is a feeling of sexual inadequacy; for this the exposure is a compensation. Exhibitionism may also be a form of masochism in which a feeling of guilt drives the person to behaviour for which he knows he will be punished. Psychotherapy is used to deal with this type of sexual deviation, but the response tends to be poor. Better responses have been claimed for behaviour therapy.

exhibitionist (ˌeksi'bishənist) a person who indulges in exhibitionism.

existentialism (ˌeksi'stenshəlizəm) an important twentieth century philosophical movement which has influenced psychology and psychiatry. The emphasis is upon personal decisions to be made in a world without reason and without purpose. Since there are no objective standards and guides to personal behaviour, the individual may, and must, actively choose his own path. The constant difficult choices of existence are made against the background of the awareness of the inevitability of death. The anxiety of making choices is rendered the more absurd by the ultimate 'nothingness' beyond life and subjective experience. Existentialism emphasises subjectivity, free will and individuality and has produced a form of psychotherapy (existential therapy) that emphasises 'authentic' existence. The existence in the world one makes for oneself should reflect the individual's subjectivity and be 'authentic' and should not be a response to what 'they', the others, either individual or institutional, expect. An existence shaped to external demand is 'inauthentic' or 'in bad faith'.

exo- word element. [Gr.] *outside of, outward.*

exocardia (ˌeksoh'kahdi·ə) congenital displacement of the heart; ectocardia.

exocardial (ˌeksoh'kahdi·əl) situated, occurring, or developed outside the heart.

exocolitis (ˌeksohkə'lietis) inflammation of the outer coat of the colon.

exocrine ('eksohˌkrin, -ˌkrien) 1. secreting externally via a duct. 2. denoting such a gland or its secretion.

exocytosis (ˌeksohsie'tohsis) 1. the discharge from a cell of particles that are too large to diffuse through the wall; the opposite of endocytosis. 2. the aggregation of migrating leukocytes in the epidermis as part of the inflammatory response.

exodeviation (ˌeksohˌdeevi'ayshən) a turning outward; in ophthalmology, exotropia.

exodontics (ˌeksoh'dontiks) that branch of dentistry dealing with extraction of teeth.

exoenzyme (ˌeksoh'enziem) an enzyme that acts outside the cell that secretes it.

exoerythrocytic (ˌeksoh·iˌrithroh'sitik) occurring or situated outside the red blood cells (erythrocytes), a term applied to a stage in the development of malarial parasites that takes place in cells other than erythrocytes.

exogamy (ek'sogəmee) 1. protozoan fertilization by union of elements that are not derived from the same cell. 2. marriage outside a particular group.

exogenous (ek'sojənəs) originating outside or caused by factors outside the organism.

exomphalos (ek'somfələs) 1. hernia of the abdominal viscera into the umbilical cord. 2. congenital umbilical hernia.

exonuclease (ˌeksoh'nyookliˌayz) a nuclease that cleaves single mononucleotides from the end of a polynucleotide chain.

exopeptidase (ˌeksoh'peptiˌdayz) a proteolytic enzyme whose action is limited to terminal peptide linkages.

exophoria (ˌeksoh'for·ri·ə) heterophoria in which there is deviation of the visual axis of an eye away from that of the other eye in the absence of visual fusional stimuli. adj. **exophoric.**

exophthalmometer (ˌeksofthal'momitə) an instrument for measuring the extent of relative protrusion of the eyeball (exophthalmos). Called also *orthometer, proptometer.*

exophthalmometry (ˌeksofthal'momitree) measurement of the extent of protrusion of the eyeball in exophthalmos.

exophthalmos (ˌeksof'thalmos) abnormal protrusion of the eye. adj. **exophthalmic.** Called also *exophthalmia.* It results in a marked stare and is often associated with HYPERTHYROIDISM. The condition may also be caused by a tumour in the orbit.

exophytic (ˌeksoh'fitik) growing outward; in oncology, proliferating externally or on the surface epithelium of an organ or other structure in which the growth originated.

exormia (ek'sormi·ə) a papular skin eruption.

exoserosis (ˌeksohsi'rohsis) an oozing of serum or exudate.

exoskeleton (ˌeksoh'skelitən) an external hard framework, as a crustacean's shell, that supports and protects the soft tissues of lower animals, derived from the ectoderm. In vertebrates the term is sometimes applied to structures produced by the epidermis, as hair, nails, hoofs, teeth, etc.

exosmosis (ˌeksoz'mohsis) osmosis or diffusion from within outward.

exostosis (ˌekso'stohsis) pl. *exostoses* [Gr.] a benign new growth projecting from a bone surface and characteristically capped by cartilage. adj. **exostotic.**

e. cartilaginea a variety of osteoma consisting of a layer of cartilage developing beneath the periosteum of a bone.

hereditary multiple e. a generally benign, hereditary disorder of enchondral growth of bone, marked by exostoses near the extremities of the diaphysis of long bones.

exothermal, exothermic (ˌeksoh'thərməl; ˌeksoh'thərmik) marked or accompanied by the evolution of heat; liberating heat or energy.

exotic (eg'zotik) pertaining to a disease occurring in a region far from where it is usually found.

exotoxin (ˌeksoh'toksin) a potent toxin formed and excreted by the bacterial cell, and found free in the surrounding medium. adj. **exotoxic.** Exotoxins are heat labile, and protein in nature. They are detoxified with retention of antigenicity by treatment with formaldehyde and are the most poisonous substances known to man. Bacteria of the genus *Clostridium* are the most frequent producers of exotoxins; diphtheria, botulism, and tetanus are all caused by bacterial toxins.

exotropia (ˌeksoh'trohpi·ə) STRABISMUS in which there is permanent deviation of the visual axis of one eye away from that of the other, resulting in diplopia. Called also *divergent strabismus* and *walleye.* adj. **exotropic.**

expander (ek'spandə) something that enlarges or prolongs; extender.

plasma volume e. a substance that can be transfused to maintain fluid volume of the blood in event of great necessity, supplementary to the use of whole blood and plasma. Called also *artificial plasma extender* and *plasma volume extender.*

expectation of life (ˌekspek'tayshən) the average length of life based on present mortality trends. Called also *life expectancy.*

expectorant (ek'spektə·rənt) 1. promoting expectoration. 2. an agent that promotes expectoration.

liquefying e. an expectorant that promotes the ejection

of mucus from the respiratory tract by decreasing its viscosity.

expectoration (ek,spektə'rayshən) 1. the coughing up and spitting out of material from the lungs, bronchi, and trachea. 2. sputum.

experiment (ek'sperimənt) a procedure done in order to discover or demonstrate some fact or general truth. adj. **experimental.**

control e. one made under standard conditions, to test the correctness of other observations.

experimental study (ek,speri'ment'l) an epidemiological study planned in a selected population to measure the effect of a therapeutic or control measure, for example a vaccine trial comparing the incidence of disease in the vaccinated persons with a control group of unvaccinated persons.

expirate ('ekspi,rayt) exhaled air or gas.

single e. the gas exhaled at a single expiration.

expiration (,ekspi'rayshən) 1. the act of breathing out, or expelling air from the lungs. 2. termination, or death. adj. **expiratory**.

expire (ek'spieə) 1. to breathe out. 2. to die.

explant ('eksplahnt, ek'splahnt) 1. to take from the body and place in an artificial medium for growth. 2. tissue taken from the body and grown in an artificial medium.

exploration (,eksplə'rayshən) investigation or examination for diagnostic purposes. adj. **exploratory**.

exposure (ek'spohzhə) 1. the act of laying open, as surgical exposure. 2. the condition of being subjected to something, as to infectious agents or extremes of weather or radiation, which may have a harmful effect. 3. in radiology, a measure of the amount of ionizing radiation reaching a particular volume of space.

expression (ek'spreshən) 1. the aspect or appearance of the face as determined by the physical or emotional state. 2. the act of squeezing out or evacuating by pressure, e.g., the removal of breast milk by hand. 3. the manifestation of a heritable trait in an individual carrying the gene or genes which determine it.

expressivity (,ekspre'sivətee) the extent to which a hereditable trait is manifested by an individual carrying the principal gene or genes that determine it.

expulsive (ek'spulsiv) driving or forcing out; tending to expel.

exsanguination (ek,sang·gwi'nayshən) extensive blood loss due to internal or external haemorrhage.

exsection (ek'sekshən) excision.

exsiccation (,eksi'kayshən) the act of drying out; in chemistry, the deprival of a crystalline substance of its water of crystallization.

exstrophy ('ekstrəfee) the turning inside out of an organ.

e. of the bladder congenital absence of a portion of the abdominal wall and bladder wall, the bladder appearing to be turned inside out, with the internal surface of the posterior wall showing through the opening in the anterior wall.

e. of cloaca, cloacal e. a developmental anomaly in which two segments of bladder (hemibladders) are separated by an area of intestine with a mucosal surface, which appears as a large red tumour in the midline of the lower abdomen.

ext. external; extract.

extender (ek'stendə) something that enlarges or prolongs; expander.

artificial plasma e., plasma volume e. plasma volume expander.

extension (ek'stenshən) 1. the movement by which the two ends of any jointed part are drawn away from each other. 2. a movement bringing the members of a limb into or toward a straight condition.

Buck's e. extension of a fractured leg by weights, the foot of the bed being raised so that the body makes counterextension.

Codivilla's e. extension for fractures made by a weight pulling on calipers or a nail passed through the lower end of the bone.

nail e., Steinmann e. traction applied to a limb by a weight attached to a nail or pin transfixing a bone, usually the calcaneus or tibia.

extensor (ek'stensə, -sor) [L.] any muscle that extends a joint.

exterior (ek'stiə·ri·ə) on the outside.

exteriorize (ek'stiə·ri·ə,riez) 1. to form a correct mental reference of the image of an object seen. 2. in psychiatry, to turn one's interest outward. 3. to transpose an internal organ to the exterior of the body.

external (ek'stərn'l) situated or occurring on the outside. In anatomy, situated toward or near the outside; lateral.

externalize (ek'stərnə,liez) to direct outwardly an internal conflict.

externus (ek'stərnəs) external; in anatomy, denoting a structure farther from the centre of an organ or cavity.

exteroception (,ekstə·roh'sepshən) the perception of stimuli originating outside or at a distance from the body.

exteroceptor (,ekstə·roh'septə) a sensory nerve ending stimulated by the immediate external environment, such as those in the skin and mucous membranes. adj. **exteroceptive**.

exterofective (,ekstə·roh'fektiv) responding to external stimuli; a term applied to the cerebrospinal nervous system.

extima ('ekstimə) outermost; the outermost coat of a blood vessel; the adventitia.

extinction (ek'stingkshən) in psychology, the disappearance of a conditioned response as a result of nonreinforcement; also, the process by which the disappearance is accomplished. See also CONDITIONING.

extirpation (,ekstər'payshən) complete removal or eradication of an organ or tissue.

extorsion (ek'stawshən) tilting of the upper part of the vertical meridian of the eye away from the midline of the face.

extra- word element. [L.] *outside, beyond the scope of, in addition.*

extra-articular (,ekstrəah'tikyuhylə) situated or occurring outside a joint.

extracapsular (,ekstrə'kapsyuhlə) situated or occurring outside a capsule.

extracellular (,ekstrə'selyuhlə) situated or occurring outside a cell or cells.

extracorporeal (,ekstrəkaw'por·ri·əl) situated or occurring outside the body.

e. circulation the circulation of blood outside the body, as through a HAEMODIALYSER for removal of substances usually excreted in the urine, or through a HEART–LUNG MACHINE for carbon dioxide–oxygen exchange.

extracorticospinal (,ekstrə,kawtikoh'spien'l) outside the corticospinal tract.

extract ('ekstrakt) a concentrated preparation of a vegetable or animal drug.

allergenic e. an extract of the protein of any substance to which a person may be sensitive.

cell-free e. the solution obtained by rupturing cells and removing all particulate matter.

extraction (ek'strakshən) 1. the process or act of pulling or drawing out. 2. the preparation of an extract.

breech e. extraction of an infant from the uterus in

cases of breech presentation.

serial e. the selective extraction of deciduous teeth during an extended period of time to allow autonomous adjustment.

vacuum e. removal of the uterine contents by application of a vacuum. (See under ABORTION, *suction curettage.*) An alternative to the forceps method of delivering a baby.

extractive (ek'straktiv) any substance present in an organized tissue, or in a mixture in a small quantity, and requiring extraction by a special method.

extractor (ek'straktə) an instrument for removing a calculus or foreign body.

extradural (,ekstrə'dyooə·rəl) situated or occurring outside the dura mater.

extraembryonic (,ekstrə,embri'onik) external to the embryo proper, as the extraembryonic coelom or the extraembryonic membranes.

extragenic (,ekstrə'jenik) occurring outside a gene, or in a gene other than the one in question.

extragenital (,ekstrə'jenit'l) not related to the genitals.

e. chancre the primary lesion of syphilis situated anywhere other than on the genital organs.

e. syphilis syphilis spread from an extragenital lesion.

extrahepatic (,ekstrəhi'patik) situated or occurring outside the liver.

extramastoiditis (,ekstrə,mastoy'dietis) inflammation of tissues adjoining the mastoid process.

extramural (,ekstrə'myooə·rəl) situated or occurring outside the wall of an organ or structure.

extraosseous (,ekstrə'ossi·əs) occurring outside a bone or bones.

extraplacental (,ekstrəplə'sent'l) outside of or independent of the placenta.

extrapleural (,ekstrə'plooə·rəl) between the chest wall and parietal layer of the pleura.

extrapolation (ek,strapə'layshən) inference of a value on the basis of that which is known or has been observed; usually applied to estimation beyond the range of observed data as opposed to interpolation between data points.

extrapsychic (,ekstrə'siekik) occurring outside the mind; taking place between the mind and the external environment.

extrapulmonary (,ekstrə'pulmənə·ree, -'puhl-) situated or occurring outside the lungs.

extrapyramidal (,ekstrəpi'ramid'l) outside the pyramidal tracts.

e. disease, e. syndrome any of a group of clinical disorders marked by abnormal involuntary movements, alterations in muscle tone, and postural disturbances; the group includes parkinsonism, chorea, athetosis, etc.

e. system, e. tract a functional, rather than anatomical, unit comprising the nuclei and fibres (excluding those of the pyramidal tract) involved in motor activities; they control and coordinate especially the postural, static, supporting, and locomotor mechanisms. It includes the corpus striatum, subthalamic nucleus, substantia nigra, and red nucleus, along with their interconnections with the reticular formation, cerebellum, and cerebrum; some authorities include the cerebellum and vestibular nuclei.

extrasensory perception (,ekstrə'sensə·ree) knowledge of, or response to, an external thought or objective event not achieved as the result of stimulation of the sense organs; abbreviated ESP.

extrasystole (,ekstrə'sistəlee) a premature cardiac contraction that is independent of the normal rhythm and arises in response to an impulse outside the sinoatrial node.

atrial e. one in which the stimulus is thought to arise in the atrium elsewhere than at the sinoatrial node.

atrioventricular e. one in which the stimulus is thought to arise in the atrioventricular node.

interpolated e. a contraction taking place between two normal heartbeats.

nodal e. atrioventricular extrasystole.

retrograde e. a premature ventricular contraction followed by a premature atrial contraction, due to transmission of the stimulus backward, usually over the bundle of His.

ventricular e. one in which either a pacemaker or a re-entry site is in the ventricular structure.

extratubal (,ekstrə'tyoob'l) situated or occurring outside a tube.

extrauterine (,ekstrə'yootə,rien) situated or occurring outside the uterus.

e. pregnancy ectopic pregnancy.

extravasation (ik,stravə'sayshən) 1. a discharge or escape, as of blood, from a vessel into the tissues; blood or other substance so discharged. 2. the process of being extravasated.

extravascular (,ekstrə'vaskyuhlə) situated or occurring outside a vessel or the vessels.

extraversion (,ekstrə'vərshən) extroversion.

extravert ('ekstrə,vərt) extrovert.

extremitas (ek'stremi,tas) pl. *extremitates* [L.] extremity.

extremity (ek'stremitee) 1. the distal or terminal portion of elongated or pointed structures. 2. the arm or leg.

extrinsic (ek'strinsik, -zik) of external origin.

e. factor a haematopoietic vitamin that combines with intrinsic factor for absorption and is needed for erythrocyte maturation; called also VITAMIN B_{12} and CYANOCOBALAMIN.

extroversion (,ekstrə'vərshən) 1. a turning inside out; exstrophy. 2. direction of one's energies and attention outward from the self.

extrovert ('ekstrə,vərt) a person whose interest is turned outward.

extrude (ek'strood) 1. to force out, or to occupy a position distal to that normally occupied. 2. in dentistry, to occupy a position occlusal to that normally occupied.

extrusion (ek'stroozhən) 1. a pushing out. 2. in dentistry, the condition of a tooth pushed too far forward from the line of occlusion.

extubation (,ekstyuh'bayshən) removal of a tube used in intubation.

exuberant (eg'zyoobə·rənt, ig-) copious or excessive in production; showing excessive proliferation.

exudate ('eksyuh,dayt) a fluid with a high content of protein and cells that has been formed by escaping from blood vessels and has been deposited in tissues or on tissue surfaces, usually as a result of inflammation.

exudation (,eksyuh'dayshən) 1. the escape of fluid, cells, or cellular debris from blood vessels as part of an inflammatory process. 2. exudate.

exudative (eg'zyoodətiv) of or pertaining to a process of exudation.

exumbilication (,eksum,bili'kayshən) 1. marked protrusion of the navel. 2. umbilical hernia.

eye (ie) the organ of vision. In the embryo the eye develops as a direct extension of the brain. To protect the eye the bones of the skull are shaped so that an orbital cavity protects the dorsal aspect of each eyeball. In addition, the conjunctiva covers part of the front of the eyeball and lines the upper and lower eyelids. Tears from the lacrimal duct constantly wash the eye to remove foreign objects, and the lids and eyelashes aid in protecting the front of the eye. In addition, the tears contain the enzyme lysozyme, which acts as a

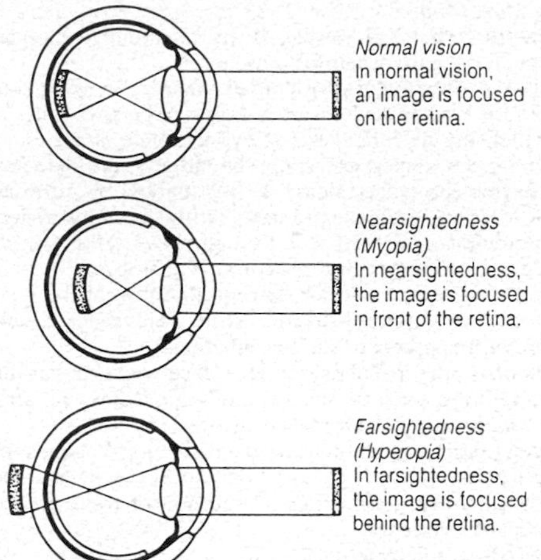

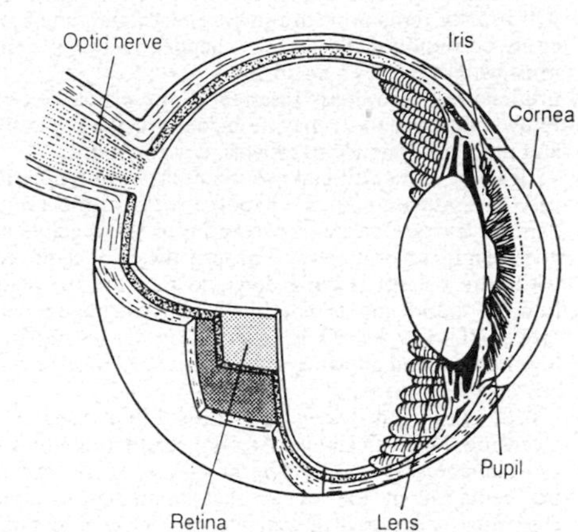

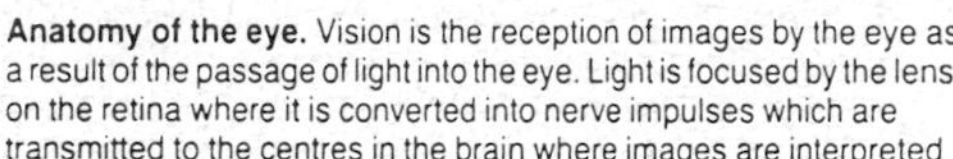

Anatomy of the eye. Vision is the reception of images by the eye as a result of the passage of light into the eye. Light is focused by the lens on the retina where it is converted into nerve impulses which are transmitted to the centres in the brain where images are interpreted

mild antiseptic.

STRUCTURE. The eyeball has three coats. The cornea is the clear transparent layer on the front of the eyeball. It is a continuation of the sclera (the white of the eye), the tough outer coat that helps protect the delicate mechanism of the eye. The choroid is the middle layer and contains blood vessels. The third layer, the retina, contains rods and cones, which are specialized cells that are sensitive to light. Behind the cornea and in front of the lens is the iris, the circular pigmented band around the pupil. The iris works much like the diaphragm in a camera, widening or narrowing the pupil to adjust to different light conditions.

FUNCTION. The refraction or bending of light rays so that they focus on the retina and can thus be transmitted to the optic nerve is accomplished by three structures: the aqueous humour, the fluid between the cornea and lens; the lens, a crystalline structure just behind the iris; and the vitreous humour, a jelly-like substance filling the space between the lens and the retina. Unlike the lens of a camera, the lens of the eye focuses by a process called accommodation. When the eye focuses for distant objects the ciliary muscle relaxes, which puts the ciliary zonule under tension and so tends to flatten the curvature of the lens. When the eye focuses for near objects the ciliary muscle contracts, allowing relaxation of the zonule, and the lens becomes thicker, and more spherical in shape due to its inherent elasticity. The lens then bends or refracts the light rays to a greater extent, focusing them on the retina.

Because the eye must function under many different circumstances, there are two different sets of nerve cells in the retina, the cone-shaped and the rod-shaped cells. They cover the full range of adaptation to light, the cones being sensitive in bright light, and the rods in dim light. The cones are responsible for colour vision. It is thought that there are three types of cones, each containing a substance that reacts to light of a different colour—one set for red, one for green, and the third for violet. These are the primary colours in light, which, when mixed together, give white. White light stimulates all three sets of colour cells; any other colour stimulates one or two. Lack of a set of colour cells causes impaired colour vision, which usually affects either the red or the green cells.

The optic nerve, which transmits the nerve impulses from the retina to the visual centre of the brain, contains nerve fibres from the many nerve cells in the retina. The small spot where it leaves the retina does not have any light-sensitive cells, and is called the blind spot.

The eyes are situated in the front of the head in such a way that human beings have stereoscopic vision, the ability to judge distances. Because the eyes are set apart, each eye sees farther around an object on its own side than does the other. The brain superimposes the two slightly different images and judges distances from the composite image. See also VISION.

DISORDERS OF THE EYE. If the eyeball is too short or too long, the lens focuses the image not on the retina, but behind or in front of it. The former condition is called hypermetropia, or longsightedness, and the latter myopia, or shortsightedness. An irregularity in the curvature of the cornea or lens can cause the impaired vision of ASTIGMATISM.

STRABISMUS, or squint, is usually caused by weakness in some of the muscles that control movement of the eyeball.

CONJUNCTIVITIS is an inflammation of the membrane that covers part of the front of the eyeball and lines the eyelids.

When the retina become detached from the underlying layers, the result is DETACHMENT OF THE RETINA. Repair by surgery can usually prevent blindness produced by retinal detachment.

PRESBYOPIA occurs in older persons and develops as the lens loses its elasticity with the passing years and thus cannot accommodate for near objects. Correction is easily made with properly prescribed glasses for reading.

Foreign bodies in the eyes are common occurrences.

Cinders, grit, or other foreign bodies are best removed by lifting the eyelid by the lashes. The foreign body will usually remain on the surface of the lid, and can easily be removed. Particles embedded in the eyeball must be removed by a doctor.

artificial e. a prosthesis inserted in the eye socket to replace the eyeball. It may be made of glass or plastic and most are designed to be worn day and night.

Cleaning of an artificial eye is similar in principle to care of dentures; both are handled with care to avoid damage and are cleansed according to the dictates of good hygienic principles. The prosthesis is removed while the patient is lying down so that the eye falls into the hand and is not likely to be dropped and broken. The prosthesis is removed by depressing the lower eyelid and allowing the artificial eye to slide out and down.

Mild soap and water are most often used for cleansing the artificial eye. Alcohol or other chemicals can damage prostheses made of plastic. If the eye is not replaced in the eye socket immediately after cleansing, it is stored in water or contact lens soaking solution.

The prosthesis is inserted by lifting the upper eyelid with the thumb or forefinger and placing the notched edge of the eye toward the nose. The prosthesis is placed as far as possible under the upper lid and then the lower lid is depressed to allow the eye to slip into place. Insertion of the eye can be made easier by moistening it with water before insertion.

The hands are washed thoroughly before removal and insertion of the prosthesis. If it is necessary to wipe the eye of the patient wearing a prosthesis, one should gently wipe toward the nose to avoid dislodging it.

eye bank an institution or agency whose primary purpose is to collect, prepare, and supply to ophthalmologists eye tissue for transplantation. Those institutions equipped with special laboratory facilities also conduct research and store eye tissue. Individuals wishing to donate their eyes may make arrangements to do so prior to their death, or the legal next-of-kin may give permission for the donation at the time of death.

eyeball ('ie,bawl) the ball or globe of the eye.

eyebrow ('ie,brow) 1. supercilium; the transverse elevation at the junction of the forehead and the upper eyelid. 2. supercilia; the hairs growing on this elevation.

eyelash ('ie,lash) cilium; one of the hairs growing on the edge of an eyelid.

eyelid ('ie,lid) either of two movable folds (upper and lower) protecting the anterior surface of the eyeball.

eyepiece ('ie,pees) the lens or system of lenses of a microscope (or telescope) nearest the user's eye, serving to further magnify the image produced by the objective.

eyestrain ('ie,strayn) eye fatigue caused by overuse of the eye or by an uncorrected defect in focus of the eye.

F

F chemical symbol, *fluorine*; Fahrenheit; field of vision; formula; French (catheter size).

F_1 first filial generation, a term used in genetics.

F_2 second filial generation, a term used in genetics.

f symbol, *femto-*.

fabella (fə'belə) pl. *fabellae* [L.] a sesamoid fibrocartilage in the gastrocnemius muscle.

Fabry's disease (syndrome) ('fabreez) a sphingolipidosis transmitted as an X-linked recessive trait, in which the glycolipid trihexosyl ceramide is deposited in various tissues, especially the kidneys; the deficient enzyme is α-galactosidase A. It is marked by purpuric skin lesions (angiokeratomas), central nervous system symptoms, and death due to progressive renal failure. Called also angiokeratoma corporis diffusum.

face (fays) 1. the anterior, or ventral, aspect of the head from the forehead to the chin, inclusive. 2. any presenting aspect or surface. adj. **facial.**

moon f. the peculiar rounded face seen in various conditions, such as in Cushing's syndrome, or after administration of adrenal corticosteroids.

facet ('fasit) a small, plane surface on a hard body, such as a bone.

facetectomy (,fasi'tektəmee) excision of the articular facet of a vertebra.

faci(o)- word element. [L.] *face.*

facial ('fayshəl) of or pertaining to the face.

f. nerve the seventh cranial nerve; its motor fibres supply the muscles of facial expression. These are a complex group of cutaneous muscles that move the eyebrows, skin of the forehead, corners of the mouth, and other parts of the face concerned with frowning, smiling, achieving a look of surprise, or any of the many and varied expressions of emotion. The sensory fibres of the facial nerve provide a sense of taste in the forward two-thirds of the tongue, and also supply the submaxillary, sublingual, and lacrimal glands for secretion.

Irritation of the facial nerve can produce a paralysis known as BELL'S PALSY. Usually the paralysis involves only one side of the face with a resulting distortion of facial expression, inability to close the mouth on one side, and difficulty in closing the eye on the affected side.

facies ('faysi,eez, 'fayshi-) pl. *facies* [L.] 1. the face. 2. a specific surface of a body structure, part, or organ. 3. the expression or appearance of the face.

adenoid f. the dull expression with open mouth, in children with adenoid growths.

f. hepatica a thin face with sunken eyeballs, sallow complexion, and yellow conjunctivae, characteristic of certain chronic liver disorders.

f. hippocratica a drawn, pinched, and livid appearance indicative of approaching death.

f. leontina a peculiar, deeply furrowed, lion-like appearance of the face seen in certain cases of advanced lepromatous leprosy.

Parkinson's f., parkinsonian f. a stolid masklike expression of the face, with infrequent blinking, which is pathognomonic of PARKINSON'S DISEASE.

facilitation (fə,sili'tayshən) hastening or assistance of a natural process; the increased excitability of a neuron after stimulation by a subthreshold presynaptic impulse. The resistance is diminished so that second application of the stimulus evokes the reaction more easily.

facilitative (fə'silitətiv) in pharmacology, denoting a reaction arising as an indirect result of drug action, as development of an infection after the normal microflora has been altered by an antibiotic.

faciobrachial (,fayshioh'brayki·əl, -'brak-) pertaining to the face and arm.

faciocervical (,fayshioh'sərvik'l, -sə'viek'l) pertaining to the face and neck.

faciolingual (,fayshioh'ling·gwəl) pertaining to the face and tongue.

facioplasty ('fayshioh,plastee) restorative or plastic surgery of the face.

facioplegia (,fayshioh'pleeji·ə) facial paralysis. adj. **facioplegic.**

facioscapulohumeral (,fayshioh,skapyuhloh-'hyoomə·rəl) pertaining to the face, scapula, and arm.

FACP Fellow of the American College of Physicians.

FACS Fellow of the American College of Surgeons.

factitial (fak'tishəl) artifically produced; produced unintentionally.

factitious (fak'tishəs) artificial; not natural.

factor ('faktə) an agent or element that contributes to the production of a result. **accelerator f.** factor V, one of the CLOTTING factors.

antihaemophilic f. AHF, factor VIII, one of the CLOTTING factors.

antihaemorrhagic f. vitamin K.

antinuclear f. (ANF) antinuclear antibody.

antirachitic f. vitamin D.

f. B a complement component (C3 proactivator) that participates in the alternate complement pathway.

C3 nephritic f. an IgG antibody which is found in the plasma of certain individuals with membranoproliferative glomerulonephritis associated with hypocomplementaemia; it is directed against the complex of C3b and factor B, which is an enzyme which splits C3 itself. The antibody stabilizes the complex against degradation so that the enzyme activity is preserved.

citrovorum f. folinic acid.

clotting f's, coagulation f's factors essential to normal blood clotting, whose absence, diminution, or excess may lead to abnormality of the clotting mechanism; at least 12 factors, commonly designated by Roman numerals (I to V and VII to XIII) have been described (factor VI is no longer considered to have a clotting function). PLATELET FACTORS, designated by Arabic numerals, also play a role in clotting (see also CLOTTING).

f. D a factor that, when activated, serves as a serine esterase in the alternate complement pathway.

extrinsic f. a haematopoietic vitamin that combines with intrinsic factor for absorption from the intestine and is needed for erythrocyte maturation; called also cyanocobalamin and vitamin B_{12}.

f. VIII inhibitory bypass activity (FEIBA) a concentrate of coagulation factors prepared from fresh human plasma which contains activated constituents which are capable of bypassing the blocking action of a factor VIII inhibitor. FEIBA is used to treat bleeding episodes in haemophiliacs who have developed a factor VIII antibody.

F f., fertility f. the plasmid that determines the mating type of conjugating bacteria, being present in the donor (male) bacterium and absent in the recipient (female).

fibrin stabilizing f. factor XIII, one of the CLOTTING factors.

Hageman f. factor XII, one of the CLOTTING factors.

intrinsic f. a glycoprotein secreted by the parietal cells of the gastric glands, necessary for the absorption of VITAMIN B_{12} (cyanocobalamin, extrinsic factor). Its absence results in pernicious anaemia.

LE f. an immunoglobulin (a 7S antibody) that reacts with nuclei, found in the serum in systemic lupus erythematosus and other conditions.

lymph node permeability f. (LNPF) a substance from normal lymph nodes which produces vascular permeability.

lymphocyte transforming f. (LTF) a lymphokine causing transformation and clonal expansion of nonsensitized lymphocytes.

osteoclast activating f. a lymphokine produced by lymphocytes which facilitates bone resorption.

platelet f's factors important in haemostasis that are contained in or attached to the platelets (see also PLATELET FACTORS).

platelet-activating f. (PAF) an immunologically produced substance which leads to clumping and degranulation of blood platelets.

R f. the bacterial plasmid (R plasmid) responsible for resistance to antibiotics; it is transmitted to other bacterial cells by conjugation, as well as to the progeny of any cell containing it.

releasing f's factors elaborated in one structure (as in the hypothalamus) that effect the release of hormones from another structure (as from the anterior pituitary gland), including corticotrophin releasing factor, melanocyte-stimulating hormone releasing factor, and prolactin inhibiting factor. Applied to substances of unknown chemical structure, while substances of established chemical identity are called *releasing hormones*.

resistance f. R f.

Rh f., Rhesus f. genetically determined antigens present on the surface of erythrocytes; incompatibility for these antigens between mother and offspring is responsible for HAEMOLYTIC disease of the newborn (see also RH FACTOR).

rheumatoid f. a protein, IgM immunoglobulin, usually detectable by serological tests, which is found in the serum of most patients with rheumatoid arthritis and in other related diseases. It also occurs after immunization of normal persons. Abbreviated RF.

Stuart f., Stuart–Prower f. factor X, one of the CLOTTING factors.

transfer f. (TF) a factor occurring in sensitized lymphocytes that has the capacity to transfer delayed hypersensitivity to a normal (nonreactive) individual.

facultative ('fakəltətiv) not obligatory; pertaining to or characterized by the ability to adjust to particular circumstances or to assume a particular role.

f. anaerobe a microorganism that can live and grow with or without molecular oxygen.

faculty ('fakəltee) 1. a normal power or function, especially of the mind. 2. the teaching staff of an institute of learning.

FAD flavin-adenine dinucleotide.

faecal ('feek'l) pertaining to or of the nature of faeces.

f. impaction accumulation of putty-like or hardened faeces in the rectum or sigmoid. The condition often occurs in patients with long-standing bowel problems and chronic constipation. It also may develop when barium is introduced into the intestinal tract and not completely removed.

Symptoms include painful defecation, feeling of fullness in the rectum, and constipation or a diarrhoeic stool. Rectal examination reveals a hard or putty-like mass. The condition can be prevented in most cases by adequate removal of barium after radiological studies, and by careful monitoring of the bowel movements of elderly patients with bowel problems.

Faecal impaction usually requires digital removal with a gloved finger to break up the mass. Prior to removal the patient is given an oil retention ENEMA to help soften the mass.

faecalith ('feekə,lith) an intestinal concretion formed around a centre of faecal material.

faecaloid ('feekə,loyd) resembling faeces.

faecaloma (,feekə'lohmə) a tumour-like accumulation of faeces in the rectum; stercoroma.

faecaluria (,feekə'lyooə·ri·ə) the presence of faecal matter in the urine.

faeces ('feeseez) [L.] plural of *faex;* body waste discharged from the intestine; called also stool, excreta, or excrement. The faeces are formed in the colon and pass down into the rectum by the process of peristalsis. When the rectum is sufficiently distended, nerve endings in its wall signal a need for evacuation, which is made possible by a voluntary relaxation of the sphincter muscles around the outer part of the anus.

The frequency of bowel movements varies according to the individual body make-up, type of intestine, eating habits, physical activity, and custom. Although one bowel movement a day is the average, a movement every 2 or 3 days may be considered normal. A balanced diet and an established routine can promote regular bowel movements.

CHARACTERISTICS. Normally the stool is soft and formed and brownish in colour. An abnormality in colour, odour, or consistency usually indicates a disorder of the intestinal tract or of the accessory organs of the digestive system. Black, tarry stools may indicate intestinal bleeding, especially in the upper portion of the tract. Some drugs, such as those containing iron or bismuth, can produce tarry stools. Bright red blood in the faeces can indicate a wide variety of disorders ranging from HAEMORRHOIDS to a malignancy of the rectum. Clay-coloured stools result from an absence or deficiency of BILE in the intestinal tract, and indicate obstruction of the biliary tract or decreased production of bile by the liver. Greenish-coloured faeces often accompany diarrhoea, especially in infants, and may be caused by growth of certain bacteria.

Bulky, fatty stools, having a foul odour, are characteristic of CYSTIC FIBROSIS. Other causes of fatty faeces include GALLBLADDER disease, pancreatic disorders, SPRUE, and excessive intake of fat in the diet. Faeces containing large amounts of mucus often occur in COLITIS and IRRITABLE BOWEL SYNDROME.

The stool of a newborn, full-term infant is called meconium. It is a dark greenish brown colour, smooth and semisolid in consistency.

DISINFECTION. In some types of communicable diseases it is necessary to decontaminate the faeces before they are flushed into the sewage system. Chlorinated lime, Lysol, or formalin may be used for this purpose. The contents of the bedpan used by the patient should be thoroughly covered with the disinfectant and allowed to stand for several hours. The contents are then disposed of in the sluice, and the bedpan is rinsed and sterilized, preferably with live steam or by autoclave.

OBSERVATIONS. Because the characteristics of the faeces can be of help in the diagnosis of various diseases, it is important to inspect the stool for colour, consistency, odour, and number of stools per day. Abnormalities should be noted on the patient's chart or reported to the doctor.

SPECIMENS. A sample of the faeces (stool specimen) may be required as a diagnostic aid. The specimen should be collected in a sterile bedpan and transferred into a sterile container, using a wooden spatula or tongue blade for this purpose. In order for certain types of intestinal parasites to be discovered in the faeces, the specimen must be fresh and kept warm until examined in the laboratory. Microorganisms that may be detected include the typhoid and paratyphoid bacilli, the anthrax bacilli, and *Entamoeba histolytica*, which causes AMOEBIC DYSENTERY.

Specimens of the faeces may be examined for occult (hidden) blood. This test is indicated when intestinal bleeding is suspected but the stools do not appear to contain blood when examined by gross inspection.

faeculent ('fekyuhlənt) 1. having dregs or sediment. 2. excrementitious.

Fahrenheit scale ('farən,hiet) a temperature scale with the ice point at 32 and the normal boiling point of water at 212 degrees (212 °F). For equivalents of Fahrenheit and Celsius temperatures, see Appendix 2.

Fahrenheit thermometer ('farən,hiet) a thermometer employing the Fahrenheit scale. The abbreviation 100 °F should be read 'one hundred degrees Fahrenheit'.

Fahr–Volhard disease (fah'fohlhaht) the malignant form of arteriolar nephrosclerosis.

failure ('faylyə) inability to perform or to function properly.

heart f. inability of the heart to maintain a circulation sufficient to meet the body's needs (see also HEART FAILURE).

kidney f., renal f. inability of the kidney to excrete metabolites at normal plasma levels under normal loading, or inability to retain electrolytes when intake is normal; in the acute form, marked by uraemia and usually by oliguria, with hyperkalaemia and pulmonary oedema.

respiratory f., ventilatory f. a life-threatening condition in which respiratory function is inadequate to maintain the body's needs for oxygen supply and carbon dioxide removal while at rest (see also RESPIRATORY FAILURE).

faint (faynt) temporary loss of consciousness due to generalized cerebral ischaemia; syncope. This may be due to a nervous reaction stemming from such causes as fear, hunger, pain, or any emotional or physical shock. Although fainting may be considered a very mild form of shock, it is not as serious and usually is not accompanied by the rapid, weak pulse and cold, clammy skin characteristic of true shock.

The person who is about to faint should be made to lie down with the legs somewhat elevated, and collar and clothing loosened. If this is not feasible, he should lower his head between his knees for about 5 minutes.

If a person has lost consciousness, he should be kept lying down with the feet and legs slightly elevated. Tight clothing should be loosened. Smelling salts (ammonium carbonate) or aromatic spirits of ammonia may be held under the patient's nose until he revives. Prolonged loss of consciousness indicates a condition more serious than simple fainting and should be treated by a doctor.

fainting ('faynting) see FAINT, SYNCOPE.

falcial ('falshəl) pertaining to a falx.

falciform ('falsi,fawm) sickle-shaped.

f. ligament a sickle-shaped sagittal fold of peritoneum that helps to attach the liver to the diaphragm and separates the right and left lobes of the liver.

falcular ('falkyuhlə) falciform.

fallopian tube (fə'lohpi·ən) uterine tube.

Fallot's tetralogy ('falohz te'traləjee) a combination of congenital cardiac defects, namely, pulmonary stenosis, ventricular septal defects, dextroposition of the aorta, so that it overrides the interventricular septum and receives venous as well as arterial blood, and right ventricular hypertrophy (see also TETRALOGY OF FALLOT).

fallout ('fawl,owt) the settling to the earth's surface of radioactive fission products from the atmosphere after a nuclear explosion.

false (fawls) not true.

f. pelvis greater pelvis; the portion of the pelvis between the brim of the true pelvis and the crest of the ilium which has no obstetrical significance.

f. joint pseudoarthrosis; a false joint formed between the fragments of a fractured bone which have failed to unite.

false-negative (,fawls'negətiv) 1. denoting a test result that wrongly excludes an individual from a diagnostic or other category. 2. an individual so excluded. 3. an instance of a false-negative result.

false-positive (ˌfawlsˈpozətiv) 1. denoting a test result that wrongly assigns a individual to a diagnostic or other category. 2. an individual so categorized. 3. an instance of a false-positive result.

falsification (ˌfawlsifiˈkayshən) a deliberate misstatement or misrepresentation.

retrospective f. unconscious distortion of past experiences to conform to present emotional needs.

falsifying (ˈfawlsiˌfie·ing) in psychology, signifying a form of facial deceit in which an individual pretends to experience a feeling not present, shows no feeling when aroused, or substitutes signs of one emotional reaction for those of another.

falx (falks) pl. *falces* [L.] a sickle-shaped structure.

f. cerebelli the fold of dura mater separating the cerebellar hemispheres.

f. cerebri a sickle-shaped fold of dura mater in the longitudinal fissure, which separates the two cerebral hemispheres.

familial (fəˈmili·əl) occurring in or affecting members of a family more than would be expected by chance.

family (ˈfamilee) 1. a group of people related by blood or marriage, especially a husband, wife, and their children. 2. a taxonomic category below an order and above a genus.

blended f. a family unit composed of a married couple and their offspring including some from previous marriages.

extended f. a nuclear family and their close relatives, such as the children's grandparents, aunts, and uncles.

extended nuclear f. a nuclear family who nevertheless make frequent social contacts with the extended family group despite geographical distance.

nuclear f. a married couple and their children by birth or adoption, who are living together and are more or less isolated from their extended family.

single-parent f. a lone parent and offspring living together as a family unit.

Fanconi's syndrome (disease) (fanˈkohneez) 1. a rare hereditary disorder, transmitted as an autosomal recessive trait, characterized by pancytopenia, hypoplasia of the bone marrow, and patchy brown discoloration of the skin due to the deposition of melanin, and associated with multiple congenital anomalies of the musculoskeletal and genitourinary systems. 2. a general term for a group of diseases marked by dysfunction of the proximal renal tubules, with generalized hyperaminoaciduria, renal glycosuria, hyperphosphaturia, and bicarbonate and water loss; the most common cause is cystinosis, but it is also associated with other genetic diseases and occurs in idiopathic and acquired forms.

Fannia (ˈfani·ə) a genus of flies whose larvae have caused both intestinal and urinary infestation in man.

fantasy (ˈfantəsee) an imagined sequence of events or mental images that serves to satisfy unconscious wishes or to express unconscious conflicts.

farad (ˈfarəd) the unit of electric capacity; capacity to hold 1 coulomb with a potential of 1 volt.

faradism (ˈfarəˌdizəm) electricity produced through induction by a rapidly alternating current.

faradization (ˌfarədieˈzayshən) treatment by the application of an induced or faradic current of electricity. The result is rapid and spasmodic contraction of the muscle to which it is applied.

Farber's disease (ˈfahbərz) a lysosomal storage disease and sphingolipidosis, transmitted as an autosomal recessive trait, due to deficiency of the enzyme ceramidase.

farcy (ˈfahsee) the more chronic and constitutional form of GLANDERS.

farinaceous (ˌfariˈnayshəs) starchy or containing starch. Refers to foods such as wheat, oats, barley and rice.

farmer's lung (ˌfahməz ˈlung) a disease occurring in those in contact with mouldy hay. It is thought to be due to a hypersensitivity, with widespread reaction in the lung tissue. It causes excessive breathlessness.

farsightedness (fahˈsietidnəs) a condition in which vision for distant objects is better than for near objects; called also HYPERMETROPIA or longsightedness.

fascia (ˈfashi·ə) pl. *fasciae* [L.] a sheet or band of fibrous tissue such as lies deep to the skin or invests muscles and various body organs. adj. **fascial.**

aponeurotic f. a dense, firm, fibrous membrane investing the trunk and limbs and giving off sheaths to the various muscles.

f. cribrosa the superficial fascia of the thigh covering the saphenous opening.

crural f. the investing fascia of the leg. **deep f.** aponeurotic fascia.

endothoracic f. that beneath the serous lining of the thoracic cavity.

extrapleural f. a prolongation of the endothoracic fascia sometimes found at the root of the neck, important as possibly modifying the auscultatory sounds at the apex of the lung.

f. lata the external investing fascia of the thigh.

Scarpa's f. the deep, membranous layer of the subcutaneous abdominal fascia.

superficial f. 1. a fascial sheet lying directly beneath the skin. 2. subcutaneous tissue.

thyrolaryngeal f. the fascia covering the thyroid gland and attached to the cricoid cartilage.

transverse f. that between the transversalis muscle and the peritoneum.

fascicle (ˈfasikˈl) a small bundle or cluster, especially of nerve or muscle fibres.

fascicular (fəˈsikyuhlə) clustered together; pertaining to or arranged in bundles or clusters; pertaining to a fascicle.

fasciculated (fəˈsikyuhˌlaytid) clustered together or occurring in bundles, or fasciculi.

fasciculation (fəˌsikyuhˈlayshən) 1. the formation of fasicles. 2. a small local involuntary muscular contraction visible under the skin, representing spontaneous discharge of a number of fibres innervated by a single motor nerve filament.

fasciculus (fəˈsikyuhləs) pl. *fasciculi* [L.] fascicle.

f. cuneatus of medulla oblongata the continuation into the medulla oblongata of the fasciculus cuneatus of the spinal cord.

f. cuneatus of spinal cord the lateral portion of the posterior funiculus of the spinal cord, composed of ascending fibres that end in the nucleus cuneatus. **f. gracilis of medulla oblongata** the continuation into the medulla oblongata of the fasciculus gracilis of the spinal cord.

f. gracilis of spinal cord the median portion of the posterior funiculus of the spinal cord, composed of ascending fibres that end in the nucleus gracilis.

fasciectomy (ˌfashiˈektəmee) excision of fascia.

fasciitis (ˌfasiˈietis) inflammation of a fascia.

necrotizing f. a gas-forming, fulminating, necrotic infection of the superficial and deep fascia, resulting in thrombosis of the subcutaneous vessels and gangrene of the underlying tissues. It is usually caused by multiple pathogens and is frequently associated with diabetes mellitus.

nodular f., proliferative f. a benign, reactive proliferation of fibroblasts in the subcutaneous tissues and commonly associated with the deep fascia.

pseudosarcomatous f. a benign soft tissue tumour occurring subcutaneously and sometimes arising from deep muscle and fascia.

fasciodesis (ˌfashi'odəsis) suture of a fascia to a skeletal attachment.

Fasciola (fə'seeələ) a genus of flukes.

F. hepatica the common liver fluke of herbivores, occasionally found in the human liver.

fascioliasis (ˌfasioh'lieəsis) infection with *Fasciola.*

fasciolopsiasis (ˌfasiohlop'sieəsis) infection with *Fasciolopsis.*

Fasciolopsis (ˌfasioh'lopsis) a genus of trematodes.

F. buski the largest of the intestinal flukes, found in the small intestines of human beings and pigs in the Far East. Enteritis and systemic toxic effects may result.

fascioplasty ('fashioh,plastee) plastic repair of a fascia.

fasciorrhaphy (ˌfashi'o·rəfee) repair of a lacerated fascia.

fasciotomy (ˌfashi'otəmee) incision of a fascia.

fast (fahst) 1. immovable, or unchangeable; resistant to the action of a specific drug, stain, or destaining agent. 2. abstention from food.

fastigium (fas'tiji·əm) [L.] 1. the highest point in the roof of the fourth ventricle of the brain. 2. the acme, or highest point. adj. **fastigial.**

fat (fat) 1. the adipose or fatty tissue of the body. 2. neutral fat; a triglyceride (or triacylglycerol), which is an ester of fatty acids and glycerol (a trihydric alcohol). Each fat molecule contains one glycerol residue connected by ester linkages to three fatty acid residues, which may be the same or different. The fatty acids may have no double bonds in the carbon chain (saturated fatty acids), one double bond (monounsaturated), or two or more double bonds (polyunsaturated).

The one essential fatty acid is linoleic acid, the absence of which will create a specific deficiency disease. It cannot be synthesized in the body, but must be obtained from the diet. Two other important fatty acids that can be synthesized in the body are linolenic acid and arachidonic acid.

About 95 per cent of the fat eaten is absorbed and utilized or stored in the body; the remainder is excreted as faecal fat. In addition to the intake of dietary fat, the body produces fat from carbohydrates and some from protein foods. Stored fat accounts for about 15 per cent of the average person's body weight.

Chemical digestion of fat is accomplished in the small intestine through the actions of agents from the gallbladder, liver, and pancreas.

The products of fat digestion are absorbed through the intestinal walls and distributed by the blood to various storage regions in the body. Some fat is used for tissue building but most of it is stored for future energy needs. These reserves are continuously being converted into carbohydrates for the body's work, and are continuously being replaced by new reserves.

When the intake of food exceeds the energy needs of the body, the food stored as fat accumulates in layers under the skin. Such fat layers provide insulation for the body against low temperatures. The insulating effect is due to the fact that there are few blood vessels in fatty tissue, and hence the heat of circulating blood is lost slowly from the body. Body fat also gives support to the viscera.

SATURATED AND UNSATURATED FATS. All of the common unsaturated fatty acids are liquid at room temperature. Through the process of hydrogenation, hydrogen can be incorporated into certain unsaturated fatty acids so that they are converted into solid fats for cooking purposes. Margarine is an example of the hydrogenation of unsaturated fatty acids into a solid substance.

Research has indicated that the unsaturated fats are less likely than saturated fats to be used by the body in ways injurious to health. The theory supporting this claim is that the body's normal supply of cholesterol and its concentration in serum are increased by saturated fats, which are found mainly in animal fats, such as meat, butter, and eggs. The unsaturated fats, found in large quantities in vegetable oils such as corn oil and sunflower oil, are thought to help reduce the amount of cholesterol in the blood. Some researchers hold that eating foods rich in cholesterol itself, such as the animal fats, will also increase the amount of cholesterol in the blood.

Although the body's own normal production of cholesterol is essential to the functioning of body systems, it is known that the formation of fatty deposits in the arteries, a condition called ATHEROSCLEROSIS, can impede the flow of blood and cause damage to the coronary arteries of the heart and other arteries. Cholesterol is recognized as an important factor in these conditions, although its exact contribution is still not clear (see also CHOLESTEROL).

fatal ('fayt'l) causing death; deadly; mortal; lethal.

fatigability (ˌfatigə'bilitee) easy susceptibility to fatigue.

fatigue (fə'teeg) a state of increased discomfort and decreased efficiency resulting from prolonged exertion; a generalized feeling of tiredness or exhaustion; loss of power or capacity to respond to stimulation. Fatigue is a normal reaction to intense physical exertion, emotional strain, or lack of rest. It is the body's way of saying that one ought to slow down, relax, and get more rest and sleep. Fatigue that is not relieved by rest may have a more serious origin. It may be a symptom of generally poor physical condition, of specific disease, or of severe emotional stress.

Poor living habits, including improper diet, lack of sleep, and insufficient fresh air and exercise, are a common cause of fatigue. Often, however, fatigue signals an oncoming illness. Fatigue is associated with a wide variety of diseases, including tuberculosis, anaemia, thyroid disorders, heart ailments, diabetes mellitus, and cancer.

Sometimes fatigue is psychological in origin. Tiredness and a loss of interest in one's work may actually result from boredom with the daily routine. If one is certain that there is nothing wrong physically, steps should be taken to vary the daily round, to seek new and more active ways to spend leisure time, perhaps to revive old interests that have been neglected.

Sometimes the demands made upon a person's nervous system are excessive and nervous exhaustion, or nervous prostration, occurs. This state of abnormal fatigue is usually brought on by the inability to cope emotionally with long periods of trouble. Insomnia combines with deep discouragement, and the person is mentally and physically exhausted. The resulting symptoms are sometimes grouped together under the descriptive term, neurasthenia, or nerve weakness. They include poor memory, irritability, aches and pains, lack of appetite, heart palpitations, and dizziness. Occasionally because of his emotional state, the person has difficulty with a particular organ and may suffer from an imaginary ailment. A cardiac neurosis (Da Costa's syndrome), in which the individual is convinced he has heart disease, is fairly common.

combat f. a gross stress reaction brought on by extended, dangerous military action. A somewhat misleading term as similar neurotic responses to stress have been reported in peacetime among civilians (civilian catastrophe reaction).

fatty ('fatee) pertaining to or characterized by fat.
f. acid an organic compound of carbon, hydrogen, and oxygen that combines with glycerol to form fat. All fats are esters of fatty acids and glycerol, the fatty acids accounting for 90 per cent of the molecule of most natural fats. A fatty acid consists of a long chain of carbon atoms with a carboxylic acid group at one end. Saturated fatty acids have no double bonds in the carbon chain. They are solid at room temperature and are the components of the common animal fats, such as butter and lard. Unsaturated fatty acids contain one or more double bonds. The unsaturated fatty acids are liquid at room temperature and are found in oils such as olive oil and linseed oil. Polyunsaturated fatty acids have two or more double bonds.

From a nutritional standpoint, some fatty acids are essential for proper growth and metabolism, and a deficiency of these fatty acids can lead to eczema and other skin disorders. Such deficiencies are rare, however, because the fatty acids occur in abundance in many foods, such as butter, whole milk, egg yolk, nuts, and vegetables.
f. degeneration deposit of fat globules in a tissue.
fauces ('fawseez) the passage from the mouth to the pharynx. adj. **faucial**.
faucitis (faw'sietis) inflammation of the fauces.
faveolate (fə'veeə,layt) honeycombed; alveolate.
faveolus (fə'veeələs) foveola.
favism ('fayvizəm) an acute haemolytic anaemia caused by ingestion of fava beans or inhalation of the pollen of the plant, usually occurring in certain individuals as a result of a genetic abnormality with a deficiency in an enzyme, glucose-6-phosphate dehydrogenase, in the erythrocytes. Called also fabism.
favus ('fayvəs) a type of tinea capitis, with formation of crusts of fungal mycelia and epithelial debris producing prominent honeycomb-like masses; due to *Trichophyton schoenleini*.
FCSP Fellow of the Chartered Society of Physiotherapists.
FDA Food and Drug Administration, Washington DC, USA.
FDS Fellow in Dental Surgery.
Fe chemical symbol, *iron* (L. *ferrum*).
fe- for words beginning thus, see also those beginning *fae-*.
fear (fiə) a normal emotional response, in contrast to anxiety and phobia, to consciously recognized external sources of danger; it is manifested by alarm, apprehension, or disquiet.
febricide ('febri,sied) lowering bodily temperature; an agent that so acts.
febrifacient (,febri'fayshənt) producing fever.
febrifuge ('febri,fyooj) an agent that reduces body temperature in fever; antipyretic.
febrile ('feebriel, 'feb-) pertaining to fever; feverish.
fecundation (,fekən'dayshən, fee-) fertilization; impregnation.
fecundity (fi'kunditee) the ability to produce offspring frequently and in large numbers. In demography, the physiological ability to reproduce, as opposed to fertility.
feeblemindedness (,feeb'l'miendidnəs) former name for MENTAL HANDICAP.
feedback ('feed,bak) the return of some of the output of a system as input so as to exert some control in the process.

Feedback controls are a type of self-regulating mechanism by which certain activities are sustained within prescribed ranges. For example, the serum concentration of oxygen is affected in part by the rate and depth of respirations and is, therefore, an output of the respiratory system. If the concentration of oxygen drops below normal, this information is transmitted as *input* to the respiratory control centre. The control centre is thereby stimulated to increase the rate of respirations in order to return the oxygen concentration in the blood to within normal range.

This series of events is an example of *negative feedback*, which always causes the controller to respond in a manner that opposes a deviation from the normal level. It is, therefore, a corrective action that returns a factor within the system to a normal range. *Positive feedback* tends to increase a deviation from normal. In other words, positive feedback reinforces and accelerates either an excess or deficit of a factor within the system. See also HOMEOSTASIS.
feedforward (,feed'faw·wəd) the anticipatory effect that one intermediate in a metabolic or endocrine control system exerts on another intermediate further along in the pathway; such effect may be positive or negative.
feeding ('feeding) the taking or giving of food.
artificial f. feeding of a baby with food other than mother's milk.
breast f. the feeding of an infant at the breast (see also BREAST FEEDING).
forced f. administration of food by force to those who cannot or will not receive it.
intravenous f. administration of nutrient fluids through a vein (see also INTRAVENOUS INFUSION).
tube f. feeding of liquids and semisolid foods through a nasogastric tube (see also TUBE FEEDING).
Feer's disease ('fay·əz) erythroedema polyneuropathy.
FEF forced expiratory flow rate.
Fehling's solution ('faylingz) (1) 34.66 g cupric sulphate in water to make 500 ml; (2) 173 g crystallized potassium and sodium tartrate and 50 g sodium hydroxide in water to make 500 ml; mix equal volumes of (1) and (2) at time of use. Used in Fehling's test for dextrose in the urine.
FEIBA factor VIII inhibitory bypassing activity.
Feldene ('feldeen) trademark for the nonsteroidal anti-inflammatory drug piroxicam.
fellatio (fə'layshioh) oral stimulation or manipulation of the penis.
felon ('felən) a purulent infection involving the pulp of the distal phalanx of a finger.
feltwork ('felt,wərk) a complex of closely interwoven fibres, as of nerve fibres.
Felty's syndrome ('feltiz) the triad of rheumatoid arthritis, splenomegaly and leukopenia. Often associated with anaemia, lymphadenopathy and vasculitic cutaneous ulceration.
female ('feemayl) 1. an individual of the sex that produces ova or bears young. 2. feminine.
feminine ('femənin) pertaining to the female sex, or having qualities normally characteristic of the female.
feminism ('femi,nizəm) the appearance or existence of female secondary sexual characteristics in the male.
feminization ('feminie'zayshən) 1. the normal induction or development of female sexual characteristics. 2. the induction or development of female secondary sexual characteristics in the male.
testicular f. a condition in which the subject is phenotypically female, but lacks nuclear sex chromatin and is of XY chromosomal sex.
femoral ('femə·rəl) pertaining to the femur or to the thigh.
f. artery the chief artery of the thigh.
f. canal the medial part of the femoral sheath lateral to the base of the lacunar ligament.
f. nerve the largest branch of the lumbar plexus.

f. triangle the area formed superiorly by the inguinal ligament, laterally by the sartorius muscle, and medially by the adductor longus muscle. Called also *Scarpa's triangle.*

f. vein the chief vein of the thigh.

femorocele ('femə·roh,seel) femoral hernia.

femorotibial (,femə·roh'tibi·əl) pertaining to the femur and tibia.

femto- ('femtoh) word element. [Scand.] *fifteen;* used in naming units of measurement to indicate 10^{-15} of the unit designated by the root with which it is combined; symbol f.

femur ('feemə) pl. *femora* [L.] 1. the thigh bone, extending from the pelvis to the knee; the longest and strongest bone in the body. Its proximal end articulates with the acetabulum, a cup-like cavity in the pelvic girdle. The greater and lesser trochanters are the two processes (prominences) at the proximal end of the femur. 2. the thigh.

fenbufen (fen'byoofen) a nonsteroidal anti-inflammatory drug (NSAID) which acts as a pro-drug. It is associated with a lower incidence of gastrointestinal haemorrhage but a higher incidence of skin rashes than other NSAIDs.

fenestra (fə'nestrə) pl. *fenestrae* [L.] a window-like opening.

f. cochleae a round opening in the inner wall of the middle ear covered by the secondary tympanic membrane; called also *round window.*

f. vestibuli an oval opening in the inner wall of the middle ear, which is closed by the stapes; called also *oval window.*

fenestrate ('feni,strayt) to pierce with one or more openings.

fenestration (,feni'strayshən) 1. the act of perforating or the condition of being perforated. 2. the surgical creation of a new opening in the labyrinth of the ear for the restoration of hearing in otosclerosis.

aortopulmonary f. aortic septal defect.

fenfluramine (fen'floo·rə,meen) an anorectic that seems to depress rather than stimulate the central nervous system, as do the amphetamines; used as the hydrochloride salt.

fenoprofen (,feenoh'prohfən) a nonsteroidal anti-inflammatory drug used for the treatment of rheumatoid arthritis and osteoarthritis.

Fenopron ('fenohpron) trademark for a preparation of fenoprofen calcium; a nonsteroidal anti-inflammatory drug.

fenoterol (fe'notərol) a β^2-adrenergic agonist which is used like salbutamol. It is available as an inhaler and a solution for use in a nebulizer.

fentanyl ('fentə,nil) a piperidine derivative; the citrate salt is used as a narcotic analgesic, and in combination with droperidol as a neuroleptanalgesic. It is widely used as an analgesic during anaesthesia.

Fentazin ('fentəzin) trademark for preparations of perphenazine, a tranquillizer and antiemetic.

Fenwick ('fenik) Ethel Gordon, 1857–1947. (Mrs. Bedford Fenwick, née Manson.) Pioneer of nursing reform, and leader of the movement for the registration of nurses.

Educated privately, the daughter of a doctor, she trained as a lady probationer at the Children's Hospital, Nottingham, spending a further year at Manchester Royal Infirmary. In 1879 she was appointed as a sister at the London Hospital. In 1881 (aged 24 years) she became matron of St. Bartholomew's Hospital, London. Miss Manson left St. Bartholomew's to marry Dr. Bedford Fenwick in 1887.

In 1887, Mrs. Bedford Fenwick formed a group of nurses, the British Nurses' Association, whose aim was the control of nursing by the statutory registration of nurses.

In 1889, a mass meeting of nurses led by Mrs. Bedford Fenwick was held at Mansion House, London, to call for an official register of nurses. Florence Nightingale was opposed to the concept of the registration of nurses and said nursing 'cannot be tested by public examination, though it may be tested by current supervision'.

In 1893, Mrs. Bedford Fenwick acquired the magazine 'The Nursing Record', later to become the British Journal of Nursing, of which she remained editor for nearly fifty years.

In 1894, Mrs. Bedford Fenwick founded the Matrons' Council of Great Britain and Ireland which was also pledged to the registration of nurses. In 1899, the Matrons' Council founded the International Council of Nurses, with the support of the International Council of Women. In 1901, the first Congress was held in Buffalo, USA, and Mrs. Bedford Fenwick was elected the first President.

Following the First World War, universal suffrage was agreed and women received 'The Vote' for the first time. The Nurses' Bill received Royal Assent in December 1919, and the General Nursing Council was founded with the duty of establishing and maintaining a Register of Nurses.

Mrs. Bedford Fenwick was entered as State Registered Nurse: Number 1 on the Register.

After Registration of nurses was achieved, Mrs. Bedford Fenwick continued to take an active interest in nursing issues, holding honorary posts in various professional organizations for many years. She died 13th. March 1947.

Fergon ('fərgon) trademark for preparations of ferrous gluconate, an iron preparation.

ferment (fə'ment) 1. to undergo fermentation. 2. any substance that causes fermentation.

fermentation (,fərmen'tayshən) the anaerobic enzymatic conversion of organic compounds, especially carbohydrates, to simpler compounds, especially to lactic acid or ethyl alcohol, producing energy in the form of ATP.

fermium ('fərmi·əm) a chemical element, atomic number 100, atomic weight 253, symbol Fm. See table of elements in Appendix 2.

Fern test (fərn) cervical cytology undertaken to determine the amount of oestrogen in cervical mucus. When oestrogen is adequate the dried cervical mucus has a fern-like appearance on low power microscopy.

ferning ('fərning) the appearance of a fernlike pattern in a dried specimen of cervical mucus, an indication of the presence of oestrogen.

-ferous word element. [L.] *bearing, producing.*

ferredoxin (,ferə'doksin) a nonhaem iron-containing protein having a very low redox potential; the ferredoxins participate in electron transport in photosynthesis, nitrogen fixation, and various other biological processes.

ferric ('ferik) containing iron in its plus-three oxidation state, Fe(III) (sometimes designated Fe^{3+}).

f. chloride $FeCl_3$, used as a reagent and topically as an astringent and antiseptic.

ferritin ('feritin) the iron–apoferritin complex, one of the forms in which iron is stored in the body.

Ferrograd ('ferəgrad) trademark for preparations of ferrous sulphate, an iron preparation.

ferrokinetics (,ferohki'netiks) the turnover or rate of change of iron in the body.

ferroprotein (,feroh'prohteen) a protein combined with an iron-containing radical; ferroproteins are respiratory carriers.

ferrous ('ferəs) containing iron in its plus-two oxidation state, Fe(II) (sometimes designated Fe^{2+}).

f. fumarate the anhydrous salt of a combination of ferrous iron and fumaric acid; used as a haematinic.

f. gluconate a haematinic that is less irritating to the gastrointestinal tract than other haematinics, and generally used as a substitute when ferrous sulphate cannot be tolerated.

f. sulphate the most widely used haematinic for the treatment of iron deficiency anaemia. It is believed to be less irritating than equivalent amounts of ferric salts and is more effective.

All iron preparations should be administered after meals, never on an empty stomach. The patient should be warned that the drugs cause stools to turn dark green or black. Overdosage may cause severe systemic reactions.

ferrule ('ferool, -rəl) a cap made of rubber or a synthetic material used on the end of walking sticks, frames and crutches to prevent slipping.

ferrum ('ferəm) [L.] *iron* (symbol Fe).

fertile period ('fərtiel) 1. the nine days surrounding ovulation when fertilization of the ovum is theoretically possible. It is usually taken to be the five days before, the day of, and the three days following ovulation, which is assessed over a period of months by recording the basal temperature. See also rhythm method of CONTRACEPTION. 2. that period of a woman's life during which she has potential for childbearing. For statistical purposes it is usually taken to be the period between the ages of 15 and 45.

fertility (fər'tilətee) the capacity to conceive and produce viable offspring. See INFERTILITY. adj. **fertile**.

fertilization (ˌfərtilie'zayshən) in human reproduction, the process by which the male's sperm unites with the female's ovum. By this event, also called conception, a new life is created and the sex and other biological traits of the new individual are determined. These traits are determined by the combined genes and chromosomes that exist in the sperm and ovum.

After injection into the vagina, the sperm cells—millions of them—make use of their whiplike tails to swim through the cervix toward the uterus. Most are destroyed along the way by secretions in the vagina, but some reach the uterus and a few may enter the UTERINE TUBES. A very small number may survive as long as 48 hours. If during this period only one sperm succeeds in entering a uterine tube and meeting there an ovum ready to be fertilized, conception can occur. This event is possible only during a period of about 4 days of the month. After the sperm lodges in the ovum, the tail disappears, but the head unites with the ovum to form the zygote. See also REPRODUCTION.

in vitro f. (IVF) artificial fertilization of the ovum in laboratory conditions. The timing and conditions for implantation into a uterus have to be perfect if successful pregnancy is to ensue.

in vivo f. that which takes place by artificial means in the living situation, i.e., within the mother's uterus. The ovum is retrieved from the ovary and placed on the endometrium when it is capable of supporting implantation. Spermatozoa are injected to achieve fertilization.

fervescence (fər'vesəns) increase of fever or body temperature.

fester ('festə) to suppurate superficially.

festinant ('festinənt) accelerating.

festination (ˌfesti'nayshən) an involuntary tendency to take short accelerating steps in walking.

fetal ('feet'l) of or pertaining to a fetus or to the period of its development.

f. alcohol syndrome (FAS) a constellation of physical and mental abnormalities due to maternal alcohol intake during pregnancy. Abnormalities may include microcephaly, growth deficiencies, mental handicap, hyperactivity, heart murmurs and skeletal malformation.

The exact amount of alcohol consumption that will produce fetal damage is unknown, but the periods of gestation during which the alcohol is most likely to result in fetal damage are three to four-and-a-half months after conception and during the last trimester.

f. assessment determination of the well-being of the fetus. Assessment techniques and procedures include: (1) medical and family histories and physical examination of the mother, (2) ULTRASONOGRAPHY, (3) assessment of fetal activity using the Cardiff kick chart, (4) chemical assessment of placental function, (5) assays of amniotic fluid obtained by AMNIOCENTESIS, and (6) electronic and ultrasonic fetal heart rate monitoring.

Extensive and thorough assessment of the health status of the fetus is indicated when maternal characteristics, obstetrical complications, and familial and genetic factors place the fetus at risk.

ULTRASONOGRAPHY is a noninvasive technique helpful in diagnosing unusual fetal presentations, placenta praevia, multiple pregnancy and fetal abnormalities such as hydrocephalus and hydronephrosis. It also can be used to trace fetal growth by periodic measurement of the biparietal diameter of the head of the fetus.

The Cardiff kick chart is a new simple method by which the mother plays an important part in checking the health of her own baby. She is required to count the number of movements made by her baby during the day. When 10 kicks have been felt, the time is noted on the chart. If less than 10 kicks are recorded in any 12 hour daytime period on two consecutive occasions the mother is advised to contact her obstetrician immediately. If no movements are felt in any day the mother is advised to contact the hospital at once. The value of this simple test is that it can highlight the potential case of fetal distress and alert medical attention before it is too late.

Chemical assessment of the nutritive and respiratory functions of the placenta can be accomplished by determining the amount of the hormone oestriol in the maternal blood or urine. Throughout gestation a normally functioning placenta produces increasing amounts of oestriol, the precursors for the production of which are provided by the fetal adrenal glands. Thus, a normal oestriol value in maternal blood or urine indicates that both the placenta and the fetus are healthy. Some centres have now stopped using these techniques because they are difficult, time-consuming, costly, and less accurate than ultrasound where this is readily available.

Amniotic fluid assay is most often done to establish the diagnosis of a genetic disorder, to monitor the Rh-sensitized fetus, or to determine fetal lung maturity. Cells floating in the amniotic fluid sample can be examined to detect genetic disorders caused by chromosomal abnormalities and to detect certain metabolic aberrations. Neural tube defects such as spina bifida and anencephaly are detected by analysing the amniotic fluid for alpha-fetoprotein (AFP). When a neural tube defect is present the amount of AFP can be increased as much as eight times the normal value.

The amniotic fluid also can be assayed for bilirubin, an indicator of the severity of Rh-incompatibility between maternal and fetal blood. Fetal lung maturity can be assessed by evaluating the presence of pulmonary surfactant, a phospholipid protein, in the amniotic fluid. In normal fetal development production of surfactant, essential to lung expansion and adequate

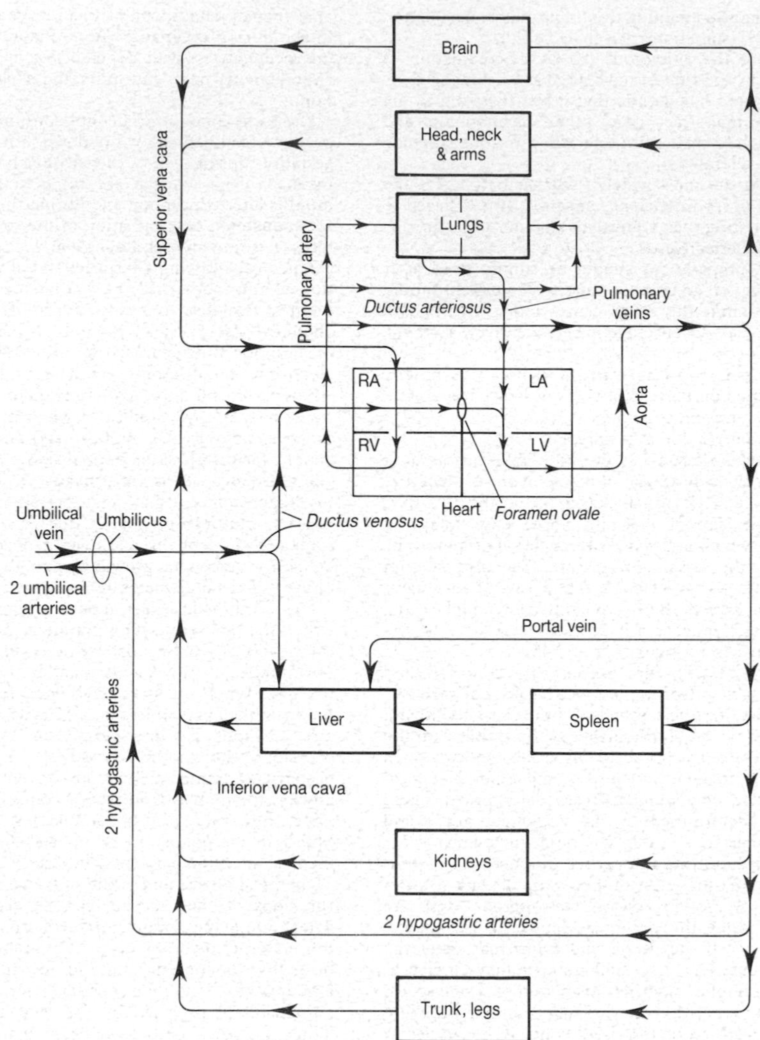

Diagrammatic representation of the pattern of fetal blood flow. The italicized headings indicate the 4 adaptations from adult circulation

ventilation after birth, begins at about the 22nd week of gestation and is not present in sufficient quantities until 35 to 36 weeks. Two principal constituents of the surfactant, lecithin (L) and sphingomyelin (S), can be evaluated by measuring the L/S ratio in a sample of amniotic fluid. In general, a ratio greater than 2:1 indicates that the fetal lungs are mature and the newborn infant is not likely to develop RESPIRATORY DISTRESS SYNDROME of the newborn.

Fetal monitoring using either ultrasound or direct electronic monitoring equipment to measure fetal heart rate and uterine contractions is discussed under FETAL MONITORING.

f. circulation the circulation of blood through the body of the fetus and to and from the placenta through the umbilical cord. Oxygenated blood from the placenta is carried to the embryo by the umbilical vein. The blood from the embryo is returned to the placenta by two umbilical arteries. Oxygenation of the fetal blood and disposal of its waste products is carried on through the placenta. When the lungs begin to function at birth some of the fetal vessels, such as the ductus arteriosus, and the fetal passages, such as the foramen ovale, begin to fall into disuse. This is a gradual process of fibrosis that takes place in the period after birth.

f. monitoring the continuous, simultaneous recording of uterine contractions (UCs) and fetal heart rate (FHR) during pregnancy or labour so that potential problems related to fetal hypoxia can be detected and corrected in order to prevent perinatal morbidity and death.

NONINVASIVE (INDIRECT) MONITORING. The fetal heart

rate is measured by ultrasonography or phonocardiotocography using an external transducer placed on the mother's abdomen over the fetal heart. A tocodynameter placed on the fundus records the amplitude and frequency of uterine contractions. Both recordings are displayed on a screen and a permanent record kept on graph paper. The quality of recording is affected by the position of the fetus, and the restlessness and relative obesity of the mother. However because the membranes remain intact it is suitable for use in pregnancy or early labour. Whenever a fetus is thought to be at risk a fetal heart trace may be performed and repeated at regular intervals, sometimes daily, as often as needed. In pregnancy the trace is said to be reactive if, in the absence of uterine contractions, the fetal heart responds to fetal movement identified by the mother. There should be a minimum of 5 beats in the base line variability, heart rate between 120 and 160 beats per minute and no abnormal accelerations or decelerations.

Ultrasonic fetal heart detectors using a Doppler effect may be used to monitor the fetal heart in isolation. Useful in early pregnancy or if fetal heart muffled with aural stethoscope. In some centres an oxytocin challenge or fetal stress test is preferred to the nonstress cardiotocograph monitoring described above. It aims to initiate the interuterine conditions produced by labour by inducing uterine contractions with intravenous Syntocinon 0.5 unit in 500 ml of 5% dextrose solution. The fetal response determines the management of labour.

INVASIVE (INTERNAL) MONITORING. An ECG electrode is attached to the fetal scalp by a spiral pin or clip once the cervix has dilated to 1 cm and the membranes have ruptured. An open-ended Teflon catheter filled with fluid is introduced into the maternal cervix through which changes in the pressure of the amniotic fluid due to maternal contractions are transmitted to a pressure transducer, which converts the signals on to the visual display unit (VDU) and cardiotocograph. The fetal heart is monitored by means of the electrode attached to the fetal scalp. The resulting ECG is transmitted audibly if required, and displayed on the VDU and graph. In addition to the fetal heart rate and base line variability, fetal condition is assessed by the presence of type 1 and type 2 dips. A type 1 dip, sometimes called an early deceleration, *accompanies* a uterine contraction, the fetal heart rate slowing by approximately 30 beats. It is not serious, but should not be ignored. It is thought to be caused by pressure on the fetal head by the bony pelvis or cervix. It may precede type 2 dips. These are serious and occur when there is a late deceleration of the fetal heart rate, when the heart rate slows by 40 or 50 beats at the end of and following a contraction. These are associated with fetal hypoxia and require urgent intervention if the fetus is to be born alive. The greater the time lapse between the height of the mother's contraction and the lowest point of the fetal deceleration, the more serious the sign.

f. telemetry a portable battery-operated transmitter may be carried by the mother who wishes to be ambulant in labour. The fetal scalp electrode transmits the fetal ECG through a radiotransmitter to the cardiotocometer where it is recorded on the cardiotocograph.

fetalization (ˌfeetəlie'zayshən) retention in the adult of characters that at an earlier stage of evolution were only infantile and were rapidly lost as the organism attained maturity.

fetation (fee'tayshən) 1. development of the fetus. 2. pregnancy.

FETC Further Education Teaching Certificate.

fetid ('fetid, 'fee-) having a rank, disagreeable smell.

fetish ('fetish) an object symbolically endowed with special meaning; e.g., an object or body part with special erotic interest.

fetography (fee'togrəfee) radiography of the fetus in utero.

fetoplacental (ˌfeetohplə'sent'l) pertaining to the fetus and placenta.

α-fetoprotein (ˌalfəˌfeetoh'prohteen) alpha-fetoprotein.

fetor ('feetə, -tor) stench or offensive odour.

hepatic f., f. hepaticus the peculiar odour of the breath characteristic of hepatic disease.

f. oris halitosis.

fetoscope ('feetəˌskohp) an endoscope for viewing the fetus in utero.

fetoscopy (fee'toskəpee) viewing of the fetus in utero by means of the fetoscope. See also AMNIOSCOPY. adj. **fetoscopic**.

fetus ('feetəs) [L.] the developing young in the uterus, specifically the unborn offspring in the postembryonic (see also EMBRYO) period, in man from eight weeks after fertilization until birth. adj. **fetal**.

calcified f. lithopedion; a fetus that has become calcified.

f. in fetu a small, imperfect fetus, incapable of independent life, contained within the body of another fetus.

harlequin f. EXFOLIATION.

mummified f. a dried-up and shrivelled fetus.

f. papyraceus a fetus flattened by being pressed against the uterine wall by a living twin.

parasitic f. an incomplete minor fetus attached to a larger, more completely developed fetus, or autosite.

FEV forced expiratory volume.

fever ('feevə) 1. an abnormally high body temperature; pyrexia. 2. any disease characterized by marked increase of body temperature.

Normal body temperature when the body is at rest is 36.8 °C (98.4 °F). This is an average or mean body temperature that varies from person to person and from hour to hour in an individual. The route by which a body temperature is measured affects the reading. The normal *oral* temperature ranges from 36 to 37.0 °C (96.8 to 98.6 °F). If the temperature is measured *rectally*, the norm would be 0.5 °C (1 °F) higher. An *axillary* temperature would be 0.5 °C (1 °F) lower. Because of these differences, the number should always be followed by the route by which the temperature was taken when the reading is recorded.

Factors that can cause a temporary elevation in body temperature include age, physical activity, emotional stress, and ovulation. If a person has a consistently elevated temperature, fever is said to exist. A *low-grade* fever is marked by temperatures between 37.0 and 38.2 °C (98.6 and 101 °F) when taken orally. A *high-grade* fever is present when the oral temperature is above 38.2 °C (101 °F).

The regulation of body temperature is under the control of the HYPOTHALAMUS. *Thermolysis*, or dissipation of body heat, is regulated by the anterior hypothalamus in conjunction with the parasympathetic nervous system. The overall effect of heat loss is accomplished by vasodilation of the peripheral blood vessels, increased sweating, and decreased metabolic and muscular activities. The production and conservation of body heat, or *thermogenesis*, is regulated by the posterior hypothalamus in conjunction with the sympathetic nervous system. The mechanisms by which body heat is produced and conserved are in opposition to those that increase heat loss; that is, by constriction of cutaneous blood vessels, decreased sweat gland activity, and increased metabolic and muscular activities.

Fever develops when there is some disturbance in the homeostatic mechanisms by which the hypothalamus maintains a balance between heat production and heat loss. Although dehydration, cerebral haemorrhage, thyroxine, and certain other drugs can cause an elevated body temperature or hyperthermia, fever, in the precise sense of the term, occurs as a result of inflammation or infection, or both. During the infectious and inflammatory processes certain substances called *pyrogens* are produced within the body. These *endogenous* pyrogens are the result of inflammatory reactions, such as those that occur in tissue damage, cell necrosis, rejection of transplanted tissues, malignancy, and antigen antibody reactions. *Exogenous* pyrogens are introduced into the body when it is invaded by bacteria, viruses, fungi, and other kinds of infectious organisms.

Both endogenous and exogenous pyrogens act directly on the hypothalamus, affecting its thermostatic functions by 'resetting' it to a higher temperature. When this happens, all of the physiological activities concerned with heat production and conservation operate to maintain body temperature at a higher level. The symptoms of chill and shivering are the result of increased muscular activity, which is an attempt by the body to raise its temperature to the higher setting. This increased muscular activity is accompanied by an elevation of the metabolic rate, which in turn increases the demand for nutrients and oxygen. Outward signs of these internal activities include a higher pulse rate, increased respirations, and thirst caused by the loss of extracellular water via the lungs and by sweating.

Once the body temperature reaches the setpoint of the hypothalamic thermostat, the mechanisms of heat production and heat loss keep it at a fairly constant level and the fever persists. This is sometimes called the *second stage of fever*. If it continues, fluid and electrolyte losses become more severe and there is evidence of cellular dehydration. During this stage DELIRIUM in older persons and CONVULSIONS in infants and children can occur. Febrile convulsions in children are believed to be closely related to cerebral damage that becomes evident as afebrile convulsions later in life.

Prolonged fever eventually brings about tissue destruction owing to the catabolism of body proteins. Because of this the patient experiences muscle aches and weakness, malaise, and the excretion of albumin in the urine. Anorexia also is present. If the body does not receive a sufficient supply of energy from dietary intake to meet its metabolic needs, it catabolizes its own fat. The patient then rapidly loses weight and can develop KETOSIS and metabolic ACIDOSIS.

Reversal of the fever-producing process is necessary in order to restore body temperature to the normal range. Antipyretic agents that lower the temperature temporarily 'break' a fever, but the temperature will rise again if the pyrogenic agents that affect the hypothalamus have not been removed.

The period during which a fever abates is called the period of *defervescence*. It may occur rapidly and dramatically, as the temperature falls from peak to normal in a matter of hours. This is called the *crisis*, that is, the critical point at which the fever is broken. A more gradual resetting of the thermostat and slow decline of the fever is called *resolution* of the fever by *lysis*.

TREATMENT. In addition to medical measures to remove the primary cause of the fever, symptomatic relief is provided by means of drugs and nursing measures. Antipyretic drugs, such as aspirin and paracetamol, may be prescribed to lower the body temperature. Anti-infective drugs are of value when the pyrogen is an infectious agent. Some of the phenothiazines, such as chlorpromazine and promethazine, may be prescribed to prevent shivering.

Fluids and electrolytes are replaced orally or intravenously as indicated by laboratory tests and signs of dehydration. Frequent, small feedings of high-calorie, high-protein foods are recommended to combat fatigue and debility caused by the increased metabolic rate. The selection of oral liquids and foods should be based on the patient's preferences. Vitamin supplements may be prescribed in prolonged, low-grade fevers.

PATIENT CARE. The patient with acute hyperpyrexia or hyperthermia will require extreme measures to lower the body temperature as quickly and safely as possible in order to prevent brain damage. Patients with sunstroke or heatstroke should be cooled rapidly by blowing cold air over exposed skin and the use of cool water sprays or wet sheets. In order to keep the temperature at a tolerable level until the thermostat is reset, a cooling blanket or hypothermia mattress may be used. Care must be taken to maintain the integrity of the skin and avoid extreme hypothermia when such a device is used.

Other measures include sponging parts of the body with cool water or a mixture of alcohol and water in order to increase heat loss through evaporation of moisture. The part being sponged should be left exposed to the air until it is almost dry, and then should be lightly covered while another part is being sponged. An ice cap or cold compress on the forehead helps to reduce the fever and relieve headache and delirium. Fanning can also be effective, especially if the patient's torso is covered with a sheet saturated with water as for heatstroke.

Chills are uncomfortable and sometimes frightening to the patient. When the patient complains of feeling chilled or cold, some form of external warmth should be provided. An extra blanket is helpful as is a hot water bottle filled with warm, *not hot*, water. As the body temperature declines the difference between body temperature and environmental temperature will decrease and the patient will begin to feel warmer. During the second stage of fever the patient may complain of feeling hot; his skin feels warm to the touch and his face is flushed. These symptoms are the result of vasodilation of surface blood vessels, an attempt by the body to prevent further escalation of the body temperature.

The patient with fever presents nursing care challenges related to fluid volume deficit, alterations in nutrition, and potential for injury during attacks of delirium and convulsive seizures. Vital signs and fluid intake and output should be monitored at frequent intervals. Laboratory values for electrolytes, albuminuria, and arterial blood gases also should be monitored, and the patient should be watched for early signs of cellular dehydration. Care should include safety precautions to prevent injury to those patients at risk for either delirium or convulsive seizures.

Because of increased metabolic activity, every effort should be made to meet the nutritional needs of the patient with prolonged fever. Broths, soups, ice cream, and milk shakes with egg are good sources of electrolytes, protein, and calories. Anorexia presents the challenge of selecting foods that are pleasing to the patient and at the same time rich in the nutrients that he needs.

For diseases characterized by fever, see the eponymic or descriptive name, as ROCKY MOUNTAIN SPOTTED FEVER or TYPHOID FEVER, respectively.
aseptic f. fever associated with aseptic wounds, presumably due to the disintegration of leukocytes or to the absorption of avascular or traumatized tissue.
f. blister an itching or stinging sore on the skin or mucous membrane, due to infection with the virus of HERPES SIMPLEX. It often accompanies fever, and is most commonly seen about the lips or nose. Called also *herpes febrilis*.
central f. sustained fever resulting from damage to the thermoregulatory centres of the hypothalamus.
continued f., continuous f. persistently elevated body temperature, showing no or little variation and never falling to normal during any 24-hour period.
intermittent f. an attack of MALARIA or other fever, with recurring paroxysms of elevated temperature separated by intervals during which the temperature is normal.
periodic f. a condition characterized by repeated febrile episodes accompanied by abdominal or pleuritic pain, occurring in precise or irregular cycles of days, weeks, or months.
remittent f. elevated body temperature showing fluctuation each day, but never falling to normal.

FFARCS Fellow of the Faculty of Anaesthetists, Royal College of Surgeons.

FFP fresh frozen plasma.

fibr(o)- word element. [L.] *fibre, fibrous*.

fibra ('fiebrə) pl. *fibrae* [L.] fibre.

fibre ('fiebə) 1. an elongated threadlike structure. 2. dietary fibre.
A f's myelinated fibres of the somatic nervous system having a diameter of 1 micrometre to 22 micrometres and a conduction velocity of 5 to 120 metres per second.
accelerating f's, accelerator f's adrenergic fibres that transmit the impulses which accelerate the heart beat.
adrenergic f's nerve fibres that liberate adrenaline-like substances at the time of passage of nerve impulses across a synapse.
alpha f's motor and proprioceptive fibres of the A type having conduction velocities of 70 to 120 metres per second and ranging from 13 to 22 micrometres in diameter.
arcuate f's any of the bow-shaped fibres in the brain, such as those connecting adjacent gyri in the cerebral cortex, or the external or internal arcuate fibres of the medulla oblongata.
association f's nerve fibres that interconnect portions of the cerebral cortex within a hemisphere. Short association fibres interconnect neighbouring gyri; long fibres interconnect more widely separated gyri and are arranged into bundles or fasciculi.
B f's myelinated preganglionic autonomic axons having a fibre diameter less than 3 micrometres and a conduction velocity of 3 to 15 metres per second.
beta f's touch and temperature fibres of the A type having conduction velocities of 30 to 70 metres per second and ranging from 8 to 13 micrometres in diameter.
C f's unmyelinated postganglionic fibres of the autonomic nervous system; also, the unmyelinated fibres at the dorsal roots and at free nerve endings having a diameter of 0.3 to 1.3 micrometres and a conduction velocity of 0.6 to 2.3 metres per second.
cholinergic f's nerve fibres that liberate acetylcholine at the synapse.
collagen f's, collagenic f's, collagenous f's the soft, flexible, white fibres that are the most characteristic constituent of all types of connective tissue, consisting of the protein collagen, and composed of bundles of fibrils that are in turn made up of smaller units (microfibrils) that show a characteristic crossbanding with a major periodicity of 65 nanometres.
depressor f's nerve fibres which, when stimulated reflexly, cause a diminished vasomotor tone and thereby a decrease in arterial pressure.
dietary f. that portion of ingested foodstuffs that cannot be broken down by intestinal enzymes and juices and, therefore, passes through the small intestine and colon undigested. It is composed of cellulose, which is the 'skeleton' of plants, hemicellulose, gums, lignin, pectin, and other carbohydrates undigestible by humans.

Dietary fibre is not to be confused with 'crude fibre', which is mainly lignin and cellulose and is the residue remaining after a food has been subjected to a standardized treatment with dilute acid and alkali. Crude fibre measurements usually underestimate actual total dietary fibre by at least 50 per cent.

Vegetables, cereals, and fruits are the main sources of dietary fibre. Although bran is advertised as an excellent source of fibre, it is not unique nor is it as nutritious as fruits and vegetables and some other whole unprocessed cereals. The typical diet in Western countries contains 10 to 30 grams of dietary fibre.

The primary effects of dietary fibre are to increase the bulk of the stool and make it softer by taking up water as it passes through the colon, and to absorb organic wastes and toxins and carry them out of the intestinal tract. The increase in stool bulk hastens the passage of faeces and may reduce the length of time the intestinal wall is exposed to toxic substances.

BENEFITS OF A HIGH-FIBRE DIET. In spite of claims that high-fibre foods, especially bran, can prevent or cure a variety of diseases, ranging from cancer of the colon to atherosclerosis, there is no conclusive evidence that this is so. Dietary fibre is helpful in the treatment and prevention of uncomplicated constipation. Unlike strong laxatives and purgatives, it presents no problems when taken on a long-term basis. Metamucil, a medicinal faecal softener, is made from seed husks and is often prescribed for persons having problems with normal bowel activity. Haemorrhoids are aggravated by straining on defecation, and so there is some basis for recommending a high-fibre diet for persons who have this condition.

The symptoms of diverticular disease, which is an outpouching of the wall of the colon with subsequent inflammation, are relieved by a high-fibre diet. There is valid evidence to support the theory that the more rapid passage of softer stools through the colon decreases the pressure exerted against its walls and thereby prevents formation of diverticula.

Spastic colon is believed by some to be relieved by increasing the bulk of the stools. However, inflammatory bowel disease in which there is a narrowing of the bowel, as in some cases of Crohn's disease, can be worsened by more roughage in the intestinal tract.

Fibre does have the capacity to unite with intestinal bile salts and dietary cholesterol, preventing their absorption from the gut and hastening their elimination via the intestinal tract. Because of these properties, fibre has been advocated as a preventive measure against the formation of gallstones and the production of atherosclerotic plaques in the blood vessels. As yet, there are no experimental data to substantiate a theory linking high intake of dietary fibre with prevention of these medical problems.
elastic f's yellowish fibres of elastic quality traversing the intercellular substance of connective tissue.
gamma f's A fibres that conduct touch and pressure impulses and innervate the intrafusal fibres of the

muscle spindle; they conduct at velocities of 15 to 40 metres per second and range from 3 to 7 micrometres in diameter.

grey f's unmyelinated nerve fibres found largely in the sympathetic nerves.

intrafusal f's modified muscle fibres which, surrounded by fluid and enclosed in a connective tissue envelope, compose the muscle spindle.

light f's muscle fibres poor in sarcoplasm and more transparent than dark fibres.

medullated f's myelinated fibres.

motor f's nerve fibres transmitting motor impulses to a muscle fibre.

muscle f. any of the cells of skeletal or cardiac muscle tissue. Skeletal muscle fibres are cylindrical multinucleate cells containing contracting myofibrils, across which run transverse striations. Cardiac muscle fibres have one or sometimes two nuclei, contain myofibrils, and are separated from one another by an intercalated disc; although striated, cardiac muscle fibres branch to form an interlacing network.

myelinated f's greyish white nerve fibres encased in a myelin sheath.

nerve f. a slender process of a neuron, especially the prolonged axon which conducts nerve impulses away from the cell; classified on the basis of the presence or absence of a myelin sheath as myelinated or unmyelinated.

nonmedullated f's unmyelinated fibres.

osteogenetic f's, osteogenic f's precollagenous fibres formed by osteoclasts and becoming the fibrous component of bone matrix.

postganglionic f's nerve fibres passing to involuntary muscle and gland cells, the cell bodies of which lie in the autonomic ganglia.

preganglionic f's nerve fibres passing to the autonomic ganglia, the cell bodies of which lie in the brain or spinal cord.

pressor f's nerve fibres which, when stimulated reflexly, cause or increase vasomotor tone.

projection f's bundles of axons that connect the cerebral cortex with the subcortical centres, brain stem, and spinal cord.

Purkinje's f's modified cardiac muscle fibres in the subendothelial tissue concerned with conducting impulses in the heart.

radicular f's fibres in the roots of the spinal nerves.

reticular f's immature connective tissue fibres, staining with silver, forming the reticular framework of lymphoid and myeloid tissue, and occurring in interstitial tissue of glandular organs, the papillary layer of the skin, and elsewhere.

Sharpey's f's 1. collagenous fibres that pass from the periosteum and are embedded in the outer circumferential and interstitial lamellae of bone. 2. terminal portions of principal fibres that insert into the cementum of a tooth.

spindle f's the microtubules radiating from the centrioles during mitosis and forming a spindle-shaped configuration.

unmyelinated f's nerve fibres that lack a myelin sheath.

fibre-illuminated (ˌfiebə·i'loomiˌnaytid) transmitting light by means of bundles of glass or plastic fibres, utilizing a lens system to transmit the image; said of endoscopes of such design.

fibrecolonoscope (ˌfiebəkoh'lonəˌskohp) a fibrescope for viewing the colon.

fibregastroscope (ˌfiebə'gastrəˌskohp) a fibrescope for viewing the stomach.

fibreoptic (ˌfiebə'roptik) pertaining to fibreoptics; coated with flexible glass or plastic fibres having special optical properties and orientation.

fibreoptics (ˌfiebə'roptiks) the transmission of an image along flexible bundles of glass or plastic fibres each of which carries an element of the image.

fibrescope ('fiebəˌskohp) a flexible endoscope whose lumen is coated with fibreoptic glass or plastic fibres having special optical properties.

fibril ('fiebril, 'fib-) a minute fibre or filament. adj. **fibrillar, fibrillary**.

fibrillation (ˌfibri'layshən, ˌfie-) 1. a small, local, involuntary, muscular contraction, due to spontaneous activation of single muscle cells or muscle fibres. 2. the quality of being made up of fibrils. 3. the initial degenerative changes in osteoarthritis, marked by softening of the articular cartilage and development of vertical clefts between groups of cartilage cells. **atrial f.** a cardiac arrhythmia marked by rapid randomized contractions of the atrial myocardium, causing a totally irregular, often rapid, ventricular rate.

ventricular f. a cardiac arrhythmia marked by fibrillary contractions of the ventricular muscle due to rapid repetitive excitation of myocardial fibres without coordinated ventricular contraction. Ventricular fibrillation is a frequent cause of CARDIAC ARREST. An apparatus called a defibrillator sometimes is used to alleviate fibrillation. The defibrillator delivers an electric shock to the heart muscle, depolarizing the muscle and ending the irregular contractions. The heart may then be able to resume normal, regular contractions.

fibrillogenesis (ˌfiebriloh'jenəsis) the formation and development of fibrils.

fibrin ('fiebrin) an insoluble protein that is essential to CLOTTING of blood, formed from fibrinogen by action of thrombin.

fibrinocellular (ˌfiebrinoh'selyuhlə) made up of fibrin and cells.

fibrinogen (fie'brinəjən) a high-molecular-weight protein in the blood plasma that by the action of thrombin is converted into fibrin; called also *clotting factor I*. In the CLOTTING mechanism, fibrin threads form a meshwork for the basis of a blood clot. Most of the fibrinogen in the circulating blood is formed in the liver. Normal quantities of fibrinogen in the plasma vary from 2 to 4 grams per litre of plasma.

Preparations containing human fibrinogen used to restore blood fibrinogen levels after extensive surgery, or to treat diseases and haemorrhagic conditions that are complicated by AFIBRINOGENAEMIA include fresh frozen plasma and cryoprecipitate. Pure fibrinogen is rarely used because of the risk of transmitting hepatitis.

f. degradation products fragments of fibrinogen or fibrin degraded by plasmin, which are found in the serum and urine of patients with disseminated intravascular coagulation (DIC) and in the urine of patients who have had renal transplants.

fibrinogenaemia (fieˌbrinəjə'neemi·ə) hyperfibrinogenaemia.

fibrinogenolysis (fieˌbrinəjə'nolisis) the proteolytic destruction of fibrinogen in the circulating blood. adj. **fibrinogenolytic**.

fibrinogenopenia (fieˌbrinəjenoh'peeni·ə) decreased fibrinogen in the blood.

fibrinoid ('fiebriˌnoyd) 1. resembling fibrin. 2. a homogeneous, eosinophilic, relatively acellular refractile substance with some of the staining properties of fibrin.

fibrinolysin (ˌfiebri'nolisin) 1. plasmin. 2. a preparation of proteolytic enzyme formed from profibrinolysin (plasminogen) by action of physical agents or by specific bacterial kinases; used to promote dissolution of thrombi.

fibrinolysis (ˌfiebri'nolisis) the dissolution of fibrin by enzymatic action. adj. **fibrinolytic.**

fibrinopenia (ˌfiebrinoh'peeni·ə) deficiency of fibrinogen in the blood.

fibrinopeptide (ˌfiebrinoh'peptied) either of two peptides (A and B) split off from fibrinogen during blood CLOTTING by the action of thrombin.

fibrinous ('fiebrinəs) pertaining to or of the nature of fibrin.

fibrinuria (ˌfiebri'nyooə·ri·ə) discharge of fibrin in the urine.

fibroadenoma (ˌfiebrohˌadə'nohmə) adenoma containing fibrous elements; usually, and most commonly, a tumour of the breast.

fibroadipose (ˌfiebroh'adipohs, -z) both fibrous and fatty.

fibroangioma (ˌfiebrohˌanji'ohmə) an angioma containing much fibrous tissue.

fibroareolar (ˌfiebroh·ə'reeələ) both fibrous and areolar.

fibroblast ('fiebrohˌblast) an immature fibre-producing cell of connective tissue. Called also *fibrocyte*. adj. **fibroblastic.**

fibroblastoma (ˌfiebrohbla'stohmə) any tumour arising from fibroblasts, now classified as fibromas and or fibrosarcomas.

fibrocalcific (ˌfiebrohkal'sifik) pertaining to or characterized by partially calcified fibrous tissue.

fibrocarcinoma (ˌfiebrohˌkahsi'nohmə) scirrhous carcinoma.

fibrocartilage (ˌfiebroh'kahtilij) cartilage made up of parallel, thick, compact collagenous bundles, separated by narrow clefts containing the typical cartilage cells (chondrocytes).

fibrochondritis (ˌfiebrohkon'drietis) inflammation of fibrocartilage.

fibrochondroma (ˌfiebrohkon'drohmə) chondroma containing areas of fibrosis.

fibrocyst ('fiebrohˌsist) cystic fibroma.

fibrocystic (ˌfiebroh'sistik) characterized by an overgrowth of fibrous tissue and the development of cystic spaces, especially in a gland.

f. disease of breast cystic disease of breast.

f. disease of pancreas cystic fibrosis.

fibrocystoma (ˌfiebrohsi'stohmə) cystic fibroma.

fibrocyte ('fiebrəˌsiet) a cell that produces fibrous tissue; called also FIBROBLAST.

fibrodysplasia (ˌfiebrohdis'playzi·ə) fibrous dysplasia.

fibroelastic (ˌfiebroh·i'lastik) both fibrous and elastic.

fibroelastosis (ˌfiebrohˌeela'stohsis) overgrowth of fibroelastic elements.

endocardial f. a condition characterized by left ventricular hypertrophy and conversion of the endocardium into a thick fibroelastic coat, with ventricular capacity sometimes reduced, but often increased.

fibroenchondroma (ˌfiebrohˌenkon'drohmə) enchondroma containing fibrous elements.

fibroepithelioma (ˌfiebrohˌepiˌtheeli'ohmə) a tumour composed of both fibrous and epithelial elements.

fibrohistiocytic (ˌfiebrohˌhistioh'sitik) having fibrous and histiocytic elements.

fibroid ('fiebroyd) 1. having a fibrous structure; resembling a fibroma. 2. fibroma. 3. LEIOMYOMA. 4. myoma; *fibroids* is a colloquial term for myoma of the uterus.

f. tumour fibroma or myoma.

fibroidectomy (ˌfiebroy'dektəmee) excision of a uterine fibroma (leiomyoma).

fibrolipoma (ˌfiebrohli'pohmə) a lipoma containing excessive fibrous tissue. adj. **fibrolipomatous.**

fibroma (fie'brohmə) a tumour composed mainly of fibrous or fully developed connective tissue.

ameloblastic f. an odontogenic fibroma, marked by simultaneous proliferation of both epithelial and mesenchymal tissue, without formation of enamel or dentine.

cementifying f. cementoblastoma; a tumour usually occurring in the mandible of older persons and consisting of fibroblastic tissue containing masses of cementum-like tissue.

chondromyxoid f. of bone a benign slowly growing tumour of chondroblastic origin, usually affecting the long bones of the leg.

cystic f. one that has undergone cystic degeneration.

f. myxomatodes myxofibroma; a fibroma containing myxomatous tissue.

nonosteogenic f. a degenerative and proliferative lesion of the medullary and cortical tissues of bone.

odontogenic f. a benign tumour of the jaw arising from the embryonic portion of the tooth germ, the dental papilla, or dental follicle, or later from the periodontal membrane.

ossifying f., ossifying f. of bone a benign, relatively slow-growing, central bone tumour, usually of the jaws, especially the mandible, which is composed of fibrous connective tissue within which bone is formed.

fibromatoid (fie'brohməˌtoyd) resembling fibroma; fibroma-like.

fibromatosis (ˌfiebrohmə'tohsis) 1. the presence of multiple fibromas. 2. the formation of a fibrous, tumour-like nodule arising from the deep fascia, with a tendency to local recurrence.

f. gingivae, gingival f. a noninflammatory fibrous hyperplasia of the gingivae and palate, manifested as a dense, smooth or nodular overgrowth of the tissues.

palmar f. fibromatosis involving the palmar fascia, and resulting in Dupuytren's contracture.

plantar f. fibromatosis involving the plantar fascia manifested as single or multiple nodular swellings, sometimes accompanied by pain but usually unassociated with contractures.

fibromatous (fie'brohmətəs) pertaining to or of the nature of fibroma.

fibromuscular (ˌfiebroh'muskyuhlə) both fibrous and muscular.

fibromyoma (ˌfiebrohmie'ohmə) a myoma containing fibrous elements, a leiomyoma.

fibromyomectomy (ˌfiebrohˌmieə'mektəmee) excision of a fibromyoma (leiomyoma).

fibromyositis (ˌfiebrohmieoh'sietis) inflammation of muscle with fibrous degeneration.

fibromyxoma (ˌfiebrohmik'sohmə) a fibroma containing myxomatous tissue; myxofibroma.

fibromyxosarcoma (ˌfiebrohˌmiksohsah'kohmə) a sarcoma containing fibrous and mucous elements.

fibronectin (ˌfiebrə'nektin) an adhesive glycoprotein: one form circulates in plasma, acting as an opsonin, another is a cell-surface protein which mediates cellular adhesive interactions.

fibroneuroma (ˌfiebrohnyuh'rohmə) neurofibroma.

fibropapilloma (ˌfiebrohˌpapi'lohmə) a papilloma containing much fibrous tissue.

fibroplasia (ˌfiebroh'playzi·ə) the formation of fibrous tissue, as in the healing of a wound. adj. **fibroplastic.**

retrolental f. a condition characterized by retinal vascular proliferation and tortuosity and by the presence of fibrous tissue behind the lens, leading to detachment of the retina and arrest of growth of the eye, generally attributed to use of excessively high concentrations of oxygen in the care of preterm infants.

fibrosarcoma (ˌfiebrohsah'kohmə) a sarcoma arising from collagen-producing fibroblasts.

odontogenic f. a malignant tumour of the jaws,

originating from one of the mesenchymal components of the tooth or tooth germ.

fibroserous (ˌfiebroh'siə·rəs) composed of both fibrous and serous elements.

fibrosis (fie'brohsis) formation of fibrous tissue; fibroid degeneration. adj. **fibrotic**.

congenital hepatic f. a developmental disorder of the liver, marked by formation of irregular broad bands of fibrous tissue containing multiple disordered terminal bile ducts, and resulting in vascular constriction and portal hypertension.

cystic f., cystic f. of pancreas a generalized hereditary disorder with widespread dysfunction of exocrine glands, chronic pulmonary disease, pancreatic deficiency, high levels of electrolytes in sweat, and sometimes biliary cirrhosis. See also CYSTIC FIBROSIS.

diffuse idiopathic interstitial f. chronic inflammatory progressive fibrosis of the pulmonary alveolar walls, with steadily progressive dyspnoea, resulting in death from oxygen lack or right heart failure. It may result from pneumoconiosis, hypersensitivity pneumonitis, scleroderma, and other diseases. About half of the cases are of unknown origin.

endomyocardial f. idiopathic myocardiopathy occurring endemically in various regions of Africa and rarely in other areas, characterized by cardiomegaly, by marked thickening of the endocardium with dense, white fibrous tissue that frequently extends to involve the inner third or half of the myocardium, and by congestive heart failure.

mediastinal f. development of whitish, hard fibrous tissue in the upper portion of the mediastinum, sometimes obstructing the air passages and large blood vessels.

periapical ossifying f. an odontogenic fibroma whose cells are developing into cementoblasts and in which there is only a small proportion of calcified tissue.

periureteric f. progressive development of fibrous tissue spreading from the great midline vessels and causing strangulation of one or both ureters. Often referred to as *retroperitoneal fibrosis*.

postfibrinous f. that occurring in tissues in which fibrin has been deposited.

proliferative f. that in which the fibrous elements continue to proliferate after the original causative factor has ceased to operate.

pulmonary f. diffuse idiopathic interstitial fibrosis.

retroperitoneal f. deposition of fibrous tissue in the retroperitoneal space, producing vague abdominal discomfort, and often causing blockage of the ureters, with resultant hydronephrosis and impaired renal function, which may result in renal failure. Called also *Ormond's disease*.

f. uteri a morbid condition characterized by overgrowth of the smooth muscle and increase in the collagenous fibrous tissue of the uterus, producing a thickened, coarse, tough myometrium.

fibrositis (ˌfiebrə'sietis) inflammatory hyperplasia of the white fibrous tissue, especially of the muscle sheaths and fascial layers of the locomotor system, causing pain and stiffness; called also *muscular rheumatism*.

fibrothorax (ˌfiebroh'thor·raks) adhesion of the two pleural layers, the lung being covered by thick nonexpansible fibrous tissue.

fibrous ('fiebrəs) composed of or containing fibres.

f. dysplasia localized overgrowth of fibrous tissue in bone (see also fibrous DYSPLASIA).

fibrovascular (ˌfiebroh'vaskyuhlə) both fibrous and vascular.

fibula ('fibyuhlə) the lateral and smaller of the two bones of the leg. adj. **fibular**.

ficin ('fiesin) a highly active, crystallizable proteinase from the sap of fig trees, which catalyses the hydrolysis of many proteins at acid (4.1) pH, the clotting of milk, and 'digestion' of some living worms, e.g., whipworms. Ficin is used as a protein digestant and to enhance the agglutination of red blood cells with IgG antibodies (e.g., Rh antibodies). It also shows esterase activity.

FICS Fellow of the International College of Surgeons.

field (feeld) 1. an area or open space, as an operative field or visual field. 2. a range of specialization in knowledge, study, or occupation. 3. in embryology, the developing region within a range of modifying factors.

auditory f. the space or range within which stimuli will be perceived as sound.

high-power f. the area of a slide visible under the high magnification system of a microscope.

individuation f. a region in which a chemical organizer influences adjacent tissue to become a part of a total embryo.

low-power f. the area of a slide visible under the low magnification system of a microscope.

morphogenetic f. an embryonic region out of which definite structures normally develop.

f. of vision the area within view, as for a camera or in an operation.

visual f. the area within which stimuli will produce the sensation of sight with the eye in a straight-ahead position.

fila ('fielə) [L.] plural of *filum*.

filaceous (fie'layshəs) composed of filaments.

filament ('filəmənt) a delicate fibre or thread.

filamentous (ˌfilə'mentəs) composed of long, threadlike structures.

filaria (fi'lair·ri·ə) pl. *filariae* [L.] a nematode worm of the superfamily Filarioidea. adj. **filarial**.

filariasis (ˌfilə'rieəsis) infection with filariae. The organism causing the most common form of filariasis is *Wuchereria bancrofti*, which is widely distributed in the tropics, and is transmitted by mosquitoes. The larvae invade lymphoid tissues and then grow to adult worms an inch or two long. The resulting obstruction of the lymphatic circulation causes swelling, inflammation, and pain. Repeated infections over many years, with impaired circulation and formation of excess connective tissue, may cause enlargement of the affected part, usually the arm, leg, or scrotum. In cases of extreme enlargement, known as ELEPHANTIASIS, the affected part may grow to many times its normal size.

The larvae can be killed by treatment with diethylcarbamazine, but it is less effective for the adult worms. Oedema of the legs can be reduced by rest and by the use of pressure bandages. The prognosis is favourable for all but the most severe cases.

filaricide (fi'lariˌsied) an agent that destroys filariae. adj. **filaricidal**.

filariform (fi'lariˌfawm) resembling filariae; threadlike.

Filarioidea (fiˌlair·ri'oydi·ə) a superfamily of nematode parasites (filariae), the adults of which are threadlike worms that invade the tissues and body cavities, where the female deposits microfilariae (prelarvae). These microfilariae are ingested by bloodsucking insects in whom they pass their developmental stage and are returned to man by the bites of such insects (see also FILARIASIS).

filiform ('filiˌfawm, fie-) 1. threadlike. 2. an extremely slender bougie.

fillet ('filit) 1. a loop, as of cord or tape, for making traction. 2. in the nervous system, a long band of nerve fibres.

film (film) 1. a thin layer or coating. 2. a thin sheet of material (e.g., gelatin, cellulose acetate) specially treated for use in photography or radiography; used also to designate the sheet after exposure to the energy to which it is sensitive.

bite-wing f. an x-ray film for radiography of oral structures, with a protruding tab to be held between the upper and lower teeth.

spot f. a radiograph of a small anatomical area obtained (1) by rapid exposure during fluoroscopy to provide a permanent record of a transiently observed abnormality, or (2) by limitation of radiation passing through the area to improve definition and detail of the image produced.

x-ray f. film sensitive to x-rays, either before or after exposure.

film badge ('film ˌbaj) a pack of radiographic film or films worn as a badge, used for the detection and approximate measurement of radiation exposure of personnel.

filopressure ('fieloh,preshə) compression of a blood vessel by a thread.

filter ('filtə) a device for eliminating certain elements, as (1) particles of certain size from a solution, or (2) rays of certain wavelength from a stream of radiant energy.

Berkefeld's f. one composed of diatomaceous earth, impermeable to ordinary bacteria.

Millipore f. trademark for a device used to filter nutrient solutions as they are administered intravenously.

Pasteur–Chamberland f. a hollow column of unglazed porcelain through which liquids are forced by pressure or by vacuum exhaustion.

Wood's f. a nickel-oxide filter that holds back all but a few violet rays and passes ultraviolet rays of about 365 nm (see also WOOD'S LIGHT).

filterable, filtrable ('filtə·rab'l; 'filtrab'l) capable of passing through the pores of a filter.

filtrate ('filtrayt) a liquid that has passed through a filter.

filtration (fil'trayshən) passage through a filter or through a material that prevents passage of certain molecules.

filum ('fieləm) pl. *fila* [L.] a threadlike structure or part.

f. terminale a slender, threadlike prolongation of the spinal cord from the conus medullaris to the back of the coccyx.

fimbria ('fimbri·ə) pl. *fimbriae* [L.] 1. a fringe, border, or edge; a fringelike structure. 2. one of the minute filamentous appendages of certain bacteria, associated with antigenic properties of the cell surface. Called also *pilus*.

f. hippocampi the band of white matter along the median edge of the ventricular surface of the hippocampus.

fimbriae of uterine tube the numerous divergent fringelike processes on the distal part of the infundibulum of the uterine tube.

fimbriate ('fimbri,ayt) fringed.

finger ('fing·gə) one of the five digits of the hand.

clubbed f. one with enlargement of the terminal phalanx with constant osseous changes.

hammer f., mallet f. permanent flexion of the distal phalanx of a finger due to avulsion of the extensor tendon.

trigger f. temporary flexion of a finger which is overcome in a sudden jerk by active or passive extension of the finger. It is caused by thickening of the flexor tendon in a narrowed tendon sheath.

webbed f's fingers more or less united by strands of tissue; syndactyly.

fingerprint ('fing·gə,print) 1. an impression of the cutaneous ridges of the fleshy distal portion of a finger. 2. in biochemistry, the characteristic pattern of a peptide after subjection to an analytical technique.

Finney's pyloroplasty ('finiz) enlargement of the pyloric canal by establishment of an inverted U-shaped anastomosis between the stomach and duodenum after longitudinal incision.

Finsen's lamp ('finsənz) a carbon arc lamp operating at 50 volts and 50 amperes, so constructed that radiation is concentrated on an area 2.5 mm square; a water-cooled quartz system is used to remove calorific radiation and a compression quartz piece to dehaematize the skin.

Finsen's light light consisting mainly of violet and ultraviolet rays given off by Finsen's lamp; used in treatment of lupus and similar diseases.

first aid (fərst ayd) emergency care and treatment of an injured person before complete medical and surgical treatment can be secured.

fission ('fishən) 1. the act of splitting. 2. asexual reproduction in which the cell divides into two (binary fission) or more (multiple fission) daughter parts, each of which becomes an individual organism. 3. nuclear fission; the splitting of the atomic nucleus, with release of energy.

fissiparous (fi'sipə·rəs) propagated by fission.

fissula ('fishyuhlə) pl. *fissulae* [L.] a small cleft.

fissura (fish'yooə·rə) pl. *fissurae* [L.] fissure.

fissure ('fishə) a narrow slit or cleft, especially one of the deeper or more constant furrows separating the gyri of the brain.

abdominal f. a congenital cleft in the abdominal wall.

anal f., f. in ano a painful lineal ulcer at the margin of the anus.

anterior median f. a longitudinal furrow along the midline of the ventral surface of the spinal cord and medulla oblongata.

f. of Bichat transverse fissure (2).

branchial f. branchial cleft.

central f. fissure of Rolando.

collateral f. a longitudinal fissure on the inferior surface of the cerebral hemisphere between the fusiform gyrus and the hippocampal gyrus.

Henle's f's spaces filled with connective tissue between the muscular fibres of the heart.

hippocampal f. one extending from the splenium of the corpus callosum almost to the tip of the temporal lobe; called also *hippocampal sulcus*.

longitudinal f. the deep fissure between the cerebral hemispheres.

palpebral f. the longitudinal opening between the eyelids.

portal f. porta hepatis.

posterior median f. 1. a shallow vertical groove in the closed part of the medulla oblongata, continuous with the posterior median sulcus of the spinal cord. 2. a shallow vertical groove dividing the spinal cord throughout its whole length in the midline posteriorly. Called also *posterior median sulcus*.

presylvian f. the anterior branch of the fissure of Sylvius.

Rolando's f., f. of Rolando a groove running obliquely across the superolateral surface of the cerebral hemisphere, separating the frontal from the parietal lobe. Called also *central fissure* and *central sulcus*.

f. of round ligament one on the visceral surface of the liver, lodging the round ligament in the adult.

sylvian f., f. of Sylvius one extending laterally between the temporal and frontal lobes, and turning posteriorly between the temporal and parietal lobes.

transverse f. 1. porta hepatis. 2. the transverse cerebral fissure between the diencephalon and the cerebral hemispheres; called also *fissure of Bichat*.

zygal f. a cerebral fissure consisting of two branches

connected by a stem.

fistula ('fistyuhlə) an abnormal passage between two epithelial surfaces. Among the many kinds of fistulas, the anal type (fistula in ano) is one of the most common. This generally develops as a result of a fissure in the wall of the anal canal or from the rectum in association with an abscess.

Difficult labour in childbirth may result in a vesicovaginal fistula, between the bladder and the vagina, with resulting leakage of urine into the vagina. In a rectovaginal fistula, faeces escape through the wall of the anal canal or rectum into the vagina. These conditions are now rare. Vesicointestinal fistulas occur in Crohn's disease and diverticulitis; when they involve the sigmoid colon pneumaturia is not uncommon.

anal f., f. in ano a fistula between the rectum or anal canal and the skin near the anus.

arteriovenous f. a fistula between an artery and a vein.

biliary f. a fistula from any part of the biliary system to the skin.

blind f. one open at one end only, opening on the skin (external blind fistula) or on an internal surface (internal blind fistula).

branchial f. a persisting branchial cleft. **craniosinus f.** one between the cerebral space and one of the sinuses, permitting escape of cerebrospinal fluid into the nose.

Eck's f. an artificial communication made between the portal vein and the vena cava.

enterocutaneous f. one in which there is communication between the intestinal tract and the skin.

enteroenteric f. an internal fistula between two parts of the intestine, common in Crohn's disease. When between the duodenum and the ascending colon it may result in severe nutritional failure with steatorrhoea.

faecal f. a colonic fistula opening on the external surface of the body and discharging faeces.

gastric f. an abnormal passage communicating with the stomach; often applied to an artificially created opening, through the abdominal wall, into the stomach.

horseshoe f. a semicircular fistulous tract running behind the anus.

incomplete f. blind fistula.

pulmonary arteriovenous f., congenital a congenital anomalous communication between the pulmonary arterial and venous systems, allowing unoxygenated blood to enter the systemic circulation.

umbilical f. an abnormal passage communicating with the gut or the urachus at the umbilicus.

fistulectomy (,fistyuh'lektəmee) excision of a fistula.

fistulization (,fistyuhlie'zayshən) 1. the process of becoming fistulous. 2. surgical creation of a fistula.

fistulotomy (,fistyuh'lotəmee) incision of a fistula.

fistulous ('fistyuhləs) pertaining to or of the nature of a fistula.

fit (fit) a commonly used term for paroxysmal motor discharges leading to sudden convulsive movements, as in epilepsy, eclampsia and hysteria. The term is sometimes applied to apoplexy.

fixation (fik'sayshən) 1. the act or operation of holding, suturing, or fastening in a fixed position, as of a fracture. 2. the condition of being held in a fixed position. 3. (a) excessive attachment to (or 'fixation' on) an object, person or situation that was appropriate to an earlier stage of development (affective fixation); (b) persistent, compulsive behaviour or preoccupation seemingly without rational motivation—usually assumed to result from affective fixation. 4. in microscopy, the treatment of material so that its structure can be examined in greater detail with minimal alteration of the normal state, and also to provide information concerning the chemical properties (as of cell constituents) by interpretation of fixation reactions. 5. in chemistry, the process which renders a substance solid or nonvolatile. 6. in ophthalmology, direction of the gaze so that the visual image of the object falls on the fovea centralis. 7. in film processing, the chemical removal of all undeveloped salts of the film emulsion, as on x-ray films.

complement f., f. of complement the combining of complement component C1 with the antigen–antibody complex (see also COMPLEMENT FIXATION).

fixative ('fiksətiv) an agent used in preserving a histological or pathological specimen so as to maintain the normal structure of its constituent elements.

flaccid ('flaksid, 'flasid) weak, lax, soft; applied especially to muscles.

flagellar (flə'jelə) of or pertaining to a flagellum.

flagellate ('flajilət) 1. any microorganism having flagella. 2. any protozoon of the subphylum Mastigophora. 3. having flagella.

flagellation (,flaji'layshən) 1. massage by tapping the part with the fingers. 2. whipping or being whipped to achieve erotic pleasure.

flagelliform (flə'jeli,fawm) shaped like a flagellum or lash.

flagellosis (,flaji'lohsis) infection with flagellate protozoa.

flagellum (flə'jeləm) pl. *flagella* [L.] a long, mobile, whiplike appendage arising from a basal body at the surface of a cell, serving as a locomotor organelle; in eukaryotic cells, flagella contain nine pairs of microtubules arrayed around a central pair; in bacteria, they contain tightly wound strands of flagellin.

Flagyl ('flagil) trademark for a preparation of metronidazole, an antibacterial and antiprotozoal.

flail (flayl) exhibiting abnormal or pathological mobility, as flail chest or flail joint.

f. chest a loss of stability of the chest wall due to multiple rib fractures or detachment of the sternum from the ribs as a result of a severe crushing chest injury. The loose chest segment moves in a direction which is the reverse of normal; that is, the segment moves inward during inspiration and outward during expiration (PARADOXICAL RESPIRATION). Other manifestations of flail chest include shortness of breath, cyanosis, and extreme pain in the area of trauma.

Emergency treatment is aimed at stabilizing the loose chest segment to reduce ineffective and exhausting chest movement, and to provide for adequate ventilation of the lungs. The segment may be immobilized by application of a weighted object, such as a sandbag, or by splinting the area using a bulky dressing and tape. The patient is transported lying on the affected side to further stabilize the chest wall. Positive pressure resuscitation is administered, using a bag-mask or the mouth-to-mouth technique.

f. joint an unusually movable joint.

Flamazine ('flaməzeen) trademark for silver sulphadiazine cream, used in the treatment of skin infections.

flame (flaym) 1. the luminous, irregular appearance usually accompanying combustion, or an appearance resembling it. 2. to render sterile by exposure to a flame.

flank (flangk) the side of the body between the ribs and ilium.

flap (flap) 1. a mass of tissue for GRAFTING, usually including skin, only partially removed from one part of the body so that it retains its own blood supply during transfer to another site. 2. an uncontrolled movement.

free f. a full-thickness skin flap detached from its

original site and reattached at a remote site by microvascular anastomosis.

island f. a flap consisting of skin and subcutaneous tissue separated at its circumference but retaining its attachment to deep tissues centrally.

jump f. a full-thickness skin flap raised in one area and moved to the recipient site by successive detachments and reattachments of its ends.

myocutaneous f. a compound flap of skin and muscle.

pedicle f. one made by elevating a full-thickness strip of skin from its bed except at one end, the cut edges then being sutured together to form a tube. One end remains attached while the other is transferred to the recipient site.

skin f. a full-thickness mass or flap of tissue containing epidermis, dermis, and subcutaneous tissue.

sliding f. a flap carried to its new position by a sliding technique.

tube f., tunnel f. pedicle flap.

flare (flair) a diffuse area of redness on the skin around the point of application of an irritant, due to vasomotor reaction.

flask (flahsk) a laboratory vessel, usually of glass and with a constricted neck.

flatfoot ('flat,fuht) a condition in which one or more arches of the foot have flattened out.

flatness ('flatnəs) a peculiar sound lacking resonance, heard on percussing an abnormally solid part.

flatulence ('flatyuhləns) excessive formation of gases in the stomach or intestine.

flatulent ('flatyuhlənt) characterized by flatulence; distended with gas.

flatus ('flaytəs) 1. gas or air in the gastrointestinal tract. 2. gas or air expelled through the anus.

flatworm ('flat,wərm) an individual organism of the phylum Platyhelminthes (see also WORMS).

flav(o)- word element. [L.] *yellow*.

flavin ('flayvin) any of a group of water-soluble yellow pigments widely distributed in animals and plants, including riboflavin and yellow enzymes. **f. adenine dinucleotide (FAD)** a coenzyme that is a condensation product of riboflavin phosphate and adenylic acid; it forms the prosthetic group of certain enzymes, including D-amino acid oxidase and xanthine oxidase, and is important in electron transport in mitochondria.

f. mononucleotide (FMN) a derivative of riboflavin consisting of a three-ring system (isoalloxazine) attached to an alcohol (ribitol); it acts as a coenzyme for a number of oxidative enzymes, including L-amino acid oxidase and cytochrome C reductase.

flavivirus ('flayvi,vierəs) a group B arbovirus, one of a subcategory of togaviruses; the type species is the yellow fever virus.

Flavobacterium (,flayvohbak'tiə·ri·əm) a genus of bacteria characteristically producing yellow, orange, red, or yellow-brown pigmentation, found in soil and water; one species, *F. meningosepticum*, is pathogenic.

flavoenzyme (,flayvoh'enziem) any enzyme containing a flavin nucleotide (FMN or FAD) as a prosthetic group.

flavoprotein (,flayvoh'prohteen) a conjugated protein containing a flavin nucleotide.

flavoxate (flay'voksayt) a smooth muscle relaxant used as a urinary tract spasmolytic for relief of symptoms associated with various urological disorders.

fl.dr. fluid dram.

flea (flee) a small, wingless, bloodsucking insect. Many fleas are ectoparasites and may act as disease carriers; they act as vectors of such diseases as plague and murine typhus.

Fleming ('fleming) Sir Alexander (1881–1955), bacteriologist and discoverer of penicillin. He was born on 6 August 1881 in Ayrshire, Scotland. In 1901 he became a student at St. Mary's Hospital medical school and took the conjoint qualification in 1906 and the MB BS of London University in 1908 with honours. In 1909 he became FRCS.

He was appointed lecturer in bacteriology in St. Mary's medical school in 1920 and eight years later he was given the title of Professor of Bacteriology in the University of London. He retired from the chair with the title emeritus in 1948, but continued until the end of 1954 as principal of the Wright–Fleming Institute of Microbiology. In 1928, Fleming made the world-famous observation which was to lead in time to the new antibiotic era. He was studying colony variation in the *Staphylococcus* in relation to the chapter he was writing on that organism for the System of Bacteriology. This necessitated frequent examination of plate cultures of the organism over a period of days when: 'It was noticed that around a large colony of a contaminating mould the *Staphylococcus* colonies became transparent and were obviously undergoing lysis'. As he himself often said, it was a chance observation which he followed up as a bacteriologist.

Fleming in his original paper, published in the *British Journal of Experimental Pathology* (June 1929), described most of the properties of what we now know as penicillin.

Innumerable honours were conferred upon Fleming in the last 10 years of his life. He was knighted in 1944, and was awarded the Nobel prize for medicine jointly with Sir Howard (later Lord) Florey and (Sir) E B Chain in 1945.

He died suddenly of a heart attack in March 1955 and is buried in St. Paul's Cathedral.

flesh (flesh) the soft muscular tissue of the animal body.

goose f. cutis anserina; erection of the papillae of the skin, as from cold or shock. Called also *goose pimples*.

proud f. exuberant granulation tissue.

flex (fleks) to bend or put in a state of flexion.

flexibilitas (,fleksi'bilitəs) [L.] *flexibility*.

f. cerea a cataleptic state in which the limbs retain any position in which they are placed; called also *waxy flexibility*.

flexibility (,fleksi'bilitee) the state of being unusually pliant.

waxy f. flexibilitas cerea.

flexion ('flekshən) the act of bending or the condition of being bent.

Flexner's bacillus ('fleksnəz) one of the group of pathogenic bacteria which cause bacillary dysentery; *Shigella flexneri*.

flexor ('fleksə) any muscle that flexes a joint.

flexura (flek'shooə·rə) pl. *flexurae* [L.] flexure.

flexure ('flekshə) a bend or fold; a curvation.

caudal f. the bend at the aboral end of the embryo.

cephalic f. the curve in the mid-brain of the embryo.

cervical f. a bend in the neural tube of the embryo at the junction of the brain and spinal cord.

colic f., left the angular junction of the transverse and descending colon.

colic f., right the angular junction of the ascending and transverse colon.

dorsal f. one of the flexures in the mid-dorsal region of the embryo.

duodenojejunal f. the bend at the junction of duodenum and jejunum.

hepatic f. right colic flexure.

lumbar f. the ventral curvature in the lumbar region of the back.

mesencephalic f. a bend in the neural tube of the embryo at the level of the mesencephalon, or midbrain.

pontine f. a flexure of the hindbrain in the embryo.

sacral f. caudal flexure.

sigmoid f. the S-shaped bend of the sigmoid colon.

splenic f. left colic flexure.

flight of ideas (fliet ov iediəz) the rapid movement of ideas and speech from one fragmentary topic to another that occurs in mania.

flint disease (flint) chalicosis.

floaters ('flohtəz) wisps or strands within the eye that are visible to the patient. Usually caused by detachment and collapse of the vitreous humour and the normal ageing process.

floating kidney ('flohting) excessive mobility of the kidney; called also *hypermobile kidney*. NEPHROPTOSIS refers to a dropping of the kidney from its normal position. Surgical correction, by NEPHROPEXY, is necessary when the condition interferes with normal kidney function.

floccillation (ˌfloksi'layshən) carphology; involuntary picking at the bedclothes, seen in grave fevers and in conditions of great exhaustion.

floccose ('flokohz) wooly; said of bacterial growth composed of short, curved chains variously oriented.

flocculation (ˌflokyuh'layshən) a colloid phenomenon in which the disperse phase separates in discrete, usually visible, particles rather than in a continuous mass, as in coagulation.

flocculent ('flokyuhlənt) containing downy or flaky shreds.

flocculus ('flokyuhləs) pl. *flocculi* [L.] 1. a small tuft or mass, as of wool or other fibrous material. 2. a small mass on the lower side of each cerebral hemisphere, continuous with the nodule of the vermis. adj. **floccular.**

flooding ('fluding) in behaviour therapy, a form of desensitization for the treatment of phobias and related disorders in which the patient is repeatedly exposed, in imagination or real life, to emotionally distressing aversive stimuli of high intensity. Called also *implosion*.

flora ('flor·rə) the collective plant organisms of a given locality.

intestinal f. the bacteria normally residing within the lumen of the intestine.

florid ('flo·rid) 1. fully developed. 2. a bright red colour.

flowmeter ('floh,meetə) an apparatus for measuring the rate of flow of liquids or gases.

fl.oz. fluid ounce.

flu (floo) popular name for INFLUENZA.

gastric f. a popular name for what may be any of several disorders of the stomach and intestinal tract.

flucloxacillin (ˌflookloksə'silin) an antibiotic drug used in the treatment of infection by penicillin-resistant bacteria.

fluctuation (ˌfluktyoo'ayshən, -chyoo-) a variation, as about a fixed variation or mass; a wavelike motion.

flucytosine (floo'sietə,seen) an antifungal used in the treatment of severe candidal and cryptococcal infections.

fludrocortisone (ˌfloodroh'kawti,sohn, -ˌzohn) a synthetic adrenal corticoid with effects similar to those of hydrocortisone and desoxycorticosterone but used for its potent mineralocorticoid activity in the treatment of adrenocortical insufficiency and in salt-losing adrenogenital syndrome.

fluid ('flooid) 1. a liquid or gas; any liquid of the body. 2. composed of molecules which freely change their relative positions without separation of the mass.

allantoic f. the fluid contained within the allantosis.

amniotic f. the fluid within the amnion that bathes the developing fetus and protects it from mechanical injury (see also AMNIOTIC FLUID).

body f's the fluids within the body, composed of water, electrolytes, and nonelectrolytes. The volume and distribution of body fluids vary with age, sex, and amount of adipose tissue. Throughout life there is a slow decline in the volume of body fluids; obesity decreases the relative amount of water in the body.

Although the body fluids are continuously in motion, moving in and out of the cells, tissue spaces, and vascular system, physiologists consider them to be 'compartmentalized'. Fluid within the cell membranes is called *intracellular* fluid and comprises about two-thirds of the total body fluids. The remaining one-third is outside the cell and is called *extracellular* fluid. The extracellular fluid can be further divided into tissue fluid (*interstitial* fluid), which is found in the spaces between the blood vessels and surrounding cells, and intravascular fluid, which is the fluid component of blood.

Intracellular fluid serves as a medium for the basic materials needed by cells for growth, repair, and performance of their various functions. Extracellular fluid circulates in the spaces between the cells and brings to them the nutrients and other substances needed for cell function.

The composition of intracellular fluid differs from that of extracellular fluid, and the difference in these components is important to the normal functioning of the cells. For example, extracellular fluid contains large amounts of the positively charged sodium ions and relatively small amounts of similarly charged potassium ions, whereas intracellular fluid contains these ions in inverse concentrations. The gain and loss of sodium is particularly important in the maintenance of FLUID BALANCE because of the ability of sodium to retain water.

The movement of body fluids and their components from one compartment to another is essential for the maintenance of constant internal conditions (HOMEOSTASIS) that allow for nutrition of the cell, excretion of waste products, and the production of energy and other specific functions of the cells. The substances passing through the cell membranes are transported by DIFFUSION and active transport. These processes are dependent on differences in the concentrations of the intracellular and extracellular fluids, the permeability of the membranes, and the effect of the positively and negatively charged ions in the fluids. The concentrations of the body fluids, particularly in regard to the amount of osmotically active particles in proportion to the amount of water (OSMOLALITY), are important to the movement of fluids in and out of their compartments. As we know from the principles of OSMOSIS, the concentration of the fluids on either side of the cell membrane directly affects the rate at which water moves in and out of the cell.

The maintenance of a proper balance between the intracellular and extracellular fluid volumes is essential to health. In patients with HEART FAILURE and renal failure the balance becomes upset, producing either localized or generalized OEDEMA. Excessive fluid loss produces FLUID VOLUME DEFICIT causing cellular dehydration and impaired cellular function.

cerebrospinal f. the fluid contained within the ventricles of the brain, the subarachnoid space, and the central canal of the spinal cord (see also CEREBROSPINAL FLUID).

f. dram a unit of liquid measure of the apothecaries' system, containing 60 minims, and equivalent to 3.697 ml.

interstitial f. the extracellular fluid bathing most tissues, excluding the fluid within the lymph and blood vessels.

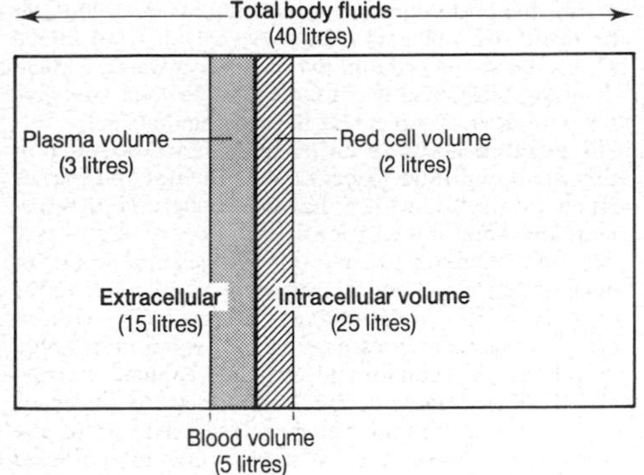

Diagrammatic representation of the body fluids, showing the extracellular fluid volume, intracellular fluid volume, blood volume and total body fluids.

f. ounce a unit of liquid measure of the apothecaries' system, being 8 fluid drams, or the equivalent of 29.57 ml.

prostatic f. the liquid secretion of the prostate, which contributes to semen formation.

seminal f. semen.

spinal f. the fluid within the spinal canal.

synovial f. synovia.

fluid balance a state in which the volume of body water and its solutes (electrolytes and nonelectrolytes) is within normal limits and there is normal distribution of fluids within the intracellular and extracellular compartments. The total volume of body fluids should be about 60 per cent of the body weight, and it should be distributed so that one-third is extracellular fluid and two-thirds intracellular fluid. Although this distribution remains constant in a healthy individual, there is continuous movement of fluid into and out of the various compartments.

Most organs are concerned in some way with the maintenance of fluid balance within the body; however, the KIDNEYS play a major role in regulating most of the constituents of the fluids. It is in the renal tubules that water is reabsorbed into the blood stream or allowed to enter the urine for excretion. The antidiuretic hormone (ADH) controls this process. It is also in the distal tubules of the kidneys that sodium reabsorption takes place and this process is influenced by the hormone aldosterone.

Water and sodium are particularly important in fluid balance because they are the components directly affecting the concentration (OSMOLALITY) of the fluids and, therefore, their distribution. The body does not tolerate differences in osmotic pressure. Thus, whenever there is an imbalance in the concentration of fluids, there is shifting of the fluids, with water moving from the less concentrated fluid to the more concentrated until an equilibrium is established. In addition to these osmotic factors, the movement of fluids in and out of compartments is affected by capillary permeability, arterial and venous blood pressure, and the rate of flow of blood through the capillaries.

The adaptive mechanisms for maintaining normal volume and distribution of fluids inside and outside the cells function only as long as there is adequate and *equal* intake and output of water and electrolytes. When either gains or losses of these components of body fluids are excessive and prolonged, a fluid imbalance exists.

A *deficit* of body fluids is manifested by either intracellular dehydration or hypovolaemia, or both. The result is an insufficient volume of fluid to meet the needs of the cells. The deficit can be made up by oral or parenteral administration of fluids. It is essential, however, that in making up the deficit overenthusiastic use of intravenous fluids does not produce an excess of water and an imbalance in the other direction. See also FLUID VOLUME DEFICIT.

An *excess* of water can be manifested as water intoxication, circulatory overload (vascular hypervolaemia), and increased volume of water within the cell or interstitial spaces (OEDEMA). See also FLUID VOLUME EXCESS.

A fluid balance record is kept on each patient who is susceptible to or already suffering from a disturbance in the balance of body fluids. This record, also called the record of intake and output, shows the amount of fluid entering the body and the amount lost from the body. Intake includes *all* routes by which water enters the body: by mouth, by rectum, via irrigation tubes, and parenterally. Output consists of all fluids lost via the urinary tract and the intestinal tract, whether by suction, vomiting and diarrhoea, or by drainage from wounds and from fistulas. An accurate measuring and recording of fluid intake and output can be a valuable aid in detecting imbalances and in determining the amount needed for fluid replacement when a fluid volume deficit is found.

In addition to measurement and recording of intake and output and evaluation of the clinical signs of fluid imbalance, certain laboratory tests are helpful in the accurate assessment of a patient's hydration status. Among these are OSMOLALITY, SODIUM, and blood UREA NITROGEN. The serum osmolality expresses the status of the concentration of dissolved particles in the serum. When the body is dehydrated by excessive fluid loss or inadequate intake, the serum is less dilute or more concentrated than it normally would be and the serum osmolality is increased. Conversely, overhydration of the body would be reflected in a less concentrated serum and a decrease in serum osmolality. Because of osmotic pressure, a state of equilibrium exists between the osmolality of serum and that of the fluid within the cells. Water moves freely across the cell membrane to maintain that equilibrium. It is possible, therefore, to determine the state of hydration within the cells by determining the osmolality of the serum. It is for this reason that serum osmolality reflects total body hydration.

Measurement of serum sodium is of value in determining the body's state of hydration because of the ability of sodium to retain water. Serum sodium concentration is not an index of sodium deficit or excess, but rather an index of water deficit or excess. An elevated level of sodium in the blood (hypernatraemia) would indicate that the loss of water from the body has exceeded the loss of sodium, as might occur, for example, in the administration of osmotic diuretics, uncontrolled diabetes insipidus, gastroenteritis, and extensive burns.

An elevated blood urea nitrogen (BUN) can be caused by hypovolaemia and is indicative of an imbalance between the rate of urea synthesis and its excretion by the kidneys. If the kidneys are functioning normally, the elevated BUN resulting from a fluid deficit can be relieved by an increased fluid intake. Fluid volume deficit also plays a major role in the development of HYPERGLYCAEMIC HYPEROSMOLAR NONKETOTIC COMA.

fluid extract a liquid preparation of a vegetable drug, containing alcohol as a solvent or preservative, or both.

fluid restriction the limitation of oral fluid intake to a prescribed amount for each 24-hour period. This therapeutic measure is indicated in patients who have oedema associated with kidney disease, such as nephrotic syndrome and glomerulonephritis, or Laënnec's cirrhosis, and also in certain patients with pulmonary oedema.

Approaches to the problem of discomfort from thirst and dryness of the mouth include careful distribution of the fluid intake over the entire 24 hours in small, frequent drinks; giving oral medications at mealtime, when not contraindicated, so as to allow sips of liquid at other times; providing cold water for rinsing the mouth without swallowing between drinks; giving hard sweets and chewing gum; and allowing the patient to choose the fluids he prefers to drink. Frequent mouth care with a refreshing mouthwash also is helpful.

fluid volume deficit an imbalance in fluid volume in which there is loss of fluid from the body not compensated for by an adequate intake of water. The major causes are: (1) insufficient fluid intake, and (2) excessive fluid loss from vomiting, diarrhoea, suctioning of gastric contents, or drainage through operative wounds, burns, or fistulas. Decreased volume in the intravascular compartment is called *hypovolaemia.* Because water moves freely between the compartments, extracellular fluid deficit causes intracellular fluid deficit (*cellular dehydration*), which leaves the cells without adequate water to carry on normal function.

When a person engages in normal physical activity and the environmental temperature is 20 °C, the body loses about 2400 ml of water a day; about 1400 ml is lost in the urine, 200 ml in faeces, and 100 ml in sweat. The remaining 700 ml are lost through what is called *insensible water loss;* that is, one does not sense that the water is being excreted. Insensible water loss occurs through the skin by diffusion, and by evaporation from the lungs. About 300 ml of water diffuse through the epithelial cells. The lungs excrete about 400 ml per day.

PATIENT CARE. There are several laboratory tests used in assessing the hydration status of the patient. It is important that all health care professionals responsible for the care of a patient with a fluid deficit be familiar with the patient's test results. The plan of care should include the monitoring of serum sodium, serum osmolality, blood urea nitrogen, blood pH, and serum bicarbonate levels.

Daily weighing of the patient gives information about the amount of body water gained or lost each day. Intake and output amounts should be maintained within normal limits. One criterion that indicates an adequate replacement of fluid is a urinary output of 50 to 100 ml per hour. Other criteria include a systolic blood pressure of 100 mmHg, which would indicate correction of hypovolaemia, and a pulse of less than 120 beats per minute.

The care plan of a patient with existing or potential fluid volume deficit should include frequent evaluation of bowel sounds and notation of the presence or absence of nausea. Notice should be given to the patient's mental acuity and orientation to person, place, and time. These latter observations are particularly important in the care of a patient who is in danger of profound and potentially fatal fluid deficit, as in a severe and extensive burn case.

Measures to improve hydration must take into account the patient's ability to drink and retain oral fluids, his preference for certain liquids, and whether he prefers hot or cold drinks. A goal for fluid intake should be about 2000 ml per day. Fresh water, a clean drinking glass, and a gracious offer to help can give the patient encouragement in reaching that goal.

fluid volume excess an overabundance of water in the interstitial fluid spaces or body cavities (*oedema*) or an excess of fluid within the blood vessels (*hypervolaemia*) and water intoxication.

Factors that contribute to the accumulation of oedematous fluid are: (1) dilation of the arteries, as occurs in the inflammatory process; (2) reduced effective osmotic pressure, as in hypoproteinaemia, lymphatic obstruction, and increased capillary permeability; (3) increased venous pressure, as in congestive heart failure, thrombophlebitis, and cirrhosis of the liver; and (4) retention of sodium due to increased reabsorption of sodium by the renal tubules.

PATIENT CARE. The plan of care for a patient with fluid volume excess will depend in large part on his specific medical diagnosis, the cause of the oedema or hypervolaemia, and the particular problems identified through assessment. The measurement of intake and output and daily weight, careful handling of oedematous tissue to maintain integrity of the skin, and restriction of sodium (and possibly fluid) intake are usually included in the care of all patients with fluid excess. Those patients who have localized oedema, as from inflammation, lymphatic obstruction, and ASCITES, will need an objective measurement of the size of the oedematous area to determine whether or not the accumulation of fluid is increasing or decreasing.

fluidrachm (ˌflooid'dram) fluid dram.

fluke (flook) an organism of the class Trematoda (phylum Platyhelminthes), characterized by a body that is usually flat and often leaflike. Trematodes can infect the blood, liver, intestines, and lungs. See also WORM.

flumen ('floomen) pl. *flumina* [L.] a stream. **flumina pilorum** the lines along which the hairs of the body are arranged.

flumethasone (floo'methəˌzohn) an anti-inflammatory glucocorticoid used topically in the treatment of certain dermatoses.

flunisolide (floo'nisəˌlied) an anti-inflammatory steroid administered as an aerosol spray to the nasal mucosa in the treatment of seasonal or perennial rhinitis when conventional treatment is unsatisfactory.

fluocinolone acetonide (ˌfloo·oh'sinəˌlohn) an anti-inflammatory glucocorticoid used topically in eczema.

fluocinonide (ˌfloo·oh'sinəˌnied) an ester of fluocinolone acetonide used topically in the treatment of certain inflammatory, pruritic, and allergic skin conditions.

fluorescein (ˌflooə'resee·in) a fluorescing dye; the sodium salt is used in solution to reveal corneal epithelial damage and in fluorescein angiography of the retinal circulation.

fluorescence (ˌflooə'res'ns) the property of emitting light while exposed to light, the wavelength of the emitted light being longer than that of the absorbed light. adj. **fluorescent**.

f. microscopy the use of techniques for conjugating antibodies with fluorescent dyes in order to identify specific microorganisms or tissue constituents using a fluorescence microscope. Fluorescent antibody (FA) techniques can be used in place of time-consuming culture methods for identifying bacteria. There are two major types of FA techniques, direct and indirect, both of which are based on the antigen–antibody reaction in which the antibody attaches itself to its specific antigen.

In the *direct* fluorescent antibody (DFA) method, the antibody coats the antigen, for example, a bacterial cell, and cannot be easily removed by elution (washing). The antibody remains attached to the cell after all nonantibody globulin has been washed away. Since the antibody has been rendered fluorescent by conjugation with fluorescein or another dye, the outline of the bacterial cell that it coats can readily be seen with a special microscope.

In the indirect method (IFA), the specific antibody is allowed to react with the antigen. The nonantibody globulin is then washed off. This is then treated with a labelled antibody to the specific antibody. For example, if the specific antibody was raised in a rabbit, it is then treated with fluorescein labelled anti-rabbit globulin, which results in a combination of this labelled antibody with the rabbit immunoglobulin already attached to the antigen.

Fluorescent antibody studies have been used in the detection of numerous bacterial, viral, fungal, and protozoan infections and in the identification of many microscopic tissue constituents.

fluorescent (ˌflooə'res'nt) capable of producing fluorescence.

f. screen a screen which becomes fluorescent when exposed to x-rays.

f. treponemal antibody test a serological test for syphilis; the first to become positive after infection.

fluoridation (ˌflooə·ri'dayshən) treatment with fluorides; the addition of fluorides to drinking water as a measure to reduce the incidence of dental caries.

Minute traces of fluoride are found in almost all food, but the quantity apparently is too small to meet the requirements of the body in building tooth enamel that resists CARIES. Drinking water containing one part fluoride to one million parts of water does meet this need. It has been found to reduce tooth decay in children by as much as 40 to 60 per cent. Since few natural water supplies contain the necessary amount of fluoride, it usually must be added if protection against tooth decay is desired.

Recent statistics indicate that 20 per cent of the teenagers who drank fluoridated water from birth have teeth that are totally free of caries. There also is evidence that topically applied fluoride solutions help alleviate periodontal disease by removing bacteria from the site and rebuilding supporting bone tissue around the teeth.

In spite of the evidence in favour of fluoridation, some authorities have hesitated to add fluoride to their water supply because of economic and moral objections. In fact in the UK only about 10 per cent of the population drink fluoridated water. This compares rather poorly with about 40 per cent in the USA and 90 per cent in Australia.

When fluoridated water is not available, it is possible to safeguard the teeth by other means. Dentists may apply fluoride solutions directly to a child's teeth, beginning as soon as the first teeth appear, and repeating this treatment every 3 or 4 years until the child is 13. This has been found to reduce caries by about 40 per cent.

Fluoridated water can be bought by the bottle or prepared at home, but both methods require special care and are far more costly to the individual than is the fluoridation of a public water supply. The dentist or doctor may prescribe sodium fluoride drops to be added to milk, water, or juice. The use of these drops must be carefully supervised, since a slight excess of fluoride causes mottling of teeth (dental FLUOROSIS) and since, like most medicines, fluoride in large amounts is a poison. Taking fluoride by drops or tablets is however widely recommended and is an important part of the work of public health dentistry in the UK. A toothpaste containing fluoride may also prove effective. A gel form of fluoride is also available for home use. A dentist should be consulted before any fluoride preparation is used.

fluoride ('flooəˌried) any binary compound of fluorine.

fluoridization (ˌflooə·ridie'zayshən) 1. application of fluoride solution to the teeth. 2. fluoridation.

fluorimeter (ˌflooə'rimitə) fluorometer.

fluorimetry (ˌflooə'rimətree) fluorometry.

fluorine ('flooə·reen) a chemical element, atomic number 9, atomic weight 18.998, symbol F. See table of elements in Appendix 2.

fluorochrome ('flooə·rəˌkrohm) a fluorescent compound, as a dye, used to mark protein with a fluorescent label.

fluorography (ˌflooə'rografee) the photographic recording of fluoroscopic images on small films, using a fast lens; a procedure used in mass radiography of the chest. Called also *photofluorography*.

fluorometer (ˌflooə'romitə) the instrument used in fluorometry, consisting of an energy source (e.g., a mercury arc lamp or xenon lamp) to induce fluorescence, monochromators for selection of the wavelength, and a detector.

fluorometholone (ˌflooə·roh'methəˌlohn) an anti-inflammatory glucocorticoid used as eye drops in non-infective inflammatory conditions.

fluorometry (ˌflooə'romətree) an analytical technique for identifying minute amounts of a substance by detection and measurement of the characteristic wavelength of the light it emits during fluorescence.

fluorophotometry (ˌflooə·rohfə'tomətree) the measurement of light given off by fluorescent substances.

vitreous f. the measurement of light given off by intravenously injected fluorescein that has leaked through the retinal vessels into the vitreous; done to detect the breakdown of the blood-retinal barrier, an early ocular change in diabetes mellitus.

fluororoentgenography (ˌflooə·rohˌrontjə'nogrəfee) fluorography.

fluoroscope (ˌflooə·rəˌskohp) an instrument for the study of moving internal organs and contrast medium in motion using x-rays. It is also used for optimal patient positioning so that better radiographs may be obtained. Radiological examination by this method is called fluoroscopy. The simplest fluoroscope uses an x-tray tube which projects its image onto a flat fluorescent screen. The visual image produced by this instrument is of such low intensity that the human eye must adapt to darkness before it can be viewed. Modern fluoroscopy uses a device called an image intensifier instead of the fluoroscopic screen and this amplifies the image so that it is bright enough to be seen in daylight. This image is usually transferred via a television camera to a television or the image intensifier can be coupled to a cine or still camera.

fluoroscopy (ˌflooə'roskəpee) examination by means of the fluoroscope.

fluorosis (ˌflooə'rohsis) a condition due to ingestion of excessive amounts of fluorine or its compounds. See also FLUORIDATION.

dental f. an enamel hypoplasia resulting from prolonged ingestion of drinking water containing high levels of fluoride, manifested by a mottled discoloration of the teeth.

endemic f., chronic that due to unusually high concentrations of fluorine in the natural drinking water supply, typically causing dental fluorosis but also combined osteosclerosis and osteomalacia.

fluorouracil (ˌflooə·roh'yooə·rəsil) an antimetabolite

used as an antineoplastic agent.

Fluothane ('floo·oh,thayn) trademark for a preparation of halothane, a general anaesthetic.

fluoxymesterone (floo,oksi'mestə,rohn) an anabolic androgenic steroid used in the treatment of male hypogonadism and the palliative treatment of certain cancers.

flupenthixol (,floopen'thiksol) a thioxanthene used in the treatment of schizophrenia.

fluphenazine (floo'fenə,zeen) a major tranquillizer, used as the enanthate, decanoate or hydrochloride salt.

flurandrenolone (,flooə·ran'drenəlohn) a topical steroid used for eczema and other inflammatory skin conditions which have not responded to weaker steroids.

flurazepam (,flooə'razipam) a hypnotic, used as the hydrochloride salt.

flurbiprofen (,flərbi'prohfen) a nonsteroidal anti-inflammatory drug which is a propionic acid derivative.

flush (flush) redness, usually transient, of the face and neck.

hectic f. a persistent or chronic flush associated with chronic debilitating disease, usually febrile.

malar f. hectic flush at the malar eminence.

flutter ('flutə) a rapid vibration or pulsation.

atrial f. cardiac arrhythmia in which the atrial contractions are rapid (200–320 per minute), but regular.

diaphragmatic f. peculiar wavelike fibrillations of the diaphragm of unknown cause.

impure f. atrial flutter in which the atrial rhythm is irregular.

mediastinal f. abnormal mobility of the mediastinum during respiration.

pure f. atrial flutter in which the atrial rhythm is regular.

ventricular f. a possible transition stage between ventricular tachycardia and ventricular fibrillation, the electrocardiogram showing rapid, uniform, and virtually regular oscillations, 250 or more per minute.

flutter-fibrillation (,flutə,fibri'layshən) impure flutters that vary from moment to moment in their resemblance to flutter or fibrillation, respectively.

flux (fluks) 1. an excessive flow or discharge. 2. matter discharged.

bloody f. dysentery.

fly (flie) a dipterous, or two-winged insect, which is often the vector of organisms causing disease.

Fm chemical symbol, *fermium*.

FMN flavin mononucleotide.

FNIF Florence Nightingale International Foundation.

focus ('fohkəs) pl. *foci* [L.] 1. the point of convergence of light rays or sound waves. 2. the chief centre of a morbid process. adj. **focal.**

Ghon f. the primary parenchymal lesion of primary pulmonary TUBERCULOSIS in children. Called also *Ghon tubercle*.

focusing ('fohkəsing) the act of converging at a point.

isoelectric f. electrophoresis in which the protein mixture is subjected to an electric field in a gel medium in which a pH gradient has been established; each protein then migrates until it reaches the site at which the pH is equal to its isoelectric point.

foe- for words beginning thus, see those beginning *fe-*.

fog (fog) a colloid system in which the dispersion medium is a gas and the dispersed particles are liquid.

fogging ('foging) in ophthalmology, a method of determining refractive error in astigmatism, the patient being first made artifically myopic by means of plus spheres, in order to relax all accommodation before using cylinders.

folate ('fohlayt) a general term used to describe a large group of compounds, i.e., the folates, which are derived from the parent compound, FOLIC ACID (pteroylglutamic acid). Chemical reactions which change folic acid to folates include (1) reduction to metabolically active forms, (2) the addition of extra glutamic acid residues and (3) the addition of single carbon units (e.g., methyl, methylene). Folates are essential for a variety of biochemical reactions in the body, the most important of which is required for DNA synthesis. Folate levels in the serum and red blood cells are measurable and are used to assess the body stores; low levels of both are found in megaloblastic anaemia secondary to folate deficiency.

fold (fohld) plica; a thin, recurved margin, or doubling.

amniotic f. the folded edge of the amnion where it rises over and finally encloses the embryo.

aryepiglottic f. a fold of mucous membrane extending on each side between the lateral border of the epiglottis and the summit of the arytenoid cartilage.

circular f's the permanent transverse folds of the luminal surface of the small intestine.

costocolic f. a fold of peritoneum passing from the left colic flexure to the adjacent part of the diaphragm. Called also *phrenicocolic ligament*.

Douglas f. a crescentic line marking the termination of the posterior layer of the sheath of the rectus abdominis muscle just below the level of the iliac crest.

gastric f's the series of folds in the mucous membrane of the stomach.

gluteal f. the crease separating the buttocks from the thigh.

head f. a fold of blastoderm at the cephalic end of the developing embryo.

lacrimal f. a fold of mucous membrane at the lower opening of the nasolacrimal duct.

mucosal f., mucous f. a fold of mucous membrane.

nail f. the fold of palmar skin around the base and sides of the nail of a finger or toe.

neural f. one of the paired folds lying on either side of the neural plate that form the neural tube.

palmate f's folds on the anterior and posterior walls of the cervical canal.

semilunar f. of conjunctiva a mucous fold at the medial angle of the eye.

spiral f. a spirally arranged elevation in the mucosa of the first part of the cystic duct.

tail f. a fold of the blastoderm at the caudal end of the developing embryo.

transverse f's three permanent transverse folds in the rectum.

ventricular f., vestibular f. a false vocal cord.

vestigial f. a pericardial fold enclosing the remnant of the embryonic left anterior cardinal vein.

vocal f. a fold of mucous membrane in the larynx, forming the inferior boundary of the ventricle of the larynx, the vocal muscle being situated deep to it; called also *true vocal chord*.

folic acid ('fohlik) one of the VITAMINS of the B complex. Folic acid is involved in the synthesis of amino acids and DNA; its deficiency causes megaloblastic anaemia. Green vegetables, liver, and yeast are major sources of folic acid in the diet. It is also produced synthetically. Folic acid deficiency may result from the inability of the body to utilize the vitamin.

acid f. a. antagonist a compound, such as methotrexate, that acts as an antimetabolite of folic acid, interfering with DNA replication and cell division by inhibiting the enzyme dihydrofolate reductase; used in the treatment of many tumours.

folie (fo'lee) [Fr.] *psychosis, insanity.*

f. à deux the occurrence of identical psychoses

simultaneously in two closely associated persons.

f. à quatre the occurrence of identical psychoses simultaneously in four closely associated persons.

f. à trois the occurrence of identical psychoses simultaneously in three closely associated persons.

f. circulaire the circular form of manic-depressive psychosis.

f. du doute pathological inability to make even the most trifling decisions.

f. du pourquoi psychopathological constant questioning.

f. gémellaire psychosis occurring simultaneously in twins.

f. musculaire severe chorea.

folinic acid (foh'linik) 5-formyltetrahydrofolic acid, a metabolically active derivative of folic acid used to treat folic acid deficiency and as an antidote to folic acid antagonists. Called also *citrovorum factor* and *leucovorin*.

folium ('fohli·əm) pl. *folia* [L.] a leaflike structure, especially one of the leaflike subdivisions of the cerebellar cortex.

follicle ('folik'l) a sac or pouchlike depression or cavity. adj. **follicular**.

atretic f. an involuted ovarian follicle.

f. centre cells (FCC) dividing lymphocytes which develop into centrocytes and centroblasts which are found within follicular germinal centres arising in lymph nodes and other lymphoid tissue in response to antigenic stimulation.

dental f. the structure within the substance of the jaws enclosing a tooth before its eruption; the dental sac and its contents.

gastric f's lymphoid masses in the gastric mucosa.

graafian f. a maturing ovarian follicle among whose cells fluid has begun to accumulate, leading to the formation of a single cavity and leaving the ovum located in the cumulus oophorus; called also vesicular ovarian follicle (see also GRAAFIAN FOLLICLE).

hair f. one of the tubular invaginations of the epidermis enclosing the hairs, and from which the hairs grow.

lymph f., lymphatic f 1. a small collection of actively proliferating lymphocytes in the cortex of a lymph node. 2. a small collection of lymphoid tissue in the mucous membrane of the gastrointestinal tract; such collections may occur singly (solitary lymphatic follicle) or closely packed together (aggregated lymphatic follicles).

Naboth's f's, nabothian f's Naboth's cysts.

ovarian f. the ovum and its encasing cells, at any stage of its development.

ovarian f., primary an immature ovarian follicle consisting of an immature ovum and the few specialized epithelial cells surrounding it.

primordial f. an ovarian follicle consisting of an ovum enclosed by a single layer of cells.

sebaceous f. a hair follicle with a relatively large sebaceous gland, producing a relatively insignificant hair.

solitary f's 1. areas of concentrated lymphatic tissue in the mucosa of the colon. 2. small lymph follicles scattered throughout the mucosa and submucosa of the small intestine. Called also *solitary glands*.

thyroid f's discrete cystlike units filled with a colloid substance, constituting the lobules of the thyroid gland.

vesicular f. graafian follicle.

follicle-stimulating hormone (ˌfolik'l'stimyoolayting) one of the gonadotrophic hormones of the anterior lobe of the PITUITARY GLAND that stimulates the growth and maturation of graafian follicles in the ovary, and stimulates spermatogenesis in the testis. Abbreviated FSH.

follicular (fo'likyuhlə) pertaining to a follicle.

f. conjunctivitis conjunctivitis associated with proliferation of lymphoid tissue in the tarsal conjunctiva. Often viral or chlamydial in origin.

f. tonsillitis tonsillitis arising from infection of the tonsillar follicles.

folliculitis (foˌlikyuh'lietis) inflammation of a follicle(s); used ordinarily in reference to hair follicles, but sometimes in relation to follicles of other kinds.

f. barbae a papulopustular folliculitis of the beard; called also *barber's itch* or SYCOSIS BARBAE and caused by staphylococci. Treatment involves not shaving and applying topical antibiotics to the anterior nares and the beard area.

keloid f. infection of hair follicles of the back of the neck and scalp, occurring chiefly in men, producing large, irregular keloid plaques and scarring.

folliculoma (foˌlikyuh'lohmə) granulosa–theca cell tumour.

folliculosis (foˌlikyuh'lohsis) an abnormal increase in the number of lymph follicles.

conjunctival f. a benign non-inflammatory overgrowth of follicles of the conjunctiva of the eyelids. Usually occurs in children.

folliculus (fo'likyuhləs) pl. *folliculi* [L.] follicle.

fomentation (ˌfohmen'tayshən) treatment by warm, moist applications; also, the substance thus applied.

fomes ('fohmeez) see FOMITES.

fomites (fə'mieteez, 'fohmə-) [L.] plural of *fomes;* inanimate objects or material on which disease-producing agents may be conveyed.

fontanelle (ˌfontə'nel) a soft spot; one of the membrane-covered spaces remaining at the junction of the sutures in the incompletely ossified skull of the fetus or infant. Actually there are two soft spots close together, representing gaps in the bone structure which will be filled in by bone during the normal process of growth. The anterior fontanelle is diamond shaped and lies at the junction of the frontal and parietal bones. This fontanelle usually fills in and closes between the eighth and fifteenth months of life. The posterior fontanelle lies at the junction of the occipital and parietal bones, is triangular in shape and usually closes by the third or fourth month of life. Though these 'soft spots' may appear very vulnerable, they may be touched gently without harm. Care should be exercised that they are protected from strong pressure or direct injury.

food (food) anything which, when taken into the body, serves to nourish or build up the tissues or to supply body heat.

f. poisoning a group of notifiable acute illnesses due to ingestion of contaminated food. It may result from toxaemia from foods, such as those inherently poisonous or those contaminated by poisons; foods containing poisons formed by bacteria, or foodborne infections. Food poisoning usually causes inflammation of the gastrointestinal tract (gastroenteritis). This may occur quite suddenly, soon after the food has been eaten. The symptoms are acute, and include tenderness, pain or cramps in the abdomen, nausea, vomiting, diarrhoea, weakness, and dizziness.

Food poisoning is often falsely attributed to ptomaines, substances that are formed when protein foods 'spoil', or decompose. Because ptomaines produce toxic reactions when injected into experimental animals, 'ptomaine poisoning' was formerly believed to be responsible for food-poisoning symptoms in human beings. It is now known that the human digestive system is well able to cope with these substances.

Although they should be avoided, spoiled foods are not necessarily harmful. When they are, it is because foods in the process of decomposition frequently harbour disease-causing bacteria.

Bacterial food poisoning may be staphylococcal in origin or it may result from other microorganisms, as in BOTULISM or salmonella infections.

Staphylococcal poisoning is a common form of food poisoning. If a food handler is afflicted with a staphylococcal infection, or if he is a carrier, one of the rare persons who carries the disease without suffering infection, he may pass the bacteria on to food. In some foods, the bacteria will multiply very quickly, especially if the food is not refrigerated. Staphylococci are toxin-producing bacteria which do not harm the body directly but produce poisonous substances in the body, causing disease symptoms. The symptoms of staphylococcal poisoning result from the effects of the toxins which have built up in the staphylococci-harbouring food. The condition does not spread throughout the body and is not infectious.

Custard-filled pastry is the food most liable to contain staphylococci. Other susceptible foods are cream, milk, cheddar cheese, potato salad, many kinds of sauces, and processed meats, especially ham. These foods should always be purchased from reliable dealers and be kept refrigerated.

Staphylococcal poisoning is characterized by a sudden, sometimes violent onset of nausea, vomiting, and weakness. There may be severe diarrhoea. It is rarely serious, except for young children, the elderly, and persons who are weakened by other illness. Symptoms may appear as soon as half an hour or as late as 4 hours after the contaminated food is eaten.

There are a number of poisonous berries and mushrooms. Every year people die or become seriously ill because they have decided that one of these looks good enough to eat. Children are frequently tempted by poisonous holly berries or the berries that grow on privet (the shrub often used for hedges). Adults often place their faith in some incorrect notion, such as the old superstition that you can tell edible mushrooms from toadstools by cooking a silver coin with them; the coin is supposed to tarnish if the variety is poisonous. These mistaken notions cause a number of deaths every year. Although it is possible to learn to identify poisonous mushrooms and berries, it is much wiser to play safe. Children should be trained not to eat things they find in the woods or fields.

Mushroom poisoning causes a sudden reduction in the concentration of sugar in the blood. There may be convulsions, severe abdominal pain, intense thirst, nausea, vomiting, diarrhoea, dimness of vision, and symptoms resembling those of alcoholic intoxication. Symptoms appear 6 to 15 hours after eating.

Mussels and clams may grow in beds contaminated by the typhoid bacillus (*Salmonella typhi*) and other pathogens. Mussels, clams, and certain other shellfish are dangerous during some seasons of the year. They become poisonous as a result of feeding on microorganisms that appear in the ocean during the warm months, particularly in the Pacific. Shellfish poisoning is characterized by paralysis of the respiratory tract. The symptoms vary. There may be trembling about the lips or loss of power in the muscles of the neck. Symptoms develop within 5 to 30 minutes after eating.

FIRST AID FOR FOOD POISONING.

1. Give the patient weak tea and, when he can tolerate them, soft foods.
2. Keep the patient warm and apply heat to the abdomen by means of an electric pad or hot water bottle.
3. The patient should be seen by a doctor as soon as possible.

Botulism and Poisoning from Mushrooms, Berries, or Shellfish. If the patient has difficulty seeing, swallowing, or breathing; or if his eyes are sunken; or if his breath has a sweet, fruity odour, his condition is serious and a doctor should be called immediately.

foot (fuht) the distal part of the primate leg, upon which the individual stands and walks.

athlete's f. a chronic, superficial fungal infection of the skin of the foot (see also ATHLETE'S FOOT, TINEA PEDIS).

dangle f., drop f. a condition in which the foot hangs in a plantar-flexed position, due to lesion of the peroneal nerve.

flat f. flatfoot.

immersion f. a condition resembling trench foot occurring in persons who have spent long periods in water.

Madura f. maduromycosis of the foot.

march f. painful swelling of the foot, usually with a stress fracture of a metatarsal bone, after excessive foot strain.

trench f. a condition of the feet resembling FROSTBITE, due to the prolonged action of water on the skin combined with circulatory disturbance due to cold and inaction.

foot-pound ('fuht,pownd) the amount of energy necessary to raise 1 pound of mass a distance of 1 foot.

footboard ('fuht,bord) a device placed at the foot of the bed and situated so that the feet rest firmly against it and are at right angles to the legs. It is used to relieve the weight of the bedclothes and to maintain proper positioning of the feet while a patient is confined to bed. Its purpose is to prevent the development of footdrop. It also helps maintain good posture because it prevents the patient from slipping down in bed.

A footboard can be made from wood or improvised from a cardboard box. When the patient is a child and immobilization of the foot, as well as correct positioning, is desired, rubber-soled tennis shoes can be nailed to the footboard and the child's feet laced into the shoes.

footdrop ('fuht,drop) dropping of the foot from paralysis of the anterior muscles of the leg.

footplate ('fuht,playt) the flat portion of the stapes, which is set into the oval window on the medial wall of the middle ear.

foramen (fo'raymən) pl. *foramina* [L.] an anatomical opening.

apical f. an opening at or near the apex of the root of a tooth.

auditory f., external the external acoustic meatus.

auditory f., internal the passage for the auditory (vestibulocochlear) and facial nerves in the pars petrosa of the temporal bone.

caecal f. 1. a blind opening between the frontal crest and the crista galli. 2. a pit on the dorsum of the tongue at the median sulcus.

condyloid f., anterior hypoglossal canal.

condyloid f., posterior condylar canal. **epiploic f.** an opening connecting the two sacs of the peritoneum, situated below and behind the porta hepatis.

ethmoidal foramina, foramina ethmoidalis small openings in the ethmoid bone at the junction of the medial wall with the roof of the orbit, the anterior transmitting the nasal branch of the ophthalmic nerve and the anterior ethmoid vessels, the posterior transmitting the posterior ethmoid vessels.

incisive f. one of the openings of the incisive canals into the incisive fossa of the hard palate.

interventricular f. a passage from the third to the

lateral ventricle of the brain. **intervertebral f.** a passage for a spinal nerve and vessels formed by notches on the pedicles of adjacent vertebrae.
jugular f. an opening in the base of the skull formed by the jugular notches of the temporal and occipital bones.
f. magnum a large opening in the anterior inferior part of the occipital bone, between the cranial cavity and spinal canal, and accommodating the brain stem.
mastoid f. an opening in the temporal bone behind the mastoid process.
f. of Monro interventricular foramen.
obturator f. the large opening between the pubic bone and the ischium.
optic f. a canal through to the orbit transmitting the optic nerve.
f. ovale 1. the septal opening in the fetal heart that provides a communication between the atria. The opening closes at birth; failure to close results in atrial septal defect (see also CONGENITAL HEART DEFECT). 2. an aperture in the great wing of the sphenoid for the trigeminal nerve.
palatine f., anterior incisive foramen.
f. rotundum a round opening in the great wing of the sphenoid for the maxillary branch of the trigeminal nerve.
sacral foramina, anterior eight passages (four on each side) on the anterior surface of the sacrum for the anterior branches of the sacral nerves.
sacral foramina, posterior eight passages (four on each side) on the dorsal surface of the sacrum for the posterior branches of the sacral nerves.
Scarpa's f. an opening behind the upper medial incisor, for the nasopalatine nerve.
sciatic f. either of two foramina, the greater and the lesser sciatic foramina, formed by the sacrotuberal and sacrospinal ligaments in the sciatic notch of the hip bone.
sphenopalatine f. a space between the orbital and sphenoidal processes of the palatine bone, opening into the nasal cavity and transmitting the sphenopalatine artery and the nasal nerves.
f. spinosum, spinous f. a hole in the great wing of the sphenoid for the middle meningeal artery.
supraorbital f. passage in the frontal bone for the supraorbital vessels and nerve; often present as a notch bridged only by fibrous tissue.
thebesian foramina minute openings in the walls of the right atrium through which the smallest cardiac veins (thebesian veins) empty into the heart.
transverse f. the passage in either transverse process of a cervical vertebra that, in the upper six vertebrae, transmits the vertebral vessels.
vena cava f. an opening in the diaphragm for the inferior vena cava and some branches of the right vagus nerve.
vertebral f. 1. the large opening in a vertebra formed by its body and its arch. 2. transverse foramen.
f. of Vesalius an occasional opening medial to the foramen ovale of the sphenoid, for passage of a vein from the cavernous sinus.
f. of Winslow epiploic foramen.

Forbes' disease (forbz) glycogenosis (type III) in which a deficiency of the debrancher enzyme dextrin-1,6-glucosidase affects the heart and liver, with hepatomegaly, hypoglycaemia, acidosis, stunted growth, and doll facies. Called also *Cori's disease* and *limit dextrinosis*.

force (faws) energy or power; that which originates or arrests motion or other activity.
electromotive f. the force that, by reason of differences in potential, causes a flow of electricity from one place to another, giving rise to an electric current.
reserve f. energy above that required for normal functioning. In the heart it is the power that will take care of the additional circulatory burden imposed by bodily exertion.
Van der Waals f's the relatively weak, short-range forces of attraction existing between atoms and molecules, which results in the attraction of nonpolar organic compounds to each other (hydrophobic bonding); see BOND.

forceps ('forseps) pl. *forcipes* [L.] a two-bladed instrument for compressing or grasping tissues in surgical operations, for handling sterile dressings, etc., or for assisting the delivery of a baby.
alligator f. strong toothed forceps having a double clamp.
artery f. forceps with a ratchet mechanism used to maintain haemostasis until ligation of a vessel can be achieved.
axis traction f. obstetric forceps which allow traction to be applied along the line of the pelvic axis.
Chamberlen f. the original form of obstetric forceps.
Cheatle f. long forceps for lifting utensils.
clamp f. a forceps-like clamp with an automatic lock, for compressing arteries, etc.
dissecting f. forceps with ridged flat blades for grasping tissues.
dressing f. forceps with scissor-like handles for grasping drainage tubes and wound dressings.
Kielland f. obstetric forceps with a sliding lock and no pelvic curve, designed to apply to the fetal head whatever its position in the pelvis.
obstetric f. forceps for extracting the fetal head from the maternal passages.
Simpson f. obstetric forceps with both a pelvic and a cephalic curve.
Spencer Wells f. artery forceps for compressing bleeding points.
vulsellum f. forceps with hinged blades used to apply traction to structures.
Wrigley f. small, light, obstetric forceps with a short shank.

Fordyce's disease ('fawdiesiz) a developmental anomaly marked by enlarged and ectopic sebaceous glands that appear as minute yellowish papules on the oral mucosa.

forearm ('for,ahm) the part of the arm between the elbow and wrist; antebrachium.

forebrain ('for,brayn) prosencephalon. 1. the portion of the brain developed from the anterior of the three primary brain vesicles in the early embryo, and comprising the diencephalon and telencephalon. 2. the most anterior of the primary brain vesicles.

foreconscious ('for,konshəs) preconscious; material not ordinarily in consciousness, but subject to voluntary recall.

forefinger ('for,fing·gə) the first or index finger.

forefoot ('for,fuht) the front part of the foot.

foregut ('for,gut) the endodermal canal of the embryo cephalic to the junction of the yolk stalk, giving rise to the pharynx, lung, oesophagus, stomach, liver, and most of the small intestine.

forehead ('for,hed, 'fo·rid) the part of the face above the eyes; the anterior portion of the cranium. Called also *frons*.

forensic (fə'renzik, -sik) pertaining to or applied in legal proceedings.

foreplay ('for,play) the sexually stimulating, usually pleasurable, play preceding intercourse.

foreskin ('for,skin) prepuce; a loose fold of skin that covers the glans penis. It is a continuation of the loose skin that covers the entire penis and scrotum.

forewaters ('for,wawtəz) the part of the amniotic sac that pouches into the uterine cervix in front of the presenting part of the fetus.

fork (fawk) a pronged instrument.

tuning f. a device that produces harmonic vibration of a particular frequency when its two prongs are struck; used to test hearing and bone conduction.

formaldehyde (faw'maldi,hied) a gaseous compound with strongly disinfectant properties. It is used in solution (formol) for disinfection of excreta and utensils and also in the preparation of toxoids from toxins.

formalin ('fawməlin) a 37 per cent solution of gaseous formaldehyde which, once suitably further diluted, is used as a fixative.

formamidase (for'mami,dayz) an enzyme that catalyses the hydrolysis of formylkynurenine to kynurenine and formate in tryptophan metabolism.

formatio (for'mayshioh) pl. *formationes* [L.] formation.

formation (for'mayshən) 1. the process of giving shape or form; the creation of an entity, or of a structure of definite shape. 2. a structure of definite shape.

reaction f. the development of mental mechanisms which hold in check and repress the components of forbidden wishes.

formic acid ('fawmik) a colourless, pungent liquid with vesicant properties, from nettles and ants and other insects; derivable from oxalic acid and from glycerin and from the oxidation of formaldehyde.

formication (,fawmi'kayshən) a sensation as if small insects were crawling on the body.

formiciasis (,fawmi'kieəsis) a morbid condition caused by ant bites.

formiminoglutamic acid (,fawmi'meenohgloo,tamik) a product of histidine metabolism; abbreviated FIGLU. The urine FIGLU concentration is elevated in some individuals with folic acid deficiency.

formol ('formol) formaldehyde solution.

formula ('fawmyuhlə) pl. *formulae,formulas* [L.] 1. an expression, using numbers or symbols, of the composition of, or of directions for preparing, a compound, such as a medicine, or of a procedure to follow to obtain a desired result, or of a single concept. 2. a mixture for feeding an infant, composed of milk and/or other ingredients.

chemical f. a combination of symbols used to express the chemical components of a substance.

empirical f. a chemical formula that expresses the proportions of the elements present in a substance.

molecular f. a chemical formula expressing the number of each element present in a substance, without indicating how they are linked.

spatial f., stereochemical f. a chemical formula giving the numbers of atoms of each element present in a molecule of a substance, which atom is linked to which, the types of linkages involved, and the relative positions of the atoms in space.

structural f. a chemical formula showing the spatial arrangement of the atoms and the linkage of every atom.

formulary ('fawmyuhlə·ree) a collection of formulae.

British National F. see BRITISH NATIONAL FORMULARY.

formyl ('formil) the radical, HCO or H·C:O–, of formic acid.

fornix ('forniks) pl. *fornices* [L.] 1. an archlike structure or the vaultlike space created by such a structure. 2. fornix of cerebrum; either of a pair of arched fibre tracts that unite under the corpus callosum, so that together they comprise two columns, a body, and two crura.

Fort Bragg fever (fort brag) pretibial fever.

Fortral ('fawtral) trademark for preparations of pentazocine; an analgesic.

Fortum ('fawtəm) trademark for ceftazidime, a broad-spectrum antibiotic.

forward-bending manoeuvre ('forwəd,bending) a method of detecting retraction signs in neoplastic changes in the breasts; the patient bends forward from the waist with chin held up and arms extended toward the examiner. If retraction is present, an asymmetry in the breast is seen.

fossa ('fosə) pl. *fossae* [L.] a trench or channel; in anatomy, a hollow or depressed area.

amygdaloid f. the depression in which the tonsil is lodged.

cerebral f. any of the depressions on the floor of the cranial cavity.

condylar f., condyloid f. either of two pits on the lateral portion of the occipital bone.

coronoid f. a depression in the humerus for the coronoid process of the ulna.

cranial f. any one of the three hollows (anterior, middle, and posterior) in the base of the cranium for the lobes of the brain.

digastric f. a depression on the inner surface of the mandible, giving attachment to the anterior belly of the digastric muscle.

epigastric f. 1. one in the epigastric region. 2. urachal fossa.

ethmoid f. the groove in the cribriform plate of the ethmoid bones, for the olfactory bulb.

glenoid f. mandibular fossa.

hyaloid f. a depression in the front of the vitreous body, lodging the lens.

hypophyseal f. a depression in the sphenoid lodging the pituitary gland; called also *pituitary fossa.*

iliac f. a concave area occupying much of the inner surface of the ala of the ilium, especially anteriorly; from it arises the iliac muscle.

incisive f. a slight depression on the anterior surface of the maxilla above the incisor teeth.

infratemporal f. an irregularly shaped cavity medial or deep to the zygomatic arch.

interpeduncular f. a depression on the inferior surface of the midbrain, between the two cerebral peduncles, the floor of which is the posterior perforated substance.

ischiorectal f. a potential space between the pelvic diaphragm and the skin below it; an anterior recess extends a variable distance between the pelvic and urogenital diaphragms.

mandibular f. a depression in the inferior surface of the pars squamosa of the temporal bone at the base of the zygomatic process, in which the condyle of the mandible rests; called also *glenoid fossa.*

mastoid f. a small triangular area between the posterior wall of the external acoustic meatus and the posterior root of the zygomatic process of the temporal bone.

nasal f. the portion of the nasal cavity anterior to the middle meatus.

navicular f. 1. the vaginal vestibule between the vaginal orifice and the frenulum of the pudendal labia. 2. the lateral expansion of the urethra of the glans penis; called also *lacuna majus*. 3. a depression on the internal pterygoid process of the sphenoid, giving attachment to the tensor veli palatini muscle.

f. ovalis cordis a fossa in the right atrium of the heart; the remains of the fetal foramen ovale.

ovarian f. a shallow pouch on the posterior surface of the broad ligament of the uterus in which the ovary is located.

pituitary f. hypophyseal fossa.

subarcuate f. a depression in the posterior inner

surface of the pars petrosa of the temporal bone.

subpyramidal f. a depression on the internal wall of the middle ear.

subsigmoid f. a fossa between the mesentery of the sigmoid flexure and that of the descending colon.

supraspinous f. a depression above the spine of the scapula.

temporal f. an area on the side of the cranium bounded posteriorly and superiorly by the temporal lines, anteriorly by the frontal and zygomatic bones, and laterally by the zygomatic arch, lodging the temporal muscle.

tibiofemoral f. a space between the articular surfaces of the tibia and femur mesial or lateral to the inferior pole of the patella.

urachal f. one on the inner abdominal wall, between the urachus and the hypogastric artery.

fossette (fo'set) 1. a small depression. 2. a small, deep corneal ulcer.

fossula ('fosyuhlə) pl. *fossulae* [L.] a small fossa.

Fothergill's neuralgia ('fodhə,gilz) tic douloureux.

Fothergill's operation Manchester operation.

foulage ('foolahzh) [Fr.] kneading and pressing of the muscles in massage.

fourchette (fooə'shet) [Fr.] the posterior junction of the labia minora.

fovea ('fohvi·ə) pl. *foveae* [L.] a small pit or depression; often used alone to indicate the central fovea of the retina.

central f. of retina, f. centralis retinae a small pit in the centre of the macula lutea, composed of slim, elongated cones; it is the area of clearest vision, because here the layers of the retina are spread aside, permitting light to fall directly on the cones.

foveate ('fohvi,ayt) pitted.

foveation (,fohvi'ayshən) formation of pits on a surface, as on the skin; a pitted condition.

foveola (,fohvi'ohlə) pl. *foveolae* [L.] a minute pit or depression.

Fowler's solution ('fowləz) potassium arsenite solution, composed of arsenic trioxide, potassium bicarbonate, and water; formerly used as an antileukaemic agent.

Fox–Fordyce disease (,foks'fordies) a condition of unknown cause characterized by plugging of the pores of the apocrine sweat glands and vesiculation of the epidermis.

FPA Family Planning Association.

FPC Family Practitioner Committee.

FPS Fellow of the Pharmaceutical Society.

Fr chemical symbol, *francium.*

FRACP Fellow of the Royal Australasian College of Physicians.

FRACS Fellow of the Royal Australasian College of Surgeons.

fractionation (,frakshə'nayshən) 1. in radiotherapy, division of the total dose of radiation into small doses given at intervals. 2. in chemistry, separation of a substance into components, as by distillation or crystallization. 3. in pathology, isolation of components of living cells by differential centrifugation.

fracture ('frakchə) 1. to break a part, especially a bone. 2. a break in the continuity of bone. Fractures are generally caused by trauma, either by a direct or an indirect force on the bone. Fractures may also be caused by muscle spasm or by disease that results in decalcification of the bone. The different types and classification of fractures are shown in the illustrations.

TREATMENT. Immediate first aid consists in splinting the bone. No attempt should be made to set the bone; it should be splinted 'as it lies'; i.e., it should be supported in such a way that the injured part will remain steady and will resist jarring if the patient is moved.

A fracture is treated by reduction, which means that the broken ends are placed in alignment. Closed reduction is performed by manipulation of the fractured bone so that the fragments are brought into proper alignment; no surgical incision is made. Open reduction is performed when closed reduction fails or is not possible, during surgery to internally fix a fracture, or when débridement is required for a compound fracture. A fracture may also require internal fixation with pins, nails, metal plates, or screws to stabilize the alignment.

Once reduction is accomplished the bone may be immobilized by application of a plaster CAST or by an apparatus exerting TRACTION on the distal end of the bone.

avulsion f. separation of a fragment of bone cortex at the site of attachment of a ligament or tendon.

Barton's f. fracture of the distal end of the radius into the wrist joint.

Bennett's f. fracture of the base of the first metacarpal bone, running into the carpometacarpal joint, complicated by subluxation of the lateral fragment.

blow-out f. fracture of the orbital floor caused by a sudden increase of intraorbital pressure due to traumatic force; the orbital contents herniate into the maxillary sinus so that the inferior rectus or inferior oblique muscle may become incarcerated in the fracture site, producing diplopia on looking up.

closed f. one that does not produce an open wound.

Colles' f. an impacted fracture of the lower end of the radius, the distal fragment being displaced backward; if the lower fragment is displaced forward, it is a reversed Colles' fracture.

comminuted f. a fracture producing several fragments.

complete f. one involving the entire cross section of the bone.

complicated f. one in which there is associated damage to vital neighbouring structures, e.g., nerves or vessels.

compound f. fracture with fragments penetrating the skin (compounded from within) or as part of an open wound (compounded from without).

condylar f. a fracture through a condyle of a long bone.

crush f. one in which the fragments are pressed into one another; usually seen in thoracolumbar vertebrae.

depressed f. fracture of the skull in which a fragment is depressed.

direct f. one at the site of injury.

f.-dislocation fracture of a bone near an articulation with concomitant dislocation of that joint.

double f. fracture of a bone in two places.

Dupuytren's f. Pott's fracture.

extracapsular f. fracture of the lower aspect of the neck of the femur which lies outside the joint capsule.

fissure f. a crack extending from a surface into, but not through, a long bone.

Galeazzi f. fracture of the shaft of the radius with dislocation of the distal radio-ulnar joint.

greenstick f. one in which one side of a bone is broken, the other being bent; occurs in children.

hairline f. a fine linear fracture with no displacement.

impacted f. fracture in which one fragment is firmly driven into the other.

incomplete f. one that does not involve the complete cross section of the bone.

indirect f. one at a point distant from the site of injury.

interperiosteal f. greenstick or incomplete fracture.

intertrochanteric f. fracture through the trochanters

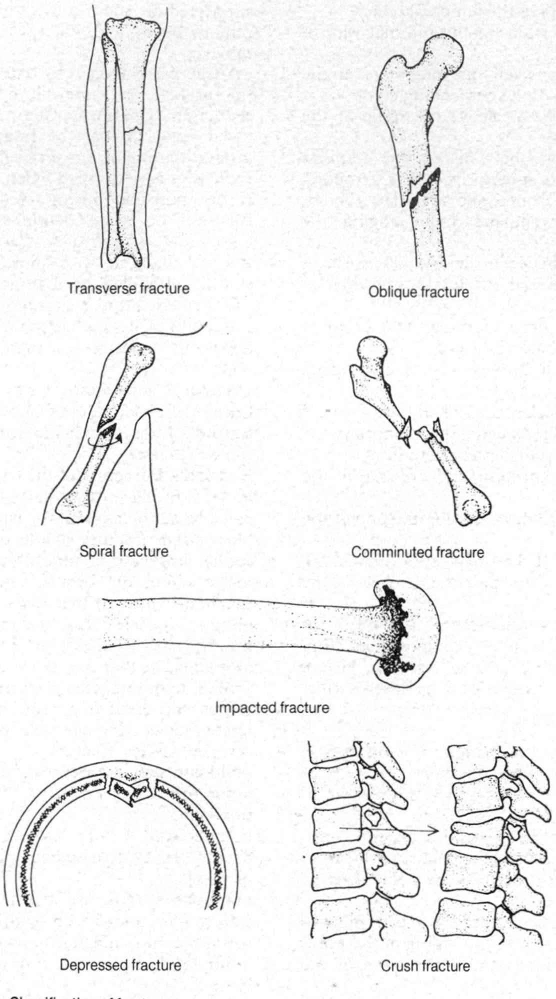

Classification of fractures

and the base of the neck of the femur.
intracapsular f. fracture of the upper aspect of the neck of the femur which lies inside the joint capsule.
intrauterine f. fracture of a fetal bone incurred in utero.
Le Fort's f. bilateral horizontal fracture of the maxilla. Le Fort fractures are classified as follows: *Le Fort I fracture*, a horizontal segmented fracture of the alveolar process of the maxilla, in which the teeth are usually contained in the detached portion of the bone. *Le Fort II fracture*, unilateral or bilateral fracture of the maxilla, in which the body of the maxilla is separated from the facial skeleton and the separated portion is pyramidal in shape; the fracture may extend through the body of the maxilla down the midline of the hard palate, through the floor of the orbit, and into the nasal cavity. *Le Fort III fracture*, a fracture in which the entire maxilla and one or more facial bones are completely separated from the craniofacial skeleton; such fractures are almost always accompanied by multiple fractures of the facial bones.
Monteggia's f. one in the proximal half of the shaft of the ulna, with dislocation of the head of the radius.
oblique f. one in which the line of the fracture is not directly across the axis of the bone.
open f. compound fracture.
pathological f. one due to weakening of the bone structure by pathological processes, such as neoplasia, osteomalacia, or osteomyelitis.
pertrochanteric f. one in which the fracture line involves the trochanters; one or both may be fractured or separated.
Pott's f. fracture of the lower end of the fibula with or without fracture of the medial malleolus of the tibia and lateral or posterior dislocation of the ankle joint. Fracture of the posterior part of the inferior articular surface of the tibia may also be present.
secondary f. pathological fracture.
simple f. closed fracture.
Smith's f. reversed Colles' fracture.
spiral f. an oblique fracture whose outline gives a spiral appearance.

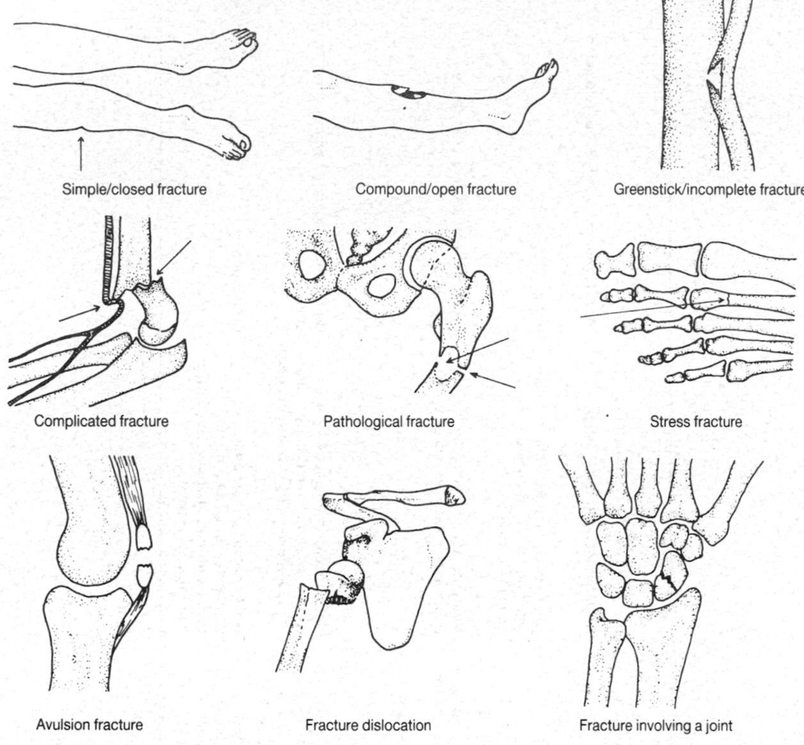

Types of fracture

spontaneous f. a fracture occurring without apparent trauma; occurs in bone disease, called also *pathological fracture*.

stellate f. one with a central point of injury, from which radiate numerous fissures, as seen in the patella.

Stieda's f. a fracture of the internal condyle of the femur.

stress f. one found in a bone subjected to persistent and excessive stress.

subcapital f. a fracture through the neck of the femur immediately distal to the head of the femur.

transcervical f. one through the neck of the femur within the joint capsule.

transverse f. one at right angles to the axis of the bone.

trimalleolar f. a fracture dislocation of the ankle involving fractures of the medial and lateral malleoli and fracture of the posterior part of the inferior articular surface of the tibia.

frae- for words beginning thus, see those beginning *fre-*.

fragilitas (frə'jilitəs) [L.] *fragility*.

f. crinium a brittleness of the hair.

f. ossium congenita osteogenesis imperfecta.

fragility (frə'jilitee) susceptibility, or lack of resistance, to influences capable of causing disruption of continuity or integrity.

f. of blood erythrocyte fragility.

capillary f. abnormal susceptibility of capillary walls to rupture.

erythrocyte f. susceptibility of erythrocytes to haemolysis when subjected to mechanical trauma (mechanical fragility) or when exposed to increasingly hypotonic saline solutions (osmotic fragility). A test of erythrocyte osmotic fragility is used in diagnosing haemolytic anaemia. Called also *fragility of blood*.

osmotic f. the ability to withstand changes in fluid and electrolyte concentrations. Red cell osmotic fragility is used to diagnose a number of haematological disorders associated with an increased or decreased susceptibility to saline concentration. The end point of the test is lysis of the red cell. In hereditary spherocytosis the red cell osmotic fragility is decreased and spherocytes will lyse at higher concentrations of saline than normal.

fragmentation (ˌfragmen'tayshən) division into small pieces.

framboesia (fram'beezi·ə) yaws.

framboesioma (fram,beezi'ohmə) mother yaw; the initial cutaneous lesion of YAWS.

frame (fraym) a rigid supporting structure or a structure for immobilizing a part.

Balkan f. BALKAN BEAM.

Braun f. a metal frame used to elevate the lower limb in fractures of the tibia and fibula.

quadriplegic standing f. a device for supporting in the upright position a patient whose four limbs are paralysed. **Stryker f.** one consisting of canvas stretched on anterior and posterior frames, on which the patient can be rotated around his longitudinal axis (see also STRYKER FRAME).

framycetin (ˌframi'seetin) an aminoglycoside antibiotic which is very similar to neomycin.

Franceschetti's syndrome (ˌfrangkə'sheteez) see mandibulofacial DYSOSTOSIS.

Possible complications from fractures

Complication	Early clinical features	Recommended nursing action	Most common fracture type — location
Pulmonary embolism (may occur without clinical symptoms)	1. Substernal pain 2. Dyspnoea 3. Rapid weak pulse 4. Expectoration of fresh blood	Notify doctor immediately of vital signs and pain, administer prescribed oxygen	Lower extremities
Fat embolism	1. Altered mental state, confusion, apprehension, restlessness due to hypoxia 2. Petechial over back, chest and conjunctival folds 3. Dyspnoea, tachypnoea, tachycardia and pyrexia	Notify doctor immediately, administer prescribed oxygen	Lower extremities and/or multiple fractures
Gas gangrene	1. Local pain and oedema 2. Gas formation with possible crepitus 3. Tachycardia, followed by pyrexia	Notify doctor immediately; take a wound swab for microscopy, culture and administer prescribed antibiotics	Compound (especially with a small open area)
Tetanus	May be none until patient has difficulty opening mouth followed by tonic rigidity involving skeletal muscles	Notify doctor immediately; administer prescribed human tetanus immunoglobulin, antibiotics and muscle relaxants	Compound

Francisella (ˌfransiˈselə) a genus of bacteria.

F. tularensis the aetiological agent of tularaemia; formerly called *Pasteurella tularensis.*

francium (ˈfransi·əm) a chemical element, atomic number 87, atomic weight 223, symbol Fr. See table of elements in Appendix 2.

Frankenhaüser's ganglion (ˈfrangkenˌhoyzəz) a ganglion near the uterine cervix; called also *cervical,* or *cervicouterine ganglion.*

FRC functional residual capacity.

FRCGP Fellow of the Royal College of General Practitioners.
FRcn Fellow of the Royal College of Nursing.
FRCOG Fellow of the Royal College of Obstetricians and Gynaecologists.
FRCP Fellow of the Royal College of Physicians.
FRCPath Fellow of the Royal College of Pathologists.
FRCPE Fellow of the Royal College of Physicians of Edinburgh.
FRCPI Fellow of the Royal College of Physicians of Ireland.
FRCPsych Fellow of the Royal College of Psychologists.
FRCR Fellow of the Royal College of Radiologists.
FRCS Fellow of the Royal College of Surgeons.
FRCSE Fellow of the Royal College of Surgeons of Edinburgh.
FRCSI Fellow of the Royal College of Surgeons of Ireland.
freckle ('frek'l) a pigmented spot on the skin due to accumulation of melanin resulting from exposure to sunlight. Called also *lentigo*.
melanotic f. of Hutchinson a noninvasive malignant melanoma occurring most often on the face of women during the fourth decade; called also *lentigo maligna*.
freeze-drying (ˌfreez'drie·ing) a method of tissue preparation in which the tissue specimen is frozen and then dehydrated at low temperature in a high vacuum.
freeze-etching (ˌfreez'eching) a method used to study unfixed cells by electron microscopy, in which the object to be studied is placed in 20 per cent glycerol, frozen at -100 °C, and then mounted on a chilled holder.
freeze-fracturing (ˌfreez'frakchə·ring) a method of preparing cells for electron-microscopical examination: a tissue specimen is frozen at -150 °C, inserted into a vacuum chamber, and fractured by a microtome; a platinum carbon replica of the exposed surfaces is made, freed of the underlying specimen, and then examined.
freeze-substitution (freezˌsubsti'tyooshən) a modification of freeze-drying in which the ice within the frozen tissue is replaced by alcohol or other solvents at a very low temperature.
freezing point ('freezing) the temperature at which a liquid begins to freeze; for water, the freezing point is 0 °C, or 32 °F.
Frei's test (friez) intracutaneous injection of antigen derived from infected chick embryos, used in the diagnosis of lymphogranuloma venereum.
Freiberg's disease ('friebərgz) osteochondrosis of the head of the second metatarsal bone.
fremitus ('fremitəs) a vibration perceptible on palpation or auscultation.
tactile f. a vibration, as in the chest wall, felt on the thorax while the patient is speaking.
tussive f. one felt on the chest while the patient coughs.
vocal f. one caused by speaking, perceived on auscultation.
French scale (french) a scale used for denoting size of catheters, sounds, and other tubular instruments, each unit being roughly equivalent to 0.33 mm in diameter.
frenectomy (fri'nektəmee) excision of a frenulum.
Frenkel's exercises ('frenkəlz) exercises used in the treatment of tabes dorsalis to teach muscle and joint sense.
frenoplasty ('freenohˌplastee) the correction of an abnormally attached frenulum by surgically repositioning it.
frenotomy (fri'notəmee) the cutting of a frenulum.
frenulum ('frenyuhləm) pl. *frenula* [L.] a small fold of integument or mucous membrane that limits the movements of an organ or part.
f. of clitoris a fold formed by union of the labia minora with the clitoris.
f. of ileocaecal valve a fold formed by the joined extremities of the ileocaecal valve, partially encircling the lumen of the colon.
f. labiorum pudendi fourchette.
f. linguae frenulum of tongue.
f. of lip a median fold of mucous membrane connecting the inside of each lip to the corresponding gum.
f. of prepuce of penis a fold under the penis connecting it with the prepuce.
f. of superior medullary velum a band lying in the superior medullary velum at its attachment to the inferior colliculi.
f. of tongue the vertical fold of mucous membrane under the tongue, attaching it to the floor of the mouth; called also *frenulum linguae*.
frenum ('freenəm) pl. *frena* [L.] a restraining structure or part; see FRENULUM.
frequency ('freekwənsee) the number of occurrences of a periodic process in a unit of time.
f. distribution a table or graph showing the frequencies of a particular measurement in a population.
urinary f. urination at short intervals without increase in daily volume of urinary output, due to reduced bladder capacity.
Freud (froyd) Sigmund (1856–1939). Clinical neurologist and founder of PSYCHOANALYSIS. Born in Freiberg in Moravia, and educated at the University of Vienna, he studied in Paris in 1885 under the neurologist J. M. Charcot, who encouraged him to investigate hysteria from a psychological point of view. Freud stressed the existence of an unconscious that exerts a dynamic influence on consciousness, and was led to develop his method of 'free association' in order to discover these buried memories. He emphasized the role of sexuality in the development of neurotic conditions, and published *Interpretation of Dreams* (1900), *Psychopathology of Everyday Life* (1901), and many more works. He was also director of the *International Journal of Psychology*. Fleeing the Nazi regime in Vienna in 1938, he died in London.
freudian ('froydi·ən) pertaining to Sigmund Freud, the founder of PSYCHOANALYSIS, and to his doctrines regarding the causes and treatment of neuroses and psychoses.
FRFPS Fellow of the Royal Faculty of Physicians and Surgeons.
friable ('frieəb'l) easily pulverized or crumbled.
friction ('frikshən) the act of rubbing; a physiotherapy technique. Small, accurately localized, penetrating movements performed in a circular or transverse direction whereby superficial tissues are moved on deeper ones. It produces (1) local hyperaemia with a local histamine response, (2) mechanical restoration of mobility in structures by the release of adhesions, (3) dispersal of blood clot, and (4) anaesthesia. Indications for use are (1) fibrositis, (2) chronic tenosynovitis, (3) chronic ligament adhesions, (4) chronic adherent scar, and (5) haematoma.
friction rub ('frikshən rub) an auscultatory sound caused by the rubbing together of two serous surfaces.
Friedländer's bacillus ('freedlendəz) *Klebsiella pneumoniae*, the cause of a rare form of pneumonia.
Friedländer's disease endarteritis obliterans.
Friedländer's pneumonia a form of pneumonia characterized by massive mucoid inflammatory exudates in a lobe of the lung, due to *Klebsiella pneumoniae*.
Friedreich's ataxia ('freedrieks) hereditary sclerosis of

the dorsal and lateral columns of the spinal cord, usually beginning in childhood or youth. It is attended by ataxia, speech impairment, scoliosis, and peculiar swaying and irregular movements, with paralysis of the muscles, especially of the lower extremities.

Friedreich's disease 1. paramyoclonus multiplex. 2. Friedreich's ataxia.

frigidity (fri'jiditee) coldness; especially, sexual unresponsiveness of the female to physical stimulation, due to psychological causes.

frigorific (ˌfrigə'rifik) producing coldness.

FRIPHH Fellow of the Royal Institute of Public Health and Hygiene.

Froben ('frohben) trademark for preparations of flurbiprofen.

Fröhlich's syndrome ('frərliks) a condition associated with lesions of the hypothalamus and pituitary gland, marked by obesity and sexual infantilism; called also *adiposogenital dystrophy*.

frolement ('frohlmonh) [Fr.] 1. a rustling sound heard on auscultation in pericardial disease. 2. a brushing movement in massage.

frons (fronz) [L.] *the forehead.*

frontad ('fruntad) toward a front, or frontal aspect.

frontal ('frunt'l) 1. pertaining to the forehead. 2. denoting a longitudinal plane passing through the body from side to side, and dividing it into front and back parts.

f. bone the unpaired bone constituting the anterior part of the skull.

f. lobe the rostral (anterior) portion of the cerebral hemisphere.

frontalis (fron'taylis) [L.] *frontal.*

frost (frost) a deposit resembling frozen dew or vapour.

frostbite ('frost,biet) injury to tissues due to exposure to cold. Usually the first areas of the body to freeze are the nose, ears, fingers, and toes. The flesh feels cold to the touch, and frozen parts become pale and feel numb. There may also be some prickly or itchy sensation. A person suffering from frostbite may feel no warning pain.

In mild cases of frostbite proper treatment can quickly restore normal circulation of blood. In more serious cases the area may become painfully inflamed, and blistering may follow. Especially severe frostbite can cause death of the injured tissues and gangrene may result.

TREATMENT. The frozen parts should be gradually and gently rewarmed. Hot water bottles or other applications of heat are contraindicated, as is rubbing or massaging, which may further damage the injured tissues. Cool or lukewarm water may be used to rewarm the frozen parts. If water is not available, the part may be rewarmed by covering it with warm clothing or by placing it in contact with any other part of the body that is warm. Contrary to a common theory, frostbite should *never* be treated by rubbing the affected area with snow or by the application of snow or ice.

frottage (fro'tahzh) [Fr.] 1. a rubbing movement in massage. 2. sexual gratification by rubbing against a person of the opposite sex.

frotteur (fro'tər) one who practices frottage (2).

frozen section ('frohzən) a specimen of tissue that has been quick-frozen, cut by microtome, and stained immediately for rapid diagnosis of possible malignant lesions. A specimen processed in this manner is not satisfactory for detailed study of the cells, but it is valuable because it is quick and gives the surgeon immediate information regarding the malignancy of a piece of tissue.

frozen shoulder adhesive capsulitis; brachial fibrositis; periarthritis of the shoulder; a stiff and painful shoulder. Treatment is by analgesics and anti-inflammatory drugs, short-wave diathermy and exercises, sometimes combined with corticosteroid injections into the joint. Manipulation under anaesthesia may be performed. The cause is unknown.

FRS Fellow of the Royal Society.

FRSE Fellow of the Royal Society of Edinburgh.

FRSH Fellow of the Royal Society of Health.

FRSM Fellow of the Royal Society of Medicine.

fructofuranose (ˌfruktoh'fyooə·rə,nohz) the combining and more reactive form of fructose.

β-fructofuranosidase (ˌbeetə,fruktohfyooə·rə'nohsidayz) an enzyme occurring in yeasts and other organisms that catalyses the hydrolysis of sugars with a terminal unsubstituted β-D-fructofuranosyl residue.

fructokinase (ˌfruktoh'kienayz) an enzyme that catalyses the transfer of a high-energy phosphate group to D-fructose.

fructosaemia (ˌfruktoh'seemi·ə) the presence of fructose in the blood, as in fructose intolerance.

fructose ('fruktohs, -tohz, 'fruhk-) a sugar found in honey and many sweet fruits; called also *laevulose* and *fruit sugar*. It is used in solution as a fluid and nutrient replenisher.

fructoside ('fruktə,sied, 'fruhk-) a compound that bears the same relation to fructose as a glucoside does to glucose.

fructosuria (ˌfruktə'syooə·ri·ə, ˌfruhk-) the presence of fructose in the urine.

essential f. a benign hereditary disorder of carbohydrate metabolism due to a defect in fructokinase and manifested only by fructose in the blood and urine.

fructosyl ('fruktə,sil, 'fruhk-) a radical of fructose.

fruit (froot) the matured ovary of a plant, including the seed and its envelopes.

frusemide ('froozəmied) a diuretic that acts by blocking reabsorption of sodium and chloride in the ascending loop of Henle; used for treatment of oedema and acute renal failure.

frustration (fru'strayshən) increased emotional tension due to failure to achieve sought gratifications or satisfactions.

FSH follicle-stimulating hormone.

FSH/LH-RH follicle-stimulating hormone and luteinizing hormone releasing hormone.

FSH-RH follicle-stimulating hormone releasing hormone.

FSR(R) Fellow of the Royal Society of Radiographers (Radiography).

FSR(T) Fellow of the Society of Radiographers (Radiotherapy).

FTA fluorescent treponemal antibody test.

fuchsin ('fooksin) any of several red to purple dyes.

acid f. a mixture of sulphonated fuchsins; used in various complex stains.

basic f. a histological stain, a mixture of pararosaniline, rosaniline, and magenta II. Also, a mixture of rosaniline and pararosaniline hydrochlorides used as a local anti-infective.

fucose ('fyookohz, -ohs) a monosaccharide occurring as L-fucose in a number of mucopolysaccharides and mucoproteins.

fucosidase (fyoo'kohzidayz) an enzyme occurring in two forms that catalyses the hydrolysis of fucoside to an alcohol and fucose.

fucoside ('fyookoh,sied) an acetal derivative of fucose.

fucosidosis (fyooˌkohzi'dohsis) a hereditary disease due to deficient enzymatic activity of fucosidase and resulting in accumulation of fucose in all tissues; marked by progressive cerebral degeneration, muscle weakness with eventual spasticity, emaciation, cardio-

megaly, thick skin, and excessive sweating.
-fugal word element. [L.] *driving away, fleeing from, repelling.*
fugue (fyoog) a dissociative reaction in which amnesia is accompanied by physical flight from customary surroundings.
Fulcin ('fuhlsin) trademark for a preparation of griseofulvin, an antibiotic used as a fungistatic in dermatophytoses.
fulgurate ('fulgyuh,rayt) 1. to come and go like a flash of lightning. 2. to destroy by contact with electric sparks generated by a high-frequency current.
fulguration (,fulgyuh'rayshən) controlled localized destruction of tissue by a high-frequency current transmitted through electrodes.
fulminate ('fulmi,nayt, -'fuh-) to occur suddenly with great intensity. adj. **fulminant.**
fumarase ('fyoomə,rayz) an enzyme that catalyses the interconversion of fumarate and malate.
fumarate ('fyoomə,rayt) a salt of fumaric acid.
ferrous f. the anhydrous salt of a combination of ferrous iron and fumaric acid; used as a haematinic.
fumaric acid (fyoo'marik) an unsaturated dibasic acid; it is the *trans*-isomer of maleic acid and an intermediate in the tricarboxylic acid cycle.
fumigation (,fyoomi'gayshən) exposure to disinfecting fumes.
function ('fungkshən) the special, normal, or proper action of any part or organ.
functional ('fungkshən'l) pertaining to or fulfilling a function; affecting the function but not the structure.
f. disease a disease involving body functions but having no known organic basis.
fundament ('fundəmənt) 1. a base or foundation, as the breech or rump. 2. the anus and parts adjacent to it.
fundectomy (fun'dektəmee) excision of the fundus of an organ, as of the stomach.
fundiform ('fundi,fawm) shaped like a loop or sling.
fundoplication (,fundohplie'kayshən) mobilization of the lower end of the oesophagus and plication of the fundus of the stomach up around it, in the treatment of oesophageal reflux.
fundus ('fundəs) pl. *fundi* [L.] the bottom or base of anything; used in anatomical nomenclature as a general term to designate the bottom or base of an organ, or the part of a hollow organ farthest from its mouth. adj. **fundal, fundic.**
f. of bladder the base or posterior surface of the urinary bladder.
f. of eye the back portion of the interior of the eyeball, visible through the pupil by use of the ophthalmoscope.
f. of gallbladder the inferior, dilated portion of the gallbladder.
f. of stomach the part of the stomach to the left and above the level of the opening between the stomach and oesophagus.
f. tympani the floor of the tympanic cavity.
f. uteri, f. of uterus the part of the uterus above the orifices of the uterine tubes.
funduscope ('fundə,skohp) ophthalmoscope. adj. **funduscopic.**
fundusectomy (,fundə'sektəmee) excision of the fundus of the stomach.
fungaemia (fun'jeemi·ə) the presence of fungi in the bloodstream.
fungal ('fung·g'l) pertaining to or caused by a fungus.
fungate ('fung·gayt) to produce fungus-like growths; to grow rapidly, like a fungus.
fungi ('fung·gi, 'funjie) [L.] plural of *fungus.*
fungicide ('funji,sied) an agent that destroys fungi. adj. **fungicidal.**
fungiform ('funji,fawm) shaped like a fungus, or mushroom.
fungistasis (,funji'staysis) inhibition of the growth of fungi. adj. **fungistatic.**
fungistat ('funji,stat) a substance that checks the growth of fungi.
fungitoxic (,funji'toksik) exerting a toxic effect upon fungi.
Fungizone ('funji,zohn) trademark for a preparation of amphotericin B, an antibiotic used in cryptococcal meningitis and systemic fungal infections.
fungoid ('fung·goyd) resembling a fungus.
chignon f. a nodular growth on the hair.
fungosity (fung'gositee) a fungoid growth or excrescence.
fungous ('fung·gəs) of the nature of, caused by, or resembling a fungus.
fungus ('fung·gəs) pl. *fungi* [L.] a general term for a group of eukaryotic organisms (mushrooms, yeasts, moulds, etc.) marked by the absence of chlorophyll, the presence of a rigid cell wall in some stage of the life cycle, and reproduction by means of spores. Fungi are present in the soil, air, and water, but only a few species can cause disease. Among the fungal diseases (mycoses) are HISTOPLASMOSIS, COCCIDIOIDOMYCOSIS, RINGWORM, ATHLETE'S FOOT, and THRUSH. Although the fungal diseases develop slowly, are difficult to diagnose, and are resistant to treatment, they are rarely fatal except for systemic mycotic infections, which can be life-threatening (see also opportunistic MYCOSIS).
funicle ('fyoonik'l) funiculus.
funiculitis (fyoo,nikyuh'lietis) 1. inflammation of the spermatic cord. 2. inflammation of that portion of a spinal nerve root which lies within the intervertebral canal.
funiculoepididymitis (fyoo,nikyuhloh,epididi'mietis) inflammation of the spermatic cord and the epididymis.
funiculus (fyoo'nikyuhləs) pl. *funiculi* [L.] a cord; a cordlike structure or part, especially one of the large bundles of nerve tracts making up the white matter of the spinal cord. adj. **funicular.**
anterior f. the white substance of the spinal cord lying on either side between the anterior median fissure and the ventral root.
lateral f., f. lateralis the lateral mass of fibres on either side of the spinal cord, between the anterolateral and posterolateral sulci.
posterior f. the white substance of the spinal cord lying on either side between the posterior median sulcus and the dorsal root.
f. spermaticus the spermatic cord.
funiform ('fyooni,fawm) resembling a rope or cord.
funis ('fyoonis) the umbilical cord.
funnel chest ('fun'l) a congenital abnormality of the anterior chest wall in which the sternum is depressed; called also PECTUS EXCAVATUM.
Furadantin (,fyooə·rə'dantin) trademark for preparations of nitrofurantoin, an antibacterial used in urinary tract infections.
furcal ('fərk'l) forked.
furfuraceous (,fərfyuh'rayshəs) fine and loose; said of scales resembling dandruff or bran.
furrow ('furoh) a groove or trench.
atrioventricular f. the transverse groove marking off the atria of the heart from the ventricles.
digital f. any one of the transverse folds across the joints on the palmar surface of a finger.
gluteal f. the furrow that separates the buttocks.
furuncle ('fyooə·rungk'l) a focal suppurative inflammation of the skin and subcutaneous tissues, enclosing a central slough or 'core'; called also BOIL. It is caused by

staphylococci, which enter through the hair follicles; formation is favoured by constitutional or digestive derangement and local irritation.

furunculoid (fyuh'rungkyuh,loyd) resembling a furuncle or boil.

furunculosis (fyuh,rungkyuh'lohsis) 1. the persistent sequential occurrence of furuncles over a period of weeks or months. 2. the simultaneous occurrence of a number of furuncles.

furunculus (fyuh'rungkyuhləs) a furuncle.

f. orientalis a protozoal infection mainly of the tropics, which causes a chronic ulceration; cutaneous leishmaniasis.

Fusarium (fyoo'sair·ri·əm) a genus of fungi; some species are plant pathogens and some are opportunistic infectious agents of man and animals.

fuscin ('fusin) a brown pigment of the retinal epithelium.

fusible ('fyoozəb'l) capable of being melted.

fusidic acid (fyoo'sidik) an antibiotic used to treat penicillin-resistant staphylococci. It is usually used in combination with another antibiotic effective against staphylococci.

fusiform ('fyoozi,fawm) spindle-shaped.

fusimotor (,fyoozi'mohtə) denoting motor nerve fibres (of gamma motor neurons) that innervate intrafusal fibres of the muscle spindle.

fusion ('fyoozhən) 1. the act or process of melting. 2. the merging or coherence of adjacent parts or bodies. 3. the coordination of separate images of the same object in the two eyes into one. 4. the operative formation of an ankylosis or arthrodesis.

diaphyseal–epiphyseal f. operative establishment of bony union between the epiphysis and diaphysis of a bone.

nerve f. nerve anastomosis done to induce regeneration for resupplying empty tracts of a nerve with new growth of fibres.

nuclear f. the fusion of two atomic nuclei to form a single heavier nucleus, resulting in the release of enormous amounts of energy.

spinal f. surgical creation of ankylosis between contiguous vertebrae; spondylosyndesis.

fusional ('fyoozhənəl) marked by fusion.

Fusobacterium (,fyoozohbak'tiə·ri·əm) a genus of anaerobic gram-negative bacteria found as normal flora in the mouth and large bowel, and often in necrotic tissue, probably as secondary invaders.

F. necrophorum a member of the family Bacteroidaceae, a pathogen of animals, causing diphtheria with abscesses in cattle, gangrenous dermatitis in horses, necrotic lesions in hogs, cattle, and sheep, and abscesses and necrotic areas in rabbits; also found in chronic ulcer of the colon in man.

F. plautivincenti a species found in necrotizing ulcerative gingivitis (trench mouth) and in necrotizing ulcerative stomatitis. Called also *F. fusiforme* and *Leptotrichia buccalis*.

fusocellular (,fyoozoh'selyuhlə) having spindle-shaped cells.

fusospirillosis (,fyoozoh,spieri'lohsis) trench mouth.

fusospirochaetal (,fyoozoh,spieroh'keetəl) of or caused by fusiform bacilli and spirochaetes.

fusospirochaetosis (,fyoozoh,spierohkee'tohsis) trench mouth.

FVC forced vital capacity.

Fybogel ('fiebohjel) trademark for preparations of ispaghula husk.

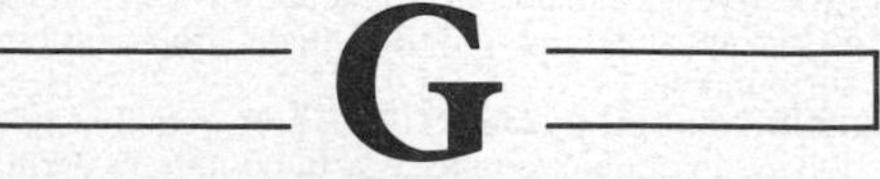

G gingival; glucose; gonidial.

g gram (formerly gramme); gravity; the unit of force exerted upon a body during acceleration and deceleration.

Ga chemical symbol, *gallium*.

gadolinium (,gadə'lini·əm) a chemical element, atomic number 64, atomic weight 157.25, symbol Gd. See table of elements in Appendix 2.

gag (gag) 1. a surgical device for holding the mouth open. 2. to retch, or strive to vomit.

g. reflex elevation of the soft palate and retching elicited by touching the back of the tongue or the wall of the pharynx; called also *pharygeal reflex*.

Gaisböck's disease ('gayzboks) a term previously used to describe a condition characterized by an apparent polycythaemia: the basic abnormality is not an increased red call mass but is due to a reduced plasma volume, i.e. a relative polycythaemia. Clinical features are hypertension, obesity and heavy smoking.

gait (gayt) the manner or style of walking. **g. analysis** evaluation of the manner or style of walking, usually done by observing the individual as he walks naturally in a straight line. The normal forward step consists of two phases: the *stance phase*, during which one leg and foot are bearing most or all of the body weight, and the *swing phase*, during which the foot is not touching the walking surface and the body weight is borne by the other leg and foot.

An analysis of each component of the three phases of ambulation is an essential part of the diagnosis of various neurological disorders and the assessment of patient progress during rehabilitation and recovery from the effects of a neurological disease, a musculoskeletal injury or disease process, or amputation of a lower extremity.

antalgic g. a limp adopted so as to avoid pain on weight-bearing structures, characterized by a very short stance phase.

ataxic g. an unsteady, uncoordinated walk, employing a wide base.

double-step g. a gait in which there is a noticeable difference in the length or timing of alternate steps.

drag-to g. a gait in which the feet are dragged (rather than lifted) toward the CRUTCHES.

equine g. a walk accomplished mainly by flexing the hip joint to lift the foot clear in the presence of dropfoot.

festinating g. one in which the patient involuntarily moves with short, shuffling, accelerating steps, often on tiptoe, due to generalized muscular rigidity and slowness of movement, as seen in Parkinson's disease; festination.

four-point g. a gait in forward motion using CRUTCHES. Most likely used by the paraplegic patient. It is the slowest and safest crutch gait, offering maximum balance and support since there are always at least three points of contact with the ground. See accompanying illustration.

gluteal g. the gait characteristic of paralysis of the gluteus medius muscle, marked by a listing of the trunk toward the affected side at each step.

helicopod g. a gait in which the feet describe half circles, as in some hysterical disorders.

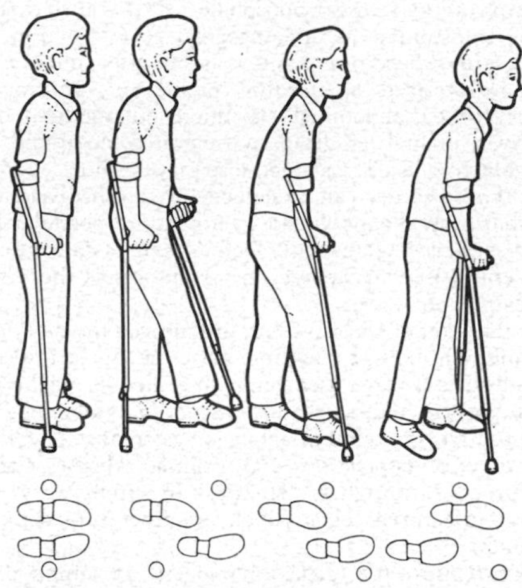
A four-point gait

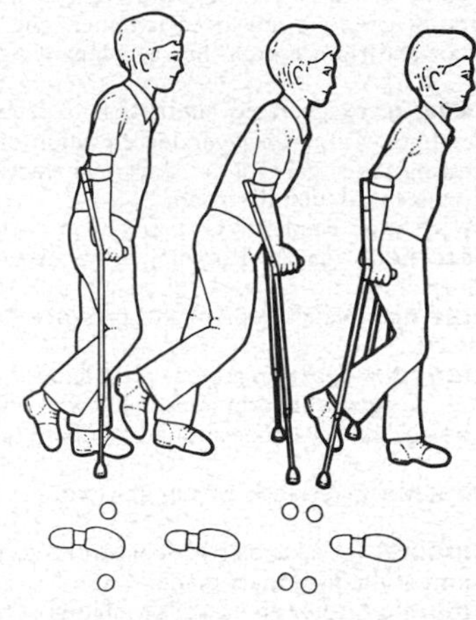
A three-point gait

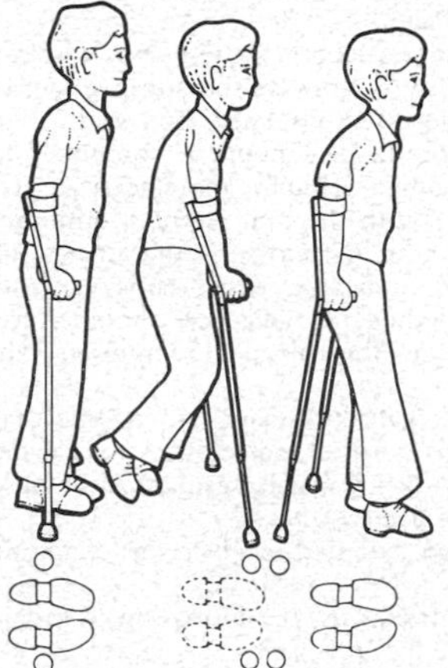
A swing-through gait

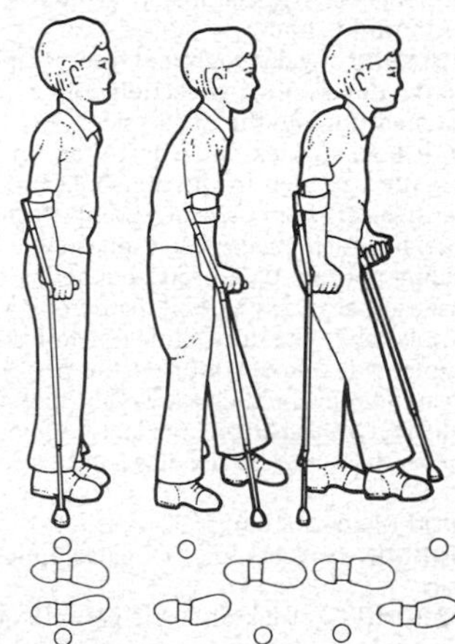
A two-point gait

hemiplegic g. a gait involving circumduction of the leg at the hip as it is swung forward, with catching of the toes because of stiffness of the leg due to spasticity.
Oppenheim's g. a gait marked by irregular oscillation of the head, limbs, and body; seen in some cases of multiple sclerosis.
spastic g. a walk in which the legs are held together and move in a stiff manner, the toes seeming to drag and catch.
steppage g. the gait which results from footdrop in which the advancing leg is lifted high in order that the toes may clear the ground. It is due to paralysis of the anterior tibial and peroneal muscles, and is seen in lesions of the lower motor neuron, such as polyneuritis, lesions of the anterior motor horn cells, and lesions of the cauda equina.
swing-through g. that in which the CRUTCHES are advanced and then the legs are swung past them. Used mainly by paraplegics and severe arthritics who have good balance and muscle power in the arms and hands. From the tripod position, both crutches are brought forward, the patient bears down on the handpieces, lifts the body and swings it through the crutches into a reversed tripod position. To maintain balance in this gait, the pelvis moves first, then the shoulders and head. See accompanying illustration.
swing-to g. that in which the CRUTCHES are advanced and the legs are swung to the same point. The swing-to gait is slower than the swing-through gait. From the tripod position, the patient places both crutches forward, either alternately or at the same time, and then swings his body ahead into a tripod position. The crutches and feet must never be even or the patient loses stability.
tabetic g. an ataxic gait in which, because of sensory loss, the feet slap the ground; in daylight the patient can avoid some unsteadiness by watching his feet.
three-point g. that in which both CRUTCHES and the affected leg are advanced together and then the normal leg is moved forward. See accompanying

illustration.

two-point g. that in which the right foot and left CRUTCH or cane are advanced together, and then the left foot and right crutch. See accompanying illustration.

waddling g. exaggerated alternation of lateral trunk movements with an exaggerated elevation of the hip, suggesting the gait of a duck; characteristic of progressive muscular dystrophy.

galact(o)- word element. [Gr.] *milk*.

galactacrasia (ˌgaləktəˈkrayzi·ə) an abnormal state of the breast milk.

galactaemia (ˌgaləkˈteemi·ə) the presence of milk in the blood.

galactagogue (gəˈlaktəˌgog) 1. promoting the flow of milk. 2. an agent that promotes the flow of milk.

galactic (gəˈlaktik) 1. pertaining to milk. 2. galactagogue.

galactischia (ˌgaləkˈtiski·ə) suppression of milk secretion.

galactoblast (gəˈlaktəˌblast) a colostrum corpuscle in the acini of the mammary gland.

galactobolic (gəˌlaktəˈbolik) of or relating to the action of neurohypophyseal peptides which contract the mammary myoepithelium and cause ejection of milk.

galactocele (gəˈlaktəˌseel) 1. a milk-containing, cystic enlargement of the mammary gland. 2. hydrocele filled with milky fluid.

galactography (ˌgaləkˈtogrəfee) radiography of the mammary ducts after injection of a radiopaque contrast medium into the duct system.

galactokinase (gəˌlaktohˈkienayz) an enzyme that catalyses the first step in the metabolism of galactose, the transfer of a phosphate group from ATP to galactose, producing galactose-1-phosphate.

g. deficiency a rare type of galactosaemia transmitted as an autosomal recessive trait, caused by a deficiency of galactokinase. The only clinical manifestation is the development of cataracts during the first year of life, which can be prevented by a low-galactose diet.

galactolipid, galactolipin (gəˌlaktohˈlipid; gəˌlaktohˈlipin) a cerebroside which yields galactose on hydrolysis.

galactoma (ˌgaləkˈtohmə) galactocele (1).

galactophore (gəˈlaktəˌfor) 1. galactophorous. 2. a milk duct.

galactophoritis (gəˌlaktohforˈrietis) inflammation of the milk ducts.

galactophorous (ˌgaləkˈtofə·rəs) conveying milk.

galactophygous (ˌgalakˈtofigəs) arresting the flow of milk.

galactoplania (gəˌlaktəˈplayni·ə) secretion of milk in some abnormal part.

galactopoiesis (gəˌlaktohpoyˈeesis) the production of milk by the mammary glands.

galactopoietic (gəˌlaktohpoyˈetik) 1. pertaining to, marked by, or promoting milk production. 2. an agent that promotes milk flow.

galactopyra (gəˌlaktəˈpierə) milk fever.

galactorrhoea (ˌgaləktəˈreeə) excessive or spontaneous milk flow; persistent secretion of milk irrespective of nursing; lactorrhoea.

galactosaemia (gəˌlaktəˈseemi·ə) a genetically determined biochemical disorder in which there is a lack of an enzyme necessary for proper metabolism of galactose. Normally the sugar derived from lactose in milk is changed by enzymatic action into glucose. When the conversion of galactose to glucose does not take place, the galactose accumulates in the tissues and blood. There are two types: classic galactosaemia and GALACTOKINASE DEFICIENCY.

Classic galactosaemia is due to a deficiency of the enzyme galactose-1-phosphate uridyl transferase, and is transmitted as an autosomal recessive trait. The disorder becomes manifest soon after birth and is characterized by feeding problems, vomiting and diarrhoea, abdominal distention, enlargement of the liver, mental handicap, and elevated blood and urine galactose levels. Cataracts also may develop.

The disorder can be detected by a sensitivity test so that early diagnosis and treatment are possible. If the disease is detected early, before there is damage to the central nervous system, the symptoms of the disorder can be prevented.

Treatment consists of exclusion from the diet of milk and all foods containing galactose or lactose. Milk substitutes are used and the diet is planned to substitute necessary nutrients normally obtained from products containing lactose or galactose. The British Dietetic Association, 103 Daimler House, Paradise Street, Birmingham B1 2BJ, can supply a list of all manufactured foods which are free from milk products.

galactosamine (gəˌlaktohˈsameen) an amino derivative of galactose.

galactose (gəˈlaktohz, -ohs) a monosaccharide derived from lactose. D-galactose is found in lactose, cerebrosides of the brain, raffinose of the sugar beet, and in many gums and seaweeds; L-galactose is found in flaxseed mucilage.

g. tolerance test a laboratory test done to determine the liver's ability to convert the sugar galactose into glycogen. Two methods may be used. The oral method requires about 5 hours to complete, and the intravenous method, which is more accurate, requires about 2 hours. With the oral method, elimination of more than 3 g of galactose in the urine during a 5-hour period indicates liver damage. With the intravenous method, all galactose should have been eliminated from the blood 45 minutes after its injection.

galactosidase (galəkˈtohsidayz) an enzyme that catalyses the conversion of galactoside to galactose; it occurs in two forms: α-galactosidase (melibiase) and β-galactosidase (lactase).

galactoside (gəˈlaktəˌsied) a glycoside containing galactose.

galactosis (ˌgaləkˈtohsis) the formation of milk by the lacteal glands.

galactostasis (ˌgaləkˈtostəsis) 1. cessation of milk secretion. 2. abnormal collection of milk in the mammary glands.

galactosuria (gəˌlaktohˈsyooə·ri·ə) the presence of galactose in the urine.

galactotherapy (gəˌlaktohˈtherəpee) treatment of a nursing infant by medication given to the mother or wet nurse.

galacturia (ˌgaləkˈtyooə·ri·ə) chyluria; the discharge of urine with a milky appearance.

galea (ˈgayli·ə) pl. *galeae* [L.] a helmet-shaped structure.

g. aponeurotica aponeurosis connecting the frontal and occipital bellies of the occipitofrontal muscle.

Galen (ˈgaylən) Claudius Galenus (AD 130–200). The celebrated Greek physician to the Roman Emperor Marcus Aurelius. Although he did not dissect the human cadaver, he made many valuable anatomical and physiological observations on animals (and applied many of them inaccurately to man), and his writings on these and other subjects were extensive. His influence on medicine was profound for many centuries—his teleology ('nature does nothing in vain') being particularly attractive to the medieval mind, although it was stultifying as regards advances in medical thought and practice.

galenicals, galenics (gə'lenik'lz, gay-; gə'leniks, gay-) medicines prepared according to the formulae of Galen. The term is now used to denote standard preparations containing one or several organic ingredients, as contrasted with pure chemical substances.

galeophobia (ˌgalioh'fohbi·ə) morbid fear of cats; ailurophobia.

gall (gawl) the bile.

gallamine ('galəˌmeen) a synthetic muscle relaxant, chemically related to curare but less potent and shorter acting.

gallbladder ('gawlˌbladə) an elongated sac located below the liver. It serves as a storage place for bile.

Acute inflammation of the gallbladder (CHOLECYSTITIS) causes severe pain and tenderness in the right upper abdomen, accompanied by fever, nausea, prostration, and sometimes jaundice.

Chronic inflammation of the gallbladder may cause recurrent pain, indigestion, flatulence and nausea. The indigestion is most evident after heavy meals or meals of fatty foods. GALLSTONES are often present. The condition may respond to conservative treatment with diet and medication. Removal of the gallbladder may be required, especially if there are gallstones.

DIAGNOSTIC STUDIES. The presence of bile in the urine is indicative of biliary tract obstruction.

Radiological investigation of gallbladder disease is most easily performed using ULTRASOUND. It is noninvasive and without known hazard. Ultrasonography will demonstrate the morphology of the gallbladder, gallstones and dilation of the biliary tree. Conventional x-ray examination of the gallbladder is by CHOLECYSTOGRAPHY in which an iodinated contrast medium is ingested and following absorption and excretion by the liver is concentrated in the gallbladder. At a serum bilirubin level between 34 and 50 μmol l^{-1} intravenous CHOLANGIOGRAPHY is more likely to opacify the gallbladder and will also outline the extrahepatic bile ducts. Ultrasonography has largely replaced these two x-ray techniques both in the nonjaundiced patient and in the presence of high serum bilirubin levels where neither of these methods is applicable.

When ultrasonography of a jaundiced patient shows dilated ducts and thus an obstructive jaundice, the level of that obstruction and its possible cause may be further evaluated by *percutaneous transhepatic cholangiography*. A fine needle is inserted through the skin into the liver and an intrahepatic bile duct located under flouroscopic guidance. Contrast medium is injected directly into the duct and the biliary tree opacified. If the patient is not intended for early surgical relief of the obstruction it is possible to drain the obstructed ducts by inserting a catheter. An alternative method of outlining the bile ducts is *endoscopic retrograde cholangiopancreatography* (ERCP). An endoscope is passed through the mouth as far as the second part of the duodenum and the ampulla of Vater is located. A cannula can be passed along the endoscope and directed into the common bile duct. Contrast medium is injected through the cannula and may be observed by fluoroscopy to outline the common bile duct.

The biliary tree and gallbladder may be demonstrated by nuclear medicine. Technetium tagged to a derivative of iminodiacetic acid (IDA), e.g. ^{99}Tc^{m}-BIDA (butyl iminodiacetic acid) is excreted by the liver into the bile following intravenous injection and its passage through the liver, down the biliary tree and out into the duodenum may be observed by a gamma camera.

Another aid to the diagnosis of gallbladder disease is the *biliary drainage test*, in which a specimen of bile is obtained by passing a Rehfuss tube orally and locating it at the site where the common bile duct empties into the duodenum. This test is especially helpful in identifying infections, parasitic infestations of the gallbladder, and other disorders not discerned by more conventional tests.

SURGERY OF THE GALLBLADDER AND BILE DUCTS. The two surgical procedures most commonly performed on the gallbladder are CHOLECYSTECTOMY and CHOLEDOCHOSTOMY.

Patient Care. During the preoperative period the patient usually receives a thorough physical examination as well as specific tests for liver function and x-ray studies of the gallbladder and bile ducts. Since nausea and flatulence are common occurrences in these patients both before and after surgery, a nasogastric tube is usually inserted prior to surgery.

When the patient returns from the operating theatre a careful check should be made for drainage tubes, which may have been inserted during surgery. Most drains are devised so that bile and serous fluid from the operative site drain directly onto the dressings applied over the wound. Other drains or tubes, such as the T tube or X tube, should be attached to a drainage apparatus so that the bile is collected in a bottle and can be measured periodically. In either case dressings over the wound are checked frequently for signs of haemorrhage or abnormalities in the drainage. When bile leakage is excessive the dressings will need frequent reinforcing and the outer layers will require frequent changing to keep the patient dry and comfortable and to avoid irritation of the skin around the incision.

The nursing care plan of a patient with either a T tube or an X tube should take into account three major potential problems: infection, obstruction, and dislodging of the tube. Monitoring should include measurement of the body temperature and inspection of the tube site for redness, warmth, swelling, and purulent drainage around the tube. The patient also must be watched for jaundice and complaints of right upper quadrant pain; drainage around the tube when it is clamped; nausea and vomiting; very dark urine; and clay-coloured stools, all of which indicate obstruction. Jaundice occurs as the result of accumulations of bile pigment in the blood. The amount of drainage through the tube should be measured and recorded periodically. A marked decrease in amount may indicate that the tube has been dislodged from the bile duct.

gallipot ('galiˌpot) a small receptacle for lotions or ointments.

gallium ('gali·əm) a chemical element, atomic number 31, atomic weight 69.72, symbol Ga. See table of elements in Appendix 2.

g.-67 a radioisotope of gallium having a half-life of 78.1 hours; used in the imaging of soft tissue tumours of Hodgkin's disease, lymphomas, and infections (abscesses).

g. scan a nuclear medicine procedure using the radioisotope gallium-67 in the form of gallium citrate. Gallium has a high affinity for certain tumours and also for non-neoplastic lesions, such as abscesses. Gallium scans are particularly useful in the staging of HODGKIN'S DISEASE and other lymphomas, and in localizing occult abscesses.

gallon ('galən) a unit of liquid measure (4 quarts, or 3.785 litres, or 3785 ml).

gallop ('galəp) a disordered rhythm of the heart. See also gallop RHYTHM.

gallstone ('gawlˌstohn) calculus forming in the gallbladder. The presence of gallstones is known medically as cholelithiasis. Their cause is unknown, although there is evidence of a connection between gallstones and obesity. They are most common in women after pregnancy, and in men and women over 35 years.

Gallstones may be present without causing trouble. Common symptoms are vague discomfort and pain in the upper abdomen. There may be indigestion and nausea, especially after eating fatty foods. X-rays will generally reveal the presence of gallstones, either directly or by use of a dye introduced into the gallbladder (CHOLECYSTOGRAPHY).

The most common complication of gallstones occurs when one of the stones from the gallbladder travels along the common bile duct, where it may lodge, blocking the flow of bile to the intestine and causing obstructive jaundice. This condition should be corrected by surgery before the liver is damaged.

When a gallstone passes through or obstructs a bile duct it can cause severe continuous pain known as biliary colic, felt in the upper right quadrant of the abdomen, and radiating through to the back. Morphine is usually not given to relieve the pain because it increases spasm of the biliary sphincters. Other drugs such as papaverine hydrochloride and atropine may be given.

Surgery is undertaken as soon as the patient is fit to withstand it. In most cases the gallbladder is removed and a tube is inserted into the common bile duct to establish drainage of bile that has been dammed up by the stone. See also surgery of the GALLBLADDER.

Drugs have not so far been as effective in dissolving gallstones as was hoped.

Over recent years it has become more common to investigate the biliary tree endoscopically, and it is possible to remove gallstones from the common bile duct. Many believe that the risks and complications are lower by exploring the common bile duct endoscopically than by the more conventional surgical route. The endoscope is used to pass a diathermy wire into the lower bile duct, and to open up the sphincter so that the stones can pass through.

PATIENT CARE. The patient has the procedure explained and the reasons for performing it before signing consent. He is not allowed food or fluids for 8–12 hours prior to the procedure. Fluids are given intravenously before the investigation, and intravenous antibiotics are used to lessen the risk of infection.

Following the procedure the patient's vital signs are regularly assessed as the problems that can occur are haemorrhage from the incision, cholangitis from the impacted stone, pancreatitis, and rarely duodenal perforation and gallstone ileus. Intravenous fluid is continued until food and fluids are given (usually after 12–18 hours). Intravenous antibiotics are normally given for 48 hours. The patient can normally go home two to three days following the procedure.

galvanic current (gal'vanik) a steady direct electric current.

galvanism ('galvə,nizəm) electrical treatment using direct current to stimulate the muscles. See also FARADIZATION.

galvanocauterization (,galvənoh,kawtə·rie'zayshən) burning by means of a wire heated by galvanic current.

galvanocontractility (,galvənoh,kontrak'tilitee) contractility in response to stimulation by galvanic current.

galvanofaradization (,galvənoh,farədie'zayshən) galvanic faradization; the application of a galvanic (direct) and faradic (induced) current simultaneously to a nerve or muscle.

galvanometer (,galvə'nomitə) an instrument for measuring current by electromagnetic action.

galvanopalpation (,galvənohpal'payshən) testing of nerves of the skin by means of galvanic current.

gamete ('gameet) 1. one of two cells, male (spermatozoon) and female (ovum), whose union is necessary in sexual reproduction to initiate the development of a new individual. 2. the malarial parasite in its sexual form in a mosquito's stomach, either male (microgamete) or female (macrogamete); the latter is fertilized by the former to develop into an ookinete. adj. **gametic**.

gametocide (gə'meetoh,sied) an agent that destroys gametes or gametocytes. adj. **gametocidal**.

gametocyte (gə'meetoh,siet) 1. an oocyte or spermatocyte; a cell that produces gametes. 2. the sexual stage of the malarial parasite in the blood which may produce gametes when taken into the mosquito host; it may be male (microgametocyte) or female (macrogametocyte).

gametogenesis (,gamitoh'jenəsis) the formation and development of the male and female sex cells (gametes). adj. **gametogenic**. Called also *gametogeny*.

gametogeny (,gami'tojənee) gametogenesis.

gametogony (,gami'togənee) the development of merozoites into male and female gametes, which later fuse to form a zygote.

Gamgee tissue ('gamjee) an absorbent dressing formed from cotton wool sandwiched between thin outer layers of gauze.

gamma ('gamə) the third letter of the Greek alphabet, γ; used in names of chemical compounds to distinguish one of three or more isomers or to indicate the position of substituting atoms or groups.

g. camera a machine for imaging nuclear medicine investigations.

g. globulin a class of plasma proteins composed almost entirely of IgG an IMMUNOGLOBULIN protein that contains most antibody activity.

Commercial preparations of gamma globulin are derived from blood serum and are used for prevention, modification, and treatment of various infectious diseases. This type of gamma globulin contains almost all the known antibodies circulating in the blood. It can provide passive immunity, usually for about 6 weeks against infections to which most of the population has antibodies. Certain specific types of gamma globulin may be used to raise the body's resistance to measles, mumps, and poliomyelitis.

The total production of gamma globulin may be increased in the body by repeated immunization by, for example, microorganisms. An increased amount of gamma globulin in the blood, a condition known as hypergammaglobulinaemia, may be indicative of a chronic infection or certain malignant blood diseases.

There is also a rare condition, AGAMMAGLOBULINAEMIA, in which the body is unable to produce gamma globulin; patients suffering from this condition are extremely susceptible to infection and must be given frequent injections of gamma globulin.

g. rays, γ-rays electromagnetic emissions from radioactive substances. Gamma rays are similar to and have the same general properties as x-rays, except that they are produced through the disintegration of certain radioactive elements. They consist of high energy photons, have short wavelengths, and have no mass and no electric charge. Gamma rays are sometimes used in the treatment of deep-seated malignancies (see RADIATION THERAPY).

gamma-aminobutyric acid (,gamə·ə,meenohbyoo'tirik, -ə'mienoh-) an amino acid that is one of the principal inhibitory neurotransmitters in the central nervous system. Abbreviated GABA.

gamma benzene hexachloride ('gamə 'benzeen ˌheksə'klor·ried) a pediculicide and scabicide.

gammacism ('gaməˌsizəm) imperfect utterance of velar consonants, especially *g* and *k* sounds.

gammaglobulinopathy (ˌgaməˌglobyuhli'nopəthee) gammopathy.

gammopathy (ga'mopəthee) abnormal proliferation of the lymphoid cells producing immunoglobulins; they may be monoclonal or polyclonal, benign or malignant. Multiple myeloma and macroglobulinaemia are examples of malignant monoclonal gammopathy. Called also *gammaglobulinopathy*.

Gamna's disease ('gamnəz) splenomegaly with thickening of the splenic capsule and the presence of small brownish areas (Gamna's nodules), iron-containing pigment being deposited in the splenic pulp.

Gamna's nodules brown or yellow pigmented nodules seen in the spleen in certain cases of enlargement, as in Gamna's disease and siderotic splenomegaly.

gamogenesis (ˌgamoh'jenəsis) sexual reproduction.

gangli(o)- word element. [Gr.] *ganglion*.

ganglial ('gang·gli·əl) pertaining to a ganglion.

gangliated ('gang·gliˌaytid) provided with ganglia; ganglionated.

gangliform ('gang·gliˌfawm) having the form of a ganglion.

gangliitis (ˌgang·gli'ietis) inflammation of a ganglion; ganglionitis.

ganglioblast ('gang·gliohˌblast) an embryonic cell of the cerebrospinal ganglia.

gangliocyte ('gang·gliohˌsiet) a ganglion cell.

gangliocytoma (ˌgang·gliohsie'tohmə) ganglioneuroma.

ganglioform ('gang·gliohˌfawm) gangliform.

ganglioglioma (ˌgang·gliohglie'ohmə) a glioma rich in mature neurons or ganglion cells.

ganglioglioneuroma (ˌgang·gliohˌglieohnyuh'rohmə) ganglioneuroma.

ganglioma (ˌgang·gli'ohmə) ganglioneuroma.

ganglion ('gang·gli·ən) pl. *ganglia,ganglions* [Gr.] 1. a knot or knotlike mass; used in anatomic nomenclature as a general term to designate a group of nerve cell bodies, located outside the central nervous system. Occasionally applied to certain nuclear groups within the brain or spinal cord, e.g., basal ganglia. 2. a form of cystic tumour occurring on an aponeurosis or tendon, such as the wrist. adj. **ganglial, ganglionic.**

Arnold's g. otic ganglion.

autonomic ganglia aggregations of cell bodies of neurons of the autonomic nervous system; the parasympathetic and the sympathetic ganglia combined.

basal ganglia subcortical masses of grey matter embedded in each cerebral hemisphere, comprising the corpus striatum (caudate and lentiform nuclei), amygdaloid body, and claustrum. Other structures have also been considered to be part of the basal ganglia. Called also *basal nuclei*.

g. blocker 1. blocking transmission of impulses through the sympathetic and parasympathetic ganglia. 2. an agent that so acts.

cardiac ganglia ganglia of the superficial cardiac plexus under the arch of the aorta.

carotid g. an occasional small enlargement in the internal carotid plexus.

coeliac ganglia two irregularly shaped ganglia, one on each crus of the diaphragm within the coeliac plexus.

cephalic ganglia parasympathetic ganglia in the head, consisting of the ciliary, otic, pterygopalatine, and submandibular ganglia.

cerebrospinal ganglia those associated with the cranial and spinal nerves.

cervical g. 1. any of the three ganglia (inferior, middle, and superior) of the sympathetic trunk in the neck region. 2. one near the cervix uteri.

cervicothoracic g. a ganglion on the sympathetic trunk anterior to the lowest cervical or first thoracic vertebra. It is formed by a union of the seventh and eighth cervical and first thoracic ganglia. Called also *stellate ganglion*.

cervicouterine g. one near the cervix uteri.

ciliary g. a parasympathetic ganglion in the posterior part of the orbit.

coccygeal g. glomus coccygeum.

Corti's g. spiral ganglion.

dorsal root g. spinal ganglion.

false g. an enlargement on a nerve that does not have a true ganglionic structure.

Frankenhäuser's g. cervical ganglion (2).

gasserian g. trigeminal ganglion.

geniculate g. the sensory ganglion of the facial nerve, on the geniculum of the facial nerve.

g. impar the ganglion commonly found in front of the coccyx, where the sympathetic trunks of the two sides unite.

inferior g. 1. the lower of two ganglia of the glossopharyngeal nerve as it passes through the jugular foramen. 2. the lower of two ganglia of the vagus nerve as it passes through the jugular foramen.

jugular g. superior ganglion (1 and 2).

Ludwig's g. a ganglion near the right atrium of the heart, connected with the cardiac plexus.

lumbar ganglia the ganglia on the sympathetic trunk, usually four or five on either side.

lymphatic g. a lymph node.

otic g. a parasympathetic ganglion next to the medial surface of the mandibular division of the trigeminal nerve, just inferior to the foramen ovale. Its postganglionic fibres supply the parotid gland. Called also *Arnold's ganglion*.

parasympathetic ganglia aggregations of cell bodies of cholinergic neurons of the parasympathetic nervous system; these ganglia are located near to or within the wall of the organs being innervated.

petrous g. inferior ganglion (1).

pterygopalatine g. a parasympathetic ganglion in a fossa in the sphenoid bone, formed by postganglionic cell bodies that synapse with preganglionic fibres from the fascial nerve via the nerve of the pterygopalatine canal. Called also *sphenopalatine ganglion*.

sacral ganglia those of the sacral part of the sympathetic trunk, usually three or four on either side.

Scarpa's g. vestibular ganglion.

semilunar g. 1. trigeminal ganglion. 2. *semilunar ganglia*, coeliac ganglia.

sensory g. any of the ganglia of the peripheral nervous system that transmit sensory impulses; also, the collective masses of nerve cell bodies in the brain subserving sensory functions.

simple g. a cystic tumour in a tendon sheath.

sphenopalatine g. pterygopalatine ganglion.

spinal ganglia ganglia on the posterior root of each spinal nerve.

spiral g. the ganglion on the cochlear nerve, located within the modiolus, sending fibres peripherally to the organ of Corti and centrally to the cochlear nuclei of the brain stem. Called also *Corti's ganglion*.

stellate g. cervicothoracic ganglion.

submandibular g., submaxillary g. a parasympathetic ganglion located superior to the deep part of the submandibular gland, on the lateral surface of the hyoglossal muscle; its postganglionic fibres supply the sublingual and submandibular glands.

superior g. 1. the upper of two ganglia on the

glossopharyngeal nerve as it passes through the jugular foramen. 2. the upper of two ganglia of the vagus nerve just as it passes through the jugular foramen. Called also *jugular ganglion*.

sympathetic ganglia aggregations of cell bodies of adrenergic neurons of the sympathetic nervous system; these ganglia are arranged in chainlike fashion on either side of the spinal cord.

thoracic ganglia the ganglia on the thoracic portion of the sympathetic trunk, 11 or 12 on either side.

trigeminal g. a ganglion on the sensory root of the fifth cranial nerve, situated in a cleft within the dura mater on the anterior surface of the pars petrosa of the temporal bone, and giving off the ophthalmic and maxillary and part of the mandibular nerve. Called also *gasserian ganglion* and *semilunar ganglion*.

tympanic g. an enlargement on the tympanic branch of the glossopharyngeal nerve.

vestibular g. the sensory ganglion of the vestibular part of the eighth cranial nerve, located in the upper part of the lateral end of the internal acoustic meatus. Called also *Scarpa's ganglion*.

Walther's g. glomus coccygeum.

Wrisberg's ganglia cardiac ganglia.

wrist g. cystic enlargement of a tendon sheath on the back of the wrist.

ganglionated ('gang·gli·ə,naytid) provided with ganglia; gangliated.

ganglionectomy, gangliectomy (,gang·gli·ə'nektəmee; gang·gli·əktəmee) excision of a ganglion.

ganglioneuroma (,gang·gliohnyuh'rohmə) a benign neoplasm composed of nerve fibres and mature ganglion cells; called also gangliocytoma, ganglioglioneuroma, and ganglioma.

ganglionic (,gang·gli'onik) pertaining to a ganglion.

g. blockade inhibition by drugs of nerve impulse transmission at autonomic ganglionic synapses.

ganglionitis (,gang·gli·ə'nietis) inflammation of a ganglion; gangliitis.

ganglionostomy (,gang·gli·ə'nostəmee) incision to a cyst on a tendon sheath or aponeurosis.

ganglioside ('gang·gli·ə,sied) a class of galactose-containing cerebrosides found in central nervous system tissues; they are glycolipids of the basic composition ceramide-glucose-galactose-*N*-acetyl neuraminic acid. The form GM_1 accumulates in tissues in generalized gangliosidosis, the form GM_2 in Tay–Sachs disease.

gangliosidosis (,gang·gliohsie'dohsis) a lipid storage disorder marked by accumulation of gangliosides in tissues due to an enzyme defect. In generalized gangliosidosis, a hereditary defect in β-galactosidase causes accumulation of galactoside GM_1, resulting in mental handicap, hepatomegaly, skeletal deformities, and, often, a cherry-red spot. In TAY–SACHS DISEASE, a defect of hexosaminidase A results in accumulation of ganglioside GM_2.

gangosa (gang'gohsə) one of the late lesions of yaws, manifested as a destructive ulceration of the nose, nasopharynx, and hard palate.

gangrene ('gang·green) death of body tissue, generally in considerable mass, either due to loss of blood supply, or to the effects of certain infections, and presenting in moist (wet) and dry forms or as gas gangrene.

TYPES OF GANGRENE. The three major types of gangrene are moist, dry, and gas gangrene. Moist and dry gangrene result from failure of the circulation. Gas gangrene develops in lacerated wounds infected by various species of *Clostridium*, which together break down muscle tissue first by toxins, then by saprophytic liquefaction and gas formation which proceeds emphysematously along tissue planes and in the bloodstream.

Moist gangrene is caused by sudden stoppage of blood, resulting from burning by heat or acid, severe freezing, physical accident that destroys the tissue, a tourniquet that has been left on too long, or a clot or other embolism. At first, tissue affected by moist gangrene has the colour of a bad bruise, is swollen, and often blistered. The gangrene is likely to spread with great speed. Toxins are formed in the affected tissues and absorbed.

Dry gangrene occurs gradually and results from slow reduction of the blood flow in the arteries. There is no subsequent bacterial decomposition; the tissues become dry and shrivelled. It occurs only in the extremities, and can occur with ARTERIOSCLEROSIS, in old age, or in advanced stages of DIABETES MELLITUS. BUERGER'S DISEASE can also sometimes cause dry gangrene. Symptoms include gradual shrinking of the tissue, which becomes cold and lacking in pulse, and turns first brown and then black. Usually a line of demarcation is formed where the gangrene stops, owing to the fact that the tissue above this line continues to receive an adequate supply of blood.

Gas gangrene results from dirty lacerated wounds infected by anaerobic bacteria, especially species of *Clostridium*. It is an acute, severe, painful condition in which muscles and subcutaneous tissues become filled with gas and a serosanguineous exudate.

Internal Gangrene. An intra-abdominal lesion when the blood supply is cut off from a loop of intestine, either by an adhesive band or a strangulated HERNIA. Acute inflammation may also impair the blood supply to the appendix (see APPENDICITIS) or the gallbladder (see CHOLECYSTITIS), causing either to become gangrenous.

PREVENTION. To prevent gangrene in an open wound, the wound should be kept as clean as possible. Special wound care is particularly important in patients with DIABETES MELLITUS, malnutrition, and immunodeficiency. FROSTBITE is especially dangerous, for the freezing impedes circulation, skin becomes tender and easily broken, and underlying cells are destroyed.

gangrenous ('gang·grinəs) pertaining to, marked by, or of the nature of gangrene.

Ganser's syndrome (state) ('ganzəz) amnesia, disturbance of consciousness, and hallucinations, associated with senseless answers to questions, and absurd acts. Usually a transient response to a troublesome situation, e.g. prisoners on remand (prison psychosis).

Gantrisin ('gantrisin) trademark for preparations of sulphafurazole, an antibacterial sulphonamide.

Garamycin (,garə'miesin) trademark for a preparation of gentamicin, an antibiotic.

Gardner's syndrome ('gahdnəz) familial polyposis of the colon associated with osseous and soft tissue tumours.

Gardnerella (,gahdnə'rellə) a genus of gram-negative, rod-shaped bacteria having one species. *G. vaginalis* (formerly called *Haemophilus vaginalis*). It is found in the normal female genital tract and is the causative organism for nonspecific vaginitis. *Gardnerella* infection is one of the most common and most infectious of the sexually transmitted diseases; the infection is thought to be caused in association with anaerobic organisms.

The major symptom is increased vaginal discharge that is thin and grey and has a fishy odour, especially after sexual intercourse. The pH of the discharge is between 5 and 5.5. There is usually no itching or sign of mucosal irritation since the organism does not invade the vaginal mucosa. The presence of the latter symptoms suggests that a concomitant infecton is present.

Treatment is with metronidazole. The sexual partner should be treated concurrently if re-infection is to be avoided.

gargle ('gahg'l) 1. a solution for rinsing the mouth and throat. 2. to rinse the mouth and throat by holding a solution in the open mouth and agitating it by expulsion of air from the lungs.

gargoylism ('gahgoy,lizəm) HURLER'S SYNDROME, the prototypical form of mucopolysaccharidosis.

Garré's osteomyelitis ('garayz) sclerosing nonsuppurative osteomyelitis.

gas (gas) any elastic aeriform fluid in which the molecules are widely separated from each other and so have free paths.

alveolar g. the gas in the alveoli of the lungs, where gaseous exchange with the capillary blood takes place.

g. gangrene a condition often resulting from dirty, lacerated wounds in which the muscles and subcutaneous tissue become filled with gas and a serosanguineous exudate. It is due to species of *Clostridium* that break down tissue by gas production and by toxins.

laughing g. nitrous oxide.

g. pains pains caused by distention of the stomach or intestines by accumulations of air or other gases. The presence of gas is indicated by the distention of the abdomen and by belching or the discharge of gas by rectum. Gas-forming foods include highly flavoured vegetables such as onions, cabbage, and turnips, and members of the bean family. Melons and raw apples are gas-forming fruits. Seasonings and other chemical irritants are also likely to produce gas in the intestinal tract.

tear g. a gas that produces severe lacrimation by irritating the conjunctivae.

Gasser's ganglion ('gasəz) the trigeminal ganglion. The ganglion of the sensory root of the fifth cranial nerve.

gasserectomy (,gasə'rektəmee) excision of the trigeminal ganglion.

gaster ('gastə) [Gr.] *stomach.*

Gasterophilus (,gastə'rofiləs) a genus of flies, the horse botflies, the larvae of which develop in the gastrointestinal tract of horses and may sometimes infect man.

gastr(o)- word element. [Gr.] *stomach.*

gastradenitis (,gastradə'nietis) inflammation of the gastric glands.

gastralgia (ga'stralji·ə) pain in the stomach; gastric colic.

gastrectomy (ga'strektəmee) excision of the stomach, partial, total or subtotal, sometimes undertaken for gastric ULCER, rarely for duodenal ulcer, and gastric cancer (see also surgery of the STOMACH).

gastric ('gastrik) pertaining to, affecting, or originating in the stomach.

g. analysis analysis of the stomach contents by microscopy and tests to determine the amount of acid present.

Procedures for a gastric analysis vary according to the type of test meal or stimulating substance given to increase the flow of gastric juices. Alcohol, caffeine, or histamine may be used as a stimulant but the synthetic hormone pentagastrin is now usually used. All gastric analyses require that the patient be in a fasting state, that he refrain from smoking, and that he remain calm and undisturbed prior to withdrawal of the stomach's contents. Measures must be taken to make the passage of the stomach tube as easy as possible for the patient under the circumstances. Once the stomach tube is in place specimens are obtained at varying intervals, depending on the stimulant administered.

g. bypass surgical creation of a small gastric pouch that empties directly into the jejunum through a gastrojejunostomy, thereby causing food to bypass the duodenum; done for the treatment of gross OBESITY.

g. flu a popular term for what may be any of several disorders of the stomach and intestinal tract. The symptoms are nausea, diarrhoea, abdominal cramps and fever.

During the acute stage all foods should be avoided. Carbonated soft drinks can be taken in moderation to relieve the nausea.

When the symptoms subside, the diet should at first be confined to liquids and soft, bland foods. Milk and dairy products, butter, and fats generally, fruits and greens, should be avoided completely until the patient is free of all symptoms. If the symptoms persist a doctor should be consulted.

g. juice the secretion of glands in the walls of the stomach for use in digestion. The essential ingredients are pepsin, an enzyme that breaks down proteins in food, and hydrochloric acid, which destroys bacteria and is of assistance in the digestive process.

At the sight and smell of food, the stomach increases its output of gastric juice. When the food reaches the stomach, it is thoroughly mixed with the juice, the breakdown of the proteins is begun and the food then passes on to the duodenum for the next stage of digestion.

Normally the hydrochloric acid in gastric juice does not irritate or injure the delicate stomach tissues. However, in certain persons the stomach produces too much gastric juice, especially between meals when it is not needed, and the gastric secretions presumably erode the stomach lining, producing a peptic ULCER, and also hinder its healing once an ulcer has formed.

g. partitioning a gastric bypass procedure undertaken for obesity in which the stomach is partitioned into two sections by two rows of staples applied across the stomach approximately 1.5 cm distal to the gastro-oesophageal junction, thus creating a small pouch approximately 50 ml in capacity. The rows of staples are deliberately interrupted at one point so that a small funnel-shaped opening permits the flow of food from the upper pouch to the remaining portion of the stomach. There is no interruption in the continuity of the intestinal tract in this procedure as there is in gastric bypass and intestinal bypass. Candidates for this procedure must meet the same criteria as for other surgical methods of treatment for OBESITY. Although less hazardous than other procedures that require severing the intestinal tube and altering its continuity, surgical partitioning of the stomach is not completely free of complications and long-term problems for the patient. Perforation of the gastric mucosa is a possibility during the immediate postoperative period, and adjustment to a strict dietary regimen and new eating habits can be frustrating and discouraging. As with other forms of surgical intervention for treatment of obesity, these patients require continued monitoring and support for the rest of their lives.

g. ulcer an ULCER of the inner wall of the stomach. It is one of the two most common types of peptic ulcer, the other type being duodenal ulcer.

gastricism ('gastri,sizəm) gastric disorder.

gastricsin (ga'striksin) a proteolytic enzyme isolated from gastric juice; its precursor is pepsinogen but it differs from pepsin in molecular weight and in the amino acid content at the *N* terminal.

gastrin ('gastrin) a polypeptide hormone secreted by certain cells of the pyloric glands, which strongly stimulates secretion of gastric acid and pepsin, and weakly stimulates secretion of pancreatic enzymes and gallbladder contraction.

gastrinoma (,gastri'nohmə) a gastrin-secreting, non-beta islet cell tumour of the pancreas, associated with Zollinger–Ellison syndrome.

gastritis (ga'strietis) inflammation of the lining of the stomach. Gastritis is one of the most common stomach disorders, and occurs in acute, chronic, and toxic forms.

acute g. severe gastritis caused by food poisoning, overeating, excessive intake of alcoholic beverages, or bacterial or viral infection, and often accompanied by enteritis. The outstanding symptom of acute gastritis is abdominal pain. There is a feeling of distention, with loss of appetite, nausea, and headache. There may be a slight fever and vomiting.

The substance causing the irritation can often be identified and it should of course be avoided. A bland diet of liquids and easily digested food should be followed for 2 or 3 days. Simply prepared solid foods in small quantities can then be added.

chronic g. an inflammation of the stomach that may occur repeatedly or continue over a period of time. Pain, especially after eating, and symptoms associated with indigestion occur in chronic gastritis. Among its possible causes are vitamin deficiencies, abnormalities of the gastric juice, ulcers, hiatus hernia, excessive use of alcohol, chronic emotional tension, or a combination of any of these.

Chronic gastritis is treated with a bland diet. Food should be taken frequently, in small amounts. Antacids may also be used in moderation to minimize stomach acidity. A tranquillizer or mild sedative may help relieve tension and thus speed the healing process.

giant hypertrophic g. Menetrier's disease.

toxic g. gastritis resulting from ingestion of a corrosive substance such as a strong acid or poison. There is an acute burning sensation and cramping stomach pain, accompanied by diarrhoea and vomiting. The vomitus may be bloody. The victim may collapse.

This condition is an emergency and immediate measures must be taken to prevent serious damage to the tissues of the stomach. First-aid measures are begun at once to flush out and neutralize the POISON.

gastrocamera (,gastroh'kamə·rə) a small camera which can be passed down the oesophagus to photograph the inside of the stomach.

gastrocardiac (,gastroh'kahdi·ak) pertaining to the stomach and the heart.

gastrocele ('gastroh,seel) hernial protrusion of the stomach or of a gastric pouch.

gastrocnemius (,gastrok'neemi·əs) the principal muscle of the calf of the leg. It is a flexor of both the ankle and the knee.

gastrocolic (,gastroh'kolik) pertaining to or communicating with the stomach and colon.

gastrocolitis (,gastrohkə'lietis) inflammation of the stomach and colon.

gastrocutaneous (,gastrohkyoo'tayni·əs) pertaining to the stomach and skin, or communicating with the stomach and the cutaneous surface of the body, as a gastrocutaneous fistula.

gastrodiaphany (,gastrohdie'afənee) examination of the stomach by transillumination of its walls with a small electric lamp passed down the oesophagus.

gastrodidymus (,gastroh'didiməs) symmetrical conjoined twins joined in the abdominal region.

gastroduodenal (,gastroh,dyooə'deenəl) pertaining to the stomach and duodenum.

gastroduodenitis (,gastroh,dyooədi'nietis) inflammation of the stomach and duodenum.

gastroduodenoscopy (,gastroh,dyooədi'noskəpee) endoscopic examination of the stomach and duodenum.

gastroduodenostomy (,gastroh,dyooədi'nostəmee) anastomosis of the stomach to part of the duodenum.

gastrodynia (,gastroh'dini·ə) pain in the stomach.

gastroenteralgia (,gastroh,entə'ralji·ə) pain in the stomach and intestines.

gastroenteric (,gastroh·en'terik) pertaining to the stomach and intestines.

gastroenteritis (,gastroh,entə'rietis) inflammation of the lining of the stomach and intestine. Psychological causes of gastroenteritis include fear, anger, and other forms of emotional upset. Allergic reactions to certain foods can cause gastroenteritis, as can irritation by excessive use of alcohol. Severe gastroenteritis, with such symptoms as headache, nausea, vomiting, weakness, diarrhoea, and gas pains, may result from various viral and bacterial infections such as INFLUENZA, and FOOD POISONING.

eosinophilic g. a disorder, commonly associated with intolerance to specific foods, marked by infiltration of the mucosa of the small intestine and frequently the stomach by eosinophils, with oedema but without vasculitis and by eosinophilia of the peripheral blood. Symptoms depend on the site and extent of the disorder.

gastroenterocolitis (,gastroh,entə·rohkə'lietis, -koh-) inflammation of the stomach, small intestine, and colon.

gastroenterologist (,gastroh,entə'roləjist) a doctor specializing in gastroenterology.

gastroenterology (,gastroh,entə'roləjee) the study of the stomach and intestine and their diseases.

gastroenteropathy (,gastroh,entə'ropəthee) any disease of the stomach and intestine.

gastroenteroptosis (,gastroh,entə·rop'tohsis) downward displacement or prolapse of the stomach and intestine.

gastroenterostomy, gastroenteroanastomosis (,gastroh,entə'rostəmee; gastroh,entə·roh·ə,nastə'mohsis) surgical anastomosis of the stomach to the intestine.

gastroenterotomy (,gastroh,entə'rotəmee) incision into the stomach and intestine.

gastrofibrescope (,gastroh'fiebə,skohp) a fibrescope for viewing the stomach.

gastrogastrostomy (,gastrohga'strostəmee) anastomosis between the pyloric and cardiac ends of the stomach, usually performed after resection of hourglass deformity of the stomach.

gastrogavage (,gastroh'ga'vahzh) artificial feeding through a tube passed into the stomach.

gastrogenic (,gastrə'jenik) originating in the stomach.

Gastrografin (,gastroh'grafin) trademark for a preparation of meglumine diatrizoate, an oral diagnostic radiopaque contrast medium.

gastrograph ('gastroh,grahf, -graf) an instrument for registering motions of the stomach.

gastrohepatic (,gastroh·hi'patik) pertaining to the stomach and liver.

gastrohepatitis (,gastroh,hepə'tietis) inflammation of the stomach and liver.

gastroileac (,gastroh'iliak) pertaining to the stomach and ileum.

gastroileitis (,gastroh,ili'ietis) inflammation of the stomach and ileum.

gastrointestinal (,gastroh·in'testin'l) pertaining to the stomach and intestine.

g. series GI series, an examination of the upper gastrointestinal tract using barium as the contrast medium for a series of x-ray films. Called also a *barium meal* (see BARIUM examination).

g. tract the stomach and intestines in continuity (see also DIGESTIVE SYSTEM).

gastrojejunocolic (ˌgastrohjiˌjoonoh'kolik) pertaining to the stomach, jejunum, and colon.

gastrojejunostomy (ˌgastrohˌjejuh'nostəmee) surgical anastomosis of the stomach to the jejunum.

gastrolienal (ˌgastroh'lieənəl) pertaining to the stomach and spleen; gastrosplenic.

gastrolith ('gastrəˌlith) a calculus in the stomach.

gastrolithiasis (ˌgastrohli'thieəsis) the presence or formation of gastroliths.

gastrology (ga'strolәjee) study of the stomach and its diseases.

gastrolysis (ga'strolisis) surgical division of perigastric adhesions to mobilize the stomach.

gastromalacia (ˌgastrohmə'layshi·ə) softening of the wall of the stomach.

gastromegaly (ˌgastroh'megəlee) enlargement of the stomach.

gastromycosis (ˌgastrohmie'kohsis) fungal infection of the stomach.

gastromyxorrhoea (ˌgastrohˌmiksə'reeə) excessive secretion of mucus by the stomach.

gastro-oesophageal (ˌgastroh·iˌsofə'jeeəl) pertaining to the stomach and oesophagus.

gastro-oesophagitis (ˌgastroh·iˌsofə'jietis) inflammation of the stomach and oesophagus.

gastro-oesophagostomy (ˌgastroh·iˌsofə'gostəmee) surgical anastomosis between the stomach and oesophagus.

gastroparalysis (ˌgastroh·pə'ralisis) paralysis of the stomach; gastroplegia.

gastropathy (ga'stropəthee) any disease of the stomach.

gastropexy ('gastrohˌpeksee) surgical fixation of the stomach.

Gastrophilus (ga'strofiləs) *Gasterophilus.*

gastrophrenic (ˌgastroh'frenik) pertaining to the stomach and diaphragm.

gastroplasty ('gastrohˌplastee) plastic repair of the stomach.

gastroplegia (ˌgastroh'pleeji·ə) gastroparalysis.

gastroplication (ˌgastrohplie'kayshən) enfolding the stomach wall by operation.

gastroptosis (ˌgastrop'tohsis) downward displacement of the stomach.

gastropulmonary (ˌgastroh'pulmənə·ree, -'puhl-) pertaining to the stomach and lungs.

gastropylorectomy (ˌgastrohˌpielə'rektəmee) excision of the pyloric part of the stomach.

gastropyloric (ˌgastrohpie'lo·rik) pertaining to the stomach and pylorus.

gastrorrhagia (ˌgastrə'rayji·ə) haemorrhage from the stomach.

gastrorrhaphy (ga'stro·rəfee) suture of the stomach.

gastrorrhoea (ˌgastrə'reeə) excessive secretion by the glands of the stomach.

gastroschisis (ga'stroskisis) a congenital fissure of the abdominal wall.

gastroscope ('gastrəˌskohp) an endoscope especially designed for passage into the stomach to permit examination of its interior. The gastroscope is a hollow, cylindrical tube fitted with special lenses and lights. The newer types of gastroscope are made of glass fibre (fibrescope) which is more flexible. Each glass fibre reflects light and creates a mirror effect, making it possible to 'go around corners', and facilitating visualization of the curvature of the stomach.

gastroscopy (ga'stroskəpee) inspection of the interior of the stomach with a gastroscope.

PATIENT CARE. A careful explanation of the procedure and the reasons for performing it should be given to the patient before obtaining his signed consent. He is not allowed to take any food or fluids for 6–8 hours prior to the procedure.

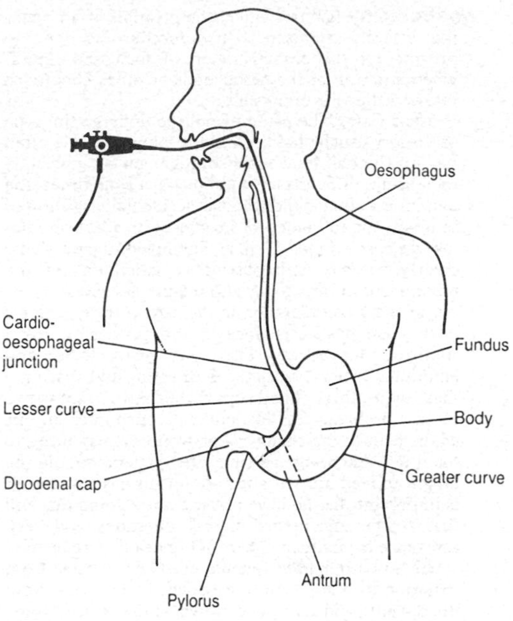

Fibreoptic gastroscope

A sedative, such as diazepam, is given just prior to the gastroscopy. A local pharyngeal anaesethetic using a lignocaine-based spray is also given, so as to depress the gag reflex and reduce local reaction to the passage of the gastroscope. The patient is observed for toxic reaction to these drugs, and an emergency tray containing naxolone hydrochloride and adrenaline should be readily available.

A gastroscope is then passed so as to visualize the oesophagus, stomach and duodenum. Biopsies may be taken.

After the procedure is completed the patient is observed until he is awake and orientated. Food and fluids are not given until the gag reflex returns, usually in 2–3 hours. If biopsies are taken the patients vital signs should be checked regularly, as there is a danger of bleeding.

Many patients have this procedure performed as outpatients. If they have been given intravenous sedatives they should not drive a car or operate dangerous machinery for 24 hours. They should be collected from hospital by a friend or relative because of the time it takes for the effects of the drugs to wear off.

gastrospasm ('gastrohˌspazəm) spasm of the stomach.

gastrosplenic (ˌgastroh'splenik) pertaining to the stomach and spleen; gastrolienal.

gastrostaxis (ˌgastroh'staksis) the oozing of blood from the stomach mucosa.

gastrostenosis (ˌgastrohstə'nohsis) contraction or shrinkage of the stomach.

gastrostogavage (gaˌstrostoh'gavahzh) feeding through a gastric fistula.

gastrostolavage (gaˌstrostoh'lavahzh) irrigation of the stomach through a gastric fistula.

gastrostomy (ga'strostəmee) the creation of an opening into the stomach. This procedure is done to provide for the administration of food and liquids when stricture of the oesophagus or other conditions make swallowing impossible.

PATIENT CARE. The patient who is to undergo this type of surgery usually has been ill for some time. He often has nutritional deficiencies brought on by a steadily increasing difficulty in swallowing. Sometimes the patient is a small child who has accidentally swallowed some caustic substance, or he may be an adult who has taken a corrosive poison in an attempted suicide. Some elderly patients with obstructive carcinoma of the oesophagus or throat may also require gastrostomy.

A primary consideration in the care of these patients is the patient's acceptance of the gastrostomy as a substitute for eating. There are many social and emotional factors associated with eating and sharing a meal with others. The hospital staff must be sensitive to the problems the patient will encounter in his adjustment to the changes a gastrostomy may bring to his life. Whenever possible the patient should be taught to feed himself and care for his gastrostomy. It is important that he have privacy while doing this and that he be encouraged to ask questions and seek assistance from the members of the health care team.

The skin around the opening must be protected from irritation by the gastric juices, which may leak from the opening and act as a corrosive on the skin. In some cases the gastrostomy tube can be removed after each feeding.

Food for a gastrostomy patient is gradually increased according to his tolerance. At first, water and glucose are given at regular intervals. If there is no leakage and the patient has no difficulty with these liquids, other liquids and puréed foods are gradually added until a full meal can be tolerated.

In order to stimulate gastric secretions and aid digestion, the patient should see, smell, and taste small amounts of food before each feeding. It is recommended that he be allowed to chew small bits of food even though he cannot swallow them. This allows for proper stimulation of the gums and teeth and helps promote the health of the mouth and teeth.

Food should be warmed before it is given through the tube. Although commercially prepared liquid foods are more convenient, they can cause diarrhoea. The foods to be given through the tube should be cooked until they are soft and then puréed in an electric blender. They can be diluted with the water in which they have been cooked, so that no vitamins are lost. The dietitian must work very closely with the patient and his family, instructing them in the planning and preparation of the patient's meals and offering suggestions for a variety of foods that will provide a well-balanced diet.

gastrothoracopagus (ˌgastrohˌthor·rə'kopəgəs) symmetrical conjoined twins joined at the abdomen and thorax.

gastrotomy (ga'strotəmee) incision into the stomach.

gastrotropic (ˌgastroh'tropik) having affinity for or exerting a special effect on the stomach.

gastrotympanites (ˌgastrohˌtimpə'nieteez) tympanitic distention of the stomach.

gastrula ('gastruhlə) an embryo in the stage following the blastula stage; the simplest type consists of two layers of cells, the ectoderm and entoderm, which have invaginated to form the archenteron and an opening, the blastopore.

gastrulation (ˌgastruh'layshən) the process by which a blastula becomes a gastrula or, in forms without a true blastula, the process by which three germ cell layers are acquired.

Gatinar ('gatinə) trademark for a preparation of lactulose, a cathartic.

Gaucher's cells ('gohshayz) a large cell characteristic of Gaucher's disease, with eccentrically placed nuclei and fine wavy fibrils parallel to the long axis of the cell.

Gaucher's disease (goh'shayz) a hereditary disorder of glucocerebroside metabolism, marked by the presence of Gaucher's cells in the marrow, and by hepatosplenomegaly and erosion of the cortices of long bones and pelvis. The adult form is associated with moderate anaemia and thrombocytopenia, and yellowish pigmentation of the skin; in the infantile form there is, in addition, marked central nervous system impairment; in the juvenile form there are rapidly progressive systemic manifestations but moderate central nervous system involvement.

Gaussian distribution ('gowsi·ən) normal distribution. A continuous symmetrical frequency distribution.

gauze (gawz) a light, open-meshed fabric of muslin or similar material.

absorbent g. white cotton cloth of various thread counts and weights, supplied in various lengths and widths and in different forms (rolls or folds).

petroleum g. a sterile material produced by saturation of sterile absorbent gauze with sterile white petroleum jelly.

zinc gelatin impregnated g. absorbent gauze impregnated with zinc gelatin.

gavage ('gəvahzh) [Fr.] 1. forced feeding, especially through a tube passed into the stomach (see also TUBE feeding). 2. superalimentation.

Gaviscon ('gaviskon) a proprietary antacid combination containing alginic acid, aluminium hydroxide, magnesium trisilicate and sodium barcarbonate.

Gay's gland (gayz) specialized sweat and sebaceous glands around the anus; called also circumanal glands.

gaze (gayz) 1. to look in one direction for a period of time. 2. the act or state of looking steadily in one direction.

Gd chemical symbol, *gadolinium*.

GDC General Dental Council.

Ge chemical symbol, *germanium*.

Gee's disease, Gee–Herter disease, Gee–Herter–Heubner disease (jeez; jee'hərtə; jeeˌhərtə'hoybnə) names previously used for the infantile form of COELIAC DISEASE.

Gee–Thaysen disease (jee'thiesən) an almost obsolete name for the adult form of COELIAC DISEASE.

gegenhalten ('gaygənˌhaltən) [Ger.] an involuntary resistance to passive movement as may occur in cerebral cortical disorders.

Geiger counter, Geiger–Müller counter ('giegə; ˌgiegə'muhlə) an amplifying device that indicates and counts the presence of ionizing particles emitted by a substance; used as a means of determining the presence of radioactivity.

gel (jel) a colloid that is firm in consistency, although containing much liquid; a colloid in a gelatinous form.

gelatin ('jelətin) a substance obtained by partial hydrolysis of collagen derived from skin, white connective tissue, and bones of animals; used as a suspending agent for various drugs or in manufacture of capsules and suppositories; suggested for intravenous use as a plasma substitute, and has been used as an adjuvant protein food. In absorbable film and sponge, it is used in surgical procedures.

zinc g. a preparation of zinc oxide, gelatin, glycerin, and purified water, applied topically as a protective.

gelatinize (jə'latiˌniez) to convert into a jelly, or to become converted into gelatin.

gelatinoid (jə'lati,noyd) resembling gelatin.

gelatinous (jə'latinəs) like jelly or softened gelatin.

gelation (ji'layshən) conversion of a sol into a gel.

Gelofusin (jeloh'fyoosin) trademark for a preparation of partially degraded gelatin used as a plasma expander.

gelosis (jə'lohsis) a hard, swollen lump in a tissue, especially in muscle.

Gelusil ('jelyuhsil) a proprietary antacid combination containing aluminium hydroxide and magnesium trisilicate.

gemellology (,jemə'loləjee) the scientific study of twins and twinning.

geminate ('jeminət, -,nayt) paired; occurring in twos.

gemmation (je'mayshən) development of a new organism from a protuberance on the cell body of the parent, a form of asexual reproduction; called also budding.

gemmule ('gemyool) 1. a reproductive bud; the immediate product of gemmation. 2. any of the little spinelike processes on the dendrites of a nerve cell.

-gen word element. [Gr.] *an agent that produces.*

genal ('jeenəl) pertaining to the cheek; buccal.

gender ('jendə) sex; the category to which an individual is assigned on the basis of sex.

g. identity a person's concept of himself or herself as being male and masculine or female and feminine, or ambivalent.

g. identity disorder a psychiatric label for those disorders marked by a sense of inappropriateness and attendant discomfort concerning one's sexual anatomy and one's sex role. This category usually includes transvestism, transsexualism and gender identity disorders in childhood.

g. role the image projected by a person that identifies him or her as being boy or girl, man or woman. It is the public expression of gender identity.

gene (jeen) one of the biological units of heredity, self-reproducing, and located at a definite position (locus) on a particular chromosome. Genes make up segments of the complex DEOXYRIBONUCLEIC ACID (DNA) molecule that controls cellular reproduction and function. There are thousands of genes in the chromosomes of each cell nucleus; they play an important role in heredity because they control the individual physical, biochemical, and physiological traits inherited by offspring from their parents. Through the genetic code of DNA they also control the day-to-day functions and reproduction of all cells in the body. For example, the genes control the synthesis of structural proteins and also the enzymes that regulate various chemical reactions that take place in a cell.

The gene is capable of replication. When a cell multiplies by mitosis each daughter cell carries a set of genes that is an exact replica of that of the parent cell. This characteristic of replication explains how genes can carry hereditary traits through successive generations without change.

allelic g's genes situated at corresponding loci in a pair of chromosomes.

complementary g's two independent pairs of nonallelic genes, neither of which will produce its effect in the absence of the other.

dominant g. one that produces an effect (the phenotype) in the organism regardless of the state of the corresponding allele. An example of a trait determined by a dominant gene is brown eye colour.

histocompatibility g. one that determines the specificity of tissue antigenicity (HLA antigens) and thus the compatibility of donor and recipient in tissue transplantation and blood transfusion.

holandric g's genes located on the Y chromosome and appearing only in male offspring.

immune response (Ir) g's genes of the major histocompatibility complex (MHC) that govern the immune response to individual immunogens.

Is g's genes that govern the formation of suppressor T-lymphocytes.

lethal g. one whose presence brings about the death of the organism or permits survival only under certain conditions.

mutant g. one that has undergone a detectable mutation.

operator g. one serving as a starting point for reading the genetic code, and which, through interaction with a repressor, controls the activity of structural genes associated with it in the operon.

recessive g. one that produces an effect in the organism only when it is transmitted by both parents, i.e., only when the individual is homozygous.

regulator g., repressor g. one that synthesizes repressor, a substance which, through interaction with the operator gene, switches off the activity of the structural genes associated with it in the operon.

sex-linked g. one that is carried on a sex chromosome, especially an X chromosome.

g. splicing the process of taking a gene from one organism and inserting it into the genome of another. See also RECOMBINANT DNA.

structural g. one that forms templates for messenger RNA and is thereby responsible for the amino acid sequence of specific polypeptides.

genera ('jenə·rə) [L.] plural of *genus.*

generation (,jenə'rayshən) 1. the process of reproduction. 2. a class composed of all individuals removed by the same number of successive ancestors from a common predecessor, or occupying positions on the same level in a genealogical (pedigree) chart.

alternate g. reproduction by alternate asexual and sexual means in an animal or plant species.

asexual g., direct g. production of a new organism not originating from union of gametes.

filial g., first the first-generation offspring of two parents; symbol F_1.

filial g., second all of the offspring produced by two individuals of the first filial generation; symbol F_2.

parental g. the generation with which a particular genetic study is begun; symbol P_1.

sexual g. production of a new organism from the zygote formed by the union of gametes.

spontaneous g. the discredited concept of continuous generation of living organisms from nonliving matter.

generative ('jenə,rətiv) pertaining to reproduction.

generator ('jenə,raytə) something that produces or causes to exist; a machine that converts mechanical to electrical energy.

pulse g. a device for supplying electrical impulses at a fixed rate or in a programmed pattern. In a cardiac pacemaker system it also supplies power to the implanted electrodes. In ultrasonic imaging systems it controls the emission of the ultrasonic pulses.

generic (ji'nerik) 1. pertaining to a genus. 2. nonproprietary; denoting a drug name not protected by a trademark, usually descriptive of the drug's chemical structure.

genesiology (ji,neezi'oləjee) the sum of what is known concerning generation.

genesis ('jenəsis) creation; origination; used as a word termination joined to an element indicating the thing created, e.g., carcinogenesis.

genetic (jə'netik) 1. pertaining to reproduction or to birth or origin. 2. inherited.

g. code the manner in which the arrangement of nucleotides in the polynucleotide chain of a chromosome governs the transmission of genetic information to proteins, i.e., determines the sequence of amino acids in the polypeptide chain making up each protein synthesized by the cell. Genetic information is coded in DNA by means of four bases (two purines: adenine and guanine; and two pyrimidines: thymine and cystosine). Each adjacent sequence of three bases (a codon) determines the insertion of a specific amino acid. In RNA, uracil replaces thymine.

g. counselling the process of support of and giving advice to persons who run the risk that any child born to them may suffer from a genetically transmitted disorder. Sometimes adoption may be preferable or antenatal diagnosis by amniocentesis may be offered. Counselling depends upon knowledge of probability of transmission found empirically and derived from information about genetic mechanisms.

g. engineering the manipulation of genetic material on the chromosome in order to reproduce desired characteristics and eliminate others. Although this has value for parents who carry genetically transmitted disorders it is also potentially open to abuse.

geneticist (jə'neti,sist) a specialist in genetics.

genetics (jə'netiks) the branch of biology dealing with the phenomena of heredity and the laws governing it.

biochemical g. the science concerned with the chemical and physical nature of genes and the mechanism by which they control the development and maintenance of the organism.

The field of biochemical genetics is relatively new and recently it has become the study of the cause of many specific diseases that are now known to be inherited. These diseases include those resulting from the improper synthesis of haemoglobins and protein, such as SICKLE CELL DISEASE and THALASSAEMIA, both of which are hereditary anemias; some 200 inborn errors of metabolism, such as PHENYLKETONURIA and GALACTOSAEMIA, in which lack or alteration of a specific enzyme prohibits proper metabolism of carbohydrates, proteins, or fats and thus produces pathological symptoms; and genetically determined variations in response to certain drugs, for example, isoniazid.

clinical g. the study of the possible genetic factors influencing the occurrence of a pathological condition. In addition to the diseases mentioned under biochemical genetics, other aspects of clinical genetics include the study of chromosomal aberrations, such as those that cause mental handicap and DOWN'S SYNDROME, and immunogenetics, or the genetic aspects of the IMMUNE RESPONSE and the transmission of genetic factors from generation to generation.

Geneva Convention (jə'neevə kən'venshən) an international agreement of 1864, whereby, among other pledges, the signatory nations pledged themselves to treat the wounded and the army medical and nursing staff as neutrals on the field of battle.

genial (jə'neeəl) pertaining to the chin.

genic ('jenik) pertaining to or caused by the genes.

-genic word element. [Gr.] *giving rise to, causing.*

genicular (je'nikyuhlə) pertaining to the knee.

geniculate (je'nikyuh,layt) bent, like a knee.

geniculum (je'nikyuhləm) pl. *genicula* [L.] a little knee; used in anatomical nomenclature to designate a sharp kneelike bend in a small structure or organ.

genioplasty ('jeenioh,plastee) plastic surgery of the chin.

genital ('jenit'l) 1. pertaining to reproduction, or the reproductive organs. 2. *genitals,* the REPRODUCTIVE ORGANS.

genitalia (,jeni'tayli·ə) the REPRODUCTIVE ORGANS; called also the genitals.

The internal female reproductive organs consist of the ovaries, uterine tubes, uterus, and vagina. The external genitalia, referred to collectively as the vulva, consist of the mons pubis, labia majora, labia minora, clitoris, vestibule of the vagina, vulvovaginal glands, and the bulb of the vestibule.

The male genitalia consist of the testes, seminiferous (semen-carrying) tubules, epididymides, ductus deferentes, ejaculatory ducts, seminal vesicles, prostate, bulbourethral glands, and glans penis.

genito- word element. [L.] relating to the organs of reproduction.

genitocrural (,jenitoh'krooə·rəl) pertaining to the genitalia and the thigh.

genitofemoral (,jenitoh'femə·rəl) genitocrural.

genitography (,jeni'tografee) radiography of the urogenital sinus and internal duct structures after injection of a contrast medium through the sinus opening.

genitoplasty ('jenitoh,plastee) plastic surgery on the reproductive (genital) organs.

genitourinary (,jenitoh'yooə·rinə·ree) pertaining to the genitalia and urinary apparatus; urogenital.

g. medicine the medical speciality concerned with the diagnosis and treatment of sexually transmitted diseases (STDs).

g. system the organs of reproduction, together with the organs concerned with production and excretion of urine; called also *urogenital system.*

genocopy ('jenoh,kopee) an individual whose phenotype mimics that of another genotype but whose character is determined by a distinct assortment of genes.

genodermatosis (,jenoh,dərmə'tohsis) a genetic disorder of the skin, usually generalized.

genome ('jeenohm) the complete set of hereditary factors contained in the haploid set of chromosomes. adj. **genomic.**

genotype ('jenoh,tiep, 'jeenoh-) 1. the entire genetic constitution of an individual; also, the alleles present at one or more specific loci. 2. the type species of a genus. adj. **genotypical.**

-genous word element. [Gr.] *arising or resulting from, produced by.*

gentamicin (,jentə'miesin) an antibiotic complex elaborated by fungi of the genus *Mircromonospora,* effective against many gram-negative bacteria, especially *Pseudomonas* species, as well as certain gram-positive bacteria, especially *Staphylococcus aureus.*

gentian ('jenshən) the dried rhizome and roots of *Gentiana lutea;* has been used as a bitter tonic.

g. violet an antibacterial, antifungal, and anthelmintic dye, applied topically in the treatment of infections of the skin and mucous membranes associated with gram-positive bacteria and moulds, and administered orally in pinworm and liver fluke infections.

gentianophilic (,jenshənoh'filik) staining readily with gentian violet.

gentianophobic (,jenshənoh'fohbik) not staining with gentian violet.

genu ('jenyoo) pl. *genua* [L.] the knee.

g. recurvatum hyperextensibility of the knee joint.

g. valgum knock-knee.

g. varum bowleg.

genupectoral (,jenyoo'pektə·rəl) relating to the knee and chest.

g. position the knee–chest position. See POSITION.

genuplasty ('jenyooplastee) surgical reconstruction of the knee by the insertion of an artificial joint.

genus ('jeenəs) pl. *genera* [L.] a taxonomic category (taxon) subordinate to a tribe (or subtribe) and superior to a species (or subgenus).

geo- word element. [Gr.] *the earth, the soil.*
geode ('jeeohd) a dilated lymph space.
geographical pathology (jeeə'grafik'l) medical geography. The study of geographical variations in health, disease and mortality.
geomedicine (,jeeoh'medisin, -'medsin) the branch of medicine dealing with the influence of climatic and environmental conditions on health.
geometric mean (jeeə'metrik) see MEAN.
geophagia, geophagism (,jiə'fayji·ə, -jə; ji'ofə,jizəm) the habit of eating clay or earth (soil); chthonophagia.
geotaxis (,jeeoh'taksis) geotropism.
geotrichosis (,jeeohtri'kohsis) a candidiasis-like infection due to *Geotrichum candidum*, which may attack the bronchi, lungs, mouth, or intestinal tract.
Geotrichum (ji'otrikəm) a genus of yeastlike fungi.
G. candidum a species found in the faeces and dairy products.
geotropism (ji'otrə,pizəm) a tendency of growth or movement toward or away from the earth; the influence of gravity on growth.
ger-, gero-, geronto- word element. [Gr.] *old age, the aged, the elderly.*
geratic (jə'ratik) pertaining to old age.
geratology, gereology (,jerə'toləjee; ,jeri'oləjee) the science dealing with old age.
geriatric nursing (,jeri'atrik) specialization in the treatment, care and welfare of elderly patients.
geriatrician (,jeri·ə'trishən) a medical specialist in geriatrics.
geriatrics (,jeri'atriks) a term first used by Nascher in 1909 for the application of orthodox medicine to the problems of ageing and disease in the elderly; became a branch of medicine in the UK in the mid 1940s. It is related to the science of gerontology, and it embodies an in-depth knowledge and understanding of the health and social problems of old people and the philosophy of a positive approach to these problems.

Its practice is based on the multidisciplinary team of specialist doctor, hospital and community nurses, physiotherapist, occupational therapist, social worker and others; care-planning is a basic principle, involving the patient, his family and the general practitioner. The services are hospital based, usually incorporating assessment and rehabilitation, continuing care, outpatient clinics and a day hospital. Domiciliary visits are undertaken when appropriate and increasingly the care of long-term patients is provided by nursing homes.

AIMS OF GERIATRICS. to promote mental and physical health and social wellbeing in old age; to restore elderly patients to optimum mental and physical functioning; to returm to and maintain elderly patients in the community, preferably in their own homes.

There are few illnesses, if any, that affect only elderly people but they tend to present differently than in younger persons, e.g., mental confusion can be the first indication of acute illness. Multiple pathology is the common characteristic and social problems often accompany illness and disability in old age hence the need for the multidisciplinary team in the practice of geriatrics.

Health care services of this kind grow increasingly important as modern medicine and a rising standard of living lengthens life expectancy and increases the proportion of aged persons in society. See also AGED.
germ (jərm) 1. a pathogenic microorganism. 2. living substance capable of developing into an organ, part, or organism as a whole; a primordium.
wheat g. the embryo of wheat, which contains tocopherol, thiamine, riboflavin, and other vitamins.
German measles ('jərmən 'meez'lz) See RUBELLA.
germanium (jər'mayni·əm) a chemical element, atomic number 32, atomic weight 72.59, symbol Ge. See table of elements in Appendix 2.
germicidal (,jərmi'sied'l) destructive to pathogenic microorganisms.
germicide ('jərmi,sied) an agent that destroys pathogenic microorganisms.
germinal ('jərmin'l) pertaining to or of the nature of a germ cell or the primitive stage of development.
germination (,jərmi'nayshən) the sprouting of a seed or spore or of a plant embryo.
germinative ('jərminətiv) pertaining to germination or to a germ cell.
germinoma (,jərmi'nohmə) a neoplasm of germ tissue (testis or ovum), e.g., a seminoma.
gerocomia (,jeroh'kohmi·ə) the care of old men; the hygiene of old age.
geroderma, gerodermia ('jeroh'dərmə; ,jeroh'dərmi·ə) dystrophy of the skin and genitals, giving the appearance of old age.
gerodontics (,jeroh'dontiks) dentistry dealing with the dental problems of older people. adj. **gerodontic**.
gerodontist (,jeroh'dontist) a dentist specializing in gerodontics.
gerodontology (,jerohdon'toləjee) study of the dentition and dental problems in the aged and ageing.
geromarasmus (,jerohmə'razməs) the emaciation sometimes characteristic of old age.
geromorphism (,jeroh'mawfizəm) premature senility.
gerontal (je'ront'l) pertaining to old age.
gerontologist (,jeron'toləjist) a doctor or social scientist specializing in gerontology.
gerontology (,jeron'toləjee) the scientific study of the problems of ageing in all its aspects.
gerontopia (,jeron'tohpi·ə) second sight; improvement of vision, especially near vision, in the aged, a sign of incipient cataract. Called also senopia.
gerontotherapeutics (je,rontoh,therə'pyootiks) the science of retarding and preventing the development of many of the aspects of senescence.
gerontoxon (,jeron'toksən) arcus senilis.
geropsychiatry (,jerohsie'kieətree) psychogeriatrics.
Gessel's developmental chart ('ges'lz) a chart which shows the expected motor, social and psychological development of children.
gestagen ('jestə,jen) any hormone with progestational activity.
gestalt (gə'shtalt) a whole perceptual configuration.
g. therapy a psychotherapeutic approach which encourages the individual to cease intellectualizing his difficulties and instead to focus on feelings and emotions and thereby to gain emotional insight and balance.
gestaltism (gə'shtaltizəm) the theory in psychology that the objects of mind, as immediately presented to direct experience, come as complete unanalysable wholes or forms (Gestalten) that cannot be split up into parts.
gestation (je'stayshən) the period of development of the young in mammals, from the time of fertilization of the ovum to birth. adj. **gestational**. See also PREGNANCY.
g. period the duration of pregnancy, in the human female about 280 days when measured from the first day of the last menstrual period.
GeV gigaelectron volt.
GFR glomerular filtration rate, used as a measure of renal function.
Ghon focus (lesion, tubercle) (gon) the initial focus of parenchymal infection in primary pulmonary TUBERCULOSIS in children; when associated with a corresponding lymph node focus, it is known as the

primary, or *Ghon complex*.

GI gastrointestinal; globin (zinc) insulin.

Giannuzzi's crescents (ja'nootseez) crescent-shaped patches surrounding the mucous tubercles in mixed glands.

giant cell tumour ('jieənt) 1. a bone tumour, ranging from benign to frankly malignant, composed of cellular spindle cell stroma containing multinucleated giant cells resembling osteoclasts. 2. a benign, small, yellow, tumour-like nodule of tendon sheath origin, most often of the wrist and fingers or ankle and toes, laden with lipophages and containing multinucleated giant cells.

giantism ('jieən,tizəm) 1. gigantism. 2. excessive size, as of cells or nuclei.

Giardia (ji'ahdi·ə) a genus of flagellate protozoa parasitic in the intestines of man and animals, which may cause protracted, intermittent diarrhoea with symptoms suggesting malabsorption.

G. lamblia a species parasitic in the intestines of man.

giardiasis (,jiah'dieəsis) infection with *Giardia*.

gibbosity (gi'bositee) see KYPHOSIS.

gibbous ('gibəs) humped; protuberant.

gibbus ('gibəs) a hump.

Gibney boot ('gibnee) an adhesive tape support used in the treatment of sprains and other painful conditions of the ankle, the tape being applied in a basket-weave fashion with strips placed alternately under the sole of the foot and around the back of the leg.

Gibson murmur (gibsən) a long rumbling sound occupying most of systole and diastole, usually localized in the second left interspace near the sternum, and usually indicative of patent ductus arteriosus.

Giemsa stain ('gyemzə) a solution containing azure II-eosin, azure II, glycerin, and methanol; used for staining protozoan parasites, *Leptospira*, *Borrelia*, viral inclusion bodies, and *Rickettsia*.

Gierke's disease ('giəkəz) glycogenosis (type I) in which deficiency of the hepatic enzyme glucose-6-phosphatase results in liver and kidney involvement, with hepatomegaly, hypoglycaemia, hyperuricaemia, and gout. Called also von Gierke's disease and hepatorenal glycogenosis.

giga- word element. [Gr.] *huge;* used in naming units of measurement to designate an amount 10^9 (one thousand million) times the size of the unit to which it is joined, e.g., gigametre (10^9 metres); symbol G.

gigantism ('jiegan,tizəm, jie'gantizəm) abnormal overgrowth of the body or a part; excessive size and stature. Generally applied to a rare abnormality of the PITUITARY GLAND that causes excessive growth in a child so that he becomes an unusually tall adult. If the abnormality is extreme, he may reach a height of 8 feet or more, although the body proportions usually are normal.

The condition is brought on by overproduction of growth hormone from a pituitary adenoma occurring before the growing ends of bone have closed. The opposite condition, DWARFISM, is caused by underproduction of the same hormone. (Overproduction of growth hormone in adults causes ACROMEGALY.) Gigantism can be corrected only by early diagnosis in childhood and removal by surgery of the pituitary adenoma or by x-ray treatment.

cerebral g. gigantism in the absence of increased levels of growth hormone, attributed to a cerebral defect; infants are large, and accelerated growth continues for the first 4 or 5 years, the rate being normal thereafter. The hands and feet are large, the head large and dolichocephalic, the eyes have an antimongoloid slant, with hypertelorism. The child is clumsy, and mental handicap of varying degree is usually present.

gigantomastia (jie,gantoh'masti·ə) extreme hypertrophy of the breast.

Gilbert's disease ('gilbəts) benign hereditary hyperbilirubinaemia marked by mild intermittent jaundice and often by fatigue, weakness, and abdominal pain.

Gilles de la Tourette's syndrome (disease) (,zheel də lah tooə'rets) multiple tics, especially of the face and upper part of the body, often associated with involuntary obscene utterances. The condition usually has its onset in childhood and often becomes chronic. The cause is unknown.

Gilliam's operation ('gili·əmz) the correction of retroversion of the uterus by drawing a loop at each round ligament through the abdominal wall and fixing them to the anterior rectus sheath thus achieving ventrosuspension.

Gillies needle-holder ('giliz) combined scissors and fine suture needle-holder used in plastic surgery.

Gimbernat's ligament (,himbər'nats) a membrane with its base just medial to the femoral ring, one side attached to the inguinal ligament and the other to the pectineal line of the pubis. Called also *lacunar ligament*.

gingiva ('jinjivə, jin'jievə) pl. *gingivae* [L.] covering the tooth-bearing border of the jaw; the gum. adj. **gingival**.

attached g. the portion overlying the alveolar process and firmly attached to it.

unattached g. the portion attached to the alveolar process by loose areolar connective tissue.

free g. the portion that surrounds the tooth and is not directly attached to the tooth surface.

gingivectomy (,jinji'vektəmee) surgical excision of all loose infected and diseased gingival tissue to eradicate periodontal infection and reduce the depth of the gingival sulcus.

gingivitis (,jinji'vietis) a general term for inflammation of the gums of which bleeding is one of the usual symptoms. Other symptoms include swelling, redness and an unpleasant taste.

Chronic gingivitis if untreated can progress to chronic PERIODONTITS. The most fundamental cause of gingivitis is the accumulation of bacterial plaque. Related environmental factors such as food impaction, carious cavities, poor fillings and malaligned teeth may contribute to the problem.

Gingivitis is therefore both treated and prevented by removing plaque and correcting related environmental factors.

necrotizing ulcerative g. TRENCH MOUTH; a gingival infection marked by redness and swelling, necrosis, pain, haemorrhage, a necrotic odour, and often a pseudomembrane. Extension to the oral mucosa is called necrotizing ulcerative gingivostomatitis.

pregnancy g. any of various gingival changes ranging from gingivitis to the so-called pregnancy tumour.

gingivo- word element. [L.] *gingival*.

gingivoglossitis (,jinjivohglo'sietis) inflammation of the gingiva and tongue.

gingivolabial (,jinjivoh'laybi·əl) pertaining to the gingivae and lips.

gingivoplasty ('jinjivoh,plastee) surgical remodelling of the gingiva.

gingivosis (,jinji'vohsis) a chronic, diffuse inflammation of the gums, with desquamation of the papillary epithelium and mucous membrane.

gingivostomatitis (,jinjivoh,stohmə'tietis) inflammation of the gingiva and oral mucosa.

herpetic g. that due to infection with herpes simplex virus, with redness of the oral tissues, formation of multiple vesicles and painful ulcers, and fever.

necrotizing ulcerative g. that due to extension to the

oral mucosa of necrotizing ulcerative gingivitis (TRENCH MOUTH) (see also VINCENT'S ANGINA).

ginglymus ('jing·glimәs) a joint that allows movement in one plane only, forward and backward, as does a door hinge; called also *hinge joint*.

girdle ('gәrd'l) an encircling or confining structure.

pectoral g. shoulder girdle.

pelvic g. the encircling bony structure supporting the lower limbs.

shoulder g., thoracic g. the encircling bony structure supporting the upper limbs.

Girdlestone's excision arthropathy of the hip ('gәrd'l,stohnz) pseudoarthrosis of the hip. A false joint made by excising the head and neck of the femur and part of the acetabulum, and suturing a muscle mass between the bones' ends. A treatment for osteoarthritis.

Girdlestone's operation 1. tendon transference of the flexor to extensor tendons of the toes for claw toes. 2. resection of part of the proximal phalanx of the great toe for hallux valgus.

glabella (glә'belә) the area on the frontal bone above the nasion and between the eyebrows.

glabrous ('glaybrәs) smooth and bare.

gladiolus (gladi'ohlәs) the main portion or body of the sternum.

glairy ('glair·ree) resembling the white of an egg.

gland (gland) an aggregation of cells specialized to secrete or excrete materials not related to their ordinary metabolic needs. Glands are divided into two main groups, endocrine and exocrine. adj. **glandular.** The ENDOCRINE glands or ductless glands, discharge their secretions (hormones) directly into the blood; they include the adrenal, pituitary, thyroid, and parathyroid glands, the islands of Langerhans in the pancreas, the gonads, the thymus, and the pineal body.

The exocrine glands, which discharge through ducts opening on an external or internal surface of the body, include the salivary, sebaceous, and sweat glands, the liver, the gastric glands, the pancreas, the intestinal, mammary, and lacrimal glands, and the prostate.

The organs sometimes called lymph glands are more accurately called lymph nodes; they are not glands in the usual sense.

acinous g. one made up of one or more oval or spherical sacs (acini).

adrenal g. a flattened body above either kidney, an endocrine gland consisting of a cortex and medulla, the former elaborating steroid hormones, and the latter adrenaline and noradrenaline; called also *suprarenal gland* (see also ADRENAL GLAND).

apocrine g. one whose discharged secretion contains part of the secreting cells.

areolar g's Montgomery's glands.

axillary g's lymph nodes situated in the axilla.

Bartholin's g's vulvovaginal glands, two minute glands, one on each side of the vagina, their ducts opening on the vulva (see also BARTHOLIN'S GLANDS).

Bowman's g's olfactory glands.

bronchial g's seromucous glands in the mucosa and submucosa of the bronchial walls.

Brunner's g's glands in the duodenum secreting intestinal juice.

buccal g's seromucous glands on the inner surface of the cheeks; called also *genal glands*.

bulbocavernous g's, bulbourethral g's two glands embedded in the substance of the sphincter of the male urethra, posterior to the membranous part of the urethra; their secretion lubricates the urethra; called also *Cowper's glands*.

cardiac g's mucus-secreting glands of the cardiac part (cardia) of the stomach.

ceruminous g's cerumin-secreting glands in the skin of the external auditory canal.

cervical g's 1. the lymph nodes of the neck. 2. compound clefts in the wall of the uterine cervix.

ciliary g's sweat glands that have become arrested in their development, situated at the edges of the eyelids; called also *Moll's glands*.

circumanal g's specialized sweat and sebaceous glands around the anus; called also *Gay's glands*.

Cobelli's g's mucous glands in the oesophageal mucosa just above the cardia.

coccygeal g. glomus coccygeum.

coeliac g's lymph nodes anterior to the abdominal aorta.

compound g. one made up of a number of smaller units whose excretory ducts combine to form ducts of progressively higher order.

conglobate g. a lymph node.

Cowper's g's bulbourethral glands.

ductless g's endocrine g's.

duodenal g's Brunner's glands.

Ebner's g's serous glands at the back of the tongue near the taste buds.

eccrine g. one of the ordinary, or simple, sweat glands, which are of the merocrine type.

fundic g's, fundus g's very numerous, tubular glands in the mucosa of the fundus and body of the stomach that contain the cells which produce acid and pepsin.

gastric g's the secreting glands of the stomach, including the fundic, cardiac, and pyloric glands.

Gay g's circumanal glands.

genal g's buccal glands.

glossopalatine g's mucous glands at the posterior end of the smaller sublingual glands.

haematopoietic g's glandlike bodies, e.g., the spleen, that take a part in blood formation.

haemolymph g's minute nodes resembling small lymph nodes but red or brown in colour and containing blood sinuses instead of or alongside lymph spaces. They occur especially in the retroperitoneal tissue near the origin of the superior mesenteric and renal arteries, but are also found elsewhere. They are believed to take part in blood destruction and formation. Two varieties are distinguished—splenolymph glands and marrow-lymph glands.

haversian g's folds on synovial surfaces regarded as secretors of synovia.

holocrine g. one whose discharged secretion contains the entire secreting cells.

intestinal g's straight tubular glands in the mucous membrane of the intestines, opening, in the small intestine, between the bases of the villi, and containing argentaffin cells. Called also *crypts* (or glands) *of Lieberkühn*.

jugular g. a lymph node behind the clavicular insertion of the sternocleidomastoid muscle.

Krause's g. an accessory lacrimal gland deep in the conjunctival connective tissue, mainly near the upper fornix.

lacrimal g's the glands that secrete tears (see also LACRIMAL APPARATUS).

g's of Lieberkühn intestinal glands.

lingual g's the seromucous glands on the surface of the tongue.

lingual g's, anterior seromucous glands near the apex of the tongue.

Littre's g's 1. preputial glands. 2. the male urethral glands.

lymph g. lymph node.

mammary g. the milk-secreting organ of female mammals, existing also in a rudimentary state in the male (see also BREAST).

marrow-lymph g's haemolymph glands having a marrow-like tissue.
meibomian g's sebaceous follicles between the cartilage and conjunctiva of the eyelids.
merocrine g. one whose discharged secretion contains no part of the secreting cells.
mixed g's 1. seromucous glands. 2. glands that have both exocrine and endocrine portions.
Moll's g's ciliary glands.
Montgomery's g's sebaceous glands in the mammary areola; called also areolar glands.
mucous g's glands that secrete mucus.
olfactory g's small mucous glands in the olfactory mucosa; called also *Bowman's glands.*
parathyroid g's small bodies in the region of the thyroid glands, developed from the entoderm of the brachial clefts, occurring in a variable number of pairs, commonly two; they secrete parathyroid hormone and are concerned chiefly with the metabolism of calcium and phosphorus (see also PARATHYROID GLANDS).
parotid g. the large salivary gland located in front of the ear (see also PAROTID GLAND).
peptic g's gastric glands that secrete pepsin.
pineal g. a small, conical structure attached by a stalk to the posterior wall of the third ventricle of the cerebrum (see also PINEAL BODY).
pituitary g. the hypophysis; the epithelial body of dual origin at the base of the brain in the sella turcica, attached by a stalk to the hypothalamus; it consists of two main lobes, the anterior lobe, secreting several important hormones which regulate the proper functioning of the thyroid, gonads, adrenal cortex, and other endocrine organs, and the posterior lobe, whose cells serve as a reservoir for hormones having antidiuretic and oxytocic action, releasing them as needed. See also PITUITARY GLAND.
preputial g's small sebaceous glands of the corona of the penis and the inner surface of the prepuce, which secrete smegma; called also *Littre's glands* and *Tyson's glands.*
prostate g. prostate.
pyloric g's the mucin-secreting glands of the pyloric part of the stomach.
salivary g's glands of the oral cavity whose combined secretion constitutes the saliva (see also SALIVARY GLANDS).
sebaceous g. holocrine glands of the corium that secrete an oily material (sebum) into the hair follicles.
sentinel g. an enlarged lymph node, considered to be pathognomonic of some pathological condition elsewhere.
seromucous g's glands that are both serous and mucous.
serous g. a gland that secretes a watery albuminous material, commonly but not always containing enzymes.
sex g's, sexual g's gonads (see OVARY and TESTIS).
simple g. one with a nonbranching duct.
Skene's g's the largest of the female urethral glands, which open into the urethral orifice; they are regarded as homologous with the prostate. Called also *paraurethral ducts.*
solitary g's solitary follicles.
splenolymph g's haemolymph glands having more of the splenic type of tissue.
sublingual g. a salivary gland on either side under the tongue.
submandibular g., submaxillary g. a salivary gland on the inner side of each ramus of the lower jaw.
sudoriferous g's, sudoriparous g's sweat glands.
suprarenal g. adrenal gland.
sweat g's glands that secrete sweat, situated in the corium or subcutaneous tissue, opening by a duct on the body surface; they promote cooling of the body by evaporation of the secretion (see also SWEAT GLANDS).
target g. one specifically affected by a pituitary hormone.
thymus g. a ductless glandlike body in the anterior mediastinal cavity, which is involved in cell-mediated immunity (see also THYMUS).
thyroid g. an endocrine gland consisting of two lobes, one on each side of the trachea, joined by a narrow isthmus, producing hormones (thyroxine and triiodothyronine), which require iodine for their elaboration and which are concerned in regulating metabolic rate; it also secretes calcitonin (see also THYROID GLAND).
tubular g. any gland made up of or containing a tubule or tubules.
Tyson's g's preputial glands.
unicellular g. a single cell that functions as a gland, e.g., a goblet cell. **urethral g's** mucous glands in the wall of the urethra; in the male, called also *Littre's glands.*
vulvovaginal g's two minute glands, one on either side of the vaginal orifice, their ducts opening on the vulva (see also BARTHOLIN'S GLANDS).
Waldeyer's g's glands in the attached edge of the eyelid.
Weber's g's the tubular mucous glands of the tongue.

glanders ('glandəz) a disease of horses communicable to man, and caused by the glanders bacillus, *Pseudomonas mallei.* It is marked by a purulent inflammation of the mucous membranes and an eruption of nodules on the skin that coalesce and break down, forming deep ulcers, which may end in necrosis of cartilage and bones. The more chronic and constitutional form is known as farcy.

glandilemma (ˌglandi'lemə) the capsule or outer envelope of a gland.

glandula ('glandyuhlə) pl. *glandulae* [L.] gland.

glandular ('glandyuhlə) 1. pertaining to or of the nature of a gland. 2. pertaining to the glans penis.
g. fever an acute infectious disease caused by the Epstein–Barr virus (see INFECTIOUS mononucleosis).

glandule ('glandyool) a small gland.

glans (glanz) pl. *glandes* [L.] a small, rounded mass or glandlike body.
g. clitoridis the erectile tissue on the free end of the clitoris.
g. penis the cap-shaped expansion of the corpus spongiosum at the end of the penis.

glanular ('glanyuhlə) pertaining to the glans penis or to the glans clitoris.

Glanzmann's disease (thrombasthenia) ('glantsmənz) thrombasthenia.

glass (glahs) 1. a hard, brittle, often transparent material, usually consisting of the fused amorphous silicates of potassium or sodium, and of calcium, with silica in excess. 2. a container, usually cylindrical, made from glass. 3. *glasses,* lenses worn to aid or improve vision (see also GLASSES and LENS).

glasses ('glahsis) spectacles; LENSES arranged in a frame holding them in the proper position before the eyes, as an aid to vision.
bifocal g. glasses with lenses having two different refracting powers, one for distant and one for near vision.
trifocal g. lenses that have three different refracting powers, one for distant, one for intermediate, and one for near vision.

glaucoma (glaw'kohmə) a group of diseases of the eye characterized by increased intraocular pressure, resulting in pathological changes in the optic disc and typical visual field defects, and eventually blindness if it is not treated successfully. adj. **glaucomatous.**

Glaucoma is responsible for about 12 per cent of all cases of blindness, and strikes more than 2 per cent of all those over 40 years of age in the UK. It rarely occurs in anyone under 40. The cause is unknown, but there is a hereditary tendency toward the development of most common forms of glaucoma. Early detection and treatment are essential to prevention of permanent loss of vision. Any person over 40 with a family history of glaucoma should have his intraocular pressure checked once a year.

The normal eye is filled with aqueous humour in an amount carefully regulated to maintain the shape of the eyeball. In glaucoma, the balance of this fluid is disturbed; fluid is formed more rapidly than it leaves the eye, and pressure builds up. The increased pressure damages the retina and disturbs the vision, for example, by the loss of side vision. If not relieved by proper treatment, the pressure will eventually damage the optic nerve, interrupting the flow of impulses and causing blindness.

Classification. Glaucoma can be divided into three major types: adult primary glaucoma, secondary glaucoma, and congenital glaucoma. The most common type of adult primary glaucoma is *open angle glaucoma*, in which there are normal 'open' chamber angles but there is resistance to the outward flow of aqueous humour. This type of glaucoma, also called chronic simple glaucoma, is characterized by very few symptoms in the early stages; thus, many people have the disease without knowing it. There may be some hazy vision and mild discomfort in the eye and later there is a barely noticed loss of peripheral vision. As the disease progresses there is reduced visual acuity and greatly increased intraocular pressure that can cause the appearance of coloured rings or halos around bright objects.

Another form of adult primary glaucoma is *angle closure glaucoma*, which can be either acute or chronic. In this type of glaucoma the chamber angle is narrowed or completely closed because of forward displacement of the final roll and root of the iris against the cornea. This closure obstructs the flow of aqueous humour from the eyeball and permits a buildup of pressure.

Secondary glaucoma occurs as a result of a variety of disorders, such as uveitis, neoplastic disease, trauma, and degenerative changes in the eye.

Treatment. Open angle, or chronic simple, glaucoma is treated medically through the use of miotics to facilitate aqueous outflow, and carbonic anhydrase inhibitors to reduce the rate at which aqueous humour is produced. β-Blockers and sympathomimetic agents also increase the facility of outflow and reduce the production of aqueous. The patient must be informed about his problem and made to understand that he must continue the prescribed medications for the rest of his life.

Angle closure glaucoma is usually treated surgically. If the condition becomes acute, a medical and surgical emergency exists. If the excessive intraocular pressure is not relieved promptly by medical and surgical means, nerve fibres in the eye are destroyed and vision is irretrievably lost. The surgical procedure is peripheral iridectomy, in which a portion of the iris is removed, thus leaving an outlet for the flow of aqueous humour. This may also require to be combined with a drainage operation (usually trabeculectomy) if permanent damage to the angle has already occurred.

congenital g. that due to defective development of the structures in and around the anterior chamber of the eye, and resulting in impairment of the aqueous humour.

infantile g. congenital glaucoma that may be fully developed at birth with enlarged eyes and hazy corneas, or may develop at any time up to two or three years of age.

juvenile g. congenital glaucoma differing from the infantile form in that it occurs in older children and young adults, and there is no gross enlargement of the eyeball.

narrow-angle g. a form of primary glaucoma in an eye characterized by a shallow anterior chamber and a narrow angle, in which filtration is compromised as a result of the iris blocking the angle. **open-angle g.** a form of primary glaucoma in an eye in which the angle of the anterior chamber remains open, but filtration is gradually diminished because of the tissues of the angle.

primary g. increased intraocular pressure occurring in an eye without previous disease.

secondary g. increased intraocular pressure due to disease or injury to the eye.

g. simplex glaucoma without pronounced symptoms, but attended with progressive loss of vision.

gleet (gleet) 1. chronic gonorrhoeal urethritis. 2. a urethral discharge, especially one that is mucous or purulent.

glenohumeral (,gleenoh'hyoomə·rəl) referring to the shoulder joint.

glenoid ('gleenoyd) resembling a pit or socket.

g. cavity a depression in the lateral angle of the scapula for articulation with the humerus.

g. fossa a depression in the temporal bone in which the condyle of the lower jaw rests; called also mandibular fossa.

g. lip a ring of fibrocartilage joined to the rim of the glenoid cavity.

glia ('glieə) neuroglia; the supporting structure of nervous tissue, consisting, in the central nervous system, of astrocytes, oligodendrocytes, and microglia.

gliacyte ('glieə,siet) a cell of the glia or neuroglia.

gliadin ('glieə,din) a protein in wheat that contains the toxic factor associated with coeliac disease.

glial ('glieəl, 'gleeəl) of or pertaining to glia or neuroglia.

glibenclamide (glie'benklə,mied) a drug of the sulphonylurea group used in the treatment of diabetes mellitus.

gliclazide ('gliklәzied) a sulphonylurea used in the treatment of diabetes mellitus.

glioblastoma (,glieohbla'stohmə) any malignant astrocytoma.

g. multiforme astrocytoma Grade III or IV; a rapidly growing tumour, usually of the cerebral hemispheres, composed of spongioblasts, astroblasts, and astrocytes.

glioma (glie'ohmə) a tumour composed of neuroglia in any of its states of development; sometimes extended to include all intrinsic neoplasms of the brain and spinal cord, as astrocytomas, ependymomas, etc. adj. **gliomatous**.

g. retinae retinoblastoma.

gliomatosis (,glieohmə'tohsis) excessive development of the neuroglia, especially of the spinal cord, in certain cases of syringomyelia.

glioneuroma (,glieohnyuh'rohmə) glioma combined with neuroma.

gliosarcoma (,glieohsah'kohmə) glioma combined with sarcoma.

gliosis (glie'ohsis) an excess of astroglia in damaged areas of the central nervous system.

glissade (gli'sahd, gli'sayd) [Fr.] a gliding involuntary movement of the eye in changing the point of fixation; it is a slower, smoother movement than is a saccade. adj. **glissadic**.

Glisson's capsule ('glisənz) a sheath of connective tissue enclosing the hepatic artery, hepatic duct, and portal vein.

glissonitis (ˌglisə'nietis) inflammation of Glisson's capsule.

globi ('glohbi, -bie) 1. plural of *globus*. 2. encapsulated globular masses containing bacilli; seen in smears of lepromatous leprosy lesions.

globin ('glohbin) the protein constituent of haemoglobin; also, any member of a group of proteins similar to the typical globin.

globoid ('glohboyd) globe-shaped; spheroid.

globoside ('glohbəˌsied) a sphingoglycolipid containing acetylated amino sugars and simple hexoses, occurring in human serum, spleen, liver, and erythrocytes, and accumulating in tissues in Sandhoff's disease.

globule ('globyool) a small spherical mass; a little globe or pellet, as of medicine. adj. **globular**.

globulin ('globyuhlin) a general term for proteins that are insoluble in water or in highly concentrated salt solutions but soluble in moderately concentrated salt solutions. All plasma proteins except albumin and prealbumin are globulins. The plasma globulins are separated into 5 fractions by serum protein electrophoresis (SPE). In order of decreasing electrophoretic mobility these fractions are the alpha$_1$-, alpha$_2$-, beta$_1$-, and beta$_2$-globulins, and the gamma globulins.

The globulins include carrier proteins, which transport specific substances; acute phase reactants, which are involved in the inflammatory process; clotting factors; complement components; and immunoglobulins. Examples are transferrin, a beta$_1$-globulin that transports iron, and alpha$_1$-antitrypsin, an acute phase reactant that inhibits serum proteases. The GAMMA GLOBULIN fraction is composed of one IMMUNOGLOBULIN class known as IgG.

accelerator g. a substance present in plasma, but not in serum, that functions in the formation of intrinsic and extrinsic thromboplastin; called also CLOTTING factor V.

antihaemophilic g. AHG, CLOTTING factor VIII.

antilymphocyte g. ALG, a substance used as an immunosuppressive agent in organ transplantation, usually in combination with immunosuppressive drugs; it is the gamma globulin fraction of antilymphocyte serum.

hepatitis B immune g. a sterile nonpyrogenic solution consisting of globulins derived from blood plasma of human donors who have high titres of antibodies against hepatitis B surface antigen; used as a passive immunizing agent.

immune g. a sterile solution containing antibodies present in blood. It is prepared from donor plasma or serum; used for passive immunization against infectious hepatitis, poliomyelitis, rubella, rubeola, and varicella.

pertussis immune g. a sterile solution of globulins derived from the blood plasma of human donors immunized with pertussis vaccine; used for the prophylaxis and treatment of pertussis.

rabies immune g. a sterile nonpyrogenic solution of globulins from blood plasma or serum of human donors who have been immunized with rabies vaccine and have high titres of rabies antibody; used as a passive immunizing agent.

serum g. the fraction of proteins precipitated from blood serum by half saturation with ammonium sulphate; the principal groups are the α-, β-, and γ-globulins.

tetanus immune g. a sterile solution of gamma globulins derived from the blood plasma of human donors who have been immunized with tetanus toxoid; used in the prophylaxis and treatment of tetanus.

vaccinia immune human g. a sterile solution of globulins derived from the blood plasma of human donors who have been immunized against vaccinia with vaccinia virus smallpox vaccine; used as a passive immunizing agent.

zoster immune g. specific immune globulin prepared from the plasma of those who have recovered from herpes zoster (shingles); used for prevention or treatment of varicella in susceptible or infected individuals, such as those with immunodeficiency.

globulinuria (ˌglobyuhli'nyooə·ri·ə) the presence of globulins in the urine.

globus ('glohbəs) pl. *globi* [L.] 1. a sphere or ball; a spherical mass. 2. a subjective sensation as of a lump or mass.

g. hystericus a feeling of a lump in the throat displayed in some hysterical conversion reactions in which the illusory lump can actually interfere with swallowing.

g. pallidus the smaller and more medial part of the lentiform nucleus of the brain.

glomangioma (glohˌmanji'ohmə) a benign, often painful tumour derived from a glomus, usually occurring on the distal portion of the fingers or toes, in the skin, or sometimes in deeper structures.

glomectomy (gloh'mektəmee) excision of a glomus.

glomera ('glomə·rə) plural of *glomus*.

glomerular (glo'meryuhlə) pertaining to or of the nature of a glomerulus, especially a renal glomerulus.

glomeruli (glo'meryuhlie) plural of *glomerulus*.

glomerulitis (gloˌmeryuh'lietis) inflammation of the glomeruli of the kidney.

glomerulonephritis (gloˌmeryuhlohnə'frietis) a bilateral, diffuse, non-infectious inflammation of the kidneys. The cause is unknown but it is associated with immunological disturbance. It may be acute, presenting rapidly but reversibly, or it may be chronic, presenting slowly and irreversibly. Glomerulonephritis may occur at any age and there are hereditary forms of the disease, such as Alport's syndrome. Some forms of glomerulonephritis may recur in a transplanted kidney.

Glomerulonephritis is characterized by inflammatory changes in the glomerular tuft. Progressive changes may cause glomerular damage, impairing the glomerular filtration rate, and may spread to include all areas of the nephron. Chronic glomerulonephritis manifests as hyaline deposits in the nephron, interstitial fibrosis and atrophy of tubular cells.

It is believed that antigen–antibody response and activity is responsible for most lesions, which may be divided broadly into immune complex disease and nephritis caused by nephrotoxic antibodies. Immune complex disease may be acute or chronic. If acute, a single large stimulus of a foreign protein such as an invading organism, e.g. streptococcus, induces the production of large amounts of antibody. Circulating antigen–antibody complexes form and are deposited in the glomeruli, causing an acute attack of glomerulonephritis. Repeated small stimuli of foreign antigens cause a different type of lesion, which often develops into chronic glomerulonephritis. Nephritis due to nephrotoxic antibodies occurs when there is an invasion of the glomerular basement membrane.

acute diffuse g., proliferative g. classically occurs 2–3 weeks after an infection, usually pharyngitis due to group A haemolytic streptococcus. It is commonest in young adults and children. The lesion is essentially an acute inflammation of the glomerulus. It presents with malaise, facial oedema, oliguria and moderate hypertension.

focal g. patchy changes are seen in some but not all glomeruli. Haematuria, sometimes severe, and proteinuria are the only signs. Often recovery is fast, but repeated recurrences may end in chronic renal failure.

membranoproliferative g., mesangiocapillary g. a chronic, slowly progressive glomerulonephritis in which the glomeruli are enlarged as a result of proliferation of mesangial cells and irregular thickening of the capillary walls, which narrows the capillary lumina; the onset is sudden, with haematuria, proteinuria, or nephrotic syndrome and a persistent reduction in serum complement levels and deposition of activated complement components in the glomerular capillaries.

minimal change g. occurs mainly in children and occasionally in adults, and is associated with nephrotic syndrome. Clinical features include albuminuria, lipid-rich protein casts in the urine, gross oedema and hyperlipidaemia.

rapidly progressive g. same presentation as acute diffuse glomerulonephritis, but focal sclerosis is more common, probably because of ischaemia induced by the glomerular lesion. Epithelial atrophy occurs and interstitial tissue increases. Symptoms are similar to acute diffuse glomerulonephritis but more severe. Malignant hypertension, sepsis and pericarditis may be fatal.

glomerulonephropathy (glo,meryuhlohnə'fropəthee) any noninflammatory disease of the renal glomeruli.

glomerulopathy (glo,meryuh'lopəthee) any disease, especially any noninflammatory disease, of the renal glomeruli.

diabetic g. intercapillary glomerulosclerosis.

glomerulosclerosis (glo,meryuhlohsklə'rohsis) progressive closure of capillaries, with fibrous obliteration of the capsular space and the whole glomerulus. Secondary tubular atrophy follows.

intercapillary g. Kimmelstiel–Wilson syndrome, a degenerative complication of DIABETES MELLITUS, manifested as albuminuria, oedema, hypertension, renal insufficiency, and retinopathy.

glomerulus (glo'meryuhləs) pl. *glomeruli* [L.] a small tuft or cluster; a small convoluted mass of capillaries, especially a network of vascular tufts encased in the Bowman's capsule of the kidney. adj. **glomerular.**

The glomerulus is an integral part of the NEPHRON, the basic unit of the KIDNEY. Each nephron is capable of forming urine by itself, and each kidney has approximately one million nephrons. The specific function of each glomerulus is to bring blood (and the waste products it carries) to the nephron. As the blood flows through the glomerulus, about one-fifth of the plasma passes through the glomerular membrane under pressure, collects in the Bowman's capsule, and then flows through the renal tubules. Much of this fluid is reabsorbed into the blood via the small capillaries around the tubules (peritubular capillaries). The continuous filtration of fluid from the glomeruli and its reabsorption into the peritubular capillaries is made possible by a high pressure in the glomerular capillary bed and a low pressure in the peritubular bed.

Any disease of the glomeruli, such as acute or chronic glomerulonephritis, must be considered serious because it interferes with the basic functions of the kidneys, that is, filtration of liquids and excretion of certain end products of metabolism and excess sodium, potassium, and chloride ions that may accumulate in the blood.

glomoid ('glohmoyd) resembling a glomus.

glomus ('glohməs) pl. *glomera* [L.] a small histologically recognizable body composed primarily of fine arterioles connecting directly with veins, and having a rich nerve supply.

g. caroticum carotid body.

g. choroideum an enlargement of the choroid plexus of the lateral ventricle.

coccygeal g., g. coccygeum a collection of arteriovenous anastomoses formed, close to the tip of the coccyx, by the median sacral artery.

gloss(o)- word element. [Gr.] *tongue.*

glossal ('glos'l) pertaining to the tongue.

glossalgia (glo'salji·ə) pain in the tongue.

glossectomy (glo'sektəmee) excision of all or a portion of the tongue.

Glossina (glo'sienə) a genus of biting flies, known as the tsetse flies, which serve as vectors of trypanosomes causing various forms of TRYPANOSOMIASIS in man and animals.

glossitis (glo'sietis) inflammation of the tongue.

rhomboid g., median a congenital anomaly of the tongue, with a flat or slightly raised reddish patch or plaque on the midline of the dorsal surface.

glossocele ('glosə,seel) swelling and protrusion of the tongue.

glossodynia (,glosə'dini·ə) pain in the tongue.

glossograph ('glosə,grahf, -graf) an apparatus for registering tongue movements in speech.

glossolalia (,glosə'layli·ə) unintelligible speech.

glossology (,glo'soləjee) 1. the sum of knowledge regarding the tongue. 2. a treatise on nomenclature.

glossopathy (glo'sopəthee) any disease of the tongue.

glossopharyngeal (,glosoh,fə'rinji·əl, -,farin'jeeəl) pertaining to the tongue and pharynx.

g. nerve the ninth cranial nerve; it supplies the carotid sinus, mucous membrane, and muscles of the pharynx, soft palate, and posterior third of the tongue, and the taste buds in the posterior third of the tongue. By serving the carotid sinus, the glossopharyngeal nerve provides for reflex control of the heart. It is also responsible for the swallowing reflex, for stimulating secretions of the parotid glands, and for the sense of taste in the posterior third of the tongue.

glossoplasty ('glosoh,plastee) reconstruction of the tongue.

glossoplegia (,glosoh'pleeji·ə) paralysis of the tongue.

glossorrhaphy (glo'so·rəfee) suture of the tongue.

glossospasm ('glosə,spazəm) spasm of the tongue.

glossotrichia (,glosə'triki·ə) hairy tongue.

glottic ('glotik) pertaining to the glottis or to the tongue.

glottis ('glotis) pl. *glottides* [Gr.] the vocal apparatus of the larynx, consisting of the true vocal cords (vocal folds) and the opening between them. adj. **glottal.**

gluc(o)- word element. [Gr.] *sweetness, glucose;* see also words beginning *glyco-*.

glucagon ('glookə,gon) a polypeptide hormone secreted by the alpha cells of the islets of Langerhans in response to hypoglycaemia or to stimulation by growth hormone. It increases blood glucose concentration by stimulating glycogenolysis in the liver and is administered to relieve hypoglycaemic coma from any cause, especially hyperinsulinism.

glucagonoma (,glookəgə'nohmə) a glucagon-secreting tumour of the alpha cells of the islets of Langerhans.

glucocerebroside (,glookoh'seribroh,sied) a cerebroside containing a glucose sugar; it accumulates in the tissues in Gaucher's disease.

glucocorticoid (,glookoh'kawti,koyd) any corticoid substance that increases gluconeogenesis, raising the concentration of liver glycogen and blood sugar, i.e., cortisol (hydrocortisone), cortisone, and corticosterone.

The release of glucocorticoids from the adrenal cortex is initially triggered by the corticotrophin-releasing factor (CRF) elaborated by the hypothalamus. The target organ for this factor is the anterior lobe of the pituitary gland, which reacts to the presence of CRF by releasing adrenocorticotrophic hormone (ACTH, or corticotrophin). ACTH, in turn, stimulates the release of the glucocorticoids from the adrenal cortex. See also ADRENAL GLAND.

The principal glucocorticoid hormone is cortisol. It regulates the metabolism of proteins, carbohydrates, and lipids. Specifically, it increases the catabolism or breakdown of protein in bone, skin, muscle, and connective tissue. Cortisol also diminishes the cellular utilization of glucose and increases the output of glucose from the liver.

Because of their effects on glucose levels and fat metabolism, all of the glucocorticoids are referred to as anti-insulin diabetogenic hormones. They increase the blood sugar level, raise the concentration of plasma lipids, and, when insulin secretion is insufficient, promote the formation of KETONE BODIES, which contributes to ketoacidosis.

Other physiological processes within the body can occur only in the presence of or with the 'permission of' the glucocorticoids. For example, the secretion of digestive enzymes by gastric cells and the normal excitability of myocardial and central nervous system neurons require a certain level of glucocorticoids.

The glucocorticoids also promote the transport of amino acids into the extracellular compartment, making them more readily available for the production of energy. In times of stress the glucocorticoids influence the effectiveness of the CATECHOLAMINES: dopamine, adrenaline, and noradrenaline. For example, the presence of cortisol is essential to noradrenaline-induced vasoconstriction and other physiological phenomena necessary for survival under stress. This particular property of cortisol demonstrates the one identifiable relationship between hormones from the adrenal cortex and those from the adrenal medullae. One of the medullary hormones is noradrenaline, which is secreted in large quantities when the gland is stimulated by the sympathetic nervous system in response to stress.

Another effect of cortisol is that of dampening the body's inflammatory response to invasion by foreign agents. When present in large amounts, cortisol inhibits the release of histamine and counteracts potentially destructive reactions, such as increased capillary permeability and the migration of leukocytes. Since the immune response can damage body cells as well as those of foreign agents, the anti-inflammatory protective mechanisms of cortisol help preserve the integrity of body cells at the site of the inflammatory response.

glucofuranose (ˌglookoh'fooə·rəˌnohz) a form of glucose in which carbon atoms 1 and 4 are bridged by an oxygen atom.

glucogenic (ˌglookoh'jenik) giving rise to or producing sugar.

glucokinase (ˌglookoh'kienayz) an enzyme that in the presence of ATP catalyses glucose to glucose-6-phosphate.

glucokinetic (ˌglookohki'netik) activating sugar so as to maintain the sugar level of the body.

gluconeogenesis (ˌglookohˌneeoh'jenəsis) the synthesis of glucose from noncarbohydrate sources, such as amino acids and glycerol. It occurs primarily in the liver and kidneys whenever the supply of carbohydrates is insufficient to meet the body's energy needs. Gluconeogenesis is stimulated by cortisol and other GLUCOCORTICOIDS and by the thyroid hormone thyroxine. Formerly called glyconeogenesis.

glucophore ('glookohˌfor) the group of atoms in a molecule that gives the compound a sweet taste.

glucopyranose (ˌglookoh'pierəˌnohz) a form of glucose in which carbon atoms 1 and 5 are bridged by an oxygen atom.

glucosamine (ˌgloo'kohsəˌmeen) an amino derivative of glucose occurring in many glycoproteins and mucopolysaccharides.

glucose ('glookohs, -kohz) D-glucose; a simple sugar, a monosaccharide in certain foodstuffs, especially fruit, and in normal blood; the chief source of energy for living organisms. See also DEXTROSE.

Glucose, whose molecular formula is $C_6H_{12}O_6$, is the end product of carbohydrate digestion; very soon after digestion the other monosaccharides (fructose and galactose) are converted into glucose. Because of this conversion, glucose is the only monosaccharide present in significant amounts in the body fluids. The metabolism of glucose produces energy for the body cells; the rate of metabolism is controlled by insulin. Glucose that is not needed for energy is stored in the form of glycogen as a source of potential energy, readily available when needed. Most of the glycogen is stored in the liver and muscle cells. When these and other body cells are saturated with glycogen, the excess glucose is converted into fat and stored as adipose tissue.

The normal fasting level for glucose in the blood is between 70 and 90 mg per 100 ml (3.9-5.6 mmol/l). Unusually high levels of glucose in the blood (hyperglycaemia) may indicate such diseases as DIABETES MELLITUS, HYPERTHYROIDISM, or hyperpituitarism. Levels of blood sugar below 40 mg per 100 ml (HYPOGLYCAEMIA) may be caused by diseases of the kidneys or liver, hypopituitarism, and hyperinsulinism, an uncommon condition in which too much insulin is produced. A GLUCOSE TOLERANCE TEST is done to assess the ability of the body to metabolize glucose.

liquid g. a thick syrupy, sweet liquid, consisting chiefly of dextrose, with dextrins, maltose, and water, obtained by incomplete hydrolysis of starch; used as a flavouring agent, as a food, and in the treatment of dehydration.

g.-1-phosphate an intermediate in carbohydrate metabolism.

g.-6-phosphate an intermediate in carbohydrate metabolism.

g. tolerance test a test of the body's ability to utilize carbohydrates. It is often used to detect abnormalities of carbohydrate metabolism such as occur in diabetes mellitus, hypoglycaemia, and liver and adrenocortical dysfunction.

There are two types of glucose tolerance tests. In the standard test, which is used most often, the patient is given a single dose of 100 g of glucose, and blood and urine specimens are collected periodically for up to 6 hours. The Exton and Rose test is also useful for the diagnosis of diabetes mellitus and is completed in 1 hour.

In the standard test the patient must be in a fasting state when the test is begun, and a blood sample is taken for measurement of fasting glucose before the test dose is given. Glucose is given dissolved in water and flavoured with lemon juice, or commercial preparations in the form of a carbonated drink or gelatin, which are more palatable and provide exactly 100 g of glucose, may be used.

One-half hour after the glucose is ingested a blood sample and urine specimen are obtained. The specimens are collected at hourly intervals for the next 4 or 5 hours as indicated. Each specimen must be labelled with the exact time it was collected. The patient may be allowed to drink water during the testing period but he may not drink anything else or eat or smoke until the test is completed.

Usually the patient experiences some weakness and perspires excessively, and he may faint during the test. These are normal reactions to a fall in the blood glucose level as insulin is secreted in response to the presence of glucose.

In both the standard test and in the Exton and Rose test the patient is usually fed a high-carbohydrate diet for 3 days before the test. In the Exton and Rose test the patient is given 50 g of glucose, and blood and urine samples are obtained 30 minutes later. Immediately after these specimens are collected he is given a second dose of 50 g of glucose. Half an hour later specimens of blood and urine are obtained.

NORMAL VALUES. *Standard test* (results given in milligrams per 100 ml of blood): fasting—80 mg; 30 min—150 mg; 60 min—135 mg; 2 hours—100 mg; 2½ hours—80 mg. *Exton and Rose test* (results given in milligrams per 100 ml of blood): fasting—80 mg, urine neg.; 30 min—150 mg, urine neg.; 1 hour—160 mg, urine neg.

glucosidase (ˌglooˈkohsiˌdayz) an enzyme of the hydrolase class that splits glucoside, occurring as α-, β-, and α-1,3-glucosidase; α-glucosidase (maltase) occurs in intestinal juice, and β-glucosidase (cellobiase) in the kidney, liver, and intestinal mucosa.

glucosuria (ˌglookohˈsyooə·ri·ə) 1. the presence of glucose in the urine. 2. dextrosuria.

glucuronic acid (ˌglookyuhˈronik) a uronic acid formed by oxidation of C-6 of glucose to a carboxy group; it occurs in proteoglycans (mucopolysaccharides), and is conjugated to many poisons and drugs by the liver, forming glucuronides, which are excreted in the urine.

β-glucuronidase (ˌbeetəˌglookəˈroniˌdayz) an enzyme that attacks glycosidic linkages in natural and synthetic glucuronides and which has been implicated in oestrogen metabolism and cell division; it occurs in the spleen, liver, and endocrine glands.

glucuronide (glooˈkyooə·rəˌnied) any glycosidic compound of glucuronic acid; glucuronides, which are generally inactive, constitute the major proportion of the metabolites of many phenols, alcohols, and carboxylic acids.

glutamate (ˈglootəˌmayt) a salt of glutamic acid; in biochemistry, the term is often used interchangeably with glutamic acid.

glutamic acid (glooˈtamik) a dibasic nonessential amino acid occurring in proteins. It is also an inhibitory neurotransmitter in the central nervous system. Its hydrochloride salt is used as a gastric acidifier. The monosodium salt (sodium glutamate) is used in treating encephalopathies associated with hepatic disease, and to enhance the flavour of foods and tobacco.

glutamic-oxaloacetic transaminase (glooˌtamikˌolsəloh·əˈseetik tranzˈamiˌnayz) abbreviated GOT; see ASPARTATE AMINOTRANSFERASE (AST).

glutamic-pyruvic transaminase (glooˌtamikpieˈroovik tranzˈamiˌnayz) abbreviated GPT; see ALANINE AMINOTRANSFERASE (ALT).

glutaminase (glooˈtamiˌnayz) an enzyme that catalyses the splitting of glutamine into glutamic acid and ammonia.

glutamine (ˈglootəˌmeen) an amide of glutamic acid, an amino acid occurring in proteins; it is an important carrier of urinary ammonia and is broken down in the kidney by glutaminase.

glutaral (ˈglootə·ral) glutaraldehyde.

glutaraldehyde (ˌglootəˈraldiˌhied) a disinfectant active against all viruses, fungi, vegetative bacteria and spores. Used in aqueous solution for sterilization of non-heat-resistant equipment; also used topically as an anhidrotic in the treatment of plantar warts and as a tissue fixative for light and electron microscopy.

glutathione (ˌglootəˈthieohn) reduced glutathione (GSH), a tripeptide of glutamic acid, cysteine, and glycine, which serves as a reducing agent in many biochemical reactions, being converted to oxidized glutathione (GSSG) in which the cysteine residues of two glutathione molecules are connected by a disulphide bridge. Reduced glutathione is important in protecting erythrocytes from oxidation and haemolysis; deficiency causes sensitivity to oxidant drugs.

glutathionuria (ˌglootəˌthieəˈnyooə·ri·ə) the excretion of excessive amounts of glutathione in the urine.

gluteal (ˈglooti·əl, glooˈti·əl) pertaining to the buttocks.

g. muscles three muscles, the greatest, middle, and least, which extend, abduct, and rotate the thigh; called also gluteus maximus, medius, and minimus muscles.

g. nerves nerves that innervate the gluteal muscles.

gluten (ˈglootən) the protein of wheat and other grains that gives dough its tough elastic character; avoidance of this substance will alleviate COELIAC DISEASE (nontropical sprue) in certain persons.

g. enteropathy coeliac disease.

glutethimide (glooˈtethiˌmied) a hypnotic and sedative.

glutinous (ˈglootinəs) adhesive; sticky.

glutitis (glooˈtietis) inflammation of the gluteal muscles.

glycaemia (glieˈseemi·ə) the presence of glucose in the blood.

glycan (ˈgliekan) polysaccharide.

glyceraldehyde (ˌglisəˈraldiˌhied) a compound, glyceric aldehyde, formed by the oxidation of glycerol.

glyceride (ˈglisəˌried) an organic acid ester of glycerin, designated, according to the number of ester linkages, as a mono-, di-, or triglyceride.

glycerin (ˈglisəˌrin) a clear, colourless, syrupy liquid, used as a humectant and as a solvent for drugs; it is a trihydric sugar alcohol, being the alcoholic component of fats. Called also glycerol.

glycerol (ˈglisəˌrol) a trihydric sugar alcohol, $CH_2OH{\cdot}CHOH{\cdot}CH_2OH$, which is a component of fats. It is an intermediate in the metabolism of fatty acids and serves as a phosphate acceptor. Pharmaceutical preparations are called glycerin.

glycerolize (ˈglisə·rəˌliez) to treat with or preserve in glycerol, as in the exposure of red blood cells to glycerol solution so that glycerol diffuses into the cells before they are frozen for preservation.

glycerophosphate (ˌglisə·rohˈfosfayt) a combination of a base with glycerin and phosphoric acid.

glycerose (ˈglisəˌrohz) a sugar formed by oxidizing glycerin; there are two glyceroses, glyceraldehyde and dihydroxyacetone.

glyceryl (ˈglisə·ril, -riel) the mono-, di-, or trivalent radical formed by the removal of hydrogen from one, two, or three of the hydroxy groups of glycerol.

glyceryl trinitrate (ˌglisə·ril trieˈnietrayt, -riel) a chemical well known as an explosive (nitroglycerin) but also possessing medical uses.

Glyceryl trinitrate is a vasodilator and is used medically to relieve certain types of pain, especially in the prophylaxis and treatment of ANGINA PECTORIS. Generally the tablet is placed under the tongue when the attack occurs; it quickly dissolves and gives relief within 1 or 2 minutes. It is not effective when swallowed. It may cause transient palpitation, flushing, faintness, and perhaps headache.

The patient who is taking glyceryl trinitrate should keep the medication with him at all times. It should be kept in a tightly closed, dark, glass container, free from heat and moisture. The drug is not addicting and there is no limit to the number that may be taken in a 24-hour period; however, no more than three tablets should be taken at 5 minute intervals during an attack. If no relief is obtained 15 minutes after the third tablet is taken, the doctor should be notified immediately.

An alternative to sublingual administration of glyceryl trinitrate is application in an ointment to a hairless site on the body surface. Rotation of sites helps eliminate minor skin irritation which is a common problem. The drug is applied by using a manufacturer-supplied measuring applicator paper. A measured amount of ointment is squeezed on to the paper (never directly on to the skin) in a thin uniform layer and the paper is placed on the site. The paper is then covered with plastic wrap and held in place with tape or an elastic bandage.

The usual dosage is a 1- to 2-inch strip, but 5-inch strips are also available. Most patients need several applications per day. The area is cleansed of any remaining ointment and a new site chosen when the next dose is due. Patients who are to use the ointment at home must be given detailed instructions on its use and should be aware of its expected results and local and systemic side-effects.

Patches of glyceryl trinitrate are also available. These deliver a fixed rate of drug through the skin. The patches are applied to the anterior chest wall and are left in place for 24 hours.

glycine ('glieseen) a nonessential amino acid, $H_2N{\cdot}CH_2{\cdot}COOH$, occurring as a constituent of proteins and functioning as an inhibitory neurotransmitter in the central nervous system; used as a gastric antacid and dietary supplement, and in the treatment of various myopathies. Called also aminoacetic acid.

glycocalyx (ˌgliekoh'kayliks) the glycoprotein-polysaccharide that covers the free surface of many cells.

glycocholate (ˌgliekoh'kohlayt) a salt of glycocholic acid.

glycocholic acid (ˌgliekoh'kohlik) a conjugated form of one of the bile acids that yields glycine and cholic acid on hydrolysis.

glycogen ('gliekəjən) a polysaccharide that is the chief carbohydrate storage material in animals. It is formed by and largely stored in the liver, and to a lesser extent in muscles; it is depolymerized to glucose and liberated as needed. Called also animal starch.

glycogen storage disease any of a group of genetically determined disorders of glycogen metabolism, marked by abnormal storage of glycogen in the body tissues. See GIERKE'S DISEASE (type I), POMPE'S DISEASE (type II), FORBES' DISEASE (type III), AMYLOPECTINOSIS (type IV), MCARDLE'S DISEASE (type V), and HERS' DISEASE (type VI). In *type VII*, a deficiency in phosphofructokinase affects muscle and erythrocytes, with temporary weakness and cramping of skeletal muscle after exercise. In *type VIII*, the enzyme deficiency is unknown, but the liver and brain are affected, with hepatomegaly, truncal ataxia, and nystagmus; the neurological deterioration progresses to hypertonia, spasticity, and death. In *type IX*, a deficiency in liver phosphorylase kinase results in marked hepatomegaly, which may disappear in early adulthood. In *type X*, a lack of activity of cyclic AMP-dependent kinase affects the liver and muscle, with mild clinical symptoms. Called also *glycogen disease* and *glycogenosis*.

glycogenase ('gliekəjəˌnayz) an enzyme that splits glycogen into dextrin and maltose.

glycogenesis (ˌgliekoh'jenəsis) the conversion of glucose to glycogen for storage in the liver. adj. **glycogenetic**.

glycogenic (ˌgliekoh'jenik) pertaining to, characterized by, or promoting glycogenesis; pertaining to glycogen.

glycogenolysis (ˌgliekəjə'nolisis) the splitting up of glycogen in the liver, yielding glucose.

glycogenosis (ˌgliekəjə'nohsis) pl. *glycogenoses;* any genetically determined disorders of glycogen metabolism, marked by abnormal storage of glycogen in the tissues of the body. See GLYCOGEN STORAGE DISEASE.

generalized g. Pompe's disease.

hepatorenal g. Gierke's disease.

myophosphorylase deficiency g. McArdle's disease.

glycogeusia (ˌgliekoh'gyoozi·ə) a sweet taste in the mouth.

glycohaemoglobin (ˌgliekohˌheemə'glohbin) glycosylated haemoglobin; see HAEMOGLOBIN A_{1c}.

glycolipid (ˌgliekoh'lipid) a lipid containing carbohydrate groups, usually galactose but also glucose, inositol, or others; the glycolipids include the cerebrosides.

glycolysis (glie'kolisis) the anaerobic enzymatic conversion of glucose to lactate or pyruvate, resulting in energy stored in the form of ATP, as occurs in muscle. adj. **glycolytic**.

glyconeogenesis (ˌgliekohˌneeoh'jenəsis) gluconeogenesis.

glyconucleoprotein (ˌgliekohˌnyooklioh'prohteen) nucleoprotein bearing carbohydrate groups.

glycopenia (ˌgliekoh'peeni·ə) a deficiency of sugar in the tissues.

glycopeptide (ˌgliekoh'peptied) any of a class of peptides that contain carbohydrates, including those that contain amino sugars.

glycopexis (ˌgliekoh'peksis) fixation or storing of sugar or glycogen. adj. **glycopectic**.

glycophorin (ˌgliekoh'for·rin) a protein that projects through the thickness of the cell membrane of erythrocytes; it is attached to oligosaccharides at the outer cell membrane surface and to contractile proteins (spectrin and actin) at the cytoplasmic surface.

glycoprotein (ˌgliekoh'prohteen) any of a class of conjugated proteins consisting of a compound of protein with a carbohydrate group.

glycoptyalism (ˌgliekoh'tieəˌlizəm) glycosialia.

glycopyrronium bromide (ˌgliekohpie'rohni·əm) an anticholinergic used to reduce gastric acid secretion and hypermotility.

glycorrachia (ˌgliekə'raki·ə, -'rayki·ə) the presence of sugar in the cerebrospinal fluid.

glycorrhoea (ˌgliekə'reeə) any sugary discharge from the body.

glycosamine (ˌglie'kohsəˌmeen) an amino sugar.

glycosaminoglycan (ˌgliekohsˌaminoh'gliekan) any of the carbohydrates containing amino sugars occurring in proteoglycans, e.g., hyaluronic acid or chondroitin sulphate.

glycosaminolipid (ˌgliekohsˌaminoh'lipid) any of a class of lipids that contain amino sugars.

glycosecretory (ˌgliekohsi'kreetə·ree) concerned in secretion of glycogen.

glycosialia (ˌgliekohsie'ayli·ə) glucose in the saliva; glycoptyalism.

glycosialorrhoea (ˌgliekohˌsieələ'reeə) excessive flow of saliva containing sugar.

glycosidase (glie'kohsiˌdayz) any of a large group of

hydrolytic enzymes acting on glycosyl compounds.

glycoside ('gliekə,sied) any compound containing a carbohydrate molecule (sugar), particularly any such natural product in plants, convertible, by hydrolytic cleavage, into a sugar and a nonsugar component (aglycone), and named specifically for the sugar contained, as glucoside (glucose), pentoside (pentose), fructoside (fructose), etc.

cardiac g. any one of a group of glycosides occurring in certain plants (*Digitalis*, etc.), having a characteristic action on the contractile force of the heart muscle.

glycosphingolipid (,gliekoh,sfing·goh'lipid) a sphingolipid containing the sugar glucose or galactose.

glycostatic (,gliekoh'statik) tending to maintain a constant sugar level.

glycosuria (,gliekoh'syooə·ri·ə) the presence of glucose in the urine.

renal g. glycosuria due to an inherited inability of the renal tubules to reabsorb glucose normally.

glycosyl ('gliekə,sil) a radical derived from a carbohydrate.

glycosylation (,gliekəsi'layshən) the formation of linkages with glycosyl groups.

glycotropic (,gliekoh'tropik) having an affinity for sugar; causing hyperglycaemia.

glycuresis (,gliekyuh'reesis) the normal increase in the glucose content of the urine that follows an ordinary carbohydrate meal.

glymidine ('gliemi,deen) a drug of the sulphonylurea group showing most of this group's properties; used in the treatment of diabetes mellitus.

gm gram.

GMC General Medical Council.

GMP guanosine monophosphate.

gnath(o)- word element. [Gr.] *jaw*.

gnathic ('nathik) pertaining to the jaw or cheeks.

gnathion ('naythi,on, 'nath-) the most outward and everted point on the profile curvature of the chin.

gnathitis (nə'thietis) inflammation of the jaw.

gnathocephalus (,nathoh'kefələs, -'sef-) a headless fetus or infant with jaws.

gnathodynamometer (,nathoh,dienə'momitə) an instrument for measuring the force exerted in closing the jaws.

gnathology (nə'tholəjee) the science dealing with the masticatory apparatus as a whole. adj. **gnathological**.

gnathoplasty ('nathoh,plastee) plastic repair of the jaw or cheek.

gnathoschisis (nə'thoskisis) congenital cleft of the upper jaw, as in cleft palate.

gnathostomiasis (,nathohstə'mieəsis) infection with the nematode *Gnathostoma spinigerum*, seen in South East Asia and acquired from eating undercooked fish infected with the larvae.

gnosia ('nohsi·ə) the faculty of perceiving and recognizing. adj. **gnostic**.

Gn-RH gonadotrophin-releasing hormone.

goblet cell ('goblit ,sel) a goblet-shaped cell, found in the intestinal epithelium, which produces mucus.

goitre ('goytə) enlargement of the thyroid gland, causing a swelling in the front part of the neck. adj. **goitrous**. Simple endemic goitre, sometimes referred to as *Derbyshire neck*, is usually caused by lack of iodine in the diet. Although the administration of iodine will not cure simple goitre, it will prevent it or stop an existing goitre from enlarging. If there is evidence of pressure against the throat, or the possibility of a malignancy, the goitre may be removed surgically.

Exophthalmic, or toxic, goitre (known also as GRAVES' DISEASE) is accompanied by excessive concentrations of thyroid hormones in the blood, which produce the symptoms of hyperthyroidism. There is protrusion of the eyeballs (exophthalmos) and there may be other ocular changes.

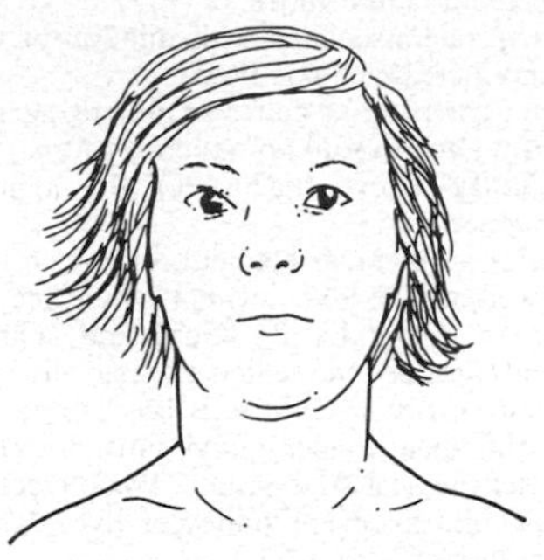

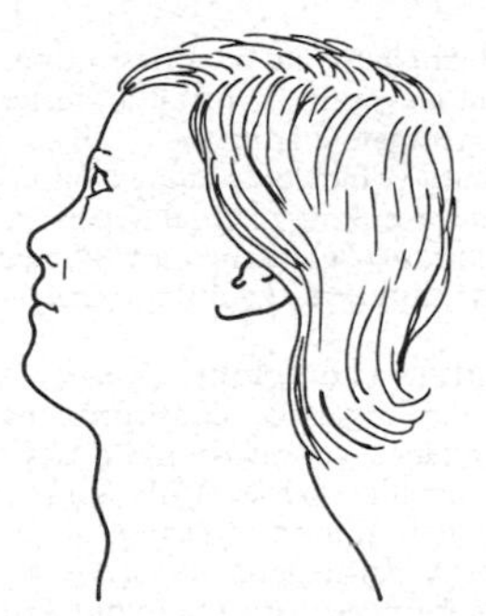

Exophthalmic goitre

aberrant g. goitre of an ectopic thyroid gland.

adenomatous g. that caused by adenoma or multiple colloid nodules of the thyroid gland.

Basedow g. a colloid goitre which has become hyperfunctioning after administration of iodine.

colloid g. a large thyroid gland with distended spaces filled with colloid.

cystic g. one with cysts formed by mucoid or colloid degeneration.

endemic g. see GOITRE.

exophthalmic g. enlargement of the thyroid with protrusion of the eyeballs; see GOITRE.

fibrous g. goitre in which the capsule and the stroma of the thyroid gland are hyperplastic.

follicular g. parenchymatous goitre.

intrathoracic g. one in which a portion of the enlarged gland is in the thoracic cavity.

iodide g. that occurring in reaction to iodides at high concentrations, due to inhibition of iodide organification.

nodular g. goitre with circumscribed nodules within the gland.

nontoxic g. that occurring sporadically and not associated with hyperthyroidism or hypothyroidism.

parenchymatous g. goitre marked by increase in follicles and proliferation of epithelium.

perivascular g. one that surrounds a large blood vessel.

retrovascular g. goitre with a process or processes behind an important blood vessel.

substernal g. goitre in which a portion of the enlarged gland is beneath the sterum.

suffocative g. one that causes dyspnoea by pressure.

toxic g. exophthalmic goitre.

vascular g. one associated with dilation of the blood vessels and increased blood flow.

goitrogen ('goytrə,jen) a goitre-producing agent.

goitrogenic (,goytrə'jenik) producing goitre.

goitrogenicity (,goytrohjə'nisitee) the tendency to produce goitre.

gold (gohld) a chemical element, atomic number 79, atomic weight 196.967, symbol Au. (See table of elements in Appendix 2.) Gold and many of its compounds are used in medicine, especially in treating rheumatoid arthritis. Gold salts are among the most toxic of therapeutic agents and must be given only under strict medical supervision. Toxic reactions may vary from mild to severe kidney or liver damage and blood dyscrasias.

g.-198 a radioisotope of gold having a half life of 2.7 days and emitting gamma and beta radiation. Symbol ^{198}Au.

g. sodium thiomalate an odourless, fine, white to yellowish powder with a metallic taste; used in treatment of rheumatoid arthritis.

Goldblatt kidney ('goldblat) a kidney with obstruction of its blood flow, resulting in renal hypertension.

Goldflam's disease ('goltflǝmz) myasthenia gravis.

Goldflam–Erb disease (,goltflam'airp) myasthenia gravis.

Golgi apparatus (complex) ('goljee, 'golgee) a complex cellular organelle consisting mainly of a number of flattened concavo-convex sacs (cisternae) arranged in parallel stacks with some associated vesicles. It is involved in the synthesis of glycoproteins and lipoproteins, particularly for secretion from the cell. The sacs form primary lysosomes and secretory vacuoles.

Golgi neurons (cells) 1. *Type I:* pyramidal cells with long axons, which leave the grey matter of the central nervous system, traverse the white matter, and terminate in the periphery. 2. *Type II:* stellate neurons with short axons in the cerebral and cerebellar cortices and in the retina.

Golgi tendon organ any of the mechanoreceptors arranged in series with muscle in the tendons of mammalian muscles, being the receptor for stimuli responsible for the lengthening reaction.

gomitoli (go'mitohlee) a network of capillaries in the upper infundibular stem (of the hypothalamus), which surround terminal arterioles of the superior hypophyseal arteries and that lead into the portal veins to the adenohypophysis.

gomphosis (gom'fohsis) a type of fibrous joint in which a conical process is inserted into a socket-like portion.

gonad ('gohnad, 'gonad) a sex gland; a gamete-producing gland; the OVARY in the female and the TESTIS in the male. adj. **gonadal, gonadial.** The ovary produces the ovum and the testis produces the spermatozoon. In addition, the gonads secrete hormones that influence the development of the reproductive organs at puberty, and they control other physical traits that differentiate men from women, such as pitch of the voice and body form and size (the secondary sexual characteristics). The hormones produced by the ovary include OESTROGEN and PROGESTERONE. The principal hormone produced by the testis is TESTOSTERONE.

gonadectomy (,gonə'dektəmee) removal of a gonad.

gonadopathy (,gonə'dopəthee) any disease of the gonads.

gonadorelin (go,nadə'relin) gonadotrophin releasing hormone.

gonadotherapy (,gonədoh'therəpee) treatment with gonadal hormones.

gonadotrope ('gonədoh,trohp) a basophilic cell of the anterior pituitary specialized to secrete follicle-stimulating hormone or luteinizing hormone.

gonadotroph ('gonədoh,trohf) gonadotrope.

gonadotrophic (,gonədoh'trohfik) stimulating the gonads; applied to hormones of the anterior PITUITARY GLAND which influence the gonads.

g. hormone one that has influence on the gonads.

gonadotrophin (,gonədoh'trohfin) any hormone having a stimulating effect on the gonads. Two such hormones are secreted by the anterior pituitary: follicle-stimulating hormone and luteinizing hormone, both of which are active, but with differing effects, in the two sexes.

chorionic g. a gonad-stimulating hormone produced by cytotrophoblastic cells of the placenta; used in treatment of underdevelopment of the gonads and to induce ovulation in infertile women. See also PREGNANCY TESTS.

gonadotropic (,gonədoh'trohpik) gonadotrophic.

gonadotropin (,gonədoh'trohpin) gonadotrophin.

gonaduct ('gonə,dukt) the duct of a gonad; an oviduct or seminal duct.

gonagra (go'nagrə) gout in the knee.

gonalgia (go'nalji·ə) pain in the knee.

gonangiectomy (,gonanji'ektəmee) vasectomy.

gonarthritis (,gonah'thrietis) inflammation of the knee joint.

gonarthrocace (,gonah'throkəsee) tuberculous arthritis of the knee joint.

gonarthrotomy (,gonah'throtəmee) incision into the knee joint.

gonecystis (,goni'sistis) a seminal vesicle.

gonecystitis (,gonisi'stietis) inflammation of a seminal vesicle.

gonecystolith (,goni'sistə,lith) a concretion in a seminal vesicle.

gonecystopyosis (,goni,sistohpie'ohsis) suppuration of a seminal vesicle.

gonidium (gə'nidi·əm) pl. *gonidia* [Gr.] 1. the algal component of the thallus of a lichen. 2. a motile reproductive unit of certain nitrogen-fixing bacteria. adj. **gonidial.**

goniometer (,gohni'omitə) an instrument for measuring angles; the instrument used in GONIOMETRY.

finger g. one for measuring the limits of flexion and extension of the joints between the phalanges of the fingers.

goniometry (,gohni'omətree) the measurement of range of motion in a joint. The technique may be used as a diagnostic or therapeutic measure to determine the functional status of a patient with a musculoskeletal or neurological disability. There is a variety of tools and techniques by which joint motion can be measured, but for most clinical purposes the simple universal goniometer is an adequate instrument. The system for recording measurements of range of motion may be somewhat complex or it may be based upon the simple technique of relating the degree of joint motion to a full circle (360 degrees). See accompanying illustration.

In this system of measurement the axis of the goniometer is placed in alignment with the axis of rotation of the joint, and the 0° position of the circle is assigned in terms of one of the bones of the joint in alignment with a point above the head of the patient. In the sagittal plane, which divides the body into right

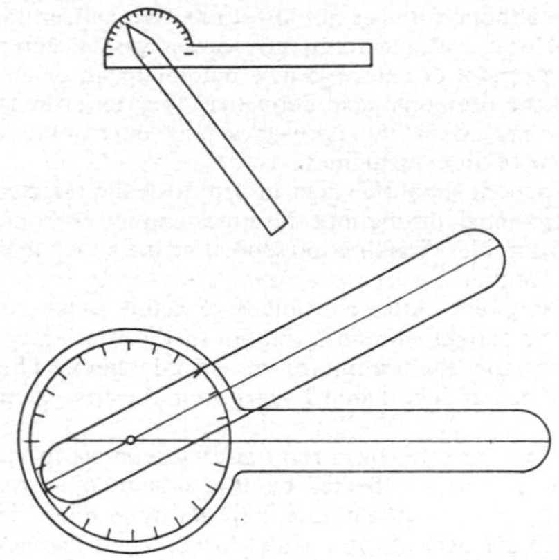

Two examples of universal goniometers commonly used by the clinician

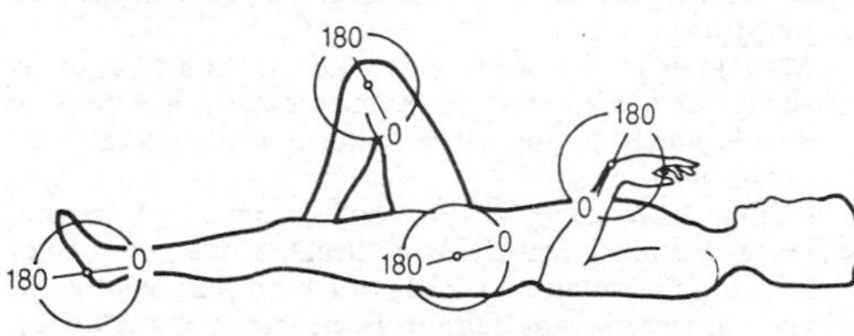

The full circle or 360° system of goniometry applied to several joints of the body, illustrating the locations of the zero degree (0°) position

and left halves, motion that rotates the distal member of the joint toward the 0° position is flexion, and motion which rotates it away from the 0° position is extension. In the frontal plane, which divides the body into ventral and dorsal portions, motion toward the 0° position is abduction (that is, toward the midline of the body), and motion away from the 0° position is adduction.

The 360° system for measurement of joint motion is relatively simple and easily understood by members of the health care team. For this reason it is frequently used. It is especially important, however, that all persons using this or any other system for joint measurement communicate with one another and come to a mutual understanding of the terms and methods to be used to maintain continuity of readings.

gonion ('gohni·ən) pl. *gonia* [Gr.] the most inferior, posterior, and lateral point on the angle of the mandible. adj. **gonial.**

goniopuncture (ˌgohnioh'pungkchə) insertion of a knife blade through the clear cornea, just within the limbus, across the anterior chamber of the eye and through the opposite corneoscleral wall, in treatment of glaucoma.

gonioscope ('gohnioh,skohp) an optical instrument for examining the angle of the anterior chamber of the eye.

gonioscopy (ˌgohni'oskəpee) examination of the angle of the anterior chamber of the eye with a gonioscope.

goniotomy (ˌgohni'otəmee) an operation for glaucoma; it consists in opening Schlemm's canal under direct vision.

gono- word element. [Gr.] *seed, semen.*

gonococcaemia (ˌgonəkok'seemi·ə) the presence of gonococci in the blood.

gonococcal (ˌgonə'kok'l) relating to gonorrhoea.

g. arthritis intractable infection of joints causing great pain and disability.

g. ophthalmia, g. conjunctivitis in the newly born (*ophthalmia neonatorum*) a notifiable disease and a potential cause of blindness.

gonococcus (ˌgonoh'kokəs) pl. *gonococci* [L.] an individual of the species *Neisseria gonorrhoeae*, the aetiological agent of GONORRHOEA. adj. **gonococcal.**

gonocyte ('gonoh,siet) the primitive reproductive cell of the embryo.

gonophore ('gonoh,for) an accessory reproductive organ, such as the oviduct.

gonorrhoea (ˌgonə'reeə) a bacterial infection of the genitourinary system. adj. **gonorrhoeal.** It is currently the second most common sexually transmitted disease (STD) in the UK (non-specific genital infection being the most common).

CAUSE. Gonorrhoea is caused by the bacterium *Neisseria gonorrhoeae*, or gonococcus. Characteristically, the gonococcus attacks the mucous membranes of the genital and urinary organs, producing inflammation and pus. In adults the disease is almost always contracted by coitus or intimate contact with an infected person.

Occasionally the gonococci may attack the membranes of the eye, resulting in blindness if untreated. This is not common in adults. The eyes of babies, however, may be infected at birth during passage through the birth canal of an infected mother. The condition that results is called OPHTHALMIA NEONATORUM (notifiable disease), and in the past it was a major cause of blindness in babies.

SYMPTOMS. The first symptoms of gonorrhoea usually appear within a week after exposure to the gonococcus, but they may take as long as 3 weeks to develop; 10–40 per cent of males and 10–80 per cent of females with gonorrhoea are asymptomatic. In men the inflammation generally causes a painful burning sensation during urination, and the infected penis discharges a whitish fluid, or pus. If the condition remains untreated, the discharge increases and continues for 2 or 3 months. As the infection spreads to other membranes, complications such as inflammation of the prostate and the testes may result and may cause sterility.

A woman infected with gonorrhoea may feel no pain and notice no early symptoms. She may, however, experience pain in the lower abdomen, with or without a burning sensation during urination or a whitish discharge from the vagina. If the infection is allowed to reach other organs of her reproductive system, the ovaries and the uterine tubes may become inflamed and sterility may result.

If uncontrolled, the gonococcal infection may continue to spread and affect other parts of the body such as the bladder, kidneys, and rectum. The disease can also cause inflammation of the joints, resulting in painful arthritis. As the infection spreads it can lead to meningitis or to peritonitis, and may even cause death if the gonococci enter the blood and lodge in the valves of the heart, causing endocarditis.

DIAGNOSIS AND TREATMENT. Diagnosis is confirmed by the presence of gonococci in the discharge from the penis or vagina or in fluid from any affected area. Gonorrhoea can be cured with comparative speed, particularly in its early stages. Penicillin and other antibiotics, as well as the sulphonamide drugs, are effective in treatment. The drug of choice is usually penicillin, administered in a single dose of the long-acting form, which provides concentrations of the drug in the blood for several weeks. In cases of allergy to penicillin, spectinomycin and tetracycline can be used. The patient cannot be considered cured until cultures taken from the discharge are negative for 3 to 4 weeks. No immunity is established and reinfection is possible.

gonycampsis (ˌgoniˈkampsis) abnormal curvature of the knee.

Goodell's sign (ˈguhdelz) softening of the cervix uteri and vagina; a sign of pregnancy.

Goodpasture's syndrome (ˈguhdˌpahschəz) an autoimmune disease in which glomerulonephritis and pulmonary haemorrhage are produced by complement-mediated tissue damage caused by antibodies directed against the glomerular and alveolar basement membranes, and characterized by proteinuria, haematuria, haemoptysis, and dyspnoea; the glomerulonephritis usually progresses to renal failure. Treatment is with plasmapheresis and/or haemodialysis. Some patients recover renal function after a prolonged period of treatment.

gorget (ˈgawjit) a grooved, guiding instrument used in lithotomy.

GOT glutamic-oxaloacetic transaminase.

gouge (gowj) a hollow chisel.

goundou (ˈgoondoo) a sequel of yaws, seen in natives of Central and South America, and also West Africa, with headache, purulent nasal discharge, and formation of bony exostoses at the side of the nose.

gout (gowt) a hereditary form of arthritis in which uric acid appears in excessive quantities in the blood and may be deposited in the joints and other tissues. During an acute attack of gout there is swelling, inflammation, and extreme pain in a joint, frequently that of the big toe. After several years of attacks, the chronic form of the disease may set in, permanently damaging and deforming joints and destroying cells of the kidney. About 95 per cent of all cases occur in men and the first attack rarely occurs before the age of 30.

Causes. The causes of gout are not fully understood. It is a disorder of the metabolism of purines. These nitrogenous substances are found in high-protein foods and the net product of their metabolism is uric acid. For unknown reasons, the uric acid, normally expelled in the urine, is retained in the blood in excess amounts. Uric acid crystals are deposited in the joints and in cartilage, where they form lumps called tophi. The uric acid crystals also predispose to the formation of calculi in the kidney (kidney stones) and lead to permanent damage of the kidney cells.

Acute Gout. The acute form of gout usually strikes without warning. The affected joint, which in 70 per cent of cases is that of the big toe, becomes swollen, inflamed, and very painful. The first attack may follow an operation, infection, or minor irritation such as tight shoes, or it may have no apparent cause. The patient may have a headache or fever, and often cannot walk because of the pain.

Without treatment, acute attacks of gout usually last a few days or weeks. The symptoms then disappear completely until the next attack. As the disease progresses, the attacks tend to last longer and the intervals between attacks become shorter.

Treatment. An acute attack of gout can be treated successfully with any of several medicines. Colchicine has long been used to treat gout. In most cases, colchicine relieves the pain and swelling in 72 hours or less, although it does not affect the high concentration of uric acid and frequently causes gastric upset. The treatment of choice is now indomethacin or any one of the propionic acid derivatives (e.g. ibuprofen). Corticotrophin or the cortisones may be combined with one of these medicines.

The patient should be kept in bed, with the affected joint protected, throughout the attack and for 24 hours after it subsides. Walking too soon after the attack may set off another one.

Chronic Gout. After a number of acute attacks of gout, the patient who goes without medical treatment may develop the symptoms of chronic gout. This seldom occurs less than 10 years after the first acute attack.

The joints affected by chronic gout degenerate in the same way as joints affected by RHEUMATOID ARTHRITIS, and they may eventually lose their ability to move. In 10 to 20 per cent of those with chronic gout, damage to the renal tubules occurs as the result of the formation of kidney stones.

Treatment. Chronic gout is usually treated with allopurinol, a xanthine oxidase inhibitor which reduces the formation of uric acid. It may also be treated with probenecid or other medicines which promote the urinary excretion of uric acid. Sometimes surgery to remove the tophi and correct deformities may be helpful.

Management Between Attacks. If acute gout is recognized at an early stage and treated correctly, the development of the chronic form can generally be prevented.

Since uric acid is the end product of purine metabolism, the patient is usually put on a diet limiting the amount of foods of a high purine content, such as sweetbreads, kidney, liver, sardines, anchovies, and meat extracts and gravies. He also should keep his weight within normal limits and is instructed to increase his daily intake of liquids to encourage the production of urine. Allopurinol, which prevents the formation of uric acid by blocking an enzyme step, is very useful in the long-term treatment of gout and medications such as probenecid, which prevents the retention of uric acid in the body and the formation of tophi, may also be prescribed.

GP general practitioner.

G6PD glucose-6-phosphate dehydrogenase.

GPT glutamic-pyruvic transaminase.

gr. grain.

graafian follicle (ˈgrahfi·ən) a cystic structure developing in the ovarian cortex during the menstrual cycle. In fetal life each ovary has a large number of immature follicles, each of which contains an undeveloped egg cell. These structures are called primordial follicles and develop into graafian follicles. About every 28 days between puberty and the onset of menopause, one of these follicles develops to maturity, or ripens.

As the follicle ripens, it increases in size. The ovum within becomes larger, the follicular wall becomes thicker, and fluid collects in the follicle and surrounds the egg. At this point, it is also known as a vesicular ovarian follicle. The follicle also secretes oestrogen, the hormone that prepares the endometrium to receive a fertilized egg. As the follicle matures, it moves to the surface of the ovary and forms a projection. When fully mature, the graafian follicle breaks open and releases the ovum, which passes into the UTERINE tubes. This release of the ovum is called OVULATION; it occurs midway in the menstrual cycle, generally about 14 days before the next expected period.

The empty graafian follicle in the ovary becomes filled with cells containing a yellow substance and becomes known as the corpus luteum, or yellow body. The corpus luteum secretes progesterone, a hormone that causes further change in the endometrium, allowing it to provide a good milieu in which a fertilized ovum can grow through the stages of gestation to become a fetus.

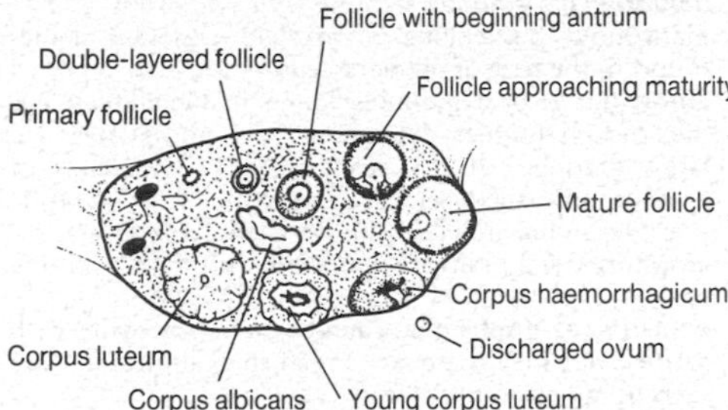

Sequence of events in origin, growth and rupture of the graafian (ovarian) follicle and the formation and retrogression of the corpus luteum. Follow clockwise around the ovary, beginning at the primary follicle

gracile ('grasiel) slender; delicate.

Gradenigo's syndrome (ˌgradə'neegohz) sixth nerve palsy and unilateral headache in suppurative disease of the middle ear, due to involvement of the abducens and trigeminal nerves by direct spread of the infection.

gradient ('graydi·ənt) rate of increase or decrease of a variable value, or its representative curve.

graduate ('gradyoo·ət, 'grajoo-) person who has received a degree from a university or college.

graduated ('gradyooˌaytid, 'grajoo-) marked by a succession of lines, steps, or degrees.

Graefe's knife ('grayfəz) a narrow pointed knife used in some older techniques of cataract surgery.

graft (grahft) 1. any tissue or organ for implantation or transplantation. 2. to implant or transplant such tissue (see also FLAP and GRAFTING).

autologous g., autoplastic g. a graft taken from another area of the patient's own body; an autograft.

cable g. a nerve graft made up of several sections of nerve in the manner of a cable.

cadaver g. a split skin graft taken from a cadaver, freeze-dried and stored; used as epithelial cover for burns, more as a dressing than in expectation of successful grafting.

cutis g. dermal graft.

dermal g. skin from which epidermis and subcutaneous fat have been removed.

epidermal g. a piece of epidermis implanted on a raw surface.

fascial g. a graft taken from the fascia lata, most often implanted in order to strengthen hernial repair.

free g. a graft of tissue completely freed from its blood supply.

full-thickness g. a skin graft consisting of the full thickness of the skin, with little or none of the subcutaneous tissue.

heterologous g., heteroplastic g. a graft of tissue transplanted between animals of different species; a heterograft or xenograft.

homologous g. a graft of tissue obtained from the body of another animal of the same species but with a genotype differing from that of the recipient; a homograft or allograft.

isologous g., isoplastic g. a graft of tissue transplanted between genetically identical individuals; an isograft.

lamellar g. replacement of the superficial layers of an opaque cornea by a thin layer of clear cornea from a donor eye.

omental g's free or attached segments of omentum.

pedicle g. see pedicle FLAP.

penetrating g. a full-thickness corneal transplant.

periosteal g. a piece of periosteum to cover a denuded bone.

pinch g. a piece of skin graft about 0.5 cm in diameter, obtained by elevating the skin with a needle and slicing it off with a knife.

sieve g. a skin graft from which tiny circular islands of skin are removed so that a larger denuded area can be covered, the sievelike portion being placed over one area, and the individual islands over surrounding or other denuded areas.

skin g. a piece of skin transplanted to replace a lost portion of skin.

split-skin g. a skin graft consisting of only a portion of the skin thickness. Called also *Thiersch graft*.

Thiersch g. a very thin skin graft in which long, broad strips of skin, consisting of the epidermis, rete, and part of the corium, are used.

graft-versus-host disease (reaction) (ˌgrahftvərsiz'hohst) a condition that occurs when immunologically competent cells or their precursors are transplanted into an immunologically incompetent recipient (host) that is not histocompatible with the donor; abbreviated GVH disease. Because the host is immunodeficient, the graft is not rejected. Immunocompetent T-lymphocytes derived from the donor tissue recognize the recipient's tissue as 'foreign' and react with it producing clinical manifestations including oedema, erythema, ulceration, loss of hair, and heart and joint lesions similar to those occurring in connective tissue disorders. GVH disease is a frequent complication of bone marrow transplants. HLA matching of the donor and recipient reduces the possibility of GVH disease.

grafting ('grahfting) the implanting or transplanting of skin or other tissue from another part of the body or from another person. Sometimes used as a synonym for organ TRANSPLANTATION.

Grafting of skin is most common, but other tissues can be grafted, such as bone, cartilage, muscle, fat, blood vessels, nerves, and certain body organs. Usually, grafts are either autologous—that is, taken from the same individual—or homologous, taken from another individual. The autologous graft (autograft) is the most commonly used and the most successful. A graft from a genetically identical individual, e.g., an identical twin, is an isologous graft (isograft), and a graft in which the donor and recipient are of different species is a heterologous graft (heterograft or xenograft).

SKIN GRAFTING. The skin to be grafted is usually cut from the chest, thigh, or abdomen, from the lower part of the neck, or from behind the ear. It may be removed in very thin strips or as a thin layer of superficial skin, and it must be placed in its new location without delay. If delay is unavoidable, it is placed in a saline solution or refrigerated.

This is a free graft and the skin is sewn into place and a pressure dressing applied. The skin must then depend for its nourishment on the surrounding tissue in the new location.

For full-thickness of skin, a pedicle graft is required, the base remaining attached at the donor site while the blood supply develops at the recipient site (see also PLASTIC SURGERY).

OTHER GRAFTS. Keratoplasty allows a diseased cornea that has become opaque to be replaced by healthy corneal tissue from an eye bank.

Cartilage and bone are other tissues that can be successfully transplanted from one individual to another. Cartilage lends itself particularly well to various shapes and is widely used in reconstructive surgery. Bone grafts are sometimes used instead of metal plates in operations to repair fractures. They are also used to replace diseased bone. See also TRANSPLANTATION.

Graham's law ('grayəmz) the rate of diffusion of a gas through porous membranes varies inversely with the square root of its density.

grain (grayn) 1. a seed, especially of a cereal plant. 2. the twentieth part of a scruple: 0.065 g; abbreviated gr.

gram (gram) formerly gramme; the basic unit of mass (weight) of the metric system, being the equivalent of 15.432 grains; symbol g; abbreviated gm. See also SI UNITS.

Gram's stain (gramz) a staining procedure in which bacteria are stained with crystal violet, treated with strong iodine solution, decolorized with ethanol or ethanol-acetone, and counterstained with a contrasting dye; those retaining the stain are gram-positive, and those losing the stain but staining with the counterstain are gram-negative.

-gram word element. [Gr.] *written, recorded.*

gram-molecule (gram'moli,kyool) mole (3).

gram-negative (gram'negətiv) losing the stain or decolorized by alcohol in Gram's method of staining (see GRAM'S STAIN), a primary characteristic of bacteria having a cell wall surface more complex in chemical composition than the gram-positive bacteria.

gram-positive (gram'pozətiv) retaining the stain or resisting decolorization by alcohol in Gram's method of staining (see GRAM'S STAIN), a primary characteristic of bacteria whose cell wall is composed of peptidoglycan and teichoic acid.

gramicidin (,grami'siedin) an antibacterial substance produced by the growth of *Bacillus brevis*, one of the two principal components of tyrothricin; called also gramicidin D. Gramicidin S is a closely related substance produced by a thermophilic strain of *B. brevis*.

grand mal (,gronh 'mal) [Fr.] a major epileptic seizure attended by loss of consciousness and convulsive movements, as distinguished from petit mal, a minor seizure (see also EPILEPSY).

grandiose ('grandiohs) in psychiatry, pertaining to exaggerated belief or claims of one's importance or identity, often manifested by delusions of great wealth, power, or fame.

granular ('granyuhlə) made up of or marked by the presence of granules or grains.

g. cell tumour a benign, circumscribed, tumour-like lesion of soft tissue, particularly of the tongue, skin, and muscle, composed of large cells with prominent granular cytoplasm; considered by some to arise from myoblasts (myoblastoma) and by others from neurogenic elements (granular cell schwannoma); still others regard it as a manifestation of lipid storage cell disease.

g. reticulum rough-surfaced endoplasmic reticulum.

granulatio (,granyuh'layshioh) pl. *granulationes* [L.] a granule, or granular mass.

granulation (,granyuh'layshən) 1. the division of a hard substance into small particles. 2. the formation in wounds of small, rounded masses of vascular tissue during healing; also the mass so formed.

arachnoid g's enlarged arachnoid villi projecting into the venous sinuses and creating slight depressions on the inner surface of the cranium.

exuberant g's excessive proliferation of granulation tissue in the healing of a wound.

g. tissue the new tissue formed in repair of wounds of soft tissue, consisting of connective tissue cells and ingrowing young vessels. It ultimately forms the cicatrix.

granule ('granyool) 1. a small particle or grain. 2. a small pill made of sucrose.

acidophil g's granules staining with acid dyes.

aleuronoid g's colourless myeloid colloidal bodies found in the base of pigment cells.

alpha g's 1. oval granules found in blood platelets; they are lysosomes containing acid phosphatase. 2. large granules in the alpha cells of the islets of Langerhans; they secrete glucagon. 3. acidophilic granules in the alpha cells of the adenohypophysis.

amphophil g's granules that stain with both acid and basic dyes.

azur g's, azurophil g's granules that stain easily with azure dyes; they are coarse, reddish granules and are seen in many lymphocytes.

Babès–Ernst g's metachromatic granules.

basophil g's granules staining with basic dyes.

beta g's 1. granules in the beta cells of the islets of Langerhans that secrete insulin. 2. basophilic granules in the beta cells of the adenohypophysis.

chromatic g's, chromophilic g's Nissl bodies.

cone g's the nuclei of the visual cells in the outer nuclear layer of the retina which are connected with the cones.

eosinophil g's those staining with eosin.

Grawitz's g's minute granules seen in the erythrocytes in the basophilia of lead poisoning.

iodophil g's granules staining brown with iodine, seen in polymorphonuclear leukocytes in various acute infectious diseases.

metachromatic g's granules present in many bacterial cells, having an avidity for basic dyes and causing irregular staining of the cell.

neutrophil g's neutrophilic granules from the protoplasm of polymorphonuclear leukocytes; called also *epsilon granules.*

Nissl's g's Nissl bodies.

oxyphil g's acidophil granules.

pigment g's small masses of colouring matter in pigment cells.

rod g's the nuclei of the visual cells in the outer nuclear layer of the retina which are connected with the rods.

Schüffner's g's small granules seen in erythrocytes infected with the malarial parasite *Plasmodium vivax* when stained by certain methods; called also *Schuffner's dots.*

seminal g's the small granular bodies in the semen.

granuloadipose (,granyuhloh'adi,pohs, -z) showing fatty degeneration containing granules of fat.

granuloblast ('granyuhlə,blast) myeloblast; an immature granulocyte.

granulocyte ('granyuhlə,siet) any cell containing granules, especially a granular leukocyte. adj. **granulocytic.**

band-form g. band cell.

granulocytopathy (,granyuhlohsie'topəthee) any disorder of the granulocytes.

granulocytopenia (,granyuhloh,sietə'peeni·ə) lack of granulocytes.

granulocytopoiesis (,granyuhloh,sietəpoy'eesis) the production of granulocytes. adj. **granulocytopoietic.**

granulocytosis (,granyuhlohsie'tohsis) an excess of granulocytes in the blood.

granuloma (,granyuh'lohmə) a tumour-like mass or

nodule of granulation tissue, with actively growing fibroblasts and capillary buds, consisting of a collection of modified macrophages resembling epithelial cells, surrounded by a rim of mononuclear cells, chiefly lymphocytes, and sometimes a centre of giant multinucleate cells; it is due to a chronic inflammatory process associated with infectious disease or invasion by a foreign body.

apical g. modified granulation tissue containing elements of chronic inflammation located adjacent to the root apex of a tooth with infected necrotic pulp.

benign g. of thyroid chronic inflammation of the thyroid gland, converting it into a bulky tumour that later becomes extremely hard.

coccidioidal g. the secondary, progressive, chronic (granulomatous) stage of coccidioidomycosis.

dental g. one usually surrounded by a fibrous sac continuous with the periodontal ligament and attached to the root apex of a tooth.

eosinophilic g. 1. a type of xanthomatosis characterized by the presence of rarefactions or cysts in one or more bones, and sometimes associated with eosinophilia. 2. a disorder similar to eosinophilic gastroenteritis, characterized by localized nodular or pedunculated lesions of the submucosa and muscle walls, especially of the pyloric area of the stomach, caused by infiltration of eosinophils, but without peripheral eosinophilia and allergic symptoms.

g. fissuratum a firm, whitish, fissured, fibrotic granuloma of the gum and buccal mucosa, occurring on an edentulous alveolar ridge and between the ridge and the cheek.

foreign body g. a localized macrophage reaction to a foreign body in the tissue.

g. inguinale a granulomatous disease that is associated with uncleanliness, and is caused by the microorganism *Calymmatobacterium granulomatis*, sometimes called a Donovan body. Although granuloma inguinale is generally considered to be a venereal disease, there is no absolute proof that it is transmitted by sexual contact. It is possible that natural resistance to the disease is very high, so that only a few of the persons exposed are affected.

Generally, 10 days to 3 months elapse after exposure before the first symptoms appear. Small painless ulcers that bleed easily may occur first. Swelling in the groin may then follow. A new ulcer or ulcers may appear as the old one heals, so that granuloma inguinale may eventually cover the reproductive organs, buttocks, and lower abdomen. The extensive sores give off a foul odour. As persons who have the disease seem to develop little immunity to it, granuloma inguinale may be present for many years.

In recent years, both streptomycin and tetracyclines have been successfully employed to treat the disease. Excellent results have been obtained with troleandomycin. There is no known prophylaxis for granuloma inguinale, although the disease is rare in areas of good sanitation.

lethal midline g. a rare, destructive necrotizing granuloma that destroys the midface, starting in the nose or palate and invariably results in death. There is longstanding nonspecific destructive inflammation of the nose or nasal sinuses, with purulent, often bloody discharge.

lipoid g. a granuloma containing lipoid cells; xanthoma.

lipophagic g. a granuloma attended by the loss of subcutaneous fat.

Majocchi's g. trichophytic granuloma.

paracoccidioidal g. paracoccidioidomycosis.

peripheral giant cell reparative g. a pedunculated or sessile lesion of the gingivae or alveolar ridge, usually due to trauma.

pyogenic g. a benign, solitary, nodule of granulation tissue, protruding from an ulcerated epithelial surface found anywhere on the body, commonly intraorally. It is usually a response of the tissues to trauma or nonspecific infection.

swimming pool g. a granulomatous lesion at the site of a swimming pool injury, attributed to *Mycobacterium balnei*; it tends to heal spontaneously in a few months or years.

g. telangiectaticum a form characterized by numerous dilated blood vessels.

trichophytic g. a form of tinea corporis, occurring chiefly on the lower legs, due to *Trichophyton* infecting the hairs at the site of involvement, marked by raised, circumscribed, rather boggy granulomas, disseminated or arranged in chains; the lesions slowly resolve, or undergo necrosis, leaving depressed scars. Called also *Majocchi's granuloma*.

g. tropicum yaws.

ulcerating g. of pudenda, venereal g., g. venereum granuloma inguinale.

granulomatosis (ˌgranyuhˌlohmə'tohsis) the formation of multiple granulomas.

g. siderotica a condition in which brownish nodules are seen in the enlarged spleen.

Wegener's g. a progressive disease, with granulomatous lesions of the respiratory tract, focal necrotizing arteriolitis with mainly glomerular renal involvement, and, finally, widespread inflammation of all organs of the body.

granulomatous (ˌgranyuh'lohmətəs) composed of granulomas. An inflammatory reaction in which macrophages and lymphocytes are the dominant cellular infiltrate.

granulomere ('granyuhləˌmiə) the centre portion of a platelet in a dry, stained blood smear, apparently filled with fine, purplish red granules.

granulopenia (ˌgranyuhloh'peeni·ə) lack of granulocytes.

granuloplastic (ˌgranyuhloh'plastik) forming granules.

granulopoiesis (ˌgranyuhlohpoy'eesis) the formation and development of granulocytes. adj. **granulopoietic**.

granulosa cell tumour (ˌgranyuh'lohsə) an ovarian tumour originating in the solid mass of cells (granulosa cells) that surrounds the ovum in a developing graafian follicle. It may be associated with excessive production of oestrogen, inducing endometrial hyperplasia with menorrhagia.

granulosa-theca cell tumour (ˌgranyuhˌlohsə'theekə) an ovarian tumour predominantly composed of either granulosa cells (follicular cells) or theca cells, and often associated with excessive production of oestrogen, with hyperplasia of the breast and endometrium and carcinoma of the endometrium. When luteinized, i.e., having cells resembling those of the corpus luteum, it is known as luteoma.

granulosis (ˌgranyuh'lohsis) the formation of granules.

g. rubra nasi redness and marked sweating confined to the nose and surrounding area of the face, with red papules and sometimes many small vesicles, seen most often in children, and usually clearing up at puberty.

granum (graynəm) [L.] *grain*.

graph (grahf, graf) a diagram or curve representing varying relationships between sets of data. Often used as a word ending denoting a recording instrument.

graphorrhoea (ˌgrafə'reeə) in psychiatry, the writing of a meaningless flow of words.

graphospasm ('grafohˌspazəm) writer's cramp.

-graphy word element. [Gr.] *writing; recording, a method of recording*. adj. **graphic**.

grattage (grə'tahzh) [Fr.] removal of granulations by scraping.
gravedo (grə'veedoh) head cold; nasal catarrh.
gravel ('grav'l) calculus occurring in small particles.
Graves' disease (grayvz) a clinical syndrome in which thyrotoxicosis is associated with diffuse GOITRE, infiltrative exophthalmos, and sometimes infiltrative dermopathy. It is probably an AUTOIMMUNE DISEASE. As in the other autoimmune thyroid diseases, Hashimoto's disease and primary thyroid atrophy, 60–80 per cent of patients have autoantibodies against thyroglobulin or thyroid microsomes. About 80 per cent of patients with Graves' disease also have autoantibodies against some components of the thyroid cell membrane that alter or block the binding sites for thyroid stimulating hormone (TSH). The first stage of treatment often uses antithyroid drugs, such as carbimazole or propylthiouracil. In severe cases, surgery or radioactive iodine therapy is used.
gravid ('gravid) pregnant; containing developing young.
gravida ('gravidə) a pregnant woman; called gravida I (primigravida) during the first pregnancy, gravida II (secundigravida) during the second, and so on. See also MULTIGRAVIDA.
gravimetric (ˌgravi'metrik) pertaining to measurement by weight; performed by weight, as the gravimetric method of drug assay.
gravity ('gravətee) weight; tendency toward the centre of the earth.
specific g. the weight of a substance compared with that of another taken as a standard (see also SPECIFIC GRAVITY).
Gravlee Jet Washer ('gravlee) a diagnostic instrument consisting of a cannula, an adjustable rubber flange, a saline reservoir, and a 30 ml syringe, and employed to obtain endometrial cells for cytological and histological examination. The procedure of endometrial washing for which the Gravlee Jet Washer is used, provides a relatively quick and easy means of screening for endometrial carcinoma in its early stages.
Grawitz's granules ('gravitsiz) minute granules seen in the erythrocytes in the basophilia of lead poisoning.
Grawitz tumour ('gravitz) renal carcinoma; see KIDNEY.
gray (gray) the SI unit of absorbed radiation dose, defined as the transfer of 1 joule of energy per kilogram of absorbing material (1 J/kg); abbreviated Gy. 1 gray equals 100 rads.
green (green) the colour of grass or of an emerald.
brilliant g. a basic dye having powerful bacteriostatic properties for gram-positive organisms; used topically as an anaesthetic.
indocyanine g. a dye used as a diagnostic aid in the determination of blood volume, cardiac output, and hepatic function.
Greenfield's disease ('greenfeeldz) the infantile form of metachromatic LEUKODYSTROPHY.
grenz rays (grents) very soft electromagnetic radiation of wavelengths about 2 angstroms.
grey matter (gray) grey areas of the nervous system, so called because the nerve fibres in these areas are not enveloped in a white fatty material called the MYELIN sheath. Called also *grey substance*. These fibres are described as unmyelinated, or nonmedullated. White matter or substance is the term used to describe the tissues composed mainly of myelinated, or medullated, fibres.

The bodies of the nerve cells are centred in the grey matter. The cerebral cortex is composed of grey matter and there are some deep-seated masses of grey matter within the diencephalon and the cerebellum. In the spinal cord there is a central core of grey matter surrounded by white matter. On a cross section of the spinal cord the grey matter follows the general pattern of the letter H.
grey scale a representation of intensities in shades of grey; as in grey scale ultrasonography.
grey substance grey matter.
grey syndrome a potentially fatal condition seen in neonates, particularly preterm infants, due to a reaction to chloramphenicol, characterized by an ashen grey cyanosis, vomiting, abdominal distention, hypothermia and shock.
GRH growth hormone releasing hormone.
grid (grid) 1. a grating; in radiology, a device consisting essentially of a series of narrow lead strips closely spaced on their edges and separated by spacers of low density material; used to reduce the amount of scattered radiation reaching the x-ray film. 2. a chart with horizontal and perpendicular lines for plotting curves.
baby g. a direct-reading chart on infant growth.
Wetzel g. a direct-reading chart for evaluating physical fitness in terms of body build, developmental level, and basal metabolism.
grip (grip) a grasping or clasping.
devil's g. epidemic pleurodynia.
grippe (grip) influenza.
griseofulvin (ˌgrizioh'fuhlvin) an antibiotic used orally for treatment of fungal infections of the skin, nails, and scalp. Treatment usually must be prolonged and the patient must be watched for signs of leukopenia, which often occurs when the drug is administered over a long period of time.
groin (groyn) the junctional region between the abdomen and thigh.
groove (groov) a narrow, linear hollow or depression.
branchial g. an external furrow lined with ectoderm, occurring in the embryo between two branchial arches.
Harrison's g. a horizontal groove along the lower border of the thorax corresponding to the costal insertion of the diaphragm; seen in advanced rickets in childhood.
medullary g., neural g. that formed by the beginning invagination of the neural plate of the embryo to form the neural tube.
gross (grohs) coarse or large; visible to the naked eye.
ground substance (grownd) the gel-like material in which connective tissue cells and fibres are imbedded.
group (groop) 1. an assemblage of objects having certain things in common. 2. a number of atoms forming a recognizable and usually transferable portion of a molecule.
azo g. the bivalent radical, –N=N–.
blood g's categories into which blood can be classified on the basis of agglutinogens (see also BLOOD GROUP).
encounter g. a small group which focuses on intensive interpersonal interactions (or 'encounters') with the aim of facilitating emotional expression and promoting personal growth and self-awareness.
g. dynamics 1. any of the collective interactions that take place within a group. 2. the study of groups with an emphasis on intragroup processes such as power, power shift, leadership, cohesiveness, decision making, etc.
prosthetic g. 1. an organic radical, nonprotein in nature, which together with a protein carrier forms an enzyme. 2. a cofactor tightly bound to an enzyme, i.e., it is an integral part of the enzyme and not readily dissociated from it. 3. a cofactor that may reversibly dissociate from the protein component of an enzyme; a coenzyme.

sensitivity g., sensitivity training g., T g., training g. a nonclinical group intended for persons without severe emotional problems, which, in an effort to develop skills in leadership, management, counselling, or other roles, focuses on self-awareness and understanding and on interpersonal interactions.

g. therapy a form of psychotherapy in which a group of patients meets regularly with the therapist, who is usually called the group leader. A typical group has six to eight patients who are similar in age, intelligence, and social outlook, and are usually of the same sex. The group should be balanced, having patients with some diversity of problems and attitudes. Groups usually meet once a week. The group leader generally has undergone personal psychotherapy and has had training in psychopathology and group dynamics and supervised clinical experience with groups.

Group therapy is particularly helpful in dealing with problems that arose from destructive sibling rivalry, separation anxiety, loneliness, or parental spoiling or exploitation. The group functions as a substitute family in which patients can unconsciously act out their expectations and fantasies that derived from their family of origin. From hearing how the group leader and other members feel about this behaviour, the patient can gain insight into his anxieties and conflicts. The group also provides emotional support for self-revelation and a structured environment for trying out new ways of relating to people.

group-transfer (ˌgroop'transfər, -'trahns-) denoting a chemical reaction (excluding oxidation and reduction) in which molecules exchange functional groups, a process catalysed by enzymes called transferases.

growing pains ('groh·ing) recurrent quasirheumatic limb pains peculiar to early youth, once believed to be caused by the growing process. It is now recognized that growth does not cause pain and that these pains can be a symptom of many different disorders.

growth (grohth) 1. the progressive development of a living thing, especially the process by which the body reaches its point of complete physical development. 2. an abnormal formation of tissue, such as a tumour.

HUMAN GROWTH. Human growth from infancy to maturity involves great changes in body size and appearance, including the development of the sexual characteristics. The growth process is not a steady one: at some times growth occurs rapidly, at others slowly. It also varies with the seasons of the years. Individual patterns of growth vary widely because of differences in heredity and environment. Children tend to have physiques similar to those of their parents or of earlier forebears; however, environment may modify this tendency. Living conditions, including nutrition, hygiene, and emotional deprivation have considerable influence on growth.

Glands and Growth. The main regulators of growth are the ENDOCRINE GLANDS. The PITUITARY GLAND secretes growth hormone, which controls general body growth, particularly the growth of the skeleton, and also influences METABOLISM.

In addition to influencing growth directly, the pituitary gland has a central role in regulating the other endocrine glands. These other glands in turn control many body functions, and they secrete the various hormones that directly regulate metabolism. Thyroid hormones are essential for normal growth.

Variations in Growth Rates. The growth of different individuals varies a great deal. It should be remembered that the rate of growth we call 'normal' is really only an average rate. The range of normal growth rates are shown best on a centile chart that displays growth measurements for a normal population of children. The individual child's measurements can be plotted on this to indicate which group of normals he follows. For example a child on the 40th centile will have 60 normals who are taller and 40 normals who are shorter.

Periods of Rapid Growth. Children in general have two periods of noticeably rapid growth. One occurs after birth, the other near puberty. In the first year of life the average baby grows about 50 per cent in height and about triples his weight. Thereafter his development proceeds more slowly until he reaches the rapid growth associated with puberty, which generally takes place between the ninth and thirteenth years in girls and between the eleventh and fifteenth years in boys.

During the pubertal period of rapid somatic growth the sexual differences become evident. The girl begins to assume the characteristics of a woman's physique, with full breasts, rounded hips, and soft deposits of fatty tissue, and she begins MENSTRUATION. The boy likewise undergoes changes associated with masculinity: enlargement of the testes and penis, broadening of shoulders, deepening of the voice, and appearance of facial hair. In both sexes the appearance of pubic hair accompanies these developments. The average girl may attain her adult size by the age of 17, the average boy by 18 or 19.

GROWTH DISORDERS. Disorders in growth are due to genetic, nutritional, infective and endocrine factors. Genetic shortness or tallness may be familial. Abnormal shortness may be due to prolonged severe illness or malnutrition. The most important endocrine influence is pituitary growth hormone. Dwarfism results from deficiency of growth hormone in childhood. Prolonged thyroxine deficiency will have the same effect. Excess of pituitary growth hormone in childhood causes gigantism; if it occurs in a grown adult it causes acromegaly with an overgrowth of skin and bone, giving large spatulate hands and feet and coarsened facial features. Disorders of growth hormone secretion are relatively rare.

g. hormone a substance that stimulates growth, especially a secretion of the anterior lobe of the PITUITARY GLAND that directly influences protein, carbohydrate, and lipid metabolism and controls the rate of skeletal and visceral growth.

grumous ('grooməs) lumpy or clotted.

gryposis (grie'pohsis) abnormal curvature, as of the nails.

GSH reduced glutathione.

GSSG oxidized glutathione.

GU genitourinary.

guanethidine (gwah'nethiˌdeen) an adrenergic-blocking agent; the sulphate salt is used as an antihypertensive.

guanidoacetic acid (ˌgwahnidoh·ə'seetik, ˌgwan-) an intermediate product in the synthesis of creatine.

guanine ('gwahneen) a purine base, one of the fundamental components of nucleic acids (DNA and RNA).

guanosine ('gwahnəˌseen, -ˌzeen) a nucleoside, guanine riboside, one of the major constituents of RNA.

cyclic g. monophosphate (cyclic GMP, cGMP) a cyclic 3′, 5′-phosphate that acts as an intercellular second messenger mediating the activity of hormones and other substances.

g. monophosphate (GMP) a nucleotide important in metabolism, and RNA synthesis.

g. triphosphate (GTP) an energy-rich compound involved in several metabolic reactions.

guar gum ('gooə gum) used to slow down the increase in blood glucose levels observed after a meal.

gubernaculum (ˌgyoobə'nakyuhləm) a cord of fibromuscular tissue attached to the lower pole of the testis. It functions only during the descent of the testis.

guidance ('giedəns) counselling, leading, directing, assisting, influencing as in educational, vocational or child guidance.

Guillain–Barré syndrome (,giyanh'baray) a relatively rare disease affecting the peripheral nervous system, especially the spinal nerves, but also the cranial nerves. Pathological changes include demyelination, inflammation, oedema, and nerve root decompression. Called also acute idiopathic polyneuritis, postinfectious polyneuritis, and Landry's paralysis.

The cause of the disease is unknown; however, it usually follows a febrile illness such as respiratory infection or gastroenteritis within 10 to 21 days and is believed by some to be related to an autoimmune mechanism. Because it is characterized by a flaccid paralysis, it is sometimes mistaken for poliomyelitis.

The early symptoms are fever, malaise, nausea, or prostration. Muscular weakness usually starts in the lower extemities and tends to go upward through the body, but it may affect the facial muscles and arms first and then move downward. The paralysis is not accompanied by loss of sensation, but rather by abnormal sensations of tingling and numbness. The classic cerebrospinal fluid findings are of an elevated protein level without an increase in the number of leukocytes. The cerebrospinal fluid pressure is within normal limits.

The progression of the paralysis may stop at any point. Once the weakness reaches its maximum, the paralysis remains unchanged for days or weeks. Improvement begins spontaneously and continues for weeks, or rarely, months. The prognosis for full recovery is good.

Guillain-Barré syndrome affects primarily the ventral roots of the spinal cord, hence the motor disturbances. The sensory counterpart of this syndrome affects the dorsal roots and is usually called Guillain-Barré-Strohl syndrome. The symptoms of this disease include severe stabbing pains at first, followed by abnormally exaggerated response to painful stimuli.

There is no specific treatment for the disease. Corticosteroids have been widely used but may in fact retard recovery. Recently, plasma exchange has been shown to be helpful, but is not generally available. The condition generally must run its course and for this reason skilled patient care is imperative, particularly in the acute phase, when respiratory failure is a very real possibility. All measures needed to prevent complications in the patient who cannot move about in bed are required for these patients. The experience of paralysis and sensory disturbances is an ordeal for the patient. He will need continued physical and psychological support throughout all stages of recovery, which may last for weeks or months.

guillotine ('gilə,teen) a surgical instrument with a sliding blade for excising a tonsil or the uvula.

guinea-worm ('gini,wərm) a nematode worm, *Dracunculus medinensis*. See DRACONTIASIS.

Gull's disease (gulz) atrophy of the thyroid gland with myxoedema.

gullet ('gulit) oesophagus.

Gullstrand's slit lamp ('gulstrandz) an apparatus for projecting a narrow flat beam of intense light into the eye (see also slit LAMP).

gum (gum) 1. a mucilaginous excretion of various plants. 2. gingiva.

karaya g., sterculia g. the dried gummy exudate from *Sterculia urens* and other *Sterculia* species; used as a bulk cathartic. It has adhesive properties and is used as a dental adhesive and in fitting ostomy appliances.

gumboil ('gum,boyl) the opening on the gum of an abscess at the root of a tooth.

gumma ('gummə) a soft nodule with central rubbery necrotic contents and a fibrosing chronic inflammatory reaction around the necrosis such as that occurring in tertiary syphilis.

gummatous ('gumətəs) of the nature of gumma.

gummy ('gumee) resembling gum or gumma.

Gunn's dots (gunz) white dots seen about the macula lutea on oblique illumination.

Günther's disease ('goontəz) congenital erythropoietic porphyria.

gustation (gu'stayshən) the act of tasting or the sense of taste. adj. **gustatory**.

gut (gut) 1. the bowel or intestine. 2. the primitive digestive tube, consisting of the fore-, mid-, and hindgut. 3. catgut.

gutta ('gutə) pl. *guttae* [L.] a drop.

gutta-percha (,gutə'pərchə) the coagulated latex of a number of tropical trees of the family Sapotaceae; used as a dental cement and in splints.

guttat. [L.] *guttatim* (drop by drop).

guttate ('gutayt) resembling a drop.

guttatim (gu'taytim) [L.] *drop by drop*.

guttering ('gutə·ring) the cutting of a gutter-like excision in bone.

guttural ('gutə·rəl) pertaining to the throat.

Gy gray.

gymnospore ('jimnə,spor) a spore without a protective envelope.

gyn-, gynae-, gynaeco-, gyno- word element. [Gr.] *woman*.

gynaecic (ji'neesik) pertaining to women.

gynaecogenic (,gienəkoh'jenik) producing female characteristics.

gynaecography (,gienə'kogrəfee) radiography of the female reproductive organs following introduction of air into the peritoneal cavity.

gynaecoid ('gienə,koyd) woman-like, or female.

gynaecologist (,gienə'kolə,jist) a specialist in gynaecology, diseases specific to women.

gynaecology (,gienə'koləjee) the branch of medicine dealing with diseases of the genital tract in women. adj. **gynaecological**.

gynaecomania (,gienəkoh'mayni·ə) satyriasis.

gynaecomastia (,gienəkoh'masti·ə) excessive development of mammary glands in the male, even to the functional state.

gynaecopathy (,gienə'kopəthee) any disease peculiar to women.

gynaephobia (,gieni'fohbi·ə) morbid aversion to women.

gynandrism (ji'nandrizəm, jie-, gie-) 1. hermaphroditism. 2. female pseudohermaphroditism.

gynandroblastoma (ji,nandrohbla'stohmə, jie-, gie-) an ovarian tumour containing elements of both arrhoenoblastoma and granulosa cell tumour; it produces both androgenic and oestrogenic effects.

gynandroid (ji'nandroyd, jie-, gie-) a hermaphrodite or a female pseudohermaphrodite.

gynandromorph (ji'nandroh,mawf, jie-, gie-) an organism exhibiting gynandromorphism.

gynandromorphism (ji,nandroh'mawfizəm, jie-, gie-) the presence of chromosomes of both sexes in different tissues of the body, which produces a mosaic of male and female sexual characteristics. adj. **gynandromorphous**.

gyneco- for words beginning thus, see those beginning *gynaeco-*.

gynogenesis (,gienoh'jenəsis) development of an egg that is stimulated by a sperm in the absence of any participation of the sperm nucleus.

gynopathic (ˌgienoh'pathik) pertaining to disease of women.

gynoplastics (ˌgienoh'plastiks) plastic or reconstructive surgery of female reproductive organs. adj. **gynoplastic.**

gypsum ('jipsəm) native calcium sulphate, which, when calcined, becomes plaster of Paris; used in making plaster casts for fractures and for taking dental impressions.

gyrate (jie'rayt) convoluted; ring- or spiral-shaped.

gyration (jie'rayshən) revolution about a fixed centre.

gyre (jieə) gyrus.

gyrectomy (jie'rektəmee) excision or resection of a cerebral gyrus, or a portion of the cerebral cortex.

Gyrencephala (ˌjieren'kefələ, -'sef-) a group of higher mammals, including man, having a brain marked by convolutions.

gyrencephalic (ˌjierenkə'falik, -sə'falik) pertaining to the Gyrencephala; having a brain marked by convolutions.

gyrospasm ('jierohˌspazəm) rotatory spasm of the head.

gyrus ('jierəs) pl. *gyri* [L.] one of the many convolutions of the surface of the brain caused by infolding of the cortex (gyri cerebri), separated by fissures or sulci.

angular g. one continuous anteriorly with the supramarginal gyrus.

annectent gyri various small folds on the cerebral surface that are too inconstant to bear specific names; called also gyri transitivi.

Broca's g. inferior frontal gyrus.

central g., anterior precentral gyrus.

central g., posterior postcentral gyrus. **cerebral gyri** the tortuous elevations (convolutions) on the surface of the cerebral hemisphere, caused by infolding of the cortex and separated by fissures or sulci.

cingulate g. an arch-shaped convolution situated just above the corpus callosum.

frontal g. any of the three (inferior, middle, and superior) gyri of the frontal lobe.

fusiform g. one on the inferior surface of the hemisphere between the inferior temporal and parahippocampal gyri, consisting of a lateral (lateral occipitotemporal gyrus) and a medial (medial occipitotemporal gyrus) part.

hippocampal g., g. hippocampi one on the inferior surface of each cerebral hemisphere, lying between the hippocampal and collateral fissures; called also parahippocampal gyrus.

infracalcarine g., lingual g. one on the occipital lobe that forms the inferior lip of the calcerinesulcus and, together with the cuneus, the visual cortex.

marginal g. the middle frontal gyrus.

occipital g. any of the three (superior, middle, and inferior) gyri of the occipital lobe.

occipitotemporal g., lateral the lateral portion of the fusiform gyrus.

occipitotemporal g., median the medial portion of the fusiform gyrus.

orbital gyri irregular gyri on the orbital surface of the frontal lobe.

parahippocampal g. hippocampal gyrus.

paraterminal g. a thin sheet of grey matter in front of and ventral to the genu of the corpus callosum.

postcentral g. the convolution of the frontal lobe immediately behind the central sulcus; the primary sensory area of the cerebral cortex. Called also posterior central gyrus.

precentral g. the convolution of the frontal lobe immediately in front of the central sulcus; the primary motor area of the cerebral cortex. Called also anterior central gyrus.

g. rectus a cerebral convolution on the orbital aspect of the frontal lobe.

supracallosal g. indusium griseum.

supramarginal g. that part of the inferior parietal convolution which curves around the upper end of the fissure of Sylvius.

temporal g. any of the gyri of the temporal lobe, including inferior, middle, superior, and transverse temporal gyri; the more prominent of the latter (anterior transverse temporal gyrus) represents the cortical centre for hearing.

gyri transitivi annectant gyri.

uncinate g. the uncus.

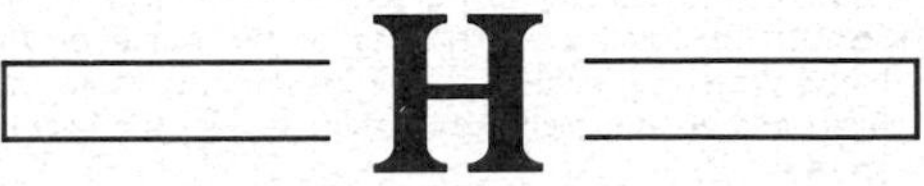

H

H chemical symbol, *hydrogen.*

H⁺ symbol, *hydrogen ion.*

h symbol, *hecto-*; *hour.*

H & E, H. and E. haematoxylin and eosin (stain).

Ha chemical symbol, *hahnium;* produced by an induced nuclear reaction, atomic weight 260. atomic number 105.

habena (hə'beenə) the peduncle of the pineal body.

habenula (hə'benyuhlə) pl. *habenulae* [L.] 1. any frenulum, especially one of a series of structures in the cochlea. 2. a triangular area in the dorsomedial aspect of the thalamus rostral to the pineal gland.

habit ('habit) 1. an action that has become automatic or characteristic by repetition. 2. predisposition; bodily temperament.

habitat ('habiˌtat) the natural surroundings of an animal or plant.

habituation (həˌbityuh'ayshən, -ˌbichuh-) 1. the gradual adaptation to a stimulus or to the environment. 2. the extinction of a conditioned reflex by repetition of the conditioned stimulus; called also negative adaptation. 3. a condition resulting from the repeated consumption of a drug, with a desire to continue its use, but with little or no tendency to increase the dose; there may be psychic but no physical dependence on the drug.

habitus ('habitəs) [L.] *habit, body conformation.*

hachement ('ash,monh) [Fr.] a hacking or chopping stroke in massage.

hacking ('haking) in massage, rhythmic beating using the lateral borders of the fingers. This increases the circulation to the part being treated.

Haelan ('heelan) trademark for preparations containing flurandrenolone, a topical glucocorticoid.

haem (heem) the nonprotein, insoluble, iron protoporphyrin constituent of haemoglobin, of various other respiratory pigments, and of many cells, both animal and vegetable. It is an iron compound of protoporphyrin and so constitutes the pigment portion or protein-free part of the haemoglobin molecule, and is responsible for its oxygen-carrying properties.

Haemaccel ('heeməsel) trademark for a gelatin-based plasma expander.

haemacytometer (ˌheeməsie'tomitə) haemocytometer.

haemadsorption (ˌheeməd'sawpshən, -'zawp-) the adherence of red cells to other cells, particles, or surfaces. adj. **haemadsorbent.**

haemadynamometer (ˌheeməˌdienə'momitə) an instrument for measuring blood pressure.

haemadynamometry (ˌheeməˌdienə'momətree) measurement of blood pressure.

haemagglutination (ˌheeməˌglooti'nayshən) agglutination of erythrocytes.

haemagglutinin (ˌheemə'glootinin) an antibody that causes agglutination of erythrocytes.

cold h. one that acts only at temperatures near 4 °C.

cold h. syndrome a group of conditions in which the development of antibody (usually IgM) against red cells acting at a low temperature gives rise to symptoms related to red cell agglutination and possibly haemolysis. The condition may be primary (chronic cold haemagglutinin disease) or secondary, for example, to mycoplasma pneumonia or malignant lymphoma. Treatment will depend on the underlying cause. Many episodes are self-limiting.

warm h. one that acts only at temperatures near 37 °C.

haemal ('heeməl) 1. pertaining to the blood or the blood vessels. 2. ventral to the spinal axis, where the heart and great vessels are located, as, e.g., the haemal arches.

haemanalysis (ˌheemə'nalisis) analysis of the blood.

haemangiectasis (heeˌmanji'ektəsis) dilation of blood vessels.

haemangioameloblastoma (heeˌmanjioh·əˌmelohbla'stohmə) a highly vascular ameloblastoma.

haemangioblast (hee'manjiohˌblast) a mesodermal cell that gives rise to both vascular endothelium and haemocytoblasts.

haemangioblastoma (heeˌmanjiohbla'stohmə) a capillary haemangioma of the brain consisting of proliferated blood vessel cells or angioblasts.

haemangioendothelioblastoma (heeˌmanjiohˌendohˌtheeliohbla'stohmə) a tumour of mesenchymal origin of which the cells tend to form endothelial cells and line blood vessels.

haemangioendothelioma (heeˌmanjiohˌendohˌtheeli'ohmə) a haemangioma in which endothelial cells are the predominant component.

haemangiofibroma (heeˌmanjiohfie'brohmə) a haemangioma containing fibrous tissue.

haemangioma (ˌheemanji'ohmə) a tumour made up of blood vessels, clustered together. Haemangiomas may be present at birth in various parts of the body, including the liver and bones. In many cases it appears as a network of small blood-filled capillaries near the surface of the skin, forming a flat red or purple birthmark (a 'strawberry' or 'raspberry' mark), which tends to disappear in childhood. The type of haemangioma known as a 'port-wine stain' tends to persist; when it occurs on the limbs the deeper tissues may be affected, leading to unequal growth, the affected side being larger. If the lesion is close to the eye and is likely to interfere with vision, radiotherapy may be used to cause the lesion to resolve.

A cavernous haemangioma presents as a spongy swelling containing large vascular spaces. It should be treated early, since it may enlarge, with the possibility of haemorrhage due to direct injury. It may also create a haemodynamic shunt, precipitating heart failure. Treatment is by curettage and cautery under local anaesthetic.

haemangiomatosis (ˌheemanjiohmə'tohsis) the presence of multiple haemangiomas.

haemangiopericytoma (heeˌmanjiohˌperisie'tohmə) a tumour with a rich vascular network composed of spindle cells. These apparently arise from pericytes.

haemangiosarcoma (heeˌmanjiohsah'kohmə) a malignant tumour of vascular tissue; called also *angiosarcoma.*

haemapheresis (ˌheemafə'reesis) any procedure in which blood is withdrawn, a portion (plasma, leukocytes, platelets, etc.) is separated and retained, and the remainder is retransfused into the donor.

haemarthros, haemarthrosis (hee'mahthros; ˌheemah'throsis) blood in a joint cavity.

haemat(o)- word element. [Gr.] *blood;* see also words beginning *haem-* and *haemo-*.

haematemesis (ˌheemə'teməsis) the vomiting of blood. The appearance of the vomitus depends on the amount and character of the gastric contents at the time blood is vomited and on the length of time the blood has been in the stomach. Gastric acids change bright red blood to a brownish colour and the vomitus is often described as 'coffee-ground' in colour. Bright red blood in the vomitus indicates a fresh haemorrhage and little contact of the blood with gastric juices.

The most common causes of haematemesis are peptic ulcer, gastritis, oesophageal lesions or varices, and cancer of the stomach. Benign tumours, traumatic postoperative bleeding, and swallowed blood from points in the nose, mouth, and throat can also produce haematemesis.

haematencephalon (ˌheemətenˈkefəlon, -'sef-) effusion of blood into the brain.

haemathermous (ˌheemə'thərməs) warm-blooded; haematothermal.

haematic (hee'matik) 1. pertaining to the blood. 2. haematinic.

haematidrosis (ˌheeməti'drohsis) excretion of bloody sweat.

haematin ('heemətin) a compound formed by the oxidation of haem from the ferrous Fe(II) to the ferric Fe(III) state; it does not combine with oxygen.

haematinaemia (ˌheeməti'neemi·ə) the presence of haem in the blood.

haematinic (ˌheemə'tinik) 1. improving the quality of the blood. 2. an agent that improves the quality of the blood, increasing the haemoglobin level and the number of erythrocytes; examples are iron preparations, liver extract, and the B complex vitamins.

haematinuria (ˌheeməti'nyooə·ri·ə) the presence of haem in the urine.

haematobilia (ˌheemətoh'bili·ə) bleeding into the biliary passages.

haematoblast ('heemətohˌblast) haemocytoblast.

haematocele ('heemətohˌseel) an effusion of blood into a cavity, especially into the tunica vaginalis testis.

haematochezia (ˌheemətoh'kezi·ə) blood in the faeces.

haematochromatosis (ˌheemətohˌkrohmə'tohsis) haemochromatosis.

haematochyluria (ˌheemətohkie'lyooə·ri·ə) the discharge of blood and chyle in the urine.

haematocolpometra (ˌheemətohˌkolpə'meetrə) accumulation of menstrual blood in the vagina and uterus.

haematocolpos (ˌheemətoh'kolpos) accumulation of menstrual blood in the vagina.

haematocrit ('heemətohˌkrit, hi'matə-) the volume percentage of erythrocytes in whole blood; also, the apparatus or procedures used in its determination. The haematocrit (which means, literally, 'to separate blood') is determined by centrifuging a blood sample to separate the cellular elements from the plasma; the results of the test indicate the ratio of cell volume to plasma volume and are expressed as a percentage of packed cells or as a volume per litre. Normal range is 0.42 to 0.53 $l \cdot l^{-1}$ for males, and 0.36 to 0.45 $l \cdot l^{-1}$ for females. The haematocrit, in conjunction with other haematological tests, provides information about the size, functioning capacity, and number of erythrocytes.

haematocyst ('heemətohˌsist) effusion of blood into the bladder or in a cyst.

haematocyturia (ˌheemətohsie'tyooə·ri·ə) the presence of erythrocytes in the urine.
haematogenic (ˌheemətoh'jenik) 1. haematopoietic. 2. haematogenous.
haematogenous (ˌheemə'tojənəs) produced by or derived from the blood; disseminated through the bloodstream or by the circulation.
haematoid ('heeməˌtoyd) like blood.
haematoidin (ˌheemə'toydin) a substance apparently chemically identical with bilirubin but formed in the tissues from haemoglobin, particularly under conditions of reduced oxygen tension.
haematologist (ˌheemə'toləjist) a specialist in haematology.
haematology (ˌheemə'toləjee) the science dealing with the morphology of blood and blood-forming tissues, and with their physiology and pathology. adj. **haematological.**
haematolymphangioma (ˌheemətohˌlimfanji'ohmə) a tumour composed of blood and lymph vessels.
haematolysis (ˌheemə'tolisis) haemolysis.
haematoma (ˌheemə'tohmə) a localized collection of extravasated blood in an organ, space, or tissue. Contusions (bruises) and black eyes are familiar forms of haematoma that are seldom serious. Haematomas can occur almost anywhere on the body; they are almost always present with a fracture and are especially serious when they occur inside the skull, where they may produce local pressure on the brain. In minor injuries the blood is absorbed unless infection develops.

CRANIAL HAEMATOMA. The two most common kinds of cranial haematomas are extradural and subdural. *Extradural haematoma* collects between the dura mater and the skull and is most often caused by a heavy blow to the head. Since the skull is rigid, the haematoma presses inward against the brain. If the pressure continues, the brain can be affected. An extradural haematoma may result from rupture of an artery, with haemorrhage, causing severe pressure that can be quickly fatal.

Subdural haematoma develops between the tough casing of the dura and the more delicate membranes covering the brain, the pia-arachnoid. It is more often caused by the head striking an immovable object than by a blow from a moving object. There may be no fracture or immediate injury of noticable severity. The blow causes the brain to move suddenly, tearing a surface vein away from its entry into the sagittal sinus. The resulting haematoma may become encapsulated, giving rise to a chronic subdural haematoma. See also HEAD INJURY.

Symptoms. The most common symptoms of extradural haematoma occur within a few hours after injury. There can be a sudden or gradual loss of consciousness, partial or full paralysis on the side opposite the injury, and dilation of the pupil of the eye on the same side as the injury.

The symptoms of chronic subdural haematoma are similar to those of a brain tumour, and may fluctuate. Diagnosis was difficult, particularly in older people, until the introduction of computed tomography.

Subdural haematoma may occasionally occur in babies as a result of injury. Unless the injury is discovered and treated at an early stage, the child's mental and physical development may be retarded, and spastic paralysis can occur. Early surgery is usually successful in preventing permanent symptoms and disabilities.

Treatment. Prompt operation is imperative for extradural haematoma. The clotted blood is removed by a combination of suction and irrigation through openings made in the skull, and the bleeding is controlled. The same approach is required for subdural haematomas.

SEPTAL HAEMATOMA. Injury to the nose sometimes causes haematoma of the nasal septum. Its symptoms include nasal obstruction and headache. The condition may be treated by incision and drainage or may clear up spontaneously in a few weeks. If the haematoma becomes infected, an abscess may result, requiring drainage and treatment with antibiotics.
haematomediastinum (ˌheemətohˌmeedi·ə'stienəm) effusion of blood into the mediastinum.
haematometra (ˌheemətoh'meetrə) an accumulation of menstrual blood in the uterus.
haematometry (ˌheemə'tomətree) measurement of haemoglobin and estimation of the percentage of various cells of the blood.
haematomphalocele (ˌheemə'tomfəlohˌseel) an umbilical hernia containing blood.
haematomyelia (ˌheemətohmie'eeli·ə) haemorrhage into the substance of the spinal cord.
haematomyelitis (ˌheemətohˌmieə'lietis) acute myelitis with bloody effusion into the spinal cord.
haematomyelopore (ˌheemətoh'mieəlohˌpor) formation of canals in the spinal cord due to haemorrhage.
haematonephrosis (ˌheemətohnə'frohsis) the presence of blood in the renal pelvis.
haematopathology (ˌheemətohpə'tholəjee) the study of diseases of the blood; haemopathology.
haematophagous (ˌheemə'tofəgəs) subsisting on blood.
haematophilia (ˌheemətə'fili·ə) haemophilia.
haematopoiesis (ˌheemətohpoy'eesis) the formation and development of blood cells, usually taking place in the bone marrow.
extramedullary h. the formation of and development of blood cells outside the bone marrow, as in the spleen, liver, and lymph nodes.
haematopoietic (ˌheemətohpoy'etik) 1. pertaining to or affecting the formation of blood cells. 2. an agent that promotes the formation of blood cells.
haematoporphyria (ˌheemətohpaw'firi·ə) a constitutional state marked by abnormal quantity of porphyrin (uroporphyrin and coproporphyrin) in the tissues and secreted in the urine, pigmentation of the face (and later of the bones), sensitivity of the skin to light, vomiting, and intestinal disturbance; see PORPHYRIA.
haematoporphyrin (ˌheemətoh'porfirin) an iron-free derivative of haem, a product of the decomposition of haemoglobin.
haematoporphyrinaemia (ˌheemətohˌporfiri'neemi·ə) haematoporphyrin in the blood.
haematoporphyrinuria (ˌheemətohˌporfiri'nyooə·ri·ə) haematoporphyrin in the urine.
haematorrhachis (ˌheemətə'rakis) haematomyelia; haemorrhage into the vertebral canal.
haematorrhoea (ˌheemətə'reeə) copious haemorrhage.
haematosalpinx (ˌheemətoh'salpingks) an accumulation of blood in the uterine tube.
haematoscheocele (ˌheemə'toski·əˌseel) an accumulation of blood within the scrotum.
haematospermatocele (ˌheemətoh'spərmətohˌseel) a spermatocele containing blood.
haematospermia (ˌheemətoh'spərmi·ə) blood in the semen.
haematosteon (ˌheemə'tosti·ən) haemorrhage into the medullary cavity of a bone.
haematotoxic (ˌheemətoh'toksik) 1. pertaining to blood poisoning. 2. poisonous to the blood and haematopoietic system.
haematotrachelos (ˌheemətohtrə'keelos) distention of

the uterine cervix with blood.

haematotropic (ˌheemətoh'tropik) having a special affinity for or exerting a specific effect on the blood or blood cells.

haematotympanum (ˌheemətoh'timpənəm) haemorrhage into the middle ear.

haematoxylin (ˌheemə'toksilin) an acid colouring matter obtained from the wood of a tree (*Haematoxylon campechianum*); used as a stain for histological specimens and as an indicator.

haematuria (ˌheemə'tyooə·ri·ə) the discharge of blood in the urine. The urine may be slightly blood tinged, grossly bloody, or a smoky brown colour.

Haematuria is symptomatic of disease, infection, or injury to a part of the urinary system. Tumours of the bladder, cystitis, urethritis, and small kidney stones passing along the ureter can cause blood in the urine. Vascular diseases and some types of kidney disorders produce haematuria. Traumatic injury to the kidney is usually accompanied by haematuria.

PATIENT CARE. When haematuria is suspected because of the outward appearance of the urine, a specimen should be saved and sent to the laboratory for microscopic analysis. An accurate record of the patient's intake and output of fluids is kept and the characteristics of the urine should be noted on the patient's chart. If haematuria occurs suddenly and unexpectedly this should be reported immediately to the doctor in charge.

haemic ('heemik) pertaining to blood.

haemo- word element. [Gr.] *blood;* see also words beginning *haem-* and *haemato-*.

haemobilia (ˌheemoh'bili·ə) haematobilia.

haemoblast ('heemohˌblast) haemocytoblast.

haemoblastosis (ˌheemohbla'stohsis) a general term for proliferative disorders of the blood-forming tissues.

haemocatheresis (ˌheemohkə'therisis) the destruction of erythrocytes.

Haemoccult ('heemohˌkult) trademark for a guaiac reagent strip test for occult blood.

haemochromatosis (ˌheemohˌkrohmə'tohsis) a disorder of iron metabolism with excess deposition of iron in the tissues, bronze skin pigmentation, cirrhosis of the liver, and diabetes mellitus. Called also *bronze diabetes* and *iron storage disease.* adj. **haemochromatotic.**

haemoclasis (hee'mokləsis) destruction of erythrocytes. adj. **haemoclastic.**

haemoconcentration (ˌheemohˌkonsən'trayshən) increase in the proportion of formed elements in the blood, as a result of a decrease in its fluid content.

haemoconia (ˌheemoh'kohni·ə) pl. *hemoconiae* [L.] small, round or dumbbell-shaped bodies exhibiting brownian movement, observed in blood platelets in darkfield microscopy of a wet film of blood.

haemoconiosis (ˌheemohˌkohni'ohsis) presence in blood of excessive amounts of haemoconia.

haemocyte ('heemohˌsiet) a blood cell.

haemocytoblast (ˌheemoh'sietohˌblast) the free stem cell from which, according to some theorists, all other blood cells are derived. Called also *haemohistioblast*.

haemocytoblastoma (ˌheemohˌsietohbla'stohmə) a tumour containing all the cells typical of bone marrow.

haemocytocatheresis (ˌheemohˌsietohkə'therisis) destruction of erythrocytes.

haemocytogenesis (ˌheemohˌsietoh'jenəsis) formation of blood cells; haematopoiesis.

haemocytology (ˌheemohsie'toləjee) the study of blood cells.

haemocytolysis (ˌheemohsie'tolisis) haemolysis.

haemocytometer (ˌheemohsie'tomitə) an instrument used in counting blood cells, commonly applied to a combination of counting chambers with coverglasses and pipettes for erythrocytes and leukocytes, all meeting established specifications.

haemocytotripsis (ˌheemohˌsietoh'tripsis) disintegration of blood cells by pressure.

haemodiagnosis (ˌheemohˌdieəg'nohsis) diagnosis by examination of the blood.

haemodialyser (ˌheemoh'dieəˌliezə) a device used for HAEMODIALYSIS (see also DIALYSIS); called also a *dialyser.* It contains a series of semipermeable membranes which separate extracorporeal blood from a specially prepared solution called dialysis fluid. Blood flows continually over one side of the membrane whilst dialysis fluid flows continually over the other side. Water and some solutes diffuse across the semipermeable membrane, removing toxic waste products from the body and restoring electrolyte and fluid balance. The rate of clearance of solutes depends on the total surface area of membrane and the rate of flow of blood and dialysis fluid. The blood and dialysis fluid usually flow in opposite directions as clearance of solutes is more efficient with a counter-current mechanism. The semipermeable membranes may be made from cuprophane, cellulose or other synthetic materials.

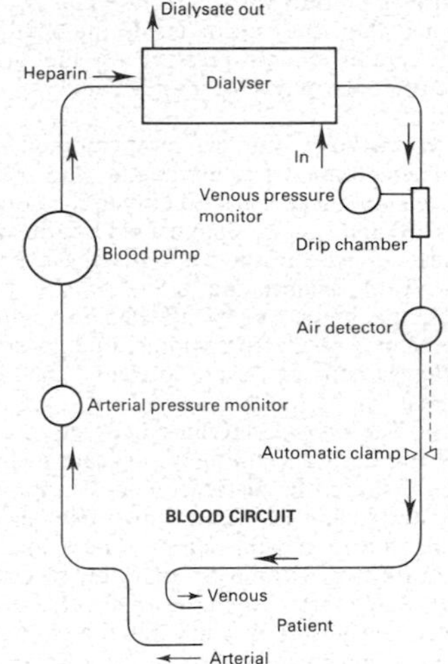

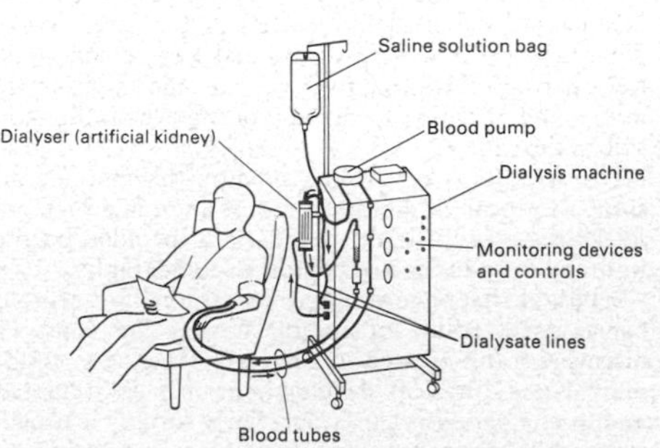

haemodialysis (ˌheemohdie'aləsis) a procedure used to remove toxic wastes from the blood of a patient with acute or chronic renal failure. See also KIDNEY.

The patient's blood is pumped at between 180 and 250 ml/min from either the arterial circulation or a large vein through the HAEMODIALYSER to the venous circulation. In the dialyser, it flows past semipermeable synthetic membranes, while dialysis fluid flows past the other side of the membranes. Water and waste products diffuse across the membrane from the blood into the dialysis fluid, which is then discarded. The blood is continuously circulated, kept warm and free from air, anticoagulated and monitored by the haemodialysis machine. The dialysis fluid contains sodium, potassium, chloride, calcium, magnesium, glucose, and either acetate or bicarbonate, and is mixed and monitored by the haemodialyser. The concentrations of the electrolytes in the dialysis fluid can be adjusted so that the serum pH and electrolytes can be either changed or maintained by the dialysis. Large molecules and blood cells cannot pass through the membrane and, therefore, stay in the blood.

Heparin is added to the blood during dialysis to prevent it clotting during the procedure.

Access to the patient's vascular system may be by *external* shunt, *internal* arteriovenous (AV) fistula or via a subclavian or internal jugular line. An external shunt requires two lengths of specially prepared tubing: one for insertion in a vein and the other in an artery, usually in the forearm or lower leg. Although the external shunt has the advantage of being immediately available for use in an emergency, it has the potential of becoming infected or obstructed with clots, and, if the integrity of the system is disrupted, rapid and copius blood loss may occur.

The internal AV fistula is surgically created by anastomosing an artery to a vein. The fistula must heal gradually and become mature before large-bore needles can be inserted. When end-stage renal disease is inevitable, the fistula can be prepared months in advance for use when symptoms of uraemia appear.

Subclavian or internal jugular lines have the advantage of being quick to insert for emergency dialysis. They may be single or double lines.

Haemodialysis treatments for chronic renal failure are usually done two to three times a week for a total of 10–18 hours. The problems that a patient on haemodialysis may experience are fluid overload (hypervolaemia), electrolyte imbalance, and alterations in blood components, leading to anaemia or platelet abnormalities resulting in a tendency to bleed excessively. Another problem is infection, either of the access site and the blood or in the urinary or respiratory tract because of urinary or pulmonary stasis.

Patients who depend on haemodialysis require extensive instruction in the care of their cannulas and access sites. If haemodialysis is to be undertaken at home patients must be fully trained and home support be available. Patients undergoing haemodialysis in hospital are trained to do as much as possible in order to retain their independence. They must also understand fluid restriction, especially if anuric, and the need for a low potassium and moderate sodium diet as these electrolytes are only excreted during dialysis.

Haemodialysis is an effective treatment. Patients are able to work and lead a relatively normal life. Support must be provided by the dialysis unit of the hospital and the patient helped to run their own dialysis as much as possible.

haemodilution (ˌheemohdie'looshən) increase in the fluid content of blood, resulting in diminution of the concentration of formed elements.

haemodynamic monitoring (ˌheemohdie'namik) continuous monitoring of the movement of blood and the pressures being exerted in the veins, arteries, and chambers of the heart. Current invasive techniques permit the monitoring of intra-arterial blood pressure, pulmonary artery pressure, left atrial pressure, and central venous pressure. Invasive pressure monitoring requires the insertion of a catheter into an artery (usually the radial, brachial, or femoral artery), vein (the antecubital, jugular, or subclavian), or a heart chamber. The SWAN–GANZ CATHETER is a pulmonary catheter that can permit measurement of pulmonary artery diastolic and systolic pressure, pulmonary-capillary wedge pressure (PCWP), left atrial filling pressure, central venous pressure, and cardiac output.

In all physiological monitoring systems the catheter is connected to a pressure extension line attached to a transducer in an airtight, solution-filled system. The transducer converts pressure into an electrical signal that is displayed on an oscilloscope or recorder. Most transducers used in clinical pressure monitoring function in a range of minus 50 to plus 300 mmHg. The amplifier enlarges the signal being produced by the transducer; it contains a digital or analogue meter to indicate pressure, controls for setting alarms, audible and visual alarm systems, and a selector switch for systolic, diastolic, and mean pressures.

Invasive haemodynamic pressure monitoring permits continuous assessment of the status of a critically ill patient and his response to ongoing therapy; thus providing information essential for more precise diagnosis and prompt correction of a problem. Measurement of intra-arterial blood pressure is especially helpful in the care of haemodynamically unstable patients, including those receiving potent drugs that affect the vascular system. Pulmonary artery pressure readings are indicated for patients in cardiogenic shock secondary to myocardial infarction, and for monitoring pulmonary congestion due to elevated pulmonary wedge pressure. Central venous pressure measures right-sided heart pressures (in the vena cava and right atrium) to determine the adequacy of central venous return.

The major risks of invasive haemodynamic pressure monitoring are sepsis, bleeding back, and the formation of thrombi and emboli.

haemodynamics (ˌheemohdie'namiks) the study of the movements of the blood and the forces concerned therein. adj. **haemodynamic**.

haemofiltration (ˌheemohfil'trayshən) the bulk transfer of water and solutes across a semipermeable membrane under hydrostatic pressure. The hydraulic permeability and surface area of the membrane, together with the transmembrane pressure, determine the amount of fluid filtered. It is of particular use in acute renal failure either to maintain fluid balance while feeding parenterally or to remove waste products by removing several litres of fluid per hour and replacing it simultaneously with physiologically suitable fluid. It is possible to maintain cardiovascular stability more easily than when using HAEMODIALYSIS.

The vascular access is almost always provided by an arteriovenous shunt, which must be observed for patency and checked for infection and haemorrhage. Care must be taken not to dehydrate the patient by excess fluid removal or to overhydrate by insufficient fluid removal or overinfusion.

haemoflagellate (ˌheemə'flajiˌlət) any flagellate protozoan parasitic in the blood.

haemofuscin (ˌheemə'fyoosin) a brownish-yellow pigment resulting from haemoglobin decomposition; it gives urine a deep ruddy colour.

haemogenesis (ˌheemə'jenəsis) the formation of blood; haematogenesis.

haemogenic (ˌheemə'jenik) pertaining to production of blood.

haemoglobin (ˌheemə'glohbin) an allosteric protein found in erythrocytes that transports molecular oxygen (O_2) in the blood. Symbol Hb.

Each haemoglobin molecule is a tetramer composed of four monomers held together by weak bonds. Each monomer consists of a polypeptide chain (apoprotein) and a prosthetic group, which is a porphyrin ring that binds an iron atom in the +2 oxidation state. The prosthetic group is referred to as *haem* and the apoprotein as *globin*.

CHEMISTRY AND PHYSIOLOGY. The iron atom has a free valency and can bind one molecule of oxygen. Thus, each haemoglobin molecule can bind four atoms of oxygen. The tetramer exhibits positive cooperativity; the binding of oxygen by one monomer increases the affinity for oxygen of the other tetramers. This makes haemoglobin a more efficient transport protein than a monomeric protein such as myoglobin.

Oxygenated haemoglobin (*oxyhaemoglobin*) is bright red in colour; haemoglobin unbound to oxygen (*deoxyhaemoglobin*) is darker. This accounts for the bright red colour of arterial blood, in which the haemoglobin is about 97 per cent saturated with oxygen. Venous blood is darker because it is only about 20–70 per cent saturated, depending on how much oxygen is being used by the tissues.

The affinity of haemoglobin for carbon monoxide is 210 times as strong as its affinity for oxygen. The complex formed (*carboxyhaemoglobin*) cannot transport oxygen. Thus, carbon monoxide poisoning results in hypoxia and asphyxiation.

Another form of haemoglobin that cannot transport oxygen is *methaemoglobin*, in which the iron atom is oxidized to the +3 oxidation state. During the 120-day life span of a red cell, haemoglobin is slowly oxidized to methaemoglobin. At least four different enzyme systems can convert methaemoglobin back to haemoglobin. When these are defective or overloaded, methaemoglobinaemia, in which high methaemoglobin levels cause dyspnoea and cyanosis, can result.

A secondary function of haemoglobin is as part of the blood buffer system. The histidine residues in the globin chains act as weak bases to minimize the change in blood pH that occurs as oxygen is absorbed and carbon dioxide released in the lungs and as oxygen is delivered and carbon dioxide taken up from the tissues.

As red cells wear out or are damaged, they are ingested by macrophages of the reticuloendothelial system. The porphyrin ring of haem is converted to the bile pigment bilirubin, which is excreted by the liver. The iron is transported to the bone marrow to be incorporated in the haemoglobin of newly formed erythrocytes.

The haemoglobin concentration of blood varies with the haematocrit. The normal values for the blood haemoglobin concentration are 8.4 to 11.2 mmol/l (13.5 to 18.0 g/dl) in males and 7.4 to 10 mmol/l (12.0 to 16.0 g/dl) in females. The normal mean corpuscular haemoglobin concentration (MCHC), which is the concentration within the red cells, is 20 to 22.3 mmol/l (32 to 36 g/dl).

VARIANT AND ABNORMAL HAEMOGLOBINS. There are six different types of globin chains, designated by the Greek letters α, β, γ, δ, ϵ, and ζ (alpha, beta, gamma, delta, epsilon and zeta, respectively). The composition of a haemoglobin is specified by a formula such as $\alpha_2\beta_2$, which indicates a tetramer containing two α chains and two β chains.

The chains are coded by different genes, which are turned on and off during development in order to produce haemoglobins with the oxygen-carrying properties required at each developmental stage. In the first three months of embryonic development, when blood cells are produced in the yolk sac, the embryonic haemoglobins Hb Gower I ($\zeta_2\epsilon_2$), Hb Gower II ($\alpha_2\epsilon_2$), and Hb Portland ($\zeta_2\gamma_2$) are produced. As erythropoiesis shifts to the liver and spleen, the fetal haemoglobin HbF ($\alpha_2\gamma_2$) appears. When erythropoiesis shifts to the bone marrow during the first year of life, the adult haemoglobins HbA ($\alpha_2\beta_2$) and HbA_2 ($\alpha_2\delta_2$) begin to be produced.

More than 250 abnormal haemoglobins arising from mutations have been discovered. Some have altered oxygen affinity, some are unstable, and in some the iron atom is oxidized, resulting in congenital methaemoglobinaemia. Some mutations result in a reduced rate of haemoglobin synthesis. All such conditions are known as *haemoglobinopathies*.

The most common haemoglobinopathy is SICKLE CELL DISEASE, caused by a mutation replacing the sixth amino acid in the β chain, normally glutamic acid, by valine. The variant haemoglobin $\alpha_2\beta^S{}_2$ is known as HbS. Mutations resulting in reduced synthesis of one of the chains are called THALASSAEMIAS. They can result from deletion of the gene for a chain or from a mutation in the regulatory gene that controls the synthesis of the chain.

h. A_{1c} haemoglobin A with a glucose moiety attached to the amino terminal valine of the beta chain. This type of haemoglobin is made at a slow constant rate during the 120-day life span of the erythrocyte. It accounts for 3 to 6 per cent of the total haemoglobin in a normal person and up to 14 per cent in persons with diabetes mellitus. Increased levels of haemoglobin A_{1c} correlate with the average blood glucose concentration over a period of 6 to 8 weeks prior to the test in diabetics; with good diabetic control the haemoglobin A_{1c} level returns to normal range. Periodic A_{1c} assays can be helpful in evaluating effective control of diabetes mellitus.

haemoglobinaemia (ˌheeməˌglohbi'neemi·ə) presence of excessive haemoglobin in the blood plasma.

haemoglobinolysis (ˌheeməˌglohbi'nolisis) the splitting up of haemoglobin.

haemoglobinometer (ˌheeməˌglohbi'nomitə) a laboratory instrument for colorimetric determination of the haemoglobin content of the blood.

haemoglobinopathy (ˌheeməˌglohbi'nopəthee) any haematological disorder due to alteration in the genetically determined molecular structure of haemoglobin, with characteristic clinical and laboratory abnormalities and often overt anaemia.

haemoglobinous (ˌheemə'glohbinəs) containing haemoglobin.

haemoglobinuria (ˌheeməˌglobi'nyooə·ri·ə) the presence of free haemoglobin in the urine. adj. **haemoglobinuric**.

march h. a benign condition in which haemolysis is produced by repeated uncushioned shocks or trauma to some body part; seen in some soldiers after long marches, in marathon runners, and in karate experts.

paroxysmal cold h. an autoimmune or postviral disease in which there is IgG immunoglobulin directed against the P blood group antigen. It is marked by episodes of haemoglobinaemia and haemoglobinuria after exposure to cold and is detected by the Donath–Landsteiner test. The condition is treated with prednisone and cyclophosphamide and by protection from exposure to cold.

paroxysmal nocturnal h. (PNH) a rare acquired blood cell dysplasia in which there is proliferation of abnormal red cells (PNH cells) with an increased susceptibility to lysis by complement. It is marked by episodes of severe haemolysis associated with the passage of dark urine and thrombosis. It is diagnosed by showing lysis of the red cells on incubation with fresh acified serum (the Ham test). The condition is treated with androgens or prednisone and, during thrombotic episodes, with heparin. It may progress to aplastic anaemia or acute leukaemia.

haemogram ('heemə,gram) a graphic representation of the differential blood count.

haemohistioblast (,heemoh'histioh,blast) the hypothetical stem cell from which all blood cells are derived. Called also *haemocytoblast*.

haemoid ('heemoyd) resembling blood.

haemokinesis (,heemohki'neesis) the flow of blood in the body. adj. **haemokinetic**.

haemolith ('heemə,lith) a concretion in the walls of a blood vessel.

haemolymph ('heemə,limf) 1. blood and lymph. 2. the blood-like fluid of invertebrates having open blood-vascular systems.

haemolymphangioma (,heemoh,limfanji'ohmə) haematolymphangioma.

haemolysate (hee'moli,sayt) the product resulting from haemolysis.

haemolyse ('heemə,liez) to subject to or to undergo haemolysis.

haemolysin (hee'molisin) a substance that liberates haemoglobin from erythrocytes by interrupting their structural integrity.

haemolysis (hee'molisis) rupture of erythrocytes with release of haemoglobin into the plasma.

Some microbes form substances called haemolysins that have the specific action of destroying red blood corpuscles; the beta-haemolytic streptococcus is an example.

Intravenous administration of a hypotonic solution or plain distilled water will cause the red cells to fill with fluid until their membranes rupture and the cells are destroyed.

In a transfusion reaction or in HAEMOLYTIC disease of the newborn, incompatibility causes the red blood cells to clump together. The agglutinated cells become trapped in the smaller vessels and eventually disintegrate, releasing haemoglobin into the plasma. Kidney damage may result as the haemoglobin crystallizes and obstructs the renal tubules, producing renal shutdown and uraemia.

Snake venoms and certain vegetable poisons, e.g., mushrooms, may cause haemolysis. A great variety of chemical agents can lead to destruction of erythrocytes if there is exposure to a sufficiently high concentration of the substance. These chemical haemolytics include arsenic, lead, benzene, acetanilide, nitrites, and potassium chlorate.

haemolytic (,heemə'litik) pertaining to, characterized by, or producing haemolysis.

h. anaemia anaemia caused by the shortened survival of mature erythrocytes and inability of the bone marrow to compensate for their decreased life span. It may result from Rh incompatibility (see RH FACTOR and haemolytic disease of the newborn below); from mismatched blood transfusions; from industrial poisons such as benzene, trinitrotoluene (TNT) or aniline; and from hypersensitivity to drugs including certain antibiotics and tranquillizers. Haemolytic anaemia may occur as a result of a disorder of the IMMUNE RESPONSE in which B-cell-produced antibodies fail to recognize erythrocytes that are 'self' and directly attack and destroy them. Haemolytic anaemia may also appear in the course of other diseases such as systemic lupus erythematosus, widespread cancer, leukaemia, Hodgkin's disease, acute alcoholism, and liver diseases. In addition to the usual symptoms of anaemia, the patient may exhibit jaundice.

Severe haemolytic anaemia may be very quickly fatal. Patients must be hospitalized immediately so that transfusions can be given and other treatment begun if the cause of the condition is to be located, and successfully treated. In some cases, surgery to remove the SPLEEN may bring about great improvement.

h. disease of the newborn a blood dyscrasia of the newborn characterized by haemolysis of erythrocytes usually due to incompatibility between the infant's blood and the mother's. The fetus has Rh-positive blood and its mother has Rh-negative blood (see RH FACTOR). Called also *erythroblastosis fetalis, Rhesus isoimmunization*, or *Rhesus disease*.

In Rh incompatibility the mother builds up antibodies against the cells of the fetus; these antibodies pass through the placenta, entering the fetal circulation. They then proceed to destroy the fetal erythrocytes very rapidly. In order to compensate for this rapid destruction of red blood cells, there is increased bone marrow production and early release of newly formed cells and immature red blood cells (erythroblasts). Thus an extremely high percentage of the fetal erythrocytes are erythroblasts; this condition is called erythroblastosis.

SYMPTOMS. If the fetus survives under these circumstances, it is usually anaemic at birth and becomes jaundiced within 24 hours. The antibodies from the mother's blood usually circulate in the baby's blood for 1 to 2 months after birth, continuing their destruction of red blood cells unless an exchange TRANSFUSION is done.

Other symptoms depend on the number of red cells destroyed and the amount of damage done to other tissues of the body, such as the brain and central nervous system.

TREATMENT. The usual treatment for haemolytic disease of the newborn is exchange transfusion in which the infant's blood is replaced with Rh-negative blood. The average amount used for transfusion of this kind is 400 ml. This measure stops the destruction of the infant's red cells, and gradually the Rh-negative blood is replaced with the baby's own blood. In about 6 weeks the antibodies left over from the mother's blood have been destroyed and are no longer a menace to the baby. Exposure to blue light from a fluorescent tube (phototherapy) breaks down the bilirubin causing the jaundice and reduces the number of transfusions that are required.

Recent developments in the management of haemolytic disease include AMNIOCENTESIS and intrauterine fetal transfusion. The former is puncture of the amniotic sac through the maternal abdomen and is done for the purpose of obtaining a sample of AMNIOTIC FLUID for analysis. This allows determination of the concentration of bilirubin pigments and protein in the amniotic fluid; a high concentration indicates excessive destruction of fetal erythrocytes. If there is a mild haemolysis the mother is watched closely and allowed to deliver at term. In more severe cases, induced labour and premature delivery are usually advised so that further destruction of the erythrocytes will not take place and an exchange transfusion can be performed as soon as possible. For cases of very severe haemolysis it has been recommended that an intrauterine transfusion be administered to the fetus. This is a very delicate procedure, not without risks, and advised only if the mother's past history and the present evidence indicate that the infant would not survive or would suffer damage from erythroblastosis. See also RH FACTOR.

PREVENTION. Immunization of Rh-negative mothers by the fetal red cells that enter the circulation at parturition can be prevented by the injection of anti-D gamma globulin immediately after delivery. Anti-D gamma globulin is also given in any other situation where it is thought that fetal red cells may have entered the maternal circulation; this can be assessed using the KLEIHAUER TEST. See also RH FACTOR.

h. jaundice a rare, chronic, and generally hereditary disease characterized by periods of excessive haemolysis due to abnormal fragility of the erythrocytes, which are small and spheroidal. It is accompanied by enlargement of the spleen and by jaundice. The hereditary or congenital form is known as hereditary spherocytosis, congenital haemolytic jaundice or familial acholuric jaundice; the acquired form is known as acquired haemolytic jaundice.

haemomediastinum (ˌheemohˌmeedi·əˈstienəm) an effusion of blood into the mediastinum.

haemometra (ˌheemohˈmeetrə) haematometra.

haemonephrosis (ˌheemohnəˈfrohsis) effused blood in the renal pelvis; haematonephrosis.

haemopathology (ˌheemohpəˈtholəjee) the study of diseases of the blood.

haemopathy (heeˈmopəthee) any disease of the blood. adj. **haemopathic.**

haemoperfusion (ˌheemohpəˈfyoozhən) the passage of blood through an extracorporeal adsorptive system to remove compounds of larger molecular size than those removed by haemodialysis.

haemopericardium (ˌheemohˌperiˈkahdi·əm) an effusion of blood in the pericardial cavity.

haemoperitoneum (ˌheemohˌperitəˈneeəm) an effusion of blood in the peritoneal cavity.

haemopexin (ˌheemohˈpeksin) a haem-binding serum protein.

haemophagocyte (ˌheemohˈfagəˌsiet) a cell that destroys blood corpuscles.

haemophil (ˈheemohˌfil) 1. thriving on blood. 2. a microorganism that grows best in media containing haemoglobin.

haemophilia (ˌheemohˈfili·ə) a condition characterized by impaired coagulability of the blood, and a strong tendency to bleed. Over 80 per cent of all patients with haemophilia have haemophilia A (classic haemophilia), which is characterized by a deficiency of clotting factor VIII. Haemophilia B (Christmas disease), which affects about 15 per cent of all haemophiliac patients results from a deficiency of factor IX. Both types of haemophilia are inherited as an X-linked recessive trait; that is, female carriers can transmit the gene for haemophilia to half their daughters, who become carriers themselves, and to half their sons, who develop the disease. Other less common types of haemophilia with similar symptoms but attributable to the absence of different clotting factors are known to exist.

SYMPTOMS. Haemophilia produces the typical symptom of abnormal bleeding from minor wounds and spontaneous haemorrhages under the skin and in the gums, joints, muscles, and gastrointestinal tract. Haemarthrosis can lead to painful stiffening of the joints and permanent crippling if the condition is not corrected. The abnormal bleeding can range from mild to severe, depending on the degree to which the factor is absent.

Haemophilia A is characterized by a factor VIII level of from 0 to 30 per cent of normal; in severe haemophilia the level is less than 1 per cent. There is a prolonged partial thromboplastin time (PTT), but the platelet count, bleeding time, and prothrombin time are normal. In haemophilia B there is a low factor IX level and the activated partial thromboplastin time is usually prolonged.

TREATMENT. In order to avoid the debilitating and crippling effects of haemophilia, treatment must raise the level of the deficient clotting factor and maintain it in order to stop local bleeding. Haemophilia A patients are given cryoprecipitated antihaemophilic factor (AHF) or lyophilized AHF in sufficient doses to raise the level of the clotting factor to 10 per cent or more depending on the nature of the bleed. Haemophilia B can be treated with fresh frozen plasma or factor IX concentrates to raise the factor IX level to within an acceptable range. Serious episodes of bleeding may require blood transfusion in addition to the above replacement therapy. Home treatment given by a relative or the patient himself has markedly improved the management and life style of the severe haemophiliac. The patient must learn to avoid trauma and to obtain prompt treatment for bleeding episodes. Before surgery or dental treatment the patient must be given an infusion of the appropriate clotting factor. Whenever these patients must receive injections, a small needle is used, pressure is applied at the site after the needle is withdrawn and the area should be inspected frequently for bleeding until the danger of hemorrhage is past.

Complications of treatment with blood concentrates include the development of hepatitis and infection with HIV, which causes the acquired immune deficiency syndome (AIDS).

h. A classical haemophilia, due to deficiency of clotting factor VIII, transmitted by the female to the male as a sex-linked recessive abnormality.

h. B a form similar to classical haemophilia but due to a deficiency of clotting factor IX; called also *Christmas disease* and *factor IX* deficiency.

h. C an autosomal dominant form due to deficiency of clotting factor XI. Called also *factor XI deficiency*.

vascular h. von Willebrand's disease.

haemophiliac (ˌheemohˈfiliˌak) a person affected with haemophilia.

haemophilic (ˌheemohˈfilik) 1. pertaining to haemophilia. 2. in bacteriology, growing well on culture media containing blood or having a nutritional requirement for constituents of fresh blood.

Haemophilus (heeˈmofiləs) a genus of haemophilic gram-negative bacteria.

H. aegyptius an organism closely related to *H. influenzae*, which is the cause of pinkeye (acute contagious conjunctivitis).

H. ducreyi the causative agent of chancroid.

H. influenzae a species once thought to be the cause of epidemic influenza; it produces a highly fatal form of meningitis, especially in infants.

haemophoric (ˌheemohˈfo·rik) conveying blood.

haemophthalmia (ˌheemofˈthalmi·ə) extravasation of blood inside the eye.

haemopleura (ˌheemohˈplooə·rə) haemothorax.

haemopneumopericardium (ˌheemohˌnyoomohˌperiˈkahdi·əm) effused blood and air in the pericardium.

haemopneumothorax (ˌheemohˌnyoomohˈthor·raks) an accumulation of blood and air in the pleural cavity.

haemopoiesis (ˌheemohpoyˈeesis) haematopoiesis. adj. **haemopoietic.**

haemoprecipitin (ˌheemohpriˈsipitin) a precipitin specific for blood.

haemoprotein (ˌheemohˈprohteen) a conjugated protein whose nonprotein portion is haem.

haemopsonin (ˌheemopˈsənin) an opsonin that renders erythrocytes more liable to phagocytosis. Called also *erythrocyto-opsonin*.

haemoptysis (hee'moptisis) coughing and spitting of blood as a result of bleeding from any part of the respiratory tract. In true haemoptysis the sputum is bright red and frothy with air bubbles; it must not be confused with the dark red or black colour of haematemesis.

Although recent developments in drug therapy have reduced the incidence of serious bleeding in tuberculous patients, tuberculosis remains a common cause of haemoptysis. Other causes may be bronchiectasis, lung abscess, or malignancy. In acute pneumonia the sputum may be bright red or it may contain old blood which gives it a characteristic rusty appearance. Vascular disorders such as congestive heart failure, pulmonary infarction, and aortic aneurysm can also cause haemoptysis.

Treatment is aimed at the primary cause of the symptom. The patient with severe haemorrhage is more likely to die from drowning in his own blood than from blood loss. Emergency measures for severe haemoptysis include application of an ice pack to the neck and chest, administration of a sedative, and absolute bed rest with the head of the bed elevated slightly. The patient may be given codeine to depress the cough reflex, and he should be instructed to cough with the glottis open, without straining.

parasitic h. a disease due to infection of the lungs with lung flukes of the genus *Paragonimus*, with cough and spitting of blood and gradual deterioration of health.

haemorrhage ('hemə·rij) the escape of blood. Haemorrhage can be external, internal, or into the tissues. Blood from an artery is bright red in colour and comes in spurts; that from a vein is dark blue/red and flows steadily.

SYMPTOMS. Aside from the obvious flow of blood from a wound or body orifice, massive internal haemorrhage can be detected by signs such as restlessness, cold and clammy skin, thirst, increased and thready pulse, rapid and shallow respirations, and a fall in blood pressure. If the haemorrhage continues unchecked, the patient may complain of visual disturbances, ringing in the ears, or extreme weakness.

FIRST AID

Bleeding from an Open Wound

(1) Apply direct pressure on the wound with a thick compress of gauze or any other available clean cloth.

(2) When bleeding has been controlled, bind the compress firmly in place with strips of cloth.

(3) If direct pressure does not control bleeding, apply digital pressure at the appropriate pressure point.

Internal Bleeding

The patient should be covered with a blanket or coat, keeping the head and chest a little lower than the feet.

capillary h. oozing of blood from minute vessels.

cerebral h. an episode of bleeding into the cerebrum; one of the three main forms of STROKE.

concealed h. internal haemorrhage.

internal h. that in which the extravasated blood remains within the body.

intracranial h. bleeding within the cranium, which may be extradural, subdural, subarachnoid, or cerebral.

petechial h. subcutaneous haemorrhage occurring in minute spots.

postpartum h. that which follows soon after labour.

primary h. that which soon follows an injury.

secondary h. that which follows an operation or injury after a lapse of time; usually associated with wound infection.

haemorrhagenic (ˌhemə·rə'jenik) causing haemorrhage.

haemorrhagic (ˌhemə'rajik) pertaining to or characterized by haemorrhage.

h. disease of newborn a self-limited haemorrhagic disorder of the first days of life, caused by deficiency of vitamin K-dependent blood clotting factors II, VII, IX, and X. It should be prevented by the prophylactic administration of vitamin K to all newborn babies.

h. fever with renal syndrome an acute haemorrhagic fever first reported in Korea in 1951, and now known to be present in China, the USSR, and northern Europe. It is caused by the Hantaan virus and is a zoonosis acquired from rodents, usually considered to be spread by mites. A few cases have been reported in the UK associated with infection in laboratory rats. The incubation period is 12–16 days. Human-to-human transmission has not been described. Called also *Korean haemorrhagic fever, epidemic haemorrhagic fever* or *nephropathia epidemica*.

viral h. fevers a group of notifiable virus diseases of diverse aetiology but with similar characteristics of fever, headache, myalgia, prostration, and haemorrhagic symptoms. They include dengue haemorrhagic fever (Southeast Asia, India, western Pacific and Caribbean), chikungunya fever (Southeast Asia, India), Crimean-Congo haemorrhagic fever (central Asia, eastern Europe, Middle East, Africa), Ebola virus disease (central Africa), haemorrhagic fever with renal syndrome (Korea, China, USSR, northern Europe), Kyasanur Forest disease (India), Lassa fever (West Africa), Marburg disease (central Africa), Omsk haemorrhagic fever (western Siberia), Rift Valley fever (Africa), and yellow fever (central Africa, central and South America).

haemorrheology (ˌhemə·ri'oləjee) the scientific study of the deformation and flow properties of cellular and plasmatic components of blood in macroscopic, microscopic, and submicroscopic dimensions and the rheological properties of vessel structure with which the blood comes in direct contact.

haemorrhoea (ˌhemə'reeə) haematorrhoea.

haemorrhoid ('hemə,royd) an enlarged vessel, usually a vein found inside or just outside the anal canal. In the plural, called also piles.

Internal haemorrhoids usually are first noticed when minor bleeding occurs with defecation. Pain occurs rarely, unless there is an associated disorder such as an anal fissure, thrombosis, or strangulation of the affected vein. External haemorrhoids produce varying degrees of pain, feelings of pressure, itching, irritation, and a palpable mass. Bleeding occurs only if the external haemorrhoid is injured or ulcerated and begins to break down.

Haemorrhoids are caused by increased pressure on the veins of the anus. Prolonged sitting, constipation, and hard, dry stools that are difficult to pass can lead to straining and sitting at stool for long periods of time, all of which add pressure on the anal veins. Failure to follow through on the urge to defecate can also lead to haemorrhoids. In women, probably the single most common cause is pregnancy.

External haemorrhoids can be treated by local applications of cold and an astringent cream, by salt baths, and by avoidance of constipation. Internal haemorrhoids may require sclerosing or cryosurgery to obliterate the affected tissue. More advanced, chronic haemorrhoids usually must be removed surgically by ligation and excision (HAEMORRHOIDECTOMY) or by BARRON'S LIGATOR.

external h. one distal to the pectinate line.

internal h. one originating above the pectinate line and covered by mucous membrane.

prolapsed h. an internal haemorrhoid that has descended below the pectinate line and protruded outside the anal sphincter.

strangulated h. a prolapsed internal haemorrhoid constricted by anal spasm.

haemorrhoidectomy (ˌhemə·roy'dektəmee) surgical excision of haemorrhoids. Although the operation is considered minor and dressings may not be needed, the patient may experience much discomfort and require analgesic drugs and frequent nursing measures to relieve discomfort.

Barron ligation (rubber band ligation) is a relatively new, conservative surgical technique for the treatment of haemorrhoids, in which the haemorrhoids are bound with rubber ligatures so that the ligated portion sloughs away after several days.

PATIENT CARE. Postoperatively the patient must be watched for signs of haemorrhage, an uncommon occurrence but one that can develop quickly. The patient may be placed on his abdomen to relieve pressure on the operative site, or he may lie on his back with a rubber air ring under the buttocks for support. Compresses of witch hazel or some other astringent agent may be applied to reduce swelling and promote healing. Difficulty in evacuating often occurs during the immediate postoperative period. Salt baths are often helpful in relieving this situation.

haemosiderin (ˌheemoh'sidə·rin) an insoluble form of storage iron, visible microscopically both with and without the use of special stains.

haemosiderinuria (ˌheemohˌsidə·ri'nyooə·ri·ə) the presence of haemosiderin in the urine.

haemosiderosis (ˌheemohˌsidi'rohsis) a focal or general increase in tissue iron stores without associated tissue damage.

pulmonary h. the deposition of abnormal amounts of haemosiderin in the lungs, due to bleeding into the lung interstitium.

haemospermia (ˌheemoh'spərmi·ə) the presence of blood in the semen.

haemostasis (ˌheemoh'staysis, hee'mostəsis) arrest of the escape of blood by either natural (clot formation or vessel spasm) or artificial (compression or ligation) means, or the interruption of blood flow to a part.

haemostat ('heemohˌstat) 1. a small surgical clamp for constricting blood vessels. 2. an antihaemorrhagic agent.

haemostatic (ˌheemoh'statik) checking blood flow.

haemostyptic (ˌheemoh'stiptik) haemostatic.

haemotherapy (ˌheemoh'therəpee) the use of blood in treating disease.

haemothorax (ˌheemoh'thor·raks) collection of blood in the pleural cavity.

haemotoxic (ˌheemə'toksik) haematotoxic.

haemotoxin (ˌheemə'toksin) an exotoxin characterized by haemolytic activity.

haemotroph ('heeməˌtrohf) the sum total of the nutritive material from the circulating blood of the maternal body, utilized by the early embryo. adj. **haemotrophic.**

hafnium ('hafni·əm) a chemical element, atomic number 72, atomic weight 178.49, symbol Hf. See table of elements in Appendix 2.

Hagedorn's needle ('hahgəˌdawnz) a needle flattened from side to side and curved on the flat.

Hageman factor ('haygəmən) clotting factor XII.

hahnium ('hahni·əm) former name for UNNILPENTIUM.

Hailey–Hailey disease ('haylee'haylee) benign familial pemphigus.

hair (hair) a threadlike structure, especially the specialized epidermal structure developing from a papilla sunk in the dermis, produced only by mammals and characteristic of that group of animals. Also, the aggregate of such hairs.

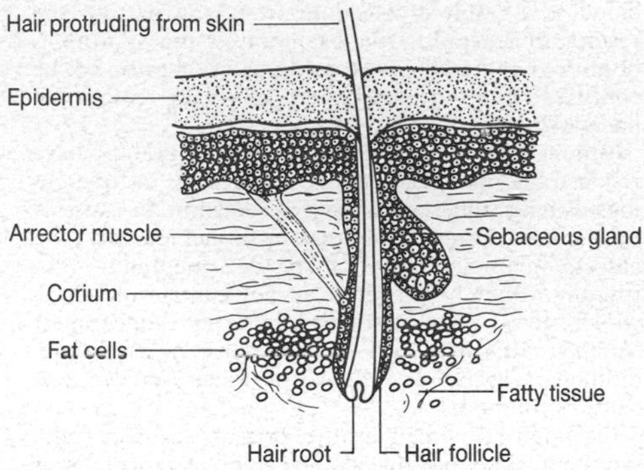

Structure of a hair. The follicle is the protective casing of the hair root. Contraction of the arrector muscle, caused by cold, fear or other stimulus, produces so-called goose flesh (cutis anserina)

auditory h's hairlike attachments of the epithelial cells of the inner ear.

bamboo h. trichorrhexis nodosa.

beaded h. hair marked with alternate swellings and constrictions; seen in monilethrix.

h. bulb the bulbous expansion at the lower end of a hair root.

burrowing h. one that grows horizontally in the skin.

club h. a hair whose root is surrounded by a bulbous enlargement composed of keratinized cells, preliminary to normal loss of the hair from the follicle.

h. follicle a pouchlike depression in the skin in which a hair develops from the matrix at its base and grows to emerge from its opening on the body surface.

Frey's h's stiff hairs mounted in a handle; used for testing the sensitiveness of pressure points of the skin.

ingrown h. one that has curved and reentered the skin.

lanugo h. the fine hair on the body of the fetus.

moniliform h. beaded hair.

pubic h. the hair on the external genitalia; called also *pubes*.

sensory h's hairlike projections on the surface of sensory epithelial cells.

tactile h's hairs sensitive to touch.

taste h's short hairlike processes projecting freely into the lumen of the pit of a taste bud from the peripheral ends of the taste cells.

terminal h. the coarse hair on various areas of the body during adult years.

twisted h. pilus tortus; a hair which at spaced intervals is twisted through an axis of 180 degrees, being abnormally flattened at the site of twisting.

hairball ('hairˌbawl) trichobezoar; a concretion of hair sometimes found in the stomach or intestines of man or other animals.

halation (hə'layshən) indistinctness of the visual image caused by strong illumination coming from the same direction as the object being viewed.

halcinonide (hal'sinəˌnied) a topical corticosteroid used in the treatment of acute and chronic dermatoses.

Haldol ('haldol) trademark for a preparation of haloperidol, an antipsychotic agent.

half-life ('hahfˌlief) the time in which the radioactivity usually associated with a particular isotope is reduced by half through radioactive decay.

half-value layer (hahf'valyoo) that thickness of a given substance (a filter) which will reduce the intensity of a beam of radiation by half.

halfway house ('hahfway,hows) a residence for patients (e.g., mental patients, drug addicts, alcoholics) who do not require hospitalization but who need an intermediate degree of care until they can return to the community.

halibut oil ('halibət ,oyl) a vitamin-rich (A and D) oil derived from the liver of halibut.

halide ('halied, 'hay-) a compound of a halogen with an element or radical.

halisteresis (,halistə'reesis) deficiency of mineral salts (calcium) in a part, as in osteomalacia.

halitosis (,hali'tohsis) offensive odour of the breath.

halitus ('halitəs) an expired breath.

Hallervorden–Spatz syndrome (,haləfordən'spatz) a hereditary disorder involving marked reduction in the number of myelin sheaths of the globus pallidus and substantia nigra, with accumulations of iron pigment, progressive rigidity beginning in the legs, choreoathetoid movements, dysarthria, and progressive mental deterioration.

hallucination (hə,loosi'nayshən) a sensory impression (sight, touch, sound, smell, or taste) that has no basis in external stimulation. Hallucinations can have psychological causes, as in mental illness, or they can result from drugs, alcohol, organic illnesses, such as brain tumour or senility, or exhaustion. When hallucinations have a psychological origin, they usually represent a disguised form of a repressed conflict.

auditory h. a hallucination of hearing; the most common type.

gustatory h. a hallucination of taste.

haptic h. tactile hallucination.

hypnagogic h. a hallucination occurring between sleeping and awakening.

olfactory h. a hallucination of smell.

tactile h. a hallucination of touch.

visual h. a hallucination of sight.

hallucinogen (hə'loosinə,jen) an agent capable of producing hallucinations or false sensory perceptions. adj. **hallucinogenic.** Drugs that have hallucinogenic properties include mescaline, LSD (lysergic acid diethylamide), and psilocybin. Certain mushrooms and seeds are also hallucinogenic. The experiences brought about by the use of hallucinogens involve a more acute 'awareness' of one's environment and a distorted response to visual, auditory, and tactile stimuli. They can also cause a person to exhibit behaviour that is symptomatic of a psychotic state of mind.

Hallucinogenic drugs have been used experimentally in research on mental illness; their value in determining brain function and the mechanisms of mental illness is yet to be proved. Abuse of the hallucinogenic compounds by persons who have obtained them through illicit channels, or taken them in medically unsupervised or socially unacceptable settings, has led to the regulation of their distribution by the Department of Health. Indiscriminate use of these compounds can bring on psychotic states and may result in permanent harm to the psyche. Synthetic hallucinogens, e.g., 'angel dust' (phencyclidine), are a particularly dangerous component of drug abouse patterns.

hallucinogenesis (hə,loosinoh'jenəsis) the production of hallucinations.

hallucinosis (hə,loosi'nohsis) the experiencing of more or less constant hallucinations.

acute h., alcoholic h. alcoholic psychosis marked by auditory hallucinations and delusions of persecution.

hallux ('haləks) the great toe.

h. dolorosa a painful disease of the great toe, usually associated with flatfoot.

h. flexus hallux rigidus.

h. malleus hammer toe affecting the great toe.

h. rigidus painful flexion deformity of the great toe with limitation of motion at the metatarsophalangeal joint.

h. valgus angulation of the great toe toward the other toes of the foot.

h. varus angulation of the great toe away from the other toes of the foot.

halo ('hayloh) a circular structure, such as a luminous circle seen surrounding an object or light.

Fick's h. a coloured circle appearing around a light, experienced by wearers of contact lenses.

glaucomatous h., h. glaucomatosus a narrow light zone surrounding the optic disc in glaucoma.

senile h. a zone of variable width around the optic disc, due to exposure of various elements of the choroid as a result of senile atrophy of the pigmented epithelium.

halogen ('halə,jen, -ləjən) an element of group VII of the periodic table, the members of which form similar (saltlike) compounds in combination with sodium. The halogens are bromine, chlorine, fluorine, iodine, and astatine.

haloperidol (,haloh'peri,dol) an antipsychotic drug of the butyrophenone group; used for the management of symptoms of pyschoses and for control of the vocal utterances and tics of Gilles de la Tourette's syndrome.

halophil ('halə,fil, -,fiel) a halophilic microorganism.

halophilic (,halə'filik) pertaining to or characterized by an affinity for salt; requiring a high concentration of salt for optimal growth.

halothane ('haloh,thayn) a colourless, nonflammable, volatile liquid whose vapour is inhaled to produce general ANAESTHESIA. Its pleasant nonirritant odour leads to a smooth induction and recovery is relatively rapid. It depresses the cardiovascular system, leading to hypotension and bradycardia, and arrhythmias, usually benign, are not uncommon. At one time the most widely used inhalational agent, its use is declining because of the rare complication of postoperative severe liver damage.

h. hepatitis hepatitis following halothane anaesthesia. It is rare (1 in 35,000) and is diagnosed by exclusion of other causes of postoperative jaundice. It appears to be associated with more than one exposure to halothane within a short interval (4–6 weeks). Middle-aged obese women seem to be particularly prone. There is no specific treatment and mortality is high.

Ham test (ham) one for paroxysmal nocturnal haemoglobinuria, performed by incubating red cells in an acid environment; a positive test may be obtained in other forms of anaemia.

hamamelis (,hamə'meelis) a soothing agent prepared from witch-hazel and used in suppository form in the treatment of haemorrhoids.

hamartia (hə'mahshi·ə) a defect of tissue combination in development.

hamartoblastoma (hə,mahtohbla'stohmə) a tumour developing from a hamartoma.

hamartoma (,hamah'tohmə) a benign tumour-like nodule composed of an overgrowth of mature cells and tissues normally present in the affected part, but in disorganized proportions and often with one element predominating.

hamartomatous (,hamah'tohmətəs) pertaining to a disturbance in growth of a tissue in which the cells of a circumscribed area outstrip those of the surrounding areas.

hamate ('hamayt) hooked, as the hamate bone.

Hamilton–Russell traction (,hamәltən'rus'l) a

method of applying traction on the leg by the use of skin traction and a sling support under the knee.

Hamman's disease ('hamənz) interstitial emphysema of the lungs due to spontaneous rupture of the alveoli.

Hamman–Rich syndrome ('hamən,rich) diffuse idiopathic interstitial fibrosis.

hammer ('hamə) the malleus, the largest of the three bones of the ear.

h. toe a condition in which the proximal phalanx of the toe—most often that of the second toe—is extended and the second and distal phalanges are flexed, causing a clawlike appearance.

hamstring ('ham,string) one of the tendons that laterally and medially bound the depression in the posterior region of the knee (popliteal space).

inner h's the tendons of the gracilis, sartorius, and two other muscles of the leg.

outer h. the tendon of the biceps muscle of the thigh.

hamulus ('hamyuhləs) pl. *hamuli* [L.] any hookshaped process.

hand (hand) the terminal part of an arm, or of the upper (anterior) extremity of a primate.

ape h. one with the thumb permanently extended.

cleft h. a malformation in which the division between the fingers extends into the metacarpus; also, a hand with the middle digits absent.

claw h. see CLAWHAND.

drop h. wristdrop.

lobster-claw h. cleft hand.

obstetrician's h. the contraction of the hand in tetany; the hand is flexed at the wrist, the fingers at the metacarpophalangeal joints but extended at the interphalangeal joints, the thumb being strongly flexed into the palm.

writing h. in Parkinson's disease, assumption of the position by which a pen is commonly held.

hand-foot-and-mouth disease (,hand,fuhtənd'mowth) a mild, infectious virus disease of children, with vesicular lesions in the mouth and on the hands and feet; caused by coxsackie A viruses.

Hand–Schüller–Christian disease (,hand,shoolə'krischən) chronic idiopathic histiocytosis with multifocal histiocytic lipogranulomas of bone and of the skin, the histiocytes containing abundant cholesterol. It affects chiefly children and young adults. Called also *Hand's disease*, *Schüller's disease*, *Schüller–Christian disease*, and *chronic idiopathic xanthomatosis*.

The three classic symptoms of the syndrome are softened areas of the skull and other flat, membranous bones, exophthalmos, and diabetes insipidus. However, all three symptoms are rarely found in one patient. Otitis frequently accompanies the disease. Skin lesions resembling those of seborrhoeic dermatitis may appear, as may xanthomas.

There is no specific treatment. X-ray therapy is sometimes helpful in treating specific local lesions and corticosteroids have been used with success in some cases. Complete recovery does occur, but about 40 per cent of the cases terminate fatally.

handedness ('handidnəs) the preferential use of the hand of one side in all voluntary motor acts.

handicap ('handi,kap) a disadvantage for a given individual, resulting from an impairment or a disability that limits or prevents the fulfilment of a role that is normal (depending on age, sex and social and cultural factors) for that individual.

hangnail ('hang,nayl) a shred of eponychium at one side of a nail. Hangnail is prevented by gently pushing the cuticle instead of cutting it, and it is treated by clipping off the shred of skin to prevent infection.

Hanot's disease ('anohz) biliary cirrhosis.

Hansen's bacillus ('hansənz) *Mycobacterium leprae*, the causative agent of leprosy.

Hansen's disease leprosy.

haphalgesia (,hafal'jeezi·ə) pain on touching objects.

haploid ('haployd) having half the number of chromosomes characteristically found in the somatic (diploid) cells of an organism; typical of the gametes of a species whose union restores the diploid number.

haploidentity (,haploh·ie'dentitee) the condition of having the same antigenic phenotype at certain specified loci; said of donor-recipient combinations in transplantation studies.

haploidy ('haploydee) the state of being haploid.

haploscope ('haplə,skohp) a stereoscope for testing the visual axis. adj. **haploscopic**.

haplotype ('haploh,tiep) the group of alleles of linked genes contributed by either parent; the haploid genetic constitution contributed by either parent.

Hapsburg jaw ('hapsbərg) a mandibular prognathous jaw, often accompanied by Hapsburg lip.

Hapsburg lip a thick, overdeveloped lower lip that often accompanies Hapsburg jaw.

hapten, haptene ('haptən; 'hapteen) the portion of an antigenic molecule or complex that determines its immunological specificity. adj. **haptenic**.

haptic ('haptik) tactile.

haptics ('haptiks) the science of the sense of touch.

haptoglobin (,haptə'glohbin) a group of serum alpha-2 globulin glycoproteins that bind free haemoglobin; the different types, genetically determined, are distinguished electrophoretically.

Harada's syndrome (hə'rahdəz) a syndrome, possibly caused by a virus, consisting of uveomeningitis associated with retinochoroidal detachment, temporary or permanent deafness and blindness, and sometimes, though often transiently, alopecia, vitiligo, and poliosis.

Harmogen ('hahmohgen) trademark for a preparation of piperazine oestrone sulphate, an oestrone used in the treatment of oestrogen deficiency associated with menopausal symptoms.

Harris's operation ('harisiz) suprapubic transvesical prostatectomy.

Harrison's groove ('haris'nz) a horizontal groove along the lower border of the thorax corresponding to the costal insertion of the diaphragm; seen in rickets.

Hartmann's operation ('hahtmənz) resection of the upper rectum and lower sigmoid colon, with the proximal colon brought out as a colostomy and the distal stump of rectum being closed by suture.

Hartmann's solution a solution containing sodium chloride, sodium lactate, and phosphates of calcium and potassium; used intravenously as a systemic alkalizer and as a fluid and electrolyte replenisher.

Hartnup disease ('hahtnup) a genetically determined disorder of intestinal and renal transport of neutral alpha-amino acids, with pellagra-like skin lesions, transient cerebellar ataxia, constant renal aminoaciduria and other biochemical abnormalities.

harvest fever ('hahvist) spirochaetosis affecting harvest workers, due to *Leptospira grippotyphosa*, with fever, diarrhoea, conjunctivitis, stupor, and vomiting.

Harvey ('hahvee) William (1578–1657). English physician and physiologist. Born at Folkestone in Kent, he attended the universities of Cambridge and Padua, and announced in 1628 his discovery of the circulation of blood, which was a model of accurate experimentation and inductive proof, and the first application of quantitative demonstration in any biological investigation. His *De generatione animalium* is important in the history of embryology, for in it Harvey rejected the doctrine of preformation of the fetus and stated that almost all animals, and man himself, are produced from eggs.

HAS Health Advisory Service.

HASAW Health and Safety at Work Act.

Hashimoto's disease (ˌhashi'mohtohz) a progressive autoimmune disease of the thyroid gland with degeneration of its epithelial elements and replacement by lymphoid and fibrous tissue; called also *struma lymphomatosa*.

hashish ('hasheesh, -ish) a preparation of the unadulterated resin scraped from the flowering tops of female hemp plants (*Cannabis sativa*), smoked or chewed for its intoxicating effects. Its possession is illegal in many countries. It is far more potent than MARIJUANA. See also CANNABIS.

Hassall's corpuscles ('has'lz) small striated bodies in the thymus gland which are the remains of tissue found in the early stages of development of this gland.

haustration (haw'strayshən) 1. the formation of a haustrum. 2. a haustrum.

haustrum ('hawstrəm) pl. *haustra* [L.] one of the pouches of the colon, produced by adaptation of its length to the taeniae coli, or by collection of circular muscle fibres at 1 or 2 cm distances, and responsible for the sacculated appearance.

HAV hepatitis A virus.

Haverhill fever ('havəˌhil) a form of RATBITE FEVER, an acute febrile disease caused by *Streptobacillus moniliformis*, transmitted by the bite of an infected rat, and characterized by an erythematous eruption and more or less generalized arthritis, with adenitis, headache, and vomiting; first described in Haverhill, Massachusetts, USA, in 1926.

haversian (hə'vərsi·ən, -shən) named after the English physician and anatomist Clopton Havers, 1650–1702.

h. canal any of the anastomosing channels of the harversian system in compact bone, containing blood and lymph vessels, and nerves.

h. glands synovial villi.

h. system a haversian canal and its concentrically arranged lamellae, constituting the basic unit of structure in compact bone (osteon).

Hawthorne effect ('hawthawn) the term given to the usual beneficial effect of a study on the persons participating in the study.

hay fever (hay) an atopic ALLERGY characterized by sneezing, itching and watery eyes, running nose, and a burning sensation of the palate and throat.

It is a localized anaphylactic reaction to an extrinsic allergen—most commonly pollens and the spores of moulds. When the allergen comes in contact with mast cell-bound IgE immunoglobulin in the tissues of the conjunctiva, nasal mucosa, and bronchial tree, the cells release mediators of ANAPHYLAXIS and produce the characteristic symptoms of hay fever.

The amount of pollen in the air varies with the season and geographical area. The most frequent cause is grass pollen in the spring and early summer. Symptoms usually cease before mid-June. Earliér symptoms are usually from tree pollens. Mould-bearing plants such as wheat, barley, and maize are prevalent in agricultural areas, and attacks of hay fever caused by mould spores are common there as these crops ripen.

Hay fever deserves to be recognized as more than a mere nuisance. By causing lack of sleep and loss of appetite, it can lower the body's resistance to disease. It can cause inflammation of the ears, sinuses, throat, and bronchi. A number of hay fever sufferers develop ASTHMA.

Hay fever can be relieved, although not cured, by antihistamines and sympathomimetic drugs such as ephedrine and phenylpropanolamine hydrochloride. Intranasal sprays have greatly improved the management of hay fever and sodium cromoglycate, delivered topically, reduces symptom severity by stabilizing the mast cells and reducing histamine release. A series of preventive injections (desensitization) may be recommended in advance of the hay fever season. This consists of administering controlled and gradually increasing amounts of the offending substance in order to develop a certain amount of immunity. In some cases it may be helpful to avoid part of the hay fever season by taking a holiday in an area that is relatively free of the annoying pollen (see also ALLERGY).

nonseasonal h. f., perennial h. f. nonseasonal allergic rhinitis.

Hb haemoglobin.

HB_cAg hepatitis B core antigen.

HB_eAg hepatitis B e antigen.

HB_sAg hepatitis B surface antigen.

HBV hepatitis B virus.

HCG, hCG human chorionic gonadotrophin. A hormone produced by the trophoblastic cells of the ovum within 7 days of fertilization. Its action on the posterior pituitary gland prevents the withdrawal of luteotrophic hormone, so that menstruation does not occur. It forms the basis of pregnancy tests. Raised levels in the urine indicate twin pregnancy. Later in the pregnancy it is produced by the placenta.

HCl hydrochloric acid.

HDL high-density lipoprotein.

He chemical symbol, *helium*.

he- for words beginning thus, see also those beginning *hae-*.

HEA Health Education Authority.

head (hed) the anterior or superior part of a structure or organism, in vertebrates containing the brain and the organs of special sense.

articular h. an eminence on a bone by which it articulates with another bone.

h. injury traumatic injury to the head resulting from a fall or violent blow. Such an injury may be open or closed and may involve a brain CONCUSSION, skull fracture, or contusions of the brain. All head injuries are potentially dangerous because there may be a slow leakage of blood from damaged blood vessels into the brain, or the formation of a blood clot which gradually increases pressure against brain tissue (see cranial HAEMATOMA). One of the most common complications of head injury is subdural haematoma, resulting from the oozing of blood from the cortical veins and the small blood vessels that lie between the arachnoid and the dura mater. A less common but more serious complication that constitutes an extreme surgical emergency is extradural haematoma, a collection of blood in the space between the skull and the dura mater. The leaking of blood into the extradural space progresses rapidly and therefore requires immediate treatment. A third complication that may occur following head injury is herniation of either the brain stem or a part of the cerebellum through the tentorial hiatus (*transtentorial herniation*). This is an extreme emergency demanding immediate relief of pressure against the blood vessels serving the brain stem and cerebellum.

Long-term effects of head injury may include chronic headache, disturbances in mental and motor function, and a host of other symptoms that may or may not be psychogenic. Organic brain damage and posttraumatic epilepsy resulting from scar formation are possible sequels to head injury.

TREATMENT. The method of treatment will depend on the kind and amount of damage inflicted on the brain and surrounding membranes. Surgical procedures to relieve intracranial pressure may include the drilling of burr holes in the skull to aspirate accumulated blood, and intracranial surgery to remove haematomas. Oedema of brain tissue may be reduced by the intravenous administration of an osmotic diuretic, e.g., mannitol. If no immediate surgery is indicated, the doctor may choose to treat the head injury conservatively, with rest and quiet and the careful monitoring of the patient for signs of change in the neurological status.

PATIENT CARE. Continuous assessment of the patient's neurological status and monitoring of the vital signs are essential to the care of the patient with a head injury. Knowledge of the neurological status and in particular, the conscious level, will indicate improvement or deterioration in the patient's condition. Two extracranial factors have been identified as contributing to secondary brain damage in the acutely head injured victim. These are hypoxia and hypotension, and patient care must aim towards the avoidance or minimization of these.

Maintenance of optimal respiratory status, especially in the unconscious patient, must be achieved. This may involve simple measures such as positioning the patient on his side or full mechanical ventilatory support. Administration of oxygen and suctioning may also be necessary. Unnecessary suctioning or applying suction for more than 15 seconds at a time will serve to increase intracranial pressure and exacerbate the patient's condition. In order to determine which measures are needed, respiratory status must be assessed initially and at frequent intervals thereafter. This will include assessment of respiratory rate, depth, volume, and colour of the patient's skin. Monitoring of arterial blood gases may also be included.

Nursing care in terms of preventing hypotension involves the monitoring of vital signs and observing for signs of hypotension and instituting simple first-aid measures to minimize the effects. Fluids and other treatment may be prescribed by the doctor. Unchecked, severe hypotension will lead to a reduction in the circulating cerebral blood volume and thus depletion of oxygen to the brain. Head injury itself rarely causes hypotension, but hypotension is usually an indication of injury elsewhere in the body.

Signs of rising intra-cranial pressure should be treated at once. These include a rising blood pressure and falling pulse, a decrease in the level of consciousness, and altered or absent pupil responses to light.

Other aspects of patient care to consider include observation of, and first-aid measures for, seizures, including protection of the patient from injury and maintaining a patent airway. Cerebrospinal fluid leaks, either via the nose (rhinorrhoea) or ear (otorrhoea) can expose the patient to the risk of meningitis. Identification of the cerebrospinal fluid with the use of glucose reagent dipstick and application of a sterile dry dressing, either under the nose or over the ear, will be necessary. The patient should be advised to try and avoid sniffing. The leak will either cease spontaneously or require surgical repair. In the interim period the patient is given a course of prophylactic antibiotics. It may be that the cerebrospinal fluid trickles down the back of the patient's throat and, if alert, he may complain of a salty taste in his mouth.

An excessive urinary output may be indicative of damage to the hypothalamus with resultant suppression of the antidiuretic hormone. This should be reported so that treatment can be instituted; usually an intramuscular injection of artificial antidiuretic hormone such as desmopressin (DDAVP) is given. A criterion is normally set to determine what is an excessive output; an example of one is voiding more than 1 litre of urine in 6 hours with a specific gravity below 1000.

Difficulty can be experienced in managing the patient with profound memory loss or a marked confusion. Alterations in behaviour are difficult for both relatives and staff to comprehend and sedation is contraindicated, lest it should mask any deterioration in the patient's neurological status. The patient needs to be handled firmly but tactfully and prevented from harming himself. Confused patients can often be abusive and offensive and it is imperative that the family is reassured that the patient does not realize or mean what he is saying. For most patients this confusional state is temporary and the nurse should always eliminate simple causes of restlessness, e.g., a full bladder or headache.

In order to assist patients and their families in the longer term with the rehabilitative problems of head injury, a support network known as Headway has now developed. It is located at 200 Mansfield Road, Nottingham NG1 3HX, and has a growing number of local brances throughout the UK.

nerve h. the optic disc.

headache ('hed,ayk) a pain or ache in the head. One of the most common ailments of man, it is a symptom rather than a disorder in itself. It accompanies many diseases and conditions, including emotional distress. See also MIGRAINE.

Although recurring headache may be an early sign of serious organic disease, relatively few headaches are caused by disease-induced structural changes. Most result from vasodilation of blood vessels in tissues surrounding the brain, or from tension in the neck and scalp muscles.

Immediate medical attention is indicated when (1) a severe headache comes on suddenly without apparent cause; (2) there are accompanying symptoms of neurological abnormality, for example, blurring of vision, mental confusion, loss of mental acuity or consciousness, motor dysfunction, or sensory loss; or (3) the headache is highly localized, as behind the eye or near the ear, or in one location in the head. Fever and stiffness of the neck accompanying the headache may indicate MENINGITIS.

Treatment of headache varies according to its severity and its tendency to recur. A mild transient headache can be relieved by the administration of an analgesic such as aspirin; however, aspirin and other drugs should not be taken habitually. It is best to determine the primary cause of the headache. BIOFEEDBACK may be useful when stress and tension are shown to be responsible for recurring headaches.

cluster h. a migraine-like disorder marked by attacks of unilateral intense pain over the eye and forehead, with flushing and watering of the eyes and nose; attacks last about an hour and occur in clusters.

histamine h. cluster headache.

tension h. a type due to prolonged overwork or emotional strain, or both, affecting especially the occipital region.

Heaf test (heef) a form of tuberculin testing. A drop of tuberculin solution on the skin is injected by means of a number of very short needles mounted on a spring-loaded device (Heaf's gun).

healing ('heeling) the restoration of structure and function of injured or diseased tissues. The healing processes include blood clotting, inflammation and repair.

BLOOD CLOTTING. In order to prevent continued bleeding, blood CLOTTING, occurs at the site of the injury. Essential clotting proteins or factors are present in plasma in their inactive precursor form.

In the BLOOD platelets come in contact with the rough edge of injured tissue, to which they attach themselves and subsequently disintegrate, thus liberating thromboplastin. The thromboplastin acts upon the clotting factors to establish a cascade in which one activated factor converts the next precursor factor into its active form. This occurs sequentially until thrombin is formed from prothrombin. Thrombin then reacts with fibrinogen to form fibrin, which is insoluble, fibrillar and has the property of being able to contract. It forms a network of threads that enmesh the erythrocytes; it pulls them together, as it contracts, to form a clot. See also PLATELET.

INFLAMMATION. When an injury occurs, the body's first-aid mechanisms automatically begin to operate. The blood vessels in the neighbourhood of the injury dilate to provide an increased blood supply. At the same time the pores in the thin walls of the capillaries also widen, letting more plasma than usual flow through to the injured tissues. The immediate result is twofold: the increased flow of blood and plasma brings the body's repair materials to the spot in large quantities, the increased blood flow raises the local temperature, and the increase in fluid at the spot distends tissues. This whole process is called INFLAMMATION. It is one of the body's protective devices. Inflammation causes pain, which impairs the function of the injured part.

REPAIR. The fibrin threads contract and pull together the edges of the wound and repair begins. Neutrophils migrate into the wound along with macrophages. These phagocytose debris, including bacteria, and slowly remove the clot. At the same time new capillaries grow into the clot accompanied by fibroblasts. These form collagen and eventually the edges of the wound will be united. When a cut is relatively clean and small the scar that results will be invisible, but if extensive, or with uneven edges, a large and sometimes unsightly scar may form.

When so much tissue has been lost that the wound must be left open or gaping, as in an abscess or ulcer, the fibroblasts must fill in the wound from the depth and sides before it can be re-epithelialized. In addition to being unsightly, the scars from extensive wounds may interfere with nerves, blood vessels, and muscles. With increasing time contracture deformities may result if these scars are formed across a joint. In such cases, PLASTIC SURGERY may be necessary or advisable to restore function or for cosmetic reasons.

There are various factors that favourably influence the healing process. The chief ones are youth (healing is slow in elderly people), rest of the injured part, adequate nutrition, with plenty of protein and vitamins, and warmth.

h. by first intention union of accurately coapted edges of a wound, with an irreducible minimum of granulation tissue.

h. by second intention union by adhesion of granulating surfaces.

h. by third intention union of a wound that is closed surgically several days after the injury. See also DELAYED PRIMARY CLOSURE.

health (helth) the World Health Organisation (WHO) states that 'Health is a state of complete physical, mental and social well-being and not merely the absence of disease or infirmity'.

h. centre a community health organization for providing ambulatory health care and coordinating the efforts of all health agencies, commonly focused around the general practitioner's services.

holistic h. a system of preventive medicine that takes into account the whole individual, his own responsibility for his well-being, and the total influences—social, psychological, environmental—that affect health, including nutrition, exercise, and mental relaxation.

public h. the field of medicine that is concerned with safeguarding and improving the health of the community as a whole.

h. services the term is usually employed to connote the system or programme by which health care is made available to the population and financed by government or private enterprise or both.

h. statistics summated data on any aspect of the health of populations, for example, mortality, morbidity, use of health services, treatment outcome, costs of health care.

health care system an organized plan of health services. The term usually is employed to denote the system or programme by which health care is made available to the population and financed by government or private enterprise or both. In a larger sense, the elements of a health care system embrace the following: (1) personal health care services available to individuals and families through hospitals and outpatient clinics, and through family practitioner services and health centres, including the care they provide in the patients' own homes; (2) the public health services needed to maintain a healthy environment; for example, control of water and food supplies, regulation of drugs, and safety regulations intended to protect a given population; and (3) teaching and research activities related to the prevention and treatment of disease.

In the UK, health care provided by the National Health Service is the responsibility of the Department of Health, which has its own Secretary of State and Ministers accountable to Parliament. It has two main sections—those controlled by local Family Practitioner Clinics, which provide medical care in the home, and those under the responsibility of Regional Health Authorities, which provide institutional care. Health care under the National Health Service is free, or heavily subsidized, at the point of delivery.

Private health care also exists outside government control and this is paid for by the consumer. Much of this payment is provided for by people contributing to private health insurance companies.

Primary care is the usual point at which an individual enters the health care system. Its major task is the early detection and prevention of disease and the maintenance of health. This level of care also encompasses the routine care of individuals with common health problems and chronic illnesses that can be managed in the home or through periodic visits to an outpatient clinic. Providers of care at the primary level include family members as well as the staff of health centres, hospital outpatient departments, doctors' surgeries, industrial health units, and school and college health units.

Secondary or *acute care* is concerned with emergency treatment and intensive care involving intense and elaborate measures for the diagnosis and treatment of a specified range of illness or pathology. Entry into the system at this level is either by direct admission to a hospital or by referral. Provider groups for secondary care include both acute and long-stay hospitals and their staff.

Tertiary care includes highly technical services for the treatment of individuals and families with complex or complicated health needs. Providers of tertiary care are health professionals who are specialists in a particular clinical area who work in units such as psychiatric hospitals and clinics, chronic disease centres, or the highly specialized units of general hospitals such as an intensive care unit. Entry into the health care system at this level is gained by referral from either the primary or secondary level.

Restorative care comprises routine follow-up care and rehabilitation in places such as nursing or convalescent homes, halfway houses, facilities for alcohol and drug abusers, and in the homes of patients.

Continuing care is provided on an ongoing basis to support those persons who are physically handicapped, elderly and suffering from a chronic and incapacitating illness, mentally or emotionally handicapped, or otherwise unable to cope unassisted with daily living. Such care is provided in places such as long-stay hospitals, nursing homes, and geriatric or psychiatric day care centres.

Health Education Authority the former Health Education Council (now reconstituted as an NHS special health authority), responsible for giving authoritative advice both nationally and locally on a wide range of health education issues through campaigns and publications. Abbreviated HEA.

As an integral part of the health service, the Authority is able to participate with other health authorities in planning health service policies and priorities.

health visitor a registered nurse who is also either a midwife or has undertaken a 12-week obstetric course and who has completed a 52-week course leading to a health visiting certificate. The main area of responsibility of health visitors is health education and preventive care of mothers and children under five, although some specialize in school health and preventive care of the elderly.

Health Visitors' Association a certificated independent trade union representing health visitors; abbreviated HVA; affiliated to the TUC since 1924. Their address is 36 Eccleston Square, London SW1V 1PF.

healthy ('helthee) pertaining to, characterized by, or promoting health.

hearing ('hiə·ring) the sense by which sounds are perceived, by conversion of sound waves into nerves impulses, which are then interpreted by the brain. Also, the capacity to perceive sound. The organ of hearing is the EAR, which is divided into three sections, the outer, middle, and inner ear. Each plays a special role in hearing. Connecting the middle ear with the nasopharynx is the pharyngotympanic tube, through which air enters to equalize the pressure on both sides of the TYMPANIC MEMBRANE (eardrum).

THE MECHANICS OF HEARING. When sound waves strike the tympanic membrane, they start it vibrating. Most of the sound waves simply bounce off; what remains may be a very tiny vibration of the drum. To be useful, the ear must be able to record very light sound, and yet survive a violent sound such as a thunderclap.

The problem of protecting the tympanic membrane is handled by two tiny muscles that damp the vibrations in the eardrum and ossicles. The main function, that of hearing, is achieved by the ear's transmitting chain of membrane-ossicles-cochlea, a mechanical transformer that converts the large-amplitude sound waves striking the drum into smaller, more concentrated vibrations.

The ossicles act as a series of levers, each one amplifying the minute movement of the eardrum as it passes it along. By the time the stirrup taps the window of the cochlea, it has 22 times the pressure of the original vibration. The thin oval window membrane vibrates in turn, setting the fluid in the cochlea in motion along its spiral course. The constricted channel of the cochlea multiplies the pressure still further, until the original vibrations reach the nerve ends in the form of powerful sideways motions rubbing against the sensitive hairlike cells of the organ of Corti. The vibrations are transformed into impulses that pass along the vestibulocochlear nerve to the brain, and the waves of pressure in the cochlea are released by way of another membrane-covered window, the round window, at the other end of the cochlea.

It is still not certain how the organ of Corti transforms the vibrations into nerve impulses. There are two major theories. One, the Helmholtz theory, points out that the organ of Corti is shaped much like a piano or harp, with long strands at one end and short ones at the other. Perhaps these strands vibrate sympathetically, each strand for a different note, just as the strings of a harp or piano will vibrate when another instrument is played nearby. The second theory, the telephone theory, holds that the frequency of notes is transmitted to the brain by nerve impulses of the same frequency. This is the principle on which the telephone is based.

There are technical objections to both theories. It is possible that the organ of Corti operates on both principles—for example, like the telephone for low notes and according to the Helmholtz theory for high notes, with the two systems overlapping in the middle range, where the ear is more sensitive.

Whatever system the ear uses, it is a remarkably versatile organ. The human ear can distinguish more than 1500 separate musical tones, can recognize thousands of different sounds and can hear clearly from the softest whisper to the roar of a factory or a battleship's guns. See also DEAFNESS for discussion of hearing loss.

PATIENT CARE FOR THE HEARING IMPAIRED. Communication with the person who has some degree of hearing loss can be helped by some simple but effective techniques. A patient in hospital or at home usually has a need for guidance and always needs support, encouragement, and a sense of being in control of what is happening to him or her. In order to meet these needs one must make an effort to communicate with the person who has impaired hearing.

In the assessment of the patient's disorder, it is important to determine the degree and kind of hearing loss the patient has. Is it limited to one ear, or more severe in one ear than the other (as is often the case in elderly persons)? Does the patient wear a hearing aid? Should he be encouraged to wear one? What can family members and others do to help communication? What does the patient want you to do to help him understand what is being said?

General guidelines that are helpful in improving communication with any patient with impaired hearing include the following:

(1) Speak slowly and distinctly, using short words and phrases.

(2) Lower your voice in volume (do not shout) and in pitch or tone. High-pitched sounds are more difficult to hear than those in the lower register.

(3) Keep down background noises as much as possible when delivering an important message.

(4) Give directions, which should be brief, one at a time, and wait for a response to each message before speaking again.

(5) Use gestures, facial expressions, and objects to clarify and emphasize the message.

(6) Do not ignore misunderstood messages; correct misinterpretations immediately.

(7) Use printed communication aids when appropriate;

for example, written instructions and precautions, signs, posters, labels, and charts.

h. aid an instrument to amplify sounds for the hard of hearing. There are two types of electronic hearing aids: the air-conduction type, which is worn in the external acoustic meatus, and the bone-conduction type, which is worn behind the ear over the mastoid process. Those who have conductive DEAFNESS can often use any one of the better aids with good results. Patients with OTOSCLEROSIS will probably need the bone-conduction type of instrument. Those with sensorineural deafness, caused by injury to the vestibulocochlear nerve, or mixed deafness may have more trouble selecting a suitable hearing aid, and may get less satisfactory results.

Those wearing a hearing aid for the first time should have special training in its proper use. A hearing aid picks up and amplifies all the sounds in the vicinity. Often a person whose hearing has declined gradually will have lost the facility to ignore background noises. When he first tries a hearing aid, his ears will be assaulted by the sounds of passing cars, of doors slamming, of telephones ringing. Training in how to filter out these noises and concentrate on the essential is necessary if the person is to get good results from his hearing aid. For best results, this should be combined with lessons in lip-reading.

hearing loss ('hiə·ring los) partial or complete loss of hearing; see also DEAFNESS.

Alexander's h. l. congenital deafness due to cochlear aplasia involving chiefly the organ of Corti and adjacent ganglion cells of the basal coil of the cochlea; high-frequency hearing loss results.

conductive h. l. that due to a defect of the sound-conducting apparatus, i.e., of the external auditory canal or middle ear.

pagetoid h. l. that occurring in osteitis deformans of the bones of the skull.

paradoxical h. l. that in which the hearing is better during loud noise.

sensorineural h. l. that due to a defect in the inner ear or the acoustic nerve.

transmission h. l. conductive h. l.

heart (haht) the hollow muscular organ lying slightly to the left of the midline of the chest. The heart serves as a pump controlling the blood flow in two circuits, the pulmonary and the systemic (see also CIRCULATORY SYSTEM).

DIVISIONS OF THE HEART. The septum, a thick muscular wall, divides the heart into right and left halves. Each half is again divided into upper and lower quarters or chambers. The lower chambers are called ventricles; the upper chambers are called atria. The right side of the heart, consisting of the right atrium and right ventricle, sends blood into the pulmonary circuit. The left side, consisting of the left atrium and left ventricle, sends blood into the systemic circuit.

VALVES OF THE HEART. Between the right atrium and right ventricle is the tricuspid valve. Similarly, the left atrium and left ventricle are connected by the mitral, or bicuspid, valve. In addition to the valves between the atrium and ventricle on each side of the heart, there are valves at the blood's exit points: the pulmonary valve opening from the right ventricle into the pulmonary artery, and the aortic valve opening from the left ventricle into the aorta. These valves, both within the heart and leading out of it, open and shut in such a way as to keep the blood flowing in one direction through the heart's two separate pairs of chambers: from atrium to ventricle and out through its appropriate artery.

LAYERS OF THE HEART. The heart wall is composed of three layers of tissues. Its chambers are lined by a delicate membrane, the endocardium. The thick muscular wall essential to normal pumping action of the heart is called the myocardium. The thin but sturdy membranous sac surrounding the exterior of the heart is called the pericardium.

THE HEART'S PACEMAKER. The heart is made up of special muscle tissue, capable of continuous rhythmic contraction without tiring. The impulse that starts the heartbeat has its origin in an area of the right atrium called the sinoatrial node; it is this special tissue that acts as a pacemaker for the heart. It transmits the impulse in a fraction of a second through the atria to another group of similarly sensitive fibres called the atrioventricular node, which conducts the stimulus via the atrioventricular bundle (bundle of His) and the bundle branches into the ventricular walls, resulting in contraction of the ventricles. See also PACEMAKER.

PUMPING ACTION. Although the right and left sides of the heart serve two separate branches of the circulation, each with its distinct function, they are coordinated so that the heart efficiently serves both sides with a single pumping action. The valve action on both sides is also coordinated with the two phases of the pumping action. Thus during diastole, the relaxation phase, oxygen-poor blood returning from the systemic circulation and accumulated in the right atrium pours into the right ventricle. At the same time, the oxygen-rich blood that has accumulated in the left atrium returning from the pulmonary circulation pours into the left ventricle. The walls of both atria contract to press blood into the relaxed ventricles. In the next contraction phase (systole) the valve between the atrium and ventricle on each side closes, and the muscular walls contract the ventricles and force the blood through the pulmonary artery and the aorta. At the end of the contraction the pulmonary and aortic valves snap shut, preventing any backward surge of the blood into the ventricles. The diastole follows, the ventricles again filling with the flow from their separate atria, and the cycle is repeated.

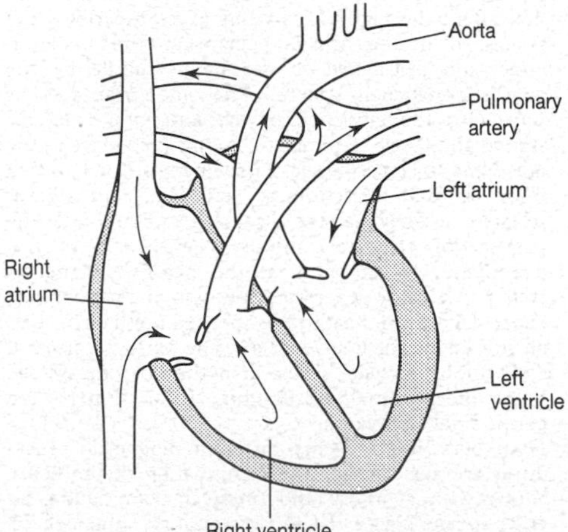

Passage of blood through heart. Blood enters the right atrium from the body and then passes into the right ventricle, where it is pumped into the lungs. It returns from the lungs into the left atrium. It enters the left ventricle and then is pumped to the body via the aorta.

DISORDERS OF THE HEART. The heart is subject to a variety of disorders. Among them are CONGENITAL HEART DEFECTS, which begin or exist at the time of birth. Disorders of this nature may interfere with the flow of the blood from the heart to the lungs. TETRALOGY OF FALLOT and PATENT DUCTUS ARTERIOSUS are examples of congenital heart defects.

In syphilitic heart disease, there is damage to the aorta or the aortic valve, interfering with the proper functioning of the valve, so that the blood may flow backward into the heart as well as forward from the ventricle.

Another heart ailment is rheumatic heart disease, associated with RHEUMATIC FEVER. The disease can injure the endocardium, the valves, or the muscle fibres. The valves may lose their original efficiency, so that passage of the blood is hindered.

Coronary insufficiency is a condition in which the coronary arteries are unable to transport an adequate supply of oxygenated blood to nourish the heart muscle itself. One form of coronary insufficiency, manifested as ANGINA PECTORIS, may be precipitated by hampered circulation of the blood caused by athero-sclerotic narrowing of the coronary artery, combined with a stepped-up demand for oxygen during exercise or some other form of exertion.

A 'heart attack' is the common description for the condition in which the formation of a blood clot within a coronary artery may shut off, or occlude, the blood flow to a section of the heart muscle. This is called a coronary occlusion or thrombosis, and can damage or cause permanent injury to the affected area of myocardium (MYOCARDIAL INFARCTION).

HEART FAILURE is the inability of the heart to perform its function of pumping sufficient blood to assure a normal flow through the circulation. The heart is unable to pump out the blood returned to it from the veins. In the condition known as congestive heart failure, one or more chambers of the heart do not empty adequately during contraction of the heart muscle. This results in shortness of breath, oedema, and abnormal retention of sodium and water in body tissues.

Cardiac arrhythmias are disturbances in the normal rate and rhythm of the heartbeat. Electrical impulses that affect the rate and rhythm of the heartbeat are generated in the heart's pacemaker—the sinoatrial node—and distributed to the heart muscle by the heart's conduction system. The sino-atrial node is subject to the influence of the autonomic nervous system and it also responds to chemical changes in the blood and to certain drugs. Tissue necrosis such as that in myocardial infarction or resulting from athero-sclerotic coronary artery disease also can block the passage of electrical impulses. When there is a disturbance in any part of the heart's conduction system or electric generating function, the patient may experience a heartbeat that is speeded up (tachycardia) or slowed down (bradycardia). The various forms of arrhythmia include sinus arrhythmia, extrasystole, heart block, atrial fibrillation, atrial flutter, and paroxysmal tachycardia.

DIAGNOSTIC TESTS. Many different diagnostic procedures are available for the examination of the heart. Along with a history and physical examination, an ELECTROCARDIOGRAM (ECG) is routinely obtained. It shows a tracing of the electrical excitation that spreads over the heart during each beat. It is the definitive source of information about cardiac arrhythmias, and also gives diagnostic information about most myocardial infarctions.

Exercise stress testing is a valuable tool for detecting persons who are at risk of developing coronary heart disease. The test subject performs maximal exercise while being monitored by ECG. A positive stress test occurs when the subject cannot sustain the exercise for the duration of the test, cannot attain a normal maximal heart rate, or shows ECG changes indicative of ischaemia. When stress testing is used for screening purposes, it is not diagnostic. However, persons with a positive stress test are 13 times more likely to develop coronary disease and should work to reduce their risk factors. Stress testing is also used to evaluate the severity of known coronary disease and to guide the rehabilitation of a patient after a myocardial infarction.

Phonocardiography is the recording of heart sounds and murmurs. It is more precise than auscultation with a stethoscope because it provides a permanent visual record that can be used to obtain precise timing information and can be used as baseline data for comparison with later findings.

Echocardiography is a type of diagnostic ULTRASONOGRAPHY. The first method to be developed was M-mode echocardiography (M stands for motion), in which a narrow stationary ultrasound beam is aimed through the heart. It reflects back from each fluid–tissue interface, and the time the echo takes to return indicates the distance of the interface from the transducer. The M-mode scan shows the motion of heart valves and chamber walls over a period of time. The M-mode scan thus provides a two-dimensional view (since time is plotted against distance). A newer development is real-time cross-sectional echocardiography, in which a computerized scanner is used to make a sequence of cross-sectional scans of the cardiac anatomy. These are viewed like a film and show the motion of the valves and walls in a two-dimensional cross-section through the heart. Echocardiography is a noninvasive technique that is safe and comfortable for the patient. It is capable of establishing a diagnosis in several types of heart disease, especially those involving the heart valves, which formerly required the use of invasive techniques.

Several types of *radioisotope examination* are used to detect heart disease. A radiopharmaceutical is injected into the patient, and a gamma camera is then used to make an image of the distribution of radioactivity.

Thallium-201, like potassium, has an affinity for heart tissue; when injected intravenously, it is carried to areas with adequate perfusion. Myocardial infarcts and areas of acute ischaemia or scarring appear as 'cold spots' on the scintigram. When the isotope is injected during maximal exercise in an exercise stress test, the scan shows areas of inadequate perfusion and is a better indicator of coronary disease than a stress test alone.

Radiopharmaceuticals that label the blood pool can be used with a computerized scintillation camera to evaluate ventricular performance. Images of the first pass of the radioisotope through the heart or gated images can be used to determine the cardiac output and ejection fraction, the size of the ventricles, and regional wall motion.

The imaging agents used for bone scans, such as technetium-99m pyrophosphate or diphosphonate, also have an affinity for areas of acute ischaemic tissue damage. 'Hot spots' on the scintigram show areas of acute infarction. Usually, the scan is negative by approximately 6 days after the infarction.

Cardiac catheterization is an invasive technique that is used primarily when a cardiac operation is being considered and definitive data are required to decide whether the operation is necessary and to plan the surgical approach. A catheter is inserted into a vein or artery, usually the right basilic vein, the brachial artery, or the femoral vein or artery, and guided into the heart. Tracings of the pressure pulses within the chambers during the heart cycle are obtained. Cardiac output, pulmonary vascular resistance, the orifice area of stenotic valves, and the degree of left-to-right shunting can be determined.

Angiocardiography is the radiological examination of the heart after injection of a radiopaque contrast medium through a catheter at various locations in the heart. The films show the size and motion of the heart chambers and can demonstrate valve stenoses or regurgitation. In *coronary arteriography* the contrast medium is injected through a catheter into the orifice of each coronary artery. The films show atherosclerotic obstructions of the arteries and are useful in planning coronary bypass surgery.

PREVENTION OF HEART DISEASE. In spite of the fact that heart disease is still the leading cause of death in the industrialized countries, the mortality rate for diseases of the heart has steadily declined in some countries (notably the United Sates) since the late 1960s, early 1970s. A major factor in this decline is thought to be the development of more effective preventive measures and modes of treatment for ischaemic heart disease. These advances include open-heart surgery to repair congenital defects and replace malfunctioning valves; vascular and intercardiac surgery to repair or bypass obstructions in the coronary arteries and aorta; newer and more accurate diagnostic tests and procedures for detecting problems involving the heart and blood vessels; chemotherapy for the treatment of rheumatic fever, syphilis, and other infectious diseases that are damaging to the heart; more sophisticated monitoring equipment and intensive care units; and aggressive medical treatment and management of heart disease and hypertension.

While these contributions to the control and correction of cardiovascular diseases are of great importance in the reduction of mortality rates and improvement in the quality of life for persons suffering from heart disease, it is important for the prevention of cardiovascular disease that there be an improvement of the general public's awareness of the causes and risk factors of cardiac disorders. Among the major risk factors that can be avoided, controlled. or corrected are elevated blood lipids, obesity, habitual dietary excesses, lack of exercise, hypertension, cigarette smoking, and personality type.

Efforts on the part of health professionals to reduce the incidence of heart disease and mitigate its effect once it has become manifest are aimed at educating the general public about high risk factors and encouraging active participation in preventive methods, particularly those requiring a change in life style. Another important aspect of prevention of heart disease is detection and control of hypertension. And, finally, skills and techniques for adapting to and coping with stress are believed to be effective in reducing the risk for serious heart disease, even though it is difficult to obtain an objective measurement of the effectiveness of these preventive measures.

MODES OF TREATMENT. Ischaemic heart disease is the most common form of heart disease in most westernized countries and is almost always caused by atherosclerotic narrowing of the blood vessels that supply the myocardium. In order to overcome problems caused by atheromatous lesions cardiac surgeons have developed techniques for bypassing the affected artery or arteries using a section of the patient's saphenous or mammary vein and grafting it onto the aorta or one of the branches of the coronary artery. The bypass around the occluded artery reinstates the blood supply to the myocardium.

A recently developed alternative to the major surgery required for coronary bypass is *percutaneous transluminal coronary angioplasty* (PTCA). This procedure involves dilation of a sclerosed artery by means of a special catheter that is introduced through the skin and into a femoral artery. Under fluoroscopy the catheter is directed to the site of the atheromatous lesion. There a balloon that is a part of the catheter is inflated to compress the plaque occluding the lumen of the artery and thereby enlarging the diameter of the artery. PTCA is an alternative to bypass surgery for patients with single vessel coronary artery stenosis.

Other surgical procedures that have been performed for many years are those for the correction of congenital and acquired defects in the structural components of the heart. These procedures include replacement of the mitral, aortic, and tricuspid valves with prosthetic devices, closure of a septal defect using a Dacron patch over the opening, and surgical correction of abnormal channels for the flow of blood into and out of the heart.

There are many drugs that are used in the management of heart disease. None are curative but they can often mitigate the effects of heart disease and provide symptomatic relief, allowing a heart patient to continue leading an active life. Among the more commonly used drugs are the DIGITALIS preparations, used to treat heart failure; antiarrhythmic drugs, such as procainamide, lignocaine, and quinidine, which block abnormal conduction of impulses in the heart; ANTIHYPERTENSIVE drugs, such as DIURETICS, BETA-BLOCKERS, (e.g., propranolol), alpha-blockers, (e.g., prazosin), centrally acting drugs (e.g., methyldopa), vasodilators, and the angiotensin-converting enzyme inhibitors (e.g., captopril); and drugs for treatment of ANGINA PECTORIS, such as glyceryl trinitrate and other nitrates, vasodilators, beta-blockers, and CALCIUM-CHANNEL BLOCKERS.

heart block impairment of conduction in heart excitation; often applied specifically to atrioventricular heart block.

When isolated impulses from the atria fail to reach the ventricles, heartbeats are missed and the block is called incomplete. When no impulses reach the ventricles from the atria the heart block is complete, with the result that the atria and the ventricles beat at separate rates. In this case the beats remain regular but the rate of the ventricular beats is greatly slowed down.

Heart block can occur with various forms of heart disease, and as a result of excessive dosage of digitalis. A particularly severe instance of heart block can be complicated by the Stokes-Adams disease, in which a sudden attack of unconsciousness results from the slowed heartbeat. It may be accompanied by convulsions.

The treatment for heart block caused by digitalis overdosage is to stop the medication temporarily and give reduced amounts thereafter. When heart block results from a form of heart disease, treatment is given for the underlying cause. An artificial PACEMAKER may be used in the treatment of complete heart block and Stokes-Adams disease.

atrioventricular (A-V) h. b. a form in which the blocking is at the atrioventricular junction. It is *first degree* when A-V conduction time is prolonged; *second degree* (partial heart block) when some but not all atrial impulses reach the ventricle; *third degree* (complete heart block) when no atrial impulses at all reach the ventricle and the atria and ventricles act independently of each other.

bundle-branch h. b. a form in which one ventricle is excited before the other because of absence of conduction in one of the branches of the bundle of His (the atrioventricular bundle).

complete h. b. see atrioventricular heart block (above).

interventricular h. b. bundle-branch heart block.

Mobitz type I h. b. second degree A-V heart block in which the P-R interval increases progressively until an atrial impulse is blocked. Called also *Wenckebach type A-V heart block.*

Mobitz type II h. b. second degree A-V heart block in which the P-R interval is fixed, with periodic blocking of an atrial impulse.

sinoatrial h. b. partial or complete impairment of conduction from the sinoatrial node to the atria, resulting in delay or absence of an atrial beat.

heart failure inability of the heart to maintain a circulation sufficient to meet the body's needs; most often applied to myocardial failure affecting the right or left ventricle.

backward h. f. a concept of heart failure emphasizing the contribution of passive engorgement of the systemic venous system as a cause.

congestive h.f. (CHF) that which occurs as a result of impaired pumping capability of the heart and is associated with abnormal retention of water and sodium. The condition ranges from mild congestion with few symptoms to life-threatening fluid overload and total heart failure.

CHF results in an inadequate supply of blood and oxygen to the body's cells. The decreased cardiac output causes an increase in the blood volume within the vascular system. Congestion within the blood vessels interferes with the movement of body fluids in and out of the various fluid compartments, and they accumulate in the tissue spaces, causing oedema.

There are three general kinds of pathological conditions that can bring about CHF: (1) *ventricular failure*, in which the contractions of the ventricles become weak and ineffective, as in myocardial ischaemia from coronary artery disease; (2) *mechanical failure* of the ventricles to fill with blood during the diastole phase of the cardiac cycle, which can occur when the mitral valve is narrowed, as in rheumatic mitral stenosis, or when there is an accumulation of fluid within the pericardial sac (cardiac tamponade) pressing against the ventricles, preventing them from accepting a full load of blood; and (3) an *overload* of blood in the ventricles during the systole phase of the cycle. High blood pressure, aortic stenosis, and aortic valvular regurgitation are some of the conditions that can cause ventricular overload.

Compensatory Mechanisms. In an attempt to compensate for inadequate pumping of the heart the body utilizes three basic adaptive mechanisms which, though they are effective for a brief period of time, will eventually become insufficient to meet the oxygen needs of the body. These mechanisms are also responsible for many of the symptoms experienced by the patient with CHF.

First, the failing heart attempts to maintain a normal output of blood by enlarging its pumping chambers so that they are capable of holding a greater volume of blood. This increases the amount of blood ejected from the heart, but it also leads to fluid overload within the blood vessels and excessive accumulation of body fluids in all of the fluid compartments.

Second, the heart begins to increase its muscle mass in order to strengthen the force of its contractions. This results in ventricular hypertrophy and a need for more oxygen to supply the additional muscle cells. Eventually, the coronary arteries can no longer meet the oxygen demands of the enlarged myocardium and the patient experiences angina pectoris owing to ischaemia.

Third, there is a response from the sympathetic nervous system. The involuntary muscle of the heart is regulated by autonomic, or involuntary, innervation. In response to failing contractility of the myocardial cells, the sympathetic nervous system activates adaptive processes that increase the heart rate, redistribute peripheral blood flow, and retain urine. These mechanisms are responsible for the symptoms of sweating, cool skin, tachycardia, cardiac arrhythmias, and oliguria.

The combined efforts of these three compensatory mechanisms achieve a fairly normal level of cardiac output for a period of time. During this phase of CHF the patient is said to have *compensated* CHF. When these mechanisms are no longer effective the disease progresses to the final stage of impaired heart function and the patient has *decompensated* CHF.

Clinical Symptoms. Left-sided heart failure produces dyspnoea of varying intensity. In the early stages, shortness of breath occurs only when the patient is physically active. Later, as the heart action becomes more seriously impaired, the dyspnoea is present even when the patient is resting. In advanced cases, the patient must sit up in order to breathe (orthopnoea). Attacks of breathlessness severe enough to wake the patient frequently occur during sleep. These attacks usually are accompanied by coughing and wheezing (cardiac asthma), and the patient seeks relief by sitting upright. Orthopnoea and cardiac asthma or paroxysmal nocturnal dyspnoea are related to congestion of the pulmonary blood vessels and oedema of the lung tissues. They are aggravated by lying down because in the prone position quantities of blood in the lower extremities move upward into the blood vessels of the lungs.

Fluid retention is another common symptom of CHF. In left-sided failure there is higher than normal pressure of blood in the pulmonary vessels. This increased pressure forces fluid out of the intravascular compartment and into the tissue spaces of the lungs causing pulmonary oedema. Right-sided failure causes congestion in the capillaries of the peripheral circulation and results in oedema and congestion of the liver, legs, and feet, and in the sacral region in bedridden patients.

Decreased cardiac output also affects the kidneys by reducing their blood supply, which in turn causes a decrease in the rate of glomerular filtration of plasma from the renal blood vessels into the renal tubules. Sodium and water not excreted in the urine are retained in the vascular system, adding to the blood volume. The diminished blood supply to the kidney also causes it to secrete renin, which indirectly stimulates the secretion of aldosterone from the adrenal gland. Aldosterone in turn acts on the renal tubules, causing them to increase reabsorption of sodium and water, and thus to further increase the volume of body fluids.

Treatment. Medical management of congestive heart failure is aimed at improving contractibility of the heart, reducing salt and water retention, and providing rest for the heart muscle. Drugs used to accomplish these goals include digitalis glycosides to slow and strengthen the heart beat, *vasodilators* to reduce resistance to the flow of blood being pumped from the heart, and diuretics to assist in the elimination of water and sodium in the urine.

Devices to boost the pumping action of the atria by means of electrical stimulation through pacemaker catheters can provide temporary relief for certain patients. Electroconversion of atrial fibrillation enlists the help of the atria to fill the ventricles to maximum capacity.

PATIENT CARE. Hospitalized patients with severe CHF present problems related to their needs for physical and mental rest, adequate aeration of the lungs and oxygenation of the tissues, prevention of circulatory stasis, maintenance of the integrity of the skin, restoration and maintenance of fluid and electrolyte balances, and adequate nutrition.

The care plan should include frequent monitoring of the vital signs, intake and output, daily weight, serum ELECTROLYTE and BLOOD GAS levels, and nutritional intake. Patients with CHF are placed on sodium-restricted diets and sometimes also on limited fluid intake. Before the patient leaves the hospital he should have a good understanding of the rationale for limiting his intake of sodium and the importance of avoiding an excess of body fluids. In addition, he should have a plan for regular exercise within the limits set by the doctor. Since it is likely that the patient will need to continue taking several kinds of medications once he returns home, he or a member of his family should be taught about the pharmacological action of each drug, the need for taking it exactly as prescribed, any precautions to be taken, and any untoward reactions that warrant notification of the doctor.

forward h. f. a concept of heart failure emphasizing the inadequacy of cardiac output as the primary cause and considering venous distention to be secondary.

high output h. f. that in which cardiac output remains high, associated with hyperthyroidism, anaemia, emphysema, etc.

left-sided h. f., left ventricular h. f. failure of the left ventricle to maintain a normal output of blood. Since the left ventricle does not empty completely, it cannot accept blood returning from the lungs via the pulmonary veins. The pulmonary veins become engorged and fluid seeps out through the veins and collects in the pleural cavity. Pulmonary oedema and pleural effusion result. In many cases heart failure begins on the left side and eventually involves both sides of the heart.

low-output h. f. that in which cardiac output is diminished, associated with cardiovascular diseases.

right-sided h. f., right ventricular h. f. failure of proper functioning of the right ventricle, with subsequent engorgement of the systemic veins, producing pitting oedema, enlargement of the liver, and ascites.

heart–lung machine (haht'lung) a mechanical device that temporarily takes over the functions of the heart and lungs; called also a *pump-oxygenator*. It is used as an aid to surgery of the heart.

A pump draws blood from the patient's great veins from where it is routed through a chamber made of plastic, where the red cells are exposed to oxygen. The oxygenated blood is then returned to the patient's vessels. This method of circulating the blood outside the patient's body is known as extracorporeal circulation.

heart murmur any sound in the heart region other than normal heart sounds (see also MURMUR). A murmur may be caused by several different factors, including changes in the valves of the heart or blood leaking through a disease-scarred valve that does not close properly.

RHEUMATIC FEVER is a common cause of heart murmur. A murmur may also indicate other types of heart disease. In many cases, however, the murmur may be of the innocent or 'functional' type, which does not indicate any heart damage at all and causes no trouble. Such murmurs vary from time to time, and often go away completely.

heart rate the number of contractions of the cardiac ventricles per unit of time.

heart sounds the sounds heard on the surface of the chest in the heart region. They are amplified by and heard more distinctly through a stethoscope. These sounds are caused by the vibrations of the normal cardiac cycle. They may be produced by muscular action, valvular actions, motion of the heart, and blood as it passes through the heart.

The first heart sound is heard as a firm but not sharp 'lubb' sound. It consists of four components: a low-frequency, indistinct vibration caused by ventricular contraction; a louder sound of higher frequency caused by closure of the mitral and tricuspid valves; a vibration caused by opening of the semilunar valves and early ejection of blood from the ventricles; and a low-pitched vibration produced by rapid ejection.

The second heart sound is shorter and higher pitched than the first, is heard as a 'dupp' and is produced by closure of the aortic and pulmonary valves. The sound splits into 2 components (A_2 and P_2) on inspiration in normal circumstances.

The third heart sound is very faint and is caused by blood rushing into the ventricles. It can be heard in most normal persons between the ages of 10 and 20 years, but is pathological in the middle-aged and elderly.

The fourth heart sound is rarely audible in a normal heart but can be demonstrated on graphic records. It is short and of low frequency and intensity, and is caused by atrial contraction. The vibrations arise from atrial muscle and from blood flow into, and distention of, the ventricles.

ABNORMALITIES IN HEART SOUNDS. Failure of the heart muscle to contract is characterized by a gallop or triple rhythm. Accentuation of the third heart sound (protodiastolic gallop) is caused by the filling of a large flabby ventricle with blood under high venous pressure. A presystolic gallop is an accentuated fourth heart sound and is also caused by blood filling a dilated and inert ventricle. Merging of the third and fourth heart sounds is called a mesodiastolic or summation gallop. A very rare abnormality in which four heart sounds are heard distinctly is called a 'locomotive' rhythm.

HEART MURMURS are sounds other than the normal heart sounds emanating from the heart region. They are often heard as blowing or hissing sounds as blood leaks through diseased and malfunctioning valves.

heartbeat ('haht,beet) the cycle of contraction of the heart muscle, during which the chambers of the heart contract. The beat begins with a rhythmic impulse in the sinoatrial node, which serves as a pacemaker for the heart (see also HEART).

heartburn ('haht,bərn) pyrosis; a burning sensation in the oesophagus, or below the sternum in the region of the heart. It is one of the common symptoms of indigestion.

Heartburn often occurs when there is distention of a part of the oesophagus, particularly the lower part. This may happen when the stomach regurgitates part of its contents, forcing them upward into the oesophagus. Since this matter is acid, it acts as an irritant, producing discomfort or pain.

Recent evidence indicates that hyperacidity in itself may not be the actual cause, and that heartburn results from excessive gastric secretions only when there is improper eating or emotional disturbance.

There is no doubt that emotional disturbance, excitement, and nervous tension are frequent causes of heartburn. The functions of the stomach, both those of motion and secretion, are controlled by the VAGUS NERVE, one of the cranial nerves. Emotional stress can stimulate this nerve, which in turn starts the churning of the stomach and the flow of the various gastric juices; it can also cause contraction and spasm of the pylorus. If some of the stomach contents are displaced into the oesophagus during this nervous activity, heartburn may result.

HEAT human erythrocyte agglutination test.

heat (heet) energy that raises the temperature of a body or substance; also, the rise of the temperature itself. Heat is associated with molecular motion, and is generated in various ways, including combustion, friction, chemical action, and radiation. The total absence of heat is absolute zero, at which all molecular activity ceases.

BODY HEAT

Heat Production. Body heat is the by-product of the metabolic processes of the body. The hormones thyroxine and adrenaline increase metabolism and consequently increase body heat. Muscular activity also produces body heat. At complete rest (basal metabolism) the amount of heat produced from muscular activity may be as low as 25 per cent of the total body heat. During exercise or shivering the percentage may rise to 60 per cent.

Body temperature is regulated by the thermostatic centre in the HYPOTHALAMUS. A body temperature above the normal range is called FEVER.

Heat Loss. Loss of body heat occurs in three main ways: by radiation (heat waves), by conduction to air or objects in contact with the body, and by evaporation of perspiration. Some body heat is also lost in expiration of air and in elimination of urine and faeces.

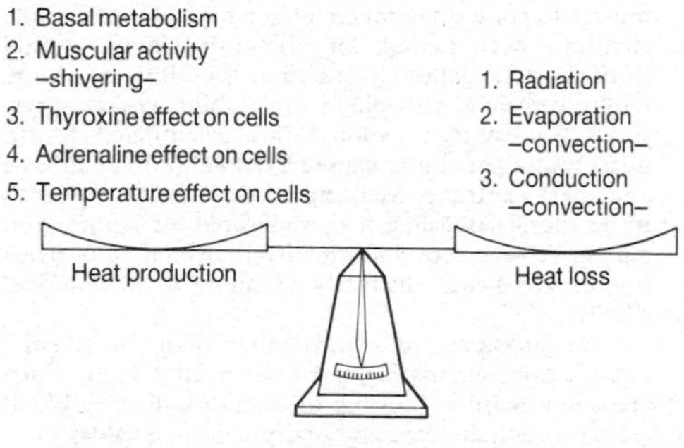

Balance between heat production and heat loss, illustrating that the body temperature remains constant as long as these two are equal

APPLICATIONS OF EXTERNAL HEAT

Purposes. Local applications of heat may be used to provide warmth and promote comfort, rest, and relaxation. Heat is also applied locally to promote suppuration and drainage from an infected area by hastening the inflammatory process; to relieve congestion and swelling by dilating the blood vessels, thereby increasing circulation; and to improve repair of diseased or injured tissues by increasing local metabolism.

Effects. Factors that determine the physiological action of heat include the type of heat used, length of time it is applied, age and general condition of the patient, and area of body surface to which the heat is applied. Moist heat is more penetrating than dry heat. Prolonged applications of heat produce an increase in skin secretions, resulting in a softening of the skin and a lowering of its resistance. Extreme heat produces constriction of the blood vessels; moderate heat produces vascular dilation. Repeated applications of heat will result in an increased tolerance to heat so that the individual may be burned without his being aware of it. Elderly persons and infants are more susceptible to burns from high temperatures.

Heat applied to an infected area can localize the infection; for this reason, external heat should not be applied to the abdomen when appendicitis is suspected, because it may lead to rupture of the inflamed appendix.

Methods. In general, applications of heat are dry or wet. Dry heat may be applied to the superficial tissues in the form of hot water bottles, electric heating pads, or an electric incandescent bulb with a heat cradle. Three modes of heat application to deeper tissues are shortwave, ultrasound, and microwave DIATHERMY.

Hot water bottles should be filled with water not exceeding 52 °C (125 °F), and should be about half full; the air is expelled before the bottle is sealed. The hot water bottle is covered with a flannel or cotton covering before it is applied and this covering should remain dry at all times, unless the hot water bottle is used over moist dressings to keep them warm. The hot water bottle should be refilled at least every 2 hours.

Electric heating pads are never used over wet dressings or in other areas where moisture may come in contact with the electricity. Those used in hospitals should have an automatic control and the thermostat should be turned to low or medium.

Heat lamps may generate heat through ultraviolet or infrared radiation. Ultraviolet rays are more penetrating than infrared rays. Moderate radiation from ultraviolet rays produces local vasodilation and stimulates growth of tissue cells. It must be used with caution because of the danger of producing deep burns.

Infrared rays provide surface heat but penetrate to a depth of only 10 mm. Prolonged and intense application can lead to burning and blistering of the skin. Before being exposed to infrared rays, the skin should be cleansed and all ointments or other medicinal preparations removed.

The heat cradle employs an ordinary bed cradle to support the top bed covers and an electric light bulb to generate heat. This type of apparatus is often used for patients with circulatory disturbances of the extremities.

Moist or wet heat can be applied in a variety of ways, including baths, hot packs, and compresses (see also HYDROTHERAPY).

Uses. Local applications of heat are used for a variety of disorders. Moderate heat is used to relax the muscles and reduce spasm that often accompanies muscle strain (see also DIATHERMY).

Heat, applied by boiling, autoclaving, flaming, or burning, is a commonly used physical antiseptic.

h. exhaustion a disorder resulting from overexposure to heat or to the sun; called also *heat prostration*. Long exposure to extreme heat or too much activity under a hot sun causes excessive sweating, which removes large quantities of salt and fluid from the body. When the amount of salt and fluid in the body falls too far below normal, heat exhaustion may result.

SYMPTOMS. The early symptoms of heat exhaustion are headache and a feeling of weakness and dizziness, usually accompanied by nausea and vomiting. There may also be cramps in the muscles of the arms, legs, or abdomen. These first symptoms are similar to the early signs of SUNSTROKE, or heat stroke, but the disorders are not the same and should be treated differently. In heat exhaustion, the person turns pale and perspires profusely. The skin is cool and moist, and the pulse and breathing are rapid. Body temperature remains at a normal level or slightly below, whereas in sunstroke the body temperature may be dangerously elevated. The person may seem confused and may find it difficult to coordinate his body movements. Usually he remains conscious.

TREATMENT. In cases of heat exhaustion, a doctor should be called, the patient should lie quietly in a cool place and should be given half a teaspoonful of salt dissolved in tomato juice or in half a glass of water every 15 minutes for 2 hours if tolerated. Tea or coffee may then be given.

If the condition is accompanied by cramps, the pain may be relieved by gentle massage of the painful area or by firm hand pressure. In cases of severe heat exhaustion and cramps, it may be necessary to keep the patient at rest in bed for a day or more.

PREVENTION. Heat exhaustion and other heat disorders may be prevented by avoiding long exposure to sun or heat. When the weather is very hot, or when working in an extremely hot place, it is essential to drink plenty of water and maintain an adequate intake of salt. Regular breaks from work are necessary, and in the event of weakness or dizziness, the victim should stop working at once and rest in a cool place. **latent h.** the heat that a body may absorb without changing its temperature. **prickly h., h. rash** MILIARIA; inflammation of the skin, due to retention of sweat, occurring during hot, humid weather.

specific h. the number of calories required to raise the temperature of 1 g of a particular substance 1 °C.

h. stroke a severe life-threatening condition resulting from prolonged exposure to heat. See SUNSTROKE.

heavy-chain disease ('hevee,chayn) a monoclonal gammopathy in which there is elaboration of immunoglobulin of IgG class from one gene product of the four which code for an IgG molecule. The resultant globulin fragment (molecular weight, 53,000), resembling the Fc fragment, is found in both serum and urine. Symptoms include recurring bacterial infections, anaemia, enlargement of lymphoid organs, and oedema of the palate. Histologically there is lymphoma, ranging from Hodgkin's disease to reticulum cell sarcoma. Heavy-chain disease involving the IgA and IgM systems has also been reported.

Heberden's nodes ('hebə,dənz) small, hard nodules, formed usually at the distal interphalangeal joints of the fingers in osteoarthritis.

hebetic (hi'betik) pertaining to puberty.

hebetude ('hebityood) mental dullness; apathy.

HEC Health Education Council, now replaced by the HEALTH EDUCATION AUTHORITY.

hecatomeric (hekətə'merik) having processes that divide in two, one going to each side of the spinal cord; said of certain neurons.

hectic ('hektik) occurring regularly.

h. fever a regularly occurring increase in temperature; it is frequently observed in pulmonary tuberculosis.

h. flush a redness of the face accompanying a sudden rise in temperature.

hecto- word element. [Fr.] *hundred;* used in naming units of measurement to designate an amount 100 times (10^2) the size of the unit to which it is joined, e.g., hectolitre (100 litres); symbol h.

hedonism ('heedə,nizəm, 'hed-) excessive devotion to pleasure.

heel (heel) the hindmost part of the foot; called also calx. By extension, a part comparable to the heel of the foot, or the hindmost portion of an elongate structure.

Thomas h. a shoe correction consisting of a heel 12 mm longer and 3 to 4 mm higher on the inside; used to bring the heel of the foot into varus and to prevent depression in the region of the head of the talus.

Heerfordt's disease ('hairforts) uveoparotid fever.

Hegar's dilators ('haygahz) a series of graduated dilators used to dilate the uterine cervix.

Hegar's sign ('haygahz) compressibility and softening of the lower uterine segment, an indication of pregnancy.

Heimlich manoeuvre ('hiemlik) a technique for removing foreign matter from the trachea of a choking victim. The manoeuvre is also recommended as a preliminary step in the emergency treatment of accident victims in need of artificial ventilation. Before administering mouth-to-mouth respiration the manoeuvre is carried out to clear material that may prevent adequate ventilation of the lungs. The technique may be carried out with the victim in a standing position or lying down.

STANDING POSITION. The rescuer stands behind the victim and wraps his arms around the victim's waist, allowing the victim's head, arms, and upper torso to hang forward. A fist is made with one hand and held with the other. The fist is then placed against the victim's abdomen at a point slightly above the umbilicus and below the rib cage. The rescuer's fist is then pressed into the victim's abdomen with a forceful upward thrust. The manoeuvre may be repeated if necessary to clear the air passages.

SUPINE POSITION. The victim is placed on his back with his head turned to one side. The rescuer kneels astride the victim's hips and places both hands on his abdomen, one hand upon the other. The heel of the lower hand is placed slightly above the umbilicus and below the rib cage. Pressure is applied to the victim's abdomen with a forceful upward thrust. The manoeuvre may be repeated if necessary to clear the air passages.

Heine-Medin disease (,hienə'maydin) the major form of POLIOMYELITIS.

Heineke–Mikulicz pyloroplasty ('hienikə-'mikyuhlich) enlargement of a pyloric stricture by incising the pylorus longitudinally and suturing the incision transversely.

HeLa cells ('heelə) cells of the first continuously cultured carcinoma strain, descended from a human cervical carcinoma (originally isolated from an American patient, Henrietta Lacks, in 1951); used in the study of life processes, including viruses, at the cell level.

helcoid ('helkoyd) like an ulcer.

heli(o)- ('heelioh) word element. [Gr.] *sun.*

helical ('helik'l) shaped like a helix.

helicine ('heli,seen) spiral.

helicoid ('heli,koyd) coiled; spiral.

helicopodia (,helikoh'pohdi·ə) helicopod GAIT.

helicotrema (,helikoh'treemə) the passage that connects the scala tympani and the scala vestibuli at the apex of the cochlea.

heliotherapy (,heelioh'therəpee) treatment of disease by exposure of the body to sunlight.

helium ('heeli·əm) a chemical element, atomic number 2, atomic weight 4.003, symbol He. See table of elements in Appendix 2.

Helium is a chemically inert element that is odourless, tasteless, and noncombustible. Because of its low density it is easily moved through the air passages and therefore requires little effort in breathing on the part of the patient who is in respiratory distress. Although helium itself has no chemical therapeutic value, when combined with oxygen it facilitates the delivery of this gas to the lungs (see HELIUM–OXYGEN THERAPY).

helium–oxygen therapy (,heeli·əm'oksijən) the administration of a mixture of helium and oxygen (commonly 80 per cent He and 20 per cent O_2 or 70 per cent He and 30 per cent O_2); used in the management of airway obstruction associated with bronchospasm or bronchial asthma. The $He\text{-}O_2$ mixture is about one-third the density of air. This reduces turbulent flow and the patient effort required for ventilation.

It should be noted that helium causes the voice to be high-pitched and the spoken word difficult to understand. This should be explained to the patient with the assurance that the effect is harmless and temporary.

helix ('heeliks) 1. a coiled structure. 2. the superior and posterior free margin of the pinna of the ear.

α-h., alpha-h. the complex structural arrangement of parts of protein molecules in which a single polypeptide chain forms a right-handed helix.

double h., Watson–Crick h. the structure of DEOXYRIBONUCLEIC ACID (DNA), consisting of two coiled chains, each of which contains information completely specifying the other chain.

Heller's operation ('heləz) an operation for the relief of cardiospasm by longitudial incision through the muscle coat at the lower end of the oesophagus and into the cardia.

Heller's syndrome disorder of infancy preceded by a few years of ostensibly normal development but involving severe disturbance of behaviour, affect, speech, and social skills. There may be overactivity and, in some cases, intellectual impairment. Sometimes precipitated by overt brain disease, e.g. encephalitis.

Heller's test a test for the presence of albumin in urine, using concentrated nitric acid.

Hellin's law ('helinz) one in about 89 pregnancies ends in the birth of twins; one in 89^2, or 7921, in the birth of triplets; one in 89^3, or 704,969, in the birth of quadruplets. This is roughly correct–the incidence of twin pregnancies ranges from 1 in 80 to 1 in 90 in the UK.

helminth ('helminth) a worm, especially a parasitic worm; a nematode, trematode, or cestode.

helminthagogue (hel'minthə,gog) anthelmintic; vermifuge; an agent that expels worms or intestinal animal parasites.

helminthemesis (,helmin'themisis) the vomiting of worms.

helminthiasis (,helmin'thieəsis) an infection with worms.

helminthology (,helmin'tholəjee) the scientific study of parasitic worms.

helminthoma (,helmin'thohmə) a tumour caused by a parasitic worm.

heloma (hi'lohmə) a corn.

h. durum hard corn, the usual type occurring over joints of the toes.

h. molle a soft corn.

helotomy (hi-lotəmee) excision or paring of a corn or callus.

hemeralopia (,hemə·rə'lohpi·ə) day blindness; defective vision in a bright light.

hemi- word element. [Gr.] *half.*

hemiacardius (,hemiə'kahdi·əs) an unequal twin in which the heart is rudimentary, its circulation being assisted by the other twin.

hemiachromatopsia (,hemi·ə,krohmə'topsi·ə) loss of the normal perception of colour in half, or in corresponding halves, of the visual field.

hemiageusia (,hemee·ə'goosi·ə) absence of the sense of taste on one side of the tongue.

hemiamyosthenia (,hemi·ə,mieəs'theeni·ə) lack of muscular power on one side of the body.

hemianacusia (,hemi,anə'kyooosi·ə) loss of hearing in one ear.

hemianaesthesia (,hemi,anəs'theezi·ə) anaesthesia of one side of the body.

crossed h., h. cruciata loss of sensation on one side of the face and loss of pain and temperature sense on the opposite side of the body.

hemianalgesia (,hemi,an'l'jeezi·ə) analgesia on one side of the body.

hemianencephaly (,hemi,anən'kefəlee, -'sef-) congenital absence of one side of the brain.

hemianopia, hemianopsia (,hemi·ə'nohpi·ə; ,hemi·a'nopsi·ə) defective vision or blindness in half of the visual field; usually applied to bilateral defects caused by a single lesion. adj. **hemianopic, hemianoptic.**

hemianosmia (,hemi·ə'nozmi·ə) absence of the sense of smell in one nostril.

hemiapraxia (,hemi·ə'praksi·ə) inability to perform coordinated movements on one side of the body.

hemiataxia (,hemi·ə'taksi·ə) ataxia on one side of the body.

hemiathetosis (,hemi,athi'tohsis) athetosis of one side of the body.

hemiatrophy (,hemi'atrəfee) atrophy of one side of the body or one half of an organ of part.

hemiaxial (,hemi'aksi·əl) at any oblique angle to the long axis of the body or a part.

hemiballism, hemiballismus (,hemi'balizəm; ,hemibə'lizməs) violent motor restlessness of half of the body, most marked in the upper extremity.

hemibladder (,hemi'bladə) a half bladder; a developmental anomaly in which the bladder is formed as two physically separated parts, each with its own ureter.

hemiblock ('hemi,blok) failure in conduction of cardiac impulse in either of the two main divisions of the left branch of the bundle of His (atrioventricular bundle); the interruption may occur in either the anterior (superior) or posterior (inferior) division.

hemicardia (,hemi'kahdi·ə) the presence of only one side of a four-chambered heart.

hemicephalia (,hemike'fayli·ə, -se-) congenital absence of the cerebrum.

hemicephalus (,hemi'kefələs, -'sef-) a fetus exhibiting hemicephalia.

hemichorea (,hemiko'reeə) chorea affecting only one side of the body.

hemichromatopsia (,hemi,krohmə'topsi·ə) defective perception of colour in half of the visual field.

hemicolectomy (,hemikoh'lektəmee) excision of approximately half of the colon.

hemicrania (,hemi'krayni·ə) 1. headache on one side of the head. 2. a developmental anomaly with absence of half of the cranium.

hemicraniosis (,hemi,krayni'ohsis) hyperostosis of one side of the cranium and face.

hemidiaphoresis (,hemi,dieəfə'reesis) sweating on one side of the body only.

hemidysaesthesia (,hemi,disis'theezi·ə) a disorder of sensation affecting only one side of the body.

hemidystrophy (,hemi'distrəfee) unequal development of the two sides of the body.

hemiectromelia (,hemi,ektrə'meeli·ə) a developmental anomaly with imperfect limbs on one side of the body.

hemiepilepsy (,hemi'epi,lepsee) epilepsy affecting one side of the body.

hemifacial (,hemi'fayshəl) affecting one side of the face.

hemigastrectomy (,hemiga'strektəmee) excision of half of the stomach.

hemiglossectomy (,hemiglo'sektəmee) excision of half of the tongue.

hemiglossitis (ˌhemiglo'sietis) inflammation of half of the tongue.
hemignathia (ˌhemi'nathi·ə) a developmental anomaly characterized by partial or complete lack of the lower jaw on one side.
hemihidrosis (ˌhemihi'drohsis) sweating on one side of the body only.
hemihypaesthesia (ˌhemiˌhiepis'theezi·ə) diminished sensitivity on one side of the body.
hemihypalgesia (ˌhemiˌhiepal'jeezi·ə) diminished sensitivity to pain on one side of the body.
hemihyperaesthesia (ˌhemiˌhiepə·ris'theezi·ə) increased sensitivity of one side of the body.
hemihyperhidrosis (ˌhemiˌhiepə·hi'drohsis) excessive sweating on one side of the body.
hemihyperplasia (ˌhemiˌhiepə'playzi·ə) overdevelopment of one side of the body or of half of an organ or part.
hemihypertonia (ˌhemiˌhiepə'tohni·ə) increased muscle tone on one side of the body.
hemihypertrophy (ˌhemihie'pərtrəfee) overgrowth of one side of the body or of a part.
hemihypoplasia (ˌhemiˌhiepoh'playzi·ə) underdevelopment of one side of the body or of half of an organ or part.
hemihypotonia (ˌhemiˌhiepoh'tohni·ə) diminished muscle tone on one side of the body.
hemilaminectomy (ˌhemiˌlami'nektəmee) removal of a vertebral lamina on one side only.
hemilaryngectomy (ˌhemiˌlarin'jektəmee) excision of one lateral half of the larynx.
hemilateral (ˌhemi'latə·rəl) affecting one side of the body only.
hemilesion (ˌhemi'leezhən) a lesion on one side of the spinal cord.
hemimaxillectomy (ˌhemiˌmaksi'lektəmee) the surgical removal of part of the maxilla—usually less than half—performed almost exclusively for malignant tumours involving the palate and/or the antrum.

This usually involves a multidisciplinary surgical approach and many patients have obturators constructed post-operatively to enable speech and eating to take place. If the tumour involves the orbital floor and enucleation of the eye is required then a further prosthesis will be required.
hemimelia (ˌhemi'meeli·ə) congenital absence of all or part of the distal half of a limb.
hemimelus (ˌhemi'meləs) an individual exhibiting hemimelia.
heminephrectomy (ˌheminə'frektəmee) excision of half of a kidney.
Heminevrin (ˌhemi'nevrin) tradename for chlormethiazole, an anticonvulsant and sedative.
hemiopia (ˌhemi'ohpi·ə) hemianopia.
hemipagus (he'mipəgəs) twin fetuses joined laterally at the thorax.
hemiparaesthesia (ˌhemiˌparis'theezi·ə) perverted sensation on one side.
hemiparalysis (ˌhemipə'ralisis) paralysis of one side of the body.
hemiparanaesthesia (ˌhemiˌparənis'theezi·ə) anaesthesia of the lower half of one side.
hemiparaplegia (ˌhemiˌparə'pleeji·ə, -jə) paralysis of the lower half of one side.
hemiparesis (ˌhemipə'reesis) paresis affecting one side of the body.
hemiparetic (ˌhemipə'retik) 1. pertaining to hemiparesis. 2. one affected with hemiparesis.
hemipeptone (ˌhemi'peptohn) a form of peptone obtained from pepsin digestion.
hemiplegia (ˌhemi'pleeji·ə, -jə) paralysis of one side of the body; usually caused by a brain lesion, such as a tumour, or by a stroke. adj. **hemiplegic.** The paralysis occurs on the side opposite the brain disorder. This is explained by the fact that motor axons from the cerebral cortex enter the medulla oblongata and form two well defined bands known at the pyramidal tracts. The majority of the fibres in these tracts cross to the opposite side; therefore damage to the right hemisphere of the brain affects motor control of the left half of the body. See also STROKE for symptoms and care of the patient with hemiplegia.
Hemiptera (he'miptə·rə) an order of arthropods (class Insecta) characterized usually by the presence of two pairs of wings; including some 30,000 species, known as the true bugs, and characterized by having mouth parts adapted to piercing or sucking.
hemirachischisis (ˌhemirə'kiskisis) fissure of the vertebral column without prolapse of the spinal cord.
hemisacralization (ˌhemiˌsaykrəlie'zayshən) fusion of the fifth lumbar vertebra to the first segment of the sacrum on only one side.
hemisection ('hemiˌsekshən) division into two equal parts; bisection.
hemispasm ('hemiˌspazəm) spasm affecting only one side.
hemisphere ('hemiˌsfiə) half of a spherical or roughly spherical structure or organ.

cerebral h. one of the paired structures constituting the largest part of the brain, which together comprise the extensive cerebral cortex, centrum semiovale, basal ganglia, and rhinencephalon, and contain the lateral ventricle. See also BRAIN.

dominant h. that cerebral hemisphere which is more concerned than the other in the integration of sensations and the control of many functions.
hemispherium (ˌhemi'sfiə·ri·əm) pl. *hemispheria* [L.] hemisphere.
hemithorax (ˌhemi'thor·raks) one side of the chest; the cavity lateral to the mediastinum.
hemithyroidectomy (ˌhemiˌthieroy'dektəmee) excision of one lobe of the thyroid.
hemivertebra (ˌhemi'vərtibrə) a developmental anomaly in which one side of a vertebra is incompletely developed.
hemizygosity (ˌhemizie'gositee) the state of having only one of a pair of alleles transmitting a specific character. adj. **hemizygous.**
hemizygote (ˌhemi'ziegoht) an individual exhibiting hemizygosity.
hemp (hemp) see CANNABIS.
henbane ('henbayn) see HYOSCYAMINE.
Henderson ('hendəˌsən) Virginia. A nursing theorist. She gained a basic Diploma in Nursing from the US Army School of Nursing, following this with a degree in Bachelor of Science and Master of Arts from Columbia University.

From 1953, Virginia Henderson has been associated with Yale University, first as a Research Associate, then as Director of Nursing Studies Index Project and, since 1971, as Research Associate Emeritus.

Virginia Henderson is a prolific writer. *Principles and Practice of Nursing* is in its sixth edition, but perhaps her best known work is *Basic Principles of Nursing Care* written for and published by the International Council of Nurses. In these publications, she makes explicit her model of nursing and her definition of the 'unique function of the nurse'. Another major work is the *Nursing Studies Index*, which covers abstracts and reports of research material published in English from 1900 to 1959.

Virginia Henderson has received many honours, including Honorary Doctorates, from many Universities. In 1977, she was awarded the Honorary Fellowship of the American Academy of Nursing, and in 1978 she was made a Fellow of The Royal College of Nursing (UK).

Henle's fissure ('henleez) spaces filled with connective tissue between the muscular fibres of the heart.

Henle's layer the outermost layer of the inner root sheath of the hair follicle.

Henle's ligament a lateral expansion of the lateral edge of the rectus abdominis which attaches to the pubic bone.

Henle's loop the U-shaped loop of the uriniferous tubule of the kidney.

Henle's membrane fenestrated membrane.

Henle's sheath the endoneurium, especially the delicate continuation around terminal branches of nerve fibres; called also *connective tissue sheath of Key and Retzius*.

Henle's tubules the straight ascending and descending portions of a renal tubule forming Henle's loop.

Henoch's disease (purpura) (henokhs) Schönlein-Henoch purpura in which abdominal symptoms predominate.

Henry's law ('henriz) the solubility of a gas in a liquid solution is proportional to the partial pressure of the gas.

hepar ('heepah) [L.] *liver*.

heparan sulphate ('hepə,ran) a sulphated mucopolysaccharide structurally related to heparin, which occurs normally in the liver, aorta, and lung; it is an accumulation product in several mucopolysaccharidoses.

heparin ('hepə·rin) an acid mucopolysaccharide present in many tissues, especially the liver and lungs, and having potent ANTICOAGULANT properties. It also has lipotrophic properties, promoting transfer of fat from blood to the fat depots by activation of lipoprotein lipase. Also, a mixture of active principles capable of prolonging blood clotting time, obtained from domestic animals; used in the prophylaxis and treatment of disorders in which there is excessive or undesirable clotting and as a preservative for blood specimens.

heparinize ('hepə·ri,niez) to treat with heparin.

hepat(o)- ('hepətoh) word element. [Gr.] *liver*.

hepatalgia (,hepə'talji·ə) pain in the liver.

hepatatrophia (,hepətə'trohfi·ə) atrophy of the liver.

hepatectomy (,hepə'tektəmee) surgical excision of liver tissue.

hepatic (hi'patik) pertaining to the liver.

h. duct the excretory duct of the liver, or one of its branches in the lobes of the liver (see also BILE DUCTS).

hepatic(o)- word element. [Gr.] *hepatic duct*.

hepaticoduodenostomy (hi,patikoh,dyooədi'nostəmee) anastomosis of the hepatic duct to the duodenum.

hepaticoenterostomy (hi,patikoh,entə'rostəmee) anastomosis of the hepatic duct to the intestine (duodenum or jejunum).

hepaticogastrostomy (hi,patikohga'strostəmee) anastomosis of the hepatic duct to the stomach.

hepaticojejunostomy (hi,patikoh,jejuh'nostəmee) anastomosis of the hepatic duct to the jejunum.

hepaticolithotomy (hi,patikohli'thotəmee) incision of the hepatic duct with removal of calculi.

hepaticolithotripsy (hi,patikoh'lithə,tripsee) the crushing of a calculus in the hepatic duct.

hepaticostomy (hi,pati'kostəmee) fistulization of the hepatic duct.

hepaticotomy (hi,pati'kotəmee) incision of the hepatic duct.

hepatin ('hepətin) glycogen.

hepatitis (,hepə'tietis) inflammation of the liver.

amoebic h. invasion of the liver parenchyma by trophozoites of *Entamoeba histolytica*, leading to amoebic abscess.

anicteric h. viral hepatitis without jaundice, tending to occur chiefly in infants and young children; symptoms include mild anorexia and gastrointestinal disturbances, slight fever, and enlargement and tenderness of the liver.

cholestatic h. inflammation of the bile ducts associated with obstructive jaundice; symptoms include progressively deepening jaundice, pruritus, dark urine, acholic stools, and a protracted course. It usually occurs as a form of viral hepatitis. Called also *cholangiolytic hepatitis*.

chronic active h. chronic inflammatory liver disease in which an expanding mesenchymal reaction in the portal triads progressively destroys adjacent liver cells. There is mononuclear and plasma cell infiltration of the liver that is particularly marked adjacent to the hepatic lobules. Progressive fibrosis leads to macronuclear cirrhosis. Hypergammaglobulinaemia is usually associated with positive serological tests (LE, antinuclear antibody, smooth muscle antibody, and rheumatic factor). This form of hepatitis may be the result of viral infection (some patients have positive tests for the hepatitis B antigen) but it also may result from sensitivity to drugs; e.g., the laxative oxyphenisatin. Most cases are thought to be autoimmune and of unknown cause. Called also *chronic aggressive hepatitis*.

The diagnosis of chronic hepatitis is established by a liver biopsy. This procedure provides an opportunity for microscopic examination to determine the extent of liver damage and to guide the doctor in the selection of drugs for treatment. Corticosteroids are sometimes prescribed to reduce the inflammatory reaction in the liver. There is some evidence that interferon can suppress the disease process for short periods of treatment, although it is not certain that the drug can be used effectively for prolonged periods of time.

chronic persistant h. low grade continued inflammation around portal tracts, not leading to cirrhosis. May become more aggressive as chronic active hepatitis (see above).

fulminant h. (acute hepatitis with coma), an acute fulminating form of hepatitis resulting from extensive hepatic necrosis. It may be due to: (1) toxic liver injury, as in carbon tetrachloride poisoning or paracetamol overdosage; (2) a hypersensitivity reaction to a drug, such as halothane; or (3) viral hepatitis. Death is usually caused by acute yellow atrophy of the liver, in which the organ becomes smaller than normal, has a soft consistency, and is reddish brown in colour. The disease is characterized by severe preicteric symptoms, an early appearance of jaundice, a sharp rise in temperature, and haemorrhages from the mucous membranes and into the skin because of prolongation of the prothrombin time. In the final stages, there is confusion, drowsiness, and stupor, followed by coma, which deepens until death occurs.

viral h. an acute, notifiable, infectious hepatitis caused by one of at least two different viral strains: hepatitis A virus (HAV) and hepatitis B virus (HBV). Type A hepatitis was formerly called *infectious hepatitis*, *epidemic hepatitis*, and *acute catarrhal jaundice*. Type B hepatitis was formerly called *serum hepatitis*, *homologous serum jaundice*, and *long incubation period hepatitis*. Standard nomenclature and definitions of terms associated with these two types of hepatitis are shown in the accompanying table.

TYPE A HEPATITIS. Infection depends on exposure to viruses from an infected person; the primary mode of

Standard nomenclature and definition of terms associated with viral hepatitis

Hepatitis A virus	
HAV	*Hepatitis A virus*: a 27 nm virus. Detectable in stool as early as 2 weeks after exposure and prior to onset of disease.
Anti-HAV	*Antibody to hepatitus A virus*: may be detected at onset of disease and before onset of jaundice. Peak levels reached 1 to 2 months later; appearance of anti-HAV in serum coincides with disappearance of HAV in stool. Remains detectable in serum for many years and apparently confers life-long immunity to reinfection.
Hepatitis B virus	
HBV	*Hepatitis B virus*: a 42-nm, double-shelled virus, originally known as the "Dane particle".
HB_sAg	*Hepatitis B surface antigen*: the antigen found on the surface of the virus, and on variable-length tubular and spherical particles (22 nm in diameter) accompanying HBV. Usually detected within 30 days of exposure, although the time interval varies with the size of inoculum and type of exposure. Hepatitis B surface antigen may persist up to 3 months after onset of jaundice. Persistence beyond this period is usually associated with a carrier state.
HB_cAg	*Hepatitis B core antigen*: the antigen found within the core of the virus.
HB_eAg	*The e antigen (closely associated with hepatitis B infectivity)*: usually detectable several days after appearance of HB_sAg. A soluble antigen found in sera containing HB_sAg: associated with presence of many circulating HBV particles, high levels of anti-HB_c, and DNA polymerase activity. Usually disappears by the time jaundice is noted.
anti-HB_s	*Antibody to hepatitis B surface antigen*: usually detectable 1 to 2 months after HB_sAg is no longer detectable. Found in about 80 per cent of patients who eventually become HB_sAg-negative.
anti-HB_c	*Antibody to hepatitis B core antigen*: detectable shortly after onset of jaundice; may be closely associated with hepatitis B infectivity.
anti-HB_e	*Antibody to the e antigen*: detection in HBV carriers indicates a relatively low degree of infectivity.
Hepatitis non-A, non-B	No virus has been specifically morphologically identified. Several studies are in progress to identify the virus and to find a reliable serological method of detection.
DNA polymerase activity	An indicator of active virus replication.
AST	*Aspartate aminotransferase*: an indicator of liver damage when present in an excessive amount.
ALT	*Alanine aminotransferase*: an indicator of liver damage when present in an excessive amount. Increased levels of AST and ALT denote hepatocellular necrosis; elevated during clinical disease and period of jaundice in all forms of viral hepatitis.
Serum bilirubin	An indicator of the extent of liver dysfunction. Values are abnormal during the period of jaundice in all forms of viral hepatitis.

From Jackson, M.M. (1980) Viral hepatitis. *Nursing Clinics of North America*, Vol. 15, p. 729.

transmission is the oral–faecal route. The peak viral excretion occurs during the two-week period before the onset of jaundice, and before the infected person becomes clinically ill. Thus, the greatest danger of infection is during the incubation period and early prodromal phase of the disease, when the person is probably not aware that he is ill. As the disease progresses and jaundice appears, the excretion of viruses declines rapidly, the person becomes less infectious, and there is less danger of cross-infection.

Type A hepatitis primarily affects children and young adults, especially in environments in which there is poor sanitation and overcrowding, as in day care centres, schools, and similar institutions. It is often a very mild disease with symptoms similar to 'flu' and, therefore, may be either misdiagnosed or ignored completely. Hepatitis A does not cause lasting damage to the liver; it can, however, produce profound fatigue, anorexia, fever, and generalized aching for weeks. Other symptoms include abdominal pain, clay-coloured stools, dark urine, and jaundice.

Treatment is primarily symptomatic and supportive. Bed rest is recommended for those patients who are icteric (jaundiced) in order to avoid complications from acute liver damage. In 98 per cent of the cases there is total recovery. Younger patients seem to have less severe symptoms than do those who are older.

Type B Hepatitis. This form of hepatitis is caused by a double-shelled virus (HBV), formerly called the 'Dane particle'. Traditionally, hepatitis B was believed to be transmitted only through contact with blood and blood products, as in blood transfusions, contaminated needles, etc. It is now known that the virus can be transmitted via such body fluids as tears, saliva, and semen, which makes it qualify as a sexually transmitted disease passed along to others by either heterosexual or homosexual intercourse. In addition to these parenteral and nonparenteral modes of transmission, there is a so-called *vertical transmission* mode by which an infant is infected by its mother either during pregnancy or after birth. Whereas the hepatitis A virus (HAV) usually has been eliminated from the body by the time jaundice appears, the body is not always able to rid itself of HBV so easily. The virus can persist in body fluids for years or even a lifetime.

Persons who are carriers of the disease are not only a threat to others, they themselves are at risk for chronic hepatitis, cirrhosis of the liver, and primary hepatocellular carcinoma. It is estimated that a carrier of HBV has about 340 times the risk of developing primary liver cancer than does a person from the same environment who is not a carrier of the virus. Because the symptoms of hepatitis B vary in their intensity, some infected individuals are not aware that they ever had the disease.

About 10 per cent of infected persons become carriers, and are a major cause of the spread of the disease. In underdeveloped countries perinatal transmission of the disease from an asymptomatic mother to her child is a major problem. In the United Kingdom and North America spread is by sexual intercourse, contaminated needles, and by blood and blood products. Transmission of hepatitis B from commercially prepared clotting concentrates derived from the plasma of commercial donors was common until serological testing for the presence of hepatitis B surface antigen (HB_sAg) in whole blood significantly decreased transfusion-related hepatitis B. Heat treatment of clotting concentrates will further reduce the risk of hepatitis transmission by this route.

The symptoms of hepatitis B can vary from asymptomatic to jaundice, joint pain, and a rash, with the potential for internal bleeding due to prolonged prothrombin time. The onset of hepatitis B is more insidious and less abrupt than for type A hepatitis. Patients who are at greatest risk for necrosis of liver cells as a result of viral hepatitis are the elderly and those who have diabetes mellitus, cancer, or some other severe illness, particularly a condition which requires surgery and transfusions.

Non-A, Non-B Hepatitis. About 85 per cent of all cases of viral hepatitis can be traced to either HAV or HBV. The remaining 10 to 15 per cent are believed to be caused by at least one and possibly several other types of viruses. At present, the causative agent(s) are lumped together under the term Non-A, Non-B for want of a more definitive term.

Clinically, Non-A, Non-B hepatitis is similar to type B hepatitis. It can develop into chronic hepatitis and often is associated with blood transfusions, particularly when the source of the blood is paid donors rather than volunteers. In fact, researchers suspected another causative agent when patients who received blood that had passed screening tests for hepatitis A and B still developed the disease one to three months after transfusion. There is evidence that Non-A, Non-B hepatitis can develop into a carrier state in some individuals. In both Non-A, Non-B and type B hepatitis abnormally high levels of AST (aspartate aminotransferase) and ALT (alanine aminotransferase) can persist for months whereas the elevation of these enzymes is only of one to three weeks' duration in type A hepatitis. Both type B and Non-A, Non-B hepatitis affect people in all age groups.

Prevention and Treatment. A vaccine can be used to provide active immunity against type B hepatitis to protect high-risk people. A hepatitis A vaccine is under development.

Until recently, Hepatitis B vaccine was prepared by isolating HB_sAg from the plasma of asymptomatic carriers. Because it does not contain intact virus particles, it is noninfectious. The vaccine is highly immunogenic, producing immunity in about 95 per cent of vaccinated individuals. It is recommended for immunization of certain high-risk groups: doctors, dentists, nurses, and laboratory technicians; immunocompromised patients and patients requiring haemodialysis or frequent transfusions; residents and staff of institutions, e.g., the mentally disabled and prisoners; household and classroom contacts of carriers; infants and young children in high-risk areas; and homosexually active males, prostitutes, and drug addicts. A new vaccine, made entirely by bioengineering using recombinant DNA technology, is now available and avoids the need to use plasma as a source of antigen.

Passive immunity to hepatitis A and hepatitis B can be conferred through the administration of immune serum globulin (ISG). Pre-exposure and postexposure prophylaxis against type A is through the administration of ISG. Both ISG and high-titre immune globulin for type B hepatitis (HBIG) are recommended for those persons who have been exposed to persons infected with HBV.

Gamma globulins provide passive immunity for three to four months and are recommended for household members and others who are known to have had close contact with a hepatitis patient. Passive immunization also is strongly suggested for those persons who are travelling to countries with poor sanitation.

Health care personnel who work in high-risk areas, such as haemodialysis units and clinical laboratories, do not need *routine* passive immunization with ISG or HBIG. Those who are known carriers of hepatitis B antigen are advised to adhere to strict principles of personal hygiene and to take measures to avoid contamination of others by their blood and body secretions.

There is no specific treatment or drug that kills the hepatitis virus and can overcome an active infection. Supportive care is given to help the patient's natural defences overcome the disease. It is important to maintain adequate hydration and nutrition and to provide sufficient rest in order to avoid complications.

Patient Care. Viral hepatitis is a notifiable disease and requires the completing of forms for the community health physician. When a hepatitis patient is admitted to the hospital the infection control nurse should be notified as soon as possible.

The patient's condition should be monitored regularly as well as his levels of AST, ALT, and serum bilirubin. Jaundice, urticaria, nausea, abdominal pain, arthralgia, and other symptoms should be noted and recorded when present. The care plan for the patient should include measures to provide rest and an adequate dietary intake to meet energy requirements. Fluid intake and output and the colour and other characteristics of urine and stools should be noted and recorded.

The patient, his family, and close contacts need instruction about isolation precautions and an explanation of why they are imposed as long as the patient is infectious. They also need guidance about being immunized when this is indicated. Although viral hepatitis can be a very mild disease, it has the potential for becoming very serious in some patients and presenting problems of silent gastrointestinal bleeding, respiratory problems, and neurological dysfunction, including mental confusion and profound coma.

hepatization (ˌhepətie'zayshən) transformation into a liver-like mass, especially the solidified state of the lung in lobar pneumonia. The early stage, in which the pulmonary exudate is blood stained, is called red hepatization. The later stage, in which the red cells disintegrate and a fibrinosuppurative exudate persists, is called grey hepatization.

hepatoblastoma (ˌhepətohbla'stohmə) a malignant intrahepatic tumour consisting chiefly of embryonic tissue, occurring in infants and young children.

hepatocarcinoma (ˌhepətohˌkahsi'nohmə) hepatocellular carcinoma; carcinoma derived from the parenchymal cells of the liver (hepatocytes).

hepatocele ('hepətohˌseel) hernia of the liver.

hepatocellular (ˌhepətoh'selyuhlə) pertaining to or affecting liver cells.

hepatocholangiocarcinoma (ˌhepətohkəˌlanjiohˌkahsi'nohmə) cholangiohepatoma.

hepatocholangitis (ˌhepətohˌkohlanjietis) inflamma-

tion of the liver and bile ducts.
hepatocirrhosis (ˌhepətohsi'rohsis) cirrhosis of the liver.
hepatocystic (ˌhepətoh'sistik) pertaining to the liver and gallbladder.
hepatocyte ('hepətohˌsiet) a hepatic cell.
hepatodynia (ˌhepətoh'dini·ə) pain in the liver.
hepatogastric (ˌhepətoh'gastrik) pertaining to the liver and stomach.
hepatogenic (ˌhepətoh'jenik) 1. giving rise to or forming liver tissue. 2. hepatogenous.
hepatogenous (ˌhepə'tojənəs) 1. originating in or caused by the liver. 2. hepatogenic.
hepatogram ('hepətohˌgram) 1. a tracing of the liver pulse in the sphygmogram. 2. a radiograph of the liver.
hepatography (ˌhepə'tografee) 1. a treatise on the liver. 2. radiography of the liver. 3. the recording of the liver pulse.
hepatojugular (ˌhepətoh'jugyuhlə) pertaining to the liver and jugular vein.
h. reflux distention of the jugular vein induced by manual pressure over the liver; it suggests insufficiency of the right heart.
hepatolenticular degeneration (ˌhepətohlen'tikyuhlə) a hereditary disorder of copper metabolism, marked by a pigmented ring at the outer margin of the cornea, degenerative changes in the brain, cirrhosis of the liver, splenomegaly, tremor, rigidity, contractures, psychic disturbances, dysphagia, and increasing weakness and emaciation. Commonly called *Wilson's disease*.
hepatolienography (ˌhepətohˌlieə'nografee) radiography of the liver and spleen.
hepatolith ('hepətohˌlith) a calculus in the liver.
hepatolithectomy (ˌhepətohli'thektəmee) removal of a calculus from the liver.
hepatolithiasis (ˌhepətohli'thieəsis) the presence of calculi in the biliary ducts of the liver.
hepatology (ˌhepə'toləjee) the scientific study of the liver and its diseases.
hepatolysin (ˌhepə'tolisin) a cytolysin destructive to liver cells.
hepatolysis (ˌhepə'tolisis) destruction of the liver cells. adj. **hepatolytic**.
hepatoma (ˌhepə'tohmə) any tumour of the liver, especially hepatocellular carcinoma (malignant hepatoma).
hepatomalacia (ˌhepətohmə'layshi·ə) softening of the liver.
hepatomegaly (ˌhepətoh'megəlee) enlargement of the liver.
hepatomelanosis (ˌhepətohˌmelə'nohsis) melanosis of the liver.
hepatomphalocele (ˌhepə'tomfəlohˌseel) umbilical hernia with liver involvement in the hernial sac.
hepatonephric (ˌhepətoh'nefrik) pertaining to the liver and kidney.
hepatopathy (ˌhepə'topəthee) any disease of the liver.
hepatopexy ('hepətohˌpeksee) surgical fixation of a displaced liver to the abdominal wall.
hepatopleural (ˌhepətoh'plooə·rəl) pertaining to the liver and pleura or pleural cavity.
hepatopneumonic (ˌhepətohnyoo'monik) pertaining to, affecting, or communicating with the liver and lungs.
hepatoportal (ˌhepətoh'pawt'l) pertaining to the portal system of the liver.
hepatopulmonary (ˌhepətoh'pulmənə·ree, -'puhl-) hepatopneumonic.
hepatorenal (ˌhepətoh'reen'l) pertaining to the liver and kidneys.
hepatorrhaphy (ˌhepə'to·rəfee) suture of the liver.
hepatorrhexis (ˌhepətoh'reksis) rupture of the liver.
hepatoscopy (ˌhepə'toskəpee) examination of the liver.
hepatosis (ˌhepə'tohsis) any functional disorder of the liver.
serous h. veno-occlusive disease of the liver.
hepatosplenitis (ˌhepətohsplə'nietis) inflammation of the liver and spleen.
hepatosplenography (ˌhepətohˌsplə'nografee) radiography of the liver and spleen.
hepatosplenomegaly (ˌhepətohˌspleenoh'megəlee) enlargement of the liver and spleen.
hepatotherapy (ˌhepətoh'therəpee) administration of liver or liver extract.
hepatotomy (ˌhepə'totəmee) incision of the liver.
hepatotoxaemia (ˌhepətohtok'seemi·ə) septicaemia originating in the liver.
hepatotoxin (ˌhepətoh'toksin) a toxin that destroys liver cells. adj. **hepatotoxic**.
hepta- word element. [Gr.] *seven*.
heptachromic (ˌheptə'krohmik) 1. pertaining to or exhibiting seven colours. 2. having vision for all seven colours of the spectrum.
heptose ('heptohs, -ohz) a sugar whose molecule contains seven carbon atoms.
herd immunity (hərd) the immunity of a population or group. When there is a high enough number of persons in a population immune to a particular infection, the infection fails to spread because of the absence of enough susceptibles. For example, in measles this could probably be achieved by vaccination of 90 to 95 per cent of the population.
hereditary (hi'reditə·ree) transmissible or transmitted from parent to offspring; genetically determined.
heredity (hi'reditee) the genetic transmission of traits from parents to offspring. The hereditary material is contained in the ovum and sperm, so that the child's heredity is determined at the moment of conception.

CHROMOSOMES AND GENES. Inside the nucleus of each germ cell are structures called *chromosomes*. A chromosome is composed of DEOXYRIBONUCLEIC ACID (DNA) on a framework of protein. Genes are segments of the DNA molecule; there are thousands of GENES in each cell. Each gene carries a specific hereditary trait. These traits are physical, biochemical, and physiological. Thus genes affect not only the physical appearance of an individual but also his physiological makeup, his tendency to develop certain diseases, and the daily activities of all the cells of his body.

The human ovum contains 23 chromosomes. The sperm also contains 23 chromosomes, and aside from the pair determining the sex, each one is similar in shape and size to one in the ovum. When the sperm penetrates the ovum, the fertilized ovum thus contains 23 pairs of chromosomes, or 46 chromosomes in all.

The fertilized ovum then begins to reproduce itself by dividing (MITOSIS). The original cell divides and forms two cells, each of these divides and forms a total of four cells and so on until a many-celled embryo begins to take form.

In the process of cell division, the chromosomes in the nucleus have the ability to make duplicates of themselves. They do not split in two, but instead each one produces another chromosome exactly like itself. When the two cells are formed from one, the chromosomes are divided so that each cell contains the same number and kind of chromosomes as the original. For this reason, all the cells in the developing embryo and in the human body, except the ovum and sperm, contain identical sets of 46 chromosomes.

The ovum and the sperm are formed by a special

process of cell division (MEIOSIS) in which each sperm or ovum receives only one member of each chromosome pair.

In the formation of the germ cells, it is a matter of chance which member of each pair of chromosomes goes to a given ovum or sperm. It is also purely a matter of chance which sperm fertilizes an ovum. Incredible as it seems, there are, all in all, about 70 billion possible combinations of chromosomes that a child can inherit.

INHERITED TRAITS. Although many of the details of human heredity are not known, in general we can say that the child receives a set of genes from his parents. These genes, or hereditary determinants, develop into characteristics which reflect those of his parents, grandparents, and other ancestors. Before birth these inherited traits are influenced by conditions within the mother's body. After birth they are shaped in various ways by environmental influences such as diet, training, and education.

Some specific aspects of human heredity are well understood, for example, the inheritance of eye colour. Remember that one member of a chromosome pair is contributed by one parent and the other by the other parent. A gene in one chromosome acts on the same trait as a gene in the same position on the other chromosome.

It has been found that one gene may be more powerful in its influence than the other gene that acts on the same trait. The more powerful gene is then said to be dominant, and the other gene is said to be recessive. A gene that produces blue eyes, for example, is recessive to a gene that produces brown eyes.

SEX DETERMINATION. Of the 23 pairs of chromosomes in each of the body cells, one pair is distinctly different from the others. The members of this pair are the sex chromosomes, and they determine the sex of offspring. In the female, they look alike and are termed X chromosomes. But in the male, one sex chromosome is an X chromosome and the other is a smaller, Y chromosome. Thus each germ cell produced by the male contains either an X or a Y chromosome. If a sperm containing a Y chromosome fertilizes an egg, the child will be male. If the sperm has an X chromosome, the child will be female.

In the development of the male embryo it is essential that fetal male hormones (androgens) be released at a certain time during early gestation. Otherwise, the infant will be born with external female genitalia even though he has the chromosomal sex pattern of a male and has no internal female reproductive organs.

SEX-LINKED TRAITS. Certain hereditary traits are known as sex-linked because they are carried on the X chromosome. Colour blindness is an example. This condition, in which colours appear as varying shades of grey, is rare in females but appears in about 8 per cent of the male population. The genes for colour vision are located on the X chromosomes, and the gene for normal vision is dominant to that for colour blindness. A female having one gene for normal vision on one X chromosome and one for colour blindness on the other will have normal vision, since the colour blindness gene is recessive. A male, however, having only one X chromosome, will be colour blind if that chromosome has the recessive gene, since there is no corresponding dominant gene to suppress it.

Another characteristic associated with sex is baldness. The gene for baldness is dominant in males and recessive in females. Thus a male need have only one gene for baldness for the trait to be expressed, but a female must have two.

HEREDITARY DISEASES. Hereditary diseases should be distinguished from congenital birth defects. A congenital defect is one that the infant is born with, such as a cleft lip, a birthmark, or congenital syphilis, but the defect can arise during conception or pregnancy and not be related to heredity. Hereditary diseases, on the other hand, are passed from generation to generation by genes. Some diseases, such as cystic fibrosis, are transmitted by recessive genes.

Classic HAEMOPHILIA is a hereditary disease transmitted by a sex-linked gene. A recessive gene carried on the X chromosome is responsible for it, and it is transmitted in the same way as colour blindness. In extremely rare cases a female carries two recessive genes for the trait.

Certain diseases are not inherited directly, but the tendency to contract them may be inherited. Epilepsy, for example, occurs more frequently in some families than in others. The tendency to develop allergy, asthma, and bronchitis also seems to run in families. Whether these conditions actually develop in a person with such a tendency depends on environmental circumstances. Strong evidence indicates that longsightedness, shortsightedness, and night blindness have a hereditary basis.

Certain mental disorders are known to be hereditary. In children afflicted with DOWN'S SYNDROME there is an abnormality in the chromosomes. This condition is classified as a trisomy, which refers to the state of having an extra chromosome per cell. Inborn errors of metabolism such as PHENYLKETONURIA and GALACTOSAEMIA are inherited.

ROLE OF MUTATION. Mutation is the term used for a spontaneous change in a chromosome or gene. Normally chromosomes duplicate themselves exactly during cell division. Occasionally, however, the new cells contain an altered gene or chromosome. If the mutation occurs in an ovum or sperm involved in reproduction, the new trait will be expressed in the offspring.

Many mutations are so minor that they have no visible effect. A mutation that is very harmful will usually result in the death of the fetus and spontaneous abortion. Occasionally a mutation is beneficial. Favourable mutations gradually tend to spread through a population. The accumulation of mutations over millions of years has contributed to evolution.

heredofamilial (ˌheridohfə'mili·əl) occurring in certain families under circumstances that implicate a hereditary basis.

Herellea (hə'reli·ə) a genus of nonmotile, paired, gram-negative, enteric bacilli, including *H. vaginicola*, a species causing various hospital-acquired infections.

Hering–Breuer reflexes (ˌhering'broyə) inflation and deflation reflexes that help regulate the rhythmic ventilation of the lungs, thereby preventing overdistention and extreme deflation. These reflexes arise outside the respiratory centre in the brain; that is, the receptor sites are located in the respiratory tract, mainly in the bronchi and bronchioles. They are activated by either a stretching or a nonstretching and compression of the lung; the impulses are transmitted from the receptor sites through the vagus nerve to the brain stem and thence to the respiratory centre.

The *inflation* reflex acts to inhibit inspiration and thereby prevents further inflation. When the lung tissue is stretched by inflation, the stretch receptors respond by sending impulses to the respiratory centre, which in turn slows down inspiration. As the expiratory phase begins, the receptors are no longer stretched, impulses are no longer sent, and inspiration can begin again. This is called the Hering–Breuer *deflation* reflex. It is also believed that in addition to the cessation of impulses from the stretch receptors, there may be an activation of compression receptors which transmit impulses that inhibit expiration, thus allowing inspiration to begin.

hermaphrodism (hər'mafrə,dizəm) hermaphroditism.

hermaphrodite (hər'mafrə,diet) an individual whose body contains tissue of both male and female gonads. The ovaries and testes may be present as separate organs, or ovarian and testicular tissue may be combined in the same organ (ovotestis). See also HERMAPHRODITISM.

hermaphroditism (hər'mafrədie,tizəm) a state characterized by the presence of both ovarian and testicular tissue and of ambiguous morphological criteria of sex, a rare condition in human beings. Hermaphroditism is not to be confused with pseudohermaphroditism, in which an individual with only one kind of gonad possesses reproductive organs that reflect some characteristics of the opposite sex, owing to improper balance of male and female hormones or other endocrine disorder.

bilateral h. that in which gonadal tissue typical of both sexes occurs on each side of the body.

false h. pseudohermaphroditism.

lateral h. presence of gonadal tissue typical of one sex on one side of the body and tissue typical of the other sex on the opposite side.

transverse h. that in which the external genital organs are typical of one sex and the gonads typical of the other sex.

true h. coexistence in the same person of both ovarian and testicular tissue, with somatic characters typical of both sexes.

unilateral h. presence of gonadal tissue typical of both sexes on one side and of only an ovary or a testis on the other.

hermetic (hər'metik) impervious to the air.

hernia ('hərni·ə) the abnormal protrusion of part of an organ or tissue through the structures normally containing it. Called also a *rupture*. adj. **hernial.** It is commonly due to a defect of the abdominal wall permitting the protrusion of the peritoneal sac together with its various contents. The term is also applied to a defect in encapsulation or ensheathment allowing the protrusion of a muscle through an aponeurosis.

Removal of the hernial sac and reconstruction of the abdominal wall is called HERNIORRHAPHY.

h. cerebri protrusion of brain substance through the skull.

crural h. femoral hernia.

diaphragmatic h. protrusion of some of the contents of the abdomen through an opening in the diaphragm into the chest cavity, hiatus hernia being one type of diaphragmatic hernia.

fat h., fatty h. protrusion of extraperitoneal fat through the abdominal wall, usually at the linea alba.

femoral h. protrusion into the femoral canal.

hiatal h., hiatus h. protrusion of a structure, usually a portion of the stomach, through the oesophageal hiatus of the diaphragm; a type of DIAPHRAGMATIC HERNIA.

incarcerated h. hernia in which the contents cannot be reduced; it may or may not become strangulated.

incisional h. hernia at the site of a surgical incision.

inguinal h. hernia occurring in the groin. A sac of peritoneum containing intestine or omentum, or both, pushes either directly outward through the external inguinal ring, the weakest point in the abdominal wall (direct inguinal hernia), or downward at an angle into the inguinal canal (indirect inguinal hernia). Indirect inguinal hernia occurs more frequently in males because it follows the tract that develops when the testes descend into the scrotum before birth, and the hernia itself may descend into the scrotum. When present in the female, the hernia follows the course of the round ligament of the uterus.

Inguinal hernia begins usually as a small breakthrough. It may be hardly noticeable, appearing as a soft lump under the skin. As time passes, the pressure of the contents of the abdomen against the weak abdominal wall may increase the size of the opening and, accordingly, the size of the hernia.

internal h. herniation occurring within the abdomen into a peritoneal pocket or loculus which may be anatomical, e.g. through the epiploic foramen, or artefactual when the pocket is created unintentionally by operation, e.g. to the left and behind the anastomosis of a partial gastrectomy.

irreducible h. incarcerated or strangulated hernia.

paraoesophageal h. hiatal hernia in which part or almost all of the stomach protrudes through the hiatus into the thorax to the left of the oesophagus, with the gastro-oesophageal junction remaining below the diaphragm.

reducible h. one that can be returned by manipulation.

scrotal h. inguinal hernia which has passed into the scrotum.

sliding h. hernia in which the wall of a viscus forms a portion of the hernial sac, the remainder of the sac being formed by parietal peritoneum.

sliding hiatal h. hiatal hernia in which the upper stomach and the cardio-oesophageal junction pass upward into the posterior mediastinum; the protrusion, which may be fixed or intermittent, is partially covered by a peritoneal sac.

strangulated h. a hernia in which the blood supply of the contents is cut off by constriction either from the neck of the sac or from an anatomical structure outside the sac.

A hernia becomes tense, tender, irreducible and loses its cough impulse when strangulated.

umbilical h. protrusion at the umbilicus (see also UMBILICAL HERNIA).

vaginal h., posterior vaginal h. hernia of the pouch of Douglas into the vagina.

herniation (,hərni'ayshən) abnormal protrusion of an organ or other body structure through a defect or natural opening in a covering membrane, muscle or bone.

h. of nucleus pulposus rupture or prolapse of the nucleus pulposus into the spinal canal, or against the spinal cord (see also prolapsed intervertebral DISC).

tonsillar h. protrusion of the cerebellar tonsils through the foramen magnum.

transtentorial h. downward displacement (caudal transtentorial herniation; uncal herniation) of the medial brain structures through the tentorial notch by a supratentorial mass, exerting pressure on the underlying structures, including the brain stem.

uncal h. transtentorial herniation.

hernioplasty ('hərnioh,plastee) surgical repair of hernia, with reconstruction of the abdominal wall after removal of the peritoneal sac.

herniorrhaphy (,hərni'o·rəfee) surgical repair of hernia by removing the sac and suturing the abdominal wall.

herniotomy (,hərni'otəmee) surgical repair of hernia by removal of the sac alone.

heroin ('heroh·in) a narcotic made from morphine by the acetylation of both the phenolic and the alcoholic hydroxyl groups. Called also *diacetylmorphine*. Used medicinally as an analgesic and abused illicitly for its euphoriant effects. The drug has a great capacity for inducing physical dependence and may be sniffed, smoked ('chasing the dragon') or injected subcutaneously or intravenously ('shooting up' or 'mainlining'). Slang terms for heoin include 'smack', 'H', and 'brown sugar'.

herpangina (ˌhərpan'jienə) an infectious febrile disease of children due to coxsackieviruses, marked by vesicular or ulcerated lesions on the fauces or soft palate.

herpes ('hərpeez) any inflammatory skin disease caused by a herpesvirus and characterized by the formation of small vesicles in clusters. When used alone the term may refer to *herpes simplex* or to *herpes zoster*.

h. simplex a viral infection which gives rise to localized vesicles in the skin and mucous membranes and is characterized by latency and subsequent recurrence. It is caused by herpes simplex viruses types 1 and 2 and has a worldwide distribution. Type 1 infection is common in children and is often symptomless. Type 2 infection is common in older age groups and is associated with sexual activity. Man is the source of infection and spread is by direct or indirect contact with saliva or genital secretions. Neonates may be infected from the birth canal. Health care staff may be infected by entry of the virus through breaks in the skin, giving rise to herpetic whitlow on the fingers. The incubation period is 2–12 days. The infection is communicable for several weeks after primary infection, and transient virus shedding occurs in symptomless infections and during reactivation.

SYMPTOMS. The commonest clinical manifestation in children is gingivostomatitis, the sudden onset of fever with sore ulcerated mouth sometimes accompanied by lesions on the face, neck, or chest. Eye infection may occur. Severe infections may occur in eczematous subjects (eczema herpeticum) and in infants, and may be fatal. Reactivation of the infection causes 'fever blisters' or 'cold sores', usually on the face or lips. Rarely ENCEPHALITIS may follow primary infection with type 1 virus, usually in older children and adults.

Genital herpes is usually caused by type 2 virus. Lesions appear on the cervix, vulva, and surrounding skin in women and on the penis in men. In homosexual men rectal lesions are common. Recurrent genital herpes may follow primary infection. Type 2 virus may cause aseptic meningitis which usually follows a benign course.

TREATMENT. Astringent lotions can be used topically at the blistering stage. Topical treatment with idoxuridine is used in severe skin lesions and eye lesions. Oral or intravenous acyclovir is used in disseminated infections and encephalitis.

PREVENTION. Prevention involves avoidance of contact with infected lesions. Health care staff should wear gloves when attending patients with lesions. Particular care should be taken to avoid infection in infants and in eczematous patients; nursing staff with lesions should be excluded from work. Caesarean section has been recommended for those who have clinical genital tract herpes within two weeks of delivery in order to prevent neonatal herpes.

Because of the widespread incidence of the disease, and the emotional trauma it provokes, patients often find it useful to talk to fellow sufferers. The Herpes Association is a well established self-help group in the UK which acts as a counselling and information centre. Information can be obtained by writing to The Herpes Association, 41 North Road, London N7 9DP.

h. zoster is a local manifestation of reactivation of infection of the varicella zoster virus, the causative agent of chickenpox, characterized by a vesicular rash in the area of distribution of a sensory nerve. Called also *shingles*. It is common in adults and the elderly and in immunocompromised persons, especially those suffering from leukaemia and other malignant diseases. Other precipitating factors are trauma and certain drugs and it is believed that exposure to chickenpox may sometimes precipitate the disease although in most cases there is no apparent cause.

Pain of segmental distribution occurs before the appearance of the rash, which evolves from macules to papules, vesicles and then pustules in the same way as chickenpox but is more dense.

Herpes zoster affecting the eye causes severe conjunctivitis and possible ulceration and scarring of the cornea if not treated successfully. Herpes zoster affecting the ear due to involvement of the geniculate ganglion (Ramsay Hunt syndrome), causes paralysis of the facial nerve with severe pain in the ear and throat.

TREATMENT. Analgesics are given to relieve the pain, which may be severe and persistent. Local applications of idoxuridine may be used, especially if the eye is involved. Acyclovir is given for severe infections in immunocompromised patients.

herpesvirus ('hərpeezˌvierəs) any of a large group of DNA viruses found in many animal species, with a nucleocapsid of about 100 nm in diameter, composed of 162 capsomers, and sometimes enclosed in a loose membrane. The viruses mature in the nucleus of the infected cell, where they induce the formation of a characteristic inclusion body; some also induce formation of a cytoplasmic inclusion body.

There are two types of herpes simplex virus (HSV) affecting man (Herpesvirus hominis), *type 1* mainly affecting children and causing stomatitis and 'cold sores' and *type 2* mainly affecting the genital tract of adults (see HERPES SIMPLEX). Other herpesvirus infections include varicella (CHICKENPOX) and HERPES ZOSTER (which are different manifestations of infection by the same virus), as well as cytomegalic inclusion disease and infectious MONONUCLEOSIS.

Herpesvirus hominis ('hominis) the herpesvirus that causes HERPES SIMPLEX, occurring in two immunological types: type 1 (primarily nongenital infections) and type 2 (primarily genital infections).

herpetic (hər'petik) pertaining to or of the nature of herpes; relating to or caused by herpesviruses.

herpetiform (hər'petiˌfawm) resembling herpes.

Hers' disease (hərz) glycogenosis (type VI) in which a deficiency in liver phosphorylase affects the liver and leukocytes, with hepatomegaly, mild hypoglycaemia, mild acidosis, and growth retardation.

hertz (hərts) a unit of frequency, equal to one cycle per second; symbol, Hz.

Herxheimer reaction ('hərks·hiemə) an inflammatory reaction in the tissues in cases of syphilis, which can occur on starting treatment.

Hess's test ('hesiz) a test used to diagnose purpura. An inflated blood pressure cuff causes an increase in capillary pressure and rupture of the walls, causing purpuric spots to develop.

hetastarch ('hetəˌstahch) an artificial colloid produced by addition of hydroxyethyl ether groups into amylopectin; used as a plasma volume expander for treatment of shock.

heter(o)- word element. [Gr.] *other, dissimilar*.

heteradelphus (ˌhetərə'delfəs) a twin fetus or infant with one twin more developed than the other.

heteraesthesia (ˌhetəris'theezi·ə) variation of cutaneous sensibility on adjoining areas.

heteroagglutination (ˌhetə·roh·əˌglooti'nayshən) agglutination of particulate antigens of one species by agglutinins derived from another species.

heteroagglutinin (ˌhetə·roh·ə'glootinin) an agglutinin

that is capable of heteroagglutination.

heteroantibody (ˌhetə·roh'antiˌbodee) an antibody combining with antigens originating from a species foreign to the antibody producer.

heteroantigen (ˌhetə·roh'antijen, -jən) an antigen originating from a species foreign to the antibody producer.

heteroblastic (ˌhetə·roh'blastik) originating in a different kind of tissue.

heterocellular (ˌhetə·roh'selyuhlə) composed of cells of different kinds.

heterocephalus (ˌhetə·roh'kefələs, -'sef-) a monster with two unequal heads.

heterochromatin (ˌhetə·roh'krohmətin) that state of chromatin in which it is dark-staining, genetically inactive, and tightly coiled.

heterochromia (ˌhetə·roh'krohmi·ə) diversity of colour in a part normally of one colour.

h. iridis difference in colour of the iris in the two eyes, or in different areas in the same iris.

heterochronia (ˌhetə·roh'krohni·ə) irregularity in time; occurrence at abnormal times.

heterochronic (ˌhetə·roh'kronik) 1. pertaining to or characterized by heterochronia. 2. existing for different periods of time; showing a difference in ages.

heterochthonous (ˌhetə'rokthənəs) originating in an area other than that in which it is found.

heterocyclic (ˌhetə·roh'sieklik) having or pertaining to a closed chain or ring formation that includes atoms of different elements.

heterocytotropic (ˌhetə·rohsietoh'tropik) having an affinity for cells from different species.

heterodermic (ˌhetə·roh'dərmik) denoting a skin graft from an individual of another species.

heterodont ('hetə·rohˌdont) having teeth of different shapes, as molars, incisors, etc.

heterodromous (ˌhetə'rodrəməs) moving or acting in other than the usual or forward direction.

heteroecious (ˌhetə'reeshəs) requiring different hosts in different stages of development; a characteristic of certain parasites.

heteroerotism (ˌhetə·roh'erəˌtizəm) sexual feeling directed toward another person.

heterogamety (ˌhetə·roh'gamitee) production by an individual of one sex (as the human male) of unlike gametes with respect to the sex chromosomes. adj. **heterogametic**.

heterogamy (ˌhetə'rogəmee) the conjugation of gametes differing in size and structure, to form the zygote from which the new organism develops.

heterogeneity (ˌhetə·rohjə'neeətee, -'nay-) the state of being heterogeneous.

heterogeneous (ˌhetəroh'jeeni·əs) not of uniform composition, quality, or structure.

heterogenesis (ˌhetə·roh'jenəsis) 1. alternation of generations; reproduction differing in character in successive generations. 2. asexual generation.

heterogenote ('hetə·rohˌjeenoht) a cell that has an additional genetic fragment, different from its intact genotype; usually resulting from transduction.

heterogenous (ˌhetə'rojənəs) of other origin; not originating in the body.

heterogony (ˌhetə'rogənee) heterogenesis.

heterograft ('hetə·rohˌgraft) a graft of tissue transplanted between individuals of different species; a xenograft.

heterography (ˌhetə'rogrəfee) writing of other than the intended words.

heterohaemagglutination (ˌhetə·rohˌheeməˌglooti'nayshən) agglutination of erythrocytes by a haemagglutinin derived from an individual of a different species.

heterohaemagglutinin (ˌhetə·rohˌheemə'glootinin) a haemagglutinin that agglutinates erythrocytes of organisms of other species.

heterohaemolysin (ˌhetə·roh·hee'molisin) a haemolysin that destroys erythrocytes of animals of other species than that of the animal in which it is formed.

heteroimmunity (ˌhetə·roh·i'myoonitee) 1. an immune state induced in an individual by immunization with cells of an animal of another species. 2. a state in which an immune response to exogenous antigen (e.g. drugs or pathogens) results in immunopathological changes. adj. **heteroimmune**.

heterokeratoplasty (ˌhetə·roh'kerətohˌplastee) grafting of corneal tissue taken from an individual of another species.

heterokinesis (ˌhetə·rohki'neesis) the differential distribution of the sex chromosomes in the developing gametes of a heterogametic organism.

heterolalia (ˌhetə·roh'layli·ə) utterance of inappropriate or meaningless words instead of those intended.

heterolateral (ˌhetə·roh'latə·rəl) relating to the opposite side; contralateral.

heterologous (ˌhetə'roləgəs) 1. made up of tissue not normal to the part. 2. derived from an individual of a different species.

heterolysin (ˌhetə'rolisin) an antibody that lyses cells of species other than the one in which it is formed.

heterolysis (ˌhetə'rolisis) destruction of cells of one species by lysin from another species. adj. **heterolytic**.

heteromeric (ˌhetə·roh'merik) sending processes through one of the commissures to the white matter of the opposite side of the spinal cord.

heterometaplasia (ˌhetə·rohˌmetə'playzi·ə) formation of tissue foreign to the part where it is formed.

heterometropia (ˌhetə·rohme'trohpi·ə) the state in which the refraction in the two eyes differs.

heteromorphosis (ˌhetə·rohmaw'fohsis) the development, in regeneration, of an organ or structure different from the one that was lost.

heteromorphous (ˌhetə·roh'mawfəs) of abnormal shape or structure.

heteronomous (ˌhetə'ronəməs) subject to different laws; in biology, subject to different laws of growth or specialized along different lines. In psychology, subject to another's will.

hetero-osteoplasty (ˌhetə·roh'ostiohˌplastee) osteoplasty with bone taken from an individual of another species.

heteropagus (ˌhetə'ropəgəs) conjoined twins consisting of unequally developed components.

heteropathy (ˌhetə'ropəthee) abnormal or morbid sensibility to stimuli.

heterophagosome (ˌhetə·roh'fagəˌsohm) an intracytoplasmic vacuole formed by phagocytosis or pinocytosis, which becomes fused with a lysosome, subjecting its contents to enzymatic digestion. Called also a *secondary lysosome* or a *phagolysosome*.

heterophagy (ˌhetə'rofəjee) the taking into a cell of exogenous material by phagocytosis or pinocytosis and the digestion of the ingested material after fusion of the newly formed vacuole with a lysosome.

heterophasia, heterophaemia (ˌhetə·roh'fayzi·ə; hetə·roh'feemi·ə) the utterance of words other than those intended by the speaker.

heterophil (ˌhetə·rohˌfil) 1. a finely granular polymorphonuclear leukocyte represented by neutrophils in man, but characterized in other mammals by granules that have variable sizes and staining characteristics. 2. heterophilic.

heterophilic (ˌhetə·roh'filik) 1. having affinity for other antigens or antibodies besides the one for which it is specific. 2. staining with a type of stain other than the usual one.

heterophonia (ˌhetə·roh'fohni·ə) any abnormality of the voice.

heterophoria (ˌhetə·roh'for·ri·ə) failure of the visual axes to remain parallel after the visual fusional stimuli have been eliminated. The various forms of heterophoria are spoken of as phorias, their direction being indicated by the appropriate prefix, as *cyclo*phoria, *eso*phoria, *exo*phoria, *hyper*phoria, and *hypo*phoria. adj. **heterophoric.**

heterophthalmia (ˌhetə·rof'thalmi·ə) difference in the direction of the axes, or in the colour, of the two eyes.

heteroplasia (ˌhetə·roh'playzi·ə) replacement of normal by abnormal tissues; malposition of normal cells. adj. **heteroplastic.**

heteroplasty ('hetə·rohˌplastee) plastic repair with tissue derived from an individual of a different species.

heteroploid ('hetə·rohˌployd) 1. characterized by heteroploidy. 2. an individual or cell with an abnormal number of chromosomes.

heteroploidy ('hetə·rohˌploydee) the state of having an abnormal number of chromosomes.

heteropsia (ˌhetə'ropsi·ə) unequal vision in the two eyes.

heteropyknosis (ˌhetə·rohpik'nohsis) 1. the quality of showing variations in density throughout. 2. a state of differential condensation observed in different chromosomes, or in different regions of the same chromosome; it may be attenuated (negative heteropyknosis) or accentuated (positive heteropyknosis). adj. **heteropyknotic.**

heterosexual (ˌhetə·roh'seksyooəl) 1. pertaining to, characteristic of, or directed toward the opposite sex. 2. a person with erotic interests directed toward the opposite sex.

heterosexuality (ˌhetə·rohˌseksyoo'alitee) sexual attraction to persons of the opposite sex.

heterosis (ˌhetə'rohsis) the existence, in the first generation hybrid, of greater vigour than is shown by either parent.

heterotaxia (ˌhetə·roh'taksi·ə) abnormal position of viscera.

heterotonia (ˌhetə·roh'tohni·ə) a state characterized by variations in tension or tone. adj. **heterotonic.**

heterotopia (ˌhetə·roh'tohpi·ə) displacement or misplacement of parts. adj. **heterotopic.**

heterotransplant (ˌhetə·roh'transplahnt, -'trahns-) tissue taken from one individual and transplanted into one of a different species; a xenograft.

heterotrichosis (ˌhetə·rohtri'kohsis) growth of hairs of different colours on the body.

heterotroph ('hetə·rohˌtrohf) a heterotrophic organism.

heterotrophic (ˌhetə·roh'trofik) unable to synthesize metabolic products from inorganic materials; requiring complex organic substances (growth factors) for nutrition.

heterotropia (ˌhetə·roh'trohpi·ə) failure of the visual axes to remain parallel when fusion is possible (see also STRABISMUS).

heterotypic (ˌhetə·roh'tipik) pertaining to, characteristic of, or belonging to a different type. adj. **heterotypical.**

heteroxenous (ˌhetə'roksinəs) requiring more than one host to complete the life cycle.

heterozygosity (ˌhetə·rohzie'gositee) the state of having different alleles in regard to a given character. adj. **heterozygous.**

heterozygote (ˌhetə·roh'ziegoht) an individual exhibiting heterozygosity.

Heubner–Herter disease (ˌhoybnə'hərtə) coeliac disease of infants.

heuristic (hyooə'ristik) encouraging or promoting investigation; conducive to discovery.

hex(a)- ('heksə) word element. [Gr.] *six.*

Hexabrix ('heksəbriks) trademark for an iodine-containing, water-soluble, radiological contrast medium containing a mixture of sodium and meglumine salts of ioxaglate.

hexachlorophane (ˌheksə'klor·rəˌfeen) a detergent and germicidal compound commonly incorporated in soaps and dermatological agents.

hexachromic (ˌheksə'krohmik) 1. pertaining to or exhibiting six colours. 2. able to distinguish only six of the seven colours of the spectrum.

hexad ('heksad) 1. a group or combination of six similar or related entities. 2. an element with a valency of six.

hexamethonium (ˌheksəme'thohni·əm) a ganglion-blocking ammonium compound used as an antihypertensive.

hexamine ('heksəˌmeen) methenamine; a urinary antiseptic which releases formaldehyde in an acid urine.

hexavalent (ˌheksə'vaylənt) having a valency of six.

hexokinase (ˌheksoh'kienayz) an enzyme that catalyses the transfer of a high-energy phosphate group of a donor to D-glucose, producing D-glucose-6-phosphate.

hexosamine (hek'sohsəˌmeen) a nitrogenous sugar in which an amino group replaces a hydroxyl group.

hexose ('heksohs, -sohz) a monosaccharide containing six carbon atoms in a molecule.

hexosephosphate (ˌheksohs'fosfayt) an ester of glucose with phosphoric acid that aids in the absorption of sugars and is important in carbohydrate metabolism.

HF Hageman factor, or clotting factor XII.

Hf chemical symbol, *hafnium.*

Hg chemical symbol, *mercury* (L. *hydrargyrum*).

Hgb haemoglobin.

HGH human growth hormone.

HHNK hyperglycaemic hyperosmolar nonketotic coma.

5-HIAA 5-hydroxyindoleacetic acid.

hiatus (hie'aytəs) pl. *hiatus* [L.] a gap, cleft, or opening. adj. **hiatal.**

aortic h., h. aorticus the opening in the diaphragm through which the aorta and thoracic duct pass.

oesophageal h., h. oesophageus the opening in the diaphragm for the passage of the oesophagus and the vagus nerves.

h. hernia protrusion of any structure through the oesophageal hiatus of the diaphragm.

hibernation (ˌhiebə'nayshən) the dormant state in which certain animals pass the winter, marked by narcosis and by sharp reduction in body temperature and metabolism.

artificial h. a state of reduced metabolism, muscle relaxation, and a twilight sleep resembling narcosis, produced by controlled inhibition of the sympathetic nervous system and causing attenuation of the homeostatic reactions of the organism.

hibernoma (ˌhiebə'nohmə) a rare benign tumour made up of large polyhedral cells with a coarsely granular cytoplasm closely resembling fetal fat cells and occurring on the back or around the hips.

hiccough, hiccup ('hikup) spasmodic involuntary contraction of the diaphragm that results in uncontrolled breathing in of air; called also *singultus.* The peculiar noise of hiccups is produced by a beginning inspiration that is suddenly checked by closure of the glottis.

Hiccups may be due to a variety of causes, such as rapid eating or irritation in the digestive system or the respiratory system, or of the diaphragm muscle itself. Hiccups sometimes occur as a complication following some kinds of surgery, and in serious diseases such as uraemia and epidemic encephalitis. They may also have emotional causes. Hiccups are serious only when they persist for a long time; usually they stop after a few minutes.

Standard home remedies for hiccups include holding the breath, swallowing sugar or a bread crust, pulling the tongue forward, applications of cold to the back of the neck, simply sipping water slowly, and breathing into a paper bag. The paper bag device has the effect of cutting off the normal exchange of air with the surrounding atmosphere. The air in the bag, after a few breaths, will have an increasingly high carbon dioxide content, and so will the air in the lungs, and finally the blood. As a consequence, the automatic respiratory centres in the brain call for stronger and deeper breathing to get rid of the carbon dioxide. This frequently makes the contractions of the diaphragm more regular and eliminates the hiccups.

In extreme cases of prolonged hiccups sedative drugs or tranquillizers may be necessary.

Hicks contractions (hiks) Braxton Hicks contractions.

HIDA an imunodiacetic acid derivative; complexed with technetium-99m it is a radiopharmaceutical used in hepatobiliary imaging.

hidr(o)- word element. [Gr.] *sweat.*

hidradenitis (ˌhidradəˈnietis) inflammation of the sweat glands.

h. suppurativa a severe, chronic, recurrent suppurative infection of the apocrine sweat glands.

hidradenoid (hiˈdradəˌnoyd) resembling a sweat gland; having components resembling elements of a sweat gland.

hidradenoma (ˌhidradəˈnohmə) a general term for tumours of the skin, the components of which resemble epithelial elements of sweat glands; they may be nodular (solid) or papillary.

hidrocystoma (ˌhidrohsiˈstohmə) a retention cyst of a sweat gland.

hidropoiesis (ˌhidrohpoyˈeesis) the formation of sweat. adj. **hidropoietic.**

hidrorrhoea (ˌhidrəˈreeə) profuse perspiration.

hidroschesis (hiˈdroskisis) suppression of perspiration.

hidrosis (hiˈdrohsis) the excretion of sweat.

hidrotic (hiˈdrotik) pertaining to, characterized by, or causing sweating.

hieralgia (ˌhieəˈralji·ə) pain in the sacrum.

hierolisthesis (ˌhieə·rohlisˈtheesis) displacement of the sacrum.

Higginson's syringe (ˈhiginsənz) a rubber catheter with a bulb in the centre which, when compressed, aspirates fluid from one end and forces it through a nozzle at the other, flow being maintained in one direction only by valves. Originally designed in leather for arm-to-arm blood transfusion; now used for introducing fluid into the rectum when performing an enema.

high-altitude sickness (hieˈaltityood) the condition resulting from difficulty in adjusting to diminished oxygen pressure at high altitudes. It may take the form of mountain sickness, high-altitude pulmonary oedema, or cerebral oedema.

high blood pressure (hie) a disorder of the circulatory system marked by persistently excessive pressure of the blood against the walls of the arteries (see also HYPERTENSION).

hilitis (hieˈlietis) inflammation of a hilus.

hillock (ˈhilək) a small prominence or elevation.

hilum (ˈhieləm) hilus.

hilus (ˈhieləs) pl. *hili* [L.] a depression or pit on an organ, giving entrance and exit to vessels and nerves. adj. **hilar.**

hindbrain (ˈhiendˌbrayn) the rhombencephalon, the portion of the brain developed from the most caudal of the three primary brain vesicles of the early embryo, comprising the metencephalon and myelencephalon.

hindfoot (ˈhiendˌfuht) the posterior portion of the foot, comprising the region of the talus and calcaneus.

hindgut (ˈhiendˌgut) a pocket formed beneath the caudal portion of the developing embryo, which develops into the distal portion of the small intestine, the colon and the rectum.

hip (hip) 1. the region of the body at the articulation of the femur and the innominate bone at the base of the lower trunk. These bones meet at the hip joint. Called also *coxa.* 2. loosely, the hip joint.

At each hip joint, the smooth, rounded head of the femur fits into the deeply recessed socket (the acetabulum) in the innominate bone, which comprises the ilium, ischium, and pubis. The joint is covered by a tough, flexible protective capsule and is heavily reinforced by strong ligaments that stretch across the joint.

As in most joints, the ends of the bones, where they meet at the hip joint, are covered with a layer of cartilage that reduces friction and absorbs shock. The synovial membrane lines the socket and lubricates the joint with synovia. Cushioning is provided by small fluid-filled sacs, or bursae.

FRACTURE AND DISLOCATION. The hip is much more susceptible to fracture than to dislocation. The hip joint is very stable and possesses great strength; severe injury is necessary to dislocate it and it will often fracture first. Hip fractures usually involve the neck or the base of the neck of the femur. A fracture usually causes the leg to appear shortened, with the foot pointing outward; usually the patient is unable to raise his leg and there is pain, swelling, and discoloration around the joint. The diagnosis is confirmed by radiological examination.

A wrench of considerable force, such as may occur in a car accident, in skiing, or in football, may dislocate the hip. Dislocation usually tears the capsule and ligaments that bind the joint together, and fragments may be torn from the rim of the hip socket.

First-aid measures are the same for a fractured hip as for a dislocated hip. In either case the injured person will probably not be able to lift his heel while lying on his back. If the patient must be moved, his legs should be gently brought together and tied at the thigh and ankle; the uninjured leg is used as a splint. If possible, a stretcher should be improvised for carrying him.

CONGENITAL DISLOCATION. Congenital dislocation of the hip occurs more frequently in females than in males. It may not be evident until the child starts to walk, when it causes limping or waddling. It is important that the condition be recognized before the child does much walking on the weakened joint. Early treatment can cure the condition, but neglect for a year or two may make reconstruction of the hip joint necessary.

OTHER HIP DISORDERS. Like most joints, the hip may be affected by ARTHRITIS and by BURSITIS, or inflammation of the bursae, which lie outside the joint.

A condition known as slipped upper femoral epiphysis occasionally occurs in growing children. It is most commonly seen in adolescent boys who are overweight or who have grown in height at an excessive rate. Hormonal factors seem to play an important part in the aetiology. The epiphysis is a cartilaginous disc found at the heads of long bones throughout the body; it is the site at which bone growth takes place and it becomes permanently united to the bone only when growth has finished. There is an epiphyseal line at the top of the femur where the head of the bone joins its neck. Injury to the femur of a child, or its subjection to unusual pressure, may cause the epiphysis to slip out of alignment. This produces shortening of the leg, limitation of movement of the hip, and pain. If the condition is diagnosed early enough it may be corrected with splints and plaster casts.

h. bone the innominate bone, which comprises the ilium, ischium, and pubis.

h. joint the ball and socket joint formed between the head of the femur and the acetabulum of the innominate bone.

total h. replacement replacement of the femoral head and acetabulum with prostheses that are cemented into the bone; called also *total hip arthroplasty*. The procedure is done to replace a severely damaged arthritic hip joint.

HIPE Hospital Inpatient Enquiry.

Hippel's disease ('hip'lz) von Hippel's disease.

hippocampus (ˌhipoh'kampəs) pl. *hippocampi* [L.] a curved elevation on the floor of the inferior horn of the lateral ventricle; it is an important functional component of the limbic system.

h. major hippocampus.

h. minor the lower of two medial elevations in the lateral cerebral ventricle (see also CALCAR AVIS).

Hippocrates (hi'pokrəˌteez) (late 5th century BC) 'Father of Medicine'. Son of a priest-physician, he was born on the Greek island of Cos. By stressing that there is a natural cause for disease he did much to dissociate the care of the sick from the influence of magic and superstition. His carefully kept records of treatment and solicitous observation of the ill provided a foundation for clinical medicine in the case report; and by reporting also unsuccessful methods of treatment he anticipated the modern scientific attitude. The way for the professional nurse was prepared by his emphasis on the importance of skilled bedside care, and his bedside example demonstrated the value of clinical instruction. A moral code for medicine has been established by his ideals of ethical conduct and practice as embodied in the Hippocratic Oath.

hippuria (hi'pyooə·ri·ə) an excess of hippuric acid in urine.

hippuric acid (hi'pyooə·rik) a compound formed by conjugation of benzoic acid and glycine; it occurs in the urine of herbivorous animals, rarely in human urine.

hippus ('hipəs) abnormal exaggeration of the rhythmic contraction and dilation of the pupil, independent of changes in illumination or in fixation of the eyes.

hirci ('hərsie) plural of *hircus*. [L.] the hairs growing in the axilla.

hircus ('hərkəs) pl. *hirci* [L.] one of the hairs growing in the axilla.

Hirschsprung's disease ('hərshspruhngz) congenital absence of the parasympathetic nerve ganglia in the anorectum or proximal rectum, resulting in the absence of peristalsis in the affected portion of the colon and a consequent massive enlargement of the colon, constipation, and obstruction. Severe cases require surgery. Called also *aganglionic megacolon* and *congenital megacolon*.

hirsute ('hərsyoot) shaggy; hairy.

hirsuties, hirsutism (hər'syooshiˌeez; 'hərsyooˌtizəm) abnormal hairiness, especially in women.

hirudicide (hi'roodiˌsied) an agent that is destructive to leeches.

hirudin (hi'roodin) the active principle of the buccal secretion of leeches; it prevents clotting of the blood.

Hirudo (hi'roodoh) a genus of leeches.

H. medicinalis the medical leech.

His's bundle ('hiziz) a band of atypical cardiac muscle fibres connecting the atria with the ventricles of the heart; called also *atrioventricular bundle*.

His's disease trench fever; called also *His–Werner disease*.

hist(io)(o)- word element. [Gr.] *tissue*.

histaminaemia (ˌhistəmi'neemi·ə) histamine in the blood.

histaminase (hi'stamiˌnayz) an enzyme that inactivates histamine.

histamine ('histəmeen) an amine, $C_5H_9N_3$, produced by decarboxylation of histidine, found in all body tissues. adj. **histaminic.** It induces capillary dilation,

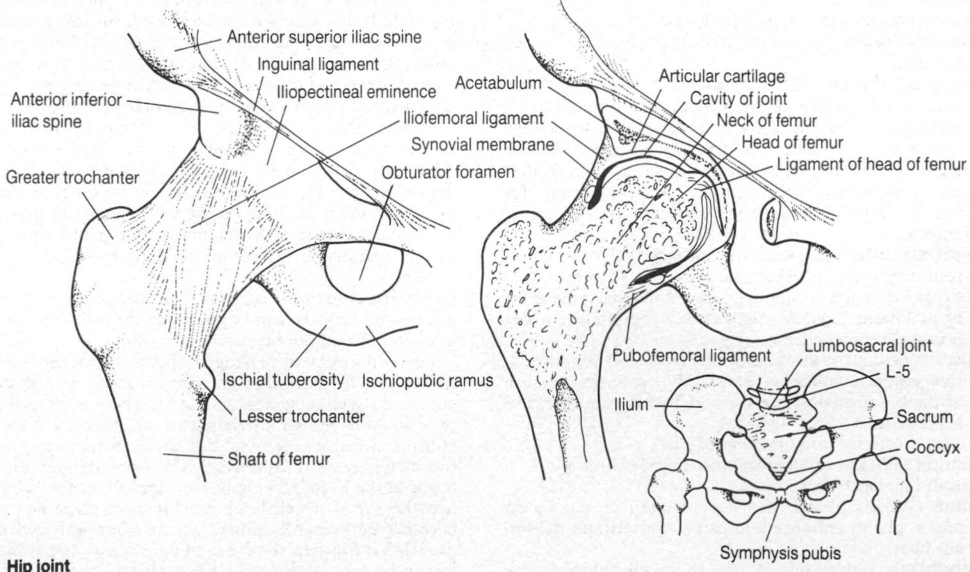

Hip joint

which increases capillary permeability and lowers blood pressure; contraction of most smooth muscle tissue; increased gastric acid secretion; and acceleration of the heart rate. It is also a mediator of immediate hypersensitivity. There are two types of cellular receptors of histamine: H_1 receptors, which mediate contraction of smooth muscle and capillary dilation; and H_2 receptors, which mediate acceleration of heart rate and promotion of gastric acid secretion. Both H_1 and H_2 receptors mediate the contraction of vascular smooth muscle. Histamine may also be a neurotransmitter in the central nervous system. It is used as a diagnostic aid in testing gastric secretion and in the diagnosis of phaeochromocytoma.

Although histamine was discovered in 1909, its role is still not fully understood. Histamine normally functions as a stimulant to the production of gastric juice. It also dilates the small blood vessels, as part of the regular adaptation of the body to changing inner and exterior conditions. An excess of histamine can dilate blood vessels to the extent that extravasation occurs. This appears as the reddening and swelling seen in inflammation. Continued extravasation causes oedema. Histamine also constricts bronchial smooth muscle.

In certain people, histamine may bring on a severe form of headache, known as histaminic cephalalgia. It usually occurs during sleep, and is caused by release of histamine into the system. It is treated by desensitizing the patient to histamine.

An excess of histamine apparently is released when the body comes in contact with certain substances to which it is sensitive. This excess histamine is believed to be the final cause of hay fever, urticaria, and most other allergies, as well as certain stomach upsets and some headaches. It is possible that histamine also causes vomiting, diarrhoea, and muscular spasm, since these reactions are seen in animals injected with histamine. The fact that a person suffering from shock has large amounts of histamine in the blood suggests that histamine also plays a role in this condition, but its presence may be an incidental side-effect.

There are two types of histamine antagonists that act at either the H_1 or the H_2 receptors. Drugs such as diphenhydramine and chlorpheniramine are referred to as ANTIHISTAMINES or H_1-blockers; they block the effects of histamine on vascular, bronchial, and gastrointestinal smooth muscle and on capillary permeability. They are used for relief of allergic and gastrointestinal disorders and in over-the-counter cold medicines. Drugs such as cimetidine are referred to as H_2-blockers; they block the stimulation of gastric acid secretion and are used to treat peptic ULCER.

histaminergic (ˌhistəmiˈnərjik) pertaining to the effects of histamine at histamine receptors of target tissues.

histidase (ˈhistiˌdayz) an enzyme of the liver that converts histidine to urocanic acid.

histidinaemia (ˌhistidiˈneemi·ə) a hereditary metabolic defect marked by excessive histidine in the blood and urine due to deficient histidase activity; many affected persons show mild mental handicap and disordered speech development.

histidine (ˈhistiˌdeen) a naturally occurring amino acid, essential for optimal growth of infants; its decarboxylation results in formation of histamine.

histidinuria (ˌhistidiˈnyooə·ri·ə) an excess of histidine in the urine (see also HISTIDINAEMIA).

histiocyte (ˈhistiohˌsiet) a large phagocytic interstitial cell of the reticuloendothelial system; a macrophage. adj. **histiocytic.**

histiocytoma (ˌhistiohsieˈtohmə) a tumour containing histiocytes.

histiocytosis (ˌhistiohsieˈtohsis) a condition marked by the abnormal appearance of histiocytes in the blood.

lipid h. Niemann–Pick disease.

h. X a generic term embracing eosinophilic granuloma, Letterer–Siwe disease, and Hand–Schüller–Christian disease.

histiogenic (ˌhistiohˈjenik) formed by the tissues.

histioid (ˈhistiˌoyd) histoid.

histoblast (ˈhistohˌblast) a tissue-forming cell.

histochemistry (ˌhistohˈkemistree) that branch of histology that deals with the identification of chemical components in cells and tissues.

histoclinical (ˌhistohˈklinikˈl) combining histological and clinical evaluation.

histocompatibility (ˌhistohkəmˌpatəˈbilitee) the quality of a cellular or tissue graft enabling it to be accepted and functional when transplanted to another organism. adj. **histocompatible.**

h. genes genes that determine the specificity of tissue antigenicity and thus the compatibility of donor and recipient in tissue transplantation (see HLA).

histodialysis (ˌhistohdieˈaləsis) disintegration or breaking down of tissue.

histodifferentiation (ˌhistohˌdifəˌrenshiˈayshən) the acquisition of tissue characteristics by cell groups during development.

histogenesis (ˌhistohˈjenəsis) differentiation of cells into the specialized tissues forming the various organs and parts of the body.

histogram (ˈhistəˌgram) a graph in which values found in a statistical study are represented by lines or symbols placed horizontally or vertically, to indicate frequency distribution.

histoid (ˈhistoyd) 1. developed from one kind of tissue. 2. resembling one of the tissues of the body.

histoincompatibility (ˌhistohˌinkəmˌpatəˈbilitee) the quality of a cellular or tissue graft preventing its acceptance or functioning when transplanted to another organism; said of the relationship between the genotypes (histocompatibility genes) of donor and host in which a graft generally will be rejected. adj. **histoincompatible.**

histokinesis (ˌhistohkiˈneesis) movement in the tissues of the body.

histological MLSO (ˌhistəˈlojikˈl) an allied health professional trained in tissue processing techniques (fixation, dehydration, embedding, sectioning, routine and special staining, and mounting of tissue specimens), and also in histology and histochemistry.

histologist (hiˈstoləjist) one who specializes in histology.

histology (hiˈstoləjee) the visualization of the minute structure, composition, and function of tissues and organs. adj. **histological.**

pathological h. the science of diseased tissues.

histolysis (hiˈstolisis) breaking down of tissues. adj. **histolytic.**

histoma (hiˈstohmə) any tissue tumour.

histone (ˈhistohn) a simple protein, soluble in water and insoluble in dilute ammonia, found combined as salts with acidic substances, such as nucleic acids or the globin of haemoglobin.

histonuria (ˌhistəˈnyooə·ri·ə) histone in the urine.

histopathology (ˌhistohpəˈtholəjee) pathological histology.

histophysiology (ˌhistohˌfiziˈoləjee) the correlation of function with the microscopic structures of cells and tissues.

Histoplasma (ˌhistohˈplazmə) a genus of fungi.

H. capsulatum a species of pathogenic fungi that cause infection (histoplasmosis) in man.

histoplasmin (ˌhistoh'plazmin) a preparation of growth products of *Histoplasma capsulatum*, injected intracutaneously as a test for histoplasmosis.

histoplasmoma (ˌhistohplaz'mohmə) a rounded granulomatous density of the lung due to infection with *Histoplasma capsulatum*; seen radiographically as a coin-shaped lesion.

histoplasmosis (ˌhistohplaz'mohsis) a systemic fungal disease caused by inhalation of dust contaminated by *Histoplasma capsulatum*. Histoplasmosis is worldwide in distribution. It is not transmitted from one person to another. The disease begins in the lungs and may spread to other organs. Infection is usually asymptomatic, but may cause acute pneumonia, or disseminated reticuloendothelial hyperplasia with hepatosplenomegaly and anaemia, or an influenza-like illness with joint effusion and erythema nodosum. Reactivated infection involves the lungs, meninges, heart, peritoneum, and adrenals in that order of frequency. Radiologically the lungs may resemble tuberculous lungs.

The specific drug used in the treatment of histoplasmosis is amphotericin, an antifungal antibiotic. In extreme cases surgery may be necessary to remove the affected portions of the lung.

ocular h. disseminated choroiditis resulting in scars in the periphery of the fundus near the optic nerve, and characteristic disciform macular lesions; *Histoplasma capsulatum* is implicated strongly as the causative agent.

historical cohort study (his'torik'l) an epidemiological study of a cohort or group of persons making use of data collected in the past. Also called a retrospective cohort study (see also INCIDENCE STUDY).

historrhexis (ˌhistə'reksis) the breaking up of tissue.

histotechnologist (ˌhistohtek'noləjist) a medical technologist that specializes in the preparation of tissue specimens.

histothrombin (ˌhistohˌthrombin) thrombin derived from connective tissue.

histotoxic (ˌhistoh'toksik) poisonous to tissue.

histotroph ('histohˌtrohf) the sum total of nutritive material derived from maternal tissue other than the blood, utilized by the early embryo.

histotrophic (ˌhistoh'trofik) 1. encouraging formation of tissue. 2. pertaining to histotroph.

histotropic (ˌhistoh'tropik) having affinity for tissue cells.

histrionism ('histri·ə'nizəm) a morbid or hysterical adoption of an exaggerated manner and gestures. adj. **histrionic**.

HIV human immunodeficiency virus. See AIDS.

HLA human leukocyte antigen; the human major histocompatibility complex (MHC), located on the short arm of chromosome 6. Five loci have been identified, designated HLA-A, HLA-B, HLA-C, HLA-D, and HLA-DR (D related), each with multiple alleles, designated by numerals (e.g., HLA-B5). Provisionally identified alleles are designated by the letter *w* (e.g., HLA-Bw22).

There are two types of MHC antigen, Class I and Class II, which differ in structure and are expressed on different cell types. The HLA-A, -B, and -C loci gene products are examples of Class I antigens and occur on the surface of almost all normal nucleated cells, although very low levels are found on liver, muscle and nerve cells and some tumours are negative. They are the most important antigens in transplant rejection, when donor and recipient HLA antigens do not match. The HLA-A, -B, and -C antigens are recognized by killer T-lymphocytes that lyse the target cells. They are also involved in the cell-mediated lysis of virus-infected cells.

The HLA-D and -DR loci gene products are examples of Class II antigens and are cell surface antigens of B-lymphocytes and macrophages. They are involved in antigen presentation and other forms of cooperation between immunocompetent cells and also in the stimulation of transplant rejection.

Transplants and platelet and leukocyte transfusions are least likely to be rejected by the recipient when the donor and recipient are HLA-identical siblings and close HLA compatibility is essential for renal and bone marrow transplants. For most platelet and granulocyte transfusions an ABO blood group compatible unrelated donor is acceptable.

A statistical association has been shown between certain HLA antigens and a number of diseases (e.g., HLA-B27 and ankylosing spondylitis). Such an association may be due to a genetic defect at a locus closely linked to the HLA locus, such as the immune response (Ir) genes or certain complement components (C2, C4, factor B), or to a defect in cell-mediated cytotoxicity or another mechanism that involves the HLA antigens.

HMSO Her Majesty's Stationery Office.

Ho chemical symbol, *holmium*.

hoarseness ('hawsnəs) a rough quality of the voice.

Hodgkin's disease ('hojkinz) a primary lymph node neoplastic disease characterized by painless, progressive enlargement of the lymph nodes, spleen, and lymphoid tissues generally, which often begins in a cervical node on the side of the neck and spreads through the body. Called also *malignant granuloma* and *lymphogranuloma*.

Hodgkin's disease, along with leukaemias and lymphomas, accounts for approximately 6% of malignancies in the UK. The disease is unusual in that there are two peaks of the incidence curve, one between 15 and 35 years of age and the other between 55 and 75. Chemotherapy and supervoltage radiation therapy have increased the survival rate, which, with early diagnosis, approaches 40% at five years for Stage 1 disease.

SYMPTOMS. The first sign of the disease usually is an enlargement of a cervical node. Occasionally there may be swelling of nodes on both sides of the neck or enlargement of nodes elsewhere in the body. Severe itching is often an early sign of the disorder.

As Hodgkin's disease progresses, it is usually marked by sweating, weakness, fever, and loss of weight and appetite. It spreads through the lymphatic system, involving other lymph nodes elsewhere in the body as well as the spleen, liver, and bone marrow. The lymph nodes and the spleen and liver may swell, and by obstructing other organs may cause coughing, breathlessness, or enlargement of the abdomen. The patient often becomes anaemic, and because of blood changes the body becomes less able to combat infections.

The disease is classified according to stages of development of the malignancy. These stages are helpful in establishing the prognosis and prescribing treatment. In Stage I only one localized lymph node region is involved. Stage IE indicates involvement of a single extralymphatic organ. Stage II indicates two or more involved nodes on the same side of the diaphragm. Stage IIE indicates involvement of an extralymphatic organ and one or more nodes on the same side of the diaphragm. Stage IIS designates splenic involvement with localization below the diaphragm. In Stage III there is disease on both sides of the diaphragm, sometimes with splenic involvement (IIIS) or extralymphatic organ involvement (IIIE), or both. In Stage IV there is diffuse involvement of one or more extralymphatic organs or tissues with or without associated lymph node involvement.

DIAGNOSIS. The diagnosis of Hodgkin's disease requires the histological identification of the characteristic malignant cell of the disease, the Reed–Sternberg cell. The accepted histopathological classification distinguishes four different disease patterns: lymphocyte predominance, mixed cellularity, lymphocyte depletion, and nodular sclerosis. The evaluation required for staging includes a history and physical examination; chest x-rays and lower extremity lymphangiography; laboratory tests, including a complete blood count, serum alkaline phosphatase, and liver and kidney function tests; and a surgical lymph node biopsy. Osseous involvement is evaluated with bone marrow biopsy and bone scans. The evaluation of abdominal involvement may require exploratory laparotomy and splenectomy.

TREATMENT. If the disease is localized (Stages IA, IIA, or IIIA), the treatment of choice is radiation of the affected nodules using a cobalt machine or a linear accelerator capable of delivering a high dose of radiation deep into the tissues. Chemotherapy is recommended for patients with systemic involvement (Stages IB, IIB, and IIIB). The chemotherapeutic agents are administered in combination and intermittently so that there is a synergistic cytotoxic effect without overlapping toxicities. Drugs are chosen according to their effect on different phases of their growth and proliferation (see also ANTINEOPLASTIC agents).

Hodgson's disease ('hojsənz) aneurysmal dilation of the proximal part of the aorta.

hodoneuromere (ˌhodoh'nyooə·rəˌmiə) a segment of the embryonic trunk with its pair of nerves and their branches.

Hoffmann's sign ('hofmənz) 1. increased mechanical irritability of the sensory nerves in tetany; the ulnar nerve is usually tested. 2. a sudden nipping of the nail of the index, middle, or ring finger produces flexion of the terminal phalanx of the thumb and of the second and third phalanx of some other finger; called also *digital reflex*.

hol(o)- word element. [Gr.] *entire*, *whole*.

holandric (ho'landrik) inherited exclusively through the male descent; transmitted through genes located on the Y chromosome.

holergasia (ˌholə'gayzi·ə) a psychiatric disorder involving the entire personality. adj. **holergastic**.

holism ('hohlizəm) a philosophy in which the person is considered as a functioning whole rather than as a composite of several systems.

holistic (hoh'listik) pertaining to totality, or to the whole. In recent years, there has been a growing interest in the concept of holistic health and the notion that the physical, mental, social, and spiritual aspects of a person's life must be viewed as an integrated whole. This leads to a broader concept of patient care in which the patient's physical, emotional and social needs are recognized as inter-dependent and he is treated as a complete person rather than as the sum of his diseases or his individual needs.

Hollander test ('holəndə) a gastric function test that measures the response of gastric secretory cells to an insulin-induced hypoglycaemia.

Hollenhorst plaques (ˌholənhorst 'plahks) atheromatous emboli containing cholesterol crystals in the retinal arterioles, a sign of impending serious cardiovascular disease.

Holmgren test ('hohmgren) test for detection of imperfect perception of colour, based on matching various strands of yarn.

holmium ('holmi·əm) a chemical element, atomic number 67, atomic weight 164.930, symbol Ho. See table of elements in Appendix 2.

holoacardius (ˌholoh·ay'kahdi·əs) an unequal twin fetus in which the heart is entirely absent.

holoblastic (ˌholə'blastik) undergoing cleavage in which the entire ovum participates; completely dividing.

holocrine ('holəkrin) wholly secretory: denoting that type of glandular secretion in which the entire secreting cell, along with its accumulated secretion, forms the secreted matter of the gland, as in the sebaceous glands; cf. apocrine and merocrine.

holodiastolic (ˌholohˌdieə'stolik) pertaining to the entire diastole.

holoendemic (ˌholoh·en'demik) affecting practically all the residents of a particular region.

holoenzyme (ˌholoh'enziem) the active compound formed by combination of a coenzyme and an apoenzyme.

holography (ho'logrəfee) a method of recording 3-dimensional images in a 2-dimensional form. A laser beam is usually used to reflect light from an object on to photographic film. After exposure and development the film (or hologram) is illuminated with a laser and the 3-dimensional image can be seen.

hologynic (ˌholoh'jienik) inherited exclusively through the female descent; transmitted through genes located on attached X chromosomes.

holoprosencephaly (ˌholohˌprosen'kefəlee, -'sef-) developmental failure of cleavage of the prosencephalon with a deficit in midline facial development and with cyclopia in the severe form; sometimes due to trisomy 13–15.

holorachischisis (ˌholohrə'kiskisis) fissure of the entire vertebral column with prolapse of the spinal cord.

holosystolic (ˌholohsi'stolik) pertaining to the entire systole.

Holthouse's hernia ('hohlt·howziz) an inguinal hernia that has turned outward into the groin.

homaluria (ˌhomə'lyooə·ri·ə) production and excretion of urine at a normal, even rate.

Homan's sign ('hohmənz) discomfort behind the knee on forced dorsiflexion of the foot; a sign of thrombosis in the leg.

homatropine (hoh'matrəˌpin) an anticholinergic alkaloid obtained by the condensation of tropine and mandelic acid having anticholinergic effects similar to but weaker than those of atropine; used to produce parasympathetic blockade and as a mydriatic.

homeo- word element. [Gr.] *similar*, *same*, *unchanging*. Sometimes spelled *homoeo-*.

homeomorphous, homoeomorphous (ˌhohmi·ə'mawfəs, ˌhom-) of like form and structure.

homeopathy, homoeopathy (ˌhohmi'opəthee, ˌhom-) a system of therapeutics founded by Samuel Hahnemann (1755–1843) in which diseases are treated by drugs that are capable of producing in healthy persons symptoms like those of the disease to be treated, the drug being administered in minute doses. adj. **hom(o)eopathic**.

homeoplasia, homoeoplasia (ˌhohmioh'playzi·ə, ˌhom-) formation of new tissue like that normal to the part. adj. **hom(o)eoplastic**.

homeostasis, homoeostasis (ˌhohmioh'stayis, ˌhom-) a tendency of biological systems to maintain stability while continually adjusting to conditions that are optimal for survival. adj. **hom(o)eostatic**.

Homeostatic mechanisms are necessary for the body to regain its balance when disease or injury occurs and to maintain that balance if it is to remain healthy. Many of the medications and treatments prescribed during illness are given to help preserve this dynamic equilibrium within the body. Without successful physiological homeostasis, in which relatively constant conditions are maintained in the internal environment, the body cannot survive.

It is through homeostatic mechanisms that body temperature is kept within normal range, the osmotic pressure of the blood and its hydrogen ion concentration (pH) is kept within strict limits, nutrients are supplied to cells as needed, and waste products are removed before they accumulate and reach toxic levels of concentration. These are but a few examples of the thousands of homeostatic control systems within the body. Some of these systems operate within the cell and others operate within an aggregate of cells (organs) to control the complex interrelationships among the various organs.

The two basic types of homeostatic regulators are: (1) *negative feedback* controls, in which the system continuously adjusts and takes corrective action in order to maintain a factor within normal range; and (2) *on-off switches*, in which a response either does or does not occur. Hormonal secretions from the ENDOCRINE GLANDS are typically regulated by closed-loop FEEDBACK control systems, while responses in the nervous system are mainly of the on-off type.

Feedback controls are those in which some product or factor, the 'output', of a system acts to regulate some process, the 'input', that influences the production of that product. In *negative feedback* the output is maintained at some level, the 'setpoint'. In some systems the setpoint is fixed, in others, like the regulation of body temperature, the setpoint is controlled by factors outside the negative feedback loop. Any deviation of the output from the setpoint is fed back to the input where it has a negative effect and moves the output in the opposite direction until it returns to the setpoint. An example is the regulation of extracellular fluid carbon dioxide concentration, the output, which affects pulmonary ventilation, the input. High CO_2 concentration causes an increase in pulmonary ventilation which lowers the CO_2 concentration.

Homeostatic feedback mechanisms tend to be slower than voluntary responses and so there is always a lag between stimulus and response in homeostasis. The nerve fibres reserved for the processes of homeostasis have a considerably slower rate of transmission than do voluntary nerve fibres, and many of the messages of homeostasis are carried by such chemical messengers as hormones and carbon dioxide in the blood.

Because of the lag, the adjustments made through homeostatic mechanisms are not always perfect. If the lag becomes too great, the compensating mechanisms may be too extreme or occur out of phase, and produce 'overshoots' of increasing magnitude each time the input enters and goes through the circuit of stimulus–response–effect. This situation can bring about collapse of the system.

Positive feedback leads to instability which can produce serious and even fatal results. In this situation the initiating stimulus produces a condition similar to the one already existing. In this way the mechanism enters a vicious and sometimes deadly cycle. A mild degree of positive feedback can be overcome by the normal negative feedback control systems of the body. If these systems fail, however, death will ensue. In some instances positive feedback and overshoots can result in overproduction of a normal body chemical and bring about such conditions as allergies, epilepsy, cirrhosis of the liver, and nephritis. In a malignancy the homeostatic mechanism has gone awry and inhibitors of cell division do not function at the point at which cell division should cease; thus the cells continue to divide and produce new growth.

homeotherapy, homoeotherapy (ˌhohmioh'therəpee, ˌhom-) treatment with a substance with effects similar to the causative agent of the disease.

homeotherm, homoeotherm ('hohmioh,thərm, ˌhom-) a warm-blooded animal, whose heat-regulating mechanism maintains a constant body temperature in spite of the environment. adj. **hom(o)eothermic, hom(o)eothermal**. Called also *homoiotherm, homotherm*.

homeothermy, homoeothermy (ˌhohmioh'thərmee, ˌhom-) maintenance of a constant body temperature despite variation in environmental temperature. Called also *homoiothermy, homothermy*.

homeotypical, homoeotypical (ˌhohmioh'tipik'l, ˌhom-) resembling the normal or usual type.

homicide ('homi,sied) the killing of a human being.

culpable h. covers murder (malice aforethought), manslaughter (without malice aforethought), causing death by reckless driving, and infanticide.

nonculpable h. covers justifiable homicide (e.g. lawful execution) and excusable homicide (misadventure or accident). See MCNAUGHTEN'S RULES.

Homo ('hohmoh, 'homo) [L.] the genus of primates containing the single living species *H. sapiens* (man).

homo- 1. word element. [Gr.] *same, similar*. 2. chemical prefix indicating the addition of one CH_2 group to the main compound.

homocystine (ˌhomoh'sisteen, ˌhohm-) a homologue of cystine which results from demethylation of methionine.

homocystinuria (ˌhomoh,sisti'nyooə·ri·ə, ˌhohm-) an inborn error of sulphur amino acid metabolism due to lack of the enzyme cystathionine synthase; it is characterized by homocystine in the urine, mental handicap, hepatomegaly, ectopia lentis, and cardiovascular and skeletal disorders.

homocytotropic (ˌhomoh,sietə'tropik, ˌhohm-) having an affinity for cells of individuals of the same species.

homodromous (ho'modrəməs) moving or acting in the same or in the usual direction.

homoeo- for words beginning thus, see those beginning *homeo-*.

homogametic (ˌhomohgə'metik, ˌhohm-) having only one kind of gamete with respect to the sex chromosomes, as in the human female.

homogenate (ho'moji,nayt) material obtained by homogenization.

homogeneity (ˌhoməjə'neeətee, ˌhohm-, -'nay-) the state of being homogeneous.

homogeneous (ˌhomə'jeeni·əs) of uniform quality, composition, or structure.

homogenesis (ˌhomə'jenəsis, ˌhohm-) reproduction by the same process in each generation.

homogenic (ˌhomə'jenik, ˌhohm-) homozygous.

homogenicity (ˌhoməjə'nisitee, ˌhohm-) homogeneity.

homogenize (ho'mojə,niez) to convert into material that is of uniform quality or consistency throughout; to render homogeneous.

homogenous (ho'mojənəs) derived from the same source.

homogentisic acid (ˌhomohjen'tisik, ˌhohm-) 2,5-dihydroxyphenyl acetic acid, an intermediate product in the metabolism of tyrosine and phenylalanine, excreted in the urine in an inborn error of metabolism (PHENYLKETONURIA).

homograft ('homə,grahft, 'homoh-) a graft of tissue transplanted between individuals of the same species, but of a different genotype; an allograft.

homoiotherm (hə'moyoh,thərm) see HOMEOTHERM.

homoiothermy (hə'moyoh,thərmee) see HOMEOTHERMY.

homolateral (ˌhomə'latə·rəl, ˌhohmoh-) ipsilateral; pertaining to or situated on the same side.

homologous (hə'moləgəs) 1. corresponding in structure, position, origin, etc. 2. derived from an animal of the same species but of different genotype; allogeneic.

homologue ('homəˌlog) 1. any homologous organ or part. 2. in chemistry, one of a series of compounds distinguished by addition of $-CH_2$ group in successive members.

homology (hə'moləjee, hohm-) the state of being homologous.

homonomous (hə'monəməs) subject to the same laws; in biology, subject to the same laws of growth or developed along the same line.

homonymous (hə'moniməs) 1. having the same or corresponding sound or name. 2. standing in the same relation.

homophilic (ˌhomə'filik, ˌhohm-) reacting only with specific antigen.

homophobia (ˌhomoh'fohbiə, hohm-) an irrational fear of homosexuality.

homoplastic (ˌhomoh'plastik, ˌhohm-) 1. pertaining to homoplasty. 2. denoting organs or parts, as the wings of birds and insects, that resemble one another in structure and function but not in origin or development.

homoplasty ('homohˌplastee, 'hohm-) 1. operative replacement of lost parts or tissues by similar parts from another individual of the same species. 2. similarity between organs or their parts not due to common ancestry.

homorganic (ˌhomaw'ganik) produced by the same or by homologous organs.

homosexual (ˌhomoh'seksyooəl, ˌhohm-) 1. sexually and emotionally oriented toward persons of the same sex. 2. a homosexual individual.

homosexual panic (ˌhomoh'seksyooəl, ˌhohm-) an acute severe episode of anxiety, due to unconscious conflicts involving gender identity, in which there is the fear or delusional conviction that the person is thought by others to be a homosexual or is in danger of sexual attack by a person of the same sex, often accompanied by agitation, guilt, hallucinations, or depression.

homosexuality (ˌhomohˌseksyoo'alitee, ˌhohm-) sexual and emotional orientation toward persons of the same sex.

homotherm ('homohˌthərm, 'hohm-) see HOMEOTHERM.

homothermy (ˌhomoh'thərmee, ˌhohm-) see HOMEOTHERMY.

homotopic (ˌhomə'topik, ˌhohm-) occurring at the same place upon the body.

homotype ('homəˌtiep, 'hohm-) a part having reversed symmetry with its mate, as the hand. adj. **homotypic**.

homozygosis (ˌhomohzie'gohsis, ˌhohmə-) the formation of a zygote by the union of gametes that have one or more identical alleles.

homozygosity (ˌhomohzie'gositee, ˌhohm-) the state of having identical alleles in regard to a given character or characters. adj. **homozygous**.

homozygote (ˌhomoh'ziegoht, ˌhohm-) an individual exhibiting homozygosity.

homunculus (hə'mungkyuhləs) 1. a dwarf without deformity or disproportion of parts. 2. a graphical representation of motor or sensory function of the strip of cortex anterior to the central fissure. The feet of the homunculus are located in the area of the longitudinal fissure and the head at the opposite end. The size of different parts of the homunculus are drawn in proportion to the amount of cortex serving each part; thus the hands and lips are disproportionately large in the motor homunculus (see accompanying illustration).

hookworm ('huhkˌwərm) a parasitic roundworm that enters the human body through the skin and migrates to the intestines, where it attaches itself to the intestinal wall and sucks blood from it for nourishment. The infection is found in temperate regions where conditions are very insanitary and in many parts of the tropics and subtropics. There are two main species: *Ancylostoma duodenale* and *Necator americanus*.

Hookworms are about one centimetre long with a muscular gullet for sucking blood. The female, slightly larger than the male, can lay more than 10,000 eggs a day, any one of which can hatch into a larva and invade the human body.

The larval hookworms enter the body by burrowing through the skin, usually that of the sole of the foot. The first sign of the disease may appear on the skin as small eruptions that develop into pus-filled blisters; this condition is sometimes called 'ground itch'.

Meanwhile the hookworms enter blood vessels and are carried by the blood into the lungs. They leave the lungs, propel themselves up the trachea, are swallowed and washed through the stomach and end up in the intestines. Here, if left alone, they will make a permanent home, using their host's body as a source of nourishment.

By the time they reach the intestines, about 6 weeks after they enter the body as larvae, the worms are full-grown adults. Each worm now attaches itself by its hooked teeth to the intestinal wall, where it sucks its host's blood by contraction and expansion of its gullet. If large numbers of worms are present, they can cause considerable loss of blood and severe anaemia. The symptoms include pallor and loss of energy; the appetite may increase.

The thousands of eggs laid every day by each female worm pass out of the body in the stool, in which they can easily be seen. If the stool is not properly disposed of, the larvae that hatch from the eggs may infect other persons.

TREATMENT AND PREVENTION. A nutritious, high-protein diet supplemented by iron is given to relieve anaemia and improve the health. Specific drugs include the anthelmintics mebendazole, bephenium hydroxynaphthoate, and tetrachloroethylene. When left untreated, hookworm can cause not only anaemia but also bronchial inflammation and, occasionally, stunting of growth, retardation of mental development, and even death.

Hookworm infection can be prevented by installation of sanitary toilets or, if that is not possible, by disposal of human faeces in deep holes so that the soil with which the human foot comes in contact is not contaminated. Shoes should be worn out of doors to protect the feet from infection.

hordeolum (hordi'ohləm) inflammation of one or more sebaceous glands of the eyelid; called also STY.

horizon (hə'riezən) a specific anatomical stage of embryonic development, of which 23 have been defined, beginning with the unicellular fertilized egg and ending 7 to 9 weeks later, with the beginning of the fetal stage.

hormesis (haw'meesis) stimulation by a subinhibitory concentration of a toxic substance.

hormonagogue (haw'mohnəˌgog) an agent that increases the production of hormones.

hormone ('hawmohn) a chemical transmitter substance produced by cells of the body and transported by the bloodstream to the cells and organs on which it has a specific regulatory effect. adj. **hormonal.** Hormones act as chemical messengers to body organs, stimulating certain life processes and retarding others. Growth, reproduction, control of metabolic processes, sexual attributes, and even mental conditions and personality traits are dependent on hormones.

Hormones are produced by various organs and body tissues, but mainly by the ENDOCRINE GLANDS, such as the pituitary, thyroid, and gonads (testes and ovaries). Each hormone has its unique function and its own chemical formula. After a hormone is discharged by its parent gland into the capillaries or the lymph, it may travel a circuitous path through the bloodstream to exert influence on cells, tissues, and organs (target organs) far removed from its site of origin.

One of the best-known hormones is INSULIN, a protein manufactured by the beta cells of the islets of Langerhans in the pancreas that is important in carbohydrate metabolism. Other important hormones are THYROXINE, an iodine-carrying amino acid produced by the thyroid gland; CORTISOL, a member of the steroid family from the adrenal glands; and the sex hormones, OESTROGEN from the ovaries and ANDROGEN from the testes.

Certain hormone substances can be synthesized in the laboratory for treatment of human disease. Animal hormones can also be used, as endocrine hormones are to some extent interchangeable among species. Extracts from the pancreas of cattle, for example, enabled diabetes sufferers to live normal lives even before the chemistry of insulin was fully understood.

Endocrine hormone synthesis and secretion is controlled and regulated by a closed-loop system. Negative FEEDBACK loops maintain optimal levels of each hormone in the body. If there are abnormally high levels of a hormone in the blood, feedback to the gland responsible for its production inhibits secretion. If there are abnormally low levels, the gland is stimulated to step up production and secretion. In this way a homeostatic balance is maintained (see also ENDOCRINE GLANDS).

Any significant imbalance in the kind and number of hormones produced by the glands must be corrected if the body and mind are to function properly. Extreme imbalances account for such forms of abnormal development as DWARFISM and CRETINISM.

adrenocortical h. any of the corticosteroids elaborated by the ADRENAL CORTEX, the major ones being the glucocorticoids and mineralocorticoids, and including some androgens, progesterone, and oestrogens.

adrenocorticotrophic h. a hormone elaborated by the anterior lobe of the PITUITARY GLAND that stimulates the action of the ADRENAL CORTEX (see also ACTH).

adrenomedullary h's substances secreted by the ADRENAL MEDULLA, including adrenaline and noradrenaline.

androgenic h's the masculinizing hormones, androsterone and testosterone.

antidiuretic h. (ADH) a polypeptide hormone from the posterior lobe of the pituitary gland that suppresses the secretion of urine; called also VASOPRESSIN.

corpus luteum h. progesterone.

cortical h. corticosteroid.

ectopic h's those secreted by tumours of nonendocrine tissues but having the same physiological effects as their normally produced counterparts. It is not known exactly how the synthesis and secretion of endocrine hormones from nonendocrine tissues occurs. Most of these tumours are derived from tissues that have a common embryonic origin with endocrine tissues. When the cells undergo neoplastic transformation, they can revert to a more primitive stage of development and begin to synthesize hormones. Examples of ectopic hormones and the kinds of tumours responsible for their production are shown in the accompanying table.

Ectopic hormones present serious problems for patients and add to the problems of caring for patients with certain kinds of neoplastic diseases. They do not respond to the feedback mechanisms that regulate normal hormonal production; hence, surgery and destruction of the tumorous tissue by radiation and chemotherapy are the treatments of choice (see accompanying table).

oestrogenic h's substances capable of producing certain biological effects, the most characteristic of which are the changes which occur in mammals at oestrus; the naturally occurring oestrogenic hormones are β-oestradiol, oestrone, and oestriol.

follicle-stimulating h. (FSH) one of the gonadotrophic hormones of the anterior pituitary, which stimulates the growth and maturity of graafian follicles in the ovary, and stimulates spermatogenesis in the male.

follicle-stimulating hormone releasing h. (FSH-RH) gonadotrophin releasing hormone.

follicle stimulating hormone and luteinizing hormone releasing h. (FSH/LH-RH) gonadotrophin releasing hormone.

gonatotrophic h. any hormone that has an influence on the gonads. Called also *gonadotrophin*.

gonadotrophin releasing h. (Gn-RH) a decapeptide hormone of the hypothalamus, which stimulates the release of follicle-stimulating hormone (FSH) and luteinizing hormone (LH) from the pituitary gland; used in the differential diagnosis of hypothalamic, pituitary, and gonadal dysfunction. Called also *follicle-stimulating hormone releasing hormone (FSH-RH)*, *luteinizing hormone releasing hormone (LH-RH)*, and *follicle stimulating hormone and luteinizing hormone releasing hormone (FSH/LH-RH)*.

growth h. (GH) a polypeptide hormone secreted by the anterior lobe of the PITUITARY GLAND that directly influences protein, carbohydrate, and lipid metabolism and controls the rate of skeletal and visceral growth. Called also *somatotrophin*.

growth hormone release inhibiting h. somatostatin.

growth hormone releasing h. (GH-RH) a hormone elaborated by the hypothalamus, which stimulates the release of growth hormone from the pituitary gland.

interstitial cell-stimulating h. luteinizing hormone.

lactation h., lactogenic h. prolactin.

luteinizing h. (LH) a gonadotrophic hormone of the anterior pituitary gland, acting with follicle-stimulating hormone to cause ovulation of mature follicles and secretion of oestrogen by thecal and granulosa cells of the ovary; it is also concerned with corpus luteum formation. In the male, it stimulates development of the interstitial cells of the testes and their secretion of testosterone. Called also *interstitial cell-stimulating hormone*.

luteinizing hormone releasing h. (LH-RH) gonadotrophin releasing hormone.

luteotrophic h. prolactin.

melanocyte-stimulating h. (MSH) a substance from the anterior pituitary that influences the formation or deposition of melanin in the body.

neurohypophyseal h's those stored and released by the neurohypophysis, i.e., oxytocin and vasopressin.

parathyroid h. (PTH) a polypeptide hormone secreted by the parathyroid glands that influences calcium and phosphorus metabolism and bone formation.

placental h. one secreted by the placenta, including chorionic gonadotrophin, relaxin, placental lactogen, and other substances having oestrogenic, progestational, or adrenocorticoid activity.

progestational h's substances, including PROGESTER-

Syndromes of ectopic hormones produced by nonendocrine tissues

Syndrome	Ectopic hormone	Responsible tumors
Dilutional hyponatraemia	Antidiuretic hormone	Carcinoma of the lung (oat cell), pancreas, or duodenum
Cushing's syndrome	Corticotrophin (adrenocorticotrophic hormone)	Thymoma; carcinoma of the lung (oat cell), pancreas, thyroid, prostate, breast, stomach, oesophagus, liver, ovary, or testis
Hyperpigmentation	Melanocyte-stimulating hormone	Thymoma; carcinoma of the lung (oat cell), pancreas, thyroid, prostate, breast, stomach, oesophagus, liver, ovary or testis
Hypercalcaemia	Parathormone	Carcinoma of the lung, pancreas, kidney, liver, colon, ovary, uterus, vagina, prostate, penis, or bladder
Hypoglycaemia	Nonsuppressible insulin-like substance	Hepatoma, sarcoma, fibroma, mesothelioma, bronchogenic carcinoma, adrenal carcinoma
Precocious puberty, menstrual irregularity, or gynaecomastia	Gonadotrophins	Hepatoma; lung carcinoma (trophoblastic tumours, not ectopic)
Polycythaemia	Erythropoietin-like hormone	Cerebellar haemangioblastoma; uterine fibroma; hepatoma; thymoma, carcinoma of the ovary, adrenals, or lung
Hyperthyroidism	Thyrotrophin	Bronchogenic carcinoma (trophoblastic tumours, not ectopic)

From Hoffman, J.T.T. (1980) Syndromes of ectopic hormone production in cancer. *Nursing Clinics of North America*, Vol. 15, p. 499.

ONE, that are concerned mainly with preparing the endometrium for nidation of the fertilized ovum if conception has occurred.

sex h's hormones having oestrogenic (female sex hormones) or androgenic (male sex hormones) activity.

somatotrophic h. growth hormone.

somatotrophin release inhibiting h. somatostatin.

somatotrophin releasing h. (SRH) growth hormone releasing hormone.

thymic h. thymosin.

thyroid-stimulating hormone (TSH) a hormone of the anterior lobe of the pituitary gland that exerts a stimulating influence on the thyroid gland; called also *thyrotrophin*.

thyrotrophin releasing h. (TRH) a tripeptide hormone of the hypothalmus, which stimulates release of thyrotrophin from the pituitary gland. In humans, it also acts as a prolactin releasing factor. It is used in the diagnosis of mild hyperthyroidism and Graves' disease and in differentiating between primary, secondary, and tertiary hypothyroidism.

hormonogen (haw'monəjən) prohormone.

hormonopoiesis (haw,mohnohpoy'eesis) the production of hormones. adj. **hormonopoietic.**

hormonotherapy (haw,mohnoh'therəpee) treatment by the use of hormones; endocrinotherapy.

horn (hawn) a pointed projection such as the paired processes on the head of various animals, or other structure resembling them in shape.

anterior h. of spinal cord the horn-shaped structure seen in transverse section of the spinal cord, formed by the anterior column of the cord.

cicatricial h. a hard, dry outgrowth from a cicatrix, commonly scaly and rarely osseous.

posterior h. of spinal cord the horn-shaped structure seen in transverse section of the spinal cord, formed by the posterior column of the cord.

sebaceous h. a hard outgrowth of the contents of a sebaceous cyst.

warty h. a hard, pointed outgrowth of a wart.

Horner's syndrome ('hawnəz) sinking in of the eyeball, ptosis of the upper eyelid, slight elevation of the lower lid, constriction of the pupil, narrowing of the palpebral fissure, and anhidrosis caused by paralysis of the cervical sympathetic nerve supply.

horopter (hor'optə) the sum of all points seen in binocular vision with the eyes fixed.

horseshoe kidney (,haws·shoo 'kidnee) see KIDNEY.

Horton's syndrome ('hawtənz) severe headache caused by the release of histamine in the body or by its administration. Called also *histamine cephalalgia*.

hospice ('hospis) originally, a medieval guest house or way station for pilgrims and travellers; currently used to designate either a place or a philosophy of care for persons in the last stages of life and their families.

Hospice care in the UK is considered to have been initiated by Cecily Saunders, a social worker, nurse and doctor, who became particularly concerned about the inadequacy of pain control in terminally ill patients. She founded St. Christopher's Hospice in the London area, where the aim is to ensure a high quality of life for both the patient and the relatives. Many hospices have an attached group of nurses which continue care in the patients' own home. Hospices have been set up in many areas of the UK. They are supported mainly by voluntary contributions, although some Health Authorities may make a contribution to help provide care for patients from their area.

A hospice programme provides palliative and supportive care for terminally ill patients and their families. The concept of hospice is that of a caring community of professional and nonprofessional people, supplemented by volunteer services. The emphasis is on dealing with emotional and spiritual problems as well as medical problems. Of primary concern is control of pain and other symptoms, on keeping the patient at home for as long as possible or desirable, and on making his or her remaining days as comfortable and meaningful as possible. After the patient dies family members are given support throughout their period of bereavement.

hospital ('hospit'l) an institution for the care and treatment of the sick and injured.

h.-acquired infection see hospital-acquired INFECTION.

h. activity analysis a system to collect, on Regional Health Authority computers, a series of data items for each patient discharged from hospital in the region, and the source of a national sample, the Hospital Inpatient Enquiry; abbreviated HIPE. HAA and HIPE were superceded in 1987 by systems based on KÖRNER DATA SETS.

teaching h. one that conducts formal educational programmes or courses of instruction that lead to granting of recognized certificates, diplomas, or degrees, or that are required for professional certification or licensure.

Hospital Inpatient Enquiry see HOSPITAL activity analysis.

hospitalization (,hospitəlie'zayshən) 1. the placing of a patient in a hospital. 2. the period of confinement in a hospital.

host (hohst) 1. an animal or plant that harbours and provides sustenance for another organism (the parasite). 2. the recipient of an organ or other tissue derived from another organism (the donor).

accidental h. one that accidentally harbours an organism that is not ordinarily parasitic in the particular species.

alternate h. intermediate host.

definitive h., final h. the organism in which a parasite passes its adult and sexual stage.

intermediate h. the organism in which a parasite passes its larval or nonsexual stage or stages.

paratenic h. an animal acting as a substitute intermediate host of a parasite, usually having acquired the parasite by ingestion of the original host.

h. of predilection the host preferred by a parasite.

primary h. definitive host.

reservoir h. an animal (or species) that is infected by a parasite, and which serves as a source of infection for man or another species.

secondary h. intermediate host.

transfer h. one that is used until the appropriate definitive host is reached, but is not necessary to completion of the life cycle of the parasite.

hot line ('hot ,lien) round-the-clock telephone assistance for those in need of crisis intervention, staffed by nonprofessionals with health professionals serving as advisers or in a back-up capacity.

Hounsfield unit ('hownzfeeld) an arbitrary unit of x-ray attenuation used for CT scans. Each voxel is assigned a value on a scale in which air has a value of -1000; water, 0; and compact bone, +1000.

hour-glass contraction ('owə,glahs kən,trakshən) a contraction near the middle of a hollow organ, such as the stomach or uterus, producing an outline resembling that shape. Specifically used to describe abnormal uterine action in third stage of labour when the spasm may trap the separated placenta and cause haemorrhage. See also tetanic or tonic CONTRACTION.

household survey ('howshold) collection of data from a representative sample of households. A continuous household survey collecting health and social data is carried out in England and Wales by the Office of Population Censuses and Surveys.

housemaid's knee ('howsmaydz) a swelling at the front of the knee, caused by enlargement of a bursa in front of the patella (kneecap), with accumulation of fluid within it.

The condition is so called because it was formerly supposed to be common among domestic workers who injured the knee by frequent kneeling.

The knee swells, is tender to the touch, and hurts when bent; if the bursa continues to be aggravated, these symptoms become acute. The injury may result in BURSITIS. Infection is possible if the knee is cut or scratched.

The condition can be treated by withdrawal of the fluid with a hollow needle and syringe. Sometimes the bursa must be removed altogether to prevent a chronic or recurrent condition.

Howell–Jolly bodies (,howəl'jolee) small, round or oval bodies, probably nuclear remnants, seen in erythrocytes when stains are added to fresh blood and found in various anemias and after splenectomy or splenic atrophy.

Hp haptoglobin, a serum protein that binds free haemoglobin.

HPG human pituitary gonadotrophin.

HPL human placental lactogen. A hormone produced by the placenta which can be measured to assess fetal well-being.

HPO hyperbaric (high-pressure) oxygenation.

hr hour.

HSA Hospital Savings Association; human serum albumin.

HSC Health and Safety Commission.

HSE Health and Safety Executive.

HSV herpes simplex virus.

5-HT (,fievaych'tee) serotonin (5-hydroxytryptamine).

Hubbard tank ('hubəd) a tank designed for full immersion of the body for the purpose of employing HYDROTHERAPY. A narrow section at the middle of the tank allows the therapist to reach the patient, and wider sections at each end permit full abduction of the patient's legs and arms. The tank is fitted with an aerator that agitates the water and provides gentle massage and débridement of wounds. An overhead crane facilitates transfer of the patient to and from the tank. The Hubbard tank is especially useful in the treatment of patients with extensive burns and those with chronic arthritic disorders in which there is involvement of several joints.

Huhner test ('hoonə) determination of the number and condition of spermatozoa in mucus aspirated from the canal of the uterine cervix within 2 hours after coitus.

hum (hum) a low, steady, prolonged sound.

venous h. a continuous blowing, singing, or humming murmur heard on auscultation over the right jugular vein in the sitting or erect position; it is an innocent sign that is obliterated on assumption of the recumbent position or on exerting pressure over the vein.

human erythrocyte agglutination test ('hyoomən) an adaptation of the sheep cell agglutination test; human Rh-positive cells coated with incomplete anti-Rh antibody are used instead of the sheep red blood cells sensitized with rabbit gamma globulin. The sera of some patients with rheumatoid arthritis will agglutinate these cells. The agglutination may be inhibited by some normal sera, and not others, and this test is the basis for the determination of the inherited gamma globulin groups (Gm system). Abbreviated HEAT.

human leukocyte antigen see HLA.

human T-cell leukaemia virus an RNA retrovirus that produces a unique enzyme, reverse transcriptase, which enables the virus to utilize host DNA to support its own replication. The human T-cell leukaemia virus I (HTLV-I) was first isolated from patients with an aggressive T-cell lymphoma/leukaemia seen in Japan and the Caribbean. Subsequently HTLV-III, now known as the human immune deficiency virus (HIV), was shown to cause AIDS.

humectant (hyoo'mektənt) 1. moistening. 2. a moistening or diluent medicine.

humeral ('hyoomə·rəl) of or pertaining to the humerus.

humeroradial (ˌhyoomə·roh'raydi·əl) pertaining to the humerus and radius.

humeroscapular (ˌhyoomə·roh'skapyuhlə) pertaining to the humerus and scapula.

humeroulnar (ˌhyoomə·roh'ulnə) pertaining to the humerus and ulna.

humerus ('hyoomə·rəs) the bone of the upper arm, extending from shoulder to elbow. It consists of a shaft and two enlarged extremities. The proximal end has a smooth round head that articulates with the scapula to form the shoulder joint. Just below the head are two rounded processes called the greater and lesser tubercles. Just below the tubercles is the 'surgical neck', so named because of its liability to fracture. The distal end of the humerus has two articulating surfaces: the trochlea, which articulates with the ulna, and the capitulum, which articulates with the radius, at the elbow.

humidifier (hyoo'midiˌfieə) an apparatus for controlling humidity by adding moisture to the air.

humidity (hyoo'miditee) the degree of moisture in the air.

h. therapy the therapeutic use of water to prevent or correct a moisture deficit in the respiratory tract. Under normal conditions the respiratory tract is kept moist by humidifying mechanisms that allow for evaporation of water from the respiratory mucosa. If these mechanisms fail to work, are bypassed as in ENDOTRACHEAL INTUBATION, or are inadequate to overcome the drying and irritating effects of therapeutic gases and mucosal crusting, some form of humidification must be provided.

The principal reasons for employing humidity therapy are: (1) to prevent drying and irritation of the respiratory mucosa, (2) to facilitate ventilation and diffusion of oxygen and other therapeutic gases being administered, and (3) to aid in the removal of thick and viscous secretions that obstruct the air passages. Another important use of water aerosol therapy is to aid in obtaining an induced sputum specimen.

Humidity therapy may be delivered in a variety of ways. Humidifiers and vaporizers increase the water content of an environment and are limited to the treatment of upper respiratory disorders because they produce particles that are too large to penetrate deeply into the lungs. Nebulizers generate clouds or mists of particles that are extremely small and thus capable of penetrating more deeply into the bronchioles and small structures of the lower respiratory tract. Examples of these include jet instruments and ultrasonic nebulizers.

humour ('hyoomə) pl. *humoures,humours* [L.] any fluid or semifluid in the body. adj. **humoral**.

aqueous h. the fluid produced in the eye and filling the spaces (anterior and posterior chambers) in front of the lens and its attachments.

ocular h. either of the humours of the eye—aqueous or vitreous.

vitreous h. the fluid portion of the vitreous body; often used to designate the entire vitreous body.

hunchback ('hunsh,bak) a rounded deformity, or hump, of the back, or a person with such a deformity. The condition is called also KYPHOSIS and is the result of an abnormal backward curvature of the spine.

hunger ('hung·gə) a craving, as for food.

air h. dyspnoea affecting both inspiration and expiration, characteristic of diabetic acidosis and coma. Called also *Kussmaul's respiration*.

Hunner's ulcer ('hunəz) an ulcer involving all layers of the bladder wall, occurring in chronic interstitial cystitis.

Hunt's neuralgia (hunts) neuralgia involving the geniculate ganglion, the pain being limited to the middle ear and external acoustic meatus; called also *geniculate neuralgia*.

Hunter's canal ('huntəz) a fascial tunnel in the middle third of the medial part of the thigh, containing the femoral vessels and saphenous nerve. Called also *adductor canal*.

Huntington's disease (chorea) ('huntingtənz) a rare hereditary disease characterized by quick involuntary movements, speech disturbances, and mental deterioration due to degenerative changes in the cerebral cortex and basal ganglia; called also *chronic progressive chorea* and *hereditary chorea*.

The disease appears in adulthood, usually between the ages of 30 to 45, and the patient's condition deteriorates over a period of 15 years or so, progressing to total incapacitation and death. There is no treatment as yet that is successful in curing this disorder. Sedatives and tranquillizers may be used to relieve the symptoms in the early stages. As the disease progresses, institutionalization in a psychiatric hospital is usually necessary.

Hurler's syndrome ('hərləz) the prototypical form of mucopolysaccharidosis, with gargoyle-like facies, dwarfism, severe somatic and skeletal changes, severe mental handicap, cloudy corneas, deafness, cardiovascular defects, hepatosplenomegaly, and joint contractures. It is due to a deficiency of the enzyme α-L-iduronidase, and is transmitted as an autosomal recessive trait. Called also *gargoylism*.

Hürthle cell tumour ('hooətlə) a tumour of the thyroid gland composed wholly or predominantly of large cells (Hürthle cells) having abundant granular, eosinophilic cytoplasm. Such tumours are usually benign (Hürthle cell adenoma) but on occasion may be locally invasive or may rarely metastasize (Hürthle cell carcinoma, or malignant Hürthle cell tumour).

Hürthle cells large eosinophilic cells sometimes found in the thyroid gland (see also HÜRTHLE CELL TUMOUR).

Hutchinson–Gilford disease (ˌhuchinsən'gilfəd) see PROGERIA.

Hutchinson's incisors ('hutchinsənz) the upper central incisor teeth with a characteristic shovel shape and a notched incisal edge; sometimes seen in congenital syphilis.

Hutchinson's pupil a pupil that is dilated while the pupil of the other eye is not.

Hutchinson's triad diffuse interstitial keratitis, labyrinthine disease, and Hutchinson's incisors, seen in congenital syphilis.

HVA Health Visitors' Association.

HVCert Health Visitor's Certificate.

HVL half-value layer.

hyal(o)- word element. [Gr.] *glassy*.

Hyalase ('hieəlayz) trademark for a preparation of hyaluronidase for injection, used as a spreading agent to promote diffusion and hasten absorption.

hyalin ('hieəlin) a structureless, amorphous, glassy, smooth eosinophilic substance when visualized under the microscope. It describes the appearance of amyloid deposition and also a form of degeneration of aged collagen.

hyaline ('hieəˌlien) glassy; pellucid.

h. cartilage cartilage with a glassy, translucent appearance, the matrix and embedded collagenous fibres having the same index of refraction.

h. membrane disease a disorder of newborn infants,

usually preterm, characterized by the formation of a hyalin-like membrane lining the terminal respiratory passages. Infants with this disease do not secrete adequate quantities of a substance called surfactant, which is secreted by the epithelium of the alveoli and decreases the surface tension of the fluids lining the alveoli and bronchioles. When the surface tension is kept low, air can pass through the fluids and into the alveoli. If the surface tension is not decreased by adequate supplies of surfactant, the alveoli cannot fill with air and there is partial or complete collapse of the lung (atelectasis). Thus the infant with hyaline membrane disease suffers from respiratory embarrassment with severe DYSPNOEA and cyanosis. Called also respiratory distress syndrome of newborn.

The cause of hyaline membrane disease is not known and at present there is no cure for it.

hyalinization (ˌhieəlinie'zayshən) conversion into a substance resembling glass.

hyalinosis (ˌhieəli'nohsis) hyaline degeneration.

hyalinuria (ˌhieəli'nyooə·ri·ə) hyalin in the urine.

hyalitis (ˌhieə'lietis) inflammation of the vitreous body.

h. punctata a form marked by small opacities.

h. suppurativa purulent inflammation of the vitreous body. See also HYALOSIS.

hyaloid ('hieəˌloyd) pellucid; like glass.

hyalomere ('hieəlohˌmiə) the pale, homogeneous portion of a blood platelet.

Hyalomma (ˌhieə'lomə) a genus of ticks occurring only in Africa, Asia, and Europe; ectoparasites of animals and man, they may transmit disease by their bite.

hyalophagia (ˌhieəloh'fayji·ə) the eating of glass.

hyaloserositis (ˌhieəlohˌsiə·roh'sietis) inflammation of serous membranes marked by conversion of the serous exudate into a pearly coating of the affected organ.

hyalosis (ˌhieə'lohsis) degenerative changes in the vitreous humour.

asteroid h. the presence of spherical or star-shaped opacities in the vitreous humour, called also BENSON'S DISEASE.

hyaluronic acid (ˌhieəlyuh'ronik) a sulphate-free mucopolysaccharide in the intercellular substance of various tissues, especially the skin; also isolated from the vitreous humour, synovial fluid, umbilical cord, etc.

hyaluronidase (ˌhieəlyuh'roniˌdayz) an enzyme that catalyses the hydrolysis of hyaluronic acid, the 'cement material' of connective tissues; it is found in leeches, snake and spider venom, in testes, and is produced by various pathogenic bacteria, enabling them to spread through tissue. A preparation from mammalian testes is used to promote absorption and diffusion of solutions injected subcutaneously. When hyaluronidase is mixed with fluids administered subcutaneously, absorption is more rapid and less uncomfortable. This is especially valuable when large amounts of fluid must be given by subcutaneous infusion instead of intravenously. The drug should be dissolved just before it is used and usually is injected with the first portion of the fluid to be given. Hyaluronidase should not be given in areas where there is infection. Since it hastens absorption, it must be given with caution when administered with toxic drugs, as the toxic reaction can occur very rapidly.

hybrid ('hiebrid) an offspring of parents of different strains, varieties, or species.

hybridization (ˌhiebridie'zayshən) the production of hybrids.

hybridoma (ˌhiebri'dohmə) a cell culture consisting of a clone of a hybrid cell formed by fusing cells of different kinds. Hybridomas formed from mouse lymphocytes and myeloma cells are immortal and produce monoclonal antibodies.

hydatid ('hiedətid) 1. a hydatid cyst. 2. any cystlike structure.

h. cyst the larval stage of the tapeworm *Echinococcus granulosus* or *E. multilocularis*, containing daughter cysts, each of which has many scolices; it is the cause of hydatid disease. Called also *echinococcus cyst* and *hydatid*.

h. disease an infection, usually of the liver, caused by larval forms (hydatid cysts) of TAPEWORMS of the genus *Echinococcus*, and characterized by the development of expanding cysts. In the infection caused by *E. granulosus*, single or multiple cysts that are unilocular in character are formed, and in that caused by *E. multilocularis*, the host's tissues are invaded and destroyed as the cyst(s) enlarge by peripheral budding. Called also *echinococcosis*.

h. mole hydatidiform mole.

h. of Morgagni a cystlike remnant of the müllerian duct attached to a testis or to a uterine tube.

sessile h. the hydatid of Morgagni connected with a testis.

stalked h. the hydatid of Morgagni connected with a uterine tube.

hydatidiform (ˌhiedə'tidiˌfawm) resembling a hydatid.

h. mole an abnormal pregnancy resulting from a pathological ovum, with proliferation of the epithelial covering of the chorionic villi and dissolution and cystic cavitation of the avascular stroma of the villi. It results in a mass of cysts resembling a bunch of grapes. Called also *hydatid mole*. See also CHORIOCARCINOMA.

hydatidocele (ˌhiedə'tidəˌseel) a tumour of the scrotum containing hydatids.

hydatidoma (ˌhiedəti'dohmə) a tumour containing hydatids.

hydatidosis (ˌhiedəti'dohsis) hydatid disease.

hydatidostomy (ˌhiedəti'dostəmee) incision and drainage of a hydatid cyst.

hydatiduria (ˌhiedəti'dyooə·ri·ə) excretion of hydatid cysts in the urine.

Hydergine ('hiedəˌjeen) trademark for a preparation of ergoloid mesylates, a cognition adjuvant.

hydr(o)- word element. [Gr.] *hydrogen, water*.

hydraemia (hie'dreemi·ə) excess of water in the blood.

hydraeroperitoneum (hiˌdrair·rohˌperitə'neeəm) water and gas in the peritoneal cavity.

hydragogue ('hiedrəˌgog) 1. increasing the fluid content of the faeces. 2. a purgative that causes evacuation of watery stools.

hydralazine hydrochloride (hie'draləˌzeen) an antihypertensive and vasodilator; used in peripheral vascular disease, essential and early malignant hypertension, thrombophlebitis, and other conditions in which dilation of the blood vessels of the extremities is desired.

The drug may be administered orally, intramuscularly, or intravenously. Dosage is adjusted to the individual patient's response. The blood pressure should be checked frequently, especially during parenteral administration of the drug. Side-effects are rare with therapeutic doses, but the drug must be administered with caution to patients with coronary artery disease, advanced kidney damage, and existing or incipient stroke.

hydramnios (hie'dramnios) excess of AMNIOTIC FLUID. See also POLYHYDRAMNIOS.

hydranencephaly (ˌhiedranen'kefəlee, -'sef-) absence of the cerebral hemispheres, their normal site being occupied by cerebrospinal fluid.

hydrargyria (ˌhiedrah'jieri·ə) chronic poisoning from mercury.

hydrargyrosis (hie'drahjir'ohsis) chronic mercurial

poisoning.

hydrargyrum (hie'drahjirəm) [L.] *mercury* (symbol Hg).

hydrarthrosis (ˌhiedrah'throhsis) an accumulation of watery fluid in the cavity of a joint. adj. **hydrarthrodial.**

hydrase, hydratase ('hiedrayz; 'hiedrəˌtayz) any enzyme that catalyses the hydration–dehydration of C–O linkages.

hydrate ('hiedrayt) 1. a compound of water with a radical. 2. a salt or other compound that contains water of crystallization.

hydration (hie'drayshən) the absorption of or combination with water.

hydraulics (hie'droliks) the science dealing with the mechanics of liquids.

hydrazine ('hiedrəˌzeen) a gaseous diamine, H_4N_2, or any of its substitution derivatives.

Hydrea (hie'dreeə) trademark for a preparation of hydroxyurea, an antineoplastic agent.

hydrencephalocele (ˌhiedren'kefəlohˌseel, -'sef-) hernial protrusion of brain tissue containing fluid.

hydrencephalomeningocele (ˌhiedrenˌkefəlohmə'ning·gohˌseel, -ˌsef-) hernial protrusion, through a cranial defect, of meninges containing cerebrospinal fluid and brain substance.

Hydrenox ('hiedrənoks) trademark for a preparation of hydroflumethiazide, a diuretic.

hydroa (hie'droh·ə) a vesicular eruption, with intense itching and burning, occurring on skin surfaces exposed to sunlight.

hydroappendix (ˌhiedroh·ə'pendiks) distention of the vermiform appendix with watery fluid.

hydrocalycosis (ˌhiedrohˌkali'kohsis) a usually asymptomatic cystic dilation of a major renal calix, lined by transitional epithelium, and due to obstruction of the infundibulum.

hydrocarbon (ˌhiedroh'kahbən) an organic compound that contains carbon and hydrogen only.

alicyclic h. one that has cyclic structure and aliphatic properties.

aliphatic h. one that does not contain an aromatic ring.

aromatic h. one that has cyclic structure and a closed conjugated system of double bonds.

hydrocele ('hiedrəˌseel) a painless swelling of the scrotum caused by a collection of fluid in the sac formed by the tunica vaginalis. The fluid can be removed by aspiration or the condition cured by surgical removal of the outer layer of the tunica.

hydrocephalocele (ˌhiedroh'kefəlohˌseel, -'sef-) hydrencephalocele.

hydrocephaloid (ˌhiedroh'kefəˌloyd, -'sef-) resembling hydrocephalus.

h. disease a condition resembling hydrocephalus, but with depressed fontanelles, following severe diarrhoea.

hydrocephalus (ˌhiedroh'kefələs, 'sef-) a condition characterized by enlargement of the cranium caused by abnormal accumulation of cerebrospinal fluid within the cerebral ventricular system; called also *water on the brain.* adj. **hydrocephalic.** Although hydrocephalus occurs occasionally in adults, it is usually associated with a congenital defect in infants.

There are two types of hydrocephalus, the distinction being based on whether there is abnormal absorption of the cerebrospinal fluid or an obstruction to its flow. In *communicating hydrocephalus* there is some abnormality in the capacity to absorb fluid from the arachnoid space. There is no obstruction to the flow of fluid between the ventricles. In *noncommunicating hydrocephalus* there is an obstruction at some point in the ventricular system. The cause of noncommunicating hydrocephalus usually is a congenital abnormality, such as stenosis of the aqueduct of Sylvius, congenital atresia of the foramina of the fourth ventricle, or spina bifida cystica. Infections, intraventricular haemorrhage, trauma, and tumours can produce acquired communicating hydrocephalus.

Medical treatment has had only limited success in controlling the secretion of cerebrospinal fluid and relieving hydrocephalus. The most effective treatment is surgical correction employing a shunting technique. The basic components of the shunt are a ventricular catheter, a valve, and a distal catheter. Multiple perforations along the ventricular catheter permit the drainage of fluid from the ventricle. The valve is constructed so that fluid will flow in one direction only, and some valves have a pumping chamber to facilitate drainage. The distal catheter may be positioned at any of a number of sites, the most common being the peritoneal cavity (ventriculoperitoneal shunt) and the right atrium (ventriculoatrial shunt).

hydrochloric acid (ˌhiedrə'klo·rik, -'klor·rik) HCl, a normal constituent of gastric juice in man and other animals. The absence of free hydrochloric acid in the stomach, called achlorhydria, may be found with chronic gastritis, gastric carcinoma, pernicious anaemia, pellagra, and alcoholism. This condition is also referred to as gastric anacidity. Hyperacidity of the gastric juice is often associated with emotional stress and tension and is believed to be a factor in the development of peptic ULCER.

hydrochloride (ˌhiedrə'klor·ried) an addition salt of hydrochloric acid with an organic base.

hydrochlorothiazide (ˌhiedrəˌklor·roh'thieəˌzied) a thiazide diuretic used as an antihypertensive agent.

hydrocholecystis (ˌhiedrohˌkohli'sistis) distention of gallbladder with watery fluid.

hydrocholeresis (ˌhiedrohˌkohlə'reesis) secretion of bile relatively low in specific gravity, viscosity, and total solid content.

hydrocholeretic (ˌhiedrohˌkohlə'retik) 1. pertaining to or producing hydrocholeresis. 2. an agent that stimulates an increased output of bile of low specific gravity.

hydrocirsocele (ˌhiedroh'sərsohˌseel) hydrocele with variocele.

hydrocolloid (ˌhiedroh'koloyd) a colloid in which water is the dispersion medium.

hydrocolpos (ˌhiedroh'kolpos) collection of watery fluid in the vagina.

hydrocortisone (ˌhiedroh'kawtiˌzohn) the pharmaceutical term for cortisol, the principal GLUCOCORTICOID secreted by the adrenal gland; it is used in the treatment of inflammations, allergies, pruritus, collagen diseases, adrenocortical insufficiency, severe status asthmaticus, shock, and certain neoplasms.

Hydrocortistab (ˌhiedroh'kawtistab) trademark for preparations of hydrocortisone, a corticosteroid.

Hydrocortisyl (ˌhiedroh'kawtizil) trademark for preparations of hydrocortisone, an adrenocortical steroid.

Hydrocortone (ˌhiedroh'kawtohn) trademark for preparations of hydrocortisone, a corticosteroid.

hydrocyanic acid (ˌhiedrohsie'anik) a volatile liquid that is extremely poisonous because it checks the oxidation process in protoplasm.

hydrocyst ('hiedrohˌsist) a cyst with watery contents.

hydroflumethiazide (ˌhiedrohˌfloomi'thieəˌzied) an antihypertensive and diuretic.

hydrogel ('hiedrəˌjel) a gel that contains water.

hydrogen ('hiedrəjən) a chemical element, atomic number 1, atomic weight 1.00797, symbol H. (See table of elements in Appendix 2.) It exists as the mass 1 isotope (protium, or light or ordinary hydrogen), mass 2 isotope (deuterium, heavy hydrogen), and mass 3 isotope (tritium).

heavy h. hydrogen having double the mass of ordinary hydrogen; deuterium.

h. ion concentration the degree of concentration of hydrogen ions (the acid element) in a solution often indicated thus [H+]. The symbol pH is $-10 \log_{10}$ of the hydrogen ion concentration and expresses the degree to which a solution is acidic or alkaline. The pH range extends from 0 to 14, pH 7 being neutral. A pH of less than 7 indicates acidity, above 7 indicates alkalinity. See also ACID–BASE BALANCE.

h. peroxide see HYDROGEN PEROXIDE.

h. sulphide an ill-smelling, colourless, poisonous gas, H_2S; much used as a chemical reagent. Called also *hydrosulphuric acid.*

hydrogen peroxide ('hiedrə,jən pər'oksied) a strong disinfectant cleansing and bleaching liquid used diluted in water.

hydrogenase ('hiedrəje,nayz, hie'drojə-) an enzyme that catalyses the reduction of various substances by combining them with molecular hydrogen.

hydrogenate ('hiedrəjə,nayt, hie'drojə-) to cause to combine with hydrogen; to reduce with hydrogen.

hydrogymnastics (,hiedrohjim'nastiks) therapeutic exercise performed in water.

hydrokinetic (,hiedrohki'netik) relating to movement of water or other fluid, as in a whirlpool bath.

hydrokinetics (,hiedrohki'netiks) the science dealing with fluids in motion.

hydrolase ('hiedrə,layz) one of the six main classes of enzymes, comprising those that catalyse the hydrolysis of a compound.

hydro-lyase (,hiedroh'lieayz) an enzyme that catalyses the removal of a hydrogen atom and a hydroxyl group from the substrate molecule as water and the formation of a double bond.

hydrolysate (hie'droli,sayt) any compound produced by hydrolysis.

protein h. a mixture of amino acids prepared by splitting a protein with acid, alkali, or enzyme. Such preparations provide the nutritive equivalent of the original material in the form of its constituent amino acids and are used in special diets or for patients unable to take the ordinary food proteins.

hydrolysis (hie'drolisis) the cleavage of a compound by the addition of water, the hydroxyl group being incorporated in one fragment and the hydrogen atom in the other. adj. **hydrolytic.**

hydroma (hie'drohmə) hygroma.

hydromeningitis (,hiedroh,menin'jietis) meningitis with serous effusion.

hydromeningocele (,hiedrohmə'ning·goh,seel) protrusion of the meninges, containing fluid, through a defect in the skull or vertebral column.

hydrometer (hie'dromitə) an instrument for determining the specific gravity of a fluid.

hydrometra (,hiedroh'meetrə) collection of watery fluid in the uterus.

hydrometrocolpos (,hiedroh,meetroh'kolpos) collection of watery fluid in the uterus and vagina.

hydrometry (hie'dromətree) measurement of specific gravity with a hydrometer.

hydromicrocephaly (,hiedroh,miekroh'kefəlee, -'sef-) smallness of the head with an abnormal amount of cerebrospinal fluid.

hydromphalus (hie'dromfələs) a cystic accumulation of watery fluid at the umbilicus.

hydromyelia (,hiedrohmie'eeli·ə) dilation of the central canal of the spinal cord with an abnormal accumulation of fluid.

hydromyelomeningocele (,hiedroh,mieəlohmə'ning·goh,seel) a defect of the spine marked by protrusion of the membranes and tissue of the spinal cord, forming a fluid-filled sac.

hydromyoma (,hiedrohmie'ohmə) a leiomyoma with cystic degeneration.

hydronephrosis (,hiedrohnə'frohsis) dilation of the renal calices and pelvis with uninfected urine due to obstruction in the ureter or beyond, first detectable by radiology in the calyx. adj. **hydronephrotic.** If it is allowed to persist, the functioning units of the kidney are destroyed. The collecting tubules dilate and the muscular walls of the renal pelvis and calices stretch, are replaced by fibrous tissue, and eventually form a large, fluid-filled, functionless sac. Persistent hydronephrosis is prone to infection when PYONEPHROSIS may supervene.

The cause of hydronephrosis is obstruction or atrophy of the urinary tract. Mechanical obstruction may result from ureteral tumours, calculi, NEPHROPTOSIS, benign or malignant hyperplasia of the prostate, or carcinoma of the bladder, urethra, or glans penis. Inflammatory obstruction is the outcome of a urinary tract infection that produces oedema and narrowing of the ureters or urethra. Rarely there occurs during pregnancy a loss of muscle tone in the urinary tract. The atony is thought to be induced by placental hormones.

The condition may be clinically silent or give rise to pain in the respective lumbar area ranging from a persistent dull ache to an acute pain almost of the intensity of renal colic. If both kidneys are involved, uraemia develops as the functional units of the kidneys are destroyed.

Hydronephrosis should be regarded as a secondary phenomenon. Treatment must depend upon establishing the primary diagnosis, finding the site of the obstruction and then removing the cause—as with ureteric stone. Permanent drainage of the kidney through pyelostomy or nephrostomy is a measure of last resort when obstruction cannot be overcome in any other way as may occur in malignancy.

Demonstration of hydronephrosis is performed by renal ultrasound or intravenous pyelography and usually identifies the underlying cause.

hydronium (hie'drohni·əm) the hydrated proton H_3O^+; it is the form in which the proton (hydrogen ion, H^+) exists in aqueous solution, a combination of H^+ and H_2O.

hydropathy (hie'dropəthee) the treatment of disease by the use of water internally and externally. Called also *hydrotherapy.*

hydropericarditis (,hiedroh,perikah'dietis) pericarditis with watery effusion.

hydropericardium (,hiedroh,peri'kahdi·əm) an excess of transudate in the pericardial cavity.

hydroperitoneum (,hiedroh,peritə'neeəm) a collection of fluid in the peritoneal cavity; ASCITES.

hydrophilia (,hiedrə'fili·ə) the property of absorbing water; having a strong affinity for water.

hydrophilic (,hiedrə'filik) readily absorbing moisture; hygroscopic; having strongly polar groups that readily interact with water.

hydrophilous (hie'drofiləs) hydrophilic.

hydrophobia (,hiedrə'fohbi·ə) 1. rabies. 2. irrational fear of water.

hydrophobic (,hiedrə'fohbik) 1. pertaining to hydrophobia (RABIES). 2. repelling water; insoluble in water; not readily absorbing water.

hydrophthalmus (,hiedrof'thalməs) distention of the eyeball in infantile glaucoma.

hydrophysometra (,hiedroh,fiesoh'meetrə) collection of fluid and gas in the uterus.

hydropic (hie'dropik) affected with dropsy, or hydrops.

hydropneumatosis (,hiedroh,nyoomə'tohsis) collection of fluid and gas in the tissues.

hydropneumopericardium (ˌhiedrohˌnyoomohˌperi'kahdi·əm) fluid and gas in the pericardium.

hydropneumoperitoneum (ˌhiedrohˌnyoomohˌperitə'neeəm) fluid and gas in the peritoneal cavity.

hydropneumothorax (ˌhiedrohˌnyoomoh'thor·raks) a collection of fluid and gas within the pleural cavity.

hydrops ('hiedrops) [L.] abnormal accumulation of serous fluid in the tissues or in a body cavity; called also dropsy.

fetal h., h. fetalis gross oedema of the entire body of the newborn infant, occurring in haemolytic disease of the newborn.

hydropyonephrosis (ˌhiedrohˌpieohnə'frohsis) urine and pus in the renal pelvis.

hydrorrhoea (ˌhiedrə'reeə) a copious watery discharge; usually called leukorrhoea.

hydrosalpinx (ˌhiedroh'salpingks) accumulation of watery fluid in a uterine tube.

HydroSaluric (ˌhiedrohsal'yuhrik) trademark for a preparation of hydrochlorothiazide, a diuretic and antihypertensive.

hydrosarcocele (ˌhiedroh'sahkohˌseel) hydrocele and sarcocele together.

hydroscheocele (hie'droskiohˌseel) a scrotal hernia containing fluid.

hydrosol ('hiedrəˌsol) a colloid in which the dispersion medium is a liquid.

hydrostatic (ˌhiedroh'statik) pertaining to a liquid in a state of equilibrium or the pressure exerted by a stationary fluid.

hydrostatics (ˌhiedroh'statiks) the science of equilibrium of fluids.

hydrosyringomyelia (ˌhiedrohsiˌring·gohmie'eeli·ə) distention of the central canal of the spinal cord, with the formation of cavities and degeneration.

hydrotaxis (ˌhiedroh'taksis) an orientation movement of motile organisms or cells in response to the influence of water or moisture.

hydrotherapy (ˌhiedroh'therəpee) the external use of water in the treatment of disease and injury.

The patient is immersed in a hydrotherapy pool, the water being at a temperature of 34–37 °C (94–98 °F). The use of warm water can help relieve pain and improve circulation, promote relaxation and reduce muscle spasms, maintain or increase joint range, re-educate paralysed muscle, strengthen muscles, develop power and endurance, and improve the functional activities of walking.

The special properties of buoyancy, cohesion, and viscosity make water a particularly useful medium in which exercises may be carried out. Buoyancy can be used to assist, support or to resist movement. The first two allow for a greater range of movement with less discomfort. This is particularly useful in exercising painful arthritic joints. The cohesion and viscosity of water account for its resistance to objects moving through it. This resistance can be used to good advantage in the progressive improvement of muscle strength and endurance by exercise. An additional benefit of exercise in water is its psychological impact on the patient who has impaired mobility. In the water he has a feeling of movement accomplished with relatively more ease than outside the water.

Hydrotherapy is particularly useful in generalized conditions, for example, osteoarthritis, rheumatoid arthritis, ankylosing spondylitis, and for those who are heavily disabled, for example, those with multiple sclerosis or spinal injuries.

hydrothermal, hydrothermic (ˌhiedroh'thərməl; ˌhiedroh'thərmik) relating to the temperature effects of water, as in hot baths.

hydrothionaemia (ˌhiedrohˌthieə'neemi·ə) hydrogen sulphide in the blood.

hydrothionuria (ˌhiedrohˌthieə'nyooə·ri·ə) hydrogen sulphide in the urine.

hydrothorax (ˌhiedroh'thor·raks) the presence of non-inflammatory serous fluid within the pleural cavity.

hydrotropism (hie'drotrəˌpizəm) a growth response of a nonmotile organism to the presence of water or moisture.

hydrotubation (ˌhiedrohtyooˌbayshən) introduction into the uterine tube of hydrocortisone in saline solution followed by chymotrypsin in saline solution to maintain its patency.

hydrotympanum (ˌhiedroh'timpənəm) a collection of serous fluid in the middle ear.

hydroureter (ˌhiedroh·yuh'reetə) distention of the ureter with fluid, due to obstruction.

hydrous ('hiedrəs) containing water.

hydrovarium (ˌhiedroh'vair·ri·əm) a collection of serous fluid in an ovary.

hydroxide (hie'droksied) the OH^- anion or a compound containing the OH^- ion.

hydroxocobalamin (hieˌdroksohkoh'baləmin) an analogue of cyanocobalamin (vitamin B_{12}) having exceptionally long-acting haematopoietic activity; used in the treatment of pernicious anaemia and other macrocytic anaemias.

hydroxy- a chemical prefix indicating the presence of the univalent radical –OH.

hydroxyapatite (hieˌdroksi'apəˌtiet) an inorganic constituent of bone matrix and teeth, imparting rigidity to these structures.

β-hydroxybutyric acid (beetəhieˌdroksibyoo'tirik) one of the KETONE BODIES, occurring in abnormal amounts in diabetic ketoacidosis and in starvation due to fatty acid oxidation.

hydroxychloroquine (hieˌdroksi'klor·rohˌkween) a drug used as the sulphate salt in the treatment of malaria, lupus erythematosus, rheumatoid arthritis, and symptomatic giardiasis.

25-hydroxycholecalciferol (ˌtwenteefievhieˌdroksiˌkohlikal'sifə·rol) a metabolically activated form of cholecalciferol synthesized in the liver.

hydroxyl (hieˌdroksil) the univalent radical –OH.

hydroxylase (hie'droksiˌlayz) any enzyme that brings about the coupled oxidation of two donors, with incorporation of oxygen into one of them.

hydroxylysine (hieˌdroksi'lieseen) a naturally occurring amino acid.

hydroxyprogesterone (hieˌdroksiproh'jestəˌrohn) a synthetic progestin used in the treatment of functional uterine bleeding, menstrual abnormalities, threatened abortion, and uterine cancer.

hydroxyprolinaemia (hieˌdroksiˌprohli'neemi·ə) a disorder of amino acid metabolism, characterized by an excess of free hydroxyproline in the plasma and urine, due to a defect in the enzyme hydroxyproline oxidase.

hydroxyproline (hieˌdroksi'prohleen) an amino acid produced in the digestion of hydrolytic decomposition of proteins, especially of collagens.

hydroxypropyl methylcellulose (hieˌdroksi'prohpiel ˌmeethiel'selyuhˌlohs, -lohz) a compound applied topically to the conjunctiva to protect the cornea during certain ophthalmic procedures and to lubricate the cornea. Also used as a tear substitute in impaired tear production.

hydroxytetracycline (hieˌdroksiˌtetrə'siekleen) oxytetracycline, a broad-spectrum antibiotic.

5-hydroxytryptamine (ˌfievhieˌdroksi'triptəˌmeen) see SEROTONIN.

hydroxyurea (hieˌdroksiyuh'reeə) an ANTINEOPLASTIC agent that blocks the conversion of ribonucleotides to deoxyribonucleotides, thus stopping DNA synthesis; used in the treatment of melanoma, resistant chronic myelocytic leukaemia, and recurrent, metastatic, or inoperable ovarian carcinoma.

hydroxyzine (hie'droksi,zeen) a central nervous system depressant having antispasmodic and antihistaminic actions; used as the hydrochloride or pamoate salt.

hydruria (hie'drooə·ri·ə) excretion of urine of low specific gravity.

hygiene ('hiejeen) 1. the science of health and its preservation. 2. a condition or practice, such as cleanliness, that is conducive to preservation of health. adj. **hygienic.**

mental h. the science dealing with development of healthy mental and emotional reactions and habits.

oral h. the proper care of the mouth and teeth.

hygienics (hie'jeeniks) a system of principles for promoting health.

hygienist (hie'jeenist) a specialist in hygiene.

dental h. a dental health specialist whose primary concern is maintenance of dental health and prevention of oral disease (see also under DENTAL).

hygro- ('hiegroh) word element. [Gr.] *moisture.*

hygroma (hie'grohmə) an accumulation of fluid in a sac, cyst, or bursa. adj. **hygromatous.**

cystic h., h. cysticum an endothelium-lined, fluid-containing lesion of lymphatic origin, encountered most often in infants and children and occurring in various regions of the body, most commonly in the posterior triangle of the neck, behind the sternocleidomastoid muscle (hygroma colli cysticum).

Fleischmann's h. enlargement of a bursa in the floor of the mouth, to the outer side of the genioglossus muscle.

hygrometer (hie'gromitə) an instrument for measuring atmospheric moisture.

hygroscopic (,hiegroh'skopik) readily absorbing moisture.

Hygroton ('hiegrohton) trademark for a preparation of chlorthalidone, a diuretic.

hymen ('hiemen) the membranous fold partly or completely closing the vaginal orifice. adj. **hymenal.**

hymenectomy (,hiemə'nektəmee) excision of the hymen.

hymenitis (,hiemə'nietis) inflammation of the hymen.

hymenolepiasis (,hiemənohlə'pieəsis) infection with *Hymenolepis* species.

Hymenolepis (,hiemə'noləpis) a genus of TAPEWORMS; *H. nana*, much the commonest, *H. diminuta*, and *H. lanceolata* have been found in man.

hymenotomy (,hiemə'notəmee) incision of the hymen.

hyoepiglottidean (,hieoh,epiglo'tidi·ən) pertaining to the hyoid bone and epiglottis.

hyoglossal (,hieoh'glos'l) pertaining to the hyoid bone and tongue or to the hyoglossal muscle.

hyoid ('hieoyd) 1. shaped like Greek letter upsilon (υ). 2. pertaining to the hyoid bone.

h. bone a horseshoe-shaped bone situated at the base of the tongue, just below the thyroid cartilage.

hyoscine ('hieə,seen) an anticholinergic drug used as an anaesthetic premedicant, antispasmodic, and in the treatment of motion sickness. Should be avoided in the elderly because of its tendency to cause restlessness and confusion (central cholinergic syndrome). Called also *scopolamine.*

hyoscyamine (,hieoh'sieə,meen) an anticholinergic alkaloid usually obtained from species of the plant *Hyoscyamus* (henbane) and other solanaceous plants. It is the laevorotatory component of atropine with actions and uses similar to those of atropine but with more potent effects.

hyp- see HYPO-.

hypacusia (,hiepə'kyoozi·ə) slightly diminished acuteness of the sense of hearing.

hypaesthesia (,hiepis'theezi·ə) abnormally diminished sensitiveness; hypoaesthesia.

hypalgesia (,hiepal'jeezi·ə) diminished sensibility to noxious stimulation. Called also *hypoalgesia.* adj. **hypalgesic.**

hypanakinesia (,hiepanəki'neezi·ə) hypokinesia.

Hypaque ('hiepayk) trademark for preparations of sodium and/or meglumine diatrizoate used as radiological contrast media.

hypaxial (hie'paksi·əl) beneath an axis, as the axis of the vertebral column.

hyper- word element. [Gr.] *abnormally increased, excessive.*

hyperabsorption (,hiepə·rəb'zawpshən, -'sawp) increased intestinal absorption of a substance.

hyperacid (,hiepə'rasid) abnormally or excessively acid.

hyperacidity (,hiepə·rə'siditee) excessive acidity.

hyperactive (,hiepə'raktiv) exhibiting hyperactivity; hyperkinetic.

hyperactivity (,hiepə·rak'tivitee) abnormally increased activity. Developmental hyperactivity of children (*hyperkinesia)* is characterized by very restless, impulsive behaviour. These children are usually inattentive and have a poor concentration span. Other features which may be associated with hyperactivity include aggression, anxiety, poor eating and sleeping patterns, and social and learning difficulties.

Patterns of behaviour vary in individual children and even in the same child from day to day, at times from hour to hour. The condition usually abates during adolescence.

A small percentage of cases of hyperactivity result from brain damage and psychoses; however, the specific causes of most cases have not been determined.

Special diets, designed around the rigid exclusion of certain foods to which the child may be allergic, have been tried. However, at the present time the efficacy of such diets has not been proven. Diets based on the exclusion of food additives and colouring continue to be used by some parents for their children.

Medications that have been tried with varying degrees of success are stimulants and antidepressants, which have the paradoxical effect of calming the child, and tranquillizers. This form of drug therapy is highly controversial and is only a palliative measure that is not without risks.

hyperacusia, hyperacusis (,hiepə·rə'kyoozi·ə; ,hiepə·rə'kyoosis) abnormal acuteness of the sense of hearing.

hyperacute (,hiepə·rə'kyoot) extremely acute.

hyperadenosis (,hiepə,radə'nohsis) enlargement of glands.

hyperadiposis (,hiepə,radi'pohsis) extreme fatness.

hyperadrenalaemia (,hiepə·rə,dreenə'leemi·ə) increased amount of adrenal secretion in the blood.

hyperadrenalism, hyperadrenia (,hiepə·rə'dreenə,lizəm; ,hiepə·rə'dreeni·ə) overactivity of the adrenal glands.

hyperadrenocorticalism, hyperadrenocorticism (,hiepə·rə,dreenoh'kawtikə,lizəm; ,hiepə·rə,dreenoh'kawti,sizəm) hypersecretion of the adrenal cortex; CUSHING'S SYNDROME.

hyperaemia (,hiepə'reemi·ə) an excess of blood in a part. adj. **hyperaemic.**

active h., arterial h. that due to local or general relaxation of arterioles.

leptomeningeal h. congestion of the pia-arachnoid.

passive h. that due to obstruction to flow of blood

from the area.
reactive h. that due to increase in blood flow after its temporary interruption.
venous h. passive hyperaemia.
hyperaesthesia (ˌhiepə·ris'theezi·ə) a state of abnormally increased sensitivity to stimuli. adj. **hyperaesthetic.**
hyperaffectivity (ˌhiepə·rafek'tivitee) abnormally increased sensibility to mild stimuli; abnormally heightened emotional reactivity.
hyperalbuminaemia (ˌhiepə·ralˌbyoomi'neemi·ə) excessive albumin content of the blood.
hyperaldosteronaemia (ˌhiepə·ralˌdostə·rə'neemi·ə) excess of aldosterone in the blood.
hyperaldosteronism (ˌhiepə·ral'dostə·rəˌnizəm) see ALDOSTERONISM.
hyperaldosteronuria (ˌhiepə·ralˌdostə·roh'nyooə·ri·ə) excess of aldosterone in the urine.
hyperalgesia (ˌhiepə·ral'jeezi·ə) excessive sensitiveness to noxious stimulation. adj. **hyperalgesic.**
hyperalimentation (ˌhiepəˌralimen'tayshən) a programme of parenteral administration of all nutrients for patients with gastrointestinal dysfunction; also called *total parenteral alimentation (TPA)* and *total parenteral nutrition (TPN)*.
Although the term *hyperalimentation* is commonly used to designate total or supplementary nutrition by intravenous feedings, it is not technically correct inasmuch as the procedure does not involve an abnormally increased or excessive amount of feeding. For more information, see parenteral NUTRITION.
hyperalkalinity (ˌhiepəˌralkə'linitee) excessive alkalinity.
hyperalphalipoproteinaemia (ˌhiepəˌalfəˌlipohˌprohti'neemi·ə) the presence of abnormally high levels of α-lipoproteins in the serum.
hyperammoniaemia (ˌhiepə·rəˌmohni'eemi·ə) a metabolic disorder marked by elevated levels of ammonia or ammonium ion in the blood.
hyperammoniuria (ˌhiepə·rəˌmohni'yooə·ri·ə) excess of ammonia in the urine.
hyperamylasaemia (ˌhiepəˌramilay'zeemi·ə) abnormally high levels of amylase in the blood serum.
hyperanakinesia (ˌhiepəˌranəki'neezi·ə) excessive motor activity.
hyperaphia (ˌhiepə'rafi·ə) abnormal acuteness of the sense of touch. adj. **hyperaphic.**
hyperarousal (ˌhiepə·rə'rowzəl) a state of increased psychological and physiological tension marked by such effects as reduced pain tolerance, insomnia, fatigue, and accentuation of personality traits.
hyperasthenia (ˌhiepə·ras'theeni·ə) extreme weakness.
hyperazotaemia (ˌhiepəˌrazoh'teemi·ə) excess of nitrogenous matter in the blood.
hyperazoturia (ˌhiepəˌrazoh'tyooə·ri·ə) excess of nitrogenous matter in the urine.
hyperbaric (ˌhiepə'barik) characterized by greater than normal pressure or weight; applied to gases under greater than atmospheric pressure, or to a solution of greater specific gravity than another taken as a standard of reference.
h. oxygenation exposure to oxygen under conditions of greatly increased pressure; abbreviated HPO, for high-pressure oxygenation. This treatment is given to patients who, for various reasons, need more oxygen than they can take in by breathing while in the ordinary atmosphere, or even in an oxygen tent.
The patient is placed in a sealed enclosure, called a hyperbaric chamber. Compressed air is introduced to raise the atmospheric pressure to several times normal. At the same time the patient is given pure oxygen through a face mask. The increase in atmospheric pressure forces enough air into the patient so that the pressure within his body equals the pressure outside. Thus all his tissues become flooded with more than the usual supply of oxygen. While the patient is in the chamber, pressure changes are controlled with extreme care to avoid injury to his lungs or other tissues.
USE OF HYPERBARIC OXYGENATION. This form of treatment may be administered in many types of disorders in which oxygen supply is deficient. If, because of injury or disease, the lungs or heart are unable to maintain good circulation, the increase in oxygen can temporarily compensate for the reduction in circulation. If injury or disease has caused the breaking or blocking of arteries, an extra supply of oxygen in the vessels that are still functioning will help.
Hyperbaric oxygenation has been used with apparent success in some cases of heart surgery and other operations during which a forced supply of oxygen to the patient is vital. During such operations, the surgeon and his assistants must work within the chamber. Since the high pressure could cause the

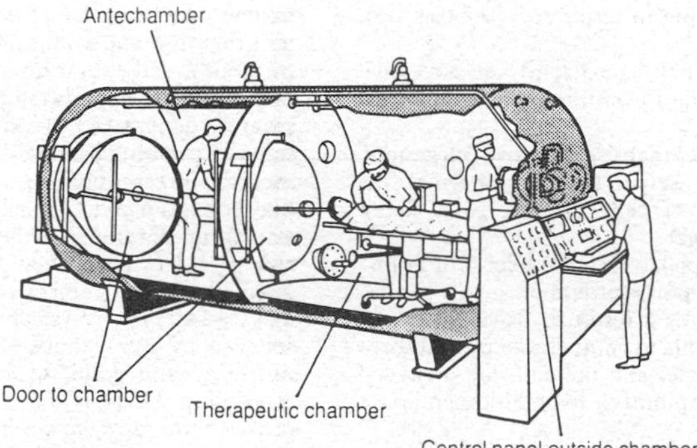

Hyperbaric chamber

physical and mental disturbances of BENDS, as sometimes happens with deep-sea divers, it must be carefully controlled. All persons must be decompressed after leaving the chamber.

Patients suffering from tetanus and gas gangrene, infections caused by bacteria that are resistant to antibiotics but vulnerable to oxygen, are helped by hyperbaric oxygenation. The technique is apparently also useful in radiotherapy for cancer. When full of oxygen, cancer cells seem more vulnerable to radiation.

Carbon monoxide poisoning can be treated by hyperbaric oxygenation. Carbon monoxide molecules, displacing the oxygen in the erythrocytes, usually cause asphyxiation, but hyperbaric oxygenation can often keep the patient alive until the carbon monoxide has been eliminated from his system.

hyperbarism (ˌhiepəˈbarizəm) a condition due to exposure to ambient gas pressure or atmospheric pressures exceeding the pressure within the body.

hyperbetalipoproteinaemia (ˌhiepəˌbeetəˌlipohˌprohtiˈneemi·ə) increased accumulation of β-lipoproteins in the blood.

hyperbilirubinaemia (ˌhiepəˌbiliˌroobiˈneemi·ə) excess of bilirubin in the blood; classified as conjugated or unconjugated according to the form of bilirubin present.

hyperbrachycephalic (ˌhiepəˌbrakikəˈfalik, -səˈfalik) having a very short, wide head.

hyperbradykininaemia (ˌhiepəˌbradiˌkiniˈneemi·ə) an excess of bradykinin in the blood.

hyperbradykininism (ˌhiepəˌbradiˈkiniˌnizəm) a syndrome in which bradykininaemia is associated with a fall in systolic blood pressure on standing, increased diastolic pressure and heart rate, and purplish discoloration and ecchymoses over the legs.

hyperbulia (ˌhiepəˈbyooli·ə) excessive wilfulness.

hypercalcaemia (ˌhiepəkalˈseemi·ə) abnormally high concentration of calcium in the blood; may be caused by overadministration of vitamin D, hyperparathyroidism, thyrotoxicosis, breakdown of bone by malignant disease, or impaired renal function.

idiopathic h. a condition of infants, associated with vitamin D intoxication, characterized by elevated serum calcium levels, increased skeletal density, mental deterioration, and nephrocalcinosis.

hypercalciuria (ˌhiepəˌkalsiˈyooə·ri·ə) excess of calcium in the urine.

hypercapnia, hypercarbia (ˌhiepəˈkapni·ə; ˌhiepəˈkahbi·ə) excess of carbon dioxide in the blood, indicated by an elevated $P\text{CO}_2$ as determined by BLOOD GAS ANALYSIS, and resulting in respiratory ACIDOSIS. adj. **hypercapnic.**

hypercatabolism (ˌhiepəkəˈtabəˌlizəm) an excessive rate of catabolism leading to wasting or destruction of a part or tissue.

hypercatharsis (ˌhiepəkəˈthahsis) excessive purgation.

hypercellularity (ˌhiepəˌselyuhˈlaritee) abnormal increase in the number of cells present, as in bone marrow. adj. **hypercellular.**

hyperchloraemia (ˌhiepəˌkloˈreemi·ə) excess of chlorides in the blood. adj. **hyperchloraemic.**

The condition occurs as a result of fluid deficit for which the kidney attempts to compensate by reabsorbing large amounts of water and the chloride dissolved in it. The signs and symptoms of hyperchloraemia are those of ACIDOSIS.

hyperchlorhydria (ˌhiepəklorˈhiedri·ə) excess of HYDROCHLORIC ACID in the gastric juice.

hypercholesteraemia, hypercholesterolaemia (ˌhiepəkəˌlestəˈreemi·ə; ˌhiepəkəˌlestə·roˈleemi·ə) excess of cholesterol in the blood.

familial h. hyperlipoproteinaemia (type II).

hypercholia (ˌhiepəˈkohli·ə) excessive secretion of bile.

hyperchromatism (ˌhiepəˈkrohməˌtizəm) 1. excessive pigmentation. 2. abnormal cell nuclei filled with particles of chromatin. 3. increased staining capacity. adj. **hyperchromatic.**

hyperchromatosis (ˌhiepəˌkrohməˈtohsis) hyperchromatism.

hyperchromia (ˌhiepəˈkrohmi·ə) 1. hyperchromatism. 2. abnormal increase in the haemoglobin content of erythrocytes. adj. **hyperchromic.**

hyperchylia (ˌhiepəˈkieli·ə) excessive secretion of gastric juice.

hyperchylomicronaemia (ˌhiepəˌkielohˌmiekrəˈneemi·ə) the presence in the blood of an excessive number of particles of fat (chylomicrons).

hypercoagulability (ˌhiepəkohˌagyuhləˈbilitee) abnormally increased coagulability of the blood.

hypercorticism (ˌhiepəˈkawtiˌsizəm) hyperadrenocorticalism.

hypercryalgesia, hypercryaesthesia (ˌhiepəˌkriealˈjeezi·ə; ˌhiepəˌkrieisˈtheezi·ə) excessive sensitiveness to cold.

hypercusis (ˌhiepəˈkyoosis) hyperacusis.

hypercyanotic (ˌhiepəˌsieəˈnotik) extremely cyanotic.

hypercytosis (ˌhiepəsieˈtohsis) an abnormally increased number of cells, especially of leukocytes.

hyperdactyly (ˌhiepəˈdaktilee) the presence of supernumerary digits on the hand or foot.

hyperdicrotic (ˌhiepədieˈkrotik) markedly dicrotic.

hyperdistention (ˌhiepədiˈstenshən) excessive distention.

hyperdiuresis (ˌhiepəˌdieyuhˈreesis) excessive secretion of urine.

hyperdontia (ˌhiepəˈdonshi·ə) a condition characterized by the presence of supernumerary teeth.

hyperdynamia (ˌhiepədieˈnami·ə) excessive muscular activity. adj. **hyperdynamic.**

hyperemesis (ˌhiepəˈreməsis) excessive vomiting. adj. **hyperemetic.**

h. gravidarum excessive and pernicious vomiting of pregnancy, usually in the first trimester. The condition is more serious than simple MORNING SICKNESS, a common discomfort during the first 3 months of pregnancy. The exact cause of hyperemesis gravidarum is not known; however, psychological factors are thought to play an important role in its development and control.

SYMPTOMS. It initially presents as morning sickness which persists beyond 14 weeks, and causes loss of weight and acetone in the urine. Eventually the patient may complain of uncontrollable nausea, persistent retching and vomiting, inability to take any food by mouth, and exhaustion due to restlessness and lack of sleep. As the condition persists the patient becomes severely dehydrated, develops a fever, and may show signs of peripheral nerve involvement and jaundice if medical intervention does not take place. The urine may contain blood, bile, albumin, and ketone bodies as starvation develops. Although hyperemesis gravidarum is rarely fatal, these latter symptoms indicate a grave illness that demands prompt treatment.

TREATMENT. The physical symptoms of the patient are relieved by intravenous administration of fluids and nutrients and mild sedation to promote rest and relaxation. There is some controversy as to the value of psychotherapy; however, it is generally agreed that the patient will need help in overcoming emotional problems and nervous tension if they contribute to the occurrence of the disorder.

Dietary treatment is aimed at avoiding dehydration and electrolyte imbalance.

PATIENT CARE. The hospitalized patient should be placed in a quiet, well ventilated room that is free from odours or sights that may cause nausea. She should be encouraged to talk about her fears and anxieties if she indicates a desire to do so. The midwifery staff should be alert to signs of depression or fears of pregnancy, labour, or the responsibilities of motherhood. Recovery is much more likely if the patient is able to vocalize her fears and seek aid in solving the mental conflicts that may be an underlying cause of her illness. Those who care for her should be sympathetic, optimistic, and reassuring in discussing her condition with her.

hyperencephalus (ˌhiepə·renˈkefələs, -ˈsef-) a fetus or infant with the cranial vault absent and the brain exposed.

hypereosinophilia (ˌhiepəˌreeəˌsinəˈfili·ə) an extreme degree of eosinophilia. adj. **hypereosinophilic.**

hypereosinophilic syndrome (ˌhiepəˌreeəˌsinəˈfilik) a massive increase in the number of eosinophils in the blood, mimicking leukaemia, and characterized by eosinophilic infiltration of the heart, brain, liver, and lungs and by a fatal course.

hyperequilibrium (ˌhiepəˌreekwiˈlibri·əm) excessive tendency to vertigo.

hypererethism (hiepəˈreriˌthizəm) extreme irritability.

hyperergasia (ˌhiepə·rərˈgayzi·ə) excessive functional activity.

hyperesophoria (ˌhiepəˌresohˈfor·ri·ə) deviation of the visual axes upward and inward.

hyperexophoria (ˌhiepəˌreksohˈfor·ri·ə) deviation of the visual axes upward and outward.

hyperextension (ˌhiepə·rekˈstenshən) extension of a limb or part beyond the normal limit.

hyperferraemia (ˌhiepəfəˈreemi·ə) excess of iron in the blood. adj. **hyperferraemic.**

hyperfibrinogenaemia (ˌhiepəfieˌbrinəjəˈneemi·ə) excessive fibrinogen in the blood; fibrinogenaemia.

hyperflexion (ˌhiepəˈflekshən) flexion of a limb or part beyond the normal limit.

hyperfunction (ˌhiepəˈfungkshən) excessive functioning of a part or organ.

hypergalactia, hypergalactosis (ˌhiepəgəˈlakti·ə; ˌhiepəˌgaləkˈtohsis) excessive secretion of milk.

hypergammaglobulinaemia (ˌhiepəˌgaməˌglobyuhliˈneemi·ə) increased gamma globulins in the blood. adj. **hypergammaglobulinaemic.**

monoclonal h. an excess of homogeneous immunoglobulin molecules of a single specificity in the blood following proliferation of a clone of immunoglobulin-producing cells.

hypergastrinaemia (ˌhiepəˌgastriˈneemi·ə) an excess of gastrin in the blood.

hypergenesis (ˌhiepəˈjenəsis) excessive development.

hypergenitalism (ˌhiepəˈjenitəˌlizəm) hypergonadism.

hypergeusaesthesia, hypergeusia (ˌhiepəˌgyoozisˈtheezi·ə; ˌhiepəˈgyoozi·ə) abnormal acuteness of the sense of taste.

hyperglandular (ˌhiepəˈglandyuhlə) marked by excessive glandular activity.

hyperglobulia (ˌhiepəgloˈbyooli·ə) excess of erythrocytes; erythrocytosis; polycythaemia.

hyperglobulinaemia (ˌhiepəˌglobyuhliˈneemi·ə) excess of globulin in the blood.

hyperglucagonaemia (ˌhiepəˌglookəgəˈneemi·ə) abnormally high levels of glucagon in the blood.

hyperglycaemia (ˌhiepəglieˈseemi·a) excess of glucose in the blood.

hyperglycaemic (ˌhiepəglieˈseemik) characterized by or causing hyperglycaemia.

h. hyperosmolar nonketotic coma (HHNK) a metabolic derangement in which there is an abnormally high serum glucose level without ketoacidosis. It can occur in DIABETES MELLITUS, even in borderline and unrecognized cases, in pancreatic disorders that interfere with the production of insulin, as a complication of extensive burns, and in conditions marked by an excess of steroids, as in steroid therapy or acute stress conditions. The condition also may develop during HYPERALIMENTATION, HAEMODIALYSIS, and PERITONEAL DIALYSIS.

SYMPTOMS. The hyperglycaemia of HHNK is usually extreme, with fasting blood sugar levels ranging from 35 to 155 mmol/l of blood. In contrast to typical diabetic coma, however, the serum acetone level is normal or only slightly elevated. This occurs because, although there is sufficient insulin available to avoid ketosis, there is not enough to metabolize the glucose and thereby relieve the hyperglycaemia. It is also believed that the glucocorticoids and dehydration inhibit the production of ketone bodies.

Hyperosmolality, resulting from the extremely high concentration of sugar in the blood, causes a shift of water from the intracellular fluid (the less concentrated solution) into the blood (the higher concentrated solution). This results in cellular dehydration. Another symptom of HHNK, polyuria, occurs because the high plasma osmolality prevents the normal osmotic return of water to the blood by the renal tubules, and it is excreted in the urine. This leads to a decreased blood volume, which severely hampers the kidney's excretion of glucose and a vicious cycle is begun.

TREATMENT. It is essential that HHNK be recognized early and treatment begun immediately to break the chain of metabolic aberrations that are occurring. It is estimated that the mortality rate of HHNK is 60 to 70 per cent, and the probable reason for this high mortality rate is failure to recognize the condition and institute prompt corrective measures.

Insulin is administered in small doses, the amount and frequency depending on periodic assessment of blood glucose levels. The objective is to avoid the extremes of hyperglycaemia and hypoglycaemia. Intravenous fluids are administered cautiously, so that the sodium and water deficits can be corrected without producing extreme shifts of water from the blood into the intracellular compartment and thus failing to correct the hyperosmolar condition of the blood. Electrolytes other than the sodium lost through diuresis also must be replaced as indicated by laboratory findings.

Dehydration plays a major role in the development of severe HHNK; thus patient care is concerned with careful monitoring of those patients susceptible to its development, especially the elderly, the debilitated, and the mild or unsuspected diabetic. Maintenance of an adequate fluid balance can do much to prevent the hyperosmolar condition and the development of a chain of events that can rapidly lead to coma and death.

hyperglyceridaemia (ˌhiepəˌglisə·riˈdeemi·ə) excess of glycerides in the blood.

hyperglycinaemia (ˌhiepəˌgliesiˈneemi·ə) a hereditary metabolic disorder involving excessive glycine in the blood and urine. One form is characterized by episodic vomiting, lethargy, dehydration, ketosis, and increased susceptibility to infection; a second form by generalized hypotonia, lethargy, absence of reflexes, and periodic myoclonic jerks.

hyperglycinuria (ˌhiepəˌgliesiˈnyooə·ri·ə) an excess of glycine in the urine (see also HYPERGLYCINAEMIA).

hyperglycogenolysis (ˌhiepəˌgliekohjiˈnolisis) excessive splitting up of glycogen (glycogenolysis).

hyperglycorrhachia (ˌhiepəˌgliekə'raki·ə, -'rayki·ə) excessive sugar in the cerebrospinal fluid.
hyperglycosuria (ˌhiepəˌgliekoh'syooə·ri·ə) extreme glycosuria.
hypergnosia (ˌhiepə'nohsi·ə) a paranoic condition marked by distortion of perception with a tendency to project psychic conflicts to the environment.
hypergonadism (ˌhiepə'gonəˌdizəm) abnormally increased functional activity of the gonads, with excessive growth and precocious sexual development.
hyperhaemoglobinaemia (ˌhiepəˌheeməˌglohbi'neemi·ə) an excess of haemoglobin in the blood.
hyperhedonia (ˌhiepəhi'dohni·ə) morbid increase of pleasure in agreeable acts.
hyperhidrosis (ˌhiepəhi'drohsis) excessive perspiration. adj. **hyperhidrotic.**
hyperhydration (ˌhiepəhie'drayshən) abnormally increased water content of the body.
hyperidrosis (ˌhiepə·ri'drohsis) hyperhidrosis.
hyperimmune (ˌhiepə·ri'myoon) possessing very large quantities of specific antibodies in the serum.
hyperimmunoglobulinaemia (ˌhiepəˌrimyuhnohˌglobyuhli'neemi·ə) abnormally high levels of immunoglobulins in the serum.
hyperinflation (ˌhiepə·rin'flayshən) excessive inflation or expansion, as of the lungs; overinflation.
hyperinsulinism (ˌhiepə'insyuhliˌnizəm) 1. excessive secretion of insulin by the pancreas, resulting in hypoglycaemia. 2. hypoglycaemia from overdosage of insulin.
hyperinvolution (ˌhiepəˌrinvə'looshən) superinvolution.
hyperirritability (ˌhiepəˌriritə'bilitee) pathological responsiveness to slight stimuli.
hyperisotonic (ˌhiepəˌiesə'tonik) denoting a solution containing more than 0.45 per cent salt, in which erythrocytes become crenated as a result of exosmosis.
hyperkalaemia (ˌhiepəkə'leemi·ə) abnormally high potassium concentration in the blood; it may be caused by decreased renal excretion, severe or extensive burns, intestinal obstruction, adrenocortical insufficiency, or overadministration of potassium. adj. **hyperkalaemic.**

Potassium levels greater than 5.5 mmol/l can produce electrocardiographic abnormalities evident first as elevated T waves and depressed P waves, and eventually by atrial asystole. Other signs and symptoms include muscular weakness, tingling of the hands, feet, and tongue, and a slow irregular pulse. As the amount of serum potassium continues to rise to above 7 mmol/l there is potential for respiratory paralysis, asystole or ventricular fibrillation, and cardiac arrest.

Treatment of hyperkalaemia consists of removing the excess potassium from the body or giving calcium gluconate to ameliorate the cardiotoxic effects.

hyperkeratinization (ˌhiepəˌkerətinie'zayshən) excessive development of keratin in the epidermis.
hyperkeratosis (ˌhiepəˌkerə'tohsis) 1. hypertrophy of the horny layer of the skin, or any disease characterized by it. 2. hypertrophy of the cornea. adj. **hyperkeratotic.**

epidermolytic h. a hereditary disease, with hyperkeratosis, blisters, and erythema; at birth, the skin is entirely covered with thick, horny, armour-like plates that are soon shed, leaving a raw surface on which the scales re-form.

hyperketonaemia (ˌhiepəˌkeetə'neemi·ə) abnormally increased concentration of ketone bodies in the blood.
hyperketonuria (ˌhiepəˌkeetə'nyooə·ri·ə) excessive ketone in the urine.
hyperketosis (ˌhiepəkee'tohsis) excessive formation of ketone.
hyperkinaemia (ˌhiepəki'neemi·ə) abnormally high cardiac output.
hyperkinesia (ˌhiepəki'neezi·ə) abnormally increased motor function or activity. See also HYPERACTIVITY.
hyperkinesis (ˌhiepəki'neesis) hyperkinesia.
hyperkinetic (ˌhiepəki'netik) pertaining to or marked by hyperkinesia.

h. syndrome a disorder of childhood, usually abating during adolescence, marked by overactivity, distractibility, restlessness, and low tolerance for frustration (see also HYPERACTIVITY).

hyperlactation (ˌhiepəlak'tayshən) lactation in greater than normal amount or for a longer than normal period.
hyperleukocytosis (ˌhiepəˌlookohsie'tohsis) excess of leukocytes in the blood.
hyperlipaemia (ˌhiepəli'peemi·ə) an excess of lipids in the blood.

carbohydrate-induced h. hyperlipoproteinaemia (type IV).

fat-induced h. hyperlipoproteinaemia (type I).

hyperlipidaemia (ˌhiepəˌlipi'deemi·ə) a general term for elevated concentrations of any or all of the lipids in the plasma.
hyperlipoproteinaemia (ˌhiepəˌlipohˌprohti'neemi·ə) an excess of lipoproteins in the blood, which is due to a disorder of lipoprotein metabolism, and may be acquired or hereditary. The *acquired* form occurs secondarily to another disorder or as a result of environmental factors (e.g., diet). The *hereditary* form is classified into five major phenotypes based on clinical features, enzymatic abnormalities, and serum lipoprotein electrophoretic patterns: *Type I* may be manifested clinically by repeated bouts of abdominal pain and vomiting, recurrent acute pancreatitis, eruptive xanthomas, hepatosplenomegaly, and lipaemia retinalis; *Type II* by tendinous and tuberous xanthomas, xanthelasmas, early onset of corneal arcus, and accelerated atherosclerosis; *Type III* chiefly by planar xanthomas; *Type IV* by increased incidence of vascular disease, abnormal glucose tolerance, and family history of diabetes mellitus; and *Type V* by diabetes mellitus, eruptive xanthomas, and recurrent acute pancreatitis.
hyperliposis (ˌhiepəli'pohsis) excess of fat in the serum or tissues.
hyperlithuria (ˌhiepəli'thyooə·ri·ə) excess of uric (lithic) acid in the urine.
hyperlysinaemia (ˌhiepəˌliesi'neemi·ə) an inborn error of amino acid metabolism characterized by elevated levels of lysine in the blood, and marked by vomiting, spasticity, coma, and mental handicap; symptoms are related to protein intake.
hypermagnesaemia (ˌhiepəˌmagni'zeemi·ə) an abnormally large magnesium content of the blood plasma.
hypermastia (ˌhiepə'masti·ə) 1. excessive size of mammary glands. 2. the presence of one or more supernumerary mammary glands; polymastia.
hypermature (ˌhiepəmə'tyooə) beyond maturity; overripe, as a cataract when the lens becomes enlarged.
hypermenorrhoea (ˌhiepəˌmenə'reeə) excessive uterine bleeding occurring at regular intervals, the period of flow being of usual duration. More usually called menorrhagia.
hypermetabolism (ˌhiepəmə'tabəˌlizəm) increased metabolism.

extrathyroidal m. abnormally elevated basal metabolism unassociated with thyroid disease.

hypermetria (ˌhiepə'meetri·ə) ataxia in which movements overreach the intended goal.
hypermetrope (ˌhiepə'metrohp) one who is hyperme-

tropic.

hypermetropia (ˌhiepəme'trohpi·ə) longsightedness; a visual defect in which parallel light rays reaching the eye come to focus behind the retina, vision being better for distant objects than for near (see also VISION).

Most children are born with some degree of longsightedness. As the child grows the condition decreases and usually disappears by the age of 8 years. If the child is excessively longsighted, however, the constant effort to focus may cause headaches and fatigue, and may also contribute to the development of a convergent strabismus with amblyopia.

The glasses used to correct hypermetropia are convex; that is, they bend the light rays toward the centre, helping the lens of the eye to focus them on the retina.

hypermnesia (ˌhiepərm'neezi·ə) extreme retentiveness of memory.

hypermorph ('hiepəˌmawf) 1. a person who is tall, but of low sitting height. 2. in genetics, a hypermorphic mutant gene, i.e. one exaggerating or increasing normal activity. adj. **hypermorphic.**

hypermotility (ˌhiepəmoh'tilitee) excessive or abnormally increased motility, as of the gastrointestinal tract.

hypermyotonia (ˌhiepəˌmieoh'tohni·ə) excessive muscular tonicity.

hypermyotrophy (ˌhiepəmie'otrəfee) excessive development of muscular tissue.

hypernasality (ˌhiepənay'zalitee) a quality of voice in which the emission of air through the nose is excessive due to velopharyngeal incompetence; it causes deterioration of intelligibility of speech.

hypernatraemia (ˌhiepənə'treemi·ə) an excess of SODIUM in the blood, indicative of water loss exceeding the sodium loss. adj. **hypernatraemic.**

hyperneocytosis (ˌhiepəˌniohsie'tohsis) leukocytosis with an excessive number of immature forms of leukocytes.

hypernephroma (ˌhiepəne'frohmə) former term for carcinoma of the kidney. Called also *Grawitz tumour.* See KIDNEY.

hypernoia (ˌhiepə'noyə) excessive mental activity.

hypernutrition (ˌhiepənyoo'trishən) overfeeding and its ill effects.

hyperonychia (ˌhiepə·rə'niki·ə) hypertrophy of the nails.

hyperorchidism (ˌhiepə'rawkiˌdizəm) abnormally increased functional activity of the testes.

hyperorexia (ˌhiepə·rə'reksi·ə) excessive appetite.

hyperorthocytosis (ˌhiepəˌrawthohsie'tohsis) leukocytosis with a normal proportion of the various forms of leukocytes.

hyperosmia (ˌhiepə'rozmi·ə) abnormal acuteness of the sense of smell.

hyperosmolality (ˌhiepəˌrozmə'lalitee) an increase in the osmolality of the body fluids.

hyperosmolarity (ˌhiepəˌrozmə'laritee) abnormally increased osmotic concentration of a solution.

hyperostosis (ˌhiepə·ro'stohsis) excessive growth of bony tissue. adj. **hyperostotic.**

frontal internal h., h. frontalis interna a new formation of bone tissue protruding in patches on the internal surface of the cranial bones in the frontal region, most commonly affecting women near menopause.

generalized cortical h. a hereditary disorder beginning during puberty, marked by osteosclerosis of the skull, mandible, clavicles, ribs, and diaphyses of long bones, associated with elevated blood alkaline phosphatase.

infantile cortical h. a disease of young infants characterized by soft tissue swellings over the affected bones, fever, and irritability, and marked by periods of remission and exacerbation.

Morgagni's h. frontal internal hyperostosis.

hyperoxaemia (ˌhiepə·rok'seemi·ə) excessive acidity of the blood.

hyperoxaluria (ˌhiepəˌroksə'lyooə·ri·ə) an excess of oxalate in the urine.

enteric h. formation of calcium oxalate calculi in the urinary tract, occurring after extensive resection or disease of the ileum, due to excessive absorption of oxalate from the colon.

primary h. a genetic disorder characterized by urinary excretion of oxalate, with nephrolithiasis, nephrocalcinosis, early onset of renal failure, and often a generalized deposit of calcium oxalate.

hyperoxia (ˌhiepə'roksi·ə) an abnormally increased supply or concentration of oxygen.

hyperparasite (ˌhiepə'parəˌsiet) a parasite that preys on a parasite. adj. **hyperparasitic.**

hyperparathyroidism (ˌhiepəˌparə'thieroyˌdizəm) abnormally increased activity of the parathyroid gland which may be primary or secondary. *Primary* hyperparathyroidism is associated with single or multiple adenomas of the parathyroid glands. In the latter case the disease may be familial. *Secondary* hyperparathyroidism, with hyperplastic parathyroid glands, develops as a compensating mechanism when the serum calcium level is persistently pushed down, as in chronic renal failure. The clinical manifestations of this frequently afflict patients on renal dialysis. The same mechanism operates without obvious clinical effect in states of vitamin D deficiency.

An excess of parathyroid hormone alters the function of bone cells, renal tubules, and gastrointestinal mucosa. Calcium is brought out of bone to raise the serum calcium above normal. Bones are weakened by demineralization and by the formation of cysts full of osteoclasts (osteitis fibrosa cystica). Excess calcium is excreted in the urine, causing renal stones to form. The majority of primary hyperparathyroid cases are to be found among patients with renal stones. Hypercalcaemia itself causes muscular weakness, anorexia, and vomiting; it may cause pancreatitis.

Primary hyperparathyroidism is treated surgically, removing the parathyroid adenoma(s). In chronic renal failure, partial parathyroidectomy may be indicated for secondary hyperparathyroidism. The level of serum calcium can be brought down towards normal by full hydration of the patient and the administration of phosphate (orally or by intravenous infusion).

hyperpepsinia (ˌhiepəpep'sini·ə) excessive secretion of pepsin in the stomach.

hyperperistalsis (ˌhiepəˌperi'stalsis) excessively active peristalsis.

hyperphagia (ˌhiepə'fayji·ə) over-eating.

hyperphalangism (ˌhiepəfə'lanjizəm) the presence of a supernumerary phalanx on a finger or toe.

hyperphasia (ˌhiepə'fayzi·ə) excessive talkativeness.

hyperphenylalaninaemia (ˌhiepəˌfeenieˌlaləni'neemi·ə) an excess of phenylalanine in the blood, as in phenylketonuria.

hyperphonesis (ˌhiepəfoh'neesis) intensification of the sound in auscultation or percussion.

hyperphoria (ˌhiepə'for·ri·ə) HETEROPHORIA in which there is permanent upward deviation of the visual axis of an eye in the absence of visual fusional stimuli.

hyperphosphataemia (ˌhiepəˌfosfə'teemi·ə) an excess of phosphates in the blood.

hyperphosphatasaemia (ˌhiepəˌfosfətə'seemi·ə) high levels of alkaline phosphatase in the blood; see HYPERPHOSPHATASIA.

hyperphosphatasia (ˌhiepəˌfosfə'tayzi·ə) a hereditary condition transmitted as an autosomal recessive trait, marked by abnormally high alkaline phosphatase levels in the serum and by macrocranium, short neck and thorax, lateral bowing of the femurs, and anterior bowing of the tibias.

hyperphosphaturia (ˌhiepəˌfosfə'tyooə·ri·ə) an excess of phosphates in the urine.

hyperphrenia (ˌhiepə'freeni·ə) 1. extreme mental excitement. 2. accelerated mental activity.

hyperpiesis (ˌhiepəpie'eesis) abnormally high blood pressure (see HYPERTENSION).

hyperpigmentation (ˌhiepəˌpigmen'tayshən) abnormally increased pigmentation.

hyperpituitarism (ˌhiepəpi'tyooitəˌrizəm) a condition due to pathologically increased PITUITARY GLAND, activity, especially increased secretion of growth hormone, resulting in acromegaly or gigantism.

hyperplasia (ˌhiepə'playzi·ə) abnormal increase in volume of a tissue or organ caused by the formation and growth of new normal cells. adj. **hyperplastic**.

hyperplasmia (ˌhiepə'plazmi·ə) 1. excess in the proportion of blood plasma to corpuscles. 2. increase in size of erythrocytes through absorption of plasma.

hyperploid ('hiepəˌployd) 1. characterized by hyperploidy. 2. a hyperploid individual or cell.

hyperploidy ('hiepəˌploydee) the state of having more than the typical number of chromosomes in unbalanced sets, as in Down's syndrome.

hyperpnoea (ˌhiepə'neeə, -pəp'neeə) abnormal increase in depth and rate of respiration. adj. **hyperpnoeic**.

hyperponesis (ˌhiepəpə'neesis) excessive action-potential output from the motor and premotor areas of the cortex. adj. **hyperponetic**.

hyperposia (ˌhiepə'pohzi·ə) abnormally increased ingestion of fluids for relatively brief periods.

hyperpotassaemia (ˌhiepəˌpotə'seemi·ə) hyperkalaemia; excess of potassium in the blood.

hyperpragic (ˌhiepə'prayjik) characterized by excessive activity.

hyperpraxia (ˌhiepə'praksi·ə) abnormal activity; restlessness.

hyperprebetalipoproteinaemia (ˌhiepəpreeˌbeetəˌlipohˌprohti'neemi·ə) an excess of prebeta-lipoproteins in the blood.

hyperprolactinaemia (ˌhiepəprohˌlakti'neemi·ə) increased levels of prolactin in the blood; in women, it is associated with infertility and may lead to galactorrhoea, and it has been reported to cause impotence in men.

hyperprolinaemia (ˌhiepəˌprohli'neemi·ə) a disorder of amino acid metabolism marked by excessive proline in the blood.

hyperprosexia (ˌhiepəproh'seksi·ə) preoccupation with one idea to the exclusion of all others.

hyperproteinaemia (ˌhiepəˌprohtiˌneemi·ə) an excess of protein in the blood.

hyperproteosis (ˌhiepəˌprohti'ohsis) a condition due to excess of protein in the diet.

hyperpselaphesia (ˌhiepəˌsela'feezi·ə) increased tactile sensitiveness.

hyperpsychosis (ˌhiepəsie'kohsis) exaggeration of the function of thought.

hyperptyalism (ˌhiepə'tieəˌlizəm) abnormally increased secretion of saliva.

hyperpyrexia (ˌhiepəpie'reksi·ə) excessively high fever; hyperthermia. adj. **hyperpyrexial, hyperpyrexic** (see also FEVER).

malignant h. malignant hyperthermia.

hyperreactive (ˌhiepə·ri'aktiv) showing a greater than normal response to stimuli.

hyperreflexia (ˌhiepə·ri'fleksi·ə) exaggeration of reflexes.

hyperreninaemia (ˌhiepəˌreeni'neemi·ə) a condition of elevated levels of renin in the blood, which may lead to aldosteronism and hypertension.

hyperresonance (ˌhiepə'rezənəns) exaggerated resonance on percussion.

hypersalaemia (ˌhiepəsə'leemi·ə) abnormally increased content of salt in the blood.

hypersalivation (ˌhiepəˌsalie'vayshən) abnormally increased secretion of saliva.

hypersarcosinaemia (ˌhiepəˌsahkohsi'neemi·ə) an inborn error of metabolism due to a defect of sarcosine dehydrogenase, and marked by elevated levels of sarcosine in the blood.

hypersecretion (ˌhiepəsi'kreeshən) excessive secretion.

hypersensitivity (ˌhiepəˌsensi'tivitee) a state of altered reactivity in which the body reacts with an exaggerated immune response to a foreign agent; ANAPHYLAXIS and ALLERGY are forms of hypersensitivity. adj. **hypersensitive**.

contact h. that produced by contact of the skin with a chemical substance having the properties of an antigen or hapten; it includes CONTACT DERMATITIS.

delayed h. a slowly developing increase in cell-mediated immune response (involving T-lymphocytes) to a specific antigen, as occurs in graft rejection, autoimmune disease, etc.

immediate h. antibody-mediated hypersensitivity characterized by lesions resulting from release of histamine and other mediators of hypersensitivity from reagin-sensitized mast cells, causing increased vascular permeability, oedema, and smooth muscle contraction; it includes anaphylaxis and atopy.

hypersensitization (ˌhiepəˌsensitie'zayshən) the induction of hypersensitivity.

hypersialosis (ˌhiepəˌsieə'lohsis) excessive secretion of the salivary glands.

hypersomnia (ˌhiepə'somni·ə) pathologically excessive sleep or drowsiness.

hypersplenism (ˌhiepə'splenizəm) a condition characterized by exaggeration of the haemolytic function of the spleen, resulting in deficiency of peripheral blood elements, and by hypercellularity of the bone marrow and splenomegaly.

hypersthenia (ˌhiepəs'theeni·ə) increased strength or tonicity. adj. **hypersthenic**.

hypertelorism (ˌhiepə'teləˌrizəm) abnormally increased distance between two organs or parts.

ocular h., orbital h. increase in the interocular distance, often associated with cleidocranial or craniofacial dysostosis and sometimes with mental handicap.

hypertensinogen (ˌhiepəten'sinəjən) angiotensinogen.

hypertension (ˌhiepə'tenshən) persistently high BLOOD PRESSURE. In adults, it is generally agreed that a blood pressure is abnormally high when the resting, supine arterial systolic pressure is equal to or greater than 140 mmHg and the diastolic pressure is equal to or greater than 90 mmHg.

A diagnosis of hypertension should be based on a series of readings rather than a single measurement that could be influenced by emotional state or physical activity. Hypertension is not a single disease entity in the usual sense, but rather a major indicator of the prognosis for future development of cardiovascular, cerebrovascular, and renal disease. Results from numerous studies indicate that a diastolic pressure above 90 mmHg reduces life expectancy in all persons of all ages and both sexes. Furthermore, studies have shown that an elevation in systolic pressure is as dangerous and likely to lead to cardiovascular disease as an elevated diastolic pressure.

The Medical Research Council trial of the treatment

of hypertension studied the effect of therapy on more than 17,000 patients with mild to moderate elevation of blood pressure. They concluded that treatment dramatically reduced the likelihood of sustaining a stroke but that there was little effect on the incidence of myocardial infarction.

Hypertension is a major threat to life and health. It is estimated that one in six adults in the UK is hypertensive. Although the disease primarily affects men over 35 and women over 45 years of age, it is not limited to older persons. In recent years, screening clinics have detected hypertension in increasing numbers of teenagers. Between 2 and 6 per cent of adolescents have persistent blood pressure elevations. Prevalence rates for prepubertal children have been reported to be as high as 1 per cent. Hypertension is more severe and more prevalent in blacks of African origin than in whites or Asians by an overall ratio of two to one. Socioeconomic status does not seem to be a factor; the disease is distributed throughout all social, economic, and educational levels.

Statistical data on causes of death do not reflect the role of hypertension as a major contributing factor. Hypertensive individuals usually die from damage to the blood vessels in such vital organs as the heart, brain, and kidney. A large proportion of deaths from strokes are thought to result from pre-existing hypertension. Immediate causes of death related to an extremely high blood pressure include cerebral haemorrhage and heart or kidney failure.

TYPES AND CAUSATIVE FACTORS. There are two major types of hypertension: essential (primary or idiopathic) and secondary hypertension. *Essential* hypertension is by far the most common, accounting for about 95 per cent of all known cases. The cause of this form of hypertension is not known and it is likely that a combination of factors contribute to its occurrence. Contributing factors include age (blood pressure tends to rise throughout life), obesity, excess alcohol consumption, and diet, but heredity seems to be the major predisposing factor. A stressful environment also can produce a tendency toward high blood pressure.

It is known that there is a direct relationship between hypertension and ATHEROSCLEROSIS. Elevated blood pressure levels speed up the atherosclerotic process, and most of the complications of essential hypertension are directly related to this accelerated disease process.

Essential hypertension is insidious and usually asymptomatic, although headaches sometimes occur. As the disease progresses the patient may experience fatigue, dizziness, and palpitations. Eventually, the effects of uncontrolled hypertension become manifest in the form of heart disease, stroke, or renal disease.

Examination of the retinal vessels with an ophthalmoscope can be a reliable index to the extent to which high blood pressure has damaged blood vessels throughout the body.

Malignant or *accelerated* hypertension is a particularly severe form of hypertension. It occurs most often in persons in the fourth or fifth decade of life. About half of its victims have an underlying chronic kidney disease. Diastolic pressures of 130 to 170 mmHg are not unusual in these patients. The most common symptoms are morning headache, blurred vision, breathlessness related to early pulmonary oedema, and symptoms of uraemia.

Malignant hypertension is treated as a medical emergency as soon as it is diagnosed because it can be fatal if not treated promptly. It causes progressive damage to blood vessels in the kidneys and can cause cerebral haemorrhage. With proper care malignant hypertension can be kept under control indefinitely. Without adequate treatment it is often fatal within two years.

Secondary hypertension is actually a sign of a variety of underlying or primary diseases, such as renal vascular disease (e.g. atherosclerosis of the renal artery) and renal parenchymal disease. Other disorders that produce secondary hypertension include dysfunction of the adrenal cortex and medulla, and coarctation of the aorta.

The most common primary disorders leading to secondary hypertension are those that interfere with the supply of blood to the kidney. The resulting ischaemia of renal tissue stimulates the secretion of renin, an enzyme that catalyses the conversion of angiotensinogen to angiotensin I. Other enzymes in the body then convert angiotensin I to angiotensin II, which is the most potent vasoconstrictor known.

Angiotensin II acts directly on the blood vessels and also acts as a physiological stimulant to the adrenal gland and the production of aldosterone. Hence, there is a two-fold effect: (1) an increase in peripheral resistance due to vasoconstriction and a resulting elevation of blood pressure, and (2) a retention of sodium and water by the renal tubules in response to increased levels of serum aldosterone. The retained sodium and water increase blood volume, since they remain in the vascular system rather than being excreted by the kidney. The result is an increased cardiac output and an elevation of blood pressure.

Although the above mechanisms are responsible for elevation of blood pressure in many patients with renal hypertension, they do not completely explain the hypertension. Other factors being studied as possible causes include failure of the kidney either to secrete vasodilators or to inactivate pressor substances produced elsewhere in the body. Another possibility is that there are factors other than the renin–angiotensin–aldosterone axis responsible for the retention of water and sodium by the renal tubules.

TREATMENT. The regimen of therapy prescribed for a patient with essential hypertension is based on the degree of elevation of blood pressure. Patients who have extreme hypertension need immediate drug therapy to bring the blood pressure down to safer levels and avoid catastrophic effects such as heart failure and cerebral haemorrhage. Those who have 'mildly' or 'moderately' high blood pressure should be advised to lose weight if they are obese, to reduce alcohol consumption if excessive, and to stop smoking to reduce the risk of vascular disease.

Drugs used in the treatment of hypertension are prescribed both singly and in combination. One approach commonly used is to begin with a thiazide diuretic or a beta-blocker. If the diuretic or beta-blocker alone does not bring the blood pressure to an acceptable level then both these drugs are combined.

If diuretic and beta-blocker therapy together are not effective, the doctor can choose from a variety of additional drugs with different pharmacological actions. Among the drugs used are calcium channel blockers such as nifedipine or angiotensin-converting enzyme inhibitors such as captopril, both of which reduce blood pressure by a dilator action on blood vessels. Alternatively a centrally acting drug such as methyldopa may be added.

Nonpharmacological modes of therapy include weight loss, limiting SODIUM intake, and limiting the dietary intake of fat. Another adjunct to drug therapy is reduction of stress and promotion of relaxation through biofeedback, relaxation techniques, and meditation.

PATIENT CARE. The greatest challenge in the continued control and management of essential hypertension is gaining the cooperation of the patient so that he will comply with the prescribed regimen of care. Hypertension is a chronic health problem that must be dealt with for the rest of the patient's life. Because the disease is often without symptoms, requires alterations in life style and changes in life-long habits, and demands continued surveillance by health care professionals, many patients become discouraged and fail to follow the advice and counsel offered to them. In order to keep the patient participating in a programme of control, he must be given a clear understanding of the pathology of his disease and the rationale for each aspect of therapy.

There are many reasons why patients do not take an active part in managing their high blood pressure and avoiding its complications. Some discontinue their medications once they begin to feel better, and others stop taking them because they experience unpleasant side-effects and do not realize that other medications can be substituted. It is difficult for some patients to accept the fact that their illness will persist throughout life and that, although there are means by which the disease can be managed, these modes of therapy are effective only insofar as each patient is willing and able to accept the responsibility for carrying out the regimen prescribed for him.

Patient and family education should include information about the factors contributing to hypertension, the changes that uncontrolled hypertension can bring about within the body, the purpose of each prescribed medication, the importance of following the prescribed diet, the expected results of weight loss and other recommendations, and the need to consult with the doctor or other health care professional on a regular basis for support and guidance.

ocular h. persistently elevated intraocular pressure in the absence of any other signs of glaucoma; it may or may not progress to chronic simple glaucoma.

portal h. abnormally increased pressure in the portal circulation.

systemic venous h. elevation of systemic venous pressure, usually detected by inspection of the jugular veins.

hypertensive (ˌhiepəˈtensiv) 1. characterized by or causing increased tension or pressure, as abnormally high blood pressure. 2. a person with hypertension.

hypertensor (ˌhiepəˈtensə) a substance that raises the blood pressure.

hyperthecosis (ˌhiepəthiˈkohsis) hyperplasia and excessive luteinization of the cells of the inner stromal layer of the ovary.

hyperthelia (ˌhiepəˈtheeli·ə) the presence of supernumerary nipples.

hyperthermaesthesia (ˌhiepəˌthərmisˈtheezi·ə) increased sensibility for heat.

hyperthermalgesia (ˌhiepəˌthərmˈlˈjeezi·ə) abnormal sensitiveness to heat.

hyperthermia (ˌhiepəˈthərmi·ə) greatly increased temperature. adj. **hyperthermal, hyperthermic.**

malignant h. a syndrome affecting patients undergoing general anaesthesia, marked by rapid rise in body temperature, signs of increased muscle metabolism, and, usually, rigidity. The sensitivity is inherited as an autosomal dominant trait. This syndrome is associated particularly with the use of suxamethoniumn and/or halothane but is extremely rare (1 in 100,000). Treatment consists of stopping the anaesthetic, cooling the patient, and giving 100 per cent oxygen, sodium bicarbonate to correct acidosis, chlorpromazine and the drug of choice, dantrolene. Since introduction of the latter drug the previous very high mortality has been substantially reduced. Susceptibility to the syndrome is diagnosed using a muscle biopsy.

hyperthrombinaemia (ˌhiepəˌthrombiˈneemi·ə) an excess of thrombin in the blood.

hyperthymia (ˌhiepəˈthiemi·ə) excessive emotionalism.

hyperthymism (ˌhiepəˈthiemizəm) excessive thymus activity.

hyperthyroidism (ˌhiepəˈthieroyˌdizəm) excessive functional activity of the thyroid gland. adj. **hyperthyroid.** It is predominantly a disease of adult women, with peak incidence between 30 and 50 years of age. The clinical state of hyperthyroidism is produced by excessive secretion of normal thyroid hormones, and is also called thyrotoxicosis. This is frequently part of a syndrome that includes goitre and exophthalmos and is known as Graves' disease or Basedow's disease.

Occasionally hyperthyroidism is due to an autonomous functioning adenoma of the thyroid. Usually the thyroid is stimulated to overactivity by thyroid-stimulating immunoglobulins produced as part of autoimmune disease attacking the thyroid. As the tendency to autoimmune thyroid disorders is familial, Graves' disease and myxoedema are often found in the same family. There is anecdotal evidence that emotionally traumatic events in the patient's life may 'trigger' the onset of Graves' disease.

SYMPTOMS. Excess thyroid hormone produces weight loss despite a good appetite. The metabolic rate is greatly accelerated, speeding up all the bodily processes and exaggerating emotional responses. Constant apprehension, fatigue, frequent bowel movements, palpitations and tachycardia are all common symptoms. Tremor of the hands and weakness of proximal limb muscles are often found. Intolerance of heat is very common. In Graves' disease the thyroid enlarges diffusely and its increased vascularity may produce an audible bruit or hum. The eyes appear to stare as the lids retract. Protrusion of one or both eyeballs may occur and may progress to extreme exophthalmos; this is not caused by excess thyroid hormone but by an autoimmune process.

TREATMENT AND PATIENT CARE. General measures of support for the patient suffering from hyperthyroidism include physical and emotional rest and a high calorific, nutritional diet. Tranquillizing drugs may be required in the short term if anxiety is overwhelming. β-Adrenergic blocking drugs, such as propranolol, are prescribed to control the symptoms of tremor, palpitations, and tachycardia. The choice of direct antithyroid treatment will depend on the age of the patient, the size of the goitre, and the patient's response to selected therapies.

It is important that the patient and his family understand the course of the disease, the patient's helplessness in controlling his emotions without medication and support from those around him, and the need to follow conscientiously the regimen prescribed. The patient's environment should be as calm and nonstimulating as possible, both at home and in the hospital.

Hormone production can be controlled with antithyroid drugs, thyroid cells can be destroyed by radioactive iodine or the bulk of the thyroid removed surgically.

Antithyroid Drugs. Carbimazole is currently the most effective and safest of the antithyroid drugs. It can be used alone for long-term treatment or to reduce thyroid hormone production prior to subtotal thyroidectomy; it can also be used in conjunction with radioiodine therapy. Initially it is required in 8-hourly doses and the patient must adhere strictly to the schedule prescribed. It is a useful long-term therapy for children, young adults and pregnant women, and all those hyperthyroid patients who have concomitant destructive autoimmune thyroiditis that will lead to spontaneous 'cure' of hyperthyroidism. Carbimazole may cause skin rashes and arthralgia. Very rarely it causes agranulocytosis, so it is important to monitor the blood count and for the patient to report immediately any sore throat or fever.

Radioactive Iodine. Iodine-131 is the radioactive isotope used; it has a physical half-life of 8 days. It is the choice of treatment for women over childbearing age, those with small goitres or who have relapsed into thyrotoxicosis following surgery. The dosage depends on the size of the thyroid and its sensitivity to radiation, factors that cannot be determined with accuracy. The aim is to 'cure' thyrotoxicosis by one dose. The eventual incidence of postradiation hypothyroidism is very high but it may take many years to develop. If one dose fails to control hyperthyroidism, the patient should receive carbimazole for some months.

Radioactive iodine is excreted in the urine and hence special precautions should be taken in its disposal. Patients receiving large doses of radioiodine are placed in isolation for 8 days. Very occasionally the immediate effect of the radiation may provoke a dramatic increase in hyperthyroidism (thyroid crisis) which requires emergency treatment.

Surgery. Subtotal thyroidectomy is the treatment of choice for patients with large goitres and for many who relapse after adequate treatment with antithyroid drugs. The patient should be made euthyroid (with carbimazole) before operation. Iodide given for 10 days prior to operation will reduce the vascularity of the gland, but the effect is transient and iodides should not be used for longer periods. The complications of thyroid surgery include damage to the vocal cords and the parathyroid glands.

hyperthyroxinaemia (ˌhiepəthieˌroksi'neemi·ə) an excess of thyroxine in the blood.

hypertonia (ˌhiepə'tohni·ə) abnormally increased tonicity or strength.

hypertonic (ˌhiepə'tonik) 1. pertaining to or characterized by an increased tonicity or tension. 2. having an osmotic pressure greater than that of the solution with which it is compared.

hypertonicity (ˌhiepətə'nisitee) the state or quality of being hypertonic.

hypertrichiasis, hypertrichosis (ˌhiepətri'kieəsis; ˌhiepətri'kohsis) excessive hairiness; hirsutism.

hypertriglyceridaemia (ˌhiepətrieˌglisə·ri'deemi·ə) an excess of triglycerides in the blood; a familial form occurs in hyperlipoproteinaemia types I and IV.

hypertrophy (hie'pərtrəfee) increase in volume of a tissue or organ produced entirely by enlargement of existing cells. adj. **hypertrophic.**

ventricular h. hypertrophy of the myocardium of a ventricle, causing undue deviation of the axis of the electrocardiogram.

hypertropia (ˌhiepə'trohpi·ə) STRABISMUS in which there is permanent upward deviation of the visual axis of one eye.

hyperuricaemia (ˌhiepəˌyooə·ri'seemi·ə) an excess of uric acid in the blood. adj. **hyperuricaemic.**

hypervalinaemia (ˌhiepəˌvali'neemi·ə) an inborn error of metabolism characterized by elevated levels of serum valine, valinuria, and failure to thrive.

hypervascular (ˌhiepə'vaskyuhlə) extremely vascular.

hyperventilation (ˌhiepəˌventi'layshən) 1. increase of air in the lungs above the normal amount. 2. abnormally prolonged and deep breathing, usually associated with acute anxiety or emotional tension. It is most commonly seen in nervous, anxious females who have other functional disturbances related to emotional problems. A transient, respiratory ALKALOSIS commonly results from hyperventilation. More prolonged hyperventilation may be caused by disorders of the central nervous system, or by drugs, such as high concentrations of salicylate, that increase the sensitivity of the respiratory centres.

Symptoms of hyperventilation include 'faintness' or impaired consciousness without actual loss of consciousness. At the outset the patient may have felt a tightness of the chest, a sensation of smothering, and some degree of apprehension. Other symptoms may be related to the heart and digestive tract, for example, palpitation or pounding of the heart, fullness in the throat, and pain over the stomach region. In prolonged attacks the patient may exhibit tetany with muscular spasm of the hands and feet.

Immediate treatment consists of having the patient rebreathe in a paper bag, to replace the carbon dioxide he has been 'blowing off' during hyperventilation. He may need to be convinced that there is nothing seriously wrong with him in the organic sense and that he can control the 'attack' by using the paper bag for rebreathing. Treatment of the underlying emotional disturbance is recommended.

hyperviscosity (ˌhiepəvis'kositee) excessive viscosity, as of the blood.

h. syndrome a syndrome produced by increased viscosity of the blood leading to stasis in the blood vessels. Increased red cells in polycythaemia and increased plasma proteins in myeloma and macroglobulinaemia are the main causes. Symptoms include headache, visual disturbances, impaired consciousness, bleeding, and thrombotic episodes. Treatment is to define and correct the underlying abnormality, if possible. Venesection to remove excess red cells and plasmapheresis to remove very high protein levels are useful early measures when the condition is severe.

hypervitaminosis (ˌhiepəˌvitəmi'nohsis) a condition produced by ingestion of excessive amounts of vitamins; symptom complexes are associated with excessive intake of vitamins A and D.

hypervolaemia (ˌhiepəvo'leemi·ə) abnormal increase in the volume of circulating fluid (plasma) in the body. See also FLUID VOLUME EXCESS.

hypha ('hiefa) pl. *hyphae* [L.] one of the filaments composing the mycelium of a fungus. adj. **hyphal.**

hyphaemia (hie'feemi·ə) 1. oligaemia, or deficiency of blood. 2. hyphema.

hyphedonia (ˌhiep·hi'dohni·ə) diminution of power of enjoyment.

hyphema (hie'feemə) haemorrhage into the anterior chamber of the eye.

hyphidrosis (ˌhiep·hi'drohsis) too scanty perspiration.

Hyphomycetes (ˌhiefohmie'seeteez) the mycelial (hyphal) fungi, i.e., the moulds.

hypn(o)- word element. [Gr.] *sleep, hypnosis.*

hypnagogic (ˌhipnə'gojik) 1. producing sleep. 2. occurring just before sleep; said of dreams.

hypnagogue ('hipnəˌgog) 1. hypnotic; inducing sleep. 2. an agent that produces sleep.

hypnalgia (hip'nalji·ə) pain during sleep.

hypnoanaesthesia (hipnohˌanəs'theezi·ə) reduction of sensitivity to pain by hypnosis.

hypnoanalysis (ˌhipnoh·ə'nalisis) psychoanalysis with use of hypnosis to help uncover unconscious material.

hypnodontics (ˌhipnoh'dontiks) the application of hypnosis and controlled suggestion in the practice of dentistry.

hypnogenic (ˌhipnoh'jenik) inducing sleep or a hypnotic state.

hypnoid ('hipnoyd) resembling hypnosis.

hypnolepsy (hipnoh'lepsee) narcolepsy.

hypnology (hip'noləjee) the scientific study of sleep or of hypnotism.

Hypnomidate (hip'nomidayt) trademark for a preparation of etomidate, an induction anaesthetic.

hypnonarcosis (,hipnohnah'kohsis) light hypnosis combined with narcosis.

hypnosis (hip'nohsis) an artificially induced passive state in which there is increased amenability and responsiveness to suggestions and commands. In hypnosis, a drowsy phase is followed by a sleep that is light or deep, depending on the cooperation of the sleeper. Although this sleep seems normal, a part of the sleeper remains aware of the outside world and of the wishes of the hypnotist. STATE OF HYPNOSIS. The nature of hypnosis and the way it works are still largely unknown. One widely accepted theory is that the person's ego—that is, the part of his mind that consciously restrains his instincts—is temporarily weakened under hypnosis at his own wish. How deeply he responds depends on many psychological and biological factors. The ability to respond to hypnosis varies from person to person; it tends to increase after successive experiences.

It is not true that a hypnotized person will do absolutely anything he is asked. Most subjects, for instance, will not respond to any suggestions they would consider immoral or illegal if they were awake. USE OF HYPNOSIS. A common medical use of hypnosis is in treating mental illness. Historically, Sigmund Freud developed his theory of the unconscious as a result of his experiments with a hypnotized patient. Out of this theory came some of the techniques of PSYCHOANALYSIS. By lessening the mind's unconscious defences, hypnosis can make some patients able to recall and even reexperience important childhood events that have long been forgotten or repressed by the conscious mind.

In certain cases when the use of anaesthetics is not advisable, hypnosis has been used successfully during dental treatment, setting of fractures, and childbirth, usually in addition to pain-killing medicines.

hypnotherapy (,hipnoh'therəpee) the therapeutic use of hypnotism.

hypnotic (hip'notik) 1. pertaining to or inducing hypnosis or sleep. 2. an agent that induces sleep.

hypnotism ('hipnə,tizəm) the method or practice of inducing hypnosis.

hypnotize ('hipnə,tiez) to put into a condition of hypnosis.

Hypnovel ('hipnəvel) trademark for a preparation of midazolam, a benzodiazepine used in anaesthetics.

hypo ('hiepoh) sodium thiosulphate, used as a photographic fixing agent.

hypo- word element. [Gr.] *abnormally decreased, deficient, beneath, under.*

hypoacidity (,hiepoh·ə'siditee) decreased acidity.

hypoacusia, hypoacusis (,hiepoh·ə'kyoozi·ə; ,hiepoh·ə'kyoosis) slightly diminished auditory sensitivity.

hypoadrenalism (,hiepoh·ə'dreenə,lizəm) deficiency of adrenal activity, as in Addison's disease.

hypoadrenocorticism (,hiepoh·ə,dreenoh'kawti,sizəm) diminished activity of the adrenal cortex; Addison's disease.

hypoaesthesia (,hiepoh·is'theezi·ə) a state of abnormally decreased sensitivity to stimuli. adj. **hypoaesthetic.**

hypoaffectivity (,hiepoh,afek'tivitee) abnormally diminished sensitivity to superficial stimuli; abnormally decreased emotional reactivity.

hypoalbuminaemia (,hiepoh·al,byoomi'neemi·ə) abnormally low levels of albumin in the blood.

hypoalbuminosis (,hiepoh·al,byoomi'nohsis) abnormally low level of albumin.

hypoaldosteronism (,hiepoh·al'dostə·rə,nizəm) deficiency of aldosterone in the body.

hypoalgesia (,hiepoh·al'jeezi·ə) hypalgesia.

hypoalimentation (,hiepoh,alimen'tayshən) insufficient nourishment.

hypoazoturia (,hiepoh,azoh'tyooə·ri·ə) diminished nitrogenous material in the urine.

hypobaric (,hiepoh'barik) characterized by less than normal pressure or weight; applied to gases under less than atmospheric pressure, or to solutions of lower specific gravity than another taken as a standard of reference.

hypobaropathy (,hiepohbə'ropəthee) the disturbances experienced at high altitudes due to reduced air pressure and lack of oxygen; altitude sickness.

hypoblast ('hiepoh,blast) the entoderm. adj. **hypoblastic.**

hypocalcaemia (,hiepohkal'seemi·ə) abnormally low concentration of calcium in the blood.

hypocalciuria (,hiepoh,kalsi'yooə·ri·ə) an abnormally diminished amount of calcium in the urine.

hypocapnia (,hiepoh'kapni·ə) diminished carbon dioxide in the blood. adj. **hypocapnic.**

hypocarbia (,hiepoh'kahbi·ə) hypocapnia.

hypocellularity (,hiepoh,selyuh'laritee) abnormal decrease in the number of cells present, as in bone marrow.

hypochloraemia (,hiepohklo'reemi·ə) an abnormally low level of chloride in the blood; signs and symptoms are those of ALKALOSIS. adj. **hypochloraemic.**

hypochlorhydria (,hiepohklor'hiedri·ə) deficiency of HYDROCHLORIC ACID in the gastric juice.

hypochlorization (,hiepoh,klor·rie'zayshən) reduction of sodium chloride in the diet.

hypochlorous acid (,hiepoh'klor·rəs) an unstable compound used as a disinfectant and bleaching agent.

hypochloruria (,hiepohklor'yooə·ri·ə) diminished chloride content in the urine.

hypocholesteraemia, hypocholesterolaemia (,hiepohkə,lestə'reemi·ə; ,hiepohkə,lestə·ro'leemi·ə) low level of cholesterol in the blood.

hypochondria (,hiepə'kondri·ə) hypochondriasis.

hypochondriac (,hiepə'kondri,ak) 1. pertaining to the hypochondrium. 2. a person affected with hypochondriasis.

hypochondriasis (,hiepohkon'drieəsis) abnormal concern about one's health. The hypochondriac exaggerates trivial symptoms and often believes that he is suffering from some serious ailment.

True hypochondriasis is a type of neurosis caused by an unresolved conflict in the patient's unconscious mind. His fears are usually related to a specific organ, such as the heart, eyes, or lungs. This organ often has a deep symbolic connection with the inner conflict causing the neurosis. In many cases, the relationship between the patient's mind and the organ on which his fears centre is so strong that he develops real symptoms, even though there is no physical disorder to explain them.

The treatment of hypochondriasis is usually difficult and of long duration. Psychotherapy is the most effective means of dealing with this disorder.

hypochondrium (,hiepoh'kondri·əm) the upper abdominal region on either side, just below the thorax. adj. **hypochondriacal.**

hypochromasia (,hiepohkrə'mayzi·ə) 1. staining less intensely than normal. 2. decrease of haemoglobin in

erythrocytes so that they are abnormally pale. adj. **hypochromatic**.
hypochromatism (ˌhiepoh'krohməˌtizəm) abnormally deficient pigmentation, especially deficiency of chromatin in a cell nucleus.
hypochromatosis (ˌhiepohˌkrohmə'tohsis) the gradual fading and disappearance of the nucleus (the chromatin) of a cell.
hypochromia (ˌhiepoh'krohmi·ə) 1. hypochromatism. 2. decrease of haemoglobin in the erythrocytes so that they are abnormally pale. adj. **hypochromic**.
hypochylia (ˌhiepoh'kieli·ə) deficiency of chyle.
hypocomplementaemia (ˌhiepohˌkomplimən'teemi·ə) diminution of complement levels in the blood.
hypocorticism (ˌhiepoh'kawtiˌsizəm) hypoadrenocorticism.
hypocrinism (ˌhiepoh'krienizəm) a state due to deficient secretion of an endocrine gland.
hypocupraemia (ˌhiepohkyoo'preemi·ə) abnormally diminished concentration of copper in the blood.
hypocyclosis (ˌhiepohsie'klohsis) insufficient accommodation in the eye.
hypocythaemia (ˌhiepohsie'theemi·ə) deficiency in the number of erythrocytes in the blood.
hypodactyly (ˌhiepoh'daktilee) less than the usual number of digits on the hand or foot.
Hypoderma (ˌhiepoh'dərmə) a genus of ox-warble or heel flies, whose larvae cause warbles in cattle and a form of larva migrans in man.
hypodermiasis (ˌhiepohdər'mieəsis) a creeping eruption of the skin in man and cattle caused by the larvae of *Hypoderma*.
hypodermic (ˌhiepə'dərmik) 1. beneath the skin; injected into subcutaneous tissues. 2. a hypodermic, or subcutaneous, injection; a hypodermic syringe.
hypodipsia (ˌhiepoh'dipsi·ə) abnormally diminished thirst.
hypodynamia (ˌhiepohdie'nami·ə) abnormally diminished power. adj. **hypodynamic**.
hypoeccrisia (ˌhiepoh·i'krizi·ə) abnormally diminished excretion. adj. **hypoeccritic**.
hypoechoic (ˌhiepoh·e'koh·ik) in ultrasonography, giving off few echoes; said of tissues or structures that reflect relatively few of the ultrasound waves directed at them.
hypoendocrinism (ˌhiepoh'endəkriˌnizəm) insufficiency of endocrine gland activity.
hypoergasia (ˌhiepoh·ər'gayzi·ə) abnormally decreased functional activity.
hypoesophoria (ˌhiepohˌesoh'for·ri·ə) deviation of the visual axes downward and inward.
hypoexophoria (ˌhiepohˌeksoh'for·ri·ə) deviation of the visual axes downward and laterally.
hypoferraemia (ˌhiepohfə'reemi·ə) deficiency of iron in the blood.
hypofertility (ˌhiepohfər'tilitee) diminished reproductive capacity. adj. **hypofertile**.
hypofibrinogenaemia (ˌhiepohfieˌbrinəjə'neemi·ə) deficiency of fibrinogen in the blood.
hypofunction (ˌhiepoh'fungkshən) diminished functioning.
hypogalactia (ˌhiepohgə'lakti·ə) deficiency of milk secretion. adj. **hypogalactous**.
hypogammaglobulinaemia (ˌhiepohˌgaməˌglobyuhli'neemi·ə) an immunological deficiency state marked by abnormally low levels of generally all classes of serum gamma globulins, with heightened susceptibility to infectious diseases. It may be congenital or secondary, or it may be physiological, occurring in normal infants and occasionally being prolonged, so-called transient hypogammaglobulinaemia (see also AGAMMAGLOBULINAEMIA).
acquired h. hypogammaglobulinaemia that becomes manifest after early childhood; the condition may be primary (that is, without discoverable underlying cause) or secondary (that is, associated with such conditions as multiple myeloma, lymphoma, and chronic lymphatic leukaemia, in which there is failure of gamma globulin synthesis).
congenital h. hypogammaglobulinaemia in which the manifestations of immunological inadequacy appear shortly after birth.
hypoganglionosis (ˌhiepohˌgang·gli·ə'nohsis) deficiency in the number of myenteric ganglion cells in the distal segment of the large bowel, resulting in constipation; a variant of congenital megacolon.
hypogastric (ˌhiepoh'gastrik) pertaining to the hypogastrium.
hypogastrium (ˌhiepoh'gastri·əm) the lowest middle abdominal region.
hypogenesis (ˌhiepoh'jenəsis) defective development.
hypogenitalism (ˌhiepoh'jenitəˌlizəm) lack of sexual development because of deficient activity of the gonads; hypogonadism.
hypogeusaesthesia, hypogeusia (ˌhiepoh'gyoozis'theezi·ə; ˌhiepoh'gyoozi·ə) abnormally diminished acuteness of the sense of taste.
hypoglossal (ˌhiepoh'glos'l) situated beneath the tongue, as the hypoglossal nerve.
hypoglottis (ˌhiepoh'glotis) 1. the under side of the tongue. 2. ranula.
hypoglucagonaemia (ˌhiepohˌglookəgə'neemi·ə) abnormally reduced levels of glucagon in the blood.
hypoglycaemia (ˌhiepohglie'seemi·ə) an abnormally low level of sugar (glucose) in the blood. The condition may result from an excessive rate of removal of glucose from the blood or from decreased secretion of glucose into the blood. Oversecretion of insulin from the islets of Langerhans or an overdose of exogenous insulin can lead to increased utilization of glucose, so that glucose is removed from the blood at an accelerated rate. By far the commonest cause of hypoglycaemia is the injection of too much insulin for the circumstances in a patient with diabetes mellitus. Some large tumours of the retroperitoneal area and tumours of the islets of Langerhans can increase the production of insulin and result in rapid removal of glucose from the blood. Because the liver is the source of most of the glucose entering the blood while a person is fasting, damage to the liver cells can result in impaired ability to convert glycogen into glucose. If secretion of the adrenocortical hormones, especially the GLUCOCORTICOIDS, is deficient, the protein precursors of glucose are not available and the blood glucose level drops as the liver's glycogen supply is depleted.
SYMPTOMS. Hypoglycaemia may be tolerated by normal persons for brief periods of time without symptoms; however, if the blood sugar level remains very low for a prolonged period of time, symptoms of cerebral dysfunction develop. These include mental confusion, hallucinations, convulsions, and eventually deep coma as the nervous system is deprived of the glucose needed for its normal metabolic activities. Other symptoms are a result of a greatly increased secretion of adrenaline, a normal response to hypoglycaemia. The patient then experiences increased pulse rate, tachycardia, a rise in blood pressure, sweating, and anxiety (see also INSULIN REACTION).
TREATMENT. An acute episode of hypoglycaemia or insulin reaction demands emergency treatment with intravenous injections of glucose. If the patient can swallow and no facilities for intravenous therapy are available, sugar, sweets, sweetened fruit juice, or honey

may be given by mouth. The intramuscular injection of glucagon will mobilize sugar from the liver and bring the patient to a level of consciousness when sugar can be given by mouth.

Specific treatment depends on the primary cause of hypoglycaemia. If hyperinsulinism is due to a tumour or hyperplasia of the islets of Langerhans, surgical intervention is necessary. The large sarcomas of the retroperitoneal or mediastinal areas that cause hyperinsulinism also must be treated surgically.

Reactive or *postprandial* hypoglycaemia is a form of low blood sugar that develops rather suddenly several hours after ingestion of a high carbohydrate meal. It is characterized by a blood sugar level of 2.8 mmol/l (50 mg/100 ml) or less, and symptoms of palpitations, sweating, anxiety, hunger, and tremulousness. The usual treatment for this form of chronic hypoglycaemia involves dietary changes that are aimed at avoiding extremes in blood glucose level and maintaining an adequate level of glucose in the blood at all times. The diet is high in protein and fat and low in carbohydrate content and is given in frequent, small feedings during the day and before retiring. This regimen avoids extreme fluctuations in blood glucose concentration by restricting carbohydrate intake, and supplies adequate precursors of glycogen through the protein intake.

hypoglycaemic (ˌhiepohglie'seemik) pertaining to, characterized by, or producing hypoglycaemia.

oral h. agents synthetic drugs that lower the blood sugar level. Those currently used are *sulphonylureas* such as chlorpropamide, tolbutamide, and glibenclamide. These drugs stimulate the synthesis and release of INSULIN from the beta cells of the islets of Langerhans in the pancreas, and are used to treat patients with non-insulin-dependent DIABETES MELLITUS (NIDDM). They have no hypoglycaemic effect in patients with insulin-dependent DIABETES MELLITUS (IDDM), who have nonfunctional beta cells that cannot produce insulin. These drugs should not be used as a substitute for adherence to a strict diet. However, they can be effective for treating patients who have NIDDM that cannot be controlled by diet alone.

hypoglycogenolysis (ˌhiepohˌgliekohji'nolisis) defective splitting up of glycogen in the body.

hypoglycorrhachia (ˌhiepohˌgliekə'raki·ə, -rayki·ə) abnormally low sugar content in the cerebrospinal fluid.

hypogonadism (ˌhiepoh'gonəˌdizəm) decreased functional activity of the gonads, with retardation of growth and sexual development.

hypogonadotrophic (ˌhiepohˌgonədə'trohfik) relating to or caused by deficiency of gonadotrophin.

hypohidrosis (ˌhiepoh·hi'drohsis) abnormally diminished secretion of sweat. adj. **hypohidrotic**.

hypoinsulinism (ˌhiepoh'insyuhliˌnizəm) a deficiency of insulin excretion caused by pancreatic failure or incorrect treatment of diabetes mellitus.

hypokalaemia (ˌhiepohkə'leemi·ə) abnormally low potassium concentration in the blood; it may result from potassium loss by renal secretion or via the gastrointestinal tract, as in vomiting and diarrhoea. Other causes include uncontrolled diabetes mellitus and attendant polyuria, increased adrenocortical secretion, steroid therapy, diuretic therapy, excessive diaphoresis, and burns or other injuries that result in loss of potassium. Called also *hypopotassaemia*.

The earliest signs of hypokalaemia are weakness and muscle cramps and numbness and tingling that usually begin in the lower extremities. Other symptoms include nausea and vomiting, which can further contribute to potassium deficit. Paralysis of the muscles of respiration can produce respiratory arrest. Neurological involvement can lead to confusion, irritability, and coma.

The heart is particularly sensitive to potassium deficiency. The electrocardiographic abnormalities presented are depression of the T wave and elevation of the U wave. Susceptibility to digitalis toxicity is increased when a patient has hypokalaemia.

Replacement of the deficient potassium can be accomplished by administration of potassium chloride, either orally or intravenously.

hypokalaemic (ˌhiepohkə'leemik) 1. pertaining to or characterized by hypokalaemia. 2. an agent that lowers blood potassium levels.

hypokinesia (ˌhiepohki'neezi·ə) abnormally diminished motor activity. adj. **hypokinetic**.

hypolactasia (ˌhiepohlak'tayzi·ə) deficiency of lactase activity in the intestines.

hypoleydigism (ˌhiepoh'liedigizəm) abnormally diminished secretion of androgens by Leydig's cells.

hypolipidaemic (ˌhiepohˌlipi'deemik) promoting the reduction of lipid concentrations in the serum.

hypomagnesaemia (ˌhiepohˌmagni'zeemi·ə) abnormally low magnesium content of the blood, manifested chiefly by neuromuscular hyperirritability.

hypomania (ˌhiepoh'mayni·ə) mania of a mild type. adj. **hypomanic**.

hypomastia (ˌhiepoh'masti·ə) abnormal smallness of mammary glands.

hypomenorrhoea (ˌhiepohˌmenə'reeə) diminution of menstrual flow or duration.

hypomere ('hiepohˌmiə) 1. one of the ventrolateral portions of the fusing myotomes in embryonic development, forming muscles innervated by the ventral rami of the spinal nerves. 2. the lateral plate of mesoderm that develops into the walls of the body cavities.

hypometabolism (ˌhiepohmə'tabəˌlizəm) decreased metabolism; low metabolic rate.

hypometria (ˌhiepoh'meetri·ə) ataxia in which movements fall short of the intended goal.

hypometropia (ˌhiepohme'trohpi·ə) myopia; shortsightedness.

hypomnesia (ˌhiepom'neezi·ə) defective memory.

hypomorph ('hiepohˌmawf) 1. a person short in standing height as compared to his sitting height. 2. in genetics, a hypomorphic mutant gene, i.e., showing only a slight reduction of the activity it influences. adj. **hypomorphic**.

hypomotility (ˌhiepohmoh'tilitee) deficient power of movement in any part.

hypomyotonia (ˌhiepohˌmieoh'tohni·ə) deficient muscular tonicity.

hypomyxia (ˌhiepoh'miksi·ə) decreased secretion of mucus.

hyponasality (ˌhiepohnay'zalitee) a quality of voice in which there is a complete lack of nasal emission of air and nasal resonance, so that the speaker sounds as if he has a cold.

hyponatraemia (ˌhiepohnə'treemi·ə) deficiency of SODIUM in the blood; salt depletion. Hyponatraemia is present when the sodium concentration is less than 135 mmol/l. It can occur as a result of inadequate sodium intake, as in a sodium-restricted diet, excessive water ingestion or retention, or excessive wasting of salt.

Symptoms include muscular weakness and twitching, progressing to convulsions if unrelieved; alterations in level of consciousness; mental confusion; and anxiety. When the cause of hyponatraemia is salt wasting there is an accompanying loss of body fluids. Treatment is based on correction of the underlying cause.

hyponeocytosis (,hiepoh,niohsie'tohsis) leukopenia with the presence of immature leukocytes in the blood.

hyponoia (,hiepoh'noyə) sluggish mental activity.

hyponychium (,hiepoh'niki·əm) the thickened epidermis beneath the free distal end of the nail of a digit. adj. **hyponychial**.

hypo-orthocytosis (,hiepoh,awthohsie'tohsis) leukopenia with a normal proportion of the various forms of leukocytes.

hypo-osmolality (,hiepoh,ozmə'lalitee) a decrease in the osmolality of the body fluids.

hypopancreatism (,hiepoh'pankri·ə,tizəm) diminished activity of the pancreas.

hypoparathyroidism (,hiepoh,parə'thieroy,dizəm) the condition produced by deficient function of the parathyroid glands or by the removal of these bodies. The lack of parathyroid hormone leads to a fall in serum calcium level, which increases neuromuscular excitability and this produces tetany. There is also a rise in the plasma phosphate level, which results in a decrease in bone resorption and an increased density of bone. There also may be dermatological, ophthalmological (cataracts), psychiatric, and dental symptoms if hypocalcaemia persists for years.

Hypoparathyroidism is usually due to inadvertent removal of parathyroid glands during thyroidectomy. Very rarely it is the result of autoimmune destruction of the glands in childhood; the resultant tetanic spasms may be mistaken for epilepsy.

Treatment consists of immediately raising the serum calcium. Calcium injections are necessary for the relief of tetany. Oral calcium is necessary for long-term treatment. As a substitute for parathyroid hormone, vitamin D is required, either in the form of calciferol or as alfacalcidol. This must be taken indefinitely and the patient's serum calcium has to be measured regularly to ensure the correct dosage.

hypoperfusion (,hiepohpə'fyoozhən) decreased blood flow through an organ, as in circulatory shock; if prolonged, it may result in permanent cellular dysfunction and death.

hypophalangism (,hiepohfə'lanjizəm) absence of a phalanx on a finger or toe.

hypopharynx (,hiepoh'faringks) laryngopharynx.

hypophonesis (,hiepohfoh'neesis) diminution of the sound in auscultation or percussion.

hypophonia (,hiepoh'fohni·ə) a weak voice due to incoordination of the vocal muscles.

hypophoria (,hiepoh'for·ri·ə) HETEROPHORIA in which there is permanent downward deviation of the visual axis of an eye in the absence of visual fusional stimuli.

hypophosphataemia (,hiepoh,fosfə'teemi·ə) deficiency of phosphates in the blood. See also HYPOPHOSPHATASIA. adj. **hypophosphataemic**.

hypophosphatasia (,hiepoh,fosfə'tayzi·ə) an inborn error of metabolism marked by abnormally low serum alkaline phosphatase activity and excretion of phosphoethanolamine in the urine. It is manifested by rickets in infants and children and by osteomalacia in adults. It is most severe in babies under six months of age.

hypophosphaturia (,hiepoh,fosfə'tyooə·ri·ə) abnormally decreased levels of urinary phosphate.

hypophrenic (,hiepoh'frenik) below the diaphragm.

hypophyseal, hypophysial (hie,pofi'zeeəl) pertaining to the hypophysis (PITUITARY GLAND).

hypophysectomy (hie,pofi'sektəmee) excision of the hypophysis, or pituitary gland. Surgical removal of all or part of the pituitary gland is indicated when there is a tumour of the gland.

Hormone-sensitive malignant tumours such as those of the breast and prostate have been treated by hypophysectomy in order to impede tumour growth and metastases and to relieve pain.

hypophyseoportal (,hiepoh,fizioh'pawt'l) denoting the portal system of the pituitary gland, in which hypothalamic venules connect with capillaries of the anterior pituitary.

hypophysioprivic (,hiepoh,fizioh'privik) due to deficiency of hormonal secretion of the hypophysis.

hypophysis (hie'pofisis) pl. *hypophyses* [Gr.] an epithelial body of dual origin at the base of the brain in the sella turcica, attached by a stalk to the hypothalamus; called also PITUITARY GLAND. It is composed of two main lobes, the anterior lobe (adenohypophysis, anterior pituitary), secreting several important hormones that regulate the proper functioning of the thyroids, gonads, adrenal cortex, and other endocrine glands, and the posterior lobe (neurohypophysis, posterior pituitary), whose cells serve as a reservoir for hormones having antidiuretic and oxytocic action, releasing them as needed.

h. cerebri hypophysis.

h. sicca posterior pituitary.

hypopiesis (,hiepohpie'eesis) abnormally low pressure, in particular, low blood pressure.

hypopigmentation (,hiepoh,pigmen'tayshən) abnormally decreased pigmentation.

hypopituitarism (,hiepohpi'tyooitə,rizəm) the condition resulting from diminution or cessation of hormonal secretion by the pituitary gland, especially the anterior pituitary. Symptoms vary with the degree of dysfunction.

hypoplasia, hypoplasty (,hiepoh'playzi·ə; 'hiepoh,plastee) incomplete development or underdevelopment of an organ or tissue. adj. **hypoplastic**.

hypopnoea (,hiepoh'neeə, -'popni·ə) abnormal decrease in depth and rate of respiration. adj. **hypopnoeic**.

hypoporosis (,hiepohpor'rohsis) deficient callus formation after bone fracture.

hypoposia (,hiepoh'pohzi·ə) abnormally diminished ingestion of fluids.

hypopotassaemia (,hiepoh,potə'seemi·ə) hypokalaemia.

hypopraxia (,hiepoh'praksi·ə) abnormally diminished activity.

hypoprosody (,hiepoh'prosədee) diminution of the normal variation of stress, pitch, and rhythm of speech.

hypoproteinaemia (,hiepoh,prohti'neemi·a) deficiency of protein in the blood.

hypoprothrombinaemia (,hiepohproh,thrombi'neemi·ə) deficiency of prothrombin in the blood.

hypopselaphesia (,hiepoh,selə'feezi·ə) dullness of tactile sensitiveness.

hypopsychosis (,hiepohsie'kohsis) diminution of the function of thought.

hypoptyalism (,hiepoh'tieə,lizəm) abnormally decreased secretion of saliva.

hypopyon (hie'pohpi·ən) pus in the anterior chamber of the eye.

hyporeactive (,hiepohri'aktiv) showing less than normal response to stimuli.

hyporeflexia (,hiepohri'fleksi·ə) diminution or weakening of reflexes.

hyporeninaemia (,hiepoh,reeni'neemi·ə) low levels of renin in the blood.

hyposalaemia (,hiepohsə'leemi·ə) diminution of salt levels in the blood.

hyposalivation (,hiepoh,sali'vayshən) hypoptyalism.

hyposcleral (,hiepoh'skliə·rəl) beneath the sclera.

hyposecretion (,hiepohsi'kreeshən) diminished secretion.

hyposensitivity (,hiepoh,sensi'tivitee) 1. abnormally decreased sensitivity. 2. the state of being less sensitive to a specific allergen after repeated and gradually increasing doses of the offending substance. adj. **hyposensitive**.

hyposensitization (,hiepoh,sensitie'zayshən) the act or process of inducing hyposensitivity; desensitization (see also IMMUNOTHERAPY).

hyposmia (hie'pozmi·ə) diminished acuteness of the sense of smell.

hyposmolarity (hie,pozmə'laritee) abnormally decreased osmolar concentration of a solution.

hyposomatotrophism (,hiepoh,sohmətoh'trohfizəm) deficient secretion of somatotrophin (growth hormone) or secretion of inactive somatotrophin, resulting in short stature.

hyposomnia (,hiepoh'somni·ə) pathologically diminished sleep; insomnia.

hypospadiac (,hiepoh'spaydiak) 1. pertaining to hypospadias. 2. a person affected with hypospadias.

hypospadias (,hiepə'spaydi·əs) a developmental anomaly in the male in which the urethra opens on the under side of the penis or on the perineum.

female h. a developmental anomaly in the female in which the urethra opens into the vagina.

hyposplenism (,hiepoh'splenizəm) diminished functioning of the spleen, resulting in an increase in peripheral blood elements.

hypostasis (,hie'postəsis) poor or stagnant circulation in a dependent part of the body or an organ.

hypostatic (,hiepoh'statik) 1. pertaining to, due to, or associated with hypostasis. 2. abnormally static; said of certain inherited traits that are liable to be suppressed by other traits.

hyposthenia (,hiepəs'theeni·ə) diminished strength or tonicity. adj. **hyposthenic**.

hyposthenuria (,hiepohsthi'nyooə·ri·ə) excretion of urine of low specific gravity.

hypostomia (,hiepoh'stohmi·ə) a developmental anomaly characterized by abnormal smallness of the mouth, the slit being vertical instead of horizontal.

hypostypsis (,hiepoh'stipsis) moderate astringency. adj. **hypostyptic**.

hyposynergia (,hiepohsi'nərji·ə) defective coordination.

hypotelorism (,hiepoh'telə,rizəm) abnormally decreased distance between two organs or parts.

ocular h., orbital h. abnormal decrease in the intraocular distance.

hypotension (,hiepoh'tenshən) diminished tension; lowered blood pressure. A consistently low blood pressure with a systolic pressure less than 100 mmHg is no cause for concern. In fact, low blood pressure often is associated with long life and an old age free of illness. An extremely low blood pressure is occasionally a symptom of a serious condition. In shock there is a disproportion between the blood volume and the capacity of the circulatory system, resulting in greatly reduced blood pressure.

Hypotension may be associated with Addison's disease but the primary disease produces so many other symptoms that the hypotension is only one aspect.

orthostatic h., postural h. a fall in blood pressure associated with dizziness, syncope, and blurred vision occurring upon standing or when standing motionless in a fixed position (see also ANTIHYPERTENSIVE).

hypotensive (,hiepoh'tensiv) 1. characterized by or causing diminished tension or pressure, as abnormally low blood pressure. 2. a person with abnormally low blood pressure.

hypotensor (,hiepoh'tensə) a substance that lowers the blood pressure.

hypothalamus (,hiepə'thaləməs) the portion of the diencephalon lying beneath the thalamus at the base of the cerebrum, and forming the floor and part of the lateral wall of the third ventricle. Anatomically, it includes the optic chiasm, mammillary bodies, tuber cinereum, infundibulum, and hypophysis (pituitary gland), but for physiological purposes, the hypophysis is considered a distinct structure. adj. **hypothalamic**.

The hypothalamic nuclei activate, control, and integrate many of the involuntary functions necessary for living. The various hypothalamic centres influence peripheral autonomic mechanisms, endocrine activity, and many somatic functions, e.g., a general regulation of water balance, body temperature, sleep, thirst, and hunger, and the development of secondary sexual characteristics.

Because of its influence on the release and inhibition of pituitary hormones, the hypothalamus indirectly plays an important role in the regulation of protein, fat, and carbohydrate metabolism, body fluid volume and electrolyte content, and internal secretion of endocrine hormones. The hormones synthesized and secreted by the special neurons of the hypothalamus are called *hypothalamic releasing* and *inhibiting hormones* or *factors* (see accompanying table). They act directly on the tissues of the pituitary gland. Some of the major hypothalamic factors are: *thyroid-stimulating hormone releasing hormone* (TRH), which activates the release of the thyroid-stimulating hormone (TSH) from the anterior lobe of the pituitary gland; *corticotrophin-releasing factor* (CRF); *growth hormone releasing factor* (GHRF); *gonadotrophin releasing hormone* (GnRH); and *prolactin-inhibiting factor* (PIF). In addition, there are other stimulating and inhibiting factors that influence the release and retention of other anterior pituitary hormones.

Hypothalamic hormones regulating pituitary function

TSH releasing hormone* (TRH)	Stimulates release of thyroid stimulating hormone (TSH)
Corticotrophin releasing factor† (CRF)	Stimulates release of corticotrophin (ACTH)
Gonadotrophin releasing hormone (GnRH)	Stimulates release of follicle stimulating hormone (FSH) and luteinizing hormone (LH)
Growth hormone regulating factors Growth hormone releasing factor (GHRF) Somatostatin (GHIF)	Dual control system, one stimulating, the other inhibiting, release of growth hormone (GH)
Prolactin inhibiting factor (PIF)	Predominant effect is inhibiting release of prolactin

* Hormone is applied to substances of established chemical identity
† Factor is applied to substances of unknown chemical nature

The hypothalamic hormones or factors are secreted directly into the veins in the lower part of the hypothalamus and are transported directly to the tissues of the pituitary gland. This transportation network is called the *hypothalamic–hypophyseal portal system*. The secretion of the hypothalamic hormones is a part of a regulatory negative FEEDBACK system that continuously operates to maintain homeostasis.

hypothenar (ˌhiepoh'theenah) 1. the fleshy eminence on the palm along the ulnar margin. 2. relating to this eminence.

hypothermia (ˌhiepoh'thərmi·ə) subnormal body temperature. adj. **hypothermal, hypothermic**. May be symptomatic of a disease or disorder or may occur accidentally or be induced deliberately as a therapeutic measure.

ACCIDENTAL HYPOTHERMIA. The main causes are diseases, drugs and exposure, or often a combination of these. Diseases include stroke, myxoedema and hypopituitarism. Drugs that have been implicated are alcohol and the phenothiazines. Exposure includes that occurring not only on mountains or at sea but also during severe winters. The latter is particularly important in the elderly but also the very young, the mentally handicapped or ill and the homeless who may have inadequte heating, be on drugs that promote heat loss, and, because of age or cerebrovascular disease, have inadequate heat-conserving mechanisms.

PREVENTION. Accidental hypothermia can be avoided by eating high energy foods, exercising when cold, wearing several layers of clothing and covering the head. For families and persons on a limited income, advice must be realistic and it may be more appropriate to heat only one room and for the family to live, eat and sleep in that.

Investigation of a suspected case should include arterial blood gases, electrolyte and sugar levels in blood, an ECG to detect arrhythmias, serum thyroxine level and a chest x-ray to exclude aspiration and trauma. Pulse, blood pressure, amd rectal temperatures are monitored regularly. The thermometer used must be able to read low temperatures and often special electronic ones are used. Patients should be connected to a cardiac monitor since arrhythmias are common, especially in severe hypothermia which is defined as a core temperature below 32 °C. Fluid intake and output are charted and to do this the patient may need to be catheterized.

Patients are nursed on their side and turned every 2 hours. The eyes may need to be irrigated frequently and covered with saline compresses if corneal reflex is absent and eye secretions reduced. Rewarming is accomplished by covering with blankets and nursing in a warm room (21–27 °C) with the aim of raising the rectal temperature by 1 °C an hour. Oxygen is given, but if the patient is not breathing or the blood gases indicate respiratory failure, mechanical ventilation will be necessary. Intravenous fluids, which should be warmed, are given to stabilize the cardiovascular system, preferably with central venous pressure monitoring. A nasogastric tube is required as paralytic ileus is common. Hydrocortisone is given 6-hourly.

INDUCED HYPOTHERMIA. This may be general, when the temperature of the whole body is reduced, or local, when it is restricted to a part of the body. Hypothermia reduces the dangers of hypoxia and cellular damage by reducing the metabolism of cells. This enables specialized tissues such as the heart and brain to withstand periods of hypoxia or ischaemia which would otherwise cause harm.

Local Hypothermia. When applied to a limb, this has in the past been used as refrigeration anaesthesia prior to, for example, an amputation, but is seldom if ever used in this way today. The main use of local hypothermia is as a preservative, for instance of severed limbs or kidneys for donation.

General Hypothermia. Generalized lowering of the body temperature is used in three main situations: (1) to control fever as in malignant hyperthermia; (2) to enable certain cardiac and neurological operations to be carried out; and (3) to protect the brain from raised intracranial pressure in patients with head injuries or following drowning.

Hypothermia is induced by surface cooling, which is appropriate for treating fevers, for reducing intracranial pressure or for neurosurgical operations, or by extracorporeal methods, which are suitable where cardiac surgery is being undertaken. Surface cooling involves placing the patient in a cold environment, either using cold water or ice-bags, or between two blankets that incorporate coils of tubing through which cold antifreeze solution circulates. Chlorpromazine has been used to promote vasodilation and heat loss and to prevent shivering. Active cooling is stopped a few degrees above the desired level as the temperature will continue to drop (the after-drop).

Extracorporeal methods involve removing blood from the circulation, cooling it in a heat exchanger and returning it to the patient. This method is used in cardiac surgery. Reducing body temperature to 30 °C allows up to 8 minutes of circulatory arrest whilst profound hypothermia to 15 °C allows about an hour. Alternatively the patient may be put on cardiopulmonary bypass with mild or moderate hypothermia and the heart perfused with ice-cold solution once it is isolated from the circulation—a combination of mild general hypothermia and profound local hypothermia.

hypothesis (hie'pothisis) a supposition that appears to explain a group of phenomena and is assumed as a basis of reasoning and experimentation.

hypothrombinaemia (ˌhiepohˌthrombi'neemi·ə) deficiency of thrombin in the blood, resulting in a tendency to bleed.

hypothymia (ˌhiepoh'thiemi·ə) abnormally diminished emotionalism.

hypothymism (ˌhiepoh'thiemizəm) diminished thymus activity.

hypothyroidism (ˌhiepohthieroydizəm) deficiency of THYROID GLAND activity, with underproduction of thyroxine, or the condition resulting from it. adj. **hypothyroid**. Hypothyroidism may be primary, due to a thyroid defect, or secondary, due to deficient pituitary thyroid-stimulating hormone (TSH). Primary hypothyroidism may be congenital, as in the child born without a thyroid, or acquired, usually caused by destructive autoimmune disease of the thyroid or following radioiodine therapy or thyroidectomy. Primary hypothyroidism in an infant is termed CRETINISM and in an adult, MYXOEDEMA. The serum thyroxine is low and the TSH high. Newborns are now screened for cretinism by measurement of TSH soon after birth.

The low levels of thyroxine cause the metabolic rate to fall, with a slowing of all bodily functions. Physical and mental sluggishness, obesity, thickened dry skin, loss of hair and constipation are common symptoms. Treatment is very effective and has to be continued for life. Thyroxine is given in amounts appropriate for the age of the patient. Most adult patients will require a maintenance dose of 0.2 mg daily.

hypotonia (ˌhiepoh'tohni·ə) abnormally decreased tonicity or strength.

hypotonic (ˌhiepoh'tonik) 1. having an abnormally reduced tonicity or tension. 2. having an osmotic pressure lower than that of the solution with which it is compared.

hypotoxicity (ˌhiepohtok'sisitee) abnormally reduced toxic quality.

hypotransferrinaemia (ˌhiepohtransˌferi'neemi·ə) deficiency of transferrin in the blood.

hypotrichosis (ˌhiepohtri'kohsis) presence of less than the normal amount of hair.

hypotrophy (hie'potrəfee) abiotrophy.

hypotropia (hiepoh'trohpi·ə) STRABISMUS in which there is permanent downward deviation of the visual axis of one eye.

hypotympanotomy (ˌhiepohˌtimpə'notəmee) surgical opening of the hypotympanum.

hypotympanum (ˌhiepoh'timpənəm) the lower part of the cavity of the middle ear, in the temporal bone.

hypo-uricaemia (ˌhiepohˌyooə·ri'seemi·ə) deficiency of uric acid in the blood, along with xanthinuria, due to deficiency of xanthine oxidase, the enzyme required for conversion of hypoxanthine to xanthine and of xanthine to uric acid.

Hypovase ('hiepohvayz) trademark for a preparation of prazosin hydrochloride; an antihypertensive.

hypoventilation (ˌhiepohˌventi'layshən) reduction in the amount of air entering the pulmonary alveoli.

hypovitaminosis (ˌhiepohˌvitəmi'nohsis) a condition produced by lack of an essential vitamin.

hypovolaemia (ˌhiepohvo'leemi·ə) abnormally decreased volume of circulating fluid (plasma) in the body. adj. **hypovolaemic**.

hypovolia (ˌhiepoh'vohli·ə) diminished water content or volume, as of extracellular fluid.

hypoxaemia (ˌhiepok'seemi·ə) deficient oxygenation of the blood. The most reliable method for measuring the degree of hypoxaemia is BLOOD GAS ANALYSIS to determine the partial pressure of oxygen in the arterial blood. Insufficient oxygenation of the blood eventually leads to HYPOXIA.

hypoxanthine (ˌhiepoh'zantheen) an intermediate product of uric acid synthesis, formed from adenylic acid and itself a precursor of xanthine.

hypoxia (hie'poksi·ə) a broad term meaning diminished availability of oxygen to the body tissues. adj. **hypoxic**. Its causes are many and varied. There may be a deficiency of oxygen in the atmosphere, as in ALTITUDE SICKNESS, or a pulmonary disorder that interferes with adequate ventilation of the lungs. Anaemia or circulatory deficiencies can lead to inadequate transport and delivery of oxygen to the tissues. Finally, oedema or other abnormal conditions of the tissues themselves may impair the exchange of oxygen and carbon dioxide between the capillaries and the tissues.

SYMPTOMS. Signs and symptoms of hypoxia vary according to its cause. Generally they include dyspnoea, rapid pulse, syncope, and mental disturbances such as delirium or euphoria. Cyanosis is not always present and in some cases is not evident until the hypoxia is far advanced. The localized pain of ANGINA PECTORIS due to hypoxia occurs because of impaired oxygenation of the myocardium. Discoloration of the skin and eventual ulceration that sometimes accompany varicose veins are a result of hypoxia of the involved tissues.

TREATMENT. The treatment of hypoxia depends on the primary cause. Administration of oxygen by inhalation may be useful in some cases and of no help in others. For example, in situations in which there is difficulty with the transport of oxygen from the lungs to other parts of the body, increasing the intake of oxygen will do little to correct the problem of distribution (see OXYGEN therapy). In some vascular diseases the administration of vasodilators may help increase circulation, hence oxygen supply, to the tissues.

hyps(o)- word element. [Gr.] *height*.

hypsarrhythmia (ˌhipsə'ridhmi·ə) a term for an electroencephalographic abnormality sometimes observed in infants, with random high-voltage slow waves and spikes arising from multiple foci and spreading to all cortical areas; the disorder is characterized by spasms or quivering spells, and is commonly associated with mental handicap.

hypsokinesis (ˌhipsohki'neesis) a backward swaying or falling in erect posture, seen in paralysis agitans and other neurological disorders.

hyster(o)- word element. [Gr.] *uterus, hysteria.*

hystera (hi'sterə) [Gr.] *the uterus.*

hysteralgia (ˌhistə'ralji·ə) pain in the uterus.

hysteratresia (ˌhistə·rə'treezi·ə) atresia of the uterus.

hysterectomy (ˌhistə'rektəmee) surgical removal of the UTERUS.

abdominal h. that performed through the abdominal wall.

caesarean h. caesarean section followed by removal of the uterus.

radical h. excision of the uterus, upper vagina, and parametrium.

subtotal h. that in which the cervix is left in place.

total h. that in which the uterus and cervix are completely excised.

vaginal h. that performed through the vagina.

Wertheim's h. radical excision of the uterine body and cervix, vagina, and as much parametrial tissue as possible. Performed to eradicate cervical cancer.

hysteresis (histə'reesis) the lack of complete reversibility of a process, such as that exhibited in the differing temperatures of gelation and of liquefaction of a reversible colloid. The area of a hysteresis curve representing a cyclic phenomenon usually indicates the energy lost per cycle.

hystereurynter (ˌhistəˌyooə'rintə) an instrument for dilating the cervical os.

hystereurysis (ˌhistə'yooə·risis) dilation of the cervical os.

hysteria (his'tiə·ri·ə) a form of psychoneurosis in which the individual converts anxiety created by emotional conflict into physical symptoms that have no organic basis; called also *conversion reaction* or *conversion hysteria*. The term hysteria is also used to describe a state of tension or excitement in which there is a temporary loss of control over the emotions. adj. **hysterical**.

The patient with conversion hysteria is mentally ill. He converts his mental distress into physical symptoms in an effort to escape severe emotional conflict. The physical symptoms may include blindness, deafness, mutism, or paralysis of an arm or leg. In most cases the symptom can be related to some aspect of the conflict. For example, a college student interested in creative writing, but studying music because her parents want her to, may attempt to solve the problem by developing a loss of hearing. She then has an excuse for not continuing with the music and can at the same time satisfy her own desires without openly defying her parents. The patient who employs such methods is unaware that he is using the physical symptom to solve his emotional problem. Treatment is by PSYCHOTHERAPY in which the patient is helped to resolve the emotional conflict in a more normal manner.

The milder form of hysteria that is characterized by such symptoms as crying, pointless laughter, shouting, aimless walking about, or a temper tantrum usually results from an incident in which a person is pushed beyond his normal endurance. It might be provoked by danger, severe fright, or the reception of bad news.

hysterocatalepsy (ˌhistə·roh'katəˌlepsee) hysteria with cataleptic symptoms.

hysterocele ('histə·rohseel) hernia of the uterus.

hysterocleisis (ˌhistə·roh'kliesis) surgical closure of the cervical os.

hysteroepilepsy (ˌhistə·roh'epiˌlepsee) severe hysteria with epileptic convulsions.
hysterogenic (ˌhistə·roh'jenik) causing hysterical phenomena or symptoms.
hysterography (ˌhistə'rografee) radiography of the uterus after instillation of a contrast medium.
hysteroid ('histəˌroyd) resembling hysteria.
hysterolith ('histə·rəˌlith) a uterine calculus.
hysterolysis (ˌhistə'rolisis) freeing of the uterus from adhesions.
hysterometer (ˌhistə'romitə) an instrument for measuring the uterus.
hysterometry (ˌhistə'romətree) measurement of the uterus.
hysteromyoma (ˌhistə·rohmie'ohmə) leiomyoma of the uterus.
hysteromyotomy (ˌhistə·rohmie'otəmee) incision of the uterus for removal of a solid tumour.
hystero-oophorectomy (ˌhistə·rohˌoh·əfə'rektəmee) excision of the uterus and one or both ovaries.
hysteropathy (ˌhistə'ropəthee) any uterine disease; metropathy.
hysteropexy ('histə·rohˌpeksee) fixation of a displaced uterus by surgery.
hysteropia (ˌhistə·rohpi·ə) a hysterical disorder of vision.
hysterorrhaphy (ˌhistə'ro·rəfee) 1. suture of the uterus. 2. hysteropexy.
hysterorrhexis (ˌhistə·rə'reksis) rupture of the uterus.
hysterosalpingectomy (ˌhistə·rohˌsalpin'jektəmee) excision of the uterus and one or both of the uterine tubes.
hysterosalpingography (ˌhistə·rohˌsalping'gografee) radiography of the uterus and uterine tubes after instillation of a contrast medium.
hysterosalpingo-oophorectomy (ˌhistə·rohsalping·gohˌoh·əfə'rektəmee) excision of the uterus, uterine tubes, and ovaries.
hysterosalpingostomy (ˌhistə·rohˌsalping'gostəmee) anastomosis of a uterine tube and the uterus.
hysteroscope ('histə·rohˌskohp) an endoscope used in direct visual examination of the canal of the uterine cervix and the cavity of the uterus.
hysterospasm ('histə·rohˌspazəm) spasm of the uterus.
hysterotomy (ˌhistə'rotəmee) incision of the uterus—usually in order to remove a fetus in midpregnancy when it is too late to perform a therapeutic abortion.
hysterotrachelorrhaphy (ˌhistə·rohˌtrakə'lo·rəfee) suture of the uterus and uterine cervix.
hysterotrachelotomy (ˌhistə·rohˌtrakə'lotəmee) incision of the uterus and uterine cervix.
hysterotraumatism (ˌhistə·roh'trawməˌtizəm) hysterical symptoms following injury.
hysterotubography (ˌhistə·rohtyoo'bografee) hysterosalpingography.
Hz hertz (cycles per second).

I

I chemical symbol, *iodine.*
-ia word element, *state; condition.*
IACVF International Association of Cancer Victims and Friends.
IAL International Association of Laryngectomees.
IAPB International Association for the Prevention of Blindness.
-iasis word element. [Gr.] *condition, state.*
iatr(o)- word element. [Gr.] *medicine, physician.*
iatric (ie'atrik) pertaining to medicine or to a doctor.
iatrogenic (ieˌatroh'jenik) resulting from the activity of a doctor; said of any adverse condition in a patient resulting from treatment by a doctor or surgeon.
ibuprofen (ie'byooprohˌfen) a nonsteroidal anti-inflammatory agent that possesses analgesic and antipyretic activities; used for symptomatic relief of rheumatoid arthritis and osteoarthritis. It is similar in action to aspirin but less apt to cause gastrointestinal side-effects.
ICAA International Council on Alcohol and Addictions; Invalid Children's Aid Association.
ICD International Classification of Diseases (of the World Health Organization).
ice (ies) water in a solid state, at or below freezing point.
dry i. carbon dioxide snow.
i. bag see BAG.
Iceland disease ('iesland) benign myalgic encephalomyelitis.
ichor ('iekor) a watery discharge from wounds or sores. adj. **ichorous.**
ichorrhoea (ˌiekə'reeə) copious discharge of ichor.
ichthammol ('ikthəˌmol) an ammoniated coal tar product, used in ointment form for certain skin diseases.
ichthyismus (ˌikthi'izməz) ichthyotoxism.
ichthyoid ('ikthiˌoyd) fishlike.
ichthyology (ˌikthi'oləjee) the study of fishes.
ichthyophagous (ikthi'ofəgəs) eating or subsisting on fish.
ichthyosarcotoxin (ˌikthiohˌsahkoh'toksin) a toxin found in the flesh of poisonous fishes.
ichthyosarcotoxism (ˌikthiohˌsahkoh'toksizəm) poisoning due to ingestion of poisonous fish, marked by various gastrointestinal and neurological disturbances.
ichthyosis (ˌikthi'ohsis) 1. any of several generalized skin disorders marked by dryness, roughness, and scaliness, due to hypertrophy of the horny layer, resulting from excessive production or retention of keratin, or a molecular defect in the keratin. 2. ichthyosis vulgaris. adj. **ichthyotic.**
i. congenita lamellar exfoliation of the newborn.
i. fetalis lamellar exfoliation of the newborn.
i. hystrix a rare form of epidermolytic hyperkeratosis marked by generalized, dark brown, linear verrucoid ridges somewhat like porcupine skin.
lamellar i. of newborn see LAMELLAR EXFOLIATION OF THE NEWBORN.
ichthyotoxin (ˌikthioh'toksin) any toxic substance derived from fish.
ichthyotoxism (ˌikthioh'toksizəm) any intoxication due to an ichthyotoxin.
ICM International Confederation of Midwives.
ICN Infection Control Nurse; International Council of Nurses.
ICNA Infection Control Nurses Association.
ICP intracranial pressure.
ICRC International Committee of the Red Cross.
ICRF Imperial Cancer Research Fund.
ICSH interstitial cell-stimulating hormone (luteinizing hormone).
ictal ('ikt'l) pertaining to, characterized by, or due to a stroke or an acute epileptic seizure.
icteric (ik'terik) pertaining to or affected with jaundice.
icterogenic (ˌiktə·roh'jenik) causing jaundice.
icterohepatitis (ˌiktə·rohˌhepə'tietis) inflammation of the liver with marked jaundice.
icteroid ('iktə·royd) resembling jaundice.
icterus ('iktə·rəs) jaundice.

i. gravis acute yellow atrophy of the liver.

i. neonatorum jaundice in newborn infants. See HAEMOLYTIC DISEASE OF THE NEWBORN.

i. praecox mild jaundice developing within the first 24 hours of life (before physiological jaundice normally occurs), due to ABO blood group incompatibility between mother and infant; it usually clears rapidly and spontaneously, only occasionally resulting in haemolytic disease.

ictus ('iktəs) a seizure, stroke, blow, or sudden attack. adj. **ictal**.

ICU intensive care unit.

ICW International Council of Women.

id (id) 1. a freudian term used to describe that part of the personality which harbours the unconscious, instinctive impulses that lead to immediate gratification of primitive needs such as hunger, the need for air, the need to move about and relieve body tension, and the need to eliminate. Id impulses produce drives aimed at the satisfaction of physiological and bodily needs, as opposed to the EGO and SUPEREGO, which are psychological and social processes. The id is dominated by the pleasure principle and some gratification of the id impulses is necessary for survival of a person's personality. 2. a rash associated with but remote from the main lesion of the disease; considered to be an allergic reaction to the causative agent of the disease; often used as a suffix of a root representing the causative factor, as syphilid.

-id 1. word element. [Gr.] having the shape of, or resembling. 2. see ID (2).

-ide (ied) word element. [Ger., Fr.] *a binary compound.*

idea (ie'diə) a mental impression or conception.

autochthonous i. a strange idea that comes into the mind in some unaccountable way, but is not a hallucination.

compulsive i. an idea that persists despite reason and will and that drives one to action, usually inappropriate.

dominant i. a morbid or other impression that controls or colours every action and thought.

fixed i. a persistent morbid impression or belief that cannot be changed by reason.

i. of reference the incorrect idea that the words and actions of others refer to one's self, or the projection of the causes of one's own imaginary difficulties upon someone else.

ideal (ie'di·əl) a pattern or concept of perfection.

ego i. the standard of perfection unconsciously created by a person for himself.

idealization (ie,diəlie'zayshən) a conscious or unconscious mental mechanism, in which the individual overestimates an admired aspect or attribute of another person.

ideation (,iedi'ayshən) the formation of ideas or images. adj. **ideational.**

idée fixe (,eeday 'feeks) [Fr.] *fixed idea.*

identical (ie'dentik'l) exactly alike.

i. twins twins developing from the same ovum.

identification (ie,dentifi'kayshən) a defence mechanism by which an individual unconsciously takes as his own the characteristics, postures, achievements, or other identifying traits of other persons or groups. Identification plays a major role in the development of the SUPEREGO and of awareness and acceptance of the standards and rules accepted by society. However, as a person matures emotionally, his own self-identity should become clearer as he relates more to his own personal achievements and less to the accomplishments and successes of others with whom he identifies.

Identification is not to be confused with imitation, which is a conscious process. It should be pointed out also that overuse of identification as a defence mechanism denies one the opportunity of enjoying the benefits and self-satisfaction derived from one's own accomplishments.

identity (ie'dentətee) the aggregate of characteristics by which an individual is recognized by himself and others.

gender i. a person's concept of himself as being male and masculine or female and feminine, or ambivalent.

ideogenetic, ideogenous (,iediohjə'netik; ,iedi'ojənəs) induced by or related to vague sense impressions rather than organized images.

ideology (,iedi'oləjee) 1. the science of the development of ideas. 2. the body of ideas characteristic of an individual or of a social unit.

ideomotion (,iedioh'mohshən) muscular action induced by a dominant idea.

idiocy ('idi·əsee) obsolete term for severe MENTAL HANDICAP.

amaurotic familial i. a group of hereditary disorders due to an inborn defect of lipid metabolism, in which sphingolipids accumulate in the brain (see also AMAUROTIC FAMILIAL IDIOCY).

idio- word element. [Gr.] *self, peculiar to a substance or organism.*

idioglossia (,idioh'glosi·ə) imperfect articulation, with utterance of meaningless vocal sounds. adj. **idioglottic**.

idiogram ('idi·ə,gram) a drawing or photograph of the chromosomes of a particular cell.

idiopathic (,idioh'pathik) self-originated; occurring without known cause.

idiopathy (,idi'opəthee) a morbid state arising without known cause.

idiosyncrasy (,idioh'singkrəsee) 1. a habit or quality of body or mind peculiar to any individual. 2. an abnormal susceptibility to an agent (e.g., a drug) that is peculiar to the individual. adj. **idiosyncratic**.

idiot ('idi·ət) an obsolete term for one who would now be designated severely mentally handicapped.

idiotrophic (,idioh'trofik) capable of selecting its own nourishment.

idioventricular (,idiohven'trikyuhlə) pertaining to the cardiac ventricle alone.

Idoxene (ie'dokseen) trademark for a preparation of idoxuridine, an antiviral used topically for herpes simplex infections.

idoxuridine (,iedoks'yooə·rideen) a pyrimidine analogue that prevents replication of DNA viruses; used topically in herpes simplex keratitis.

IDU idoxuridine.

Iduridin (i'dyooə·ridin) trademark for a preparation of idoxuridine, an antiviral used topically for herpes simplex infections.

IDV intermittent demand ventilation.

ifosfamide (ie'fosfəmied) an alkylating agent used as an antineoplastic.

Ig immunoglobulin of any of the five classes: IgA, IgD, IgE, IgG, and IgM.

ignis ('ignis) [L.] *fire.*

i. sacer 1. ergotism. 2. herpes zoster.

IHF International Hospitals Federation.

ile(o)- word element. [L.] *ileum.*

ileac ('ili,ak) 1. of the nature of ileus. 2. pertaining to the ileum.

ileal ('ili·əl) pertaining to the ileum.

i. conduit use of a segment of the ileum for the diversion of urinary flow from the ureters to the abdominal wall. The segment is resected from the intestine with blood supply intact. The proximal end of the segment is closed, forming a pouch, and the proximal ends of the divided ureters are inserted into it. The distal end of the ileum is brought to the outside of the abdominal wall and everted to form a stoma. The remaining ends of the small intestine are anastomosed to reestablish bowel continuity, the ileal loop no longer being a part of the intestinal tract. Known also as urinary ileostomy or the Bricker procedure.

Indications for an ileal conduit include surgical removal of the bladder for malignancy, ectopia vesicae and neurogenic nonfunctioning bladder in which other devices to maintain urinary flow are unsatisfactory.

Prior to surgery, the placement of the stoma is determined by a thorough examination of the abdomen while the patient assumes various body positions. The site is selected so that old scar tissue, skin folds, bony prominences, and the umbilicus are avoided. Paraplegics or others wearing braces for ambulation must have the stoma placed so that there is no pressure on it from the appliance.

PATIENT CARE. The diversion of urinary flow to a collection pouch outside the body presents a very real challenge to the patient and those responsible for helping him develop a positive attitude about himself and his ability to achieve the goal of independence and rehabilitation. Psychologically he must adjust to a new body image, and he must deal with the most personal and intimate problems associated with the collection and disposal of urine. He will be concerned with the physical, social, and recreational limitations imposed by the stoma and with his acceptance socially. He will fear embarrassment from odours and leakage of urine, with his appearance and mode of dress, and with the amount of time involved in emptying and caring for the collection apparatus. With adequate instruction and continued support and reassurance, each of his concerns can be dealt with in a positive and helpful manner.

Because there is continuous drainage of urine down the ureters from the kidneys, the appliance for collection of urine must be worn at all times. In most cases the appliance must be emptied every 3 to 4 hours, depending on the amount of fluid intake and whether a leg bag is also used. These pouches are reusable for a short period of time and are discarded at the patient's discretion. They are cleaned with soap and water and may be rinsed in white vinegar to help eliminate odour. Commercial deodorizers are also available.

Skin irritation and infection around the stoma is always a danger because the moisture that collects under the faceplate of the appliance provides an ideal environment for the development of fungus (yeast or mould) infections. Soap and water are used to clean the area, which is then thoroughly dried and treated with topical medications to protect the skin.

It is especially important that the patient receives coordinated care from all available members of the health care team. The certified ostomy care specialist is an invaluable source of help and guidance for the patient and his family. In many communities there is an ostomy club whose members have some type of stoma and who meet regularly to share their experiences and to learn about self-care. Information about these and other local resources can be obtained by contacting the Ileostomy Advisory Service, Saltair House, Lord Street, Nechells, Birmingham B7 4OS; this service has a number of centres in other parts of the UK. See also STOMA.

ileectomy (ˌili'ektəmee) excision of the ileum.

ileitis (ˌili'ietis) inflammation of the ileum, or distal portion of the small intestine. It may result from infection, obstruction, severe irritation, or faulty absorption of material through the intestinal walls.

A specific type of inflammation of unknown cause involving the small and large intestines is known as regional ileitis, regional enteritis, or CROHN'S DISEASE. The advanced stage is marked by hardening, thickening, and ulceration of parts of the bowel lining. An obstruction may cause the development of a fistula.

A common symptom of ileitis is pain in the lower right quandrant of the abdomen or around the umbilicus. Other symptoms include loss of appetite, loss of weight, anaemia, and diarrhoea, which may alternate with periods of constipation. Treatment may require medication to remove any source of infection, special diet or surgery if there is obstruction.

ileocaecal (ˌilioh'seek'l) pertaining to the ileum and caecum.

i. valve the valve guarding the opening between the ileum and caecum; called also ileocolic valve.

ileocaecostomy (ˌiliohsee'kostəmee) surgical anastomosis of the ileum to the caecum.

ileocolic (ˌilioh'kolik) pertaining to the ileum and colon.

i. valve ileocaecal valve.

ileocolitis (ˌiliohkə'lietis) inflammation of the ileum and colon.

i. ulcerosa chronica chronic ileocolitis with fever, rapid pulse, anaemia, diarrhoea, and right iliac pain.

ileocolostomy (ˌiliohkə'lostəmee) surgical anastomosis of the ileum to the colon.

ileocolotomy (ˌiliohkə'lotəmee) incision of the ileum and colon.

ileocystoplasty (ˌilioh'sistohˌplastee) repair of the wall of the urinary bladder with an isolated segment of the ileum.

ileocystostomy (ˌiliohsi'stostəmee) use of an isolated segment of ileum to create a passage from the urinary bladder to an opening in the abdominal wall.

ileoileostomy (ˌiliohˌili'ostəmee) surgical anastomosis between two parts of the ileum.

ileoproctostomy (ˌiliohprok'tostəmee) surgical anastomosis between the ileum and the rectum. Ileorectal anastomosis.

ileorectal (ˌilioh'rekt'l) pertaining to or communicating with the ileum and rectum.

ileorrhaphy (ˌili'o·rəfee) suture of the ileum.

ileosigmoidostomy (ˌiliohˌsigmoy'dostəmee) surgical anastomosis of the ileum to the sigmoid colon.

ileostomy (ˌili'ostəmee) an artificial opening (stoma) created from the ileum and brought to the surface of the abdomen for the purpose of evacuation. Ileostomy is an inevitable part of proctocolectomy. ULCERATIVE COLITIS, CROHN'S DISEASE (regional ileitis), congenital defects of the bowel, CANCER and trauma are other conditions which may necessitate ileostomy to deflect the faecal stream.

An ileostomy may be temporary or permanent. When the ileostomy is done in conjunction with partial or complete removal of the colon and anus, it is always permanent. The stoma created by ileostomy is usually located in the right lower quadrant of the abdomen.

PATIENT CARE. The patient with an ileostomy requires care similar to that of the patient with a COLOSTOMY. Attention must be paid to the physical and psychological adjustments demanded of the patient as he works through his problems and strives to lead a normal and productive life.

The appliance for collection of faeces must be worn continuously and emptied every 4 to 5 hours because there is continuous flow of faeces through the ileostomy. The pouch should be changed at least once every week and more often if skin irritation, leakage, or persistent odour become a problem. The patient's main concerns will be obstruction and diarrhoea. He must be taught the signs of developing obstruction and the technique for gentle irrigation and massage around the stoma to remove material obstructing the movement of intestinal contents. If either irrigation or massage will not relieve the obstruction, he is instructed to report to his doctor.

Diarrhoea is a more frequent problem in a patient with an ileostomy and is more likely to result in serious difficulties arising from fluid and electrolyte loss and an upset in the ACID–BASE BALANCE. The patient must be aware of the early signs and symptoms of these difficulties and report to his doctor should they occur.

The patient's diet need not be restricted, but he should be warned to avoid foods that produce flatus and those which might lead to obstruction of the stoma, such as the indigestible skins of plums and tomatoes. He is instructed to chew all of his food thoroughly in order to facilitate digestion of the food before it passes through the ileostomy.

Skin irritations are a constant threat, as are topical fungus (yeast and mould) infections that may develop around the stoma. Because of the liquidity of the faeces there is always danger of leakage around the pouch where it fits over the stoma. The skin must be cleansed frequently and protected with a skin barrier such as Stomahesive and karaya gum.

The patient requires continued support as he learns to care for and live with his ileostomy. Fortunately, there are many sources of assistance for him, his family, and members of the health care team responsible for his care and rehabilitation (see also STOMA). Further information may be obtained from the Ileostomy Advisory Service, Saltair House, Lord Street, Nechells, Birmingham B7 4OS.

urinary i. use of a segment of the ileum as a stoma for the diversion of urinary flow from the ureters (see also ILEAL CONDUIT).

ileotomy (ˌili'otəmee) incision of the ileum.

ileum ('ili·əm) the distal portion of the small intestine, extending from the jejunum to the caecum.

duplex i. congenital duplication of the ileum.

ileus ('ili·əs) intestinal obstruction, especially failure of peristalsis. The condition frequently accompanies peritonitis and usually results from disturbances in neural stimulation of the bowel. It also may occur in many painful conditions involving the thoracolumbar region, for example, the colicky pains of GALLSTONES or KIDNEY stones and spinal injuries.

SYMPTOMS. The principal symptoms of ileus are abdominal pain and distention, vomiting (the vomitus may contain faecal material), and constipation. If the intestinal obstruction is not relieved, the circulation in the wall of the intestine is impaired and the patient appears extremely ill with symptoms of SHOCK and DEHYDRATION.

TREATMENT. Distention of the abdomen is relieved by decompression of the gut with a tube—e.g. Ryle's tube on regular aspiration—rather than constant suction. Because of the disruption in absorption of fluids and nutrients from the intestinal tract, fluids, electrolytes, and glucose are given intravenously. Surgical intervention to remove the cause of ileus is usually necessary when the obstruction is complete or the bowel is likely to become gangrenous. The type of surgical procedure will depend on the condition of the bowel and the cause of the obstruction. In some cases ILEOSTOMY or COLOSTOMY, either temporary or permanent, may be necessary (see also INTESTINAL OBSTRUCTION).

adynamic i. ileus resulting from inhibition of bowel motility, which may be produced by various causes, most frequently peritonitis.

dynamic i., hyperdynamic i. spastic ileus.

mechanical i. that due to mechanical causes, such as hernia, adhesions, volvulus, etc.

meconium i. ileus in the newborn due to blocking of the bowel with thick meconium.

paralytic i. adynamic ileus.

spastic i. that due to persistent contracture of a bowel segment.

i. subparta ileus due to pressure of the gravid uterus on the pelvic colon.

ili(o)- word element. [L.] *ilium.*

iliac ('iliˌak) pertaining to the ilium.

iliacus (i'lieəkəs) a muscle arising from the ilium and acting with the psoas muscle to flex the hip joint.

iliadelphus (ˌili·ə'delfəs) symmetrical conjoined twins united in the iliac region; iliopagus.

iliofemoral (ˌilioh'femə·rəl) pertaining to the ilium and femur.

ilioinguinal (ˌilioh'ing·gwin'l) pertaining to the iliac and inguinal regions.

iliolumbar (ˌilioh'lumbə) pertaining to the iliac and lumbar regions.

iliopagus (ˌili'opəgəs) symmetrical conjoined twins united in the iliac region.

iliopectineal (ˌiliohpek'tini·əl) pertaining to the ilium and pubes.

iliopsoas (ˌilioh'soh·əs) a flexor muscle of the hip comprising the iliacus and the psoas.

iliotrochanteric (ˌiliohˌtrohkan'terik) pertaining to the ilium and femoral trochanter.

ilium ('ili·əm) pl. *ilia* [L.] the lateral, flaring portion of the hip bone. adj. **iliac**.

illness ('ilnəs) a condition marked by pronounced deviation from the normal healthy state; sickness.

illumination (i'loomi'nayshən) the lighting up of a part, cavity, organ, or object for inspection.

darkfield i., dark-ground i. the casting of peripheral light rays upon a microscopical object from the side, the centre rays being blocked out; the object appears bright on a dark background.

illuminator (i'loomiˌnaytə) the source of light for viewing an object.

illusion (i'loozhən) a mental impression derived from misinterpretation of an actual sensory stimulus. adj. **illusional**.

Ilosone ('ilohˌsohn) trademark for preparations of erythromycin estolate, an antibiotic.

IM, i.m. intramuscular(ly).

im- a prefix, replacing *in-* before words beginning *b*, *m*, and *p*.

image ('imij) a picture or concept with more or less likeness to an objective reality.

body i. the three-dimensional concept of one's self, recorded in the cortex by the perception of ever changing postures of the body, and constantly changing with them.

mirror i. 1. the image of light made visible by the reflecting surface of the cornea and lens when illuminated through the slit lamp. 2. an image with right and left relations reversed, as in the reflection of an object in a mirror.

motor i. the organized cerebral model of the possible movements of the body.

imaging ('imijing) the production of diagnostic images, e.g., radiography, ultrasonography, or scintigraphy.

electrostatic i. a method of visualizing deep structures of the body, in which an electron beam is passed through the patient and the emerging beam strikes an electrostatically charged plate, dissipating the charge according to the strength of the beam. A film is then made from the plate.

imago (i'maygoh, i'mahgoh) pl. *imagoes,imagines* [L.] 1. the adult or definitive form of an insect. 2. in psychoanalysis, a childhood memory or fantasy of a loved person that persists in adult life.

imbalance (im'baləns) lack of balance; especially lack of balance between muscles, as in insufficiency of ocular muscles.

autonomic i. defective coordination between the sympathetic and parasympathetic nervous systems, especially with respect to vasomotor activities.

sympathetic i. vagotonia.

vasomotor i. autonomic imbalance.

imbecile ('imbə,seel, -,siel) an obsolete term for a person suffering from a moderate to severe degree of MENTAL HANDICAP.

imbecility (,imbə'silətee) MENTAL HANDICAP less severe than idiocy but more severe than moronity.

imbibition (,imbi'bishən) absorption of a liquid.

imbricated ('imbri,kaytid) overlapping.

Imferon ('imfəron) trademark for a preparation of iron dextran solution, an iron replacement used parenterally.

imidazole (,imi'dayzohl) a base found combined with alanine in histidine.

imide ('imied) any compound containing the bivalent group >NH (-CONHCO-).

imino acid (,iminoh'asid, i'meen-) proline or hydroxyproline, the two amino acids in which the amino group is part of a closed ring.

iminoglycinuria (,iminoh,gliesi'nyooə·ri·ə) a benign hereditary disorder of renal tubular reabsorption of glycine and the imino acids, marked by excessive levels of all three substances in the urine.

imipramine (i'miprə,meen) an antidepressant, used as the hydrochloride salt.

immature (,imə'tyooə) unripe or not fully developed.

immersion (i'mərshən) 1. the plunging of a body into a liquid. 2. the use of the microscope with the object lens and underlying portion of the microscope glass slide both covered with a liquid.

i. foot a condition resembling trench foot occurring in persons who have spent long periods in water.

immiscible (i'misəb'l) not susceptible to being mixed.

immobilization (i,mohbilie'zayshən) the rendering of a part incapable of being moved.

immobilize (i'mohbi,liez) to render incapable of being moved, as by a plaster of Paris cast.

immune (i'myoon) 1. being highly resistant to a disease because of the formation of humoral antibodies or the development of immunologically competent cells, or both, or as a result of some other mechanism, as interferon activities in viral infections. 2. characterized by the development of humoral antibodies or cellular IMMUNITY, or both, following antigenic challenge. 3. produced in response to antigenic challenge, as immune serum globulin.

i. reaction 1. immune response. 2. formation of a papule and areola without development of a vesicle following smallpox vaccination.

i. response the reaction to and interaction with substances interpreted by the body as not-self, the result being humoral and cellular IMMUNITY. Called also immune reaction. The immune response depends on a functioning THYMUS and the conversion of stem cells to B- and T-lymphocytes. These B- and T-cells contribute to ANTIBODY production, cellular immunity, and immunological memory.

DISORDERS OF THE IMMUNE RESPONSE. Pathological conditions associated with an abnormal immune reponse (immunopathy) may result from: (1) immunodepression, that is, an absence or deficient supply of the components of either humoral or cellular immunity, or both; (2) excessive production of gamma globulins; (3) overreaction to antigens of extrinsic origin, that is, antigens from outside the body; and (4) abnormal response of the body to its own cells and tissues.

Those conditions arising from immunosuppression include agammaglobulinaemia (the absence of gamma globulins) and hypogammaglobulinaemia (a decrease of circulating antibodies). Factors that may cause or contribute to suppression of the immune response include: (1) congenital absence of the thymus or of the stem cells that are precursors of B- and T-lymphocytes; (2) malnutrition, in which there is a deficiency of the specific nutrients essential to the life of antibody-synthesizing cells; (3) cancer, viral infections, and extensive burns, all of which overburden the immune response mechanisms and rapidly deplete the supply of antigen-specific antibody; (4) certain drugs, including alcohol and heroin, some antibiotics, antipsychotics, and the antitumour drugs used in the treatment of CANCER.

Overproduction of gamma globulins is a result of an excessive proliferation of plasma cells (multiple myeloma).

Hypersensitivity is the result of an overreaction to substances entering the body. Examples of this kind of inappropriate immune response include HAY FEVER, drug and food ALLERGIES, extrinsic ASTHMA, serum sickness, and ANAPHYLAXIS.

AUTOIMMUNE DISEASES are manifestations of the body's abnormal response to and inability to tolerate its own cells and tissues. For reasons not yet fully understood, the body fails to interpret its own cells as *self* and, as it would with other foreign (*not- self*) substances, utilizes antibodies and immunologically competent cells to destroy and contain them.

immunifacient (i,myooni'fayshənt) producing immunity; said of diseases, such as diphtheria and typhoid, that produce immunity against reinfection, which lasts for some time after an infection.

immunity (i'myoonitee) 1. the condition of being immune; security against a particular disease; nonsusceptibility to the invasive or pathogenic effects of foreign microorganisms or to the toxic effect of antigenic substances. Called also functional or protective immunity. 2. heightened responsiveness to antigenic challenge that leads to more rapid binding or elimination of antigen than in the nonimmune state; it includes both humoral and cell-mediated immunity (see below). 3. the capacity to distinguish foreign material from *self*, and to neutralize, eliminate, or metabolize that which is foreign (*not-self*) by the physiological mechanisms of the IMMUNE RESPONSE.

The mechanisms of immunity are essentially concerned with the body's ability to recognize and dispose of substances which it interprets as foreign and harmful to its well-being. When such a substance enters the body, complex chemical and mechanical activities are set into motion to defend and protect the body's cells and tissues. The foreign substance, usually a protein, is called an ANTIGEN, that is, one which generates the production of an antagonist. The most common response to the antigen is the production of ANTIBODY. The antigen–antibody reaction is an essential component of the overall immune response. The cellular response is another essential component.

The various and complex mechanisms of immunity are basic to the body's ability to protect itself against specific infectious agents and parasites, to accept or reject cells and tissues from other individuals, as in blood transfusions and organ transplants, and to protect against cancer, as when the immune system recognizes malignant cells as not-self and destroys them.

In recent years there has been extensive research into the body's ability to differentiate between cells, organisms, and other substances that are self, and therefore not alien to the body, and those which are not self and therefore must be eliminated. A major motivating force behind these research efforts has been the need for more information about rejection of transplanted tissues, the growth and proliferation of malignant cells, the inability of certain individuals to develop normal immunological responses, as in immune deficient diseases, and the failure of the body to recognize its own tissues, as in AUTOIMMUNE DISEASE.

IMMUNOLOGICAL RESPONSES. Immunological responses in humans can be divided into two broad categories: humoral immunity, which takes place in the body fluids (humours) and is concerned with antibody and complement activities; and cell-mediated or cellular immunity, which involves a variety of activities designed to destroy or at least contain cells that are recognized by the body as alien and harmful. Both types of responses are instigated by lymphocytes that originate in the bone marrow as stem cells and later are converted into mature cells having specific properties and functions.

The two kinds of lymphocytes that are important to establishment of immunity are T-lymphocytes (T-cells) and B-lymphocytes (B-cells). The T-LYMPHOCYTES differentiate in the THYMUS and are therefore called thymus-dependent. There are several types of T-cells involved in cell-mediated immunity, delayed hypersensitivity, the production of lymphokines, and the regulation of the immune response of other T- and B-cells.

The B-LYMPHOCYTES are so named because they were first identified during research studies involving the immunological activity of the bursa of Fabricius, a lymphoid organ in the chicken. Humans have no analogous organ. B-lymphocytes mature into plasma cells that are primarily responsible for forming antibodies, thereby providing humoral immunity.

Humoral Immunity. At the time that a substance enters the body and is interpreted as foreign, antibodies are released from plasma cells and enter the body fluids where they can react with the specific antigens for which they were formed. This release of antibodies is stimulated by antigen-specific groups (clones) of B-lymphocytes. Each B-lymphocyte has IgM IMMUNOGLOBULIN receptors which play a major role in capturing its specific antigen and in launching production of the immunoglobulins (which are antibodies) that are capable of neutralizing and destroying that particular type of antigen.

Most of the B-lymphocytes activated by the presence of their specific antigen become plasma cells, which then synthesize and export antibodies. The activated B-lymphocytes that do not become plasma cells continue to reside as 'memory' cells in the lymphoid tissue, where they stand ready for future encounters with antigens that may enter the body. It is these memory cells that provide continued immunity after initial exposure to the antigens.

There are two types of humoral immune response: primary and secondary. The primary response begins immediately after the initial contact with an antigen; the resulting antibody appears 48 to 72 hours later. The antibodies produced during this primary response are predominantly of the IgM class of immunoglobulins.

A secondary response occurs within 24 to 48 hours. This reaction produces large quantities of immunoglobulins that are predominantly of the IgG class. The secondary response persists much longer than the primary response and is the result of repeated contact with the antigens. This phenomenon is the basic principle underlying consecutive IMMUNIZATIONS.

The ability of the antibody to bind with or 'stick to' antigen renders it capable of destroying the antigen in a number of ways; for example, agglutination and opsonization. Antibody also 'fixes' or activates COMPLEMENT, which is the second component of the humoral immune system. Complement is the name given to a complex series of enzymatic proteins which are present but inactive in normal serum. When complement fixation takes place, the antigen, antibody, and complement become bound together. The cell membrane of the antigen (which usually is a bacterial cell) then ruptures, resulting in dissolution of the antigen cell and a leakage of its substance into the body fluids. This destructive process is called lysis.

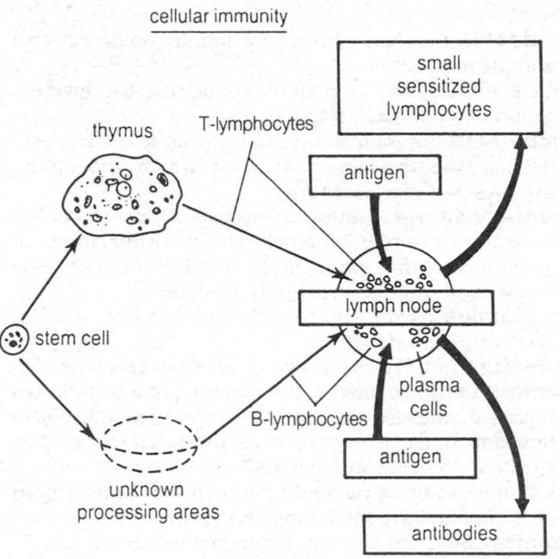

Formation of antibodies and sensitized lymphocytes by a lymph node in response to antigens. This figure also shows the origin of *thymic* ('T') and *bursal* ('B') lymphocytes that are responsible for the cellular and humoural immune processes of the lymph nodes

Cellular Immunity. This type of immune response is dependent upon T-lymphocytes, which are primarily concerned with a delayed type of immune response. Examples of this type of response include the rejection of transplanted organs, defence against slowly developing bacterial diseases that result from intracellular infections, delayed hypersensitivity reactions, certain autoimmune diseases, some allergic reactions, and recognition and rejection of self cells undergoing alteration, for example, those infected with viruses, and cancer cells that have tumour-specific antigens on their surfaces. These responses are called cell-mediated immune (CMI) responses.

The T-lymphocyte becomes sensitized by its first contact with a specific antigen. Subsequent exposure to the antigen stimulates a host of chemical and mechanical activities, all designed to either destroy or inactivate the offending antigen. Some of the sensitized T-lymphocytes combine with the antigen to deactivate it, while others set about to destroy the invading organism by direct invasion or the release of chemical factors. These chemical factors, through their influence on macrophages and unsensitized lymphocytes, enhance the effectiveness of the immune response.

Among the more active chemical factors are lymphokines, which are potent and biologically active proteins. The names of the lymphokines are somewhat descriptive of their functions. Factors that directly affect the macrophages are: the macrophage chemotactic factor (MCF), which attracts macrophages to the invasion site; macrophage migration inhibiting factor (MIF), which causes macrophages to remain at the invasion site; and macrophage activating factor (MAF), which stimulates the metabolic activities of these large cells, thereby improving their ability to ingest the foreign invaders.

Another factor, a protein called INTERFERON, is produced by the body cells, especially T-lymphocytes, following viral infection or in response to a wide variety of inducers, such as certain nonviral infectious agents and synthetic polymers.

A portion of the population of T-lymphocytes is transformed into 'killer cells' by the lymphocyte transforming factor (LTF). These activated lymphocytes produce a lymphotoxin or cytotoxin, which damages the cell membranes of the antigens, causing them to rupture.

In order to ensure an ample supply of T-lymphocytes, additional factors are at work. The blastogenic factor stimulates lymphocytes that have already undergone conversion to sensitized T-lymphocytes to increase their number by repeated cell division and the formation of clones.

It is apparent that the immune response brings about intensive activity at the site of invasion; it is not only the pathogen that is destroyed, but invariably, there is death and damage to some normal tissues.

Interactions Between the Two Systems. There are several areas in which the cellular and humoral systems interact and thereby improve the efficiency of the overall immune response. For example, a by-product of the enzymatic activity of the complement system acts as a chemotactic factor, attracting T-lymphocytes and macrophages to the invasion site. In another example, although T-lymphocytes are not required for the production of antibody, there is optimal antibody production after interaction between T-cells and B-cells. Abnormalities of the immune response system are discussed under disorders of the IMMUNE RESPONSE.

TYPES OF IMMUNITY. An individual may be naturally immune to certain pathological conditions, or he may acquire immunity through either active or passive means.

Natural immunity is a genetic characteristic of an individual and is due to the particular species and race to which he belongs, to his sex, and to his individual ability to produce immune bodies. All humans are immune to certain diseases that affect animals of the lower species; males are more resistant to some disorders than are females, and vice versa. Persons of one race are more susceptible to some diseases than those of another race that has had exposure to the infectious agents through successive generations. An individual's ability to produce immune bodies, and thereby ward off pathogens, is influenced by his state of physical health, his nutritional status, and his emotional response to stress.

In order for an individual to acquire immunity his body must be stimulated to produce its own immune response components (active immunity) or these substances must be produced by other persons or animals and then passed on to him (passive immunity). *Active immunity* can be established in two ways: by having the disease or by receiving modified pathogens and toxins. When an individual is exposed to a disease and the pathogenic organisms enter his body, the production of antibody is initiated. After recovery from the illness, memory cells remain in his body and stand ready as a defence against future invasion. It is possible, through the use of vaccines, bacterins, and modified toxins (toxoids) to stimulate the production of specific antibodies without having an attack of the disease. These are artificial means by which an individual can acquire active immunity.

Sometimes it is desirable to provide 'ready-made' immune bodies, as in cases in which the patient has already been exposed to the antigen, is experiencing the symptoms of the disease, and needs reinforcements to help mitigate its harmful effects. Examples of conditions for which an individual may be given such *passive immunity* include tetanus, diphtheria, and a venomous snake bite. The patient is given immune serum, or *gamma globulin*, which contains antibodies (including antitoxin) produced by the animal from which the serum was taken.

It is not always necessary that the patient actually suffer from the disease and exhibit its symptoms before passive immunity is provided. In some instances in which exposure to an infectious agent is suspected, immune bodies may be given to ward off a full-blown attack or at least to lessen its severity.

Another way in which immunity can be passively acquired is across the placental barrier from mother to fetus. The maternal antibody thus acquired serves as protection for the newborn until he can actively establish immunity on his own. Although IgG antibody can be acquired in this way, other antibodies and cellular immunity cannot.

acquired i. specific immunity attributable to the presence of antibody and to a heightened reactivity of antibody-forming cells, specifically immune lymphoid cells (responsible for cell-mediated immunity), and of phagocytic cells, following prior exposure to an infectious agent or its antigens, or passive transfer of antibody or immune lymphoid cells (adoptive immunity).

active i. acquired immunity attributable to the presence of antibody or of immune lymphoid cells formed in response to antigenic stimulus.

adoptive i. passive immunity of the cell-mediated type conferred by the administration of sensitized lymphocytes from an immune donor.

artificial i. acquired (active or passive) immunity produced by deliberate exposure to an antigen, such as a vaccine.

immunization (ˌimyuhnie'zayshən) the process of rendering a subject immune, or of becoming immune. Called also inoculation and vaccination; the word vaccine originally referred to the substance used to immunize against SMALLPOX, the first immunization developed. Now, however, the term is used for any preparation used in active immunization.

active i. stimulation with a specific antigen to promote antibody formation in the body. The immunity develops slowly after one or more doses of vaccine and lasts for many years. The antigenic substance may be either killed or inactivated agents, or live and suitably attenuated organisms.

Killed or inactivated vaccines are of three types: (1) suspensions of killed organisms such as inactivated (Salk) poliovaccine or Pol/Vac (Inact), typhoid and whooping cough vaccines; (2) components of organisms such as in influenza, meningococcal and pneumococcal vaccines; (3) toxoids which are altered toxins detoxicated by formalin as in diphtheria and tetanus toxoids.

Live attenuated vaccines are of two types: (1) a strain of the living organism attenuated so that it loses its disease producing capacity but retains its ability to promote antibody formation, such as tuberculosis vaccine (BCG), measles, oral poliovaccine (Sabin) or Pol/Vac (Oral), and rubella vaccine; (2) a related organism which produces immunity but little or no disease, such as vaccinia virus used in the vaccination against smallpox.

contraindications to i. immunization is usually an elective procedure and should be postponed if the person has any febrile or acute illness. Live vaccines should not normally be administered to pregnant women because of the theoretical possibility of fetal damage. Nor should they normally be given to immunocompromised persons. Specific contraindications are given on each vaccine pack and details are also given in 'Immunization against infectious disease' issued by the Departments of Health in the UK. Copies are obtainable from the Department of Health and Social Security, London, the Scottish Home and Health Department, Edinburgh, the Department of Health and Social Services, Belfast, and the Welsh Office, Cardiff.

passive i. transient immunity resulting from the injection of antibody preformed in human beings (human immunoglobulin) or in animals, usually horses (antisera). The immunity is rapidly acquired but lasts only a limited period of weeks or months until the foreign sera are eliminated from the body.

Immunoglobulins are of two types: (1) human normal immunoglobulin (HNIG) prepared from large donor pools and used for protection against hepatitis A and in the treatment of congenital disorders of gamma globulin production; (2) human specific immunoglobulins made from plasma of selected donors with high antibody levels against the particular diseases, such as human tetanus immunoglobulin (HTIG) (Humotet) and human rabies immunoglobulin (HRIG).

Antisera are not now often used because of the serum sickness and other allergic reactions they produce. However, botulinum antitoxin is available for the treatment of botulism, and diphtheria antitoxin for the treatment of diphtheria.

schedule of i. the recommended schedule of immunization in childhood is available from the above health departments.

side-effects of i. all vaccines and immunological products carry some risk of side-effects but serious reactions are very rare. Some cause virtually no reactions, such as poliovaccine, others may cause a very mild form of the disease, such as measles and rubella vaccines; inactivated vaccines may cause pain and swelling at the site of injection with fever. Occasionally more severe reactions occur and these should always be reported to the Committee on Safety of Medicines in the UK on yellow cards available in the BRITISH NATIONAL FORMULARY.

Because of their potential for causing sensitivity reactions, including anaphylaxis in hypersensitive subjects, all immunization procedures should only be given after a full medical history to assess contraindications. Emergency equipment and appropriate drugs should be available at all immunization sessions.

immunize ('imyuh,niez) to render immune.

immunoabsorbent (,imyuhnoh·əb'sawbənt, -'zaw-) immunosorbent.

immunoadjuvant (,imyuhnoh'ajəvənt) a nonspecific stimulator of the immune response, e.g., BCG vaccine or Freund's complete and incomplete adjuvants.

immunoadsorbent (,imyuhnoh·ad'sawbənt, -'zaw-) a preparation of antigen attached to a solid support or antigen in an insoluble form, which adsorbs homologous antibodies from a mixture of immunoglobulins.

immunoassay (,imyuhnoh'asay) the quantitative determination of antigenic substances, e.g., hormones, drugs, vitamins, specific proteins by means of antigen–antibody interaction, as by immunofluorescent techniques, radioimmunoassay, etc.

immunobiology (,imyuhnohbie'oləjee) that branch of biology dealing with immunological effects on such phenomena as infectious disease, growth and development, recognition phenomena, hypersensitivity, heredity, ageing, cancer, and transplantation.

immunoblast ('imyuhnoh,blast) lymphoblast.

immunoblastic (,imyuhnoh'blastik) pertaining to or involving the stem cells (immunoblasts) of lymphoid tissue.

immunochemistry (,imyuhnoh'kemistree) the study of the chemical basis of immune phenomena and their interactions.

immunochemotherapy (,imyuhnoh,keemoh-'therəpee, -,kem-) a combination of immunotherapy and chemotherapy.

immunocompetence (,imyuhnoh'kompitəns) the capacity to develop an immune response following exposure to antigen. adj. **immunocompetent**.

immunocomplex (,imyuhnoh'kompleks) antibody combined with its specific antigen and frequently with the first complement component; deposition of immunocomplexes that fix complement in tissues may lead to inflammation and tissue injury, as in immune complex glomerulonephritis.

immunocompromised (,imyuhnoh'komprə,miezd) having the immune response attenuated by administration of immunosuppressive drugs, by irradiation, by malnutrition, and by certain disease processes (e.g., cancer).

immunoconglutinin (,imyuhnohkən'glootinin) antibody formed against complement components that are part of an antigen–antibody complex, especially C3.

immunocyte ('imyuhnoh,siet) any cell of the lymphoid series which can react with antigen to produce antibody or to participate in cell-mediated immunity or delayed hypersensitivity reactions; called also immunologically competent cell.

immunocytoadherence (,imyuhnoh,sietoh·əd-'hiə·rəns) the aggregation of red cells to form rosettes around lymphocytes with surface immunoglobulins.

immunodeficiency (,imyuhnohdi'fishənsee) a deficiency of the immune response, either that mediated by humoral antibody or that mediated by immune lymphoid cells. adj. **immunodeficient**.

common variable i. a term encompassing a heterogeneous group of syndromes, which may be inherited or acquired, characterized by recurring persistent infections and deficiencies of some of the immunoglobulin classes.

immunodermatology (,imyuhnoh,dərmə'toləjee) the study of immunological phenomena as they affect skin disorders and their treatment or prophylaxis.

immunodiffusion (,imyuhnohdi'fyoozhən) the diffusion of antigen and antibody from separate reservoirs to form concentration gradients in hydrophilic gels.

immunoelectrophoresis (,imyuhnoh·i,lektrohfə-'reesis) a method of distinguishing proteins and other materials on the basis of their electrophoretic mobility and antigenic specificities.

rocket i. electrophoresis in which antigen migrates

THE FIVE CLASSES

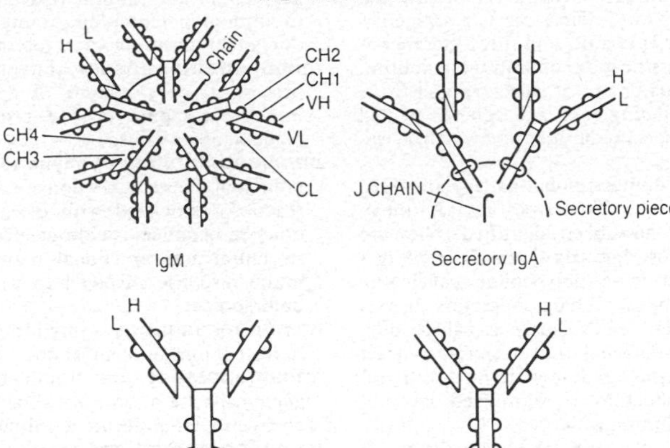

STRUCTURE OF IMMUNOGLOBULIN G AND A SUBCLASSES

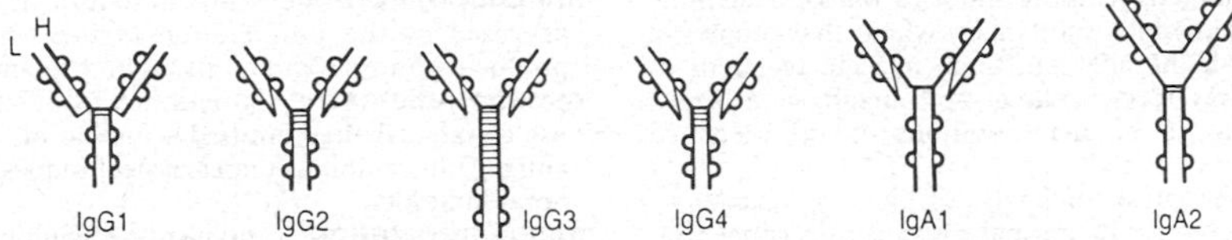

Molecular structure of immunoglobulins. Schematic representation of the basic four polypeptide chain, monomeric unit structure of immunoglobulin molecules. Heavy (H) chains determine *class*. Those in IgG are gamma, in IgM are mu, in IgA are alpha, in IgD are delta, and in IgE are epsilon. The two *types* of light (L) chains (kappa and lambda) are shared in common by all five immunoglobulin classes, although only one *type* is present in any individual molecule. Both heavy and light chains have looped structures referred to as domains or regions. Heavy chains possess one variable (VH) (wherein the antigen-binding site resides) and three constant (CH1, CH2, CH3) regions, with the exception of IgM and IgE which contain one variable (VH) and four constant regions (CH1, CH2, CH3, CH4). Light chains contain one variable (VL) and one constant (CL) region each. The heavy and light chains are fastened together by disulphide bonds as well as noncovalent forces. The disulphide bonds differ in number at the *hinge* (inter-H chain) region according to immunoglobulin subclass. Antigen-binding sites are located in the variable (amino-terminus) regions of each immunoglobulin monomer. IgM and dimeric or multimeric IgA molecules have J chains which are associated with the ability of these molecules to form polymers. Secretory IgA contains a secretory piece made by epithelial cells and believed to protect the molecule from enzymatic cleavage in the hinge region. Serum IgA2 has no heavy to light chain disulphide bonds, whereas IgA1 has a classic structure

from a well through agar gel containing antiserum, forming cone-shaped (rocket) precipitin bands.

immunofiltration (ˌimyuhnohfilˈtrayshən) the extraction of antibodies in pure form by subjection of serum to insoluble specific antigen, the antigen then being removed from the antibody by treatment with soluble carriers.

immunofluorescence (ˌimyuhnohˌflooəˈresəns) a method of determining the location of antigen (or antibody) in a tissue section or smear using a specific antibody (or antigen) labelled with a fluorochrome, usually fluorescein. In the direct methods, the fluorochrome is chemically linked to the specific antibody. In indirect methods, a labelled anti-immunoglobulin that binds to the specific antibody is used.

immunogen (iˈmyoonəˌjen) any substance capable of eliciting an immune response.

immunogenetics (ˌimyuhnohjəˈnetiks) the study of the genetic factors controlling the individual's immune response and the transmission of those factors from generation to generation. adj. **immunogenetic**.

immunogenic (ˌimyuhnohˈjenik) producing immunity; evoking an immune response.

immunogenicity (ˌimyuhnohjəˈnisitee) the ability of a substance to provoke an immune response or the degree to which it provokes a response. adj. **immunogenic**.

immunoglobulin (ˌimyuhnohˈglobyuhlin) a protein of animal origin with known ANTIBODY activity. Immunoglobulins are major components of the humoral IMMUNE RESPONSE system. They are synthesized by lymphocytes and plasma cells and found in the serum and in other body fluids and tissues, including the urine, spinal fluid, lymph nodes, and spleen. See also IMMUNITY.

Each immunoglobulin molecule consists of four

polypeptide chains: two heavy chains (H-chains) and two light chains (L-chains). There are five antigenically different kinds of H-chains, and this difference is the basis for the classification of immunoglobulins. Each class varies in its chemical structure and in its number of antigen-binding sites and adheres to and reacts only with the specific antigen for which it was produced.

The five classes of immunoglobulins (Ig) are: IgA, IgD, IgE, IgG, and IgM. Two types of IgA (mean concentration 2.5 g/l) have been identified. They are serum IgA and secretory IgA (sIgA). In sIgA two IgA molecules are linked by a polypeptide called the secretory piece and by a J chain. Secretory IgA is present in nonvascular fluids, such as saliva, bile, synovial fluid, and intestinal and respiratory tract secretions. Both IgA types are known to have antiviral properties; their production is stimulated by oral vaccines and aerosol immunizations.

IgD is found in trace quantities in the serum. It serves as a B-lymphocyte surface receptor.

IgE is called the reaginic antibody and may be increased in persons with allergy. When IgE attaches itself to cells within the body, for example, those of the mucous membrane and skin, the cells become sensitized to allergens, causing them to release histamine and histamine-like substances when they come in contact with the allergen. Such allergic reactions as urticaria, hay fever, asthma, and anaphylactic shock are thought to be manifestations of IgE-mediated reactions.

IgG is the most abundant of the five classes of immunoglobulins. Its normal mean serum concentration is 12 g/l. It is the major antibody in the secondary humoral response of immunity, serves to activate the complement system, and is frequently involved in opsonization. IgG is the only immunoglobulin that can cross the placental barrier.

IgM is principally concerned with the primary antibody response, appearing soon after initial invasion by an antigen and capable of destroying the antigen when it is first introduced. Its normal mean serum concentration is 1 g/l. Like the IgG, IgM activates the complement system and together these two classes of immunoglobulins serve as specific antitoxins against the toxins of diphtheria, tetanus, botulism, and anthrax microorganisms, and snake venins.

surface i. immunoglobulins are produced by plasma cells and other B-lymphocytes and can be detected on the surface of these cells by techniques such as immunofluorescence using specific antibodies. Tumours such as myeloma and B-cell lymphomas arise from one clone of cells (i.e., are monoclonal). All produce the same class of Ig with single light chain and can be identified as such by their surface Ig. A reactive (as opposed to neoplastic) proliferation of B-cells will have more than one species of Ig, i.e., is polyclonal.

immunohistochemical (ˌimyuhnohˌhistoh'kemik'l) denoting the application of antigen–antibody interactions to histochemical techniques, as in the use of immunofluorescence.

immunoincompetent (ˌimyuhnoh·in'kompitənt) lacking the ability or capacity to develop an immune response to antigenic challenge.

immunologist (ˌimyuh'noləjist) a specialist in immunology.

immunology (ˌimyuh'noləjee) the scientific study of all aspects of immunity, including allergy, hypersensitivity, etc. adj. **immunological.**

immunomodulation (ˌimyuhnohˌmodyuh'layshən) adjustment of the immune response to a desired level, as in immunopotentiation, immunosuppression, or induction of immunological tolerance.

immunopathogenesis (ˌimyuhnohˌpathə'jenəsis) the process of development of a disease in which an immune response or the products of an immune reaction are involved.

immunopathology (ˌimyuhnohpə'tholəjee) 1. that branch of biomedical science concerned with immune reactions associated with disease, whether the reactions be beneficial, without effect, or harmful. 2. the structural and functional manifestations of the immune response involved in a disease. adj. **immunopathological.**

immunophysiology (ˌimyuhnohˌfizi'oləjee) the physiology of immunological processes.

immunopotency (ˌimyuhnoh'pohtənsee) the immunogenic capacity of an individual antigenic determinant on an antigen molecule to initiate antibody synthesis.

immunopotentiation (ˌimyuhnohpəˌtenshi'ayshən) accentuation of the response to an immunogen by administration of another substance.

immunoprecipitation (ˌimyuhnohpriˌsipi'tayshən) precipitation resulting from interaction of specific antibody and antigen.

immunoproliferative (ˌimyuhnohprə'lifə·rətiv) characterized by the proliferation of the lymphoid cells producing immunoglobulins, as in the gammopathies.

immunoradiometry (ˌimyuhnohˌraydi'omətree) the use of radiolabelled antibody (instead of radiolabelled antigen) in radioimmunoassay techniques. adj. **immunoradiometric.**

immunoregulation (ˌimyuhnohˌregyuh'layshən) the control of specific immune responses and interactions between B- and T-lymphocytes and macrophages.

immunoresponsiveness (ˌimyuhnohri'sponsivnəs) the capacity to react immunologically.

immunosorbent (ˌimyuhnoh'sawbənt, -'zaw-) an insoluble support for antigen or antibody used to absorb homologous antibodies or antigens, respectively, from a mixture; the antibodies or antigens so removed may then be eluted in pure form.

immunostimulant (ˌimyuhnoh'stimyuhlənt) 1. stimulating an immune response. 2. an agent that stimulates the immune response.

immunostimulation (ˌimyuhnohˌstimyuh'layshən) stimulation of an immune response, e.g., by use of BCG vaccine.

immunosuppressant (ˌimyuhnohsə'presənt) immunosuppressive.

immunosuppression (ˌimyuhnohsə'preshən) inhibition of the formation of antibodies to antigens that may be present; used in transplantation procedures to prevent rejection of the transplanted organ or tissue.

immunosuppressive (ˌimyuhnohsə'presiv) 1. pertaining to or inducing immunosuppression. 2. an agent that induces immunosuppression.

immunosurveillance (ˌimyuhnohsə'vayləns) the monitoring function of the immune system whereby it recognizes and reacts against aberrant cells arising within the body.

immunotherapy (ˌimyuhnoh'therəpee) passive immunization of an individual by administration of preformed antibodies (serum or gamma globulin) actively produced in another individual; by extension, the term has come to include the use of immunopotentiators, replacement of immunocompetent lymphoid tissue (e.g., bone marrow or thymus), etc. Because the immune response is a process of surveillance, recognition, and attack of foreign cells, immunotherapy has emerged as a promising mode of treatment for cancer. In general, there are three basic approaches to immunotherapy: active (specific and nonspecific), passive, and adoptive. See also CANCER.

Nonspecific immunotherapy relies on general immune stimulants to activate the whole immune system. In the past decade, immunotherapy against cancer has involved the use of the BCG VACCINE, which is evolved from strains of *Mycobacterium tuberculosis*, and is used to provide some immunity to tuberculosis. Recently, INTERFERON has been considered as a good prospect for converting inactive immune cells into active 'natural killers' that attack tumour cells directly.

One drawback to the use of general immune stimulants is that there is a limit to the extent to which the immune system can be forced to respond. At some point there is an automatic dampening of the response which controls immunological activities so as to protect the body from attack by its own destructive immune cells.

Specific immunotherapy is still experimental but it has promise. Particularly promising is the technique that involves the use of specific antibodies for a type of tumour cell that has been 'loaded' with either antineoplastic drugs or radioactive materials. When injected into the bloodstream of a patient with that particular kind of tumour, the 'loaded' antibodies attach to the surface of the malignant cells. Thus, the antitumour drug or radiation does more damage to the malignant cells than to nonmalignant cells to which the antibody does not bind.

Immunotherapy is also used in the desensitization or hyposensitization of individuals allergic to specific allergens. Minute amounts of allergen to which the person is allergic are administered by injection in increasing doses over prolonged periods of time, in order to provoke production of large quantities of *blocking antibody* (predominantly IgG), which prevents an immediate hypersensitivity reaction from occurring. Presumably, the blocking antibody prevents the reaction by competing locally or in the circulation for the antigen.

immunotoxin (i,myoonoh'toksin) an antitoxin.

immunotransfusion (i,myoonohtrans'fyoozhən, -trahns-) transfusion of blood from a donor previously rendered immune to the disease affecting the patient.

Imodium (i'mohdiəm) trademark for preparations of loperamide hydrochloride, an antidiarrhoeal.

impacted (im'paktid) being wedged in firmly. In obstetrics, denoting twins so situated during delivery that the pressure of one against the other prevents complete engagement of either. Also called locked twins. Management usually requires decapitation of one twin. The condition may be fatal to both infants. Also refers to obstructed labour in a singleton pregnancy when the breech or shoulder becomes impacted within the pelvis.

impaction (im'pakshən) the condition of being wedged in firmly.

faecal i. a collection of putty-like or hardened faeces in the rectum or sigmoid (see also FAECAL IMPACTION).

impairment (im'pairmənt) any loss or abnormality of psychological, physiological, or anatomical structure or function.

impalpable (im'palpəb'l) not detectable by touch.

impar ('impah) not even; unequal; unpaired.

impatent (im'paytənt) not open; closed.

impedance (im'peedəns) obstruction or opposition to passage or flow, as of an electric current or other form of energy.

acoustic i. an expression of the opposition to passage of sound waves, being the ratio of the acoustic pressure and the particle velocity in the wave. For a plane wave it is equal to the product of the density of a substance and the velocity of sound in it. Sometimes called the *characteristic* acoustic impedance of the material.

imperforate (im'pərfə·rət) not open; abnormally closed.

impermeable (im'pərmi·əb'l) not permitting passage, as for fluid.

impetigo (,impə'tiegoh) a streptococcal or staphylococcal skin infection marked by vesicles or bullae that become pustular, rupture, and form yellow crusts, called also impetigo contagiosa or impetigo vulgaris. The disease occurs most frequently in children. It is spread by direct contact with the moist discharges of the lesions. If not properly treated, it can be serious or even fatal to newborn infants.

Treatment consists of cleansing the lesions with soap and water before the application of topical antibiotics such as fusidic acid or neomycin. Care should be taken to avoid spreading the infection and children should be kept away from school. The lesions should be kept dry and open to the air as much as possible. Systemic administration of antibiotics is rarely recommended.

implant (im'plahnt, 'implahnt) 1. to insert or to graft (tissue or radioactive material) into intact tissues or a body cavity. 2. any material inserted or grafted into the body.

implantation (,implahn'tayshən) 1. the insertion of an organ or tissue in a new site in the body. 2. the attachment and embedding of the fertilized ovum in the endometrium. 3. the insertion or grafting into the body of biological, living, inert, or radioactive material.

implantology (,implahn'toləjee) the science dealing with implants.

implosion (im'plohzhən) in behaviour therapy, a form of desensitization used in the treatment of phobias and related disorders; the patient is repeatedly exposed, in imagination or real life, to emotionally distressing stimuli while the therapist makes verbal interpretation of the psychological meaning of the stimuli in order to intensify the patient's emotional arousal. Called also flooding.

impotence ('impətəns) inability of the male to achieve or maintain a penile erection of sufficient rigidity to perform sexual intercourse successfully. adj. **impotent**.

Impotence is related to infertility only in that the condition prevents coitus with and impregnation of the female partner. An impotent man may produce sufficient numbers of normal spermatozoa. While underlying emotional problems can cause inability to have and maintain an erection and probably account for a large percentage of cases of impotence, abnormally low levels of testosterone can be the primary cause. Occasionally successful functioning and early morning erections do not preclude the possibility of endocrine dysfunction. Impotence may also be due to vascular and neuropathic disorders.

impregnation (,impreg'nayshən) 1. the act of fertilizing or rendering pregnant. 2. saturation.

impressio (im'presioh) pl. *impressiones* [L.] impression (1).

impression (im'preshən) 1. a slight indentation or depression, as one produced in the surface of one organ by pressure exerted by another. 2. a negative imprint of an object made in some plastic material that later solidifies. 3. an effect produced upon the mind, body, or senses by some external stimulus or agent.

imprinting ('imprinting) a species-specific, rapid kind of learning during a critical period of early life in which social attachment and identification are established.

impulse ('impuls) 1. a sudden pushing force. 2. a sudden uncontrollable act. 3. nerve impulse.

cardiac i. movement of the chest wall caused by the heart beat.

nerve i. the electrochemical process propagated along nerve fibres.

impulsion (im'pulshən) an abnormal impulse to perform certain acts, usually of a disagreeable nature.

Imunovir ('imyoonohvi·ə) trademark for a preparation of inosine pranobex, an antiviral agent.

Imuran ('imyuhran) trademark for a preparation of azathioprine, an immunosuppressant.

IMV intermittent mandatory ventilation.

In chemical symbol, *indium*.

in- 1. a prefix, *in*, *within*, or *into*. 2. an intensive prefix. 3. a negative or privative prefix.

in extremis (ˌin ek'streemis) [L.] *at the point of death*.

in situ (in'sityoo) [L.] *in its normal place*, *confined to the site of origin*.

in tela (ˌin 'teelə) [L.] *in tissue;* relating especially to stained histological preparations.

in utero (in 'yootə·roh) [L.] *within the uterus*.

in vitro (in'veetroh, -'vit-) [L.] *within a glass*, *observable in a test tube*, *in an artificial environment*.

in vivo (in'veevoh) [L.] *within the living body*.

inactivation (inˌakti'vayshən) the destruction of activity, as of a virus, by the action of heat or other agent.

inanimate (in'animət) 1. without life. 2. lacking in animation.

inanition (ˌinə'nishən) the exhausted state due to prolonged undernutrition; starvation.

inappetence (in'apitəns) lack of appetite or desire.

inarticulate (ˌinah'tikyuhlət) 1. not having joints; disjointed. 2. uttered so as to be unintelligible; incapable of articulate speech.

inassimilable (ˌinə'similəb'l) not susceptible of being utilized as nutriment.

inborn ('inbawn) congenital; inherited or acquired before birth.

inbreeding ('inˌbreeding) the mating of closely related individuals or of individuals having closely similar genetic constitutions.

incarceration (inˌkahsə'rayshən) unnatural retention or confinement of a part.

incentive spirometry (in'sentiv) a goal-oriented inspiratory manoeuvre in which the patient is encouraged by visual feedback from an incentive spirometer to execute sustained maximal inspiration. The patient usually performs 10 to 20 sustained deep breaths an hour until he can achieve his predicted inspiratory reserve volume.

incest ('insest) sexual activity between persons so closely related that marriage between them is legally or culturally prohibited.

incidence ('insidəns) the number of particular new events which occur in a population in a given period of time. For example, the number of new cases of a disease such as measles expressed per 1000 of population per year.

i. study, cohort study an epidemiological study carried out over a period of time to determine the incidence of disease in a defined population group in persons exposed and not exposed to possible causative factors.

incident ('insidənt) impinging upon, as incident radiation.

incineration (inˌsinə'rayshən) the act of burning to ashes.

incipient (in'sipi·ənt) beginning to exist; coming into existence.

incision (in'sizhən) 1. a cut or a wound made by a sharp instrument. 2. the act of cutting.

incisive (in'siesiv) 1. having the power of cutting; sharp. 2. pertaining to the incisor teeth.

i. bone the portion of the maxilla bearing the incisors; developmentally, it is the premaxilla, which in humans later fuses with the maxilla, but in most other vertebrates persists as a separate bone.

incisor (in'siezə) 1. adapted for cutting. 2. any one of the four front teeth of either jaw.

Hutchinson's i's see HUTCHINSON'S INCISORS.

incisure (in'siezhə) a cut, notch, or incision.

Rivinus i. tympanic notch; a defect in the upper tympanic part of the temporal bone, filled by the upper portion of the tympanic membrane.

inclination (ˌinkli'nayshən) a sloping or leaning; the angle of deviation from a particular line or plane of reference.

i. of the pelvis the angle between the plane of the pelvic inlet and the horizontal plane.

inclusion (in'kloozhən) 1. the act of enclosing or the condition of being enclosed. 2. anything that is enclosed; a cell inclusion.

i. bodies round, oval, or irregular shaped bodies in the cytoplasm and nuclei of cells, as in diseases due to viral infection, such as rabies, smallpox, etc.

cell i. a usually lifeless, often temporary, constituent in the cytoplasm of a cell.

i. conjunctivitis conjunctivitis affecting mainly newborn infants, caused by a strain of *Chlamydia trachomatis*, which resides in the genital tract and is primarily a cause of SEXUALLY TRANSMITTED DISEASE. The infection is contracted by the infant during delivery. It begins as an acute purulent conjunctivitis and can lead to papillary hypertrophy of the palpebral conjunctiva.

dental i. a tooth so surrounded with bony material that it is unable to erupt.

fetal i. a partially developed fetus enclosed within the body of another.

incoagulability (ˌinkohˌagyuhlə'bilitee) the state of being incapable of coagulation. adj. **incoagulable**.

incompatibility (ˌinkəmpatə'bilitee) the quality of being incompatible.

incompatible (ˌinkəm'patəb'l) not suitable for combination, simultaneous administration, or transplantation; mutually repellent.

incompetence (in'kompitəns) 1. inability to function properly. 2. the legal status of an incompetent.

incompetent (in'kompitənt) 1. not able to function properly. 2. a person determined by the courts to be unable to manage his own affairs.

incontinence (in'kontinəns) 1. inability to control excretory functions. 2. immoderation or excess. adj. **incontinent**.

Faecal incontinence may result from disorders of the nervous system or weakening of the anal sphincters in elderly persons. Anal or rectal surgery and anal tears resulting from childbirth also may impair control.

Urinary incontinence has many possible causes. Brain and spinal cord injuries may remove or impair both the sensation and the control of the bladder. Urinary infection, especially in the elderly, increases the desire to void and may result in incontinence. Incontinence sometimes occurs after surgery or in connection with irritation of the urinary tract by inflammation or injury. In some instances incontinence is due to an obstruction that prevents normal emptying of the urinary bladder, resulting in constant dribbling of the overflow. Stress incontinence is involuntary urine loss when a sudden increase in intra-abdominal pressure and intravesicular pressure occurs, such as during a cough or a sneeze. The angle between the urethra and the bladder wall is found to be 90° in continent women, allowing the circular muscles around the urethra and the tight pelvic muscles to control urine flow. At micturition the angle is obliterated by increased intra-abdominal pressure and lowering of the bladder. In stress incontinence the angle may be relieved by the effort of a cough or sneeze, thereby allowing urine to escape. This is thought to explain 90 per cent of cases.

PATIENT CARE. The ultimate goal in the care of an incontinent patient is to keep him dry, comfortable, and odour-free, and to help him achieve some degree of independence and social acceptability. Loss of control of urine and faeces can be a devastating blow emotionally and can present multiple problems because of complications that can develop (see BLADDER TRAINING).

URETEROSTOMY and ILEAL CONDUIT may be considered for certain patients having problems with control of urinary flow. Indwelling CATHETERS must be used with restraint because of the dangers of infection. And in some cases there is no other choice but to use some type of protective pants that can be worn over an absorbent pad for women; penile sheaths are often effective for men.

Finding a way to keep the incontinent patient clean and dry can be a very real challenge. It requires knowing the patient and making no assumptions about his ability to cooperate and achieve control until an effort has been made to involve him in a plan for control. It demands ingenuity, perseverance, and patience and a very real desire to help the patient cope with his problem.

continuous i. uninhibited urination that occurs whenever the micturition reflex is stimulated.

paradoxical i. retention of urine with overflow when urination is involuntary.

stress i. involuntary escape of urine due to strain on the orifice of the bladder, as in coughing or sneezing.

urgency i. inability to hold back urination when feeling the urge to void; a major complaint of patients with urinary tract infections; also present in some women two or three days before onset of the menstrual period.

incoordination (ˌinkohˌawdi'nayshən) lack of normal adjustment of muscular motions; failure to work harmoniously.

incorporation (inˌkawpə'rayshən) 1. the union of one substance with another, or with others, in a composite mass. 2. an unconscious mental mechanism in which a person figuratively ingests the psychic representation of another person, or parts of him.

increment ('ingkrimənt) an increase or addition; the amount by which a value or quantity is increased. adj. **incremental.**

incrustation (ˌinkru'stayshən) 1. the formation of a crust. 2. a crust, scab, or scale.

incubate ('ingkyuhˌbayt) to subject to or to undergo incubation.

incubation ('ingkyuh'bayshən) 1. the provision of proper conditions for growth and development, as for bacterial or tissue cultures. 2. the development of an infectious disease from time of the entrance of the pathogen to the appearance of clinical symptoms. 3. the development of the embryo in the egg of oviparous animals. 4. the maintenance of an artificial environment for an infant, especially a preterm infant.

i. period the interval of time required for development; especially the time between invasion of the body by an infectious agent and appearance of the first sign or symptom of the disease.

incubator ('ingkyuhˌbaytə) a warmed, perspex box for nursing preterm and ill babies. The first infant incubator was used in 1880 by Dr. Tamier, a Paris obstetrician. His successor, Professor Pierre Budin routinely used incubators for nursing preterm infants and thereby improved their chances of survival. Modern incubators allow warmed, humidified oxygen to be given to babies whose temperature is servo-controlled using a probe attached to the baby. Care must be taken not to provide excessive oxygen to preterm babies as this may cause retinopathy of prematurity (RETROLENTAL FIBROPLASIA).

Incubators are also used to encourage bacterial growth in specimens sent to the microbiology laboratory.

incubus ('ingkyuhbəs) 1. nightmare. 2. a heavy mental burden.

incudal ('ingkyuhdəl) pertaining to the incus.

incudectomy (ˌingkyuh'dektəmee) excision of the incus.

incudiform (ing'kyoodiˌfawm) anvil-shaped.

incudomalleal (ingˌkyoodoh'mali·əl) pertaining to the incus and malleus.

incudostapedial (ingˌkyoodohstə'peedi·əl) pertaining to the incus and stapes.

incurable (in'kyooə·rəb'l) 1. not susceptible of being cured. 2. a person with a disease that cannot be cured.

incus ('ingkəs) the middle of the three ossicles of the ear; called also *anvil.*

indanedione (ˌindayn'die·ohn) any of a group of synthetic anticoagulants derived from 1,3-indanedione, e.g., phenindione, which interfere with the synthesis of the vitamin K-dependent coagulation factors (prothrombin, factors VII, IX, and X).

Inderal ('indəˌral) trademark for a preparation of propranolol hydrochloride, a β-adrenergic blocking agent.

index ('indeks) pl. *indexes, indices* [L.] 1. the second digit of the hand, the forefinger. 2. the numerical ratio of measurement of any part in comparison with a fixed standard.

i. case the first case of a disease reported in a population, a group of persons, or a family.

Colour I. a publication of the Society of Dyers and Colorists and the American Association of Textile Chemists and Colorists containing an extensive list of dyes and dye intermediates. Each chemically distinct compound is identified by a specific number, the CI number, avoiding the confusion of trivial names used for dyes in the dye industry.

diagnostic i. a record system to categorize and list patients by their disease(s).

I. Medicus a monthly publication of the US National Library of Medicine in which the world's leading biomedical literature is indexed by author and subject.

opsonic i. a measure of opsonic activity determined by the ratio of the number of microorganisms phagocytized by normal leukocytes in the presence of serum from an individual infected by the microorganism, to the number phagocytized in serum from a normal individual.

phagocytic i. the average number of bacteria ingested per leukocyte of the patient's blood.

refractive i. the refractive power of a medium compared with that of air (assumed to be 1).

short increment sensitivity i. (SISI) a hearing test in which randomly spaced, 0.5-second tone bursts are superimposed at 1 to 5-decibel increments in intensity on a carrier tone having the same frequency and an intensity of 20 decibels above the speech recognition threshold; the fraction of responses in which a given level is distinguished from the carrier level is compared with a normal response.

therapeutic i. originally, the ratio of the maximum tolerated dose to the minimum curative dose; now defined as the ratio of the median lethal dose (LD_{50}) to the median effective dose (ED_{50}). It is used in assessing the safety of a drug.

indican ('indikən) 1. a substance formed by decomposition of tryptophan in the intestines and excreted in the urine. 2. a yellow indoxyl glycoside from indigo plants.

indicanuria (,indikə'nyooə·ri·ə) an excess of indican in the urine.

indication (,indi'kayshən) a sign or circumstance that points to or shows the cause, treatment, etc., of a disease.

indicator ('indi,kaytə) 1. the index finger, or the extensor muscle of the index finger. 2. any substance that indicates the appearance or disappearance of a chemical by a colour change or attainment of a certain pH.

indigenous (in'dijənəs) occurring naturally in a certain locality.

indigestion (,indi'jeschən) lack or failure of digestive function; commonly used to denote vague abdominal discomfort after meals. Among the symptoms of indigestion are heartburn, nausea, flatulence, cramps, a disagreeable taste in the mouth, belching, and sometimes vomiting or diarrhoea. Ordinary indigestion can result from eating too much or too fast; from eating when tense, tired, or emotionally upset; from food that is too fatty or spicy; and from heavy food or food that has been badly cooked or processed.

Indigestion and its symptoms may also accompany other disorders such as allergy, migraine, influenza, typhoid fever, food poisoning, peptic ulcer, inflammation of the gallbladder (chronic cholecystitis), appendicitis, and coronary occlusion ('heart attack').

indigitation (in,diji'tayshən) INTUSSUSCEPTION (1).

indium ('indi·əm) a chemical element, atomic number 49, atomic weight 114.82, symbol In. See table of elements in Appendix 2.

i.-111 a cyclotron-produced isotope of indium which has a half-life of 2.8 days and decays by emitting gamma rays of 173 and 247 keV. When tagged to human white blood cells or platelets it is used as a nuclear medicine imaging agent to detect and monitor inflammatory conditions, e.g., abscesses. Symbol ^{111}I.

i.-113m a generator-produced radionuclide with a half-life of 1.7 hours and which decays by isomeric transition by emitting gamma rays of 393 keV. It can be used instead of ^{99}Tc^{m} in some nuclear medicine investigations but because of the high energy of its photon emissions a rectilinear scanner must be used instead of a gamma camera. Symbol ^{113}In^{m}.

individual variation (indi'vidyooəl) 1. variation of biological values within individuals at different times; for example, temperature variation at different times of the day. 2. biological variation between individuals, for example, height, weight.

individuation (,indi,vidyoo'ayshən, -,vijoo-) 1. the process of developing individual characteristics. 2. differential regional activity in the embryo occurring in response to organizer influence. 3. in Jungian psychology, the process of maturation and development and realization of the individual personality. In immature personalities, the process of individuation and self-realization is delayed. See also JUNG.

Indocid ('indohsid) trademark for a preparation of indomethacin, a nonsteroidal anti-inflammatory agent.

indocyanine green (,indoh'sieə,neen) a dye used intravenously as a diagnostic aid in the determination of blood volume, cardiac output, and hepatic function.

indole ('indohl) a compound obtained from coal tar and indigo and produced by decomposition of tryptophan in the intestine, where it contributes to the peculiar odour of faeces. It is excreted in the urine in the form of indican.

indolent ('indələnt) causing little pain; slow growing.

indomethacin (,indoh'methəsin) an anti-inflammatory, analgesic, and antipyretic agent, used in arthritic disorders and degenerative joint disease.

indoramin (in'dorəmin) a postsynaptic α-adrenergic receptor blocker, used as an oral antihypertensive.

indoxyl (in'doksil) an oxidation product of indole formed in tryptophan decomposition, and excreted in the urine as indican.

indoxyluria (in,doksi'lyooə·ri·ə) an excess of indoxyl in the urine.

inducer (in'dyoosə) in biosynthesis, a compound that induces synthesis of a specific enzyme or sequence of enzymes, by antagonizing the corresponding repressor, or by some other mechanism.

induction (in'dukshən) 1. the process or act of inducing, or causing to occur, especially the production of a specific morphogenetic effect in the embryo through evocators or organizers, or the production of anaesthesia or unconsciousness by use of appropriate agents. 2. the generation of an electric current or magnetic properties in a body because of its proximity to an electrified or magnetized object.

inductor (in'duktə) a tissue elaborating a chemical substance that acts to determine the growth and differentiation of embryonic parts.

indurated ('indyuh,raytid) hardened; abnormally hard.

induration (,indyuh'rayshən) the quality of being hard; the process of hardening; an abnormally hard spot or place. adj. **indurative**.

black i. the hardening and pigmentation of the lung tissue, as in pneumonia.

brown i. increase in the pulmonary connective tissue and excessive pigmentation by large numbers of haemosiderin-laden macrophages due to chronic congestion from valvular heart disease—classically mitral stenosis.

cyanotic i. hardening of an organ from chronic venous congestion.

granular i. cirrhosis.

grey i. induration of lung tissue in or after pneumonia, without pigmentation.

red i. interstitial pneumonia in which the lung is red and congested.

indusium griseum (in'dyoozi·əm 'grizi·əm) [L.] a thin layer of grey matter on the dorsal surface of the corpus callosum.

industrial (in'dustri·əl) referring to industry.

i. diseases those that are caused by the nature of the work.

prescribed i. diseases those for which sickness benefit is payable, including those that are notifiable under the Factories Act.

inebriant (i'neebri·ənt) 1. causing drunkenness. 2. an agent that causes drunkenness.

inelastic (,ini'lastik) lacking elasticity.

inert (i'nərt) inactive.

inertia (i'nərshə) [L.] *inactivity, inability to move spontaneously*.

colonic i. weak muscular activity of the colon, leading to distention of the organ and constipation.

i. time the time required to overcome the inertia of a muscle after reception of a stimulus from a nerve.

uterine i. weak and/or infrequent uterine contractions in labour. It may be *primary*, when the contractions are abnormal throughout labour, or *secondary* to obstruction or maternal exhaustion in the late first or second stage.

infancy ('infənsee) the first year of life.

infant ('infənt) a young child from birth to 1 year of age.

NEEDS OF THE INFANT. Emotional and physical needs include love and security, a sense of trust, warmth and comfort, feeding and sucking pleasure.

GROWTH AND DEVELOPMENT. Development is a continuous process, and each child progresses at his own rate. There is a developmental sequence, which means that the changes leading to maturity are specific and orderly. The various types of growth and development and the accompanying changes in appearance and behaviour are interrelated; that is, physical, emotional, social, and spiritual developments affect one another in the progress toward maturity.

Development of muscular control proceeds from the head downward (cephalocaudal development). The infant controls the head first and gradually acquires the ability to control the neck, then the arms, and finally the legs and feet. Movements are general and random at first, beginning with use of the larger muscles and progressing to specific smaller muscles, such as those needed to handle small objects.

Factors that influence growth and development are: hereditary traits, sex, environment, cultural, nationality and race, and physical makeup.

floppy i., floppy i. syndrome a congenital myopathy of infants, marked clinically by myotonia and muscle weakness.

i. mortality rate the number of deaths of children under one year of age per 1000 live births in any one year.

premature i. one born before the state of maturity (see also PRETERM INFANT).

preterm i. see PRETERM INFANT.

infanticide (in'fanti,sied) the killing of a child by its mother during the first year of its life.

infantile ('infən,tiel) relating to infancy; having features or traits characteristic of early childhood.

i. paralysis poliomyelitis.

infantilism (in'fanti,lizəm) persistence of the characters of childhood into adult life, marked by underdevelopment of the reproductive organs, and often dwarfism.

infarct ('infahkt) a localized area of necrosis produced by sudden occlusion of the arterial supply or the venous drainage of the part.

anaemic i. one due to sudden interruption of flow of arterial blood to the area. Also referred to as a pale infarct because of the lack of blood in the infarcted zone. It implies lack of a collateral circulation.

haemorrhagic i. one that is red owing to oozing of erythrocytes into the injured area. This may be from collateral circulation with an arterial occlusion or from congestion with venous occlusion.

infarctectomy (,infahk'tektəmee) surgical removal of an infarct.

infarction (in'fahkshən) 1. the formation of an infarct. 2. an infarct.

cardiac i. myocardial infarction.

cerebral i. an ischaemic condition of the brain, causing a persistent focal neurological deficit in the area affected.

myocardial i. gross necrosis of the myocardium, due to interruption of the blood supply to the area (see also MYOCARDIAL INFARCTION).

pulmonary i. localized necrosis of lung tissue, due to obstruction of the arterial blood supply.

infection (in'fekshən) 1. invasion and multiplication of microorganisms in body tissues, especially that causing local cellular injury due to competitive metabolism, toxins, intracellular replication, or antigen–antibody response. 2. an infectious disease.

The infectious process is similar to a circular chain with each link representing one of the factors involved in the process. An infectious disease occurs only if each link is present and in proper sequence. These links are: (1) the causative agent, which must be of sufficient number and virulence or capable of destroying normal tissue; (2) reservoirs in which the organism can thrive and reproduce; for example, body tissues and the wastes of humans, animals, and insects, and contaminated food and water; (3) a portal through which the pathogen can leave the host; for example, via the respiratory tract and intestinal tract; (4) a mode of transfer, that is, the hands, air currents, vectors, fomites, or other means by which the pathogens can be moved from one place or person to another; and (5) a portal of entry through which the pathogens can enter the body of a (6) susceptible host. Open wounds, the respiratory, intestinal, and reproductive tracts are examples of portals of entry. The host must be susceptible to the disease, not having any immunity to it, or lacking adequate resistance to overcome the invasion by the pathogens. The body responds to the invading organisms by the formation of ANTIBODIES and by a series of physiological changes known as INFLAMMATION.

The spectrum of infectious agents changes with the passage of time and the introduction of drugs and chemicals designed to destroy them. The advent of antibiotics and the resultant development of resistant strains of bacteria have introduced new types of pathogens little known or not previously thought to be significantly dangerous to man. The gram-positive organisms were the most common infectious agents in the 1950s. Today the gram-negative microorganisms, *Proteus*, *Pseudomonas*, and *Serratia* are particularly troublesome, especially in the development of hospital-acquired infections. It can safely be predicted that within the next two or three decades other lesser known pathogens and new strains of bacteria will emerge as the most common causes of infections.

The development of resistant strains of pathogens can be limited by the judicious use of antibiotics. This requires culturing and sensitivity testing for a specific antibiotic to which the identified causative organism has been found to be sensitive. If the patient has been receiving a broad-spectrum antibiotic prior to culture and sensitivity testing, this should be discontinued as soon as the specific antibiotic for the organism has been found. It would be helpful, too, if the general public understood that antibiotics are not cure-alls and that there is danger in using them indiscriminately. In some instances an antibiotic can upset the normal flora of the body, thus compromising the body's natural resistance and making it more susceptible to a second infection (called a *superinfection*) by a microorganism resistant to the antibiotic. Although antibacterials have greatly reduced mortality and morbidity rates for many infectious diseases, the ultimate outcome of an infectious process depends on the effectiveness of the host's IMMUNE RESPONSES. The antibacterial drugs provide a holding action, keeping the growth and reproduction of the infectious agent in check until the interaction between the organism and the immune bodies of the host can subdue the invaders.

Intracellular infectious agents include viruses, mycobacteria, *Brucella*, *Salmonella*, and many others. Infections of this type are overcome primarily by T-lymphocytes and their products, which are the components of cell-mediated IMMUNITY. Extracellular infectious agents live outside the cell; these include pneumococcus, streptococcus, and haemophilus. These microorganisms have a carbohydrate capsule that acts as an antigen to stimulate the production of antibody, an essential component of humoral IMMUNITY.

Infection may be transmitted by direct contact, by indirect contact, or by vectors. Direct contact may be with body excreta such as urine, faeces, or mucus, or with drainage from an open sore, ulcer, or wound. Indirect contact refers to transmission via inanimate objects such as bed linens, bedpans, drinking glasses, or eating utensils. Vectors are flies, mosquitoes, or other insects capable of harbouring and spreading the infectious agent.

aerobic i. infection caused by AEROBES.

airborne i. infection by inhalation of organisms suspended in air on water droplets, droplet nuclei, or dust particles.

anaerobic i. infection caused by ANAEROBES.

i. control the utilization of procedures and techniques in the surveillance, investigation, and compilation of statistical data in order to reduce the spread of infection, particularly hospital-acquired infections.

Practitioners in infection control are frequently nurses who are employed by Health Authorities. They have titles such as Infection Control Officer and Infection Control Nurse, and they function as liaison between staff nurses, doctors, department heads, the infection control committee, and the health authority. Such practitioners also assume some responsibility for teaching patients and their families, as well as employees of the Health Authority.

cross i. infection transmitted between patients infected with different pathogenic microorganisms.

droplet i. infection due to inhalation of respiratory pathogens suspended on liquid particles exhaled by someone already infected.

droplet nuclei i. small droplets from the respiratory tract evaporate within seconds, leaving behind droplet nuclei which contain any microorganisms present in the original droplet. Droplet nuclei may travel considerable distances.

dustborne i. infection by inhalation of pathogens that have become affixed to particles of dust.

endogenous i. 1. that due to reactivation of organisms present in a dormant focus, as occurs in tuberculosis, etc. 2. that caused by organisms present in or on the body, e.g. surgical wound infection due to organisms from the GI tract.

exogenous i. that caused by organisms not normally present in the body but which have gained entrance from the body surface of others or from the environment.

hospital-acquired i's those acquired during hospitalization; called also *nosocomial infections*. A prevalence survey showed that 10 per cent of patients in hospitals in England and Wales in 1982 acquired an infection whilst in hospital. The most common causative agents are *E. coli*, *Proteus*, *Pseudomonas*, and *Klebsiella*, among the gram-negative organisms, and *Staphylococcus* and *Enterococcus* among the gram-positive organisms. See also infection control (above).

mixed i. infection with more than one kind of organism at the same time.

nosocomial i. see hospital-acquired infections (above).

pyogenic i. infection by pus-producing organisms.

secondary i. infection by a pathogen following an infection by a pathogen of another kind.

subclinical i. infection associated with no detectable symptoms but caused by microorganisms capable of producing easily recognizable diseases, such as poliomyelitis or mumps; it is detected by the production of antibody, or by delayed hypersensitivity exhibited in a skin test reaction to such antigens as tuberculoprotein.

terminal i. an acute infection occurring near the end of a disease and often causing death.

waterborne i. infection by microorganisms transmitted in water.

Infection Control Nurses Association founded in 1970 as a professional association, its aims include the promotion of increased awareness of infection control issues, together with the development of specialist professional education for its practitioners. Further information may be obtained from the Chairperson, Mrs. J. Sedgwick, Wycombe General Hospital, High Wycombe, Bucks. HP11 2TT.

infectious (in'fekshəs) caused by or capable of being communicated by infection.

i. disease disease resulting from multiplication of microorganisms in the body. Most are communicable but not all (see also COMMUNICABLE DISEASE).

i. mononucleosis (glandular fever) an acute virus infection characterized by sore throat and glandular enlargement, caused by the Epstein–Barr (EB) virus. Worldwide common infection particularly prevalent in older children and young adults in western countries. The source of infection is man and spread is by oropharyngeal secretions, for example, during kissing. The incubation period is 4 to 6 weeks and infectivity after the disease may be prolonged. Other causes of the syndrome of sore throat, fever, and glandular enlargement are cytomegalovirus, toxoplasmosis, and human immune deficiency virus (HIV) infection.

CLINICAL FEATURES. In children may be symptom free, or mild sore throat and glandular enlargement. May present with vague malaise and fever. In young adults, acute sore throat (anginose type of disease) is more common and the course may be prolonged. Enlargement of liver and spleen common. Jaundice and aseptic meningitis may occur. Drug-induced rashes are frequent, particularly after ampicillin therapy. Laboratory diagnosis by Paul–Bunnel (Monospot) test, EB virus antibodies and typical blood count. EB virus infection is associated with the development of the malignant disease Burkitt's lymphoma in Africa where it is linked with hyperendemic malaria.

TREATMENT. No specific treatment available. Antibiotics of no value. Convalescence may be prolonged.

infective (in'fektiv) infectious, capable of producing infection; pertaining to or characterized by the presence of pathogens.

inferior (in'fiə·ri·ə) situated below, or directed downward; in anatomy, used in reference to the lower surface of a structure, or to the lower of two (or more) similar structures.

inferiority feelings (in,fiə·ri'oritee) a term introduced by Alfred ADLER for the child's feelings of inadequacy in relation to his parents and to society.

infertility (,infər'tilətee) difficulty in conceiving and producing viable offspring (cf. sterility: inability to conceive). adj. **infertile.**

The diagnosis of infertility is not usually considered valid until after one year of engaging in sexual relations without contraception. About 35 per cent of the cases of infertility are due to male factors, about 35 per cent to female factors, and the remaining 30 per cent to a combination of male and female factors. Most specialists subject both partners to an infertility study.

Feelings of anger, helplessness, grief, and other emotions can be very intense and may require great understanding and support. Either partner may feel that infertility is a threat to his or her sexuality and sexual self-image.

If the infertility cannot be corrected, as in women who fail to ovulate or men who have no sperm-producing cells, there are alternatives. Adoption is becoming more difficult because of the availability of birth control methods and the fact that more than 70 per cent of single mothers now choose to keep and raise their children themselves. Artificial insemination by husband (AIH) or donor (AID) is an alternative for couples who have no moral or religious objection to the procedure. Recently in vitro fertilization has achieved successful pregnancy for suitable couples.

infestation (ˌinfeˈstayshən) parasitic attack or subsistence on the skin and/or its appendages, as by insects, mites, or ticks; sometimes used to denote parasitic invasion of the organs and tissues, as by helminths.

infiltrate (ˈinfilˌtrayt) 1. to penetrate the interstices of a tissue or substance. 2. material deposited by infiltration.

infiltration (ˌinfilˈtrayshən) the diffusion or accumulation in a tissue or cells of substances not normal to it or in amounts in excess of the normal; also, the material so accumulated.

adipose i. fatty infiltration.

calcareous i. deposit of lime and magnesium salts in the tissues.

cellular i. the migration and accumulation of cells within the tissues.

fatty i. 1. a deposit of fat in tissues, especially between cells. 2. the presence of fat vacuoles in the cell cytoplasm.

urinous i. the extravasation of urine into a tissue.

infirm (inˈfərm) weak; feeble, as from disease or old age.

infirmary (inˈfərmə·ree) a hospital or place where the sick or infirm are maintained or treated.

inflammagen (inˈflaməˌjen) an irritant that elicits both oedema and the cellular response of inflammation.

inflammation (ˌinfləˈmayshən) a localized protective response elicited by injury or destruction of tissues, which serves to destroy, dilute, or wall off both the injurious agent and the injured tissue. adj. **inflammatory**. See also HEALING.

The inflammatory response can be provoked by physical, chemical, and biological agents, including mechanical trauma, exposure to excessive amounts of sunlight, x-rays and radioactive materials, corrosive chemicals, extremes of heat and cold, and infectious agents such as bacteria, viruses, and other pathogenic microorganisms. Although these infectious agents can produce inflammation, infection and inflammation are not synonymous.

The classic signs of inflammation are *heat*, *redness*, *swelling*, *pain*, and *loss of function*. These are manifestations of the physiological changes that occur during the inflammatory process. The three major components of this process are: (1) changes in the calibre of blood vessels and the rate of blood flow through them (haemodynamic changes); (2) increased capillary permeability; and (3) leukocytic exudation (see also *leukocyte* CHEMOTAXIS).

Haemodynamic changes begin soon after injury and progress at varying rates, according to the extent of injury. This series of events starts with dilation of the arterioles and the opening of new capillaries and venular beds in the area. With these changes comes an accelerated flow of blood, accounting for the signs of heat and redness. Next follows *increased permeability* of the microcirculation, which permits leakage of protein-rich fluid out of small blood vessels and into the extravascular fluid compartment, accounting for the inflammatory oedema.

Leukocytic migration occurs in the following sequence. First, the leukocytes move to the endothelial lining of the small blood vessels (*margination*) and line the endothelium in a tightly packed formation (*pavementing*). Eventually, these leukocytes move through the endothelium—usually between the cells—and escape into the extravascular space (*emigration*). Once they are outside the blood vessels they move on the chemotactic gradient to the site of injury. Accumulations of neutrophils and macrophages at the area of inflammation act to neutralize foreign particles including bacteria by phagocytosis.

Chemical mediators of the inflammatory process include a variety of substances originating in the plasma, the cells of uninjured tissue, and possibly from the damaged tissue. The major kinds of mediators are: (1) *vasoactive amines*, such as histamine and serotonin; (2) *plasma proteases* that comprise three interrelated systems, the kinin system that produces bradykinin, the complement system that produces proteins that interact with antigen–antibody complexes and mediate immunological injury and inflammation, and the clotting system that increases vascular permeability and chemotactic activity for the leukocytes; (3) prostaglandins, which can reproduce several aspects of the inflammatory process; (4) neutrophil products; (5) lymphocyte factors; and (6) other mediators, such as slow-reacting substance (SRS-A) and endogenous pyrogen.

Hormonal Response. Some hormones, such as cortisol, have an anti-inflammatory action that limits inflammation to a local reaction while others, such as aldosterone, are proinflammatory. Thus, the endocrine system has a regulatory effect on the process of inflammation so that it can be balanced and beneficial in the body's attempts to recover from injury.

acute i. inflammation, usually of sudden onset, marked by the classical signs of heat, redness, swelling, pain and loss of function, and in which vascular and exudative processes predominate.

catarrhal i. a form affecting mainly a mucous surface, marked by a copious discharge of mucus and epithelial debris.

chronic i. prolonged and persistent inflammation marked chiefly by new connective tissue formation and an inflammatory infiltrate in which lymphocytes and macrophages dominate; it may be a continuation of an acute form or a prolonged low-grade form.

exudative i. one in which the prominent feature is an exudate.

fibrinous i. one marked by an exudate of fibrin.

granulomatous i. a form, usually chronic, attended by formation of granulomas.

interstitial i. inflammation affecting chiefly the stroma of an organ.

parenchymatous i. inflammation affecting chiefly the essential tissue elements of an organ.

productive i., proliferative i. one leading to the production of new connective tissue fibres.

pseudomembranous i. an acute inflammatory response to a powerful necrotizing toxin, e.g., diphtheria toxin, characterized by formation on a mucosal surface of a false membrane composed of precipitated fibrin, necrotic epithelium, and inflammatory leukocytes.

purulent i. suppurative inflammation.

serous i. one producing a serous exudate.

specific i. one due to a particular microorganism.

subacute i. a condition intermediate between chronic and acute inflammation, exhibiting some of the characteristics of each.

suppurative i. one marked by pus formation.

toxic i. one due to a poison, e.g., a bacterial product.

traumatic i. one that follows a wound or injury.

ulcerative i. that in which necrosis on or near the surface leads to loss of tissue and creation of a local defect (ulcer).

inflation (inˈflayshən) distention or the act of distending, with air, gas, or fluid.

inflection, inflexion (inˈflekshən) the act of bending inward, or the state of being bent inward.

influenza (ˌinflooˈenzə) an acute viral infection of the respiratory tract, occurring in isolated cases, epidemics, and pandemics. Called also flu. adj. **influenzal.** Transmission is by droplet inhalation and the period of infectivity lasts from 1 day before the onset of symptoms until up to 7 days later. In Britain, most cases occur between December and May, with the peak incidence being in February.

Three main types of the virus have been recognized, types A (with many subgroups, labelled A_1, A_2, etc.), B, and C. Influenza B virus is chiefly associated with epidemics among children and young adults, usually in schools or other closed communities.Influenza C is rare. Most older adults carry antibodies against the disease because of repeated exposure to these viruses. Influenza A viruses are responsible for epidemics and pandemics of influenza. Influenza A undergoes periodic antigenic 'shift', with a major change in its surface structure so that antibodies devloped following previous infection are not protective. Such 'shifts' are associated with the major pandemics which occurred in 1890, 1918, 1957, 1968 and 1977 when millions died worldwide. Each pandemic strain tends to acquire a nickname, hence Asian (1957), Hong Kong (1968) and Russian (1977). Less marked antigenic changes in influenza A virus are called 'drift'.

SYMPTOMS. Influenza has a brief incubation period (1-4 days). The symptoms appear suddenly and though the virus enters the respiratory tract it soon affects the entire body. The symptoms include fever, chills, headache, sore throat, cough, gastrointestinal disturbances, muscular pain, and neuralgia. Acute symptoms last about 4 days and then gradually resolve. Complications include convulsions (especially in children and the elderly) from hyperpyrexia, bronchitis, pneumonia, myocarditis, and sudden death.

TREATMENT. There is no drug that will cure influenza. An antibiotic may be prescribed to ward off complications of secondary bacterial infections such as pneumonia and bronchitis. Bed rest, increasing the intake of fluids, and aspirin to relieve aches and discomfort and help control fever are prescribed.

PREVENTION. Vaccination with influenza vaccine, the formulation of which is changed annually to include recently circulating strains of viruses on recommendation of the WHO. Annual vaccination is advised for persons with chronic heart, lung or renal disease, those with diabetes, and patients on immunosuppressive therapy. It should also be considered for residents of old people's homes. Other precautions include avoiding contact with others who have influenza, avoiding crowded places when there is a local epidemic, and observing good personal hygiene to increase the body's resistance.

information system (ˌinfə'mayshən) a system for collecting, analysing and interpreting health data.

informed consent (in'fawmd) see CONSENT.

infra- word element. [L.] *beneath.*

infra-axillary (ˌinfrə·ak'silə·ree) below the axilla.

infraclavicular (ˌinfrəklə'vikyuhlə) below the clavicle.

infraclusion (ˌinfrə'kloozhən) a condition in which the occluding surface of a tooth does not reach the normal occlusal plane and is out of contact with the opposing tooth.

infracostal (ˌinfrə'kost'l) below a rib.

infraction (in'frakshən) incomplete bone fracture without displacement.

infradian (ˌinfrə'di·ən) pertaining to a period longer than 24 hours; applied to the cyclic behaviour of certain phenomena in living organisms (infradian rhythm).

infrahyoid (ˌinfrə'hieoyd) below the hyoid bone.

inframaxillary (ˌinfrəmak'silə·ree) beneath the maxilla.

infranuclear (ˌinfrə'nyookli·ə) below a nucleus.

infraorbital (ˌinfrə'awbit'l) lying under or on the floor of the orbit.

infrapatellar (ˌinfrəpə'telə) beneath the patella.

infrared rays (ˌinfrə'red) denoting electromagnetic radiation of wavelength greater than that of the red end of the spectrum, having wavelengths of 0.75-1000 μm. Infrared rays are sometimes subdivided into long-wave or far infrared (about 3.0-1000 μm) and short-wave or near infrared (about 0.75-3.0 μm). They are capable of penetrating body tissues to a depth of 10 mm. Sources of infrared rays include heat lamps, hot water bottles, steam radiators, and incandescent light bulbs.

Infrared rays are used therapeutically to promote muscle relaxation, to speed up the inflammatory process, and to increase circulation to a part of the body. See also HEAT.

infrascapular (ˌinfrə'skapyuhlə) below the scapula.

infrasonic (ˌinfrə'sonik) below the frequency range of sound waves.

infraspinous (ˌinfrə'spienəs) beneath the spine of the scapula.

infrasternal (ˌinfrə'stərnəl) beneath the sternum.

infratentorial (ˌinfrəten'tor·ri·əl) beneath the tentorium of the cerebellum.

infratrochlear (ˌinfrə'trokli·ə) beneath the trochlea.

infraversion (ˌinfrə'vərshən) 1. downward deviation of the eye. 2. infraclusion.

infundibuliform (ˌinfun'dibyuhliˌfawm) shaped like a funnel.

infundibulum (ˌinfun'dibyuhləm) pl. *infundibula* [L.] 1. any funnel-shaped passage. 2. conus arteriosus, the anterosuperior portion of the right ventricle of the heart. adj. **infundibular**.

ethmoidal i. 1. a passage connecting the nasal cavity with the anterior ethmoidal cells and frontal sinus. 2. a sinuous passage connecting the middle meatus of the nose with the anterior ethmoidal cells and often with the frontal sinus.

i. of hypothalamus a hollow, funnel-shaped mass in front of the tuber cinereum, extending to the posterior lobe of the pituitary gland.

i. of uterine tube the distal, funnel-shaped portion of the uterine tube.

infusion (in'fyoozhən) 1. the steeping of a substance in water to obtain its soluble principles. 2. the product obtained by this process. 3. the slow therapeutic introduction of fluid other than blood into a vein (see also INTRAVENOUS INFUSION).

NOTE: An *infusion* flows in by gravity, an *injection* is forced in by a syringe, an *instillation* is dropped in, and an *insufflation* is blown in.

subcutaneous i. the introduction into the subcutaneous tissues of fluids, especially physiological sodium chloride solution, in large quantity; particularly useful in the administration of fluids to small children and elderly persons not suited to intravenous infusion but now only infrequently used. The most common sites for insertion of the needles for subcutaneous infusion are the anterior aspect of the thighs and the loose tissue below each breast. Two needles are used to deliver the fluid; one in each thigh or on each side of the chest. This method of introducing fluids into the body is contraindicated in cases of oedema, and it may be complicated by abscess formation, puncture of a large blood vessel, and necrosis and sloughing of the tissues due to poor absorption. The enzyme hyaluronidase is injected into the tubing at each injection site at the start of infusion, and sometimes an additional 1 ml is added to the solution to facilitate absorption.

ingesta (in'jestə) material taken into the body by mouth.

ingestant (in'jestənt) a substance that is or may be taken into the body by mouth or through the digestive system.

ingestion (in'jeschən) the taking of food, drugs, etc., into the body by mouth.

ingravescent (ˌingrə'ves'nt) gradually becoming more severe.

ingrowing nail ('inˌgrohing) aberrant growth of a toenail, with one or both lateral margins pushing deeply into adjacent soft tissue, causing pain, inflammation, and possible infection. The condition occurs most frequently in the great toe, and is often caused by pressure from tight-fitting shoes. Another common cause is improper cutting of the toenails, which should be cut straight across or with a curved toenail scissors so that the sides are a little longer than the middle.

inguen ('ing·gwən) pl. *inguina* [L.] the groin.

inguinal ('ing·gwin'l) pertaining to the groin. **i. canal** the oblique passage in the lower anterior abdominal wall, through which passes the round ligament of the uterus in the female, and the spermatic cord in the male.

i. hernia hernia occurring in the groin; protrusion of intestine or omentum, or both, either directly through a weak point in the abdominal wall (direct inguinal hernia) or downward into the inguinal canal (indirect inguinal hernia). See also inguinal HERNIA.

inhalant (in'haylənt) a substance that is or may be taken into the body by way of the nose and trachea (through the respiratory system).

inhalation (ˌinhə'layshən) 1. the drawing of air or other substances into the lungs. 2. any drug or solution of drugs administered (as by means of nebulizers or aerosols) by the nasal or oral respiratory route.

inhaler (in'haylə) an apparatus for administering vaporized or volatilized agents by inhalation, or for protecting the lungs from harmful substances in the air.

inherent (in'hiə·rənt, -'her-) pertaining to a characteristic that is innate or natural and essentially a part of the person.

inheritance (in'heritəns) 1. the acquisition of characters or qualities by transmission from parent to offspring. 2. that which is transmitted from parent to offspring. See also GENE, DEOXYRIBONUCLEIC ACID, and HEREDITY.

intermediate i. inheritance in which the phenotype of the heterozygote falls between that of either homozygote.

maternal i. the transmission of characters that are dependent on peculiarities of the egg cytoplasm produced, in turn, by nuclear genes.

inhibition (ˌinhi'bishən) arrest or restraint of a process; in psychiatry, the unconscious restraining of an instinctual drive. adj. **inhibitory**.

competitive i. inhibition of enzyme activity by an inhibitor (a substrate analogue) that competes with the substrate for binding sites on the enzymes.

contact i. inhibition of cell division and cell motility in normal animal cells when in close contact with each other.

noncompetitive i. inhibition of enzyme activity by substances that combine with the enzyme at a site other than that utilized by the substrate.

inhibitor (in'hibitə) 1. any substance that interferes with a chemical reaction, growth, or other biological activity. 2. a chemical substance that inhibits or checks the action of a tissue organizer or the growth of microorganisms. 3. an effector that reduces the catalytic activity of an enzyme.

inion ('ini·ən) the external occipital protuberance. adj. **inial.**

iniopagus (ˌini'opəgəs) a twin fetus or infant joined at the occiput.

initis (i'nietis) inflammation of the substance of a muscle.

injected (in'jektid) 1. introduced by injection. 2. congested.

injection (in'jekshən) 1. the forcing of a liquid into a part, as into the subcutaneous tissues, the vascular tree, or an organ. 2. a substance so forced or administered; in pharmacy, a solution of a medicament suitable for injection. 3. prominence of small blood vessels on the surface of an organ or tissue, frequently indicating the vascular phase of an inflammatory response.

Immunizing substances, or inoculations, are generally given by injection. When a patient is unconscious, injection may be the only means of administering medication, and in some cases nourishment. Some medicines cannot be given by mouth because chemical action of the digestive juices would change or reduce their effectiveness, or because they would be removed from the body too quickly to have any effect. Certain potent medicines must be injected because they would irritate body tissues if administered any other way. Occasionally a medication is injected so that it will act more quickly.

In addition to the most common types of injections described below, injections are sometimes made into arteries, bone marrow, the spine, the sternum, the pleural space of the chest region, the peritoneal cavity, and joint spaces. In sudden heart failure, heart-stimulating drugs may be injected directly into the heart (intracardiac injection).

hypodermic i. subcutaneous injection.

intracutaneous i., intradermal i. injection of small amounts of material into the corium or substance of the skin. This method is used in diagnostic procedures and in administration of regional anaesthetics, as well

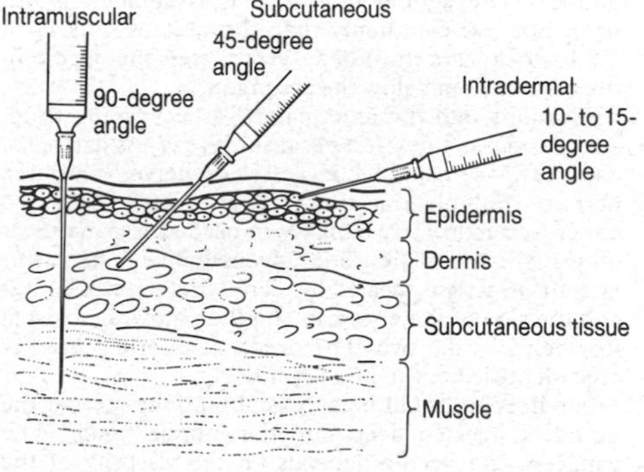

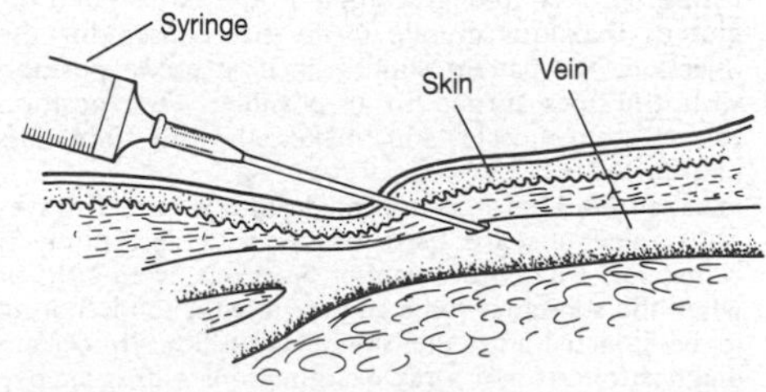

Intramuscular, subcutaneous, intradermal and intravenous injections.

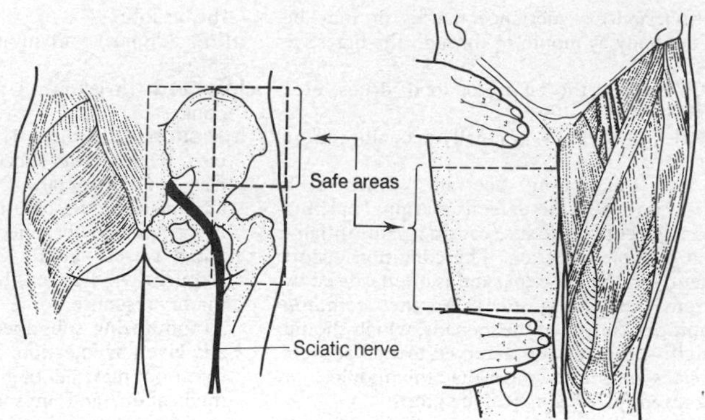

Safe sites for intramuscular injection

as in treatment procedures. In certain allergy tests, the allergen is injected intracutaneously. These injections are given in an area where the skin and hair are sparse, usually on the inner part of the forearm. A 25-gauge needle, 1 to 1.25 cm long, is recommended. The needle is inserted at a 10- to 15-degree angle to the skin.

intramuscular i. injection into the substance of a muscle, usually the muscle of the upper arm, thigh, or buttock. Intramuscular injections are given when the substance is to be absorbed quickly. They should be given with extreme care, especially in the buttock, because the sciatic nerve may be injured or a large blood vessel may be entered if the injection is not made correctly into the upper, outer quadrant of the buttock. The deltoid muscle at the shoulder is also used, but less commonly than the gluteus muscle of the buttock; care must be taken to insert the needle in the centre, 2 cm below the acromion.

Injections into the anterolateral aspect of the thigh are considered the safest because there is less danger of damage to a major blood vessel or nerve. The area permits multiple injections, is more accessible, and easier to stabilize, particularly in paediatric patients or others who are restless and uncooperative. The vastus lateralis muscle is located by identifying the trochanter and the side of the knee cap and then drawing a visual line between the two. The needle is inserted into the area identified as the middle third.

The needle should be at least 4 cm long so that the liquid is injected deep into the muscle tissue. The gauge of the needle depends on the viscosity of the fluid being injected. As a general rule, not more than 5 ml is given in an intramuscular injection. The needle is inserted at a 90-degree angle to the skin. When the gluteus maximus muscle is the site chosen for the injection, the patient should be in a prone position with the toes turned in if possible. This position relaxes the muscle and makes the injection less painful.

intravenous i. an injection made into a vein. Intravenous injections are used when rapid absorption is called for, when fluid cannot be taken by mouth, or when the substance to be administered is too irritating to be injected into the skin or muscles. In certain diagnostic tests and x-ray examinations a drug or dye may be administered intravenously. Blood transfusions also are given by this route. See also INTRAVENOUS INFUSION.

subcutaneous i. injection made into the subcutaneous tissues; called also hypodermic injection. Although usually fluid medications are injected, occasionally solid materials, such as steroid hormones, are administered subcutaneously in small, slowly absorbed pellets to prolong their effect. Subcutaneous injections may be given wherever there is subcutaneous tissue, usually in the upper, outer arm or thigh. A 25-gauge needle 2 cm long is usually used, and the amount injected should not exceed 2 ml. The needle is held at a 45-degree angle to the skin.

injury ('injə·ree) harm or hurt; a wound or maim; usually applied to damage inflicted on the body by an external force.

non-accidental i. the non-accidental, or deliberate, use of physical force or non-accidental class of omission. Usually applied to child abuse.

inlay ('in,lay) material laid into a defect in tissue; in dentistry, a filling made outside the tooth to correspond with the cavity form and then cemented into the cavity.

inlet ('in,let) a means or route of entrance. **pelvic i.** the upper limit of the pelvic cavity.

INN International Nonproprietary Names, the designations recommended by the World Health Organization for pharmaceuticals.

innate (i'nayt) inborn; hereditary; congenital.

innervation (,inə'vayshən) 1. the distribution or supply of nerves to a part. 2. the supply of nervous energy or of nerve stimulation sent to a part.

innidiation (i,nidi'ayshən) development of cells in a part to which they have been carried by metastasis.

innocent ('inəsənt) not malignant; benign.

innocuous (i'nokyooəs) harmless.

innominate (i'nominət) nameless.

i. artery brachiocephalic trunk, the first branch of the arch of the aorta.

i. bone the HIP bone.

i. veins the brachiocephalic veins, which unite to form the superior vena cava.

Innovace ('inəvays) trademark for a preparation of enalapril, an angiotensin-converting enzyme inhibitor used in hypertension and congestive heart failure.

inochondritis (,inohkon'drietis) inflammation of a fibrocartilage.

inoculability (i,nokyuhlə'bilitee) the state of being inoculable.

inoculable (i'nokyuhləb'l) 1. susceptible of being inoculated; transmissible by inoculation. 2. not immune against a transmissible disease.

inoculation (i,nokyuh'layshən) introduction of pathogenic microorganisms, injected material, serum, or other substances into tissues of living organisms or into culture media; introduction of a disease agent (usually a live infectious agent) into a healthy individual to produce a mild form of the disease, followed by IMMUNITY.

inoculum (i'nokyuhləm) material used in inoculation.

inogenous (i'nojənəs) produced from or forming tissue.

inoperable (in'opə·rəb'l) not susceptible to treatment by surgery.

inorganic (,inaw'ganik) 1. having no organs. 2. not of organic origin.

i. chemistry that branch of chemistry which deals with inorganic compounds, those not containing carbon and also carbides, oxides of carbon, and carbonates.

inosaemia (,inoh'seemi·ə) 1. the presence of inositol in the blood. 2. an excess of fibrin in the blood.

inoscopy (i'noskəpee) the diagnosis of disease by artificial digestion and examination of the fibres or fibrinous matter of the sputum, blood, effusions, etc. Called also fibrinoscopy.

inosine ('inoh,seen) a purine nucleoside containing the base hypoxanthine and the sugar ribose, which occurs in transfer RNAs.

i. monophosphate (IMP) a nucleotide produced by the deamination of adenosine monophosphate (AMP) in the metabolism of purine nucleotides.

inosinic acid (,inoh'sinik) a mononucleotide constituent of muscle, made up of hypoxanthine, ribose, and phosphoric acid.

inositol (i'nohsi,tol) a cyclic sugar alcohol, $C_6H_{12}O_6$; usually referring to the most abundant isomer, *myo*-inositol, which is found in many plant and animal tissues.

inosituria (i,nohsi'tyooə·ri·ə) the presence of inositol in the urine.

inotropic (,ienə'trohpik, -tropik) affecting the force of muscular contractions.

inquest ('inkwest) a legal inquiry before a coroner or medical examiner, and sometimes a jury, into the manner of death.

INR Index of Nursing Research.

insalubrious (,insə'loobri·əs) injurious to health.

insanity (in'sanətee) a legal term for mental illness, roughly equivalent to PSYCHOSIS and implying inability to be responsible for one's acts. adj. **insane**.

inscriptio (in'skripshi·oh) pl. *inscriptiones* [L.] inscription; a mark or line.

i. tendinea intersectio tendinea.

insect ('insekt) any individual of the class Insecta.

i. bites and stings injuries caused by the mouth parts and venom of insects and of certain related creatures, known as arachnids—spiders, scorpions, ticks—but popularly classified with insects. Bites and stings can be the cause of much discomfort. Usually there is no real danger, although a local infection can develop from scratching. Some insects, however, establish themselves on the skin as parasites, others inject poison, and still others transmit disease. A knowledge of first-aid measures for bites and stings can do much to relieve discomfort, to prevent infection and, in some cases, even to save a life. See also BEE STINGS.

First Aid Treatment for Insect Bites:

(1) Clean with soap and water.

(2) Apply a cold compress to reduce oedema and relieve itching.

(3) Apply calamine lotion.

(4) Avoid scratching the bite, which can lead to secondary infection.

Insecta (in'sektə) a class of arthropods whose members are characterized by division of the body into three distinct regions: head, thorax, and abdomen.

insecticide (in'sekti,sied) an agent that kills insects. adj. **insecticidal**.

insemination (in,semi'nayshən) the deposit of seminal fluid within the vagina or cervix.

artificial i. that done by artificial means.

insensible (in'sensəb'l) 1. devoid of sensibility or consciousness. 2. not perceptible to the senses.

insertion (in'sərshən, -'zər-) 1. the act of implanting, or condition of being implanted. 2. the site of attachment, as of a muscle to the bone that it moves.

velamentous i. attachment of the umbilical cord to the fetal membranes.

insidious (in'sidi·əs) coming on stealthily; of gradual and subtle development.

insight ('in,siet) self-understanding; in psychiatry, referring to the extent to which the patient is aware of his illness and understands its nature.

insolation (,insoh'layshən) exposure to sun's rays.

insoluble (in'solyuhb'l) not susceptible of being dissolved.

insomnia (in'somni·ə) abnormal wakefulness; an inability to fall asleep easily or to remain asleep throughout the night. The frequency of persistent insomnia is high.

The causes of insomnia may be physical or psychological or, most often, a combination of both. Some persons are more sensitive to conditions around them than others, and may be kept awake by slight noises, light, or sharing their bed. Beverages that contain caffeine, such as coffee, tea, and cola drinks, keep some people awake. A heavy meal shortly before bedtime may prevent sleep. Drinking large quantities of fluids may cause an uncomfortable feeling of distention of the bladder.

The type of bedding may be a cause of insomnia. Changing to a firmer or softer mattress, doing without a pillow, or making other changes in the bedding may help. Those who are bothered by the weight of blankets may sleep better under lightweight blankets, or with a device that supports the bedclothes at the foot of the bed.

Elderly persons are particularly prone to sleep disturbances because of chronic sleep-induced respiratory problems and nocturnal myoclonus which causes painful cramping of the legs. Others who suffer from insomnia are often experiencing some disturbing or traumatic event in their lives, such as personal problems arising from financial loss or the death of a family member. Frequently, the insomnia persists long after the traumatic event has passed, and the condition becomes chronic and self-perpetuating as the person becomes more anxious and worried about not being able to sleep.

Initial (early) insomnia refers to insomnia characterized by difficulty in falling asleep.

Early morning waking occurs in depressive disorders and the term refers to a type of insomnia where the patient falls asleep without much difficulty but awakens in the early hours of the morning and is thereafter unable to get back to sleep.

Most experts agree that sleeping pills do not help and may add dependence and addiction to the problems of the insomniac. In recent years behavioural techniques have been used with some measure of success. The patient is urged to try to avoid focusing his or her thoughts on the problem of insomnia, and to learn and practise relaxation techniques. Another form of behaviour therapy 'deconditions' the patient, breaking old nonproductive habits that reinforce sleeplessness and substituting more effective ones that assure an adequate night's sleep.

insomniac (in'somni,ak) a person suffering from insomnia.

insonate (in'sohnayt) to expose to ultrasound waves.

insorption (in'sawpshən, -'zaw-) movement of a substance into the blood, especially from the gastrointestinal tract into the circulating blood.

inspection (in'spekshən) visual examination for detection of features or qualities perceptible to the eye.

inspirate ('inspi,rayt) the air inhaled at a single inspiration.

inspiration (,inspi'rayshən) the drawing of air into the lungs. adj. **inspiratory**.

inspissated (in'spisaytid) being thickened, dried, or made less fluid by evaporation.

instep ('in,step) the dorsal part of the arch of the foot.

instillation (,insti'layshən) administration of a liquid drop by drop.

instinct ('instingkt) a complex of unlearned responses characteristic of a species. adj. **instinctive**.

death i. in psychoanalysis, the latent instinctive impulse toward death; the drive to reduce tensions by reaching the ultimate tensionless state of death.

herd i. the instinct or urge to be one of a group and to conform to its standards of conduct and opinion.

sex i. in psychoanalysis a generic term to cover the impetus generating pleasure seeking behaviour—now rarely used.

instrumentarium (,instrəmen'tair·ri·əm) the equipment or instruments required for any particular operation or purpose; the physical adjuncts with which a doctor combats disease.

instrumentation (,instrəmen'tayshən) 1. the use of an instrument; an operation. 2. the provision and selection of instruments in preparation for operation or other medical procedures.

insudation (,insyuh'dayshən) 1. the accumulation, as in the kidney, of a substance derived from the blood. 2. the substance so accumulated.

insufficiency (,insə'fishənsee) inability to perform properly an allotted function.

adrenal i. hypoadrenalism.

aortic i. inadequacy of the aortic valve, permitting blood to flow back into the left ventricle of the heart.

cardiac i. inability of the heart to perform its function properly; heart failure.

coronary i. decrease in flow of blood through the coronary blood vessels.

ileocaecal i. inability of the ileocaecal valve to prevent backflow of contents from the caecum into the ileum.

pulmonary i. insufficiency of the pulmonary valve, permitting blood to flow into the right ventricle of the heart.

respiratory i. a condition in which respiratory function is inadequate to meet the body's needs when increased physical activity places extra demands on it (see also RESPIRATORY INSUFFICIENCY).

thyroid i. hypothyroidism.

valvular i. failure of a cardiac valve to close perfectly, causing the blood to flow back through the orifice (valvular regurgitation); named, according to the valve affected, aortic, mitral, pulmonary, or tricuspid insufficiency.

velopharyngeal i. failure of velopharyngeal closure due to cleft palate, muscular dysfunction, etc., resulting in defective speech.

venous i. inadequacy of the venous valves with impairment of venous drainage, resulting in oedema.

insufflation (,insu'flayshən) 1. the blowing of a powder, vapour, or gas into a body cavity. 2. a drug administered by this method, especially a powder or aerosol carried into the respiratory passages.

perirenal i. injection of air around the kidney for x-ray examination of the adrenal glands.

tubal i. insufflation of carbon dioxide gas through the uterus into the uterine tubes as a test of their patency. Called also Rubin's test.

insufflator ('insu,flaytə) an instrument used in insufflation.

insula ('insyuhlə) pl. *insulae* [L.] a triangular area of the cerebral cortex that forms the floor of the lateral cerebral fossa; called also island of Reil.

insular ('insyuhlə) pertaining to the insula or to an island.

insulation (,insyuh'layshən) 1. the surrounding of a space or body with material designed to prevent the entrance or escape of radiant energy. 2. the material so used.

insulin ('insyuhlin) a double-chain protein hormone formed from proinsulin in the beta cells of the pancreatic islets of Langerhans. The major fuel-regulating hormone, it is secreted into the blood in response to a rise in concentration of blood glucose or amino acids. Insulin promotes the storage of glucose and the uptake of amino acids, increases protein and lipid synthesis, and inhibits lipolysis and gluconeogenesis.

The secretion of endogenous insulin is a response of the beta cells to a stimulus. The primary stimulus is glucose; others are amino acids and the 'gut hormones', such as secretin, pancreozymin, and gastrin. These chemicals play an important role in maintaining normal blood glucose levels by triggering the release of insulin after ingestion of a meal.

When insulin is released from the beta cells it enters the bloodstream and is transported first to cells of the liver and then to cells throughout the body. The cell membranes possess insulin receptors to which the insulin becomes bonded or 'fixed'. An interaction between the insulin and its receptors leads to biochemical processes that include: (1) the transport of glucose, amino acids, and certain ions across the membrane and into the cell body; (2) the storage of glycogen in liver and muscle cells; (3) the synthesis of triglycerides and storage of fat; and (4) the synthesis of protein, RNA, and DNA. Although insulin increases the transport of glucose across the cell membrane of most cells, in the brain glucose enters the cells by simple diffusion through the blood–brain barrier.

TYPES OF EXOGENOUS INSULIN. Commercially prepared insulin is available in various types which are absorbed at different rates and therefore differ in the speed with which they act and in the duration of their effectiveness. There are three main groups: rapid acting, intermediate acting, and long acting. (See accompanying table.) Diabetic patients react differently in the rate at which they absorb and utilize exogenous insulin; therefore, the duration of action varies from patient to patient. Moreover, the site of injection and the condition of the tissues into which the insulin is injected can alter its rate of absorption and peak action times.

STRENGTHS OF EXOGENOUS INSULIN. Insulin is measured in units and was available in various strengths; for example, 40 units per ml (U40), 80 units per ml (U80), and 100 units per ml (U100). The concentration used now is U100. This strength allows for more accurate measurement of dosage and reduces the possibility of error in calculating an individual dose. *When measuring the drug in an insulin syringe, one must be careful to use the calibrations on the syringe that correspond with the strength of the insulin being measured.* If the insulin bottle is labelled U100, then the calibrations on the

Examples of commonly used insulins

Category	Preparations	Molecular species	Onset (hours)	Peak (hours)	Duration (hours)
Short acting	Actrapid	Pork	0.5	2–5	8–10
	Human Actrapid	Human	0.5	2–5	8–10
	Humulin S	Human	0.5	2–5	8–10
	Velosulin	Pork	0.5	2–5	8–10
	Human Velosulin	Human	0.5	2–5	8–10
	Semitard M C	Pork	1	3–8	12–14
Intermediate	Humulin I	Human	1	4–10	16–24
	Insulatard	Pork	1	4–10	16–24
	Human Insulatard	Human	1	4–10	16–24
	Monotard M C	Pork	1	4–10	16–24
	Human Monotard	Human	2	6–16	24
	Humulin Zinc	Human	2	6–16	24
Long acting	Ultratard M C	Beef	4	8–30	36
Mixture of short and intermediate acting insulins	Initard 50/50	Pork	0.5	3–8	16–24
	Human Initard 50/50	Human	0.5	3–8	16–24
	Mixtard 30/70	Pork	0.5	3–8	16–24
	Human Mixtard 30/70	Human	0.5	3–8	18–24
	Rapitard M C	Pork and beef	1	3–15	20
	Lentard M C	Pork and beef	3	8–18	24

Time course of action of insulin may vary in different patients, at various times of the day and according to molecular species of the insulin. Human insulins can have a more rapid onset than pork or beef.
From Shuldham, C. (1985) Diabetic ketoacidosis—an endocrine emergency. *Nursing*, Vol. 2, Series 2, p. 1248.

syringe must be for U100 insulin.

PROBLEMS OF INSULIN THERAPY. The problem of either too much or too little insulin is always a potential hazard for the person on insulin therapy. The causes, symptoms, and treatment of hypoglycaemic or insulin reaction and hyperglycaemia are discussed under DIABETES MELLITUS.

Other problems of insulin therapy include insulin allergy, insulin resistance, insulin rebound due to the SOMOGYI EFFECT, and lipodystrophies or localized tissue changes at injection sites.

Insulin allergy is usually due to hypersensitivity to the protein components of insulin. The newer insulins on the market are purer than the older products and, therefore, less likely to cause an allergic reaction and other complications. There are three main types of insulin available commercially: bovine, porcine, or human. The bovine or porcine insulins are excreted from the pancreas of cattle and pigs. Human insulin is made biosynthetically by recombinant DNA technology using *Escherichia coli* or semisynthetically by enzymatic modification of porcine insulin. In theory human insulin should be less immunogenic, but this has not been proven in trials.

The exact cause of *insulin resistance* is not known, but it is suspected that patients with this problem have either circulating anti-insulin antibodies in their blood or they produce specific insulin antagonists that are destructive to insulin. Patients who have insulin resistance require more than 100 units daily. Some may need as much as 500 or 1000 units daily.

Insulin rebound is characterized by extreme fluctuations in blood sugar levels owing to overreaction of the body's homeostatic feedback mechanisms for control of glucose metabolism. When exogenous insulin is given, the hypoglycaemia triggers an outpouring of glucagon and adrenaline, both of which raise the blood sugar concentration markedly. Although the patient may actually have periods of hypoglycaemia, his urine may be loaded with sugar and blood tests will show hyperglycaemia. Treatment is aimed at modifying the extremes by gradually lowering the insulin dosage so as to reduce stimulation of the feedback system of glucose regulation. The patient may need to take smaller doses of insulin or take it at more frequent intervals and at different times during the day.

Lipodystrophies are localized manifestations of disordered fat metabolism at the sites of insulin injection. Tissue *hypertrophy* can be seen as a mass of fibrous scar tissue and is sometimes called 'insulin tumour'. *Atrophy* of the tissues at the injection site appears as dimpling and pitting of the skin and underlying tissues. These problems are more common in adult females and in children. Atrophy of the tissues is a relatively harmless nuisance but hypertrophy can cause malabsorption of the insulin and a possible misdiagnosis of insulin resistance.

Some measures that can help prevent lipodystrophies are: (1) systematic rotation of injection sites; (2) warming insulin to room temperature before injection; and (3) pinching the skin when injecting the insulin so that it is deposited between fat and muscle tissue.

i. pump a device consisting of a syringe filled with a predetermined amount of short-acting insulin, a plastic cannula and a needle, and a pump that periodically delivers the desired amount of insulin.

insulin sensitivity test a test used to determine the body's response to hypoglycaemia induced by a small intravenous dose of insulin. It is used to test anterior pituitary function, particularly the ability to secrete growth hormone.

insulinaemia (ˌinsyuhli'neemi·ə) the presence of insulin in the blood.

insulinase ('insyuhliˌnayz) an enzymatic activity in body tissues that destroys or inactivates insulin; this effect is probably due to several nonspecific proteases.

insulinogenesis (ˌinsyuhlinoh'jenəsis) the formation and release of insulin by the islets of Langerhans.

insulinogenic (ˌinsyuhlinoh'jenik) relating to insulinogenesis.
insulinoma (ˌinsyuhli'nohmə) a tumour of the beta cells of the islets of Langerhans; although usually benign, it is one of the chief causes of organic hypoglycaemia.
insulitis (ˌinsyuh'lietis) cellular infiltration of the islands of Langerhans, possibly in response to invasion by an infectious agent.
insuloma (ˌinsyuh'lohmə) insulinoma.
insulopenic (ˌinsyuhloh'peenik) diminishing, or pertaining to a decrease in, the level of circulating insulin.
insusceptibility (ˌinsəˌseptə'bilitee) the state of being unaffected or uninfluenced; immunity.
intake ('intayk) the substances, or the quantities thereof, taken in and utilized by the body. The record of liquid intake and output is called the FLUID BALANCE record.
Intal ('intal) trademark for preparations of sodium cromoglycate.
integration (ˌinti'grayshən) 1. assimilation; anabolic action or activity. 2. the combining of different acts so that they cooperate toward a common end; coordination. 3. assimilation into the personality, as of knowledge and experience, as reflected in distinctive behaviour patterns. 4. in bacterial genetics, assimilation of genetic material from one bacterium (donor) into the chromosome of another (recipient).

primary i. the recognition by a child that his or her body is a unit apart from the environment; it is probably not achieved before the second half of the first year of life.

secondary i. the sublimation of the separate elements of the early sexual instinct into the mature psychosexual personality.

integument (in'tegyuhmənt) a covering or investment; the skin.
integumentary (inˌtegyuh'mentə·ree) 1. pertaining to or composed of skin. 2. serving as a covering.
integumentum (inˌtegyuh'mentəm) [L.] *integument*.
intellect ('intə'lekt) the mind, thinking faculty, or understanding.
intellectualization (ˌintəˌlektyooəlie'zayshən) the mental process in which reasoning is used as a defence against confronting unconscious conflict and its stressful emotions.
intelligence (in'telijəns) the ability to comprehend or understand. It is basically a combination of reasoning, memory, imagination, and judgement. Each of these faculties relies upon the others.

The brain may store up many memories, but they are useful only when brought to surface consciousness at the right time and in the right connection. Imagination is the faculty of associating several memories—they may be of facts, images, or sensations—to produce another fact or image. In general, the more efficiently the brain combines memories in an orderly fashion, the greater the intelligence. Imagination, however, must be governed by reason and judgement. Reason is the ability to draw logical conclusions by relating memories and observations. Judgement relies on experience to choose between different forms of reasoning. All these factors are controlled by the cerebral cortex (see also BRAIN).

In speaking of general intelligence, authorities often distinguish between a number of different kinds of basic mental ability. One of these is verbal aptitude, the ability to understand the meaning of words and to use them effectively in writing or speaking. Another is skill with numbers, the ability to add, subtract, multiply, and divide and to use these skills in problems. The capacity to work with spatial relationships, that is, with visualizing how objects take up space, is still another (for example, how two triangles can fit together to make a square). Perception, memory, and reasoning may also be considered different basic abilities. Often a person is more proficient in some of these areas than he is in others. Commonly, for example, a child may excel in using words but have some difficulty with arithmetic, or the opposite may be true.

Schoolgirls often achieve verbal skills more quickly than boys, while boys are often more skilful in spatial relations and number work. As a person grows older and as his interests and need develop and change, his aptitudes may change as well.

These abilities are the ones that are usually examined by intelligence tests. There are others, however, that may be as important or more important. Determination and perseverance make intelligence effective and useful. Artistic talent, such as proficiency in art or music, and creativity, the ability to use thought and imagination to produce original ideas, are difficult to measure but are certainly part of intelligence.

i. quotient (IQ) a numerical expression of intellectual capacity obtained by multiplying the mental age of the subject, ascertained by testing, by 100 and dividing by his chronological age.

intensimeter (ˌinten'simitə) a device for measuring intensity of x-rays.
intensionometer (inˌtensi·ə'nomitə) an ionometric instrument for measuring the intensity of x-rays. Two series of plates, separated by an air gap that serves as the dielectric, are connected to opposite terminals in a closed chamber. An electric circuit is completed when the air becomes ionized by the x-rays, and the difference in electric potential is registered by deflection of a galvanometer needle.
intensive care unit (in'tensiv) a hospital unit in which is concentrated special equipment and specially trained personnel for the care of seriously ill patients requiring immediate and continuous monitoring and treatment. Abbreviated ICU. Called also *critical care unit (CCU)*, *intensive therapy unit*.
intensive therapy unit see INTENSIVE CARE UNIT.
intention (in'tenshən) a manner of HEALING.
inter- word element. [L.] *between*.
interaction (ˌintə'rakshən) the quality, state, or process of (two or more things) acting on each other.

drug i. the action of one drug upon the effectiveness or toxicity of another (or others).

interarticular (ˌintə·rah'tikyuhlə) between articulating surfaces.
interatrial (ˌintə'raytri·əl, -'ratri·əl) between the atria of the heart.
interbrain ('intəˌbrayn) 1. thalamencephalon. 2. diencephalon.
intercalary (in'tərkələ·ree) inserted between; interposed.
intercalated (in'tərkəˌlaytid) inserted between.
intercartilaginous (ˌintəˌkahti'lajinəs) between, or connecting, cartilages.
intercellular (ˌintə'selyuhlə) between the cells.
interchondral (ˌintə'kondrəl) intercartilaginous.
intercilium (ˌintə'sili·əm) the space between the eyebrows.
interclavicular (ˌintəklə'vikyuhlə) between the clavicles.
intercondylar (ˌintə'kondilə) between two condyles.
intercostal (ˌintə'kost'l) between two ribs.
intercourse ('intəˌkaws) mutual exchange.

sexual i. coitus.

intercricothyrotomy (ˌintəˌkriekohthie'rotəmee) incision of the larynx through the lower part of the fibroelastic membrane of the larynx (cricothyroid membrane); inferior laryngotomy.

intercritical (ˌintə'kritik'l) denoting the period between attacks, as of gout.

intercurrent (ˌintə'kurənt) occurring during the course of, as a disease occurring during the course of an already existing disease.

interdigital (ˌintə'dijit'l) between two digits (fingers or toes).

interdigitation (ˌintəˌdiji'tayshən) 1. an interlocking of parts by finger-like processes. 2. one of a set of finger-like processes.

interface ('intəˌfays) in chemistry, the boundary between two systems or phases.

interfascicular (ˌintəfə'sikyuhlə) between adjacent fascicles.

interfemoral (ˌintə'femə·rəl) between the thighs.

interferon (ˌintə'fiə·ron) a natural glycoprotein released by cells invaded by viruses. Interferon is not itself an antiviral agent but rather acts as a stimulant to noninfected cells causing them to synthesize another protein with antiviral characteristics, probably by initiating DNA-directed RNA synthesis and, thus, protein synthesis.

The natural production of interferon is not restricted to viral infections; it can be released in response to a wide variety of inducers, including certain nonviral and infectious agents such as rickettsiae, bacteria, and synthetic polymers.

Interferon acts as a regulator of cell growth and has a variety of effects on the immune system by either activating or suppressing selected components of the immune system. For example, interferon can activate macrophages and thereby increase phagocytosis, enhance some primary antibody responses and inhibit others, and affect the specific cytotoxicity of lymphocytes. In regard to cell growth, interferon has the ability to inhibit the proliferation of certain cells. The combined effects of interferon on cell growth and the immune response have motivated scientists to conduct experimental studies on its usefulness in the treatment of various types of cancer.

Several types of interferon have become commercially available. These are either extracted from cell cultures or made biosynthetically by recombinant DNA technology.

interfibrillar (ˌintə'fiebrilə, -'fib-) between fibrils.

interfilar (ˌintə'fielə) between or among the fibrils of a reticulum.

interictal (ˌintə'rikt'l) occurring between attacks or paroxysms.

interkinesis (ˌintəki'neesis) the period between the first and second divisions in meiosis.

interlobar (ˌintə'lohbə) between lobes.

interlobitis (ˌintəloh'bietis) inflammation of the pleura between lobes of the lung; called also interlobular pleurisy.

interlobular (ˌintə'lobyuhlə) between lobules.

intermaxillary (ˌintəmak'silə·ree) between the maxillae.

intermediate (ˌintə'meedi·ət) 1. between; intervening; resembling, in part, each of two extremes. 2. a substance formed in a chemical process that is essential to formation of the end product of the process.

intermedin (ˌintə'meedin) melanocyte-stimulating hormone.

intermedius (ˌintə'meedi·əs) [L.] *intermediate;* in anatomy, denoting a structure lying between a lateral and a medial structure.

intermeningeal (ˌintəmə'ninji·əl) between the meninges.

intermenstrual (ˌintə'menstrooəl) occurring between two menstrual periods.

intermission (ˌintə'mishən) a temporary interruption, particularly of a feverish condition.

intermittent (ˌintə'mitənt) marked by alternating periods of activity and inactivity.

i. claudication a group of symptoms characterized by pain in the calf muscles of one or both legs, brought on by walking and relieved by resting for a few minutes. It is caused by atherosclerotic lesions in the femoral artery which diminish blood supply to the muscles of the lower leg.

Treatment has traditionally involved vascular reconstructive surgery to bypass the diseased portion of the vessel. More recent modes of therapy include stopping smoking (which can produce dramatic results), reducing excess weight, and following a graduated walking and exercise programme.

i. mandatory ventilation (IMV) a type of mechanical ventilation in which the VENTILATOR is set to deliver a prescribed tidal volume at specified intervals and a high-flow gas system permits the patient to breathe spontaneously between cycles. The ventilator rate is set to maintain the patient's P_aco_2 at normal levels and is reduced gradually to zero as the patient's condition improves.

i. positive-pressure ventilation (IPPV) a form of respiratory therapy utilizing a VENTILATOR for the treatment of patients with inadequate breathing. As the name implies, the treatment involves application of pressure only during the inspiratory phase, its purpose being to assist the patient to breathe more deeply. Among the types of ventilators used in IPPV therapy are the Bird Mark VII, the Bennett PR-2, and the RETIC automatic respirator. The RETIC is an example of the newer, more simply designed units that are generally smaller in size and are portable.

IPPV may be prescribed for a patient who is unable to cough effectively (as during the postoperative period), and for one who is suffering from a chronic obstructive or restrictive airways disease and whose breathing is further impaired by either infection or trauma. IPPV is frequently used as a means of providing deep pulmonary AEROSOL therapy, in the relief of bronchospasms and in the removal of bronchial secretions.

Overenthusiastic use of IPPV at the time ventilators made their debut on the medical scene has led some to question the superiority of this treatment over such less expensive and more conservative measures as POSTURAL DRAINAGE and instruction of the patient in effective deep breathing and coughing techniques. It is now generally agreed that IPPV offers an acceptable alternative to these techniques when the patient is unable or unwilling to make the necessary effort to ventilate his lungs adequately. There remain, however, inherent risks in IPPV and no one should attempt to administer assisted ventilation without extensive knowledge and operational skill in the use of a ventilator.

intermural (ˌintə'myooə·rəl) between the walls of an organ or organs.

intermuscular (ˌintə'muskyuhlə) between muscles.

internal (in'tərn'l) situated or occurring within or on the inside; in anatomy, many structures formerly called internal are now termed medial.

internalization (inˌtərnəlie'zayshən) a mental mechanism whereby certain external attributes, attitudes, or standards are unconsciously taken as one's own.

internatal (ˌintə'nayt'l) between the nates, or buttocks.

International Council of Nurses (ˌintəˈnashənˈl) a federation of National Nurses' Associations founded in 1899 by Mrs Bedford Fenwick; abbreviated ICN. Present membership 90. Aims to: (1) promote the development of strong nurses' associations; (2) assist such associations to improve the standard of nursing education and competency; (3) assist the associations to improve the economic and social standing of nurses; and (4) serve as an international voice for nurses and nursing.

Provides professional advice to member organizations; runs a 'Nursing Abroad' programme to facilitate education and experience outside the individual's own country; provides two 3Ms Fellowships per year; produces a number of publications, including the *International Nursing Review*, which is its official journal.

ORGANIZATION. The Council of National Representatives (CNR) is the governing body and comprises Presidents of the member associations. It meets biannually to determine policy matters. Every fourth year the meeting is held in conjunction with the Quadrennial Congress.

The Board of Directors consists of the ICN President, three Vice Presidents and eleven members of the CNR elected at the time of the Quadrennial Congress. The Board meets at least once a year and has several committees.

The Board also governs the Florence Nightingale International Foundation which is an endowed Trust devoted to educational purposes.

International System of Units see SI UNITS.

interneuron (ˌintəˈnyooə·ron) a neuron between the primary afferent neuron and the final motor neuron (motoneuron). Also any neuron whose processes lie entirely within a specific area, such as the olfactory lobe.

internode (ˈintəˌnohd) a space between two nodes.

internuclear (ˌintəˈnyookli·ə) situated between nuclei or between nuclear layers of the retina.

internuncial (ˌintəˈnunshəl) transmitting impulses between two different parts.

internus (inˈtərnəs) [L.] *internal;* in anatomy, denoting a structure nearer to the centre of an organ or part.

interoceptor (ˌintə·rohˈseptə) a sensory nerve terminal located in and transmitting impulses from the viscera. adj. **interoceptive**.

interofective (ˌintə·rohˈfektiv) affecting the interior of the organism—a term applied to the autonomic nervous system.

interolivary (ˌintəˈrolivə·ree) between the olivary bodies.

interorbital (ˌintəˈrawbit'l) between the orbits.

interosseous (ˌintəˈrosi·əs) between two bones.

interpalpebral (ˌintəˈpalpibrəl) between the eyelids.

interpandemic (ˌintəpanˈdemik) denoting outbreaks of an infectious disease (e.g., influenza) occurring between major pandemics of the same disease.

interparietal (ˌintəpəˈrieət'l) 1. intermural. 2. between the parietal bones.

interparoxysmal (ˌintəˌparokˈsizməl) between paroxysms.

interphalangeal (ˌintəfəˈlanji·əl) situated between two contiguous phalanges.

interphase (ˈintəˌfayz) the interval between two successive cell divisions, during which the chromosomes are not individually distinguishable.

interplant (ˈintəˌplahnt) an embryonic part isolated by transference to an indifferent environment provided by another embryo.

interpolation (inˌtərpəˈlayshən) 1. surgical insertion or transplantation of tissue. 2. the insertion of intermediate values in a series of known values.

interpretation (inˌtərpriˈtayshən) in psychotherapy, the therapist's explanation to the patient of the latent or hidden meanings of what he says, does, or experiences.

interproximal (ˌintəˈproksiməl) between two adjoining surfaces.

interpubic (ˌintəˈpyoobik) between the pubic bones.

interpupillary (ˌintəˈpyoopilə·ree) between the pupils.

interscapular (ˌintəˈskapyuhlə) between the scapulae.

intersectio (intəˈsekshioh) pl. *intersectiones* [L.] intersection.

i. tendinea a fibrous band traversing the belly of a muscle, dividing it into two parts; called also inscriptio tendinea.

intersection (ˌintəˈsekshən) a site at which one structure crosses another.

intersex (ˈintəˌseks) 1. intersexuality. 2. an individual who exhibits intersexuality.

female i. a female pseudohermaphrodite.

male i. a male pseudohermaphrodite.

true i. a true hermaphrodite.

intersexuality (ˌintəˌseksyooˈalitee) an intermingling, in varying degrees, of the characters of each sex, including physical form, reproductive tissue, and sexual behaviour, in one individual, as a result of some flaw in embryonic development (see also HERMAPHRODITISM and PSEUDOHERMAPHRODITISM). adj. **intersexual**.

interspace (ˈintəˌspays) a space between similar structures.

interspinal (ˌintəˈspien'l) between two spinous processes.

interstice (inˈtərstis) an interval, space, or gap in a tissue or structure.

interstitial (ˌintəˈstishəl) pertaining to or situated betweeen parts or in the interspaces of a tissue.

i. cell-stimulating hormone luteinizing hormone.

i. cells the cells of the connective tissue of the ovary or the testis (Leydig's cells), which furnish the internal secretion of those structures.

i. fluid the extracellular fluid bathing most tissues, excluding the fluid within the lymph and blood vessels.

i. pneumonia a form of pneumonia characterized by a thickening of alveolar walls and septa by a chronic inflammatory infiltrate of lymphocytes, macrophages, and plasma cells. An exudate into the alveoli is scanty and any intra-alveolar infiltrate is usually of macrophages. There are many causes, particularly viruses, and many cases remain of uncertain aetiology.

i. tissue connective tissue between the cellular elements of a structure.

interstitium (ˌintəˈstishi·əm) 1. interstice. 2. interstitial tissue.

intertransverse (ˌintəˈtranzvərs, -ˈtrahnz-) situated between or connecting the transverse processes of the vertebrae.

intertrigo (ˌintəˈtriegoh) an erythematous skin eruption occurring on apposed surfaces of the skin, as the creases of the neck, folds of the groin and armpit, and beneath pendulous breasts. It is caused by moisture, warmth, friction, sweat retention, and infectious agents. Symptoms include burning, itching, moistness, redness, maceration, and sometimes erosions, fissures, and exudations. It is most likely to occur in obese persons, and particularly in those with diabetes mellitus. Intertrigo is most prevalent in hot and humid regions.

In treatment of intertrigo, the apposing body surfaces should be thoroughly cleansed and dried, and then sprinkled with talcum powder containing zinc oxide. Sometimes gauze strips between the adjacent skin surfaces will keep the area dry and exposed to air.

intertubular (,intə'tyoobyuhlə) between tubules.

interureteral, interureteric (,intəyuh'reetə·rəl; ,intə-,yooə·ri'terik) between the ureters.

intervaginal (,intəvə'jien'l) between sheaths.

interval ('intəvəl) the space between two objects or parts; the lapse of time between two events.

atrioventricular i., A-V i. P-R i.

c.-a. i., cardioarterial i. the time between the apex beat and arterial pulsation.

lucid i. a brief period of remission of symptoms in a psychosis.

postsphygmic i. the short period (0.08 seconds) of ventricular diastole, after the sphygmic period, and lasting until the atrioventricular valves open. Called also postsphygmic period.

P-R i. in electrocardiography, the time between the onset of the P wave (atrial activity) and the QRS complex (ventricular activity).

presphygmic i. the first phase of ventricular systole, being the period (0.04–0.06 seconds) immediately after closure of the atrioventricular valves and lasting until the semilunar valves open. Called also presphygmic period.

QRST i., Q-T i. the duration of ventricular electrical activity.

intervalvular (,intə'valvyuhlə) between valves.

intervascular (,intə'vaskyuhlə) between blood vessels.

intervention study (intə'venshən) an epidemiological study to test the relationship between a particular factor and disease by removing or modifying the factor.

interventricular (,intəven'trikyuhlə) between the ventricles of the heart.

intervertebral (,intə'vərtibrəl) between two vertebrae.

i. disc the layer of fibrocartilage between the bodies of adjoining vertebrae (see also slipped DISC).

intervillous (,intə'viləs) between or among villi.

intestinal (,inte'sticnəl, in'testin'l) pertaining to the intestine.

i. bypass a surgical procedure in which all but a few inches of the proximal jejunum and terminal ileum are occluded from circuit in order to correct OBESITY. Also called jejunoileal bypass or shunt. Patients having this type of surgery must be meticulously managed so that severe nutritional CIRRHOSIS and serious loss of water and electrolytes are avoided.

i. obstruction any hindrance to the passage of the intestinal contents. Causes may be mechanical or neural or both. Some of the more common mechanical causes are HERNIA, ADHESIONS of the peritoneum, volvulus, INTUSSUSCEPTION, malignant or benign tumour, congenital defect, and local inflammation. Failure of peristalsis (adynamic ileus) is usually due to PERITONITIS; it also may occur with GALLSTONES, uraemia, heavy metal poisoning, infection, and spinal injury.

SYMPTOMS. The characteristic symptoms are colicky abdominal pain, vomiting, cessation of bowel movements and flatus, and ultimately, distention. The symptoms may be mild at first and in its early stages the condition may be mistaken for less serious disorders of the intestinal tract. Under no circumstances should a patient with suspected obstruction be given a laxative or purgative because it will aggravate the situation. If the obstruction continues the patient suffers from dehydration and shock because of inadequate absorption of fluids, electrolytes, and nutrients from the intestinal tract. If the bowel is also strangulated and circulation to the bowel wall is obstructed, the patient's condition will be more acute and the abdominal pain continuous. Tenderness is extreme over the affected loop with rigidity of the abdomen and peritonitis develops.

TREATMENT. The basic steps of treatment are decompression of the intestine, replacement of fluids and electrolytes and laparotomy to relieve the obstruction.

Decompression of the gut is accomplished by passing a Ryle's tube and aspirating at regular intervals.

Fluids, sodium chloride, and glucose are administered intravenously. Transfusions of whole blood plasma may be given as necessary to restore normal blood values.

Surgical removal of the cause of obstruction is usually necessary in cases of complete obstruction. If there is no evidence of strangulation of the bowel, the surgeon may choose to postpone surgery until dehydration and shock have been overcome and a normal electrolyte balance is restored. The type of surgical procedure performed depends on the cause of the obstruction and whether or not the intestine is gangrenous. In some cases a COLOSTOMY may be necessary before the damaged portion of the bowel is removed. A surgical incision into the caecum with insertion of a drainage tube (caecostomy) may be done when decompressing the bowel is not successful in relieving distention.

PATIENT CARE. Assessment of the patient with intestinal obstruction includes noting the location and character of abdominal pain, degree of distention, character of the bowel sounds, and occurrence or absence of bowel movements or passing of flatus. Should defecation occur a specimen is saved for examination and laboratory analysis. If there is vomiting, the amount and special characteristics of the vomitus should be noted and recorded. In severe cases of obstruction of the small bowel the vomitus may contain faecal material because of the reversal of peristalsis and forcing of the intestinal contents backward into the stomach.

Foods and fluids by mouth are restricted. If a tube has been inserted it should be irrigated as necessary to keep the lumen open so that intestinal decompression by aspiration is achieved. Frequent mouth care is necessary to relieve the dryness and foul taste that accompanies intestinal obstruction and vomiting.

Urinary output is measured and recorded because there is a possibility that pressure on the bladder will produce urinary retention. In some cases catheterization may be necessary.

Preoperative Care. If conservative measures fail to relieve the obstruction, or if the bowel has become strangulated, surgery is indicated. Before the operation the surgeon may order a low enema. Aspiration and free drainage is continued and the intestinal tube is left in place when the patient goes to the operating room.

Postoperative Care. Routine postoperative care of the patient with abdominal surgery is indicated. Specific measures depend on the type of surgical procedure done. Aspiration and free drainage is usually continued until peristalsis resumes. Results of the assessment of bowel sounds and the passing of flatus or faeces should be noted as they indicate a return of normal peristaltic movements of the bowel. In some cases a caecostomy tube or rectal tube is inserted during surgery; the tube is attached to a drainage bottle and the amount and type of material collected in the bottle are recorded. If there is evidence that the tube has become obstructed the surgeon should be notified. The skin around the site of insertion of a caecostomy tube should be protected. The area must be washed frequently to avoid erosion of the skin by intestinal contents leaking around the tube.

See also COLOSTOMY for patient care after that

procedure.

i. tract the small and large intestines in continuity. The long, coiled tube of the intestine is the part of the DIGESTIVE SYSTEM where most of the digestion of food takes place.

Among the disorders of the intestinal tract are the disturbances of function, such as DIARRHOEA, CONSTIPATION, and IRRITABLE BOWEL SYNDROME; the organic diseases, ULCERATIVE COLITIS, APPENDICITIS, and ILEITIS; and communicable diseases, such as DYSENTERY. Irritable bowel syndrome is characterized by constipation, sometimes alternating with diarrhoea. Ulcerative colitis is a disorder in which ulcers may appear in the wall of the large intestine. Ileitis is a disorder of the ileum, or lower portion of the small intestine. A symptom of both is diarrhoea. Dysentery, which is characterized by diarrhoea, is the result of infection by bacteria, viruses, or various parasites.

intestine (in'testin) the part of the alimentary tract extending from the pyloric opening of the stomach to the anus. It is a membranous tube, comprising the small intestine and large intestine; called also bowel and gut (see also INTESTINAL TRACT).

intestinum (ˌinte'stienəm) pl. *intestina* [L.] intestine.

intima ('intimə) the innermost coat of a blood vessel; called also tunica intima. adj. **intimal**.

intimitis (ˌinti'mietis) endarteritis; inflammation of the innermost coat of an artery.

intolerance (in'tolə·rəns) inability to withstand or consume; inability to absorb or metabolize nutrients.

drug i. the state of reacting to the normal pharmacological doses of a drug with the symptoms of overdosage.

intorsion (in'tawshən) tilting of the upper part of the vertical meridian of the eye toward the midline of the face.

intoxication (inˌtoksi'kayshən) 1. poisoning; the state of being poisoned. 2. the condition produced by excessive use of alcohol.

Intoxication in the sense of poisoning can be caused by carbon monoxide, lead, or other toxic agents. Some medications can be poisonous in excessive doses. Intoxication can also occur in persons who have an allergy to medications such as penicillin, to various serums, and to other substances. Any type of drug addiction is medically recognized as a state of intoxication. In addition to those mentioned there are the commonly recognized types of poisoning, such as those caused by chemicals and food contaminants.

Intoxication in the sense of drunkenness is legally defined as a concentration of alcohol in the blood of 80 mg/100 ml. See also ALCOHOLISM.

intra- word element. [L.] *inside, within.*

intra vitam (ˌintrə 'vietam) [L.] *during life.*

intra-abdominal (ˌintrə·əb'domin'l) within the abdomen.

intra-aortic balloon pump (ˌintrəay'awtik) a mechanical aid to the circulatory function of the heart that acts to provide internal COUNTERPULSATION; abbreviated IABP. The basic components of the device are a catheter tipped with a 10-inch balloon and a pump machine that inflates the balloon with either helium or carbon dioxide. The balloon is inserted via a femoral artery cutdown and guided under fluoroscopic control to a position in the descending thoracic aorta just distal to the left subclavian artery. In some models, the balloon is tri-segmented. When inflation begins in a tri-segmented balloon, the middle segment is inflated first, then the distal ends inflate simultaneously; there is no occlusion of the aorta. An alternative type of balloon catheter consists of only one segment with a second small balloon just distal to the main one; the smaller balloon partially occludes the aorta only during diastole, thus providing directional flow.

The pump console contains signal processing, drive, and timing and control mechanisms for appropriate inflation and deflation. The system also contains a display and diagnostic unit.

The physiological effect of the IABP is to improve coronary blood flow and systemic circulation. It does this by: (1) augmenting aortic root pressure during ventricular diastole at the time of maximum blood flow, and (2) reducing the workload of the heart by decreasing the amount of residual blood in the aortic arch, thereby decreasing resistance to the flow of blood from the ventricle. Inflation of the balloon during diastole just after aortic valve closure, and deflation just prior to ventricular systole reduces the pressure workload of the left ventricle and lessens oxygen demand and consumption by the myocardium. Timing of the inflation–deflation cycle is based on the arterial pulse wave configuration seen on the console's display screen. Adjustments to the cycle are made according to the site of arterial wave sampling, heart rate, and the depth of diastolic dip.

Indications for employment of the IABP include cardiogenic shock or severe pump failure secondary to acute myocardial infarction or following open-heart surgery, unstable angina resistant to drug therapy, and refractory ventricular irritability after myocardial infarction. The effect of improved oxygenation of the myocardium can result in reversal of ischaemic damage resulting from infarction, and limitation of the size of the myocardial infarction.

Following insertion of the IABP catheter and initiation of the pumping action nursing care is focused on proper administration of medications, monitoring the patient's response and the function of the equipment for evidence of safe and effective pumping, observation for ischaemia of the limb in which the catheter is inserted, and observation for side-effects and complications, such as excessive bleeding from the insertion site or formation of a haematoma, wound inflammation and infection, abdominal or back pain, reduction in platelet count and haematocrit and other signs of clotting abnormalities, and thrombus formation.

Nursing care problems associated with IABP include patient anxiety involving fear of the procedure, concerns about coronary angiography and surgery, or lack of knowledge about the procedure and its purpose; the need for cardiovascular and respiratory support; physical discomfort; and patient dependency.

intra-arterial (ˌintrəah'tiə·ri·əl) within an artery.

intra-articular (ˌintrəah'tikyuhlə) within a joint.

intra-atrial (ˌintrə'aytri·əl) within the atrium.

i.-a. thrombosis a blood clot formed in the atrium of the heart.

intracanalicular (ˌintrəˌkanə'likyuhlə) within canaliculi.

intracapsular (ˌintrəˌkapsyuhlə) within a capsule.

intracardiac (ˌintrə'kahdiˌak) within the heart.

intracartilaginous (ˌintrəˌkahti'lajinəs) within a cartilage.

intracellular (ˌintrə'selyuhlə) within a cell or cells.

intracerebral (ˌintrə'seribrəl) within the brain substance.

i. haemorrhage an escape of blood in the cerebrum, most often arising from the middle cerebral artery or from an aneurysm.

intracervical (ˌintrə'sərvik'l, -sə'vie-) within the canal of the cervix uteri.

intracisternal (ˌintrəsi'stərnəl) within a subarachnoid cistern.

intracranial (ˌintrəˈkrayni·əl) within the cranium.

i. pressure (ICP) the pressure exerted by the cerebrospinal fluid within the subarachnoid space and ventricles of the brain. The normal range for intracranial pressure is between 50 and 180 mmH_2O (approximately 4 to 13 mmHg). A reading above 200 mmH_2O (about 15 mmHg) is considered abnormally high; however, intracranial pressure, like arterial blood pressure, can fluctuate markedly and quickly during certain activities. For example, a transient elevation of pressure occurs during the Valsalva manoeuvre. Straining at stool, isometric exercises, and similar activities can momentarily raise the intracranial pressure to as high as 1360 mmH_2O. While signs of sustained increased intracranial pressure can be significant in the assessment of a patient with a neurological disorder, momentary increases in intracranial pressure are not in themselves necessarily detrimental.

The level of intracranial pressure can be inferred by determining the pressure of lumbar spinal fluid during a spinal tap, but this is not the most accurate method and it can be dangerous. Removal of even a small amount of spinal fluid from a patient with a significantly high intracranial pressure can alter the pressure difference between the spinal column and the cranial cavity and cause herniation of the midbrain downward into the foramen magnum. A more accurate and continuous measurement of intracranial pressure can be obtained by monitoring pressure within the cerebral ventricles (cerebral ventricular pressure).

CAUSES OF INCREASE IN PRESSURE. The skull is a rigid container that holds the brain, blood vessels, and cerebrospinal fluid. There is room for some expansion within the skull, but not much, and any condition that causes an increase in volume in one or more of the structures within the cranium will cause an increase of pressure within the contained area. A tumour or swelling of brain tissue can increase the volume, as can extravascular leakage of blood and the formation of clots, dilation of the cerebral vessels, and excess production, impeded outflow, or insufficient absorption of cerebrospinal fluid, as in HYDROCEPHALUS.

Increased fluid volume creates pressure against the structures inside the cranium, disrupting the blood and oxygen supply, and resulting in cellular hypoxia. As the pressure increases the brain mass shifts or is distorted, causing compression of the neurons and nerve tracts or of the cerebral arteries. The effect of increased volume can be generalized, as in brain oedema from lead poisoning, or focal. Cellular hypoxia resulting from direct pressure on the brain cells, distortion of the brain mass, or occlusion of cerebral blood vessels accounts for the signs and symptoms of increased intracranial pressure. A sustained increase in the pressure causes persistent hypoxia, irreversible damage to the brain cells, and eventually death.

SIGNS AND SYMPTOMS. The four classic groups of intracranial signs of increased intracranial pressure are: (1) altered levels of consciousness; (2) changes in sensory and motor function; (3) changes in pupil size, equality, and reaction to light, and extraocular movements; and (4) changes in vital signs and patterns of respiration. However, only a few of these signs occur early in the process and usually only then at peak pressures.

Altered levels of consciousness occur as a result of compression of the ascending reticular activating system (ARAS) pathways and the resulting hypoxia of the cells of these tissues as well as the cells of the cortex. Decreased sensory input by way of the ARAS causes a decrease in wakefulness. As compression increases the patient becomes more difficult to arouse. Assessment of the patient is based on the extent to which he is oriented and able to respond to stimuli. See also levels of CONSCIOUSNESS.

Motor and sensory dysfunction are the result of pressure on the cortex and the upper motor and sensory pyramidal pathways. The motor fibres descend through the brain stem where most of them cross over (decussate) in the medulla oblongata and then extend into the spinal cord. Sensory fibres ascend from the spinal cord to the brain stem and from there to the sensory areas in the parietal lobe of the brain. These fibres also decussate in either the spinal cord or the medulla. Assessment of the patient for motor and sensory dysfunction would include an evaluation of movement and strength of the extremities and a comparison of right side to left; perception of touch, pressure, and deep pain; and the presence or absence of BABINSKI'S REFLEX.

Changes in pupil size, equality, and reaction to light, and extraocular movements are indicative of compression of the third, fourth, and sixth cranial nerves. Assessment of these changes should be as accurate and objective as possible. Unilateral and bilateral evaluations are important and usually are recorded by comparing the size of the pupil with a pupil size scale (measured in millimetres).

Vital sign changes come very late in the process of cellular hypoxia and indicate that pressure is being exerted on the lower brain stem and medulla. If not relieved, these changes quickly accelerate and death ensues. Compression of the brain stem causes a rise in the systolic blood pressure and a widening of the pulse pressure followed by a sharp drop in blood pressure. The pulse rate slows and then rises sharply owing to blocking of the parasympathetic impulses. As pressure on the respiratory centre builds up there are changes in the rate, rhythm, and ratio of inspiration to expiration, and periods of apnoea.

Earlier in the process, more subtle changes in the neurological status of the patient can be detected by an experienced practitioner and are extremely important for prompt intervention and correction of the problem before irreversible damage is done. Signs and symptoms frequently noted early in the process and at peak pressure include increased restlessness, mental dullness, disorganized and unfocused behaviour, such as plucking at the bedclothes, and increasingly severe headache. Another significant event is a *transient* worsening of the neurological status as indicated by changes in the four classic signs and symptoms. These transient changes reflect a situation in which a critical volume of intracranial contents has been reached; small increases beyond that point are likely to lead to rapid and sustained increases in pressure. This situation demands immediate intervention for relief of compression on vital neuronal structures.

PATIENT CARE. In addition to a thorough understanding of the pathophysiological changes brought on by increased intracranial pressure and the signs and symptoms they produce, health professionals should be aware of factors that can precipitate increases in intracranial pressure. It is known, for example, that hypercapnia, profound hypoxia, and certain anaesthetics can cause vasodilation of cerebral vessels and an increase in intracranial pressure. Patients who are known to be at risk for increases in pressure should not be given vasodilating drugs whenever such therapy can be avoided. The blood gases and chest sounds of these patients should be monitored periodically to determine whether there is adequate ventilation and oxygenation. Maintenance of a patent airway and adequate oxygenation by means of oxygen therapy, if necessary, are essential to the prevention of an escalating intracranial pressure.

Other protective measures for patients at risk for sudden increases in intracranial pressure include careful positioning to avoid flexion of the neck, extreme flexion of the hip, and the prone position. Elevating the head 15 to 30 degrees decreases baseline pressure. The patient also should avoid the VALSALVA MANOEUVRE when moving about in bed and when defecating. Isometric exercises to avoid the hazards of immobility are contraindicated but passive range-of-motion exercises are not.

i. pressure monitoring continuous monitoring of pressure within the skull. The three basic techniques for intracranial monitoring are intraventricular, subarachnoid (subdural), and extradural. Ventricular-fluid pressures are recorded from a zero baseline; the normal range is 0 to 15 mmHg. Pressures are usually expressed in mmHg rather than mmH_2O in order to facilitate comparison with mean systemic arterial pressures. The difference between mean ventricular pressure and mean arterial pressure indicates the pressure at which the brain is being perfused with blood (cerebral perfusion pressure).

ICP monitoring gives a far more accurate picture of forces at work within the closed cranial cavity than does clinical observation of the patient for signs of increased INTERCRANIAL PRESSURE. Most authorities agree that dangerously high levels of intracranial pressure exist well before clinical symptoms become evident. Invasive ICP monitoring also provides access for cerebrospinal fluid drainage to relieve pressure, for procurement of samples of cerebrospinal fluid for laboratory evaluations, and for observation of volume–pressure responses to therapeutic intervention.

To obtain a reading, an intraventricular catheter is inserted into the nondominant lateral ventricle or a bolt or screw is inserted, via a burr hole in the frontal area, with its tip lying in the subarachnoid space. A third option is the insertion of an implantable subdural pressure transducer. Whichever of the first two methods is used, each is then connected via fluid-filled tubing to a transducer, which in turn is connected to a paper recorder or oscilloscope. Readings or changes in intracranial pressure can thus be obtained by observing the oscilloscope screen or graph display. Through the use of intracranial pressure monitoring, elevations in intracranial pressure can be detected before changes in the vital signs and other symptoms of increased pressure become apparent. In this way measures can be taken to reduce the pressure before irreversible damage is done to the brain tissue.

Risks associated with intracranial pressure monitoring vary with the type of equipment used. The intraventricular and subarachnoid bolt method carry the risk of infection and the possibility of disconnection and subsequent leakage of cerebrospinal fluid. The intraventricular method also carries the very rare risk of catheter tract haemorrhage.

intractable (in'traktəb'l) not able to be relieved, controlled or cured.

intracutaneous (,intrəkyoo'tayni·əs) within the substance of the skin.

i. injection an injection into the corium or substance of the skin; called also intradermal injection (see also intracutaneous INJECTION).

intracystic (,intrə'sistik) within the bladder or a cyst.

intradermal (,intrə'dərməl) within the dermis.

i. injection intracutaneous injection.

intraductal (,intrə'dukt'l) within a duct.

intradural (,intrə'dyooə·rəl) within or beneath the dura mater.

intrafusal (,intrə'fyooz'l) pertaining to the striated fibres within a muscle spindle.

intragastric (,intrə'gastrik) within the stomach.

i. tube feeding artificial feeding, usually by nasogastric tube.

intrahepatic (,intrəhi'patik) within the liver.

intralesional (,intrə'leezhən'l) occurring in or introduced directly into a localized lesion.

Intralipid (,intrə'lipid) trademark for an intravenous fat emulsion used to prevent or correct deficiency of essential fatty acids and to provide calories in high density form during total parenteral nutrition.

intralobar (,intrə'lohbə) within a lobe.

intralobular (,intrə'lobyuhlə) within a lobule.

i. veins veins which collect blood from within the lobules of the liver.

intralocular (,intrə'lokyuhlə) within the loculi of a structure.

intraluminal (,intrə'loominəl) within the lumen of a tubular structure.

intramedullary (,intrəmə'dulə·ree) within 1. the spinal cord, 2. the medulla oblongata, or 3. the marrow cavity of a bone.

intramural (,intrə'myooə·rəl) within the wall of an organ.

intramuscular (,intrə'muskyuhlə) within the muscular substance.

i. injection an injection made into the substance of a muscle (see also intramuscular INJECTION).

intranasal (,intrə'nayz'l) within the nose.

intraocular (,intrə'okyuhlə) within the eye.

intraoperative (,intrə'opə·rətiv) occurring during a surgical operation.

intraoral (,intrə'or·rəl) within the mouth.

intraorbital (,intrə'awbit'l) within the orbit.

intraosseous (,intrə'osi·əs) within a bone.

intraparietal (,intrəpə'rieət'l) 1. intramural. 2. within the parietal region of the brain.

intrapartum (,intrə'pahtəm) occurring during childbirth or during delivery.

intraperitoneal (,intrə,peritə'neeəl) within the peritoneal cavity.

intrapleural (,intrə'plooə·rəl) within the pleura.

intrapsychic (,intrə'siekik) taking place within the mind.

intrapulmonary (,intrə'pulmənə·ree, -'puhl-) within the substance of the lung.

intraspinal (,intrə'spien'l) within the substance of the spinal column.

intrasternal (,intrə'stərnəl) within the sternum.

intrathecal (,intrə'theek'l) within a sheath; through the theca of the spinal cord into the subarachnoid space.

intrathoracic (,intrəthor'rasik) within the thorax.

intratracheal (,intrə'traki·əl, -trətrə'keeəl) endotracheal.

intratubal (,intrə'tyoob'l) within a tube.

intratympanic (,intrətim'panik) within the tympanic cavity.

intrauterine (,intrə'yootə·rien) within the uterus.

i. contraceptive device (IUCD) a mechanical device inserted into the uterine cavity for the purpose of contraception. These devices are made of metallic, plastic, or other substances and are manufactured in various sizes and shapes. Examples include the Hall–Stone ring, Lippes loop, Brinberg bow, and Margulies coil. Their exact effect is not known but it is believed that they increase mobility of the ovum through the uterine tube and interfere with implantation of the fertilized ovum.

After the IUCD has been inserted, the patient is instructed to have yearly follow-up examinations.

Contraindications to insertion include recent pelvic infection, suspected pregnancy, cervical stenosis, myoma of the uterus, and abnormal uterine bleeding. They are not recommended for women who have never been pregnant because of the severe pain and bleeding that they produce in the majority of these patients.

The IUCD is not 100 per cent effective and its use carries some risks. The increased risk for pelvic inflammatory disease (PID) is from three to five times that of women who do not use an IUCD. Because PID frequently leads to an inability to conceive as a result of scarring and narrowing of the uterine tubes, the IUCD also increases the chances for infertility. Many experts advise against the use of IUCD's in women under 25 years of age and in those who hope to have children later in life.

Other possible adverse effects associated with the use of IUCD's include uterine perforation, which is rare, and severely increased menstrual flow, increased dysmenorrhoea, and intermenstrual bleeding are common in women who have an IUCD in place.

Intraval Sodium ('intrəval 'sohdi·əm) trademark for a preparation of thiopentone sodium, used as an anaesthetic.

intravasation (in,travə'sayshən) the entrance of foreign material into vessels.

intravascular (,intrə'vaskyuhlə) within a vessel or vessels.

intravenous (,intrə'veenəs) within a vein.

i. infusion the therapeutic introduction of a fluid, such as saline, into a vein. The infusion works by gravity in that the container of fluid is higher than the blood vessel into which the fluid is being introduced. It is important that aseptic conditions are maintained in order to prevent the introduction into the body of infection. The apparatus must also be airtight and the reservoir container not allowed to run dry as entry of air into the blood vessel as an air embolus could block a major vessel with fatal results.

A third important precaution is to ensure that the needle or catheter remains in the vein so that the fluid does not seep into surrounding tissue, causing tissue necrosis. Fluids to be used are prescribed by the doctor and may be for the purpose of combating dehydration, replacing body electrolytes or administering medication. The rate of infusion is also prescribed and must be carefully followed. Control may be by a simple clip or a more sophisticated flowmeter.

During the infusion, the patient's pulse and blood pressure are monitored and observations made of any abnormal reactions, including pain at the site of infusion. If an arm or leg is being used it is important that the needle or cannula is securely fixed so that the limb can be moved without fear of its being dislodged.

See also parenteral NUTRITION.

i. flow rate the rate at which fluids, medications, and blood products flow into the bloodstream during intravenous infusion. The flow rate is usually ordered by the doctor as total volume (ml) per total hours or, in the case of drugs, total dose per total hours. Manufacturers of intravenous fluid administration sets offer devices for monitoring flow rates, e.g. electronic drop counters or devices such as a burette. Alternatively one can use a flow rate conversion chart that shows the number of drops to be administered per minute when using different kinds of intravenous sets with different drop factors. The drop factor is printed on the set and is stated in terms of drops per ml. For example, a paediatric microdrip set might be labelled 60 drops/ml, while a macrodrop set for the administration of blood would be labelled 10 drops/ml.

A simple formula for determining the number of drops to be administered per minute can be used if neither a flowmeter nor a conversion chart is available. The formula is as follows:

$$\frac{\text{total volume of}}{\text{fluid to be given}} \times \frac{\text{drop factor}}{\text{time in min}} = \text{drops/min}$$

For example, if the doctor orders 1000 ml of dextrose 5% every 8 hours and the drop factor is 10 drops/ml, the problem is written:

$$\frac{1000\text{ml}}{480\text{min}} \times 10 \text{ drops/ml} = 20.80\ (21) \text{ drops/min}$$

i. regional anaesthesia Bier's block.

intraventricular (,intrəven'trikyuhlə) within a ventricle.

intravital (,intrə'viet'l) occurring during life.

intrinsic (in'trinsik, -zik) situated entirely within, or pertaining exclusively to, a part.

i. factor a glycoprotein secreted by the gastric glands, which is necessary for the assimilation and absorption of cyanocobalamin (extrinsic factor, vitamin B_{12}) contained in food, an essential for the production of the antianaemia factor. It is absent in PERNICIOUS ANAEMIA.

introitus (in'troh·itəs) pl. *introitus* [L.] the entrance to a cavity or space.

introjection (,intrə'jekshən) a mental mechanism in which loved or hated external objects are unconsciously and symbolically taken within oneself.

intromission (,intrə'mishən) the entrance of one part or object into another.

Intropin ('intrəpin) trademark for a preparation of dopamine.

introspection (,intrə'spekshən) contemplation or observation of one's thoughts and feelings; self-analysis. adj. **introspective**.

introsusception (,introhsəs'sepshən) intussusception.

introversion (,intrə'vərshən) 1. the turning outside in, more or less completely, of an organ. 2. pre-occupation with oneself, with reduction of interest in the outside world.

introvert ('intrə,vərt) a person whose interests are turned inward upon himself.

intubate ('intyuh,bayt) to perform intubation.

intubation (,intyuh'bayshən) the insertion of a tube, as into the trachea. The purpose of intubation varies with the location and type of tube inserted; generally the procedure is done to allow for drainage, to maintain an open airway, or for the administration of anaesthetics or OXYGEN.

Intubation into the stomach or intestine is done to remove gastric or intestinal contents for the relief or prevention of distention, or to obtain a specimen for analysis. A plastic nasogastric tube is introduced through the nose and into the stomach. Shorter tubes (e.g. LEVIN TUBE) are designed for intubation into the stomach, whereas longer tubes are designed to pass through the stomach and into the small intestine. The tubes may be attached to a suction apparatus so that gas and liquids can be removed. A nasogastric tube also may be inserted for the purpose of providing nourishment (see also TUBE FEEDING).

The SENGSTAKEN–BLAKEMORE TUBE is a four-lumen tube with an oesophageal balloon, a gastric balloon, pharyngeal aspiration channel, and gastric tubes with sucking ports at its tip. It is used to stop haemorrhage from gastric and oesophageal varices.

A T-tube may be inserted in the common bile duct to allow for drainage of bile from the ducts that drain the

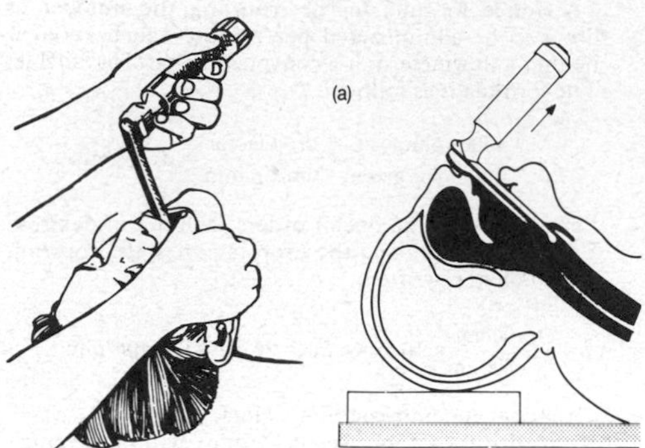

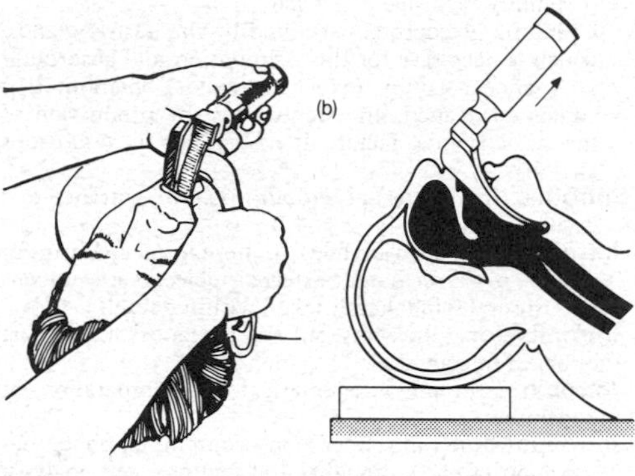

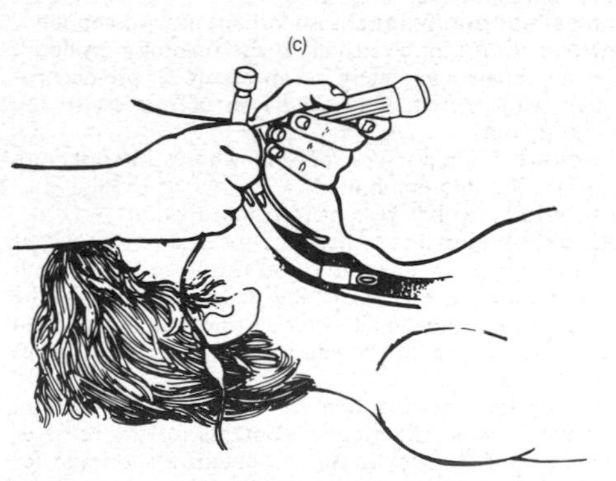

Technique of orotracheal intubation. (a) Laryngoscopy for endotracheal intubation with straight laryngoscope blade. Left, insertion of blade; right, larynx exposed. Note the elevated occiput with the head tilted backward (sniffing position), and the direct elevation of the epiglottis with the tip of the blade. Do not use the teeth as a fulcrum. Keep pressure off the upper teeth and lip! See text. (b) Laryngoscopy for endotracheal intubation with curved laryngoscope blade. Left, insertion of blade; right, larynx exposed. Note the indirect elevation of the epiglottis by the tip of the blade elevating the base of the tongue. Note also the direction of lift, which is anteriorly and inferiorly at 45° to the vertical (coronal) plane. See text. (c) Exposure of the larynx with a curved blade and insertion of a cuffed tube through the right corner of the mouth, while looking along the laryngoscope blade. See text.

liver after surgery on the gallbladder or the common bile duct.

Endotracheal intubation can be achieved by insertion of an ENDOTRACHEAL TUBE via the mouth or nose. It is done for the purpose of assuring patency of the upper airway. The tube is inserted (usually after a laryngoscope has been used to explore the larynx) between the vocal cords, through the larynx, and far enough into the trachea that the cuff is beyond the larynx. TRACHEOSTOMY is also a form of endotracheal intubation. See accompanying illustration.

intumescence (ˌintyuh'mesəns) 1. a swelling, normal or abnormal. 2. the process of swelling. adj. **intumescent**.

intussusception (ˌintəsə'sepshən) 1. prolapse of one part of the intestine into the lumen of an immediately adjacent part, causing INTESTINAL OBSTRUCTION. 2. the reception into an organism of matter, such as food, and its transformation into new protoplasm.

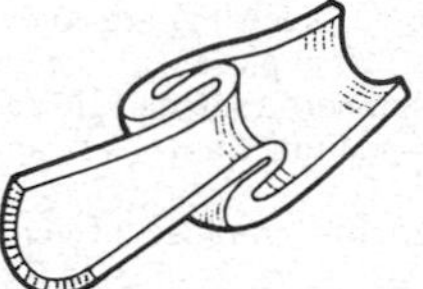

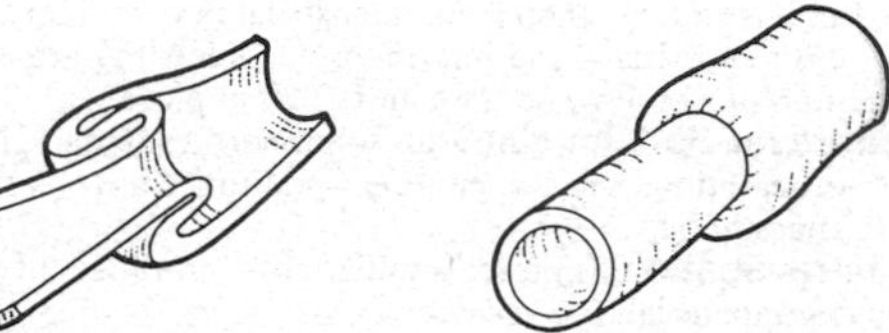

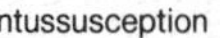

Intussusception

Intussusception is a rather rare disorder. Most cases occur in children during the first year of life, and some cases occur in the second year, but very few thereafter. The condition may be caused by a growth in the intestine or by any condition that causes the intestine to contract strongly. Frequently there is no obvious cause. The child seems healthy, yet paroxysms of abdominal pain begin, with vomiting and restlessness. Within 12 to 24 hours bloody mucus is passed by rectum. On the second day a high fever may appear. Death can occur within 2 to 4 days after the onset unless the condition is remedied by surgery.

The diagnosis may be confirmed by BARIUM TEST in the form of a barium enema. This examination will frequently reduce the intussusception and in some cases will completely correct the condition. Treatment by surgery may be advised and ordinarily gives a permanent cure.

intussusceptum (ˌintəsə'septəm) the portion of intestine that has prolapsed in intussusception.

intussuscipiens (ˌintəsə'sipi·ənz) the portion of the intestine containing the intussusceptum.

inulin ('inyuhlin) a starch occurring in the rhizome of certain plants, which on hydrolysis yields fructose. It is sometimes used as a measure of glomerular function in tests of renal function.

inunction (in'ungkshən) 1. the act of anointing or applying an ointment by friction. 2. an ointment made with lanolin as a solvent.

invaginate (in'vajiˌnayt) to infold one portion of a structure within another portion.

invagination (inˌvaji'nayshən) 1. the infolding of one part within another part of a structure, as of the blastula during gastrulation. 2. intussusception.

invasive (in'vaysiv, -ziv) 1. having the quality of invasiveness. 2. involving puncture or incision of the skin or insertion of an instrument or foreign material into the body; said of diagnostic techniques.

invasiveness (in'vaysivnəs) 1. the ability of microorganisms to enter the body and spread in the tissues. 2.

the ability to infiltrate and actively destroy surrounding tissue, a property of malignant tumours. adj. **invasive.**

inversion (in'vərshən) 1. a turning inward, inside out, or other reversal of the normal relation of a part. 2. homosexuality. 3. a chromosomal aberration due to the inverted reunion of the middle segment after breakage of a chromosome at two points, resulting in a change in sequence of genes or nucleotides.

invert ('invərt) a homosexual.

invertase (in'vərtayz, 'in-) a ferment of intestinal juice which hydrolyses cane sugar.

invertebrate (in'vərti,brət, -brayt) 1. having no vertebral column. 2. any animal that has no vertebral column.

investment (in'vestmənt) material in which a denture, tooth, crown, or model for a dental restoration is enclosed for curing, soldering, or casting, or the process of such enclosure.

inveterate (in'vetə·rət) confirmed and chronic; long-established and difficult to cure.

involucrum (,invo'lookrəm) pl. *involucra* [L.] a covering or sheath. It is classically used to describe the sheath of new bone formed from the periosteum of a bone affected by chronic osteomyelitis and which surrounds the original bone.

involuntary (in'volantə·ree) performed independently of the will.

involution (,invə'looshən) 1. a rolling or turning inward. 2. one of the movements involved in the gastrulation of many animals. 3. a retrograde change of the entire body or in a particular organ, such as the retrograde changes in the female genital organs that result in normal size after delivery. 4. the progressive degeneration occurring naturally with advancing age, resulting in shrivelling of organs or tissues. adj. **involutional.**

Io chemical symbol, *ionium.*

iocetamic acid (,ieohsi'tamik) an iodinated radiopaque radiological contrast medium used for oral cholecystography. Called also *cholebrin.*

iodamide (ie'ohdəmied) a water-soluble, radiopaque, iodinated radiological contrast medium; used mainly for intravenous excretory urography. Trademark Uromiro.

Iodamoeba (,ieədə'meebə) a genus of amoebas, including *I. buetschlii*, parasitic in the large intestine of man, though probably non-pathogenic, and *I. suis*, found in pigs.

iodide ('ieə,died) a binary compound of iodine or the I^- anion. Iodide inhibits the release of thyroxine from the thyroid gland.

iodination (,ieədi'nayshən) the incorporation or addition of iodine in a compound.

iodine ('ieə,deen) a chemical element, atomic number 53, atomic weight 126.904, symbol I. (See table of elements in Appendix 2.) Iodine is essential in nutrition, being especially prevalent in the colloid of the THYROID GLAND. It is used in the treatment of HYPOTHYROIDISM and as a topical antiseptic. Iodine is a frequent cause of poisoning (see also IODISM).

Since iodine is opaque to x-rays, it can be combined with other compounds and used as *contrast media* in diagnostic radiology.

protein-bound i. test a test of thyroid function (see also PROTEIN-BOUND IODINE TEST).

i.-123 a cyclotron-produced isotope of iodine with a half-life of 13.3 hours and which decays by emitting gamma rays of 159 and 28 keV. Its principal use is in imaging the kidney in nuclear medicine when used as ^{123}I-ortho iodohippurate. Symbol ^{123}I.

i.-125 a radioisotope of iodine having a half-life of 60 days and a principal gamma ray photon energy of 28 keV; used as a label in radioimmunoassays and other in vitro tests. Symbol ^{125}I.

i.-131 a radioisotope of iodine having a half-life of 8.1 days and a principal gamma ray photon energy of 364 keV; used in treatment of hyperthyroidism and carcinoma of the thyroid. Because of the high radiation dose its role in diagnosis of thyroid disease has been replaced by ^{99}Tc^m except when there is the possibility of a retrosternal thyroid. Symbol ^{131}I.

iodinophilous (,ieədi'nofiləs) easily stainable with iodine.

iodism ('ieə,dizəm) chronic poisoning by iodine or iodides, causing coryza, ptyalism, frontal headache, emaciation, weakness, and skin eruptions.

iodochlorhydroxyquin (,ieədohklorhie'droksi,kwin) a spongy yellowish powder used as a topical anti-infective in the treatment of amoebiasis, *Trichomonas vaginalis* infection, and eczema.

iododerma (,ieədoh'dərmə) any skin lesion resulting from iodism.

iodohippurate (,ieədoh'hipyuh,rayt) an iodine-containing compound which, when labelled with radioactive ^{123}I, is sometimes used in nuclear medicine to image the kidneys.

iodophilia (,ieədoh'fili·ə) a reaction shown by leukocytes in certain pathological conditions, as in toxaemia and severe anaemia, in which the polymorphonuclear cells show diffuse brownish coloration when treated with iodine or iodides.

iodopsin (,ieə'dopsin) a violet pigment found in the retinal cones of the eye.

iodoquinol (ie,ohdə'kwinol) an amoebicide used in the treatment of intestinal amoebiasis and (formerly) *Trichomonas* vaginitis.

Iodosorb (ie'ohdohzawb) trademark for a preparation of cadexomer iodide used to cleanse venous leg ulcers and pressure sores.

iodotherapy (,ieədoh'therəpee) treatment with iodine or iodides.

iodoxamate (,ieə'doksəmayt) an iodine-containing radiological contrast medium used in intravenous cholangiography. Meglumine iodoxamate, trademark Endobil.

iodum (ie'ohdəm) [L.] *iodine.*

ioglycamate (,ieə'glykəmayt) an iodine-containing radiological contrast medium used in intravenous cholangiography. Meglumine ioglycamate, trademark Biligram.

iohexol (,ieə'heksol) an iodine-containing radiological contrast medium used for intravenous urography, arteriography, venography, and myelography. Trademark Omnipaque.

ion ('ieən) an atom or group of atoms having a positive (cation) or negative (anion) electric charge by virtue of having gained or lost one or more electrons. Substances forming ions are ELECTROLYTES. adj. **ionic.**

dipolar i. zwitterion.

hydrogen i. the positively charged hydrogen atom (H^+), present to excess in acid solutions.

ion-exchange resin (,ieəniks'chaynj) a high-molecular-weight, insoluble polymer of simple organic compounds with the ability to exchange its attached ions for other ions in the surrounding medium. They are classified as cation- or anion-exchange resins, depending on which ions the resin exchanges. Cation-exchange resins are used to restrict sodium absorption in oedematous states; anion-exchange resins are used as antacids in the treatment of ulcers. Ion-exchange resins may also be classified as carboxylic, sulphonic, etc., depending on the nature of the active groups.

Ionamin (ie'ohnəmin) trademark for a preparation of phentermine, an anorexic.

ionization (,ieənie'zayshən) 1. the dissociation of a substance in solution into ions. 2. iontophoresis.

i. chamber an enclosure containing two or more electrodes between which an electric current may be passed when the enclosed gas is ionized by radiation; used for determining the intensity of x-rays and other rays.

ionophore (ie'onə,for) any molecule, as of a drug, that increases the permeability of cell membranes to a specific ion.

ionophose (ie'onə,fohz) a violet phose.

iontophoresis (ie,ontohfə'reesis) the introduction of ions of soluble salts into the body by an electric current. adj. **iontophoretic**.

iopamidol (,ieə'pamidol) an iodine-containing radiological contrast medium used for intravenous urography, arteriography, venography, and myelography. Trademark Niopam.

iopanoic acid (,ieohpə'noh·ik) an acid used as a radiopaque contrast medium in oral cholecystography. Trademark Telepaque.

iophendylate (ieoh'fendi,layt) an oily radiopaque contrast medium used in myelography. Trademark Myodil.

iothalamate (ieoh'thalə,mayt) a water-soluble, iodine-containing, radiopaque contrast medium used in urography and angiography. Trademark Conray. May also be used as an oral contrast medium; trademark Gastrografin.

iotroxate (,ieə'troksayt) an iodine-containing radiological contrast medium used in intravenous cholangiography. Meglumine iotroxate, trademark Biliscopin.

ioxaglate (,ie'oksəglayt) an iodine-containing radiological contrast medium used for intravenous urography, arteriography, and venography.

ipecacuanha (,ipi,kakyoo'ahnə) the dried rhizome and roots of *Cephaëlis ipecacuanha* or *Cephaëlis acuminata*; used as an emetic or expectorant.

ipodate ('iepoh,dayt) a radiopaque contrast medium used in oral cholecystography. Trademarks Biloptin and Solu-Biloptin.

IPPV intermittent positive-pressure ventilation.

Ipral ('ipral) trademark for a preparation of trimethoprim, an antibacterial agent.

iproniazid (,ieprə'nieəzid) an antidepressant drug that belongs to the group of monoamine oxidase inhibitors.

ipsi- word element. [L.] *same*, *self*.

ipsilateral (,ipsi'latə·rəl) situated on or affecting the same side.

IQ intelligence quotient.

Ir chemical symbol, *iridium*.

irid(o)- word element. [Gr.] *iris of the eye*, *a coloured circle*.

iridaemia (,iri'deemi·ə) haemorrhage from the iris.

iridal ('iridal) pertaining to the iris.

iridalgia (,iri'dalji·ə) pain in the iris.

iridauxesis (,iridawk'seesis) thickening of the iris.

iridectomy (,iri'dektəmee) excision of part of the iris.

iridencleisis (,iriden'kliesis) surgical incarceration of a slip of the iris within a corneal or limbal incision to act as a wick for aqueous drainage in glaucoma.

irideremia (iridə'reemi·ə) congenital absence of the iris.

irides ('iri,deez) [Gr.] plural of *iris*.

iridescence (,iri'des'ns) the condition of gleaming with bright and changing colours. adj. **iridescent**.

iridesis (,iri'deesis) repositioning of the pupil by fixation of a sector of iris in a corneal or limbal incision.

iridic (i'ridik) pertaining to the iris.

iridium (i'ridi·əm) a chemical element, atomic number 77, atomic weight 192.2, symbol Ir. See table of elements in Appendix 2.

iridoavulsion (,iridoh·ə'vulshən) complete tearing away of the iris from its periphery.

iridocapsulitis (,iridoh,kapsyuh'lietis) inflammation of the iris and lens capsule.

iridocele (i'ridoh,seel) hernial protrusion of part of the iris through the cornea.

iridochoroiditis (,iridoh,ko·roy'dietis) inflammation of the iris and choroid.

iridocoloboma (,iridoh,kolə'bohmə) congenital fissure or coloboma of the iris.

iridocyclectomy (,iridohsie'klektəmee) excision of part of the iris and of the ciliary body.

iridocyclitis (,iridohsie'klietis) inflammation of the iris and ciliary body.

heterochromic i. a low-grade form leading to depigmentation of the iris of the affected eye; called also *Fuchs' heterochromic cyclitis*.

iridocyclochoroiditis (,iridoh,siekloh,ko·roy'dietis) inflammation of the iris, ciliary body, and choroid.

iridodesis (,iridoh'deesis) iridesis.

iridodialysis (,iridohdie'aləsis) separation by tearing of the iris from its root, usually due to trauma.

iridodonesis (,iridohdə'neesis) tremulousness of the iris on movement of the eye, occurring in subluxation of the lens.

iridokeratitis (,iridoh,kerə'tietis) inflammation of the iris and cornea.

iridokinesia, iridokinesis (,iridohki'neezi·ə; ,iridohki'neesis) contraction and expansion of the iris. adj. **iridokinetic**.

iridoleptynsis (,iridohlep'tinsis) thinning or atrophy of the iris.

iridology (,iri'doləjee) the study of the iris as associated with disease.

iridomalacia (,iridohmə'layshi·ə) softening of the iris.

iridomotor (,iridoh'mohtə) pertaining to movements of the iris.

iridoncus (,iri'dongkəs) tumour or swelling of the iris.

iridoparalysis (,iridohpə'ralisis) iridoplegia.

iridoperiphakitis (,iridohperifa'kietis) inflammation of the iris and the lens capsule.

iridoplegia (,iridoh'pleeji·ə) paralysis of the sphincter of the iris, with lack of contraction or dilation of the pupil; called also *iridoparalysis*.

iridoptosis (,iridop'tohsis) prolapse of the iris.

iridopupillary (,iridoh'pyoopilə·ree) pertaining to the iris and pupil.

iridorhexis (,iridə'reksis) 1. rupture of iris. 2. the tearing away of the iris.

iridoschisis (,iri'doskisis) splitting of the mesodermal stroma of the iris into two layers, with fibrils of the anterior layer floating in the aqueous.

iridosclerotomy (,iridohsklə'rotəmee) incision of the sclera and of the edge of the iris in glaucoma.

iridosteresis (,iridohstə'reesis) removal of all or part of the iris.

iridotomy (,iri'dotəmee) incision of the iris.

iris ('ieris) pl. *irides* [Gr.] the circular pigmented membrane behind the cornea, perforated by the pupil; the most anterior portion of the vascular tunic of the eye, it is made up of a flat bar of circular muscular fibres surrounding the pupil, a thin layer of plain muscle fibres by which the pupil is dilated, and, posteriorly, of two layers of pigmented epithelial cells.

iritis (ie'rietis) inflammation of the iris. adj. **iritic.** The condition may be acute, occurring suddenly with pronounced symptoms, or chronic, with less severe but longer-lasting symptoms.

SYMPTOMS. Iritis is characterized by pain, which may

radiate to the forehead and become worse at night, and photophobia. The eye is usually red and the pupil contracts and may be irregular in shape; there is extreme sensitivity to light, together with blurring of vision and tenderness of the eyeball. The iris becomes swollen and discoloured. If not treated promptly, iritis can be dangerous because of scarring and adhesions that may cause secondary cataract and glaucoma.

TREATMENT. This includes dilation of the pupil with atropine drops to prevent adhesions between the iris and the lens (posterior synechiae). Topical steroids may be used to reduce the inflammation quickly.

With proper treatment, acute iritis usually clears up fairly quickly, although it may recur. For permanent relief, elimination or control of the underlying cause, if one can be identified, is necessary.

serous i. iritis with a serous exudate.

iritomy (ie'ritəmee) iridotomy.

iron ('ieən) a chemical element, atomic number 26, atomic weight 55.847, symbol Fe. (See table of elements in Appendix 2.) Iron is chiefly important to the human body because it is the main constituent of haemoglobin, cytochrome, and other components of respiratory enzyme systems. A constant although small intake of iron in food is needed to replace erythrocytes that are destroyed in the body processes.

Most iron reaches the body in food, where it occurs naturally in the form of iron compounds. These are converted for use in the body by the action of the hydrochloric acid produced in the stomach. This acid separates the iron from the food and combines with it in a form that is readily assimilable by the body. Vitamin C enhances the absorption of food iron. The administration of alkalis hampers iron absorption.

IRON DEFICIENCIES. The amount of new iron needed every day by the adult body is about 15 mg. A child needs a bit more in proportion to his weight. Although these amounts are very small, iron deficiencies may cause serious disorders.

The most common form of anaemia results from iron deficiency. A great loss of blood, such as may result from bleeding ulcers, haemorrhoids, or injury, may cause a deficiency of iron. Women who lose much blood in menstruation may have to supplement their diet with iron-rich food. Iron deficiency sometimes occurs in pregnancy as a result of increased demands on the mother's blood. Iron deficiency may also occur in infants, since milk contains little iron. Although babies are born with an extra supply of haemoglobin, by the age of 2 or 3 months they need iron-rich food to supplement milk.

Iron preparations, such as ferrous sulphate, are necessary for the treatment of iron deficiency anaemia; they should be administered after meals, never on an empty stomach. The patient should be warned that the drugs cause stools to turn dark green or black. Overdosage may cause severe systemic reactions.

Malabsorption of iron due to gastrointestinal disorders may warrant parenteral administration of an iron supplement. Intramuscular injections of iron are given using the Z-track technique; however, no more than 2 ml (100 mg) can be administered in one site. Intravenous administration of iron avoids some of the problems of intramuscular injections but can increase the risk of phlebitis. Not all brands of iron preparations can be given intravenously. Multiple dose vials of iron dextran contain phenol as a preservative and are toxic when administered parenterally. Imferon in 2-ml and 5-ml ampoules without preservatives is safe.

Hypersensitivity to iron supplements is not uncommon and the parenteral administration of iron can cause vomiting, chills, fever, headache, joint pain, and urticaria.

FOOD SOURCES OF IRON. Liver is the richest source of iron, containing enough in 150 g for a whole day's supply for an adult. Other iron-rich foods include lean meat, oysters, kidney beans, wholewheat bread, egg yolk, green vegetables, carrots, apricots, and raisins.

i.-59 a radioisotope of iron having a half-life of 45 days; used in ferrokinetics tests to determine the rate at which iron is cleared from the plasma and incorporated in red cells. Symbol ^{59}Fe.

i. lung a popular name for a Drinker respirator, a type of VENTILATOR that provides controlled, automatic breathing for a patient whose respiratory muscles are paralysed; it consists of a metal tank, enclosing the patient's body with his head outside, and within which artificial respiration is maintained by alternating negative and positive pressure.

i. storage disease haemochromatosis.

iron dextran a complex of ferric hydroxide with dextrans used as a parenteral iron replacement solution.

iron sorbitol a complex of iron, sorbitol, and citric acid used as a parenteral iron replacement solution.

irotomy (ie'rotəmee) iridotomy.

irradiate (i'raydi,ayt) to expose to radiant energy.

irradiation (i,raydi'ayshən) exposure to radiant energy (heat, x-rays, etc.) for therapeutic or diagnostic purposes (see also RADIATION).

There are many kinds of rays, all travelling at the speed of light. Every living thing is subject to some irradiation by cosmic rays, ultraviolet rays in sunlight, and other natural radiation in the environment. Such radiation is usually slight and harmless. In large amounts, certain kinds of radiation—those rays with a greater frequency and producing more energy—cause direct harm to living cells. USES. Irradiation of certain foods, including milk, kills harmful bacteria and prevents spoilage. X-ray photography is used in industrial research and in diagnosis of disorders within the body.

RADIATION THERAPY usually refers to treatment by x-rays and gamma rays. X-rays are produced by bombarding a tungsten target with high-speed electrons in a vacuum tube; gamma rays are emitted during the decay of radioisotopes. X-rays may be employed to kill organisms causing skin diseases, for example, or to destroy the abnormal cells that form tumours. Gonads, blood cells, and cancer cells are especially sensitive to radiation, particularly to x-rays and gamma rays. These rays are used principally for the treatment of cancer, and the radiotherapist attempts to destroy diseased cells without producing other ill effects.

Other rays are also used medically. Infrared rays produce a radiant heat used for the treatment of sprains and bursitis; tissues such as muscles and joints are relaxed and soothed by the penetration of these rays. Ultraviolet rays are used in sun lamps to treat skin diseases, such as acne and psoriasis.

PROTECTION AGAINST HARMFUL EFFECTS. Excessive radiation can cause RADIATION SICKNESS in the person exposed; sterility or genetic mutations in offspring are other possible results of excessive exposure to radiation. Hence the great danger from the blasts of nuclear or thermonuclear explosions and from the radioactive materials (fallout) scattered by these blasts.

The harmful effects of radiation are determined by both the degree of exposure and the type of radiation. Prevention must take into account time, distance, and shielding of both areas and people. Persons who are employed in nuclear power plants or other places where radioactive materials are accumulated must be properly shielded, and should wear or carry a dosimeter on which the amount of radiation received is recorded. Proper shielding is necessary also for radiologists, nurses, and others who spend much time near radiation emitted from either machinery or materials. See also RADIATION protection.

Since radiation effects, such as those of x-rays, build up in the body, a person should not be exposed to any more radiation during his lifetime than is necessary, and all radiotherapy must be under the control of a competent medical practitioner.

Radiologists reduce harmful effects by limiting the field of exposure, by means of fast films, filters, and other technical devices. This shortens measurably the length of exposure of patients receiving medical and dental x-rays.

irreducible (ˌiri'dyoosəb'l) not susceptible to reduction, as a fracture, hernia, or chemical substance.

irrigation (ˌiri'gayshən) washing of a body cavity or wound by a stream of water or other fluid.

GENERAL PRINCIPLES. A steady, gentle stream is used in irrigation. The pressure should be sufficient to reach the desired area, but not enough to force the fluid beyond the area to be irrigated. The greater the height of the container of solution, the greater will be the pressure exerted by the stream of solution. Return flow of solution must always be allowed for. Directions about the type of solution to be used, the strength desired, and correct temperature should be followed carefully. Aseptic technique must be observed if sterile irrigation is ordered.

BLADDER. The purpose is to cleanse the bladder or to apply medication to the bladder lining. Aseptic technique must be used. The amount and type of solution will be ordered by the doctor.

EAR. The stream is kept flowing steadily but with very low pressure; excessive pressure is painful and may spread infection to the middle ear. The patient usually is seated for this procedure, but he may lie on his side, with the ear to be irrigated uppermost while the solution is entering the ear. The head is turned to allow for return flow. The output flow of solution must never be obstructed.

EYE (CONJUNCTIVAL SAC). The patient's head is turned to the side so that the eye to be irrigated is lower than the other eye. The solution is allowed to run over the eyelids to cleanse them and to accustom the patient to the flow of the solution. The flow of solution is directed from the inner to outer corner of the eye. The eyelids are separated by exerting pressure on the facial bones, not on the eyeball.

PERINEUM. The purpose of the procedure is to cleanse the vulva. Flow of the solution prescribed is from front to back. The patient is instructed to wipe from the front to back to avoid contamination from the anal region.

THROAT (ORAL PHARYNX). This type of irrigation reaches a more extensive area than does gargling. The temperature of the solution may be slightly higher than for other irrigations because the mouth and throat are more accustomed to hot liquids. The patient may be more comfortable sitting, with his head bent forward slightly. The patient is instructed to hold his breath while the solution is flowing.

irritability (ˌiritə'bilətee) 1. ability of an organism or a specific tissue to react to the environment. 2. the state of being abnormally responsive to slight stimuli, or unduly sensitive.

myotatic i. the ability of a muscle to contract in response to stretching.

irritable ('iritəb'l) 1. capable of reacting to a stimulus. 2. abnormally sensitive to stimuli.

i. bowel syndrome a group of symptoms that represent the most common disorder presented by patients consulting a specialist in gastrointestinal disorders. The characteristics of the disorder are: (1) altered bowel habits, manifested by diarrhoea, constipation, or alternating diarrhoea and constipation; (2) abdominal pain and intolerance to flatus; and (3) absence of detectable organic disease. Many terms including mucous colitis, nervous colon, spastic colon, and irritable colon have been used to describe this disorder, but they are inappropriate. Irritable bowel syndrome should not be confused with colitis and other inflammatory diseases of the intestinal tract; there is no inflammation. Futhermore, irritable bowel syndrome is not necessarily limited to the colon.

Because of psychological factors that usually contribute to the disorder and its tendency to be chronic in nature, treatment should be holistic and individualized to meet the needs of each patient. In most cases, treatment is needed for an extended period of time. Patients should be assured that there is no relationship between their disorder and malignancy of the bowel. Modes of therapy include psychotherapy, biofeedback training, medications such as antidepressants, antispasmolytics, and analgesics, and a diet that is high in bran and fibre.

irritant ('iritənt) 1. causing irritation. 2. an agent that causes irritation.

irritation (ˌiri'tayshən) 1. the act of stimulating. 2. a state of overexcitation and undue sensitivity. adj. **irritative**.

ischaemia (is'keemi·ə) deficiency of blood in a part, due to functional constriction or actual obstruction of a blood vessel. adj. **ischaemic**.

myocardial i. deficiency of blood supply to the heart muscle, due to obstruction or constriction of the coronary arteries.

ischi(o)- word element. [Gr.] *ischium*.

ischiadic, ischial (ˌiski'adik; 'iski·əl) ischiatic.

ischialgia (ˌiski'alji·ə) pain in the ischium.

ischiatic (ˌiski'atik) pertaining to the ischium.

ischidrosis (ˌiski'drohsis) anhidrosis.

ischiobulbar (ˌiskioh'bulbə) pertaining to the ischium and the bulb of the urethra.

ischiocapsular (ˌiskioh'kapsyuhlə) pertaining to the ischium and the capsular ligament of the hip joint.

ischiocele ('iskioh,seel) hernia through the sacrosciatic notch.

ischiococcygeal (ˌiskiohkok'siji·əl) pertaining to the ischium and coccyx.

ischiodidymus (ˌiskioh'didiməs) conjoined twins united at the pelvis.

ischiodynia (ˌiskioh'dini·ə) pain in the ischium.

ischiofemoral (ˌiskioh'femə·rəl) pertaining to the ischium and femur.

ischiohebotomy (ˌiskioh·hi'botəmee) surgical division of the ischiopubic ramus and ascending ramus of the pubes.

ischioneuralgia (ˌiskiohnyuh'ralji·ə, -jə) sciatica.

ischiopagus (ˌiski'opəgəs) conjoined twins fused at the ischial region.

ischiopubic (ˌiskioh'pyoobik) pertaining to the ischium and pubes.

ischiorectal (ˌiskioh'rekt'l) pertaining to the ischium and rectum.

ischium ('iski·əm) the inferior, dorsal portion of the hip bone.

ischuria (is'kyooə·ri·ə) retention or suppression of the urine. adj. **ischuretic**.

iseikonia (iesie'kohni·ə) iso-iconic. adj. **iseikonic**.

Ishihara colour charts (ˌishi'hahrə) patterns of dots of the primary colours on similar backgrounds. The patterns can be seen by a normal-sighted person, but one whose colour vision is impaired will only be able to identify some of the patterns.

island ('ieland) a cluster of cells or an isolated piece of tissue.

blood i's aggregations of mesenchymal cells in the angioblast of the embryo, developing into vascular endothelium and blood cells.

i's of Langerhans see ISLETS of Langerhans.

i. of Reil insula.

islet ('ielət) an island.

i's of Langerhans irregular microscopic structures scattered throughout the pancreas and comprising its endocrine portion. They contain the *alpha cells*, which secrete the hyperglycaemic factor glucagon; the *beta cells*, which secrete insulin, and whose degeneration is one of the causes of DIABETES MELLITUS; and the *delta cells*, which secrete somatostatin.

Walthard's i's microscopic inclusions of the ovarian germinal epithelium, which have been implicated in the development of Brenner tumours.

Ismelin ('isməlin) trademark for a preparation of guanethidine, an antihypertensive.

iso- word element. [Gr.] *equal*, *alike*, *same*.

isoagglutinin (,iesoh·ə'glootinin) an isoantibody that acts as an agglutinin.

isoallele (,iesoh·ə'leel) an allelic gene that is considered as being normal but can be distinguished from another allele by its differing phenotypic expression when in combination with a dominant mutant allele.

isoamylase (,iesoh'ami,layz) 1. any of the several isoenzymes of α-amylase. 2. a hydrolase that catalyses the hydrolysis of 1,6-α-glycosidic branch linkages in glycogen and amylopectin.

isoanaphylaxis (,iesoh,anəfi'laksis) anaphylaxis produced by serum from an individual of the same species.

isoantibody (,ieso'anti,bodee) an antibody produced by one individual that reacts with isoantigens of another individual of the same species; called also *alloantibody*.

isoantigen (,iesoh'antijən) an antigen existing in alternative (allelic) forms in a species, thus inducing an immune response when one form is transferred to members of the species who lack it; typical isoantigens are the blood group antigens; called also *alloantigen*.

isobar ('iesoh,bah) 1. one of two or more chemical species with the same atomic weight but different atomic numbers. 2. a line on a map or chart joining the points of constant atmospheric pressure.

isocarboxazid (,iesohkah'boksə,zid) a monoamine oxidase inhibitor used as an antidepressant.

isocellular (,iesoh'selyuhlə) made up of identical cells.

isochromatic (,iesohkrə'matik) of the same colour throughout.

isochromatophil (,iesohkrə'matəfil) staining equally with the same stain.

isochromosome (,iesoh'krohmə,sohm) an abnormal chromosome having a median centromere and two identical arms, formed by transverse, rather than normal longitudinal, splitting of a replicating chromosome.

isochronic, isochronous (,iesoh'kronik; ie'sokrənəs) performed in equal times; said of motions and vibrations occurring at the same time and being equal in duration.

isocitric acid (,iesoh'sitrik) an intermediate in the tricarboxylic acid cycle, formed from oxaloacetic acid and itself converted to ketoglutaric acid.

isocoria (,iesoh'kor·ri·ə) equality of size of the pupils of the two eyes.

isocortex (,iesoh'kawteks) neopallium.

isocytolysin (,iesohsie'tolisin) an isoantibody that acts as a cytolysin.

isocytosis (,iesohsie'tohsis) equality in size of cells, especially of erythrocytes.

isodactylism (,iesoh'dakti,lizəm) relatively even length of the fingers.

isodiametric (,iesoh,dieə'metrik) measuring the same in all diameters.

isodontic (,iesoh'dontik) having all the teeth alike.

isodose ('iesoh,dohs) a radiation dose of equal intensity to more than one body area.

isoelectric (,iesoh·i'lektrik) showing no variation in electric potential.

i. period the moment in muscular contraction when no deflection of the galvanometer is produced.

isoenzyme (,iesoh'enziem) any of the several forms of an enzyme, all of which catalyse the same reaction, but which may differ in reaction rate, inhibition by various substances, electrophoretic mobility, or immunological properties. Several enzymes, particularly alkaline phosphatase, lactate dehydrogenase, and creatine kinase, have clinically important isoenzymes. Isoenzymes are separated by electrophoresis, and the pattern indicates which damaged organ has released the enzymes.

isoetharine (,iesoh'ethə·reen) a sympathomimetic amine having more effect on the β_2-adrenergic receptors of the bronchi and vascular smooth muscle than the β_1-adrenergic receptors of the heart; used as a bronchodilator in bronchial asthma and for relief of bronchospasm in chronic obstructive airways disease.

isoflurane (,iesoh'flooə·rayn) a modern inhalational anaesthetic agent being the isomer of enflurane. A substituted ether, it is as potent as halothane but recovery is more rapid. Induction would be faster if it was not for its pungent smell. Notable for maintaining cardiac output, although blood pressure falls in a dose-related manner due to peripheral vasodilation. Depresses respiration less than enflurane but more than halothane. Broken down in the body to a much lesser extent, its potential for toxicity is less and is the agent of choice when a patient requires frequent anaesthetics. Likely to overtake halothane as the most used inhalational agent.

isogamety (,iesoh'gamətee) production by an individual of one sex of gametes identical with respect to the sex chromosome. adj. **isogametic**.

isogamy (ie'sogəmee) reproduction resulting from union of two gametes identical in size and structure, as in protozoa. adj. **isogamous**.

isogeneic (,iesohjə'nee·ik, -'nayik) having the same genetic constitution; syngeneic.

isogeneric (,iesohjə'nerik) of the same kind; belonging to the same species.

isogenesis (,iesoh'jenəsis) similarity in the processes of development.

isograft ('iesoh,grahft) a graft between genetically identical individuals.

isohaemagglutination (,iesoh,heemə,glooti'nayshən) agglutination of erythrocytes caused by an isohaemagglutinin.

isohaemagglutinin (,iesoh·heemə'glooti,nin) an isoantigen that agglutinates erythrocytes.

isohaemolysin (,iesoh·hee'molisin) an isoantigen that causes haemolysis.

isohaemolysis (,iesoh·hee'molisis) haemolysis produced by isohaemolysin. adj. **isohaemolytic**.

isohypercytosis (,iesoh,hiepəsie'tohsis) increase in the number of leukocytes, with normal proportions of neutrophil cells.

isohypocytosis (,iesoh,hiepohsie'tohsis) decrease in the number of leukocytes with normal relation between the number of various forms.

iso-iconia (ˌiesoh·ie'kohni·ə) a condition in which the image of an object is the same in both eyes. adj. **iso-iconic.**

isoimmunization (ˌiesohˌimyuhnie'zayshən) development of antibodies in response to isoantigens; called also *alloimmunization.*

Isoket ('iezohket) trademark for an intravenous preparation of isosorbide dinitrate used in the treatment of congestive cardiac failure.

isolate ('iesəˌlayt) 1. to separate from others, or set apart. In infection control, to separate from others during the period of infectivity. 2. a group of individuals prevented by geographic, genetic, ecological, or social barriers from interbreeding with others of their kind.

isolation (ˌiesə'layshən) the act of isolating or state of being isolated, such as (a) the physiological separation of a part, as by tissue culture or by interposition of inert material; (b) the segregation of patients with a communicable disease; (c) the successive propagation of a growth of microorganisms until a pure culture is obtained; (d) the chemical extraction of an unknown substance in pure form from a tissue; (e) an unconscious defence mechanism in which there is a failure to connect behaviour with motives, or contradictory attitudes and behaviour with each other.

i. nursing the use of special precautionary measures and procedures when caring for a patient with an infection or who is at risk of catching infection from others.

Recommended techniques take into account the site of infection and mode of transmission so that strict isolation of the patient is avoided unless essential. Local infection control personnel will advise as to precautions necessary and these should be communicated and adhered to by all staff and visitors coming into contact with the patient. Known also as barrier nursing.

General Principles of Patient Care. In addition to the specific measures taken to prevent the spread of certain types of infectious diseases, there are general principles that are basic to the care of any patient who is a source of infection to others or likely to become infected by those who are in contact with him. The factors most important in preventing the spread of infection are proper disinfection techniques and conscientious handwashing. The hands are used for many tasks in patient care and are an excellent source of infection if they are not washed properly before and after each contact with the patient or with articles in his environment.

Disinfection can be concurrent or terminal. *Concurrent disinfection* refers to immediate destruction of infectious agents as they leave the body, or after they have contaminated linen, eating utensils, hospital equipment, and other objects that have come in contact with the patient, his excreta, or discharge from wounds. Concurrent disinfection is a continuous process in the daily care of the patient.

Terminal disinfection refers to destruction of pathogenic microorganisms remaining in the patient's environment after he is no longer considered to be a source of infection.

The spread of microorganisms can be kept at a minimum if it is always kept in mind that one must touch only 'clean' to 'clean' and 'contaminated' to 'contaminated'. Once a clean article comes in contact with a contaminated article, both must be considered contaminated. In this context the word 'clean' does not mean unsoiled; it means that an object is free from the organisms causing the patient's illness. Unsoiled linen, for example, might be contaminated with infectious agents and therefore could not be considered clean.

While carrying out the multitude of special procedures and precautionary measures necessary in strict isolation technique, one must not forget their psychological impact on the patient, who should be told the reason for the precautions with special emphasis on concern for his well-being as well as for the protection of others. Unless very seriously ill some provision should be made for diversional activities that will help relieve the loneliness and boredom that result from isolation from other human beings.

Visitors are limited to a very few persons and they should be instructed in the ways in which the patient's disease can be spread and the precautions necessary to prevent infection of others. If the patient is a child, parents are allowed to stay; they should wear protective clothing as prescribed by local policy. Toys, books, and other items brought into the unit for the child's amusement must be of the type that can be thoroughly disinfected; otherwise it will be necessary to dispose of them when he is no longer ill.

isoleucine (ˌiesoh'looseen) an amino acid produced by hydrolysis of fibrin and other proteins; essential for optimal infant growth and for nitrogen equilibrium in adults.

isologous (ie'sologəs) characterized by an identical genotype.

isolysin (ie'solisin) a lysin acting on cells of animals of the same species as that from which it is derived.

isolysis (ie'solisis) lysis of cells by isolysins. adj. **isolytic.**

isomer ('iesəmə) any compound exhibiting, or capable of exhibiting isomerism. adj. **isomeric.**

isomerase (ie'somə·rayz) a major class of enzymes comprising those that catalyse the process of isomerization, such as the interconversion of aldoses and ketoses.

isomerism (ie'somə·rizəm) the possession by two or more distinct compounds of the same molecular formula, each molecule having the same number of atoms of each element, but in different arrangement.

isomerization (ieˌsomə·rie'zayshən) the process whereby any isomer is converted into another isomer, usually requiring special conditions of temperature, pressure, or catalysts.

isometric (ˌiesoh'metrik) maintaining, or pertaining to, the same length; of equal dimensions.

i. contraction muscle contraction without appreciable shortening or change in distance between its origin and insertion.

i. exercise active exercise performed against stable resistance, without change in the length of the muscle.

isometropia (ˌiesohme'trohpi·ə) equality in refraction of the two eyes.

isomorphism (ˌiesoh'mawfizəm) identity in form; in genetics, referring to genotypes of polypoid organisms that produce similar gametes even though containing genes in different combinations on homologous chromosomes. adj. **isomorphic.**

isoniazid (ˌiesoh'nieəzid) an antibacterial compound used in treatment of tuberculosis.

isopathy (ie'sopəthee) the treatment of disease by means of products of the disease or with material from the affected organ. adj. **isopathic.**

isophoria (ˌiesoh'for·ri·ə) correspondence of the visual axes of the two eyes; equality in the tension of the vertical muscles of the two eyes.

isoprecipitin (ˌiesohpri'sipitin) an isoantibody that acts as a precipitin.

isoprenaline (ˌiesoh'prenəlin) a sympathomimetic used as a bronchodilator and cardiac stimulant.

isopropanol (ˌiesoh'prohpəˌnol) isopropyl alcohol, used as a solvent and as a rubefacient.

isopter (ie'soptə) a curve representing areas of equal visual acuity in the field of vision.
Isopto-Carpine (ie'soptoh,kahpeen) trademark for a preparation of pilocarpine hydrochloride, an ophthalmic cholinergic.
isopyknosis (,iesohpik'nohsis) the quality of showing uniform density throughout, especially the uniformity of condensation observed in comparison of different chromosomes or in different areas of the same chromosome. adj. **isopyknotic.**
Isordil (ie'sordil) trademark for a preparation of isosorbide, a coronary vasodilator.
isorrhoea (,iesə'reeə) an equilibrium between the intake and output, by the body, of water and/or solutes. adj. **isorrhoeic.**
isosensitization (,iesoh,sensitie'zayshən) allosensitization.
isosexual (,iesoh'seksyooəl) pertaining to or characteristic of the same sex.
isosmotic (,iesoz'motik) having the same osmotic pressure.
isosorbide (,iesoh'sorbied) an osmotic diuretic; the dinitrate and mononitrate of isosorbide are used as coronary vasodilators in treatment of coronary insufficiency and angina pectoris.
Isospora (ie'sospə·rə) a genus of sporozoan parasites (order Coccidia), found in birds, amphibians, reptiles, and various mammals, including man; *I. belli* and *I. hominis* are aetiological agents of coccidiosis in man.
isospore ('iesoh,spor) 1. an isogamete of organisms that reproduce by spores. 2. an asexual spore produced by a homosporous organism.
isosthenuria (,iesohsthə'nyooə·ri·ə) maintenance of a constant osmolality of the urine, regardless of changes in osmotic pressure of the blood.
isotherm ('iesoh,thərm) a line on a map or chart joining the points at which the temperature is the same.
isothermal, isothermic (,iesoh'thərməl; ,iesoh'thərmik) having the same temperature.
isotone ('iesoh,tohn) one of several nuclides having the same number of neutrons, but differing in number of protons in their nuclei.
isotonia (,iesoh'tohni·ə) 1. a condition of equal tone, tension, or activity. 2. equality of osmotic pressure between two elements of a solution or between two different solutions.
isotonic (,iesoh'tonik) 1. of equal tension. 2. denoting a solution in which body cells can be bathed without net flow of water across the semipermeable cell membrane; also, denoting a solution having the same tonicity as another solution with which it is compared.
i. contraction muscle contraction without appreciable change in the force of contraction; the distance between the muscle's origin and insertion becomes lessened.
i. exercise active exercise without appreciable change in the force of muscular contraction, with shortening of the muscle.
isotope ('iesoh,tohp) a chemical element having the same atomic number as another (i.e., the same number of nuclear protons), but having a different atomic mass (i.e., a different number of nuclear neutrons).
radioactive i. one having an unstable nucleus and which emits characteristic radiation during its decay to a stable form. See also RADIOISOTOPE.
stable i. one that does not transmute into another element with emission of corpuscular or electromagnetic radiations.
isotretinoin (,iesoh'tretinoh·in) a vitamin A derivative used in the treatment of acne.
isotropic (,iesoh'tropik) 1. having the same value of a property, such as refractive index, in all directions, as in a cubic crystal or a piece of glass. 2. being singly refractive.
isotropy (ie'sotrəpee) the quality or condition of being isotropic.
isotypical (,iesoh'tipik'l) of the same kind.
isoxsuprine (ie'soksyuh,preen) a beta-adrenergic stimulant used as a vasodilator in peripheral vascular disease and cerebrovascular insufficiency.
isozyme ('iesoh,ziem) isoenzyme.
issue ('ishoo) a discharge of pus, blood, or other matter; a suppurating lesion emitting such a discharge.
isthmectomy (is'mektəmee) excision of an isthmus, especially of the isthmus of the thyroid.
isthmoparalysis, isthmoplegia (,ismohpə'ralisis; ,ismoh'pleeji·ə) paralysis of the isthmus faucium.
isthmus ('isməs) a narrow connection between two larger bodies or parts. adj. **isthmian.**
i. of auditory tube, i. of pharyngotympanic tube the narrowest part of the pharyngotympanic tube at the junction of its bony and cartilaginous parts.
i. of fauces, i. faucium the constricted aperture between the cavity of the mouth and the pharynx.
i. of rhombencephalon the narrow segment of the fetal brain, forming the plane of separation between the rhombencephalon and cerebrum.
i. of thyroid the band of tissue joining the lobes of the thyroid.
i. of uterine tube the narrower, thicker-walled portion of the uterine tube closest to the uterus.
i. of uterus the constricted part of the uterus between the cervix and the body of the uterus.
isuria (ie'syooə·ri·ə) excretion of urine at a uniform rate.
itch (ich) a skin disease attended with itching.
bakers' i. any of several inflammatory dermatoses of the hands, especially chronic candidal paronychia, seen with special frequency in bakers.
barber's i. infection and irritation of the hair follicles of the beard region (see also SYCOSIS BARBAE).
dhobie i. 1. allergic contact dermatitis, caused by catechols in the marking fluid used on laundry by native washermen (dhobie) in India. 2. a term for ringworm of the groin.
grain i. itching dermatitis due to a mite, *Pyemotes ventricosus*, which preys on certain insect larvae which live on straw, grain, and other plants.
grocers' i. a vesicular dermatitis caused by certain mites found in stored hides, dried fruits, grain, dried coconut, and cheese.
ground i. the itching eruption caused by the entrance into the skin of the larvae of the hookworm *Ancylostoma duodenale* or *Necator americanus* (see also HOOKWORM DISEASE).
seven-year i. scabies.
winter i. itching of the skin in cold weather, unassociated with structural lesions.
itching ('iching) pruritus; an unpleasant cutaneous sensation, provoking the desire to scratch or rub the skin.
-itis pl. *itides;* word element. [Gr.] inflammation.
ITP idiopathic thrombocytopenic purpura.
ITU intensive therapy unit.
IU International Unit.
IUCD intrauterine contraceptive device.
IUD intrauterine death.
IV, i.v. intravenous(ly).
IVP intraveous pyelogram.
IVS International Voluntary Service.
Ixodes (ik'sohdeez) a genus of hard-bodied ticks (family Ixodidae); some species are vectors of disease.
ixodiasis (,iksoh'dieəsis) any disease or lesion due to

tick bites; infestation with ticks.

ixodic (ik'sodik) pertaining to, or caused by, ticks.

Ixodidae (ik'sodi,dee) a family of ticks (superfamily Ixodoidea), comprising the hard-bodied ticks.

Ixodides (ik'sodi,deez) the ticks, a suborder of Acarina, including the superfamily Ixodoidea.

Ixodoidea (,iksoh'doydi·ə) a superfamily of arthropods (suborder Ixodides), comprising both the hard- and soft-bodied ticks.

J

J symbol for *joule.*

jacket ('jakit) an encasement or covering for the trunk, especially the thorax.

plaster-of-Paris j. a casing of plaster of Paris enveloping the body, for the purpose of giving support or correcting deformities (see also CAST).

Sayre's j. a plaster-of-Paris jacket used as a support for the vertebral column.

strait j. straitjacket.

jacksonian epilepsy (jak'sohni·ən) a form of EPILEPSY marked by clonic movements that start in one muscle group and spread systematically to adjacent groups.

jactitation (,jakti'tayshən) restless tossing to and fro in acute illness.

janiceps ('jani,seps) a double fetus or infant with one head and two opposite faces.

jaundice ('jawndis) yellowness of skin, sclerae, mucous membranes, and excretions due to hyperbilirubinaemia and deposition of BILE pigments. Called also *icterus.* It is usually first noticeable in the eyes, although it may come on so gradually that it is not immediately noticed by those in daily contact with the jaundiced person.

Jaundice is not a disease. It is a symptom of one of a number of different diseases and disorders of the LIVER, GALLBLADDER, and blood. One such disorder is the presence of a gallstone in the common bile duct, which carries bile from the liver to the intestine. This may obstruct the flow of bile, causing it to accumulate and enter the bloodstream. The obstruction of bile flow may cause bile to enter the urine, making it dark in colour, and also decrease the bile in the stool, making it light and clay-coloured. This condition requires surgery to remove the gallstone before it causes serious liver injury.

Certain diseases of the blood, such as haemolytic anaemia, increase the amount of yellow pigment in the bile, causing jaundice.

The pigment causing jaundice is called BILIRUBIN. It is derived from haemoglobin that is released when erythrocytes are haemolysed and therefore is constantly being formed and introduced into the blood as worn-out or defective erythrocytes are destroyed by the body. Normally the liver cells absorb the bilirubin and secrete it along with other bile constituents. If the liver is diseased, or if the flow of bile is obstructed, or if destruction of erythrocytes is excessive, the bilirubin accumulates in the blood and eventually will produce jaundice. Determination of the level of bilirubin in the blood is of value in detecting elevated bilirubin levels at the earliest stages before jaundice appears, when liver disease or haemolytic anaemia is suspected.

acholuric j. jaundice without bilirubinaemia, associated with elevated unconjugated bilirubin that is not excreted by the kidney.

breast milk j. elevated unconjugated bilirubin in some breast-fed infants due to the presence of 5-β-pregnane-3-α-20-β-diol, which inhibits glucuronyl transferase conjugating activity.

cholestatic j. that resulting from abnormality of bile flow in the liver.

haematogenous j. haemolytic jaundice.

haemolytic j. jaundice associated with HAEMOLYTIC ANAEMIA.

haemorrhagic j. leptospiral jaundice.

hepatocellular j. jaundice caused by injury to or disease of the liver cells.

homologous serum j. serum hepatitis.

infectious j., infective j 1. infectious hepatitis. 2. leptospiral jaundice.

leptospiral j. severe leptospirosis with fever, jaundice, myalgia, and occasionally with nephritis and meningitis. The symptoms last from 10 days to 2 weeks and recovery is usually uneventful. Called also *Weil's disease.*

nonhaemolytic j. that due to an abnormality in bilirubin metabolism.

obstructive j. that due to blockage of the flow of bile.

physiological j. mild icterus neonatorum during the first few days after birth.

jaw (jor) either of the two opposing bony structures (maxilla and mandible) of the mouth of vertebrates; they bear the teeth and are used for seizing prey, for biting, or for masticating food.

j. bone the mandible or maxilla, especially the mandible.

Hapsburg j. a mandibular prognathous jaw, often accompanied by Hapsburg lip.

phossy j. phosphonecrosis.

jaw-winking ('jaw,wingking) elevation of a congenitally ptotic eyelid when the mouth is opened, giving the appearance of constant winking.

JCA juvenile chronic arthritis.

Jeanselme's nodules (zhonh'selmz) gummata of tertiary syphilis and of nonvenereal treponemal diseases, located on joint capsules, bursae, or tendon sheaths.

Jectofer ('jektəfə) trademark for a preparation of iron sorbitol.

jejunectomy (,jejuh'nektəmee) excision of the jejunum.

jejunitis (,jejuh'nietis) inflammation of the jejunum.

jejunocaecostomy (ji,joonohsi'kostəmee) anastomosis of the jejunum to the caecum.

jejunocolostomy (ji,joonohkə'lostəmee) anastomosis of the jejunum to the colon.

jejunoileal (ji,joonoh'ili·əl) pertaining to the jejunum and ileum; connecting the proximal jejunum with the distal ileum.

jejunoileitis (ji,joonoh,ili'ietis) inflammation of the jejunum and ileum.

jejunoileostomy (ji,joonoh,ili'ostəmee) surgical creation of an anastomosis between the proximal jejunum and the terminal ileum; anastomosis of the jejunum to the ileum.

jejunojejunostomy (ji,joonoh,jejuh'nostəmee) surgical anastomosis between two portions of the jejunum.

jejunorrhaphy (,jejuh'no·rəfee) operative repair of the jejunum.

jejunostomy (,jejuh'nostəmee) surgical creation of a permanent opening between the jejunum and the surface of the abdominal wall.

jejunotomy (,jejuh'notəmee) incision of the jejunum.

jejunum (ji'joonəm) that part of the small intestine extending from the duodenum to the ileum. adj. **jejunal.**

jelly ('jelee) a soft, coherent, resilient substance; generally, a colloidal semisolid mass.

cardiac j. a gelatinous substance present between the endothelium and myocardium of the embryonic heart that transforms into the connective tissue of the endocardium.

contraceptive j. a nongreasy jelly used in the vagina for prevention of conception (see also CONTRACEPTION).

petroleum j. a purified mixture of semisolid hydrocarbons obtained from petroleum (called also PETROLATUM).

Wharton's j. the soft, jelly-like intracellular substance of the umbilical cord, which insulates the vein and arteries preventing occlusion and fetal hypoxia.

Jenner ('jenə) Edward (1749–1823). English physician. Born at Berkeley, Gloucestershire, he discovered the principle of smallpox vaccination in 1796. By experimental demonstration, Jenner turned a local country tradition that dairymaids who had contracted cowpox did not acquire smallpox into a permanent working principle in science.

jennerian (je'niə·ri·ən) relating to Edward Jenner, who developed vaccination.

jerk (jərk) a sudden reflex or involuntary movement.

Achilles j., ankle j. plantar extension of the foot elicited by a tap on the Achilles tendon, preferably while the patient kneels on a bed or chair, the feet hanging free over the edge; called also Achilles reflex, and triceps surae jerk or reflex.

biceps j. biceps reflex. Involuntary flexion of the elbow elicited by tapping the lower end of the radius causing contraction of the biceps muscle.

jaw j. jaw-jerk reflex.

knee j. contraction of the quadriceps muscle and extension of the leg elicited by tapping the patellar ligament when the leg hangs loosely flexed at a right angle (see also KNEE JERK).

tendon j. tendon reflex.

triceps j. involuntary extension of the forearm, elicited by tapping triceps tendon just above the olecranon causing contraction of the triceps brachii muscle.

triceps surae j. ankle jerk.

jigger ('jigə) a sand flea found in the tropics (see CHIGOE).

joint (joynt) the site of the junction or union of two or more bones of the body. The primary function of a joint is to provide motion and flexibility to the human frame.

Some joints are immovable, such as certain fixed joints where segments of bone are fused together in the skull. Other joints, such as those between the vertebrae, have extremely limited motion. However, most joints allow considerable motion.

Many joints have an extremely complex internal structure. They are composed not merely of ends of bones but also of ligaments, which are tough whitish fibres binding the bones together; cartilage, which is connective tissue, covering and cushioning the bone ends; the articular capsule, a fibrous tissue that encloses the ends of the bones; the synovial membrane, which lines the capsule and secretes a lubricating fluid (synovia); and sometimes bursae, which are fluid-filled sacs that cushion the movements of muscles and tendons.

Joints are classified by variations in structure that make different kinds of movement possible. The movable joints are usually subdivided into hinge, pivot, gliding, ball-and-socket, condyloid, and saddle joints.

DISEASES AND DISORDERS. Joints are often subject to great stress in day-to-day living; likewise they are exposed daily to injuries of all kinds because of their prominent location on the body. Wrenches and SPRAINS are fairly common. DISLOCATIONS are only slightly less frequent and they may be the aftermath of disease as well as accident. Joints can also be subject to inflammation. The two most prevalent types are OSTEOARTHRITIS, a degenerative joint disorder common to elderly people, and rheumatoid ARTHRITIS, which may occur in even the very young and the cause of which is largely unknown. BURSITIS is inflammation of one or more bursae. It may cause pain and partial or complete immobility of the adjacent joint; it may be either acute or chronic. Synovitis, painful inflammation of the lining of the synovial membrane, may be caused by external injury or by disease, for example, tuberculosis or syphilis. ANKYLOSIS is immobility and solidification of a joint.

arthrodial j. gliding joint.

ball-and-socket j. a synovial joint in which the rounded or spheroidal surface of one bone ('ball') moves within a cup-shaped depression ('socket') on another bone, allowing greater freedom of movement than any other type of joint. Called also *spheroidal joint.*

cartilaginous j. one in which the bones are united by cartilage, providing slight flexible movement; it includes symphysis and synchondrosis.

condyloid j. one in which an ovoid head of one bone moves in an elliptical cavity of another, permitting all movements except axial rotation. Such a joint is found at the wrist, connecting the radius and carpal bones, and at the base of the index finger.

diarthrodial j. synovial joint.

facet j's the articulations of the vertebral column.

fibrous j. one in which the bones are connected by fibrous tissue and no or very little motion is possible; it includes suture, syndesmosis, and gomphosis. Called also *synarthrodial joint.*

flail j. an unusually mobile joint.

gliding j. a synovial joint in which the opposed surfaces are flat or only slightly curved, so that the bones slide against each other in a simple and limited way. The intervertebral joints are gliding joints, and many of the small bones of the wrist and ankle meet in gliding joints. Called also *arthrodial joint* and *plane joint.*

hinge j. a synovial joint that allows movement in only one plane, forward and backward. Examples are the elbow and the interphalangeal joints of the fingers. The jaw is primarily a hinge joint but it can also move somewhat from side to side. The knee and ankle joints are hinge joints that also allow some rotary movement. Called also *ginglymus.*

hip j. the joint formed at the head of the femur and the acetabulum of the hip bone; loosely called hip.

knee j. the compound joint between the femur, patella, and tibia.

pivot j. a joint in which one bone pivots within a bony or an osseoligamentous ring, allowing only rotary movement; an example is the joint between the first and second cervical vertebrae (the atlas and axis).

plane j. gliding joint.

saddle j. a joint whose movement resembles that of a rider on horseback, who can shift in several directions at will; there is a saddle joint at the base of the thumb, so that the thumb is more flexible and complex than the other fingers, and more difficult to treat if injured.

spheroidal j. ball-and-socket joint.

synarthrodial j. fibrous joint.

synovial j. a specialized form of articulation permitting more or less free movement, the union of the bony elements being surrounded by an articular capsule enclosing a cavity lined by synovial membrane. Called also *diarthrosis* and *diarthrodial joint.*

joule (jool) the SI unit of energy, being the work done

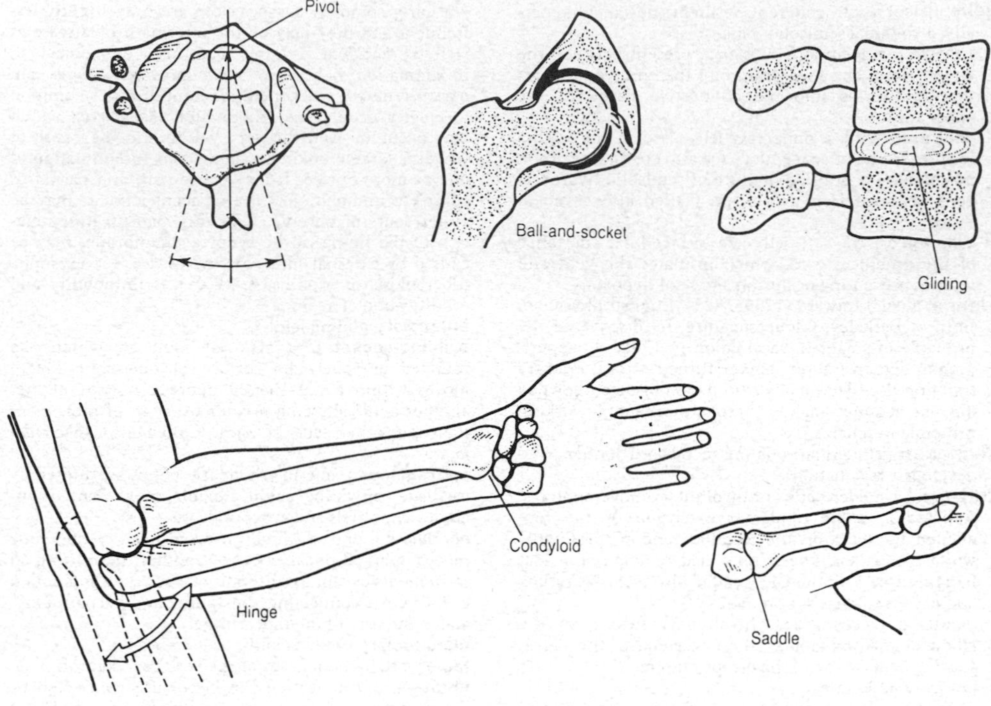

Synovial joints

by a force of 1 newton acting over a distance of 1 metre. Symbol J.

judgement ('jujmənt) the ability of an individual to estimate a situation, to arrive at reasonable conclusions, and to decide on a course of action.

jugal ('joog'l) pertaining to the cheek or zygomatic (cheek) bone.

j. point the point at the angle formed by the masseteric and maxillary edges of the zygomatic bone. Called also *jugale*.

jugale (joo'gaylee) jugal point.

jugular ('jugyuhlə) 1. pertaining to the neck. 2. one of the jugular veins.

j. veins large veins that return blood to the heart from the head and neck.

Each side of the neck has two sets of jugular veins, external and internal. The external jugular carries blood from the face, neck, and scalp and has two branches, posterior and anterior. The internal jugular vein receives blood from the brain, the deeper tissues of the neck and the interior of the skull. The external jugular vein empties into the subclavian vein, and the internal jugular vein joins it to form the brachiocephalic vein, which carries the blood to the superior vena cava, where it continues to the heart.

If one of these veins is severed, rapid loss of blood will result and air bubbles may enter the circulatory system unless preventive measures are taken. If such an event should occur, a compress should be applied to the wound with pressure. Under no circumstance is a tourniquet used.

jugum ('joogəm) pl. *juga* [L.] a depression or ridge connecting two structures.

j. penis a forceps for compressing the penis.

juice (joos) any fluid from animal or plant tissue.

gastric j. the liquid secretion of the gastric glands (see also GASTRIC JUICE).

intestinal j. the liquid secretion of glands in the intestinal lining.

pancreatic j. the enzyme-containing secretion of the pancreas, conducted through its ducts to the duodenum.

junction ('jungkshən) the place of meeting or coming together. adj. **junctional**.

neuromuscular j. the point of junction of a nerve fibre with the motor endplate of the skeletal muscle that it innervates.

sclerocorneal j. the line of union of the sclera and cornea.

junctura (jungk'tyoo·rə) pl. *juncturae* [L.] a junction or joint.

Jung (yuhng) Carl Gustav (1875–1961). Swiss-born psychologist and psychiatrist; the founder of analytical psychology. He received his medical degree from the University of Basel and continued his education at the University of Zurich, where he worked as research assistant and lecturer and later served on the staff of the university psychiatric clinic under the direction of Eugen Bleuler, another important Swiss psychologist.

Analytical psychotherapy as formulated by Jung

attaches more importance to analysis and interpretation of certain aspects of the subject's dreams and fantasies and far less emphasis on free association than does freudian psychoanalysis.

Jung's view of the dynamics of personality represents an attempt to interpret human behaviour from a philosophical, religious, and mystical, as well as scientific, viewpoint. The whole personality (psyche) consists of these three interacting systems: the *collective unconscious*, the *personal unconscious*, and the *conscious mind (ego)*.

The *ego* is the centre of the conscious, comprising the conscious perceptions, thoughts, and feelings, and is the focal point for individual identity. The *personal unconscious* consists of the individual's experiences, wishes, and impulses, which were once conscious but have been repressed or forgotten, but can be brought to consciousness once again. The *collective unconscious* is that part of the psyche which retains and transmits the cumulative experience of all previous generations. The structural components of the collective unconscious are the ARCHETYPES, the universal patterns of behaviour, the inherited dispositions which dispose an individual to experience and behave in eternally recurrent situations (birth, death, marriage, war, religious customs, initiations, etc.) as his ancestors experienced and behaved in them. The primary archetype from which all others come is the *self*, the organizing centre from which all the regulatory forces of the psyche emanate, expressed in the innate striving of each person toward psychic wholeness through INDIVIDUATION.

jurisprudence (ˌjooə·ris'prood'ns) the science of the law.

medical j. the science of the law as applied to the practice of medicine.

juvenile ('joovəˌniel) 1. pertaining to youth or childhood; young or immature. 2. a youth or child; a young animal. 3. a cell or organism intermediate between the immature and mature forms.

juxta- word element. [L.] *situated near, adjoining.*

juxta-articular (ˌjukstə·ah'tikyuhlə) near or in the region of a joint.

juxtaglomerular (ˌjukstəglo'meryuhlə) near to or adjoining a glomerulus of the kidney.

juxtaposition (ˌjukstəpə'zishən) apposition; a placing side by side or close together; the condition of being side by side or close together.

juxtapyloric (ˌjukstəpie'loorik) near the pylorus.

juxtaspinal (ˌjukstə'spien'l) near the vertebral column.

juxtavesical (ˌjukstə'vesik'l) situated near or adjoining the urinary bladder.

K

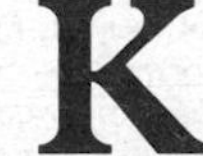

K chemical symbol, *potassium* (L. *kalium*); symbol for *kelvin.*

k symbol, *kilo-.*

Kabikinase (kabi'kienayz) trademark for a preparation of streptokinase used in the treatment of life-threatening venous thrombosis and pulmonary embolism.

Kahler's disease ('kahləz) multiple myeloma.

Kahn test (kahn) an agglutination test for syphilis.

kak- for words beginning thus, see also those beginning *cac-.*

kakosmia (ka'kozmi·ə) cacosmia.

kala-azar (ˌkahlə·ə'zah) an infectious disease, highly fatal if untreated, endemic in the tropics and subtropics, caused by the protozoon *Leishmania donovani.* Sandflies of the genus *Phlebotomus* are the vectors. Called also *visceral leishmaniasis.*

SYMPTOMS. Symptoms are usually vague, resembling those of incipient pulmonary tuberculosis. The disease is often confused with malaria. There may be fever, chills, malaise, cough, anorexia, anaemia, and wasting. The *Leishmania* organisms multiply in the cells of the reticuloendothelial system, eventually causing hyperplasia of the cells, especially those of the liver and spleen. Diagnosis is confirmed by demonstration of the parasite.

TREATMENT. Two groups of compounds are recommended: pentavalent organic antimonials, such as sodium antimony gluconate, and aromatic diamidines, such as pentamidine.

kalaemia, kaliaemia (kə'leemi·ə; ˌkali'eemi·ə) the presence of potassium in the blood.

kaliopenia (ˌkaylioh'peeni·ə) hypokalaemia.

kalium ('kayli·əm) [L.] *potassium* (symbol K).

kaliuresis (ˌkayliyuh'reesis) excretion of potassium in the urine.

kaliuretic (ˌkayliyuh'retik) 1. pertaining to or promoting kaliuresis. 2. an agent that promotes kaliuresis.

kallidin ('kalidin) kinin liberated by the action of kallikrein on a globulin of blood plasma. Kallidin I is the same as bradykinin; kallidin II is composed of bradykinin with a lysine added at the *N*-terminal.

kallikrein (ˌkali'kree·in) any of a group of enzymes present in various glands, lymph, urine, blood plasma, etc., the major action of which is the liberation of kinins from α-2-globulins, and hence which have vasodilator and whealing actions.

kallikreinogen (ˌkali'krienəjən) the inactive precursor of kallikrein which is normally present in blood.

kanamycin (ˌkana'miesın) a broad-spectrum antibiotic derived from *Streptomyces kanamyceticus*; effective against many gram-negative bacteria, and some gram-positive bacteria and acid-fast bacteria.

Kanner's syndrome, Kannerian psychosis ('kanəz; kə'niə·ri·ən) early infantile autism.

Kantrex ('kantreks) trademark for preparations of kanamycin, an antibiotic.

kaolin ('kayəlin) native hydrated aluminium silicate, powdered and freed from gritty particles by elutriation; used externally (in a poultice) as an adsorbent and protective, and internally (in a mixture) as a gastrointestinal adsorbent and demulcent in mild diarrhoea.

kaolinosis (ˌkayəli'nohsis) pneumoconiosis from inhaling particles of kaolin.

Kaposi's sarcoma ('kapohˌzeez) a multifocal, metastasizing, malignant reticulosis with angiosarcoma-like features, involving chiefly the skin. Rarely seen in the developed world until the outbreak of AIDS. Kaposi's sarcoma is a major feature of this disease, particularly in homosexuals.

Kaposi's varicelliform eruption a generalized and serious vesiculopustular eruption of viral origin, superimposed on preexisting atopic dermatitis; it may be due to the herpes simplex virus (eczema herpeticum) or the vaccinia virus (eczema vaccinatum). Called also *Kaposi's spots.*

karaya gum (kə'rie·ə) the dried gummy exudation from *Sterculia urens* or other species of *Sterculia*, which becomes gelatinous when moisture is added. It is available in rings that can be moulded into any desired shape. Products containing karaya gum are often used as protective skin barriers in the care of COLOSTOMY and other conditions in which there is a

STOMA. Called also *sterculia gum*.

Kartagener's syndrome (kah'taginərz) a hereditary syndrome consisting of dextrocardia, bronchiectasis, and sinusitis.

karyo- word element. [Gr.] *nucleus*.

karyocyte ('karioh,siet) a nucleated cell.

karyogenesis (,karioh'jenəsis) the formation of a cell nucleus. adj. **karyogenic**.

karyokinesis (,kariohki'neesis) division of the nucleus, usually an early stage in the process of cell division, or mitosis. adj. **karyokinetic**.

karyolymph ('karioh,limf) the fluid portion of the nucleus of a cell, in which the other elements are dispersed.

karyolysis (,kari'olisis) the dissolution of the nucleus of a cell. adj. **karyolytic**.

karyomegaly (,karioh'megəlee) abnormal enlargement of the nucleus of a cell.

karyomorphism (,karioh'mawfizəm) the shape of a cell nucleus.

karyon ('karion) the nucleus of a cell.

karyophage ('karioh,fayj) a protozoon that phagocytizes the nucleus of the cell it infects.

karyoplasm ('karioh,plazəm) nucleoplasm.

karyopyknosis (,kariohpik'nohsis) shrinkage of a cell nucleus, with condensation of the chromatin. adj. **karyopyknotic**.

karyorrhexis (,kari·ə'reksis) rupture of the cell nucleus in which the chromatin disintegrates into formless granules. adj. **karyorrhectic**.

karyotheca (,karioh'theekə) the nuclear membrane.

karyotype ('karioh,tiep) the chromosomal constitution of the cell nucleus; by extension, the photomicrograph of chromosomes arranged in numerical order.

Kashin–Beck disease (,kashin'bek) a disabling degenerative disease of the peripheral joints and spine, endemic in eastern Siberia, northern China, and Korea; believed to be caused by ingestion of cereal grains infected with the fungus *Fusarium sporotrichiella*.

kat katal.

kat(a)- word element. [Gr.] *down, against;* see also words beginning *cat(a)-*.

katal ('katəl) a unit of measurement proposed to express activities of all catalysts, including enzymes, being that amount of a catalyst that catalyses a reaction rate of 1 mole of substrate per second. Symbol kat.

katathermometer (,katətha'momitə) a thermometer with a wet bulb and a dry bulb, for detecting cooling rates.

Katayama fever (,katə'yəmə) fever resulting from a sensitivity reaction to severe schistosomal infections, accompanied by hepatosplenomegaly and by eosinophilia.

Kawasaki's disease (,kahwə'sahkeez) an illness of unknown aetiology characterized by high fever, macroerythematous rash, cervical lymph node swelling, and pain; called also mucocutaneous lymph node syndrome. Treatment is largely supportive; however, corticosteroids are contraindicated. If the disease is fatal, death occurs as a result of cardiomyopathy and vasculitis.

Kayser–Fleischer ring (,kiezə'flieshə) a grey-green to red-gold pigmented ring at the outer margin of the cornea, seen in progressive lenticular degeneration and pseudosclerosis.

kcal kilocalorie.

Kefadol ('kefədol) trademark for a preparation of cefamandole, a broad-spectrum cephalosporin antibiotic.

Keflex ('kefleks) trademark for preparations of cephalexin, an oral cephalosporin.

Keflin ('keflin) trademark for a preparation of cephalothin, an analogue of cephalosporin C.

Kefzol ('kefzol) trademark for a preparation of cephazolin, a cephalosporin antibiotic.

Kegel exercises ('kaygəl) specific exercises named after Dr. Arnold H. Kegel, a gynaecologist who first developed the exercises to strengthen the pelvic–vaginal muscles as a means of controlling stress incontinence in women. He later learned from patients who had been performing the exercises that strengthening of the pubococcygeus muscle, a sphincteric muscle that surrounds the vagina, also improved feminine sexual response and contributed to the attainment of orgasm. Research has since demonstrated that this muscle contains specialized nerve endings which contribute to a satisfactory sexual experience.

A third area in which the Kegel exercises are important is in NATURAL CHILDBIRTH. The exercises strengthen the pelvic floor and therefore are helpful in reducing discomfort and congestion during pregnancy and in providing support for the pelvic organs before and after birth. During delivery the mother who has developed good tone and conscious control over the pubococcygeus muscle is able to release the muscle and thereby facilitate the passage of the infant through the birth canal. After delivery the exercises maintain the strength of the muscle and greatly diminish the possibility of rectocele and cystocele, dyspareunia, and other after-effects of delivery.

Most patients must be taught an awareness of the muscle and how to control it. This usually can be done by having the woman shut off urine flow while sitting with the knees widely separated. After a few trials the sensation of control is recognized and the patient is able to perform the exercise on her own. Usually the exercises are begun with five or ten contractions before arising in the morning and also during each voiding of urine. Gradually the number of sessions and the number of contractions are increased until ultimately a pattern of three hundred daily contractions is reached. The exercises require concentration but a small expenditure of energy. Once the muscle has been strengthened it tends to maintain its strength and state of partial contraction at all times. Sexual activity helps preserve the muscle tone.

Keith's bundle (keeths) a bundle of fibres in the wall of the right atrium between the openings of the venae cavae; called also *sinoatrial bundle*.

Keith–Flack node (,keeth'flak) sinoatrial node.

Keith's node (keeths) sinoatrial node.

Keith–Wagener–Barker classification (,keeth-,wagənə'bahkə) a classification of hypertension and arteriolosclerosis based on retinal changes.

Keller's arthroplasty (operation) ('keləz) excision arthroplasty of the first metatarsophalangeal joint for correcting hallux valgus.

keloid ('keeloyd) a protuberant, prominent scar, due to excessive collagen formation in the corium during connective tissue repair. It is common in pigmented skin and not infrequent in pregnancy. adj. **keloidal**.

Keloids are generally considered harmless and noncancerous, although they may produce contractures. Ordinarily they cause no trouble beyond an occasional itching sensation.

Surgical removal is not effective because of a high rate of recurrence.

kelvin ('kelvin) the SI unit of absolute temperature, equal to 1/273.15 of the absolute temperature of the triple point of water. Symbol K.

Kelvin scale ('kelvin) a scale of temperature in which measurements are made from absolute zero. The unit of measurement corresponds to that of the CELSIUS (centigrade) SCALE, but the ice point is at 273.15 K.

Kelvin thermometer ('kelvin) a thermometer employing the KELVIN SCALE.

Kemadrin ('kemədrin) trademark for a preparation of procyclidine, an antiparkinsonism drug.

Kemicetine (kemee'seteen, -in) trademark for a preparation of chloramphenicol, an antibiotic.

Kenalog ('kenəlog) trademark for a preparation of triamcinolone acetonide, a prednisolone derivative used as an anti-inflammatory steroid administered by deep intramuscular injection. See also TRIAMCINOLONE.

Kennedy's syndrome ('kenədiz) ipsilateral optic atrophy caused by a frontal lobe tumour which involves one of the optic nerves.

Kenny treatment ('kenee) treatment of poliomyelitis by wrapping the patient in woollen cloths wrung out of hot water and re-educating muscles by passive exercises after pain has subsided.

keno- word element. [Gr.] *empty.*

kerasin ('kerəsin) a cerebroside from brain tissue, yielding galactose, sphingosine, and lignoceric acid on hydrolysis.

kerat(o)- word element. [Gr.] *horny tissue, cornea.*

keratalgia (ˌkerə'talji·ə) pain in the cornea.

keratan sulphate ('kerətan) either of two sulphated mucopolysaccharides (I and II). Keratan sulphate is an important component of the proteoglycan of cartilage, and occurs in the cornea and the nucleus pulposus.

keratectasia (ˌkerətek'tayzi·ə) protrusion of a thin, scarred cornea.

keratectomy (ˌkerə'tektəmee) excision of a portion of the cornea; kerectomy.

keratic (kə'ratik) 1. pertaining to keratin. 2. pertaining to the cornea.

keratin ('kerətin) a scleroprotein that is the principal constituent of epidermis, hair, nails, horny tissues, and the organic matrix of the enamel of the teeth. Its solution is sometimes used in coating pills when the latter are desired to pass through the stomach unchanged.

keratinase (kə'ratiˌnayz) a proteolytic enzyme that hydrolyses keratin.

keratinization (ˌkerətinie'zayshən) the development of or conversion into keratin.

keratinocyte (kə'ratinohˌsiet) the cell of the epidermis that synthesizes keratin, known in its successive stages in the various layers of the skin as basal cell, prickle cell, and granular cell.

keratinous (kə'ratinəs) containing or of the nature of keratin.

keratitis (ˌkerə'tietis) inflammation of the cornea. Keratitis may be deep, when the infection causing it is carried in the blood or spreads to the cornea from other parts of the eye, or superficial, caused by bacterial or viral infection or by allergic reaction. Agents causing the inflammation can be introduced into the cornea during the removal of foreign bodies from the eye. All infections of the eye are potentially serious because opaque fibrous tissue or scar tissue may form on the cornea during the healing process and cause partial or total loss of vision.

CAUSES. There are several kinds of keratitis. Dendritic patterns of corneal ulceration are caused by the herpes simplex virus; they usually affect only one eye. A bacterial form, acute serpiginous keratitis, may result from infection by pneumococci, streptococci, or staphylococci.

Burns of the cornea, such as those produced by chemicals or ultraviolet rays, also give rise to a form of keratitis. In TRACHOMA, an infectious disease of the conjunctiva, the eyes become inflamed, and small, gritty particles develop on the cornea. Herpetic keratitis may accompany HERPES ZOSTER.

Interstitial keratitis is very rarely caused by congenital syphilis, although occasionally it may also result from acquired SYPHILIS. When caused by congenital syphilis, the disease usually appears when the child is between the ages of 5 and 15. In other cases, interstitial keratitis may also be associated with tuberculosis or rheumatic infection in other parts of the body.

SYMPTOMS. Symptoms vary somewhat among the different forms of keratitis, but pain, which may be severe, and inability to tolerate light (photophobia) are usual. There may also be considerable effusion of tears and a conjunctival discharge.

TREATMENT. Antibiotics are the usual treatment for keratitis caused by an infectious organism. Cortisone is used for other forms, but may be dangerous in some patients. Antiviral agents, such as idoxuridine, have been used to treat herpes simplex (dendritic) keratitis. In cases of syphilitic interstitial keratitis, the syphilis is treated. Congenital interstitial keratitis can be prevented if syphilis is detected early in pregnancy by means of blood tests, and the mother is treated.

keratoacanthoma (ˌkerətohˌakən'thohmə) a rapidly growing, benign papular lesion, with a superficial crater filled with a keratin plug, usually on the face; it resolves spontaneously.

keratoconjunctivitis (ˌkerətohkənˌjungkti'vietis) inflammation of the cornea and conjunctiva.

epidemic k. a highly infectious form, commonly with regional lymph node involvement, occurring in epidemics; an adenovirus has been repeatedly isolated from affected patients.

phlyctenular k. a form marked by formation of a small, grey, circumscribed lesion at the corneal limbus.

k. sicca a condition marked by hyperaemia of the conjunctiva, thickening and drying of the corneal epithelium, and itching and burning of the eye.

keratoconus (ˌkerətoh'kohnəs) conical protrusion of the central part of the cornea, resulting in an irregular astigmatism.

keratocyst (ˌkerətoh'sist) a type of cyst occurring in the jaws which is keratinized and distinct from most other odontogenic cysts in that it has an exceedingly high recurrence rate.

keratoderma (ˌkerətoh'dərmə) hypertrophy of the horny layer of the skin.

k. blennorhagica pustular psoriasis associated with gonorrhoea.

k. climactericum, endocrine k. circumscribed hyperkeratosis of palms and soles, occurring in menopausal women.

keratodermia (ˌkerətoh'dərmi·ə) keratoderma.

keratogenous (ˌkerə'tojənəs) giving rise to a growth of horny material.

keratoglobus (ˌkerətoh'glohbəs) a bilateral anomaly in which the cornea is enlarged and globular in shape.

keratohaemia (ˌkerətoh'heemi·ə) deposition of blood in the cornea.

keratohelcosis (ˌkerətoh·helkohsis) ulceration of the cornea.

keratohyalin (ˌkerətoh'hieəlin) the substance in the granules in the stratum granulosum of the epidermis. adj. **keratohyaline.**

keratoid ('kerəˌtoyd) resembling horn or corneal tissue.

keratoiritis (ˌkerətoh·ie'rietis) inflammation of the cornea and iris, corneoiritis.

keratoleptynsis (ˌkerətohlep'tinsis) removal of the anterior portion of the cornea and replacement with bulbar conjunctiva.

keratoleukoma (ˌkerətohloo'kohmə) leukoma.

keratolysis (ˌkerəˈtolisis) loosening or separation of the horny layer of the epidermis.

pitted k., k. plantare sulcatum a tropical disease marked by thickening and deep fissuring of the skin of the soles, occurring during the rainy season.

keratolytic (ˌkerətohˈlitik) 1. pertaining to or promoting keratolysis. 2. an agent that promotes keratolysis.

keratoma (ˌkerəˈtohmə) keratosis.

keratomalacia (ˌkerətohməˈlayshi·ə) softening and necrosis of the cornea associated with vitamin A deficiency.

keratome (ˈkerəˌtohm) a knife for incising the cornea.

keratometer (kerəˈtomitə) an instrument for measuring the curvature of the cornea.

keratometry (ˌkerəˈtomətree) measurement of corneal curves. adj. **keratometric**.

keratomileusis (ˌkerətohmiˈlyoosis) keratoplasty in which a slice of the patient's cornea is removed, shaped to the desired curvature, and then sutured back on the remaining cornea to correct optical error.

keratomycosis (ˌkerətohmieˈkohsis) fungal disease of the cornea.

keratopathy (ˌkerəˈtopəthee) noninflammatory disease of the cornea.

band k. a condition characterized by an abnormal grey circumcorneal band.

keratophakia (ˌkerətohˈfayki·ə) keratoplasty in which a slice of donor's cornea is shaped to a desired curvature and inserted between layers of the recipient's cornea to change its curvature.

keratoplasty (ˈkerətohˌplastee) plastic surgery of the cornea; corneal grafting.

optic k. transplantation of corneal material to replace scar tissue that interferes with vision.

refractive k. removal of a section of cornea from a patient or donor, which is shaped to the desired curvature and inserted either between (keratophakia) layers of or on (keratomileusis) the patient's cornea to change its curvature and correct optical errors.

tectonic k. transplantation of corneal material to replace tissue that has been lost.

keratorhexis, keratorrhexis (ˌkerətəˈreksis) rupture of the cornea.

keratoscleritis (ˌkerətohskləˈrietis) inflammation of cornea and sclera.

keratoscope (ˈkerətohˌskohp) an instrument for examining the cornea.

keratoscopy (ˌkerəˈtoskəpee) inspection of the cornea.

keratosis (ˌkerəˈtohsis) any horny growth, such as a wart or callosity.

actinic k. a sharply outlined verrucous or keratotic growth, which may develop into a cutaneous horn, and may become malignant; it usually occurs in the middle aged or elderly and is due to excessive exposure to the sun. Called also *senile*, or *solar*, *keratosis*.

k. follicularis a rare hereditary condition manifested by areas of crusting, verrucous papular growths, usually occurring symmetrically on the trunk, axillae, neck, face, scalp, and retroauricular areas. Called also *Darier's disease*.

k. palmaris et plantaris congenital, hereditary thickening of the skin of the palms and soles, sometimes with painful lesions resulting from fissuring; often associated with other anomalies.

k. pharyngea horny projections from the tonsils and pharyngeal walls.

k. pilaris hyperkeratosis limited to the hair follicles.

k. punctata a hereditary hyperkeratosis in which the lesions are localized in multiple points on the palms and soles. **seborrhoeic k., k. seborrhoeica** a benign, noninvasive tumour of epidermal origin, marked by numerous yellow or brown, sharply marginated, oval, raised lesions.

k. senilis, solar k. actinic keratosis.

keratotomy (ˌkerəˈtotəmee) incision of the cornea.

radial k. an operation in which a series of incisions is made in the cornea from its outer edge toward its centre in a spoke-like fashion; done to flatten the cornea and thus to correct myopia.

Kerecid (ˈkerəsid) trademark for a preparation of idoxuridine, an antiviral used topically for herpes simplex infections.

kerion (ˈkeeri·ən) a boggy, exudative tumefaction covered with pustules, as may occur in tinea infections.

kernicterus (kərˈniktə·rəs) a condition in the newborn marked by severe neural symptoms, associated with high levels of bilirubin in the blood; it is commonly a sequela of icterus gravis neonatorum.

Kernig's sign (ˈkərnigz) in the supine position the patient can easily and completely extend the leg; in the sitting posture or when lying with the thigh flexed upon the abdomen the leg cannot be completely extended; it is a sign of meningitis.

Ketalar (ˈketəlah) trademark for preparations of ketamine, an anaesthetic agent.

ketamine (ˈketəˌmeen) a nonbarbiturate anaesthetic related to phencyclidine (PCP) administered intravenously or intramuscularly to produce analgesia in low doses and dissociative anaesthesia in higher doses. Useful in poor-risk patients as it tends to increase the blood pressure and heart rate; to cover short painful procedures such as burns dressing; and as an induction agent given intramuscularly in children. Is associated in a proportion of patients with emergence delirium in the immediate postoperative period and hallucinations in the first 24 hours. These can be reduced by the use of benzodiazepines during anaesthesia and by talking gently to patients as they emerge from the anaesthesia. Also useful as an analgesic for casualties in the field.

keto- word element, *ketone group*.

keto acids (ˈkeetoh) compounds containing the groups =CO (carbonyl) and -COOH (carboxyl).

Keto-Diastix (ˌkeetohˈdieəstiks) trademark for a reagent strip for detection of ketones and glucose in the urine.

ketoacidosis (ˌkeetohˌasiˈdohsis) the accumulation of ketone bodies in the blood which results in metabolic acidosis. See also KETOSIS.

ketoaciduria (ˌkeetohˌasiˈdyooə·ri·ə) the presence of keto acids in the urine.

ketoconazole (ˌkeetohˈkohnəˌzohl) a synthetic imidazole that is a broad-spectrum antifungal agent used for treatment of chronic mucocutaneous candidiasis and systemic fungal infections due to *Candida* species, dermatophytes (*Trichophyton* species, *Microsporum* species, *Epidermophyton floccosum*), *Histoplasma capsulatum*, *Coccidioides immitis*, *Blastomyces dermatitidis*, and *Paracoccidioides brasiliensis*.

ketogenesis (ˌkeetohˈjenəsis) the production of ketone bodies. adj. **ketogenetic**.

ketogenic (ˌkeetohˈjenik) forming or capable of being converted into ketone bodies.

k. diet one containing large amounts of fat, with minimal amounts of protein and carbohydrate. The object of such a diet is to produce KETOSIS; it is occasionally used in the treatment of certain types of epilepsy in young children.

α-ketoglutarate (ˌalfəˌkeetohˈglootə·rayt) a salt or anion of α-ketoglutaric acid.

α-ketoglutaric acid (ˌalfəˌkeetohglooˈtarik) a metabolic intermediate involved in the tricarboxylic acid cycle, in amino acid metabolism, and as an amino group acceptor in transamination reactions.

ketolysis (kee'tolisis) the splitting up of ketone bodies. adj. **ketolytic.**

ketonaemia (ˌkeetə'neemi·ə) an excess of ketone bodies in the blood.

ketone ('keetohn) any compound containing the carbonyl group, CO, and having hydrocarbon groups attached to the carbonyl carbon, i.e., the carbonyl group is within a chain of carbon atoms.

k. bodies the substances acetone, acetoacetic acid, and β-hydroxybutyric acid; except for acetone (which may arise spontaneously from acetoacetic acid), they are normal metabolic products of lipid and pyruvate within the liver, and are oxidized by muscles; excessive production leads to urinary excretion of these bodies, as in diabetes mellitus. Called also *acetone bodies*. See also KETOSIS.

ketonuria (ˌkeetoh'nyooə·ri·ə) an excess of ketone bodies in the urine.

ketoprofen (ˌkeetoh'prohfen) a nonsteroidal anti-inflammatory agent used in the treatment of arthritic conditions.

ketose ('keetohz) any sugar that contains a ketone group.

ketosis (kee'tohsis) accumulation in the blood and tissues of large quantities of the KETONE BODIES: β-hydroxybutyric acid, acetoacetic acid, and acetone. Because the first two are acids, this results in metabolic acidosis. Thus, the condition is often referred to as ketoacidosis. adj. **ketotic.**

When fatty acids are metabolized in the liver, an intermediate, acetylcoenzyme A (acetyl CoA), is produced. Normally, acetyl CoA is condensed with oxaloacetic acid, a product of carbohydrate metabolism, to form citric acid. This then enters the tricarboxylic acid cycle, the final common pathway of cellular energy metabolism.

When oxaloacetate is not present, acetyl CoA is converted by another pathway to ketone bodies. These compounds cannot be metabolized by the liver and are released into the blood stream. Other tissues, including muscle, brain, heart, and kidneys, can convert ketone bodies back to acetyl CoA and metabolize them as an energy source.

In acute starvation or in uncontrolled DIABETES MELLITUS, there is a great increase in fatty acid metabolism and impaired or absent carbohydrate metabolism, which results in a greatly increased production of ketone bodies. This can also occur when the diet is composed almost entirely of fat. The production of ketone bodies is reduced to the normal low level and the ketoacidosis is reversed when adequate carbohydrate metabolism is restored.

The patient with ketosis often has a sweet or 'fruity' odour to his breath. This is produced by acetone, a ketone body that is highly volatile and is blown off in small amounts with air expired from the lungs.

ketosteroid (ˌkeetoh'stiə·royd) a steroid having ketone groups on functional carbon atoms.

17-k's steroids found in normal urine and in excess in certain tumours, which have a ketone group on the 17th carbon atom, and include certain androgenic and adrenocortical hormones.

Ketostix ('keetoh,stiks) trademark for a reagent strip for detection of ketone bodies in the urine.

ketotifen (kee'totifen) a drug with anti-allergenic properties used in the prophylactic treatment of asthma.

keV kilo electron-volt (3.82×10^{-17} calorie, or 1.6×10^{-9} erg).

Kew Gardens spotted fever (kyoo 'gahdənz) rickettsialpox.

KFC King's Fund Centre; King's Fund College.

kg kilogram.

kHz kilohertz.

kidney ('kidnee) either of the two bean-shaped organs in the lumbar region that filter the blood, excreting the end-products of body metabolism in the form of urine, and regulating the concentrations of hydrogen, sodium, potassium, phosphate, and other ions in the extracellular fluid.

ANATOMY AND PHYSIOLOGY. In an average adult each kidney is about 11–13 cm long, 5–7.5 cm wide and 2.5 cm thick, and weighs 150 g. In this small area the kidney contains over a million microscopic filtering units, the NEPHRONS. Blood arrives at the kidney via the renal artery, and is distributed through arterioles into many millions of capillaries which lead into the nephrons. Fluids and dissolved salts in the blood pass through the walls of the capillaries of the glomeruli and are collected within the central capsule of each nephron, the Bowman's capsule. The glomerulus, a tuft of capillaries within the capsule, acts as a semipermeable membrane permitting a protein-free ultrafiltrate of plasma to pass through. This filtrate is forced into convoluted collecting channels in the nephrons, called tubules. Capillaries in the walls of the tubules reabsorb the water and the solutes required by the body and deliver them to a system of peritubular capillaries and then to small renal veins which, in turn, carry them into the renal vein and return them to the general circulation. Excess water and other waste materials remain in the tubules to be passed as urine. The urine contains, besides water, a quantity of urea, uric acid, yellow pigments, amino acids, and trace metals. The urine moves through a system of ducts into a collecting funnel (renal pelvis) in each kidney, whence it is led into the two ureters.

Filtering Capacity. About 1500 ml of urine are excreted daily by the average adult. The efficiency of the normal kidney is one of the most remarkable aspects of the body. It has a filtering capacity of 1200 ml of blood per minute—that is, 72 l per hour, or 1728 l per day. Ordinarily it draws off from the blood about 180 litres of fluid daily, and returns usually 98 to 99 per cent of the water plus the useful dissolved salts, according to the body's changing needs. *Maintaining Acid–Base Balance.* The kidneys help control the body's acidity by reabsorbing filtered bicarbonate ions in exchange for chloride and by secreting hydrogen ions. When alkalosis is present the kidney compensates by reabsorbing less bicarbonate ions and more hydrogen ions.

Regulation of Sodium–Water Balance. Normal osmolality and volume of body fluids are preserved by the normally functioning kidney. It does this by actively reabsorbing sodium and, by osmosis, reabsorbing more water; thus varying the urine concentration. The regulation of the sodium level in the blood is influenced by aldosterone, which increases sodium reabsorption and is secreted by the cortex of the adrenal gland in response to low serum sodium levels and the presence of angiotensin II. Detection of low sodium levels is by the juxtaglomerular cells in the afferent arteriolar wall and stimulates the production of renin. The reabsorption of water is affected not only by the reabsorption of sodium but also by antidiuretic hormone, which is secreted by the posterior pituitary gland in response to high serum osmolality.

Endocrine Functions. Blood pressure regulation by the kidneys involves the RENIN–angiotensin–aldosterone mechanisms. The kidney responds to ischaemia by secreting a proteolytic enzyme called renin. This acts on a plasma protein (renal substrate) in the blood to

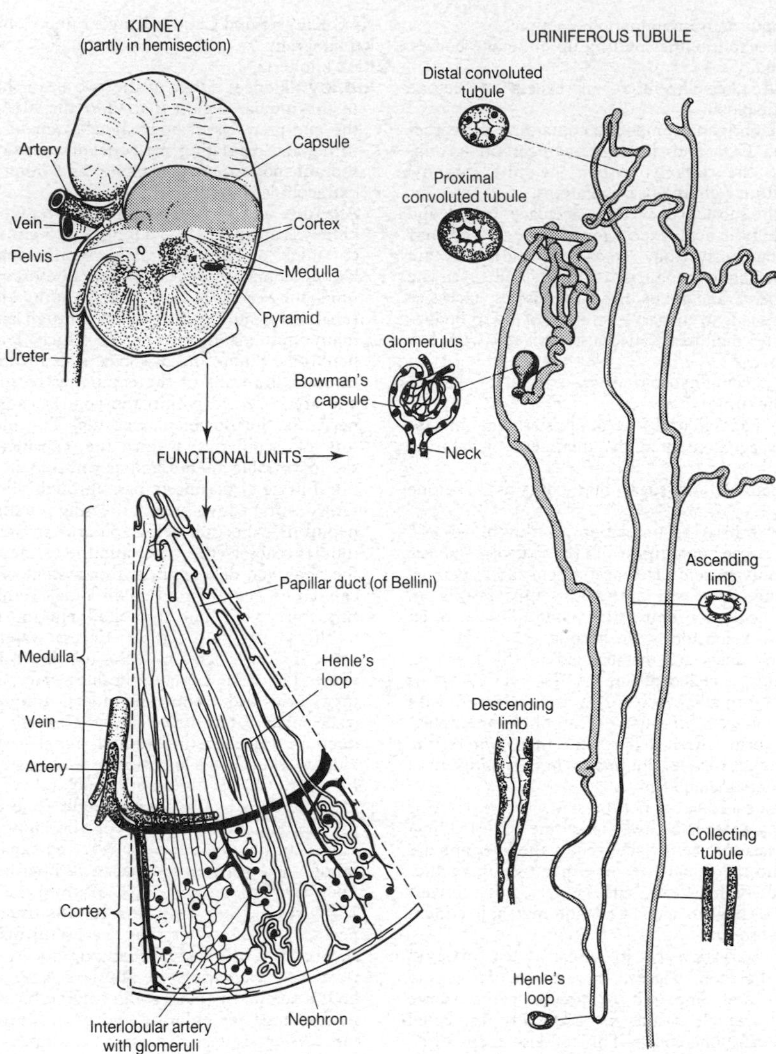

Details of structure of the kidney

produce angiotensin I. A converting enzyme from the lungs converts angiotensin I to II, which causes widespread arteriolar vasoconstriction, increases peripheral resistance and raises the blood pressure. Angiotensin II also effects an increase in blood pressure through its influence on sodium and water retention, by increasing the secretion of aldosterone from the adrenal cortex. Additionally, when kidney cells become hypoxic they release an enzyme called *renal erythropoietic factor*, which stimulates the maturation of oxygen-bearing red blood cells in the bone marrow. The kidneys also are involved in the conversion of inactive vitamin D to the active form (1,25-dihydrocholecalciferol), which increases calcium absorption in the intestine and calcium uptake by the bones.

Disorders of the Kidneys. Disorders of the kidney include inflammation, infection, obstruction, structural defects, injuries, calculus formation, and tumours.

PYELITIS is an inflammation of the renal pelvis. When the inflammation reaches deeper portions of the kidneys, it is called pyelonephritis.

NEPHRITIS is widespread inflammation of the kidney, usually affecting the glomeruli. See also **GLOMERULONEPHRITIS.**

NEPHROTIC SYNDROME presents as gross oedema due to excess (greater than 4 g/day) protein loss through the kidney as a complication of various diseases, including glomerulonephritis, renal vein thrombosis and amyloid.

KIDNEY STONES (renal calculi) form in the pelvis or calyx of the kidney or in the bladder when salts in solution in the urine precipitate and form crystals. Ninety per cent of these contain calcium and are radiopaque. Ten per cent of renal stones are mainly composed of uric acid or cysteine. Prevention of recurrence is important. Health education plays a vital role and often is simple dietary advice. About 90 per cent of kidney stones that are small enough to enter the ureter are passed in the urine.Those too large to traverse the ureter require surgical removal.

Kidney infection can be completely cured if treated early. Unchecked infection can destroy the organs and lead to uraemia. One intact kidney or even less than half a kidney is capable of maintaining renal function. Failure of both kidneys will necessitate substitution therapy for their role. This may be HAEMODIALYSIS or PERITONEAL DIALYSIS, in hospital or at home, or a kidney transplant (see also TRANSPLANTATION). It should not be necessary for a dramatic change in lifestyle to occur. After a period of training and adjustment, the patient should be able to return to work (some never stop working) and resume normal life.

Kidney disease caused by infection may be treated by antibiotics, but for a disorder caused by diseases such as tuberculosis or diabetes mellitus, the underlying disease must also be treated.

Primary and secondary malignancies are found in the kidney. Renal carcinoma is the commonest tumour of the kidney and was formerly called hypernephroma since it was wrongly thought to arise from the adrenal gland. Called also *Grawitz tumour*. It most frequently presents with haematuria and blood clots causing renal colic, but may present with metastatic foci in the lungs, liver or bones. Surgical removal offers the only hope of cure. See also NEPHROBLASTOMA.

Acute RENAL FAILURE occurs when there is sudden and severe impairment of kidney function as a result of disease, physical trauma, toxic damage and acute or prolonged hypotension or hypovolaemia. Chronic renal failure may occur as a result of unresolved acute disease or it may be a slow progressive process that develops as a sequel to glomerulonephritis, chronic pyelonephritis, hypertensive nephrosclerosis, polycystic kidney disease, diabetes mellitus or other causes. Presentation may be with deterioration of renal function over several years with progressive symptoms of uraemia or there may be sudden acute illness and end-stage kidney disease without progressive symptoms.

Structural defects in kidneys may be congenital or acquired. A kidney may be displaced, fused, malformed, or totally absent. Floating kidney, or NEPHROPTOSIS, is a condition in which the kidney is displaced, usually to a position somewhat lower than normal. This condition may be corrected by a surgical procedure called NEPHROPEXY.

SURGERY OF THE KIDNEY. Surgical removal of the kidney is called nephrectomy. It is done when the kidney is unable to function because of severe disease or injury and is causing pain, recurrent infection or hypertension by remaining in situ. An elective nephrectomy may be performed in a healthy person with two functioning kidneys in order to transplant one into a relation who has renal failure.

When obstruction prevents an adequate flow of urine from the kidney, nephrostomy may be performed. This procedure involves percutaneous puncture into the pelvis of the kidney and usually includes the insertion of a tube or catheter so that drainage can be established. Removal of large kidney stones may entail a surgical incision and a 'splitting' of the kidney; that is, an incision is made from one end of the kidney to the other. Removal of a calculus from the pelvis of the kidney is known as a pyelolithotomy. If the stone is located in the upper ureter it is removed by a procedure known as a ureterolithotomy. This operation may involve an abdominal incision but the kidney is not incised.

Patient Care. The site of the incision for surgery of the kidney creates special problems. The incision is referred to as a flank incision and, because it is directly below the diaphragm, deep breathing, coughing, and other measures necessary to prevent pulmonary complications are extremely painful and difficult for the patient. Narcotic drugs that relieve pain are usually ordered to be given every 4 hours so that coughing and deep breathing can be done. In addition to these measures, the patient should be turned from side to side and encouraged to get out of bed as soon as possible.

If a nephrostomy tube has been inserted, care must be taken that it does not kink while the patient is lying in bed. When he moves about there should be enough slack in the connecting tubes so that there is no tension exerted on the nephrostomy tube. CATHETERS or drainage tubes inserted during surgery of the kidney or ureters are used specifically to facilitate and monitor drainage. Care must be taken to avoid obstruction or their accidental removal. In either case the surgeon should be notified immediately so that steps can be taken to reestablish drainage and prevent serious damage to the kidney.

In most cases when a nephrectomy has been done, a corrugated or low-suction self-contained system drain is left in place to facilitate removal of serous material collecting in the space left by the kidney. There will not be urine in this drainage. The drainage may be blood-stained at first, but should it continue to be bright red in colour, it may indicate haemorrhage and should be reported immediately. The amount, colour, consistency, and odour of drainage should be noted and recorded. Dressings may be changed or reinforced as necessary to keep the patient dry and comfortable. A sterile safety pin may be attached to the end of the drain to keep it in place. The drain must not be compressed by the weight of the patient's body. Small pillows may be used to support the area around the drain when the patient is lying on the operative side.

Abdominal distention frequently occurs after renal surgery. Fluids by mouth should be given slowly at first until there is evidence that peristalsis is normal.

Haemorrhage is likely to occur after kidney surgery, especially when the highly vascular parenchyma has been incised. The times at which haemorrhage is most likely to occur are the day of surgery and 8 to 12 days after surgery when there is sloughing of tissue during the healing process. Dressings should be observed frequently and any undue drainage of bright red blood must be reported immediately.

amyloid k. one marked by deposition of amyloid; called also *waxy kidney*, *renal amyloidosis*.

artificial k. see HAEMODIALYSER.

contracted k. an atrophic kidney that may be scarred and granular.

k. failure see RENAL failure.

floating k. one that is freely movable; called also *hypermobile kidney* (see also NEPHROPTOSIS).

fused k. a single anomalous organ developed as a result of fusion of the renal anlagen.

horseshoe k. an anomalous organ resulting from fusion of the corresponding poles of the renal anlagen by an isthmus of renal parenchyma.

hypermobile k. one that is freely movable; called also *floating kidney* (see also NEPHROPTOSIS).

polycystic k. disease a hereditary disease in which there is an enlargement of both kidneys due to the formation of cortical cysts. It occurs in two forms, distinguished by age of onset and other characteristics.

Childhood polycystic kidney disease (CPKD) is inherited as an autosomal recessive trait, and is diagnosed at birth or in the first ten years of life. It is not as common as the adult form of the disease. Both the kidney and the liver are involved, causing renal failure and liver failure with portal hypertension. Characteristic symptoms early in the process include pain, haematuria, urinary tract infection, KIDNEY STONES, or obstructive uropathy with anuria.

Adult polycystic kidney disease (APKD) is the most common type of renal cystic disease. The kidneys may have single cysts or be multicystic. They are greatly enlarged and often exceed 1 kg in weight. It is transmitted as an autosomal dominant trait in 4 per cent of cases and is usually manifested during the third to fifth decades of life. Onset is slow and renal failure may not be apparent for many years. Although there is rarely any liver dysfunction accompanying this disorder, cyst formation in the liver does occur.

Treatment of both types of polycystic kidney disease is symptomatic. Dialysis and kidney transplant during end-stage renal failure can provide a good quality of life but offer no cure. Families with histories of polycystic kidney disease require genetic counselling and may need help in coping with the prospect of future offspring afflicted with the disease.

sponge k. a usually asymptomatic congenital condition in which multiple small cystic dilations of the collecting tubules of the medullary portion of the renal pyramids give the organ a spongy, porous feeling and appearance.

k. stones calculi in the kidney, which are composed of crystals precipitated from the urine on a particulate nidus of bacteria, cells or inspirational mucus. The vast majority of stones (about 90 per cent) are composed of either calcium or magnesium in combination with phosphate or oxalate. The remaining 10 per cent contain urate, cystine, or xanthine. Stones are more common in men between the ages of 30 and 50. Areas such as southeast Asia have a high incidence of the disease, but it is virtually unknown in some African tribes. These differences in incidence are believed to be due to dietary differences.

The formation of kidney stones can be attributed to various factors although idiopathic stones are attributed to an affluent society and diet. In many cases the cause can be traced to persistent urinary tract infection (phosphate stones) or stasis of urine due to obstruction of the flow of urine or to immobility. Inborn errors of metabolism of cystine and purine can also cause renal calculi. Recurrent stone formation is commonly due to hyperparathyroidism.

Radiopaque stones are easily located by an intravenous pyelogram, which will also show whether the calculi are causing obstruction to the flow of urine and resulting hydronephrosis.

Kidney stones do not always produce symptoms. However, they can lead to an infection or inflammation requiring medical attention. If a calculus is dislodged from the renal pelvis and begins to pass down the ureter, it can cause the classic symptoms of renal colic-pain and haematuria. Renal colic is characterized by waves of flank pain that usually radiates to the groin and the testes or genital labia. Obstruction by stones may cause acute renal failure until the obstruction is removed.

In general, treatment consists of efforts to avoid dehydration and to maintain a dilute urine continuously. This requires an intake of about 4 litres of fluid every 24 hours. If present infection must be treated promptly, not only to relieve current problems but also to avoid the future formation of stones. Analgesia may be necessary to relieve the acute pain. The patient's urine should be sieved and any debris or stones sent for analysis.

Whenever possible the stone should be passed without surgical intervention. Lithotripsy may be used to shatter the stone with ultrasound waves so that it can be passed in the urine. Where this is unavailable surgical removal is necessary.

Prevention of renal calculi in immobilized paralytic patients is usually very difficult because of urinary stasis and susceptibility to urinary tract infection. All persons prone to urinary stone formation should be encouraged to drink large quantities of fluid to remove precipitate matter from the renal pelvis. Dietary restrictions of red meat and other high-purine foods can help prevent the formation of urate stones.

waxy k. amyloid kidney.

Kiel classification (keeəl) a classification of the nonHodgkin's malignant lymphona, based on the concept that the tumour arises from a clone of lymphocytes at different stages seen in normal lymphocyte development (centroblast, centrocyte, etc.). They may be follicular (nodular) or diffuse in their histological pattern.

Kienböck's disease ('keenbeks) 1. slowly progressive osteochondrosis of the lunate bone; it may affect other wrist bones. 2. traumatic cavitation of the spinal cord.

Kienböck's unit a unit of x-ray exposure equal to 0.1 erythema dose; symbol X.

kilo- word element. [Gr.] *one thousand;* used to indicate a quantity 1000 (10^3) times the unit with which it is combined, e.g., kilometre (10^3 metres); symbol k.

kilocalorie ('kiloh,kalə·ree) a unit of heat equal to 1000 calories; symbol kcal.

kilogram ('kilə,gram) the SI unit of mass (weight), 1000 grams; equivalent to 15,432 grains, or 2.205 pounds (avoirdupois) or 2.679 pounds (apothecaries' weight); abbreviated kg.

kilohertz ('kilə,hərts) 1000 (10^3) hertz; abbreviated kHz.

kilometre (ki'lomitə, 'kilə,meetə) 1000 metres; 3280.83 feet; five-eighths of a mile; abbreviated km.

kilovolt ('kilə,vohlt) 1000 volts; abbreviated kV.

k. peak the maximal amount of voltage that an x-ray machine is using; abbreviated kVp.

kilovoltage (,kilə'vohltij) in radiography, the x-ray tube peak voltage during an exposure, measured in kilovolts.

Kimmelstiel–Wilson syndrome (,kiməlsteel'wilsən) a degenerative complication of DIABETES MELLITUS, with albuminuria, oedema, hypertension, renal insufficiency, and retinopathy. Called also *intercapillary glomerulosclerosis*.

kinaesthesia (,kinis'theezi·ə) the sense by which position, weight, and movement are perceived. adj. **kinaesthetic.**

kinaesthesiometer (,kinis,theezi'omitə) an apparatus for testing kinaesthesia.

kinaesthesis (,kinis'theesis) kinaesthesia.

kinanaesthesia (,kinanəs'theezi·ə) loss of the power of perceiving sensations of movement.

kinase ('kienayz) 1. a subclass of the transferases, comprising the enzymes that catalyse the transfer of a high-energy group from a donor (usually ATP) to an acceptor, and named, according to the acceptor, as creatine kinase, fructokinase, etc. 2. an enzyme that activates a zymogen, and named, according to its source, as enterokinase, streptokinase, etc.

kine- word element. [Gr.] *movement;* see also words beginning *cine-*.

kinematics (ˌkini'matiks) that branch of mechanics which deals with the possible motions of a material body.
kineplasty ('kiniˌplastee) plastic amputation; amputation in which the stump is so formed as to be utilized for producing motion of the prosthesis.
kinesalgia (ˌkini'salji·ə) pain on muscular exertion.
kinesi(o)- word element. [Gr.] *movement.*
kinesia (ki'neezi·ə) motion sickness.
kinesialgia (kiˌneezi'alji·ə) kinesalgia.
kinesics (ki'neesiks) the scientific study of the role of body movements, such as facial expressions, gestures, and eye movements, in interpersonal communication.
kinesimeter (ˌkini'simitə) 1. an instrument for quantitative measurement of motions. 2. an instrument for exploring the body surface to test cutaneous sensibility.
kinesiology (kiˌneezi'oləjee) scientific study of movement of body parts.
kinesis (ki'neesis) [Gr.] 1. *movement*, e.g., the activity of an organism in response to a stimulus; the direction of the response is not controlled by the direction of the stimulus (in contrast to a taxis). 2. a word termination denoting movement or motion, e.g., cytokinesis.
kinesitherapy (kiˌneezi'therəpee) treatment of disease by movements or exercise.
kinetic (ki'netik) pertaining to or producing motion.
kinetics (ki'netiks) the branch of dynamics investigating the relationship between the motions of bodies and the forces acting upon them.
chemical k. the scientific study of the rates and mechanisms of chemical reactions.
kinetocardiogram (kiˌneetoh'kahdiohˌgram) the record produced by kinetocardiography.
kinetocardiography (kiˌneetohˌkahdi'ogrəfee) the graphic recording of the slow vibrations of the anterior chest wall in the region of the heart, representing the absolute motion at a given point on the chest.
kinetochore (ki'neetohˌkor) a centromere.
kinetogenic (kiˌneetoh'jenik) causing or producing movement.
kinetoplast (ki'neetohˌplast) an accessory body found in many protozoa, primarily the Mastigophora; it contains DNA and replicates independently.
kinetosis (ˌkini'tohsis) any disorder due to unaccustomed motion (see also MOTION SICKNESS).
kinetotherapy (kiˌneetoh'therəpee) kinesitherapy.
King's Fund (kingz fund) King Edward's Hospital Fund for London was founded in 1897 for the support, by the giving of grants, of voluntary hospitals in London and was incorporated by an Act of Parliament in 1907. Since the inception of the NHS in 1948, its grant-making activity has been less for general maintenance and more concerned with funding of experimental schemes, particularly relating to the management of services.

Educational function has varied over the years and now focuses on Health Service Management based in the King's Fund College.

In 1963 a Hospital Centre was opened to provide an information and advisory service based on a large library, to initiate and support research projects (e.g. the development of bed design); to provide a venue for exhibitions of equipment and materials and to organize lectures, study days and conferences for all grades of hospital staff.

K. F. bed a bed fitted with jointed springs which may be adjusted to various positions, developed as the result of research undertaken on behalf of and funded by the King's Fund.
kingdom ('kingdəm) one of the three major categories into which natural objects are usually classified: the animal (including all animals), plant (including all plants), and mineral (including all substance and objects without life). A fourth, the Protista, includes all single-celled organisms.
kinin ('kienin) any of a group of endogenous peptides that increase vascular permeability, elevate blood pressure, and induce smooth muscle contraction.
venom k. a peptide found in the venom of insects.
kininogen (kie'ninəjən) an α_2-globulin of plasma that is a precursor of the kinins.
kinocilium (ˌkienoh'sili·əm) pl. *kinocilia;* a motile, protoplasmic filament on the free surface of a cell.
kinship ('kin·ship) a group of individuals of varying degrees of descent from a common ancestor.
Kirschner wire ('kiəshnə) a steel wire for skeletal transfixing of fractured bones and for obtaining skeletal traction in fractures. It is inserted through the soft parts and the bone and is held tight in a clamp.
kiss of life (ˌkis əv 'lief) the expired-air method of artificial respiration, by either mouth-to-nose or mouth-to-mouth breathing.
Klebsiella (ˌklebsi'elə) a genus of gram-negative bacteria (family Enterobacteriaceae).
K. friedländeri, K. pneumoniae the aetiological agent of Friedländer's pneumonia and other respiratory infections.
K. rhinoscleromatis a species isolated from the nasal secretions of patients with rhinoscleroma.
Klebs–Löffler bacillus (ˌklebz'lərflə) *Corynebacterium diphtheriae*, the causative agent of diphtheria.
kleeblattschädel (ˌklayblat'shaydel) [Ger.] *cloverleaf skull;* a congenital anomaly in which there is intrauterine synostosis of multiple or all cranial sutures.
Kleihauer test ('kliehowə) a test based on the different susceptibility of fetal haemoglobin (HbF) and adult haemoglobin (HbA) to treatment with acids and alkalis. It is used to detect the presence of fetal cells in the maternal circulation after delivery, of importance in the prevention of Rhesus disease of the newborn. Also used in the investigation of the haemoglobinopathies, e.g., thalassaemia.
kleptomania (ˌkleptə'mayni·ə) an abnormal, uncontrollable desire to steal. This should not be confused with the stage children naturally go through before they understand the concept of ownership. Repeated stealing by an older child may be done simply for the sake of adventure, or it may be an indication of emotional disturbance.

In an adult, the uncontrollable impulse to steal arises from a serious psychological problem, or neurosis. Since the impulse is an irrational one rooted in subconscious needs of which the person who steals is not aware, he often does not actually covet the object he steals. Sometimes the impulse is expressed by ostensibly borrowing an object and not returning it.

kleptomaniac (ˌkleptə'mayniˌak) a person exhibiting kleptomania.
Klinefelter's syndrome ('klienfeltəz) a condition characterized by the presence of small testes, with fibrosis and hyalinization of the seminiferous tubules, impairment of function and clumping of Leydig cells, and an increase in urinary gonadotrophins, associated with an abnormality of the sex chromosomes. It is associated typically with an XXY chromosome complement.
Klippel's disease ('klip'lz) arthritic general pseudoparalysis.
Klippel–Feil syndrome (ˌklip'l'fiel) shortness of the neck due to reduction in the number of cervical vertebrae or the fusion of multiple hemivertebrae into one osseous mass, with limitation of neck motion and low hairline.

Klumpke–Dejerine paralysis (ˌkloompkəˌdayzhə'reen) Klumpke's paralysis.

Klumpke's paralysis ('kloompkəz) atrophic paralysis of the lower arm and hand; due to lesion of the eighth cervical and first dorsal nerves. Called also *Klumpke–Dejerine paralysis*.

km kilometre.

kneading ('needing) a method used in massage. Pétrissage.

knee (nee) a complex hinge joint, one of the largest joints of the body, and one that sustains great pressure. The knee is formed by the head of the tibia, the lower end of the femur, and the patella, or kneecap. The bones are jointed by ligaments, and the patella is secured to the adjacent bones by powerful tendons. The fibula is attached at the side of the knee to the tibia. Crescent-shaped pads of cartilage lying on top of the tibia cushion it from the femur and form the gliding surfaces of the joint in motion.

Further cushioning is supplied by bursae, which are located around the main joint, between it and the patella and on the outside of the patella. A capsule of ligaments binds the whole assembly together. The capsule is lined with synovial membrane, which secretes a lubricating fluid (synovial fluid) that makes possible a smooth, gliding motion.

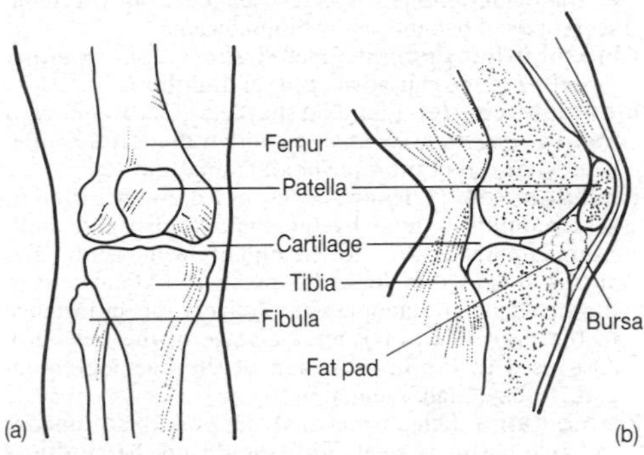

Knee joint.(a) Front view. (b) Flexed, in profile

DISORDERS OF THE KNEE. Twists and wrenches of the knee may result from a blow or from pressure. If the injury is followed by swelling and soreness, rest and heat are usually helpful. An elastic bandage may be helpful to bolster the knee against further stress and strain. If symptoms are severe or persistent, they should be reported to a doctor.

HOUSEMAID'S KNEE results from frequent kneeling on hard surfaces, causing injury to the front of the knee and inflammation of the bursa in front of the patella, with fluid accumulating within it.

Water on the knee is an excessive accumulation of synovial fluid within the knee joint. The condition may follow a knee injury or result from an infection or acute arthritis. The patella is raised or 'floats' on the accumulated fluid, and there is general swelling around the knee. In most cases, the effusion subsides if the joint is rested.

The knee is subject to many joint inflammations that come under the general heading of ARTHRITIS. When the knee is severely inflamed, the patient is confined to bed, and the knee is bound and splinted to rest the joint.

The knee is subject to bone and joint injuries, including DISLOCATION, SPRAIN, and FRACTURE. A fractured patella without wide separation of the parts is often treated by immobilization of the leg for several weeks with a cast or splint, so that the parts can grow together. The surgeon extracts with a needle or syringe the excess blood or fluid that has accumulated in the knee. If the injury is a complicated one, with wide separation of the parts, the parts may be bound together surgically with fine steel wire or similar material. Torn soft tissues are sewn together, and the knee is immobilized in a plaster cast for 4 or 5 weeks.

Recently developed techniques in the surgical restoration of a joint now permit total or partial replacement of the knee. Surgery of this kind is indicated when there has been severe joint damage due to rheumatoid and degenerative arthritis or a severely traumatic fracture.

Another condition that interferes with free knee movement may be caused by loose fragments in the knee resulting from tuberculosis of the bone, arthritis, torn meniscus, or inflammation of the synovial membrane that lines the knee joint.

KNOCK-KNEE, an inward curving of the knees, is usually caused by irregular bone growth or by weak ligaments; rickets may still be a common cause; called also *genu valgum*.

k. jerk, k. reflex a kick reflex produced by sharply tapping the patellar liagment. To test this reflex, the lower part of the leg is allowed to hang relaxed, usually by crossing the legs at the knees. The doctor taps the ligament below the patella with a small rubber hammer. The normal reaction is contraction of the quadriceps muscle, causing involuntary extension of the lower leg. Called also *patellar reflex* and *quadriceps reflex*.

The knee jerk is a stretch reflex; striking the patellar ligament stretches the quadriceps muscle at the front of the thigh and causes it to contract. Two nerves are involved; one receives the stimulus and transmits the impulse to the spinal cord, and the other, a motor nerve, receives the impulse and relays it to the quadriceps muscle.

Inadequate response to the knee jerk test may mean that the reflex mechanism involved is in some way impaired. In some people the knee jerk is normally so light that it is nearly imperceptible, and the doctor makes other tests to check the reflex mechanism.

kneecap ('neeˌkap) patella.

knock-knee ('nokˌnee) a childhood deformity, developing gradually, in which the knees rub together or 'knock' in walking and the ankles are far apart; called also *genu valgum*. At one time, knock-knee and bowleg were common symptoms of rickets. Knock-knee is now more often caused by an irregularity in the growth of the leg bones, sometimes stemming from injury to the bone ends at the knee, or by weak ligaments. The weight of the body, which is not supported properly, turns the knees in and the weak lower legs buckle until the ankles are spread far apart.

Knock-knee in young children varies in seriousness. Milder cases frequently disappear after early childhood as bones, ligaments, and muscles strengthen and coordination improves. More serious cases can often be corrected by strengthening exercises and by proper manipulation of the joints. Sometimes braces are used to ensure the proper alignment of growing legs.

In a very young child, knock-knee involves only the soft bone ends where the bone grows. If allowed to continue for a number of years, the condition can lead to abnormal developments in body structure. The sooner corrective measures are taken, the more effective the treatment is likely to be.

knot (not) 1. an intertwining of the ends or parts of one or more threads, sutures, or strip of cloth. 2. in anatomy, a knob-like swelling or protuberance. 3. a disorderly entanglement.

surgeon's k., surgical k. a knot in which the thread is passed twice through the first loop.

knuckle ('nuk'l) the dorsal aspect of any interphalangeal joint, or any similarly bent structure.

Koch's law (postulates) in order for a given microorganism to be established as the cause of a given disease, the following conditions must be fulfilled: (1) the microorganism must be present in every case of the disease; (2) it must be isolated and cultivated in pure culture; (3) inoculation of such culture must produce the disease in susceptible animals; (4) it must be observed in, and recovered from, the experimentally diseased animal.

Köhler's bone disease ('kərləz) 1. osteochondrosis of the tarsal navicular bone in children. 2. thickening of the shaft of the second metatarsal bone and changes about its articular head, with pain in the second metatarsophalangeal joint on walking or standing.

koilo- word element. [Gr.] *hollowed, concave.*

koilonychia (ˌkoylə'niki·ə) dystrophy of the nails in which they are abnormally thin and concave from side to side, with the edges turned up.

koilorrhachic (ˌkoylə'rakik) having a vertebral column in which the lumbar curvature is anteriorly concave.

koilosternia (ˌkoylə'stərni·ə) pectus excavatum (funnel chest).

kolp- for words beginning thus, see those beginning *colp-*.

kolypeptic (ˌkohli'peptik) hindering or checking digestion.

Konakion (kə'nakeeon) trademark for preparations of phytomenadione, a vitamin K preparation.

Koplik's spots ('kopliks) small, irregular, bright red spots on the buccal and lingual mucosa, with a minute bluish white speck in the centre of each; they are pathognomonic of beginning measles.

Korean haemorrhagic fever (kə'ree·ən) see HAEMORRHAGIC FEVER WITH RENAL SYNDROME.

Körner data sets information items for England recommended in a series of reports published from 1982 by the Steering Group on Health Services Information (chaired by Mrs E. Körner). The data sets cover a wide range of hospital and community activity and are designed for use by local managers in planning and monitoring services, and from them data to meet central requirements are derived. Implementation was generally in April 1987, but some items, notably those relating to maternity and community services, were not collected before April 1988.

koro ('koroh) a form of acute anxiety state, with hysterical features, occurring in S.E. Asia and associated with a belief that the penis will retract into the abdomen causing death.

Korotkoff's method (ko'rotkofs) a method of finding the systolic and diastolic blood pressure by listening to the sounds produced in an artery while the pressure in a previously inflated cuff is gradually reduced.

Korotkoff's sounds sounds heard during auscultatory determination of BLOOD PRESSURE, thought to be produced by vibratory motion of the arterial wall as the artery suddenly distends when compressed by a pneumatic blood pressure cuff. Origin of the sound may be within the blood passing through the vessel or within the wall itself.

Korsakoff's syndrome (psychosis) ('kawsəkofs) a psychosis associated with chronic ALCOHOLISM and caused by vitamin B_1 (thiamine) deficiency; characteristics include disturbances of orientation, memory defect, susceptibility to external stimulation and suggestion, hallucinations, and, usually, the signs of polyneuritis (wristdrop, etc.). There is irreversible brain damage; confinement to an institution is a frequent outcome of this condition. See also WERNICKE–KORSAKOFF SYNDROME.

Kr chemical symbol, *krypton.*

Krabbe's disease ('krabeez) a familial form of leukoencephalopathy beginning in infancy, in which the sphingolipid ceramide galactoside accumulates in the tissues due to a deficiency of β-galactosidase, marked pathologically by cerebral demyelination and by the presence of large globoid bodies in the white substance.

kraurosis (kror'rohsis) a dried, shrivelled condition.

k. vulvae atrophy of the female external genitalia, resulting in drying and shrivelling, with leukoplakic patches on the mucosa and intense itching.

Krause's bulbs ('krowzəz) Krause's corpuscles.

Krause's corpuscles ('krowzəz) small encapsulated bodies at the end of sensory nerve fibres in skin, mucous membranes, muscles, and other areas. Called also *end-bulbs* and *Krause's bulbs.*

Krause's glands ('krowzəz) mucous glands in the middle portion of the conjunctiva.

Krebs cycle (krebz) tricarboxylic acid cycle.

Kromayer lamp ('krohmieə) a mercury-vapour lamp used for ultraviolet radiation. It is water-cooled and is used in contact with the skin, and within cavities, using a quartz-rod applicator.

Krukenberg's tumour ('krookenbərgz) a type of carcinoma of the ovary, usually metastatic from cancer of the gastrointestinal tract, especially of the stomach. It is characterized by areas of mucoid degeneration and the presence of signet-ring-like cells.

krypton ('kriptən) a chemical element, atomic number 36, atomic weight 83.80, symbol Kr. (See table of elements in Appendix 2.) Used in isotope lung scanning.

k-81m a radioactive gas which decays to krypton-81 by emitting gamma rays of 190 keV and has a half-life of 13 s. It is used in nuclear medicine to assess lung ventilation. Symbol $^{81}Kr^{m}$.

KStJ Knight Commander, Order of St. John of Jerusalem.

Kufs' disease (kuhfs) the late juvenile, or adult, form of AMAUROTIC FAMILIAL IDIOCY, occurring between 15 and 26 years of age, differing from the infantile form (TAY–SACHS DISEASE) in that it shows no racial predilection, and from the infantile, late infantile (BIELSCHOWSKY–JANSKY DISEASE), and juvenile (SPIELMEYER–VOGT DISEASE) forms in that ocular lesions are absent; clinical findings are those of cerebellar or basal ganglia disorders.

Kugelberg–Welander disease (ˌkoog'lbərgvee'landə) a hereditary juvenile form of muscular atrophy, due to lesions of the anterior horns of the spinal cord, with onset principally between 2 and 17 years of age; it is marked by atrophy and weakness of the proximal muscles of the lower extremities and pelvic girdle, followed by involvement of the distal muscles and muscular twitchings.

Kümmell's disease (spondylitis) ('koom'lz) compression fracture of vertebra, with symptoms occurring a few weeks after injury, including spinal pain, intercostal neuralgia, motor disturbances of the legs, and kyphosis that is painful on pressure and easily reduced by extension. Called also *post-traumatic spondylitis.*

Küntscher nail ('koontshə) an intramedullary nail used in treating fractures of long bones, especially the shaft of the femur.

Kupffer's cells ('kuhpfəz) large, stellate or pyramidal, intensely phagocytic cells lining the walls of the hepatic sinusoids and forming part of the reticuloendothelial system.

kuru ('kuhroo) a chronic, progressive, uniformly fatal central nervous system disorder thought to be due to a slow virus and transmissible to subhuman primates; seen only in the Fore tribe and neighbouring peoples of New Guinea.

Kussmaul's disease ('kuhsmowlz) an inflammatory disease of the coats of the small and medium-sized arteries, marked by a variety of systemic symptoms (see also COLLAGEN DISEASES). Called also *periarteritis nodosa.*

Kussmaul's respiration a distressing dyspnoea occurring in paroxysms, characteristic of diabetic acidosis and coma. Called also *air hunger*.

kV kilovolt.

Kveim test ('kvaym) a test for sarcoidosis where antigen from the lymph nodes or spleen of a sarcoidosis patient is injected intradermally.

kVp kilovolt peak.

kwashiorkor (ˌkwashi'awkə) a syndrome occurring in infants and young children soon after weaning. It is due to severe protein deficiency, and the symptoms include oedema, pigmentation changes of skin and hair, impaired growth and development, distention of the abdomen (pot belly), and pathological liver changes.

Kyasanur Forest disease (ˌkieəsənaw 'fo·rist) a highly fatal virus disease of monkeys in the Kyasanur Forest of India, communicable to man, in whom it produces haemorrhagic symptoms.

kymatism ('kiemə,tizəm) myokymia; quivering of muscles.

kymogram ('kiemə,gram) the graphic record (tracing or film) produced by the kymograph.

kymograph ('kiemə,grahf, -ˌgraf) an instrument for recording variations or undulations, arterial or other.

kymography (kie'mogrəfee) the use of the kymograph.

kynocephalus (kienoh'kefələs, -'sef-) a fetus or infant with a head like that of a dog.

kynurenine (ˌkie'nyooə·rəneen) a metabolite of tryptophan found in microorganisms and in the urine of normal animals; it is a precursor of kynurenic acid and an intermediate in the conversion of tryptophan to niacin.

kyphos ('kiefos) the hump in the spine in kyphosis.

kyphoscoliosis (ˌkiefoh,skohli'ohsis) backward (kyphosis) and lateral (scoliosis) curvature of the spine, in vertebral osteochondrosis (Scheuermann's disease).

kyphosis (kie'fohsis) abnormally increased convexity in the curvature of the thoracic spine as viewed from the side; called also *hunchback*. adj. **kyphotic.** The condition may be the result of an acquired disease, an injury, or a congenital disorder or disease. It never develops from poor posture.

This spinal deformity usually is caused by vertebral tuberculosis (POTT'S DISEASE), or by some other destructive inflammation of the vertebrae (spondylitis). Kyphosis sometimes occurs with certain forms of poliomyelitis and with diseases that cause bone destruction, as happens in osteitis deformans (Paget's disease). An injury, such as a fracture of the spine, treated improperly or not at all, may also result in hunchback. There are some rare cases of kyphosis caused by congenital deformities and diseases. One example, achondroplasia, or fetal rickets, is a congenital bone disorder that affects growth and bone formation.

There are no specific symptoms of kyphosis besides back pain and increasing immobility of the spine. Symptoms vary with the cause, and any back pain or injury should be investigated.

kyrtorrhachic (ˌkərtə'rakik) having a vertebral column in which the lumbar curvature is anteriorly convex.

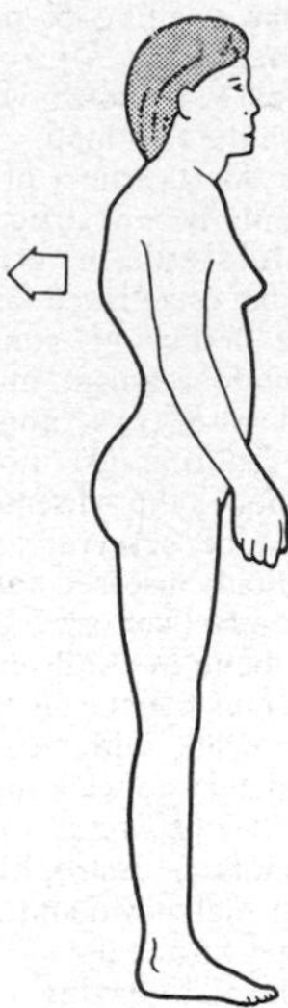

Kyphosis

kyto- for words beginning thus, see those beginning *cyto-*.

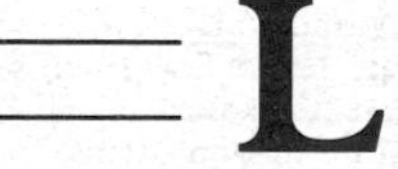

L

L Latin; left; length; libra (*pound*, *balance*); licentiate; light sense; limes (*boundary*); litre; lumbar; coefficient of induction.

L_0 Ehrlich's symbol for a toxin–antitoxin mixture that is completely neutralized and will not kill an animal.

L+ Ehrlich's symbol for a toxin–antitoxin mixture that contains one fatal dose in excess and will kill the experimental animal.

L- chemical prefix (written as small capital) that specifies that the substance corresponds in chemical configuration to the standard substance L-glyceraldehyde. Carbohydrates are named by this method to distinguish them by their chemical composition. The opposite prefix is D-.

L-dopa (el'dohpə) L-3,4-dihydroxyphenylalanine, a precursor of the neurotransmitter dopamine; used in the treatment of Parkinson's disease. Called also *levodopa*. See also DOPA.

l litre.

l- chemical abbreviation, *laevo-* (i.e., left or anticlockwise).

λ lambda, the eleventh letter of the Greek alphabet; symbol for *decay constant*.

La chemical symbol, *lanthanum*.

label ('layb'l) something that identifies; an identifying mark, tag, etc.

radioactive l. radioactive tracer.

labetalol (lə'beetəlol) an alpha and beta adrenergic receptor blocker used in the treatment of hypertension.

labia ('laybi·ə) [L.] plural of *labium*.

labial ('laybi·əl) pertaining to a lip, or labium.

labialism ('laybi·ə,lizəm) defective speech with use of labial sounds.

labile ('laybiel) 1. gliding; moving from point to point over the surface; unstable; fluctuating. 2. chemically unstable.

lability (lə'bilətee) the quality of being labile. In psychiatry, emotional instability; a tendency to show alternating states of gaiety and sombreness.

labio- word element. [L.] *lip*.

labioglossolaryngeal (,laybioh,glosohlə'rinji·əl, -,larin'jeeəl) pertaining to the lips, tongue, and larynx.

labioglossopharyngeal (,laybioh,glosohfə'rinji·əl, -,farin'jeeəl) pertaining to the lips, tongue, and pharynx.

labiograph ('laybioh,grahf, ,graf) an instrument for recording movements of the lips in speaking.

labiomental (,laybioh'ment'l) pertaining to the lips and chin.

labionasal (,laybioh'nayz'l) pertaining to the lip and nose.

labiopalatine (,laybioh'palə,tien) pertaining to the lips and palate.

labioplasty ('laybioh,plastee) plastic repair of a lip; cheiloplasty.

labium ('laybi·əm) pl. *labia* [L.] a fleshy border or edge; a lip. adj. **labial.**

l. majus pl. *labia majora;* an elongated fold in the female, one on either side of the rima pudendi.

l. minus pl. *labia minora;* the small fold of skin on either side, between the labia majora and the opening of the vagina.

labia oris the lips of the mouth.

laboratory (lə'bo·rətree) a place equipped for making tests or doing experimental work.

clinical l. one for examination of materials derived from the human body for the purpose of providing information on diagnosis, prevention, or treatment of disease.

labour ('laybə) parturition or childbirth. Literally, the process by which the products of conception are expelled from the uterus via the birth canal. May also be referred to as *confinement* or (in USA) *accouchement*.

NORMAL LABOUR. Said to occur spontaneously, at term (i.e. between 37 and 42 weeks of pregnancy). The fetus should present by the vertex, and, once started, contractions should increase in length, strength, and frequency without interruption or artificial stimulation until the baby, placenta, and membranes have been completely expelled by maternal effort via the vagina. The process should be completed without undue trauma to either mother or baby within 18 hours from the onset of regular, painful contractions.

Labour is described in three distinct stages. The *first stage*, usually the longest, begins with the onset of regular, painful uterine contractions and ends when the cervical canal is completely obliterated and the external os fully dilated to a diameter of 10 centimetres. The *second, expulsive stage* lasts from full dilation until the baby has been completely expelled from the birth canal. The *third stage*, usually the shortest, is concluded by the separation and complete expulsion of the placenta and membranes, and the control of bleeding by a well contracted uterus.

Onset of labour. This is thought to be initiated by the interaction of several hormonal and mechanical factors. During pregnancy, high levels of progesterone inhibit the action of oxytocin, produced by the posterior lobe of the pituitary gland. A fall in progesterone allows oxytocin to stimulate activity in uterine muscle. High levels of oestrogen, possibly influenced by changes in fetal pituitary–adrenal activity, sensitize the uterus, particulaly the cervix, to enable it to respond to oxytocin. Prostaglandins, probably synthesized in the decidua at term in response to the release of oestrogens from the fetoplacental unit, are thought to be the major factor initiating the onset of labour. The mechanical effect of the growing fetus pressing on the internal os and paracervical ganglia, and relative overdistention of the uterus by the fetus, liquor and placenta at term, combine with the hormonal factors to induce labour.

Signs of the onset of labour include one or more of the following: (1) *a show*—passage of the operculum or mucus plug from the lumen of the cervical canal; this may appear blood-stained due to the rupture of small capillaries; (2) *rupture of the membranes*—a distinct gush, or more usually a sensation of dampness, which represents the escape of amniotic fluid, particularly the forewaters, from a break in the membranes, particularly those in front of the presenting part of the fetus; (3) *onset of regular, rhythmic, painful uterine contractions*, sometimes perceived initially as backache; these may occur with or without the other two signs and constitute the only reliable evidence that labour is imminent. Painful uterine contractions may be distinguished from the painless BRAXTON HICKS CONTRACTIONS, which occur throughout pregnancy, by their regularity and because they cause increased pressure within the amniotic sac, which eventually causes rupture of the membranes.

Progress in labour. This is effected by the unique quality of uterine muscle in that when it relaxes following a contraction the fibres also retract, that is, become permanently decreased in length and increased in thickness. The longitudinal fibres which are inserted at the margin of the internal os and pass over the top of the fundus before reaching the other edge of the os thus bring about dilation of the os. The increasing thickness of the uterine wall in the fundus presses the fetus onto the cervix, also encouraging dilation. The circular muscle fibres, concentrated in the lower uterine segment, stretch and thin, while the upper segment fibres contract and retract. This harmonious working together of the upper and lower segments of the uterus is called *polarity*, and allows the fetus to be pushed downwards within the uterus until full dilation is achieved.

First stage of labour. The length of the first stage is related to size and presentation of the fetus, the quality and duration of the uterine contractions, and the contours of the birth canal. Maternal discomfort may be relieved by various types of analgesia. The condition of mother and fetus should be monitored regularly in order to detect and correct any adverse effect from labour.

Second stage of labour. This may be preceded by nausea or a small vomit, and the urge to 'push' or bear down. Pushing should not be allowed until full dilation of the cervix has been confirmed because premature pushing can be harmful to both mother and baby. The nature of the contractions changes and they become expulsive; the mother assists the descent of the fetus though the birth canal by use of her abdominal muscles. During the second stage the fetus negotiates the curves of the birth canal, a phenomenon called the *mechanism of labour*. The presenting part, usually the vertex, appears at the vulva and eventually the head is crowned when the biparietal diameter is delivered. There is usually a pause after the birth of the head before the trunk is expelled.

Third stage of labour. Once the baby is expelled, the

uterus retracts firmly until the fundus is at the level of the mother's umbilicus. This has the effect of reducing the area of the placental site, which is consequently shorn off the inner uterine wall. The weight of the placenta causes it to sink into the lower uterine segment, and the membanes peel off the uterine wall behind it. A few moments after the birth of the baby, the uterus contracts strongly to expel the placenta and its attached membranes. When the fetal surface appears first it is called a Schultz method of separation; in a Matthews Duncan method of separation, the maternal surface of the placenta is seen at the vulva. Normally the uterus contracts and retracts once the placenta is delivered, reducing the placental site still further in an attempt to control bleeding. The possibility of haemorrhage is further reduced by the action of 'living ligatures', the figure-of-eight, oblique uterine muscle fibres which intertwine around individual blood vessels and by their contraction effectively occlude them. The process is completed by the normal blood clotting mechanism. It is important that the placenta and membranes are checked for completeness following delivery, and blood loss measured.

MANAGEMENT OF LABOUR. This may be active or passive. In *passive management* (see NATURAL CHILDBIRTH) the course of nature is allowed to proceed without interference and the baby, placenta and membranes are delivered by maternal effort and minimal assistance from a midwife or other attendant. In *active labour*, contractions may be induced or accelerated during the first stage of labour and the third stage speeded up by the administration of an oxytocic drug with the birth of the anterior shoulder or following the birth of the baby. Other details of care and management depend on hospital policy. See also FETAL MONITORING and CERVICAL OS.

dry l. that in which the amniotic fluid escapes before contraction of the uterus begins, or labour in a mother with oligohydramnios where liquor volume is reduced in pregnancy.

false l. ineffective pains resembling labour pains, not accompanied by cervical dilation; called also *false pains* or *spurious labour*. These sometimes accompany 'taking up of the cervix' in primigravidae, which allows the fetal head to sink into the pelvic cavity. They are more commonly experienced by multigravidae where a high head provides ineffective stimulation of the paracervical ganglion.

induced l. that which is induced artificially, to safeguard the health of fetus or mother, by rupture of the membranes and/or administration of oxytocic drugs or prostaglandins to stimulate uterine contractions.

obstructed l. labour in which there is a mechanical hindrance due to a fault in the fetus or the birth canal which produces an impassable barrier preventing progress of labour in spite of strong uterine contractions. May occur in the first or second stage and if untreated is potentially fatal to mother and fetus.

precipitate l. one in which the first, second or third stages are completed in unusually short time. A form of abnormal uterine action which may produce extremely powerful but frequently painless uterine contractions. The speed of labour and force of delivery may cause severe trauma to mother and baby.

premature l., preterm l. expulsion of a viable infant before the normal end of gestation; usually applied to the spontaneous interruption of pregnancy between the twenty-eighth and thirty-seventh weeks.

spontaneous l. that which occurs without being artificially induced or accelerated.

spurious l. labour pains which sometimes precede true labour pains and are ineffective in achieving progress in labour. Called also *false labour*.

labrum ('laybrəm, 'labrəm) pl. *labra* [L.] an edge, rim, or lip.

labyrinth ('labə·rinth) the internal ear, consisting of the vestibule, cochlea, and SEMICIRCULAR CANALS. adj. **labyrinthine**. The cochlea is concerned with hearing, and the vestibule and semicircular canals with equilibrium (sense of balance).

The bony portion of the labyrinth (osseous labyrinth) is composed of a series of canals tunnelled out of the temporal bone. Inside the osseous labyrinth is the membranous labyrinth, which conforms to the general shape of the osseous labyrinth but is much smaller. A fluid called perilymph fills the space between the osseous and membranous labyrinths. Fluid inside the membranous labyrinth is called endolymph. These fluids play an important role in the transmission of sound waves and the maintenance of body balance.

Disorders of the inner ear, such as labyrinthitis and MENIÈRE'S DISEASE, are characterized by episodes of dizziness, ringing in the ears, and hearing loss.

ethmoid l., ethmoidal l. either of the paired lateral masses of the ethmoid bone, consisting of numerous thin-walled cellular cavities, the ethmoidal cells.

labyrinthectomy (ˌlabə·rin'thektəmee) excision of the labyrinth.

labyrinthitis (ˌlabə·rin'thietis) inflammation of the labyrinth; otitis interna.

labyrinthotomy (ˌlabə·rin'thotəmee) incision of the labyrinth.

lac (lak) pl. *lacta* [L.] milk.

laceration (ˌlasə'rayshən) 1. the act of tearing. 2. a wound with irregular edges, as distinguished from a cut or incision.

A laceration may be a ragged tear with many tag ends of skin or a torn flap of skin and muscle. Although the amount of bleeding may be less than that caused by a cut, the danger of infection is greater. In a laceration there is likely to be more damage to surrounding tissue, with a greater area exposed and areas of potential necrosis due to impairment of blood supply.

Because of the danger of infection, cleaning the laceration is the first and most important step in treatment. If the wound is no more than skin deep, cleaning is a simple task, after which the wound is covered with dry sterile gauze. If parts of the wound are deep, surgical débridement will be required. Immunity against tetanus is established and antibiotic prophylaxis may be given.

Internal lacerations occur when an organ is compressed or displaced by an external force. This kind of laceration may result from a blow that does not penetrate the skin. Surgical repair is usually necessary for internal lacerations in order to achieve haemostasis and to repair any hollow organs that have been ruptured.

lacertus (lə'sərtəs) pl. *lacerti* [L.] a name given certain fibrous attachments of muscles.

lacrimal ('lakriməl) pertaining to tears.

l. apparatus a group of organs concerned with the production and drainage of tears. Its function is to protect the eye and to keep it moist and free of dust and other irritating particles. The lacrimal gland, which secretes tears, lies over the upper, outer corner of the eye; its excretory ducts branch downward toward the eye. A constant stream of tears washes down over the front of the eye and is drained off through two small openings, the lacrimal puncta, located in the medial part of the eyelid margin on either side of the *lacrimal* LAKE. Through these openings the tears pass into the lacrimal canaliculus, then through the lacrimal sac into the nasolacrimal duct and finally into the nasal cavity.

lacrimation (ˌlakri'mayshən) secretion and discharge of tears.

lacrimonasal (ˌlakrimoh'nayz'l) pertaining to the lacrimal sac and nose.

lact(o)- word element. [L.] *milk*.

lactacidaemia (ˌlaktasi'deemi·ə) an excess of lactic acid in the blood; lacticaemia.

lactaciduria (ˌlaktasi'dyooə·ri·ə) lactic acid in the urine.

lactagogue ('laktəˌgog) an agent that promotes the flow of milk; galactagogue.

lactalbumin (lak'talbyuhmin) an albumin of milk.

lactam ('laktam) a cyclic amide formed from aminocarboxylic acids by elimination of water; lactams are isomeric with lactims, which are enol forms of lactams.

β-lactamase (ˌbeetə'laktəˌmayz) either of two enzymes: β-lactamase I is penicillinase; β-lactamase II is cephalosporinase.

lactase ('laktayz) D-galactosidase; an enzyme in the intestinal mucosa that hydrolyses lactose, producing glucose and galactose.

l. deficiency a deficiency of intestinal lactase, which causes abdominal distention and cramping and often diarrhoea when milk is drunk. The condition is usually hereditary with an onset between infancy and early adulthood. It may also occur secondary to massive small bowel resection or to diseases involving the mucosa, such as coeliac disease, Crohn's disease, tropical sprue, and ulcerative colitis.

lactate ('laktayt) 1. any salt of lactic acid or the anion of lactic acid. 2. to secrete milk.

l. dehydrogenase (LD, LDH) an enzyme that catalyses the interconversion of lactate and pyruvate. It is widespread in tissues and is particularly abundant in kidney, skeletal muscle, liver, and myocardium. It has five isoenzymes denoted LD_1 to LD_5. The 'flipped' pattern in which the serum LD_1 level is greater than the LD_2 level is indicative of an acute myocardial infarction. This pattern occurs within 12 to 24 hours after the attack.

lactation (lak'tayshən) the secretion of milk by the breasts. The word is also used to describe the period of weeks or months during which a child is breast-fed.

Lactation is thought to be brought about by action of progesterone and oestrogen and specific pituitary hormones, such as prolactin (lactogenic hormone). Lactation does not begin until at least 3 days after the birth of the baby. Before that the breast secretes colostrum, a fluid containing substances valuable to the baby until milk is formed. **l. hormone** lactogenic hormone, or prolactin.

lacteal ('lakti·əl) 1. pertaining to milk. 2. any of the intestinal lymphatics that transport chyle.

lactescence (lak'tes'ns) resemblance to milk.

lactic ('laktik) pertaining to milk.

l. acid a compound formed in the body in anaerobic metabolism of carbohydrate, and also produced by bacterial action on milk. The sodium salt of racemic or inactive lactic (sodium lactate) acid is used as an electrolyte and fluid replenisher.

lacticaemia (ˌlakti'seemi·ə) an excess of lactic acid in the blood; lactacidaemia.

lactiferous (lak'tifə·rəs) conveying milk.

lactifuge ('laktifyooj) checking or stopping milk secretion; an agent that so acts.

lactigenous (lak'tijənəs) producing milk.

lactigerous (lak'tijə·rəs) lactiferous.

lactim ('laktim) see LACTAM.

lactivorous (lak'tivə·rəs) feeding or subsisting upon milk.

Lactobacillus (ˌlaktohbə'siləs) a genus of bacteria, some of which are considered to be aetiologically related to dental caries, but are otherwise nonpathogenic. They produce lactic acid by fermentation. See also DÖDERLEIN'S BACILLUS and VAGINA.

lactobacillus (ˌlaktohbə'siləs) pl. *lactobacilli;* any individual organism of the genus *Lactobacillus.*

lactocele ('laktohˌseel) galactocele.

lactoferrin (ˌlaktoh'ferin) an iron-binding protein found in neutrophils and bodily secretions (milk, tears, saliva, bile, etc.), having bactericidal activity, and acting as an inhibitor of colony formation by granulocytes and macrophages.

lactoflavine (ˌlaktoh'flayveen) riboflavin.

lactogen ('laktəˌjen) any substance that enhances lactation.

human placental l. (hPL, HPL) a hormone secreted by the placenta, which disappears from the blood immediately after delivery. It has lactogenic, luteotrophic, and growth-promoting activity, and inhibits maternal insulin activity during pregnancy.

lactogenic (ˌlaktə'jenik) stimulating the production of milk.

l. hormone one of the gonadotrophic hormones of the anterior pituitary; it stimulates and sustains lactation in postpartum animals, and shows luteotrophic activity in certain mammals. Called also *prolactin.*

lactoglobulin (ˌlaktoh'globyuhlin) a globulin occurring in milk.

immune l's antibodies (immunoglobulins) occurring in the colostrum of mammals.

lactometer (lak'tomitə) an instrument for measuring the specific gravity of milk.

lactone ('laktohn) 1. an aromatic liquid from lactic acid. 2. a cyclic organic compound in which the chain is closed by ester formation between a carboxyl and a hydroxyl group in the same molecule.

lactorrhoea (ˌlaktə'reeə) excessive or spontaneous milk flow; persistent secretion of milk irrespective of nursing; galactorrhoea.

lactose ('laktohz, -tohs) a sugar derived from milk, which on hydrolysis yields glucose and galactose. Many persons are intolerant to lactose as a result of hereditary lactase deficiency.

lactoside ('laktəˌsied) glycoside in which the sugar constituent is lactose.

lactosuria (ˌlaktə'syooə·ri·ə) lactose in the urine.

lactotherapy (ˌlaktoh'therəpee) treatment by milk diet.

lactotrophe ('laktohˌtrohf) an acidophilic cell of the anterior pituitary that secretes prolactin.

lactotrophin (ˌlaktoh'trohfin) prolactin.

lactovegetarian (ˌlaktohˌveji'tair·ri·ən) 1. a person who subsists on a diet of milk or milk products and vegetables. 2. pertaining to such a diet.

lactulose ('laktyuhlohz) a synthetic disaccharide used as a cathartic and to enhance the excretion of ammonia in the treatment of portosystemic encephalopathy.

lacuna (lə'kyoonə) pl. *lacunae* [L.] 1. a small pit or hollow cavity. 2. a defect or gap, as in the field of vision (scotoma). adj. **lacunar**.

absorption l. a pit or groove in developing bone that is undergoing resorption; frequently found to contain osteoclasts.

bone l. a small cavity within the bone matrix, containing an osteocyte, and from which slender canaliculi radiate and penetrate the adjacent lamellae to anastomose with the canaliculi of neighbouring lacunae, thus forming a system of cavities interconnected by minute canals.

cartilage l. any of the small cavities within the cartilage matrix, containing a chondrocyte.
intervillous l. one of the blood spaces of the placenta in which the fetal villi are found.
l. magna the lateral expansion of the urethra of the glans penis; called also *navicular fossa.*
osseous l. bone lacuna.
l. pharyngis a depression of the pharyngeal end of the pharyngotympanic tube.

lacunule (lə'kyoonyool) a minute lacuna.

lacus ('laykəs) pl. *lacus* [L.] lake.
l. lacrimalis lacrimal lake.

Laënnec (,la·e'nek) René Théophile Hyacinthe (1781–1826). French physician. He is known for the invention of the stethoscope in 1819 and his *De l'auscultation médiate,* from which much of our knowledge of chest diseases is derived.

Laënnec's cirrhosis (,la·e'neks) cirrhosis of the liver associated with chronic excessive alcohol ingestion (see also Laënnec's CIRRHOSIS).

Laënnec's pearls soft casts of the smaller bronchial tubes expectorated in bronchial asthma.

Laetrile ('laytriel) American trademark for a substance derived from apricot stones, alleged to have antineoplastic activity.

laevo- word element. [L.] *left;* see also those words beginning *levo-*.

laevocardia (,leevoh'kahdi·ə) a term denoting normal position of the heart associated with transposition of other viscera (situs inversus). Called also *sinistrocardia.*

laevoclination (,leevohkli'nayshən) rotation of the upper poles of the vertical meridians of the two eyes to the left.

laevoduction (,leevoh'dukshən) movement of an eye to the left.

laevogyration (,leevohjie'rayshən) laevorotation.

laevorotary (,leevoh'rohtə·ree) laevorotatory.

laevorotation (,leevohroh'tayshən) a turning to the left; laevogyration.

laevorotatory (,leevoh'rohtətə·ree) turning the plane of polarization, or rays of light, to the left.

laevoversion (,leevoh'vərshən) a turning toward the left.

laevulose ('levyuh,lohz) a sugar from honey and many sweet fruits, used in solution as a fluid and nutrient replenisher; called also *fructose* and *fruit sugar.*

Lafora's bodies (la'for·rəz) intracytoplasmic inclusions consisting of a complex of glycoprotein and acid mucopolysaccharide; widespread deposits are found in myoclonus epilepsy.

Lafora's disease myoclonus epilepsy.

lag (lag) 1. the time elapsing between application of a stimulus and the resulting reaction. 2. the early period after inoculation of bacteria into a culture medium, in which the growth or cell division is slow.

lagena (lə'jeenə) the curved, flask-shaped organ of hearing in vertebrates lower than mammals, corresponding to the cochlear duct.

lageniform (lə'jeni,fawm) flask-shaped.

lagophthalmos (,lagof'thalmos) inability to shut the eyelids completely.

lake (layk) 1. to undergo separation of haemoglobin from erythrocytes. 2. a lacuna; a circumscribed collection of fluid in a hollow or depressed cavity.
lacrimal l. *lacus lacrimalis* [L.] the triangular space at the medial angle of the eye, where the tears collect. See also LACRIMAL APPARATUS.

lal(o)- word element. [Gr.] *speech, babbling.*

LaLeche League (la'lesh) an organization formed in 1957 for the purpose of helping women to breast-feed their infants. Information about the organization and the services it provides can be obtained from local groups or from LaLeche League of Great Britain, P.O. Box BM 3424, London WC1V 6XX.

laliatry (la'lieətree) the study and treatment of disorders of speech.

lallation (la'layshən) a babbling, infantile form of speech.

lalognosis (,lalog'nohsis) the understanding of speech.

lalopathology (,lalohpə'tholəjee) the branch of medicine dealing with disorders of speech.

lalopathy (la'lopəthee) any speech disorder.

laloplegia (,laloh'pleeji·ə) paralysis of the organs of speech.

lalorrhoea (,lalə'reeə) excessive flow of words.

Lamarck's theory (la'mahks) the theory that acquired characteristics may be inherited.

Lamaze method (la'mayz) a method of preparations for NATURAL CHILDBIRTH developed by the French obstetrician Fernand Lamaze, and based on the Russian psychoprophylactic technique of training the mind and body for the purpose of modifying the perception of pain during labour and delivery. The Lamaze method of prepared childbirth involves class sessions for both parents in which they learn about the birth process and the mechanisms of labour, are taught what to expect and what is expected of them during the birth of their child, and are trained in special exercises that develop neuromuscular control, promote physical conditioning, and eliminate or reduce the need for drugs and instruments during delivery. Advocates of the Lamaze method do not claim complete absence of pain during labour and delivery in every case, but they do feel that the method enriches the lives of the parents in many ways and provides for them a means of sharing the birth experience that is denied to them in the more conventional method of hospital deliveries.

lambda ('lamdə) the point of union of the lambdoid and sagittal sutures.

lambdacism ('lamdəsizəm) inability to utter the *l* sound.

lambdoid ('lamdoyd) shaped like the Greek letter lambda, Λ or λ.

lambliasis (lam'blieəsis) giardiasis.

lame (laym) incapable of normal locomotion; deviation from the normal gait.

lamella (lə'melə) pl. *lamellae* [L.] 1. a thin scale or plate, as of bone. adj. **lamellar.** 2. a thin medicated disc or wafer intended to be applied to the eye ball.
circumferential l. one of the bony plates that underlie the periosteum and endosteum.
concentric l. haversian lamella.
endosteal l. one of the bony plates lying beneath the endosteum.
ground l. interstitial lamella.
haversian l. one of the concentric bony plates surrounding a haversian canal.
intermediate l., interstitial l. one of the bony plates that fill in between the haversian systems.

lamellipodia (lə,meli'pohdi·ə) plural of *lamellipodium,* delicate sheet-like extensions of cytoplasm that form transient adhesions with the cell substrate and wave gently, enabling the cell to move along the substrate.

lamina ('laminə) pl. *laminae* [L.] a thin, flat plate or layer; used in anatomical nomenclature to designate such a structure, or a layer of a composite structure. Often used alone to mean a vertebral lamina.
l. basilaris the posterior wall of the cochlear duct, separating it from the scala tympani.
l. choroidocapillaris the inner layer of the choroid, composed of a single-layered network of small capillaries.
l. cribrosa 1. fascia cribrosa. 2. (of ethmoid bone) the

horizontal plate of ethmoid bone forming the roof of the nasal cavity, and perforated by many foramina for passage of olfactory nerves. 3. (of sclera) the perforated part of the sclera through which pass the axons of the retinal ganglion cells.

epithelial l. the layer of ependymal cells covering the choroid plexus.

l. fusca the pigmentary layer of the sclera.

l. propria 1. the connective tissue layer of mucous membrane. 2. the middle fibrous layer of the tympanic membrane.

spiral l., l. spiralis 1. a double plate of bone winding spirally around the modiolus, dividing the spiral canal of the cochlea into the scala tympani and scali vestibuli. 2. a bony projection on the outer wall of the cochlea in the lower part of the first turn.

terminal l. of hypothalamus the thin plate derived from the telencephalon, forming the anterior wall of the third ventricle of the cerebrum.

vertebral l. either of the pair of broad plates of bone flaring out from the pedicles of the vertebral arches and fusing together at the midline to complete the dorsal part of the arch and provide a base for the spinous process.

laminagraphy (ˌlami'nagrəfee) a special technique of body-section RADIOGRAPHY.

laminar ('laminə) made up of laminae or layers; pertaining to a lamina.

l. airflow room a special room with controlled airflow to maintain a protected 'infection-free' environment for the treating of patients at particular risk, e.g. patients undergoing a bone marrow transplant for acute leukaemia.

Laminaria (ˌlamin'ari·ə) a genus of seaweeds, the kelps, various species of which are used as sources of alginates. The dried stems of *L. digitata* are used to dilate the uterine cervix in induced ABORTION. See also Laminaria TENT.

laminated ('lamiˌnaytid) made up of laminae or thin layers.

lamination (ˌlami'nayshən) a laminar structure or arrangement.

laminectomy (ˌlami'nektəmee) surgical excision of the posterior arch of a vertebra. The procedure is most often performed to relieve the symptoms of a prolapsed intervertebral DISC. During laminectomy the spinal cord is exposed and the portion of the nucleus pulposus that has herniated through the prolapsed disc is removed. Laminectomy is indicated when conservative treatment is not effective and nerve damage is becoming progressively worse or when the patient is suffering from repeated attacks of pain. Laminectomy is sometimes followed by fusion of the adjacent vertebrae (spinal fusion) as a means of stabilizing that part of the spinal column in a fixed position. Bone grafts, usually taken from the iliac crest, are applied to fuse the affected vertebrae permanently, resulting in limitation of movement of this portion of the spine. Laminectomy is also performed for the removal of an intervertebral or spinal cord tumour.

PATIENT CARE. Before surgery the patient will receive treatment for prolapsed intervertebral disc. It should be remembered that when the patient is transported to other departments for various preoperative diagnostic tests, special care must be taken to keep the spine in good alignment.

Postoperatively the patient is placed in a bed with bed boards and a firm mattress. His position is changed by 'log-rolling' to prevent motion of the vertebral column. In addition he is observed for signs of haemorrhage or leakage of cerebrospinal fluid on the surgical dressing. Should such signs appear, the surgeon should be notified at once. If necessary the dressing may be reinforced but great care must be exercised in the handling of the operative area lest an infection develop and lead to meningitis.

Pain usually persists for some time after surgery, until the local oedema and muscle spasms subside. Analgesic medications are given as ordered. Special 'bicycle' exercises for the legs may be ordered to relieve muscle pains of the legs. Early ambulation depends on the desires of the surgeon. If the patient is confined to bed, his position must be changed often to avoid respiratory and pulmonary complications.

laminotomy (ˌlami'notəmee) transection of a vertebral lamina.

lamp (lamp) an apparatus for furnishing heat or light.

Finsen's l. a carbon arc lamp operating at 50 V and 50 A and so constructed that radiation is concentrated on an area of about 6 cm^2; a water-cooled quartz system is used to remove calorific radiation and a compression quartz piece to dehaematize the skin.

slit l. one embodying a diaphragm containing a slitlike opening, by means of which a narrow, flat beam of intense light may be projected into the eye. It gives intense illumination so that microscopic study may be made of the conjunctiva, cornea, iris, lens, and vitreous, the special feature being that it illuminates a section through the substance of these structures.

sun l. ultraviolet lamp.

ultraviolet l. an electric light source that transmits ultraviolet rays; used as a therapeutic device and as a means of obtaining an artificial sun tan. See also ULTRAVIOLET THERAPY.

lamprophonia (ˌlamproh'fohni·ə) clearness of voice.

lanatoside C (la'natohsied ˌsee) a glycoside obtained from *Digitalis lanata*, used as a cardiotonic like digitalis.

lance (lahns) 1. lancet. 2. to cut or incise with a lancet.

Lancefield classification ('lansfeeld) the classification of haemolytic streptococci into groups on the basis of serological action.

lancet ('lahnsət) a small, pointed, two-edged surgical knife.

lancinating ('lahnsiˌnayting) tearing, darting, or sharply cutting; used to describe pain.

Landouzy–Déjérine dystrophy (lanˌdoozeeˌdezhə'reen) a type of MUSCULAR DYSTROPHY.

Landry's paralysis (lan'dreez) Guillain-Barré syndrome.

Landsteiner's classification ('landstienəz) a classification of blood types in which they are designated O, A, B, and AB, depending on the presence or absence of agglutinogens A and B in the erythrocytes; called also *International classification*.

Lange colloidal gold test ('langə) a test made on cerebrospinal fluid to detect syphilis, disseminated sclerosis, meningitis and other neurological conditions.

Langerhans' islets (islands) ('langəˌhanz) irregular microscopic structures scattered throughout the pancreas, composed of alpha cells, which secrete glucagon; beta cells, which secrete insulin; and delta cells, which secrete gastrin.

Langhans' cell ('langhanz) see Langhans' giant CELL.

lanolin ('lanəlin) wool fat or wool grease that is refined and incorporated into many commercial preparations. Lanolin is a by-product of the process that accompanies the removal of sheep's wool from the pelt. In its crude form it is a greasy yellow wax of unpleasant odour. This odour disappears when the lanolin is emulsified and made into salves, creams, ointments, and cosmetics. Although lanolin is slightly antiseptic, it has no other medicinal benefits and is valuable principally because of the ease with which it penetrates the skin, and because it does not turn rancid.

Lanoxin (la'noksin) trademark for preparations of digoxin, a cardiotonic.

lanthanum ('lanthənəm) a chemical element, atomic number 57, atomic weight 138.91, symbol La. See table of elements in Appendix 2.

lanugo (lə'nyoogoh, -noo-) the fine hair that covers the body of the fetus. Called also *down*.

Lanvis ('lanvis) trademark for a preparation of thioguanine, an antineoplastic agent.

laparo- word element. [Gr.] *loin* or *flank*, *abdomen*.

laparoscope ('lapə·rə,skohp) an endoscope for examining within the peritoneal cavity.

laparoscopy (,lapə'roskəpee) examination by means of the laparoscope. adj. **laparoscopic**.

laparotomy (,lapə'rotəmee) incision through any part of the abdominal wall to enter the peritoneal cavity.

lapinization (,lapinie'zayshən) serial passage of a virus or vaccine through rabbits to modify its characteristics.

lapinize ('lapi,niez) to attenuate (as a virus or vaccine) by serial passage through rabbits.

lard (lahd) the purified internal fat of the pig; used as a basis for ointments.

lardaceous (lah'dayshəs) 1. resembling lard. 2. containing amyloid.

Largactil (,lah'gaktil) trademark for preparations of chlorpromazine, an antiemetic and tranquillizer.

larva ('lahvə) pl. *larvae* [L.] an independent, immature stage in the life cycle of an animal, in which it is markedly unlike the parent and must undergo changes in form and size to reach the adult stage.

l. currens a variant of larva migrans caused by *Strongyloides stercoralis*, in which the progression of the linear lesions is much more rapid.

l. migrans creeping eruption; a convoluted threadlike skin eruption that appears to migrate, caused by the burrowing beneath the skin of roundworm larvae, particularly the larvae of *Ancylostoma* species that parasitize dogs and cats. Similar lesions are caused by the larvae of botflies.

l. migrans, ocular infection of the eye with larvae of the roundworm *Toxocara canis* or *T. cati*, which may lodge in the choroid or retina or migrate to the vitreous; on the death of the larvae, a granulomatous inflammation occurs, the lesion varying from a translucent elevation of the retina to massive retinal detachment and pseudoglioma.

l. migrans, visceral a condition due to prolonged migration by larvae of animal nematodes in human tissue other than skin commonly caused by larvae of the roundworms *Toxocara canis* and *T. cati*.

larval ('lahv'l) 1. pertaining to larvae. 2. larvate.

larvate ('lahvayt) masked; concealed: said of a disease or of a symptom of a disease.

larvicide ('lahvi,sied) an agent that kills insect larvae.

laryng(o)- word element. [Gr.] *larynx*.

laryngalgia (,larin'galji·ə) pain in the larynx.

laryngeal (lə'rinji·əl, ,larin'jeeəl) pertaining to the larynx.

laryngectomee (,larin'jektəmee) a person whose larynx has been removed.

laryngectomy (,larin'jektəmee) partial or total removal of the larynx by surgery. It is usually performed as treatment for cancer of the larynx.

There are three methods of speaking without use of the larynx. Oesophageal speech, the simplest method, is usually the first one the patient learns. He is taught to swallow air and then to form simple sounds and words while belching. With careful instruction and persistent practice, he can make sustained belches that cause a column of air to vibrate in his throat and pharynx. This air column substitutes for vocal cords as he forms words with his mouth. Oesophageal speech is not smooth, and once the patient has mastered it he begins to learn the smoother, more advanced pharyngeal method.

In pharyngeal speech, a person uses only the limited amount of air that enters the nose and mouth when he breathes through the tracheostomy tube. Sound is generated by blocking this air with quick tongue actions, forcing it to vibrate against the roof of the pharynx. By controlling the air and expelling it slowly, it is possible to approach the rhythm and phrasing of normal, fluent speech. As he grows in skill and confidence, the pharyngeal speaker sounds like a person with an ordinary, slightly hoarse voice.

The third method is use of an electronic voice box which connects the opening of the trachea in the neck to the mouth. It can be removed when the patient desires.

Patient Care. Because of the physical and emotional adjustments that the patient and his family must make to the surgical procedure and its aftermath, it is especially important that they receive instruction and counselling prior to surgery. They will need help in coping with their fears and anxieties about the patient's ability to communicate after surgery, and they must know that the members of the health care team are available to listen to them uncritically and answer their questions honestly. The patient should be given an explanation about the type of equipment to be used in the immediate postoperative period and the purpose of each procedure. He should be assured that a pencil and paper or other means of communicating by writing will be at his bedside at all times after surgery and that he will not be left without some means of summoning help. It is understandable that one of the greatest fears of these patients is that, since they will be unable to cry out or speak, they will be left alone and might suffocate.

There is some justification for the patient's fear of suffocation; this is the major hazard during the immediate postoperative period. Suction is usually ordered every hour and whenever necessary to keep the airway open. Should this not relieve the symptoms of extreme dyspnoea and tachycardia, the inner *and outer* cannula may be removed to relieve obstruction. The stoma will not collapse as it might in a tracheostomy patient because the stoma is sutured open. An extra laryngectomy tube is kept at the bedside in case an emergency arises and for daily changing of the outer tube if the surgeon so chooses. It is usually possible to remove the tube permanently after the third or fourth postoperative day. At this time the patient will also be able to swallow liquids.

In preparation for his return home, the patient is taught self-care of his laryngectomy. He is warned against aspirating water into the lungs during bathing or showering. Although a dressing is not necessary for covering the tracheal opening in the neck, the patient may wish to conceal it with a small square of cotton material or wear a collar or scarf of porous material to hide the wound. These types of covering are useful in that they act as filters and remove dust and other irritants from the air being inhaled through the stoma.

Printed material about self-care is available from the local cancer societies and many communities have a laryngectomee club which offers much moral support and information that are valuable to the patient as he adjusts to his new way of life. Information regarding these laryngectomee clubs and other aspects of postlaryngectomy rehabilitation can be obtained from the hospital prior to discharge.

laryngemphraxis (ˌlarinjem'fraksis) obstruction or closure of the larynx.

laryngismus (ˌlarin'jizməs) spasm of the larynx. adj. **laryngismal**.

l. stridulous sudden laryngeal spasm with crowing inspiration.

laryngitis (ˌlarin'jietis) inflammation of the mucous membrane of the larynx, characterized by dryness and soreness of the throat, hoarseness, cough, and dysphagia.

ACUTE LARYNGITIS. Acute laryngitis may be caused by overuse of the voice, allergies, irritating dust or smoke, hot or corrosive liquids, or even violent weeping. It also occurs in viral or bacterial infections, and is frequently associated with other diseases of the respiratory tract.

In adults, a mild case of acute laryngitis begins with a dry, tickling sensation in the larynx, followed quickly by partial or complete loss of the voice. There may be a slight fever, minor discomfort, and poor appetite, with recovery after a few days. Other and more uncomfortable symptoms can include a feeling of heat and pain in the throat, difficulty in swallowing, and dry cough followed by expectoration; the voice may be either painful to use or absent. Swelling of the larynx and epiglottis may impair breathing. Increasing difficulty in breathing may be a sign of oedematous laryngitis, or CROUP.

Treatment for acute laryngitis requires that the patient rest in bed and refrain from talking. The room temperature should be even and warm. The air is kept moist with a humidifier or vaporizer. An ice bag on the throat often is soothing. In some cases, antibiotics may be necessary.

Children are especially vulnerable to laryngitis because of the smallness of their air passages. Most cases in children subside within a few days, but if inflammation and swelling continue to increase, severe dyspnoea occurs.

CHRONIC LARYNGITIS. After repeated attacks of the acute type, chronic laryngitis may develop. This is caused mostly by continual irritation from overuse of the voice, tobacco smoke, dust, or chemical vapours, or by a chronic nasal or sinus disorder. Often the moist mucous membrane lining the larynx becomes granulated. The granulation can proceed to thickening and hardening of the mucous membrane, which changes the voice or makes it hoarse. There is little or no pain, though there may be tickling in the throat and a slight cough.

Chronic laryngitis that has persisted for a number of years may result in chronic hypertrophic laryngitis, a condition in which there is a permanent change in the voice because of hypertrophy of the membrane lining the larynx.

Treatment for chronic laryngitis is the same as for the acute form, with elimination of all sources of irritation and reinfection. Hoarseness that lasts longer than 2 weeks may be a warning of tumour or cancer of the larynx, or of a tumour in the thorax that presses on the recurrent laryngeal nerve, which controls the larynx.

OTHER FORMS OF LARYNGITIS. Paroxysmal laryngitis is a nervous disorder affecting infants that seems to be associated with enlarged adenoids and rickets. It consists of unexplained spasms in which the larynx closes, cutting off the air passage, and then suddenly opens. Sometimes the condition may be fatal. Treatment of this form of laryngitis calls for removal of adenoids.

Other types include diphtheritic laryngitis, tuberculous laryngitis, traumatic laryngitis, and allergic laryngitis. Treatment of diphtheritic laryngitis often involves intubation or tracheostomy in order to admit air. Traumatic laryngitis also often requires tracheostomy. Allergic laryngitis, often caused by smoking or other irritants, is treated in the same way as other allergies.

laryngocele (lə'ring·gohˌseel) a congenital anomalous air sac communicating with a cavity of the larynx; it may produce a tumour-like lesion visible on the outside of the neck.

laryngocentesis (ləˌring·gohsen'teesis) surgical puncture of the larynx, with aspiration.

laryngofissure (ləˌring·goh'fishə) median laryngotomy.

laryngogram (lə'ring·gohˌgram) a radiograph of the larynx.

laryngography (ˌlaring'gogrəfee) radiography of the larynx following instillation of a contrast medium.

laryngology (ˌlaring'goləjee) that branch of medicine which has to do with the throat, pharynx, larynx, nasopharynx, and tracheobronchial tree.

laryngopathy (ˌlaring'gopəthee) any disorder of the larynx.

laryngophantom (ləˌring·goh'fantəm) an artificial model of the larynx.

laryngopharyngeal (ləˌring·gohfə'rinji·əl, -ˌfarin'jeeəl) pertaining to the larynx and pharynx.

laryngopharyngectomy (ləˌring·gohˌfarin'jektəmee) excision of the larynx and pharynx.

laryngopharyngitis (ləˌring·gohˌfarin'jietis) inflammation of the larynx and pharynx.

laryngopharynx (ləˌring·goh'faringks) the portion of the pharynx below the upper edge of the epiglottis, opening into the larynx and oesophagus.

laryngophony (ˌlaring'gofənee) the vocal sound heard in auscultating the larynx.

laryngoplasty (lə'ring·gohˌplastee) plastic repair of the larynx.

laryngoplegia (ləˌring·goh'pleeji·ə) paralysis of the larynx.

laryngoptosis (ləˌring·goh'tohsis) a lowering and mobilization of the larynx, as sometimes seen in the aged.

laryngorhinology (ləˌring·gohrie'noləjee) the branch of medicine that deals with the larynx and nose.

laryngoscleroma (ləˌring·gohsklia'rohmə) scleroma of the larynx.

laryngoscope (lə'ring·gohˌskohp) an endoscope equipped with a light and mirrors for illumination and examination of the larynx.

laryngoscopy (ˌlaring'goskəpee) direct visual examination of the larynx with a laryngoscope. adj. **laryngoscopic**.

Before direct examination the patient is given a mild sedative to promote relaxation during the procedure which, though not uncomfortable, may be frightening and exhausting for the patient. Immediately before the laryngoscope is passed, the throat is anaesthetized locally with cocaine spray. The patient lies on his back on the examining table with his head extending over the edge. An attendant stands at his head, holding it in position and supporting its weight.

Following the laryngoscopy, fluids and foods are withheld until the effects of the local anaesthetic have worn off and the gag reflex has returned.

Indirect laryngoscopy is examination of the larynx by observation of the reflection of it in a laryngeal mirror.

laryngospasm (lə'ring·gohˌspazəm) spasmodic closure of the larynx.

laryngostenosis (ləˌring·gohstə'nohsis) narrowing or stricture of the larynx.

laryngostomy (ˌlaring'gostəmee) surgical creation of an artificial opening into the larynx.

laryngotomy (ˌlaring'gotəmee) incision of the larynx.
inferior l. incision of the larynx through the lower part of the fibroelastic membrane of the larynx (cricothyroid membrane).
median l. incision of the larynx through the thyroid cartilage.
subhyoid l., superior l. incision of the larynx through the fibroelastic membrane attached to the hyoid bone and the thyroid cartilage (thyrohyoid membrane).

laryngotracheal (ləˌring·goh'traki·əl, -trə'keeəl) pertaining to the larynx and trachea.

laryngotracheitis (ləˌring·gohˌtraki'ietis) inflammation of the larynx and trachea.

laryngotracheobronchitis (ləˌring·gohˌtrakiohbrong'kietis) an acute viral infection of the respiratory tract which occurs particularly in young children.

laryngotracheotomy (ləˌring·gohˌtraki'otəmee) incision of the larynx and trachea.

laryngoxerosis (ləˌring·gohzə'rohsis) dryness of the larynx.

larynx ('laringks) pl. *larynges* [Gr.] the muscular and cartilaginous structure, lined with mucous membrane, situated at the top of the trachea and below the root of the tongue and the hyoid bone. The larynx contains the vocal cords, and is the source of the sound heard in speech; it is called also the *voice box.* It is part of the respiratory system, and air passes through the larynx as it travels from the pharynx to the trachea and back again on its way to and from the lungs.

The larynx is composed of nine cartilages (thyroid, cricoid, and epiglottis and the paired arytenoid, corniculate, and cuneiform) held together by muscles and ligaments. The largest of these cartilages, the thyroid cartilage, forms the Adam's apple, which protrudes in the front of the neck. Two flexible vocal cords reach from the back to the front wall of the larynx and are manipulated by small muscles to produce sound. The epiglottis, a flap or lid at the base of the tongue, closes the larynx as it is lifted up during swallowing and so prevents passage of food or drink into the larynx and trachea.

DISORDERS OF THE LARYNX. Hoarseness is often the result of inflammation of the mucous membrane of the larynx, or LARYNGITIS. Persistent hoarseness or a change of voice without apparent cause may, however, be a warning signal, an indication of tuberculosis, syphilis, or a tumour.

In cancer of the larynx the first symptom may be persistent hoarseness or the feeling of a lump in the throat, although this feeling, like other laryngeal symptoms, may be caused by emotional stress. Early diagnosis of laryngeal cancer is essential to effective treatment.

Lasègue's sign (la'saygz) in sciatica, aggravation of pain in the back and leg elicited by passive raising of the heel from the bed with the knee straight; no pain is produced when the knee is flexed.

laser ('layzə) a device that transfers electromagnetic radiation of various frequencies into an extremely intense, small, and nearly nondivergent beam of monochromatic radiation in the visible region, with all the waves in phase; from *l*ight *a*mplification by *s*timulated *e*mission of *r*adiation. Capable of mobilizing immense heat and power when focused at close range, it is used as a tool in surgery, in diagnosis, and in physiological studies. Called also *optical maser*.

Lasix ('laysiks) trademark for preparations of frusemide, a diuretic.

Lassa fever ('lasə) a West African viral haemorrhagic fever with insidious onset and an incubation period of 6–21 days. It is a zoonosis, the reservoir of infection of which is the multimammate rat, *Mastomys natalensis.* Transmission to man occurs by contamination of broken skin or mucous membrane with the urine of infected rats. Devastating outbreaks of person-to-person transmission have occurred in hospital by accidental inoculation of blood and tissue fluid from infected patients. At least 10 importations into the UK have occurred.

TREATMENT. This consists of nursing under strict security precautions, antiviral drugs, convalescent serum and general supportive care.

PREVENTION. In the UK prevention is dependent on the early detection of cases and their isolation, and strict precautions to protect health care staff caring for febrile patients from Africa from inoculation or other accidents.

Lassar's paste ('lasəz) a soothing paste used in skin diseases, containing salicylic acid, zinc oxide, starch and soft paraffin. A common base for dithrand, etc. Widely used in dermatology.

lassitude ('lasiˌtyood) weakness; exhaustion.

latamoxef sodium ('moksəˌlaktam) a third generation cephalosporin antibiotic having an oxa-β-lactam ring and a broad spectrum of activity, effective against β-lactamase-producing strains of *Haemophilus influenzae* and gram-negative enteric bacilli, including multiple drug-resistant strains.

latency ('laytənsee) a state of being latent.
l. period 1. latent period. 2. the period from the ages of five to seven years to adolescence, when there is cessation of psychosexual development.

latent ('laytənt) dormant or concealed; not manifest; potential.
l. period a seemingly inactive period, as that between exposure of tissue to an injurious agent and the manifestations of response, or that between the instant of stimulation and the beginning of response.

laterad ('latə·rad) toward the lateral aspect.

lateral ('latə·rəl) 1. denoting a position further from the median plane or midline of the body or a structure. 2. pertaining to a side.

lateralis (ˌlatə'raylis) [L.] *lateral.*

laterality (ˌlatə'ralitee) a tendency to use preferentially the organs (hand, foot, ear, eye) of the same side in voluntary motor acts.
crossed l. the preferential use of contralateral members of the different pairs of organs in voluntary motor acts, e.g. right eye and left hand.
dominant l. the preferential use of ipsilateral members of the different pairs of organs in voluntary motor acts, e.g. right (dextrality) or left (sinistrality) ear, eye, hand, and leg.

lateroduction (ˌlatə·roh'dukshən) movement of an eye to either side.

lateroflexion (ˌlatə·roh'flekshən) flexion to one side.

laterotorsion (ˌlatə·roh'tawshən) twisting of the vertical meridian of the eye to either side.

lateroversion (ˌlatə·roh'vərshən, -zhən) abnormal turning to one side.

lathyrism ('lathiˌrizəm) a morbid condition marked by spastic paraplegia, pain, hyperaesthesia, and paraesthesia, due to ingestion of the seeds of leguminous plants of the genus *Lathyrus*, which includes many kinds of peas. adj. **lathyritic**.

latissimus (la'tisiməs) [L.] *widest;* in anatomy, denoting a broad structure.

Latrodectus (ˌlatroh'dektəs) a genus of poisonous spiders.
L. mactans a species found in the United States; commonly known as the black widow. Its bite may cause severe symptoms or even death.

LATS long-acting thyroid stimulator.

LATS protector an antibody found in hyperthyroid

patients with the capacity to block LATS (long-acting thyroid stimulator) from combining with thyroid microsomes.

latus ('laytəs, 'lat-) [L.] 1. *broad, wide.* 2. *the side* or *flank.*

laudanum ('lawd'nəm) tincture of opium; a preparation formerly used as a narcotic.

laughing gas ('lahfing) nitrous oxide.

Laurence–Moon–Biedl syndrome (ˌlo·rənsˌmoon-'beed'l) a hereditary syndrome transmitted as an autosomal recessive trait characterized by degeneration of the retina, obesity and mental handicap. Called also *retinodiencephalic degeneration.*

lavage ('lavij, la'vahzh) 1. irrigation or washing out of an organ or cavity, as of the stomach or intestine. 2. to wash out, or irrigate.

Gastric lavage, or irrigation of the stomach, is usually done to remove ingested poisons. The only time gastric lavage is done prior to anaesthesia is in babies with congenital pyloric stenosis. The solutions used for gastric lavage are physiological saline, 1 per cent sodium bicarbonate, plain water or a specific antidote for a poison. A nasogastric tube is passed and then the irrigating fluid is funneled into the tube. It is allowed to flow into the stomach by gravity. The solution is removed by siphonage; when the funnel is lowered, the fluid flows out, bringing with it the contents of the stomach.

Lavoisier (lə'vwaziay) Antoine Laurent (1743–1794). French chemist, born in Paris and later guillotined by the French Revolutionists. Lavoisier demolished the phlogiston theory (a theory of combustion) and explained the true nature of respiration by his introduction of quantitative relations in chemistry. He was secretary and treasurer of a committee seeking the uniformity of weights and measures in France, which led to the establishment of the metric system.

law (lor) a uniform or constant fact or principle.

l. of independent assortment the members of gene pairs segregate independently during meiosis (see also MENDEL'S LAW).

l. of segregation in each generation the ratio of (a) pure dominants, (b) dominants giving descendants in the proportion of three dominants to one recessive, and (c) pure recessives is 1:2:1. This ratio follows from the fact that the two alleles of a gene cannot be a part of a single gamete, but must segregate to different gametes (see also MENDEL'S LAW).

lawrencium (lor'rensi·əm, lo'ren-) a chemical element, atomic number 103, atomic weight 257, symbol Lr. See table of elements in Appendix 2.

laxative ('laksətiv) a medicine that loosens the bowel contents and encourages evacuation. A laxative with a mild or gentle effect on the bowels is also known as an aperient; one with a strong effect is referred to as a cathartic or a purgative.

Bland laxatives may be used temporarily in the treatment of CONSTIPATION along with other measures. Mineral oil, or liquid petrolatum, and olive oil act as lubricants. Sometimes liquid paraffin is used in combination with agar, which is bulk-producing. Cascara and milk of magnesia are two other mild laxatives. Psyllium, which is prepared from a plant seed, helps elimination by encouraging peristaltic movements.

Saline purges, such as sodium phosphate and magnesium sulphate (Epsom salts), flush the intestinal tract. They do this by preventing the intestines from absorbing water; evacuation takes place as soon as water accumulates.

Castor oil is a strong cathartic that effects complete evacuation of the bowels. Its administration is followed by temporary constipation.

DANGERS OF LAXATIVES. Laxatives should be employed only with the advice of a doctor. Constipation may be a symptom of serious organic illness as well as the result of improper diet and habits. Also, laxatives taken regularly tend to deprive the colon of its natural muscle tone. In this way laxatives can be the cause of chronic constipation rather than its cure.

Liquid paraffin taken regularly tends to dilute certain vitamins derived from the food one eats. It can also seep into the lungs, causing a reaction resembling PNEUMONIA, especially in older people.

Purgative salts can produce DEHYDRATION. Laxatives that produce bulk may cause stonelike balls (bezoars) to develop.

A strong cathartic, such as castor oil, can have fatal results if used when there is nausea, vomiting, abdominal pain, or other symptoms of APPENDICITIS. It is also dangerous to use during pregnancy.

Children, in particular, cannot use the same dosage or the strong laxatives taken by adults.

laxator (lak'saytə) that which slackens or relaxes.

layer ('layə) stratum; a sheetlike mass of tissue of nearly uniform thickness, several of which may be superimposed, one above the other, as in the epidermis.

ameloblastic l. the inner layer of cells of the enamel organ, which forms the enamel prisms of the teeth.

bacillary l. layer of rods and cones.

basal l. 1. the deepest layer of the epidermis. 2. the deepest layer of the uterine mucosa.

blastodermic l. germ layer.

clear l. stratum lucidum; the clear translucent layer of the epidermis, just beneath the horny layer.

columnar l. 1. layer of rods and cones. 2. mantle layer.

compact l. the layer of the endometrium nearest the surface, containing the necks of the uterine glands.

enamel l. the outermost layer of cells of the enamel organ.

functional l. the compact and spongy layers of the endometrium considered together, the cells of which are cast off at menstruation and parturition; known as the *decidua* during pregnancy.

ganglionic l. of cerebellum the thin middle grey layer of the cortex of the cerebellum, consisting of a single layer of Purkinje cells.

germ l. any of the three primary layers of cells formed in the early development of the embryo (ectoderm, entoderm, and mesoderm), from which the organs and tissues develop.

germinative l. the basal layer of the epidermis; reproductive layer of the skin, providing new cells for the upper layers of the epidermis and also, by invagination and differentiation, the cells for hair follicles, sweat glands and other structures in the dermis.

granular l. 1. the layer of epidermis between the clear and prickle-cell layers; called also *stratum granulosum.* 2. the deep layer of the cortex of the cerebellum. 3. the layer of follicle cells lining the theca of the vesicular ovarian follicle.

half-value l. the thickness of a given substance which, when introduced in the path of a given beam of radiation, will reduce its intensity by one half.

Henle's l. the outermost layer of the inner root sheath of the hair follicle.

horny l. 1. stratum corneum; the outermost layer of the epidermis, consisting of dead and desquamating cells. 2. the outer, compact layer of the nail.

keratohyaline l. granular layer (1).

malpighian l. the basal layer and the prickle-cell layer considered together.

mantle l. the middle layer of the wall of the primitive

neural tube, containing primitive nerve cells and later forming the grey matter of the central nervous system.

nervous l. all of the retina except the pigment layer; the inner layer of the optic cup.

odontoblastic l. the epithelioid layer of odontoblasts in contact with the dentine of teeth.

Ollier's l., osteogenetic l. the innermost layer of the periosteum.

prickle-cell l. stratum spinosum; the layer of the epidermis between the granular and basal layers, marked by the presence of prickle cells.

l. of rods and cones a layer of the retina immediately beneath the pigment epithelium, between it and the external limiting membrane, containing the rods and cones.

spinous l. prickle-cell layer.

spongy l. the middle layer of the endometrium, containing the tortuous portions of the uterine glands.

subendocardial l. the layer of loose fibrous tissue uniting the endocardium and myocardium.

zonal l. of thalamus a layer of myelinated fibres covering the dorsal surface of the thalamus.

lazy leukocyte syndrome ('layzee) a syndrome occurring in children, marked by recurrent low-grade infections, associated with a defect in neutrophil chemotaxis and deficient random mobility of neutrophils.

lb [L.] *libra* (pound).

LBW low birth weight.

LD lactate dehydrogenase; lethal dose.

LD_{50} median lethal dose; the quantity of an agent that will kill 50 per cent of the test subjects; in radiology, the dose of radiation which when absorbed by members of the population will result in the death of 50 per cent of that population.

LDH lactate dehydrogenase.

LDL low-density lipoprotein.

LDS Licentiate in Dental Surgery.

LE lupus erythematosus.

LE cell a mature neutrophilic polymorphonuclear leukocyte, which has phagocytized a large spherical, homogeneous-appearing inclusion, itself derived from another neutrophil; a characteristic of lupus erythematosus, but also found in analogous connective tissue disorders.

LE phenomenon, LE test the formation of LE cells on incubation of normal neutrophils with the serum of patients with lupus erythematosus.

Le Fort's fracture (lə 'for) bilateral horizontal fracture of the maxilla (see also Le Fort's FRACTURE).

lead[1] (led) a chemical element, atomic number 82, atomic weight 207.19, symbol Pb. See table of elements in Appendix 2.

l. poisoning a form of poisoning caused by the presence of lead or lead salts in the body. Lead poisoning affects the brain, nervous system, blood, and digestive system. It can be either chronic or acute.

Chronic lead poisoning (plumbism) was once fairly common among painters, and was called 'painter's colic'. It became less frequent as paints composed of other chemicals were substituted for lead-based paints and as plastic toys replaced lead ones. Replacement of lead piping by copper and plastic has also greatly reduced the incidence of lead poisoning. The disease is still seen among children with pica (a craving for unnatural articles of food) who may eat lead paint or coatings.

Symptoms include weight loss, anaemia, stomach cramp (lead colic), a bluish black line at the edge of the gums, and constipation. Other symptoms may be mental depression and, in children, irritability and convulsions. In addition to the poisoning, the anaemia and weight loss must also be treated, usually by providing an adequate diet. In serious cases, EDTA (ethylenediamine tetraacetate) may be prescribed.

Acute lead poisoning, which is rare, can be caused in two ways. Lead may accumulate in the bones, liver, kidneys, brain, and muscles and then be released suddenly to produce an acute condition; or large amounts of lead may be inhaled or ingested at one time. Symptoms are a metallic taste in the mouth, vomiting, bloody or black diarrhoea, and muscle cramps. Diagnosis is made by examination of the blood and urine. Treatment consists of immediate removal of unabsorbed lead in the intestinal tract through the administration of mild saline cathartics and enemas. EDTA is given and in most cases measures must be taken to reduce the increased intracranial pressure that accompanies acute lead poisoning.

PREVENTION. Workers exposed to lead are required to undergo regular medical examination and monitoring under the Control of Lead at Work Regulations Act 1980, with reporting to the Chief Employment Medical Adviser as a notifiable industrial disease. Levels up to 60 μg/dl in blood samples are considered safe but above this, treatment with chelating agents may be required.

An important aspect of prevention of lead poisoning is determination of sources of lead in the environment and efforts to remove them. Sources include peeling paint from window sills, walls, floors, and bannisters, and from soil around old houses that have shed exterior paint through the years. A vital factor in coping with the problem of lead contamination is public education and development of a community awareness of possible sources and of the need for elimination of these hazards from the environment. The levels of lead in petrol are one area of particular current concern.

lead[2] (leed) a specific array (pair) of electrodes used in recording changes in electric potential, created by activity of an organ, such as the heart (electrocardiography) or brain (electroencephalography); applied also to the particular segment of the tracing produced by the potential registered through the specific electrodes; in electrocardiography, lead I records the potential differences between the two arms, lead II between the right arm and left leg, lead III between the left arm and left leg, and a fourth lead (V) from various sites over the heart (see accompanying table and illustration).

bipolar l. an array involving two electrodes placed at different body sites.

oesophageal l. one attached to an electrode inserted in the oesophagus.

limb l's electrodes placed on the arms and left leg.

precordial l's leads recording electric potential from various sites over the heart, designated V with a subscript numeral indicating the exact site: V_1, fourth intercostal space immediately to the right of the sternum; V_2, fourth intercostal space immediately to the left of the sternum; V_3, midway between V_2 and V_4; V_4, fifth intercostal space in the midclavicular line (the imaginary vertical line on the anterior surface of the body), passing through the centre of the nipple; V_5, at the same horizontal level as V_4, in the left anterior axillary line (the imaginary vertical line passing through the middle of the axilla); V_6, left midaxillary line at the same horizontal level as V_4 and V_5 (see accompanying table and illustration).

unipolar l. an array of two electrodes, only one of which transmits potential variations..

Leber's optic atrophy (laybərz) hereditary bilateral

ECG leads

	ECG lead	Connection	Orientation
Standard leads of Einthoven	I	LA v. RA	Lateral
(bipolar)	II	LL v. RA	Inferior/lateral
	III	LL v. LA	Inferior/cavity
Augmented leads of Goldberger	AVR	RA v. LA+LL	Cavity
('unipolar')	AVL	LA v. RA+LL	Lateral
	AVF	LL v. RA+LA	Inferior
Chest leads of Wilson	V_1	4th RICS PS v. RA+LL+LA	Cavity
(unipolar)	V_2	4th LICS PS v. RA+LL+LA	Septum/anterior
	V_3	4th/5th LICS PS-MCL v. RA+LL+LA	Septum/anterior
	V_4	5th LICS MCL v. RA+LL+LA	Anterior
	V_5	5th LICS AAL v. RA+LL+LA	Anterior/lateral
	V_6	5th LICS MAL v. RA+LL+LA	Lateral

LA = left arm
RA = right arm
LL = left leg

RA+LL+LA = Wilson's common terminal
RICS = right intercostal space

LICS = left intercostal space
PS = parasternal
MCL = mid-clavicular line
AAL = anterior axillary line
MAL = mid-axillary line
PS-MCL = midway between PS and MCL

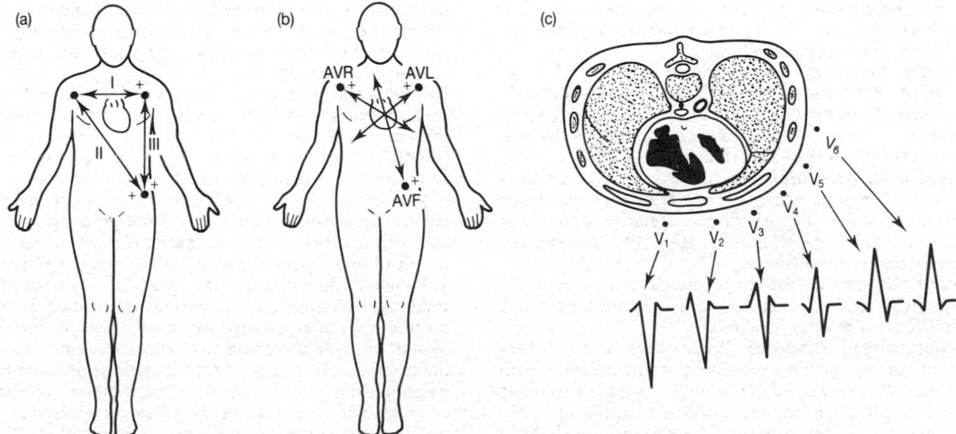

The connections or directions which comprise the 12-lead electrocardiogram. (a) The bipolar leads. (b) The unipolar leads. (c) The chest leads.

atrophy of the optic nerve affecting postpubertal males; there is rapid loss of vision resulting in permanent central scotoma. Called also *Leber's disease*.

lecithin ('lesithin) any of a group of phospholipids found in animal tissues, especially nerve tissue, the liver, semen, and egg yolk, consisting of esters of glycerol with two molecules of long-chain aliphatic acids and one of phosphoric acid, the latter being esterified with the alcohol group of choline.

lecithin–sphingomyelin ratio (ˌlesithinˌsfing·goh-'mieəlin) the ratio of lecithin to sphingomyelin in amniotic fluid, the determination of which is helpful in establishing the maturity of the fetus and its susceptibility to *hyaline membrane disease* after birth. Abbreviated L/S ratio.

lecithinase ('lesithiˌnayz) an enzyme that splits up lecithin. Called also *phospholipase*.

lecitho- word element. [Gr.] *the yolk of an egg* or *ovum*.

lecithoblast ('lesithohˌblast) the primitive entoderm of a two-layered blastodisc.

lectin ('lektin) a term applied to haemagglutinating substances present in saline extracts of certain plant seeds, which specifically agglutinate erythrocytes of certain blood groups or stimulate lymphocyte proliferation.

Lederfen ('ledərfen) trademark for a preparation of fenbufen, a nonsteroidal anti-inflammatory agent.

leech ('leech) any of the annelids of the class Hirudinea, especially *Hirudo medicinalis*; some species are bloodsuckers, and in rare occasions may be used for drawing blood.

Leeuwenhoek ('layvən,huhk) Antony van (1632–1723). Dutch microscopist. Born in Delft, Holland, he made many interesting discoveries through his careful observations even though his work was not conducted on a definite scientific plan. He gave the first accurate description of the red blood corpuscles in 1674, and in 1677 he described and illustrated the spermatozoa in animals, although he had been anticipated in this discovery by several months. He investigated the structure of muscle, the crystalline lens, and teeth, and was the first to see protozoa and bacteria under the microscope.

left ventricular assist device (left) a circulatory support device consisting of a pump with afferent and efferent conduits attached to the left ventricular apex and the ascending aorta, respectively, each conduit containing a porcine valve to ensure unidirectional blood flow; the pump rests on the external chest wall and is connected to an external pneumatic power source and control circuit.

leg (leg) the lower limb, especially the part between the knee and foot.

bayonet l. ankylosis of the knee after backward displacement of the tibia and fibula.

bow l. genu varum.

milk l. phlebitis of the femoral vein, with swelling of the leg (see also PHLEGMASIA ALBA DOLENS). Called also *white leg*.

restless l's syndrome a disagreeable, creeping, irritating sensation in the legs, usually the lower legs, relieved only by walking or keeping the legs moving. Called also Ekbom's syndrome.

Legg's disease, Legg–Calvé disease, Legg–Calvé–Perthes disease, Legg–Calvé–Waldenström disease (legz; legkal'vay; leg,kalvay'pərtayz; leg,kalvay'valdenstrohm) osteochrondrosis of the epiphysis of the head of the femur.

Legionella pneumophila (,leejə'nelə nyoo'mofilə) a species of gram-negative, non-acid-fast, rod-shaped bacteria which require both cysteine and iron for growth; it is the causative agent of LEGIONNAIRES' DISEASE and PONTIAC FEVER.

legionellosis (,leejəne'lohsis) disease caused by infection with *Legionella* species, such as *L. pneumophila*. A notifiable disease in Scotland.

legionnaires' disease (leegən'airz) a pulmonary form of legionellosis, resulting from infection with *Legionella pneumophila*. The disease acquired its name as a result of an outbreak of illness during the 1976 convention of the American Legion that was held in Philadelphia. The gram-negative bacillus causing the disease was isolated from the lungs of four persons who attended the convention, contracted the disease, and succumbed to the infection.

The prevalence of legionnaires' disease is not certain but it is estimated that between 5 and 10 per cent of the annual cases of pneumonia in the UK are caused by *L. pneumophila*. Approximately 70 per cent of those cases occur in epidemic form, while the remainder are sporadic infections. The disease is seen most often in middle-aged to elderly men who are cigarette smokers or are immunosuppressed. There is evidence of an increased incidence in the late summer months in temperate climates, and roughly one-third of all cases diagnosed in the UK appear to contract the disease while on holiday in southern European countries.

Specific diagnostic tests for legionnaires' disease include both direct and indirect fluorescent testing for antibodies against the organism. Other laboratory tests reveal mild leukocytosis; elevated erythrocyte sedimentation rate; increased liver enzymes, especially lactate dehydrogenase; elevated blood urea nitrogen; and abnormal blood gases showing hypoxaemia and hypocarbia.

Pulmonary symptoms of legionnaires' disease are typical of pneumonia; however, patients do not respond to the usual therapy for pneumonia and there can be permanent lung damage. Possible nonpulmonary complications include liver damage, altered levels of consciousness owing to neuronal involvement, and renal abnormalities that can require renal dialysis.

Treatment consists of erythromycin and, in patients who do not respond to erythromycin alone, rifampicin plus erythromycin. Severe hypoxia requires mechanical ventilation and oxygen therapy. Isolation of the patient is not considered to be necessary; however, respiratory precautions are indicated. Supportive measures to help the patient cope with high FEVER, nausea and vomiting, and RENAL FAILURE are essential components of patient care. See also PNEUMONIA.

legume ('legyoom) the pod or fruit of a leguminous plant, such as peas and beans.

legumin (le'gyoomin) a protein of peas, beans, and all pulses.

Leiner's disease ('lienəz) erythroderma desquamativum.

leiodermia (,lieoh'dərmi·ə) abnormal smoothness and glossiness of the skin.

leiomyoblastoma (,lieoh,mieohblas'tohmə) epithelioid leiomyoma.

leiomyofibroma (,lieoh,mieohfie'brohmə) epithelioid leiomyoma with a prominent fibrous component.

leiomyoma (,lieohmie'ohmə) a benign tumour derived from smooth muscle, most often of the uterus (leiomyoma uteri).

epithelioid l. leiomyoma, usually of the stomach or small intestine, in which the cells are polygonal rather than spindle shaped.

l. uteri leiomyoma of the UTERUS; called also *myoma uteri* and, colloquially, *fibroids*. It is the most common of all tumours found in women. It may occur in any part of the uterus, although it is most frequently in the body of the organ. Leiomyomas usually occur during the third and fourth decades, and are often multiple, although a single tumour may occur. They are usually small but may grow quite large and occupy most of the uterine wall; after menopause, growth usually ceases. Symptoms vary according to the location and size of the tumours. As they grow they may cause pressure on neighbouring organs, painful menstruation, profuse and irregular menstrual bleeding, vaginal discharge, or frequent urination, as well as enlargement of the uterus.

In pregnancy, the tumours may interfere with natural enlargement of the uterus with the growing fetus. They may also cause spontaneous abortion and death of the fetus.

Small leiomyomas are usually left undisturbed and are checked at frequent intervals. Larger tumours may be removed surgically. In some instances, hysterectomy is performed.

leiomyosarcoma (,lieoh,mieohsah'kohmə) a sarcoma in which the cells are of smooth muscle origin or differentiation.

Leishman–Donovan bodies (,leeshman'donəvən) round or oval bodies found in the reticuloendothelial cells, especially those of the spleen and liver, in kala-azar; they are nonflagellate intracellular forms of *Leishmania donovani*. The term is also used to designate similar forms of *L. tropica* found in macrophages in lesions of cutaneous leishmaniasis.

Leishmania (leesh'mayni·ə) a genus of parasitic protozoa, including *L. braziliensis*, the cause of mucocutaneous leishmaniasis; *L. braziliensis* and *L. aethiopica*, the cause of diffuse cutaneous leishmaniasis; *L. donovani*, the cause of kala-azar; and *L. tropica*, the main cause of cutaneous leishmaniasis of the Old World.

leishmaniasis (ˌleeshmə'nieəsis) any disease due to infection with *Leishmania*.

American l. mucocutaneous leishmaniasis.

cutaneous l., dermal l. chronic ulcerative granulomatous disease caused in the Old World by *Leishmania tropica*, *L. major*, and *L. aethiopica*, and in the New World by *L. mexicana* and *L. braziliensis* and transmitted by the sandfly. It is endemic in the tropics and subtropics, and has various names such as Aleppo boil, Delhi sore, Baghdad sore, and oriental sore (Old World) and chiclero sore (New World). Treatment consists of injections of pentavalent antimonial compounds. Antibiotics are employed to combat secondary infection. Simple lesions may be cleaned, curetted, and left to heal.

diffuse cutaneous l., disseminated cutaneous l. a generalized cutaneous disease endemic in South America and Mexico, caused by *Leishmania braziliensis pifanoi*, in which the lesions resemble those of nodular leprosy or of keloid. Pentavalent antimonial compounds are useful in some forms, while others are antimony-resistant. The prognosis for a complete cure is not good; relapses are common.

mucocutaneous l., naso-oral l., nasopharyngeal l. a disease endemic in South and Central America caused by *Leishmania braziliensis*, marked by ulceration of the mucous membranes of the nose, mouth, and pharynx; widespread destruction of soft tissues in nasal and oral regions may occur. Called also *American leishmaniasis*, *uta* or *espundia*. Treatment consists of injections of pentavalent antimonial compounds.

visceral l. kala-azar.

Lembert's suture (lanh'bairz) an inverting continuous suture used to invaginate intestinal edges without penetrating the mucosa so the peritoneal surfaces are in contact.

lemmoblastic (ˌlemoh'blastik) forming or developing into a neurolemma cell.

lemmocyte ('lemohˌsiet) a cell that develops into a neurolemma cell.

lemniscus (lem'niskəs) pl. *lemnisci* [L.] a ribbon or band; in anatomy, a band or bundle of nerve fibres in the central nervous system.

length (length) an expression of the longest dimension of an object, or of the measurement between its two ends. The internationally accepted (SI) unit of length is the metre (m).

crown–heel l. the distance from the crown of the head to the heel in embryos, fetuses, and infants; the equivalent of standing height in older persons.

crown–rump l. the distance from the crown of the head to the breech in embryos, fetuses, and infants; the equivalent of sitting height in older subjects. Measured by B-mode ultrasound during the first 14 weeks of pregnancy to assess fetal maturity; accurate to within 3 to 4 days.

focal l. the distance between a lens and an object from which all rays of light are brought to a focus.

lens (lenz) 1. a piece of glass or other transparent material so shaped as to converge or diverge light rays. See also GLASSES. 2. crystalline lens; the transparent, biconvex body separating the anterior chamber and the vitreous body of the eye. The crystalline lens refracts (bends) light rays so that they are focused on the RETINA. In order for the eye to see objects close at hand, light rays from the objects must be bent more sharply to bring them to focus on the retina; light rays from distant objects require much less refraction. It is the function of the lens to 'accommodate' or make some adjustment for viewing near objects and objects at a distance. To accomplish this the lens must be highly elastic so that its shape can be changed and made more or less convex. The more convex the lens, the greater the refraction. The ciliary muscle is responsible for altering the shape of the lens, its contraction making the lens more convex.

With increasing age the lens loses its elasticity; thus its ability to focus near objects on the retina becomes impaired. This condition is called PRESBYOPIA. In longsightedness (HYPERMETROPIA) the image is focused behind the retina because the refractive power of the lens is too weak or the eyeball axis is too short. Shortsightedness (MYOPIA) occurs when the refractive power of the lens is too strong or the eyeball is too long, so that the image is focused in front of the retina.

achromatic l. a lens corrected for chromatic aberration.

apochromatic l. one corrected for chromatic and spherical aberration.

biconcave l. one concave on both faces.

biconvex l. one convex on both faces.

bifocal l. one made up of two segments, the upper for far vision and the lower for near vision.

concave l. one with one or both (biconvex) faces curved like a section of the interior of a hollow sphere; it disperses light rays.

contact l. a thin, curved shell of plastic that is applied directly to the cornea to correct refractive errors (see also CONTACT LENSES). Many different materials are used, producing 'hard', 'soft', or 'semi-soft' lenses.

converging l., convex l. one curved like the exterior of a hollow sphere; it brings light to a focus.

convexoconcave l. one that has one convex and one concave face.

crystalline l. see LENS (2).

dispersing l. concave lens.

honeybee l. a magnifying eyeglass lens designed to resemble the multifaceted eye of the honeybee. It consists of three or six small telescopes mounted in the upper portion of the spectacles and directed toward the centre and right and left visual fields. Prisms are included to provide a continuous, unbroken magnified field of view.

omnifocal l. a lens whose power increases continuously and regularly in a downward direction, avoiding the discontinuity in field and power inherent in bifocal and trifocal lenses.

orthoscopic l. one that gives a flat and undistorted field of vision.

trial l's lenses used in determining visual acuity.

trifocal l. one made up of three segments, the upper for distant, the middle for intermediate, and the lower for near vision (see also GLASSES).

varilux l. omnifocal lens.

lenticonus (ˌlenti'kohnəs) a congenital conical bulging, anteriorly or posteriorly, of the lens of the eye.

lenticular (len'tikyuhlə) 1. pertaining to or shaped like a lens. 2. pertaining to the lens of the eye. 3. pertaining to the lenticular nucleus.

lenticulostriate (lenˌtikyuhloh'strieayt) pertaining to the lenticular nucleus and corpus striatum.

lenticulothalamic (lenˌtikyuhlohthə'lamik) relating to the lenticular nucleus and the thalamus.

lentiform ('lentiˌfawm) lens-shaped.

lentiglobus (ˌlenti'glohbəs) exaggerated curvature of the lens of the eye, producing an anterior spherical bulging.

lentigo (len'tiegoh) pl. *lentigines* [L.] a flat, brownish pigmented spot on the skin due to increased deposition of melanin and an increased number of melanocytes; a freckle.

l. maligna, malignant l. melanotic freckle of Hutchinson.

Lentizol ('lentizol) trademark for a sustained release preparation of amitriptyline, an antidepressant.

leontiasis (ˌliən'tieəsis) the leonine facies of lepromatous leprosy, due to nodular invasion of the subcutaneous tissue.

leper ('lepə) a person with leprosy; a term now in disfavour.

lepidic (lə'pidik) pertaining to scales.

lepidosis (ˌlepi'dohsis) a scaly eruption.

lepothrix ('lepoh·thriks) infection of the axillary and sometimes the pubic hairs, with development of clumps of bacteria on the hairs (see also TRICHOMYCOSIS AXILLARIS).

lepra ('leprə) leprosy.

leprechaunism ('lepriˌkawnizəm) a lethal familial congenital condition in which the infant is small and has elfin facies and severe endocrine disorders, as indicated in females by an enlarged clitoris.

leprid ('leprid) the cutaneous lesion or lesions of tuberculoid leprosy: hypopigmented or erythematous maculae or plaques, lacking bacilli.

leproma (lep'rohmə) a superficial granulomatous nodule, rich in bacilli, the characteristic lesion of lepromatous leprosy. adj. **lepromatous.**

lepromin ('leprohmin) a repeatedly boiled, autoclaved, gauze-filtered suspension of finely ground lepromatous tissue and leprosy bacilli, used in the skin test for tissue resistance to leprosy.

leprosarium (ˌleproh'sair·ri·əm) a hospital or colony for treatment and isolation of patients with leprosy.

leprostatic (ˌleproh'statik) 1. inhibiting the growth of the leprosy bacillus, *Mycobacterium leprae.* 2. a leprostatic agent.

leprosy ('leprəsee) inflammatory disease caused by *Mycobacterium leprae* (Hansen's bacillus), and manifested in various ways, depending on the host's ability to develop cell-mediated IMMUNITY. It is a chronic communicable disease characterized by the production of granulomatous lesions of the skin, upper respiratory mucous membranes, and peripheral nervous system. Called also *Hansen's disease.* Not readily transmissible, it often results in severe disability but is rarely fatal.A notifiable disease except in Scotland. adj. **leprous**.

FREQUENCY AND TRANSMISSION. Leprosy is essentially a disease of the tropics and subtropics, although it has occurred in every country. It is estimated that about 12 million cases of leprosy exist worldwide. There is a fear that the incidence of leprosy may increase within the next few years because of the increasing prevalence of resistance to dapsone, the drug of choice for many years in the treatment of leprosy.

Leprosy is not inherited, but the actual means of transmission of the disease have not yet been established. It is known that the main source of infection is the nasal discharge from lesions of persons with the lepromatous type. It is believed that the bacillus enters the body through cuts or abrasions of the skin or, more likely, through the mucous membranes of the nose and throat. Leprosy is considered one of the least infectious diseases; it has been estimated only 3–5 per cent of those at risk, because of prolonged close exposure, ever develop it.

SYMPTOMS. The incubation period of leprosy is often 5 years or more. Early symptoms consist of the development of 'indeterminate' lesions on the skin, which are slightly hypopigmented macules. In the *tuberculoid* type, these lesions become better defined, with a papular edge, clearly hypopigmented; tactile sensation is reduced or lost from the affected areas. Damage to one or more peripheral nerves may result in weakness and wasting of muscles; characteristic sequelae are 'claw hand' and 'drop foot' and also gradual loss of fingers and toes.

In the *lepromatous* type, numerous new lesions appear all over the body and become nodular. These sometimes ulcerate, discharging vast numbers of leprosy bacilli. Similar lesions develop in the nose and mouth. Body hair tends to fall out. Polyneuritis, arthritis, iritis and orchitis are well-known complications.

In the *borderline* (dimorphous) type, there are features of both the other types, and there is a tendency to shift towards lepromatous in the untreated, and towards tuberculoid in the treated, patient. In all types acute adverse episodes, 'reactions', may occur and may result in irreversible damage to nerves.

TREATMENT. Until a few years ago, leprosy was effectively and inexpensively treated with dapsone, which was developed around 1950; this had to be given for at least 2 years, often much longer. Nowadays, because of widespread resistance, dapsone alone can no longer be recommended. In tuberculoid leprosy, the daily dose of dapsone is reinforced by a monthly dose of rifampicin and normally 6 months is considered an adequate period for treatment to last. In the lepromatous type, and many cases of borderline type, daily dapsone and monthly rifampicin have to be reinforced by a monthly dose of clofazimine. Treatment should continue until skin smears become negative and in any case for at least 2 years. Infectivity is lost within a few days of commencing treatment with rifampicin, a point of great public health importance.

In addition to specific medical therapy, adequate diet and exercise are important. Physiotherapy is employed to retrain affected muscles, and various surgical procedures may be required. Psychiatric help, not only for leprosy patients but for their close contacts and those who only imagine they have been exposed, may relieve the anxieties arising from the age-old misconceptions about the disease.

PREVENTION. Early diagnosis (on the biopsy of a skin lesion and nasal swabs) and correct therapy, wherever possible on an outpatient basis, are the cornerstones of modern prevention. Many patients are soon completely free of symptoms; this is most likely in cases diagnosed and treated at an early stage, especially among the young. BCG vaccination of child contacts has had varying success, and drug prophylaxis may have a place in certain circumstances. A leprosy vaccine is currently under development, but several years must elapse before this becomes available.

lepto- word element. [Gr.] *slender, delicate.*

leptocephalus (ˌleptoh'kefələs, -'sef-) a person with an abnormally tall, narrow skull.

leptocyte ('leptohˌsiet) an erythrocyte characterized by a haemoglobinated border surrounding a clear area containing a centre of pigment; called also *target cell.*

leptocytosis (ˌleptohsie'tohsis) leptocytes in the blood.

leptodactyly (ˌleptoh'daktilee) abnormal slenderness of the digits. adj. **leptodactylous.**

leptomeninges (ˌleptohmə'ninjeez) (plural of *leptomeninx*) the two more delicate components of the meninges: the pia mater and arachnoid considered together; the pia-arachnoid. adj. **leptomeningeal.**

leptomeningitis (ˌleptohˌmenin'jietis) inflammation of the leptomeninges.

leptomeningopathy (ˌleptohˌmening·gopəthee) any disease of the leptomeninges.

leptomonad (ˌleptoh'mohnad) 1. of or pertaining to *Leptomonas*, a genus of protozoa parasitic in the digestive tract of insects. 2. denoting the leptomonad form; see also PROMASTIGOTE. 3. a protozoon exhibiting the leptomonad (promastigote) form.

leptopellic (ˌleptoh'pelik) having a narrow pelvis.

leptophonia (ˌleptoh'fohni·ə) weakness or feebleness of the voice. adj. **leptophonic**.

Leptospira (ˌleptoh'spierə) a genus of bacteria (family Treponemataceae), certain serotypes of which cause leptospirosis.

leptospirosis (ˌleptohspie'rohsis) any of a group of notifiable infectious diseases due to certain serotypes of *Leptospira*. The best known is Weil's disease, or leptospiral jaundice; others are mud fever, autumn fever, and swineherd's disease.

The aetiological agent is a spiral organism that infects the kidneys of cattle, swine, dogs, cats, rats, and other animals. The organisms are spread through the animals' urine.

Usually they are inhaled with the air or taken in food or drink by mouth. The disease is most common among people who handle infected animals or the kidneys and other infected tissues of such animals.

SYMPTOMS. Leptospirosis is usually a short illness which produces a variety of symptoms. It begins with fever, acute headache, chills, and sometimes nausea and vomiting. Later, other symptoms may be caused by the effects of the disease upon the kidneys, liver, skin, blood, and other organs. These symptoms can include jaundice, skin rashes, haemorrhages of the skin and mucous membranes, inflammation of the eye, haematuria, and oliguria.

Diagnosis is often difficult because the symptoms resemble those of several other diseases. Jaundice is a key symptom that, when present, aids in diagnosis.

Most cases are mild, consisting only of the early symptoms and having a duration of 1 to 2 weeks. In a few cases, a severe infection may cause damage to the kidneys, liver, or heart. Only rarely is the disease fatal.

TREATMENT AND PREVENTION. Treatment is basically symptomatic. Penicillin or other antibiotics may be prescribed.

Sanitation measures can reduce the spread of the disease in both man and animals. Vaccines for animals are available, but provide only partial immunity to the disease. At the present time there are no vaccines of established value for human beings.

leptotene ('leptohˌteen) the stage of meiosis in which the chromosomes are threadlike in shape.

leptothricosis (ˌleptohthri'kohsis) leptotrichosis.

Léri's pleonosteosis ('layreez) a hereditary syndrome of premature and excessive ossification of the epiphyses of long bones, with short stature, limitation of movement, broadening and deformity of digits, and mongolian facies.

Leriche's syndrome (lə'reeshiz) fatigue in the hips, thighs, or calves on exercising, absence of pulsation in femoral arteries, impotence, and often pallor and coldness of the legs, usually affecting males and due to obstruction of the terminal aorta.

lesbian ('lezbi·ən) 1. pertaining to lesbianism. 2. a female homosexual.

lesbianism ('lezbi·ənizəm) homosexuality between women.

Lesch–Nyhan syndrome (ˌlesh'niehan) a hereditary disorder of purine metabolism transmitted as an X-linked recessive trait with physical and mental handicap, compulsive self-mutilation of fingers and lips by biting, choreoathetosis, spastic cerebral palsy, and impaired renal function.

lesion ('leezhən) any pathological or traumatic discontinuity of tissue or loss of function of a part. Lesion is a broad term, including wounds, sores, ulcers, tumours, cataracts, and any other tissue damage. They range from the skin sores associated with eczema to the changes in lung tissue that occur in tuberculosis.

lethal ('leethəl) deadly; fatal.

lethargy ('lethəjee) a condition of drowsiness or indifference. adj. **lethargic**.

Letterer–Siwe disease (ˌletə·rə'seevə) a nonlipid reticuloendotheliosis of early childhood, marked by a haemorrhagic tendency, eczematoid skin eruption, hepatosplenomegaly with lymph node involvement, and progressive anaemia.

leucine ('looseen) a naturally occurring amino acid, essential for growth in infants and for nitrogen equilibrium in adults.

leuco- for words beginning thus, see also those beginning *leuko-*.

leucovorin (ˌlookoh'vor·rin) folinic acid; used as an antidote for folic acid antagonists, e.g. methotrexate, and in the treatment of megaloblastic anaemias due to folic acid deficiency.

leuk(o)- word element. [Gr.] *white, leukocyte*.

leukaemia (loo'keemi·ə) a progressive, malignant disease of the blood-forming organs, marked by abnormal proliferation and development of leukocytes and their precursors in the blood and bone marrow. It is accompanied by a reduced number of erythrocytes and blood platelets, resulting in anaemia and increased susceptibility to infection and haemorrhage. Other typical symptoms include fever, pain in the joints and bones, and swelling of the lymph nodes, spleen, and liver. adj. **leukaemic**.

TYPES OF LEUKAEMIA. Leukaemia is classified clinically on the basis of (1) the duration and character of the disease—acute or chronic; (2) the cell line involved—myeloid (myelocytic, myeloblastic, granulocytic), or lymphoid (lymphatic, lymphoblastic, lymphocytic). A widely used classification of acute leukaemia based on cell type is the French American British (FAB) classification.

In acute leukaemia the white cells in the bone marrow and usually the blood consist of increased numbers of blasts, which are precursor, or immature, cells. They are larger than mature cells, and they accumulate, preventing the production of normal functioning blood cells. In chronic leukaemia the white cells are more mature, resembling normal cells, and have some capacity to oppose invading organisms.

Different types of leukaemia dominate in various age groups. Acute lymphoblastic (lymphoid) leukaemia (ALL) occurs in young children, particularly those 3 and 4 years of age. Acute myeloid leukaemia (AML) is seen at all ages and is the commonest acute leukaemia in adults. Chronic lymphocytic (lymphoid) leukaemia is found chiefly in persons 50 to 70 years old, and chronic myeloid leukaemia (also known as chronic granulocytic leukaemia) in those 30 to 50 years old. Leukaemias account for the highest number of cancer deaths in children under14 years of age in the United Kingdom.

The incidence of the disease is growing, and the increase is only partially explained by increased efficiency of detection.

CAUSE. The precise cause of leukaemia is unknown. Much research has been directed toward exploring the possibility of a virus or a genetic defect as the cause. Experiments have produced findings that confirm the viral origin in animals. Evidence of possible viral origin in humans is inconclusive.

Radiation is an established factor in myeloid leukaemia; there is a statistical correlation between the size of the dose of radiation beyond a certain point and the occurrence of leukaemia.

It is also known that heredity plays a role in some types of the disease. Leukaemia frequency is increased in Down's syndrome and other rare hereditary diseases associated with chromosomal abnormalities, and among persons who have an identical twin with leukaemia.

Clinical Manifestations. The acute form of leukaemia is usually of fairly sudden onset, and is characterized by symptoms relating to anaemia, thrombocytopenia and neutropenia (for example, pallor, fatigue and dyspnoea), stomatitis, bleeding from the mucous membranes of the mouth, alimentary canal, and rectum, and acute infections such as septicaemia. Pain in the bones and joints is a common presenting symptom in acute lymphoblastic leukaemia. Enlargement of the lymph nodes, liver, and spleen may be found on examination.

Chronic leukaemia, particularly chronic lymphocytic leukaemia, can cause no symptoms at all for months or years after onset, and may be found accidentally during a routine physical examination and blood testing. Lymphadenopathy is often prominent. The *Roi classification*, a staging classification of chronic lymphatic leukaemia, was described by Roi and colleagues in 1975. The disease is graded from 0 to IV and features of importance are lymphadenopathy, hepatosplenomegaly, anaemia and thrombocytopenia. Stages III and IV carry the worst prognosis. Chronic myeloid leukaemia may present with marked splenomegaly, loss of weight and general malaise, and has a median survival of about 3 years. Common to all leukemias are anaemia, the tendency to bleed and increased susceptibility to infection.

Treatment. With new aggressive chemotherapy regimens about one-third of children with acute lymphoblastic leukaemia can be cured. The prognosis for acute myeloid leukaemia remains poor long term and only about 10 per cent of treated patients survive five years. Transfusion and replacement of blood cells relieve the symptoms, and various ANTINEOPLASTIC agents temporarily destroy the leukaemic cells, prolonging the life of many patients.

Often no treatment is necessary for chronic lymphatic leukaemia; steroids, alkylating agents such as chlorambucil, or splenic irradiation are treatment options to reduce the large lymph nodes or spleen. The patient may live a normal life. Chronic myeloid leukaemia requires treatment with chemotherapeutic agents to relieve the symptoms, but the prognosis is poor and in about half the patients the disease transforms to an acute leukaemia. Selected patients may benefit from bone marrow transplantation in the controlled phase of the disease.

Treatment of acute leukaemia is both supportive and definitive. Supportive treatment involves giving transfusions of red cells, platelets, possibly white cells, and antibiotics, the correction of metabolic abnormalities, and a high standard of nursing care (see below). Definitive antileukaemia treatment aims to achieve complete remission, i.e. to rid the blood, bone marrow, and tissues of leukaemic cells; to control or prevent the proliferation of malignant cells in the brain and cerebrospinal fluid; and to maintain a leukaemic cell-free status within the body. Once remission is achieved chemotherapy is continued to consolidate and maintain the remission. Central nervous system prophylaxis is given to children with acute lymphoblastic leukaemia. Bone marrow transplantation is a recent advance in the treatment of acute leukaemia, particularly for acute myeloid leukaemia in first remission.

Patient Care. Leukaemia affects almost every system within the body and can present a variety of patient care problems. Of primary concern are those symptoms resulting from suppression of normal bone marrow function, particularly susceptibility to infection due to the predominance of immature and abnormally functioning white blood cells, bleeding tendency owing to decreased platelet count, and anaemia due to decreased erythrocyte count. Electrolyte abnormalities are common in acute leukaemia and many of the drugs used are toxic to the liver, kidneys, heart and normal bone marrow, and intensive comprehensive nursing and medical supervision is necessary to enable these patients to achieve complete remission and survive.

Because of the malignant nature of leukaemia and the fear and anxiety created by the knowledge that one has a form of cancer, the patient and his family will need help in coping with anxiety, mental depression, and realistic fears about dying and death. The financial burden of the illness and disruption of the life of the individual and his family also impose a special burden on them. Referral to appropriate persons and supportive services that can help meet their needs is an essential part of the care of the patient with leukaemia.

aleukaemic l. leukaemia in which the leukocyte count is normal or below normal, and blasts are not seen in the peripheral blood.

basophilic l., basophilocytic l. leukaemia in which basophilic granulocytes predominate.

l. cutis leukaemia with leukocytic invasion of the skin marked by pink, reddish brown, or purple macules, papules, and tumours.

embryonal l. stem cell leukaemia.

eosinophilic l. leukaemia in which eosinophils are the predominating cells.

granulocytic l. myelocytic leukaemia.

hairy-cell l. leukaemic reticuloendotheliosis. The 'hairy cells' are mononuclear cells with very fine processes (hairs) visible on the cell surface using scanning electron microscopy.

leukopenic l. aleukaemic leukaemia.

lymphatic l., lymphoblastic l., lymphocytic l., lymphogenous l., lymphoid l. leukaemia associated with hyperplasia and overactivity of the lymphoid tissue, in which the leukocytes are lymphocytes or lymphoblasts.

lymphosarcoma cell l. a form of malignant lymphoma marked by large numbers of abnormal lymphocytes (lymphoma cells) in the peripheral blood indicating marked bone marrow involvement.

mast cell l. a form marked by overwhelming numbers of tissue mast cells in the peripheral blood.

megakaryocytic l. haemorrhagic thrombocythaemia.

micromyeloblastic l. a form marked by the presence of large numbers of micromyeloblasts.

monocytic l. leukaemia in which the predominating leukocytes are monocytes.

myeloblastic l. leukaemia in which myeloblasts predominate.

myelocytic l., myelogenous l., myeloid l. a form arising from myeloid tissue in which the granular polymorphonuclear leukocytes and their precursors, especially myelocytes, predominate.

plasma cell l., plasmacyte l. a form in which the predominating cell in the peripheral blood is the plasma cell.

promyelocytic l. a form in which the predominant cells are promyeloblasts, rather than myeloblasts, often associated with abnormal bleeding secondary to disseminated intravascular coagulation with thrombocytopenia and hypofibrinogenaemia.

Rieder cell l. myeloblastic leukaemia in which the blood contains asynchronously developed cells with immature cytoplasm and a lobulated, relatively more mature nucleus.

smouldering l. a subacute or preleukaemic state which can eventually transform into acute leukaemia; also referred to as 'refactory anaemia with excess of blasts'; one of the variants of the myelodysplastic syndrome.

stem cell l. leukaemia in which the predominating cell is so immature and primitive that its classification is difficult.

subleukaemic l. aleukaemic leukaemia.

leukaemid (loo'keemid) any of the polymorphic skin eruptions associated with leukaemia; clinically, they may be nonspecific, i.e., papular, macular, purpuric, etc., but histopathologically they may represent true leukaemic infiltrations.

leukaemogen (loo'keeməjən) any substance that produces leukaemia. adj. **leukaemogenic**.

leukaemogenesis (loo,keemoh'jenəsis) the induction or development of leukaemia.

leukaemoid (loo'keemoyd) exhibiting blood counts, particularly leukocytosis, and sometimes other clinical findings resembling those of leukaemia, but not due to uncontrolled proliferation of leukocytes; it can be extremely difficult to differentiate from leukaemia.

leukapheresis, leucapheresis (,lookafə'reesis) the selective removal of leukocytes from withdrawn blood, which is then retransfused into the donor.

Leukeran ('lookə·ran) trademark for preparation of chlorambucil, and antineoplastic agent.

leukoagglutinin, leucoagglutinin (,lookohə'glootinin) an agglutinin that acts upon leukocytes.

leukoblast, leucoblast ('lookoh,blast) an immature granular leukocyte.

granular l. promyelocyte.

leukoblastosis, leucoblastosis (,lookohbla'stohsis) a general term for proliferation of leukocytes.

leukocidin, leucocidin (,lookoh'siedin) a substance produced by some pathogenic bacteria that is toxic to polymorphonuclear leukocytes (neutrophils).

leukocrit, leucocrit ('lookoh,krit) the volume percentage of leukocytes in whole blood.

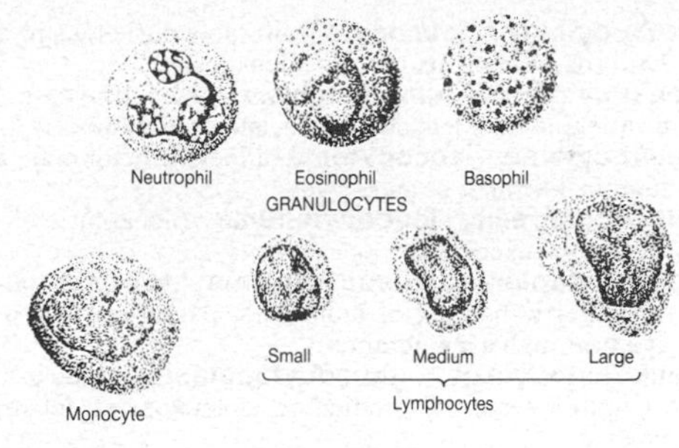

Types of leukocytes

leukocyte, leucocyte ('lookə,siet) a colourless blood corpuscle capable of amoeboid movement, whose chief function is to protect the body against microorganisms causing disease and which may be classified in two main groups: granular (basophils, eosinophils, neutrophils) and nongranular (lymphocytes, monocytes). adj. **leukocytic**. The leukocytes act by moving through blood vessel walls in order to reach a site of injury. Foreign particles such as bacteria may be engulfed or phagocytosed by the leukocytes, especially the neutrophils and monocytes. It is this process that causes the increase in the number of leukocytes in the blood during infection, and one of the laboratory determinations to diagnose infectious states is based on it. The leukocytes also play some role in the repair of injured tissue, removing debris and preparing the inflammatory site for healing.

granular l's granulocytes; leukocytes containing abundant granules in their cytoplasm, including neutrophils, eosinophils, and basophils.

polymorphonuclear l. any of the fully developed, segmented cells of the granulocyte series, especially a neutrophil, whose nuclei contain three or more lobes joined by filamentous connections.

leukocytogenesis, leucocytogenesis (,lookoh,sietoh'jenəsis) the formation of leukocytes.

Categories of white blood cells and their functions

White cell type	% in normal WBC	Function
Granulocytes		
Neutrophils		Phagocytosis and killing of bacteria; release of pryogen that produces fever
Segmented	56	
Band	3	
Eosinophils	2.7	Phagocytosis of antigen–antibody complexes; killing of parasites
Basophils	0.3	Release of chemical mediators of immediate hypersensitivity
Lymphocytes	34	
B lymphocytes		Humoral immunity; production of specific antibodies against viruses, bacteria, and other proteins
T lymphocytes		Cell-mediated immunity, including delayed hypersensitivity and graft rejection; regulation of immune response
Monocytes	4	Phagocytosis of microorganisms and cell debris; cooperation in immune response

Adapted from Waserkitz, M. and Heyn, R.M. (1981) Potential stresses during the preschool years. In Tackett, J.J.M. and Hunsberger, M. *Family-Centered Care of Children and Adolescents*, W.B. Saunders.

leukocytolysin, leucocytolysin (ˌlookohsie'tolisin) a lysin that leads to disruption of leukocytes.

leukocytolysis, leucocytolysis (ˌlookohsie'tolisis) disintegration of leukocytes. adj. **leukocytolytic**.

leukocytoma, leucocytoma (ˌlookohsie'tohmə) a tumour-like mass of leukocytes.

leukocytopenia, leucocytopenia (ˌlookohˌsietoh'peeni·ə) leukopenia.

leukocytoplania, leucocytoplania (ˌlookohˌsietoh'playni·ə) wandering of leukocytes; passage of leukocytes through a membrane.

leukocytopoiesis, leucocytopoiesis (ˌlookohˌsietohpoy'eesis) the production of leukocytes; leukopoiesis.

leukocytosis, leucocytosis (ˌlookohsie'tohsis) a transient increase in the number of leukocytes in the blood, due to various causes.

basophilic l. basophilia (3).

mononuclear l. mononucleosis.

pathological l. that due to some morbid reaction, e.g. infection or trauma.

leukocytotaxis, leucocytotaxis (ˌlookohˌsietoh'taksis) leukotaxis.

leukocytotoxin, leucocytotoxin (ˌlookohˌsietoh'toksin) a toxin that destroys leukocytes.

leukocyturia, leucocyturia (ˌlookohsie'tyooə·ri·ə) leukocytes in the urine.

leukoderma, leucoderma (ˌlookoh'dərmə) an acquired condition with localized loss of pigmentation of the skin.

l. acquisitum centrifugum a pigmented naevus surrounded by a ring of depigmentation (see also halo NAEVUS).

syphilitic l. indistinct, coarsely mottled hypopigmentation, usually on the sides of the neck, in late secondary syphilis.

leukodystrophy, leucodystrophy (ˌlookoh'distrəfee) disturbance of the white substance of the brain. See also LEUKOENCEPHALOPATHY.

metachromatic l. a hereditary leukoencephalopathy, marked by accumulation of a sphingolipid (sulphatide) in tissues, with diffuse loss of myelin in the central nervous system and progressive dementia and paralysis; classified according to age of onset as infantile, juvenile, and adult.

leukoencephalitis, leucoencephalitis (ˌlookoh·enˌkefə'lietis, -ˌsef-) inflammation of the white substance of the brain.

leukoencephalopathy, leucoencephalopathy (ˌlookoh·enˌkefə'lopəthee, -ˌsef-) any of a group of diseases affecting the white substance of the brain. The term *leukodystrophy* is used to denote such disorders due to defective formation and maintenance of myelin in infants and children.

leukoerythroblastic reaction, leucoerythroblastic reaction (ˌlookoheˌrithroh'blastik) a response noted in the peripheral blood and characterized by the presence of immature white cells and nucleated red cells. It may be caused by bone marrow infiltration (e.g., metastatic cancer) or by a brisk bone marrow response (e.g., following acute severe blood loss).

leukoerythroblastosis, leucoerythroblastosis (ˌlookoh·iˌrithrohbla'stohsis) an anaemic condition which may be caused by space-occupying lesions of the bone marrow, marked by a variable number of immature erythroid and myeloid cells in the circulation.

leukokeratosis, leucokeratosis (ˌlookohˌkerə'tohsis) leukoplakia.

leukokoria, leucokoria (ˌlookoh'kor·ri·ə) any condition marked by the appearance of a whitish reflex or mass in the pupillary area behind the lens.

leukolymphosarcoma, leucolymphosarcoma (ˌlookohˌlimfohsah'kohmə) lymphosarcoma cell leukaemia.

leukolysin, leucolysin (loo'kolisin) leukocytolysin.

leukolysis, leucolysis (loo'kolisis) leukocytolysis.

leukoma, leucoma (loo'kohmə) 1. a dense, white corneal opacity. 2. leukoplakia of the buccal mucosa.

l. adhaerens a white tumour of the cornea enclosing a prolapsed adherent iris.

leukomyelitis, leucomyelitis (ˌlookohˌmieə'lietis) inflammation of white matter of the spinal cord.

leukomyelopathy, leucomyelopathy ('lookoh'mieə'lopəthee) disease of the white matter of the spinal cord.

leukonecrosis, leuconecrosis (ˌlookohnə'krohsis) gangrene with formation of a white slough.

leukonychia, leuconychia (ˌlookoh'niki·ə) abnormal whiteness of the nails, either total or in spots or streaks.

leuko-oedema, leuco-oedema (ˌlookoh·i'deem·ə) an abnormality of the buccal mucosa, consisting of an increase in thickness of the epithelium, with intracellular oedema of the malpighian layer.

leukopathia, leucopathia (ˌlookoh'pathi·ə) 1. leukoderma. 2. any disease of the leukocytes.

l. unguium leukonychia.

leukopedesis, leucopedesis (ˌlookohpe'deesis) diapedesis of leukocytes through blood vessel walls.

leukopenia, leucopenia (ˌlookoh'peeni·ə) reduction of the number of leukocytes in the blood. adj. **leukopenic**.

malignant l., pernicious l. agranulocytosis.

leukoplakia, leucoplakia (ˌlookoh'playki·ə) a disease marked by the development on the mucous membranes of the cheeks (leukoplakia buccalis), gums, or tongue (leukoplakia lingualis) of white thickened patches which sometimes show a tendency to fissure and have a pronounced tendency to become malignant. They tend to grow into larger patches, or they may take the form of ulcers. Those in the mouth may in time cause pain during the swallowing of food or in speaking.

Leukoplakia affects mostly elderly or middle-aged men, often as a result of prolonged irritation of the mouth from such varying factors as badly fitting dentures or immoderate use of tobacco.

Treatment is aimed at removing any possible cause of physical or chemical irritation. The patient with leukoplakia should give up tobacco and possibly also alcohol and extremely hot food. Dental attention may be necessary if the patient's teeth are uneven or his dentures do not fit properly. A special mouthwash may be prescribed to be used after each meal.

Surgical removal of the affected area is relatively simple and is frequently the best means of preventing its further development.

l. vulvae the presence of hypertrophic greyish-white infiltrated patches on the vulvar mucosa.

leukopoiesis, leucopoiesis (ˌlookohpoy'eesis) the production of leukocytes; leukocytopoiesis.

leukorrhagia, leucorrhagia (ˌlookə'rayji·ə) profuse leukorrhoea.

leukorrhoea, leucorrhoea (ˌlookə'reeə) a whitish or yellowish, viscid discharge from the vagina or uterine cavity; see CONTRACEPTION, ovulation method.

The glands of the cervix normally secrete a certain amount of mucus-like fluid that moistens the membranes of the vagina. This discharge is frequently increased at the time of ovulation, before a menstrual period and throughout pregnancy. It is also stimulated by sexual excitement, whether or not coitus takes place. It should be white, inoffensive and nonirritating. Otherwise infection should be suspected and investigated for.

leukosarcoma, leucosarcoma (ˌlookohsah'kohmə) the development of spillover of lymphoma cells in the blood in patients with malignant lymphoma.

leukosis, leucosis (loo'kohsis) proliferation of leukocyte-forming tissue.

leukotaxine, leucotaxine (ˌlookoh'taksin) a polypeptide that appears in injured tissue and inflammatory exudates; it promotes leukocytosis and leukotaxis and increases capillary permeability.

leukotaxis, leucotaxis (ˌlookoh'taksis) cytotaxis of leukocytes; the tendency of leukocytes to collect in regions of injury and inflammation. adj. **leukotactic.**

leukotomy cutting of nerve fibres connecting a lobe of the brain with the thalamus. In most cases the affected parts are the prefrontal or frontal lobes, the areas of the brain involved with emotion; thus the operation is referred to as prefrontal, or frontal, leukotomy.

Leukotomy is a form of psychosurgery—a field in which the purpose of the operation is not to remove a growth or repair an injury to the body but to change the patient's mental and emotional state. Today most doctors regard leukotomy as a last resort and use the operation either for certain violent cases when all else has failed or for people with severe and otherwise untreatable anxiety. Although it can make formerly violent and uncontrollable patients calm and docile, it often seems to lead to emotional emptiness. Prefrontal leukotomy has been largely replaced by a variety of sterotactic surgical techniques, where carefully controlled and very small lesions are made in one or more of the pathways of the limbic system.

Furthermore, in recent years, drugs have been developed that have revolutionized the treatment of severe mental illnesses. Among these are the NEUROLEPTICS, which suppress the violent symptoms of psychosis.

leukotoxic, leucotoxic (ˌlookoh'toksik) destructive to leukocytes.

leukotoxin, leucotoxin (ˌlookoh'toksin) a toxin that destroys leukocytes.

leukotrichia, leucotrichia (ˌlookoh'triki·ə) whiteness of the hair.

levallorphan (ˌlevə'lorfan) an analogue of levorphanol, which acts as an antagonist to analgesic narcotics.

levarterenol (ˌlevah'terənol) noradrenaline.

levator (lə'vaytə) pl. *levatores* [L.] 1. a muscle that elevates an organ or structure. 2. an instrument for raising depressed osseous fragments in fractures.

LeVeen shunt (lə'veen) a peritoneal-venous shunt used in the control of ASCITES. It routes excess ascitic fluid out of the peritoneal cavity and into the superior vena cava or the jugular vein. See also peritoneal-venous SHUNT.

levels of care ('lev'lz) the six divisions of the HEALTH CARE SYSTEM: preventive care, primary care, secondary or acute care, tertiary care, restorative care, and continuing care.

levigation (ˌlevi'gayshən) the grinding to a powder of a moist or hard substance.

Levin tube ('levən) a gastroduodenal catheter of sufficiently small calibre to permit transnasal passage.

levo- for words beginning thus, see also those beginning *laevo-*.

levodopa (ˌleevoh'dohpə) the pharmaceutical name for L-dopa, used as an antiparkinsonian drug. See also DOPA.

levonorgestrel (ˌleevohnor'jestrel) a potent progestin used in combination with an oestrogen as an oral contraceptive.

levorphanol (le'vorfənol) a potent synthetic narcotic analgesic.

Leydig's cells ('liedigz) interstitial cells of the testis, which secrete testosterone.

LH luteinizing hormone.

LH-RH luteinizing hormone releasing hormone (gonadotrophin releasing hormone).

Lhermitte's sign ('lairmeets) a sensation like an electric shock coursing down the spine when the neck is flexed; a fairly common sign in MULTIPLE SCLEROSIS.

Li chemical symbol, *lithium.*

libido (li'beedoh) pl. *libidines* [L.] 1. sexual desire. 2. the psychic energy derived from instinctive biological drives; in psychoanalysis, the energy of the sex drive. adj. **libidinal.**

Freud postulated that libido development occurs in distinct stages: *oral, anal,* and *genital.* According to him, mental illnesses are disturbances of libido development and regression to an earlier, disturbed phase. Jung proposed that libido can be conceived according to the freudian pattern, but also can be desexualized, and viewed as an undifferentiated energy that is at the basis of such mental processes as thinking, feeling, sensation, and intuition. See also FREUD and JUNG.

Libman–Sacks disease (endocarditis) (ˌlibmən'saks) verrucous endocarditis associated with systemic lupus erythematosus; called also *atypical verrucous endocarditis.*

Librium ('libri·əm) trademark for preparations of chlordiazepoxide, an anxiolytic (minor tranquillizer).

lice (lies) plural of *louse.*

licentiate (lie'senshiˌayt) one holding a licence from an authorized agency entitling him to practice a particular profession.

lichen ('liekən, 'lichən) 1. any of certain plants formed by the mutual combination of an alga and a fungus. 2. any of various papular skin diseases in which the lesions are typically small, firm papules set very close together, the specific kind being indicated by a modifying term.

l. amyloidosus a condition characterized by localized cutaneous amyloidosis.

l. chronicus simplex lichen simplex chronicus.

l. fibromucinoidosus, l. myxoedematosus a condition resembling myxoedema but unassociated with hypothyroidism, marked by mucinosis and a widespread eruption of asymptomatic, soft, pale red or yellowish, discrete papules.

l. nitidus a skin eruption consisting of many, pinhead-sized, pale, flat, sharply marginated, glistening, discrete papules, scarcely raised above the skin level.

l. pilaris lichen spinulosus.

l. planopilaris a variant of lichen planus characterized by formation of acuminate horny papules around the hair follicles, in addition to the typical lesions of ordinary lichen planus.

l. planus an inflammatory skin disease with wide, flat, violaceous, shiny papules in circumscribed patches; it may involve the hair follicles, nails, and buccal mucosa; called also *lichen ruber planus.*

l. ruber moniliformis a variant of lichen simplex chronicus with papules arranged in linear beaded bands.

l. ruber planus lichen planus.

l. sclerosus et atrophicus a chronic atrophic skin disease marked by white papules with an erythematous halo and keratotic plugging. It sometimes affects the vulva (kraurosis vulvae) or penis (balanitis xerotica obliterans).

l. scrofulosorum, l. scrofulosus any eruption of minute reddish lichenoid follicular papules in children and young adults with tuberculosis.

l. simplex chronicus a dermatosis of psychogenic origin, marked by a pruritic discrete, or more often, confluent lichenoid papular eruption, usually confined to a localized area. Called also *circumscribed* or *localized neurodermatitis* and *lichen chronicus simplex*.

l. spinulosus a condition in which there is a horn or spine in the centre of each hair follicle; called also *lichen pilaris*.

l. striatus a self-limited condition characterized by a linear lichenoid eruption, usually in children.

l. urticatus papular urticaria.

lichenification (lie,kenifi'kayshən) thickening and hardening of the skin, with exaggeration of its normal markings. Can be caused by excessive scratching.

lichenoid ('liekə,noyd, 'lichə,noyd) resembling lichen.

Lichtheim's syndrome ('likht·hiemz) subacute combined degeneration of spinal cord.

lid (lid) eyelid.

granular l. trachoma.

l. lag failure of the upper lid to lower in time with the downward rotation of the eyeball. A sign of dysthyroid eye disease.

lie (lie) the relationship of the long axis of the fetus with respect to that of the uterus (see also POSITION, PRESENTATION).

transverse l. the situation during labour when the long axis of the fetus crosses the long axis of the uterus. See also table under POSITION.

longitudinal l. that in which the long axis of the fetus lies parallel to that of the mother's uterus, with either the head or the breech the presenting part.

oblique l. that in which the long axis of the fetal body lies obliquely to that of the mother's uterus; the shoulder presents first.

lie detector (lie di'tektə) polygraph.

Lieberkühn's glands ('leebə,koonz) tubular glands of the small intestine.

lien ('lie·en) [L.] *spleen*. adj. **lienal**.

l. accessorius an accessory spleen.

l. mobilis floating spleen.

lien(o)- word element. [L.] *spleen;* see also words beginning *splen(o)-*.

lienculus (lie'engkyuhləs) an accessory spleen.

lienitis (lieə'nietis) inflammation of the spleen; splenitis.

lienocele (lie'enoh,seel) hernia of the spleen.

lienography (,lieə'nogrəfee) radiography of the spleen; splenography.

lienomalacia (,lieənohmə'layshi·ə) abnormal softness of the spleen; splenomalacia.

lienomedullary (,lieənohmə'dulə·ree) pertaining to the spleen and bone marrow; splenomedullary.

lienomyelogenous (,lieənoh,mieə'lojənəs) formed in the spleen and bone marrow; splenomyelogenous.

lienomyelomalacia (,lieənoh,mieəlohmə'layshi·ə) softening of the spleen and bone marrow; splenomyelomalacia.

lienorenal (,lieənoh'reen'l) relating to the spleen and kidneys; splenorenal; splenonephric.

lienotoxin (,lieənoh'toksin) splenotoxin.

lientery ('lieəntə·ree) diarrhoea with passage of undigested food. adj. **lienteric**.

lienunculus (,lieə'nungkyuhləs) a detached mass of splenic tissue; an accessory spleen.

life expectancy (lief) see EXPECTATION OF LIFE.

life lie term to cover one's use of rationalization about what one cannot do or what one will surely fail at if attempted, owing to one's personal weaknesses and negative feelings about self (coined by ADLER).

life table a statistical method of summarizing in tabular form, the mortality and survival of groups of individuals in a population.

ligament ('ligəmənt) 1. a band of fibrous tissue connecting bones or cartilages, serving to support and strengthen joints. 2. a double layer of peritoneum extending from one visceral organ to another. 3. cordlike remnants of fetal tubular structures that are nonfunctional after birth. adj. **ligamentous**. The injury suffered when a joint is wrenched with sufficient violence to stretch or tear the ligaments is called a SPRAIN.

accessory l. one that strengthens or supports another.

arcuate l's the arched ligaments that connect the diaphragm with the lowest ribs and the first lumbar vertebra.

broad l. of uterus a broad fold of peritoneum supporting the uterus, extending from the side of the uterus to the wall of the pelvis.

capsular l. the fibrous layer of a joint capsule.

conoid l. the posteromedial portion of the coracoclavicular ligament, extending from the coracoid process to the inferior surface of the clavicle.

coracoclavicular l. a band joining the coracoid process of the scapula and the acromial extremity of the clavicle, consisting of two ligaments, the conoid and trapezoid.

costotransverse l. three ligaments (lateral, middle, and superior) that connect the neck of a rib to the transverse process of a vertebra.

cruciate l's of knee more or less cross-shaped ligaments, one anterior and one posterior, which arise from the femur and pass through the intercondylar space to attach to the tibia.

crural l. inguinal ligament.

deltoid l. medial ligament.

falciform l. of liver a sickle-shaped sagittal fold of peritoneum that helps to attach the liver to the diaphragm and separates the right and left lobes of the liver. Called also *broad ligament of liver*.

Gimbernat's l. a membrane with its base just lateral to the femoral ring, one side attached to the inguinal ligament and the other to the pectineal line of the pubis. Called also *lacunar ligament*.

glenohumeral l's bands, usually three, on the inner surface of the articular capsule of the humerus, extending from the glenoid lip to the anatomical neck of the humerus.

Henle's l. a lateral expansion of the lateral edge of the rectus abdominis muscle which attaches to the pubic bone.

inguinal l. a fibrous band running from the anterior superior spine of the ilium to the spine of the pubis; called also *Poupart's ligament*.

lacunar l. Gimbernat's ligament.

Lisfranc's l. a fibrous band extending from the medial cuneiform bone to the second metatarsal.

Lockwood's l. a suspensory sheath supporting the eyeball.

medial l. a large fan-shaped ligament on the medial side of the ankle.

meniscofemoral l's two small fibrous bands of the knee joint attached to the lateral meniscus, one (the anterior) extending to the anterior cruciate ligament and the other (the posterior) to the medial femoral condyle.

nephrocolic l. fasciculi from the fatty capsule of the kidney passing down on the right side to the posterior wall of the ascending colon and on the left side to the posterior wall of the descending colon.

nuchal l. a broad, fibrous, roughly triangular sagittal septum in the back of the neck, separating the right and left sides.

patellar l. the continuation of the central portion of the tendon of the quadriceps femoris muscle distal to

the patella, extending from the patella to the tuberosity of the tibia; called also *patellar tendon*.
pectineal l. a strong aponeurotic lateral continuation of the lacunar ligament along the pectineal line of the pubis.
periodontal l. the connective tissue structure that surrounds the roots of the teeth and holds them in place in the dental alveoli.
Petit's l. uterosacral ligament.
phrenicocolic l. costocolic fold.
Poupart's l. inguinal ligament.
pulmonary l. a vertical fold extending from the hilus to the base of the lung.
rhomboid l. the ligament connecting the cartilage of the first rib to the undersurface of the clavicle.
round l. of femur a broad ligament arising from the fatty cushion of the acetabulum and inserted on the head of the femur.
round l. of liver a fibrous cord from the navel to the anterior border of the liver.
round l. of uterus a fibromuscular band attached to the uterus near the uterine tube, passing through the abdominal ring, and into the labium majus.
suspensory l. of axilla a layer ascending from the axillary fascia and ensheathing the smaller pectoral muscle. **suspensory l. of lens** ciliary zonule.
sutural l. a band of fibrous tissue between the opposed bones of a suture or immovable joint.
tendinotrochanteric l. a portion of the capsule of the hip joint.
transverse humeral l. a band of fibres bridging the intertubercular groove of the humerus and holding the tendon in the groove.
trapezoid l. the anterolateral portion of the coracoclavicular ligament, extending from the upper surface of the coracoid process to the trapezoid line of the clavicle.
umbilical l., medial a fibrous cord, the remains of the obliterated umbilical artery, running cranialward beside the bladder to the umbilicus.
uteropelvic l's expansions of muscular tissue in the broad ligament of the uterus, radiating from the fascia over the internal obturator muscle to the side of the uterus and the vagina.
uterosacral l. a part of the thickening of the visceral pelvic fascia beside the cervix and vagina; called also *Petit's ligament*.
ventricular l. vestibular ligament.
vesicouterine l. a ligament that extends from the anterior aspect of the uterus to the bladder.
vestibular l. the membrane extending from the thyroid cartilage in front to the anterolateral surface of the arytenoid cartilage behind; called also *ventricular ligament*.
vocal l. the elastic tissue membrane extending from the thyroid cartilage in front to the vocal process of the arytenoid cartilage behind.
Weitbrecht's l. a small ligamentous band extending from the ulnar tuberosity to the radius.

ligamentopexy (ˌligəˌmentoh'peksee) fixation of the uterus by shortening the round ligament.

ligamentum (ˌligə'mentəm) pl. *ligamenta* [L.] ligament.

ligand ('liegənd, 'li-) an organic molecule that donates the necessary electrons to form coordinate covalent bonds with metallic ions. Also, an ion or molecule that reacts to form a complex with another molecule.

ligase ('ligayz, -gays) any of a class of enzymes that catalyse the joining together of two molecules coupled with the breakdown of a pyrophosphate bond in ATP or a similar triphosphate.

ligate ('liegayt) to apply a ligature.

ligation (lie'gayshən) application of a ligature.

ligature ('ligəchə) any material, such as catgut, thread or wire, used in SURGERY to tie off blood vessels.

light (liet) electromagnetic radiation with a range of wavelength between 390 (violet) and 770 (red) nanometres, capable of stimulating the subjective sensation of sight; sometimes considered to include ultraviolet and infrared radiation as well.
l. adaptation adaptation of the eye to vision in the sunlight or in bright illumination (photopia), with reduction in the concentration of the photosensitive pigments of the eye.
Finsen's l. light consisting mainly of violet and ultraviolet rays given off by FINSEN'S LAMP; used in treatment of lupus and similar diseases.
intrinsic l. the sensation of light in the complete absence of external stimuli.
polarized l. light of which the vibrations are made over one plane or in circles or ellipses.
Wood's l. ultraviolet radiation from a mercury vapour source, transmitted through a nickel-oxide filter (Wood's filter or glass), which holds back all but a few violet rays and passes ultraviolet wavelengths of about 365 nanometres; used in diagnosis of fungal infections of the scalp and erythrasma, and to reveal the presence of porphyrins and fluorescent minerals.

lightening ('lietəning) the sensation of decreased abdominal distention caused by descent of the fetal head into the pelvic cavity, 2 or 3 weeks before labour begins.

Lignac–Fanconi disease (leen,yakfan'kohnee) Fanconi syndrome.

lignocaine ('lignohˌkayn) a local anaesthetic of the amide group which is used in all types of local anaesthetic procedures—surface application, regional blocks, local infiltration, spinal and epidural blocks. Also used intravenously as an anti-arrhythmic agent, particularly against ventricular arrhythmias and those associated with myocardial infarction.

lignoceric acid (ˌlignoh'siə·rik) a saturated fatty acid found in wood tar, various cerebrosides, and in small amounts in most natural fats.

limb (lim) 1. one of the paired appendages of the body used in locomotion and grasping; in man, an arm or leg, with all its component parts. 2. a structure or part resembling an arm or leg.
anacrotic l. the ascending portion of an arterial pulse tracing.
catacrotic l. the descending portion of an arterial pulse tracing.
pectoral l. the arm, or a homologous part.
pelvic l. the leg, or a homologous part. **phantom l.** the sensation, after amputation of a limb, that the absent part is still present; there may also be paraesthesias, transient aches, and intermittent or continuous pain perceived as originating in the absent limb.
thoracic l. pectoral limb.

limbic ('limbik) pertaining to a limbus, or margin.
l. system a group of brain structures common to all mammals, comprising the cortex and related nuclei (see also limbic SYSTEM).

limbus ('limbəs) pl. *limbi* [L.] an edge, fringe, or border; used in anatomical nomenclature to designate the edge of the cornea, where it joins the sclera (limbus corneae), and other margins in the body.

lime (liem) 1. calcium oxide, a corrosively alkaline earth, used for absorbing carbon dioxide from air. 2. the acid fruit of *Citrus aurantifolia*.

limen ('liemən) pl. *limina* [L.] a threshold or boundary.
l. of insula, l. insulae the point at which the cortex of the insula is continuous with the cortex of the frontal lobe.
l. nasi the ridge marking the boundary between the

vestibule of the nose and the nasal cavity proper.

liminal ('limin'l) barely perceptible; pertaining to a threshold.

liminometer (ˌlimi'nomitə) an instrument for measuring the strength of a stimulus that just induces a tendon reflex.

limitans ('limitanz) [L.] *limiting*.

Lincocin ('lingkohsin) trademark for a preparation of lincomycin, an antibiotic.

lincomycin (ˌlinkoh'miesin) an antibiotic produced by *Streptomyces lincolnensis*; used as the hydrochloride salt in infections with gram-positive cocci and gram-negative bacilli.

linctus ('lingktəs) a thick syrup given to soothe and allay coughing.

lindane ('lindayn) the gamma isomer of benzene hexachloride used as a topical pediculicide and scabicide.

Lindau's disease ('lindowz) Lindau–von Hippel disease.

Lindau–von Hippel disease (ˌlindowvon'hip'l) a hereditary condition marked by angiomatosis of the retina and cerebellum, which may be associated with similar lesions of the spinal cord and cysts of the viscera; neurological symptoms, including seizures and mental handicap, may be present. Called *also von Hippel–Lindau disease.*

line (lien) a stripe, streak, mark, or narrow ridge; often an imaginary line connecting different anatomical landmarks (linea). adj. **linear.**

absorption l's dark lines in the spectrum due to absorption of light by the substance through which the light has passed.

Beau's l's transverse furrows on the fingernails, usually a sign of systemic disease but also due to other causes.

bismuth l. a thin blue-black line along the gingival margin in bismuth poisoning. **blue l.** a characteristic line on the gums showing chronic lead or bismuth poisoning.

cement l. a line visible in microscopic examination of bone in cross-section, marking the boundary of an osteon (haversian system).

l. of Douglas a crescentic line marking the termination of the posterior layer of the rectus sheath.

epiphyseal l. one on the surface of an adult long bone, marking the junction of the epiphysis and diaphysis.

gingival l. 1. a line determined by the level to which the gingiva extends on a tooth; called also *gum line*. 2. any linear mark visible on the surface of the gingiva.

gluteal l. any of the three rough curved lines (anterior, inferior, and posterior) on the gluteal surface of the ala of the ilium.

gum l. gingival line (1).

iliopectineal l. the ridge on the ilium and pubes showing the brim of the true pelvis.

intertrochanteric l. one running obliquely from the greater to the lesser trochanter on the anterior surface of the femur.

lead l. a bluish line at the edge of the gums in lead poisoning; called also *blue line*.

median l. an imaginary vertical line dividing the body equally into right and left parts.

milk l. the line of thickened epithelium in the embryo along which the mammary glands are developed and on which accessory nipples are formed.

mylohyoid l. a ridge on the inner surface of the lower jaw from the base of the symphysis to the ascending rami behind the last molar tooth.

nuchal l's three lines (inferior, superior, and highest) on the outer surface of the occipital bone.

pectinate l. the junction between the stratified squamous epithelium and the columnar epithelium in the anus.

Schwalbe's l. a circular ridge composed of collagenous fibres surrounding the outer margin of Descemet's membrane.

semilunar l. a curved line along the lateral border of each rectus abdominis muscle, marking the edge of the rectus sheath. Called also *linea semilunaris*.

Shenton's l. a line seen in radiographs of the hip which forms a natural curve from the inferior border of the superior pubic ramus to the medial border of the femoral neck when the femoral head and neck are in the normal anatomical relationship with the acetabulum and pelvis.

temporal l's inferior and superior ridges on the external surface of the parietal bone, the latter being continuous with the temporal line of the frontal bone, extending forwards to run down to the zygomatic process.

terminal l. one on the inner surface of each pelvic bone, from the sacroiliac joint to the iliopubic eminence anteriorly, separating the false from the true pelvis.

visual l. a line from the point of vision of the retina to the object of vision; called also *visual axis*.

linea ('lini·ə) pl. *lineae* [L.] a narrow ridge or streak on a surface, as of the body or a bone or other organ; a line.

l. alba white line; the tendinous median line on the anterior abdominal wall between the two rectus muscles.

lineae albicantes white or colourless lines on the abdomen, breasts, or thighs caused by mechanical stretching of the skin, with weakening of the elastic tissue (see also atrophic STRIAE).

l. aspera a rough longitudinal line on the back of the femur for muscle attachments.

lineae atrophicae atrophic striae.

l. nigra the linea alba when it has become pigmented in pregnancy.

linear ('lini·ə) pertaining to line.

l. accelerator a megavoltage machine for accelerating electrons so that powerful x-rays are given off for use in the treatment of deep-seated tumours.

lingua ('ling·gwə) pl. *linguae* [L.] tongue.

l. geographica geographical tongue.

l. nigra black tongue.

lingual ('ling·gwəl) pertaining to or near the tongue.

lingula ('ling·gyuhlə) pl. *lingulae* [L.] a small, tongue-like structure, such as the projection from the lower portion of the upper lobe of the left lung (lingula pulmonis sinistra), or the bony ridge between the body and great wing of the sphenoid (lingula sphenodalis). adj. **lingular**.

lingulectomy (ˌling·gyuh'lektəmee) excision of the lingula of the left lung.

linguo- word element. [L.] *tongue*.

linguopapillitis (ˌling·gwohˌpapi'lietis) inflammation or ulceration of the papillae of the edges of the tongue.

liniment ('linimənt) a medicinal preparation in an oily, soapy, or alcoholic vehicle, intended to be rubbed on the skin as a counterirritant or analgesic.

linitis (li'nietis) inflammation of gastric cellular tissue.

l. plastica diffuse fibrous proliferation of the submucous connective tissue of the stomach, resulting in thickening and fibrosis so that the organ is constricted, inelastic, and rigid (like a leather bottle). Called also *leather bottle stomach*.

linkage ('lingkij) 1. the connection between different atoms in a chemical compound, or the symbol representing it in structural formulas (see also BOND). 2. in genetics, the association of genes having loci on the same chromosome, which results in the tendency of a group of such nonallelic genes to be associated in inheritance.

linseed ('lin,seed) seed of the common flax, which contains an oil with a demulcent action.

lint (lint) an absorbent surgical dressing material made from cotton cloth with a raised nap.

Lioresal (,lieoh'reesal) trademark for a preparation of baclofen, a skeletal muscle relaxant.

liothyronine (,lieoh'thierə,neen) the pharmaceutical name for the thyroid hormone triiodothyronine (T_3); used in the treatment of hypothyroidism.

lip (lip) 1. the upper or lower fleshy margin of the mouth. 2. any liplike part; labium.

cleft l. congenital fissure of the upper lip; harelip (see also CLEFT LIP).

double l. redundancy of the submucous tissue and mucous membrane of the lip on either side of the median line.

glenoid l. a ring of fibrocartilage joined to the rim of the glenoid cavity.

Hapsburg l. a thick, overdeveloped lower lip that often accompanies Hapsburg jaw.

l. reading understanding of speech through observation of the speaker's lip movements.

lip(o)- word element. [Gr.] *fat, lipid.*

lip reading (lip 'reeding) understanding of speech through observation of the speaker's lip movements; called also *speech reading.*

lipacidaemia (,lipasi'deemi·ə) an excess of fatty acids in the blood.

lipaciduria (,lipasi'dyooə·ri·ə) fatty acid in the urine.

lipaemia (li'peemi·ə) an excess of lipids in the blood; hyperlipidaemia.

alimentary l. that occurring after ingestion of food.

l. retinalis that manifested by a milky appearance of the veins and arteries of the retina.

lipase ('lipayz, -pays) fat-splitting enzyme; any enzyme that catalyses the splitting of fats into glycerol and fatty acids. Measurement of the serum lipase level is an important diagnostic test for acute and chronic pancreatitis.

lipectomy (li'pektəmee) excision of a mass of fat.

lipid ('lipid) a group of substances comprising fatty, greasy, oily, and waxy compounds that are insoluble in water and soluble in nonpolar solvents, such as hexane, ether, and chloroform.

Simple lipids are the triglycerides or neutral fats. Each triglyceride molecule is composed of one molecule of glycerol joined by ester linkages to three fatty acid molecules. They are an important source of fuel to the body and a much lighter form of energy storage than carbohydrate.

Compound lipids are important structural components of cell membranes. Phospholipids include lecithin and the cephalins, which are composed of fatty acids linked to phosphatidic acid, and the sphingomyelins, which are composed of fatty acids linked to sphingosine. Glycolipids are composed of a carbohydrate chain and fatty acids linked to sphingosine or ceramide. Cholesterol is a steroid alcohol. Another important function of the phospholipids is as lung surfactants.

lipidosis (,lipi'dohsis) any disorder of lipid metabolism involving abnormal accumulation of lipids, including Hand-Schüller-Christian disease, Niemann-Pick disease, Tay-Sachs disease, Gaucher's disease, etc.

lipiduria (,lipi'dyooə·ri·ə) the presence of lipids in the urine.

lipoarthritis (,lipoh·ah'thrietis) inflammation of the fatty tissue of a joint.

lipoatrophy (,lipoh'atrəfee) atrophy of subcutaneous fatty tissues of the body.

lipoblast ('lipoh,blast) a connective tissue cell that develops into a fat cell.

lipocardiac (,lipoh'kahdi,ak) pertaining to fatty degeneration of the heart.

lipochondrodystrophy (,lipoh,kondroh'distrəfee) Hurler's syndrome.

lipochondroma (,lipohkon'drohmə) a tumour composed of mature lipomatous and cartilaginous elements.

lipochrome ('lipoh,krohm) any one of a group of fat-soluble hydrocarbon pigments, such as carotene, lutein, chromophane, and the natural yellow colouring material of butter, egg yolk, and yellow corn. They are also known as *carotenoids.*

lipocyte ('lipoh,siet) a fat cell.

lipodystrophy (,lipoh'distrəfee) 1. any disturbance of fat metabolism. 2. progressive lipodystrophy.

congenital generalized l. an autosomal recessive condition marked by the virtual absence of subcutaneous adipose tissue, macrosomia, visceromegaly, hypertrichosis, acanthosis nigricans, and reduced glucose tolerance in the presence of high insulin levels. The loss of fat may be confined to the upper part of the body—partial lipodystrophy.

intestinal l. a malabsorption syndrome marked by diarrhoea, steatorrhoea, skin pigmentation, arthralgia and arthritis, lymphadenopathy, central nervous system lesions, and infiltration of the intestinal mucosa with macrophages containing PAS-positive material. Called also *Whipple's disease.*

progressive l. progressive and symmetrical loss of subcutaneous fat from the parts above the pelvis, facial emaciation, and abnormal accumulation of fat about the thighs and buttocks.

lipoedema (,lipi'deemə) an accumulation of excess fat and fluid in subcutaneous tissues.

lipofibroma (,lipohfie'brohmə) a lipoma containing fibrous elements.

lipofuscin (,lipoh'fusin) any of a class of fatty pigments formed by the solution of a pigment in fat.

lipofuscinosis (,lipoh,fusi'nohsis) any disorder due to abnormal storage of lipofuscins.

neuronal ceroid l. a group of hereditary autosomal recessive diseases marked by the accumulation in neurons and other tissues of ceroid and lipofuscin; clinically, there is central nervous deterioration, optic atrophy, macular degeneration, retinitis pigmentosa, and seizures.

lipogenesis (,lipoh'jenəsis) the formation of fat; the transformation of nonfat food materials into body fat. adj. **lipogenetic.**

lipogenic (,lipoh'jenik) producing, forming, or caused by fat.

lipogenous (li'pojənəs) producing fatness.

lipogranuloma (,lipoh,granyuh'lohmə) a nodule of extracellular lipoid material associated with or inducing granulomatous inflammation.

lipogranulomatosis (,lipoh,granyuh,lohmə'tohsis) a condition of faulty lipid metabolism in which yellow nodules of lipoid material are deposited in the skin and mucosae, giving rise to granulomatous reactions.

lipoid ('lipoyd) 1. fat-like. 2. lipid.

l. cell tumour a rare, usually benign ovarian tumour composed of eosinophilic cells or cells with lipoid vacuoles. It may cause virilization. Called also *masculinovoblastoma.*

lipoidaemia (,lipoy'deemi·ə) lipids in the blood; lipaemia.

lipoidosis (,lipoy'dohsis) a disturbance of lipid metabolism with abnormal deposit of lipids in the cells.

lipoiduria (,lipoy'dyooə·ri·ə) lipids in the urine; lipiduria.

lipolysis (li'polisis) the splitting up or decomposition of fat. adj. **lipolytic.**

lipoma (li'pohmə) a benign encapsulated tumour usually composed of mature fat cells.

lipomatosis (,lipohmə'tohsis) a condition characterized by abnormal localized, or tumour-like, accumulations of fat in the tissues.

lipomatous (li'pohmətəs) affected with, or of the nature of, lipoma.

lipomeningocele (,lipohmə'ning·goh,seel) meningocele associated with an overlying lipoma, as in spina bifida.

lipomeria (,lipoh'miə·ri·ə) congenital absence of a limb.

lipometabolism (,lipohmə'tabə,lizəm) metabolism of fat. adj. **lipometabolic.**

lipomyxoma (,lipohmik'sohmə) a myxoma containing fatty elements.

lipopenia (,lipoh'peeni·ə) deficiency of lipids in the body.

lipophage ('lipoh,fayj) a cell that absorbs or ingests fat.

lipophagia (,lipoh'fayji·ə) lipophagy.

l. granulomatosis intestinal lipodystrophy.

lipophagy (li'pofəjee) the absorption of fat; lipolysis. adj. **lipophagic.**

lipophilia (,lipoh'fili·ə) affinity for fat. adj. **lipophilic.**

lipopolysaccharide (,lipoh,poli'sakə·ried) a molecule in which lipids and polysaccharides are linked.

lipoprotein (,lipoh'prohteen) any of the macromolecular complexes that are the form in which lipids are transported in the blood. They consist of a core of hydrophobic lipids covered by a layer of phospholipids and apoproteins, which make the complex water soluble. There are four main classes of lipoproteins: *chylomicrons*, in which lipids are transported after a meal from the intestine to tissues where they are stored or used; *very low density lipoproteins* (VLDL); *low density lipoproteins* (LDL); and *high density lipoproteins* (HDL). VLDL and HDL are produced by both the liver and intestine; LDL is produced by the metabolism of VLDL.

LDL transports 60 to 75 per cent of the serum cholesterol, and is believed to carry cholesterol from the liver to body cells, including those of the blood vessels. HDL transports 20 to 25 per cent of the plasma cholesterol, and is believed to collect excess cholesterol from the body cells and carry it to the liver to be excreted.

It has long been known that high levels of serum cholesterol are associated with an increased risk of coronary heart disease (CHD). Because LDL carries most of the cholesterol, the serum LDL level is directly associated with CHD risk. The higher the LDL level, the greater the incidence of heart attacks or angina pectoris.

Clinical findings indicate that the HDL level is inversely related to CHD risk. This suggests that HDL may in some way protect against the development of atherosclerosis and heart disease. It is also possible that there is no cause-and-effect relationship between CHD risk and HDL because other factors that increase the risk of heart disease, including lack of exercise, obesity, smoking, poor control of diabetes, and use of oral contraceptives, are also correlated with HDL levels. LDL levels are directly related to the ingestion of saturated fats and cholesterol and inversely related to ingestion of polyunsaturated fats. Therefore, stopping smoking, taking regular exercise, losing weight, and reducing the consumption of animal fat and cholesterol can reduce the risk of developing heart disease.

lipoproteinaemia (,lipoh,prohti'neemi·ə) the presence of excessive lipoproteins in the blood.

liposarcoma (,lipohsah'kohmə) a malignant tumour characterized by large anaplastic lipoblasts, sometimes with foci of normal fat cells.

liposis (li'pohsis) lipomatosis.

liposoluble (,lipoh'solyuhb'l) soluble in fats.

lipothymia (,lipoh'thiemi·ə) syncope.

lipotrophic (,lipoh'trohfik) 1. acting on fat metabolism by hastening removal, or decreasing the deposit, of fat in the liver. 2. a lipotrophic agent.

β-lipotrophin (,beetə,lipoh'trohfin) a polypeptide synthesized by cells of the adenohypophysis (anterior pituitary), which promotes fat mobilization and skin darkening by stimulation of melanocytes. It contains β-endorphin and methionine enkephalin.

lipotrophism (li'potrə,fizəm) the condition of being lipotrophic.

lipotrophy (li'potrəfee) increase of bodily fat. adj. **lipotrophic.**

lipovaccine (,lipoh'vakseen) a vaccine in a vegetable oil vehicle.

lipoxidase (li'poksi,dayz) lipoxygenase.

lipoxygenase (li'poksijə,nayz) an enzyme that catalyses the oxidation of polyunsaturated fatty acids to form a peroxide of the acid.

Lippes loop ('lipeez) a form of intrauterine contraceptive device.

lipping ('liping) the development of a bony overgrowth in osteoarthritis (an osteophyte).

lipuria (li'pyooə·ri·ə) lipids in the urine.

liquefacient (,likwi'fayshənt) 1. producing or pertaining to liquefaction. 2. an agent that produces liquefaction.

liquefaction (,likwi'fakshən) conversion into a liquid form.

liquescent (li'kwesənt) tending to become liquid or fluid.

liquid ('likwid) 1. a substance that flows readily in its natural state. 2. flowing readily; neither solid nor gaseous.

l. diet a diet limited to the intake of liquids or foods that can be changed to a liquid state. A liquid diet may be restricted to clear liquids or it may be a full liquid diet.

CLEAR LIQUID DIET. This is a temporary diet of clear liquids without residue. It is not nutritionally adequate, and is used in some acute illnesses and infections, postoperatively (especially after gastrointestinal surgery), and to reduce faecal matter in the colon. Foods allowed include water, tea, coffee, fat-free broth, carbonated beverages, synthetic fruit juices, ginger ale, plain gelatin, and sugar.

FULL LIQUID DIET. This diet can be nutritionally adequate with careful planning. It is used for acute gastritis, as a transition between clear liquid and soft diet, and in conditions in which there is intolerance to solid food. Milk, strained soups, and fruit juices are allowed. Foods that liquefy at body temperature, such as ice cream, flavoured gelatin, and soft custards, can be included. Cereal gruels and egg nogs are allowed. When a full liquid diet is used as a TUBE FEEDING it must be of a consistency that will allow easy passage through the tube. Most full liquid diets are given in feedings every 2 to 4 hours.

liquor ('likə, 'liekwor) 1. a liquid, especially an aqueous solution, containing medicinal substances. 2. a term applied to certain body fluids.

l. amnii amniotic fluid.

l. cerebrospinalis cerebrospinal fluid.

l. folliculi the fluid in the cavity of a developing graafian follicle.

liquorice ('likərish) glycyrrhiza; used as a flavouring in some medicines.

Lisfranc's ligament (lis'franks) a fibrous band extending from the medial cuneiform bone to the second metatarsal.

Liskonum (lis'kohnəm) trademark for a preparation of lithium carbonate, a psychotropic drug.

lisping ('lisping) faulty enunciation of *s* and *z* sounds. Called also *parasigmatism*.

lissencephaly (,lisen'kefəlee, -'sef-) agyria. adj. **lissencephalic.**

Lister ('listə) Baron Joseph (1827–1912). Founder of modern antiseptic surgery. Born at Upton, Essex, England, Lister set out in a scientific manner to apply Pasteur's discoveries to the prevention of the development of microorganisms in wounds. His research was on the early stages of inflammation and blood coagulation, and in 1865 he successfully used carbolic acid in the treatment of compound fractures. Next he turned his attention to the arrest of haemorrhage in aseptic wounds, which led him to adopt a sulphochromic catgut for tying arteries, a material capable of more speedy absorption than silk or flax, which had long been employed. He wrote articles on amputation and anaesthetics.

Listeria (lis'tiə·ri·ə) a genus of gram-negative bacteria (family Corynebacterium); the single species, *L. monocytogenes*, is found chiefly in lower animals. In man, it produces upper respiratory disease, septicaemia, and encephalitic disease.

listeriosis (lis,tiə·ri'ohsis) infection with organisms of the genus *Listeria*.

Litarex ('litə·reks) trademark for a preparation of lithium citrate, a psychotropic drug.

lith(o)- word element. [Gr.] *stone, calculus*.

lithaemia (li'theemi·ə) an excess of uric (lithic) acid in the blood.

lithagogue ('lithə,gog) 1. expelling calculi. 2. an agent that promotes expulsion of calculi.

lithectasy (li'thektəsee) extraction of calculi through a mechanically dilated urethra.

lithiasis (li'thieəsis) 1. a condition marked by formation of calculi and concretions. 2. gouty diathesis.

lithium ('lithi·əm) a chemical element, atomic number 3, atomic weight 6.939, symbol Li. See table of elements in Appendix 2.

l. carbonate a psychotropic drug used to treat acute manic attacks and, when given on a maintenance basis, to prevent the recurrence of manic-depressive episodes. The desired serum levels are in the range 0.5–1.5 mmol/l. Life-threatening central nervous system effects and kidney damage occur at levels above 3.0 mmol/l. It is very important that the levels be carefully controlled. Lithium should not be given to patients with severe renal or cardiovascular disease or taken with diuretics because the potential for toxicity is very high. It is suspected of causing birth defects and should not be used during pregnancy.

lithoclast ('lithoh,klast) lithotrite.

lithocystotomy (,lithohsi'stotəmee) incision of the bladder for removal of stone.

lithodialysis (,lithohdie'aləsis) 1. the solution of calculi in the bladder by injected solvents. 2. litholapaxy.

lithogenesis (,lithoh'jenəsis) formation of calculi, or stones. adj. **lithogenous.**

litholapaxy (li'tholə,paksee) the removal of fragments of stone from the bladder after lithotrity.

litholysis (li'tholisis) dissolution of calculi.

lithonephritis (,lithohnə'frietis) inflammation of the kidney due to irritation by calculi.

lithonephrotomy (,lithohnə'frotəmee) excision of a renal calculus.

lithopedion (,lithoh'peedi·ən) a fetus calcified in utero.

lithophone ('lithoh,fohn) a device for detecting calculi in the bladder by sound.

lithoscope ('lithoh,skohp) an instrument for detecting calculi in the bladder.

lithotome ('lithə,tohm) a knife used in lithotomy.

lithotomy (li'thotəmee) incision of a duct or organ for removal of calculi.

l. position the patient lies on his back, and the lower limbs are flexed and abducted and supported in stirrups.

lithotripsy ('lithoh,tripsee) the crushing of vesical calculi in situ.

lithotrite ('lithoh,triet) an instrument for crushing calculi.

lithotrity (li'thotritee) the operation at which lithotripsy is achieved.

lithous ('lithəs) pertaining to or of the nature of a calculus.

lithuresis (,lithyuh'reesis) passage of gravel in the urine.

litmus ('litməs) a blue pigment prepared from *Rocella tinctoria* and other lichens. **l. paper** absorbent paper impregnated with a solution of litmus, dried and cut into strips. It is used to indicate the acidity or alkalinity of solutions. If dipped into alkaline solution it remains blue; acid solution turns it red. It is used to test urine and other body fluids; it has a pH range of 4.5 to 8.3.

litre ('leetə) the unit of capacity of the metric system, being equal to 1 cubic decimetre (1.76 pints) or 1000 mls. Defined as the volume occupied by a mass of 1 kilogram of pure water at its maximum density and at standard atmospheric pressure. Abbreviated l.

Little's disease ('lit'lz) congenital spastic stiffness of the limbs, a form of cerebral spastic paralysis due to lack of development of the pyramidal tracts.

Littré's glands ('leetrayz) 1. small sebaceous glands on the corona of the penis and the inner surface of the prepuce, which secrete smegma; called also *preputial glands*. 2. mucous glands in the wall of the male urethra.

Littré's hernia a Meckel's diverticulum in a hernia sac.

livedo (li'veedoh) a discoloured patch on the skin. adj. **livedoid.**

l. annularis, l. racemosa, l. reticularis reddish-blue, netlike mottling of the skin.

liver ('livə) the large, dark-red gland located in the upper right portion of the abdomen, just beneath the diaphragm. Its manifold functions include storage and filtration of blood; secretion of bile; conversion of sugars into glycogen; the synthesis and breakdown of fats and the temporary storage of fatty acids; and the synthesis of serum proteins such as certain of the alpha and beta globulins, albumin, which helps regulate blood volume, and fibrinogen and prothrombin, which are essential clotting factors.

STORAGE FUNCTIONS. The liver can store up to 20 per cent of its weight in glycogen and up to 40 per cent of its weight in fats. The basic fuel of the body is a simple form of sugar called glucose. This comes to the liver as one of the products of digestion, and is converted into glycogen for storage. It is reconverted to glucose, when necessary, to keep up a steady level of blood glucose. This is normally a slow, continuous process, but in emergencies the liver, responding to adrenaline in the blood, releases large quantities of this fuel into the blood for use by the muscles.

As the chief supplier of glucose in the body, the liver is sometimes called on to convert other substances into glucose. The liver cells can make glucose out of protein and fat. This may also work in reverse: the liver cells can convert excess glucose into fat and send it for storage to other parts of the body.

In addition to these functions, the liver builds many

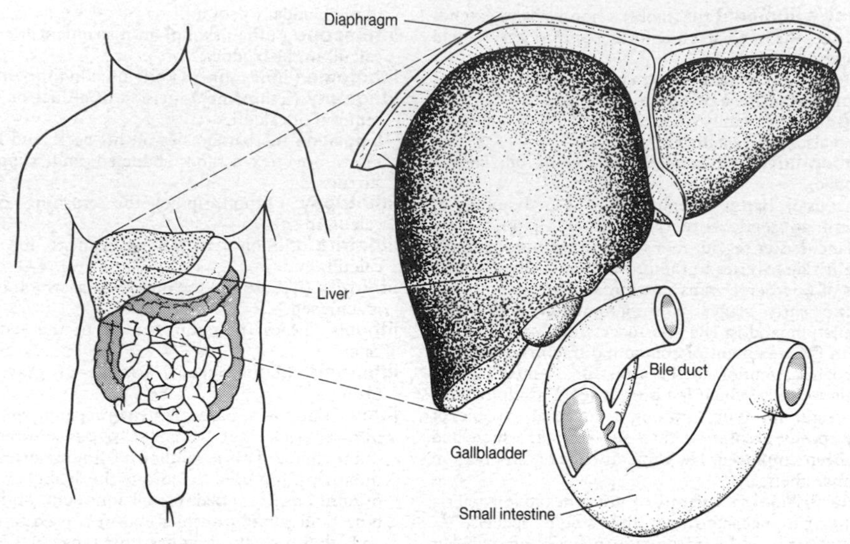

Liver. Bile, manufactured in the liver, is stored in the gallbladder; it passes through the bile duct into the duodenum, the upper end of the small intestine, where it aids in digestion

essential proteins and stores up certain necessary vitamins until they are needed by other organs in the body.

PROTECTIVE FUNCTIONS. The liver disposes of worn-out blood cells by breaking them down into their different elements, storing some and sending others to the kidneys for disposal in the urine. It also filters and destroys bacteria. One of the most important functions of the liver is the detoxification of drugs, alcohol, and environmental poisons.

The liver also metabolizes steroid hormones. In liver failure oestrogens are not broken down at the usual rate and the consequent high blood levels affect both male and female. Certain drugs enhance the rate of liver metabolism of oestrogens so that an oestrogen-containing contraceptive pill will no longer be effective.

Finally, the liver regulates the proteins that have passed through the digestive system. Some of the amino acids derived from protein metabolism cannot be used by the body; the liver rejects and neutralizes these acids and sends them to the kidneys for disposal.

LIVER FUNCTION TESTS. There are many laboratory procedures that measure some aspect of liver functions. Serum BILIRUBIN and urine bilirubin and urobilinogen levels provide information about the metabolism and excretion of bile pigments. Albumin and many of the alpha and beta globulins are synthesized by the liver. Disease that impairs their synthesis is shown by serum protein electrophoresis. Blood-clotting tests, such as one-stage prothrombin time, demonstrate a reduced synthesis of vitamin K-dependent clotting factors by the liver.

There are many enzymes that occur in the liver and are released into the blood when there is liver damage or biliary obstruction. The ones most commonly determined in the laboratory are alkaline phosphatase, aspartate aminotransferase (AST), and alanine aminotransferase (ALT). AST and ALT are also sometimes called *serum glutamic-oxaloacetic* transaminase (SGOT) and *serum glutamic-pyruvic transaminase* (SGPT). Alkaline phosphatase is elevated in patients with intrahepatic or extrahepatic obstruction of bile flow, as in cholestatic jaundice or in primary or metastatic carcinoma. AST and ALT are elevated in patients with hepatocellular injury as in acute viral or toxic hepatitis.

Both ULTRASONOGRAPHY and radioisotope scans (scintiscans) are useful in demonstrating space-occupying lesions of the liver, such as cysts, abscesses, and tumours. Ultrasonography is an excellent tool for evaluating ascites or preparing for a liver biopsy. The scintiscans use technetium-99m sulphur colloid, which is taken up by the reticuloendothelial cells of the liver and spleen, or gallium-67, which has an affinity for abscesses and certain tumours. On a colloid scan, abscesses and tumours appear as filling defects or 'cold spots'; on the gallium scan, they appear as 'hot spots'.

A needle biopsy of the liver is useful in demonstrating the presence of cirrhosis, steatosis, alcoholic hepatitis, chronic hepatitis, and carcinoma. Liver biopsy is contraindicated in patients who have clotting defects, severe anaemia, or a bacterial infection in an area to be traversed by the biopsy needle, for example, right lower lobar pneumonia.

DISORDERS OF THE LIVER. The liver, with its many complex functions, can be damaged by various disorders and diseases. Often such damage first manifests itself as JAUNDICE. This is a yellowish tinge, best seen in the eyes, that is caused by an excess of bile pigment in the blood. Jaundice is not a disease, it is a symptom of any one of a number of liver disorders or blood dyscrasias.

Besides jaundice, other symptoms of liver disease may be a gradual, unexplained swelling in the legs, or abdomen (ASCITES), uncontrolled bleeding resulting from a decrease of clotting factors, and increased sensitivity to drugs.

Inflammation of the liver (HEPATITIS) can be caused

by many different aetiological agents, including viruses, drugs, excessive amounts of alcohol, and exposure to environmental poisons such as carbon tetrachloride. Obstructive disorders of the GALLBLADDER also can damage the liver.

Through the work of Nobel Prize winner Baruch S. Blumberg and his colleagues it is now known that there is a direct link between primary cancer of the liver and type B hepatitis virus (HBV). Primary hepatocellular carcinoma (PHC) is one of the most common cancers in humans throughout the world. In parts of Asia and Africa the frequency is estimated to be as high as 50 per 100,000 population. The high rate of incidence is related to the prevalence of HBV, particularly in carriers of type B hepatitis. It is predicted that through the use of an HBV vaccine there will be a major decrease in chronic liver disease and PHC.

CIRRHOSIS of the liver is a chronic inflammation marked by degeneration of the liver cells and thickening of the surrounding tissue; it is the final stage of many kinds of liver damage. The condition often accompanies ALCOHOLISM because of the poor dietary habits of the alcoholic and the toxicity of alcohol. Although alcoholism is the most common cause of cirrhosis, it may also occur as a result of damage from toxins and infections.

Abscess of the liver usually occurs as a complication of peritonitis or abdominal cellulitis, or as an amoebic abscess following infection with *Entamoeba histolytica*.

fatty l. one affected with fatty infiltration.

l. spots a lay term for the small brownish patches that appear on the face, neck, or back of the hands of many older people. It is a misleading term because these spots have little or nothing to do with the liver. The spots, smooth, flat, irregularly spaced, and roundish or oval in shape, are caused by an increase in pigmentation and are entirely harmless. Although liver spots are associated with the process of ageing, it is actually not age that is the principal cause but many years of exposure to sun and wind. Hyperpigmentation may also occur in primary adrenal insufficiency (see also ADDISON'S DISEASE).

livid ('livid) discoloured, as from a contusion or bruise; black and blue.

lividity (li'vidətee) the quality of being livid; discoloration, as of dependent parts, by gravitation of blood.

livor ('lievor) discoloration.

l. mortis discoloration of dependent parts of the body after death due to the gravitation of blood.

lixiviation (lik,sivi'ayshən) separation of soluble from insoluble material by use of an appropriate solvent, and drawing off the solution.

LMA left mentoanterior (position of the fetus).

LML left mentolateral (position of the fetus).

LMP last menstrual period (first day of); left mentoposterior (position of the fetus).

LMRCP Licentiate in Midwifery of the Royal College of Physicians.

LMSSA Licentiate in Medicine and Surgery of the Society of Apothecaries, London.

LOA left occipitoanterior (position of the fetus).

Loa ('loh·ə) a genus of filarial nematodes. **L. loa** a threadlike worm of West Africa, 2.5–5 centimetres long, that inhabits the subcutaneous connective tissue of the body, which it traverses freely. It is seen especially about the orbit and even under the conjunctiva. It causes itching and occasionally oedematous swellings (Calabar swellings). The immature forms, or microfilariae, are diurnal, being found in the peripheral circulation in greatest concentrations during the day. Flies of the genus *Chrysops* are the intermediate hosts and vectors.

loading ('lohding) administering sufficient quantities of a substance to test a subject's ability to metabolize or absorb it.

loaiasis (loh'ieəsis) infection with nematodes of the genus *Loa*; loiasis.

lobar (lohbə) pertaining to a lobe.

l. atrophy a progressive atrophy of the cerebral convolutions in a limited area (lobe) of the brain; called also *Pick's disease*.

l. pneumonia pneumonia affecting one or more lobes of the lungs (see also PNEUMONIA).

lobate ('lohbayt) divided into lobes.

lobe (lohb) 1. a more or less well defined portion of an organ or gland. 2. one of the main divisions of a tooth crown.

azygos l. a small accessory or anomalous lobe at the apex of the right lung.

caudate l. a small lobe of the liver between the inferior vena cava on the right and the left lobe.

ear l. the lower fleshy, noncartilaginous portion of the external ear.

frontal l. the rostral (anterior) portion of the grey matter of the cerebral hemisphere.

hepatic l. one of the lobes of the liver, designated the right and left and the caudate and quadrate.

occipital l. the most posterior portion of the cerebral hemisphere, forming a small part of its dorsolateral surface.

parietal l. the upper central portion of the grey matter of the cerebral hemisphere, between the frontal and occipital lobes, and above the temporal lobe (see also PARIETAL LOBE).

polyalveolar l. a congenital disorder characterized in early infancy by the presence of far more than the normal number of alveoli in a lobe of the lungs; thereafter, normal multiplication of alveoli does not take place and they become enlarged, i.e., emphysematous.

prefrontal l. the part of the frontal lobe of the brain anterior to the ascending convolution.

quadrate l. 1. precuneus. 2. a small lobe of the liver, between the gallbladder on the right, and the left lobe.

Riedel's l. an anomalous tongue-shaped mass of tissue projecting from the right lobe of the liver in some individuals.

spigelian l. caudate lobe.

temporal l. a long, tongue-shaped process constituting the lower lateral portion of the cerebral hemisphere.

lobectomy (loh'bektəmee) excision of a lobe, as of the lung, brain, or liver.

lobitis (loh'bietis) inflammation of a lobe, as of the lung.

lobotomy (lə'botəmee) incision into a lobe; in psychosurgery, surgical incision of all the fibres of the brain. See also LEUKOTOMY.

Lobstein's disease ('lohbstienz) see OSTEOGENESIS IMPERFECTA.

lobulated ('lohbyuh,laytid) made up of lobules.

lobule ('lobyool) a small segment or lobe, especially one of the smaller divisions making up a lobe. adj. **lobular.**

l's of epididymis the wedge-shaped parts of the head of the epididymis, each comprising an efferent ductule of the testis.

hepatic l. one of the small vascular units comprising the substance of the liver.

l. of lung one of the smaller subdivisions of the lobes of the lungs served by bronchi of less than 1mm in diameter (see also BRONCHOPULMONARY SEGMENT).

paracentral l. a lobe on the medial surface of the cerebral hemisphere, continuous with the pre- and postcentral gyri, limited below by the cingulate sulcus.

parietal l. one of two divisions, inferior and superior, of the parietal lobe of the brain.

portal l. a polygonal mass of liver tissue containing portions of three adjacent hepatic lobules, and having a portal vein at its centre and a central vein peripherally at each corner.

primary l. of lung, respiratory l. the functional unit of the lung, including a respiratory bronchiole, alveolar ducts and sacs, and alveoli.

lobulus ('lobyuhləs) pl. *lobuli* [L.] lobule.

lobus ('lohbəs) pl. *lobi* [L.] lobe.

local ('lohk'l) restricted to or pertaining to one spot or part; not general.

localization (,lohkəlie'zayshən) 1. restriction to a circumscribed or limited area. 2. the determination of a site or place of any process or lesion.

cerebral l. determination of areas of the cortex involved in performance of certain functions.

germinal l. the location on a blastoderm of prospective organs.

lochia ('lohki·ə) the uterine discharge per vaginam occurring during the puerperium, consisting of placental debris and other waste products following delivery. Its colour, amount and odour indicate the healing process of the placental site. See PUERPERIUM. A plural word meaning 'bits and pieces'. adj. **lochial**.

l. alba the final vaginal discharge after childbirth, appearing on the tenth day and lasting until the fifteenth day, when the amount of blood is decreased and the leukocytes are increased; creamy white in appearance.

l. rubra that occurring immediately after childbirth, consisting almost entirely of blood and decidual fragments, and shreds of chorion tissue, amniotic fluid, lanugo, vernix, and meconium. It is deep red in colour and normally lasts from the first to the fourth day.

l. sanguinolenta, l. serosa a serous vaginal discharge, brownish-pink in colour, which appears after lochia rubra from the fifth to ninth day following delivery; contains less blood and many leukocytes.

lochiocolpos (,lohkioh'kolpos) distention of the vagina by retained lochia.

lochiometra (,lohkioh'meetrə) distention of the uterus by retained lochia.

lochiometritis (,lohkiohmi'trietis) puerperal METRITIS.

lochiopyra (,lohkioh'pierə) puerperal fever.

lochiorrhagia, lochiorrhoea (,lohki·ə'rayji·ə, ,lohki·ə'reeə) an abnormally profuse lochia.

lochioschesis (,lohki'oskisis) retention of the lochia.

loci ('lohsie, 'lokee) [L.] plural of *locus*.

Locke's solution (loks) an aqueous solution of sodium chloride, calcium chloride, potassium chloride, sodium bicarbonate, and dextrose adjusted to pH 7.4; used in physiological experiments to keep the excised heart beating.

lockjaw ('lok,jor) 1. tetanus. 2. trismus.

Lockwood's ligament ('lokwuhdz) a suspensory sheath supporting the eyeball.

locomotion (,lohkə'mohshən) movement, or the ability to move, from one place to another. adj. **locomotive**.

locomotor (,lohkə'mohtə) of or pertaining to locomotion.

l. ataxia inability to walk properly as a result of damage to the spinal cord by syphilis (called also TABES DORSALIS).

loculus ('lokyuhləs) pl. *loculi* [L.] 1. a small space or cavity. 2. a local enlargement of the uterus in some mammals, containing an embryo. adj. **locular**.

locus ('lohkəs) pl. *loci* [L.] place; site; in genetics, the specific site of a gene on a chromosome.

l. ceruleus a pigmented eminence in the superior angle of the floor of the fourth ventricle of the brain.

Loestrin (loh'estrin) trademark for a combination preparation of norethisterone and ethinyloestradiol, and oral contraceptive.

lofepramine (loh'feprəmin) a tricyclic antidepressant.

Löffler's endocarditis (disease) ('lərfləz) endocarditis associated with eosinophilia (see also Löffler's ENDOCARDITIS).

logagnosia (,logag'nohzi·ə) central word defect, as aphasia or alogia.

logagraphia (,logə'grafi·ə) inability to express ideas in writing.

logamnesia (,logam'neezi·ə) receptive aphasia.

logaphasia (,logə'fayzi·ə) expressive aphasia.

logasthenia (,logas'theeni·ə) disturbance of the mental processes necessary to the comprehension of speech.

logo- word element. [Gr.] *words, speech.*

logoclonia (,logə'klohni·ə) spasmodic repetition of the end-syllables of words.

logokophosis (,logohkə'fohsis) word deafness, or auditory aphasia.

logopaedia, logopaedics (,logə'peedi·ə; ,logə'peediks) the study and treatment of speech defects.

logopathy (lo'gopəthee) any disorder of speech due to derangement of the central nervous system.

logoplegia (,logə'pleeji·ə) paralysis of the speech organs.

logorrhoea (,logə'reeə) excessive or abnormal talkativeness.

logospasm ('logə,spazəm) the spasmodic utterance of words.

-logy word element. [Gr.] *science, treatise, sum of knowledge in a particular subject.*

Logynon (loh'gienon) trademark for a combination preparation of ethinyloestradiol and levonorgestrel, and oral contraceptive.

loiasis (loh'ieəsis) infection with nematodes of the genus *Loa*; loaiasis.

loin (loyn) the part of the back between the thorax and pelvis.

LOL left occipitolateral (position of the fetus).

Lomotil ('lomətil) trademark for preparations of diphenoxylate, an antidiarrhoeal.

lomustine (loh'musteen) CCNU; a nitrosourea used as an antineoplastic in the treatment of Hodgkin's disease and brain tumours.

long-acting thyroid stimulator (long'akting 'thieroyd 'stimyuhlaytə) a substance occurring in the blood in hyperthyroidism, which exerts a stimulating effect on the thyroid of longer duration than does thyrotrophin; abbreviated LATS; it is an IgG immunoglobulin and an autoantibody.

longissimus (lon'jisiməs) [L.] *longest.*

longitudinal study (,long·gi'tyoodin'l, ,lonji-) cohort or INCIDENCE STUDY.

longitudinalis (,lonji,tyoodi'naylis) lengthwise; in official anatomical nomenclature it designates a structure that is parallel to the long axis of the body or an organ.

longsightedness (,long'sietidnəs) hypermetropia.

longus ('long·gəs) [L.] *long.*

loop (loop) a turn or sharp curve in a cordlike structure.

capillary l's minute endothelial tubes that carry blood in the papillae of the skin.

closed l. a system in which the input to one or more of the subsystems is affected by its own output.

Henle's l. the U-shaped loop of the uriniferous tubule of the kidney.

Lippes l. a form of intrauterine contraceptive device.

open l. a system in which an input alters the output, but the output has no effect on the input.

loosening ('loosəning) in psychiatry, a disorder of thinking in which associations of ideas become so shortened, fragmented, and disturbed as to lack logical relationship.

LOP left occipitoposterior (position of the fetus).

loperamide (loh'perə,mied) an antiperistaltic used as an antidiarrhoeal and to reduce the volume of discharge from ileostomies.

lophotrichous (loh'fotrikəs) having two or more flagella at one end (of a bacterial cell).

Lopresor (loh'presə) trademark for preparations of metoprolol tartrate, an antihypertensive.

lorazepam (lo'razipam, -ayzipam) a benzodiazepine derivative used as an antianxiety agent.

lordoscoliosis (ˌlordohˌskohli'ohsis) lordosis complicated with scoliosis.

lordosis (lor'dohsis) forward curvature of the lumbar spine (see accompanying illustration). adj. **lordotic**.

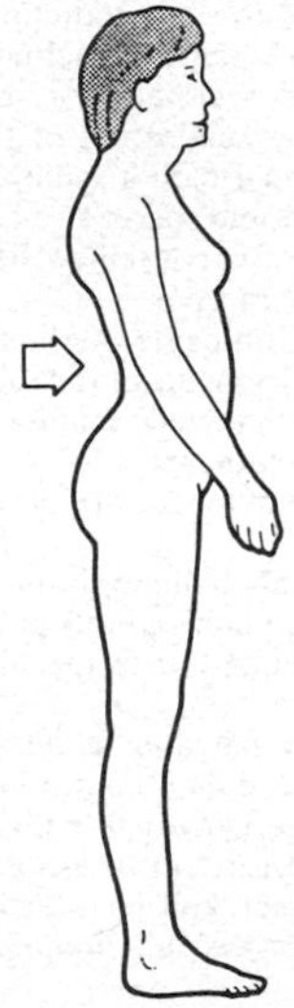

Lordosis

lotio ('lohshioh) [L.] *lotion.*

lotion ('lohshən) a medicinal liquid suspension or dispersion for external application to the body. Lotions usually have a soothing or antiseptic effect.

calamine l. a mixture of calamine, zinc oxide, glycerin, bentonite magma, and calcium hydroxide solution; used as a protectant, and antipruritic.

evaporating l. a dilute alcoholic solution applied to bruises.

Louis-Bar syndrome (ˌlooee'bah) ataxia-telangiectasia.

loupe (loop) a magnifying lens.

louse (lows) pl. *lice;* a general name for various host-specific parasitic insects, the true lice, which infest mammals and belong to the order Anoplura. They are greyish, wingless, and dorsoventrally flattened. Human lice vary in length from 1 to 3 mm. Those that are parasitic on man are *Pediculus humanus capitis*, the head louse, which attaches itself to the hairs of the head; *P. humanus humanus*, the body or clothing louse; and *Phthirus pubis*, the crab louse, which lives in coarse hair including pubic hair, eyelashes, beards and underarm hair.

Louse infestation is called pediculosis. Lice live on the host's blood, obtained by piercing the skin and sucking the blood through the mouth parts. The area bitten itches once sensitization has developed. The time that this takes varies from one individual to another. Bites may then become infected from scratching. Not only are lice an annoyance, but they can also transmit diseases, including typhus and relapsing fever.

TREATMENT. Head lice hatch from silvery oval-shaped envelopes (nits) that are glued to the shafts of the hairs. Neither hatched nor unhatched eggs can be removed by chemotherapy, this being effected if required for cosmetic purposes by use of a very fine toothed comb, or by drawing off by hand, after treatment with an ovicidal insecticide. Evidence that head lice had developed resistance to the insecticides DDT and HCH (lindane) led to their replacement in the UK with malathion and carbaryl during the mid 1970s. Lotion preparations containing 0.5% w/v, applied to dry hair, were found to be effective against lice and eggs in a 12 hour treatment for malathion and 24 hour treatment for carbaryl. The absence of consistent monitoring frustrates substantiation of fears that resistance to malathion and carbaryl is now emerging.

Clothing lice attach their eggs to cloth fibres and visit the skin to feed. Frequent changing of clothing is helpful in their control. When infestation is discovered it is necessary to raise the temperature of the clothing and bed linens used by the infected person to 52 °C for 10 minutes to kill the eggs. This can be achieved by tumble drying *dry* clothing in a drier with an exhaust temperature above 60 °C. Clothing that cannot be boiled, autoclaved or tumble dried as described should be dry cleaned. Dusting with a powder containing carbaryl or pyrethroids may be effective in destroying lice on bedclothing, mattresses and other inanimate objects. Vacuum cleaning offers a mechanical method of disposal. Crab lice are cured by same preparations as are available for head lice, a water-based product being most comfortable. All the hairy parts of the body including the head hair should be treated. Eyelashes can be treated by smearing a finger dipped in the lotion along the closed lid. There is no need to remove the eggs.

In dealing with lice it is essential to treat all infested contacts simultaneously to avoid reinfection. Eradication programmes are often defeated by the difficulty of early diagnosis. It is thought modern shampoos, conditioners and shower gels may loosen the louse's gripping power by lubricating hairs and facilitating its detachment from the hose during rinsing. This probably prolongs the period during which infestation remains at a low level, postponing detection unless a watch is kept on the rinsing water for washed-out lice.

Lowe's disease (lohz) oculocerebrorenal syndrome.

loxoscelism (lok'sosəˌlizəm) a morbid condition resulting from the bite of the brown spiders, *Loxosceles reclusa* and *L. laeta*, beginning with a painful erythematous vesicle and progressing to a gangrenous slough of the affected area; first recognized in South America, but a few cases have been diagnosed in North America, Australia, and the Middle East.

lozenge ('lozinj) 1. a medicated tablet or disc; a troche. 2. a triangular area of tissue marked for excision in plastic surgery.

Lr chemical symbol, *lawrencium*.

LRCP Licentiate of the Royal College of Physicians.

LRCPE Licentiate of the Royal College of Physicians of Edinburgh.

LRCS Licentiate of the Royal College of Surgeons.

LRFPS Licentiate of the Royal Faculty of Physicians and Surgeons.

LSA left sacroanterior (position of the fetus); Licentiate of the Society of Apothecaries.

LSD a hallucinogenic compound (lysergic acid diethylamide), derived from lysergic acid, a constituent of ergot alkaloids; called also *lysergide*.

LSD has consciousness-expanding effects and is capable of producing a state of mind in which there is false sense perception (hallucination). (See also HALLUCINOGEN.) The perceptual changes brought about by LSD in normal persons are extremely variable and depend on factors such as age, personality, education, physical make-up, and state of health. The danger of the drug lies in the fact that it loosens control over impulsive behaviour and may lead to a full-blown psychosis or less serious mental disorder in persons with latent mental illness. The production, supply and possession of LSD are regulated by the Home Office.

LSD was first developed in 1938 and was believed to be potentially useful in the treatment of mental illness. This theory was based on the belief that the drug could produce a schizophrenic syndrome and that psychiatrists and other persons concerned with mental illness could observe the manifestations of a psychosis under controlled conditions. However, competent investigators have shown that the effect of LSD is more closely related to a toxic psychosis such as that produced by fever, stress, or drugs of many kinds and is of doubtful use in understanding the mechanism of a true psychosis resulting from severe personality disorder.

Abuse of LSD by semiscientific investigators and lay persons has led to much publicity, with the result that a black market now operates to make the drug available to those who wish to 'increase their awareness' or attain a state of euphoria. Although LSD is not addictive, the greatest number of persons abusing the drug also have been found to be users of marijuana, amphetamines, and barbiturates, and are extremely likely to develop a drug dependence. They apparently use the drug to escape reality rather than for the purpose of helping themselves cope with reality.

The controversy concerning chromosomal damage caused by abuse of LSD is yet to be resolved. Is also called Acid.

LSL left sacrolateral (position of the fetus).

LSP left sacroposterior (position of the fetus).

LT lymphotoxin.

LTF lymphocyte transforming factor.

LTH luteotrophic hormone (prolactin).

Lu chemical symbol, *lutetium*.

lubb (lub) a syllable used to represent, or mimic, the first sound of the heart in auscultation (see also HEART SOUNDS).

lubb-dupp (lub'dup) syllables used to represent, or mimic, the combination of the first (lubb) and second (dupp) HEART SOUNDS.

lucidity (loo'sidətee) clearness of mind. adj. **lucid**.

lucifugal (loo'sifyuhg'l) avoiding, or repelled by, bright light.

lucipetal (loo'sipit'l) seeking, or attracted to, bright light.

Ludiomil ('loodioh,mil) trademark for a preparation of maprotiline hydrochloride, an antidepressant.

Ludwig's angina ('luhdvigz) see under ANGINA.

Ludwig's ganglion a ganglion near the right atrium of the heart, connected with the cardiac plexus.

lues ('looeez) syphilis. adj. **luetic**.

Lugol's solution ('loogolz) strong iodine solution, each 100 ml containing 4.5 to 5.5 g of iodine and 9.5 to 10.5 g of potassium iodide; a source of iodine.

lumb(o)- word element. [L.] *loin*.

lumbago (lum'baygoh) pain in the lower part (lumbar region) of the back. Lumbago is a popular term for lower back pain. It embraces a number of illnesses. Such pain may be caused by injury, such as back strain, by arthritis, by abuse of the back muscles (from poor posture, a sagging mattress, or ill-fitting shoes, for example), or by a number of other disorders.

lumbar ('lumbə) pertaining to the loins.

l. plexus one formed by the ventral branches of the second to fifth lumbar nerves in the psoas major muscle (the branches of the first lumbar nerve often are included).

l. puncture insertion of a hollow needle into the subarachnoid space between the third and fourth lumbar vertebrae; called also SPINAL PUNCTURE. A lumbar puncture may be done to obtain a specimen of CEREBROSPINAL FLUID for examination and to measure the pressure within the cerebrospinal cavities. As a therapeutic measure it is sometimes done to remove blood or pus from the subarachnoid space. A lumbar puncture also is necessary for injection of a spinal anaesthetic. For visualization of the spinal canal and course of the spinal cord a radiopaque dye is injected into the subarachnoid space.

l. vertebrae the five vertebrae between the thoracic vertebrae and the sacrum.

lumbarization (,lumbə·rie'zayshən) nonfusion of the first and second segments of the sacrum so that there is one additional articulated vertebra, the sacrum consisting of only four segments.

lumbocostal (,lumboh'kost'l) pertaining to the loin and ribs.

lumbodynia (,lumboh'dini·ə) lumbago.

lumbosacral (,lumboh'saykrəl) pertaining to the lumbar and sacral region, or to the lumbar vertebrae and sacrum.

l. plexus the lumbar and sacral plexuses considered together, because of their continuous nature.

lumbricoid ('lumbri,koyd) resembling the earthworm; designating the ascaris, or intestinal roundworms.

lumbricosis (,lumbri'kohsis) infection with lumbrici.

lumbricus ('lumbrikəs) pl. *lumbrici* [L.] 1. the earthworm. 2. ascaris.

lumbus ('lumbəs) [L.] *loin*.

lumen ('loomin) pl. *lumina* [L.] 1. the cavity or channel within a tube or tubular organ, as a blood vessel or the intestine. 2. the SI unit of light flux. adj. **luminal**.

luminescence (,loomi'nes'ns) the property of giving off light without a corresponding degree of heat.

luminophore ('loominəfor) a chemical group that gives the property of luminescence to organic compounds.

lumirhodopsin (,loomiroh'dopsin) an intermediate product of exposure of rhodopsin to light.

lumpectomy (,lump'ektəmee) the surgical excision of only the local lesion (benign or malignant) of the BREAST.

lunate ('loonayt) 1. moon-shaped or crescentic. 2. the lunate bone.

Lund and Browder chart (luhnd ənd 'browdə) a chart that has been adopted by many burn centres in Britain for calculation of the surface area of a burn in a child. This chart is based on tables prepared by Charles C. Lund and Newton C. Browder in 1944 and takes into account the areas of the body affected by growth (see accompanying illustration).

At birth the size and area of the head is large compared with the adult, and the legs and thighs constitute a much smaller proportion of the total body surface. On admission to a Burns Unit or ward the area of the body burned is mapped onto the Lund and Browder chart and the area of the burn affecting each portion of the body surface is calculated.

 Lund and Browder chart

Name ______________ Age ______ Number ______________

Burn record Ages – Birth – 7½. Date of observation ______________

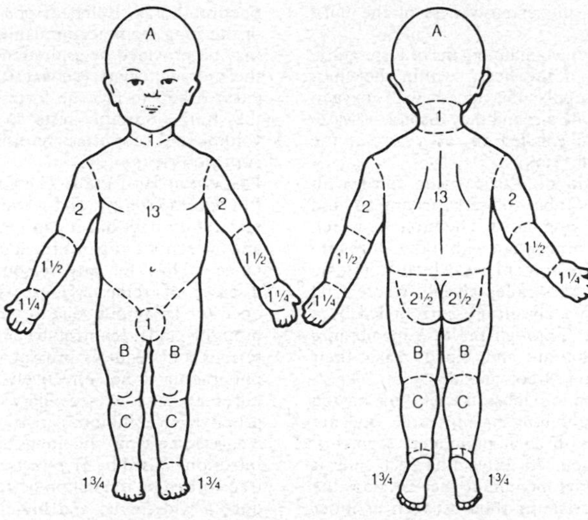

RELATIVE PERCENTAGES OF AREAS AFFECTED BY GROWTH

Area	Age 0	1	5
A = ½ of head	9½	8½	6½
B = ½ of one thigh	2¾	3¼	4
C = ½ of one leg	2½	2½	2¾

% BURN BY AREAS

Name ______________ Age ______ Number ______________

Burn record. Ages 7½ to Adult. Date of observation ______________

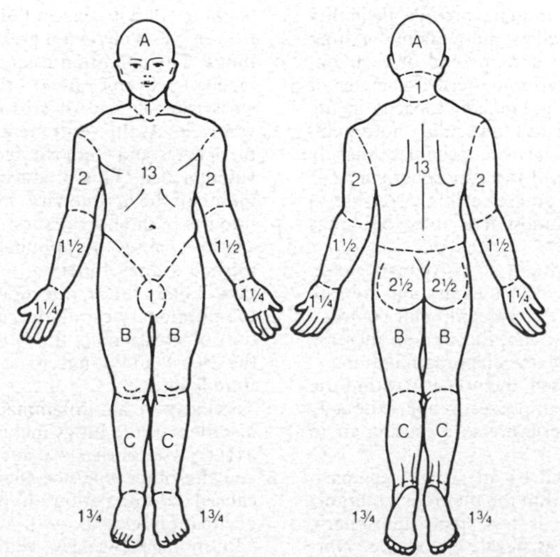

RELATIVE PERCENTAGES OF AREAS AFFECTED BY GROWTH

Area	Age 10	15	Adult
A = ½ of head	5½	4½	3½
B = ½ of one thigh	4¼	4½	4¾
C = ½ of one leg	3	3¼	3½

% BURN BY AREAS

Lund and Browder chart: estimation of extent of burn

The Lund and Browder chart eliminates some of the errors produced by the earlier BERKOW FORMULA because changes in the growth of the head, thighs and legs are incorporated into the table, which makes the overall assessment of the extensiveness of the burn more accurate.

lung (lung) either of the two main organs of respiration, lying on either side of the heart, within the chest cavity. The lungs supply the blood with oxygen inhaled from the outside air, and they dispose of waste carbon dioxide in the exhaled air, as a part of the process known as RESPIRATION.

The lungs are made of elastic tissue filled with interlacing networks of tubes and sacs carrying air, and with blood vessels carrying blood. The bronchi, which bring air to the lungs, branch out within the lungs into many smaller tubes, the bronchioles, which culminate in clusters of tiny air sacs called alveoli, whose total runs into millions. The alveoli are surrounded by a network of capillaries. Through the thin membranes of the capillaries, the air and blood make their exchange of oxygen and carbon dioxide.

The lungs are divided into lobes, the left lung having two lobes and the right lung having three, and are further subdivided into bronchopulmonary segments, of which there are about 20. Protecting each lung is the pleura, a two-layered membrane that envelops the lung and contains lubricating fluid between its inner and outer layers.

MECHANICS OF INFLATION AND DEFLATION. The lungs are inflated and deflated because of the alteration of the intra-alveolar pressure caused by the movement of respiratory muscles. Inspiration is active and caused by the contraction of the diaphragm and intercostal muscles. The diaphragm, a large dome-shaped muscle, forms the bottom of the thoracic cage. As it contracts it flattens, increasing the diameter of the thorax and elevating the lower ribs. Both of these actions increase the space for expansion of the lungs.

The external intercostal muscles provide flexibility to the thoracic cage and allow more room for lung expansion by elevating the anterior end of each rib, thereby increasing the anterior–posterior diameter of the chest wall. Because of the greater capacity in the thoracic cavity created by this muscular movement, the air pressure in the alveoli becomes slightly negative in relation to that of the atmospheric air (−3 mmHg). As air flows from an area of high pressure to low, it flows from the atmosphere into the lungs (inspiration).

Deflation of the lungs is chiefly a passive manoeuvre. The major muscles involved in expiration are the abdominal muscle group. As these muscles contract, they depress the lower ribs, and, through an increase in abdominal pressure, move the diaphragm upward.

As the lungs are compressed, the pressure within the alveoli (intra-alveolar pressure) rises to approximately +3 mmHg above atmospheric pressure causing air to flow outward (expiration).

The lungs are surrounded by an airtight compartment, the pleural space, within the pleural membrane. The intrapleural pressure is less than atmospheric pressure and is expressed as negative pressure. Normally the intrapleural pressure is about −4 mmHg. When the lungs are fully expanded this pressure may be as great as −9 mmHg. Under normal conditions, however, the intrapleural pressure fluctuates between −4 and −6 mmHg.

If anything should penetrate the walls of the pleura, the negative pressure is lost as air rushes into the pleural cavity in response to atmospheric pressure. This condition is called PNEUMOTHORAX. The walls of the alveoli also must remain intact in order to maintain normal intrapleural pressure. If a lesion causes a break in the alveolar membranes, air enters the pleural cavity through the break and produces pneumothorax. Relief of pneumothorax and collapse of the lung from accumulations of either air or fluids may be provided by aspiration of the air or fluid from the thoracic cavity (THORACENTESIS) or by insertion of CHEST drains to provide for a gradual re-expansion of the lung. Specific tests to determine pulmonary volume and capacities are discussed under PULMONARY FUNCTION TESTS.

DISEASES OF THE LUNGS. The air brought to the lungs is filtered, moistened, and warmed on its way along the respiratory tract but it can nevertheless bring irritants and infectious organisms, and when the body resistance is low for any reason the lungs may suffer diseases of some seriousness. Bacterial PNEUMONIA, once a dangerous disease, is now usually quickly brought under control by antibiotics, but it is still serious and requires prompt medical attention. Viral pneumonia is not effectively treated with antibiotics but may lead to secondary bacterial infection and prophylactic antibiotics are sometimes appropriate.

TUBERCULOSIS of the lungs is a chronic pulmonary infection caused by *Mycobacterium tuberculosis*, usually transmitted by inhalation of infectious material. It was once a widespread and highly fatal disease, but now the prevalence and mortality rate have been reduced drastically because of the improvement in the standard of living and nutrition in many areas, detection of the disease in its earliest stages, and the development of tuberculostatic drugs. There has been some success in inducing specific immunity against tuberculosis by vaccination with BCG (bacille Calmette–Guérin) vaccine, a live attenuated strain of bovine tubercle bacilli.

Oedema of the lung, or pulmonary OEDEMA, is a condition in which the alveoli and interstitial spaces begin to fill with excess fluid. It occurs when the fluid load of the body is too great for the heart, kidneys, or lungs. The condition frequently is a complication of a type of chronic heart disease in which there is weakness of and decreased output from the left ventricle. As the ventricle weakens it becomes less able to accept and remove blood from the pulmonary vascular bed. This produces congestion and engorgement of the pulmonary vessels with escape of fluid into the pulmonary tissues.

Other causes of pulmonary oedema include diminished kidney function, which allows for accumulation of body fluids, infections of the lungs which affect the pulmonary capillaries, and a too-rapid administration of intravenous fluids in relation to the ability of the heart and lungs to accommodate an additional fluid load.

PLEURISY is an inflammation of the pleura. Other disorders of the lungs include ASTHMA, BRONCHIECTASIS, ATELECTASIS, EMPHYSEMA, and fungal infections. SILICOSIS and the other PNEUMOCONIOSES are pulmonary diseases caused by inhalation of particulates and are often occupation related.

Pulmonary EMBOLISM, while not a primary disease of the lung, does involve an obstruction of the pulmonary artery or one of its branches. The source of obstruction usually is a blood clot that has entered the blood stream from a distant point and been carried by blood flow to the pulmonary artery. The condition can be fatal if not treated promptly.

CHRONIC OBSTRUCTIVE AIRWAYS DISEASE (COAD) is a classification of lung disease indicating a long-term illness in which there are structural and functional changes in the bronchi and bronchioles, and in the lungs and the blood vessels that serve them. These changes bring about an obstruction of bronchial air flow and loss of elasticity of the lungs. Called also *chronic obstructive lung disease* (COLD), *chronic obstructive pulmonary disease* (COPD) and *diffuse obstructive lung disease* (DOLD).

Lung Abscess. Lung abscess is an infection of the lung, characterized by a localized accumulation of pus and destruction of tissue. It may be a complication of pneumonia or tuberculosis. A lung abscess may also follow a period of excessive drinking by an alcoholic. Infected matter that has been aspirated may lodge in a bronchiole and produce inflammation. Lung cancer may also be responsible for formation of an abscess.

The first symptoms of lung abscess include a dry cough and chest pain. Later these may be followed by fever, rigors, productive cough, headache, perspiration, foul-smelling sputum, and sometimes dyspnoea. If the abscess is a complication of pneumonia, the symptoms tend to be moderated to an exaggeration of the pneumonia symptoms.

When a lung abscess forms, it is in the acute stage and treatment with antibiotics usually is effective. POSTURAL DRAINAGE may be prescribed to assist in drainage of exudate from lungs and bronchioles. In most cases, this treatment produces a cure. If the abscess becomes chronic, surgery may be necessary and usually involves removal of the portion of the lung containing the abscess.

Lung Cancer. Malignant growths of the lung are among the most common types of CANCER. Although the exact cause of lung cancer is not known, irritants that are inhaled over a period of time are known to be important predisposing causes. Years ago it was realized that miners of certain ores developed lung cancer much more often than men in other occupations. Later, other irritants of lung tissue, such as air polluted by fumes from burning fuels or motor exhausts, were singled out as probable causes of the increasing number of cases of the disease in urban and industrial areas. The irritant most widely encountered is tobacco smoke, especially cigarette smoke, which is much more frequently and deeply inhaled than the smoke of pipes or cigars.

A study based on autopsies of the lungs of individuals who had died from many varied causes, but whose smoking history was known, showed that unrecognized cancer and precancerous changes in tissue were numerous among smokers and rare among nonsmokers. Tobacco causes about 90 per cent of all British lung cancer.

The search for other possible causes of lung cancer has not been neglected. However, no definite findings have been reported thus far.

Since the factors causing lung cancer act slowly and may produce a tumour near the periphery of the lung, early symptoms are vague or may not appear at all, and nearly a third of the cases are in an advanced stage when they are discovered.

The earliest and most common symptom is a cough. Dry at first, this cough later produces sputum which eventually becomes blood-streaked. A wheeze in the chest is frequently a symptom and indicates a partial obstruction in a bronchus. Chest pains, weakness, and loss of weight are later symptoms, as is dyspnoea.

Diagnosis depends on a careful physical examination, including a chest x-ray. If a suspicious density is seen on the x-ray, samples of sputum will be examined microscopically for the presence of malignant cells. BRONCHOSCOPY is also done, and at the same time a specimen for biopsy can be obtained or the bronchial secretions can be washed out and the cells stained and examined.

When examination indicates lung cancer, prompt treatment is essential. This may involve the surgical removal of the lobe of the lung containing the cancer or of an entire lung if the malignant cells have spread. A significant number of persons affected by lung cancer can be cured by such operations if the surgery is performed in time. In some cases of widespread involvement surgery is not possible; these patients are treated with x-rays or radium or ANTINEOPLASTIC drugs.

Further information about lung disease and its prevention can be obtained from: The Chest, Heart and Stroke Association (Tavistock House North, Tavistock Square, London WC1H 9JE); The Asthma Research Council (12 Pembridge Square, London W2 4EH); and the Asthma Society and Friends of the Asthma Research Council (300 Upper Street, London N1 2XX).

SURGERY OF THE LUNG. Surgical procedures performed on the lung include removal of the entire lung (pneumonectomy), removal of a lobe of the lung (lobectomy), and removal of only a bronchopulmonary segment (segmental resection). The procedure done depends on the size of the area involved and the type of lesion present.

Pneumonectomy is usually necessary for treatment of cancer, multiple abscesses of the lung, or severe bronchiectasis. In this procedure a thoracotomy incision is made and one or two ribs are resected. The large pulmonary vessels (the artery and vein leading to and from the lung) are ligated and cut and the main bronchus serving the lung is closed with sutures. One or more tubes may be inserted to provide for drainage of blood and fluid from the cavity (see also CHEST drain).

Cysts, abscesses, or benign tumours that involve only a lobe of the lung are treated by lobectomy. A thoracotomy incision is made and the lung is collapsed before the lobe is removed. The remaining lobes are then re-expanded and chest drains are inserted for removal of air and fluid. See also COLLAPSE therapy.

Patient Care. Before surgery the patient is given an explanation of the procedure to be done and the purpose of the CHEST drains, oxygen therapy, and other apparatus to be used postoperatively. Special exercises of the arms, shoulders, and chest muscles are often started before surgery and resumed postoperatively. Their purpose is to strengthen the muscles and provide for continued motion of the shoulder and arm and normal functioning of the remaining lung tissue.

Immediately after surgery the patient's pulse, respirations, and blood pressure are checked and recorded every 15 minutes until they become stabilized. Oxygen is administered and the patient is watched closely for signs of respiratory difficulty. Positioning of the patient depends on the specific orders of the surgeon. Generally, the patient is allowed to lie only on his back or the operative side. Lying on the operative side facilitates drainage, and enhances ventilation of the unaffected lung. When turning a patient to the operative side, care must be taken that the tube(s) is not kinked and the patient's weight is adequately supported with pillows so that the tubes are not obstructed. An exception to the turning routine for patients having lung surgery is the pneumonectomy patient. Such patients should be placed in the high Fowler position and should not be turned for 24 hours.

Dressings are reinforced but usually not changed until the drainage tubes have been removed and the incision is closed and healing.

Coughing is encouraged although it may be painful

for the patient during the first few postoperative days. Discomfort can be reduced by splinting the chest with the hands or a pillow, or turning the patient onto the operative side during episodes of coughing.

The convalescent period after lung surgery is often long and difficult for the patient. He will need encouragement in continuing his exercises and in other procedures necessary for adequate ventilation and normal function of the remaining lung tissue.

brown l. byssinosis.

l. calculus a concretion formed in the bronchi by accretion about an inorganic nucleus, or from calcified portions of lung tissue or adjacent lymph nodes.

l. compliance a measure of the ability of the lung to distend without disruption in response to pressure; expresses the unit volume of change in the lung per unit of pressure. Compliance or distensibility of the lung is increased in conditions such as emphysema, in which the lung distends more readily, and is decreased in fibrotic conditions in which the lung distends with difficulty. See also COMPLIANCE.

iron l. a popular name for a Drinker respirator, a type of negative pressure VENTILATOR that provides controlled, automatic breathing for a patient whose respiratory muscles are paralysed, consisting of a metal tank, enclosing the patient's body with the head outside, and within which artificial respiration is maintained by alternating negative and positive pressure.

l. reflexes Hering–Breuer reflexes.

shock l. adult respiratory distress syndrome.

lungmotor ('lung,mohtə) an apparatus for forcing air, or air and oxygen, into the lungs.

lungworm ('lung,wərm) any parasitic worm that invades the lungs, e.g., *Paragonimus westermani* in man.

lunula ('loonyuhlə) pl. *lunulae* [L.] a small, crescentic or moon-shaped area or structure, e.g., the white area at the base of the nail of a finger or toe, or one of the segments of the semilunar valves of the heart.

lupiform ('loopi,fawm) resembling lupus.

lupoid ('loopoyd) 1. pertaining to lupus vulgaris. 2. a variant of sarcoidosis marked by small papular lesions.

lupus ('loopəs) a name originally given to a destructive type of skin lesion. The original term included quite different conditions which have now been designated lupus vulgaris and lupus erythematosus. The Latin word *lupus* means wolf; erythematosus refers to redness. The name lupus erythematosus has been used since the 13th century because doctors thought the shape and colour of the skin lesions resembled the bite of a wolf. Currently, there are at least two recognized manifestations of the disease: discoid lupus erythematosus and systemic lupus erythematosus.

discoid l. erythematosus (DLE) a superficial inflammation of the skin, marked by red macules up to 3 to 4 cm in width, and covered with scanty adherent scales, which extend into patulous follicles that fall off, leaving scars. The lesions typically form a butterfly pattern over the bridge of the nose and cheeks, but other areas may be involved, notably the scalp. It is exacerbated by sunlight, which should be avoided. Topical steroids used in short courses can suppress the disorder. **drug-induced l.** a syndrome closely resembling systemic lupus erythematosus, precipitated by prolonged use of certain drugs, most commonly hydralazine, isoniazid, various anticonvulsants, and procainamide.

systemic l. erythematosus (SLE) a chronic, inflammatory disease, often febrile, and characterized by injury to the skin, joints, kidneys, nervous system, and mucous membranes. It can, however, affect any organ of the body and is usually characterized by periods of remissions and exacerbations.

It was once thought that SLE was a fairly rare disease, but improved immunological testing procedures have shown that its prevalence rate is approximately 1 per 800 population. It is primarily a disease of women, occurring five to ten times more frequently among females than among males. Although the peak incidence is between 30 and 40 years of age, it has been diagnosed in the very young and the very old.

SLE is the classic prototype of autoimmune connective tissue disease. Its aetiology is unknown, but the high level of autoantibodies in persons with SLE indicates a defect in the regulatory mechanisms that sustain self-tolerance and prevent the body from attacking its own cells, cell constituents, and proteins. Patients with SLE can have a wide variety of autoantibodies against nuclear and cytoplasmic cellular components. The presence of high levels of antinuclear antibody (ANA) in SLE patients with glomerulonephritis indicates a *pathogenic* role for ANA. Antinuclear antibodies are directed against deoxyribonucleoprotein, DNA, histone, and a soluble non-nucleic acid molecule (Sm antigen).

Factors that appear to contribute to the development of SLE include exposure to sunlight or ultraviolet radiation from sunlamps, a genetic predisposition to the disease, certain drugs, viral and bacterial infections, and hormonal influences.

Clinical manifestations of SLE are confusingly diverse owing to the involvement of connective tissue throughout the body. Typically, the patient seeks medical help for relief of fever, weight loss, joint pain, the characteristic butterfly rash, pleural effusion and pleuritic pain, and nephritis. The detection of ANA by microscopic immunofluorescence is virtually diagnostic of SLE.

Either glomerulonephritis, which is usually mild, or cardiovascular manifestations such as myocarditis, endocarditis, or pericarditis, are found in about half the patients with SLE. Pulmonary disease, especially pleurisy, is also relatively common, as are gastrointestinal disturbances and lymph node involvement. Organic neurological disturbances produce behavioural aberrations and frank psychosis in some patients; in a few others, there are peripheral neuropathies, motor aphasia, and diplopia.

There is no specific treatment for the underlying pathologies of SLE. Supportive measures are employed to prevent or minimize acute relapses and exacerbations of symptoms. The patient is instructed to avoid exposure to sunlight and ultraviolet radiation from other sources, blood transfusions, penicillin, and the sulphonamides. Active disease is treated with topical steroids, salicylates for fever and joint pain, corticosteroids, and immunosuppressive agents. Physiotherapy may be required to alleviate muscle weakness and prevent orthopaedic deformities.

l. pernio 1. soft, violaceous skin lesions on the cheeks, forehead, nose, ears, and digits, frequently associated with bone cysts, which may be the first manifestation of sarcoidosis or occur in the chronic stage of the disease. 2. a form of discoid lupus erythematosus aggravated by cold, initially resembling chilblains, in which the lesions consist of erythematous infiltrated patches on the exposed areas of the body, especially the finger knuckles.

l. vulgaris the most common and severe form of tuberculosis of the skin, most often affecting the face, marked by the formation of reddish brown patches of nodules in the corium, which progressively spread peripherally with central atrophy, causing ulceration and scarring and destruction of cartilage in involved sites.

Lurselle (lər'sel) trademark for a preparation of probucol, an antihyperlipoproteinaemic.

luteal ('looti·əl) pertaining to or having the properties of the corpus luteum or its active principle.

lutein ('lootee·in) 1. a lipochrome from the corpus luteum, fat cells, and egg yolk. 2. any lipochrome.

luteinic (ˌlootee'inik) pertaining to the corpus luteum, to lutein, or to luteinization.

luteinization (ˌlootee·inie'zayshan) the process taking place in the follicle cells of graafian follicles that have matured and discharged their egg: the cells become hypertrophied and there is vascularization and lipid accumulation (the latter in some species giving a yellow colour), the follicles becoming corpora lutea.

luteinizing hormone ('lootee·iˌniezing) a gonadotrophic hormone of the anterior pituitary gland acting, with follicle-stimulating hormone, to cause ovulation of mature follicles and secretion of oestrogen by thecal and granulosa cells of the ovary; it is also concerned with corpus luteum formation. In the male, it stimulates development of the interstitial cells of the testes and their secretion of testosterone.

Lutembacher's syndrome ('lootəmˌbakəz) mitral stenosis (usually rheumatic) associated with atrial septal defect.

luteohormone (ˌlootioh'hawmohn) progesterone.

luteoma (ˌlooti'ohmə) 1. a luteinized granulosa–theca cell tumour. 2. nodular hyperplasia of ovarian lutein cells sometimes occurring in the last trimester of pregnancy.

luteotrophe ('lootiohtrohf) lactotrophe.

luteotrophic (ˌlootioh'trohfik) stimulating formation of the corpus luteum.

l. hormone luteotrophin.

luteotrophin (ˌlootioh'trohfin) a hormone of the anterior pituitary which stimulates formation of the corpus luteum in women; identical with prolactin. Called also *luteotrophic hormone* (LTH).

lutetium (loo'teeshi·əm) a chemical element, atomic number 71, atomic weight 174.97, symbol Lu. See table of elements in Appendix 2.

Lutz–Splendore–Almeida disease (ˌluhts-ˌsplendawal'maydə) paracoccidioidomycosis.

lux (luks) the SI unit of illumination, being 1 lumen per metre squared.

luxation (luk'sayshən) dislocation.

luxus ('luksəs) [L.] *excess.*

lyase ('lieayz) any of a class of enzymes that remove groups from their substrates (other than by hydrolysis), leaving double bonds, or that conversely add groups to double bonds.

lycoperdonosis (ˌliekohˌpərdə'nohsis) a respiratory disease due to inhalation of spores of the puffball fungus, *Lycoperdon.*

lye (lie) an alkaline percolate from wood ashes; household lye is a crude mixture of sodium hydroxide with some sodium carbonate.

lying-in (ˌlieing'in) 1. puerperal. 2. puerperium.

l.-i. period postnatal period.

Lyme disease (liem) a zoonosis transmitted by ticks and characterized by rash—erythema chronicum migrans—arthritis and aseptic meningitis, caused by the spirochaete *Borrelia burgdorferi.* It was originally described in an outbreak in Lyme, Connecticut, USA in the 1970s, but the skin condition was previously regonized in Sweden early in the twentieth century. Few cases have been reported in the UK. The highest incidence is in the summer months. The reservoir of infection is probably deer and wild rodents. The incubation period is 3–32 days after the tick bite; there is no evidence of human-to-human transmission.

Following the tick bite, which may or may not be noticed, the disease begins with an annular extending rash and sometimes malaise and fever. The disease may spontaneously regress and several weeks or months later, joint involvement, especially the knees, and neurological manifestations, particulary aseptic meningitis, may follow and persist for several years if untreated.

Treatment involves giving penicillin or tetracycline.

lymph (limf) a transparent, usually slightly yellow, often opalescent liquid found within the lymphatic vessels, and collected from tissues in all parts of the body and returned to the blood via the lymphatic system. It is about 95 per cent water; the remainder consists of plasma proteins and other chemical substances contained in the blood plasma, but in slightly smaller percentage than in plasma. Its cellular component consists chiefly of lymphocytes.

The body contains three main kinds of fluid: blood, tissue fluid, and lymph. The blood consists of the blood cells and platelets, the plasma, or fluid portion, and a variety of chemical substances dissolved in the plasma. When the plasma, without its solid particles and some of its dissolved substances, seeps through the capillary walls and circulates among the body tissues, it is known as tissue fluid. When this fluid is drained from the tissues and collected by the lymphatic system, it is called lymph. The LYMPHATIC SYSTEM eventually returns the lymph to the blood, where it again becomes plasma. This movement of fluid through the body is described under CIRCULATORY SYSTEM.

l. node any of the accumulations of lymphoid tissue organized as definite lymphoid organs along the course of lymphatic vessels, consisting of an outer cortical and an inner medullary part; they are the main source of lymphocytes of the peripheral blood and, as part of the reticuloendothelial system, serve as a defence mechanism by removing noxious agents, e.g., bacteria and toxins, and probably play a role in antibody formation. Sometimes called, incorrectly, lymph glands.

lymph(o)- word element. [L.] *lymph, lymphoid tissue, lymphatics, lymphocytes.*

lymph-vascular (limf'vaskyuhlə) pertaining to lymphatic vessels.

lympha ('limfə) [L.] *lymph.*

lymphadenectasis (ˌlimfadə'nektəsis) enlargement of a lymph node.

lymphadenectomy (ˌlimfadə'nektəmee) excision of one or more lymph nodes.

lymphadenia (ˌlimfə'deeni·ə) hypertrophy of lymph nodes.

lymphadenitis (ˌlimfadə'nietis) inflammation of lymph nodes.

lymphadenocele (lim'fadənohˌseel) a cyst of a lymph node.

lymphadenogram (lim'fadənohˌgram) the film produced by lymphadenography.

lymphadenography (ˌlimfadə'nogrəfee) radiography of lymph nodes after injection of a contrast medium into a lymphatic vessel.

lymphadenoid (lim'fadəˌnoyd) resembling the tissues of the lymph nodes. Lymphadenoid tissue includes the spleen, bone marrow, tonsils, and the lymphoid tissues of the organs and mucous membranes.

lymphadenoma (ˌlimfadə'nohmə) lymphoma.

lymphadenopathy (ˌlimfadə'nopəthee) enlargement of the lymph nodes.

angioimmunoblastic l. immunoblastic lymphadenopathy.

dermatopathic l. regional lymph node enlargement associated with melanoderma and other dermatoses

marked by chronic erythroderma.
giant follicular l. nodular well-differentiated lymphocytic malignant lymphoma, microscopically characterized by multiple, proliferative, follicle-like nodules which disturb the normal architecture of the lymph nodes. Called also *Brill–Symmers disease* and *giant follicular lymphoma.*
immunoblastic l. a hyperimmune disorder resembling Hodgkin's disease, characterized by malaise, and generalized lymphadenopathy, constitutional symptoms, and proliferation of immunoblasts and small vessels.
lymphadenosis (ˌlimfadə'nohsis) hypertrophy or proliferation of lymphoid tissue.
l. benigna cutis a benign inflammatory hyperplasia of lymphocytes in the skin, principally on the face or ears, in the form of solitary or disseminated yellowish brown to bluish red nodules that usually involute spontaneously.
lymphadenotomy (ˌlimfadə'notəmee) incision of a lymph node.
lymphaemia (lim'feemi·ə) the presence of an undue number of lymphocytes or their precursors in the blood.
lymphagogue ('limfəˌgog) an agent promoting the production of lymph.
lymphangial (lim'fanji·əl) pertaining to a lymphatic vessel.
lymphangiectasia, lymphangiectasis (ˌlimfanjiek'tayzi·ə; ˌlimfanji'ektasis) dilation of the lymphatic vessels. adj. **lymphangiectatic.**
lymphangiectomy (ˌlimfanji'ektəmee) excision of one or more lymphatic vessels.
lymphangiitis (ˌlimfanji'ietis) lymphangitis.
lymphangioendothelioma (limˌfanjiohˌendohˌtheeli'ohmə) lymphangioma in which endothelial cells are the main component.
lymphangiofibroma (limˌfanjiohfie'brohmə) a fibrosing lymphangioma.
lymphangiogram (lim'fanjiohˌgram) the film produced by lymphangiography.
lymphangiography (ˌlimfanji'ografee) radiography of lymphatic channels and lymph glands after introduction of a contrast medium.
lymphangiology (ˌlimfanji'oləjee) the scientific study of the lymphatic system.
lymphangioma (ˌlimfanji'ohmə) a tumour composed of new-formed lymph spaces and channels. adj. **lymphangiomatous.**
cavernous l. dilation of the lymphatic vessels, resulting in cavities filled with lymph.
cystic l., l. cysticum a cystic growth usually found in the neck or groin, thought to originate from a developmental anomaly of the primitive lymphatic spaces; symptoms are largely due to compression of adjoining structures by the mass.
lymphangiomyomatosis (limˌfanjiohˌmieohmə'tohsis) a progessive disorder of women of child-bearing age, marked by nodular and diffuse interstitial proliferation of smooth muscle in the lungs, lymph nodes, and thoracic duct.
lymphangiophlebitis (limˌfanjiohfli'bietis) inflammation of lymphatic vessels and veins.
lymphangioplasty (lim'fanjiohˌplastee) surgical restoration of lymphatic channels.
lymphangiosarcoma (limˌfanjiohsah'kohmə) a malignant tumour of lymphatic vessels, usually arising in a limb that is the site of chronic lymphoedema.
lymphangiotomy (ˌlimfanji'otəmee) incision of a lymphatic vessel.
lymphangitis (ˌlimfan'jietis) inflammation of a lymphatic vessel.

lymphapheresis (limfˌafə'reesis) lymphocytapheresis.
lymphatic (lim'fatik) 1. pertaining to lymph or to a lymphatic vessel. 2. a lymphatic vessel.
l. ducts the two larger vessels into which all lymphatic vessels converge. The right lymphatic duct joins the venous system at the junction of the right internal jugular and subclavian veins and carries lymph from the upper right side of the body. The left lymphatic duct, or thoracic duct, enters the circulatory system at the junction of the left internal jugular and subclavian veins; it returns lymph from the upper left side of the body and from below the diaphragm.
l. system the lymphatic vessels and lymphoid tissue, considered collectively. See also CIRCULATORY SYSTEM.

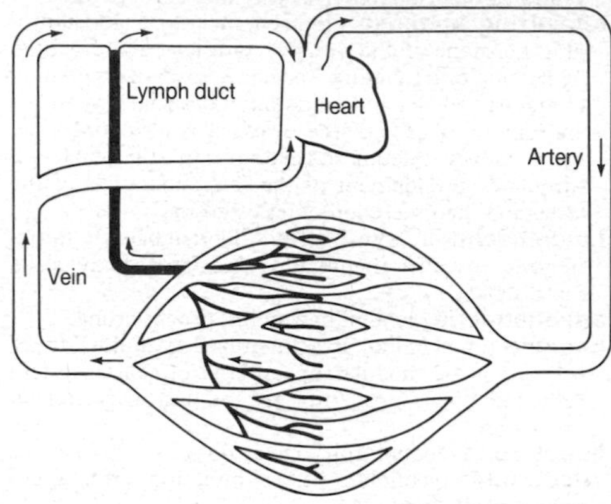

Diagram of lymphatic system, showing its relationship to the circulatory system.

DISORDERS OF THE LYMPHATIC SYSTEM. Several diseases affect the lymphatic system. LYMPHOGRANULOMA VENEREUM is a viral disease that attacks lymph nodes in the groin and usually is transmitted by sexual contact.

Lymphadenitis is an inflammation of the lymph nodes, particularly in the neck; swollen tonsils is an example. Generalized lymphadenitis can be a symptom of the secondary stage of syphilis.

Cancer attacks the lymphatic system, as it does other systems of the body. A tumour of the lymphoid tissue is known as a lymphoma. The general term lymphosarcoma refers to malignant neoplastic disorders of lymphoid tissue.
l. vessels the capillaries, collecting vessels, and trunks that collect lymph from the tissues and carry it to the blood stream; called also *lymphatics.*
lymphaticostomy (ˌlimfati'kostəmee) surgical creation of a permanent opening into a lymphatic duct, usually the thoracic duct.
lymphatolysis (ˌlimfə'tolisis) destruction of lymphoid tissue. adj. **lymphatolytic.**
lymphectasia (ˌlimfek'tayzi·ə) distention with lymph.
lymphenteritis (ˌlimfentə'rietis) enteritis with serous infiltration.
lymphnoditis (ˌlimfnoh'dietis) inflammation of a lymph node.
lymphoblast ('limfohˌblast) the immature, nucleolated precursor of the mature lymphocyte. adj. **lymphoblastic.**
lymphoblastic (ˌlimfoh'blastik) pertaining to a lymphoblast; producing lymphocytes.
lymphoblastoma (ˌlimfohbla'stohmə) poorly-differentiated lymphocytic malignant LYMPHOMA.

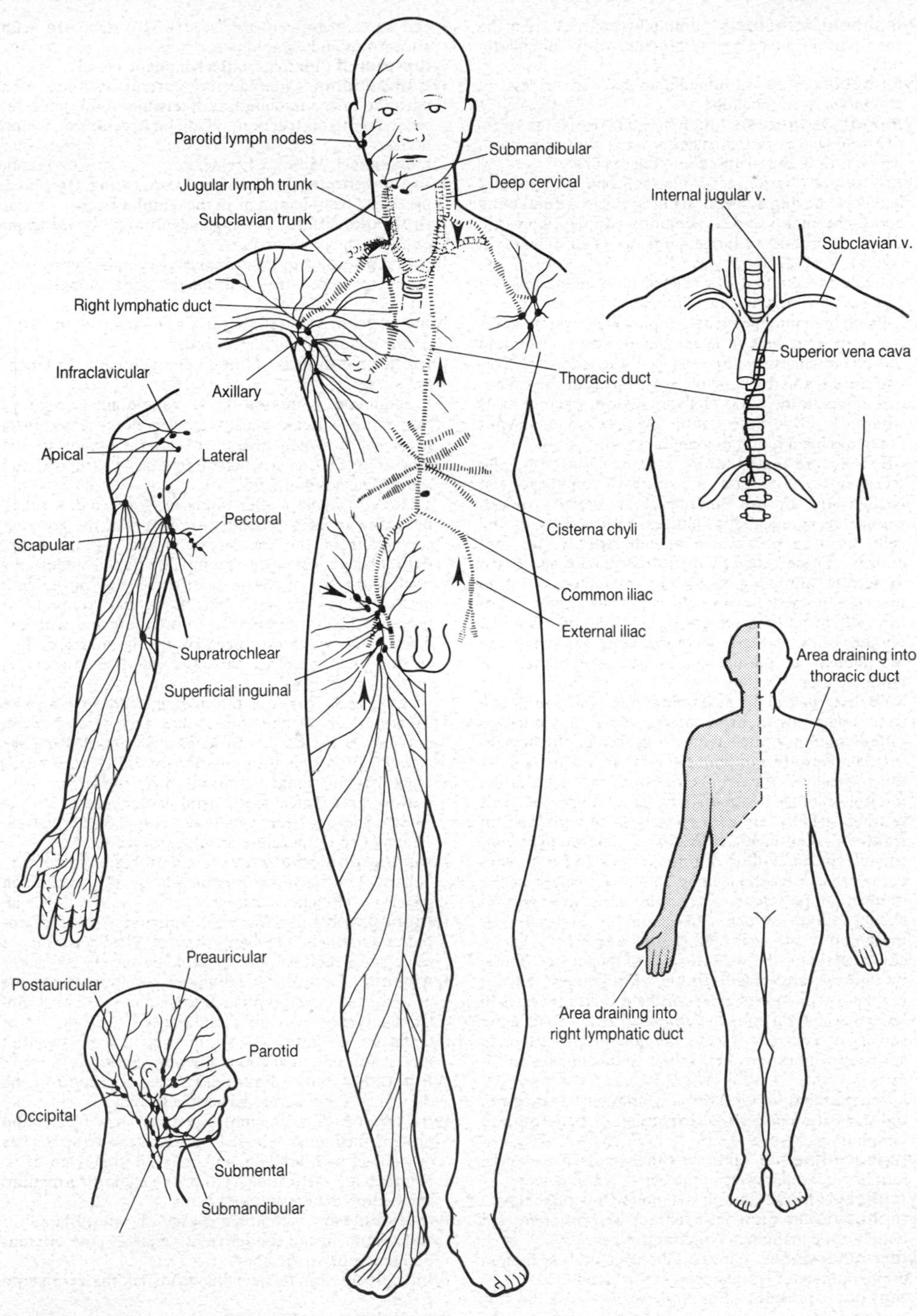

Lymphatic system

lymphoblastomatosis (ˌlimfohˌblastohmə'tohsis) the condition produced by the presence of lymphoblastomas.

lymphoblastosis (ˌlimfohbla'stohsis) an excess of lymphoblasts in the blood.

lymphocytapheresis (ˌlimfohsieˌtafə'reesis) the selective removal of lymphocytes from withdrawn blood, which is then retransfused into the donor.

lymphocyte ('limfohˌsiet) a mononuclear, nongranular leukocyte having a deeply staining nucleus containing dense chromatin and a pale-blue-staining cytoplasm. Chiefly a product of lymphoid tissue, it participates in IMMUNITY. adj. **lymphocytic**.

activated l. one that has reacted immunologically on exposure to antigen or to a mitogen.

B-l's thymus-independent lymphocytes, which develop from stem cells in haemopoietic tissue, including the blood islands of the fetal yolk sac, the fetal liver and spleen, and the bone marrow. The *B* in B-lymphocyte refers to the bursa of Fabricius, an organ in birds where B cell differentiation occurs. No analogous organ has been found in mammals.

B cells are involved in humoral IMMUNITY, the secretion of ANTIBODIES. A mature B-lymphocyte can be activated by the binding of an antigen to cell surface receptors. This induces proliferation of the cell, resulting in a clone of cells specific for that antigen. These cells can then differentiate and begin to secrete immunoglobulin (Ig) molcules; this step involves interaction with helper T-lymphocytes. All of the cells of a clone secrete Ig with identical antigen binding sites. Antigen-secreting cells can have the morphology of plasma cells, large lymphocytes, or lymphoblasts.

T-l's thymus-dependent lymphocytes, which originate from stem cells in haemopoietic tissue and undergo differentiation in the thymus triggered by thymopoietin. There are five different T-lymphocyte subpopulations. *Cytotoxic T cells*, or *killer cells*, are responsible for cell-mediated cytotoxicity, the killing of cells bearing specific antigens, which is the mechanism involved in cell-mediated IMMUNITY, delayed hypersensitivity, and the killing of tumour cells and transplant tissue cells. A second subpopulation is involved in the production of *lymphokines*, substances that are released into the blood and cause the activation or inhibition of macrophages, destroy target cells, or are chemotactic for the various types of leukocytes. These two groups are called *effector cells*; the rest have a regulatory function. *Helper cells* help B-lymphocytes to recognize certain antigens. *Amplifier cells* enhance the activity of cytotoxic T cells. *Suppressor cells* suppress antibody synthesis by their action on helper cells and B cells.

l. transforming factor (LTF) a lymphokine that causes transformation and clonal expansion of nonsensitized lymphocytes.

lymphocythaemia (ˌlimfohsie'theemi·ə) an excessive number of lymphocytes in the blood; lymphocytosis.

lymphocytoblast (ˌlimfoh'sietohblast) a lymphoblast.

lymphocytoma (ˌlimfohsie'tohmə) well-differentiated lymphocytic malignant lymphoma.

lymphocytopenia (ˌlimfohˌsietoh'peeni·ə) reduction of the number of lymphocytes in the blood.

lymphocytopoiesis (ˌlimfohˌsietohpoy'eesis) the formation of lymphocytes. adj. **lymphocytopoietic**.

lymphocytosis (ˌlimfohsie'tohsis) increase in the number of normal lymphocytes in the blood or in an effusion.

lymphocytotoxicity (ˌlimfohˌsietohtok'sisitee) the quality or capability of lysing lymphocytes, as in procedures in which lymphocytes having a specific cell surface antigen are lysed when incubated with antiserums and complement.

lymphoduct ('limfohˌdukt) a lymphatic vessel.

lymphoedema (ˌlimfi'deemə) chronic swelling of a part due to accumulation of interstitial fluid (oedema) secondary to obstruction of lymphatic vessels or lymph nodes.

congenital l. Milroy's disease.

lymphogenous (lim'fojənəs) 1. producing lymph. 2. produced from lymph or in the lymph vessels.

lymphoglandula (ˌlimfoh'glandyuhlə) pl. *lymphoglandulae* [L.] a lymph node.

lymphogonia (ˌlimfə'gohni·ə) large lymphocytes with a large nucleus, little chromatin, and nongranular cytoplasm.

lymphogram ('limfohˌgram) a radiogram of the lymphatic channels and lymph nodes.

lymphogranuloma (ˌlimfohˌgranyuh'lohmə) Hodgkin's disease.

l. inguinale, venereal l., l. venereum a sexually transmitted disease caused by a strain of *Chlamydia trachomatis*, which affects the lymph organs in the genital area. It occurs most frequently in tropical and semitropical regions.

Three to 21 days after the body is infected, a small, hard sore appears in the genital area. The disease soon spreads from the local sore to the lymph nodes, particularly those in the groin. The lymph nodes may swell to the size of a walnut. As these swellings seldom break open and drain pus, they may remain for months unless aspirated. In women infected with the disease, the vulva may become greatly enlarged. The rectum may become narrowed, so that surgery is necessary for relief.

In the early stages of the disease, there may also be inflammation of the joints, skin rashes, and fever. Sometimes the brain and its covering membrane are affected. It is thought that after the initial sore heals, men may no longer transmit the disease. Women, however, may infect sexual partners for years.

Lymphogranuloma venereum may be successfully treated with tetracycline or sulphafurazole.

lymphogranulomatosis (ˌlimfohˌgranyuhlohmə'tohsis) 1. infectious granuloma of the lymphatic system. 2. Hodgkin's disease.

lymphography (lim'fogrəfee) radiography of the lymphatic channels and lymph nodes, after injection of radiopaque material into a lymphatic vessel.

lymphoid ('limfoyd) resembling or pertaining to lymph or to tissue of the lymphatic system.

l. cells lymphocytes and plasma cells.

l. tissue a lattice work of reticular tissue, the interspaces of which contain lymphocytes.

lymphoidectomy (ˌlimfoy'dektəmee) excision of lymphoid tissue, such as tonsils and adenoids.

lymphokine ('limfohˌkien) a general term for soluble protein mediators released by sensitized lymphocytes on contact with antigen, and believed to play a role in macrophage activation, lymphocyte transformation, and cell-mediated IMMUNITY.

lymphokinesis (ˌlimfohki'neesis) 1. movement of endolymph in the semicircular canals. 2. the circulation of lymph in the body.

lymphology (lim'foləjee) the study of the lymphatic system.

lympholytic (ˌlimfoh'litik) causing destruction of lymphocytes.

lymphoma (lim'fohmə) any neoplastic disorder of lymphoid tissue, including Hodgkin's disease and nonHodgkin's malignant lymphoma (NHML), classifications of which are based on predominant cell type and degree of differentiation; NHML may be subdivided into nodular (follicular) and diffuse types depending on the predominant pattern of cell arrangement. The majority of the NHMLs are of B-cell origin and lymphoid cell markers are useful to define a monoclonal, usually malignant clone. The NHMLs are difficult to classify and several different schemes exist, e.g. Rappaport, Lukes-Collins, and Kiel. All the classifications have some prognostic and therapeutic implications; in general, large cells and a diffuse pattern of node involvement are associated with a poor prognosis.

The *Rappaport classification,* developed before the use of cell markers to define cell origins and the B- and T-cell nature of lymphocytes, is incorrect in histopathological terms but remains clinically useful. On the basis of cell morphology it recognizes two cell types—lymphocytes and histiocytes, both of which are in fact lymphoid. Subgroups within this classification include well and poorly differentiated lymphocytic and histiocytic, and tumours of mixed lineage. Larger cell tumours are presumed to be less well differentiated and to carry a poorer prognosis. Diffuse and nodular patters of tissue involvement are also important in prognosis, the former being associated with shorter survival.

The *Lukes-Collins classification* is based on the B- and T-cell lineage of the predominant tumour cell and the site of origin of the cell within the node (medullery centre, follicular centre, or paracortical region).

The *Kiel classification* subdivides lymphomas according to their cell type—B-cell, T-cell or macrophage-/monocyte—and then subdivides each of these into morphologically determined subgroups.

B-CELL LYMPHOMAS. B-cell lymphomas are further subdivided according to the cell type into lymphocytic and follicle centre cell varieties.

Lymphocytic lymphomas. These lymphomas have tumour cells closely resembling small lymphocytes and may be categorized according to the degree of maturity—lymphocytic or prolymphocytic, and the degree of differentiation towards the plasma cell series—lymphoplasmacytoid, lymphoplasmacytic and plasmacytic. Splenomegaly is characteristic of the prolymphocytic variety, and dysproteinaemias (including Waldenström's macroglobulinaemia) are found in association with those lymphomas showing plasmacytoid differntiation.

Follicle centre cell lymphomas. These lymphomas have tumour cells derived from cells in the follicle centre of lymph nodes. Centrocytic tumours have small tumour cells, slightly larger then lymphocytes, with an irregular contorted nuclear structure and an inconspicuous nucleolus. They have been designated as poorly differentiated lymphocytic tumours in other classifications. Centroblastic tumours have large vesicular irregular nuclei with prominent nucleoli attached to the nuclear membrane. Immunoglobulin is demonstrable on the surface of the centrocytic tumour cells and within the cytoplasm of the centroblasts. This immunoglobulin is monomorphic and its specific characterization may further subcategorize these tumours. It is probable that lymphomas producing predominantly a heavy chain component of immunoglobulin are variants of follicle centre cell and of lymphoplasmacytoid lymphomas. Variants of centroblastic lymphoma include immunoblastic lymphoma, which is also known as immunoblastic sarcoma.

T-CELL LYMPHOMAS. T-cell lymphomas are further subdivided by their morphology and partly by their clinical manifestations, including their skin manifestations. Nodal T-cell lymphomas have an interfollicular infiltrate of tumour cells with many epithelioid macrophages, plasma cells and high endothelial-lined venules. According to the type of tumour cell they may then be subclassified into pleomorphic or monomorphic, and the monomorphic variety into blast and nonblast forms. Those with a high content of epithelioid cells are sometimes referred to as Lennert's lymphoma. T-cell lymphomas also include MYCOSIS FUNGOIDES and SÉZARY'S SYNDROME.

T-Cell Lymphomas with Hypercalcaemia. This group of T-cell lymphomas is characteristically associated with hypercalcaemia and shows a striking geographical distribution. It is common in Japan and the West Indies. An association with an HTLV retrovirus has been described.

T-Lymphocytic Lymphoma. This is a rare tumour forming a small proportion (2 per cent) of all cases of chronic lymphocytic leukaemia. It is characterized by splenomegaly, severe neutropenia and skin involvement. Lymph node enlargement is rare. The tumour cells are more pleomorphic than their B-cell counterparts and have lysosomal enzymes (ß-glucuronidase and acid phosphatase) in the cytoplasm. In the spleen they show a periarteriolar distribution.

HISTIOCYTIC LYMPHOMA. This is a malignant lymphoma derived from the cells of the monocyte/macrophage series. It is difficult to define by morphological criteria alone but the presence of granules of alpha-1-antitrypsin in the cytoplasm is one of the more reliable immunological markers. These tumours may present as nodal lymphomas closely resembling some other nonHodgkin's lymphomas or as a diffuse leukaemic infiltrate of various solid organs (malignant histiocytosis). One specialized form (malignant histiocystosis of the intestine) arises in the small intestine as a complication of long-standing coeliac disease. This form may present with intestinal perforation. Histiocytic lymphomas may be difficult to separate from centroblastic follicle centre cell lymphomas on the one hand and secondary carcinoma on the other.

EXTRANODAL LYMPHOMAS. These are lymphomas that arise in primary sites other than lymph nodes, spleen or thymus. Such sites include the gastrointestinal tract, testis, thyroid and central nervous system. They may remain confined to the primary site for some considerable periods of time. Their classification is similar to that of nodal lymphomas but spread of nodal lymphomas to extranodal sites should be excluded. It may be difficult to distinguish these primary extranodal lymphomas from chronic inflammatory or reactive conditions. Such difficulty has resulted in confusion and employment of the term *pseudolymphoma.*

African l. Burkitt's lymphoma.

Burkitt's l. a lymphoma first described by Burkitt in 1959 that occurs predominantly in young children in parts of Africa, especially East Africa. Presentation with jaw tumours is characteristic but retroperitoneal masses and kidney involvement is common. The tumour is composed of sheets of monomorphic blast cells. There is no immunoglobulin synthesis so that the cells may be of B-lymphoblast lineage but an origin from follicular centre cells has also been proposed. In many cases, especially in Africa, Epstein-Barr virus DNA is present in the genome of the tumour cell.

Mediterranean l. a gastrointestinal lymphoma occurring in the Middle East and characterized by a diffuse plasmacytic infiltrate in affected parts of the small intestine. Clinically there is malabsorption. An abnormal alpha heavy chain is produced by the tumour cells in some cases. It is possible to regard this lymphoma as a variant of follicle centre cell lymphoma with plasmacytic differentiation. Also called *alpha chain disease* and *immunoproliferative small intestinal disease (IPSID)*.

lymphomatosis (,limfohmə'tohsis) the formation of multiple lymphomas in the body.

lymphomatous (lim'fohmətəs) pertaining to, or of the nature of, lymphoma.

lymphopathia (,limfoh'pathi·ə) lymphopathy.

l. venereum lymphogranuloma venereum.

lymphopathy (lim'fopəthee) any disease of the lymphatic system.

lymphopenia (,limfoh'peeni·ə) decrease in the number of lymphocytes of the blood.

lymphopoiesis (,limfohpoy'eesis) the development of lymphocytes or of lymphoid tissue. adj. **lymphopoietic**.

lymphoproliferative (,limfohprə'lifə·rətiv) pertaining to or characterized by proliferation of lymphoid tissue.

l. syndrome a general term applied to a group of diseases characterized by proliferation of lymphoid tissue, such as lymphocytic leukaemia and malignant lymphoma.

lymphoreticular (,limfohre'tikyuhlə) pertaining to the reticuloendothelial cells of lymph nodes.

lymphoreticulosis (,limfohre'tikyuh'lohsis) proliferation of the reticuloendothelial cells of the lymph nodes.

benign l. cat-scratch disease.

lymphorrhagia, lymphorrhoea (,limfə'rayji·ə; ,limfə'reeə) flow of lymph from cut or ruptured lymphatic vessels.

lymphorrhoid ('limfə,royd) a localized dilation of a perianal lymph channel, resembling a haemorrhoid.

lymphosarcoma (,limfohsah'kohmə) a general term applied to malignant neoplastic disorders of lymphoid tissue, but not including Hodgkin's disease.

lymphosarcomatosis (,limfoh,sahkohmə'tohsis) a condition characterized by the presence of multiple lesions of lymphosarcoma.

lymphostasis (lim'fostəsis) stoppage of lymph flow.

lymphotaxis (,limfoh'taksis) the property of attracting or repulsing lymphocytes.

lymphotomy (lim'fotəmee) the anatomy of the lymphatic system.

lymphotoxin (,limfoh'toksin) a chemical mediator released by sensitized lymphocytes and involved in target-cell injury and inhibition of cell division.

lynoestrenol (li'neestrə,nol) a synthetic drug similar in action to progesterone, used chiefly in oral contraceptives.

Lyon hypothesis ('lieən) the random and fixed inactivation (in the form of sex chromatin) of all X chromosomes in excess of one in mammalian cells at an early stage of embryogenesis, leading to mosaicism for X-linked genes in the female, since the paternal X chromosome is inactivated in some cells and the maternal one in the remainder.

lyonization (,lieənie'zayshən) the process by which or the condition in which all X chromosomes of the cells in excess of one are inactivated on a random basis.

lyophil ('lieoh,fil) a lyophilic substance.

lyophile ('lieoh,fiel) 1. lyophil. 2. lyophilic.

lyophilic (,lieoh'filik) having an affinity for, or stable in, solution.

lyophilization (lie,ofilie'zayshən) the creation of a stable preparation of a biological substance by rapid freezing and dehydration of the frozen product under high vacuum.

lyophobe ('lieoh,fohb) a lyophobic substance.

lyophobic (,lieoh'fohbik) not having an affinity for, or unstable in, solution.

lyotropic (,lieoh'tropik) readily soluble.

lypressin (lie'presin) a synthetic preparation of lysine vasopressin used as an antidiuretic and vasoconstrictor in the treatment of diabetes insipidus due to deficiency of endogenous posterior pituitary antidiuretic hormone (vasopressin).

lyse (liez) 1. to cause or produce disintegration of a compound, substance, or cell. 2. to undergo lysis.

lysergic acid diethylamide (lie'sərjik 'asid die,ethil'amied) a hallucinogenic drug better known as LSD.

lysergide (lie'sərjied) LSD.

lysin ('liesin) an ANTIBODY capable of causing dissolution of cells, including haemolysin, bacteriolysin, etc.

lysine ('lieseen) a naturally occurring amino acid, essential for optimal growth in human infants and for maintenance of nitrogen equilibrium in adults.

lysinogen (lie'sinəjen) lysogen.

lysis ('liesis) 1. destruction or decomposition, as of a cell or other substance, under the influence of a specific agent. 2. mobilization of an organ by division of restraining adhesions. 3. gradual abatement of the symptoms of a disease.

-lysis word element. [Gr.] *dissolution*. adj. **-lytic**.

lysogen ('liesəjen) an antigen causing the formation of lysin; called also *lysinogen*.

lysogenesis (,liesoh'jenəsis) 1. the production of lysis or lysins. 2. lysogenicity.

lysogenicity, lysogeny (,liesəjə'nisətee; lie'sojənee) 1. the ability to produce lysins or cause lysis. 2. the potentiality of a bacterium to produce bacteriophage. 3. the specific association of the phage genome (prophage) of a temperate phage and the bacterial host cell. The phage particles may be liberated from the bacterial cell, which is lysed.

lysokinase (,liesoh'kienayz) a general term for substances of the fibrinolytic system that activate plasma proactivators.

Lysol ('liesol) trademark for a solution containing phenol derivatives; used as a disinfectant and antiseptic.

lysosome ('liesə,sohm) one of the minute membrane-bound vacuoles occurring in many types of cells, containing various hydrolytic enzymes and normally involved in the process of localized intracellular digestion. adj. **lysosomal**.

lysotype ('liesə,tiep) phage type.

lysozyme ('liesə,ziem) a crystalline, basic protein present in saliva, tears, egg white, and many animal fluids, which functions as an antibacterial enzyme.

lysozymuria (,liesohzie'myooə·ri·ə) urinary excretion of elevated levels of lysozyme.

lyssa ('lisə) rabies. adj. **lyssic**.

lyssoid ('lisoyd) resembling rabies.

lyssophobia (,lisoh'fohbi·ə) morbid fear of rabies.

lytic ('litik) pertaining to lysis or a lysin.

l. cycle the synthesis of bacteriophages in a bacterial cell and their subsequent release with lysis of the bacterial cell; occurs with both temperate and virulent bacteriophages.

lyze (liez) lyse.

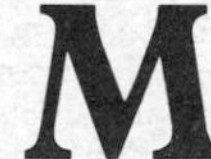

M

M [L.] *mil* or *mille;* (thousand); symbol, *mega;* symbol, *molar* (solution)—the expressions M/10, M/100, etc., denote the strength of a solution in comparison with the molar, as tenth molar, hundredth molar, etc.; minim.

M-R measles-rubella (vaccine).
m symbol, *metre;* symbol, *milli-*.
m- symbol, *meta-*.
μ symbol, *micro-*; sometimes incorrectly used as symbol, *micron*.
MA Master of Arts.
mA milliampere.
Maalox ('mayloks) trademark for preparations of magnesium hydroxide and aluminium hydroxide, an antacid.
McArdle's disease (mə'kahd'lz) glycogenosis (type V) in which a deficiency of muscle phosphorylase results in accumulation of glycogen in skeletal muscles, with muscle cramps and a depressed blood lactate level during exercise. Called also *myophosphorylase deficiency glycogenosis*.
McBurney's point (mək'bərniz) the point of special tenderness in acute appendicitis; situated about 2 inches from the right anterior superior spine of the ilium, on a line between this spine and the umbilicus. It corresponds with the normal position of the appendix.
McBurney's sign special tenderness at McBurney's point; indicative of appendicitis.
McMurray's sign (mək'muriz) occurrence of a cartilage click during manipulation of the knee; indicative of menisceal injury.
McMurray's test as the patient lies supine with one knee fully flexed, the examiner rotates the patient's foot fully outward and the knee is slowly extended; a painful 'click' indicates a tear of the medial meniscus of the knee joint; if the click occurs when the foot is rotated inward, the tear is in the lateral meniscus.
McNaghten's Rules on Insanity at Law (mək'nawtənz) the rules which define the factors on which a defence to a charge of murder on grounds of insanity may be established. These were evolved after Sir Robert Peel's Secretary was killed by McNaghten in 1843. He was suffering from delusions and the judge ordered that he be found not guilty. The Homicide Act 1957 provided for a defence based on 'diminished responsibility', i.e. the accused was suffering from such abnormality of mind as to impair his mental responsibility for his actions. See also DURHAM RULE.
macerate ('masə,rayt) to soften by wetting or soaking.
maceration (,masə'rayshən) the softening of a solid by soaking. In histology, the softening of a tissue by soaking, especially in acids, until the connective tissue fibres are dissolved so that the tissue components can be teased apart. In obstetrics, the degenerative changes with discoloration and softening of tissues, and eventual disintegration, of a fetus retained in the uterus after its death. It indicates that a stillbirth has been dead in utero before the commencement of labour, and may lead to hypofibrinogenaemia.
macies ('maysi·eez) [L.] *wasting*.
Mackenrodt's ligaments ('maken,rohts) the transverse or cardinal ligaments that support the uterus in the pelvic cavity.
macr(o)- word element. [Gr.] *large, long*.
macrencephalia (,makrenkə'fayli·ə, -sə'fay-) hypertrophy of the brain.
macroamylasaemia (,makroh,amilay'seemi·ə) the presence of macroamylase in the blood. adj. **macroamylasaemic**.
macroamylase (,makroh'ami,layz) a complex in which normal serum amylase is bound to a variety of specific binding proteins, forming a complex too large for renal excretion. It is not correlated with any specific disease state; however, in hyperamylasaemia or pancreatitis, it can result in urinary amylase levels not rising concomitantly with serum levels.
macroblast ('makroh,blast) an abnormally large, nucleated erythrocyte; a large young normoblast with megaloblastic features.
macroblepharia (,makrohble'fair·ri·ə) abnormal largeness of the eyelid.
macrocardius (,makroh'kahdi·əs) a fetus with an extremely large heart.
macrocephalous (,makroh'kefələs, -'sef-) having an abnormally large head.
macrocephaly (,makroh'kefəlee, -'sef-) abnormal enlargement of the cranium.
macrocheilia (,makroh'kieli·ə) excessive size of the lip.
macrocheiria (,makroh'kieri·ə) excessive size of the hands.
macrocolon (,makroh'kohlon) megacolon.
macrocrania (,makroh'krayni·ə) abnormal increase in size of the skull in relation to the face.
macrocyte ('makroh,siet) an abnormally large erythrocyte. adj. **macrocytic**.
macrocythaemia, macrocytosis (,makrohsie'theemi·ə; ,makrohsie'tohsis) the presence of macrocytes in the blood.
macrodactyly (,makroh'daktilee) abnormal largeness of the fingers or toes.
Macrodantin (,makroh'dantin) trademark for a preparation of nitrofurantoin; an antibacterial agent.
macrodontia (,makroh'donshi·ə) abnormal increase in size of one or more teeth. adj. **macrodont, macrodontic**.
macroelement (,makroh'elimənt) a chemical element that has a minimal daily requirement greater than 100 mg; calcium, phosphorus, magnesium, potassium, sodium, and chloride are macroelements.
macrogamete (,makroh'gameet) the larger, less active female gamete in anisogamy, which is fertilized by the smaller male gamete (microgamete).
macrogametocyte (,makrohgə'meetoh,siet) 1. a cell that produces macrogametes. 2. the female gametocyte of certain Sporozoa, such as malarial plasmodia, which matures into a macrogamete.
macrogenitosomia (,makroh,jenitoh'sohmi·ə) excessive bodily development, with unusual enlargement of the genital organs.
m. praecox macrogenitosomia occurring at an early age.
macroglia (mə'krogli·ə) large neuroglial cells, including the astrocytes and oligodendrocytes.
macroglobulin (,makroh'globyuhlin) a protein (globulin) of unusually high molecular weight, in the range of 1,000,000; observed in the blood in a number of diseases.
macroglobulinaemia (,makroh,globyuhli'neemi·ə) increased levels of macroglobulins (IgM) in the blood.
macroglossia (,makroh'glosi·ə) excessive size of the tongue.
macrognathia (,makroh'nathi·ə) abnormal overgrowth of the jaw. adj. **macrognathic**.
macrogyria (,makroh'jieri·ə) moderate reduction in the number of sulci of the cerebrum, sometimes with increase in the brain substance, resulting in excessive size of the gyri.
macrolide ('makroh,lied) any antibiotic with molecules having many-membered lactone rings.
macromastia (,makroh'masti·ə) excessive size of the breasts.
macromelia (,makroh'meeli·ə) enlargement of one or more limbs.
macromelus (mə'kroməlas) a fetus with abnormally large or long limbs.
macromere ('makroh,miə) one of the larger cells (blastomeres) formed in unequal cleavage of the fertilized ovum (at the vegetal pole).

macromolecule (ˌmakroh'moliˌkyool) a very large molecule having a polymeric chain structure, as in proteins, polysaccharides, etc. adj. **macromolecular**.

macromyeloblast (ˌmakroh'mieəlohˌblast) a large myeloblast.

macronormoblast (ˌmakroh'nawmohˌblast) a very large nucleated erythrocyte; macroblast.

macronutrient (ˌmakroh'nyootri·ənt) an essential nutrient that has a large minimal daily requirement (greater than 100 mg); calcium, phosphorus, magnesium, potassium, sodium, and chloride are macronutrients.

macronychia (ˌmakroh'niki·ə) abnormally enlarged nails.

macrophage ('makrohˌfayj) any of the large, mononuclear, highly phagocytic cells derived from monocytes that occur in the walls of blood vessels (adventitial cells) and in loose connective tissue (histiocytes, phagocytic reticular cells). They are components of the reticuloendothelial system. Macrophages are usually immobile but become actively mobile when stimulated by inflammation; they also interact with lymphocytes to facilitate antibody production. See also IMMUNITY.

m. activating factor (MAF) a lymphokine that induces in macrophages an increased content of lysosomal enzymes, more aggressive phagocytosis, and increased mitotic activity.

alveolar m's rounded, granular, mononuclear phagocytes within the alveoli of the lungs that ingest inhaled particulate matter.

armed m's those capable of inducing cytotoxicity as a consequence of antigen-binding by cytophilic antibodies on their surfaces or by factors derived from T-lymphocytes.

m. chemotactic factor (MCF) a lymphokine that attracts macrophages to the invasion site.

m. migration inhibiting factor (MIF) a lymphokine that inhibits migration of macrophages, causing them to accumulate at the site of antigen.

macrophthalmia (ˌmakrof'thalmi·ə) abnormal enlargement of the eyeball.

macropodia (ˌmakroh'pohdi·ə) excessive size of the feet.

macropolycyte (ˌmakroh'poliˌsiet) a hypersegmented polymorphonuclear leukocyte of greater than normal size.

macroprosopia (ˌmakrohproh'sohpi·ə) excessive size of the face.

macropsia (mə'kropsi·ə) a disorder of visual perception in which objects appear larger than their actual size.

macroradiography (ˌmakrohraydi'ogrəfee) the technique of producing a magnified radiographic image in diagnostic radiology to improve spatial resolution.

macrorrhinia (ˌmakroh'rieni·ə) excessive size of the nose.

macroscopic (ˌmakroh'skopik) of large size; visible to the unaided eye.

macroscopy (mə'kroskəpee) examination with the unaided eye.

macrosigmoid (ˌmakroh'sigmoyd) excessive size of the sigmoid colon.

macrosomatia, macrosomia (ˌmakrohsə'mayshi·ə, ˌmakrə'sohmi·ə) great bodily size.

macrostomia (ˌmakroh'stohmi·ə) excessive width of the mouth.

macrotia (mə'krohshi·ə) abnormal enlargement of the pinna of the ear.

macula ('makyuhlə) pl. *maculae* [L.] 1. a stain, spot, or thickening; in anatomy, an area distinguishable by colour or otherwise from its surroundings. Often used alone to refer to the macula retinae. 2. a macule: a discoloured spot on the skin that is not raised above the surface. 3. a corneal scar that can be seen without special optical aids; presenting as a grey spot intermediate between a nebula and a leukoma. 4. macula lutea. adj. **macular, maculate**.

maculae acusticae terminations of the vestibulocochlear nerve in the utricle and saccule.

m. atrophica a white atrophic patch on the skin.

m. cerulea a blue patch on the skin seen in pediculosis.

m. corneae a circumscribed opacity of the cornea.

m. cribrosa a perforated spot or area; one of three perforated areas (inferior, medial, and superior) in the wall of the vestibule of the ear through which branches of the vestibulocochlear nerve pass to the saccule, utricle, and semicircular canals.

m. densa a zone of heavily nucleated cells in the distal renal tubule.

m. flava a yellow nodule at one end of a vocal cord.

m. folliculi the point on the surface of a vesicular ovarian follicle where rupture occurs; follicular stigma.

m. germinativa germinal area; the part of the ovum where the embryo is formed.

m. lutea, m. retinae an irregular yellowish depression on the retina, lateral to and slightly below the optic disc.

m. sacculi a thickening on the wall of the saccule where the epithelium contains hair cells that receive and transmit vestibular impulses.

m. solaris a freckle.

m. utriculi a thickening in the wall of the utricle where the epithelium contains hair cells that are stimulated by linear acceleration and deceleration and by gravity.

maculate ('makyuhlayt) spotted or blotched.

macule ('makyool) a macula.

maculocerebral (ˌmakyuhloh'seribrəl) pertaining to the macula lutea and the brain.

maculopapular (ˌmakyuhloh'papyuhlə) both macular and papular.

madarosis (ˌmadə'rohsis) loss of eyelashes or eyebrows.

Maddox rod test ('madəks) a test for muscle balance of the eyes using a lens comprised of red glass cylinders.

Maddox wing test a method of measuring the amount of heterophoria.

Madelung's deformity ('madəluhngz) radical deviation of the hand secondary to overgrowth of the distal ulna or shortening of the radius.

Madelung's disease 1. Madelung's deformity. 2. Madelungs's neck.

Madelung's neck diffuse symmetrical lipomas of the neck.

Madopar ('madohpah) trademark for fixed combination preparations of levodopa and benserazide used in parkinsonism.

Madura foot (mə'dyooə·rə) maduromycosis of the foot.

Madurella (ˌmadyuh'relə) a genus of fungi causing mycetoma.

maduromycosis (məˌdyooə·rohmie'kohsis) a chronic disease due to various fungi or actinomycetes, affecting various body tissues, including the hands, legs and feet; called also *mycetoma*. The most common form affects the foot (Madura foot) and is characterized by sinus formation, necrosis, and swelling.

mafenide ('mafənied) a compound used in the topical treatment of superficial infections.

MAFF Ministry of Agriculture, Fisheries and Food.

Magendie's foramen (ˌmazhon'deez) aperture in the roof of the fourth ventricle of the brain through which cerebrospinal fluid passes into the subarachnoid space.

magenta (mə'jentə) fuchsin or other salt of rosaniline.

maggot ('magət) the soft-bodied larva of an insect, especially one living in decaying flesh.

magma ('magmə) 1. a suspension of finely divided material in a small amount of water. 2. a thin, paste-like substance composed of organic material.

Magnapen ('magnəpen) trademark for a fixed combination preparation of ampicillin and flucloxacillin, an antibiotic.

magnesia (mag'neeshi·ə) magnesium oxide; an aperient and antacid.

magnesium (mag'neezi·əm) a chemical element, atomic number 12, atomic weight 24.312, symbol Mg. (See table of elements in Appendix 2.) Its salts are essential in nutrition, being required for the activity of many enzymes, especially those concerned with oxidative phosphorylation. It is found in the intra- and extracellular fluids and is excreted in urine and faeces. The normal serum level is approximately 1 mmol/l. Magnesium deficiency causes irritability of the nervous system with tetany, vasodilation, convulsions, tremors, depression, and psychotic behaviour.

m. carbonate an odourless, stable compound used as an antacid.

m. citrate a mild cathartic.

m. gluconate a magnesium replenisher.

m. hydroxide a bulky white powder used as an antacid and cathartic.

m. oxide a white powder used as an antacid.

m. phosphate a white, odourless, tasteless powder used as an antacid.

m. salicylate the magnesium salt of salicylic acid used as an antiarthritic.

m. sulphate Epsom salt; used as an electrolyte replenisher, cathartic, and local anti-inflammatory.

m. trisilicate a combination of magnesium oxide and silicon dioxide with varying proportions of water; used as a gastric antacid.

magnet ('magnit) an object having polarity and capable of attracting iron.

magnetic resonance imaging (mag'netik) an imaging technique based on the NUCLEAR MAGNETIC RESONANCE properties of the hydrogen nucleus. Abbreviated MRI. Cross-sectional images in any plane may be obtained and the images may represent one or more of several properties—hydrogen distribution in the body (proton density), or time constants of the return to equilibrium following disturbance by the radiofrequency pulse. MRI is without hazard to the patient.

magnetism ('magnə,tizəm) magnetic attraction or repulsion.

magnetropism (,magnə'trohpizəm, mag'netrə,pizəm) a growth response in a nonmotile organism under the influence of a magnet.

magnification (,magnifi'kayshən) 1. apparent increase in size, as under the microscope. 2. the process of making something appear larger, as by use of lenses. 3. the ratio of apparent (image) size to real size.

main (manh) [Fr.] *hand.*

m. en griffe clawhand.

Majocchi's disease (ma'yokeez) annular telangiectatic purpura.

Majocchi's granuloma a form of tinea corporis, occurring chiefly on the lower legs due to *Trichophyton* infecting the hairs at the site of involvement, marked by raised, circumscribed, rather boggy granulomas, disseminated or arranged in chains; the lesions are slowly absorbed, or undergo necrosis, leaving depressed scars. Called also *trichophytic granuloma.*

mal (mal) [Fr.] *illness, disease.*

grand m. a generalized convulsive seizure attended by loss of consciousness (see also EPILEPSY).

m. de Meleda symmetrical keratosis of the palms and soles associated with an ichthyotic thickening of the wrists and ankles.

m. de mer seasickness.

petit m. momentary loss of consciousness without convulsive movements (see also EPILEPSY).

mala ('maylə) the cheek or cheek bone. adj. **malar.**

malabsorption (,maləb'sawpshən, -'zaw-) impaired intestinal absorption of nutrients.

m. syndrome a group of disorders marked by subnormal intestinal absorption of dietary constituents, and thus excessive loss of nutrients in the stool; it may be due to a digestive defect, a mucosal abnormality, or lymphatic obstruction.

malacia (mə'layshi·ə) 1. morbid softening or softness of a part or tissue; also used as a word termination, as in osteomalacia. 2. morbid craving for highly spiced foods.

malacoma (,malə'kohmə) a morbidly soft part or spot.

malacoplakia (,maləkoh'playki·ə) a circumscribed area of softening on the membrane lining a hollow organ, as the ureter, urethra, or renal pelvis.

m. vesicae a soft, yellow, fungus-like growth on the mucosa of the bladder and ureters.

malacosis (,malə'kohsis) malacia.

malacosteon (,malə'kosti·ən) softening of the bones; osteomalacia.

malacotic (,malə'kotik) soft.

maladjustment (,malə'justmənt) in psychiatry, defective adaptation to the environment, marked by anxiety.

malady ('malədee) a disease or illness.

malaise (ma'layz) [Fr.] a feeling of uneasiness or indisposition.

malalignment (,malə'lienmənt) displacement, especially of the teeth from their normal relation to the line of the dental arch.

malaria (mə'lair·ri·ə) a serious,notifiable, infectious illness characterized by periodic chills, fever, sweating and splenomegaly. Serious and often fatal complications may arise in falciparum malaria. adj. **malarial.**

It is endemic in parts of Africa, Asia, and Central and South America, and is estimated to occur at the rate of 100 million cases each year throughout the world. Some 2,000 imported cases per year are reported in the UK, with up to 10 deaths. Epidemics usually occur in areas where mosquitoes persist in large numbers and the parasite is introduced into a region that is populated with persons who are not immune to malaria. Acute cases of malaria occur when nonimmune persons travel to regions where the disease is endemic.

A worldwide cooperative eradication programme has met with limited success. Some difficulties encountered have been resistance of mosquitoes to insecticides, insufficient funding in some developing countries, and resistance of plasmodia to antimalarial drugs. In view of these difficulties recent efforts have been toward malaria control rather than eradication.

CAUSE. Malaria is caused by a protozoan parasite, *Plasmodium*, which is passed on by infected *Anopheles* mosquitoes. When the mosquito bites an infected person, it sucks in the parasites, which reside in the blood. In the mosquito the plasmodia multiply and travel to the salivary glands from which they are transmitted to the human bloodstream by the mosquito bite. Inside the human host they develop in the liver, later emerging into the blood and penetrating the erythrocytes, where they mature, reproduce and at complete maturity burst out of the blood cells. The cycle varies according to the species of *Plasmodium*. For *P. vivax* it lasts 48 hours, *P. malariae* 72 hours, and *P. falciparum* 36 to 48 hours.

SYMPTOMS. There may be no symptoms until several

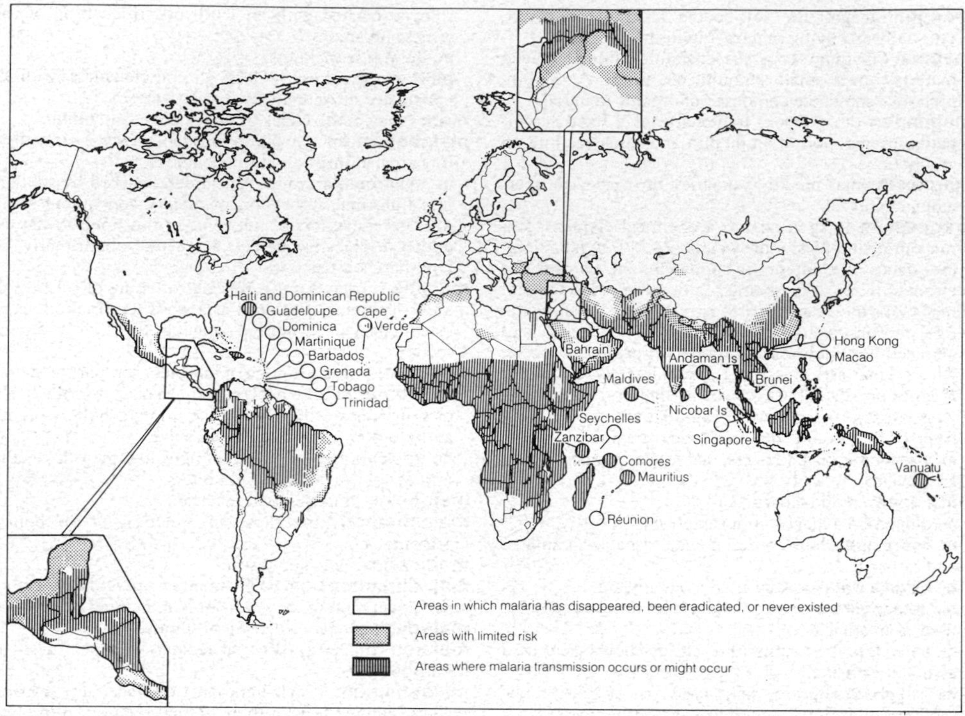

cycles have been completed. Then there is a simultaneous rupturing of erythrocytes by the entire brood, causing the characteristic chills followed in a few hours by fever. The temperature may rise to 40 to 40.5 °C (104 to 105 °F). As it subsides, there is profuse sweating. Other symptoms are headache, nausea, body pains and, after the attack, exhaustion. The symptoms last from 4 to 6 hours and recur at regular intervals, depending upon the parasitic species and its cycle. If the attack occurs every other day, the disease is called tertian malaria (*P. vivax*); if it occurs at 3 day intervals, it is quartan malari (*P. malariae*). In *P. falciparm* malaria peaks of fever tend to be less regular, particuarly at first. In *P. vivax* and *P. malariae* infections, the attacks occur less frequently as the disease progresses. Bouts of malaria last from 1 to 4 weeks but usually about 2 weeks. Relapses are common, with attacks ceasing and recurring at irregular intervals for several years, especially if untreated. Malaria due to these species is not usually fatal.

In *P. falciparum* malaria severe anaemia is common and splenomegaly rapidly develops. Complications such as cerebral malaria, hyperpyrexia, gastointesinal, hepatic and renal damage, and blackwater fever may all cause a fatal outcome. Speedy appropriate treatment is therefore vital in this form of the disease.

Treatment. For many years, quinine was the standard treatment for malaria. The intensive research carried on since World War II has provided synthetic medicines such as chloroquine and amodiaquine that can either relieve the attack promptly or cure the infection. Quinine is still important in the treatment of infections with drug-resistant plasmodia, and may be life-saving in grave cases.

Prevention. There is no effective inoculation against malaria, but antimalarial drugs, e.g. chloroquine, proguanil, should be given prophylactically to persons travelling to areas where the disease is widespread. Preventive measures are concentrated on destroying the mosquito. This is done by filling in pools, swamps, and places containing stagnant water where mosquitoes breed, and by intensive use of DDT and other insecticides. Personal protection against anopheline bites is also important.

airport m. a term sometimes used to describe malaria occuring at or near an airport, in a country normally free of the disease, and spread by infected mosquitoes brought in on an aeroplane from an endemic area. Control measures include disinsectization of aircraft where appropriate.

malariacidal (mə,lair·ri·ə'sied'l) destructive to malarial plasmodia.

malariotherapy (mə,lair·rioh'therəpee) form of cure in which a hyperpyrexia is induced by infecting a patient with malaria. Once used in the treatment of neurosyphilis.

Malassezia (,malə'seezi·ə) *Pityrosporon*.

M. furfur *Pityrosporon orbiculare*.

malassimilation (,malə'simi'layshən) 1. imperfect, faulty, or disordered assimilation. 2. the inability of the gastrointestinal tract to take up one or more ingested nutrients, whether due to faulty digestion (maldigestion) or to impaired intestinal mucosal transport (malabsorption).

malate ('malayt) a salt of malic acid.

malaxate ('malak,sayt) to knead, as in making pills.

malaxation (,malak'sayshən) an act of kneading.

maldevelopment (,maldi'veləpmənt) abnormal growth or development.

male (mayl) an individual of the sex that produces spermatozoa.

maleruption (ˌmali'rupshən) eruption of a tooth out of its normal position.

malformation (ˌmalfaw'mayshən) defective or abnormal formation; deformity; an anatomical aberration, especially one acquired during development.

malic acid (ˌmakik) a compound that is found in the juices of many fruits and plants, and is an intermediate in the tricarboxylic acid cycle.

malignancy (mə'lignənsee) a tendency to progress in virulence. In popular usage, any condition that, if uncorrected, tends to worsen so as to cause serious illness or death. Cancer is the best known example.

malignant (mə'lignənt) tending to become progressively worse and to result in death; having the properties of anaplasia, invasiveness, and metastasis; said of tumours.

malignin (mə'lignin) a protein fragment present in the serum of patients with malignant glial tumours.

malingerer (mə'ling·gə·rə) one who is guilty of malingering.

malingering (mə'ling·gə·ring) wilful, deliberate, and fraudulent feigning or exaggeration of the symptoms of illness or injury to attain a consciously desired end.

malleable ('mali·əb'l) susceptible to being beaten out into a thin plate.

malleoincudal (ˌmalioh'ingkyuhdəl) pertaining to the malleus and incus.

malleolus (mə'leeələs) pl. *malleoli* [L.] a rounded process, especially either of the two rounded prominences on either side of the ankle joint, at the lower end of the fibula (external, lateral, or outer malleolus) or of the tibia (inner, internal, or medial malleolus). adj. **malleolar**.

malleotomy (ˌmali'otəmee) 1. operative division of the malleus. 2. operative separation of the malleoli.

malleus ('mali·əs) the largest of the three ossicles of the ear; called also *hammer*.

malnutrition (ˌmalnyoo'trishən) poor nourishment resulting from improper diet or from some defect in metabolism that prevents the body from using its food properly. Extreme malnutrition may lead to starvation.

CAUSES. Although poverty is still the major cause of malnutrition, the condition is by no means confined to the underdeveloped parts of the world. Anyone can become undernourished if he seriously neglects his diet. A well balanced diet, the requirements of which vary slightly with a person's age, should include adequate amounts of protein, vitamins, minerals, and carbohydrates. For an explanation of the value of properly balanced diets, see NUTRITION.

Ignorance of the basic principles of nutrition is probably almost as great a cause of undernourishment as poverty. Misplaced faith in vitamin pills as a substitute for food, for example, can, if carried to extremes, cause undernourishment. So can over-reliance on excessively processed foods. Modern methods of processing and refining foods can sometimes cause a loss of valuable nutrients, as happens in the refining of certain grains, such as rice. However, this danger is recognized by both the government and the manufacturers who try to retain or restore the nutritional value of many foods. ALCOHOLISM, which frequently leads a person to rely on alcohol at the expense of food, is another cause of malnutrition.

People who want to gain or lose weight, or who, like vegetarians, avoid certain foods, may endanger their health by following an unbalanced diet that lacks essential nutrients. Anyone who plans to follow a special diet should talk the matter over with his doctor.

Malnutrition can also stem from disease. If the organs of the digestive system that transform food into bone, tissue, blood, and energy fail to function properly, the body will not receive adequate nourishment. Such deficiencies can cause diabetes mellitus, certain liver diseases, and some anaemias. The ENDOCRINE GLANDS and enzymes are also vital to the proper use of food by the body, and defects in their functioning may cause forms of malnutrition.

SYMPTOMS. In general, the symptoms of malnutrition are physical weakness, lassitude, and an increasing sense of detachment from the world. There are also specific symptoms that vary according to the essential substance lacking in the diet. For example, lack of vitamin A can result in NIGHT BLINDNESS, or poor vision in dim light. In the absence of adequate exposure to sunlight, a lack of vitamin D can cause RICKETS, which results in malformed limbs in infants and children because the bones fail to harden properly. A lack of vitamin C causes SCURVY, with symptoms of bleeding gums and easily bruised skin. Other vitamin deficiency diseases are BERIBERI and PELLAGRA. If there is not enough iron in the diet, iron deficiency ANAEMIA develops. Malnutrition can also result from allergic reactions to foods, as in COELIAC DISEASE.

In starvation there are signs of multiple vitamin deficiency. There may be oedema, abdominal distention, and excessive loss of weight. As starvation progresses, fat cells become small and accumulations of fat are depleted. The liver is reduced in size, the muscles shrivel, and the lymphoid tissue, gonads, and blood deteriorate.

Because the stomach and the intestinal tract may no longer be capable of digesting food of any bulk, treatment of starvation should begin by feeding the patient easily digested liquids, such as soups, in small quantities. If he is unable to eat or drink, the necessary nutrients can be supplied by intravenous infusion.

malocclusion (ˌmalə'kloozhən) malposition of the teeth resulting in the faulty meeting of the teeth or jaws. The condition should be corrected because it predisposes to dental caries, may lead to digestive disorders and inadequate nutrition because of difficulty in chewing, and can cause serious psychological effects if there is facial distortion. Corrective treatment is provided by an orthodontist, who may apply appropriate dental braces to improve the position of the teeth.

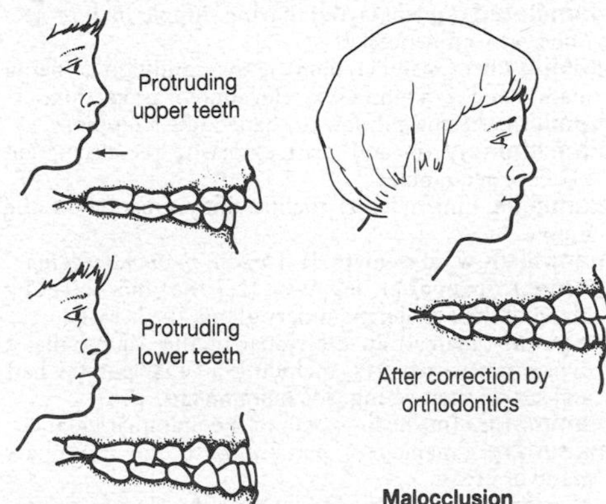

Malocclusion

Maloprim ('malohprim) trademark for a fixed combination preparation of pyrimethamine and dapsone, an antimalarial.

malpighian corpuscle (mal'pigi·ən) the funnel-like structure constituting the beginning of the structural unit of the kidney (nephron) and comprising the

Bowman's capsule and its partially enclosed glomerulus. Called also *renal corpuscle*.

malpighian layer the basal layer and the prickle-cell layer of the skin considered together.

malposition (ˌmalpəˈzishən) abnormal placement.

malpractice (malˈpraktis) any professional misconduct, unreasonable lack of skill or fidelity in professional duties, or illegal or immoral conduct. Malpractice is one form of negligence, which in legal terms can be defined as the omission to do something that a reasonable man, guided by those ordinary considerations which ordinarily regulate human affairs, would do, or the doing of something that a reasonable and prudent man would not do. In medical and nursing practice, malpractice means bad, wrong, or injudicious treatment of a patient professionally; it results in injury, unnecessary suffering, or death to the patient. The court may hold that malpractice has occurred even though the physician or nurse acted in good faith. Also, malpractice and negligence may occur through omission to act as well as commission of an unwise or negligent act.

malpresentation (ˌmalprezənˈtayshən) faulty fetal presentation, i.e. not a well flexed vertex presentation.

malrotation (ˌmalrohˈtayshən) abnormal or pathological rotation, as of the vertebral column; failure of normal rotation of an organ, as of the gut, during embryological development.

malt (mawlt) grain which has been soaked, made to germinate, and dried. It is used as a nutrient in wasting diseases.

m. sugar maltose.

Malta fever (ˈmawltə) brucellosis.

maltase (ˈmawltayz) a sugar-splitting enzyme which converts maltose to glucose. Present in pancreatic and intestinal juice.

maltose (ˈmawltohz, -tohs) a sugar (disaccharide) formed when starch is hydrolysed by amylase.

malum (ˈmaləm) [L.] *a disease*.

m. articulorum senilis a painful degenerative state of a joint as a result of ageing.

m. coxae senilis osteoarthritis of the hip joint.

m. perforans pedis perforating ulcer of the foot.

malunion (malˈyooni·ən) faulty union of the fragments of a fractured bone.

mamilla (məˈmilə) pl. *mamillae* [L.] 1. the nipple of the breast. 2. any nipple-like prominence. adj. **mamillary**.

mamillated (ˈmamiˌlaytid) having nipple-like projections or prominences.

mamillation (ˌmamiˈlayshən) 1. the condition of being mamillated. 2. a nipple-like elevation or projection.

mamilliform (məˈmiliˌfawm) shaped like a nipple.

mamilliplasty (məˈmiliˌplastee) plastic reconstruction of depressed nipples.

mamillitis (ˌmamiˈlietis) thelitis; inflammation of the nipple.

mamm(o)- word element. [L.] *breast, mammary gland*.

mamma (ˈmamə) pl. *mammae* [L.] the milk-secreting gland of the female; mammary gland; the breast.

mammal (ˈmaməl) an individual of the Mammalia, a division of vertebrates, including all that possess hair and suckle their young. adj. **mammalian**.

mammalgia (məˈmalji·ə) pain in the mammary gland.

mammary (ˈmamə·ree) pertaining to the mammary gland or breast.

m. gland the specialized gland of the skin of female mammals, which secretes milk for nourishment of the young, existing in a rudimentary state in the male (see also BREAST).

mammatrope (ˈmaməˌtrohp) mammotrope.

mammectomy (məˈmektəmee) mastectomy.

mammilla (məˈmilə) mamilla.

mammiplasia (ˌmamiˈplayzi·ə) mammoplasia.

mammitis (məˈmietis) mastitis.

mammogram (ˈmamohˌgram) a radiograph of the breast.

mammography (məˈmogrəfee) radiography of the breast with or without injection of an opaque substance into its ducts. Simple mammography, without the use of a contrast medium, is a routine screening procedure for the diagnosis of cancer and other disorders of the breast.

mammoplasia (ˌmamohˈplayzi·ə) development of breast tissue.

mammoplasty (ˈmamohˌplastee) plastic surgery of the breast.

augmentation m. an operation to increase the size of the breast.

reduction m. an operation to decrease the size of the breast.

mammose (ˈmamohz) 1. having unusually large breasts. 2. mamillated.

mammothermography (ˌmamohthərˈmogrəfee) an examination of the breast that depends on the more active cells producing heat that can be shown on a thermograph, and may indicate abnormalities of the breast tissue.

mammotomy (məˈmotəmee) mastotomy.

mammotrophe (ˈmamohˌtrohf) one of the acidophils of the adenohypophysis that secrete prolactin.

mammotrophin (ˌmamohˈtrohfin) prolactin.

mammotropic (ˌmamohˈtropik) having a stimulating effect on the mammary gland.

Manchester operation (ˈmanchestə) amputation of the cervix, with anterior and posterior colporrhaphy.

mandelic acid (manˈdelik) a keto acid used as a urinary antiseptic in nephritis, pyelitis, and cystitis. It must be excreted in the urinary tract unchanged in order to have a bacteriostatic effect and it is therefore not effective in anuria. A strongly acid urine should be maintained during its administration. To accomplish this, fluids may be limited and an acidifying agent given. Citrus fruits and other foods producing an alkaline ash must be restricted. The average dose of mandelic acid or preparations containing this substance depends on the type of preparation used.

mandible (ˈmandibˈl) the horseshoe-shaped bone forming the lower jaw. adj. **mandibular.** It consists of a central portion, which forms the chin and supports the lower teeth, and two perpendicular portions, or rami, which point upward from the back of the chin on either side and articulate with the temporal bones.

mandrin (ˈmandrin) a guide for a flexible catheter.

manganese (ˈmang·gəˌneez) a chemical element, atomic number 25, atomic weight 54.938, symbol Mn. (See table of elements in Appendix 2.) Its salts occur in the body tissue in very small amounts and serve as activators of liver arginase and other enzymes.

m. poisoning a condition usually caused by inhalation of manganese dust; symptoms include mental disorders accompanying a syndrome resembling paralysis agitans, and inflammation throughout the respiratory system.

mange (maynj) a skin disease of domestic animals, due to mites.

mania (ˈmayni·ə) a disordered mental state of extreme excitement; specifically, the manic type of manic-depressive psychosis. Also used as a word termination to denote obsessive preoccupation with something, as in tomomania. adj. **maniacal, manic**.

maniac (ˈmayniˌak) one affected with mania.

manic-depressive (ˌmanikdiˈpresiv) marked by alternating periods of mania and depression. Called also *bipolar disorder*.

manipulation (mə,nipyuh'layshən) skillful or dexterous treatment by the hands. In physiotherapy, the forceful passive movement of a joint beyond its active limit of motion.

mannitol ('mani,tol) a sugar alcohol occurring widely in nature, especially in fungi; an osmotic diuretic used for forced diuresis and in cerebral oedema.

mannosidosis (,manohsi'dohsis) an inborn error of metabolism marked by a defect in alpha-mannosidase activity that results in lysosomal accumulation of mannose-rich substrates. Clinically, there are coarse features, upper respiratory congestion and infections, profound mental handicap, hepatosplenomegaly, cataracts, radiographic signs of dysostosis multiplex, and gibbus deformity. A much milder clinical form also occurs. It is thought to be an autosomal recessive trait.

manometer (mə'nomitə) an instrument for ascertaining the pressure of liquids or gases.

Mansonella (,mansə'nelə) a genus of nematode parasites of the superfamily Filarioidea.

M. ozzardi a species found in the mesentery and visceral fat of man in Central and South America; symptomatic infections are rare.

Mansonia (man'sohni·ə) a genus of mosquitoes comprising some 55 species, distributed primarily in tropical regions, important as vectors of microfilariae and viruses.

mantle ('mant'l) an enveloping structure or layer, especially the brain mantle, or pallium.

Mantoux test (man'too) a tuberculin skin test in which a solution of 0.1 ml of PPD-tuberculin containing 5 tuberculin units is injected intradermally into either the anterior or posterior surface of the forearm. The test is read 48 to 72 hours after injection. It is considered positive when the induration at the site of injection is more than 10 mm in diameter.

manubrium (mə'nyoobri·əm) pl. *manubria* [L.] 1. the uppermost portion of the sternum (manubrium sterni). 2. the largest process of the malleus, giving attachment to the tendon of the tensor muscle of the tympanum (manubrium mallei).

manus ('manəs, 'may-) pl. *manus* [L.] hand.

MAO Master of the Art of Obstetrics; monoamine oxidase.

MAOI monamine oxidase inhibitor.

MAOT Member of the Association of Occupational Therapists.

maple bark disease ('mayp'l bahk) a granulomatous interstitial pneumonitis due to inhalation of the spores from *Cryptostroma corticale*, a mould found beneath the bark of maple logs.

maple syrup urine disease ('mayp'l 'sirəp 'yooə·rin) a genetic disorder involving deficiency of an enzyme necessary in the metabolism of branched-chain amino acids, marked clinically by mental and physical handicap, feeding difficulties, and a characteristic odour of the urine.

maprotiline (ma'prohti,leen) a tetracyclic ANTIDEPRESSANT used for relief of symptoms of depression. It acts by blocking the re-uptake of noradrenaline at nerve terminals; unlike tricyclic antidepressants, it has no effect on serotoninergic transmission.

marasmus (mə'razməs) a form of protein–calorie malnutrition occurring chiefly in the first year of life, with growth retardation and wasting of subcutaneous fat and muscle, but usually with retention of appetite and mental alertness. It is considered to be related to KWASHIORKOR. adj. **marantic, marasmic.**

marble bones (mahb'l 'bohnz) see ALBERS-SCHÖNBERG DISEASE.

Marburg virus disease ('mahbərg) a Central African viral haemorrhagic fever with acute onset and characteristic morbilliform rash. It is clinically identical to Ebola virus disease but is due to an antigenically different virus. The incubation period is 3 to 7 days. It was first reported in an outbreak in Europe in 1967 associated with the importation of green monkeys from Uganda. Since then several isolated incidents have occurred in Africa. The reservoir of infection is not known. Person-to-person transmission by inoculation of blood and tissue fluid and by sexual intercourse has been reported.

march foot (mahch) painful swelling of the foot, usually with fracture of a metatarsal bone, after excessive foot strain.

Marchiafava–Micheli syndrome (,mahki·ə-,fahvə·mi'kaylee) paroxysmal nocturnal haemoglobinuria.

Marevan ('mareevan) trademark for preparations of warfarin, an anticoagulant.

Marfan's syndrome (mah'fanhz) a hereditary disorder of connective tissue characterized by abnormal length of the extremities, especially of the fingers and toes, subluxation of the lens, congenital anomalies of the heart, and other deformities.

margination (,mahji'nayshən) accumulation and adhesion of leukocytes to the endothelial cells of blood vessel walls at the site of injury in the early stages of inflammation.

marginoplasty ('mahjinoh,plastee) surgical restoration of a border, as of the eyelid.

margo ('mahgoh) pl. *margines* [L.] border; margin.

Marie's disease (mə'reez) acromegaly.

Marie–Bamberger disease (mə,ree'bambərgə) hypertrophic pulmonary osteoarthropathy.

Marie–Strümpell disease (mə,ree'stroompel) ankylosing spondylitis.

Marie–Tooth disease (mə,ree'tooth) progressive neuropathic (peroneal) muscular atrophy.

marijuana, marihuana ('mariyuh'ahnə, -hwahnə) a preparation of the leaves and flowering tops of *Cannabis sativa*, the hemp plant, which contains a number of pharmacologically active principles (cannabinoids—see CANNABIS). HASHISH, also derived from the hemp plant, is obtained from the clear resin secreted by the flowering tops of the plant. Hashish is thought to be four to eight times more potent than marijuana. Both drugs are used for their euphoric properties and are three to four times more potent when smoked and inhaled than when ingested. Its possession is illegal in many countries.

Controversy over the legalization of marijuana continues. It is known that the use of marijuana as a recreational drug in this country is exceeded only by the the use of alcohol and tobacco. Unfortunately, many years of widespread use are usually required for the full implications of the use of a drug to become apparent. Such has been the case with alcohol and tobacco, which many defenders of marijuana cite as examples of legal drugs that are 'no better and no worse' than marijuana. Those opposed to marijuana agree that alcohol and tobacco are similar in some ways, but they too are detrimental to health. Their deleterious effects are well documented, but the search for evidence of the effects of marijuana must continue before it can be declared more or less harmful than the other two drugs.

Tetrahydrocannabinol (THC), the most active ingredient of marijuana can, with heavy smoking, narrow the bronchi and bronchioles and produce inflammation of the mucous membranes. In addition, marijuana smoke contains many of the same chemicals and 'tars' of tobacco smoke and, therefore, increases the risk of lung cancer.

There is some evidence that marijuana increases the risk for miscarriage and birth defects. Even though these dangers have not been completely documented, it is recommended that both men and women who plan to have children should avoid marijuana as they would any other unnecessary drug.

One beneficial effect of THC is the lowering of intraocular pressure, which might, in theory, be helpful in the control of glaucoma. However, because it causes tachycardia and increased work for the heart, it cannot be used in most elderly persons, the age group in which glaucoma is most prevalent. Another use of THC is for relief of extreme nausea and vomiting in patients undergoing cancer chemotherapy. Not every patient responds favourably to the THC, but it does benefit some.

marrow ('maroh) the soft, organic, sponge-like material in the cavities of bones. Bone marrow is a network of blood vessels and special connective tissue fibres that hold together a composite of fat and blood-producing cells.

The chief function of marrow is to manufacture erythrocytes, leukocytes, and platelets. These blood cells normally do not enter the bloodstream until they are fully developed, so that the marrow contains cells in all stages of growth. If the body's demand for white cells is increased because of infection, the marrow responds immediately by stepping up production. The same is true if more red blood cells are needed, as in haemorrhage or anaemia.

There are two types of marrow, red and yellow. The former produces the blood cells; the latter, which is mainly formed of fatty tissue, normally has no blood-producing function.

During infancy and early childhood all bone marrow is red. But gradually, as one gets older and less blood cell production is needed, the fat content of the marrow increases as some of the marrow turns from red to yellow. Red marrow continues to be present in adulthood only in the flat bones of the skull, the sternum, ribs, vertebral column, clavicle, humerus, pelvic bones, and part of the femur. However, under certain conditions, as after haemorrhage, yellow marrow in other bones may again be converted to red and resume its cell-producing functions.

The marrow is occasionally subject to disease, as in aplastic anaemia, which may be caused by destruction of the marrow by chemical agents or excessive x-ray exposure. Other diseases that affect the bone marrow are leukaemia, pernicious anaemia, myeloma, and metastatic tumours.

marsupialization (mah,soopi·əlie'zayshən) conversion of a closed cavity, such as an abscess or cyst, into an open pouch, by incising it and suturing the edges of its wall to the edges of the wound.

marsupium (mah'soopi·əm) pl. *marsupia* [L.] pouch; the scrotum.

masculine ('maskyuhlin) pertaining to the male sex.

masculinity (,maskyuh'linitee) the possession of masculine qualities.

masculinization (,maskyuhlinie'zayshən) the normal induction or development of male sexual characteristics in the male; also, the induction or development of male secondary sexual characteristics in the female.

masculinize ('maskyuhli,niez) to produce masculine qualities in women.

masculinovoblastoma (,maskyuhlin,ohvohbla-'stohmə) lipoid cell tumour.

maser ('mayzə) a device that produces an extremely intense, small and nearly nondivergent beam of monochromatic radiation in the microwave region, with all the waves in phase.

optical m. see LASER.

mask ('mahsk) 1. to cover or conceal, as the masking of the nature of a disorder by the presence of unassociated signs, organisms, etc.; in audiometry, to obscure or diminish a sound by the presence of another sound of different frequency. 2. an appliance for shading, protecting, or medicating the face.

luetic m. a brownish, blotchy pigmentation over the forehead, temples, and cheeks, sometimes occurring in tertiary syphilis.

m. of pregnancy brown pigmentation of the forehead, cheeks and nose, sometimes seen in pregnancy; melasma gravidarum.

Venturi m. any of three types of masks used to administer controlled amounts of oxygen (see also OXYGEN THERAPY); each of these masks provides a constant concentration above that of the atmospheric concentration (21 per cent).

masochism ('masə,kizəm) a perversion in which infliction of physical or psychological pain gives sexual gratification to the recipient. adj. **masochistic**.

masochist ('masəkist) a person exhibiting or characterized by masochism.

mass (mas) 1. a lump or collection of cohering particles. 2. that characteristic of matter which gives it inertia. The internationally accepted (SI) unit of mass is the kilogram.

inner cell m. an internal cluster of cells at the embryonic pole of the blastocyst which develops into the body of the embryo.

lean body m. that part of the body including all its components except neutral storage lipid; in essence, the fat-free mass of the body.

m. number the number expressive of the mass of a nucleus, being the total number of nucleons—protons and neutrons—in the nucleus of an atom or nuclide; symbol A.

massa (,masə) pl. *massae* [L.] MASS (1).

massage ('masahzh, -sahj) systematic therapeutic stroking or kneading of the body.

cardiac m. intermittent compression of the heart by pressure applied over the sternum (closed cardiac massage) or directly to the heart through an opening in the chest wall (open cardiac massage). See also CARDIAC MASSAGE.

vibratory m. massage by rapidly repeated light percussion with a vibrating hammer or sound.

masseter muscle (ma'seetə) the muscle that closes the jaws.

masseur (ma'sər) [Fr.] a man who performs massage.

masseuse (ma'sərz) [Fr.] a woman who performs massage.

massotherapy (masoh'therəpee) treatment of disease by massage.

mast cell (mahst) a connective tissue cell whose specific physiological function is unknown. It elaborates granules that contain histamine, heparin, and, in the rat and mouse, serotonin.

m. c. disease urticaria pigmentosa.

m. c. tumour a local aggregation of mast cells forming a nodular tumour. It may be benign or malignant.

mastadenitis (,mastadə'nietis) inflammation of a mammary gland; mastitis.

mastalgia (ma'stalji·ə) pain in the breast.

mastatrophy (ma'statrəfee) atrophy of the breast.

mastectomy (ma'stektəmee) surgical removal of the breast. Mastectomy is usually performed to remove a malignant breast tumour; rarely it may be advised for a benign tumour and for other diseases of the breast, such as chronic cystic mastitis. See also BREAST.

modified radical m. a term covering a variety of surgical techniques for removal of breast cancers. All these procedures involve removal of the breast; variations in technique depend on the extent to which the axillary lymph nodes and pectoral muscles are removed.

radical m. surgical removal of the breast with the underlying pectoral muscles and full clearance of lymphatic tissue from the relevant axilla. This more extensive surgery offers no better prognosis than the modified radical mastectomy in stage I and stage II breast cancers.

simple m. surgical removal of the breast; usually the procedure of choice for noninvasive breast cancer that is clearly confined to breast tissue. It may be followed by radiation therapy and sometimes requires later removal of lymph nodes in the axilla if metastases develop there.

subcutaneous m. excision of breast tissue with preservation of overlying skin, nipple, and areola so that the breast form may be reconstructed.

Master '2-step' exercise test (mahstə) a test of coronary circulation, electrocardiographic tracings being recorded while the subject repeatedly ascends and descends two steps, each 9 inches high, then immediately after and 2 and 6 minutes after cessation of the climbs. The amount of work (number of trips) is standardized for age, weight, and sex.

mastication (ˌmasti'kayshən) the act of chewing.

masticatory (ˌmasti'kaytə·ree, 'mastikəˌtree) 1. pertaining to mastication. 2. a substance to be chewed, but not swallowed.

Mastigophora (ˌmasti'gofə·rə) a subphylum of protozoa, including all those that have one or more flagella throughout most of their life cycle, and a simple, centrally located nucleus; many are parasitic in both invertebrates and vertebrates, including man.

mastigote ('mastiˌgoht) any member of the Mastigophora.

mastitis (ma'stietis) inflammation of the BREAST, occurring in a variety of forms and in varying degrees of severity.

Chronic cystic mastitis, called also *fibrocystic disease* of the breast and *cystic disease* of the breast, is the most common disorder of the breast resulting from hormonal imbalance. This condition generally occurs in women between the ages of 35 and 50. It is probably related to the activity of the ovaries and is rare after the menopause.

The disease is characterized by the formation of cysts which give a lumpy appearance to the breast. Symptoms may include pain and tenderness, which are usually aggravated before the menstrual period, at which time the cysts tend to enlarge. There may also be discharge from the nipple. Periodic change in the size of a lump or its rapid appearance and disappearance is common in cystic mastitis. Since there are times when it may be difficult to distinguish this condition from cancer of the breast, biopsy may be necessary. It is especially important for women with chronic cystic breast disease to have examinations every four to six months because there is a risk of developing carcinoma of the breast.

Chronic cystic mastitis is a benign disease that can usually be treated by aspiration of fluid from the cysts. If this is not effective, surgical excision of the cysts is necessary.

To help relieve the pain associated with cystic mastitis a good supporting brassiere that fits well and is not constricting should be worn day and night. Care should be taken to avoid injury to the breasts.

Young girls whose breasts are maturing sometimes experience a painful swelling and hardness of the breast, known as puberty mastitis. Occasionally a cloudy liquid may be squeezed from the nipples. The condition, rarely serious, usually subsides within a few weeks. It is best to wear a brassiere that gives mild support but does not irritate.

Enlargement of one or both breasts, gynaecomastia, is sometimes found in adolescent boys and old men. The condition is usually due to transient excessive oestrogenic activity. Secretions may be extruded from the nipple.

A mild inflammation known as stagnation mastitis, or caked breast, may occur during the early lactation period. Glands of the breast can become congested with milk, with formation of painful lumps.

Acute mastitis may occur after childbirth, when it is known as puerperal mastitis. It is an infection resulting usually from the presence of staphylococci and, occasionally, streptococci, which enter through cracks in the skin of the breast, particularly of the nipples. In puerperal mastitis, the breasts are tender, red, and warm. They become swollen and painful, and the inflammation responds quickly to one of the antibiotics, but in some cases an abscess may develop which must be incised and drained.

A milk cyst, galactocele, sometimes develops during lactation. It is probably caused by obstruction of a duct. The cyst can be removed after the baby has been weaned.

There are other types of infectious mastitis not related to lactation. Inflammation of the breast sometimes accompanies mumps, particularly in adults.

Tuberculous mastitis usually occurs in young women and accompanies tuberculosis of the lungs or of the cervical lymph nodes. Treatment is with antibiotics, although surgery is sometimes necessary.

A condition that may occur at the time of the menopause or later in women who have had children is comedomastitis, which is distention of the milk-producing ducts caused by the caking of secretions. Some of the material may be discharged from the nipple. Eventually the condition may develop into plasma cell mastitis. The breast may be tender and painful, with lump formation, nipple retraction, change in the breast contour, and possibly a cloudy discharge from the nipple.

Some cases of mastitis may require mastectomy.

masto- word element. [Gr.] *mammary gland, breast.*

mastocyte ('mastohˌsiet) a mast cell.

mastocytoma (ˌmastohsie'tohmə) a benign, local aggregation of mast cells forming a nodular tumour.

mastocytosis (ˌmastohsie'tohsis) an accumulation, local or systemic, of mast cells in the tissues; known as urticaria pigmentosa when widespread in the skin.

mastodynia (ˌmastoh'dini·ə) pain in the breast.

mastography (ma'stogrəfee) radiography of the breast; mammography.

mastoid ('mastoyd) 1. breast or nipple-shaped. 2. the mastoid process. 3. pertaining to the mastoid process.

m. antrum an air space in the mastoid portion of the temporal bone communicating with the middle ear and the mastoid cells.

m. bone mastoid process.

m. cells hollow spaces of various size and shape in the mastoid process of the temporal bone, communicating with the mastoid antrum and lined with a continuation of its mucous membrane.

m. process the conical projection at the base of the mastoid portion of the temporal bone.

mastoidalgia (ˌmastoy'dalji·ə) pain in the mastoid region.

mastoidectomy (ˌmastoy'dektəmee) surgical removal of mastoid cells. The most frequent indication for mastoidectomy is chronic infection in the mastoid process occurring as a complication of chronic OTITIS MEDIA. The extent of surgery depends on extent of destruction. A radical mastoidectomy involves removal of diseased portions of the mastoid process as well as the incus and malleus of the middle ear and the tympanic membrane. The degree of hearing loss following mastoidectomy depends on the extent of surgery. In some cases tympanoplasty (plastic reconstruction of the middle ear) can preserve much of the hearing. For nursing care after ear surgery, see EAR.

mastoideocentesis (ma,stoydiohsen'teesis) paracentesis of the mastoid cells.

mastoiditis (,mastoy'dietis) inflammation of the mastoid antrum and cells. It is usually the result of an infection of the middle ear, with which the mastoid cells communicate. Mastoiditis most commonly follows sore throat and respiratory infection, but it can also be caused by such diseases as diphtheria, measles, and scarlet fever.

The symptoms include earache and a ringing in the ears. The mastoid process may become painful and swollen.

Treatment formerly was limited to mastoidectomy, in which infected cells are removed surgically. However, the development of antibiotics has made it possible to check most cases of mastoiditis at an early stage, so that surgery usually is avoided.

mastoidotomy (,mastoy'dotəmee) incision of the mastoid process of the temporal bone.

mastology (ma'stoləjee) study of the mammary gland.

mastoncus (ma'stongkəs) a tumour or swelling of the breast.

masto-occipital (,mastoh·ok'sipit'l) pertaining to the mastoid process and occipital bone.

mastoparietal (,mastohpə'rieət'l) pertaining to the mastoid process and parietal bone.

mastopathy (ma'stopəthee) any disease of the mammary gland.

mastopexy ('mastoh,peksee) surgical correction of a pendulous breast.

mastoplasia (,mastoh'playzi·ə) mammoplasia.

mastoplasty ('mastoh,plastee) mammoplasty.

mastoptosis (,mastop'tohsis) a pendulous condition of the breast.

mastorrhagia (,mastə'rayji·ə) haemorrhage from the mammary gland.

mastoscirrhus (,mastoh'sirəs) hardening of the mammary gland.

mastosquamous (,mastoh'skwayməs) pertaining to the mastoid and squama of the temporal bone.

mastotomy (ma'stotəmee) incision of a mammary gland.

masturbation (,mastə'bayshən) sexual gratification by self-manipulation of the genitalia. Masturbation is too often thought of as shameful and unwholesome. Many harmful effects have mistakenly been attributed to it. The desire to masturbate is now known to be part of the normal process of sexual development. Unless excessive, masturbation at any age may be normal. Many infants and children masturbate as a form of self-gratification analogous to thumb-sucking. For older children and adolescents, it may serve as an expression of their newly developing awareness of their sexual capabilities, and may also help to gain control over sexual urges.

matching ('maching) comparison for the purpose of selecting objects having similar or identical characteristics.

m. of blood comparing the blood of a contemplated donor with that of the recipient to ascertain whether their bloods belong to the same group.

cross m. determination of the compatibility of the blood or tissue of a donor and that of a recipient before transfusion by placing erythrocytes or leukocytes of the donor in the recipient's serum and erythrocytes or leukocytes of the recipient in the donor's serum. Absence of agglutination, haemolysis, and cytotoxicity indicates that the two blood or tissue samples belong to the same group and are compatible.

materia medica (mə'tiə·ri·ə 'medikə) pharmacology.

maternal (mə'tərn'l) pertaining to the female parent.

m. deprivation see maternal DEPRIVATION syndrome.

m. mortality rate the number of deaths associated with childbirth per 1000 total births in any one year.

maternity (mə'tərnətee) motherhood.

mathematical model (,mathə'matik'l) a mathematical representation of a system to predict the outcome of various actions, for example, models of infectious disease to determine the likely effect of different vaccination policies.

matrix ('maytriks) pl. *matrices* [L.] 1. the intercellular substance of a tissue, as bone matrix, or the tissue from which a structure develops, as hair or nail matrix. 2. a metal band used to provide proper form to a dental restoration, such as amalgam in a prepared cavity.

bone m. the intercellular substance of bone, consisting of collagenous fibres, ground substance, and inorganic salts.

cartilage m. the intercellular substance of cartilage consisting of cells and extracellular fibres embedded in an amorphous ground substance rich in acid mucopolysaccharides and proteoglycans.

nail m., m. unguis the nail bed.

matter ('matə) physical material having form and weight under ordinary conditions of gravity.

maturation (,matyuh'rayshən, ,machuh-) 1. the stage or process of attaining maximal development; attainment of maximal intellectual and emotional development. In biology, a process of cell division during which the number of chromosomes in the germ cell is reduced to one-half the number characteristic of the species. 2. the formation of pus.

Maurer's dots ('mowrərz) irregular dots, staining red with Leishman's stain, seen in erythrocytes infected with *Plasmodium falciparum*.

Maxidex ('maksideks) trademark for a fixed combination preparation of dexamethasone and hypromellose, an anti-inflammatory eye drop.

maxilla (mak'silə) pl. *maxillae,maxillas* [L.] one of two identical bones that form the upper jaw. The maxillae meet in the midline of the face and often are considered as one bone. They have been described as the architectural key of the face because all bones of the face except the mandible touch them. Together the maxillae form the floor of the orbit for each eye, the sides and lower walls of the nasal cavities, and the hard palate. The lower border of the maxilla supports the upper teeth. Each maxilla contains an air space called the maxillary sinus.

maxillectomy (,maksi'lektəmee) surgical removal of a maxilla.

maxilloethmoidectomy (,maksiloh,ethmoy'dektəmee) excision of the portion of the maxilla surrounding the maxillary sinus and of the cribriform plate and anterior ethmoid cells.

maxillofacial (,maksiloh'fayshəl) pertaining to the maxilla and the face.

maxillomandibular (,maksilohman'dibyuhlə) pertaining to the upper and lower jaws.

maxillotomy (,maksi'lotəmee) surgical sectioning of the maxilla which allows movement of all or part of the maxilla into the desired position.

maximum ('maksiməm) the greatest quantity, effect, or value possible or achieved under given circumstances.

adj. **maximal.**
tubular m. the highest rate in milligrams per minute at which the renal tubules can transfer artificially administered test substances; the maximal tubular excretory capacity. Abbreviated Tm.

Maxolon ('maksəlon) trademark for a preparation of metoclopramide, an antiemetic.

May–Hegglin anomaly (ˌmay'heglin) a rare dominantly inherited disorder of blood cell morphology, characterized by RNA-containing cytoplasmic inclusions (similar to Döhle bodies) in granulocytes, by large, poorly granulated platelets, and by thrombocytopenia.

maze (mayz) a complicated system of intersecting paths used in intelligence tests and in demonstrating learning in experimental animals.

mazindol ('mayzindohl) an adrenergic having amphetamine-like actions; used as an anorexic.

MB Bachelor of Medicine (other than from Oxford).

MC, MCh, MChir [L.] *Magister Chirurgiae* (Master of Surgery).

mcg microgram.

MCH mean corpuscular haemoglobin, an expression of the average haemoglobin content of a single cell in picograms, obtained by multiplying the haemoglobin in grams by 10 and dividing by the number of erythrocytes (in millions). Normal range 27–33 pg.

MCHC mean corpuscular haemoglobin concentration, an expression of the average haemoglobin concentration in grams per decilitre (g/dl), obtained by multiplying the haemoglobin in grams by 100 and dividing by the haematocrit determination. Normal range 32–35 g/dl.

MChOrth Master of Orthopaedic Surgery.

MChS Member of the Society of Chiropodists.

mCi millicurie.

μCi microcurie.

MCSP Member of the Chartered Society of Physiotherapists.

MCT mean circulation time.

MCV mean corpuscular volume, an expression of the average volume of individual red cells in femtolitres (cubic microns), obtained by multiplying the haematocrit determination by 10 and dividing by the number of erythrocytes (in millions).

MD Doctor of Medicine (other than from Oxford).

Md chemical symbol, *mendelevium.*

meal (meel) a portion of food or foods taken at some particular and usually stated or fixed time.

mean (meen) an average; a numerical value intermediate between two extremes.
geometric m. the *n*th root of the product of *n* numbers.

measles ('meezəlz) a highly infectious statutorily notifiable disease, caused by a virus; called also *rubeola* or *morbilli*. It occurs worldwide. Infection is commonest in childhood. Prior to infant immunization, epidemics occurred every other year in England and Wales, but immunization interrupted this regular pattern. Vaccine acceptance is only about 70 per cent in England and Wales, where over 80,000 cases were reported in 1988.

The source of infection is man and spread is by droplet infection or by direct contact with nasal or pharyngeal secretions. The incubation period is usually 10 to 14 days, and the disease is communicable from the fifth day of incubation to the first 5 to 7 days of the rash. It is most infectious during the prodromal period before the rash appears. One attack of measles usually gives a lifetime immunity.

SYMPTOMS. Measles symptoms generally appear in two stages. In the prodromal stage the patient feels tired and uncomfortable, and may have a running nose, a cough, a slight fever, and pains in the head and back. The eyes may become reddened and sensitive to light. The fever rises a little each day.

The second stage begins at the end of the third or beginning of the fourth day. The patient's temperature is generally between 39.5 and 40 °C (103 and 104 °F). Koplik's spots, small white dots like grains of salt surrounded by inflamed areas, can often be seen on the gums and the inside of the cheeks. A rash appears, starting at the hairline and behind the ears and spreading downward, covering the body in about 36 hours.

The most serious complication of measles is encephalitis, which occurs in about 0.1 per cent of all cases. Other complications include pneumonia, otitis media, and mastoiditis.

TREATMENT. This involves bed rest while the fever and rash persist. Analgesics are given, but aspirin should be avoided because of its relationship with Reye's syndrome. Antibiotics are of no value in uncomplicated measles. Broad-spectrum antibiotics, e.g. ampicillin, are given for secondary pneumonia and otitis media.

PREVENTION. Routine immunization with live attenuated vaccine (in combination with mumps and rubella vaccines) is given in the UK in the second year of life. In an outbreak, vaccination should be offered to susceptible contacts within 48 hours of exposure. Normal human immune globulin may provide some protection to susceptible contacts if given within 5 days of exposure. Children should be excluded from school until 7 days after the onset of the rash.

measure ('mezhə) 1. to determine the quantity of a substance. 2. a specified quantity of a substance. 3. an implement with which a specified quantity of a substance can be determined.

meatorrhaphy (ˌmi·ə'to·rəfee) suture of the cut end of the urethra to the glans penis after incision for enlarging the urinary meatus.

meatoscopy (ˌmi·ə'toskəpee) visual examination of any meatus, especially the urinary meatus or the ureteral orifices.

meatotomy (ˌmi·ə'totəmee) incison of the urinary meatus in order to enlarge it.

meatus (mi'aytəs) pl. *meatus* [L.] an opening or passage. adj. **meatal.**
acoustic m., m. acusticus, m. auditorius, auditory m. a passage in the ear, one leading to the eardrum (external acoustic meatus) and one for passage of nerves and blood vessels (internal acoustic meatus).
m. nasi, m. of nose one of the three portions of the nasal cavity on either side of the septum, inferior, middle, or superior (meatus nasi inferior, medius, superior).
m. urinarius, urinary m. the opening of the urethra on the body surface through which urine is discharged.

mebendazole (mi'bendəˌzohl) an anthelmintic used in the treatment of trichuriasis, enterobiasis, ascariasis, and hookworm disease.

mebeverine (me'bevərin) an antispasmodic used in irritable bowel syndrome.

mechanics (mə'kaniks) the science dealing with the motions of material bodies.
body m. the application of kinesiology to use of the body in daily life activities and to the prevention and correction of problems related to posture.

mechanism ('mekəˌnizəm) 1. a machine or machine-like structure. 2. the manner of combination of parts, processes, etc., which subserve a common function. 3. the theory that the phenomena of life are based on the same physical and chemical laws that govern inorganic matter, as opposed to *vitalism*.

defence m., escape m. a mental mechanism by which psychic tension is diminished, e.g. repression, denial, overcompensation, rationalization, etc. See also DEFENCE MECHANISM.

mental m. 1. the organization of mental operations. 2. an unconscious and indirect manner of gratifying a repressed desire.

mechanoreceptor (ˌmekənohri'septə) a nerve ending sensitive to mechanical pressures or distortions, as those responding to touch and muscle contractions.

mechanotherapy (ˌmekənoh'therəpee) use of mechanical apparatus in treatment of disease or its results, especially in therapeutic exercises.

Meckel's cartilage ('mekəlz) the ventral cartilage of the first branchial arch.

Meckel's diverticulum a congenital sac or appendage occasionally found in the ileum; a relic of a fetal structure that connects the yolk sac with the intestinal cavity of the embryo.

meclozine ('meklohzeen, -in) an antinauseant, used as the hydrochloride salt.

meconium (mi'kohni·əm) dark green mucilaginous material in the intestine of the full-term fetus; it constitutes the first stools passed by the newborn infant. Indicates fetal distress when present in the liquor. See meconium ASPIRATION.

m. ileus intestinal obstruction in the newborn due to the blocking of the bowels with thick meconium.

MED minimal erythema dose.

media ('meedi·ə) [L.] 1. plural of *medium*. 2. middle, especially the middle coat of a blood vessel, or tunica media.

medial ('meedi·əl) pertaining to or situated toward the midline.

medialis (ˌmeedi'aylis) [L.] *medial*.

median ('meedi·ən) 1. situated in the median plane or in the midline of a body or structure. 2. the perpendicular line that divides the area of a frequency curve into two equal halves.

m. nerve a nerve that originates in the brachial plexus and innervates muscles of the wrist and hand.

m. plane an imaginary plane passing longitudinally through the body from front to back and dividing it into right and left halves.

mediastinal (ˌmeedi·ə'stien'l) of or pertaining to the mediastinum.

m. flutter movement of the tissues and organs of the mediastinum back and forth with each movement of air in and out of an open sucking wound in the thoracic cavity. The condition can produce serious impairment of cardiopulmonary function and is fatal if not treated promptly. Symptoms are similar to those of mediastinal shift.

m. shift a shifting or moving of the tissues and organs that comprise the mediastinum (heart, great vessels, trachea, and oesophagus) to one side of the chest cavity. The condition occurs when a severe injury to the chest causes the entrapment of air in the pleural space (tension PNEUMOTHORAX). As the volume of air increases on the affected side, the lung collapses and the organs and tissues of the mediastinum are crowded to the opposite side of the chest. This can produce compression of the other lung and kinking or twisting of one or more of the great blood vessels, which in turn seriously impairs blood flow to and from the heart.

Symptoms of mediastinal shift include severe dyspnoea, cyanosis, displacement of the trachea to one side, and distended neck veins. The immediate treatment is insertion of a hollow needle or trochar into the pleural space (THORACENTESIS) to provide an outlet for the escape of air and fluid. After the trapped air is released, closed chest drainage is initiated to allow for re-expansion of the lung.

mediastinitis (ˌmeedi·asti'nietis) inflammation of the mediastinum.

mediastinography (ˌmeedi·asti'nogrəfee) radiography of the structures of the mediastinum.

mediastinopericarditis (ˌmeedi·əˌstienohˌperikah'dietis) inflammation of the mediastinum and pericardium.

mediastinoscope (ˌmeedi·ə'stienohˌskohp) a specially designed endoscope used in mediastinoscopy.

mediastinoscopy (ˌmeedi·asti'noskəpee) examination of the mediastinum by means of an endoscope inserted through an anterior midline incision just above the thoracic inlet.

mediastinotomy (ˌmeedi·asti'notəmee) incision of the mediastinum.

mediastinum (ˌmeedi·ə'stienəm) pl. *mediastina* [L.] 1. a median septum or partition. 2. the mass of tissues and organs separating the sternum in front and the vertebral column behind, containing the heart and its large vessels, trachea, oesophagus, thymus, lymph nodes, and other structures and tissues. It is divided into anterior, middle, posterior, and superior regions.

m. testis a partial septum of the testis formed near its posterior border by a continuation of the tunica albuginea.

medical ('medik'l) pertaining to medicine.

m. audit an evaluative process applied to the quality of clinical practice, often by peer review of routine or specially collected records of individual cases. Judgements are frequently made on the appropriateness of the processes carried out during the management of the case, in the light of the outcome. Deaths are frequently the subject of medical audit, two established examples being the Confidential Enquiry into Maternal Deaths (carried out at National level), and local reviews of perinatal deaths.

m. jurisprudence medical science as applied to aid the law, e.g. in the case of death by poisoning, violence, etc.

M. Laboratory Scientific Officer (MLSO) an allied health professional skilled in the theory and practice of clinical laboratory procedures that provide data used to determine the presence, extent, and course of disease. The MLSO has the knowledge to perform complex laboratory procedures, to recognize errors or physiological conditions that invalidate test results, to carry out quality control procedures and to implement new procedures. The specialist fields in which MLSOs work include clinical chemistry, haematology, transfusion science, immunology, histopathology, cytology, bacteriology and virology.

Further information about MLSOs may be obtained from the Institute of Medical Laboratory Sciences, 12 Queen Anne Street, London W1M 0AU.

m. records traditionally written, but increasingly a computer, file containing information relating to individual patients. The term is also used to designate departments and personnel responsible for the safekeeping and retrieval of such files.

m. record administrator one who is responsible for the indexing, recording, and storage of medical records and reports of patients admitted to hospitals and other health care agencies.

m. social worker a professionally qualified worker who looks after the patients' socio-economic and welfare needs.

m. statistics that branch of statistics concerned with data relating to health and health services. Traditionally these include the use of routine data relating to death, illness and use of hospitals, clinics etc. The term is often also used to encompass statistics derived from aspects of medical research such as the conduct of trials of new drugs or procedures.

medicament (mə'dikəmənt) a medicinal agent.

medicated ('medi,kaytid) imbued with a medicinal substance.

medication (,medi'kayshən) 1. administration of remedies. 2. a medicinal agent. 3. impregnation with a medicine.

medicinal (mə'disin'l) having healing qualities; pertaining to a medicine.

medicine ('medisin, 'medsin) 1. any drug or remedy. 2. the art and science of the diagnosis and treatment of disease and the maintenance of health. 3. the nonsurgical treatment of disease.

aviation m. that branch of medicine which deals with the physiological, medical, psychological, and epidemiological problems involved in flying.

clinical m. 1. the study of disease by direct examination of the living patient. 2. the last three years of the usual curriculum in a medical school.

community m. that speciality which deals with all aspects of medical care in the community, including notification and control of infectious diseases, preschool and school health care, and factors affecting the health of the population as a whole.

emergency m. that speciality which deals with the acutely ill or injured who require immediate medical treatment.

experimental m. study of the science of healing diseases based on experimentation in animals.

family m. family practice; the medical speciality concerned with the provision of comprehensive primary health care.

forensic m. the application of medical knowledge to questions of law; medical jurisprudence. Called also *legal medicine*.

group m. the practice of medicine by a group of doctors, usually representing various specialities, who are associated together for the cooperative diagnosis, treatment, and prevention of disease.

legal m. forensic medicine.

nuclear m. that branch of medicine concerned with the use of radionuclides in the diagnosis and treatment of disease.

physical m. that branch of medicine using physical agents in the diagnosis and treatment of disease. It includes the use of heat, cold, light, water, electricity, manipulation, massage, exercise, and mechanical devices.

preclinical m. the subjects studied in medicine before the student observes actual diseases in patients.

preventive m. science aimed at preventing disease.

proprietary m. any chemical, drug, or similar preparation used in the treatment of diseases, if such article is protected against free competition as to name, product, composition, or process of manufacture by secrecy, patent, trademark, or copyright, or by other means.

psychosomatic m. the study of the interrelations between bodily processes and emotional life.

space m. that branch of aviation medicine concerned with conditions to be encountered in space.

sports m. the field of medicine concerned with injuries sustained in athletic endeavours, including their prevention, diagnosis, and treatment.

tropical m. medical science as applied to diseases occurring primarily in the tropics and subtropics.

veterinary m. the diagnosis and treatment of the diseases of animals.

medicochirurgical (,medikohkie'rərjik'l) applying to both medicine and surgery.

medicolegal (,medikoh'leeg'l) pertaining to medicine and law, or to forensic medicine.

medicosocial (,medikoh'sohshəl) having both medical and social aspects.

medionecrosis (,medikohnə'krohsis) focal areas of destruction of the elastic tissue and smooth muscle of the tunica media of a blood vessel, especially of the aorta or its major branches.

mediotarsal (,meedioh'tahs'l) pertaining to the centre of the tarsus.

meditation (,medi'tayshən) a state of extended reflection or contemplation which is experienced by the subject as relaxing and refreshing. It is achieved by a variety of learned techniques and accompanied by physiological changes, e.g. the EEG pattern shows alpha waves, oxygen consumption drops and energy expenditure is reduced. It is reported to be effective in relieving tension and anxiety.

Mediterranean anaemia (disease) (,meditə'rayni·ən) the homozygous form of beta-THALASSAEMIA.

Mediterranean fever (familial) a hereditary disease usually occurring in Armenians and Sephardic Jews, and marked by short recurrent attacks of fever with pain in the abdomen, chest, or joints, and erythema resembling that seen in erysipelas; it is sometimes complicated by amyloidosis.

medium ('meedi·əm) pl. *media,mediums* [L.] 1. an agent by which something is accomplished or an impulse is transmitted. 2. a substance providing the proper nutritional environment for the growth of microorganisms; called also *culture medium*.

contrast m. a substance, usually radiopaque but which may be radiolucent, used in radiology to permit visualization of body structures.

culture m. a substance used to support the growth of microorganisms or other cells.

dioptric media refracting media.

disperse m., dispersion m. the continuous phase of a colloid system; the medium in which a colloid is dispersed, corresponding to the solvent in a true solution.

refracting media the transparent tissues and fluid in the eye through which light rays pass and by which they are refracted and brought to a focus on the retina.

medius ('meedi·əs) [L.] *situated in the middle*.

MEDLARS ('medlahz) acronym for *Med*ical *L*iterature *A*nalysis and *R*etrieval *S*ystem, a computerized bibliographic system of the National Library of Medicine (Bethesda, Md., USA), from which the *Index Medicus* is produced. The system is available in major national libraries.

MEDLINE ('medlien) acronym for *MED*LARS on-*line*, a computerized bibliographical retrieval system, an on-line segment of MEDLARS.

Medrone ('medrohn) trademark for a preparation of methylprednisolone, an anti-inflammatory steroid.

medroxyprogesterone (med,roksiproh'jestə,rohn) a compound used as a progestational agent.

medulla (mə'dulə) pl. *medullae,medullas* [L.] the central or inner portion of an organ. adj. **medullary**.

adrenal m. the inner portion of the ADRENAL GLAND, where adrenaline is produced.

m. of bone bone MARROW, contained in the medullary canal of bone.

m. oblongata that part of the hindbrain continuous with the pons above and the spinal cord below; it houses nerve centres for both motor and sensory nerves, where such functions as breathing and the beating of the heart are controlled (see also BRAIN).

m. ossium bone marrow.

renal m. the inner part of the substance of the kidney,

composed chiefly of collecting tubules, and organized into a group of structures called the renal pyramids.

spinal m., m. spinalis spinal cord.

m. of thymus the central portion of each lobule of the thymus; it contains many more reticular cells and far fewer lymphocytes than does the surrounding cortex.

medullated ('medə,laytid) myelinated; equipped with myelin sheaths.

medullization (,medəlie'zayshən) the enlargement of the haversian canals in rarefying osteitis followed by their conversion into marrow channels; also the replacement of bone by marrow cells.

medulloadrenal (mə,duloh·ə'dreen'l) pertaining to the adrenal medulla.

medulloblast (mə'duloh,blast) an undifferentiated cell of the neural tube that may develop into either a neuroblast or spongioblast.

medulloblastoma (mə,dulohbla'stohmə) a brain tumour composed of medulloblasts.

medulloepithelioma (mə,duloh,epi,theeli'ohmə) a brain tumour composed of primitive neuroepithelial cells lining the tubular spaces.

mefenamic acid (,mefə'namik) a nonsteroidal anti-inflammatory agent with analgesic and antipyretic activity, used for relief of mild to moderate pain.

Mefoxin (me'foksin) trademark for a preparation of cefoxitin, an antibiotic.

mega- ('megə) word element. [Gr.] *large;* used in naming units of measurement to designate an amount 10^6 (one million) times the size of the unit to which it is joined, as in megacuries (10^6 curies); abbreviation M.

megabladder (,megə'bladə) permanent overdistention of the bladder.

megacalycosis (,megə,kali'kohsis) nonobstructive dilation of the renal calices due to malformation of the renal papillae.

Megace (me'gays) trademark for a preparation of megestrol acetate, an antineoplastic steroid.

megacolon (,megə'kohlon) dilation and hypertrophy of the colon.

acquired m. colonic enlargement associated with chronic constipation, but with normal ganglion cell innervation.

aganglionic m., congenital m. that due to congenital absence of myenteric ganglion cells in a distal segment of the large bowel, with resultant loss of motor function in the aganglionic segment and massive hypertrophic dilation of the normal proximal colon. Called also *Hirschsprung's disease.*

megacystis–megaureter syndrome (,megə,sistis-,megəyuh'reetə) chronic ureteral dilation (megaureter) associated with hypotonia and dilation of the bladder (megacystis) and gaping of the ureteral orifices, permitting vesicoureteral reflux of urine, and resulting in chronic pyelonephritis.

megaduodenum (,megə,dyooə'deenəm) a gross enlargement of the duodenum.

megahertz ('megə,hərts) one million (10^6) hertz; abbreviated MHz.

megakaryoblast (,megə'karioh,blast) the earliest cytologically identifiable precursor in the thrombocytic series, which matures to form the promegakaryocyte.

megakaryocyte (,megə'karioh,siet) the giant cell of bone marrow; it is a large cell with a greatly lobulated nucleus, and gives rise to blood platelets.

megakaryocytopoiesis (,megə,karioh,sietohpoy-'eesis) the production of megakaryocytes.

megakaryocytosis (,megə,kariohsie'tohsis) the presence of megakaryocytes in the blood or of excessive numbers in the bone marrow.

megal(o)- ('megəloh) word element. [Gr.] *large, abnormal enlargement.*

megalencephaly (,megəlen'kefəlee, -'sef-) macrencephalia; hypertrophy of the brain.

megalgia (me'galji·ə) a severe pain.

megaloblast ('megəloh,blast) a large, nucleated immature progenitor of an abnormal erythrocytic series; megaloblasts are present in the blood in certain anaemias. See also ANAEMIA. adj. **megaloblastic.**

megalocardia (,megəloh'kahdi·ə) cardiomegaly; enlargement of the heart.

megalocephaly (,megəloh'kefəlee, -'sef-) abnormally increased size of the head.

megalocheiria (,megəloh'kieri·ə) abnormal largeness of the hands.

megalocornea (,megəloh'kawni·ə) a developmental anomaly of the cornea, which is of abnormal size at birth and continues to grow, sometimes reaching a diameter of 14 or 15 mm in the adult.

megalocystis (,megəloh'sistis) an abnormally enlarged bladder.

megalocyte ('megəloh,siet) an extremely large erythrocyte.

megalodactyly (,megəloh'daktilee) excessive size of the fingers or toes.

megaloenteron (,megəloh'entə·ron) enlargement of the intestine.

megalogastria (,megəloh'gastri·ə) enlargement of the stomach.

megaloglossia (,megəloh'glosi·ə) macroglossia; hypertrophy of the tongue.

megalohepatia (,megəloh·hi'pati·ə) enlargement of the liver; hepatomegaly.

megalomania (,megəloh'mayni·ə) a mental state characterized by delusions of exaggerated personal importance, wealth, power, etc.

megalomaniac (,megəloh'mayni,ak) a person exhibiting megalomania.

megalomelia (,megəloh'meeli·ə) abnormal largeness of the limbs.

megalonychosis (,megəloni'kohsis) hypertrophy of the nails and their matrices.

megalo-oesophagus (,megəloh·i'sofəgəs) megaoesophagus.

megalopenis (,megəloh'peenis) abnormal largeness of the penis.

megalophthalmos (,megəlof'thalmos) abnormally large size of the eyes; buphthalmos.

megalopodia (,megəloh'pohdi·ə) abnormal largeness of the feet.

megalopsia (,megə'lopsi·ə) macropsia.

megalosplenia (,megəloh'spleeni·ə) enlargement of the spleen; splenomegaly.

megalosyndactyly (,megəlohsin'daktilee) a condition in which the digits are large and more or less webbed together.

megaloureter (,megəloh·yuh'reetə) congenital ureteral dilation without demonstrable cause.

-megaly word element. [Gr.] *enlargement.*

megaoesophagus (,megə·i'sofəgəs) dilation and muscular hypertrophy of most of the oesophagus, above a constricted, often atrophied, distal segment. See also ACHALASIA.

megarectum (,megə'rektəm) a greatly dilated rectum.

megavitamin (,megə'vitəmin) a term denoting massive doses of vitamins far exceeding the recommended daily allowances.

megavolt ('megə,vohlt) one million volts.

megestrol (mi'jestrol) a synthetic progestational agent.

meglumine ('megloo,meen) a crystalline base used in preparing salts of certain acids for use as diagnostic radiopaque media, e.g., meglumine diatrizoate and meglumine iothalamate. Called also *methylglucamine.*

megohm ('megohm) one million ohms.

megophthalmos (,megof'thalmos) abnormally large eyes.

meibomian cyst (mie'bohmi·ən) a small retention cyst of the meibomian gland.

meibomianitis (mie,bohmi·ə'nietis) a bilateral chronic inflammation of the meibomian glands.

Meigs's syndrome ('megziz) a fibroma or benign solid tumour of the ovary causing ascites and pleural effusion.

meiogenic (,mieoh'jenik) promoting meiosis.

meiosis (mie'ohsis) the process of cell division by which reproductive cells (gametes) are formed. There are two successive divisions, meiosis I and meiosis II, in which four daughter cells that have the haploid chromosome number (23 in humans) are formed. As in MITOSIS (somatic cell division), meiosis I and II are each divided into four phases: *prophase*, *metaphase*, *anaphase*, and *telophase*. adj. **meiotic.**

The first meiotic prophase is a complex process separated into five stages. During *leptotene* the chromosomes coil and contract; each consists of two chromatids joined along their length. During *zygotene* pairs of homologous chromosomes come into point-to-point contact along their length. This process is called *synapsis* and the structure formed is called a *bivalent*. The X and Y chromosomes synapse only at the ends of the short arms. During *pachytene* the chromosomes thicken, and the chromatids of each chromosome separate except at the centromeres. The bivalent is now a tetrad of four chromatids. During this stage crossing over occurs, in which the chromatids of homologous chromosomes break and rejoin, resulting in chromatids that contain sections derived from both the mother and the father. During *diplotene* the two chromosomes of each bivalent separate except for Y-shaped chiasmata where crossover has occurred. In the female, this stage (called *dictyotene*) is prolonged; the oocyte remains in this stage from late fetal life until the time of ovulation. In the last stage, *diakinesis*, the chiasmata move to the ends of the chromosomes.

The other phases of meiosis I and II resemble those of mitosis, except that in meiosis I the two chromosomes of each bivalent separate and move to opposite poles. Thus, each daughter cell receives the haploid number of chromosomes, each with two chromatids. The assortment is random; either the maternal or the paternal chromosome can go to a daughter cell. Meiosis II then follows immediately without DNA replication. Both daughter cells formed by meiosis I divide again and the two chromatids of each chromosome separate and go to separate daughter cells. This produces four haploid daughter cells with chromosomes composed of single chromatids.

Meissner's plexus ('miesnəz) the submucous plexus; a network of autonomic nerve fibres in the wall of the intestines.

melaena (mə'leenə) darkening of the faeces by blood pigments.

melalgia (mə'lalji·ə) pain in the limbs.

melan(o)- word element. [Gr.] *black, melanin*.

melancholia (,melən'kohli·ə) a mental state characterized by extreme sadness or depression, with inhibition of mental and physical activity. adj. **melancholic.**
involutional m. a major DEPRESSION occurring in late middle life, with agitation, worry, anxiety, somatic preoccupations, insomnia, and sometimes paranoid reactions.

mélangeur (,maylonh'zhər) [Fr.] an instrument for drawing and diluting specimens of blood for examination.

melaniferous (,melə'nifə·rəs) containing melanin or other black pigment.

melanin ('melənin) a dark, sulphur-containing pigment normally found in the hair, skin, ciliary body, choroid of the eye, pigment layer of the retina, and certain nerve cells. It occurs abnormally in certain tumours, known as melanomas, and is sometimes excreted in the urine when such tumours are present (melanuria).

melanism ('melə,nizəm) excessive deposit of melanin in the skin.

melanoameloblastoma (,melənoh·ə,melohbla'stohmə) melanotic neuroectodermal tumour.

melanoblast ('melənoh,blast) a cell that develops into a melanocyte.

melanoblastoma (,melənohbla'stohmə) melanotic neuroectodermal tumour.

melanocarcinoma (,melənoh,kahsi'nohmə) malignant melanoma.

melanocyte ('melənoh,siet) any of the dendritic clear cells of the epidermis, found particularly in the basal layers, that synthesize tyrosinase and, within their melanosomes, the pigment melanin; the melanosomes are then transferred from melanocytes to keratinocytes. adj. **melanocytic.**
m.-stimulating hormone (MSH) a peptide from the anterior pituitary that influences the formation or deposition of melanin in the body.

melanoderma (,melənoh'dərmə) an abnormally increased amount of melanin in the skin due to either an increase in production of melanin by the melanocytes normally present or to an increase in the number of melanocytes, with production of hyperpigmented patches.

melanodermatitis (,melənoh,dərmə'tietis) dermatitis with a deposit of melanin in the skin.

melanogen (mə'lanəjən) a colourless chromogen, convertible into melanin, which may occur in the urine in certain diseases.

melanogenesis (,melənoh'jenəsis) the production of melanin.

melanoglossia (,melənoh'glosi·ə) blackening and elongation of the papillae of the tongue; black tongue.

melanoid ('melə,noyd) 1. resembling melanin. 2. a substance resembling melanin.

melanoleukoderma (,melənoh,lookoh'dərmə) a mottled appearance of the skin.
m. colli a mottled appearance of the skin of the neck

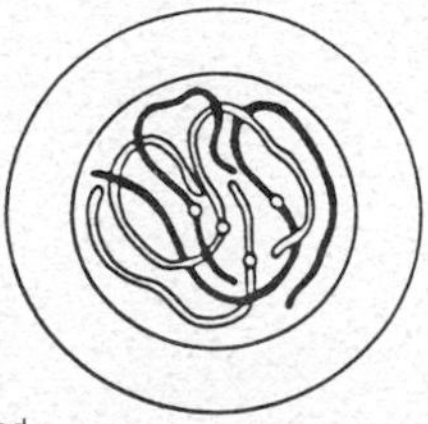

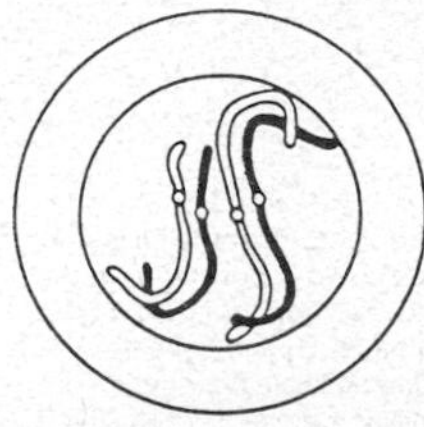

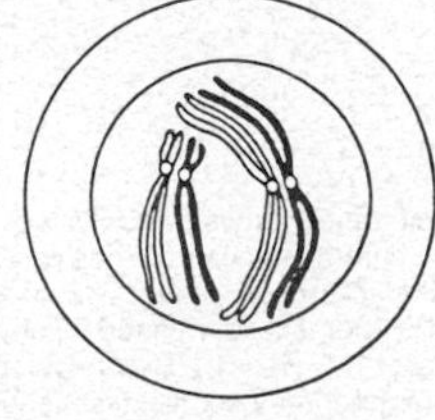

The first meiotic division. Continued on page 580.

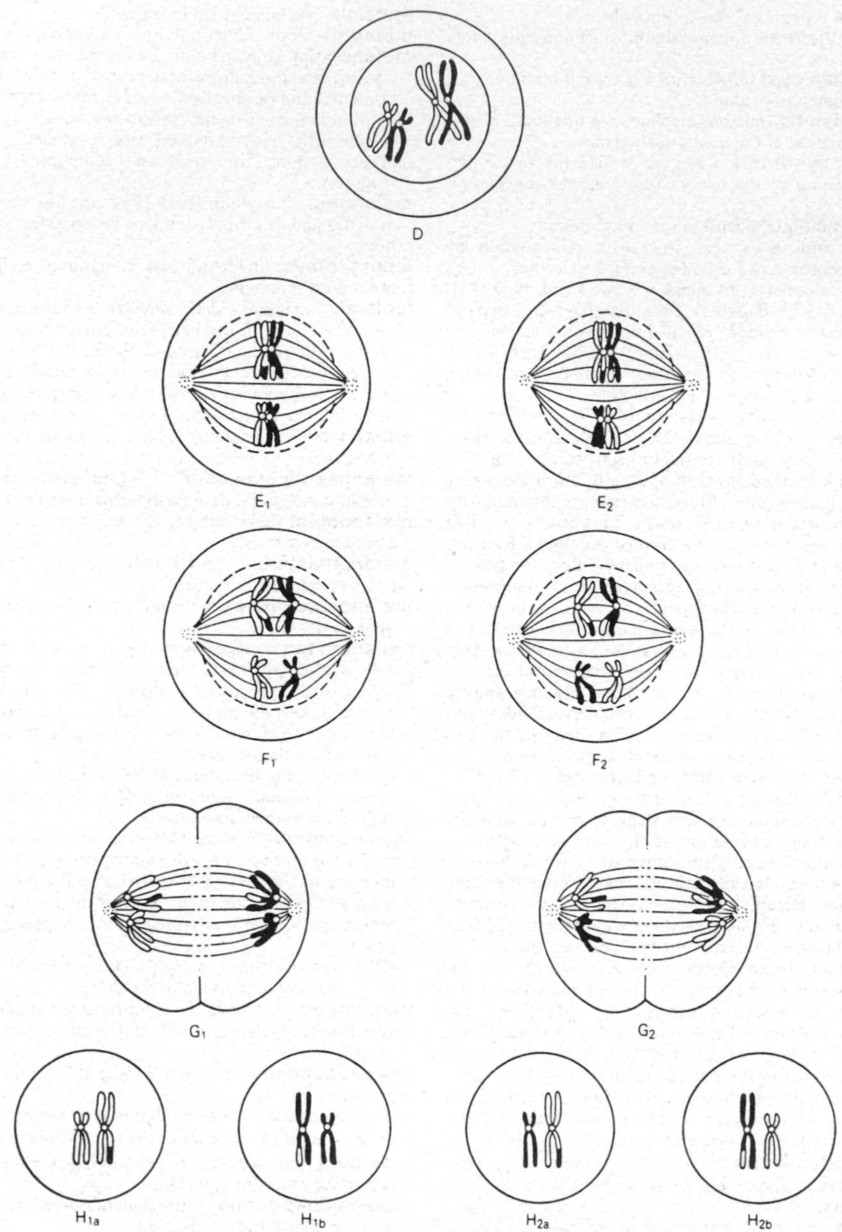

The first meiotic division. Only two of the 23 chromosome pairs are shown: chromosomes from one parent are shown in outline, from the other in black. A. Leptotene; B. Zygotene; C. Pachytene; D. Diplotene; E_1 and E_2 Metaphase; F_1 and F_2. Early anaphase; G_1 and G_2. Late anaphase; H_{1a}, H_{1b}, H_{2a}, H_{2b}, Telophase. One possible distribution of the parental chromosome pairs is shown in illustrations E_1 to H_1, the alternative combination in illustrations E_2 to H_2

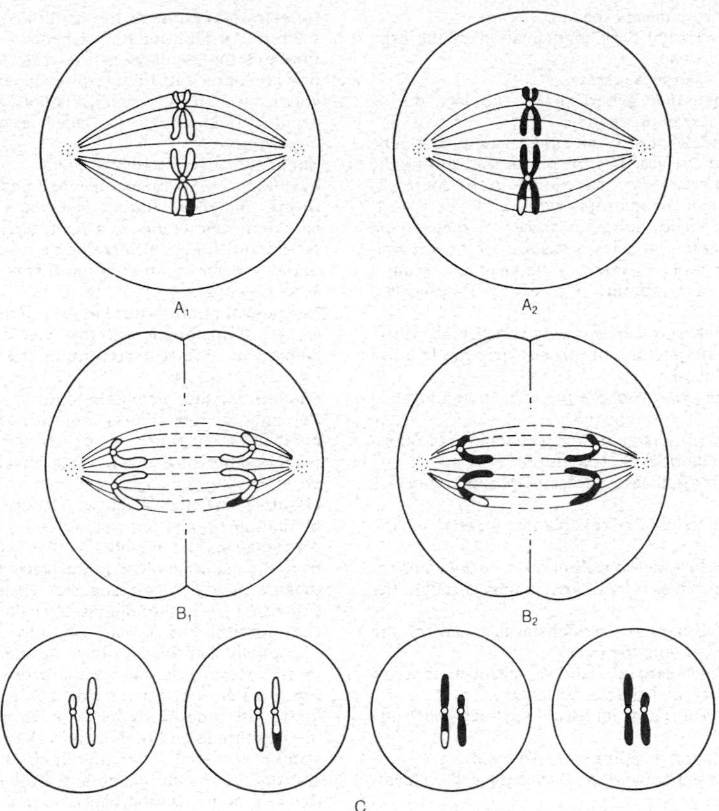

The second meiotic division. A. Metaphase; B. Anaphase; C. Telophase. A_1 and A_2 represent H_{1a} and H_{1b} of figure of first meiotic division

and adjacent regions, a rare manifestation of syphilis.

melanoma (ˌmelə'nohmə) 1. any tumour composed of melanin-pigmented cells. 2. malignant melanoma.

juvenile m. a benign, pink to purplish red papule, usually on the face, especially the cheeks, most commonly originating before puberty; histologically, it suggests and has been mistaken for malignant melanoma.

malignant m. a malignant tumour of melanocytes, usually developing from a naevus, with a marked tendency to metastasis; increasing in incidence in caucasian populations, especially those resident in sunny climes.

melanomatosis (ˌmelənohmə'tohsis) the formation of melanomas throughout the body.

melanonychia (ˌmelənoh'niki·ə) blackening of the nails by melanin pigmentation.

melanophage ('melənoh,fayj) a histiocyte laden with phagocytosed melanin.

melanophore ('melənoh,for) a pigment cell containing melanin, especially such a cell from fishes, amphibians, and reptiles.

melanoplakia (ˌmelənoh'playki·ə) pigmented patches on the mucous membrane of the mouth.

melanosarcoma (ˌmelənohsah'kohmə) malignant melanoma.

melanosis (ˌmelə'nohsis) 1. a condition characterized by dark pigmentary deposits. 2. a disorder of pigment metabolism.

m. coli brown-black discoloration of the mucosa of the colon.

melanosome ('melənoh,sohm) any of the granules that contain melanin. The melanin is synthesized within melanocytes; then the melanosomes are transferred to keratinocytes.

melanotic (ˌmelə'notik) characterized by the presence of melanin; pertaining to melanosis.

m. neuroectodermal tumour a benign, rapidly growing, dark tumour of the jaw and occasionally of other sites; almost always seen in infants. Called also *melanoameloblastoma.*

melanotrichia (ˌmelənoh'triki·ə) abnormally increased pigmentation of the hair.

melanotroph ('melənoh,trohf) a pituitary cell that elaborates melanocyte-stimulating hormone (MSH).

melanuria (ˌmelə'nyooə·ri·ə) the discharge of darkly stained urine.

melarsoprol (me'lahsoh,prol) an antiprotozoal effective against *Trypanosoma* species.

melasma (me'lazmə) dark pigmentation of the skin; called also *chloasma*.

m. addisonii Addison's disease.

m. gravidarum that occurring on the face during pregnancy (mask of pregnancy).

melatonin (,melə'tohnin) an indoleamine hormone synthesized and released by the pineal body during the hours of darkness; it may have a role in the control of the regulation of gonadotropin release.

melioidosis (,melioy'dohsis) a disease of rodents and many other animal species, transmissible in contaminated soil or water to man, in whom it can cause a wide range of symptoms. Caused by *Pseudomonas pseudomallei*.

melitagra (,meli'tagrə) eczema with honeycomb crusts.

melitoptyalism (,melitoh'tieə,lizəm) secretion of saliva containing glucose.

melituria (,meli'tyooə·ri·ə) the presence of any sugar in the urine.

Melleril ('melə·ril) trademark for preparations of thioridazine hydrochloride, a tranquillizer.

melomelus (mə'loməlas) a fetus with supernumerary limbs.

meloplasty ('meloh,plastee) plastic surgery of the cheek.

melorheostosis (,meloh,rio'stohsis) a form of osteosclerosis, with linear tracks extending through the long bones.

melotia (mə'lohshi·ə) congenital displacement of the auricle of the ear onto the cheek.

melphalan ('melfəlan) a cytotoxic nitrogen mustard alkylating agent used as an antineoplastic.

member ('membə) a distinct part of the body, especially a limb.

membra ('membrə) [L.] plural of *membrum*.

membrana (mem'braynə) pl. *membranae* [L.] membrane.

membrane ('membrayn) a thin layer of tissue that covers a surface, lines a cavity, or divides a space or organ. adj. **membranous**.

alveolocapillary m. a thin tissue barrier through which gases are exchanged between the alveolar air and the blood in the pulmonary capillaries.

alveolodental m. periodontium.

arachnoid m. arachnoid; one of the layers of the meninges.

basement m. the delicate layer underlying the epithelium of mucous membranes and secreting glands.

basilar m. the lower boundary of the scala media of the ear.

Bowman's m. a thin layer of basement membrane between the outer layer of stratified epithelium and the substantia propria of the cornea.

Bruch's m. the inner layer of the choroid, separating it from the pigmented layer of the retina.

cell m. plasma membrane.

decidual m's, deciduous m's see DECIDUA.

Descemet's m. the posterior lining membrane of the cornea; it is a thin hyaline membrane between the substantia propria and the endothelial layer of the cornea.

diphtheritic m. the peculiar false membrane characteristic of diphtheria, formed by coagulation necrosis.

drum m. tympanic membrane.

extraembryonic m's those that protect the embryo or fetus and provide for its nutrition, respiration, and excretion; the yolk sac (umbilical vesicle), allantois, amnion, chorion, decidua, and placenta.

false m. a membranous exudate, like the diphtheritic membrane.

fenestrated m. one of the perforated elastic sheets of the tunica intima and tunica media of arteries.

fetal m's the membranes that protect the embryo and provide for its nutrition, respiration, and excretion: the yolk sac (umbilical vesicle), allantois, amnion, chorion, decidua, and placenta. Called also *extraembryonic membranes*.

Henle's m. fenestrated membrane.

hyaline m. 1. a membrane between the outer root sheath and inner fibrous layer of a hair follicle. 2. basement membrane. 3. a homogeneous eosinophilic membrane lining alveolar ducts and alveoli, frequently found at necropsy in preterm infants (see also HYALINE MEMBRANE DISEASE).

hyoglossal m. a fibrous lamina connecting the under surface of the tongue with the hyoid bone.

limiting m. one that constitutes the border of some tissue or structure.

mucous m. the membrane covered with epithelium that lines the tubular organs of the body.

nuclear m. 1. either of the membranes, inner and outer, comprising the nuclear envelope. 2. nuclear envelope.

olfactory m. the olfactory portion of the mucous membrane lining the nasal fossa.

placental m. the membrane that separates the fetal from the maternal blood in the placenta.

plasma m. the membrane that encloses a cell; it is composed of phospholipids, glycolipids, cholesterol, and proteins. The primary structure is a lipid bilayer. Phospholipid molecules have an electrically charged 'head' that attracts water and a hydrocarbon 'tail' that repels water; they line up side by side in two opposing layers with their heads on the inner or outer surface of the membrane and their tails in the core, from which water is excluded. The other lipids affect the structural properties of the membrane. Proteins embedded in the membrane transport specific molecules across the membrane, act as hormone receptors, or perform other functions.

Reissner's m. the thin anterior wall of the cochlear duct, separating it from the scala vestibuli.

Scarpa's m. tympanic membrane, secondary.

semipermeable m. one permitting passage through it of some but not all substances.

serous m. the membrane lining the walls of the body cavities and enclosing the contained organs; it consists of mesothelium lying upon a connective tissue layer and it secretes a watery fluid.

synovial m. the inner of the two layers of the articular capsule of a synovial joint; composed of loose connective tissue and having a free smooth surface that lines the joint cavity.

tympanic m. the eardrum; the membrane marking the inner termination of the external acoustic meatus, separating it from the middle ear (see also TYMPANIC MEMBRANE).

tympanic m., secondary the membrane enclosing the fenestra cochlearis; called also *Scarpa's membrane*.

unit m. the trilaminar structure of all cellular membranes (such as the plasma membrane, nuclear membranes, mitochondrial membranes, endoplasmic reticulum, lysosomes) as they appear in electron micrographs. The biochemical structure is a lipid bilayer.

virginal m. hymen.

vitelline m. the external envelope of the ovum.

vitreous m. 1. Descemet's membrane. 2. hyaline membrane (1). 3. Bruch's membrane. 4. a delicate boundary layer investing the vitreous body.

membraniform (mem'brayni,fawm) resembling a membrane.

membranocartilaginous (ˌmembrənohˌkahti'lajinəs) 1. developed in both membrane and cartilage. 2. partly cartilaginous and partly membranous.

membranoid ('membrəˌnoyd) resembling a membrane.

membrum ('membrəm) pl. *membra* [L.] a limb or member of the body; an entire arm or leg.

m. muliebre clitoris.

m. virile penis.

memory ('meməˑree) the mental faculty that enables one to retain and recall previously experienced sensations, impressions, information, and ideas.

The ability of the brain to retain and to use knowledge gained from past experience is essential to the process of learning. Although the exact way in which the brain remembers is not completely understood, it is believed that a portion of the temporal lobe of the brain, lying in part under the temples, acts as a kind of memory centre, drawing on memories stored in other parts of the brain.

There are many theories about the way memories are stored. Millions of nerve cells in special patterns are probably involved. One possible explanation for the vast number of memories and the ways the mind has access to them is the chemical one. Brain cells, like other cells in the body, are made up of giant protein molecules. Each living cell contains great numbers of these molecules.The impulses that run along the nerves can change these molecules into new combinations, and each cell constantly reproduces these molecules exactly. This, then, could be a chemical way by which memories are stored: the nerve impulses of the experience leave traces in the minutely changed molecules within the cells. These molecules, as they disappear, are steadily reproduced, each according to its pattern. And so the memory trace would, theoretically, remain.

MEMORY THROUGH SENSE IMPRESSIONS. Much of memory is based on the brain's ability to record impressions, images, and sensations received by the sense organs. A person remembers only a small portion of the sense impressions he receives; he is more apt to remember impressions that are pleasing to him, but this is only a general rule, and everyone remembers much that is unpleasant as well. But though the brain probably retains only about a tenth of the impressions it receives, even this amount adds up to an enormous store of memories. These memories of touch, taste, smell, sound, and sight become raw material that the brain can draw upon in many ways—to recall past experience, to apply it to present situations, to anticipate the nature of future events or to form new thoughts or concepts. As a person continues to have experiences and store up memories, the brain's association of memories becomes increasingly complex.

Sometimes a person may retain certain kinds of sense impressions more efficiently than others. Some persons, for example, have very accurate memories of things they hear, such as conversations or melodies. Others recall visual images more clearly. An extreme example of such aptitude is eidetic memory, in which a person is able to reproduce exact visual images of things he has seen.

OTHER KINDS OF REMEMBERING. The term 'memory' is a general one, and it includes other kinds of remembering besides the collection of simple sense impressions. One of these is the ability to remember events that have just occurred and to add them to one's storehouse of memories. It is thought that this process begins when a new event stimulates a circular chain of electrical impulses in the brain. These impulses then stimulate each other, keeping the event part of one's conscious knowledge. Thinking about the event or mulling it over accentuates the impulses. Eventually the brain turns its attention to something new, but the impulses have left a record and made the event an enduring memory that can be clearly recalled. The ability to form memories of new events seems to be strongest in younger persons. Older persons may recall recent events poorly or with difficulty, while they are still able to remember the past clearly.

Memories of events, actions, or facts become stronger if the remembered thing is repeatedly experienced or used. This is why 'cramming' may get students through an examination for a day but leave little residue of knowledge. Too much information at once cannot be effectively handled by memory. The repetition of actions contributes to the kind of memory that enables one to perform acts automatically. Many everyday actions and skills are performed in this way.

DISTORTION OF MEMORY. Memories can easily be distorted. Experiments have shown that when a number of people observe an event and are later asked to describe it, no two persons describe it in exactly the same way. When a person has strong emotional feeling about an event, his memory of it is apt to be coloured by his emotions. He may remember those aspects of the event that fit in with his own emotions and attitudes, and forget those that do not. Or he may unconsciously add to his recollection details that did not really happen. All of us have probably unconsciously altered the truth in this way at one time or another.

Another distortion of memory that may occur is the feeling that some situation is familiar and has previously been experienced, when in reality the situation is a completely new one. The person may feel he knows exactly what someone to whom he is talking will say next. It is not known exactly why one suddenly has the feeling, called *déja vu* (literally, 'already seen'). Some psychologists suggest that this feeling may be because of some coincidental similarity between the new situation and a past experience.

LOSS OF MEMORY. Loss of memory, or AMNESIA, may be a symptom of damage to some area of the brain, or of a decrease in the brain's blood supply. It may also result from psychological causes; certain experiences may be so distressing to recall that the brain relegates them to the subconscious mind.

Only rarely is all memory lost in amnesia. Sometimes an incident or a certain period in the patient's life is forgotten. Or he may recall events in the wrong order but remember each separate event accurately. Amnesia may take different forms, depending on what area of the brain has been injured; in amnesia of hearing, for example, the patient cannot remember spoken language, while in visual amnesia he has forgotten his written language.

screen m. a consciously tolerable memory serving as a 'screen' for another memory that may be disturbing or emotionally painful if recalled.

menacme (me'nakmee) the period of a woman's life which is marked by menstrual activity.

menadiol (ˌmenə'dieol) a vitamin K analogue; its sodium diphosphate salt is used as a prothrombinogenic vitamin.

menaphthone (me'nafthohn) a synthetic preparation of vitamin K; menadione.

menaquinone (ˌmenə'kwinohn) any of a series of compounds having vitamin K activity, in which the phytyl side chain of phytonadione (vitamin K_1) is replaced by a side chain of prenyl units.

menarche (me'nahkee) establishment or beginning of the menstrual function. adj. **menarcheal.**

MENCAP ('menkap) the Royal Society for Mentally Handicapped Children and Adults. A voluntary organization, founded in 1946, with the aims of providing help for mentally handicapped persons and of increasing public awareness of the problems faced by mentally handicapped persons and their families. MENCAP has a network of 450 local societies and 12 regional offices and organizes symposia and conferences in addition to funding research into the causes of mental handicap. MENCAP also organizes holiday and leisure activities (including sports) for the mentally handicapped and almost all are dependent on the participation of nonhandicapped volunteers.

Publications include *Parents' Voice*, *Journal of Mental Deficiency* and a wide range of books and pamphlets, which are available from MENCAP National Centre, 123 Golden Lane, London EC1 0RT.

Mendel–Bechterew reflex (ˌmend'l'bektə·roo) dorsal flexion of the second to fifth toes on percussion of the dorsum of the foot; in certain organic nervous disorders, plantar flexion occurs.

Mendel's law ('mend'lz) in the inheritance of certain traits or characters, offspring are not intermediate in type between the parents, but inherit from one or the other parent in this respect. Thus, if a plant with the factor tallness (TT) is mated with one with the factor shortness (SS), then the offspring will inherit these factors in the ratio TT, 2TS, SS. This law is usually expressed as the law of independent assortment and the law of segregation. Called also *mendelian law*.

mendelevium (ˌmendə'leevi·əm) a chemical element, atomic number 101, atomic weight 256, symbol Md. See table of elements in Appendix 2.

mendelian law (men'deeli·ən) Mendel's law.

mendelian rate an expression of the numerical relations of the occurrence of distinctly contrasted mendelian characteristics in succeeding generations of hybrid offspring.

Mendelson's syndrome ('mend'lˌsənz) chemical pneumonitis due to aspiration of acid stomach contents (pH <2.5) into the lung; first described in 1946 by Mendelson, an American obstetrician. It is a leading cause of death in obstetric patients undergoing general anaesthesia. The syndrome consists of cyanosis, bronchospasm hypotension, pulmonary oedema and heart failure and is accompanied by significant mortality. Treatment is entirely symptomatic and usually includes mechanical ventilation, maintenance of oxygenation and blood pressure until the lung heals itself. Prevention consists of the use of antacids and/or H_2-receptor antagonists such as ranitidine preoperatively in order to raise and keep the gastric acidity above a pH of 2.5.

Ménétrier's disease (ˌme'naytreeˌayz) excessive proliferation of the gastric mucosa, producing diffuse thickening of the wall; inflammatory changes may be associated. Called also *giant hypertrophic gastritis*.

Menière's disease ('meniˌairz) a disorder of the labyrinth of the inner ear; called also *Menière's syndrome* and sometimes spelled *Meniere* and *Ménière*. It is believed to result from dilation of the lymphatic channels in the cochlea. In about 90 per cent of cases only one ear is affected. The usual symptoms are tinnitus, heightened sensitivity to loud sounds, progressive loss of hearing, headache, and vertigo. In the acute stage there may be severe nausea with vomiting, profuse sweating, disabling dizziness, and nystagmus. Some attacks last only minutes, and others continue for hours; they may occur frequently or only several weeks apart.

The disease usually lasts a few years, with progressive loss of hearing in the affected ear; sometimes the symptoms stop before all hearing is lost. If loss of hearing in the affected ear does become complete, nausea symptoms are likely to disappear.

Menière's disease sometimes develops after an injury to the head or infection of the middle ear. Many cases, however, have no apparent cause. The disorder is most common among men between the ages of 40 and 60.

Sedatives are usually ordered to promote sleep and rest. If the ringing sensation becomes too disturbing to the patient, it may be masked (for example, by music piped in through earphones) to make sleeping easier.

Surgical treatment involves relief from accumulation of inner ear fluid in the endolymphatic sac. Procedures may be directed toward relief of pressure by the bony structures surrounding the sac, or toward opening the sac and diverting the flow of endolymph by means of a shunt to the mastoid bone or to the subarachnoid space.

mening(o)- word element. [Gr.] *meninges*, *membrane*.

meningeal (mə'ninji·əl) pertaining to the meninges.

meningeorrhaphy (məˌninji'o·rəfee) suture of membranes, especially the meninges.

meninges (mə'ninjeez, 'menin-) plural of *meninx*. [Gr.] the three membranes covering the brain and spinal cord: the dura mater, arachnoid, and pia mater. adj. **meningeal**.

meningioma (məˌninji'ohmə) a hard, usually vascular tumour occurring mainly along the meningeal vessels and superior longitudinal sinus, invading the dura and skull and leading to erosion and thinning of the skull.
angioblastic m. angioblastoma.

meningism ('meninˌjizəm) 1. the symptoms and signs of meningitis associated with acute febrile illness or dehydration but without actual inflammation of the meninges. 2. a hysterical simulation of meningitis.

meningitis (ˌmenin'jietis) inflammation of the meninges. When the inflammatory process affects the dura mater, the disease is termed *pachymeningitis*; when the arachnoid and pia mater are involved, it is called *leptomeningitis* or *meningitis proper*.

The term *meningitis* does not refer to a specific disease entity but rather to the pathological condition of inflammation of the tissues of the meninges. The aetiological agent can be anything that activates the inflammatory process, including both pathogenic and nonpathogenic organisms, such as bacteria, viruses, and fungi; chemical toxins such as lead and arsenic; contrast media used in myelography; and metastatic malignant cells.Meningitis, and its causal organism if known, is a notifiable disease.

Bacterial Meningitis. This form of meningitis occurs when pathogenic bacteria enter the subarachnoid space and cause a pyogenic inflammatory response. The most common causes are *Streptococcus pneumoniae* (pneumococcus), *Neisseria meningitidis* (meningococcus), and *Haemophilus influenzae*, which are responsible for approximately 70 per cent of all cases. The incidence is age-related. In adults, *S. pneumoniae* and *N. meningitidis* cause most of the cases; in children aged 1 month to 15 years, *N. meningitidis* and *H. influenzae* predominate; in neonates less than 1 month old, the disease is usually a hospital-acquired infection with gram-negative enteric bacilli.

Almost all bacterial infections of the meninges enter the nervous system after having invaded and infected another region of the body and then are spread by local extension, as from the sinuses, or through the blood, as in septicaemia. The organisms gain access to the ventriculosubarachnoid spaces and the cerebrospinal fluid where they cause irritation of the tissues bathed by the fluid.

Bacterial meningitis typically begins with headache,

nausea and vomiting, stiff neck (nuchal rigidity), and chills and fever. Irritability and confusion occur early in the course of the disease, and convulsive seizures occur in about 25 per cent of patients. As the disease progresses the patient becomes less rational, has decreasing levels of consciousness, and lapses into coma. Inability to straighten the knee when the hip is flexed (a positive Kernig's sign) and involuntary flexing of the hip and knee when the neck is flexed forward (a positive Brudzinski's sign) are indicative of meningeal irritation.

A diagnosis of bacterial meningitis is verified by isolation of the organism from a specimen of cerebrospinal fluid obtained by lumbar puncture. Treatment with the appropriate antibacterial agent is begun at once to reduce the numbers of proliferating bacteria attacking the central nervous system. Supportive measures include rest, maintenance of fluid and electrolyte balance, and avoidance or control of convulsions with anticonvulsant drugs.

The prognosis is generally good, especially for meningococcal meningitis in which residual neurological deficits and persisting convulsive seizures are rare. Pneumococcal meningitis and meningitis due to *Haemophilus influenzae* are more likely to be complicated by these sequelae as well as by septic shock and hydrocephalus.

BENIGN VIRAL MENINGITIS. This term encompasses a group of disorders in which there is some meningeal irritation but no pyogenic organism can be found in the cerebrospinal fluid. It is, therefore, called also *aseptic meningitis complex*, which is somewhat misleading because the meningeal irritation often follows infection with the mumps virus or with one of the picornaviruses.

The patient with this disorder typically complains of headache and signs characteristic of meningeal irritation, intolerance to light, and pain when the eyes are moved from side to side. Most of the symptoms are mild, and treatment is largely supportive and symptomatic; the disease is self-limiting.

PATIENT CARE. Assessment of the patient with meningitis includes monitoring vital signs, neurological status, and fluid and electrolyte status. The plan of care should include provisions for rest and relief from discomfort, a quiet and nonstimulating environment, protection from injury during convulsions, control of elevated body temperature, and isolation precautions as indicated by the specific causative organism. Antibiotics must be given precisely as ordered so as to avoid further damage to the central nervous system. Early signs of increased INTRACRANIAL PRESSURE from brain oedema are reported promptly so that measures to reduce pressure can be taken as soon as possible. During the acute phase and convalescence the patient is watched for signs of complications such as septic shock, vascular collapse, and hydrocephalus. Nutritional status must be maintained throughout the course of illness to reinforce the patient's natural resources for combating infection and recovering from its deleterious effects.

cerebrospinal m. an inflammation of the brain and spinal cord; it may be caused by many different organisms.

epidemic cerebrospinal m. an acute infectious disease attended by seropurulent inflammation of the membranes of the brain and spinal cord, which is due to infection by *Neisseria meningitidis* (meningococcus). The disease usually occurs in epidemics, and the symptoms are those of acute cerebral and spinal meningitis. In addition, an eruption of erythematous, herpetic, or haemorrhagic spots on the skin are usually present. The fulminating or malignant form is known as *Waterhouse–Friderichsen syndrome*.

spinal m. inflammation of the meninges of the spinal cord.

meningocele (mə'ning·goh,seel) hernial protrusion of meninges through a defect in the skull or vertebral column.

meningocerebritis (mə,ning·goh,seri'brietis) inflammation of the brain and meninges.

meningococcaemia (mə,ning·gohkok'seemi·ə) the presence of meningococci in the blood, producing an acute fulminating disease or an insidious disorder persisting for months or years. It is a notifiable disease.

acute fulminating m. Waterhouse–Friderichsen syndrome.

meningococcidal (mə,ning·gohkok'sied'l) destroying meningococci.

meningococcus (mə,ning·goh'kokəs) pl. *meningococci* [Gr.] a microorganism of the species *Neisseria meningitidis*, the cause of some types of meningitis. adj. **meningococcal.**

meningocortical (mə,ning·goh'kawtik'l) pertaining to the meninges and cortex of the brain.

meningocyte (mə'ning·goh,siet) a histiocyte of the meninges.

meningoencephalitis (mə,ning·goh·en,kefə'lietis, -,sef-) encephalomeningitis; inflammation of the brain and its meninges.

meningoencephalocele (mə,ning·goh·en'kefəloh-,seel, -'sef-) hernial protrusion of the meninges and brain substance through a defect in the skull.

meningoencephalomyelitis (mə,ning·goh·en-,kefəloh,mieə'lietis, -,sef-) inflammation of the meninges, brain, and spinal cord.

meningoencephalopathy (mə,ning·goh·en,kefə'lopəthee, -,sef-) noninflammatory disease of the cerebral meninges and brain.

meningogenic (mə,ning·goh'jenik) arising in the meninges.

meningomalacia (mə,ning·gohmə'layshi·ə) softening of a membrane.

meningomyelitis (mə,ning·goh,mieə'lietis) inflammation of the spinal cord and its meninges.

meningomyelocele (mə,ning·goh'mieəloh,seel) hernial protrusion of the meninges and spinal cord through a defect in the vertebral column.

meningomyeloradiculitis (mə,ning·goh,mieəlohrə-,dikyuh'lietis) inflammation of the meninges, spinal cord, and spinal nerve roots.

meningopathy (,menin'gopəthee) any disease of the meninges.

meningoradicular (mə,ning·gohrə'dikyuhlə) pertaining to the meninges and the cranial or spinal nerve roots.

meningoradiculitis (mə,ning·gohrə,dikyuh'lietis) inflammation of the meninges and spinal nerve roots.

meningorhachidian (mə,ning·gohrə'kidi·ən) pertaining to the spinal cord and meninges.

meningorrhagia (mə,ning·gə'rayji·ə) haemorrhage from cerebral or spinal membranes.

meningorrhoea (mə,ning·gə'reeə) effusion of blood between or upon the meninges.

meninx ('meningks) pl. *meninges* [Gr.] a membrane, especially one of the membranes of the brain or spinal cord—the dura mater, arachnoid, and pia mater. adj. **meningeal.**

meniscectomy (,meni'sektəmee) excision of a meniscus, as of the knee joint.

meniscitis (,meni'sietis) inflammation of a meniscus of the knee joint.

meniscocyte (mə'niskoh,siet) a sickle cell.

meniscocytosis (mə,niskohsie'tohsis) sickle cell anaemia.

meniscosynovial (mə,niskohsie'nohvi·əl, -si-) pertaining to a meniscus and the synovial membrane.

meniscus (mə'niskəs) pl. *menisci* [L.] something of crescent shape, as the concave or convex surface of a column of liquid in a pipette or burette, or a crescent-shaped fibrocartilage (semilunar cartilage) in the knee joint. adj. **meniscal**.

Menkes' disease ('menkeez) a hereditary abnormality in copper absorption marked by severe cerebral degeneration and arterial changes resulting in death in infancy and by sparse, brittle scalp hair. It is transmitted as an X-linked recessive trait.

meno- word element. [Gr.] *menstruation*.

menolipsis (,menoh'lipsis) temporary cessation of menstruation.

menometrorrhagia (,menoh,metrə'rayji·ə) excessive uterine bleeding at and between menstrual periods.

menopause ('menə,pawz) the span of time during which the menstrual cycle wanes and gradually stops; called also *change of life* and *climacteric*. It is the period when ovaries stop functioning and therefore menstruation and childbearing cease. adj. **menopausal**.

The menopause is a natural physiological process that results from the normal ageing of the ovaries. It occurs when the ovaries can no longer perform the function of ovulation and production of hormones (oestrogen and progesterone). Because oestrogen secretion stops, physiological changes occur in the woman's body. The uterine (fallopian) tubes shrink in size and become less capable of movement. The uterus, the cavity of the uterus and the cervix also decrease in size. The vagina becomes dry. It contracts and its folds become shallower. The clitoris and external sexual organs become smaller. There may be some thinning of the pubic and axillary hair. The breasts usually become less full and firm.

Menopause normally takes place between the ages of 35 and 58. If it occurs before the age of 35 it is *premature menopause*; after 58 it is called *delayed menopause*. Both premature and delayed menopause should be evaluated by a gynaecologist because they can be inherited or be indicative of a primary endocrine disorder or gynaecological dysfunction.

The menopause can last from 6 months to 3 years or more. Some investigators believe that a women whose menarche was at a relatively early age will experience menopause later than the average age, while other findings indicate that there is little relation between the date of onset of the menarche and the age at which menopause occurs. If for medical reasons surgery or radiation of the reproductive organs becomes necessary, *artificial menopause* can occur if both ovaries are rendered dysfunctional or surgically removed. The symptoms usually are more severe than in natural menopause because of the sudden rather than gradual diminution of hormonal secretion.

SYMPTOMS AND TREATMENT. Approximately 15 per cent of all menopausal women experience no symptoms at all. Of the remaining 85 per cent, only about one-fourth are uncomfortable enough to seek relief by consulting a doctor.

The most frequent symptoms are hot flushes (flashes) of the face, neck, and upper body, and excessive perspiration, especially at night. Emotional instability, depression, irritability, and anxiety are probably related to hormonal imbalance and to other physiological changes. A woman who is physically active, well nourished without being overweight, and engaged in meaningful activity is less likely to suffer serious emotional upheavals than the one who sees herself as useless and physically unattractive. There is no truth in the notion that a woman who has experienced the menopause must necessarily be less attractive sexually or that she no longer has interest in sexual activities. In fact, many women find sexual intercourse more enjoyable after menopause because they are free of the fear of pregnancy and the inconvenience of contraceptive devices.

The first and most obvious sign of the menopause is change in the menstrual flow. In the majority of women, bleeding decreases with each period, and the periods are spaced farther apart. In some cases, there may be excessive bleeding during the regular period.

Bleeding may also occur between periods, either as a full flow, or in drops. Vaginal bleeding that occurs after menstruation has definitely stopped is not a normal part of the menopause.

Oestrogen replacement therapy is now available by implant, dermal patches, or oral administration. It is effective in removing the side-effects of the menopause, preventing osteoporosis, but the association with uterine cancer and thromboembolic disorders cannot be excluded. See also OESTROGEN.

menorrhagia (,menə'rayji·ə) excessive menstruation. Its causes include uterine tumours, pelvic inflammatory disease, and abnormal conditions of pregnancy. Endocrine disturbances may produce functional menorrhagia. Excessive menstruation may cause anaemia.

menorrhalgia (,menə'ralji·ə) pain during menstruation (see also DYSMENORRHOEA).

menoschesis (mə'noskisis) suppression of menstruation.

menostasis (mə'nostəsis) amenorrhoea.

menostaxis (,menoh'staksis) a prolonged menstrual period.

menotrophin (,menoh'trohfin) a purified preparation of gonadotrophins extracted from the urine of postmenopausal women, containing follicle-stimulating hormone (FSH) and luteinizing hormone (LH); used in the treatment of infertility.

menses ('menseez) menstruation.

menstrual ('menstrooəl) pertaining to menstruation.

m. cycle the period of the regularly recurring physiological changes in the endometrium that culminate in its shedding (MENSTRUATION).

Menstrual cycles vary in length; the average is approximately 28 days. The menstrual flow generally lasts about 5 days, although this too varies from person to person. Women menstruate from puberty to menopause, except during pregnancy.

Fourteen days before the next expected menstruation, a follicle containing an ovum develops in the ovaries. As the menstrual flow ceases, the lining of the uterus is stimulated by oestrogen and begins to increase in thickness to prepare for reproduction.

On about the fourteenth day of the cycle, OVULATION takes place and the ovary discharges the ovum. At the time of ovulation, the ruptured follicle is transformed into a yellowish material called the corpus luteum, which in turn secretes progesterone. Progesterone acts on the endometrium, building up tissues with an enriched supply of blood to nourish the future embryo.

If conception does not take place, the oestrogen level in the blood falls, the endometrium is no longer stimulated, and the uterus again becomes thinner. Blood circulation slows, blood vessels contract and the unused tissue breaks down into the bloody discharge known as menstruation. With its onset, the cycle starts again.

menstruation (,menstroo'ayshən) the functional periodic discharge from the vagina of blood and tissues

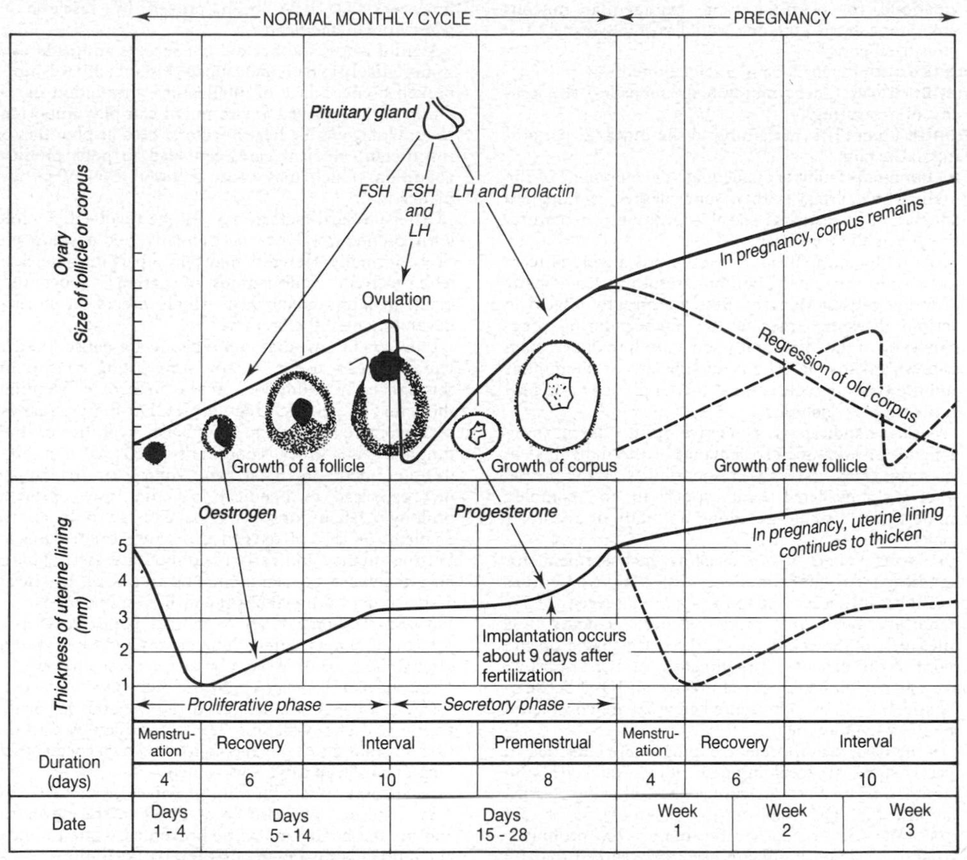

Average 28-day menstrual cycle. The cycle begins when hormones from the pituitary gland stimulate the development of an egg in a follicle inside one of the ovaries. About the fourteenth day, ovulation occurs. The follicle bursts, and the egg is discharged from the ovary. If the egg is not fertilized, the cycle ends in menstruation on the twenty-eighth day. If the egg is fertilized, pregnancy begins.

from a nonpregnant uterus; the culmination of the MENSTRUAL CYCLE. Menstruation occurs every 28 days or so between puberty and menopause, except during pregnancy, and the flow lasts about 5 days, the times varying from woman to woman.

MENSTRUAL DIFFICULTIES. Some menstrual discomfort is common, but acute discomfort is usually indicative of some disorder. Among the disorders sometimes causing DYSMENORRHOEA are myoma of the uterus, endometrial cysts, or displacement of the uterus. Menstrual pain may, in some cases, be related to tension or anxiety.

Excessive bleeding, or prolonged periods, called menorrhagia, is sometimes an indication of tumours, polyps, cancer, or inflammation.

Menstruation usually starts between the ages of 11 and 14 and continues into the forties. At first the periods may be irregular, but once they are established they usually occur in a fairly definite rhythm, at intervals of 21 to 35 days. In these regular cycles, there may be monthly variations of a few days, which are considered to be quite normal. These cycles may be influenced by changes in climate or living conditions, or by emotional factors. Slight irregularities, especially if they occur over a period of time, may be warnings of disturbance of either the thyroid or pituitary glands, or of tumours of the uterus or ovaries.

Occasionally menstruation does not occur at puberty. This condition is known as primary AMENORRHOEA. It may be caused by underdevelopment or malformation of the reproductive organs, or by glandular disturbances, which generally can be corrected by the administration of hormones.

General ill health, a change in climate or living conditions, emotional shock or, frequently, either the hope or fear of becoming pregnant can sometimes stop menstruation after it has begun. This is called secondary amenorrhoea. If this cessation is of short duration, it is not a cause for alarm. If it continues over a long period of time, and there is also the problem of infertility, hormone treatments may be necessary.

anovular m., anovulatory m. periodic uterine bleeding without preceding ovulation.

vicarious m. bleeding from extragenital mucous membrane at the time one would normally expect the menstrual period.

menstruum ('menstrooəm) a solvent medium.

mensuration (ˌmensyuh'rayshən, ˌmenshə-) the process of measuring.

mental ('ment'l) 1. pertaining to the mind. 2. pertaining to the chin.

m. handicap faulty or inadequate development of the brain which brings with it some degree of impaired adaptation in learning, social adjustment, or maturation, or in all three areas.

Mental handicap is not a disease; it is a general term for a wide range of conditions, resulting from many different causes. Many of these are directly related to various diseases, either in the mother during pregnancy, or in the infant; only some are hereditary, such as DOWN'S SYNDROME. The general health of the mother and the economic situation of the family may also play a role in this condition.

Mental handicap is a relative term. Its meaning depends on what society demands of the individual in learning, skills, and social responsibility. Many people who are considered handicapped in the complex modern world would get along normally in a simpler society.

DIAGNOSIS. There is no absolute measurement for handicap. At one time the different types were classified only according to the apparent severity of the handicap. Since the most practical standard was intelligence, the degree of handicap was based on the score of the patient on intelligence, or IQ, tests. The average person is considered to have an IQ of between 90 and 110. Those who score below 70 are considered mentally handicapped.

In the past, the different groupings were classified in terms such as feebleminded, idiot, imbecile and moron. Today, most doctors use the following classifications: for IQs from 50 to 70, mild; 35 to 50, moderate; 20 to 35, severe; under 20, profound. Whatever classifications are used, it is agreed that IQ measurements are only one of the factors to be considered in determining mental handicap. Others, such as the person's adaptability to his surroundings, the services and training available to him, and the amount of control he has over his emotions, are also very important.

About 85 per cent of the people who are considered mentally handicapped are in the least severe, or mild group. Those in this group do not usually have any obvious physical defects and for this reason are not always easy to identify as mentally handicapped while they are still infants. Sometimes such a child's mental handicaps do not show up until he enters school, where he has difficulty in learning and keeping up with others in his age group.

Many of those in the mild category, when they grow up, find employment or a place in society suitable to their abilities, and are no longer identified as mentally handicapped. In general, most of those who are mildly handicapped are much closer to being normal than abnormal.

Many conditions that can cause severe handicap can be diagnosed during pregnancy, and in some cases proper treatment can lessen or even prevent handicap. Proper care for the mother during pregnancy and for the baby in his first months of life are also important.

CAUSES. There are many causes of mental handicap. Many are known, many are simply suspected. No apparent defect can be found in the vast majority of the mentally handicapped. The specific cause of their handicap cannot be pinpointed. There are factors, however, that have been proved by research to contribute to handicap.

A child whose mother did not receive antenatal care is more likely to be handicapped. Financial hardship, a broken home, a lack of intellectual stimulation in the family, or a deprived environment can play important roles. Unfavourable health factors, such as poor diet or insufficient medical care, can lead to poor physical condition, which may cause a lower level of performance.

Other physical factors may also be involved. A child born prematurely may occasionally not develop entirely normally. Heredity may play a part in some cases when certain combinations of parents' genes may result in faulty metabolism which affects the normal development of the brain.

The conditions that are known to cause mental handicap can occur at any time from conception through early childhood. At the time of conception, there may be genetic irregularities. During pregnancy, certain infections, such as rubella, syphilis, or meningitis, and other conditions such as glandular disorder, poor antenatal care, injury, or inadequate diet can lead to handicap. At the time of birth, prolonged labour, unusual stress, damage in the course of birth, or lack of oxygen can cause brain damage. During infancy and early childhood diseases, glandular imbalances, accidents such as a blow on the head, and disorders of metabolism may be responsible.

PREVENTION. Some types of mental handicap can be prevented; others cannot. The causes and diseases that offer some hope of prevention are discussed below.

Metabolic or Hormonal Disorders. PHENYLKETONURIA, or PKU, is a congenital defect in the metabolism of the amino acid phenylalanine. If PKU is diagnosed in the first few months of life and controlled by a special diet, mental handicap can be prevented.

GALACTOSAEMIA is a disorder of galactose metabolism. This condition can also be detected in the newborn, and mental handicap can be prevented if the infant is given no milk during the first few weeks of life.

A deficiency in a hormone that has a specific effect on the activities of other organs can have various consequences. The best known condition of this kind is hypothyroidism, which results in CRETINISM. Hormone imbalances can often be treated by injections of artificial hormones to correct the imbalance.

Haemolytic Disease of the Newborn. Occasionally the blood of the mother and that of her unborn child may be incompatible because of a difference in the RH FACTOR. The infant suffering from haemolytic disease of the newborn can be treated by exchange or intrauterine fetal transfusion.

Infections. If the mother contracts RUBELLA during pregnancy, especially during the first 3 months, it may result in defects of the baby's heart and eyes as well as damage to the brain.

SYPHILIS (but not gonorrhoea) in the mother can cause mental handicap. This disease can be discovered by blood tests, and if it is treated soon enough, it may not damage the child.

MENINGITIS in childhood can result in severe damage to the brain. Fortunately, modern drugs can usually cure the disease and prevent mental handicap.

TREATMENT. Some types of mental handicap can be prevented or lessened by proper medical treatment; most, however, cannot. Almost all handicapped children can benefit from special education and training which can lead to greater independence.

Parents who believe that their child is not developing at a proper rate or that he shows symptoms of handicap should consult their family doctor or local child care clinic at once. It may be very difficult to face the fact that a child may be mentally handicapped, but the sooner it is faced the better chance there is of developing a programme to help the child make the best adjustment possible. A complete study of the child's condition can be arranged. From this, it will be possible to say how severe the handicap is and what improvement can be expected; a programme of education and training for him will be planned. The doctor or agency will also be familiar with the kinds of help that are available in the community. Many school systems now have special programmes for mentally handicapped children, and help is available from other agencies, both public and private.

MENCAP (Royal Society for Mentally Handicapped Children and Adults) provides community support to sufferers and their families via a network of 450 local societies and 12 regional offices.

Today health authorities liaise with local authorities and voluntary organizations to provide a network of day centres, sheltered workshops, special schools and other facilities for the mentally handicapped and their families.

INSTITUTIONS. A very small percentage of children are mentally handicapped to such a degree that they cannot learn to care for themselves. In these cases, the child can usually be better cared for in a residential school or other institution.

A decision of this sort should be made by the parents with the help and advice of a professionally qualified person in the community who is familiar with the various alternatives available. Among the factors that must be seriously considered are how disruptive the child is to the home and other children, whether the family can give the child the care and attention he needs, whether an institution could better meet the child's needs, and whether the type and location of the institution are suitable.

It is always a difficult decision for parents to send a mentally handicapped child to an institution, but with professional guidance all factors can be taken into consideration, and the decision is likely to be one that brings the most benefit to everyone in the family.

m. hygiene the science that deals with the development of healthy mental and emotional reactions.

m. mechanism an unconscious and indirect manner of gratifying a repressed desire.

mentha ('menthə) mint.

m. piperata peppermint oil.

menthol ('menthol) an alcohol from various mint oils or produced synthetically, used locally to relieve itching and by inhalation for treatment of upper respiratory tract disorders.

mentoplasty ('mentoh,plastee) plastic surgery of the chin; surgical correction of deformities and defects of the chin.

mentum ('mentəm) [L.] *chin.*

mepacrine ('mepə,krin) a synthetic drug used as an antimalarial agent and in the treatment of giardiasis. Its use as an antimalarial has largely been replaced by chloroquine. It is a yellow fluorescent dye also used in chromosome banding. Called also *quinacrine.*

mepenzolate (mə'penzoh,layt) an anticholinergic used in the form of the bromide to relieve abdominal pain, gaseous distention, and diarrhoea associated with colonic disease.

meperidine (mə'peri,deen) pethidine.

mephitic (mə'fitik) noxious; foul smelling.

meprobamate (mə'prohbə,mayt) a minor tranquillizer and skeletal muscle relaxant.

meptazinol (mep'tazinol) a newer narcotic analgesic claimed to cause less respiratory depression. It has a relatively quick onset of action but a short duration of action of 2 to 4 hours. Nausea and vomiting are quite common and the drug appears not to have any great advantage over more established agents.

Meptid ('meptid) trademark for a preparation of meptazinol.

mepyramine (me'pierə,meen) an antihistamine drug used as the maleate salt in the treatment of allergic reactions.

mEq milliequivalent.

meralgia (mi'ralji·ə) pain in the thigh.

m. paraesthetica a condition of numbness and tingling on the anterolateral aspect of the thigh, rarely accompanied by pain; it is due to entrapment of the lateral femoral cutaneous nerve at the inguinal ligaments.

Merbentyl (mər'bentil) trademark for preparations of dicyclomine hydrochloride, an anticholinergic.

mercaptan (mər'kaptan) an alcohol in which oxygen is replaced by sulphur.

mercaptopurine (mə,kaptoh'pyooə·reen) a yellow crystalline compound used as an antineoplastic agent, primarily in acute leukaemia.

mercurial (mər'kyooə·ri·əl) 1. pertaining to mercury. 2. a preparation containing mercury.

mercurialism (mər'kyooə·ri·ə,lizəm) chronic mercury poisoning.

mercuric (mər'kyooə·rik) pertaining to mercury as a bivalent element; containing bivalent mercury.

mercurous ('mərkyuhrəs) pertaining to mercury as a monovalent element; containing monovalent mercury.

mercury ('mərkyə·ree) a chemical element, atomic number 80, atomic weight 200.59, symbol Hg. (See table of elements in Appendix 2.) A heavy liquid; called also *quicksilver*. Mercury forms two sets of classes of compounds: mercurous, in which a single atom of mercury combines with a monovalent radical, and mercuric, in which a single atom of mercury combines with a bivalent radical. Mercury and its salts have been employed therapeutically as purgatives; as alternatives in chronic inflammations; and as antisyphilitics, intestinal antiseptics, disinfectants, and astringents. They are absorbed by the skin and mucous membranes, causing chronic mercurial poisoning, or hydrargyria. The mercuric salts are more soluble and irritant than the mercurous.

ammoniated m. a compound used as an antiseptic skin and ophthalmic ointment.

m. poisoning acute or chronic disease caused by mercury and its salts. The *acute* form, due to ingestion, is marked by severe abdominalgia, metallic taste in the mouth, vomiting, bloody diarrhoea with watery stools, oliguria or anuria (usually at onset), and corrosion and ulceration of the entire digestive tract. The *chronic* form, due to absorption by the skin and mucous membranes, inhalation of vapours, or ingestion of mercury salts, is marked by stomatitis, metallic taste in the mouth, a blue line along the border of the gum, sore hypertrophied gums that bleed easily, loosening of the teeth, erethism, excessive secretion of saliva, tremors, and incoordination. Called also *mercurialism* and *hydrargyrism*.

m.-vapour lamp one in which air is exhausted from the tube and replaced by mercury vapour, through which passes a strong electric current, resulting in a powerful ultraviolet light. Quartz glass permits the ultaviolet rays to pass though.

meridian (mə'ridi·ən) an imaginary line on the surface of a globe or sphere, connecting the opposite ends of its axis. adj. **meridional**.

mero- word element. [Gr.] 1. *part.* 2. *thigh.*

meroblastic (,meroh'blastik) partially dividing; undergoing cleavage in which only part of the egg participates.

merocele ('miə·roh,seel) femoral hernia.

merocrine ('meroh,krien, -krin) partly secreting: denoting that type of glandular secretion in which the secreting cell remains intact throughout the process of formation and discharge of the secretory products, as in the salivary and pancreatic glands; see also APOCRINE and HOLOCRINE.

merogenesis (,meroh'jenəsis) cleavage of an ovum.

merogony (mə'rogənee) the development of only a portion of an ovum. adj. **merogonic.**

meromelia (,meroh'meeli·ə) congenital absence of a part, but not all, of a limb.

meromicrosomia (,meroh,miekroh'sohmi·ə) unusual smallness of some part of the body.

meromyosin (,meroh'mieəsin) a fragment of the myosin molecule isolated by treatment with proteolytic enzyme; there are two types, heavy (H-meromyosin) and light (L-meromyosin).

merorachischisis (,merohrə'kiskisis) fissure of part of the spinal cord.

merosmia (mə'rozmi·ə) inability to perceive certain odours.

merotomy (mə'rotəmee) a cutting into segments.

merozoite (,meroh'zoh·iet) one of the organisms formed by multiple fission (schizogony) of a sporozoite within the body of the host.

mersalyl ('mərsəlil) an obsolete mercurial diuretic which prevents reabsorption of water in the renal tubules, so reducing oedema in heart failure and renal insufficiency.

mes(o)- word element. [Gr.] *middle.*

mesalazine (mə'salizeen) 5-aminosalicylic acid, used in the treatment and prophylaxis of patients intolerant to sulphasalazine.

mesangiocapillary (me,sanjiohkə'pilə·ree) pertaining to or affecting the mesangium and the associated capillaries.

mesangium (me'sanji·əm) the thin membrane supporting the capillary loops in renal glomeruli. adj. **mesangial.**

mesaortitis (,mesay·aw'tietis) inflammation of the tunica media of the aorta.

mesarteritis (,mesahtə'rietis) inflammation of the tunica media of an artery.

mesatipellic (mes,ati'pelik) having a round pelvis.

mescaline ('meskə,leen) a poisonous alkaloid derived from the flowering heads (mescal buttons) of a Mexican cactus, which produces hallucinations of sound and colour (see also HALLUCINOGEN and DRUG ABUSE).

mescalism ('meskə,lizəm) intoxication due to mescal buttons or mescaline.

mesencephalitis (,mesen,kefə'lietis, -,sef-) inflammation of the mesencephalon, or midbrain.

mesencephalon (,mesen'kefə,lon, -'sef-) 1. the midbrain. 2. the middle of the three primary brain vesicles of the embryo. adj. **mesencephalic.**

mesencephalotomy (,mesen,kefə'lotəmee, -,sef-) surgical production of lesions in the midbrain for the relief of intractable pain.

mesenchyma (me'sengkimə) the meshwork of embryonic connective tissue in the mesoderm from which are formed the connective tissues of the body and also the blood vessels and lymph vessels. adj. **mesenchymal.**

mesenchyme ('meseng,kiem) mesenchyma.

mesenchymoma (,mesengkie'mohmə) a mixed mesenchymal tumour composed of two or more cellular elements that are not commonly associated, exclusive of fibrous tissue.

mesenterectomy (,mesentə'rektəmee) resection of the mesentery.

mesenteriopexy (,mesen'terioh,peksee) fixation or suspension of a torn mesentery.

mesenteriorrhaphy (,mesenteri'orəfee) suture of the mesentery.

mesenteriplication (,mesen,teriplie'kayshən) the operation of taking a tuck in the mesentery to shorten it.

mesenteritis (,mesentə'rietis) inflammation of the mesentery.

mesenterium (,mesen'teeri·əm) mesentery.

mesenteron (me'sentə,ron) the midgut.

mesentery ('mesənta·ree, 'mez-) a membranous fold attaching various organs to the body wall, especially the peritoneal fold attaching the small intestine to the dorsal body wall. adj. **mesenteric.**

mesiad ('meezi,ad) toward the middle or centre.

mesial ('meezi·əl) situated in the middle; median; nearer the middle line of the body or nearer the centre of the dental arch.

mesially ('meezi·əlee) toward the median line.

mesiobuccal (,meezioh'buk'l) pertaining to or formed by the mesial and buccal surfaces of a tooth, or the mesial and buccal walls of a tooth cavity.

mesiocervical (,meezioh'sərvik'l, -sə'vie-) pertaining to the mesial surface of the neck of a tooth.

mesioclusion (,meezi·ə'kloozhən) anteroclusion; malrelation of the dental arches with the mandibular arch anterior to the maxillary arch (prognathism).

mesiodistal (,meezioh'dist'l) pertaining to the mesial and distal surfaces of a tooth.

mesiolabial (,meezioh'laybi·əl) pertaining to the mesial and labial surfaces of a tooth or a tooth cavity.

mesion ('meezi·ən) the plane dividing the body into right and left symmetrical halves.

mesmerism ('mezmə,rizəm) hypnotism.

mesna ('meznə) an agent that reacts with the acrolein metabolite of cyclophosphamide and ifosfamide, preventing urinary tract toxicity.

mesoappendix (,mesoh·ə'pendiks) the peritoneal fold connecting the appendix to the ileum.

mesoblast ('mesoh,blast) the mesoderm, especially in the early stages.

mesobronchitis (,mesohbrong'kietis) inflammation of middle coat of the bronchi.

mesocaecum (,mesoh'seekəm) the occasionally occurring mesentery of the caecum.

mesocardia (,mesoh'kahdi·ə) location of the apex of the heart in the midline of the thorax.

mesocardium (,mesoh'kahdi·əm) the part of the embryonic mesentery which connects the embryonic heart with the body wall in front and the foregut behind.

mesocephalon (,mesoh'kefə,lon, -'sef-) mesencephalon, or midbrain.

mesococcus (,mesoh'kokəs) pl. *mesococci* [L.] a spherical microorganism of medium size.

mesocolon (,mesoh'kohlon) the peritoneal process attaching the colon to the posterior abdominal wall, and called ascending, descending, or transverse, according to the portion of the colon to which it attaches.

pelvic m., sigmoid m. the peritoneum attaching the sigmoid colon to the posterior abdominal wall.

mesocolopexy (,mesoh'kohloh,peksee) suspension or fixation of the colon.

mesocoloplication (,mesoh,kohlohplie'kayshən) plication of the mesocolon to limit its mobility.

mesocord ('mesoh,kawd) an umbilical cord adherent to the placenta.

mesoderm ('mesoh,dərm) the middle of the three

primary germ layers of the embryo, lying between the ectoderm and entoderm; from it are derived the connective tissue, bone, cartilage, muscle, blood and blood vessels, lymphatics, lymphoid organs, notochord, pleura, pericardium, peritoneum, kidneys, and gonads. adj. **mesodermal, mesodermic**.

somatic m. the outer layer of the developing mesoderm.

splanchnic m. the inner layer of the developing mesoderm.

mesodiastolic (ˌmesohˌdieə'stolik) pertaining to the middle of the diastole.

mesoduodenum (ˌmesohˌdyooə'deenəm) the mesenteric fold that in early fetal life encloses the duodenum.

mesoepididymis (ˌmesohˌepi'didiməs) a fold of tunica vaginalis connecting the epididymis and testis.

mesogastrium (ˌmesoh'gastri·əm) the portion of the primitive mesentery that encloses the stomach and from which the greater omentum develops. adj. **mesogastric**.

mesoileum (ˌmesoh'ili·əm) the mesentery of the ileum.

mesojejunum (ˌmesohji'joonəm) the mesentery of the jejunum.

mesolymphocyte (ˌmesoh'limfohˌsiet) a medium-sized lymphocyte.

mesomere ('mesohˌmiə) 1. a blastomere of size intermediate between a macromere and a micromere. 2. a midzone of the mesoderm between the epimere and hypomere.

mesometrium (mesoh'meetri·əm) the portion of the broad ligament below the mesovarium.

mesomorph ('mesohˌmawf) 1. an individual having the type of body build in which mesodermal tissues predominate: there is relative preponderance of muscle, bone, and connective tissue, usually with heavy, hard physique of rectangular outline. 2. a well-proportioned individual.

mesomorphy ('mesohˌmawfee) the condition of being a mesomorph. adj. **mesomorphic**.

meson ('meson, 'meez-) 1. mesion. 2. any elementary particle having a mass intermediate between the mass of the electron and that of the proton.

mesonephroma (ˌmesohnə'frohmə) a malignant tumour of the female genital tract, usually the ovary, formerly thought to arise from mesonephric rests. Two types are recognized: one of müllerian duct derivation, the other an embryonal tumour occurring chiefly in children; the latter may also arise in the testis.

mesonephron (ˌmesoh'nefron) mesonephros.

mesonephros (ˌmesoh'nefros) pl. *mesonephroi* [Gr.] the excretory organ of the embryo, arising caudad to the pronephros and using its duct. adj. **mesonephric**.

mesopexy ('mesohˌpeksee) repair of the mesentery; mesenteriopexy.

mesophile ('mesohˌfiel) a microorganism that grows best at 20 to 55 °C.

mesophlebitis (ˌmesohfli'bietis) inflammation of the tunica media of a vein.

mesorchium (me'sawki·əm) the portion of the primitive mesentery enclosing the fetal testis, represented in the adult by a fold between the testis and epididymis. adj. **mesorchial**.

mesorectum (ˌmesoh'rektəm) the fold of peritoneum connecting the upper portion of the rectum with the sacrum.

mesoropter (ˌmesə'roptə) the normal position of the eyes with their muscles at rest.

mesorrhaphy (me'so·rəfee) suture of the mesentery.

mesosalpinx (ˌmesoh'salpingks) the part of the broad ligament above the mesovarium, investing the uterine tube.

mesosigmoid (ˌmesoh'sigmoyd) the peritoneal fold by which the sigmoid flexure is attached to the abdominal wall.

mesosigmoidopexy (ˌmesohsig'moydohˌpeksee) fixation of the mesosigmoid in prolapse of the rectum.

mesosome ('mesohˌsohm) an invagination of the bacterial cell membrane, forming organelles thought to be the site of cytochrome enzymes and the enzymes of oxidative phosphorylation and the citric acid cycle.

mesosternum (ˌmesoh'stərnəm) the middle piece or body of the sternum.

mesotendineum, mesotendon (ˌmesohten'dini·əm; ˌmesoh'tendən) the connective tissue sheath attaching a tendon to its fibrous sheath.

mesothelial (ˌmesoh'theeli·əl) pertaining to the mesothelium.

mesothelioma (ˌmesohˌtheeli'ohmə) a malignant tumour made up of cells derived from the mesothelium. Often associated with asbestosis.

mesothelium (ˌmesoh'theeli·əm) the layer of flat cells, derived from the mesoderm, that lines the body cavity of the embryo. In the adult it forms the simple squamous epithelium that covers the surface of all true serous membranes (peritoneum, pericardium, pleura).

mesotympanum (ˌmesoh'timpənəm) the portion of the middle ear medial to the tympanic membrane.

mesovarium (ˌmesoh'vair·ri·əm) the portion of the broad ligament between the mesometrium and mesosalpinx, enclosing and holding the ovary in place.

Mestinon ('mestinon) tradename for pyridostigmine, an anticholinesterase drug.

mestranol ('mestrəˌnol) an oestrogenic agent, used in combination with various progestogens as an oral contraceptive.

meta- word element. [Gr.] 1. *change, transformation, exchange*. 2. *after, next*. 3. the 1,3-position in derivatives of benzene.

metabasis (mə'tabəsis) change in the manifestations or course of a disease.

metabiosis (ˌmetəbie'ohsis) the dependence of one organism upon another for its existence; commensalism.

metabolism (mə'tabəˌlizəm) the sum of the physical and chemical processes by which living organized substance is built up and maintained (anabolism), and by which large molecules are broken down into smaller molecules to make energy available to the organism (catabolism). adj. **metabolic.** Essentially these processes are concerned with the disposition of the nutrients absorbed into the blood following digestion.

There are two phases of metabolism: the anabolic and the catabolic phase. The anabolic, or constructive, phase is concerned with the conversion of simpler compounds derived from the nutrients into living, organized substances that the body cells can use. In the catabolic, or destructive, phase these organized substances are reconverted into simpler compounds, with the release of energy necessary for the proper functioning of the body cells. The rate of metabolism can be increased by exercise; by elevated body temperature, as in a high fever, which can more than double the metabolic rate; by hormonal activity, such as that of thyroxine, insulin, and adrenaline; and by specific dynamic action that occurs following the ingestion of a meal.

The basal metabolic rate refers to the lowest rate obtained while an individual is at complete physical and mental rest. Metabolic rate usually is expressed in terms of the amount of heat liberated during the chemical reactions of metabolism. About 25 per cent of all energy from nutrients is utilized by the body to carry on its normal function; the remainder becomes heat.

basal m. the minimal energy expended for the maintenance of respiration, circulation, peristalsis, muscle tonus, body temperature, glandular activity, and the other vegetative functions of the body.

inborn error of m. a genetically determined biochemical disorder in which a specific enzyme defect produces a metabolic block that may have pathological consequences at birth, as in phenylketonuria, or in later life.

metabolite (mə'tabə,liet) any substance produced during metabolism.

metabolize (mə'tabə,liez) to subject to or be transformed by metabolism.

metacarpal (,metə'kahp'l) 1. pertaining to the metacarpus. 2. a bone of the metacarpus.

metacarpectomy (,metəkah'pektəmee) excision or resection of a metacarpal bone.

metacarpophalangeal (,metə,kahpohfə'lanji·əl) pertaining to the metacarpus and phalanges of the fingers.

metacarpus (,metə'kahpəs) the part of the hand between the wrist and fingers, its skeleton being five bones (metacarpals) extending from the carpus to the phalanges.

metacentric (,metə'sentrik) having the centromere almost at the middle of the replicating chromosome.

metacercaria (,metəsər'kair·ri·ə) pl. *metacercariae;* the encysted resting or maturing stage of a trematode parasite in the tissues of an intermediate host.

metachromasia (,metəkroh'mayzi·ə) 1. failure to stain true with a given stain. 2. the different coloration of different tissues produced by the same stain. 3. change of colour produced by staining. adj. **metachromatic.**

metachromatism (,metə'krohmə,tizəm) metachromasia.

metachromophil (,metə'krohmə,fil) not staining normally.

metagenesis (,metə'jenəsis) alteration of generations.

Metagonimus (,metə'gonimәs) a genus of trematodes, including *M. yokogawai*, which is parasitic in the small intestine of fish-eating mammals, and occasionally of man, in Japan, China, Indonesia, the Balkans, and Israel.

metal ('met'l) any chemical element marked by lustre, malleability, ductility, and conductivity of electricity and heat, and which will ionize positively in solution. adj. **metallic.**

alkali m. one of a group of monovalent elements including lithium, sodium, potassium, rubidium, and caesium.

m. fume fever an occupational disorder with malaria-like symptoms occurring in those engaged in welding and other metallic operations and due to the volatilized metals. It includes brassfounder's fever (brass chill, brazier's chill) and spelter's fever (zinc chill, zinc fume fever).

metalloenzyme (mə,taloh'enziem) any enzyme containing tightly bound metal atoms, e.g., the cytochromes.

metalloid ('metə,loyd) 1. any element with both metallic and nonmetallic properties. 2. any metallic element that has not all the characters of a typical metal.

metalloporphyrin (mə,taloh'pawfirin) a combination of a metal with porphyrin, as in haem.

metalloprotein (mə,taloh'prohteen) a protein molecule bound to a metal ion, e.g., haemoglobin.

metallurgy (me'taləjee) the science and art of using metals.

metamere ('metə,miə) one of a series of homologous segments of the body of an animal.

metamorphopsia (,metəmaw'fopsi·ə) defective vision, with distortion of the shape of objects looked at.

metamorphosis (,metə'mawfəsis) change of structure or shape; particularly, transition from one developmental stage to another, as from larva to adult form. adj. **metamorphic.**

fatty m. any normal or pathological transformation of fat, including fatty infiltration and fatty degeneration.

Metamucil (,metə'myoosil) trademark for preparations of ispaghula, a bulk laxative.

metamyelocyte (,metə'mieəloh,siet) a precursor in the granulocytic series, being a cell intermediate in development between a myelocyte and the mature, segmented (polymorphonuclear) granular leukocyte, and having a U-shaped nucleus.

metanephrine (,metə'nefreen) a urinary metabolite of adrenaline.

metanephros (,metə'nefros) pl. *metanephroi* [Gr.] the permanent embryonic kidney, developing later than and caudad to the mesonephros. adj. **metanephric.**

metaphase ('metə,fayz) the second stage of cell division (mitosis or meiosis), in which the chromosomes, each consisting of two chromatids, are arranged in the equatorial plane of the spindle prior to separation.

metaphysis (mə'tafisis) pl. *metaphyses* [Gr.] the wider part at the end of the shaft of a long bone, adjacent to the epiphyseal disc. adj. **metaphyseal.**

metaplasia (,metə'playzi·ə) the change in the type of adult cells in a tissue to a mature form abnormal for that tissue. adj. **metaplastic.**

agnogenic myeloid m. a condition characterized by foci of extramedullary haemopoiesis and by splenomegaly, immature red and white cells in the peripheral blood, and mild to moderate anaemia.

metapneumonic (,metənyoo'monik) succeeding or following pneumonia.

metapsychology (,metəsie'koləjee) the branch of speculative psychology that deals with the significance of mental processes that are beyond empirical verification.

metaraminol (,metə'rami,nol) an ephedrine compound used as a sympathomimetic and pressor agent.

metarubricyte (,metə'roobri,siet) an orthochromatic normoblast.

metastasis (mə'tastəsis) pl. *metastases* [Gr.] 1. the transfer of disease from one organ or part to another not directly connected with it. It may be due either to the transfer of pathogenic microorganisms (e.g., tubercle bacilli) or to transfer of cells, as in malignant tumours. 2. *metastases*, a growth of pathogenic microorganisms or of abnormal cells distant from the site primarily involved by the morbid process. adj. **metastatic.** See also CANCER.

metastasize (mə'tastə,siez) to form new foci of disease in a distant part by metastasis.

metasternum (,metə'stərnəm) the xiphoid process.

metatarsal (,metə'tahs'l) 1. pertaining to the metatarsus. 2. a bone of the metatarsus.

metatarsalgia (,metətah'salji·ə) pain and tenderness in the metatarsal region.

metatarsectomy (,metətah'sektəmee) excision or resection of a metatarsal bone.

metatarsophalangeal (,metə,tahsohfə'lanji·əl) pertaining to the metatarsus and the phalanges of the toes.

metatarsus (,metə'tahsəs) the part of the foot between the ankle and the toes, its skeleton being the five bones (metatarsals) extending from the tarsus to the phalanges.

m. primus varus angulation of the first metatarsal

bone toward the midline of the body, producing an angle sometimes of 20 degrees or more between its base and that of the second metatarsal bone.

metathalamus (,metə'thaləməs) the part of the diencephalon composed of the medial and lateral geniculate bodies; often considered to be part of the thalamus.

metathesis (mə'tathəsis) 1. artificial transfer of a morbid process. 2. a chemical reaction in which an element or radical in one compound exchanges places with another element or radical in another compound.

metatrophic (,metə'trofik) utilizing organic matter for food.

Metazoa (,metə'zoh·ə) the division of the animal kingdom that includes the multicellular animals, i.e., all animals except the Protozoa. adj. **metazoal, metazoan.**

metazoon (,metə'zoh·on) pl. *metazoa* [Gr.] an individual organism of the Metazoa.

Metchnikoff theory ('mechnikof) the theory that bacteria and other harmful elements in the body are attacked and destroyed by cells called phagocytes, and that the contest between such harmful elements and the phagocytes produces inflammation. Named after Elie Metchnikoff (1845–1916), Russian zoologist in Paris and winner, with Ehrlich, of the Nobel prize for medicine and physiology in 1908.

metencephalon (,meten'kefə,lon, -'sef-) pl. *metencephala* [Gr.] 1. the part of the central nervous system comprising the pons and cerebellum. 2. the anterior of two brain vesicles formed by specialization of the rhombencephalon in the developing embryo.

Metenix S (,metəniks 'es) trademark for a preparation of metolazone; a diuretic.

meteorism ('meeti·ə,rizəm) tympanites; drumlike distention of the abdomen caused by the presence of gas in the abdomen or intestines.

meteorotropism (,meeti·ə'rotrə,pizəm) the response to influence by meteorological factors noted in certain biological events, such as sudden death, attacks of angina, joint pain, insomnia, and traffic accidents. adj. **meteorotropic.**

-meter word element. [Gr.] *instrument for measuring.*

metformin (met'fawmin) a biguanide hypoglycaemic used in the treatment of diabetes mellitus.

methacycline (,methə'siekleen) a tetracycline analogue used as an oral broad-spectrum antibiotic.

methadone ('methə,dohn) a synthetic compound with pharmacological properties qualitatively similar to those of morphine and heroin.

methaemalbumin (,met·heem'albyoomin) a brownish pigment formed in the blood by the binding of albumin with haem; indicative of intravascular haemolysis.

methaemalbuminaemia (,met·heemal,byoomi'neemi·ə) the presence of methaemalbumin in the blood.

methaemoglobin (,met·heemə'glohbin) a compound formed from haemoglobin by oxidation of the iron atom from the ferrous to the ferric state. A small amount of methaemoglobin is present in the blood normally, but injury or toxic agents convert a larger proportion of haemoglobin into methaemoglobin, which does not function as an oxygen carrier.

methaemoglobinaemia (,met·heemə,glohbi'neemi·ə) methaemoglobin in the blood, usually due to toxic action of drugs or other agents, or to haemolytic processes.

methaemoglobinuria (,met·heemə,glohbi'nyooə·ri·ə) methaemoglobin in the urine.

methamphetamine (,metham'fetə,meen, -min) a central nervous system stimulant and pressor drug; used as the hydrochloride salt. Abuse may lead to dependence. See also AMPHETAMINE.

methandienone (,methan'dieə,nohn) an anabolic steroid used to build up body tissues in wasting diseases.

methane ('meethayn) an inflammable, explosive gas from decomposition of organic matter.

methanol ('methə,nol) a mobile, colourless liquid widely used as a solvent; methyl alcohol.

methaqualone (me'thakwə,lohn) a nonbarbiturate hypnotic similar to barbituates in its effects; no longer commercially available in the UK.

methenamine (me'thenə,meen) a white crystalline powder used as a urinary antiseptic; called also *hexamine.*

m. hippurate a salt of methenamine and hippuric acid, used in infections of the urinary tract.

m. mandelate a salt of methenamine and mandelic acid, used in infections of the urinary tract.

methicillin (,methi'silin) a semisynthetic penicillin which is highly resistant to inactivation by penicillinase; its sodium salt is used parenterally.

methionine (me'thieoh,neen) 1. a sulphur-containing amino acid occurring in proteins, which is an essential component of the diet. 2. a drug used orally in the treatment of paracetamol poisoning.

methocarbamol (,methoh'kahbə,mol) a compound used as a skeletal muscle relaxant.

methodology (,methə'doləjee) the science dealing with principles of procedure in research and study.

methohexitone (,methoh'heksitohn) an ultra-short-acting barbiturate.

methotrexate (,methoh'treksayt) folic acid antagonist used as an antineoplastic agent; it is also used in the treatment of psoriasis.

methotrimeprazine (,methohtrie'meprəzeen) a phenothiazine with sedative and analgesic properties.

methoxamine (me'thoksə,meen) a sympathomimetic amine used for its vasopressor effects.

methoxyphenamine (me,thoksi'fenə,meen) a sympathomimetic drug used as a bronchodilator and nasal decongestant.

methoxypsoralen an acrylic acid compound which induces melanin production on exposure of the skin to ultraviolet light; used in the treatment of idiopathic vitiligo and as a suntan accelerator and protectant.

methyclothiazide (,methikloh'thieə,zied) an orally effective diuretic and antihypertensive.

methyl ('methil, 'meethiel) the monovalent radical, $-CH_3$.

m. alcohol a clear, colourless, inflammable liquid, CH_3OH, used as a solvent and fuel; it is poisonous if taken internally. Called also *methanol* and *wood alcohol.*

m. orange an orange-yellow aniline dye, used as an indicator with a pH range of 3.2–4.4 and a colour change from pink to yellow.

m. salicylate a natural or synthetic wintergreen oil, used as a topical analgesic in rheumatic disorders, lumbago, and sciatica, and as a flavouring agent.

methylamphetamine (,methilam'fetə,meen) a synthetic drug which stimulates the central nervous system and raises the blood pressure. Its usage can be habit forming.

methylate ('methi,layt) 1. a compound of methyl alcohol and a base. 2. to add a methyl group to a substance.

methylated spirit (,methi,laytid 'spirit) a mixture of 95% ethanol and 5% methanol. An industrial spirit which, taken as a drink, is poisonous.

methylation (,methi'layshən) the addition of methyl groups.

methylcellulose (,methil'selyuhlohs, -lohz) a methyl ester of cellulose; used as a bulk laxative and applied topically to the cornea as an artificial tear preparation in impaired tear production. May also be used during certain ophthalmic procedures to protect and lubricate the cornea.

methylcytosine (ˌmethil'sietohˌseen) a pyrimidine occurring in deoxyribonucleic acid.

methyldopa (ˌmethil'dohpə) an oral antihypertensive agent.

methyldopate hydrochloride (ˌmethil'dohpayt) an ethyl ester of methyldopa given by intravenous infusion for acute hypertensive crisis.

methylene blue ('methiˌleen) a synthetic organic compound, in dark green crystals or lustrous crystalline powder, used in treatment of methaemoglobinaemia, as an antidote in cyanide poisoning, as a stain in pathology and bacteriology, and as an antiseptic.

methylglucamine (ˌmethil'glookəˌmeen) meglumine.

methylmalonic acidaemia (ˌmethilmə'lonik) an inborn error of metabolism characterized by excretion of excessive amounts of methylmalonic acid, a structural isomer of succinic acid, in the urine, developmental retardation, hepatomegaly, intermittent neutropenia, thrombocytopenia, and severe metabolic acidosis. It is due to an inability to convert D- to L-methylmalonyl-CoA or the latter to succinyl-CoA or to a defect in the metabolism of vitamin B_{12}.

methylmalonic aciduria (ˌmethilmə'lonik) excretion of excessive amounts of methylmalonic acid in the urine; a characteristic symptom of methylmalonic acidaemia.

methylphenidate (ˌmethil'feniˌdayt) a central nervous system stimulant used in the treatment of attention deficit disorder (childhood hyperactivity) and narcolepsy. Only available through hospitals.

methylphenobarbitone (ˌmethilˌfenoh'bahbitohn) a white crystalline powder used as an anticonvulsant with a slight hypnotic action.

methylprednisolone (ˌmethilpred'nisəˌlohn) a corticosteroid of the glucogenic type, having an anti-inflammatory action similar to that of prednisolone.

methyltestosterone (ˌmethilte'stostə·rohn) an orally effective, synthetic form of testosterone.

methyltransferase (ˌmethil'transfəˌrayz, -'trahnz) any enzyme that catalyses transmethylation.

methyprylone (me'thiprilohn) a white, crystalline powder used as a sedative and hypnotic.

methysergide (ˌmethi'sərjied) a potent serotonin antagonist used in the prophylaxis of migraine; also available as the maleate salt.

metmyoglobin (metˌmieoh'glohbin) a compound formed from myoglobin by oxidation of the ferrous to the ferric state with essentially ionic bonds.

metoclopramide (ˌmetoh'klohprəmied) a dopamine antagonist that stimulates motility of the upper gastrointestinal tract; used for treatment of diabetic gastric stasis (gastroparesis), to facilitate small bowel intubation, to stimulate gastric emptying in barium studies, and as an antiemetic.

metolazone (me'toləˌzohn) a diuretic and saluretic used in the treatment of hypertension and oedema.

metopic (me'topik) pertaining to the forehead.

metoprolol (me'tohprəˌlol) a cardioselective BETA—BLOCKER having a greater effect on β_1-adrenergic receptors of the heart than on the β_2-adrenergic receptors of the bronchi and blood vessels; used for treatment of hypertension.

Metosyn ('metəsin) trademark for preparations of fluocinonide, a synthetic glucocorticoid used topically.

metoxenous (mə'toksənəs) requiring two hosts for the entire life cycle; said of parasites.

metra ('meetrə) the uterus.

metra-, metro- word element. [Gr.] *uterus*.

metralgia (mi'tralji·ə) pain in the uterus.

metratonia (ˌmeetrə'tohni·ə) uterine atony.

metratrophia (ˌmeetrə'trohfi·ə) atrophy of the uterus.

metre ('meetə) the basic unit of linear measure of the metric system, being the equivalent of 39.371 inches; abbreviated m.

metrectasia (ˌmeetrek'tayzi·ə) dilation of the nonpregnant uterus.

metreurynter (ˌmeetrooə'rintə) an inflatable bag for dilating the cervical canal of the uterus.

metreurysis (mi'trooə·risis) dilation of the uterine cervix by means of the metreurynter.

metric ('metrik) 1. pertaining to measures or measurement. 2. having the metre as a basis.

m. system the system of units of measurement that is based on the metre, gram, and litre and in which new units are formed by prefixes denoting multiplication by a power of ten. See also SI UNITS.

metritis (mi'trietis) inflammation of the uterus.

m. dissecans metritis with necrosis of portions of the uterine wall.

puerperal m. infection of the uterus of the puerperal woman, called also *lochiometritis*.

metrizamide (mə'trizəˌmied) a nonionic, water-soluble, iodinated radiographic contrast medium used in myelography and cisternography.

metrocele ('meetrohˌseel) hernia of the uterus.

metrocolpocele (ˌmeetroh'kolpohˌseel) hernia of the uterus with vaginal prolapse.

metrocystosis (ˌmeetrohsi'stohsis) formation of cysts in the uterus.

metrodynia (ˌmeetroh'dini·ə) pain in the uterus.

metroleukorrhoea (ˌmeetrohˌlookə'reeə) leukorrhoea of uterine origin.

metrolymphangitis (ˌmeetrohˌlimfan'jietis) inflammation of the uterine lymphatic vessels.

metromalacoma (ˌmeetrohˌmalə'kohmə) abnormal softening of the uterus.

metronidazole (ˌmetroh'nidaˌzohl) a compound used as a trichomonacide and amoebicide, and in the treatment of anaerobic infections.

metroparalysis (ˌmeetrohpə'ralisis) paralysis of the uterus.

metropathia (meetroh'pathi·ə) any disorder of the uterus.

m. haemorrhagica a disease characterized by excessive, painless menstrual and intermenstrual bleeding. Associated with failure of ovulation and nondevelopment of the corpus luteum.

metropathy (mi'tropəthee) any uterine disorder. adj. **metropathic.**

metroperitoneal (ˌmeetrohˌperitə'neeəl) pertaining to the uterus and peritoneum.

metroperitonitis (ˌmeetrohˌperitə'nietis) inflammation of the peritoneum about the uterus.

metrophlebitis (ˌmeetrohfli'bietis) inflammation of the uterine veins.

metroplasty (ˌmeetrohˌplastee) reconstructive surgery on the uterus.

metroptosis (ˌmeetrop'tohsis) prolapse of the uterus.

metrorrhagia (ˌmeetrə'rayji·ə) uterine bleeding, occurring at completely irregular intervals and independent of menstruation.

metrorrhexis (ˌmeetrə'reksis) rupture of the uterus.

metrorrhoea (ˌmeetrə'reeə) abnormal uterine discharge.

metrosalpingitis (ˌmeetrohˌsalpin'jietis) inflammation of the uterus and uterine tubes.

metrosalpingography (ˌmeetrohˌsalping'gogrəfee) hysterosalpingography; radiography of the uterus and uterine tubes.

metroscope ('meetrohˌskohp) an instrument for examining the uterus.

metrostaxis (ˌmeetroh'staksis) slight but persistent uterine bleeding.

metrostenosis (ˌmeetrohstə'nohsis) stenosis of the uterus.

-metry word element. [Gr.] *measurement.*

metyrapone (me'tirəˌpohn) a compound that selectively inhibits the synthesis of cortisol; used in a test of pituitary reserve.

MeV megaelectron volt.

mexiletine (mek'siliteen) an antiarrhythmic agent used to treat ventricular arrhythmias.

Mexitil ('meksitil) trademark for preparations of mexiletine, an antiarrhythmic.

mezlocillin (ˌmezloh'silin) an extended-spectrum penicillin used parenterally for treatment of serious infections due to susceptible organisms.

Mg chemical symbol, *magnesium.*

mg milligram.

μg microgram.

MGDS Member in General Dental Surgery.

MHC major histocompatibility complex.

mho (moh) the S.I. unit for conductivity. See also SIEMENS.

mianserin (mie'ansərin) a tetracyclic antidepressant.

mication (mie'kayshən) a quick motion, such as winking.

micelle (mie'sel) a supermolecular colloid particle, most often a packet of chain molecules in parallel arrangement.

Michel's suture clips (mi'shelz) small metal clips used for opposing and fixing the skin edges of a wound.

miconazole (mie'konəˌzohl) an antifungal agent used topically for dermatophytic infections such as athlete's foot or vulvovaginal candidiasis, orally for candidiasis of the mouth and gastrointestinal tract, and systemically by intravenous infusion for systemic fungal infections.

micr(o)- word element. [Gr.] *small;* used in naming units of measurement to designate an amount 10^{-6} (one-millionth) the size of the unit to which it is joined, e.g. microgram; symbol μ.

micrencephaly (ˌmiekren'kefəlee, -'sef-) abnormal smallness and underdevelopment of the brain.

microabscess (ˌmiekroh'abses) an abscess visible only under a microscope.

microaerophilic (ˌmiekroh·air·roh'filik) requiring oxygen for growth but at lower concentration than is present in the atmosphere; said of bacteria.

microaggregate (ˌmiekroh'agrigət) a microscopic collection of particles, as of platelets, leukocytes, and fibrin, that occurs in stored blood.

microanalysis (ˌmiekroh·ə'nalisis) the chemical analysis of minute quantities of material.

microanatomy (ˌmiekroh·ə'natəmee) histology.

microaneurysm (ˌmiekroh'anyəˌrizəm) a minute aneurysm occurring on a vessel of small size, as one in the retina of the eye or as occurs in thrombotic purpura.

microangiopathy (ˌmiekrohˌanji'opəthee) a disorder involving the small blood vessels. adj. **microangiopathic.**

thrombotic m. formation of thrombi in the arterioles and capillaries.

microbe ('miekrohb) a microorganism, especially a pathogenic bacterium. adj. **microbial, microbic.**

microbicidal (ˌmiekrohbi'sied'l) destroying microbes.

microbicide (mie'krohbiˌsied) an agent that destroys microbes.

microbiologist (ˌmiekrohbie'oləjist) a specialist in microbiology.

microbiology (ˌmiekrohbie'oləjee) the study of microorganisms, including bacteria, fungi, viruses, and pathogenic protoza; bacteriology. adj. **microbiological.**

microbiota (ˌmiekrohbie'ohtə) the microscopic living organisms of a region. adj. **microbiotic.**

microblast ('miekrohˌblast) a blast of 5 μm or less in diameter.

microblepharia (ˌmiekrohble'fair·ri·ə) abnormal shortness of the vertical dimensions of the eyelids.

microbody ('miekrohˌbodee) any of the cytoplasmic particles found in kidney and liver cells and in certain other cells, surrounded by a limiting membrane, and containing dense crystalline-like inclusions and oxidases.

microbrachius (ˌmiekroh'brayki·əs) a fetus with abnormally small arms.

microcardia (ˌmiekroh'kahdi·ə) abnormal smallness of the heart.

microcephalus (ˌmiekroh'kefələs, -'sef-) an individual with a very small head.

microcephaly (ˌmiekroh'kefəlee, -'sef-) a congenital defect in brain development leading to an abnormally small brain and skull; usually with mental handicap. adj. **microcephalic.**

microcheilia (ˌmiekroh'kieli·ə) abnormal smallness of the lip.

microcheiria (ˌmiekroh'kieri·ə) abnormal smallness of the hands.

microcirculation (ˌmiekrohˌsərkyuh'layshən) the flow of blood through the fine vessels (arterioles, capillaries, and venules). adj. **microcirculatory.**

Micrococcaceae (ˌmiekrohkok'aysi·ee) a family of gram-positive, aerobic or facultatively anaerobic bacteria containing *Staphylococcus* and *Micrococcus.*

Micrococcus (ˌmiekroh'kokəs) a genus of gram-positive bacteria of the family Micrococcaceae found in soil, water, etc.

micrococcus (ˌmiekroh'kokəs) pl. *micrococci* [Gr.] 1. any organism of the genus *Micrococcus.* 2. a very small, spherical microorganism.

microcolon (ˌmiekroh'kohlon) abnormal smallness of the colon.

microcoria (ˌmiekroh'kor·ri·ə) smallness of the pupil.

microcornea (ˌmiekroh'kawni·ə) unusual smallness of the cornea, usually bilateral.

microcrystalline (ˌmiekroh'kristəˌlien) made up of minute crystals.

microcurie (ˌmiekroh'kyooə·ree) one-millionth (10^{-6}) curie; abbreviated μCi.

microcurie-hour (ˌmiekroh'kyooə·reeˌowə) a unit of dose equivalent to that obtained by exposure for one hour to radioactive material disintegrating at the rate of 3.7×10^4 atoms per second; abbreviated μCi-h.

microcyst ('miekrohˌsist) a cyst visible only under a microscope.

microcyte ('miekrohˌsiet) an erythrocyte 5 μm or less in diameter. adj. **microcytic.**

microcythaemia, microcytosis (ˌmiekrohsie'theemi·ə; ˌmiekrohsie'tohsis) a condition in which the erythrocytes are smaller than normal.

microdactyly (ˌmiekroh'daktilee) abnormal smallness of the fingers or toes.

microdissection (ˌmiekrohdie'sekshən, -di-) dissection of tissue or cells under the microscope.

microdontia (ˌmiekroh'donshi·ə) abnormal smallness of the teeth.

microdrepanocytic (ˌmiekrohˌdrepənoh'sitik) containing microcytic and drepanocytic elements, as in sickle cell-thalassaemia disease.

microembolus (ˌmiekroh'embələs) pl. *microemboli* [L.] an embolus of microscopic size.

microerythrocyte (ˌmiekroh·i'rithrohˌsiet) microcyte.

microfarad (ˌmiekroh'farəd) one-millionth (10^{-6}) farad; abbreviated μF.

microfibril (ˌmiekroh'fiebril, -'fib-) an extremely small fibril.

microfilament (ˌmiekroh'filəmənt) any of the submicroscopic filaments found in the cytoplasmic matrix of almost all cells, often in close association with the microtubules. Most cells have some actin microfilaments but other microfilaments exist which are related to the specificity of the cell type. Thus epithelial cells contain cytokeratin microfilaments of which at least 20 exist. Combinations of different numbers of these cytokeratin microfilaments are related to specific epithelial cell types.

microfilaraemia (ˌmiekrohˌfilə'reemi·ə) the presence of microfilariae in the circulating blood.

microfilaria (ˌmiekrohfi'lair·ri·ə) the prelarval stage of Filaroidea in the blood of man and in the tissues of the vector.

microgamete (ˌmiekroh'gameet) the smaller, actively motile male gamete which fertilizes the macrogamete in anisogamy.

microgametocyte (ˌmiekrohgə'meetohˌsiet) 1. a cell that produces microgametes. 2. the male gametocyte of certain Sporozoa, such as malarial plasmodia.

microgastria (ˌmiekroh'gastri·ə) congenital smallness of the stomach.

microgenia (ˌmiekroh'jeeni·ə) abnormal smallness of the chin.

microgenitalism (ˌmiekroh'jenit'lizəm) smallness of the external genitalia.

microglia (mie'krogli·ə) non-neural cells forming part of the adventitial structure of the central nervous system. They are migratory and act as phagocytes of waste products of the nervous system. adj. **microglial.**

microglioma (ˌmiekrohglie'ohmə) a tumour composed of microglial cells.

microglobulin (ˌmiekroh'globyuhlin) any globulin, or any fragment of a globulin, of low molecular weight.

microglossia (ˌmiekroh'glosi·ə) abnormal smallness of the tongue.

micrognathia (ˌmiekroh'nathi·ə) abnormal smallness of the jaws, especially the lower jaw. adj. **micrognathic**.

microgram ('miekrohˌgram) one-millionth (10^{-6}) gram, or one-thousandth (10^{-3}) milligram; abbreviated μg.

micrograph ('miekrohˌgrahf, -ˌgraf) 1. an instrument for recording very minute movements by making a greatly magnified photograph of the minute motions of a diaphragm. 2. a photograph of a minute object or specimen as seen through a microscope.

electron m. a graphic reproduction of an object as viewed with an electron microscope.

Microgynon (ˌmiekroh'gienon) trademark for a fixed combination preparation of ethinyloestradiol and levonorgestrel, an oral contraceptive.

microgyria (ˌmiekroh'jieri·ə) abnormal smallness of convolutions of the brain.

microgyrus (ˌmiekroh'jierəs) an abnormally small, malformed convolution of the brain.

microinfarct (ˌmiekroh'infahkt) a very small infarct due to obstruction of circulation in capillaries, arterioles, or small arteries.

microinjector (ˌmiekroh·in'jektə) an instrument for infusion of very small amounts of fluids or drugs.

microinvasion (ˌmiekroh·in'vayzhən) microscopic extension of malignant cells into adjacent tissue in carcinoma in situ. adj. **microinvasive**.

microlesion (ˌmiekroh'leezhən) a minute lesion.

microlith ('miekrohˌlith) a minute concretion or calculus.

microlithiasis (ˌmiekrohli'thiəsis) the formation of minute concretions in an organ.

m. alveolaris pulmonum, pulmonary alveolar m. a condition simulating pulmonary tuberculosis, with deposition of minute calculi in the alveoli of the lungs.

microlitre ('miekrohˌleetə) one-millionth (10^{-6}) part of a litre, or one-thousandth (10^{-3}) of a millilitre; abbreviated μl.

micromanipulation (ˌmiekrohmə'nipyuh'layshən) the performance of surgery, injections, dissections, etc., by means of micromanipulators.

micromanipulator (ˌmiekrohmə'nipyuhˌlaytə) an instrument for the moving, dissecting, etc., of minute specimens under the microscope.

micromastia (ˌmiekroh'masti·ə) abnormal smallness of the breast.

micromelia (ˌmiekrohmeeli·ə) abnormal smallness of one or more extremities.

micromelus (ˌmie'kroməlәs) an individual with abnormally small limbs.

micromere ('miekrohˌmiə) one of the small blastomeres formed by unequal cleavage of a fertilized ovum.

micrometer (mie'kromitə) an instrument for making minute measurements.

micromethod ('miekrohˌmethəd) a technique dealing with exceedingly small quantities of material.

micrometre ('miekrohˌmeetə) one-thousandth (10^{-3}) of a millimetre or one-millionth (10^{-6}) of a metre; abbreviated μm. Formerly called *micron.*

micrometry (mie'kromətree) measurement of microscopic objects.

micromicro- word element. [Gr.] designating 10^{-12} (one-billionth) part of the unit to which it is joined; now supplanted by the prefix *pico-*.

micromyelia (ˌmiekrohmie'eeli·ə) abnormal smallness of spinal cord.

micromyeloblast (ˌmiekroh'mieəlohˌblast) a small myeloblast. adj. **micromyeloblastic**.

micron ('miekron) pl. *micra,microns* [Gr.] MICROMETRE.

microneedle (ˌmiekroh'need'l) a fine glass needle used in micromanipulation.

microneurosurgery (ˌmiekrohˌnyooə·roh'sərjə·ree) surgery conducted under high magnification with miniaturized instruments on structures of the nervous system.

micronodular (ˌmiekroh'nodyuhlə) marked by the presence of small nodules.

Micronor ('miekrohnor) trademark for a preparation of norethisterone, an oral contraceptive.

micronucleus (ˌmiekroh'nyookli·əs) 1. in ciliate protozoa, the kinetoplast, the smaller of two types of nucleus in each cell, which functions in sexual reproduction. 2. a small nucleus. 3. nucleolus.

micronutrient (ˌmiekroh'nyootri·ənt) a dietary element essential only in small quantities.

micronychia (ˌmiekroh'niki·ə) abnormal smallness of the nails of the fingers or toes.

microorganism (ˌmiekroh'awgəˌnizəm) a microscopic organism; those of medical interest include bacteria, rickettsiae, viruses, fungi, and protozoa.

micropathology (ˌmiekrohpə'tholəjee) 1. the sum of what is known about minute pathological change. 2. pathology of diseases caused by microorganisms.

microphage ('miekrohˌfayj) a small phagocyte; an actively motile neutrophilic leukocyte capable of phagocytosis.

microphakia (ˌmiekroh'fayki·ə) abnormal smallness of the crystalline lens.

microphallus (miekroh'faləs) abnormal smallness of the penis.

microphone ('miekrohˌfohn) a device to pick up sound for purposes of amplification or transmission.

microphonia (ˌmiekroh'fohni·ə) marked weakness of

voice.
microphonic (ˌmiekroh'fonik) 1. serving to amplify sound. 2. cochlear microphonic.
cochlear m. any of the electrical potentials generated in the hair cells of the organ of Corti in response to acoustic stimulation.
microphotograph (ˌmiekroh'fohtəˌgrahf, -ˌgraf) a photograph of small size.
microphthalmia (ˌmiekrof'thalmi·ə) microphthalmos.
microphthalmos (ˌmiekrof'thalmos) abnormal smallness in all dimensions of an eye.
micropinocytosis (ˌmiekrohˌpienohsie'tohsis) the taking up into a cell of specific macromolecules by invagination of the plasma membrane, which is then pinched off, resulting in small vesicles in the cytoplasm. Usually referred to simply as *pinocytosis*.
micropipette (ˌmiekrohpi'pet) a pipette for handling small quantities of liquids (up to 1 ml).
microplethysmography (ˌmiekrohˌplethiz'mogrəfee) the recording of minute changes in the size of a part as produced by circulation of blood.
micropodia (ˌmiekroh'pohdi·ə) abnormal smallness of the feet.
microprobe ('miekrohˌprohb) a minute probe, as used in microsurgery.
micropsia (mie'kropsi·ə) a disorder of visual perception in which objects appear smaller than their actual size.
micropyle ('miekrohˌpiel) an opening through which a spermatozoon enters certain ova.
microradiography (ˌmiekrohˌraydi'ogrəfee) radiography under conditions that permit subsequent microscopic examination or enlargement of the radiograph up to several hundred linear magnifications.
microrespirometer (ˌmiekrohˌrespi'romitə) an apparatus for investigating oxygen utilization in isolated tissues.
microscope ('miekrəˌskohp) an instrument used to obtain an enlarged image of small objects and reveal details of structure not otherwise distinguishable.
acoustic m. one using very high frequency ultrasound waves, which are focused on the object; the reflected or transmitted beam is converted to an image by electronic processing.
binocular m. one with two eyepieces, permitting use of both eyes simultaneously.
compound m. one consisting of two lens systems whereby the image formed by the system near the object is magnified by the one nearer the eye.
darkfield m. one so constructed that illumination is from the side of the field so that details appear light against a dark background.
electron m. a transmission electron microscope or a scanning electron microscope.
fluorescence m. one used for the examination of specimens stained with fluorochromes or fluorochrome complexes, e.g., a fluorescein-labelled antibody, which fluoresces in ultraviolet light.
light m. one in which the specimen is viewed under ordinary illumination.
operating m. one designed for use in performance of delicate surgical procedures, e.g., on the middle ear or small vessels of the heart.
phase m., phase-contrast m. a microscope that alters the phase relationships of the light passing through and that passing around the object, the contrast permitting visualization of the object without the necessity for staining or other special preparation.
scanning electron m. (SEM) an electron microscope that produces a high magnification image of the surface of a metal-coated specimen by scanning an electron beam and building an image from the electrons reflected at each point.
simple m. one that consists of a single lens.
slit lamp m. a corneal microscope with a special attachment that permits examination of the endothelium on the posterior surface of the cornea.
stereoscopic m. a binocular microscope modified to give a three-dimensional view of the specimen.
transmission electron m. (TEM) an electron microscope that produces highly magnified images of ultrathin tissue sections or other specimens. An electron beam passes through the metal-impregnated specimen and is focused by magnetic lenses into an image.
x-ray m. one in which x-rays are used instead of light, the image usually being reproduced on film.
microscopic (ˌmiekrə'skopik) 1. of extremely small size; visible only by aid of a microscope. 2. pertaining to a microscope or to microscopy.
microscopist (mie'kroskəpist) a person skilled in using the microscope.
microscopy (mie'kroskəpee) examination with a microscope.
microsecond ('miekrohˌsekənd) one-millionth (10^{-6}) of a second; abbreviated μs.
microsome ('miekrohˌsohm) any of the vesicular fragments of endoplasmic reticulum produced during disruption and centrifugation of cells. adj. **microsomal.**
microsomia (ˌmiekrə'sohmi·ə) abnormally small size of the body.
microspectroscope (ˌmiekroh'spektrəˌskohp) a spectroscope and microscope combined.
microspherocyte (ˌmiekroh'sfiə·rohˌsiet) an erythrocyte whose diameter is less than normal, but whose thickness is increased.
microspherocytosis (ˌmiekrohˌsfiə·rohsie'tohsis) the presence in the blood of an excessive number of microspherocytes.
microsphygmia (ˌmiekroh'sfigmi·ə) that condition of the pulse in which it is perceived with difficulty by the finger.
microsplenia (ˌmiekroh'spleeni·ə) smallness of the spleen.
microsporid (ˌmiekroh'spor·rid) a secondary skin eruption which is an expression of hypersensitivity to *Microsporum* infection.
Microsporum (ˌmiekroh'spor·rəm) a genus of fungi that cause various diseases of the skin and hair, including the species *M. audouini*, *M. canis (lanosum)*, and *M. fulvum (gypseum)*.
microstomia (ˌmiekroh'stohmi·ə) abnormally decreased size of the mouth.
microsurgery (ˌmiekroh'sərjə·ree) dissection of minute structures under the microscope, with the use of extremely small instruments. With increasingly sophisticated operating microscopes surgeons are now able to perform tissue transfers without the cumbersome standard transfer procedures such as tubed pedicle graft and cross-leg flap that were once necessary to ensure adequate blood supply to the grafted part. Today, microvascular surgery permits anastomosis of peripheral blood vessels less than 2 mm in diameter. Similarly, microneural techniques allow the surgeon to re-establish sensation by repairing or replacing severed and damaged peripheral nerves. Because of the advances in microsurgery, it is possible to reattach amputated parts, provided the health status of the patient and the condition of the amputated part are favourable.
microsyringe (ˌmiekrohsi'rinj) a syringe fitted with a screw-threaded micrometer for accurate measurement of minute quantities.
microtia (mie'krohshi·ə) abnormal smallness of the

pinna of the ear.

microtitre (ˌmiekroh'tietə, -'tee-) a titre of minute quantity.

microtome ('miekroh,tohm) an instrument for making thin sections for microscopic study.

freezing m. one for cutting frozen tissues.

rotary m. one in which wheel action is translated into a back-and-forth movement of the specimen being sectioned.

sliding m. one in which the specimen being sectioned is made to slide on a track.

microtomy (mie'krotəmee) the cutting of thin sections.

microtrauma (ˌmiekroh'trawmə) a microscopic lesion or injury.

microtubule (ˌmiekroh'tyoobyool) any of the slender, tubular structures, composed chiefly of tubulin, found in the cytoplasmic ground substance of nearly all cells; they are involved in maintenance of cell shape and in the movements of organelles and inclusions, are a major structural component in cilia, and form the spindle fibres of mitosis.

Microval ('miekrohval) trademark for a preparation of levonorgestrel, an oral contraceptive.

microvasculature (ˌmiekroh'vaskyuhləchə) the finer vessels of the body, as the arterioles, capillaries, and venules. adj. **microvascular.**

microvillus (ˌmiekroh'viləs) pl. *microvilli;* a minute finger-like process protruding from the free surface of a cell, especially cells of the proximal convoluted renal tubules, of the intestinal epithelium, and of the sinusoidal surface of hepatocytes.

microvolt ('miekroh,vohlt) one-millionth of a volt; abbreviated μV.

microwave ('miekroh,wayv) a wave typical of electromagnetic radiation between far infrared and radiowaves.

micrurgy (mie'krərjee) manipulative technique in the field of a microscope. adj. **micrurgic.**

micturate ('miktyuh,rayt) urinate.

micturition (ˌmiktyuh'rishən) urination.

Midamor ('miedə,mor) trademark for a preparation of amiloride hydrochloride; a potassium-sparing diuretic.

midazolam (mi'dayzəlam, -dazə-) a water-soluble benzodiazepine given intravenously either to induce anaesthesia or as a sedation to cover local anaesthetic blocks or diagnostic procedures such as gastroscopy. Has the advantage over diazepam of not causing pain on injection and having a shorter duration of action. Doses should be reduced in the elderly. It can be given intramuscularly as a premedication.

midbrain ('mid,brayn) the short part of the brain stem just above the pons. It contains the nerve pathways between the cerebral hemispheres and the medulla oblongata, and also contains nuclei (relay stations or centres) of the third and fourth cranial nerves. The centre for visual reflexes, such as moving the head and eyes, is located in the midbrain. Called also *mesencephalon.*

middle lobe syndrome (mid'l lohb) atelectasis of the middle lobe of the right lung, with chronic pneumonitis, due to compression of the bronchus by tuberculous hilar lymph nodes.

midgut ('mid,gut) the region of the embryonic digestive tube into which the yolk sac opens; ahead of it is the foregut and caudal to it is the hindgut.

midline ('mid,lien) the imaginary line that divides the body into right and left halves.

midwife ('mid,wief) 'a person who, having been regularly admitted to a midwifery education programme, duly recognized in the country in which it is located, has successfully completed the prescribed course of studies in midwifery and has acquired the requisite qualifications to be registered and/or legally licensed to practise midwifery. She must be able to give the necessary supervision, care and advice to women during pregnancy, labour and the postpartum period, to conduct deliveries on her own responsibility and to care for the newborn and the infant. This care includes preventative measures, the detection of abnormal conditions in mother and child, the procurement of medical assistance and the execution of emergency measures in the absence of medical help. She has an important task in health counselling and health education, not only for the patients, but also within the family and the community. The work should involve antenatal education and preparation for parenthood and extends to certain areas of gynaecology, family planning and child care. She may practise in hospitals, clinics, health units, domiciliary conditions or in any other service.' Definition adopted by the International Confederation of Midwives and International Federation of Gynaecologists and Obstetricians, in 1972 and 1973 respectively, following amendment of the definition formulated by the World Health Organization.

midwifery (mid'wifə·ree, 'mid,wifə·ree) the practice of assisting at childbirth. See also MIDWIFE.

migraine ('meegrayn, 'mie-) a headache, usually severe, often limited to one side of the head, and sometimes accompanied by nausea and vomiting; called also a *sick headache.* adj. **migrainous.**

Those who suffer from frequent and persistent migraine headaches should have a complete medical evaluation, including a thorough history, to identify, if possible, personal and environmental factors that trigger an attack. Although emotional stress is related to many attacks of headache, the stereotype of migraine sufferers as rigid, compulsive, perfectionists is not applicable to everyone with a migraine headache. Those who do have headache problems related to stress are often helped by BIOFEEDBACK techniques and do not require medication.

Other contributing factors include dietary substances, particularly cheese, chocolate, alcohol, excessive caffeine or sudden withdrawal from caffeine-rich foods, and some food preservatives and artificial flavourings. Skipping meals and fasting can also trigger a headache in certain people. Drugs that are known to precipitate migraine headaches include hormonal contraceptives and the antihypertensive agent reserpine.

The selection of medications for relief of migraine headaches should be based on the individual patient's history, symptoms, and needs. Analgesics may or may not be effective and there is the danger of habituation with prolonged use. Ergotamine tartrate and other ergot alkaloids have been used as specifics for migraine headache for many years. These drugs prevent dilation of the cerebral blood vessels and are most effective when taken in the beginning phase of the headache before throbbing is evident. However, ergot preparations can be habit forming, and they have some unpleasant side-effects. In recent years, propranolol, a beta-adrenergic blocking agent, has been used to control migraine headache in a large number of people. If the migraine is associated with fluid retention during menstruation, a mild diuretic may help avoid attacks.

Information about migraine headaches and doctors who specialize in the treatment of headache problems can be obtained by writing to the British Migraine Association, 178A High Road, Byfleet, Surey or the Migraine Trust, 45 Great Ormond Street, London WC1.

abdominal m. migraine in which abdominal symptoms are prominent.

Migravess ('miegrəves) trademark for combination preparations containing aspirin and metoclopramide, used in migraine.

Migril ('miegril) trademark for a combination preparation containing ergotamine, cyclizine and caffeine, used in migraine attacks.

Mikulicz's disease ('mikoo,lichiz) a benign, chronic lymphocytic infiltration and enlargement of the lacrimal and salivary glands, of unknown origin.

Miles' operation (mielz) rectosigmoidectomy to achieve rectal amputation in the treatment of rectal prolapse, as advocated by Ernest Miles in 1904.

milestone ('miel,stohn) see DEVELOPMENTAL MILESTONES.

miliaria (,mili'air·ri·ə) a cutaneous condition with retention of sweat, which is extravasated at different levels in the skin; called also *prickly heat* or *heat rash*. Treatment of miliaria is directed at reducing sweating generally by reducing the external heat load and avoiding irritating agents and tight clothing. Bland powders may be helpful.

miliary ('milyə·ree) 1. like millet seeds. 2. characterized by the formation of lesions resembling millet seeds.

m. fever an acute infectious disease characterized by fever, profuse sweating and the formation of a great many papules, succeeded by a crop of pustules; called also *sweating sickness*.

m. tuberculosis an acute form of tuberculosis in which minute tubercles are formed in a number of organs of the body, owing to dissemination of the bacilli throughout the body by the bloodstream.

milieu ('meelyər) [Fr.] *surroundings, environment*.

m. extérieur external environment.

m. intérieur internal environment; the blood and lymph in which the cells are bathed.

milium ('mili·əm) pl. *milia* [L.] a whitish nodule in the skin, especially of the face, usually 1 to 4 mm in diameter. Milia are spheroidal epithelial cysts of lamellated keratin lying just under the epidermis, often associated with vellus hair follicles. Popularly called *whitehead*.

milk (milk) 1. a nutrient fluid produced by the mammary gland of many animals for nourishment of young mammals. 2. a liquid (emulsion or suspension) resembling the secretion of the mammary gland.

acidophilus m. milk fermented with cultures of *Lactobacillus acidophilus*; used in gastrointestinal disorders to modify the bacterial flora of the intestinal tract.

m.-alkali syndrome ingestion of milk and absorbable alkali in excess amounts, resulting in kidney damage and elevated blood calcium levels.

casein m. a prepared milk containing very little salts and sugars and a large amount of fat and casein.

condensed m. milk that has been partly evaporated and sweetened with sugar.

dialysed m. milk from which the sugar has been removed by dialysis through a parchment membrane.

evaporated m. milk prepared by evaporation of half of its water content.

m. fever 1. an endemic fever said to be due to the use of unwholesome cow's milk. 2. a form of paralysis due to a metabolic disorder affecting cows near delivery, and usually accompanied by hypocalcaemia.

fortified m. milk made more nutritious by addition of cream, egg white, or vitamins.

homogenized m. milk treated so the fats form a permanent emulsion and the cream does not separate.

m. of magnesia a suspension containing 7 to 8.5 per cent of magnesium hydroxide, used as an antacid and laxative.

modified m. cow's milk made to correspond to composition of human milk.

protein m. milk modified to have a relatively low content of carbohydrate and fat and a relatively high protein content.

witch's m. milk secreted in the breast of a newborn infant.

Milkman's syndrome ('milkmənz) a generalized bone disease marked by multiple transparent stripes of absorption in the long and flat bones.

milli- word element. [Fr.] *one-thousandth;* used in naming units of measurement to designate an amount 10^{-3} the size of the unit to which it is joined, e.g. milligram (0.001 g); symbol m.

milliamperage (,mili'ampə·rij) in radiography, the x-ray tube current during an exposure, measured in milliamperes.

milliampere (,mili'ampair) one-thousandth of an ampere; abbreviated mA.

milliampere-second (,mili,ampair'sekənd) a unit of radiographic exposure equal to the product of the milliamperage and the exposure time in seconds. Abbreviated mAs.

millicurie-hour (,mili'kyooə·ree,owə) a unit of dose equivalent to that obtained by exposure for one hour to radioactive material disintegrating at the rate of 3.7×10^7 atoms per second; abbreviated mCi-h.

milliequivalent (,mili·i'kwivələnt) one-thousandth of a chemical equivalent; abbreviated mEq.

milligram ('mili,gram) one-thousandth of a gram; abbreviated mg.

millilitre ('mili,leetə) one-thousandth of a litre; abbreviated ml.

millimetre ('mili,meetə) one-thousandth of a metre; equivalent of 0.039 inch; abbreviated mm.

millimicro- word element. [Fr., Gr.] formerly used to designate 10^{-9} part of the unit to which it is joined; now supplanted by the prefix *nano-*.

millimole ('mili,mohl) one-thousandth part of a mole; abbreviated mmol.

milliosmole (,mili'ozmohl) one-thousandth of an osmole; abbreviated mosmol.

Millipore filter ('mili,por) trademark for a device used to filter nutrient solutions as they are administered intravenously.

millivolt ('mili,vohlt) one-thousandth of a volt; abbreviated mV.

milphae, milphosis ('milfee; mil'fohsis) the falling out of the eyelashes.

Milroy's disease ('milroyz) hereditary permanent lymphoedema of the legs due to lymphatic obstruction; called also *congenital lymphoedema*.

Milwaukee brace (mil'wawkee) a brace consisting of a leather girdle and neck ring connected by metal struts; used to brace the spine in the treatment of SCOLIOSIS.

Mima ('meemə) a genus of nonmotile, paired, gram-negative, enteric bacilli, causing a variety of hospital-acquired infections, including meningitis, pneumonia, and urinary tract infections.

MIMS (mimz) Monthly Index of Medical Specialities.

min. minim; minimum; minute.

Minamata disease (,minə'mahtə) a severe neurological disorder due to alkyl mercury poisoning, leading to severe permanent neurological and mental disabilities or death; once prevalent among those who ate contaminated seafood from Minamata Bay, Japan.

MIND (miend) National Association for Mental Health. A voluntary organization founded as a charity in 1946 with the aims of promoting improvements in the field of mental health care, of pressing for improvements in statutory mental health services, and of promoting better understanding of the nature and causes of mental disorder. The association has also promoted research and educational activities and operates courses and short conferences in addition to many pilot projects in community care. MIND also offers a legal and welfare rights service to safeguard the rights of patients and mental health workers and to draw attention to legislative anomalies which tend to disadvantage patients. A lawyers' group has brought test cases on selected issues involving mental health and associated legislation.

In addition to a bimonthly journal (*Open Mind*) MIND, 22 Harley Street, London W1N 2ED, produces a wide range of publications and educational material and there are almost 200 local mental health organizations throughout the country.

mind (miend) the psyche; the faculty by which one is aware of surroundings and by which one is able to experience emotions, remember, reason, and make decisions.

mineral ('minə·rəl) any naturally occurring nonorganic homogeneous solid substance. There are 19 or more minerals forming the mineral composition of the body; at least 13 are essential to health. These minerals must be supplied in the diet and generally can be supplied by a varied or mixed diet of animal and vegetable products which meet the energy and protein needs. The Department of Health includes calcium and iron in their recommended daily amounts of food, energy and nutrients for population groups in the United Kingdom.

m. oil a mixture of liquid hydrocarbons from petroleum. Mineral oil is available in both light (light liquid petrolatum) and heavy (liquid, or heavy liquid, petrolatum) grades. Light mineral oil is used chiefly as a vehicle for drugs, but it may also be used as a cathartic and to cleanse the skin. Heavy mineral oil is used as a cathartic, solvent, and oleaginous vehicle. Prolonged use of mineral oil as a cathartic should be avoided because it prevents absorption of the fat-soluble vitamins. Lipid pneumonia caused by aspiration of the oil has been shown to occur in those who habitually take it, especially the elderly.

mineralization (ˌminə·rəlie'zayshən) the addition of mineral matter to the body.

mineralocorticoid (ˌminə·rəloh'kawtiˌkoyd) any of a group of hormones elaborated by the cortex of the ADRENAL GLAND, so called because of their effects on sodium, chloride, and potassium concentrations in the extracellular fluid. They are the adrenocortical hormones that are essential to the maintenance of adequate fluid volume in the extracellular and intravascular fluid compartments, normal cardiac output, and adequate levels of blood pressure. Without sufficient supply of the mineralocorticoids fatal shock from diminished cardiac output can occur very quickly.

The principal mineralocorticoid is *aldosterone*, which accounts for most of the activities of this group of hormones. The primary effects of the mineralocorticoids are increasing the reabsorption of sodium and the secretion of potassium in the renal tubules. Secondary effects are related to the reabsorption of water, serum levels of sodium and potassium, anion reabsorption, and secretion of hydrogen ions. The net result of these activities is maintenance of fluid and electrolyte balance and, therefore, adequate cardiac output.

minim ('minim) a unit of volume (liquid measure) in the apothecaries system, equivalent to 0.0616 ml.

Minims (minimz) trademark for eye drops packaged in single use containers.

Ministry of Agriculture, Fisheries and Food ('minisˌtree) a government department which undertakes research and takes advice from scientific bodies into topics relating to agriculture, fisheries and food; abbreviated MAFF. The Ministry can make recommendations and introduce legislation for changes in policy relating to food and nutrition in the United Kingdom.

Minocin (mi'nohsin) trademark for preparations of minocycline hydrochloride; a tetracycline antibiotic.

minocycline (ˌminoh'siekleen) a semisynthetic broad-spectrum antibiotic of the tetracycline group.

Minovlar (mi'novlah) trademark for combination preparations containing norethisterone and ethinyloestradiol, an oral contraceptive.

minoxidil (mi'noksidil) a potent, long-acting vasodilator, acting primarily on arterioles, used as an antihypertensive.

Mintezol ('mintizol) trademark for a preparation of thiabendazole, an anthelmintic.

miocardia (ˌmioh'kahdi·ə) the contraction of the heart; systole.

miopus (mie'ohpəs) a fetus or infant with two fused heads, one face being rudimentary.

miosis (mie'ohsis) contraction of the pupil.

miotic (mie'otik) 1. pertaining to, characterized by, or causing miosis. 2. an agent that causes contraction of the pupil.

miracidium (mierə'sidi·əm) pl. *miracidia* [Gr.] the free-swimming larva of a trematode parasite which emerges from an egg and penetrates the body of a snail host.

mire (meeə) [Fr.] a figure on the arm of an ophthalmometer, the image of which is reflected on the cornea; used to measure corneal astigmatism.

miscarriage ('miskarij) the lay term used to designate loss of the fetus before it is viable; spontaneous abortion. See also ABORTION.

miscible ('misib'l) susceptible of being mixed.

misogamy (mi'sogəmee) morbid aversion to marriage.

misogyny (mi'sojinee) aversion to women.

misopedia (ˌmisoh'peedi·ə) morbid dislike of children.

Mitchell's disease ('michəlz) erythromelalgia.

mite (miet) any arthropod of the order Acarina except the ticks; they are characterized by minute size, usually transparent or semitransparent body, and other features distinguishing them from the ticks. They may be free living or parasitic on animals or plants, and may produce various irritations of the skin or act as vectors of disease such as scrub typhus.

harvest m. a six-legged red larva of mites of the family Trombiculidae. Its bites produce severe dermatitis.

itch m. *Sarcoptes scabiei.*

Mithracin ('mithrəsin) trademark for preparations of mithramycin.

mithramycin (ˌmithrə'miesin) an antineoplastic antibiotic produced by *Streptomyces argillaceus* and *S. tanashiensis*. Used in the treatment of severe hypercalcaemia due to malignant disease.

mithridatism ('mithrədayˌtizəm) acquisition of immunity to a poison by ingestion of gradually increasing amounts of it.

miticide ('mietiˌsied) an agent destructive to mites.

mitochondria (ˌmietoh'kondri·ə) plural of *mitochondrion* [Gr.] small, spherical to rod-shaped, membrane-bounded cytoplasmic organelles that are the principal sites of ATP synthesis; they also contain enzymes of the citric acid cycle and for fatty acid oxidation, oxidative phosphorylation, and other biochemical pathways. Mitochondria also contain DNA, RNA, and ribosomes; they replicate independently and synthesize some of their own proteins. adj. **mitochondrial.**

mitogen ('mietohˌjen) an agent that induces mitosis and lymphocyte transformation. adj. **mitogenic.**

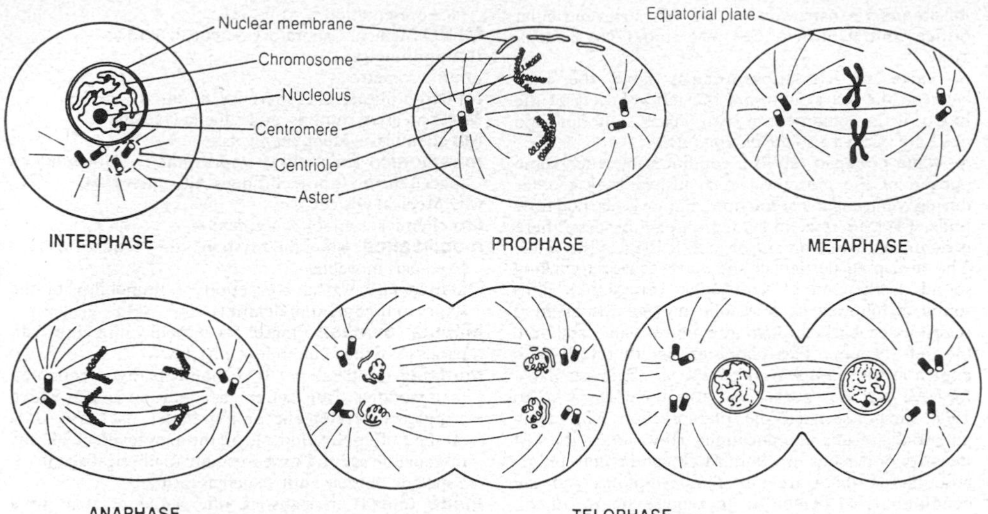

Mitosis, showing details of division. Shown are a pair of identical (homologous) chromosomes. Prior to the onset of mitosis, DNA replicates, giving rise to the double-stranded chromosomes that become apparent during mitosis. In prophase the two strands of each chromosome, attached to a common centromere, can be clearly seen. In metaphase the centromeres of the double-stranded chromosomes are lined up along the equatorial plate. The centromeres divide and, during anaphase, the single strands move toward the centrioles at opposite poles of the cell. The end results of mitosis are two daughter cells with the same genetic composition as the original parent cell.

mitogenesis (ˌmietoh'jenəsis) the induction of mitosis in a cell.

mitomycin (ˌmietoh'miesin) a group of highly toxic antineoplastics (mitomycin A, B, and C) produced by *Streptomyces caespitosus*, indicated for palliative treatment of certain neoplasms that do not respond to surgery, radiation, and other drugs.

mitosis (mie'tohsis) the ordinary process of cell division which results in the formation of two daughter cells, and by which the body replaces dead cells. The two daughter cells receive identical diploid complements of chromosomes (46 in humans), which are characteristic of somatic cells. Cell division that results in haploid reproductive cells is known as MEIOSIS. The period between mitotic divisions is called *interphase*. Mitosis itself occurs in four phases: *prophase*, *metaphase*, *anaphase*, and *telophase*. adj. **mitotic**.

During *interphase* the chromosomes are extended long threads that cannot be visibly identified. The DNA of the chromosomes is replicated during this phase, resulting in duplication of the genetic material.

During *prophase* the chromosomes coil up and contract, becoming short rods. Each chromosome consists of a pair of strands, called *chromatids*, held together at the centromere. At the same time the nuclear envelope disappears, and the centriole divides and the two daughter centrioles move toward opposite poles of the cell.

During *metaphase* the chromosomes move so that their centromeres are aligned in the equatorial plane of the cell (the metaphase plate), and the mitotic spindle forms. The mitotic spindle is formed of fibres composed of microtubules, which extend from the centrioles to the metaphase plate and to the centromeres of the chromosomes.

During *anaphase* the chromatids of each chromosome separate, becoming new daughter chromosomes, which are drawn to opposite poles of the cell by the spindle fibres.

During *telophase* the daughter chromosomes arrive at the poles of the cell, where they are surrounded by two new nuclear envelopes as they begin to uncoil and extend. During this phase, *cytokinesis*, division of the cytoplasm occurs. A furrow forms around the cell in the equatorial plane and deepens until the two daughter cells are separated.

Originally, the term *mitosis* referred only to the division of the nucleus, which can occur without cytokinesis in certain fungi and in the fertilized eggs of insects. As used now, it usually refers to mitotic cell division..

Mitoxana (ˌmietok'sahnə) trademark for preparations of ifosfamide, an antineoplastic.

mitozantrone (ˌmietoh'zantrohn) an antineoplastic agent structurally related to doxorubicin.

mitral ('mietrəl) shaped like a mitre; pertaining to the mitral valve.

m. commissurotomy surgical incision of thickened leaflets of a stenotic mitral valve (see also mitral COMMISSUROTOMY).

m. stenosis a narrowing of the left atrioventricular orifice (mitral orifice). See also mitral COMMISSUROTOMY.

m. valve the left atrioventricular valve, the valve between the left atrium and the left ventricle of the heart; it is composed of two cusps, anterior and posterior. Called also the *bicuspid valve*.

m. valve prolapse (MVP) a condition in which some portion of the mitral valve is pushed back too far during ventricular contraction. For reasons not fully understood (there is no evident disease process) there is redundant tissue on one or both leaflets of the valve. The prolapsed portion of the valve causes a clicking sound at the end of ventricular contraction. This sound is followed by a systolic murmur as blood is regurgitated back through the mitral valve and into the left atrium. The condition is, therefore, also known as the *click–murmur syndrome*. Another name for MVP is *Barlow's syndrome*, after the doctor who, in 1968, first associated the phenomenon with some potentially serious complications. However, in the vast majority of persons in whom MVP can be detected by auscultation there are no other symptoms and the condition is so benign as to require no treatment.

MVP is found in persons of all ages and is fairly common. The few who have problems usually experience some chest pain, dyspnoea, palpitations, and fatigue. Syncope and anxiety also occur, though less commonly. Many patients become less anxious when they understand the difference between MVP and coronary heart disease. Electrocardiographic studies may show some premature ventricular contractions (PVCs) but, unlike those in coronary heart disease, the PVCs are not harmful nor do they indicate injury to the heart muscle.

Persons who suffer from the above symptoms may require administration of a beta-adrenergic blocking agent, such as propranolol, restriction of caffeine intake, and avoidance of heavy meals.

Long-term effects of MVP have not been thoroughly documented owing to the relatively short time that it has been recognized as a disease entity. There are sufficient data to show that almost all persons with MVP can lead normal and full lives.

mitralization (ˌmietrəlie'zayshən) a straightening of the left border of the cardiac shadow, commonly seen radiographically in mitral stenosis.

mittelschmerz ('mit'lˌshmərts) [Ger.] pain midway between the menstrual periods, associated with ovulation.

Mittendorf's dot ('mitənˌdawfs) a congenital anomaly of the eye manifested as a small grey or white opacity just inferior and nasal to the posterior pole of the lens, representing the remains of the lenticular attachment of the hyaloid artery; it does not affect vision.

mixed connective tissue disease (mikst) a combination of scleroderma, myositis, systemic lupus erythematosus, and rheumatoid arthritis, and marked serologically by the presence of antibody against extractable nuclear antigen.

mixture ('mikschə) a combination of different drugs or ingredients, as a fluid with other fluids or solids, or of a solid with a liquid.

Miyagawanella (ˌmieyəˌgahwə'nelə) a genus of organisms, the species of which are now assigned to the genus *Chlamydia* as follows: *M. lymphogranulomatosis* and *M. bronchopneumoniae* are assigned to *C. trachomatis*, and *M. bovis*, *M. felis*, *M. illinii*, *M. louisianae*, *M. opossumi*, *M. ornithosis*, *M. ovis*, *M. pecoris*, *M. pneumoniae*, and *M. psittaci* are assigned to *C. psittaci*.

ml millilitre.

MLA in obstetrics, mentolaevoanterior position of the face presentation.

MLSO Medical Laboratory Scientific Officer.

mm millimetre.

μm micrometre.

mmHg millimetres of mercury; a unit of pressure.

MMR measles, mumps, and rubella (vaccine).

Mn chemical symbol, *manganese*.

mnemonics (ni'moniks) improvement of memory by special methods or techniques. adj. **mnemonic**.

MO Medical Officer.

Mo chemical symbol, *molybdenum*.

mobilization (ˌmobilie'zayshən) the rendering of a fixed part movable.

stapes m. surgical correction of immobility of the stapes in treatment of deafness.

Möbius' disease ('mərbi·əs) periodic migraine with paralysis of the oculomotor muscles.

modality (moh'dalitee) 1. in homeopathy, a condition that modifies drug action; a condition under which symptoms develop, becoming better or worse. 2. a method of application of, or the employment of, any therapeutic agent; limited usually to physical agents. 3. a specific sensory entity, such as taste.

mode (mohd) in statistics, the value or item in a variations curve that shows the maximal frequency of occurrence.

Modecate ('modikayt) trademark for a preparation of fluphenazine, an antipsychotic.

modiolus (moh'dieələs) the central pillar or columella of the cochlea.

Moditen ('moditen) trademark for preparations of fluphenazine, an antipsychotic.

modulation (ˌmodyuh'layshən) the normal capacity of cell adaptability to its environment.

antigenic m. the alteration of antigenic determinants in a living cell surface membrane following interaction with antibody.

Moduretic (ˌmodyuh'retik) trademark for combination preparations of amiloride and hydrochlorothiazide, a diuretic.

Mogadon ('mogədon) trademark for a preparation of nitrazepam, a hypnotic.

MOH Medical Officer of Health.

moiety ('moyətee) any equal part; a half; also any part or portion, as a portion of a molecule.

mol (mohl) mole (2).

mol.wt molecular weight.

molal ('mohləl) containing one mole of solute per kilogram of solvent. See also MOLAR.

molality (moh'lalətee) the number of moles of a solute per kilogram of solvent.

molar ('mohlə) 1. massive; pertaining to a mass; not molecular. 2. pertaining to an amount of substance specified in moles rather than mass units. 3. adapted for grinding (see also TOOTH). 4. containing 1 mole of solute per litre of solution. Symbol M. NOTE: *molal* refers to the mass of *solvent*, *molar* to the volume of the *solution*.

mulberry m. a first molar tooth with a characteristically globular shape, sometimes seen in congenital syphilis.

molarity (moh'larətee) the number of moles of a solute per litre of solution.

mole (mohl) 1. a fleshly mass formed in the uterus by abortive development of an ovum. 2. the amount of a substance that contains as many elementary entities (atoms, ions, molecules, or free radicals) as there are atoms in 12 g of pure carbon-12, i.e., Avogadro's number, 6.023×10^{23}, of elementary entities; equivalent to the amount of a chemical compound having a mass in grams equal to its molecular weight. 3. a fleshy growth or blemish on the skin; a NAEVUS.

carneous m. see CARNEOUS mole.
hairy m. hairy naevus.
hydatid m., hydatidiform m. an abnormal pregnancy resulting from a pathological ovum, with proliferation of the epithelial covering of the chorionic villi and dissolution and cystic cavitation of the avascular stroma of the villi. It results in a mass of cysts resembling a bunch of grapes.
pigmented m. naevus pigmentosus.

molecular (mə'lekyuhlə) of, pertaining to, or composed of molecules.
m. biology study of the biochemical and biophysical aspects of structure and function of genes and other subcellular entities, and of such specific proteins as haemoglobins, enzymes, and hormones; it provides knowledge of cellular differentiation and metabolism and of comparative evolution.
m. weight the weight of a molecule of a chemical compound as compared with the weight of an atom of carbon-12; it is equal to the sum of the weights of its constituent atoms.

molecule ('moli,kyool) a group of atoms joined by chemical bonds; the smallest amount of a substance that possesses its characteristic properties.

molimen ('mohlimen, moh'liemen) pl. *molimina* [L.] a laborious effort made for the performance of any normal body function, especially that manifested by a variety of unpleasant symptoms preceding or accompanying menstruation.

Molipaxin (,moli'paksin) trademark for trazodone hydrochloride, an antidepressant drug.

Moll's glands (molz) sweat glands that have become arrested in their development, situated at the edges of the eyelids; called also *ciliary glands*.

mollities (mo'lishi·eez) abnormal softening.
m. ossium osteomalacia.

molluscum (mo'luskəm) 1. any of various skin diseases marked by the formation of soft rounded cutaneous tumours. 2. molluscum contagiosum. adj. **molluscous.**
m. contagiosum a viral disease of the skin marked by the formation of firm, rounded, translucent, crateriform papules containing caseous matter and peculiar encapsulated bodies (molluscum bodies). The disease is spread by contact and is common in young children. In adults, lesions in the pubic area indicate sexual transmission.

Treatment consists of curettage or light cauterization with an electric cautery.

molybdenum (mə'libdənəm) a hard, silvery-white, metallic element, atomic number 42, atomic weight 95.94, symbol Mo. (See table of elements in Appendix 2.) It is an essential trace element, being a component of the enzymes xanthine oxidase, aldehyde oxidase, and nitrate reductase.

momentum (mə'mentəm, moh-) the quantity of motion; the product of mass by velocity.

monad ('mohnad, 'mo-) 1. a single-celled protozoon or coccus. 2. a univalent radical or element. 3. in meiosis, one member of a tetrad.

monaesthetic (,monis'thetik) affecting a single sense or sensation.

monarthric (mon'ahthrik) pertaining to a single joint.

monarthritis (monah'thrietis) inflammation of a single joint.

monarticular (,monah'tikyuhlə) pertaining to a single joint.

monathetosis (,monathi'tohsis) athetosis of one limb.

monatomic (,monə'tomik) 1. containing one atom. 2. univalent.

Mönckeberg's arteriosclerosis ('mərngkə,bərgz) ARTERIOSCLEROSIS involving the middle coat of the arteries, with destruction of the muscle and elastic fibres and calcium deposits. Called also *medial calcific sclerosis*.

Mondor's disease ('mondawz) phlebitis affecting the large subcutaneous veins normally crossing the lateral chest wall and breast from the epigastric or hypochondriac region to the axilla.

mongolian spot (mong'gohli·ən) a smooth, brown to grayish blue naevus consisting of an excess of melanocytes, sometimes found at birth in the sacral region. It usually disappears during childhood.

mongolism ('mong·gə,lizəm) a congenital condition involving some degree of mental handicap and various physical malformations. The name is based on characteristic facial traits resembling somewhat those of persons of the Mongolian race. The term mongolism is now considered to be inaccurate and undesirable and is being replaced by the term DOWN'S SYNDROME or trisomy 21. The latter name refers to the presence of three twenty-first chromosomes, found in those with Down's syndrome, instead of the usual pair.

mongoloid ('mong·gə,loyd) 1. pertaining to or resembling the Mongols. 2. an individual with Down's syndrome (see MONGOLISM).

monilethrix (mo'nili,thriks) a hereditary condition in which the hair is brittle and beaded.

Monilia (mo'nili·ə) former name of a genus of parasitic fungi, now called *Candida*.

monilial (mo'nili·əl) pertaining to or caused by *Monilia* (*Candida*).

moniliasis (,moni'lieəsis) candidiasis.

moniliform (mo'nili,fawm) beaded; having the appearance of a string of beads.

Monistat ('mohni,stat) trademark for a preparation of miconazole nitrate; an antifungal.

Monit ('monit) trademark for a preparation of isosorbide mononitrate.

Monitor ('monitor) an adaptation for the UK of the USA Rush Medicus system of assessing quality of nursing care. It consists of 'checklists' for quality leading to a scoring system. The closer the score to 100 per cent the better the care being given. The master list has over 200 criteria which are divided into four categories based on patient dependency levels.

monitor ('monitə) 1. to check constantly on a given condition or phenomenon, e.g., blood pressure or heart or respiration rate. 2. an apparatus by which such conditions or phenomena can be constantly observed and recorded.

mono- ('monoh) word element. [Gr.] *one, single, limited to one part, combined with one atom.*

monoamine (,monoh'ameen) an amine containing only one amino group.
m. oxidase (MAO) a cuproprotein enzyme that deaminates monoamines such as serotonin, adrenaline, noradrenaline, dopamine, tyramine and tryptamine.
m. oxidase inhibitors, MAO inhibitors substances that inhibit the activity of monoamine oxidase, increasing catecholamine and serotonin levels in the brain; they are used as antidepressants and antihypertensives.

monoaminergic (,monoh,ami'nərjik) of or pertaining to neurons that secrete the monoamine neurotransmitters dopamine, noradrenaline, and serotonin.

monoamniotic (,monoh,amni'otik) having or developing within a single amniotic cavity; said of monozygotic twins.

monobasic (,monoh'baysik) having but one atom of replaceable hydrogen.

monoblast ('monoh,blast) the earliest precursor in the monocytic series, which develops into the promonocyte.

monoblastoma (,monohbla'stohmə) a tumour containing monoblasts and monocytes.

monoblepsia (ˌmonoh'blepsi·ə) 1. a condition in which vision is better when only one eye is used. 2. blindness to all colours but one.

monobrachius (ˌmonoh'brayki·əs) a fetus with only one arm.

monocephalus (ˌmonoh'kefələs, -'sef-) a fetus or infant with two bodies and one head.

monochorea (ˌmonohko'reeə) chorea affecting but one part.

monochorionic (ˌmonohˌko·ri'onik) having or developing in a common chorionic sac; said of monozygotic twins.

monochromat (ˌmonoh'krohmat) a person affected by monochromatism.

monochromatic (ˌmonohkroh'matik) 1. existing in or having only one colour. 2. pertaining to or affected by monochromatism. 3. staining with only one dye at a time.

monochromatism (ˌmonoh'krohməˌtizəm) complete colour blindness; inability to discrimate hues, all colours of the spectrum appearing as neutral grays with varying shades of light and dark.

cone m. that in which there is some cone function.

rod m. that in which there is complete absence of cone function.

monoclonal (ˌmonoh'klohn'l) derived from a single cell; pertaining to a single clone.

monococcus (ˌmonoh'kokəs) a form of coccus consisting of single cells.

monocontaminated (ˌmonohkən'tamiˌnaytid) infected by only one species of microorganisms or a single contaminating agent.

monocular (mo'nokyuhlə) 1. pertaining to one eye. 2. having but one eyepiece, as in a microscope.

m. diplopia double vision in one eye.

monocyte ('monohˌsiet) a mononuclear, phagocytic leukocyte, 13 μm to 25 μm in diameter, having an ovoid or kidney-shaped nucleus and azurophilic cytoplasmic granules. Monocytes are derived from promonocytes in the bone marrow. They circulate in the blood for about 24 hours before migrating to the tissues, as in the lung and liver, where they develop into macrophages. adj. **monocytic**.

monocytopenia (ˌmonohˌsietoh'peeni·ə) deficiency of monocytes in the blood.

monocytosis (ˌmonohsie'tohsis) excess of monocytes in the blood.

monodactyly (ˌmonoh'daktilee) the presence of only one finger or toe on a hand or foot.

monodermoma (ˌmonohdər'mohmə) a tumour developed from one germinal layer.

monoecious (mo'neeshəs) having reproductive organs typical of both sexes in a single individual.

monogerminal (ˌmonoh'jərmin'l) developed from one ovum; said of identical twins.

monolayer (ˌmonoh'layə) pertaining to or consisting of a single layer of molecules.

monolocular (ˌmonoh'lokyuhlə) having but one cavity, as a cyst.

monomania (ˌmonoh'mayni·ə) psychosis on a single subject or class of subjects.

monomelic (ˌmonoh'melik) affecting one limb.

monomer ('monəmə) 1. a simple molecule of relatively low molecular weight, which is capable of reacting chemically with other molecules to form a polymer, in which the monomers are linked by covalent bonds. 2. a single protein molecule that combines with other monomers by hydrogen bonds to form a larger protein.

fibrin m. the material resulting from the action of thrombin on fibrinogen, which then polymerizes to form fibrin.

monomeric (ˌmonə'merik) 1. pertaining to a single segment. 2. in genetics, determined by a gene or genes at a single locus. 3. consisting of monomers.

monomolecular (ˌmonohmə'lekyuhlə) pertaining to a single molecule or to a layer one molecule thick.

monomorphic (ˌmonoh'mawfik) existing in only one form.

monomphalus (mo'nomfələs) twins conjoined at the navel.

monomyoplegia (ˌmonohˌmieoh'pleeji·ə) paralysis of a single muscle.

monomyositis (ˌmonohˌmieoh'sietis) inflammation of a single muscle.

mononeural (ˌmonoh'nyooə·rəl) supplied by a single nerve.

mononeuritis (ˌmonohnyuh'rietis) inflammation of a single nerve.

m. multiplex simultaneous inflammation of several nerves remote from one another.

mononuclear (ˌmonoh'nyookli·ə) having only one nucleus.

mononucleosis (ˌmonohˌnyookli'ohsis) excess of mononuclear leukocytes (monocytes) in the blood.

infectious m. see INFECTIOUS mononucleosis and GLANDUALR FEVER.

monoparaesthesia (ˌmonohˌparis'theezi·ə) paraesthesia of a single part.

monoparesis (ˌmonohpə'reesis) paresis of a single part.

monopathy (mə'nopəthee) a disease affecting a single part.

monophasia (ˌmonoh'fayzi·ə) aphasia in which speech is limited to one word or phrase.

monophthalmus (monof'thalməs) a fetus with one eye; cyclops.

monophyletic (ˌmonohfie'letik) descended from a common ancestor or stem cell.

monoplegia (ˌmonoh'pleeji·ə) paralysis of a single part. adj. **monoplegic**.

monopoiesis (ˌmonohpoy'eesis) the development of monocytes.

monopolar (ˌmonoh'pohlə) having a single pole.

monops ('monops) a fetus with a single eye.

monopus ('monəpəs) a fetus with only one foot.

monorchid (mon'awkid) a person having only one testis in the scrotum.

monorchidism, monorchism (mon'awkidizəm; 'monawkizəm) the condition of having only one testis or one descended testis.

monosaccharide (ˌmonoh'sakəˌried) a simple sugar; a carbohydrate that cannot be broken down to simpler substances by hydrolysis.

monosomy (ˌmonoh'sohmee) existence in a cell of only one instead of the normal diploid pair of a particular chromosome. adj. **monosomic**.

monospecific (ˌmonohspə'sifik) having an effect only on a particular kind of cell or tissue, or reacting with a single antigen, as a monospecific antiserum.

Monosporium (ˌmonoh'spor·ri·əm) a genus of fungi.

M. apiospermum a fungus that is one of the causative organisms of maduromycosis.

monospot test ('monoˌspot) see PAUL–BUNNELL TEST.

monostotic (ˌmonoh'stotik) affecting a single bone.

monosymptomatic (ˌmonohˌsimptə'matik) manifested by only one symptom.

monosynaptic (ˌmonohsi'naptik) pertaining to or passing through a single synapse.

monothermia (ˌmonoh'thərmi·ə) a condition in which the body temperature remains the same throughout the day.

monotrichous (mo'notrikəs) having a single flagellum; applied to a bacterial cell.

monovalent (ˌmonoh'vaylənt) 1. having a valency of one. 2. capable of binding with only one antigenic or antibody specificity.

monoxenous (mo'noksənəs) requiring only one host to complete the life cycle.

monozygotic (ˌmonohzie'gotik) pertaining to or derived from a single zygote (fertilized ovum); said of TWINS.

Monro's foramen (mun'rohz) the communication between the lateral and third ventricles of the brain.

mons (monz) pl. *montes* [L.] a prominence.

m. pubis the rounded fleshy prominence over the symphysis pubis in the female.

m. veneris mons pubis.

Monteggia's fracture (mon'tejəz) a fracture in the proximal half of the shaft of the ulna, with dislocation of the head of the radius (see also illustration accompanying FRACTURE).

Montgomery's glands (mənt'guməˑriz) sebaceous glands in the mammary areola; called also *areolar glands*.

monticulus (mon'tikyuhləs) pl. *monticuli* [L.] a small eminence.

m. cerebelli the projecting part of the superior vermis cerebelli.

mood (mood) a prevailing emotional tone or feeling.

moon face ('moon ˌfays) one of the features occurring in Cushing's syndrome and as a result of prolonged treatment with steroid drugs.

Mooren's ulcer ('morˑrənz) a progressive ulceration of the peripheral (marginal) cornea.

MOPP a regimen of mustine, Oncovin (vincristine), procarbazine, and prednisone, used in cancer chemotherapy.

Moraxella (moˑrak'selə) a genus of bacteria found as parasites and pathogens in warm-blooded animals.

morbid ('mawbid) 1. pertaining to, affected with, or inducing disease; diseased. 2. unhealthy; unwholesome.

morbidity (maw'biditee) the condition of being diseased.

morbific (mor'bifik) causing or inducing disease.

morbilli (mor'bilie) [L.] *measles*.

morbilliform (mor'biliˌfawm) resembling measles.

morbus ('mawbəs) [L.] *disease*.

morcellation (ˌmawsə'layshən) division into small pieces, or piecemeal removal.

mordant ('mawdənt) 1. a substance capable of intensifying or deepening the reaction of a specimen to a stain. 2. to subject to the action of a mordant before staining.

Morgagni's hyperostosis (mor'ganyeez) frontal internal hyperostosis.

Morgagni's ventricle the space between the true and false vocal cords; called also *ventricle of larynx*.

moria ('morˑriˑə) a morbid tendency to joke.

moribund ('moˑriˌbund) in a dying state.

Morison's pouch ('morisənz) a fold of the peritoneum below the liver.

Morita therapy (mo'reetə) a therapy based on Zen Buddhism in which strict internal and external discipline, intensive work and repeated denial of symptoms are coupled with frank examination of self. The therapy was developed by Dr. Shoma Morita who found it effective with many of his Japanese patients suffering from neurosis or personality disorder.

morning sickness ('morning) nausea or vomiting occurring during pregnancy, usually before 14 weeks. Between 50 and 65 per cent of all women experience some degree of morning sickness at some time during pregnancy, and about one-third are affected to the point of vomiting. Morning sickness usually begins during the fifth or sixth week of pregnancy but may precede the first missed menstrual period. Some cases may clear up in 1 to 3 weeks; others may persist until the fourteenth week.

In most cases, morning sickness begins with a feeling of nausea on arising. Despite its name, however, morning sickness is not always limited to the morning. It should not cause marked loss of weight, acetone in the urine or undue interference with the daily routine.

In rare cases—affecting about one woman in 200—HYPEREMESIS GRAVIDARUM, or pernicious vomiting of pregnancy, may develop. If unchecked, it may result in such symptoms as dehydration and weight loss, and may threaten the life of both mother and the unborn child.

CAUSES. Morning sickness is thought to be due to a disturbance in the metabolism of glucose or as a result of the increased metabolism of pregnancy causing a low blood sugar and accompanying feeling of nausea on rising. It is sometimes more apparent in women who are 'highly strung'. There is an undisputed psychological component to hyperemesis gravidarum. Morning sickness is less pronounced where the mother has been eating regular well-balanced meals and has not been dieting prior to or during early pregnancy.

TREATMENT. Morning sickness is little more than a discomfort, and usually requires no treatment. If a woman can be diverted from thinking about it, the condition tends to lessen or to pass away entirely. If possible, a woman should have something light to eat before getting out of bed in the morning. This could be biscuits and/or weak tea, possibly left on the bedside table at night, the tea in a vacuum flask; or better still, she should have breakfast in bed. After eating, she should rest for about 15 minutes before getting up.

Excessive fluid intake should be avoided. At meals, it is best to eat dry foods first. Liquids should be taken last and should be sipped in small quantities. Instead of three large meals, small meals should be eaten at more frequent intervals. It is also advisable to rest after each meal. Dry foods, such as crackers, or soft foods eaten every 2 hours until the nausea is over can also be helpful.

Sights, smells, and foods that may be disturbing should be avoided, as should greasy foods, fats, and butter. Also to be avoided are those vegetables which are hard to digest, such as cabbage, cauliflower, cucumbers, and onions. In certain cases, the doctor may prescribe an antiemetic.

Moro reflex ('moˑroh) flexion of an infant's thighs and knees, fanning and then clenching of fingers, with arms first thrown outward and then brought together as though embracing something; produced by a sudden stimulus, such as striking the table on either side of the child, and seen normally in the newborn. Called also *embrace reflex*.

moron ('morˑron) a term previously used to describe a mentally handicapped person whose mental age is between 8 and 12 years, usually requiring special training and supervision. The term is no longer acceptable as an expression of degree of MENTAL HANDICAP.

morphea (maw'feeə) [Gr.] a condition in which there is connective tissue replacement of the skin and sometimes of the subcutaneous tissues, marked by the formation of ivory white or pinkish patches, bands, or lines that are sometimes bordered by a purplish areola. The lesions are firm, but not hard, and are usually depressed; they may remain localized or may involute, leaving atrophy and scarring. Called also *circumscribed* or *localized scleroderma*.

morphine ('mawfeen) the principal and most active opium alkaloid, a narcotic analgesic and respiratory depressant, usually used as morphine sulphate. The use of morphine carries with it the dangers of addiction (see DRUG ADDICTION) and tolerance, so that increasingly larger doses are needed to achieve the desired effect. Since morphine is a powerful respiratory depressant, the drug should be withheld and the doctor notified when the patient's respirations are less than 12 per minute.

morphinism ('mawfi,nizəm) a morbid state due to habitual misuse of morphine.

morphium ('mawfi·əm) morphine.

morphogenesis (,mawfoh'jenəsis) the developmental changes of growth and differentiation occurring in the organization of the body and its parts. adj. **morphogenetic.**

morphology (maw'foləjee) the science of the forms and structure of organisms; the form and structure of a particular organism, organ, tissue, or cell. adj. **morphological.**

morphometry (maw'fomətree) the measurement of forms.

-morphous word element. [Gr.] *shape, form.*

Morquio's disease (syndrome) (maw'keeohz) a form of mucopolysaccharidosis becoming evident when the affected infant starts to walk, marked by severe dwarfism, prominent sternum, short neck, kyphosis, genu valgum, and waddling gait; mental handicap is absent or slight. Called also *osteochondrodystrophy* and *familial osteochondrodystrophy.*

Morquio–Ullrich disease (maw,keeoh'uhlrik) Morquio's disease.

morrhuate ('mor·roo,ayt) the fatty acids of cod liver oil used as a sclerosing agent, especially for the treatment of varicose veins and haemorrhoids.

mors (morz) [L.] *death.*

morsus ('mawsəs) [L.] *bite.*

m. diaboli the fimbriated end of a uterine tube.

mortal ('mawt'l) 1. destined to die. 2. causing or terminating in death; fatal.

mortality (maw'talitee) 1. the quality of being mortal. 2. mortality rate. See death RATE.

mortar ('mawtə) a vessel with a rounded internal surface, used with a pestle, for reducing a solid to a powder or producing a homogeneous mixture of solids.

mortification (,mawtifi'kayshən) gangrene.

Morton's toe ('mawtənz) tenderness or pain in the metatarsal area of the foot and in the third and fourth toes caused by pressure on a neuroma of the branch of the medial plantar nerve supplying these toes. The neuroma is produced by chronic compression of the nerve between the metatarsal heads. Called also *plantar neuroma* and *Morton's disease, foot,* or *neuralgia.*

mortuary (mawg) a place where dead bodies may be temporarily kept, for identification or until claimed for burial.

morula ('mo·ryuhlə) a solid mass of cells (blastomeres) resembling a mulberry, formed by cleavage of a fertilized ovum.

Morvan's disease ('mawvanhz) a form of syringomyelia, with painless ulceration of the fingertips and analgesic paralysis and atrophy of the forearms and hands.

mosaic (moh'zayik) a pattern made of numerous small pieces fitted together; in genetics, occurrence in an individual of two or more cell populations each having a different chromosome complement.

mosaicism (moh'zayi,sizəm) the presence in an individual of cells derived from the same zygote, but differing in chromosomal constitution.

mosmol milliosmole.

mosquito (mo'skeetoh) a blood-sucking winged insect. Genera of importance medically include *Aedes, Anopheles, and Culex.* Certain species are responsible for the transmission of disease, including yellow fever and MALARIA.

motile ('mohtiel) having spontaneous but not conscious or volitional movement.

motilin (moh'tilin) a polypeptide hormone secreted by enterochromaffin cells of the gut; it causes increased motility of several portions of the gut and stimulates pepsin secretion. Its release is stimulated by the presence of acid and fat in the duodenum.

motility (moh'tilitee) the ability to move spontaneously.

Motilium (moh'tiliəm) trademark for preparations of domperidone, an antiemetic.

motion sickness ('mohshən) discomfort felt by some people on a moving boat, train, plane, or car, or even in a lift or on a swing. Called also *travel sickness.* The discomfort is caused by irregular and abnormal motion that disturbs the organs of balance located in the inner ear. There may be mild symptoms of nausea, dizziness, or headache, as well as pallor and cold perspiration. In more acute cases, there may be vomiting and sometimes prostration.

Though most people quickly adapt to travel by plane, ship, and car, few are wholly immune to motion sickness. Even astronauts become ill if the inner ear organs of balance are continuously stimulated by unusual motion. Fortunately, most cases of motion sickness vanish quickly once the journey is over, leaving no ill-effects.

CAUSES. The inner ear possesses three semicircular canals, located at right angles in three different planes. Man is accustomed to movement in the horizontal plane, which stimulates certain semicircular canals; but he is not accustomed to vertical movements, such as the motion of a lift or a ship pitching at sea. These vertical movements stimulate the semicircular canals in an unusual way, producing the sensation of nausea, or motion sickness. Anxiety, grief, or other emotions can also cause motion sickness. A person unaccustomed to travelling by boat or airplane may be apprehensive or nervous and therefore may develop symptoms of nausea. Some individuals with previous experience of motion sickness become ill on a boat at dock or on an airplane prior to take-off.

Airsickness usually occurs during a bumpy flight caused by stormy weather or turbulent air. However, it may also be triggered by poorly ventilated cabins, hunger, digestive upset, overindulgence in food and drink, and unpleasant odours, particularly tobacco smoke.

TREATMENT. Certain antihistamines have proved highly effective in treating symptoms of seasickness. Like nerve depressants, they may be used alone or in combination with mild sedatives. Those who suffer from motion sickness should ask their general practioner what he recommends before they embark on a trip. Symptoms may also be reduced if the seasick person rests lying down, with his head low, in a comfortable, well aired place.

PREVENTION. Being rested and in good health prior to a journey helps to prevent motion sickness. A cup of strong coffee taken just before departure may also be helpful. Alcoholic beverages in moderation make some people less nervous and thus help ward off motion sickness; however, in excess they can encourage the condition.

During a voyage by boat, it is advisable for the passenger to remain near the centre of the ship, where there will be the least motion. Ample fresh air and exercise and avoidance of stuffy rooms and disagreeable smells are also good precautions. The traveller should keep comfortably warm and avoid overeating and rich foods.

For those travelling by air, a sedative or tranquillizer taken a half hour before departure, and small, easily digested meals taken during the flight help to prevent airsickness. The passenger who experiences motion sickness may benefit from reclining in his seat as far as possible and closing his eyes.

Carsickness is often relieved if the journey is interrupted for short walks in the fresh air and by keeping a window open. Children will frequently find it helpful to glance down, to refrain from reading, but being kept occupied with diversional is often helpful. Tobacco smoke can be an aggravating factor.

Motival ('mohtival) trademark for a fixed combination preparation of fluphenazine and nortriptyline, an antidepressant.

motivate ('mohti,vayt) to provide an incentive or purpose for a course of action.

motivation (,mohti'vayshən) the reason or reasons, conscious or unconscious, behind a particular attitude or behaviour.

motive ('mohtiv) the incentive that determines a course of action or its direction.

motoceptor ('mohtoh,septə) any muscle sense receptor.

motoneuron, motoneurone (,mohtoh'nyooə·ron; -rohn) motor neuron; a neuron having a motor function; an efferent neuron conveying motor impulses.

lower m's peripheral neurons whose cell bodies lie in the ventral grey columns of the spinal cord and whose terminations are in skeletal muscles.

peripheral m's neurons in a peripheral reflex arc that receive impulses from interneurons and transmit them to voluntary muscles.

upper m's neurons in the cerebral cortex that conduct impulses from the motor cortex to the motor nuclei of the cerebral nerves or to the ventral grey columns of the spinal cord.

motor ('mohtə) 1. pertaining to motion. 2. a muscle, nerve, or centre that effects movements.

mottling ('motling) discoloration in irregular areas.

moulage (moo'lahzh) [Fr.] a wax model of a structure or lesion.

mould (mohld) any of a group of parasitic and saprophytic fungi causing a cottony growth on organic substances; also, the deposit of growth produced by such fungi.

moulding ('mohlding) the change in shape of the vault of the fetal skull brought about by pressure from the birth canal over a period of time once the membranes have ruptured in labour. The engaging (presenting) diameter is reduced by up to 1.25 cm, while the diameter at right angles to it is correspondingly increased. Moulding is possible because, at term, the membranous bones of the vault of the fetal skull are not completely ossified. The presence of sutures and fontanelles between them allow overlapping of the bones. The frontal and occipital bones slide under the parietal bones, which slide under and on top of each other. By examination of the baby's head following delivery it is possible to diagnose the presentation and method of delivery. The head returns to its normal shape within 3 days of birth. Moulding which is abnormal in direction, excessive in amount, or extremely rapid may cause tearing of the falx cerebri and tentorium cerebellum, leading to intracranial haemorrhage and possible death..

mounding ('mownding) the rising in a lump of a wasting muscle when struck.

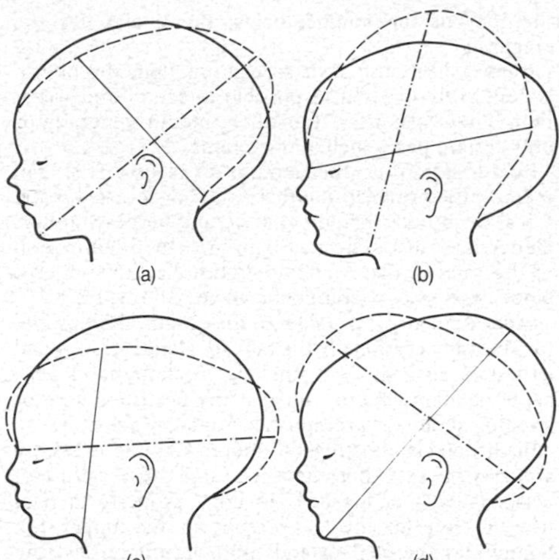

Moulding of the fetal head. (a) Vertex presentation with good flexion (suboccipitobregmatic decreased, biparietal decreased, mentovertical increased). (b) Persistent occipitoposterior position of the vertex (occipitofrontal decreased, biparietal decreased, submentobregmatic increased). (c) Face presentation (submentobregmatic decreased, biparietal decreased, occipitofrontal increased). (d) Brow presentation (mentovertical decreased, biparietal probably decreased, suboccipitobregmatic increased)

mount (mownt) to prepare specimens and slides for study.

mountain fever ('mowntin) 1. Colorado tick fever. 2. Rocky Mountain spotted fever. 3. brucellosis.

mountain sickness disturbances due to poor adjustment to high altitude. Symptoms include fatiguability, shortness of breath, polycythaemia, cyanosis and epistaxis.

mouse (mows) 1. small rodent, various species of which are used in laboratory experiments. 2. a small loose body.

joint m. a movable fragment of synovial membrane, cartilage, or other body within a joint; usually associated with degenerative osteoarthritis and osteochondritis dissecans.

peritoneal m. a free body in the peritoneal cavity, probably a small detached mass or omentum, sometimes visible radiographically.

mouth (mowth) an opening, especially the oral cavity, which forms the beginning of the DIGESTIVE SYSTEM and in which the chewing of food takes place. The mouth is also the site of the organs of taste and the teeth, tongue, and lips. Not only is the mouth the entrance to the body for food and sometimes air, but it is a major organ of speech and emotional expression.

STRUCTURE. Except for the teeth, the interior of the mouth is covered with mucous membrane. This thin lining extends out from the front of the mouth to form the lips. Salivary glands lie in the upper and lower parts of the mouth and produce saliva, a liquid that protects the delicate membranes and mixes with food in the first step of digestion of food.

The palate forms the roof of the mouth. The front two-thirds of the palate comprises the hard palate, and the back third, the soft palate. The soft palate is hinged to the hard palate and is flanked on both sides by the tonsils. In the middle of the soft palate is the uvula, a projection pointing down to the tongue. At the root of the tongue, below the uvula, lies the epiglottis.

DISORDERS. Because of its special functions the mouth is constantly exposed to possible infection and irritation. These can affect the whole mouth generally or only certain parts, such as the tongue.

Inflammation of the mouth, or STOMATITIS, can indicate the presence of either a mild or severe disease. Local conditions include THRUSH, and herpes simplex. Generalized diseases can also give rise to inflammation of the mouth; these include diphtheria, tuberculosis, blood dyscrasias, vitamin deficiencies, and syphilis.

CANCER can afflict the sides of the mouth, the lips, the tongue and occasionally the salivary glands. Continued irritation, such as pipe smoking, is thought to be a cause of many mouth cancers. Any persistent sore or swelling should be promptly examined by a doctor.

Birth defects affecting the mouth include CLEFT LIP and CLEFT PALATE. Both have the same cause: failure of adjacent parts of the body to unite properly in fetal life. A cleft lip involves a split in the upper lip. Sometimes the cleft extends into the upper jaw, the floor of the nose and the palate. The resulting deformity of nose and mouth interferes with sucking and speech unless corrected by surgery. A cleft palate, which may cause difficulties in speaking and eating, signifies a cleavage in the uvula and the soft palate. Both conditions are successfully corrected by surgery.

mouth-to-mouth resuscitation (ˌmowthtə'mowth) a method of ARTIFICAL RESPIRATION in which the rescuer covers the patient's mouth with his own and exhales vigorously.

mouthwash ('mowthwosh) a solution for rinsing the mouth.

movement ('moovmənt) 1. an act of moving; motion. 2. an act of defecation.

active m. movement produced by the person's own muscles.

amoeboid m. movement like that of an amoeba, accomplished by protrusion of cytoplasm of the cell.

associated m. movement of parts that act together, as the eyes.

brownian m., molecular m. the peculiar, rapid, oscillatory movement of fine particles suspended in a fluid medium.

passive m. a movement of the body or of the extremities of a patient performed by another person without voluntary motion on the part of the patient.

vermicular m's the worm-like movements of the intestines in peristalsis.

Moxalactam (ˌmoksə'laktam) trademark for a preparation of latamoxef sodium.

MPD maximum permissible dose.

MPS Member of the Pharmaceutical Society.

mR milliroentgen.

mrad millirad.

MRC Medical Research Council.

MRCOG Member of the Royal College of Obstetricians and Gynaecologists.

MRCP Member of the Royal College of Physicians.

MRCPath Member of the Royal College of Pathologists.

MRCPsych Member of the Royal College of Psychiatrists.

MRCS Member of the Royal College of Surgeons.

MRCVS Member of the Royal College of Veterinary Surgeons.

MRI magnetic resonance imaging.

mRNA messenger RNA (ribonucleic acid).

MRSH Member of the Royal Society for the Promotion of Health.

MS Master of Surgery; Master of Science (in the USA); multiple sclerosis.

MSA Member of the Society of Apothecaries.

MSc Master of Science.

MSH melanocyte-stimulating hormone.

MSR(R) Member of the Society of Radiographers (Radiography).

MSR(T) Member of the Society of Radiographers (Radiotherapy).

MSRG Member of the Society of Remedial Gymnasts.

MST continus (ˌemestee 'continəs) trademark for preparations of a sustained release tablet of morphine sulphate, an opiate analgesic.

MSU midstream specimen of urine.

MTD Midwife Teacher's Diploma.

Mucaine ('myookayn) trademark for a combination preparation of aluminium hydroxide, magnesium hydroxide and oxethazaine, an antacid.

muciferous (myoo'sifə·rəs) secreting mucus.

muciform ('myoosiˌfawm) resembling mucus.

mucigen ('myoosijən) a substance present in mucous cells, convertible into mucin and mucus.

mucilage ('myoosilij) an aqueous solution of a gummy substance, used as a vehicle or demulcent. adj. **mucilaginous.**

mucilloid ('myoosiˌloyd) a preparation of a mucilaginous substance.

mucin ('myoosin) a viscous secretion composed of glycoproteins and/or mucopolysaccharides that is the chief constituent of mucus.

mucinase ('myoosiˌnayz) an enzyme that acts upon mucin.

mucinogen (myoo'sinəjən) a precursor of mucin.

mucinoid ('myoosiˌnoyd) 1. resembling mucin. 2. mucoid (2).

mucinosis (ˌmyoosi'nohsis) a state with abnormal deposits of mucin in the skin, often associated with hypothyroidism (myxoedema).

follicular m. a disease of unknown cause, characterized by plaques of folliculopapules and usually alopecia.

muciparous (myoo'sipə·rəs) secreting mucin.

mucocele ('myookohˌseel) 1. dilation of a cavity with accumulated mucous secretion. 2. a mucous polyp.

mucocutaneous (ˌmyookohkyoo'tayni·əs) pertaining to mucous membrane and skin.

mucocutaneous lymph node syndrome (ˌmyookohkyoo'tayni·əs) a multisystem disease of unknown aetiology, occurring in children, and characterized by fever and a macular erythematous skin rash. Aneurysms and coronary thrombosis may occur in severe cases. Called also KAWASAKI'S DISEASE.

mucoenteritis (ˌmyookohˌentə'rietis) mucous colitis.

mucoepidermoid (ˌmyookohˌepi'dərmoyd) composed of both mucus-producing and squamous epithelial cells.

Mucogel ('myookohjel) trademark for a combination preparation of aluminium hydroxide, magnesium hydroxide and oxethazaine, an antacid.

mucoid ('myookoyd) 1. resembling mucus. 2. a mucus-like conjugated protein of animal origin, differing from mucin in solubility.

mucolipidosis (ˌmyookohˌlipi'dohsis) any of a group of genetic disorders in which both glycosaminoglycans (GAGs) and lipids accumulate in tissues, but without excess of GAGs in the urine.

m. I a hereditary congenital disorder characterized by Hurler-like manifestations with skeletal dysplasias, cherry-red macular spots, progressive ataxia, speech impairment, and mental handicap, peculiar inclusions in the fibroblasts, and normal urinary GAG levels. It is due to an isolated deficiency of neuraminidase.

m. II a rapidly progressing disease of young children, histologically characterized by abnormal fibroblasts containing a large number of dark inclusions which fill the central part of the cytoplasm except for the juxtanuclear zone (I-cells), and clinically by severe growth impairment, minimal hepatic enlargement, extreme mental handicap and motor retardation, and clear corneas; inherited as an autosomal recessive trait, it is due to deficiency of multiple lysosomal hydrolases. Called also *I-cell disease*.

m. III a disorder similar to but milder than mucolipidosis II, and thought to be due to the same enzyme deficiency but to a lesser extent. Called also *pseudo-Hurler polydystrophy*.

m. IV a form marked by early corneal clouding, psychomotor retardation, and the presence of lysosomal storage bodies; thought to be transmitted as an autosomal recessive trait.

mucolytic (ˌmyookoh'litik) destroying or dissolving mucus; an agent that so acts.

mucomembranous (ˌmyookoh'membrənəs) pertaining to or composed of mucous membrane.

mucoperiosteum (ˌmyookohˌperi'osti·əm) periosteum having a mucous surface, as in parts of the auditory apparatus. adj. **mucoperiosteal**.

mucopolysaccharide (ˌmyookohˌpoli'sakə·ried) a group of polysaccharides that contain hexosamine, that may or may not be combined with protein and that, dispersed in water, form many of the mucins.

mucopolysaccharidosis (ˌmyookohpoliˌsakə·ri'dohsis) any of a group of genetically determined disorders due to a defect in mucopolysaccharide metabolism, marked by skeletal changes, mental handicap, visceral involvement, corneal clouding, with widespread tissue deposits and mucopolysacchariduria. HURLER'S SYNDROME is the prototype of this disorder.

mucopolysacchariduria (ˌmyookohˌpoliˌsakə·ri'dyooə·ri·ə) an excess of mucopolysaccharides in the urine.

mucoprotein (ˌmyookoh'prohteen) a compound present in all connective and supporting tissues, containing, as prosthetic groups, mucopolysaccharides; soluble in water and relatively resistant to denaturation.

mucopurulent (ˌmyookoh'pyooə·rələnt) marked by an exudate containing both mucus and pus.

mucopus ('myookohˌpus) mucus blended with pus.

Mucor ('myookor) a genus of saprophytic mould fungi; some species cause mucormycosis.

mucormycosis (ˌmyookormie'kohsis) mycosis due to fungi of the order Mucorales, including species of *Absidia*, *Mucor*, and *Rhizopus*, usually occurring in debilitated patients, often beginning in the upper respiratory tract or lungs, from which mycelial growths metastasize to other organs.

mucosa (myoo'kohsə) pl. *mucosae* [L.] mucous membrane. adj. **mucosal**.

mucosanguineous (ˌmyookohsang'gwini·əs) composed of mucus and blood.

mucoserous (ˌmyookoh'siə·rəs) composed of mucus and serum.

mucosocutaneous (myooˌkohsohkyoo'tayni·əs) pertaining to a mucous membrane and the skin.

mucous ('myookəs) pertaining to or resembling mucus; secreting mucus.

m. membrane the membrane covered with epithelium that lines the tubular organs of the body.

mucoviscidosis (ˌmyookohˌvisi'dohsis) a condition characterized by accumulation of extremely thick, tenacious mucus in the important mucus-secreting glands, involving especially the exocrine glands of the pancreas; called also CYSTIC FIBROSIS.

mucus ('myookəs) the free slime of the mucous membrane, composed of the glycoprotein and mucopolysaccharide-rich secretion of its glands, various salts, desquamated cells, and leukocytes.

fertile m. see ovulation method of CONTRACEPTION.

Müller's manoeuvre ('muhləz) an inspiratory effort with a closed glottis after expiration, used during fluoroscopic examination to cause a negative intrathoracic pressure with engorgement of intrathoracic vascular structures.

müllerian duct (muh'liə·ri·ən) either of the paired embryonic ducts developing into the vagina, uterus, and uterine tubes in the female, and becoming largely obliterated in the male. Called also *paramesonephric duct*.

multi- word element. [L.] *many*.

multiallelic (ˌmultee·ə'lelik) pertaining to or occupied by many different genes affecting the same or different hereditary characters.

multiarticular (ˌmultee·ah'tikyuhlə) pertaining to or affecting many joints.

Multibionta (ˌmultibie'ontə) trademark for an injectable multivitamin preparation for addition to infusion solutions.

multicapsular (ˌmulti'kapsuhlə) having many capsules.

multicellular (ˌmulti'selyuhlə) composed of many cells.

multicultural (ˌmulti'kulchə·rəl) an adjective relating to a society, community or country consisting of a number of different cultural and/or ethnic groups. See also CULTURE.

multicuspidate (ˌmulti'kuspiˌdayt) having numerous cusps.

multicystic (ˌmulti'sistik) polycystic.

multifactorial (ˌmultifak'tor·ri·əl) 1. of or pertaining to, or arising through the action of, many factors. 2. in genetics, arising as the result of the interaction of several genes.

multifocal (ˌmulti'fohk'l) arising from or pertaining to many foci.

multiform ('multiˌfawm) occurring in many forms; polymorphic.

multiglandular (ˌmulti'glandyuhlə) affecting several glands.

multigravida (ˌmulti'gravidə) a woman pregnant for the third (or more) time.

grand m. a pregnant woman who has had four or more previous pregnancies.

multilobar (ˌmulti'lohbə) having numerous lobes.

multilobular (ˌmulti'lobyuhlə) having many lobules.

multilocular (ˌmulti'lokyuhlə) having many compartments.

multinodular (ˌmulti'nodyuhlə) having many nodules.

multinucleate (ˌmulti'nyookli·ət, -kliˌayt) having many nuclei.

multipara (mul'tipə·rə) a woman who has had two or more pregnancies resulting in viable offspring. adj. **multiparous**.

grand m. a woman who has had five or more pregnancies that resulted in viable offspring.

multiparity (ˌmulti'parətee) the condition of being a multipara.

multiple ('multip'l) manifold; occurring in various parts of the body at once.

m. myeloma a malignant neoplasm of plasma cells in which the plasma cells proliferate and invade the bone marrow, causing destruction of the bone and resulting in pathological fracture and bone pain. It is characterized by the presence of an immunoglobulin recognized as a single protein (monoclonal immunoglobulin), Bence Jones proteinuria, anaemia, and lowered resistance to infection. Called also *Kahler's disease*, *myelopathic albumosuria*, *Bence Jones albumosuria*, and *lymphadenia ossea*.

Diagnostic procedures to confirm suspected multiple myeloma include blood analyses, quantitative immunological assay, urinalysis, bone marrow aspiration and biopsy, and radiography. Findings indicative of the disease are an increased number of plasma cells in the bone marrow (usually over 10 per cent of the total), anaemia, hypercalcaemia due to release of calcium from deteriorating bone tissue, an elevated blood urea nitrogen, Bence Jones protein in the urine, and osteolytic lesions that give the bone a honeycomb appearance on radiographs and lead to vertebral collapse.

Treatment of multiple myeloma involves chemotherapy and the use of radiation to relieve pain and improve the acute lesions of the spinal column when present.

Patient Care. Major problems presented by the patient with multiple myeloma are related to anaemia, hypercalcaemia, bone pain and pathological fractures, and emotional distress created by trying to cope with the day-to-day physiological and emotional aspects associated with the diagnosis of a malignant disease. The more common complications arising are infection, and renal failure; spinal cord compression is rare but presents major problems in management.

Transfusions with packed red cells can help alleviate the symptoms of anaemia. It is important that the patient be adequately hydrated to improve viscosity of the blood and circulation, to help avoid hypercalcaemia, and to maintain kidney function and the excretion of the products of protein metabolism. Continued ambulation and moderate exercise help slow down the loss of minerals, especially calcium, from the bones.

Other problems are related to the administration of highly toxic ANTINEOPLASTIC drugs.

m. sclerosis (MS) a chronic neurological disease in which there are patches of demyelination scattered throughout the white matter of the central nervous system (CNS), sometimes extending into the grey matter. The disease primarily affects the myelin and not the nerve cells themselves; any damage to the neurons is secondary to destruction of the myelin covering the axon (the long process of the neuron that transmits electrical impulses from one nerve cell to the next).

Typically, the symptoms caused by these lesions of the CNS are weakness, incoordination, paraesthesias, speech disturbances, and visual disturbances, particularly diplopia. More specific signs and symptoms depend on the location of the lesions and the severity and destructiveness of the inflammatory and sclerotic processes.

The course of MS is usually prolonged with remissions and relapses over a period of many years. Brief exacerbations, even with acute and severe symptoms, are thought to be the result of a transient inflammatory depression of neural transmission. Recovery occurs when there has been no permanent damage to the myelin sheath during the attack. Repeated attacks can, however, eventually permanently denude the axons and leave the yellow sclerotic plaques that are characteristic of the disease. Once the disease process reaches the stage of sclerosis the affected axons cannot recover and there is permanent damage.

The prevalence of MS is not certain because the disease is not one that is reported, and mild cases can be either misdiagnosed or never brought to the attention of a doctor. It is far more common in most of the countries of the temperate zones than in tropical and subtropical climates. The onset of symptoms most often occurs between the ages of 20 and 40 years, and the disease affects both sexes about equally.

The cause of MS remains uncertain, but a viral aetiology has always been attractive. Antimeasles antibodies can be found in serum and CSF but the measles antigen has not been found in the nervous system, and a direct connection has never been established. It is possible that an inherited immune response is somehow responsible for the production of autoantibodies that attack the myelin sheath. Some authorities believe that infection by one of the 'slow' viruses occurs during childhood and after some years of latency the virus triggers an antoimmune response.

The diagnosis of MS is difficult because of the wide variety of possible clinical manifestations and the resemblance they bear to other neurological disorders, hysteria, and alcohol intoxication. There is no definitive diagnostic test for MS, but persons with objectively measured CNS abnormalities, a history of episodes of exacerbation and remission of symptoms, and demonstrable delayed blink reflex and evoked visual response are diagnosed as having either possible or probable MS. With time and progressive worsening of symptoms the diagnosis can become definite.

Treatment. A multidisciplinary approach is required to identify with the patient and help him and his family cope with the problems attendant to MS. Stress due to trauma, infection, overexertion, surgery, and emotional upset can aggravate the condition and precipitate a flare-up of symptoms. Supportive measures include a regimen of rest and exercise, a well-balanced diet, avoidance of extremes of heat and cold, and known sources of infection, and adaptation of a productive but relatively unstressful life style. Therapeutic measures include medications to diminish muscle spasticity; measures to overcome urinary retention, for example, CREDÉ'S TECHNIQUE and self-catheterization; speech therapy; and physical therapy to maintain muscle tone and avoid orthopaedic deformities. Because of the impact of the disease on the patient's physical activity and life style and on his relationships with his family and associates, counseling is often advised. It is important that the patient with severe disability maintain a positive attitude toward his illness and that he focus on what he can do rather than dwell on what he is no longer able to do. Regeneration of the damaged neural tissue is not possible but retraining and adaptation are.

Many MS patients and their families receive valuable support and encouragement from continued communication with other MS victims and their families. The Multiple Sclerosis Society of Great Britain and Northern Ireland, 25 Effie Road, Fulham, London SW6 1EE, provides a welfare and support service for patients and their families.

multipolar (ˌmulti'pohlə) having more than two poles or processes.

multisynaptic (ˌmultisi'naptik) pertaining to or relayed through two or more synapses.

multivalent (ˌmulti'vaylənt) 1. combining with several univalent atoms. 2. active against several strains of an organism.

multivitamin (ˌmulti'vitəmin) brown sugar-coated tablet containing vitamin A 2500 units, thiamine hydrochloride 500 μg, ascorbic acid 12.5 mg, and vitamin D 250 units.

mumps (mumps) a communicable paramyxovirus disease, which is statutorily notifiable, that attacks one or both of the parotid glands, the largest of the three pairs of salivary glands; called also *epidemic parotitis* or *epidemic parotiditis*. Occasionally the submaxillary glands are also affected. Although older people may contract the disease, mumps is most common in children.It is rare in infants who are usually protected by maternal antibody.

Mumps is spread by droplet infection. The disease is infectious from 1 to 2 days before symptoms appear until 1 or 2 days after they disappear. The incubation period is usually 18 days, although it may vary from 12 to 26 days. One attack usually gives immunity.

SYMPTOMS. Often the first noticeable symptom of mumps is a swelling of one of the parotid glands. The swelling is frequently accompanied by pain and tenderness. In the first stage of mumps, the patient may have a fever of 37.8 to 40 °C (100 to 104 °F). Other common symptoms include loss of appetite, headache, and back pain.

The swelling increases for the first 2 or 3 days and then diminishes, disappearing by the sixth or seventh day. The swelling usually appears first on one side and then on the other, with as many as 12 days intervening. Sometimes both sides swell at once; occasionally the second side does not swell at all.

Sometimes the disease occurs virtually without symptoms. This mild form of mumps is responsible for the presence of antibodies and immunity in persons who cannot recall having had the disease and yet seem to be immune to it.

COMPLICATIONS. Mumps may affect other parts of the body as well as the salivary glands. In the male, when the testes are affected, the infection is known as orchitis. It strikes about one-third of those who contract mumps after the age of puberty. Orchitis may occur before the swelling of the parotid glands, but usually does not develop until about 7 to 10 days thereafter.

Involvement of the gonads in females is less common and more difficult to detect. Lower abdominal pain and enlargement of the ovaries are symptoms indicating involvement of the ovaries. The breasts may also be affected.

Mumps may affect the central nervous system. Acute meningoencephalitis is a complication in about 10 per cent of cases. It causes dizziness, vomiting, and headache. It may occur before the parotid glands swell or in the absence of other signs of mumps. No specific treatment is required, and the condition disappears without causing permanent damage.

Other less common complications are involvement of the auditory nerve (resulting in deafness), myelitis, and facial neuritis.

TREATMENT. Most children with mumps do not feel ill enough to be confined to bed, and it is sufficent if they remain quietly at home, unless there is a rise in temperature or a complication develops. When the swelling of the parotid glands disappears, the child may return to school. If both glands are involved, this time interval is approximately 7 days. A soft diet with plenty of fluids is recommended until fever and swelling vanish.

PREVENTION. Total isolation of the child is not essential. Males over the age of puberty should avoid contact with the patient. The mumps virus cannot survive for any length of time in open air, so it is unnecessary to take special precautions with the patient's clothing, bedding, dishes, or utensils.

Routine immunization in the first two years of life (with measles and rubella—MMR) has almost eliminated mumps in the USA. It was introduced in the UK in 1988.

iodine m. swelling of the salivary and lacrimal glands as a toxic reaction to iodine therapy.

Munchausen's syndrome ('muhnchowzənz) habitual seeking of hospital treatment for apparent acute illness, the patient giving a plausible and dramatic history, all of which is false.

M. s. by proxy an uncommon situation in which a parent (usually the mother) or both parents fabricate symptoms or signs in a child which is then presented for hospital treatment; overlaps with other forms of child abuse, and fatal outcomes have been reported.

mupirocin (myoo'pierohsin) a topical antibacterial agent, active against staphylococci and streptococci.

mural ('myooə·rəl) pertaining to or occurring in a wall of an organ or cavity.

muramidase (myooə'ramidayz) lysozyme.

Murchison–Pel–Ebstein fever (ˌmərchisənˌpel-'ebstien) a type of fever typical of Hodgkin–s disease, marked by irregular episodes of pyrexia of several days duration, with intervening periods in which the temperature is normal.

murine ('myooə·rien, -rin) pertaining to or affecting mice or rats.

murmur ('mərmə) an auscultatory sound, particularly a periodic sound of short duration of cardiac or vascular origin.

aortic m. a sound indicative of disease of the aortic valve.

apical m. one heard over the apex of the heart.

arterial m. one in an artery, sometimes aneurysmal and sometimes constricted.

Austin Flint m. a loud presystolic murmur at the apex heard in aortic regurgitation.

blood m. one due to an abnormal, commonly anaemic, condition of the blood.

cardiac m. any adventitious sound heard over the region of the heart.

cardiopulmonary m. one produced by the impact of the heart against the lung.

Carey Coombs m. a rumbling mid-diastolic murmur occurring in the early stages of rheumatic fever.

continuous m. a humming murmur heard throughout systole and diastole.

crescendo m. one marked by progressively increasing loudness.

Cruveilhier–Baumgarten m. one heard at the abdominal wall over veins connecting the portal and caval systems.

diastolic m. one at diastole, due to mitral obstruction or to aortic or pulmonic regurgitation.

Duroziez's m. a double murmur over the femoral or other large peripheral artery; due to aortic insufficiency.

ejection m. systolic murmurs heard predominantly in mid-systole, when ejection volume and velocity of blood flow are at their maximum.

Flint's m. Austin Flint murmur.

friction m. friction rub.

functional m. a cardiac murmur occurring in the absence of structural changes in the heart.

Gibson m. a long, rumbling sound occupying most of systole and diastole, usually localized in the second left interspace near the sternum, and usually indicative of patent ductus arteriosus.

Graham Steell m. one due to pulmonary regurgitation in patients with pulmonary hypertension and mitral stenosis.

haemic m. blood murmur.

heart m. any adventitious sound heard over the region of the heart.

machinery m. Gibson murmur.

mitral m. one due to disease of the mitral valve.

musical m. a cardiac murmur having a periodic harmonic pattern.

organic m. one due to structural change in the heart.

pansystolic m. one heard throughout systole.

prediastolic m. one occurring just before and with diastole, due to mitral obstruction or to aortic or pulmonary regurgitation.

presystolic m. one shortly before the onset of ventricular ejection, usually associated with a narrowed atrioventricular valve.

pulmonic m. one due to disease of the valves of the pulmonary artery.

regurgitant m. one due to a dilated valvular orifice with consequent regurgitation of blood through the valve. **seagull m.** a raucous murmur resembling the call of a seagull, frequently heard in aortic insufficiency.

Still's m. a functional cardiac murmur of childhood, heard in mid-systole.

systolic m. one occurring at systole, usually due to mitral or tricuspid regurgitation, or to aortic or pulmonary obstruction.

tricuspid m. one caused by disease of the tricuspid valve.

vascular m. one heard over a blood vessel.

vesicular m. the normal breath sounds heard over the lungs.

Murphy's sign ('mərfeez) a sign of gallbladder disease consisting of pain on taking a deep breath when the examiner's fingers are on the approximate location of the gallbladder.

Musca ('muskə) a genus of flies, including the common housefly, *M. domestica.*

musca ('muskə) pl. *muscae* [L.] a fly.

muscae volitantes specks seen as floating before the eyes.

muscarine ('muskə·reen) a deadly alkaloid from various mushrooms, e.g., *Amanita muscaria* (the fly agaric), and also from rotten fish.

muscarinic (ˌmuskə'rinik) pertaining to the transmission of nerve impulses mediated by muscarinic receptors.

m. receptors cholinergic receptors of autonomic effector cells (and also on some autonomic ganglion cells and in some central neurons) that are stimulated by muscarine and parasympathomimetic drugs and blockaded by atropine.

muscle ('mus'l) a bundle of long slender cells, or fibres, that have the power to relax and contract and hence to produce movement. Muscles are responsible for locomotion and play an important part in performing vital body functions. They also protect the contents of the abdomen against injury and help support the body.

Muscle fibres range in length from a few millimetres to several centimetres. They also vary in shape, and in colour from white to deep red. Each muscle fibre receives its own nerve impulses, so that fine and varied motions are possible. Each has its small stored supply of glycogen, which, when converted to glucose, it uses as fuel for energy. Muscles, especially the heart, also use free fatty acids as fuel. At the signal of an impulse traveling down the nerve, the muscle fibre changes chemical energy into mechanical energy, and the result is muscle contraction.

Some muscles are attached to bones by tendons. Others are attached to other muscles, and to skin—producing the smile, the wink and other facial expressions, for example. All or part of the walls of hollow internal organs, such as the heart, stomach, intestines, and blood vessels, are composed of muscles. The last stages of swallowing and of peristalsis are actually series of contractions followed by relaxations of the muscles in the walls of the organs involved.

TYPES OF MUSCLE. There are three types of muscle—involuntary, voluntary, and cardiac. They are composed respectively of smooth, striated (or striped), and mixed smooth and striated tissue.

Muscles that are not under the control of the conscious part of the brain are called involuntary muscles. They respond to the nerve impulses of the autonomic nervous system. These involuntary muscles are the countless short-fibred, or smooth, muscles of the internal organs. They power the digestive tract, the pupils of the eyes, and all other involuntary mechanisms.

The muscles controlled by the conscious part of the brain are called voluntary muscles, and are striated. These are the skeletal muscles that enable the body to move, and there are more than 600 of them in the human body. The fibres of voluntary muscles are grouped together in a sheath of muscle cells. Groups of fibres are bundled together into fascicles and the bundles are surrounded by a tough sheet of connective tissue to form a muscle group like the biceps.

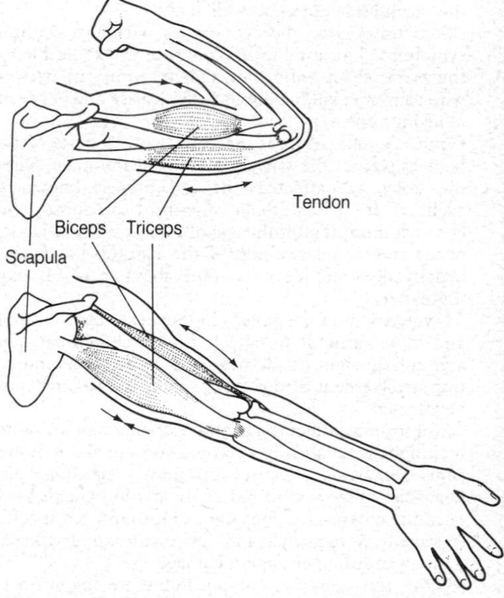

Voluntary muscles. These extend from one bone to another, effect movements by contraction and work on the principle of leverage. For every direct action made by a muscle, an antagonistic muscle effects an opposite movement. To flex the arm, the biceps contracts and the triceps relaxes; to extend the arm, the triceps contracts and the biceps relaxes

Unlike the involuntary muscles, which can remain in a state of contraction for long periods without tiring and are capable of sustained rhythmic contractions, the voluntary muscles are readily subject to fatigue.

The third kind of muscle, cardiac muscle, or the muscle of the heart, is involuntary and consists of striated fibres different from voluntary muscle fibres. The contraction and relaxation of cardiac muscle continue at a rhythmic pace from the fetal period until death unless the muscle is injured in some way. See also HEART.

PHYSIOLOGY OF MUSCLES. No muscle stays completely relaxed, and as long as a person is conscious, it remains slightly contracted. This condition is called tonus, or tone. It keeps the bones in place and enables a posture to be maintained. It allows a person to remain standing, sitting up straight, kneeling, or in any other natural position. Muscles also have elasticity. They are capable of being stretched and of performing reflex actions. This is made possible by the motor and

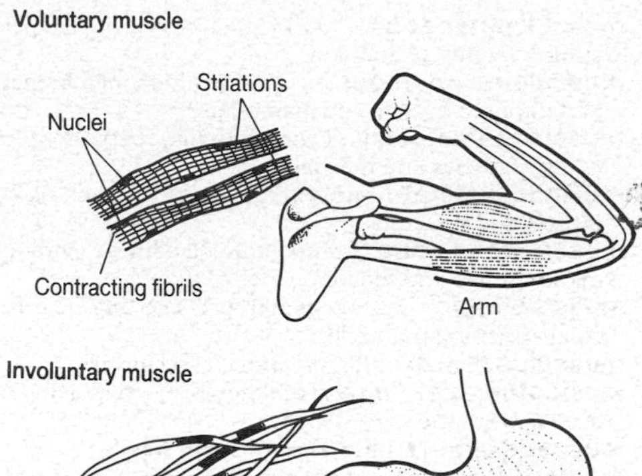

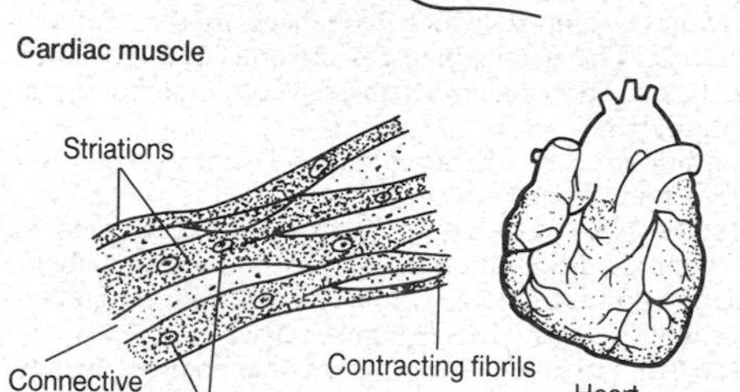

Types of muscle

sensory nerves which serve the muscles.

Muscles enable the body to perform different types of movement. Those that bend a limb at a joint, raising a thigh or bending an elbow, are called flexors. Those that straighten a limb are called extensors. There are others, the abductors, that make possible movement away from the midline of the body, whereas the adductors permit movement toward the midline. Muscles always act in opposing groups. In bending an elbow or flexing a muscle, for example, the biceps (flexor) contracts and the triceps (extensor) relaxes. The reverse happens in straightening the elbow.

A muscle that has contracted many times, and has exhausted its stores of glycogen and other substances, and accumulated too much lactic acid, becomes unable to contract further and suffers from what is called muscle fatigue. In prolonged exhausting work, fat in the muscles can also be used for energy, and as a consequence the muscles become leaner.

MUSCULAR DISORDERS AND DISEASES. Strenuous physical activity that strains and tears the fibres can cause muscular disorders such as strain and muscle cramps.

Muscles may become infected or inflamed by the invasion of organisms, such as the parasite *Trichinella spiralis*, which is taken into the body by eating uncooked or poorly cooked pork. It causes the disease called trichinosis. Another type of muscular inflammation is fibrositis.

In poliomyelitis and other diseases of the nervous system, the muscles are disabled because the nerves leading to them have been injured or destroyed. The muscles are not directly harmed, but because they can no longer be stimulated they eventually waste away from disuse. The group of diseases called the progressive muscular atrophies result from wasting.

MYASTHENIA GRAVIS involves primarily the muscles of the face, eyelids, larynx, and throat. The cause is an impairment of the conduction of nerve impulses to the muscles.

Some diseases directly disable the muscles. MUSCULAR DYSTROPHY weakens the muscles of the trunk and limbs. The muscles sometimes enlarge or they may weaken and atrophy.

Benign and malignant tumours may (rarely) develop in muscles, producing myomas.

agonistic m. one opposed in action by another muscle, called the antagonist.

antagonistic m. one that counteracts the action of another muscle (the agonist).

appendicular m. one of the muscles of a limb.

articular m. one that has one end attached to the capsule of a joint.

cutaneous m. striated muscle that inserts into the skin.

extraocular m's the six voluntary muscles that move the eyeball: superior, inferior, middle, and lateral recti, and superior and inferior oblique muscles.

extrinsic m. one that originates in another part than that of its insertion, as those originating outside the eye, which move the eyeball.

fixation m's, fixator m's accessory muscles that serve to steady a part.

hamstring m's the muscles of the back of the thigh.

intraocular m's the intrinsic muscles of the eyeball.

intrinsic m. one whose origin and insertion are both in the same part or organ, as those entirely within the eye.

orbicular m. one that encircles a body opening, e.g., the eye or mouth.

m. relaxant an agent that specifically aids in reducing muscle tension.

skeletal m's striated muscles that are attached to bones and typically cross at least one joint.

sphincter m. a ringlike muscle that closes a natural orifice; called also *sphincter*.

synergic m's, synergistic m's those that assist one another in action.

thenar m's the abductor and flexor muscles of the thumb.

yoked m's those that normally act simultaneously and equally, as in moving the eyes.

muscular ('muskyuhlə) 1. pertaining to a muscle. 2. having well developed muscles.

m. dystrophy a group of genetically determined, painless, degenerative myopathies that are progressively crippling because muscles are gradually weakened and eventually atrophy. At present there is no specific cure. The disease can sometimes be arrested temporarily; not all forms of it are totally disabling.

The word dystrophy means faulty or imperfect nutrition. In muscular dystrophy the muscles suffer a vital loss of protein, and muscle fibres are replaced gradually by fat and connective tissue until, in the late stages of the disease, the voluntary muscle system becomes virtually useless. In muscular dystrophy all visible damage occurs in the muscles themselves, and thus the disease is markedly different from MULTIPLE SCLEROSIS, in which the muscles are rendered impotent by damage to the nerves that control them.

Muscular dystrophy is hereditary, although the way it is inherited is not the same for all types of the disease. The disease (or a propensity for the disease) seems to be carried mainly by women who, while not suffering from it themselves, may pass it on to their offspring, usually their sons. A woman who has conceived a dystrophic child is likely to be a carrier, as may be a woman who has had a dystrophic relative such as an uncle.

Childhood Muscular Dystrophy. Muscular dystrophy cannot be detected at birth. In most cases the symptoms begin to be noticeable about the second or third year. The child gradually finds it more difficult to play and get about. Then, as the weakening process of the disease continues, he relies on a wheelchair, and later must spend most of his time in bed. In many cases death comes before the age of 20 from respiratory ailments or heart failure.

This childhood type of disease—unfortunately the most common type—is known as the *Duchenne type* or *progressive muscular dystrophy*. It is also called *pseudohypertrophic muscular dystrophy* because at the beginning the muscles, especially those in the calves, appear healthy and bulging when actually they are already weakened and their size is due to an excess of fat.

Other Types. Another type of the disease sometimes begins in childhood but is much more likely to appear during the teens or twenties. When the first symptom is a failure of the musculature of the pelvic girdle, this type is referred to as *limb-girdle muscular dystrophy*. It usually proceeds more slowly than does the childhood form.

This same type may take the form of facioscapulohumeral muscular dystrophy (affecting the face, shoulder, and upper arm muscles), which is likely to manifest itself first in an almost imperceptible weakening of the facial muscles. It is also known as *Landouzy-Déjérine muscular dystrophy*. Muscle deterioration starts in childhood or early adulthood but it may proceed very gradually over a number of years, sometimes until late in life. Some patients may only be slightly handicapped.

Other, rarer types of muscular dystrophy have been identified, including a distal type that begins in the peripheral muscles of the extremities. Still another type affects only muscles of the eye. Sometimes two or more forms are present in the same patient.

Management of Muscular Dystrophy. There is almost never any pain in muscular dystrophy. The mind is not affected; patients have normal intelligence. As the small muscles often are the last to be damaged, patients may continue to use their fingers. Children with muscular dystrophy are able to enjoy many recreations, even when they must rely on crutches or wheelchairs. The disease is not infectious.

Recent experiments hold out some hope that the progress of the disease can be slowed down, at least temporarily, by the use of certain medications that contribute to a build-up of protein in the patient's body or strengthen his muscle-cell membranes to prevent excessive escape of protein. Physiotherapy exercises, including exercise of the lungs by deep breathing, can sometimes bolster the delaying action against muscular weakness. The aim of such exercise is not to restore muscle power (which cannot be done) but to ensure that the patient makes the best use of the good muscle tissue remaining.

The more active the patient is, the better he will be physically and mentally. Obesity should be avoided.

The Muscular Dystrophy Group of Great Britain, Nattrass House, 35 Macavlay Road, London SW4 0QP, is concerned not only with research but with every aspect of the care and comfort of dystrophic patients and can offer many valuable suggestions.

muscularis (ˌmuskyuh'lair·ris) [L.] relating to muscle, specifically a muscular layer or coat.

musculature ('muskyuhləchə) the muscular system of the body, or the muscles of a particular region.

musculocutaneous (ˌmuskyuhlohkyoo'tayni·əs) pertaining to muscle and skin.

musculomembranous (ˌmuskyuhloh'membrənəs) pertaining to muscle and membrane.

musculophrenic (ˌmuskyuhloh'frenik) pertaining to (chest) muscles and the diaphragm.

musculoskeletal (ˌmuskyuhloh'skelit'l) pertaining to muscle and skeleton.

musculotendinous (ˌmuskyuhloh'tendinəs) pertaining to muscle and tendon.

musculotropic (ˌmuskyuhloh'tropik) exerting its principal effect upon muscle.

musculus ('muskyuhləs) pl. *musculi* [L.] muscle.

musicotherapy (ˌmyoozikoh'therəpee) treatment of disease by music.

Musset's sign ('muhsayz) de Musset's sign.

mustard ('mustəd) an irritant compound derived from dried ripe seed of *Brassica nigra* or *B. juncea*.

nitrogen m. mustine.

nitrogen m's a group of toxic, blistering alkylating agents homologous to dichlorodiethyl sulphide (mustard gas), some of which have been used as antineoplastics. The group includes mustine (nitrogen mustard), cyclophosphamide, thiotepa, chlorambucil, and melphalan.

sulphur m. a synthetic compound with vesicant and other toxic properties.

mustine hydrochloride (ˌmusteen) nitrogen mustard; a cytotoxic drug which may be given intravenously for malignant disease of lymph glands and reticuloendothelial cells, such as Hodgkin's disease.

mutagen ('myootəˌjen) an agent that induces genetic mutation.

mutagenesis (ˌmyootə'jenəsis) the induction of genetic mutation.

mutagenic (ˌmyootə'jenik) inducing genetic mutation.

mutagenicity (ˌmyootəjə'nisitee) the property of being able to induce genetic mutation.

mutant ('myootənt) 1. in genetics, a variation that breeds true, owing to genetic changes. 2. produced by mutation.

mutase ('myootayz) any of a group of enzymes (transferases) that catalyse the intramolecular shifting of a chemical group from one position to another.

mutation (myoo'tayshən) a permanent transmissible change in the genetic material. Also, an individual exhibiting such change; a sport.

point m. a mutation resulting from a change in a single base pair in the DNA molecule.

somatic m. a genetic mutation occurring in a somatic cell, providing the basis for mosaicism.

suppressor m. the correction of the effect of a mutation at one locus by a mutation at another locus.

mute (myoot) 1. unable or unwilling to speak. 2. a person who cannot speak. In most cases, mutes are also deaf (deaf-mute).

mutilation (ˌmyooti'layshən) deliberate infliction of bodily injury.

mutism ('myootizəm) inability or refusal to speak. In almost all cases, mutes are unable to speak because deafness has prevented them from hearing the spoken word. Speech is learned by imitating the speech of others. Even the child who is born with normal hearing and then loses it may lose part or all of his power of speech through loss of contact with the speech of others. In certain cases, mutism occurs because the voice organs themselves have been damaged or removed. This is particularly true in the case of cancer of the throat, in which LARYNGECTOMY is performed.

akinetic m. a state in which the person makes no spontaneous movement or vocal sound, because of either neurological or psychological reasons.

hysterical m. hysterical inability to utter words.

muton ('myooton) a gene when specified as the smallest hereditary element that can be altered by mutation.

mutualism ('myootyooə,lizəm) the biological association of two individuals or populations of different species, both of which are benefited by the relationship and sometimes unable to exist without it.

mutualist ('myootyooə,list) one of the organisms or species living in a state of mutualism.

mV millivolt.

μV microvolt.

my(o)- word element. [Gr.] *muscle.*

myaesthesia (,mie·is'theezi·ə) muscle sensibility.

myalgia (mie'alji·ə) muscular pain.

epidemic m. epidemic pleurodynia.

Myambutol (mie'ambyuhtol) trademark for preparations of ethambutol, an antituberculous drug.

myasthenia (,mieəs'theeni·ə) muscular debility or weakness. adj. **myasthenic.**

angiosclerotic m. excessive muscular fatigue due to vascular changes; intermittent claudication.

m. gastrica weakness and loss of tone in the muscular coats of the stomach; atony of the stomach.

m. gravis an AUTOIMMUNE DISEASE manifested by a syndrome of fatigue and exhaustion of the muscles that is aggravated by activity and relieved by rest, the weakness ranging from being very mild to being life-threatening. There is no muscular atrophy or loss of sensation. The disorder characteristically affects the ocular and other cranial muscles, tends to fluctuate in severity, and responds to cholinergic drugs.

The muscular weakness is believed to be caused by the presence of circulating antibodies which are directed against the postsynaptic acetylcholine receptors at the neuromuscular junction. It is not clear what events initiate the formation of the antibodies. There also is some evidence of altered cellular immunity, but the role of the sensitized lymphocytes is not fully understood.

Symptoms of myasthenia gravis include ptosis, diplopia, difficulty in chewing, and dysphagia. Weakness of the legs and arms usually is first noted when the patient tries to walk upstairs, gets up from a sitting position, raises his arms over his head, or lifts a heavy object. Ventilatory deficiency due to weakness of the respiratory muscles occurs in patients who have a severe form of the disease. About 20 per cent of all cases have only ocular myasthenia; the remaining cases have some form of generalized weakness. Diagnosis is established when there is a favourable response to cholinergic drugs. These drugs are inhibitors of the enzyme acetylcholinesterase, which breaks down acetylcholine. They permit acetylcholine levels to become high enough to stimulate the postsynaptic receptors.

Children born of mothers with the disease exhibit a transient weakness that is evident at birth or may appear in the first day or so, with feeding difficulties manifested by poor sucking and swallowing abilities. These children rarely have bulbar involvement, and usually recover in a week or so after birth. This condition is called *neonatal myasthenia*, and is related to circulating antibodies acquired from the mother while the fetus was in utero. *Congenital myasthenia* is also present at birth, but it may not be evident until after the first year of life. The child produces antibodies against acetylcholine receptor sites and experiences symptoms similar to those presented by myasthenia gravis patients of all ages.

There are two general modes of therapy: one is purely symptomatic, and the other entails the use of measures to induce remission of the disease itself. The patient is started on cholinergic drugs, such as neostigmine or pyridostigmine, as soon as the diagnosis is confirmed. The steroid prednisone and other immunosuppressive drugs such as azathioprine provide some relief of symptoms and longer periods of remission. Thymectomy is an alternative treatment for those patients whose weakness and debility do not respond adequately to cholinergic drug therapy. Plasma exchange to remove the circulating autoantibodies is a relatively new therapy that may provide some clinical improvement.

Myasthenic crisis can develop suddenly after a systemic infection, surgery, or some other stressful event. The crisis usually is transient, but during the critical phase assisted VENTILATION and intensive care are needed to assure survival of the patient with respiratory failure.

neonatal m. a transient (a week to a month) myasthenia affecting offspring of myasthenic women.

myatonia (,mieə'tohni·ə) defective muscular tone.

m. congenita amyotonia congenita.

myatrophy (mie'atrəfee) atrophy of a muscle.

myc(o)- word element. [Gr.] *fungus.*

mycelium (mie'seeli·əm) pl. *mycelia;* the mass of threadlike processes (hyphae) constituting the fungal thallas. adj. **mycelial.**

mycetismus (,miesi'tizməs) mushroom poisoning.

mycetoma (,miesi'tohmə) 1. a chronic disease caused by a variety of fungi, affecting the foot, hands, legs, and other parts; called also *maduromycosis*. The most common form is that of the foot (Madura foot), characterized by sinus formation, necrosis and swelling. 2. a tumour-like tangled mass of fungal mycelia.

Mycobacterium (,miekohbak'tiə·ri·əm) a genus of gram-positive bacteria characterized by acid-fast staining.

M. balnei the cause of swimming pool granuloma.

M. bovis the bovine variety of tubercle bacillus, most commonly infecting cattle but can be acquired by man by ingestion of infected milk.

M. kansasii the aetiological agent of a tuberculosis-like disease in man.

M. leprae the aetiological agent of leprosy.

M. tuberculosis the causative agent of tuberculosis in man.

mycobacterium (,miekohbak'tiə·ri·əm) pl. *mycobacteria* [L.] 1. an individual organism of the genus *Mycobacterium*. 2. a slender, acid-fast microorganism resembling the bacillus that causes tuberculosis.

mycodermatitis (,miekoh,dərmə'tietis) fungal infection of the skin.

mycologist (mie'koləjist) a specialist in mycology.

mycology (mie'koləjee) the study of fungi and fungus diseases.

mycomyringitis (,miekoh,mirin'jietis) fungus inflammation of the eardrum.

Mycoplasma (,miekoh'plazmə) a genus of highly pleomorphic, gram-negative, aerobic or facultatively anaerobic bacteria that lack cell walls, including the pleuropneumonia-like organisms (PPLO) and separated into 15 species.

M. hominis a species found associated with nongonococcal urethritis and reported to cause mild pharyngitis in humans.

M. pneumoniae a cause of primary atypical pneumonia; called also *Eaton agent*.

mycosis (mie'kohsis) any disease caused by fungi.

m. fungoides a T-cell LYMPHOMA presenting with skin rashes due to tumour infiltration of the epidermis. As the disease progresses the skin infiltrates become more tumour-like and lymph nodes become involved. Characterization of the tumour infiltrate suggests that the tumour cells are derived from helper T-cells.

opportunistic m. a fungal or fungus-like disease occurring in a person with a compromised immune system. Opportunistic organisms are normal resident flora that become pathogenic only when the host's immune defences are altered, as in immunosuppressive therapy, in a chronic disease, such as diabetes mellitus, or during steroid or antibacterial therapy that upsets the balance of bacterial flora in the body.

True pathogenic fungi include species of *Aspergillus*, *Candida*, *Mucor*, and *Cryptococcus*. Opportunistic mycoses are caused by the actinomycetes, which are actually bacteria that produce diseases similar to true systemic fungal infections. Successful treatment of opportunistic mycoses depends on identification of the specific organism causing the infection. Without effective therapy a systemic infection of this type can be fatal.

mycostasis (mie'kostəsis) prevention of growth and multiplication of fungi.

mycostat ('miekoh,stat) an agent that inhibits the growth of fungi.

mycotic (mie'kotik) pertaining to a mycosis; caused by fungi.

mycotoxicosis (,miekohtoksi'kohsis) 1. poisoning due to a fungal or bacterial toxin. 2. poisoning due to ingestion of fungi.

mydriasis (mi'drieəsis, mie-) dilation of the pupil.

mydriatic (,midri'atik) 1. pertaining to, characterized by, or causing mydriasis. 2. a drug that dilates the pupil.

myectomy (mie'ektəmee) excision of all or part of a muscle.

myectopia (mie·ek'tohpi·ə) displacement of a muscle.

myel(o)- word element. [Gr.] *marrow* (often with specific reference to the spinal cord).

myelalgia (,mieə'lalji·ə) pain in the spinal cord.

myelapoplexy (,mieə'lapə,pleksee) haematomyelia; haemorrhage in the spinal cord.

myelatelia (,mieələ'teeli·ə) imperfect development of the spinal cord.

myelatrophy (,mieə'latrəfee) atrophy of the spinal cord.

myelencephalon (,mieəlen'kefə,lon, -'sef-) 1. the part of the central nervous system comprising the medulla oblongata and lower part of the fourth ventricle. 2. the posterior of the two brain vesicles formed by specialization of the rhombencephalon in the developing embryo.

myelin ('mieəlin) 1. the lipid substance forming a sheath around the axons of certain nerve fibres; these nerve fibres are spoken of as myelinated or medullated fibres. 2. lipoid substance found in various normal and pathological tissues, which differs from fats in being doubly refractive. adj. **myelinic.**

Myelinated nerve fibres occur predominantly in the cranial and spinal nerves and compose the white matter of the brain and spinal cord. In fact, it is the myelin sheath that gives the whitish colour to the areas of white matter. Unmyelinated fibres are abundant in the autonomic nervous system. The term 'grey matter' refers to areas in the nervous system in which the nerve fibres are unmyelinated.

The myelin sheath is formed by a glial cell, either an oligodendrocyte (in the central nervous system) or a Schwann cell (in the peripheral nervous system). An arm of the glial cell is wrapped around the axon, making a sheath composed of many layers of cell membrane. Between the segments of the sheath formed by different glial cells are spaces called *nodes of Ranvier*, which are about 1 mm apart.

In unmyelinated nerves impulses are conducted by the propagation of the action potential along the membrane of the axon. In myelinated nerves impulses are transmitted by an entirely different process, called *saltatory conduction*, in which the impulse jumps from one node of Ranvier to the next. Impulses in myelinated nerves are transmitted hundreds of times faster and require much less energy than in unmyelinated nerves.

myelinated ('mieəli,naytid) having a myelin sheath.

myelination, myelinization (,mieəli'nayshən; ,mieəlinie'zayshən) production of myelin around an axon.

myelinolysis (,mieəli'nolisis) destruction of myelin; demyelination.

myelinosis (,mieəli'nohsis) fatty degeneration, with formation of myelin.

myelinotoxic (,mieəlinoh'toksik) having a deleterious effect on myelin; causing demyelination.

myelitis (,mieə'lietis) inflammation of the spinal cord (see also POLIOMYELITIS) or bone marrow (see also OSTEOMYELITIS). adj. **myelitic.**

bulbar m. that involving the medulla oblongata.

myeloblast ('mieəloh,blast) an immature cell of bone marrow, not normally found in peripheral blood; it is the most primitive precursor in the granulocytic series, which develops into the promyelocyte and eventually into a granulocyte.

myeloblastoma (,mieəlohbla'stohmə) a focal malignant tumour composed of myeloblasts, observed in acute myelocytic leukaemia.

myelocele ('mieəloh,seel) protrusion of the spinal cord through a defect in the vertebral column.

myelocyst ('mieəloh,sist) a cyst developed from rudimentary medullary canals.

myelocystocele (,mieəloh'sistoh,seel) hernial protrusion of spinal cord through a defect in the vertebral column.

myelocystomeningocele (,mieəloh,sistohmə'ning·goh,seel) protrusion of cystic spinal cord and meninges through a defect in the vertebral column.

myelocyte ('mieəloh,siet) 1. a precursor in the granulocytic series intermediate between a promyelocyte and a metamyelocyte, normally occurring only in the bone marrow. In this stage, differentiation into specific cytoplasmic granules has begun. 2. any cell of the grey matter of the nervous system. adj. **myelocytic.**

myelodysplasia (,mieəlohdis'playzi·ə) defective development of the spinal cord.

myelodysplastic syndrome (,mieəlohdis'plastik) a group of conditions which have in common abnormalities in the blood and bone marrow indicating disturbed maturation of myeloid cell lines (including red cells, white cells and platelets). Lymphoid abnormalities are not a feature of these disorders. Well-defined conditions within this group include refractory anaemia, sideroblastic anaemia, and chronic myelomonocytic leukaemia. Called also *dysmyelopoietic syndrome*.

myeloencephalic (,mieəloh,enkə'falik, -sə-) pertaining to the spinal cord and brain.

myeloencephalitis (,mieəloh·en,kefə'lietis, -,sef-) inflammation of the spinal cord and brain.

myelofibrosis (,mieəlohfie'brohsis) replacement of bone marrow by fibrous tissue; a myeloproliferative disorder of elderly people characterized by anaemia and marked splenomegaly.

myelogenesis (,mieəloh'jenəsis) 1. development of the central nervous system. 2. the deposition of myelin around the axon.

myelogenic, myelogenous (,mieəloh'jenik; ,mieə'lojənəs) produced in the bone marrow.

myelogeny (ˌmieə'lojənee) development of the myelin sheaths of nerve fibres.

myelogone ('mieəloh,gohn) a white blood cell of the myeloid series having a reticulate violaceous nucleus, well-stained nucleolus, and deep blue rim of cytoplasm. adj. **myelogonic.**

myelogram ('mieəloh,gram) 1. the film produced by myelography. 2. a graphic representation of the differential count of cells found in a stained representation of bone marrow.

myelography (ˌmieə'lografee) radiography of the spinal cord after injection of a contrast medium into the subarachnoid space.

myeloid ('mieə,loyd) 1. pertaining to, derived from or resembling bone marrow. 2. pertaining to the spinal cord. 3. having the appearance of myelocytes, but not necessarily derived from bone marrow.

m. tissue red bone marrow.

myeloidosis (ˌmieəloy'dohsis) formation of myeloid tissue, especially hyperplastic development of such tissue.

myelolipoma (ˌmieəlohli'pohmə) a rare benign tumour of the adrenal gland composed of adipose tissue, lymphocytes, and primitive myeloid cells.

myeloma (ˌmieə'lohmə) a tumour composed of plasma cells. See also MULTIPLE myeloma.

multiple m. a primary malignant tumour of plasma cells usually arising in bone marrow, and usually associated with anaemia and with a paraprotein in the blood or Bence Jones protein in the urine. Called also *Kahler's disease*, *myelopathic albumosuria*, *Bence Jones albumosuria*, and *lymphadenia ossea*. See also MULTIPLE myeloma.

osteosclerotic m. multiple myeloma associated with osteosclerosis (rather than bone destruction) and often with peripheral neuropathy.

plasma cell m. multiple myeloma.

myelomalacia (ˌmieəlohmə'layshi·ə) morbid softening of the spinal cord.

myelomatosis (ˌmieəlohmə'tohsis) multiple myeloma.

myelomenia (ˌmieəloh'meeni·ə) vicarious menstruation into the spinal cord.

myelomeningitis (ˌmieəloh,menin'jietis) inflammation of the spinal cord and meninges.

myelomeningocele (ˌmieəlohmə'ning·goh,seel) hernial protrusion of the spinal cord and its meninges through a defect in the vertebral column.

myeloneuritis (ˌmieəlohnyuh'rietis) inflammation of the spinal cord and peripheral nerves.

myelopathy (ˌmieə'lopəthee) 1. any functional disturbance or pathological change in the spinal cord; often used to denote nonspecific lesions, as opposed to myelitis. 2. pathological bone marrow changes. adj. **myelopathic.**

spondylotic cervical m. myelopathy secondary to encroachment of cervical spondylosis upon a congenitally small cervical spinal canal.

myeloperoxidase (ˌmieəlohpə'roksi,dayz) a haemoprotein having peroxidase activity, occurring in the primary granules of promyelocytes, myelocytes, and neutrophils, and which exhibits bactericidal, fungicidal, and viricidal properties.

myelopetal (ˌmieə'lopit'l) moving toward the spinal cord.

myelophthisis (ˌmieə'lofthisis) 1. wasting of the spinal cord. 2. reduction of the cell-forming functions of bone marrow.

myelopoiesis (ˌmieəlohpoy'eesis) the formation of marrow or the cells arising from it.

ectopic m., extramedullary m. formation of myeloid tissue outside bone marrow.

myeloproliferative (ˌmieəlohprə'lifə·rətiv) pertaining to or characterized by abnormal proliferation of bone marrow constituents.

m. syndrome a group of diseases related histogenetically and marked, at varying times in varying degrees, by medullary and extramedullary proliferation (in the spleen or liver, for example) of one or more lines of bone marrow constituents, including myelocytic, erythroblastic, and megakaryocytic forms, in addition to various cells derived from the reticulum and mesenchymal elements.

myeloradiculitis (ˌmieəlohrə,dikyuh'lietis) inflammation of the spinal cord and posterior nerve roots.

myeloradiculodysplasia (ˌmielohrə,dikyuhlohdis'playzi·ə) abnormal development of the spinal cord and spinal nerve roots.

myeloradiculopathy (ˌmieəlohrə,dikyuh'lopəthee) disease of the spinal cord and spinal nerve roots.

myelorrhagia (ˌmieələ'rayji·ə) haematomyelia; spinal haemorrhage.

myelosarcoma (ˌmieəlohsah'kohmə) a sarcomatous growth made up of myeloid tissue or bone marrow cells.

myelosclerosis (ˌmieəlohsklə'rohsis) 1. sclerosis of the spinal cord. 2. obliteration of the marrow cavity by small spicules of bone. 3. myelofibrosis.

myelosis (ˌmieə'lohsis) 1. proliferation of bone marrow tissue, producing the blood changes of myelocytic leukaemia. 2. formation of a tumour of the spinal cord.

erythraemic m. a malignant blood dyscrasia, one of the myeloproliferative disorders, with progressive anaemia, megaloblastic erythroid hyperplasia, myeloid dysplasia, hepatosplenomegaly, and haemorrhagic phenomena.

myelospongium (ˌmieəloh'spunji·əm) a network developing into the neuroglia.

myelosuppressive (ˌmieəlohsə'presiv) 1. inhibiting bone marrow activity, resulting in decreased production of blood cells and platelets. 2. an agent having such properties.

myelotomy (ˌmieə'lotəmee) severance of nerve fibres in the spinal cord.

myelotoxin (ˌmieəloh'toksin) a toxin that destroys bone marrow cells. adj. **myelotoxic.**

myenteron (mie'entə·ron) the muscular coat of the intestine. adj. **myenteric.**

Myerson's sign ('mieəsənz) in Parkinson's disease, repeated blinking of the eyes on tapping the forehead.

myiasis (mie'ieəsis, 'mieəsis) invasion of the body by the larvae of flies, characterized as cutaneous (subdermal tissue), gastrointestinal, nasopharyngeal, ocular, or urinary, depending on the region invaded.

myko- for words beginning thus, see those beginning *myco-*.

Myleran ('mielərən) trademark for preparations of busulphan, an antineoplastic.

mylohyoid (ˌmieloh'hieoyd) pertaining to the hyoid bone and molar teeth.

Mynah ('mienə) trademark for combination preparations of ethambutol and isoniazid, antituberculous drugs.

myo- word element. [Gr.] *muscle.*

myoatrophy (ˌmieoh'atrəfee) muscular atrophy.

myoblast ('mieoh,blast) an embryonic cell that becomes a cell of muscle fibre. adj. **myoblastic.**

myoblastoma (ˌmieohbla'stohmə) a benign circumscribed tumour-like lesion of soft tissue.

myobradia (ˌmieoh'braydi·ə) slow reaction of muscle to stimulation.

myocardial (ˌmieoh'kahdi·əl) pertaining to the muscular tissue of the heart (the myocardium).

m. infarction (MI) necrosis of the cells of an area of the heart muscle (myocardium) occurring as a result of oxygen deprivation, which in turn is caused by obstruction to the blood supply; commonly referred to as a 'heart attack'.

The myocardium receives its blood supply from the two large coronary arteries and their branches. Occlusion of one or more of these blood vessels (coronary occlusion) is one of the major causes of myocardial infarction. The occlusion may result from the formation of a clot that develops suddenly when an atheromatous plaque ruptures through the sublayers of a blood vessel, or when the narrow, roughened inner lining of a sclerosed artery leads to thrombosis. Coronary artery disease is the most common type of heart disease in many countries. The risk rises rapidly with age, women tending to develop the disease 15 to 20 years later than men.

Other causes of MI are related to a sudden increased need for blood supply to the heart, as in shock, haemorrhage, and severe physical exertion, and to restriction of blood flow through the aorta, as in aortic stenosis, which predisposes to the formation of emboli.

PATHOLOGY. The most common sites of MI are in the left ventricle, that chamber of the heart which has the greatest work load. Tissue changes that occur in the myocardium are related to the extent to which the cells have been deprived of oxygen. Total deprivation results in an *area of infarction*, in which the cells die and the tissue becomes necrotic. Necrosis in this area is evident within 5 to 6 hours after the occlusion. In response to this necrosis the body increases its production of leukocytes, which aid in removal of the dead cells. As collateral circulation enlarges, it brings fibroblasts, which form connective tissues within the area of infarction. Usually, the formation of fibrous scar tissue is complete within 2 to 3 months.

Immediately surrounding the area of infarction is a less seriously damaged *area of injury*. It may deteriorate and thus extend the area of infarction or, with adequate collateral circulation, it may regain its function within 2 to 3 weeks.

The outermost area of damage is the *zone of ischaemia*, which borders the area of injury. The cells in this area are weakened by decreased oxygen supply, but function can return usually within 2 to 3 weeks after the onset of occlusion.

All of the pathological changes described above can be identified by electrocardiography. The information thus obtained is used to prescribe the varying degrees of physical activity allowed the patient as he convalesces.

RISK FACTORS. Unavoidable traits that increase a person's chances for coronary artery disease include racial and genetic susceptibility, sex, and increasing age. Factors that can be controlled to some extent in order to ameliorate the risk include hypertension, cigarette smoking, and elevated serum lipids. Almost half of the persons who have suffered heart attacks have a history of one or more of these latter three risk factors. Minimizing or eliminating these avoidable factors can reduce the incidence and severity of ischaemic heart disease. Preventive measures are discussed more fully under HEART.

SYMPTOMS. The most outstanding symptom of acute MI is a sudden painful sensation of pressure, often described as a 'crushing pain' in the chest, occasionally radiating to the arms, throat, and back, and persisting for hours. Pallor, profuse perspiration, and other signs of shock are present. There may be nausea and vomiting, leading to the mistaken impression that the victim is suffering from acute indigestion. In almost all cases of severe MI the patient is extremely apprehensive and has a sense of impending death.

Severity of symptoms depends on the size of the artery at the point of occlusion and the amount of myocardial tissue served by the artery. In some instances the artery may be small and the symptoms mild. In other cases the extent of damage is large and the attack is fatal.

Within 24 hours of the initial attack there is an elevated temperature and increased white cell count in response to the inflammatory process arising from necrosis of myocardial tissue. Death of the cells also brings about the release of certain enzymes which enter the general circulation. The levels of these enzymes in the blood can be determined by clinical laboratory tests. Within 2 to 4 hours after infarction the level of creatine kinase (CK) is increased. It reaches its peak in 24 to 36 hours and subsides to normal level in 3 days. The level of serum aspartate aminotransferase (AST) increases rapidly in 4 to 6 hours, reaches its peak in 24 to 48 hours, and returns to normal in 5 days. In contrast to the rapid rise and decline of these two enzyme levels, lactate dehydrogenase (LD) levels begin to increase the first day after attack and persist at high levels for 10 to 20 days. These tests can be made more specific by measuring the LD_1 and CK_2 isoenzymes, which are found in the heart. Diagnosis of MI is based on the presenting symptoms and evidence of impaired heart function found by physical examination and electrocardiography and on abnormal serum enzyme levels.

TREATMENT AND PATIENT CARE. Immediate care of acute MI is concerned with combatting shock, relieving respiratory difficulty, and preventing further circulatory collapse. The victim should be kept lying down, and all tight clothing should be loosened to relieve dyspnoea and promote comfort. Without delay, but in a calm, unhurried manner, the patient is transported to a hospital. If the victim shows signs of CARDIAC ARREST, CARDIOPULMONARY RESUSCITATION efforts are begun immediately.

Medical treatment includes administration of an analgesic such as diamorphine or morphine with an antiemetic; on occasion the doctor may order atropine sulphate with morphine to prevent serious bradycardia. Oxygen therapy may be of help.

A new surgical procedure that shows promise in preventing the destruction of heart muscle from infarction was first used in West Germany in the late 1970s. The treatment, called *intracoronary thrombolysis*, involves insertion of a cardiac catheter into the occluded coronary artery and injection of streptokinase, an enzyme that breaks down thrombi and thereby enlarges the diameter of the artery. This procedure is done as soon as possible after a definitive diagnosis of MI has been established. When injections are made within a few hours of an attack, the obstructed artery resumes its job of supplying blood to the heart muscle and massive destruction of myocardial cells is avoided.

Rest is essential to the repair of damaged myocardial cells, but this does not usually mean absolute bed rest. Whether the patient is placed on bed rest or allowed up in a chair depends on his condition.

Adequate rest can only be achieved by the patient if he is free from mental anxiety and is attended by personnel who anticipate his needs and meet them cheerfully and willingly. The amount of rest needed and the degree of physical activity allowed depends on how extensive the area of infarction is thought to be, whether cardiac arrhythmias and other complications develop, and the response of the patient to increased physical activity. Careful monitoring of the pulse rate and blood pressure before and after each activity can provide information on which to evaluate the patient's tolerance for exercise and self-care activities.

Many patients with a myocardial infarction are cared for in a coronary care unit during the acute stage. It is important that the patient and his family be given a brief explanation of the various kinds of monitoring equipment in use and that they be reassured of each staff member's concern for the patient's welfare. There is always the danger that health care personnel become so engrossed in the operating of electronic gadgetry in the unit that they forget the patient's need to be recognized as a fellow human being.

As the patient's physical state improves he is gradually weaned away from intensive care and encouraged to do more for himself in preparation for the day when he will go home. For some patients this is a traumatic experience and they become very apprehensive about leaving the security of the monitors and the attention of the staff. It is possible that the stress of leaving the unit can cause development of complications. In some hospitals the transition from coronary care unit to home is made easier by transfer to a convalescent unit where the patient's response to activities is monitored and he is given instruction regarding his own care after discharge. Information about local coronary clubs, assistance in patient education and physical rehabilitation can be provided by the hospital or local voluntary groups.

myocardiograph (ˌmieohˈkahdiohˌgrahf, -ˌgraf) an instrument for making tracings of heart movements.

myocardiopathy (ˌmieohˌkahdiˈopəthee) any noninflammatory disease of the myocardium.

myocarditis (ˌmieohkahˈdietis) inflammation of the muscular walls of the heart (the myocardium). The condition may result from bacterial or viral infections or it may be a toxic inflammation caused by drugs or toxins from infectious agents. Other systemic diseases that may be accompanied by myocarditis are TRICHINOSIS, SERUM SICKNESS, RHEUMATIC FEVER, and COLLAGEN DISEASES. In many cases the aetiology is unknown.

SYMPTOMS. The most common symptoms of acute myocarditis are pain in the epigastric region or under the sternum, dyspnoea, and cardiac arrhythmias. If the condition persists and becomes chronic, there is pain in the right upper quadrant of the abdomen, owing to hepatic congestion. The latter symptom is a sign of left ventricular failure and often is accompanied by oedema and other signs of congestive heart failure.

TREATMENT. Acute myocarditis usually subsides when the primary illness improves. It is considered incidental to the systemic disease and, though it may be a serious manifestation of a systemic illness, acute myocarditis often does not require specific treatment. Steroids and pressor agents such as noradrenaline may be used to reduce the inflammatory process and maintain adequate arterial pressure.

If the heart involvement becomes chronic, treatment then must be aimed at management of the chronic heart failure. See also congestive HEART FAILURE.

myocardium (ˌmieohˈkahdi·əm) the middle and thickest layer of the heart wall, composed of cardiac muscle. adj. **myocardial**.

myocardosis (ˌmieohkahˈdohsis) any degenerative, noninflammatory disease of the myocardium.

myocele (ˈmieohˌseel) hernia of muscle through its sheath.

myocellulitis (ˌmieohˌselyuhˈlietis) myositis with cellulitis.

myoceptor (ˈmieohˌseptə) the end-plate.

myocerosis (ˌmieohsiˈrohsis) waxy degeneration of muscle.

myoclonus (ˌmieohˈklohnəs) shocklike contractions of part of a muscle, an entire muscle, or a group of muscles; usually a manifestation of a convulsive disorder. adj. **myoclonic**.

m. epilepsy slowly progressive hereditary epilepsy beginning in childhood, with intermittent or continuous clonus of muscle groups, resulting in difficulties in voluntary movements; there is mental deterioration and the presence of Lafora bodies in various cells. Called also *Lafora's disease* and *Unverricht's disease* or *syndrome*.

palatal m. a condition characterized by a rapid rhythmic movement of one or both sides of the palate.

Myocrisin (mieohˈkriezin) trademark for preparations of sodium aurothiomalate.

myocyte (ˈmieohˌsiet) a cell of muscular tissue.

myocytoma (ˌmieohsieˈtohmə) a tumour composed of myocytes.

myodemia (ˌmieohˈdeemi·ə) fatty degeneration of muscle.

myodystonia (ˌmieohdiˈstohni·ə) disorder of muscular tone.

myoelectric (ˌmieoh·iˈlektrik) pertaining to the electric properties of muscle.

myoendocarditis (ˌmieohˌendohkahˈdietis) combined myocarditis and endocarditis.

myoepithelioma (ˌmieohˌepiˌtheeliˈohmə) a tumour composed of outgrowths of myoepithelial cells from a sweat gland.

myoepithelium (ˌmieohˌepiˈtheeli·əm) tissue made up of contractile epithelial cells. adj. **myoepithelial**.

myofascitis (ˌmieohfəˈsietis) inflammation of a muscle and its fascia.

myofibril (ˌmieohˈfiebril, -ˈfib-) a muscle fibril, one of the slender threads of a muscle fibre, composed of numerous myofilaments. adj. **myofibrillar**.

myofibroblast (ˌmieohˈfiebrohˌblast) a modified fibroblast combining the ultrastructural features of a fibroblast and a smooth muscle cell, and containing many actin-rich microfilaments.

myofibroma (ˌmieohfieˈbrohmə) myoma combined with fibroma.

myofibrosis (ˌmieohfieˈbrohsis) replacement of muscle tissue by fibrous tissue.

myofibrositis (ˌmieohˌfibrəˈsietis) inflammation of the sheath of muscle fibre.

myofilament (ˌmieohˈfiləmənt) any of the ultramicroscopic threadlike structures composing the myofibrils of striated muscle fibres.

myogenesis (ˌmieohˈjenəsis) the formation of muscle fibres and muscles in embryonic development. adj. **myogenetic**.

myogenic (ˌmieohˈjenik) giving rise to or forming muscle tissue.

myogenous (mieˈojənəs) originating in muscular tissue.

myoglobin (ˌmieəˈglohbin) the oxygen-transporting pigment of muscle, a conjugated protein resembling a single subunit of haemoglobin, being composed of one globin polypeptide chain and one haem group.

myoglobinuria (ˌmieohˌglohbiˈnyooə·ri·ə) the presence of myoglobin in the urine.

myoglobulin (ˌmieohˈglobyuhlin) a globulin from muscle serum.

myogram (ˈmieohˌgram) a record produced by myography.

myograph (ˈmieohˌgrahf, -ˌgraf) an apparatus for recording the effects of muscular contraction.

myography (mieˈogrəfee) 1. the use of a myograph. 2. description of muscles. 3. radiography of muscle tissue after injection of a radiopaque medium. adj. **myographic**.

myohaemoglobinuria (ˌmieohˌheeməˌglohbi-

'nyooə·ri·ə) the presence of myohaemoglobin in the urine.

myoid ('mieoyd) resembling muscle.

myoischaemia (,mieoh·is'keemi·ə) local deficiency of blood supply in muscle.

myokinesimeter (,mieoh,kini'simitə) an apparatus for measuring muscular contraction induced by electrical stimulation.

myokinetic (,mieohki'netik) pertaining to the motion or kinetic function of muscle, as contrasted with the myotonic or tonic function.

myokymia (,mieoh'kimi·ə) a benign condition in which there is persistent quivering of the muscles.

myolipoma (,mieohli'pohmə) myoma with fatty elements.

myology (mie'oləjee) scientific study or description of the muscles and accessory structures (bursae and synovial sheath).

myolysis (mie'olisis) degeneration of muscle tissue.

myoma (mie'ohmə) a tumour formed of muscle tissue. adj. **myomatous.**

m. uteri, m. of uterus a benign tumour of the smooth muscle fibres of the uterus (see LEIOMYOMA UTERI).

myomalacia (,mieohmə'layshi·ə) morbid softening of a muscle.

myomatosis (,mieohmə'tohsis) the formation of multiple myomas.

myomectomy (,mieə'mektəmee) 1. excision of a myoma. 2. myectomy.

myomelanosis (,mieoh,melə'nohsis) melanosis of muscle.

myomere ('mieoh,miə) myotome; the muscle plate or portion of a somite that develops into voluntary muscle.

myometer (mie'omitə) an apparatus for measuring muscle contraction.

myometritis (mieohmi'trietis) inflammation of the myometrium.

myometrium (,mieoh'meetri·əm) the smooth muscle coat of the uterus. adj. **myometrial.**

myonecrosis (,mieohnə'krohsis) necrosis or death of individual muscle fibres.

myoneural (,mieoh'nyooə·rəl) pertaining to nerve terminations in muscles.

m. junction the point of junction of a nerve fibre with the muscle that it innervates.

myoneuralgia (,mieohnyuh'ralji·ə) neuralgic pain in a muscle.

myo-oedema (,mieoh·i'deemə) 1. mounding. 2. oedema of a muscle.

myopalmus (,mieoh'palməs) muscle twitching.

myoparalysis (,mieohpə'ralisis) paralysis of a muscle.

myoparesis (,mieohpə'reesis) slight muscle paralysis.

myopathy (mie'opəthee) any disease of a muscle. adj. **myopathic.**

centronuclear m. myotubular myopathy. **late distal m.** hereditary muscular dystrophy starting in the hands and feet and spreading proximally.

myotubular m. a form marked by myofibres resembling those of early fetal muscle, i.e., myotubules.

nemaline m. a congenital abnormality of myofibrils in which small threadlike fibres are scattered through the muscle fibres; marked by hypotonia and proximal muscle weakness.

ocular m. a slowly progressive form affecting the extraocular muscles, with ptosis and progressive immobility of the eyes.

myope ('mieohp) a person affected with myopia.

myopericarditis (,mieoh,perikah'dietis) inflammation of both the myocardium and pericardium.

myopia (mie'ohpi·ə) that error of refraction in which rays of light entering the eye parallel to the optic axis are brought to a focus in front of the retina, as a result of the eyeball being too long from front to back, so that vision for near objects is better than for far; called also *near-sightedness* and *short-sightedness* (see also VISION). adj. **myopic.**

Myopia generally appears before the age of 8, often becoming gradually worse until about the age of 20, when it ceases to change very much. In later years the myopic person may find he can read comfortably without his glasses.

curvature m. myopia due to changes in curvature of the refracting surfaces of the eye.

index m. myopia due to abnormal refractivity of the media of the eye.

progressive m. myopia that continues to increase in adult life.

myoplasm ('mieoh,plazəm) the contractile part of the muscle cell.

myoplasty ('mieoh,plastee) plastic surgery on muscle whereby portions of detached muscles are used, especially in the field of defects or deformities. adj. **myoplastic.**

myoreceptor (,mieohri'septə) a receptor situated in skeletal muscle that is stimulated by muscular contraction, providing information to higher centres regarding muscle position.

myorrhaphy (mie'o·rəfee) suture of a muscle.

myorrhexis (,mieə'reksis) rupture of a muscle.

myosarcoma (,mieohsah'kohmə) a malignant tumour derived from myogenic cells.

myosclerosis (,mieohsklə'rohsis) hardening of muscle tissue.

myosin ('mieəsin) one of the two main proteins of muscle. Myosin and actin are the proteins involved in contraction of muscle fibres.

myositis (,mieoh'sietis) inflammation of a voluntary muscle.

epidemic m. epidemic pleurodynia.

m. fibrosa a type in which there is a formation of connective tissue in the muscle.

multiple m. polymyositis.

m. ossificans myositis marked by bony deposits in muscle.

trichinous m. that which is caused by the presence of *Trichinella spiralis.*

myospasm ('mieoh,spazəm) spasm of a muscle.

myotactic (,mieoh'taktik) pertaining to the proprioceptive sense of muscles.

myotasis (mie'otəsis) stretching of muscle. adj. **myotatic.**

myotenositis (,mieoh,tenoh'sietis) inflammation of a muscle and tendon.

myotenotomy (,mieohtə'notəmee) surgical division of the tendon of a muscle.

myotome ('mieə,tohm) 1. an instrument for dividing muscles. 2. a segmented embryonic mass, derived from a somite, which gives rise to a group of muscles innervated by one specific nerve root. adj. **myotomic.**

myotomy (mie'otəmee) 1. cutting or dissection of muscular tissue or of a muscle. 2. cutting of an ocular tendon in treatment of strabismus.

myotonia (,mieə'tohni·ə) any disorder involving tonic spasm of muscle. adj. **myotonic.**

m. atrophica myotonia dystrophica.

m. congenita a hereditary disease marked by tonic spasm and rigidity of certain muscles when attempts are made to move them. The stiffness tends to disappear as the muscles are used.

m. dystrophica a rare, slowly progressive, hereditary disease, marked by myotonia followed by muscular atrophy (especially of the face and neck), cataracts, hypogonadism, frontal balding, and cardiac disorders.

Called also *dystrophia myotonica*.

myotonus (,mieə'tohnəs) tonic spasm of a muscle or a group of muscles.

myotrophic (,mieoh'trofik) 1. increasing the weight of muscle. 2. pertaining to myotrophy.

myotrophy (mie'otrəfee) nutrition of muscle.

myotropic (,mieoh'tropik) having a special affinity for muscle.

myotube, myotubule ('mieoh,tyoob; ,mieoh'tyoobyool) a developing skeletal muscle fibre with a centrally located nucleus. adj. **myotubular**.

myovascular (,mieoh'vaskyuhlə) pertaining to muscle and blood vessels.

Myriapoda (,miri'apədə) a class of arthropods, including the millipedes and centipedes.

myring(o)- (mi'ring·goh) word element. [L.] *tympanic membrane.*

myringa (mi'ring·gə) the tympanic membrane.

myringectomy (,mirin'jektəmee) excision of the tympanic membrane; called also *myringodectomy*.

myringitis (,mirin'jietis) inflammation of the tympanic membrane.

m. bullosa, bullous m. a form of viral otitis media in which serous or haemorrhagic blebs appear on the tympanic membrane and adjacent wall of the acoustic meatus.

myringodectomy (mi,ring·gə'dektəmee) myringectomy.

myringomycosis (mi,ring·gohmie'kohsis) fungus disease of the tympanic membrane.

myringoplasty (mi'ring·goh,plastee) surgical reconstruction of the tympanic membrane.

myringostapediopexy (mi,ring·gohstə'peedioh,peksee) fixation of the large lower portion of the tympanic membrane to the head of the stapes.

myringotomy (,miring'gotəmee) tympanotomy; incision of the tympanic membrane. Called also *tympanocentesis*.

The procedure usually is performed to relieve pressure and allow for drainage of either serous or purulent fluid in the middle ear behind the tympanic membrane. Sometimes, as in the case of serous otitis media or 'fluid ear', a ventilating tube (e.g. a grommet) is inserted to permit continuous drainage and avoid a chronic middle ear problem with fluid accumulation, pain, and loss of hearing.

When a simple myringotomy is done for purposes of draining purulent material resulting from suppurative otitis media, care should be taken to avoid contamination by the fluid. Absorbent materials and dressings used to collect the drainage must be disposed of properly. The outer ear and canal should be protected against prolonged contact with the discharge from the ear. Frequent cleansing with a mild antiseptic and use of a protective salve to act as a skin barrier may be necessary. These precautions are not necessary when myringotomy is done to alleviate and prevent accumulation of sterile serous or mucoid fluid in the middle ear. See also OTITIS MEDIA.

Mysoline ('miesohleen, -in) trademark for preparations of primidone, an anticonvulsant.

mysophilia (,miesoh'fili·ə) a form of paraphilia in which there is a lustful attitude toward excretions.

mysophobia (,miesoh'fohbi·ə) morbid dread of contamination and filth.

mythomania (,mithə'mayni·ə) morbid tendency to lie or exaggerate.

myx(o)- word element. [Gr.] *mucus, slime.*

myxadenitis (,miksadə'nietis) inflammation of a mucus-secreting gland.

myxadenoma (,miksadə'nohmə) an epithelial tumour with the structure of a mucous gland.

myxasthenia (,miksəs'theeni·ə) deficient secretion of mucus.

myxochondroma (,miksohkon'drohmə) chondroma with stroma resembling primitive mesenchymal tissue.

myxocyte ('miksoh,siet) one of the cells of mucous tissue.

myxoedema (,miksi'deemə) a condition resulting from advanced hypothyroidism, or deficiency of thyroxine due to destruction of the thyroid. It is the adult form of the disease known as CRETINISM in its congenital form. adj. **myxoedematous.**

Caused by atrophy, surgical removal, or a disorder of the thyroid gland, or its destruction by radioactive iodine, or by deficient excretion of thyrotrophin by the pituitary gland, myxoedema is marked primarily by a growing puffiness and sogginess of the skin, involving a dry, waxy type of swelling (nonpitting oedema) with abnormal deposits of mucin in the skin and distinctive facial changes (swollen lips and thickened nose).

Because thyroxine plays such an important role in the body's metabolism, lack of this hormone seriously upsets the balance of body processes. Among the symptoms associated with myxoedema are excessive fatigue and drowsiness, headaches, weight gain, dryness of the skin, sensitivity to cold, and increasing thinness and brittleness of the nails. In women, menstrual bleeding may become irregular and excessive. Medical tests reveal slow relaxation of tendon reflexes, low serum thyroxine, below-normal metabolism, and a high serum TSH if the thyroid itself is destroyed.

In myxoedema the body's defences against infection are weakened. If the patient has heart disease, this is likely to worsen. Upset of the functions of the adrenal glands may become critical. In time, if myxoedema is not brought under control, progressive mental deterioration may result in a psychosis marked by paranoid delusions.

Myxoedema is treated by administration of thyroxine. If treatment is begun soon after the symptoms appear, recovery may be complete. Delayed or interrupted treatment may mean permanent deterioration. Treatment must be continued throughout the patient's lifetime.

pretibial m. a localized myxoedema associated with preceding hyperthyroidism occurring typically on the anterior surface of the legs.

myxoedematoid (,miksi'deemə,toyd) resembling myxoedema.

myxofibroma (,miksohfie'brohmə) a fibroma containing myxomatous tissue; called also *fibroma myxomatodes* and *fibromyxoma*.

myxofibrosarcoma (,miksoh,fiebrohsah'kohmə) fibrosarcoma with myxomatous areas.

myxoid ('miksoyd) having a large acellular stromal component in which connective tissue mucins are present.

myxolipoma (,miksohli'pohmə) lipoma with foci of myxomatous degeneration.

myxoma (mik'sohmə) a tumour composed of primitive connective tissue cells and stroma resembling mesencyhma. adj. **myxomatous**.

myxomatosis (,miksəmə'tohsis) 1. the development of multiple myxomas. 2. myxomatous degeneration.

myxomyoma (,miksohmie'ohmə) a myoma with myxomatous degeneration.

myxopoiesis (,miksohpoy'eesis) the formation of mucus.

myxorrhoea (,miksə'reeə) a flow of mucus.

m. intestinalis excessive secretion of intestinal mucus.

myxosarcoma (,miksohsah'kohmə) a sarcoma containing myxomatous tissue.

myxovirus (ˌmiksoh'vierəs) any of a group of RNA viruses, including the viruses of influenza, parainfluenza, mumps, and Newcastle disease, characteristically causing agglutination of chicken erythrocytes.

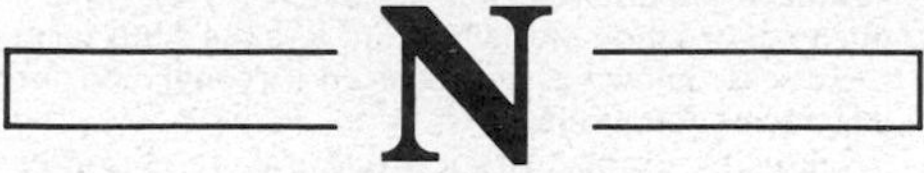

N 1. symbol, *newton*. 2. chemical symbol, *nitrogen*. 3. symbol, *normal* (solution); the expressions 2N (double normal), 0.5N (half-normal), 0.1N (tenth-normal), etc., denote the strength of a solution in comparison with the normal.

n 1. symbol, *refractive index*. 2. symbol, *nano-*.

NA Nomina Anatomica, the internationally approved official body of anatomical nomenclature.

Na chemical symbol, *sodium* (L. *natrium*).

nabilone ('nabilohn) a synthetic cannabinoid used as an antiemetic.

Naboth's cysts (follicles) ('naybohths) cyst-like formations due to occlusion of the lumina of glands in the mucosa of the uterine cervix, causing them to be distended with retained secretion. Called also *nabothian cysts* or *follicles*.

nabothian cysts (follicles) (nə'bohthi·ən) Naboth's cysts.

nacreous ('naykri·əs) having a pearl-like lustre.

NAD nicotinamide-adenine dinucleotide; no abnormality detected.

nadolol ('naydoh,lol) a β-adrenergic blocking agent that affects both β_1- and β_2-receptors; used for the treatment of hypertension.

NADP nicotinamide-adenine dinucleotide phosphate.

naevocarcinoma (ˌneevoh,kahsi'nohmə) malignant melanoma.

naevoid ('neevoyd) resembling a naevus.

naevoxanthoendothelioma (ˌneevoh,zanthoh-ˌendoh,theeli'ohmə) a condition in which groups of yellow-brown papules or nodules occur on the extensor surfaces of the extremities of infants.

naevus ('neevəs) pl. *naevi* [L.] a general term for a birthmark or mole. Most birthmarks are haemangiomata, most moles are pigmented spots or plaques. They vary in size and thickness, and occur in groups or singly. Naevi seldom become cancerous; but malignant melanoma can develop, particularly at puberty. Change in size, colour, or texture of a mole, any itching or bleeding may be significant.

n. arachnoideus, n. araneosus, n. araneus one composed of dilated, radiating capillaries sometimes resembling the legs of a spider, hence spider naevus. They occur most often on the upper arms and chest, usually in children and pregnant women, but also in persons with liver disease. These forms are various and include Campbell de Morgan's spots.

blue n. a dark blue nodular lesion composed of closely grouped melanocytes and melanophages situated in the mid-dermis.

n. comedonicus a rare epidermal naevus marked by one or more patches 2 to 5 cm or more in diameter, in which there are collections of large comedones or comedo-like lesions.

connective tissue n. any naevus occurring in the dermal connective tissue and characterized by nodules, papules, or plaques, or by combinations of such lesions. Histologically, there is irregular focal or diffuse thickening and abnormal staining of collagen.

epidermal naevi congenital skin tumours that do not contain melanocytes, which vary widely in appearance, size, and distribution, and which are commonly hyperkeratotic.

n. flammeus a diffuse, flat, poorly defined area varying from pink to dark bluish red, usually on the neck or face, involving otherwise normal skin; port-wine stain.

hairy n. a more or less pigmented mole with hairs growing from its surface.

halo n. a pigmented naevus surrounded by a ring of depigmentation; called also *leukoderma acquisitum centrifugum* and *Sutton's disease or naevus*.

intradermal n. a naevus in which the cells occur in nests in the upper part of the dermis, with no evidence of the proliferative process by which they orginated.

junction n. a pigmented, flat or slightly raised naevus; histologically, there are nests of melanin-containing cells at the dermoepidermal junction.

n. lipomatosus one that contains much fibrofatty tissue.

melanocytic n. any naevus, usually pigmented, composed of melanocytes.

naevocytic n., naevus-cell n. the common mole; a usually more or less hyperpigmented naevus, initially flat but soon becoming elevated, composed of nests of naevus cells.

pigmented n., n. pigmentosus one containing melanin; the term is usually restricted to naevocytic naevi (moles), but may be applied to other pigmented naevi.

n. pilosus a hairy naevus.

sebaceous n. yellow naevus of the scalp or less often the face containing sebaceous elements, frequently growing larger during puberty or early adult life, and rarely giving rise to a variety of new growths, including basal cell carcinoma.

spider n. see naevus arachnoideus (above).

n. spongiosus albus a white sponge naevus.

strawberry n. a cavernous haemangioma, usually congenital. Tends to grow bigger initially, then fades and disappears in early years of life.

n. unius lateris a verrucous epidermal naevus occurring as a warty band, patch, or streak, usually along the margin between two neuromeres on the side of the trunk.

n. vascularis, n. vasculosus a reddish swelling or patch on the skin due to hypertrophy of the skin capillaries: the term includes naevus flammeus, the elevated strawberry marks, blue rubber bleb naevus, vascular spider, and cavernous haemangioma.

Naffziger's operation ('nafzigəz) decompression of the orbit transfrontally to reduce intraorbital pressure, e.g. in dysthyroid eye disease.

naftidrofuryl (naf,tidroh'fyooəril) an agent used in the treatment of peripheral and cerebral vascular disorders.

Nägele's pelvis ('naygələz) one contracted in an oblique diameter, with complete ankylosis of the sacroiliac synchondrosis of one side and imperfect development of the sacrum and coxa on the same side.

Nägele's rule a rule for calculating the estimated date of labour: subtract 3 months from the first day of the last menstrual period and add 7 days.

NAHA National Association of Health Authorities.

nail (nayl) 1. a rod of metal, bone, or other material used for fixation of the ends of fractured bones. 2. a hardened or horny cutaneous plate overlying the dorsal surface of the distal end of a finger or toe, called also an unguis. The nails are part of the outer layer of the skin. They are composed of hard tissue formed of keratin, the substance that gives skin its toughness.

CARE OF THE NAILS. The main care of the fingernails consists in keeping them trimmed and clean. Trimming may be done with nail scissors or clippers or by filing. With certain types of delicate nail, an emery board is preferable to a metal file. Hand lotion or cream applied to the cuticle helps to keep it soft and avoid hangnails. Wearing rubber gloves for housework and dishwashing helps to protect the nails from breaking.

Toenails seldom give trouble if they are cleaned and trimmed regularly and if shoes fit well. It is advisable to bathe the feet at least once a day and to clean dirt from under the toenails with a nailbrush. The toenails should be trimmed every 2 weeks or so by cutting them straight across rather than rounding them by cutting off their corners. This helps prevent ingrowing toenails.

Disorders of the Nails. Any change in the basic structure, shape, or appearance of the nails—such as softness, brittleness, furrowing, or speckling—may be a symptom of a systemic disease.

Certain disorders affect the nails themselves. They are readily exposed to outside sources of infection and are particularly vulnerable to injury in the course of daily life. Many of the diseases that afflict the skin may also affect the nail bed and be aggravated by the confining presence of the nail. Congenital defects and metabolic disturbances may affect the nails.

Infections. Most infections involving the nails originate in the folds of tissue around them. Inflammation of this area is called paronychia. It is a fairly common infection by staphylococci, streptococci, or other bacteria or by fungi, and causes painful swelling around the nail, with red, shiny skin. If untreated, paronychia may spread to the nail bed and cause inflammation there. This condition is known as onychia, and is more serious. The bacteria grow under the nail and can cause severe inflammation and pain. Onychia may also arise when the nail is injured and bacteria or fungi gain entrance to the tissue underneath. If the organisms that penetrate the nail produce pigments, the nail may change colour as a result. In extreme cases onychia may also cause the nail to separate from its bed. Among the diseases from which paronychia and onychia may result are tuberculosis, diphtheria, and syphilis, and also skin diseases such as psoriasis, fungal diseases, and contact dermatitis.

Dermatitis is the most common disorder that involves the nails and often leads to the complete loss of the nail. After treatment the nail will generally grow back, but if the matrix is severely damaged a new nail may be deformed or may fail to grow.

Occasionally toenails become infected with the fungi that cause athlete's foot.

Injuries. A bruise on the nail can be extremely painful and may cause the nail to turn black and blue. Both effects are due to the accumulation of blood underneath. The nail may become detached from its bed or may fall off. The pain of such an injury can be relieved by releasing the accumulated blood by a small incision under the nail.

Burns and frostbite can injure the nails and in severe cases may destroy the matrix, so that regrowth is impossible. Radiotherapy may cause atrophy of the nail.

Nutritional and Metabolic Disturbances. The general condition of the body is readily reflected in the condition of the nails. Poor circulation may result in weak nails. Digestive disturbances may impair their growth, and vitamin deficiencies may cause them to become inflamed and sometimes to fall out.

Brittle nails may also be caused by metabolic disorders, for example, hypothyroidism.

Hereditary Defects. The shape and thickness of nails may be an inherited family trait. A child is sometimes born without nails or with one or more missing. In this case he will remain without them for life.

Minor Disorders. Hangnails (shreds of skin at one side of a nail) are unsightly and can best be prevented from forming by gently pushing the cuticle instead of cutting it. A hangnail should be clipped off to avoid the slight danger of infection.

n. extension extension exerted on the distal fragment of a fractured bone by means of a nail or pin (Steinmann pin) driven into the bone distal to the fragment. Called also *Steinmann extension.*

ingrowing n. aberrant growth of a toenail, with one or both lateral margins pushing deeply into adjacent soft tissue (see also INGROWN NAIL).

Smith-Petersen n. a flanged nail for fixing the head of the femur in fracture of the femoral neck.

spoon n. a nail with a concave surface.

nalbuphine ('nalbyoo,feen) a potent synthetic narcotic agonist–antagonist used for relief of moderate-to–severe pain.

Nalcrom ('nalkrom) trademark for a preparation of sodium cromoglycate.

NALGO ('nalgoh) National Association of Local Government Officers.

nalidixic acid (,nali'diksik) a naphthylidine derivative used for the treatment of urinary tract infections due to susceptible gram-negative bacteria including most strains of *Escherichia coli*, *Proteus* species, and *Klebsiella–Aerobacter* species.

nalorphine ('nalawfeen) a semisynthetic congener of morphine used as an antagonist to morphine and related narcotics and in the diagnosis of narcotic addiction.

naloxone (na'loksohn) a narcotic antagonist structurally related to oxymorphone used as an antidote to narcotic overdosage and as an antagonist for pentazocine overdosage.

NAMCW National Association for Maternal and Child Welfare.

NAMH National Association for Mental Health.

nandrolone ('nandrə,lohn) an androgenic, anabolic steroid; used for the control of metastatic breast cancer and for adjunctive therapy of senile and postmenopausal osteoporosis.

nanism ('nanizəm) dwarfism or marked small size from any cause.

nano- word element. [Gr.] *dwarf, small size;* used in naming units of measurement to designate an amount 10^{-9} (one-thousand-millionth) the size of the unit to which it is joined, e.g. nanocurie; symbol n.

nanocephaly (,nanoh'kefəlee, -'sef-) microcephaly. adj. **nanocephalous.**

nanocormia (,nanoh'kawmi·ə) abnormal smallness of the body or trunk.

nanocurie ('naynoh,kyooə·ree, 'nanoh-) a unit of radioactivity, being 10^{-9} curie, or the quantity of radioactive material in which the number of nuclear disintegrations is 3.7 × 10, or 37, per second; abbreviated nCi.

nanogram ('naynoh,gram, 'nanoh-) one billionth (10^{-9}) gram.

nanoid ('nanoyd) dwarfish.

nanomelus (na'noməlэs) micromelus.

nanometre ('naynoh,meetə, 'nanoh-) abbreviated nm; one thousand millionth of a metre.

nanophthalmia (,nanof'thalmi·ə) nanophthalmos.

nanophthalmos (,nanof'thalmos) abnormal smallness in all dimensions of one or both eyes in the absence of other ocular defects; pure microphthalmos.

nanophthalmus (,nanof'thalməs) 1. nanophthalmos. 2. a person affected with nanophthalmos.

nanosecond ('naynoh,sekənd, 'nanoh-) one thousand millionth (10^{-9}) second, abbreviated ns or nsec.
nanosomia (,nanə'sohmi·ə) dwarfism.
nanous ('naynəs) dwarfed; stunted.
nanus ('naynəs) a dwarf.
nape (nayp) the back of the neck.
naphthalene ('nafthə,leen) a hydrocarbon from coal tar oil; used as an antiseptic.
naphthol ('nafthol) a phenol occurring in coal tar: α-naphthol (1-hydroxynaphthalene) or β-naphthol (2-hydroxynaphthalene).
napkin rash ('napkin) an erythematous rash which may occur in infants in the napkin area. Often caused by the passage of frequent loose stools containing fatty acids which cause breakdown of urea in the urine, producing ammonia which burns the skin.
Naprosyn (na'prohsin) trademark for a preparation of naproxen; a nonsteroidal anti-inflammatory agent.
naproxen (na'proksen) a propionic acid derivative with analgesic, antipyretic, and anti-inflammatory activity (a nonsteroidal anti-inflammatory agent); used for treatment of rheumatoid arthritis and osteoarthritis.
Narcan ('nahkan) trademark for preparations of naloxone, an opiate antagonist.
narcissism ('nahsi,sizəm) dominant interest in one's self; self-love. adj. **narcissistic.**

The term is derived from *Narcissus*, a character in Greek mythology who fell in love with his own image reflected in water. Narcissism may or may not be associated with genital excitation. In psychoanalysis, *primary* narcissism is the original energy embodied in the infantile ego; *secondary* narcissism denotes libidinous attachments withdrawn from others and attached to elements of the ego, such as ideas of grandeur.

narco- word element. [Gr.] *stupor, stuporous state.*
narcoanalysis (,nahkoh·ə'nalisis) psychoanalysis with use of sedative drugs to help uncover unconscious material. Called also *narcosynthesis.*
narcohypnia (,nahkoh'hipni·ə) numbness felt on waking from sleep.
narcohypnosis (,nahkoh·hip'nohsis) hypnotic suggestions made while the patient is narcotized.
narcolepsy ('nahkoh,lepsee) recurrent attacks of uncontrollable desire for sleep. adj. **narcoleptic.**
narcosis (nah'kohsis) a reversible state of cental nervous system depression induced by a drug.
narcosynthesis (,nahkoh'sinthəsis) narcoanalysis.
narcotic (nah'kotik) 1. pertaining to or producing narcosis. 2. a drug that produces insensibility or stupor.

Medically, the term narcotic includes any drug that has this effect. By legal definition, however, the term refers to habit-forming drugs—for example, opiates such as morphine and heroin and synthetic drugs such as pethidine. Narcotics can be legally obtained only with a doctor's prescription. The sale or possession of narcotics for other than medical purposes is strictly prohibited by the Misuse of Drugs Act 1971. See also DRUG ABUSE.

narcotize ('nahkə,tiez) to put under the influence of a narcotic.
Nardil ('nahdil) trademark for a preparation of phenelzine, an antidepressant.
nares ('nair·reez) plural of *naris.* [L.] the nostrils; the external openings of the nasal cavity.
Narphen ('nahfen) trademark for a preparation of phenazocine, an opiate analgesic.
nasal ('nayz'l) pertaining to the nose.
n. concha see nasal CONCHA.
n. septum a plate of bone and cartilage covered with mucous membrane that divides the cavity of the nose (see also SEPTUM).
nascent ('nas'nt, 'nay-) 1. being born; just coming into existence. 2. just liberated from a chemical combination, and hence more reactive because uncombined.
Naseptin (nay'septin) trademark for a combination preparation containing chlorhexidine and neomycin, a nasal cream for the treatment of staphyloccal infections.
nasion ('nayzi·ən) the middle point of the junction of the frontal and the two nasal bones (frontonasal suture).
naso- word element. [L.] *nose.*
nasoantral (,nayzoh'antrəl) pertaining to the nose and maxillary antrum.
nasoantrostomy (,nayzoh·an'trostəmee) surgical formation of a nasoantral window for drainage of an obstructed maxillary sinus.
nasociliary (,nayzoh'sili·ə·ree) pertaining to the eyes, brow, and root of the nose.
nasofrontal (,nayzoh'frunt'l) pertaining to the nasal and frontal bones.
nasogastric tube (,nayzoh'gastrik) a tube of soft rubber or plastic that is inserted through a nostril and into the stomach. The tube may be inserted for the purpose of instilling liquid foods or other substances, or as a means of withdrawing gastric contents.

Prior to insertion of the nasogastric tube a measurement is made to assure that the distal end of the tube will be positioned in the stomach. This is done by placing the tip of the tube on the bridge of the patient's nose and then marking on the tube the point at which it touches the tip of the xiphoid process. Once the tube is inserted its position should be checked to be sure it is in the stomach and not the trachea or bronchi. This is done by aspirating for stomach contents, using an aspirating syringe. Alternatively, the syringe can be used to inject air into the tube while at the same time listening through a stethoscope for a 'whooshing' sound made by the air being injected.

The nasogastric tube should be anchored so that it points downward away from the nares. It is *not* brought up over the nose and anchored by tape over the bridge of the nose. This increases irritation of the nasal mucosa, impedes circulation, and causes unnecessary discomfort. To avoid tension and drag on the tube a pin and rubber band can be used to secure the tube to the shoulder of the patient's gown or pajama top.

Gentle rotation of the tube once or twice daily can help prevent adherence of the sucking parts to the gastric mucosa. Either advancing or retracting the tube 3–5 cm can also help restore patency. However, if the tube has been positioned during surgery for a specific purpose, it should not be moved at all without first consulting the surgeon.

Mouth care is of particular importance while a tube is in place. Medications and feedings can be given through the tube. If possible, the patient should be in a sitting position when medications, water, and feedings are being instilled and this position should be maintained for 30 minutes after the procedure to avoid regurgitation. The patient also sits upright while the tube is being removed. See also TUBE FEEDING.

nasolabial (,nayzoh'laybi·əl) pertaining to the nose and lip.
nasolacrimal (,nayzoh'lakriməl) pertaining to the nose and lacrimal apparatus.
naso-oral (,nayzoh'or·rəl) pertaining to the nose and mouth.
nasopalatine (,nayzoh'palətien) pertaining to the nose and palate.
nasopharyngitis (,nayzoh,farin'jietis) inflammation of

the nasopharynx.

nasopharyngogram (ˌnayzohfə'ringohgram) the film obtained by nasopharyngography.

nasopharyngography (ˌnayzohˌfaring'gogrəfee) radiography of the nasopharynx following the instillation of a radiopaque contrast medium into the nose.

nasopharyngolaryngoscope (ˌnayzohfəˌring·gohlə-'ring·gohˌskohp) a flexible fibreoptic endoscope for examining the nasopharynx and larynx.

nasopharynx (ˌnayzoh'faringks) the part of the pharynx above the soft palate. adj. **nasopharyngeal**.

nasosinusitis (ˌnayzohˌsienə'sietis) inflammation of the paranasal sinuses.

nasus ('nayzəs) [L.] *nose*.

natal ('nayt'l) 1. pertaining to birth. 2. pertaining to the nates (buttocks).

natality (nay'talitee) the birth rate.

nates ('nayteez) [L.] *the buttocks*.

National Association of Theatre Nurses (nashən'l) a professional association for qualified nurses (RGN and SEN) who are actively engaged in nursing duties in operating theatres or central supply departments. Abbreviated NATN. Provides legal advice, film library, professional conferences and study days, scholarships, and research grants.

National Boards for Nursing, Midwifery and Health Visiting set up in England, Northern Ireland, Scotland and Wales by the 1979 Nurses, Midwives and Health Visitors' Act. Functions as described in the Act are to: (1) provide, or arrange for others to provide, at institutions approved by the board (i) courses of training with a view to enabling persons to qualify for registration as nurses, midwives or health visitors or for the recording of additional qualifications in the register and (ii) courses of further training for those already registered; (2) ensure that such courses meet the requirements of the Central Council as to their content and standard; (3) hold, or arrange for others to hold, such examinations as are necessary to enable persons to satisfy requirements for registration or to obtain additional qualifications; (4) collaborate with the Council in the promotion of improved training methods; and (5) carry out investigations of cases of alleged misconduct, with a view to proceedings before the Central Council or a committee of the Council for a person to be removed from the register.

National Childbirth Trust a charitable organization concerned with education for pregnancy, birth and parenthood, with over 300 branches and groups in the UK; abbreviated NCT. Primarily through these local groups, it runs antenatal classes, breastfeeding counselling and postnatal support. For further information contact: NCT, 9 Queensborough Terrace, London W2 3TB.

NATN National Association of Theatre Nurses.

natraemia (nə'treemi·ə) hypernatraemia.

Natrilix ('natriliks) trademark for a preparation of indapamide, a diuretic.

natrium ('natri·əm) [L.] *sodium* (symbol Na).

natriuresis (ˌnatriyuh'reesis) the excretion of abnormal amounts of sodium in the urine.

natriuretic (ˌnatriyuh'retik) 1. pertaining to or promoting natriuresis. 2. an agent that promotes natriuresis.

natural childbirth (nachər'l) a term used to describe an approach to LABOUR and delivery in which the parents are prepared for the event so that the mother is awake and cooperative and the father is able to assume an active and supportive role during the birth of their child.

The underlying concept for all methods of natural childbirth is avoidance of medical interference and analgesia in labour, and education of the parents so that they can actively participate in and share the experience of childbirth. The methods of instruction may vary, but all proponents advocate a family-centred maternity care programme. The benefits of this approach are believed to be a more comfortable pregnancy, a shorter period of labour, less trauma during birth, and a decrease in the morbidity and mortality rates among newborn infants.

Among the most widely used methods of childbirth is the LAMAZE METHOD, named after the French obstetrician Fernand Lamaze, who adapted the Russian psychoprophylactic method to his practice. The overall goal of psychoprophylaxis is use of the mind in the prevention of pain and, more specifically, the modification of the perception of pain. The Read method of preparation, based on the teaching and philosophy of Dr. Grantly Dick-Read, had its beginning earlier than the Lamaze method. The emphasis in the Read-based classes is on passivity of the mother and an interruption of the fear–tension–pain cycle. Other methods include the Erna Wright method, which originated in England, and the psychosexual method of Sheila Kitzinger, which includes marriage counselling and encompasses all family interrelationships and their effect on childbirth and feminine sexual response.

Although there are variations in the underlying philosophies and the specific techniques that are characteristic of each method, all are concerned with helping both parents understand the birth process and become familiar with their expected roles during labour and delivery, instruction in exercises that develop neuromuscular control, and physical conditioning exercises and specific breathing patterns that are employed during the three stages of labour. The father is given instruction in the ways in which he can support his partner and promote her comfort during labour. Many of the techniques learned in natural childbirth classes can be used to reduce the effects of stress and to relieve the discomfort associated with tension in many situations not related to childbirth. Most parents who have chosen natural childbirth describe it as an exhilarating and emotionally satisfying experience, provided complications do not arise.

natural experiment naturally occurring circumstances which expose populations to different levels of intensity of a possible causal factor of a disease and in which the incidence of that disease can be studied.

natural history of disease the description of the stages in the development of a disease.

naturopath ('naychə·rohˌpath) a practitioner of naturopathy.

naturopathy (ˌnaychə'ropəthee) a drugless system of healing by a combination of diet, fasting, exercise, hydrotherapy, and positive thinking.

nausea ('nawzi·ə) an unpleasant sensation vaguely referred to the epigastrium and abdomen, with a tendency to vomit. Nausea may be a symptom of a variety of disorders, some minor and some more serious.

Nausea is usually felt when nerve endings in the stomach and other parts of the body are irritated. The irritated nerves send messages to the centre in the brain that controls the vomiting reflex. When the nerve irritation becomes intense, vomiting results.

Nausea and vomiting may be set off by nerve signals from many other parts of the body besides the stomach. For example, intense pain in almost any part of the body can produce nausea. The reason is that the nausea–vomiting mechanism is part of the involuntary autonomic nervous system. Nausea can also be precipitated by strong emotions.

nauseant ('nawzi·ənt) 1. inducing nausea. 2. an agent causing nausea.
nauseate ('nawzi,ayt) to affect with nausea.
nauseous ('nawzi·əs) pertaining to or producing nausea or disgust.
navel ('nayv'l) the umbilicus, the scar marking the site of entry of the umbilical cord in the fetus.
navicular (nə'vikyuhlə) boat-shaped; applied to certain bones, as the navicular bone.
Navidrex ('navidreks) trademark for preparations of cyclopenthiazide, a diuretic.
NAWCH (nawch) National Association for the Welfare of Children in Hospital.
NB [L.] *nota bene* (note well).
Nb chemical symbol, *niobium*.
nCi nanocurie.
NCT National Childbirth Trust.
NCW National Council for Women.
Nd chemical symbol, *neodymium*.
Ne chemical symbol, *neon*.
nearsightedness (niə'sietidnəs) called also MYOPIA.
Nebcin ('nebsin) trademark for preparations of tobramycin sulphate, an aminoglycoside antibiotic.
Nebuhaler (,nebyuh'haylə) a plastic conical device used as a chamber for inhalation of several drugs in obstructive airways disease.
nebula ('nebyuhlə) 1. slight corneal opacity. 2. an oily preparation for use in an atomizer.
nebulization (,nebyuhlie'zayshən) 1. conversion into a spray. 2. treatment by a spray.
nebulizer ('nebyuh,liezə) an atomizer; a device for throwing a spray.
Necator (ne'kaytə) a genus of HOOKWORMS.
N. americanus a species widely distributed in tropical and subtropical America, Africa and Asia; HOOKWORM.
necatoriasis (ne,kaytə'rieəsis) infection with organisms of the genus *Necator*; hookworm disease.
neck (nek) a constricted portion, such as the part connecting the head and trunk of the body, or the constricted part of an organ, as of the uterus (cervix uteri) or other structure.
anatomic n. of humerus the constriction of the humerus just below its proximal articular surface.
n. of femur the heavy column of bone connecting the head of the femur and the shaft.
surgical n. of humerus the constricted part of the humerus just below the tuberosities.
n. of a tooth the narrowed part of a tooth between the crown and the root.
uterine n., n. of uterus cervix uteri.
webbed n. a thick skin fold on the side of the neck, from the mastoid region to the acromion. Called also *pterygium colli*.
wry n. torticollis.
necrectomy (nə'krektəmee) excision of necrotic tissue.
necro- word element. [Gr.] *death*.
necrobiosis (,nekrohbie'ohsis) the physiological death of cells; a normal mechanism in the constant turnover of many cell populations. Sometimes a feature of iron deficiency anaemia. adj. **necrobiotic**.
n. lipoidica diabeticorum a dermatosis characterized by patchy degeneration of the elastic and connective tissue of the skin with degenerated collagen occurring in irregular patches, especially in the dermis, most often on the mid or lower shins; usually associated with diabetes.
necrocytosis (,nekrohsie'tohsis) death and decay of cells.
necrogenic (,nekroh'jenik) productive of necrosis or death.
necrogenous (nə'krojənəs) originating or arising from dead matter.
necrolysis (nə'krolisis) separation or exfoliation of necrotic tissue.
toxic epidermal n. an exfoliative skin disease in which erythema spreads rapidly over the body, followed by blisters much like those seen in a second degree burn. Staphylococci of phage Type 71 (in infants) and a toxic reaction to various drugs (in adults) are the usual causes.
necromania (,nekroh'mayni·ə) necrophilia.
necroparasite (,nekroh'parə,siet) an organism that lives in dead tissue.
necrophagous (nə'krofəgəs) feeding upon dead flesh.
necrophilia (,nekroh'fili·ə) morbid attraction to death or to dead bodies; coitus with a dead body; necromania.
necrophilic (,nekroh'filik) 1. pertaining to necrophilia. 2. necrophilous.
necrophilous (nə'krofiləs) showing a preference for dead tissue; said of microorganisms.
necrophobia (,nekroh'fohbi·ə) morbid dread of death or of dead bodies.
necropneumonia (,nekrohnyoo'mohni·ə) gangrene of the lung.
necropsy ('nekropsee) examination of a body after death (see also AUTOPSY).
necrose (nə'krohz) to become necrotic or to undergo necrosis.
necrosis (nə'krohsis) pl. *necroses* [Gr.] the morphological changes indicative of cell or tissue death.
acidophilic n. necrosis applied usually to single cells where the residual cytoplasm is stained more intensely by acidophilic dyes, e.g. eosin.
aseptic n. necrosis without infection or inflammation; sometimes called *dry necrosis*, as demonstrated in separation of the unbilical cord stump following birth.
Balser's fatty n. gangrenous pancreatitis with omental bursitis and disseminated patches of necrosis of fatty tissues.
caseous n. necrosis in which the material is soft, dry, structureless, and cheesy, occurring typically in tuberculosis.
central n. necrosis affecting the central portion of an affected bone, cell, or lobule of the liver.
cheesy n. that in which the tissue resembles cottage cheese; most often seen in tuberculosis and syphilis.
coagulation n. death of cells, the protoplasm of the cells becoming fixed and opaque by coagulation of the protein elements, the cellular outline persisting for a long time.
colliquative n. liquefactive necrosis.
dry n. the process by which the umbilical cord separates from its stump at 7 to 10 days; sometimes called *dry gangrene*.
fat n. necrosis in which fat is broken down into fatty acids and glycerol, usually occurring in subcutaneous tissue as a result of trauma.
liquefactive n. necrosis in which the necrotic material becomes softened and liquefied, usually by neutrophil leukocyte enzymic digestion.
moist n. necrosis in which the dead tissue is wet and soft.
postpartum pituitary n. necrosis of the pituitary gland during the postpartum period, often associated with shock and excessive uterine bleeding during delivery, and leading to variable patterns of hypopituitarism. Called also *Sheehan's syndrome*.
subcutaneous fat n. of newborn a benign condition seen in the first few weeks of life, in which there is induration of the subcutaneous fat.
Zenker's n. hyaline degeneration and necrosis of striated muscle; called also *Zenker's degeneration*.
necrospermia (,nekroh'spərmi·ə) a condition in which

the spermatozoa of the semen are dead or motionless.

necrotizing ('nekrə,tiezing) causing necrosis.

necrotomy (nə'krotəmee) 1. dissection of a dead body. 2. removal of a sequestrum.

necrotoxin (,nekroh'toksin) a factor or substance produced by certain staphylococci that kills tissue cells.

need (need) something that is required or necessary. Basic human needs are those things that are required for complete physical and mental well-being. Needs vary greatly in the degree to which they are necessary for survival. For this reason, they can be classified into a hierarchy according to their relative urgency. Those on lower levels must be met before attention can be paid to needs on higher levels. The most widely used classification is one devised by Abraham H. Maslow.

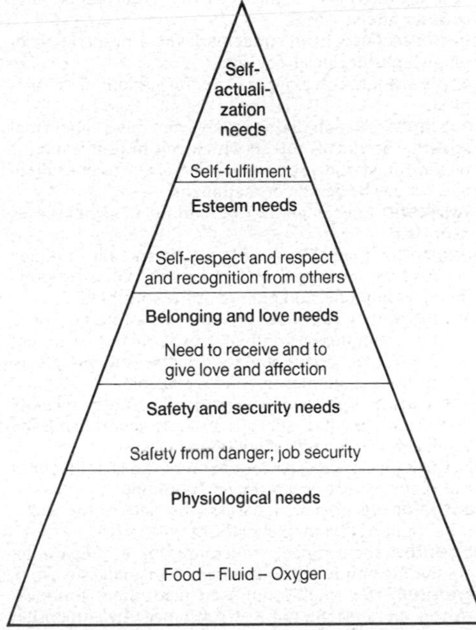

Maslow's hierarchy of needs

Physiological Needs. These are the needs that are essential for the maintenance of biological homeostasis and the survival of the individual and the species. They include needs for oxygen, water, food, elimination of wastes, temperature regulation, avoidance of pain, rest and sleep, exercise and sex.

Needs for Safety and Security. These include needs for protection from physical harm, for order, consistency, and familiarity in one's surroundings, and for some degree of control over matters concerning oneself.

Needs for Love and Belonging. These include needs for giving and receiving love and affection and for sexual intimacy, for friendship and companionship, and to identify with a group.

Needs for Esteem and Self-Esteem. These are the needs that are necessary for a person to have a basic sense of self-respect and self-acceptance and to be self-sufficient. Self-esteem requires an understanding of oneself and one's limitations and the ability to face and cope with stress and painful realities. Persons in whom these needs have been met are relatively free of feelings of inferiority or inadequacy. This level also includes needs for approval and recognition from others.

The Need for Self-Actualization. This is the need to make full use of one's talents, capabilities, and potential. Self-actualizing persons tend to be dedicated, realistic, autonomous, creative, and open. They are not in conflict with themselves and are motivated by their own values and goals.

Maslow's hierarchy has been modified by Richard A. Kalish, who proposed an additional level, *Needs for Stimulation*, which he placed between the levels of physiological needs and needs for safety and security. This level includes the need to explore and manipulate the environment, which is especially important in the growth and development of the individual. Kalish also puts needs for sex, activity, and novelty on this level.

needle ('need'l) 1. a sharp instrument for suturing or puncturing. 2. to puncture or separate with a needle.

aneurysm n. a blunt curved instrument with an eye used in ligating blood vessels in continuity. Called also *ligature needle.*

aspirating n. a long, hollow needle for removing fluid from a cavity.

cataract n. one used in removing a cataract.

discission n. a form of cataract needle. **Hagedorn's n.** a form of flat suture needle.

hypodermic n. a hollow, sharp-pointed needle to be attached to a syringe for injection beneath the skin.

Jamshidi n. a bone marrow trephine needle which safely enables a long core (up to 4 cm) of bone marrow to be taken, usually from the posterior iliac crest. Useful in the diagnosis of malignant infiltrations of the bone marrow and other conditions, e.g. aplastic anaemia.

knife n. a slender knife with a needle-like point, used in cataract operations.

ligature n. see aneurysm needle (above).

Reverdin's n. a curved needle with an eye that can be opened and closed by means of a slide or a long handle.

Salah n. a commonly used needle for bone marrow aspiration.

Silverman's n. an instrument for taking tissue specimens.

stop n. one with a shoulder that prevents too deep penetration.

needling ('needling) discission; the procedure of cutting the lens capsule so that the cortical lens material may be absorbed.

nefopam ('nefohpam) an analgesic claimed to have no respiratory effects or addiction potential.

negative ('negətiv) having a value of less than zero; indicating lack or absence, as chromatin-negative or Wassermann-negative; characterized by denial or opposition.

negativism ('negəti,vizəm) a tendency to manifest or produce the opposite response to that requested. The individual may do the opposite of what he is asked to do. May occur in schizophrenia as a form of resistance to what is seen as an imposed demand.

negatron ('negə,tron) a negatively charged electron.

negligence ('neglijəns) in law, the failure to do something that a reasonable person of ordinary prudence would do in a certain situation or the doing of something that such a person would not do. Negligence may provide the basis for a lawsuit when there is a legal duty, as the duty of a doctor or nurse to provide reasonable care to patients and when the negligence results in damage to the patient.

Negram ('neg,gram) trademark for preparations of nalidixic acid, an antibacterial.

Negre antibody ('negray) an antigen prepared from

dead, dried, and triturated tubercle bacilli by means of acetone and methyl alcohol; used in serum tests for tuberculosis.

Negri bodies ('negree) oval or round bodies in the nerve cells of animals who have died of rabies.

Neisseria (nie'siə·ri·ə) a genus of gram-negative bacteria (family Neisseriaceae). **N. gonorrhoeae** the aetiological agent of gonorrhoea.

N. meningitidis a prominent cause of meningitis and the specific aetiological agent of meningococcal meningitis.

Neisseriaceae (nie,siə·ri'aysi·ee) a family of parasitic bacteria (order Eubacteriales).

neisserial (nie'siə·ri·əl) of, relating to, or caused by *Neisseria.*

Nelson's syndrome ('nelsənz) the development of an ACTH-producing pituitary tumour after bilateral adrenalectomy in Cushing's syndrome; it is characterized by aggressive growth of the tumour and hyperpigmentation of the skin.

nem (nem) a unit of nutrition equivalent to the nutritive value of 1 g of breast milk.

Nemathelminthes (,nemət·hel'mintheez) in some classifications, a phylum including the Acanthocephala and Nematoda.

nematocide ('nemətoh,sied) 1. destroying nematodes. 2. an agent that destroys nematodes.

Nematoda (,nemə'tohdə) a class of helminths (phylum Aschelminthes), the roundworms, many of which are parasites; in some classifications, considered to be a phylum, and sometimes known as Nemathelminthes, or a class of that phylum. See also WORM.

nematode ('nemə,tohd) a roundworm; any individual organism of the class Nematoda.

Nembutal ('nembyuhtal) trademark for preparations of pentobarbitone, a hypnotic and barbiturate.

neo- word element. [Gr.] *new, recent.*

Neo-Cortef (neeoh'kawtef) trademark for fixed combination preparations of neomycin and hydrocortisone.

neoantigen (,neeoh'antijən) an intranuclear antigen, e.g. a T antigen, present in cells infected by oncogenic viruses.

neoblastic (,neeoh'blastik) originating in or of the nature of new tissue.

neocerebellum (,neeoh,seri'beləm) phylogenetically (see also PHYLOGENY), the newer parts of the cerebellum, consisting of those parts predominately supplied by corticopontocerebellar fibres.

neocortex (,neeoh'kawteks) neopallium.

neodymium (,neeoh'dimi·əm) a chemical element, atomic number 60, atomic weight 144.24, symbol Nd. See table of elements in Appendix 2.

neogenesis (,neeoh'jenəsis) tissue regeneration. adj. **neogenetic.**

neoglottis (,neeoh'glotis) a glottis created by suturing the pharyngeal mucosa over the superior end of the transected trachea above the primary tracheostoma and making a permanent stoma in the mucosa; done to permit phonation after laryngectomy. adj. **neoglottic.**

neoglycogenesis (,neeoh,glieko'jenəsis) the formation of liver glycogen from non-carbohydrate sources. Glyconeogenesis.

neokinetic (,neeohki'netik) pertaining to the nervous motor mechanism regulating voluntary muscular control.

neologism (nee'olə,jizəm) in psychiatry, a word whose meaning may be known only to the patient using it. Classically described in schizophrenia, but may occur in dreams.

neomembrane (,neeoh'membrayn) a false membrane.

neomycin (,neeoh'miesin) a broad-spectrum antibiotic produced by *Streptomyces fradiae*; used as an intestinal antiseptic.

neon ('neeon) a chemical element, atomic number 10, atomic weight 20.183, symbol Ne. See table of elements in Appendix 2.

neonatal (,neeə'nayt'l) pertaining to the first 4 weeks after birth.

n. mortality rate the number of deaths of infants up to 4 weeks old per 1000 live births in any one year.

neonate ('neeə,nayt) a newborn infant up to 4 weeks old.

neonatologist (,neeənay'toləjist) a doctor who specializes in neonatology.

neonatology (,neeənay'toləjee) the branch of medicine dealing with disorders of the newborn infant.

neopallium (,neeoh'pali·əm) that part of the pallium (cerebral cortex) showing stratification and organization of the most highly evolved type; called also *isocortex* and *neocortex.*

Neophryn ('neeohfrin) trademark for a preparation of phenylephrine, an adrenergic.

neoplasia (,neeoh'playzi·ə) the formation of a neoplasm.

neoplasm ('neeoh,plazəm) any new and abnormal growth, specifically one in which cell multiplication is uncontrolled and progressive. See also TUMOUR. Neoplasms may be benign or malignant.

neoplastic (,neeoh'plastik) pertaining to neoplasia or neoplasm.

Neosporin (,neeoh'spor·rin) trademark for a fixed combination preparation of neomycin sulphate, polymyxin B sulphate, and gramicidin; an antibiotic.

neostigmine (,neeoh'stigmeen) a cholinergic drug (acetylcholinesterase inhibitor) used in the treatment of myasthenia gravis and to reverse the effects of curare used as an intraoperative relaxant.

neostriatum (,neeohstrie'aytəm) the more recently developed part of the corpus striatum, comprising the caudate nucleus and the putamen.

neoteny (nee'otənee) prolongation of the larval form in a sexually mature organism. adj. **neotenic.**

neothalamus (,neeoh'thaləməs) the part of the thalamus connected to the neopallium.

Nepenthe (nə'penthee) trademark for a preparation containing opium alkaloids, used as an analgesic.

nephelometer (,nefə'lomitə) an instrument for measuring the concentration of substances in suspension by the amount of light that is scattered by the suspended particles.

nephelometry (,nefə'lomətree) measurement of the concentration of a suspension by means of a nephelometer. adj. **nephelometric.**

nephelopia (,nefə'lohpi·ə) a visual defect due to cloudiness of the cornea.

nephr(o)- word element. [Gr.] *kidney.*

nephralgia (nə'fralji·ə) pain in a kidney.

nephralgic (nə'fraljik) relating to pain arising from the kidney.

n. crises spasms of pain in the lumbar region in tabes dorsalis.

nephrectasia (,nefrek'tayzi·ə) distention of the kidney.

nephrectomy (nə'frektəmee) removal of a kidney. Usually undertaken when the organ is irreparably damaged by infection or injury, or for tumour. A single kidney can carry on the functions formerly done by both kidneys. An elective nephrectomy may be performed from a healthy person with two functioning kidneys for transplantation to a related person with renal failure. See also surgery of the KIDNEY.

nephric ('nefrik) pertaining to the kidney.

nephridium (nə'fridi·əm) pl. *nephridia* [L.] either of the paired excretory organs of certain invertebrates, having the inner end of the tubule opening into the coelomic cavity.

nephritic (nə'fritik) 1. pertaining to or affected with nephritis. 2. pertaining to the kidneys; renal. 3. an agent useful in kidney disease.

nephritis (nə'frietis) inflammation of the kidney; a focal or diffuse proliferative or destructive disease that may involve the glomerulus, tubule, or interstitial renal tissue. Called also *Bright's disease.* The most usual form is glomerulonephritis, that is, inflammation of the glomeruli, which are clusters of renal capillaries. Damage to the membranes of the glomeruli results in impairment of the filtering process, so that blood and proteins such as albumin pass out into the urine. Depending on the symptoms it produces, nephritis is classified as acute nephritis, chronic nephritis, or nephrotic syndrome.

ACUTE NEPHRITIS. Acute nephritis occurs most frequently in children and young people. The disease seems to strike those who have recently suffered from sore throat, scarlet fever, and other infections that are caused by streptococci, and it is believed to originate as an immune response on the part of the kidney.

An attack of acute nephritis may produce no symptoms. More often, however, there are headaches, a rundown feeling, back pain, and perhaps slight fever. The urine may look smoky, bloody, or wine-coloured. Analysis of the urine shows the presence of erythrocytes, albumin, and casts. Another symptom is oedema. If this occurs, the face or ankles are swollen, more so in the morning than in the evening. The blood pressure usually rises during acute nephritis, and in severe cases hypertension may be accompanied by convulsions.

Recovery is usually complete. Penicillin is often used if an earlier streptococcal infection is still lingering. In a small percentage of cases, however, acute nephritis resists complete cure. It may subside for a time and then become active again, or it may develop into chronic nephritis.

CHRONIC NEPHRITIS. Chronic nephritis, generally known as GLOMERULONEPHRITIS, may follow a case of acute nephritis, or may occur with no apparent precipitating cause. Most cases of glomerulonephritis occur in people who have never had the acute form of the disease.

The symptoms of glomerulonephritis are often unpredictable, with great variations in different cases. But in almost every case of the disease there is steady, progressive, permanent damage to the kidneys.

Glomerulonephritis generally moves through three stages. In the first stage, the latent stage, there are few outward symptoms, if any. There may be slight malaise, but often the only indication of the disease is the presence of albumin and other abnormal substances in the urine. If a blood count is made during this stage, anaemia may be found. There is no special treatment during the latent stage of glomerulonephritis. The patient can live a perfectly normal life. He should avoid extremes of fatigue and exposure, and should eat a well balanced diet.

There may be a second stage of glomerulonephritis in which oedema occurs. Excess body fluids collect in the face, legs, or arms. The main treatment in this stage consists of a high-protein, low-sodium diet. Steroid hormones may be helpful.

It is particularly important, at any stage of glomerulonephritis, to avoid other infections, which will aggravate the condition.

At the final stage of glomerulonephritis is URAEMIA. At this point damage to the kidneys is so extensive that they begin to fail.

There is no known cure for glomerulonephritis, although the progress of the disease can be delayed, so that the patient can live an almost normal life for years. HAEMODIALYSIS or peritoneal dialysis may be used as a replacement for this renal function providing a good quality of life. Transplantations of a healthy kidney may be done and 80–90 per cent are successful.

glomerular n. glomerulonephritis.

interstitial n. nephritis with increase of interstitial tissue and thickening of vessel walls and malpighian corpuscles; sometimes due to alcohol, lead poisoning, gout, analgesia or some drugs, e.g. nonsteroidal anti-inflammatory agents such as indomethacin, and some antibiotics.

lupus n. glomerulonephritis associated with systemic lupus erythematosus.

parenchymatous n. nephritis affecting the parenchyma of the kidney.

salt-losing n. intrinsic renal disease causing abnormal urinary sodium loss in persons ingesting normal amounts of sodium chloride, with vomiting, dehydration, and vascular collapse.

scarlatinal n. an acute nephritis due to scarlet fever.

suppurative n. a form accompanied by abscess of kidney.

transfusion n. nephropathy following transfusion from an incompatible donor.

nephritogenic (nə͵fritoh'jenik) causing nephritis.

nephroblastoma (͵nefrohbla'stohmə) a rapidly developing malignant mixed tumour of the kidneys, made up of embryonic cells, and occurring chiefly in children before the fifth year; called also *Wilms' tumour*.

nephrocalcinosis (͵nefroh͵kalsi'nohsis) deposition of calcium phosphate in the renal tubules, resulting in renal insufficiency.

nephrocapsulectomy (͵nefroh͵kapsyuh'lektəmee) excision of the renal capsule.

nephrocardiac (͵nefroh'kahdi͵ak) pertaining to the kidney and the heart.

nephrocele ('nefroh͵seel) hernia of a kidney.

nephrocolic (͵nefroh'kolik) 1. pertaining to the kidney and the colon. 2. renal colic.

nephrocoloptosis (͵nefrohkohlop'tohsis) downward displacement of the kidney and colon.

nephrocystitis (͵nefrohsi'stietis) inflammation of the kidney and bladder.

nephrogenic (͵nefroh'jenik) producing kidney tissue.

nephrogenous (nə'frojənəs) arising in a kidney.

nephrogram ('nefroh͵gram) a radiograph of the kidney with contrast medium in the renal tubules. Usually the immediate film in an excretion urogram.

nephrography (nə'frogrəfee) radiography of the kidney (see also PYELOGRAPHY).

nephroid ('nefroyd) resembling a kidney.

nephrolith ('nefroh͵lith) a calculus in a kidney.

nephrolithiasis (͵nefrohli'thieəsis) a condition marked by the presence of renal calculi.

nephrolithotomy (͵nefrohli'thotəmee) incision of kidney for removal of stones.

nephrology (nə'froləjee) the branch of medicine dealing with the kidneys.

nephrolysin (nə'frolisin) nephrotoxin, a toxin destructive to kidney tissue.

nephrolysis (nə'frolisis) 1. freeing of a kidney from adhesions. 2. destruction of kidney substance. adj. **nephrolytic.**

nephroma (ne'frohmə) a tumour of kidney tissue.

nephromegaly (͵nefroh'megəlee) enlargement of the kidney.

nephron ('nefron) the structural and functional unit of the KIDNEY, each nephron being capable of forming urine by itself. The nephron consists of the renal corpuscle, the proximal convoluted tubule, the descending and ascending limbs of the loop of Henle, the distal convoluted tubule, and the collecting tubule. Each kidney is an aggregation of about a million nephrons. The specific function of the nephron is to remove from the blood plasma certain end products of metabolism, such as urea, uric acid, and creatinine, and also any excess sodium, chloride, and potassium ions. By allowing for reabsorption of water and some electrolytes back into the blood, the nephron also plays a vital role in the maintenance of normal fluid balance in the body.

The nephron is a complex system of arterioles, capillaries, and tubules. Blood is brought to the nephron via the afferent arteriole. As the blood flows through the glomerulus (a network of capillaries), about one-fifth of the plasma is filtered through the glomerular membrane and collects in the Bowman's capsule, which encases the glomerulus. The fluid then passes through the proximal tubule, from there into the loop of Henle, then into the distal tubule, and finally into the collecting tubule. As the fluid is making its tortuous journey through these various tubules, most of its water and some of the solutes are reabsorbed into the blood via the peritubular capillaries. The water and solutes remaining in the tubules become urine.

nephronophthisis (ˌnefrəˈnofthisis) tuberculosis of the kidney substance.

familial juvenile n. a progressive hereditary kidney disease marked by anaemia, polyuria, renal loss of sodium, progressing to chronic renal failure, tubular atrophy, interstitial fibrosis, glomerular sclerosis, and medullary cysts.

nephropathy (nəˈfropəthee) any disease of the kidneys. adj. **nephropathic**.

IgA n. a chronic form marked by haematuria and proteinuria and by deposits of IgA immunoglobulin in the mesangial areas of the renal glomeruli, with subsequent reactive hyperplasia of mesangial cells. Called also *Berger's disease* and *IgA glomerulonephritis*.

reflux r. childhood pyelonephritis in which the renal scarring results from vesicoureteric reflux, with radiological appearance of intrarenal reflux.

nephropexy (ˈnefrohˌpeksee) operation to fix the position of a nephroptopic or hypermobile kidney (NEPHROPTOSIS), now almost obsolete. The care of a patient having this type of surgery is generally the same as that for any type of surgery of the kidney (see also KIDNEY). One important point is that after nephropexy the patient is positioned so that his chest is lower than his hips; this position relieves strain on the sutures and helps to maintain the kidney in a normal position.

nephroptosis (ˌnefropˈtohsis) downward displacement of a kidney; called also *floating*, *hypermobile*, or *wandering kidney*. This is found most often in young adult women, especially those who are thin and long waisted. Displacement can occur when the kidney supports are weakened by a sudden strain or blow, or are congenitally defective.

Although the condition may not produce symptoms of a serious nature, it can lead to difficulties if there is kinking of the ureters, producing an obstruction to urinary flow from the kidneys to the bladder. In addition, the patient may have an increased susceptibility to infection.

Correction of nephroptosis is usually by NEPHROPEXY, surgical fixation of the floating kidney.

nephropyelitis (ˌnefrohˌpieəˈlietis) inflammation of the kidney and its pelvis; pyelonephritis.

nephropyelography (ˌnefrohˌpieəˈlogrəfee) radiography of the kidney (see also PYELOGRAPHY).

nephropyeloplasty (ˌnefrohˈpieəlohˌplastee) a plastic operation on the pelvis of the kidney performed in cases of hydronephrosis.

nephrorrhaphy (nefˈro·rəfee) suture of the kidney.

nephrosclerosis (ˌnefrohskləˈrohsis) hardening of the kidney associated with hypertension and disease of the renal arterioles. It is characterized as benign or malignant depending on the severity and rapidity of the hypertension and arteriolar changes.

arteriolar n. that involving chiefly the arterioles, with degeneration of the renal tubules and fibrotic thickening of the glomeruli; the benign form is often associated with benign hypertension and hyaline arteriolosclerosis, the malignant with malignant hypertension and hyperplastic arteriolosclerosis.

benign n. arteriolar nephrosclerosis usually occurring in patients 60 years of age or older, and frequently associated with benign hypertension and hyaline arteriosclerosis. In younger persons, it may occur in diabetics with a predisposition to arteriosclerosis and in those who have hypertension resulting from an apparent underlying disease, such as phaeochromocytoma.

nephroscope (ˈnefrəˌskohp) an instrument inserted into an incision in the renal pelvis for viewing the inside of the kidney, equipped with three channels for telescope, fibreoptic light input, and irrigation.

nephroscopy (nəˈfroskəpee) visualization of the kidney by means of the nephroscope.

nephrostoma (ˌnefrohˈstohmə) one of the ciliated funnel-shaped orifices of the excretory tubules that open into the coelom in the embryo; best seen in lower vertebrates.

nephrostomy (nəˈfrostəmee) creation of a permanent opening into the renal pelvis.

nephrotic syndrome (nəˈfrotik) any kidney disease, especially disease marked by purely degenerative lesions of the renal tubules. adj. **nephrotic**. It probably represents one stage of NEPHRITIS. It is marked by excessive accumulation of fluid in the body, due to a great loss of protein in the urine and decreased serum albumin. The disease may last for many years in children, without fatal result if serious infections and other disorders do not occur. In adults the disease is less common and more likely to become chronic.

The exact cause of nephrotic syndrome is not known. The disease may follow acute nephritis, either directly or after an interval as long as a number of years. It may follow or accompany some other disease of the kidneys, e.g. systemic lupus erythematosus. It may also occur without preceeding primary or secondary renal impairment (idiopathic). It is suggested that it may be the result of an immunological antigen–antibody reaction.

The chief symptoms are oedema, usually settling in the legs at first but then affecting the arms, face, and torso, and proteinuria, hypoproteinaemia and often hyperlipidaemia.

Treatment of the patient involves albumin infusion and intravenous diuretics to resolve oedema. A high protein diet is indicated to maintain the total protein. Steroids are often very effective in reducing the oedema, especially in children. There has also been success with certain immunosuppressive drugs, e.g. cyclophosphamide and azathioprine.

amyloid n. s. chronic nephrotic syndrome with amyloid degeneration of the median coat of the arteries and glomerular capillaries. Usually presents with heavy proteinuria.

lipid n. s. nephrotic syndrome marked by oedema, albuminuria, and changes in the protein and lipids of the blood and accumulation of globules of cholesterol esters in the tubular epithelium of the kidney.

lower nephron n. s. renal insufficiency leading to uraemia, due to necrosis of the lower nephron cells, blocking the tubular lumens of this region; seen after severe injuries, especially crushing injury to muscles (see also CRUSH SYNDROME).

nephrotome ('nefroh,tohm) one of the segmented divisions of the embryonic mesoderm connecting the somite with the lateral plates of unsegmented mesoderm; the source of much of the urogenital system.

nephrotomogram (,nefroh'tohmə,gram) a tomogram of the kidney obtained by nephrotomography.

nephrotomography (,nefrohtə'mogrəfee) radiological visualization of the kidney by tomography after introduction of a contrast medium. adj. **nephrotomographic**.

nephrotomy (nə'frotəmee) incision of a kidney.

nephrotoxic (,nefroh'toksik) destructive to kidney cells.

nephrotoxin (,nefroh'toksin) a toxin having a specific destructive effect on kidney tissue.

nephrotropic (,nefroh'tropik) having a special affinity for kidney tissue.

nephrotuberculosis (,nefrohtyuh,bərkyuh'lohsis) renal disease due to *Mycobacterium tuberculosis*.

nephroureterectomy (,nefroh·yuh,reetə'rektəmee) surgical removal of the kidney and the ureter.

neptunium (nep'tyooni·əm) a chemical element, atomic number 93, atomic weight 237, symbol Np. See table of elements in Appendix 2.

NERU Nursing Education Research Unit.

nerve (nərv) a macroscopic cordlike structure of the body, comprising a collection of nerve fibres that convey impulses between a part of the central nervous system and some other body region.

Depending on their function, nerves are known as sensory, motor, or mixed. Sensory nerves, or afferent nerves, carry information from the outside world to the brain and spinal cord. Sensations of heat, cold, and pain are conveyed by the sensory nerves. Motor nerves, or efferent nerves, transmit impulses from the brain and spinal cord to the muscles. Mixed nerves are composed of both motor and sensory fibres, and transmit messages in both directions.

Together, the nerves make up the peripheral nervous system, as distinguished from the central nervous system, which consists of the brain and spinal cord. There are 12 pairs of CRANIAL NERVES, which carry messages to and from the brain. Spinal nerves arise from the spinal cord and pass out between the vertebrae; there are 31 pairs, 8 cervical, 12 thoracic, 5 lumbar, 5 sacral, and 1 coccygeal. The various nerve fibres and cells that make up the autonomic nervous system innervate the glands, heart, blood vessels, and involuntary muscles of the internal organs.

accelerator n's the cardiac sympathetic nerves, which, when stimulated, accelerate the action of the heart.

n. block regional anaesthesia secured by injection of an anaesthetic in close proximity to the appropriate nerve.

depressor n. 1. an inhibitory nerve whose stimulation depresses a motor centre. 2. a nerve that lessens activity of an organ.

excitor n. one that transmits impulses resulting in an increase in functional activity.

excitoreflex n. a visceral nerve that produces reflex action.

fusimotor n's those that innervate the intrafusal fibres of the muscle spindle.

gangliated n. any nerve of the sympathetic nervous system.

inhibitory n. one that transmits impulses resulting in a decrease in functional activity.

medullated n. myelinated nerve.

myelinated n. one whose axons are encased in a myelin sheath.

peripheral n. any nerve outside the central nervous system.

pilomotor n's those that supply the arrector muscles of hair.

pressor n. an afferent nerve whose irritation stimulates a vasomotor centre and increases intravascular tension.

secretory n. an efferent nerve whose stimulation increases vascular activity. **somatic n's** the sensory and motor nerves supplying skeletal muscle and somatic tissues.

splanchnic n's those of the blood vessels and viscera, especially the visceral branches of the thoracic, lumbar, and pelvic parts of the sympathetic trunks.

sudomotor n's those that innervate the sweat glands.

sympathetic n's 1. see sympathetic TRUNK. 2. any nerve of the sympathetic nervous system.

trophic n. one concerned with regulation of nutrition.

unmyelinated n. one whose axons are not encased in a myelin sheath.

vasoconstrictor n. one whose stimulation causes contraction of blood vessels.

vasodilator n. one whose stimulation causes dilation of blood vessels.

vasomotor n. one concerned in controlling the calibre of vessels, whether as a vasoconstrictor or vasodilator.

vasosensory n. any nerve supplying sensory fibres to the vessels.

nervimotor (,nərvi'mohtə) pertaining to a motor nerve.

nervone ('nərvohn) a cerebroside isolated from nerve tissue.

nervous ('nərvəs) 1. pertaining to a nerve or nerves. 2. unduly excitable.

n. breakdown a popular and misleading term for any type of mental illness that interferes with a person's normal activities. The term does not refer to a specific disturbance; a so-called 'nervous breakdown' can include any of the mental disorders, including NEUROSIS, PSYCHOSIS, or DEPRESSION, but is usually used to describe neurosis.

n. system the organ system which, along with the endocrine system, correlates the adjustments and reactions of an organism to internal and environmental conditions. It is composed of the BRAIN, the spinal cord, and the NERVES, which act together to serve as the communicating and coordinating system of the body, carrying information to the brain and relaying instructions from the brain. The system has two main divisions: the central nervous system, composed of the brain and spinal cord; and the peripheral nervous system, which is subdivided into the voluntary and autonomic systems.

THE NERVE CELL. The basic unit of the nervous system is the nerve cell, or NEURON. This highly specialized cell has many fibres extending from it which carry messages in the form of electrical charges and chemical changes. The fibres of some cells are only a fraction of an inch long, but those of others—for example, the sciatic nerve—extend for 2 or 3 feet. These fibres reach into muscles and organs throughout the body, to the ends of the fingers and toes, and cluster by the thousands in areas of the skin no larger than the head of a pin.

The nerve fibres come together from the extremities of the body and gather into cables running to and from the brain. Along the length of the spinal cord are a number of junctions where impulses or messages are

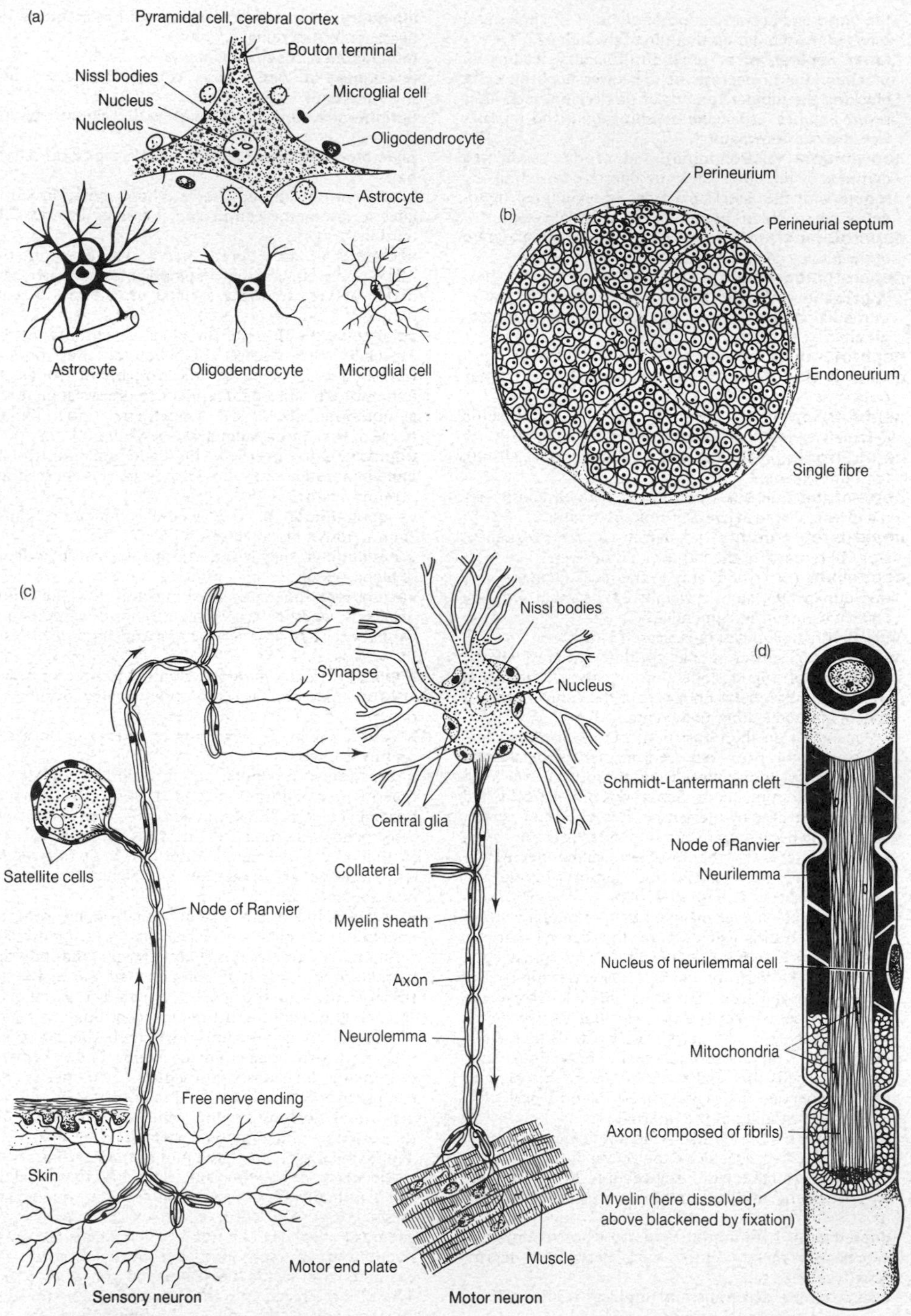

Details of structure of components of nerve tissue. (a) Three types of human neuroglial cell. (b) Transverse section of a nerve. (c) Diagrammatic representation of two types of neurones. (d) Longitudinal section of a nerve fibre

sorted or relayed to higher centres.

The fibres of connecting nerve cells do not touch each other. Impulses are relayed from one to another by chemical means across the gap or synapse between them. In most cases an impulse must cross more than one synapse to cause the desired action.

In a REFLEX, the impulse is relayed from one nerve to another by a shortcut that produces a reaction without involving the brain. The knee jerk is an example of the simplest sort of reflex reaction. When the knee is tapped, the impulse travels through the sensory nerve that receives the tap, crosses a single synapse, and activates the motor nerve that controls the quadriceps muscle in the thigh, causing the leg to jerk up automatically.

A very different sort of reflex is the conditioned reflex. Conditioning is the process of building links or paths in the nervous system. When an action is done repeatedly the nervous system becomes familiar with the situation and learns to react automatically. A new reflex has been built into the system. Hundreds of daily actions are conditioned reflexes. Walking, running, going up and down stairs, and even buttoning a shirt all involve great numbers of complex muscle coordinations that have become automatic.

AUTONOMIC AND VOLUNTARY SYSTEMS. The peripheral nervous system in man evolved over many millennia, developing the ability to perform more and more complicated functions. It is divided into two specialized subsystems. The autonomic nervous system operates without conscious control as the caretaker of the body. The voluntary nervous system, which includes both motor and sensory nerves, controls the muscles and carries information to the brain.

The autonomic system is further specialized into two subsidiary systems: the sympathetic and the parasympathetic. The control centres of these systems lie in the hypothalamus. The sympathetic and parasympathetic nervous systems are continuously operative, functioning to adjust body processes to external and internal demands.

The sympathetic nervous system has in general an excitatory effect, and in response to danger or some other challenge, almost instantly puts body processes into high gear. This is done by the discharge of stimulating secretions at nerve junctions. These secretions, along with adrenaline discharged into the blood by the adrenal medulla, help start muscle action quickly. Glucose is released from the liver into the blood and thus is made available to all the body's muscles as a source of quick energy. The rates of heart and lung action increase, digestive activity slows down, blood vessels constrict, and sweating begins so that the body will be kept cool while under stress. Thus the body is prepared for an extraordinary effort.

The parasympathetic nervous system prevents body processes from accelerating to extremes. Acting more slowly than the sympathetic system, it causes the discharge of secretions that slow the heartbeat and lung action, restore digestive functioning, and limit the constriction of the blood vessels. Generally it acts as a damper, so that unless the challenge demands a prolonged effort, body processes will begin returning to normal.

The voluntary nervous system has nerves of two kinds, sensory and motor. The sensory nerves bring messages to the brain from all parts of the body. They are sorted in the spinal cord and sent on to the brain to be analysed, acted upon, associated with other information and stored as memory.

Messages from the brain, often in response to information received by way of the sensory nerves, are delivered to the muscles by the motor nerves. One motor nerve with its branching fibres may control thousands of muscle fibres.

The different parts of the nervous system are constantly interacting, and are so well coordinated that man can think, feel, and act on many different levels and without serious confusion, all at the same time. See also NEUROLOGICAL ASSESSMENT.

DISORDERS OF THE NERVOUS SYSTEM. The various organs of the nervous system may be affected by inflammatory processes, neoplastic disease, degenerative disease, and injury. These are referred to as neurological disorders and may be manifested by paralysis, sensory malfunction, and convulsive seizures.

Inflammation of the meninges, the membranes covering the brain and spinal cord, is called MENINGITIS. The brain tissue itself may become inflamed (ENCEPHALITIS), may be deprived of adequate blood supply (cerebral thrombosis, cerebral haemorrhage, STROKE), or may be damaged by a violent blow to the head (HEAD INJURY, concussion, contusion). Malignant or benign tumours of the BRAIN can produce varying degrees of sensory and motor disorders.

The spinal cord may be affected by viral infections, as POLIOMYELITIS, or bacterial infections. In its late stage SYPHILIS may involve the brain and spinal cord. Accidental injury to the spinal cord can produce paralysis below the site of injury. A ruptured, or slipped, intervertebral DISC causes neurological symptoms because it presses on the spinal cord.

Degenerative diseases affecting the nervous system include MYASTHENIA GRAVIS, MULTIPLE SCLEROSIS, and PARKINSON'S DISEASE.

EPILEPSY, which may or may not be traced to a brain lesion, is another disorder that affects the nervous system.

nervousness ('nərvəsnəs) a state of excitability, with great mental and physical unrest.

nervus ('nərvəs) pl. *nervi* [L.] nerve.

nesidiectomy (ni,sidi'ektəmee) excision of the islet cells of the pancreas.

nesidioblast (ni'sidioh,blast) any of the cells giving rise to islet cells of the pancreas.

Netillin (nə'tilin) trademark for preparations of netilmicin, an aminoglycoside antibiotic.

netilmicin (netil'misin) an aminoglycoside antibiotic.

nettle rash ('net'l ,rash) a vascular reaction characterized by sudden outbreaks of itching and burning swellings on the skin; called also URTICARIA.

Nettleship's dilator ('net'l,ships) an instrument for dilating the lacrimal puncta.

network ('net,wərk) a mesh-like structure of interlocking fibres or strands.

neur(o)- word element. [Gr.] *nerve.*

neurad ('nyooə·rad) toward the neural axis or aspect.

neural ('nyooə·rəl) pertaining to a nerve or to the nerves.

neuralgia (nyuh'raljə, -ji·ə) pain in a nerve or along the course of one or more nerves. adj. **neuralgic.** Neuralgia is usually a sharp, spasm-like pain that may recur at intervals. It is caused by inflammation of or injury to a nerve or group of nerves.

Inflammation of a nerve, or NEURITIS, may affect different parts of the body, depending upon the location of the nerve. TIC DOULOUREUX (called also *trigeminal neuralgia*) is due to involvement of the trigeminal nerve, with neuralgic pain over the jaw, cheek, and forehead.

Another form of neuralgia is SCIATICA, or pain occurring along the sciatic nerve. This pain is felt in the back and down the back of the thigh to the ankle. It may result from inflammation of or injury to the sciatic nerve, and is often associated with conditions such as arthritis of the spine, prolapsed intervertebral disc, diabetes mellitus, and gout.

n. facialis vera geniculate neuralgia.

Fothergill's n. tic douloureux (trigeminal neuralgia).

geniculate n., Hunt's n. neuralgia involving the geniculate ganglion, producing pain in the middle ear and external acoustic meatus. Called also *Ramsay Hunt syndrome.*

glossopharyngeal n. that affecting the petrosal and jugular ganglion of the glossopharyngeal nerve, marked by severe paroxysmal pain originating on the side of the throat and extending to the ear.

idiopathic n. neuralgia of unknown aetiology, not accompanied by any structural change.

intercostal n. neuralgia of the intercostal nerves, causing pain in the side.

mammary n. neuralgic pain in the breast.

Morton's n. pain in the metatarsus of the foot.

nasociliary n. pain in the eyes, brow, and root of the nose.

postherpetic n. persistent burning pain and hyperaesthesia along the distribution of a cutaneous nerve following an attack of herpes zoster.

trifacial n., trigeminal n. tic douloureux.

neuraminidase (ˌnyooə·rə'mini,dayz) an enzyme of the surface coat of myxoviruses that destroys the neuraminic acid of the cell surface during attachment, thereby preventing haemagglutination.

neuranagenesis (ˌnyooə·ranə'jenəsis) regeneration of nerve tissue.

neurapophysis (ˌnyooə·rə'pofisis) a structure forming either side of the neural arch; also, the part supposedly homologous with this structure in a so-called cranial vertebra.

neurapraxia (ˌnyooə·rə'praksi·ə) failure of nerve conduction in the absence of structural changes, due to blunt injury, compression, or ischaemia.

neurarthropathy (ˌnyooə·rah'thropəthee) neuroarthropathy.

neurasthenia (ˌnyooə·rəs'theeni·ə) neurasthenic neurosis; a neurosis marked by chronic abnormal fatiguability, lack of energy, feelings of inadequacy, moderate depression, inability to concentrate, loss of appetite, insomnia, etc. Popularly called nervous prostration. adj. **neurasthenic.**

neuratrophia (ˌnyooə·rə'trohfi·ə) impaired nutrition of the nervous system.

neuratrophic (ˌnyooə·rə'trofik) characterized by atrophy of the nerves; also, a person so affected.

neuraxis (nyuh'raksis) 1. axon. 2. central nervous system. adj. **neuraxial.**

neuraxon (nyuh'rakson) axon.

neurectasia, neurectasis (ˌnyooə·rek'tayzi·ə; nyuh'rektəsis) the surgical stretching of a nerve; neurotony.

neurectomy (nyuh'rektəmee) excision of a part of a nerve.

neurectopia (ˌnyooə·rek'tohpi·ə) displacement or abnormal situation of a nerve.

neurenteric (ˌnyooə·ren'terik) pertaining to the neural tube and archenteron of the embryo.

neurergic (nyuh'rərjik) pertaining to or dependent on nerve action.

neurexeresis (ˌnyooə·rek'serisis) avulsion of a nerve.

neurilemma (ˌnyooə·ri'lemə) the plasma membrane of a Schwann cell, forming the sheath of Schwann of a myelinated or unmyelinated peripheral nerve. adj. **neurilemmal.**

neurilemmitis (ˌnyooə·rilə'mietis) inflammation of the neurilemma.

neurilemoma (ˌnyooə·rilə'mohmə) a tumour of a peripheral nerve sheath (neurilemma); called also *schwannoma.*

neurinoma (ˌnyooə·ri'nohmə) neurilemoma.

neuritis (nyuh'rietis) pl. *neuritides;* inflammation of a nerve; also used to denote noninflammatory lesions of the peripheral nervous system (see also NEUROPATHY). adj. **neuritic.** There are many forms with different effects. Some increase or decrease the sensitivity of the body part served by the nerve; others produce paralysis; some cause pain and inflammation. The cases in which pain is the chief symptom are generally called NEURALGIA.

Neuritis and neuralgia attack the peripheral nerves, the nerves that link the brain and spinal cord with the muscles, skin, organs, and all other parts of the body. These nerves usually carry both sensory and motor fibres; hence both pain and some paralysis may result. Treatment varies with the specific form of neuritis involved.

GENERALIZED NEURITIS. Certain toxic substances such as lead, arsenic, and mercury may produce a generalized poisoning of the peripheral nerves, with tenderness, pain, and paralysis of the limbs. Other causes of generalized neuritis include alcoholism, vitamin-deficiency diseases such as beriberi, and diabetes mellitus, thallium poisoning, some types of allergy, and some viral and bacterial infections, such as diphtheria, syphilis, and mumps.

Some attacks of generalized neuritis begin with fever and other symptoms of an acute illness. However, neuritis caused by lead or alcohol poisoning comes on very slowly over the course of weeks or months.

Usually an attack of generalized neuritis will subside by itself when the toxic substance is eliminated. Rest and a nutritious diet containing extra vitamins, especially of the B group, are helpful. Physiotherapy may relieve the pain and paralysis. Generalized neuritis may be prevented through knowledge of the dangers of poor nutrition, industrial hazards, chronic alcoholism, and infections.

SPECIAL TYPES OF NEURITIS. Frequently, instead of a generalized irritation of the nerves, only one nerve is affected. BELL'S PALSY, or facial paralysis, results when the facial nerve is affected. It usually lasts only a few days or weeks. Sometimes, however, the cause is a tumour pressing on the nerve, or injury to the nerve by a blow, cut, or bullet. In that event, recovery depends on the success in treating the tumour or injury.

Sciatica. The sciatic nerve, which runs from the spinal cord down each leg, is the widest nerve in the body and one of the longest. It is exposed to many different kinds of injury in the back, in the pelvis, and along its course in the leg.

Inflammation of or injury to the sciatic nerve, with resultant SCIATICA, causes pain that travels down from the back or thigh into the feet and toes. Certain muscles of the leg may be partly or completely paralysed, so that it is difficult to move the thigh or leg. A back injury, irritation from arthritis of the spine, or pressure on the nerve that occurs during certain types of work may be the cause. Certain diseases such as diabetes mellitus or gout may be the inciting factor. The most common cause is probably a herniated or prolapsed intervertebral disc.

Neuritis of the Spinal Nerves. Injury or disease may affect any of the many nerves travelling out from the spine. For example, inflammation of the nerves between the ribs causes pain in the chest that may resemble pleurisy or even coronary occlusion (heart attack). This is called intercostal neuritis or intercostal neuralgia. Similarly, the nerves traveling down the neck to the arm may be subject to various injuries or diseases. For example, too vigorous pulling on the nerves in the newborn infant's neck, as might occur in difficult obstetrical deliveries, causes the condition known as brachial paralysis.

Neuritis of the Cranial Nerves. Bell's palsy results from inflammation of the seventh cranial, or facial nerve. Another nerve, the fifth cranial, or trigeminal, nerve, also ends in the face and jaws, and may be the source of a neuralgia that causes spasms of pain on one side of the face. This is called TIC DOULOUREUX or trigeminal neuralgia. It may be set off by a draught of cold air, by chewing, or by other factors. Medicines and, if necessary, surgery can relieve this painful malady.

The nerves leading to the retina of the eye may be involved in various ailments. This condition, optic neuritis, is potentially dangerous to vision and requires immediate treatment. Any of the other cranial nerves may be affected by infections, tumours, and toxins. The antibiotic streptomycin occasionally causes damage to the eighth cranial nerve, which helps control the sense of balance in the inner ear. Any disturbance of vision, hearing, balance, swallowing, taste, or speech may be a sign of trouble in the cranial nerves, and should be brought to a doctor's attention at once.

endemic n. beriberi.

interstitial n. inflammation of the connective tissue of a nerve trunk.

multiple n. neuritis affecting several nerves at once; polyneuritis.

optic n. inflammation of the optic nerve, affecting the part of the nerve within the eyeball (neuropapillitis) or the part behind the eyeball (retrobulbar neuritis).

parenchymatous n. neuritis affecting primarily the axons and the myelin of the peripheral nerves.

retrobulbar n. optic neuritis affecting the part of the optic nerve behind the eyeball.

toxic n. neuritis due to some poison.

traumatic n. neuritis following and due to injury.

neuroanastomosis (ˌnyooə·roh·əˌnastə'mohsis) surgical anastomosis of one nerve to another.

neuroanatomy (ˌnyooə·roh·ə'natəmee) anatomy of the nervous system.

neuroarthropathy (ˌnyooə·roh·ah'thropəthee) any disease of joint structures associated with disease of the central or peripheral nervous system.

neuroastrocytoma (ˌnyooə·rohˌastrohsie'tohmə) a glioma composed mainly of astrocytes, found mostly in the floor of the third ventricle and the temporal lobes of the brain.

neurobehavioural (ˌnyooə·rohbi'hayvyə·rəl) relating to neurological status as assessed by observation of behaviour.

neurobiologist (ˌnyooə·rohbie'olәjist) a specialist in neurobiology.

neurobiology (ˌnyooə·rohbie'oləjee) biology of the nervous system.

neuroblast ('nyooə·rohˌblast) an embryonic cell from which nervous tissue is formed.

neuroblastoma (ˌnyooə·rohbla'stohmə) sarcoma of nervous system origin, composed chiefly of neuroblasts, affecting mostly infants and children up to 10 years of age, usually arising in the autonomic nervous system (sympathicoblastoma) or in the adrenal medulla.

neurocanal (ˌnyooə·rohkə'nal) vertebral canal.

neurocardiac (ˌnyooə·roh'kahdiˌak) pertaining to the nervous system and the heart.

neurocentrum (ˌnyooə·roh'sentrəm) one of the embryonic vertebral elements from which the spinous processes of the vertebrae develop. adj. **neurocentral**.

neurochemistry (ˌnyooə·roh'kemistree) that branch of neurology dealing with the chemistry of the nervous system.

neurochorioretinitis (ˌnyooə·rohˌko·riohˌreti'nietis) inflammation of the optic nerve, choroid, and retina.

neurochoroiditis (ˌnyooə·rohˌko·roy'dietis) inflammation of the optic nerve and choroid.

neurocirculatory (ˌnyooə·rohˌsərkyuh'laytə·ree) pertaining to the nervous and circulatory systems.

neurocladism (nyuh'rokləˌdizəm) the formation of new branches by the process of a neuron; especially the force by which, in regeneration of divided nerves, the newly formed axons become attracted by the peripheral stump, so as to form a bridge between the two ends.

neuroclonic (ˌnyooə·roh'klonik) marked by nervous spasm.

neurocommunications (ˌnyooə·rohkəˌmyooni'kayshənz) the branch of neurology dealing with the transfer and integration of information within the nervous system.

neurocranium (ˌnyooə·roh'krayni·əm) the part of the cranium enclosing the brain. adj. **neurocranial**.

neurocrine ('nyooə·rohˌkrien) 1. denoting an endocrine influence on or by the nerves. 2. pertaining to neurosecretion.

neurocristopathy (ˌnyooə·rohkri'stopəthee) any disease arising from maldevelopment of the neural crest.

neurocutaneous (ˌnyooə·rohkyoo'tayni·əs) pertaining to nerves and skin, or the cutaneous nerves.

neurocyte ('nyooə·rohˌsiet) a nerve cell of any kind.

neurocytoma (ˌnyooə·rohsie'tohmə) a brain tumour consisting of undifferentiated cells of nervous origin, i.e., cells resembling medullary neural epithelium. Called also *neuroepithelioma*.

neurodendrite, neurodendron (ˌnyooə·roh'dendriet; ˌnyooə·roh'dendron) dendrite.

neurodermatitis (ˌnyooə·rohˌdərmə'tietis) a general term for a dermatosis presumed to be caused by itching due to emotional causes. The term is also used to refer to LICHEN SIMPLEX CHRONICUS (circumscribed or localized neurodermatitis) and sometimes atopic DERMATITIS (disseminated neurodermatitis).

neurodynamic (ˌnyooə·rohdie'namik) pertaining to nervous energy.

neurodynia (ˌnyooə·roh'dini·ə) pain in a nerve.

neuroectoderm (ˌnyooə·roh'ektohˌdərm) the portion of the ectoderm of the early embryo which gives rise to the central and peripheral nervous systems, including some glial cells. adj. **neuroectodermal**.

neuroeffector (ˌnyooə·roh·i'fektə) of or relating to the junction between a neuron and the effector organ it innervates.

neuroencephalomyelopathy (ˌnyooə·roh·enˌkefəlohˌmieə'lopəthee; -ˌsef-) disease involving the nerves, brain, and spinal cord.

neuroendocrine (ˌnyooə·roh'endohˌkrin, -ˌkrien) pertaining to neural and endocrine influence, and particularly to the interaction between the nervous and endocrine systems.

neuroendocrinology (ˌnyooə·rohˌendəkri'noləjee) the study of the interactions of the nervous and endocrine systems.

neuroepithelioma (ˌnyooə·rohˌepiˌtheeli'ohmə) neurocytoma.

neuroepithelium (ˌnyooə·rohˌepi'theeli·əm) 1. epithelium made up of cells specialized to serve as sensory cells for reception of external stimuli. Called also *sense*, or *sensory*, *epithelium*. 2. the ectodermal epithelium, from which the central nervous system develops.

neurofibril (ˌnyooə·roh'fiebril, -'fib-) one of the delicate threads running in every direction through the cytoplasm of a nerve cell, extending into the axon and dendrites.

neurofibroma (ˌnyooə·rohfie'brohmə) a tumour of peripheral nerves due to abnormal proliferation of Schwann cells. Called also *fibroneuroma*.

neurofibromatosis(ˌnyooə·rohˌfiebrohmə'tohsis) a familial condition characterized by developmental changes in the nervous system, muscles, bones, and skin, and marked by the formation of neurofibromas over the entire body associated with patches of pigmentation; called also *von Recklinghausen's disease*.

neurofilament (ˌnyooə·roh'filəmənt) any of the slender, fibrillar elements which, along with the neurotubules, forms a neurofibril.

neurogenesis (ˌnyooə·roh'jenəsis) the development of nervous tissue.

neurogenic (ˌnyooə·rə'jenik) 1. forming nervous tissue, or stimulating nervous energy. 2. originating in the nervous system.

neurogenous (nyuh'rojənəs) arising from the nervous system, or from some lesion of the nervous system.

neuroglia (nyuh'rogli·ə) the supporting structure of nervous tissue, consisting, in the central nervous system, of astrocytes, oligodendrocytes, and microglia; called also *glia*. adj. **neuroglial**.

neurogliocyte (nyuh'roglioh,siet) one of the cells composing the neuroglia.

neuroglioma (ˌnyooə·rohglie'ohmə) a tumour composed of neuroglial tissue.

n. ganglionare ganglioneuroma.

neurogliosis (ˌnyooə·rohglie'ohsis) a condition marked by numerous neurogliomas.

neurohistology (ˌnyooə·roh·hi'stoləjee) histology of the nervous system.

neurohormone (ˌnyooə·roh'hawmohn) a hormone stimulating the neural mechanism.

neurohumour (ˌnyooə·roh'hyoomə) a chemical substance formed in a neuron and able to activate or modify the function of a neighbouring neuron, muscle, or gland. adj. **neurohumoural**.

neurohypophysis (ˌnyooə·roh·hie'pofisis) the posterior lobe of the PITUITARY GLAND. adj. **neurohypophyseal**.

neuroid ('nyooə·royd) resembling a nerve.

neuroimmunology (ˌnyooə·rohˌimyuh'noləjee) that branch of science which deals with the interaction of the nervous and immune systems in health and disease, as in the effect of autonomic nervous activity on the immune response and the role of antibodies in myasthenia gravis. adj. **neuroimmunological**.

neuroinduction (ˌnyooə·roh·in'dukshən) mental suggestion.

neurolemma (ˌnyooə·roh'lemə) neurilemma.

neurolemmitis (ˌnyooə·rohlə'mietis) neurilemmitis.

neurolemmoma (ˌnyooə·rohlə'mohmə) neurilemoma.

neuroleptic (ˌnyooə·roh'leptik) 1. modifying psychotic behaviour. 2. any drug that favourably modifies psychotic symptoms; the main categories of neuroleptics include the phenothiazines, butyrophenones, and thioxanthenes. Called also *antipsychotic* and *major tranquillizer*.

Drugs of this type stabilize mood and reduce anxiety, tension, and hyperactivity. They are also effective in helping to control agitation and aggressiveness. Delusions and hallucinations are often modified and may be eliminated by a neuroleptic drug, but once the drug is discontinued, the delusions and hallucinations frequently return within a short while.

Neuroleptic drugs are thought to block dopamine receptors in the brain, a physiological effect that exerts an antipsychotic action and also produces their neurological side-effects. The drugs are contraindicated in patients who are suffering from central nervous system depression, severe allergy, Parkinson's disease, or a blood dyscrasia. There also is the possibility of drug–drug interaction when neuroleptic drugs are given concurrently with barbiturates, alcohol, tricyclic antidepressants, antihypertensives, pethidine, anticonvulsants, or levodopa. Many neuroleptic drugs have alarming side-effects and, therefore, require frequent monitoring of the patient and individualized adjustments in dosage. The side-effects can usually be minimized by gradually increasing the dosage until the optimum for the individual patient is reached. Side-effects such as a discomforting restlessness and agitation (*akathisia*), involuntary rhythmic movements of the trunk and limbs, parkinsonism, and sucking, chewing, licking, and pursing movements of the lips are often misinterpreted as symptoms of some unrelated disorder; they are frequently responsible for noncompliance on the part of the patient who refuses to continue taking his prescribed medication once he is aware of the side-effects.

Approximately 20 per cent of the patients treated with neuroleptics for long periods develop tardive dyskinesia, a syndrome of choreoathetoid movements of the tongue, mouth, face, neck, extremities, and trunk, which may continue after the drug is stopped.

Neuroleptic drugs are sometimes prescribed for conditions other than mental disorders. They can be beneficial in the control of nausea, in the treatment of intractable hiccoughs, and, in combination with other drugs, for the control of pain.

neurological assessment (ˌnyooə·roh'lojik'l) evaluation of the health status of a patient with a nervous system disorder or dysfunction. Purposes of the assessment include establishing a *medical diagnosis* to guide the doctor in prescribing medical and surgical treatments, and *nursing goals* to guide the nurse in planning and implementing nursing measures to help the patient cope effectively with daily living activities.

Responsibilities of the doctor in a neurological assessment include conducting a general physical examination and a detailed neurological examination, obtaining a neurological history, and requesting special neurological diagnostic studies. The neurological physical examination involves evaluation of the patient's level of consciousness, mood, orientation, speech, content of thought, and memory; his gait while walking and ability to stand quietly with feet together; the physical status of his head, neck, and spine as determined by palpation, inspection, and auscultation; function of the cranial nerves; sensory and motor function; and reflex activity.

Nursing assessment of a patient's neurological status is concerned with identifying functional disabilities that interfere with the person's ability to care for himself and lead an active life. A functionally oriented nursing assessment includes: (1) consciousness, (2) mental functions, (3) motor function, and (4) sensory function. Evaluation of these functions gives the nurse information about the patient's ability to perform everyday activities such as thinking, remembering, seeing, eating, speaking, moving, smelling, feeling, and hearing.

A patient with an acute and life-threatening alteration in neurological function is evaluated and monitored in four general areas: (1) level of consciousness, (2) sensory and motor function, (3) pupillary changes, and (4) vital signs and pattern of respiration. See also INTRACRANIAL PRESSURE.

neurologist (nyuh'roləjist) a medical practitioner specializing in neurology.

neurology (nyuh'roləjee) that branch of medical science which deals with the nervous system, both normal and in disease. adj. **neurologic**.

clinical n. that especially concerned with the diagnosis and treatment of disorders of the nervous system.

neurolysin (nyuh'rolisin) a cytolysin with a specific destructive action on neurons.

neurolysis (nyuh'rolisis) 1. release of a nerve by cutting the sheath longitudinally. 2. dissolution or stretching of perineural adhesions. 3. destruction or dissolution of nerve tissue. adj. **neurolytic.**

neuroma (nyuh'rohmə) a tumour or new growth largely made up of nerve cells and nerve fibres. adj. **neuromatous.**

acoustic n. a benign tumour (neurofibroma) within the auditory canal arising from the eighth cranial (vestibulocochlear) nerve.

amputation n. traumatic neuroma occurring after amputation of an extremity or part.

n. cutis neuroma in the skin.

false n. one that does not contain nerve elements.

plexiform n. one made up of contorted nerve trunks.

n. telangiectodes one containing an excess of blood vessels.

traumatic n. an unorganized bulbous or nodular mass of nerve fibres and Schwann cells produced by hyperplasia of nerve fibres and their supporting tissues after accidental or purposeful sectioning of the nerve.

neuromalacia (,nyooə·rohmə'layshi·ə) morbid softening of the nerves.

neuromatosis (,nyooə·rohmə'tohsis) condition characterized by the presence of many neuromas.

neuromere ('nyooə·roh,miə) 1. any of a series of transitory segmental elevations in the wall of the neural tube in the developing embryo; also, such elevations in the wall of the mature rhombencephalon. 2. a part of the spinal cord to which a pair of dorsal roots and a pair of ventral roots are attached.

neuromuscular (,nyooə·roh'muskyuhlə) pertaining to the nerves and muscles.

neuromyelitis (,nyooə·roh,mieə'lietis) inflammation of nervous and medullary substance; myelitis attended with neuritis.

n. optica combined demyelination of the optic nerve and spinal cord, with diminution of vision and possible blindness, flaccid paralysis of extremities, and sensory and genitourinary disturbances.

neuromyositis (,nyooə·roh,mieoh'sietis) neuritis blended with myositis.

neuron, neurone ('nyooə·ron; 'nyooə·rohn) nerve cell; any of the conducting cells of the nervous system, consisting of a cell body, containing the nucleus and its surrounding cytoplasm, and the axon and dendrites. adj. **neuronal.** Neurons are highly specialized cells having two characteristic properties: irritability, which means they are capable of being stimulated; and conductivity, which means they are able to conduct impulses. They are composed of a cell body (neurosome or perikaryon), containing the nucleus and its surrounding cytoplasm and one or more processes (nerve fibres) extending from the body.

The processes or nerve fibres are actually extensions of the cytoplasm surrounding the nucleus of the neuron. A nerve cell may have only one such slender fibre extending from its body, in which case it is classified as unipolar. A neuron having two processes is bipolar, and one with three or more processes is multipolar. Most neurons are multipolar, this type of neuron being widely distributed throughout the central nervous system and autonomic ganglia. The multipolar neurons have a single process called an axon and several branched extensions called dendrites. The dendrites receive stimuli from other nerves or from a receptor organ, such as the skin or ear, and transmit them through the neuron to the axon. The axon conducts the impulses to the dendrite of another neuron or to an effector organ that is thereby stimulated to action.

Many processes are covered with a layer of lipid material called MYELIN. Peripheral nerve fibres have a thin outer covering called neurilemma.

TYPES OF NEURONS. Neurons that receive stimuli from the outside environment and transmit them toward the brain are called afferent or sensory neurons. Neurons that carry impulses in the opposite direction, away from the brain and other nerve centres to muscles, are called efferent or motor neurons, or motoneurons. Another type of nerve cell, the association or internuncial neuron, or interneuron, is found in the brain and spinal cord; these neurons conduct impulses from afferent to efferent neurons.

SYNAPSES. The point at which an impulse is transmitted from one neuron to another is called a synapse. The transmission is chemical in nature; that is, there is no direct contact between the axon of one neuron and the dendrites of another. The cholinergic nerves (parasympathetic nervous system) liberate at their axon endings a substance called acetylcholine, which acts as a stimulant to the dendrites of adjacent neurons. In a similar manner, the adrenergic nerves (sympathetic nervous system) liberate sympathin, a substance that closely resembles adrenaline and probably is identical to noradrenaline.

The synapse may involve one neuron in chemical contact with many adjacent neurons, or it may involve the axon terminals of one neuron and the dendrites of a succeeding neuron in a nerve pathway. There are many different patterns of synapses.

RECEPTOR END-ORGANS. The dendrites of the sensory neurons are designed to receive stimuli from various parts of the body. These dendrites are called receptor end-organs and are of three general types: exteroceptors, interoceptors, and proprioceptors. Their names give a clue to their specific function. The exteroceptors are located near the external surface of the body and receive impulses from the skin. They transmit information about the senses of touch, heat, cold, and other factors in the external environment. The interoceptors are located in the internal organs and receive information from the viscera, e.g. pressure, tension, and pain. The proprioceptors are found in muscles, tendons, and joints and transmit 'muscle sense', by which one is aware of the position of the body in space.

NEURONS AND EFFECTORS. The axons of motor neurons form synapses with skeletal fibres to produce motion. These junctions are called motor end-plates or neuromuscular junctions. The axon of a motor neuron divides just before it enters the muscle fibres and forms synapses near the nuclei of muscle fibres. These motor neurons are called somatic efferent neurons. Visceral efferent neurons form synapses with smooth muscle, cardiac muscle, and glands.

Golgi n's 1. *type I,* pyramidal cells with long axons, which leave the grey matter of the central nervous system, traverse the white matter, and terminate in the periphery. 2. *type II,* stellate neurons with short axons in the cerebral and cerebellar cortices and in the retina.

motor n. motoneuron.

postganglionic n's neurons whose cell bodies lie in the autonomic ganglia and whose purpose is to relay impulses beyond the ganglia.

preganglionic n's neurons whose cell bodies lie in the central nervous system and whose efferent fibres terminate in the autonomic ganglia.

neuronaevus (,nyooə·roh'neevəs) a cellular or naevocytic naevus, especially a mature one with differentiation toward neural skin structures.

neuronophage (nyuh'ronoh,fayj) a phagocyte that destroys nerve cells.

neuronophagia (,nyooə·ronoh'fayji·ə) phagocytic destruction of nerve cells.

neuro-ophthalmology (,nyooə·roh,ofthal'moləjee) that branch of ophthalmology dealing with portions of the nervous system related to the eye.

neuropapillitis (,nyooə·roh,papi'lietis) optic NEURITIS affecting the part of the optic nerve within the eyeball.

neuroparalysis (,nyooə·rohpə'ralisis) paralysis due to disease of a nerve or nerves.

neuropathogenicity (,nyooə·roh,pathəjə'nisitee) the quality of producing or the ability to produce pathological changes in nerve tissue.

neuropathology (,nyooə·rohpə'tholəjee) pathology of the nervous system.

neuropathy (nyuh'ropəthee) a general term denoting functional disturbances and pathological changes in the peripheral nervous system. The aetiology may be known (e.g. arsenical, diabetic, ischaemic, or traumatic neuropathy) or unknown. Encephalopathy and myelopathy are corresponding terms relating to involvement of the brain and spinal cord, respectively. The term is also used to designate noninflammatory lesions in the peripheral nervous system, in contrast to inflammatory lesions (neuritis). adj. **neuropathic.**

alcoholic n. neuropathy due to thiamine deficiency in chronic alcoholism.

diabetic n. a chronic symmetrical sensory polyneuropathy affecting first the nerves of the lower limbs and often affecting autonomic nerves. Pathologically, there is segmental demyelination of the peripheral nerves. An uncommon, acute form is marked by severe pain, weakness, and wasting of proximal and distal muscles, peripheral sensory impairment, and loss of tendon reflexes. With autonomic involvement there may be orthostatic hypotension, nocturnal diarrhoea, retention of urine, impotence, and small diameter of the pupils with sluggish reaction to light.

entrapment n. any of a group of neuropathies, e.g. carpal tunnel syndrome, due to mechanical pressure on a peripheral nerve.

hereditary sensory radicular n. a dominantly inherited disorder characterized by signs of radicular sensory loss in both the upper and lower extremities; shooting pains; chronic, indolent, trophic ulceration of the feet; and sometimes deafness.

progressive hypertrophic interstitial n. a slowly progressive familial disease beginning in early life, marked by hyperplasia of interstitial connective tissue, causing thickening of peripheral nerve trunks and posterior roots, and by sclerosis of the posterior columns of the spinal cord, with atrophy of distal parts of the legs and diminution of tendon reflexes and sensation. Called also *Déjérine's disease* and *Déjérine-Sottas disease.*

serum n. a neurological disorder, usually involving the cervical nerves or brachial plexus, occurring 2 to 8 days after the injection of foreign protein, as in immunization or serotherapy for tetanus, diphtheria, or scarlet fever, and characterized by local pain followed by sensory disturbances and paralysis. Called also *serum neuritis.*

neuropeptide (,nyooə·roh'peptied) any of the molecules composed of short chains of amino acids (endorphins, enkephalins, vasopressin, etc.) found in brain tissue.

neuropharmacology (,nyooə·roh,fahmə'koləjee) scientific study of the effects of drugs on the nervous system.

neurophthisis (,nyooə·roh'thiesis) wasting of nerve tissue.

neurophysin (,nyooə·roh'fiesin) any of a group of soluble proteins secreted in the hypothalamus that serve as binding proteins for vasopressin and oxytocin, playing a role in their transport in the neurohypophyseal tract and their storage in the posterior pituitary.

neurophysiology (,nyooə·roh,fizi'oləjee) physiology of the nervous system.

neuropil ('nyooə·roh,pil) a dense feltwork of interwoven cytoplasmic processes of nerve cells (dendrites and axons) and of neuroglial cells in the central nervous system and some parts of the peripheral nervous system.

neuroplasm ('nyooə·roh,plazəm) the protoplasm of a nerve cell. adj. **neuroplasmic.**

neuroplasty ('nyooə·roh,plastee) plastic repair of a nerve.

neuropodium (,nyooə·roh'pohdi·əm) a bulbous termination of an axon in one type of synapse.

neuropore ('nyooə·roh,por) an opening in the anterior or posterior end of the neural tube of the developing embryo that closes eventually.

neuropsychiatrist (,nyooə·rohsie'kieətrist) a specialist in neuropsychiatry.

neuropsychiatry (,nyooə·rohsie'kieətree) a branch of medicine combining neurology and psychiatry.

neuroradiology (,nyooə·roh,raydi'oləjee) radiology of the nervous system.

neuroretinitis (,nyooə·roh,reti'nietis) inflammation of the optic nerve and retina.

neuroretinopathy (,nyooə·roh,reti'nopəthee) pathological involvement of the optic disc and retina.

neurorrhaphy (nyuh'ro·rəfee) suture of a divided nerve.

neurosarcocleisis (,nyooə·roh,sahkoh'kliesis) an operation to relieve pressure upon a nerve by removal from a bony canal through which it passes and transplantation to soft tissue.

neurosarcoma (,nyooə·rohsah'kohmə) a sarcoma with neuromatous elements.

neuroscience (,nyooə·roh'sieəns) the embryology, anatomy, physiology, biochemistry, and pharmacology of the nervous system.

neurosclerosis (,nyooə·rohsklə'rohsis) hardening of nerve tissue.

neurosecretion (,nyooə·rohsi'kreeshən) 1. secretory activities of nerve cells. 2. a substance secreted by nerve cells. adj. **neurosecretory.**

neurosis (nyuh'rohsis) pl. *neuroses;* an emotional disorder that can interfere with a person's ability to lead a normal, useful life, or can impair his physical health; sometimes called psychoneurosis. adj. **neurotic.**

A neurosis is generally a milder form of mental illness than a PSYCHOSIS. Those persons with neurotic symptoms are usually in contact with reality; they are able to function in society even though they may feel uncomfortable or their efficiency may be impaired. By contrast, psychotic persons tend to withdraw from the real world into one of their own, or to act in strange, even bizarre, ways, and are often not aware of their illness.

CAUSES. Current theories agree that neuroses arise from mental conflicts rooted in a person's childhood. The budding personality handles these ever present conflicts by means of mental and DEFENCE MECHANISMS, including identification, rationalization, repression, projection, and others.

How each child uses these defence mechanisms in the process of maturing determines whether he will be healthy or neurotic. Symptoms such as obsessions, compulsions, phobias, and other behaviour represent unsuccessful attempts to master these conflicts. These symptoms can be so mild as to be barely noticeable. They can sometimes even be useful: a compulsion for neatness makes a good craftsman. It is a rare person who does not at some time show some trace of neurotic symptoms or behaviour. At the other extreme, neurotic patterns can be severe enough to warrant intensive treatment.

TYPES OF NEUROSES. Psychiatrists today prefer to call neuroses 'reactions' because these conditions result from, or are reactions to, psychological factors. At the time the word 'neurosis' came into use, it was thought that disorders of the nervous system were responsible for neurotic symptoms.

Types of neurosis include the neurotic character and the various specific neuroses. Specific neuroses may take a number of different forms, which are not necessarily clearly defined as separate. A person may have several different neurotic symptoms but usually one tends to dominate.

Neurotic Character. Practically everyone has unconscious conflicts to some extent. Most people take them in their stride. Some people, however, develop a neurotic character, and suffer from a general maladjustment to society. In most cases the neurotic cannot sustain satisfactory relationships in the world around him, though some of them are charming, attractive people. A neurotic character is more difficult to treat than a specific neurotic symptom. The patient with a specific neurosis usually senses that there is something wrong with him, but the patient with a neurotic character structure may not, since he has convinced himself his ways of behaviour are reasonable.

Anxiety Neurosis. In this condition, the patient has periods of anxiety which can vary from mild uneasiness ('free-floating anxiety') to blind panic. The anxiety can produce a variety of physical symptoms such as sweating, dizziness, and shortness of breath.

Everyone occasionally experiences anxiety as a normal response to a dangerous or unusual situation. In anxiety neurosis the person feels the same emotion without any apparent reason. He cannot identify the source of the threat that produces his anxiety. The symptoms are the result of unconscious fears, which often are triggered by an apparently harmless stimulus that the patient unconsciously links with a deeply buried anxiety-producing experience.

Phobic Neurosis (Phobias). Phobic neurosis is an exaggerated fear. The feared objects, ideas, or situations are often symbolic of the unconscious conflict. They divert attention from the conflict, and thus help to keep it unconscious. The neurotic may make elaborate changes in his life to avoid the object of his fear, often with severe effects on his family and friends.

Before the roots of neurosis in psychological conflicts were discovered, it was believed that the different phobias were separate conditions. Names were assigned to an almost endless list of fears. Some of these, such as claustrophobia, fear of enclosed spaces, have become fairly common words. Behaviour therapy (desensitization or flooding) is now widely used in the treatment of monosymptomatic phobias, but more diffuse phobias may respond better to interpretive psychotherapy.

Obsessive–Compulsive Neurosis. There are actually two different symptoms in this neurosis, although they are closely related and are often found in the same person. The obsessive symptom is an overwhelming intrusion of certain thoughts or desires into the mind. The patient does not know why these thoughts or desires keep intruding, but it is very difficult for him to eliminate them from his mind. The compulsive symptom is an uncontrollable urge to act in certain patterns. He does not know why he follows these patterns, but he is very uncomfortable if he does not.

The mild forms of these symptoms are familiar to most people. For example, most children play the game of avoiding the cracks on a pavement. As adults, they may find themselves doing this occasionally, perhaps when they are thinking over a problem. The neurotic who follows this pattern, however, will feel real anxiety if he steps on a crack in the pavement.

In phobias and obsessive–compulsive neurosis, the patient deflects, or displaces, the unresolved conflict onto an external object or action as a substitute. By doing this, the person tries to control the conflict magically and to eliminate his anxiety. The obsession or ritual probably represents a smokescreen which the mind throws up to keep the inner conflict from becoming conscious.

Depressive Neurosis. This is an excessively deep and long-lasting depression. It may be set off by an external event, such as the death of a loved one, or there may be no apparent cause.

Depression as such is not abnormal. The well-adjusted person, however, works out and absorbs his grief. He is soon able to resume his activities and re-establish social relationships. The neurotic is not able to escape his depression for any length of time.

The depressive neurotic suffers from a general slowing down of mental and physical activity. He may have symptoms such as insomnia, loss of appetite and lack of interest in outside activities. The condition can vary from very mild to extremely severe; in severe cases, the person may even attempt suicide.

Neurotic depression is closely associated with a lack of confidence and self-esteem and with an inability to express strong feelings. Repressed anger is thought to be a powerful contributor to depression. The person feels inadequate to cope with the situations that arise in everyday life and feels that he is insecure.

Dissociative Neurosis (Dissociative Hysteria). In this condition, parts of the personality and memory become cut off from each other. At times, anxiety causes the person to forget who he is or what he is doing. When he regains his self-awareness, he does not recall what has taken place. An example of this is amnesia; a less severe form is sleepwalking.

A dissociative neurosis is very likely an attempt by the mind to shield itself from anxiety caused by an unresolved conflict. When the patient encounters a situation that may be symbolic of his inner conflict, he goes into a form of trance to avoid experiencing the conflict.

In a few extreme cases, dissociative neurosis may take the form of multiple personality. The change from one personality to another, with no conscious awareness of the other, takes place in situations of extreme emotional stress.

Conversion Neurosis (Conversion Hysteria). Conversion neurosis, or conversion reaction, is a severe form of hysteria, in which the person unconsciously converts his anxiety into a physical symptom. This symptom may be blindness, deafness, inability to speak, or paralysis of one or several limbs. The symptom is real, but there is no physical explanation for it. The symptom may disappear with as little apparent cause as it appeared.

The symptom in a conversion neurosis serves to spare the patient from dealing with an anxiety-producing situation that is too difficult to face. The best-known examples of this are shell shock and combat fatigue, in which the soldier becomes paralysed and cannot participate in battle. The part of the body affected by conversion neurosis often has an important symbolic relationship to the patient's unconscious conflict. It may also be a part of the body which the patient considers weak.

Because the symptom is so obvious, a conversion neurosis is easily detected and diagnosed. It is a comparatively rare condition today.

PREVENTION. The formation of neurotic symptoms can be prevented to some extent. There is no doubt that a warm, secure home life, parental affection, and the proper balance between understanding and discipline promote a healthy soil for the sound development of the child. The overall solidity of the parents' relationship to their child is of enormous importance. However, other elements also play a role: each child is born with different possibilities of reaction to the world around him. School and community influences are also meaningful. All these are also responsible to some degree for the mental health of everyone.

PSYCHOSOMATIC DISORDERS. Illnesses that result from the interaction of mind and body are known as psychosomatic disorders. They are an exaggerated physical reaction to emotional stress. Psychosomatic disorders usually affect only organs under the control of the autonomic nervous system, such as the digestive tract, the endocrine glands, the heart, the genitourinary, circulatory and respiratory systems, and the skin. Among illnesses known to be partly or completely psychosomatic illnesses are MIGRAINE, IRRITABLE BOWEL SYNDROME, ULCERATIVE COLITIS, peptic ULCER, SKIN allergies, and perhaps ASTHMA. Treatment must be directed at both the physical symptoms and the underlying psychological cause. See also PSYCHOSOMATIC ILLNESS.

TREATMENT. All neuroses are in part or entirely the result of unconscious conflicts and can be treated, even though the neurotic is entirely unaware of the conflicts. The form of treatment, PSYCHOTHERAPY, tries through many different methods to make the patient conscious of his unresolved conflict. Once he is aware of it, the therapist can help him resolve it.

neurospasm ('nyooə·roh,spazəm) nervous twitching of a muscle.

neurosplanchnic (,nyooə·roh'splangknik) pertaining to the cerebrospinal and sympathetic nervous systems.

neurospongioma (,nyooə·roh,spunji'ohmə) neuroglioma.

neurospongium (,nyooə·roh'spunji·əm) 1. the fibrillar component of neurons. 2. a meshwork of nerve fibrils, especially the inner reticular layer of the retina.

Neurospora (nyuh'rospə·rə) a genus of fungi, comprising the bread moulds, capable of converting tryptophan to niacin; used in genetic and enzyme research.

neurosurgeon (,nyooə·roh'sərjən) a surgeon who specializes in neurosurgery.

neurosurgery (,nyooə·roh'sərjə·ree) surgery of the nervous system.

neurosyphilis (,nyooə·roh'sifilis) a manifestation of third stage syphilis in which the nervous system is involved. The three commonest forms are: (1) meningovascular syphilis, affecting the blood vessels to the meninges, (2) tabes dorsalis (see ATAXIA), and (3) general paralysis of the insane.

neurotendinous (,nyooə·roh'tendinəs) pertaining to both nerve and tendon.

neurotensin (,nyooə·roh'tensin) a tridecapeptide that induces vasodilation and hypotension; present in human brain tissue and postulated to be a neurotransmitter.

neurotic (nyuh'rotik) 1. pertaining to or affected with a neurosis. 2. pertaining to the nerves. 3. a nervous person in whom emotions predominate over reason.

neuroticism (nyuh'roti,sizəm) a neurotic condition or trait.

neurotization (,nyooə·rətie'zayshən) 1. regeneration of a nerve after its division. 2. the implantation of a nerve into a paralysed muscle.

neurotmesis (,nyooə·rot'meesis) partial or complete severance of a nerve, with disruption of the axon and its myelin sheath and the connective tissue elements.

neurotome ('nyooə·roh,tohm) 1. a needle-like knife for dissecting nerves. 2. neuromere.

neurotomy (nyuh'rotəmee) dissection or cutting of nerves.

neurotony (nyuh'rotənee) the surgical stretching of a nerve; neurectasia; neurectasis.

neurotoxicity (,nyooə·rohtok'sisitee) the quality of exerting a destructive or poisonous effect upon nerve tissue. adj. **neurotoxic.**

neurotoxin (,nyooə·roh'toksin) a substance that is poisonous or destructive to nerve tissue.

neurotransmitter (,nyooə·rohtranz'mitə, -trahnz-) a substance (e.g. noradrenaline, acetylcholine, dopamine) that is released from the axon terminal of a presynaptic neuron on excitation, and that travels across the synaptic cleft to either excite or inhibit the target cell.

neurotrauma (,nyooə·roh'trawmə) mechanical injury to nerve.

neurotripsy ('nyooə·roh,tripsee) the surgical bruising or crushing of a nerve.

neurotrophy (nyuh'rotrəfee) nutrition and maintenance of tissues as regulated by nervous influence. adj. **neurotrophic.**

neurotropic (,nyooə·roh'tropik) having an affinity for nerve tissue.

n. viruses those that particularly attack the nervous system.

neurotropism (nyuh'rotrə,pizəm) 1. the quality of having a special affinity for nervous tissue. 2. the alleged tendency of regenerating nerve fibres to grow toward specific portions of the periphery. adj. adj. **neurotropic.**

neurotubule (,nyooə·roh'tyoobyool) any of the long, straight, parallel tubules within neurons, which along with neurofilaments form neurofibrils.

neurovaccine (,nyooə·roh'vakseen) vaccine virus prepared by growing the virus in the brain of a rabbit.

neurovascular (,nyooə·roh'vaskyuhlə) pertaining to both nervous and vascular elements, or to nerves controlling the calibre of blood vessels.

neurovisceral (,nyooə·roh'visə·rəl) neurosplanchnic.

neurula ('nyooə·rələ) the early embryonic stage following the gastrula, marked by the first appearance of the nervous system.

neurulation (,nyooə·rə'layshən) formation in the early embryo of the neural plate, followed by its closure with development of the neural tube.

neutral ('nyootrəl) neither basic nor acid.

neutralize ('nyootrə,liez) to render neutral.

neutrino (nyoo'treenoh) a subatomic particle with an extremely small mass and no electric charge.

neutrocyte ('nyootrə,siet) neutrophil (2).

neutron ('nyootron) an electrically neutral or uncharged particle of matter existing along with protons in the atoms of all elements except the mass 1 isotope of hydrogen.

neutropenia (,nyootrə'peeni·ə) diminished number of neutrophils in the blood.

cyclic n. periodic neutropenia.

malignant n. agranulocytosis.

periodic n. a chronic form marked by regular, periodic episodic recurrences, associated with malaise, fever, stomatitis, and various infections.

neutrophil ('nyootrə,fil) 1. a granular leukocyte having a nucleus with three to five lobes connected by threads of chromatin, and cytoplasm containing very fine granules; called also *polymorphonuclear leukocyte*. See also HETEROPHIL. 2. any cell, structure, or histological element readily stainable with neutral dyes.

stab n. a neutrophilic leukocyte whose nucleus is not divided into segments.

neutrophilia (,nyootrə'fili·ə) increase in the number of neutrophils in the blood.

neutrophilic (,nyootrə'filik) 1. pertaining to neutrophils. 2. stainable by neutral dyes.

newborn ('nyoo,bawn) 1. recently born. 2. a human infant during the first 4 weeks after birth.

Newcastle disease ('nyoo,kahs'l) a viral disease of birds, including domestic fowl, characterized by respiratory and gastrointestinal or pneumonic and encephalitic symptoms; also transmissible to man.

newton ('nyootən) the SI unit of force; the force that, when acting continuously upon a mass of 1 kilogram, will impart to it an acceleration of 1 metre per second squared. Symbol N.

nexus ('neksəs) 1. a bond, as between members of a series or group. 2. gap junction.

ng nanogram.

NHS (,enaych'əs) National Health Service.

NHSR National Hospital Service Reserve.

Ni chemical symbol, *nickel*.

niacin ('nieəsin) a water-soluble vitamin of the B complex found in various animal and plant tissues, especially liver, yeast, bran, peanuts, lean meats, fish, and poultry. A well balanced diet usually supplies more than the daily requirement. It is required by the body for the synthesis of the coenzymes NAD and NADP, which are required for many oxidation–reduction reactions. Deficiency of niacin produces pellagra. Niacin is used for the prophylaxis and treatment of pellagra. Called also *nicotinic acid*.

niacinamide (,nieə'sinə,mied) the amide of niacin, occurring naturally in the body and interconvertible with niacin; used in the prophylaxis and treatment of pellagra.

niche (neesh, nich) 1. a small recess, depression or indentation. 2. in radiology, a recess in the wall of a hollow organ that tends to retain contrast media, particularly a gastric or duodenal ulcer.

nickel ('nik'l) a chemical element, atomic number 28, atomic weight 58.71, symbol Ni. See table of elements in Appendix 2.

nicking ('niking) localized constriction of the retinal blood vessels.

niclosamide (ni'klohsəmied) an anthelmintic, used in tapeworm infestations.

Nicolas–Favre disease (,nikohlas'fahvrə) lymphogranuloma venereum.

nicotinamide (,nikə'tinə,mied, -'teen-) niacinamide.

n.-adenine dinucleotide (NAD) a coenzyme that is involved in many biochemical oxidation–reduction reactions. The symbols for the oxidized and reduced forms are NAD^+ and NADH.

n.-adenine dinucleotide phosphate (NADP) a coenzyme similar to nicotinamide-adenine dinucleotide but involved in fewer reactions. The symbols for the oxidized and reduced forms are $NADP^+$ and NADPH.

nicotine ('nikə,teen) a very poisonous alkaloid that in its pure state is a colourless, pungent, oily liquid, having an acrid burning taste. It is a constituent of tobacco, and is produced synthetically. In water solution, it is sometimes used as an insecticide and plant spray.

Although nicotine is highly toxic, the amount inhaled while smoking tobacco is too small to cause death. The nicotine in tobacco can, however, cause indigestion and increase in blood pressure, and dull the appetite. It also acts as a vasoconstrictor. SMOKING, especially of cigarettes, is closely linked with heart disease, lung cancer, and some other tumours.

nicotinic (,nikə'tinik) pertaining to the transmission of nerve impulses mediated by nicotinic receptors.

n. receptors cholinergic receptors of autonomic ganglion cells and motor end-plates of skeletal muscle that are stimulated by low doses of nicotine and blockaded by high doses or by tubocurarine.

nicotinic acid (,nikə'tinik) NIACIN, the antipellagra factor of the vitamin B complex.

nicotinism ('nikətee,nizəm, -ti-) nicotine poisoning, marked by stimulation and subsequent depression of the central and autonomic nervous systems, with death due to respiratory paralysis.

nicotinyl alcohol ('nikoh,tinil) a compound that is oxidized to nicotinic acid (niacin) in the body and acts as a weak vasodilator; used in conditions associated with deficient circulation.

nicoumalone (nie'koomәlohn) an orally administered anticoagulant.

nictitation (,nikti'tayshən) the act of winking.

nidation (nie'dayshən) implantation of the fertilized ovum (zygote) in the endometrium of the uterus in pregnancy.

nidus ('niedəs) pl. *nidi* [L.] 1. a nest; point of origin or focus of a morbid process. 2. nucleus (2). adj. **nidal**.

Niemann–Pick disease (,neemən'pik) a rare hereditary disease with massive enlargement of the liver and spleen, brownish-yellow discoloration of the skin, and nervous system dysfunction. Foamy reticular cells containing phospholipids infiltrate the liver, spleen, lungs, lymph nodes, and bone marrow. It occurs chiefly in Jewish chidren.

nifedipine (nie'fedi,peen) a calcium channel blocker used as a coronary vasodilator in the treatment of angina pectoris, and in the treatment of hypertension.

Niferex ('nifəreks) trademark for preparations of a polysaccharide-iron complex, an iron supplement.

night blindness (niet) inability or a reduced ability to see in dim light. In night blindness, the eyes not only see more poorly in dim light, but are slower to adjust from brightness to dimness. Called also *nyctalopia*.

Depending on its brightness, light is perceived by either of two sets of visual cells located in the retina of the eye. One set, the cones, perceive bright light primarily; the other set, the rods, perceive dim light primarily. Dim light produces a change in a pigment called rhodopsin in the rods. This change causes nerve impulses to travel to the brain, where they register as visual impressions. Night blindness occurs when the rods lack rhodopsin.

night sweat ('niet ,swet) profuse perspiration during sleep, especially typical of tuberculosis.

Nightingale ('nieting,gayl) Florence (1820–1910). Founder of modern nursing. Born in Florence, Italy, of wealthy English parents, Miss Nightingale in 1854 led a group of nurses to the Crimea to care for English troops, and proceeded to reorganize military nursing and sanitation in England and later in India. She contributed to the field of dietetics, and her skill as a statistician in gathering data won her election to the Royal Statistical Society and honorary membership in the American Statistical Association.

She founded The Nightingale School at St Thomas' Hospital in 1860. The newly built hospital was re-sited to the southern approach to Westminster Bridge from its original position in Southwark by an ancient religious foundation, St Mary Overie. The 'new' hospital was built on the pavilion plan to allow maximum ventilation at a time when cross-infection was not yet fully understood. The 'Nightingale Ward' with its open plan design was incorporated into hospitals throughout the country.

Schools of nursing in the UK and worldwide were subsequently founded by 'Nightingale nurses'. The Nightingale School has a museum of Nightingale memorabilia and it continues to play a leading role in nursing education.

Miss Nightingale was bedridden following her pioneer work at Crimea but nevertheless was the driving force for nurse training, keeping in touch personally with her 'probationers', and the improvement of conditions in the army. She had far-reaching political influence both at home and abroad. Her understanding and use of statistics and data gathering made her the first nurse researcher.

nightmare ('niet,mair) a frightening dream, especially one that is so terrifying or disturbing that it causes the sleeper to wake up.

nigra ('niegrə) [L.] *black;* see SUBSTANTIA nigra. adj. **nigral.**

nigrities (nie'grishi·eez) [L.] *blackness.*

n. linguae black tongue.

nigrostriatal (,niegrohstrie'ayt'l) projecting from the substantia nigra to the corpus striatum; said of a bundle of nerve fibres.

nihilism ('nieə,lizəm) in psychiatry, the delusion of nonexistence of the self, part of the self, or of some object in external reality. adj. **nihilistic.**

nikethamide (ni'kethə,mied) a central and respiratory stimulant.

Nikolsky's sign (ni'kolskiz) in pemphigus vulgaris and some other bullous diseases, the outer epidermis separates easily from the basal layer on exertion of firm sliding manual pressure.

niobium (nie'ohbi·əm) a chemical element, atomic number 1, atomic weight 92.906, symbol Nb. See table of elements in Appendix 2.

Niopam ('nieohpam) trademark for a preparation of iopamidol, a radiological contrast medium used in excretion urography, arterography, venography and myelography.

niphablepsia (,nifə'blepsi·ə) see SNOWBLINDNESS.

nipple ('nip'l) the pigmented projection at the tip of each BREAST, which gives outlet to milk from the breast. Also, any similarly shaped structure. The nipples are located slightly to the side rather than in the middle of the breasts. Usually, the size of the nipple is in proportion to the size of the breast, but large nipples may be found on small breasts and vice versa. In men, the nipple is smaller than in women.

Surrounding the nipple is a pigmented area called the areola. The colour of the areola varies with the complexion. In childless women, it is usually reddish. During pregnancy it increases in size and darkens in colour, becoming almost black in brunettes. The colour fades after the milk-producing period ends.

The tip of the female nipple contains tiny depressions that are openings of the lactiferous ducts. During pregnancy special care should be given the nipples. Any secretion that accumulates should be gently washed off.

PAGET'S DISEASE of the breast, a rare type of breast cancer, causes ulceration and itching of the nipple.

Nissl bodies (granules) ('nis'l) large granular bodies that stain with basic dyes, forming the substance of the reticulum of the cytoplasm of a nerve cell. Ribonucleoprotein is one of the main constituents.

nisus ('niesəs) [L.] an effort, strong tendency, or molimen.

nit (nit) the egg of a louse.

nitraemia (nie'treemi·ə) excess of nitrogen in the blood.

nitrate ('nietrayt) any salt of nitric acid; organic nitrates are used in the treatment of angina pectoris.

nitrazepam (nie'trazi,pam) a hypnotic and sedative drug used to treat insomnia with early morning wakening.

nitric ('nietrik) pertaining to or containing nitrogen in one of its higher valencies.

n. acid. a highly caustic, fuming acid that has a characteristic choking odour. It is sometimes used as a cauterizing agent in the eradication of various kinds of warts. It can be fatal if swallowed, and large amounts of nitric acid applied to the skin can cause necrosis.

nitride ('nietried) a binary compound of nitrogen with a metal.

nitrification (,nietrifi'kayshən) the bacterial oxidation of ammonia and organic nitrogen to nitrites and nitrates in the soil.

nitrifying ('nietri,fie·ing) oxidizing ammonia into nitrites and then into nitrates; said of certain bacteria.

nitrile ('nietriel) an organic compound containing trivalent nitrogen attached to one carbon atom, $-C{\equiv}N$.

nitrite ('nietriet) any salt of nitrous acid; organic nitrites are used in the treatment of angina pectoris.

Nitrocine ('nitrohseen, -in) trademark for a preparation of glyceryl trinitrate; a coronary vasodilator.

Nitrocontin Continus (,nietroh,kontin 'kontinəs) trademark for a preparation of glyceryl trinitrate; a coronary vasodilator.

nitrofuran (,nietroh'fyooə·ran) any of a group of antibacterials, including nitrofurantoin, nitrofurazone, etc., that are effective against a wide range of bacteria.

nitrofurantoin (,nietrohfyooə'rantoh·in) an antibacterial agent used in treatment of urinary tract infections.

nitrofurazone (,nietroh'fyooə·rə,zohn) an antibacterial, used topically as a local anti-infective.

nitrogen ('nietrəjən) a chemical element, atomic number 7, atomic weight 14.007, symbol N. (See table of elements in Appendix 2.) It is a gas constituting about four-fifths of common air; chemically it is almost inert. It is not poisonous but is fatal if breathed alone because of oxygen deprivation. It is soluble in the blood and body fluids, and can cause serious symptoms when released as bubbles of gas by rapid decompression. (See also BENDS.) Nitrogen occurs in proteins and amino acids and is thus present in all living cells.

n. balance the state of the body in regard to the rate of protein intake and protein utilization. When protein is metabolized, about 90 per cent of the protein nitrogen is excreted in the urine in the form of urea, uric acid, creatinine, and other nitrogen end-products. The remaining 10 per cent of the nitrogen is eliminated in the faeces.

A *negative* nitrogen balance occurs when more protein is utilized by the body than is taken in. A *positive* nitrogen balance implies a net gain of protein in the body. Negative nitrogen balance can be caused by such factors as malnutrition, debilitating diseases, blood loss, and glucocorticoids. A positive balance can be caused by exercise, growth hormone, and testosterone.

n. mustards a group of toxic, blistering alkylating agents, including nitrogen mustard itself (mechlorethamine hydrochloride) and related compounds; some have been used as antineoplastics in certain forms of cancer. Nitrogen mustards do not cure these conditions, but ease their effects by destroying mitotic cells—those newly formed by division—thereby affecting malignant tissue in its early stage of development, and leaving normal tissue unaffected. They are especially useful in the treatment of leukaemia, in which they reduce the leukocyte count, and in cases in which the malignant disease is widespread throughout the body and therefore cannot be effectively treated locally by surgery or radiotherapy. In cases of lung cancer, mechlorethamine hydrochloride is usually injected directly into the lungs via the pulmonary circulation. Side-effects, which tend to limit the usefulness of these drugs, include nausea, vomiting, and a decrease in bone marrow production.

nonprotein n. NPN, the nitrogenous constituents of the blood exclusive of the protein bodies, consisting of the nitrogen of urea, uric acid, creatine, creatinine, amino acids, polypeptides, and an undetermined part known as rest nitrogen.

Measurement of nonprotein nitrogen is used as a test of renal function, but has been largely replaced by measurement of specific substances, e.g., urea and creatinine.

nitrogenous (nie'trojənəs) containing nitrogen.

nitroglycerin (ˌnietroh'glisərin) see GLYCERYL TRINITRATE.

nitrosourea (nieˌtrohsohyuh'reeə) any of a group of lipid-soluble biological alkylating agents, including carmustine and lomustine, which cross the blood–brain barrier and are used as antineoplastic agents.

nitrous ('nietrəs) pertaining to or containing nitrogen in its lowest valency.

n. oxide a gas used by inhalation as a general anaesthetic; called also *laughing gas*. See also ANAESTHETIC.

Nivaquine ('nivəkwin) trademark for preparations of choloroquine sulphate, an antimalarial.

Nizoral (ni'zor·rəl) trademark for a preparation of ketoconazole, an antifungal.

NMR nuclear magnetic resonance.

NNEB National Nursery Examination Board.

No chemical symbol, *nobelium*.

nobelium (noh'beeli·əm) a chemical element, atomic number 102, atomic weight 253, symbol No. See table of elements in Appendix 2.

Nocardia (noh'kahdi·ə) a genus of bacteria (family Actinomycetaceae), including *N. asteroides*, which produces a tuberculosis-like infection in man, and *N. farcina* (probably identical with *N. asteroides*), which produces a tuberculosis-like infection in cattle.

nocardial (noh'kahdi·əl) pertaining to or caused by *Nocardia.*

nocardiosis (nohˌkahdi'ohsis) infection with *Nocardia.*

noci- word element. [L.] *harm, injury.*

nociassociation (ˌnohsi·əˌsohsi'ayshən) unconscious discharge of nervous energy under the stimulus of trauma.

nociceptor (ˌnohsi'septə) a receptor that is stimulated by injury; a receptor for pain. adj. **nociceptive**.

noci-influence (ˌnohsi'inflooəns) injurious or traumatic influence.

nociperception (ˌnohsipə'sepshən) the perception of traumatic stimuli.

noctalbuminuria (ˌnoktalˌbyoomi'nyooə·ri·ə) excess of albumin in the urine secreted at night.

noctambulation (ˌnoktambyuh'layshən) sleepwalking; somnambulism.

Noctec ('noktek) trademark for preparations of chloral hydrate, a hypnotic and sedative.

noctiphobia (ˌnokti'fohbi·ə) morbid dread of night.

nocturia (nok'tyooə·ri·ə) excessive urination at night.

nocturnal (nok'tərn'l) referring to the night.

n. enuresis bed wetting; incontinence of urine during sleep. See also ENURESIS.

node (nohd) a small mass of tissue in the form of a swelling, knot, or protuberance, either normal or pathological. adj. **nodal**.

n. of Aschoff and Tawara atrioventricular node.

atrioventricular (AV) n. a collection of cardiac fibres at the base of the interatrial septum that transmits the cardiac impulse initiated by the sinoatrial node (see also ATRIOVENTRICULAR NODE).

Bouchard's n's cartilaginous and bony enlargements of the proximal interphalangeal joints of the fingers in degenerative joint disease.

Delphian n. a lymph node encased in the fascia in the midline just above the thyroid isthmus, so called because it is exposed first at operation and, if diseased, is indicative of disease of the thyroid gland.

Flack's n. sinoatrial node.

Haygarth's n's joint swellings in rheumatoid arthritis.

Heberden's n's nodular protrusions on the phalanges at the distal interphalangeal joints of the fingers in osteoarthritis.

haemal n's nodes with a rich content of erythrocytes within sinuses, found near large blood vessels along the ventral side of the vertebrae and near the spleen and kidneys in various mammals, especially ruminants, having functions probably like those of the spleen; their presence in man is doubtful.

Keith's n., Keith–Flack n. sinoatrial node.

Legendre's n's Bouchard's nodes.

lymph n. any of the accumulations of lymphoid tissue organized as definite lymphatic organs along the course of lymphatic vessels, consisting of an outer cortical and inner medullary part (see also LYMPH NODE).

Meynet's n's nodules in the capsules of joints and in tendons in rheumatic conditions, especially in children.

Osler's n's small, raised, swollen, tender areas, bluish or sometimes pink or red, occurring commonly in the pads of the fingers or toes, in the thenar or hypothenar eminences or the soles of the feet; they are practically pathognomonic of subacute bacterial endocarditis.

Parrot's n. bony nodes on the outer table of the skull of infants with congenital syphilis.

n's of Ranvier constrictions of myelinated nerve fibres at regular intervals at which the myelin sheath is absent and the axon is enclosed only by Schwann cell processes.

Schmorl's n. an irregular or hemispherical bone defect in the upper or lower margin of the body of a vertebra into which the nucleus pulposus of the intervertebral disc herniates.

sentinel n., signal n. an enlarged supraclavicular lymph node usually on the node close to the junction of the thoracic duct with the subclavian vein; often the first sign of a malignant abdominal tumour.

singer's n. a small, white nodule on the vocal cord. The condition results from a degenerative change in the stroma of the cord and occurs in persons who use their voices excessively.

sinoatrial (SA) n. a collection of atypical muscle fibres in the wall of the right atrium where the rhythm of cardiac contraction is usually initiated; therefore also referred to as the pacemaker of the heart.

syphilitic n. a swelling on a bone due to syphilitic periostitis.

n. of Tawara atrioventricular node. Called also TAWARA'S NODE.

teacher's n. singer's node.

Troisier's n., Virchow's n. sentinel node.

nodi ('nohdie) plural of *nodus.*

nodose ('nohdohs) having nodes or projections.

nodosity (noh'dositee) 1. a node. 2. the quality of being nodose.

nodular ('nodyuhlə) marked with, or resembling, nodules.

nodulation (ˌnodyuh'layshən) the formation of or presence of nodules.

nodule ('nodyool) a small boss or node that is solid and can be detected by touch.

Albini's n's grey nodules of the size of small grains, sometimes seen on the free edges of the atrioventricular valves of infants; they are remains of fetal structures.

apple jelly n's minute, yellowish or reddish-brown, translucent nodules, seen on diascopic examination of the lesions of lupus vulgaris.

Aschoff's n's Aschoff's bodies.

Gamna n's brown or yellow pigmented nodules seen in the spleen in certain cases of enlargement, such as Gamna's disease and siderotic splenomegaly.

Jeanselme's n's, juxta-articular n's gummata of tertiary syphilis and of nonvenereal treponemal diseases, located on joint capsules, bursae, or tendon sheaths.

lymphatic n. 1. lymph node. 2. lymph follicle.

milker's n's hard circumscribed nodules on the hands of those who milk cows affected with cowpox.

rheumatic n's small, round or oval, mostly subcutaneous nodules made up chiefly of a mass of Aschoff bodies and seen in rheumatic fever.

Schmorl's n. see SCHMORL'S NODE.

typhus n's minute skin nodules formed by perivascular infiltration of mononuclear cells in typhus.

n. of vermis the part of the vermis of the cerebellum, on the ventral surface, where the inferior medullary velum attaches.

nodulus ('nodyuhləs) pl. *noduli* [L.] nodule.

nodus ('nohdəs) pl. *nodi* [L.] node.

Noludar ('nolyuhdah) trademark for preparations of methyprylon, a sedative.

Nolvadex ('nolvədeks) trademark for a preparation of tamoxifen citrate, an anti-oestrogen used for treatment of advanced breast cancer.

noma ('nohmə) gangrenous processes of the mouth or genitalia. In the mouth (cancrum oris, gangrenous stomatitis, stomatitis gangrenosa, stomatonecrosis, stomatonoma), it begins as a small gingival ulcer and results in gangrenous necrosis of surrounding facial tissues; on the genitalia (cancrum pudendi, noma pudendi, noma vulvae), it affects one labium majus and then the other.

nomenclature (noh'menkləchə) terminology; a classified system of technical names, as of anatomical structures, organisms, etc.

binomial n. the system of designating plants and animals by two latinized words signifying the genus and species.

Nomina Anatomica ('nominə ˌanə'tomikə) the internationally approved official body of anatomic nomenclature; abbreviated NA.

nomogram ('noməˌgram, 'noh-) a graph with several scales arranged so that a ruler laid on the graph intersects the scales at related values of the variables; the values of any two variables can be used to find the values of the others.

nomotopic (ˌnohmoh'topik) occurring at a normal place.

non compos mentis (non 'kompəs 'mentis) [L.] *not of sound mind.*

non-accidental injury (ˌnonaksi'dent'l) injuries inflicted upon children or infants by those looking after them, usually the parents. The injuries are usually physical (beatings, burnings, biting) but the term includes the giving of poisons and dangerous drugs, sexual abuse, starvation and any other form of physical assault. The persons inflicting the injuries are often, but not invariably, psychologically disturbed.

nonan ('nohnan) recurring on the ninth day (every eight days).

nonconductor (ˌnonkən'duktə) a substance that does not readily transmit electricity, light, or heat.

nondisjunction (ˌnondis'jungkshən) failure (a) of two homologous chromosomes to pass to separate cells during the first division of meiosis, or (b) of the two chromatids of a chromosome to pass to separate cells during mitosis or during the second meiotic division. As a result, one daughter cell has two chromosomes or two chromatids, and the other has none.

nonelectrolyte (ˌnoni'lektrəˌliet) a compound which, dissolved in water, does not separate into charged particles and is incapable of conducting an electric current.

non-neuronal (ˌnon·nyuh'rohnəl) pertaining to or composed of nonconducting cells of the nervous system, e.g. neuroglial cells.

nonoxynol (noh'noksiˌnol) a group of compounds of the general composition, $C_{15}H_{24}O(C_2H_4O)_n$, which are assigned a number according to the value of *n*. Nonoxynol 4, 15, and 30 are nonionic surfactants; nonoxynol 9 is a spermaticide.

nonpolar (non'pohlə) not having poles; not exhibiting dipole characteristics.

nonsecretor (ˌnonsi'kreetə) a person with A or B type blood whose body secretions do not contain the particular (A or B) substance.

nonspecific (ˌnonspə'sifik) 1. not due to any single known cause. 2. not directed against a particular agent, but rather having a general effect.

nonsteroidal anti-inflammatory agents (nonˌstiə'royd'l, -ˌster-) a group of drugs having analgesic, antipyretic, and anti-inflammatory activity due to their ability to inhibit the synthesis of prostaglandins. It includes aspirin, phenylbutazone, indomethacin, tolmetin, ibuprofen, and related drugs.

nonunion (non'yooni·ən) failure of the ends of a fractured bone to unite.

nonviable (non'vieəb'l) not capable of living.

Noonan's syndrome ('noonənz) the male phenotype of Turner's syndrome, with short stature, webbed neck, low nuchal hairline, low-set ears, and cubitus valgus; valvular pulmonary stenosis, rather than coarctation of the aorta, is often present.

nor- chemical prefix denoting 1. a compound of normal structure (having an unbranched chain of carbon atoms) that is isomeric with one having a branched chain. 2. a compound whose chain or ring contains one less methylene (CH_2) group than does that of its homologue.

noradrenalin (ˌnor·rə'drenəlin) noradrenaline.

noradrenaline (ˌnor·rə'drenəlin) a catecholamine which is the neurotransmitter of most sympathetic postganglionic neurons and also of certain tracts in the central nervous system. It is also a neurohormone stored in the chromaffin granules of the adrenal medulla and released in response to sympathetic stimulation, primarily in response to hypotension. It produces vasoconstriction, an increase in heart rate, and elevation of blood pressure. It is used as a vasopressor, administered by intravenous infusion, to restore blood pressure in certain cases of acute hypotension and as an adjunct in the treatment of cardiac arrest.

noradrenergic (norˌradrə'nərjik) activated by or secreting noradrenaline.

norethandrolone (ˌnor·rə'thandrəˌlohn) an anabolic steroid that aids in the utilization of protein. May be used to treat severe wasting and in osteoporosis.

norethindrone (nor'rethin,drohn) US name for norethisterone.

norethisterone (,nor·re'thistə,rohn) an anabolic steroid similar in action to progesterone. Used in the treatment of abnormal uterine bleeding, amenorrhoea, and endometriosis and, in combination with an oestrogen, as an oral contraceptive.

Norgesic (nor'jeezik) trademark for a combination preparation of paracetamol with orphenadrine citrate; used for relief of muscle pain.

Norinyl-1 (,no·rinil'wun) trademark for a preparation of norethisterone with mestranol; used as an oral contraceptive.

norm (nawm) a fixed or ideal standard.

norm(o)- word element. [L.] *normal*, *usual*, *conforming to the rule.*

normal ('nawm'l) 1. agreeing with the regular and established type. When said of a solution, it denotes one containing one chemical equivalent of solute per litre of solution; e.g. a 0.5 normal (0.5 N) solution has a concentration of 0.5 Eq/l. The use of standard units (Eq/l) is now preferred. 2. in bacteriology, not immunized or otherwise bacteriologically treated.

normetanephrine (naw,metə'nefreen) metabolite of noradrenaline excreted in the urine and found in certain tissues.

normoblast ('nawmoh,blast) a nucleated precursor cell in the erythrocytic series. adj. **normoblastic.** Four developmental stages are recognized: the PRONORMOBLAST; the *basophilic normoblast* (basophilic erythroblast), in which the cytoplasm is basophilic, the nucleus is large with clumped chromatin, and the nuclei have disappeared; the *polychromatic normoblast* (polychromatic erythroblast), in which the nuclear chromatin shows increased clumping and the cytoplasm begins to acquire haemoglobin and take on an acidophilic tint; and the *orthochromatic normoblast* (acidophilic normoblast; orthochromatic erythroblast), the final stage before nuclear loss, in which the nucleus is small and ultimately becomes a blue-black homogeneous structureless mass.

normoblastosis (,nawmohbla'stohsis) excessive production of normoblasts by the bone marrow.

normocalcaemia (,nawmohkal'seemi·ə) a normal level of calcium in the blood. adj. **normocalcaemic.**

normochromia (,nawmoh'krohmi·ə) normal colour of erythrocytes.

normocyte ('nawmoh,siet) an erythrocyte that is normal in size, shape, and colour.

normoglycaemia (,nawmohglie'seemi·ə) normal glucose content of the blood. adj. **normoglycaemic.**

normokalaemia (,nawmohkə'leemi·ə) a normal level of potassium in the blood. adj. **normokalaemic.**

normospermic (,nawmoh'spərmik) producing spermatozoa normal in number and motility.

normotensive (,nawmoh'tensiv) 1. characterized by normal tension, tone, or pressure, as by normal blood pressure. 2. a person with normal blood pressure.

normothermia (,nawmoh'thərmi·ə) a normal state of temperature. adj. **normothermic.**

normotonia (,nawmoh'tohni·ə) normal tone or tension. adj. **normotonic.**

normovolaemia (,nawmohvo'leemi·ə) normal blood volume.

Norpace ('norpays) trademark for a preparation of disopyramide, an antiarrhythmic.

Norrie's disease ('no·riz) a hereditary disorder consisting of bilateral blindness from retinal malformation, mental handicap, and deafness.

Norton score ('nortən) a pressure sore risk assessment scale devised by Norton, McLaren and Exton Smith and used primarily in the care of elderly patients. It comprises five health state components, each with a four-point descending scale. Maximum points are 20 and the minimum five; a 'score' of 14 and below indicates that the patient is at risk of developing pressure sores and needs 1–2 hourly changes of posture and the use of pressure-relieving aids. The system requires weekly application and whenever a change occurs in the patient's condition and/or circumstances of care (see also PRESSURE SORE).

nortriptyline (naw'tripti,leen) an antidepressant, used as the hydrochloride salt.

nos(o)- word element. [Gr.] *disease.*

noscapine ('noskə,peen) an alkaloid present in opium; used as a nonaddictive antitussive.

nose (nohz) the specialized structure of the face that serves both as the organ of smell and as a means of bringing air into the lungs. Air breathed in through the nose is warmed, filtered, and moistened; that breathed through the mouth is warmed and moistened to a lesser extent.

The nostrils, which form the external entrance of the nose, lead into the two nasal cavities, which are separated from each other by a partition (the nasal septum) formed of cartilage and bone. Three bony ridges project from the outer wall of each nasal cavity and partially divide the cavity into three air passages. At the back of the nose these passages lead into the pharynx. The passages are also connected by openings with the paranasal sinuses. One of the functions of the nose is to drain fluids discharged from the sinuses. The nasal cavities also have a connection with the ears by the pharyngotympanic tubes, and with the region of the eyes by the nasolacrimal ducts.

The interior of the nose is lined with mucous membrane. Most of this membrane is covered with minute hair-like projections called cilia. Moving in waves these cilia sweep out from the nasal passages the nasal mucus, which may contain pollen, dust, and bacteria from the air. The mucous membrane also acts to warm and moisten the inhaled air. High in the interior of each nasal cavity is a small area of mucous membrane that is not covered with cilia. In this pea-sized area are located the endings of the nerves of smell, the olfactory receptors. These receptors sort out odours. Unlike the taste buds of the tongue, which distinguish between only four different tastes (salt, sweet, sour, and bitter), the olfactory receptors can detect innumerable different odours. This ability to smell contributes greatly to what we usually think of as taste, because much of what we consider flavour is really odour. See also SMELL.

DISORDERS OF THE NOSE. The mucous membrane of the nose is subject to inflammation; any such inflammation is called RHINITIS, a term derived from the Greek word *rhinos*, meaning nose. Rhinitis is often caused by an infection, as in the COMMON COLD, or by an allergy, particularly HAY FEVER. In both cases the symptoms are similar, including runny eyes, sneezing, a nasal discharge, and temporary stopping-up of the nasal passages. In such an infection, the nasal mucus is white or yellow in colour.

Nasal polyps may obstruct the nasal passages and limit breathing through the nose. Enlarged adenoids also may interfere with nasal breathing.

Nosebleed may be caused by injury to the nose, or it may be a symptom of various diseases. See also EPISTAXIS.

The nasal septum may grow irregularly or be deflected to one side by an injury. This condition is known as deviated SEPTUM. The surgical procedure to correct deviations of the septum is called a submucous resection (SMR).

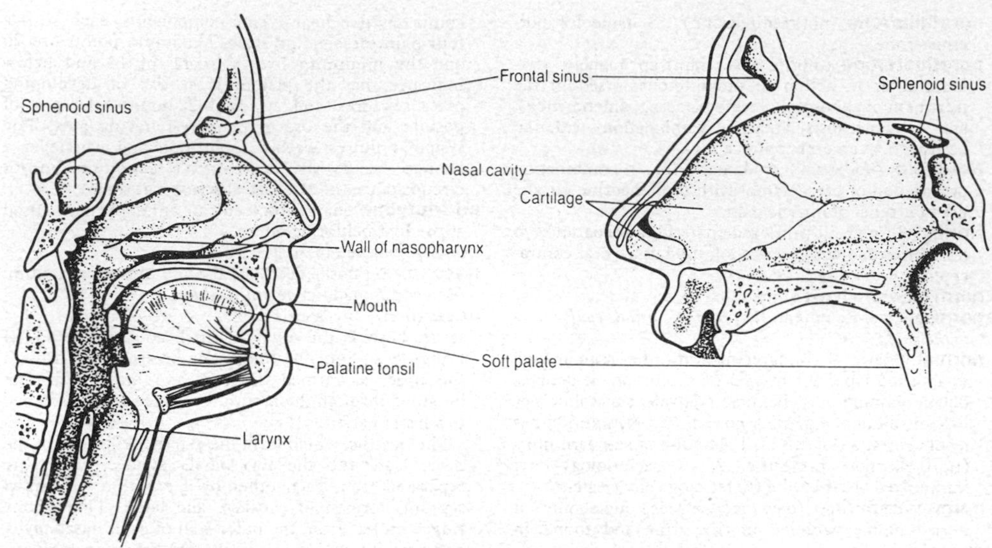

Nose and related structures

SURGERY OF THE NOSE. Nasal surgery is indicated in disorders of the nasal septum, polyps and other growths, and traumatic injury to the structures that interfere with normal nasal breathing. Cosmetic plastic surgery is also done to correct disfigurement that is disturbing to the patient.

Patient Care. Prior to surgery the patient is instructed in the kind of surgery anticipated and is informed of the immediate after-effects of swelling and discoloration. He is told that the residual swelling may last for several weeks and success of the operation cannot be assessed until after that time.

Immediately after surgery the greatest danger is haemorrhage. If the patient swallows repeatedly or spits up blood, excessive bleeding should be suspected. A Teflon splint or intranasal packing is often used to support the nasal structures and prevent the formation of haematoma, another complication that may develop.

Ice compresses may be applied for 24 hours after surgery to reduce swelling and minimize bleeding. The patient is placed in semi-Fowler position during this time.

During convalescence the patient should avoid blowing his nose and picking at crusts. A lubricant may be used to soften the crusts, but no swabs or other objects should be used to clean the nose. A humidifier in the room may help reduce drying and irritation of the mucous membranes during healing.

nosebleed ('nohz,bleed) bleeding from the nose (called also EPISTAXIS).

FIRST AID FOR NOSEBLEED

Have the person sit up and tilt the head forward to avoid aspiration or swallowing of blood.

(1) Grasp nose firmly between the thumb and forefinger and gently squeeze nose closed for 10 to 15 minutes by the clock.

(2) Once bleeding stops, have the person rest quietly for an hour or so, and for the next several hours avoid stooping, lifting, and vigorously blowing the nose.

(3) If bleeding persists, consult a doctor. Blood loss from a nosebleed can be considerable and there is a danger of haemorrhagic shock from uncontrolled nosebleed.

nosocomial (,nosoh'kohmi·əl) pertaining to or originating in a hospital.

n. infections those acquired during hospitalization, usually referred to as hospital-acquired INFECTIONS.

nosogeny (no'sojənee) the development of a disease; pathogenesis.

nosology (no'soləjee) the scientific classification of diseases.

nosoparasite (,nosoh'parə,siet) an organism found in a disease that it is able to modify, but not to produce.

nosophilia (,nosoh'fili·ə) morbid desire to be sick.

nosophobia (,nosoh'fohbi·ə) morbid dread of sickness or of a specific disease.

nosopoietic (,nosohpoy'etik) causing disease.

nosotaxy ('nosoh,taksee) the classification of disease.

nostril ('nostrəl) one of the two apertures (or nares) of the nose.

nostrum ('nostrəm) a quack, patent, or secret remedy.

not(o)- word element. [Gr.] *the back.*

not-self ('not,self) a term denoting antigenic constituents foreign to the organism (self), which are eliminated through humoral or cell-mediated IMMUNITY.

notalgia (noh'talji·ə) pain in the back.

notch (noch) an indentation, especially one on the edge of a bone or other organ.

aortic n., dicrotic n. a small downward deflection in the arterial pulse or pressure contour immediately following the closure of the semilunar valves, sometimes used as a marker for the end of systole or the ejection period.

parotid n. the notch between the ramus of the mandible and the mastoid process of the temporal bones.

tympanic n. Rivinus' incisure.

notencephalocele (,nohten'kefəloh,seel, -'sef-) her-

nial protrusion of brain at the back of the head.
notencephalus (ˌnohten'kefələs, -'sef-) a fetus affected with notencephalocele.
notifiable ('nohtiˌfieəb'l) in relation to disease; those designated diseases, the occurrence of which by law must be reported to health authorities; see notifiable DISEASE.
notochord ('nohtohˌkawd) a cylindrical cord of cells on the dorsal aspect of an embryo, marking its longitudinal axis; the common factor of all chordates. It is the centre of development of the axial skeleton.
noxious ('nokshəs) hurtful; injurious; pernicious.
Np chemical symbol, *neptunium*.
NPRU Nursing Practise Research Unit.
NREM non-rapid eye movements (see under SLEEP).
ns nanosecond.
NSC National Staff Committee.
nsec. nanosecond.
NSPCC (ˌenesˌpeesee'see) National Society for the Prevention of Cruelty to Children.
Nubain ('nyoobayn) trademark for a preparation of nalbuphine hydrochloride; a narcotic analgesic.
nucha ('nyookə) the nape, or back, of the neck. adj. **nuchal**.
nuclear ('nyookli·ə) pertaining to a nucleus.
n. medicine that branch of medicine concerned with the use of radionuclides in the diagnosis and treatment of disease.
nuclear magnetic resonance a phenomenon exhibited by atomic nuclei having a magnetic moment, i.e. those nuclei that behave as if they are tiny bar magnets. In the absence of a magnetic field these magnets are arranged randomly but when a strong magnetic field is applied they align with the field. When disturbed from equilibrium by a radiofrequency pulse their alignment changes but at the termination of the pulse the nuclei return to their position of equilibrium. Return to the equilibrium state induces a signal in a coil wrapped around the sample being studied. These signals can be analysed and used for chemical analysis (NMR spectroscopy) or for imaging (MAGNETIC RESONANCE IMAGING).
nuclease ('nyookliˌayz) any of a group of enzymes that split nucleic acids into nucleotides and other products.
nucleated ('nyookliˌaytid) having a nucleus or nuclei.
nuclei ('nyookli·ie) plural of *nucleus*.
nucleic acids (nyoo'klee·ik, -'klay-) extremely complex, long-chain compounds of high molecular weight that occur naturally in the cells of all living organisms. They form the genetic material of the cell and direct the synthesis of protein within the cell.

Nucleic acids are composed of repeating smaller units, called *nucleotides*, which are made up of a pentose sugar, a nitrogenous base, and a phosphate group. There are two major classes of nucleic acids: DEOXYRIBONUCLEIC ACID (DNA) whose pentose sugar is deoxyribose, and RIBONUCLEIC ACID (RNA) whose pentose sugar is ribose. The major purine and pyrimidine bases in the nucleic acids are adenine (A), guanine (G), and cytosine (C), which occur in both, and thymine (T) in DNA and uracil (U) in RNA.

RNA is present in both the nucleus and the cytoplasm of many cells. Most of the cytoplasmic RNA is associated with ribosomes, which are the site of protein synthesis. RNA molecules perform several functions in the cell, depending on the type of RNA molecule and its specific properties. DNA is a major constituent of chromosomes in the nuclei of all cells. Its chief function is to provide a genetic message that is encoded in the sequence of bases.
nucleocapsid (ˌnyooklioh'kapsid) a unit of viral structure, consisting of a capsid with the enclosed nucleic acid.
nucleofugal (ˌnyookli'ofyuhgəl) moving away from a nucleus.
nucleohistone (ˌnyookliohˈhistohn) the nucleoprotein complex made up of deoxyribonucleic acid (DNA) and histones. It is the principal constituent of chromatin.
nucleoid ('nyookliˌoyd) 1. resembling a nucleus. 2. a nucleus-like body sometimes seen in the centre of an erythrocyte. 3. the genetic material (nucleic acid) of a virus situated in the centre of the virion.
nucleolonema (ˌnyookliˌohlə'neemə) a network of strands formed by organization of a finely granular substance, perhaps containing RNA, in the nucleolus of a cell.
nucleolus (ˌnyookli'ohləs, nyoo'kleeələs) pl. *nucleoli* [L.] a rounded refractile body in the nucleus of most cells, which is the site of synthesis of ribosomal RNA, becoming enlarged during periods of synthesis and smaller during quiescent periods; multiple nucleoli occur in some cells.
nucleon ('nyookliˌon) a particle of an atomic nucleus; a proton or neutron, the total number of which constitutes the mass number of the isotope.
nucleonics (ˌnyookli'oniks) the study of nucleons or of atomic nuclei and their reactions; nuclear physics.
nucleopetal (ˌnyookli'opit'l) moving toward a nucleus.
nucleophile ('nyooklioh,fiel) an electron donor in chemical reactions involving covalent catalysis in which the donated electrons bond other chemical groups (electrophiles). adj. **nucleophilic**.
nucleoplasm ('nyooklioh,plazəm) karyoplasm; the protoplasm of the nucleus of a cell.
nucleoprotein (ˌnyooklioh'prohteen) any of a class of conjugated proteins, consisting of nucleic acids and simple proteins (e.g. a histone).
nucleosidase (ˌnyookli'ohsidayz) an intracellular enzyme that is capable of causing the decomposition of nucleosides.
nucleoside ('nyooklioh,sied) any of a class of compounds produced by hydrolysis of nucleotides, consisting of a sugar (a pentose or a hexose) and a purine or pyrimidine base.
nucleosome ('nyooklioh,sohm) any of the complexes of histone and DNA in eukaryotic cells, seen under the electron microscope as bead-like bodies on a string of DNA.
nucleotidase (ˌnyookli'ohti,dayz) an enzyme that splits nucleotides into nucleosides and phosphoric acid.
nucleotide ('nyooklioh,tied) any of a group of compounds obtained by hydrolysis of nucleic acids, consisting of a purine or pyrimidine base linked to a sugar (ribose or deoxyribose), which in turn is esterified with phosphoric acid.
cyclic n's those in which the phosphate group bonds to two atoms of the sugar forming a ring, as in cyclic AMP and cyclic GMP, which act as intracellular second messengers.
nucleotidyl (ˌnyooklioh'tiedil) a nucleotide residue.
nucleotoxin (ˌnyooklioh'toksin) a toxin from cell nuclei, or one that affects cell nuclei.
nucleus ('nyookli·əs) pl. *nuclei* [L.] 1. cell nucleus; a spheroid body within a cell, contained in a double membrane, the nuclear envelope, and containing the CHROMOSOMES and one or more nucleoli. The contents are collectively referred to as *nucleoplasm*. The chromosomes contain DEOXYRIBONUCLEIC ACID (DNA), which is the genetic material that codes for the structure of all the proteins of the cell. 2. a mass of grey matter in the central nervous system, especially such a mass marking the central termination of a cranial nerve. 3. in organic chemistry, the combina-

tion of atoms forming the central element or basic framework of the molecule of a specific compound or class of compounds. 4. the dense core of an atom; called also *atomic nucleus*. It is made of protons and neutrons held together by the strong nuclear force. Travelling in orbit around the nucleus is a cloud of negatively charged particles called ELECTRONS. The number of protons in the atomic nucleus gives a substance its identity as a particular ELEMENT. adj. **nuclear.**

n. ambiguus the nucleus of origin of motor fibres of the glossopharyngeal, vagus, and accessory nerves in the medulla oblongata.

arcuate nuclei, nuclei arcuati small irregular areas of grey substance on the ventromedial aspect of the pyramid of the medulla oblongata.

atomic n. nucleus (3).

caudate n., n. caudatus an elongated, arched grey mass closely related to the lateral ventricle throughout its entire extent, which, together with the putamen, forms the neostriatum.

cochlear nuclei, dorsal and ventral the nuclei of termination of sensory fibres of the cochlear part of the vestibulocochlear (eighth cranial) nerve, which partly encircle the inferior cerebellar peduncle at the junction of the medulla oblongata and pons.

dentate n., n. dentatus the largest of the deep cerebellar nuclei lying in the white matter of the cerebellum.

fastigial n., n. fastigii the most medial of the deep cerebellar nuclei, near the midline in the roof of the fourth ventricle.

lenticular n., lentiform n. the part of the corpus striatum just lateral to the internal capsule, comprising the putamen and globus pallidus.

motor n. any collection of cells in the central nervous system giving origin to a motor nerve.

n. olivaris, olivary n. 1. a folded band of grey matter enclosing a white core and producing the elevation (olive) on the medulla oblongata. 2. olive (2).

n. of origin any collection of nerve cells giving origin to the fibres, or a part of the fibres, of a peripheral nerve.

paraventricular n., n. paraventricularis a band of cells in the wall of the third ventricle in the supraoptic part of the hypothalamus; many of its cells are neurosecretory in function and project to the neurohypophysis, where they secrete oxytocin (and, to a lesser extent, antidiuretic hormone).

pontine nuclei, nuclei pontis groups of nerve cell bodies in the part of the pyramidal tract within the ventral part of the pons, upon which the fibres of the corticopontine tract synapse, and whose axons in turn cross to the opposite side and form the middle cerebellar peduncle.

n. pulposus, pulpy n. a semifluid mass of fine white elastic fibres forming the centre of an intervertebral disc.

red n. see nucleus ruber (below).

n. ruber an oval mass of grey matter (pink in fresh specimens) in the anterior part of the tegmentum and extending into the posterior part of the hypothalamus; it receives fibres from the cerebellum. Called also *red nucleus*.

sensory n. the nucleus of termination of the afferent (sensory) fibres of a peripheral nerve.

supraoptic n., n. supraopticus one just above the lateral part of the optic chiasm; many of its cells are neurosecretory in function and project to the neurohypophysis, where they secrete antidiuretic hormone (ADH) and, to a lesser extent, oxytocin; other cells are osmoreceptors that stimulate ADH release in response to increased osmotic pressure.

tegmental nuclei several nuclear masses of the reticular formations of the pons and midbrain, especially of the latter, where they are in close approximation to the superior cerebellar peduncles.

thoracic n., n. thoracicus a column of cells in the posterior grey column of the spinal cord, extending from the 7th or 8th cervical segments to the 2nd or 3rd lumbar level.

vestibular nuclei, nuclei vestibularis the four cellular masses (superior, lateral, medial, and inferior) in the floor of the fourth ventricle, in which the branches of the eighth cranial (vestibulocochlear) nerve terminate.

nuclide ('nyooklied) a species of atom characterized by the charge, mass, number, and quantum state of its nucleus, and capable of existing for a measurable lifetime (usually more than 10^{-10} s).

Nuelin ('nyooəlin) trademark for preparations of theophylline, a bronchodilator.

null hypothesis (nul hie'pothisis) an epidemiological term meaning that the results observed in an experiment do not differ from those which could have occurred by chance.

nullipara (nu'lipə·rə) a woman who has not produced a viable offspring; PARA 0. adj. **nulliparous.**

nulliparity (,nuli'parətee) the state of being a nullipara.

number ('numbə) a symbol, as a figure or word, expressive of a certain value or a specified quantity determined by count.

atomic n. a number expressive of the number of protons in an atomic nucleus, or the positive charge of the nucleus expressed in terms of the electronic charge; symbol A.

Avogadro's n. the number of particles in one mole of a substance; the value assigned to the number is 6.023×10^{23}.

mass n. the number expressive of the mass of a nucleus, being the total number of nucleons—protons and neutrons—in the nucleus of an atom or nuclide.

numbness ('numnəs) a lack or diminution of sensation in a part.

numerator ('nyoomərayta) the upper part of a fraction of a rate or ratio. See also DENOMINATOR.

nummular ('numyuhlə) 1. coin-sized and coin-shaped. 2. made up of round, flat discs. 3. arranged like a stack of coins.

nunnation (nu'nayshən) the too frequent use of *n* sounds.

NUPE ('nyoopee) National Union of Public Employees.

nurse (nərs) 1. a person who is qualified in the art and science of nursing and meets certain prescribed standards of education and clinical competence (see also NURSING PRACTICE). 2. to provide services that are essential to or helpful in the promotion, maintenance, and restoration of health and well-being. 3. to nourish at the breast (see also BREAST FEEDING).

enrolled n. a nurse who has undertaken a 2-year apprenticeship in nurse training (in Scotland 18 months) meant to provide a practical nurse who works under the supervision of the registered nurse. An enrolled nurse may undertake further training to become a registered nurse.

registered n. in the UK, one whose name is on the Register held by the United Kingdom Central Council for Nurses, Midwives and Health Visitors (UKCC).

wet n. a woman who breast-feeds the infant of another.

nursing ('nərsing) the profession of performing the functions of a NURSE.

n. audit a systematic procedure for assessing the quality of nursing care rendered to a specific patient population. The nursing audit developed partly in response to public demand for accountability for the kind of health care being provided, and partly as the result of a growing recognition among nurses of the need for professional self-regulation.

As in any type of audit, the nursing audit involves a thorough and systematic examination of patient records and other sources of information for the purpose of acquiring specific and relevant data. The observable data related to nursing activities are then applied to previously established criteria stated in terms of patient-centred outcomes. Deficiencies in patient care can thus be identified by comparing the actual nursing practice and the effects of the NURSING PROCESS to the established criteria. If deficiencies are identified, appropriate correction can then be made. This may involve a change in staffing patterns, in service education programmes for members of the nursing staff, patient education programmes, a change in available resources (both human and material), and a host of other actions designed to cope with the specific problems identified through the nursing audit.

The nursing audit provides a means of evaluating both the nursing process and the changes in the patient's health status that are a result of the nursing process. Because the implementation of an audit is greatly facilitated by the development of a database, the identification of major problems the patient is experiencing, the recording of a plan of action, and the maintenance of progress notes to determine whether the plan of action is effectively achieving desired outcomes, it is clear that a PROBLEM-ORIENTED RECORD is essential to the assessment and improvement of patient care through nursing audits. See also EVALUATION and MONITOR.

n. history a written record providing data for assessing the nursing care needs of a patient.

n. models a conceptual framework of nursing practice based on knowledge, ideas and beliefs. A model of nursing clarifies the meaning of nursing, provides criteria for policy, gives direction to team nursing thereby obviating conflicts in approach and giving the framework for continuity of care. It identifies the nurse's role, highlights areas of practice where research is needed and can be a basis for the nursing curriculum.

Among current nursing models which now supersede the biomedical model are: (1) a Developmental Model for Nursing by Peplau (USA) 1952; (2) the Adaptation Model described by Roy (USA), developed in the 1960s; (3) the Interaction Model for Nursing proposed by King (USA) in 1971; (4) the Health Care Systems Model by Neuman (USA) 1972; (5) the Self Care Model developed by Orem (USA) 1980—a popular model in American nursing; (6) the Activities of Living Model developed by Roper, Logan and Tierney (UK) 1980 from Virginia Henderson's authoritative definition of nursing in 1966. This model is now widely used by British nurses.

Models of nursing have common components and some are specific to certain groups of patients. Orem's Self Care Model would be unsuitable for the unconscious or totally dependent patient, for example. Models of nursing place the patient at the centre of a democratically agreed plan of adaptation to illness or rehabilitation and education. The structural framework is provided by the stages of the nursing process and the model of care is the practical ideal, e.g. building an image or a model of a redevelopment area would serve to focus an architect's mind on the site, its existing characteristics and potential, giving all the participants something tangible to work towards. In terms of nursing, the model is imaginary and intellectual, the nurse's mental tool to enable the patient to fulfil his potential.

n. practice the performance or compensation of any act in the observation, care, and counsel of the ill, injured, or infirm, or in the maintenance of health or prevention of illness of others, or in the supervision and teaching of other personnel, or in the administration of medications and treatments as prescribed by a doctor or dentist, requiring substantial specialized judgement and skill and based on knowledge and application of the principles of biological, physical, and social sciences.

In the United Kingdom nursing practice is governed first by primary legislation, that is the 1979 Nurses, Midwives and Health Visitors' Act, and then by Rules approved by Parliament. Nurses on parts 1, 3, 5 or 8 of the United Kingdom Central Council (UKCC) Register must demonstrate competencies as laid down in the 1983 Nurses, Midwives and Health Visitors' Rules. There are: (1) advise on the promotion of health and the prevention of illness; (2) recognize situations that may be detrimental to the health and well-being of the individual; (3) carry out those activities involved when conducting the comprehensive assessment of a person's nursing requirements; (4) recognize the significance of the observations made and use these to develop an initial nursing assessment; (5) devise a plan of nursing care based on the assessment with the cooperation of the patient, to the extent that this is possible, taking into account the medical prescription; (6) implement the planned programme of nursing care and, where appropriate teach and coordinate other members of the caring team who may be responsible for implementing specific aspects of the nursing care; (7) review the effectiveness of the nursing care provided and, where appropriate, initiate any action that may be required; (8) work in a team with other nurses and with medical and paramedical staff and social workers; (9) undertake the management of the care of a group of patients over a period of time and organize the appropriate support services related to the care of the particular type of patient with whom she is likely to come in contact when registered in that part of the Register for which the student intends to qualify.

For nurses on Parts 2, 4, 6 or 7 of the Register (enrolled nurses) the competencies are to: (1) assist in carrying out comprehensive observation of the patient and help in assessing the patient's care requirements; (2) develop skills to enable the nurse to assist in the implementation of nursing care under the direction of a person registered in Part 1, 3, 5 or 8 of the Register; (3) accept delegated nursing tasks; (4) assist in reviewing the effectiveness of the care provided; (5) work in a team with other nurses and with medical and paramedical staff and social workers; related to the care of the particular type of patients with whom she is likely to come into contact when registered in that Part of the Register for which the student intends to qualify.

In addition, nursing practice is expected to conform to the UKCC Code of Professional Conduct.

n. process a systematic approach to nursing care derived from many occupational groups. The system itself is not specific to nursing. It has been used as a framework for nursing care by American nurses and subsequently its principles have been adapted to the UK's culture and health care system by British nurses. It is the vehicle for a NURSING MODEL.

It is an organized approach to the identification of a patient's nursing care problems and the utilization of nursing actions that effectively alleviate, minimize, or prevent the specific problems being presented or likely to develop. The nursing process begins with a search for data on which to base a nursing diagnosis and is completed only after the process has been evaluated for effectiveness. It has been described as the essence of nursing.

There are certain assumptions that are basic to an understanding of the goals of the nursing process, and upon which the acceptance and successful employment of the process will depend. First, it is assumed that nurses recognize each patient as an individual with worth, dignity, and basic human needs. Each person has a right to service of high quality regardless of his socioeconomic status, cultural background, and religious beliefs.

The second assumption is that the patient or client and his family prefer a client-centred approach that actively seeks their input and respects their feelings and needs. Such an approach encourages them to enter into a partnership with members of the health care professions. It is also assumed that the focus of care will be on maintenance of health and prevention of disease.

Another assumption is that those nurses who engage in the nursing process will have current knowledge in their particular discipline and in such related fields as the physical and behavioural sciences. This implies, of course, continued informal study and formal education.

COMPONENTS OF THE PROCESS. Although the nursing process does follow a logical and systematic pattern, it also has a cyclical nature which sometimes demands that two or more components may be operating simultaneously. The components are not separate steps that must always follow a preordained sequence; there often is movement between and among the components.

The four major components of the nursing process are generally agreed to be: (1) assessment, (2) planning, (3) implementation, and (4) evaluation.

Assessment. The assessment phase of the process begins with data gathering and concludes with identification of client/patient problems. Sources of data other than physical examination include a nursing history, observation of and interviewing the patient and his family, reviewing the patient's medical records, and communication with other members of the health care team.

With the accumulated data at hand the nurse then organizes the information, analysing it, finding relationships and patterns, and drawing inferences about the nature of the client's/patient's problems. While she is formulating inferences or conclusions about the client's problems and needs, she provides him with an opportunity to present his point of view in order to confirm the inferences drawn from the data. Throughout the nursing process it is essential that inferences be validated; otherwise much time and effort can be wasted in planning and implementing nursing activities which are of no use because they are not central to the client's real problems. If there is confirmation of the conclusions drawn from the data, the nursing problem is identified. This provides the basis for formulation of a plan of care and should be shared with other nurses as well as with other members of the interdisciplinary health care team.

Planning. If no problems have been found during the assessment phase, the nurse and client sit down together to discuss plans for maintenance of wellbeing. It is the client's responsibility to implement the plan and to return for periodic assessments and identification of either new problems or the potential for them.

When problems are present and have been identified, priorities are set and specific actions are planned to meet the problems having the highest priorities. The nursing care plan should include all pertinent information about the client, the ordering of his problems, and expected outcomes of the prescribed nursing orders. The plan is shared with others who are appropriately concerned with the care of the client and the resolution of his problems.

The nursing care plan is not an inflexible and unchanging prescription for action. It is revised as often as necessary according to the reordering of priorities as indicated by the status of the patient.

Implementation. Nursing actions which implement the nursing care plan should include all aspects of patient care for which the nurse is prepared and willing to accept responsibility. In some instances implementation may include delegated medical therapy, and the implementation most certainly cannot ignore the nurse's attitude toward unplanned immediate intervention should the patient's condition warrant prompt and decisive action on the part of the nurse.

During implementation the nursing care plan is tested for effectiveness and accuracy. Data gathering continues and plans may change on the basis of new information obtained.

The implementation phase concludes with the recording of the activities performed and the response of the patient.

Evaluation. The first three major components of the nursing process are all client-centred and so, too, must the phase of evaluation be concerned with the client's judgement about resolution of the identified problems. EVALUATION is conducted for the purpose of determining the effectiveness of the process in light of accepted standards, and making decisions about whether the nursing actions taken should be employed in the same way in the future.

By accepting responsibility for evaluation of the process, the nurse demonstrates a professional attitude toward her clients and her own actions. She shows a willingness to be held accountable for what she does and to seek ways in which she can assure her clients of the optimum care that can be reasonably expected.

Criteria by which the nursing process can be measured include the following: (1) The collection of data about the health status of the client/patient is systematic and continuous. The data are accessible, communicated, and recorded. (2) Identification of nursing problems or potential problems is based on the data gathered in formulating a nursing history. (3) The nursing care plan includes goals derived from the identification of nursing problems in order of priority. (4) The nursing care plan includes the nursing measures needed to achieve goals derived from the nursing problems. (5) Nursing actions provide for client/patient participation in health promotion, maintenance, and restoration. (6) Nursing actions help the client/patient to realize his health potential. (7) The client/patient's progress or lack of progress in achieving the goals is reassessed continuously by the nurse and the client/patient. The nursing care plan is revised, priorities reordered and new goals set.

n. prognosis see under PROGNOSIS.

theories of n. proposed explanations of the way in which nursing achieves its aims. They require a definition of the nurse's perception of the patient and his needs, the nurse's own role and the context in which nursing care is being performed. The understanding of the relationship of these variables enables nursing care to be planned in such a way that the outcome may be predicted and set goals achieved.

Well known theories of nursing are those described by Henderson, Roper, Orem, Roy and others. See nursing models (above).

nutation (nyoo'tayshən) the act of nodding, especially involuntary nodding.

nutrient ('nyootri·ənt) 1. nourishing; aiding nutrition. 2. a nourishing substance, food, or component of food.

nutriment ('nyootrimənt) nourishment; nutritious material; food.

nutrition (nyoo'trishən) 1. the sum of the processes involved in taking in nutriments and assimilating and utilizing them. 2. nutriment. adj. **nutritional**. It includes all the processes by which the body uses food for energy, maintenance, and growth. Nutrition is particularly concerned with those properties of food that build sound bodies and promote health. Good nutrition means a balanced diet containing adequate amounts of the essential nutritional elements that the body must have to function normally.

THE BALANCED DIET. The essential ingredients of a balanced diet are proteins, vitamins, minerals, fats, and carbohydrates. The body can manufacture sugars from fats, and fats from sugars and proteins, depending on the need. But it cannot manufacture proteins from sugars and fats.

The most important constituents of proteins are the AMINO ACIDS. These complex organic compounds of nitrogen play a vital role in nutrition. The best sources of complete proteins—that is, proteins containing all the essential amino acids—are meat, fish, eggs, and dairy products. The amount of protein that a person actually needs, however, is much smaller than many people suppose.

Vitamins are special substances that are present, in varying amounts, in all food. Their absence from the diet can cause such diseases as beriberi (lack of vitamin B_1, or thiamine), pellagra (lack of the B vitamin niacin) and scurvy (lack of vitamin C, or ascorbic acid). See also VITAMINS.

The principal minerals needed by the body are calcium and phosphorus (to build bones and teeth) and iron (to assure a sufficient supply of erythrocytes). All three are plentiful in eggs, dairy products, lean meat, and enriched flour. Some sources of calcium are cheese, molasses, turnip tops, and greens; of phosphorus, cereals, meat, and fish; of iron, kidney beans, liver and other meats, spinach, and whole-wheat bread.

The trace of iodine needed to prevent goitre is easily provided by iodized table salt. The minute amounts of magnesium, manganese, and copper that are necessary are found in any balanced diet.

For quick energy, the body should have sugars (carbohydrates) and starches (which the body converts into sugars). Fats and proteins can also provide energy and can be stored for future use, whereas complex sugars and starches cannot. Since the body can manufacture most of its own fat, fats are of secondary importance in a balanced diet.

AGE AND NUTRITION. Because the body's needs change as it grows and develops, good nutrition for a child or teenager is not the same as good nutrition for a mature or older person. Growing bodies need plentiful supplies of calcium, phosphorus, and other minerals to build strong bones and teeth, and abundant protein for firm muscles, energy, and stamina.

For children especially, breakfast is the key meal of the day. Expending as much energy as they do, children need a hearty morning meal, rich in vitamin C, calcium, iron, and thiamine, in order to offset the physical and mental fatigue that they usually feel before lunch time.

SPACING AND SERVING OF MEALS. Nutritionists generally consider breakfast the most important meal of the day because it ends the body's overnight fast and supplies the 'fuel' for a person to get under way at top efficiency. If possible, meals should be spaced at regular intervals. They should never be rushed. This is especially true of the main daily meal.

DIETARY RECOMMENDATIONS. The high incidence of diseases which are prevalent in western society such as coronary heart disease, cerebrovascular disease, hypertension, cancer, diabetes and dental decay, is thought to be linked to the diet consumed by the population. Adoption of a diet which would contain less sugar, fat, salt and alcohol, and more fibre, cereals and fresh fruit and vegetables is recommended. However, it is difficult to influence people to eat less of the foods they prefer in favour of foods which may initially be less acceptable to them. Although some countries, including N. America, have stated dietary goals for the nation they remain a controversial issue. In the UK it is hoped to influence the public to alter eating habits in favour of a healthier diet by promoting health education. Legislation in the UK at present relates to topics such as correct labelling of manufactured goods, and to hygiene in food production industries. Scientific groups and departments such as the Foods Standards Committee, the Medical Research Council, and the Department of Scientific and Industrial Research act as advisors to the Government about issues related to the national diet. More detailed information about dietary recommendations can be found in publications by the National Advisory Committee on Nutrition Education, and the Department of Health.

DIETARY SODIUM RESTRICTION. Dietary sodium is mainly taken in the form of salt which contains 40 per cent sodium. The daily dietary salt intake in the UK is approximately 7 to 10 g per person. Such a salt intake exceeds the body requirements and the effects of an excessive salt intake are widely debated. In countries such as Japan where the people are known to consume very large amounts of salt the incidence of hypertension is correspondingly great, and salt intake was thought to be instrumental in the development of hypertension. However a mechanism whereby salt could lead to the development of essential hypertension has not been established, and there is some support for the argument that it may be the chloride content of salt that has an effect upon blood pressure.

Conversely salt restriction has been found to have a beneficial effect upon people with hypertension and it would therefore be reasonable to aim to reduce the salt intake of the population until further information is available. Most of the salt consumed is added to food during manufacture, only about 30 per cent being added during cooking or on served food. Avoidance of obviously salty foods and a reduction of the amount of salt added to cooking and cooked food would cause an appreciable reduction in salt consumption. For hypertensive people a therapeutic low-salt diet may be indicated which could reduce salt intake to a specified amount, usually approximately 2.5 g of salt per day.

n. disease one that is due to the continued absence of a necessary food factor.

enteral n. the provision of nutrients in fluid form to the alimentary tract by mouth, nasogastric tube, or via an opening into the tract such as through a gastrostomy.

parenteral n. a technique for meeting a patient's nutritional needs by means of intravenous feedings; sometimes called *hyperalimentation*, even though it does not provide excessive amounts of nutrients.

Nutrition by intravenous feeding may be total parenteral nutrition (TPN) or supplemental. TPN provides all of the carbohydrates, proteins, fats, water, electrolytes, vitamins. and minerals needed for the building of tissue, expenditure of energy, and other physiological activities.

The procedure originated as an emergency lifesaving technique following surgery for severe and massive trauma of the gastrointestinal tract. It has become a relatively common means of providing bowel rest and nutrition in a variety of conditions in spite of inherent risks. Although primarily employed as a short-term temporary measure until either surgical or medical treatment corrects the gastrointestinal dysfunction, it has also been used with some success as a long-term therapy for selected patients on an outpatient basis.

Parenteral nutrition may be employed in the following conditions: malnutrition from such acute and chronic inflammatory bowel diseases as regional ileitis (CROHN'S DISEASE) and ULCERATIVE COLITIS, partial or total obstruction of the gastrointestinal tract that cannot be relieved immediately by surgery, congenital anomalies in the newborn prior to surgery, massive burns that produce critical protein loss, and other disorders in which malnutrition is a threat to the life of the patient who cannot receive nutrients via the digestive tract.

The nutrient mix is tailored to the individual needs and tolerance of the patient. There is not complete agreement among the experts as to the ideal mix, especially of amino acids. The nutrient solutions usually are prepared in clean-air rooms in the pharmacy of a hospital under aseptic conditions to avoid contamination.

Administration of the nutrients is accomplished via a CENTRAL VENOUS CATHETER, usually inserted in the superior vena cava. The route of administration, constant rate of flow required, and potential patient sensitivity to the elements administered, all contribute to the potential complications of parenteral nutrition.

Of the many complications that may develop, the most common are febrile reactions arising from patient intolerance to the required rate of flow, reactions due to individual sensitivity to some of the elements in the nutrient mix, and infection from contamination of either the site of insertion of the catheter or the apparatus used to administer the nutrients. Other complications that may develop include phlebitis and thrombosis of the vena cava, electrolyte imbalance, hyperglycaemia, cardiac overload, dehydration, metabolic acidosis, and mechanical trauma to the heart.

PATIENT CARE. The patient receiving parenteral nutrition requires nearly continuous monitoring and assessment of his status by skilled members of the health care team who are fully aware of the hazards of the procedure. The doctor, nurse, and pharmacist are essential members of the team, and must work cooperatively to meet the needs of the patient and avoid complications. During the first 24 hours the patient is watched closely for signs of pneumothorax, haemothorax, internal bleeding, and cardiac complications.

Principles of strict aseptic technique must be followed in the changing of dressings and in handling the nutrient solution and the administration equipment. The catheter through which the nutrients are administered should not be used for administration of medication, blood, or any other substance that may induce clotting in the vein.

Vital signs are usually checked every 4 hours and any indication of a developing infection is attended to immediately. Intake and output are measured and the patient is weighed daily. The urine is usually checked 6-hourly throughout the day for sugar and acetone as a means of assessing the body's ability to utilize available carbohydrate. Daily blood sugar tests may be done for the same reason. See also HYPERGLYCAEMIC HYPEROSMOLAR NONKETOTIC COMA.

The rate of flow is checked regularly every half-hour to assure that the rate is constant. If, for any reason, the rate falls behind, no effort is made to increase the rate to catch up. If the nutrient mix is used up before a fresh supply is available, 5 per cent dextrose may be given to keep the catheter and vein patent. Any unused nutrient remaining after a 24-hour period is discarded to reduce the danger of contamination.

nutritious (nyoo'trishəs) affording nourishment.

nutritive ('nyootritiv) pertaining to or promoting nutrition.

nutriture ('nyootrichə) the status of the body in relation to nutrition.

nux (nuks) a nut.

n. vomica the seed of an East Indian tree, from which strychnine is derived.

nyct(o)- word element. [Gr.] *night, darkness*.

nyctalgia (nik'talji·ə) pain that occurs only in sleep.

nyctalope ('niktə,lohp) a person affected with nyctalopia.

nyctalopia (,niktə'lohpi·ə) see NIGHT BLINDNESS.

nycterine ('niktə,rien) occurring at night.

nyctohemeral (,niktoh'hemə·rəl) pertaining to both day and night.

nyctophilia (,niktoh'fili·ə) a preference for darkness or for night.

nyctophobia (,niktoh'fohbi·ə) morbid dread of darkness.

nyctophonia (,niktoh'fohni·ə) loss of voice during the day but not at night.

nyctotyphlosis (,niktohti'flohsis) called also NIGHT BLINDNESS, or nyctalopia.

nycturia (nik'tyooə·ri·ə) incontinence of urine at night. Nocturnal enuresis.

nymph (nimf) a developmental stage in certain arthropods (e.g. ticks) between the larval form and the adult, and resembling the latter in appearance.

nymph(o)- word element. [Gr.] *nymphae* (labia minora).

nympha ('nimfə) pl. *nymphae* [L.] labium minus.

nymphectomy (nim'fektəmee) excision of the nymphae (labia minora).

nymphitis (nim'fietis) inflammation of the nymphae (labia minora).

nymphomania (,nimfə'mayni·ə) a contentious diagnostic category once widely used to describe women driven by excessive sexual desire. The term has largely fallen into disuse and this may reflect the fact that it incorporated a moral rather than a medical judgement insofar as it was used to describe sexually active women whose sexual behaviour happened to exceed clinicians' conceptions of what was right and proper. Many of today's 'liberated women' would have been described as nymphomaniacs in the repressive climate of Edwardian times which suppressed women's sexuality by the illicit use of medical language.

nymphoncus (nim'fongkəs) swelling or enlargement of the nymphae (labia minora).

nymphotomy (nim'fotəmee) surgical incision of the nymphae (labia minora) or clitoris.

nystagmiform (ni'stagmi,fawm) resembling nystagmus.

nystagmograph (ni'stagmoh,grahf, -,graf) an instrument for recording the movements of the eyeball in nystagmus.

nystagmoid (ni'stagmoyd) resembling nystagmus.

nystagmus (ni'stagməs) involuntary, rapid, rhythmic movement (horizontal, vertical, rotatory, or mixed, i.e., of two types) of the eyeball. adj. **nystagmic**.

aural n. labyrinthine nystagmus.

Cheyne's n. a peculiar rhythmical eye movement resembling Cheyne–Stokes respiration in rhythm.

dissociated n. that in which the movements in the two eyes are dissimilar.

end-position n. that occurring only at extremes of gaze.

fixation n. that occurring only on gazing fixedly at an object.

gaze n. nystagmus made apparent by looking to the right or to the left.

labyrinthine n. vestibular nystagmus due to labyrinthine disturbance.

latent n. that occurring only when one eye is covered.

lateral n. involuntary horizontal movement of the eyes.

optokinetic n. nystagmus induced by looking at objects moving across the field of vision.

pendular n. that which consists of to-and-fro movements of equal velocity.

positional n. that which occurs, or is altered in form or intensity, on assumption of certain positions of the head.

retraction n., n. retractorius a spasmodic backward movement of the eyeball occurring on attempts to move the eye; a sign of midbrain disease.

rotatory n. involuntary rotation of the eyes about the visual axis.

spontaneous n. that occurring without specific stimulation of the vestibular system.

vertical n. involuntary up-and-down movement of the eyes.

vestibular n. nystagmus due to disturbance of the labyrinth or of the vestibular nuclei; the movements are usually jerky.

Nystan ('niestan) trademark for a preparation of nystatin, an antifungal agent.

nystatin (nie'statin, ni'-) an antifungal antibiotic produced by *Streptomyces noursei*; used in treatment of infections due to *Candida albicans*.

nystaxis (ni'staksis) nystagmus.

nyxis ('niksis) puncture, or paracentesis.

O

O chemical symbol, *oxygen;* [L.] *oculus* (eye); [L.] *octarius* (pint); opening.

Ω symbol for *ohm*.

o- symbol, *ortho-*.

oasthouse urine disease ('ohst·hows) Smith-Strang disease.

ob- word element. [L.] *against, in front of, toward.*

obcaecation (ˌobsi'kayshən) incomplete blindness.

obesity (oh'beesətee) excessive accumulation of fat in the body; increase in weight beyond that considered desirable with regard to age, height, and bone structure. adj. **obese**.

One must take into account what is meant by 'excessive' body fat. An overweight person is not obese, even though his body weight is in excess of the normal range according to a weight chart, if he does not have excess body fat. A large body frame and dense musculature, as in an athlete, can contribute to a person's weighing more than the weight indicated as optimal on a weight chart. In an effort to establish more precise guidelines, authorities suggest the following standards: *Overweight* persons weigh 10 per cent more than their optimum weight; *obese* persons weigh 15 per cent more, and *grossly obese* persons 20 per cent or more above their optimum weight.

A popular method by which obesity can be determined is the so-called *pinch test*. This is a measurement of subcutaneous fat reserves. The 'pinch' can be done in various places on the body but the most common site is the upper arm over the triceps muscle. A fold of skin and subcutaneous fat is lifted free, between the thumb and forefinger, from the underlying structures. An accurate measurement can be obtained by using a pair of calipers. Since the skin fold is a double thickness, one-half the total measurement is the thickness of the layer of excess fat. In general, a fold that measures ½ to 1 inch (¼ to ½ actual thickness) is considered normal. A fold significantly greater than one inch indicates excessive body fat.

EFFECTS OF OBESITY. Being obese can affect physical and mental health. Too many extra pounds are a strain on the body, and can eventually shorten the span of life. Obesity is also unattractive, and this may create psychological problems.

The obese person is inviting a number of unnecessary complications. Some of these are an overworked heart; shortness of breath; a tendency to arteriosclerosis and high blood pressure or to diabetes mellitus; chronic back and joint pains from increased strain on joints and ligaments; a greater tendency to contract infectious diseases; and a reduced ability to exercise or enjoy sports. Carefully compiled statistics show that mortality from circulatory conditions is about 45 per cent higher in grossly obese men than in those whose weight is reasonably close to normal, and death from such conditions is apt to occur sooner. Because of this increased risk, life insurance companies are reluctant to grant insurance to people who are obese.

Psychologically, too, the obese person is at a disadvantage. The show of good cheer sometimes associated with obese people usually masks unconscious—or even conscious—unhappiness and disappointment. Obesity can cause personality problems; in turn, emotional difficulties such as those caused by persistent loneliness, tension, or boredom sometimes find an outlet in compulsive overeating.

CAUSES. Most cases of obesity are due to an excessive intake of calories in proportion to expenditure of calories. Cultural factors, such as the abundance in Western cultures of purified high-calorific foods (fast foods) of low nutrient value, are among the most important contributing factors in the incidence of moderate overweight. Extreme obesity seems to be familial; in families in which both parents are obese, the children are also very likely to be overweight. Overweight children usually become overweight adults.

Endocrine and metabolic disturbances have been used by many persons as an excuse for their obesity, but these causes are relatively rare among the obese and most are probably secondary to the obesity.

Lack of exercise frequently is associated with obesity. Changes in eating patterns (excessive weight gain or loss) can be a symptom of major depression. In many very obese persons the major calorie intake occurs during the evening meal or 'bedtime snack'. Early life patterns of eating and emotional responses to food are considered a major factor in obesity. Especially significant are the responses learned from the mother who rewarded good behaviour with food, particularly food that is high in calories.

MANAGEMENT. Among the techniques currently in use in the management of obesity are: hospitalization with fasting, self-help groups, behavioural techniques, and drugs to suppress the appetite or increase metabolism, or both, and surgical intervention (as a last resort).

Hospitalization with fasting usually is confined to select groups of patients with massive obesity that is resistant to other weight reducing measures and is not caused by endocrine dysfunction. It is essential that the clients be carefully supervised in a follow-up management programme because many have a tendency to regain the lost pounds when they return home.

Surgical intervention for the management of obesity should be reserved for persons who are grossly obese and at risk for life-threatening consequences of their obesity. These surgical procedures carry grave risks. Their purpose is either to manipulate the absorption of food elements from the small intestine or to modify the intake of food. Candidates for surgical intervention should meet the following criteria: (1) twice the ideal body weight or 100 pounds overweight; (2) unable to lose weight or maintain weight losses after having faithfully tried other methods of management of the problem, and (3) willing to comply with a strict postoperative regimen and programme of lifetime physiological and psychological monitoring. Very few meet these criteria.

One form of surgical intervention is INTESTINAL BYPASS, or jejunoileal shunt, which is a procedure in which a length of intestine is bypassed by anastomosing the proximal end of the jejunum to the distal end of the ileum. This procedure is not without danger; the operative mortality rate is about 4 per cent. Those patients who survive the immediate postoperative period are likely to suffer from persistent and prolonged diarrhoea and electrolyte imbalance, postoperative wound infection and dehiscence, thrombophlebitis, hepatitis and liver failure, malnutrition, and urinary calculi.

A less drastic surgical procedure for control of obesity is GASTRIC PARTITIONING or stapling. In this procedure, a small gastric pouch is created by applying two rows of staples across the stomach, markedly diminishing its capacity to approximately 50 ml. Over time the stomach wall will stretch so that it can hold 120 to 180 ml. The expected outcome of gastric partitioning is assurance of satisfaction after the intake of a very small amount of food.

Patients who are treated by surgical intervention for control of obesity need lifetime follow-up to monitor their physiological and psychological health status and to forestall serious complications attending this kind of therapy.

Self-help groups are considered by many health professionals to offer some of the best available techniques in weight reduction. The combination of low calorie diet and increased exercise, in conjunction with peer pressure and group interest, seems to be the most effective in bringing about gradual and permanent weight loss. Among the better known and more successful groups are Weight Watchers and Slimming Magazine Clubs.

The emphasis in *behaviour modification programmes* is on understanding and changing behaviour, stimuli, and REINFORCEMENT. The goal of the programme is to alter gradually the maladaptive eating patterns and to increase the expenditures of calories through exercise. Results of studies have shown these techniques to be consistently better than other more conventional plans for medical management of obesity.

Drugs that inhibit appetite and increase metabolic rate have come under criticism in recent years. There is an increasing awareness of the dangers of drug dependency and abuse, and the deleterious side-effects of some of these drugs.

adult-onset o. that beginning in adulthood and characterized by increase in size (hypertrophy) of adipose cells with no increase in number.

lifelong o. that beginning in childhood and characterized by an increase both in number (hyperplasia) and in size (hypertrophy) of adipose cells.

obex ('ohbeks) the ependyma-lined junction of the teniae of the fourth ventricle of the brain at the inferior angle.

objective (əb'jektiv) 1. perceptible by the external senses. 2. a result for whose achievement an effort has been made. 3. the lens or system of lenses of a microscope nearest the object that is being examined.

achromatic o. one in which the chromatic aberration is corrected for two colours and the spherical aberration for one colour.

apochromatic o. one in which chromatic aberration is corrected for three colours and the spherical aberration for two colours.

immersion o. one designed to have its tip and the coverglass over the specimen connected by a liquid instead of air.

obligate ('obligət, -gayt) not facultative; necessary; compulsory; pertaining to or characterized by the ability to survive only in a particular environment or to assume only a particular role, as an obligate anaerobe.

oblique (ə'bleek) slanting; inclined.

obliquity (ə'blikwitee) the state of being oblique or slanting.

obliterate (ə'blitərayt) to remove completely; to obscure.

oblongata (oblong'gahtə) medulla oblongata (see also BRAIN). adj. **oblongatal**.

observational study (obzər'vayshən'l) an epidemiological study of events without the intervention of the investigator.

observer variation (əb'zərvə) an epidemiological term meaning variations over time in the observations of one investigator, or variations between two or more investigatiors.

obsession (əb'seshən) an unwanted idea or impulse that repeatedly intrudes into consciousness. Morbid obsession may dominate the mind and lead to irrational actions that are an attempt to escape the obsessional thoughts. adj. **obsessive**.

obsessive–compulsive (əb,sesivkəm'pulsiv) marked by a compulsion to repeatedly perform certain acts or carry out certain rituals. Obsessive-compulsive reaction is a type of NEUROSIS in which there is the intrusion of insistent, repetitious, and unwanted ideas or impulses to perform certain acts. The patient may feel compelled to wash his hands repeatedly, to utter certain words or phrases over and over again, or to carry out ritualistically other acts that interfere with his normal daily activities.

obstetric pulsar (əb'stetrik) an appliance used for TENS.

obstetrician (,obstə'trishən) a doctor who specializes in obstetrics.

obstetrics (ob'stetriks) the branch of medicine dealing with pregnancy, labour, and the puerperium. adj. **obstetric, obstetrical**.

obstipation (obsti'payshən) intractable constipation.

obstruction (əb'strukshən) the act of blocking or clogging; state of being clogged.

intestinal o. any hindrance to the passage of faeces

(see also INTESTINAL OBSTRUCTION).

obstruent ('obstrooənt) 1. causing obstruction. 2. any agent or agency that causes obstruction.

obtund (ob'tund) to render dull or blunt.

obtundent (ob'tundənt) 1. having the power to dull sensibility or to soothe pain. 2. a soothing or partially anaesthetic agent.

obturator ('obtyuh,raytə) a disc or plate that closes an opening.

o. foramen the large opening between the pubic bone and the ischium.

o. muscles the muscles that rotate the thighs laterally.

o. sign pain on outward pressure on the obturator foramen as a sign of inflammation in the sheath of the obturator nerve, probably caused by appendicitis.

obtusion (ob'tyoozhən) a deadening or blunting of sensitivity.

occipital (ok'sipit'l) pertaining to the occiput; located near the occipital bone, as the occipital lobe.

o. bone the unpaired bone constituting the back and part of the base of the skull.

o. lobe the most posterior portion of the cerebral hemisphere, forming a small part of its dorsolateral surface. The centre of sight.

occipitalization (ok,sipit'lie'zayshən) synostosis of the atlas with the occipital bone.

occipitoanterior (ok,sipitoh·an'tiə·ri·ə) referring to the position of the child's head when the occiput is to the front of the maternal pelvis when the fetal head comes through the birth canal. *Occipitoposterior* is the reverse position.

occipitocervical (ok,sipitoh'sərvik'l, -sə'vie-) pertaining to the occiput and neck.

occipitofrontal (ok,sipitoh'frunt'l) pertaining to the occiput and the face.

occipitomastoid (ok,sipitoh'mastoyd) pertaining to the occipital bone and mastoid process.

occipitomental (ok,sipitoh'ment'l) pertaining to the occiput and chin.

occipitoparietal (ok,sipitohpə'rieət'l) pertaining to the occipital and parietal bones or lobes of the brain.

occipitoposterior (ok,sipitohpos'tiə·ri·ə) see OCCIPITOANTERIOR.

occipitotemporal (ok,sipitoh'tempə·rəl) pertaining to the occipital and temporal bones.

occipitothalamic (ok,sipitohthə'lamik) pertaining to the occipital lobe and thalamus.

occiput ('oksi,puht) the back part of the head.

occlude (ə'klood) to fit close together; to close tight; to obstruct or close off.

occlusal (ə'klooz'l) pertaining to closure; applied to the masticating surfaces of the premolar and molar teeth, or to the contacting surfaces of opposing occlusion rims, or designating a position toward the hypothetical plane passing between the mandibular and maxillary teeth when the jaws are brought into approximation.

occlusion (ə'kloozhən) 1. the act of closure or state of being closed; an obstruction or a closing off. 2. the relation of the teeth of the upper to the lower jaw when the jaws are shut.

central o., centric o. occlusion of the teeth when the mandible is centered upon the maxilla, with both occlusal surfaces fitting normally.

coronary o. obstruction to the flow of blood through an artery of the heart usually from progressive ATHEROSCLEROSIS (sometimes complicated by thrombosis), rarely from embolism, arteritis, or dissecting aneurysm (see also CORONARY OCCLUSION and MYOCARDIAL INFARCTION).

eccentric o. occlusion of the teeth when the lower jaw is displaced.

functional o. the apposition of the maxillary to the mandibular teeth which provides the greatest efficiency for mastication.

occlusive (ə'kloosiv) pertaining to or effecting occlusion.

occult ('okult) obscure or hidden from view.

o. blood test examination, microscopically or by a chemical test, of a specimen of faeces, urine, gastric juice, etc., to determine the presence of blood not otherwise detectable. Faeces are tested when intestinal bleeding is suspected but there is no visible evidence of blood in the stools.

occupational diseases (okyuh'payshən'l) diseases caused by various factors involved in one's occupation. The diseases vary with the type of work involved.

Dusts are a common cause of occupational diseases. Fine particles of silica can lead to SILICOSIS among miners, glassworkers, and persons involved in the manufacture of cement and similar materials. Another cause of occupational disease is poisonous gases and vapours, which can result in respiratory disorders and may also involve the blood and other body systems. Certain kinds of chemicals can affect the skin, causing some forms of DERMATITIS. Working conditions, such as high temperatures or humidity, excessive noise, changes in air pressure, or continuous exposure to sun and wind, can cause varied disorders such as HEAT EXHAUSTION, impaired hearing or vision, BENDS, or skin conditions.

Control and prevention of occupational diseases is very much a major concern of the individual worker, management, the community health service, and local and central governments. It involves education of the worker on how to protect himself against occupational hazards; management's cooperation in supplying proper equipment and conditions; inspection and testing services performed by the government; the existence of adequate medical and first-aid services at the location of the work; adequate hospitalization facilities, insurance and compensation; and research into methods to provide safety and good health.

occupational therapist a professional trained in the skills of occupational therapy. They complete a 3-year training programme to gain a diploma of the College of Occupational Therapists (20 Rede Place, Bayswater, London W2).

occupational therapy the evaluation and planning of a rehabilitation programme to maintain or increase function in all aspects of daily living following disability or debilitating illness, taking into consideration the patient's psychological, intellectual, emotional, and social needs.

occupational therapy assistant works under the supervision of a qualified occupational therapist. Assistants have no special training or qualifications.

occurrence (ə'kurəns) the frequency of an event in a population.

ochrometer (oh'kromitə) an instrument for measuring capillary blood pressure.

ochronosis (,ohkrə'nohsis) a peculiar discoloration of body tissues caused by deposit of alkapton bodies as the result of the metabolic disorder, alkaptonuria.

ocular o. brown or grey discoloration of the sclera, sometimes involving also the conjunctivae and eyelids.

octa- word element. [Gr., L.] *eight*.

octan ('oktan) occurring on the eighth day (every seven days).

octavalent (,oktə'vaylənt) having a valency of eight.

ocul(o)- word element. [L.] *eye*.

ocular ('okyuhlə) 1. pertaining to the eye. 2. eyepiece (of a microscope).

oculentum (,okyuh'lentəm) an eye ointment (old term).

oculist ('okyuhlist) ophthalmologist.

oculocerebrorenal syndrome (ˌokyuhlohˌseribroh'reen'l) a hereditary syndrome of males, with vitamin D-refractory rickets, hydrophthalmia, congenital glaucoma and cataracts, mental handicap, and renal tubule dysfunction as evidenced by hypophosphataemia, acidosis, and aminoaciduria. Called also *Lowe's disease.*

oculocutaneous (ˌokyuhlohkyoo'tayni·əs) pertaining to or affecting both the eyes and the skin.

oculofacial (ˌokyuhloh'fayshəl) pertaining to the eyes and face.

oculogyration (ˌokyuhlohjie'rayshən) the movement of the eyeball about the anteroposterior axis. adj. **oculogyric.**

oculogyric (ˌokyuhloh'jierik) causing movements of the eyes.

o. crisis involuntary, violent movements of the eye, usually upwards.

oculomotor (ˌokyuhloh'mohtə) pertaining to or affecting eye movements.

o. nerve the third cranial nerve; it is mixed, that is, it contains both sensory and motor fibres. Various branches of the oculomotor nerve provide for muscle sense and movement in most of the muscles of the eye, for constriction of the pupil, and for accommodation of the eye.

oculomotorius (ˌokyuhlohmoh'tor·ri·əs) the oculomotor nerve.

oculomycosis (ˌokyuhlohmie'kohsis) any fungal disease of the eye.

oculonasal (ˌokyuhloh'nayz'l) pertaining to the eye and the nose.

oculoplastic (ˌokyuhloh'plastik) denoting plastic surgery of the eye, eyelids, ocular muscles, lacrimal apparatus, or orbit.

oculopupillary (ˌokyuhloh'pyoopilə·ree) pertaining to the pupil of the eye.

oculozygomatic (ˌokyuhlohziegə'matik) pertaining to the eye and the zygoma.

oculus ('okyuhləs) pl. *oculi* [L.] eye.

OD [L.] oculus dexter (right eye).

ODA Operating Department Assistant.

odont(o)- word element. [Gr.] *tooth.*

odontalgia (ˌohdon'talji·ə) toothache.

odontic (oh'dontik) pertaining to the teeth.

odontoblast (oh'dontohˌblast) one of the connective tissue cells that deposit dentine and form the outer surface of the dental pulp adjacent to the dentine.

odontoblastoma (ohˌdontohbla'stohmə) a tumour made up of odontoblasts.

odontoclast (oh'dontohˌklast) an osteoclast associated with absorption of the roots of deciduous teeth.

odontogenesis (ohˌdontoh'jenəsis) the origin and development of the teeth. adj. **odontogenetic.**

o. imperfecta dentinogenesis imperfecta.

odontogenic (ohˌdontoh'jenik) 1. forming teeth. 2. arising in tissues that give origin to the teeth.

odontoid (oh'dontoyd) like a tooth.

odontolith (oh'dontohˌlith) tartar, the calcareous matter deposited upon teeth.

odontology (ˌohdon'toləjee) 1. scientific study of the teeth. 2. dentistry.

odontolysis (ˌohdon'tolisis) the resorption of dental tissue.

odontome (ˌohdon'tohmə) any odontogenic tumour, but usually applied to developmental anomalies of enamel and dentine.

ameloblastic o. a rare neoplasm composed of enamel, dentine, and an odontogenic epithelium like that seen in ameloblastoma.

complex o. a solid mass of dental tissue.

composite o. one consisting of both enamel and dentine in an abnormal pattern.

compound o. a mass of tiny denticles lying in connective tissue.

invaginated o. a malformation in which the enamel organ is folded inwards.

radicular o. one associated with a tooth root, or formed when the root was developing.

odorant ('ohdə·rənt) any substance capable of stimulating the sense of smell.

odynacusis (ˌohdinə'koosis) painful hearing.

-odynia word element. [Gr.] *pain.*

odynometer (ˌohdi'nomitə) an instrument for measuring pain.

odynophagia (ˌohdinoh'fayji·ə) painful swallowing of food.

oedema (i'deemə) an abnormal accumulation of fluid in the intercellular spaces of the body. If the finger is pressed upon an affected part, the surface pits and regains slowly its original contour. adj. **oedematous.**

Oedema can be caused by a variety of factors, including hypoproteinaemia, in which a lowered concentration of plasma proteins decreases the osmotic pressure, thereby permitting passage of abnormal amounts of fluid out of the blood vessels and into the tissue spaces. Some other causes are poor lymphatic drainage, increased capillary permeability (as in inflammation), and congestive HEART FAILURE.

Factors contributing to oedema formation

I. Arteriolar dilation
   A. Inflammation
   B. Heat
   C. Toxins
   D. Neurohemoral excess or deficit
II. Reduced effective osmotic pressure
   A. Hypoproteinaemia
      1. Malnutrition
      2. Cirrhosis
      3. Nephrotic syndrome
      4. Protein-losing gastroenteropathy
   B. Leaky vascular endothelium
      1. Inflammation
      2. Burns
      3. Trauma
      4. Allergic or immunological reaction
   C. Lymphatic obstruction
III. Increased venous pressure
   A. Congestive heart failure
   B. Thrombophlebitis
   C. Cirrhosis of liver
IV. Sodium retention
   A. Excessive salt intake
   B. Increased tabular reabsorption of sodium
      1. Reduced renal perfusion
      2. Increased renin–angiotensin–aldosterone secretion

From Leaf, A. and Cotran, R. S. (1976) *Renal Pathophysiology,* Oxford University Press, New York.

Local oedema due to inflammation or poor drainage through the lymph vessels may be relieved by elevation of the part and application of cold to the area. Generalized oedema is treated by the administration of DIURETICS, which increase the loss of certain salts and thereby increase removal of tissue fluids, which are eliminated as urine. Sodium, which enhances retention of fluid in the tissues, is usually restricted in the diet of patients with oedema.

angioneurotic o. temporary oedema suddenly appearing in areas of skin or mucous membrane and occasionally in the viscera (see also ANGIONEUROTIC

OEDEMA).
brain o. an excessive accumulation of fluid in the brain substance (wet brain).
cardiac o. a manifestation of congestive heart failure, due to increased venous and capillary pressures and often associated with renal sodium retention.
dependent o. oedema affecting most severely the lowermost parts of the body.
famine o. that due to protein deficiency.
lymph o. that due to blockage of the lymph vessels.
o. neonatorum a disease of preterm and feeble infants resembling sclerema, marked by spreading oedema with cold, livid skin.
pitting o. oedema in which pressure leaves a persistent depression in the tissues.
pulmonary o. diffuse extravascular accumulation of fluid in the tissues and air spaces of the LUNG due to changes in hydrostatic forces in the capillaries or to increased capillary permeability.
renal o. that occurring due to kidney malfunction.
vasogenic o. that characterized by increased permeability of capillary endothelial cells; the most common form of brain oedema.

oedemagen (i'deeməjən) an irritant that elicits oedema by causing capillary damage but not the cellular response of true inflammation.

oedematogenic (i,deemətə'jenik) producing or causing oedema.

oedipal ('eedip'l) pertaining to the Oedipus complex.

Oedipus complex ('eedipəs) a term used originally in PSYCHOANALYSIS to signify the complicated conflicts and emotions felt by a child when, during a stage of his normal development as a member of the family circle, he becomes aware of a particularly strong, sexually tinged attachment to his mother; the term also applies to a similar attachment felt by a girl to her father (called also *Electra complex*). At the same time, the child tends to view the other parent as a rival and yearns to take that parent's place. This pattern, which was described by Sigmund Freud, is named from the legend of the mythical Greek hero, King Oedipus of Thebes, who was raised by foster parents, unknowingly killed his real father in a quarrel, and later married his mother. When he learned of his unwitting incestuous relationship with his wife he blinded himself.

According to psychoanalysts, a child enters the oedipal phase at about the third year and usually has solved his largely unconscious conflicts in a satisfactory way by the age of 5 or 6. He does this by turning his feelings of possessiveness toward one parent and competitiveness toward the other into a wish to be liked by both of them. Eventually, a child who has worked out his conflicts well can focus his affection on members of the opposite sex outside the family circle and can establish satisfactory marital relationships as an adult.

Freud's theory is generally accepted by psychiatrists, although many have developed supplementary theories for the behaviour pattern he described.

oesophageal (i,sofə'jeeəl) of or pertaining to the oesophagus.
o. atresia a congenital abnormality in which the oesophagus is not continuous between the pharynx and the stomach. May be associated with a fistula into the trachea.
o. varices varicose veins of the lower oesophagus secondary to portal hypertension.

oesophagectasia (i,sofəjek'tayzi·ə) dilation of the oesophagus.

oesophagectomy (i,sofə'jektəmee) excision of a portion of the oesophagus.

oesophagism (i'sofə,jizəm) spasm of the oesophagus.

oesophagitis (i,sofə'jietis) inflammation of the oesophagus.
peptic o., reflux o. inflammation of the oesophagus due to a reflux of acid and pepsin from the stomach.

oesophagobronchial (i,sofəgoh'brongki·əl) pertaining to or communicating with the oesophagus and a bronchus.

oesophagocele (i'sofəgoh,seel) abnormal distention of the oesophagus; protrusion of the oesophageal mucosa through a rupture in the muscular coat.

oesophagocoloplasty (i,sofəgoh'kohloh,plastee) excision of a portion of the oesophagus and its replacement by a segment of the colon.

oesophagodynia (i,sofəgoh'dini·ə) pain in the oesophagus.

oesophagoenterostomy (i,sofəgoh,entə'rostəmee) formation of an anastomosis between the oesophagus and the small intestine.

oesophagogastrectomy (i,sofəgohga'strektəmee) excision of the oesophagus and stomach.

oesophagogastric (i,sofəgoh'gastrik) pertaining to the oesophagus and the stomach.

oesophagogastroanastomosis (i,sofəgoh-,gastroh·ə,nastə'mohsis) oesophagogastrostomy.

oesophagogastroduodenoscopy (i,sofəgoh-,gastroh,dyooədi'noskəpee) endoscopic examination of the oesophagus, stomach, and duodenum. During the procedure the patient is watched for signs of respiratory difficulty, excessive diaphoresis, and laryngospasm.

oesophagogastroplasty (i,sofəgoh'gastroh,plastee) reconstruction of the cardia of the stomach.

oesophagogastroscopy (i,sofəgohga'stroskəpee) endoscopic inspection of the oesophagus and stomach.

oesophagogastrostomy (i,sofəgohga'strostəmee) anastomosis of the oesophagus to the stomach.

oesophagography (i,sofə'gogrəfee) radiography of the oesophagus.

oesophagojejunostomy (i,sofəgoh,jejuh'nostəmee) anastomosis of the oesophagus to the jejunum.

oesophagomalacia (i,sofəgohmə'layshi·ə) softening of the walls of the oesophagus.

oesophagometer (i,sofə'gomitə) an instrument for measuring the oesophagus.

oesophagomyotomy (i,sofəgohmie'otəmee) incision through the muscular coat of the oesophagus.

oesophagooesophagostomy (i,sofəgoh·i,sofə-'gostəmee) anastomosis between two formerly remote parts of the oesophagus.

oesophagoplasty (i'sofəgoh,plastee) plastic repair of the oesophagus.

oesophagoplication (i,sofəgohplie'kayshən) infolding of the wall of an oesophageal pouch.

oesophagoptosis (i,sofəgop'tohsis) prolapse of the oesophagus.

oesophagorespiratory (i,sofəgohri'spiritə·ree) pertaining to or communicating with the oesophagus and respiratory tract (trachea or a bronchus).

oesophagoscope (i'sofəgoh,skohp) an endoscope for examination of the oesophagus.

oesophagoscopy (i,sofə'goskəpee) direct visual examination of the oesophagus with an oesophagoscope. Oesophagoscopy usually is done as a diagnostic procedure for the purpose of locating and inspecting a disorder of the oesophagus. After the oesophagoscope has been inserted it is possible to obtain samples of tissue for microscopic study. In some instances the oesophagoscope can be used to remove a foreign object that has become lodged in the oesophagus.

PATIENT CARE. Food and liquids are withheld for at least 6 hours prior to the procedure so that the stomach will be empty and there will be no regurgitation during the procedure. Rigid oesophagoscopy is performed under general anaesthetic as a surgical procedure. Fibreoptic oesophagoscopy, using a flexible endoscope, is done with minimal sedation. The throat may be anaesthetized with a local anaesthetic such as Xylocaine spray to depress the gag reflex and reduce local reaction to the passage of the instrument.

After use of a local anaesthetic spray, food and fluids are withheld until the gag reflex has returned (usually about 1 hour). This is necessary because there is danger of aspiration as long as the gag reflex is depressed. Hoarseness and a sore throat may remain for a few days after the examination.

oesophagostenosis (iˌsofəgohstə'nohsis) stricture of the oesophagus.

oesophagostomy (iˌsofə'gostəmee) the creation of an artificial opening into the oesophagus.

oesophagotomy (iˌsofə'gotəmee) incision of the oesophagus.

oesophagotracheal (iˌsofəgohtrə'keeəl, -'traki·əl) pertaining to or communicating with the oesophagus and trachea.

oesophagus (i'sofəgəs) the musculomembranous passage extending from the pharynx to the stomach, consisting of an outer fibrous coat, a muscular layer, a submucous layer, and an inner mucous membrane. The junction between the stomach and oesophagus is closed by a muscular ring known as the cardiac sphincter, which opens to allow the passage of food into the stomach. In an adult the oesophagus is usually 25 to 30 cm long. See also DIGESTIVE SYSTEM.

Disorders of the oesophagus often involve either an obstruction or a reflux (backward flow) of food and gastric juices. Foreign bodies, accidentally swallowed and lodged in the oesophageal passage, can obstruct the flow of foods and fluids, as can malignant or benign tumours. The term ACHALASIA is used to describe a particular disturbance in motility which leads to obstruction at the level of the cardiac sphincter.

Oesophagitis, inflammation of the mucous membrane lining the oesophagus, may occur in conjunction with gastroenteritis, or as a result of a backward flow of the gastric contents upward into the oesophagus. The symptoms of hiatal hernia are due in large part to this type of reflux. Hiatal hernia is a protrusion of the stomach, colon, or other intestinal organs through the oesophageal hiatus, a narrow opening in the diaphragm through which the oesophagus normally passes. When the herniation occurs the normal downward passage of food is interrupted.

Oesophageal varices are varicose veins of the oesophagus and occur most often as a result of obstruction in the portal circulation, especially in portal hypertension. These varices are potentially dangerous since they tend to rupture easily and may result in serious haemorrhage.

Visual examination of the interior lining of the oesophagus is accomplished by OESOPHAGOSCOPY.

oestradiol (ˌeestrə'dieol) the most potent naturally occurring OESTROGEN in humans; pharmacologically, it is usually used in the form of its esters (e.g. oestradiol benzoate, cyprionate, and valerate), or as a semisynthetic derivative (ethinyl oestradiol).

oestrin ('eestrin) an oestrogen.

oestrinization (ˌeestrinie'zayshən) production of the cellular changes in the vaginal epithelium characteristic of oestrus.

oestriol ('eestriol) a relatively weak human OESTROGEN, being a metabolic product of oestradiol and oestrone found in high concentration in the urine.

oestrogen ('eestrəjən, -trəˌjen) a generic term for oestrus-producing compounds; the female sex hormones, including oestradiol, oestriol, and oestrone.

In humans, the oestrogens are formed in the ovary (see GRAAFIAN FOLLICLE), adrenal cortex, testis, and fetoplacental unit, and are responsible for female secondary sexual characteristic development, and during the menstrual cycle act on the female genitalia to produce an environment suitable for fertilization, implantation, and nutrition of the early embryo.

Oestrogen is used as a palliative in post-menopausal cancer of the breast and in prostatic cancer, in oral contraceptives, for relief of menopausal discomforts, etc (see MENOPAUSE). There is evidence from controlled studies that oestrogen therapy (given without a progestogen) for menopausal symptoms is closely linked to cancer of the endometrium. The degree of risk is closely related to the dosage and the length of time it is taken.

The risk of endometrial cancer, gallstones, and possibly cardiovascular disease in women who take oestrogenic drugs poses a dilemma for doctors wishing to prescribe oestrogens for the prevention of OSTEOPOROSIS in postmenopausal women. While there is widespread agreement that the demineralization of bones after menopause can be prevented and the incidence of fractures greatly reduced by oestrogen therapy, the decision to use this form of therapy must be based on each patient's need and her response to a vitamin D supplement, exercise, and other alternative measures for prevention of osteoporosis.

conjugated o's a mixture of sulphate esters of oestrogenic substances, principally oestrone and equilin; the uses are those of oestrogens.

esterified o's a mixture of esters of oestrogenic substances, principally oestrone; the uses are those of oestrogens.

oestrogenic (ˌeestrə'jenik) oestrus-producing; having the properties of, or properties similar to, an oestrogen.

oestrone ('eestrohn) an OESTROGEN isolated from pregnancy urine, the human placenta, and palm kernel oil, and also prepared synthetically.

oestrophilin (ˌeestrə'filin) a cell protein that acts as a receptor for oestrogen, found in oestrogenic target tissue and in oestrogen-dependent tumours and metastases.

oestropipate (ˌeestroh'piepayt) a preparation of piperazine oestrone sulphate administered orally in the treatment of oestrogen deficiency associated with moderate to severe vasomotor symptoms of menopause, atrophic vaginitis, kraurosis vulvae, female hypogonadism, female castration, and primary ovarian failure; and topically for the treatment of atrophic vaginitis and kraurosis vulvae.

oestruation (ˌeestroo'ayshən) oestrus.

oestrum ('eestrəm) oestrus.

Oestrus ('eestrəs) a genus of botflies.

O. ovis a widespread species that deposits its larvae on the nostrils of sheep and goats, and which may cause ocular myiasis in man.

oestrus ('eestrəs) the recurrent, restricted period of sexual receptivity in female mammals other than human females, marked by intense sexual urge. See also oestrous CYCLE. adj. **oestrual, oestrous**.

official (ə'fishəl) inferring that the drug, medicament or substance is controlled or authorised by an official publication. In the UK this means the British Pharmacopoeia or the British Pharmaceutical Codex.

Oguchi's disease (oh'goocheez) a form of hereditary night blindness occurring in Japan.

ohm (ohm) the SI unit of electrical resistance, being

that of a resistor in which a current of 1 ampere is produced by a potential difference of 1 volt. Symbol Ω.

Ohm's law (ohmz) the electric current flowing through a conductor is equal to the voltage divided by the resistance.

ohmmeter ('ohm,meetə) an instrument that measures electrical resistance in ohms.

OHNC Occupational Health Nursing Certificate.

oil (oyl) 1. an unctuous, combustible substance that is liquid, or easily liquefiable, on warming, and is not miscible with water, but is soluble in ether. Such substances, depending on their origin, are classified as animal, mineral, or vegetable oils. Depending on their behaviour on heating, they are classified as volatile or fixed. For specific oils, see the specific name, as CASTOR OIL. 2. a fat that is liquid at room temperature.

essential o., ethereal o. volatile oil.

fixed o. an oil that does not evaporate on warming and occurs as a solid, semisolid, or liquid.

volatile o. an oil that evaporates readily; such oils occur in aromatic plants, to which they give odour and other characteristics.

ointment ('oyntmənt) a semisolid preparation for external application to the body. Official ointments consist of medicinal substances incorporated in suitable vehicles (bases).

OL [L.] oculus laevus (left eye).

-ol word element; indicating an alcohol or a phenol.

oleaginous (,ohli'ajinəs) oily; greasy.

oleate ('ohli,ayt) 1. a salt of oleic acid. 2. a solution of a substance in oleic acid.

olecranarthritis (oh,lekrənah'thrietis) inflammation of the elbow joint.

olecranarthrocace (oh,lekrənah'throkəsee) tuberculosis of the elbow joint.

olecranarthropathy (oh,lekrənah'thropəthee) disease of the elbow joint.

olecranoid (oh'lekrə,noyd) resembling the olecranon.

olecranon (oh'lekrə,non, ,ohli'kraynən) the bony projection of the ulna at the elbow. adj. **olecranal**.

oleic acid (oh'lee·ik) a long-chain unsaturated fatty acid found in animal and vegetable fats.

oleo- word element. [L.] *oil*.

oleoresin (,ohlioh'rezin) 1. a compound of a resin and a volatile oil, such as exudes from pines, etc. 2. a compound extracted from a drug by percolation with a volatile solvent, such as acetone, alcohol, or ether, and evaporation of the solvent.

oleotherapy (,ohlioh'therəpee) treatment by injections of oil.

oleothorax (,ohlioh'thor·raks) intrapleural injection of oil to compress the lung in pulmonary tuberculosis.

oleovitamin (,ohlioh'vitəmin) a preparation of fat-soluble vitamins in fish liver or edible vegetable oil.

oleum ('ohli·əm) pl. *olea* [L.] oil.

olfact ('olfakt) a unit of odour, the minimal perceptible odour, being the minimal concentration of a substance in solution that can be perceived by a large number of normal individuals, expressed in terms of grams per litre.

olfaction (ol'fakshən) 1. the act of smelling. 2. the sense of smell.

olfactology (,olfak'toləjee) the science of the sense of smell.

olfactometer (,olfak'tomitə) an instrument for testing the sense of smell.

olfactory (ol'faktə·ree) pertaining to the sense of smell.

o. bulb the bulb-like extremity of the olfactory nerve on the undersurface of each anterior lobe of the cerebrum.

o. nerve the first cranial nerve: it is purely sensory and is concerned with the sense of smell. The nerve cell bodies are situated in the olfactory area of the mucous membrane of the nose. The nerve fibres lead upward through openings in the ethmoid bone and connect with the cells of the olfactory bulb. From there the fibres pass inward to the cerebrum.

olig(o)- word element. [Gr.] *few, little, scanty*.

oligaemia (,oli'geemi·ə) deficiency in volume of the blood. adj. **oliagaemic**.

oligochymia (,oligoh'kiemi·ə) deficiency of chyme.

oligodactyly (,oligoh'daktilee) congenital absence of one or more fingers or toes.

oligodendrocyte (,oligoh'dendroh,siet) a cell of oligodendroglia.

oligodendroglia (,oligohden'drogli·ə) 1. the non-neural cells of ectodermal origin forming part of the adventitial structure of the central nervous system. 2. the tissue composed of such cells.

oligodendroglioma (,oligoh,dendrohglie'ohmə) a neoplasm derived from and composed of oligodendroglia.

oligodipsia (,oligoh'dipsi·ə) abnormally diminished thirst.

oligodontia (,oligoh'donshi·ə) congenital absence of some of the teeth.

oligodynamic (,oligohdie'namik) active in a small quantity.

oligogalactia (,oligohgə'lakshi·ə) deficient secretion of milk.

oligohaemia (,oligoh'heemi·ə) oligaemia.

oligohydramnios (,oligoh·hie'dramnios) deficiency in the amount of amniotic fluid.

oligohydruria (,oligoh·hie'drooə·ri·ə) abnormally high concentration of urine.

oligomeganephronia (,oligoh,megənə'frohni·ə) congenital renal hypoplasia in which there is a reduction in the number of lobes and of the total number of nephrons, and hypertrophy of the nephrons. adj. **oligomeganephronic**.

oligomenorrhoea (,oligoh,menə'reeə) abnormally infrequent menstruation.

oligonucleotide (,oligoh'nyookli·ə,tied) a polymer made up of a few (2–10) nucleotides.

oligophosphaturia (,oligoh,fosfə'tyooə·ri·ə) deficiency of phosphates in the urine.

oligoplasmia (,oligoh'plazmi·ə) deficiency of blood plasma.

oligopnoea (,oligop'neeə) hypoventilation.

oligoptyalism (,oligoh'tieə,lizəm) diminished secretion of saliva.

oligospermia (,oligoh'spərmi·ə) deficiency of spermatozoa in the semen.

oligotrophia, oligotrophy (,oligoh'trohfi·ə; ,oli'gotrəfee) a state of poor (insufficient) nutrition.

oliguria (,oli'gyooə·ri·ə) diminished urine secretion in relation to fluid intake.

olivary ('olivə·ree) shaped like an olive.

o. body, o. nucleus olive (2).

olive ('oliv) 1. the tree *Olea europaea* and its fruit. 2. olivary body; a rounded elevation lateral to the upper part of each pyramid of the medulla oblongata.

olivifugal (,oli'vifyuhg'l) moving or conducting away from the olive.

olivipetal (,oli'vipit'l) moving or conducting toward the olive.

olivopontocerebellar (,olivoh,pontoh,seri'belə) pertaining to the olive, the middle peduncles, and the cerebellar cortex.

Ollier's disease ('oli,ayz) enchondromatosis.

Ollier's layer the innermost layer of the periosteum; called also *osteogenetic layer*.

Ollier–Thiersch graft (,oliay'teeəsh) a very thin split-skin graft in which long, broad strips of skin, consisting of the epidermis, rete, and part of the corium, are used. Called also Thiersch graft.

olophonia (,olə'fohni·ə) defective speech due to malformed vocal organs.

-oma word element. [Gr.] *tumour, neoplasm.*

omagra (oh'magrə) gout in the shoulder.

omalgia (oh'malji·ə) pain in the shoulder.

omarthritis (,ohmah'thrietis) inflammation of the shoulder joint.

omentectomy (,ohmen'tektəmee) excision of all or part of the omentum.

omentitis (,ohmen'tietis) inflammation of the omentum.

omentofixation, omentopexy (oh,mentohfik'sayshən; oh'mentə,peksee) implantation of the omentum, to or within the interstices of the abdominal wall to establish collateral circulation in portal obstruction.

cardio-o. attachment of the omentum to the heart to establish a collateral circulation when there is coronary occlusion.

omentorrhaphy (,ohmen'to·rəfee) suture or repair of the omentum.

omentum (oh'mentəm) pl. *omenta* [L.] a fold of peritoneum extending from the stomach to adjacent abdominal organs. adj. **omental.**

gastrocolic o. greater omentum.

gastrohepatic o. lesser omentum.

greater o. a peritoneal fold attached to the anterior surface of the transverse colon.

lesser o. a peritoneal fold joining the lesser curvature of the stomach and the first part of the duodenum to the porta hepatis.

o. majus greater omentum.

o. minus lesser omentum.

omitis (oh'mietis) inflammation of the shoulder.

Omnipaque ('omnipayk) trademark for a preparation of iohexol, a radiological contrast medium used in excretion urography, arteriography, venography and myelography.

omnivorous (om'nivə·rəs) eating both plant and animal foods.

Omnopon ('omnəpon) tradename for preparations of papaveretum, an opiate analgesic.

O.-scopolamine tradename for a fixed combination preparation of papaveretum and hyoscine, used as a premedication prior to surgery.

omoclavicular (,ohmohklə'vikyuhlə) pertaining to the shoulder and clavicle.

omodynia (,ohmoh'dini·ə) pain in the shoulder.

omohyoid (,ohmoh'hieoyd) pertaining to the shoulder and the hyoid bone.

omphal(o)- word element. [Gr.] *umbilicus.*

omphalectomy (,omfə'lektəmee) excision of the umbilicus.

omphalelcosis (,omfəlel'kohsis) ulceration of the umbilicus.

omphalic (om'falik) pertaining to the umbilicus.

omphalitis (,omfə'lietis) inflammation of the umbilicus.

omphaloangiopagus (,omfəloh'anji'opəgəs) twin fetuses, one of which derives its blood supply from the umbilicus or placenta of the other.

omphalocele ('omfəloh,seel) protrusion, at birth, of part of the intestine through a defect in the abdominal wall at the umbilicus.

omphalomesenteric (,omfəloh,mesən'terik, -,mez-) pertaining to the umbilicus and mesentery.

omphalophlebitis (,omfəlohfli'bietis) inflammation of the umbilical veins.

omphaloproptosis (,omfəlohprop'tohsis) excessive protusion of the umbilicus.

omphalorrhagia (,omfələ'rayji·ə) haemorrhage from the umbilicus.

omphalorrhoea (,omfələ'reeə) effusion of lymph at the umbilicus.

omphalorrhoexis (,omfələ'reksis) rupture of the umbilicus.

omphalosite ('omfəloh,siet) the underdeveloped member of allantoidoangiopagous twins, joined to the more developed member (autosite) by the vessels of the umbilical cord.

omphalotomy (,omfə'lotəmee) the cutting of the umbilical cord.

omphalus ('omfələs) the umbilicus.

onanism ('ohnə,nizəm) 1. coitus interruptus. 2. masturbation.

ONC Orthopaedic Nursing Certificate.

Onchocerca (,ongkoh'sərkə) a genus of nematode parasites (superfamily Filarioidea).

O. volvulus a species causing human infection by invading the skin, subcutaneous tissues, and other tissues, producing fibrous nodules; blindness occurs after ocular invasion. It is spread by blackflies of the genus *Simulium* in Africa and Central and South America.

onchocerciasis (,ongkohsər'kieəsis) infection by nematodes of the genus *Onchocerca.*

onco- word element. [Gr.] *tumour, swelling, mass.*

oncofetal antigen (,ongkoh'feet'l) a fetal antigen that is also produced by some type of cancer cells, such as carcinoembryonic antigen (CEA) or alpha-fetoprotein (AFP) (see also oncofetal ANTIGEN).

oncogenesis (,ongkoh'jenəsis) the production or causation of tumours. adj. **oncogenetic.**

oncogenic (,ongkoh'jenik) giving rise to tumours or causing tumour formation; said especially of tumour-inducing viruses.

oncogenous (ong'kojənəs) arising in or originating from a tumour.

oncology (ong'koləjee) the sum of knowledge regarding tumours; the study of tumours.

oncolysate (ong'koli,sayt) any agent that lyses or destroys tumour cells.

oncoma (ong'kohmə) a tumour.

oncometer (ong'komitə) an instrument for measuring the size of the spleen, kidneys and other organs. See PLETHYSMOGRAPHY.

oncosis (ong'kohsis) a morbid condition marked by the development of tumours.

oncosphere ('ongkoh,sfiə) the larva of the tapeworm contained within the external embryonic envelope and armed with six hooks.

oncotic (ong'kotik) pertaining to swelling.

oncotomy (ong'kotəmee) incision of a tumour or swelling.

oncotropic (,ongkoh'tropik) having special affinity for tumour cells.

Oncovin ('onkohvin) trademark for a preparation of vincristine sulphate; an antineoplastic.

oncovirus ('onkoh,vierəs) any virus that causes cancer.

OND Ophthalmic Nursing Diploma.

Ondine's curse ('undeenz) a condition in which patients have lost autonomic control of respiration and become apnoeic upon falling asleep, due to lesions or surgery of the high spinal cord or brain stem; named after Ondine, a water nymph in Greek mythology who caused a mortal who loved her to sleep forever.

oneir(o)- word element. [Gr.] *dream.*

oneiric (oh'nieə·rik) pertaining to dreams.

oneirism (oh'nieə,rizəm) a dream-like state occurring while the person is awake.

oneirology (,ohnieə'roləjee) the science of dreams.

oneiroscopy (,ohnieə'roskəpee) analysis of dreams for diagnosis of a patient's mental state.

onlay ('on,lay) a graft applied or laid on the surface of an organ or structure.
onomatology (,onohmə'toləjee) the science of names and nomenclature.
onomatomania (,onə,matə'mayni·ə) mental derangement with regard to words or names.
onomatophobia (,onə,matə'fohbi·ə) morbid aversion to a certain word or name.
ontogeny (on'tojənee) the complete developmental history of an individual organism. adj. **ontogenetic, ontogenic.**
onyalai, onyalia (,ohni'aylayee; ,onhi'ayli·ə) a form of thrombopenic purpura due to a nutritional disorder occurring in Africa, marked by blebs on the buccal and palatal mucosa which contain semicoagulated blood.
onych(o)- word element. [Gr.] *the nails.*
onychalgia (,oni'kalji·ə) pain in the nails.
onychatrophia (,onikə'trohfi·ə) atrophy of a nail or the nails.
onychauxis (,oni'kawksis) hypertrophy of the nails.
onychectomy (,oni'kektəmee) excision of a nail or nail bed.
onychia (o'niki·ə) inflammation of the nail bed, resulting in loss of the nail. See also infections of the NAIL.
onychitis (,oni'kietis) inflammation of the matrix of a nail.
onychocryptosis (,onikohkrip'tohsis) ingrowing nail.
onychodystrophy (,onikoh'distrəfee) malformation of a nail.
onychogenic (,onikoh'jenik) producing nail substance.
onychograph (o'nikoh,grahf, -,graf) an instrument for observing and recording the nail pulse and capillary circulation.
onychogryphosis, onychogryposis (,onikohgri'fohsis; ,onikohgri'pohsis) abnormal hypertrophy and curving of the nails, giving a claw-like appearance.
onychoheterotopia (,onikoh,hetə·roh'tohpi·ə) abnormal location of the nails.
onychoid ('oni,koyd) resembling a fingernail.
onycholysis (,oni'kolisis) loosening or separation of a nail from its bed; onychoschizia.
onychomadesis (,onikohmə'deesis) complete loss of the nails.
onychomalacia (,onikohmə'layshi·ə) softening of the fingernail.
onychomycosis (,onikohmie'kohsis) fungal disease of the nails; the nails become opaque, white, thickened, and friable.
onychopathy (,oni'kopəthee) any disease of the nails.
onychophagia, onychophagy (,onikoh'fayji·ə; ,oni'kofəjee) biting of the nails.
onychorrhexis (,onikə'reksis) spontaneous splitting or breaking of the nails.
onychoschizia (,onikoh'skitsi·ə) onycholysis.
onychosis (,oni'kohsis) disease or deformity of a nail or the nails.
onychotillomania (,onikoh,tilə'mayni·ə) neurotic picking or tearing at the nails.
onychotomy (,oni'kotəmee) incision into a fingernail or toenail.
onyx ('oniks) a fingernail or toenail.
oo- word element. [Gr.] *egg, ovum.*
ooblast ('oh·ə,blast) a primitive cell from which an ovum ultimately develops.
oocyst ('oh·ə,sist) the encysted or encapsulated ookinete in the wall of a mosquito's stomach; also, the analogous stage in the development of any sporozoon.
oocyte ('oh·ə,siet) an immature ovum; it is derived from an oogonium, and is called a primary oocyte prior to completion of the first maturation division, and a secondary oocyte between the first and second maturation division.

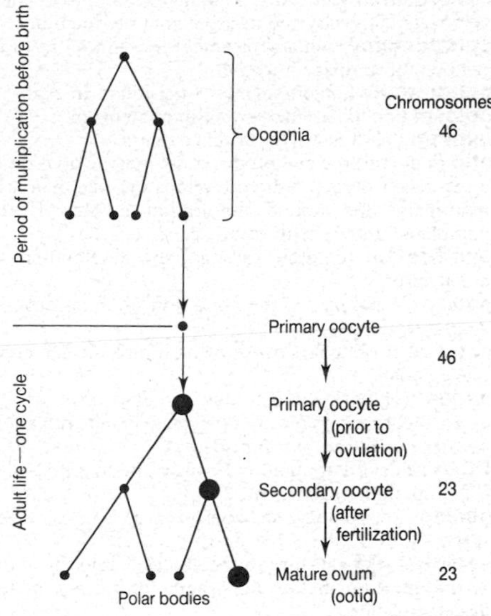

Summary of ovum development. Each primitive ovum produces only 1 mature ovum containing 23 chromosomes

oogamous (oh'ogəməs) pertaining or relating to or produced by oogamy; heterogamous.
oogamy (oh'ogəmee) 1. fertilization of a large nonmotile egg by a small, motile male gamete or sperm, as seen in certain algae. 2. conjugation of two dissimilar gametes; heterogamy.
oogenesis (,oh·ə'jenəsis) the development of mature ova from oogonia. adj. **oogenetic.**
oogonium (,oh·ə'gohni·əm) pl. *oogonia* [Gr.] an ovarian egg during fetal development; near the time of birth it becomes a primary oocyte.
ookinesis (,oh·əki'neesis) the mitotic movements of an ovum during maturation and fertilization.
ookinete (,oh·ə'kineet) the fertilized form of the malarial parasite in a mosquito's body, formed by fertilization of a macrogamete by a microgamete and developing into an oocyst.
oolemma (,oh·ə'lemə) zona pellucida (1).
oophor(o)- word element. [Gr.] *ovary.*
oophoralgia (,oh·əfə'ralji·ə) pain in an ovary.
oophorectomy (,oh·əfə'rektəmee) excision of one or both ovaries; called also *ovariectomy.* The procedure is done for tumours, severe infection, or other disorders of the ovary. Removal of the ovaries from a girl who has not yet reached puberty prevents the development of secondary sexual characteristics. If both ovaries are removed from an adult woman, reproduction is not possible and the female sex hormones oestrogen and progesterone are no longer produced.
oophoritis (,oh·əfə'rietis) inflammation of an ovary; ovaritis.
oophorocystectomy (oh,ofə·rohsi'stektəmee) excision of an ovarian cyst.
oophorocystosis (oh,ofə·rohsi'stohsis) the formation of an ovarian cyst.
oophorohysterectomy (oh,ofə·roh,histə'rektəmee) excision of the ovaries and uterus.
oophoron (oh'ofə·ron) an ovary.
oophoropexy (oh'ofə·roh,peksee) ovariopexy.

oophoroplasty (oh'ofə·roh,plastee) plastic repair of an ovary.
oophorosalpingectomy (oh,ofə·roh,salpin'jektəmee) removal of an ovary and its associated uterine tube.
oophorostomy (,oh·əfə'rostəmee) incision of an ovarian cyst for drainage purposes.
oophorotomy (,oh·əfə'rotəmee) incision of an ovary.
ooplasm ('oh·ə,plazəm) cytoplasm of an ovum.
oosperm ('oh·ə,spərm) a fertilized ovum.
ootid ('oh·ə,tid) the cell produced by meiotic division of a secondary oocyte, which develops into the ovum. In mammals, this second maturation division is not completed unless fertilization occurs.
opacification (oh,pasifi'kayshən) the development of an opacity.
opacity (oh'pasitee) 1. the condition of being opaque. 2. an opaque area.
opalescent (,ohpə'les'nt) showing a milky iridescence, like an opal.
opaque (oh'payk) impervious to light rays or, by extension, to x-rays or other electromagnetic radiation; neither translucent nor transparent.
OPCS Office of Population Censuses and Surveys.
OPD outpatient department.
opening ('ohpəning) an aperture, orifice, or open space.
aortic o. 1. the aperture of the ventricle into the aorta. 2. the aperture in the diaphragm for passage of the descending aorta.
cardiac o. the opening from the oesophagus into the stomach.
pyloric o. the opening between the stomach and duodenum.
operable, operability ('opə·rəb'l; ,opə·rə'bilitee) the feasibility of an operation taking into account the fitness of the patient and therefore the risk involved, and the likelihood of achieving cure or palliation. Operability is used more to refer to the case as a whole, operable to the lesion.
operant ('opə·rənt) see instrumental (operant) CONDITIONING.
o. conditioning a form of behaviour therapy in which a reward is given when the subject performs the action required of him. The reward serves to encourage repetition of the action.
operate ('opə,rayt) to perform an operation.
operating department assistant a paramedical trained to aid surgeons and anaesthetists in the operating theatre.
operation (,opə'rayshən) any action performed with instruments or by the hands of a surgeon; a surgical procedure.
Any effect produced by a therapeutic agent. For specific operations, see the specific name, as BLALOCK–TAUSSIG OPERATION.
operational research (,opə·rayshən'l) the study of the functioning of a system.
operative ('opə·rətiv) 1. pertaining to an operation. 2. effective; not inert.
operculum (oh'pərkyuhləm) pl. *opercula* [L.] 1. a lid or covering; the folds of pallium from the frontal, parietal, and temporal lobes of the cerebrum overlying the insula. 2. the mucous plug which fills the cavity of the cervical canal during PREGNANCY and which is referred to as the 'show' when it is shed prior to LABOUR. adj. **opercular**.
dental o. the hood of gingival tissue overlying the crown of an erupting tooth. **trophoblastic o.** the plug of trophoblast that helps close the gap in the endometrium made by the implanting blastocyst.
operon ('opə·ron) a segment of a chromosome comprising an operator gene and closely linked structural genes having related functions, the activity of the latter being controlled by the operator gene through its interaction with a regulator gene.
ophiasis (oh'fieəsis) a form of alopecia areata involving the temporal and occipital margins of the scalp in a continuous band.
ophidism ('ohfi,dizəm) poisoning by snake venom.
ophryosis (,ofri'ohsis) spasm of the eyebrow.
ophthalm(o)- word element. [Gr.] *eye*.
ophthalmagra (,ofthal'magrə) sudden pain in the eye.
ophthalmalgia (,ofthal'malji·ə) pain in the eye.
ophthalmencephalon (,ofthalmen'kefəlon, -'sef-) the retina, optic nerve, and visual apparatus of the brain.
ophthalmia (of'thalmi·ə) severe inflammation of the eye or of the conjunctiva or deeper structures of the eye.
Egyptian o. trachoma.
gonorrhoeal o. acute and severe purulent conjunctivitis due to gonorrhoeal infection.
o. neonatorum any hyperacute purulent conjunctivitis which may be due to the gonococcus, *Escherichia coli*, staphylococci or *Chlamydia trachomatis*, occurring within the first 21 days of life, usually contracted during birth from infected vaginal discharge of the mother. This condition is notifiable except in Scotland.
phlyctenular o. phlyctenular keratoconjunctivitis.
sympathetic o. granulomatous inflammation of the uveal tract of the uninjured eye following a wound involving the uveal tract of the other eye, resulting in bilateral granulomatous inflammation of the entire uveal tract. Called also *sympathetic uveitis*.
ophthalmic (of'thalmik) pertaining to the eye.
ophthalmitis (,ofthal'mietis) inflammation of the eyeball. adj. **opthalmitic.**
ophthalmoblennorrhoea (of,thalmoh,blenə'reeə) gonorrhoeal ophthalmia.
ophthalmocele (of'thalmoh,seel) exophthalmos.
ophthalmodonesis (of,thalmohdə'neesis) trembling motion of the eyes.
ophthalmodynamometry (of,thalmoh,dienə'momətree) determination of the blood pressure in the retinal artery.
ophthalmoeikonometer (of,thalmoh,iekə'nomitə) an instrument used to determine both the refraction of the eye and the relative size and shape of the ocular images.
ophthalmogyric (of,thalmoh'jierik) oculogyric.
ophthalmolith (of'thalmoh,lith) a lacrimal calculus.
ophthalmologist (,ofthal'moləjist) a professional who specializes in diagnosing and prescribing medical and surgical treatment for defects, injuries, and diseases of the EYE.
ophthalmology (,ofthal'moləjee) that branch of medicine dealing with the eye, its anatomy, physiology, pathology, etc. adj. **ophthalmological**.
ophthalmomalacia (of,thalmohmə'layshi·ə) abnormal softness of the eyeball.
ophthalmometer (,ofthal'momitə) an instrument used in ophthalmometry.
ophthalmometry (,ofthal'momətree) determination of the refractive powers and defects of the eye.
ophthalmomycosis (of,thalmohmie'kohsis) any disease of the eye caused by a fungus.
ophthalmopathy (,ofthal'mopəthee) any disease of the eye.
ophthalmoplegia (of,thalmoh'pleeji·ə) paralysis of the eye muscles. adj. **ophthalmoplegic.**
o. externa paralysis of the extraocular muscles.
o. interna paralysis of the iris and ciliary apparatus.
nuclear o. that due to a lesion of nuclei of motor nerves of eye.

Parinaud's o. paralysis of conjugate upward movement of the eyes without paralysis of convergence, associated with midbrain lesions.

partial o. that affecting some of the eye muscles.

progressive o. gradual paralysis of all the eye muscles.

total o. paralysis of all the eye muscles, both intraocular and extraocular.

ophthalmoptosis (of,thalmop'tohsis) exophthalmos.

ophthalmoreaction (of,thalmohri'akshən) local reaction of the conjunctiva after instillation into the eye of toxins or organisms causing typhoid fever and tuberculosis, being more severe in those affected with these diseases. Called also *ophthalmic reaction*.

ophthalmorrhagia (of,thalmə'rayji·ə) haemorrhage from the eye.

ophthalmorrhoea (of,thalmə'reeə) oozing of blood from the eye.

ophthalmorrhoexis (of,thalmə'reksis) rupture of an eyeball.

ophthalmoscope (of'thalmə,skohp) an instrument for examining the interior of the eye. It sends a bright, narrow beam of light through the lens of the eye, and contains a perforated mirror and lenses through which the doctor can examine interior parts of the eye. It is helpful in detecting possible disorders of the eyes, as well as disorders of other organs that are reflected in the condition of the eyes.

direct o. one that produces an upright, or unreversed, image of approximately 15 times magnification.

indirect o. one that produces an inverted, or reversed, direct image of two to five times magnification.

ophthalmoscopy (,ofthal'moskəpee) examination of the eye by means of the ophthalmoscope.

ophthalmosteresis (of,thalmohstə'reesis) loss of an eye.

ophthalmosynchysis (of,thalmoh'singkisis) effusion into the eye.

ophthalmotomy (,ofthal'motəmee) incision of the eye.

ophthalmotonometer (of,thalmohtə'nomitə) an instrument for measuring the intraocular pressure. Called also *tonometer*.

ophthalmotrope (of'thalmoh,trohp) a mechanical eye that moves like a real eye.

ophthalmoxerosis (of,thalmohzə'rohsis) xerophthalmia; abnormal dryness and thickening of the conjunctiva and cornea due to vitamin A deficiency or to local disease.

opiate ('ohpi·ət, -,ayt) a class of drugs including (1) the naturally occurring opiates, all of which are derived from the opium poppy (*Papaver somniferum*).This group includes opium and its alkaloids (morphine and codeine); (2) the semi-synthetic opiates including heroin (diacetylmorphine or diamorphine) and various other preparations including dihydromorphinone; (3) the synthetic opiates including methadone, meperidine and phenazocine, all of which are wholly synthetic but have morphine-like characteristics; (4) the narcotic antagonists which when used in conjunction with an opiate block its effects but when used alone have opiate-like properties (note however that naloxone is an important exception, being an opiate antagonist but having no narcotic properties).

The opiates have powerful analgesic and narcotic effects and also produce (often rapidly) both drug tolerance and drug dependence.

These drugs are sometimes called opioids.

opioid ('ohpi,oyd) 1. any synthetic narcotic that has OPIATE-like activities. 2. denoting naturally occurring peptides, e.g. enkephalins, that exert opiate-like effects by interacting with opiate receptors of cell membranes.

opisthorchiasis (,ohpisthor'kieəsis) infection of the biliary tract by the liver flukes *Opisthorchis felineus* or *O. viverrini*.

Opisthorchis (,ohpis'thawkis) a genus of flukes parasitic in the liver and biliary tract of various birds and mammals, including man. Infection results from eating raw fish.

O. felineus a species prevalent in the Philippines, India, Japan, Vietnam, the Soviet Union, and Eastern Europe.

O. viverrini a species prevalent in Laos and Thailand.

opisthotonos (,ohpis'thotənəs) a form of spasm in which the head and heels are bent backward and the body bowed forward. adj. **opisthotonic**.

opium ('ohpi·əm) the air-dried milky exudation from unripe capsules of the opium poppy *Papaver somniferum* or its variety *album*. Opium contains some 25 alkaloids, the most important being morphine (from which heroin is derived), narcotine, codeine, papaverine, thebaine, and narceine; the alkaloids are used for their narcotic and analgesic effect. It is poisonous in large doses. As it is highly addictive, opium production and cultivation of opium poppies is prohibited by most nations by international agreement, and its sale or possession for other than medical uses is strictly prohibited by law. See also DRUG ABUSE.

opocephalus (,ohpoh'kefələs, -'sef-) a fetus or infant with ears fused to the head, one orbit, no mouth, and no nose.

opodidymus (,ohpoh'didiməs) a fetus or infant with two fused heads and sense organs partly fused.

Oppenheim's disease ('opən,hiemz) amyotonia congenita.

Oppenheim's gait a gait marked by irregular oscillation of the head, limbs, and body; seen in some cases of multiple sclerosis.

opponens (o'pohnənz) opposing, a term applied to certain muscles controlling the movements of the fingers.

o. pollicis a muscle that adducts the thumb so that it and the little finger can be brought together.

opportunistic (,opətyoo'nistik) 1. denoting a microorganism which does not ordinarily cause disease but becomes pathogenic under certain circumstances. 2. denoting a disease or infection caused by such an organism.

opsinogen (op'sinə,jen) a substance (antigen) capable of producing the formation of opsonins. adj. **opsinogenous**.

opsiuria (opsi'yooə·ri·ə) excretion of urine more rapidly during fasting than after a meal.

opsoclonia, opsoclonus (,opsoh'klohni·ə; ,opsoh'klohnəs) involuntary, nonrhythmic horizontal and vertical oscillations of the eyes.

opsogen ('opsə,jen) opsinogen.

opsomania (,opsə'mayni·ə) an abnormal craving for some special food.

opsonic index (op,sonik 'indeks) a measurement of the bactericidal power of the phagocytes in the blood of an individual.

opsonin ('opsənin) an antibody that renders bacteria and other cells susceptible to phagocytosis. adj. **opsonic**.

immune o. an antibody that sensitizes a particulate antigen to phagocytosis, after combination with the homologous antigen in vivo or in vitro.

opsoninopathy (,opsəni'nopəthee) a condition marked by reduced levels of serum opsonins, leading to increased susceptibility to infection.

opsonization (,opsənie'zayshən) the rendering of bacteria and other cells subject to phagocytosis.

opsonize ('opsə,niez) to subject to opsonization.

opsonocytophagic (,opsənoh,sietoh'fayjik) denoting

the phagocytic activity of blood in the presence of serum opsonins and homologous leukocytes.

opsonotherapy (,opsənoh'therəpee) treatment by use of bacterial vaccines to increase the opsonic index.

optaesthesia (,optis'theezi·ə) visual sensibility; ability to perceive visual stimuli.

optic ('optik) of or pertaining to the eye.

o. nerve the second cranial nerve; it is purely sensory and is concerned with carrying impulses for the sense of sight. The rods and cones of the RETINA are connected with the optic nerve which leaves the eye slightly to the nasal side of the centre of the retina. The point at which the optic nerve leaves the eye is called the blind spot because there are no rods and cones in this area. The optic nerve passes through the optic foramen of the skull and into the cranial cavity. It then passes backward and undergoes a division; those nerve fibres leading from the nasal side of the retina cross to the opposite side while those from the temporal side continue to the thalamus uncrossed. After synapsing in the thalamus the neurons convey visual impulses to the occipital lobe of the brain.

optical ('optik'l) pertaining to vision.

optician (op'tishən) a professional trained in the detection of refractive errors and the dispensing of appropriate spectacles or contact lenses.

opticociliary (,optikoh'sili·ə·ree) pertaining to the optic and ciliary nerves.

opticopupillary (,optikoh'pyoopilə·ree) pertaining to the optic nerve and pupil.

Opticrom ('optikrom) trademark for a preparation of sodium cromoglycate.

optics ('optiks) the science of light and vision.

optimum ('optiməm) the best and most favourable.

opto- word element. [Gr.] *visible, vision, sight.*

optogram ('optoh,gram) the visual image formed on the retina by bleaching of visual purple under the influence of light.

optokinetic (,optohki'netik) pertaining to movement of the eyes, as in nystagmus.

optometer (op'tomitə) a device for measuring the power and range of vision.

optometrist (op'tomətrist) a specialist in optometry; a professional person trained to examine the eyes and prescribe glasses or contact lenses to correct irregularities in the vision.

optometry (op'tomətree) measurement of the powers of vision and the adaptation of lenses for the aid thereof, utilizing any means other than drugs.

optomyometer (,optohmie'omitə) a device for measuring the power of ocular muscles.

ora[1] ('ohrə) pl. *orae* [L.] an edge or margin.

o. serrata retinae the most anterior part of the retina of the eye.

ora[2] ('ohrə) [L.] plural of *os*, mouth.

orad ('or·rad) toward the mouth.

oral ('or·rəl) 1. pertaining to the mouth; taken through or applied in the mouth, as an oral medication or an oral thermometer. 2. denoting that aspect of the teeth which faces the oral cavity or tongue.

orality (or'ralitee) a term embracing all of the aspects and components (sucking, mouthing, etc.) of the oral stage of psychosexual development.

orange ('o·rinj) 1. the tree *Citrus aurantium* and its edible yellow fruit; the peel of two varieties is used in making various pharmaceuticals. 2. a colour between yellow and red.

Orap ('awrap) trademark for a preparation of pimozide, an antipsychotic.

Orbenin (aw'benin) trademark for a preparation of cloxacillin, an antibiotic.

orbicular (aw'bikyuhlə) circular; rounded.

orbit ('awbit) 1. the bony cavity containing the eyeball and its associated muscles, vessels, and nerves; the ethmoid, frontal, lacrimal, nasal, palatine, sphenoid, and zygomatic bones and the maxilla contribute to its formation. 2. the path of an electron around the nucleus of an atom. adj. **orbital**.

orbitonasal (,awbitoh'nayz'l) pertaining to the orbit and nose.

orbitonometer (,awbitə'nomitə) an instrument for measuring backward displacement of the eyeball produced by a given pressure on its anterior aspect.

orbitotomy (,awbi'totəmee) incision into the orbit.

orbivirus ('awbi,vierəs) a group of RNA viruses, a subgroup of the diplornavirus.

orcein ('awsee·in) a brownish-red colouring substance obtained from orcinol; used as a stain for elastic tissue.

orchi(d)(o)- word element. [Gr.] *testis.*

orchidalgia, orchialgia (,awki'dalji·ə; ,awki'alji·ə) pain in a testicle.

orchidectomy, orchiectomy (,awki'dektəmee; ,awki-'ektəmee) excision of one or both testes. This procedure is sometimes necessary when a testis is seriously diseased or injured. It may be performed, also, in order to control cancer of the prostate through diminution in the production of the hormone testosterone. Removal of the testes usually reduces sexual desire.

orchidic (aw'kidik) pertaining to a testis.

orchiditis (,awki'dietis) see ORCHITIS.

orchidopexy, orchiopexy ('awkidoh,peksee; 'awkioh-,peksee) fixation of an undescended testis in the scrotum. Called also orchidorrhaphy. An incision is made over the inguinal canal and the testis is brought down into the scrotum. In most cases the surgeon applies traction by placing a suture in the lower scrotum and attaching the suture to the inner thigh by a piece of adhesive tape. This traction is continued for about 1 week.

orchidoplasty, orchioplasty ('awkidoh,plastee; 'aw-kioh,plastee) plastic surgery of a testis.

orchidorrhaphy (,awki'do·rəfee) see ORCHIDOPEXY.

orchidotomy, orchiotomy (,awki'dotəmee; ,awki-'otəmee) incision and drainage of a testis.

orchiectomy (,awki'ektəmee) see ORCHIDECTOMY.

orchiepididymitis (,awki,epididi'mietis) inflammation of a testis and epididymis.

orchiocele, orchidocele ('awkioh,seel; 'awkidoh,seel) 1. hernial protrusion of a testis. 2. scrotal hernia. 3. tumour of a testis.

orchiomyeloma, orchidomyeloma (,awkioh,mieə-'lohmə; ,awkidoh,mieə'lohmə) plasmacytoma of a testis.

orchiopathy, orchidopathy (,awki'opəthee; ,awki-'dopəthee) any disease of the testes.

orchiopexy ('awkioh,peksee) see ORCHIDOPEXY.

orchioscheocele, orchidoscheocele (,awki'oskioh-,seel; ,awki'doskioh,seel) scrotal tumour with scrotal hernia.

orchis ('awkis) a testicle.

orchitis, orchiditis (aw'kietis; ,awki'dietis) inflammation of a testis. adj. **orchitic**. Orchitis is not a common disorder, but it can occur in a variety of infectious diseases, including syphilis, tuberculosis, glanders, leprosy, and certain of the parasitic diseases. It usually accompanies EPIDIDYMITIS. Acute orchitis may also occur in such diseases as typhoid fever, pneumonia, or mumps in adult males.

The symptoms of acute orchitis are swelling of one or both testes with pain and sensitivity to touch. In chronic orchitis there is no pain but the testes swell slowly and become hard.

orciprenaline (,awsi'prenəlin) a bronchodilator indicated in treatment of bronchial asthma, reversible bronchospasm of bronchitis, and emphysema. It is closely related to isoprenaline but is of longer duration and has fewer cardiovascular side-effects.

order ('awdə) a taxonomic category subordinate to a class and superior to a family (or suborder).

ordinate ('awdinət) the vertical line in a graph along which is plotted one of the factors considered in the study, as temperature in a temperature–time study. The other line is called the abscissa.

orexigenic (ə,reksi'jenik) increasing or stimulating the appetite.

orf (awf) an infectious pustular viral dermatitis of sheep, communicable to man.

organ ('awgən) a body part that performs a specific function or functions.

o. of Corti the organ lying against the basilar membrane in the cochlear duct, containing special sensory receptors for hearing, and consisting of neuroepithelial hair cells and several types of supporting cells.

effector o. a muscle or gland that contracts or secretes, respectively, in direct response to nerve impulses.

enamel o. a process of epithelium forming a cap over a dental papilla and developing into the enamel.

Golgi tendon o. any of the mechanoreceptors arranged in series with muscle in the tendons of mammalian muscles, being the receptor for stimuli responsible for the lengthening reaction.

reproductive o's those concerned with reproduction (see also REPRODUCTIVE ORGANS).

sense o's, sensory o's organs that receive stimuli that give rise to sensations, i.e. organs that translate certain forms of energy into nerve impulses which are perceived as special sensations.

spiral o. organ of Corti.

target o. the organ affected by a particular hormone.

vestigial o. an undeveloped organ that, in the embryo or in some remote ancestor, was well developed and functional.

o's of Zuckerkandl para-aortic bodies.

organ-specific (,awgənspə'sifik) restricted to, or having an effect only on, a particular organ, as an organ-specific antigen.

organelle (,awgə'nel) a specialized structure of a cell, such as a mitochondrion, Golgi complex, lysosome, endoplasmic reticulum, ribosome, centriole, chloroplast, cilium, or flagellum.

organic (aw'ganik) 1. pertaining to an organ or organs. 2. having an organized structure. 3. arising from an organism. 4. pertaining to substances derived from living organisms. 5. denoting chemical substances containing carbon. 6. pertaining to or cultivated by use of animal or vegetable fertilizers, rather than synthetic chemicals.

o. brain syndrome any mental disorder, psychotic or nonpsychotic, caused by or associated with impairment of brain tissue function; it may be *acute* and reversible, arising in one previously psychologically normal and due to injury, infection, exogenous or endogenous intoxications, nutritional deficiency, etc., or *chronic*, resulting from or associated with relatively permanent and more or less irreversible diffuse organic impairment of brain tissue function.

o. chemistry the scientific study of compounds containing carbon.

o. disease a disease due to or accompanied by structural changes.

organism ('awgə,nizəm) an individual animal or plant.

organization (,awgənie'zayshən) 1. the process of organizing or being organized. 2. the replacement of blood clots by fibrous tissue. 3. an organized body, group, or structure.

organizer ('awgə,niezə) a special region of the embryo that is capable of determining the differentiation of other regions.

primary o. the dorsal lip region of the blastopore.

organo- word element. [Gr.] *organ.*

organogenesis, organogeny (,awgənoh'jenəsis; ,awgə'nojənee) the origin or development of organs.

organoid ('awgə,noyd) 1. resembling an organ. 2. a structure that resembles an organ.

organology (,awgə'noləjee) the sum of what is known regarding the body organs.

organomegaly (,awgənoh'megəlee) enlargment of the viscera; visceromegaly.

organomercurial (,awgənohmər'kyooə·ri·əl) any mercury-containing organic compound, e.g. the diuretic mersalyl.

organometallic (,awgənohmə'talik) consisting of a metal combined with an organic radical.

organon ('awgə,non) pl. *organa* [Gr.] organ.

organophosphate (,awgənoh'fosfayt) an organic ester of phosphoric or thiophosphoric acid; such compounds are powerful acetylcholinesterase inhibitors and are used as insecticides and nerve gases. adj. **organophosphorous.**

organotherapy (,awgənoh'therəpee) therapeutic administration of animal endocrine organs or their extracts.

organotrophic (,awgənoh'trofik) 1. relating to the nutrition of organs of the body. 2. deriving energy from the oxidation of organic compounds; said of bacteria.

organotropism (,awgə'notrə,pizəm) the special affinity of chemical compounds or pathogenic agents for particular tissues or organs of the body. adj. **organotropic.**

organum ('awgənəm) pl. *organa* [L.] an organ; a part of the body that performs a special function.

orgasm ('awgazəm) the apex and culmination of sexual excitement.

orientation (,or·rien'tayshən) the recognition of one's position in relation to time and space.

orifice ('o·rifis) 1. the entrance or outlet of any body cavity. 2. any foramen, meatus, or opening. adj. **orificial.**

orificium (,o·ri'fishi·əm) pl. *orificia* [L.] orifice.

origin ('o·rijin) the source or beginning of anything, especially the more fixed end or attachment of a muscle (as distinguished from its insertion), or the site of emergence of a peripheral nerve from the central nervous system.

Orimeten (o·ri'metin) tradename for a preparation of aminoglutethimide.

Ormond's disease ('awməndz) retroperitoneal fibrosis.

ornithine ('awni,theen) an amino acid obtained from arginine by splitting of urea; it is an intermediate in urea biosynthesis.

Ornithodoros (,awnithoh'dor·rəs) a genus of soft-bodied ticks, many species of which are reservoirs and vectors of the spirochetes (*Borrelia*) of relapsing fevers.

ornithosis (,awni'thohsis) a disease of birds and domestic fowl, transmissible to man, caused by a strain of *Chlamydia psittaci*; the human disease is called PSITTACOSIS.

orofaciodigital syndrome (,or·roh,fayshioh'dijit'l) a syndrome occurring only in females, with mental handicap and anomalies of the mouth and tongue, the fingers, and frequently the face.

orolingual (,or·roh'ling·gwəl) pertaining to the mouth and tongue.

oronasal (,or·roh'nayz'l) pertaining to the mouth and nose.

oropharynx (ˌor·roh'faringks) the part of the pharynx between the soft palate and the upper edge of the epiglottis.

orosomucoid (ˌor·rəsoh'myookoyd) α_1-acid glycoprotein, a glycoprotein occurring in blood plasma.

orotic acid (oh'rotik) an intermediate in the biosynthesis of pyrimidine nucleotides.

orotic aciduria (oh'rotik) a hereditary defect of pyrimidine metabolism associated with excessive urinary excretion of orotic acid, and characterized by megaloblastic anaemia, crystalluria, and frequently physical and mental handicap.

Oroya fever (oh'rohyə) the acute febrile anaemic stage of Carrión's disease, bartonellosis.

orphenadrine (aw'fenəˌdrin) an anticholinergic agent and analgesic used in treatment of muscle spasm, especially that secondary to muscle injury, and in the treatment of Parkinson's disease.

orth(o)- word element. [Gr.] *straight, normal, correct.* In chemistry, *ortho-* indicates an isomer; also, a cyclic derivative having two substitutes in adjacent positions.

orthesis (aw'theesis) pl. *ortheses* [Gr.] orthosis.

orthetics (aw'thetiks) orthotics.

orthetist ('awthətist) orthotist.

orthocephalic (ˌawthohkə'falik, -sə-) having a head with a vertical index of 70.1 to 75.

orthochorea (ˌawthohko'reeə) choreic movements in the erect posture.

orthochromatic (ˌawthohkrə'matik) staining normally.

orthodeoxia (ˌawthohdi'oksi·ə) accentuation of arterial hypoxaemia in the erect position.

orthodontia, orthodontics (ˌawthoh'donshi·ə; ˌawthoh'dontiks) that branch of dentistry concerned with irregularities of teeth and malocclusion, and associated facial problems.

orthodontist (ˌawthoh'dontist) a dentist who specializes in orthodontics.

orthodromic (ˌawthoh'dromik) conducting impulses in the normal direction; said of nerve fibres.

orthognathics (ˌawthoh'nathiks) the science deaing with the cause and treatment of malposition of the bones of the jaw. adj. **orthognathic**.

orthograde ('awthohˌgrayd) carrying the body upright in walking.

orthomolecular (ˌawthohmə'lekyuhlə) pertaining to the theory that certain diseases are associated with biochemical abnormalities resulting in increased needs for certain nutrients, e.g. vitamins, and can be treated by administration of large doses of these substances.

orthomyxovirus (ˌawthohˌmiksoh'vierəs) a subgroup of myxoviruses that includes the viruses of human and animal influenza.

Ortho-Novin 1/50 (ˌawthoh'novin wun fiftee) trademark for preparations of norethisterone with mestranol; used as an oral contraceptive.

orthopaedic (ˌawthə'peedik) pertaining to the correction of deformities of the musculoskeletal system; pertaining to orthopaedics.

orthopaedics (ˌawthə'peediks) that branch of surgery dealing with the preservation and restoration of the function of the skeletal system, its articulations, and associated structures.

orthopaedist (ˌawthə'peedist) an orthopaedic surgeon.

orthopantomogram (ˌawthohpan'tohməgram) the film obtained by orthopantomography.

orthopantomography (ˌawthohpantə'mogrəfee) radiography of the mandible and maxilla using a moving x-ray tube and a curved film cassette.

orthopercussion (ˌawthohpə'kushən) percussion with the distal phalanx of the finger held perpendicularly to the body wall.

orthophoria (ˌawthoh'for·ri·ə) normal equilibrium of the eye muscles, or muscular balance. adj. **orthophoric**.

orthopnoea (ˌawthop'neeə) ability to breathe easily only in the upright position.

orthopnoeic position (ˌawthop'nee·ik) a position assumed to relieve orthopnoea, in which the patient sits upright in a chair, or in an upright or semivertical position that is achieved by using two or more pillows to support his head and thorax.

orthopraxis, orthopraxy (ˌawthoh'praksis; 'awthohˌpraksee) mechanical correction of deformities.

orthopsychiatry (ˌawthohsie'kieətree) that branch of psychiatry that deals with mental and emotional development, embracing child psychiatry and mental hygiene. The term is now falling into disuse.

orthoptic (aw'thoptik) correcting obliquity of one or both visual axes.

orthoptics (aw'thoptiks) assessment and treatment of strabismus and related disorders of ocular mobility.

orthoptist (aw'thoptist) one who specializes in the assessment and management of strabismus.

orthoscopic (ˌawthoh'skopik) affording a correct and undistorted view.

orthosis (aw'thohsis) pl. *orthoses* [Gr.] an orthopaedic appliance or apparatus used to support, align, prevent or correct deformities, or to improve function of movable parts of the body. See also SPLINT.

orthostatic (ˌawthoh'statik) pertaining to or caused by standing erect.

orthostatism (ˌawthoh'statizəm) an erect standing position of the body.

orthotast ('awthohˌtast) an apparatus for straightening curvatures of bone.

orthotic (aw'thotik) serving to protect or to restore or improve function; pertaining to the use or application of an orthosis.

orthotics (aw'thotiks) the field of knowledge relating to orthoses and their use.

orthotist ('awthəˌtist) a person skilled in orthotics and practicing its application in individual cases.

orthotonos, orthotonus (ˌaw'thotənos; aw'thotənəs) tetanic spasm that fixes the head, body, and limbs in a rigid straight line.

orthotopic (ˌawthoh'topik) occurring at the normal place.

orthovoltage (ˌawthoh'vohltij) in radiotherapy, voltage in the range of 140 to 400 kV.

Ortolani's sign (ˌawtoh'lahniz) a test performed soon after birth to detect possible congenital dislocation of the hip. A 'click' or popping sensation is felt on reversing the movements of abduction and rotation of the hip while the child is lying with knees flexed.

Orudis ('or·roodis) trademark for a preparation of ketoprofen.

OS [L.] *oculus sinister* (left eye).

Os chemical symbol, *osmium*.

os[1] (ohs) pl. *ora* [L.] 1. any body orifice. 2. the mouth. See also CERVICAL OS.

os[2] (os) pl. *ossa* [L.] a bone.

osche(o)- word element. [Gr.] *scrotum*.

oscheitis (ˌoski'ietis) inflammation of the scrotum.

oscheocele ('oskiohˌseel) a swelling or tumour of the scrotum.

oscheoma (ˌoski'ohmə) tumour of the scrotum.

oscheoplasty ('oskiohˌplastee) plastic surgery of the scrotum.

oscillation (ˌosi'layshən) a backward and forward motion, like that of a pendulum; also vibration, fluctuation, or variation.

oscillo- word element. [L.] *oscillation*.

oscillometer (ˌosi'lomitə) an instrument for measuring oscillations.

oscillometry (ˌosi'lomətree) the measurement of oscillations.

oscillopsia (ˌosi'lopsi·ə) a visual sensation that stationary objects are swaying back and forth.

oscilloscope (ə'siləˌskohp) an instrument that displays a visual representation of electrical variations on the fluorescent screen of a cathode-ray tube.

oscitation (ˌosi'tayshən) the act of yawning.

osculum ('oskyuhləm) a small aperture or minute opening.

Osgood–Schlatter disease (ˌozguhd'shlatə) osteochondrosis of the tuberosity of the tibia; called also Schlatter–Osgood disease.

-osis word element. [Gr.] *disease, morbid state, abnormal increase.*

Osler's disease ('ohsləz) 1. polycythaemia vera. 2. hereditary haemorrhagic telangiectasia.

Osler's nodes small, raised, swollen, tender areas, bluish or sometimes pink or red, occurring commonly in the pads of the fingers or toes, in the thenar or hypothenar eminences, or on the soles of the feet; they are practically pathognomonic of subacute bacterial endocarditis.

Osler–Vaquez disease (ˌohslə'vakez) polycythaemia vera.

osmatic (oz'matik) pertaining to the sense of smell.

osmics ('ozmiks) the science dealing with the sense of smell.

osmidrosis (ˌozmi'drohsis) the secretion of foul-smelling sweat; bromhidrosis.

osmium ('ozmi·əm) a chemical element, atomic number 76, atomic weight 190.2, symbol Os. See table of elements in Appendix 2.

osmolality (ˌozmoh'lalitee) the concentration of a solution in terms of osmoles of solutes per kilogram of solvent.

serum o. a measure of the number of dissolved particles per unit of water in serum. In a solution, the fewer the particles of solute in proportion to the number of units of water (solvent), the less concentrated the solution. A low serum osmolality would be indicative of a higher than usual amount of water in relation to the amount of particles dissolved in it. It would be expected, then, that a low serum osmolality would accompany overhydration, or OEDEMA, and an increased serum osmolality would be present in a state of FLUID VOLUME DEFICIT.

Measurement of the serum osmolality gives information about the hydration status within the cells because of the osmotic equilibrium that is constantly being maintained on either side of the cell membrane (HOMEOSTASIS). Water moves freely back and forth across the membrane in response to the osmotic pressure being exerted by the molecules of solute in the intracellular and extracellular fluids. Serum osmolality reflects the status of hydration of the intracellular as well as the extracellular compartments and thus describes total body hydration. The normal value for serum osmolality is 270–300 mOsm/kg water.

urine o. a measure of the number of dissolved particles per unit of water in the urine. A more accurate measure of urine concentration than specific gravity, urine osmolality is useful in diagnosing renal disorders of urinary concentration and dilution and in assessing status of hydration.

osmolar (oz'mohlə) pertaining to the concentration of osmotically active particles in solution.

osmolarity (ˌozmoh'laritee) the concentration of a solution in terms of osmoles of solutes per litre of solution.

osmole ('ozmohl) a unit of osmotic pressure equivalent to the amount of solute substances that dissociates in solution to form one mole (Avogadro's number) of particles (molecules and ions). Abbreviated Osm.

osmometer (oz'momitə) 1. a device for testing the sense of smell. 2. an instrument for measuring osmotic pressure.

osmophilic (ˌozmoh'filik) having an affinity for solutions of high osmotic pressure.

osmophore ('ozmohˌfor) the group of atoms in a molecule of a compound that is responsible for its odour.

osmoreceptor (ˌozmohri'septə) 1. a specialized sensory nerve ending sensitive to stimulation giving rise to the sensation of odours. 2. any of a group of specialized neurons of the supraoptic nuclei of the thalamus that are stimulated by increased extracellular fluid osmolality to cause the release of antidiuretic hormone (ADH) from the posterior pituitary.

osmoregulation (ˌozmohˌregyuh'layshən) adjustment of internal osmotic pressure of a simple organism or body cell in relation to that of the surrounding medium. adj. **osmoregulatory**.

osmose ('ozmohs, -mohz, 'os-) to diffuse by osmosis.

osmosis (oz'mohsis, os-) [Gr.] the passage of pure solvent from a solution of lesser to one of greater solute concentration when the two solutions are separated by a membrane which selectively prevents the passage of solute molecules, but is permeable to the solvent. adj. **osmotic.**

The process of osmosis and the factors that influence it are important clinically in the maintenance of adequate body fluids and in the proper balance between volumes of extracellular and intracellular fluids.

The term 'osmotic pressure' refers to the amount of pressure necessary to stop the flow of water across the membrane. The hydrostatic pressure of the water exerts an opposite effect; that is, it exerts pressure in favour of the flow of water across the membrane. The osmotic pressure of the particles in a solute depends on the relative concentrations of the solutions on either side of the membrane, and on the area of the membrane. The osmotic pressure exerted by the nondiffusible particles in a solution is determined by the numbers of particles in a unit of fluid and not by the mass of the particles.

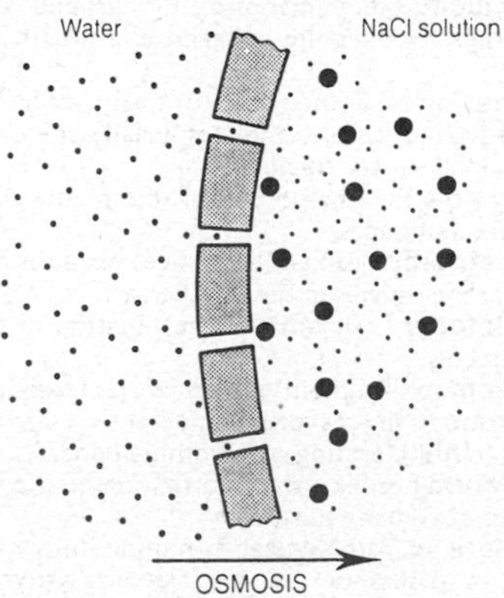

Osmosis at a cell membrane when a sodium chloride solution is placed on one side of the membrane and water on the other side

osmostat ('ozmohˌstat) the regulatory centres that control the osmolality of the extracellular fluid.

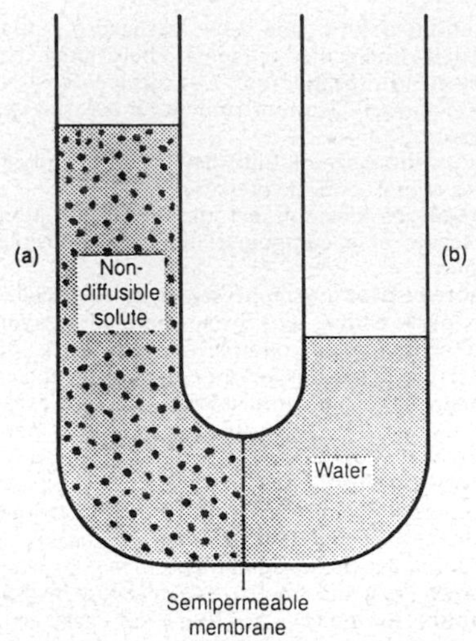

Demonstration of osmotic pressure on the two sides of a semipermeable membrane

osmotic fragility susceptibility of erythrocytes to haemolysis when exposed to increasingly hypotonic solutions.

osphresiology (os,freezi'olajee) the science of odours and sense of smell.

osphresiometer (os,freezi'omita) an instrument for measuring acuteness of the sense of smell.

osphresis (os'freesis) the sense of smell. adj. **osphretic**.

Ospolot ('ospalot) tradename for sulthiame, an anticonvulsant.

ossein ('osee·in) the collagen of bone.

osseocartilaginous (,osioh,kahti'lajinas) composed of bone and cartilage.

osseofibrous (,osioh'fiebras) made up of fibrous tissue and bone.

osseomucin (,osioh'myoosin) the ground substance that binds together the collagen and elastin fibrils of bone.

osseous ('osi·as) of the nature or quality of bone; bony.

ossicle ('osik'l) a small bone, especially one of those in the middle ear. adj. **ossicular**.

auditory o's the small bones of the middle ear: incus, malleus, and stapes.

ossiculectomy (,osikyuh'lektamee) excision of one or more of the ossicles of the middle ear.

ossiculotomy (,osikyuh'lotamee) incision of the auditory ossicles.

ossiculum (o'sikyuhlam) pl. *ossicula* [L.] ossicle.

ossiferous (o'sifa·ras) producing bone.

ossific (o'sifik) forming or becoming bone.

ossification (,osifi'kayshan) formation of or conversion into BONE or a bony substance.

ectopic o. a pathological condition in which bone arises in tissues not in the osseous system and in connective tissues usually not manifesting osteogenic properties.

endochondral o. ossification that occurs in and replaces cartilage.

intramembranous o. ossification of bone that occurs in and replaces connective tissue.

ossify ('osi,fie) to change or develop into bone.

Ossopan ('osohpan) trademark for preparations of hydroxyapatite, a calcium supplement.

oste(o)- word element. [Gr.] *bone*.

ostealgia (,osti'alji·a) pain in the bones; osteodynia.

ostearthritis (,ostiah'thrietis) osteoarthritis.

ostearthrotomy (,ostiah'throtamee) excision of an articular end of a bone.

ostectomy (o'stektamee) excision of a bone or part of a bone.

osteectopia (,ostiek'tohpi·a) displacement of a bone.

ostein ('ostee·in) ossein.

osteitis (,osti'ietis) inflammation of bone. The term is used to describe a number of conditions; for instance, advanced cases of syphilis can lead to syphilitic osteitis.

condensing o. osteitis with hard deposits of earthy salts in affected bone.

o. deformans rarefying osteitis of unknown cause resulting in deformed bones of increased mass leading to bowing of the long bones and deformation of the flat bones. The bones most commonly affected are the long bones of the legs, the lower spine, the pelvis, and the skull. Called also *Paget's disease of bone*.

The disease is relatively common, particularly in the United States, United Kingdom, Australia, France, and Germany, occurring in 3 per cent of the population over the age of 40 and 10 per cent of those over the age of 70. It occurs more often in males than in females. Once thought to be a rare form of localized bone disease, the disorder is now diagnosed more frequently because of newer diagnostic techniques, such as bone scanning, and routine testing of plasma alkaline phosphatase.

Symptoms of osteitis deformans depend on the site of the bone lesions and their severity. In 20 per cent of diagnosed cases there are no symptoms at all, and in others the symptoms are very mild. Lesions in the long bones seem to cause the most difficulty. The disease disturbs the growth of new bone tissue with the result that the bones often thicken, become soft, and coarsen in texture. In an advanced case, the weakened bone may be fractured by even a light blow, or, as in the case of the vertebrae, may collapse.

Lesions in the long bones can cause pain, deformity from bowing, and disability due to the arthritic changes that are a complication of the disease. When the disease process affects the skull the patient may complain of headaches, intermittent ringing in the ears and dizziness, and hearing loss. Severe involvement of the occipital region can cause pressure on the pons and cerebellum and compression of the spinal cord. These pathological changes produce loss of coordination, muscle weakness, diplopia, ataxia, and other signs of neurological dysfunction.

Diagnosis of osteitis deformans is verified by radiological studies of the affected bones and by laboratory tests. The serum alkaline phosphatase and urinary hydroxyproline levels are elevated.

Drugs of choice in the treatment of osteitis deformans are calcitonin, mithramycin, and etidronate disodium.

o. fibrosa cystica rarefying osteitis with fibrous degeneration and the formation of cysts and the presence of fibrous nodules on the affected bones, due to osteoclastic activity secondary to HYPERPARATHYROIDISM. If a tumour of the parathyroid gland is the cause of the hyperparathyroidism, treatment includes removal of the tumour. When the disease is generalized, all the bones are affected (von Recklinghausen's disease). Orthopaedic surgery may be necessary to correct severe bone deformities.

o. fragilitans osteogenesis imperfecta.

o. fungosa chronic osteitis in which the haversian

canals are dilated and filled with granulation tissue.

rarefying o. a bone disease in which the inorganic matter is diminished and the hard bone becomes cancellated.

sclerosing o. 1. sclerosing nonsuppurative osteomyelitis. 2. condensing osteitis.

ostempyesis (ˌostempie'eesis) suppuration within a bone.

osteoarthritis (ˌostioh·ah'thrietis) non-inflammatory joint disease characterized by loss of articular cartilage, eburnation (sclerosis) of underlying bone and formation of new bone (osteophytosis) at articular margins. Probably represents 'joint failure' arising from a variety of causes of which one is the 'worn-out' joint of old age. Primary osteoarthritisis where no pre-existing, underlying cause can be defined. Primary generalized osteoarthritis typically presents in women in the fourth and fifth decades with terminal bony swelling of proximal interphalangeal joints and 1st carpometacarpal joints of the hands, cervical and lumbar spondylosis and involvement of knees and 1st metatarsophalangeal joints of the feet. Bony swellings of terminal (Heberden's nodes) and proximal interphalangeal joints (Bouchard's nodes) are characteristic of this disorder. Symptoms of primary osteoarthritis are pain and stiffness which is usually much milder than that associated with rheumatoid arthritis. Primary osteoarthritis localized to one or two weight-bearing joints such as the hip or knee is common in the elderly. Symptoms include pain, particularly on weight bearing, and loss of joint function. Secondary osteoarthritis may follow preexisting severe inflammatory joint disease or any condition which alters the normal biomechanical integrity of a joint.

Treatment of osteoarthritis is aimed at relieving pain and maintaining or restoring joint function. Primary generalized osteoarthritis is usually a mild condition treated largely on a symptomatic basis with general advice and simple analgesics or low doses of NSAIDs. Localized osteoarthritis of weight-bearing joints is treated with analgesics or low doses of NSAIDs where necessary, physiotherapy and where necessary surgery which includes joint replacement (see also treatment of ARTHRITIS).

Further information on services available can be obtained from the Arthritis and Rheumatism Council, 41 Eagle Street, London WC1R 4AR.

osteoarthropathy (ˌostioh·ah'thropəthee) any disease of the joints and bones.

hypertrophic pulmonary o., secondary hypertrophic o. symmetrical osteitis of the four limbs, chiefly localized to the phalanges and terminal epiphyses of the long bones of the forearm and leg; it is often secondary to chronic lung and cyanotic heart conditions.

osteoarthrosis (ˌostioh·ah'throhsis) chronic noninflammatory bone disease.

osteoarthrotomy (ˌostioh·ah'throtəmee) ostearthrotomy.

osteoblast ('ostioh,blast) a cell arising from a fibroblast, which, as it matures, is associated with bone production.

osteoblastoma (ˌostiohbla'stohmə) a benign, painful, rather vascular tumour of bone marked by formation of osteoid tissue and primitive bone.

osteocampsia (ˌostioh'kampsi·ə) curvature of a bone.

osteochondral (ˌostioh'kondrəl) pertaining to bone and cartilage.

osteochondritis (ˌostiohkon'drietis) inflammation of bone and cartilage.

o. deformans juvenilis osteochondritis of the head of the femur.

o. deformans juvenillis dorsi osteochondrosis of vertebrae.

o. dissecans osteochondritis resulting in partial or complete detachment of a fragment of articular cartilage and underlying bone, particularly the knee or shoulder joint. The fragment of cartilage is called a joint mouse.

osteochondrodysplasia (ˌostiohˌkondrohdis'playzi·ə) disease or abnormal development of bony cartilaginous structures.

osteochondrodystrophy (ˌostiohˌkondroh'distrəfee) Morquio's disease.

familial o. a familial form of mucopolysaccharidosis becoming evident when the affected infant begins to walk (see also MORQUIO'S DISEASE).

osteochondrolysis (ˌostiohkon'drolisis) osteochondritis dissecans.

osteochondroma (ˌostiohkon'drohmə) a benign bone tumour consisting of projecting adult bone capped by cartilage.

osteochondromatosis (ˌostiohˌkondrohmə'tohsis) the occurrence of multiple osteochondromas.

osteochondromyxoma (ˌostiohˌkondrohmik'sohmə) osteochondroma blended with myxoma.

osteochondrosarcoma (ˌostiohˌkondrohsah'kohmə) sarcoma blended with osteoma and chondroma.

osteochondrosis (ˌostiohkon'drohsis) a disease of the growth ossification centres in children, beginning as a degeneration or necrosis followed by regeneration or recalcification; known by various names, depending on the bone involved.

o. deformans tibiae aseptic necrosis of the medial tibial condyle, with lateral bowing of the leg.

osteoclasis (ˌosti'okləsis) 1. surgical fracture or refracture of a bone. 2. the breaking down and absorption of bone tissue by osteoclasts.

osteoclast ('ostiohˌklast) 1. a large, multinuclear cell frequently associated with resorption of bone. 2. a surgical instrument used for osteoclasis. adj. **osteoclastic.**

osteoclastoma (ˌostiohkla'stohmə) giant cell tumour of bone.

osteocope ('ostiohˌkohp) severe pain in a bone. adj. **osteocopic.**

osteocranium (ˌostioh'krayni·əm) the fetal skull during the period of ossification, from early in the third month of gestation.

osteocystoma (ˌostiohsi'stohmə) a bone cyst.

osteocyte ('ostiohˌsiet) an osteoblast that has become embedded within the bone matrix, occupying a bone lacuna, and sending through canaliculi cytoplasmic processes that connect with other osteocytes in developing bone.

osteodentine (ˌostioh'denteen) dentine that resembles bone.

osteodermia (ˌostioh'dərmi·ə) osteoma cutis.

osteodiastasis (ˌostiohdie'astəsis) the separation of two adjacent bones.

osteodynia (ˌostioh'dini·ə) pain in a bone; ostealgia.

osteodystrophy (ˌostioh'distrəfee) abnormal development of bone.

renal o. a condition due to chronic renal disease, marked by impaired kidney function, elevated serum phosphorus levels, and low or normal serum calcium levels, and by stimulation of parathyroid function, resulting in a variable admixture of bone disease, including osteitis fibrosa cystica, osteomalacia, osteoporosis, and sometimes osteosclerosis; if the onset is in childhood, renal dwarfism may result.

osteoectomy (ˌostioh'ektəmee) surgical excision of bone.

osteoepiphysis (ˌostioh·i'pifisis) any bony epiphysis.

osteofibroma (,ostiohfie'brohmə) osteoma blended with fibroma.
osteogen ('ostioh,jen) the substance composing the inner layer of the periosteum, from which bone is formed.
osteogenesis (,ostioh'jenəsis) the formation of bone; the development of the bones.
o. imperfecta an inherited condition marked by abnormally brittle bones that are subject to fracture; osteogenesis imperfecta congenita occurs during intrauterine life and the child is born with deformities; in osteogenesis imperfecta tarda, the fractures occur when the child begins to walk. It is usually attended by blue coloration of the sclera (Lobstein's disease) and sometimes by otosclerotic deafness (van der Hoeve's syndrome).
osteogenic (,ostioh'jenik) derived from or composed of any tissue concerned in bone growth or repair.
osteogeny (,osti'ojənee) osteogenesis.
osteography (,osti'ogrəfee) description of the bones.
osteohalisteresis (,ostioh,halistə'reesis) deficiency in mineral elements of bone.
osteoid ('osti,oyd) 1. resembling bone. 2. the organic matrix of bone; young bone that has not undergone calcification.
osteolipochondroma (,ostioh,lipohkon'drohmə) osteochondroma with fatty elements.
osteologist (,osti'oləjist) a specialist in osteology.
osteology (,osti'oləjee) scientific study of the bones.
osteolysis (,osti'olisis) dissoluton of bone; applied especially to the removal or loss of calcium from the bone. adj. **osteolytic.**
osteoma (,osti'ohmə) a tumour, benign or malignant, composed of bony tissue; a hard tumour of bone-like structure developing on a bone (homoplastic osteoma) or other structures (heteroplastic osteoma).
BENIGN OSTEOMA. Benign tumours of bone are slow growing and often cause no symptoms. They frequently are first noticed as a swelling in the area; if they involve the joints symptoms result from decreased mobility. As the tumour develops, the patient experiences pain and tenderness, and pathological fractures are not uncommon with large tumours. Treatment includes surgical removal of the tumour and repair of the affected bone. Some benign tumours require no treatment.
MALIGNANT OSTEOMA. Malignant bone tumours that arise from bone (sarcoma) are rare, only about 15 occurring per million persons. They are found most often in children and young adults.

Cancer that spreads to bone tissue from other parts of the body usually is carcinoma rather than sarcoma.

Cancer of the bone can spread to other organs of the body through the blood and lymph channels. It tends to metastasize to the lungs, and from the lungs to the brain or the organs of the abdomen.
Symptoms. Symptoms of bone cancer are pain, swelling, and disability in the area of the diseased bones. The pain at first is mild, stops and starts again, and then becomes increasingly severe. Swelling may appear soon after the first signs of pain, but often it cannot be seen until later. The disability may affect a nearby joint, such as the knee, shoulder, or hip. There may also be a hard, painful lump over which the skin moves freely. The skin temperature in the area may be slightly elevated.
Diagnosis and Treatment. Diagnosis of bone tumour is made after examination of radiographs and a microscopic study of the suspected tissue. Malignant tumours can be treated by radiotherapy and surgery during the early stage of development. The prognosis for these tumours is grave, however. Hormone therapy and medication can also be helpful in certain types of the disease.
o. cutis a condition in which bone-containing nodules form in the skin; called also *osteodermia* and *osteosis cutis*.
o. durum, o. eburneum one containing hard bony tissue.
o. medullare one containing marrow spaces.
osteoid o. a small, benign but painful, circumscribed tumour of spongy bone, occurring especially in the bones of the extremities and vertebrae, most often in young persons.
o. spongiosum one containing cancellated bone.
osteomalacia (,ostiohmə'layshi·ə) softening of the bones, resulting from impaired mineralization, with excess accumulation of osteoid, caused by a vitamin D deficiency in adults. adj. **osteomalacic.** A similar condition in children is called RICKETS. The deficiency may be due to lack of exposure to ultraviolet rays, inadequate intake of vitamin D in the diet, or failure to absorb or utilize vitamin D.

The disease is characterized by decalcification of the bones, particularly those of the spine, pelvis, and lower extremities. Radiological examination reveals transverse, fracture-like lines in the affected bones and areas of demineralization in the matrix of the bone. As the bones soften they become bent, flattened, or otherwise deformed.

Treatment consists of administration of large daily doses of vitamin D and dietary measures to insure adequate calcium and phosphorus intake.
osteomatoid (,osti'ohmə,toyd) resembling an osteoma.
osteomere ('ostioh,miə) one of a series of similar bony structures, such as the vertebrae.
osteometry (,osti'omətree) measurement of the bones.
osteomyelitis (,ostioh,mieə'lietis) inflammation of bone, localized or generalized, due to a pyogenic infection. It may result in bone destruction, in stiffening of joints if the infection spreads to the joints, and, in extreme cases occurring before the end of the growth period, in the shortening of a limb if the growth centre is destroyed.

Acute osteomyelitis is caused by bacteria that enter the body through a wound, spread from an infection near the bone, or come from a skin or throat infection. The infection usually affects the long bones of the arms and legs and causes acute pain and fever. It most often occurs in children and adolescents, particularly boys.

The onset may be quite sudden, with chills, high fever and severe pain. Signs and symptoms include a marked increase in leukocytes, tenderness, swelling, redness of the skin over the bone involved, and bacteraemia. About 10 to 14 days after the onset of symptoms, radiographs show signs of the bone infection.

Usually, antibiotic treatment will clear the infection. If not, the infection destroys areas of the bone involved and an abscess forms. Acute osteomyelitis may become chronic, especially if the patient has a low resistance to infection. Tuberculous osteomyelitis is caused by tubercle bacilli that enter the bloodstream and settle in a bone. The disease progresses slowly and is chronic. Any bone may be infected but those most commonly involved are the vertebrae. Spinal tuberculosis, or POTT'S DISEASE, causes bone destruction and often spinal deformities. Other bones that may be affected are the long bones of the hands or feet.
TREATMENT. Treatment of acute osteomyelitis consists of administration of antibiotics and sometimes surgical drainage of the abscess. Fragments of dead bone (sequestra) that remain and prevent healing must be

removed surgically. If the blood supply to the bone is not obstructed, the bone can grow back. Treatment of chronic osteomyelitis is similar to that for the acute type.

Tuberculous osteomyelitis is treated like other forms of TUBERCULOSIS and sometimes by surgical drainage and immobilization of the bones involved.

PATIENT CARE. Absolute rest of the affected part is essential to proper healing and prevention of deformity. Because of pain and local tenderness one must be very gentle in handling the patient. Proper positioning with pillows and sandbags helps relieve the discomfort and also keeps the affected limb in good alignment. When a cast has been applied to ensure immobilization, the nursing care is the same as for any patient in a cast (see CAST). Drainage from the infected bone must be considered grossly contaminated and requires special precautions so that the infection is not spread to others.

Since most patients with osteomyelitis are children, schooling, occupational therapy, play or diversionary activities must be devised to ensure adequate rest for the affected bone. The parents must also be cautioned against letting the child indulge in strenuous exercise during the convalescent period at home. At all times during both the acute stage and the convalescent period the patient must be protected from other infections, which may result in a recurrence of symptoms. A well balanced diet, adequate periods of rest and other measures to promote the general well-being of the patient are important in overcoming the infection and preventing complications.

Garré's o., sclerosing nonsuppurative o. a chronic form involving the long bones, especially the tibia and femur, marked by a diffuse inflammatory reaction, increased density and spindle-shaped sclerotic thickening of the cortex, and an absence of suppuration.

osteomyelodysplasia (ˌostioh,mieəlohdis'playzi·ə) a condition characterized by thinning of the osseous tissue of bones, increase in size of the marrow cavities, and associated leukopenia and fever.

osteomyxochondroma (ˌostioh,miksohkon'drohmə) an osteochondroma with myxoid elements.

osteon ('ostion) the basic unit of structure of compact bone, comprising a haversian canal and its concentrically arranged lamellae.

osteonecrosis (ˌostiohnə'krohsis) necrosis of a bone.

osteoneuralgia (ˌostiohnyuh'ralji·ə, -jə) neuralgia of a bone.

osteopath ('ostioh,path) a practitioner of OSTEOPATHY.

osteopathia (ˌostioh'pathi·ə) osteopathy (1). **o. condensans disseminata** osteopoikilosis.

o. striata an asymptomatic condition characterized radiographically by multiple condensations of cancellous bone tissue, giving a striated appearance.

osteopathology (ˌostiohpə'tholəjee) any disease of bone.

osteopathy (ˌosti'opəthee) 1. any disease of a bone. 2. a system of therapy utilizing generally accepted physical, medicinal, and surgical methods of diagnosis and therapy, and emphasizing the importance of normal body mechanics and manipulative methods of detecting and correcting faulty structure. adj. **osteopathic.**

Osteopathy is founded on the theory that the body is capable of producing the remedies necessary to protect itself against disease and other toxic conditions when it is in normal structural relationship and has favourable environmental conditions and adequate nutrition.

During the past few decades, many changes have been made in the practice of osteopathy, bringing it closely into line with conventional medical practices. While still holding to the tenet that the body is a unit that possesses the inherent ability to overcome most curable diseases, osteopaths recognize that physical, chemical, and nutritional factors influence the state of health and that medicines and surgery are necessary in the treatment of disease. Disorders that can be recognized are treated as distinct diseases, and manipulation may or may not be used as an adjunct to other treatment.

osteopenia (ˌostioh'peeni·ə) reduced bone mass due to a decrease in the rate of osteoid synthesis to a level insufficient to compensate for normal bone lysis. The term is also used to refer to any decrease in bone mass below the normal. adj. **osteopenic.**

osteoperiosteal (ˌostioh,peri'osti·əl) pertaining to bone and its periosteum.

osteoperiostitis (ˌostioh,perio'stietis) inflammation of a bone and its periosteum.

osteopetrosis (ˌostiohpe'trohsis) a hereditary disease marked by abnormally dense bone, and by the common occurrence of fractures of affected bone. It may lead to obliteration of the marrow spaces, causing anaemia. Called also *Albers-Schönberg disease* and *marble bones.*

osteophage ('ostioh,fayj) osteoclast.

osteophlebitis (ˌostiohfli'bietis) inflammation of the veins of a bone.

osteophony (ˌosti'ofənee) bone conduction.

osteophore ('ostioh,for) a bone-crushing forceps.

osteophyma, osteophyte (ˌostioh,fiemə; 'ostioh,fiet) a bony excrescence or outgrowth.

osteoplasty ('ostioh,plastee) plastic surgery of the bones.

osteopoikilosis (ˌostioh,poyki'lohsis) a mottled condition of bones, apparent radiographically, due to the presence of multiple sclerotic foci and scattered stippling. adj. **osteopoikilotic.**

osteoporosis (ˌostiohpor'rohsis) abnormal rarefaction of bone which may be idiopathic or secondary to other conditions. adj. **osteoporotic.**

The disorder leads to thinning of the skeleton and decreased precipitation of lime salts. There also may be inadequate calcium absorption into the bone and excessive bone resorption.

The principal causes are lack of physical activity, lack of oestrogens or androgens, and nutritional deficiency. There is almost always some degree of osteoporosis that occurs with ageing.

Symptoms include pathological fractures and collapse of the vertebrae without compression of the spinal cord. The latter is often discovered 'accidentally' on radiological examination made for some other reason. Treatment varies with the cause but hormone therapy is helpful in most cases. Measures are taken to improve the nutritional status, and a diet high in protein and calcium is recommended. Patients should be kept active and those confined to bed must be given passive and active exercises. Prognosis usually is good when treatment is carried out diligently.

o. circumscripta demineralization occurring in localized areas of bone, especially in the skull.

o. of disuse that occurring when the normal laying down of bone is slowed because of lack of the normal stimulus of functional stress on the bone.

post-traumatic o. loss of bone substance after an injury in which there is nerve damage, sometimes due to decreased blood supply caused by the neurogenic insult, or to disuse secondary to pain. Called also *Sudeck's disease.*

osteoradionecrosis (ˌostioh,raydiohnə'krohsis) necrosis of bone as a result of excessive exposure to radiation.

osteorrhagia (ˌosti·ə'rayji·ə) haemorrhage from bone.

osteorrhaphy (ˌosti'o·rəfee) fixation of fragments of bone with sutures or wires; called also *osteosuture*.

osteosarcoma (ˌostiohsah'kohmə) osteogenic sarcoma. adj. **osteosarcomatous.**

osteosclerosis (ˌostiohsklə'rohsis) the hardening, or abnormal density, of bone. adj. **osteosclerotic.**

o. congenita achondroplasia.

o. fragilis osteopetrosis; so called because of frequency of pathological fracture of affected bones.

o. fragilis generalisata osteopoikilosis.

osteosis (ˌosti'ohsis) the formation of bony tissue.

o. cutis osteoma cutis.

osteostixis (ˌostioh'stiksis) surgical puncture of a bone.

osteosuture (ˌostioh'soochə) osteorrhaphy.

osteosynovitis (ˌostiohˌsienoh'vietis) synovitis with osteitis of neighbouring bones.

osteosynthesis (ˌostioh'sinthəsis) surgical fastening of the ends of a fractured bone.

osteotabes (ˌostioh'taybeez) a disease, chiefly of infants, in which bone marrow cells are destroyed and the marrow disappears.

osteothrombosis (ˌostiohthrom'bohsis) thrombosis of the veins of a bone.

osteotome ('ostiohˌtohm) a chisel-like knife for cutting bone.

osteotomoclasis (ˌostiohtə'mokləsis) correction of bone curvature by partial division with the osteotome, followed by forcible fracture.

osteotomy (ˌosti'otəmee) incision or transection of a bone.

cuneiform o. removal of a wedge of bone.

displacement o. surgical division of a bone and shifting of the divided ends to change the alignment of the bone or to alter weight-bearing stresses.

ostitis (o'stietis) osteitis.

ostium ('osti·əm) pl. *ostia* [L.] a mouth or orifice; used in anatomical nomenclature as a general term to designate an opening into a tubular organ, or between two distinct body cavities. adj. **ostial.**

o. abdominale the fimbriated end of the uterine tube.

coronary o. either of the two openings in the aortic sinus which mark the origin of the (left and right) coronary arteries.

o. internum ostium uterinum tubae.

o. pharyngeum the nasopharyngeal end of the pharyngotympanic tube.

o. primum an opening in the lower portion of the membrane dividing the embryonic heart into right and left sides. See also CONGENITAL HEART DEFECT.

o. secundum an opening in the upper portion of the membrane dividing the embryonic heart into right and left sides, appearing later than the ostium primum. See also CONGENITAL HEART DEFECT.

tympanic o., o. tympanicum the opening of the pharyngotympanic tube on the carotid wall of the tympanic cavity.

o. uteri the external opening of the cervix of the uterus into the vagina.

o. uterinum tubae the point where the cavity of the uterine tube becomes continuous with that of the uterus.

o. vaginae the external orifice of the vagina.

OStJ Officer of the Order of St. John of Jerusalem.

OT occupational therapy; old tuberculin.

ot(o)- word element. [Gr.] *ear*.

otalgia (oh'talji·ə) pain in the ear; earache; otodynia.

OTC over the counter; applied to drugs not required by law to be sold on prescription only.

otectomy (oh'tektəmee) excision of tissues of the internal and middle ear.

othelcosis (ˌoht·hel'kohsis) 1. ulceration of the auricle or external meatus of the ear. 2. suppuration of the middle ear.

Othello syndrome (complex) (ə'theloh) a state of delusional jealousy arising in some paranoid states and occasionally in alcoholism.

othemorrhoea (ˌoht·hemə'reeə) otorrhagia.

otic ('ohtik) pertaining to the ear; aural.

otitis (oh'tietis) inflammation of the ear. adj. **otitic.**

aviation o. a symptom complex resulting from fluctuations between atmospheric pressure and air pressure in the middle ear; called also *barotitis media*.

o. externa inflammation of the external ear.

furuncular o. the formation of furuncles in the external ear.

o. interna, o. labyrinthica labyrinthitis.

o. mastoidea inflammation of the mastoid spaces.

o. media inflammation of the middle ear, occurring most often in infants and young children, and classified as *serous*, *secretory*, and *suppurative*. All three types characteristically result in accumulations of fluid behind the tympanic membrane with some degree of hearing loss.

SEROUS OTITIS MEDIA. In this condition the pharyngotympanic tube fails to maintain equality of the barometric pressure within and outside the middle ear; when the tube fails to open and close as it should air within the middle ear is under negative pressure. This causes inward retraction of the ear drum and movement of serous fluid from the mucosal capillaries into the middle ear space. The serous fluid can fill up the space and cause conductive hearing loss.

Acute serous otitis media usually follows an upper respiratory infection or trauma to the ear or is associated with an allergy or enlarged adenoids or both. Symptoms are mild and may consist only of a feeling of fullness in the ear and some evidence of hearing loss.

Although chronic otitis media also causes hearing loss, a young child may not be aware of this and offer no complaints. Treatment consists of removal of the primary cause by elimination of infection, therapy for allergy, and removal of enlarged adenoids. If the accumulation of serous fluid persists, MYRINGOTOMY and insertion of a ventilatory tube may be necessary.

SECRETORY OTITIS MEDIA. In this condition it is not the pharyngotympanic tube that is involved but rather the structures in the middle ear itself. Probably because of a primary allergic response, the mucosae secrete large amounts of an amber, mucoid, or greyish fluid, as in serous otitis media. Antihistamines and decongestants are administered, and a myringotomy and placement of ventilating tubes may be necessary to permit drainage of the excess fluid.

SUPPURATIVE OTITIS MEDIA. Purulent bacteria in the middle ear cause suppurative otitis media, gaining access from the nasopharynx with an upper respiratory infection.

Symptoms may include acute pain, irritability, difficulty in sleeping, and loss of hearing. If sufficient pressure builds up behind the tympanic membrane it may rupture spontaneously and exude a purulent discharge. If the pus-laden fluid breaks through internally it can result in intracranial abscess, meningitis, and mastoiditis. Acute suppurative otitis media is treated aggressively with antibiotics and tympanocentesis (MYRINGOTOMY) to relieve pressure and obtain fluid for bacterial culture. When the condition becomes chronic there is continuous otorrhoea and hearing loss. In addition to antibiotics, treatment includes topical therapy with ear drops, tympanoplasty to repair a ruptured ear drum and damaged ossicles, and, sometimes, mastoidectomy to eliminate all sources of infection.

o. media sclerotica sclerosis of the structures of the middle ear due to chronic inflammation.

otoantritis (ˌohtoh·an'trietis) inflammation of the attic of the tympanum and the mastoid antrum.

Otobius (oh'tohbi·əs) a genus of soft-bodied ticks whose larvae are parasitic in the ears of various animals and known also to infest man.

otoblennorrhea (ˌohtohˌblenə'reeə) mucous discharge from the ear.

otocephalus (ˌohtoh'kefələs, -'sef-) an individual exhibiting otocephaly.

otocephaly (ˌohtoh'kefəlee, -'sef-) a congenital malformation characterized by lack of a lower jaw and by ears that are united below the face.

otocleisis (ˌohtoh'kliesis) closure of the auditory passages.

otoconia (ˌohtoh'kohni·ə) statoconia.

otocranium (ˌohtoh'krayni·əm) 1. the chamber in the petrous bone lodging the internal ear. 2. the auditory portion of the cranium. adj. **otocranial.**

otocyst ('ohtohˌsist) 1. the auditory vesicle of the embryo. 2. the organ of hearing in some lower animals.

otodynia (ˌohtoh'dini·ə) pain in the ear; earache; otalgia.

otoencephalitis (ˌohtoh·enˌkefə'lietis, -ˌsefə-) inflammation of brain extending from an inflamed middle ear.

otoganglion (ˌohtoh'gang·gli·ən) the otic ganglion.

otogenic, otogenous (ˌohtoh'jenik; oh'tojənəs) originating within the ear.

otography (oh'tografee) description of the ear.

otolaryngology (ˌohtohˌlaring'goləjee) that branch of medicine dealing with disease of the ear, nose and throat; called also *otorhinolaryngology*.

otolith ('ohtohˌlith) statolith.

otologist (oh'toləjist) a specialist in otology.

otology (oh'toləjee) the branch of medicine dealing with the ear and its anatomy, physiology, and pathology. adj. **otological.**

otomassage (ˌohtoh'masahzh, -sahj) massage of the middle ear and ossicles.

otomucormycosis (ˌohtohˌmyookawmie'kohsis) mucormycosis of the ear.

otomycosis (ˌohtohmie'kohsis) a fungal infection of the external auditory meatus and ear canal. The infection thrives in warm, moist climates and is encouraged by poor local hygiene and swimming. Symptoms include itching, which may be intense, pain, and a stinging sensation in the external acoustic meatus.

The condition is treated with antibiotics to prevent secondary infection and the administration of ear drops containing neomycin or polymyxin B sulphate. The area should be cleaned locally with dilute aluminium acetate solution combined with acetic acid before ear drops are applied.

otoneurology (ˌohtohnyuh'roləjee) that branch of otology dealing especially with those portions of the nervous system related to the ear. adj. **otoneurological.**

otopathy (oh'topəthee) any disease of the ear.

otopharyngeal (ˌohtohfə'rinji·əl, -ˌfarin'jeeəl) pertaining to the ear and pharynx.

otoplasty ('ohtohˌplastee) plastic sugery of the ear.

otopolypus (ˌohtoh'polipəs) a polyp in the ear.

otopyorrhoea (ˌohtohˌpieə'reeə) a copious purulent discharge from the ear.

otorhinolaryngology (ˌohtohˌrienohˌlaring'goləjee) the branch of medicine dealing with disease of the ear, nose, and throat; called also *otolaryngology*.

otorhinology (ˌohtohrie'noləjee) the branch of medicine dealing with ear and nose.

otorrhagia (ˌohtə'rayji·ə) haemorrhage from the ear.

otorrhoea (ˌohtə'reeə) a discharge from the ear.

otosclerosis (ˌohtohsklə'rohsis) the formation of spongy bone in the capsule of the labyrinth of the ear, often causing the auditory ossicles to become fixed and less able to pass on vibrations when sound enters the ear. adj. **otosclerotic.** The ossicle chiefly involved in the condition is the stirrup or stapes, which becomes fixed to the oval window.

The cause of otosclerosis is still unknown. It may be hereditary, or perhaps related to vitamin deficiency or otitis media. An early symptom is ringing in the ears, but the most noticeable symptom is progressive loss of hearing.

This disease usually begins in the teens or early twenties. It strikes women about twice as often as men, and may be worsened by pregnancy.

Although no cure is known, recently developed surgical techniques can often restore hearing by freeing the stirrup or replacing it with other tissue. In this operation, STAPEDECTOMY, the stirrup is removed and replaced with grafted body tissue attached to a stainless steel wire or plastic tube.

In some cases of otosclerosis the hearing loss may be relieved by the use of a hearing aid.

otoscope ('ohtohˌskohp) an instrument for inspecting or auscultating the ear.

otoscopy (oh'toskəpee) examination of the external acoustic meatus with an otoscope.

otospongiosis (ˌohtohˌspunji'ohsis) the formation of spongy bone in the bony labyrinth of the ear.

Otosporin (ohtə'sporin) trademark for a combination preparation containing hydrocortisone, neomycin and polymyxin.

otosteal (oh'tosti·əl) pertaining to the ossicles of the ear.

ototomy (oh'totəmee) dissection of the ear.

ototoxic (ˌohtoh'toksik) having a deleterious effect upon the eighth cranial (vestibulocochlear) nerve or on the organs of hearing and balance.

ototoxicity (ˌohtohtok'sisitee) the property of being ototoxic.

Otrivine ('otrivin) trademark for preparations of xylometazoline, a nasal decongestant.

Otto pelvis ('otoh) a pelvis in which the acetabulum is depressed, with protrusion of the femoral head into the pelvis.

ouabain (wah'bah·in, 'wahbayn) a cardiac glycoside obtained chiefly from the plant *Strophanthus gratus*; its effect is similar to that of digitalis, but digitalization is achieved more rapidly.

ounce (owns) a measure of weight in both the avoirdupois and the apothecaries' system; abbreviation oz. The ounce avoirdupois is 1/16 lb, or 437.5 gr, or 28.3495 g. The apothecaries' ounce is 1/12 lb, or 480 gr, or 31.103 g; symbol ℥.

fluid o. a unit of liquid measure of the apothecaries' system, being 8 fluid drams, or the equivalent of 29.57 ml.

outlet ('owtlet) a means or route of exit or egress.

pelvic o. the inferior opening of the pelvis; literally that bounded by the ischial spines, lower border of the symphisis pubis and the sacrococcygeal joint.

outpatient ('owtˌpayshənt) a patient who comes to the hospital, clinic, or dispensary for diagnosis and/or treatment but does not occupy a bed overnight.

outpocketing (owt'pokiting) evagination.

output ('owtˌpuht) the yield or total of anything produced by any functional system of the body.

cardiac o. the effective volume of blood expelled by either ventricle of the heart per unit of time (usually volume per minute); it is equal to the stroke output multiplied by the number of beats per the time unit used in the computation.

energy o. the energy a body is able to manifest in work or activity.

stroke o. the amount of blood ejected by each ventricle at each beat of the heart.

urinary o. the amount of urine secreted by the kidneys (see also FLUID BALANCE).

ova ('ohvə) plural of *ovum.*

ovalocyte ('ohvəloh,siet) elliptocyte, an elliptical erythrocyte.

ovalocytosis (,ohvəlohsie'tohsis) elliptocytosis.

ovari(o)- word element. [L.] *ovary;* see also words beginning *oophor(o)-*.

ovarialgia (,ohvə·ri'alji·ə) pain in an ovary.

ovarian (oh'vair·ri·ən) pertaining to an ovary.

ovarian vein syndrome obstruction of the ureter due to compression by an enlarged or varicose ovarian vein; typically the vein becomes enlarged during pregnancy, the symptoms being those of obstruction or infection of the upper urinary tract. The right side is usually affected.

ovariectomy (,ohvə·ri'ektəmee) excision of an ovary (see also OOPHORECTOMY).

ovariocele (oh'vair·rioh,seel) hernia of an ovary.

ovariocentesis (oh,vair·riohsen'teesis) surgical puncture of an ovary.

ovariocyesis (oh,vair·riohsie'eesis) ovarian pregnancy.

ovariopexy (oh,vair·rioh'peksee) the operation of elevating and fixing an ovary to the abdominal wall.

ovariorrhexis (oh,vair·ri·ə'reksis) rupture of an ovary.

ovariosalpingectomy (oh,vair·rioh,salpin'jektəmee) excision of an ovary and uterine tube.

ovariostomy (oh,vair·ri'ostəmee) incision of an ovary, with drainage; oophorostomy.

ovariotomy (oh,vair·ri'otəmee) surgical removal of an ovary, or removal of an ovarian tumour.

ovariotubal (oh,vair·rioh'tyoob'l) pertaining to an ovary and uterine tube.

ovaritis (,ohvə'rietis) inflammation of an ovary; oophoritis.

ovarium (oh'vair·ri·əm) pl. *ovaria* [L.] ovary.

ovary ('ohvə·ree) the female gonad; either of the sex glands in the female in which the ova are formed. adj. **ovarian.** Almond-shaped and about the size of large walnuts, the two ovaries are located in the lower abdomen one on either side of the uterus.

FUNCTIONS OF THE OVARIES. The ovaries have two basic functions: ovulation and the production of hormones, chiefly oestrogen and progesterone, which influence a woman's feminine physical characteristics and affect the reproductive process. See also OVULATION and REPRODUCTION.

DISORDERS OF THE OVARIES. One of the commonest disorders of the ovary is a cyst. Not all so-called ovarian cysts are true cysts; many are tumours. Ovarian cysts occur frequently and in a variety of sizes and types.

The commonest ovarian cysts are simple follicle retention cysts, small and frequently numerous cysts containing a clear fluid. Ordinarily follicle cysts disappear without treatment within 2 months. They do not change into malignant growths.

Another type of ovarian cyst, the mucinous cystadenoma, is in reality a tumour. These tumours may reach enormous size, creating pressure within the abdominopelvic cavity. Although these tumours are benign, they may become malignant.

DERMOID CYSTS of the ovary are usually benign although they may be subject to malignant change. They grow slowly and when opened after removal are found to be filled with a thick, yellow sebaceous fluid.

Oophoritis (inflammation of an ovary) may be caused by infection reaching the ovary by way of the uterine tube. Tuberculous and streptococcal infections of the ovary are common, and the ovary may also become infected in GONORRHOEA. Fever and pain, sometimes accompanied by swelling, are the usual symptoms. Sulphonamides and antibiotics usually can eliminate the infection, but if it fails to respond to treatment, surgery may become necessary. Surgical removal of an ovary is called OOPHORECTOMY, or ovariectomy.

Tumours of the ovary are generally classified as malignant or benign. They may arise from misplaced endometrial tissue or from the ovarian tissues. Malignant cells from other organs may travel to the ovary and set up a secondary malignant tumour in the ovary; an example is Krukenberg's tumour, which usually originates in the stomach.

Symptoms of an ovarian tumour usually do not present themselves until the tumour is fairly well advanced. Tumours in the early stage are usually found during a routine examination. Treatment of these tumours in all stages involves surgical removal or the use of radiotherapy or a combination of the two.

overbite ('ohvə,biet) 1. extension of incisal edges of the upper anterior teeth below the incisal edges of the anterior teeth in the lower jaw when the jaws are closed normally. 2. a measure of the vertical overlap between the upper and lower incisor teeth when in occlusion.

overcompensation (,ohvə,kompən'sayshən) a term introduced by Alfred ADLER for exaggerated and pathological striving for power and dominance in compensation for overpowering feelings of inferiority.

overdenture (,ohvə'denchə) a complete denture supported both by mucosa and by a few remaining natural teeth that have been altered, as by insertion of a long or short coping, to permit the denture to fit over them.

overdosage (,ohvə'dohsij) 1. the administration of an excessive dose. 2. the condition resulting from an excessive dose.

overdose ('ohvə,dohs) 1. to administer an excessive dose. 2. an excessive dose.

overhydration (,ohvə·hie'drayshən) a state of excess fluids in the body.

overjet ('ohvə,jet) 1. extension of the incisal or buccal cusp edges of the upper teeth labially or buccally to the edges of the teeth in the lower jaw when the jaws are closed normally. 2. a measure of the horizontal overlap between the upper and lower incisor teeth when in occlusion.

overlay ('ohvə,lay) a later component superimposed on a preexisting state or condition.

psychogenic o. an emotionally determined increment to a preexisting symptom or disability of organic or physically traumatic origin.

overventilation (,ohvə,venti'layshən) hyperventilation.

ovi- word element. [L.] *egg, ovum.*

ovicide ('ohvi,sied) an agent destructive to the ova of certain organisms.

oviduct ('ohvi,dukt, 'ovi-) a passage through which ova leave the maternal body or pass to an organ communicating with the exterior of the body (see also UTERINE TUBE). adj. **oviducal, oviductal.**

oviferous (oh'vifə·rəs) producing ova.

oviform ('ohvi,fawm) egg-shaped.

ovigenesis (,ohvi'jenəsis) oogenesis. adj. **ovigenetic.**

ovine ('ohvien) pertaining to, characteristic of, or derived from sheep.

oviparous (oh'vipə·rəs) producing eggs in which the embryo develops outside of the maternal body, as in birds.

oviposition (,ohvipə'zishən) the act of laying or

depositing eggs.

ovipositor (ˌohviˈpozitə) a specialized organ by which many female insects deposit their eggs.

ovo- word element. [L.] *egg, ovum.*

ovoplasm (ˈohvohˌplazəm) the cytoplasm of an unfertilized ovum.

ovotestis (ˌohvohˈtestis) a gonad containing both testicular and ovarian tissue.

ovoviviparous (ˌohvohviˈvipə·rəs) bearing living young that hatch from eggs inside the maternal body, the embryo being nourished by food stored in the egg; said of lizards, etc.

Ovran (ˈovran) trademark for a preparation of levonorgestrel with ethinyloestradiol, an oral contraceptive.

Ovranette (ovrəˈnet) trademark for a combination preparation of levonorgestrel and ethinyloestradiol, an oral contraceptive.

ovular (ˈovyuhlə, ˈoh-) pertaining to an ovule or an ovum.

ovulation (ˌovyuhˈlayshən, ˌoh-) the discharge of the ovum from the GRAAFIAN FOLLICLE. adj. **ovulatory.** Normally, in an adult woman, ovulation occurs at intervals of about 28 days and alternates between the two ovaries. As a rule, only one ovum is produced, but occasionally ovulation produces two or more ova; if such ova subsequently become fertilized, the result may be multiple births, such as twins or triplets.

Ovulation takes place approximately at the midpoint of the menstrual cycle, 14 days before onset of the next menstruation. During the preceding weeks, a graafian follicle, or cell cluster in the ovary containing the ovum, grows from the size of a pinhead to that of a pea. At the moment of ovulation, the follicle bursts open and the ovum is discharged.

ovule (ˈovyool, ˈohv-) 1. the ovum within the graafian follicle. 2. any small, egg-like structure.

ovum (ˈohvəm) pl. *ova* [L.] egg; the female reproductive or germ cell which, after fertilization, is capable of developing into a new member of the same species; sometimes applied to any stage of the fertilized germ cell during cleavage and even until hatching or birth of the new individual. The human ovum consists of protoplasm that contains some yolk, enclosed by a cell wall consisting of two layers, an outer one (zona pellucida, zona radiata) and an inner, thin one (vitelline membrane). There is a large nucleus (germinal vesicle) within which is a nucleolus (germinal spot). adj. **ovular**.

centrolecithal o. one with the yolk concentrated at the centre of the egg, surrounded by a peripheral shell of cytoplasm, and with an island of cystoplasm surrounding the nucleus.

holoblastic o. one that undergoes total cleavage.

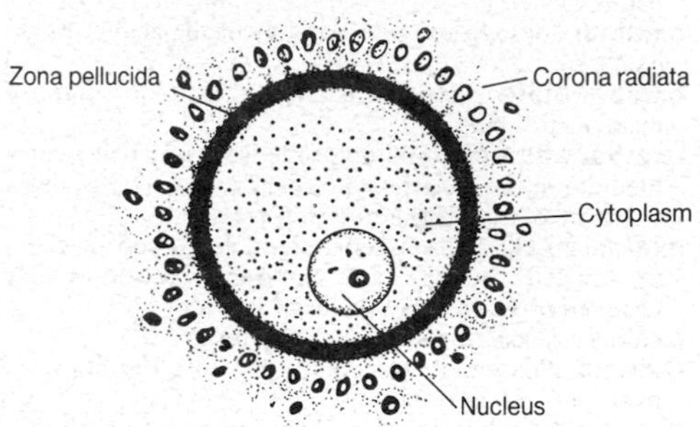

Human ovum.

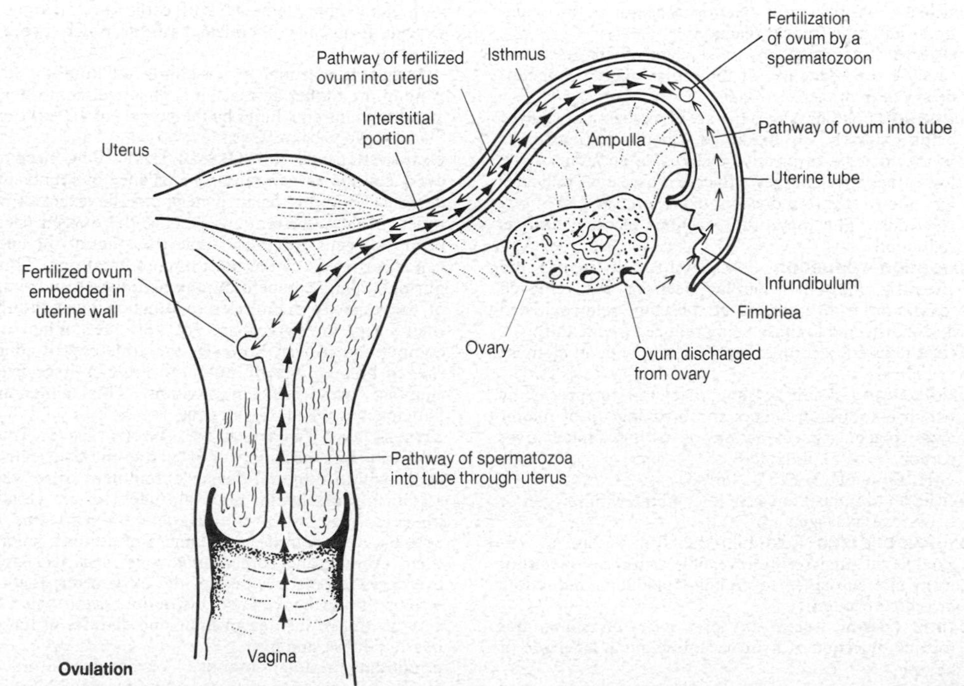

Ovulation

isolecithal o. one with a small amount of yolk evenly distributed throughout the cytoplasm.

meroblastic o. one that undergoes partial cleavage.

primitive o., primordial o. any egg cell very early in its development.

telolecithal o. one with a comparatively large amount of yolk massed at one pole.

Owren's disease ('owrenz) factor V deficiency.

oxalaemia (,oksə'leemi·ə) excess of oxalates in the blood.

oxalate ('oksə,layt) any salt of oxalic acid.

oxalic acid (ok'salik) a poisonous, dibasic acid found in various fruits and vegetables, and formed in the metabolism of ascorbic acid. It is highly toxic and if ingested should be neutralized by the administration of lime water (calcium hydroxide solution) or other convenient source of calcium, which reacts with the acid to form insoluble calcium oxalate. High urinary oxalate concentrations may cause the deposition of urinary calculi.

oxalism ('oksə,lizəm) poisoning by oxalic acid or by an oxalate.

oxaloacetate (,oksəloh'asitayt) a salt or ester of oxaloacetic acid.

oxaloacetic acid (,oksəloh·ə'seetik) a metabolic intermediate in the tricarboxylic acid cycle, which is also a substrate of aspartate aminotransferase.

oxalosis (,oksə'lohsis) generalized deposition of calcium oxalate, in renal and extrarenal tissues, as may occur in primary hyperoxaluria.

oxaluria (,oksə'lyooə·ri·ə) hyperoxaluria.

Oxamid ('oksəmid) trademark for a preparation of oxazepam; an anxiolytic.

oxazepam (ok'sazi,pam) a benzodiazepine tranquillizer, used as an antianxiety agent, especially in the elderly, and may be used as an adjunct for acute withdrawal symptoms in chronic alcoholics.

oxethazaine (ok'sethə,zayn) a topical anaesthetic, used orally to relieve gastric distress.

oxidant ('oksidənt) the electron acceptor in an oxidation–reduction (redox) reaction.

oxidase ('oksi,dayz) any of a class of enzymes that catalyse the reduction of molecular oxygen independently of hydrogen peroxide.

oxidation (,oksi'dayshən) the act of oxidizing or state of being oxidized. adj. **oxidative**. Chemically it consists in the increase of positive charges on an atom or the loss of negative charges. Univalent oxidation indicates loss of one electron; divalent oxidation, the loss of two electrons. The opposite reaction to oxidation is reduction.

oxidation–reduction (,oksi,dayshənri'dukshənn) the chemical reaction whereby electrons are removed (oxidation) from atoms of the substance being oxidized and transferred to those being reduced (reduction).

oxide ('oksied) a compound of oxygen with an element or radical.

oxidization (,oksidie'zayshən) oxidation; the process by which combustion occurs and breaking up of matter takes place; e.g. oxidation of carbohydrates gives carbon dioxide and water: $C_6H_{12}O_6 + 6O_2 = 6CO_2 + 6H_2O$.

oxidize ('oksi,diez) to cause to combine with oxygen or to remove hydrogen.

oxidoreductase (,oksidohri'duktayz) a class of enzymes that catalyse the reversible transfer of electrons from one substance to another (oxidation–reduction, or redox reaction).

oxime ('oksim, -seem) any of a series of compounds formed by action of hydroxylamine on an aldehyde or ketone.

oximeter (ok'simitə) a device for measuring oxygen concentration.

5-oxoproline (,fiev,oksoh'prohleen) a modified amino acid occurring in several proteins. Called also *pyroglutamic acid.*

5-oxoprolinuria (,fiev,oksoh,prohli'nyooə·ri·ə) an inborn error of metabolism marked by abnormally increased levels of 5-oxoproline in the urine, metabolic acidosis, and an increase in the rate of haemolysis. Called also *pyroglutamic aciduria.*

oxprenolol (oks'prenoh,lol) a beta-blocking drug used in the treatment of angina, hypertension and cardiac arrhythmias.

oxy- word element. [Gr.] *sharp, quick, sour, presence of oxygen in a compound.*

oxyaesthesia (,oksi·is'theezi·ə) abnormal acuteness of the senses.

oxybenzone (,oksi'benzohn) a topical sunscreening agent.

oxybuprocaine (be'noksi,nayt) a short-acting surface anaesthetic for the eye; used as drops.

oxycephaly (,oksi'kefəlee, -'sef-) a condition in which the top of the skull is pointed or conical owing to premature closure of the coronal and lambdoid sutures. adj. **oxycephalic**.

oxychlorosene (,oksi'klor·roh,seen) a stabilized organic complex of hypochlorous acid used as a topical antiseptic in the treatment of localized infections.

oxycinesia (,oksisi'neezi·ə) pain on motion.

oxycodone (,oksi'kohdohn) a semisynthetic narcotic analgesic derived from morphine.

oxygen ('oksijən) a chemical element, atomic number 8, atomic weight 15.999, symbol O. (See table of elements in Appendix 2.) It is a colourless and odourless gas that makes up about 20 per cent of the atmosphere. In combination with hydrogen, it forms water; by weight, 90 per cent of water is oxygen. It is the most abundant of all the elements of nature. Large quantities of it are distributed throughout the solid matter of the earth, because the gas combines readily with many other elements. With carbon and hydrogen, oxygen forms the chemical basis of much organic material.

Oxygen is essential in sustaining all kinds of life. Among the higher animals, it is obtained from the air and drawn into the lungs by the process of RESPIRATION. See also BLOOD GAS ANALYSIS.

OXYGEN BALANCE AND 'OXYGEN DEBT'. The need of every cell for oxygen requires a balance in supply and demand. But this balance need not be exact at all times. In fact, in strenuous exercise the oxygen needs of muscle cells are greater than the amount the body can absorb even by the most intense breathing. Thus, during athletic competition, the participants make use of the capacity of muscles to function even though their needs for oxygen are not fully met. When the competition is over, however, the athletes will continue to breathe heavily until the muscles have been supplied with sufficient oxygen. This temporary deficiency is called oxygen debt.

EFFECTS AND TREATMENT OF OXYGEN LACK. Total deprivation of the supply of oxygen to the body causes death within minutes. Severe curtailment of oxygen, as during ascent to high altitudes or in certain illnesses, may bring on a variety of symptoms of HYPOXIA, or oxygen lack. A number of poisons, among them cyanide and carbon monoxide, and also large overdoses of sedatives disrupt the oxygen distribution system of the body. Such disruption occurs also in various illness, such as anaemia and diseases of lungs, heart, kidneys, and liver.

o. content the total amount of oxygen in 100 ml of blood. Consists of oxygen bound to haemoglobin plus

oxygen in solution in the plasma. Its value is ascertained by measuring the amount of oxygen released from a sample of blood using either a fuel cell or the traditional Van Slyke apparatus.
o. saturation the amount of oxygen bound to haemoglobin in the blood expressed as a percentage of the maximal binding capacity. Oxygen saturation is measured with an oximeter which uses a spectrophotometric technique to assess the amount of deoxygenated haemoglobin in the blood. **o. tension** the partial pressure of oxygen in blood or a gas mixture measured in units of kilopascals or mmHg. It can be measured using a polarographic (Clark) electrode which uses electrochemical measurement like other blood gas analysers. Oxygen tension in gases can also be measured with either the paramagnetic analyser which makes use of the magnetic properties of oxygen or the galvanic fuel cell analyser.
o. tent a large plastic canopy that encloses the patient in a controlled environment; used for oxygen therapy, humidity therapy, or aerosol therapy.
o. therapy supplementary oxygen administered for the purpose of relieving hypoxaemia and preventing damage to the tissue cells as a result of oxygen lack (HYPOXIA). Oxygen can be toxic and therefore, as with a drug, its dosage and mode of administration are based on an assessment of the needs of the individual patient. Although many types of hypoxia can be treated successfully by the administration of oxygen, not all cases respond to this therapy. There is also the possibility that the injudicious use of oxygen can produce serious and permanent damage to the body tissues. The administration of oxygen should never be considered a 'routine' or harmless procedure.
ADVERSE EFFECTS OF OXYGEN. Although it is true that all living organisms require oxygen to maintain life, excessive amounts can be detrimental. For example, an environment of 100 per cent oxygen inhibits the growth of living tissue cultures, and laboratory experiments have shown that hyperoxygenation of the body tissues can cause irreversible damage. It is now known that inhaling 100 per cent oxygen can result in collapse of alveoli because of the displacement of nitrogen by the oxygen. RETROLENTAL FIBROPLASIA in preterm infants was found to be caused by excessively high levels of oxygen in the blood.

Another serious complication of oxygen therapy is high pressure resulting in the development of pulmonary oxygen toxicity. The pathological changes produced are not specific but resemble adult respiratory distress syndrome, that is hyaline membrane formation in alveoli, pulmonary oedema, cellular infiltration and, later, fibrosis. For this reason patients on long-term oxygen and especially those on mechanical ventilators are kept as far as possible on percentages of oxygen of less than 50 per cent.

The danger of oxygen toxicity can be minimized by careful assessment of each patient's need for oxygen therapy and the systematic monitoring of blood gases to determine patient response and effectiveness of treatment. See also BLOOD GAS ANALYSIS.

Symptoms of oxygen toxicity in the conscious patient are tracheitis, substernal distress due to tracheobronchitis, nausea and vomiting, malaise, fatigue, and numbness and tingling of the extremities.
INDICATIONS FOR OXYGEN THERAPY. In theory oxygen should be given whenever arterial oxygen tension (P_ao_2) falls below normal. As mild hypoxaemia does little damage to the patient and oxygen therapy carries its own risks, oxygen therapy should be reserved for patients with a potentially harmful degree of hyperaemia. The oxygen dissociation curve (see accompanying illustration) describes the relationship between oxygen saturation and oxygen tension and is sigmoid in shape. This shows that a fall in oxygen tension from the normal 100 mmHg (13.3 kPa) to 60 mmHg (8 kPa) is accompanied by a very small fall in oxygen saturation from 97 per cent to 90 per cent. Once the P_ao_2 reaches 60 mmHg (8 kPa) it is at the top of the steep portion of the curve and any further fall will cause a significant drop in saturation and therefore the amount of oxygen carried by the blood.

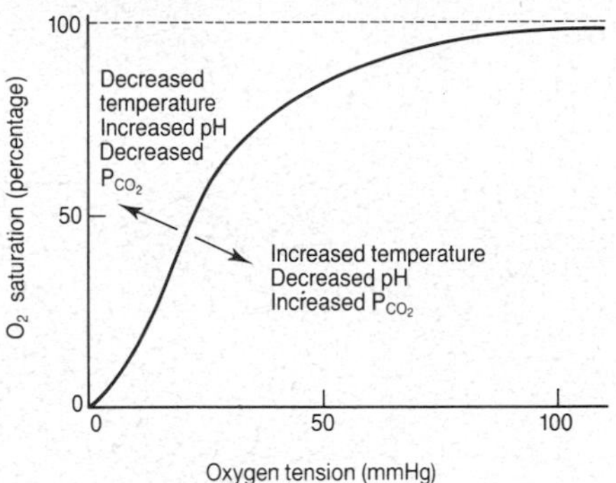

Oxygen – haemoglobin dissociation curve

Specific indications for oxygen therapy include the following: (1) Hypoventilation, due to either temporary depression of ventilation from drugs, or upper respiratory tract obstruction. The correct treatment of both is restoration of normal ventilation either by use of assisted or mechanical ventilation or by relief of the obstruction, but oxygen is used as a temporary expedient to maintain the P_ao_2. (2) Apnoea. Oxygen given to an apnoeic patient will obviously be ineffective but a period of apnoea can be tolerated if the patient breathes 100 per cent oxygen for several minutes prior to an apnoeic episode. This technique is used during general anaesthesia prior to intubation and in anaesthesia for laryngoscopy and bronchoscopy. Apnoea occurring from cardiovascular and/or respiratory arrest, or after endotracheal intubation, requires resuscitation with 100 per cent oxygen using self-inflating bag and mask. (3) Patients with circulatory failure from, for example, congestive cardiac failure, myocardial infarction and pulmonary embolism should be given oxygen to increase the oxygen supply to the tissues. Although haemoglobin is almost completely saturated with oxygen at normal arterial oxygen tension, patients breathing 100 per cent oxygen can increase the amount of oxygen carried in solution in the plasma by six times. (4) Postoperative patients have a reduced arterial P_ao_2, the degree and magnitude of which depend on the type of operation performed. Thoracic and upper abdominal operations are followed by hypoxaemia that lasts 6 to 10 days. Although oxygen is not given for this length of time, these patients particularly should receive oxygen in the postoperative period. (5) Patients with carbon monoxide poisoning.

In the above examples oxygen is given in moderate to high concentration. There is one situation—the patient with chronic obstructive airways disease—where the oxygen therapy must be strictly controlled. This is because these patients rely on hypoxia for their

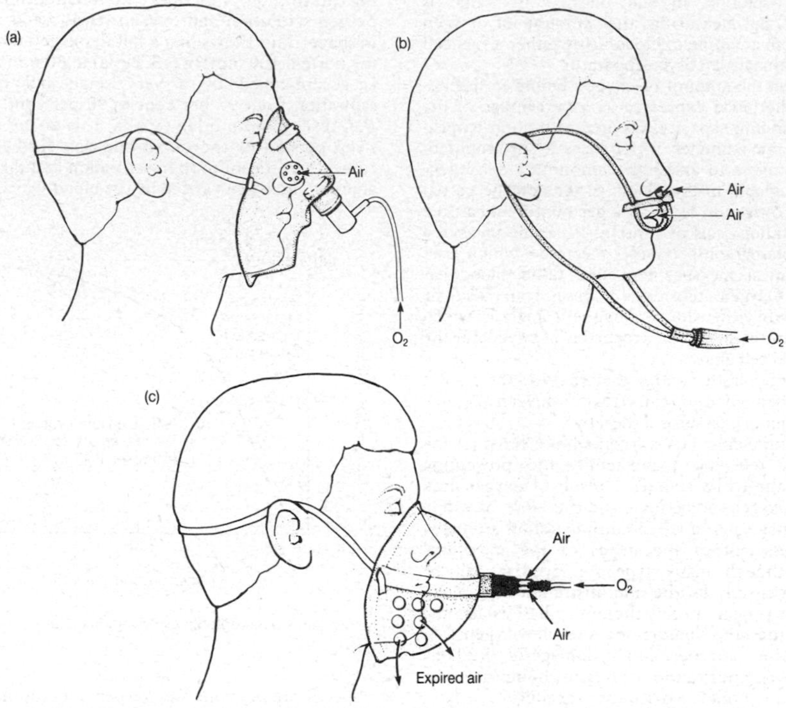

Devices for oxygen administration. (a) Simple face mask; (b) Nasal cannula; (c) Venturi mask

respiratory drive. Suddenly relieving their hypoxia leads to further hypoventilation and carbon dioxide narcosis. These patients often have arterial oxygen tensions toward the bottom of the steep part of the oxygen dissociation curve. Giving them low concentrations of oxygen will slightly increase their P_ao_2 but this will be accompanied by a marked increase in their oxygen saturation and a significant increase in the amount of oxygen carried in the blood.

The delivery of appropriate and effective oxygen therapy requires frequent monitoring of arterial blood gases. An initial BLOOD GAS ANALYSIS at the time the therapy is started provides baseline data with which to evaluate changes in the patient's status.

In addition to monitoring blood gases to assess the patient's need for and response to supplementary oxygen, it is helpful to observe the patient closely for signs of hypoxaemia. However, these signs are not as reliable as blood gas analysis because the clinical manifestations of hypoxaemia vary widely in individual patients. The typical clinical manifestations are confusion, impaired judgement, restlessness, tachycardia, central cyanosis, and loss of consciousness.

DOSAGE AND METHOD OF ADMINISTRATION. There must be specific written orders for flow rate and mode of administration of oxygen. Decisions about the initial dosage, as well as any changes in mode of administration and dosage, including the discontinuance of oxygen therapy, should be based on evaluation of the Po_2, the Pco_2, and the blood pH (BLOOD GAS ANALYSIS).

Oxygen is delivered to the patient through either a fixed performance or a variable performance device. Fixed performance devices deliver oxygen of a known percentage that does not vary in response to alterations in the patient's ventilation. Gases are premixed: either metered flows are delivered to a mask and reservoir bag system, or oxygen is delivered to a venturi device that entrains air to produce the final oxygen percentage. The former device is used to deliver close to 100 per cent oxygen, though it does depend on ensuring a tightly fitting mask while the latter is used for controlled oxygen therapy. By altering the entrainment ratio the percentage of oxygen delivered to the patient can be altered. Common values are 24, 28, 35 and 40 per cent.

In variable performance devices such as the Edinburgh, MC, and Hudson masks, the oxygen percentage delivered depends on oxygen flow to the mask and the patient's breathing pattern. It may vary therefore from breath to breath but this does not matter where moderately high concentrations of oxygen are required. These devices deliver anything from 24 to 80 per cent oxygen and are suitable for most situations where oxygen therapy is required.

Other methods of oxygen administration include: (1) The nasal catheter, a soft rubber or plastic tube inserted through the nose into the nasopharynx. Simple and efficient oxygen flows of one to four times a minute will produce percentages of 25 to 60 per cent. The oxygen should be humidified and the catheter changed to the opposite nostril every 4 to 6 hours. (2) Nasal spectacles are two short nasal cannulae inserted into the external nares of both nostrils. This is less efficient than the nasal catheter. The oxygen delivered to the lungs is dependent on the extent of nose breathing but flows of six times per minute produce 30 to 40 per cent. (3) Oxygen tents. These are not satisfactory for high concentration oxygen therapy: high oxygen flows are required, mixing is poor, it takes a long time for the oxygen concentration to build up, and the concentration falls whenever the tent is opened. Oxygen tents are occasionally used for children who cannot tolerate other forms of oxygen therapy.

Patient Care. No matter what mode of administration is used, it is essential that the inspired air be moisturized. This is necessary to prevent drying of the respiratory mucosa, inhibition of the action of the cilia, and thickening of secretions that can further inhibit the flow of air through the air passages. Humidity may be provided by humidifying the oxygen with water, or by nebulizing the water into fine particles and adding it to the oxygen. Most patients need 60 to 65 per cent relative humidity at room temperature. Patients with endotracheal tubes require as close to 100 per cent humidity as possible.

Oxygen is not an explosive gas, but it does support combustion and presents a serious fire hazard. All electrical equipment should be checked for defects that could produce sparks. All appliances that transmit house current must be kept outside an oxygen tent, and all equipment with exposed switches and meters must be considered potential sources of fire. Static electricity is a minimal risk which can be further reduced by maintaining a relatively high humidity in the oxygen tent. Smoking in the immediate area of oxygen administration is prohibited and there should be signs informing visitors and others of this restriction.

When the patient is wearing a mask for an extended period of time, his discomfort can be minimized by removing the mask and washing and drying his face every few hours. To be effective the mask must fit snugly and follow the contour of the face. This means that reddened areas will appear where the mask has pressed against the skin. These areas should be gently massaged and the skin lightly powdered to reduce friction.

Nasal catheters have a tendency to produce irritation of the nasal mucosa and therefore require frequent changing, using alternate nostrils. The patient may be more comfortable if some type of nonoily lubricant is applied to the nasal mucosa. Patients who have suffered stroke, are very elderly, or are deeply comatose may have diminished or absent epiglottal reflexes. In these cases the flow of oxygen may be directed into the stomach via the oesophagus. This presents the very real danger of gastric rupture at worst, and severe distention which may further aggravate breathing difficulties at best. For such patients it is suggested that a mode of oxygen administration other than nasal catheter be chosen.

A programme of infection control is especially important in the prevention of cross-infection from the equipment that is used to administer oxygen. Some humidifiers and nebulizers heat the water to 53 °C (127 °F) so as to increase water vapour and facilitate humidification. These may serve as sources of infection because they provide an excellent medium for the growth of bacteria and moulds. There is less danger of this happening when disposable equipment is used, but this does not preclude the need for a systematic development of policies and procedures to prevent and control the spread of infection. Each and every person involved in the care of the patient must be aware of this programme and cooperate in its implementation.

The termination of oxygen therapy is never done abruptly. The patient is gradually weaned from the oxygen administration by alternating periods of oxygen supplemented inspiration with periods of breathing without the additional oxygen.

oxygenase ('oksijə,nayz) any enzyme of the oxidoreductase class that catalyses the incorporation of both atoms of molecular oxygen into the substrate.

oxygenation (,oksijə'nayshən) saturation with oxygen.

hyperbaric o. exposure to oxygen under conditions of greatly increased pressure (see also HYPERBARIC OXYGENATION).

oxygenator ('oksijə,naytə) an apparatus by which oxygen is introduced into the blood during circulation outside the body, as during open-heart surgery. See also HEART–LUNG MACHINE.

bubble o. a device in which pure oxygen is bubbled through an extracorporeal reservoir of blood, either directly or through a filter.

film o. a device, encased in a container of oxygen, that makes possible reduction of a thin film of blood to facilitate the exchange of gases.

screen o. a type of film oxygenator in which the venous blood is passed over a series of screens in a container of oxygen, gaseous exchange taking place in the thin film of blood produced on the screens.

oxygeusia (,oksi'gyoozi·ə) extreme acuteness of the sense of taste.

oxyhaemoglobin (,oksi,heemə'glohbin) haemoglobin combined with molecular oxygen, the form in which oxygen is transported in the blood.

oxylalia (,oksi'layli·ə) rapidity of speech.

oxymetazoline (,oksimə'tazoh,leen) a vasoconstrictor used topically as the hydrochloride salt in nasal congestion.

oxymetholone (,oksi'methə,lohn) an anabolic steroid compound.

oxymyoglobin (,oksi,mieoh'glohbin) myoglobin charged with oxygen.

oxyntic (ok'sintik) secreting acid, as the parietal (oxyntic) cells.

oxypertine (,oksi'pərteen) an antipsychotic tranquillizing drug used in the treatment of schizophrenia and related psychoses, and of mania and hyperactivity.

oxyphil ('oksi,fil) 1. Hürthle cell. 2. oxyphilic.

oxyphilic, oxyphilous (,oksi'filik; ok'sifiləs) stainable with an acid dye.

oxyphonia (,oksi'fohni·ə) an abnormally sharp quality or pitch of the voice.

oxytalan (ok'sitə,lan) a connective tissue fibre found in the periodontal membrane.

oxytetracycline (,oksi,tetrə'siekleen) a broad-spectrum antibiotic of the tetracycline group produced by *Streptomyces rimosus*.

oxytocia (,oksi'tohsi·ə) rapid labour.

oxytocic (,oksi'tohsik) 1. pertaining to, marked by, or promoting oxytocia. 2. an agent that promotes rapid labour by stimulating contractions of the myometrium.

oxytocin (,oksi'tohsin) a hypothalamic hormone stored in and released from the posterior pituitary, or prepared synthetically. It acts as a powerful stimulant to the pregnant uterus, especially toward the end of gestation. The hormone also causes milk to be expressed from the alveoli into the lactiferous ducts during suckling.

Injection of oxytocin may be used to induce labour or strengthen the uterine contractions during labour, to contract uterine muscle after delivery of the placenta, and to control postpartum haemorrhage. It is administered with care so as to avoid trauma to the mother or infant by hyperactivity of the uterine muscles during labour. Oxytocin also may be administered intravenously by slow drip and it is sometimes applied to the mucous membranes of the nasal cavity and absorbed into the bloodstream.

oxyuriasis (ˌoksiyuh'rieəsis) infection with *Enterobius vermicularis* (in humans) or with other oxyurids; enterobiasis.

oxyuricide (ˌoksi'yooə·riˌsied) an agent that kills oxyurids.

oxyurid (ˌoksi'yooə·rid) a pinworm, seatworm, or threadworm; an individual organism of the superfamily Oxyuroidea.

Oxyuroidea (ˌoksiyuh'roydi·ə) a superfamily of small nematodes—the pinworms, seatworms, or threadworms—usually parasitic in the caecum and colon of vertebrates, but may infect invertebrates.

oz. ounce.

ozena (oh'zeenə) an atrophic rhinitis marked by a thick mucopurulent discharge, mucosal crusting, and fetor.

ozone ('ohzohn) a bluish explosive gas or blue liquid, being an allotropic form of oxygen, O_3; it is antiseptic and disinfectant, and irritating and toxic to the pulmonary system.

ozostomia (ˌohzoh'stohmi·ə) foulness of the breath.

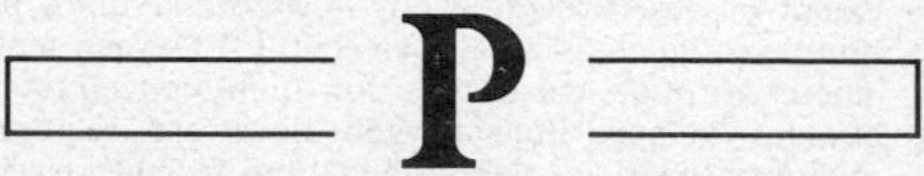

P chemical symbol, *phosphorus*; symbol *peta-*.

P probability.

P_1 parental generation.

P_2 pulmonic second sound (see HEART SOUNDS).

P_{CO_2} carbon dioxide partial pressure or tension; also written P_{CO_2}, pCO_2, or pCO_2 (see RESPIRATION and BLOOD GAS ANALYSIS).

P_{O_2} oxygen partial pressure (tension); also written P_{O_2}, pO_2, and pO_2 (see also BLOOD GAS ANALYSIS).

P_{aCO_2} symbol for partial pressure of carbon dioxide in the arterial blood (see also BLOOD GAS ANALYSIS).

P_{aO_2} symbol for partial pressure of oxygen in arterial blood (see also BLOOD GAS ANALYSIS).

p symbol for (1) the short arm of a chromosome; or (2) the frequency of the more common allele of a pair; (3) pico-.

p- symbol, *para-*.

Pa chemical symbol, *protactinium*; symbol, *pascal.*

PAB, PABA para-aminobenzoic acid, used as a sunscreen and in bacterial culture media.

pabulum ('pabyuhləm) food or aliment.

pacemaker ('paysˌmaykə) an object or substance that controls the rate at which a certain phenomenon occurs; often used alone to indicate an artificial cardiac pacemaker; however, there are other natural and artificial pacemakers. In biochemistry, a pacemaker is a substance whose rate of reaction sets the pace for a series of interrelated reactions.

CARDIAC PACEMAKER. The natural pacemaker of the heart is the sinoatrial (SA) node, a small mass of specialized muscle tissue in the heart near the junction with the superior vena cava. It sets a rhythm of contraction and relaxation that is followed by the rest of the heart. Thus the heartbeat is established.

The normal rhythm, 60 to 100 contractions per minute, is increased by physical or emotional stress, and decreases during rest. The rate varies from person to person and is affected by acute infection, cardiac disorder, drugs and many other conditions. If the natural pacemaker fails to function, its regulating task may be taken over by another small mass of special muscular tissue, the atrioventricular node.

ELECTRONIC CARDIAC PACEMAKERS. In some types of heart disease in which the SA node is malfunctioning, an electronic device known as an *artificial cardiac pacemaker* may be employed to regulate the heart beat. The electronic pacemaker contains batteries, transistors, and other components designed to send a very brief stimulus to the heart via a soft plastic cable attached to the heart muscle. The pacemaker regulates the beat of the heart causing the myocardium to contract at a rate of 60 to 70 beats per minute.

Indications. Any person who has had one or more attacks of Stokes-Adams syndrome caused by heart block or tachycardia and does not respond to drug therapy is a candidate for a pacemaker. Other indications include extremely slow heart rates due to sinus bradycardia, or the carotid sinus syndrome.

Types. The *temporary* or *external* pacemaker is very similar to a small transistor radio. Its components are a pulse generator and an electrode catheter. The pulse generator remains outside the body and the leads from it are directed to the heart through the catheter, usually inserted transvenously through a large systemic vein. Other methods, used less frequently, are insertion of the electrodes through the chest wall into the myocardium and the direct application of the electrodes to the external chest wall. The latter technique is painful and can cause burns of the chest. External pacemakering is used as an emergency or semiemergency procedure.

Temporary pacemakers are also routinely used after cardiac surgery. In this instance two tiny wires are loosely sewn to the epicardium and a third is sewn into subcutaneous tissue. The wires exit through an incision in the chest wall and are attached to the pulse generator, and are easily removed when no longer needed.

The *permanent* or *implantable* pacemaker is small, about half the size of a pack of cigarettes. The pulse generator is sewn into a subcutaneous pocket located beneath the clavicle or under the axilla. The wires that connect the pulse generator to the heart muscle are inserted transvenously. Permanent cardiac pacemakers may be used for months to years.

Pacemakers may be designed to send impulses at a fixed rate or only on demand, the simplest being the *fixed rate* or asynchronous type. It sends electrical stimuli to the heart at a predetermined rate regardless of demands upon the heart. Because it may compete with the SA node and initiate ventricular tachycardia or fibrillation, this type of device is less acceptable than the *demand* pacemaker, which avoids competition by stimulating the heart at a pre-fixed rate only if the patient's rate falls below a predetermined level.

Patient Care. Patients should be informed prior to surgery that the pacemaker will not be silent and that it may take a little while for them to get used to the constant ticking.

During the immediate postoperative period and after insertion of a cardiac pacemaker the patient must be closely monitored for complications. The operative site must be stabilized to avoid displacement of the electrodes and breaking of electrical connections, especially when the pacemaker is a temporary one and the wires are taped to an extremity.

Pacemaker failure does not often occur, but when it does the ECG monitor will show an increased rate and decreased amplitude. Another problem to watch for is *cardiac tamponade*, manifested by distended neck veins and muffled heart sounds. As with any surgery involving a break in the skin, infection at the insertion sites is a possibility. Another potential hazard is phlebitis in the vein, when the catheter of an external pacemaker is left in place for a week or more.

asynchronous p. an implanted cardiac pacemaker in which the induced ventricular rhythm is independent of the atrium; it is usually set at a fixed rate of ventricular stimulation.

gastric p. a saddle-shaped area of the greater curvature of the stomach at the junction of its proximal and middle thirds, which regulates the frequency of gastric contractions.

phrenic p. a device designed to facilitate respiration by converting radiofrequency signals into electrical impulses to stimulate the phrenic nerve, resulting in contraction of the diaphragm and improved inspiration of air. It is an adaptation of a cardiac pacemaker and can be used for many patients who are dependent on VENTILATORS for adequate respiration; for example, those whose involuntary respiratory centre in the brain is no longer functioning normally, and for patients with spinal cord injury above the level of the third cervical vertebra. Candidates for a phrenic pacemaker must have normal phrenic nerves, lungs, and diaphragm.

uterine p. either of the two regulating centres controlling uterine contractions located near the uterine CORNUA and uterine tubes. When birth is imminent, the pacemakers set off a series of rhythmic contractions in the uterine muscle. The contractions start at the cornua and spread over the fundus in waves of decreasing strength called fundal dominance. When the pacemakers do not work properly, uncoordinated uterine action occurs, with ectopic, irregular, ineffective contractions. Fundal dominance is sometimes reversed.

wandering p. a condition in which the site of origin of the impulses controlling the heart rate shifts from the head of the sinoatrial node to a lower part of the node or to another part of the atrium.

pachy- word element. [Gr.] *thick.*

pachyacria (,paki'akri·ə) enlargement of the soft parts of the extremities.

pachyblepharon (,paki'blefə·ron) thickening of the eyelids.

pachycephaly (,paki'kefəlee, -'sef-) abnormal thickness of the bones of the skull. adj. **pachycephalic.**

pachycheilia (,paki'kieli·ə) thickening of the lips.

pachychromatic (,pakikroh'matik) having the chromatin in thick strands.

pachydactyly (,paki'daktilee) enlargement of the fingers and toes.

pachydermatocele (,pakidər'matoh,seel) plexiform neuroma attaining large size, producing an elephantiasis-like condition.

pachydermia, pachyderma (,paki'dərmi·ə; ,paki'dərma) abnormal thickening of the skin. adj. **pachydermatous.**

p. circumscripta, p. laryngis localized warty epithelial thickenings on the vocal cords.

p. vesicae thickening of the mucous membrane of the bladder.

pachydermoperiostosis (,paki,dərmoh,perio'stohsis) pachyderma affecting the face and scalp, thickening of the bones of the distal extremities, and clubbing of the fingers and toes.

pachyglossia (,paki'glosi·ə) abnormal thickness of the tongue.

pachygyria (,paki'jieri·ə) macrogyria.

pachyhaematous (,paki'heemətəs) pertaining to or having thickened blood.

pachyleptomeningitis (,paki,leptoh,menin'jietis) inflammation of the dura mater and pia mater.

pachymeningitis (,paki,menin'jietis) inflammation of the dura mater; perimeningitis.

pachymeningopathy (,paki,mening'gopəthee) noninflammatory disease of the dura mater.

pachymeninx (,paki'meningks) the dura mater.

pachynsis (pə'kinsis) an abnormal thickening. adj. **pachyntic.**

pachyonychia (,pakio'niki·ə) abnormal thickening of the nails.

p. congenita a hereditary congenital dominantly inherited disorder marked by great thickening of the nails, hyperkeratosis of palms and soles, and leukoplakia.

pachyperiostitis (,paki,perio'stietis) periostitis of long bones resulting in abnormal thickness of affected bones.

pachyperitonitis (,paki,peritə'nietis) inflammation and thickening of the peritoneum.

pachypleuritis (,pakiplooə'rietis) fibrothorax.

pachysalpingitis (,paki,salpin'jietis) chronic interstitial inflammation of the muscular coat of the oviduct, producing thickening; called also mural salpingitis and parenchymatous salpingitis.

pachysalpingo-ovaritis (ˌpakisalˌping·gohˌohvə'rietis) chronic inflammation of the ovary and oviduct, with thickening.

pachysomia (ˌpaki'sohmi·ə) thickening of parts of the body.

pachytene ('pakiˌteen) in prophase of meiosis, the stage following zygotene during which the chromosomes shorten, thicken, and separate into two sister chromatids joined at their centromeres. Paired homologous chromosomes, which were joined by synapsis, now form a tetrad of four chromatids. Where crossing over has occurred between nonsister chromatids, they are joined by Y-shaped chiasmata.

pachyvaginalitis (ˌpakiˌvajinə'lietis) inflammation and thickening of the tunica vaginalis of the testis.

pachyvaginitis (ˌpakiˌvaji'nietis) chronic vaginitis with thickening of the vaginal walls.

Pacini's corpuscles (pa'cheeniz) specialized sensory nerve end-organs, situated in the subcutaneous tissue of the extremities and near joints, which react to firm pressure.

pack (pak) 1. a large swab used to control abdominal contents during operation, or to control bleeding in any wound. 2. a tampon.

packer ('pakə) an instrument for introducing a dressing into a cavity or a wound.

packing ('paking) 1. the filling of a wound or cavity with gauze, sponge, or other material. 2. the material used for this purpose.

pad (pad) a cushion-like mass of soft material.

abdominal p. a pad for the absorption of discharges from abdominal wounds, or for packing off abdominal viscera to improve exposure during surgery.

dinner p. a pad placed over the stomach before a plaster jacket is applied; the pad is then removed to leave space under the jacket to take care of expansion of the stomach after eating.

knuckle p's nodular thickenings of the skin on the dorsal surface of the interphalangeal joints.

Mikulicz's p. a pad made of folded gauze, for packing off viscera in surgical procedures.

sucking p., suctorial p. a lobulated mass of fat that occupies the space between the masseter muscle and the external surface of the buccinator muscle. It is well developed in infants.

padimate ('padiˌmayt) an ultraviolet screen.

paediatrician (ˌpeedi·ə'trishən) a specialist in paediatrics.

paediatrics (ˌpeedi'atriks) that branch of medicine dealing with the child and its development and care and with the diseases of children and their treatment. adj. **paediatric**.

paedodontics (ˌpeedoh'dontiks) that branch of dentistry dealing with the teeth and mouth conditions of children.

paedodontist (ˌpeedoh'dontist) a dentist who specializes in paedodontics.

paedophilia (ˌpeedə'fili·ə) abnormal fondness for children; sexual activity of adults with children. adj. **paedophilic**.

PAF platelet activating factor.

Paget's disease ('pajits) any of three diseases named after Sir James Paget (1814–1889).

Paget's disease of bone is a localized bone disorder that is called also OSTEITIS DEFORMANS.

Paget's disease of the breast is an erythematous scaling lesion of the breast, involving the nipple and areola unilaterally, and associated with an underlying malignancy. It usually appears around the age of 55 in women, but can also affect males.

Extramammary Paget's disease is characterized by similar lesions occurring in middle-aged women and men, but the lesions are located in the anogenital area. The skin disorder is not always associated with malignancy, as it is when affecting the breast, but in almost half the cases there is an underlying carcinoma.

pagetoid ('pajiˌtoyd) resembling Paget's disease.

-pagus word element. [Gr.] *conjoined twins*.

PAH, PAHA para-aminohippuric acid.

pain (payn) a feeling of distress, suffering, or agony, caused by stimulation of specialized nerve endings. Its purpose is chiefly protective; it acts as a warning that tissues are being damaged and induces the sufferer to remove or withdraw from the source.

PAIN RECEPTORS AND STIMULI. All receptors for pain stimuli are free nerve endings of groups of small myelinated or unmyelinated nerve fibres abundantly distributed in the superficial layers of the skin and in certain deeper tissues such as the periosteum, surfaces of the joints, arterial walls, and the falx and tentorium of the cranial cavity. The distribution of pain receptors in the gastrointestinal mucosa apparently is similar to that in the skin; thus, the mucosa is quite sensitive to irritation and other painful stimuli. Although the parenchyma of the liver is almost insensitive to pain, the liver capsule and bile ducts are extremely sensitive. Similarly, the alveoli of the lungs are insensitive but the bronchi and parietal pleura are very sensitive.

Some pain receptors are selective in their response to stimuli, but most are sensitive to more than one of the following types of excitation: (1) mechanical stress of trauma; (2) extremes of heat and cold; and (3) chemical substances, such as histamine, potassium ions, acids, prostaglandins, bradykinin, and acetylcholine.

Pain receptors, unlike other sensory receptors in the body, do not adapt or become less sensitive to repeated stimulation. Under certain conditions the receptors become more sensitive over a period of time. This accounts for the fact that as long as a traumatic stimulus persists the person will continue to be aware that damage to the tissues is occurring.

The body is able to recognize tissue damage because when cells are destroyed they release the chemical substances previously mentioned. These substances can stimulate pain receptors or cause direct damage to the nerve endings themselves. A lack of oxygen supply to the tissues can also produce pain by causing the release of chemicals from ischaemic tissue. Muscle spasm is another cause of pain; probably because it has the indirect effect of causing ischaemia and stimulation of chemosensitive pain receptors.

TRANSMISSION AND RECOGNITION OF PAIN. When superficial pain receptors are excited the impulses are transmitted from these surface receptors to synapses in the grey matter (*substantia gelatinosa)* of the dorsal horns of the spinal cord. They then travel upward along the sensory pathways to the thalamus, which is the main sensory relay station of the brain. The dorsomedial nucleus of the thalamus projects to the prefrontal cortex of the brain. The conscious perception of pain probably takes place in the thalamus and lower centres; interpretation of the quality of pain is probably the role of the cerebral cortex.

The perception of pain by an individual is highly complex and individualized, and is subject to a variety of external and internal influences. The cerebral cortex is concerned with the appreciation of pain, its quality, location, type, and intensity; thus, an intact sensory cortex is essential to the perception of pain. In addition to neural influences that transmit and modulate sensory input, the perception of pain is affected by psychological and cultural responses to pain-related stimuli. A person can be unaware of pain at the time of an acute injury or other very stressful situation, when in a state of depression, or when experiencing an emotional crisis. Cultural influences also precondition the perception of and response to painful stimuli. The reaction to similar circumstances can range from complete stoicism to histrionic behaviour.

Pain Control. There have been several theories to explain the physiological control of pain, of which the '*Gate control*' theory of Melzack and Wall, first propounded in 1965, is the most famous. This theory proposes that the substantia gelatinosa of the dorsal horn of the spinal cord acts as a 'gate' that controls the entry of pain impulses into central pathways. The gate is opened by activity in small nerve fibres that carry pain signals, but can be closed by activity in larger nerve fibres that carry tactile and pressure signals. The onward passage of pain impulses therefore depends on the relative activity in small and large nerve fibres feeding the dorsal horn of the spinal cord. In addition, there are descending influences from sites higher up the central nervous system.

Melzack and Wall's theory appeared before the discovery of the brain's own analgesic substances known as endorphins and enkephalins. These morphine-like substances have differing distributions; endorphins are found in the pituitary gland and the hypothalamus, whereas enkephalins are distributed much more widely and in areas known to be associated with pain perception and the transmission of pain signals. For instance, enkephalin is found in the substantia gelatinosa, concentrated in small interneurons that synapse with the endings of small nerve fibres thought to be involved in pain transmission. Stimulation of these interneurons releases the enkephalin that inhibits transmission in these small nerve fibres.

It may be that these enkephalinergic interneurons are stimulated by activity in larger nerve fibres, thus explaining the suppressive effect of activity in large nerve fibres on smaller pain transmitting nerve fibres. Furthermore, signals from groups of neurons in the midbrain and brain stem are known to attenuate or abolish pain impulses in the substantia gelatinosa, again perhaps by acting through the enkephalinergic interneurons.

The discovery of endorphins and the inhibition of pain transmission by tactile signals has provided a scientific explanation for the effectiveness of such techniques as relaxation, massage, application of liniments, and acupuncture in the control of pain and discomfort.

Reactions to Pain. There are two general types of individual reaction to pain: physical and psychological. The physical reaction is usually an automatic response to superficial pain resulting from stimulation of the sympathetic nervous system and an outpouring of adrenaline. There is a shift of blood from the skin, brain, and intestinal tract toward the muscles; the blood pressure increases and the pulse rate rises. This reaction soon subsides if the pain persists and remains intense. The person then becomes weak, shows signs of shock, and may become nauseated and vomit. He or she most often seeks rest and quiet and becomes withdrawn. These signs and symptoms are significant in the assessment of pain and the need for relief.

The psychological aspects of pain are more complex and difficult to identify. An individual's reaction to pain is subject to a variety of psychological and cultural influences. These would include previous experience with pain, training in regard to proper and acceptable responses to pain and discomfort, state of health, and the presence or absence of fatigue. One's degree of attention to and distraction from the presence of painful stimuli can also affect one's perception of pain.

Management of Pain. Pain is a subjective symptom that is based on perception. If a person thinks he is experiencing pain, then he is suffering and in need of help. Denying or expressing doubt that the pain actually exists or implying by speech and manner that a person is not acting in an acceptable way when something is causing him to suffer only serves to increase his discomfort.

Among the measures employed to provide relief from pain, administration of analgesic drugs is probably the one that is most often misunderstood and abused. Analgesic needs must be carefully assessed in consultation with the patient and should be prescribed on a regular basis so that pain onset is prevented. Prescription of analgesia on an 'as needed' (p.r.n.) basis is to be avoided as it implies that the patient must experience pain before the analgesia is administered. Habituation and addiction to analgesics probably result as much from the failure to use other measures along with analgesics for the control of pain as from giving prescribed analgesics when they are ordered.

When analgesics are not appropriate or sufficient, there are several noninvasive techniques that can be used as alternatives or adjuncts to analgesic therapy. The selection of a particular technique for the management of pain depends on the cause of the pain, its intensity and duration, whether it is acute or chronic, and whether the patient perceives the technique as effective.

Distraction techniques provide a kind of sensory shielding to make the person less aware of discomfort. Distraction can be effective in the relief of brief periods of acute pain, such as that associated with minor surgical procedures under local anaesthesia, wound débridement, and venepuncture.

Massage and gentle pressure activate the thick-fibre impulses and produce a preponderance of tactile signals to compete with pain signals. It is interesting that stimulation of the large sensory fibres leading from superficial sensory receptors in the skin can relieve pain at a site distant from the area being rubbed or otherwise stimulated. Since ischaemia and muscle spasm can both produce discomfort, massage to improve circulation and frequent repositioning of the body and limbs to avoid circulatory stasis and promote muscle relaxation can be effective in the prevention and management of pain.

Specific relaxation techniques can help relieve physical and mental tension and stress and reduce pain. They have been especially effective in mitigating discomfort during labour and delivery but can be used in a variety of situations. Learning proper relaxation techniques is not easy for some people, but once these techniques have been mastered they can be of great benefit in the management of chronic pain.

The intensity of pain also can be reduced by stimulating the skin through applications of either heat or cold, menthol ointments, and liniments. Contralateral stimulation involves stimulating the skin in an area on the side opposite a painful region. Stimulation can be done by rubbing, massaging, or applying heat or cold.

Many of the comfort measures traditionally taught to nurses and others concerned with the reduction of mental anxiety and the promotion of rest are now known to have physiological benefits as well as psychological effects.

Since pain is a symptom and therefore of value in diagnosis, it is important to keep accurate records of the observations of the patient having pain. These observations should include the following: the nature of the pain, that is, whether it is described by the patient as being sharp, dull, burning, aching, etc.; the location of the pain, if the patient is able to determine this; the time of onset and the duration, and whether or not certain nursing measures and drugs are successful in obtaining relief; and the relation to other circumstances, such as the position of the patient, occurrence before or after eating, and stimuli in the environment such as heat or cold that may trigger the onset of pain.

bearing-down p. pain accompanying uterine contractions during the second stage of LABOUR.

false p's ineffective pains during pregnancy that resemble labour pains, not accompanied by cervical dilation; called also false labour. See also BRAXTON HICKS CONTRACTIONS.

gas p's pains caused by distention of the stomach or intestine by accumulations of air or other gases (see also GAS PAINS).

hunger p. pain coming on at the time for feeling hunger for a meal; a symptom of gastric disorder.

intermenstrual p. pain accompanying ovulation, occurring during the period between the menses, usually about midway. Also called mittelschmerz.

labour p's the rhythmic pains of increasing severity and frequency due to contraction of the uterus at childbirth. See also LABOUR.

lancinating p. sharp, darting pain.

phantom p. pain felt as if it were arising in an absent (amputated) limb. See also AMPUTATION.

referred p. pain in a part other than that in which the cause that produced it is situated. Referred pain usually originates in one of the visceral organs but is felt in the skin or sometimes in another area deep inside the body. Referred pain probably occurs because pain signals from the viscera travel along the same neural pathways used by pain signals from the skin. The person perceives the pain but interprets it as having originated in the skin rather than in a deep-seated visceral organ.

rest p. a continuous burning pain due to ischaemia of the lower leg, which begins or is aggravated after reclining and is relieved by sitting or standing.

root p. pain caused by disease of the sensory nerve roots and occurring in the cutaneous areas supplied by the affected roots.

painful bruising syndrome ('paynf'l 'broozing) autoerythrocyte sensitization syndrome.

palae(o)- word element. [Gr.] *old.*

palaeencephalon (,palee·enkefəlon) the (phylogenetically) old brain; all of the brain except the cerebral cortex and its dependences.

palaeocerebellum (,palioh,seri'beləm) originally, the phylogenetically older parts of the cerebellum; the term is now applied specifically to those parts whose afferent inflow is predominantly supplied by spinocerebellar fibres. adj. **palaeocerebellar**.

palaeocortex (,palioh'kawteks) palaeopallium.

palaeogenetic (,paliohjə'netik) originated in the past; not newly acquired; said of traits, structures, etc., of species.

palaeokinetic (,paliohki'netik) old kinetic; a term applied to the nervous motor mechanism concerned in automatic associated movements.

palaeopallium (,palioh'pali·əm) that part of the pallium (cerebral cortex) developing with the archipallium in association with the olfactory system; it is phylogenetically older and less stratified than the neopallium, and composed chiefly of the piriform cortex and parahippocampal gyrus. Called also *palaeocortex*.

palaeopathology (,paliohpə'tholəjee) study of disease in bodies that have been preserved from ancient times.

palaeostriatum (,paliohstrie'aytəm) the phylogenetically older portion of the corpus striatum, represented by the globus pallidus. adj. **palaeostriatal.**

palaeothalamus (,palioh'thaləməs) the phylogenetically older part of the thalamus, i.e., the medial portion which lacks reciprocal connections with the neopallium.

palat(o)- word element. [L.] *palate.*

palate (–palət) the roof of the mouth. adj. **palatal.** The front portion braced by the upper jaw bones (maxillae) is known as the hard palate and forms the partition between the mouth and the nose. The fleshy part arching downward from the hard palate to the throat is called the soft palate and separates the mouth and the upper throat cavity, or pharynx. When one swallows, the rear of the soft palate swings up against the back of the pharynx and blocks the passage of food and air to the nose. A fleshy lobe called the uvula hangs from the middle of the soft palate.

cleft p. congenital fissure of median line of palate (see also CLEFT LIP).

palatine bone ('palə,tien) one of a pair of bones which form a part of the nasal cavity and the hard palate.

palatitis (,palə'tietis) inflammation of the palate.

palatoglossal (,palətoh'glos'l) pertaining to the palate and tongue.

palatognathous (,palə'tognəthəs) having a congenitally cleft palate.

palatomaxillary (,palətohmak'silə·ree) pertaining to the palate and maxilla.

palatopharyngeal (,palətohfə'rinji·əl, -,farin'jeeəl) pertaining to the palate and pharynx.

palatoplasty ('palətoh,plastee) plastic reconstruction of the palate.

palatoplegia (,palətoh'pleeji·ə) paralysis of the palate.

palatorrhaphy (,palə'to·rəfee) surgical correction of a cleft palate.

palatoschisis (,palə'toskisis) cleft palate.

palatum (pə'laytəm) [L.] *palate.*

Palfium (palfi·əm) trademark for preparations of dextromoramide, an analgesic.

pali(n)- word element. [Gr.] *again, pathological repetition.*

palikinesia (,paliki'neezi·ə) pathological repetition of movements.

palilalia (,pali'layli·ə) a condition in which a phrase or word is repeated with increasing rapidity.

palindromia (,palin'drohmi·ə) a recurrence or relapse. adj. **palindromic.**

palingraphia (,palin'grafi·ə) pathological repetition of words or phrases in writing.

palinopsia (,pali'nopsi·ə) visual perseveration; the continuance of a visual sensation after the stimulus is gone.

palinphrasia (,palin'frayzi·ə) pathological repetition of words or phrases in speaking.

palladium (pə'laydi·əm) a chemical element, atomic number 46, atomic weight 106.4, symbol Pd. See table of elements in Appendix 2.

pallaesthesia (,palis'theezi·ə) sensibility to vibrations; the peculiar vibrating sensation felt when a vibrating tuning-fork is placed against a subcutaneous bony prominence of the body. adj. **pallaesthetic.**

pallanaesthesia (,palanəs'theezi·ə) loss or absence of pallaesthesia.

palliate ('pali,ayt) to relieve symptoms.

palliative ('pali·ətiv) affording relief; also, a drug that so acts.

pallidectomy (,pali'dektəmee) extirpation of the globus pallidus.

pallidotomy (ˌpali'dotəmee) creation of lesions by stereotaxic surgery in the globus pallidus for treatment of extrapyramidal disorders.
pallidum ('palidəm) the globus pallidus of the brain. adj. **pallidal**.
pallium ('pali·əm) the cerebral cortex viewed in its entirety, i.e., the mantle of grey matter covering both cerebral hemispheres. Also, the cerebral cortex during its development.
pallor ('palə) paleness, as of the skin.
palm (pahm) the hollow or flexor surface of the hand. adj. **palmar**.
palma ('palmə) pl. *palmae* [L.] palm.
palmar ('pahmə) relating to the palm of the hand.
p. fascia the arrangement of tendons in the palm of the hand.
deep and superficial p. arches the chief arterial blood supply to the hand formed by the junction of the ulnar and radial arteries.
palmaris (pal'mayris) palmar.
palmitic acid (pal'mitik) a saturated fatty acid from animal and vegetable fats.
palmus ('palməs) 1. palpitation. 2. clonic spasm of leg muscles, producing a jumping motion.
palpable ('palpəb'l) perceptible by touch.
palpate ('palpayt) to perform palpation.
palpation (pal'payshən) the act of feeling with the hand; the application of the fingers with light pressure to the surface of the body for the purpose of determining the condition of the parts beneath in physical diagnosis.
palpebra ('palpibrə) pl. *palpebrae* [L.] eyelid. adj. **palpebral**.
palpebral ('palpibrəl) referring to the eyelids.
p. ligaments a band of fibrous tissue which stretches from the junction of the upper and lower lid to the orbital bones, both medially and laterally.
palpitation (ˌpalpi'tayshən) a heartbeat that is unusually rapid, strong or irregular enough to make a person aware of it—usually over 120 per minute, as opposed to the normal 60 to 100 per minute. In most cases, palpitation is the result of excitement or nervousness, of strong exertion or of taking certain medications. There are also palpitations that result from various types of heart disorders such as paroxysmal tachycardia and flutter, abnormal rhythms in which the heart executes runs of rapid beats. Another is atrial fibrillation, in which the beats are rapid but irregular, seeming to occur at random.

These palpitations may be caused by organic heart disease, but they also can result from other factors. Similarly, emotional pressures rather than organic changes may cause the so-called 'nervous heart', or functional heart disease.
palsy ('pawlzee) paralysis.
Bell's p. facial paralysis due to lesion of the facial nerve, resulting in characteristic facial distortion (see also BELL'S PALSY).
birth p. birth paralysis.
cerebral p. a persisting qualitative motor disorder appearing before age 3, due to nonprogressive damage of the brain (see also CEREBRAL PALSY).
Erb's p. Erb–Duchenne paralysis.
facial p. Bell's palsy.
Saturday night p. paralysis of the extensor muscles of the wrist and fingers, so called because of its frequent occurrence in alcoholics. It is most often due to prolonged compression of the radial (musculospiral) nerve, and, depending upon the site of nerve injury, sometimes accompanied by weakness and extension of the elbow. Called also musculospiral or radial paralysis.
shaking p. paralysis agitans.
paludism ('palyuhˌdizəm) malaria.
Paludrine ('palədrin, 'palyoo-) trademark for a preparation of proguanil, an antimalarial.
pampiniform (pam'piniˌfawm) shaped like a tendril.
pan- word element. [Gr.] *all.*
panacea (ˌpanə'seeə) a remedy for all diseases.
Panadol ('panədol) trademark for preparations of paracetamol, an analgesic and antipyretic.
panaesthesia (ˌpanis'theezi·ə) the sum of the sensations experienced. adj. **panaesthetic**.
panagglutinin (ˌpanə'glootinin) an agglutinin that agglutinates the erythrocytes of all human blood groups.
panangiitis (ˌpananji'ietis) inflammation involving all the coats of a vessel.
panarthritis (ˌpanah'thrietis) inflammation of all the joints.
panatrophy (pa'natrəfee) atrophy of several parts; diffuse atrophy.
panautonomic (paˌnawtə'nomik) pertaining to or affecting the entire autonomic (sympathetic and parasympathetic) nervous system.
pancarditis (ˌpankahdi'ietis) diffuse inflammation of the heart.
Pancoast's syndrome ('pankohsts) 1. radiographic shadow at the apex of the lung, neuritic pain in the arm, atrophy of the muscles of the arm and hand, and Horner's syndrome, observed in tumour near the apex of the lung, due to involvement of the brachial plexus. 2. osteolysis in the posterior part of one or more ribs and sometimes involving also the corresponding vertebra.
pancolectomy (ˌpankə'lektəmee) excision of the entire colon, with creation of an outlet, an ileostomy.
pancreas ('pangkri·əs) a large, elongated, racemose gland located transversely behind the stomach, between the spleen and duodenum.

The pancreas is composed of both exocrine and endocrine tissue. The *acini* secrete digestive enzymes, and small ductules leading from the acini secrete sodium bicarbonate solution. The combined product, *pancreatic juice*, enters a long pancreatic duct and from there is transported through the hepatic duct to the duodenum. The pancreatic juice contains enzymes for the breakdown of proteins, carbohydrates, and fats. The bicarbonate ions in the pancreatic secretion help neutralize the acidic chyme that is passed along from the stomach to the duodenum.

Regulation of pancreatic secretion of enzymes and bicarbonate ions is both neural and hormonal; however, the influences of the hormones *secretin* and *cholecystokinin* are more important than vagal stimulation. The entry of chyme into the small intestine causes the transformation of an inactive proenzyme, *prosecretin*, into active *secretin* that is released from the mucosa of the upper portion of the duodenum. The composition of the partially digested food entering the duodenum influences the amount of each hormone that is released and, therefore, the characteristics of the pancreatic juice.

The endocrine functions of the pancreas are related to the islets of Langerhans located on the surface of the pancreas. These small islands contain three major types of cells: the *alpha*, *beta*, and *delta* cells. The alpha cells secrete the hormone *glucagon*, which elevates blood glucose. The beta cells secrete *insulin*, which affects the metabolism of carbohydrates, proteins, and fats. The delta cells secrete *somatostatin*, the functions of which are not fully understood, but it is known that it can inhibit the secretion of both glucagon and insulin and may act as a controller of metabolic

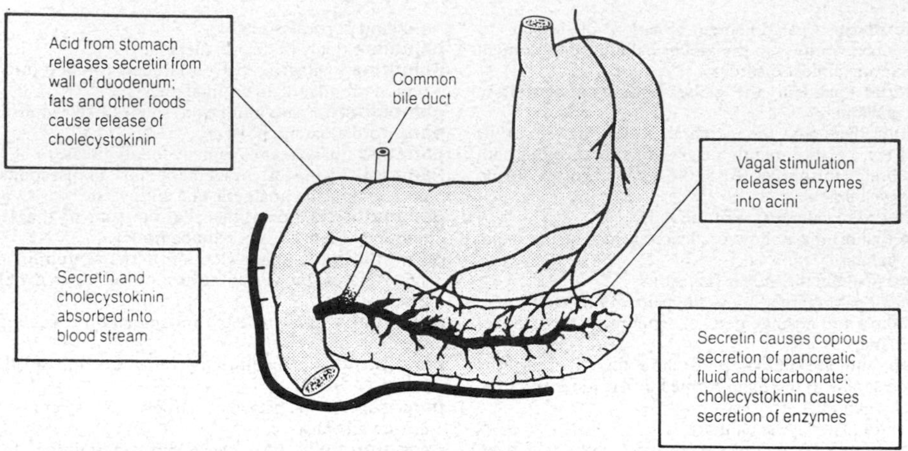

Regulation of pancreatic secretion

processes. The somatostatin produced by the delta cells of the pancreas is the same as that produced by the hypothalamus as an inhibitor of the release of growth hormone from the pituitary gland.

DISORDERS OF THE PANCREAS. Failure of the islands of Langerhans to produce sufficient amounts of insulin results in DIABETES MELLITUS. Disturbances in the exocrine functions of the pancreas produce serious digestive disorders. The pancreas can also be the seat of cancerous growth, and occasionally the pancreatic ducts are blocked by stones; either condition may require surgery. Various factors, not yet fully understood, may result in acute PANCREATITIS, a condition in which the fluids digest the tissue of the organ itself. This self-digesting may also be set off if the flow in the ducts is reversed and bile enters the pancreas, activating the enzymes in its secretions. Excessive alcohol intake also may be implicated in pancreatitis. Sudden severe abdominal pain, vomiting, and fever can accompany pancreatitis. Treatment may involve surgery, though bed rest and antibiotics are frequently prescribed. Chronic PANCREATITIS, a less serious disorder, sometimes occurs after gallbladder diseases.

CYSTIC FIBROSIS, a serious congenital disease, is characterized by a deficiency in the secretion of pancreatic juice, and an increase in its viscosity.

annular p. a developmental anomaly in which the pancreas forms a ring entirely surrounding the duodenum.

pancreatalgia (ˌpangkri·əˈtalji·ə) pain in the pancreas.

pancreatectomy (ˌpangkri·əˈtektəmee) excision of the pancreas.

pancreatic (ˌpangkriˈatik) pertaining to the pancreas.

p. duct the main excretory duct of the pancreas, which usually unites with the common bile duct before entering the duodenum at the major duodenal papilla (see also BILE DUCTS).

pancreatico- word element. [Gr.] *pancreatic duct.*

pancreaticoduodenal (ˌpangkriˌatikohˌdyooəˈdeenəl) pertaining to the pancreas and duodenum.

pancreaticoduodenostomy (ˌpangkriˌatikohˌdyooədiˈnostəmee) anastomosis of the pancreatic duct to a different site on the duodenum.

pancreaticoenterostomy (ˌpangkriˌatikohˌentəˈrostəmee) anastomosis of the pancreatic duct to the intestine.

pancreaticogastrostomy (ˌpangkriˌatikohgaˈstrostəmee) anastomosis of the pancreatic duct to the stomach.

pancreaticojejunostomy (ˌpangkriˌatikohˌjejuhˈnostəmee) anastomosis of the pancreatic duct to the jejunum.

pancreatin (ˈpangkri·ətin, panˈkreeə-) a substance from the pancreas of the hog or ox containing enzymes, principally amylase, protease, and lipase; used as a digestive aid.

pancreatitis (ˌpangkri·əˈtietis) inflammation of the PANCREAS, which is due to autodigestion of pancreatic tissue by its own enzymes.

Acute pancreatitis can arise from a variety of aetiological factors, but in most cases the specific cause is unknown. In some instances chronic alcoholism or toxicity from some other agent, such as glucocorticoids, thiazide diuretics, or paracetamol, can bring on an acute attack of pancreatitis. In about half the patients a mechanical obstruction of the biliary tract is present, usually because of gallstones in the bile ducts. Viral infections also can cause an acute inflammation of the pancreas.

The patient with acute pancreatitis typically complains of epigastric pain that is accompanied by fever, malaise, nausea, and vomiting. Very mild cases can be overlooked or misdiagnosed quite easily. There is no specific laboratory diagnostic test for acute pancreatitis.

Treatment is largely symptomatic and designed to provide rest for the organ. Oral intake may be restricted and intravenous fluids given to maintain an adequate blood volume. Analgesics and other noninvasive techniques are necessary for the management of pain, which can be quite severe in some patients. Surgical removal of gallstones can provide an excellent prognosis for acute pancreatitis related to obstruction of the biliary system by the stones. Alcoholic pancreatitis responds relatively well to conservative treatment if the patient stops drinking; however, there is a tendency toward recurrent attacks. Surgical removal of the pancreas is a drastic measure usually reserved for the severe form of the disease with life-threatening complications.

Chronic pancreatitis is characterized by progressive loss of the exocrine functions of the pancreas; that is, the production of pancreatic enzymes essential for normal digestion. There is relative preservation of the organ's endocrine functions until late in the disease. .The specific cause of chronic pancreatitis can rarely be identified, but most of the factors that produce the acute form of the disease can also cause the chronic form. Alcoholism is considered by many to be one of the primary causes now that prompt diagnosis and treatment of biliary obstruction has reduced the incidence of pancreatitis secondary to obstruction.

Chronic pancreatitis can lead to pancreatic insufficiency as a result of the replacement of acinar tissue with fibrous tissue. Because the acini secrete pancreatic enzymes necessary for the digestion of proteins, carbohydrates, and fats, dysfunction of acinar tissue results in malabsorption of nutrients from the small intestine. The patient may complain of bulky, fatty, foul-smelling stools, weight loss, fever, malaise, and nausea and vomiting. There also can be a negative nitrogen balance resulting in wasting of the muscles, and malabsorption of the fat-soluble vitamins resulting in easy bruising and bleeding from mild injury. Inadequate absorption of calcium and vitamin B_{12} also can occur. Glucose intolerance due to insulin lack resulting from degeneration of the islets of Langerhans is a late manifestation of chronic pancreatitis.

Treatment is chiefly substitutive and palliative. Pancreatic insufficiency can be treated with the administration of pancreatic extract with each meal. Relief of pain is not so easily accomplished and often necessitates the use of addictive narcotic analgesics such as codeine, morphine, and pethidine. Symptomatic relief can make the patient more comfortable and substitutive therapy can help maintain adequate nutrition and strengthen the patient's resources so that he can continue most everyday activities of living, but there is no cure for chronic pancreatitis and the long-term prognosis is not good.

acute haemorrhagic p. a condition due to autolysis of pancreatic tissue caused by escape of enzymes into the substance, resulting in haemorrhage into the parenchyma and surrounding tissues.

pancreato- word element. [Gr.] *pancreas.*

pancreatoduodenectomy (ˌpangkri·ətohˌdyooədi'nektəmee) excision of the head of the pancreas along with the encircling loop of the duodenum, performed for carcinoma of the head of the pancreas. Most of the pancreas, the pylorus, duodenum and the common bile duct are excised. Gastrojejunostomy is perfomed with anastomosis of the tail of the pancreas and gallbladder to the jejunum. Called also *Whipple's operation.*

pancreatogenous (ˌpangkri·ə'tojinəs) arising in the pancreas.

pancreatogram (ˌpangkri'atəˌgram) the radiograph produced by pancreatography.

pancreatography (ˌpangkri·ə'togrəfee) radiology of the pancreas, performed during surgery by injecting contrast medium into the pancreatic duct.

endoscopic retrograde p. that in which the radiopaque medium is injected into the pancreatic duct at the ampulla of Vater via a cannula introduced through a fibreoptic endoscope. See also GALLBLADDER.

pancreatolithectomy (ˌpangkriˌatohli'thektəmee) excision of a calculus from the pancreas.

pancreatolithiasis (ˌpangkriˌatohli'thieəsis) the presence of calculi in the ductal system or parenchyma of the pancreas.

pancreatolithotomy (ˌpangkriˌatohli'thotəmee) incision of the pancreas for the removal of calculi.

pancreatolysis (ˌpangkri·ə'tolisis) destruction of pancreatic tissue. adj. **pancreatolytic.**

pancreatotomy (ˌpangkri·ə'totəmee) incision of the pancreas.

pancreatotropic (ˌpangkri·ətoh'tropik) having a special affinity for the pancreas.

pancreolithotomy (ˌpangkriohli'thotəmee) pancreatolithotomy.

pancreolysis (ˌpangkri'olisis) pancreatolysis.

pancreozymin (ˌpangkrioh'ziemin) a hormone of the duodenal mucosa that stimulates the external secretory activity of the pancreas, especially its production of amylase; identical with cholecytokinin.

pancuronium (ˌpangkyuh'rohni·əm) a neuromuscular blocking agent of the nerve depolarizing type used as a muscle relaxant during surgery. The molecule is based on a steroid nucleus. It has a relatively long duration of action, a single intravenous dose lasting 45–60 minutes. The drug does not cause hypotension but does produce significant tachycardia. It is often used in poor risk patients.

pancystitis (ˌpansi'stietis) cystitis involving the entire thickness of the wall of the urinary bladder, as occurs in interstitial cystitis.

pancytopenia (ˌpansietoh'peeni·ə) abnormal depression of all the cellular elements of the blood.

pandemic (pan'demik) a widespread epidemic disease; over a wide area, worldwide.

panencephalitis (ˌpanenˌkefə'lietis, -ˌsef-) encephalitis, probably of viral origin, which produces intranuclear or intracytoplasmic inclusion bodies that result in parenchymatous lesions of both the grey and white matter of the brain.

panendoscope (pan'endəˌskohp) a cystoscope that gives a wide-angle view of the bladder.

panhypopituitarism (panˌhiepohpi'tyooitəˌrizəm) generalized hypopituitarism due to absence or damage to the pituitary gland, which in its complete form leads to absence of gonadal function and insufficiency of thyroid and adrenal function. When cachexia is a prominent feature, it is called SIMMONDS' DISEASE or pituitary cachexia.

panhysterectomy (ˌpanhistə'rektəmee) total hysterectomy.

panhysterosalpingectomy (panˌhistə·rohˌsalpin'jektəmee) excision of the uterus, cervix, and oviducts.

panhysterosalpingo-oophorectomy (panˌhistə·rohˌsalping·gohˌoh·əfə'rektəmee) excision of the uterus, cervix, oviducts, and ovaries.

panic ('panik) extreme and unreasoning fear and anxiety.

panimmunity (ˌpani'myoonitee) immunity to several bacterial and viral infections.

panleukopenia (ˌpanlookoh'peeni·ə) a deficiency of all the white blood cells.

panmyeloid (pan'mieəˌloyd) pertaining to all elements of the bone marrow.

panmyelopathy (ˌpanmieə'lopəthee) a disease affecting all the cells formed in the bone marrow.

panmyelosis (ˌpanmieə'lohsis) proliferation of all the elements of the bone marrow.

panniculectomy (pəˌnikyuh'lektəmee) surgical excision of the abdominal apron of superficial fat in the obese.

panniculitis (peˌnikyuh'lietis) inflammation of the panniculus adiposus, especially of the abdomen.

nodular nonsuppurative p., relapsing febrile nonsuppurative p. a disease marked by fever and the formation of crops of tender nodules in the subcutaneous fatty tissues. Called also Weber-Christian or Christian–Weber disease.

panniculus (pə'nikyuhləs) pl. *panniculi* [L.] a layer of membrane.

p. adiposus the subcutaneous fat; a layer of fat underlying the corium.

p. carnosus a muscular layer in the superficial fascia of certain lower animals; represented in man mainly by the platysma.

pannus ('panəs) 1. superficial vascularization of the cornea with infiltration of granulation tissue. 2. an inflammatory exudate overlying synovial cells on the inside of a joint capsule, usually occurring in rheumatoid arthritis or related articular rheumatism. 3. panniculus adiposus.

panophobia (,panə'fohbi·ə) fear of everything; vague and persistent dread of an unknown evil.

panophthalmia (,panof'thalmi·ə) panophthalmitis; inflammation of all the tissues of the eyeball.

panophthalmitis (,panofthal'mietis) inflammation of all the eye structures or tissues.

panosteitis (,panosti'ietis) inflammation of every part of a bone.

panotitis (,panoh'tietis) inflammation of all the parts or structures of the ear.

panphobia (pan'fohbi·ə) panophobia.

panproctocolectomy (pan,proktohkoh'lektəmee) total excision of the large bowel at one operation.

pansinusitis (,pansienə'sietis) inflammation involving all the paranasal sinuses.

pansystolic murmur (,pansi,stolik 'mərmə) a heart murmur heard throughout the time when the heart is in systole. See MURMUR.

pant(o)- word element. [Gr.] *all, the whole.*

pantalgia (pan'talji·ə) pain over the whole body.

panthenol ('panthə,nol) nonproprietary name for pantothenyl alcohol.

pantothenate (pan'tothə,nayt, ,pantə'thenayt) any salt of pantothenic acid.

pantothenic acid (,pantə'thenik) a vitamin of the B complex present in all living tissues, almost entirely in the form of coenzyme A (CoA). This coenzyme has many metabolic roles in the cell, and a lack of pantothenic acid can lead to depressed metabolism of both carbohydrates and fats. The daily requirement for this vitamin is not known and no definite deficiency syndrome has been recognized in man, perhaps because of its wide occurrence in almost all foods. However, some symptoms attributed to deficiency of other B-complex vitamins may be due to a lack of pantothenic acid.

pantothenyl alcohol (,pantoh'thenil) a compound that is oxidized in the body to pantothenic acid.

pantotropic, pantropic (,pantə'tropik; pan'tropik) having affinity for tissues derived from all three of the germ layers (ectoderm, endoderm, and mesoderm).

panzootic (,panzoh'otik) occurring pandemically among animals.

papain (pə'payin, pə'pie·in) a proteolytic enzyme from the latex of papaw, *Carica papaya.* It has been used for enzymatic débridement of a sloughing wound.

Papanicolaou test (smear) (,papə,nikə'layoo) a simple, painless test used most commonly to detect cancer of the uterus and cervix; often called the smear test. The test is based on the discovery by Dr. George N. Papanicolaou (1883–1962) that malignant uterine tumours slough off cancerous cells into surrounding vaginal fluid.

The Papanicolaou technique, an exfoliative cytological staining procedure, is used also in diagnosis of lung, stomach, and bladder cancers. The test can be performed on any body excretion (urine, faeces), secretion (sputum, prostatic fluid, vaginal fluid), or tissue scraping (as from the uterus or the stomach). The sample is removed from the area being examined, placed on a glass slide, stained, and then studied under a microscope for evidence of abnormal or cancerous cells.

In 5 minutes, the Pap test can reveal uterine or cervical cancer at a stage in which it produces no visible symptoms, has done no damage and usually can be completely cured.

papaveretum (pə'pahvə'reetəm) a mixture of opium alkaloids used as an analgesic.

papaverine (pə'pavə·reen) an alkaloid obtained from opium and prepared synthetically; the hydrochloride salt is used as a smooth muscle relaxant.

papilla (pə'pilə) pl. *papillae* [L.] a small, nipple-shaped projection or elevation. adj. **papillary.**

circumvallate p. vallate papilla.

conical p. one of the sparsely scattered elevations on the tongue, often considered to be modified filiform papillae.

papillae of corium conical extensions of the fibres, capillary blood vessels, and sometimes nerves of the corium into corresponding spaces among downward- or inward-projecting rete ridges on the undersurface of the epidermis.

dental p., dentinal p. the small mass of condensed mesenchyme capped by each of the enamel organs.

duodenal p. either of the small elevations (major and minor) on the mucosa of the duodenum, the major at the entrance of the conjoined pancreatic and common bile ducts, the minor at the entrance of the accessory pancreatic duct.

filiform p. one of the threadlike elevations covering most of the tongue surface.

foliate p. one of the parallel mucosal folds on the tongue margin at the junction of its body and root.

fungiform p. one of the knoblike projections of the tongue scattered among the filiform papillae.

gingival p. the triangular pad of the gingiva filling the space between the proximal surfaces of two adjacent teeth. **hair p.** the fibrovascular mesodermal papilla enclosed within the hair bulb.

incisive p. an elevation at the anterior end of the raphe of the palate.

lacrimal p. an elevation on the margin of either eyelid, near the medial angle of the eye.

lingual papillae elevations on the surface of the tongue, containing the taste buds; the conical, filiform, foliate, fungiform, and vallate papillae.

mammary p. the nipple of the breast.

optic p. optic disc.

palatine p. incisive papilla.

p. pili hair papilla.

renal p. the blunted apex of a renal pyramid.

tactile papillae tactile corpuscles.

urethral p. a slight elevation in the vestibule of the vagina at the external orifice of the uretha.

vallate p. one of the 8 to 12 large papillae arranged in a V near the base of the tongue.

p. of Vater, Vater's p. major duodenal papilla.

papillectomy (,papi'lektəmee) excision of a papilla.

papillitis (,papi'lietis) inflammation of the optic nerve disc.

papillocarcinoma (,papiloh,kahsi'nohmə) papillary carcinoma.

papilloedema (,papili'deemə) oedema and hyperaemia of the optic disc, usually associated with increased intracranial pressure; called also choked disc.

papilloma (,papi'lohmə) a benign tumour derived from epithelium. Papillomas may arise from skin, mucous membranes, or glandular ducts. adj. **papillomatous.**

papillomatosis (,papi,lohmə'tohsis) development of multiple papillomas.

papilloretinitis (,papiloh,reti'nietis) inflammation of

the optic nerve and disc.

papillotomy (ˌpapi'lotəmee) incision of a papilla, as of a duodenal papilla.

papovavirus (pə'pohvəˌvierəs) a group of relatively small, ether-resistant DNA viruses, containing papilloma viruses and polyoma viruses, many of which are oncogenic or potentially oncogenic.

papulation (ˌpapyuh'layshən) the formation of papules.

papule ('papyool) a small circumscribed, solid, elevated lesion of the skin. adj. **papular**.

papulopustular (ˌpapyuhloh'pustyuhlə) marked by papules and pustules.

papulosis (ˌpapyuh'lohsis) the presence of multiple papules.

papulosquamous (ˌpapyuhloh'skwayməs) both papular and scaly.

papulovesicular (ˌpapyuhlohve'sikyuhlə) marked by papules and vesicles.

papyraceous (ˌpapi'rayshəs) like paper.

par (pah) [L.] *pair*.

para ('parə) [L.] used to describe a woman who has produced one or more viable offspring. adj. **parous**.

Numerals designate the number of pregnancies that have resulted in the birth of viable offspring, as para 0 (none = nullipara), para I, para II, para III, para IV. The number is not indicative of the number of offspring produced in the event of a multiple birth, or synonymous with the number of pregnancies. See GRAVIDA.

para- word element. [Gr.] *beside, beyond, accessory to, apart from, against*. In chemistry, a prefix indicating the substitution in a derivative of the benzene ring of two atoms linked to opposite carbon atoms in the ring; abbreviated *p-*.

para-aminobenzoic acid (ˌparəˌaminohben'zoh·ik) PAB or PABA; a compound that is a growth factor for certain bacteria that use it to synthesize folic acid. Sulphonamides act by blocking a step in this synthesis. PABA absorbs ultraviolet light and is used in sunscreens.

para-aminohippuric acid (ˌparəˌaminoh·hi'pyooə·rik) PAH or PAHA; a derivative of para-aminobenzoic acid used to measure the effective renal plasma flow and to determine the functional capacity of the renal tubular excretory mechanism. Called also aminohippuric acid.

para-aminosalicylic acid (ˌparəˌaminohˌsali'silik) PAS or PASA; a derivative of benzoic acid used in treatment of tuberculosis. Called also aminosalicylic acid. It enhances the potency of streptomycin and delays development of bacilli resistant to streptomycin. Gastrointestinal irritation accompanied by anorexia, nausea, and vomiting may be reduced by administering the drug together with food at mealtimes.

para-anaesthesia (ˌparəˌanəs'theezi·ə) anaesthesia of the lower part of the body.

para-aortic bodies (ˌparə·ay'awtik) small masses of chromaffin cells near the sympathetic ganglia along the abdominal aorta that secrete noradrenaline. They reach their maximum size during fetal life and then degenerate during childhood as the adrenal medulla matures. Tumours of these structures produce symptoms similar to those of PHAEOCHROMOCYTOMA. Called also organs of Zuckerkandl.

parabiosis (ˌparəbie'ohsis) 1. the union of two individuals, as conjoined twins, or of experimental animals by surgical operation. 2. temporary suppression of conductivity and excitability. adj. **parabiotic**.

parablepsia (ˌparə'blepsi·ə) false or perverted vision.

parabulia (ˌparə'byooli·ə) perversion of will.

paracenaesthesia (ˌparəˌseenəs'theezi·ə) any disturbance of the general sense of well-being.

paracentesis (ˌparəsen'teesis) surgical puncture of a cavity for the aspiration of fluid. adj. **paracentetic**. Called also tapping.

abdominal p. insertion of a trocar through a small incision and into the abdominal cavity, to remove ascitic fluid or inject a therapeutic agent.

Before the procedure the patient is instructed to empty his bladder to reduce the danger of accidental puncture of the bladder. The skin in the midline below the umbilicus is cleansed with an antiseptic. A local anaesthetic is used to anaesthetize the skin and underlying tissues at the site of insertion of the trocar. During the procedure the patient may be placed in a sitting position with his feet resting on a foot stool or on the floor. His back and arms should be well supported. The container for collecting the drainage is placed at the patient's feet. As the fluid is being withdrawn the patient is observed for symptoms of fainting or shock.

The amount and character of the fluid obtained is recorded and a specimen is saved if the doctor requests laboratory examination of the fluid. After the trocar is removed a sterile dressing is applied to the site. A more permanent procedure for relief of accumulations of excess fluid in the peritoneal cavity is insertion of a peritoneal-venous SHUNT.

thoracic p. surgical puncture and drainage of the thoracic cavity (called also THORACENTESIS).

paracephalus (ˌparə'kefələs, -'sef-) a fetus with a defective head and imperfect sense organs.

paracetamol (ˌparə'seetəˌmol, -'setə-) an analgesic and antipyretic drug commonly used instead of aspirin for relief of moderate pain and reduction of fever, particularly for children or patients who are allergic to aspirin, who are taking anticoagulants, or who have peptic ulcer or gastritis. Unlike aspirin, it has only weak anti-inflammatory effects and is not used to treat rheumatoid arthritis.

Acute paracetamol overdosage can cause severe and potentially fatal hepatic necrosis, when a large amount of the drug is accidentally ingested. One of the ways that the liver detoxifies the drug is by conjugation of a metabolite with glutathione, and when the glutathione stores are used up, the metabolite attacks the liver tissues. Treatment is symptomatic and supportive. Two drugs, methionine and acetylcysteine, can reduce the liver damage by serving as substitutes for glutathione.

parachlorometacresol (ˌparəˌklor·rohˌmetə'kreesol) chlorocresol. A coal-tar antiseptic preparation.

paracholera (ˌparə'kolə·rə) a disease resembling true cholera clinically, but not caused by *Vibrio cholerae*.

parachordal (ˌparə'kawd'l) beside the notochord.

parachromatopsia (ˌparəˌkrohmə'topsi·ə) colour blindness.

paraclinical (ˌparə'klinik'l) pertaining to abnormalities (e.g., morphological or biochemical) underlying clinical manifestations (e.g., chest pain or fever).

Paracoccidioides (ˌparəkokˌsidi'oydeez) a genus of fungi that proliferate by multiple budding yeast cells in the tissues.

P. brasiliensis the aetiological agent of paracoccidioidomycosis. Called also *Blastomyces brasiliensis*.

paracoccidioidomycosis (ˌparəkoksidiˌoydohmie'kohsis) an often fatal, chronic granulomatous disease caused by *Paracoccidioides brasiliensis*. The disease is endemic in Brazil and occurs in other parts of South America, in Central America, and in the arid southwestern regions of the United States. Infection primarily involves the lungs, but spreads to the skin, mucous membranes, lymph nodes, and internal organs. Amphotericin B is the specific drug used for treatment. Called also *South American blastomycosis*.

paracolitis (ˌparəkə'lietis, -koh-) inflammation of the outer coat of the colon.

paracusis (ˌparə'kyoosis) any perversion of hearing.

paracystic (ˌparə'sistik) situated near the bladder.

paracystitis (ˌparəsi'stietis) inflammation of tissues around the bladder.

paradidymis (ˌparə'didimis) a small, vestigial structure found occasionally in the adult in the anterior part of the spermatic cord.

paradipsia (ˌparə'dipsi·ə) a perverted appetite for fluids.

paradontal (ˌparə'dont'l) periodontal.

paradoxical respiration (ˌparə'doksik'l) a type of breathing in which all or part of a lung inflates during inspiration and balloons out during expiration; the opposite of normal chest motion. Called also paradoxical motion. The condition seriously inhibits the movement of gases during respiration and can produce severe and even fatal cardiovascular disturbances and respiratory insufficiency if not quickly relieved by emergency treatment.

Paradoxical respiration or paradoxical motion of the lung usually results from traumatic injury to the thorax (FLAIL CHEST) in which several ribs are fractured in two or more places and are no longer attached by bony cartilage to the rest of the rib cage. The condition can also be seen following surgical removal of several ribs and in paralysis of the diaphragm.

paraesthesia (ˌparis'theezi·ə) morbid or perverted sensation; an abnormal sensation, as burning, prickling, formication, etc.

paraffin ('parəfin) 1. a purified hydrocarbon wax used for embedding histological specimens. 2. formerly, a saturated hydrocarbon (alkane).

liquid p. liquid petrolatum (mineral oil). See PETROLEUM.

paraffinoma (ˌparəfi'nohmə) a chronic granuloma produced by prolonged exposure to paraffin.

paraformaldehyde (ˌparəfaw'maldiˌhied) paraform; a preparation of formaldehyde used as an antiseptic and also for fumigating rooms.

paragammacism (ˌparə'gaməˌsizəm) faulty enunciation of *g*, *k*, and *ch* sounds.

paraganglioma (ˌparəˌgangli'ohmə) a tumour of the tissue composing the paraganglia.

paraganglion (ˌparə'gang·gli·ən) pl. *paraganglia* [Gr.] a collection of chromaffin cells derived from neural ectoderm, occurring outside the adrenal medulla, usually near the sympathetic ganglia and in relation to the aorta and its branches. Most secrete adrenaline or noradrenaline.

parageusia (ˌparə'gyoozi·ə) perversion of the sense of taste. adj. **parageusic**.

paraglossia (ˌparə'glosi·ə) inflammation of the oral tissues under the tongue.

paragonimiasis (ˌparəˌgoni'mieəsis) infection with flukes of the genus *Paragonimus*.

Paragonimus (ˌparə'gonimәs) a genus of trematode parasites, having two invertebrate intermediate hosts, the first a snail, the second a crab or crayfish.

P. westermani the lung fluke, occurring especially in Asia; it is found in cysts in the lungs, and sometimes the pleura, abdominal cavity, liver, and elsewhere in man and lower animals that ingest infected freshwater crayfish and crabs.

paragrammatism (ˌparə'graməˌtizəm) a disorder of speech, with confusion in the use and order of words and grammatical forms.

paragranuloma (ˌparəˌgranyuh'lohmə) the most benign form of Hodgkin's disease, largely confined to the lymph nodes.

paragraphia (ˌparə'grafi·ə) impairment of ability to express thoughts in writing.

parahaemophilia (ˌparəˌheemoh'fili·ə) a hereditary haemorrhagic tendency due to deficiency of CLOTTING factor V.

parahormone (ˌparə'hawmohn) a substance, not a true hormone, that has a hormone-like action in controlling the functioning of some distant organ.

parainfluenza virus (ˌparəˌinfloo'enzə) one of a group of viruses isolated from patients with upper respiratory tract disease of varying severity.

parakeratosis (ˌparəˌkerə'tohsis) persistence of the nuclei of keratinocytes as they rise into the horny layer of the skin; it occurs normally in the epithelium of the true mucous membrane of the mouth and vagina.

parakinesia (ˌparəki'neezi·ə) perversion of motor powers; in ophthalmology, irregular action of an individual ocular muscle.

paralalia (ˌparə'layli·ə) a disorder of speech, especially the production of a vocal sound different from the one desired, or the substitution in speech of one letter for another.

paralambdacism (ˌparə'lamdəˌsizəm) faulty enunciation of the *l* sound.

paraldehyde (pə'raldiˌhied) a sedative and hypnotic and anticonvulsant that has an unpleasant taste and imparts an unpleasant odour to the breath. Because of its low therapeutic index, it is now little used, except in the treatment of status epilepticus.

paralexia (ˌparə'leksi·ə) impairment of reading ability, with transposition of words and syllables into meaningless combinations.

paralgesia (ˌparal'jeezi·ə) an abnormal and painful sensation.

parallagma (ˌparə'lagmə) displacement of a bone or of the fragments of broken bone.

parallax ('parəˌlaks) an apparent displacement of an object due to change in the observer's position.

parallergy (pə'raləjee) a condition in which an allergic state, produced by specific sensitization, predisposes the body to react to other allergens with clinical manifestations that differ from the original reaction. adj. **parallergic**.

paralogia (ˌparə'lohji·ə) derangement of the reasoning faculty, marked by illogical or delusional speech.

paralysant ('parəˌliezənt) 1. causing paralysis. 2. a drug that causes paralysis.

paralysis (pə'ralisis) loss or impairment of motor function in a part due to a lesion of the neural or muscular mechanism; also, by analogy, impairment of sensory function (sensory paralysis). Called also palsy. Paralysis is a symptom of a wide variety of physical and emotional disorders rather than a disease in itself.

TYPES OF PARALYSIS. Paralysis results from damage to parts of the nervous system. The kind of paralysis resulting, and the degree, depend on whether the damage is to the central nervous system or the peripheral nervous system.

If the central nervous system is damaged, paralysis frequently affects the movement of a limb as a whole, not the individual muscles. The more common forms of central paralysis are HEMIPLEGIA, in which the whole of one side of the body, including the face, arm, and leg, is affected, and PARAPLEGIA, in which both legs and possibly the trunk are affected. In central paralysis the tone of the muscles is increased (spasticity).

If the peripheral nervous system is damaged, individual muscles or groups of muscles in a particular part of the body, rather than a whole limb, are more likely to be affected. The muscles are flaccid, and there is often impairment of sensation.

CAUSES OF CENTRAL PARALYSIS. STROKE is one of the

commonest causes of central paralysis. Although there is usually some permanent disability, much can be done to rehabilitate the patient.

Paralysis produced by damage to the spinal cord can be the result of direct injuries, tumours, and infectious diseases.

Paralysis in children may be a result of failure of the brain to develop properly in intrauterine life or of injuries to the brain, as in the case of CEREBRAL PALSY. Congenital SYPHILIS may also leave a child partially paralysed.

There is no organic basis for the paralysis resulting from hysteria. This type of paralysis is a result of emotional disturbance or mental illness.

CAUSES OF PERIPHERAL PARALYSIS. Until the recent development of immunizing vaccines, the most frequent cause of peripheral paralysis in children was POLIOMYELITIS. NEURITIS, inflammation of a nerve, can produce paralysis. Causes can be physical, as with cold or injury; chemical, as in lead poisoning; or disease states, such as diabetes mellitus or infection. Paralysis caused by neuritis frequently disappears when the disorder causing it is corrected.

p. of accommodation paralysis of the ciliary muscles of the eye so as to prevent accommodation.

p. agitans a form of parkinsonism of unknown aetiology; it is a slowly progressive disease usually occurring in late life, marked by masklike facies, tremor, slowing of voluntary movements, festinating gait, peculiar posture, and muscle weakness (see also PARKINSON'S DISEASE).

ascending p. spinal paralysis that progresses upward.

birth p. that due to injury received at birth.

brachial p. paralysis of an arm from damage to the brachial plexus.

bulbar p. that due to changes in motor centres of the medulla oblongata; the chronic form is marked by progressive paralysis and atrophy of the lips, tongue, pharynx, and larynx, and is due to degeneration of the nerve nuclei of the floor of the fourth ventricle.

central p. any paralysis due to a lesion of the brain or spinal cord.

cerebral p. paralysis caused by some intracranial lesion (see also CEREBRAL PALSY).

compression p. that caused by pressure on a nerve.

conjugate p. loss of ability to perform some parallel ocular movements.

crossed p. paralysis affecting one side of the face and the other side of the body.

decubitus p. paralysis due to pressure on a nerve from lying for a long time in one position.

diver's p. decompression sickness (BENDS).

Duchenne's p. 1. Erb–Duchenne paralysis. 2. progressive bulbar paralysis.

Erb–Duchenne p. paralysis of the upper roots of the brachial plexus due to destruction of the fifth and sixth cervical roots, without involvement of the small muscles of the hand. Called also Erb's palsy.

facial p. weakening or paralysis of the facial nerve, as in BELL'S PALSY.

familial periodic p. a hereditary disease with recurring attacks of rapidly progressive flaccid paralysis, associated with a fall in (hypokalemic type), a rise in (hyperkalemic type), or normal (normokalemic type) serum potassium levels; all three types are inherited as autosomal dominant traits.

flaccid p. paralysis with loss of muscle tone of the paralysed part and absence of tendon reflexes.

immunological p. the absence of immune response to a specific antigen.

infantile p. the major form of poliomyelitis.

infantile cerebral ataxic p. a congenital condition due to defective development of the frontal regions of the brain, affecting all extremities.

ischaemic p. local paralysis due to stoppage of circulation.

Klumpke's p., Klumpke-Dejerine p. atrophic paralysis of the lower arm and hand, due to lesion of the eighth cervical and first dorsal nerves.

Landry's p. Guillain-Barré syndrome.

lead p. wristdrop due to lead poisoning.

mixed p. combined motor and sensory paralysis.

motor p. paralysis of the voluntary muscles.

musculospiral p. Saturday night palsy.

obstetric p. birth paralysis.

progressive bulbar p. the chronic form of bulbar paralysis; called also Duchenne's disease or paralysis.

pseudobulbar muscular p. pseudohypertrophic muscular dystrophy.

pseudohypertrophic muscular p. pseudohypertrophic muscular dystrophy. **radial p.** Saturday night palsy.

sensory p. loss of sensation resulting from a morbid process.

spastic p. paralysis with rigidity of the muscles and heightened deep muscle reflexes.

spastic spinal p. lateral sclerosis.

tick p. progressive ascending flaccid motor paralysis following the bite of certain ticks, usually *Dermacentor andersoni*, in children.

Volkmann's p. ischaemic paralysis.

paralytic (ˌparə'litik) 1. pertaining to paralysis. 2. a person affected with paralysis.

p. ileus adynamic ileus.

paramania (ˌparə'mayni·ə) parathymia in which the patient manifests joy by complaining.

paramastigote (ˌparə'masti,goht) having an accessory flagellum by the side of a larger one.

paramastitis (ˌparəma'stietis) inflammation of tissues around the mammary gland.

parameatal (ˌparəmi'aytəl) situated near or around a meatus.

Paramecium (ˌparə'meesi·əm) a genus of ciliate protozoa.

paramecium (ˌparə'meesi·əm) pl. *paramecia;* any organism of the genus *Paramecium.*

paramedian (ˌparə'meedi·ən) situated to the side of the median line.

paramedical, paramedic (ˌparə'medik'l; ˌparə'medik) having some connection with or relation to the science or practice of medicine; adjunctive to the practice of medicine in the maintenance or restoration of health and normal functioning. The paramedical services include physiotherapy, and occupational and speech therapy, etc., and the activity of social workers.

paramenia (ˌparə'meeni·ə) disordered or difficult menstruation.

parameter (pə'ramitə) 1. in mathematics and statistics, an arbitrary constant, such as a population mean or standard deviation. 2. a property of a system that can be measured numerically.

parametric (ˌparə'metrik) 1. situated near the uterus; parametrial. 2. pertaining to or defined in terms of a parameter.

parametritis (ˌparəmi'trietis) inflammation of the parametrium.

parametrium (ˌparə'meetri·əm) the extension of the subserous coat of the supracervical portion of the uterus laterally between the layers of the broad ligament.

paramimia (ˌparə'mimi·ə) the use of improper or inappropriate gestures when speaking.

paramnesia (ˌparam'neezi·ə) 1. perversion of memory in which the person believes he remembers events or circumstances that never happened; called also retrospective falsification. 2. a state in which words are remembered, but are used without a comprehension of their meaning.

paramyloidosis (pə,ramiloy'dohsis) accumulation of an atypical form of amyloid in tissues.

paramyoclonus (,parəmie'oklənəs) a condition characterized by myoclonic contractions of various muscles.

p. multiplex a condition characterized by sudden shocklike contractions.

paramyotonia (,parə,mieə'tohni·ə) a disease marked by tonic spasms due to disorder of muscular tonicity, especially a hereditary and congenital affectation.

p. congenita myotonia congenita.

paramyxovirus (,parə,miksoh'vierəs) any of a subgroup of myxoviruses, including the viruses of human and animal parainfluenza, mumps, and Newcastle disease.

paranaesthesia (,paranəs'theezi·ə) para-anaesthesia.

paranasal sinuses (,parə'nayz'l) mucosa-lined air cavities in bones of the skull, communicating with the nasal cavity (see also SINUS).

paraneoplastic syndrome (,parə,neeoh'plastik) a collective term for disorders arising from metabolic effects of cancer on tissues remote from the tumour; such disorders may, for example, appear as primary endocrine, haematological, or neuromuscular disorders.

paranephric (,parə'nefrik) 1. near the kidney. 2. pertaining to the adrenal gland.

paranephritis (,parənə'frietis) 1. inflammation of the adrenal gland. 2. inflammation of the connective tissue around the kidney.

paranephros (,parə'nefros) pl. *paranephroi* [Gr.] an adrenal gland.

paraneural (,parə'nyooə·rəl) alongside a nerve.

paranoia (,parə'noyə) a mental disorder characterized by well systematized delusions of persecution, illusions of grandeur, or a combination of both. adj. **paranoic.**

It is a chronic disease that develops over months and years and for which there is usually no cure.

In the acute stage of the disease, the paranoiac regards himself as being very important and distinguished, or he believes he is being plotted against by others, and in his imagination he builds up an elaborate system of 'evidence' to support this belief. This imaginary system is kept separate from the paranoiac's everyday attitudes and activities; hence his outward behaviour may appear normal. The extent of his illness remains mostly hidden, though it may erupt occasionally into crimes of violence.

Symptoms of paranoia sometimes appear in lesser degrees in SCHIZOPHRENIA. In slight to moderate form, paranoid personality traits are found in many neurotic persons who are excessively suspicious of other people's motives and are quick to take offense at imagined wrongs. See also PSYCHOSIS.

paranoiac (,parə'noyak) a person affected with paranoia.

paranoid ('parə,noyd) 1. resembling paranoia. 2. paranoiac.

paranomia (,parə'nohmi·ə) aphasia marked by inability to name objects felt (myotactic paranomia) or seen (visual paranomia).

paranormal (,parə'nawm'l) pertaining to phenomena lying outside the range of current scientific knowledge, e.g. extra-sensory perception.

paranosis (,parə'nohsis) the primary advantage that is to be gained by illness.

paranucleus (,parə'nyookli·əs) a body sometimes seen in cell protoplasm near the nucleus. adj. **paranuclear.**

paraparesis (,parəpə'reesis) a partial paralysis of the lower extremities.

paraphaemia (,parə'feemi·ə) aphasia marked by the employment of the wrong words.

paraphasia (,parə'fayzi·ə) partial aphasia in which the patient employs wrong words, or uses words in wrong and senseless combinations (*choreic paraphasia).*

paraphia (pə'rafi·ə) perversion of the sense of touch; parapsis.

paraphilia (,parə'fili·ə) expression of the sexual instinct in practices that are socially prohibited or unacceptable, or biologically undesirable. Called also sexual deviation.

paraphimosis (,parəfie'mohsis) retraction of a phimotic foreskin, causing swelling of the glans.

paraphrasia (,parə'frayzi·ə) disorderly arrangement of spoken words.

paraplasm ('parə,plazəm) any abnormal growth.

paraplastic (,parə'plastik) exhibiting a perverted formative power; of the nature of a PARAPLASM.

paraplectic (,parə'plektik) paraplegic.

paraplegia (,parə'pleeji·ə) paralysis of the legs and, in some cases, the lower part of the body. adj. **paraplegic.** Paraplegia is a form of central nervous system paralysis, in which the paralysis affects all the muscles of the parts involved.

In the majority of cases, paraplegia results from disease or injury of the spinal cord that causes interference with nerve paths connecting the brain and the muscles. Conditions that may result in such interference include physical injuries, haemorrhage, tuberculosis, tumour, and syphilis.

In paraplegia, the loss of ability to use the legs may be accompanied by a loss of sensation in them and, in some cases, by loss of control over the bowels and bladder. Fortunately, much has been learned about the techniques of restoring paraplegics to normal activity, and today many are able to resume useful and productive lives.

PATIENT CARE. Because rehabilitation is the ultimate goal for a paraplegic patient, the patient care during the early stages of the disorder must be particularly concerned with preventing complications that may stand in the way of successful rehabilitation. These complications include PRESSURE SORES, DECUBITUS ulcer, respiratory disorders, orthopaedic deformities, urinary infections or calculi, and gastrointestinal disorders.

The psychological and emotional aspects of paraplegia also must be considered. The paraplegic patient may have been suddenly thrust into the role of dependence because of accidental injury to the spinal cord. This means that he must make a tremendous adjustment to his condition in a short time. His mental attitude and emotional response to paralysis will greatly affect the success of attempts at rehabilitation.

During the early stages of his illness the patient may not be able to assist in his daily personal care, but as his condition improves and the doctor allows more physical activity he must be encouraged to do as much as possible for himself. As he learns to become less dependent on others, his attitude toward his future will improve.

If it is anticipated that the patient will be confined to a wheelchair or will use crutches, he is taught transfer techniques so that he can move himself from bed to chair and from chair to other surfaces. Wheelchairs and crutches are prescribed according to the individual patient's body build and weight, and the purpose for which they are to be used. The patient is instructed in correct CRUTCH walking if he will be using them; if he is to be using a wheelchair, he is taught how to operate the chair to receive maximum benefit from it. Mastering these techniques can enhance his mobility, increase his independence, and give him a certain degree of confidence that can greatly improve his outlook.

Care of the Skin. The type of bed used and the positioning of the patient with paraplegia will depend on the cause and extent of the paralysis and the preference of the doctor. Patients with spinal cord injuries may be placed in traction or the spinal cord may be hyperextended by placing the patient's head at the foot of the bed and adjusting the bed. In some cases the doctor may request a special orthopaedic frame such as the STRYKER FRAME or CircOlectric bed. These devices facilitate daily care but the patient still must be turned frequently and receive special skin care to avoid the development of pressure sores (decubitus ulcers).

Since the patient has no feeling below the point of damage to the spinal cord, he will not be aware of discomfort or other signs of pressure. Injections should not be given in the area of paralysis because of limited absorption of the drug and decreased circulation to the part.

Respiratory Disorders. Hypostatic pneumonia and other respiratory problems are guarded against by deep breathing exercises. Coughing and frequent changing of position may be contraindicated and the doctor must be consulted before these measures are taken. The patient should be protected from respiratory infections, such as the COMMON COLD, which can have serious complications in a paraplegic who is confined to bed.

Orthopaedic Deformities. Until the patient is allowed out of bed and can engage in some form of physical activity, a range of passive movement EXERCISES for all joints should be performed at least once a day. Proper positioning of the feet and legs will help prevent contractures, footdrop, and ankylosis.

A therapeutic EXERCISE programme, including passive and active exercises, is initiated to maintain any remaining muscle function and to restore as much muscle activity in the affected parts as possible. If the patient is to use crutches or wheelchair he must strengthen his arm and shoulder muscles in preparation for transfer techniques. HYDROTHERAPY and DIATHERMY may be utilized to promote relaxation of muscle spasms and tension and to facilitate implementation of the exercise programme.

Urinary Problems. Urinary infections and the formation of calculi, particularly in the bladder, present very real problems for the patient with paralysis in the lumbosacral area. If he has no control over urination, an indwelling catheter may seem to be the technique of choice for keeping him dry, but it also predisposes him to infection. A thorough assessment of the patient's status and his potential for achieving bladder control should be made before a final choice is made.

Ideally, the patient learns to achieve bladder control through an intensive BLADDER TRAINING programme designed to fit his individual needs. Whether this can be accomplished depends on the extent of nerve damage suffered and the degree of success in avoiding such complications as infection and calculi. The achievement of bladder control is more difficult than that of bowel control, but every effort must be made to help the patient accomplish as much as possible and to avoid, whenever feasible, the use of artificial collecting and drainage devices.

Patients with neurogenic or cord bladder are unaware of the need to void and therefore require training to initiate voiding. In some patients the bladder empties by reflex, and training involves techniques to make reflex emptying more effective. If the lesion causing paralysis is at the 2nd, 3rd, or 4th sacral segment, the bladder is flaccid and training must be aimed at avoiding overdistention and dribbling. Some patients may never be able to achieve bladder control to any appreciable degree, requiring the use of catheters, penile clamps, or other collecting devices. URETEROSTOMY and ureteroileostomy may be required in some cases.

The formation of bladder stones results from incomplete emptying of the bladder, with pooling of urine and inadequate elimination of wastes. To minimize the formation of stones it is recommended that the patient receive between 2500 and 3000 ml of fluid every 24 hours. Since an alkaline urine supports the growth of bacteria and the formation of stones, an excess of citrus fruit juices should be avoided. The high calcium content of milk also may foster stone formation and carbonated drinks irritate the bladder. A wide variety of liquids can be most effective in avoiding the formation of stones.

Gastrointestinal Complications. A flaccid bowel produces abdominal distention and predisposes the patient to faecal impaction. If the bowel paralysis is temporary, the distention may be relieved by a rectal tube and injections of neostigmine or other drugs to stimulate peristalsis. If the lumbar region is permanently paralysed, the patient will have faecal incontinence as well as frequent accumulations of flatus and faecal material in the lower intestine. Rehabilitation of the patient then necessitates working out some method of bowel control so that regularity of defecation can be accomplished.

As in bladder training, the programme for BOWEL TRAINING is designed according to the individual needs of the patient and his ability to work with those who are trying to help him. It is essential that an assessment be made of the patient's status in regard to nerve damage and potential for rehabilitation. In addition, it is important to know about the patient's previous bowel habits in regard to frequency and time of day for a movement.

The training programme also should include attention to fluid and food intake. The patient learns to avoid foods that produce diarrhoea and flatus, and to rely upon a daily intake of fluids sufficient to ensure soft, formed stools. Adequate physical exercise is also helpful in establishing regularity of defecation. Rectal suppositories and digital stimulation at regular intervals may be necessary to stimulate evacuation at a time convenient for the patient.

Sexual Counselling. Frequently there is impairment of normal sexual function; the patient and partner will need help in alternative methods of obtaining sexual satisfaction.

paraplegiform (ˌparə'pleejiˌfawm) resembling paraplegia.

parapoplexy (pə'rapəˌpleksee) a condition resembling apoplexy.

parapraxia (ˌparə'praksi·ə) parapraxis.

parapraxis (ˌparə'praksis) a lapse of memory or mental error, such as a slip of the tongue or misplacement of an object, which, in psychoanalytic theory, is due to unconscious associations and motives; commonly called a 'freudian slip'.

paraprofessional (ˌparəprə'feshən'l) 1. a person who is specially trained in a particular field or occupation to assist a professional. 2. allied health professional. 3. pertaining to a paraprofessional.

paraprotein (ˌparə'prohteen) immunoglobulin produced by a clone of neoplastic plasma cells proliferating abnormally, e.g., myeloma proteins and cryoglobulins.

paraproteinaemia (ˌparəˌprohti'neemi·ə) the presence in the blood of paraproteins.
parapsis (pə'rapsis) perversion of the sense of touch; paraphia.
parapsoriasis (ˌparəsə'rieəsis) a group of slowly developing, persistent, maculopapular scaly erythrodermas, devoid of subjective symptoms and resistant to treatment.
parapsychology (ˌparəsie'koləjee) the branch of psychology dealing with psychical effects and experiences that appear to fall outside the scope of physical law, e.g., telepathy and clairvoyance.
paraquat ('parəˌkwat) a poisonous dipyridilium compound whose dichloride and dimethylsulphate salts are used as a contact herbicide. Contact with concentrated solutions causes irritation of the skin, cracking and shedding of the nails, and delayed healing of cuts and wounds. After ingestion of large doses, renal and hepatic failure may develop, followed by pulmonary insufficiency and death.
parareflexia (ˌparə·ri'fleksi·ə) any disorder of the reflexes.
pararhotacism (ˌparə'rohtəˌsizəm) faulty enunciation of *r* sound.
pararosaniline (ˌparə·roh'zaniˌleen) a basic dye; a triphenylmethane derivative, one of the components of basic fuchsin.
pararrhythmia (ˌparə'ridhmi·ə) parasystole.
pararthria (pa'rahthri·ə) imperfect utterance of words.
parasacral (ˌparə'saykrəl) situated near the sacrum.
parasigmatism (ˌparə'sigməˌtizəm) lisping.
parasinoidal (ˌparəsie'noydəl) situated along the course of a sinus.
parasitaemia (ˌparəsi'teemi·ə) the presence of parasites, especially malarial plasmodia, in the blood.
parasite ('parəˌsiet) a plant or animal that lives upon or within another living organism at whose expense it obtains some advantage (see also SYMBIOSIS). adj. **parasitic.** Among the many parasites in nature, a few feed upon human hosts, causing diseases ranging from the mildly annoying to the severe and even fatal. Parasites include multicelled and single-celled animals, fungi, and bacteria. Viruses are sometimes considered to be parasites.
accidental p. one that parasitizes an organism other than the usual host.
facultative p. one that may be parasitic upon another organism but can exist independently.
incidental p. accidental parasite.
malarial p. *Plasmodium.*
obligate p., obligatory p. one that is entirely dependent upon a host for its survival.
periodic p. one that parasitizes a host for short periods.
temporary p. one that lives free of its host during part of its life cycle.
parasiticide (ˌparə'sitiˌsied) destructive to parasites; also, an agent that is destructive to parasites.
parasitism ('parəsieˌtizəm) 1. symbiosis in which one population (or individual) adversely affects another, but cannot live without it. 2. infection or infestation with parasites.
parasitize ('parəsiˌtiez) to live on or within a host as a parasite.
parasitogenic (ˌparəˌsietoh'jenik) due to parasites.
parasitologist (ˌparəsie'toləjist) a person skilled in parasitology.
parasitology (ˌparəsie'toləjee) the scientific study of parasites and parasitism.
parasitotropic (ˌparəˌsietoh'tropik) having affinity for parasites.
paraspadias (ˌparə'spaydi·əs) a congenital condition in which the urethra opens on one side of the penis.
parasternal (ˌparə'stərnəl) beside the sternum.
parasuicide (ˌparə'sooiˌsied) an act of deliberate self-harm. Formerly called attempted suicide, a term now increasingly regarded as inappropriate as the intention is often not to end life but elicit concern and love when all other methods have failed.
parasympathetic nervous system (ˌparəˌsimpə'thetik) part of the autonomic NERVOUS SYSTEM, the preganglionic fibres of which leave the central nervous system with cranial nerves III, VII, IX, and X and the first three sacral nerves; postganglionic fibres are distributed to the heart, smooth muscles, and glands of the head and neck, and thoracic, abdominal, and pelvic viscera. Almost three-fourths of all parasympathetic nerve fibres are in the VAGUS NERVES, which serve the entire thoracic and abdominal regions of the body.

The predominant secretion of the nerve endings of the parasympathetic nervous system is *acetylcholine*, which acts on the various organs of the body to either excite or inhibit certain activities. For example, stimulation of the parasympathetic system causes constriction of the pupil of the eye and contraction of the ciliary muscle; increase of the glandular secretion of enzymes, as in the case of the pancreas; increased peristalsis; and a slowed heart rate. It often happens that excitation of the sympathetic nervous system results in an effect opposite that caused by excitation of the parasympathetic system; however, most organs are under the almost exclusive control of either one or the other of the two nervous systems that compose the autonomic nervous system.
parasympatholytic (ˌparəˌsimpəthoh'litik) anticholinergic: producing effects resembling those of interruption of the parasympathetic nerve supply of a part; having a destructive effect on the parasympathetic nerve fibres or blocking the transmission of impulses by them. Also, an agent that produces such effects.
parasympathomimetic (ˌparəˌsimpəthohmi'metik) cholinergic: producing effects resembling those of stimulation of the parasympathetic nerve supply of a part. Also, an agent that produces such effects.
parasynapsis (ˌparəsi'napsis) the union of chromosomes side by side during meiosis.
parasynovitis (ˌparəˌsienoh'vietis) inflammation of the tissues about a synovial sac.
parasystole (ˌparə'sistəlee) a cardiac irregularity attributed to the interaction of two foci independently initiating cardiac impulses at different rates. Called also pararrhythmia.
paratenon (ˌparə'tenon) the fatty areolar tissue filling the interstices of the fascial compartment in which a tendon is situated.
parathion (ˌparə'thieon) an agricultural insecticide highly toxic to humans and animals.
parathormone (ˌparə'thawmohn) parathyroid hormone.
parathymia (ˌparə'thiemi·ə) perverted, contrary, or inappropriate emotions.
parathyroid (ˌparə'thieroyd) 1. situated beside the thyroid gland. 2. one of the parathyroid glands. 3. a preparation containing parathyroid hormone from animal parathyroid glands; used for diagnosis and treatment of hypoparathyroidism.
p. glands small bodies in the region of the thyroid gland, occurring in a variable number of pairs, commonly two. The parathyroid contains two types of cells: chief cells and oxyphils. Chief cells are the major source of parathyroid hormone (PTH), the secretion of which is dependent on the serum calcium level. Through a closed-loop feedback mechanism a low serum calcium level stimulates secretion of PTH;

Some animal parasites harmful to man

Parasite Areas of occurrence	Condition caused	Usual source of infection	Prevention
AMOEBA Tropics and subtropics	Amoebic dysentery	Contaminated food and drink	Avoiding unsanitary food and drink
MALARIA PARASITE Tropics	Malaria	Mosquito bites	Mosquito control; protection against bites; chemoprophylaxis
BLOOD FLUKE Tropics	Schistosomiasis (disease of liver, intestine, bladder)	Water (organism can penetrate skin)	Avoiding contaminated water
TAPEWORM Most countries (in UK mainly beef tapeworm)	Tapeworm (in intestine)	Raw or poorly cooked beef, pork or fish	Cooking meat and fish thoroughly
HOOKWORM Warm regions	Hookworm disease (ancylostomiasis)	Contaminated soil	Wearing shoes; avoiding direct contact with infected soil
ASCARIS ROUNDWORM Wherever sanitation is poor	Intestinal disorder (ascariasis)	Raw vegetables and fruits; contaminated soil	Cooking fruits and vegetables; avoid ingestion of soil
THREADWORM Throughout world	Threadworm infection (enterobiasis)	Contact with infected person directly or through food	Personal cleanliness
TRICHINA WORM Throughout world, wherever raw or undercooked pork is eaten	Trichinosis	Poorly cooked pork	Thorough cooking of pork products
FILARIA WORM Tropics	Filariasis	Mosquito bites	Avoiding mosquito bites
Skin parasites			
ITCH MITE Most countries	Scabies	Contact with infected person	Cleanliness of body and clothing; avoiding contact with infected person
LICE Most countries	Itching of skin (pediculosis); also may carry disease germ	Contact with human carrier, clothing, bedding	Cleanliness of body and clothing; avoiding contact with infected person; louse control
TICKS Most countries	Skin infestation; also may carry rabbit fever, other diseases	Tick-infested areas	Avoiding tick-infested areas or wearing heavy tight-fitting clothing
FLEAS Most countries	Skin irritation; also may carry disease germs	Animal and human carriers	Cleanliness; avoid close contact with carriers

conversely, a high serum calcium level inhibits its secretion.

The essential role of PTH is maintenance of a normal serum calcium level in association with vitamin D and calcitonin. It does this by exerting its effects on bone, kidney, and gastrointestinal tract. In bone, it enhances bone resorption by increasing digestion of the bone matrix by osteoclasts. This effects the release of calcium from the bone into the blood stream. In the kidney, PTH increases the excretion of phosphate and the reabsorption of filtered calcium. In the intestine, it increases intestinal absorption of calcium.

The parathyroid glands are subject to two major types of disorder: HYPERPARATHYROIDISM and HYPOPARATHYROIDISM.

parathyroidectomy (ˌparəˌthieroy'dektəmee) excision of a parathyroid gland.

parathyrotrophic (ˌparəˌthieroh'trohfik) having an affinity for the parathyroid glands.

paratrophy (pə'ratrəfee) dystrophy.

paratuberculosis (ˌparətyuhˌbərkyuh'lohsis) a tuberculosis-like disease not due to *Mycobacterium tuberculosis.*

paratyphoid (ˌparə'tiefoyd) a notifiable infection caused by *Salmonella* of all groups except *S. typhosa.* The disease is usually milder and has a shorter incubation period, more abrupt onset, and a lower mortality rate than does typhoid. Clinically and pathologically, the two diseases cannot be distinguished. Called also *paratyphoid fever.* See also TYPHOID FEVER.

paraurethral (ˌparəyuh'reethrəl) near the urethra.

paravaginitis (ˌparəˌvaji'nietis) inflammation of the

tissues alongside the vagina.

paravertebral (,parə'vərtibrəl) near the vertebrae.

parencephalous (,paren'kefələs, -'sef-) having a congenital malformation of the brain.

parenchyma (pə'rengkimə) the essential or functional elements of an organ, as distinguished from its stroma or framework. adj. **parenchymal, parenchymatous.**

parenchymatitis (pə,rengkimə'tietis) inflammation of a parenchyma.

parenteral (pə'rentə·rəl) not through the alimentary canal, e.g., by subcutaneous, intramuscular, intrasternal, or intravenous injection. See also parenteral NUTRITION.

parepididymis (,parepi'didimis) paradidymis.

paresis (pə'reesis, 'parəsis) 1. slight or incomplete paralysis. 2. dementia paralytica. adj. **paretic.**

general p. a chronic syphilitic meningoencephalitis called also dementia paralytica.

paries ('pair·ri·eez) pl. *parietes* [L.] a wall, as of an organ or cavity.

parietal (pə'rieət'l) 1. of or pertaining to the walls of an organ or cavity. 2. pertaining to or located near the parietal bone.

p. bone one of two quadrilateral bones forming the sides and roof of the cranium.

p. lobe the upper central portion of the cerebral hemisphere, between the frontal and occipital lobes, and above the temporal lobe. It is the receptive area for fine sensory stimuli, and the highest integration and coordination of sensory information is carried on in this area. Damage to the parietal lobe can produce defects in vision and aphasia.

parietofrontal (pə'rieətoh'frunt'l) pertaining to the parietal and frontal bones, gyri, or fissures.

parietography (pə,rieə'togrəfee) radiographic visualization of the walls of an organ.

Parinaud's oculoglandular syndrome ('pari,nohz) a general term applied to conjunctivitis, usually unilateral and of the follicular type, followed by tenderness and enlargement of the preauricular lymph nodes; often due to leptotrichosis but may be associated with other infections. Called also leptothricosis conjunctivae.

Parinaud's ophthalmoplegia paralysis of conjugate upward movement of the eyes without paralysis of convergence, associated with midbrain lesions.

parity ('parətee) 1. para; the condition of a woman with respect to her having borne viable offspring. 2. equality; close correspondence or similarity.

Parkinson's disease ('pahkinsənz) a slowly progressive disease usually occurring in later life, characterized pathologically by degeneration within the nuclear masses of the extrapyramidal system, and clinically by masklike facies (PARKINSON'S FACIES), a characteristic tremor of resting muscles, a slowing of voluntary movements, a festinating gait, peculiar posture, and muscular weakness. When this symptom complex occurs secondarily to another disorder, the condition is called PARKINSONISM.

SYMPTOMS. Parkinson's disease usually appears gradually and progresses slowly. At first the victim may be troubled by mild tremors of the hands and nodding of the head. He may notice that his movements are somewhat slower and more difficult than usual. Then loss of mobility in the face produces the characteristic masklike facies. As the disease advances, the tremors increase and may involve the whole body, although generally they are not apparent with intentional movements. The muscles become stiffer, making movement increasingly difficult. The gait becomes shuffling and festinating. The back tends to become bent forward in a stooped position. Parkinson's disease does not affect the mental capacity.

TREATMENT. In general, treatment is symptomatic, supportive, and palliative. Most patients require lifelong management consisting of drug therapy, supportive psychotherapy, physiotherapy, and rarely, surgical intervention. Newer forms of treatment now give hope for freedom from the progressive disability that once was the expected outcome.

The biochemical basis of parkinsonism is a loss or inhibition of dopamine activity in the corpus striatum, resulting from degeneration of the dopaminergic nigrostriatal pathway. Normally, the two opposing neurotransmitters, *dopamine* and *acetylcholine*, in this structure are in balance. When dopamine is depleted, the functional overactivity of acetylcholine produces the symptoms of parkinsonism. In patients with mild symptoms and little functional impairment, some relief from symptoms can be obtained with anticholinergic agents, such as trihexylphenidyl, or with antihistamines with anticholinergic properties, such as diphenhydramine. These drugs block the muscarinic effects of acetylcholine in the central nervous system. Tricyclic antidepressants, such as imipramine or amitriptyline, are also effective; they block the reuptake of dopamine from nerve synapses and also have anticholinergic effects.

In patients with more severe symptoms and some difficulty with routine daily activities, it is necessary to augment the dopamine level in the brain. This is accomplished by administering the drug levodopa (L-dopa), which crosses the blood-brain barrier and is converted to dopamine by decarboxylation. This reaction also occurs in the peripheral tissues, and the dopamine produced may cause side-effects such as cardiac stimulation (tachycardia and arrhythimas) and also nausea and vomiting. A newer drug that combines a chemical called carbidopa with L-dopa is now being used to counteract the undesirable effects that may occur when L-dopa is used alone. Carbidopa inhibits production of dopamine outside the brain and, therefore, allows more effective relief of symptoms. A disadvantage of the combination drug is that it sometimes has only a limited span of effectiveness in some patients; therefore, it is usually reserved for more severe cases.

Patients receiving levodopa alone or in combination with carbidopa require nutritional counselling because dietary habits can greatly affect the action of the drug. Protein intake requires special attention because levodopa, an amino acid, must compete with the dietary amino acids for transport through the intestinal epithelium and across the blood-brain barrier. Alcohol intake also must be limited because in large amounts it can antagonize the effects of dopamine. Although the newer combined form of medication offers relief to many persons with Parkinson's disease, it must be given with caution and under continued supervision.

Since the patient's mental outlook and motivation can affect the extent to which he can successfully cope with his disability, it is important that he receive psychological support. He should know the nature of the disease affecting him and be given realistic hopes for forestalling or preventing its more serious effects.

Some benefits can be derived from physical therapy in the form of applications of heat and massage to alleviate muscle cramps and relieve the tension headaches that often accompany rigidity of the cervical muscles. The patient also is instructed in simple EXERCISES that he can perform at home.

The best candidates for surgical treatment are those who exhibit unilateral involvement. The procedure involves either electrocoagulation or freezing of tissues to interrupt the neural pathways in the ventrolateral nucleus of the thalamus which appear essential for the production of symptoms, and at a site where normal sensory and motor function will not be affected. The advent of newer pharmacological modes of therapy that have produced satisfying results has decreased the number of cases requiring surgery.

Parkinson's facies a stolid masklike expression of the face, with infrequent blinking; it is pathognomonic of PARKINSON'S DISEASE.

parkinsonian (ˌpahkin'sohni·ən) pertaining to parkinsonism.

p. syndrome any disorder manifesting the symptoms of PARKINSON'S DISEASE.

parkinsonism ('pahkinsəˌnizəm) any disorder manifesting the symptoms of PARKINSON'S DISEASE. Any such symptom complex occurring secondarily to another disorder, such as encephalitis, cerebral arteriosclerosis, poisoning with certain toxins, and neurosyphilis.

Parlodel ('pahlohˌdel) trademark for a preparation of bromocriptine mesylate, a dopamine receptor agonist.

Parnate ('pahnayt) trademark for a preparation of tranylcypromine, an antidepressant.

paroccipital (ˌparok'sipit'l) beside the occipital bone.

paromphalocele (pə'romfəlohˌseel) hernia near the navel.

paronychia (ˌparo'niki·ə) inflammation involving the folds of tissue surrounding the fingernail. The causative organisms may be bacteria or fungi, which usually gain entrance through a hangnail or break in the skin due to improper manicuring. Acute infections are treated with hot compresses and the application of an antibiotic or fungicidal ointment. A pocket of purulent material may require incision with a scalpel to promote drainage and healing. Chronic infections are more difficult to cure. If the infection is widespread and difficult to treat topically, removal of the nail may be necessary. See also NAIL.

paroophoron (ˌparoh'ofə·ron) an inconstantly present, small group of coiled tubules between the layers of the mesosalpinx, being a remnant of the excretory part of the mesonephros.

parophthalmia (parof'thalmi·ə) inflammation of the connective tissue around the eye.

paropsis (pa'ropsis) a disorder of vision.

parorchidium (ˌparaw'kidi·əm) displacement of a testis or testes.

parorexia (ˌparə'reksi·ə) nervous perversion of the appetite, with craving for special articles of food or for articles not suitable for food.

parosmia (pa'rozmi·ə) perversion of the sense of smell.

parostosis (ˌparo'stohsis) ossification of tissues outside of the periosteum.

parotid (pə'rotid) near the ear.

p. glands the largest of the three main pairs of salivary glands, located on either side of the face, just below and in front of the ears. From each gland a duct, the parotid duct (sometimes called Stensen's duct), runs forward across the cheek and opens on the inside surface of the cheek opposite the second molar of the upper jaw.

The parotid glands are made up of groups of cells clustered around a globular cavity, resembling a bunch of grapes. Small ducts draining each cavity join the ducts of neighbouring cavities to form large ducts, which in turn join the parotid duct.

From the system of ducts flows the thin, watery secretion of the parotid glands called saliva, which plays an important role in the process of digestion. As food is chewed the saliva with which it is mixed and moistened makes it possible for the food to be reduced to a substance that can be swallowed.

Controlled by the autonomic nervous system, the secretion of the salivary glands begins whenever the sensory nerves of the mouth, or in some cases nerves located elsewhere in the body, are stimulated.

Salivation may be an involuntary reflex, as when food or even inedible material placed in the mouth starts the flow of the secretion from the glands, or it may be a conditioned reflex, as when the flow is started by the sight, smell, or thought of food.

DISORDERS OF THE PAROTID GLANDS. The most common disease affecting the parotid glands is MUMPS, or epidemic parotitis.

Swelling and tenderness may also result from infections caused by other viruses or bacteria in the glands. Less often, these symptoms indicate a blockage of a duct by either infection or a calculus, in which case the swelling is likely to fluctuate, especially at mealtimes. Though stubborn or recurring cases sometimes require surgery, stones often can be removed by massage. For infections, antibiotics and warm compresses are the usual treatment.

Occasionally additional glandular masses grow in or near a parotid gland. The majority of such growths are mixed tumours, so called because they contain cartilage or other material as well as the usual glandular material. Usually they are benign; occasionally they may be malignant and require surgery.

parotidectomy (pəˌroti'dektəmee) excision of a parotid gland.

parotiditis, parotitis (pəˌroti'dietis; ˌparə'tietis) inflammation of the parotid gland.

epidemic p. MUMPS; an acute, communicable viral disease involving chiefly the parotid gland, but frequently affecting other oral glands or the pancreas or gonads.

parous ('parəs) having borne one or more viable children.

parovarian (ˌparoh'vairi·ən) 1. beside the ovary. 2. pertaining to the parovarium (epoophoron).

parovarium (ˌparoh'vairi·əm) epoophoron; a vestigial structure associated with the ovary.

paroxysm ('parokˌsizəm) 1. a sudden recurrence or intensification of symptoms. 2. a spasm or seizure. adj. **paroxysmal.**

paroxysmal (ˌparok'sizməl) occurring in paroxysms.

p. cardiac dyspnoea cardiac asthma. Recurrent attacks of dyspnoea associated with pulmonary oedema and left-sided heart failure.

p. tachycardia recurrent attacks of rapid heart beats that may occur without heart disease.

Parrot's node ('parohz) bony nodes on the outer table of the skull of infants with congenital syphilis.

Parrot's pseudoparalysis pseudoparalysis of one or more extremities in infants, due to syphilitic osteochondritis of an epiphysis.

parrot fever ('parət) an infection transmitted to man by birds; called also PSITTACOSIS.

Parry's disease ('pariz) Graves' disease.

pars (pahz) pl. *partes* [L.] a division or part.

p. mastoidea the mastoid portion of the temporal bone, being the irregular, posterior part.

p. petrosa the petrous portion of the temporal bone, containing the inner ear and located at the base of the cranium.

p. plana the thin part of the ciliary body; the ciliary disc.

p. squamosa the flat, scalelike, anterior and superior portion of the temporal bone.

p. tympanica the tympanic portion of the temporal bone, forming the anterior and inferior walls and part of the posterior wall of the external acoustic meatus.

parthenogenesis (ˌpahthənoh'jenəsis) asexual reproduction in which an egg develops without being fertilized by a spermatozoon, as in certain lower animals, especially arthropods; it may occur as a natural phenomenon or be induced by chemical or mechanical stimulation (artificial parthenogenesis). adj. **parthenogenetic**.

particle ('pahtik'l) an extremely small mass of material. See also ALPHA PARTICLES and BETA PARTICLES.

Dane p. an intact hepatitis B virion.

elementary p. any of the subatomic particles, including electrons, protons, neutrons, positrons, neutrinos, and muons.

particulate (pah'tikyuhlət) composed of separate particles.

parturient (pah'tyooə·ri·ənt) giving birth or pertaining to birth; by extension, a woman in LABOUR.

parturiometer (pah,tyooə·ri'omitə) a device used in measuring the expulsive power of the uterus.

parturition (,pahtyuh'rishən) the act or process of giving birth to a child. See also LABOUR.

parumbilical (,pahrum'bilik'l, -bi'liek'l) alongside the navel.

parvicellular (,pahvi'selyuhlə) composed of small cells.

parvovirus (,pahvoh'vierəs) a group of extremely small, morphologically similar, ether-resistant DNA viruses, including the adeno-associated viruses.

PAS para-aminosalicylic acid, used in treatment of tuberculosis.

pascal (pa'skal, 'pask'l) the SI unit of pressure, which corresponds to a force of one newton per square metre; symbol, Pa.

Paschen bodies ('pashən) small granules demonstrable in the fluid of the vesicles of smallpox.

passive ('pasiv) not active.

p. immunity see IMMUNITY.

p. movements manipulation by a physiotherapist without the help of the patient.

Pasteur (pa'stər) Louis (1822–1895). French chemist and bacteriologist, founder of microbiology and developer of the method of vaccination by attenuated virus. He was born at Dôle, Jura.

By optical investigation of racemic acid, he discovered a new class of isomeric substances which led to work by others on stereochemistry and for which he received the ribbon of the Legion of Honour. Pasteur came to the rescue of the wine industry by his interest in fermentation, and showed that spoiling of wine caused by microorganisms could be prevented by partial heat sterilization (pasteurization), a process now applied to many perishable foods. Experimental foundation was given to his ideas of fermentation and the long-accepted theory of spontaneous generation was disposed of once and for all. Later he came to the rescue of the silkworm industry and found methods for detecting and preventing pébrine and flâcherie, the two diseases that were destroying it. He turned his attention then to anthrax, chicken cholera, and hydrophobia (rabies), and developed preventive inoculations against them. The Pasteur Institute was opened shortly thereafter. Other institutions were founded all over the world to promote inoculation against rabies.

Pasteur effect the decrease in the rate of glucose utilization and the suppression of lactate accumulation by tissues or microorganisms in the presence of oxygen.

Pasteur–Chamberland filter (,pastər'shanhbə,lanh) a hollow column of unglazed porcelain through which liquids are forced by pressure or by vacuum exhaustion.

Pasteurella (,pahstə'relə) a genus of gram-negative bacteria (family Brucellaceae).

P. multocida (Septica) the aetiological agent of the haemorrhagic septicaemias in cattle and buffaloes. May cause infections in humans, including those following cat and dog bites.

P. pestis *Yersinia pestis*.

P. tularensis *Francisella tularensis*.

pasteurellosis (,pastə·re'lohsis) infection with organisms of the genus *Pasteurella*.

pasteurization (,pastə·rie'zayshən, ,pahstyə-) heating of milk or other liquids to a temperature of 60 °C (140 °F) for 30 minutes, killing pathogenic bacteria and considerably delaying other bacterial development.

Patau's syndrome ('patohz) trisomy 13 syndrome.

patch (pach) a small area differing from the rest of a surface.

Peyer's p's whitish, oval, elevated patches of closely packed lymph follicles in mucous and submucous layers of the small intestine.

p. test a test for hypersensitivity in which filter paper or gauze saturated with the substance in question is applied to the skin, usually on the forearm or back. A positive reaction is reddening or swelling at the site. See also SKIN TEST.

patella (pə'telə) pl. *patellae* [L.] a triangular bone at the knee; the kneecap.

patellar (pə'telə) of or pertaining to the patella.

p. ligament the continuation of the central portion of the tendon of the quadriceps femoris muscle distal to the patella, extending from the patella to the tuberosity of the tibia; called also patellar tendon.

p. reflex involuntary contraction of the quadriceps muscle and jerky extension of the leg when the patellar ligament is sharply tapped. It is often used as a test of nervous system function. Called also KNEE JERK and quadriceps reflex.

patellectomy (,pate'lektəmee) excision of the patella.

patelliform (pə'teli,fawm) shaped like the patella.

patellofemoral (pə,teloh'femə·rəl) pertaining to the patella and femur.

patency ('paytənsee) the condition of being wide open.

patent ('paytənt) 1. open, unobstructed, or not closed. 2. apparent, evident.

p. ductus arteriosus abnormal persistence of an open lumen in the ductus arteriosus, between the aorta and the pulmonary artery, after birth. The ductus arteriosus is open during prenatal life, allowing most of the blood of the fetus to bypass the lungs, but normally this channel closes shortly before birth. When the ductus arteriosus remains open, it places special burdens on the left ventricle and causes a diminished blood flow in the aorta.

The symptoms of patent ductus arteriosus are usually so slight they are not noticed until the child is older and more active. He then begins to experience dyspnoea on exertion. If the ductus is large there may be retardation of growth.

Treatment is surgical, preferably when the child is from 4 to 10 years of age. The open ductus arteriosus is ligated. Prognosis for this condition, when not accompanied by other congenital heart defects, is excellent.

Closure of a patent ductus arteriosus can be produced in preterm infants by administration of an inhibitor of prostaglandin formation, such as indomethacin. Conversely, in neonates suffering from severe complex congenital heart defects in which an open ductus arteriosus could be beneficial, injections of prostaglandins are used to keep the channel open.

p. medicine a drug or remedy protected by a trademark, available without a prescription.

Paterson–Kelly syndrome (,patəsən'kelee) Plummer–Vinson syndrome.

path(o)- word element. [Gr.] *disease*.

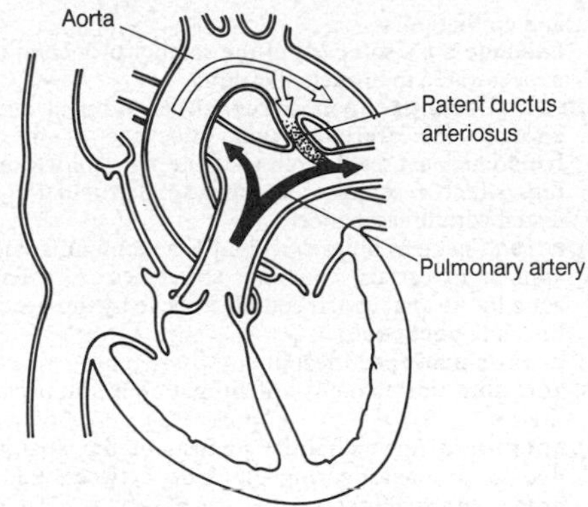

Patent ductus arteriosus.

pathergy ('pathəjee) 1. a condition in which the application of a stimulus leaves the organism unduly susceptible to subsequent stimuli of a different kind. 2. a condition of being allergic to several antigens. adj. **pathergic.**

pathfinder ('pahth,fiendə) an instrument for locating urethral strictures.

pathobiology (,pathohbie'oləjee) pathology.

pathoclisis (,pathoh'klisis) a specific sensitivity to specific toxins, or a specific affinity of certain toxins for certain systems or organs.

pathogen ('pathə,jen) any disease-producing agent or microorganism. adj. **pathogenic.**

pathogenesis (,pathə'jenəsis) the processes involved in development of disease; more specifically the cellular events and reactions and other pathological mechanisms occurring in the development of disease. adj. **pathogenetic.**

pathogenicity (,pathəjə'nisitee) the quality of producing or the ability to produce pathological changes or disease.

pathogeny (pə'thojənee) pathogenesis.

pathognomonic (,pathəgnə'monik) specifically distinctive or characteristic of a disease or pathological condition; denoting a sign or symptom on which a diagnosis can be made.

pathological (,pathə'lojik'l) 1. pertaining to pathology. 2. causing or arising from disease. 3. indicating a diseased state or condition.

p. fracture a fracture occurring in diseased bone where there has been little or no external trauma. See also spontaneous FRACTURE.

pathologist (pə'tholəjist) a specialist in pathology.

pathology (pə'tholəjee) 1. the branch of medicine treating of the essential nature of disease, especially of the changes in body tissues and organs which cause or are caused by disease. 2. the structural and functional manifestations of a disease. adj. **pathologic, pathological.**

clinical p. pathology applied to the solution of clinical problems, especially the use of laboratory methods in clinical diagnosis.

comparative p. that which considers human disease processes in comparison with those of other animals.

experimental p. the study of artificially induced pathological processes.

oral p. that which treats of conditions causing or resulting from morbid anatomic or functional changes in the structures of the mouth.

speech-language p. a field of the health sciences dealing with the evaluation of speech, language, and voice disorders and the rehabilitation of patients with such disorders not amenable to medical or surgical treatment.

surgical p. the pathology of disease processes that are surgically accessible for diagnosis or treatment.

pathomimesis (,pathohmi'meesis) malingering.

pathomorphism (,pathoh'mawfizəm) perverted or abnormal morphology.

pathonomia (,pathə'nohmi·ə) the science of the laws of disease.

pathophobia (,pathə'fohbi·ə) an exaggerated dread of disease.

pathophysiology (,pathoh,fizi'oləjee) the physiology of disordered function.

pathopsychology (,pathohsie'koləjee) the psychology of mental disease.

pathosis (pə'thohsis) a diseased condition.

pathway ('pahth,way) a course usually followed. In neurology, the nerve structures through which a sensory impression is conducted to the cerebral cortex (afferent pathway), or through which an impulse passes from the brain to the skeletal musculature (efferent pathway). Also used alone to indicate a sequence of reactions that convert one biological material to another (metabolic pathway).

alternative complement p. one in which complement components C3 and C5 through C9 are activated without participation by C1, C2, and C4.

biosynthetic p. the sequence of enzymatic steps in the synthesis of a specific end-product in a living organism.

classical complement p. the one in which all of the complement components C1 through C9 participate.

Embden–Meyerhof p. (of glucose metabolism) the series of enzymatic reactions in the anaerobic conversion of glucose to lactic acid, resulting in energy in the form of adenosine triphosphate (ATP).

final common p. 1. the motor neurons by which nerve impulses from many central sources pass to a muscle or gland in the periphery. 2. any mechanism by which several independent effects exert a common influence.

pentose phosphate p. a pathway of hexose oxidation in which glucose-6-phosphate undergoes two successive oxidations by NADP, the final forming a pentose phosphate.

properdin p. alternative complement pathway.

-pathy word element. [Gr.] *morbid condition* or *disease*; generally used to designate a noninflammatory condition.

patient ('payshənt) a person who is ill or is undergoing treatment for disease.

patient's rights ('payshəns riets) patients have three basic rights, namely, the right to know, the right to privacy and the right to treatment. The first two are moral rights while the third is, in the UK, both a moral and legal right.

The right to know is not absolute, in as much as health professionals are allowed to exercise professional judgement over the extent to which an individual patient should be informed of his/her diagnosis and prognosis. The patient too has the right to choose not to be fully informed. It is, however, fairly generally accepted that patients have the right to be told their diagnosis, the treatment options and possible outcomes of treatment. In some specific instances, when it is necessary for the patient to sign a consent form, then they clearly have the right to information which will enable them to give informed consent.

The right to privacy is also not absolute. The patient entering open ward in a hospital clearly gives up a degree of privacy in so doing. Patients do, however, have a right to expect that any treatment or care will be given to them in reasonable privacy. Additionally, they have the right to expect that information about them, their diagnosis and treatment, will be treated in a confidential manner by health professionals; and that while it may be necessary for information to be shared between the professionals involved in their care, it will not be shared with other patients, nor any other person not involved in their care, without their prior consent.

The right to treatment is a right in law as well as being a moral right. It is enshrined in the legislation under which the National Health Service was set up. Patients have a right to treatment on request irrespective of age, gender, ethnicity, mental and physical capacity. They also have the right to choose not to seek treatment and to refuse the treatment offered. They have a right to expect that treatment and care will be given in a considerate and respectful manner. See also ETHICS.

Patrick's test ('patriks) the thigh and knee of the supine patient are flexed, the external malleolus rests on the patella on the opposite leg, and the knee is depressed; production of pain indicates arthritis of the hip. Also known as *fabere sign*, from the initial letters of movements necessary to elicit it, i.e.,*f*lexion, *ab*duction, *e*xternal *r*otation, and *e*xtension.

patrilineal (,patri'lini·əl) descended through the male line.

patulous ('patyuhləs) spread widely apart; open; distended.

Paul–Bunnell test (,pawlbə'nel) a method of testing for the presence of heterophil antibodies in the blood for the diagnosis of infectious mononucleosis, based on the agglutination of sheep erythrocytes by the inactivated serum of patients with the disease. Heterophil antibodies are present in other conditions, e.g. serum sickness. In infectious mononucleosis, the antibody is not absorbed by guinea pig kidney but is absorbed by ox red cells. These absorption tests are incorporated in the commercially available monospot test, widely used to diagnose mononucleosis.

pause (pawz) an interruption, or rest.

compensatory p. the pause after a premature ventricular systole, related to blockage of one beat of the basic pacemaker of the heart.

Pb chemical symbol, *lead* (L. *plumbum*).

PBB polybrominated biphenyl.

PBI protein-bound iodine.

p.c. *post cibum* (after meals).

PCB polychlorinated biphenyl.

PCG phonocardiogram.

PCP PHENCYCLIDINE, a central nervous system depressant with unpredictable side-effects. Popularly called 'angel dust' and 'animal tranquillizer', it is one of the most abused illicit drugs in the US, but so far has not played a major role in illegal drug use in the UK.

PCV packed-cell volume, the volume of packed red cells in litres per litre of blood.

Pd chemical symbol, *palladium*.

p.d. potential difference; prism diopter.

pe- for words beginning thus, see also those beginning with *pae-*.

peanut oil ('pee,nut) a refined fixed oil from seed kernels of cultivated varieties of *Arachis hypogaea*; used as a solvent for drugs.

pearl (pərl) 1. a small medicated granule, or a glass globule with a single dose of volatile medicine, as amyl nitrite. 2. a rounded mass of tough sputum, as seen in the early stages of an attack of bronchial asthma.

epidermic p's, epithelial p's rounded concentric masses of epithelial cells found in certain papillomas and epitheliomas.

Laënnec's p's soft casts of the smaller bronchial tubes expectorated in bronchial asthma.

peau d'orange (,poh do'ronhzh) a dimpled appearance of the overlying skin. Blockage of the skin lymphatics causes dimpling of the hair follicle openings which resembles orange skin. Particularly associated with breast cancer.

pecten ('pekten) pl. *pectines* [L.] 1. a comb; in anatomy, applied to certain comblike structures. 2. a narrow zone in the anal canal, bounded above by the pectinate line. adj. **pectineal**.

p. ossis pubis pectineal line.

pectenitis (,pektə'nietis) inflammation of the pecten of the anus.

pectenosis (,pektə'nohsis) stenosis of the anal canal due to an inelastic ring of tissue between the anal groove and anal crypts.

pectin ('pektin) a homosaccharidic polymer of sugar acids of fruit that forms gels with sugar at the proper pH; a purified form obtained from the acid extract of the rind of citrus fruits or from apple pomace is used as a protectant and in cooking. adj. **pectic**.

pectinate ('pekti,nayt) comb-shaped.

p. line the line marking the junction of the zone of the anal canal lined with stratified squamous epithelium and the zone lined with columnar epithelium.

pectineal (pek'tini·əl) pertaining to the os pubis.

pectiniform (pek'tini,fawm) comb-shaped.

pectoral ('pektə·rəl) 1. of or pertaining to the chest or breast. 2. relieving disorders of the respiratory tract, as an expectorant.

p. muscles four muscles of the chest.

pectoralis (,pektə'raylis) [L.] *pertaining to the chest or breast, pectoral*.

pectoriloquy (,pektə'riləkwee) transmission of the sound of spoken words through the chest wall, indicating the presence of a cavity or solidification of pulmonary structures.

pectus ('pektəs) the breast, chest, or thorax.

p. carinatum a malformation of the chest wall in which the sternum is abnormally prominent; called also pigeon chest or chicken breast.

Moderate cases cause no difficulties and require no treatment. In severe cases, the deformity of the chest may interfere with lung and heart action, causing dyspnoea on exercise and increased susceptibility to respiratory infections. Serious malformations can usually be corrected by surgery.

p. excavatum a congenital malformation of the chest wall characterized by a pronounced funnel-shaped depression with its apex over the lower end of the sternum; called also funnel chest.

The condition is caused by a shortening of the central portion of the diaphragm, which pulls the sternum backward during inhalation, and by the growth of ribs. Except in mild cases, it decreases the ability of the child to engage in sustained exercise. It delays recovery from coughs and colds, reduces the ability to eat a full meal, so that most patients are underweight, and often produces a functional heart murmur. Noisy breathing may occur during sleep. A child may also develop an emotional problem because of embarrassment over the deformity.

The deformity can be satisfactorily corrected by surgery.

ped(o)- word element. 1. [Gr.] *child*. 2. [L.] *foot*.

pedal ('peed'l) pertaining to the foot or feet.

pederast ('pedə,rast) one who practices pederasty.

pederasty ('pedə,rastee) homosexual anal intercourse between men and boys, with the latter as the passive partners.

pedia- word element. [Gr.] *child.*

pedicellation (,pedisə'layshən) the development of a pedicle.

pedicle ('pedik'l) a footlike, stemlike, or narrow basal part or structure, such as a narrow strip by which a graft of tissue remains attached to the donor site.

vertebral p. one of the paired parts of the vertebral arch that connect a lamina to the vertebral body.

pediculation (pə,dikyuh'layshən) 1. the process of forming a pedicle. 2. infestation with lice.

pediculicide (pə'dikyuhli,sied) 1. destroying lice. 2. an agent that destroys lice.

pediculosis (pə,dikyuh'lohsis) infestation with lice. See also LOUSE.

pediculous (pə'dikyuhləs) infested with lice.

Pediculus (pə'dikyuhləs) a genus of lice.

P. humanus a species that feeds on human blood and is an important vector of relapsing fever, typhus, and trench fever; two subspecies are recognized: *P. humanus* var. *capitis* (head louse) found on the scalp hair, and *P. humanus* var. *corporis* (body, or clothes, louse) found elsewhere on the body.

pedigree ('pedi,gree) a table, chart, diagram, or list of an individual's ancestors, used in genetics in the analysis of mendelian inheritance.

pedodynamometer (,pedoh,dienə'momitə) an instrument for measuring leg strength.

pedorthics (pə'dawthiks) the design, manufacture, fitting, and modification of shoes and related foot appliances as prescribed for the amelioration of painful or disabling conditions of the foot and leg. adj. **pedorthic.**

pedorthist (pə'dawthist) a person skilled in pedorthics and practising its application.

peduncle (pə'dungk'l) a stemlike connecting part, especially, (a) a collection of nerve fibres coursing between different regions in the central nervous system, or (b) the stalk by which a nonsessile tumour is attached to normal tissue. adj. **peduncular.**

cerebellar p's three sets of paired bundles (superior, middle, and inferior) connecting the cerebellum to the midbrain, pons, and medulla oblongata, respectively.

cerebral p. the ventral half of the midbrain, divisible into a dorsal part (*tegmentum*) and a ventral part (*crus cerebri*), which are separated by the substantia nigra.

pineal p. HABENULA (2).

pedunculated (pə'dungkyuh,laytid) having a peduncle.

pedunculotomy (pə,dungkyuh'lotəmee) incision of a cerebral peduncle.

pedunculus (pə'dungkyuhləs) peduncle.

PEEP positive-end-expiratory pressure.

peer review (piə ri'vyoo) a basic component of a QUALITY ASSURANCE programme in which the results of health and/or nursing care given to a specific patient population are evaluated according to defined criteria established by the peers of the professionals delivering the care. Peer review is focused on the patient and on the results of care given by a group of professionals rather than on individual professional practitioners.

Review by peer groups is promoted by professional organizations as a means of maintaining standards of care. (In 1974, the American Nurses' Association issued 'Guidelines for Peer Review'. Throughout the United States professional nurses have utilized these guidelines to initiate systems for formal peer review and NURSING AUDIT).

Retrospective review critically evaluates the results of work that has been completed; it is done for purposes of improving future practice. The source of data is medical records which document the full continuum of care provided and each patient's response to that care.

Concurrent review takes place at the time the care is being given. It critically examines each patient's progress toward desired health-wellness outcomes. Sources of data for concurrent review are the patient's record and interview, observation, and inspection of the patient. A major advantage of concurrent review is that it provides the opportunity to improve care so that patients benefit from the review and recommended changes in ongoing care.

peg (peg) a projecting structure.

rete p's inward projections of the epidermis into the dermis, as seen histologically in vertical sections.

pelage ('pelij) [Fr.] the hairy coat of mammals; the hairs of the body, limbs, and head, collectively.

Pel–Ebstein fever (pel'ebstien) a cyclic fever occasionally seen in HODGKIN'S DISEASE and other diseases, characterized by irregular episodes of fever of several days duration.

peliosis (,peli'ohsis) purpura.

pellagra (pə'lagrə, -'lay-) a syndrome caused by a diet seriously deficient in niacin (or by failure to convert tryptophan to niacin). Most persons with pellagra also suffer from deficiencies of vitamin B_2 (riboflavin) and other essential vitamins and minerals. The disease also occurs in persons suffering from alcoholism and drug addiction. adj. **pellagrous.**

SYMPTOMS. Chief symptoms of pellagra are various skin, digestive, and mental disturbances. The mouth becomes inflamed and the tongue red and sore; cracks and sores appear in the skin around the mouth. The skin on the back of the hands may become red, thick, and scaly, as may that of the neck and chest-areas exposed to sunlight and the chafing of clothes.

Vomiting and loss of appetite occur. Diarrhoea often appears early and becomes worse as the disease progresses, thus hampering treatment by preventing effective absorption of essential vitamins.

Mental symptoms are variable. In some cases, there may be only insomnia and minor depression. In other cases, the sufferer may become stuporous, or on the contrary become violent and irrational. Headache, irritability, and general anxiety may also be present.

TREATMENT. Treatment of pellagra consists of an improved diet, often combined with large doses of niacinamide. In acute cases, niacinamide must be administered by injection and must be accompanied by large doses of other vitamins.

The patient's diet should include meat (particularly liver), whole-grain cereals, and peanuts, all of which are especially good sources of niacin. In severe cases of pellagra, bed rest is required. Skin lesions are treated with antibiotics.

pellagroid (pə'lagroyd) resembling pellagra.

Pellegrini's disease, Pellegrini–Stieda disease (,peli,greeniz; ,peli,greenee'steedə) calcification of the medial collateral ligament of the knee due to trauma.

pellet ('pelit) a small pill or granule.

pellicle ('pelik'l) a thin scum forming on the surface of liquids.

pellucid (pe'loosid) translucent.

pelvic ('pelvik) pertaining to the pelvis.

p. bone hip bone, comprising the ilium, ischium and pubis.

p. diameter any diameter of the pelvis, such as the diagonal conjugate, joining the posterior surface of the pubis to the tip of the sacral promontory; the external conjugate, joining the depression under the last lumbar spine to the upper margin of the pubis; the true (internal) conjugate, the anteroposterior diameter of the pelvic inlet, measured from the upper margin of the pubic symphysis to the sacrovertebral angle; the oblique, joining the one sacroiliac articulation to the iliopubic eminence of the other side; the transverse (of inlet), joining the two most widely separated points of the pelvic inlet; the transverse (of outlet), joining the medial surfaces of the ischial tuberosities.

As the true PELVIS forms the birth canal, precise measurement of the internal diameters is desirable, but difficult to achieve. The smallest diameters, called the essential diameters, are the anteroposterior diameter at the brim and the transverse diameter at the outlet. The anteroposterior diameter at the brim is also called the *true conjugate* and is measured between the central point of the sacral promontory and the upper inner border of the symphysis pubis. It should be 11.5 cm or more. It can only be accurately measured by ultrasound scan or radiography, but this would only be undertaken for breech delivery or suspected CEPHALOPELVIC disproportion. Usually the true conjugate is assessed by measuring the diagonal conjugate, i.e. the distance between the sacral promontory and the lower border of the symphysis pubis. In practice, if the sacral promontory is not felt by the examining finger on vaginal examination, the anteroposterior diameter of the brim is said to be adequate.

The transverse diameter of the outlet is measured between the two ischial spines and should also be 11.5 cm. In practice, the distance between the two ischial tuberosities is assessed by a fist placed between the two landmarks.

The sub-pubic angle should be greater than 90°. This is assessed on vaginal examination by placing the two fingers of the examining hand against the lower border of the symphysis pubis. If the fist is flushed, the angle is adequate. If the fingers will not fit snugly and there is a space left (waste space of Morris), cephalopelvic disproportion should be suspected.

p. inflammatory disease (PID) infection involving the uterine tubes, ovaries, and parametrium. Other organs in the pelvis, especially the gut, may also be involved.

The infection may follow delivery or abortion, may be secondary to infection elsewhere in the pelvis or abdomen (e.g., appendicitis), or in the genital tract (e.g., gonorrhoea), or may be due to blood-borne infection (e.g., tuberculosis).

Acute PID causes lower abdominal pain, fever and vaginal discharge. Treatment involves antibiotics, bed rest, and analgesia. Early diagnosis and treatment is important in order to prevent blockage of the uterine tubes by fibrous adhesions.

Chronic PID may follow an inadequately treated acute attack or may develop insidiously. Symptoms may include lower abdominal pain or backache, vaginal discharge, menorrhagia, and dyspareunia. Acute exacerbations are treated with antibiotics, but surgery may eventually be required. If the uterine tubes become blocked, operations to restore fertility may be performed, but are often unsuccessful.

p. inlet the superior opening of the pelvis.

p. outlet the inferior opening of the pelvis.

pelvicaliceal, pelvicalyceal (ˌpelviˌkali'seeəl; ˌpelviˌkali'seeəl) pertaining to the renal pelves and calices.

pelvicephalometry (ˌpelviˌkefə'lomətree, -ˌsef-) measurement of the fetal head in relation to the maternal pelvis.

pelvifixation (ˌpelvifik'sayshən) surgical fixation of a displaced pelvic organ.

pelvimeter (pel'vimitə) an instrument for measuring the pelvis.

pelvimetry (pel'vimətree) measurement of the capacity and diameter of the pelvis, either internally or externally or both, with the hands, with a pelvimeter, or by radiography.

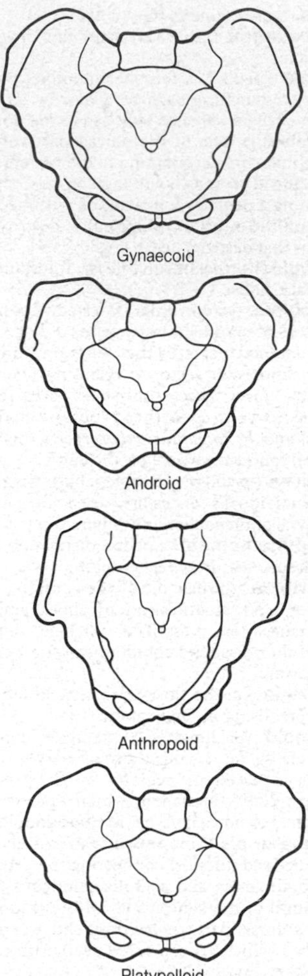

Various types of pelvic inlet

pelviostomy (ˌpelvi'ostəmee) drainage of the renal pelvis by a tube or by reimplantation of the ureter.

pelviotomy (ˌpelvi'otəmee) 1. incision or transection of a pelvic (hip) bone. 2. pyelotomy; incision of the renal pelvis.

pelviperitonitis (ˌpelviˌperitə'nietis) inflammation of the pelvic peritoneum.

pelvirectal (ˌpelvi'rekt'l) pertaining to the pelvis and rectum.

pelvis ('pelvis) pl. *pelves;* the lower (caudal) portion of the trunk of the body, forming a basin bounded anteriorly and laterally by the ilium, ischium and pubis and posteriorly by the sacrum and coccyx. Also applied to any basin-like structure, e.g., the renal pelvis.

The bony pelvis is formed by the sacrum, the coccyx, and the ilium, pubis, and ischium, bones that form the hip and pubic arch. These bones are separate in the child, but become fused by adulthood.

The pelvis is subjected to more stress than any other

body structure. The upper part of the pelvic girdle, which is somewhat flared, supports the weight of internal organs in the upper part of the body.

Pelvic structures in men and women differ both in shape and in relative size. The male pelvis is heart-shaped and narrow and proportionately heavier and stronger than the female, so that it is better suited for lifting and running. The female pelvis is constructed to accommodate the fetus during pregnancy and to facilitate its downward passage through the pelvic cavity in childbirth. The most obvious difference between the male and female pelvis is in the shape. A woman's hips are wider and her pelvic cavity is round and relatively large. Even among women, moreover, there are differences in the shape of the pelvis, and these differences must be taken into account in childbirth. During pregnancy the capacity of the pelvis and the PELVIC diameters may be measured, so that possible complications during labour can be avoided.

android p. one with a wedge-shaped inlet and narrow anterior segment; a typically male pelvis, which in the female predisposes to occipitoposterior position of the fetus.

anthropoid p. a female pelvis whose anteroposterior diameter at the brim equals or exceeds the transverse diameter, so that rotation of the fetus during its passage through the birth canal is not needed.

assimilation p. one in which the ilia articulates with the vertebral column higher (high assimilation pelvis) or lower (low assimilation pelvis) than normal, the number of lumbar vertebrae being correspondingly decreased or increased.

beaked p. one with the pelvic bones laterally compressed and their anterior junction pushed forward.

contracted p. one showing a decrease of 1.5 to 2 cm in an important diameter; when all dimensions are proportionately diminished, it is a generally contracted pelvis, or justo minor pelvis.

cordate p. a heart-shaped pelvis.

dolichopellic p. a long, oval pelvis with the anteroposterior diameter greater than the transverse diameter.

extrarenal p. see renal PELVIS.

flat p. platypellic pelvis, platypelloid pelvis.

frozen p. a condition, due to infection or carcinoma, in which the adnexa and uterus are fixed in the pelvis.

funnel p. one with a normal inlet but a greatly narrowed outlet.

gynecoid p. the normal female pelvis: a rounded oval brim with well rounded anterior and posterior segments, facilitating easy rotation and delivery of the fetus. See PELVIC diameters.

infantile p. a generally contracted pelvis with an oval shape, a high sacrum, and inclination of the walls; called also *juvenile pelvis*.

p. justo major an unusually large gynaecoid pelvis, with all dimensions increased.

p. justo minor a small gynecoid pelvis, with all dimensions symmetrically reduced.

juvenile p. infantile pelvis.

kyphotic p. a deformed pelvis marked by increase of the conjugate diameter at the brim with decrease of the transverse diameter at the outlet.

p. major false pelvis.

mesatipellic p. a round type of pelvis, in which the transverse diameter is equal to the anteroposterior diameter or exceeds it by no more than 1 cm.

p. minor true pelvis.

Nägele's p. one contracted in an oblique diameter, with complete ankylosis of the sacroiliac synchondrosis on one side and imperfect development of the sacrum and coxa on the same side.

Otto p. one in which the acetabulum is depressed, accompanied by protrusion of the femoral head into the pelvis.

platypellic p., platypelloid p. one shortened in the anteroposterior aspect, with an enlarged transverse diameter and kidney-shaped brim, may be caused by a sub-clinical form of rickets. Delivery is straightforward once the head has engaged, but caesarean section may be needed.

rachitic p. one distorted as a result of rickets.

renal p. the funnel-shaped expansion of the upper end of the ureter into which the renal calices open; it is usually within the renal sinus, but under certain conditions, a large part of it may be outside the kidney (*extrarenal pelvis*).

Robert's p. a transversely contracted pelvis caused by osteoarthritis affecting both sacroiliac joints, the inlet becoming a narrow wedge.

scoliotic p. a congenitally deformed pelvis in which there are no wings to the sacrum. The brim consists of a narrow opening which makes vaginal delivery impossible.

split p. one with a congenital separation at the symphysis pubis or subluxation of the symphysis as a complication of pregnancy or childbirth.

spondylolisthetic p. one in which the last, or rarely the fourth or third, lumbar vertebra is dislocated in front of the sacrum, more or less occluding the pelvic brim and making vaginal delivery impossible.

true p. the pelvic cavity or basin which lies below the pelvic brim. It encloses and provides protection for the pelvic organs and dictates the contours and diameters of the birth canal.

pelviureteral (ˌpelviyuh'reetə·rəl) relating to the renal pelvis and the ureter.

pelvospondylitis (ˌpelvohˌspondi'lietis) inflammation of the pelvic portion of the spine.

p. ossificans rheumatoid spondylitis.

pemoline ('pemohˌleen) a central nervous system stimulant.

pemphigoid ('pemfiˌgoyd) 1. resembling pemphigus. 2. a group of skin disorders similar to but clearly distinguishable from pemphigus.

benign mucosal p. a chronic bullous disease of elderly persons, involving primarily the mucous membranes, particularly the conjunctiva and oral mucosa, with scarring.

bullous p. a chronic, generalized, usually nonfatal, bullous skin eruption usually seen in elderly persons. IgE antibodies are found at the basement membrane.

localized chronic p. a form in which bulla formation is confined for many years to a circumscribed region, with scarring but without affecting the mucous membranes.

mucous membrane p. tense subepidermal blisters initially involving any mucous membrane, including those of the conjunctivae, nose, larynx, pharynx, oesophagus, penis, vulva, vagina and anus. Local steroids are effective if only one site is involved. On healing, scarring of the affected areas can be seen.

pemphigus ('pemfigəs) a distinctive group of diseases characterized by successive crops of large bullae ('water blisters'); the name is derived from the Greek word for blister: *pemphix.* A rare disease, it is also a serious one that requires prompt treatment. It can occur in acute or chronic form. The term pemphigus generally refers to pemphigus vulgaris. Clusters of blisters usually appear first near the nose and mouth—sometimes inside them—and then gradually spread over the skin of the rest of the body. When the blisters burst, they leave round patches of raw and tender skin.

The skin itches, burns and gives off an offensive odour. The patient loses appetite and weight. If the disease is allowed to progress, it may cause extreme weakness, prostration and shock, accompanied by chills, sweating, fever, and often pneumonia.

Pemphigus is considered to be an auto-immune disorder. Antibodies have been identified which act against the intercellular substance of the epidermal cells. Thus the epidermal cells separate, causing the formation of blisters and destruction of the epidermis.

The patient must be hospitalized from the beginning and given antibiotics and sometimes blood transfusions. He suffers intense discomfort and may need to suck anaesthetic tablets to allay pain around the mouth while eating.

Progress has been made in the treatment of this disease through the persistent use of prednisolone, used in high doses initially and gradually reduced to a maintenance dose of 5-40 mg daily. The disease is difficult to control, however, and therapy sometimes must be maintained for years to prevent continuing attacks, which can lead to complications of long-term steroid therapy.

benign familial p. a hereditary, recurrent vesiculobullous dermatitis, usually involving the axillae, groin, and neck, with crops of lesions that regress over several weeks or months. Called also *Hailey–Hailey disease*.

p. erythematosus a chronic form in which the lesions, limited to the face and chest, resemble those of disseminated lupus erythematosus.

p. foliaceus a chronic, generalized, vesicular and scaling eruption resembling dermatitis herpetiformis or, later in its course, exfoliative dermatitis. **p. vegetans** a variant of pemphigus vulgaris in which the bullae are replaced by verrucoid hypertrophic vegetative masses.

p. vulgaris a rare relapsing disease with suprabasal, intraepidermal bullae of the skin and mucous membranes; invariably fatal if untreated (see PEMPHIGUS).

Penbritin (pen'britin) trademark for preparations of ampicillin; an antibiotic.

pendulous ('pendyuhləs) hanging loosely; dependent.

penetrance ('penitrəns) the frequency with which a heritable trait is manifested by individuals carrying the principal gene or genes conditioning it.

penetrometer (ˌpeni'tromitə) an instrument for measuring the penetrating power of x-rays; qualimeter.

-penia word element. [Gr.] *deficiency*.

penicillamine (ˌpeni'siləˌmeen) D-penicillamine; a product of penicillin which chelates copper and other metals; used mainly to remove excess copper from the body in hepatolenticular degeneration, and also used in the treatment of rheumatoid arthritis.

penicillic acid (ˌpeni'silik) an antibiotic substance isolated from cultures of various species of *Penicillium* and *Aspergillus*.

penicillin (ˌpeni'silin) any of a large group of natural or semisynthetic antibacterial antibiotics derived directly or indirectly from strains of fungi of the genus *Penicillium* and other soil-inhabiting fungi grown on special culture media. Penicillins exert a bactericidal as well as a bacteriostatic effect on susceptible bacteria by interfering with the final stages of the synthesis of peptidoglycan, a substance in the bacterial cell wall. Despite their relatively low toxicity for the host, they are active against many bacteria, especially gram-positive pathogens (streptococci, staphylococci, pneumococci); clostridia; certain gram-negative forms (gonococci and meningococci); certain spirochetes (*Treponema pallidum* and *T. pertenue*); and certain fungi. Certain strains of some target species, for example staphylococci, secrete the enzyme *penicillinase*, which inactivates penicillin and confers resistance to the antibiotic. Some of the newer penicillins, for example flucloxacillin, are more effective against penicillinase-producing organisms. A new class of extended-spectrum penicillins, called the ureidopenicillins, includes piperacillin, azlocillin and mezlocillin.

Penicillin is administered intramuscularly and orally, in liquid or tablet form. Oral administration requires larger doses of the drug because absorption is incomplete.

Allergic reaction to penicillin occurs in some persons. The reaction may be slight—a stinging or burning sensation at the site of injection—or it can be more serious—severe dermatitis or even anaphylactic shock, which may be fatal. **p. G** benzylpenicillin; the most widely used penicillin; used principally in the treatment of infections due to gram-positive bacteria, *Treponema pallidum* and *Actinomyces israeli*.

p. G procaine a compound of penicillin G and procaine used as a long-acting antibacterial.

p. V a biosynthetically or semisynthetically produced antibiotic, similar to penicillin G, used orally for mild to moderately severe infections due to susceptible gram-positive bacteria.

penicillinase (ˌpeni'siliˌnayz) an enzyme produced by bacteria that inactivates penicillin, thus increasing resistance to the antibiotic; a purified form from *Bacillus cereus* is used in the treatment of reactions to penicillin.

penicilloyl-polylysine (ˌpeniˌsiloylˌpoli'lieseen) an agent prepared from polylysine and a penicillic acid; intradermal reaction elicits a wheal and erythema response in those sensitive to penicillin.

penicillus (ˌpeni'siləs) pl. *penicilli* [L.] any of the brushlike groups of arterial branches in the lobules of the spleen.

penile ('peeniel) of or pertaining to the penis.

penis ('peenis) the external male organ of urination and copulation.

The body of the penis consists of three cylindrical-shaped masses of erectile tissue which run the length of the penis. Two of the masses lie alongside each other and end behind the head of the penis. The third mass lies underneath them. This latter mass contains the urethra. The penis terminates in an oval or cone-shaped body, the glans penis, which contains the exterior opening of the urethra.

The glans penis is covered by a loose skin, the foreskin or prepuce, which enables it to expand freely during erection. The skin ends just behind the glans penis and folds forward to cover it. The inner surface of the foreskin contains glands that secrete a lubricating fluid called smegma which makes it easy for the penis to expand and retract past the foreskin.

DISORDERS OF THE PENIS. Disorders of the penis are rare. One of the most common complaints is phimosis, due to tight foreskin, which may make erection painful. This condition can be easily remedied by circumcision.

Among the most common diseases of the penis are sexually transmitted diseases such as HERPES GENITALIS, SYPHILIS, and GONORRHOEA. Cancer of the penis is rare and rarely occurs in a man who has been circumcised.

p. envy in psychoanalytic theory a common component of the genital stage of psychosexual development when the penis allegedly becomes a focus of interest to children of both sexes. Often extended as a metaphor to describe personality traits in women related to envy of the male role.

penitis (pee'nietis) inflammation of the penis.

penniform ('peniˌfawm) shaped like a feather.

Penrose drain ('penrohz) a drain made by drawing a strip of gauze or surgical sponge into a tube of gutta-percha, rubber or other plastic material; called also *cigarette drain*.

pent(a)- word element. [Gr.] *five*.

pentaerythritol tetranitrate (ˌpentə·i'rithri,tol ˌtetrə-'nietrayt) a vasodilator used in angina pectoris and coronary insufficiency; because of its explosiveness it must be diluted with lactose or a similar diluent.

pentagastrin (ˌpentə'gastrin) a synthetic pentapeptide consisting of β-alanine and C-terminal tetrapeptide of gastrin; used as a test of gastric secretory function.

pentamidine (pen'tamideen) an antiprotozoal drug used mainly in the treatment of *Pneumocystis carinii* infections.

pentasomy (ˌpentə'sohmee) the presence of three additional chromosomes of one type (e.g., 5 X chromosomes) in an otherwise diploid cell (2n + 3).

pentavalent (ˌpentə'vaylənt) having a valency of five.

pentazocine (pen'tazoh,seen) a synthetic narcotic analgesic developed as an attempt to produce a narcotic without abuse potential. It is used orally as a mild analgesic and by infusion for more severe pain. It has both agonist and antagonist properties. Respiratory depression is less than with morphine and not dose related. However, it occasionally causes hallucinations and the infusion is irritant. It should not be used in patients with myocardial infarction, as it increases pulmonary artery pressure.

pentetic acid (pen'teetik) diethylenetriamine penta-acetic acid.

pentobarbitone (ˌpentoh'bahbi,tohn) a short- to intermediate-acting basal narcotic of the barbiturate group; used in the treatment of severe insomnia and as a hypnotic and sedative in the form of the sodium salt.

pentose ('pentohz) a monosaccharide containing five carbon atoms in a molecule.

pentoside ('pentoh,sied) a compound (glycoside) of pentose with another substance.

pentosuria (ˌpentoh'syooə·ri·ə) a benign inborn error of metabolism due to a defect in the activity of the enzyme L-xylulose dehydrogenase, resulting in high levels of L-xylulose in the urine.

peotillomania (ˌpeeoh,tilə'mayni·ə) constant but non-masturbatory pulling at the penis.

peplomer ('pepləmə) a subunit of a peplos.

peplos ('peplos) the lipoprotein envelope of some types of virions, assembled in some cases from subunits (peplomers).

pepsin ('pepsin) a proteolytic enzyme that is the principal digestive component of gastric juice. It acts as a catalyst in the chemical breakdown of protein to form a mixture of polypeptides; it is formed from pepsinogen in the presence of acid or, autocatalytically, in the presence of pepsin itself. Pepsin also has milk-clotting action similar to that of rennin and thereby facilitates the digestion of milk protein.

pepsinogen (pep'sinəjən) a zymogen secreted by the chief cells of the gastric glands and converted into pepsin in the presence of gastric acid or of pepsin itself.

peptic ('peptik) pertaining to pepsin or to digestion or to the action of gastric juices.

p. ulcer an ulceration of the mucous membrane of the oesophagus, stomach, or duodenum, caused by the action of the acid gastric juice. There are two kinds of peptic ulcers: *gastric* ulcers occur in the stomach; *duodenal* ulcers occur in the duodenum, the part of the small intestine nearest the stomach.

It is estimated that 3 out of every 1000 people have peptic ulcers. Ulcers develop at any age, though rarely in children under ten. They occur in people of all races and occupations; in men more than in women; and most frequently in tense, hard-driving, or anxious persons. See also ULCER.

peptidase ('pepti,dayz) any of a subclass of proteolytic enzymes that catalyse the hydrolysis of peptide linkages.

peptide ('peptied) any of a class of compounds of low molecular weight which yield two or more amino acids on hydrolysis; known as di-, tri-, tetra-, (etc.) peptides, depending on the number of amino acids in the molecule. Peptides form the constituent parts of proteins.

peptidergic (ˌpepti'dərjik) of or pertaining to neurons that secrete peptide hormones.

peptidoglycan (ˌpeptidoh'gliekan) a glycan (polysaccharide) attached to short cross-linked peptides; found in bacterial cell walls.

peptidolytic (ˌpeptidə'litik) capable of splitting up peptide bonds.

Peptococcus ('peptohkokəs) a genus of gram-positive, anaerobic, coccoid bacteria. As commensal organisms they form part of the flora of the mouth, upper respiratory tract, and large intestine, but as pathogens they also cause soft tissue infection and bacteraemias.

peptogenic (ˌpeptə'jenik) 1. producing pepsin or peptones. 2. promoting digestion.

peptolysis (pep'tolisis) the splitting up of peptone. adj. **peptolytic**.

peptone ('peptohn) a substance produced by the action of pepsin on protein.

peptonuria (ˌpeptə'nyooə·ri·ə) the presence of peptones in the urine.

Peptostreptococcus (ˌpeptoh'streptohkokəs) a genus of obligate anaerobic streptococci occurring as parasitic inhabitants of the intestinal tract, and occasionally found in gangrenous and necrotic lesions, probably as secondary invaders.

per- word element. [L.] 1. *throughout*, *completely*, *extremely*. 2. in chemistry, a *large amount*, *combination of an element in its highest valency*.

per anum (pər 'aynəm) [L.] *through the anus*.

per os (pər os) [L.] *by mouth*.

per primam (intentionem) (pər 'priemam in,tenshi-'ohnem) [L.] *by first intention;* see HEALING.

per rectum (pər 'rektəm) [L.] *by way of the rectum*.

per secundam (intentionem) (pər se'kuhndam in-,tenshi'ohnem) [L.] *by second intention;* see HEALING.

per tertiam (intentionem) (pər 'tərshi·am in,tenshi-'ohnem) [L.] *by third intention;* see HEALING.

per tubam (pər 'tyoobam) [L.] *through a tube*.

per vaginam (pər və'jienəm) [L.] *through the vagina*.

peracid (pər'rasid) an acid containing more than the usual quantity of oxygen.

peracute (pər·rə'kyoot) very acute.

percept ('pərsept) the object perceived; the mental image of an object in space perceived by the senses.

perception (pə'sepshən) the conscious mental registration of a sensory stimulus. adj. **perceptive**.

depth p. the ability to recognize depth or the relative distances to different objects in space.

extrasensory p. knowledge of, or response to, an external thought or objective event not achieved as the result of stimulation of the sense organs; abbreviated ESP.

perceptive (pə'septiv) related to or important in the function of perception.

perceptivity (ˌpərsep'tivitee) ability to receive sense impressions.

percolate ('pərkə,layt) 1. to strain; to submit to percolation. 2. a liquid that has been submitted to percolation. 3. to trickle slowly through a substance.

percolation (ˌpərkə'layshən) the extraction of soluble

parts of a drug by passing a solvent liquid through it.

percolator ('pərkə,laytə) a vessel used in percolation.

percuss (pə'kus) to perform percussion.

percussible (pə'kusəb'l) detectable on percussion.

percussion (pə'kushən) in medical diagnosis, striking a part of the body with short, sharp blows of the fingers in order to determine the size, position, and density of the underlying parts by the sound obtained. Percussion is most commonly used on the chest and back for examination of the heart and lungs. For example, since the heart is not resonant and the adjacent lungs are, when the examiner's fingers strike the chest over the heart the sound waves will change in pitch. This serves as a guide to the precise location and size of the heart.

auscultatory p. auscultation of the sound produced by percussion.

immediate p. that in which the blow is struck directly against the body surface.

mediate p. that in which a pleximeter is used.

palpatory p. a combination of palpation and percussion, affording tactile rather than auditory impressions.

percussor (pə'kusə) an instrument for performing percussion.

percutaneous (,pərkyoo'tayni·əs) performed through the skin.

p. transluminal coronary angioplasty (PTCA) a procedure intended to enlarge the lumen of a sclerotic coronary artery by using a balloon-tipped catheter that is guided under fluoroscopy to the site of an atheromatous lesion. It is currently an investigative procedure that may provide an alternative to by-pass cardiac surgery for selected patients with ischaemic heart disease. See also HEART.

Percutol ('pərkyootol) trademark for a preparation of glyceryl trinitrate.

perencephaly (,pər·ren'kefəlee, -'sef-) porencephaly.

perfectionism (pə'fekshə,nizəm) the setting of impossible high standards for oneself.

perforans ('pərfə,ranz) [L.] *penetrating;* a term applied to various muscles and nerves.

perforation (,pərfə'rayshən) a hole or break in the containing walls or membranes of an organ or structure of the body. Perforation occurs when erosion, infection, or other factors create a weak spot in the organ and internal pressure causes a rupture. It also may result from a deep penetrating wound.

A perforated ULCER is a complication of duodenal and gastric ulceration. It requires immediate surgical correction to prevent shock and peritonitis.

Perforation of the eardrum occurs when an infectious process of the middle ear leads to increased pressure behind the tympanic membrane. Although perforation may occur spontaneously in OTITIS MEDIA, allowing adequate drainage of exudate and relieving pain, it is not desirable because the ragged edges of the perforation may not heal as they should for the eardrum to remain intact. Surgical incision of the eardrum (myringotomy) is preferred to spontaneous perforation. The eardrum also may be perforated when a sharp object is inserted into the external acoustic meatus or when extreme pressure from the outside, such as occurs when swimming or diving in deep water, or with bomb blast, causes the tympanic membrane to rupture.

Gallbladder perforation sometimes occurs as a complication of ACUTE CHOLECYSTITIS, usually secondary to GALLSTONES. When the gallbladder is infected, necrosis may progress to the point of destroying the wall of the gallbladder, so that the bile spills out into the abdominal cavity, causing biliary PERITONITIS. Gallstones may cause complete obstruction of the cystic duct so that the flow of bile is dammed up and the gallbladder becomes inflamed and eventually ruptures. Treatment of gallbladder perforation usually involves cholecystectomy.

Intestinal perforation is a complication of typhoid fever, ULCERATIVE COLITIS, INTESTINAL OBSTRUCTION, and other disorders in which there is inflammation of the intestinal wall or obstruction of the intestinal lumen. The condition is treated surgically with resection of the affected portion of intestine.

Perforation of the OESOPHAGUS may arise from inadvertent damage during endoscopy, especially during the dilation of strictures. It is less likely to occur if a flexible oesophagoscope is used rather than a rigid instrument. Small tears may seal, but larger tears require emergency thoracotomy and repair.

performance indicators 'package' of routine statistics derived nationally and visually presented in ways which highlight the relative efficiency of health services in each Health Authority compared with other Authorities. Performance Indicators are intended to identify aspects which merit further scrutiny locally with a view to changes in organization or practice.

perfusate (pə'fyoozayt) a liquid that has been subjected to perfusion.

perfusion (pə'fyoozhən) 1. the act of pouring through or over; especially the passage of a fluid through the vessels of a specific organ. 2. a liquid poured through or over an organ or tissue.

peri- word element. [Gr.] *around*, *near;* see also words beginning *para-*.

periacinal, periacinous (,peri'asinəl; ,peri'asinəs) around an acinus.

Periactin (,peri'aktin) trademark for preparations of cyproheptadine, an antihistamine and antiserotonin.

periadenitis (,peri,adə'nietis) inflammation of tissues around a gland.

p. mucosa necrotica recurrens the more severe form of aphthous stomatitis, marked by recurrent attacks of aphtha-like lesions that begin as small, firm nodules, which enlarge, ulcerate, and heal by scar formation, leaving numerous atrophied scars on the oral mucosa. Called also Sutton's disease.

periampullary (,peri·am'puhlə·ree) situated around an ampulla.

perianal (,peri'ayn'l) around the anus.

periangiitis (,peri,anji'ietis) inflammation of the tissue around a blood or lymph vessel.

periangiocholitis (,peri,anjiohkoh'lietis) inflammation of tissues around the bile ducts; pericholangitis.

periaortitis (,peri,ay·aw'tietis) inflammation of tissues around the aorta.

periapical (,peri'aypik'l) surrounding the apex of the root of a tooth.

periappendicitis (,peri·ə,pendi'sietis) inflammation of the vermiform appendix and surrounding tissues.

periarterial (,periah'tiə·ri·əl) around an artery.

periarteritis (,peri,ahtə'rietis) inflammation of the outer coat of an artery and of the tissues surrounding it.

p. gummosa accumulation of gummas in the blood vessels in syphilis.

p. nodosa an inflammatory disease of the coats of small and medium-sized arteries, marked by a variety of systemic symptoms (see also COLLAGEN DISEASES). Called also Kussmaul's disease.

periarthritis (,periah'thrietis) inflammation of the tissues around a joint.

periarticular (,periah'tikyuhlə) situated around a joint.

periaxial (,peri'aksi·əl) around an axis.

periaxillary (ˌperiak'silə·ree) around the axilla.
periblast ('periˌblast) the portion of the blastoderm of telolecithal eggs, the cells of which lack complete cell membranes.
peribronchial (ˌperi'brongki·əl) around a bronchus or bronchi.
peribronchiolar (ˌperiˌbrongki'ohlə) around the bronchioles.
peribronchiolitis (ˌperiˌbrongkioh'lietis) inflammation of the tissues around the bronchioles.
peribronchitis (ˌperibrong'kietis) a form of bronchitis consisting of inflammation and thickening of the tissues around the bronchi.
pericaecal (ˌperi'seek'l) around the caecum.
pericaliceal, pericalyceal (ˌperiˌkali'seeəl) situated near or around a renal calix.
pericallosal (ˌperikə'lohs'l) situated around the corpus callosum.
pericardiac (ˌperi'kahdiˌak) pertaining to the pericardium; around the heart.
pericardial (ˌperi'kahdi·əl) pertaining to the pericardium.
p. rub a scraping or grating noise heard with the heart beat, usually a to-and-fro sound, associated with an inflamed pericardium.
pericardiectomy (ˌperiˌkahdi'ektəmee) excision of a portion of abnormal pericardium.
pericardiocentesis, pericardicentesis (ˌperiˌkahdiohsen'teesis; ˌperiˌkahdisen'teesis) surgical puncture of the pericardial cavity with aspiration of fluid.
pericardiolysis (ˌperiˌkahdi'olisis) freeing of adhesions between the visceral and parietal pericardium.
pericardiophrenic (ˌperiˌkahdioh'frenik) pertaining to the pericardium and diaphragm.
pericardiopleural (ˌperiˌkahdioh'plooə·rəl) pertaining to the pericardium and pleura.
pericardiorrhaphy (ˌperiˌkahdi'o·rəfee) suture of the pericardium.
pericardiostomy (ˌperiˌkahdi'ostəmee) creation of an opening into the pericardium, usually for drainage of effusions.
pericardiotomy (ˌperiˌkahdi'otəmee) incision of pericardium.
pericarditis (ˌperikah'dietis) inflammation of the pericardium. adj. **pericarditic.**
Types of Pericarditis. There are many forms of pericarditis. Acute pericarditis is usually secondary to some other bacterial infection, for example, osteomyelitis, lung abscess, or pneumonia. It may also occur without bacterial infection, resulting from a tumour, rheumatic heart disease, uraemia, or coronary thrombosis, or it may be the aftermath of a chest wound in which the pericardium is pierced. Acute pericarditis may be dry, or fibrinous, in which a fibrinous exudate forms on the serous membrane, or it may occur with effusion, that is, with accumulation of fluid in the pericardial cavity.

Occasionally the pericardium is affected directly by what appears to be a virus; this condition is called acute nonspecific pericarditis. Another form, chronic pericarditis, is usually adhesive—that is, the heart is anchored to surrounding tissues by adhesions. It sometimes follows acute pericarditis, but often the cause is unknown. In the constrictive form of chronic pericarditis, which may be tuberculous in origin, calcium and fibrous deposits may form around the heart and interfere with its movements. This form may be extremely serious and difficult to cure.
Symptoms and Treatment. The symptoms of acute pericarditis vary with the cause but usually include chest pain and dyspnoea, an increase in the pulse rate, and a rise in temperature. In dry pericarditis distinct sounds of friction caused by deposits of fibrin may be heard through a stethoscope. In the effusive form, the excess accumulation of pericardial fluid can be detected by radiography or electrocardiography. The excess fluid is sometimes drained by pericardicentesis.

Treatment of acute pericarditis is directed mainly at curing its original cause. Antibiotics have proved successful in treating bacterial pericarditis. Many patients with nonspecific pericarditis with effusion are helped dramatically by cortisone medications.

In the constrictive form of chronic pericarditis there may be dyspnoea and pain in the heart region, plus symptoms elsewhere in the body, such as oedema, enlargement of the liver, or distention of the neck veins. The best means of treatment is surgery to remove the constrictions and permit free heart action.
pericardium (ˌperi'kahdi·əm) the fibroserous sac enclosing the heart and the roots of the great vessels, composed of external (fibrous) and internal (serous) layers.
adherent p. one abnormally connected with the heart by dense fibrous tissue.
fibrous p. the external layer of the pericardium, consisting of dense fibrous tissue.
parietal p. the parietal layer of the serous pericardium, which is in contact with the fibrous pericardium.
serous p. the inner, serous portion of pericardium, consisting of two layers, visceral and parietal; the space between the layers is the pericardial cavity.
visceral p. the inner layer of the serous pericardium, which is in contact with the heart and roots of the great vessels. Called also epicardium.
pericecitis (ˌperisee'sietis) inflammation of the tissues around the caecum.
pericellular (ˌperi'selyuhlə) surrounding a cell.
pericholangitis (ˌperiˌkohlan'jietis) inflammation of tissues surrounding the bile ducts; periangiocholitis.
pericholecystitis (ˌperiˌkohlisi'stietis) inflammation of tissues around the gallbladder.
perichondritis (ˌperikon'drietis) inflammation of the perichondrium.
perichondrium (ˌperi'kondri·əm) the layer of fibrous connective tissue investing all cartilage except the articular cartilage of synovial joints. adj. **perichondral.**
perichordal (ˌperi'kawd'l) surrounding the notochord.
perichoroidal (ˌperiko'royd'l) surrounding the choroid coat of the eye.
pericolic (ˌperi'kolik) around the colon.
pericolitis, pericolonitis (ˌperikə'lietis, -koh-; ˌperiˌkohlə'nietis) inflammation around the colon, especially of its peritoneal coat.
pericolpitis (ˌperikol'pietis) inflammation of the tissues around the vagina; perivaginitis.
periconchal (ˌperi'kongk'l) around the concha.
pericorneal (ˌperi'kawni·əl) around the cornea.
pericoronal (ˌperikə'rohn'l) around the crown of a tooth.
pericranitis (ˌperikray'nietis) inflammation of the pericranium.
pericranium (ˌperi'krayni·əm) the periosteum of the skull. adj. **pericranial.**
pericystitis (ˌperisi'stietis) inflammation of tissues about the bladder.
pericyte ('periˌsiet) one of the peculiar elongated, contractile cells found wrapped about precapillary arterioles outside the basement membrane.
pericytial (ˌperi'sishəl) around a cell.
periderm ('periˌdərm) the outer layer of the bilaminar fetal epidermis, generally disappearing before birth.
peridesmitis (ˌperidez'mietis) inflammation of the peridesmium.
peridesmium (ˌperi'dezmi·əm) the areolar membrane

that covers the ligaments.

peridіdymis (ˌperi'didimis) the tunica vaginalis testis, the membrane covering the front and sides of the testis and epididymis.

perididymitis (ˌperiˌdidi'mietis) inflammation of the tunica vaginalis testis.

peridiverticulitis (ˌperiˌdievəˌtikyuh'lietis) inflammation around an intestinal diverticulum.

periductal (ˌperi'duktəl) around a duct.

periduodenitis (ˌperiˌdyooədi'nietis) inflammation around the duodenum.

periencephalitis (ˌperi·enˌkefə'lietis, -ˌsef-) inflammation of the surface of the brain.

periencephalomeningitis (ˌperi·enˌkefəlohˌmenin'jietis, -ˌsef-) inflammation of the cerebral cortex and meninges.

perienteritis (ˌperiˌentə'rietis) inflammation of the peritoneal coat of the intestines.

perifistular (ˌperi'fistyuhlə) around a fistula.

perifollicular (ˌperifo'likyuhlə) surrounding a follicle.

perifolliculitis (ˌperifoˌlikyuh'lietis) inflammation around the hair follicles.

perigangliitis (ˌperiˌgang·gli'ietis) inflammation around a ganglion.

perigastric (ˌperi'gastrik) around the stomach; pertaining to the peritoneal coat of the stomach.

perigastritis (ˌperiga'strietis) inflammation of the peritoneal coat of the stomach.

perihepatic (ˌperihi'patik) around the liver.

perihepatitis (ˌperiˌhepə'tietis) inflammation of the peritoneal coat of the liver and the surrounding tissue.

peri-islet (ˌperi'ielət) situated around the islets of Langerhans.

perijejunitis (ˌperiˌjejuh'nietis) inflammation around the jejunum.

perikaryon (ˌperi'karion) the cell body of a neuron.

perilabyrinthitis (ˌperiˌlabə·rin'thietis) inflammation of the tissues around the labyrinth.

perilaryngitis (ˌperiˌlarin'jietis) inflammation of the tissues around the larynx.

perilesional (ˌperi'leezhən'l) located or occurring around a lesion.

perilymph, perilympha ('periˌlimf; ˌperi'limfə) the fluid contained in the space separating the membranous and osseous labyrinths of the ear.

perilymphangitis (ˌperiˌlimfan'jietis) inflammation around a lymphatic vessel.

perimeningitis (ˌperiˌmenin'jietis) pachymeningitis; inflammation of the dura mater.

perimeter (pə'rimitə) 1. the boundary of a two-dimensional figure. 2. an apparatus for determining the extent of the peripheral visual field.

perimetritis (ˌperimi'trietis) inflammation of the perimetrium.

perimetrium (ˌperi'meetri·əm) the serous membrane enveloping the uterus.

perimetry (pə'rimətree) determination of the extent of the peripheral visual field. adj. **perimetric**.

perimyelitis (ˌperiˌmieə'lietis) inflammation of (a) the pia of the spinal cord, or (b) the endosteum.

perimyositis (ˌperiˌmieoh'sietis) inflammation of connective tissue around a muscle.

perimysiitis (ˌperiˌmizi'ietis) inflammation of the perimysium; myofibrositis.

perimysium (ˌperi'mizi·əm) connective tissue demarcating a fascicle of skeletal muscle fibres. adj. **perimysial**.

perinatal (ˌperi'nayt'l) relating to the period shortly before and 7 days after birth.

p. mortality rate the number of stillbirths plus deaths of babies under 7 days old per 1000 total births in any one year.

perinatologist (ˌperinay'toləjist) a specialist in perinatology.

perinatology (ˌperinay'toləjee) the branch of medicine (obstetrics and paediatrics) dealing with the fetus and infant during the perinatal period.

perineal (ˌperi'neeəl) pertaining to the perineum.

perineocele (ˌperi'neeohˌseel) a hernia between the rectum and the prostate or between the rectum and the vagina.

perineoplasty (ˌperi'neeohˌplastee) plastic repair of the perineum.

perineorrhaphy (ˌperini'o·rəfee) suture of the perineum.

perineotomy (ˌperini'otəmee) incision of the perineum.

perineovaginal (ˌperiˌneeohvə'jien'l) pertaining to or communicating with the perineum and vagina.

perinephric (ˌperi'nefrik) around the kidney.

perinephritis (ˌperinə'frietis) inflammation of the perinephrium.

perinephrium (ˌperi'nefri·əm) the peritoneal envelope and other tissues around the kidney. adj. **perinephrial**.

perineum (ˌperi'neeəm) the pelvic floor and associated structures occupying the pelvic outlet, bounded anteriorly by the pubic symphysis, laterally by the ischial tuberosities, and posteriorly by the coccyx. During childbirth the perineum may be torn, resulting in possible damage to the urinary meatus and anal sphincter. To avoid a perineal tear, the midwife may cut the perineum just before delivery and sutures the incision after delivery of the infant and the placenta. This procedure is called an episiotomy. Surgical repair of a torn or lacerated perineum is called perineorrhaphy.

perineuritis (ˌperinyuh'rietis) inflammation of the perineurium.

perineurium (ˌperi'nyooə·ri·əm) the connective tissue sheath surrounding each bundle of nerve fibres (fascicle) in a peripheral nerve. adj. **perineurial**.

periocular (ˌperi'okyuhlə) around the eye.

periodic (ˌpiə·ri'odik) repeated or recurring at intervals.

periodic syndrome (ˌpiə·ri'odik) recurrent head, limb or abdominal pains in children for which no organic cause can be found. It often leads to migraine in adult life.

periodicity (ˌpiə·ri·ə'disitee) recurrence at regular intervals of time.

periodontal (ˌperi·ə'dont'l) around a tooth; pertaining to the periodontium.

p. disease any disease or disorder of the periodontium. See also PERIODONTITIS and PERIODONTOSIS.

periodontics (ˌperi·ə'dontiks) the branch of dentistry dealing with the study and treatment of diseases of the periodontium.

periodontist (ˌperi·ə'dontist) a dentist who specializes in periodontics.

periodontitis (ˌperi·ədon'tietis) inflammation of the periodontium. The condition is the inevitable sequel to chronic gingivitis if this is allowed to progress unchecked. Once true periodontitis is present and the infection spreads deeper, the alveolar bone starts to be resorbed and the problem becomes a self-perpetuating one. Periodontitis is the major cause of tooth loss after the age of 35. Treatment must be based around eliminating the progressive lesion and preventing its recurrence. In general, this will include scaling and plaque control, and surgery if required. As in the treatment of chronic gingivitis, the most important aspect is oral hygiene control.

periodontium (ˌperi·ə'donshi·əm) pl. *periodontia* [L.] the tissues investing and supporting the teeth, including the cementum, periodontal ligament, alveolar bone, and gingiva. In NA, restricted to the periodontal ligament.

periodontosis (ˌperiohdon'tohsis) a degenerative, non-inflammatory condition of the periodontium, characterized by destruction of the tissues.

perioesophagitis (ˌperi·iˌsofə'jietis) inflammation of the tissues around the oesophagus.

periomphalic (ˌperiom'falik) situated around the umbilicus.

perionychium (ˌperi·ə'niki·əm) the epidermis bordering a nail.

perioophoritis (ˌperiˌoh·əfə'rietis) inflammation of the tissues around the ovary.

perioophorosalpingitis (ˌperiohˌofə·rohˌsalpin'jietis) inflammation of the tissues around the ovary and oviduct.

perioperative (ˌperi'opə·rətiv) pertaining or relating to the period immediately before or after an operation, as perioperative care.

periophthalmic (ˌperiof'thalmik) around the eye.

perioptometry (ˌperiop'tomətree) measurement of acuity of peripheral vision or of the limits of the visual field.

perioral (ˌperi'or·rəl) around the mouth.

periorbita (ˌperi'awbitə) the periosteum of the bones forming the orbit, or eye socket. adj. **periorbital**.

periorbitis (ˌperi·aw'bietis) inflammation of the periorbita.

periorchitis (ˌperi·aw'kietis) inflammation of the tunica vaginalis testis; vaginalitis.

periosteal (ˌperi'ostiəl) pertaining to the periostium.

p. reaction a radiological sign of bone repair, infection or tumour.

periosteitis (ˌperiˌosti'ietis) periostitis.

periosteoma (ˌperiˌosti'ohmə) a morbid bony growth surrounding a bone.

periosteomyelitis (ˌperiˌostiohˌmieə'lietis) inflammation of the entire bone, including periosteum and marrow.

periosteophyte (ˌperi'ostiohˌfiet) a bony growth on the periosteum.

periosteotomy (ˌperiˌosti'otəmee) incision of the periosteum.

periosteum (ˌperi'osti·əm) a specialized connective tissue covering all bones of the body, and possessing bone-forming potentialities. Periosteum also serves as a point of attachment for certain muscles. The connective tissues of the muscle fuse with the fibrous layers of periosteum. adj. **periosteal**.

periostitis (ˌperio'stietis) inflammation of the periosteum.

dental p. periodontitis.

diffuse p. widespread periostitis of the long bones.

periostosis (ˌperio'stohsis) abnormal deposition of periosteal bone; the condition manifested by the growth of periosteomas.

periotic (ˌperi'ohtik) 1. situated about the ear, especially the internal ear. 2. the petrous and mastoid portions of the temporal bone, at one stage a distinct bone.

peripachymeningitis (ˌperi·pakiˌmenin'jietis) inflammation of the substance between the dura mater and the bony covering of the central nervous system.

peripancreatitis (ˌperiˌpangkri·ə'tietis) inflammation of tissues around the pancreas.

peripapillary (ˌperipə'pilə·ree) around the optic papilla.

periphacitis (ˌperifə'sietis) inflammation of the capsule of the eye lens.

peripherad (pə'rifəˌrad) toward the periphery.

peripheral (pə'rifə·rəl) pertaining to or situated at or near the periphery.

p. nervous system the portion of the NERVOUS SYSTEM consisting of the nerves and ganglia outside the brain and spinal cord.

p. vision vision produced by stimulation of receptors in the retina outside the macula lutea; called also indirect vision.

periphery (pə'rifə·ree) an outward structure or surface; the portion of a system outside the central region.

periphlebitis (ˌperifli'bietis) inflammation of the tissues around a vein, or the external coat of a vein.

periplasmic (ˌperi'plazmik) around the plasma membrane; between the plasma membrane and the cell wall of a bacterium.

periportal (ˌperi'pawt'l) situated around the portal vein.

periproctitis (ˌperiprok'tietis) inflammation of tissues around the rectum and anus.

periprostatic (ˌperipro'statik) around the prostate.

periprostatitis (ˌperiˌprostə'tietis) inflammation of the tissues around the prostate.

peripylephlebitis (ˌperiˌpielifli'bietis) inflammation of tissues around the portal vein.

peripyloric (ˌperipie'lo·rik) around the pylorus.

perirectal (ˌperi'rekt'l) around the rectum.

perirectitis (ˌperirek'tietis) periproctitis.

perirenal (ˌperi'reen'l) around the kidney.

perirhinal (ˌperi'rien'l) around the nose.

perisalpingitis (ˌperiˌsalpin'jietis) inflammation of tissues around the uterine tube.

periscopic (ˌperi'skopik) affording a wide range of vision.

perisigmoiditis (ˌperiˌsigmoy'dietis) inflammation of the peritoneum of the sigmoid flexure.

perisinusitis (ˌperiˌsienə'sietis) inflammation of the tissues around a sinus.

perispermatitis (ˌperiˌspərmə'tietis) inflammation of tissues around the spermatic cord.

perisplanchnic (ˌperi'splangknik) around a viscus or the viscera.

perisplanchnitis (ˌperisplangk'nietis) inflammation of tissues around the viscera.

perisplenic (ˌperi'splenik) around the spleen.

perisplenitis (ˌperisplə'nietis) inflammation of the peritoneal surface of the spleen.

perispondylitis (ˌperiˌspondi'lietis) inflammation of tissues around a vertebra.

peristalsis (ˌperi'stalsis) the wormlike movement by which the alimentary canal or other tubular organs with both longitudinal and circular muscle fibres propel their contents, consisting of a wave of contraction passing along the tube. adj. adj. **peristaltic**.

When food is swallowed, it passes into the oesophagus. Muscular contractions in the wall of the oesophagus work the food downward, pushing it into the stomach. Here peristaltic contractions not only move the food in small amounts into the intestine but also aid in the disintegration of the food and help mix it with gastric juice. Peristalsis forces the food into and through the intestine for further digestion until the food waste finally reaches the rectum, from which it is periodically discharged from the body. The waves of peristalsis are irregular; they are stronger at some times than others. They are also weaker in some people, notably the elderly.

Although the normal peristaltic wave is downward, it is sometimes reversed. Reverse peristaltic action may be triggered by mild digestive upsets or more serious disorders, such as an obstruction in the stomach or intestines.

peristaphyline (ˌperi'stafiˌlien) around the uvula.

perisynovial (ˌperisie'nohvi·əl, -si-) around a synovial structure.

peritectomy (ˌperi'tektəmee) excision of a ring of conjunctiva around the cornea in treatment of pannus.

peritendineum (ˌperiten'dini·əm) connective tissue

investing larger tendons and extending between the fibres composing them.

peritendinitis, peritenonitis (ˌperiˌtendiˈnietis; ˌperiˌtenəˈnietis) inflammation of the sheath of a tendon; TENOSYNOVITIS.

perithelioma (ˌperiˌtheeliˈohmə) haemangiopericytoma.

perithelium (ˌperiˈtheeli·əm) the connective tissue layer surrounding the capillaries and smaller vessels.

perithyroiditis (ˌperiˌthieroyˈdietis) inflammation of the capsule of the thyroid.

peritomy (peˈritəmee) 1. surgical incision of the conjunctiva and subconjunctival tissue about the whole circumference of the cornea. 2. circumcision.

peritoneal (ˌperitəˈneeəl) pertaining to the peritoneum.

p. cavity the space between the parietal and visceral layers of the peritoneum.

p. dialysis use of the peritoneum surrounding the abdominal cavity as a dialysing membrane for the purpose of removing waste products or toxins accumulated as a result of renal failure. See also DIALYSIS. Certain crystalloids, such as urea, creatinine, electrolytes, and some drugs, such as the salicylates, bromides, and barbiturates, can be removed. The exchange of substances across a semipermeable membrane, such as the peritoneal membrane, involves three physical processes: diffusion, osmosis, and solvent drag. In *diffusion* the random motion of the molecules of solids, liquids, or gases in solution causes a flow of each solute from regions of high concentration to regions of low concentration. Diffusible solutes, those with molecules small enough to pass through the pores of the membrane, flow from the side on which the concentration is high to the side on which it is low. *Osmosis* is a flow of water molecules (or some other solvent) through the membrane. The flow moves from the side on which the concentration of nondiffusible solutes, those with molecules too large to pass through the membrane pores, is low (and thus there is more water) to the side on which the concentration is high (and there is less water). Solutes with molecules of intermediate size are retarded in their flow through the membrane, but their flow is subject to *solvent drag.* The rate at which a solute flows through the membrane is increased by a solvent flow in the same direction and decreased by a solvent flow in the opposite direction.

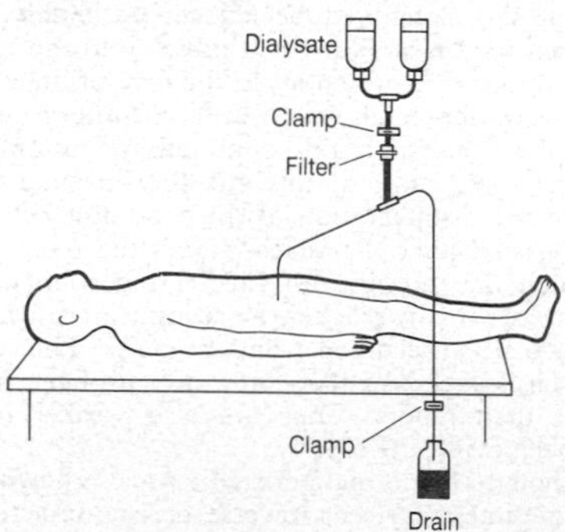

Peritoneal dialysis. Manual, three-way method.

INDICATIONS AND CONTRAINDICATIONS. Peritoneal dialysis may be used for acute or chronic renal failure. For acute renal failure where haemodialysis is available, it is often the treatment of choice as insertion and management of a temporary rigid peritoneal catheter may be difficult and hazardous. Advantages of peritoneal dialysis are that chemical and fluid exchanges occur more slowly, vascular access is not required and anticoagulants are unnecessary.

For long-term treatment, peritoneal dialysis is easy to learn and the procedure is safe and simple. Expensive and intricate equipment is not required and the patient has great flexibility about place and time of exchanges.

Peritoneal dialysis cannot be employed when there is severe abdominal trauma, multiple abdominal surgical procedures, adhesions, severe coagulation defects, paralytic ileus, or previous diffuse peritonitis.

THE PROCEDURE. Sterile fluid equal in osmolarity and similar in chemical composition to normal body fluid is introduced into the peritoneal cavity via a catheter. The fluid infuses by gravity or pump; its rate of flow can be controlled by lowering or raising the container of dialysate, by manipulating the occlusive clamp on the tubing or changing the pump speed.

The length of time the dialysing solution is left in the peritoneal cavity depends on the molecular weight of the substance to be removed and the amount of dialysing solution used. Substances with low molecular weights equilibrate in two to three hours, while those with high molecular weight can take more than 12 hours to move across the membrane and equalize the concentrations of the two solutions. This period of equalization is sometimes called the 'dwell time'. It is followed by a period of drainage to complete the dialysis or to prepare for instillation of fresh dialysate.

Peritoneal dialysis can be accomplished by a number of methods. Intermittent dialysis can be done manually with the dialysis achieved with short cycles of about one hour. The dialysate is allowed to flow in, it is left in the peritoneal cavity for about 30 minutes, and then allowed to flow out by gravity flow. Intermittent peritoneal dialysis also can be done using an automated device that performs the procedure at prescribed lengths of time. Timing devices or volume control devices control the instillation, dwell time, and drainage time.

With the development of newer equipment it is possible for a patient to have either intermittent or continuous ambulatory dialysis. The patient can be taught to operate a portable, manual device and to perform his own dialysis three to five times a day or as often as necessary. The patients are educated about fluid and dietary restrictions which, though minimal, as water and electrolyte clearance is constant, must be understood. A high protein diet is prescribed as protein is lost in the dialysis.

Because HAEMODIALYSIS was developed first and efficiently removes toxins from the blood and body fluids, it has always been the treatment of choice for end-stage renal disease. Peritoneal dialysis is now successful for a wide range of patients to use at home. There has been rapid growth in the UK as it is quick and easy for patients of variable abilities and skills to manage safely.

COMPLICATIONS. The most obvious complication of peritoneal dialysis is peritonitis, which is a real danger to any patient receiving this treatment. Contamination of some part of the system, a malfunctioning piece of equipment, contamination of the fluid, and infection of the catheter site are all possible sources of peritonitis. The catheter itself can cause complications through leakage at the site of insertion, infection, and occlusion of the perforations on the catheter. Respiratory difficulty can occur as a result of fluid retention that increases pressure against the diaphragm, and fluid overload that requires the more frequent use of hypertonic solutions. Fluid depletion and hypotension are also possible complications.

PATIENT CARE. To avoid complications strict adherence to aseptic technique is essential. If there is any break in the tubing connections during the procedure the peritoneal cavity must be considered contaminated.

An *exchange record* is kept of the fluid that is introduced into and withdrawn from the peritoneal cavity. If isotonic fluid is used, the volume drained should equal the volume introduced and perhaps a little more. If a hypertonic bag is used, it should drain considerably more. The exchange record contains information about the starting time of infusion, amount infused, concentration of fluid and drugs added, finishing time of infusion, starting time of drainage, volume of drainage, and total patient fluid loss (-) or retention (+) up to the time of recording. Since this last item is frequently a source of error, it is essential that all personnel involved in the dialysis procedure know how the recording is done. Daily weight is essential for calculation of fluid loss or gain. Constipation is a common problem affecting drainage of fluid. A high fibre diet should be encouraged and stool softeners may be necessary.

The peritoneal drainage fluid is observed for cloudiness and the presence of blood or other abnormal constituents. The vital signs are recorded at frequent intervals so hypervolaemia or hypovolaemia may be quickly detected and rectified, and the development of peritonitis can be detected. Respiratory difficulty should not develop as a result of pressure of the fluid against the diaphragm. If dyspnoea develops, fluid should be drained immediately and the doctor notified.

peritonealgia (ˌperiˌtohni'alji·ə) pain in the peritoneum.

peritoneocentesis (ˌperitəˌneeohsen'teesis) aspiration of the abdominal (peritoneal) cavity by puncture.

peritoneoclysis (ˌperitəˌneeə'kliesis) injection of fluid into the peritoneal cavity.

peritoneopathy (ˌperitəni'opəthee) any disease of the peritoneum.

peritoneopericardial (ˌperitohˌneeohˌperi'kahdi·əl) pertaining to the peritoneum and pericardium.

peritoneoscope (ˌperitə'neeəˌskohp) an endoscope for use in peritoneoscopy.

peritoneoscopy (ˌperitəni'oskəpee) visual examination of the organs of the abdominal (peritoneal) cavity through a peritoneoscope.

peritoneotomy (ˌperitəni'otəmee) incision into the peritoneum.

peritoneovenous (ˌperitəˌneeoh'veenəs) communicating with the peritoneal cavity and the venous system. See also peritoneal-venous SHUNT.

peritoneum (ˌperitə'neeəm) the serous membrane lining the walls of the abdominal and pelvic cavities (parietal peritoneum) and investing contained viscera (visceral peritoneum), the two layers enclosing a potential space, the peritoneal cavity.

peritonitis (ˌperitə'nietis) inflammation of the peritoneum.

ACUTE PERITONITIS. Acute peritonitis may be produced by inflammation of abdominal organs, by irritating substances from a perforated gallbladder or gastric ulcer, by rupture of a cyst, or by irritation from blood, as in cases of internal bleeding.

Symptoms and Diagnosis. Immediate and intense pain is felt at the site of infection, followed usually by fever, vomiting, and extreme weakness. The abdomen becomes rigid and sensitive to the touch. The patient may suffer mental confusion, fever, prostration, or shock. Although antibiotics have greatly reduced the mortality rate of acute peritonitis, the infection should be treated and controlled immediately; it can be fatal if neglected.

Diagnosis is based on manual examination, radiographs, and blood tests.

Treatment. The basic treatment for acute peritonitis is a combination of surgery, antibiotics, and other measures. The peritoneal cavity often must be opened and the toxic material removed. The original source of infection, such as an inflamed appendix, may have to be removed, or an abscess caused by the peritonitis may have to be drained. Antibiotics such as penicillin, streptomycin, or tetracycline are used to fight the infection itself.

The patient usually takes nothing by mouth. Fluids are given intravenously. Narcotics and sedatives are often used to relieve pain and ensure rest. Treatment may also include blood transfusions and suction through a nasogastric tube to relieve abdominal pressure and to prevent accumulation of gas in the intestines.

CHRONIC PERITONITIS. The chronic form of this disease is comparatively rare, and is often associated with tuberculosis. Less frequently it may result from longstanding irritation caused by the presence in the abdomen of a foreign body such as gunshot, or by chronic peritoneal dialysis.

In general, symptoms of chronic peritonitis are milder than those of acute peritonitis. Symptoms of tuberculous peritonitis are abdominal pain, lowgrade fever, constipation, and general ill health, including loss of weight and appetite. Treatment depends on the underlying cause and the severity of the condition.

adhesive p. peritonitis characterized by adhesions between adjacent serous structures.

bile p., biliary p. that due to the presence of bile in the peritoneum; choleperitoneum.

silent p. asymptomatic peritonitis.

peritonsillar (ˌperi'tonsilə) around a tonsil.

peritonsillitis (ˌperiˌtonsi'lietis) inflammation of peritonsillar tissues.

peritracheal (ˌperi'traki·əl, -trə'keeəl) around the trachea.

Peritrate ('periˌtrayt) trademark for a preparation of pentaerythritol, a vasodilator used in treatment of angina pectoris.

peritrichous (pə'ritrikəs) 1. having flagella around the entire surface; said of bacteria. 2. having flagella around the cytostome only; said of Ciliophora.

periumbilical (ˌperium'bilik'l, -umbi'liek'l) around the umbilicus.

periureteral (periyuh'reetə·rəl) around the ureter.

periureteritis (ˌperiˌrioyuhˌreetə'rietis) inflammation of tissues around the ureter.

periurethral (ˌperiyuh'reethrəl) around the urethra.

periuterine (ˌperi'yootəˌrien) around the uterus.

perivaginal (ˌperivə'jien'l) around the vagina.

perivaginitis (ˌperiˌvaji'nietis) inflammation of tissues around the vagina; pericolpitis.

perivascular (ˌperi'vaskyuhlə) around a vessel.

perivasculitis (ˌperiˌvaskyuh'lietis) inflammation of a perivascular sheath and surrounding tissue.

perivesical (ˌperi'vesik'l) around the bladder.

perivesiculitis (ˌperiveˌsikyuh'lietis) inflammation of tissues around the seminal vesicles.

perlèche (pər'lesh) inflammation with exudation, maceration, and fissuring at the labial commissures.

permeability (ˌpərmi·ə'bilitee) the property or state of being permeable.

permeable ('pərmi·əb'l) not impassable; pervious; permitting passage of a substance.

permease ('pərmi,ayz) any carrier protein involved in transporting substances across cell membranes.

permeate ('pərmi,ayt) 1. to penetrate or pass through, as through a filter. 2. the constituents of a solution or suspension that pass through a filter.

pernicious (pə'nishəs) tending to a fatal issue.

p. anaemia a form of anaemia caused by vitamin B_{12} deficiency secondary to lack of the intrinsic factor normally produced by the stomach mucosa. The deficiency results in inadequate and abnormal formation of erythrocytes. Some persons with pernicious anaemia show only mild symptoms and are not particularly aware of the illness; in others the condition becomes serious and, if it remains untreated, can be fatal. SYMPTOMS. A pale, colourless complexion is typical of all anaemias, including pernicious anaemia. Mild jaundice also occurs in pernicious anaemia, with soreness and reddening of the tongue, difficulty in swallowing, and digestive disturbances, including diarrhoea. Other symptoms may include fatigue, palpitations, and dyspnoea. Changes in the nerves and spinal cord may produce numbness and tingling in the fingers and toes, and the gait may become unsteady. The involvement of the nerves can be completely cured if it has existed for less than 6 months, but may be incurable if it is of long standing. In advanced cases, mental disturbances may also occur. Laboratory tests reveal abnormalities in the erythrocytes in the blood and megaloblastic change in the bone marrow. Gastric analysis shows an absence of hydrochloric acid and intrinsic factor secretion.

TREATMENT. Pernicious anaemia is successfully treated by regular injections of vitamin B_{12}, given several times a week at first and at 3-monthly intervals once the condition has been brought under control. This treatment must be lifelong to prevent relapse. The injections do not restore intrinsic factor secretion but provide the body directly with the necessary vitamin that it fails to absorb from the digestive tract. Special diets, liver extract, and other medications taken by mouth are not required since the basic defect is a failure of vitamin B_{12} absorption.

Pernicious anaemia runs in families. with other autoimmune disorders. The disease usually occurs after the age of 35, and it is more common in persons of Scandinavian, Irish, and English descent. Although no cure is known, patients who continue with treatment can look forward to a normal life span with good health and normal activities.

See also ANAEMIA for patient care.

pernio ('pərnioh) chilblain.

perniosis (,pərni'ohsis) a condition resulting from persistent exposure to cold which produces vascular spasm in the superficial arterioles of the hands and feet, causing thrombosis and necrosis. Perniosis includes chilblains and Raynaud's disease.

pero- word element. [Gr.] *deformity, maimed.*

perobrachius (,peeroh'brayki·əs) a fetus with deformed arms.

perocephalus (,peeroh'kefələs, -'sef-) a fetus with a deformed head.

perochirus (,peeroh'kierəs) a fetus with deformed hands.

peromelia (,peeroh'meeli·ə) congenital deformity of the limbs.

peromelus (pi'roməlǝs) a fetus with deformed limbs.

peroneal (,peroh'neeəl) pertaining to the fibula or to the outer side of the leg; fibular.

p. nerve, common a nerve originating in the sciatic nerve and innervating the calf and foot.

peropus (pi'rohpəs) a fetus with malformed legs and feet.

peroral (pər'ror·rəl) performed or administered through the mouth.

peroxidase (pə'roksi,dayz) any of a group of iron-porphyrin enzymes that catalyse the oxidation of some organic substrates in the presence of hydrogen peroxide.

peroxide (pə'roksied) that oxide of any element containing more oxygen than any other; more correctly applied to compounds having such linkage as -O-O-.

hydrogen p. H_2O_2, an antiseptic with a mildly antibacterial action. A 3 per cent solution foams on touching skin or mucous membrane and appears to have a mechanical cleansing action.

peroxisome (pə'roksi,sohm) small, membrane-found microbody found in the cytoplasm of vertebrate animal cells, especially kidney and liver cells, that contains urate oxidase, amino acid oxidase, catalase, and other enzymes.

perphenazine (pər'fenə,zeen) a phenothiazine compound used as a tranquillizer and antiemetic.

Persantin (pər'santin) trademark for preparations of dipyridamole, a coronary vasodilator and antithrombotic agent.

perseveration (pər,sevə'rayshən) persistent repetition of the same verbal or motor response to varied stimuli; continuance of activity after cessation of the causative stimulus.

persona (pər'sohnə) Jung's term for the personality 'mask' or facade presented by a person to the outside world, as opposed to the anima, the unconscious, or inner being, of a person.

personality (,pərsə'nalitee) that which constitutes, distinguishes, and characterizes a person as an entity over a period of time; the total reaction of a person to his environment. Many factors that determine personality are inherited; they are shaped and modified by the individual's environment. Students of human behaviour have long debated whether inherited traits or life experiences play the greater role in moulding personality. They all agree, however, on the influence of the early years on personality development.

EARLY LIFE AND PERSONALITY. The infant comes into the world completely dependent on others for his basic needs. His feelings of security in a relationship with his mother, or an adequate substitute, is the cornerstone of his mental health in later years.

As a child develops, he needs to learn and to meet the day-to-day problems of life, and to master them. In resolving these challenges, he chooses his solutions from many possibilities. He must substitute other ways of behaviour for his many natural antisocial impulses. Psychologists have studied how these choices are made and use technical terms to describe them, such as repression and sublimation. The behaviour patterns chosen result in certain character traits which will influence a child's way of meeting the world—whether he will lead or follow, be conscientious or reckless, imitate his parents or prefer to be as different from them as possible, or take a realistic, flexible path between these extremes. The sum total of these traits represents the personality.

THE WELL ADJUSTED PERSONALITY. A well adjusted individual is one who adjusts himself to his surroundings, the world he lives in, and the people in it. If he cannot, he makes realistic efforts to change the situation. He also uses his abilities constructively and successfully.

The well adjusted person is realistic. He faces facts whether they are pleasant or unpleasant and deals with them instead of merely worrying about them or denying them.

The mature person is independent. He forms reasoned opinions and then acts on them. He seeks a reasonable amount of information and advice before making a decision. Once the decision is made, he is willing to face the consequences of it. He does not attempt to force others to make decisions for him.

An ability to love others is typical of the well adjusted individual. On the other hand, the mature person is also able to enjoy receiving love and affection. He can accept a reasonable dependence on others.

The well adjusted individual has the ability to make long-range choices and to forego immediate pleasures for the sake of these long-range goals. He is also able to reevaluate these goals and change them if necessary.

The mature person can get angry, but his anger is directed at rational targets. When the occasion demands, he can be stirred to fierce anger, but he never loses sight of the reason for his anger or of what he hopes to accomplish with it. He is not a chronic worrier. He usually likes his work and does it well, but it is not his entire life.

Finally, the mature person has the capacity for continued emotional growth. He continues to deepen his understanding of others throughout his life.

Naturally, few people meet all these qualifications of the ideally developed personality, just as few people are in perfect physical health, and many descriptions of 'adjustment' are thought to reflect middle class values rather than medical norms.

DISORDERS OF PERSONALITY. In addition to specific types of mental illness, such as NEUROSIS and PSYCHOSIS, there are a number of what are known as personality or character disorders. In general these are difficult both to diagnose and to treat.

Terms that are often used to describe persons with disturbed personalities are neurotic or neurotic character. Such persons are able to function in their daily life, but are emotionally and psychologically 'crippled' by inadequate or unstable personalities, and their chances of forming good relationships and fulfilling their potentialities are poor. Among the patterns often encountered in such persons are either passive or aggressive reactions to life, in which the person is excessively dependent on other people or hostile to them. Sometimes his behaviour represents a combination of both attitudes. Other personality types have traits that show some similarity to the symptoms of the three major types of psychosis—schizophrenia, paranoia, and affective psychosis—although these people are not psychotic. They are referred to as schizoid, paranoid, or cyclothymic personalities.

A special form of personality disorder is the SOCIOPATHIC personality, or psychopathic personality. A person with this disorder shows abnormal behaviour patterns, although they differ from the patterns observed in neurosis and psychosis. He may have a greatly exaggerated sense of self-importance, and his emotions are often very shallow. Some of the problems of the sociopathic personality can include sexual deviation, alcoholism, and drug addiction. Certain kinds of criminals belong in this group.

Although personality disorders are more difficult to treat than other forms of mental illness, a great deal can be done in many cases. Since these disorders are the result of unresolved emotional conflicts, often dating back to childhood, the treatment attempts to uncover the roots of these conflicts and to help the patient resolve them. The various techniques for doing this are included under the term PSYCHOTHERAPY.

alternating p. multiple personality. Now thought to be a rather dubious diagnostic category, as so-called 'multiple personality' may be the result of psychotherapeutic suggestion.

anankastic p. see ANANKASTIC.

antisocial p. a personality disorder in which repetitive antisocial behaviour is associated with ego eccentricity, lack of guilt or anxiety, and imperviousness to punishment. Called also *sociopathic (psychopathic) personality.*

cyclothymic p. a personality marked by alternate moods of elation and dejection. **double p., dual p.** multiple personality.

multiple p. a dissociative reaction in which an individual adopts two or more personalities alternatively, in none of which is he aware of the experiences of the other(s).

psychopathic p. antisocial personality, sociopathic personality.

schizoid p. a personality disorder marked by timidness, self-consciousness, introversion, feelings of isolation and loneliness, and failure to form close interpersonal relationships; the individual is frequently ambitious, meticulous, and a perfectionist.

perspiration (ˌpərspiˈrayshən) 1. sweating; the excretion of moisture through the pores of the skin. 2. sweat; the salty fluid, consisting largely of water, excreted by the sweat glands in the skin.

The body has approximately 2 million sweat glands. The secretory portion is located in the corium and is connected to the epidermis by a long straight duct. The largest of these glands are in the armpits and groin, but the greatest number per square inch is found on the soles of the feet and the palms of the hands.

In midsummer temperatures—or during strenuous exertion or unusual emotional stress—the body's perspiration output may exceed several quarts per day. On a cool day without exertion or emotional stress, the body loses well over a pint of perspiration. This kind of sweating is known medically as 'insensible' perspiration because it is virtually unnoticeable; as the sweat reaches the surface of the skin, it evaporates immediately. When sweating becomes noticeable, it is known as 'sensible' perspiration.

FUNCTIONS. The chief role of sweat glands and perspiration is to maintain the body temperature at a constant level. Thus the skin is cooled as perspiration evaporates. The blood in the capillaries of the skin likewise is cooled before it courses back into the body.

The sweat glands have a minor excretory function. Perspiration contains water, sodium chloride, and small amounts of urea, lactic acid, and potassium ions. It also contains antibacterial substances that defend the body against infection.

ABNORMAL PERSPIRATION. Malfunctioning of the sweat glands is somewhat unusual and seldom is cause for alarm unless accompanied by another disease. For example, profuse sweating (diaphoresis) may accompany such diseases as tuberculosis, rickets, and malaria. Night sweats may be a sign of serious disease. Excessive perspiration may also be generated temporarily by shock or by motion sickness or hormonal changes during menopause.

The commonest serious problem from excessive sweating is probably the temporary loss of salt, resulting in a sodium deficiency.

Excessive sweating, or hyperhidrosis, that is not accompanied by disease is sometimes hereditary and is difficult to treat. Diminished or total absence of sweating, or anhidrosis, may occur in the elderly and in those with pronounced thyroid deficiency or severe skin disease. In treating anhidrosis the primary step is to try to cure the condition causing it.

In CYSTIC FIBROSIS the sweat contains an abnormally

high sodium chloride content, and excessive sweating in these patients must be guarded against. In the rare malady called chromhidrosis, the perspiration turns black, blue, green, red, yellow, or a combination of colours. The cause is unknown although certain bacteria may be responsible.

Perthes' disease ('pərtayz) osteochondrosis of the epiphysis of the head of the femur.

Pertofran ('pərtoh,fran) trademark for a preparation of desipramine, an antidepressent.

pertussis (pə'tusis) an infectious disease due to *Bordetella pertussis*, and characterized by coryza, bronchitis, and a typical explosive cough ending in crowing or whooping inspiration (see also WHOOPING COUGH).

pertussoid (pə'tusoyd) 1. resembling whooping cough. 2. an influenzal cough resembling that of whooping cough.

perversion (pə'vərshən) deviation from the normal course.

sexual p. sexual deviation, or paraphilia.

pervert ('pərvərt) a deviant person, especially a paraphiliac.

pes (payz, peez) pl. *pedes* [L.] foot; the terminal organ of the leg, or lower limb; any footlike part.

p. abductus a deformity in which the anterior part of the foot is displaced and lies laterally to the vertical axis of the leg.

p. adductus a deformity in which the anterior part of the foot is displaced and lies medially to the vertical axis of the leg.

p. cavus a foot with an abnormally high longitudinal arch, either congenital or caused by contractures or disturbed muscle balance.

p. hippocampi a formation of two or three elevations on the ventricular surface of the hippocampus.

p. planus flatfoot.

p. valgus flatfoot: deviation of the foot outwards at the talocalcanean joint.

p. varus a permanent toeing-in position of the foot; pigeon toe; talipes varus.

pessary ('pesə·ree) 1. an instrument placed in the vagina to support the uterus or rectum or as a contraceptive device. 2. a medicated vaginal suppository.

pesticide ('pesti,sied) a poison used to destroy pests of any sort.

pestilence ('pestilens) a term used in the past to describe an infectious epidemic disease. adj. **pestilential**.

pestis ('pestis) plague.

pestle ('pes'l) an instrument with a rounded end, used in a mortar to reduce a solid to a powder or produce a homogeneous mixture of solids.

PET positron emission TOMOGRAPHY, a nuclear medicine technique that combines computed tomography and radioisotope brain scanning.

peta- ('petə) a word element used in naming units of measurement to designate a quantity 10^{15} (a quadrillion, or thousand million million) times the unit to which it is joined. Symbol P.

-petal word element. [L.] *directed* or *moving toward*.

petechia (pə'teeki·ə) pl. *petechiae* [L.] a minute, pinpoint, nonraised, perfectly round, purplish red spot caused by intradermal or submucous haemorrhage, which later turns blue or yellow. adj. **petechial**.

pethidine ('pethi,deen, -in) a synthetic narcotic analgesic, less potent than morphine with quicker onset but shorter duration of action used in obstetrics and pre- and postoperative medication. Particularly useful, as it relaxes smooth muscle, in patients with ureteric and biliary colic and as an analgesic in patients with asthma. Under the Misuse of Drugs Regulations 1973, a Registered Midwife who has notified the local supervisory authority of her intention to practise is authorized to be in possession of pethidine as long as it is necessary for the practice of her profession and has been obtained in the recognized manner. This applies only to midwives working in the community or in independent practice. Because of depression of the fetal respiratory centre, and its effect on breast feeding, pethidine is now less popular for use in labour.

petiole ('peti,ohl) a stem, stalk, or pedicle.

epiglottic p. the pointed lower end of the epiglottic cartilage, attached to the thyroid cartilage.

petiolus (pə'teeələs) petiole.

Petit's ligament (pə'teez) uterosacral ligament.

petit mal (,peti 'mal) a relatively mild epileptic attack occurring in children, contrasting with grand mal, a major attack. In petit mal, the affected person loses consciousness only momentarily. Often the only outward signs of the attack are twitching of the eyes and mouth and a brief lapse of attention. The facial expression is blank and empty. See also EPILEPSY.

Petri dish ('petree) a round shallow glass or plastic dish with a lid, in which bacteria are grown on a culture medium.

pétrissage (paytri'sahzh) [Fr.] *foulage*.

petrol sniffing ('petrəl) a form of SOLVENT abuse in which petrol vapours are inhaled. Carries the long-term hazard of lead poisoning as well as the immediate hazards of inhalation asphyxia.

petrolatum (,petrə'laytəm) petroleum jelly.

petroleum (pə'trohli·əm) a thick natural oil obtained from beneath the earth. It consists of a mixture of various hydrocarbons of the alkane and alkene series.

p. jelly a purified mixture of hydrocarbons obtained from petroleum; used as a base for ointments, protective dressings, and soothing applications to the skin. Called also *petrolatum*.

p. sniffing see PETROL SNIFFING.

petromastoid (,petroh'mastoyd) 1. pertaining to the petrous portion of the temporal bone and its mastoid process. 2. OTOCRANIUM (2).

petrosal (pe'trohs'l) pertaining to the pars petrosa, or petrous portion of the temporal bone.

petrositis (,petroh'sietis) inflammation of the pars petrosa or petrous portion of the temporal bone.

petrosphenoid (,petroh'sfeenoyd) pertaining to the petrous portion of the temporal bone and to the sphenoid bone.

petrosquamous (,petroh'skwayməs) pertaining to the petrous and squamous portions of the temporal bone.

petrous ('petrəs) resembling rock or stone; stony.

p. bone the pars petrosa, or petrous portion of the temporal bone.

Peutz-Jeghers syndrome (,pərts'jaygəz) familial gastrointestinal polyposis, especially in the small bowel, associated with mucocutaneous pigmentation.

pexis ('peksis) 1. the fixation within a tissue. 2. surgical fixation, usually by suturing. adj. **pexic**.

-pexy word element. [Gr.] *surgical fixation*. adj. **-pectic**.

Peyer's patches ('pieəz) whitish, oval, elevated patches of closely packed lymph follicles in mucous and submucous layers of the small intestine.

peyote (pay'ohtee) a stimulant drug from mescal buttons, the flowering heads of the cactus *Lophophora williamsii*, whose active principle is mescaline; used by North American Indians in certain ceremonies to produce an intoxication marked by feelings of ecstasy (see also HALLUCINOGEN).

Peyronie's disease ('payrəneez) induration of the corpora cavernosa of the penis, producing a fibrous chordee.

Pezzer's catheter ('petsəz) a self-retaining catheter with a bulbous extremity.

PF3 platelet factor 3; a phospholipid released from platelets. Once activated, it forms a lipoprotein surface on which coagulation factors interact, leading to the production of a thrombus. See also PLATELET.

Pfeiffer's disease ('fiefəz) infectious mononucleosis.

PG prostaglandin.

pg picogram.

pH the negative logarithm of the hydrogen ion concentration $[H^+]$ a measure of the degree to which a solution is acidic or alkaline. An acid is a substance that can give up a hydrogen ion (H^+); a base is a substance that can accept H^+. The more acidic a solution the greater the hydrogen ion concentration and the lower the pH; a pH of 7.0 indicates neutrality; a pH of less than 7 indicates acidity, and a pH of more than 7 indicates alkalinity. The pH is used as a measure of whether the body is maintaining a normal ACID–BASE BALANCE. A favourable pH is essential to the functioning of enzymes and other biochemical systems. The body's fluids are normally somewhat alkaline, the pH being between 7.35 and 7.45. A pH above 7.8 or below 6.8 is generally fatal.

PHA phytohaemagglutinin.

phac(o)- word element. [Gr.] *lens;* see also words beginning *phako-*.

phacoanaphylaxis (ˌfakohˌanəfi'laksis) hypersensitivity to the protein of the crystalline lens of the eye, induced by leakage of this material through the lens capsule.

phacocele ('fakohˌseel) hernia of the eye lens.

phacocystectomy (ˌfakohsi'stektəmee) excision of part of the lens capsule for cataract.

phacocystitis (ˌfakohsi'stietis) inflammation of the capsule of the eye lens.

phacoemulsification (ˌfakohiˌmulsifi'kayshən) a technique of CATARACT extraction, utilizing high-frequency ultrasonic vibrations to fragment the lens nucleus combined with controlled irrigation to maintain normal pressure in the anterior chamber, and suction to remove lens fragments and irrigating fluid.

phacoerysis (ˌfakoh·e'reesis) removal of the eye lens in cataract by suction.

phacoid ('fakoyd) shaped like a lens.

phacolysis (fə'kolisis) dissolution or discission of the crystalline lens. adj. **phacolytic**.

phacoma (fə'kohmə) a congenital tumour of the lens of the eye.

phacomalacia (ˌfakohmə'layshi·ə) softening of the eye lens; a soft cataract, that is, one without a hard nucleus.

phacometachoresis (ˌfakohˌmetəkə'reesis) displacement of the eye lens.

phacosclerosis (ˌfakohsklə'rohsis) hardening of the eye lens; a hard cataract, that is, one with a hard nucleus.

phacoscope ('fakohˌskohp) an instrument for viewing accommodative changes of the eye lens.

phacotoxic (ˌfakoh'toksik) exerting a deleterious effect upon the crystalline lens.

phaeochrome ('feeohˌkrohm) chromaffin.

phaeochromoblast (ˌfeeoh'krohməˌblast) any of the embryonic structures that develop into chromaffin (pheochrome) cells.

phaeochromocyte (ˌfeeoh'krohməˌsiet) a chromaffin cell.

phaeochromocytoma (ˌfeeohˌkrohmohsie'tohmə) a chromaffin cell tumour, usually located in the adrenal medulla but occasionally occurring in chromaffin tissue of the sympathetic paraganglia. It is relatively rare and has a tendency to occur in families. The tumour is potentially fatal, but the condition can be cured if diagnosed early, before there has been irreparable damage to the cardiovascular system.

SYMPTOMS. Because the tumour is composed of cells similar to the secreting cells of the adrenal medulla, it is capable of secreting adrenaline and noradrenaline. The symptoms of the tumour are therefore directly related to excessive amounts of these two hormones in the tissues and blood.

The cardinal symptom is hypertension. In some cases the blood pressure is consistently high with slight fluctuations, and in others the hypertension is intermittent with periods of normal blood pressure. Other symptoms include severe headache, sweating, visual blurring, apprehension, tachycardia, and postural hypotension.

DIAGNOSIS. Phaeochromocytoma must be differentiated from several other disorders such as essential hypertension and thyrotoxicosis, which it closely resembles. Diagnosis is based on the patient's symptoms and the findings of specific chemical and pharmacological tests. The test considered most reliable is direct assay of adrenaline and noradrenaline in the plasma and urine following an attack. Another test involving measurement of vanillylmandelic acid (VMA) and of metanephrine and normetanephrine in urine is considered satisfactory. The level of these substances in the urine in patients with phaeochromocytoma is almost twice the upper limits of normal.

Two types of pharmacological tests may be used; one provokes an increase in blood pressure, the other causes a fall in blood pressure. The provocative test uses histamine or methacholine to stimulate action of the tumour and thereby provoke an attack. This test must be given with extreme caution and only when the patient is between attacks and the blood pressure is near normal (less than 170/110 mmHg).

For the patient with sustained hypertension the test of choice involves the administration of an adrenolytic agent such as phentolamine, which will produce hypotension. If, after administration of the drug, the blood pressure decreases to near normal within 3 to 4 minutes and remains depressed for several minutes more, the diagnosis of phaeochromocytoma is confirmed.

The pharmacological tests have largely been replaced by the more reliable and less hazardous hormonal assays. The presence of phaeochromocytoma often can be confirmed by radiological studies or a CAT scan.

TREATMENT. Surgical removal of the tumour, or tumours, is necessary for complete remission of symptoms. There are two possible complications of surgery: a sudden rise in blood pressure and development of tachycardia due to discharge of pressor agents as the tumour is being manipulated, and severe hypotension and shock following removal of the tumour. These hazards have been substantially reduced in recent years by the preoperative administration of sedatives and antihypertensive drugs, and the use of blood or plasma to maintain adequate blood volume.

If surgery has involved resection of a portion of the adrenal cortex, it may be necessary for the patient to receive adrenocortical hormones by injection.

PATIENT CARE. Once the diagnosis of phaeochromocytoma has been established, the patient is prepared for surgery. The preoperative period may extend for several weeks while attempts are made to stabilize the blood pressure and hormonal imbalances. The patient should be kept in a quiet atmosphere and usually is given sedatives, such as phenobarbitone, to promote rest. His blood pressure is taken at frequent intervals and recorded. These readings are used later as a basis for comparison during the postoperative period. They also alert the doctor to extremes in blood pressure that are characteristic in this disorder.

A day or two before surgery the patient may be given repeated doses of drugs such as phenoxybenzamine to block the vasoconstricting effects of adrenaline and noradrenaline. The blood pressure may be drastically affected and therefore must be monitored frequently for signs of instability and dangerous extremes.

Postoperatively the patient must again be watched for the development of severe hypertension, which can lead to stroke and for extreme hypotension with circulatory collapse and profound shock.

If the adrenal cortex has been resected during surgery, hormonal imbalances are likely to occur. These include HYPOGLYCAEMIA, Addisonian crisis and extreme diuresis, and electrolyte and fluid imbalance. The hypoglycaemia is most likely to occur in patients who have had symptoms of diabetes mellitus prior to surgery, and is treated with infusions of glucose solution. Adrenocortical hormones may be administered by slow intravenous drip, the rate of flow being adjusted according to blood pressure readings and other reactions of the patient. The patient's status is closely monitored so that disturbances in ELECTROLYTE and FLUID BALANCE, extremes in BLOOD PRESSURE, and disorders of metabolism can be recognized early and treated promptly.

phaeohyphomycosis (ˌfeeohˌhiefohmie'kohsis) any opportunistic infection caused by fungi of the family Dematium.

phag(o)- word element. [Gr.] *eating, ingestion*.

phage (fayj, fahzh) bacteriophage.

p. type an intraspecies type of bacterium demonstrated by phage typing.

p. typing characterization of bacteria, extending to strain differences, by demonstration of susceptibility to one or more (a spectrum) bacteriophage; widely applied to staphylococci, typhoid bacilli, etc., for epidemiological purposes.

phagedena (ˌfaji'deenə) rapidly spreading and sloughing ulceration.

-phagia, -phagy word element. [Gr.] *eating, swallowing*.

phagocyte ('fagəˌsiet) any cell that ingests microorganisms or other cells and foreign particles. adj. **phagocytic**.

phagocytin (ˌfagə'sietin) a bactericidal substance from neutrophilic leukocytes.

phagocytize ('fagəsieˌtiez) phagocytose.

phagocytoblast (ˌfagə'sietohˌblast) a cell giving rise to phagocytes.

phagocytolysis (ˌfagəsie'tolisis) destruction of phagocytes. adj. **phagocytolytic**.

phagocytose ('fagəsieˌtohz) to envelop and engulf bacteria and other foreign material for the purpose of enzymic digestion, if necessary by first killing live microorganisms; phagocytize.

phagocytosis (ˌfagəsie'tohsis) the engulfing of microorganisms or other cells and foreign particles by phagocytes. adj. **phagocytotic**.

phagokaryosis (ˌfagohˌkari'ohsis) phagocytosis allegedly effected by the cell nucleus.

phagomania (ˌfagoh'mayni·ə) an insatiable craving for food or an obsessive preoccupation with the subject of eating.

phagosome ('fagəˌsohm) a membrane-bound vesicle in a phagocyte containing the phagocytized material as well as endogenous cell products designed to kill and digest the engulfed material.

phagotype ('fagohˌtiep) phage type.

phak(o)- see *phac(o)-*.

phakitis (fə'kietis) inflammation of the crystalline lens of the eye.

phakoma (fə'kohmə) 1. an occasional small, greyish-white tumour seen in the retina in tuberous sclerosis. 2. a patch of myelinated nerve fibres seen very infrequently in the retina in neurofibromatosis.

phakomatosis (ˌfakohmə'tohsis) any of four hereditary syndromes (neurofibromatosis, tuberous sclerosis, Sturge–Weber syndrome, and von Hippel–Lindau disease) marked by disseminated hamartomas of the eye, skin, and brain.

phalangeal (fə'lanji·əl) pertaining to a phalanx.

phalangectomy (ˌfalən'jektəmee) excision of a phalanx.

phalangitis (ˌfalən'jietis) inflammation of one or more phalanges.

phalanx ('falangks) pl. *phalanges* [Gr.] any bone of a finger or toe. adj. **phalangeal.**

Phalen's manoeuvre ('falənz) (for detection of carpal tunnel syndrome), the size of the carpal tunnel is reduced by holding the affected hand with the wrist fully flexed or extended for 30 to 60 seconds, or by placing a sphygmomanometer cuff on the involved hand and inflating to a point between diastolic and systolic pressure for 30 to 60 seconds.

phallectomy (fə'lektəmee) amputation of the penis.

phallic ('falik) pertaining to the penis.

phallitis (fə'lietis) penitis.

phallocampsis (ˌfaloh'kampsis) curvature of the penis during erection.

phalloidin, phalloidine (fə'loydin; fə'loydeen) a hexapeptide poison from the mushroom *Amanita phalloides*, which causes asthenia, vomiting, diarrhoea, convulsions, and death.

phalloplasty ('falohˌplastee) a plastic operation on the penis to repair deformity or after injury.

phallus ('faləs) the penis. adj. **phallic**.

phanerosis (ˌfanə'rohsis) the process of becoming visible.

phantasm ('fantazəm) PHANTOM (1).

phantom ('fantəm) 1. an image or impression not evoked by actual stimuli. 2. a model of the body or of a specific part thereof. 3. a device for simulating the in vivo interaction of radiation with tissues.

p. pain pain felt as if it were arising in an absent (amputated) limb. See also AMPUTATION.

phar., pharm. pharmacy; pharmaceutical; pharmacopoeia.

pharmac(o)- word element. [Gr.] *drug, medicine*.

pharmaceutical (ˌfahmə'syootik'l) 1. pertaining to pharmacy or drugs. 2. a medicinal drug.

pharmaceutics (ˌfahmə'syootiks) 1. PHARMACY (1). 2. pharmaceutical preparations.

pharmacist ('fahməsist) an individual who is licensed to prepare, compound, and dispense drugs upon written order (prescription) from a licensed practitioner, such as a general practitioner or dentist. (See also CHEMIST.) A pharmacist is a health care professional who cooperates and consults with and sometimes advises the licensed practitioner concerning drugs.

A pharmacist's education gives him or her advanced knowledge of the chemical and physical properties of drugs and their available dosage forms. By virtue of this training, the pharmacist is qualified to play a key role in supplying information about drugs, both prescription and over-the-counter, to those to whom such information is most important—the patients. Since the pharmacist may be the last health care professional to communicate with the patient or his significant others before the medication is taken, he or she is therefore in the best position to discuss the drug with those concerned. The discussion may include any side-effects associated with the drug that may concern the patient, the stability of the drug under various conditions, its toxicity and dosage, and its route of administration, all of which may be reassuring to the patient and benefit him by helping to ensure his compliance with the drug regimen.

pharmacoangiography (ˌfahməkohˌanji'ogrəfee) the use of drugs in angiography either to enhance the imaging process or in the treatment of pathology.

pharmacodiagnosis (ˌfahməkohˌdieəg'nohsis) use of drugs in diagnosis.

pharmacodynamics (ˌfahməkohdie'namiks) the study of the mechanisms of action of drugs and other biochemical and physiological effects. adj. **pharmacodynamic**.

pharmacogenetics (ˌfahməkohjə'netiks) the study of the relationship between genetic factors and the nature of responses to drugs.

pharmacognosy (ˌfahmə'kognəsee) the branch of pharmacology dealing with natural drugs and their constituents.

pharmacokinetics (ˌfahməkohki'netiks) the study of the movement of drugs in the body, including the processes of absorption, distribution, localization in tissues, biotransformation, and excretion. adj. **pharmacokinetic**.

pharmacologist (ˌfahmə'koləjist) a specialist in pharmacology.

pharmacology (ˌfahmə'koləjee) the science that deals with the origin, nature, chemistry, effects, and uses of drugs; it includes pharmacognosy, pharmacokinetics, pharmacodynamics, pharmacotherapeutics, and toxicology. adj. **pharmacological**.

pharmacomania (ˌfahməkoh'mayni·ə) uncontrollable desire to take or to administer drugs.

pharmacophobia (ˌfahməkoh'fohbi·ə) morbid dread of medicines or drugs.

pharmacophore ('fahməkohˌfor) the group of atoms in the molecule of a drug responsible for the drug's action.

pharmacopoeia (ˌfahməkə'pee·ə) authoritative treatise on drugs and their preparations. adj. **pharmacopoeial**.

pharmacopsychosis (ˌfahməkohsie'kohsis) a group of mental diseases due to alcohol, drugs, or poisons.

pharmacotherapy (ˌfahməkoh'therəpee) treatment of disease with medicines.

pharmacy ('fahməsee) 1. the branch of the health sciences dealing with the preparation, dispensing, and proper utilization of drugs. 2. a place where drugs are compounded or dispensed.

pharyng(o)- word element. [Gr.] *pharynx*.

pharyngalgia (ˌfaring'galji·ə) pain in the pharynx.

pharyngeal (ˌfarin'jeeəl, fə'rinji·əl) pertaining to the pharynx.

p. reflex gag reflex.

pharyngectomy (ˌfarin'jektəmee) excision of part of the pharynx.

pharyngemphraxis (ˌfarinjem'fraksis) obstruction of the pharynx.

pharyngismus (ˌfarin'jizməs) muscular spasm of the pharynx.

pharyngitis (ˌfarin'jietis) inflammation of the pharynx. adj. **pharyngitic**. Acute pharyngitis usually appears suddenly and runs its course in a few days or a week. Symptoms, more severe in children, are dry, sore throat, fatigue, and mild fever. Often, swallowing is painful, the head aches, and there is a harsh cough and a persistent desire to clear the throat. The throat frequently becomes swollen and covered with a thick mucous material. Sometimes there is pain in the ears, or hoarseness. In most cases, treatment is similar to that for a cold: rest, liquids, analgesia, and, when prescribed, antibiotics.

Chronic pharyngitis is the result of continuous reinfection or chronic irritation of exposed parts of the throat. It is similar to acute pharyngitis, but less severe. The simple catarrhal form can be caused by smoking, dust, smog, or constant breathing through the mouth.

Symptomatic treatment includes hot saline gargles, liquid diet, and an increase in fluid intake. Sulphonamides or antibiotics may be prescribed when a bacterial infection is present.

The symptoms of pharyngitis can occur during the early stages of such diseases as scarlet fever, measles, and whooping cough.

pharyngocele (fə'ring·gohˌseel) a herniation or cystic deformity of the pharynx.

pharyngoconjunctival fever (fəˌring·gohˌkonjungk'tiev'l) an epidemic disease due to an adenovirus, occurring chiefly in school children, with fever, pharyngitis, conjunctivitis, rhinitis, and enlarged cervical lymph nodes.

pharyngodynia (fəˌring·goh'dini·ə) pain in the pharynx.

pharyngoglossal (fəˌring·goh'glos'l) pertaining to the pharynx and tongue.

pharyngokeratosis (fəˌring·gohˌkerə'tohsis) keratosis of the pharynx.

pharyngolaryngitis (fəˌring·gohˌlarin'jietis) inflammation of the pharynx and larynx.

pharyngomycosis (fəˌring·gohmie'kohsis) any fungal infection of the pharynx.

pharyngonasal (fəˌring·goh'nayz'l) pertaining to the pharynx and nose.

pharyngooesophageal (fəˌring·goh·iˌsofə'jeeəl) pertaining to the pharynx and oesophagus.

pharyngoparalysis (fəˌring·gohpə'ralisis) paralysis of the pharyngeal muscles; pharyngoplegia.

pharyngoperistole (fəˌring·gohpə'ristəlee) pharyngostenosis.

pharyngoplasty (fə'ring·gohˌplastee) plastic repair of the pharynx.

pharyngoplegia (fəˌring·goh'pleeji·ə) pharyngoparalysis.

pharyngorhinitis (fəˌring·gohrie'nietis) inflammation of the nasopharynx.

pharyngorrhoea (fəˌring·gə'reeə) mucous discharge from the pharynx.

pharyngoscleroma (fəˌring·gohsklia'rohmə) scleroma of the pharynx.

pharyngoscope (fə'ring·gohˌskohp) an instrument for inspecting the pharynx.

pharyngoscopy (ˌfaring'goskəpee) direct visual examination of the pharynx.

pharyngospasm (fə'ring·gohˌspazəm) spasm of the pharyngeal muscles.

pharyngostenosis (fəˌring·gohstə'nohsis) narrowing of the pharynx; pharyngoperistole.

pharyngotomy (ˌfaring'gotəmee) incision of the pharynx.

pharyngotympanic tube (fəˌring·gohtim'panik) the narrow channel that connects the tympanum with the nasopharynx. The pharyngotymphanic tube serves to equalize pressure on either side of the tympanic membrane (eardrum). In children this tube is wider and shorter than in adults, and thus children are especially prone to infections of the middle ear that originate in the pharynx and travel through the tube. Called also *eustachian tube, auditory tube*.

pharynx ('faringks) the throat; the musculomembranous cavity, about 5 inches long, behind the nasal cavities, mouth, and larynx, communicating with them and with the oesophagus.

The pharynx includes many individual structures and may be divided into three areas: the nasopharynx (top), oropharynx (centre, behind the mouth), and laryngopharynx (bottom). The nasopharynx, connected with the nasal cavities, provides a passage for air during breathing; it also contains the openings of the pharyngotympanic tubes through which air enters the middle ear. The oropharynx and laryngopharynx provide passageways for both air and food. The pharynx also functions as a resonating organ in speech.

The pharynx is separated from the mouth by the soft palate and its fleshy V-shaped extension or flap, the uvula, which hangs from the top of the back of the mouth, above the root of the tongue. In swallowing, the uvula lifts up, closing off the nasopharynx as food passes from the mouth through the lower parts of the pharynx to the oesophagus. On each side of the entrance to the pharynx from the mouth, and behind the nasal passage, are the TONSILS and ADENOIDS, masses of lymphoid tissue.

The most common disorders of the pharynx are PHARYNGITIS and the inflammation and discomfort resulting from TONSILLITIS.

phase (fayz) 1. one of the aspects or stages through which a varying entity may pass. 2. In physical chemistry, a component that is homogeneous of itself, bounded by an interface, and mechanically separable from other phases of the system.

continuous p. in a heterogeneous system, the component in which the disperse phase is distributed, corresponding to the solvent in a true solution.

disperse p. the discontinuous portion of a heterogeneous system, corresponding to the solute in a true solution.

phasmid ('fazmid) 1. either of the two caudal chemoreceptors occurring in certain nematodes (Phasmidia). 2. any nematode containing phasmids.

PhD (ˌpeeaych'dee) Doctor of Philosophy.

phenanthrene (fə'nanthreen) a colourless, crystalline hydrocarbon.

phenazocine (fe'nazohˌseen) an analgesic drug used to relieve severe pain. It is a drug of addiction.

phenazopyridine (ˌfenəzoh'piriˌdeen) a urinary analgesic, used as the hydrochloride salt.

phencyclidine (fen'siekliˌdeen) a central nervous system depressant originally introduced as an anaesthetic in the early 1950s, but later abandoned because of unpredictable side-effects such as agitation, disorientation, and hallucination. The drug is easily synthesized by anyone with a basic knowledge of chemistry and has become one of the drugs most frequently used by drug abusers. It has a variety of street names, including 'angel dust', 'animal tranquillizer', 'PCP' or 'peace pill', 'crystal joints', and 'peace weed'. The name often reflects the form in which the drug is taken. It can be smoked, 'snorted' through the nose, ingested, or taken intravenously. There is great danger from the poor and erratic quality of the product that is illegally sold on the streets. It can produce a schizophrenia-like syndrome, neurological and cognitive dysfunction, coma, convulsions, and respiratory arrest.

phenelzine (fe'nelzeen) a monoamine oxidase inhibitor, used as an ANTIDEPRESSANT.

Phenergan ('fenəˌgan) trademark for preparations of promethazine, an antihistamine.

phenethicillin (feˌnethi'silin) a semisyr. hetic acid-resistant penicillin, which is a methyl analogue of penicillin V.

phenformin (fen'fawmin) a synthetic hypoglycaemic drug whose action is not yet completely understood; it is not related to other hypoglycaemic agents such as tolbutamide or chlorpropamide in activity and chemical structure. Phenformin can produce lactic acidosis, and the use of this drug is not approved.

phenindamine (fe'nindəˌmeen) an antihistaminic, used as the tartrate salt.

phenindione (ˌfenin'dieohn) an anticoagulant.

phenobarbitone (ˌfeenoh'bahbiˌtohn) a long-lasting barbiturate drug used as an anticonvulsant drug in the treatment of epilepsy.

phenocopy ('feenohˌkopee) 1. an environmentally induced phenotype mimicking one usually produced by a specific genotype. 2. an individual exhibiting such a phenotype; the simulated trait in a phenocopy.

phenodeviant (ˌfeenoh'deevi·ənt) an individual whose phenotype differs significantly from that of the typical phenotype in the population.

phenol ('feenol) 1. an extremely poisonous compound obtained by distillation of coal tar or produced synthetically; used as an antibiotic. Called also *carbolic acid*. Ingestion or absorption of phenol through the skin causes colic, weakness, collapse, and local irritation and corrosion. Phenol should be properly labelled and stored to avoid accidental poisoning. 2. any organic compound containing one or more hydroxyl groups attached to an aromatic or carbon ring.

p. coefficient a measure of the bactericidal activity of a chemical compound in relation to phenol under specified conditions.

phenolphthalein (ˌfeenol'thalee·in, -leen, -'thay-) a cathartic.

phenomenology (fiˌnomin'oləjee) in psychiatry the psychotherapeutic approach which gives precedence to the patient's actual experiences and his communications about his subjective state. The antitheseis of approaches derived from preconceived theories.

phenomenon (fi'nominən) pl. *phenomena;* any sign or objective symptom; any observable occurrence or fact.

phenoperidine (ˌfeenoh'perideen) synthetic narcotic analgesic used intraoperatively to supplement general anaesthesia. It has longer duration of action than fentanyl and a greater tendency to reduce the blood pressure. It is also used in the intensive care unit to facilitate patients accepting mechanical ventilation. Called also *Operidine*.

phenothiazine (ˌfeenoh'thieəzeen) a veterinary anthelmintic; also used to denote a group of major tranquillizers, the phenothiazine derivatives.

phenotype ('feenohˌtiep) 1. the outward, visible expression of the hereditary constitution of an organism. 2. an individual exhibiting a certain phenotype; a trait expressed in a phenotype. adj. **phenotypic**.

phenoxybenzamine (feeˌnoksi'benzəmeen) an adrenergic blocking agent; the hydrochloride salt is used as a vasodilator and sometimes as an antihypertensive.

phenoxymethylpenicillin (feˌnoksiˌmethilˌpeni'silin) a penicillinase-sensitive antibiotic similar in action to benzylpenicillin. Used mainly against streptococcal infections in children, it is taken orally. Penicillin V.

phenozygous (fə'nozigəs) having the calvaria narrower than the face, so that the zygomatic arches are visible when the head is viewed from above.

phentermine ('fentəˌmeen) an anorexic.

phentolamine (fen'toləˌmeen) a potent alpha-adrenergic blocking agent; it blocks the hypertensive action of adrenaline and noradrenaline and most responses of smooth muscles that involve alpha-adrenergic cell receptors. Its hydrochloride and mesylate salts are used in the diagnosis of hypertension due to phaeochromocytoma.

Phenurone ('fenyuhˌrohn) trademark for a preparation of phenacemide, an anticonvulsant.

phenyl ('feenil, -niel, 'fenil) the monovalent radical, C_6H_5. adj. **phenylic.**

p. salicylate a salicylic acid ester used as an analgesic.

phenylalanine (ˌfeenil'alәneen) a naturally occurring amino acid essential for optimal growth in infants and for nitrogen equilibrium in human adults.

phenylbutazone (ˌfeenil'byootәzohn) a nonsteroidal anti-inflammatory drug; formerly available for use in the treatment of gout, rheumatoid arthritis, and other rheumatoid conditions. Now only available in hospitals for the treatment of ankylosing spondylitis.

phenylephrine (ˌfeeni'lefrin) an adrenergic used as the hydrochloride salt for its potent vasoconstrictor properties.

phenylketonuria (ˌfeenilˌkeetә'nyooә·ri·ә) PKU, a congenital disease due to a defect in the metabolism of the amino acid phenylalanine. adj. **phenylketonuric.**

The condition is hereditary and is transmitted recessively through apparently healthy parents who, if tested, will show signs of the disease. It results from lack of an enzyme, phenylalanine hydroxylase, necessary for the conversion of the amino acid phenylalanine into tyrosine. Thus there is accumulation of phenylalanine in the blood with eventual excretion of phenylpyruvic acid in the urine. If untreated, the condition results in mental handicap and other abnormalities.

Persons with phenylketonuria are usually blue-eyed and blond, with defective pigmentation, the skin being excessively sensitive to light and tending to eczema. Other manifestations besides mental handicap are tremors, poor muscular coordination, excessive perspiration, a mousy odour, and perhaps convulsions.

DIAGNOSIS. Mass screening of newborns for PKU entails a simple blood test. (The detection of urinary abnormalities is unreliable for several weeks after birth, and in some cases may never become positive.) A sample of blood is taken from infants' heels at approximately 2 weeks and phenylalanine levels are assessed.

The current criteria for establishment of a diagnosis of classic PKU are: (1) a rise in plasma phenylalanine during the first few weeks of life from a level of 1 to 4 mg/100 ml at birth to 20 mg/100 ml or higher; (2) a normal serum tyrosine level; and (3) urine that contains ortho-hydroxyphenylacetic acid during the newborn period, and later contains phenylketones. Diagnosis of variants of the disease depends in part on values of plasma phenylalanine, family history, clinical course, and the infant's response to ingestion of natural protein.

TREATMENT. A normal diet contains more phenylalanine than can be tolerated by the child with PKU. Treatment therefore consists of a diet containing only the amount of phenylalanine which is essential for normal growth and development.

Natural protein foods are given in small measured quantities so that the blood phenylalanine, which should be measured regularly, is kept within safe limits. Meat, fish, cheese and egg, which are rich in phenylalanine, are usually omitted but measured quantities of milk, cereal, cream and potato can be included. These measured foods should be spread out between the day's meals. The quantities permitted will vary from child to child and from time to time in the same child.

The high protein foods, which cannot be eaten safely, are replaced by a protein substitute such as Minafen, Lofenalac, Albumaid XP, Aminogran, PK Aid or Maxamaid XP. A paediatrician or dietitian should advise which is best for the child, the amount required and how it is to be given.

The child need not be hungry. High energy ingredients are included in some of the protein substitutes. Alternatively, they can be given as household items (sugar, jam, honey, boiled sweets, barley sugar, pure fats, vegetable or cooking oil, sago, tapioca), or as special low protein flour, bread, biscuits or pasta. A variety of low protein fruit and vegetables can also be given.

Vitamins and minerals must be included in the diet either with the protein substitute or as a medicine.

Further information about the phenylalanine content of manufacturers' foods, and about phenylketonuria, can be obtained from The National Society for Phenylketonuria and Allied Disorders, 26 Towngate Grove, Mirfield, West Yorkshire, UK.

Although PKU cannot be cured, its effects can be counteracted by proper management. Research has shown that the mean intelligence quotient of children treated within the first month of life is about 28 points higher than that of either siblings or matched pairs who were treated after the first month or who were never treated.

phenylmercuric (ˌfeenilmә'kyooә·rik) denoting a compound containing the radical C_6H_5Hg–, forming various antiseptic, antibacterial, and fungicidal salts; compounds of the acetate and nitrate salts are used as bacteriostatics, and the former is also used as a herbicide.

phenylpropanolamine (ˌfeenilˌprohpә'nolәmeen) an adrenergic used chiefly as a nasal and sinus decongestant in the form of the hydrochloride salt.

phenylpyruvic acid (ˌfeenilpie'roovik) an intermediate product of the metabolism of phenylalanine in the body.

phenyltoloxamine (ˌfeeniltә'loksәmeen) an antihistaminic.

phenytoin (ˌfeni'toh·in) an anticonvulsant used in the treatment of tonic-clonic and psychomotor seizures. It is also used for the control of cardiac arrhythmias, especially those caused by digitalis intoxication. Formerly called diphenylhydantoin.

pheresis (fә'reesis) any procedure in which blood is withdrawn from a donor, a portion (plasma, leukocytes, etc.) is separated and retained, and the remainder is retransfused into the donor. It includes plasmapheresis, leukapheresis, etc.

pheromone ('ferәˌmohn) a substance secreted to the outside of the body and perceived (as by smell) by other individuals of the same species, releasing specific behaviour in the percipient.

PHI Public Health Inspector.

phial ('fieәl) a small glass container or bottle for drugs.

Philadelphia (Ph^1) chromosome (filә'delfiә) see Philadelphia CHROMOSOME.

-philia word element. [Gr.] *affinity for*, *morbid fondness of*. adj. **-philic.**

philtrum ('filtrәm) the vertical groove in the median portion of the upper lip.

phimosis (fie'mohsis) constriction of the orifice of the prepuce so that it cannot be drawn back over the glans. adj. **phimotic.**

pHisoHex ('fiesohˌheks) trademark for an emulsion containing chlorhexidine; used as a skin cleanser.

phleb(o)- word element. [Gr.] *vein.*

phlebangioma (ˌflebanji'ohmә) a venous aneurysm.

phlebarteriectasia (ˌflebahtiә·ri·ek'tayzi·ә) general dilation of veins and arteries.

phlebectasia (ˌflebek'tayzi·ә) dilation of a vein or veins; a varicosity.

phlebectomy (fli'bektәmee) excision of a vein, or a segment of a vein.

phlebemphraxis (ˌflebem'fraksis) stoppage of a vein

by a plug or clot.

phlebismus (fli'bizməs) obstruction and consequent turgescence of veins.

phlebitis (fli'bietis) inflammation of a vein. adj. **phlebitic.** It is relatively common, especially in the veins of the lower limbs.

Phlebitis is not serious when the inflammation is located in a superficial vein since these veins are numerous enough to permit the flow of blood to be rechannelled, so that the inflamed vein is bypassed. Phlebitis in a deep vein can be a cause of THROMBOSIS and EMBOLISM. It can also have serious consequences if it occurs in certain areas such as the veins of the cranium, where it may lead to cerebral abscess.

CAUSES. The causes of phlebitis are uncertain although it is thought to be one of the rheumatoid conditions. The disease sometimes occurs for no apparent reason; at other times, it seems to follow a variety of other disorders—for example, circulatory difficulties, blood disorders, and obesity. Phlebitis may be a complication of pneumonia, typhoid fever, or other general infections, and may occur in those taking oestrogens. It may also result from injury to a vein, either after an accident or occasionally as an aftermath of surgery. Superficial phlebitis may be a harbinger of occult cancer.

Phlebitis may also develop when circulation is sluggish after long periods of staying in bed without proper exercising of the limbs and frequent changing of position.

SYMPTOMS AND TREATMENT. When phlebitis occurs in a superficial vein, there is usually pain and tenderness. This may be so slight at first that the tenderness is felt only when pressure is applied to the painful area. As the inflammation increases, the pain becomes more acute, especially during walking or other exercise.

The inflamed area swells and becomes red and warm. A tender cordlike mass may form under the skin; it may grow smaller as the condition subsides, but occasionally lasts for some time.

When the inflammation occurs in a deep vein and affects the vein's inner lining, there may be formation of a thrombus on the vein wall. This condition is known as thrombophlebitis. When clots in the veins interfere with the normal flow of blood, fluid accumulates and causes oedema.

If phlebitis is superficial, the patient usually does not have to be confined to bed. Frequently, a supportive elastic dressing is used until the vein is healed.

When deeper veins are affected, however, or if the inflammation is severe, bed rest is required to prevent any clot that may have formed from being dislodged. Antibiotics are sometimes prescribed to combat infection. Anticoagulants are used and the extremity is elevated to prevent further clots or propagation of the existing clot. In some extreme cases, or when an embolism is likely to occur, surgery may be necessary as a preventive measure.

In persons prone to thrombophlebitis, anticoagulation is used as a preventive measure, particularly when long periods of bed rest are required, such as after surgery.

phleboclysis (fli'boklisis) injection of fluid into a vein; venoclysis (see also INTRAVENOUS INFUSION).

phlebogram ('flebə,gram) 1. a radiogram of a vein filled with contrast medium. 2. a phlebographic or sphygmographic tracing of the venous pulse.

phlebograph ('flebə,grahf, -,graf) an instrument for recording the venous pulse.

phlebography (fli'bogrəfee) 1. radiography of a vein filled with contrast medium. 2. the graphic recording of the venous pulse. 3. a description of the veins.

phlebolith ('fleboh,lith) a venous calculus or concretion.

phlebolithiasis (,flebohli'thieəsis) the development of phleboliths.

phlebomanometer (,flebohmə'nomitə) an instrument for the direct measurement of venous blood pressure.

phlebophlebostomy (,flebohfli'bostəmee) anastomosis of one vein to another, as of the portal vein and inferior vena cava.

phleboplasty ('fleboh,plastee) plastic repair of a vein.

phleborrhaphy (fli'bo·rəfee) suture of a vein.

phleborrhexis (,flebə'reksis) rupture of a vein.

phlebosclerosis (,flebohsklə'rohsis) fibrous thickening of the walls of veins.

phlebostasis (fli'bostəsis) 1. retardation of blood flow in veins. 2. temporary sequestration of a portion of blood from the general circulation by compressing the veins of an extremity.

phlebothrombosis (,flebohthrom'bohsis) the development of venous thrombi in the absence of associated inflammation of the vessel wall, as opposed to thrombophlebitis, in which there are inflammatory changes in the vessel wall.

Phlebotomus (flə'botəməs) a genus of biting flies, called sandflies, the females of which are blood sucking. They are vectors of various diseases, including kala-azar (*P. argentipes*, *P. chinensis*, *P. martini*, *P. perniciosus*), Carrión's disease (*P. noguchi*, *P. verrucarum*), cutaneous leishmaniasis (*P. sergenti*), and phlebotomus fever (*P. papatasii*).

phlebotomus fever (flə'botəməs) a febrile viral disease of short duration, transmitted by the sandfly *Phlebotomus papatasii*, with dengue-like symptoms, occurring in Mediterranean and Middle East countries. Called also *sandfly fever*.

phlebotomy (fli'botəmee) venesection.

phlegm (flem) viscid mucus excreted in abnormally large quantities from the respiratory tract.

phlegmasia (fleg'mayzi·ə) inflammation.

p. alba dolens phlebitis of the femoral vein, with swelling of the leg, usually without redness, occasionally following parturition or an acute febrile illness. Called also white leg, or *milk* LEG.

p. alba dolens puerperarum phlebitis of the femoral vein in puerperal women, known as 'painful white leg'.

p. cerulea dolens an acute fulminating form of deep venous thrombosis, with pronounced oedema and severe cyanosis of the extremity.

phlegmatic (fleg'matik) of dull and sluggish temperament.

phlegmon ('flegmon) diffuse inflammation of the soft or connective tissue due to infection. adj. **phlegmonous.**

phlog(o)- word element. [Gr.] *inflammation.*

phlogogenic (,flohgə'jenik) producing inflammation.

phlyctena, phlycten (flik'teenə; 'fliktən) 1. a small blister caused by a burn. 2. a small inflammatory nodule containing lymph occurring on the conjunctiva or cornea of the eye in certain conditions such as tuberculosis. adj. **phlyctenar.**

phlyctenoid ('fliktə,noyd) resembling a phlyctena.

phlyctenular (flik'tenyuhlə) associated with the formation of phlyctenules, or of vesicle-like prominences.

phlyctenule ('fliktən,yool) a minute vesicle; an ulcerated nodule of the cornea or conjunctiva.

phlyctenulosis (flik,tenyuh'lohsis) a condition marked by formation of phlyctenules.

phobia (fohbi·ə) any persistent abnormal dread or fear that appears to result from repressed inner conflicts of which the affected person is not aware. Used as a word ending designating abnormal or morbid fear of or aversion to the subject indicated by the stem to which it is affixed. adj. **phobic**.

A person with a phobia reacts uncontrollably and unreasonably to the situation of which he is afraid. A wide variety of exaggerated fears can exist in neurotic persons (see also NEUROSIS).

Some typical phobias are: acrophobia—fear of heights; agoraphobia—fear of open or public places; astraphobia—fear of lightning; cenotophobia—morbid fear of new things or new ideas; claustrophobia—morbid fear of closed places; haemophobia—fear of blood; xenophobia—morbid dread of strangers.

phobophobia (ˌfohboh'fohbi·ə) morbid fear of being afraid.

phocomelia (ˌfohkə'meeli·ə) congenital absence of the proximal portion of a limb or limbs, the hands or feet being attached to the trunk by a small, irregularly shaped bone. adj. **phocomelic**.

phocomelus (foh'koməlәs) an individual exhibiting phocomelia.

pholcodine ('folkohˌdeen) a linctus for the suppression of a dry or painful cough.

phon(o)- word element. [Gr.] *sound, voice, speech.*

phonal ('fohnəl) pertaining to the voice.

phonasthenia (ˌfohnəs'theeni·ə) weakness of the voice; difficult phonation from fatigue.

phonation (foh'nayshən) the utterance of vocal sounds.

phonatory (ˌfohnətə·ree) subserving or pertaining to phonation.

phoneme ('fohneem) the smallest distinct unit of sound in speech; the basic unit of spoken language.

phonendoscope (foh'nendəˌskohp) a stethoscopic device that intensifies auscultatory sounds.

phonetic (fə'netik) pertaining to the voice or to articulate sounds.

phonetics (fə'netiks) the science of vocal sounds.

phoniatrics (ˌfohni'atriks) the treatment of speech defects.

phonic ('fohnik, 'fonik) pertaining to the voice.

phonism ('fohnizəm) a sensation of hearing produced by the effect of something seen, felt, tasted, smelled, or thought of.

phonoangiography (ˌfohnohˌanji'ogrəfee) the recording and analysis of arterial bruits to estimate the extent of arterial stenosis.

phonocardiogram (ˌfohnoh'kahdiohˌgram) the record produced by phonocardiography.

phonocardiograph (ˌfohnoh'kahdiohˌgrahf, -graf) the instrument used in phonocardiography.

phonocardiography (ˌfohnohˌkahdi'ogrəfee) the graphic recording of heart sounds and murmurs; by extension, the term includes pulse tracings (carotid, apex, and venous pulse). adj. **phonocardiographic**.

Phonocardiography involves picking up, through a highly sensitive microphone, sonic vibrations from the heart which are then converted into electrical energy and fed into a galvanometer, where they are recorded on paper. The procedure is most useful when there is evidence of heart murmurs or unusual heart sounds, such as gallops, that are difficult to discern by the human ear.

phonocatheter (ˌfohnoh'kathitə) a catheter with a device in its tip for picking up and transmitting sound.

phonogram ('fohnəˌgram) a graphic record of a sound.

phonology (fə'noləjee) the study of speech sounds, their production and the relationship between sounds as elements of language.

phonomassage (ˌfohnoh'masahzh, -sahj) the treatment of ear disease by an apparatus which carries a more or less musical vibration into the auditory canal, stimulating the ossicles.

phonometer (foh'nomitə) a device for measuring the intensity of sounds.

phonomyoclonus (ˌfohnoh'mieoh'klohnəs) myoclonus in which a sound is heard on auscultation of an affected muscle, indicating fibrillar contractions.

phonomyogram (ˌfohnoh'mieəˌgram) a record produced by phonomyography.

phonomyography (ˌfohnohmie'ogrəfee) the recording of sounds produced by muscle contraction.

phonopathy (foh'nopəthee) any disease of the organs of speech.

phonophobia (ˌfohnoh'fohbi·ə) morbid dread of sounds or of speaking aloud.

phonophotography (ˌfohnohfə'togrəfee) photographic recording of the movements of a diaphragm set up by sound waves.

phonopneumomassage (ˌfohnohˌnyoomoh'masahzh, -sahj) air massage of the middle ear.

phonopsia (foh'nopsi·ə) a visual sensation caused by the hearing of sounds.

phonoreceptor (ˌfohnohri'septə) a receptor for sound stimuli.

phonorenogram (ˌfohnoh'reenəˌgram) a record of the sounds produced by pulsation of the renal artery obtained by a phonocatheter passed through a ureter into the renal pelvis.

phonostethograph (ˌfohnoh'stethəˌgrahf, -ˌgraf) an instrument by which chest sounds are amplified, filtered, and recorded.

-phore word element. [Gr.] *a carrier.*

-phoresis word element. [Gr.] *transmission.*

phoria ('for·ri·ə) any tendency to deviation of the eyes from the normal when fusional stimuli are absent or fusion is otherwise prevented; a latent or usually unmanifested tropia. See also HETEROPHORIA.

phorometer (fə'romitə) an instrument for measuring heterophoria, and more generally the relative strength of the ocular muscles.

phose (fohz) a subjective visual sensation, as of light or colour.

phosgene ('fozjeen, 'fos-) a suffocating and highly poisonous war gas, carbonyl chloride, $COCl_2$.

phosphataemia (ˌfosfə'teemi·ə) an excess of phosphates in the blood.

phosphatase ('fosfəˌtayz) any of a group of enzymes capable of catalysing the hydrolysis of esterified phosphoric acid, with liberation of inorganic phosphate, found in practically all tissues, body fluids, and cells, including erythrocytes and leukocytes.

acid p. a type showing optimal activity at a pH between 3 and 6; found in erythrocytes, prostatic tissue, spleen, kidney, and other tissues.

alkaline p. a type showing optimal activity at a pH of about 9.3; found in bone, liver, kidney, leukocytes, adrenal cortex, and other tissues.

phosphate ('fosfayt) any salt or ester of phosphoric acid. adj. **phosphatic**.

Phosphates are widely distributed in the body, the largest amounts being in the bones and teeth. They are continually excreted in the urine and faeces, and must be replaced in the diet. Inorganic phosphates function as buffer salts to maintain the ACID–BASE BALANCE in blood, saliva, urine, and other body fluids. The principal phosphates in this buffer system are monosodium and disodium phosphate. Organic phosphates, in particular adenosine triphosphate (ATP), take part in a series of reversible reactions involving phosphoric acid, lactic acid, glycogen, and other substances, which furnish the energy expended in muscle contraction. This is thought to occur through the hydrolysis of the so-called high-energy phosphate bond present in ATP, phosphocreatine, and certain other body compounds.

phosphaturia (ˌfosfə'tyooə·ri·ə) an excess of phosphates in the urine.

phosphene ('fosfeen) an objective visual sensation that occurs with the eyes closed, and in the absence of retinal stimulation by visible light.

phosphoamidase (ˌfosfoh'amidayz) an enzyme that catalyses the conversion of phosphocreatine to creatine and orthophosphate.

phosphocreatine (ˌfosfoh'kreeəˌteen, -tin) a compound of creatine and phosphoric acid occurring in muscle, being the most important storage form of high-energy phosphate, the energy source in muscle contraction.

phosphofructokinase (ˌfosfohˌfruhktoh'kienayz) an enzyme of the glycolytic (Embden–Meyerhof) pathway that catalyses the conversion of fructose-6-phosphate to fructose-1,6-bisphosphate.

phosphoglyceride (ˌfosfə'glisəˌried) a class of phospholipids, including lecithin and cephalin, consisting of a glycerol backbone, two fatty acids, and a phosphorylated alcohol, e.g., choline, ethanolamine, serine, or inositol. They are a major component of cell membranes.

phosphokinase (ˌfosfə'kienayz) kinase.

phospholipase (ˌfosfə'lipayz) any of four enzymes (phospholipase A to D) which catalyse the hydrolysis of a phospholipid.

phospholipid (ˌfosfə'lipid) any lipid that contains phosphorus, including those with a glycerol backbone (phosphoglycerides and plasmalogens) or a backbone of sphingosine or a related substance (sphingomyelins). They are the major lipids in cell membranes.

phosphonecrosis (ˌfosfənə'krohsis) necrosis of the jaw bone due to exposure to phosphorus; called also phossy jaw.

phosphoprotein (ˌfosfə'prohteen) a conjugated protein in which phosphoric acid is esterified with a hydroxy amino acid.

phosphorated ('fosfəˌraytid) charged or combined with phosphorus.

phosphorescence (ˌfosfə'res'ns) the emission of light without appreciable heat; it is characterized by the emission of absorbed light after a delay and at a considerably longer wavelength than that of the absorbed light. adj. **phosphorescent.**

phosphoribulokinase (ˌfosfəˌriebyooloh'kienayz) an enzyme that catalyses the conversion of ATP and D-ribulose-5-phosphate to ADP and D-ribulose-1,5-diphosphate.

phosphoric acid (fos'fo·rik) a crystalline acid formed by oxidation of phosphorus; its salts are called phosphates.

phosphorism ('fosfəˌrizəm) chronic PHOSPHORUS poisoning.

phosphorolysis (ˌfosfə'rolisis) cleavage of a chemical bond with simultaneous addition of the elements of phosphoric acid to the residues.

phosphorus ('fosfə·rəs) a chemical element, atomic number 15, atomic weight 30.974, symbol P. (See table of elements in Appendix 2.) Phosphorus is an essential element in the diet. In the form of phosphates it is a major component of the mineral phase of bone and is involved in almost all metabolic processes. It also plays an important role in cell metabolism. It is obtained by the body from milk products, cereals, meat, and fish, and its use by the body is controlled by vitamin D and calcium.

Phosphorus is very inflammable and exceedingly poisonous. Inhalation of its vapour by workers in chemical industries may cause necrosis of the mandible (phosphonecrosis or phossy jaw). Free phosphorus causes fatty degeneration of the liver and other viscera. adj. **phosphorous.**

p.-32 a radioisotope of phosphorus having a half-life of 14.3 days and emitting only beta rays; used in the form of sodium [^{32}P] phosphate for treatment of polycythaemia vera, chronic myelocytic leukaemia, and chronic lymphocytic leukaemia. Symbol ^{32}P.

phosphorylase (fos'fo·riˌlayz) an enzyme that, in the presence of inorganic phosphate, catalyses the conversion of glycogen into glucose-1-phosphate.

phosphorylation (fosˌfo·ri'layshən) the process of introducing a phosphate group into an organic molecule.

oxidative p. the final common pathway of aerobic energy metabolism in which high-energy phosphate bonds are formed by phosphorylation of ADP to ATP coupled with the transfer of electrons along a chain of carrier proteins with molecular oxygen as the final acceptor. It occurs in mitochondria.

phosphotransacetylase (ˌfosfohˌtranzə'setiˌlayz) an enzyme which catalyses the transfer of an acetyl group between acetylphosphate and acetylcoenzyme A.

phosphotransferase (ˌfosfoh'transfəˌrayz, -'trahn) any of a class of enzymes that catalyse the transfer of a phosphate group.

phot(o)- word element. [Gr.] *light.*

photalgia (foh'talji·ə) pain, as in the eye, caused by light.

photic ('fohtik) pertaining to light.

photism ('fohtizəm) a visual sensation produced by the effect of something heard, felt, tasted, smelled, or thought of.

photoactive (ˌfohtoh'aktiv) reacting chemically to sunlight or ultraviolet radiation.

photobiology (ˌfohtohbie'oləjee) the branch of biology dealing with the effect of light on organisms. adj. **photobiological.**

photobiotic (ˌfohtohbie'otik) living only in the light.

photocatalysis (ˌfohtohkə'talisis) promotion or stimulation of a chemical reaction by light. adj. **photocatalytic.**

photocatalyst (ˌfohtoh'katəlist) a substance, e.g., chlorophyll, that brings about a chemical reaction on exposure to light.

photochemistry (ˌfohtoh'kemistree) the branch of chemistry that deals with the chemical properties or effects of light rays or other radiation. adj. **photochemical.**

photochemotherapy (ˌfohtohˌkeemoh'therəpee, -ˌkem-) treatment by means of drugs (e.g., methoxsalen) that react to ultraviolet radiation or sunlight. Used in the treatment of psoriasis.

photochromogen (ˌfohtoh'krohməjən) a microorganism whose pigmentation develops as a result of exposure to light. adj. **photochromogenic.**

photocoagulation (ˌfohtohkohˌagyuh'layshən) destruction of intraocular tissue by the use of an intense burn of light (e.g., xenon arc; krypton laser; argon laser; and ruby laser). Used in the treatment of certain forms of glaucoma, destruction of abnormal blood vessels, and prevention of retinal detachment.

photoconvulsive (ˌfohtohkən'vulsiv) photoparoxysmal.

photodermatitis, photodermatosis (ˌfohtohˌdərmə'tietis; ˌfohtohˌdərmə'tohsis) an abnormal state of the skin in which light is an important causative factor.

photodynia (ˌfohtoh'dini·ə) photalgia.

photofluorography (ˌfohtohflooə'rogrəfee) fluorography.

photogenic (ˌfohtoh'jenik) 1. produced by light. 2. emitting or producing light.

photokinetic (ˌfohtohki'netik) moving in response to the stimulus of light.

photolysis (foh'tolisis) chemical decomposition by

light. adj. **photolytic**.

photolyte ('fohtoh,liet) a substance decomposed by light.

photometer (foh'tomitə) a device for measuring the intensity of light.

photometry (foh'tomətree) measurement of the intensity of light.

photomicrograph (,fohtoh'miekrə,grahf, -,graf) a photograph of an object as seen through an ordinary light microscope.

photomyoclonic (,fohtoh,mieoh'klonik) photomyogenic.

photomyogenic (,fohtoh,mieoh'jenik) photomyoclonic; denoting an electroencephalographic response to photic stimulation (brief flashes of light) marked by myoclonus of the facial muscles.

photon ('fohton) a particle (quantum) of radiant energy.

photo-onycholysis (,fohtoh,oni'kolisis) onycholysis resulting from exposure to sunlight or ultraviolet rays, as after treatment with tetracyclines or methoxypsoralen.

photo-ophthalmia (,fohtoh·of'thalmi·ə) ophthalmia caused by exposure to intense light, as in snow blindness.

photoparoxysmal (,fohtoh,parok'sizməl) photoconvulsive; denoting an abnormal electroencephalographic response to photic stimulation (brief flashes of light), marked by diffuse paroxysmal discharge recorded as spike-wave complexes; the response may be accompanied by minor seizures.

photoperceptive (,fohtohpə'septiv) able to perceive light.

photoperiod (,fohtoh'piə·ri·əd) the period of time per day that an organism is exposed to daylight (or to artificial light). adj. **photoperiodic**.

photoperiodism (,fohtoh'piə·ri·ə,dizəm) the physiological and behavioural reactions brought about in organisms by changes in the duration of daylight and darkness.

photophilic (,fohtoh'filik) thriving in light.

photophobia (,fohtoh'fohbi·ə) abnormal visual intolerance to light. adj. **photophobic**.

photophthalmia (,fohtof'thalmi·ə) photo-ophthalmia.

photopia (foh'tohpi·ə) day vision. adj. **photopic**.

photopsia (foh'topsi·ə) an appearance as of sparks or flashes, in retinal irritation.

photoptarmosis (,fohtoptah'mohsis) sneezing caused by the influence of light.

photoptometer (,fohtop'tomitə) an instrument for measuring visual acuity by determining the smallest amount of light that will render an object just visible.

photoreactivation (,fohtohri,akti'vayshən) reversal of the biological effects of ultraviolet radiation on cells by subsequent exposure to visible light.

photoreceptive (,fohtohri'septiv) sensitive to stimulation by light.

photoreceptor (,fohtohri'septə) a nerve end-organ or receptor sensitive to light.

photoretinitis (,fohtoh,reti'nietis) retinitis due to exposure to intense light.

photosensitive (,fohtoh'sensitiv) exhibiting abnormally heightened sensitivity to sunlight.

photosensitization (,fohtoh,sensitie'zayshən) the development of abnormally heightened reactivity of the skin to sunlight. The reaction can be caused by a wide variety of drugs and chemicals.

Phototoxic reactions occur when the photosensitizing drug absorbs ultraviolet light from the sun and a sunburn-like response occurs in a very short period of time. Within hours there is a burning sensation of the exposed skin, followed by redness and swelling. Within a day or two the skin becomes heavily pigmented and begins to peel; a severe reaction can cause scarring. Phototoxic reactions are more likely to occur in light-skinned persons than in those with darkly pigmented skin that can block harmful radiation.

Photoallergic reactions occur after an initial exposure to the drug or chemical which triggers the production of antibodies. On second exposure a skin eruption appears and there may be intense itching. It is possible for the eruption to appear on unexposed areas of skin as well as exposed areas.

There is a long list of drugs that can cause photosensitization reactions. Antineoplastics, antibiotics, diuretics, hypoglycaemic agents, and even antihistamines are capable of triggering photosensitivity reactions in certain individuals.

photostable ('fohtoh,stayb'l) unchanged by the influence of light.

photosynthesis (,fohtoh'sinthəsis) a chemical combination caused by the action of light; specifically the formation of carbohydrates from carbon dioxide and water in the chlorophyll tissue of plants under the influence of light. adj. **photosynthetic**.

phototaxis (,fohtoh'taksis) the movement of cells and microorganisms under the influence of light. adj. **phototactic**.

phototherapy (,fohtoh'therəpee) treatment of disease by exposure to light as, for example, bilirubinaemia in the newborn.

phototoxic (,fohtoh'toksik) having a toxic effect triggered by exposure to light.

phototrophic (,fohtoh'trofik) capable of deriving energy from light.

phototropism (fohtoh'tropizəm) 1. the tendency of an organism to turn or move toward (positive phototropism) or away from (negative phototropism) light. 2. change of colour produced in a substance by the action of light. adj. **phototropic**.

photuria (foh'tyooə·ri·ə) excretion of urine having a luminous appearance.

phren(o)- word element. [Gr.] 1. *diaphragm*. 2. *mind*.

phrenalgia (frə'nalji·ə) pain in the diaphragm.

phrenemphraxis, phrenicotripsy (,frenem'fraksis; ,frenikoh'tripsee) surgical crushing of the phrenic nerve.

phrenetic (frə'netik) maniacal.

phrenic ('frenik) pertaining to the diaphragm or to the mind.

p. nerve a major branch of the cervical plexus. It extends through the thorax to provide innervation of the diaphragm. Nerve impulses from the inspiratory centre in the brain travel down the phrenic nerve, causing contraction of the diaphragm, and inspiration occurs.

phrenicectomy (,freni'sektəmee) resection of the phrenic nerve.

phrenicoexeresis (,frenikoh·ek'serisis) avulsion of the phrenic nerve.

phrenicotomy (,freni'kotəmee) surgical division of the phrenic nerve.

phrenitis (frə'nietis) 1. delirium or frenzy. 2. diaphragmitis.

phrenocolic (,frenoh'kolik) pertaining to the diaphragm and colon.

phrenogastric (,frenoh'gastrik) pertaining to the diaphragm and stomach.

phrenohepatic (,frenoh·hi'patik) pertaining to the diaphragm and liver.

phrenoplegia (,frenoh'pleeji·ə) paralysis of the diaphragm.

phrenosin ('frenohsin) a cerebroside containing cerebronic acid attached to the sphingosine.

phrynoderma (ˌfrinəˈdərmə) a follicular hyperkeratosis probably due to deficiency of vitamin A or of essential fatty acids.

phthalylsulphathiazole (ˌthalilsulfəˈthieəˌzohl) an insoluble sulphonamide, poorly absorbed in the intestine. It was thus used to kill intestinal bacteria prior to surgery, before the introduction of METRONIDAZOLE.

phthalylsulphonazole (ˌthalilsulˈfonəˌzohl) a sulphonamide.

phthiriasis (thiˈrieəsis) infestation with lice of the species *Pthirus pubis*, the crab louse, which is most often found in the pubic hairs but sometimes involves other hairy areas of the body, such as the eyelashes, chest hair, axillae, beard and leg hair. Crab lice are usually transmitted sexually but may be passed on in any intimate contact.

Phthirus (ˈthirəs) a genus of lice.

P. pubis the pubic, or crab, LOUSE, a species of louse that infests the pubic hair and sometimes other hairy areas of the body.

phthisis (ˈthiesis) 1. a wasting of the body. 2. tuberculosis.

p. bulbi shrinkage of the eyeball.

grinder's p. a combination of tuberculosis and pneumoconiosis occurring in grinders in the cutlery trade.

miner's p. pneumoconiosis of coal workers.

phyco- word element. [Gr.] *seaweed, algae.*

phycology (fieˈkoləjee) the scientific study of algae.

Phycomycetes (ˌfiekohmieˈseeteez) a group of fungi comprising the common water, leaf, and bread moulds.

phycomycosis (ˌfiekohmieˈkohsis) any of a group of acute fungal diseases caused by members of the Phycomycetes.

Phyllocontin Continus (ˌfielohˈkontin ˈkontinəs) trademark for a preparation of aminophylline.

phylogeny (fieˈlojənee) the complete developmental history of a race or group of organisms. adj. **phylogenetic, phylogenic.**

phylum (ˈfieləm) pl. *phyla* [L., Gr.] a primary division of the plant or animal kingdom, including organisms that are assumed to have a common ancestry.

phyma (ˈfiemə) pl. *phymata* [Gr.] a skin tumour or tubercle.

Physeptone (fieˈseptohn) trademark for preparations of methadone.

physic (ˈfizik) 1. the art of medicine and therapeutics. 2. a medicine, especially a cathartic.

physical (ˈfizikˈl) pertaining to the body, to material things, or to physics.

p. examination examination of the bodily state of a patient by ordinary physical means, as inspection, palpation, percussion, and auscultation.

physician (fiˈzishən) a DOCTOR who practises medicine as distinct from surgery.

community p. a doctor who practises community MEDICINE.

consultant p. senior doctor in overall charge of patients under his/her care and responsible for directing junior medical staff.

house p. a junior doctor, resident in hospital whilst on duty acting under the orders of a consultant physician.

physicochemical (ˌfizikohˈkemikˈl) pertaining to both physics and chemistry.

physics (ˈfiziks) the study of the laws and phenomena of nature, especially of forces and general properties of matter and energy.

physio- word element. [Gr.] *nature, physiology, physical.*

physiochemical (ˌfiziohˈkemikˈl) pertaining to both physiology and chemistry.

physiognomy (ˌfiziˈonəmee) 1. the determination of mental or moral character and qualities by the face. 2. the countenance, or face. 3. the facial expression and appearance as a means of diagnosis.

physiological (ˌfizi·əˈlojikˈl) pertaining to physiology; normal; not pathological.

physiologist (ˌfiziˈoləjist) a specialist in physiology.

physiology (ˌfiziˈoləjee) 1. the science which treats of the functions of the living organism and its parts, and of the physical and chemical factors and processes involved. 2. the basic processes underlying the functioning of a species or class of organism, or any of its parts or processes.

cell p. the scientific study of phenomena involved in cell growth and maintenance, self-regulation and division of cells, interactions between nucleus and cytoplasm, and general behaviour of protoplasm.

morbid p., pathological p. the study of disordered functions or of function in diseased tissues.

physiopathological (ˌfiziohˌpathəˈlojikˈl) pertaining to pathological physiology.

physiotherapist (ˌfiziohˈtherəpist) a professionally trained person skilled in the techniques of rehabilitation. Physiotherapists train at a School of Physiotherapy attached either to a Teaching Hospital or a College of Higher Education. The course lasts 3–4 years, leading to a Diploma or Degree in Physiotherapy. Minimum entry requirements of two A levels are necessary. Further information is available from the Chartered Society of Physiotherapy, 14 Bedford Row, London WC1R 4ED.

Physiotherapy aides have no special training, but work under the direct supervision of a trained physiotherapist. They do not give patients treatment, but aid the physiotherapist as required.

physiotherapy (ˌfiziohˈtherəpee) the use of physical means for the treatment and prevention of injury and disease, for the restoration of function including the ability to perform the activities of daily living, and to assist in rehabilitation. Methods used include exercise, massage, mobilization and manipulation, hydrotherapy and electrical stimulation.

physique (fiˈzeek) the body organization, development, and structure.

physo- word element. [Gr.] *air, gas.*

physohaematometra (ˌfiesohˌheemətohˈmetrə) gas and blood in the uterine cavity.

physohydrometra (ˌfiesohˌhiedrohˈmeetrə) gas and serum in the uterine cavity.

physometra (ˌfiesohˈmeetrə) gas in the uterine cavity.

physopyosalpinx (ˌfiesohˌpieohˈsalpingks) gas and pus in the oviduct.

physostigmine (ˌfiesohˈstigmeen) an alkaloid usually obtained from the dried seed of *Physostigma venenosum;* used as a topical miotic in the form of the base and of the salicylate and sulphate salts. Now only very rarely used.

phyt(o)- word element. [Gr.] *plant, an organism of the vegetable kingdom.*

phytoagglutinin (ˌfietoh·əˈglootinin) an agglutinin of plant origin.

phytobezoar (ˌfietohˈbeezor) a bezoar composed of vegetable fibres.

phytogenous (fieˈtojənəs) derived from plants, or caused by a vegetable growth.

phytohaemagglutinin (ˌfietohˌheeməˈglootinin) a haemagglutinin of plant origin; abbreviated PHA.

phytoid (ˈfietoyd) resembling a plant.

phytomenadione (ˌfietohˌmenəˈdieohn) an intravenous preparation of vitamin K, effective in treating haemorrhage occurring during anticoagulant therapy, and due to vitamin K deficiency.

phytoparasite (ˌfietohˈparəˌsiet) any parasitic vegetable organism.

phytophotodermatitis (ˌfietohˌfohtohˌdərmə'tietis) phototoxic dermatitis due to contact with certain plants and subsequent exposure to sunlight.

phytoprecipitin (ˌfietohpri'sipitin) a precipitin formed in response to vegetable antigen.

phytosis (fie'tohsis) any disease caused by a phytoparasite.

phytosterol (ˌfietoh'stiə·rol) a sterol of vegetable origin.

phytotoxic (ˌfietoh'toksik) 1. pertaining to phytotoxin. 2. poisonous to plants.

phytotoxin (ˌfietoh'toksin) an exotoxin produced by certain species of higher plants; any toxin of plant origin.

pia-arachnitis (ˌpieəˌarək'nietis) leptomeningitis; inflammation of the leptomeninges, or pia mater and arachnoid.

pia-arachnoid (ˌpieə·ə'raknoyd) the pia mater and arachnoid considered together as one functional unit; the leptomeninges.

pia mater (ˌpieə 'maytə) [L.] the innermost of the three meninges covering the brain and spinal cord.

pial ('pieəl) pertaining to the pia mater.

piarachnitis (ˌpieə·rak'nietis) leptomeningitis; pia-arachnitis.

piarachnoid (ˌpieə'raknoyd) pia-arachnoid.

pica ('piekə) craving for unnatural articles of food such as dirt, sometimes seen during pregnancy and in mentally handicapped children.

Pick's cells (piks) round, oval, or polyhedral cells with foamy, lipid-containing cytoplasm, found in the bone marrow and spleen in Niemann–Pick disease.

Pick's disease a form of presenile brain failure (dementia) with an age of onset between 50 and 60. There is shrinkage of the brain and loss of cortical cells.

pickwickian syndrome (pik'wiki·ən) the specific association of extreme obesity, hypersomnia, polycythaemia, chronic alveolar hypoventilation, and excessive appetite; named after a character, Fat Joe, in Charles Dickens' *Pickwick Papers.* Respiratory problems are caused by the increased work of ventilation in moving the ponderous thorax and abdomen.

pico- a word element used in naming units of measurement to designate a quantity 10^{-12} (one trillionth) times the unit to which it is joined. Symbol p.

picogram ('piekohˌgram) one trillionth (10^{-12}) gram. Abbreviated pg.

Picolax ('pikəlaks, 'pie-) trademark for a combination preparation of sodium picosulphate and magnesium citrate, a laxative.

picometre ('piekohˌmeetə) a unit of length, 10^{-12} metre. Abbreviated pm.

picornavirus (pie'kawnəˌvierəs) an extremely small, ether-resistant RNA virus, one of the group comprising the enteroviruses and the rhinoviruses.

picric acid ('pikrik) a substance used as dye, tissue fixative, antiseptic, astringent, and stimulant of epithelialization; it can be detonated on percussion or by heating above 300 °C. Called also trinitrophenol.

picrocarmine (ˌpikroh'kahmeen) a histological stain consisting of a mixture of carmine, ammonia, distilled water, and aqueous solution of picric acid.

pie chart (pie chaht) a circular diagram divided into segments showing the proportional distribution of observations of particular events.

piebaldism ('piebawldizəm) a condition in which the skin is partly brown and partly white, as in partial albuminism and vitiligo.

piedra (pie'aydrə) a fungal disease of the hair in which white or black nodules of fungi form on the shafts.

Pierre Robin syndrome (peeˌair ro'banh) micrognathia occurring in association with cleft palate, glossoptosis, and absent gag reflex.

piesaesthesia (pieˌeezis'theezi·ə) the sense by which pressure stimuli are felt.

piesimeter (ˌpiei'zimitə) an instrument for testing the sensitiveness of the skin to pressure.

-piesis word element. [Gr.] *pressure.* adj. **-piesic.**

pigeon chest ('pijən) prominence of the sternum and rib cartilage; called also PECTUS CARINATUM, chicken or pigeon breast.

pigeon toe a foot condition in which the toes turn inward; called also pes varus. Severe cases are considered a form of CLUBFOOT.

pigment ('pigmənt) 1. any colouring matter of the body. 2. a stain or dyestuff. 3. a paintlike medicinal preparation applied to the skin. adj. **pigmentary.**

bile p. any one of the colouring matters of the bile, derived from haem, including bilirubin, biliverdin, etc.

blood p. any one of the pigments derived from haemoglobin, including haem, haematoidin, etc.

respiratory p's substances, e.g., haemoglobin, myoglobin, or cytochromes, which take part in the oxidative processes of the animal body.

pigmentation (ˌpigmen'tayshən) the deposition of colouring matter; the coloration or discoloration of a part by a pigment.

haematogenous p. pigmentation produced by accumulation of haemoglobin derivatives, such as haematoidin or haemosiderin.

pigmented ('pigmentid) coloured by deposit of pigment.

pigmentolysin (ˌpigmen'tolisin) a lysin that destroys pigment.

pigmentophage (pig'mentohˌfayj) any pigment-destroying cell, especially such a cell of the hair.

piitis (pie'ietis) inflammation of the pia mater.

pilar, pilary ('pielə; 'pilə·ree) pertaining to the hair.

pile (piel) 1. a haemorrhoid. 2. in nucleonics, a chain-reacting fission device for producing slow neutrons and radioisotopes.

sentinel p. a haemorrhoid-like thickening of the mucous membrane at the lower end of an anal fissure.

piles (pielz) haemorrhoids.

pileus ('pieli·əs) caul.

pili ('pielie) plural of *pilus.*

pill (pil) a small globular or oval medicated mass to be swallowed; a tablet.

enteric-coated p. one enclosed in a substance that dissolves only when it has reached the intestines.

pillar ('pilə) a supporting column, usually occurring in pairs.

p's of the fauces folds of mucous membrane at the sides of the fauces.

pillion ('pilyən) a temporary artificial leg.

pilo- word element. [L.] *hair, composed of hair.*

pilocarpine (ˌpieloh'kahpeen) a cholinergic alkaloid from leaves of *Pilocarpus jaborandi* and *P. microphyllus*; used as an ophthalmic miotic in the form of its hydrochloride and nitrate salts.

pilocystic (ˌpieloh'sistik) hollow or cystlike, and containing hair; said of dermoid tumours.

piloerection (ˌpieloh·i'rekshən) erection of the hair.

pilomatrixoma (ˌpielohˌmaytrik'sohmə) a benign, circumscribed, calcifying epithelial neoplasm derived from hair matrix cells, manifested as a small firm intracutaneous spheroid mass, usually on the face, neck, or arms.

pilomotor (ˌpieloh'mohtə) causing movement of the hairs; pertaining to the arrector muscles, the contraction of which produces cutis anserina (goose flesh) and piloerection.

p. nerves the nerves supplying the arrector muscles of the hair.

pilonidal (ˌpieloh'nied'l) having a nest of hairs.

p. cyst an implantation dermoid in the natal cleft. The cyst results from penetration of hairs in the natal cleft through the skin of the fold thus causing a sinus (pilonidal sinus) and epithelial cell implantation. Prone to recurrent infection.

pilose ('pielohz) hairy; covered with hair.

pilosebaceous (ˌpielohsi'bayshəs) pertaining to the hair follicles and sebaceous glands.

pilosis (pie'lohsis) an abnormal growth of hair.

pilot study ('pielət 'studee) a preliminary study to test the feasibility of a larger study.

pilule ('pilyool) a small pill.

pilus ('pieləs) pl. *pili* [L.] 1. a hair. adj. **pilial**. 2. one of the minute filamentous appendages of certain bacteria associated with antigenic properties of the cell surface. adj. **piliate**.

p. cuniculatus pl. *pili cuniculati;* burrowing hair.

p. incarnatus pl. *pili incarnati;* ingrown hair.

p. tortus pl. *pili torti;* twisted hair.

pimelitis (ˌpimə'lietis) inflammation of the adipose tissue.

pimelopterygium (ˌpiməlohtə'riji·əm) a fatty outgrowth on the conjunctiva.

pimelosis (ˌpimə'lohsis) 1. conversion into fat. 2. obesity.

pimozide ('piməzied) an antipsychotic drug.

pimple ('pimp'l) a papule or pustule.

pin (pin) a slender, elongated piece of metal used for securing fixation of parts. **Denham's p.** a metal pin, with a thread in its centre part, which is inserted into a bone to allow the attachment of a weight by way of a stirrup to exert traction on the bone.

Steinmann p. a metal pin which is inserted into the bone to allow the attachment of a weight by way of a stirrup to exert traction on the bone. See also STEINMANN EXTENSION.

Pinard's stethoscope a metal trumpet-shaped instrument which can be placed on the abdomen over the fetal shoulders to hear the heart sounds. Called also *fetal* or *monoaural* stethoscope.

pincement ('pansmonh) [Fr.] pinching of the flesh in massage.

pineal ('pini·əl, 'pie-) 1. shaped like a pine cone. 2. pertaining to the pineal body.

p. body, p. gland a small, conical structure attached by a stalk to the posterior wall of the third ventricle of the cerebrum, believed by many to be an endocrine gland. In certain amphibians and reptiles the gland is thought to function as a light receptor. In most mammals, including man, it appears to be the major or unique site of melatonin biosynthesis. The effect of melatonin on the body and the exact function of the pineal body remain obscure.

pinealectomy (ˌpini·ə'lektəmee) excision of the pineal body.

pinealism ('pini·əˌlizəm) the condition due to deranged secretion of the pineal body.

pinealoblastoma (ˌpini·əlohbla'stohmə) pinealoma in which the pineal cells are not well differentiated.

pinealocyte ('pini·əlohˌsiet) an epithelioid cell of the pineal body.

pinealoma (ˌpini·ə'lohmə) a tumour of the pineal body composed of neoplastic nests of large epithelial cells; it may cause hydrocephalus, precocious puberty, and gait disturbances.

pinguecula (ping'gwekyuhlə) pl. *pingueculae* [L.] a small, benign, yellowish spot on the bulbar conjunctiva, seen usually in the elderly. Caused by degeneration of elastic tissue of conjunctiva.

piniform ('piniˌfawm) conical or cone-shaped.

Pink disease (pink) acrodynia.

pinkeye ('pingkˌie) an infectious inflammation of the conjunctiva caused by *Haemophilus aegypticus;* called also acute contagious CONJUNCTIVITIS.

pinna ('pinə) the projecting part of the ear lying outside the head; auricle. adj. **pinnal**.

pinocyte ('pienohˌsiet) a cell that exhibits pinocytosis.

pinocytosis (ˌpienohsie'tohsis) a mechanism by which cells ingest extracellular fluid and its contents; it involves the formation of invaginations by the cell membrane, which close and break off to form fluid-filled vacuoles in the cytoplasm. adj. **pinocytotic**.

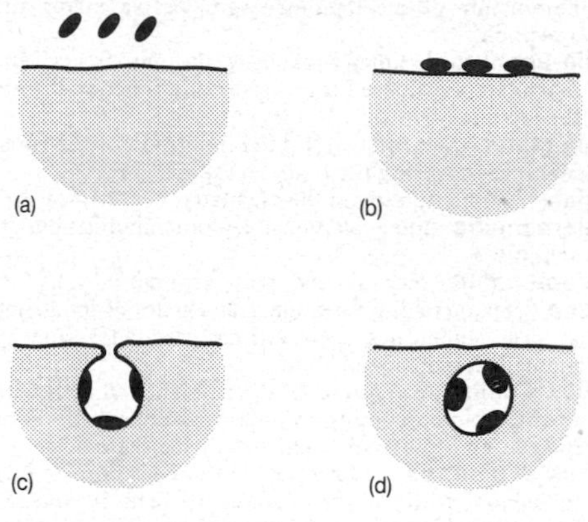

Mechanism of pinocytosis

pinosome (ˌpienohˌsohm) the intracellular vacuole formed by pinocytosis.

pint (pient) a unit of liquid measure in the apothecaries' system, 16 fluid ounces or equivalent to 473.17 millilitres.

pinta ('pintə) a treponemal infection characterized by bizarre pigmentary changes in the skin occurring in tropical America; it is effectively treated by penicillin.

pinworm ('pinˌwərm) an individual of the species *Enterobius vermicularis* (see also WORM). Called also THREADWORM.

piperacillin (pieˌperə'silin, pi-) a broad-spectrum semi-synthetic penicillin active against a wide variety of gram-negative, gram-positive, and anaerobic bacteria.

piperazine (pie'perəˌzeen, pi-) a compound, various salts of which are used as anthelmintics.

pipette (pi'pet) [Fr.] 1. a glass or transparent plastic tube used in measuring or transferring small quantities of liquid or gas. 2. to dispense by means of a pipette.

Pipril ('pipril) trademark for a preparation of piperacillin sodium, an antibacterial.

piriform ('piriˌfawm) pear-shaped.

Piriton ('piriton) trademark for chlorpheniramine maleate; a preparation used for the relief of allergy and the emergency treatment of anaphylactic reactions.

piroxicam (pi'roksikam) a nonsteroidal anti-inflammatory drug used in the treatment of rheumatic diseases.

Pirquet's reaction (peeər'kayz) appearance of a papule with a red areola 24–48 hours after introduction of two small drops of Old tuberculin by slight scarification of the skin; a positive test indicates previous infection with tubercle bacilli.

pisiform ('piesiˌfawm) resembling a pea in size and shape.

pit (pit) 1. a hollow fovea or indentation. 2. a pockmark. 3. to indent, or to become and remain for a few minutes indented, by pressure.

anal p. proctodeum.

auditory p. a distinct depression in each auditory placode, marking the beginning of the embryonic development of the internal ear.

lens p. a pitlike depression in the fetal head where the lens develops.

nasal p., olfactory p. a depression appearing in the olfactory placodes in the early stages of development of the nose.

p. of stomach the epigastric fossa or epigastric region.

pitch (pich) 1. a dark, more or less viscous residue from distillation of tar and other substances. 2. natural asphalt of various kinds. 3. the quality of sound dependent on the frequency of vibration of the waves producing it.

pitchblende ('pich,blend) a black mineral containing uranium oxide; from it are obtained radium, polonium, and uranium.

pithecoid ('pithi,koyd) apelike.

pithing ('pithing) destruction of the brain and spinal cord by thrusting a blunt needle into the vertebral canal and cranium, done on animals to destroy sensibility preparatory to experimenting on their living tissue.

Pitressin (pi'tresin) trademark for a preparation of arginine vasopressin.

pitting ('piting) 1. the removal from erythrocytes, by the spleen, of such structures as iron granules, without destruction of the cells. 2. remaining indented for a few minutes after removal of firm-finger-pressure, distinguishing fluid oedema from myxoedema.

pituicyte (pi'tyooi,siet) any of the distinctive fusiform cells composing most of the neurohypophysis.

pituitary (pi'tyooitə·ree) 1. pertaining to the pituitary gland. 2. pituitary gland. 3. a preparation of the pituitary glands of animals, used therapeutically.

p. gland an endocrine gland located at the base of the brain in a small recess of the sphenoid bone called the *sella turcica.* It is attached by the hypophyseal stalk to the HYPOTHALAMUS. The pituitary gland (called also the hypophysis) is divided into two regions that differ in function and embryological origin.

The *adenohyphophysis* originates from epithelial tissue and consists of the anterior lobe, which secretes six important hormones–growth hormone (GH), thyroid-stimulating hormone (TSH), adrenocorticotrophic hormone (ACTH), prolactin, follicle-stimulating hormone (FSH), and lutenizing hormone (LH); and of the middle lobe (*pars intermedia*), which secretes melanocyte-stimulating hormone (MSH). Most of the hormones of the anterior lobe are trophic hormones, which regulate the growth, development, and proper functioning of other endocrine glands and are of vital importance to the growth, maturation, and reproduction of the individual.

The secretion of anterior pituitary hormones is controlled by releasing and inhibiting hormones produced by the hypothalamus. Information about the well-being of an individual that is gathered by the

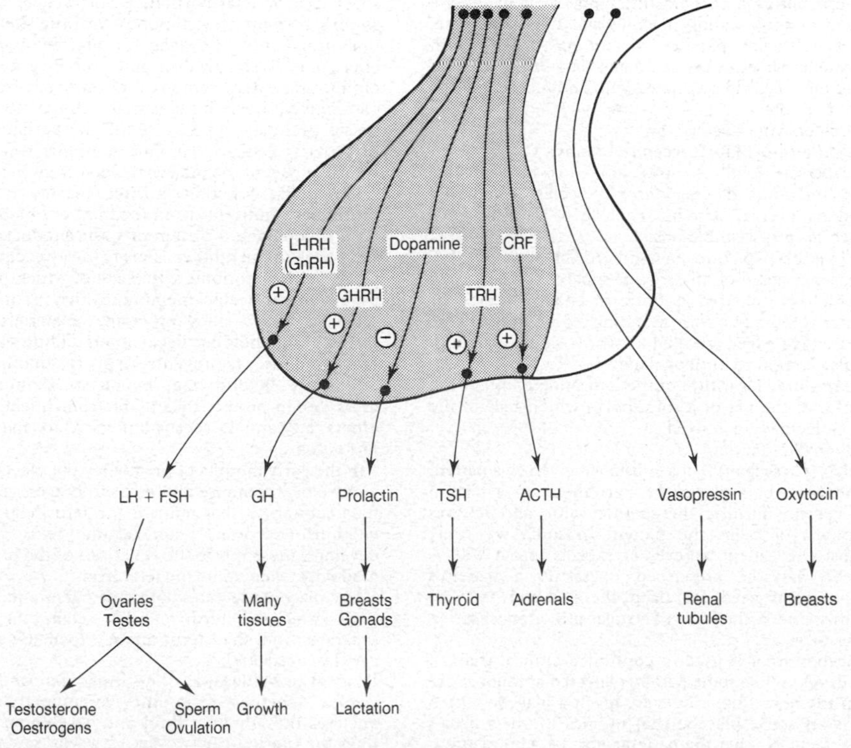

Hypothalamic releasing hormones and the pituitary trophic hormones

nervous system is collected in the hypothalamus and used to control the secretion of hormones by the pituitary gland. The hypothalamic releasing and inhibiting hormones are transported to the pituitary gland by way of the hypothalamic–hypophyseal portal system in which the hypothalamic venules connect with the capillaries of the anterior pituitary.

The *neurohypophysis* (posterior lobe) originates from neural tissue; it stores and secretes two hormones, oxytocin and antidiuretic hormone (ADH), or vasopressin. These hormones are synthesized in the cell bodies of neurons located in the hypothalamus and transported along the axons to the terminals located in the neurohypophysis. They are released in response to neural stimulation.

Surgical removal of part or all of the pituitary gland (HYPOPHYSECTOMY) is sometimes performed in the treatment of a pituitary tumour, and occasionally to control the pain associated with metatastic carcinoma of the breast and prostate gland.

posterior p. 1. the posterior lobe of the pituitary gland; the neurohypophysis. 2. a preparation of animal posterior pituitary having the pharmacological actions of its hormones, oxytocin and vasopressin; used mainly as an antidiuretic in the treatment of diabetes inspidus and as a vasoconstrictor..

pityriasis (ˌpitiˈrieəsis) originally, a group of skin diseases marked by the formation of fine, branny scales, but now used only with a modifier.

p. alba a chronic condition with patchy scaling and hypopigmentation of the skin of the face.

p. rosea a dermatosis marked by scaling pink oval macules arranged with the long axes parallel to the cleavage lines of the skin.

p. rubra pilaris a chronic inflammatory skin disease marked by pink scaling macules and fine acuminate, horny, follicular papules, beginning usually with severe seborrhoea of the scalp and seborrhoeic dermatitis of the face, and associated with keratoderma of the palms and soles.

p. versicolor tinea versicolor.

pityroid (ˈpitiˌroyd) furfuraceous; branny.

Pityrosporon (ˌpitiˈrospə·ron) a genus of yeast-like fungi, including *P. orbiculare*, a species customarily found on normal skin but capable of causing tinea versicolor in susceptible hosts.

pixel (ˈpiksel) a picture element. A CT scan or PET scan is composed of an array of squares (pixels), each of which is coloured a uniform shade of grey or another colour. The corresponding region in the tissue slice that is imaged is called a *voxel* (volume element). See also computed TOMOGRAPHY.

pK the negative logarithm of the ionization constant (K) of an acid; the pH of a solution in which half of the acid molecules are ionized.

PKU phenylketonuria.

placebo (pləˈseeboh) [L.] a substance given to a patient as medicine or a procedure performed on a patient that has no intrinsic therapeutic value and relieves symptoms or helps the patient in some way only because the patient believes or expects that it will. A placebo may be prescribed to satisfy a patient's psychological need for drug therapy and may be administered in the form of a sugar pill or an injection of sterile water.

Placebos are also used in controlled clinical trials of new drugs. While some patients selected at random are given the new drug, others are given a placebo. Often this is an active placebo that mimics the new drug's side-effects. Neither the patients nor the administrator of the drug know who is receiving the real drug. The patients taking the new drug must have significantly more relief of symptoms than the control group taking the placebo for the new drug to be considered to be effective. Placebos can produce an effect that is either positive, with improvement of symptoms, or negative, with worsening of symptoms or the appearance of adverse side-effects.

The origin of the word 'placebo' is the Latin word meaning 'I will please'. The term can be used to cover all nonspecific aspects of treatment, particularly the patient's beliefs and expectations, the doctor, nurse or therapist's beliefs and expectations, and the psychological interaction between patient and therapist. The patient's anticipation that a placebo will produce a physiological effect can lead to the realization of that effect. This is not a case of gullibility, emotional instability, or deception of the patient, although these often have been given credit for the positive effects of a placebo. Rather, it is an example of mind–body interaction that has been observed from the earliest days of medical practice when ancient healers used anything from crocodile dung to powdered buffalo horn to cure the ills of clients. Today, the placebo effect is being reconsidered and respected as a legitimate therapeutic tool that can be used without deception to enhance the practice of modern health care.

placenta (pləˈsentə) pl. *placentas,placentae* [L.] an organ characteristic of true mammals during pregnancy, joining mother and offspring, providing endocrine secretion and selective exchange of soluble bloodborne substances through apposition of uterine and chorionic tissues. Called also *afterbirth*. adj. **placental**.

In anatomical nomenclature the placenta consists of a uterine and a fetal portion. The amnion, the superficial or fetal portion, is surfaced by a smooth, shining membrane continuous with the sheath of the umbilical cord. The deep, or uterine, portion, the chorion, is divided by deep sulci into lobes of irregular outline and extent composed of millions of branching chorionic villi which lie bathed in the maternal blood spaces (the cotyledons). Around the periphery of the placenta is a large vein (the marginal sinus), which returns a part of the maternal blood from the organ.

The major function of the placenta is to allow diffusion of nutrients from the mother's blood into the fetus's blood and diffusion of waste products from the fetus back to the mother. This two-way exchange takes place via the chorionic villi, each of which is bounded by a semipermeable membrane; that is, it acts as a selective filter, allowing some materials to pass through and holding back others. Thus some drugs cross and are teratogenic, e.g. THALIDOMIDE, while others are helpful, e.g. PENICILLIN. Antibodies also cross. Some protect the infant from infection, while others, e.g. anti D rhesus antibody, are harmful. See RH FACTOR.

In the early months of pregnancy the placenta acts as a nutrient storehouse and helps to process some of the food substances that nourish the fetus, e.g. glycogen, vitamins and iron. Later, as the fetus grows and develops, these metabolic functions of the placenta are gradually taken on by the fetal liver.

The placenta secretes both oestrogens and progesterone. After the birth of the infant the placenta separates from the uterus and is expelled via the birth canal (see LABOUR).

PLACENTAL MEMBRANES. The inner *amnion* and outer *chorion* together form the gestational sac which encloses the amniotic fluid and developing fetus and lines the uterine cavity after 12 weeks' gestation. The amnion is formed from the inner cell mass of the blastocyst, and is continous with the epithelium of the umbilical cord and the fetal epidermis. A tough, transparent membrane, the amnion is thought to secrete and absorb amniotic fluid. Following delivery, it may be stripped back as far as the insertion of the cord in the placenta.

The outer chorion develops from the trophoblastic layer of the blastocyst. It is an opaque, friable membrane continuous with the placenta. Following delivery, the chorion will strip only to the placental margin. Part or all of the chorion and the amnion may sometimes be retained in the uterus and become a source of haemorrhage or infection.

The membranes should always be checked for completeness following delivery.

abruptio placentae premature separation of a normally situated placenta.

Serious abruptio placentae occurs most often before the onset of labour. Symptoms include sudden, severe pain in the region of the uterus, some external bleeding, and indications of fetal distress. Three types are described, related to the degree of evident blood loss per vaginam: revealed, concealed and mixed. Treatment is conservative unless there is an indication of severe haemorrhage or fetal death, in which case a caesarean section is indicated.

p. accreta one abnormally adherent to the myometrium, with partial or complete absence of the decidua basalis.

battledore p. one with the umbilical cord inserted at the edge.

p. circumvallata one encircled with a dense, raised, white nodular ring, the attached membranes being doubled back over the edge of the placenta.

p. fenestrata one that has one or more spots where placental tissue is lacking.

haemochorial p. a stage of early placental development when placental or chorionic tissue is in direct contact with maternal blood.

haemoendothelial p. a stage of early placental development when maternal blood comes in contact with the endothelium of chorionic vessels.

p. increta placenta accreta with penetration of the myometrium.

p. membranacea one that is abnormally thin and spread over an unusually large area of the myometrium.

p. percreta placenta accreta with invasion of the myometrium to the peritoneal covering, sometimes causing rupture of the uterus.

p. previa one located in the lower uterine segment, so that it partially or entirely covers the internal os, instead of in the proper position in the fundus. Four degrees are described. Type 1: placenta dips into lower uterine segment but does not reach the os. Type 2: placenta margin reaches the os but does not cover it. Type 3: placenta covers the os up to 3 cm dilation. Type 4: placenta is centrally situated, completely covering the cervical os. Any expansion of the cervix may cause tearing of placental tissue and bleeding. This condition is life threatening to both mother and fetus, and may require delivery by caesarean section.

p. reflexa one in which the margin is thickened, appearing to turn back on itself.

p. spuria an accessory portion without blood vessels connecting it with the main placenta.

p. succenturiata an accessory portion with an artery and a vein connecting it with the main placenta. It may be retained following delivery, and should always be checked for when placental membranes are examined.

placentation (ˌplasen'tayshən) the series of events following implantation of the embryo and leading to development of the placenta.

placentitis (ˌplasen'tietis) inflammation of the placenta.

placentography (ˌplasen'tografee) radiological visualization of the placenta after injection of a contrast medium.

placentoid (plə'sentoyd) resembling the placenta.

placidity (pla'siditee) a calm state, the opposite of rage, in which it takes a strong stimulus to evoke a response.

Placido's disc ('plasidohz) a disc marked with black and white circles used in the assessment of corneal distortion.

placode ('plakohd) a platelike structure, especially a thickening of the ectoderm marking the site of future development in the early embryo of an organ of special sense, e.g., the *auditory placode* (ear), *lens placode* (eye), and *olfactory placode* (nose).

placoid ('plakoyd) platelike or plaquelike.

plagiocephaly (ˌplayjioh'kefəlee, -'sef-) bizarre distortion of the shape of the skull resulting from irregular closure of the cranial sutures. adj. **plagiocephalic**.

plague (playg) an acute febrile, infectious, highly fatal disease caused by the bacillus *Yersinia pestis*. It is primarily a disease of rats and other rodents, and is usually spread to human beings by fleas. The more common form of plague is the bubonic. There is also a pneumonic type, which can be spread directly from man to man by droplet infection.

Plague can be a devastating disease. Three pandemics of plague in history were especially so. The first of these spread over Europe in the sixth century A.D. in a tremendous cycle of pestilence that lasted for more than 50 years. The second, called the Black Death, was perhaps the most deadly outbreak the world has known. It swept over Europe in the 14th century, when at least one-quarter of Europe's population died within 2 years. It then disappeared from Western Europe in the late 17th century, by which time it had become largely restricted to urban areas. A third great pandemic raged in the Orient at the turn of the 20th century. The greatest toll was in India, where there were more than 12 million deaths from 1896 to 1933.

Nowadays urban plague is under control almost everywhere in the world, but wild rodent plague is still present in parts of North and South America, Africa and Asia, and human plague is reported from time to time as sporadic cases or (usually) small outbreaks. In the USA small numbers of cases associated with wild rodents are reported in the southern half of the country. The last case reported in the UK was in 1918, apart from a single laboratory infection in 1962.

BUBONIC PLAGUE. Bubonic plague is characterized by acutely inflamed and painful swellings of the lymph nodes, or buboes, usually in the groin.

The disease strikes suddenly with chills and fever. Children may have convulsions. There is vomiting and thirst, generalized pain, headache, and mental dullness. Delirium may also be present.

Tender, enlarged lymph nodes are usually seen between the second and fifth days. Some cases of bubonic plague are mild, but the more virulent cases are usually fatal unless treated. If the patient survives past the tenth or twelfth day, there is a good chance of recovery.

The mortality rate for untreated cases varies between 25 and 50 per cent, but has reached as high as 90 per cent. Until recently, little could be done for the disease. Today, however, streptomycin, when used early enough, has cut the mortality rate to 5 per cent. Tetracycline is also effective.

PNEUMONIC PLAGUE. Pneumonic plague usually occurs during outbreaks of bubonic plague and may be a direct complication of it. There is extensive involvement of the lungs; the sputum contains many organisms and is highly infective. At one time, pneumonic plague was always fatal. Now, with streptomycin, the chances of recovery are good if treatment is begun within 24 hours.

SEPTICAEMIC PLAGUE usually occurs in conjunction with bubonic plague as an acute illness which may be fatal before bubonic or pulmonary manifestations predominate.

PREVENTION. The most important measure in controlling plague is the extermination of rats. This is especially necessary around shipping areas, in warehouses, and on docks. Rat control for ships arriving from plague areas is vital.

Plague is a notifiable disease.Where there is an outbreak, strict quarantine measures are called for, as well as the use of insecticides to protect inhabitants of the stricken area against fleas. Immunization with plague vaccine gives some protection. Persons who have been in contact with active cases of plague are given prophylactic tetracycline.

plane (playn) 1. a flat surface determined by the position of three points in space. 2. a specified level, as the plane of anaesthesia or dissection. 3. to rub away or abrade (see also PLANING and PLASTIC SURGERY).

coronal p. frontal plane.

datum p. a given horizontal plane from which craniometric measurements are made.

frontal p. any vertical plane at right angles to the median plane and dividing the body into front and back parts. Called also *coronal plane*.

horizontal p. any plane through the body at right angles to the median and frontal planes, and dividing the body into upper and lower parts.

median p. any vertical plane through the body situated upon the midline.

sagittal p. a vertical plane through the body parallel to the median plane and dividing the body into left and right portions.

transverse p. any horizontal plane at right angles to the sagittal and frontal planes, and dividing the body into upper and lower portions.

vertical p. one perpendicular to a horizontal plane, dividing the body into left and right, or front and back portions.

planigraphy (plə'nigrəfee) a method of body-section radiology that shows in detail structures lying in a predetermined plane of the body while blurring structures in other planes, produced by movement of the film and x-ray tube in certain specified directions. adj. **planigraphic**. See TOMOGRAPHY.

planing ('playning) abrasion of disfigured skin to promote reepithelization with minimal scarring; done by mechanical means (dermabrasion) or by application of a caustic (chemabrasion). See also PLASTIC SURGERY.

planned parenthood (pland pair·rənt·huhd) birth control.

planoconcave (ˌplaynoh'konkayv) flat on one side and concave on the other.

planoconvex (ˌplaynoh'konveks) flat on one side and convex on the other.

planography (plə'nogrəfee) planigraphy.

planta pedis (ˌplantə 'peedis) the sole of the foot.

Plantago (plan'taygoh) a genus of herbs, including *P. indica*, *P. psyllium* (Spanish psyllium), and *P. ovata* (blond psyllium).

plantalgia (plan'talji·ə) pain in the sole of the foot.

plantar ('plantə) pertaining to the sole of the foot.

p. wart a common WART located on the sole of the foot. Plantar warts are epidermal tumours caused by a virus which may be picked up by going barefoot. Unlike other warts, this type is usually sensitive to pressure; it may feel tender when touched and may be painful during walking. Called also verruca plantaris.

plantaris (plan'tair·ris) [L.] *plantar*.

plantigrade ('plantiˌgrayd) walking or running flat on the full sole of the foot; characteristic of man and of such quadrupeds as the bear.

planula ('planyuhlə) a larval coelenterate.

planum ('playnəm) pl. *plana* [L.] plane.

plaque (plak, plahk) any patch or flat area.

atheromatous p. a deposit of predominantly fatty material in the lining of blood vessels occurring in atherosclerosis.

bacterial p., dental p. a mass adhering to the enamel surface of a tooth, composed of a mixed colony of bacteria in an intercellular matrix of bacterial and salivary polymers and remnants of epithelial cells and leukocytes. It may cause caries, dental calculi, and periodontal disease.

Hollenhorst p's atheromatous emboli containing cholesterol crystals in the retinal arterioles, a sign of impending serious cardiovascular disease.

Plaquenil ('playkwenil) trademark for a preparation of hydroxychloroquine, used especially as a lupus erythematosus suppressant, and in rheumatoid arthritis.

plasm ('plazəm) 1. plasma. 2. formative substance, e.g. cytoplasm, hyaloplasm, etc.

plasma ('plazmə) the fluid portion of the blood in which corpuscles are suspended. Plasma is to be distinguished from serum, which is plasma from which the fibrinogen has been separated in the process of clotting. adj. **plasmatic**.

Of the total volume of blood, 55 per cent is made up of plasma. It is a clear, straw-coloured liquid, 92 per cent water, in which are contained plasma proteins, inorganic salts, foods, gases, waste materials from the cells, and various hormones, secretions, and enzymes. These substances are transported to or from the tissues of the body by the plasma.

Plasma obtained from blood donors is given to those suffering from loss of blood or from shock to help maintain adequate blood pressure. It can be deep frozen (fresh frozen plasma, FFP) or it can be dried and stored in bottles, ready for immediate use after addition of the appropriate fluid. Cross matching is not required but blood group compatibility is necessary. See also BLOOD, SERUM, and TRANSFUSION.

antihaemophilic human p. normal human plasma that has been processed promptly to preserve the antihaemophilic properties of the original blood; used for temporary correction of bleeding tendency in haemophilia.

p. exchange the removal of plasma from withdrawn blood (plasmapheresis) and retransfusion of the formed elements and type-specific fresh-frozen plasma into the donor; done for removal of circulating antibodies or abnormal plasma components.

p. protein fraction (PPF) a freeze-dried blood product prepared from fresh plasma; mainly consists of albumin and globulin. It can be reconstituted and used to maintain blood volume in acute situations, e.g. shock, severe burns. Unlike fresh frozen plasma, it is free from hepatitis.

p. viscosity depends mainly on the concentrations of the plasma proteins, including fibrinogen, a stress reactive protein. Measurement of the plasma viscosity is a sensitive index of protein levels, and will be increased in inflammatory conditions and paraproteinuraemias such as myeloma. The normal range is 1.50–1.72 cp.

p. volume expander a solution transfused instead of blood to increase the volume of fluid circulating in the blood vessels. Called also artificial plasma extender.

plasmablast ('plazmə,blast) the immature precursor of a plasmacyte, or plasma cell.

plasmacyte ('plazmə,siet) a spherical or ellipsoidal cell with a single nucleus containing chromatin, an area of perinuclear clearing, and generally abundant, sometimes vacuolated cytoplasm. Plasmacytes are involved in the synthesis, storage, and release of antibody. Called also plasmocyte and plasma cell. adj. **plasmacytic**.

plasmacytoma (,plazməsie'tohmə) any focal neoplasm of plasmacytes, including those of multiple myeloma. Isolated plasmacytomas may occur outside the bone marrow (extramedullary plasmacytomas), affecting such tissues as the nasal, oral, and pharnygeal mucosa and the viscera.

plasmacytosis (,plazməsie'tohsis) an excess of plasmacytes in the blood.

plasmalemma (,plazmə'lemə) plasma membrane.

plasmapheresis (,plazməfə'reesis) the removal of plasma from extracorporeal blood, with retransfusion of the formed elements into the donor; generally, type-specific fresh frozen plasma or albumin is used to replace the withdrawn plasma. The procedure may be done for purposes of collecting plasma components or for therapeutic purposes, such as removal of antibodies in diseases such as Goodpasture's syndrome or occasionally to prevent antibody destruction of a transplanted kidney.

plasmatorrhexis (,plazmətə'reksis) bursting of a cell from internal pressure.

plasmic ('plazmik) plasmatic; pertaining to or of the nature of plasma.

plasmid ('plazmid) any extrachromosomal self-replicating genetic element of a cell. In bacteria, plasmids are circular DNA molecules that reproduce themselves and are thus conserved, apart from the chromosome, through successive cell divisions; they include the F factor and R factor. Plasmids that may also become integrated into the chromosome are sometimes called episomes.

plasmin ('plazmin) the active principle of the fibrinolytic or clot-lysing system, a proteolytic enzyme with a high specificity for fibrin and the particular ability to dissolve formed fibrin clots.

plasminogen (plaz'minəjən) the inactive precursor of plasmin, occurring in plasma and converted to plasmin by the action of activators such as urokinase; called also *profibrinolysin*.

plasmocyte ('plazmoh,siet) plasmacyte.

plasmocytoma (,plazmohsie'tohmə) plasmacytoma.

plasmodesma (,plazmoh'dezmə) pl. *plasmodesmata;* a bridge of cytoplasm connecting adjacent cells.

plasmodicidal (plaz,mohdi'sied'l) destructive to plasmodia; malariacidal.

Plasmodium (plaz'mohdi·əm) a genus of sporozoa (family Plasmodiidae) parasitic in the red blood cells of animals and man; the malarial parasite. The organism is transmitted to the bloodstream of man by the bite of anopheline mosquitoes. The sporozoites migrate directly to the liver, where they develop and multiply within the parenchymal cells as merozoites, which then burst the liver cells and invade erythrocytes. Some of the merozoites develop into gametocytes, which are ingested by mosquitoes, beginning the sexual stage, which ends with the development of sporozoites. Four species, *P. falciparum*, *P. malariae*, *P. ovale*, and *P. vivax*, cause the four specific types of human malaria.

plasmodium (plaz'mohdi·əm) pl. *plasmodia* [Gr.] 1. a parasite of the genus *Plasmodium.* 2. a multinucleate continuous mass of protoplasm. adj. **plasmodial**.

plasmogen ('plazməjən) bioplasm; the more vital or essential part of the cytoplasm.

plasmolysis (plaz'molisis) contraction of cell protoplasm due to loss of water by osmosis. adj. **plasmolytic**.

plasmoma (plaz'mohmə) plasmacytoma.

plasmon ('plazmon) the hereditary factors of the egg cytoplasm.

plasmorrhexis (,plazmə'reksis) a morphological change in erythrocytes, consisting in the escape from the cells of round, shiny granules and splitting off of particles; called also erythrocytorrhexis.

plasmoschisis (plaz'moskisis) the splitting up of cell protoplasm.

plaster ('plahstə, 'plastə) 1. a mixture of materials that hardens; used for immobilizing or making impressions of body parts. 2. an adhesive substance spread on fabric or other suitable backing material, for application to the skin.

p. of Paris calcium sulphate dihydrate, reduced to a fine powder; the addition of water produces a porous mass used in making casts and bandages to support or immobilize body parts, and in dentistry for taking dental impressions.

plastic ('plastik) 1. capable of being moulded. 2. a substance produced by chemical condensation or by polymerization. 3. material that can be moulded.

p. surgery surgery concerned with the restoration, reconstruction, correction, or improvement in the shape and appearance of body structures that are defective, damaged, or misshapened by injury, disease, or anomalous growth and development.

SKIN GRAFTING. The most common procedure of plastic surgery is skin GRAFTING. This is the loss of severely damaged skin in one area being replaced with healthy skin obtained from another area of the patient's body. Grafting is also undertaken to prevent the formation of disfiguring scars, such as those that may form on the face from severe burns. Grafting can also prevent skin contractures.

A skin graft can sometimes be made by the simple procedure of cutting a piece of healthy skin from one part of the body, such as the back or the thigh, and stitching it to the injured area. If the area to be covered is large, a number of separate patches may be stitched to it, forming islands of skin that will enlarge with healing until the entire area is covered. This is called 'postage stamp' or pinch grafting.

In order to ensure a good blood supply to a large patch, a pedicle graft may be needed. See GRAFTING.

With the advent of MICROSURGERY much of the inconvenience and lengthy waiting necessary for successful grafting of skin flaps has been eliminated. It is now possible for a surgeon to perform what are called *free-tissue transfers.* The skin flap is removed from the donor site and transferred directly to the distant recipient site where circulation to the free flap is reestablished by microvascular anastomoses.

REPAIRING MOUTH AND OTHER DEFECTS. Among common defects that can be corrected by plastic surgery are CLEFT LIP and CLEFT PALATE. Others are webbed fingers or toes, protruding or missing ears, receding chins, and disfigured noses.

FACIAL RECONSTRUCTION. In facial reconstruction, missing bone and muscle, and sometimes skin, are replaced by substitutes. Sometimes the reconstruction is made with bone or cartilage taken from another part of the body, or sometimes it is made by artificial means.

Use of Prostheses. Often the substitute for missing tissue may be a prosthesis. A prosthesis may be inserted beneath the skin (to build out a receding chin, for instance) or attached to the skin surface (for example, to replace an ear). *Use of Cartilage, Skin and Bone.* Noses and ears are reconstructed with rib cartilage and skin grafts. Eyebrows can be made using skin grafts from the scalp, and chest deformities repaired by the use of bone chips from other parts of the body.

Dermabrasion. Skin blemishes such as acne scars and pits can be 'sandpapered' or planed. This technique, called dermabrasion, seeks to correct superficial blemishes and to remove superficial accumulations of pigment. However, as dermabrasion can occasionally cause increased scarring or introduce variation in skin colour and texture, such treatment is infrequently performed.

FACE LIFTING. This operation is performed to make an ageing face look younger. The technical term for this is rhytidoplasty, or plastic surgery for the removal of wrinkles. Such an operation performed by an experienced surgeon can be successful, but only temporarily. Reoperation is often necessary. The operation is usually done by opening skin flaps in the region around the ears and undermining the skin of the cheeks and jaws. The eyelids and the area of the eyebrows may be operated on in association with the primary operation.

plasticity (pla'stisitee) the quality of being plastic, or capable of being moulded.

plastid ('plastid) 1. any elementary constructive unit, as a cell. 2. any specialized organ of the cell other than the nucleus and centrosome, such as chloroplast or amyloplast.

-plasty ('plastee) word element. [Gr.] *formation* or *plastic repair of.*

plate (playt) 1. a flat structure or layer, as a flat layer of bone. 2. dental plate. 3. to apply a culture medium to a glass plate. 4. to cultivate bacteria on such plates.

axial p. the primitive streak of the embryo.

bite p. biteplate.

deck p. roof plate.

dental p. a plate of acrylic resin, metal, or other material that is fitted to the shape of the mouth, and serves for the support of artificial teeth.

dorsal p. roof plate.

epiphyseal p. the thin plate of cartilage between the epiphysis and the shaft of a long bone; it is the site of growth in length and is obliterated by epiphyseal closure.

equatorial p. the collection of chromosomes at the equator of the spindle in mitosis.

floor p. the unpaired ventral longitudinal zone of the neural tube; called also ventral plate.

foot p. the flat portion of the stapes.

medullary p. neural plate.

muscle p. myotome (2).

neural p. a thickened band of ectoderm in the midbody region of the developing embryo, which develops into the neural tube; called also medullary plate.

roof p. the unpaired dorsal longitudinal zone of the neural tube; called also dorsal plate and deck plate.

sole p. a mass of protoplasm in which a motor nerve ending is embedded.

tarsal p. one of the plates of connective tissue forming the framework of either (upper or lower) eyelid.

ventral p. floor plate.

platelet ('playtlət) a small disc or platelike structure, the smallest of the formed elements in blood. Blood platelets (called also thrombocytes) are disc-shaped, non-nucleated blood elements with a very fragile membrane; they tend to adhere to uneven or damaged surfaces. They average about 250×10^9 per litre of blood and are formed in the red bone marrow by fragmentation of megakaryocytes, the largest of the bone marrow cells. The rate of their formation seems to be governed by a humoral factor in the blood called thrombopoietin, and other nonspecific stimuli. At any given time about one-third of the total blood platelets can be found in the spleen; the remaining two-thirds are in the circulating blood.

The functions of platelets are related to coagulation and the clotting of blood. Because of their adhesion and aggregation capabilities platelets can occlude small breaks in blood vessels and prevent the escape of blood. Platelets also are able to take up, store, transport, and release serotonin and platelet factor 3.

Abnormally high numbers of platelets occur in the post-operative state in the presence of malignancy, splenectomy, asphyxiation, polycythaemia vera, and in inflammatory conditions. A very low count of platelets can occur as a result of autoimmune thrombocytopenic purpura, viral infections, bone marrow infiltration and disorders, and during cancer chemotherapy. There are many drugs that can cause a toxic decrease in the number of platelets.

p. factors factors important in haemostasis which are contained in or attached to the platelets: platelet factor 1 is adsorbed CLOTTING factor V from the plasma; platelet factor 2 is an accelerator of the thrombin-fibrinogen reaction; platelet factor 3 plays a role in the generation of intrinsic prothrombin converting principle (see also PF3); platelet factor 4 is capable of inhibiting the activity of heparin.

p. function disorders a group of disorders characterized by abnormal platelet function leading to a long bleeding time and a bleeding diathesis (easy bruising, bleeding from the nose, etc.). Hereditary disorders are rare, e.g. thrombasthenia. Acquired defects are more common and may be secondary to drugs, e.g. aspirin; examples are myeloma and myeloproliferative disorders.

plateletpheresis (ˌplaytlətfə'reesis) thrombocytapheresis.

platinum ('platinəm) a chemical element, atomic number 78, atomic weight 195.09, symbol Pt. See table of elements in Appendix 2.

platy- word element. [Gr.] *broad, flat.*

platybasia (ˌplati'bayzi·ə) malformation of the base of the skull, with upward displacement of the upper cervical vertebrae and bony impingement on the brain stem. It is accompanied by neurological signs referable to the medulla oblongata, cervical spinal cord, and cranial nerves. Called also basilar impression.

platycelous (ˌplati'seeləs) having one surface flat and the other concave, referring to vertebrae.

platycephalic, platycephalous (ˌplatikə'falik, -sə-; ˌplati'kefələs, -'sef-) having a wide, flat head.

platycoria (ˌplati'kor·ri·ə) a dilated condition of the pupil of the eye.

platyhelminth (ˌplati'helminth) one of the Platyhelminthes; a flatworm.

Platyhelminthes (ˌplatihel'mintheez) a phylum of acoelomate, dorsoventrally flattened, bilaterally symmetrical animals, commonly known as flatworms; it includes the classes Cestoidea (tapeworms) and Trematoda (flukes). See also WORM.

platyhieric (ˌplatihie'erik) having a wide sacrum, with a sacral index above 100.

platypellic, platypelloid (ˌplati'pelik; ˌplati'peloyd) having a broad pelvis. See platypellic PELVIS.

platypodia (ˌplati'pohdi·ə) flatfoot.

platyrrhine ('platiˌrien) having a broad nose, with a nasal index above 53.

platysma (plə'tizmə) a subcutaneous neck muscle extending from the neck to the clavicle; it acts to wrinkle the skin of the neck and to depress the jaw.

play therapist (play) one trained in the skills of play therapy.

play therapy a technique used in child psychotherapy in which play is used to reveal unconscious material. Play is the natural way in which children express and work through unconscious conflicts; thus play therapy is analogous to the technique of free association used in PSYCHOANALYSIS of adults. The therapy is done in a playroom containing toys such as dolls, a dollhouse, and furniture; blocks; art materials; toy animals, cars, trucks, guns, soldiers, and telephone; and games. As the child plays he expresses his fantasies and gives the therapist clues about his family relationships and unconscious conflicts. For example, the child may be unable to verbally express hostile feelings about a parent or sibling but be able to act out these feelings playing with a doll. The role of the therapist is nondirective. The therapist provides an accepting, understanding adult relationship that allows the child to work through his conflicts and to experiment with new ways of relating to himself and other people.

pledget ('plejit) a small compress or tuft.

-plegia word element. [Gr.] *paralysis, a stroke.*

pleiotropism, pleiotropy (plie'otrə,pizəm; plie-'otrəpee) the production by a single gene of multiple phenotypic effects.

pleocytosis (,pleeohsie'tohsis) the presence of a greater than normal number of cells, as of more than the normal number of lymphocytes in cerebrospinal fluid.

pleomastia (,pleeoh'masti·ə) the presence of supernumerary mammary glands or nipples; polymastia.

pleomorphism (,pleeoh'mawfizəm) the assumption of various distinct forms by a single organism or within a species. adj. **pleomorphic, pleomorphous**.

pleonasm ('pleeə,nazəm) an excess of parts.

pleonectic (,pleeə'nektik) characterized by having a higher than normal O_2 content at a given Po_2; said of blood.

pleonexia (,pleeə'neksi·ə) 1. morbid desire for acquisition; morbid greediness. 2. the condition of being pleonectic.

pleonosteosis (,pleeə,nosti'ohsis) abnormally increased ossification.

Léri's p. a hereditary syndrome of premature and excessive ossification, with short stature, limitation of movement, broadening and deformity of digits, and mongolian facies.

pleoptics (pli'optiks) an orthoptic method of improving the sight in cases of strabismus by stimulating the use of the macular part of the retina.

plessaesthesia (,plesis'theezi·ə) palpatory percussion.

plessimeter (plə'simitə) pleximeter.

plessor ('plesə) plexor.

plethora ('plethə·rə) a general term denoting a red florid complexion, or specifically, an excessive amount of blood. adj. **plethoric**.

plethysmograph (plə'thizmoh,grahf, -,graf) any device for measuring and recording variations in the volume of an organ, part, or limb.

body p. a device used in PULMONARY FUNCTION TESTS to measure parameters such as functional residual capacity (FRC) and lung-thorax compliance (C_{LT}). It consists of a large box in which the subject can be sealed so that volume of the thorax can be determined from pressure changes in the box while the lung volume and gas pressure in the lungs are measured by spirometry.

plethysmography (,plethiz'mogrəfee) the determination of changes in volume by means of a plethysmograph.

pleur(o)- word element. [Gr.] *pleura, rib, side.*

pleura ('plooə·rə) pl. *pleurae* [Gr.] the serous membrane investing the lungs (pulmonary pleura) and lining the walls of the thoracic cavity (parietal pleura), the two layers enclosing a potential space, the pleural cavity. adj. **pleural**.

pleuracotomy (,plooə·rə'kotəmee) incision into the pleural cavity.

pleuralgia (plooə'ralji·ə) pain in the pleura or in the side. adj. **pleuralgic**.

pleurapophysis (,plooə·rə'pofisis) a rib, or a vertebral process corresponding to a rib.

pleurectomy (plooə'rektəmee) excision of a portion of abnormal pleura.

pleurisy, pleuritis ('plooə·riseey; plooə'rietis) inflammation of the pleura; it may be caused by infection, injury, or tumour. It may be a complication of lung diseases, particularly of pneumonia, or sometimes of tuberculosis, lung abscess, or influenza. The symptoms are cough, fever, chills, sharp, sticking pain that is worse on inspiration, and rapid shallow breathing. adj. **pleuritic**.

TYPES OF PLEURISY. The membranous pleura that encases each lung is composed of two close-fitting layers; between them is a lubricating fluid. If the fluid content remains unchanged by the disease, the pleurisy is said to be dry. If the fluid increases abnormally, it is a wet pleurisy, or pleurisy with effusion. See also pleural EFFUSION.

In dry pleurisy the two layers of membrane may become congested and swollen and rub against each other with a grating effect as the lungs inflate and deflate with breathing. This can be painful. Although only the outer layer causes pain (the inner layer has no pain nerves), the pain may be severe enough to necessitate the use of a strong analgesic.

Wet pleurisy is less likely to cause pain, because there usually is no chafing. But the fluid may interfere with breathing by compressing the lung. In some cases the lung is permanently displaced, failing to return to full capacity because of thickening of the pleura.

If the excess fluid of wet pleurisy becomes infected, with formation of pus, the condition is known as purulent pleurisy or EMPYEMA.

Inflammation of the part of the pleura that covers the diaphragm is called diaphragmatic pleurisy.

TREATMENT. The most effective measures against pleurisy are antibiotics, heat applications, and bed rest. When there is intense pain on breathing, the doctor may strap the chest to limit its movement.

pleurocele ('plooə·roh,seel) hernia of lung tissue or of pleura.

pleurocentesis (,plooə·rohsen'teesis) thoracentesis; paracentesis of the pleural cavity.

pleurocentrum (,plooə·roh'sentrəm) the lateral element of the vertebral column.

pleuroclysis (plooə'roklisis) injection of fluids into the pleural cavity.

pleurodynia (,plooə·roh'dini·ə) paroxysmal pain in the intercostal muscles.

epidemic p. an epidemic disease due to cocksackievirus B, marked by a sudden attack of violent pain in the chest, fever, and a tendency to recrudescence on the third day; called also devil's grip and Bornholm disease.

pleurogenic, pleurogenous (,plooə·roh'jenik; plooə-'rojənəs) originating in the pleura.

pleurography (plooə'rogrəfee) radiology of the pleural cavity.

pleurohepatitis (,plooə·roh,hepə'tietis) hepatitis with inflammation of a portion of the pleura near the liver.

pleurolith ('plooə·roh,lith) a concretion in the pleura.

pleurolysis (plooə'rolisis) surgical separation of the

pleura from its attachments.

pleuroparietopexy (ˌplooə·rohpəˈrieətohˌpeksee) fixation of the visceral pleura to the parietal pleura, thus binding the lung to the chest wall.

pleuropericardial (ˌplooə·rohˌperiˈkahdi·əl) pertaining to the pleura and pericardium.

pleuropericarditis (ˌplooə·rohˌperikahˈdietis) inflammation involving the pleura and the pericardium.

pleuroperitoneal (ˌplooə·rohˌperitəˈneeəl) pertaining to the pleura and peritoneum.

pleuropneumonia (ˌplooə·rohnyooˈmohni·ə) 1. pneumonia accompanied by pleurisy. 2. an infectious disease of cattle, combining pneumonia and pleurisy, due to *Mycoplasma mycoides* (see also PLEUROPNEUMONIA-LIKE ORGANISMS).

pleuropneumonia-like organisms (ˌplooə·rohnyooˈmohni·əliek) PPLO, a term applied to a group of filtrable microorganisms similar to *Mycoplasma mycoides*, the cause of pleuropneumonia in cattle.

pleurothotonos (ˌplooə·rohˈthotənəs) tetanic bending of the body to one side.

pleurotomy (plooəˈrotəmee) incision of the pleura.

pleurovisceral (ˌplooə·rohˈvisə·rəl) pertaining to the pleura and viscera.

plexectomy (plekˈsektəmee) excision of a plexus.

plexiform (ˈpleksiˌfawm) resembling a plexus or network.

pleximeter (plekˈsimitə) 1. a plate to be struck in mediate percussion. 2. diascope.

plexitis (plekˈsietis) inflammation of a nerve plexus.

plexopathy (plekˈsopəthee) any disorder of a plexus, especially of nerves.

lumbar p. neuropathy of the lumbar plexus.

plexor (ˈpleksə) a hammer used in diagnostic percussion; plessor.

plexus (ˈpleksəs) pl. *plexus*, *plexuses* [L.] a network or tangle, chiefly of veins or nerves. adj. **plexal**.

brachial p. a nerve plexus originating from the ventral branches of the last four cervical and the first thoracic spinal nerves. It gives off many of the principal nerves of the shoulder, chest, and arms.

cardiac p. the plexus around the base of the heart, chiefly in the epicardium, formed by cardiac branches from the vagus nerves and the sympathetic trunks and ganglia, and made up of sympathetic, parasympathetic, and visceral afferent fibres that innervate the heart.

carotid p's nerve plexuses surrounding the common, external, and internal carotid arteries.

coeliac p. solar plexus.

cervical p. a nerve plexus formed by the ventral branches of the first four cervical spinal nerves and supplying the structures in the region of the neck. One important branch is the phrenic nerve, which supplies the diaphragm.

choroid p. infoldings of blood vessels of the pia mater covered by a thin coat of ependymal cells that form tufted projections into the third, fourth, and lateral ventricles of the brain; they secrete the cerebrospinal fluid.

coccygeal p. a nerve plexus formed by the ventral branches of the coccygeal and fifth sacral nerve and by a communication from the fourth sacral nerve, giving off the anococcygeal nerves.

cystic p. a nerve plexus near the gallbladder.

dental p. either of two plexuses (inferior and superior) of nerve fibres, one from the inferior alveolar nerve, situated around the roots of the lower teeth, and the other from the superior alveolar nerve, situated around the roots of the upper teeth.

lumbar p. one formed by the ventral branches of the second to fifth lumbar nerves in the psoas major muscle (the branches of the first lumbar nerve often are included).

lumbosacral p. the lumbar and sacral plexuses considered together, because of their continuous nature.

myenteric p. a nerve plexus situated in the muscular layers of the intestines.

nerve p. a plexus composed of intermingled nerve fibres.

pampiniform p. 1. a plexus of veins from the testis and the epididymis, constituting part of the spermatic cord. 2. a plexus of ovarian veins in the broad ligament of the uterus.

sacral p. a plexus arising from the ventral branches of the last two lumbar and first four sacral spinal nerves.

solar p. a network of ganglia and nerves supplying the abdominal viscera (see also SOLAR PLEXUS); called also coeliac plexus.

tympanic p. a network of nerve fibres supplying the mucous lining of the tympanum, mastoid air cells, and pharyngotympanic tube.

plica (ˈpliekə) pl. *plicae* [L.] a ridge or fold.

plicate (ˈpliekayt) plaited or folded.

plication (plieˈkayshən) the taking of tucks in a structure to shorten it; a folding.

plicotomy (plieˈkotəmee) surgical division of the posterior fold of the tympanic membrane.

plombage (plomˈbahzh) [Fr.] the packing of a cavity with inert material.

plug (plug) an obstructing mass.

epithelial p. mass of ectodermal cells that temporarily closes the external nares of the fetus.

mucous p. a plug formed by secretions of the mucous glands of the cervix uteri and closing the cervical canal during pregnancy. Called also OPERCULUM.

plumbic (ˈplumbik) pertaining to lead.

plumbism (ˈplumbizəm) a chronic form of poisoning caused by absorption of lead or lead salts (see also LEAD POISONING).

plumbum (ˈplumbəm) [L.] *lead* (symbol Pb).

Plummer–Vinson syndrome (ˌpluməˈvinsən) dysphagia with iron deficiency anaemia, and its associated tissue changes, such as glossitis. Difficulty in swallowing is caused by a fibrous band (web) in the postcricoid region of the oesophagus. Also called Paterson–Kelly syndrome.

pluri- word element. [L.] *many*.

pluriglandular (ˌplooə·riˈglandyuhlə) pertaining to several glands or their secretions.

plurilocular (ˌplooə·riˈlokyuhlə) multilocular; having many cells or compartments.

pluripotentiality (ˌplooə·ripəˌtenshiˈalitee) ability to develop in any one of several different ways, or to affect more than one organ or tissue. adj. **pluripotent, pluripotential**.

plutonium (plooˈtohni·əm) a chemical element, atomic number 94, atomic weight 242, symbol Pu. See table of elements in Appendix 2.

Pm chemical symbol, *promethium*.

PMRAFNS Princess Mary's Royal Air Force Nursing Service.

pneo- word element. [Gr.] *breath*, *breathing*.

pneum(o)- word element. [Gr.] *air* or *gas*, *lung*.

pneumarthrogram (ˌnyooˈmahthrohˌgram) a film obtained by pneumarthrography.

pneumarthrography (ˌnyoomahˈthrogrəfee) radiology of a joint after it has been injected with air as a contrast medium; pneumoarthrography.

pneumarthrosis (ˌnyoomahˈthrohsis) gas or air in a joint.

pneumat(o)- word element. [Gr.] *air* or *gas,lung*.

pneumatic (nyooˈmatik) pertaining to air or respiration.

pneumatization (ˌnyoomətie'zayshən) the formation of air cavities in tissue, especially such formation in the temporal bone.

pneumatocele (nyoo'matohˌseel) 1. hernia of lung tissue. 2. a usually benign, thin-walled, air-containing cyst of the lung. 3. a tumour or sac containing gas, especially a gaseous swelling of the scrotum.

pneumatorrhachis (ˌnyoomə'to·rəkis) the presence of gas in the vertebral canal.

pneumatosis (ˌnyoomə'tohsis) air or gas in an abnormal location in the body.

p. coli a condition marked by accumulation of gas under the tunica serosa of the intestine.

p. cystoides intestinalis a condition characterized by the presence of thin-walled, gas-containing cysts in the wall of the intestines.

pneumaturia (ˌnyoomə'tyooə·ri·ə) gas or air in the urine.

pneumectomy (nyoo'mektəmee) pneumonectomy.

pneumoangiogram (ˌnyoomoh'anjiohˌgram) a composite of radiographs obtained by pneumoencephalography and cerebral angiography.

pneumoarthrography (ˌnyoomohah'throgrəfee) radiology of a joint after injection of air or gas as a contrast medium; pneumarthrography.

pneumocephalus (ˌnyoomoh'kefələs, -'sef-) air in the intracranial cavity.

pneumococcaemia (ˌnyoomohkok'seemi·ə) pneumococci in the blood.

pneumococcidal (ˌnyoomohkok'sied'l) destroying pneumococci.

pneumococcosis (ˌnyoomohko'kohsis) infection with pneumococci.

pneumococcosuria (ˌnyoomohˌkokoh'syooə·ri·ə) pneumococci in the urine.

pneumococcus (ˌnyoomoh'kokəs) pl. *pneumococci;* an individual organism of the species *Streptococcus pneumoniae*, which is the commonest cause of lobar pneumonia; it is a small, slightly elongated, encapsulated coccus, one end of which is pointed or lance-shaped, and commonly occurs in pairs; 80 serological strains or types have been differentiated. adj. **pneumococcal**.

pneumoconiosis (ˌnyoomohˌkohni'ohsis, -ˌkon-) any of a group of lung diseases resulting from inhalation of particles of industrial substances, such as the dust of iron ore or coal, and permanent deposition of substantial amounts of such particles in the lungs. The diseases vary in severity but all are occupational diseases, acquired by workers in the course of their jobs.

Symptoms of the pneumoconioses include shortness of breath, chronic cough, and expectoration of mucus containing the offending particles.

SILICOSIS is probably the best known and most severe of these diseases. Asbestosis, caused by inhalation of asbestos fibres, is probably second only to silicosis in severity. Prevention and early diagnosis are important, for no effective treatment is available. Anthracosilicosis is caused by the inhalation of coal dust and silica and is similar in its development and its effects to silicosis. Beryllium lung disease or berylliosis is found in workers exposed to beryllium in the manufacture of fluorescent lamps, and in members of their families who are contaminated by the chemicals in the worker's clothing. Other types of pneumoconiosis include aluminium pneumoconiosis, cadmium worker's disease, ANTHRACOSIS, and siderosis.

Pneumocystis (ˌnyoomoh'sistis) a genus of organisms of uncertain status, but considered to be protozoa. *P. carinii* is the causative agent of interstitial plasma cell pneumonia.

pneumoderma (ˌnyoomoh'dərmə) subcutaneous emphysema; air or gas in subcutaneous tissues.

pneumodynamics (ˌnyoomohdie'namiks) the dynamics of the respiratory process.

pneumoencephalogram (ˌnyoomoh·en'kefələˌgram, -'sef-) the film produced by pneumoencephalography.

pneumoencephalography (ˌnyoomoh·enˌkefə'logrəfee, -ˌsef-) radiological visualization of the fluid-containing structures of the brain after cerebrospinal fluid is intermittently withdrawn by lumbar puncture and replaced by air.

pneumoenteritis (ˌnyoomohˌentə'rietis) inflammation of the lungs and intestine.

pneumogastric (ˌnyoomoh'gastrik) pertaining to lungs and stomach.

p. nerve the tenth cranial nerve to the lungs, stomach, etc. The vagus nerve.

pneumography (nyoo'mogrəfee) 1. an anatomical description of the lungs. 2. graphic recording of the respiratory movements. 3. radiography of a part after injection of a gas.

pneumohaemopericardium (ˌnyoomohˌheemohˌperi'kahdi·əm) air or gas and blood in the pericardium.

pneumohaemothorax (ˌnyoomohˌheemoh'thor·raks) gas or air and blood in the pleural cavity.

pneumohydrometra (ˌnyoomohˌhiedroh'meetrə) gas and fluid in the uterus.

pneumohydropericardium (ˌnyoomohˌhiedrohˌperi'kahdi·əm) air or gas with fluid in the pericardium.

pneumohydrothorax (ˌnyoomohˌhiedroh'thor·raks) air or gas with fluid in the thoracic cavity.

pneumolith ('nyoomohˌlith) a pulmonary concretion.

pneumolithiasis (ˌnyoomohli'thieəsis) the presence of concretions in the lungs.

pneumolysis (nyoo'molisis) the operation of detaching the pleura from the chest wall in order to collapse the lung when the two pleural layers are adherent. Called also *pleurolysis*.

pneumomediastinum (ˌnyoomohˌmeedi·ə'stienəm) the presence of air or gas in tissues of the mediastinum, occurring pathologically or introduced intentionally.

pneumomycosis (ˌnyoomohmie'kohsis) any fungal disease of the lungs.

pneumomyelography (ˌnyoomohˌmieə'logrəfee) radiography of the spinal canal after withdrawal of cerebrospinal fluid and injection of air or gas.

pneumonectomy (ˌnyoomə'nektəmee) excision of part of or an entire lung. See also surgery of the LUNG.

pneumonia (nyoo'mohni·ə) inflammation of the lung with consolidation and exudation. Pneumonia was once a common cause of death and killed one out of four victims. It is still a serious disease, especially in infants and the elderly, who are most vulnerable. In spite of the advent of antibiotic therapy in the 1940s and a reduction in the mortality rate for all infectious diseases, pneumonia currently accounts for about 15,000 deaths in NHS hospitals in England and Wales (OCPS, 1984) each year.

TYPES AND SYMPTOMS. Infectious pneumonia may be caused by either bacteria or viruses. It may be primary or secondary (a complication of another disease) and may involve one or both lungs. It is most frequently caused by the pneumococcus (*Streptococcus pneumoniae*), which is responsible for 90 per cent of all bacterial pneumonias. Other causative agents are staphylococci and gram-negative enteric bacilli. The microorganisms that give rise to pneumonia are always present in the upper respiratory tract. They cause no harm unless resistance is severely lowered by some other factor, such as a severe cold, disease, alcoholism, or general poor health. Age is also a factor. When resistance is lowered or the conditions are favourable, the infectious agents invade the lungs.

Lobar Pneumonia. Pneumonia that affects a segment or an entire lobe of the lung is called lobar pneumonia. When both lungs are affected, the disease is called bilateral, or double, pneumonia. Whole sections of the lung tissue become solidified by inflammatory material, so that air cannot enter the alveoli. A chest radiograph is usually made to confirm the diagnosis and determine the extent of the disease.

Lobar pneumonia strikes suddenly. The symptoms are a cough, sharp chest pains (due to accompanying PLEURISY), blood-streaked or brownish sputum, and a high fever that generally starts with a chill. Pulse and respiration increase to almost twice their normal rates.

Bronchial Pneumonia (Bronchopneumonia). Bronchopneumonia is a less dramatic form of pneumonia that is more prevalent than lobar pneumonia. The area affected is usually smaller than in the lobar type. The inflammation is localized in or around the bronchi, and causes the lung to be spotted with clusters of infected tissue. The symptoms appear gradually and are usually milder than in lobar pneumonia. The temperature rises more slowly and does not go as high, and there is no crisis as in lobar pneumonia.

Bronchopneumonia is rarely fatal except in patients with heart disease or other complications. It is often more difficult to treat, however; relapses are common and can be serious. Diagnosis is also more difficult because the causes are varied.

Staphylococcal pneumonia is a very serious form of the disease and is occasionally fatal.

Primary Atypical Pneumonia. This type of pneumonia occurs chiefly in young adults who are otherwise healthy. It is often found in military camps and is due to various viruses or to *Mycoplasma pneumoniae.*

In the past this type of pneumonia often went undetected. The symptoms are similar to those of a cold. There may be headache, fever, a dry cough, generalized aches, and a feeling of extreme fatigue. Radiographic examination of the lungs will reveal evidence of infection.

Other Types. Other kinds of pneumonia are caused by inhalation of poisonous gases (chemical pneumonia), accidental inhalation of food or liquids while unconscious (aspiration pneumonia), a blow or injury to the chest that interferes with normal respiration (traumatic pneumonia), or inhalation of oily substances (lipid or lipoid pneumonia). Hypostatic pneumonia, which is due to lying on the back, frequently occurs in elderly bedridden patients. Interstitial pneumonia is a chronic form in which there is an increase of the interstitial tissue and a decrease of the proper lung tissue, with induration.

PREVENTION. Many debilitated and elderly patients are prime candidates for the development of pneumonia, as are those who are physically inactive and immobile and those who suffer from acute and chronic pulmonary disease. It is possible to prevent pneumonia in many susceptible persons by being aware of factors that predispose one to the disease and by taking precautionary measures.

In the postoperative period it is important to position the patient properly and watch him closely while he is recovering from anaesthesia so that he does not aspirate vomitus or other material into his lungs. The same precautions are essential for all patients in varying stages of unconsciousness and coma and in those who have poorly functioning gag reflexes. Early ambulation is another preventive measure to be used in postoperative and postpartal patients unless contraindicated. All patients who are immobilized for any reason should be turned regularly to avoid hypostatic pneumonia. Oversedation and overenthusiastic use of cough depressants can make a person more susceptible to pneumonia. The infectious agents that can cause pneumonia must be considered a constant hazard; vigorous adherence to the principles of cleanliness and personal hygiene are necessary to avoid the introduction of these agents into the respiratory tract of the susceptible person.

A vaccine can provide protection for three to five years in 80 per cent of vaccinated persons. Those who can benefit most from a pneumonia vaccine are the elderly; persons suffering from chronic disorders of the lungs, heart, liver, or kidneys; patients with poorly controlled diabetes mellitus; and those whose immune system has been impaired by disease or the loss of a spleen.

PATIENT CARE. Rest is of primary importance in assisting the body to combat the infection and in preventing unnecessary strain on the lungs and respiratory system. The fever presents problems of dehydration. Fluids are given frequently by mouth, or intravenously if necessary. An accurate record must be kept of the patient's intake and output. Bowel elimination must be checked regularly since the peristaltic action of the intestines may be affected in severe pneumonia. Delirium is not uncommon because of the high fever and requires careful observation of the patient and measures to prevent self-injury (see also DELIRIUM).

Mouth care is given regularly to combat dryness and cracking of the lips, which occur as a result of fever and dehydration.

To relieve the chest pain caused by PLEURISY in pneumonia, it may help to have the patient lie on the affected side so that the side is splinted during coughing episodes. It is also helpful to place the hands on the patient's chest and apply pressure as a means of splinting the chest as the patient coughs.

The temperature, pulse, and respiration are checked and recorded at least every 4 hours. When the temperature falls the patient usually perspires profusely, requiring frequent changing of clothing and bed linen. He must be protected from drafts and kept warm during this time.

p. alba a fatal desquamative pneumonia of the newborn due to congenital syphilis, with fatty degeneration of the lungs, which appear pale and virtually airless.

desquamative p. chronic pneumonia with hardening of the fibrous exudate and proliferation of the interstitial tissue and epithelium.

desquamative interstitial p. chronic pneumonia with desquamation of large alveolar cells and thickening of the walls of distal air passages; marked by dyspnoea and nonproductive cough.

Friedländer's p., Friedländer's bacillus p. a form characterized by massive mucoid inflammatory exudates in a lobe of the lung, due to *Klebsiella pneumoniae.*

influenzal p., influenza virus p. an acute, severe, usually fatal disease due to influenza virus, with high fever, prostration, sore throat, aching pains, profound dyspnoea and anxiety, and massive oedema and consolidation. The term is also applied to influenza complicated by bacterial pneumonia.

interstitial plasma cell p. a form affecting infants and debilitated persons, including those receiving certain drugs, in which cellular detritus containing plasma cells appears in lung tissue; it is caused by *Pneumocystis carinii.*

rheumatic p. a rare, usually fatal complication of acute rheumatic fever, characterized by extensive pulmonary consolidation and rapidly progressive functional deterioration and by alveolar exudate, interstitial infiltrates, and necrotizing arteritis.

varicella p. that developing after the skin eruption in varicella (chickenpox) and apparently due to the same virus; symptoms may be severe, with violent cough, haemoptysis, and severe chest pain.

pneumonic (nyoo'monik) pertaining to the lung or to pneumonia.

p. plague a form of PLAGUE with extensive involvement of the lungs.

pneumonitis (,nyoomə'nietis) inflammation of lung tissue.

pneumono- word element. [Gr.] *lung*.

pneumonocentesis (,nyoomənohsen'teesis) surgical puncture of a lung for aspiration.

pneumonocyte (nyoo'monoh,siet) collective term for the alveolar epithelial cells (great alveolar cells and squamous alveolar cells) and alveolar phagocytes of the lungs.

pneumonolysis (,nyoomə'nolisis) pneumolysis.

pneumonopathy (,nyoomə'nopəthee) any lung disease.

pneumonopexy ('nyoomənoh,peksee) pneumopexy.

pneumonorrhaphy (,nyoomə'no·rəfee) pneumorrhaphy.

pneumonosis (,nyoomə'nohsis) any lung disease.

pneumonotomy (,nyoomə'notəmee) pneumotomy.

pneumopericardium (,nyoomoh,peri'kahdi·əm) the presence of air or gas in the pericardial cavity.

pneumoperitoneum (,nyoomoh,peritə'neeəm) the presence of air or gas in the peritoneal cavity, occurring pathologically or introduced intentionally.

pneumoperitonitis (,nyoomoh,peritə'nietis) peritonitis with accumulation of air or gas in the peritoneal cavity.

pneumopexy (,nyoomoh'peksee) fixation of the lung to the thoracic wall.

pneumopleuritis (,nyoomohplooə'rietis) inflammation of the lungs and pleura.

pneumopyopericardium (,nyoomoh,pieoh,peri'kahdi·əm) air or gas and pus in the pericardium.

pneumopyothorax (,nyoomoh,pieoh'thor·raks) air or gas and pus in the pleural cavity.

pneumoradiogrphy (,nyoomoh,raydi'ografee) radiography of a part after injection of oxygen or other gas as contrast material.

pneumoretroperitoneum (,nyoomoh,retroh,peritə'neeəm) the presence of air or gas in the retroperitoneal space.

pneumorrhagia (,nyoomə'rayji·ə) haemorrhage from the lungs; severe haemoptysis.

pneumorrhapy (,nyoo'mo·rəfee) suture of the lung.

pneumotachograph (,nyoomoh'takə,grahf, -,graf) an instrument for recording the velocity of respired air.

pneumotachometer (,nyoomohta'komitə) a transducer for measuring expired air flow.

pneumotaxic (,nyoomoh'taksik) regulating the respiratory rate.

pneumotherapy (,nyoomoh'therəpee) treatment of disease of the lungs.

pneumothorax (,nyoomoh'thor·raks) accumulation of air or gas in the pleural cavity, resulting in collapse of the lung on the affected side. The condition may occur spontaneously, as in the course of a pulmonary disease, or it may follow trauma to, and perforation of, the chest wall. *Artificial pneumothorax* is a surgical procedure sometimes used in the treatment of tuberculosis or following pneumonectomy; it involves the injection of measured amounts of air into the pleural cavity to collapse the lung and immobilize it while healing takes place (see also surgery of the LUNG).

SPONTANEOUS PNEUMOTHORAX. This condition sometimes occurs when there is an opening on the surface of the lung allowing leakage of air from the bronchi into the pleural cavity. Most often it occurs when an emphysematous bulla or other weakened area on the lung ruptures. Normally the pleural cavity is an airtight compartment with a negative pressure. When air enters the pleural cavity the lung collapses, producing shortness of breath, and mediastinal shift toward the unaffected side (see also MEDIASTINAL SHIFT).

Other symptoms of spontaneous pneumothorax are a sudden sharp chest pain, fall in blood pressure, weak and rapid pulse, and cessation of normal respiratory movements on the affected side of the chest.

Spontaneous pneumothorax may require no specific treatment beyond bed rest and the administration of oxygen to relieve dyspnoea. The patient usually is more comfortable if he is allowed to sit up. In some cases THORACENTESIS and aspiration of air from the pleural cavity may be necessary. This allows for reexpansion of the lung. If air continues to leak from the defect in the lung surface a continuous closed-drainage apparatus is set up (see also CHEST drains). As soon as the lung lesion heals and the lung is reexpanded, the patient is allowed to resume his usual activities.

Tension pneumothorax is a particularly dangerous form of pneumothorax that occurs when air escapes into the pleural cavity from a bronchus but cannot regain entry into the bronchus. As a result, continuously increasing air pressure in the pleural cavity causes progressive collapse of the lung tissue. Emergency treatment—aspiration of air from the pleural cavity—is necessary in this disorder. If untreated, increased pressure within the pleural cavity will cause lung collapse and MEDIASTINAL SHIFT.

pneumotomy (nyoo'motəmee) incision of the lung.

pneumoventriculography (,nyoomohven,trikyuh'logrəfee) pneumoencephalography.

-pnoea word element. [Gr.] *respiration, breathing*. adj. **-pneic**.

PO [L.] *per os* (by mouth; orally).

Po chemical symbol, *polonium*.

pock (pok) a pustule, especially of smallpox.

pockmark ('pok,mahk) a depressed scar left by a pustule.

pod(o)- word element. [Gr.] *foot*.

podagra (pə'dagrə) gouty pain in the great toe.

podalgia (pə'dalji·ə) pain in the feet.

podalic (pə'dalik) accomplished by means of the feet, as podalic version.

podarthritis (,podah'thrietis) inflammation of the joints of the feet.

podencephalus (,poden'kefələs, -'sef-) a fetus without a cranium, the brain hanging by a pedicle.

podiatrist (po'dieətrist, -'deeə-) chiropodist; a specialist in podiatry.

podiatry (po'dieətree, -'deeə-) chiropody; the specialized field dealing with the study and care of the foot, including its anatomy, pathology, medical and surgical treatment, etc. adj. **podiatric**.

podium ('pohdi·əm) pl. *podia* [L.] a footlike process, such as an extension of the protoplasm of a cell.

podocyte ('podoh,siet) an epithelial cell of the visceral layer of a renal glomerulus, having a number of footlike radiating processes (pedicles).

pododynamometer (,podoh,dienə'momitə) a device for determining the strength of the leg muscles.

pododynia (,podoh'dini·ə) neuralgic pain of the heel

and sole; burning pain without redness in the sole of the foot.

podology (pə'doləjee) podiatry.

podophyllum (ˌpodoh'filəm) the dried rhizome and roots of *Podophyllum peltatum*.

p. resin a mixture of resins from podophyllum, used as a topical caustic in the treatment of certain papillomas.

pogoniasis (ˌpohgə'nieəsis) excessive growth of the beard, or growth of a beard on a woman.

pogonion (pə'gohni·ən) the anterior midpoint of the chin.

-poiesis word element. [Gr.] *formation*. adj. **-poietic**.

poikilo- word element. [Gr.] *varied*, *irregular*.

poikilocyte ('poykiloh,siet) an abnormally shaped erythrocyte.

poikilocythaemia (ˌpoykilohsie'theemi·ə) poikilocytosis.

poikilocytosis (ˌpoykilohsie'tohsis) the presence of poikilocytes in the blood.

poikiloderma (ˌpoykiloh'dərmə) a condition characterized by pigmentary and atrophic changes in the skin, giving it a mottled appearance.

poikilotherm ('poykiloh,thərm, poy'kiloh,thərm) an animal that exhibits poikilothermy; a cold-blooded animal.

poikilothermy (ˌpoykiloh'thərmee) the state of having a body temperature that varies with that of the environment. adj. **poikilothermal, poikilothermic**.

point (poynt) 1. a small area or spot; the sharp end of an object. 2. to approach the surface, like the pus of an abscess, at a definite spot or place.

p. A a radiological, cephalometric landmark, determined on the lateral head film; it is the innermost part of the concavity of the curved bony outline from the anterior nasal spine to the crest of the maxillary alveolar process.

auricular p. the centre of the opening of the external acoustic meatus.

p. B a radiological, cephalometric landmark, determined on the lateral head film; it is the most posterior midline point in the concavity between the infradentale and pogonium.

boiling p. the temperature at which a liquid will boil: at sea level, 100 °C, or 212 °F.

cardinal p's 1. the points on the different refracting media of the eye that determine the direction of the entering or emerging light rays. 2. four points within the pelvic inlet—the two sacroiliac articulations and the two iliopectineal eminences.

craniometric p's the established points of reference for measurement of the skull.

dew p. the temperature at which moisture in the atmosphere is deposited as dew.

far p. the remotest point at which an object is clearly seen when the eye is at rest.

fixation p. the point on which the vision is fixed.

freezing p. the temperature at which a liquid begins to freeze; for water, 0 °C, or 32 °F.

ice p. the temperature of equilibrium between ice and air-saturated water under one atmosphere pressure.

isobestic p. the wavelength at which two substances have the same absorptivity.

isoelectric p. (pI) the pH of a solution in which molecules of a specific substance, such as a protein, have equal numbers of positively and negatively charged groups and therefore do not migrate in an electric field.

jugal p. the point at the angle formed by the masseteric and maxillary edges of the zygomatic bone; called also jugale.

lacrimal p. punctum lacrimale.

p. of maximal impulse the point on the chest where the impulse of the left ventricle is felt most strongly, normally in the fifth costal interspace inside the mamillary line.

McBurney's p. a point of special tenderness in appendicitis, about 1–5 cm from the right anterior iliac spine on a line between the spine and the navel.

melting p. the minimum temperature at which a solid begins to liquefy.

near p. the nearest point of clear vision, the absolute near point being that for either eye alone with accommodation relaxed, and the relative near point that for the two eyes together with employment of accommodation.

nodal p's two points on the axis of an optical system situated so that a ray falling on one will produce a parallel ray emerging through the other.

pressure p. 1. a point of extreme sensibility to pressure. 2. one of various locations on the body at which digital pressure may be applied for the control of haemorrhage.

trigger p. a spot on the body at which pressure or other stimulus gives rise to specific sensations or symptoms.

triple p. the temperature and pressure at which the solid, liquid, and gas phases of a substance are in equilibrium. **Valleix's p's** tender points along the course of certain nerves in neuralgia; called also puncta dolorosa.

point source outbreak (poynt saws) see COMMON SOURCE OUTBREAK.

pointillage (ˌpwanhti'ahzh) [Fr.] massage with the points of the fingers.

poison ('poyzən) a substance that, on ingestion, inhalation, absorption, application, injection, or development within the body, in relatively small amounts, may cause structural damage or functional disturbance.

Corrosives are poisons that destroy tissues directly. They include the mineral acids, such as nitric acid, sulphuric acid, and hydrochloric acid; the caustic alkalis, such as ammonia, sodium hydroxide (lye), sodium carbonate, and sodium hypochlorite; and carbolic acid (phenol).

Irritants are poisons that inflame the mucous membranes by direct action. These include arsenic, copper sulphate, salts of lead, zinc, and phosphorus, and many others.

Nerve toxins act on the nerves or affect some of the basic cell processes. This large group includes the narcotics, such as opium, heroin, and cocaine, and the barbiturates, anaesthetics, and alcohols.

Blood toxins act on the blood and deprive it of oxygen. They include carbon monoxide, carbon dioxide, hydrocyanic acid, and the gases used in chemical warfare. Some blood toxins destroy the blood cells or the platelets.

See also POISONING and names of individual poisons.

poisoning ('poyzəning) the morbid condition produced by a poison. The poison may be swallowed, inhaled (as in CARBON MONOXIDE POISONING), injected by a stinging insect as in a BEE STING, or spilled or otherwise brought into contact with the skin.

SYMPTOMS. The symptoms of poisoning vary greatly according to the poison taken and the time that has elapsed. Some poisons cause no immediate symptoms. In general, poisoning should be suspected in the following instances: (1) a revealing odour such as alcohol on the breath; (2) discoloration of the mouth or lips; (3) evidence of eating leaves or wild berries; (4) severe pain or a burning sensation in the mouth and throat; (5) nausea or vomiting; (6) convulsions; (7) confusion or disturbance of sight; (8) unconsciousness or deep sleep; (9) sudden illness, when an open bottle or container of medicine or poisonous chemicals is found nearby.

FIRST AID. In all cases of poisoning, speed in treatment is an essential, but deliberate speed and calm thinking will avoid hasty decisions that may result in ineffective if not harmful treatment.

It is not advisable to force the victim to drink a large amount of water or other liquid in an effort to neutralize an ingested poison. This may only serve to increase absorption. The victim of an inhaled poison does require immediate removal to fresh air and artificial respiration to restore breathing. When the skin has been contaminated by a poison, immediate and repeated drenching of the area with cool water is necessary to remove the poison.

Supportive measures that can be beneficial to any poison victim include maintenance of an open AIRWAY, keeping the victim quiet (especially if he is likely to have convulsions, as in strychnine poisoning), and maintaining body heat to avoid SHOCK.

Swallowed Poisons. In general, the rule of thumb is to induce vomiting except under the following conditions: (1) if the victim has swallowed a corrosive poison, such as a strong acid or alkali, in which case there is severe pain, a burning sensation in the mouth and throat, and vomiting, (2) if the victim has swallowed a petroleum product, such as gasoline, kerosene, or cigarette lighter fluid, (3) if the victim has swallowed iodine or strychnine, and (4) if the victim has convulsions, is in a coma, or is unconscious.

The administration of an emetic, usually syrup of ipecac followed by a glass of warm water, is the best way to induce vomiting. If no ipecac can be obtained, the victim should be taken immediately to a hospital or doctor's surgery. Efforts to induce vomiting by putting a finger or a spoon at the back of the throat are usually not successful, but may be tried if no emetic drug is available. When induced vomiting is unsuccessful or undesirable, gastric LAVAGE is employed to remove the stomach contents and wash out the remaining poison.

Some poisons have a specific antidote that can effectively counteract the action of the poison or neutralize it. Activated charcoal is another product that should be kept in the households where small children live. It is an adsorbent that is given when there is no specific antidote or when the nature of the poison is unknown. This substance is given in doses of 10 times the estimated ingested dose of poison, mixing 2–4 tablespoons to an 8 ounce glass of water. It is given after the syrup of ipecac, but is not useful in alcohol and insecticide poisoning.

Inhaled Poisons. General first-aid treatment for poisoning by such gases as carbon monoxide, hydrocyanic acid, and methane consists of dragging or carrying the victim to fresh air and administering artificial respiration, if breathing is irregular or has stopped. The rescuer should be careful not to risk being overcome himself. In telephoning the hospital, police, or fire service for help, one should specify the nature of the accident so that the proper emergency equipment may be brought. The victim should be wrapped in blankets to maintain body temperature, and be kept quiet. If he has convulsions, he should be kept in a semidark room and care should be taken to avoid jarring him.

External Poisons. If the skin has been contaminated by a chemical, the poison should be washed off immediately with running water, and any contaminated clothing should be removed at the same time.

If the poison is in the eye, the eyelids should be held open while a gentle, continuous stream of water is poured into the eye.

PREVENTION OF POISONING. *In poisoning, prevention is far better than any treatment.* To prevent poisoning, the following precautions should be followed:

(1) Keep all medicines, household chemicals, and other poisonous substances locked up. There is no place 'out of reach of children'.

(2) Never transfer poisonous substances to unlabelled containers, or food containers such as milk or lemonade bottles, or cereal boxes.

(3) Never reuse containers of chemical products.

(4) Never store poisonous substances on the same shelves used for storing food. Confusion might be fatal.

(5) Never leave discarded medicines within the reach of children or pets. Pour contents down the drain or toilet or incinerator. Rinse the container.

(6) Always read the label before using any chemical product.

(7) Do not give or take medicines in the dark.

(8) Never tell children the medicine you are giving them is a sweet.

(9) When preparing infant feed formula at home, taste the ingredients. Never store boric acid, salt, or talcum near the formula ingredients.

In case of poisoning, information concerning antidotes and treatment can be obtained by telephone from the nearest Poison Control centre. There are several in the UK and other countries.

blood p. septicaemia.

food p. a group of acute illnesses due to ingestion of contaminated food (see also FOOD POISONING).

Poisson distribution ('pwasonh) a statistical equation of the distribution of rare events in time or place.

polarimeter (ˌpohlə'rimitə) a device for measuring the rotation of plane polarized light.

polarimetry (ˌpohlə'rimətree) measurement of the rotation of plane polarized light.

polarity (poh'laritee) the condition of having poles or of exhibiting opposite effects at the two extremities.

polarization (ˌpohlə·rie'zayshən) the production of that condition in light in which its vibrations are parallel to each other in one plane, or in circles and ellipses.

polarizer ('pohləˌriezə) an appliance for polarizing light.

polarography (ˌpohlə'rografee) an electrochemical technique for identifying and estimating the concentration of reducible elements in an electrochemical cell by means of the dual measurement of the current flowing through the cell and the electrical potential at which each element is reduced. adj. **polarographic.**

pole (pohl) 1. either extremity of any axis, as of a body organ. 2. either one of two points that have opposite physical qualities (electric or other). adj. **polar.**

cephalic p. the end of the fetus at which the head is situated.

frontal p. the most prominent part of the anterior end of each hemisphere of the brain.

occipital p. the posterior end of the occipital lobe of the brain.

pelvic p. the end of the fetus at which the breech is situated.

temporal p. the prominent anterior end of the temporal lobe of the brain.

poli(o)- word element. [Gr.] *grey matter.*

polio ('pohlioh) poliomyelitis.

polioclastic (ˌpohlioh'klastik) destroying the grey matter of the nervous system.

poliodystrophia (ˌpohliohdis'trohfi·ə) poliodystrophy.

p. cerebri a rare disease of young children, marked by neuron degeneration of the cerebral cortex and elsewhere, with progressive mental deterioration, motor disturbances, sometimes cortical deafness and blindness, and early death. Called also Alper's disease.

poliodystrophy (ˌpohlioh'distrəfee) atrophy of the cerebral grey matter.

polioencephalitis (ˌpohlioh·enˌkefə'lietis, -ˌsef-) inflammatory disease of the grey matter of the brain.

inferior p. bulbar paralysis.

polioencephalomeningomyelitis (ˌpohlioh·enˌkefəlohməˌning·gohˌmieə'lietis, -ˌsef-) inflammation of the grey matter of the brain and spinal cord and of the meninges.

polioencephalomyelitis (ˌpolioh·enˌkefəlohˌmieə'lietis, -ˌsef-) inflammation of the grey matter of the brain and spinal cord.

polioencephalopathy (ˌpohlioh·enˌkefə'lopəthee, -ˌsef-) any disease of the grey matter of the brain.

poliomyelitis (ˌpohliohˌmieə'lietis) an acute, notifiable, infectious viral disease that attacks the central nervous system, injuring or destroying the nerve cells that control the muscles and sometimes causing paralysis; called also *polio, infantile paralysis* and HEINE–MEDIN DISEASE. Paralysis most often affects the limbs but can involve any muscles, including those that control breathing and swallowing. Since the development and the use of vaccines against poliomyelitis, the disease has been virtually eliminated in Western countries, where vaccination rates are high, but is still common in many other parts of the world.

Poliomyelitis is a very serious disease, but it is not often fatal. Paralysis develops in about half of all patients with polio, and of these about half recover completely. Only a small percentage of patients have serious symptoms; many cases are so mild that they are undiagnosed and never reported.

There are three known types of poliovirus. Most paralytic cases are caused by type 1. Poliovirus is found in the throat of a patient for the first few days of the disease, and in his intestines for a longer period, sometimes as long as 17 weeks. The disease can spread by means of droplets of moisture from an infected person's throat but usually by the faecal–oral route. The infectious period is 7 or more days from the time of onset of the disease.

The poliovirus is short-lived, and cannot survive long in the air. The incubation period of polio is usually from 1 to 2 weeks, and occasionally as long as 3 weeks. Members of the family or other contacts may be carriers, but only for a short period of time.

SYMPTOMS. The early symptoms of polio include fever, headache, vomiting, sore throat, pain and stiffness in the back and neck, and drowsiness. In the nonparalytic type, the fever usually lasts about 7 days, and the stiffness fades away in 3 to 5 days. In paralytic polio, some weakness or paralysis of the arms or legs begins 1 to 7 days after the first symptoms. The first sign of bulbar polio, which affects the muscles of swallowing and breathing, is difficulty in swallowing, speaking, and breathing. This usually occurs in the first 3 days of the disease.

TREATMENT. There is at present no cure for polio; once the disease begins it must be allowed to run its course. Supportive care is important, however, and proper symptomatic treatment can reduce discomfort and prevent some crippling aftereffects. Applications of HEAT in the form of hot wet packs, DIATHERMY, warm baths in the form of HYDROTHERAPY, and gentle exercising can reduce pain caused by muscle spasms and prevent deformities. During the acute stage of the disease bed rest is essential and the patient is kept warm and quiet.

PREVENTION. The principal method of prevention is by vaccination. Two types of vaccine are available, inactivated poliovaccine (Salk) or Pol/Vac (Inact), given by injection, and attenuated oral poliovaccine (Sabin), or Pol/Vac (Oral).In the USA and the UK, trivalent Pol/Vac (Oral), that is containing all three types of attenuated poliovirus is used for the routine immunization of the population, although in several northern European countries Pol/Vac (Inact) is used. Pol/Vac (Inact) is available in the UK for persons in whom Pol/Vac (Oral) is contraindicated, for example during pregnancy.

The Departments of Health in the UK recommend that infants be given Pol/Vac (Oral) at 3 months, then 6–8 weeks later, then 4–6 months after that, with reinforcing doses on entry to and on leaving school (see also IMMUNIZATION and immunization schedule in Appendix 12). A single reinforcing dose is recommended for adults before travelling to areas where polio is endemic or if they live in a community that experiences an outbreak.

In the control of an outbreak of poliomyelitis, close contacts should be given Pol/Vac (Oral) after faecal specimens have been obtained for laboratory examination. The case or cases should normally be isolated until their stools are shown by laboratory tests not to contain poliovirus.

poliomyelopathy (ˌpohliohˌmieə'lopəthee) any disease of the grey matter of the spinal cord.

poliosis (ˌpohli'ohsis) premature greyness of the hair.

poliovirus (ˌpohlioh'vierəs) the causative agent of poliomyelitis, separable, on the basis of specificity of neutralizing antibody, into three serotypes designated types 1, 2, and 3.

Politzer's bag ('politsəz) a rubber bag attached to a pharyngotympanic catheter, for forcing air into the pharyngotympanic tube to clear it.

politzerization (ˌpolitsə·rie'zayshən) insufflation of the middle ear and the pharyngotympanic tube by a Politzer bag.

pollen ('polən) the male fertilizing element of flowering plants.

pollenosis (ˌpolə'nohsis) pollinosis.

pollex ('poleks) [L.] *thumb.*

pollinosis (ˌpoli'nohsis) an allergic reaction to pollen; hay fever.

pollution (pə'looshən) defiling or making impure, especially contamination by noxious substances.

polonium (pə'lohni·əm) a chemical element, atomic number 84, atomic weight 210, symbol Po. See table of elements in Appendix 2.

polus ('pohləs) pl. *poli* [L.] pole.

Pol/Vac (Inact) poliomyelitis vaccine, inactivated.

Pol/Vac (Oral) poliomyelitis vaccine, live (oral).

poly- word element. [Gr.] *many, much.*

polyadenitis (ˌpoliˌadə'nietis) inflammation of several glands.

polyadenosis (ˌpoliˌadə'nohsis) disorder of several glands, particularly endocrine glands.

polyaemia (ˌpoli'eemi·ə) excessive blood in the body.

polyaesthesia (ˌpoli·is'theesi·ə) a sensation as if several points were touched on application of a stimulus to a single point.

polyangiitis (ˌpoliˌanji'ietis) inflammation involving multiple blood or lymph vessels.

polyarteritis (ˌpoliˌahtə'rietis) a condition marked by multiple sites of inflammatory and destructive lesions in the arterial system.

polyarthralgia (ˌpoliah'thralji·ə) pain in several joints.

polyarthric (ˌpoli'ahthrik) polyarticular.

polyarthritis (ˌpoliah'thrietis) inflammation of several joints.

chronic villous p. chronic inflammation of the synovial membrane of several joints.

p. rheumatica rheumatic fever.

polyarticular (ˌpoliah'tikyuhlə) affecting many joints;

polyarthric.
polyatomic (ˌpoli·əˈtomik) made up of several atoms.
Polybactrin (ˌpoliˈbaktrin) trademark for combination preparations of polymysin, neomycin and bacitracin.
polybasic (ˌpoliˈbaysik) having several replaceable hydrogen atoms.
polychemotherapy (ˌpoliˌkeemohˈtherəpee, -ˌkem-) simultaneous administration of several chemotherapeutic agents.
polycholia (ˌpoliˈkohli·ə) excessive flow or secretion of bile.
polychondritis (ˌpolikonˈdrietis) inflammation of many cartilages of the body.
chronic atrophic p., p. chronica atrophicans, relapsing p. an acquired disease of unknown origin, chiefly involving various cartilages and showing both chronicity and a tendency to recurrence; it is marked by inflammatory and degenerative lesions of various cartilaginous structures.
polychromasia (ˌpolikrohˈmayzi·ə) 1. variation in the haemoglobin content of erythrocytes. 2. polychromatophilia.
polychromatic (ˌpolikrohˈmatik) many-coloured.
polychromatocyte (ˌpolikrohˈmatəˌsiet) a cell stainable with various kinds of stains.
polychromatophil (ˌpolikrohˈmatəˌfil) a structure stainable with many kinds of stains.
polychromatophilia (ˌpolikrohˌmatəˈfili·ə) 1. the property of being stainable with various stains; affinity for all sorts of stains. 2. a condition in which the erythrocytes, on staining, show various shades of blue combined with tinges of pink. adj. **polychromatophilic**.
polyclinic (ˌpoliˈklinik) a hospital and school where diseases and injuries of all kinds are studied and treated.
polyclonal (ˌpoliˈklohnəl) derived from different cells; pertaining to several clones.
polyclonia (ˌpoliˈklohni·ə) a disease marked by many clonic spasms; called also polymyoclonus.
polycoria (ˌpoliˈkor·ri·ə) more than one pupil in an eye.
polycrotism (pəˈlikrəˌtizəm) the quality of having several secondary waves to each beat of the pulse. adj. **polycrotic**.
polycyesis (ˌpolisieˈeesis) multiple pregnancy.
polycystic (ˌpoliˈsistik) containing many cysts.
p. ovary disease Stein–Leventhal syndrome.
p. renal disease a hereditary disease in which there is massive enlargement of the kidney with the formation of many cysts (see also polycystic KIDNEY disease). Severe bleeding into cysts can occur. End stage renal disease can affect many members of one family.
polycythaemia (ˌpolisieˈtheemi·ə) an increase in the total red cell mass of the blood.

There are two distinct forms of the disease. Primary polycythaemia (called also polycythaemia vera) is a myeloproliferative disorder of unknown aetiology. There is hyperplasia of the cell-forming tissues of the bone marrow, with resultant elevation of the erythrocyte count and haemoglobin level, and an increase in the number of leukocytes and platelets. Renal tumours may give rise to this picture and should be excluded.

Secondary polycythaemia is a physiological condition resulting from a decreased oxygen supply to the tissues. The body attempts to compensate for the oxygen deficiency by manufacturing more haemoglobin and red blood cells. Living at high altitudes can produce polycythaemia, as can severe chronic lung and heart disorders, especially congenital heart defects.

Absolute polycythaemia refers to an increase in red cell mass from any cause. Relative polycythaemia refers to a loss of plasma volume causing an elevated haematocrit.

SYMPTOMS. The symptoms of both primary and secondary polycythaemia are much the same. The increased erythrocyte production results in thickening of the blood and an increased tendency toward clotting. The viscosity of the blood limits its ability to flow properly, diminishing the supply of blood to the brain and to other vital tissues. This may cause mental sluggishness, irritability, headache, dizziness, fainting, disturbances of sensation in the hands and feet, and a feeling of fullness in the head. There may be episodes of acute pain as spontaneous clots occur in the blood vessels.

The spleen becomes enlarged. The smaller veins become more prominent, so that the skin has a bluish hue. The secondary form is often accompanied by enlargement of the tips of the fingers (clubbing).

GAISBÖCK'S DISEASE is a relative polycythaemia associated with hypertension.

TREATMENT. Treatment of polycythaemia vera is aimed at reducing the red cell count and decreasing the blood volume. Mild cases can be managed by periodic phlebotomy. More serious cases require myelosuppressive therapy with radioactive phosphorus or with cytotoxic alkylating agents, such as chlorambucil, melphelan, or busulphan.

In secondary polycythaemia, successful treatment of the causative illness will relieve the polycythaemia.
polydactylism, polydactyly (ˌpoliˈdaktiˌlizəm; ˌpoliˈdaktilee) the presence of supernumerary fingers or toes.
polydipsia (ˌpoliˈdipsi·ə) excessive thirst.
polydysplasia (ˌpolidisˈplayzi·ə) faulty development of several tissues, organs, or systems.
polyendocrine (ˌpoliˈendohˌkrin, -ˌkrien) pertaining to several endocrine glands.
polyethylene (ˌpoliˈethiˌleen) polymerized ethylene, $(CH\text{-}CH_2)_n$, a synthetic plastic material, forms of which have been used in reparative surgery.
p. glycol a polymer of ethylene oxide and water, available in liquid form (polyethylene glycol 300 or 400) or as waxy solids (polyethylene glycol 1540 or 4000), used in various pharmaceutical preparations as a water-soluble ointment base.
polygalactia (ˌpoligəˈlakshi·ə) excessive secretion of milk.
polygene (ˈpoliˌjeen) a group of nonallelic genes that interact to influence the same character with additive effect.
polygenic (ˌpoliˈjenik) pertaining to or determined by several different genes.
polyglandular (ˌpoliˈglandyuhlə) pertaining to or affecting several glands.
polyglycolic acid (ˌpoliglieˈkolik) a polymer of glycolic acid used as an absorbable suture material.
polygnathus (ˌpoliˈnathəs) a double fetus in which a parasitic twin is attached to the autosite's jaw.
polygram (ˈpoliˌgram) a tracing made by a polygraph.
polygraph (ˈpoliˌgrahf, -ˌgraf) an apparatus for simultaneously recording several mechanical or electrical impulses, such as blood pressure, pulse, and respiration, and variations in electrical resistance of the skin; popularly known as a lie-detector.
polygyria (ˌpoliˈjieri·ə) a condition in which there is more than the normal number of convolutions in the brain.
polyhedral (ˌpoliˈheedrəl) having many sides or surfaces.
polyhidrosis (ˌpolihiˈdrohsis) hyperhidrosis.
polyhydramnios (ˌpolihieˈdramnios) HYDRAMNIOS.
polyhydric (ˌpoliˈhiedrik) containing more than two hydroxyl groups.

polyinfection (ˌpoli·in'fekshən) infection with more than one organism.
polyleptic (ˌpoli'leptik) having many remissions and excerbations.
polymastia (ˌpoli'masti·ə) the presence of supernumerary mammary glands or nipples; pleomastia.
polymelus (po'liməlәs) an individual with supernumerary limbs.
polymenorrhoea (ˌpoliˌmenə'reeə) abnormally frequent menstruation.
polymer ('polimə) a compound, usually of high molecular weight, formed by combination of simpler molecules (monomers).
polymer fume fever ('polimə fyoom) an occupational disorder due to exposure to the products of combustion of polymers such as Teflon; the manifestations are quite similar to those of metal fume fever.
polymerase ('poliməˌrayz) an enzyme that catalyses polymerization.
polymeric (ˌpoli'merik) exhibiting the character of a polymer.
polymerization (ˌpolimə·rie'zayshən, pəˌlimə·rie'zayshən) the combining of several simpler compounds to form a polymer.
polymicrobial (ˌpolimie'krohbi·əl) marked by the presence of several species of microorganisms.
polymicrogyria (ˌpoliˌmiekroh'jieri·ə) a brain malformation marked by development of numerous microgyri.
polymorph ('poliˌmawf) a colloquial term for a polymorphonuclear leukocyte.
polymorphic (ˌpoli'mawfik) occurring in several or many forms; appearing in different forms in different developmental stages.
polymorphism (ˌpoli'mawfizəm) the quality of existing in several different forms.
balanced p. an equilibrium mixture of homozygotes and heterozygotes maintained by natural selection against both homozygotes.
polymorphocellular (ˌpoliˌmawfoh'selyuhlə) having cells of many forms.
polymorphonuclear (ˌpoliˌmawfoh'nyookli·ə) 1. having a nucleus so deeply lobed or so divided as to appear to be multiple. 2. a polymorphonuclear leukocyte.
polymorphous (ˌpoli'mawfəs) polymorphic.
polymyalgia (ˌpolimie'alji·ə) pain involving many muscles.
p. rheumatica an inflammatory disease of the elderly causing stiffness in shoulders and thighs and often associated with temporal arteritis. There is a risk of retinal artery and other intracranial vessel involvement and the condition is best treated with corticosteroids.
polymyoclonus (ˌpoliˌmieoh'klohnəs) 1. a fine or minute muscular tremor. 2. polyclonia.
polymyopathy (ˌpolimie'opəthee) any disease affecting several muscles simultaneously.
polymyositis (ˌpoliˌmieoh'sietis) inflammation of several or many muscles at once, along with degenerative and regenerative changes, and marked by muscle weakness out of proportion to the loss of muscle bulk.
polymyxin (ˌpoli'miksin) a generic term for antibiotics derived from various strains of *Bacillus polymyxa*, several closely related compounds being designated by letters.
polynesic (ˌpoli'neesik) occurring in many foci.
polyneural (ˌpoli'nyooə·rəl) pertaining to or supplied by many nerves.
polyneuralgia (ˌpolinyuh'ralji·ə) neuralgia of several nerves.
polyneuritis (ˌpolinyuh'rietis) inflammation of many nerves simultaneously.
acute febrile p., acute idiopathic p., acute infectious p., acute postinfectious p. an acute, rapidly progressive, ascending paralysis, beginning in the feet and ascending to the other muscles, often occurring after an enteric or respiratory infection (see also GUILLAIN-BARRÉ SYNDROME).
polyneuromyositis (ˌpoliˌnyooə·rohmieoh'sietis) inflammation involving the muscles and peripheral nerves, with loss of reflexes, sensory loss, and paraesthesias.
polyneuropathy (ˌpolinyuh'ropəthee) a disease involving several nerves.
erythroedema p. a condition occurring in infants, marked by swollen bluish red hands and feet and disordered digestion, followed by multiple arthritis and muscular weakness; called also acrodynia.
polyneuroradiculitis (ˌpoliˌnyooə·rohrəˌdikyuh'lietis) inflammation of spinal ganglia, nerve roots, and peripheral nerves.
polynuclear (ˌpoli'nyookliə) 1. polynucleate. 2. polymorphonuclear.
polynucleate (ˌpoli'nyookliayt) having many nuclei.
polynucleotide (ˌpoli'nyooklioh,tied) any polymer of mononucleotides.
polyodontia (ˌpoli'donshi·ə) the presence of supernumerary teeth.
polyoestradiol phosphate (ˌpoleeˌeestrə'dieol) a polymer of oestradiol phosphate havng oestrogenic activity similar to that of oestradiol; used in the palliative therapy of prostatic carcinoma.
polyonychia (ˌpolio'niki·ə) the presence of supernumerary nails.
polyopia (ˌpoli'ohpi·ə) visual perception of several images of a single object.
polyorchidism (ˌpoli'awkiˌdizəm) the presence of more than two testes.
polyorchis (ˌpoli'awkis) a person exhibiting polyorchidism.
polyorchism (ˌpoli'awkizəm) polyorchidism.
polyostotic (ˌpolio'stotik) affecting several bones.
polyotia (ˌpoli'ohshi·ə) the presence of more than two ears.
polyovulatory (ˌpoliˌovyuh'laytə·ree) discharging several ova in one ovarian cycle.
polyp ('polip) a mass with a stalk protruding from a mucous membrane or the skin, though sometimes sessile.They are usually an overgrowth of normal tissue, but sometimes polyps are true tumours—that is, masses of new tissue separate from the supporting membrane. Usually benign, they may lead to complications or eventually become malignant.

Polyps may develop from any mucous membrane: in the nose, ears, mouth, lungs, heart, stomach, intestines, urethra, uterus, and cervix.

Polyps are most commonly found in the uterus, where they may cause excessive menstrual flow and sometimes sterility. They are often removed by surgery.

Cervical polyps are more dangerous than uterine polyps since they are more likely to become malignant.

Nasal polyps grow in the nasal cavity or in the sinuses. They are produced by local irritation, sometimes as a result of an allergy. They are not dangerous, but if they grow large enough to extend into the nose, they sometimes cause stuffiness and headaches. It is necessary to treat the allergy or any other source of irritation responsible for the growth of polyps. If the polyps continue to be troublesome, surgery may be necessary.

Polyps occasionally occur on the gingiva between the teeth. Such polyps are more commonly known as epulides. Here again, the only problem is discomfort; they may easily be removed. Much the same is true of the raspberry-shaped polyp occasionally found in the ear.

Polyps in the stomach are rarer but more serious. A polyp can cause pain if the stalk is sufficiently long for the polyp to be drawn into the duodenum. Usually, however, no pain is felt. When stomach polyps are discovered, they should be removed by surgery. Although usually benign, they may become malignant in time.

Polyps also form in the intestines. Usually they appear there in middle age, but some infants are born with polyps in the large intestine. Multiple intestinal polyps may be a hereditary disorder. In most cases they cause no symptoms unless they become large enough to obstruct the intestine or become ulcerated so that they bleed. When they do, symptoms may include cramping pains in the lower abdomen, diarrhoea, and the passage of blood and mucus.

Whether or not they cause symptoms, intestinal polyps should be removed by surgery, since any one of them may become malignant. Although all causes of intestinal cancer have not yet been discovered, it is believed that polyps are often a contributing factor.

In males, polyps sometimes occur in the urethra, usually as the result of some disorder of the prostate. They are not likely to develop into cancer, but they may cause a discharge from the urethra and make urination difficult or frequent. They do not affect sexual potency or vigour. Although these polyps can be removed by surgery, they are more often removed by fulguration.

In women, a urethral polyp, or caruncle, is a small growth on the mucous membrane of the urethra. It may cause pain on urination, vaginal discharge, or bleeding. Caruncles are easily removed by fulguration.

polyparesis (,polipə'reesis) dementia paralytica.

polypathia (,poli'pathi·ə) the presence of several diseases at one time.

polypectomy (,poli'pektəmee) removal of a polyp.

polypeptidaemia (,poli,pepti'deemi·ə) the presence of polypeptides in the blood.

polypeptide (,poli'peptied) a compound containing two or more amino acids linked by a peptide bond; called dipeptide, tripeptide, etc., depending on the number of amino acids present.

polyphagia (,poli'fayji·ə) excessive ingestion of food.

polyphalangia, polyphalangism (,polifə'lanji·ə; ,polifə'lanjizəm) excess of phalanges in a finger or toe.

polypharmacy (,poli'fahməsee) 1. the administration of many drugs together. 2. administration of excessive medication.

polyphobia (,poli'fohbi·ə) abnormal fear of many things.

polyphrasia (,poli'frayzi·ə) morbid volubility.

polyplastic (,poli'plastik) 1. containing many structural or constituent elements. 2. undergoing many changes of form.

polyplegia (,poli'pleeji·ə) paralysis of several muscles.

polyploid ('poli,ployd) 1. characterized by polyploidy. 2. an individual or cell characterized by polyploidy.

polyploidy ('poli,ploydee) the state of having more than two sets of homologous chromosomes.

polypnoea (,polip'neeə) hyperpnoea.

polypodia (,poli'pohdi·ə) the presence of supernumerary feet.

polypoid ('poli,poyd) resembling a polyp.

polyporous (po'lipə·rəs) having many pores.

polyposia (,poli'pohzi·ə) ingestion of abnormally increased amounts of fluids for long periods of time.

polyposis (,poli'pohsis) the formation of numerous polyps.

familial p. a hereditary condition marked by multiple adenomatous polyps with high malignant potential, lining the intestinal mucosa, especially that of the colon, beginning at about puberty. Multiple intestinal polyps occur in Gardner's, Peutz–Jeghers, Canada-Cronkhite, and Turcot's syndromes.

polypous ('polipəs) polyp-like.

polyptychial (,poli'tiki·əl) arranged in several layers.

polypus ('polipəs) pl. *polypi* [L.] polyp.

polyradiculitis (,polirə,dikyuh'lietis) inflammation of the nerve roots.

polyradiculoneuritis (,polirə,dikyuhlohnyuh'rietis) acute infectious polyneuritis that involves the peripheral nerves, the spinal nerve roots, and the spinal cord.

polyribosome (,poli'riebə,sohm) a cluster of ribosomes connected with messenger RNA; they play a role in peptide synthesis.

polysaccharide (,poli'sakə,ried) a carbohydrate which, on acid hydrolysis, yields many monosaccharides.

polyscelia (,poli'seeli·ə) the presence of more than two legs.

polyserositis (,polisiə·roh'sietis) general inflammation of serous membranes, with effusion.

polysinusitis (,poli,sienə'sietis) inflammation of several sinuses.

polysome ('poli,sohm) polyribosome.

polysomia (,poli'sohmi·ə) doubling or tripling of the fetal body.

polysomus (,poli'sohməs) a fetus or infant exhibiting polysomia. adj. **polysomic**.

polysomy (,poli'sohmee) an excess of a particular chromosome.

polyspermia (,poli'spərmi·ə) 1. excessive secretion of semen. 2. polyspermy.

polyspermy (,poli'spərmee) fertilization of an ovum by more than one spermatozoon; occurring normally in certain species (physiological polyspermy) and sometimes abnormally in others (pathological polyspermy).

polystichia (,poli'stiki·ə) two or more rows of eyelashes on an eyelid.

polystyrene (,poli'stiereen) the resin produced by polymerization of styrol, a clear resin of the thermoplastic type, used in the construction of denture bases.

polysynaptic (,polisi'naptik) pertaining to or relayed through two or more synapses.

polysyndactyly (,polisin'daktilee) hereditary association of polydactyly and syndactyly.

polytenosynovitis (,poli,tenoh,sienoh'vietis) inflammation of several or many tendon sheaths at the same time.

polythelia (,poli'theeli·ə) the presence of supernumerary nipples.

polythiazide (,poli'thieə,zied) a diuretic and antihypertensive.

polytocous (po'litəkəs) giving birth to several offspring at one time.

polytomogram (,poli'tohməgrəm) the record produced by polytomography.

polytomography (,politə'mogrəfee) tomography of tissue at several predetermined planes.

polytrichia (,poli'triki·ə) hypertrichosis; excessive hairiness.

polyunsaturated (,poliun'satyuh,raytid) denoting a fatty acid, e.g., linoleic acid, having more than one double bond in its hydrocarbon chain.

polyuria (,poli'yooə·ri·ə) excessive excretion of urine.

polyvalent (,poli'vaylənt) multivalent; having more than one valency.

p. vaccine one prepared from more than one strain or species of microorganisms.

polyvinylpyrrolidone (,poli,vien'lpi'roli,dohn) PVP,

povidone.

Pompe's disease (pomps) glycogenosis (type II) in which the deficiency of the enzyme α-1,4-glucosidase results in generalized glycogen accumulation, with cardiomegaly, cardiorespiratory failure, and death. Children affected with this disease appear imbecilic and hypotonic. Called also generalized glycogenosis.

pompholyx ('pomfəliks) an intensely pruritic skin eruption on the sides of the digits or on the palms and soles, consisting of small, discrete, round vesicles, typically occurring in repeated self-limited attacks. Called also dyshidrosis and cheiropompholyx.

POMR Problem-Oriented Medical Record (see PROBLEM-ORIENTED RECORD).

pomum ('pohməm) pl. *poma* [L.] apple.

p. adami the prominence on the throat caused by thyroid cartilage; Adam's apple.

pons (ponz) 1. that part of the metencephalon lying between the medulla oblongata and the midbrain, ventral to the cerebellum (see also brain stem, under BRAIN). 2. any slip of tissue connecting two parts of an organ.

p. varolii pons (1).

Ponstan ('ponstan) trademark for a preparation of mefenamic acid, an analgesic and anti-inflammatory.

Pontiac fever ('ponti,ak) an influenza-like illness with little or no pulmonary involvement, caused by *Legionella pneumophila.* It is not life-threatening as is the pulmonary form known as LEGIONNAIRES' DISEASE. The name Pontiac fever comes from an outbreak of the disease in Pontiac, Michigan.

The syndrome appears within 2 to 3 hours of contact with an infected person and lasts 2 to 5 days. There is complete recovery without residual effects, whether or not any antibiotic therapy has been instituted.

ponticulus (pon'tikyuhləs) pl. *ponticuli* [L.] delicate plates of white matter passing across the anterior end of the pyramid, just below the pons. adj. **ponticular**.

pontine ('pontien) pertaining to the pons.

pontobulbar (,pontoh'bulbə) pertaining to the pons and the region of the medulla oblongata dorsal to it.

pontocerebellar (,pontoh,seri'belə) pertaining to the pons and cerebellum.

pontomesencephalic (,pontoh,mesenkə'falik, -sə-'falik) pertaining to or involving the pons and the mesencephalon.

popliteal (,popli'teeəl, pop'liti·əl) pertaining to the area behind the knee.

popliteus (,popli'teeəs, pop'liti·əs) the flat triangular muscle in the floor of the popliteal fossa. It medially rotates the tibia and helps to flex the knee.

POR Problem-Oriented Record.

poradenitis (,por·radə'nietis) inflammation of lymph nodes with formation of small abscesses.

porcine ('pawsien) pertaining to swine.

pore (por) a small opening on an epithelial surface, or a small communication between adjacent cavities.

porencephalia (,por·renkə'fayli·ə, -sə-) porencephaly.

porencephalitis (,por·ren,kefə'lietis, -,sef-) porencephaly with inflammation of the brain.

porencephalous (,por·ren'kefələs, -'sef-) characterized by porencephaly.

porencephaly (,por·ren'kefəlee, -'sef-) development or presence of abnormal cysts or cavities in the brain tissue, usually communicating with a lateral ventricle. adj. **porencephalic, porencephalous**.

porocele ('por·roh,seel) scrotal hernia with thickening of the coverings of the testes.

porokeratosis (,por·roh,kerə'tohsis) a hereditary dermatosis marked by a centrifugally spreading hypertrophy of the stratum corneum around the sweat pores, followed by atrophy. Also known as porokeratosis of Mibelli. adj. **porokeratotic**.

poroma (por'rohmə) a tumour arising in a pore.

eccrine p. a benign tumour arising from the intradermal portion of an eccrine sweat duct, usually on the sole.

porosis (por'rohsis) 1. formation of the callus in repair of a fractured bone. 2. cavity formation.

porosity (por'rositee) the condition of being porous; a pore.

porous ('por·rəs) penetrated by pores and open spaces.

porphin ('pawfin) the fundamental ring structure of four linked pyrrole nuclei around which porphyrins, haemin, cytochromes, and chlorophyll are built.

porphobilinogen (,pawfohbi'linəjən) an intermediary product in the biosynthesis of haem.

porphyria (paw'firi·ə) a genetic disorder characterized by a disturbance in porphyrin metabolism with resultant increase in the formation and excretion of porphyrins (uroporphyrin and coproporphyrin) or their precursors; called also haematoporphyria. Porphyrins, in combination with iron, form haems, which in turn combine with specific proteins to form haemoproteins. Haemoglobin is a haemoprotein, as are many other substances that are essential to normal functioning of the cells and tissues of the body.

Two general types of porphyria are known: erythropoietic porphyrias, which are concerned with the formation of erythrocytes in the bone marrow; and hepatic porphyrias, which are responsible for liver dysfunction.

The manifestations of porphyria include gastrointestinal, neurological and psychological symptoms, cutaneous photosensitivity, pigmentation of the face (and later of the bones), and anaemia with enlargement of the spleen. Large amounts of porphyrins are excreted in the urine and faeces.

Treatment of this condition has been primarily symptomatic and varies in its effectiveness. Photosensitivity may be controlled by avoiding exposure to light. Removal of the spleen is useful in some cases of the erythropoietic type of porphyria. Drug therapy includes the use of phenothiazines, chlorpromazine and promazine in particular. These drugs allay pain and nervousness and apparently allow a period of remission from symptoms. Corticotropin has been successful in some cases.

Patients with porphyria must not be given barbiturates, sulphonamides, alcohol, or chloroquine as these chemicals may precipitate or intensify attacks. It is recommended that patients with this disease carry with them at all times some means of identifying themselves as having porphyria so that in an emergency they will not be given a drug that may precipitate an attack, and possibly cause death.

acute intermittent p. hereditary hepatic porphyria manifested by recurrent attacks of abdominal pain, gastrointestinal dysfunction, and neurological disturbances, and by excessive amounts of δ-aminolevulinic acid and porphobilinogen in the urine; it is due to an abnormality of pyrrole metabolism, transmitted as an autosomal dominant trait.

erythropoietic p. porphyria in which excessive formation of porphyrin or its precursors occurs in bone marrow normoblasts; it includes congenital erythropoietic porphyria and erythropoietic protoporphyria.

hepatic p. porphyria in which the excess formation of porphyrin or its precursors is found in the liver; it includes acute intermittent porphyria, variegate porphyria, and hereditary coproporphyria.

variegate p., p. variegata hereditary hepatic porphyria characterized by chronic cutaneous manifestations, notably extreme mechanical fragility of the skin, particularly areas exposed to the sunlight, and by episodes of abdominal pain and neuropathy. There is typically an excess of coproporphyrin and protoporphyrin in the bile and faeces. It is transmitted as an autosomal dominant trait.

porphyrin ('pawfirin) any of a group of iron- or magnesium-free cyclic tetrapyrrole derivatives, occurring universally in protoplasm, and forming the basis of the respiratory pigments of animals and plants. Porphyrins, in combination with iron, form haems.

porphyrinuria (ˌpawfiri'nyooə·ri·ə) an excess of porphyrin in the urine.

port-wine stain ('pawtwien) naevus flammeus.

porta ('pawtə) pl. *portae* [L.] an entrance or gateway, especially the site where blood vessels and other supplying or draining structures enter an organ.

p. hepatis the transverse fissure on the visceral surface of the liver, where the portal vein and hepatic artery enter and the hepatic ducts leave. Called also portal fissure and transverse fissure.

portacaval (ˌpawtə'kayv'l) pertaining to or connecting the portal vein and inferior vena cava.

portal ('pawt'l) 1. an avenue of entrance; porta. 2. pertaining to an entrance, especially the porta hepatis.

p. circulation a general term denoting the circulation of blood through larger vessels from the capillaries of one organ to those of another; applied especially to the passage of blood from the gastrointestinal tract and spleen through the portal vein to the liver. See also CIRCULATORY SYSTEM.

p. of entry the pathway by which bacteria or other pathogenic agents gain entry to the body.

p. vein a short, thick trunk formed by the union of the superior mesenteric and splenic veins behind the neck of the pancreas; it ascends to the right end of the porta hepatis, where it divides into successively smaller branches, following branches of the hepatic artery, until it forms a capillary system of sinusoids that permeates the entire substance of the liver.

portio ('pawshioh) pl. *portiones* [L.] a part or division.

p. dura the facial nerve.

p. intermedia intermediate nerve.

p. mollis vestibulocochlear nerve.

p. vaginalis the portion of the uterus that projects into the vagina.

portogram ('pawtoh,gram) the film obtained by portography.

portography (paw'togrəfee) radiography of the portal vein after injection of opaque material.

portal p. portography after injection of opaque material into the superior mesenteric vein or one of its branches, the abdomen being opened.

splenic p. portography after percutaneous injection of opaque material into the substance of the spleen.

portosystemic (ˌpawtohsi'stemik) connecting the portal and systemic venous circulation.

porus ('por·rəs) pl. *pori* [L.] an opening or pore.

p. acusticus externus the outer end of the external acoustic meatus.

p. acusticus internus the opening of the internal acoustic meatus in the cranial cavity.

p. opticus the opening in the sclera for passage of the optic nerve.

-posia word element. [Gr.] *intake of fluids*.

position (pə'zizhən) 1. a bodily posture or attitude. 2. the relationship of a given point on the presenting part of the fetus to a designated point of the maternal pelvis; see accompanying table. See also PRESENTATION.

anatomical p. that of the human body, standing erect, with arms by the side and palms facing forward, used as the position of reference in designating the site of structures of the body or the direction of movements.

Positions of the fetus in various presentations

Cephalic presentation
Vertex – occiput the point of direction
- Left occipitoanterior (LOA)
- Left occipitotransverse (LOT)
- Left occipitoposterior (LOP)
- Right occipitoposterior (ROP)
- Right occipitotransverse (ROT)
- Right occipitoanterior (ROA)

Face – chin the point of direction
- Right mentoposterior (RMP)
- Left mentoanterior (LMA)
- Right mentotransverse (RMT)
- Right mentoanterior (RMA)
- Left mentotransverse (LMT)
- Left mentoposterior (LMP)

Breech or pelvic presentation
Complete breech – sacrum, the point of direction (feet crossed and thighs flexed on abdomen)
- Left sacroanterior (LSA)
- Left sacrotransverse (LST)
- Left sacroposterior (LSP)
- Right sacroposterior (RSP)
- Right sacroanterior (RSA)
- Right sacrotransverse (RST)

Incomplete breech – sacrum the point of direction
- Same designations as above, adding the qualifications footling, knee, etc.

batrachian p. a lying position of infants in which the lower limbs are flexed, abducted, and resting on the bed on their outer aspects, somewhat resembling the legs of a frog.

Bonner's p. flexion, abduction, and outward rotation of the thigh in coxitis. **Bozeman's p.** the knee–elbow position with straps used for support.

Brickner p. the wrist is tied to the head of the bed to obtain abduction and external rotation for shoulder disability.

decubitus p. that of the body lying on a horizontal surface, designated according to the aspect of the body touching the surface as dorsal decubitus (back), left or right lateral decubitus (left or right side), and ventral decubitus position (anterior surface).

froglike p. batrachian position.

genucubital p. knee–elbow position.

knee–chest p., genupectoral p. the patient rests on his knees and chest. The head is turned to one side, and the arms are extended on the bed, the elbows flexed and resting so that they partially bear the weight of the patient. The abdomen remains unsupported, though a small pillow may be placed under the chest.

knee–elbow p. the patient resting on his knees and elbows with his chest elevated.

lithotomy p. the patient lies on his back with the legs well separated, the thighs acutely flexed on the abdomen and the legs on the thighs. Stirrups may be used to support the feet and legs.

orthopnoeic p. the patient assumes an upright or semivertical position by using two or more pillows to support his head and chest from the recumbent position, or he sits upright in a chair. Used when the patient has difficulty in breathing except in the upright position (orthopnoea).

Rose's p. a supine position with the head over the table edge in full extension.

Sims' p. the patient lies on his left side with the left thigh slightly flexed, and the right thigh acutely flexed on the abdomen. The left arm is drawn behind the body with the body inclined forward. The right arm may be positioned according to the patient's comfort.

Trendelenburg's p. the patient lies on his back, on a plane inclined 45 degrees with the head lower than the rest of the body. The legs and knees are flexed over the adjustable lower section of the table or bed, which is lowered. The patient is well supported to prevent slipping.

positive ('pozətiv) having a value greater than zero; indicating existence or presence, as chromatin-positive or Wassermann-positive; characterized by affirmation or cooperation.

positive end-expiratory pressure in mechanical ventilation, a positive airway pressure maintained until the end of expiration; abbreviated PEEP. A PEEP higher than the critical closing pressure holds alveoli open until the end of expiration and can markedly improve the arterial Po_2 in patients with a lowered functional residual capacity (FRC), as in acute respiratory failure.

positron ('pozitron) the antiparticle of the electron. When a positron is emitted by a radionuclide it combines with an electron and both undergo annihilation, producing two 511 keV gamma rays travelling in opposite directions. This effect is used in positron emission TOMOGRAPHY (PET), a nuclear medicine imaging technique similar to the radiological technique computed tomography (CT), which produces a cross-sectional image of the distribution of radioactivity in a 'slice' through the subject a few centimetres thick. Because the most useful positron-emitting isotopes have very short half-lives, they must be produced in an on-site cyclotron and attached chemically to a tracer substance. This need for a cyclotron as well as a PET scanner makes the procedure expensive and it is currently available only in a few research centres. Useful positron-emitting isotopes used in PET are ^{15}O, ^{13}N, ^{11}C, ^{18}F, and ^{81}Rb.

posology (pə'soləjee) the science of dosage or a system of dosage. adj. **posologic**.

Possum ('posəm) Patient-Operated Selector Mechanism; a machine that can be operated with a very slight degree of pressure, or suction, using the mouth, if no other muscle movement is possible. It may transmit messages from a lighted panel or be adapted for typing, telephoning, or working certain machinery.

post- word element. [L.] *after, behind.*

post mortem (pohst 'mawtəm) [L.] *after death.*

post partum (pohst 'pahtəm) [L.] *after parturition.*

postauricular (ˌpohstor'rikyuhlə) located or performed behind the auricle of the ear.

postaxial (pohst'aksi·əl) behind an axis; in anatomy, referring to the medial (ulnar) aspect of the upper arm, and the lateral (fibular) aspect of the lower leg.

postbrachial (pohst'brayki·əl, -'brak-) on the posterior part of the upper arm.

postcapillary (ˌpohstkə'pilə·ree) a venous capillary.

postcava (pohst'kayvə) the inferior vena cava. adj. **postcaval**.

postcibal (pohst'sieb'l) postprandial; after eating.

postclavicular (ˌpohstklə'vikyuhlə) behind the clavicle.

postcoital (pohst'koyt'l, -'koh·it'l) after coitus.

postcommissurotomy syndrome (pohstˌkomisyooə'rotəmee) fever, chest pain, pleuritis, pericarditis, and pneumonia, occurring frequently in patients who have undergone mitral commissurotomy, and sometimes related to cytomegalic inclusion disease.

postconcussional syndrome (ˌpohstkən'kushən'l) constant headaches with mental fatigue, difficulty in concentration and insomnia that may persist after head injury.

postcordial (pohst'kawdi·əl) behind the heart.

postcornu (pohst'kawnyoo) the posterior horn of the lateral ventricle.

postdiastolic (pohstˌdieə'stolik) after diastole.

postdicrotic (ˌpohstdie'krotik) after the dicrotic elevation of the sphygmogram.

postencephalitic (ˌpohstenˌkefə'litik, -ˌsef-) occurring after or as a consequence of encephalitis.

postepileptic (ˌpohstepi'leptik) following an epileptic attack.

posterior (po'stiə·ri·ə) directed toward or situated at the back; opposite of anterior.

postero- word element. [L.] *the back, posterior to.*

posteroanterior (ˌpostə·roh·an'tiə·ri·ə) directed from the back toward the front.

posteroexternal (ˌpostə·roh·ek'stərn'l) situated on the outside of a posterior aspect.

posteroinferior (ˌpostə·roh·in'fiə·ri·ə) behind and below.

posterolateral (ˌpostə·roh'latə·rəl) situated on the side and toward the posterior aspect.

posteromedian (ˌpostə·roh'meedi·ən) situated on the middle of a posterior aspect.

posterosuperior (ˌpostə·rohsoo'piə·ri·ə) situated behind and above.

postganglionic (ˌpohstgang·gli'onik) distal to a ganglion.

postgastrectomy syndrome (ˌpohstga'strektəmee) see DUMPING.

posthepatitic (ˌpohst·hi'patik) occurring after or as a consequence of hepatitis.

posthioplasty ('pos·thioh,plastee) plastic repair of the prepuce.

posthitis (pos'thietis) inflammation of the prepuce.

posthumous ('postyuhməs) occurring after death.

p. birth one occurring after the death of the father, or by caesarean section after the death of the mother.

posthypnotic (ˌpohst·hip'notik) following the hypnotic state.

postictal (pohst'ikt'l) following a seizure.

postmaturity (ˌpohstmə'tyooə·ritee) overdevelopment, the condition of an infant after a prolonged gestation period. adj. **postmature**.

postmenopausal (ˌpohstmenə'pawz'l) after the menopause.

postmitotic (ˌpohstmie'totik) occurring after or pertaining to the time following mitosis.

postmortem (pohst'mawtəm) [L.] performed or occurring after death.

Care of the body after death (postmortem care) is an essential component of the total care of the patient and surviving family members and friends. Specific policies and procedures for postmortem care are a matter of hospital policy, local customs, cultural and religious ritual.

Physical care of the body is based on certain changes that take place at a fairly predictable rate, depending on body temperature at the time of death, and environmental temperature once death has taken place. The size of the body and the presence or absence of bacterial infection also influence these changes.

Rigor mortis is the first of these changes after cessation of circulation and respiration. Within two to four hours after death depletion of glycogen stores prevents synthesis of adenosine triphosphate (ATP). Without ATP the muscle fibres do not relax, resulting in rigid contraction of the fibres and immobilization of the joints. The rigor first occurs in the involuntary muscles and then involves the voluntary musculature, starting with the head and neck and descending gradually to the trunk and lower extremities. The process usually takes about 45 hours and continues for about 96 hours.

Another noticeable change is cooling of the body, which occurs rather rapidly once circulation stops and the heat-regulating centre in the brain no longer is functioning. This postmortem loss of body heat is called *algor mortis*.

Decomposition of the tissues begins almost as soon as blood supply stops. With the deoxygenation of haemoglobin, discoloration, or *livor mortis*, appears as mottled, reddened areas that can be mistaken for bruises, particularly in the extremities or other parts of the body where there is a pooling of blood. As deterioration of tissues continues and bacterial fermentation occurs the tissues soften and then liquefy. Refrigeration or some other method of cooling the body inhibits this process.

p. examination autopsy.

postnatal (pohst'nayt'l) occurring after birth.

p. period defined in law as a period of not less than 10 days and not more than 28 days after the end of labour, during which the continued attendance of a midwife on the mother and baby is requisite.

postoesophageal (ˌpohstiˌsofə'jeeəl) behind the oesophagus; retroesophageal.

postoperative (pohst'opə·rətiv) relating to the period following a surgical operation.

p. care care of the patient following a surgical procedure. Immediately after surgery the patient usually is transferred to a recovery room. This is a special unit within the operating theatre suite, designed to facilitate management of the patient recovering from anaesthesia, and staffed with personnel experienced in this type of patient care.

Immediately after surgery, the patient requires constant attendance. A patent AIRWAY must be maintained so that respiration is adequate and of normal character. An endotracheal tube and VENTILATOR may be used to assist the patient with respiratory difficulties. The skin is observed for colour, turgor, and dryness. A flaccid, parchment-like skin indicates dehydration; cold clammy skin may be symptomatic of shock, and cyanosis and local discoloration are indicative of oxygen deficiency as a result of an obstructed airway or impaired circulation. The pulse, respirations, and blood pressure are checked at least every 15 minutes; a record is kept of their quality, rate, and rhythm.

The position of the patient may be governed by the type of surgery performed, but ideally the patient should be placed on his side with a pillow to his back for support. The uppermost leg is slightly flexed to relieve tension on the abdominal muscles and may be supported with a small pillow. The side position allows for drainage of mucus or other material in the mouth and lessens the danger of aspirations of vomitus. During vomiting the head is kept turned to the side and suction is used as necessary to clear the air passages. The patient's position should be changed at least every 2 hours unless there is a contraindication. When repositioning the patient, all movements should be gentle and slow, as sudden overstimulation can cause a drop in blood pressure.

While the patient is awakening from anaesthesia the hospital personnel must use particular caution in their conversations and statements made about the patients in the unit. With his senses dulled and his reasoning hampered by drugs and anaesthesia, the patient may misinterpret the sounds and statements he hears. Noise must be kept at a minimum, voices should be kept low, and whispering is especially disturbing to the patient recovering from anaesthesia.

The patient should be called by name and repeatedly told where he is and that his operation is completed. Information will need to be repeated several times until the patient is fully conscious.

In many cases a catheter, nasogastric tube, or drainage tube is inserted during surgery. The purposes of these should be understood by the nurse and it is usually the nurse's responsibility to connect them to drainage and suction apparatus. Dressings around drainage tubes should be observed for excess drainage or bleeding and reinforced as necessary.

See also specific operative procedures (e.g., COLOSTOMY) and specific organs (e.g., surgery of the KIDNEY or LUNG). For complications that may arise during the postoperative period, see also SHOCK, HAEMORRHAGE, THROMBOSIS, EMBOLISM, and CARDIAC ARREST.

postoral (pohst'or·rəl) in the back part of the mouth.

postparalytic (ˌpohstparə'litik) following an attack of paralysis.

postpartum (pohst'pahtəm) [L.] occurring after childbirth, with reference to the mother.

p. haemorrhage bleeding from the birth canal following childbirth. It may be *primary*, which is defined as blood loss of 500 ml or more within 24 hours of delivery, or *secondary*, which covers bleeding occurring in the period after 24 hours of delivery until the end of the puerperium. Causes include retained placenta, lacerations, and infection.

p. pituitary necrosis necrosis of the pituitary during the postpartum period, often associated with shock and excessive uterine bleeding during delivery, and leading to variable patterns of hypopituitarism. Called also Sheehan's syndrome.

postprandial (pohst'prandi·əl) postcibal; after a meal.

postpuberal, postpubertal (pohst'pyoobə·rəl; pohst'pyoobət'l) after puberty.

postpubescent (ˌpohstpyoo'bes'nt) after puberty.

postradiation (ˌpohst·raydi'ayshən) following exposure to radiation.

postsphygmic (pohst'sfigmik) after the pulse wave.

p. interval, p. period the short period (0.08 second) of ventricular diastole, after the sphygmic period, and lasting until the atrioventricular valves open.

poststenotic (ˌpohst·stə'notik) located or occurring distal to or beyond a stenosed segment.

postsynaptic (ˌpohst·si'naptik) distal to or occurring beyond a synapse.

posttraumatic (ˌpohst·traw'matik) following injury.

postulate ('postyuhlət) anything assumed or taken for granted.

Koch's p's a statement of the kind of experimental evidence required to establish the causative relation of a given microorganism to a given disease. The conditions are: 1, the microorganism is present in every case of the disease; 2, it is to be cultivated in pure culture; 3, inoculation of such culture must produce the disease in susceptible animals; 4, it must be obtained from such animals, and again grown in a pure culture.

postural ('postyuhrəl) pertaining to posture or position.

p. drainage a technique in which the patient assumes one or more positions that will facilitate the drainage of secretions from the bronchial airways. The procedure utilizes the force of gravity to move secretions toward the trachea, where they can be coughed up more easily. See accompanying illustration.

The choice of position is based on radiological studies and auscultatory evidence of pooled secretions. Variations of the most effective position are adapted to the patient's general physical condition, his tolerance, and pulmonary status.

Before postural drainage is attempted the patient

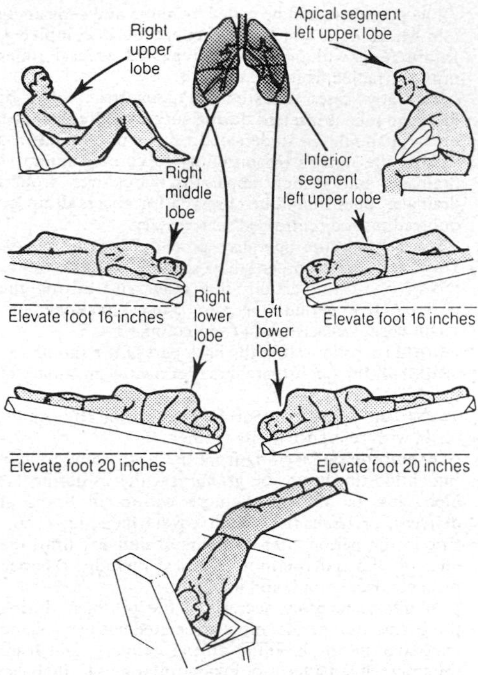

Postural drainage. Position for drainage of various portions of the lung. At bottom, a less specific position that is frequently used.

should understand and be able to perform diaphragmatic breathing and effective coughing. (See also CHRONIC OBSTRUCTIVE AIRWAYS DISEASE.) If he has difficulty in removing secretions, a suction machine should be on hand to remove secretions the patient cannot expectorate. When severe dyspnoea or exhaustion occur during the postural drainage the treatment should not be continued. Other contraindications are a full stomach (the procedure is never done immediately after a meal) and unstable vital signs. Mouth care is given after each treatment to remove the foul taste frequently accompanying removal of the stagnant mucus from the bronchial tree.

Percussion or 'clapping', and vibration are often done in conjunction with postural drainage. *Percussion* involves a rhythmic striking of the chest wall over the area being drained. It is done with the hands cupped; the fingers are flexed and the thumbs are held tightly against the index fingers. If done properly, a hollow sound is heard and there is no discomfort to the patient.

Vibration is done immediately after percussion and is directed to the same area. While the patient performs a prolonged exhalation through pursed lips, the therapist presses the flat of her hands against the thorax in a downward movement toward the midline of the body. This is repeated four or five times. While neither percussion nor vibration are difficult techniques to master, anyone attempting to assist the patient in this manner should have instruction and practice before attempting them. The purpose of both activities is to dislodge plugs of mucus, allowing air to penetrate behind them and thus aid in their removal.

posture ('poschə) an attitude of the body. Good posture cannot be defined by any rigid formula. It is usually considered to be the natural and comfortable bearing of the body in normal, healthy persons. This generally means that in a standing position the body is naturally, but not rigidly, straight, and that in a sitting position the back is comfortably straight.

Good standing and sitting posture helps promote normal functioning of the body's organs and increases the efficiency of the muscles, thereby minimizing fatigue. Good posture is also important to good appearance. Clothes fit better, movements become more graceful, and an impression of poise is achieved. See accompanying illustration.

Maintenance of good posture for a patient confined to bed or wheelchair is essential to the patient's general well-being and also is important in the prevention of deformities of the muscles and bones. The patient should be observed for evidence of 'slumping', in which the normal curves of the spine are exaggerated. The rib cage should be supported so that the ribs are elevated and there is no constriction of the chest wall. Pillows are arranged under the shoulders and head so that the chin is not forced downward on the chest. Excessive extension of the ankles should be avoided by adequate support against the soles of the feet. The legs should be supported so that the weight of one does not fall on the other. The arms are supported so that they do not lie across the chest or pull the shoulders into a 'rounded' position. Frequent changing of position and adequate exercise of the limbs are also essential to the maintenance of good posture and the prevention of deformities.

postuterine (pohst'yootə·rien) behind the uterus.

postvaccinal (pohst'vaksinəl) occurring after inoculation for smallpox.

potable ('pohtəb'l) fit to drink.

potassaemia (,potə'seemi·ə) hyperkalaemia.

potassium (pə'tasi·əm) a chemical element, atomic number 19, atomic weight 39.102, symbol K. (See table of elements in Appendix 2.) In combination with other minerals in the body, potassium forms alkaline salts that are important in body processes and play an essential role in maintenance of the acid–base and water balance in the body. All body cells, especially muscle tissue, require a high content of potassium. A proper balance between sodium, calcium, and potassium in the blood plasma is necessary for proper cardiac function.

Since most foods contain a good supply of potassium, potassium deficiency (hypokalaemia) is unlikely to be caused by an unbalanced diet. Possible causes include Cushing's syndrome (due to an adrenal gland disorder) and Fanconi's syndrome (the result of a congenital renal defect). The cause could also be an excessive dose of cortisone, prolonged vomiting or diarrhoea, or thiazide diuretics, which are administered for treatment of hypertension. Signs of potassium deficiency can include weakness and lethargy, rapid pulse, nausea, diarrhoea, and tingling sensations.

If the body absorbs enough potassium but the element is not distributed properly, various disorders may develop. Thus an abnormally low content of potassium in the blood may result in an intermittent temporary paralysis of the muscles, known as familial periodic paralysis.

Potassium deficiency can be treated by administration of potassium supplements. There are a large variety of these preparations. Some are liquids, some are powders to be dissolved in liquids, and some are

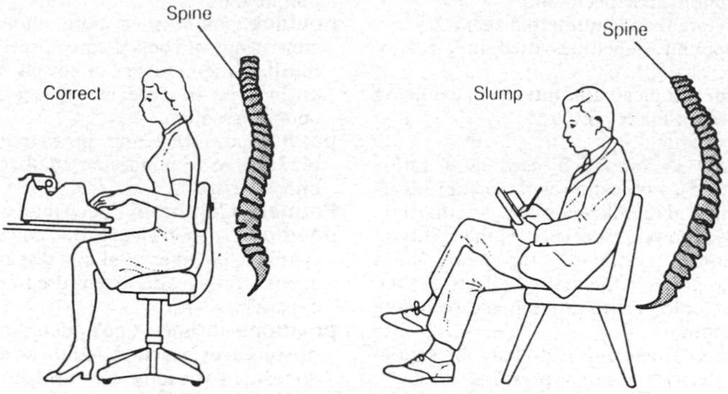

Left, good sitting **posture,** the spine and feet are in normal positions and the weight of the body is equally distributed. Right, slouching puts too much weight on the end of the spine, compresses internal organs, strains muscles and interferes with the circulation in the legs

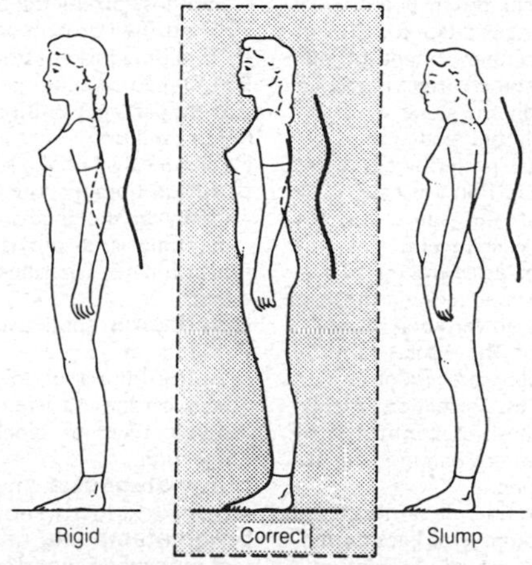

Correct standing **posture,** centre, is easy and natural. The chest is slightly raised and the buttocks are tucked in. Left, too-rigid posture. Keeping the spine unnaturally straight can cause strain on the knees and back muscles. Right, slumping can lead to backache and round shoulders

slow-release tablets that dissolve in the intestine. All can cause gastrointestinal irritation. For many persons on diuretic therapy for hypertension, potassium deficiency can be avoided by increasing their consumption of potassium-containing foods, such as bananas, dates, prunes, and raisins, and potassium supplements are not needed. Potassium supplements are never given to patients receiving potassium-sparing diuretics (amiloride, spironolactone, or triamterene). If the difficulty lies in the body's use of potassium, treatment is concerned with the primary cause of the deficiency.

Potassium excess (HYPERKALAEMIA) occurs in acute and chronic renal failure, after massive tissue breakdown (e.g., muscle crush injury, burns), in hypoadrenalism and may occur during treatment with potassium sparing diuretics. Hyperkalaemia is potentially dangerous by inducing changes in cardiac rhythm and can be treated by oral or rectal administration of ion-exchange resins, by intravenous glucose and insulin, and by long-term dietary restriction of potassium in chronic renal failure.

p. acetate a systemic and urinary alkalizer.

p. bicarbonate an electrolyte replenisher, antacid, and urinary alkalizer.

p. chloride a compound used orally or intravenously as an electrolyte replenisher.

p. citrate a diuretic, expectorant, and systemic alkalizer.

p. gluconate an electrolyte replenisher used in the prophylaxis and treatment of hypokalaemia.

p. guaiacolsulphonate an expectorant.
p. iodide an expectorant and antithyroid agent.
p. nitrite a compound sometimes used in place of potassium nitrate.
p. permanganate a topical anti-infective, oxidizing agent, and antidote for many poisons.
p. phosphate a cathartic.
p. sodium tartrate a compound used as a saline cathartic and also in combination with sodium bicarbonate and tartaric acid (Seidlitz powders, a cathartic).

potency ('poht'nsee) power; especially (1) the ability of the male to perform coitus; (2) the power of a medicinal agent to produce the desired effects; (3) the ability of an embryonic part to develop and complete its destiny. adj. **potent.**

potential (pə'tenshəl) 1. existing and ready for action, but not active. 2. electric tension or pressure.
action p. the electrical activity developed in a muscle or nerve cell during activity.
after-p. the period following termination of the spike potential.
membrane p. the electric potential that exists on the two sides of a membrane or across the wall of a cell.
resting p. the potential difference across the membrane of a normal cell at rest.
spike p. the initial, very large change in potential of an excitable cell membrane during excitation.

potentiation (pə,tenshi'ayshən) enhancement of one agent by another so that the combined effect is greater than the sum of the effects of each one alone.

potion ('pohshən) a large dose of liquid medicine.

Pott's curvature (pots) abnormal posterior curvature of the spine occurring as a result of Pott's disease.

Pott's disease tuberculosis of the spine, usually beginning as a tuberculous osteomyelitis of the vertebrae and progressing to damage of the intervertebral discs. If erosion continues unchecked, there is complete destruction of the affected vertebrae.

Symptoms include stiffness of the back, pain on motion, prominence of the spinous process of certain vertebrae, and occasionally abscess formation, paralysis, and abdominal pain. Diagnosis is confirmed by demonstration of *Mycobacterium tuberculosis* (the tubercle bacillus) in the affected bone.

Treatment includes administration of antibacterial drugs such as isoniazid and streptomycin. Para-aminosalicylic acid (PAS) may be used instead of streptomycin if streptomycin is contraindicated. Surgical fixation of the affected vertebrae (spinal fusion) may be required for correction of orthopaedic deformities such as KYPHOSIS (hunchback) which may occur as a result of Pott's disease.

Pott's fracture see Pott's FRACTURE.

pouch (powch) a pocket-like space, cavity, or sac, e.g., one formed by bending back of the peritoneum on the surfaces of adjoining organs.
abdominovesical p. the pouchlike reflection of the peritoneum from the abdominal wall to the anterior surface of the bladder.
Douglas' p. see DOUGLAS' POUCH.
Prussak's p. a recess in the tympanic membrane between the flaccid part of the membrane and the neck of the malleus.
Rathke's p. a diverticulum from the embryonic buccal cavity from which the anterior lobe of the pituitary gland is developed.
rectouterine p. Douglas' cul-de-sac.
Seesel's p. an outpouching of the embryonic pharynx rostrad to the pharyngeal membrane and caudal to Rathke's pouch.

poudrage ('poodrahzh) [Fr.] application of a powder to a surface, as done to promote fusion of serous membranes.

poultice ('pohltis) a soft, moist, mass about the consistency of cooked cereal, spread between layers of muslin, linen, gauze, or towels and applied hot to a given area in order to create moist local heat or counterirritation.

pound (pownd) a unit of weight in the avoirdupois (453.6 g, or 16 ounces) or apothecaries' (373.2 g, or 12 ounces) system.

Poupart's ligament ('poopahts) inguinal ligament.

povidone (poh'viedohn) polyvinylpyrrolidone, a synthetic polymer used as a dispersing and suspending agent; it has also been used as a plasma volume expander.

povidone-iodine (,pohvidohn'ieə,deen) a complex produced by reacting iodine with the polymer povidone; used as a topical anti-infective.

powder ('powdə) an aggregation of particles obtained by grinding or triturating a solid.
dusting p. a fine powder used as a talc substitute.

pox (poks) any eruptive or pustular disease, especially one caused by a virus, e.g., chickenpox, cowpox, etc.

poxvirus (poks'vierəs) any of a group of morphologically similar and immunologically related DNA viruses, including the virus of vaccinia (cowpox), smallpox, and those producing pox diseases in lower animals.

PPD purified protein derivative (tuberculin).

PPF plasma protein fraction; see PLASMA.

PPLO pleuropneumonia-like organisms.

p.p.m. parts per million.

PR per rectum.

Pr chemical symbol, *praseodymium.*

practice ('praktis) the exercise of a profession.
family p. the medical speciality concerned with the planning and provision of comprehensive primary health care, regardless of age or sex, on a continuing basis.

practitioner (prak'tishənə) a person who practices a profession.

practolol ('praktoh,lol) a drug used in the treatment of tachycardia and irregular heart rhythms. It is β-adrenergic receptor blocker and can only be given by injection.

pragmatagnosia (,pragmətag'nohzi·ə) inability to recognize formerly known objects.

pragmatamnesia (,pragmətam'neezi·ə) loss of power of remembering the appearance of objects.

pralidoxime (,prali'dokseem) a cholinesterase reactivator, whose salts are used in treatment of organophosphate poisoning; it also has limited value in counteracting carbamate-type cholinesterase inhibitors.

prandial ('prandi·əl) pertaining to a meal.

praseodymium (,praysioh'dimi·əm, -zioh-) a chemical element, atomic number 59, atomic weight 140.907, symbol Pr. See table of elements in Appendix 2.

Prausnitz–Küstner reaction (,prowsnits'koostnə) a local hypersensitivity reaction induced by intradermal injection into a normal person of serum from a hypersensitive individual; injection 24 hours later of the antigen to which the donor is allergic results in a wheal-and-flare response.

praxiology (,praksi'oləjee) the science or study of conduct.

prazosin ('prayzohsin) a postsynaptic α-adrenergic receptor blocker that acts as a peripheral vasodilator; used as an oral antihypertensive.

pre- word element. [L.] *before* (in time or space).

preagonal (pree'agənəl) immediately before the death agony.

preantiseptic (,preeanti'septik) pertaining to the time before the discovery of antisepsis.

preauricular (,preeor'rikyuhlə) in front of the auricle

of the ear.

preaxial (pree'aksi·əl) situated before an axis; in anatomy, referring to the lateral (radial) aspect of the upper arm, and the medial (tibial) aspect of the lower leg.

prebetalipoprotein (ˌpreebeetəˌlipoh'prohteen) very low-density lipoprotein.

prebetalipoproteinaemia (ˌpreebeetəˌlipohˌprohti'neemi·ə) hyperprebetalipoproteinaemia.

precancer (pree'kansə) a condition that tends to become malignant (see CANCER). adj. **precancerous**.

precapillary (ˌpreekə'pilə·ree) a vessel lacking complete coats, intermediate between an arteriole and a capillary.

precava (pree'kayvə) the superior vena cava. adj. **precaval**.

prechordal (pree'kawd'l) in front of the notochord.

precipitant (pri'sipitənt) a substance that causes precipitation.

precipitate (pri'sipiˌtayt) 1. to cause settling in solid particles of a substance in solution. 2. a deposit of solid particles settled out of a solution. 3. occurring with undue rapidity, as precipitate labour.

precipitation (priˌsipi'tayshən) the act or process of precipitating.

precipitin (pri'sipitin) an antibody to soluble antigen that specifically aggregates the macromolecular antigen in vivo or in vitro to give a visible precipitate.

p. reaction a reaction involving the specific serological precipitation of an antigen in solution with its specific antiserum in the presence of electrolytes. The reaction is used in the typing of pneumococcus strains, in testing whether blood is human or animal, and for diagnostic purposes.

precipitinogen (priˌsipi'tinəjən) a soluble antigen that stimulates the formation of and reacts with a precipitin.

preclinical (pree'klinik'l) before a disease becomes clinically recognizable.

precocity (pri'kositee) unusually early development of mental or physical traits. adj. **precocious**.

precognition (ˌpreekog'nishən) the extrasensory perception of a future event.

precoma (pree'kohmə) the neuropsychiatric state preceding coma, as in hepatic encephalopathy. adj. **precomatose**.

preconscious (pree'konshəs) not present in consciousness, but readily recalled into it; foreconscious.

preconvulsive (ˌpreekən'vulsiv) preceding convulsions.

precordia, precordium (pree'kawdi·ə; pree'kawdi·əm) the region over the heart and lower thorax. adj. **precordial**.

precostal (pree'kost'l) in front of the ribs.

precuneus (pree'kyooniəs) pl. *precunei* [L.] a small convolution on the medial surface of the parietal lobe of the cerebrum.

precursor (pri'kərsə) something that precedes. In biological processes, a substance from which another, usually more active or mature substance is formed. In clinical medicine, a sign or symptom that heralds another.

prediabetes (preeˌdieə'beetis, -teez) a state of latent impairment of carbohydrate metabolism in which the criteria for diabetes mellitus are not all satisfied.

prediastole (ˌpreedie'astəlee) the interval immediately preceding diastole. adj. **prediastolic**.

predicrotic (ˌpreedie'krotik) occurring before the dicrotic wave of the sphygmogram.

predictive value (pri'diktiv) a term used to mean the probability of a positive or negative test result being valid.

predigestion (ˌpreedie'jeschən, -di-) partial artificial digestion of food before its ingestion into the body.

predisposition (ˌpreedispə'zishən) a latent susceptibility to disease which may be activated under certain conditions.

prediverticular (preeˌdievə'tikyuhlə) denoting a condition of thickening of the muscular wall of the colon and increased intraluminal pressure without evidence of diverticulosis.

prednisolone (pred'nisəlohn) a glucocorticoid used as an anti-inflammatory and antiallergic agent.

prednisone ('predniˌsohn) a glucocorticoid used like prednisolone.

Predsol ('predzol) trademark for topical preparations of prednisolone, a glucocorticoid.

preeclampsia (ˌpree·i'klampsi·ə) a complication of late pregnancy, characterized by hypertension, albuminuria, and oedema, but without convulsions (see also ECLAMPSIA).

prefrontal (pree'frunt'l) 1. situated in the anterior part of the frontal region or lobe. 2. the central part of the ethmoid bone.

preganglionic (ˌpreegang·gli'onik) proximal to a ganglion.

pregenital (pree'jenit'l) antedating the emergence of genital interests.

pregnancy ('pregnənsee) the condition of having a developing embryo or fetus in the body, after union of an ovum and spermatozoon. See also CONCEPTION, OVULATION, REPRODUCTION.

The average pregnancy lasts about 266 days, or 38 weeks, from the date of conception to childbirth. Since the exact date of conception may not be known, the duration of the pregnancy (also known as the gestational age of the fetus) is calculated from the first day of the last normal menstrual period and is usually given in weeks. Measured in this way, the duration of the pregnancy is approximately two weeks greater than the length of time from conception, and so the length of the whole pregnancy is given as 280 days, or 40 weeks. The expected date of delivery (EDD) is calculated by taking the date of the first day of the last normal menstrual period and adding 9 months and 7 days. However, this is only an approximate calculation since pregnancy may be shorter or longer than the average. Adjustment is needed if the woman's normal menstrual cycle is not 28 days and regular. Ultrasonic scan is usually used to confirm gestation and the EDD where necessary.

GROWTH OF THE FETUS. The stages of growth of the fetus are fairly well defined. At a gestational age of 4 weeks implantation has occurred and the embryo has grown beyond microscopic size. By 8 weeks, the fetus is 2–2.5 cm long, its face is formed, and its limbs are partly formed. By 12 weeks the fetus is 8 cm long and weighs about 15 g. The limbs, fingers, toes, and ears are fully formed, and the sex can be distinguished.

By 16 weeks, the fetus is about 16 cm long and weighs over 100 g. The mother may be able to feel its movements, and the heartbeat can be heard using Doppler ultrasound. The eyebrows and eyelashes are forming. By the end of 20 weeks, the fetus is 25 cm long. It now has hair on its head and its skin is covered with fine hair called lanugo. By 24 weeks the fetus is 30 cm long and its heartbeat is audible with a stethoscope. By 28 weeks it is 35 cm long and weighs about 1250 g. Its skin is very wrinkled.

At 32 weeks, the fetus is about 40 cm long and weighs about 1500 g, with more fat under its skin. In the male, the testes have descended into the scrotum. By the end of 36 weeks the fetus is 45 cm long, weighs about 2500 g, and has a good chance of survival if it is born at that time. At the end of 40 weeks, the average length of the fetus is 50 cm, and the average weight is 3 kg.

Care of the Unborn Infant. A host of influences can adversely affect the growth and development of the unborn and his chances for survival and good health after birth. The diet of the mother should be nutritious and well-balanced so that the infant receives the necessary food elements for development and maturity of the body structures. Supplementary iron and vitamins may be recommended during pregnancy.

There is now less emphasis on severe restriction of the mother's dietary intake to maintain a limited weight gain. It is generally agreed that the average gain should be about 11 kg during pregnancy. Ideally, the mother should achieve normal weight before she becomes pregnant because obesity increases the possibility of ECLAMPSIA and other serious complications of pregnancy by at least 60 per cent. Mothers who are underweight are more likely to deliver low birth weight babies who, by virtue of their physiological immaturity, are more likely to suffer from birth defects, HYALINE MEMBRANE DISEASE, and other developmental disorders of the newborn.

Other factors affecting the unborn child include certain drugs taken by the mother during pregnancy. A well known example is thalidomide, which inhibits the growth of the extremities of the fetus and results in gross deformities. Many drugs, including prescription as well as nonprescription medications, are now believed to be capable of causing fetal abnormalities. In addition, consumption of alcohol during pregnancy may result in FETAL ALCOHOL SYNDROME. Most obstetricians recommend that all drugs be avoided during pregnancy excepting those essential to the control of disease in the mother.

Diseases that increase the risk of obstetrical complications include diabetes, heart disease, hypertension, kidney disease, and anaemia. Rubella (German measles) can be responsible for many types of birth defects, particularly if the mother contracts it in the first 3 months of pregnancy. Sexually transmitted diseases can have tragic effects on the baby, even though the symptoms in the mother are minor at the time of pregnancy. SYPHILIS is particularly dangerous because it is one of the few diseases that can be transmitted to the fetus in the uterus, but can be cured if treated in time, because penicillin crosses the placenta.

During the birth process the infant may be infected with GONORRHOEA as it passes through the birth canal. Gonorrhoeal infection of the eyes can cause blindness. HERPES SIMPLEX Type II involving the genitals of the mother can also be transmitted to the infant at birth. The mortality and morbidity rate for such infected infants is extremely high.

The age of the mother is also an important factor in the well-being of the unborn infant. The mortality and morbidity rate for infants born of mothers below the age of 15 and above 40 are much higher than for those of mothers between these age limits.

Tests to monitor fetal health have taken much of the guesswork out of predicting the chances of survival and health status of the fetus after birth. Such tests and evaluation techniques include AMNIOCENTESIS, chemical and hormonal assays, ultrasound examinations, electronic surveillance of fetal vital signs and reaction to uterine contractions (see FETAL MONITORING and CARDIOTOCOGRAPHY), and analyses of the infant's blood during labour.

Antenatal Care. The care of the mother during her entire pregnancy is important to her well-being and that of her unborn infant. It will help provide ease and safety during pregnancy and childbirth. The obstetrician learns about the mother's physical condition and medical history, and can detect possible complications before they become serious.

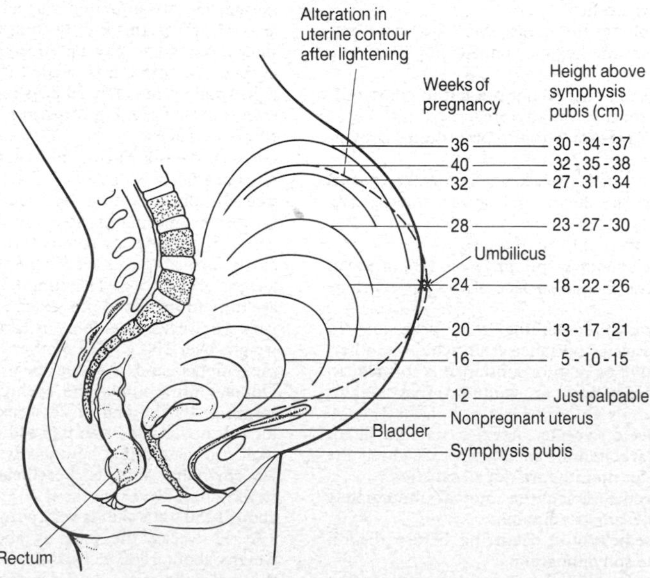

Uterine levels in pregnancy. Height above the symphysis pubis is given as the normal range with the mean figure in the centre

On the first antenatal visit the mother's medical history is taken in considerable detail, including any diseases or operations she has had, the course of previous pregnancies, if any, and whether there is a family history of multiple births or of diabetes mellitus or other chronic diseases. The first visit may also include a thorough physical examination and measurement of the pelvis. Blood samples are taken for a serological test for syphilis and for laboratory tests such as full blood count, haemoglobin determination, and blood typing. Urine is tested for albumin, sugar and acetone, and examined microscopically for asymptomatic bacteriuria. On subsequent visits the mother brings a urine specimen, collected upon arising that morning, to be tested for albumin, acetone and glucose. At each antenatal visit her blood pressure is taken and recorded and she is weighed.

Mothers who are considered 'high-risk' are usually sent to a specialist and the infant is delivered at a regional hospital where sophisticated monitoring equipment and laboratory tests are available, and specially trained personnel can attend to the needs of the mother and her infant. However, most mothers are cared for throughout their pregnancy by a combination of an obstetrician at a local hospital and their own general practitioner.

DISCOMFORTS AND COMPLICATIONS. MORNING SICKNESS usually appears in the early months of pregnancy and rarely lasts beyond the third month. Often it requires no treatment, or can be relieved by such simple measures as eating dry biscuits or toast and tea before rising. Indigestion and heartburn are best prevented by avoiding foods that are difficult to digest, such as cucumbers, cabbage, cauliflower, spinach, and onions, and rich foods. Milk of magnesia may provide relief. Constipation usually can be corrected by diet or a mild laxative like milk of magnesia. Stronger laxatives should not be used unless prescribed by the obstetrician or general practitioner.

A visit to a dentist early in pregnancy is a good idea to forestall any possibility of infection arising from tooth decay. Pregnancy does not encourage tooth decay.

HAEMORRHOIDS sometimes occur in pregnancy because of pressure from the enlarged uterus on the veins in the rectum. The obstetrician or general practitioner should be consulted for treatment.

VARICOSE VEINS also result from pressure of the uterus, which restricts the flow of blood from the legs and feet. Lying flat with the feet raised on a pillow several times a day will help relieve swelling and pain in the legs. In more difficult cases the obstetrician or general practitioner may prescribe support stockings or tights.

Backache during pregnancy is caused by bad posture and subluxation of the pelvic joints and can be relieved by rest and sensible shoes.

Swelling of the feet and ankles usually is relieved by rest and by remaining off the feet for a day or two. If the swelling does not disappear, the obstetrician or general practitioner should be informed since it may be an indication of a more serious complication.

Shortness of breath is common in the later stages of pregnancy. If at any time it becomes so extreme that the woman cannot climb a short flight of stairs without discomfort, the obstetrician or general practitioner should be consulted. If a mild shortness of breath interferes with sleep, lying in a half-sitting position, supported by several pillows, may help.

The more serious complications of pregnancy include PYELITIS, HYPEREMESIS GRAVIDARUM, ECLAMPSIA, PLACENTA PREVIA, abruptio PLACENTAE and ANAEMIA.

abdominal p. ectopic pregnancy within the peritoneal cavity.

ampullar p. ectopic pregnancy in the ampulla of the uterine tube.

cervical p. ectopic pregnancy within the cervical canal.

combined p. simultaneous intrauterine and extrauterine pregnancies.

cornual p. pregnancy in a horn (cornu) of the uterus.

ectopic p., extrauterine p. development of the fertilized ovum outside the cavity of the uterus. The site of implantation usually is one of the uterine tubes. As the fetus grows the tube ruptures, presenting the danger of haemorrhage. Symptoms include vaginal bleeding and severe pain on one side of the abdomen. Prompt surgery is necessary to remove the tube and control bleeding.

false p. development of all the signs of pregnancy without the presence of an embryo.

interstitial p. pregnancy in that part of the uterine tube within the wall of the uterus.

intraligamentary p., intraligamentous p. ectopic pregnancy within the broad ligament.

multiple p. the presence of more than one fetus in the uterus at the same time.

mural p. interstitial pregnancy.

ovarian p. pregnancy occurring in an ovary.

phantom p. false pregnancy due to psychogenic factors.

p. tests laboratory procedures for early determination of pregnancy. Within one week after the first missed menstrual period human CHORIONIC GONADOTROPHIN (hCG), a hormone secreted initially by the trophoblast and later by the placenta, is present in the blood and urine of a pregnant woman. It was formerly determined by bioassay in which a urine or serum specimen was injected into a laboratory animal and the response of ovarian tissue was noted.

All testing now uses immunological techniques based on antigen–antibody binding between hCG and anti-hCG antibody. There are several commercial kits based on the agglutination of hCG-coated latex particles by anti-hCG serum, which is inhibited if the urine specimen added to the serum contains hCG. Clinical laboratories generally use radioimmunossay (RIA) or radioreceptorassay (RRA) to determine serum hCG levels. These methods are more accurate and less likely to produce false positive results.

tubal p. ectopic pregnancy within a uterine tube.

tuboabdominal p. ectopic pregnancy occurring partly in the fimbriated end of the uterine tube and partly in the abdominal cavity.

tubo-ovarian p. ectopic pregnancy at the fimbria of the uterine tube..

pregnane ('pregnayn) a crystalline saturated steroid hydrocarbon; *β-pregnane* is the form from which several hormones, including progesterone, are derived; *α-pregnane* is the form excreted in the urine.

pregnanediol (ˌpregnayn'dieol) a crystalline, biologically inactive dihydroxy derivative of pregnane, formed by reduction of progesterone and found especially in urine of pregnant women.

pregnanetriol (ˌpregnayn'trieol) a metabolite of 17-hydroxyprogesterone; its excretion in the urine is greatly increased in certain disorders of the adrenal cortex.

pregnant ('pregnənt) with child; gravid; having a developing embryo or fetus within the uterus.

prehallux (pree'haləks) a supernumerary bone of the foot growing from the medial border of the scaphoid.

prehemiplegic (ˌpreehemi'pleejik) preceding hemiplegia.

prehensile (pri'hensiel) adapted for grasping or seizing.

prehension (pri'henshən) the act of grasping.
prehormone (pree'hawmohn) prohormone.
prehypophysis (ˌpree·hie'pofisis) the anterior lobe of the hypophysis, or pituitary gland.
preictal (pree'ikt'l) occurring before a stroke, seizure, or attack.
preicteric (ˌpree·ik'terik) preceding the appearance of jaundice (icterus).
preinvasive (ˌpree·in'vaysiv, -ziv) not yet invading tissues outside the site of origin.
preleukaemia (ˌpreeloo'keemi·ə) a stage of bone marrow dysfunction preceding the development of acute myelogenous leukaemia. adj. **preleukaemic**.
prelimbic (pree'limbik) in front of a limbus.
premalignant (ˌpreemə'lignənt) precancerous.
Premarin ('premə·rin) trademark for preparations of conjugated oestrogens.
premature (ˌpremə'tyooə) interrupted before the state of maturity; occurring before the proper time. See also PRETERM INFANT.
prematurity (ˌpremə'tyooə·ritee) underdevelopment; the condition of a premature infant.
premaxilla (ˌpreemak'silə) a separate element derived from the median nasal processes in the embryo, which later fuses with the maxilla.
premaxillary (ˌpreemak'silə·ree) 1. situated in front of the maxilla proper. 2. incisive bone.
p. bone premaxilla.
premedication (ˌpreemedi'kayshən) drugs given prior to anaesthesia and surgery in order to reduce fear and anxiety and to facilitate the induction and maintenance of, and recovery from, anaesthesia. It is usually given by an intramuscular route, but where time is limited the intravenous route can be used. Occasionally, the most suitable route is the rectal one. However, fear and anxiety are equally well if not better relieved by a preoperative visit from the anaesthetist.
premenarchal (ˌpreeme'nahk'l) occurring before establishment of menstruation.
premenstrual (pree'menstrooəl) preceding menstruation.
p. tension a complex of symptoms sometimes occurring in the 10 days before menstruation, including emotional instability and irritability, pain in the breasts, headache, nausea, anorexia, constipation, pelvic discomfort, oedema, and abdominal distention.

The causes of these symptoms are not fully understood but are believed to be associated with a disturbed salt balance, resulting in the accumulation of water in the tissues just before menstruation. Psychogenic factors may contribute. Emotional and physical symptoms usually disappear with the onset of menstruation. If symptoms are habitually troublesome, restriction of fluid and salt intake and a diuretic may be prescribed. Tranquillizers and reassurance that the condition is not serious are also helpful.
premenstruum (pree'menstrooəm) the period immediately before menstruation.
premolar (pree'mohlə) in front of the molar teeth (see also TOOTH).
premorbid (pree'mawbid) occurring before the development of disease.
premunition (ˌpreemyoo'nishən) resistance to infection by the same or closely related pathogen established after an acute infection has become chronic, and lasting as long as the infecting organisms are in the body. Usually refers to parasitic infections. adj. **premunitive**.
premyeloblast (pree'mieəlohˌblast) a precursor of a myeloblast.
premyelocyte (pree'mieəlohˌsiet) promyelocyte.
prenatal (pree'nayt'l) preceding birth.
p. care care of the pregnant woman before delivery of the infant (see also PREGNANCY).
preneoplastic (ˌpreeneeoh'plastik) before the formation of a tumour.
preoperative (pree'opə·rətiv) preceding an operation.
p. care the psychological and physiological preparation of a patient before operation. The preoperative period may be extremely short, as with an emergency operation, or it may encompass several weeks during which diagnostic tests, specific medications and treatments, and measures to improve the patient's general well-being are employed in preparation for surgery.
PSYCHOLOGICAL ASPECTS. Although each patient reacts in his own unique way to the news that he is going to have surgery, all patients experience some degree of anxiety and fear—fear of the unknown, worry over disability or death, and apprehension about the insecurity of their family's future.

Much of this anxiety can be relieved if the various aspects of his preoperative and postoperative care and the type of surgery planned are explained to the patient. Research has shown that this information and relief of anxiety may help reduce postoperative pain and hasten recovery. The surgeon usually explains the surgical procedure and assists the patient in planning rehabilitation. The anaesthetist usually reviews the type of anaesthesia to be used and the general effects it will have on the patient. The nursing staff explains the hospital routine, specific nursing procedures necessary, the purpose of diagnostic tests required, and the types of equipment that will be used during the preoperative and postoperative periods. The nurse can demonstrate interest in the patient and his family by answering questions (or referring them to the surgeon), and giving them a general idea of how long the patient will be away from the ward during surgery and recovery from anaesthesia. It is reassuring for them to know, for example, that oxygen administration, blood transfusions, and the use of a nasogastric tube or catheter do not necessarily indicate a critical situation. The use of various pieces of equipment that seem 'routine' to the hospital staff may be extremely upsetting to the patient and his family if they do not understand why the equipment is necessary.

Spiritual reinforcement during this period may be very important to some patients, and though the nurse must be careful not to give the impression of prying into the patient's private affairs, she must also show a willingness to assist him and his family in obtaining a spiritual advisor if they indicate a desire for her to do so. The nurse must always respect the individual patient's beliefs and convictions even though she may not share them, and must support the patient in his search for spiritual reassurance and guidance.
LEGAL ASPECTS. Any patient undergoing surgery, whether it is expected to be major or minor surgery, must give informed consent and sign the appropriate form according to district health policy. He has the right to know the type of surgery intended and its expected outcome, aftereffects, and possible complications. If he is underage, mentally incompetent, or unconscious, the form is signed by a relative or guardian. The form protects the patient against unwanted surgery and operative procedures he does not understand. It protects the hospital staff and surgeon from legal claims that the surgery was done without the patient's permission or knowledge of what was to be done. The signed consent form is placed in the patient's notes and is sent to the operating theatre with him. See also CONSENT.
PREVENTIVE ASPECTS. During the preoperative period

the patient should be instructed in coughing, turning, deep breathing, and exercises of the extremities. These techniques can be most effective in preventing many of the complications of surgery. Exercises to strengthen specific muscles in preparation for rehabilitation, as following AMPUTATION, for example, are begun well in advance so that the patient is in optimal condition to begin a programme of rehabilitation as soon after surgery as possible. Other topics of instruction will depend on the anticipated needs of the patient during his recovery from surgery.

PHYSIOLOGICAL ASPECTS. Except in emergency situations every effort is made to have the patient in a state of optimal health before surgery is performed. Specific diets, protein and vitamin supplements, and other measures to improve the nutritional status may be employed. Intravenous infusions and transfusions of whole blood or plasma may be necessary to improve the fluid and electrolyte status and blood volume. Infections should be brought under control before surgery if they cannot be eliminated completely. Accurate records of the patient's vital signs, to include blood pressure, pulse, respiration and urinary output, will assist the surgeon in diagnosing and correcting conditions that may adversely affect the patient's physiological response to an operative procedure.

PHYSICAL PREPARATION. The skin and hair are possible sources of infection and require special attention before surgery. The particular area to be shaved and cleansed will depend on the wishes of the surgeon and the accepted hospital procedure. An exception may be the head or face, especially the eyebrows, which are rarely shaved. If large amounts of hair must be removed from the head, provision may be made for a wig if the patient so desires.

A depilatory cream may be substituted for shaving, depending on hospital policy. Some surgeons do not require removal of the hair at all, especially in some types of gynaecological surgery.

Restriction of food and fluids varies. On a morning list the patient is allowed an evening meal then nothing by mouth after midnight. On an afternoon list a light breakfast may be allowed. Young children and babies should be allowed fluids up to 4 hours preoperatively.

PREOPERATIVE MEDICATIONS. Generally there are three types of drugs used prior to surgery: *anxiolytics*, almost always of the benzodiazepine group, which also provide amnesia—usually given orally 1–2 hours preoperatively, although with those that have a long duration of action, such as lorazepam, the timing is not critical; *anticholinergic drugs*, such as atropine and scopolamine, which decrease salivary and bronchial secretions—these also have vagolytic activity, hyoscine, in addition, having amnesic and anti-emetic effects; and *analgesics*, such as morphine and pethidine, which will relieve pain if present and also smooth the induction of anaesthesia.

Other drugs are occasionally used in specific cases: an anti-emetic in patients with a history of nausea and vomiting associated with a previous anaesthetic; antacids in patients at greater risk of regurgitation, such as those with hiatus hernia; and antihistamines in patients with multiple allergies, who may react to an anaesthetic drug.

Preoperative medications must be given at the exact time ordered because their strength, action, and duration are planned according to the type of anaesthesia used.

IMMEDIATE PREOPERATIVE CARE. Most institutions use a check list or clearance record for surgical procedures. This eliminates the danger of overlooking some aspect of the immediate preoperative preparation. Such an omission might delay surgery or result in legal problems. The consent form must be signed by the patient or his guardian or legal representative. This form is necessary to protect the surgeon against claims of unauthorized surgery, and to protect the patient against surgery to which he would not willingly agree.

The preoperative check list includes such items as laboratory tests and their findings, history and physical examination records, disposal of valuables, removal of dentures and their disposition, pulse and blood pressure of the patient immediately before he goes to the operating theatre and other specific information such as consultation for sterilization and consent form.

Unless a urinary catheter has been inserted, the patient is offered the bedpan just before he is taken to the operating room. Hairpins, clips, and combs are removed from the hair and the head is covered with a cap. As the patient leaves the unit he is reassured that everything is in order and that everyone concerned with his care is interested in him and the outcome of his operation.

preoral (pree'or·rəl) in front of the mouth.

preparalytic (ˌpreeparə'litik) preceding paralysis.

prepatellar (ˌpreepə'telə) in front of the patella.

preprandial (pree'prandi·əl) before meals.

preproinsulin (ˌpreeproh'insyuhlin) the precursor of proinsulin, containing an additional polypeptide sequence at the N-terminal.

preproprotein (ˌpreeproh'prohteen) any precursor of a proprotein.

prepuberal, prepubertal (pree'pyoobə·rəl; pree'pyoobət'l) before puberty; pertaining to the period of accelerated growth preceding gonadal maturity.

prepubescent (ˌpreepyoo'bes'nt) prepubertal.

prepuce ('preepyoos) foreskin; a cutaneous fold over the glans penis. adj. **preputial. p. of clitoris** a fold capping the clitoris formed by union of the labia minora and the clitoris.

preputiotomy (preeˌpyooshi'otəmee) incision of the prepuce of the penis to relive phimosis.

preputium (pree'pyooshi·əm) prepuce.

prepyloric (ˌpreepie'lo·rik) just proximal to the pylorus.

presacral (pree'saykrəl) anterior to the sacrum.

presby- word element. [Gr.] *old age.*

presbyatrics (ˌpresbi'atriks) geriatrics.

presbycardia (ˌpresbi'kahdi·ə) impairment of cardiac function attributed to ageing, with senescent changes in the body and no evidence of other cause of heart disease.

presbycusis (ˌpresbi'koosis) progressive, bilaterally symmetrical perceptive hearing loss occurring with age.

presbyope ('presbiˌohp) one who is affected with presbyopia.

presbyophrenia (ˌpresbioh'freeni·ə) loss of memory, disorientation, and confabulation, occurring in old age; called also Wernicke's syndrome.

presbyopia (ˌpresbi'ohpi·ə) diminution of accommodation of the lens of the eye occurring normally with ageing, and usually resulting in hyperopia, or farsightedness. adj. **presbyopic.**

Presbyopia is caused by a loss of elasticity in the crystalline lens of the eye. The lens focuses images on the retina with the aid of the ciliary muscle which contracts it to make it more convex or relaxes it to make it less spherical. As it ages, the lens may lose its ability to become convex enough to accommodate to nearby objects. This condition usually begins around the age of 40. Presbyopia can most often be comfortably corrected through the use of glasses.

prescription (pri'skripshən) a written directive, as for the compounding or dispensing and administration of drugs, or for other service to a particular patient.

Medicines are divided into two main classes: prescription medicines and over-the-counter medicines. Dangerous, powerful, or habit-forming medicines to be used under a doctor's supervision can be obtained only by prescription written and signed by a doctor.

Historically there are four parts to a drug prescription. The first is the symbol ℞ from the Latin *recipe*, meaning 'take'. This is the superscription. The second part is the inscription, specifying the ingredients and their quantities. The third part is the subscription, which tells the pharmacist how to compound the medicine. The signature is the last part, and it is usually preceded by an S to represent the Latin *signa*, meaning 'mark'. The signature is where the doctor indicates what instructions are to be put on the outside of the package to tell the patient when and how to take the medicine and in what quantities. In practice, with modern medicines it is usual to give the name of the drug, its dosage, timing method and frequency of administration, and the total quantity to be provided.

The pharmacist keeps a file of all the prescriptions dispensed.

presenile (pree'seeniel) pertaining to a condition resembling senility, but occurring in early or middle life. See also ALZHEIMER'S DISEASE.

presentation (ˌprezən'tayshən) that part of the fetus which is lowest in the uterus. Normally the head but may be the breech, a shoulder or a foot. See also POSITION, LIE.

breech p. presentation of the fetal buttocks or feet in labour; the feet may be alongside the buttocks (complete breech or flexed breech presentation); the legs may be extended against the trunk and the feet lying against the face (frank breech or incomplete, extended breech presentation); or one or both feet or knees may be prolapsed into the maternal vagina (footling or knee presentation).

cephalic p. presentation of any part of the fetal head in labour, whether the vertex, face, or brow.

compound p. prolapse of an extremity of the fetus alongside the head in cephalic presentation or of one or both arms alongside a presenting breech at the beginning of labour.

footling p. presentation of the fetus with one foot (single footling) or two feet (double footling) prolapsed into the maternal vagina.

funic p. presentation of the umbilical cord in labour. Cord presentation, i.e. before rupture of the membranes. Cord prolapse, when the membranes rupture and the cord prolapses into the vagina.

placental p. placenta praevia.

shoulder p. oblique presentation or transverse lie of the fetus when the shoulder lies over the cervical os.

preservative (pri'zərvətiv) a substance added to a product to destroy or inhibit multiplication of micro-organisms.

presomite (pree'sohmiet) referring to embryos before the appearance of somites.

presphenoid (pree'sfeenoyd) the anterior portion of the body of the sphenoid bone.

presphygmic (pree'sfigmik) preceding the pulse wave.

p. interval, p. period the first phase of ventricular systole, being the period (0.04–0.06 seconds) immediately after closure of the atrioventricular valves and lasting until the semilunar valves open.

prespinal (pree'spien'l) in front of the spine.

pressor ('presə) tending to increase blood pressure.

pressoreceptive (ˌpresoh·ri'septiv) sensitive to stimuli due to vasomotor activity; pressosensitive.

pressoreceptor (ˌpresoh·ri'septə) a receptor or nerve ending sensitive to stimuli of vasomotor activity.

pressosensitive (ˌpresoh'sensitiv) pressoreceptive.

pressure ('preshə) stress or strain, by compression, expansion, pull, thrust, or shear.

arterial p. the blood pressure in the arteries.

atmospheric p. the pressure exerted by the atmosphere, 760 mmHg at 0 °C at sea level (101.3 kPa, 14.7 p.s.i.).

blood p. the pressure of the blood on the walls of the arteries, dependent on the energy of the heart action, elasticity of the arterial walls, and volume and viscosity of the blood; the maximum or systolic pressure occurs near the end of the stroke output of the left ventricle, and the minimum or diastolic late in ventricular diastole (see also BLOOD PRESSURE).

capillary p. the blood pressure in the capillaries.

central venous p. the pressure of blood in the right atrium (see also CENTRAL VENOUS PRESSURE).

cerebrospinal p. the pressure of the cerebrospinal fluid, normally 100 to 150 mmHg.

continuous positive airway p. (CPAP) administration of gases at a pressure above ambient pressure (see also CONTINUOUS POSITIVE AIRWAY PRESSURE).

intracranial p. the pressure of the subarachnoidal fluid.

intraocular p. the pressure exerted against the outer coats by the contents of the eyeball.

mean circulatory filling p. a measure of the average (arterial and venous) pressure necessary to cause filling of the circulation with blood; it varies with blood volume and is directly proportional to the rate of venous return and thus to cardiac output.

negative p. pressure less than that of the atmosphere.

oncotic p. the osmotic pressure of a colloid in solution.

osmotic p. the potential pressure of a solution directly related to its solute osmolar concentration; it is the maximum pressure developed by osmosis in a solution separated from another by a semipermeable membrane, i.e., the pressure that will just prevent OSMOSIS between two such solutions.

partial p. pressure exerted by each of the constituents of a mixture of gases.

p. areas those parts of the body overlying bone prominences where tissue may be compressed by pressure from an external surface, common sites being the sacrum, greater trochanters and heels; the area may become ischaemic and prolonged or severe pressure may result in tissue damage and an ulcer may develop. See also PRESSURE SORE.

p. points 1. various locations on the body at which digital pressure may be applied for the control of haemorrhage. See accompanying illustration. 2. those parts of the body where tissue is compressed between an underlying bone prominence and an external surface, leading to likely interference with its blood supply.

positive p. pressure greater than that of the atmosphere.

positive end-expiratory p. (PEEP) in mechanical ventilation, a positive airway pressure maintained until the end of expiration (see also POSITIVE END-EXPIRATORY PRESSURE).

pulse p. the difference between the systolic and diastolic pressures.

p. sore see PRESSURE SORE.

venous p. the blood pressure in the veins.

wedge p. intravascular pressure as measured by a SWAN-GANZ CATHETER introduced into the pulmonary artery; it permits indirect measurement of the mean left atrial pressure..

pressure sore a lesion of surface body tissues due to

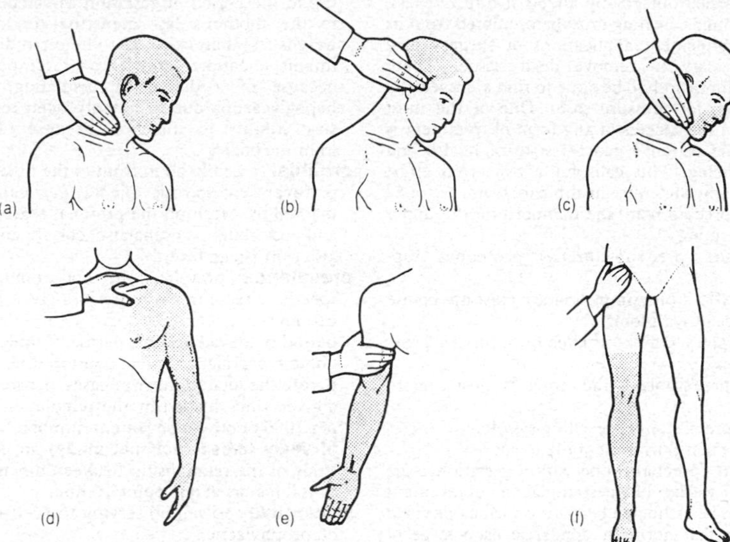

Digital pressure points. The shaded areas are those within which haemorrhage may be controlled by pressure on the specific artery. (a) Carotid artery; (b) Temporal artery; (c) External maxillary artery; (d) Subclavian artery; (e) Brachial artery; (f) Femoral artery

prolonged or severe pressure inhibiting the local circulation, usually occurring where tissues are compressed between underlying bone and an external surface. Called also *bedsore* and *decubitus ulcer*. Commonest sites are over the sacrum, hips, heels and elbows, but also often occur on the buttock. Prolonged periods of minimal pressure are just as harmful as intense pressure of short duration. Primary indication of harmful pressure is erythema of the area, and its relief at this stage may allow perfusion of the tissue and removal of toxic by-products. If unrelieved, the skin blisters and sloughs and an ulcer develops surrounded by an erythematous halo (cellulitis), and eventually a waxy greyish eschar forms and becomes a blackened area of necrosis. Invariably, the visible lesion is merely the 'tip of the iceberg', the major part of the wound being below the skin surface. Other factors which may contribute to the development of a pressure sore include wrinkling or unevenness of bedding, shearing forces and friction, accummulation of perspiration, and incontinence; pressure from apparatus or a plaster cast can be a direct cause.

Research surveys have shown that the vast majority of patients who develop pressure sores are aged 70 and over, and that prevalence increases with age and the presence of incontinence. An equally high risk group are patients with paralysis, i.e., hemiplegia, paraplegia and tetraplegia. Potential is also present in emaciated and diabetic patients, those confined to bed in traction or wearing a cast, those with generalized oedema and patients with rheumatic conditions receiving anti-inflammatory drugs. A prolonged period of immobility on an operating table or firm stretcher can be the cause of a pressure ulcer appearing several days later in vulnerable patients, such as the elderly.

Prevention of pressure sores is far simpler and less distressing and costly than treatment and cure. Normally, discomfort from prolonged or severe pressure on body tissues initiates movement to relieve it, even during sleep. When, for whatever reason, this spontaneous protective mechanism cannot operate it is necessary to apply extrinsic means to give relief. The first essential, however, is the early detection of patients at risk since this is when preventative measures are the most effective. In some cases this is obvious, as with coma and paralysis, but for others its onset is obscure or insidious. Discerning observation of body movements, nutritional intake and of any decline in general condition are therefore essential and professional judgement is aided by monitoring patients using a risk assessment system, which is usually in the form of a rating scale. See also NORTON SCORE.

The foremost preventive measure of patients at risk is frequent changing of the body's position (at least every 2 hours), day and night, and skin hygiene. Massage of the pressure areas is comforting and aids prevention mainly by the relief of pressure during its administration. Pressure-relieving aids are legion in their design and materials, ranging from special beds and mattresses, special cushions, pads and foam wedges to sheepskin and synthetic fleece. Appropriate selection for the particular patient is important, but not so much as the timeliness of their use and recognition that they are supplements to judicious nursing attention and not substitutes for it.

Treatment of a pressure sore is aimed at restoring circulation to the area as quickly and efficiently as possible, controlling secondary bacterial infection, and initiating measures to promote healing. The patient should be positioned so that the pressure sore and surrounding area are completely relieved of pressure, but regular changing of position remains paramount.

Topical applications vary widely, depending on preference. The diligence with which the prescribed regimen is carried out greatly affects it effectiveness. As with all wounds, healing must be promoted from its base, and débridement applications or surgery may first be necessary to remove dead tissue. There remains much research to be done to find a universally successful cure for pressure sores. One of the most vital factors in the success of any form of treatment is to improve the patient's general state of health and mental well-being. This calls for a concerted effort and dedication by the entire health care team.

presternum (pree'stərnəm) the manubrium; the upper part of the sternum.

presuppurative (pree'supyuhrətiv) preceding suppuration.

presymptomatic (ˌpreesimptə'matik) existing before the appearance of symptoms.

presynaptic (preesi'naptik) situated or occurring proximal to a synapse.

presystole (pree'sistəlee) the interval just before systole.

presystolic (ˌpreesi'stolik) preceding systole.

pretarsal (pree'tahs'l) in front of the tarsus.

preterm infant ('preetərm) one with a gestational age of less than 37 weeks. The gestational age of an infant after birth can be estimated by noting various physical characteristics that normally appear at each stage of gestation. For example, as the preterm infant emerges from the birth canal he will be covered with a rather heavy coating of *vernix caseosa*; the full-term infant has only a small amount of this cheeselike substance in body creases and the hair. By the 40th to 42nd week of gestation the skin of the infant is pale and opaque; the skin of an infant born before this period of gestation is thin and transparent; venules can be seen under the skin on the abdomen. At about 20 weeks the body of the infant is covered with fine hair called *lanugo*. It begins to disappear as the infant matures in the uterus; first from the face, then the trunk, and finally from the extremities. At nine months gestation it usually is seen only over the shoulders. Wrinkling of the soles of the feet is another indication of the infant's gestational stage. It first occurs near the toes and progresses toward the heel so that by 40 weeks the entire sole is covered with creases. The preterm infant will have smooth soles with only one or two creases. 'Cotton wool' hair that tends to stick together in small bunches so that it is difficult to distinguish one strand from another is common until the 38th week of gestation. This sign is of less significance in black infants. Cartilage of the ear can also be used to estimate the gestational age. Until about 32 or 33 weeks the pinnae stay folded when bent inward; by 36 weeks they spring back when released; and at term they are firm enough to stand erect from the sides of the head.

Care of the preterm infant is concerned with helping him cope with life outside the uterus until he has matured sufficiently and is able to function on his own.

The care of the preterm infant requires specialized training in the specific needs of these infants and the therapeutic procedures and techniques that their care demands.

Some infants of normal gestational age weigh much less at birth than expected because of failure to thrive and to gain weight within the uterus. They appear undernourished and many have suffered neurological damage from hypoxia during the prenatal period or at the time of birth. These infants do not present the same problems as do preterm infants. To avoid confusion between preterm infants and those who weigh less than expected at birth, the term 'small-for-dates' infant is used. This simply implies that according to the period of gestation as calculated according to the mother's last menstrual period, the infant weighs less than expected. The main difficulties these infants encounter are (1) poor temperature control because of a deficit of insulating body fat, (2) hypoglycaemia due to low glycogen reserves, and (3) susceptibility to infection because of a deficit of immune bodies.

pretibial (pree'tibi·əl) in front of the tibia.

p. fever leptospirosis due to *Leptospira autumnalis*, marked by a rash on the pretibial region, with lumbar and postorbital pain, malaise, coryza, and fever. Called also Fort Bragg fever.

prevalence ('prevələns) the total number of cases of a specific disease in existence in a given population at a certain time.

period p. prevalence in a period of time.

point p. prevalence at one point in time.

p. rate the total number of cases of a specific disease at a given time divided by the population and expressed per 1000 or other convenient number.

p. study (cross-sectional study) an epidemiological study of the relationship between disease and possible causal factors at one point in time.

preventive (pri'ventiv) serving to avert the occurrence of; prophylactic.

p. care the level of care in the HEALTH CARE SYSTEM that consists of school health education and public health services.

p. medicine science aimed at preventing disease.

prevertebral (pree'vərtibrəl) in front of a vertebra.

prevesical (pree'vesik'l) anterior to the bladder.

prezygotic (ˌpreezie'gotik) occurring before completion of fertilization.

Priadel ('priədel) trademark for a preparation of lithium carbonate.

priapism ('prieəˌpizəm) persistent abnormal erection of the penis, accompanied by pain and tenderness. It is seen in diseases and injuries of the spinal cord, and may be caused by vesical calculus and certain injuries to the penis.

Price precipitation reaction (pries) a serological test for syphilis; abbreviated PPR.

prickle cell ('prik'l) a cell with delicate radiating processes connecting with similar cells, being a dividing keratinocyte of the prickle-cell layer of the epidermis.

prickly heat ('priklee) miliaria.

prilocaine ('prilohˌkayn) a local anaesthetic of the amide group, equipotent with lignocaine but with a longer duration of action. Its lower toxicity makes it the drug of choice for intravenous regional anaesthesia (Biers Block). Very large doses (greater than 600 mg) are associated with methaemoglobinaemia.

primaquine ('priməˌkween) a compound used in the treatment of vivax and ovale malaria to produce radical cure, i.e. to prevent relapses.

primary care ('priemərее) the level of care in the HEALTH CARE SYSTEM that consists of initial care outside institutions.

p. health care the care given to individuals in the community at the first point of contact with the primary health care team. First contact may be the general practitioner, a health visitor or a district nurse.

p. health care team usually made up of a general practitioner, district nurses, health visitors and possibly paramedical staff, such as a physiotherapist. They may serve a geographical area and be based in a health centre or a general practice area.

primate ('priemayt) an individual belonging to the highest order of mammals, Primates, which includes man and the apes, monkeys, and lemurs.

primidone ('primi,dohn) an anticonvulsant.
primigravida (,priemi'gravidə) a woman pregnant for the first time; GRAVIDA I.
primipara (prie'mipə·rə) unipara; a woman who has had one pregnancy that resulted in viable offspring, PARA I. adj. **primiparous.**
primiparity (,priemi'parətee) the state of being a primipara.
primitive ('primitiv) first in point of time; existing in a simple or early form; showing little evolution.
primordial (prie'mawdi·əl) original or primitive; of the simplest and most undeveloped character.
primordium (prie'mawdi·əm) the first beginnings of an organ or part in the developing embryo.
Primperan ('primpə,ran) trademark for preparations of metoclopramide hydrochloride, a gastrointestinal promotility agent.
principle ('prinsip'l) 1. a chemical component. 2. a substance on which certain of the properties of a drug depend. 3. a law of conduct.
active p. any constituent of a drug that helps to confer upon it a medicinal property.
pleasure p. the automatic instinct or tendency to avoid pain and secure pleasure.
reality p. in freudian terminology, the mental activity that develops to control the pleasure principle under the pressure of necessity or the demands of reality.
Prinzmetal's angina (prints'met'lz) a variant of angina pectoris in which the attacks occur during rest, exercise capacity is well preserved, and attacks are associated electrocardiographically with elevation of the ST-segment.
p.r.n. [L.] *pro re nata* (according to circumstances; where necessary).
pro- word element. [L., Gr.] *before, in front of, favouring.*
Pro-Banthine (proh'bantheen) trademark for preparations of propantheline, an anticholinergic.
pro re nata (,proh ray 'naytə) [L.] *according to circumstances;* abbreviated p.r.n.
proaccelerin (,proh·ak'selə·rin) clotting factor V.
proactivator (proh'akti,vaytə) a precursor of an activator; a factor that reacts with an enzyme to form an activator.
proatlas (proh'atləs) a rudimentary vertebra which in some animals lies in front of the atlas; sometimes seen in many as an anomaly.
probability (,probə'bilitee) a statistical term meaning the likelihood of an association between variables being due to chance, indicated by the letter *P*.
proband ('prohband) propositus.
probang ('prohbang) a flexible rod of whalebone with a ball, tuft, or sponge at the end which was used to locate oesophageal strictures or to direct an impacted bolus or foreign body from the oesophagus into the stomach. Now obsolete. The word has come to be used for an applicator.
probe (prohb) a blunt, malleable instrument for exploring sinus tracks, wounds, cavities or passages.
probenecid (proh'benisid) a white, crystalline compound, used in the treatment of GOUT to promote excretion of uric acid; also used to increase serum concentration of certain antibiotics and other drugs.
Problem-Oriented Record ('probləmorientid) an approach to patient care record keeping that focuses on the patient's specific health problems requiring immediate attention, and the structuring of a health care plan designed to cope with the identified problems. Abbreviated POR. POR uses progress sheets that integrate all written notes under labelled problems. Called also *Problem-Oriented Medical Record (POMR)*.

The purpose of the system is to improve patient care by employing the systematic analysis and logical documentation of the care rendered by various members of the health care team. When properly implemented, the problem-oriented approach is expected to provide a more effective means of communication among the members of the health care team (including the patient), and to facilitate the coordination of preventive care, health maintenance, and continuity of care.

Although the details of implementing a POR system may vary according to the setting in which it is to be used and the type of clientele being served, there are four components that are basic to the problem-oriented record. These are the *assessment*, *problem list*, *plan*, and *notes*. All health care personnel participating in the care of the patient use the same documentation so that assessment, plans and patient management are co-ordinated.
probucol (proh'byookol) a bis-phenol compound taken orally to lower elevated serum cholesterol levels.
procainamide (proh'kaynə,mied) a cardiac depressant used as the hydrochloride salt in the treatment of cardiac arrhythmias.
Procainamide Durules (proh'kaynə,mied dyooə'roolz) trademark for a sustained-release preparation of procainamide hydrochloride, a cardiac antiarrhythmic.
procaine ('prohkayn) a local anaesthetic; the hydrochloride salt is used in solution for infiltration.
procarbazine (proh'kahbə,zeen) an antineoplastic that acts by inhibiting the synthesis of DNA, RNA, and protein; used in the treatment of Hodgkin's disease.
procarboxypeptidase (,prohkah,boksi'pepti,dayz) the inactive precursor of carboxypeptidase, which is converted to the active enzyme by the action of trypsin.
procarcinogen (,prohkah'sinəjən) a chemical substance that becomes carcinogenic only after it is altered by metabolic processes.
Procaryotae (proh,kari'ohtee) a kingdom comprising all prokaryotic organisms.
procelous (,proh'seeləs) having the anterior surface concave; said of vertebrae.
procentriole (proh'sentri,ohl) the immediate precursor of centrioles and ciliary basal bodies.
procephalic (prohkə'falik, -sə-) pertaining to the anterior part of the head.
procercoid (proh'sərkoyd) a larval stage of fish tapeworms.
process ('prohses) 1. a prominence or projection, as from a bone. 2. a series of operations or events leading to achievement of a specific result; also, to subject to such a series to produce desired changes.
acromial p. acromion.
alveolar p. the part of the bone in either the maxilla or mandible that surrounds and supports the teeth.
basilar p. a quadrilateral plate of the occipital bone projecting superiorly and anteriorly from the foramen magnum.
caudate p. the right of the two processes on the caudate lobe of the liver.
ciliary p's meridionally arranged ridges or folds projecting from the crown of the ciliary body.
clinoid p. any of the three (anterior, medial, and posterior) processes of the sphenoid bone.
coracoid p. a curved process arising from the upper neck of the scapula and overhanging the shoulder joint; called also coracoid.
coronoid p. 1. the anterior part of the upper end of the ramus of the mandible. 2. a projection at the proximal end of the ulna.
ensiform p. xiphoid process.
ethmoid p. a bony projection above and behind the

maxillary process of the inferior nasal concha.
frontonasal p. an expansive facial process in the embryo that develops into the forehead and bridge of the nose.
malar p. zygomatic process of the maxilla.
mamillary p. a tubercle on each superior articular process of a lumbar vertebra.
mastoid p. a conical projection at the base of mastoid portion of temporal bone.
nursing p. a systematic, problem-solving approach to the task of meeting the nursing needs and health care problems of clients/patients (see also NURSING PROCESS).
odontoid p. a toothlike projection of the axis that articulates with the atlas.
pterygoid p. one of the wing-shaped processes of the sphenoid bone.
spinous p. of vertebrae a part of the vertebrae projecting backward from the arch, giving attachment to muscles of the back.
styloid p. a long, pointed projection, particularly a long spine projecting downward from the inferior surface of the temporal bone.
uncinate p. any hooklike process, as of vertebrae, the lacrimal bone, or the pancreas.
xiphoid p. the pointed process of cartilage, supported by a core of bone, connected with the lower end of the sternum; called also xiphoid.
zygomatic p. a projection from the frontal or temporal bone, or from the maxilla, by which they articulate with the zygoma.

processus (proh'sesəs) pl. *processus* [L.] process.

prochlorperazine (,prohklor'perə,zeen) a phenothiazine derivative used as a major tranquillizer and antiemetic.

prochondral (proh'kondrəl) occurring before the formation of cartilage.

procidentia (,prohsi'denshi·ə) a state of prolapse, especially a severe prolapse of the uterus.

procoagulant (,prohkoh'agyuhlənt) 1. tending to promote coagulation. 2. a precursor of a natural substance necessary to coagulation of the blood.

proconvertin (,prohkən'vərtin) clotting factor VII.

procreation (,prohkri'ayshən) the act of begetting or generating.

proct(o)- word element. [Gr.] *rectum;* see also words beginning *rect(o)-*.

proctalgia (prok'talji·ə) pain in the rectum; proctodynia.

proctatresia (,proktə'treezi·ə) imperforate anus.

proctectasia (,proktek'tayzi·ə) dilation of the rectum or anus.

proctectomy (prok'tektəmee) excision of the rectum.

procteurynter (,proktyooə'rintə) a hydrostatic or pneumatic device to dilate the rectum.

proctitis (prok'tietis) inflammation of the rectum.

proctocele ('proktoh,seel) hernial protrusion of part of the rectum into the vagina; rectocele.

proctoclysis (prok'toklisis) slow introduction of large quantities of liquid into the rectum.

proctocolectomy (,proktohkə'lektəmee) removal of the rectum and colon.

proctocolonoscopy (,proktoh,kohlə'noskəpee) inspection of the interior of the rectum and colon.

proctocolpoplasty (,proktoh'kolpoh,plastee) repair of a rectovaginal fistula.

proctocystotomy (,proktohsi'stotəmee) removal of a bladder calculus through the rectum.

proctodeum (,proktoh'deeəm) the ectodermal depression of the caudal end of the embryo, which becomes the anal canal; called also anal pit.

proctodynia (,proktoh'dini·ə) pain in the rectum; proctalgia.

proctology (prok'toləjee) the branch of medicine concerned with disorders of the rectum and anus. adj. **proctologic**.

proctoparalysis (,proktohpə'ralisis) paralysis of the anal and rectal muscles; proctoplegia.

proctoplasty ('proktoh,plastee) plastic repair of the rectum and anus.

proctoplegia (,proktoh'pleeji·ə) proctoparalysis.

proctoptosis (,proktop'tohsis) prolapse of the rectum.

proctorrhaphy (prok'to·rəfee) suture of the rectum.

proctorrhoea (,proktə'reeə) a mucous discharge from the anus.

proctoscope ('proktə,skohp) a speculum or tubular instrument with illumination for inspecting the rectum.

proctoscopy (prok'toskəpee) inspection of the rectum with a proctoscope. The examination is usually done prior to rectal surgery, and it may be a part of the physical examination of a patient with haemorrhoids, rectal bleeding, or other symptoms of a rectal disorder.

proctosigmoidectomy (,proktoh,sigmoy'dektəmee) excision of the rectum and sigmoid colon; rectosigmoidectomy.

proctosigmoiditis (,proktoh,sigmoy'dietis) inflammation of the rectum and sigmoid colon.

proctosigmoidoscopy (,proktoh,sigmoy'doskəpee) examination of the rectum and sigmoid colon with the sigmoidoscope.

proctospasm ('proktoh,spazəm) spasm of the rectum.

proctostenosis (,proktohstə'nohsis) stricture of the rectum.

proctostomy (prok'tostəmee) creation of a permanent artificial opening from the rectum.

proctotomy (prok'totəmee) incision into the rectum.

proctovalvotomy (,proktohval'votəmee) incision of the rectal valves.

procumbent (proh'kumbənt) prone; lying on the face.

procursive (proh'kərsiv) tending to run forward.

procyclidine (proh'siekli,deen) a skeletal muscle relaxant used as the hydrochloride salt in the treatment of parkinsonism.

prodrome ('prohdrohm) a premonitory symptom; a symptom indicating the onset of a disease. adj. **prodromal, prodromic**.

pro-drug ('proh,drug) a compound that, on administration, must undergo chemical conversion by metabolic processes before becoming an active pharmacological agent; a precursor of a drug.

productive (prə'duktiv) producing or forming; said especially of an inflammation that produces new tissue or of a cough that brings forth sputum or mucus.

proencephalus (,proh·en'kefələs, -'sef-) a fetus with a protrusion of the brain through a frontal fissure.

proenzyme (proh'enziem) zymogen; an inactive precursor of an enzyme.

proerythroblast (,proh·i'rithroh,blast) pronormoblast.

proestrogen (proh'eestrəjən) a substance without oestrogenic activity but which is metabolized in the body to active oestrogen.

profession (prə'feshən) 1. an avowed, public declaration or statement of intention or purpose. 2. a calling or vocation requiring specialized knowledge, methods, and skills, as well as preparation, in an institution of higher learning, in the scholarly, scientific, and historical principles underlying such methods and skills. A profession continuously enlarges its body of knowledge, functions autonomously in formulation of policy, and maintains by force of organization or concerted opinion high standards of achievement and conduct. Members of a profession are committed to continuing study, place service above personal gain, and are committed to providing practical services vital to human and social welfare.

professional (prə'feshən'l) 1. pertaining to one's profession or occupation. 2. one who is a specialist in a particular field or occupation.

allied health p. a person with special training and licensed when necessary, who works under the supervision of a health professional with responsibilities bearing on patient care.

profibrinolysin (proh,fiebri'nolisin) plasminogen, the precursor of fibrinolysin.

profile ('prohfiel) a simple outline, as of the side view of the head or face; by extension, a graph representing quantitatively a set of characteristics determined by tests.

proflavine (proh'flayveen) a constituent of acriflavine, $C_{13}H_{11}N_3$, used as a topical antiseptic in the form of the hemisulphate salt.

profundaplasty, profundoplasty (proh'fundə,plastee; proh'fundoh,plastee) reconstruction of an occluded or stenosed deep femoral artery (profunda femoris artery).

profundus (proh'fundəs) [L.] *deep*.

progastrin (proh'gastrin) an inactive precursor of gastrin.

progeria (proh'jeeri·ə) premature old age, a condition occurring in childhood marked by small stature, absence of facial and pubic hair, wrinkled skin, grey hair, and eventual development of atherosclerosis. Called also Hutchinson–Gilford disease.

progestagen (proh'jestəjən) progestogen.

progestational (,prohje'stayshən'l) preceding gestation; referring to changes in the endometrium preparatory to implantation of the developing ovum should fertilization occur.

p. agent a group of hormones secreted by the corpus luteum and placenta and, in small amounts, by the adrenal cortex, including progesterone, pregn-4-ene-3,20-dione; agents having progestational activity are also produced synthetically. **p. hormones** substances, including PROGESTERONE, that are concerned mainly with preparing the endometrium for nidation of the fertilized ovum if conception has occurred.

progesterone (proh'jestə,rohn) a steroid sex hormone that is the principal progestational hormone. Used medically in the treatment of functional uterine bleeding, menstrual cycle abnormalities, and threatened abortion.

Progesterone plays a major part in the menstrual cycle. During the maturation of the ovum, oestrogen, the principal female sex hormone, is produced at a high rate. At ovulation oestrogen production is sharply reduced, and the ovary then creates within itself a special endocrine structure called the corpus luteum whose sole function is to produce progesterone. Unless fertilization takes place, the corpus luteum disappears when it has performed its function.

The progesterone produced by the corpus luteum is promptly carried by the blood to the uterus, as was the oestrogen that preceded it. Both hormones now work to prepare the uterus for possible conception.

In pregnancy, progesterone acts in a way that protects the embryo and fosters growth of the placenta. By decreasing the frequency of uterine contractions it helps to prevent expulsion of the implanted ovum. It also promotes secretory changes in the mucosa of the uterine tubes, thereby helping to provide nutrition for the fertilized ovum as it travels through the tube on its way to the uterus.

Another function of progesterone is promotion of the development of the mammary glands in preparation for lactation. Prolactin, from the anterior lobe of the PITUITARY GLAND, stimulates production of the milk, and progesterone is one of the hormones that prepares the glands for secretion.

Progesterone also has an indirect effect on the fluid and electrolyte balance of the body by blocking the effect of aldosterone.

Diminished secretion of progesterone can lead to menstrual difficulties in nonpregnant women and spontaneous abortion in pregnant women.

progestin (proh'jestin) originally, the crude hormone of the corpus luteum; it has since been isolated in pure form and is now known as PROGESTERONE. Certain synthetic and natural progestational agents are called progestins or progestogens.

progestogen (proh'jestəjən) any substance having progestational activity.

proglossis (proh'glosis) the tip of the tongue.

proglottid, proglottis (proh'glotid; proh'glotis) one of the segments making up the body of a tapeworm.

prognathism ('prognə,thizəm) abnormal protrusion of one or both jaws, especially the lower jaw, the gnathic index being above 103. adj. **prognathic, prognathous.**

prognathous (prog'naythəs, 'prognəthəs) having projecting jaws.

prognose (prog'nohz) to give a prognosis.

prognosis (prog'nohsis) a forecast of the probable course and outcome of an attack of disease and the prospects of recovery as indicated by the nature of the disease and the symptoms of the case. adj. **prognostic.**

dental p. an evaluation of the results to be achieved from any dental treatment.

medical p. an evaluation of the results to be achieved from any medical treatment.

nursing p. the application of information obtained during a nursing assessment in order to determine the prospect for altering, through nursing intervention, a client's/patient's response to illness or injury. The prognosis provides a rationale for setting priorities for meeting a particular client's/patient's nursing care needs and enhances continuity of nursing care by clearly indicating the agreed upon priorities.

progranulocyte (proh'granyuhloh,siet) promyelocyte.

progravid (proh'gravid) denoting the phase of the endometrium in which it is prepared for pregnancy.

progressive (prə'gresiv) advancing; increasing in scope or severity.

proguanil (proh'gwahnil) a malaria prophylactic, taken daily to prevent malarial infection.

prohormone (proh'hawmohn) a precursor of a hormone, such as a polypeptide that is cleaved to form a shorter polypeptide hormone or a steroid that is converted to an active hormone by peripheral metabolism.

proinsulin (proh'insyuhlin) a precursor of insulin, having low biological activity.

Project 2000 ('projekt too'thowzənd) Project 2000 (1986) is the title of the proposal of the United Kingdom Central Council (UKCC) to the Government to alter radically the process of nursing education.

Summary of major recommendations: (1) There should be a new registered practitioner competent to assess the need for care, provide care, monitor and evaluate and to do this in institutional and non-institutional settings.

(2) Preparation for the new registered practitioner should normally be completed within three years.

(3) All preparation for registration should begin with a common foundation programme followed by branch programmes.

(4) The common foundation programme should be a substantial part of preparation, lasting up to two years.

(5) Branch programmes should be available, in mental

illness, mental handicap, nursing of adults and nursing of children, with experimentation in a branch for midwifery.
(6) In the case of midwifery, there should also be an 18 month post registration preparation.
(7) There should be a new, single list of competencies applicable to all registered practitioners at the level of registration and set out in Training Rules.
(8) All future practitioners should register with Council. The area of practice should be indicated on the register.
(9) Midwives should debate the new registered practitioner outcomes in the light of their special needs.
(10) There should be a coherent, comprehensive, cost-effective framework of education beyond registrations.
(11) There should be specialist practitioners, some of whom will also be team leaders, in all areas of practice in hospital and community settings. The requisite specialist qualifications will be recordable on Council's register.
(12) Health visiting, occupational health nursing and school nursing should be specialist qualifications in health promotion which are recordable on Council's register.
(13) District nursing, community psychiatric nursing and community mental handicap nursing should be specialist qualifications which are recordable on Council's register.
(14) Students should be supernumerary to NHS staffing establishments throughout the whole period of preparation.
(15) There should be a new helper, directly supervised and monitored by a registered practitioner.
(16) Students should receive training grants which are primarily NHS-controlled. These should be administered via National Boards and should derive from a separately identified education budget.
(17) The position of teaching staff should be improved with a view to enhancing performance and allowing teachers opportunities for further training and for full participation in wider educational activities.
(18) The full range of means to achieve the appropriate concentrations of educational resources should be considered, including re-establishments, partnerships, consortia etc.
(19) Educational costs should be clearly identified and heads of educational institutions should be given responsibility for management of a more comprehensive and clearly delineated education budget.
(20) Practitioners should have formal preparation for teaching roles in practice settings.
(21) Moves should be made to establish teaching qualifications at degree level for teachers of nursing, midwifery and health visiting.
(22) Joint professional and academic validation should be pursued from the very outset of change, in order to achieve academic recognition for professional qualifications.
(23) Programmes of training for entry to the EN parts of the register should cease as soon as is practicable.
(24) The enhancement of opportunities for ENs to enter RGN, RMN, RNMH and RSCN parts of the register should now be given priority.
(25) Urgent consideration should be given to creating a new organization structure to implement the proposals of Project 2000.

projection (prə'jekshən) 1. a throwing forward, especially the reference of impressions made on the sense organs to their proper source, so as to locate correctly the objects producing them. 2. a connection between the cerebral cortex and other parts of the nervous system or organs of special sense. 3. the act of extending or jutting out, or a part that juts out. 4. a mental mechanism whereby emotionally unacceptable traits are denied by a person as his own and regarded (projected) as belonging to the external world or to someone else. It is often called the 'blaming' mechanism because in using it one seeks to place the blame for his inadequacies upon someone else. In its extreme form projection can lead to hostility and physical attack upon others when the person mistakenly perceives these persons as responsible for his mental anguish.

prokaryon (proh'karion) 1. nuclear material scattered in the cytoplasm of the cell, rather than bounded by a nuclear membrane; found in some unicellular organisms, such as bacteria. 2. prokaryote.

Prokaryotae (proh,kari'ohtee) Procaryotae.

prokaryote (proh'karioht) a unicellular organism lacking a true nucleus and nuclear membrane, having genetic material composed of a single loop of naked double-stranded DNA. Prokaryotes with the exception of mycoplasmas have a rigid cell wall. adj. **prokaryotic**.

prolabium (proh'laybi·əm) the prominent central part of the upper lip.

prolactin (proh'laktin) a hormone secreted by the anterior pituitary that stimulates and sustains milk production in postpartum mammals, and shows luteotrophic activity in certain mammals; called also lactogenic hormone, luteotrophic hormone, LTH, and mammotrophin. It is identical with luteotrophin.

prolactinoma (proh,lakti'nohmə) a pituitary tumour that secretes prolactin.

prolapse ('prohlaps) 1. the falling down, or downward displacement, of a part or viscus. 2. to undergo such displacement.

p. of cord protrusion of the umbilical cord ahead of the presenting part of the fetus in labour.

p. of the iris protrusion of the iris through a wound in the cornea.

rectal p., p. of rectum protrusion of the rectal mucous membrane through the anus.

p. of uterus downward displacement of the uterus so that the cervix is within the vaginal orifice (first-degree prolapse), the cervix is outside the orifice (second-degree prolapse), or the entire uterus is outside the orifice (third-degree prolapse).

prolapsus (proh'lapsəs) [L.] *prolapse.*

prolepsis (proh'lepsis) recurrence of a paroxysm before the expected time. adj. **proleptic**.

prolidase ('prohli,dayz) an enzyme that catalyses the hydrolysis of the imide bond between an α-carboxyl group and proline or hydroxyproline.

proliferation (prə,lifə'rayshən) the reproduction or multiplication of similar forms, especially of cells. adj. **proliferative, proliferous**.

proligerous (proh'lijə·rəs) producing offspring.

prolinase ('prohli,nayz) an enzyme that catalyses the hydrolysis of dipeptides containing proline or hydroxyproline as *N*-terminal groups.

proline ('prohleen) a cyclic amino acid occurring in proteins; it is a major constituent of collagen.

prolymphocyte (proh'limfoh,siet) a cell of the lymphocytic series intermediate between the lymphoblast and lymphocyte.

promastigote (proh'masti,goht) the morphological stage in the development of certain protozoa, characterized by a free anterior flagellum and resembling the typical adult form of *Leptomonas*.

promazine ('prohmə,zeen) a phenothiazine derivative used as a major tranquillizer in the form of the hydrochloride salt.

promegakaryocyte (,prohmegə'karioh,siet) a precursor in the thrombocytic series that is a developmental form intermediate between the megakaryoblast and the megakaryocyte.

promegaloblast (proh'megəloh,blast) the earliest form in the abnormal erythrocyte maturation sequence occurring in vitamin B_{12} and folic acid deficiencies; it corresponds to the pronormoblast, and develops into a megaloblast.

promethazine (proh'methə,zeen) a phenothiazine derivative used as an antihistaminic, antiemetic, and tranquillizer in the form of the hydrochloride salt.

promethium (proh'meethi·əm) a chemical element, atomic number 61, atomic weight 147, symbol Pm. See table of elements in Appendix 2.

prominence ('prominəns) a protrusion or projection.

promonocyte (proh'monoh,siet) a cell of the monocytic series intermediate between the monoblast and monocyte, with coarse chromatin structure and one or two nucleoli.

promontory ('promənta·ree) a projecting process or eminence.

promyelocyte (proh'mieəloh,siet) a precursor in the granulocytic series, intermediate between myeloblast and myelocyte, containing a few, as yet undifferentiated, cytoplasmic granules.

pronate (proh'nayt) to subject to pronation.

pronation (proh'nayshən) the act of assuming the prone position, or the state of being prone. Applied to the hand, turning the palm backward (posteriorly) or downward, performed by medial rotation of the forearm. Applied to the foot, a combination of eversion and abduction movements taking place in the tarsal and metatarsal joints and resulting in lowering of the medial margin of the foot, and hence of the longitudinal arch.

pronator (proh'naytə) a muscle that pronates.

prone (prohn) lying face downward, or on the ventral surface.

pronephros (proh'nefros) pl. *pronephroi* [Gr.] the primordial kidney; an excretory structure or its rudiments developing in the embryo before the mesonephros; its duct is later used by the mesonephros, which arises caudal to it.

Pronestyl (proh'nestil) trademark for preparations of procainamide, an antiarrhythmic.

pronormoblast (proh'nawmoh,blast) the earliest erythrocyte precursor, having a relatively large nucleus containing several nucleoli, surrounded by a small amount of cytoplasm (see also NORMOBLAST). Called also proerythroblast and rubriblast.

pronucleus (proh'nyookli·əs) the haploid nucleus of a sex cell.

female p. the haploid nucleus of the fully mature ovum which loses its nuclear envelope and liberates its chromosomes to meet the synapsis with those from the male pronucleus.

male p. the nuclear material of the head of a spermatozoon, after it has penetrated the ovum and acquired a pronuclear membrane.

pro-oestrus (proh'eestrəs) the period of heightened follicular activity preceding oestrus.

prootic (proh'ohtik) in front of the ear.

propagation (,propə'gayshən) reproduction. adj. **propagative.**

propantheline (proh'panthə,leen) an anticholinergic used as the bromide salt, especially in the treatment of peptic ulcer.

propepsin (proh'pepsin) pepsinogen; the inactive precursor of pepsin.

properdin (proh'pərdin) a relatively heat-labile, normal serum protein (a euglobulin) that, in the presence of COMPLEMENT component C3 and magnesium ions, acts nonspecifically against gram-negative bacteria and viruses and plays a role in lysis of erythrocytes. It migrates as a beta-globulin, and although not an antibody, may act in conjunction with complement-fixing ANTIBODY.

prophage ('prohfayj) the latent stage of a BACTERIOPHAGE in a lysogenic bacterium, in which the viral genome becomes inserted into a specific portion of the host chromosome and is duplicated into each cell generation.

prophase ('prohfayz) the first stage of cell replication in either meiosis or mitosis.

prophylactic (,profi'laktik) 1. tending to ward off disease; pertaining to prophylaxis. 2. an agent that tends to ward off disease.

prophylaxis (,profi'laksis) prevention of disease; preventive treatment.

propiolactone (,prohpioh'laktohn) a disinfectant.

propionic acid (prohpi'onik) CH_3CH_2COOH, found in chyme and sweat, and one of the products of bacterial fermentation of wood pulp waste; its salts (calcium and sodium propionate) are used as local antifungals, and to inhibit mould growth in bakery and dairy products.

proplexus (proh'pleksəs) the choroid plexus of the lateral ventricle of the brain.

propofol ('prohpəfol) trademark Diprivan, a non-barbiturate anaesthetic induction agent with rapid onset and short duration of action. It is presented as a milky solution due to being made up in soya bean oil. The rapidity of recovery with little hangover makes it suitable for day care surgery. However, it does cause pain on injection in a significant percentage of patients and a fall in blood pressure accompanies its use. It may also find a use, as a continuous infusion, as a sedative, in the intensive care unit.

propositus (proh'pozitəs) pl. *propositi* [L.] the original person presenting a mental or physical disorder who serves as the basis for a hereditary or genetic study; called also proband.

propoxycaine (proh'poksikayn) a topical anaesthetic used as the hydrochloride salt.

propoxyphene (proh'poksi,feen) an analgesic used as the hydrochloride and napsylate salts. Called also *dextropropoxyphene*.

propranolol (proh'pranə,lol) a β-adrenergic blocking agent used in the treatment of hypertension, cardiac arrhythmias, and angina pectoris, and in the prophylaxis of migraine, and for reducing the long-term risk of mortality and reinfarction after the acute phase of a myocardial infarction.

proprietary medicine (prə'prieətə·ree) any chemical, drug, or similar preparation used in the treatment of diseases, if such article is protected against free competition as to name, product, composition, or process of manufacture by secrecy, patent, trademark, or copyright, or by other means.

proprioception (,prohprioh'sepshən) perception mediated by proprioceptors or proprioceptive tissues.

proprioceptive neuromuscular facilitation (,prohprioh'septiv) the use of co-ordinated patterns of movement to strengthen a muscle group or increase the range of movement at a joint.

The movement patterns are performed in a straight line in a diagonal direction with a rotary component acting as the stabilizing component. The correct diagonal must be used as the muscles are stronger in pattern (in the groove) than out of pattern. Patterns exist for the head, trunk, arm and leg.

The starting position is one of maximum length of the muscle groups to be activated. A stretch stimulus is then applied at the beginning of the movement to ensure maximum stimulation of the muscle spindles. Maximal resistance is applied throughout the range of movement, to ensure maximal muscle contraction. This will cause overflow or irradiation from stronger to weaker muscle groups within a pattern, or from a stronger to weaker pattern. The physiotherapist must position her hands correctly to ensure the patient receives sensory stimulation to the skin in the direction of the movement.

Techniques used are: repeated contractions and slow reversals for strengthening; hold-relax and contract relax for relaxation/lengthening to gain increased range of movement; rhythmical stabilization to achieve either.

proprioceptor (ˌprohprioh'septə) any of the sensory nerve endings that give information concerning movements and position of the body; they occur chiefly in muscles, tendons, and the labyrinth. adj. **proprioceptive.**

proprotein (proh'prohteen) a protein that is cleaved to form a smaller protein, e.g., proinsulin, the precursor of insulin.

proptosis (prop'tohsis) forward displacement or bulging, especially of the eye.

propulsion (prə'pulshən) 1. a tendency to fall forward in walking. 2. festination.

propyl ('prohpil, -iel) the univalent radical $CH_3CH_2CH_2$– from propane.

propylthiouracil (ˌprohpilˌthieoh'yooə·rəsil) a thyroid inhibitor used in the treatment of thyrotoxicosis.

prorennin (proh'renin) the zymogen (proenzyme) in the gastric glands that is converted to rennin.

prorubricyte (proh'roobriˌsiet) basophilic normoblast.

pros(o)- word element. [Gr.] *forward*, *anterior*.

prosecretin (ˌprohsi'kreetin) the precursor of secretin.

prosection (ˌproh'sekshən) carefully programmed dissection for demonstration of anatomic structure.

prosector (proh'sektə) one who performs prosection.

prosencephalon (ˌprosen'kefəlon, -'sef-) the forebrain.

prosodemic (ˌprosoh'demik) passing directly from one person to another instead of reaching a large number at once, through such means as water supply: said of a disease progressing in that way.

prosop(o)- word element. [Gr.] *face*.

prosopagnosia (ˌprosohpag'nohzi·ə) inability to recognize the faces of other people or one's own features in a mirror, due to damage to the underside of both occipital lobes.

prosopalgia (ˌprosoh'palji·ə) trigeminal neuralgia (TIC DOULOUREUX). adj. **prosopalgic.**

prosopectasia (ˌprosohpek'tayzi·ə) oversize of the face.

prosoplasia (ˌprosoh'playzi·ə) 1. abnormal differentiation of tissue. 2. development into a higher state of organization or function.

prosopodiplegia (ˌprosəpohdie'pleeji·ə) paralysis of the face and one lower extremity.

prosoponeuralgia (ˌprosəpohnyuh'ralji·ə) facial neuralgia.

prosopoplegia (ˌprosəpoh'pleeji·ə) facial paralysis. adj. **prosopoplegic.**

prosoposchisis (ˌprosoh'poskisis) congenital fissure of the face.

prosopospasm (pro'sohpohˌspazəm) spasm of the facial muscles.

prosoposternodymia (ˌprosəpohˌstərnoh'dimi·ə) twins conjoined at the face and sternum.

prosopothoracopagus (ˌprosəpohˌthor·rə'kopəgəs) twin fetuses fused from the face to the thorax.

prospective study (prə'spektiv) see INCIDENCE study.

prostacyclin (ˌprostə'sieklin) an intermediate in the metabolic pathway of arachidonic acid, formed from prostaglandin endoperoxides in the walls of arteries and veins; it is a potent vasodilator and a potent inhibitor of platelet aggregation.

prostaglandin (ˌprostə'glandin) a group of naturally occurring, chemically related, long-chain hydroxy fatty acids that stimulate contractility of the uterine and other smooth muscle and have the ability to lower blood pressure, regulate acid secretion of the stomach, regulate body temperature and platelet aggregation, and control inflammation and vascular permeability. They also affect the action of certain hormones. First found in semen, they have since been found in cells throughout the body and in menstrual fluid. There are six types, A, B, C, D, E, and F, the degree of saturation of the side chain of each being designated by subscripts 1, 2, and 3.

Prostaglandin injections, commonly combined with urea, into the amniotic sac have been used as a recognized ABORTION technique in pregnancies after the 16th week. About 30 minutes after an injection of prostaglandin $F_2\alpha$, contractions begin, and abortion normally takes place within 19–20 hours. Prostaglandins may also be used to induce labour at term.

prostatalgia (ˌprostə'talji·ə) pain in the prostate.

prostate ('prostayt) a gland in the male which surrounds the neck of the bladder and the prostatic urethra. adj. **prostatic.** The prostate consists of a median lobe, an anterior and posterior lobe, and two lateral lobes, and is made up of glandular matter, the ducts from which empty into the prostatic portion of the urethra, and partly of muscular fibres which encircle the urethra. It contributes to the seminal fluid a secretion containing acid phosphatase, citric acid, and proteolytic enzymes, which account for the liquefaction of the coagulated semen. The rate of secretion increases greatly during sexual stimulation.

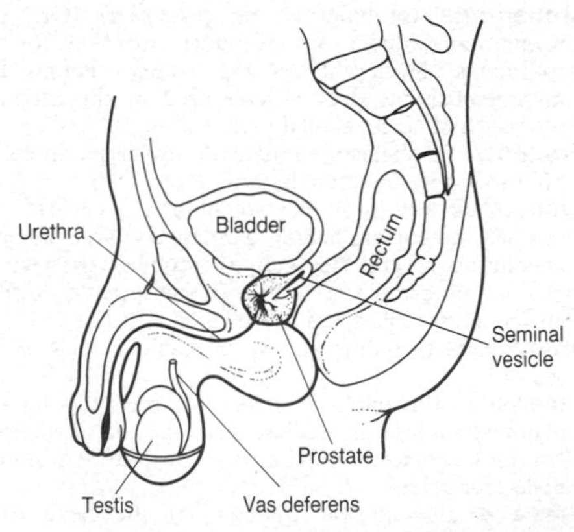

Prostate

DISORDERS OF THE PROSTATE. Enlargement of the prostate (benign prostatic hypertrophy) is a common complaint in men over 50 years of age. Because of its position around the urethra, enlargement of the prostate quickly interferes with the normal passage of urine from the bladder. Urination becomes increasingly difficult, and the bladder never feels completely emptied. If left untreated, continued enlargement of the prostate eventually obstructs the bladder outlet completely, and emergency catheterization becomes necessary to empty the bladder. The usual remedy is prostatectomy.

Cancer of the prostate may occur, usually in men over 60 years of age. The symptoms are similar to those of prostatic enlargement. If the malignancy is discovered in time, the gland can be totally removed, hopefully before the cancer has a chance to spread. Symptoms of metastatic cancer of the prostate usually respond to oestrogens or to orchidectomy, though hormonal treatment will not cure the disease.

Prevention of metastic cancer of the prostate depends on early detection and prompt treatment. In many European countries and in the USA it is recommended that all men over the age of 50 have an annual rectal examination to detect hypertrophy of the gland in its earliest stages. A blood test has been used as an indicator of the extent to which prostatic cancer has spread; however, its value as an early screening technique is doubtful. The test involves evaluation of serum prostatic acid phosphatase, a substance found in prostatic tissue and occurring at higher levels in the blood stream when the malignancy has metastasized.

Prostatitis is a relatively common inflammation of the prostate gland, which occurs as either an acute or chronic and low-grade infection. *Acute* prostatitis is characterized by an abrupt onset of fever, pain at the base of the penis, in the perineum or in the low back, dysuria, and urethral discharge. The causative agent usually is a bacterium that responds to antibiotic therapy. *Chronic* prostatitis is more difficult to eradicate. It tends to recur and may eventually require treatment by transurethral resection.

SURGERY OF THE PROSTATE. Malignancy of the prostate and intractable prostatic infection may be treated by total *prostatectomy*, which is removal of the entire gland and its capsule. In most patients however relief of symptoms is obtained by transurethral resection. Benign prostatic hypertrophy can be treated by either a closed or open approach to the gland, removing the hyperplastic tissue. In the open operation the benign adenoma is enucleated.

The closed method of treatment (*transurethral resection*, TUR) is preferred when there is relatively small enlargement of the gland and the patient is elderly and a poor surgical risk. A resectoscope is inserted through the penis along the urethra and into the bladder in a manner similar to cystoscopy. When the instrument is in the bladder an electrical cutting loop is inserted, excess tissue is resected, and bleeding vessels are cauterized. Other techniques that can be used transurethrally are the cold punch technique, using a hollow sliding knife to scoop out tissue, and cryosurgery, in which the tissue is frozen and thereby destroyed. A TUR removes the hypertrophied tissue; some normal prostatic tissue and the prostatic capsule are left intact. The transurethral approach is usually quicker and less traumatic and requires a shorter postoperative recovery period than the open methods of surgery.

There are three operative approaches to the prostate that involve a surgical incision. In the *suprapubic* (transvesical) approach, an incision is made through the abdominal wall and the bladder, and the prostatic tissue is enucleated. In the *retropubic* approach, a low abdominal incision is made and the prostate is approached between the pubic arch and the bladder. The bladder is left intact but the prostatic capsule is incised and the glandular tissue removed. The *perineal* approach requires an incision between the anus and scrotum. The prostatic capsule is opened and the prostatic tissue removed.

Total prostatectomy can result in sexual impotency, but most patients who have the other procedures can resume normal sexual function after surgery.

PATIENT CARE. The patient may be admitted to hospital because of symptoms of difficulty in micturition or with retention of urine. If this is acute retention the bladder will be distended and painful and an indwelling catheter will need to be inserted to overcome this problem.

A full general assessment of all patients admitted for prostatic surgery is mandatory as many are elderly and have other associated diseases. It is important to know of these and of the treatment which they are receiving prior to operation. Assessment of haemoglobin, blood urea and electrolytes, an EEG, chest X-ray and a plain film of the abdomen or intravenous pyelogram are desirable.

Following operating the main hazard is that of bleeding and it is usual for the patient to return to the ward with an intravenous infusion, and an indwelling catheter, either with irrigation or with systemic diuretics to increase urine flow, dilute any blood and minimise the danger of clot formation which may lead to obstruction of the catheter. As the bleeding decreases it often becomes somewhat darker in colour. The catheter must be checked at intervals to ensure that adequate drainage is occurring. If not, a bladder washout should be carried out using an aseptic technique. Usually it is possible for the patient to manage without his drip on the day after the operation and for the catheter to be removed one to two days later, A high fluid intake is desirable for the first few days after operation but care must be observed in those with cardio-respiratory problems. Wound care is of course essential after the open operations.

Infection of the urine or wound is the next major complication following prostatectomy. Later hazards include the possibility of urethral stricture formation, recurrent hypertrophy, retrograde ejaculation and sexual impotence, which is seen in up to 5 per cent of patients following transurethral resection and more than twice that number following open procedures.

prostatectomy (ˌprostəˈtektəmee) surgical removal of the PROSTATE. It may be retropubic, transurethral of transvesical/suprapubic.

prostatism (ˈprostəˌtizəm) a symptom complex resulting from compression or obstruction of the urethra, due most commonly to hyperplasia of the prostate; symptoms include diminution in the calibre and force of the urinary stream, hesitancy in initiating voiding, inability to terminate micturition abruptly (with postvoiding dribbling), a sensation of incomplete bladder emptying, and occasionally, urinary retention.

prostatitis (ˌprostəˈtietis) inflammation of the PROSTATE. adj. **prostatitic**.

allergic p., eosinophilic p. a condition seen in certain allergies, characterized by diffuse infiltration of the prostate by eosinophils, with small foci of fibrinoid necrosis.

nonspecific granulomatous p. prostatitis characterized by focal or diffuse tissue infiltration by peculiar, large, pale macrophages.

prostatocystitis (ˌprostətohsiˈstietis) inflammation of the neck of the bladder (prostatic urethra) and the bladder cavity.

prostatocystotomy (ˌprostətohsiˈstotəmee) incision of the bladder and prostate.

prostatodynia (ˌprostətohˈdini·ə) pain in the prostate.

prostatolith (proˈstatohˌlith) a calculus in the prostate.

prostatolithotomy (ˌprostətohliˈthotəmee) incision of the prostate for removal of a calculus.

prostatomegaly (ˌprostətohˈmegəlee) hypertrophy of

the prostate.

prostatorrhoea (ˌprostatəˈreeə) catarrhal discharge from the prostate.

prostatotomy (ˌprostəˈtotəmee) surgical incision of the prostate.

prostatovesiculectomy (ˌprostətohveˌsikyuhˈlektəmee) excision of the prostate and seminal vesicles.

prostatovesiculitis (ˌprostətohveˌsikyuhˈlietis) inflammation of the prostate and seminal vesicles.

prosthesis (ˈpros·theesis) pl. *prostheses* [Gr.] 1. the replacement of an absent part by an artifical substitute. 2. an artificial substitute for a missing part. adj. **prosthetic**.

ARTIFICIAL LIMB. Recent advances in the field of surgical amputation and the art of designing artificial limbs have made it possible for a person who has lost a limb to be equipped with a prosthesis that functions so efficiently, and so closely resembles the original in appearance, that he is able to resume normal activities with his handicap passing virtually unnoticed.

Fitting an Artificial Limb. The patient may be fitted with a prosthesis immediately after the lower limb is removed and before he leaves the operating theatre. He awakens from anaesthesia to find the stump encased in a rigid dressing similar to a cast and designed to accommodate a temporary prosthesis. With this device he can begin ambulation the first postoperative day and avoid many of the complications connected with inactivity. Not all patients can begin ambulation this early, however, and not all amputees are good candidates for immediate fitting of a prosthesis. Another disadvantage of immediate fitting is the hazard of wound disruption and skin breakdown, and slippage of the rigid dressing from the stump. This latter situation can cause rapid development of oedema of the stump, with resultant stress on the suture line and disruption of the wound.

Delayed fitting involves conventional wrapping of the stump and delay in using a temporary prosthesis until the 2nd or 3rd week after surgery, when the stump has healed sufficiently to allow partial weight-bearing. By the 6th week, if all goes well, the patient begins full weight-bearing and by the 10th week he is fitted with a permanent prosthesis. See also AMPUTATION.

Prosthetic fitting following amputation of an upper extremity also may be delayed or immediate, depending on the needs and status of the patient.

Powering the Limb. Most artificial limbs are powered by the muscles, either those remaining in the stump or other available muscles. The muscles of a stump often can be considerably strengthened by physiotherapy. Muscle power can be reinforced by means of springs, straps, gears, locks, levers, or, in some cases, hydraulic mechanisms.

The Artificial Leg. The most commonly fitted artificial limb is the knee-jointed leg, used by persons whose legs have been amputated above the knee. This prosthesis is powered by the hip and remaining thigh muscles, which kick the leg forward. The key points in such a limb are the socket, where it fits onto the stump, the knee, and the ankle. The possibility of walking with a normal gait depends primarily on the successful alignment of the socket joint; the knee usually consists of a joint centred slightly behind that of the natural leg, as this has been found to afford greater stability; sometimes the ankle joint is omitted and flexibility of the ankle achieved by the use of a rubber foot.

The Artificial Arm. The choice of a particular artificial arm depends largely on the person's occupation. There is a wide variety of types, ranging from the purely functional, which will enable a person to perform heavy work, to the purely cosmetic, which aims only at looking as natural as possible. Those persons whose work requires them to do heavy lifting are often fitted with a 'pegarm', a short arm without an elbow joint, which is easily controlled and has great leverage.

The Artificial Hand. There are a great many different types of artificial hands. Many artificial arms are so constructed that they can be fitted with a selection of different hands, depending on the type of work to be done. It is generally agreed by experts that the various types of hooks offer the greatest functional efficiency. These reproduce the most powerful function of natural hands—the pressure between thumb and forefinger. But there are hands that combine a certain amount of utility with cosmetic value, often by means of a cosmetic glove covering a mechanical hand; and there are also hands designed simply for appearance, though these usually offer some support as well.

Most hooks and hands are mechanically connected to the opposite shoulder and operated by a shrugging motion. However, a procedure known as kineplasty employs the person's own arm and chest muscles to work the device. In this method, selected muscles are tunnelled under by surgery and lined by skin. Pegs adapted to the tunnels can then be made to move an artificial hand mechanism. Kineplasty is employed when skill rather than strength is desired.

PROTECTING THE STUMP. In a person with an artificial limb, there is always a danger that the stump will become irritated or infected. He will probably wear a sock to cover the stump, and this should be washed daily; the stump itself should also be washed regularly and carefully, particularly between skin folds. And when the artificial limb is not being used the stump should, if possible, be exposed to the fresh air.

prosthetic (prosˈthetik) serving as a substitute; pertaining to prostheses or to prosthetics.

prosthetics (prosˈthetiks) the field of knowledge relating to prostheses, their design, use, etc.

prosthetist (prosˈtheetist) a person skilled in prosthetics and practising its application.

prosthodontics (ˌpros·thəˈdontiks) that branch of dentistry concerned with the construction of artificial appliances designed to restore and maintain oral function by replacing missing teeth and sometimes other oral structures or parts of the face.

prosthodontist (ˌpros·thəˈdontist) a specialist in prosthodontics.

prostholith (ˈpros·thohˌlith) a preputial concretion or calculus.

Prostigmin (prohˈstigmin) tradename for neostigmine, a cholinesterase inhibitor used in the treatment of myasthenia gravis.

prostration (proˈstrayshən) extreme exhaustion or lack of energy or power.

heat p. a condition caused by exposure to excessive heat (see also HEAT EXHAUSTION).

nervous p. neurasthenia.

protactinium (ˌprohtakˈtini·əm) a chemical element, atomic number 91, atomic weight 231, symbol Pa. See table of elements in Appendix 2.

protamine (ˈprohtəˌmeen) any of a class of simple proteins, soluble in water, not coagulated by heat, and precipitated from aqueous solution by addition of alcohol, found combined with nucleic acids in the sperm of certain fish, and having the property of neutralizing heparin. Protamine sulphate is used as an antidote to heparin overdosage.

protanope (ˈprohtəˌnohp) a person exhibiting protanopia.

protanopia (ˌprohtəˈnohpi·ə) red blindness; imperfect perception of red, with confusion of reds and greens. adj. **protanopic.**

protean (ˈprohti·ən, prohˈteeən) changing form or assuming different shapes.

protease (ˈprohtiˌayz) any proteolytic enzyme.

protectant, protective (prəˈtektənt; prəˈtektiv) 1. affording defence or immunity. 2. an agent affording defence against harmful influence.

protective isolation (prəˈtektiv ˌiesəˈlayshən) a type of ISOLATION designed to prevent contact between potentially pathogenic microorganisms and uninfected persons who have seriously impaired resistance. Called also *reverse isolation.*

Those entering the room should wear gowns, masks, and under some circumstances, booties and caps. The hands must be washed with an antibiotic soap or detergent and water on entering and leaving the room. Gloves are worn by all persons having direct contact with the patient. In some cases the linen is sterilized prior to use in the patient's immediate environment.

It is essential that all health care personnel, visitors, and the patient himself understand the purpose of protective isolation and the need for conscientious adherence to the precautionary rules in order to protect the patient from an infection.

protein (ˈprohteen) any large organic compound made from one or more polypeptides, which are chains of AMINO ACIDS joined by peptide linkages between the amino group of one amino acid and the carboxylic acid group of the next. The primary structure of a polypeptide chain (the sequence of amino acids) is determined by the sequence of bases in the DNA of the gene for that polypeptide (see DEOXYRIBONUCLEIC ACID).

The genetic code of the gene is first transcribed into messenger RNA (mRNA). Then the mRNA is 'read' (translated) by a ribosome to produce the polypeptide. The genetic code contains 20 different α-amino acids that can be incorporated into polypeptides by ribosomes. In some proteins other amino acids are produced by posttranslational enzymatic modification.

As the protein is synthesized it folds up into a unique 3-dimensional structure with polar (hydrophilic) side chains of amino acids on the surface and nonpolar (hydrophobic) side chains in the interior. In this way the structure and function of a protein are entirely determined by the genes.

Protein substances in the body are essential to its structure and function. For example, such structures as cell walls, various membranes, connective tissue, and muscles are mainly protein. None of the cells of the body can survive without an adequate supply of protein; in fact, proteins constitute about 20 per cent of the cell mass. Some hormones, which are important in the regulation of metabolism, are proteins, as are the ENZYMES that act as catalysts in the chemical reactions of metabolism.

The proteins in blood plasma are divided into four major classes: specific *carrier proteins*, that are involved in the transport of hormones and other substances; *acute phase reactants*, such as alpha$_1$-antitrypsin or FIBRINOGEN, that are involved in INFLAMMATION or in CLOTTING; COMPLEMENT components; and IMMUNOGLOBULINS. Albumin plays an important role in the maintenance of normal distribution of water in the various compartments of the body by exerting osmotic pressure at the capillary membrane. This pressure prevents fluid of the plasma from leaking out of the capillaries and into the space between the tissue cells. See also body FLUIDS.

Food proteins are of great nutritional importance since they are necessary for the building and repair of all kinds of body tissues, especially of muscles and organs such as the heart, liver, and kidneys. Major sources of protein are animal products such as meat, eggs, fish, and milk. Also found in nuts, peas, beans and lentils.

The digestion of protein foods begins in the stomach, is continued in the duodenum, and is completed in the small intestine. The end products of protein digestion, amino acids, pass into the blood, some to be used as structural proteins for the building of body tissues, others to be used as enzymes, and the rest to be carried to various parts of the body as a reserve. If a ready supply of carbohydrates is not available, some proteins may be converted into needed energy.

SYMPTOMS OF PROTEIN DEFICIENCY. Severe protein deficiency undermines general health, and is usually manifested in weakness, poor resistance, and swelling of body tissues (nutritional oedema) due to accumulation of fluid in the tissue spaces. Protein starvation can result from lack of protein in the diet—in persons who, from lack of available supplies of protein foods or through ignorance, satisfy their hunger with large amounts of carbohydrates and little else. Kwashiorkor is a disorder of infants and young children whose diet is deficient in protein. The illness develops soon after weaning when the child no longer receives a protein supply from his mother's milk.

Sometimes deficiency develops when digestive disorders or infections interfere with proper digestion. A congenital defect in metabolism such as PHENYLKETONURIA may lead to inability to make proper use of the protein that is available in the diet.

The first step in treatment of protein deficiency is correction of the deficiency in the diet. If the protein deficiency is secondary to another disorder, treatment is aimed at relief of the primary cause of the deficiency.

Bence Jones p. a low-molecular weight, heat-sensitive urinary protein found in multiple myeloma; it coagulates when heated to 45–55 °C. and redissolves partially or wholly on boiling.

carrier p. one which, when coupled to a hapten, renders it capable of eliciting an immune response.

complete p. one containing all the essential amino acids required in the human diet.

conjugated p's those in which the protein molecule is united with nonprotein molecules or prosthetic groups, e.g., glycoproteins, lipoproteins, and metalloproteins.

C-reactive p. a globulin that forms a precipitate with the C-polysaccharide of the pneumonococcus; its demonstration in the serum is an indicator of inflammation of infectious or noninfectious origin (see also C-REACTIVE PROTEIN).

myeloma p. a homogeneous monoclonal immunoglobulin produced by a plasmacytoma, or partial immunoglobulin molecules, such as Bence Jones protein, produced by plasma cells that have undergone neoplastic transformation.

partial p. one having a ratio of essential amino acids different from that of the average body protein.

plasma p's all the proteins present in the blood plasma, including the immunoglobulins.

serum p. proteins in the blood serum, including immunoglobulins, albumin, complement, coagulation factors, and enzymes.

protein-bound iodine test (ˈprohteenˌbownd) a laboratory test done to determine thyroid function by measuring the amount of iodine contained in compounds bound to plasma proteins. It has been largely replaced by radioimmunoassay for the thyroid hormones thyroxine (T_4) and triiodothyronine (T_3).

proteinaceous (ˌprohti'nayshəs) pertaining to or of the nature of protein.

proteinaemia (ˌprohti'neemi·ə) excess of protein in the blood.

proteinase ('prohtiˌnayz) any enzyme that catalyses the splitting of interior peptide bonds in a protein; an endopeptidase.

proteinosis (ˌprohti'nohsis) the accumulation of excess protein in the tissues.

lipid p. a hereditary defect of lipid metabolism marked by yellowish deposits of hyaline lipid carbohydrate mixture on the inner surface of the lips, under the tongue, on the oropharynx and larynx, and skin lesions.

pulmonary alveolar p. a chronic lung disease in which the distal alveoli become filled with a bland, eosinophilic, probably endogenous proteinaceous material that prevents ventilation of affected areas.

proteinuria (ˌprohti'nyooə·ri·ə) an excess of serum proteins in the urine.

proteoglycan (ˌprohtioh'gliekan) any of a group of glycoproteins found primarily in connective tissue and formed of subunits of glycosaminoglycans (long polysaccharide chains containing amino sugars) linked to a protein core like bristles on a bottle brush. Hydrated proteoglycans form the highly viscous fluid of mucus and the matrix of the intercellular ground substance of connective tissue. Called also mucopolysaccharide.

proteolipid (ˌprohtioh'lipid) a combination of a peptide or protein with a lipid, having the solubility characteristics of lipids.

proteolysis (ˌprohti'olisis) the splitting of proteins by hydrolysis of the peptide bonds, with formation of smaller polypeptides.

proteolytic (ˌprohtioh'litik) 1. pertaining to, characterized by, or promoting proteolysis. 2. a proteolytic enzyme.

proteometabolism (ˌprohtiohmə'tabəˌlizəm) the metabolism of protein.

proteopeptic (ˌprohtioh'peptik) digesting protein.

proteose ('prohtiˌohz) one of the first products in the breakdown of proteins.

Proteus ('prohti·əs) a genus of gram-negative, motile bacteria usually found in faecal and other putrefying matter, including *P. morganii*, found in the intestines and associated with summer diarrhoea of infants, and *P. vulgaris*, often found as a secondary invader in various localized suppurative pathological processes; it is a cause of cystitis.

Prothiaden (proh'thieəden) trademark for preparations of dothiepin, an antidepressant.

prothrombin (proh'thrombin) a glycoprotein present in the plasma that is converted into thrombin by extrinsic thromboplastin during the second stage of blood CLOTTING; called also clotting factor II.

p. consumption a clinical laboratory test done to determine thromboplastin generating capacity, which provides information about the first stage of coagulation. When clotting of a normal blood sample occurs, prothrombin is converted to thrombin, thus there should be little or no prothrombin in the serum after the clot is formed. If, however, there is deficiency of blood coagulation, some of the prothrombin will not be utilized. Abnormal results of the test are found in deficiencies of the first-stage factors of coagulation (factors VIII and IX), and in the presence of circulating anticoagulants, thrombocytopenia, and any other condition leading to inadequate generation of thromboplastin. **p. time** a test to measure the activity of clotting factors V, VII, and X, prothrombin, and fibrinogen; abbreviation Pro time or PT. Deficiency of any of these factors leads to a prolongation of the one-stage prothrombin times, as will circulating anticoagulants that are active against factors V, VII, or against thromboplastin.

The test is considered basic to any study of the coagulation process and is also widely used for guidance in establishing and maintaining anticoagulant therapy. Test results are best understood when both the patient's and the control times are reported. The therapeutic range for coagulation therapy is usually 2 to 4 times that of the normal (12 to 15 second) control.

prothrombinase (proh'thrombiˌnayz) thromboplastin.

prothrombinogenic (prohˌthrombinoh'jenik) promoting the production of prothrombin.

protirelin (proh'tierəlin) thyrotrophin releasing hormone.

protist ('prohtist) any member of the Protista.

Protista (proh'tistə) a kingdom comprising bacteria, algae, slime moulds, fungi, and protozoa; it includes all single-celled organisms.

protium ('prohti·əm) the mass 1 isotope of hydrogen, symbol ^{1}H; ordinary, or light, hydrogen.

proto- word element. [Gr.] *first*.

protoblast ('prohtohˌblast) a blastomere from which a particular organ or part develops. adj. **protoblastic**.

protocol ('prohtəˌkol) the original notes made on a necropsy, an experiment, or on a case of disease.

protodiastolic (ˌprohtohˌdieə'stolik) pertaining to early diastole, i.e., immediately following the second heart sound.

protoduodenum (ˌprohtohˌdyooə'deenəm) the first or proximal portion of the duodenum, extending from the pylorus to the duodenal papilla.

protofibril (ˌprohtoh'fiebril) the first elongated unit appearing in formation of any type of fibre.

protogaster ('prohtohˌgastə) archenteron.

proton ('prohton) an elementary particle of mass number 1, with a positive charge equal to the negative charge of the electron; a constituent particle of every nucleus, the number of protons in the nucleus of each ATOM of a chemical element being indicated by its atomic number.

protoneuron (ˌprohtoh'nyooə·ron) the first neuron in a peripheral reflex arc.

protoplasm ('prohtəˌplazəm) the viscid, translucent colloid material, the essential constituent of the living cell, including cytoplasm and nucleoplasm. adj. **protoplasmic**.

protoplast ('prohtəˌplast) a bacterial or plant cell deprived of its rigid wall but with its plasma membrane intact; the cell is dependent for its integrity on an isotonic or hypertonic medium.

protoporphyria (ˌprohtohpaw'firi·ə) porphyria marked by excessive protoporphyrin in erythrocytes, plasma, and faeces, and by intense itching, erythema, and oedema on short exposure to sunlight; skin lesions usually fade without scarring or pigmentation but a chronic weatherbeaten appearance is characteristic. Called also erythropoietic protoporphyria.

protoporphyrin (ˌprohtoh'pawfirin) a porphyrin whose iron complex united with protein occurs in haemoglobin, myoglobin, and certain respiratory pigments.

protoporphyrinuria (ˌprohtohˌpawfiri'nyooə·ri·ə) protoporphyrin in the urine.

prototroph ('prohtəˌtrohf) an organism with the same growth factor requirements as the ancestral strain; said of microbial mutants. adj. **prototrophic**.

prototype ('prohtəˌtiep) the original type or form that is typical of later individuals or species.

protovertebra (ˌprohtoh'vərtibrə) 1. somite. 2. the caudal half of a somite forming most of the vertebra.

Protozoa (ˌprohtəˈzoh·ə) a phylum comprising the unicellular eukaryotic organisms; most are free-living, but some lead commensalistic, mutualistic, or parasitic existences. Protozoa are usually divided into four subphyla: Sarcodina (amoebae), having pseudopodia during most of the life cycle; Mastigophora (flagellates), having one or more flagella during most of the life cycle; Ciliophora (ciliates and suctorians), having cilia during some stages of development; and Sporozoa, having no locomotor organs in the adult stages and reproducing by sporulation.

Pathogenic protozoa include *Plasmodium* species, the cause of human malaria; *Trypanosoma gambiense*, the cause of African trypanosomiasis (African sleeping sickness); *Toxoplasma gondii*, of which house cats are the reservoir and humans the intermediate host; *Entamoeba histolytica*, the cause of amoebic dysentery; and *Balantidium coli* and *Isospora belli*, both of which cause diarrhoea in man.

Certain protozoa can be ingested and transmitted through contaminated faeces. Prevention of transmission is extremely important; handwashing and stool precautions are recommended. Other protozoa, such as those causing malaria and trypanosomiasis, are transmitted through insect vectors, and control is a more complex matter.

protozoacide (ˌprohtəˈzoh·əˌsied) destructive to protozoa; an agent destructive to protozoa.

protozoal (ˌprohtəˈzoh·əl) pertaining to or caused by protozoa.

protozoan (ˌprohtəˈzoh·ən) 1. of or pertaining to protozoa. 2. an organism belonging to the Protozoa.

protozoiasis (ˌprohtohzohˈieəsis) any disease caused by protozoa.

protozoology (ˌprohtohzohˈoləjee) the scientific study of protozoa.

protozoon (ˌprohtəˈzoh·on) pl. *protozoa* [Gr.] any member of the protozoa.

protozoophage (ˌprohtohˈzoh·əˌfayj) a cell having phagocytic action on protozoa.

protraction (prəˈtrakshən) a forward projection of a facial structure; in mandibular protraction the gnathion is anterior to the orbital plane; in maxillary protraction the subnasion is anterior to the orbital plane.

protractor (prəˈtraktə) an instrument for extracting foreign bodies from wounds.

protransglutaminase (prohˌtranzglooˈtamiˌnayz) the inactive precursor of transglutaminase; called also coagulation Factor XIII.

protriptyline (prohˈtriptəˌleen) a tricyclic ANTIDEPRESSANT.

protrusion (prəˈtroozhən) extension beyond the usual limits, or above a plane surface.

protuberance (prəˈtyoobə·rəns) a projecting part, or prominence.

protuberantia (prohˌtyoobəˈranshi·ə) pl. *protuberantiae* [L.] protuberance.

proud flesh (prowd flesh) exuberant amounts of soft, oedematous, granulation tissue developing during healing of large surface wounds.

Provera (prohˈverə) trademark for preparations of medroxyprogesterone, a progestational agent. It is an i.m. contraceptive, effective for 8–12 weeks.

provertebra (prohˈvərtibrə) protovertebra.

provirus (prohˈvierəs) the genome of an animal virus integrated (by crossing over) into the chromosome of the host cell, and thus replicated in all of its daughter cells.

provitamin (prohˈvitəmin) a substance, e.g., ergosterol, from which the animal organism can form a vitamin.

proximad (ˈproksimad) in a proximal direction.

proximal (ˈproksiməl) nearest to a point of reference, as to a centre or median line or to the point of attachment or origin.

proximalis (ˌproksiˈmaylis) [L.] *proximal*.

proximate (ˈproksimət) immediate; nearest.

proximoataxia (ˌproksimoh·əˈtaksi·ə) ataxia of the proximal part of an extremity.

proximobuccal (ˌproksimohˈbukˈl) pertaining to the proximal and buccal surfaces of a posterior tooth.

prozone (ˈprohzohn) the phenomenon exhibited by some sera, in which agglutination or precipitation occurs at higher dilution ranges, but is not visible at lower dilutions or when undiluted.

pruriginous (prooəˈrijinəs) of the nature of prurigo or tending to cause prurigo.

prurigo (prooəˈriegoh) [L.] any of several itchy skin eruptions in which the characteristic lesion is dome-shaped with a small transient vesicle on top, followed by crusting or lichenification.

p. mitis prurigo of a mild type.

p. nodularis a form of neurodermatitis, usually occurring on the extremities in middle-aged women, marked by discrete, firm, rough-surfaced, dark brownish-grey, intensely itchy nodules.

p. simplex papular urticaria.

pruritogenic (ˌprooə·ritohˈjenik) causing pruritus, or itching.

pruritus (prooəˈrietis) itching. adj. **pruritic.** It is common in many types of skin disorders, especially allergic inflammation and parasitic infestations. Systemic diseases that may cause pruritus include DIABETES MELLITUS (pruritus vulvae) and liver disorders with jaundice. Haemorrhoids are often accompanied by rectal pruritus. Emotional distress plays an important role in the development and control of this disturbing symptom. Unless pruritus is relieved the patient may become exhausted from lack of sleep.

Cleanliness, soothing ointments or lotions, baths, and sometimes tranquillizing drugs are used in the relief of pruritus. Since it is a symptom of some other disorder, complete cure of pruritus depends on cure of the primary illness.

p. ani intense chronic itching in the anal region.

essential p. that occurring without known cause.

p. senilis itching in the aged, due to degeneration of the skin.

symptomatic p. that which occurs secondarily to another condition.

uraemic p. generalized itching associated with chronic renal failure and not attributable to other internal or skin disease.

p. vulvae intense itching of the external genitalia in the female.

Prussak's pouch (ˈproosahks) a recess in the tympanic membrane between the flaccid part of the membrane and the neck of the malleus.

prussic acid (ˈprusik) hydrocyanic acid.

psammoma (saˈmohmə) a tumour, especially a meningioma, which contains psammoma bodies. See BODY.

psammosarcoma (ˌsamohsahˈkohmə) a sarcoma containing the granular psammoma bodies.

pseud(o)- word element. [Gr.] *false*.

pseudaesthesia (ˌsyoodisˈtheezi·ə) a subjective sensation occurring in the absence of the appropriate stimuli; an imaginary sensation.

pseudarthrosis (ˌsyoodahˈthrohsis) a pathological entity characterized by deossification of a weight-bearing long bone, followed by bending and pathological fracture, with inability to form normal callus leading to existence of the 'false joint' that gives the condition its name.

pseudencephalus (ˌsyooden'kefələs, -'sef-) a fetus with a tumour in place of the brain.

pseudoacanthosis nigricans (ˌsyoodohˌakən'thohsis 'niegriˌkanz) a benign form of acanthosis nigricans associated with obesity; the obesity is sometimes linked to endocrine disturbance.

pseudoagraphia (ˌsyoodoh·ay'grafi·ə) a condition in which the patient can copy writing, but cannot write except in a meaningless and illegible manner.

pseudoallele (ˌsyoodoh'aleel, -ə'leel) one of two or more genes that are seemingly allelic, but which can be shown to have distinctive but closely linked loci. adj. **pseudoallelic**.

pseudoanaemia (ˌsyoodoh·ə'neemi·ə) marked pallor with no evidence of anaemia.

pseudoaneurysm (ˌsyoodoh'anyəˌrizəm) an appearance resembling an aneurysm, but due to enlargement and tortuosity of a vessel.

pseudoangina (ˌsyoodoh·an'jienə) a nervous disorder resembling angina.

pseudoankylosis (ˌsyoodohˌangki'lohsis) a false ankylosis.

pseudoapoplexy (ˌsyoodoh'apəˌpleksee) a condition resembling apoplexy, but without cerebral haemorrhage.

pseudobulbar (ˌsyoodoh'bulbə) apparently, but not really, due to a bulbar lesion.

pseudocartilaginous (ˌsyoodohˌkahti'lajinəs) resembling cartilage.

pseudocast ('syoodohˌkahst) an accidental formation of urinary sediment resembling a true cast.

pseudocele ('syoodohˌseel) pseudocoele.

pseudochancre (ˌsyoodoh'shangkə) an indurated lesion resembling chancre.

pseudocholesteatoma (ˌsyoodohˌkohliˌsteeə'tohmə) a horny mass of epithelial cells resembling cholesteatoma in the tympanic cavity in chronic middle ear inflammation.

pseudochorea (ˌsyoodohko'reeə) a state of general incoordination resembling chorea.

pseudochromaesthesia (ˌsyoodohˌkrohmis'theezi·ə) a false sensation of colour.

pseudochromhidrosis (ˌsyoodohˌkrohmi'drohsis) discoloration of sweat by surface contaminants, such as pigment-producing bacteria or chemical substances on the skin.

pseudocirrhosis (ˌsyoodohsi'rohsis) a condition suggestive of, but not due to cirrhosis; often due to pericarditis (pericardial pseudocirrhosis). Called also Pick's disease.

pseudocoarctation (ˌsyoodohˌkoh·ahk'tayshən) a condition radiographically resembling coarctation but without compromise of the lumen, as occurs in a congenital anomaly of the aortic arch.

pseudocoele ('syoodohˌseel) the fifth ventricle of the brain.

pseudocolloid (ˌsyoodoh'koloyd) a mucoid substance sometimes found in ovarian cysts.

p. of lips Fordyce's disease.

pseudocoloboma (ˌsyoodohˌkoloh'bohmə) a line or scar on the iris resembling a coloboma.

pseudocoxalgia (ˌsyoodohkok'salji·ə) osteochondrosis of the capitular epiphysis of the femur.

pseudocrisis (ˌsyoodoh'kriesis) sudden but temporary abatement of febrile symptoms.

pseudocroup (ˌsyoodoh'kroop) laryngismus stridulus; sudden laryngeal spasm with crowing inspiration.

pseudocyesis (ˌsyoodohsie'eesis) false pregnancy; development of all the signs of pregnancy without the presence of an embryo.

pseudocylindroid (ˌsyoodoh'silinˌdroyd) a shred of mucin in the urine resembling a cylindroid, sometimes of spermatic origin.

pseudocyst ('syoodohˌsist) an abnormal dilated space resembling a cyst but not lined with epithelium.

pseudodementia (ˌsyoodohdi'menshi·ə) a state of general mental impairment resembling dementia, but with no actual defect of intelligence, the symptoms being emotional in origin.

pseudodiphtheria (ˌsyoodohdif'thiə·ri·ə, -dip-) the presence of a false membrane not due to *Corynebacterium diphtheriae.*

pseudodominant (ˌsyoodoh'dominənt) the rarely observed pattern of inheritance of a recessive genetic trait in the offspring of parents one of whom is homozygous and the other heterozygous for the gene. Half the offspring are affected as in the common pattern of dominant inheritance seen when only one parent, who is heterozygous, carries the gene.

pseudoemphysema (ˌsyoodohˌemfi'seemiə, -fie-) a condition resembling emphysema, but due to temporary obstruction of the bronchi.

pseudoephedrine (ˌsyoodoh'efiˌdreen) one of the optical isomers of ephedrine; the hydrochloride salt is used as a nasal decongestant.

pseudoexstrophy (ˌsyoodoh'ekstrəfee) a developmental anomaly marked by the characteristic musculoskeletal defects of exstrophy of the bladder, but with no major defect of the urinary tract.

pseudofolliculitis (ˌsyoodohfoˌlikyuh'lietis) a chronic disorder occurring chiefly in Afro-Caribbeans, most often in the submandibular region of the neck, the characteristic lesions of which are erythematous papules, less commonly pustules, containing buried hairs whose tips can easily be freed up; in contrast to sycosis barbae, it affects exclusively those who shave.

pseudofracture (ˌsyoodoh'frakchə) appearance on x-ray of a thickened periosteum and new bone formation over what looks like an incomplete fracture.

pseudoganglion (ˌsyoodoh'gang·gli·ən) an enlargement on a nerve resembling a ganglion.

pseudogeusaesthesia (ˌsyoodohˌgyoosis'theezi·ə) a false sensation of taste associated with a sensation of another modality.

pseudogeusia (ˌsyoodoh'gyoozi·ə) a sensation of taste occurring in the absence of a stimulus or inappropriate to the exciting stimulus.

pseudoglioma (ˌsyoodohglie'ohmə) any condition mimicking retinoblastoma, e.g., retrolental fibroplasia or exudative retinopathy.

pseudoglottis (ˌsyoodoh'glotis) 1. the aperture between the false vocal cords. 2. neoglottis. adj. **pseudoglottic**.

pseudogout (ˌsyoodoh'gowt) an apparently hereditary, arthritic condition marked by attacks of goutlike symptoms, usually affecting a single joint (particularly the knee), and associated with chondrocalcinosis.

pseudogynaecomastia (ˌsyoodohˌgienəkoh'masti·ə) the deposition of adipose tissue in the male breast that may give the appearance of enlarged mammary glands.

pseudohaematuria (ˌsyoodohˌheemə'tyooə·ri·ə) the presence in the urine of pigments that impart a pink or red colour, but with no detectable haemoglobin or blood cells.

pseudohaemophilia (ˌsyoodohˌheemoh'fili·ə) von Willebrand's disease.

pseudohermaphrodite (ˌsyoodoh·hər'mafrəˌdiet) an individual exhibiting pseudohermaphroditism.

pseudohermaphroditism (ˌsyoodoh·hər'mafrədiˌtizəm) a state in which the gonads are of one sex but one or more contradictions exist in the morphological criteria of sex. In female pseudohermaphroditism, the individual is a genetic and gonadal female with partial masculinization; in male pseudohermaphroditism, the individual is a genetic and gonadal male with incomplete masculinization. Pseudohermaphroditism is not to be confused with hermaphroditism, in which the individual possesses both ovarian and testicular tissue.

pseudohernia (ˌsyoodoh'hərni·ə) an inflamed sac or gland simulating strangulated hernia.

pseudohypertrophy (ˌsyoodoh·hie'pərtrəfee) increase in size without true hypertrophy. adj. **pseudohypertrophic.**

pseudohypoaldosteronism (ˌsyoodohˌhiepoh·al-'dostə·rəˌnizəm) a hereditary disorder of infancy, characterized by severe salt loss by the kidneys despite elevated secretion and urinary excretion of aldosterone; it is thought to be due to unresponsiveness of the distal renal tubule to aldosterone.

pseudohypoparathyroidism (ˌsyoodohˌhiepohˌparə-'thieroyˌdizəm) a hereditary condition clinically resembling hypoparathyroidism, but caused by failure of response to, rather than deficiency of, parathyroid hormone; it is marked by hypocalcaemia and hyperphosphataemia and commonly by short stature, obesity, short metacarpals, and ectopic calcification.

pseudoisochromatic (ˌsyoodohˌiesohkrə'matik) seemingly of the same colour throughout: applied to solutions for testing colour blindness, containing two pigments or colours which will be distinguished by the normal eye, but not by the colour blind.

pseudojaundice (ˌsyoodoh'jawndis) yellowness of the skin due to blood changes and not to liver disease.

pseudologia (ˌsyoodoh'lohji·ə) the writing of anonymous letters to people of prominence, to one's self, etc.

p. fantastica a tendency to tell extravagant and fantastic falsehoods centred about one's self.

pseudomania (ˌsyoodoh'mayni·ə) 1. false or pretended mental disorder. 2. pathological lying.

pseudomelanosis (ˌsyoodohˌmelə'nohsis) pigmentation of tissues after death by blood pigments.

pseudomembrane (ˌsyoodoh'membrayn) false membrane.

Pseudomonas (ˌsyoodoh'mohnəs) a genus of gram-negative, strictly aerobic bacteria, some species of which are pathogenic for plants and vertebrates.

P. aeruginosa this produces the blue-green pigment, pyocyanin, which gives the colour to 'blue pus', and causes various human diseases.

P. mallei the causative agent of glanders, a disease of horses that is communicable to man.

P. pseudomallei the causative agent of melioidosis, a disease of rodents occasionally transmitted to man.

pseudomucin (ˌsyoodoh'myoosin) a mucin-like substance found in ovarian cysts. adj. **pseudomucinous**.

pseudomyopia (ˌsyoodohmie'ohpi·ə) spasm of the ciliary muscle causing increased refraction power of the lens and hence myopia.

pseudomyxoma (ˌsyoodohmik'sohmə) a mass of epithelial mucus resembling a myxoma.

p. peritonei the presence in the peritoneal cavity of mucoid material from a ruptured ovarian cyst or a ruptured mucocele of the appendix.

pseudoneuritis (ˌsyoodohnyuh'rietis) a congenital hyperemic condition of the optic papilla.

pseudo-oedema (ˌsyoodoh·i'deemə) a puffy state resembling oedema.

pseudopapilloedema (ˌsyoodohˌpapili'deemə) anomalous elevation of the optic disc, mimicking papilloedema.

pseudoparalysis (ˌsyoodohpə'ralisis) apparent loss of muscular power without real paralysis.

arthritic general p. a condition resembling dementia paralytica, dependent on intracranial atheroma in arthritic patients. Called also Klippel's disease.

Parrot's p., syphilitic p. pseudoparalysis of one or more extremities in infants, due to syphilitic osteochondritis of an epiphysis.

pseudoparaplegia (ˌsyoodohˌparə'pleeji·ə) spurious paralysis of the lower limbs, as in hysteria or malingering.

pseudoparesis (ˌsyoodohpə'reesis) a hysterical or nonorganic condition simulating paresis.

pseudopelade (ˌsyoodoh'peelayd) patchy alopecia roughly simulating alopecia areata; it may be due to various diseases of the hair follicles, some of which are associated with scarring.

pseudoplegia (ˌsyoodoh'pleeji·ə) hysterical paralysis.

pseudopodium (ˌsyoodoh'pohdi·əm) a temporary protrusion of the cytoplasm of an amoeba, serving for purposes of locomotion or to engulf food.

pseudopolyp (ˌsyoodoh'polip) a hypertrophied tab of mucous membrane resembling a polyp, but caused by ulceration surrounding intact mucosa.

pseudopolyposis (ˌsyoodohˌpoli'pohsis) numerous pseudopolyps in the colon and rectum, due to longstanding inflammation.

pseudopregnancy (ˌsyoodoh'pregnənsee) false pregnancy; development of all the signs of pregnancy without the presence of an embryo.

pseudopseudohypoparathyroidism (ˌsyoodoh-ˌsyoodohˌhiepohˌparə'thieroyˌdizəm) an incomplete form of pseudohypoparathyroidism, marked by the same constitutional features but by normal levels of calcium and phosphorus in the blood serum.

pseudopterygium (ˌsyoodohtə'riji·əm) an adhesion of the conjunctiva to the cornea following a burn or other injury.

pseudoptosis (ˌsyoodop'tohsis) decrease in the size of the palpebral aperture.

pseudoreaction (ˌsyoodohri'akshən) a false or deceptive reaction; in intradermal skin tests, a reaction not due to the specific test substance but to protein in the medium employed in producing the toxin.

pseudorickets (ˌsyoodoh'rikits) renal osteodystrophy.

pseudoscarlatina (ˌsyoodohˌskahlə'teenə) a septic condition with fever and eruption resembling scarlet fever.

pseudosclerosis (ˌsyoodohsklə'rohsis) a condition with the symptoms but without the lesions of multiple sclerosis.

Westphal–Strümpell p. hepatolenticular degeneration.

pseudosmia (syoo'dozmi·ə) a sensation of odour without the appropriate stimulus.

pseudotetanus (ˌsyoodoh'tetənəs) persistent muscular contractions resembling tetanus but not associated with *Closdridium tetani.*

pseudotruncus arteriosus (ˌsyoodoh'trungkəs ahˌtiə·ri'ohsəs) the most severe form of tetralogy of Fallot.

pseudotumour (ˌsyoodoh'tyoomə) phantom tumour.

p. cerebri cerebral oedema and raised intracranial pressure without neurological signs except occasional sixth-nerve palsy.

pseudoxanthoma elasticum (ˌsyoodohzan'thohmə i'lastikəm) a dermatosis marked clinically by small yellowish macules and papules, individual or confluent, or massed into plaques, and histologically by masses of swollen, calcified elastic fibres with degeneration of the collagen fibres in the lower and middle dermis and in the gastrointestinal tract and heart.

pseudulcus (syoo'dulkəs) a sore which appears like, but is not, an ulcer.

p. ventriculus a form of neurosis in which sensations in the stomach simulate symptoms of a gastric ulcer.

p.s.i. pounds per square inch.

psilocin ('sielohsin) a hallucinogenic substance closely related to psilocybin.

psilocybin (ˌsieloh'siebin) a HALLUCINOGEN having indole characteristics, isolated from the mushroom *Psilocybe mexicana.*

psilosis (sie'lohsis) 1. loss or falling of the hair. 2. sprue.

p. pigmentosa pellagra.

psittacosis (ˌsitə'kohsis) a disease due to a strain of *Chlamydia psittaci*, first seen in parrots and later found in other birds and domestic fowl (in which it is called *ornithosis*). It is transmissible to man.

The aetiological organism is inhaled into the body and attacks the respiratory tract. The first symptoms appear after an incubation period of 6 to 15 days and include fever, sore throat, headache, loss of appetite, chills, and profuse sweating. Later there may be coughing, difficulty in breathing, abdominal distress, and often splenomegaly. Prostration may occur. Infiltrates may appear in the chest radiograph. Special laboratory tests are necessary for accurate diagnosis.

Psittacosis usually runs its course in 2 or 3 weeks. Complications may be avoided by the administration of such antibiotics as tetracycline and penicillin. Fatalities are uncommon.

psoas ('soh·əs) a muscle forming part of the posterior abdominal wall.

p. abscess one that arises in the lumbar region and is due to spinal caries as a result of tuberculus infection.

p. major, p. magnus greater psoas muscle, originating at the lumbar vertebrae with the insertion at the lesser trochanter of the femur. Its action is to flex the trunk and flex and medially rotate the thigh.

p. minor, p. parvus smaller psoas muscle, originating at T12 and L1 vertebrae with the insertion at the iliopectineal prominence. Its action is to flex the trunk on the pelvis.

psoitis (soh'ietis) inflammation of a psoas muscle or its sheath.

psoralen ('sor·rəlen) any of the constituents of certain plants (e.g., *Psoralea corylifolia*) that have the ability to produce photoxic dermatitis when an individual is first exposed to it and then to sunlight; certain perfumes and drugs (e.g., methoxsalen) contain psoralens. Can be used in the treatment of psoriasis.

psoriasis (sə'rieəsis) a usually chronic, recurrent skin disease marked by discrete bright red macules, papules, or patches covered with lamellated silvery scales. adj. **psoriatic.**

The lesions appear most often on the scalp, knees, and elbows, and on the chest, back, and buttocks. It can also be widespread. Sometimes the nails are affected, causing pitting and scaling of the base, or ridging and furrowing with an alteration in the transparency of the nail. Emotional response to the persistence and cosmetically disfiguring effects of psoriasis can be so severe as to cause some sufferers to contemplate suicide.

The disorder can occur in either sex at any age, but is most often seen in persons 20 to 50 years of age. It affects about 3 per cent of white adults and is uncommon in Afro-Caribbeans. It sometimes occurs in association with rheumatoid arthritis but the connection between the two disorders is not clear.

The cause of psoriasis is not known. It is not an infectious disease and cannot be transmitted from one person to another. It tends to occur in families; about one-third of the cases are believed to be related to a hereditary factor. Its onset may be initiated by severe emotional or physical trauma, or a severe infection. Scratching and inflammation, or a secondary infection, can lead to the development of more lesions.

Most cases of the disorder are chronic and recurrent. Early attacks respond well to treatment, only to reappear within weeks or months. Complete and permanent remission is very rare.

TREATMENT. There is at present no curative agent available; all treatments currently in use must be prescribed with caution to avoid permanent damage to the skin. Recommended topical agents include coal tar, dithranol, and steroids. Exposure to the sun and artificial ultraviolet light can be helpful. The oldest form of therapy is the Goeckerman routine which combines coal tar with increasing exposure to ultraviolet light.

Radiotherapy is currently under investigation. It includes phototherapy with ultraviolet light and the administration of photochemotherapeutic agents which potentiate ultraviolet light (psoralens). When used with psoralens, ultraviolet light prevents the rapidly proliferating epithelial cells from replicating by interfering with production of DNA.

A folic acid antagonist, methotrexate, seems to control psoriasis by inhibiting cell reproduction. It is a systemic drug that has potentially serious side-effects and, therefore, usually is given only to those patients who have serious psoriasis that is not controlled by other forms of treatment.

guttate p. widespread pin-point areas of psoriatic lesions.

pustular p. psoriatic lesions which have become infected and contain pus.

PSP phenolsulphonphthalein, a dye used in testing kidney function.

PSW Psychiatric Social Worker.

psych(o)- word element. [Gr.] *mind.*

psychalgia (sie'kalji·ə) pain of mental or hysterical origin; pain attending or due to mental effort. adj. **psychalgic.**

psychanopsia (ˌsiekə'nopsi·ə) psychic blindness.

psychataxia (ˌsiekə'taksi·ə) a disordered mental state with confusion, agitation, and inability to fix the attention.

psyche ('siekee) the mind; the human faculty for thought, judgement, and emotion; the mental life, including both conscious and unconscious processes. adj. **psychic.**

psychedelic (ˌsiekə'delik) mind-altering, a term applied to hallucinatory or psychotomimetic drugs capable of profound effects upon the nature of perception and conscious experience. See also HALLUCINOGEN.

psychiatrist (sie'kieətrist) a doctor who specializes in psychiatry.

psychiatry (sie'kieətree) the branch of medicine that deals with the study, treatment, and prevention of mental illness. adj. **psychiatric.**

biological p. that which emphasizes physical, chemical, and neurological causes and treatment approaches.

descriptive p. that based on observation and study of external factors that can be seen, heard, or felt.

dynamic p. the study of emotional processes, their origins and the mental mechanisms underlying them.

forensic p. that dealing with the legal aspects of mental disorders.

organic p. 1. that dealing with the psychological aspects of organic brain disease. 2. biological psychiatry.

preventive p. a broad term referring to the amelioration, control, and limitation of psychiatric disability.

social p. that concerned with the cultural and social factors that engender, precipitate, intensify, or prolong maladaptive patterns of behaviour and complicate treatment.

psychic ('siekik) pertaining to the mind or psyche.

psychoactive (ˌsiekoh'aktiv) affecting the mind or behaviour, as psychoactive drugs.

psychoanaleptic (ˌsiekohˌanə'leptik) exerting a stimulating effect on the mind.

psychoanalysis (ˌsiekoh·ə'nalisis) 1. a method of investigating mental processes, developed by Sigmund Freud, which uses the techniques of free association, interpretation, and dream analysis. 2. a system of theoretical psychology formulated by Freud based on the recognition of unconscious mental processes, such as resistance, repression, and transference, and of the importance of infantile experience as a determinant of adult behaviour. 3. a method of psychotherapy based on the psychoanalytic method and psychoanalytic psychology. adj. **psychoanalytic**.

Psychoanalytic theory has increased our understanding of the causes of neurosis and personality disorders. Neurotic patterns of behaviour have their origin in conflicts, feelings, and attitudes that arise in childhood.

A child has many desires, impulses, and thoughts that are in conflict with the expectations of his parents. In order to avoid the unbearable anxiety of direct conflict with his parents which he fears would result in loss of affection or other forms of punishment, these conflicts are *repressed*; the anxiety-producing thoughts or feelings are excluded from conscious awareness. Normally, the conflict is resolved unconsciously by acting out the repressed wish in a disguised form in play, fantasy, or dreams and coming to terms with it.

When unconscious conflicts are not resolved, the repressed wishes and fantasies may continue to be acted out in daily life, producing neurotic symptoms. A neurotic adult will tend to respond to people in terms of childhood feelings toward members of his family, even though these responses are not appropriate to the situation. Without realizing it, he is going through adult life still acting out fantasies of childhood. His unresolved conflicts prevent him from seeing others as they are and reacting to them in an appropriate way.

Psychoanalytic Psychotherapy. Psychoanalysis is an insight-oriented type of PSYCHOTHERAPY. Its goal is to uncover unconscious psychological patterns and enable the patient to discover the influence of these patterns in daily life. As the patient acquires self-knowledge, the unconscious patterns are undone and areas of behaviour come under conscious control. For a person who has the required maturity and intelligence and who is motivated to accomplish a thorough reconstruction of the personality, psychoanalysis is the psychotherapy of choice.

The treatment is usually prolonged and expensive. In classic treatment, the patient has four or five analytic sessions lasting 45 minutes to an hour each week. Many analysts also conduct less intensive treatment with two or three sessions a week. An analysis usually takes two or three years.

Free Association. In this technique the patient simply says whatever comes to mind without censoring or withholding anything, no matter how distressing and embarrassing or trivial and irrelevant it seems. The analyst forms tentative explanations of the patient's associations and experiences but withholds them until they are validated by more material and until the patient is in a receptive frame of mind. Often the analyst is silent for long periods, sometimes for most of a session. In order to facilitate this process, which would be interrupted by the patient's need to respond to the analyst's facial expressions and conversational responses, the patient usually lies on a couch facing away from the analyst.

Interpretation. At appropriate times, the analyst makes interpretations, which are explanations of the connection between the patient's mental phenomena as revealed by free association and his behaviour and neurotic symptoms. Interpretations are not forced on the patient; even cautious interpretations arouse some anxiety and meet some resistance. An experienced analyst can often present an interpretation so that it seems to be an obvious inference from what the patient has just said; however, the patient still needs to work out his own conclusions and arrive at his own understanding of his psychology.

Dreams. The interpretation of dream material is an important part of the psychoanalytic process. The *manifest content* of a dream as it appears to the dreamer is a distorted and disguised form of the *latent* content, which expresses the patient's repressed wishes, thoughts, feelings, and fantasies. The patient's free associations are used to discover the latent content and to discover how these repressed patterns affect the patient's waking life.

Resistance. Neither free association nor the patient's assimilation of interpretations proceeds smoothly; both are interrupted by various forms of resistance. The associations are interrupted by forgetfulness, evasions, embarrassment, or mental blocks and the interpretations may be met with various forms of resistance, such as denial, anger, or misunderstanding. Resistance occurs because the blocked association or understanding would be too threatening to face at that point in the therapy and is in itself an important indication of the patient's unconscious patterns.

Transference. This refers to the emotional reaction of the patient to the analyst in ways that reproduce unconscious emotional attitudes toward the parents or other important persons that developed in the patient's childhood. The patient may exhibit affection, hostility, or ambivalence toward the analyst that is a projection of unconscious images onto the analyst. The analyst must remain objective about the patient's transference. Having made sure that it is not a reaction to the analyst's own behaviour, the transference can be interpreted to help the patient understand these childhood attitudes.

An emotional response of the analyst to the patient's transference is known as *countertransference.* Any overt response to the patient, such as anger, impatience, resentment, or seductive behaviour, may cause serious problems and result in a therapeutic failure.

psychoanalyst (ˌsiekoh'anəˌlist) a practitioner of psychoanalysis.

psychobiology (ˌsiekohbie'oləjee) study of the interrelations of body and mind in the formation and functioning of personality. adj. **psychobiological**.

psychocortical (ˌsiekoh'kawtik'l) pertaining to the mind and the cerebral cortex.

psychodelic (ˌsiekoh'delik) psychedelic.

psychodiagnosis (ˌsiekohˌdieəg'nohsis) the diagnostic use of psychological testing.

psychodrama (ˌsiekoh'drahmə) group PSYCHOTHERAPY in which patients dramatize their individual conflicting situations of daily life.

psychodynamics (ˌsiekohdie'namiks) the science of human behaviour and motivation.

psychogenesis (ˌsiekoh'jenəsis) 1. mental development. 2. the production of a symptom or illness by psychic, as opposed to organic, factors.

psychogenic (ˌsiekoh'jenik) having an emotional or

psychological origin.
psychogeriatrician (ˌsiekohˌjeri·əˈtrishən) medical specialist in psychogeriatrics, usually a psychiatrist.
psychogeriatrics (ˌsiekohˌjeriˈatriks) the study and treatment of the psychological and psychiatric disorders of the aged. It is a combination of the specialities of geriatrics and psychiatry.
psychogram, psychograph (ˈsiekohˌgram; ˈsiekohˌgrahf, -ˌgraf) 1. a chart for recording graphically the personality traits of an individual. 2. a written description of the mental functioning of an individual.
psychokinesis (ˌsiekohkiˈneesis) the production or alteration of motion by directed thought processes.
psycholepsy (ˈsiekohˌlepsee) a condition characterized by sudden changes of mood.
psycholeptic (ˌsiekohˈleptik) a drug that affects the mental state.
psycholinguistics (ˌsiekohlingˈgwistiks) the study of factors affecting activities involved in communicating and comprehending verbal information.
psychology (sieˈkoləjee) the science dealing with the mind and mental processes, especially in relation to human and animal behaviour. adj. **psychological**.
analytic p. psychology by introspective methods, as opposed to experimental psychology.
clinical p. the use of psychological knowledge and techniques in the treatment of persons with emotional difficulties.
community p. a broad term referring to the organization of community resources for the prevention of mental disorders.
criminal p. the study of the mentality, the motivation, and the social behaviour of criminals.
depth p. psychoanalysis.
dynamic p. psychology stressing the element of energy in mental processes.
experimental p. the study of the mind and mental operations by the use of experimental methods.
genetic p. psychology dealing with the development of the mind in the individual and with its evolution in the race.
gestalt p. gestaltism; the theory that the objects of mind, as immediately presented to direct experience, come as complete unanalysable wholes or forms that cannot be split into parts.
physiological p. the branch of psychology that studies the relationship between physiological processes and behaviour.
social p. psychology treating of the social aspects of mental life.
psychometrician (ˌsiekohməˈtrishən) a person skilled in psychometry.
psychometrics, psychometry (ˌsiekohˈmetriks; sieˈkomətree) the testing and measuring of mental and psychological ability, efficiency, potentials, and functioning. adj. **psychometric**.
psychomotor (ˌsiekohˈmohtə) pertaining to motor effects of cerebral or psychic activity.
p. epilepsy EPILEPSY manifested by impaired consciousness of variable degree, the patient carrying out a series of coordinated acts that are out of place, bizarre, and serve no useful purpose and for which he is amnesic.
psychoneural (ˌsiekohˈnyooə·rəl) relating to the totality of neural events initiated by a sensory input and leading to storage, to discrimation, or an output of any kind.
psychoneurosis (ˌsiekohnyuhˈrohsis) neurosis. adj. **psychoneurotic**.
psychonomy (sieˈkonəmee) the science of the laws of mental activity.
psychopath (ˈsiekohˌpath) see SOCIOPATHIC.
psychopathic (ˌsiekoˈpathik) see SOCIOPATHIC.
psychopathology (ˌsiekohpəˈtholəjee) the branch of medicine dealing with the causes and processes of mental disorders.
psychopathy (sieˈkopəthee) any disease of the mind.
psychopharmacology (ˌsiekohˌfahməˈkoləjee) 1. the study of the action of drugs on psychological functions and mental states. 2. the use of drugs to modify psychological functions and mental states. adj. **psychopharmacological**.
psychophysical (ˌsiekohˈfizikʼl) pertaining to the mind and its relation to physical manifestations.
psychophysics (ˌsiekohˈfiziks) scientific study of the quantitative relations between characteristics or patterns of physical stimuli and the sensations induced by them.
psychophysiology (ˌsiekohˌfiziˈoləjee) scientific study of the interaction and interrelations of psychic and physiological factors. adj. **psychophysiological**.
psychoplegic (ˌsiekohˈpleejik) an agent lessening cerebral activity or excitability.
psychoprophylaxis (ˌsiekohˌprofiˈlaksis) psychophysical training aimed at preventing pain and modifying the perception of painful sensations associated with normal uncomplicated childbirth. See also NATURAL CHILDBIRTH.
psychosensory (ˌsiekohˈsensə·ree) perceiving and interpreting sensory stimuli.
psychosexual (ˌsiekohˈseksyooəl) pertaining to the psychic or emotional aspects of sex.
psychosis (sieˈkohsis) pl. *psychoses;* any major mental disorder of organic or emotional origin, marked by derangement of the personality and loss of contact with reality, often with delusions, hallucinations, or illusions. adj. **psychotic**.

A psychotic person may live in his own private world, completely out of touch with reality. He cannot cope with the demands of the real world, and he withdraws from it. In general, this loss of contact with reality is one of the more obvious differences between psychosis and NEUROSIS.

TYPES OF PSYCHOSIS. Psychoses are usually classified as functional psychoses, those for which no physical cause has been discovered, and organic psychoses, which are the result of organic damage to the brain.

The main types of functional psychosis are schizophrenia, paranoia, and affective psychosis.

Schizophrenia. This is the most widespread form of psychosis. About half of all patients hospitalized for mental illness are schizophrenics. This condition was formerly called dementia praecox, or 'early insanity', because it usually appears between the ages of 15 and 30.

The schizophrenic is apt to be shy, dreamy, bored, and lacking in physical and mental energy. When he becomes unable to find a solution for a painful situation, he retreats into a world he imagines as he would like it to be. The schizophrenic becomes unable to distinguish fact from imagination and uninterested in doing so. As a result, his actions may seem very strange unless they are understood as the product of a dream world. For example, one symptom of schizophrenia is the use of neologisms, or made-up words that are meaningless to the listener. Hallucinations and delusions may also occur (see also SCHIZOPHRENIA).

Certain types of schizophrenia respond more readily to treatment than do others. In all types, early treatment is extremely important, as the prospects for recovery seem to be closely connected with the duration of the condition.

Paranoia. This psychosis, which is much less common than schizophrenia, is characterized by delusions of persecution or grandiose delusions. A person suffering from it becomes more and more deluded, seeing hidden meanings to support his conviction that others are plotting against him, or to substantiate his belief that he is a person of great importance. He often uses an intricate form of logic to try to explain his delusions.

There are many degrees of paranoid reaction. Paranoid attitudes also appear in one type of schizophrenia.

In paranoia, unlike other psychoses, the entire personality is not affected; the patient does not lose contact with reality, but tends rather to misinterpret reality in terms of his delusion.

Affective Psychosis. This is a general term used to refer to psychoses in which the most prominent feature is a disturbance of mood, such as manic-depressive psychosis (bipolar disorder) and involutional psychosis (involutional melancholia). In current terminology, these are called affective disorders.

Manic-depressive illness is characterized by conspicuous mood swings. Although there are two possible phases, manic and depressive, the disorder takes many forms, sometimes entirely manic, or entirely depressive, with many variations. In an extremely mild form the affective reaction is not a true psychosis.

During the manic phase, the patient's energy and optimism seem boundless, mental activity and talking are accelerated, physical activity becomes greatly increased; lack of judgement, combined with over-enthusiasm, may make the patient dangerous to himself and to others. During the depressive phase, the patient's mental activity is greatly retarded, he may sit or lie inert, scarcely able to move or speak (see also CATALEPSY). The danger of suicide may be present. In some cases the patient appears greatly agitated even though he is extremely depressed.

Affective psychosis tends to recur. Many patients seem to recover spontaneously and then exhibit symptoms again after a period of more or less normal behaviour.

Involutional psychosis is a major DEPRESSION with an onset in late middle age. It was formerly thought to be related to the menopause in women and its emotional counterpart, the climacteric, in men. Characteristics of this type of psychosis include agitation, depression, feelings of guilt, paranoia, preoccupation with minor symptoms of physical disorders, severe insomnia, and suicidal tendencies. The course of the illness tends to be prolonged.

CAUSES. There is still much to be learned about the causes of functional psychoses. The roots of these conditions may be in the patient's early emotional experiences, or in his physical make-up, or in his environment. The high incidence of psychosis in certain families with a history of mental illness suggests that heredity may also play some role. However, it should be remembered that children whose parents are mentally disturbed and untreated may absorb psychotic ways of responding emotionally and viewing reality, in the same way that young children learn healthy ways of dealing with the real world from their environment.

The causes of organic psychoses are much better understood. Among the physical causes that can lead to psychosis are infectious diseases which involve the brain, certain deficiency diseases, lead poisoning, tumours, interference with the brain's blood supply, and wounds and blows that injure the brain. In a very few cases, epilepsy may lead to some mental deterioration. These organic psychoses are more resistant to treatment than are those with a functional basis.

TREATMENT. In most cases, patients with psychosis must be treated in a psychiatric department or hospital. The major form of treatment is PSYCHOTHERAPY, in which the patient is helped to understand and deal with his condition. However, this method will not work when the patient is out of contact with reality, and completely absorbed in his own fantasies and hallucinations.

In such cases, chemotherapy, the use of drugs to control the patient's emotions and behaviour, may be very helpful. Important among these drugs are NEUROLEPTICS, such as chlorpromazine and other phenothiazine derivatives. They act to calm the patient and often to help him become more rational. LITHIUM CARBONATE is used for the prevention and treatment of manic episodes.

Another type of treatment that is sometimes used is ELECTROCONVULSIVE THERAPY (ECT). The patient is rendered unconscious briefly by electric shock or drugs. This treatment can in some cases bring patients with melancholia or schizophrenia back to reality, thus making it possible to use the techniques of psychotherapy.

In a very few cases that are not helped by any other form of treatment, psychosurgery may be used. In this treatment, the connection between different parts of the brain is surgically severed. The result is a lessening of emotional reactions and tensions. Many doctors object to psychosurgery because of the negative aspects of its results, and the operation is used as a last resort.

alcoholic p. mental disorder caused by excessive use of alcohol.

depressive p. one characterized by mental depression, melancholy, despondency, inadequacy, and feelings of guilt.

exhaustion p. a psychosis due to some exhausting or depressing occurrence, as a surgical operation.

Korsakoff's p. a syndrome marked by amnesia, confabulation, and peripheral neuritis, usually associated with alcoholism and believed to be a chronic form of Wernicke's syndrome (see also WERNICKE-KORSAKOFF SYNDROME).

puerperal p. a psychosis arising during the puerperium.

polyneuritic p. Korsakoff's psychosis.

senile p. mental deterioration in old age, with organic brain changes, the symptoms including impaired memory for recent events, confabulation, irritability, etc. Called also senile dementia.

situational p. one caused by an unbearable situation over which the patient has no control.

symbiotic p., symbiotic infantile p. a condition seen in two- to four-year-old children having an abnormal relationship to the mothering figure, characterized by intense separation anxiety, severe regression, giving up of useful speech, and autism.

toxic p. psychosis due to the ingestion of toxic agents or to the presence of toxins within the body.

psychosocial (ˌsiekoh'sohshəl) pertaining to or involving both psychic and social aspects.

psychosolytic (sieˌkohsoh'litik) relieving or abolishing psychotic symptoms.

psychosomatic (ˌsiekohsə'matik) pertaining to the interrelations of mind and body; having bodily symptoms of psychic, emotional, or mental origin.

p. illness traditionally, an illness that can be traced to an emotional cause. It is becoming increasingly more recognized, however, that emotional factors play a role in the development of nearly all organic illnesses and that the physical symptoms experienced by the patient are related to many interdependent factors, including the psychological and cultural. The physical manifestations of an illness, unless caused by mechanical trauma, cannot be divorced from a person's emotional life. He responds in his own unique way to stress; his emotions affect his sensitivity to trauma and to irritating elements in his environment, his susceptibility to infection, and his ability to recover from the effects of his illness. It is believed by some behavioural scientists that regardless of their origin, many psychosomatic symptoms are useful in some way to the patient, perhaps as a means of getting attention from others or as a way of finding relief from the pressures of a stressful situation.

Among the illnesses recognized to be precipitated or exacerbated by emotional stimuli are ASTHMA, MIGRAINE headache, ANOREXIA NERVOSA, INSOMNIA, neurodermatitis, HYPERTENSION, and some urinary and intestinal disorders, such as ENURESIS, IRRITABLE BOWEL SYNDROME, and CROHN'S DISEASE. In recent years attempts to utilize the techniques of behaviour therapy to treat these and other illnesses whose symptoms are related to the autonomic system have met with some degree of success. Clients are taught new ways of coping with stress and new patterns of behaviour. Among the techniques used by behaviour therapists are BIOFEEDBACK, relaxation training, classical CONDITIONING, and operant conditioning using social and material reinforcements.

psychostimulant (ˌsiekoh'stimyuhlənt) 1. producing a transient increase in psychomotor activity. 2. a drug that produces such effects.

psychosurgery (ˌsiekoh'sərjə·ree) brain surgery to relieve mental and psychic symptoms.

psychotherapy (ˌsiekoh'therəpee) any of a number of related techniques for treating mental illness by psychological methods. These techniques are similar in that they all rely mainly on establishing communication between the therapist and the patient as a means of understanding and modifying the patient's behaviour. On occasion, drugs may be used, but only in order to make this communication easier.

FORMS OF PSYCHOTHERAPY. Perhaps the best known form of psychotherapy is PSYCHOANALYSIS, the technique developed by Dr. Sigmund Freud. Psychoanalysis attempts, through free association and dream interpretation, to reveal and resolve the unconscious conflicts that are at the root of mental illness.

Closely related to psychoanalysis is analytically oriented therapy, or 'brief therapy'. This uses some of the techniques of psychoanalysis, but tends to concentrate on the patient's present-life difficulties rather than on the unconscious roots of these difficulties.

One widely used technique is group therapy. Six to ten patients meet regularly to discuss their problems under the guidance of a group therapist. Group therapy is based on the principle of transference—that is, a patient tends to react to others in terms of his childhood attitudes toward family members. During group therapy, he may react to one member of the group as a hated rival brother, and to another as a dominating mother. In the give-and-take of discussion, he will begin to recognize the distortions in these reactions, and to see similar distortions in his day-to-day relationships with other people. Group therapy is generally combined with individual therapy and can help reduce the cost to each patient.

Adjunctive therapy, such as occupational therapy and music therapy, is helpful in relieving tensions and emotional problems that are associated with a feeling of uselessness. Psychodrama, in which patients act out fantasies or real-life situations, may provide a means of communication for patients who are not capable of expressing their problem by speech.

Play therapy is a form of psychotherapy adapted to children. It is very difficult to induce an emotionally disturbed or even a normal child to talk about his problems. Play therapy provides an alternative. The child reveals himself when he plays with toys provided by the therapist and acts out his fantasies. The therapist helps him 'get things out of his system', accepting him warmly as he is, and guiding him toward a solution to his problems. Since these are closely related to the way he is treated at home, play therapy is usually combined with some form of therapy for the parents. Experiments have been made with family therapy, in which the entire family meets regularly with the therapist, in an attempt to isolate those forces operating within the family system which may have produced 'illness' in one or more family members.

focal p. a form of psychotherapy in which one particular problem is singled out and made the focus of the theray. Called also *focal therapy*.

psychotic (sie'kotik) 1. pertaining to, characterized by, or caused by psychosis. 2. a person exhibiting psychosis.

psychotogenic (sieˌkotoh'jenik) producing a psychosis.

psychotomimetic (sieˌkotohmi'metik) characterized by or producing symptoms similar to those of a psychosis.

psychotrophic (ˌsiekoh'trohfik) exerting an effect on the mind; capable of modifying mental activity; a drug that affects the mental state.

There are several classes of psychotrophic drugs. ANTIDEPRESSANTS are used for the relief of symptoms of major depression. LITHIUM CARBONATE is used for the treatment of manic episodes of manic-depressive illness (bipolar disorder). NEUROLEPTICS (called also antipsychotic agents or major tranquillizers) are used for management of the manifestations of psychotic disorders, e.g., schizophrenia. Antianxiety agents (called also minor tranquillizers), such as diazepam (Valium), are used for relief of symptoms of anxiety and tension associated with disorders such as phobias or anxiety neurosis. While none of these drugs can effect a cure, they can reduce the severity of symptoms and permit the patient to resume more normal activity.

Also included in the catagory of psychotrophic drugs are many other drugs that affect the mind but are not used to treat mental disorders. These include stimulants, such as caffeine, amphetamines, and cocaine; opiates, such as morphine, heroin, and methadone; and hallucinogens, such as marijuana, mescaline, LSD, and phencyclidine (PCP).

psychr(o)- word element. [Gr.] *cold*.

psychralgia (sie'kralji·ə) a painful sensation of cold.

psychrometer (sie'kromitə) an instrument for measuring the moisture of the atmosphere.

psychrophile ('siekrohˌfiel) a psychrophilic organism.

psychrophilic (ˌsiekroh'filik) fond of cold; said of bacteria that grow best in the cold (15–20 °C).

psychrophore ('siekrohˌfor) a double catheter for applying cold to the urethra.

psychrotherapy (ˌsiekroh'therəpee) treatment of disease by applying cold.

psyllium ('sili·əm) a plant of the genus *Plantago* (see also psyllium hydrophilic MUCILLOID and plantago (psyllium) SEED).

Pt chemical symbol, *platinum*.

pt part; pint.

PTA plasma thromboplastin antecedent, clotting factor XI.

ptarmic ('tahmik) causing sneezing.

ptarmus ('tahməs) spasmodic sneezing.
PTC plasma thromboplastin component, clotting factor IX.
PTCA percutaneous transluminal coronary angioplasty.
pteroylglutamic acid (ˌteroh·ilgloo'tamik) folic acid.
pterygium (tə'riji·əm) a winglike structure, especially an abnormal triangular fold of membrane in the interpalpebral fissure, extending from the conjunctiva to the cornea.
p. colli webbed neck; a thick skin fold on the side of the neck, from the mastoid region to the acromion.
pterygoid ('teriˌgoyd) shaped like a wing.
p. bone pterygoid process.
p. process either of the two processes of the sphenoid bone descending from the points of junction of the great wings and body of the bone, and each consisting of a lateral and medial plate.
pterygomandibular (ˌterigohman'dibyuhlə) pertaining to the pterygoid process and the mandible.
pterygomaxillary (ˌterigohmak'silə·ree) pertaining to a pterygoid process and the maxilla.
pterygopalatine (ˌterigoh'paləˌtien) pertaining to a pterygoid process and the palatine bone.
ptilosis (ti'lohsis) falling out of the eyelashes.
ptomaine ('tohmayn) any of an indefinite class of toxic bases, usually considered to be formed by the action of bacterial metabolism on proteins.
p. poisoning a term commonly misapplied to FOOD POISONING. Contrary to popular belief, ptomaines are not injurious to the human digestive system, which is quite capable of reducing them to harmless substances. Decomposed foods are often responsible for food poisoning, however, because they may harbour certain forms of poison-producing bacteria.
ptosed (tohzd) affected with ptosis.
ptosis ('tohsis) 1. prolapse of an organ or part. 2. drooping of the upper eyelid due to congenital or acquired defect of the third nerve. adj. **ptotic.**
-ptosis word element. [Gr.] *downward displacement.* adj. **-ptotic.**
ptyal(o)- word element. [Gr.] *saliva.*
ptyalagogue (tie'aləˌgog, 'tieləˌgog) sialagogue, an agent that promotes the flow of saliva.
ptyalectasis (ˌtieə'lektəsis) 1. abnormal dilation of a salivary duct. 2. surgical dilation of a salivary duct.
ptyalin ('tiəlin) α-amylase occurring in saliva.
ptyalism ('tieəˌlizəm) excessive secretion of saliva.
ptyalocele ('tieəlohˌseel) a cystic tumour containing saliva.
ptyalogenic (ˌtieəloh'jenik) formed from or by the action of saliva.
ptyalography (ˌtieə'lografee) radiological examination of the salivary glands after the introduction of a radiopaque medium into the salivary ducts. Sialography.
ptyalolith ('tieəlohˌlith) a salivary calculus. A sialith.
ptyaloreaction (ˌtieəlohri'akshən) a reaction occurring in or performed on the saliva.
ptyalorrhoea (ˌtieələ'reeə) ptyalism.
Pu chemical symbol, *plutonium.*
pubarche (pyoo'bahkee) the first appearance of pubic hair.
puberty ('pyoobətee) the period during which the secondary sexual characteristics begin to develop and the capability of sexual reproduction is attained. Puberty in a girl is marked by broadening of the hips, development of the breasts, the appearance of pubic hair, and the onset of menstruation. At puberty a boy's shoulders broaden, his voice deepens, and pubic and facial hair appears. Girls usually reach puberty between the ages of 11 and 13, and boys between 13 and 15; the timing varies widely among individuals, however.
precocious p. unusually early sexual maturation, either idiopathic or pathological.
pubes ('pyoobeez) plural of *pubis.* [L.] 1. the hairs growing over the pubic region. 2. the pubic region.
pubescence (pyoo'bes'ns) the state of being pubescent.
pubescent (pyoo'bes'nt) 1. arriving at the age of puberty. 2. covered with down or lanugo.
pubic ('pyoobik) pertaining to or lying near the pubes.
pubiotomy (ˌpyoobi'otəmee) surgical separation of the pubis (pubic bone) lateral to the symphysis.
pubis ('pyoobis) pl. *pubes* [L.] the anterior portion of the hip bone, a distinct bone in early life; called also pubic bone.
public health ('publik) the field of medicine that is concerned with safeguarding and improving the physical, mental, and social well-being of the community as a whole.

Environmental aspects are the responsibility of the district local authority, whereas communicable disease control is supervised by the Medical Officer for Environmental Health, from the District Health Authority. Central government formulates national policy and is responsible for international aspects. See also HEALTH VISITOR.

pubofemoral (ˌpyooboh'femə·rəl) pertaining to the pubis and femur.
puboprostatic (ˌpyoobohpro'statik) pertaining to the pubis and prostate.
pubovesical (ˌpyooboh'vesik'l) pertaining to the pubis and bladder.
pudendum (pyoo'dendəm) pl. *pudenda* [L.] the external genitalia of humans, especially of the female, including the mons pubis, labia majora and minora, vestibule, and clitoris. Called also pudendum femininum, pudendum muliebre, and VULVA. adj. **pudendal, pudic.**
puerperal (pyoo'ərpə·rəl) pertaining to a puerpera or to the puerperium.
p. fever an infectious disease of childbirth; called also puerperal sepsis and childbed fever.

Until the mid-19th century, this dreaded, then mysterious illness sometimes swept through a hospital maternity ward, killing many of the mothers (see SEMMELWEISS). Today strict aseptic hospital techniques have made the disease uncommon in most parts of the world, except in unusual circumstances such as illegally induced abortion.

Puerperal fever results from an infection, usually streptococcal, originating in the birth canal and affecting the endometrium. This infection can spread throughout the body, causing septicaemia. The preliminary symptoms are fever, chills, excessive bleeding, foul lochia, and abdominal and pelvic pain. In acute stages, the pain spreads to the legs and chest; complications may be serious or even fatal.

Treatment consists mainly of administration of antibiotics, and in most instances they promptly clear up the infection. If the disease has progressed to an acute stage before treatment begins, blood transfusions may be necessary.

p. metritis infection of the uterus in a puerperal woman.
p. psychosis a psychotic reaction arising during the puerperium. Usually of a schizo-affective type in major disorder of mood accompanied by schizophrenia-like symptoms. Onset is usually abrupt; symptomatology is florid but prognosis is usually good. There is a risk of recurrence after subsequent births.
puerperalism (pyoo'ərpə·rəˌlizəm) a morbid condition incident to childbirth.

puerperium (ˌpyooə'piə·ri·əm) the period of 6–8 weeks following childbirth, when the body, particularly the genital tract, returns almost completely to its pre-pregnant state.

Pulex ('pyooleks) a genus of fleas.

P. irritans a widely distributed species, known as the human flea, which infests domestic animals as well as man, and may act as an intermediate host of certain helminths.

pulicide, pulicicide ('puhlisied; puh'lisi,sied) an agent destructive to fleas.

pullulation (ˌpulyuh'layshən) development by sprouting, or budding.

Pulmadil ('pulmədil) trademark for preparations of rimiterol, a bronchodilator.

pulmo ('pulmoh, 'puhlmoh) pl. *pulmones* [L.] lung.

pulmo- word element. [L.] *lung*.

pulmoaortic (ˌpulmoh·ay'awtik, ˌpuhl-) pertaining to the lungs and aorta.

pulmonary ('pulməˌnə·ree, 'puhl-) pertaining to the lungs, or to the pulmonary artery.

p. alveolar proteinosis a disease of unknown aetiology marked by chronic filling of the alveoli with a proteinaceous, lipid-rich, granular material consisting of surfactant and the debris of necrotic cells. Some patients have a history of exposure to irritating dusts or fumes. The condition is treated by whole lung lavage with balanced salt solution; most patients need repeated lavage.

p. artery the large artery originating from the superior surface of the right ventricle of the heart and passing diagonally upward to the left across the route of the aorta. The pulmonary trunk divides between the fifth and sixth thoracic vertebrae, forming the right pulmonary artery, which enters the right lung, and the left pulmonary artery, which enters the left lung.

p. circulation the circulation of blood to and from the lungs. Unoxygenated blood from the right ventricle flows through the right and left pulmonary arteries to the right and left lung. After entering the lungs, the branches subdivide, finally emerging as capillaries which surround the alveoli and release the carbon dioxide in exchange for a fresh supply of oxygen. The capillaries unite gradually and assume the characteristics of veins. These veins join to form the pulmonary veins, which return the oxygenated blood to the left atrium. See also CIRCULATORY SYSTEM.

p. embolism obstruction of the pulmonary artery or one of its branches by an embolus (see also pulmonary EMBOLISM).

p. function tests tests used to evaluate lung mechanics, gas exchange, pulmonary blood flow, and blood acid–base balance. Pulmonary function testing is used to screen high-risk patients, such as cigarette smokers and workers exposed to industrial dusts, in order to detect pneumoconiosis, emphysema, and chronic obstructive bronchitis at an early stage. It is also used to evaluate patients in the diagnosis of pulmonary disease, assessment of disease development, or evaluation of the risk of pulmonary complications from surgery.

LUNG VOLUMES AND CAPACITIES. The total lung capacity (TLC) is divided into four volumes. The tidal volume (V_T) is the volume inhaled and exhaled in normal quiet breathing. The inspiratory reserve volume (IRV) is the maximum volume that can be inhaled following a normal quiet inhalation. The expiratory reserve volume (ERV) is the maximum volume that can be exhaled following a normal quiet inhalation. The residual volume (RV) is the volume remaining in the lungs following a maximal exhalation. The vital capacity (VC) is the maximum volume that can be inhaled following a maximal exhalation; $VC = IRV + V_T + ERV$. The inspiratory capacity (IC) is the maximum volume that can be inhaled following a normal quiet exhalation; $IC = IRV + V_T$. The functional residual capacity (FRC) is the volume remaining in the lungs following a normal quiet exhalation; $FRC = ERV + RV$.

The vital capacity and its components (V_T, IRV, ERV, IC) are measured using a SPIROMETER, which is a device that measures the volumes of air inhaled and exhaled. The FRC is usually measured by the helium dilution method using a closed spirometry system. A known amount of helium is introduced into the system at the end of a normal quiet exhalation. When the helium equilibrates throughout the volume of the system, which is equal to the FRC plus the volume of the spirometer and tubing, the FRC is determined from the helium concentration. This test is time consuming and may underestimate the FRC of patients with emphysema. The FRC can be determined quickly and more accurately by body PLETHYS-

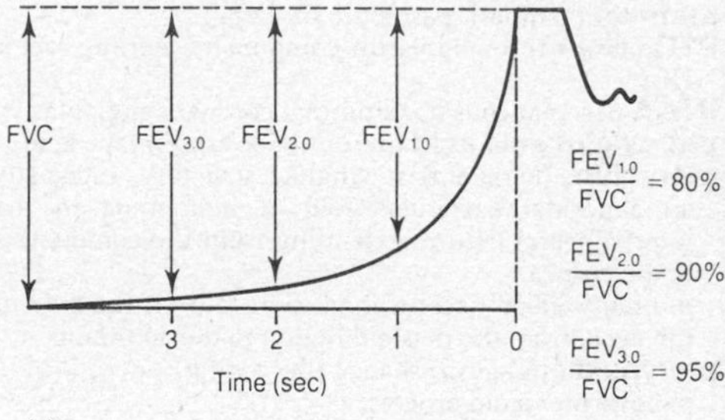

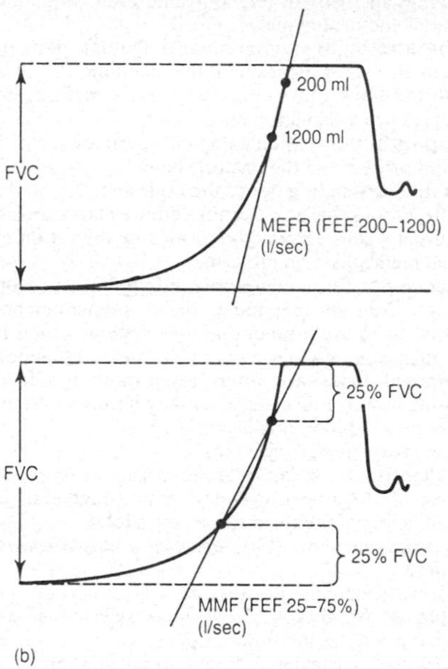

Forced expiratory spirogram. (a) Forced expiratory volumes. (b) Flow rates.

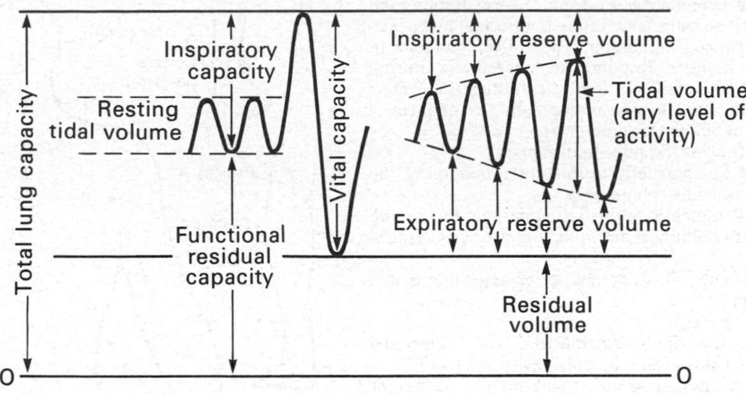

Subdivisions of the lung volume

MOGRAPHY. The residual volume and total lung capacity are determined from the FRC.

FORCED VITAL CAPACITY (FVC). In the forced vital capacity manoeuvre, the patient exhales as forcefully and rapidly as possible, beginning at maximal exhalation. Several parameters are determined from the spirogram. The FVC is the total volume of air exhaled during the manoeuvre; it is normally equal to the vital capacity. The forced expiratory volume (FEV) is the volume expired during a specified time period from the beginning of the test. The times used are 0.5, 1, 2, and 3 seconds; the corresponding parameters are $FEV_{0.5}$, $FEV_{1.0}$, $FEV_{2.0}$, and $FEV_{3.0}$. The maximal expiratory flow rate (MEFR) is the slope of the line connecting the points where 200 ml and 1200 ml have been exhaled; it is also called $FEF_{200-1200}$ (forced expiratory flow). The maximal midexpiratory flow rate (MMFR, MMF) is the slope of the line connecting the points where 25 per cent and 75 per cent of the FVC have been exhaled; it is also called $FEF_{25-75\%}$.

MAXIMAL VOLUNTARY VENTILATION (MVV). This is the maximal volume of air that can be exhaled by the patient, expressed in litres per minute; it was formerly called maximal breathing capacity (MBC). The patient breathes as rapidly and deeply as possible for 12 to 15 seconds and the volume exhaled is determined by spirometry.

PREDICTED VALUES. Because the results of pulmonary function tests vary with size and age, the normal values are calculated using prediction equations or nomograms, which give the normal value for a specific age, height, and sex. The prediction equations are derived using linear regression on the data from a population of normal subjects. The observed values are usually reported as a percentage of the predicted value.

INTERPRETATION. These tests provide evidence of impairment of ventilatory function; they do not point to specific disease processes. Abnormal test results may show either an obstructive or restrictive pattern. Sometimes, both patterns are present.

The Obstructive Pattern. This pattern occurs when there is airway obstruction from any cause, as in asthma, bronchitis, emphysema, and advanced bronchiectasis; these conditions are grouped together in the nonspecific term CHRONIC OBSTRUCTIVE AIRWAYS DISEASE (COAD). In this pattern, the residual volume is increased and the RV/TLC ratio is markedly increased. Owing to increased airway resistance, the flow rates are decreased. The FEV/FVC ratios, MMFR, and MEFR are all decreased; $FEV_{1.0}$/FVC is less than 80 per cent. The two earliest signs of obstructive airway disease are increased RV and decreased MMFR.

The Restrictive Pattern. This pattern occurs when there is a loss of lung tissue or when lung expansion is limited as a result of decreased compliance of the lung or thorax or of muscular weakness. The conditions in which this pattern can occur include pectus excavatum, myasthenia gravis, diffuse idiopathic interstitial fibrosis, and spacc occupying lesions (tumours, effusions). In this pattern, the vital capacity and FVC are less than 80 per cent of the predicted value, but the FEV/FVC ratios are normal. The TLC is decreased and the RV/TLC ratio is normal or increased.

p. oedema an effusion of serous fluid into the pulmonary interstitial tissues and air sacs (see also pulmonary OEDEMA).

p. valve the pocket-like structure that guards the orifice between the right ventricle and the pulmonary artery.

p. vein the large vein (right and left branches) that carries oxygenated blood from the lungs to the left atrium of the heart.

pulmonary artery flotation catheter a soft, flow-directed catheter with a balloon at the tip for measuring pulmonary arterial pressures, right atrial pressures, left atrial pressure, and reflected left ventricular end-diastolic pressure. It is introduced into the basilic vein and is guided by blood flow into the subclavian vein, the superior vena cava, through the right atrium and ventricle, and into the pulmonary artery where it floats freely with the movement of blood. Called also *Swan-Ganz catheter.*

The catheter permits evaluation of cardiac function by assessing the effectiveness of right and left pumping action of the heart and providing a quantitative measurement of cardiac output, and by allowing for sampling of mixed arterial-venous oxygen levels and calculation of differences between the two.

The catheter provides vital information in cases of heart failure resulting from myocardial infarction and cardiogenic shock, in the care of patients critically ill from hypovolaemic shock, and in the diagnosis and treatment of cardiac tamponade. It also is useful in preventive monitoring to avoid overhydration and pulmonary oedema, and often is inserted preoperatively in patients undergoing open-heart surgery in order to monitor response to anaesthesia during surgery. The catheter is used diagnostically to inject radiopaque dye during angiography to confirm a diagnosis of pulmonary embolism.

pulmonic (pul'monik, puhl-) pulmonary.

pulmonitis (ˌpulmə'nietis, ˌpuhl-) inflammation of the lung; pneumonitis; pneumonia.

pulmotor ('pulmohtə, 'puhl-) an apparatus for forcing oxygen into the lungs, and inducing artificial respiration.

pulp (pulp) any soft, juicy animal or vegetable tissue. adj. **pulpal.**

p. canal root canal.

dental p. the richly vascularized and innervated connective tissue inside the pulp cavity of a tooth.

digital p. a cushion of soft tissue on the palmar or plantar surface of the distal phalanx of a finger or toe.

red p., splenic p. the dark reddish brown substance filling the interspaces of the splenic sinuses.

tooth p. dental pulp.

white p. sheaths of lymphatic tissue surrounding the arteries of the spleen.

pulpa ('pulpə) pl. *pulpae* [L.] pulp.

pulpectomy (pul'pektəmee) removal of dental pulp.

pulpefaction (ˌpulpi'fakshən) conversion into pulp.

pulpitis (pul'pietis) pl. *pulpitides* [L.] inflammation of dental pulp.

pulpy ('pulpee) soft; of the consistency of pulp.

pulsatile ('pulsəˌtiel) characterized by a rhythmic pulsation.

pulsation (pul'sayshən) a throb, or rhythmic beat, as of the heart.

pulse (puls) the beat of the heart as felt through the walls of the arteries. What is usually meant by pulse is the pulsation felt in the radial artery at the wrist. Other sites of pulsation include the side of the neck (carotid artery), the elbow (brachial artery), the temple (temporal artery), the anterior side of the hip bone (femoral artery), the back of the knee (popliteal artery), and the instep (dorsalis pedis artery).

What is felt is not the blood pulsing through the arteries (as is commonly supposed) but a shock wave that travels along the fibres of the arteries as the heart contracts. This shock wave is generated by the pounding of the blood as it is ejected from the heart under pressure. It is analogous to the hammering sound heard in steampipes as the steam is admitted into the pipes under pressure. A pulse in the veins is too weak to be felt, although sometimes it is measured by sphygmograph; the tracing obtained is called a phlebogram.

The pulse is usually felt just inside the wrist below the thumb by placing two or three fingers lightly upon the radial artery. The thumb is never used to take a pulse because its own pulse is likely to be confused with the one being taken. Pressure should be light; if the artery is pressed too hard, the pulse will disappear entirely. The number of beats felt in exactly 1 minute is the pulse rate.

In taking a pulse, the rate, rhythm, and force of the pulse are noted. The average rate in an adult is between 50 and 100 beats per minute. The rhythm is checked for possible irregularities, which may be an indication of the general condition of the heart and the circulatory system. The amplitude of a pulse can range from totally impalpable to bounding and full; however, such terms are vague and subject to misinterpretation. To provide a more standardized description of pulse amplitude some agencies and hospitals use a scale that provides a more objective evaluation and reporting of the force of a pulse. On such a scale zero might mean that the pulse cannot be felt; +1 would indicate a thready, weak pulse that is difficult to palpate, fades in and out, and is easily obliterated with slight pressure; a +2 pulse would require light palpation, but once located it would be stronger than a +1; a +3 pulse would be considered normal; and a +4 would be one that is strong, bounding, easily palpated, and perhaps hyperactive, and could indicate a pathological condition such as aortic regurgitation.

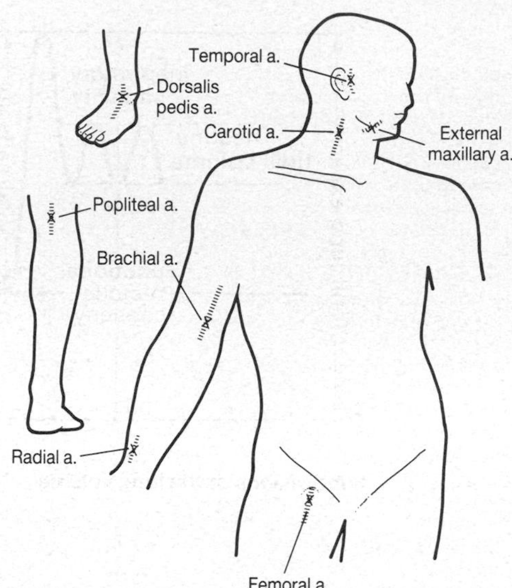

Pressure points where the pulse can be felt.

If a pulse is noted to be weaker during inspiration and stronger during expiration (*pulsus paradoxus*), this could indicate either greater reduction in the flow of blood to the left ventricle than is normal, as in constricted pericarditis or pericardial effusion, or a grossly exaggerated inspiratory manoeuvre as in tracheal obstruction, asthma, or emphysema.

An instrument for registering the movements, form, and force of the arterial pulse is called a sphygmograph. The sphygmographic tracing (or pulse tracing) consists of a curve having a sudden rise (primary elevation) followed by a sudden fall, after which there is a gradual descent marked by a number of secondary elevations.

abdominal p. that over the abdominal aorta.

alternating p. pulsus alternans; one with regular alteration of weak and strong beats without changes in cycle length.

anacrotic p. one in which the ascending limb of the tracing shows a transient drop in amplitude, or a notch.

anadicrotic p. one in which the ascending limb of the tracing shows two small additional waves or notches.

anatricrotic p. one in which the ascending limb of the tracing shows three small additional waves or notches.

atrial venous p. atriovenous pulse, a cervical pulse having an accentuated 'a' wave during atrial systole, owing to increased force of contraction of the right atrium; a characteristic of tricuspid stenosis.

bigeminal p. one in which two beats occur in rapid succession, the groups of two being separated by a

longer interval; usually related to regularly occurring ventricular premature beats.
brachial p. that which is felt over the brachial artery at the inner aspect of the elbow; palpated before taking blood pressure to determine location of the stethoscope.
capillary p. Quincke's pulse.
carotid p. the pulse felt over the carotid artery, which lies between the larynx and the sternocleidomastoid muscle in the neck; frequently used to assess effectiveness of cardiac massage during cardiopulmonary respiration (CPR). It can be felt by pushing the muscle to the side and pressing against the larynx, or, if the patient is dyspnoeic, by palpating the pulse at the groove in the muscle.
catadicrotic p. one in which the descending limb of the tracing shows two small notches.
catatricrotic p. one in which the descending limb of the tracing shows three small additional waves or notches. **Corrigan's p.** a jerky pulse with full expansion and sudden collapse occurring in aortic regurgitation; called also water-hammer pulse.
p. deficit the difference between the apical pulse and the radial pulse. Obtained by having one person count the apical pulse as heard through a stethoscope over the heart and a second person counting the radial pulse at the same time.
dicrotic p. a pulse characterized by two peaks, the second peak occurring in diastole and being an exaggeration of the dicrotic wave.
dorsalis pedis p. the pulse felt on the top of the foot, between the first and second metatarsal bones. In 8 to 10 per cent of the population this pulse cannot be detected.
entoptic p. a subjective sensation of seeing a flash of light in the dark occurring with each heart beat.
femoral p. that which is located at the site where the femoral artery passes through the groin in the femoral triangle.
funic p. the arterial tide in the umbilical cord.
hard p. one characterized by high tension.
jerky p. one in which the artery is suddenly and markedly distended.
paradoxical p. one that markedly decreases in amplitude during inspiration, as often occurs in constrictive pericarditis.
pistol-shot p. one in which the arteries are subject to sudden distention and collapse.
plateau p. one that is slowly rising and sustained.
popliteal p. the pulse palpated at the indentation in the back of the knee. Most easily detected when the patient is lying in the prone position with the knee flexed about 45 degrees.

pulse generator the power source for a cardiac pacemaker system, usually powered by a lithium battery. It supplies electrical impulses to the implanted electrodes, either at a fixed rate or in some programmed pattern. See also PACEMAKER.

pulseless disease ('pulsləs) progressive obliteration of the brachiocephalic trunk and left subclavian and left common carotid arteries above their origin in the aortic arch, leading to loss of the pulse in both arms and carotids and to symptoms associated with ischaemia of the brain, eyes, face, and arms. Called also Takayasu's arteritis or disease.

pulsion ('pulshən) a pushing outward.

pulsus ('pulsəs) [L.] *pulse.*
p. alternans alternating pulse.
p. bigeminus bigeminal pulse.
p. bisferiens a pulse characterized by two strong systolic peaks separated by a midsystolic dip, most commonly occurring in pure aortic regurgitation and in aortic regurgitation with stenosis.
p. celer a swift, abrupt pulse.
p. differens inequality of the pulse observable at corresponding sites on either side of the body.
p. paradoxus paradoxical pulse.
p. parvus et tardus a small hard pulse that rises and falls slowly.
p. tardus an abnormally slow pulse.

pultaceous (pul'tayshəs) like a poultice; pulpy.

pulverulent (pul'veryuhlənt) powdery; dusty.

pulvinar (pul'vienah) the posterior medial part of the posterior end of the thalamus.

pumice ('pumis) a substance consisting of silicates of aluminium, potassium, and sodium; used in dentistry as an abrasive.

pump (pump) 1. an apparatus for drawing or forcing liquid or gas. 2. to draw or force liquids or gases.
blood p. a machine used to propel blood through the tubing of extracorporeal circulation devices.
breast p. a pump for taking milk from the breast.
calcium p. the mechanism of active transport of calcium (Ca^{2+}) across a membrane, as of the sarcoplasmic reticulum of muscle cells, against a concentration gradient; the mechanism is driven by hydrolysis of ATP.
intra-aortic balloon p. circulatory support provided by a balloon inserted into the thoracic aorta, which is inflated during diastole and deflated during systole (see also INTRA-AORTIC BALLOON PUMP).
p. oxygenator heart–lung machine.
sodium p., sodium–potassium p. the mechanism of active transport driven by hydrolysis of ATP, by which sodium (Na^+) is extruded from a cell and potassium (K^+) is brought in, so as to maintain the low concentration of Na^+ and the high concentration of K^+ within the cell with respect to the surrounding medium.
stomach p. a pump for removing the contents from the stomach.

punchdrunk ('punch,drunk) a traumatic encephalopathy of prizefighters resulting from cumulative cerebral concussions, with general slowing of mental functions, bouts of confusion, and scattered memory loss.

punctate ('pungktayt) spotted; marked with points or punctures.

punctiform ('pungkti,fawm) like a point.

punctograph ('pungktoh,grahf, -,graf) an instrument for radiographic localization of foreign bodies.

punctum ('pungktəm) pl. *puncta* [L.] a point or small spot.
p. caecum blind spot.
puncta dolorosa Valleix's points.
p. lacrimale pl. *puncta lacrimalia;* a small aperture situated on a slight elevation at the medial end of the eyelid margin, through which tears from the lacrimal lake enter the lacrimal canaliculi. See also LACRIMAL APPARATUS.
p. proximum near point.
p. remotum far point.
puncta vasculosa minute red spots that mark the cut surface of white matter of the brain.

puncture ('pungkchə) the act of piercing or penetrating with a pointed object or instrument; a wound so made.
cisternal p. puncture of the cisterna cerebellomedullaris just below the occipital bone to obtain a specimen of cerebrospinal fluid (see also CISTERNAL PUNCTURE).
lumbar p. puncture of the subarachnoid space in the region of the lumbar vertebrae (see also LUMBAR PUNCTURE).
spinal p. puncture of the spinal canal (see also SPINAL PUNCTURE).

sternal p. removal of bone marrow from the manubrium of the sternum through a sternal puncture needle (see also STERNAL PUNCTURE).

PUO pyrexia of unknown origin.

pupa ('pyoopə) pl. *pupae* [L.] the second stage in the development of an insect, between the larva and the imago. adj. **pupal**.

pupil ('pyoop'l) the opening in the centre of the iris through which light enters the eye.

Adie's p. tonic pupil.

Argyll Robertson p. one that is miotic and responds to accommodation effort, but not to light.

fixed p. a pupil that does not react either to light or on convergence, or in accommodation.

Hutchinson's p. one that is dilated while the other is not.

tonic p. a usually unilateral condition of the eye in which the affected pupil is larger than the other, responds to accommodation and convergence in a slow, delayed fashion, and reacts to light only after prolonged exposure to dark or light. Called also Adie's pupil. See also ADIE'S SYNDROME.

pupilla (pyoo'pilə) [L.] *pupil.*

pupillometer (ˌpyoopi'lomitə) an instrument for measuring the width or diameter of the pupil.

pupillometry (ˌpyoopi'lomətree) measurement of the diameter or width of the pupil of the eye.

pupilloplegia (ˌpyoopiloh'pleeji·ə) Adie's pupil.

pupilloscopy (ˌpyoopi'loskəpee) skiametry; retinoscopy.

pupillostatometer (ˌpyoopilohstə'tomitə) an instrument for measuring the distance between the pupils.

purgation (pər'gayshən) catharsis; purging effected by a cathartic medicine.

purgative ('pərgətiv) 1. CATHARTIC (1); causing bowel evacuation. 2. a cathartic, particularly one stimulating peristaltic action.

purge (pərj) 1. a purgative medicine or dose. 2. to cause free evacuation of faeces.

Puri-Nethol (ˌpyuhi'neethol) trademark for a preparation of mercaptopurine, an antineoplastic agent.

purine ('pyooə·reen) a heterocyclic compound that is the nucleus of the purine bases (or purines) such as adenine and guanine, which occur in DNA and RNA, and xanthine and hypoxanthine.

p.-free diet a diet sometimes used in the treatment of GOUT, omitting meat, fowl, and fish, but using eggs, cheese, and vegetables. The following foods are especially high in purines: kidney, liver, sweetbreads, sardines, anchovies, and meat extracts.

Purkinje's cells (pər'kinjeez) large, branched cells of the middle layer of the brain.

Purkinje's fibres modified cardiac muscle fibres in the subendothelial tissue, concerned with conducting impulses to the heart.

purple ('pərp'l) 1. a colour between blue and red. 2. a substance of this colour used as a dye or indicator.

visual p. rhodopsin.

purpura ('pərpyuhrə) a haemorrhagic state characterized by extravasation of blood into the tissues, under the skin and through the mucous membranes, and producing spontaneous ecchymoses (bruises) and petechiae (small red patches) on the skin. When the disorder is accompanied by a decrease in the circulating platelets, it is called thrombocytopenic purpura; when there is no decrease in the platelet count, it is called nonthrombocytopenic purpura. adj. **purpuric**.

There are two general types of purpura: primary or idiopathic (usually autoimmune) thrombocytopenic purpura, in which the cause is unknown, and secondary or symptomatic thrombocytopenic purpura, which may be associated with exposure to drugs or other chemical agents, systemic diseases such as systemic lupus erythematosus, diseases affecting the bone marrow, such as leukaemia, and infections such as septicaemia and viral infections.

SYMPTOMS. The outward manifestations and laboratory findings of purpura are similar. There is evidence of bleeding under the skin, with easy bruising and the development of petechiae. In the acute form symptoms may be severe with bleeding from any of the body orifices, such as haematuria, nosebleed, vaginal bleeding, and bleeding gums. In thrombocytopenic purpura, the PLATELET count is reduced, and in severe conditions may be less than 10×10^9 litre (normal count is about 250×10^9 litre). The bleeding time is prolonged and clot retraction is poor. Coagulation tests are normal.

TREATMENT. Investigations to establish the type of purpura present and its underlying cause are required so that this may be eliminated if necessary. General measures include protection of the patient from trauma, elective surgery, and tooth extractions, any one of which may lead to severe or even fatal haemorrhage. In the thrombocytopenic form, corticosteroids may be administered when the purpura is moderately severe and of short duration. Splenectomy is indicated when other, more conservative measures fail and is successful in a majority of cases. In some instances, especially in children, there may be spontaneous and permanent recovery from idiopathic purpura.

allergic p., anaphylactic p. Schönlein–Henoch purpura; also called Henoch–Schönlein.

annular telangiectatic p. a rare form in which punctate erythematous lesions coalesce to form an annular or serpiginous pattern. Called also Majocchi's disease.

fibrinolytic p. purpura associated with increased fibrinolytic activity of the blood.

p. fulminans a form of purpura seen mainly in children, usually after an infectious disease, marked by fever, shock, anaemia, and sudden, rapidly spreading symmetrical skin haemorrhages of the lower limbs, often associated with extensive intravascular thromboses and gangrene.

p. haemorrhagica idiopathic thrombocytopenic purpura.

Henoch's p. Schönlein–Henoch purpura in which abdominal symptoms predominate.

idiopathic thrombocytopenic p. (ITP) an acquired thrombocytopenia which may be acute or chronic in its course. Acute ITP is common in young children, and in about half there is a history of preceding viral infection. The disorder is usually self-limiting and rarely fatal. Chronic ITP is more insidious in onset, and is commoner in young adult women; it is diagnosed by excluding other causes of thrombocytopenia on clinical grounds and on bone marrow examination. Initial treatment is usually with steroids, and about 80 per cent of patients will respond.

nonthrombocytopenic p. purpura without any decrease in the platelet count of the blood. In such cases the cause of purpura is either abnormal capillary fragility or a clotting factor deficiency.

Schönlein's p. Schönlein–Henoch purpura in which articular systems predominate; called also Schönlein's disease.

Schönlein–Henoch p. nonthrombocytopenic purpura of unknown cause, most often seen in children, associated with various clinical symptoms, such as urticaria and erythema, arthropathy and arthritis, gastrointestinal symptoms, and renal involvement. Called also Schönlein–Henoch disease.

p. senilis dark purplish red ecchymoses occurring on the forearms and backs of the hands in the elderly; the platelet count is normal.
steroid p. purpura secondary to prolonged use of steroids. The platelet count is normal, the basic defect being the loss of supporting connective tissue. **thrombocytopenic p.** purpura associated with a decrease in the number of platelets in the blood.
thrombotic thrombocytopenic p. a disease marked by thrombocytopenia, haemolytic anaemia, neurological manifestations, azotaemia, fever, and thromboses in terminal arterioles and capillaries.

purulence ('pyooə·rələns) the formation or presence of pus.

purulent ('pyooə·rələnt) containing or forming pus.

puruloid ('pyooə·rə,loyd) resembling pus.

pus (pus) a protein-rich liquid inflammation product made up of cells (leukocytes), a thin fluid (liquor puris), and cellular debris.
blue p. pus with a bluish tint, seen in certain suppurative infections, the colour occurring as a result of the presence of a pigment (pyocyanin) produced by *Pseudomonas aeruginosa.*

pustula ('pustyuhlə) pl. *pustulae* [L.] pustule.

pustular ('pustyuhlə) pertaining to or of the nature of a pustule; consisting of pustules.

pustulation (,pustyuh'layshən) the formation of pustules.

pustule ('pustyool) a small, elevated, circumscribed, pus-containing lesion of the skin.

pustulosis (,pustyuh'lohsis) a condition marked by an eruption of pustules.

putamen (pyoo'taymen) the larger and more lateral part of the lenticular nucleus.

Putnam–Dana syndrome (,putnəm'daynə) subacute combined degeneration of spinal cord.

putrefaction (,pyootri'fakshən) enzymatic decomposition, especially of proteins, with the production of foul-smelling compounds, such as hydrogen sulphide, ammonia, and mercaptans. adj. **putrefactive**.

putrefy ('pyootri,fie) to undergo putrefaction.

putrescence (pyoo'tres'ns) the condition of undergoing putrefaction. adj. **putrescent**.

putrescine (pyoo'treseen) a polyamine first found in decaying meat; small quantities occur in most cells.

putrid ('pyootrid) rotten; putrified.

PV per vaginam.

PVP polyvinylpyrrolidone (see POVIDONE).

PVP-I povidone-iodine.

pyaemia (pie'eemi·ə) septicaemia in which secondary foci of suppuration occur and multiple abscesses are formed. adj. **pyaemic**.
arterial p. a form due to the dissemination of septic emboli from the heart.
cryptogenic p. that in which the source of infection is in an unidentified tissue.
portal p. pylephlebitis.

pyarthrosis (,pieah'throhsis) suppuration within a joint cavity; acute suppurative arthritis.

pycn(o)- for words beginning thus, see those beginning *pykn(o)-*.

pyel(o)- word element. [Gr.] *renal pelvis.*

pyelectasis (,pieə'lektəsis) dilation of the renal pelvis.

pyelitis (,pieə'lietis) inflammation of the renal pelvis, the outer basin-like portion of the kidney at the attachment of the ureter. adj. **pyelitic**.

Pyelitis is a fairly common disease, and usually can be diagnosed and cured without great difficulty. Prompt and effective treatment is necessary to prevent the spread of infection and the development of pyelonephritis, a severely disabling disease in the chronic form, in which damage to the kidney cells may lead to high blood pressure and uraemia.

CAUSE. Pyelitis is usually caused by a microorganism such as *Escherichia coli* or (less often) streptococcus or staphylococcus, which may invade the kidneys by way of the blood. Pyelitis may also arise from an infection of the bladder (CYSTITIS).

The disease is most common among young children, affecting females far more often than males because the urethra is considerably shorter in the female than in the male. This favours ascending infections from the outside to enter the bladder. Female children not properly trained in their toilet habits will, after bowel movements, rub the toilet tissue from the anus forward toward the vagina rather than vice versa. In this way the bacteria so commonly found in faecal matter find their way into the urinary bladder and from there to the pelvis of the kidney.

Any urinary obstruction can sharply increase the chances of the development of pyelitis, since obstruction interferes with the normal ability of the kidney to rid the body of harmful bacteria.

SYMPTOMS. Probably the most common symptoms of pyelitis are frequency and urgency of urination and dysuria. Other possible symptoms include fever, chills, headache, and pain in one or both sides of the lower back. Pyelitis may also be present without any outward symptoms, but urinalysis will reveal many pus cells and occasionally erythrocytes.

TREATMENT. Pyelitis and pyelonephritis can usually be treated quite successfully with sulphonamides. Certain antibiotics are also helpful, and so are the urinary antiseptics. If the disease is treated promptly, the patient can look forward to early and complete recovery.
cystic p. pyelitis with formation of multiple submucosal cysts.

pyelocaliectases (,pieəloh,kali'ektəsis) dilation of the renal pelvis and calices.

pyelocystis (,pieəloh'sistis) inflammation of the renal pelvis and bladder.

pyelogram ('pieəloh,gram) the film produced by pyelography.

pyelography (,pieə'lografee) radiology of the renal pelvis after the injection of radiopaque contrast medium.

Preparation of the patient for pyelography includes clearing the intestinal tract of as much faecal material and gas as possible so that there can be adequate visualization of the urinary tract structures. Usually this is accomplished by administration of aperients. Care must be taken to avoid dehydrating patients in renal failure by either vigorous aperients or fluid restriction. The evening before the examination the patient is given a light meal and then all foods and fluids are restricted after midnight.

The possibility of an allergic reaction to the contrast medium must always be considered. Drugs such as adrenaline and hydrocortisone must be available should ANAPHYLAXIS occur. The patient may experience a mild transitory sensation of warmth, flushing of the face, or a salty taste in the mouth, but these should last only a few moments.
antegrade p. the renal pelvis is punctured with a needle and a water-soluble, iodine-containing contrast medium injected. This method of pyelography is used to further delineate a possible obstructive uropathy when other less invasive methods have failed. It may be combined with pressure/flow studies, the Whittaker test.
intravenous p. (IVP), intravenous urography (IVU) a water-soluble, iodine-containing contrast medium is injected intravenously and radiographs are exposed as

the contrast medium is excreted by the kidneys and passes down the ureters into the bladder.
retrograde p. a water-soluble, iodine-containing contrast medium is injected via a catheter inserted into the ureter during cystoscopy. Retrograde pyelography is indicated when intravenous pyelography has failed to demonstrate the ureter or pelvicalyceal system satisfactorily.

pyelointerstitial (ˌpieəlohˌintə'stishəl) pertaining to the interstitial tissue of the renal pelvis.

pyelolithotomy (ˌpieəlohli'thotəmee) incision of the renal pelvis for removal of calculi.

pyelonephritis (ˌpieəlohnə'frietis) inflammation of the kidney and renal pelvis (see also PYELITIS and NEPHRITIS). Called also *nephropyelitis*.

pyelonephrosis (ˌpieəlohnə'frohsis) any disease of the kidney and its pelvis.

pyelopathy (ˌpieə'lopəthee) any disease of the renal pelvis.

pyeloplasty ('pieəlohˌplastee) plastic repair of the renal pelvis.

pyeloplication (ˌpieəlohplie'kayshən) reduction in size of a renal pelvis by surgical infolding of its walls.

pyelostomy (ˌpieə'lostəmee) 1. an opening in the renal pelvis. 2. operation to introduce an opening in the renal pelvis for the purpose of temporarily diverting the urine from the ureter.

pyelotomy (ˌpieə'lotəmee) incision of the renal pelvis.

pyelovenous (ˌpieəloh'veenəs) pertaining to the renal pelvis and renal veins.

pyemesis (pie'eməsis) the vomiting of pus.

pyencephalus (ˌpie·en'kefələs, -'sef-) abscess of the brain.

pygal ('piegəl) pertaining to the buttocks.

pygalgia (pie'galji·ə) pain in the buttocks.

pygoamorphus (ˌpiegoh·ə'mawfəs) asymmetrical conjoined twins, in which the parasite is an amorphous mass attached to the sacral region of the autosite.

pygodidymus (ˌpiegoh'didiməs) a fetus with double hips and pelvis.

pygomelus (pie'goməlәs) a fetus with a supernumerary limb or limbs attached to or near the buttocks.

pygopagus (pie'gopəgəs) conjoined twins fused in the sacral region.

pykn(o)- word element. [Gr.] *thick*, *compact*, *frequent*.

pyknic ('piknik) having a short, thick, stocky build.

pyknocyte ('piknohˌsiet) a distorted and contracted, occasionally spiculed erythrocyte.

pyknocytosis (ˌpiknohsie'tohsis) conspicuous increase in the number of pyknocytes.

pyknodysostosis (ˌpiknohˌdiso'stohsis) a hereditary syndrome of dwarfism, osteopetrosis, and skeletal anomalies of the cranium, digits, and mandible.

pyknometer (pik'nomitə) an instrument for determining the specific gravity of fluids.

pyknomorphous (ˌpiknoh'mawfəs) having the stained portions of the cell body compactly arranged.

pyknophrasia (ˌpiknoh'frayzi·ə) thickness of speech.

pyknosis (pik'nohsis) a thickening, especially degeneration of a cell in which the nucleus shrinks in size and the chromatin condenses to a solid, structureless mass or masses. adj. **pyknotic**.

pyle- word element. [Gr.] *portal vein*.

pylephlebectasis (ˌpielifli'bektəsis) dilation of the portal vein.

pylephlebitis (ˌpielifli'bietis) inflammation of the portal vein.

pylethrombophlebitis (ˌpieliˌthrombohfli'bietis) thrombosis and inflammation of the portal vein.

pylethrombosis (ˌpielithrom'bohsis) thrombosis of the portal vein.

pylor(o)- word element. [Gr.] *pylorus*.

pyloralgia (ˌpielə'ralji·ə) pain in the region of the pylorus.

pylorectomy (ˌpielə'rektəmee) excision of the pylorus.

pyloric (pie'lo·rik) pertaining to the pylorus or to the pyloric part of the stomach.
p. stenosis obstruction of the pyloric orifice of the stomach; it may be congenital as in hypertrophic pyloric stenosis, or acquired, due to peptic ulceration or prepyloric carcinoma.
The initial symptom is vomiting, mild at first but becoming increasingly more forceful. It can occur both during and after feedings. Diagnosis may be confirmed by radiographical examination using a barium meal.
Treatment is usually surgical, involving longitudinal splitting of the muscle (pyloromyotomy).

pylorochesis (pieˌlo·roh'cheesis) pyloric obstruction.

pyloroduodenitis (pieˌlo·rohˌdyooədi'nietis) inflammation of the pyloric and duodenal mucosa.

pylorogastrectomy (ˌpieˌlo·rohga'strektəmee) excision of the pylorus and adjacent portion of the stomach.

pyloromyotomy (pieˌlo·rohmie'otəmee) incision of the longitudinal and circular muscles of the pylorus.

pyloroplasty (pie'lo·rohˌplastee) reconstruction of the pylorus to enlarge the communication between the stomach and duodenum.
Finney p. enlargement of the pyloric canal by establishment of an inverted U-shaped anastomosis between the stomach and duodenum after longitudinal incision.
Heineke–Mikulicz p. enlargement of a pyloric stricture by incising the pylorus longitudinally and suturing the incision transversely.

pyloroscopy (ˌpielə'roskəpee) endoscopic inspection of the pylorus.

pylorospasm (pie'lo·rohˌspazəm) spasm of the pylorus or of the pyloric portion of the stomach.

pylorostenosis (pieˌlo·rohstə'nohsis) pyloric stenosis.

pylorostomy (ˌpielə'rostəmee) formation of an opening through the abdominal wall into the stomach near the pylorus.

pylorotomy (ˌpielə'rotəmee) incision into the pylorus.

pylorus (pie'lor·rəs) the distal aperture of the stomach, opening into the duodenum. The term pylorus is variously used to mean the pyloric part of the stomach, and the pyloric antrum, canal, opening, or sphincter. A ring of muscles, the pyloric sphincter, serves as a 'gate', closing the opening from the stomach to the intestine. It opens periodically, allowing the contents of the stomach to move into the duodenum. The pylorus contains many glands that help produce hydrochloric acid.
Occasionally, in infants, the pyloric muscle is greatly enlarged and thickened, so that emptying of the stomach is prevented. This condition, hypertrophic pyloric obstruction or PYLORIC STENOSIS, can be corrected by surgery.

pyo- word element. [Gr.] *pus*.

pyocele ('pieohˌseel) a collection of pus, as in the scrotum.

pyocephalus (ˌpieoh'kefələs, -'sef-) the presence of purulent fluid in the cerebral ventricles.

pyochezia (ˌpieoh'keezi·ə) the presence of pus in the faeces.

pyococcus (ˌpieoh'kokəs) a pus-forming coccus.

pyocolpocele (ˌpieoh'kolpəˌseel) a vaginal tumour containing pus.

pyocolpos (ˌpieoh'kolpos) pus in the vagina.

pyocyanase (ˌpieoh'sieəˌnayz) an antibacterial substance from cultures of *Pseudomonas aeruginosa* (*pyocyanea*); bactericidal for many bacteria and lytic for some (*Vibrio cholerae*).

pyocyanic (ˌpieohsie'anik) pertaining to blue pus, or to *Pseudomonas aeruginosa.*

pyocyanin (ˌpieoh'sieənin) a blue-green antibiotic pigment produced by *Pseudomonas aeruginosa*; it gives the colour to 'blue pus'.

pyocyst ('pieohˌsist) a cyst containing pus.

pyoderma (ˌpieoh'dərmə) any purulent skin disease.

p. gangrenosum a rapidly evolving cutaneous ulcer or ulcers, with undermining of the border. Once regarded as a complication peculiar to ulcerative colitis, it is now known to occur in other wasting diseases.

pyodermia (ˌpieoh'dərmi·ə) pyoderma.

pyogenesis (ˌpieoh'jenəsis) the formation of pus.

pyogenic (ˌpieoh'jenik) producing pus.

pyohaemia (ˌpieoh'heemi·ə) pyaemia.

pyohaemothorax (ˌpieohˌheemoh'thor·raks) pus and blood in the pleural cavity.

pyohydronephrosis (ˌpieohˌhiedrohnə'frohsis) the accumulation of pus and urine in the kidney.

pyoid ('pieoyd) resembling or like pus.

pyolabyrinthitis (ˌpieohˌlabə·rin'thietis) inflammation of the labyrinth of the ear, with suppuration.

pyometra (ˌpieoh'meetrə) an accumulation of pus within the uterus.

pyometritis (ˌpieohmi'trietis) purulent inflammation of the uterus.

pyonephritis (ˌpieohnə'frietis) purulent inflammation of the kidney.

pyonephrolithiasis (ˌpieohˌnefrohli'thieəsis) pus and calculi in the kidney.

pyonephrosis (ˌpieohnə'frohsis) suppurative destruction of the renal parenchyma, with total or almost complete loss of kidney function.

pyo-ovarium (ˌpieoh·oh'vair·ri·əm) an abscess of the ovary.

Pyopen ('pieohpen) trademark for preparations of carbenicillin, an antibiotic.

pyopericarditis (ˌpieohˌperikah'dietis) purulent pericarditis.

pyopericardium (ˌpieohˌperi'kahdi·əm) pus in the pericardium.

pyoperitoneum (ˌpieohˌperitə'neeəm) pus in the peritoneal cavity.

pyoperitonitis (ˌpieohˌperitə'nietis) purulent inflammation of the peritoneum.

pyophthalmitis (ˌpieofthal'mietis) purulent inflammation of the eye.

pyophysometra (ˌpieohˌfiesoh'meetrə) pus and gas in the uterus.

pyopneumocholecystitis (ˌpieohˌnyoomohˌkohlisi'stietis) distention of the gallbladder, with the presence of pus and gas.

pyopneumohepatitis (ˌpieohˌnyoomohˌhepə'tietis) abscess of the liver with pus and gas in the abscess cavity.

pyopneumopericardium (ˌpieohˌnyoomohˌperi'kahdi·əm) pus and gas in the pericardium.

pyopneumoperitonitis (ˌpieohˌnyoomohˌperitə'nietis) peritonitis with the presence of pus and gas.

pyopneumothorax (ˌpieohˌnyoomoh'thor·raks) pus and air or gas within the pleural cavity.

pyoptysis (pie'optisis) expectoration of purulent matter.

pyopyelectasis (ˌpieohˌpieə'lektəsis) dilation of the renal pelvis with pus.

pyosalpingitis (ˌpieohˌsalpin'jietis) purulent salpingitis.

pyosalpingo-oophoritis (ˌpieohsalˌping·gohˌoh·əfə'rietis) purulent inflammation of the uterine tube and ovary.

pyosalpinx (ˌpieoh'salpingks) an accumulation of pus in a uterine tube.

pyosis (pie'ohsis) suppuration; the formation of pus.

pyostatic (ˌpieoh'statik) arresting suppuration; an agent that arrests suppuration.

pyothorax (ˌpieoh'thor·raks) an accumulation of pus in the thorax (see also EMPYEMA).

pyoureter (ˌpieoh·yuh'reetə) pus in the ureter.

pyramid ('pirəmid) a pointed or cone-shaped structure or part.

p. of cerebellum pyramid of vermis.

p. of light a triangular reflection seen upon the tympanic membrane.

malpighian p's renal pyramids.

p's of the medulla oblongata either of two rounded masses, one on either side of the median fissure of the medulla oblongata.

renal p's the conical masses constituting the medulla of the kidney, the base toward the cortex and culminating at the summit in the renal papilla.

p. of thyroid an occasional third lobe of the thyroid gland, extending upward from the isthmus.

p. of tympanum the hollow elevation in the inner wall of the middle ear that contains the stapedius muscle.

p. of vermis the part of the vermis cerebelli between the tuber vermis and the uvula.

pyramidal (pi'ramid'l) shaped like a pyramid.

p. tracts collections of motor nerve fibres arising in the brain and passing down through the spinal cord to motor cells in the anterior horns.

pyramis ('pirəmis) pl. *pyramides* [Gr.] pyramid.

pyran ('pieran) a cyclic compound in which the ring consists of 5 carbon atoms and 1 oxygen atom.

pyranose ('pierəˌnohz) a six-membered ring structure formed by the reaction of the carbonyl group and a hydroxy group of a sugar to form a hemiacetal.

pyrantel (pie'rantel) an anthelminthic, used as the embonate salt.

pyrazinamide (ˌpirə'zinəmied) an agent used in the treatment of tuberculosis.

pyrectic (pie'rektik) 1. pertaining to fever; feverish. 2. a fever-inducing agent.

pyretic (pie'retik) pertaining to fever.

pyretogenesis (ˌpierətoh'jenəsis) the origin and causation of fever.

pyretogenous (ˌpierə'tojənəs) 1. caused by high fever. 2. pyrogenic.

pyretotherapy (ˌpierətoh'therəpee) 1. treatment by artificially increasing the patient's body temperature. 2. the treatment of fever.

pyrexia (pie'reksi·ə) a fever, or febrile condition. adj. **pyrexial.**

pyridine ('piriˌdeen) 1. a substance derived from coal tar and also from tobacco and various organic matter. 2. any of a group of substances homologous with normal pyridine.

Pyridium (pi'ridi·əm) trademark for preparations of phenazopyridine hydrochloride; a urinary tract analgesic.

pyridostigmine (ˌpiridoh'stigmeen) a cholinesterase inhibitor; used in the treatment of myasthenia gravis and as an antidote to nondepolarizing muscle relaxants, e.g., tubocurarine.

pyridoxal (ˌpiri'doksəl) a form of vitamin B_6. **p. phosphate** a major coenzyme involved in amino acid metabolism.

pyridoxamine (ˌpiri'doksəmeen) one of the three active forms of vitamin B_6.

p. phosphate a coenzyme involved in amino acid metabolism.

pyridoxine (ˌpiri'dokseen) one of the forms of vitamin B_6, chiefly used, as the hydrochloride salt, in the prophylaxis and treatment of vitamin B_6 deficiency. It is also used in counteracting the neurotoxic effects of isoniazid, and sometimes in the treatment of myasthenia gravis.

pyrimethamine (ˌpieri'methəmeen) a folic acid antagonist used as an antimalarial, especially for suppressive prophylaxis, and also used concomitantly with a sulphonamide in the treatment of toxoplasmosis.

pyrimidine (pie'rimiˌdeen) an organic compound that is the fundamental form of the pyrimidine bases, including uracil, cytosine, and thymine.

pyro- word element. [Gr.] *fire*, *heat* (in chemistry) *produced by heating*.

pyrogen ('pierohˌjen) an agent that causes fever. adj. **pyrogenic**.

pyroglobulinaemia (ˌpierohˌglobyuhli'neemi·ə) the presence in the blood of an abnormal globulin constituent that is precipitated by heat.

pyromania (ˌpieroh'mayni·ə) obsessive preoccupation with fire; a morbid compulsion to set fires.

pyronin ('pierohnin) a red aniline histological stain.

pyrophobia (ˌpieroh'fohbi·ə) morbid dread of fire.

pyrophosphatase (ˌpieroh'fosfəˌtayz) any enzyme that catalyses the hydrolysis of central pyrophosphate linkages.

pyrophosphate (ˌpieroh'fosfayt) any salt of pyrophosphoric acid.

pyrophosphoric acid (ˌpierohfos'forik) a dimer of phosphoric acid, $H_4P_2O_7$.

pyrosis (pie'rohsis) HEARTBURN; a burning sensation in the oesophagus and stomach, with sour eructation.

pyrotic (pie'rotik) caustic; burning.

pyroxylin (pie'roksilin) a product of the action of a mixture of nitric and sulphuric acids on cotton, consisting chiefly of cellulose tetranitrate; a necessary ingredient of collodion.

pyrrole ('pirohl) a basic, cyclic substance, obtained by destructive distillation of various animal substances.

pyrrolidine (pi'roliˌdeen) a simple base obtained from tobacco or prepared from pyrrole.

pyruvate (pie'roovayt) a salt, ester, or anion of pyruvic acid. Pyruvate is the end product of glycolysis and may be metabolized to lactate or to acetyl CoA.

pyruvic acid (pie'roovik) a compound formed in the body in aerobic metabolism of carbohydrate; also formed by dry distillation of tartaric acid.

pyuria (pie'yooə·ri·ə) pus in the urine.

PZI protamine zinc insulin.

Q

Q quadrant.

q symbol for (1) the long arm of a chromosome or (2) the frequency of the rarer allele of a pair.

Q fever a febrile rickettsial infection caused by *Coxiella burnetii*. The causative microorganisms are found on the hides of sheep and cattle, and it is thought that human beings contract the disease by breathing in the dried microorganisms carried in dust particles in the air. In Australia, where the disease was first described, it is transmitted by ticks. Symptoms include sudden high fever, chills, headache, muscle pains, and coughing. The disease is usually quickly brought under control by antibiotics. The Q stands for query.

q-sort ('kyooˌsawt) a technique of personality assessment in which the subject (or an observer) indicates the degree to which a standardized set of descriptive statements applies to the subject.

QARANC Queen Alexandra's Royal Army Nursing Corps.

QARNNS Queen Alexandra's Royal Naval Nursing Service.

q.d. [L.] *quaque die* (every day).

q.h. [L.] *quaque hora* (every hour).

q.i.d. [L.] *quater in die* (four times a day).

QIDN Queen's Institute of District Nursing.

QNI Queen's Nursing Institute.

q.q.h. [L.] *quaque quarta hora* (every 4 hours).

QRS complex a group of waves depicted on an electrocardiogram; called also the QRS wave. It actually consists of three distinct waves created by the passage of the cardiac electrical impulse through the ventricles and occurs at the beginning of each contraction of the ventricles. In a normal ELECTROCARDIOGRAM the R wave is the most prominent of the three; the Q and S waves may be extremely weak and sometimes are absent.

One abnormality of the QRS complex is increased voltage resulting from enlargement of heart muscle, which produces increased quantities of electric current. This enlargement is caused by an excessive work load for some part of the heart and usually is due to a defect in the heart valves or great vessels near the heart.

A low-voltage QRS complex may result from local intraventricular block, toxic conditions of the heart, and fluid in the pericardium. Pleural effusion and emphysema also can cause a decrease in the voltage of the QRS complex.

q.s. [L.] *quantum satis* (a sufficient amount).

qt quart.

quack (kwak) one who misrepresents his ability and experience in diagnosis and treatment of disease or the effects to be achieved by his treatment.

quackery ('kwakə·ree) the practice or methods of a quack.

quadr(i)- word element. [L.] *four*.

quadrangular (kwo'drangyuhlə) having four angles.

quadrant ('kwodrənt) 1. one-fourth of the circumference of a circle. 2. one of four corresponding parts, or quarters, as of the surface of the abdomen or of the field of vision.

quadrantanopia (ˌkwodrantə'nohpi·ə) defective vision or blindness in one fourth of the visual field.

quadrate ('kwodrət, -drayt) square or squared.

quadratus (kwod'raytəs) four-sided. The term is used to describe a number of four-sided muscles.

quadriceps ('kwodriˌseps) having four heads.

q. muscle a name applied collectively to four muscles, the rectus of the thigh and intermediate lateral and medial great muscles, inserting by a common tendon that surrounds the patella and ends on the tuberosity of the tibia, and acting to extend the leg upon the thigh.

quadrigemina (ˌkwodri'jeminə) the corpora quadrigemina.

quadrigeminal (ˌkwodri'jeminəl) fourfold; in four parts; forming a group of four.

quadrilateral (ˌkwodri'latə·rəl) having four sides.

quadrilocular (ˌkwodri'lokyuhlə) having four cavities.

quadripartite (ˌkwodri'pahtiet) divided into four.

quadriplegia (ˌkwodri'pleeji·ə) paralysis of all four limbs; tetraplegia. adj. **quadriplegic**.

PATIENT CARE. The quadriplegic patient is paralysed from the neck down and is, therefore, subject to the many problems associated with immobility and loss of sensation. The immediate goal of care is the prevention of infection and the maintenance of the integrity of the body systems so that optimum rehabilitation can be achieved. The extent to which the patient may eventually achieve mobility in a wheelchair and some degree of independence can be affected by the calibre of care received and the motivation and drive of the individual patient.

Mechanical devices such as braces and crutches are helpful in compensating for the loss of muscular function. PHYSIOTHERAPY procedures and techniques and OCCUPATIONAL THERAPY are essential aspects of patient care and are vital to the attainment of the goals of REHABILITATION. See also PARAPLEGIA.

Patient education is especially important to the long-range goal of prevention of serious complications. The patient and his family should be aware of the early signs and symptoms of breakdown of the skin (PRESSURE SORE), FAECAL IMPACTION, a developing infection, and urinary difficulties. As with any type of long-term care, the patient should be medically evaluated periodically and his care should be under the supervision of a visiting nurse. In spite of the many difficulties that may be encountered by the paralysed patient, it is possible for these patients to lead full and personally rewarding lives.

quadrisect ('kwodri,sekt) to cut into four parts.

quadritubercular (,kwodrityuh'bərkyuhlə) having four tubercles or cusps.

quadrivalent (,kwodri'vaylənt) having a valency of four.

quadruped ('kwodruh,ped) 1. four-footed. 2. an animal having four feet.

quadruplet ('kwodruhplət, kwo'drooplət) one of four offspring produced at one birth.

qualifying (,kwoli'fie·ing) in psychology, signifying a form of facial deceit in which an individual adds another facial expression to one that has just been shown, e.g., a smile may be shown after an angry expression as a sign that the individual is not as angry as he may seem.

qualimeter (kwo'limitə) an instrument for measuring the penetrating power of x-rays; penetrometer.

qualitative data ('kwolitətiv) observations of mutually exclusive events such as death or survival.

quality assurance ('kwolitee) in the health care field, a pledge to the public by those within the various health disciplines that they will work toward the goal of an optimal achievable degree of excellence in the services rendered to every patient. Since the 1960s there has been an increasing emphasis on the individual citizen's right to health and the obligation of individual members of the health care team to hold themselves accountable to the public for the calibre of care they provide.

A quality assurance programme takes into account the need to define that which is to be measured. Quality assurance implies a clear understanding of what is meant by 'quality' and a valid and reliable method for evaluating the care that is provided. (See also EVALUATION.) In the health care field, evaluation of practice operates within the parameters of *outcome*, *cost-benefit*, and *access* to the health care delivery system. Outcome represents a measurable change in the health/illness status of the patient that is the end result of the care the patient received. Cost-benefit refers to the expenditure of money, time, and effort in providing health care and the relationship this cost bears to the actual benefits to the recipient. Access to health care refers to its availability, the ease with which one can obtain the kind of health care he needs.

Implementation of a quality assurance programme involves the development of criteria based on acceptable standards of care and norms of professional behaviour. The norms are established by members of the profession who are expert in the care of specific patient populations. The health/illness criteria should be patient-centred: they must express in positive terms what it is a patient should be able to do as a direct result of the care he has received. For example, in the area of nursing care, an elderly patient with 'night incontinence' should remain dry throughout the night as a result of an individualized BLADDER TRAINING programme, or a patient who is bedridden should be able to maintain joint motion as a result of a daily range-of-motion exercise programme.

The development of outcome criteria is an essential first step in a quality assurance programme. The criteria are then used as the 'yardstick' against which actual practice and its results can be evaluated. Evaluation is conducted by a review committee, preferably one composed of practitioners in the area of health care being evaluated. A *retrospective review* measures actual documented outcomes against desirable and valued outcomes. Data for documentation of actual outcomes are obtained from the medical and nursing records of a specific patient population after the patients have been discharged. A *concurrent review* evaluates patient care while it is in progress. Documentation of the calibre of care being delivered is obtained through review of the patient's charts, interview, observation, and examination of the patient. The advantage of concurrent review is that it can provide opportunities for improvement of patient care while it is in progress.

The ultimate goal of both retrospective and concurrent review is improvement of patient care. If, at the time of review, a deficiency is detected in either the health care process or the health/illness status of the patient, an effort is made to correct the difference between 'what should be' and 'what actually is'. It is this promise to evaluate thoroughly and to employ the results of the evaluation for continuous improvement of patient care that is the essence of quality assurance.

quantimeter (kwon'timitə) an instrument for measuring the quantity of x-rays generated by a Coolidge tube.

quantitative data ('kwontitətiv) observations of continuous variables such as height or weight.

quantity ('kwontətee) 1. a characteristic, as of energy or mass, susceptible to precise physical measurement. 2. a measurable amount. adj. **quantitative**.

quantivalency (,kwonti'vaylənsee) VALENCY (1).

quantum ('kwontəm) pl. *quanta* [L.] an elemental unit of energy; the amount emitted or absorbed at each step when energy is emitted or absorbed by atoms or molecules.

q. theory radiation and absorption of energy occur in quantities (quanta) which vary in size with the frequency of the radiation.

quarantine ('kwo·rən,teen) 1. a place or period of detention of ships coming from infected or suspected ports. 2. restrictions placed on entering or leaving premises where a case of communicable disease exists.

quart (kwawt) one-fourth of a gallon (946 ml); abbreviated qt.

quartan ('kwawtan) 1. recurring in 4-day cycles (every third day). 2. a variety of intermittent fever of which the paroxysms recur on every third day (see MALARIA).

double q. a quartan fever in which the paroxysms occur on two successive days followed by one day free of fever.

triple q. a fever in which the paroxysms occur every day because of infection with three different groups of quartan parasites.

quartile ('kwawtiel) one of the values establishing the division of a series of variables into fourths, or the range of items included in such a segment.

quartz (kwawts) rock crystal. Ultraviolet rays can penetrate it. Its piezoelectric properties make it suitable for use in ultrasonic transducers.

q. lamp a mercury-vapour lamp which produces ultraviolet rays.

quater in die (ˌkwaytə in 'dee·ay) [L.] *four times a day.*

quaternary (kwə'tərnə·ree) 1. fourth in a series. 2. made up of four elements or groups.

Queckenstedt's test ('kweken,stets) when the veins in the neck are compressed on one or both sides there is a rapid rise in the pressure of the cerebrospinal fluid of healthy persons, and this rise quickly disappears when pressure is taken off the neck. But when there is a block in the spinal canal the pressure of the cerebrospinal fluid is affected little or not at all by the manoeuvre.

Quellada (kwe'lahdə) trademark for preparation of lindane, a pediculicide and scabicide.

quenching ('kwenching) to put out, extinguish, or suppress; to cool (as hot metal) by immersing in water. In liquid scintillation counting, any process taking place within the sample container which results in a decrease in number or intensity of the light flashes produced, thus lowering the amount of energy recorded.

quercetin ('kwərsətin) a form of rutin and other glycosides, used to reduce abnormal capillary fragility.

Quervain's disease (kair'vanhz) inflammation of the long abductor and short extensor tendons of the thumb, with swelling and tenderness. Called also de Quervain's disease.

questionnaire (ˌkweschən'air) a specially designed set of questions used to collect data in epidemiological studies. May be self-completed, or completed by the interviewer by telephone or in face-to-face conversation.

Questran ('kwestran) trademark for a preparation of cholestyramine.

Quick one-stage prothrombin time test (kwik) a method of determining the integrity of the prothrombin complex in the blood; used in controlling anticoagulant therapy.

Quick tourniquet test (kwik) estimation of capillary fragility by counting the number of petechiae appearing in a limited area on the flexor surface of the forearm after obstruction to the circulation by a blood pressure cuff applied to the upper arm.

quickening ('kwikəning) the first perceptible movement of the fetus in the uterus, appearing usually in the sixteenth to eighteenth week of pregnancy.

quicklime ('kwik,liem) calcium oxide.

quiescent (kwi'es'nt) inactive or at rest; descriptive of a time when the symptoms of a disease are not evident.

quinalbarbitone (ˌkwinal'bahbi,tohn) a short to intermediate-acting barbiturate drug sometimes used in the treatment of severe insomnia.

Quincke's disease ('kwingkəz) angioneurotic oedema.

Quincke's pulse alternate blanching and flushing of the nail bed due to pulsation of subpapillary arteriolar and venous plexuses, as seen in aortic insufficiency.

quinestrol (kwi'neestrol) a long-acting oestrogen.

Quinicardine (kwini'kahdeen) trademark for a preparation of quinidine sulphate, a cardiac antiarrhythmic.

quinidine ('kwini,deen) the dextrorotatory isomer of quinine, used in treatment of cardiac arrhythmias.

quinine ('kwineen, kwi'neen) an alkaloid of cinchona which suppresses the asexual erythrocytic forms of malarial parasites and has a slight effect on the gametocytes. Quinine also has analgesic, antipyretic, mild oxytocic, cardiac depressant, and sclerosing properties, and it decreases the excitability of the motor endplate.

quininism ('kwini,nizəm) cinchonism; poisoning from cinchona bark or its alkaloids.

quinone ('kwinohn, kwi'nohn) a principle obtained by oxidizing quinic acid.

quinquevalent (ˌkwingkwi'vaylənt, kwin'kwevələnt) pentavalent; having a valency of five.

quinsy ('kwinzee) peritonsillar abscess.

quint- word element. [L.] *five.*

quintan ('kwintən) recurring every 5 days (every fourth day).

q. fever trench fever.

quintuplet ('kwintyuhplət, kwin'tyooplət) one of five offspring produced at one birth.

quotid. [L.] *quotidie* (every day).

quotidian (kwo'tidi·ən) 1. recurring every day. 2. a form of intermittent malarial fever with daily recurrent paroxysms.

double q. a fever having two daily paroxysms.

quotient ('kwohshənt) a number obtained by division.

achievement q. the achievement age divided by the mental age, indicating progress in learning.

calorific q. the heat evolved (in calories or joules) divided by the oxygen consumed (in milligrams) in a metabolic process.

intelligence q. I.Q., a numerical expression of intellectual capacity obtained by multiplying the mental age of the subject, ascertained by testing, by 100 and dividing by his chronological age.

respiratory q. the ratio of the volume of carbon dioxide given off by the body tissues to the volume of oxygen absorbed by them; usually equal to the corresponding volumes given off and taken up by the lungs. Abbreviated RQ.

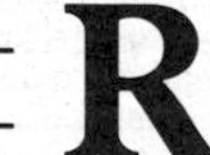

R

R symbol, *roentgen;* a symbol used in general chemical formulae to represent an organic radical; Rankine (scale); Réaumur (scale); [L.] *remotum* (far); respiration; *Rickettsia;* right.

℞ symbol. [L.] *recipe* (take); prescription; treatment.

r symbol for ring chromosome.

Ra chemical symbol, *radium.*

rabbit fever ('rabit) tularaemia.

rabiate, rabid ('raybi·ət; 'rabid) affected with rabies; pertaining to rabies.

rabies ('raybeez) *hydrophobia*; an acute, notifiable, infectious disease of the central nervous system, which may affect all warm-blooded animals, including humans. It is caused by an RNA virus belonging to the rhabdovirus group. The virus is often present in the host's saliva, and infection is usually transmitted to humans by the bite or lick of a rabid animal, such as a bat, wolf, dog, cat, fox, or other mammal; it is sometimes, though rarely, transmitted by the respiratory route. The incubation period in humans is from one to three months, being shorter following bites near the brain.

The earliest symptoms are intermittent pain, numbness, tingling, or burning around the site of infection; soon afterward, in the commoner form, generalized hyperexcitability occurs, followed by fever, paralysis of the muscles of swallowing, and glottal spasm brought on by the sight of fluids or the drinking of fluids, and by maniacal behaviour and convulsions. In the less frequent form there is an ascending flaccid paralysis, and sensory disturbances occur. Rabies is almost invariably fatal, death resulting from respiratory paralysis. The diagnosis can be determined by viral isolation (from saliva, cerebrospinal fluid, urine) or by demonstration of neutralizing antibody, and after death by the appearance of cytoplasmic inclusion bodies (Negri bodies) in degenerated neurons.

RABIES IN ANIMALS. The first sign of the disease in a rabid animal is often a change of temperament. Some, especially wild, animals may become unusually friendly. The rabid animal may next enter a 'furious' stage, in which it wanders about biting everything that moves, and even sticks and stones. It then develops paralysis of the throat, which makes swallowing difficult.

Some animals pass directly from the anxiety stage to paralysis without becoming violent. This is called the 'dumb' form of rabies. The animal may appear to have something caught in his throat. Usually, a dog with something in his throat tries to remove it himself, but a rabid dog will not. Eventually all of the rabid animal's muscles become paralysed and it dies.

OCCURENCE OF RABIES. Rabies occurs in many species of animals in many parts of mainland Europe and in all other continents except Australia and Antarctica. The UK is free of rabies, and this condition is maintained by the compulsory quarantine of imported animals.

TREATMENT. When a person is bitten by an animal in a country where rabies is endemic, the wound should be washed thoroughly with soap and water, and then treated like any other wound. It is extremely important to go to a doctor immediately. If at all possible, steps should be taken to find out if the biting animal has rabies. The animal should be confined for observation. When the biting animal must be killed in order to capture it, care must be taken to see that the head is not damaged, so that the brain can be examined to establish a diagnosis. There are times when the biting animal cannot be caught for observation. If so, the bitten person must be given antirabies treatment immediately.

Preventive post-exposure treatment is based on immunization by a series of vaccine and immune globulin injections. When bites are in areas close to the head or in areas with many nerve endings, such as the hands, the virus may reach the brain very quickly. In such cases treatment should start immediately, even though the suspected animal is still being observed.

The agent used to confer passive immunity is human rabies immune globulin (HRIG). Allergic reactions to HRIG are rare. Active immunity to rabies is conferred by the administration of human diploid cell vaccine (HDCV). For post-exposure treatment, 1.0 ml is given by deep subcutaneous or intramuscular injection on days 0, 3, 7, 14, 30 and 90. Local reactions sometimes occur but systemic side-effects are very uncommon.

Pre-exposure prophylaxis is recommended in the United Kingdom for persons who, because of their occupations, are at special risk of contracting rabies, e.g. employees at animal quarantine premises. Such people are offered a shortened course of HDCV.

There is no cure for rabies and once symptoms appear treatment can only be palliative. This includes sedation of the patient and provision of a quiet environment to reduce anxiety and relieve pain, administration of a powerful muscle relaxant (curare-like drugs) to reduce muscular contractions, and supportive measures to maintain urinary and respiratory function. Death usually occurs in 2 to 6 days, but occasionally not until 10–14 days have elapsed.

race (rays) a class or breed of animals; a group of individuals having certain characteristics in common, owing to a common inheritance.

racemase ('raysi,mayz) an enzyme that catalyses the racemization of an optically active substance, such as L-lactic acid.

racemate ('raysi,mayt) a racemic compound.

racemic (rə'seemik, -'sem-) optically inactive, being composed of equal amounts of dextrorotatory and laevorotatory isomers.

racemization (,rasimie'zayshən) the transformation of one-half of the molecules of an optically active compound into molecules that possess exactly the opposite (mirror-image) configuration, with complete loss of rotatory power because of the statistical balance between equal numbers of dextrorotatory and laevorotatory molecules.

racemose ('rasi,mohz) shaped like a bunch of grapes.

rachi(o)- word element. [Gr.] *spine*.

rachialgia (,rayki'alji·ə) pain in the spine.

rachianaesthesia (,rayki,anəs'theezi·ə) loss of sensation produced by injection of an anaesthetic into the spinal canal.

rachicentesis (,raykisen'teesis) puncture into the lumbar spinal canal (see also SPINAL PUNCTURE).

rachidial, rachidian (rə'kidi·əl; rə'kidi·ən) pertaining to the spine.

rachigraph ('rayki,grahf, -,graf) an instrument for recording the outlines of the spine and back.

rachilysis (rə'kilisis) correction of lateral curvature of the spine by combined traction and pressure.

rachiocampsis (,raykioh'kampsis) spinal curvature.

rachiometer (,rayki'omitə) an apparatus for measuring spinal curvature.

rachiomyelitis (,raykioh,mieə'lietis) inflammation of the spinal cord.

rachiotomy (,rayki'otəmee) incision through the lamina of a vertebra or the laminae of several vertebrae of the vertebral column.

rachipagus (rə'kipəgəs) twin fetuses joined at the vertebral column.

rachis ('raykis) the vertebral column.

rachischisis (rə'kiskisis) congenital fissure of the vertebral column.

r. posterior spina bifida.

rachitic (rə'kitik) pertaining to rickets.

rachitis (rə'kietis) 1. rickets. 2. inflammatory disease of the vertebral column.

rachitogenic (,raykitə'jenik) causing rickets.

rachitomy (rə'kitəmee) the surgical or anatomic opening of the spinal canal.

rad (rad) acronym for *r*adiation *a*bsorbed *d*ose; a superseded, non-SI unit of measurement of the absorbed dose of ionizing radiation. It corresponds to an energy transfer of 100 ergs per gram of any absorbing material (including tissue). The biological effect of 1 rad of radiation varies with the type of radiation. When the dose is in REMS, all types have the same biological effect. Replaced by the GRAY.

rad. [L.] *radix* (root).

RADC Royal Army Dental Corps.

radiability (,raydi·ə'bilitee) the property of being readily penetrated by x-rays or other rays.

radiad ('raydi,ad) toward the radius or radial side.

radial ('raydi·əl) 1. pertaining to the radius of the arm or to the radial (lateral) aspect of the arm as opposed to the ulnar (medial) aspect; pertaining to a radius. 2. radiating; spreading outward from a common centre.

r. artery an artery in the forearm, wrist, and hand; the one usually used for taking the PULSE.

radialis (,raydi'aylis) [L.] *radial*.

radiant ('raydi·ənt) 1. diverging from a centre. 2.

emitting rays, as of light or heat.

radiate ('raydi,ayt) 1. to diverge or spread from a common point. 2. arranged in a radiating manner.

radiathermy (,raydieə'thərmee) short wave diathermy.

radiatio (,raydi'ayshioh) pl. *radiationes* [L.] a radiating structure. In anatomy, a collection of nerve fibres connecting different portions of the brain.

radiation (,raydi'ayshən) 1. divergence from a common centre. 2. a structure made up of diverging elements, especially a tract of the central nervous system made up of diverging fibres. 3. energy carried by waves or a stream of particles. One type is *electromagnetic radiation*, which consists of wave motion of electric and magnetic fields. The *quantum theory* is based on the fact that electromagnetic waves consist of discrete particles, called *photons*, that have an energy inversely proportional to the wavelength of the wave. In order of increasing photon energy and decreasing wavelength, the electromagnetic spectrum is divided into radio waves, infrared light, visible light, ultraviolet light, and x-rays.

Another type is the radiation emitted by radioactive materials. *Alpha particles* are high-energy helium-4 nuclei consisting of two protons and two neutrons, which are emitted by radioisotopes of heavy elements, such as uranium. *Beta particles* are high-energy electrons, which are emitted by radioisotopes of lighter elements. *Gamma rays* are high-energy photons, which are emitted alone or with alpha and beta particles and are also emitted alone by metastable radionuclides, such as technetium-99m. Gamma rays have energies in the x-ray region of the spectrum and differ from x-rays only in that they are produced by radioactive decay rather than by x-ray machines.

Radiation with enough energy to knock electrons out of atoms and produce ions is called *ionizing radiation*. This includes alpha and beta particles and x-rays and gamma rays. Ionizing radiation can produce tissue damage directly by striking a vital molecule, such as DNA, or indirectly by striking a water molecule and producing highly reactive free radicals that chemically attack vital molecules. The effects of radiation can kill cells, make them unable to reproduce, or cause nonlethal mutations, producing cancer cells or birth defects in offspring. The radiosensitivity of normal tissues or cancer cells increases with their rate of cell division and decreases with their rate of cell specialization. Highly radiosensitive cells include lymphocytes, bone marrow haematopoietic cells, germ cells, and intestinal epithelial cells. Radiosensitive cancers include leukaemias and lymphomas, seminoma, dysgerminoma, granulosa cell carcinoma, adenocarcinoma of the gastric epithelium, and squamous cell carcinoma of skin, mouth, nose and throat, cervix, and bladder.

The application of radiation, whether by x-ray or radioactive substances, for treatment of various illnesses is called RADIOTHERAPY.

Three types of units are used to measure ionizing radiation. The *roentgen* (R) is a unit of exposure dose applicable only to x-rays and gamma rays. It is the amount of radiation that produces 2.58×10^{-4} coulomb of positive and negative ions passing through 1 kilogram of dry air. The *rad* (from *r*adiation *a*bsorbed *d*ose) is a unit of absorbed dose equal to 100 ergs of energy absorbed per 1 g of absorbing material. The absorbed dose depends both on the type of radiation and on the material in which it is absorbed. The *rem* (from *r*oentgen *e*quivalent *m*an) is a unit of absorbed dose equivalent, which produces the same biological effect as 1 rad of high-energy x-rays. For beta and gamma radiation, 1 rem is approximately equal to 1 rad; for alpha radiation, 1 rad is approximately 20 rem.

Previously, doses administered in radiotherapy were commonly specified as measured exposure doses in roentgens. It is more useful to specify the absorbed dose in the tissue or organ of interest in rads. Many personnel monitoring devices read out in rems. The rad and rem have been replaced by the new SI units, the grey and sievert; 1 grey equals 100 rad, and 1 sievert equals 100 rem.

The activity of a radioactive source is measured in terms of the curie (Ci) (3.7×10^{10} disintegrations per second). The equivalent SI unit is the becquerel (Bq) (1 disintegration per second). Thus, 1 mCi = 37 mBq.

RADIATION HAZARDS. The harmful effects of radiation may be considered in three main groups. The first are *somatic non-stochastic* effects, i.e. those which are dose-dependent. These include skin erythema, cataracts, nausea, aplastic anaemia and sterility. For each effect there is a threshold below which no effect occurs, and although recovery may be possible successive doses show only partial recovery. Severity of the effect is dependent on dose rate.

The second group of *somatic stochastic* effects includes the risk of carcinogenesis, especially leukaemia and the increased mutation rate in the developing fetus. The induction of tumours by radiation takes place over many years, even decades. Stochastic dose–effect curves relate the probability of an effect to the dose received. There is no threshold for these effects as there is a normal background rate of mutations and tumour formation even in the absence of radiation, and there is no recovery from these dose effects—they accumulate additively. The probability of a stochastic effect rises theoretically to 100 per cent but in practice this point is seldom reached because other serious somatic non-stochastic effects take their toll first.

The third group of *genetic* effects are expressed in future generations.

Exposure to large radiation doses over a short period produces RADIATION sickness.

RADIATION PROTECTION. In order to avoid the radiation hazards mentioned above, one must be aware of three basic principles of time, distance, and shielding involved in protection from radiation. Obviously, the longer one stays near a source of radiation the greater will be the exposure. The same is true of proximity to the source; the closer one gets to a source of radiation the greater the exposure.

Shielding is of special importance when, as in the case of hospital personnel involved in radiotherapy, time and distance cannot be completely utilized as safety factors. In such instances lead, which is an extremely dense material, is utilized as a protective device. The walls of diagnostic x-ray rooms are lined with lead, and lead containers are used for radium, cobalt-60, and other radioactive materials used in radiotherapy. Radiotherapists, radiologists and other personnel concerned with use of x-rays can obtain additional protection by wearing lead aprons and gloves.

Monitoring devices such as the film badge or pocket monitor are worn by persons working near sources of radiation. These devices contain special photographic film that is sensitive to radiation and thus serve as a guide to the amount of radiation to which a person has been exposed. For monitoring large areas in which radiation hazards may pose a problem, survey meters such as the Geiger counter may be used. The survey meter also is useful in finding sources of radiation such as a radium implant, which might be lost.

Sensible use of these protective and monitoring devices can greatly reduce unnecessary exposure to

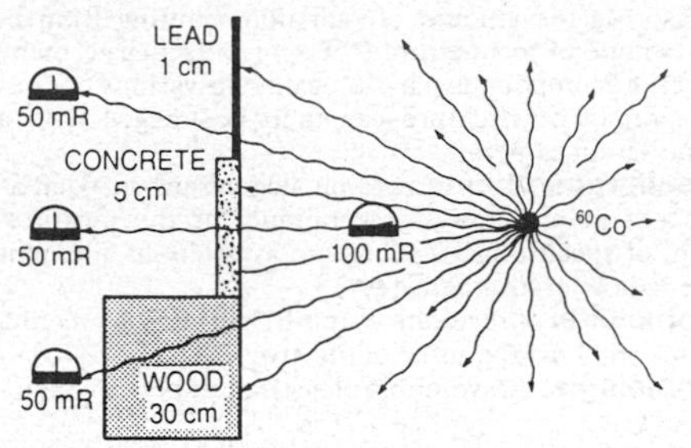

Comparison of efficacy of various materials for radiation shielding

radiation and allow for full realization of the many benefits of radiation.

corpuscular r. particles emitted in nuclear disintegration, including alpha and beta particles, protons, neutrons, positrons, and deuterons.

electromagnetic r. energy, unassociated with matter, that is transmitted through space by means of waves (electromagnetic waves) traveling in all instances at 3×10^{10} cm or 186,284 miles per second, but ranging in length from 10^{11} cm (electrical waves) to 10^{-12} cm (cosmic rays) and including radio waves, infrared, visible light and ultraviolet, x-rays, and gamma rays. See also radiation (above).

infrared r. the portion of the spectrum of electromagnetic radiation of wavelengths ranging between 0.75 and 1000 μm (see also INFRARED RAYS).

interstitial r. energy emitted by radium or radon inserted directly into the tissue. **ionizing r.** corpuscular or electromagnetic radiation that is capable of producing ions, directly or indirectly, in its passage through matter.

pyramidal r. fibres extending from the pyramidal tract to the cortex.

r. sickness a condition sometimes occurring in patients who have received therapeutic doses of radiation or in those individuals accidentally exposed to high doses. Its severity varies with the individual, the body areas exposed and the amount, kind and intensity of the exposure. Small doses will go unnoticed whereas an extremely high dose (150,000 rads; 1500 Gy) will produce very rapid death.

The events following a large radiation exposure are as follows. Within a few hours there may be a prodromal phase of gastrointestinal disturbances—nausea, vomiting, diarrhoea, abdominal pain and anorexia. The time of onset of symptoms is earliest with high doses and short exposure times, and occurs within a few hours. This is followed by a variable latent period in which the patient is well but mitosis ceases. The most rapidly mitotic cells, e.g., spermatogonia and haemopoietic cells, are the first to be affected. The main phase of the illness follows and its nature depends on the radiation dose received. 200–800 rads produces bone marrow depression. 150 rads will kill 50 per cent of stem cells; 500 rads kills 100 per cent. The white blood cell count falls at approximately 5 days, reaching its lowest point at 35 days. Death due to gastrointestinal damage occurs with doses of 1–10,000 rads, and with maximal damage occurs at 3 days. 10–15,000 rads result in death in 1–2 days from CNS damage—an acute vasculitis with haemorrhage and oedema.

r. striothalamica a fibre system joining the thalamus and the hypothalamic region.

tegmental r. fibres radiating laterally from the nucleus ruber.

thalamic r. fibres streaming out through the lateral surface of the thalamus, through the internal capsule to the cerebral cortex.

ultraviolet r. the portion of the spectrum of electromagnetic radiation of wavelengths ranging between 0.39 and 0.18 μm (see also ULTRAVIOLET RAYS).

radiation physicist a physicist who is responsible for certain technical aspects of radiotherapy, e.g. computer estimations, preparation of isodose curves, preparation of wedge and compensating filters, and calibration of teletherapy equipment and for supervision of radiation safety procedures.

radiation therapist radiotherapist.

radical ('radik'l) 1. directed to the cause; going to the root or source of a morbid process. 2. a group of atoms that enters into and goes out of chemical combination without change and that forms one of the fundamental constituents of a molecule.

free r. a radical, extremely reactive, and having a very short half-life (10^{-5} seconds less in an aqueous solution), which carries an unpaired electron.

radicle ('radik'l) one of the smallest branches of a vessel or nerve.

radicotomy (ˌradi'kotəmee) rhizotomy; division or transection of a nerve root.

radiculalgia (rəˌdikyuh'lalji·ə) pain due to disorder of the spinal nerve roots.

radicular (rə'dikyuhlə) pertaining to a root or radicle.

radiculectomy (rəˌdikyuh'lektəmee) removal of a spinal nerve root.

radiculitis (rəˌdikyuh'lietis) inflammation of a spinal nerve root, especially of the portion of the root that lies between the spinal cord and the spinal canal.

radiculoganglionitis (rəˌdikyuhlohˌgang·gli·ə'nietis) inflammation of the posterior spinal nerve roots and their ganglia.

radiculogram (rə'dikyuhlohgram) the radiograph made during radiculography.

radiculography (rəˌdikyuh'logrəfee) the study by radiography of the spinal nerve roots and their sheaths following the injection of a water-soluble radiopaque contrast medium into the subarachnoid space.

radiculomedullary (rəˌdikyuhlohmə'dulə·ree) affecting the nerve roots and spinal cord.

radiculomeningomyelitis (rəˌdikyuhlohməˌning·gohˌmieə'lietis) inflammation of the nerve roots, meninges, and spinal cord.

radiculomyelopathy (rəˌdikyuhlohˌmieə'lopəthee) disease of the nerve roots and spinal cord.

radiculoneuritis (rəˌdikyuhlohnyuh'rietis) acute febrile polyneuritis.

radiculoneuropathy (rəˌdikyuhlohnyuh'ropəthee) disease of the nerve roots and spinal nerves.

radiculopathy (rəˌdikyuh'lopəthee) disease of the nerve roots.

spondylotic caudal r. compression of the cauda equina due to encroachment upon a congenitally small spinal canal by spondylosis, resulting in neural disorders of the lower limbs.

radio- word element. [L.] *ray, radiation, emission of radiant energy, radium, radius* (bone of the forearm); affixed to the name of a chemical element to designate a radioactive isotope of that element.

radioactive (ˌraydioh'aktiv) characterized by radioactivity.

radioactivity (ˌraydioh·ak'tivitee) the quality of emitting or the emission of particulate or electromagnetic radiation as a consequence of the decay of the nuclei of unstable elements, a property of all chemical elements of atomic number above 83, and possible of induction in all other known elements.

The chemical elements are made up of atoms, each of which consists of a nucleus around which orbits a cloud of negatively charged electrons. The nucleus itself is made up of two kinds of particles: *neutrons*, which have no electrical charge; and *protons*, each of which has a single positive charge. A neutral atom has an equal number of protons and electrons and no electric charge. The *atomic number* of an element is the number of protons in the nucleus of each of its atoms. The *mass number* of an element is the sum of the number of protons and neutrons in the nucleus.

All of the atoms of a particular element have the same atomic number, but can have different numbers of protons. An *isotope* of a chemical element consists of atoms having the same number of neutrons. When an atomic nucleus is unstable it decomposes or decays spontaneously, emitting high-energy particles. The emissions from radioactive decay can consist of electrons (beta particles), or electromagnetic energy in the form of photons, or helium ions (alpha particles). (See also RADIATION.) The process of decay can produce a product that is itself unstable, in which case it too will decay. The process continues until a stable nuclide is finally formed.

The radioactivity of a substance can be measured by determining the rate at which atoms decay in a given period of time. The basic unit of measurement of radioactivity was the *curie* (Ci), which equals 37 billion disintegrations per second. One-thousandth of a curie is a *millicurie;* one-millionth is a *microcurie.* These units of measure were used to calculate the amounts of radioactivity administered for various therapeutic procedures in much the same way that units of measure such as the gram and milligram are used to measure dosages of medications. The curie has been replaced by a new SI unit of radioactivity, the *becquerel* (Bq), which is equal to 1 disintegration per second. One microcurie equals 37 kilobecquerel.

The *half-life* of an element is the time necessary for one-half of a given amount of the isotope to decay. Half-lives can range from billions of years to fractions of a second. The rate at which atomic decay occurs in a particular isotope cannot be altered by any outside force such as temperature, pressure, or chemical reaction. The knowledge of the half-life of a particular isotope is essential to the proper handling of the substance for the protection of the medical staff and the patient who is receiving some form of radiotherapy.

Both particulate and electromagnetic radiations are capable of penetrating matter and interacting with it by indiscriminately knocking out the electrons from atoms and molecules. The process of ionizing radiation produces ions (charged particles) and complex radicals (a group of charged atoms), which may combine to form different molecules. Radiation damage to the nuclei of cells interferes with their reproduction by changing their genetic structure. This ability to penetrate matter and change the basic structure and function of cells is used beneficially in the treatment of malignant tumours. See also RADIOTHERAPY.

Rendering an element radioactive by artificial means does not alter its chemical behaviour within the body; therefore, the body's systems respond to a radioactive element as if it were stable. This phenomenon makes it possible to use radioactive elements for diagnostic as well as therapeutic purposes. For example, the isotope of iodine (^{131}I) is readily taken up by the thyroid gland, permitting evaluation of iodine uptake of the gland by measuring the amount of radiation emitting from it. An isotope of technetium ($^{99}Tc^{m}$) is attached to many different compounds which localize in various organs. The organ or structure can then be imaged with a scintillation camera.

radioallergosorbent (ˌraydiohˌaləgoh'sawbənt) denoting a radioimmunoassay technique for the measurement of specific IgE antibody to a variety of allergens (see radioallergosorbent TEST).

radiobicipital (ˌraydiohbie'sipit'l) pertaining to the radius and biceps muscle of the arm.

radiobiologist (ˌraydiohbie'oləjist) an expert in radiobiology.

radiobiology (ˌraydiohbie'oləjee) the branch of science concerned with effects of light and of ultraviolet and ionizing radiations on living tissue or organisms. adj. **radiobiological**.

radiocarpal (ˌraydioh'kahp'l) pertaining to the radius and carpus.

radiochemistry (ˌraydioh'kemistree) the branch of chemistry dealing with radioactive materials.

radiocolloid (ˌraydioh'koloyd) a radioactive isotope in the form of a large molecule solution used in nuclear medicine scanning techniques for diagnosis. It can also be instilled into the body cavities to treat malignant ascites or malignant pleural effusion.

radiocurable (ˌraydioh'kyooə·rəb'l) curable by radiation.

radiocystitis (ˌraydiohsi'stietis) inflammatory tissue changes in the urinary bladder caused by irradiation.

radiodense (ˌraydioh'dens) radiopaque.

radiodensity (ˌraydioh'densitee) the property of being relatively resistant to the passage of radiant energy.

radiodermatitis (ˌraydiohˌdərmə'tietis) a cutaneous inflammatory reaction to exposure to biologically effective levels of ionizing radiation; x-ray dermatitis.

radiodiagnosis (ˌraydiohˌdieəg'nohsis) diagnosis by means of x-rays or gamma rays.

radioelectrocardiogram (ˌraydioh·iˌlektroh'kahdiohˌgram) the tracing obtained by radioelectrocardiography.

radioelectrocardiograph (ˌraydioh·iˌlektroh'kahdiohˌgrahf, -ˌgraf) the apparatus used in radioelectrocardiography.

radioelectrocardiography (ˌraydioh·iˌlektrohˌkahdi'ogrəfee) the recording of alterations in the electric potential of the heart, with impulses beamed by radio waves from the subject to the recording device by means of a small transmitter attached to the patient.

radioencephalography (ˌraydioh·enˌkefə'logrəfee, -ˌsef-) the recording of changes in the electric potential of the brain without direct attachment between the recording apparatus and the subject, the impulses being beamed by radio waves from the subject to the receiver.

radiogold (ˌraydioh'gohld) a radioisotope of gold, especially ^{198}Au, which has a half-life of 2.7 days and emits gamma and beta radiation. See GOLD-198.

radiogram ('raydiohˌgram) radiograph.

radiograph ('raydiohˌgrahf, -ˌgraf) the film produced by radiography.

panoramic r. a type of extraoral radiograph on which both maxillae and mandible are depicted on a single film.

radiographer (ˌraydi'ogrəfə) a professional health care worker in a diagnostic x-ray department (diagnostic radiographer) or in a radiotherapy department (therapy radiographer). The duties of a diagnostic radiographer include the positioning of patients for radiographic examinations; determining the proper exposure factors for each radiograph and assisting the radiologist in special procedures. Qualified diagnostic radiographers hold the Diploma of the College of Radiographers (Radiodiagnosis); DCR(R).

The duties of the therapy radiographer include delivery of courses of radiotherapy prescribed by the radiotherapist, care of the patient in the radiotherapy department and preparation of equipment and radioactive materials. Qualified therapy radiographers hold the Diploma of the College of Radiographers (Therapy); DCR(T).

radiography (ˌraydi'ogrəfee) the making of film records (radiographs) of internal structures of the body by exposure of film specially sensitized to x-rays or gamma rays. adj. **radiographic.**

body-section r. a special technique to show in detail images and structures lying in a predetermined plane of tissue, while blurring or eliminating detail in images in other planes; various mechanisms and methods for such radiography have been given various names, e.g., laminagraphy, tomography, etc.

double contrast r. a technique for revealing any abnormality of the intestinal mucosa, involving injection and evacuation of a barium enema, followed by inflation of the intestine with air under light pressure. The light coating of barium on the inflated intestine in the radiograph reveals clearly even small abnormalities.

neutron r. that in which a narrow beam of neutrons from a nuclear reactor is passed through tissues; especially useful in visualizing bony tissue.

serial r. the making of several exposures of a particular area at arbitrary intervals.

spot-film r. the making of localized instantaneous radiographic exposures during fluoroscopy.

radiohumeral (ˌraydioh'hyoomə·rəl) pertaining to the radius and humerus.

radioimmunity (ˌraydioh·i'myoonitee) diminished sensitivity to radiation.

radioimmunoassay (ˌraydiohˌimyuhnoh'asay) a sensitive assay method that can be used for the measurement of minute quantities of specific antibodies or any antigen, such as a hormone or drug, against which specific antibodies can be raised. An assay for a specific hormone uses antihormone antibody produced by injecting the human hormone into an animal, such as a rabbit, and hormone that has been labelled with a radioisotope. These are mixed with the assay specimen and the antigen (hormone) bound to antibody is separated from the unbound antigen by chromatography or other means. Because any hormone in the assay specimen competes with the radiolabelled hormone for antibody binding sites, the amount of hormone in the specimen is inversely proportional to the radioactivity of the bound fraction or directly proportional to the activity of the free fraction.

In 1977, Rosalyn S. Yalow was one of the recipients of the Nobel Prize for Physiology or Medicine, for her work in endocrinology and development of the radioimmunoassay technique. This technique has greatly facilitated research in endocrinology, pharmacology, and many other branches of medicine. It is the standard method for clinical laboratory measurements of hormones and is also used for therapeutic drug monitoring, drug abuse screening, and other laboratory tests. Abbreviated RIA.

radioimmunodiffusion (ˌraydiohˌimyuhnohdi'fyoozhən) immunodiffusion conducted with radioisotope-labelled antibodies or antigens.

radioimmunoelectrophoresis (ˌraydiohˌimyuhnoh·iˌlektrohfə'reesis) electrophoresis in which any layer of precipitate is identified by adding the corresponding radioactive-labelled antigen or antibody and subjecting it to autoradiography.

radioimmunosorbent (ˌraydiohˌimyuhnoh'sawbənt, -'zaw-) denoting a radioimmunoassay technique for measuring IgE in samples of serum.

radioiodine (ˌraydioh'ieəˌdeen) any radioactive isotope of IODINE.

radioisotope (ˌraydioh'iesəˌtohp) a radioactive form of an element. A radioisotope consists of unstable atoms that undergo radioactive decay emitting alpha, beta, or gamma radiation. Radioisotopes occur naturally, as in the cases of radium and uranium, or may be created artificially.

Scientists create artificial radioisotopes by bombarding stable atoms of an element with subatomic particles in a nuclear reactor or in an atom smasher, or cyclotron. When the nucleus of a stable atom is charged by bombarding particles, the atom usually becomes unstable, or radioactive, and is said to be 'labelled' or 'tagged'.

radioligand (ˌraydioh'liegənd, -'li-) a radioisotope-labelled substance, e.g., an antigen, used in the quantitative measurement of an unlabelled substance by its binding reaction to a specific antibody or other receptor site.

radiologist (ˌraydi'oləjist) a doctor specializing in radiology.

radiology (ˌraydi'oləjee) the branch of medical science dealing with use of x-rays, radioactive substances, and other forms of radiant energy, and ultrasound, in diagnosis. adj. **radiological.**

radiolucent (ˌraydioh'loos'nt) permitting the passage of radiant energy, such as x-rays, yet offering some resistance to it, the representative areas appearing dark on the exposed film.

radiometer (ˌraydi'omitə) 1. an instrument for estimating x-ray quantity. 2. an instrument in which radiant heat and light may be directly converted into mechanical energy. 3. an instrument for measuring the penetrating power of radiant energy.

radiomimetic (ˌraydiohmi'metik) producing effects similar to those of ionizing radiations.

radionecrosis (ˌraydiohnə'krohsis) tissue destruction due to radiant energy.

radioneuritis (ˌraydiohnyuh'rietis) neuritis from exposure to radiant energy.

radionuclide (ˌraydioh'nyooklied) a radioactive nuclide; one that disintegrates with the emission of corpuscular or electromagnetic radiations.

radiopacity (ˌraydioh'pasitee) the quality or property of obstructing the passage of radiant energy, such as x-rays, the representative areas appearing light or white on the exposed film. adj. **radiopaque.**

radiopaque, radio-opaque (ˌraydioh'payk; ˌraydioh·oh'payk) capable of obstructing the passage of x-rays.

radiopathology (ˌraydiohpə'tholəjee) the pathology of radiation effects on tissues.

radiopharmaceutical (ˌraydiohˌfahmə'syootik'l) a radioactive pharmaceutical used for diagnostic or therapeutic purposes.

radiophosphorus (ˌraydioh'fosfə·rəs) a radioactive isotope of phosphorus, ^{32}P a pure beta emitter, has a half-life of 14.3 days and is used in solution or colloidal form in erythrocyte studies and in the treatment of polycythaemia vera and chronic leukaemia.

radiopotentiation (ˌraydiohpəˌtenshi'ayshən) the action of a drug in enhancing the effects of irradiation.

radioreceptor (ˌraydiohri'septə) a receptor for the stimuli that are excited by radiant energy, such as light and heat.

radioresistance (ˌraydiohri'zistəns) resisting the effects of radiation, especially in reference to the treatment of malignancy. adj. **radioresistant**.

radioresponsive (ˌraydiohri'sponsiv) reacting favourably to irradiation.

radioscopy (ˌraydi'oskəpee) fluoroscopy.

radiosensitivity (ˌraydioh,sensi'tivitee) sensitivity, as of the skin, tumour tissue, etc., to radiant energy, such as x-ray or other radiations. adj. **radiosensitive**.

radiotelemetry (ˌraydiohtə'lemətree) measurement based on data transmitted by radio waves from the subject to the recording apparatus.

radiotherapist (ˌraydioh'therəpist) a doctor specializing in radiotherapy.

radiotherapy (ˌraydioh'therəpee) the treatment of disease by ionizing radiation such as x-rays, beta rays and gamma rays; it is mainly used in malignant disease. The purpose of radiotherapy is to deliver an optimal dose of either particulate or electromagnetic radiation to a particular area of the body with minimal damage to normal tissues. The source of radiation may be outside the body of the patient (external radiotherapy) or it may be an isotope that has been implanted or instilled into abnormal tissue or a body cavity. Called also *radiation therapy*.

Because of improvements in tumour localization, beam direction, planning and prescribing the field to be irradiated, and determining the precise dosage needed, radiotherapy is far more effective and less harmful now than when it was first introduced.

External Radiotherapy. Modern radiotherapy primarily uses high-energy x-rays or gamma rays with peak photon energies above 1 MeV. This is called 'supervoltage' or 'megavoltage' therapy. These high voltages are produced by linear accelerators or by cobalt-60 teletherapy units. Megavoltage radiation is more penetrating than lower energy radiation. It produces less damage to the skin at the entry port, is absorbed less in bone, and is scattered less, thus reducing the exposure to tissues outside the x-ray beam. Low-energy x-rays that do not penetrate are used for treatment of superficial skin lesions.

Internal Radiotherapy. This can involve the implantation of sealed radiation sources in or near cancerous tissue. Isotopes, such as radium-226, caesium-137, iridium-192, and iodine-125, are introduced either temporarily or permanently into body tissues (interstitial application) or body cavities (intercavitary application). Permanent sources have a short half-life so that the dose received by the patient is limited.

Another form of internal radiotherapy is the administration of radioactive materials into the bloodstream or a body cavity. Iodine-131 is given orally in certain cases of hyperthyroidism and cancer of the thyroid; it is absorbed by the digestive system and concentrated in the thyroid. Phosphorus-32, a pure beta emitter, is injected intravenously for the treatment of various myeloproliferative diseases, leukaemias, and lymphomas. Colloidal suspensions of radioisotopes, such as gold-198 and phosphorus-32, are administered by instillation into body cavities for the palliative treatment of malignant effusions.

Precautions. Hospital personnel concerned with the care of patients receiving radiotherapy must be aware of the hazards of radiation and the protective policies and procedures established to reduce these hazards. Since radiation cannot be seen or felt, it is extremely important to observe all such rules.

Sources of radiation that may be of particular concern to health care personnel include: radioactive substances such as radium and cobalt-60 that are used as implants and serve as internal sources of radiation; external sources of radiation such as x-ray machines and cobalt-60 therapy units; and liquid radioisotopes such as iodine-131 and suspensions of radioactive gold or phosphorus.

Generally speaking, the degree of exposure to radiation depends on three factors: (1) the distance between the source of radiation and the individual, (2) the amount of time an individual is exposed to radiation, and (3) the type of shielding provided. See also RADIATION.

When a therapist must remain with a patient while he receives diagnostic or therapeutic x-rays, the therapist should wear a lead apron and lead gloves. The therapist must be aware of, and observe carefully, the policies and procedures established for personnel in and around x-ray rooms and the rooms that house teletherapy units. After the treatment is finished the patient will not serve as a source of radiation.

Internal implants can present certain hazards to those involved in bedside care of patients receiving this type of radiation therapy. The hospital staff should be instructed in the amount of time it is safe to remain close to the patient.

Another factor to be considered is accidental removal or dislodgement of a radioactive implant. Most patients are confined to bed and refused bathroom privileges, but it is still possible for a radium needle or radon seeds, for example, to be accidentally removed from the body. Should an implant become dislodged the radiologist must be notified immediately. Under no circumstances should a radioactive substance be handled with the bare hands. A lead container and long-handled forceps should be kept at the patient's bedside in the event of an implant becoming dislodged. It can then be picked up immediately and placed in the container. Dressings, bed linen, bedpans, and emesis basins should be checked with a radiation detection instrument after each use or before disposal.

Liquid radioactive substances require additional precautions since these substances can enter the body of a worker through the skin, or by ingestion or inhalation. Not all types of radioactive materials require the same precautions. For example, iodine-131 is excreted in the urine for several days after it has been administered to the patient. In addition it appears in the patient's sweat, tears and saliva; thus all articles such as bed linens and toothbrush used by the patient must be considered a possible radiation hazard. Phosphorus-32 acts in the same way. Colloidal gold-98 usually is instilled into a body cavity and is not absorbed as are iodine and phosphorus. However, the radioactive gold emits gamma rays that penetrate beyond the patient's body and present a radiation hazard.

It is essential that the patient receives a full explanation of the need for all these precautions prior to the insertion of radioactive material. Staff must ensure that they spend adequate time with the patient within the limits set by policy guidelines.

Patient Care. The two major goals of care of a patient receiving external radiotherapy are: (1) maintaining integrity of the skin and mucous membranes over the area exposed to radiation, and (2) symptomatic relief of systemic side-effects. The skin should be protected according to established procedure; topical application of alcohol, lotions, and salves are prohibited during the course of treatment, unless specifically ordered by the radiologist. Systemic reactions to radiation include anorexia, nausea, vomiting, diarrhoea, and frequency and urgency of urination. These symptoms usually abate once the series of radiation treatments is completed.

Care of the skin is of particular importance when a

patient is receiving radiation from x-ray or teletherapy unit. Before the series of treatments is begun, the skin is washed with soap and water to remove all traces of ointments or lotions from the skin. Powders, ointments, and other applications containing metals such as zinc absorb x-rays and increase damage to the skin.

Once the treatments are begun, the areas marked as 'ports' or areas of entry for radiation are washed gently using warm water and pure soap. Alcohol, lotions, ointments and talcum powder should not be used. These ports of entry are extremely sensitive and subject to breakdown as would be a minor burn. It is important to avoid any friction or pressure on the area. No medications, lotions, or powders should be applied to the area.

Local reactions to radiation from internal sources include irritation of mucous membranes lining the mouth, pharynx, vagina, or bladder. The affected area becomes inflamed and tender. If the irritation continues, a greyish white membrane may form over the area. Bleeding also may occur as the underlying tissues become irritated.

In most cases the oral and pharyngeal mucosa heals rapidly once the radiation is discontinued. During radiotherapy frequent mouth washes, good oral hygiene, and soothing gargles may help to eliminate the distressing symptoms.

If the vaginal mucosa is irritated, the doctor may order douches to cleanse the area and promote healing. Because the area is easily irritated, douching must be done with extreme gentleness. The occurrence of bleeding is usually a contraindication to douching and should be reported to the doctor.

Irritation of the bladder mucosa may result in difficulty in voiding and painful urination. This should be reported so that urinary antiseptics may be ordered to relieve the symptoms and reduce the danger of infection.

Diarrhoea, constipation, or blood in the stool indicates irritation of the bowel mucosa in patients receiving radiotherapy for conditions of the lower abdomen or pelvis. An oil retention enema or analgesic suppository may be ordered to relieve the irritation.

The distressing side-effects of radiotherapy may be aggravated by the patient's mental attitude toward this type of treatment. It is often helpful to allow the patient and his family to discuss their feelings and express their anxieties about radiation. They should be given a simple explanation of the purpose of the treatment and helped to understand that the discomforts associated with radiotherapy are not indicative of a lack of success or an unusual reaction to radiotherapy.

radiothermy (ˌraydioh'thərmee) short-wave diathermy.

radiotoxaemia (ˌraydiohtok'seemi·ə) toxaemia produced by a radioactive substance, or resulting from radiotherapy.

radiotracer (ˌraydioh'traysə) a radioactive tracer.

radiotransparent (ˌraydiohtrans'parənt, -trahn-) permitting the passage of x-rays or other forms of radiation.

radiotropic (ˌraydioh'tropik) influenced by radiation.

radioulnar (ˌraydioh'ulnə) pertaining to the radius and ulna.

radium ('raydi·əm) a chemical element, atomic number 88, atomic weight, 226, symbol Ra. (See table of elements in Appendix 2.) Radium is highly radioactive and is found in uranium minerals. Radium-226 has a half-life of 1622 years. It and its short-lived decay products emit alpha particles, beta particles, and gamma rays. One of the decay products, radon-222, is a radioactive gas. In clinical use, radium is contained in a metal container that stops alpha and beta particles and traps radon.

Radium is used in the treatment of malignant diseases, particularly those that are readily accessible, for example, tumours of the cervix uteri, mouth, or tongue. In the form of needles or pellets, it can be inserted in the tumorous tissue (interstitial implantation) and left in place until its rays penetrate and destroy malignant cells. It can also be used in the form of plaques applied to the diseased tissue. Large amounts of radium are used as a source of GAMMA RAYS, which are capable of deep penetration of matter. Radium rays have been used in the treatment of lupus, eczema, psoriasis, xanthoma, mycosis fungoides, and other skin diseases; for the removal of papillomas, granulomas, and naevi; for palliative treatment in carcinoma and sarcoma; and in myelogenous and lymphatic leukaemia. See also RADIATION THERAPY.

radius ('raydi·əs) pl. *radii* [L.] 1. a line radiating from a centre, or a circular limit defined by a fixed distance from an established point or centre. 2. in anatomy, the bone on the outer or thumb side of the forearm.

radix ('raydiks) pl. *radices* [L.] root.

radon ('raydon) a chemical element, atomic number 86, atomic weight 222, symbol Rn. (See table of elements in Appendix 2.) Radon is a colourless, gaseous, radioactive element produced by the disintegration of radium.

rage (rayj) a state of violent anger.

sham r. an outburst of motor activity resembling the outward manifestations of fear and anger, occurring in decorticated animals and in certain pathological conditions in man.

ragocyte ('ragohˌsiet) a cell found in the joints in rheumatoid arthritis. Such cells are produced when polymorphonuclear leukocytes ingest aggregated IgG immunoglobulin, rheumatoid factor, fibrin, and complement.

rale (rahl) an abnormal respiratory sound heard in auscultation and indicating some pathological condition. Rales are distinguished as *dry* or *moist*, according to the absence or presence of fluid in the air passages, and are classified according to their site of origin as *bronchial*, *cavernous*, *laryngeal*, *pleural*, *tracheal*, and *vesicular* (*crepitant*).

amphoric r. a coarse, musical, and tinkling rale due to the splashing of fluid in a cavity connected with a bronchus.

atelectatic r. a nonpathological rale which is dissipated by deep breathing or coughing. Such rales are frequently heard in those who breathe feebly and superficially, when on deep inspiration the moist walls of the unexpanded alveoli are suddenly forced apart by the entering air; after a few deep inspirations such rales become lost.

bubbling r. a moist rale, finer than a subcrepitant rale, heard in bronchitis, in the resolving stage of croupous pneumonia, and over small cavities.

cavernous r. a hollow and metallic rale caused by the alternate expansion and contraction of a pulmonary cavity during respiration.

cellophane r. a dry, crackling chest sound, as heard in interstitial pulmonary fibrosis.

clicking r. a small sticky sound heard on inspiration, due to the passage of air through secretions in the smaller bronchi.

collapse r. a fine crepitant rale heard over collapsed lung tissue, also at the base of the healthy lung of a bedridden patient, due to incomplete expansion of the air vesicles.

consonating r. a clear, ringing sound produced in

bronchial tubes that are surrounded by consolidation tissue.

crepitant r. a very fine rale, resembling the sound produced by rubbing a lock of hair between the fingers or by particles of salt thrown on fire; heard at the end of inspiration.

dry r. a rale produced by the presence of viscid secretion in the bronchial tubes, or by spastic contraction of the walls of the tubes; it has a whistling, musical, or squeaking quality.

gurgling r. a very coarse rale resembling the bursting of large bubbles; in pulmonary oedema, heard over large cavities that contain fluid, and in the trachea in the 'death rattle'.

sibilant r. a hissing sound resembling that produced by suddenly separating two oiled surfaces. It is produced by the presence of a viscid secretion in the bronchial tubes or by thickening of the walls of the tubes; heard in asthma and bronchitis.

subcrepitant r. a fine, moist rale associated with fluid in the bronchioles.

ramal ('raymәl) pertaining to a ramus.

RAMC Royal Army Medical Corps.

rami ('raymie) [L.] plural of *ramus*.

ramification (ˌramifi'kayshәn) 1. distribution in branches. 2. a branch or set of branches.

ramify ('ramifie) 1. to branch; to diverge in different directions. 2. to traverse in branches.

ramisection (ˌrami'sekshәn) section of the appropriate rami communicantes of the sympathetic nervous system.

ramitis (ra'mietis) inflammation of a ramus.

ramose ('raymohz) branching; having many branches.

Ramsay Hunt syndrome (ˌramzi 'hunt) facial paralysis accompanied by otalgia and a vesicular eruption involving the external canal of the ear, sometimes extending to the auricle, due to herpes zoster virus infection of the geniculate ganglion.

Ramstedt's operation ('ramshtets) operation for congenital stricture of the pylorus in which the fibres of the sphincter muscle are divided leaving the mucous lining intact.

ramulus ('ramyuhlәs) pl. *ramuli* [L.] a small branch or terminal division.

ramus ('raymәs) pl. *rami* [L.] a branch, as of a nerve, vein, or artery.

r. communicans pl. *rami communicantes;* a branch connecting two nerves or two arteries.

rancid ('ransid) having a musty, rank taste or smell; applied to fats that have undergone decomposition, with the liberation of fatty acids.

random ('randәm) events influenced only by chance.

r. sample a method of sampling which ensures that each person or unit in the population has an equal chance of selection into the sample.

randomized controlled trial ('randәmˌiezd kәn-'trohld trie·әl) an epidemiological study in which the participants are randomly allocated to treatment and control groups.

range (raynj) the difference between the upper and lower limits of a variable or of a series of values.

r. of accommodation the alteration in the refractive state of the eye produced by accommodation. It is the difference in diopters between the refraction by the eye adjusted for its far point and that when adjusted for its near point. Called also amplitude of accommodation.

r. of audibility the range between the extreme frequencies of sound waves beyond which the human ear perceives no sound: lower limit, 16 to 20 cycles per second; upper limit, 18,000 to 20,000 cycles per second.

r. of movement the range, measured in degrees of a circle, through which a joint can be extended and flexed. See also range of movement EXERCISES.

ranine ('raynien) pertaining to (a) a frog; (b) a ranula, or to the lower surface of the tongue; (c) the sublingual vein.

ranitidine (ra'nitideen) an H_2 receptor antagonist, used in the treatment of gastric and duodenal ulcers.

ranula ('ranyuhlә) a cystic tumour beneath the tongue due to obstruction and dilation of the sublingual or submaxillary gland or of a mucous gland. adj. **ranular**.

pancreatic r. a retention cyst of the pancreatic duct.

Ranvier's node ('ronhviˌayz) see NODE.

rape (rayp) sexual assault or abuse; criminal forcible sexual intercourse (i.e., penetration) without the consent of the adult or child, either forcibly or by intimidation or deception as to the nature of the act. Many cases are not reported because of feelings of shame, guilt, embarrassment, or fear.

Although rape or sexual assault can occur between men (homosexual rape), it is usually associated with victims who are women.

If the woman refuses to seek medical, legal, or psychological help, she has a right to make such a choice, but she should be encouraged to consult a doctor as soon as possible. If she decides to report the crime, she is advised not to change clothes, bathe, douche, or urinate because she may destroy legal evidence needed to arrest and convict her attacker.

The physical examination of the woman has a two-fold purpose: (1) to protect her against disease, pregnancy, and psychological trauma, and (2) to aid in the collection of legal evidence that could be used later in court.

Many organizations now have on call a sympathetic and knowledgeable person who can stay with the victim through emergency treatment and provide guidance and referral for a follow-up programme of care. Rape is a crime of violence in which the sexual act is secondary to the brutality of the attack.

raphe ('rayfee) a seam; used in anatomic nomenclature as a general term to designate the line of union of the halves of various symmetrical parts.

abdominal r. linea alba.

Rappaport classification ('rapәpor) see LYMPHOMA.

rapport (ra'por) a relation of harmony and accord, as between patient and doctor.

rarefaction (ˌrair·ri'fakshәn) the condition of being or becoming less dense.

rash (rash) a temporary eruption on the skin.

butterfly r. a skin eruption across the nose and adjacent areas of the cheeks in the pattern of a butterfly, as in lupus erythematosus and seborrhoeic dermatitis.

nappy r. a cutaneous reaction in an infant, localized in areas ordinarily covered by, and in contact with, the nappy, and sparing the folds of skin. It is due to various primary irritants, such as ammonia in decomposed urine, with histopathological changes varying with the causative factor; improperly washed nappies and other contact factors may also be responsible for such irritation.

drug r. dermatitis medicamentosa.

heat r. miliaria.

nettle r. urticaria.

Rashkind catheter ('rashkint) a balloon catheter used to increase the size of the atrial septal defect in children who have transposition of the great vessels.

raspatory ('raspәtә·ree) an instrument used to scrape the periosteum from bone.

raspberry mark (rahzbәree, razbree) congenital haemangioma.

RAST radioallergosorbent test.

Rastelli's operation (ra'steliz) surgical procedure used in the treatment of transposition of the great vessels. The circulation of blood through the heart is diverted to effect adequate oxygenation.

Rastinon ('rastinon) trademark for a preparation of tolbutamide, an oral hypoglycaemic agent.

ratbite fever ('ratbiet) either of two distinct rare diseases (Haverhill fever, caused by *Streptobacillus moniliformis*, and sodoku, caused by *Spirillum minus*) that may be transmitted to man by the bite of an infected rat (and less commonly by the bite of an infected squirrel, weasel, dog, cat, or pig).

The organisms are commensals in the nasopharynx of the rat and are also excreted in the urine. Milkborne and waterborne outbreaks have been described, due to contamination by rats (the epidemic at Haverhill, USA, was considered to be milkborne).

Treatment for both forms is with penicillin, streptomycin, or other antibiotics.

rate (rayt) the speed or frequency with which an event or circumstance occurs per unit of time, population, or other standard of comparison.

attack r. the rate at which new cases of a specific disease occur. Usually refers to disease in a population in a short period of time, such as in an outbreak of infectious disease.

basal metabolic r. an expression of the rate at which oxygen is utilized in a fasting subject at complete rest as a percentage of a value established as normal for such a subject. Abbreviated BMR.

birth r. the number of live births in a population in a specified period of time (crude birth rate), for the female population (refined birth rate), or for the female population of childbearing age (true birth rate), usually expressed per year per 1000 of the estimated mid-yearspopulation.

case r. the number of cases of a specific disease occurring in a year, expressed as a proportion of a particular population. Called also *morbidity rate*.

case fatality r. the number of deaths due to a specific disease expressed as a proportion of the total number of cases of the disease in the same period of time. Usually given as a percentage.

death r. the number of deaths per stated number of persons (1000 or 10,000 or 100,000) in a certain region in a certain time period (crude death rate). The death rate calculated with allowances made for age and sex distribution in the population is termed the *standardized death rate*. Called also *mortality rate*.

dose r. the amount of any therapeutic agent administered per unit of time.

erythrocyte sedimentation r. an expression of the extent of settling of erythrocytes in a vertical column of blood per unit of time (see also SEDIMENTATION RATE).

forced expiratory flow r. (FEF) see maximal expiratory flow rate and maximal midexpiratory flow rate.

glomerular filtration r. an expression of the quantity of glomerular filtrate formed each minute in the nephrons of both kidneys, calculated by measuring the clearance of specific substances, e.g., inulin or creatinine.

growth r. an expression of the increase in size of an organic object per unit of time.

heart r. the number of contractions of the cardiac ventricles per unit of time.

maximal expiratory flow r. (MEFR) the slope of the line connecting the points 200 ml and 1200 ml on the forced expiratory volume curve (see also PULMONARY FUNCTION TESTS). Called also $FEF_{200\text{-}1200}$.

maximal mid-expiratory flow r. (MMFR, MMF) the slope of the line connecting the points on the forced expiratory volume curve at 25 and 75 per cent of the forced vital capacity (see also PULMONARY FUNCTION TESTS). Called also $FEF_{25\text{-}75\%}$.

metabolic r. an expression of the amount of oxygen consumed by the body cells.

morbidity r. case rate.

mortality r. death rate.

pulse r. the number of pulsations noted in a peripheral artery per unit of time; normally between 60 and 80 per minute in an adult.

respiration r. the number of movements of the chest wall per unit of time, indicative of inspiration and expiration; normally 16 to 20 per minute in an adult.

sedimentation r. the rate at which a sediment is deposited in a given volume of solution, especially when subjected to the action of a centrifuge. See also SEDIMENTATION RATE.

survival r. an expression of the number of survivors with no trace of disease a given number of years after each has been diagnosed or treated for the same disease.

Rathke's pouch ('rathkayz powch) a diverticulum from the embryonic buccal cavity from which the anterior pituitary is developed.

ratio ('rayshioh) [L.] an expression of the quantity of one substance or entity in relation to that of another; the relationship between two quantities expressed as the quotient of one divided by the other.

A–G r., albumin–globulin r. the ratio of albumin to globulin in blood serum, plasma, cerebrospinal fluid, or urine.

arm r. a figure expressing the relation of the length of the longer arm (chromatid) of a mitotic chromosome to that of the shorter arm.

cardiothoracic r. the ratio of the transverse diameter of the heart to the internal diameter of the chest at its widest point just above the dome of the diaphragm.

lecithin–sphingomyelin r. the ratio of lecithin to sphingomyelin in amniotic fluid (see also LECITHIN–SPHINGOMYELIN RATIO). **sex r.** the number of males in a population per number of females, usually stated as the number of males per 100 females.

urea excretion r. the ratio of the amount of urea in the urine excreted in one hour to the amount in 100 ml of blood. The normal ratio is 50.

rational ('rashən'l) based upon reason; characterized by possession of one's reason.

rationalization (ˌrashənəlie'zayshən) an unconscious defence mechanism in which a person finds logical reasons (justification) for his behaviour while ignoring the real reasons. It is a form of self-deception unconsciously employed to make tolerable certain feelings, behaviour, and motives that would otherwise be intolerable. Everyone employs rationalization at some time or other and in most instances it is a relatively harmless behaviour pattern; the danger lies in deceiving oneself habitually so that eventually harmful or destructive behaviour can be justified in one's mind.

rauwolfia (raw'wuhlfi·ə, row-) any member of the genus *Rauwolfia*; the dried root, or extract of the dried root, of *Rauwolfia*.

r. serpentina the dried root of *Rauwolfia serpentina*, sometimes with fragments of rhizome and other parts, used as an antihypertensive and sedative.

RAWP Resource Allocation Working Party.

ray (ray) a line emanating from a centre, as a more or less distinct portion of radiant energy (light or heat), proceeding in a specific direction.

alpha r's, α-r's high-speed helium nuclei ejected from radioactive substances; they have less penetrating power than beta rays. See also ALPHA PARTICLES.

beta r's, β-r's electrons ejected from radioactive substances with velocities as high as 0.98 of the velocity of light; they have more penetrating power than alpha rays, but less than gamma rays. See also BETA PARTICLES.
cosmic r's very penetrating radiations that apparently move through interplanetary space in every direction.
digital r. a digit of the hand or foot and corresponding metacarpal or metatarsal bone, regarded as a continuous unit.
gamma r's, γ-r's electromagnetic radiation of short wavelengths emitted by an atomic nucleus during a nuclear reaction, consisting of high energy photons, having no mass and no electric charge, and travelling with the speed of light and with great penetrating power. See also GAMMA RAYS.
grenz r's very soft electromagnetic radiation of wavelengths of about 0.2 nm.
infrared r's radiations just beyond the red end of the spectrum, having wavelengths of 0.75–1000 μm (see also INFRARED RAYS).
medullary r. a cortical extension of a bundle of tubules from a renal pyramid.
roentgen r's x-rays.
ultraviolet r's radiant energy beyond the violet end of the visible spectrum, of 0.39 to 0.18 μm wavelength (see also ULTRAVIOLET RAYS).
x-r's electromagnetic radiation of wavelengths ranging between 5.0×10^{-6} and 5.0×10^{-4} μm (including grenz rays). See also X-RAYS.

Raynaud's phenomenon (disease) ('raynohz) Raynaud's phenomenon is characterized by episodic digital ischaemia provoked by stimuli such as emotion, cold, trauma, hormones and drugs. Raynaud's phenomenon includes both Raynaud's disease, where no underlying cause can be found, and Raynaud's syndrome, where there is an associated underlying disorder. These disorders include scleroderma, mixed connective tissue disease, systemic lupus erythematosus (SLE), polymyositis, rheumatoid arthritis, neurovascular entrapment syndromes, occlusive arterial disease and certain drugs.

Clinically, a classic attack of Raynaud's is manifested by pallor of the affected digit followed by cyanosis and then redness; these changes reflect arterial ischaemia, venostasis and reactive hyperaemia, respectively. However, they do not always all occur and in addition the changes may be accompanied by pain and/or numbness. Women are affected nine times more commonly than men.

Treatment tends to be derived from a logical extension of the accepted theories of the phenomenon and is used on a 'try and see' basis.

Much can be done for patients with mild disease without the need for drugs. Advice on keeping warm by the use of thermal underwear, charcoal handwarmers and electrically heated gloves and socks can produce immediate symptomatic benefits, as can stopping smoking, change of occupation, avoidance of mental stress and withdrawal of drugs such as beta blockers which aggravate the response.

There is a profusion of drugs for the treatment of Raynaud's, including vasodilators, prostaglandins and calcium channel blockers. Patients vary in their response to these, Sympathectomy has a very limited place in treatment today.

For futher information about Raynaud's contact The Raynaud's Association, 112 Crewe Road, Alsager, Cheshire ST7 2JA. Telephone (0270) 872776.

razoxane (rə'zoksayn) an antineoplastic agent.

Razoxin (rə'zoksin) trademark for preparations of razoxane, an antineoplastic agent.

Rb chemical symbol, *rubidium*.

RBC red blood cells; red blood (cell) count (see BLOOD COUNT).

RBE relative biological effectiveness; effectiveness of other types of radiation compared with that of one roentgen of gamma rays or x-rays. See also REM.

RCGP Royal College of General Practitioners.

RCM Royal College of Midwives.

RCN Rcn,Royal College of Nursing.

RCR Royal College of Radiologists.

RCT Registered Clinical Teacher.

RDS respiratory distress syndrome (infants).

Re chemical symbol, *rhenium*.

reabsorb (ˌreeəb'sawb, -'zawb) to absorb again; to undergo or to subject to reabsorption; to resorb.

reabsorption (ˌreeəb'sawpshən, -'zaw-) 1. the act or process of absorbing again, as the absorption by the kidneys of substances (glucose, proteins, sodium, etc.) already secreted into the renal tubules. 2. resorption.

react (ri'akt) 1. to respond to a stimulus. 2. to enter into chemical action.

reaction (ri'akshən) 1. opposite action or counteraction; the response of a part to stimulation. 2. the phenomena caused by the action of chemical agents; a chemical process in which one substance is transformed into another substance or substances. 3. in psychology, the mental or emotional state that develops in any particular situation. For specific reactions, see under the specific name, as PIRQUET'S REACTION.
adjustment r. one elicited by a change in situation or environment, sometimes evidenced as a transient personality disorder.
alarm r. all of the nonspecific phenomena elicited by exposure to stimuli affecting large portions of the body and to which the organism is not adapted; rapid involution of lymphoid tissues due to hormonal action is a striking manifestation (see also ALARM REACTION).
allergic r. a local or general reaction characterized by altered reactivity of the animal body to an antigenic substance (see also ALLERGY).
antigen–antibody r. the specific combination of antigen with homologous antibody resulting in the reversible formation of antigen–antibody complexes that differ in solubility according to the antigen–antibody ratio (see also ANTIGEN).
anxiety r. a neurotic reaction characterized by abnormal apprehension or uneasiness.
Arthus r. see ARTHUS REACTION.
biuret r. see BIURET.
catastrophic r. emotional overreaction associated with failure to perform some simple task and almost always confined to brain damaged or brain failed patients.
chain r. one that is self-propagating; a chemical process in which each time a free radical is destroyed a new one is formed.
conversion r. a condition in which motor or sensory symptoms are used to symbolize intrapsychic conflict (see also CONVERSION REACTION).
cross r. interaction between an antibody and an antigen that is closely related to the one which specifically stimulated synthesis of the antibody.
defence r. a mental reaction that shuts out from consciousness ideas not acceptable to the ego.
r. of degeneration the reaction to electrical stimulation of muscles whose nerves have degenerated, consisting of loss of response to a faradic stimulation in a muscle, and to galvanic and faradic stimulation in the nerve.
delayed r. a reaction, such as an allergic reaction, occurring hours to days after exposure to an inducer.
dissociative r. a neurotic reaction in which such dissociated behaviour as amnesia, fugues, somnambul-

ism, and dream states occur.

false negative r. an erroneously negative reaction to a test.

false positive r. an erroneously positive reaction to a test.

gross stress r. an acute emotional reaction to severe environmental stress.

hemianopic pupillary r. in certain cases of hemianopia, light thrown upon one side of the retina causes the iris to contract, while light thrown upon the other side arouses no response.

immune r. 1. immune response. See IMMUNITY and IMMUNE RESPONSE. 2. formation of a papule and areola without development of a vesicle following smallpox vaccination.

Jones-Mote r. a mild skin reaction of the delayed hypersensitivity type occurring after challenge with protein antigens.

lengthening r. reflex elongation of extensor muscles that permits flexion of a limb.

leukaemic r., leukaemoid r. a peripheral blood picture resembling leukaemia or indistinguishable from it on the basis of morphological appearance alone, characterized by immature leukocytes in the blood.

ophthalmic r. ophthalmoreaction.

Prausnitz–Küstner r. a local hypersensitivity reaction induced by intradermal injection into a normal person of serum from a hypersensitive individual; injection 24 hours later of the antigen to which the donor is allergic results in a wheal-and-flare response.

precipitin r. a reaction involving the specific serological precipitation of an antigen in solution with its specific antiserum in the presence of electrolytes. The reaction is used in the typing of pneumococcus strains, in testing whether blood is human or animal, and for diagnostic purposes.

startle r. the various psychophysiological phenomena, including involuntary motor and autonomic reactions, evidenced by an individual in reaction to a sudden, unexpected stimulus, as a loud noise. Called the Moro reflex in the neonate.

Stella-Arias r. nuclear and cellular hypertrophy of the endometrial epithelium associated with ectopic pregnancy.

stress r. 1. alarm reaction. 2. gross stress reaction.

r. time the time elapsing between the application of a stimulus and the resulting reaction.

transfusion r. a group of symptoms due to agglutination of the recipient's blood cells when blood for transfusion is incorrectly matched, or when the recipient has a hypersensitivity to some element of the donor blood (see also TRANSFUSION).

Wassermann r. a test for syphilis based upon fixation of complement, now largely replaced by the TREPONEMAL IMMOBILIZATION TEST.

wheal-flare r. a cutaneous sensitivity reaction to skin injury or administration of antigen, due to histamine production and marked by oedematous elevation and erythematous flare.

reaction-formation (ri,akshənfaw'mayshən) a psychic mechanism by which a person unconsciously assumes an attitude which is the reverse of, and a substitute for, a repressed antisocial impulse.

reactivity (,reeak'tivitee) the process or property of reacting.

reading ('reeding) understanding of written or printed symbols representing words.

lip r., speech r. understanding of speech through observation of the speaker's lip movements.

reagent (ri'ayjənt) a substance used to produce a chemical reaction so as to detect, measure, produce, etc., other substances.

reagin ('reeəjin) 1. antibody of a specialized immunoglobulin class (IgE) which attaches to tissue cells of the same species from which it is derived, and which interacts with its antigen to induce the release of histamine and other vasoactive amines. A form of cytotrophic antibody, it is present in the serum of naturally hypersensitive individuals and can confer specific immediate hypersensitivity in nonreactive individuals. 2. a complement-fixing antibody interacting with cardiolipin in the Wassermann reaction. adj. **reaginic.**

atopic r. the antibody responsible for hypersensitivity reactions to specific substances with manifestations such as asthma and eczema.

reality orientation (ri'alitee) a technique employed to rehabilitate those suffering from a moderate to severe degree of disorientation.

reality testing the ability to objectively evaluate the external world and differentiate between it and the ego or self. Impaired reality testing is seen in psychological defence mechanisms that falsify reality, such as projection and denial.

reamer ('reemə) an instrument for enlarging root canals in dentistry.

recall (ri'kawl, 'reekawl) 1. to remember or recollect. 2. the process of bringing a memory into consciousness.

recapitulation theory (,reekə,pityuh'layshən) ontogeny recapitulates phylogeny, i.e., an organism, in the course of its development, goes through the same successive stages (in abbreviated form) as did the species in its evolutionary development.

receptaculum (,reesep'takyuhləm) pl. *receptacula* [L.] a vessel or receptable.

r. chyli cisterna chyli.

receptor (ri'septə) 1. a molecule on the surface or within a cell that recognizes and binds with specific molecules, producing some effect in the cell; e.g., the cell-surface receptors of immunocompetent cells that recognize antigens, complement components, or lymphokines, or those of neurons and target organs that recognize neurotransmitters or hormones. 2. a sensory nerve ending that responds to various stimuli.

adrenergic r's receptors for adrenaline or noradrenaline, such as those on effector organs innervated by postganglionic adrenergic fibres of the sympathetic nervous system. Classified as α-adrenergic receptors, which are stimulated by noradrenaline, and β-adrenergic receptors, which are stimulated by adrenaline. See also ADRENERGIC RECEPTORS.

cholinergic r's receptor sites on effector organs innervated by cholinergic nerve fibres and which respond to the acetylcholine secreted by these fibres. There are two types: MUSCARINIC RECEPTORS and NICOTINIC RECEPTORS.

complement r. a cell-surface receptor structure capable of binding activated complement components. For example, component C3b is bound to neutrophils, B-lymphocytes, and macrophages.

histamine r's receptors for histamine, classified as *H_1-receptors,* which produce bronchoconstriction and contraction of the gut and are blocked by antihistamines, such as mepyramine or chlorpheniramine, and *H_2-receptors,* which produce gastric acid secretion and are blocked by H_2-receptor blockers, such as cimetidine.

recess (ri'ses) a small, empty space or cavity.

recessive (ri'sesiv) tending to recede; in genetics, incapable of expression unless the responsible allele is carried by both members of a set of homologous chromosomes; a recessive allele or trait. **r. gene** one that produces an effect in the organism only when it is transmitted by both parents. See also HEREDITY.

recessus (ri'sesəs) pl. *recessus* [L.] a recess.
recidivation (ˌreesidi'vayshən) 1. the relapse or recurrence of a disease. 2. the repetition of an offence or crime.
recidivism (ri'sidiˌvizəm) a tendency to relapse, especially the tendency to return to a life of crime.
recidivist (ri'sidivist) a person who tends to relapse, especially one who tends to return to criminal habits after treatment or punishment.
recipe ('resipee) 1. [L.] *take;* used at the head of a prescription, indicated by the symbol ℞. 2. a formula for the preparation of a combination of ingredients.
recipient (ri'sipi·ənt) one who receives, as a blood transfusion, or a tissue or organ graft.
universal r. a person thought to be able to receive blood of any 'type' without agglutination of the donor cells.
Recklinghausen's disease ('rekling,howzənz) [Friedrich Daniel von *Recklinghausen*, German pathologist, 1833–1910] called also *von Recklinghausen's disease.* 1. neurofibromatosis. 2. see OSTEITIS FIBROSA CYSTICA.
recognin (ri'kognin) any of a group of protein fragments produced from cancer cells that are capable of recognizing specific cells; they include astrocytin and malignin.
recognition (ˌrekəg'nishən) 1. the act of recognizing or state of being recognized. 2. in immunology, a term used to describe the functional changes occurring in immunologically competent cells on contact with antigen, involving antigen binding with a receptor on the cell surface. Called also antigen recognition.
recombinant (ri'kombinənt) 1. the new cell or individual that results from genetic recombination. 2. pertaining or relating to such cells or individuals.
r. DNA technology the process of taking a gene from one organism and inserting it into the DNA of another; called also gene splicing. One commonly used technique involves the insertion of a new fragment of DNA that codes for a specific protein such as human insulin into a bacterium such as *Escherichia coli.* The gene is first inserted into a plasmid, a self-replicating ring of DNA involved in the transfer of genes between bacteria. The plasmid is cut at a specific site by using a special cutting enzyme called a *restriction endonuclease.* The same procedure is used to cut out a segment of DNA from another organism, for example, the gene for human insulin. This fragment of insulin DNA is inserted into the plasmid and then sealed into place by an annealing enzyme. The altered plasmid is then taken up by bacteria and incorporated into the genome. When the bacterial cells divide they pass on the new information to the next generation. This produces clones of bacteria that produce large quantities of the new protein, in this example, insulin.
The process of gene splicing has had great impact in the field of medicine. It has revolutionized the manufacture of pharmaceutical products, and within the decade the process may be used to manufacture hormones, vaccines, interferon, blood clotting factor VIII, enzymes, and a host of other proteins used in the treatment of disease.
recombination (ˌreekombi'nayshən) the reunion, in the same or different arrangement, of formerly united elements that have been separated; in genetics, the formation of new gene combinations due to crossing over by homologous chromosomes.
recompression (ˌreekəm'preshən) return to normal environmental pressure after exposure to greatly diminished pressure.
recon ('reekon) the smallest unit of genetic material capable of recombination.
reconstruction (ˌreekən'strukshən) to reassemble or re-form from constituent parts, such as the mathematical process by which an image is assembled from a series of projections in computed TOMOGRAPHY.
record ('rekawd) a permanent or long-lasting account of something (as on film, in writing, etc.); in dentistry, a registration.
recrement ('rekrimənt) saliva, or other secretion, that is reabsorbed into the blood. adj. **recrementitous**.
recrudescence (ˌreekroo'des'ns) recurrence of symptoms after temporary abatement; a recrudescence occurs after some days or weeks, a relapse after weeks or months. adj. **recrudescent**.
recruitment (ri'krootmənt) 1. the gradual increase to a maximum in a reflex when a stimulus of unaltered intensity is prolonged. 2. in audiology, an abnormal increase in loudness caused by a very slight increase in sound intensity, as in Menière's disease.
rect(o)- word element. [L.] *rectum;* see also words beginning *proct(o)-*.
rectal ('rekt'l) pertaining to the rectum.
rectalgia (rek'talji·ə) proctalgia; pain in the rectum.
rectectomy (rek'tektəmee) excision of the rectum.
rectification (ˌrektifi'kayshən) 1. the act of making straight, pure, or correct. 2. redistillation of a liquid to purify it. 3. the processing of an alternating electrical signal to make it unipolar.
rectified ('rektiˌfied) refined; made straight.
rectitis (rek'tietis) proctitis; inflammation of the rectum.
rectoabdominal (ˌrektoh·ab'domin'l) pertaining to the rectum and abdomen.
rectocele ('rektohˌseel) hernial protrusion of part of the rectum into the vagina.
rectocolitis (ˌrektohkə'lietis) coloproctitis; inflammation of the rectum and colon.
rectocutaneous (ˌrektohkyoo'tayni·əs) pertaining to the rectum and the skin.
rectolabial (ˌrektoh'laybi·əl) relating to the rectum and a labium majus.
rectoperineorrhaphy (ˌrektohˌperini'o·rəfee) the operation for repair of the perineum and rectal wall.
rectopexy ('rektohˌpeksee) fixation of the rectum; proctopexy.
rectoplasty ('rektohˌplastee) plastic operation to rectum and anus; proctoplasty.
rectoscope ('rektəˌskohp) proctoscope.
rectosigmoid (ˌrektoh'sigmoyd) the lower portion of the sigmoid colon and the upper portion of the rectum.
rectosigmoidectomy (ˌrektohˌsigmoy'dektəmee) removal of the rectum and sigmoid colon; proctosigmoidectomy.
rectostomy (rek'tostəmee) 1. a permanent opening into the rectum. 2. operation to achieve opening into the rectum.
rectourethral (ˌrektohyuh'reethrəl) pertaining to or communicating with the rectum and urethra.
rectouterine (ˌrektoh'yootəˌrien) pertaining to the rectum and uterus.
rectovaginal (ˌrektohvə'jien'l) pertaining to the rectum and vagina.
rectovesical (ˌrektoh'vesik'l) pertaining to or communicating with the rectum and bladder.
rectovestibular (ˌrektohve'stibyuhlə) pertaining to or communicating with the rectum and the vestibule of the vagina.
rectovulvar (ˌrektoh'vulvə) pertaining to or communicating with the rectum and vulva.
rectum ('rektəm) the distal portion of the large intestine, beginning anterior to the third sacral vertebra as a continuation of the sigmoid and ending

at the anal canal. The faeces, the solid waste products of digestion, are formed in the large intestine and are gradually pushed down into the rectum by the muscular action of the intestine. Distention of the rectum by the accumulating faeces sets up nerve impulses that indicate to the brain the need to empty the bowels.

The rectum is between 6 and 8 inches long, with the anal canal making up the last inch. The anus is kept closed—except during the evacuation process—by muscular rings, the anal sphincters.

In a rectal examination, the examiner palpates the rectum by inserting a gloved and lubricated finger into the rectum. The examination helps in determining whether there are masses in the rectum or pelvic region, and in determining the size and texture of the prostate in men. More extensive examination of the interior surface of the rectum may be done by proctoscopy.

rectus ('rektəs) [L.] *straight*.

recumbent (ri'kumbənt) lying down.

recuperation (ri,koopə'rayshən) recovery of health and strength.

recurrence (ri'kurəns) the return of symptoms after a remission.

recurrent (ri'kurənt) returning after a remission; reappearing.

r. fever relapsing fever.

recurvation (,reekər'vayshən) a backward bending or curvature.

red (red) 1. one of the primary colours, produced by the longest waves of the visible spectrum. 2. a red dye or stain.

r. blood cell erythrocyte.

Congo r. a dark red or brownish powder used as a diagnostic aid in amyloidosis.

phenol r. phenolsulphonphthalein.

scarlet r. an azo dye having some power to stimulate cell proliferation; once used to enhance wound healing.

vital r. a dye injected into the circulation to estimate blood volume by determining the concentration of the dye in the plasma.

redia ('reedi·ə) pl. *rediae* [L.] a larval stage of certain trematode parasites, which develops in the body of a snail host and gives rise to daughter rediae, or to the cercariae.

redintegration (re,dinti'grayshən) 1. the restoration or renewal of a lost or damaged part. 2. a psychic process in which part of a complex stimulus provokes the complete reaction that was previously made only to the complex stimulus as a whole. 3. restoration to a previous state or condition.

redox ('reedoks) oxidation-reduction.

reduce (ri'dyoos) 1. to restore to the normal place or relation of parts, as to reduce a fracture. 2. to undergo reduction. 3. to decrease in weight or size.

reducible (ri'dyoosəb'l) permitting of reduction.

reductant (ri'duktənt) the electron donor in an oxidation-reduction (redox) reaction.

reductase (ri'duktayz) an enzyme that catalyses a chemical reduction.

5α-r. an enzyme that catalyses the irreversible reduction of testosterone to dihydrotestosterone.

reduction (ri'dukshən) 1. the correction of a fracture, dislocation or hernia. 2. the addition of hydrogen to a substance, or more generally, the gain of electrons; the opposition of oxidation.

closed r. the manipulative reduction of a fracture without incision.

open r. reduction of a fracture after incision into the fracture site.

reduplication (ree,dyoopli'kayshən) 1. a doubling back. 2. the recurrence of paroxysms of a double type. 3. a developmental anomaly resulting in the doubling of an organ or part, with a connection between them at some point and the excess part usually a mirror image of the other.

reef (reef) 1. an infolding or tuck of tissue, as a tuck made in plication. 2. a double tie, the second being in line with the first.

reentry (ree'entree) in cardiology, a postulated mechanism by which a premature beat can be coupled to the normal beat.

refection (ri'fekshən) recovery; repair.

referred pain (ri,fərd 'payn) that which occurs at a distance from the place of origin due to the sensory nerves entering the cord at the same level, e.g. the phrenic nerve supplying the diaphragm enters the cord in the cervical region, as do the nerves from the shoulder, and so an abscess on the diaphragm may cause pain in the shoulder. Synalgia.

refine (ri'fien) to purify or free from foreign matter.

reflection (ri'flekshən) a turning or bending back, as the folds produced when a membrane passes over the surface of an organ and then passes back to the body wall that it lines.

reflector (ri'flektə) a device for reflecting light or sound waves.

reflex ('reefleks) a reflected action or movement; the sum total of any particular automatic response mediated by the nervous system.

A reflex is built into the nervous system and does not need the intervention of conscious thought to take effect.

The knee jerk is an example of the simplest type of reflex. When the knee is tapped, the nerve that receives this stimulus sends an impulse to the spinal cord, where it is relayed to a motor nerve. This causes the quadriceps muscle at the front of the thigh to contract and jerk the leg up. This reflex, or simple reflex arc, involves only two nerves and one synapse. The leg begins to jerk up while the brain is just becoming aware of the tap.

Other simple reflexes, the stretch reflexes, help the body maintain its balance. Every time a muscle is stretched, it reacts with a reflex impulse to contract. As a person reaches or leans, the skeletal muscles tense and tighten, tending to hold him and keep him from falling. Even in standing still, the stretch reflexes in the skeletal muscles make many tiny adjustments to keep the body erect.

The 'hot-stove' reflex is more complex, calling into play many different muscles. Before the hand is pulled away, an impulse must go from the sensory nerve endings in the skin to a centre in the spinal cord, from there to a motor centre, and then out along the motor nerves to shoulder, arm, and hand muscles. Trunk and leg muscles respond to support the body in its sudden change of position, and the head and eyes turn to look at the cause of the injury. All this happens while the person is becoming aware of the burning sensation. A reflex that protects the body from injury, as this one does, is called a nociceptive reflex. Sneezing, coughing, and gagging are similar reflexes in response to foreign bodies in the nose and throat, and the wink reflex helps protect the eyes from injury.

A conditioned reflex is one acquired as the result of experience. When an action is done repeatedly the nervous system becomes familiar with the situation and learns to react automatically, and a new reflex is built into the system. Walking, running, and typewriting are examples of activities that require large numbers of complex muscle coordinations that have

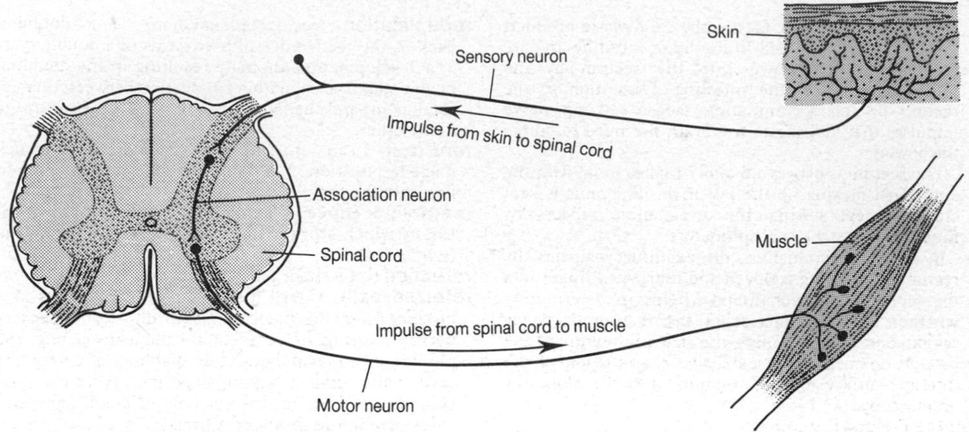

Nerve pathway of a simple reflex. When the sensory nerve ending is stimulated, a nerve impulse travels along a sensory (afferent) neuron to the spinal cord. Here an association neuron transfers the impulse to a motor (efferent) neuron. The motor neuron carries the impulse to a muscle, which contracts and moves a body part

become automatic.

abdominal r's contractions of the abdominal muscles about the navel on stimulating the abdominal skin. It indicates that the spinal cord from the eighth to the twelfth dorsal nerve is intact.

accommodation r. the coordinated changes that occur when the eye adapts itself for near vision; they are constriction of the pupil, convergence of the eyes, and increased convexity of the lens.

Achilles r. plantar extension of the foot elicited by a tap on the Achilles tendon, preferably while the patient kneels on a bed or chair, the feet hanging free over the edge; called also ankle jerk and triceps surae reflex.

acoustic r. contraction of the stapedius muscle in response to intense sound.

anal r. contraction of the anal sphincter on irritation of the anal skin.

ankle r. Achilles reflex.

auditory r. any reflex caused by stimulation of the auditory nerve; especially momentary closure of both eyes produced by a sudden sound.

Babinski's r. dorsiflexion of the big toe and fanning of the other toes when the sole of the foot is scraped (see also BABINSKI REFLEX).

Babkin r. pressure on the palms of both hands results in opening of an infant's mouth (see also BABKIN REFLEX).

biceps r. contraction of the biceps muscle when its tendon is tapped.

Brain's r. quadrupedal extensor reflex.

carotid sinus r. slowing of the heart beat on pressure on the carotid artery at the level of the cricoid cartilage (see also CAROTID SINUS SYNDROME).

Chaddock's r. in lesions of the pyramidal tract, stimulation below the external malleolus causes extension of the great toe (see also CHADDOCK'S REFLEX).

chain r. a series of reflexes, each serving as a stimulus to the next, making a complete activity.

ciliary r. the movement of the pupil in accommodation.

ciliospinal r. dilation of the ipsilateral pupil on painful stimulation of the skin at the side of the neck.

clasp-knife r. lengthening reaction; reflex elongation of extensor muscles which permits flexion of a limb.

conditioned r. conditioned response. See also CONDITIONING.

conjunctival r. closure of the eyelid when the conjunctiva is touched.

corneal r. reflex closure of the eyelids on irritation of the cornea (see also CORNEAL REFLEX).

cough r. the sequence of events initiated by the sensitivity of the lining of the passageways of the lung and mediated by the medulla as a consequence of impulses transmitted by the vagus nerve, resulting in coughing, i.e., the clearing of the passageways of foreign matter.

cremasteric r. contraction of the ipsilateral cremaster muscle, drawing the testis upward, when the upper inner aspect of the thigh is stroked longitudinally.

deep r. one elicited by a sharp tap on the appropriate tendon or muscle to induce brief stretch of the muscle.

digital r. HOFFMANN'S SIGN (2).

embrace r. Moro reflex.

gag r. elevation of the soft palate and retching which is elicited by touching the back of the tongue or the wall of the pharynx; called also pharyngeal reflex.

gastrocolic r. increase in intestinal peristalsis after food enters the empty stomach.

gastroileal r. increase in ileal motility and opening of the ileocaecal valve when food enters the empty stomach.

grasp r. flexion or clenching of the fingers or toes on stimulation of the palm of the hand or sole of the foot.

Hering–Breuer r's inflation and deflation reflexes that help regulate the rhythmic ventilation of the lungs, thereby preventing overdistention and extreme deflation (see also HERING–BREUER REFLEXES).

Hoffmann's r. HOFFMANN'S SIGN (2).

jaw r., jaw-jerk r. closure of the mouth caused by a downward blow on the passively hanging chin; rarely seen in health but very noticeable in corticospinal tract lesions.

knee r. see KNEE JERK.

light r. constriction of the pupil when a light is shown into the same (direct light reflex) or the opposite eye (indirect or consensual light reflex).

lung r's Hering–Breuer reflexes.

Magnus and de Kleijn neck r's extension of both ipsilateral limbs, or one, or part of a limb, and increase of tonus on the side to which the chin is turned when the head is rotated to the side, and flexion with loss of tonus on the side to which occiput points. Essentially a sign of decerebrate rigidity.

Mayer's r. opposition and adduction of the thumb combined with flexion at the metacarpophalangeal

joint and extension at the interphalangeal joint, on downward pressure of the index finger.
Mendel–Bechterew r. dorsal flexion of the second to fifth toes on percussion of the dorsum of the foot; in certain organic nervous disorders, plantar flexion occurs.
Moro r. flexion of an infant's thighs and knees, fanning and then clenching of fingers, with arms first thrown outward and then brought together as though embracing something; produced by a sudden stimulus and seen normally in the newborn (see also MORO REFLEX).
myotatic r. stretch reflex.
neck righting r. rotation of the trunk in the direction in which the head of the supine infant is turned; this reflex is absent or decreased in infants with spasticity.
nociceptive r's reflexes initiated by painful stimuli.
orbicularis oculi r. normal contraction of the orbicularis oculi muscle, with resultant closing of the eye, on percussion at the outer aspect of the supraorbital ridge, over the glabella, or around the margin of the orbit.
palatal r. swallowing caused by stimulation of the palate.
patellar r. knee jerk.
pharyngeal r. gag reflex.
pilomotor r. the production of goose flesh on stroking the skin.
placing r. flexion followed by extension of the leg when the infant is held erect and the dorsum of the foot is drawn along the under edge of a table top; it is obtainable in the normal infant up to the age of six weeks.
plantar r. plantar flexion of the foot when the ankle is grasped firmly and the lateral border of the sole is stroked or scratched from the heel toward the toes.
proprioceptive r. a reflex that is initiated by stimuli arising from some function of the reflex mechanism itself.
psychogalvanic r. decreased electrical resistance of the body due to emotional or mental agitation.
pupillary r. 1. contraction of the pupil on exposure of the retina to light. 2. any reflex involving the iris, resulting in change in the size of the pupil, occurring in response to various stimuli, e.g., change in illumination or point of fixation, sudden loud noise, or emotional stimulation.
quadriceps r. contraction of the quadriceps muscle and extension of the leg elicited by tapping the patellar ligament when the leg hangs loosely flexed at a right angle (see also KNEE JERK).
quadrupedal extensor r. extension of a hemiplegic flexed arm on assumption of the quadrupedal position.
red r. a luminous red appearance seen upon the retina in retinoscopy.
righting r. the ability to assume an optimal position when there has been a departure from it.
Rossolimo's r. in pyramidal tract lesions, plantar flexion of the toes on tapping their plantar surface.
spinal r. any reflex action mediated through a centre of the spinal cord.
startle r. Moro reflex.
stepping r. movements of progression elicited when the infant is held upright and inclined forward with the soles of the feet touching a flat surface; it is obtainable in the normal infant up to the age of six weeks.
stretch r. reflex contraction of a muscle in response to passive longitudinal stretching.
sucking r. sucking movements of the lips of an infant elicited by touching the lips or the skin near the mouth.
superficial r. any withdrawal reflex elicited by noxious or tactile stimulation of the skin, cornea, or mucous membrane, including the corneal, pharyngeal, and cremasteric reflexes.
swallowing r. swallowing caused by stimulation of the palate; called also palatal reflex.
tendon r. contraction of a muscle caused by percussion of its tendon.
tonic neck r. extension of the arm and sometimes of the leg on the side to which the head is forcibly turned, with flexion of the contralateral limbs; seen normally in the newborn.
triceps r. contraction of the belly of the triceps muscle and slight extension of the arm when the tendon of the muscle is tapped directly, with the arm flexed and fully supported and relaxed.
triceps surae r. Achilles reflex.
vestibular r's the reflexes for maintaining the position of the eyes and body in relation to changes in orientation of the head.
vestibulo-ocular r. nystagmus or deviation of the eyes in response to stimulation of the vestibular system by angular acceleration or deceleration or by irrigation of the ears with warm or cool water or air (calorific test).

reflexogenic, reflexogenous (ri,fleksə'jenik; ,reeflek'sojənəs) producing or increasing reflex action.

reflexograph (ri'fleksə,grahf, -,graf) an instrument for recording a reflex.

reflexometer (,reeflek'somitə) an instrument for measuring the force required to produce myotactic contraction.

reflux ('reefluks) a backward or return flow.
oesophageal r., gastroesophageal r. reflux of the stomach contents into the oesophagus.
hepatojugular r. distention of the jugular vein induced by applying manual pressure over the liver; it suggests insufficiency of the right heart.
intrarenal r. reflux of urine into the renal parenchymal tissue.
vesicoureteral r., vesicoureteric r. backward flow of urine from the bladder into a ureter.

refract (ri'frakt) 1. to cause to deviate. 2. to ascertain errors of ocular refraction.

refraction (ri'frakshən) 1. the act or process of refracting; specifically, the determination of the refractive errors of the eye and their correction with glasses. 2. the deviation of light or sound in passing obliquely from one medium to another of different density.
double r. refraction in which incident rays are divided into two refracted rays. **dynamic r.** refraction of the eye during accommodation.
ocular r. the refraction of light produced by the media of the normal eye and resulting in the focusing of images upon the retina.
static r. refraction of the eye when its accommodation is paralysed.

refractive (ri'fraktiv) pertaining to or subserving a process of refraction; having the power to refract.

refractometer (,reefrak'tomitə) 1. an instrument for measuring the refractive power of the eye. 2. an instrument for determining the indexes of refraction of various substances, particularly for determining the strength of lenses for spectacles.

refractory (ri'fraktə·ree) not readily yielding to treatment.
r. period the period of depolarization and repolarization of the cell membrane after excitation; during the first portion (absolute refractory period), the nerve or muscle fibre cannot respond to a second stimulus, whereas during the relative refractory period, it can respond only to a strong stimulus.

refrangible (ri'franjəb'l) susceptible of being refracted.

refrigerant (ri'frijə·rənt) 1. relieving fever and thirst. 2.

a cooling remedy.

refrigeration (ri,frijə'rayshən) therapeutic application of low temperature (see also induced HYPOTHERMIA).

refusion (ree'fyoozhən) the temporary removal and subsequent return of blood to the circulation.

regeneration (ri,jenə'rayshən) the natural renewal of a structure, as of a lost tissue or part.

regimen ('reji,men) a strictly regulated scheme of diet, exercise, or other activity designed to achieve certain ends.

regio ('reejioh) pl. *regiones* [L.] region; a plane area with more or less definite boundaries; used in anatomic nomenclature as a general term to designate certain areas on the surface of the body within certain defined boundaries.

region ('reejən) a plane with more or less definite boundaries; called also regio.

abdominal r's the areas into which the anterior surface of the abdomen is divided, including the epigastric, hypochondriac (right and left), inguinal (right and left), lateral (right and left), pubic, and umbilical.

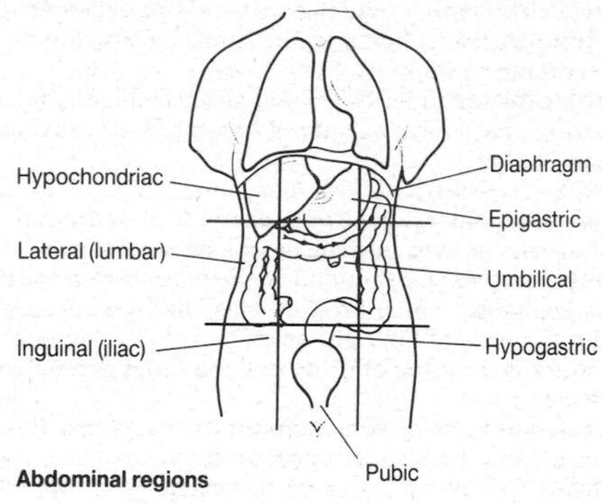

Abdominal regions

facial r's the areas into which the face is divided, including the buccal (side of oral cavity), infraorbital (below the eye), mental (chin), nasal (nose), oral (lips), orbital (eye), parotideomasseter (angle of the jaw), and zygomatic (cheek bone).

homology r's looped structures, comprising approximately 100 amino acid residues and fastened by disulphide bonds, that show similarities in primary structure from one region to another. They represent the building blocks or units of immunoglobulin molecules.

I r. that part of the major histocompatiblity complex where immune response genes are present.

lumbar r. the region of the back lying lateral to the lumbar vertebrae.

pectoral r. the areas into which the anterior surface of the chest is divided, including the axillary, infraclavicular, and mammary.

perineal r. the region underlying the pelvic outlet, including the anal and urogenital.

precordial r. the part of the anterior surface of the body covering the heart and the pit of the stomach.

pubic r. the middle portion of the most inferior region of the abdomen, located below the umbilical region and between the inguinal regions.

regional ('reejən'l) pertaining to a certain region or regions.

r. anaesthesia insensibility caused by interrupting the sensory nerve conductivity of any region of the body.

r. enteritis inflammation of the terminal portion of the ileum; called also regional ileitis and CROHN'S DISEASE.

register ('rejistə) an epidemiological term meaning an index on file of all cases with a particular disease or condition in a defined population.

registrar (,reji'strah) 1. an official keeper of records. 2. in British hospitals, a doctor training to be a specialist.

registration (,reji'strayshən) the act of recording; in dentistry, the making of a record of the jaw relations present or desired, in order to transfer them to an articulator to facilitate proper construction of a dental prosthesis.

r. of births and deaths since 1837 in England and Wales and 1855 in Scotland it has been a legal requirement to register births and deaths with a General Register Office. In England and Wales the Office comes under the Office of Population and Census Surveys, which also regulates and records civil marriages, conducts demographic research, including the 10-year census, and analyses demographic material.

Local registry offices are available in most towns.

Births should be registered within six weeks in England (21 days in Scotland).

Without a death certificate which indicates that the death has been registered it is illegal to dispose of the body.

regression (ri'greshən) 1. return to a former or earlier state. 2. subsidence of symptoms or of a disease process. 3. in biology, the tendency in successive generations toward the mean. 4. a mental mechanism utilized to resolve conflict or frustration by returning to a behaviour that was successful in earlier years. adj. **regressive.** Everyone uses this mechanism at some time, usually when under stress, resorting to tears, tantrums, or other childish behaviour to obtain certain goals or relieve frustrations. Some degree of regression frequently accompanies physical illness and can be expected in patients who are hospitalized for a physical disorder. Patients who are mentally ill may exhibit regression to an extreme degree, reverting all the way back to infantile behaviour (atavistic regression).

Regulan ('regyuhlan) trademark for a preparation of ispaghula husk, a bulk laxative.

regulation (,regyuh'layshən) 1. the act of adjusting or state of being adjusted to a certain standard. 2. in biology, the adaptation of form or behaviour of an organism to changed conditions. 3. the power of a pregastrula stage to form a whole embryo from a part. 4. the biochemical mechanisms that control the expression of genes.

regurgitant (ri'gərjitənt) flowing back.

regurgitation (ri,gərji'tayshən) a backward flowing, as the casting up of undigested food, or the backflow of blood through a defective heart valve.

valvular r. backflow of blood through the orifices of the heart valves owing to imperfect closing of the valves (valvular insufficiency); named, according to the valve affected, aortic, mitral, pulmonic, or tricuspid regurgitation.

rehabilitation (,reeə,bili'tayshən) the process of restoring a person's ability to live and work as normally as possible after a disabling injury or illness. It aims to help the patient achieve maximum possible physical and psychological fitness and regain the ability to care for himself. It offers assistance with the learning or relearning of skills needed in everyday activities, with occupational training and guidance and with psychological readjustment.

Rehabilitation is an integral part of convalescence. Proper food, medication, and hygiene and suitable exercise provide the physical basis for recovery. The patient is encouraged to be active physically and mentally to the extent recommended by the doctor. PHYSIOTHERAPY, OCCUPATIONAL THERAPY, and vocational training are used extensively in the rehabilitation of the severely handicapped.

rehalation (ˌreehəˈlayshən) rebreathing.

rehydration (ˌreehieˈdrayshən) the restoration of water or fluid content to a body or to a substance that has become dehydrated.

Reichert's cartilage (ˈriekəts) the dorsal cartilage of the second branchial arch.

reimplantation, replantation (ˌree·implahnˈtayshan; ˌreeplahnˈtayshən) replacement of tissue or a structure in the site from which it was previously lost or removed.

reinfection (ˌree·inˈfekshən) a second infection by the same agent.

reinforcement (ˌree·inˈfawsmənt) the increasing of force or strength. In behavioural science, the process of presenting a reinforcing stimulus so as to strengthen a response. Reinforcement is central in operant CONDITIONING.

A positive reinforcer is a stimulus that is added to the environment immediately after the desired response has been exhibited. It serves to strengthen the response, that is, to increase the likelihood of its occurring again. Examples of a positive reinforcer are food, money, a special privilege, or some other reward that is satisfying to the subject.

A negative reinforcer is a stimulus that is withdrawn (subtracted) from the environment immediately after the response, and the withdrawal serves to strengthen the response.

r. of reflex strengthening of a reflex response by the patient's performance of some unrelated action during elicitation of the reflex.

reinforcer (ˌree·inˈfawsə) anything that produces reinforcement; a reinforcing stimulus.

reinfusate (ˌree·inˈfyoozayt) fluid for reinfusion into the body, usually after being subjected to a treatment process.

reinfusion (ˌree·inˈfyoozhən) infusion of body fluid that has previously been withdrawn from the same individual, e.g., reinfusion of ascitic fluid after ultrafiltration.

reinnervation (reeˌinərˈvayshən) the grafting of a live nerve to restore the nerve supply of an organ or paralysed muscle.

reintegration (ˌree·intiˈgrayshən) 1. biological integration. 2. the resumption of normal mental and physical activity after disappearance of the catatonic state or other psychic disturbance.

Reiter's protein complement fixation (ˈrietəz) a serological test used to aid the diagnosis of syphilis; abbreviated RPCF.

Reiter's syndrome primarily occurs in males and is marked by initial diarrhoea or non-specific urethritis followed by conjunctivitis and arthritis and frequently accompanied by keratotic lesions of the skin. The arthritis may affect peripheral joints and/or sacro-iliac joints and the spine and is one of the seronegative arthritides.

rejection (riˈjekshən) the immune reaction of the recipient to foreign tissue cells (antigens) after allograft or xenograph TRANSPLANTATION, with the production of antibodies and ultimate destruction of the transplanted organ. In *hyperacute rejection*, there is an immediate response against the graft because of the presence of preformed antibody, resulting in fibrin deposition, platelet aggregation, neutrophilic infiltration, and eventual graft failure. In *acute rejection*, the response occurs after the sixth day and then proceeds rapidly. It is characterized by loss of function of the transplanted organ, with leukocytosis and thrombocytopenia. In *chronic rejection*, there is gradual progressive loss of function of the transplanted organ with less severe symptoms than in the acute form.

relapse (riˈlaps, ˈreeˌlaps) the return of a disease weeks or months after its apparent cessation.

relapsing fever (riˈlapsing) any one of a group of similar notifiable infectious diseases transmitted to man by the bites of ticks, and marked by alternating periods of normal temperature and periods of fever relapse. The diseases in the group are caused by several different species of spirochetes belonging to the genus *Borrelia.* Called also recurrent fever.

SYMPTOMS AND DIAGNOSIS. Generally, relapsing fever starts with a sudden high fever of 40.0–40.5 °C (104 to 105 °F), accompanied by chills, headache, muscle aches, nausea, and vomiting. There may also be jaundice and a rash. The attack lasts 2 or 3 days, after which the symptoms disappear by crisis, with profuse sweating accompanying the rapid drop in temperature. In elderly people this may be accompanied by collapse, in which the heart and respiratory system function poorly. After 3 or 4 days there is a relapse and the symptoms return in their former severity. The cycle may continue through four or more attacks before the disease has run its course. Relapsing fevers are rarely fatal, except in malnourished patients during epidemics, but they can be serious.

TREATMENT AND PREVENTION. Treatment is with antibiotics. Sponge baths and aspirin help to control the fever and comfort the patient.

Although tick-borne relapsing fever has a widespread distribution in tropical Africa, America and elsewhere (more sporadically), the louse-borne fever is now largely confined to limited areas in underdeveloped parts of Asia, Africa, and Latin America. Improved public sanitation and louse and tick control account for the decline in the incidence of the disease.

relation (riˈlayshən) the condition or state of one object or entity when considered in connection with another.

object r's the emotional bonds existing between an individual and another person, as contrasted with his interest in, and love for, himself; usually described in terms of his capacity for loving and reacting appropriately to others.

relative risk (ˈrelətiv) see under RISK.

relaxant (riˈlaksˈnt) 1. causing relaxation. 2. an agent that causes relaxation.

muscle r. an agent that either acts at the neuromuscular junction, causing muscle paralysis, and used in anaesthesia, or relieves muscle spasticity and tension by acting on muscle itself, or more commonly on the central nervous system.

relaxation (ˌreelakˈsayshən) a lessening of tension.

relaxin (riˈlaksin) a factor that produces relaxation of the symphysis pubis and dilation of the cervix uteri in certain animal species. A pharmaceutical preparation, extracted from the ovaries of pregnant sows, has been used in treatment of dysmenorrhoea and premature labour, and to facilitate labour at term.

releasing factor (riˈleesing) a substance produced in the hypothalamus which causes the anterior pituitary gland to release hormones.

REM rapid eye movement, a phase of SLEEP associated with dreaming and characterized by rapid movements of the eyes.

rem (rem) acronym for *r*oentgen *e*quivalent *m*an; the amount of any ionizing radiation which has the same biological effect as 1 rad of x-rays; 1 rem = 1 rad × RBE (relative biological effectiveness).

remedy (ˈremədee) anything that cures or palliates

disease. adj. **remedial**.

specific r. one that is invariably effective in treatment of a certain condition.

remineralization (ree,minə·rəlie'zayshən) restoration of mineral elements, as of calcium salts to bone.

reminiscence therapy (remi'nisəns) measures to stimulate long-term elderly patients with memorabilia, films and songs meaningful to their generation. Used in conjunction with or as a prelude to reality orientation therapy.

remission (ri'mishən) diminution or abatement of the symptoms of a disease; the period during which such diminution occurs.

remittence (ri'mitəns) temporary abatement, without actual cessation, of symptoms.

remittent (ri'mitənt) having periods of abatement and of exacerbation.

remotivation (ree,mohti'vayshən) in psychiatry, a group therapy technique administered by the nursing staff in a psychiatric hospital or department, which is used to stimulate the communication skills and an interest in the environment of long-term, withdrawn patients.

ren (ren) pl. *renes* [L.] kidney.

r. mobilis hypermobile kidney; nephroptosis.

renal ('reen'l) pertaining to the kidney.

r. clearance tests laboratory tests that determine the ability of the kidney to remove certain substances from the blood.

r. dialysis the application of the principles of dialysis for treatment of renal failure (see below). See also HAEMODIALYSIS and PERITONEAL DIALYSIS.

r. failure inability of the kidney to maintain normal function. Impairment of kidney function affects most of the body's systems because of its important role in maintaining fluid balance, regulating the electrochemical composition of body fluids, providing constant protection against acid-base imbalance, and controlling blood pressure. See also KIDNEY.

Acute renal failure is a sudden, severe interruption of kidney function. It is normally the complication of another disorder and is reversible. Possible causes may be inadequate renal perfusion associated with hypotension due to heart failure, sepsis, trauma, hypovolaemia associated with extravasation of plasma in burns, dehydration or haemorrhage, or renal atery occlusion. Nephrotoxic agents which may cause acute renal failure include sulphonamide and penicillin preparations, salicylates, aminoglycosides, nonsteroidal anti-inflammatory agents (e.g. indomethacin), antifungal agents (e.g. amphotericin B), cyclosporin A when poorly monitored, a variety of poisons ingested accidentally or deliberately (e.g. antifreeze), radiographic iodine contrast materials; and heavy metals. These agents inflict damage on the renal tubules, causing tubular necrosis. They also may indirectly harm the tubules by producing severe vasoconstriction of renal blood vessels and causing ischaemia of kidney tissue.

Oliguria is the hallmark of tubular necrosis, but it is not always present. Other symptoms beside a marked decrease in urinary output are related to fluid and electrolyte imbalances, anaemia, hypertension, and URAEMIA.

Dialysis will be needed to maintain fluid and electrolyte balances until kidney function improves. Acute renal failure is often accompanied by catabolism so enteral or parenteral feeding is necessary usually with haemofiltration to maintain 24-hour fluid balance. Vigilance and prompt treatment of infection is essential.

Chronic renal failure is a progressive loss of kidney function. In its early stage, renal function can remain adequate, but the glomerular filtration rate (GFR) is depressed to about 30 ml per minute and plasma chemistry begins to show abnormalities as waste products accumulate. In the later stage, the GFR drops to between 10 and 15 ml per minute; in the terminal stage it is less than 5 ml per minute. When URAEMIA becomes evident and the patient becomes symptomatic, dialysis is commenced or the patient transplanted.

Causes of renal failure are defined as:

(1) *Pre-renal.* Factors affecting the internal environment which have an effect on the kidney. These include hypertension, atheroma and stenosis of or trauma to the renal artery, recurrent infection.

(2) *Renal.* Disease of the renal tissue. These include glomerulonephritis, interstitial nephritis and infiltration of the renal substance such as amyloid and myeloma.

(3) *Post-renal.* Obstructions in the urinary tract which affect renal function. These include ureteric stones or blood-clots, invasion of tumour, papillae in the wall and outside ureter and retroperitoneal fibrosis.

The treatment of chronic renal failure is highly complex owing to its impact on systems throughout the body. It involves prevention of imbalances in water and electrolytes whenever possible and correction when they do occur. Treatment may include phosphate binders to prevent absorption of phosphorus from the intestinal tract. If blood pressure, fluid balance and heart failure are not controlled with moderate medication and the blood urea is rising, dialysis is urgently indicated. Fluids are often restricted to 500 ml and the volume of any output during each 24-hour period.

Virtually every system within the body is adversely affected in some way. Pathophysiological changes involve the gastrointestinal tract, the skin, the cardiovascular system, the lungs, bone, and blood, and the metabolism of glucose and protein.

r. pelvis the funnel-shaped expansion of the upper end of the ureter into which the renal calices open; it is usually the renal sinus, but under certain conditions, a large part of it may be outside the kidney (*extrarenal pelvis*).

Rendu–Weber–Osler disease (,rondoo,webə'ohslə) hereditary haemorrhagic telangiectasia.

reniform ('reni,fawm) kidney-shaped.

renin ('reenin) a proteolytic enzyme synthesized, stored, and secreted by the juxtaglomerular cells of the kidney; it plays a role in regulation of blood pressure by catalysing the conversion of the plasma glycoprotein angiotensinogen to angiotensin I. This, in turn, is converted to angiotensin II by an enzyme that is present in relatively high concentrations in the lung. Angiotensin II is one of the most potent vasoconstrictors known, and also is a powerful stimulator of aldosterone secretion.

Stimuli to the secretion of renin include sodium depletion, dehydration, serum albumin depletion, cirrhosis of the liver, cardiac failure, renal artery stenosis, and renal nerve stimulation.

Whenever blood flow to the kidney diminishes, renin is secreted and angiotensin is formed. The angiotensin causes widespread vasoconstriction and elevation of blood pressure consequent to greatly increased total peripheral resistance. A second effect, the increased secretion of aldosterone, results in retention of salt and water by the kidneys and therefore increased extracellular fluid volume, cardiac output, and arterial pressure. Additionally, the angiotensin acts *directly* on the kidneys to cause salt and water retention, which causes a longterm increase in arterial blood pressure.

big r. a relatively inactive protein with a higher molecular weight than normal renin, which is activated after exposure to low pH or to proteolytic enzymes.

reninism ('reeni,nizəm) a condition marked by overproduction of renin.

primary r. a syndrome of hypertension, hypokalaemia, hyperaldosteronism, and elevated plasma renin activity, due to proliferation of juxtaglomerular cells.

renipelvic (,reni'pelvik) pertaining to the pelvis of the kidney.

reniportal (,reni'pawt'l) pertaining to the portal system of the kidney.

renipuncture ('reni,pungkchə) surgical incision of the capsule of the kidney.

rennin ('renin) the milk-curdling enzyme found in the gastric juice of human infants (before pepsin formation) and abundantly in that of the calf and other ruminants; a preparation from the stomach of the calf is used to coagulate milk protein to facilitate its digestion. Rennin catalyses the conversion of casein from a soluble to an insoluble form (paracasein or curd).

renninogen (re'ninəjən) prorennin; the proenzyme in the gastric glands that is converted into rennin.

renogastric (,reenoh'gastrik) pertaining to the kidney and stomach.

renogram ('reenə,gram) a nuclear medicine investigation of renal excretion using $^{99}Tc^{m}$-DTPA (diethylenetriaminepentacetic acid). The radiopharmaceutical is injected as a rapid intravenous bolus and its uptake and excretion by the kidneys is monitored by a gamma camera.

renography (ree'nogrəfee) renogram.

renointestinal (,reenoh·in'testin'l) pertaining to the kidney and intestine.

renopathy (ree'nopəthee) any disease of the kidneys; nephropathy.

renoprival (,reenoh'prievəl) pertaining to or caused by lack of kidney function.

renotropic (,reenoh'tropik) having a special affinity for kidney tissue.

renule ('renyool) an area of the kidney supplied by a branch of the renal artery, usually consisting of three or four medullary pyramids and their corresponding cortical substance.

reorganization (,ri·awgənie'zayshən) healing by formation of new tissue identical to that which was injured or destroyed.

reovirus (,reeoh'vierəs) any of a group of ether-resistant RNA viruses isolated from healthy children, children with febrile and afebrile upper respiratory disease, children with diarrhoea, and many animals.

reoxygenation (ree,oksijə'nayshən) in radiobiology, the phenomenon in which hypoxic (and thus radioresistant) tumour cells become more exposed to oxygen (and thus more radiosensitive) by coming into closer proximity to capillaries after death and loss of other tumour cells due to previous irradiation.

rep (rep) acronym for *r*oentgen *e*quivalent *p*hysical, a unit of radiation equivalent to the absorption of 93 ergs per gram of water or soft tissue.

repair (ri'pair) the physical or mechanical restoration of the integrity and function of damaged tissues. The dead or damaged cells in a body tissue or organ may be replaced by healthy new cells or by new connective tissue.

plastic r. restoration of anatomical structure by means of tissue transferred from other sites or derived from other individuals, or by other substance.

repellent (ri–pelənt) able to repel or drive off; also, an agent that repels.

repercussion (,reepə'kushən) 1. the driving in of an eruption or the scattering of a swelling. 2. ballottement.

repetitive strain injury (re'petitiv) a soft tissue rheumatic disorder produced by repetitive use of muscle or tendon. Includes lateral epicondylitis of elbow (tennis elbow), medial epicondylitis (golfer's elbow), tenosynovitis of abductor pollicus longus and extensor policis brevis (de Quervain's syndrome), achilles tendinitis. These disorders are important in particular occupations as well as in sport.

replication (,repli'kayshən) 1. a turning back of a part so as to form a duplication. 2. repetition of an experiment to ensure accuracy. 3. the process of duplicating or reproducing, as replication of an exact copy of a polynucleotide strand of DNA or RNA.

repolarization (ree,pohlə·rie'zayshən) the reestablishment of polarity, especially the return of cell membrane potential to resting potential after depolarization.

repositor (ri'pozitə) an instrument used in returning displaced organs to the normal position.

representative sample (repri'zentətiv) a sample of a population which is representative of the characteristics of that population as a whole.

repression (ri'preshən) 1. the act of restraining, inhibiting, or suppressing. 2. in molecular genetics, inhibition of gene transcription by a repressor. 3. in psychiatry, a defence mechanism whereby a person unconsciously banishes unacceptable ideas, feelings or impulses from consciousness. A person using repression to obtain relief from mental conflict is unaware that he is 'forgetting' unpleasant situations as a way of avoiding them (motivated forgetting). If employed to extremes, repression may lead to increased tension and irresponsible behaviour that the person himself cannot understand or explain. Psychoanalysis frequently is employed to explore the causes and relieve tension resulting from repressed feelings of guilt, hostility, or rejection.

enzyme r. interference, usually by the end product of a pathway, with synthesis of the enzymes of that pathway.

repressor (ri'presə) that which restrains or inhibits; a specific protein molecule coded for by a regulatory gene, which acts through the cytoplasm to repress the synthesis of a specific protein.

reproduction (,reeprə'dukshən) 1. the process by which a living entity or organism produces a new individual of the same kind. 2. the creation of a similar object or situation; duplication; replication.

The gonads, or reproductive organs–the ovaries in the female and the testes in the male–produce the ova and spermatozoa that unite and grow into a new individual. This process, called fertilization, initiates reproduction. See also GRAAFIAN FOLLICLE.

The mature ovum is a comparatively large round cell that is just visible to the naked eye. Spermatozoa can be seen only under a microscope, where each appears as a small, flattened head with a long whiplike tail used for locomotion.

During the first 2 weeks of the menstrual cycle, one of the ova becomes mature enough to be released from the ovary.

At ovulation, the ovum is discharged into the abdominal cavity and enters the uterine tube (see also UTERINE TUBE).

Mature spermatozoa are constantly being made in the testes of the adult male and stored there in the duct system.

FERTILIZATION, OR CONCEPTION. During coitus, semen

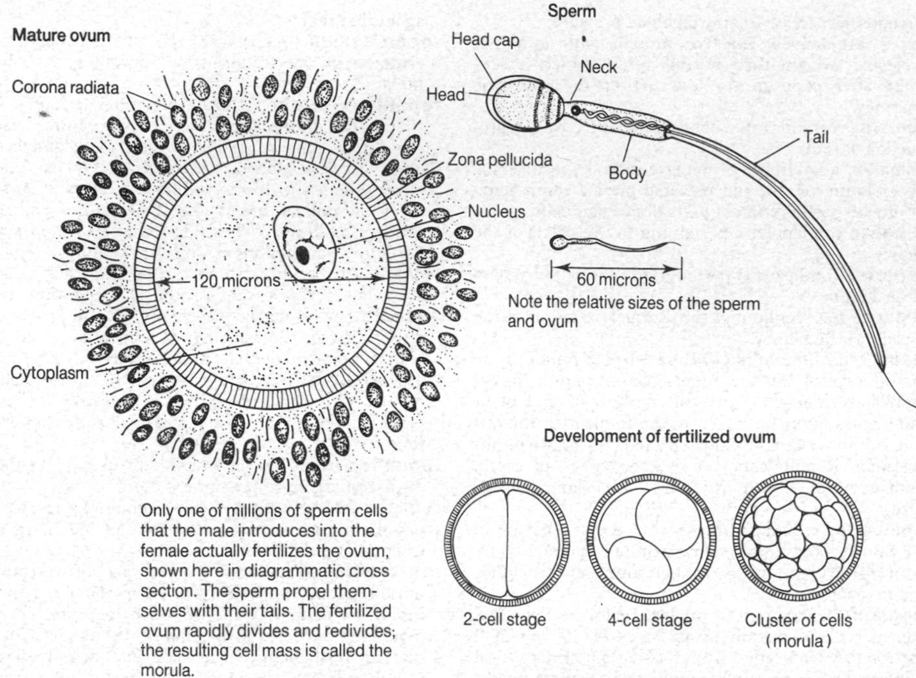

Only one of millions of sperm cells that the male introduces into the female actually fertilizes the ovum, shown here in diagrammatic cross section. The sperm propel themselves with their tails. The fertilized ovum rapidly divides and redivides; the resulting cell mass is called the morula.

Reproduction

is ejaculated from the penis into the back of the vagina near the cervix uteri. About a teaspoonful of semen is discharged with each ejaculation, containing several hundred millions of spermatozoa. Of this enormous number of spermatozoa, only one is needed to fertilize the ovum.

When one or more spermatozoan is able to reach the ovum, which is normally in the outer half (ampulla) of the uterine tube, fertilization occurs. The head end of the spermatozoan plunges through the thick wall of the ovum, leaving its tail outside. The genetic materials, the 23 chromosomes, are injected into the ovum, where they unite with the 23 chromosomes inherited from the mother (see HEREDITY). The sex of the child is determined at this instant and it depends on the nature of the sex chromosome carried by the spermatozoon (either X or Y).

If by chance two ova have been released and are fertilized by two spermatozoa, fraternal TWINS are formed. Identical twins are produced by a single fertilized ovum that divides into two early in its development.

Ovulation and Fertilization. To fertilize the ovum, coitus must take place within the period that begins 1 or 2 days before ovulation and lasts until 1 or 2 days after ovulation.

PREGNANCY. The ovum begins to change immediately after fertilization. The membrane surrounding the ovum becomes impenetrable to other spermatozoa. Soon the ovum is dividing into a cluster of two, then four, then more cells, called a MORULA, as it makes its way down the uterine (fallopian) tube toward the uterus. By the time the ovum reaches the uterus, in 3 to 5 days, the cells are formed in the shape of a minute ball, called a BLASTOCYST, hollow on the inside with an inner cell mass on one side from which the embryo will form. The blastocyst quickly buries itself in the lining of the uterus (implantation). On rare occasions, implantation takes place not in the uterine lining, but elsewhere in an ectopic, or abnormal, site. This produces an ECTOPIC PREGNANCY.

As soon as the blastocyst is implanted, its wall, called the TROPHOBLAST, begins to change into a structure that eventually develops into the placenta, while the embryo matures into a fetus. Through the placenta the fetus secures nourishment from the mother and rids itself of waste products. Growth continues until term, when birth is initiated by the onset of labour, and the baby becomes a new individual with a separate, independent existence from the mother.

asexual r. reproduction without the fusion of germ cells.

cytogenic r. production of a new individual from a single germ cell or zygote.

sexual r. reproduction by the fusion of a female germ cell with a male sexual cell or by the development of an unfertilized ovum.

somatic r. production of a new individual from a multicellular fragment by fission or budding.

reproductive (ˌreeprəˈduktiv) subserving or pertaining to reproduction.

r. organs, female the ovaries, which produce the ova, or eggs; the uterine tubes; the uterus; the vagina, or birth canal; and the vulva, comprising the external genitalia. The breasts are a secondary sexual characteristic, enclosing the mammary glands.

The reproductive system is linked to the body's system of endocrine glands by the ovaries. Besides producing the ova, the ovaries secrete the female sex hormones OESTROGEN and PROGESTERONE, which influence the body's development and general functioning as well as the sexual function.

The two ovaries, each about the size of a small plum, lie one on each side of the pear-shaped uterus at its wide upper part. When a female is born, her undeveloped ovaries already contain the specialized cells that can eventually become ova. At puberty these ova begin to ripen, one a month; usually the ovaries alternate in producing them. As the undeveloped ovum, contained in a follicle, begins to ripen, it makes its way to the ovary's surface, breaks through its own outer covering, and is released. Release of an ovum, called OVULATION, occurs about once in 28 days. After its separation from the ovary the ovum is drawn into the nearby uterine tube through its fringed, flared opening, and is moved along by rhythmic contractions of the tube's walls and by the cilia of its mucous membrane lining. In the course of its passage the ovum ripens fully, and if fertilization occurs it usually takes place while the ovum is moving through the uterine tube.

The other end of the tube opens directly into the uterus. This muscular organ is capable of stretching to contain a fertilized ovum as it grows through the 9 months of pregnancy. Its lining membrane is also specially adapted to hold the unborn infant securely and to nourish it. When the ovum arrives, the hormones oestrogen and progesterone produced in the ovary have previously stimulated the uterus to prepare its lining with extra blood vessels. If the ovum has not been fertilized, it loses its vitality, the hormone supply ceases, and the extra blood and tissues are discharged from the body through the vagina, in the menstrual flow. If fertilization, or conception, has taken place, the growth of a new life has begun; menstruation does not occur, and in fact ceases entirely during the 9 months (approximately 280 days) of pregnancy.

The lower end of the uterus forms an opening called the cervix, or neck, which protrudes into the birth canal, or vagina. Enclosed by muscles and lined with mucous membrane, the vagina measures on the average about 3 inches in length. In coitus it receives the male copulatory organ, the penis, and the discharge of spermatozoa during ejaculation. Like the uterus, the vagina undergoes changes during pregnancy that enable it to stretch to many times its usual size, allowing the infant to pass through it in childbirth.

The exterior opening of the vagina and the surrounding organs make up the vulva. The vulva consists of the labia majora (the major lips), the labia minora (the minor lips), the vestibule, and the clitoris. Somewhat anterior to the vulva lies a triangular fatty pad covered with pubic hair, the mons veneris. Between the clitoris and the entry to the vagina is the opening of the urethra, from which urine is excreted. The anus lies to the rear of the vaginal opening. In a virgin, a membrane called the hymen usually closes off a part of the opening to the vagina.

The labia majora envelop the labia minora, and these join together at the clitoris, a rudimentary, diminutive, penis-like organ that has a purely erotic function. Like the penis, the clitoris has a foreskin and many nerve endings. The area that surrounds the entry to the vagina and lies within the labia minora is the vestibule. At each side of the vaginal opening and elsewhere in the vestibule, glands secrete lubricating fluids to facilitate coitus.

A woman's breasts serve to provide milk for the newborn infant. At puberty the breasts increase in size; during pregnancy they become much larger and start to secrete milk shortly after childbirth.

DISORDERS OF THE FEMALE REPRODUCTIVE ORGANS. Bacterial and other infections, tumours, and birth injuries can affect the female reproductive organs. Growths, or tumours, can develop in all parts of the female reproductive tract. These are most often benign and may not require treatment, but they should be examined periodically in case they grow large and affect the organs, or become malignant.

In the OVARY, cysts or tumours can develop without symptoms. When diagnosed, an ovarian tumour is usually removed surgically; cysts, however, often remain without excessive harm or pain. The uterine tubes may also be the site of growths, though such tumours usually result from the involvement of some other organ. The UTERUS, particularly the cervix, is one of the most frequent locations of tumours. In the uterus they are usually leiomyomas (fibroids), which may attain considerable size. These are, however, quite readily diagnosed and, when found early enough, are treated successfully by surgery.

In the reproductive system, the BREASTS are the most common site of growths of all kinds, both cysts and tumours, the latter both benign and malignant. A variety of sores and abscesses may afflict the breasts, especially in their milk-producing periods. Any lump or other irregularity within or on a breast should receive prompt medical attention.

r. organs, male the external genitalia, accessory glands that secrete special fluids and the ducts through which these organs and glands are connected to each other and through which the spermatozoa are ejaculated during coitus.

EXTERNAL GENITALIA. The penis, testes, and scrotum (the sac that contains the testes) are together known as the external genitalia. The penis is the organ through which semen is transferred into the female during coitus. Semen is a carrier for the spermatozoa, which are produced in the testes. The testes also produce the male hormone testosterone, which gives a sexually mature male his distinctively masculine characteristics and his sexual energy and drive.

The testes are suspended from the spermatic cord, which also connects the testes with the other parts of the reproductive system. This cord consists of blood vessels, nerves and ducts, all enclosed in connective tissue.

ACCESSORY GLANDS. The accessory reproductive glands include the prostate, two seminal vesicles, and two bulbourethral glands, known also as Cowper's glands.

The PROSTATE is located below and against the urinary bladder. It completely surrounds the urethra. It produces a thin, clear, slightly alkaline fluid that neutralizes the normal acidity of the urethra caused by the continual passage of urine. This fluid enables the spermatozoa to pass through the urethra unharmed.

The seminal vesicles are two glands located just above and to the rear of the prostate. These glands consist of many small sacs, or pockets, in which is produced and stored the thick, milky fluid that is ejaculated during the male orgasm. The fluid serves as the carrier for the spermatozoa and is the major constituent of the semen.

The two bulbourethral glands, which are about the size of peas, secrete a clear, sticky fluid that lubricates the urethra, thus making it easier for the semen to pass through it during the process of ejaculation.

DUCTS. The spermatozoa are led from the testes to the urethra through a system of ducts. First, there are two convoluted tubes, one lying on top of each testis and connected directly to it. Each tube is called an epididymis. Mature spermatozoa produced in the testes are stored in each epididymis.

Each epididymis is connected to a vas deferens, a part of the spermatic cord that conducts the spermatozoa to the duct lying close to the bladder.

The vasa deferentia join with ducts leading from the seminal vesicles just before the urethra. The combined duct is called the ejaculatory duct. This duct passes through the prostate and joins with the urethra. The urethra then conducts the semen through the penis.

DISCHARGE OF SEMEN. The tissues that form the mass of the penis are called erectile tissue. This tissue is spongy in nature and filled with innumerable hollow spaces. There is also a network of veins and arteries within the penis. Sexual excitement causes the muscles surrounding the veins to contract, thereby restricting the flow of blood from the penis. At the same time, the muscles surrounding the arteries relax, permitting the free flow of blood into the penis at the full pressure of the circulatory system. The result is that the spongy tissue fills with blood and the penis swells in size and becomes stiff and erect.

Sexual excitement also stimulates the accessory glands to secrete larger amounts of their fluids. When the sexual tension becomes acute enough, as a result of coitus, masturbation, or purely mental stimulation (as in 'wet dreams'), there is a series of reflex contractions of the reproductive organs. The muscles surrounding the seminal ducts, the prostate, and the seminal vesicles contract convulsively; this causes the semen to be ejaculated forcibly from the penis. There is first an ejaculation of the fluid from the prostate, followed immediately by the semen. About 2 or 3 ml of semen is ejaculated. This volume of semen is believed to contain between 200 and 500 million spermatozoa, only one of which is necessary to fertilize the ovum.

DISORDERS OF THE MALE REPRODUCTIVE ORGANS. For disorders that affect particular organs, see PENIS, PROSTATE, and CRYPTORCHIDISM. Since the male reproductive organs are connected so closely with each other, an infection in one is likely to spread throughout the entire reproductive system. This is particularly true of venereal diseases, such as SYPHILIS and GONORRHOEA, which are contracted almost always through coitus.

reptilase ('repti,layz) an enzyme from Russell's viper venom used in determining blood clotting time.

repulsion (ri'pulshən) 1. the act of driving apart or away; a force that tends to drive two bodies apart. 2. in genetics, the occurrence on opposite chromosomes in a double heterozygote of the two mutant alleles of interest.

RES reticuloendothelial system.

resect (ri'sekt) to excise part of an organ or other structure.

resection (ri'sekshən) excision of a portion of an organ or other structure with closure of the gap in the case of hollow organs.

gastric r. partial gastrectomy.

transurethral r. resection of the prostate by means of an instrument passed through the urethra.

wedge r. removal of a triangular mass of tissue, as from the ovary.

resectoscope (ri'sektə,skohp) an endoscope with a wide-angle telescope and an electrically activated wire loop for transurethral removal or biopsy of lesions of the bladder, prostate, or urethra.

resectoscopy (,reesek'toskəpee) resection or biopsy of lesions by means of the resectoscope.

reserpine ('rezə,peen) an active alkaloid from various species of *Rauwolfia*, used rarely as an antihypertensive, tranquillizer, and sedative.

reserve (ri'zərv) 1. to hold back for future use. 2. a supply, beyond that ordinarily used, that may be utilized in emergency. **alkali r., alkaline r.** the amount of buffer compounds in the blood that are capable of neutralizing acids, such as sodium bicarbonate and proteins. See also ALKALI RESERVE.

cardiac r. the potential ability of the heart to perform work beyond that necessary under basal conditions.

reservoir ('rezə,vwah) 1. a storage place or cavity. 2. the host or environment in which an organism lives and from which it is able to infect susceptible individuals.

residual (ri'zidyooəl) remaining or left behind.

r. urine urine remaining in the bladder after voiding; seen with bladder outlet obstruction and disorders affecting nerves controlling bladder function.

residue ('rezidyoo) a remainder; that which remains after the removal of other substances; in organic chemistry a portion of a molecule that is incorporated into another molecule, e.g., an amino acid residue of a polypeptide.

residuum (ri'zidyooəm) pl. *residua* [L.] a residue or remainder.

resilience (ri'zili·əns) the ability to return to a normal shape after stretching or compression.

resin ('rezin) 1. a solid or semisolid, amorphous organic substance of vegetable origin or produced synthetically. True resins are insoluble in water, but are readily dissolved in alcohol, ether, and volatile oils. 2. rosin. adj. **resinous**.

acrylic r's products of the polymerization of acrylic or methacrylic acid or their derivatives, used in fabrication of medical prostheses and dental restorations and appliances.

anion-exchange r. see ion-exchange resin (below).

cation-exchange r. see ion-exchange resin (below).

cholestyramine r. a synthetic, strongly basic anion-exchange resin in the chloride form which chelates bile salts in the intestine, thus preventing their reabsorption; used in the symptomatic relief of pruritus associated with bile stasis.

ion-exchange r. a high-molecular-weight insoluble polymer of simple organic compounds capable of exchanging its attached ions for other ions in the surrounding medium; classified as (a) cation- or anion-exchange resins, depending on which ions the resin exchanges (the former are used to restrict intestinal sodium absorption in oedematous states, and the latter as antacids in ulcer treatment); and (b) carboxylic, sulphonic, etc., depending on the nature of the active groups.

podophyllum r. a mixture of resins from podophyllum, used as a topical caustic in the treatment of certain papillomas.

resistance (ri'zistəns) 1. opposition, or counteracting force, as opposition of a conductor to passage of electricity or other energy or substance. The measure of electrical resistance is the OHM. 2. the natural ability of a normal organism to remain unaffected by noxious agents in its environment (see also IMMUNITY). 3. in studies of respiration, an expression of the opposition to flow of air produced by the tissues of the air passages, in terms of pressure per amount of air per unit of time. 4. in psychoanalysis, opposition to the coming into consciousness of repressed material.

drug r. the ability of a microorganism to withstand the effects of a drug that are lethal to most members of its species.

peripheral r. resistance to the passage of blood through the small blood vessels, especially the arterioles.

resolution (,rezə'looshən) 1. subsidence of a pathological state, as the subsidence of an inflammation, or the softening and disappearance of a swelling. 2. perception as separate of two adjacent points; in microscopy, the smallest distance at which two adjacent objects can be distinguished as separate.

resolvent (ri'zolvənt) promoting resolution or the dissipation of a pathological growth; an agent that promotes resolution.

resolving power (ri'zolving) the ability of the eye or of a lens to make small objects that are close together separately visible, thus revealing the structure of an object.

resonance ('rezənəns) 1. the prolongation and intensification of sound produced by transmission of its vibrations to a cavity, especially such a sound elicited by percussion. Decrease of resonance is called *dullness*; its increase, *flatness*. 2. a vocal sound heard on auscultation. 3. mesomerism.

amphoric r. a sound resembling that produced by blowing over the mouth of an empty bottle.

skodaic r. increased percussion resonance at the upper part of the chest, with flatness below it.

tympanic r. drumlike reverberation of a cavity filled with air.

tympanitic r. the peculiar sound elicited by percussing a tympanitic abdomen.

vesicular r. normal pulmonary resonance.

vocal r. the sound of ordinary speech as heard through the chest wall.

resonant ('rezənənt) giving an intense, rich sound on percussion; exhibiting resonance.

resonator ('rezə,naytə) 1. an instrument used to intensify sound at a particular frequency. 2. an electric circuit in which oscillations of a certain frequency are set up by oscillations of the same frequency in another circuit.

resonium (ri'zohniəm) see CALCIUM resonium.

resorb (ri'sawb) to take up or absorb again; to undergo resorption.

resorcinism (ri'zawsi,nizəm) chronic poisoning by resorcinol, resulting in methaemoglobinaemia, paralysis, and damage to the capillaries, kidneys, heart, and nervous system.

resorcinol (ri'zawsi,nol) a phenol with bactericidal, fungicidal, keratolytic, exfoliative, and antipruritic activity; used especially as a topical keratolytic in the treatment of acne.

resorption (ri'sawpshən) 1. the lysis and assimilation of a substance, as of bone. 2. reabsorption.

respirable ('respirəb'l) suitable for respiration.

respiration (,respi'rayshən) 1. the exchange of oxygen and carbon dioxide between the atmosphere and the body cells, including inspiration and expiration, diffusion of oxygen from the pulmonary alveoli to the blood and of carbon dioxide from the blood to the alveoli, and the transport of oxygen to and carbon dioxide from the body cells. 2. cellular respiration, the metabolic processes by which living cells break down carbohydrates, amino acids, and fats to produce energy in the form of ATP (adenosine triphosphate).

THE RESPIRATORY SEQUENCE. The sequence of the respiration process begins as air enters the corridors of the nose or mouth, where it is warmed and moistened. The air then passes through the pharynx, larynx, and trachea and into the bronchi.

The bronchi branch in the lungs into smaller and smaller bronchioles, ending in clusters of tiny air sacs. There are 750 million of these alveoli, as these sacs are called, in the lungs. The blood flows through the lungs in the pulmonary circulation. Through the thin membrane of the network of capillaries around the alveoli, the air and the blood exchange oxygen and carbon dioxide. The carbon dioxide molecules migrate from the erythrocytes in the capillaries through the porous membrane into the air in the alveoli, while the oxygen molecules cross from the air into the red blood cells.

The erythrocytes proceed through the circulatory system, carrying the oxygen in loose combination with HAEMOGLOBIN and giving it up to the body cells that need it. In cellular respiration the blood cells release oxygen and pick up carbon dioxide. The lungs dispose of the carbon dioxide, left there by the red blood cells, in the process of breathing. With each breath, about one-sixth of the air in the lungs is exchanged for new air.

BREATHING. The lungs inflate and deflate 15–17 times per minute in adults, 12–20 times per minute in teenagers, 20–30 times per minute in 2-12 year olds, and 30–50 times per minute in newborns. Their elastic tissue allows them to expand and contract like a bellows worked by the diaphragm and the intercostal muscles. The diaphragm contracts, flattening itself downward, and thus enlarges the thoracic cavity. At the same time the ribs are pulled up and outward by the action of the narrow but powerful intercostal muscles that expand and contract the rib cage. As the chest expands, the air rushes in.

Exhalation occurs when the respiratory muscles relax and the chest returns automatically to its minimum size, expelling the air (see also LUNG).

Automatic Breathing Controls. The automatic control of breathing stems from poorly defined areas known as the respiratory centres, located in the medulla oblongata and pons. From there, impulses are sent down the spinal cord to the nerves that control the diaphragm, and to the intercostal muscles. Chemical and reflex signals control these nerve centres. See HERING–BREUER REFLEXES.

The chemical controls of breathing are mainly dependent on the level of carbon dioxide in the blood. The response is so sensitive that if the carbon dioxide in the blood increases two-tenths of 1 per cent, the respiratory rate increases automatically to double the amount of air taken in, until the excess of carbon dioxide is eliminated. It is not lack of oxygen but excess of carbon dioxide that causes this instant and powerful reaction.

The $P\text{CO}_2$, or carbon dioxide tension, of arterial blood normally is 38 to 40 mmHg. When the $P\text{CO}_2$ increases, the respiratory centres are stimulated and breathing becomes more rapid; conversely, decrease of the $P\text{CO}_2$ slows the rate of respiration. The $P\text{CO}_2$ acts both directly on the respiratory centres of the brain and on the carotid and aortic bodies, chemoreceptors that are responsive to changes in blood $P\text{CO}_2$, $P\text{O}_2$, and pH (see also BLOOD GAS ANALYSIS).

PROTECTIVE RESPIRATORY MECHANISMS. The lungs are constantly exposed to the surrounding atmosphere. Twenty times a minute, more or less, they take in a gaseous mixture, along with whatever foreign particles happen to be floating in it and at whatever temperature it may be. To compensate, the lungs have some remarkable protective devices.

On its way through the nasal passage, the cold air from outside is preheated by a large supply of blood, which gives off warmth through the thin mucous membrane that lines the respiratory tract. This same mucous lining is always moist, and dry air picks up moisture as it passes.

Dust, soot, and bacteria are filtered out by a barrier of cilia, tiny threadlike growths that line the passageways of the respiratory tract. The cilia catch not only foreign particles but also mucus produced by the respiratory passages themselves. Since the movement of the cilia is always toward the outside, they push the interfering matter upward, away from the delicate lung tissues, so that it can be expectorated or swallowed. Particles that are too large for the cilia to dispose of usually stimulate a sneeze or a cough, which forcibly expels them.

Sneezing and coughing are reflex acts in response to stimulation of nerve endings in the respiratory passages. The stimulus for a cough comes from the air passages in the throat; for a sneeze, from those in the nose.

abdominal r. inspiration and expiration accomplished mainly by the abdominal muscles and diaphragm.

aerobic r. oxidative transformation of certain substrates into secretory products, the released energy being used in the process of assimilation.

anaerobic r. respiration in which energy is released by chemical reactions in which free oxygen takes no part.

artificial r. that maintained by force applied to the body (see also ARTIFICIAL RESPIRATION).

Biot's r's rapid, deep respirations with abrupt pauses in breathing (see also BIOT'S RESPIRATIONS).

cell r. the processes in the living cell by which organic substances are oxidized and chemical energy is released.

Cheyne–Stokes r. breathing characterized by rhythmic waxing and waning of respiration depth, with regularly recurring apnoeic periods (see also CHEYNE-STOKES RESPIRATION).

cogwheel r. breathing with jerky inspiration.

diaphragmatic r. that performed mainly by the diaphragm.

electrophrenic r. induction of respiration by electric stimulation of the phrenic nerve.

external r. the exchange of gases between the lungs and the blood.

internal r. the exchange of gases between the body cells and the blood.

Kussmaul's r. air hunger.

paradoxical r. that in which a lung, or a portion of a lung, is deflated during inspiration and inflated during expiration (see also PARADOXICAL RESPIRATION).

tissue r. internal respiration.

respirator ('respi,raytə) an apparatus to qualify the air breathed through it, or a device for giving artificial respiration or to assist in pulmonary ventilation (see also VENTILATOR).

r. shock circulatory SHOCK due to interference with the flow of blood through the great vessels and chambers of the heart, causing pooling of blood in the veins and the abdominal organs and a resultant vascular collapse. The condition sometimes occurs as a result of increased intrathoracic pressure in patients who are being maintained on a mechanical VENTILATOR.

respiratory (ri'spiritə·ree, 'rəspirətree) pertaining to respiration.

adult r. distress syndrome (ARDS) a group of signs and symptoms resulting in acute respiratory failure; characterised clinically by tachypnoea, dyspnoea, tachycardia, cyanosis, and low P_aO_2 that persists even with oxygen therapy; called also shock lung, wet lung, stiff lung, and many other names descriptive of aetiology or clinical manifestations. Many aetiological factors have been associated with ARDS, including shock, fat embolism, fluid overload, oxygen toxicity, fluid aspiration, narcotic overdose, disseminated intravascular coagulation, multiple transfusions, inhalation of toxic gases, diffuse pulmonary infection, and systemic reactions to sepsis, pancreatitis, and massive trauma or burns.

r. distress syndrome of newborn (RDS), idiopathic r. distress syndrome, infant r. distress syndrome (IRDS) hyaline membrane disease; a condition occurring in preterm infants, full-term infants of diabetic mothers, and infants delivered by caesarean section and associated with pulmonary maturity and inability to produce sufficient lung surfactant. See HYALINE MEMBRANE DISEASE.

r. failure a life-threatening condition in which respiratory function is inadequate to maintain the body's need for oxygen supply and carbon dioxide removal while at rest; called also acute ventilatory failure. The condition usually occurs when a patient with CHRONIC OBSTRUCTIVE AIRWAYS DISEASE develops an infection or otherwise suffers an additional strain on his already seriously impaired respiratory functions. Inadequate or unsuccessful treatment of RESPIRATORY INSUFFICIENCY from a variety of causes can lead to respiratory failure.

Early symptoms include dyspnoea, wheezing, and apprehension; cyanosis is rarely present. As the condition worsens the patient becomes drowsy and mentally confused and may slip into coma. BLOOD GAS ANALYSIS is an important tool in diagnosing respiratory failure and assessing effectiveness of treatment. The condition is a medical emergency that can rapidly progress to irreversible cardiopulmonary failure and death.

r. insufficiency a condition in which respiratory function is inadequate to meet the body's needs when increased physical activity places extra demands on it. Insufficiency occurs as a result of progressive degenerative changes in the alveolar structure and the capillary tissues in the pulmonary bed, as, for example, in CHRONIC OBSTRUCTIVE AIRWAYS DISEASE and pulmonary fibrosis. Treatment is essentially supportive and symptomatic.

r. quotient the ratio of the volume of expired carbon dioxide to the volume of oxygen absorbed by the lungs per unit of time.

r. syncytial virus a virus isolated from children with bronchopneumonia and bronchitis, characteristically causing syncytium formation in tissue culture.

r. system the group of specialized organs whose specific function is to provide for the transfer of oxygen from the air to the blood and of waste carbon dioxide from the blood to the air. The organs of the system include the NOSE, the PHARYNX, the LARYNX, the TRACHEA, the bronchi, and the LUNGS. See also RESPIRATION.

r. therapy the technical speciality concerned with the treatment, management and care of patients with respiratory problems including administration of medical gases (OXYGEN THERAPY, CARBON DIOXIDE–OXYGEN THERAPY, and HELIUM–OXYGEN THERAPY), AEROSOL THERAPY, HUMIDITY THERAPY, mechanical ventilation (see VENTILATOR), INTERMITTENT POSITIVE-PRESSURE VENTILATION (IPPV) therapy, INCENTIVE SPIROMETRY, PULMONARY FUNCTION TESTING, and arterial BLOOD GAS ANALYSIS.

respirometer (,respi'romitə) an instrument for determining the nature of the respiration.

response (ri'spons) any action or change of condition evoked by a stimulus.

anamnestic r. the rapid reappearance of antibody in the blood following introduction of an antigen to which the subject had previously developed a primary immune response.

autoimmune r. the immune response in which antibodies or immune lymphoid cells are produced against the body's own tissues.

conditioned r. an acquired response developed by regular association of some physiological function with an unrelated outside event (see also CONDITIONED REPONSE and CONDITIONING).

galvanic skin r. the alteration in the electrical resistance of the skin associated with sympathetic nerve discharge.

immune r. specifically altered reactivity of the animal body after exposure to antigen, manifested as antibody production, cell-mediated immunity, or as immunological tolerance. Called also *immune reaction*. See also IMMUNE RESPONSE.

r. rate the number of returned questionnaires or other completed survey enquiries expressed as a proportion of the total.

reticulocyte r. increase in the formation of reticulocytes in reponse to a bone marrow stimulus.

triple r. (of Lewis) a physiological reaction of the skin to stroking with a blunt instrument: first a red line develops at the site of stroking, owing to the release of histamine or a histamine-like substance, then a flare develops around the red line, and lastly a wheal is formed as a result of local oedema.

unconditioned r. an unlearned response, i.e., one that occurs naturally (see also CONDITIONING).

rest (rest) 1. repose after exertion. 2. a fragment of embryonic tissue retained within the adult organism.

restenosis (ˌreestə'nohsis) recurrent stenosis, especially of a cardiac valve after surgical correction of the primary condition.

false r. stenosis recurring after failure to divide either commissure of a cardiac valve beyond the area of incision of the papillary muscles.

restibrachium (ˌresti'brayki·əm) the inferior peduncle of the cerebellum.

restiform ('restiˌfawm) shaped like a rope.

restis ('restis) the inferior peduncle of the cerebellum.

restitution (ˌresti'tyooshən) the spontaneous realignment of the fetal head with the fetal body, after delivery of the head.

restoration (ˌrestə'rayshən) 1. induction of a return to a previous state, as a return to health or replacement of a part to normal position. 2. partial or complete reconstruction of a body part, or the device used in its place.

restorative (ri'sto·rətiv, -'stor-) 1. promoting a return to health or to consciousness. 2. a remedy that aids in restoring health, vigour, or consciousness.

resuscitation (riˌsusi'tayshən) restoration to life or consciousness of one apparently dead, or whose respirations have ceased (see also ARTIFICIAL RESPIRATION).

cardiopulmonary r. an emergency technique used in cardiac arrest to reestablish heart and lung function until more advanced life support is available (see also CARDIOPULMONARY RESUSCITATION).

resuscitator (ri'susiˌtaytə) an apparatus for initiating respiration in persons whose breathing has stopped.

retainer (ri'taynə) an appliance or device that keeps a tooth or partial denture in proper position.

retardation (ˌreetah'dayshən) delay; hindrance; delayed development.

mental r. subnormal general intellectual development, associated with impairment either of learning and social adjustment or of maturation, or of both (see also MENTAL HANDICAP).

retching ('reching) a strong involuntary effort to vomit.

rete ('reetee) pl. *retia* [L.] a network or meshwork, especially of blood vessels.

arterial r., r. arteriosum an anastomotic network of minute arteries, just before they become capillaries.

articular r. a network of anastomosing blood vessels in or around a joint.

r. malpighii the innermost stratum of epidermis.

r. mirabile a vascular network formed by division of an artery or vein into many smaller vessels that reunite into a single vessel.

r. testis the network of channels formed in the mediastinum of the testis by the seminiferous tubules.

r. venosum an anastomotic network of small veins.

retention (ri'tenshən) the process of holding back or keeping in a position, as persistence in the body of material normally excreted.

r. of urine accumulation of urine within the bladder because of inability to urinate.

reticulaemia (rəˌtikyuh'leemi·ə) the presence in the blood of increased numbers of immature erythrocytes.

reticular (rə'tikyuhlə) resembling a net.

r. activating system the system of cells of the reticular formation of the medulla oblongata that receive collaterals from the ascending sensory pathways and project to higher centres; they control the overall degree of central nervous system activity, including wakefulness, attentiveness, and sleep; abbreviated RAS.

reticulated (rə'tikyuhˌlaytid) reticular.

reticulation (rəˌtikyuh'layshən) the formation or presence of a network.

reticulin (rə'tikyuhlin) a scleroprotein present in the connective fibres of reticular tissue, closely related to collagen in composition.

reticulocyte (rə'tikyuhlohˌsiet) a young erythrocyte showing a basophilic reticulum under vital staining.

reticulocytopenia (rəˌtikyuhlohˌsietoh'peeni·ə) a deficiency of reticulocytes in the peripheral blood.

reticulocytosis (rəˌtikyuhlohsie'tohsis) an excess of reticulocytes in the peripheral blood.

reticuloendothelial (rəˌtikyuhlohˌendə'theeli·əl) pertaining to the reticuloendothelium or to the reticuloendothelial system.

r. system a network of cells and tissues found throughout the body, especially in the blood, general connective tissue, spleen, liver, lungs, bone marrow, and lymph nodes. They have both endothelial and reticular attributes and the ability to take up colloidal dye particles. Some of the reticuloendothelial cells found in the blood and in the general connective tissue are unusually large in size. These cells are concerned with blood cell formation and destruction, storage of fatty materials, and metabolism of iron and pigment, and they play a role in inflammation and immunity. Some of the cells are motile—that is, capable of spontaneous motion—and phagocytic—they can ingest and destroy unwanted foreign material.

The reticuloendothelial cells of the SPLEEN possess the ability to dispose of disintegrated erythrocytes. They do not, however, destroy haemoglobin, which is liberated in the process.

The reticuloendothelial cells located in the blood cavities of the LIVER are called Kupffer cells. These cells, together with the cells of the general connective tissue and bone marrow, are capable of transforming into bile pigment the haemoglobin released by disintegrated erythrocytes.

reticuloendothelioma (rəˌtikyuhlohˌendəˌtheeli'ohmə) an outdated term for malignant lymphoma.

reticuloendotheliosis (rəˌtikyuhlohˌendəˌtheeli'ohsis) hyperplasia of reticuloendothelial tissue.

leukaemic r. leukaemia marked by splenomegaly and by an abundance of large, mononuclear abnormal cells with numerous, irregular cytoplasmic projections that give them a flagellated or hairy appearance in the bone marrow, spleen, liver, and peripheral blood; called also hairy-cell leukaemia.

reticuloendothelium (rəˌtikyuhlohˌendə'theeli·əm) the tissue of the reticuloendothelial system.

reticulohistiocytoma (rəˌtikyuhlohˌhistiohsie'tohmə) a granulomatous nodular aggregation of lipid-laden histiocytes and multinucleated giant cells frequently seen in subcutaneous sites or around joints.

reticuloma (rəˌtikyuh'lohmə) an outdated term for histiocytic malignant lymphoma.

reticulopenia (rəˌtikyuhloh'peeni·ə) reticulocytopenia.

reticulopodium (rəˌtikyuhloh'pohdi·əm) a threadlike, branching pseudopodium.

reticulosarcoma (rəˌtikyuhlohsah'kohmə) an outdated

term for malignant lymphoma, histiocytic or undifferentiated.

reticulosis (rə,tikyuh'lohsis) an abnormal increase in cells derived from or related to the reticuloendothelial cells.

familial histiocytic r., histiocytic medullary r. a fatal hereditary disorder marked by anaemia, granulocytopenia, thrombocytopenia, phagocytosis of blood cells, diffuse proliferation of histiocytes, and enlargement of the liver, spleen, and lymph nodes.

midline malignant r. lethal midline granuloma thought to be due to lymphoma.

reticulum (rə'tikyuhləm) pl. *reticula* [L.] 1. a small network, especially a protoplasmic network in cells. 2. reticular tissue.

endoplasmic r. an ultramicroscopic organelle of nearly all higher plant and animal cells, consisting of a system of membrane-bound cavities in the cytoplasm, occurring in two types, granular or rough-surfaced, bearing large numbers of ribosomes on its outer surface, and agranular or smooth-surfaced.

sarcoplasmic r. a form of agranular reticulum in the sarcoplasm of striated muscle, comprising a system of smooth-surfaced tubules surrounding each myofibril.

retiform ('reeti,fawm, 'ret-) reticular.

Retin-A (,retin'ay) trademark for preparations of tretinoin.

retina ('retinə) the innermost of the three tunics of the eyeball, surrounding the vitreous body and continuous posteriorly with the optic nerve. The retina is composed of light-sensitive neurons together with their axons, and other neural cells. The retina is responsible for the conversion of light to electrical impulses and the transmission of them to the OPTIC NERVE. The rods are sensitive in dim light, and the cones are sensitive in bright light and are responsible for colour vision. See also EYE.

Retinopathy is a general term denoting pathological conditions of the retina; they may occur in conjunction with certain systemic disorders, such as hypertension, toxaemia of pregnancy, and diabetes mellitus.

DETACHMENT OF THE RETINA. This is complete or partial separation of the retina from the underlying retinal pigment epithelium. Untreated, vision will almost always be lost, but surgery may often restore vision at least partially.

retinaculum (,reti'nakyuhləm) pl. *retinacula* [L.] 1. a structure that retains an organ or tissue in place. 2. an instrument for retracting tissues during surgery.

flexor r. of hand a fibrous band forming the carpal tunnel, through which pass the tendons of the flexor muscles of the hand and fingers and the median nerve.

r. morgagni a ridge formed by the coming together of segments of the ileocaecal valve.

r. tendinum a tendinous restraining structure, such as an annular ligament.

retinal ('retinəl) 1. pertaining to the retina. 2. the aldehyde of retinol, having vitamin A activity. One isomer (11-*cis*-retinal) combines with opsin in the retinal rods (scotopsin) to form rhodopsin (visual purple); another, all-*trans*-retinal, or visual yellow, results from the bleaching of rhodopsin by light, in which the 11-*cis*-form is converted to the all-*trans*-form. Retinal also combines with opsins in the retinal cones to form the three pigments responsible for colour vision.

r. detachment detachment of the RETINA.

retinene ('reti,neen) an ocular pigment derived from vitamin A and formed by the bleaching action of light on rhodopsin. It occurs in two forms: retinene$_1$ is RETINAL (2), and retinene$_2$ is dehydroretinal.

retinitis (,reti'nietis) inflammation of the retina.

r. pigmentosa a group of diseases, frequently hereditary, marked by progressive loss of retinal function, especially associated with contraction of the visual field and impairment of scotopic vision. On examination attenuation of retinal vessels, clumping of the retinal pigment epithelium and optic atrophy may be noted. It may be transmitted as an autosomal dominant, recessive, or X-linked trait and is sometimes associated with other genetic defects.

The disorder often follows a slow course over a period of many years, but there is considerable variation in the progression of the disease. There is no successful treatment or cure for the condition. Early diagnosis may allow genetic counselling to be given.

r. proliferans advanced retinal neovascularization extending forwards from the optic disc and/or retina. May occur with conditions such as proliferative diabetic retinopathy, retinal venous occlusion and sickle cell disease.

suppurative r. retinitis due to pyaemic infection.

retinoblastoma (,retinohbla'stohmə) a malignant tumour arising from retinal cells. Occurs in infancy and may be hereditary. Treatment includes cryosurgery, irradiation and photocoagulation, but enucleation may be required.

retinochoroiditis (,retinoh,ko·roy'dietis) inflammation of the retina and choroid.

r. juxtapapillaris a small area of inflammation on the fundus of the eye near the papilla; seen in young healthy individuals.

retinoid ('reti,noyd) 1. resembling the retina. 2. any derivative of retinal.

retinol ('reti,nol) vitamin A_1; the form of vitamin A found in mammals, which is reversibly dehydrogenated by enzymatic action into its aldehyde, retinal.

retinomalacia (,retinohmə'layshi·ə) softening of the retina.

retinopapillitis (,retinoh,papi'lietis) inflammation of retina and optic disc (papilla).

retinopathy (,reti'nopəthee) any noninflammatory disease of the retina.

central serous r. a usually self-limiting condition marked by acute localized detachment of the neural retina or retinal pigment epithelium in the region of the macula.

circinate r. the appearance of retinal haemorrhages and hard exudates in a circular pattern. Associated with conditions such as diabetic retinopathy, branch vein occlusion and senile macular degeneration.

diabetic r. the retinal manifestation of diabetes mellitis may be classified as follows: (1) *Background diabetic retinopathy*. The presence of microaneurysms, haemorrhages and hard exudates. Visual acuity is unaffected in this condition but may progress to the following stages. (2) *Diabetic maculopathy*. May be thought of as a progression of background retinopathy, with marked increase in capillary permeability, giving rise to oedema of the macular retina, in addition to the features of background diabetic retinopathy. Visual acuity may be considerably reduced in this condition, but peripheral vision remains unaffected. (3) *Proliferative diabetic retinopathy*. Here new blood vessels grow from the optic disc and/or retina, and vitreous haemorrhages may occur from these vessels, so causing severe reduction of vision. As this condition progresses, contraction of fibrous tissue associated with the neovascularization may cause the retina to detach.

Laser photocoagulation can often arrest the progress of diabetic maculopathy and proliferative retinopathy, and vitreous surgery may be of value in advanced stage of proliferative diabetic retinopathy.

hypertensive r. that associated with essential hypertension; changes may include irregular narrowing of the retinal arterioles, haemorrhages in the nerve fibre layers and the outer plexiform layer, hard exudates and cotton-wool spots, arteriosclerotic changes, and, in malignant hypertension, papilloedema.

leukaemic r. a condition occurring in leukaemia, with paleness of the fundus resulting from infiltration of the retina and choroid with accumulations of the abnormal leukocytes, and swelling of the disc with blurring of its margin.

r. of prematurity see RETROLENTAL fibroplasia.

proliferative r. the proliferative type of diabetic retinopathy.

retinoschisis (ˌreti'noskisis) splitting of the retina, occurring in the nerve fibre layer (in juvenile form), or in the external plexiform layer (in adult form).

retinoscope ('retinəˌskohp) skiascope; an instrument used in retinoscopy.

retinoscopy (ˌreti'noskəpee) an objective method of investigating, diagnosing, and evaluating refractive errors of the eye, by projection of a beam of light into the eye and observation of the movement of the illuminated area on the retina surface and of the refraction by the eye of the emergent rays. Called also pupilloscopy, shadow test, skiametry, and skiascopy.

retinotopic (ˌretinoh'topik) relating to the organization of the visual pathways and visual area of the brain.

retort (ri'tawt) a globular, long-necked vessel used in distillation.

retothelium (ˌreetoh'theeli·əm) reticuloendothelium.

retractile (ri'traktiel) susceptible of being drawn back.

retraction (ri'trakshən) the act of drawing back, or condition of being drawn back.

clot r. the drawing away of a blood clot from a vessel wall, a function of blood platelets.

retractor (ri'traktə) 1. an instrument for holding open the edges of a wound. 2. a muscle that retracts.

retrieval (ri'treev'l) in psychology, the process of obtaining memory information from wherever it has been stored.

retro- word element. [L.] *behind*, *backward*.

retroaction (ˌretroh'akshən) action in a reversed direction; reaction.

retroauricular (ˌretroh·or'rikyuhlə) behind the auricle of the ear.

retrobulbar (ˌretroh'bulbə) 1. behind the pons. 2. behind the eyeball.

retrocaecal (ˌretroh'seek'l) behind the caecum.

retrocervical (ˌretroh'sərvik'l, -sə'vie-) behind the cervix uteri.

retrocession (ˌretroh'seshən) a going backward; backward displacement.

retrocochlear (ˌretroh'kokli·ə) 1. behind the cochlea. 2. denoting the eighth cranial nerve and cerebellopontine angle as opposed to the cochlea.

retrocolic (ˌretroh'kolik) behind the colon.

retrocollic (ˌretroh'kolik) pertaining to the back of the neck; nuchal.

retrocollis (ˌretroh'kolis) spasmodic torticollis in which the head is drawn back.

retrocursive (ˌretroh'kərsiv) marked by stepping backward.

retrodeviation (ˌretrohˌdeevi'ayshən) a general term including retroversion, retroflexion, retroposition, etc.

retrodisplacement (ˌretrohdis'playsmənt) backward or posterior displacement.

retroesophageal (ˌretroh·iˌsofə'jeeəl) behind the oesophagus.

retroflexion (ˌretroh'flekshən) the bending of an organ so that its top is thrust backward: specifically, the bending backward of the body of the uterus upon the cervix.

retrogasserian (ˌretrohga'siə·ri·ən) pertaining to the sensory (posterior) root of the trigeminal (gasserian) ganglion.

retrognathia (ˌretroh'nathi·ə) underdevelopment of the maxilla and/or mandible. adj. **retrognathic**.

retrograde ('retrəˌgrayd) going backward; retracting a former course.

r. pyelography radiography of the kidney after introduction of contrast medium through the ureter, usually at cystography.

retrogression (ˌretrə'greshən) degeneration; deterioration; regression; return to an earlier, less complex condition.

retroinsular (ˌretroh'insyuhlə) behind the island of Reil of the cerebral cortex.

retrolental (ˌretroh'lent'l) behind the lens of the eye.

r. fibroplasia retinopathy of prematurity (ROP); a disease of the developing retinal vasculature of the premature newborn. Incidence correlates with the degree of maturity; that is, the shorter the gestational period the greater the possibility it will occur. The cause of the disorder is vasoconstriction of retinal capillaries due to the presence of very high concentrations of oxygen in these blood vessels. This produces the development of an overgrowth of blood vessels in the retina. The vascular proliferation and exudation of blood and serum detaches the retina and produces scarring and inevitable blindness. To prevent retrolental fibroplasia it is recommended that oxygen be administered to premature newborns in as low a concentration and for as short a time as feasible. Careful monitoring of the newborn and evaluation of oxygen tension level is essential because no totally safe dosage of oxygen that will prevent the retinal changes has been found.

retrolingual (ˌretroh'ling·gwəl) behind the tongue.

retromammary (ˌretroh'mamə·ree) behind the mammary gland.

retromandibular (ˌretrohman'dibyuhlə) behind the lower jaw.

retromastoid (ˌretroh'mastoyd) behind the mastoid process.

retromorphosis (ˌretrohmaw'fohsis) retrograde metamorphosis.

retronasal (ˌretroh'nayz'l) pertaining to the back part of the nose.

retro-ocular (ˌretroh'okyuhlə) behind the eye.

retroparotid (ˌretrohpə'rotid) behind the parotid gland.

retroperitoneal (ˌretrohˌperitə'neeəl) behind the peritoneum.

r. fibrosis deposition of fibrous tissue in the retroperitoneal space, producing vague abdominal discomfort, and often causing blockage of the ureters, with resultant hydronephrosis and impaired renal function, which may result in renal failure. Called also *Ormond's disease*.

retroperitoneum (ˌretrohˌperitə'neeəm) the retroperitoneal space; the space between the peritoneum and the posterior abdominal wall.

retroperitonitis (ˌretrohˌperitə'nietis) inflammation in the retroperitoneal space.

retropharyngeal (ˌretrohfə'rinji·əl, -ˌfarin'jeeəl) behind the pharynx.

retropharyngitis (ˌretrohˌfarin'jietis) inflammation of posterior part of the pharynx.

retroplasia (ˌretroh'playzi·ə) retrograde metaplasia; degeneration of a tissue or cell into a more primitive type.

retroposed ('retrohˌpohzd) displaced backward.

retroposition (ˌretrohpə'zishən) backward displacement.

retropubic (ˌretroh'pyoobik) behind the pubic bone.

retropulsion (ˌretroh'pulshən) 1. a driving back, as of the fetal head in labour. 2. tendency to walk backward, as in some cases of tabes dorsalis. 3. an abnormal gait in which the body is bent backward.

retrospective study (ˌretrə'spektiv) see CASE control study and INCIDENCE study.

retrosternal (ˌretroh'stərnəl) behind the sternum.

retrotarsal (ˌretroh'tahs'l) behind the tarsus of the eye.

retrouterine (ˌretroh'yootəˌrien) behind the uterus.

retroversion (ˌretroh'vərshən) the tipping backward of an entire organ, as of the uterus.

retrovesical (ˌretroh'vesik'l) behind the urinary bladder.

retrovirus (ˌretroh'vierəs) a large group of RNA viruses, including human T-cell leukaemia viruses, lentiviruses, and the causative virus of AIDS, HIV (human immunodeficiency virus).

Reuss's colour charts ('roysiz) charts with coloured letters printed on coloured backgrounds; used for testing colour vision.

revascularization (reeˌvaskyuhlə·rie'zayshən) the restoration of blood supply either by natural means or by a blood vessel graft.

Reverdin's graft ('revərdanhz) a form of skin graft in which pieces of skin are placed as islands over the raw area. See also GRAFT and GRAFTING.

Reverdin's needle a curved needle with an eye that can be opened by means of a slide on a long handle.

reversal (ri'vərs'l) a turning or change in the opposite direction.

sex r. a change in characteristics from those typical of one sex to those typical of the other.

reverse isolation (ri'vərs) see PROTECTIVE ISOLATION.

reverse transcriptase an enzyme of RNA viruses that catalyses the transcription of RNA to DNA, which is then incorporated into the genome of the host cell. It is characteristic of retroviruses. See also CANCER.

reversion (ri'vərshən) 1. a returning to a previous condition; regression. 2. in genetics, inheritance from some remote ancestor of a character that has not been manifest for several generations.

revulsant (ri'vulsənt) revulsive.

revulsion (ri'vulshən) the drawing of blood from one part to another, as in counterirritation; the diminution of morbid action in any part of the body by irritation in another.

revulsive (ri'vulsiv) 1. causing revulsion. 2. an agent causing revulsion; a counterirritant.

Reye's syndrome (riez) an acute, potentially fatal disease of childhood, characterized by severe oedema of the brain and increased intracranial pressure, hypoglycaemia, and fatty infiltration and dysfunction of the liver. The cause of Reye's syndrome is unknown but administration of salicylates in children under the age of 12 is not recommended unless specifically indicated. This follows evidence that aspirin may be a contributory factor in the development of Reye's syndrome in some children.

Further information can be obtained from the National Reye's Syndrome Foundation of the UK, 55 High Street, Banbury, Oxfordshire OX16 8FF.

Rf chemical symbol, *rutherfordium*; a transuranic element, atomic number 104, atomic weight 261, symbol Rf, produced by an induced nuclear reaction.

RGN Registered General Nurse.

Rh 1. chemical symbol, *rhodium*. 2. symbol for Rhesus factor (see RH FACTOR).

Rh$_{null}$ symbol for a rare blood type in which all Rh factors are lacking; see RH-NULL SYNDROME.

Rh factor (ˌahaych faktə) antigens present on the surfaces of erythrocytes of 83 per cent of Caucasian people and 99–100 per cent of other races. These individuals are said to be Rhesus positive. Individuals without the antigens are said to be Rhesus negative (about 17 per cent in the UK). The term comes from the Rhesus monkey, on which initial experiments were carried out. There are three pairs of Rh antigens, Cc, Dd and Ee. The D antigen is responsible for Rh immunity in the majority of cases. A capital letter indicates that a person is Rh positive to factors C, D or E, and a small letter indicates that a person is Rh negative to factors c, d or e.

The Rh factor assumes importance during blood transfusion or pregnancy. Rh negative blood may be transfused into anyone, whether their blood is Rh positive or Rh negative. However, if Rh positive blood is given to a person with Rh negative blood an autoimmune response is initiated. There will be no apparent reaction, as is the case with an ABO incompatible transfusion, and the blood cells with not clump or agglutinate. Instead, anti-D antibodies are produced by the recipient. In the event of a subsequent exposure to Rh D positive blood, these antibodies will react against the erythrocytes carrying the Rh antigen and haemolyse them. The extent of the reaction is determined by the number of antibodies produced in response to the initial immunization and the size of the subsequent transfusion.

During pregnancy, under normal circumstances, the fetal circulation remains completely separate from that of the mother. However, during the third stage of labour (transplacental haemorrhage) abortion, placenta praevia or placental abruption, or because of other trauma or sometimes for no known cause, fetal erythrocytes enter the maternal bloodstream. Under normal circumstances this is not a problem, but if the fetal blood is Rh positive and the mother's blood is Rh negative, an autoimmune response is triggered. This is called iso-immunization, Rhesus disease or HAEMOLYTIC disease of the newborn, and was formerly called erythroblastosis fetalis. The response is identical to that described in the adult for Rh incompatible blood transfusion, but the problem may not become apparent until the second or subsequent pregnancy. Anti-D antibodies are small enough to pass freely across the placenta and enter the fetal circulation, where they destroy the fetal Rh positive erythrocytes, causing anaemia, oedema (HYDROPS FETALIS) and, if not arrested, fetal death by cardiac failure. The fetus in utero does not demonstrate jaundice, because bilirubin, the end product of erythrocyte destruction, is excreted by the placenta and detoxified by the mother.

The possibility of Rhesus incompatibility is screened for during pregnancy by regular checks on the mother's antibody titres, and amniocentesis, which enables measurement of the degree of bilirubin in the liquor. Nowadays, the majority of babies can be given an interuterine transfusion of Rh *negative* blood to maintain their haemoglobin levels, and so prevent hydrops fetalis, until such time as it is possible to care for them outside the uterus.

Jaundice which develops within 24 hours of birth is suggestive of Rh incompatibility, and serum bilirubin levels should be monitored regularly. High levels of unconjugated, fat-soluble bilirubin lodge in fatty tissues, pigmenting the skin. Kernicterus is a potentially fatal condition which results from excessive levels of serum bilirubin, the immature infant being most susceptible. Exchange blood transfusion may be required to keep the serum bilirubin at a safe level, until such time as the baby's own liver can conjugate the bilirubin into a water-soluble form which can be safely excreted.

Prevention of Rhesus iso-immunization is now standard practice. A specimen of maternal blood is taken within one hour of delivery or other exposure to risk, for the KLEIHAUER TEST, which will demonstrate whether any fetal cells have entered the maternal bloodstream. If the test is positive, the fetal cells are Rh positive, and the mother is Rh negative, and intramuscular injection of Rh and anti-D immunoglobulin (IgG) is given to the mother within the next 72 hours. The effect is to coat the offending Rh positive fetal cells, making them inert, i.e. no longer capable of eliciting antibody reaction by the maternal reticuloendothelial system. Immunization must be repeated in the Rh negative woman after the birth of every Rh positive fetus, and following every termination of pregnancy.

Rh-null syndrome chronic haemolytic anaemia affecting individuals who lack all Rh factors (Rh_{null}); it is marked by spherocytosis, stomatocytosis, and increased osmotic fragility.

RHA Regional Health Authority.

rhabd(o)- word element. [Gr.] *rod, rod-shaped.*

Rhabditis (rab'dietis) a genus of minute nematodes found mostly in damp earth, and as an accidental parasite in man.

rhabdocyte ('rabdoh,siet) metamyelocyte.

rhabdoid ('rabdoyd) resembling a rod; rod-shaped.

rhabdomyoblastoma (ˌrabdohˌmieohbla'stohmə) rhabdomyosarcoma.

rhabdomyolysis (ˌrabdohmie'olisis) disintegration of striated muscle fibres with excretion of myoglobin in the urine.

rhabdomyoma (ˌrabdohmie'ohmə) a tumour containing striated muscle fibres.

rhabdomyosarcoma (ˌrabdohˌmieohsah'kohmə) a highly malignant tumour arising in striated muscle or in embryonal mesenchymal cells, and exhibiting differentiation along rhabdomyoblastic lines, including but not limited to the presence of cells with recognizable cross striations. The pleomorphic form affects predominantly the skeletal muscles of adults; the embryonal-alveolar form occurs mainly in the skeletal muscles of children and young adults, and the embryonal-botryoid form occurs predominantly in tissues of the head, neck, orbit, and urogenital tract of children and young adults.

rhabdosarcoma (ˌrabdohsah'kohmə) rhabdomyosarcoma.

rhabdovirus (ˌrabdoh'vierəs) any of a group of morphologically similar bullet-shaped or bacilliform RNA viruses.

rhachi- for words beginning thus, see those beginning *rachi-*.

rhagades ('ragəˌdeez) fissures, cracks, or fine scars in the skin, especially such lesions around the mouth or other regions subjected to frequent movement.

rhaphe ('rayfee) raphe.

RHB Regional Health Board.

rhegma ('regmə) a rupture, rent, or fracture.

rhegmatogenous (ˌregmə'tojənəs) arising from a rhegma, as in rhegmatogenous detachment of the retina, i.e. where the detachment is caused by a retinal tear.

rhenium ('reeni·əm) a chemical element, atomic number 75, atomic weight 186.2, symbol Re. See table of elements in Appendix 2.

rheo- word element. [Gr.] *electric current, flow* (as of fluids).

rheobase ('reeoh,bays) the minimum electric current necessary to produce stimulation. adj. **rheobasic.**

rheology (ri'oləjee) the science of the deformation and flow of matter, such as the flow of blood through the heart and blood vessels.

rheostat ('ri·ə,stat) an apparatus for regulating resistance in an electric circuit.

rheostosis (ˌreeo'stohsis) a condition of hyperostosis marked by the presence of streaks in the bones; melorheostosis.

rheotaxis (ˌri·ə'taksis) orientation of an organism in a stream of liquid, with its long axis parallel with the direction of flow, designated negative (moving in the same direction) or positive (moving in the opposite direction).

Rhesus blood group system ('reesəs) a complex antigenic system restricted to red cells. It is clinically important because Rh negative people readily form anti-Rh antibodies after a transfusion of Rh positive blood. Subsequent transfusions of Rh positive blood could lead to a reaction. Pregnancy in a Rh negative mother carrying a Rh positive child can result in HAEMOLYTIC DISEASE OF THE NEWBORN. The three main antigens are designated CDE, and their alternative alleles are cde. Eighty-three per cent of white populations are Rh positive. Commonly recognized genotypes include CDe/cde, CDe/CDe, CDe/cDE. Rh negative subjects are cde/cde.

rheum (room) any watery or catarrhal discharge.

rheumarthritis (ˌroomah'thrietis) rheumatoid arthritis.

rheumatalgia (ˌroomə'talji·ə) chronic rheumatic pain.

rheumatic (roo'matik) pertaining to or affected with rheumatism.

r. fever a disease associated with the presence of haemolytic streptococci in the body. It is called rheumatic fever because two of the commonest symptoms are fever and pain in the joints similar to that of rheumatism. Rheumatic fever is becoming less common; it occurs particularly among children between 5 and 15 years of age. Young adults in the early twenties are also susceptible, although less so.

CAUSES. Rheumatic fever is a delayed sequela of an upper respiratory infection caused by the Group A haemolytic streptococcus that causes such common childhood illnesses as scarlet fever, tonsillitis, 'strep throat', and ear infections. Rheumatic fever is only one of several complications that can result from a streptococcal infection.

The connection between rheumatic fever and a previous streptococcal infection has been proved only indirectly. That is, in almost all cases of rheumatic fever there is evidence of a previous streptococcal infection; and when these infections have been treated promptly, the occurrence of rheumatic fever has declined sharply. There is evidence that the symptoms of rheumatic fever may result from an antigen–antibody reaction to one or more of the products of the haemolytic streptococcus, but the exact way in which this occurs is not known. Rheumatic fever has been classified as an AUTOIMMUNE DISEASE.

Rheumatic fever tends to run in families, and there may be a hereditary predisposition to the disease. Economic and environmental conditions such as damp, cold climate and poor health habits may be contributing factors.

SYMPTOMS. The initial symptoms usually appear 1 to 4 weeks after the streptococcal infection has occurred. The actual onset of the disease may be either gradual or sudden. The symptoms vary widely and may be of any degree of severity.

The commonest initial complaints are a slight fever, a feeling of tiredness, a vague feeling of pain in the limbs, and nosebleeds. If the disease takes an acute form, the fever may reach 40 °C (104 °F) by the second day and continue for several weeks, although the usual course of the fever is about 2 weeks. On the other hand, the fever may be quite mild.

Joint pain develops at any stage of the disease and lasts from a few hours to several weeks. The joints swell and are tender to the touch. The pain and swelling often subside in one group of joints and arise in another. As the pain subsides, the joints return to normal.

Other symptoms may include spasmodic twitching movements known as Sydenham's chorea, often called St. Vitus's dance; it is most common in girls between the ages of 6 and 11. A rash caused by the fever may appear upon the body. Nodules may be seen or felt under the skin at the elbow, knee, and wrist joints, and along the spine. Among the most serious signs is the development of a heart murmur and cardiac decompensation.

HEART DAMAGE. The seriousness of rheumatic fever lies primarily in the permanent damage it can do to the heart. The disease tends to recur; and these recurrent attacks may further weaken the heart.

The usual cardiac complication of rheumatic fever is endocarditis—inflammation of the inner lining of the heart, including the membrane over the valves. As a valve heals, its edges may become so scarred and stiff that they fail to close properly. As a result, blood leaks through the valve when it is closed, producing the sound characteristic of a heart murmur. The valves may become thickened with scar tissue, so that the amount of blood that can flow through the heart is restricted. If there is severe stenosis of the mitral valve and the patient develops symptoms of congestive heart failure, surgery to enlarge the valve (mitral COMMISSUROTOMY) may be indicated.

TREATMENT. The main purposes of treatment are reduction of fever and pain and promotion of the natural healing processes; no means have yet been discovered for fighting the disease directly. Until the introduction of antibiotics, the chief medications were aspirin and other salicylates. Penicillin is prescribed if there is evidence of a ongoing streptococcal infection or the chance of exposure to streptococcal infection. Prednisone may be prescribed to reduce the pain and swelling in the joints, but it has little or no effect on the ultimate course of the disease. If pain is severe, analgesic drugs may be given.

Bed rest is an important part of the treatment, particularly if the disease has caused heart damage. Depending upon the severity of the disease, the patient may be kept in bed for months, and prolonged convalescence may be needed.

PATIENT CARE. In the acute phase of rheumatic fever rest is most important to reduce the work load of the heart. The patient should be made as comfortable as possible and disturbed only when necessary. The care should be planned so that long periods of complete rest are possible. Proper positioning with adequate support of the limbs and maintenance of good body alignment is essential to rest and the prevention of complications.

The temperature, pulse, and respirations are checked and recorded frequently. The volume and rhythm as well as the rate of the pulse should be noted. Fluid intake may be restricted if there is oedema, and sodium intake may also be limited; in either case the reason for the restriction should be explained to the patient. A record is kept of the intake and output.

Frequent turning and good oral hygiene are needed to promote comfort and relaxation. When turning the patient, one should be gentle and slow, avoiding unnecessary handling of the joints, which may be tender and swollen.

During the convalescence period the patient is allowed a gradual return to physical activities. The amount of activity is based on the patient's pulse rate, erythrocyte sedimentation rate, and C-reaction protein test. Measures must be taken to avoid respiratory infections, which will retard the progress of the patient. Small, frequent feedings that provide a well-balanced diet are usually preferred to three meals a day, which may be only partially eaten by a patient who is not engaging in a normal amount of physical activity.

As the need for rest is decreased, some provision must be made for diversional activities that will help eliminate boredom and keep the child content. The psychological effects of a prolonged period of enforced dependence on others must also be considered. The parents and the child will need encouragement and help in the transition from total dependence to relative independence.

PREVENTION. Preventive care is extremely important, especially when rheumatic fever has once occurred, since it tends to return unless precautionary steps are taken. The patient is given penicillin, orally every day or by intramuscular injection once a month, for many years in order to prevent streptococcal infection. A good nutritious diet and sufficient sleep are important. Administration of antibiotics to all patients with history of rheumatic fever undergoing even minor surgery, including tooth extraction, is important in preventing bacterial endocarditis.

Prompt and effective treatment of 'strep throat' among the general population has reduced the incidence of rheumatic fever.

r. heart disease the most important and constant manifestation of rheumatic fever, consisting of inflammatory changes with valvular deformities.

rheumatid ('roomətid) any skin lesion aetiologically associated with rheumatism.

rheumatism ('roomə,tizəm) any of a variety of disorders marked by inflammation, degeneration, or metabolic derangement of the connective tissue structures, especially the joints and related structures, and attended by pain, stiffness, or limitation of motion; a term applied by laymen to such disorders as ARTHRITIS, OSTEOARTHRITIS, BURSITIS, and SCIATICA.

acute articular r. rheumatic fever.

muscular r. fibrositis.

palindromic r. repeated attacks of arthritis and periarthritis without fever and without causing irreversible joint changes.

rheumatoid ('roomə,toyd) resembling rheumatism.

r. arthritis a chronic systemic disease with inflammatory changes occurring throughout the body's connective tissues, which lead to progressive deforming arthritis (see also rheumatoid ARTHRITIS).

r. disease rheumatoid arthritis with emphasis on nonarticular changes, e.g., pulmonary interstitial fibrosis, pleural effusion, and lung nodules.

r. factor a protein of high molecular weight in the serum of most patients with rheumatoid arthritis, detectable by serological tests.

rheumatologist (,roomə'toləjist) a specialist in rheumatology.

rheumatology (,roomə'toləjee) the branch of medicine dealing with rheumatic disorders, their causes, pathology, diagnosis, treatment, etc.

rhexis ('reksis) the rupture of a blood vessel or of an organ.

rhigosis (ri'gohsis) the perception of cold.

rhin(o)- word element. [Gr.] *nose, noselike structure.*

rhinaesthesia (,rienistheezi·ə) the sense of smell.

rhinal ('rien'l) pertaining to the nose.

rhinalgia (rie'nalji·ə) pain in the nose.

rhinencephalon (ˌrienen'kefəlon, -'sef-) 1. the part of the brain once thought to be concerned entirely with olfactory mechanisms, including olfactory nerves, bulbs, tracts, and subsequent connections (all olfactory in function) and the limbic system (not primarily olfactory in function); homologous with olfactory portions of the brain in lower animals. 2. one of the parts of the embryonic telencephalon.
rhineurynter (ˌrienyooə'rintə) a dilatable rubber bag for distending a nostril.
rhinion ('rienion) the lower end of the suture between the nasal bones.
rhinitis (rie'nietis) inflammation of the mucous membrane of the nose. It may be mild and chronic, or acute. See COMMON COLD.

Chronic rhinitis may result in a permanent thickening of the nasal mucosa.

allergic r., anaphylactic r. any allergic reaction of the nasal mucosa, occurring perennially (nonseasonal allergic rhinitis) or seasonally (HAY FEVER).
atrophic r. chronic rhinitis with wasting of the mucous membrane and glands.
r. caseosa that with a caseous, gelatinous, and fetid discharge.
fibrinous r. rhinitis with development of a false membrane.
hypertrophic r. that with thickening and swelling of the mucous membrane.
membranous r. chronic rhinitis with a membranous exudate.
nonseasonal allergic r. allergic rhinitis occurring continuously or intermittently all year round, due to exposure to a more or less ever-present allergen, marked by sudden attacks of sneezing, swelling of the nasal mucosa with profuse watery discharge, itching of the eyes, and lacrimation. Called also nonseasonal, or perennial, hay fever.
purulent r. chronic rhinitis with formation of pus.
vasomotor r. 1. nonallergic rhinitis in which transient changes in vascular tone and permeability (with the same symptoms of allergic rhinitis) are brought on by such stimuli as mild chilling, fatigue, anger, and anxiety. 2. any condition of allergic or nonallergic rhinitis, as opposed to infectious rhinitis.
rhinoantritis (ˌrienoh·an'trietis) inflammation of the nasal cavity and maxillary sinus.
rhinocanthectomy (ˌrienohkan'thektəmee) rhinommectomy.
rhinocephalus (ˌrienoh'kefələs, -'sef-) a fetus exhibiting rhinocephaly.
rhinocephaly (ˌrienoh'kefəlee) a developmental anomaly characterized by the presence of a proboscis-like nose above eyes partially or completely fused into one.
rhinocheiloplasty (ˌrienoh'kieloh,plastee) plastic surgery of the nose and lip.
rhinocleisis (ˌrienoh'kliesis) obstruction of the nasal passage.
rhinodacryolith (ˌrienoh'dakrioh,lith) a lacrimal concretion in the nasal duct.
rhinodynia (ˌrienoh'dini·ə) pain in the nose.
rhinogenous (rie'nojənəs) arising in the nose.
rhinokyphosis (ˌrienohkie'fohsis) an abnormal hump on the ridge of the nose.
rhinolalia (ˌrienoh'layli·ə) a nasal quality of speech from some disease or defect of the nasal passages.
r. aperta that due to too great opening of the nasal passages.
r. clausa that due to undue closure of the nasal passages.
rhinolaryngitis (ˌrienoh,larin'jietis) inflammation of the mucosa of the nose and larynx.
rhinolith ('rienoh,lith) a nasal calculus.
rhinolithiasis (ˌrienohli'thieəsis) a condition associated with formation of rhinoliths.
rhinologist (rie'noləjist) a specialist in rhinology.
rhinology (rie'noləjee) the sum of knowledge about the nose and its diseases.
rhinomanometer (ˌrienohmə'nomitə) a manometer used in rhinomanometry.
rhinomanometry (ˌrienohmə'nomətree) measurement of the airflow and pressure within the nose during respiration; nasal resistance or obstruction can be calculated from the figures obtained.
rhinometer (rie'nomitə) an instrument for measuring the nose or its cavities.
rhinommectomy (ˌrienə'mektəmee) excision of the inner canthus of the eye.
rhinomycosis (ˌrienohmie'kohsis) fungal infection of the nasal mucosa.
rhinonecrosis (ˌrienohnə'krohsis) necrosis of the nasal bones.
rhinopathy (rie'nopəthee) any disease of the nose.
rhinopharyngitis (ˌrienoh,farin'jietis) inflammation of the nasopharynx.
rhinophonia (ˌrienoh'fohni·ə) a nasal twang or quality of voice.
rhinophore ('rienoh,for) a nasal cannula to facilitate breathing.
rhinophycomycosis (ˌrienoh,fiekohmie'kohsis) a fungal disease caused by *Entomophora coronata*, marked by formation of large polyps in the subcutaneous tissues of the nose and paranasal sinuses; orbital involvement and unilateral blindness may follow. Cerebral involvement is common.
rhinophyma (ˌrienoh'fiemə) a form of rosacea marked by redness, sebaceous hyperplasia, and nodular swelling and congestion of the skin of the nose.
rhinoplasty ('rienoh,plastee) plastic surgery of the nose.
rhinopolypus (ˌrienoh'polipəs) a nasal polyp.
rhinorrhagia (ˌrienoh'rayji·ə) nosebleed; epistaxis.
rhinorrhoea (ˌrienə'reeə) the free discharge of a thin nasal mucus.
cerebrospinal r. discharge of cerebrospinal fluid through the nose, usually due to skull fracture.
rhinosalpingitis (ˌrienoh,salpin'jietis) inflammation of the mucosa of the nose and pharyngotympanic tube.
rhinoscleroma (ˌrienohskliə'rohmə) a granulomatous disease involving the nose and nasopharynx. The growth forms hard patches or nodules, which tend to enlarge and are painful to the touch. The disease occurs in Egypt, eastern Europe, and Central and South America. It is ascribed to the presence of *Klebsiella rhinoscleromatis*.
rhinoscope ('rienoh,skohp) a speculum for use in nasal examination.
rhinoscopy (rie'noskəpee) examination of the nose with a speculum, through either the anterior nares or the nasopharynx.
rhinosporidiosis (ˌrienohspə,ridi'ohsis) a fungal disease caused by *Rhinosporidium seeberi*, marked by large polyps on the mucosa of the nose, eyes, ears, and sometimes the penis and vagina.
rhinotomy (rie'notəmee) incision into the nose.
rhinovirus (ˌrienoh'vierəs) a subgroup of the picornaviruses, considered to be aetiologically associated with the common cold and certain other upper respiratory ailments. Over 90 antigenically different strains are known to cause the common cold. Called also coryzavirus.
Rhipicephalus (ˌriepi'kefələs, -'sef-) a genus of hard ticks which can transmit the rickettsiae which cause typhus.
rhizo- ('riezoh) word element. [Gr.] *root*.

rhizoid ('riezoyd) resembling a root.
rhizolysis (rie'zolisis) interruption of spinal nerve roots by coagulation with radiofrequency waves.
rhizomelic (ˌriezoh'melik) pertaining to the hips and shoulders (the roots of the limbs).
rhizomeningomyelitis (ˌriezohməˌning·gohˌmieə-'lietis) radiculomeningomyelitis; inflammation of the nerve roots, meninges, and spinal cord.
rhizoneure ('riezohˌnyooə) a nerve cell forming a nerve root.
Rhizopoda (rie'zopədə) a class of protozoa of the subphylum Sarcodina, having pseudopodia, and including the amoebae.
rhizopodium (ˌriezoh'pohdi·əm) pl. *rhizopodia* [Gr.] a filamentous pseudopodium, characterized by branching and anastomosis of the branches.
rhizotomy (rie'zotəmee) division or transection of a nerve root, either within the spinal canal or outside it.
rhod(o)- ('rohdoh) word element. [Gr.] *red.*
rhodium ('rohdi·əm) a chemical element, atomic number 45, atomic weight 102.905, symbol Rh. See table of elements in Appendix 2.
rhodogenesis (ˌrohdoh'jenəsis) regeneration of rhodopsin after its bleaching by light.
rhodophylaxis (ˌrohdohfi'laksis) the property of the retinal epithelium of facilitating rhodogenesis. adj. **rhodophylactic.**
rhodopsin (roh'dopsin) visual purple: a photosensitive purple-red chromoprotein in the retinal rods that is bleached to visual yellow (all-*trans* retinal) by light, thereby stimulating retinal sensory endings. Lack of rhodopsin results in NIGHT BLINDNESS. Vitamin A is the primary source of rhodopsin.
rhombencephalon (ˌromben'kefəlon, -'sef-) 1. the hindbrain, including the medulla oblongata, pons, and cerebellum. 2. the most caudal of the three primary vesicles formed in embryonic development of the brain, which later divides into the metencephalon and the myelencephalon.
rhombocoele ('rombohˌseel) the terminal expansion of the canal of the spinal cord.
rhomboid ('romboyd) shaped like a rectangle that has been skewed to one side so that the angles are oblique.
rhonchus ('rongkəs) pl. *rhonchi* [L.] a rattling in the throat; also, a dry, coarse rale in the bronchial tubes, due to a partial obstruction. adj. **rhonchal, rhonchial.**
RHV Registered Health Visitor.
rhythm ('ridhəm) a measured movement; the recurrence of an action or function at regular intervals. adj. **rhythmic, rhythmical.**

alpha r. a uniform rhythm of waves in the normal electroencephalogram, showing an average frequency of 10 per second, typical of a normal person awake in a quiet resting state. Called also *Berger's rhythm.* See also ELECTROENCEPHALOGRAPHY.

beta r. a rhythm in the electroencephalogram consisting of waves smaller than those of the alpha rhythm, having an average frequency of 25 per second, typical during periods of intense activity of the nervous system. See also ELECTROENCEPHALOGRAPHY.

biological r's the cyclic changes that occur in physiological processes of living organisms; called also biorhythms. These rhythms are so persistent throughout the living kingdom that they probably should be considered a fundamental characteristic of life, as are growth, reproduction, metabolism, and irritability. Many of the physiological rhythms occurring in humans about every 24 hours (circadian rhythm) have been known for centuries. Examples include the peaks and troughs that are manifested in body temperature, vital signs, brain function, and muscular activity. Biochemical analyses of urine, blood enzymes, and plasma serum also have demonstrated rhythmic fluctuations in a 24-hour period.

It has long been believed that the cyclic changes observed in plants and animals were totally in response to environmental changes and, as such, were exogenous or of external origin. This hypothesis is now being rejected by some chronobiologists who hold that the biological rhythms are intrinsic to the organisms, and that the organisms possess their own physiological mechanism for keeping time. This mechanism has been called the 'biological clock'. An example of adjustment of the biological clock in humans is recovery from 'jet lag'. This phenomenon, also known as jet syndrome, occurs when humans are transported by jet plane across time zones. It is characterized by fatigue and lowered efficiency, which persist until the 'biological clock' adjusts to the new environmental cycle.

Biological rhythms are responsive to, or synchronous with, environmental cycles, but it is generally agreed among chronobiologists that the rhythmic changes in environmental factors do not create biological rhythms, even though they are capable of influencing them. Even in the absence of such environmental stimuli as light, darkness, temperature, gravity, and electromagnetic field, biological rhythms continue to maintain their cyclic nature for a period of time. Seasonal changes in morbidity and mortality in humans were formerly considered to be exclusively related to environmental changes; however, this hypothesis is now being challenged by chronobiologists, who contend that circannual (yearly) biological rhythms can and do have an effect on the incidence of heart attacks, insulin needs in diabetics, and other endocrine and related disorders.

It is expected that with continued research in the fields of the physical and behavioural sciences and pharmacology, additional information on the biological rhythms in humans and the enzymatic activity in drug metabolism will greatly influence future modes of treatment and the scheduling of all forms of therapy, including elective surgery and psychotherapy.

circadian r. the regular recurrence in cycles of about 24 hours from one stated point to another, as certain biological activities which occur at that interval, regardless of constant darkness or other environmental conditions.

circannual r. the recurrence of a phenomenon in cycles of about one year. **circamensual r.** that which occurs in cycles of about one month (30 days).

circaseptan r. that which occurs in cycles of about seven days (one week).

coupled r. heart beats occurring in pairs, the second beat of the pair usually being a ventricular premature beat.

delta r. 1. electroencephalographic waves having a frequency of 2–3 hertz, typical in deep sleep, in infancy, and in serious brain disorders (see also ELECTROENCEPHALOGRAPHY). 2. delta waves.

escape r. a heart rhythm initiated by lower centres when the sinoatrial node fails to initiate impulses, its rhythmicity is depressed, or its impulses are completely blocked.

gallop r. an auscultatory finding of three or four heart sounds, the extra sounds by convention being in diastole and related to atrial contraction (fourth sound, presystolic gallop), to early rapid filling of a ventricle with an altered ventricular compliance (protodiastolic gallop), or to concurrence of atrial contraction and ventricular early rapid filling (summation gallop).

gamma r. a rhythm in the waves in the electroencephalogram having a frequency of 50 per second. See also ELECTROENCEPHALOGRAPHY.

infradian r. the regular recurrence in cycles of more than 24 hours, as certain biological activities which occur at such intervals, regardless of conditions of illumination.

nodal r. heart rhythm initiated in the specialized junctional tissue, i.e., the atrioventricular node and the main (His) bundle.

nyctohemeral r. a day and night rhythm.

pendulum r. alternation in the rhythm of the heart sounds in which the diastolic sound is equal in time, character, and loudness to the systolic sound, the beat of the heart resembling the tick of a watch.

sinus r. normal heart rhythm originating in the sinoatrial node.

theta r. electroencephalographic waves having a frequency of 4 to 7 per second, occurring mainly in children but also in adults under emotional stress. See also ELECTROENCEPHALOGRAPHY.

ultradian r. the regular recurrence in cycles of less than 24 hours, as certain biological activities which occur at such intervals, regardless of conditions of illumination.

ventricular r. the ventricular contractions which occur in cases of complete heart block.

rhythmicity (ridh'misitee) in cardiology, the ability to beat, or the state of beating, rhythmically without external stimuli.

rhytidectomy (ˌriti'dektəmee) excision of skin for elimination of wrinkles.

rhytidoplasty ('ritidohˌplastee) plastic surgery for the elimination of wrinkles.

rhytidosis (ˌriti'dohsis) a wrinkling, as of the cornea.

RIA radioimmunoassay.

rib (rib) any one of the paired bones, 12 on either side, extending from the thoracic vertebrae toward the median line on the ventral aspect of the trunk, forming the major part of the thoracic skeleton. Called also costa.

abdominal r's, asternal r's false ribs.

cervical r. a supernumerary rib arising from a cervical vertebra.

false r's the five lower ribs on either side, not attached directly to the sternum.

floating r's the two lower false ribs on either side, usually without ventral attachment.

slipping r. one whose attaching cartilage is repeatedly dislocated.

true r's the seven upper ribs on either side, attached to both vertebrae and sternum.

vertebral r's floating ribs.

vertebrocostal r's the three upper false ribs on either side, attached to vertebrae and costal cartilages.

vertebrosternal r's true ribs.

riboflavin (ˌrieboh'flayvin) vitamin B_2, a component of FAD and FMN, which are coenzymes or prosthetic groups for certain enzymes (flavoproteins) that catalyse many oxidation-reduction reactions.

Symptoms of riboflavin deficiency (ariboflavinosis) include general weakness, weight loss, lesions at the corners of the mouth, on the lips and around the nose, reddening and soreness of the tip and edges of the tongue, corneal and other eye changes, and seborrhoeic dermatitis.

Foods with the highest content of riboflavin are liver, kidney, heart, brewer's yeast, milk, eggs, greens, and enriched cereals. Riboflavin deficiency is most common among people of the southeastern United States and other regions, such as Asia and the West Indies, where the diet is likely to contain relatively large quantities of corn, potatoes, and rice, which lack riboflavin. A well-balanced diet will prevent riboflavin deficiency; it will also correct the disorder, with the help of supplementary doses of riboflavin and other vitamins.

r. kinase an enzyme (a phosphotransferase) that catalyses the conversion of free riboflavin and ATP to flavin mononucleotide (FMN) and ADP.

ribonuclease (ˌrieboh'nyookliˌayz) an enzyme that catalyses the depolymerization of ribonucleic acid.

ribonucleic acid (ˌriebohnyoo'klee·ik, -'klay-) RNA, a NUCLEIC ACID present in all living cells which controls cellular protein synthesis and replaces DNA as a carrier of genetic codes in some viruses. RNA is similar in composition to DNA with two exceptions. The sugar in RNA is ribose; in DNA it is deoxyribose. In RNA the pyrimidine uracil replaces the thymine in DNA.

The structure of RNA varies from helical to uncoiled strands of varying lengths, depending on the number of nucleotide units forming the strand. This variance in structure is evident in the different types of RNA. For example, transfer RNA (tRNA) contains only about 75 nucleotide units, while other types may contain thousands of units.

Messenger RNA (mRNA) receives its name from its function of carrying the genetic code from the nucleus of the cell to the cytoplasm, where most cellular functions take place. The transfer of the genetic code from DNA to mRNA is called transcription. Molecules of mRNA migrate to the ribosomes, where the manufacture of proteins occurs. The strands of RNA contain codons, some of which signal when formation of a particular protein should stop and the formation of another start.

Transfer RNA (tRNA), also called soluble RNA, brings about the transfer of specific amino acid molecules to protein molecules during the synthesis of proteins. Each of the 20 common amino acids found in protein molecules has a corresponding type of transfer RNA. Thus, a specific tRNA carries the appropriate amino acid to its appropriate place in the chain of the protein molecule being synthesized.

Ribosomal RNA (rRNA) is so called because it is found in the ribosomes and in some way affects the linking of amino acids into protein molecules. See also DEOXYRIBONUCLEIC ACID.

ribonucleoprotein (ˌriebohˌnyookliohˈprohteen) a substance composed of both protein and ribonucleic acid.

ribonucleoside (ˌrieboh'nyookliohˌsied) a nucleoside in which the purine or pyrimidine base is combined with ribose.

ribonucleotide (ˌrieboh'nyookliohˌtied) a nucleotide in which the purine or pyrimidine base is combined with ribose.

ribose ('riebohz) 5-carbon sugar present in ribonucleic acid (RNA).

ribosome ('riebəˌsohm) any of the intracellular ribonucleoprotein particles concerned with protein synthesis; they consist of reversibly dissociable units and are found either bound to cell membranes or free in the cytoplasm. They may occur singly or occur in clusters (polyribosomes).

ribosyl ('riebəsil) a glycosyl radical formed from ribose.

Richter's hernia ('rikhtəz) incarcerated or strangulated hernia in which only a portion of the circumference of the bowel wall is involved.

ricin ('riesin) a phytotoxin in the seeds of the castor oil plant (*Ricinus communis*), inhalation or ingestion of which causes intoxication, producing superficial inflammation of the respiratory mucosa with haemorrhages into the lungs, or oedema of the gastrointestinal tract with haemorrhages.

rickets ('rikits) a condition of infancy and childhood

caused by deficiency of vitamin D, which leads to altered calcium and phosphorus metabolism and consequent disturbance of ossification of bone.

Since the action of sunlight on the skin produces vitamin D in the human body, rickets often occurs in parts of the world where the winter is especially long, and where smoke and fog constantly intercept the sun. Dark-skinned people are somewhat more susceptible to the disease if they live in areas with little sunlight, since the pigment in the skin blocks absorption of the sun's rays.

adult r. osteomalacia; a rickets-like disease affecting adults.

fetal r. achondroplasia.

late r. OSTEOMALACIA, that occurring in older children.

renal r. renal osteodystrophy.

tardy r. late rickets.

vitamin D-resistant r. a condition almost indistinguishable from ordinary rickets clinically but resistant to unusually large doses of vitamin D; it is often familial but may occur sporadically. In hypophosphataemic vitamin D-resistant rickets, hypophosphataemia is the main characteristic, while in hypocalcaemic vitamin D-resistant rickets, the serum concentration of phosphate is within normal limits or nearly so, and the concentration of calcium is abnormally low.

Rickettsia (ri'ketsi·ə) a genus of small, rod-shaped to round microorganisms found in the cytoplasm of tissue cells of lice, fleas, ticks, and mites, and transmitted to man by their bites.

The diseases caused by rickettsiae can be classified in groups: the spotted fever group (ROCKY MOUNTAIN SPOTTED FEVER, boutonneuse fever, and rickettsialpox); the TYPHUS group (epidemic typhus and endemic typhus); a tsutsugamushi group (scrub TYPHUS); and a miscellaneous group, including Q FEVER and trench fever.

Rickettsial diseases are not common in communities with high sanitary standards, since prevention depends on controlling the rodent and insect populations. Major epidemics have occurred, especially in times of war when standards of sanitation drop.

rickettsia (ri'ketsi·ə) pl. *rickettsiae;* an individual organism of the family Rickettsiaceae.

Rickettsiaceae (ri,ketsi'aysi·ee) a family of the order Rickettsiales.

rickettsial (ri'ketsi·əl) pertaining to or caused by rickettsiae.

Rickettsiales (ri,ketsi'ayleez) an order of microorganisms occurring as elementary bodies that typically multiply only inside host cells. Parasitic for vertebrates and invertebrates, which serve as vectors, they may be pathogenic for man and other animals.

rickettsialpox (ri'ketsi·əl,poks) a febrile disease marked by a vesiculopapular eruption, resembling chickenpox clinically, caused by *Rickettsia akari* and transmitted by mites. Called also Kew Gardens spotted fever.

rickettsicidal (ri,ketsi'sied'l) destructive to rickettsiae.

ridge (rij) a linear projection or projecting structure; a crest.

dental r. any linear elevation on the crown of a tooth.

dermal r's cristae cutis, ridges of the skin produced by the projecting papillae of the corium on the palm of the hand and sole of the foot, producing a fingerprint and footprint characteristic of the individual; called also dermal ridges.

genital r. the more medial part of the urogenital ridge, giving rise to the gonad.

healing r. an indurated ridge that normally forms deep to the skin along the length of a healing wound.

interureteric r. a fold on mucous membrane extending across the bladder between the ureteric orifices.

mammary r. milk line; an ectodermal thickening in early embryos, along which the mammary glands subsequently develop.

mesonephric r. the more lateral portion of the urogenital ridge, giving rise to the mesonephros.

oblique r. a variable linear elevation obliquely crossing the occlusive surface of a maxillary molar.

urogenital r. a longitudinal ridge in the embryo, lateral to the mesentery.

Riedel's lobe ('reedəlz) an anomalous tongue-shaped mass of tissue projecting from the right lobe of the liver.

Riegel's pulse ('reegəlz) a pulse that is smaller during respiration.

Rifadin ('rifədin) trademark for a preparation of rifampicin, an antituberular drug.

rifampicin (ri'fampisin) a semisynthetic antibacterial derived from rifamycin SV, used in treatment of pulmonary tuberculosis and carriers of *Neisseria meningitidis*. Rifampicin is also used in the treatment of leprosy.

Rifinah (ri'fienə) trademark for combination preparations of rifampicin and isoniazid, antitubercular drugs.

Rift Valley fever (rift 'valee) a febrile disease with dengue-like symptoms, due to an arbovirus transmitted by mosquitoes or by contact with diseased animals; first observed in the Rift Valley, Kenya.

rigidity (ri'jiditee) inflexibility or stiffness. **clasp-knife r.** increased tension in the extensor of a joint when it is passively flexed, giving way suddenly on exertion of further pressure; seen especially in upper motor neuron disease.

cogwheel r. tension in a muscle that gives way in little jerks when the muscle is passively stretched; seen in paralysis agitans.

decerebrate r. rigid extension of the limbs as a result of decerebration; in man it also occurs as a result of lesions in the upper brain stem.

rigor ('riegor) rigidity; a sensation of cold, with convulsive shaking of the body; a chill. Rigor results from an increase in chemical activity within the body and usually ushers in a considerable rise in body temperature. The pallor and coldness of rigor, and the goose flesh that often accompanies it, are caused by constriction of the peripheral blood vessels. Rigor is symptomatic of a wide variety of diseases. It usually does not accompany well-localized infections.

PATIENT CARE. During rigor sufficient heat should be applied to maintain normal body temperature. Since the patient will most likely begin to have a sharp rise in body temperature immediately after or during rigor, it is best to use only a light blanket and several hot water bottles of moderate temperature to alleviate the sensation of cold. In addition to this the patient's temperature should be taken every 30 minutes until it is stabilized or further treatment prescribed.

r. mortis the stiffening of a dead body accompanying depletion of adenosine triphosphate in the muscle fibres.

rima ('riemə) pl. *rimae* [L.] a cleft or crack.

r. glottidis the elongated opening between the true vocal cords and between the arytenoid cartilages.

r. oris the opening of the mouth.

r. palpebrarum palpebral fissure.

r. pudendi the space between the labia majora; called also pudendal fissure.

Rimactane (ri'maktayn) trademark for a preparation of rifampicin, an antitubercular drug.

Rimactazid (ri'maktəzid) trademark for combination preparations of rifampicin and isoniazid, antitubercular drugs.

rimiterol (ri'mitərol) a beta-adrenergic receptor agonist used as a bronchodilator.

rimula ('rimyuhlə) pl. *rimulae* [L.] a minute fissure, as of the spinal cord or brain.

ring (ring) 1. any annular or circular organ, structure, or area. 2. in chemistry, a collection of atoms united in a continuous or closed chain.

abdominal r., external an opening in the aponeurosis of the external oblique muscle for the spermatic cord or round ligament.

abdominal r., internal an aperture in the transverse fascia for the spermatic cord or round ligament.

Albl's r. a ring-shaped shadow in radiographs of the skull, caused by aneurysm of a cerebral artery.

Bandl's r. pathological retraction ring. See retraction ring (below).

benzene r. the hexagon representing the arrangement of carbon atoms in a molecule of benzene, different compounds being derived by replacement of the hydrogen atoms by different elements or compounds.

Cannon's r. a focal contraction seen radiographically at the mid-third of the transverse colon, marking an area of overlap between the superior and inferiór nerve plexuses.

conjunctival r. a ring at the junction of the conjunctiva and cornea.

constriction r. localized spasm of circular muscle fibres in the uterus, resulting from incoordinate uterine action. May occur in either upper or lower segment, frequently at the junction of both. It may present in any stage of labour and may constrict the fetus around the neck or the placenta. In the third stage of labour it is referred to as 'hour-glass constriction ring'.

deep inguinal r. an aperture in the transverse fascia for the spermatic cord or the round ligament.

Kayser-Fleischer r. a grey-green to red-gold pigmented ring at the outer margin of the cornea, seen in progressive lenticular degeneration and pseudosclerosis.

retraction r. normally the physiological demarcation between upper and lower uterine segments in labour. In obstructed labour this becomes visible on the abdominal wall and is known as a *pathological* ring or BANDL'S RING.

retraction r., physiological the demarcation between the upper, contracting portion of the uterus in labour and the lower, dilating part.

Schatzki's r. a sign of hiatus hernia.

Schwalbe's r. Called also Schwalbe's LINE.

superficial inguinal r. an opening in the aponeurosis of the external oblique muscle for the spermatic cord or the round ligament.

tympanic r. the bony ring forming part of the temporal bone at birth and developing into the tympanic plate.

umbilical r. called also *annulus umbilicus*, the orifice in the abdominal wall of the fetus for transmission of the umbilical vein and arteries. After birth it is felt for some time as a distinct fibrous ring surrounding the umbilicus; these fibres later shrink progressively. See UMBILICAL HERNIA and EXOMPHALOS.

vascular r. a congenital anomaly of the aortic arch and its tributaries, the vessels forming a ring about the trachea and oesophagus and causing varying degrees of compression.

Ringer's solution ('ringəz) a sterile solution of sodium chloride, potassium chloride, and calcium chloride in purified water, a physiological salt solution for topical use.

ringworm ('ring,wərm) the popular name for a fungal infection of the skin, even though it is not caused by a worm and is not always ring-shaped in appearance. Called also TINEA.

Ringworm is caused by a group of related fungi of different types. These parasites feed on the body's waste products of dead skin and perspiration. They attack the skin in various areas, especially in body folds, such as the armpit and crotch. One type found between the toes is called ATHLETE'S FOOT; another affects the soles and toenails.

Some forms of ringworm, usually found in children and frequently traced to exposure to infected pets, attack the scalp and exposed areas of the body, particularly the arms and legs. These infections appear as reddish patches, often scaly or blistered, and may cause destruction of the hair shaft. They sometimes become ring-shaped as the infection spreads out while its centre heals or seems to heal. There is itching and soreness.

The fungi are highly infectious and are spread by humans, animals, and even objects, such as combs or towels handled by infected persons. Scratching is almost certain to pass the infection from one part of the body to another.

Ringworm is treated with an antifungal agent, griseofulvin, given orally for at least one month. Topical antifungal preparations can be used but are not 100 per cent effective. Prevention is largely a matter of cleanliness. All parts of the body should be washed with soap and water, expecially hairy areas and body folds where perspiration is likely to collect. Thorough drying is as important as bathing, for the fungi thrive in warm dampness.

Rinne test ('rinəz) a test of hearing made with tuning forks, comparing the duration of perception by bone conduction and by air conduction. In the normal ear, the fork is heard twice as long by air conduction as by bone conduction.

risk (risk) hazard, or chance of developing a disease or of complications following or during treatment. This may arise because of inherent problems with the treatment itself (e.g., drug side-effects) or because of the frailty of the patient.

absolute r. an epidemiological term for the annual rate at which a disease occurs in a given population.

acceptable r. favourable balance between possibility of complications of treatment and certainty of poor outcome if treatment not undertaken. Low probability of developing disease after exposure.

attributable r. an epidemiological term, used to reflect the likelihood of disease in a given population. Calculated as incidence rate in exposed group minus incidence rate in non-exposed group (see also relative risk below).

r. factor a factor which when added to others increases the likelihood of a disease or complication (e.g., smoking and obesity are risk factors for the development of coronary artery disease).

relative r. the likelihood of developing a disease after a given exposure; in epidemiological terms, calculated as: incidence rate of disease in an exposed group divided by incidence rate in the nonexposed group.

RIST radioimmunosorbent test.

risus ('riesəs) [L.] *laughter*.

r. sardonicus a grinning expression produced by spasm of the facial muscles.

Ritalin ('ritəlin) trademark for preparations of methylphenidate, a mild central nervous system stimulant and antidepressant.

ritodrine ('ritoh,dreen) a β_2-adrenergic receptor stimulant used to decrease uterine activity and prolong gestation in the management of premature labour.

Ritter's disease ('ritəz) dermatitis exfoliativa neonatorum.

Rivinus' incisure (ri'veenəsiz) a defect in the upper tympanic part of the temporal bone, filled by the upper portion of the tympanic membrane.
Rivotril ('rievohtril) tradename for a preparation of clonazepam, an anticonvulsant.
riziform ('rizi,fawm) resembling grains of rice.
RLL right lower lobe (of lung).
RLQ right lower quadrant (of abdomen).
RM Registered Midwife.
RMA right mentoanterior (position of the fetus).
RML right mentolateral (position of the fetus).
RMN Registered Mental Nurse.
RMO Regional Medical Officer; Resident Medical Officer.
RMP right mentoposterior (position of the fetus).
RN Registered Nurse (USA).
Rn chemical symbol, *radon.*
RNA ribonucleic acid.
RNase ribonuclease.
RNMD Registered Nurse for Mental Defectives.
RNMH Registered Nurse for the Mentally Handicapped.
RNMS Registered Nurse for the Mentally Subnormal.
RNO Regional Nursing Officer.
RNT Registered Nurse Tutor.
ROA right occipitoanterior (position of the fetus).
Roaccutane (roh'akyuhtayn) trademark for preparations of isotretinoin.
Robaxin (roh'baksin) trademark for preparations of methocarbamol, a skeletal muscle relaxant.
Robert's pelvis ('rohbairts) a transversely contracted pelvis caused by osteoarthritis affecting both sacroiliac joints, the inlet becoming a narrow wedge.
Rocaltrol (roh'kaltrohl) trademark for a preparation of calcitriol (a calcium regulator), one of the D vitamins.
Rochalimaea (,rohshəlie'meeə) a genus of the family Rickettsiaceae resembling the genus *Rickettsia*, but usually found extracellularly in the arthropod host, including *R. quintana*, the aetiological agent of trench fever, transmitted by the body louse *Pediculus humanus.*
Rocky Mountain spotted fever ('rokee 'mowntən, -tayn) an insect-borne infectious disease marked by fever, headache, muscle pain, rash, and mental symptoms. It is caused by microscopic parasites known as rickettsiae, which attack the cells lining small blood vessels. The species, *Rickettsia rickettsii* is transmitted from rodent to man by various ticks. It occurs in North and South America. Called also *tick fever*, and it is also known by various names according to the geographical area.
It responds readily to treatment with tetracyclines and chloramphenicol. If untreated, it can be extremely serious and often fatal. Preventive measures are directed mainly against the disease-carrying ticks and rodents.
rod (rod) a straight, slim mass of substance; specifically, one of the retinal rods.
Auer r. a small, stick-like inclusion seen in the cytoplasm of blast cells in acute myeloid leukaemia.
Corti's r's pillar cells; rodlike bodies in a double row in the inner ear, having their heads joined and their bases on the basilar membrane widely separated so as to form a spiral tunnel.
olfactory r. the slender apical portion of an olfactory bipolar neuron, a modified dendrite extending to the surface of the epithelium.
retinal r's highly specialized cylindrical segments of the visual cells containing rhodopsin; together with the retinal cones, they form the light-sensitive elements of the retina.
rodenticide (roh'denti,sied) 1. destructive to rodents. 2. an agent destructive to rodents.
Roentgen ('rontjən) Wilhelm Conrad (1845–1923). German physicist, born at Lennep (Rhineland). For his accidental discovery of x-rays in 1895, while experimenting with a cathode-ray tube, he received the first Nobel prize for physics in 1901.
roentgen ('rontjən) a superseded international unit of x- or γ-radiation; it is the quantity of x- or γ-radiation such that the associated corpuscular emission per 0.001293 g of air produces, in air, ions carrying 1 electrostatic unit of electrical charge of either sign. Abbreviated R. Now replaced by coulomb/kg (C/kg); see COULOMB. $1\ R = 2.58 \times 10^{-4}$ C/kg; 1 C/kg = 3876 R.
r. ray x-ray.
roentgen- for words beginning thus, see those beginning *radio-*.
Roger's disease (ro'zhairz) a ventricular septal defect; the term is usually restricted to small, asymptomatic defects.
Rogitine ('roji,teen) trademark for a preparation of phentolamine, an adrenolytic used to test for the presence of PHAEOCHROMOCYTOMA.
Rokitansky's disease (,roki'tanskiz) acute yellow atrophy of the liver.
ROL right occipitolateral (position of the fetus).
Rolando's fissure (roh'landohz) fissure of Rolando.
role (rohl) a pattern of behaviour developed in response to the demands or expectations of others; the pattern of responses to the persons with whom an individual interacts in a particular situation.
gender r. the image projected by a person that identifies his or her sex. It is the public expression of gender identity.
impaired r. the role played by a person who is disabled or chronically ill and who is experiencing a state of wellness and realization of potential commensurate with his handicap. Unlike the sick person, the impaired person cannot be expected to 'want to get well' but is expected to resume as much normal behaviour as is possible.
r. playing a technique used in family therapy and group therapy in which members of the group act out the behaviour of others in specific roles in order to recognize the roles and to clarify role responses and choices.
sick r. the role played by a person who has defined himself as ill, with or without validation of the role by doctors, nurses, or family members. Adoption of the sick role changes the behavioural expectations of others toward the sick person. He is exempted from normal social responsibilities and is not held responsible for his condition; he is obliged to 'want to get well' and to seek competent medical help. The sick role also involves behavioural changes, which include an increased attention to the body and bodily functions, regression and an increase in dependent behaviour, a narrowing of interests, and emotional overreactions.
Romberg's sign ('rombərgz) inability to stand erect without swaying if the eyes are closed. A sign of tabes dorsalis.
rombergism ('rombərg,izəm) the tendency of a patient to sway when he stands still with feet close together and eyes closed; associated with loss of position sense.
rongeur (ronh'zhər) [Fr.] forceps for cutting away tissue, particularly bone.
room (ruhm) a place in a building enclosed and set apart for occupancy or for the performance of certain procedures.
operating r. operating theatre.
recovery r. an area adjoining operating theatres, with special equipment and personnel for the care of patients immediately after operation.

root (root) 1. the descending and subterranean part of a plant. 2. that portion of an organ, such as a tooth, hair, or nail, that is buried in the tissues, or by which it arises from another structure, or the part of a nerve that is adjacent to the centre to which it is connected.

anterior r. ventral root.

r. canal that part of the pulp cavity extending from the pulp chamber to the apical foramen. Called also pulp canal.

dorsal r. the posterior, or sensory, division of each spinal nerve, attached centrally to the spinal cord and joining peripherally with the ventral root to form the nerve before it emerges from the intervertebral foramen.

motor r. ventral root.

nerve r's the series of paired bundles of nerve fibres which emerge at each side of the spinal cord, termed dorsal (or posterior) or ventral (or anterior) according to their position. There are 31 pairs (8 cervical, 12 thoracic, 5 lumbar, 5 sacral, and 1 coccygeal), each corresponding dorsal and ventral root joining to form a spinal nerve. Certain cranial nerves, e.g., the trigeminal, also have nerve roots.

posterior r. dorsal root.

sensory r. dorsal root.

ventral r. the anterior, or motor, division of each spinal nerve, attached centrally to the spinal cord and joining peripherally with the dorsal root to form the nerve before it emerges from the intervertebral foramen.

ROP right occipitoposterior (position of the fetus).

Rorschach test ('rorshahk) one for disclosing personality traits and conflicts by the patient's interpretation of 10 cards bearing symmetrical ink blots in various colours and shading.

rosacea (roh'zayshi·ə) acne rosacea.

rosaniline (roh'zani,leen) a substance from coal tar, the basis of various dyes and stains.

rosary ('rohzə·ree) a structure resembling a string of beads.

rachitic r. a succession of beadlike prominences along the costal cartilages, in rickets.

Rosenbach test ('rohzənbahkhs) detection of cold haemolysins by haemoglobinuric response to immersion of the hands or feet in ice water.

roseola (roh'zeeələ) [L.] 1. any rose-coloured rash. 2. roseola infantum.

r. infantum a fairly common acute viral disease that usually occurs in children less than 24 months old; called also exanthem subitum, it attacks suddenly but disappears in a few days, leaving no permanent marks.

syphilitic r. an eruption of rose-coloured spots in early secondary syphilis.

r. typhosa rose spots.

rosette (roh'zet) any structure or formation resembling a rose, such as (1) the clusters of polymorphonuclear leukocytes around a globule of lipid nuclear material, as observed in the test for disseminated lupus erythematosus, or (2) a figure formed by the chromosomes in an early stage of mitosis.

rosin ('rozin) the solid resin obtained from species of *Pinus*, a genus of trees; used in preparation of ointments and plasters.

RoSPA Royal Society for the Prevention of Accidents.

Rossolimo's reflex (,rosə'leemohz) in pyramidal tract lesions, plantar flexion of the toes on tapping their plantar surface.

rostellum (ro'steləm) a small protuberance or beak, especially the fleshy protuberance of the scolex of a tapeworm, which may or may not bear hooks.

rostrad ('rostrad) 1. toward a rostrum; nearer the rostrum in relation to a specific point of reference. 2. cephalad.

rostral ('rostrəl) 1. pertaining to or resembling a rostrum; having a rostrum or beak. 2. situated toward a rostrum or toward the beak (oral and nasal region), which may mean superior (in relationships of areas of the spinal cord) or anterior or ventral (in relationships of brain areas).

rostrate ('rostrayt) beaked.

rostrum ('rostrəm) pl. *rostra* [L.] a beak-shaped process.

rot (rot) decay.

rotation (roh'tayshən) the process of turning around an axis. In obstetrics, the turning of the fetal head (or presenting part) for proper orientation to the pelvic axis. It should occur naturally, but if it does not it must be accomplished manually or instrumentally by the obstetrician.

rotenone ('rohtə,nohn) a poisonous compound from derris root and other roots; used as an insecticide and as a scabicide.

Roth's spot (rohts) round or oval white spots sometimes seen in the retina early in the course of subacute bacterial endocarditis.

Rothera's test ('rodhə·rəz) a test for the presence of acetone in urine.

rotula ('rotyuhlə) 1. the patella. 2. any disclike bony process. 3. a lozenge or troche.

rotular ('rotyuhlə) patellar.

roughage ('rufij) coarse, largely indigestible material, such as bran, cereals, fruit, and vegetable fibres, that acts as an irritant to stimulate intestinal evacuation.

rouleau ('rooloh) pl. *rouleaux* [Fr.] a roll of red blood cells resembling a pile of coins.

roundworm ('rownd,wərm) any of various types of parasitic nematode worms, somewhat resembling the common earthworm, which sometimes invade the human intestinal tract and multiply there. Very common among them is the pinworm, or threadworm. Others include the ascarids, the hookworm, and trichinella, which causes TRICHINOSIS. These worms can all impair health to varying degrees, but proper treatment will generally eliminate them. See also WORMS.

Roux-en-Y (,roo·onh'wie) a Y-shaped anastomosis involving the small intestine so that after section the proximal end is anastomosed end to side at a lower level to allow the distal end to drain another viscus.

Rovsing's sign ('rohvsingz) a test for acute appendicitis in which pressure in the left iliac fossa causes pain in the right iliac fossa.

Royal College of Midwives ('roy'l ,kolij) founded in 1881 as the professional body concerned with education and standards of the professional practice of midwives. Abbreviated RCM. It is the only professional organization solely for midwives either as students or as qualified practitioners. The RCM is now concerned primarily with: (1) standards of professional practice; (2) statutory and other postbasic education for midwives; and (3) negotiation of conditions of service and salaries. Headquarters: 15 Mansfield Street, London W1M 0BE.

Royal College of Nursing founded in 1916 as the professional body for nurses. Incorporated by Royal Charter in 1928. Its main aim is to promote both the art and science of nursing. It is both a professional organisation and an independent trade union, but it is not affiliated to the Trade Union Congress (TUC). Abbreviated RCN and Rcn. The Royal College of Nursing also maintains the Institute of Advanced Nursing Education which offers a wide variety of postbasic courses. Its library is the foremost nursing library in Europe. Headquarters: 20 Cavendish Square, London W1M 0AB.

RPCF see REITER.

RPF renal plasma flow.
rpm revolutions per minute.
RQ respiratory quotient.
RRC Royal Red Cross.
-rrhage, -rrhagia word element. [Gr.] *excessive flow.* adj. **-rrhagic.**
-rrhoea word element. [Gr.] *profuse flow.* adj. **-rrhoeic.**
rRNA ribosomal RNA (ribonucleic acid).
RSA right sacroanterior (position of the fetus).
RScA right scapuloanterior (positon of the fetus).
RSCN Registered Sick Children's Nurse.
RScP right scapuloposterior (position of the fetus).
RSL right sacrolateral (position of the fetus).
RSP right sacroposterior (position of the fetus).
Ru chemical symbol, *ruthenium.*
rub (rub) friction rub, an auscultatory sound caused by the rubbing together of two serous surfaces.

pericardial r. a scraping or grating noise heard with the heart beat, usually a to-and-fro sound, associated with an inflamed pericardium.

pleural r., pleuritic r. a rub produced by friction between the visceral and costal pleurae.

rubber-band ligation (rubə'band) treatment of haemorrhoids by binding them with rubber ligatures so that the ligated portion sloughs off. Called also *Barron ligation.*

rubber-dam (ˌrubə'dam) a sheet of thin latex rubber used by dentists to isolate a tooth from the fluids of the mouth during dental treatment, and occasionally in surgical procedures to isolate certain tissues or structures. Called also dam.

rubefacient (ˌroobi'fayshənt) 1. reddening the skin. 2. an agent that reddens the skin.

rubella (roo'belə) German measles; a mild systemic, statutorily notifiable disease, caused by a virus and characterized by a fever and a transient rash; arthritis may occur in adult females and encephalitis is a rare complication. The most serious hazard is infection during the first four months of pregnancy; this may result in infection of the fetus and cause the congenital *rubella syndrome*, called also EMBRYOPATHY. This consists of congenital heart defects, cataract, mental handicap, and deafness.

Rubella is not as infectious as chickenpox or measles, but there are frequent epidemics among school children, usually during the spring and early summer. The virus is spread by direct contact and by droplet infection. The patient can transmit the disease from the first appearance of symptoms until the rash disappears, usually a total of 3 or 4 days. The incubation period of rubella is usually 16 to 18 days.

Rubella begins with a slight cold, some fever, and a sore throat. The lymph nodes just behind the ears and at the back of the neck may swell, causing some soreness or pain when the head is moved. The rash appears first on the face and scalp, and spreads to the body and arms the same day. Rubella rash is similar to that of measles, although the spots usually do not run together. The rubella rash fades after 2 or 3 days, although in a few cases the disease may last as long as a week.

TREATMENT. The patient may be kept in bed for the duration of the illness, but no special treatment, medicine, or diet is necessary unless the patient has a high fever. One attack of German measles usually gives lifetime immunity to the disease, although a second attack does occasionally occur.

PREVENTION. The main objective is to prevent congenital rubella by vaccination, to ensure that all mothers are immune before pregnancy. Two methods have been adopted to achieve this.

(1) Vaccination of all school girls between the ages of 11 and 14 years. This method allows rubella infection to continue in the male population, and reinfection of females to occur to reinforce their immunity. This method has the disadvantage that never are 100 per cent of girls immunized, and inevitably a few cases of congenital rubella continue to occur. (2) Vaccination of all children in infancy, with a booster immunization being given to girls aged 11–14 years, with the object of completely eliminating the disease from the community. The disadvantage of this method is that for it to be effective over 90 per cent of infants need to be immunized.

The first method was initially used with some success in the UK, but was augmented by vaccination of children of both sexes in the first years of life in 1988, using MMR vaccine.

When a woman is exposed to rubella during the first four months of pregnancy, serum should be taken to test for immunity to rubella. If this shows immunity and no infection, reassurance can be given to continue the preganancy. The second serum should be taken four weeks later, if the first showed no immunity. Only if this shows evidence of infection should termination be considered.

rubeola (roo'beeələ) a synonym of measles in English and of German measles in French and Spanish.

rubeosis (ˌroobi'ohsis) redness.

r. iridis a condition characterized by new formation of vessels on the surface of the iris. May be seen in diabetics with proliferative retinopathy or following retinal vein occlusion.

ruber ('roobə) [L.] *red.*
rubescent (roo'bes'nt) growing red; reddish.
rubidium (roo'bidi·əm) a chemical element, atomic number 37, atomic weight 85.47, symbol Rb. See table of elements in Appendix 2.
Rubin test ('roobin) a test for patency of the uterine tubes, made by transuterine inflation with carbon dioxide gas. Called also *tubal insufflation.*
rubor ('roobor) [L.] redness, one of the cardinal signs of inflammation.
rubriblast ('roobriˌblast) pronormoblast.
rubric ('roobrik) red; specifically, pertaining to the red nucleus.
rubricyte ('roobriˌsiet) polychromatic normoblast.
rubrospinal (ˌroobroh'spien'l) pertaining to the red nucleus and the spinal cord.
rubrothalamic (ˌroobrohthə'lamik) pertaining to the red nucleus and the thalamus.
rubrum ('roobrəm) [L.] *red.*
rudiment ('roodimənt) 1. an organ or part having little or no function but which has functioned at an earlier stage of the same individual or in his ancestors. 2. primordium.
rudimentary (ˌroodi'mentə·ree) 1. imperfectly developed. 2. vestigial.
rudimentum (ˌroodi'mentəm) rudiment; in NA, the first indication of a structure in the course of its embryonic development.
ruga ('roogə) pl. *rugae* [L.] a ridge or fold.
rugoscopy (roo'goskəpee) the study of the patterns of the grooves and ridges (rugae) of the palate to identify individual patterns.
rugose ('roogohs, -gohz) marked by ridges; wrinkled.
rugosity (roo'gositee) 1. the condition of being rugose. 2. a fold, wrinkle, or ruga.
RUL right upper lobe (of lung).
rule (rool) a statement of conditions commonly observed in a given situation, or of a prescribed procedure to obtain a given result. For specific rules, see specific name, as M'NAGHTEN RULE.
ruminant ('roominənt) 1. chewing the cud. 2. an animal

that has a stomach with four complete cavities, and that characteristically regurgitates undigested food from the rumen, the first stomach, and masticates it when at rest.

rumination (ˌroomi'nayshən) 1. in man, the regurgitation of food after almost every meal, part of it being vomited and the rest swallowed; a condition seen in infants. 2. persistent meditation on a certain subject.

rump (rump) the buttock or gluteal region.

runt disease (runt) a syndrome produced by immunologically competent cells in a foreign host that is unable to reject them, resulting in gross retardation of host development and in death.

rupia ('roopi·ə) thick, dark, raised, lamellated, adherent crusts on the skin, somewhat resembling oyster shells, as in late recurrent secondary syphilis. adj. **rupial.**

rupture ('rupchə) 1. tearing or disruption of tissue. 2. hernia.

RUQ right upper quadrant (of abdomen).

rush (rush) peristaltic rush; a powerful wave of contractile activity that travels very long distances down the small intestine, caused by intense irritation or unusual distention.

Russell's viper venom ('rus'lz) the venom of Russell's viper (*Vipera russelli*), which acts in vitro as an instrinsic thromboplastin and is useful in defining deficiencies of blood clotting factor X.

ruthenium (roo'theeni·əm) a chemical element, atomic number 44, atomic weight 101.07, symbol Ru. See table of elements in Appendix 2.

rutherford ('rudhəfəd) a unit of radioactive disintegration, representing one million disintegrations per second.

rutherfordium (ˌrudhə'fawdi·əm) former name for UNNILQUADIUM.

RV residual volume.

Rx, ℞ [L.] symbol *recipe* (take); prescription; treatment.

rye (rie) the cereal plant *Secale cereale*, and its nutritious seed.

Rynacrom ('rienəkrom) trademark for a preparation of sodium cromoglycate.

Rythmodan ('ridhmədan) trademark for a preparation of disopyramide, an antiarrythmic.

S

S chemical symbol, *sulphur;* symbol for *siemens* and *svedberg;* [L.] *semis* (half); sight; [L.] *signa* (mark); [L.] *sinister* (left).

s second.

Sa_{O_2} symbol for percentage of available haemoglobin that is saturated with oxygen (see BLOOD GAS ANALYSIS).

Sabin vaccine ('saybin) an oral vaccine against POLIOMYELITIS consisting of three types of live, attenuated polioviruses. It may be given in a capsule, on a lump of sugar, or by medicine dropper, and is especially convenient for administration to children and large groups of people.

A unique advantage of the Sabin vaccine is its potential effectiveness in checking the transmission of paralytic viruses from one person to another. Polioviruses reside first in the intestinal tract, from which they spread to other areas, eventually reaching the nervous system and causing paralysis. In a person who has been vaccinated by injection (with Salk vaccine), the viruses are destroyed by antibodies before they reach the nervous system but after they have moved out of the intestine; viruses in the intestine are not destroyed and, still infectious, pass out of the body.

Sabin vaccine, taken orally, stimulates the production of antibodies in the digestive system as well as in other systems of the body; viruses in the intestine are destroyed, not passed on. Thus persons who have received the Sabin vaccine become neither infected nor carriers, whereas those who have received the Salk vaccine can be carriers of the viruses even though they are not themselves infected.

sabulous ('sabyuhləs) gritty or sandy.

saburra (sa'byooə·rə) sordes; foulness of the mouth or stomach.

saburral (sa'byooə·rəl) 1. pertaining to saburra. 2. gritty, gravelly.

sac (sak) a pouch; a baglike organ or structure.

air s. alveolar sac.

alveolar s's the spaces into which the alveolar ducts open distally, and with which the alveoli communicate.

amniotic s. the sac enclosing the fetus suspended in the amniotic fluid; the amnion.

conjunctival s. the potential space, lined by conjunctiva, between the eyelids and the eyeball.

endolymphatic s. the blind, flattened cerebral end of the endolymphatic duct.

heart s. the pericardium.

hernial s. the peritoneal pouch that encloses protruding intestine.

lacrimal s. the dilated upper end of the nasolacrimal duct. See also LACRIMAL APPARATUS.

yolk s. the extraembryonic membrane connected with the midgut; in vertebrates below true mammals, it contains a yolk mass.

saccade (sa'kahd) the series of involuntary, abrupt, rapid, small movements or jerks of both eyes simultaneously in changing the point of fixation. adj. **saccadic.**

saccate ('sakayt) 1. shaped like a sac. 2. contained in a sac.

saccharide ('sakəˌried) one of a series of carbohydrates, including the sugars; they are divided into monosaccharides, disaccharides, trisaccharides, and polysaccharides according to the number of saccharide groups composing them.

sacchariferous (ˌsakə'rifə·rəs) containing sugar.

saccharin ('sakə·rin) a white, crystalline compound several hundred times sweeter than sucrose; used as a noncalorific sweetening agent, but now proved to be carcinogenic in test animals.

saccharogalactorrhoea (ˌsakə·rohˌgaləktə'reeə) secretion of milk containing an excess of sugar.

saccharolytic (ˌsakə·roh'litik) capable of splitting up sugar.

saccharometabolic (ˌsakə·rohˌmetə'bolik) pertaining to the metabolism of sugar.

saccharometabolism (ˌsakə·rohmə'tabəˌlizəm) the metabolism of sugar.

Saccharomyces (ˌsakə·roh'mieseez) a genus of fungi, of which yeast is an example.

saccharum ('sakə·ruhm) [L.] *sugar*, especially sucrose.

sacciform ('saksiˌfawm) shaped like a bag or sac.

saccular ('sakyuhlə) pertaining to or resembling a sac.

sacculated ('sakyuhˌlaytid) containing saccules.

sacculation (ˌsakyuh'layshən) 1. a saccule, or pouch. 2. the quality of being sacculated. 3. the formation of pouches.

saccule ('sakyool) a little bag or sac; a small, pouch-like cavity, especially the smaller of the two divisions of the membranous labyrinth of the vestibule, which communicates with the cochlear duct by way of the ductus reuniens.

laryngeal s. sacculus laryngis.
sacculus ('sakyuhləs) pl. *saculi* [L.] a saccule.
s. laryngis a diverticulum extending upward from the front of the ventricle of the larynx.
saccus ('sakəs) pl. *sacci* [L.] a sac.
sacr(o)- word element. [L.] *sacrum*.
sacrad ('saykrad) toward the sacrum.
sacral ('saykrəl) pertaining to the sacrum.
sacralgia (say'kralji·ə) pain in the sacrum.
sacralization (ˌsaykrəlie'zayshən) anomalous fusion of the fifth lumbar vertebra with the first segment of the sacrum.
sacrectomy (say'krektəmee) excision or resection of the sacrum.
sacrococcygeal (ˌsaykrohkok'siji·əl) pertaining to the sacrum and coccyx.
sacrocoxalgia (ˌsaykrohkok'salji·ə) a painful condition of the sacrum and coccyx.
sacrocoxitis (ˌsaykrohkok'sietis) inflammation of the sacroiliac joint.
sacrodynia (ˌsaykroh'dini·ə) pain in the sacral region.
sacroiliac (ˌsaykroh'iliˌak) pertaining to the sacrum and the ilium, or the joint formed by these two bones, or to the lower part of the back where these bones meet on both sides of the back. The ilium is the upper part of the hip bone. The sacrum, near the end of the spine, forms a wedge-shaped joint within the open portion of the ilium.

The tight joint allows little motion and is subject to great stress, as the body's weight pushes downward and the legs and pelvis push upward against the joint. The sacroiliac joint must also bear the leverage demands made by the trunk of the body as it turns, twists, pulls, and pushes. When these motions, especially during weight lifting, place an excess of stress on the ligaments that bind the joint and on the connecting muscles, strain may result.

s. disease chronic tuberculous inflammation of the sacroiliac joint.
sacroiliitis (ˌsaykrohˌili'ietis) inflammation of the sacroiliac joint.
sacrolumbar (ˌsaykroh'lumbə) pertaining to the sacrum and loins.
sacrosciatic (ˌsaykrohsie'atik) pertaining to the sacrum and ischium.
sacrospinal (ˌsaykroh'spien'l) pertaining to the sacrum and vertebral column.
sacrouterine (ˌsaykroh'yootəˌrien) pertaining to the sacrum and uterus.
sacrovertebral (ˌsaykroh'vərtibrəl) pertaining to the sacrum and vertebrae.
sacrum ('saykrəm) the triangular-shaped bone at the base of the spine formed usually by five fused vertebrae that are wedged dorsally between the two hip bones.
sadism ('saydizəm) a form of sexual perversion in which sexual satisfaction is gained by inflicting physical or psychological pain or humiliation on others. adj. **sadistic.** It can manifest itself in many ways other than during the sexual act. Sadism is a mental disturbance and should be treated by psychotherapy.
sadist ('saydist) a person who practises sadism.
sadomasochism (ˌsaydoh'masəˌkizəm) a state characterized by both sadistic and masochistic tendencies. adj. **sadomasochistic.**
sadomasochist (ˌsaydoh'masəˌkist) a person exhibiting sadomasochism.
sagittal ('sajit'l) 1. shaped like an arrow. 2. situated in the direction of the sagittal suture; said of an anteroposterior plane or section parallel to the median plane of the body.
sagittalis (ˌsaji'taylis) [L.] *sagittal*.
Saint Anthony's fire (sənt 'antəneez) 1. ergotism. 2. an infection of the skin and subcutaneous tissues; called also ERYSIPELAS.
Saint's triad (saynts) hiatus hernia, colonic diverticula, and cholelithiasis.
Saint Vitus dance (sənt 'veetəs) Sydenham's chorea.
sal (sal) [L.] *salt*.
Sala's cells ('saləz) star-shaped cells of connective tissue in the fibres that form the sensory nerve endings situated in the pericardium.
Salah needle ('sala) sternal puncture needle with adjustable guard.
Salazopyrin (səˌlayzoh'pierin) trademark for a preparation of sulphasalazine, used in the treatment of chronic ulcerative colitis.
salbutamol (sal'byootəmol) a relatively selective beta$_2$-adrenergic bronchodilator used for relief of bronchospasm in patients with reversible obstructive airways disease.
salicylamide (ˌsalisil'amied) an amide of salicylic acid; used as an analgesic and antipyretic.
salicylate (sə'lisəˌlayt) any salt or ester of salicylic acid. The salicylates used as drugs for their analgesic, antipyretic, and anti-inflammatory effects include aspirin (acetylsalicylic acid, ASA), methyl salicylate, and sodium salicylate. Low dosages of salicylates are used primarily for the relief of mild-to-moderate pain or fever; high dosages are particularly useful for treatment of rheumatoid arthritis and other rheumatoid disorders.

The mechanism of most of the effects of aspirin and other salicylates is inhibition of prostaglandin synthesis, thus blocking pyretic and inflammatory processes that are mediated by prostaglandins. Aspirin also prolongs the bleeding time through its effects on platelets owing to both inhibition of prostaglandin synthesis and acetylation of platelet structures. Salicylates also cause ulceration and haemorrhagic lesions of the gastric mucosa; the same mechanisms involved in the anti-inflammatory effects increase the production of stomach acid, decrease the secretion of protective mucus, and increase bleeding. Aspirin should not be taken with alcohol, because this increases gastrointestinal damage. Aspirin should be avoided by persons with gastric ulcers, haemophilia, or haemorrhagic states, and should not be given to children under the age of 12 years.

Another problem associated with the use of salicylates is hypersensitivity. This most commonly occurs with aspirin and is less common with other salicylates. Aspirin-sensitive individuals often also react to other anti-inflammatory agents, such as indomethacin, and to a yellow dye used to colour foods and drugs called tartrazine.

The allergic reaction usually takes the form of oedema of the face and intestinal tract and asthma. Aspirin sensitivity occurs in about 0.25–1.0 per cent of the population and is more common in persons with a history of asthma or other allergic disorders.

SALICYLATE POISONING. Mild salicylate toxicity, which can occur from high dosage therapy, has symptoms that include headache, dizziness, tinnitus, deafness, nausea, vomiting, and acid–base disturbances. Large overdoses produce acute poisoning that is a medical emergency. Aspirin poisoning is the most common form of poisoning of children and there is evidence that aspirin may contribute to REYE'S SYNDROME in some children.

Treatment consists of emesis or gastric lavage, intravenous fluids to correct dehydration and acid–base imbalance, and body sponging with cool water for hyperpyrexia. Blood salicylate levels and blood gases and electrolytes are periodically determined by laboratory tests. Life-threatening poisoning may require exchange transfusion or renal dialysis.

salicylic acid (ˌsali'silik) 2-hydroxybenzoic acid; used as a keratolytic. See SALICYLATE.

salicylism ('salisiˌlizəm) toxic symptoms caused by salicylic acid.

saline ('saylien) salty; of the nature of a salt.

s. bath see SALT bath.

s. solution a solution of salt (sodium chloride) in purified water. Physiological saline solution is a 0.9 per cent solution of sodium chloride and water and is isotonic, i.e., of the same osmotic pressure as blood serum. It may be given intravenously to replace lost sodium and chloride. Excessive quantities may cause oedema, elevated blood sodium levels, and loss of potassium from the tissue fluid.

saliva (sə'lievə) the enzyme-containing secretion of the salivary glands.

salivant ('salivənt) causing flow of saliva.

salivary (sə'lievə·ree, 'salivə·ree) pertaining to the saliva.

s. gland any of the glands in the mouth that secrete saliva. The major ones are the three pairs of glands known as the parotid, submaxillary, and sublingual glands. There are other smaller salivary glands within the cheeks and tongue.

The largest of the salivary glands are the parotids, located below and in front of each ear. Saliva secreted by these is discharged into the mouth through openings in the cheeks on each side opposite the upper teeth. The submaxillary glands, located inside the lower jaw, discharge saliva upward through openings into the floor of the mouth. The sublingual glands, beneath the tongue, also discharge saliva into the floor of the mouth.

The saliva is needed to moisten the mouth, to lubricate food for easier swallowing, and to provide the enzyme (ptyalin) necessary to begin food breakdown in the preliminary stage of digestion. The salivary glands produce about 3 pints of saliva daily.

The salivary glands are controlled by the nervous system. Normally they respond by producing saliva within 2 or 3 seconds after being stimulated by the sight, smell, or taste of food. This quick response is a reflex action.

In mumps (parotitis), the parotids become inflamed and swollen. Occasionally, salivary glands produce too much saliva; this condition is called ptyalism, and is the result of local irritation from dental appliances or of disturbances of digestion or of the nervous system or other causes. Certain diseases, drugs such as morphine or atropine, and nutritional deficiency of vitamin B can result in decreased secretion of saliva.

s. gland inclusion disease cytomegalic inclusion disease.

salivation (ˌsali'vayshən) 1. the secretion of saliva. 2. ptyalism.

Salk vaccine (sawlk) Pol/Vac(inact) a preparation of killed polioviruses of three types given in a series of intramuscular injections to immunize against POLIOMYELITIS.

Salmonella (ˌsalmə'nelə) a genus of gram-negative bacteria named after Dr. Daniel E. Salmon, an American veterinary surgeon who first isolated the bacterium in the late 19th century. It includes the typhoid-paratyphoid bacilli and bacteria usually pathogenic for lower animals which are often transmitted to man.

S. enteritidis a common cause of gastroenteritis in man.

S. paratyphi the usual aetiological agent of paratyphoid.

S. typhi, S. typhosa the causative organism of typhoid fever, occurring only in man.

S. typhimurium the causative agent of mouse typhoid and of food poisoning in man.

salmonella (ˌsalmə'nelə) pl. *salmonellae;* any organism of the genus *Salmonella.* adj. **salmonellal.**

salmonellosis (ˌsalmone'lohsis) infection with certain species of the genus *Salmonella*, usually caused by the ingestion of food containing salmonellae or their products. The organisms can be found in raw meats, raw poultry, eggs, and dairy products; they multiply rapidly at temperatures between 7 and 46 °C.

Symptoms of salmonellosis include violent diarrhoea attended by abdominal cramps, nausea and vomiting, and fever. It is rarely fatal and can be prevented by adequate cooking. Normal cooking temperatures, even in rare roast beef, destroy bacteria. In order to avoid salmonellosis, frozen meat should be thawed in the refrigerator rather than at room temperature, leftovers should be refrigerated promptly, and raw eggs should be avoided, especially for infants and elderly persons.

salping(o)- word element. [Gr.] *tube; (pharyngotympanic tube* or *uterine tube).*

salpingectomy (ˌsalpin'jektəmee) excision of a uterine tube.

salpingemphraxis (ˌsalpinjem'fraksis) obstruction of a pharyngotympanic tube.

salpingian (sal'pinji·ən) pertaining to the pharyngotympanic or the uterine tube.

salpingion (sal'pinjion) a point at the apex of the petrous bone on the lower surface.

salpingitis (ˌsalpin'jietis) 1. inflammation of a uterine tube. 2. inflammation of the pharyngotympanic tube.

mural s. pachysalpingitis.

parenchymatous s. pachysalpingitis.

salpingocele (sal'ping·gohˌseel) hernial protrusion of a uterine tube.

salpingocyesis (salˌping·gohsie'eesis) development of the embryo within a uterine tube; tubal pregnancy.

salpingography (ˌsalping'gogrəfee) radiography of the uterine tubes after intrauterine injection of a radiopaque medium.

salpingolithiasis (salˌping·gohli'thieəsis) the presence of calcareous deposits in the wall of the uterine tubes.

salpingolysis (ˌsalpin'golisis) surgical separation of adhesions involving the uterine tubes.

salpingo-oophorectomy (salˌping·gohˌoh·əfə'rektəmee) excision of a uterine tube and ovary.

salpingo-oophoritis (salˌping·gohˌoh·əfə'rietis) inflammation of a uterine tube and ovary.

salpingo-oophorocele (salˌping·goh·oh'ofə·rohˌseel) hernia of a uterine tube and ovary.

salpingopexy (sal'ping·gohˌpeksee) fixation of a uterine tube.

salpingopharyngeal (salˌping·gohfə'rinji·əl, -farin'jeeəl) pertaining to the auditory tube and the pharynx.

salpingoplasty (sal'ping·gohˌplastee) plastic repair of a uterine tube.

salpingostomy (ˌsalping'gostəmee) 1. formation of an opening or fistula into a uterine tube for the purpose of drainage. 2. surgical restoration of the patency of a uterine tube.

salpingotomy (ˌsalping'gotəmee) surgical incision of a uterine tube.

salpinx ('salpingks) 1. a uterine tube. 2. a pharyngotympanic tube.

salsalate ('salsəˌlayt) an ester formed from two molecules of salicylic acid; used as an analgesic and anti-inflammatory.

salt (sawlt) 1. sodium chloride, or common salt. 2. any

compound of a base and an acid. 3. *salts*, a saline purgative. **s. bath** immersion in salt water of only the hips and buttocks for the relief of pain and discomfort following rectal surgery, cystoscopy, or vaginal surgery; they also may be ordered for patients with cystitis or infections within the pelvic cavity. Temperature for a hot salt bath is started at 35 °C and gradually increased to 41 to 43 °C; the patient must be watched for fatigue and faintness, and an attendant must remain within calling distance. Cool compresses to the head or cool drinks during the bath promote comfort and relieve faintness. Called also *saline bath*, *sitz bath*.

bile s's glycine or taurine conjugates of bile acids, which are formed in the liver and secreted in the bile. They are powerful detergents which break down fat globules, enabling them to be digested.

buffer s. a salt in the blood that is able to absorb slight excesses of acid or alkali with little or no change in the hydrogen ion concentration.

Epsom s. magnesium sulphate, a cathartic.

Glauber's s. sodium sulphate.

Rochelle s. potassium sodium tartrate, a cathartic.

smelling s's aromatic ammonium carbonate, a stimúlant and restorative.

salt-losing crisis (syndrome) ('sawltloozing) vomiting, dehydration, hypotension, and sudden death due to very large sodium losses from the body. It may be seen in abnormal losses of sodium into the urine (as in congenital adrenal hyperplasia, adrenocortical insufficiency, or one of the forms of salt-losing NEPHRITIS) or in large extrarenal sodium losses, usually from the gastrointestinal tract.

saltation (sal'tayshən) the action of leaping, especially (1) chorea, or the dancing which sometimes accompanies it; (2) conduction along myelinated nerves; (3) in genetics, an abrupt variation in species; a mutation. adj. **saltatory**.

salting out ('sawlting owt) the separation of protein fractions in the serum or plasma by precipitation in increasing concentrations of neutral salts.

salubrious (sə'loobri·əs) conducive to health; wholesome.

saluresis (ˌsalyuh'reesis) excretion of sodium and chloride in the urine.

saluretic (ˌsalyuh'retik) 1. pertainig to saluresis. 2. an agent that promotes saluresis.

Saluric (sal'yuhrik) trademark for preparations of chlorothiazide, a diuretic.

salutary ('salyuhtə·ree) healthful.

salve (salv, sahv) ointment.

samarium (sə'mair·ri·əm) a chemical element, atomic number 62, atomic weight 150.35, symbol Sm. See table of elements in Appendix 2.

sample ('sahmp'l) a selected group of a population.

San Joaquin Valley fever (san 'yohəkin valee) the primary form of COCCIDIOIDOMYCOSIS.

sanative ('sanətiv) curative; healing.

sanatorium (ˌsanə'tor·ri·əm) an institution for treatment of sick persons, especially a private hospital for convalescents or patients who are not extremely ill; often applied to an institution for the treatment of tuberculosis.

sanatory ('sanətə·ree) conducive to health.

sand (sand) material occurring in fine gritty particles.

brain s. acervulus cerebri; sandy matter about the pineal gland and other parts of the brain.

sandfly ('sandˌflie) various two-winged flies, especially those of the genus *Phlebotomus*, which are important vectors in the transmission of leishmaniasis and phlebotomus fever; called also *sandfly fever*.

Sandhoff's disease ('sandhofs) a variant of Tay-Sachs disease not restricted to particular ethnic groups marked by a progressively more rapid course, due to a defect in the enzymes hexosaminidase A and B.

Sandimmun ('sandimyoon) trademark for a preparation of cyclosporin, an immunosuppressant.

sane (sayn) sound in mind.

Sanfilippo's syndrome (san'filiˌpohz) a form of mucopolysaccharidosis, transmitted as an autosomal recessive trait, resembling Hurler's syndrome, except that most of the somatic and skeletal changes are less severe. It occurs in two clinically indistinguishable types: type A, due to deficiency of heparan sulphate sulphamidase, and type B, due to deficiency of *N*-acetyl-α-D-glucosaminidase.

sangui- word element. [L] *blood*.

sanguifacient (ˌsang·gwi'fayshənt) forming blood.

sanguine ('sang·gwin) 1. abounding in blood. 2. ardent; hopeful.

sanguineous (sang'gwini·əs) bloody; abounding in blood.

sanguinolent (sang'gwinələnt) of a bloody tinge.

sanguinopurulent (ˌsang·gwinoh'pyooə·rələnt) containing both blood and pus.

sanguis ('sang·gwis) [L.] *blood*.

sanguivorous (sang'gwivə·rəs) blood-eating; said of female mosquitoes that prefer blood to other nutrients.

sanies ('sayni·eez) a fetid ichorous discharge containing serum, pus, and blood. adj. **sanious**.

saniopurulent (ˌsaynioh'pyooə·rələnt) partly sanious and partly purulent.

sanioserous (ˌsaynioh'siə·rəs) partly sanious and partly serous.

sanitarium (ˌsani'teri·əm) sanatorium.

sanitary ('sanitə·ree) promoting or pertaining to health.

sanitation (ˌsani'tayshən) the establishment of conditions favourable to health.

sanitization (ˌsanitie'zayshən) the process of making or the quality of being made sanitary.

sanitize ('saniˌtiez) to clean and sterilize.

sanity ('sanitee) soundness, especially soundness of mind.

saphena (sə'feenə) the small saphenous or the great saphenous vein.

saphenous (sə'feenəs) pertaining to or associated with a saphena; applied to certain arteries, nerves, veins, etc.

great s. vein the longest vein in the body, extending from the dorsum of the foot to just below the inguinal ligament, where it opens into the femoral vein.

small s. vein a vein in the back of the ankle passing up the back of the leg to the knee joint.

sapo ('saypoh) [L.] *soap;* a compound of fatty acids with an alkali.

saponaceous (ˌsapə'nayshəs) soapy; of soaplike feel or quality.

saponification (səˌponifi'kayshən) conversion of an oil or fat into a soap by combination with an alkali. In chemistry, the term now denotes the hydrolysis of an ester by an alkali, resulting in the production of a free alcohol and an alkali salt of the ester acid.

saponin ('sapənin) a group of glycosides widely distributed in the plant world and characterized by (1) their property of forming durable foam when their watery solutions are shaken, (2) their ability to dissolve erythrocytes even in high dilutions and (3) their having the compound sapogenin as their aglycones.

sapophore ('sapəˌfor) the group of atoms in the molecule of a compound that gives the substance its characteristic taste.

sapphism ('safizəm) homosexual behaviour in the female; lesbianism.

sapr(o)- word element. [Gr] *rotten*, *putrid*, *decay*, *decayed material*.

sapraemia (sa'preemi·ə) a form of toxaemia. The toxins are produced by saprophytes and circulate in the blood.

saprophyte ('saproh,fiet) any organism, such as a bacterium, living upon dead or decaying organic matter. adj. **saprophytic.**

saprozoic (,saproh'zoh·ik) living on decayed organic matter; said of animals, especially protozoa.

sarc(o)- word element. [Gr] *flesh.*

sarcoblast ('sahkoh,blast) a primitive cell that develops into a muscle cell.

sarcocele ('sahkoh,seel) any fleshy swelling or tumour of the testis.

sarcocyst ('sahkoh,sist) any member of, or any cyst formed by, *Sarcocystis.*

Sarcocystis (,sahkoh'sistis) a genus of parasitic sporozoa (order Sarcosporidia), found in cysts (sarcosporidian cysts, or sarcocysts) in the muscle tissue of mammals, birds, and reptiles. *S. lindeman-ni* is the species that infects man, though rarely.

Sarcodina (,sahkoh'dienə) a subphylum of Protozoa, including all the amoebae, both free-living and parasitic, characterized by the ability to produce pseudopodia during most of the life cycle; flagella, when present, develop only during the early stages.

sarcoid ('sahkoyd) 1. tuberculoid; characterized by noncaseating epithelioid cell tubercles. 2. pertaining to or resembling sarcoidosis. 3. sarcoidosis.

Boeck's s. a type of multiple benign sarcoid characterized by its superficial nature and showing a predilection for the face, arms and shoulders.

sarcoidosis (,sahkoy'dohsis) a chronic, progressive, generalized granulomatous reticulosis that may affect any part of the body but most frequently involving the lymph nodes, liver, spleen, lungs, skin, eyes, and small bones of the hands and feet, characterized by the presence in all affected organs or tissues of epithelioid cell tubercles, which become converted, in the older lesions, into a rather hyaline featureless fibrous tissue. Laboratory findings may include hypercalcaemia and hypergammaglobulinaemia; there is usually diminished or absent reactivity to tuberculin, and, in most cases, a positive Kveim reaction.

s. cordis involvement of the heart in sarcoidosis, with lesions ranging from a few asymptomatic granulomas to widespread infiltration of the myocardium by large masses of sarcoid tissue.

muscular s. sarcoidosis involving the skeletal muscles, with sarcoid tubercles, interstitial inflammation with fibrosis, and disruption and atrophy of the muscle fibres.

sarcolemma (,sahkoh'lemə) the delicate elastic sheath covering every striated muscle fibre. adj. **sarcolemmic, sarcolemmous.**

sarcoma (sah'kohmə) a tumour, often highly malignant, composed of cells derived from connective tissue such as bone and cartilage, muscle, blood vessel, or lymphoid tissue. These tumours usually develop rapidly and metastasize through the lymph channels. adj. **sarcomatous.**

The different types of sarcomas are named for the specific tissue they affect: fibrosarcoma—in fibrous connective tissue; lymphosarcoma—in lymphoid tissues; osteosarcoma—in bone; chondrosarcoma—in cartilage; rhabdosarcoma—in muscle; liposarcoma—in fat cells.

Abernethy's s. a malignant fatty tumour occurring mainly on the trunk.

alveolar soft part s. one with a reticulated fibrous stroma enclosing groups of sarcoma cells enclosed in alveoli walled with connective tissue.

botryoid s., s. botryoides an embryonal rhabdomyosarcoma arising in submucosal tissue, usually in the upper vagina, cervix uteri, or neck of the urinary bladder in young children and infants, presenting grossly as a polypoid grapelike structure.

endometrial stromal s. a pale, polypoid, fleshy, malignant tumour of the endometrial stroma.

Ewing's s. a rare malignant tumour of the bone occurring only in childhood and adolescence which arises in the medulla, occurring more often in cylindrical bones, with pain, fever, and leukocytosis as prominent symptoms. An identical tumour arises in connective tissue but is even more rare.

giant cell s. a malignant form of giant cell tumour of bone.

Kaposi's s. a multifocal, metastasizing, malignant reticulosis with features resembling those of angiosarcoma, principally involving the skin, although visceral lesions may be present; it usually begins on the distal parts of the extremities, most often on the toes or feet, as reddish-blue or brownish soft nodules and tumours. It is viral in origin and is frequently seen in AIDS.

osteogenic s. a malignant primary tumour of bone composed of a malignant connective tissue stroma with evidence of osteoid, bone, and/or cartilage formation; depending upon the dominant component, classified as osteoblastic, fibroblastic, or chondroblastic.

reticulum cell s. a form of malignant lymphoma in which the dominant cell type is derived from the reticuloendothelium.

sarcomatoid (sah'kohmə,toyd) resembling a sarcoma.

sarcomatosis (,sahkohmə'tohsis) a condition characterized by development of many sarcomas.

sarcomatous (sah'kohmətəs) pertaining to or of the nature of a sarcoma.

sarcomere ('sahkoh,miə) the contractile unit of a myofibril; sarcomeres are repeating units, delimited by the Z bands along the length of the myofibril.

sarcomphalocele (sah'komfəloh,seel) a fleshy tumour of the umbilicus.

sarcoplasm ('sahkoh,plazəm) the interfibrillary matter of striated muscle. adj. **sarcoplasmic.**

sarcoplast ('sahkoh,plast) an interstitial cell of a muscle, itself capable of being transformed into a muscle.

sarcopoietic (,sahkohpoy'etik) forming muscle.

Sarcoptes (sah'kopteez) a widely distributed genus of mites, including the species *S. scabiei*, the itch mite, the cause of scabies in man; different varieties of the organism cause mange in different animals.

sarcosis (sah'kohsis) abnormal increase of flesh.

Sarcosporidia (,sahkohspə'ridi·ə) an order of sporozoa parasitic in the cardiac and striated muscles of vertebrates. It includes the genus *Sarcocystis*, an occasional cause of human infection.

sarcosporidiosis (,sahkohspə,ridi'ohsis) infection with sporozoa of the genus *Sarcocystis.*

sarcostosis (,sahko'stohsis) ossification of fleshy tissue.

sarcotubules (,sahkoh'tyoobyoolz) the membrane-limited structures of the sarcoplasm, forming a canalicular network around each myofibril.

sarcous ('sahkəs) pertaining to flesh or muscle tissue.

sardonic (sah'donik) noting a kind of spasmodic or satanic grin or involuntary smile, the risus sardonicus.

sartorius (sah'tor·ri·əs) a long muscle of the thigh, which flexes both the thigh and the lower leg.

sat. saturated.

satellite ('satə,liet) 1. in genetics, a knob of chromatin connected by a stalk to the short arm of certain chromosomes. 2. a minor, or attendant, lesion situated near a large one. 3. a vein that closely accompanies an

artery. 4. exhibiting satellitism.
satellitism ('satəlie,tizəm) the phenomenon in which certain bacterial species grow more vigorously in the immediate vicinity of colonies of other unrelated species, owing to the production of an essential metabolite by the latter species.
satellitosis (,satəlietohsis) accumulation of neuroglial cells about neurons; seen whenever neurons are damaged.
saturated ('sachə,raytid) 1. denoting an organic compound that has only single bonds between carbon atoms. 2. holding all of a solute that can be held in solution by the solvent (saturated solution).
saturation (,sachə'rayshən) the state of being saturated, or the act of saturating.
saturnine ('satə,nien) pertaining to lead.
saturnism ('satə,nizəm) lead poisoning; plumbism.
satyriasis (,sati'rieəsis) pathological or exaggerated sexual desire in the male.
saucerization (,sawsə·rie'zayshən) 1. the excavation of tissue to form a shallow shelving depression, usually performed to facilitate drainage from infected areas. 2. the shallow saucer-like depression on the upper surface of a vertebra which has suffered a compression fracture.
Saventrine (sə'ventreen) trademark for preparations of isoprenaline.
Savlon ('savlon) trademark for combination preparations of chlorhexidine and cetrimide, used as a skin disinfectant.
saxitoxin (,saksi'toksin) a neurotoxin from poisonous mussels, clams, and plankton.
Sayre's jacket ('sayərz) a plaster-of-Paris jacket used as a support for the vertebral column.
Sb chemical symbol, *antimony* (L. *stibium)*.
SC, s.c. subcutaneous(ly).
Sc chemical symbol, *scandium*.
scab (skab) 1. the crust of a superficial sore. 2. to become covered with a crust or scab.
scabicide ('skaybi,sied) 1. lethal to *Sarcoptes scabiei*, the cause of scabies. 2. an agent effective against scabies. Called also *antiscabietic*.
scabies ('skaybeez) an infectious skin disease caused by the itch mite, *Sarcoptes scabiei*. Scabies, sometimes called 'the itch', is most likely to erupt in folds of the skin, as in the groin, beneath the breasts, or between the toes or fingers.

The adult itch mite has a rounded body about one-fiftieth of an inch long. Scabies is caused by the female, which burrows beneath the skin and digs a short tunnel parallel to the surface, in which it lays its eggs. The eggs hatch in a few days, after which the baby mites find their way to the skin surface, where they live their brief lives until they too are ready to burrow and lay their eggs.

SYMPTOMS. During the initial tunnel-digging and egg-laying, the human host may be oblivious to what is happening. There is little itching. The very slight skin discoloration may be mistaken for any one of numerous other skin disorders.

In about a week, the itching becomes intense because of hypersensitivity to the mite. The itch is much worse at night. The tunnels in the skin, often found between the fingers, can now be discerned as slightly elevated greyish-white lines. The mite itself can often be seen—with the aid of a magnifying glass—as an infinitesimal white speck at the end of the tunnel. Blisters and pustules also may develop on the skin near the tunnel.

TRANSMISSION. Scabies is easily transmitted from person to person by direct skin contact or to a limited extent by contact with clothing of infected persons. Epidemics are fairly common in such places as camps, barracks, and institutions. It is unusual for one member of a family not to communicate it to the others. The commonest way to acquire the infection is by sharing a bed with an infected person.

The period of communicability lasts until the itch mites and eggs are totally destroyed, a period of 1 to 2 weeks, depending on the effectiveness of the treatment used.

TREATMENT AND PREVENTION. The patient washes and dries himself. Lotion or cream is applied over the whole body from the neck down, left on overnight (6 to 12 hours) and washed off. The lotion should be applied again 24 hours later and washed off after a further 24 hours. Bathing before the application is no longer recommended because this may increase skin absorption and CNS toxicity.

The patient's underwear and sheets must be changed and laundered daily until all the itch mite eggs are hatched out and the mites eliminated.

Outer clothing and blankets need not be treated.

Norwegian s. a variety characterized by immense numbers of mites and marked scaling of the skin.
scabietic (,skaybi'etik) pertaining to scabies.
scabieticide (,skaybi'eti,sied) scabicide.
scala ('skaylə) pl. *scalae* [L.] a ladder-like structure, applied especially to various passages of the cochlea.
s. media the cochlear duct: a space in the ear between Reissner's membrane and the basilar membrane.
s. tympani the part of the cochlea below the spiral lamina.
s. vestibuli the part of the cochlea above the spiral lamina.
scald ('skawld) a burn caused by a hot liquid or a hot, moist vapour; to burn in such fashion.
scale (skayl) 1. a thin flake or compacted platelike body, as of cornified epithelial cells. 2. a scheme or device by which some property may be measured (as hardness, weight, linear dimension). 3. to remove calculus or other material from a surface, as from the enamel of teeth.
absolute s. a temperature scale with zero at the absolute zero of temperature.
Celsius s. a temperature scale with zero at the freezing point of water and the normal boiling point of water at 100 degrees. For equivalents of Celsius and Fahrenheit temperatures, see Appendix 2.
centigrade s. one with 100 gradations or steps between two fixed points, as the Celsius scale.
Fahrenheit s. a temperature scale with the freezing point of water at 32 and the normal boiling point of water at 212 degrees. For equivalents of Fahrenheit and Celsius temperatures, see Appendix 2.
French s. one used for denoting the size of catheters, sounds, and other tubular instruments, each unit being approximately 0.33 mm. in diameter.
Kelvin s. an absolute scale on which the unit of measurement corresponds to that of the Celsius (centigrade) scale, but the ice point is at 273.15 °K.
scalene muscles ('skayleen) four muscles (anterior, middle, posterior, smallest) of the upper thorax that raise the first and second ribs and thus aid in respiration.
scalenectomy (,skaylə'nektəmee) resection of a scalene muscle.
scalenotomy (,skaylə'notəmee) division of the scalene muscles.
scalenus (anticus) syndrome (skə'leenəs) cervical rib syndrome.
scaler ('skaylə) a dental instrument for removal of calculus from teeth.
scalp (skalp) that part of the skin of the head (exclusive

of the face) which is usually covered by a growth of hair.

scalpel ('skalp'l) surgical knife usually having a convex edge.

scaly ('skaylee) characterized by scales; scalelike.

scan (skan) an image produced using a moving detector or a sweeping beam of radiation, as in scintiscanning, B-mode ultrasonography, scanography, or computed tomography.

scandium ('skandi·əm) a chemical element, atomic number 21, atomic weight 44.956, symbol Sc. See table of elements in Appendix 2.

scanner ('skanə) scintiscanner; called also *CT scanner*.

scanning ('skaning) 1. close visual examination of a small area or of different isolated areas. 2. a manner of utterance characterized by somewhat regularly recurring pauses.

radioisotope s. production of a two-dimensional record of the gamma rays emitted by a radioactive isotope concentrated in a specific organ or tissue of the body, as brain, kidney, or thyroid gland.

CT s. utilization of computed TOMOGRAPHY (CT) to examine a cross section of the entire body. The CT scanner produces an image of tissue density in a complete cross section of the part of the body being scanned.

scanogram ('skanə,gram) the film ontained by scanography.

scanography (ska'nogrəfee) a method of making radiographs by the use of a narrow slit beneath the tube, so that, as the x-ray tube moves over the target, all the rays of the central beam pass through the part being radiographed at the same angle.

scapha ('skayfə) pl. *scaphae* [L.] the curved depression separating the helix and anthelix.

scaphocephaly (,skafoh'kefəlee, -'sef-) abnormal length and narrowness of the skull as a result of premature closure of the sagittal suture; usually accompanied by mental handicap. adj. **scaphocephalic, scaphocephalous.**

scaphoid ('skafoyd, 'skay-) shaped like a boat.

scaphoiditis (,skafoy'dietis) inflammation of the scaphoid bone.

scapula ('skapyuhlə) pl. *scapulae* [L.] the flat triangular bone in the back of the shoulder; the shoulder blade.

winged s. one having a prominent vertebral border usually owing to weakness of one of the muscles holding the scapula in place.

scapulalgia (,skapyuh'lalji·ə) pain in the scapular region.

scapular ('skapyuhlə) pertaining to the scapula.

scapulectomy (,skapyuh'lektəmee) excision or resection of the scapula.

scapuloclavicular (,skapyuhlohklə'vikyuhlə) pertaining to the scapula and clavicle.

scapulohumeral (,skapyuhloh'hyoomə·rəl) pertaining to the scapula and humerus.

scapulopexy ('skapyuhloh,peksee) surgical fixation of the scapula.

scapulothoracic (,skapyuhlohthor'rasik) pertaining to the scapula and thorax.

scar (skah) cicatrix; a mark remaining after the healing of a wound, caused by injury, illness, smallpox vaccination, or surgery. It is a zone of dense relatively avascular collagen fibres which at the surface of a tissue or organ is covered by a thinned layer of epithelium. See also HEALING and KELOID.

scarification (,skarifi'kayshən, ,skair·ri-) production in the skin of many small superficial scratches or punctures, as for introduction of vaccine. Erroneously used to mean scarring.

scarificator ('skarifi,kaytə, 'skair·ri-) scarifier.

scarifier ('skari,fieə, 'skair·ri-) an instrument with many sharp points, used in scarification.

scarlatina (,skahlə'teenə) scarlet fever. adj. **scarlatinal.**

scarlatinella (,skahləti'nelə) Duke's disease.

scarlatiniform (,skahlə'tini,fawm) resembling scarlet fever.

scarlet fever ('skahlət) a notifiable acute infectious rare childhood disease caused by Group A beta-haemolytic streptococci and rarely other serotypes of beta-haemolytic streptococci; called also scarlatina. Scarlet fever usually affects the pharynx but may also affect the skin or the birth canal (puerperal scarlet fever). It only differs from streptococcal pharyngitis in the characteristic rash. The disease is most common in late winter and spring.

Streptococcal pharyngitis is spread by droplet infection and, rarely, by fomites. Occasionally a widespread outbreak may be caused by milk or food that has been infected by a person carrying the streptococcus.

Scarlet fever was formerly a very common and serious disease. In recent years, the number and severity of cases have greatly decreased. Complications are much less common, probably due to a decline in the virulence of the organism and the use of antibiotics.

SYMPTOMS. The incubation period is usually 2 to 7 days. In some patients there is only sore throat and swelling of the lymph nodes of the neck. The tonsils may be covered by a patchy purulent discharge. The bright red rash from which the disease takes its name appears on the second day. There may be nausea and vomiting, headache and chills, with pyrexia.

If there are no complications, the temperature will slowly return to normal. The rash may last only a few hours, but typically lasts two to three days before fading. There is superficial flaking of the skin over much of the involved area; this peeling is usually most pronounced on the palms and soles. The active stage of the disease lasts about 7 days.

Scarpa's fascia ('skahpəz) the deep, membranous layer of the subcutaneous abdominal fascia.

Scarpa's foramen an opening behind the upper medial incisor, for the nasopalatine nerve.

Scarpa's ganglion vestibular ganglion.

Scarpa's membrane secondary tympanic membrane.

Scarpa's triangle femoral triangle.

SCAT SHEEP CELL AGGLUTINATION TEST, a test for infectious mononucleosis.

scataemia (ska'teemi·ə) alimentary toxaemia in which the chemical poisons are absorbed through the intestine.

scatology (ska'toləjee) study and analysis of faeces, as for diagnostic purposes. adj. **scatological.**

scatoscopy (ska'toskəpee) examination of the faeces.

scatter ('skatə) the diffusion or deviation of x-rays produced by a medium through which the rays pass.

back s. backward diffusion of x-rays.

scattergram, scatter diagram ('skatə,gram; 'skətə 'dieagram) a graph in which the values found in a statistical study are represented by disconnected, individual symbols.

scattering ('skatə·ring) a change in the direction of motion of a photon or subatomic particle as the result of a collision or interaction.

ScD Doctor of Science.

Schatzki's ring ('shatskeez) a radiological sign of a hiatus hernia seen on a barium swallow examination. It shows as an indentation on the column of barium and represents the gastro-oesophageal junction.

Scheie's syndrome (shayz) a type of mucopolysaccharidosis considered to be an atypical form of Hurler's syndrome, in which the principal sign is marked progressive corneal clouding; hirsutism, joint stiffness, mild deformities of the bones that may only affect the hands, disease of the aorta, and wide-mouthed facies occur, but there is no mental handicap.

schema ('skeemə) a plan, outline, or arrangement.

Scheuermann's disease ('shoyə,manz) osteochondrosis of the vertebral epiphyses in juveniles.

Schick test (shik) intracutaneous injection of diluted diphtheria toxin equal to one-fiftieth of the minimum lethal dose. Lack of immunity to diphtheria is indicated by redness and oedema at the injection site on the fifth to seventh day.

Schilder's disease ('shildəz) a subacute or chronic leukoencephalopathy of children and adolescents, with massive destruction of the white substance of the cerebral hemispheres; clinical symptoms include blindness, deafness, bilateral spasticity, and mental deterioration. Called also *encephalitis periaxialis diffusa* and *progressive subcortical encephalopathy*.

Schilling test ('shiling) a test for gastrointestinal absorption of vitamin B_{12}; a measured amount of radioactive vitamin B_{12} (cyanocobalamin ^{57}Co) is given orally, followed by a parenteral flushing dose of the nonradioactive vitamin, and the percentage of radioactivity is determined in the urine excreted over a 24-hour period. A low urinary excretion that becomes normal after the test is repeated with intrinsic factor is diagnostic of primary pernicious anaemia.

Schimmelbusch's disease ('shiməl,buhshiz) cystic disease of the breast.

schindylesis (,skindi'leesis) an articulation in which a thin plate of one bone is received into a cleft in another, as in the articulation of the perpendicular plate of the ethmoid bone with the vomer.

Schirmer's test ('shiəməz) a test for keratoconjunctivitis sicca; a piece of filter paper is inserted into the conjunctival sac over the lower eyelid with the end of the paper hanging down on the outside. If the projecting paper remains dry after 15 minutes, deficient tear formation is indicated.

schist(o)- word element. [Gr.] *cleft*, *split*.

schistocephalus (,shistoh'kefələs, -'sef-) a fetus with a cleft head.

schistocoelia (,shistoh'seeli·ə) congenital fissure of the abdomen.

schistocormus (,shistoh'kawməs)) a fetus with a cleft trunk.

schistocyte ('shistoh,siet) a fragment of an erythrocyte, commonly observed in the blood in haemolytic anaemia.

schistocytosis (,shistohsie'tohsis) an accumulation of schistocytes in the blood.

schistoglossia (,shistoh'glosi·ə) cleft (bifid) tongue.

schistomelus (shi'stoməlǝs) a fetus with a cleft limb.

schistometer (shi'stomitə) an instrument for measuring the aperture between the vocal cords.

schistoprosopus (,shistoh'prosəpəs) a fetus with a cleft face.

Schistosoma (,shistoh'sohmə) a genus of trematodes, including several species parasitic in the blood of man and domestic animals. The organisms are called schistosomes or blood flukes. Larvae (cercariae) enter the body of the host through the skin, after contact with contaminated water, or possibly by way of the digestive tract, or through the skin from contact with contaminated water, and migrate in the blood to small blood vessels of organs of the intestinal or urinary tract; they attach themselves to the blood vessel walls and mature and reproduce. The intermediate hosts are snails of various species.

S. haematobium a species endemic in much of Africa and the Middle East; the organisms are found in the venules of the urinary bladder wall, and eggs may be found in urine.

S. japonicum a species geographically confined to the Far East, and found chiefly in the venules of the intestine.

S. mansoni a species widely distributed in Africa and parts of South America; the organisms are found in the host's mesenteric veins, and eggs may be found in the faeces.

schistosome dermatitis ('shistoh,sohm) dermatitis caused by penetration of the skin by larvae (cercariae) of organisms of the genus *Schistosoma*.

schistosomiasis (,shistəsoh'mieəsis) infection with flukes of the genus *Schistosoma*; called also bilharziasis. It is a significant health problem in much of the tropics and subtropics, including the Middle East, Africa, the Far East, and parts of South America and the West Indies. The various species cause different forms of the disease; *S. mansoni* and *S. japonicum* produce intestinal symptoms, with damage to the liver in heavy infections and *S. haematobium* produces haematuria and other urinary symptoms, with damage to the bladder and, in heavy infections, to the kidneys.

Treatment includes correction of anaemia and other nutritional disorders caused by the parasites, and destruction of adult worms by administration of praziquantel (all 3 species), metriphonate (*S. haematobium* only), or oxamniquine (*S. mansoni* only). Improvements in sanitation and snail control are the chief preventive measures.

schistosomicide (,shistoh'sohmi,sied) an agent that destroys schistosomes.

schistosomus (,shistoh'sohməs) a fetus with a cleft abdomen.

schistothorax (,shistoh'thor·raks) congenital fissure of the chest or sternum.

schiz(o)- word element. [Gr] *divided*, *division*.

schizaxon (skits'akson) an axon that divides into two nearly equal branches.

schizoaffective disorder (,skitsoh·ə'fektiv) a nonspecific term for conditions with some characteristics of schizophrenia and some characteristics of affective disorders.

schizogenesis (,skitsoh'jenəsis) reproduction by fission.

schizogony (skit'sogənee) the asexual reproduction of a sporozoan parasite (sporozoite) by multiple fission within the body of the host, giving rise to merozoites, as in malaria. adj. **schizogonic**.

schizogyria (,skitsoh'jieri·ə) a condition in which the cerebral convolutions have wedge-shaped cracks.

schizoid ('skitsoyd) 1. resembling schizophrenia: a term applied to a shut-in, unsocial, introspective personality. 2. a person of schizoid personality.

schizomycete (,skitsoh'mieseet) an organism of the class Schizomycetes.

Schizomycetes (,skitsohmie'seeteez) a taxonomic class comprising the bacteria; they are typically unicellular organisms, considered plants which commonly multiply by cell division, and which may be free living, saprophytic, parasitic, or even pathogenic, the last causing disease in plants or animals.

schizont ('skitsont) the stage in the development of the malarial parasite following the trophozoite whose nucleus divides into many smaller nuclei.

schizonychia (,skitso'niki·ə) splitting of the nails.

schizophrenia (,skitsoh'freeni·ə) a general term encompassing a large group of mental disorders (the schizophrenic disorders) characterized by mental deterioration from a previous level of functioning and characteristic disturbances of multiple psychological processes, including delusions, loosening of associations, poverty of the content of speech, auditory hallucinations, inappropriate affect, disturbed sense of self, and withdrawal from the external world. adj. **schizophrenic.** Because the onset is usually in adolescence or early adulthood schizophrenia was formerly called *dementia praecox*. The term *schizophrenia* literally means 'split personality', referring to portions of the psyche that are contradictory; it does not mean multiple personality, which is the presence of distinct, autonomous subpersonalities.

TYPES. Schizophrenia is sometimes classified according to probable cause and expected prognosis. *Process* or *nuclear* schizophrenia is thought to be due to an organic or chemical predisposition, characterized by a prolonged deterioration of behaviour, and having a poor prognosis. *Reactive schizophrenia* is thought to be of environmental origin, having occurred as a reaction to some events in the patient's life, and presenting less severe thought disorders. The prognosis for recovery from reactive schizophrenia is much better than that of process schizophrenia.

CLASSIFICATION. The current nomenclature classifies schizophrenia into five types. *Hebephrenic (disorganized)* schizophrenia is characterized by disorganized, incoherent thinking; shallow, inappropriate, and silly affect; and regressive behaviour without systematized delusions. *Catatonic* schizophrenia is characterized by psychomotor disturbance which may involve stupor, rigidity, excitement, or posturing, or an alteration among these behaviours; associated features include mutism, stereotypy, and waxy flexibility (flexibilitas cerea). This type of schizophrenia is now rare. *Paranoid* schizophrenia is characterized by persecutory or grandiose delusions, delusional jealousy, or hallucinations with persecutory or grandiose content. The *undifferentiated* type refers to cases in which there are prominent psychotic symptoms, such as delusions, hallucinations, or incoherence, and which cannot be classified as one of the first three types. The *residual* type refers to cases in which the prominent psychotic symptoms of a previous episode have disappeared but signs of the illness, such as inappropriate affect, social withdrawal, or loosening of associations, persist.

TREATMENT. A variety of therapeutic measures may be used to help the schizophrenic patient cope with reality and the demands of everyday living. The combination of therapies will depend on the needs of the individual patient, his age and family background, the environment in which he must live, and the preferences of the attending psychiatrist and psychologist. One kind of therapy utilized is treatment with one of the neuroleptics (antipsychotic agents), such as chlorpromazine. Depot neuroleptic drugs, e.g. flupenthixol or fluphenazine decanoate allow valuable maintenance drug therapy and enable many chronic schizophrenics to tbe returned to the community. Other kinds of therapy are intensive psychotherapy for outpatients and various forms of group therapy and milieu therapy for hospitalized patients.

Social skills training and behaviour therapy will help to restore and develop atrophied or underdeveloped areas of interpersonal functioning.

childhood s. schizophrenia with onset before the age of puberty; formerly, this type was not differentiated from infantile autism.

schizoaffective s. a subtype of schizophrenia with prominent mood disorder, either manic or depressive.

schizosis (skits'ohsis) a mental state with a marked tendency to avoid contact with the outside world, and to shun social responsibilities.

schizotrichia (,skitsoh'triki·ə) splitting of the hairs at the ends.

Schlatter's disease ('shlatəz) Osgood–Schlatter disease.

Schlatter–Osgood disease (,shlatə'ozguhd) Osgood–Schlatter disease.

Schlemm's canal (shlemz) a circular canal at the junction of the sclera and cornea, within the drainage angle of the eye. Aqueous enters this canal after passing through the trabecular meshwork.

Schmorl's disease (shmorlz) herniation of the nucleus pulposus.

Schmorl's node (nodule) an irregular or hemispherical bone defect in the upper or lower margin of the body of a vertebra into which the nucleus pulposus of the intervertebral disc herniates.

Schönlein–Henoch purpura (disease) (,shərnlien'henok) nonthrombocytopenic purpura of unknown cause, most often seen in children, associated with various clinical symptoms, such as urticaria and erythema, arthropathy and arthritis, gastrointestinal symptoms, and renal involvement.

Schönlein's purpura (disease) ('shərnlienz) Schönlein–Henoch purpura in which articular symptoms predominate.

Schüffner's dots ('shoofnəz) very fine stippling seen in erythrocytes infected with *Plasmodium vivax* when stained by certain methods.

Schüller–Christian disease (,shoolə'krischən) Hand–Schüller–Christian disease.

Schüller's disease (,shooləz) Hand–Schüller–Christian disease.

Schultz–Charlton test ('shuhlts,chahltən) a test in which an intradermal injection of scarlet fever antitoxin is made into an area of rash. Blanching will occur at the injection site if the patient has scarlet fever.

Schwabach test ('shvahbak) a hearing test made, with the opposite ear masked, with tuning forks of 256, 512, 1024, and 2048 cycles, alternately placing the stem of the vibrating fork on the mastoid process of the temporal bone of the patient and that of the examiner. The result is expressed as 'Schwabach prolonged' if heard longer by the patient (indicative of conductive hearing impairment), as 'Schwabach shortened or diminished' if heard longer by the examiner (indicative of sensorineural hearing impairment), and as 'Schwabach normal' if heard for the same time by both.

Schwalbe's ring ('shvahlbəz) a circular ridge composed of collagenous fibres surrounding the outer margin of Descemet's membrane.

schwannoma (shwo'nohmə) a neoplasm originating from Schwann cells (of the myelin sheath) of neurons; schwannomas include neurofibromas and neurilemomas.

Schwartze's operation ('shwawtsəz) opening of the mastoid cells, without involvement of the middle ear, in order to drain a mastoid abscess.

sciage (see'ahzh) [Fr.] a sawing movement in massage.

sciatic (sie'atik) pertaining to the ischium.

s. nerve a nerve extending from the base of the spine down the thigh, with branches throughout the lower leg and foot. It is the widest nerve of the body and one of the longest. Inflammation of the sciatic nerve causes pain along its course, referred to as SCIATICA.

sciatica (sie'atikə) neuralgia along the course of the sciatic nerve. The term is popularly used to describe a number of disorders directly or indirectly affecting the sciatic nerve. Because of its length, the nerve is exposed to many different kinds of injury, and inflammation of the nerve or injury to it causes pain that travels down from the back or thigh along its course in the leg and into the foot and toes. Certain muscles of the legs may be partly or completely paralysed by such a disorder.

True sciatic neuritis is comparatively rare. It can be caused by certain toxic substances, such as lead and alcohol, and occasionally by various other factors. Sciatic pain can be produced by a number of conditions other than inflammation of the nerve. Probably the most common cause is a slipped, or herniated, DISC. A back injury, irritation from arthritis of the spine, or pressure on the nerve from certain types of exertion may also be the cause. Occasionally certain diseases such as diabetes mellitus, gout, and vitamin deficiencies may be the inciting factor. In rare cases, pain may be referred over connected nerve pathways to the sciatic nerve from a disorder in another part of the body. Some cases are idiopathic. Because of the long, painful, and disabling course of severe sciatica, the underlying cause should be investigated and corrected when possible.

SCID severe combined immunodeficiency disease.

scieropia (ˌsieə'rohpi·ə) a defect of vision in which objects appear in a shadow.

scintigram ('sintiˌgram) an image produced by scintigraphy.

scintigraphy (sin'tigrəfee) the production of two-dimensional images of the distribution of radioactivity in tissues after the internal administration of a radiopharmaceutical imaging agent, the images being obtained by a scintillation camera. adj. **scintigraphic**.

scintillation (ˌsinti'layshən) 1. the emission of sparks. 2. the sensation of sparks before the eyes. 3. a particle emitted in disintegration of a radioactive element.

scintiphotography (ˌsintifə'togrəfee) scintigraphy.

scintiscan ('sintiˌskan) a two-dimensional representation (map) of the gamma rays emitted by a radioisotope, revealing its concentration in a specific organ or tissue.

scintiscanner ('sintiˌskanə) the system of equipment used to make a scintiscan.

scirrho- word element. [Gr.] *hard*.

scirrhoid ('siroyd) resembling scirrhous carcinoma.

scirrhous ('sirəs) hard or indurated.

s. carcinoma carcinoma with a hard structure owing to the formation of dense connective tissue in the stroma.

scirrhus ('sirəs) scirrhous carcinoma.

scissor-gait ('sizəgayt) a spastic gait in which the legs are adducted, crossing alternately in front of one another during walking. Characteristic of spastic diplegia, paraplegia or bilateral hip disease. See LITTLE'S DISEASE.

scissura (si'syooə·rə) pl. *scissurae* [L.] an incisure; a splitting.

scler(o)- word element. [Gr.] *hard, sclera*.

sclera ('skliə·rə) pl. *sclerae* [L.] the tough, white outer coat of the eyeball, covering approximately the posterior five-sixths of its surface, continuous anteriorly with the cornea and posteriorly with the external sheath of the optic nerve. adj. **scleral**.

blue s. abnormal blueness of the sclera, a prominent feature of osteogenesis imperfecta; also seen in certain other conditions.

scleradenitis (ˌskliə·radə'nietis) inflammation and hardening of a gland.

sclerectasia (ˌskliə·rek'tayzi·ə) a bulging state of the sclera.

sclerectoiridectomy (skləˌrektoh·iri'dektəmee) excision of part of the sclera and of the iris.

sclerectomy (sklə'rektəmee) 1. excision of part of the sclera. 2. removal of sclerosed parts of the middle ear after otitis media.

sclerema (sklə'reemə) induration of the subcutaneous fat.

s. adiposum, s, neonatorum an often fatal condition characterized by diffuse, rapidly spreading, nonoedematous, tallow-like hardening of the subcutaneous tissues in the first few weeks of life.

scleriritomy (ˌskliə·rie'ritəmee) incision of the sclera and iris in anterior staphyloma.

scleritis (sklə'rietis) inflammation of the sclera. It may be superficial (episcleritis) or deep.

anterior s. inflammation of the sclera adjoining the limbus of the cornea.

posterior s. scleritis involving the post-equatorial sclera. Can be associated with serous retinal detachment.

scleroblastema (ˌskliə·rohbla'steemə) the embryonic tissue from which bone is formed.

sclerochoroiditis (ˌskliə·rohˌko·roy'dietis) inflammation of the sclera and choroid.

sclerodactyly (ˌskliə·roh'daktilee) scleroderma of the fingers and toes.

scleroderma (ˌskliə·roh'dərmə) an uncommon connective tissue disease in which both hardening of the connective tissues of many organs of the body, including the skin, heart, oesophagus, kidney and lung, and damage to the blood vessels may occur. The skin may be thickened, hard and rigid, and pigmented patches may occur. It may be generalized (systemic or diffuse scleroderma), limited to the distal parts of the extremities and face (acrosclerosis) or to the fingers and toes (sclerodactyly), or localized to oval or linear areas a few centimetres in width (morphea).

Occurring in both children and adults, the milder forms of scleroderma are most often seen in persons in the 30 to 50 year age group, and affect women three times as often as men. The most severe forms usually affect men, Afro-Caribbeans, and older persons.

The cause of scleroderma is not known. Current theories suggest three possibilities: an immunological reaction in which the white blood cells may produce factors which stimulate the production of collagen; hereditary factors; and environmental agents such as polyvinyl chloride which may also predispose towards the disease. The condition may be related to previous bacterial infection. Because the symptoms of scleroderma often mimic those of other diseases such as rheumatoid arthritis, systemic lupus erythematosus, mixed connective tissue disease, and polymyositis, it is difficult to diagnose.

There is no test specific for confirmation of a diagnosis of scleroderma but skin biopsies, tests for special antinuclear antibodies, and x-rays can be helpful in making the diagnosis.

Treatment includes drugs such as penicillamine, immunosuppressives, and anti-inflammatory agents. Ulcers that form on the knuckles, elbows, and other bony prominences as a result of calcium deposits are treated topically with ointments. Physiotherapy to restore and maintain musculoskeletal function is vital. Adequate nutrition including small, frequent meals can help relieve the gastrointestinal problems. See also RAYNAUD'S PHENOMENON. Further information about the disease can be obtained from The Raynaud's Association, 112 Crewe Road, Alsager, Cheshire, ST7 2BG.

scleroedema (ˌskliə·ri'deemə) a self-limiting disorder occurring in both children and adults, characterized by progressive thickening and induration of the dermis. Called also *scleroedema adultorum* and *Buschke's scleroedema*. See also SCLERODERMA.

s. neonatorum sclerema neonatorum.

sclerogenous (sklə'rojənəs) producing sclerosis or a hard tissue or material.

sclerokeratitis (ˌskliə·rohˌkerə'tietis) inflammation of the sclera and cornea.

scleroma (sklə'rohmə) a hardened patch or induration of skin or mucous membrane.

respiratory s. rhinoscleroma.

scleromalacia (ˌskliə·rohmə'layshi·ə) degeneration (softening) of the sclera, occurring in patients with rheumatoid arthritis.

scleromyxoedema (ˌskliə·roh,miksi'deemə) a variant of lichen myxoedematosus characterized by a generalized eruption of the nodules and diffuse thickening of the skin.

sclero-oophoritis (ˌskliə·roh,oh·əfə'rietis) sclerosing inflammation of the ovary.

sclerophthalmia (ˌskliə·rof'thalmi·ə) encroachment of the sclera upon the cornea so that only a portion of the central part remains clear.

scleroplasty ('skliə·roh,plastee) plastic repair of the sclera.

scleroprotein (ˌskliə·roh'prohteen) a simple protein characterized by its insolubility and its fibrous structure; it usually serves a supportive or protective function in the body.

sclerosant (sklə'rohzənt) a chemical irritant injected into a vein to produce inflammation and eventual fibrosis and obliteration of the lumen; used in the treatment of varicose veins.

sclerose (sklə'rohz) to become, or cause to become, hardened.

sclerosis (sklə'rohsis) an induration or hardening, especially hardening of a part from inflammation and in disease of the interstitial substance. The term is used chiefly for such a hardening of the nervous system due to hyperplasia of the connective tissue or for hardening of the blood vessels. adj. **sclerotic**.

amyotrophic lateral s. degeneration of the anterior horn cells and pyramidal tract, with muscular atrophy (see also AMYOTROPHIC LATERAL SCLEROSIS).

arteriolar s. arteriolosclerosis.

disseminated s. multiple sclerosis.

familial centrolobar s. a progressive familial form of leukoencephalopathy, marked by nystagmus, ataxia, tremor, parkinsonian facies, dysarthria, and mental deterioration.

lateral s. a form seated in the lateral columns of the spinal cord. It may be primary, with spastic paraplegia, rigidity of the limbs, and increase of the tendon reflexes but no sensory disturbances, or secondary to myelitis, with paraplegia and sensory disturbance.

medial calcific s. Mönckeberg's arteriosclerosis.

multiple s. demyelination of the white matter of the brain and spinal cord occurring in scattered patches, and resulting in a chronic disabling condition characterized by visual disturbances, weakness, tremors, and finally paralysis (see also MULTIPLE SCLEROSIS).

systemic s. see SCLERODERMA and RAYNAUD'S PHENOMENON.

tuberous s. a congenital hereditary disease with tumours on the surfaces of the lateral ventricles of the brain and sclerotic patches on its surface, and marked by mental deterioration and epileptic attacks.

scleroskeleton (ˌskliə·roh'skelitən) the part of the bony skeleton formed by ossification in ligaments, fasciae and tendons.

sclerostenosis (ˌskliə·rohstə'nohsis) induration or hardening combined with contraction.

sclerostomy (sklə'rostəmee) surgical creation of an opening through the sclera for the relief of glaucoma.

sclerotherapy (ˌskliə·roh'therəpee) injection of sclerosing solutions in the treatment of haemorrhoids or other varicose veins.

sclerothrix ('skliə·roh,thriks) abnormal hardness and dryness of the hair.

sclerotica (sklə'rotikə) [L.] *sclera*.

sclerotium (sklə'rohshi·əm) a hard blackish mass formed by certain fungi, as ergot.

sclerotome ('skliə·roh,tohm) 1. the area of a bone innervated from a single spinal segment. 2. one of the paired masses of mesenchymal tissue, separated from the ventromedial part of a somite, which develop into vertebrae and ribs.

sclerotomy (sklə'rotəmee) incision of the sclera.

sclerous ('skliə·rəs) hard; indurated.

SCM State Certified Midwife.

scolex ('skohleks) pl. *scolices* [Gr.] the attachment organ of a tapeworm, generally considered the anterior, or cephalic, end.

scoli(o)- word element. [Gr] *crooked*, *twisted*.

Scoline ('skohleen) trademark for a preparation of suxamethonium, a depolarizing skeletal muscle relaxant.

scoliokyphosis (ˌskohliohkie'fohsis) combined lateral (scoliosis) and posterior (kyphosis) curvature of the spine.

sclioorachitic (ˌskohliohrə'kitik) affected with scoliosis and rickets.

scoliosiometry (ˌskohliohsi'omətree) measurement of spinal curvature.

scoliosis (ˌskohli'ohsis) lateral deviation of the spine; it may or may not include rotation or result from deformity of the vertebrae. adj. **scoliotic**.

Scoliosis occurs in both sexes, with a preponderance in females. Although it can occur at any age, it is most often noticed during adolescence when there is an accelerated growth rate and the deformity can progress to a marked curvature in a very short period of time.

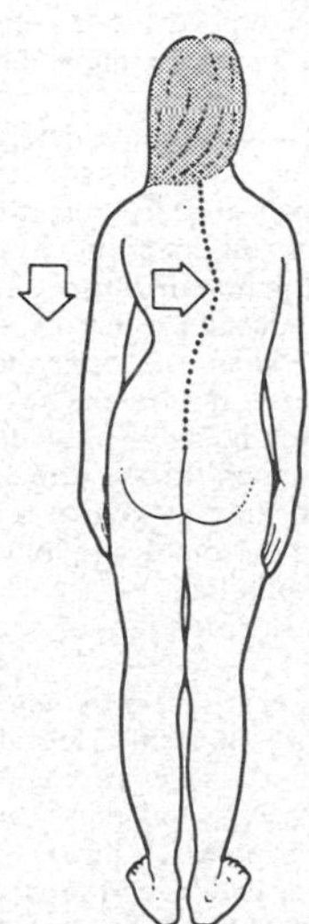

Scoliosis

CLASSIFICATION. There are two major types of scoliosis: postural and structural. *Postural* scoliosis does not involve fixed rotation of the vertebrae, is not usually pronounced, and can be corrected by exercise. *Structural* scoliosis is the result of changes in the body structure with fixed rotation of the vertebrae in the direction of the convexity of the curve. This type is further divided into three categories based on the cause and kind of deformity presented, and it may be congenital, neuromuscular, or idiopathic.

Congenital scoliosis results from improper development of the spine during the third and fifth weeks of fetal life. Congenital abnormalities, such as hemivertebra, can interfere with normal growth of the trunk. Congenital defects of the spine may be associated with other abnormalities in the newborn.

Neuromuscular scoliosis results from muscular weakness, localized muscle imbalance, or neurological dysfunction and paralysis, as from poliomyelitis. The curvature is flexible at first, with little rotation, but as the disease progresses, the curves become more pronounced and more rigid.

Idiopathic scoliosis has no known cause. The most severe cases usually appear before puberty, but it can appear at any time from infancy to adulthood. It tends to run in families; the mode of inheritance is thought to be either multifactorial with incomplete penetrance or X-linked dominant.

PREVENTION. Most cases of scoliosis can be corrected if detected early and treated promptly before inflexible structural changes occur and and cardiopulmonary complications develop.

The signs of scoliosis include: (1) one shoulder higher than the other or one shoulder blade more prominent, (2) abnormal waistline tilt with more indentation on one side, (3) a tilting of the hips with one hip more prominent, (4) a prominence of the posterior chest or the shoulder when the child bends over. Inspection of the adolescent child for the above signs should be made every few months.

TREATMENT. Milder forms of scoliosis respond well to active and passive exercise, but the more severe structural defects require either nonsurgical immobilization, with the use of a metal or plastic brace, or surgical correction.

Various surgical techniques, determined by the type of structural defects present, are employed to realign the spine through the use of external or internal fixation and instrumentation in combination with spinal fusion to maintain normal curvature. Surgical intervention is indicated when the curve is more than 40 degrees or when a congenital curvature will inevitably progress if not treated by early stabilization.

scopolamine (skoh'polə,meen) see HYOSCINE.

scopophilia (,skohpoh'fili·ə) 1. the derivation of sexual pleasure from looking at genitalia; voyeurism (active scopophilia). 2. a morbid desire to be seen; exhibitionism (passive scopophilia).

scopophobia (,skohpoh'fohbi·ə) morbid dread of being seen.

-scopy word element. [Gr] *examination of.*

scoracratia (,skor·rə'krayshi·ə) faecal incontinence.

scorbutic (skaw'byootik) pertaining to scurvy.

scorbutigenic (skaw,byooti'jenik) causing scurvy.

scorbutus (skaw'byootəs) [L.] *scurvy.*

scordinaemia (,skawdi'neemi·ə) yawning and stretching with a feeling of lassitude.

score (skor) a rating, usually expressed numerically, based on specific achievement or the degree to which certain qualities are manifest.

Apgar s. a numerical expression of an infant's condition at birth, based on heart rate, respiratory effort, muscle tone, reflex irritability, and colour. See also APGAR SCORE.

Bishop s. a gauge of cervical 'ripeness' indicating whether induction of labour is likely to be successful. See also BISHOP SCORE.

scoto- word element. [Gr.] *darkness.*

scotochromogen (,skohtoh'krohməjən) a microorganism whose pigmentation develops in the dark as well as in the light; specifically, a member of a group of the anonymous mycobacteria. adj. **scotochromogenic**.

scotodinia (,skohtoh'dini·ə) dizziness with headache and dimness of vision.

scotoma (skoh'tohmə) pl. *scotomata* [Gr.] an area of depressed vision within the visual field, surrounded by an area of less depressed or of normal vision. adj. **scotomatous**.

absolute s. an area within the visual field in which perception of light is entirely lost.

annular s. a circular area of depressed vision surrounding the point of fixation.

arcuate s. an arc-shaped defect of vision arising in an area near the blind spot and extending toward it. Typically found in chronic simple glaucoma.

central s. an area of depressed vision corresponding with the fixation point and interfering with or abolishing central vision.

centrocaecal s. a horizontal oval defect in the visual field situated between and embracing both the fixation point and the blind spot.

colour s. an isolated area of depressed or defective vision for colour in the visual field.

mental s. in psychiatry, a figurative blind spot in a person's psychological awareness, the patient being unable to gain insight into and to understand his mental problems; lack of insight.

negative s. one which appears as a blank spot or hiatus in the visual field.

peripheral s. an area of depressed vision toward the periphery of the visual field.

physiological s. that area of the visual field corresponding with the optic disc, in which the photosensitive receptors are absent.

positive s. one which appears as a dark spot in the visual field.

relative s. an area of the visual field in which perception of light is only diminished, or loss is restricted to light of certain wavelengths.

ring s. annular s.

scintillating s. blurring of vision with the sensation of a luminous appearance before the eyes, with a zigzag, wall-like outline; called also teichopsia.

scotomization (,skohtəmie'zayshən) the development of scotomata, especially mental scotomata, the patient attempting to deny existence of anything that conflicts with his ego.

scotophilia (,skohtoh'fili·ə) love of darkness.

scotophobia (,skohtoh'fohbi·ə) morbid fear of darkness.

scotopia (skoh'tohpi·ə) 1. night vision. 2. the adjustment of the eye for darkness; dark adaptation. adj. **scotopic**.

scotopsin (skoh'topsin) the protein moiety in the retinal rods that combines with 11-*cis*-retinal to form rhodopsin.

scr. scruple.

scratch test (skrach) a test for hypersensitivity in which a minute amount of the substance in question is inserted in small scratches made in the skin. A positive reaction is swelling and reddening at the site within 30 minutes. Used in allergy testing and in testing for tuberculosis (Pirquet's reaction). See also SKIN TEST.

screen (skreen) 1. a framework or agent used as a shield or protector. 2. to examine.

Bjerrum s. tangent screen, as used in perimetry.

fluorescent s. a plate in the fluoroscope coated with crystals of a substance that fluoresces, permitting visualization of internal body structures by x-ray.

tangent s. a large square of black cloth with a central mark for fixation; used in mapping the field of vision.

screening ('skreening) 1. examination of a large

number of individuals to disclose certain characteristics, or an unrecognized disease, as tuberculosis or diabetes mellitus. 2. fluoroscopy.

multiphasic s., multiple s. simultaneous examination of a population for several different diseases.

scrobiculate (skroh'bikyuhlət, -,layt) marked with pits.

scrobiculus (skroh'bikyuhləs) [L.] *pit.*

s. cordis the pit of the stomach.

scrofula ('skrofyuhlə) primary tuberculosis of the cervical lymph nodes, the inflamed structures being subject to a cheesy degeneration.

scrofuloderma (,skrofyuhloh'dərmə) suppurating abscesses and fistulous passages opening on the skin, secondary to tuberculosis of the lymph nodes, especially those of the neck (scrofula).

scrofulous ('skrofyuhləs) pertaining to or characterized by scrofuloderma or scrofula.

scrotectomy (skroh'tektəmee) excision of part of the scrotum.

scrotitis (skroh'tietis) inflammation of the scrotum.

scrotocele ('skrohtoh,seel) scrotal hernia.

scrotoplasty ('skrotoh,plastee) plastic reconstruction of the scrotum.

scrotum ('skrohtəm) the pouch that contains the testes and their accessory organs. It is composed of skin, the dartos, fascia, and the tunica vaginalis. adj. **scrotal.** Each TESTIS is connected to a cremaster muscle descending from the abdominal wall. During cold weather these muscles draw the testes closer to the body to maintain their temperature. In hot weather the reverse occurs. The scrotum usually follows this movement.

The scrotum is subject to the same diseases as the rest of the skin, including cysts and cancer. Oedema, whether caused by heart disease or the tropical disease ELEPHANTIASIS, can cause great enlargement of the scrotum by filling its loose tissues with fluid.

scrub typhus (,skrub 'tiefəs) tsutsugamushi disease, a form of typhus transmitted by larval mites.

scrumpox ('skrum,poks) skin infection of the face associated with rugby football and usually due to *Streptococcus pyogenes* (IMPETIGO), less often to *Staphylococcus aureus*, herpes simplex, and herpes zoster.

scruple ('skroop'l) a unit of weight of the apothecaries' system, equal to 20 grains; the equivalent of 1.296 g.

scultetus bandage (binder) (skul'teetəs) a many-tailed bandage applied with the tails overlapping each other and held in position by safety pins.

scurf (skərf) dandruff.

scurvy ('skərvee) a condition due to deficiency of ASCORBIC ACID (vitamin C). Symptoms of infantile scurvy include poor appetite, digestive disturbances, failure to gain weight, and increasing irritability. Black and blue spots are scattered over the skin. Severe deficiency may cause changes in bone structure.

The adults most likely to develop scurvy are older people who live alone and neglect their diet. In adults, scurvy causes swollen and bleeding gums, looseness of the teeth, rupture of small blood vessels, and small black and blue spots on the skin. Later symptoms may include anaemia, extreme weakness, soreness of the arms and legs, tachycardia, and dyspnoea.

Treatment of scurvy consists of supplying the missing vitamin in prescribed doses, and supplying the proper diet, including fresh fruits and vegetables. When this is done, the symptoms quickly disappear.

Fruits and vegetables that are rich sources of vitamin C include the following: grapefruit, oranges, lemons, limes, cantaloupes, strawberries, raspberries, turnips, raw cabbage, potatoes (baked), and tomatoes.

scute (skyoot) any squama or scalelike structure, especially the bony plate separating the upper part of the middle ear from the mastoid cells.

scutiform ('skyooti,fawm) shaped like a shield.

scutulum ('skyootyuhləm) pl. *scutula* [L.] one of the disc- or saucer-like crusts characteristic of favus.

scutum ('skyootəm) 1. scute. 2. a protective covering or shield, e.g., a chitin plate in the exoskeleton of hard-bodied ticks.

scybalous ('sibələs) of the nature of a scybalum.

scybalum ('sibələm) pl. *scybala* [Gr.] a hard mass of faecal matter in the intestine.

scyphoid ('siefoyd) shaped like a cup or goblet.

SD streptodornase.

s.d. standard deviation.

Se chemical symbol, *selenium.*

Seacole ('seekohl) Mary (1805–1881). Born in Kingston, Jamaica, the daughter of a Scotsman and a free black woman. Her mother was highly skilled in Creole medical art based on herbal medicine and midwifery knowledge brought from Africa to the Caribbean. These skills she passed on to her daughter. Mary Seacole helped to care for patients in the Panama cholera epidemic in 1850. When the Crimean War broke out in 1853 Mary Seacole journeyed to England, arriving in 1854. She applied to the War Office for the post of hospital nurse in the Crimea but was rejected. Mary Seacole finally set out for the Crimea, establishing a canteen for the British regiments at Balaclava. Besides running the canteen for the army, Mary Seacole entered the battlefields, often under gun fire, dressing wounds, giving out medicines and drugs, and comforting dying men. Reports in *The Times* by Sir William Russell described her skills in glowing terms.

The Crimean War ended in March 1856 and Mary Seacole was left with stores and supplies she could not sell and was declared bankrupt. *The Times* set up an Appeal Fund and her debts were finally discharged. She spent the rest of her life between Kingston, Jamaica and London, becoming the Princess of Wales' masseuse. She died in Paddington, London, in 1881.

sealed radiation sources (seeld) see internal RADIATION THERAPY.

searcher ('sərchə) an instrument (a sound) used in examining the bladder for calculi; called also *stone searcher*.

seasickness ('see,siknəs) discomfort caused by the motion of a boat under way, a form of MOTION SICKNESS. The unusual motion disturbs the organs of balance located in the inner ear. The symptoms are nausea and vomiting, dizziness, headache, pallor, and cold perspiration.

There are a number of ways to help ward off seasickness. It is best to stay in the fresh air instead of in a stuffy room, to eat lightly, and to avoid fatty, fried, or spicy foods. Antinausea medicines may be effective. If seasickness occurs, the sufferer should rest lying down with his head low, in a comfortable well ventilated place.

seatworm ('seet,wərm) pinworm; an individual of the species *Enterobius vermicularis* (see also WORMS).

sebaceous (si'bayshəs) pertaining to or secreting sebum.

s. cyst a benign retention cyst of a sebaceous gland containing the fatty secretion of the gland; called also wen. Sebaceous cysts may occur anywhere on the body except the palms of the hands and soles of the feet; they are most common on the scalp, back, and scrotum. A cyst may be a source of irritation or infection, and should be excised.

s. gland one of the thousands of minute holocrine glands in the skin that secrete an oily, colourless, odourless fluid (sebum) through the hair follicles.

sebiferous, sebiparous (sə'bifə·rəs; sə'bipə·rəs)

secreting or producing a fatty substance.

sebolith ('seboh,lith) a calculus in a sebaceous gland.

seborrhoea (,sebə'reeə) excessive discharge from the sebaceous glands, forming greasy scales or cheesy plugs on the body; it is generally attended with itching or burning.

s. sicca dry, scaly seborrhoeic dermatitis.

seborrhoeic (,sebə'ree·ik) affected with or of the nature of seborrhoea.

s. dermatitis an inflammatory condition of the skin of the scalp, with yellowish greasy scaling of the skin; commonly known as dandruff. It may spread to other areas about the face, neck, central part of the trunk and axillae.

The underlying cause is not known but there is often a family history. The sebaceous glands become overactive and the hair and scalp are excessively oily. The scales are greasy, yellowish and crusty. Burning or itching and erythema of the involved areas may occur.

There is also a dry form of the condition, in which the scales are hard, dry and whitish grey in colour and the hair is dry and brittle.

Although there is no specific cure for dandruff, various measures are used to control and relieve it. The most imperative point is cleanliness of the hair, scalp, combs and brushes. There are some helpful medical preparations which are prescribed for persistent cases. There usually contain sulphur, tar, salicylic acid, selenium sulphide, or steroids.

seborrhoeid (,sebə'ree·id) a seborrhoeic eruption.

sebotropic (,sebə'tropik) having an affinity for or a stimulating effect on sebaceous glands; promoting the excretion of sebum.

sebum ('seebəm) the oily secretion of the sebaceous glands, whose ducts open into the hair follicles. It is composed of fat and epithelial debris from the cells of the malpighian layer, and it lubricates the skin.

sec. second.

Seconal ('sekonal) trademark for preparations of secobarbital.

second ('sekənd) the SI unit of time. Symbol s.

second-set phenomenon (,sekənd'set) the accelerated and intensified rejection by the recipient of a second graft of tissue from the same donor as a consequence of the primary IMMUNE RESPONSE (i.e., antibody production and cell-mediated IMMUNITY) induced by the first graft.

secondary care ('sekəndree) the level of care in the HEALTH CARE SYSTEM that consists of emergency treatment and care. Called also *acute care*.

secreta (si'kreetə) [L.] *secretion products*.

secretagogue (si'kreetə,gog) 1. causing a flow of secretion. 2. an agent that stimulates secretion.

secrete (si'kreet) to synthesize and release a substance.

secretin (si'kreetin) a hormone secreted by the mucosa of the duodenum and jejunum when acid chyme enters the intestine; carried by the blood, it stimulates the secretion of pancreatic juice and, to a lesser extent, bile and intestinal secretion.

s. test an examination of the gastric and duodenal contents after intravenous administration of exogenous secretin; useful in the diagnosis of disorders affecting pancreatic exocrine function, for example, pancreatitis and neoplastic disease. Specimens are obtained via a double lumen tube having a metal weight at one end to carry it past the stomach into the duodenum. At the other end are two tails, one used to collect gastric specimens and the other to collect specimens from the duodenum. Fluid is analysed for output (secretory rate), bicarbonate concentration, and amylase activity.

secretinase (si'kreeti,nayz) a substance in the serum that inactivates secretin.

Actions of secretin

Pancreas
- Increase in secretion of H_2O, HCO_3^- and enzymes
- Increase in secretion of insulin; decreased secretion of glucagon

Biliary system
- Increase in contractions of gallbladder and flow of bile. H_2O and electrolytes
- Increase in level of cAMP in the bile

Stomach
- Decrease in secretion of HCl, but increase in pepsin
- Decrease in gastrin
- Decrease in motility, but increase in pyloric tone
- Inhibition of gastrin-induced parietal cell hyperplasia
- Increase in mucosal thickness

Intestine
- Decrease in muscle tone and duodenal motility
- Increase absorption of Na^+ and water
- Increase in secretion by Brunner's glands, but not much increase in total secretion of water and electrolytes

Other hormones
- Increase in secretion of somatostatin, pancreatic polypeptide and parathyroid hormone

From Williams, R. H. (1981) *Textbook of Endocrinology*, 6th edn, W. B. Saunders.

secretion (si'kreeshən) 1. the cellular process of elaborating a specific product. This activity may range from separating a specific substance of the blood to the elaboration of a new chemical substance. 2. any substance produced by secretion. One example is the fatty substance produced by the sebaceous glands to lubricate the skin. Saliva, produced by the salivary glands, and gastric juice, secreted by specialized glands of the stomach, are both used in digestion. The secretions of the endocrine glands include various hormones and are important in the overall regulation of body processes.

secretoinhibitory (si,kreetoh·in'hibitə·ree) inhibiting secretion; antisecretory.

secretomotor (si,kreetoh'mohtə) stimulating secretion; said of nerves.

secretor (si'kreetə) in genetics, one who secretes the ABH antigens of the ABO blood group in the saliva and other body fluids; also, the gene determining this trait.

secretory (si'kreetə·ree) pertaining to secretion.

sectio ('sekshioh) pl. *sectiones* [L.] section.

section ('sekshən) 1. an act of cutting. 2. a cut surface. 3. a segment or subdivision of an organ. 4. in histology, a thin slice of a specimen prepared for microscopic preparation.

abdominal s. laparotomy.

caesarean s. delivery of a fetus by incision through the abdominal wall into the uterus; see also CAESAREAN SECTION.

frontal s. a section through the body passing at right angles to the median plane, dividing the body into dorsal and ventral parts.

frozen s. a specimen cut by microtome from tissue that has been frozen; see also FROZEN SECTION.

perineal s. surgical dissection of the perineum, usually to expose the urethra.

sagittal s. a section through the body coinciding with the sagittal suture, thus dividing the body into right and left halves.

serial s's histological sections of a specimen made in

consecutive order and so arranged for the purpose of microscopic examination.

sectorial (sek'tor·ri·əl) cutting.

Securopen (si'kyuhrohpen) trademark for preparations of azlocillin, an antibiotic.

sedation (si'dayshən) 1. the allaying of irritability or excitement, especially by administration of a sedative. 2. the state so induced.

sedative ('sedətiv) 1. allaying irritability and excitement. 2. an agent that calms nervousness, irritability, and excitement. In general, sedatives depress the central nervous system and tend to cause lassitude and reduced mental activity. They may be classified, according to the organ most affected, as cardiac, gastric, etc.

The degree of relaxation produced varies with the kind of sedative, the dose, the means of administration, and the mental state of the patient. By causing relaxation, a sedative may help a patient go to sleep, but it does not put him to sleep. Medicines that induce sleep are known as hypnotics. A drug may act as a sedative in small amounts and as a hypnotic in large amounts.

The BARBITURATES such as phenobarbitone are the best-known sedatives. They are also widely used as hypnotics.

Sedatives are useful in the treatment of any condition in which rest and relaxation are important to recovery. Some sedatives are also useful in treatment of convulsive disorders or epilepsy and in counteracting the effect of convulsion-producing drugs. They are used to calm patients before childbirth or surgery. Restlessness in invalids, profound grief in adults, and overexcitement in children can be controlled by medically supervised sedation. Because many sedatives are habit-forming, they should be used only with caution.

Among drugs related to sedatives are the anxiolytics which also have a calming effect but, unlike sedatives, usually do not suppress body reactions. Anxiolytics are habit forming.

sedentary ('sed'nt·ə·ree) of inactive habits; pertaining to a sitting posture.

sediment ('sedimənt) a precipitate, especially that formed spontaneously.

sedimentation (ˌsedimen'tayshən) the settling out of sediment.

s. rate the rate at which a sediment is deposited in a given volume of solution, especially when subjected to the action of a centrifuge. The *erythrocyte sedimentation rate* is the rate at which erythrocytes settle out of unclotted blood in an hour. Abbreviated sed. rate or ESR. The test is based on the fact that inflammatory processes cause an alteration in blood proteins, resulting in aggregation of the red cells, which makes them heavier and more likely to fall rapidly when placed in a special vertical test tube. Normal ranges vary according to the type of tube used, each type being of a different size. The most common methods and the normal range for each are: Wintrobe method—0 to 6.5 mm per hour for men, 0 to 15 mm per hour for women; Westergren method—0 to 15 mm per hour for men, 0 to 20 mm per hour for women.

The sedimentation rate is often inconclusive and is not considered specific for any particular disorder. It is most often used as gauge for determining the progress of an inflammatory disease such as rheumatic fever, rheumatoid arthritis, and respiratory infections. The information provided by this test must be used in conjunction with results from other tests and clinical evaluations.

seed (seed) 1. the mature ovule of a flowering plant. 2. semen. 3. a small cylindrical shell of gold or other suitable material, used in application of radiation therapy. 4. to inoculate a culture medium with microorganisms.

radon s. a small sealed container for radon, for insertion into the tissues of the body in radiotherapy.

seeker (seekə) a blunt flexible probe used to explore a sinus or fistula and determine its direction.

Seessel's pouch ('zayselz) an outpouching of the embryonic pharynx rostrad to the pharyngeal membrane and caudal to Rathke's pouch.

segment ('segmənt) a demarcated portion of a whole. adj. **segmental.**

bronchopulmonary s. one of the smaller subdivisions of the lobe of a lung, separated from others by a connective tissue septum and supplied by its own branch of the bronchus leading to the particular lobe.

hepatic s's subdivisions of the hepatic lobes based on arterial and biliary supply and venous drainage.

uterine s. either of the two portions into which the uterus becomes differentiated early in labour; the upper contractile portion (corpus uteri) becomes thicker as labour approaches, and the lower noncontractile portion (the isthmus) is thin walled and passive in character.

segmentation (ˌsegmən'tayshən) 1. division into similar parts. 2. cleavage.

segregation (ˌsegri'gayshən) the separation of allelic genes during meiosis as homologous chromosomes begin to migrate toward opposite poles of the cell, so that eventually the members of each pair of allelic genes go to separate gametes.

segregator ('segriˌgaytə) an instrument for obtaining the urine from the ureter of each kidney separately.

seismotherapy (ˌsiezmoh'therəpee) treatment of disease by mechanical vibration.

seizure ('seezhə) 1. the sudden attack or recurrence of a disease. 2. a CONVULSION or attack of EPILEPSY.

absence s. an epileptic seizure marked by a momentary break in the stream of thought and activity, accompanied by a symmetrical 3-Hz spike and wave activity on the electroencephalogram.

audiogenic s. a seizure brought on by sound.

cerebral s. an attack of EPILEPSY.

febrile s. convulsions associated with high fever.

jack-knife s. a severe myoclonus appearing in the first 18 months of life, and associated with general cerebral deterioration; it is marked by severe flexion spasms of the head, neck, and trunk and extension of the arms and legs. Called also *infantile massive spasms*.

photogenic s. a seizure brought on by light.

Seldinger technique ('seldingə) the technique of percutaneous insertion of a catheter into a vessel. The vessel is punctured with a needle and a guide wire threaded through the needle into the vessel. The needle is removed, keeping the wire in the vessel. The catheter is threaded over the wire, and when safely in the vessel, the wire is removed.

selectivity (ˌsilek'tivitee) in pharmacology, the degree to which a dose of a drug produces the desired effect in relation to adverse effects. adj. **selective.**

selenium (si'leeni·əm) a chemical element, atomic number 34, atomic weight 78.96, symbol Se. (See table of elements in Appendix 2.) It is an essential mineral nutrient.

s.-75 a radioisotope of selenium having a half-life of 120 days and a principal gamma ray photon energy of 265 keV; used in the radiopharmaceutical selenomethionine Se 75. Symbol ^{75}Se.

s. sulphide a bright orange, insoluble powder; used topically in solution in the treatment of seborrhoeic dermatitis.

self (self) 1. a term used to denote an animal's own antigenic constituents, in contrast to 'not-self', denoting foreign antigenic constituents. The 'self' constituents are metabolized without antibody formation, whereas the antigens which are 'not-self' are eliminated through the immune response mechanism. It has been postulated that there exists some mechanism of 'self recognition' which enables the organism to distinguish between 'self' and 'not self'. See also IMMUNITY. 2. the complete being of an individual, comprising both physical and psychological characteristics, and including both conscious and unconscious components. The concept of self is central to the jungian personality theory. See also JUNG.

self-actualization (self,aktyooəlie'zayshən) a level of psychological development in which innate potential is realized to the full, allowing transcendance of the environment. The term is used both to describe this ideal state and to describe the motive to achieve it. The concept of 'self-actualization' has enjoyed considerable vogue within the humanistic psychotherapies but remains both elusive and controversial.

self-antigen (self'antijən) any constituent of the body's own tissues capable of stimulating autoimmunity. See also IMMUNITY.

self-awareness (selfə'wairnəs) a state of objective and accepting consciousness of one's true personal nature. Many psychotherapeutic approaches aim to increase self-awareness.

self-consciousness generally the uneasy state of tension or embarrassment arising from the suspicion that others may be aware of one's inadequacies (real or imagined).

self-esteem the extent to which one values oneself, and, to some extent, a product of how one is valued by others.

self-limited (self'limitid) limited by its own peculiarities, and not by outside influence; said of a disease that runs a definite limited course.

self-perception (selfpə'sepshən) a theoretical viewpoint which suggests that we infer or determine our attitudes and beliefs by observing our own behaviour.

self-suspension (,selfsə'spenshən) suspension of the body by the head and axillae for the purpose of stretching the vertebral column.

self-tolerance (self'tolə·rəns) immunological tolerance to self-antigens.

sella ('selə) pl. *sellae* [L.] a saddle-shaped depression. adj. **sellar**.

empty s. see EMPTY-SELLA SYNDROME.

s. turcica a depression on the upper surface of the sphenoid bone, lodging the pituitary gland.

Sellick's manoeuvre ('seliks) the application of backward pressure on the cricoid cartilage in the throat in order to occlude the oesophagus and prevent regurgitation of stomach contents into the pharynx with consequent risk of aspiration into the lung. Described by Sellick in 1961 it is applied by the anaesthetist's assistant (who may be a nurse or an operating department assistant) as the patient is going to sleep, and is not released until an endotracheal tube has been inserted and the repiratory tract sealed off. It is used in all emergency and obstetric anaesthetics. It is important to tell the patient that he will feel pressure as he is going to sleep. In the presence of active vomiting the manoeuvre should be released because of the risk of oesophageal rupture.

semantics (sə'mantiks) study of the meanings of words and the rules of their use; study of the relation between language and significance.

semeiography (,semi'ogrəfee) a description of the signs and symptoms of a disease.

semeiology (,semi'oləjee) symptomatology.

semeiotic (,semi'otik) 1. pertaining to symptoms. 2. pathognomonic.

semelincident (,seme'linsidənt) affecting a person only once.

semen ('seemen) fluid discharged at ejaculation in the male, consisting of spermatozoa in their nutrient plasma, secretions from the prostate, seminal vesicles, and various other glands, epithelial cells and minor constituents. adj. **seminal**.

semi- word element. [L.] *half*.

semicanal (,semikə'nal) a trench or furrow open at one side.

semicircular (,semi'sərkyuhlə) shaped like a half-circle.

s. canals the passages in the inner ear, in the bony labyrinth, which control the sense of balance. Each ear has three semicircular canals (anterior, lateral, and posterior) situated approximately at right angles to each other. The canals are filled with fluid and have enlarged portions at one end, called ampullae, which contain nerve endings.

The semicircular canals respond to movement of the head. When the head changes position in any direction, the fluid in the canal that lies in the plane of movement also moves but, because of its inertia, the fluid flow lags behind the head movement. Thus the fluid presses against the delicate hairs of the nerves in the ampulla, and these nerves then register the fact that the head is turning in such a direction. This helps the body maintain its equilibrium. See also EAR and HEARING.

It is the fluid movement in the semicircular canals that causes the feeling of dizziness or vertigo after spinning. When the spinning stops, the fluid in the horizontal canal continues to move for a moment in the direction of the spin, giving a temporary false reading that the head is turning in the other direction. Motion sickness is caused by the unusual and erratic motions of the head in an airplane, car, or ship, and the resulting stimulation of the semicircular canals.

semicoma (,semi'kohmə) a stupor from which the patient may be aroused. adj. **semicomatose**.

semiflexion (,semi'flekshən) the position of a limb midway between flexion and extension; the act of bringing to such a position.

semilunar (,semi'loonə) shaped like a half-moon or crescent.

s. valves valves guarding the entrances into the aorta and pulmonary trunk from the cardiac ventricles.

seminal ('semin'l) relating to the semen.

semination (,semi'nayshən) insemination.

seminiferous (,semi'nifə·rəs) producing or carrying semen.

seminin ('seeminin) a proteolytic enzyme of human semen.

seminoma (,semi'nohmə) a malignant tumour of the testis thought to arise from primordial germ cells of the sexually undifferentiated embryonic gonad.

seminuria (,seemi'nyooə·ri·ə) discharge of semen in the urine.

semipermeable (,semi'pərmi·əb'l) permitting passage only of certain molecules.

semiprone (,semi'prohn) partly prone. Applied to a position in which the patient is lying face down but the knees are turned to one side.

semiquantitative (,semi'kwontitətiv) yielding an approximation of the quantity or amount of a substance; falling short of a quantitative result.

semis ('seemis) [L.] *half;* abbreviated *ss*.

semisulcus (,semi'sulkəs) a depression that, with an adjoining one, forms a sulcus.

semisupination (ˌsemiˌsoopiˈnayshən) a position halfway toward supination.

semisynthetic (ˌsemisinˈthetik) produced by chemical manipulation of naturally occurring substances.

Semmelweiss (ˈsemelˌvies) Ignaz Philipp (1818–1865). Hungarian physician and pioneer of antisepsis in obstetrics. He was born at Buda and educated at the universities of Pest and Vienna. As assistant in an obstetrics ward of Allgemeines Krankenhaus in Vienna, where the mortality rate from puerperal fever was extremely high, Semmelweiss recognized that the infection was carried from patient to patient by the physicians, and he instituted preventive measures, such as cleansing of the physicians' hands with chlorinated lime. He met such fierce opposition from many of his colleagues that he left Vienna and returned to Pest, as physician in the maternity department.

SEN State Enrolled Nurse.

senescence (səˈnesˈns) the process of growing old. adj. **senescent**.

Sengstaken–Blakemore tube (ˌsengztaykənˈblaykmor) a device used for the tamponade of bleeding oesophageal varices, consisting of four conjoined tubes; one leading to a balloon that is inflated in the stomach, to retain the instrument in place and compress the vessels around the cardia; one leading to a long narrow balloon by which pressure is exerted against the wall of the oesophagus; one attached to a suction apparatus for aspirating the contents of the stomach; and one through which pharyngeal suction can be applied (see accompanying illustration).

Patient Care. Prior to insertion the tube is held under water to check for leaks. It is then chilled to make it more firm, and lubricated to facilitate passage. After the tube is in place, the doctor may circulate ice water through the stomach balloon to help control haemorrhage.

Mild traction is applied to the tubing at the point at which it enters the nose. Because of the danger of tissue erosion and necrosis of the gastric and oesophageal mucosa, it is recommended that the tube be deflated for 5 minutes every 1 to 2 hours. The tubing is removed in 24 hours if bleeding is controlled.

The patient must be watched continuously for signs of either injury to or rupture of the oesophagus, respiratory distress, and shock. It is possible that the tube may be pulled upward into the oropharyngeal area, causing acute respiratory distress and asphyxiation. A pair of scissors are kept readily at hand so that the tube may be cut if this happens.

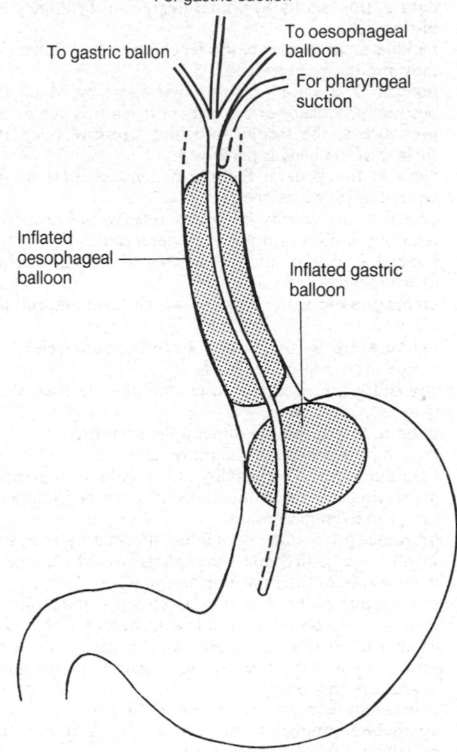

Sengstaken–Blakemore tube

senile (ˈseeniel) pertaining to old age; manifesting senility.

senilism (ˈseeniˌlizəm) premature old age.

senility (siˈnilitee) old age; denoting pronounced deterioration in mental and physical abilities in old age. Use of the term is now discouraged as being deprecatory and having no scientific value as a diagnosis. See also BRAIN FAILURE, DEMENTIA.

senna (ˈsenə) the dried leaflets of *Cassia acutiflora;* used in a syrup, fluid extract, or compound powder as a cathartic.

Senokot (ˈsenəkot) trademark for preparations of senna, a laxative.

senopia (siˈnohpi·ə) second sight; improvement of vision, especially near vision, in the aged, a sign of incipient cataract. Called also gerontopia.

sensation (senˈsayshən) an impression produced by impulses conveyed by an afferent nerve to the sensorium.

girdle s. zonaesthesia.

gnostic s's sensations perceived by the more recently developed senses, such as those of light touch and the epicritic sensibility to muscle, joint, and tendon vibrations.

primary s. that resulting immediately and directly from application of a stimulus.

referred s., reflex s. one felt elsewhere than at the site of application of a stimulus.

subjective s. one originating with the organism and not occurring in response to an external stimulus.

sense (sens) a faculty by which the conditions or properties of things are perceived. Hunger, thirst, malaise, and pain are varieties of sense; a sense of equilibrium or of well-being (euphoria) and other senses are also distinguished. The five major senses comprise VISION, HEARING, SMELL, TASTE, and TOUCH.

The operation of all senses involves the reception of stimuli by sense organs. Each sense organ is sensitive to a particular kind of stimulus. The eyes are sensitive to light; the ears, to sound; the olfactory organs of the nose, to odour; and the taste buds of the tongue, to taste. Various sense organs of the skin and other tissues are sensitive to touch, pain, temperature, and other sensations.

On receiving stimuli, the sense organ translates them into nerve impulses that are transmitted along the sensory nerves to the brain. In the cerebral cortex, the impulses are interpreted, or perceived, as sensations. The brain associates them with other information, acts upon them, and stores them as memory. See also NERVOUS SYSTEM and BRAIN.

kinaesthetic s. muscle sense.
light s. the faculty by which degrees of brilliancy are distinguished.
muscle s., muscular s. the faculty by which muscular movements are perceived.
posture s. a variety of muscular sense by which the position or attitude of the body or its parts is perceived.
pressure s. the faculty by which pressure upon the surface of the body is perceived.
sixth s. the general feeling of consciousness of the entire body; coenaesthesia.
space s. the faculty by which relative positions and relations of objects in space are perceived.
special s. one of the five senses of seeing, feeling, hearing, taste, and smell.
stereognostic s. the sense by which form and solidity are perceived.
temperature s. the faculty by which differences of temperature are appreciated.

sensibility (ˌsensi'bilitee) susceptibility of feeling; ability to feel or perceive.
deep s. the sensibility of deep tissue (muscle, tendon, etc.) to pressure, pain, and movement.
epicritic s. the sensibility to gentle stimulations permitting fine discriminations of touch and temperature, localized in the skin.
proprioceptive s. the sensibility afforded by receptors in muscles, joints, and other parts, by which one is made aware of their position and state.
protopathic s. the sensibility to strong stimulations of pain and temperature; it is low in degree and poorly localized, existing in the skin and in the viscera, and acting as a defensive agency against pathological changes in the tissues.
somaesthetic s. proprioceptive sensibility.
splanchnaesthetic s. the sensibility to stimuli received by splanchnic receptors.

sensible ('sensib'l) perceptible to the senses; capable of sensation.

sensitive ('sensitiv) 1. able to receive or respond to stimuli. 2. unusually responsive to stimulation, or responding quickly and acutely.

sensitivity (ˌsensi'tivitee) the state or quality of being sensitive.

sensitization (ˌsensitie'zayshən) 1. the initial exposure of an individual to a specific antigen, resulting in an IMMUNE RESPONSE, subsequent exposure then inducing a much stronger immune response; said especially of such exposure resulting in a hypersensitivity reaction. 2. the coating of cells with antibody as a preparatory step in eliciting an immune reaction. 3. the preparation of a tissue or organ by one hormone so that it will respond functionally to the action of another.
active s. the sensitization that results from the injection of a dose of antigen into the animal.
autoerythrocyte s. see AUTOERYTHROCYTE SENSITIZATION SYNDROME.
passive s. that which results when blood serum of a sensitized animal is injected into a normal animal.
protein s. that bodily state in which the individual is sensitive or hypersusceptible to some foreign protein, so that when there is absorption of that protein a typical reaction is set up.

sensitized ('sensiˌtiezd) rendered sensitive.

sensitogen ('sensitəˌjen) any antigen that elicits sensitizing antibody formation in an atopic individual.

sensomobile (ˌsensoh'mohbiel) moving in response to a stimulus.

sensomotor (ˌsensoh'mohtə) sensorimotor.

sensorial (sen'sor·ri·əl) pertaining to the sensorium.

sensorimotor (ˌsensə·ri'mohtə) both sensory and motor.

sensorineural (ˌsensə·ri'nyooə·rəl) of or pertaining to a sensory nerve or sensory mechanism, as sensorineural deafness.

sensorium (sen'sor·ri·əm) 1. the part of the cerebral cortex that receives and coordinates all the impulses sent to individual nerve centres. 2. the state of an individual as regards consciousness or mental awareness.
s. commune the part of the cerebral cortex that receives and coordinates all the impulses sent to individual nerve centres.

sensory ('sensə·ree) pertaining to sensation.
s. nerve a peripheral nerve that conducts impulses from a sense organ to the spinal cord or brain; called also afferent nerve.

sentient ('senti·ənt) able to feel; sensitive.

sepsis ('sepsis) the presence in the blood or other tissues of pathogenic microorganisms or their toxins; the condition associated with such presence.
puerperal s. sepsis occurring after childbirth, originating in the birth canal (see also PUERPERAL FEVER).

septa ('septə) plural of *septum.*

septal ('septəl) pertaining to a septum.

septan ('septən) recurring on the seventh day (every six days).

septate ('septayt) divided by a septum.

septectomy (sep'tektəmee) excision of part of the nasal septum.

septic ('septik) pertaining to sepsis.

septicaemia (ˌsepti'seemi·ə) BLOOD POISONING; systemic disease associated with the presence and persistence of pathogenic microorganisms in the blood. adj. **septicaemic.**
cryptogenic s. septicaemia in which the focus of infection is not evident during life.
puerperal s. that in which the focus of infection is a lesion of the mucous membrane received during childbirth.

septicophlebitis (ˌseptikohfli'bietis) septicaemic inflammation of veins.

septicopyaemia (ˌseptikohpie'eemi·ə) septicaemia with pyaemia.

septomarginal (ˌseptoh'marjin'l) pertaining to the margin of a septum.

septonasal (ˌseptoh'nayz'l) pertaining to the nasal septum.

septoplasty ('septohˌplastee) surgical reconstruction of the nasal septum.

septotomy (sep'totəmee) incision of the nasal septum.

Septrin ('septrin) trademark for a preparation of trimethoprim and sulphamethoxazole; an antibacterial.

septulum ('septyuhləm) pl. *septula* [L.] a small separating wall or partition.

septum ('septəm) pl. *septa* [L.] a wall or partition dividing a body space or cavity. adj. **septal.** Some septa are membranous, some are composed of bone, and some of cartilage, and each is named according to its location. The wall separating the atria (upper chambers) of the heart, for instance, is called the septum atriorum, atrial septum, or interatrial septum.

Usually, however, the term septum is used to refer to the nasal septum, a plate of bone and cartilage covered with mucous membrane that divides the nasal cavity. An injury or malformation of this septum can produce a deviated septum, so that one part of the nasal cavity is smaller than the other. Occasionally the deviation may handicap breathing, block the normal flow of mucus from the sinuses during a cold, and prevent proper drainage of infected sinuses. Deviated septum is fairly common and seldom causes complications. In some cases surgery may be necessary to relieve the obstruction and reduce irritation and infection in the nose and sinuses. The surgical procedure is called a partial or complete submucous resection.

An opening, or defect, in the septum dividing the right and left sides of the heart sometimes is present at birth. The most common type is ventricular septal defect, an opening between the ventricles, often described by laymen as 'a hole in the heart'. See also CONGENTITAL HEART DEFECT.

atrioventricular s. the part of the membranous portion of the interventricular septum between the left ventricle and the right atrium.

interatrial s. the partition separating the right and left atria of the heart.

interventricular s. the partition separating the right and left ventricles of the heart.

s. lucidum septum pellucidum.

pellucid s., s. pellucidum the triangular double membrane separating the anterior horns of the lateral ventricles of the brain. Called also *septum lucidum*.

s. primum a septum in the embryonic heart, dividing the primitive atrium into right and left chambers. See also CONGENTIAL HEART DEFECT.

rectovaginal s. the membranous partition between the rectum and vagina. **rectovesical s.** a membranous partition separating the rectum from the prostate and urinary bladder.

septuplet ('septyuhplət, sep'tyooplət) one of seven offspring produced at one birth.

sequel ('seekwəl) sequela.

sequela (si'kweelə) pl. *sequelae* [L.] a morbid condition following or occurring as a consequence of another condition or event.

sequester (si'kwestə) to detach or separate abnormally a small portion from the whole.

sequestrant (si'kwestrənt) a sequestering agent, as, for example, cholestyramine resin which binds bile acids in the intestine, thus preventing their absorption.

sequestration (,seekwe'strayshən) 1. abnormal separation of a part from a whole, as a portion of a bone by a pathological process, or a portion of the circulating blood in a specific part occurring naturally or produced by application of a tourniquet. 2. isolation of a patient.

pulmonary s. loss of connection of lung tissue with the bronchial tree and the normal pulmonary vasculature.

sequestrectomy (,seekwe'strektəmee) excision of a sequestrum.

sequestrum (si'kwestrəm) pl. *sequestra* [L.] a piece of dead bone that has become separated during the process of necrosis from sound bone.

sera ('siə·rə) plural of *serum*.

Serenace ('serənays) trademark for a preparation of haloperidol, an antipsychotic agent.

Serenid-D (,serənid'dee) trademark for a preparation of oxazepam; an anxiolytic.

sericeps ('seri,seps) a silken bag used to apply traction on the fetal head.

series ('siə·riz) a group or succession of events, objects, or substances arranged in regular order or forming a kind of chain; in electricity, parts of a circuit connected successively end to end to form a single path for the current. adj. **serial.**

erythrocytic s. the succession of developing cells that ultimately culminates in the erythrocyte. The morphologically distinguishable forms are: pronormoblast, basophilic normoblast, polychromatophilic normoblast, orthochromatic normoblast, reticulocyte, and erythrocyte.

granulocytic s. the succession of developing cells that ultimately culminates in mature granulocytes (neutrophils, eosinophils, or basophils). The morphologically distinguishable forms are: myeloblast, promyelocyte, metamyelocyte, band granulocyte, and segmented granulocyte. Stem cells are committed to become either neutrophils or eosinophils before the myelocyte stage. This may also be true for basophils.

lymphocytic s. the succession of developing cells that ultimately culminates in mature lymphocytes. The morphologically distinguishable forms are: lymphoblast, prolymphocyte, and lymphocyte.

monocytic s. the succession of developing cells that ultimately culminates in the monocyte. The morphologically distinguishable forms are monoblast, promonoblast, and monocyte.

thrombocytic s. the succession of developing cells that ultimately culminates in platelets (thrombocytes). The morphologically distinct cell types are: megakaryoblast, promegakaryocyte, and megakaryocyte, which fragments to form platelets.

serine ('sereen, 'siə-) a naturally occurring amino acid.

serocolitis (,siə·rohkə'lietis) inflammation of the serous coat of the colon.

seroconversion (,siə·rohkən'vərshən) the development of antibodies in response to administration of a vaccine.

seroculture ('siə·roh,kulchə) a bacterial culture on blood serum.

serodiagnosis (,siə·roh,dieəg'nohsis) diagnosis of disease based on serum reactions. adj. **serodiagnostic**.

seroenteritis (,siə·roh'entə'rietis) inflammation of the serous coat of the intestine.

seroepidemiology (,siə·roh,epi,deemi'oləjee) the epidemiological study of infectious disease by determining the levels of antibody to particular diseases in different age groups of a population.

serofibrinous (,siə·roh'fiebrinəs) marked by both a serous exudate and precipitation of fibrin.

serologist (si'roləjist) a specialist in serology.

serology (si'roləjee) the study of antigen–antibody reactions in vitro. adj. **serological**.

serolysin (si'rolisin) a lysin of the blood serum.

seroma (si'rohmə) a collection of serum in the body, producing a tumour-like mass.

seromembranous (,siə·roh'membrənəs) pertaining to or composed of serous membrane.

seromucous (,siə·roh'myookəs) both serous and mucous.

seromuscular (,siə·roh'muskyuhlə) pertaining to the serous and muscular coats of the intestine.

seronegative (,siə·roh'negətiv) showing a negative serum reaction.

seropositive (,siə·roh'pozətiv) showing positive results on serological examination.

seroprognosis (,siə·rohprog'nohsis) prognosis of disease based on serum reactions.

seroprophylaxis (,siə·roh,profi'laksis) the injection of immune serum or convalescent serum for protective purposes.

seropurulent (,siə·roh'pyooə·rələnt) both serous and purulent.

seropus ('siə·roh,pus) serum mingled with pus.

seroreaction (,siə·rohri'akshən) any reaction taking place in serum, or as a result of the action of a serum.

seroresistant (,siə·rohri'zistənt) showing a seropositive reaction to a pathogen after treatment.

serosa (si'rohsə) any serous membrane. adj. **serosal**.

serosanguineous (,siə·roh'sang·gwinəs) composed of serum and blood.

seroserous (,siə·roh'siə·rəs) pertaining to two serous surfaces.

serositis (,siə·roh'sietis) inflammation of a serous membrane.

serosity (si'rositee) the quality of serous fluids.

serosurvey (ˌsiə·roh'sərvay) a screening test of the serum of groups of persons to determine susceptibility to particular diseases.
serosynovitis (ˌsiə·rohˌsienoh'vietis) synovitis with effusion of serum.
serotherapy (ˌsiə·roh'therəpee) the treatment of infectious disease by the injection of serum from immune individuals.
serotonergic (ˌsiə·rohtə'nərjik, ˌserə-) containing or activated by serotonin.
serotonin (ˌsiə·roh'tohnin, ˌserə-) a hormone and neurotransmitter, 5-hydroxytryptamine (5-HT), found in many tissues, including blood platelets, intestinal mucosa, pineal body, and central nervous system; it has many physiological properties, including inhibition of gastric secretion, stimulation of smooth muscles, and production of vasoconstriction.
serotoninergic (ˌsiə·rohˌtohni'nərjik, ˌserə-) pertaining to neurons that release serotonin as a neurotransmitter, as those of the raphe nuclei of the brain stem, or that secrete serotonin as a hormone.
serotype ('siə·rohˌtiep) the type of a microorganism determined by its constituent antigens, or a taxonomic subdivision based thereon.
serous ('siə·rəs) 1. pertaining to serum; thin and watery, like serum. 2. producing or containing serum.
serovaccination (ˌsiə·rohˌvaksi'nayshən) injection of serum combined with bacterial vaccination to produce passive and active immunity.
Serpasil ('sərpəsil) trademark for preparations of reserpine, an antihypertensive and tranquillizer.
Serpasil-Esidrex (ˌsərpəsil'ezidreks) trademark for a fixed combination preparation of hydrochlorothiazide and reserpine, an antihypertensive.
serpiginous (sər'pijinəs) creeping from part to part; having a wavy border.
serrated (se'raytid) having a sawlike edge or border.
serration (se'rayshən) 1. the state of being serrated. 2. a serrated structure or formation.
Sertoli cell (sər'tohlee) any of the elongated cells in the tubules of the testes to which the spermatids become attached; they provide support, protection, and, apparently, nutrition until the spermatids are transformed into mature spermatozoa.
Sertoli-cell-only syndrome congenital absence of the germinal epithelium of the testes, the seminiferous tubules containing only Sertoli cells, marked by testes slightly smaller than normal, azoospermia, and elevated titres of follicle-stimulating hormone.
serum ('siə·rəm) pl. *sera,serums* [L.] the clear portion of any animal or plant fluid that remains after the solid elements have been separated out. The term usually refers to blood serum, the clear, straw-coloured, liquid portion of the plasma that does not contain fibrinogen or blood cells, and remains fluid after clotting of blood.

Blood serum from persons or animals whose bodies have built up antibodies is called antiserum or immune serum. Inoculation with such an antiserum provides temporary, or passive, immunity against the disease, and is used when a person has already been exposed to or has contracted the disease. Diseases in which passive immunization is sometimes used include diphtheria, tetanus, botulism, and gas gangrene.

antilymphocyte s. ALS, serum from animals immunized with lymphocytes from a different species, used as an immunosuppressive agent, especially in organ transplantation. The gamma globulin fraction, antilymphocytic globulin (ALG), is now more commonly used.
s. glutamic-oxaloacetic transaminase (SGOT) ASPARTATE AMINOTRANSFERASE (AST).
s. glutamic-pyruvic transaminase (SGPT) ALANINE AMINOTRANSFERASE (ALT).
immune s. serum from an immunized individual, containing specific antibody or antibodies.
s. osmolality a measure of the number of dissolved particles per unit of water in serum (see also serum OSMOLALITY).
pooled s. the mixed serum from a number of individuals.
s. sickness a hypersensitivity reaction following the administration of foreign serum or other antigens. It is marked by urticarial rashes, oedema, adenitis, joint pains, high fever, and prostration.

Reactions to tetanus antitoxin derived from horse serum are especially common. When the serum-sensitive person is injected for the first time, the reaction usually occurs after a period of 8 to 12 days. Once a person has had a serum reaction, the serum responsible should be avoided, since a second reaction will be more severe.

It is customary to test a patient's sensitivity with a small amount of serum before injecting the full dose. This precaution is especially important for patients who have other allergic susceptibilities.

s. sickness syndrome a serum sickness-like hypersensitivity reaction occurring after the administration of certain drugs. It is marked clinically by low-grade fever, urticaria, facial oedema, pain and swelling of the joints, and lymphadenopathy, and occasionally may be associated with neuritis of the brachial plexus, Guillain–Barré syndrome, periarteritis nodosa, and nephritis.
serum-fast ('siə·rəmˌfahst) resistant to the effects of serum.
serumal ('siə·rəməl) pertaining to or formed from serum.
sesamoid ('sesəˌmoyd) 1. denoting a small nodular bone embedded in a tendon or joint capsule. 2. a sesamoid bone.
sesqui- word element. [L.] *one and a half.*
sessile ('sesiel) not pedunculated; attached by a broad base.
setaceous (si'tayshəs) bristle-like.
severe combined immunodeficiency disease (sə'viə) any of several rare genetic diseases in which both humoural and cell-mediated immunity fail to develop normally and B- and T-lymphocytes are absent or have very low levels. Abbreviated SCID. Untreated patients usually die early in life; complete immune function has been restored in some patients by bone marrow transplants from matched sibling donors. Some forms have autosomal recessive inheritance; others are X-linked recessive.
sex (seks) 1. the fundamental distinction, found in most species of animals and plants, based on the type of gametes produced by the individual or the category to which the individual fits on the basis of that criterion. Ova, or macrogametes, are produced by the female, and spermatozoa, or microgametes, are produced by the male. The union of these distinctive germ cells results in the production of a new individual in sexual reproduction. 2. to determine the sex of an organism.
s. chromatin the persistent mass of chromatin situated at the periphery of the nucleus in cells of normal females; it is the material of the inactivated sex chromosome. Called also *Barr body.*
chromosomal s. sex as determined by the presence of the XX (female) or the XY (male) genotype in somatic cells, without regard to phenotypic manifestations; called also genetic sex.
s. chromosomes chromosomes that are associated with the determination of sex, in mammals constitu-

ting an unequal pair, called the X and the Y chromosome.

endocrinological s. the phenotypic manifestations of sex determined by endocrine influences, such as breast development, etc.

genetic s. chromosomal sex.

gonadal s. the sex as determined on the basis of the gonadal tissue present (ovarian or testicular).

s. hormones glandular secretions involved in the regulation of sexual functions. The principal sex hormone in the male is TESTOSTERONE, produced by the testes. In the female the principal sex hormones are the OESTROGENS and PROGESTERONE, produced by the ovaries.

These hormones influence the secondary sexual characteristics, such as the shape and contour of the body, the distribution of body hair and the pitch of the voice. The male hormones aid production of spermatozoa in men, and the female hormones control ovulation, pregnancy, and the menstrual cycle in women.

morphological s. sex determined on the basis of the morphology of the external genitals.

nuclear s. the sex as determined on the basis of the presence or absence of sex chromatin in somatic cells, its presence normally indicating the XX (female) genotype, and its absence the XY (male) genotype.

psychological s. the self-image of the gender role of an individual.

social s. the complex of attitudes, expectations, etc., that a society attaches to the male and female roles.

sex-conditioned (ˌsekskən'dishənd) sex-influenced.

sex-influenced (ˌseks'inflooənst) denoting an autosomal trait that is expressed differently, either in frequency or degree, in males and females, as for example, male-pattern baldness.

sex-limited (ˌseks'limitid) affecting individuals of one sex only.

sex-linked (ˌseks'lingkt) determined by a gene located on a sex chromosome. Although a trait may be X-linked or Y-linked, virtually all clinically significant sex-linked traits are transmitted by genes located on the X-chromosome; therefore, the terms sex-linked and X-linked are used synonymously.

sexduction (seks'dukshən) in bacterial genetics, the process whereby part of the bacterial chromosome is attached to the autonomous F factor (sex factor), and thus is transferred with high frequency from the donor (male) to the recipient (female); called also F-duction.

sexology (sek'soləjee) the scientific study of sex and sexual relations.

sextan ('sekstən) recurring on the sixth day (every five days).

sextuplet ('sekstyuhplət, seks'tyooplət) any one of six offspring produced at the same birth.

sexual ('seksyooəl) pertaining to sex.

s. development the biological and psychosocial changes that lead to sexual maturity. (Biological changes in humans are discussed under REPRODUCTIVE ORGANS.) The basis for current study of the child's normal psychosexual development is a series of essays on sexuality published by Sigmund Freud in 1905. Although Freud failed to recognize differences in the sexual development of males and females and some parts of this theory have been questioned, his essays on sexuality, in which he describes three phases or stages of human sexual development (oral, anal, phallic), are considered to be classics in the fields of psychology and psychiatry.

The *oral* stage of psychosexual development is the infantile period lasting from birth to 12 months, or even to 24 months of age, in which sensual pleasure is derived and sexual tensions are released through oral activities. It is followed by the *anal* phase at about the age of 18 months to 3 years, which is characterized by the libidinous experience of anal function. In this stage, the boy begins to identify with his father, brothers, and male peers and, after learning to stand and walk, can further fixate the image of his penis and control its urinary function; and the girl becomes aware of the differences between the sexes but is still unaware of her vagina. The female develops penis envy during the anal stage, which may be manifested through feelings of shame, inferiority, jealousy, and perhaps rage. The anal stage is followed by the *phallic* stage, which usually is seen in boys between the ages of 3 to 4½ years and in girls a short time later. During this stage, sexual interest, curiosity, and pleasurable experiences centre about the penis in boys, and in girls, to a lesser extent, the clitoris. Boys may develop castration anxiety during the phallic stage.

The *latency period* in sexual development extends from about 6 years to 9 or 10 years of age. Children in this period form close relationships with those of the same sex. Masturbation is not uncommon, and is considered by some authorities to be useful in reinforcing the child's awareness of sexuality, to discharge sexual and aggressive impulses, and to contribute to continued sexual development.

Adolescence is a time of rapid change in sexual development; puberty brings on the appearance of secondary sexual characteristics, and is the final step of a child's sexual development. In mid-adolescence both sexes become more interested in members of the opposite sex and seek heterosexual experiences.

s. deviation aberrant sexual activity; expression of the sexual instinct in practices which are socially prohibited or unacceptable, or biologically undesirable. Among the practices of sexual deviation are transsexualism, transvestism, and sadomasochism.

sexuality (ˌseksyoo'alitee) 1. the characteristic quality of the male and female reproductive elements. 2. the constitution of an individual in relation to sexual attitudes and behaviour.

sexually transmitted disease ('seksyooəlee) an infectious disease that is usually transmitted by means of sexual intercourse, either between heterosexual or homosexual individuals, or by intimate contact with the genitals, mouth, and rectum. Abbreviated STD. Within the category of STD are the three legally defined VENEREAL DISEASES (VDs), plus HUMAN IMMUNODEFICIENCY VIRUS infection, HERPES GENITALES, nonspecific URETHRITIS (NSU), TRICHOMONIASIS, pediculosis pubis (crab lice, see LOUSE), SCABIES, genital or venereal WARTS (condyloma acuminatum), HEPATITIS B infection, molluscum contagiosum, VAGINITIS caused by either *Corynebacterium vaginale* or *Haemophilus vaginalis*, and AIDS.

Sézary syndrome (ˌsayzah'ree) a variant of MYCOSIS FUNGOIDES that has peripheral blood involvement, although marrow infiltration is unusual.

SGOT serum glutamic-oxaloacetic transaminase.

SGPT serum glutamic-pyruvic transaminase.

shadow-casting ('shadohˌkahsting) application of a coating of gold, chromium, or other metal for the purpose of increasing the visibility of ultramicroscopic specimens under the microscope. Called also *sputter coating*.

shaft (shahft) a long slender part, such as the portion of a long bone between the wider ends or extremities.

shank (shangk) the tibia or shin; a leglike part.

shaping ('shayping) a technique in BEHAVIOUR THERAPY in which new behaviour is produced by providing reinforcement for progressively closer approximations of the final desired behaviour. Called also successive approximation.

Sharpey's fibres ('shahpiz) fibres that pass from the periosteum and embed in the periosteal lamellae.

sheath (sheeth) a tubular case or envelope.

arachnoid s. the delicate membrane between the pial sheath and the dural sheath of the optic nerve.

carotid s. a portion of the cervical fascia enclosing the carotid artery, internal jugular vein, and vagus nerve.

connective tissue s. of Key and Retzius Henle's sheath.

crural s. femoral sheath.

dural s. the external investment of the optic nerve.

femoral s. the fascial sheath of the femoral vessels.

Henle's s. the endoneurium, especially the delicate continuation around the terminal branches of nerve fibres; called also connective tissue sheath of Key and Retzius.

lamellar s. the perineurium.

medullary s., myelin s. the sheath surrounding the axon of myelinated nerve cells, consisting of concentric layers of myelin formed in the peripheral nervous system by the plasma membrane of Schwann cells, and in the central nervous system by the plasma membrane of oligodendrocytes. It is interrupted at intervals along the length of the axon by gaps known as *nodes of Ranvier.* Myelin is an electrical insulator that serves to speed the conduction of nerve impulses.

pial s. the innermost of the three sheaths of the optic nerve.

root s. the epidermic layer of a hair follicle.

s. of Schwann neurilemma.

synovial s. synovial membrane lining the cavity of a bone through which a tendon moves.

Sheehan's syndrome ('sheeənz) postpartum pituitary necrosis.

sheep cell agglutination test (sheep) a laboratory test for infectious mononucleosis; abbreviated SCAT. When the antibody level of a person with this disease reaches a certain level, a sample of his blood will cause agglutination of sheep erythrocytes. If there is agglutination of these cells in concentrations up to 1:28, the findings are considered positive for infectious mononucleosis.

Shenton's line ('shentənz) a curved line seen in radiographs of the normal hip, formed by the top of the obturator foramen.

SHHD Scottish Home and Health Department.

shield (sheeld) any protecting structure.

shift (shift) a change or deviation.

chloride s. the exchange of chloride and carbonate between the plasma and the erythrocytes that takes place when the blood gives up oxygen and receives carbon dioxide. It serves to maintain ionic equilibrium between the cell and surrounding fluid.

s. to the left a change in the blood picture, with a preponderance of young neutrophils.

s. to the right a preponderance of older neutrophils in the blood picture.

Shigella (shi'gelə) a genus of bacteria that cause dysentery. They are gram-negative, rod-shaped bacteria.

S. boydii the cause of an acute diarrhoeal disease in man, especially in the tropics.

S. dysenteriae a species that produces a neurotropic exotoxin in addition to the endotoxin common to all members of the *Shigella* group; it is more common in tropical regions and produces severe dysentery. Called also Shiga bacillus.

S. flexneri a common agent of acute diarrhoeal disease of man.

S. sonnei one of the commonest causes of bacillary dysentery in temperate climates.

shigella (shi'gelə) pl. *shigellae;* any individual organism of the genus *Shigella.*

shigellosis (ˌshigə'lohsis) infection with *Shigella*; bacillary dysentery.

shin (shin) the prominent anterior edge of the tibia and leg.

s. bone tibia.

sabre s. marked anterior convexity of the tibia, seen in congenital syphilis.

s. splints strain of the long flexor muscle of the toes occurring in athletes, marked by pain along the shin bone.

shingles ('shing·g'lz) herpes zoster.

Shirodkar's suture (shi'rodkəz) a 'purse-string' suture that is placed round an incompetent cervix during pregnancy to prevent abortion. It is usually removed at the thirty-eighth week or in labour if this occurs prematurely. See also CERCLAGE.

shiver ('shivə) 1. a slight tremor. 2. to tremble slightly, as from cold.

shivering ('shivə·ring) involuntary shaking of the body, as with cold. It is caused by contraction or twitching of the muscles, and is a physiological method of heat production in man and other mammals.

shock (shok) 1. a sudden disturbance of mental equilibrium. 2. a condition of acute peripheral circulatory failure due to derangement of circulatory control or loss of circulating fluid. It is marked by hypotension and coldness of the skin, and often by tachycardia and anxiety. Untreated shock can be fatal.

MECHANISMS OF CIRCULATORY SHOCK. The essentials of circulatory shock are easier to understand if the circulatory system is thought of as a four-part mechanical device made up of a pump (the heart), a complex system of flexible tubes (the blood vessels), a circulating fluid (the blood), and a fine regulating system or 'computer' (the nervous system) designed to control fluid flow and pressure. The diameter of the blood vessels is controlled by impulses from the nervous system which cause the muscular walls to contract. The nervous system also affects the rapidity and strength of the heartbeat, and thereby the blood pressure as well.

Shock, which is associated with a dangerously low blood pressure, can be produced by factors that attack the strength of the heart as a pump, decrease the volume of the blood in the system, or permit the blood vessels to increase in diameter.

TYPES OF CIRCULATORY SHOCK. There are five main types of circulatory shock. Low-volume shock occurs whenever there is insufficient blood to fill the circulatory system. Neurogenic shock is due to disorders of the nervous system. Two types of shock, allergic shock and septic shock, are due to reactions that impair the muscular functioning of the blood vessels. Cardiac shock is caused by impaired function of the heart.

Low-Volume (Hypovolaemic) Shock. This is a common form of shock that occurs when blood or plasma is lost in such quantities that the remaining blood cannot fill the circulatory system despite constriction of the blood vessels. The blood loss may be external, as when a vessel is severed by an injury, or the blood may be 'lost' into spaces inside the body where it is no longer accessible to the circulatory system, as in severe gastrointestinal bleeding from ulcers, fractures of large bones with haemorrhage into surrounding tissues, or major burns that attract large quantities of blood fluids to the burn site outside blood vessels and capillaries. The treatment of low-volume shock requires replacement of the lost blood.

Neurogenic Shock. This form of shock, often called fainting, may be brought on by severe pain, fright, unpleasant sights, or other strong stimuli that overwhelm the usual regulatory capacity of the nervous system. The diameter of the blood vessels increases, the heart slows, and the blood pressure falls to the point where the supply of oxygen carried by the blood to the brain is insufficient. The patient then faints. Placing the head lower than the body is usually sufficient to relieve this form of shock.

Allergic Shock. Allergic shock, commonly called anaphylactic shock (see ANAPHYLAXIS), is a rare phenomenon that occurs when a person receives an injection of a foreign protein to which he is highly sensitive. The blood vessels and other tissues are affected directly by the allergic reaction. Within a few minutes, the blood pressure falls and severe dyspnoea develops. The sudden deaths that in rare cases follow bee stings or injection of certain medicines are due to anaphylactic reactions.

Septic Shock. Septic shock, resulting from bacterial infection, is being recognized with increasing frequency. Certain organisms activate the alternative complement pathway and act on the blood vessels when released into the bloodstream. The permeability change causes a fall in blood volume, resulting in the blood pressure dropping sharply. Gram-negative shock is a form of septic shock due to infection with gram-negative bacteria.

Cardiac Shock. Cardiac shock may be caused by conditions that interfere with the function of the heart as a pump, such as severe myocardial infarction, severe heart failure and certain disorders of rate and rhythm.

THE PATIENT IN SHOCK. The precise progression to a state of shock depends upon the cause of the disorder and the speed of onset. In haemorrhagic shock, for example, as blood is lost the patient with gradually progressing shock feels very restless at first. He becomes thirsty. His skin takes on a pallor and feels cold. Often he perspires profusely. The pulse speeds up but is weak and indistinct. He gradually feels lethargic and faint, and may show signs of air hunger (laboured and difficult breathing). The nail beds and lips take on a bluish hue. As shock deepens and the blood pressure falls, the patient becomes comatose and eventually dies if untreated.

TREATMENT. Some relatively simple measures can be taken to reduce the effects of shock and slow its progress toward life-threatening proportions. In hypovolaemic shock and endotoxic shock the patient is placed in supine position with the lower extremities elevated unless there is severe injury to the head, back, and neck. Patients in cardiogenic shock are placed in a sitting position. Measures are taken to minimize pain, but care must be taken not to administer a dosage of medication that may predispose the patient to arterial hypotension. Only small sips of water to relieve thirst are allowed in order to decrease the possibility of vomiting and aspiration.

More severe cases of shock require administration of oxygen to prevent tissue anoxia, and administration of intravenous fluids and possibly whole blood to restore blood volume and blood pressure.

ACIDOSIS frequently accompanies severe shock and thus requires administration of sodium bicarbonate intravenously. .Other specific measures will depend on the type of shock that is manifested and the responsiveness of the patient to selected treatments. Fluid replacement, especially in hypovolaemic shock, is most accurately guided by CENTRAL VENOUS PRESSURE measurements.

There is some controversy over the use of drugs that either constrict or dilate the blood vessels. It is generally the practice to administer vasoconstrictors first if the blood volume is normal or slightly expanded. These agents are used only briefly, however, and in as small doses as possible because, although they do increase blood flow to the brain and heart, they do so at the expense of other organs, particularly the kidneys. When blood volume expansion and efforts at peripheral vasoconstriction have not proved effective, vasodilators may be used. Serious renal injury that is a threat in unrelieved shock may be avoided by the use of diuretics.

Corticosteroids, such as hydrocortisone, are administered in large doses in the treatment of septic shock and other types of complement-mediated shock. They specifically block the release reactions of platelets and phagocytic cells when reacting with C3b.

allergic s., anaphylactic s. a violent attack of symptoms produced by a second injection of serum or protein and due to anaphylaxis.

colloidoclastic s. colloidoclasia.

electric s. shock caused by electric current passing through the body (see ELECTRIC SHOCK).

insulin s. a condition of circulatory insufficiency resulting from overdosage with insulin, which causes too sudden reduction of blood sugar. It is marked by tremor, sweating, vertigo, diplopia, convulsions, and collapse.

respirator s. circulatory shock due to interference with the flow of blood through the great vessels and chambers of the heart, causing pooling of blood in the veins and the abdominal organs and a resultant vascular collapse. The condition sometimes occurs as a result of increased intrathoracic pressure in patients who are being maintained on a mechanical VENTILATOR.

shell s. condition of lost nervous control with numerous psychiatric symptoms, ranging from extreme fear to actual dementia, produced in soldiers under fire by the noise and concussion of bursting shells.

spinal s. the loss of spinal reflexes after injury of the spinal cord that appears in the muscles enervated by the cord segments situated below the site of the lesion.

s. therapy any somatic therapy that produces some type of shock to the central nervous system; used for treatment of depression and other mental disorders. The most commonly used form is ELECTROCONVULSIVE THERAPY (ECT) or ELECTROPLEXY. In other forms various pharmacological agents are used to produce a coma or convulsion, e.g., insulin shock therapy.

Shohl's solution (shohlz) a solution containing 140 g citric acid and 98 g hydrated crystalline salt of sodium citrate, distilled water to make 1000 ml; used to correct electrolyte imbalance in the treatment of renal tubular acidosis.

short-bowel syndrome ('shawt,bowəl) any of the malabsorption conditions following massive resection of the small bowel.

short-sightedness (,shawt'sietidnəs) see MYOPIA.

shoulder ('shohldə) the large joint where the humerus joins the scapula. The shoulder is a shallow ball-and-socket joint, similar to the hip joint.

At the shoulder, the smooth, rounded head of the humerus rests against the socket in the scapula. The joint is covered by a tough, flexible protective capsule and is heavily reinforced by ligaments that stretch across the joint. The ends of the bones where they meet at the joint are covered with a layer of cartilage that reduces friction and absorbs shock. A thin membrane, the synovial membrane, lines the socket and lubricates the joint with synovia. Further cushion-

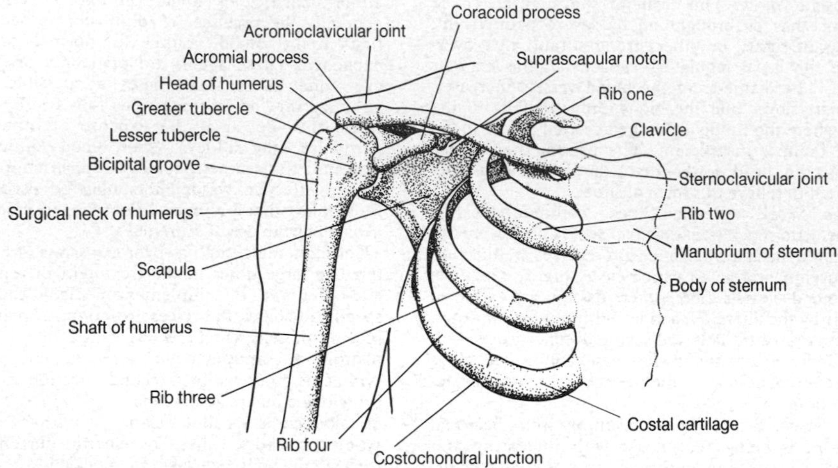

Shoulder

ing and lubrication are provided by fluid-filled sacs called bursae.

DISORDERS OF THE SHOULDER. One of the most common disorders of the shoulder is BURSITIS, or inflammation of the bursa, often caused by excessive use of the joint. The joint becomes painful and difficult to move.

The shoulder is one of the most common sites for a DISLOCATION, in which the ball of the humerus is dislodged from its socket in the scapula. This injures the ligaments and the capsule, and may cause temporary paralysis of the arm as well as pain and swelling. A dislocated shoulder is usually caused by a blow or fall, but sometimes an unusual physical effort may pull the arm from the shoulder socket. A first dislocation often makes the joint more susceptible to future dislocations. Only a doctor should set a dislocated shoulder; inexpert efforts may do far more damage than the original injury.

Frozen shoulder is a disability of the shoulder joint due to chronic inflammation in and around the joint and characterized by pain and limitation of motion.

shoulder–hand syndrome (ˌshohldəˈhand) a disorder of the upper extremity characterized by pain and stiffness in the shoulder, with puffy swelling and pain in the ipsilateral hand, sometimes occurring after myocardial infarction, but also produced by other causes.

show (shoh) appearance of blood-stained mucus preceding labour. See also OPERCULUM.

shunt (shunt) 1. to turn to one side; to divert; to bypass. 2. a passage or anastomosis between two natural channels, especially blood vessels, either by natural means or operation.

arteriovenous (A-V) s. a U-shaped plastic tube inserted between an artery and a vein (usually between the radial artery and cephalic vein), bypassing the capillary network; commonly done to allow repeated access to the arterial system for the purpose of HAEMODIALYSIS.

cardiovascular s. an abnormality of the blood flow between the sides of the heart or between the systemic and pulmonary circulation; see left-to-right SHUNT and right-to-left SHUNT.

jejunoileal s. an INTESTINAL BYPASS performed to control obesity.

left-to-right s. diversion of blood from the left side of the heart to the right side, or from the systemic to the pulmonary circulation through an anomalous opening such as a septal defect or patent ductus arteriosus.

LeVeen s. peritoneal-venous shunt.

peritoneal-venous s. a device whose purpose is to remove excess ascitic fluid from the peritoneal cavity and return it to the venous system. Called also *LeVeen shunt*.

The shunt consists of a peritoneal tube, a one-way valve, and a tube leading to a large vein, usually the superior vena cava or the jugular vein. The perforated peritoneal tube is placed in the peritoneal cavity and attached to the one-way valve which opens at a pressure of 3 cm H_2O. The valve controls the direction of the flow of ascitic fluid and prevents a backflow of blood from the vein. A tube leading from the valve empties into the venous system.

The shunt is triggered into action by the patient's breathing. Upon inspiration, the diaphragm descends toward the abdominal cavity and causes a rise in fluid pressure in the thoracic superior vena cava. The difference in pressure, usually about 5 cm H_2O, opens the shunt valve, allowing the flow of ascitic fluid into the large vein. The action of the shunt can be enhanced by the patient's inspiring against pressure, as when using a blow bottle.

A disadvantage of the shunt is dilution of the blood and a resultant drop in haematocrit, which necessitates transfusion of packed cells and perhaps a slowing of the rate of flow of ascitic fluid into the venous system. Other risks inherent in the procedure are infection, leakage of ascitic fluid from the operative site, elevated bilirubin, gastrointestinal bleeding, and disseminated intravascular coagulation.

portacaval s., postcaval s. surgical anastomosis of the portal vein to the vena cava.

reversed s. right-to-left shunt.

right-to-left s. diversion of blood from the right side of the heart to the left side or from the pulmonary to the systemic circulation through an anomalous opening such as septal defect or patent ductus arteriosus.

ventriculoatrial s. the surgical creation of a communication between a cerebral ventricle and a cardiac atrium by means of plastic tube; done for relief of HYDROCEPHALUS.

ventriculoperitoneal s. a communication between a cerebral ventricle and the peritoneum by means of plastic tubing; done for the relief of HYDROCEPHALUS.

ventriculovenous s. a communication between a lateral ventricle and the venous system by means of a plastic tube; done for relief of HYDROCEPHALUS.

Shwartzman phenomenon ('shwawtsmən) a local tissue reaction characterized by haemorrhagic necrosis due to an antigen–antibody reaction to certain bacterial substances. Its occurrence in humans is largely theoretical.

Si chemical symbol, *silicon.*

SI units (ˌesie 'yoonits) the units of measurement generally accepted for all scientific and technical uses. Together they make up the International System of Units. The abbreviation SI, from the French *Système International d'Unités*, is used in all languages. There are seven base SI units, defined by specified physical measurements and two supplementary units. Units are derived for any other physical quantities by multiplication and division of the base and supplementary units. The base units and the prefixes used for multiples are shown in the tables in Appendix 2.

SI is a *coherent* system. This means that units are always combined without conversion factors. The derived unit of velocity is the metre per second ($m \cdot s^{-1}$ or m/s); the derived unit of volume is the cubic metre (m^3). If you know that pressure is force per unit area, then you know that the SI unit of pressure (the pascal) is the unit of force divided by the unit of area and is therefore equal to 1 newton per square metre ($N \cdot m^{-2}$ or N/m^2).

The metric prefixes can be attached to any unit in order to make a unit of a more convenient size. The symbol for the prefix is attached to the symbol for the unit, e.g., nanometre (nm) = 10^{-9} m. The units of mass are specified in terms of the gram, e.g., microgram (μg) = 10^{-6} g.

Only one prefix is used with a unit. The use of units such as the millimicrometre is no longer acceptable. When a unit is raised to a power, the power applies to the prefix as well, e.g., a cubic millimetre (mm^3) = 10^{-9} m^3. When a prefix is used with a ratio unit, it should be in the numerator rather than in the denominator, e.g., kilometres/second (km/s) rather than metres/millisecond (m/ms). Only prefixes denoting powers of 10^3 are normally used. Hecto-, deka-, deci-, and centi- are usually attached only to the metric system units, gram, meter, and litre.

Owing to the force of tradition, one noncoherent unit, the litre, equal to 0.001 m^3 or 1 dm^3, is generally accepted for use with SI. The internationally accepted abbreviation for litre is the letter l; however, this can be confused with the numeral 1, especially in typescript. For this reason, the capital letter L is sometimes used as a symbol for litre. The lower case letter is generally used with prefixes, e.g., dl, ml, fl. The symbols for all other SI units begin with a capital letter if the unit is named after a person and with a lower case letter otherwise. The name of a unit is never capitalized.

SIADH syndrome of inappropriate secretion of antidiuretic hormone.

sial(o)- word element. [Gr] *saliva, salivary glands.*

sialadenitis (ˌsieəˌladə'nietis) inflammation of a salivary gland.

sialadenosis (ˌsieəˌladə'nohsis) noninflammatory swelling of the salivary glands.

sialagogue (sie'aləˌgog, 'sieələ-) an agent that stimulates the flow of saliva.

sialectasia (ˌsieəlek'tayzi·ə) dilation of a salivary duct.

sialine ('sieəˌlien) pertaining to the saliva.

sialismus (ˌsieə'lizməs) ptyalism.

sialitis (sieə'lietis) inflammation of a salivary gland or duct.

sialoadenectomy (ˌsieəlohˌadə'nektəmee) excision of a salivary gland.

sialoadenitis (ˌsieəlohˌadə'nietis) inflammation of a salivary gland.

sialoadenotomy (ˌsieəlohˌadə'notəmee) incision into a salivary gland.

sialoaerophagia (ˌsieəlohˌair·roh'fayji·ə) the swallowing of saliva and air.

sialoangiectasis (ˌsieəlohˌanji'ektəsis) dilation of a salivary duct.

sialoangiography (ˌsieəlohˌanji'ogrəfee) radiography of the ducts of the salivary glands after injection of radiopaque material.

sialocele ('sieəlohˌseel) a salivary cyst.

sialodochitis (ˌsieəlohdo'kietis) inflammation of a salivary duct.

sialodochoplasty (ˌsieəloh'dohkohˌplastee) plastic repair of a salivary duct.

sialoductitis (ˌsieəlohduk'tietis) sialoangiitis.

sialogen (sie'aləjən) an agent that induces salivation.

sialogenous (ˌsieə'lojənəs) producing saliva.

sialogogue (sie'aləˌgog, 'sieələ-) sialagogue.

sialogram (sie'aləˌgram) a film obtained by sialography.

sialography (ˌsieə'logrəfee) roentgen demonstration of the salivary ducts by means of the injection of substances opaque to x-rays.

sialolith ('sieəlohˌlith) a salivary calculus.

sialolithiasis (ˌsieəlohli'thieəsis) the formation of salivary calculi.

sialolithotomy (ˌsieəlohli'thotəmee) removal of a salivary calculus.

sialomucin (ˌsieəloh'myoosin) an acid mucopolysaccharide containing sialic acid, a component of airway secretions of the lungs.

sialorrhoea (ˌsieələ'reeə) ptyalism.

sialoschesis (ˌsieə'loskisis) suppression of secretion of saliva.

sialosis (ˌsieə'lohsis) 1. the flow of saliva. 2. ptyalism. adj. **sialotic.**

sialostenosis (ˌsieəlohstə'nohsis) stenosis of a salivary duct.

sialosyrinx (ˌsieəloh'siringks) 1. salivary fistula. 2. a syringe for washing out the salivary ducts, or a drainage tube for the salivary ducts.

Siamese twins ('sieəmeez) identical (monozygotic) twins joined together at birth. The connection may be slight or extensive. It involves skin and usually muscles or cartilage of a limited region, such as the head, chest, hip, or buttock. The twins may share a single organ, such as an intestine, or occasionally may have parts of the spine in common.

If joined superficially, the twins are easily separated by surgery soon after birth. If more deeply united, they may have to go through life, if they survive, with their handicap. New techniques in surgery, however, are making it possible to separate some Siamese twins whose physical links are highly complex.

sib (sib) 1. a blood relative; one of a group of persons all descended from a common ancestor. 2. sibling.

sibilant ('sibilənt) shrill, whistling, or hissing.

sibling ('sibling) any of two or more offspring of the same parents; a brother or sister.

half s. an individual one of whose parents was also a parent of the person of reference.

s. rivalry emotional conflict between siblings that

arises from a competition for the love, attention, and approval of one or both parents.

sibship ('sibship) a group of individuals born of the same parents.

siccative ('sikətiv) 1. drying; removing moisture. 2. an agent that produces drying.

siccus ('sikəs) [L.] *dry*.

sick (sik) 1. not in good health; ill; afflicted with disease. 2. vomit.

s. sinus syndrome a complex cardiac arrhythmia manifested as severe sinus bradycardia alone, sinus bradycardia alternating with tachycardia, or sinus bradycardia with atrioventricular block.

sicklaemia (sik'leemi·ə) sickle cell anaemia.

sickle cell ('sik'l) a crescentic or sickle-shaped erythrocyte, the abnormal shape caused by the presence of varying proportions of haemoglobin S.

s.c. anaemia sickle cell disease.

s.c. disease any of the diseases associated with the presence of haemoglobin S, including sickle cell anaemia, sickle cell-haemoglobin C or D disease, and sickle cell-thalassaemia disease.

About 8 to 10 per cent of all Afro-Caribbean people in the UK carry the sickle cell gene. About 90 per cent of these are carriers of the sickle cell trait (are heterozygous for the haemoglobin S gene) and usually are without symptoms. The remainder or about 1 in 500 are homozygous for haemoglobin S and actually have sickle cell disease and suffer from the effects of haemolysis.

Sickle cell disease is a serious, hereditary, chronic disease in which the red blood cells are rigid and crescent- or sickle-shaped. The misshapen erythrocytes are the result of an abnormality in the haemoglobin molecule that alters the electrical charge. Because of their distorted shape the red blood cells have difficulty passing through arterioles and capillaries and have a tendency to clump together, thus occluding the blood vessel.

Sickle cell disease can also occur in persons of Mediterranean ancestry; that is, Greeks, Italians, Spaniards, Turks, and North Africans. Those of Middle Eastern and Asian Indian ancestry also may be affected.

Some scientists believe that sickle cell disease developed as a defence against malaria. Malarial parasites do not grow in erythrocytes containing haemoglobin S. Therefore, carriers (heterozygotes) have an evolutionary advantage in areas where malaria is prevalent.

Reduction in the incidence of sickle cell disease and its consequences depends in large measure on adequate instruction of the public, proper screening of persons likely to have the disease or carry the trait, and continued research into effective forms of prevention and treatment.

s.c. trait the condition, usually asymptomatic, of being heterozygous for haemoglobin S. Further information may be obtained from the following agencies: Sickle Cell Society, c/o Brent Community Health Council, 16 High Street, Harlesden, London NW1D 4LX, or Organisation for Sickle Cell Anaemia Research (OSCAR), 200A High Road, Wood Green, London N22 4HH.

sickling ('sikling) the development of sickle cells in the blood.

sickness ('siknəs) 1. a condition of deviation from the normal healthy state. 2. nausea or vomiting.

side-effect ('sied i,fekt) a consequence other than that for which an agent is used, especially an adverse effect on another organ system.

sidero- word element. [Gr.] *iron*.

sideroblast ('sidə·roh,blast) a nucleated erythrocyte containing iron granules in its cytoplasm. adj. **sideroblastic**.

ring s. a sideroblast in which the iron granules lie around the perimeter of the nucleus, forming a partial or complete ring.

sideroblastic anaemia see under ANAEMIA.

siderocyte ('sidə·roh,siet) a red blood cell containing nonhaemoglobin iron.

sideroderma (,sidə·roh'dərmə) bronzed coloration of the skin due to disordered iron metabolism.

siderofibrosis (,sidə·rohfie'brohsis) fibrosis associated with deposits of iron. adj. **siderofibrotic**.

sideropenia (,sidə·roh'peeni·ə) deficiency of iron in the body or blood. adj. **sideropenic**.

siderophil ('sidə·roh,fil) 1. siderophilous. 2. a siderophilous cell or tissue.

siderophilous (,sidə'rofiləs) tending to absorb iron.

siderophore ('sidə·roh,for) a macrophage containing haemosiderin.

siderosis (,sidə'rohsis) 1. a form of PNEUMOCONIOSIS due to the inhalation of iron or other metallic particles. 2. excess of iron in the blood. 3. the deposit of iron in the tissues.

hepatic s. the deposit of an abnormal quantity of iron in the liver.

urinary s. the presence of haemosiderin granules in the urine.

SIDS sudden infant death syndrome.

siemens ('seemənz) the SI unit of conductivity, equal to one reciprocal ohm (Ω^{-1}). Called also *mho*. Symbol S.

sievert ('seevərt) the SI unit of radiation absorbed dose equivalent, defined as that producing the same biological effect in a specified tissue as 1 gray of high-energy x-rays; 1 sievert equals 100 rem.

sig. [L.] *signa* (mark).

sight (siet) 1. the act or faculty of VISION, involving the EYE itself, the visual centre in the brain, and the optic nerve and nerve fibres in the brain that connect the two. 2. a thing seen.

far s. hypermetropia.

near s. myopia.

night s. hemeralopia; day blindness.

sigmatism ('sigmə,tizəm) faulty enunciation or too frequent use of *s* sounds.

sigmoid ('sigmoyd) 1. shaped like the letter C or S. 2. the sigmoid colon, the distal part of the colon from the level of the iliac crest to the rectum.

sigmoidectomy (,sigmoy'dektəmee) excision of part of the sigmoid colon.

sigmoiditis (,sigmoy'dietis) inflammation of the sigmoid colon.

sigmoidopexy (sig'moydoh,peksee) fixation of the sigmoid colon.

sigmoidoproctostomy, sigmoidorectostomy (sig-,moydohprok'tostəmee; sig,moydohrek'tostəmee) anastomosis of the sigmoid colon to the rectum.

sigmoidoscope (sig'moydə,skohp) an endoscope for viewing the sigmoid colon and rectum.

sigmoidoscopy (,sigmoy'doskəpee) direct examination of the interior of the sigmoid colon and rectum.

sigmoidosigmoidostomy (sig,moydoh,sigmoy-'dostəmee) anastomosis of two previously remote portions of the sigmoid colon.

sigmoidostomy (,sigmoy'dostəmee) surgical creation of an opening from the surface of the body into the sigmoid colon.

sigmoidotomy (,sigmoy'dotəmee) incision into the sigmoid.

sigmoidovesical (sig,moydoh'vesik'l) pertaining to or communicating with the sigmoid colon and the urinary bladder.

sign (sien) 1. any objective evidence of disease or dysfunction. 2. an observable physical phenomenon so frequently associated with a given condition as to be considered indicative of its presence. **vital s's** the signs of life, namely pulse, respiration, and temperature.

signa ('signə) [L.] *mark* or *write;* abbreviated S or sig. in prescriptions, followed by the signature.

significant other (sig'nifikənt 'odhə) a person who plays an important role in the life of an individual, such as a member of the immediate family, a lover, a close friend, or a role model.

Silastic (si'lastik, sie-) trademark for polymeric silicone substances having the properties of rubber; it is biologically inert.

silica ('silikə) silicon dioxide, a compound occurring naturally as quartz and in other forms, some of which are used in dental materials.

silicoanthracosis (ˌsilikohˌanthrə'kohsis) silicosis combined with pneumoconiosis of coal workers.

silicon ('siliˌkən) a chemical element, atomic number 14, atomic weight 28.086, symbol Si. See table of elements in Appendix 2.

silicone ('siliˌkohn) any organic compound in which all or part of the carbon has been replaced by silicon.

silicosis (ˌsili'kohsis) a lung disease caused by the prolonged inhalation of silica dust. adj. **silicotic.** In the past it was called such colourful names as potter's asthma, stonecutter's cough, miner's mould, and grinder's rot, according to the occupation in which it was acquired. Besides silicosis, various other lung diseases result from inhaling industrial substances; together, these 'dust diseases' are called the PNEUMOCONIOSES.

Today silicosis is most likely to be contracted in such industrial jobs as sandblasting in tunnels and hardrock mining, but it can occur in anyone who is habitually exposed to the dust of silica, one of the commonest minerals. All types of miners, for example, may be subject to it, from gold miners to coal miners.

Silicosis usually takes about 10 years of fairly constant exposure to develop. It may give few warning symptoms. As time goes on, an affected person experiences progressive shortness of breath, along with steady coughing which in the early stages is dry and unproductive of mucus. Later there may be mucus tinged with blood, loss of appetite, pain in the chest, and general weakness. The silica produces a nodular fibrotic reaction that scars the lungs and makes them receptive to the further complications of bronchitis and emphysema; persons with silicosis are also more susceptible to tuberculosis.

Since silicosis is a serious disease, those who must work near silica should take precautions to breathe as little of it as possible. This can usually be effected by the use of face masks, proper ventilation, and other safety devices. The cooperation of industry, labour, and government in developing various protective measures has made silicosis a much less common disease today than it used to be.

Regular chest x-rays are recommended for all workers exposed to silica as the quickest and easiest way to detect silicosis. If discovered in its early stages, the disease can usually be arrested by a change of occupation and appropriate therapy. Once fully developed, the disease rarely yields to treatment.

silicotuberculosis (ˌsilikohtyuhˌbərkyuh'lohsis) tuberculous infection of the lung affected with silicosis.

silo-filler's disease ('sielohfiləz) pulmonary inflammation, often with acute pulmonary oedema, due to inhalation of the irritant gases (especially oxides of nitrogen) which collect in recently filled silos.

silver ('silvə) a chemical element, atomic number 47, atomic weight 107.870, symbol Ag. (See table of elements in Appendix 2.) It is used in medicine for its caustic, astringent and antiseptic effects.

s. nitrate colourless or white crystals, moulded as pencils or cones, used as a caustic for reducing excessive granulation tissue.

s. protein silver made colloidal by the presence of, or combination with, protein; an active germicide with a local irritant and astringent effect.

s. sulphadiazine the silver salt of sulphadiazine, having bactericidal activity against many gram-positive and gram-negative organisms, as well as being effective against yeasts; used as a topical anti-infective for the prevention and treatment of wound sepsis in patients with second and third degree burns.

Silverman–Andersen score (ˌsilvəmən'andəsən) a system for evaluation of breathing performance of preterm infants. It consists of five items: (1) chest retraction as compared with abdominal retraction during inspiration; (2) retraction of the lower intercostal muscles; (3) xiphoid retraction; (4) flaring of the nares with inspiration; and (5) expiratory grunt. Each of the five factors is graded 0, 1, or 2. The sum of these factors yields the score. Adequate ventilation is indicated by a 0, severe respiratory distress is indicated by a score of 10.

Simmonds' disease ('simәndz) panhypopituitarism in which cachexia is a prominent feature; called also pituitary cachexia. It follows the destruction of the pituitary gland by surgery, infection, injury, or tumour; it may also occur after difficult labour in childbirth.

Simmonds' disease was first described by Dr. Morris Simmonds of Hamburg, Germany, in 1914. Symptoms, which vary in intensity, are extreme weight loss, general debility, pallor, dry and yellowish skin, a slow pulse, hypotension, and atrophy of the genitalia and breasts, progressing to premature senility and apathy. Treatment is by regular administration of the various hormones whose release is normally dependent on pituitary function.

Sims' position (simz) the patient on his left side and chest, the right knee and thigh drawn up, the left arm along the back.

simulation (ˌsimyuh'layshən) 1. the act of counterfeiting a disease; malingering. 2. the imitation of one disease by another.

simulator ('simyuhˌlaytə) something that simulates, such as an apparatus that simulates conditions that will be encountered in real life.

SIMV synchronized intermittent mandatory ventilation.

sincalide ('sinkəˌlied) the synthetic C-terminal octapeptide of cholecystokinin, used to stimulate gallbladder contraction in order to be able to aspirate a bile specimen from the duodenum or to obtain postevacuation films in cholecystography.

sinciput ('sinsiˌput) the upper and front part of the head. adj. **sincipital.**

Sinemet ('siniˌmet) trademark for a combination of carbidopa and levodopa, used in the treatment of Parkinson's disease.

Sinequan ('siniˌkwan) trademark for a preparation of doxepin hydrochloride, an anxiolytic.

sinew ('sinyoo) a tendon of a muscle.

weeping s. an encysted ganglion, chiefly on the back of the hand, containing synovial fluid.

singultation (ˌsing·gəl'tayshən) the hiccupping reaction.

singultous (sing'gultəs) pertaining to or affected with hiccups.

singultus (sing'gultəs) [L.] *hiccup.*

sinister ('sinistə) [L.] *left, on the left side.*
sinistr(o)- word element. [L.] *left, left side.*
sinistrad (si'nistrad) to or toward the left.
sinistral ('sinistrəl) pertaining to the left side.
sinistrality (ˌsini'stralitee) the preferential use, in voluntary motor acts, of the left member of the major paired organs of the body, as ear, eye, hand, and leg.
sinistraural (ˌsini'stror·rəl) hearing better with the left ear.
sinistrocardia (ˌsinistroh'kahdi·ə) laevocardia.
sinistrocerebral (ˌsinistroh'seribrəl) situated in the left hemisphere of the brain.
sinistrocular (ˌsini'strokyuhlə) having the left eye dominant.
sinistrocularity (ˌsiniˌstrokyuh'laritee) dominance of the left eye.
sinistrogyration (ˌsinistrohjie'rayshən) a turning to the left.
sinistromanual (ˌsinistroh'manyooəl) left-handed.
sinistropedal (ˌsini'stropid'l) using the left foot in preference to the right.
sinistrotorsion (ˌsinistroh'tawshən) a twisting toward the left, as of the eye.
sinoatrial (ˌsienoh'aytri·əl) pertaining to the sinus venosus and the atrium of the heart.
s. node a collection of specialized muscle fibres in the wall of the right atrium where the rhythm of cardiac contraction is usually established; therefore also referred to as the pacemaker of the heart.
sinobronchitis (ˌsienohbrong'kietis) chronic paranasal sinusitis with recurrent episodes of bronchitis.
sinography (si'nogrəfee) radiographic examination of the extent of a sinus using a radiopaque dye.
sinuitis (ˌsienyoo'ietis) sinusitis.
sinuotomy, sinusotomy (ˌsienyoo'otəmee; ˌsienə'sotəmee) incision of a sinus.
sinuous ('sinyooəs) bending in and out; winding.
sinus ('sienəs) 1. a recess, cavity, or channel, as (a) one in bone or (b) a dilated channel for venous blood. 2. an abnormal channel or fistula, permitting escape of pus. In common usage, the word sinus refers to any of the eight cavities in the skull that are connected with the nasal cavity—the paranasal sinuses.

The paranasal sinuses are arranged in four pairs, with members of each pair on the left and right sides of the head. The pairs are the maxillary sinuses, located in the maxillae; the frontal sinuses, in the frontal bone; the sphenoid sinuses, in the sphenoid bone behind the nasal cavity; and the ethmoid sinuses, in the ethmoid bone, behind and below the frontal sinuses.

The functions of the sinuses are not certain. They are believed to help the nose in circulating, warming, and moistening the air as it is inhaled, thereby lessening the shock of cold, dry air to the lungs. They also are thought to have a minor role as resonating chambers for the voice.

anal s's furrows, with pouchlike recesses at the distal end, separating the rectal columns; called also anal crypts.
aortic s's pouchlike dilations at the root of the aorta, one opposite each semilunar cusp of the aortic valve, from which the coronary arteries originate.
s. arrhythmia the physiological cyclic variation in heart rate related to vagal impulses to the sinoatrial node; it occurs commonly in children (juvenile arrhythmia) and in the aged, and requires no treatment.
carotid s. a dilation of the proximal portion of the internal carotid or distal portion of the common carotid artery, containing in its wall pressure receptors that are stimulated by changes in blood pressure. See also CAROTID SINUS SYNDROME.
cavernous s. an irregularly shaped venous channel between the layers of dura mater of the brain, one on either side of the body of the sphenoid bone and communicating across the midline. Several cranial nerves course through this sinus.
cerebral s. one of the ventricles of the brain.
cervical s. a temporary depression in the neck of the embryo containing the branchial arches.
circular s. the venous channel encircling the pituitary gland, formed by the two cavernous sinuses and the anterior and posterior intercavernous sinuses.
coccygeal s. a sinus or fistula just over or close to the tip of the coccyx.
coronary s. the dilated terminal portion of the great cardiac vein, receiving blood from other veins draining the heart muscle and emptying into the right atrium.
dermal s. a congenital sinus tract extending from the surface of the body, between the bodies of two adjacent lumbar vertebrae, to the spinal canal.
ethmoidal s. that paranasal sinus consisting of the ethmoidal cells collectively, and communicating with the nasal meatuses.
frontal s. one of the paired paranasal sinuses in the frontal bone, each communicating with the middle meatus of the ipsilateral nasal cavity.
intercavernous s's channels connecting the two cavernous sinuses, one passing anterior and the other posterior to the stalk of the pituitary gland.
lymphatic s's irregular, tortuous spaces within lymphoid tissues through which lymph flows.
maxillary s. one of the paired paranasal sinuses in the body of the maxilla on either side, opening into the middle meatus of the ipsilateral nasal cavity.
occipital s. a venous sinus between the layers of dura mater, passing upward along the midline of the cerebellum.
paranasal s's mucosa-lined air cavities in bones of the skull, communicating with the nasal cavity and including ethmoidal, frontal, maxillary, and sphenoidal sinuses.
petrosal s., inferior a venous channel arising from the cavernous sinus and draining into the internal jugular vein.
petrosal s., superior one arising from the cavernous sinus and draining into the transverse sinus of the dura mater.
pilonidal s. a suppurating sinus containing hair, occurring chiefly in the coccygeal region.
prostatic s. the posterolateral recess between the seminal colliculus and the wall of the urethra.
s's of pulmonary trunk spaces between the wall of the pulmonary trunk and cusps of the pulmonary valve at its opening from the right ventricle.
renal s. a recess in the substance of the kidney, occupied by the renal pelvis, calices, vessels, nerves, and fat.
sagittal s., inferior a small venous sinus of the dura mater, opening into the straight sinus.
sagittal s., superior a venous sinus of the dura mater that ends in the confluence of sinuses.
sigmoid s. a venous sinus of the dura mater on either side, continuous with the straight sinus and draining into the internal jugular vein of the same side.
sphenoidal s. one of the paired paranasal sinuses in the body of the sphenoid bone, opening into the highest meatus of the ipsilateral nasal cavity.
sphenoparietal s. one of the venous sinuses of the dura mater, emptying into the cavernous sinus.
s's of spleen dilated venous channels in the substance of the spleen.
straight s. a venous sinus of the dura mater formed by

junction of the great cerebral vein and inferior sagittal sinus, and ending in the confluence of sinuses.

tarsal s. a space between the calcaneus and talus.

tentorial s. straight sinus.

transverse s. of dura mater a large venous sinus on either side of the skull.

transverse s. of pericardium a passage within the pericardial sac, behind the aorta and pulmonary trunk and in front of the left atrium and superior vena cava.

tympanic s. a deep recess on the medial wall of the middle ear.

urogenital s. an elongated sac that is formed by division of the cloaca in the early embryo, which ultimately forms most of the vestibule, urethra, and vagina in the female, and some of the urethra in the male.

uterine s's venous channels in the wall of the uterus in pregnancy.

uteroplacental s's blood spaces between the placenta and uterine sinuses.

s. of venae cavae the posterior portion of the right atrium into which the inferior and the superior vena cava open.

venous s., s. venosus 1. the common venous receptacle in the early embryo attached to the posterior wall of the primitive atrium. 2. sinus of venae cavae.

venous s's of dura mater large channels for venous blood forming an anastomosing system between the layers of the dura mater of the brain, receiving blood from the brain and draining into the veins of the scalp or deep veins at the base of the skull.

venous s. of sclera a circular channel at the junction of the sclera and cornea, into which aqueous humour filters from the anterior chamber of the eye. Called also *Schlemm's* CANAL.

sinusitis (ˌsienə'sictis) inflammation of one or more of the paranasal SINUSES, often occurring when upper respiratory infection spreads from the nose to the sinuses (sometimes encouraged by excessively strong blowing of the nose). Sinusitis may also complicate tooth infection, allergy, or certain infectious diseases, such as pneumonia and measles. There are many other causes of sinusitis, including air pollution, diving and underwater swimming, sudden extremes of temperature, and structural defects of the nose that interfere with breathing, such as deviated SEPTUM.

As the mucous membranes of the sinus become inflamed and swollen, the openings which drain each sinus into the nasal passages become partially or wholly blocked. The mucopus accumulates causing pressure within the sinus with discomfort, fever, pain, and difficulty with breathing.

SYMPTOMS. The common symptoms of sinusitis are headache, usually located near the sinuses most involved, and nasal discharge. These may be accompanied by a rise in temperature, dizziness and discomfort.

The diagnosis can be confirmed by transillumination. Radiological tests also are used to confirm the diagnosis and locate the extent of involvement. Specialized techniques such as tomography and CT scanning are sometimes used to pinpoint the nature and scope of a sinus disorder.

TREATMENT. Acute sinusitis usually responds to antibiotic therapy and increased drainage from the sinuses through the use of decongestants, which are applied locally in the form of nosedrops and also taken by mouth. Inhalation of steam or warm moisturized air, and local applications of heat encourage drainage and relieve discomfort through decongestion. When the pain is severe analgesics may be needed.

Chronic sinusitis develops when the mucous membranes in the sinuses thicken and normal drainage is obstructed. If medical management such as that described for acute sinusitis does not relieve the condition, surgical intervention may be necessary. In some cases, repair of a deviated nasal septum or removal of nasal polyps may be all that is necessary. Others may need to have a new outlet created from the sinus for drainage into the nose.

Sinusitis can lead to more serious infections nearby, for example the bones of the ear and mastoid and the brain.

Though a change of climate can be beneficial for chronic sinusitis, it is rarely a necessity. Creating a better indoor climate with air conditioners and humidifiers can be equally beneficial in reducing the number and severity of attacks of sinusitis.

sinusoid ('sienəˌsoyd) 1. resembling a sinus. 2. a form of blood channel consisting of an irregular, anastomosing channel of large diameter, having a lining of endothelium but little or no adventitia. Sinusoids are found in the liver, spleen, adrenals, heart, parathyroids, carotid bodies and lymph nodes.

Siopel ('sieohpel) trademark for preparations of dimethicone, a skin protective.

siphon ('siefən) 1. a bent tube with arms of unequal length, for drawing liquid from a higher to a lower level by force of atmospheric pressure. 2. to draw liquid by means of a siphon.

siphonage ('siefənij) the use of the siphon, as in gastric lavage or in draining the bladder.

Sipple's syndrome ('sip'lz) a hereditary syndrome of phaeochromocytoma, medullary carcinoma of the thyroid, and a tendency to hyperparathyroidism due to hyperplasia or multiple parathyroid adenomas; transmitted as an autosomal dominant trait.

sirenomelus (ˌsierə'nomələs) a fetus with fused legs and no feet.

-sis word element. [Gr] *state, condition*.

sister ('sistə) a senior female nurse in a position of responsibility related to patient care, working in either a hospital ward or in the community nursing services.

sitiology, sitology (ˌsieti'oləjee; sie'toləjee) the science of food and nourishment.

sitomania (ˌsietoh'mayni·ə) excessive hunger, or morbid craving for food.

β-sitosterolaemia (ˌbeetəsieˌtostə·rə'leemi·ə) the presence of excessive levels of plant sterols, especially β-sitosterol, in the blood. A rare form is associated with xanthomatosis, with tuberous and tendon xanthomas appearing in childhood.

sitotherapy (ˌsietoh'therəpee) treatment by food; dietotherapy.

sitotropism (sie'totrəˌpizəm) tropism in response to the influence of food.

situs ('sietəs) pl. *situs* [L.] site or position.

s. inversus total or partial transposition of the body organs to the side opposite the normal.

sitz bath (sits) see SALT bath.

Sjögren's syndrome (shərgrenz) a symptom complex usually occurring in middle-aged or older women, marked by keratoconjunctivitis sicca with pharyngitis sicca, enlargement of parotid glands, xerostomia, and chronic polyarthritis.

skatole ('skatohl) a compound formed in the putrefaction of proteins which contributes to the characteristic odour of the faeces.

skatoxyl (ska'toksil) an oxidation product of skatole found in the urine in certain diseases of the large intestine.

skelalgia (skə'lalji·ə) pain in the leg.

skeletal ('skelit'l) pertaining to the skeleton.

s. system the body's framework of bones; called also the skeleton. The skeleton of an average adult consists of 206 distinct bones.

FUNCTIONS OF THE SKELETAL SYSTEM. The bones of the skeleton give support and shape to the body and protect delicate internal organs. Muscles attached to the skeleton make motion possible. In addition to supporting the body, the bones store and help maintain the correct level of calcium (see also BONE). The bone marrow manufactures blood cells.

MAIN PARTS OF THE SKELETON. There are two main parts of the skeleton: the axial skeleton, including the bones of the head and trunk, and the appendicular skeleton, including the bones of the limbs. The axial skeleton has 80 bones; the appendicular skeleton, 126 bones.

Axial Skeleton. The axial skeleton includes the skull, the spine, and the ribs and sternum. The most important of these is the spine, called also the backbone and the vertebral column; it consists of 26 separate bones. Twenty-four vertebrae have holes through them, and the holes are lined up vertically, forming a hollow tube. The spinal cord runs through this bony tube and is protected by it.

The seven topmost spinal bones, the cervical vertebrae, are the neck bones. They support the skull, which encloses and protects the brain and provides protection for the eyes, the inner ears, and the nasal passages. The skull includes the cranium, the facial bones, and the auditory ossicles. Of the 28 bones of the skull, only one—the mandible—is movable.

Below the seven cervical vertebrae of the spine are 12 thoracic vertebrae; attached to them are 12 pairs of ribs, one pair to a vertebra. The ribs curve around to the front of the body, where most of them attach directly to the sternum or are indirectly attached to it by means of cartilage. The two bottom pairs of ribs remain unattached in front and so are called floating ribs. Together, the thoracic vertebrae, the ribs, and the sternum form a bony basket, called the thoracic (or rib) cage, that prevents the chest wall from collapsing and protects the heart and the lungs.

The remaining bones of the spine include five lumbar vertebrae, which support the small of the back, and the sacrum and coccyx.

The axial skeleton also includes a single bone in the neck, the hyoid bone, to which muscles of the mouth are attached. This is the only bone of the body that does not join with another bone.

Appendicular Skeleton. The appendicular skeleton includes the shoulder girdle, arm bones, pelvic girdle and leg bones. The shoulder (or pectoral) girdle, from which the arms hang, consists of the two clavicles (collarbones) and two scapulae (shoulder blades).

The arm has three long bones. One end of the upper arm bone, the humerus, fits into a socket in the shoulder girdle; the other end is connected at the elbow to the ulna and the radius, the two long bones of the lower arm. Eight small bones, the carpals, comprise the wrist. Five metacarpals form the palm of the hand, and the finger bones are made up of 14 phalanges in each hand.

At the lower end of the spine is the pelvic (or hip) girdle. This girdle and the last two bones of the spine, the sacrum and the coccyx, form the pelvis. This part of the skeleton encircles and protects the internal organs of the genitourinary system. In each side of the pelvis is a socket into which a femur fits.

Leg bones are similar in construction to arm bones, but are heavier and stronger. The thigh bone, or femur, which is the longest bone in the body, extends from the pelvis to the knee, and the tibia and fibula go from knee to ankle. The kneecap is a single bone, the patella. In each leg there are seven ankle bones, or tarsals; five foot bones, or metatarsals; and 14 toe bones, or phalanges.

JOINTS AND MOVEMENT. Any place in the skeleton where two or more bones come together is known as a JOINT. The way these bones are joined determines whether they can move and how they move. The elbow, for example, is a hinge joint, which allows bending in only one direction. In contrast, both bending and rotary movements are possible in the hip joint, a ball-and-socket joint. Many joints, such as most of those in the skull, are rigid and permit no movement whatsoever.

The force needed to move the bones is provided by MUSCLES, which are attached to the bones by tendons. A muscle typically spans a joint so that one end is attached by a tendon to one bone, and the other end to a second bone. Usually one bone serves as an anchor for the muscle, and the second bone is free to move. When the muscle contracts, it pulls the second bone. Actually, two sets of muscles that pull in opposite directions take part in any movement. When one set contracts, the opposing set relaxes.

skeletization (ˌskelitie'zayshən) 1. extreme emaciation. 2. removal of soft parts from the skeleton.

skeletogenous (ˌskeli'tojənəs) producing skeletal structures or tissues.

skeleton ('skelitən) the hardened tissues forming the supporting framework of an animal body (see SKELETAL SYSTEM).

Skene's glands (skeenz) the largest of the female urethral glands, which open within the urethral orifice; they are regarded as homologous with the prostate. Called also *paraurethral ducts*.

skenitis (skee'nietis) inflammation of Skene's glands.

skeptophylaxis (ˌskeptohfi'laksis) 1. a condition in which a minute dose of a substance poisonous to animals will produce immediate temporary immunity to the action of the poison, although the blood of the animal may be highly toxic during that period of immunity. 2. the method of allergic desensitization by the preliminary injection of a small amount of the allergen, as is commonly done before the injection of an antiserum.

skia- word element. [Gr.] *shadow;* (especially as produced by x-rays).

skiagram ('skeeəgram) radiograph.

skin (skin) the outer covering of the body. The skin is the largest organ of the body, and it performs a number of vital functions. It serves as a protective barrier against microorganisms. It helps shield the delicate, sensitive tissues underneath from mechanical and other injuries. It acts as an insulator against heat and cold, and helps eliminate body wastes in the form of perspiration. It guards against excessive exposure to the ultraviolet rays of the sun by producing a protective pigmentation, and it helps produce the body's supply of vitamin D. Its sense receptors enable the body to feel pain, cold, heat, touch, and pressure.

The skin consists of two main parts: an outer layer, the epidermis, and an inner layer, the dermis (corium, true skin).

EPIDERMIS. The epidermis is thinner than the corium, and is made up of several layers of different kinds of cells, greatest where the skin is thickest in the palms of the hands and soles of the feet. The cells in the outer or horny layer of the epidermis are constantly being shed and replaced by new cells from its bottom layers in the lower epidermis. The cells of the protective, horny layer are nonliving and require no supply of blood for nourishment. As long as the horny outer layer remains intact, microorganisms cannot enter.

DERMIS. Underneath the epidermis is the thicker part of the skin, the dermis, or corium, which is made up of connective tissue that contains blood vessels and nerves. The dermis projects into the epidermis in ridges called papillae of the dermis.

The nerves that extend through the dermis end in the papillae. The various skin sensations, such as touch, pain, pressure, heat, and cold, are felt through these nerves. The reaction to heat and cold causes the expansion and contraction of the blood capillaries of the corium. This in turn causes more or less blood to flow through the skin, resulting in greater or smaller loss of body heat (see TEMPERATURE).

The sweat glands are situated deep in the dermis. They collect fluid containing water, salt, and waste products from the blood and carry it away in canals that end in pores on the skin surface, where it is deposited as sweat. Perspiration helps regulate body temperature as well, because cooling of the skin occurs when sweat evaporates. The sebaceous glands are also in the dermis. They secrete the oil that keeps the skin surface lubricated.

Beneath the dermis is a layer of subcutaneous tissue. This tissue helps insulate the body against heat and cold, and cushions it against shock.

The hair and nails are outgrowths of the skin. The roots of the hair lie in follicles, or pockets of epidermal cells situated in the dermis. Hair grows from the roots, but the hair cells die while still in the follicles, and the closely packed remains that are pushed upward form the hair shaft that is seen on the surface of the skin.

The nails grow in much the same way as the hair. The nail bed, like the hair root, is situated in the dermis. The pink colour of the nails is due to their translucent quality which allows the blood capillaries of the dermis to show through.

DISORDERS OF THE SKIN. The skin reflects the general physical and emotional health. A skin disorder, for instance, may indicate disease within the body. For this reason, it is important that a particular skin condition be diagnosed and treated by a dermatologist rather than by home treatments that may be unnecessary or actually harmful.

It is important to remember that the skin, given the opportunity, tends to heal itself. Overtreatment may be worse than no treatment at all. For common skin ailments, bland treatments, such as cool or warm compresses, lotions, and ointments, are usually recommended. Under no circumstances should one scratch, pick, or rub an incipient skin irritation or inflammation.

Inflammation of the skin is termed DERMATITIS, and any itching of the skin PRURITUS. Dermatitis may occur without pruritus and vice versa, but they often occur together.

Allergic reactions that may be manifested by skin disorders include URTICARIA (hives), ECZEMA, and various forms of CONTACT DERMATITIS. Fungus infections of the skin include RINGWORM and ATHLETE'S FOOT.

BOILS and CARBUNCLES occur when bacteria gain entrance into the skin and cause the formation of pus. A related condition of the eyelid is a STY.

Streptococci or staphylococci cause IMPETIGO, which

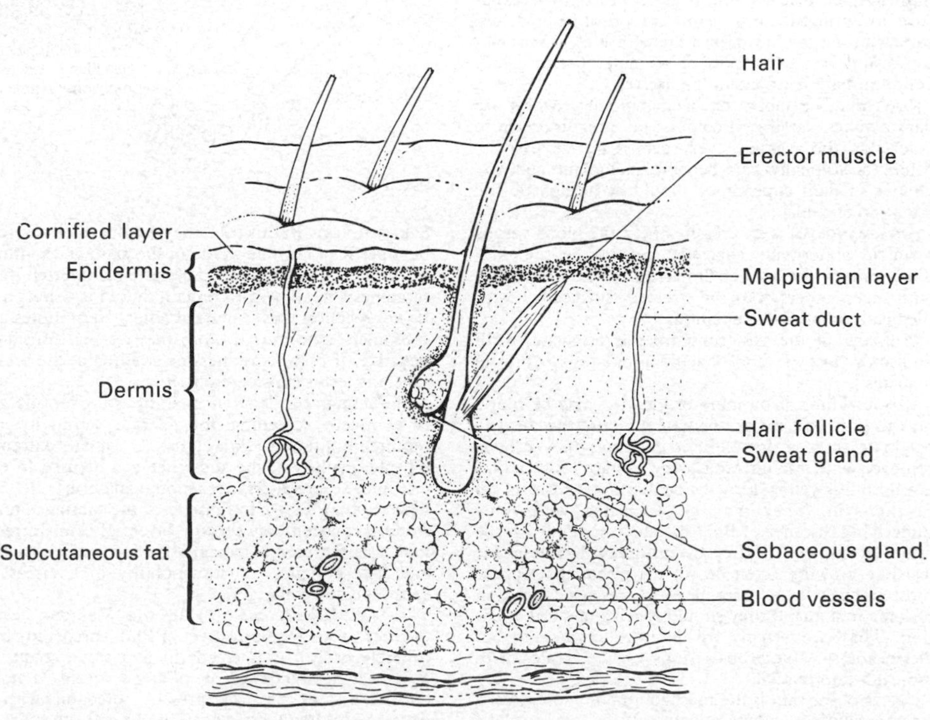

Skin

is marked by blisters and yellowish crusts and occurs most often in children.

A similar infection that affects the hair follicles at the pore openings of the skin is FOLLICULITIS. When such infection affects the follicles of the beard, it is called SYCOSIS BARBAE, or barber's itch.

ERYSIPELAS, or St. Anthony's fire, is a streptococcal infection of the skin and underlying tissues that can be very serious if not treated. This condition is one of several forms of CELLULITIS that may affect the skin.

COLLAGEN DISEASES, which cause deterioration of the connective tissues, may affect the skin. They include the relatively uncommon systemic LUPUS ERYTHEMATOSUS and SCLERODERMA.

PEMPHIGUS is a rare and serious disease that usually begins as a cluster of blisters on the nose or mouth and gradually involves the whole body.

Fever blisters, or coldsores, are caused by the virus of herpes simplex. Another virus disease affecting the skin is HERPES ZOSTER, or shingles, in which infection of a nerve root results in a skin eruption. WARTS are often also caused by a virus.

The skin is subject to a number of pigmentary disorders. Some are congenital; others occur as the result of exposure to sunlight, heat, heavy metals, and other products, or as a result of local injury, or in association with various diseases.

Some persons lack pigmentation partially or completely. This condition, which is hereditary, is known as albinism. Vitiligo and leukoderma appear as white areas of skin that occur because of localized decreased pigmentation. The cause is unknown. Leukoderma may accompany certain infections, or may result from injury or exposure to rubber products.

Excessive pigmentation includes the freckles that light-skinned persons tend to develop from overexposure to sunlight. LIVER SPOTS are brownish patches, somewhat larger and darker than freckles, that sometimes appear on the skin of an older person. Both conditions are harmless in themselves.

NAEVI may be moles or haemangiomas. Moles are dark patches, varying in colour from grey to brown to black. On the average, every person has at least 20. Moles occasionally can become malignant and any change in their appearance should be brought to the attention of a doctor.

A HAEMANGIOMA is an area in which the blood vessels form an abnormally excessive network in the skin. They usually occur as birthmarks and some disappear with age; others can be treated surgically, with medications or with irradiation.

Bronzing of the skin sometimes is associated with ADDISON'S DISEASE and haemochromatosis ('bronze diabetes').

Various kinds of tumours or growths may be found on the skin. KELOIDS are benign tumours that usually originate in scar tissue. In many cases they can be removed with radium and x-ray therapy. XANTHOMAS are harmless yellow growths caused by deposits of fat in the skin. They may be associated with some underlying disorder of lipid metabolism. They can be removed surgically if they are unsightly. Keratoses are wartlike growths, often brown in colour, that appear most frequently in older persons. Because they can become malignant, they should receive medical attention. They are usually treated with cryotherapy or elctrocautery. Numerous lesions can be treated with topical 5-fluorouracil.

CANCER of the skin is the most common of all cancers. Fortunately it is comparatively easy to treat successfully, especially if it is diagnosed early. As protection against skin cancer, sores that persist for more than 2 or 3 weeks and any patches, lumps or growths that suddenly begin to enlarge or change colour should be brought to a doctor's attention.

s. graft a piece of skin implanted to replace a lost part of the integument (see also GRAFTING and PLASTIC SURGERY).

s. test application of a substance to the skin, or intradermal injection of a substance, to permit observation of the body's reaction to it. Such a test may detect a person's sensitivity to such allergens as dust and pollen, or to preparations of microorganisms believed to be the cause of a disorder.

There are several types of skin tests, including the patch test, the scratch test, and the intradermal test.

PATCH TEST. This is the simplest type of skin test. A small piece of gauze or filter paper is impregnated with a minute quantity of the substance to be tested and is applied to the skin; the forearm is used for a single test and the back of the arm for multiple tests. After a certain length of time the patch is removed and the reaction observed. If there is no reaction, the test result is said to be negative; if the skin is reddened or swollen, the result is positive.

The patch test is used most often in testing for skin allergies, especially CONTACT DERMATITIS.

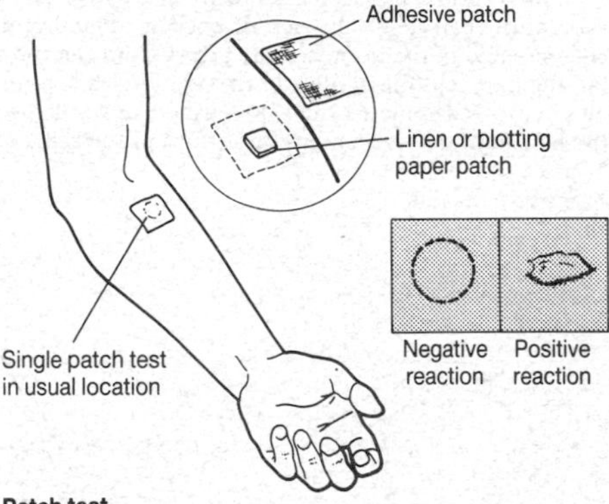

Patch test.

SCRATCH TEST. In this test, one or more small scratches or superficial cuts are made in the skin, and a minute amount of the substance to be tested is inserted in the scratches and allowed to remain there for a short time. If no reaction has occurred after 30 minutes, the substance is removed and the test is considered negative. If there is redness or swelling at the scratch sites, the test is considered positive.

The scratch test is often used in testing for allergies. A complete screening for allergic sensitivity may require numerous skin tests. Only an extremely minute quantity of the substance can be used in each test since severe allergic reactions can occur.

INTRADERMAL TESTS. In these tests, the substance under study is injected between the layers of skin. Intradermal tests are used for diagnosis of infectious diseases and determination of susceptibility to a disease or sensitivity to an allergen.

Tests for Tuberculosis. (1) In the Mantoux test, a purified protein derivative (PPD), prepared from tubercle bacilli, is injected. In a positive result, the area becomes reddened or inflamed within 72 hours. This indicates past or present infection with or exposure to the tubercle bacillus. An infection that has been present for at least 2 to 8 weeks will usually be revealed by the test. (2) In the HEAF TEST, a multiple

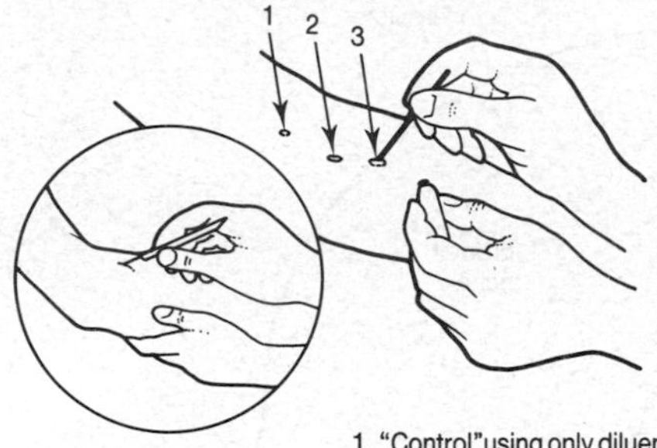

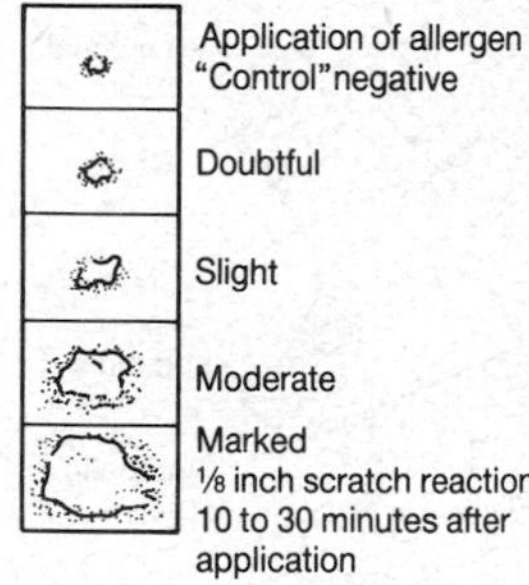

Scratch test

puncture 'gun' is used to inject PPD. This method is used mostly prior to giving routinized vaccination with BCG VACCINE.

The Schick test, used to determine susceptibility to diphtheria, is one of the best-known intradermal skin tests. A very small dose of diphtheria antitoxin is injected into the forearm. In a positive reaction the area becomes red and remains so for about a week. If no reaction occurs, the person is considered to be immune to the disease.

Skinner box ('skinə) an experimental enclosure for testing animal conditioning, in which the subject animal performs (e.g., presses a bar or lever) to obtain a reward (see also instrumental CONDITIONING).

skler(o)- for words beginning thus, see those beginning *scler(o)-*.

skot(o)- for words beginning thus, see those beginning *scot(o)-*.

skull (skul) the bony framework of the head, enclosing and protecting the brain. The skull consists of two parts, the cranium and the facial section.

The cranium is the domed top, back, and sides of the skull. It is formed by comparatively large, smooth and gently curved bones connected to each other by dovetailed joints called sutures, which permit no movement and make the mature skull rigid. At birth, however, the skull joints are flexible, so that the infant's head can be compressed as it emerges from the birth canal. The joints remain flexible to allow expansion until the cranial bones are fully formed, around the second year of life. An infant's skull contains soft areas, or FONTANELLES, where the bones of the cranium do not meet. See accompanying illustration.

The facial bones are smaller and more complex than the cranial bones. None of them are movable, except the mandible, which is hinged to the rest of the skull.

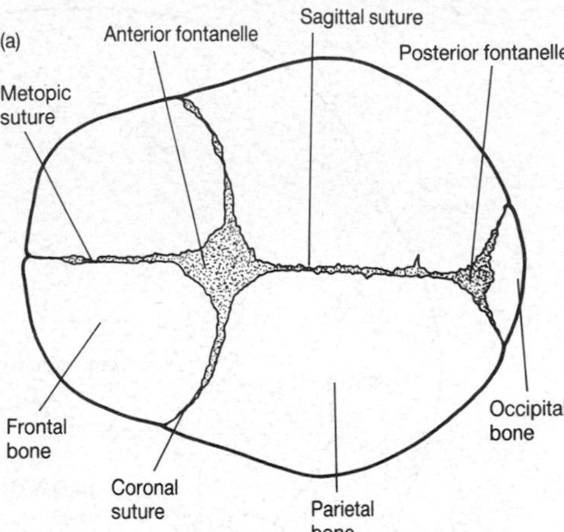

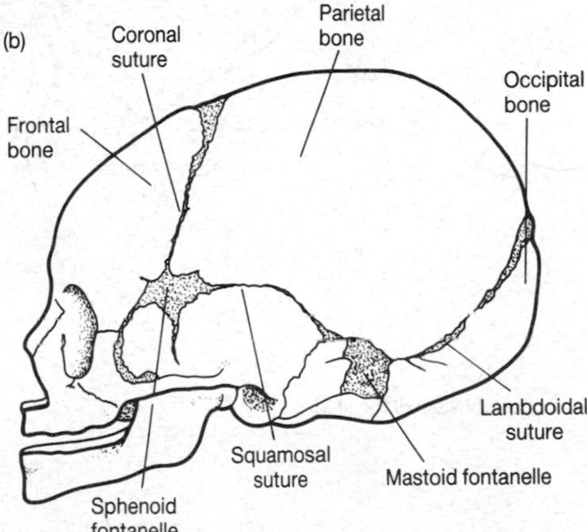

Skull at birth. (a) Showing anterior and posterior fontanelles. (b) Lateral view.

The skull protects the brain, the curve of the cranium serving to deflect blows, and it also protects the eyes, ears, and nose, which are surrounded by bone and recessed in the skull.

The skull is supported by the highest vertebra, called the atlas. This joint permits a back-and-forth, nodding motion. The atlas turns on the vertebra below it, the axis, which allows the skull to turn from side to side.

DISORDERS OF THE SKULL. The skull is rarely affected by disease. Uncommon ones like OSTEITIS DEFORMANS and ACROMEGALY cause the bones to increase in size. Like other bones, the skull may be fractured by blows, falls, or other accidents, but skull fracture can be far more dangerous because of its proximity to the brain. Concussion is almost always present with such fractures. If the fracture is simple, it will usually heal itself. There may be complications, however. If the fracture crosses an artery, surgery may be necessary. Another danger is that a bone or fragment of bone may be pushed in and exert pressure on the brain, possibly causing convulsions. Such a bone intrusion must be corrected by surgery. Open or compound fractures of the skull present the additional danger of

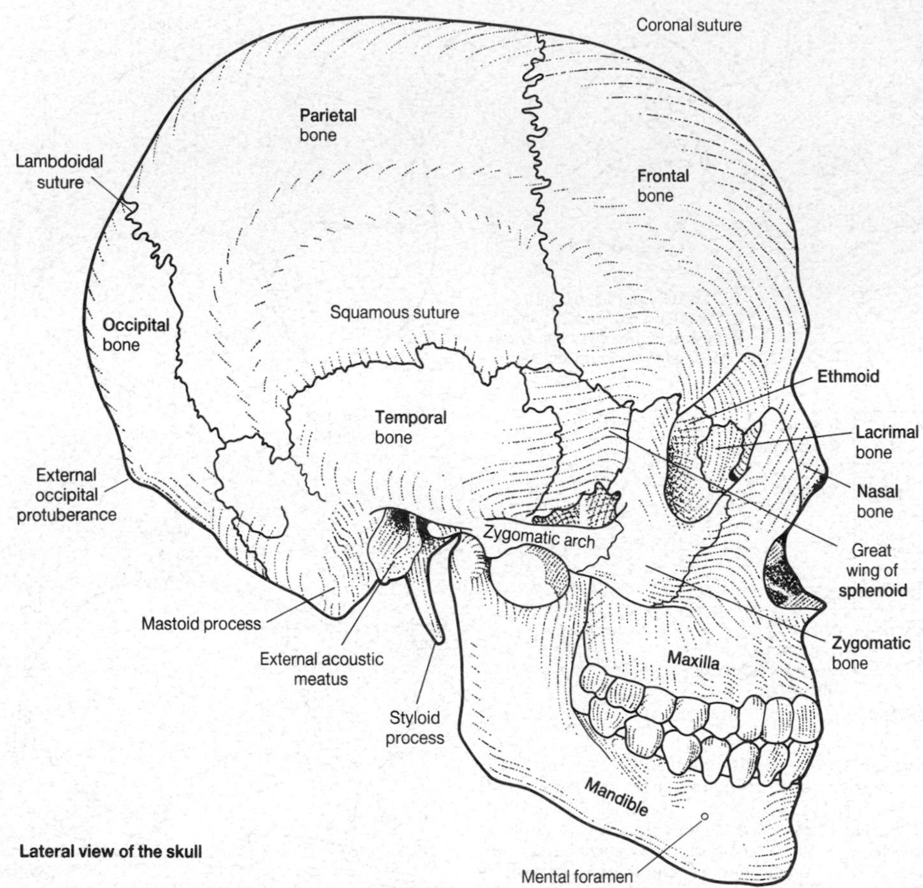

Lateral view of the skull

infection to the brain. See also HEAD INJURY.

During infancy the bones of the skull may unite prematurely, causing the head to be misshapen and sometimes resulting in brain damage because of pressure effects on the growing brain.

sleep (sleep) a period of rest for the body and mind, during which volition and consciousness are in partial or complete abeyance and the bodily functions partially suspended. Sleep has also been described as a behavioural state marked by characteristic immobile posture and diminished but readily reversible sensitivity to external stimuli.

NREM AND REM SLEEP. Prior to the discovery and reporting of rapid eye movements (REM) during sleep, it was thought that sleep was a single state of passive recuperation in which the central nervous system was deactivated. Studies reported by Eugene Aserinsky and Nathaniel Kleitman in 1953, and subsequent studies by others concerned with the measurement of central and autonomic activities during sleep have led to the dividing of sleep into two categories: NREM, or non-rapid eye movement sleep, also called orthodox or synchronized (S) sleep; and REM, or rapid eye movement sleep, so called because of the rapid eye movements that are manifested during this stage of sleep. REM sleep is also called paradoxical or desynchronized (D) sleep.

On the basis of electroencephalographic (EEG) criteria, NREM sleep is subdivided into four stages. *Stage 1* is observed immediately after sleep begins or after momentary arousals and is characterized by low-voltage, mixed-frequency EEG tracing, with predominantly theta-wave activity (four to seven hertz, that is, cycles per second). *Stage 2* is characterized by intermittent waves of 12 to 16 hertz known as 'sleep spindles'. *Stages 3 and 4* consist of relatively high voltage EEG tracings with a predominance of delta wave activity (one to two hertz).

The EEG patterns of NREM sleep suggest that this kind of sleep is the kind of apparently restful state that supports the recuperative functions assigned to sleep. NREM sleep is increased after physical activity and has a relatively high priority among humans in the recovery sleep following extended periods of wakefulness.

Within 90 minutes after sleep begins, an adult progresses through all four stages of NREM sleep and then proceeds into the first of a series of REM periods of sleep. Brief cycles of about 10 to 30 minutes of REM sleep recur throughout the night, alternating with various stages of NREM sleep. With each cycle, NREM sleep decreases and REM sleep increases so that during the last few hours of the night most of the sleep is REM sleep, which is when dreams occur. While everyone dreams every night, many do not remember dreaming; most people are aware, however, that they dream more during the early morning hours just before rising.

In addition to the rapid eye movements that can be observed through closed eyelids, REM sleep can be recognized by complete relaxation of the lower jaw. Convulsions, myocardial infarction, and cardiac arrhythmias are more likely to occur during REM sleep. This is probably because of increased autonomic activity, irregular pulse, and fluctuations in blood pressure, which are all typical of REM sleep.

PATTERNS OF SLEEP. Although the average adult spends approximately 25 per cent of total accumulated sleep in REM sleep and 75 per cent in NREM sleep, the cyclic changes vary with individuals. The pattern of sleep, in addition to the REM and NREM states, also includes the periods of sleep and wakefulness within a 24-hour period.

Factors affecting the total sleep pattern include age, state of physical health, psychological state, and certain drugs. Newborn infants follow a pattern of several hours of sleep followed by a period of wakefulness. REM sleep occurs at the onset of sleep in infants; it rarely does in adults. As the child matures there is an increasing tendency toward longer periods of nocturnal sleep. Elderly persons sometimes return to the shorter periods of sleep that are typical of infants.

SLEEP REQUIREMENTS. There is a great variability in sleep requirements among individuals. Infants usually require 16 to 20 hours of total sleep during a 24-hour period, with the number of hours decreasing as they mature. An adult usually requires 6 to 9 hours of total sleep.

The effects of *sleep deprivation* have been the subject of much research, including deprivation of total sleep, of REM sleep, and of NREM sleep. Total sleep deprivation usually leads to irritability and fatigue, difficulty in concentrating and remembering, poor muscle coordination, and visual or tactile hallucinations and illusions. There is no evidence that total sleep deprivation induces psychosis. Some bizarre behaviours may be manifested after an extended period of sleep loss, but these symptoms do not recur in most subjects once they have slept through a recovery period. It is suspected that when inappropriate behaviour does persist after recovery sleep, the subject already had a tendency toward such behaviour before sleep deprivation.

Selective sleep deprivation studies have shown that there is a need for both stage 4 NREM and REM sleep. REM sleep deprivation can produce such symptoms as irritability, apathy, decrease in alertness, poor judgement, and increased sensitivity to pain. Most sedatives and tranquillizers, antidepressants, and alcohol interfere with REM sleep.

BENEFITS OF SLEEP. Most theorists agree that sleep has value as a recuperative and adaptive function in the lives of humans. The relatively high metabolic needs of mammals and birds to maintain a constant body temperature in a wide range of environmental temperatures suggests that the periodic decreases in metabolic rate and body temperature that occur in NREM sleep allow for recuperation and restitution of body tissues. For example, even though the function of stage 2 NREM sleep is not clear, approximately half of human sleep time is spent in this stage.

It is also theorized that REM sleep provides a period of recuperation of mental activities and preparation for wakefulness. During REM sleep it is believed that there is increased metabolic activity in the brain so that during waking hours it is more receptive to new information and can assimilate it more easily.

SLEEP DISORDERS. Among the minor disorders of sleep are sleepwalking, sleep talking, ENURESIS, tooth-grinding (which is probably an orthodontic problem), and nightmares. Sleepwalking is not considered serious if it occasionally occurs in childhood. It should be considered pathological, however, if it persists into adulthood. Sleep talking is common to many persons and, while it may annoy others whose sleep it may disturb, it is not considered pathological.

A sleep disorder occurring in early childhood, and not to be confused with nightmares, is *night terrors* (pavor nocturnus). In this event, the child awakens with a scream, is in panic and cannot be consoled, and often is incoherent. There is poor recall of the event the following morning. Treatment usually involves reassurance of the parents. Adults who experience night terrors often have some psychological problem requiring treatment.

More serious disorders of sleep include persistent INSOMNIA, narcolepsy, and chronic hypersomnia. Hypersomnia can occur with central nervous system damage and it may be secondary to some physical and mental illnesses, particularly depression.

sleeping disease ('sleeping) narcolepsy.

sleeping sickness see African TRYPANOSOMIASIS.

sleepwalking ('sleep,wawking) walking while asleep; called also somnambulism. Much mystery has been attached to sleepwalking, although it is no more mysterious than dreaming. The chief difference between the two is that the sleepwalker, besides dreaming, is also using the part of his brain that stimulates walking.

Sleepwalking is most likely to happen during periods of emotional stress. Usually it ceases when the source of anxiety is removed. Often it occurs only once or twice and does not happen again. If sleepwalking recurs frequently, it may stem from serious emotional distress. See also SLEEP.

slide (slied) a piece of glass or other transparent substance on which material is placed for examination under the microscope.

sling (sling) a bandage or suspensory for supporting a part.

slipped disc (slipt) the popular name for a rupture of a disc, or pad of cartilage, between vertebrae (see PROLAPSED INTERVERTEBRAL DISC).

slit lamp ('slit ,lamp) a special light source so arranged with a microscope that examination of the interior of the eye can be carried out at the level of each layer.

slough (sluf) 1. a mass of dead tissue in, or cast out from, living tissue. 2. to shed or cast off.

Slow-K ('slohkay) trademark for a sustained release preparation of potassium chloride.

slow-reacting substance ('slohri,akting) a substance released in the anaphylactic reaction that induces slow, prolonged contraction of certain smooth muscles. Symbol SRS or SRS-A.

slow virus (sloh) a group of infections caused by agents (possibly viruses) which have very long incubation periods and show no antibody response. See also CREUTZFELDT–JAKOB DISEASE.

sludge (sluj) a suspension of solid or semisolid particles in a fluid.

sludging ('slujing) settling out of solid particles from solution.

s. of blood intravascular agglutination of erythrocytes into irregular masses, interfering with circulation of blood.

Sm chemical symbol, *samarium*.

smallpox ('smawl,poks) a highly infectious, often fatal disease caused by a poxvirus; called also *variola*. Its most noticeable symptom is the appearance of blisters and pustules on the skin.

Smallpox was eradicated from the world in 1977, the last naturally acquired infection being reported in Somalia in November 1977. Despite intensive worldwide surveillance no cases have since been detected except for two cases in Birmingham, England, associated with a poxvirus laboratory.It remains a notifiable disease.

Because of the eradication of the disease, vaccination is no longer required for travellers to any part of the world.

smear (smiə) a specimen for microscopic study, the material being spread thinly and unevenly across the slide with a swab or loop, or with the edge of another slide.

s. test see PAPANICOLAOU TEST.

smegma ('smegmə) the secretion of sebaceous glands, especially the cheesy secretion, consisting principally of desquamated epithelial cells, found chiefly beneath the prepuce. adj. **smegmatic.**

smell (smel) the sense that enables one to perceive odours. The sense of smell depends on the stimulation of sense organs in the nose by small particles carried in inhaled air. It is important not only for the detection of odours, but also for the enjoyment of food. Flavour is a blend of taste and smell. Taste registers only four qualities: salt, sour, bitter, and sweet; other qualities of flavour depend on smell.

The organs of smell are small patches of special (olfactory) cells in the nasal mucosa. One patch is located in each of the two main compartments of the back of the nose. The olfactory cells are connected to the brain by the first cranial (olfactory) nerve. Air currents do not flow directly over the patches in breathing; this is why one must sniff to detect a faint odour or to enjoy a fragrance to the fullest.

When one sniffs, air currents carrying molecules of odourous chemicals enter special compartments, called olfactory chambers, where the chemicals are dissolved in mucus. There they can act on the organs of smell in much the same way that solutions act on the taste buds of the tongue. The endings of the sensory nerves that detect odours, the olfactory receptors, can quickly adapt to an odour and cease to be stimulated by it after a few minutes of full exposure.

The sense of smell may be diminished or lost entirely, usually temporarily, as a result of an obstruction of the nose, a nasal infection, injury or deterioration of the nasal tissue, brain tumour, or mental illness. In rare instances, injury or disease causes such damage to the olfactory nerve that loss of the sense of smell is permanent. The complete absence of the sense of smell is known as anosmia.

Smith's fracture (smiths) reversed Colles' fracture.

Smith–Lemli–Opitz syndrome (ˌsmithˌlemli'ohpits) a hereditary syndrome, transmitted as an autosomal recessive trait, characterized by microcephaly, mental handicap, hypotonia, incomplete development of male genitalia, short nose with anteverted nostrils, and syndactyly of the second and third toes.

Smith-Petersen nail (ˌsmith'peetəsən) a flanged nail for fixing the head of the femur in fracture of the femoral neck.

Smith–Strang disease (ˌsmith'strang) a hereditary defect in methionine absorption, in which the urine has a characteristic odour resembling that of the interior of an oasthouse due to alpha-hydroxybutyric acid formed by bacterial action on the unabsorbed methionine; it is marked by white hair, mental handicap, convulsions, and attacks of hyperpnoea. Called also *oasthouse urine disease*.

smoking ('smohking) the act of drawing into the mouth and puffing out the smoke of tobacco contained in a cigarette, cigar, or pipe. For centuries, tobacco smoking has been suspected of being a health hazard. In recent years a close relationship between smoking and lung cancer and heart disease has definitely been established. While smoking is not the only cause of these diseases, its relationship to them and also to other diseases has been so strongly established that no smoker can afford to ignore the evidence. Parents especially owe it to their children to educate them in order that the cigarette habit will never begin.

In 1985 a report ('The Big Kill') on smoking, death, and disease was published by the Health Education Council and the British Medical Association. The report makes the following points.

Smoking kills 77,774 people each year in England and Wales.

The cost to the NHS of treating the 108,218 people admitted with smoking-related diseases is estimated at over £111,000,000. Each day, on average, 4009 beds are occupied by patients with these diseases—1,463,400 bed days a year.

GENERAL EFFECTS ON HEALTH. Tobacco smoke contains a number of harmful substances, including poisons such as NICOTINE, various irritants, and carcinogenic compounds. Because cigarette smokers usually inhale this smoke, they are much more subject to its harmful effects than pipe and cigar smokers, who generally do not inhale. In pipe and cigar smoking, however, there is some danger to the heart because of the nicotine that is absorbed by the mouth. There is also the possibility of cancer of the lips, tongue, and mouth. Statistically, there is no question that nonsmokers are far less subject to the diseases that affect smokers.

Among the respiratory diseases closely related to cigarette smoking are lung cancer, cancer of the larynx, chronic bronchitis, and emphysema. Coronary artery disease and hypertensive heart disease are also closely related to smoking, as are peptic ulcer, Buerger's disease (thromboangiitis obliterans), and cancer of the bladder. Other diseases have been linked with smoking. The risk of incurring any of these diseases increases with the number of cigarettes smoked daily, the length of each cigarette consumed, and the length of time the smoking habit has persisted. In general, heavy smokers as a group die younger than do nonsmokers.

smouldering leukaemia ('smohldə·ring) see smouldering LEUKAEMIA.

Sn chemical symbol, *tin* (L. *stannum*).

snake (snayk) a limbless reptile, many species of which are poisonous.

snakebite ('snaykˌbiet) injury caused by the mouth parts of a snake. It is estimated that throughout the world the number of deaths resulting from venomous snakebites is between 20,000 and 25,000 per year. The greatest number of reported snakebite deaths is in the subcontinent of India.

In addition to local wound treatment, which may require skin grafting at a later date, treatment is concerned with administration of an immune serum (antisera or antivenin), counteraction of the specific pharmacological effects of the venom, symptomatic relief, and prevention of complications. See also TOURNIQUET.

snap (snap) a short, sharp sound.
opening s. a short, sharp, high-pitched click occurring in early diastole caused by opening of the mitral cusps, a characteristic sound in mitral stenosis.

snare (snair) a wire loop for removing polyps.

sneeze (sneez) 1. an involuntary, sudden, violent, and audible expulsion of air through the mouth and nose. 2. to expel air in such a manner. Sneezing is usually caused by the irritation of sensitive nerve endings in the mucous membrane that lines the nose. Allergies, drafts of cold air, and even bright light can produce sneezing.

Sneezing and coughing are similar in that both are reflex actions and are preceded by quick inhalations. (However, a cough may also be deliberate, to clear the throat or bronchi.) Sneezing and coughing both involve the glottis. The power for a cough is achieved by closing the glottis and holding the air under pressure for a moment, then suddenly forcing it out by action of the diaphragm and of the muscles of the chest wall and abdomen.

In a sneeze, the glottis is momentarily closed after air is inhaled and the tongue is pressed against the roof of the mouth. When the glottis is suddenly opened, part of the air goes through the nose and, when the tongue is released, part goes through the mouth; in this way mucus and other irritants are expelled from the nose.

Snellen chart ('snelən) a chart printed with block letters in gradually decreasing sizes, used in testing visual acuity.

snoring ('snor·ring) breathing during sleep accompanied by harsh sounds. It occurs when inhaled air causes the soft palate to vibrate. Snoring is common among persons who sleep with their mouths open.

Although snoring is a sign of sound sleep, it is sometimes desirable to eliminate or reduce it. If the mouth-breathing is stopped, the snoring will also stop. An obvious reason for mouth-breathing is lying on the back, in which position the mouth tends to hang open. Further, when a person is in deep sleep and lying on his back, his tongue may rest back in his throat, partly blocking the air passage and helping to make the snoring sounds. Gently rolling the snorer on his side can sometimes eliminate the snoring in these cases.

There may be some functional reason for mouth-breathing, such as a common cold or allergy, causing mucus to stop up the nose. Growths, called polyps, may obstruct the nasal passages. A deformity of the nasal SEPTUM, the bony portion that divides the nasal cavity into two compartments, may make nose-breathing difficult.

Correction of sleeping habits and of nose or throat troubles may lessen snoring or reduce it to a minimum. However, if an elderly person has been snoring regularly for many years, there is little that can be done to change his sleeping habits.

snow (snoh) a freezing or frozen mixture consisting of discrete particles or crystals.
carbon dioxide s. the solid formed by rapid evaporation of liquid carbon dioxide, giving a temperature of about -79 °C (-110 °F); used locally in various skin conditions. See also CARBON DIOXIDE SNOW.

snowblindness ('snoh,bliendnəs) temporary impairment of vision due to injury to the epithelial cells of the cornea caused by ultraviolet rays of the sun reinforced by those reflected by snow. Called also *niphablepsia.*

snuffles ('snuf'lz) catarrhal discharge from the nasal mucous membrane in congenital syphilis in infants.

soap (sohp) any compound of one or more fatty acids, or their equivalents, with an alkali. Soap is a detergent and is employed in liniments and enemas and in making pills. It is also a mild aperient, antacid, and antiseptic.

social breakdown syndrome ('sohshəl) a term used to express the concept that some of the mental patient's symptomatology, especially in large, understaffed institutions, is a result of treatment conditions and facilities and not part of the primary illness.

social class a category arising from the division of society into economic or occupational groupings. Since 1911, the office of the Registrar General in the UK (since 1969 the Office of Population Censuses and Surveys) has used a five-category measurement of social class based on occupational groupings (see accompanying table).

Scale showing measurement of social class

Social class	Occupation (examples)
1. Professional	Doctors, dentists, lawyers, architects, university teachers
2. Intermediate	Nurses, pharmacists, members of parliament, school teachers
3. Skilled	Clerical workers, police, shop assistants, sales representatives
4. Semi-skilled	Agricultural workers, barmen/maids, telephone operators, postmen
5. Unskilled	Porters, labourers, cleaners, bus conductors, packers, messengers

From Lyttle, J.R. (1986) *Mental Disorder: Its Care and Treatment,* 1st edn, Baillière Tindall, p. 22.

social worker a professional trained in the treatment of individual and social problems of patients and their families. See also MEDICAL *social worker.*

socialization (,sohshəlie'zayshən) the process by which society integrates the individual, and the individual learns to behave in socially acceptable ways.

sociobiology (,sohsiohbie'oləjee) the branch of theoretical biology which proposes that all animal (including human) behaviour has a biological basis, which is controlled by the genes. adj. **sociobiological.**

sociogenic (,sohsioh'jenik) arising from or imposed by society.

sociologist (,sohsi'oləjist) a specialist in sociology.

sociology (,sohsi'oləjee) the scientific study of social relationships and phenomena.

sociometry (,sohsi'omətree) the branch of sociology concerned with the measurement of human behaviour.

sociopath ('sohsioh,path) a person with an antisocial personality; a psychopath. adj. **sociopathic.**

sociopathic (,sohsioh'pathik) antisocial; pertaining to a sociopath; called also *psychopathic.*
s. personality a type of personality disorder, characterized by a conspicuous disregard for the rights or needs of others; called also *psychopathic personality.* The behaviour patterns of the sociopath are not typical of either NEUROSIS or PSYCHOSIS, and differ somewhat from those of other types of personality disorders.

There is no sharp dividing line between the normal and the sociopathic personality. The sociopath shows a lack of emotional maturity, an unwillingness to take responsibility and emotional instability. Unlike the neurotic person, he expresses his conflict in antisocial acts so that society suffers, rather than the sociopath himself.

CHARACTERISTICS. The chief characteristic of a sociopath is an apparent lack of conscience. He expresses his conflicts in various ways, including compulsive lying, stealing, and certain other types of antisocial or criminal activity. He may suffer from alcoholism or drug addiction; sexual deviation may also be an expression of sociopathic personality.

Like other types of mental illness, a sociopathic personality probably has many roots in the emotions and experiences of early childhood, but their form of expression is different. A sociopathic personality affects the entire structure of the character, so that the person feels that everyone else is out of step. If the patient is a criminal, he may honestly believe that anyone who is not a criminal is merely stupid. Those with sociopathic personalities often seem to be unable to learn from experience.

TREATMENT. Unfortunately, it is extremely difficult to treat a patient with a sociopathic personality. The techniques of PSYCHOTHERAPY depend on the cooperation of the patient, and this in turn depends on his willingness to admit that something is wrong with him. This is an admission that those with sociopathic personalities are rarely willing or able to make. They seldom accept psychiatric help, and since they are legally sane, they cannot be compelled to undergo treatment.

sociopathy (ˌsohsi'opəthee) the condition of being antisocial (sociopathic).

sociotherapy (ˌsohsioh'therəpee) any treatment emphasizing socioenvironmental and interpersonal rather than intrapsychic factors.

socket ('sokit) a hollow into which a corresponding part fits.

dry s. a condition sometimes occurring after tooth extraction, with exposure of bone, inflammation of an alveolar crypt, and severe pain.

soda ('sohdə) sodium carbonate.

baking s. sodium bicarbonate.

sodium ('sohdi·əm) a chemical element, atomic number 11, atomic weight 22.990, symbol Na. (See table of elements in Appendix 2.) Sodium is the major cation of the extracellular fluid (ECF), constituting 90 to 95 per cent of all cations in the blood plasma and interstitial fluid; it thus determines the osmolality of the ECF. The serum sodium concentration is normally about 140 mEq/l. If the sodium level and osmolality fall, osmoreceptors in the HYPOTHALAMUS are stimulated and cause the release of ANTIDIURETIC HORMONE (ADH) from the posterior lobe of the PITUITARY GLAND. ADH increases the absorption of water in the collecting ducts of the kidneys so that water is conserved while sodium and other electrolytes are excreted in the urine. If the sodium level and osmolality rises, neurons in the thirst centre of the hypothalamus are stimulated. The thirsty person then drinks enough water to restore the osmolality of the ECF to the normal level.

A decrease in the serum sodium concentration below normal levels (*hyponatraemia*) can occur in a variety of conditions. It is often associated with FLUID VOLUME DEFICIT due to diarrhoea or vomiting when water is replaced faster than sodium. Hyponatraemia can also occur in *syndrome of inappropriate secretion of antidiuretic hormone* (SIADH), in the late stages of congestive HEART FAILURE or CIRRHOSIS of the liver, in acute or chronic RENAL FAILURE, and in DIURETIC therapy. An increase in the serum sodium concentration above normal levels (*hypernatraemia*) occurs when insensible water loss is not replaced by drinking, as in a comatose patient with diabetes insipidus.

DIETARY SODIUM RESTRICTION. The average British diet has a salt intake of 3.5 grams per day.

For a discussion of the role of dietary salt and cardiovascular disease, consult the Department of Health and Social Security's Report Number 28 *Diet and Cardiovascular Disease* (HMSO, 1984).

s. ascorbate an antiscorbutic vitamin for parenteral administration.

s. aurothiomalate a gold salt used in the treatment of rheumatoid arthritis and nondisseminated lupus erythematosus, administered intramuscularly.

s. bicarbonate a white powder found in most households in the form of baking soda; called also bicarbonate of soda. Taken in water, it is a popular remedy for acid indigestion. It has a rapid and soothing effect on the stomach, but should not be used regularly since when taken in excess it tends to cause ALKALOSIS. It should never be taken by those who have a heart condition or who are on salt-restricted diet, because it is a source of sodium. A teaspoonful of milk of magnesia will usually prove equally effective and is less harmful.

Sodium bicarbonate can also be mixed with water and applied as a paste for the relief of pain in the treatment of minor BURNS and insect stings. A cupful of bicarbonate of soda in the bath water will sometimes help to relieve itching caused by an allergic reaction. Applied in powder form, bicarbonate of soda is often a more effective deodorant than many commercial preparations.

s. carbonate $Na_2CO_3 \cdot H_2O$, used as an alkalizing agent in pharmaceuticals, and has been used as a lotion or bath in the treatment of scaly skin, and as a detergent.

s. chloride a white, crystalline compound, a necessary constituent of the body and therefore of the diet; sometimes used parenterally in solution to replenish electrolytes in the body; called also *salt*.

s. cromoglycate an antiallergic agent used in the prophylaxis of bronchial asthma and allergic rhinitis. It inhibits the release of chemical mediators of immediate sensitivity from basophils and mast cells, and is administered as an aerosol. It has the advantage of reducing or eliminating the need for steroids and sympathomimetics.

s. fluoride a white, odourless powder used in fluoridation of drinking water or applied locally to teeth, in 1 to 2 per cent solution, to reduce the incidence of dental caries.

s. glutamate the monosodium salt of L-glutamic acid; used in treatment of encephalopathies associated with liver diseases. Also used to enhance the flavour of foods.

s. hypochlorite a compound having germicidal, deodorizing, and bleaching properties; used in solution to disinfect utensils, and in diluted form (Dakin's solution) as a local antibacterial and to irrigate wounds.

s. iodide a compound used as a source of iodine and as an expectorant.

s. lactate a compound used in solution to replenish body fluids and electrolytes.

s. monofluorophosphate a dental caries prophylactic.

s. nitroprusside sodium nitroferricyanide, an antihypertensive used in the treatment of hypertensive crisis and to produce controlled hypotension during surgery; also used as a reagent.

s. phosphate a colourless or white granular salt, used as a cathartic.

s. salicylate an analgesic, antipyretic compound (see SALICYLATE).

s. thiosulphate a compound used intravenously as an antidote for cyanide poisoning, in the prophylaxis of ringworm (added to foot baths), and as a topical application in tinea versicolor. Also used in measuring the volume of extracellular body fluid and the renal glomerular filtration rate.

s. valproate an anticonvulsant.

sodoku ('sohdohkoo) a relapsing type of infection due to *Spirillum minus*, an organism transmitted by the bite of an infected rat; a form of RATBITE FEVER.

sodomy ('sodəmee) anal intercourse; also used to denote bestiality and fellatio.

soft palate (soft) the fleshy structure at the back of the mouth, which, together with the hard palate, forms the roof of the mouth. From the middle of the free border of the soft palate hangs the fleshy conical body called the uvula. In swallowing, the soft palate is drawn upward against the back of the pharynx and prevents food and fluids from straying into the nasal passage while they pass through the throat.

softening ('sof'ning) a change of consistency, with loss of firmness or hardness.

sol (sol) a liquid colloid solution.

sol. solution.

solar plexus ('sohlə) a network of ganglia and nerves in the centre of the abdomen; it is part of the autonomic nervous system. It is important in the control of the function of the liver, stomach, kidneys, and adrenal glands. A blow to it may knock a person out or cause great pain because the organs are momentarily thrown out of gear. Although the plexus recovers quickly, the effects on the body as a whole last longer.

solarium (sə'lair·ri·əm) 1. a room designed to admit as much sunlight as possible. 2. a room in which artificial sunlight treatment is given.

solarization (ˌsohlə·rie'zayshən) exposure to sunlight and the effects produced thereby.

solation (so'layshən) the liquefaction of a gel.

sole (sohl) the bottom of the foot.

solid ('solid) 1. not fluid or gaseous; not hollow. 2. a substance or tissue not fluid or gaseous.

Solu-Biloptin (ˌsolyuhbie'loptin) trademark for a preparation of calcium ipodate (an oral cholecystographic contrast medium).

solubility (ˌsolyuh'bilitee) the quality of being soluble.

soluble ('solyuhb'l) susceptible of being dissolved.

solum ('sohləm) pl. *sola* [L.] the bottom or lowest part.

solute ('solyoot) the substance that is dissolved in a liquid (solvent) to form a solution.

solution (sə'looshən) 1. in pharmacology, a liquid preparation of one or more soluble chemical substances usually dissolved in water. 2. the process of dissolving or disrupting.

PREPARATION OF SOLUTIONS. Formula for preparing solutions from a pure drug:

$$\text{pure drug} : \text{finished solution} = \text{strength of solution}$$

(expressed as a ratio or percentage). For example, to prepare 2000 ml of a 2 per cent solution from boric acid crystals, the proportion would be:

$$x\text{g}: 2000\text{ml} = 2\text{g} : 100\text{ml}$$

$$x = 40\text{g pure drug}$$

Formula for preparing solutions from stock solutions:

$$\frac{\text{lesser amount}}{\text{stock solution}} : \frac{\text{greater amount}}{\text{stock solution}} = \frac{\text{lesser}}{\text{strength}} : \frac{\text{greater}}{\text{strength}}$$

For example, to prepare 1000 ml of a 2 per cent solution from a 4 per cent stock solution, the proportion would be:

$$x\text{ml} : 1000\text{ml} = 2\% : 4\%$$

$$x = 500\text{ml of 4 per cent stock solution}$$

aqueous s. one in which water is the solvent.

buffer s. one that resists appreciable change in its hydrogen ion concentration (pH) when acid or alkali is added to it.

colloid s., colloidal s. a suspension of particles in a fluid.

hyperbaric s. one having a greater specific gravity than a standard of reference.

hypertonic s. one having an osmotic pressure greater than that of a standard of reference.

hypobaric s. one having a specific gravity less than that of a standard of reference.

hypotonic s. one having an osmotic pressure less than that of standard of reference.

iodine s. a transparent, reddish brown liquid, each 100 ml of which contains 1.8 to 2.2 g of iodine and 2.1 to 2.6 g of sodium iodide; a local anti-infective.

iodine s., strong Lugol's solution.

isobaric s. a solution having the same specific gravity as a standard of reference.

isotonic s. one having an osmotic pressure the same as that of a standard of reference.

molar s. a solution each litre of which contains 1 mole of the dissolved substance; designated 1 M. The concentration of other solutions may be expressed in relation to that of molar solutions, e.g. one-tenth molar (0.1 M).

normal s. a solution each litre of which contains 1 chemical equivalent of the dissolved substance; designated 1 N.

ophthalmic s. a sterile solution, free from foreign particles, for instillation into the eye.

physiological saline s., physiological salt s., physiological sodium chloride s. an aqueous solution of sodium chloride and other components, having an osmotic pressure identical to that of blood serum.

saline s. a solution of sodium chloride, or common salt, in purified water.

saturated s. a solution in which the solvent has taken up all of the dissolved substance that it can hold in solution.

sclerosing s. one containing an irritant substance that will cause an inflammatory response.

standard s. one containing a fixed amount of solute.

supersaturated s. one containing a greater quantity of the solute than a given solvent would dissolve and hold in solution at a given temperature.

volumetric s. one that contains a specific quantity of solvent per stated unit of volume.

solvent ('solvənt) 1. capable of dissolving other material. 2. the liquid in which another substance (the solute) is dissolved to form a solution.

s. abuse the deliberate inhalation of volatile chemicals with the aim of inducing intoxication. The practice is still sometimes referred to as 'glue sniffing', a misleading term as a wide range of substances other than glues are also abused and the vapours are not sniffed but are deeply inhaled. See also PETROL SNIFFING.

The range of substances abused is very diverse but

Commonly abused solvents

Product	Main solvent
Impact adhesives	Toluene, acetone and other ketones
Lighter refills	Butane, propane
Hair lacquers	Ethanol, methanol, fluorocarbons and propellant gases
Aerosols	Fluorocarbons and propellant gases
Petrol	Benzene and other aromatic compounds
Nail varnish remover	Acetone and amyl acetate
Rubber solution	Benzene
Fire extinguishers	Halogenated hydrocarbons
Cleaning fluids	Halogenated hydrocarbons
Dyes	Acetone, methylene chloride
Industrial solvents/cleaners/degreasers	Trichloroethylene, benzene, carbon tetrachloride

the accompanying table lists some commonly abused products.

As a group, organic solvents are lipophilic, easily absorbed and are cerebral depressants. Intoxication is achieved within a few minutes, is often gross and may be accompanied by hallucinations and uncontrolled or impulsive behaviour. Intoxication usually lasts for 30–40 minutes and the solvent is excreted by lungs and kidneys.

Risks are many and include suffocation, inhalation of vomitus, liver, kidney or myocardial damage, and bone marrow depression. Status epilepticus and solvent encephalopathy have also been reported. If aerosols are sprayed directly into the mouth there is a risk of freezing injury to the larynx followed by inhalation of body fluids and asphyxia. The risk of antisocial, criminal or self-injuring behaviour whilst intoxicated is high.

Most solvent abusers are adolescent working-class males, though atypical instances of abuse occur (e.g. the reported abuse of the anaesthetic gas Trilene by some anaesthetists).

Signs of solvent abuse include a rash around the mouth and nostrils (the substance to be abused is often placed in a plastic or paper bag to concentrate its vapours, and the bag is then placed over the mouth and nostrils and held firmly in place while the vapours are deeply inhaled), a strong smell of solvent from breath and clothing, reddened conjunctivae, rhinorrhoea, dried glue on clothing or hair, a history of truancy and episodes of disturbed behaviour.

There is evidence that many solvent abusers will go on to experiment with illicit drugs as they grow older, though most make the transition to the legal intoxicant, alcohol, which they have an increased tendency to misuse.

soma ('sohmə) 1. the body as distinguished from the mind. 2. the body tissue as distinguished from the germ cells. 3. the cell body. adj. **somal, somatic**.

somaesthesia (,sohmis'theezi·ə) sensibility to bodily sensations. adj. **somaesthetic**.

somasthenia (,sohməs'theeni·ə) bodily weakness with poor appetite and poor sleep.

somat(o)- word element. [Gr.] *body*.

somataesthesia (,sohmətis'theezi·ə) body consciousness or awareness.

somatalgia (,sohmə'talji·ə) bodily pain.

somatic (soh'matik) pertaining to or characteristic of the body (soma).

somatization (,sohmətie'zayshən) the conversion of mental experiences or states into bodily symptoms.

somatochrome (soh'matə,krohm) any neuron which has a well marked cell body completely surrounding the nucleus, its colourable protoplasm having a distinct contour; used also adjectively.

somatogenic (,sohmətoh'jenik) originating in the body.

somatology (,sohmə'toləjee) the sum of what is known about the body.

somatome ('sohmə,tohm) 1. an appliance for cutting the body of a fetus. 2. a somite.

somatomedin (,somətoh'medin) any of a group of peptides found in the liver and in plasma which mediate the effect of growth hormone (somatotropin) on cartilage; they are responsible for uptake of sulphate and increased synthesis of collagen and other proteins by cartilage.

somatometry (,sohmə'tomətree) measurement of the dimensions of the entire body.

somatopagus (,sohmə'topəgəs) a double fetus united at the trunks.

somatopathy (,sohmə'topəthee) a bodily disorder rather than a mental one. adj. **somatopathic**.

somatoplasm (soh'matə,plazəm) the protoplasm of the body cells exclusive of the germ cells.

somatopsychic (,sohmətoh'siekik) pertaining to both mind and body; denoting a physical disorder that produces mental symptoms.

somatopsychosis (,sohmətohsie'kohsis) any mental disease symptomatic of bodily disease.

somatoschisis (,sohmə'toskisis) splitting of the bodies of the vertebrae.

somatoscopy (,sohmə'toskəpee) examination of the body.

somatosexual (,sohmətoh'seksyooəl) pertaining to both physical and sex characteristics or to physical manifestations of sexual development.

somatostatin (,sohmətoh'statin) a cyclic tetradecapeptide hormone and neurotransmitter that inhibits the release of peptide hormones in many tissues. It is released by the hypothalamus to inhibit the release of growth hormone (GH, somatotrophin) and thyroid

Biological actions of somatostatin outside the central nervous system

Inhibits hormone secretion of:	Other gastrointestinal actions
Pituitary gland	*Inhibits:*
TSH, GH	Gastric acid secretion
Gastrointestinal tract	Gastric secretion
Gastrin	Gastric emptying
Secretin	Pancreatic bicarbonate
Gastrointestinal polypeptide	Pancreatic enzyme secretion
Motilin	Intestinal absorption
Enteroglucagon	Gastrointestinal blood flow
Vasoactive intestinal peptide (VIP)	Genitourinary tract inhibits renin
Pancreas	VP-stimulated water transport (to bladder)
Insulin	
Glucagon	

From Reichlin, S. (1981) Neuroendocrinology. In Williams, R. H. *Textbook of Endocrinology*, 6th edn, W. B. Saunders.

stimulating hormone (TSH) from the anterior pituitary; it is also released by the delta cells of the islets of Langerhans in the pancreas to inhibit the release of glucagon and insulin and by the similar D cells in the gastrointestinal tract (see accompanying table).

somatotherapy (ˌsohmətoh'therəpee) treatment aimed at relieving or curing ills of the body.

somatotonia (ˌsohmətoh'tohni·ə) a group of traits characterized by dominance of muscular activity and vigorous body assertiveness; considered typical of a mesomorph.

somatotopic (ˌsohmətoh'topik) related to particular areas of the body; describing the organization of the motor area of the brain, specific regions of the cortex being responsible for the motor control of different areas of the body.

somatotrope (soh'matəˌtrohp) any of the cells of the adenohypophysis that secrete growth hormone (GH, somatotrophin).

somatotroph (soh'matəˌtrohf) somatotrope.

somatotrophin (ˌsohmətoh'trohfin) growth hormone (see also PITUITARY GLAND). adj. **somatotrophic**.

somatotropin (ˌsomətoh'trohpin) somatotrophin.

somatotype (soh'matəˌtiep) a particular type of body build.

somatotyping (ˌsohmətoh'tieping) objective classification of individuals according to type of body build.

somite ('sohmiet) one of the paired segments along the neural tube of a vertebrate embryo, formed by transverse subdivision of the thickened mesoderm next to the midplane, that develop into the vertebral column and muscles of the body.

somnambule (som'nambyool) one who sleepwalks.

somnambulism (som'nambyuhˌlizəm) sleepwalking; noctambulation.

somnifacient (ˌsomni'fayshənt) causing sleep.

somniferous (som'nifə·rəs) producing sleep.

somniloquism (som'niləˌkwizəm) habitual talking in one's sleep.

somnipathy (som'nipəthee) any disorder of sleep; a condition of hypnotic trance.

somnolence ('somnələns) sleepiness; also, unnatural drowsiness.

somnolentia (ˌsomnə'lenshi·ə) 1. incomplete sleep; drowsiness. 2. sleep drunkenness; a condition of incomplete sleep marked by loss of orientation and by excited or violent behaviour.

Somogyi effect (soh'mohgee) a rebound phenomenon occurring in diabetes mellitus; overtreatment with insulin induces hypoglycaemia, which initiates the release of adrenaline, ACTH, glucagon, and growth hormone, which stimulate lipolysis, gluconeogenesis, and glycogenolysis, which, in turn, result in rebound hyperglycaemia and ketosis.

Indications that the Somogyi effect may be taking place include the following: (1) the appearance of strongly positive tests for sugar and acetone in the urine within a few hours after a period in which the urine had been negative for both tests, (2) a 2 per cent glycosuria all day preceded by nocturnal sweating, headaches, and other symptoms of hypoglycaemia, (3) unresponsiveness of insulin during the period of rebound hyperglycosuria, (4) wide fluctuations in blood glucose levels, over several hours, and unrelated to meals, and (5) improved control of blood sugar levels and ketonuria with gradual reduction in the amount of insulin taken. Treatment consists of gradual reduction of the insulin dose until the optimum dose is reached.

sonicate ('soniˌkayt) 1. to expose to sound waves; to disrupt bacteria by exposure to high-frequency sound waves. 2. the products of such disruption.

sonication (ˌsoni'kayshən) exposure to sound waves; disruption of bacteria by exposure to high-frequency sound waves.

sonitus ('sonitəs) tinnitus.

Sonne dysentery (soni) a mild form of bacillary dysentery which is common in Britain and other countries with temperate climates. The symptoms are diarrhoea and abdominal pain. (There may be some vomiting early on, but it is not a marked feature.) The causative agent is *Shigella sonnei*.

sonogram ('sonəˌgram) a record or display obtained by ultrasonic scanning.

sonography (sə'nogrəfee) ultrasonography. adj. **sonographic**.

sonolucent (ˌsohnoh'loos'nt) in ultrasonography, permitting the passage of ultrasound waves without reflecting them back to their source (without giving off echoes).

sonometer (soh'nomitə) an instrument for measuring the acuity of heating or the frequency and pitch of sound waves.

sonorous ('sonə·rəs) resonant; sounding.

sopor ('sohpə) [L.] *deep or profound sleep.*

soporific (ˌsopə'rifik) 1. producing deep sleep. 2. an agent that induces sleep.

soporous ('sohpə·rəs) associated with coma or deep

sleep.

sorb (sawb) to attract and retain substances by absorption or adsorption.

sorbefacient (ˌsawbiˈfayshənt) 1. promoting absorption. 2. an agent that promotes absorption.

sorbent (ˈsawbənt) an agent that sorbs.

sorbitol (ˈsawbiˌtol) a sugar alcohol found in various berries and fruits; in mammals, sorbitol is an intermediate in the conversion of glucose to fructose. It is found in lens deposits in diabetes mellitus. A 50 per cent solution is used as an osmotic diuretic. Sorbitol is used as a sweetener in some dietetic foods; it has the same calorific value as other sugars.

Sorbitrate (ˈsawbiˌtrayt) trademark for a preparation of isosorbide dinitrate; a coronary vasodilator.

sordes (ˈsawdeez) foul matter collected on the lips and teeth in low fevers, consisting of food, microorganisms, and epithelial elements.

s. gastricae undigested food, mucus, etc., in the stomach.

sore (sor) a popular term for any lesion of the skin or mucous membrane.

bed s. pressure sore (decubitus ulcer).

cold s. one around the mouth or lips due to herpes simplex virus. See HERPES SIMPLEX.

Delhi s. cutaneous leishmaniasis.

desert s. a form of tropical ulcer occurring in desert areas of Africa, Australia, and the Near East.

oriental s. cutaneous leishmaniasis.

pressure s. see PRESSURE SORE.

sorption (ˈsawpshən) the process or state of being sorbed; absorption or adsorption.

SOS [L.] *si opus sit* (if necessary).

souffle (ˈsoofˈl) a soft, blowing auscultatory sound.

aneurysmal s. a blowing sound heard over an aneurysm.

cardiac s. any heart murmur of a blowing quality.

fetal s. a murmur sometimes heard over the pregnant uterus, supposed to be due to compression of the umbilical cord.

funic s. a soft, rhythmic murmur heard (on auscultation) as fetal blood passes along the umbilical cord; called also *funic bruit*.

placental s. a soft, blowing auscultatory sound supposed to be produced by the blood current in the placenta; called also *placental bruit*.

uterine s. a sound made by the blood within the arteries of the gravid uterus.

sound (sownd) 1. percept resulting from stimulation of the ear by mechanical radiant energy of frequency between 20 and 20,000 Hz. 2. a slender instrument to be introduced into body passages or cavities, especially for the dilation of strictures or detection of foreign bodies. 3. a noise, normal or abnormal, emanating from within the body.

ejection s's high-pitched clicking sounds heard very shortly after the first heart sound, attributed to sudden distention of a dilated pulmonary artery or aorta or to forceful opening of the pulmonic or aortic cusps.

friction s. one produced by rubbing of two surfaces.

heart s's the sounds produced by the functioning of the heart (see HEART SOUNDS).

Korotkoff's s's those heard during auscultatory blood pressure determination (see also KOROTKOFF'S SOUNDS).

percussion s. any sound obtained by percussion.

physiological s's those heard when the external acoustic meatus are plugged, caused by the rush of blood through blood vessels in or near the inner ear and by adjacent muscles in continuous low-frequency vibration.

respiratory s. any sound heard on ausculation over the respiratory tract.

succussion s's splashing sounds heard on succussion over a distended stomach or in hydropneumothorax.

to-and-fro s. a peculiar friction sound or murmur heard in pericarditis and pleurisy.

urethral s. a long, slender instrument for exploring and dilating the urethra.

white s. that produced by a mixture of equal energies of all frequencies of mechanical vibration perceptible as sound.

sp. gr. specific gravity.

space (spays) 1. a delimited area. 2. an actual or potential cavity of the body. 3. the areas of the universe beyond the earth and its atmosphere. adj. **spatial**.

dead s. 1. space remaining in tissues as a result of failure of proper closure of surgical or other wounds, permitting accumulation of blood or serum. 2. the portions of the respiratory tract (passages and space in the alveoli) occupied by gas not concurrently participating in oxygen–carbon dioxide exchange.

epidural s. the space between the dura mater and the lining of the spinal canal.

intercostal s. the space between two adjacent ribs.

interpleural s. mediastinum.

intervillous s. the space of the placenta into which the chorionic villi project and through which the maternal blood circulates.

lymph s's open spaces filled with lymph in connective or other tissue, especially in the brain and meninges.

Meckel's s. a recess in the dura mater that lodges the trigeminal ganglion.

mediastinal s. mediastinum.

medullary s. the central cavity and the intervals between the trabeculae of bone that contain the marrow.

palmar s. a large fascial space in the hand, divided by a fibrous septum into a midpalmar and a thenar space.

parasinoidal s's spaces in the dura mater along the superior sagittal sinus which receive the venous blood.

perivascular s. a lymph space within the walls of an artery.

plantar s. a fascial space on the sole of the foot, divided by septa into the lateral, middle, and median plantar spaces.

pneumatic s. a portion of bone occupied by air-containing cells, especially the spaces constituting the paranasal sinuses.

retroperitoneal s. the space between the peritoneum and the posterior abdominal wall.

retropharyngeal s. the space behind the pharynx, containing areolar tissue.

subarachnoid s. the space between the arachnoid and the pia mater, containing cerebrospinal fluid.

subdural s. the space between the dura mater and the arachnoid.

subphrenic s. the space between the diaphragm and subjacent organs.

subumbilical s. somewhat triangular space in the body cavity beneath the umbilicus.

Tenon's s. a lymph space between the sclera and Tenon's capsule.

Spanish fly (ˌspanish ˈflie) a species of beetle from which cantharidin, a blistering agent, is derived.

sparganosis (ˌspahgəˈnohsis) infection with spargana, which invade the subcutaneous tissues, causing inflammation and fibrosis. If the lymphatics are involved, elephantiasis may result.

sparganum (ˈspahgənəm) pl. *spargana* [Gr.] a migrating larva of a tapeworm, belonging to the genus *Diphyllobothrium*.

spasm (ˈspazəm) 1. a sudden involuntary contraction of a muscle or group of muscles. 2. a sudden but transitory constriction of a passage, canal, or orifice. Spasms usually occur when the nerve supplying muscles are irritated, and are commonly accompanied by pain. Occasionally a spasm may occur in a blood vessel, and is then called vasospasm.

Spasms vary from mild twitches to severe CONVULSIONS and may be the symptoms of any number of disorders. Usually, spasms will cease when the cause is corrected, although sometimes the only treatment is to suppress the symptoms, as in EPILEPSY.

CLONIC SPASMS. Spasms in which contraction and relaxation of the muscle alternate are called clonic. This is the more common type of spasm and usually is not severe. A typical clonic spasm is the hiccup. Hiccups usually occur when the diaphragm is irritated, as by indigestion; very occasionally they may result from a serious condition, such as a brain tumour. Hiccups generally disappear by themselves or after a drink of water.

Spasms may be repetitive twitching motions, some of which are called tics. Tics often accompany other types of spasm, as in such diseases as cerebral palsy and Sydenham's chorea. They may also be seen in neuralgia. In tic douloureux (trigeminal neuralgia) the nerves of the face are involved.

Other types of repetitive twitching movements seem to be purposeless or without a cause and are called habit spasms. They include twitching of the face, blinking of the eyes, and grimacing. The movements are rapid and always repeated in the same way, unlike the spasms associated with chorea. The motions are carried out automatically in response to a stimulus that once may have existed but no longer does.

Spasms may also stem from emotional stress. Stuttering that continues after the age of 5 years is generally considered a habit spasm that is caused by emotional conflict or difficulty.

In a convulsive spasm the entire body is jerked by sudden violent movements that may involve almost all the muscles. These spasms may last from a fraction of a second to several seconds, or even minutes. Spasms accompanying epilepsy are usually convulsive. Treatment includes sedatives and any one of several anticonvulsants. In small children convulsions usually indicate a high fever and the onset of infection, or any general illness; at times they may be a symptom of severe disease.

TONIC SPASMS. If the contraction of a spasm is sustained or continuing, it is called tonic, or tetanic, spasm. Tonic spasms are generally severe because they are caused by diseases that affect the central nervous system or brain, as tetanus, rabies, and cerebral palsy. Severe tonic spasms can be fatal if not treated in time. Continued spasms can bring on exhaustion or asphyxiation. Treatment varies with the cause. If the disease is caused by a microorganism present in the system, as in tetanus, antiserum must be administered immediately. Antibiotics are also used to help curb infection. In many cases, tranquillizers, sedatives, and narcotics must be administered to help ease the spasms.

bronchial s. bronchospasm; spasmodic contraction of the muscular coat of the smaller divisions of the bronchi, as occurs in asthma.

nodding s. clonic spasm of the sternomastoid muscles, causing a nodding motion of the head.

spasmodic (spaz'modik) of the nature of a spasm; occurring in spasms.

spasmolysis (spaz'molisis) the arrest of spasm.

spasmolytic (ˌspazmə'litik) 1. arresting or checking spasms. 2. an agent that arrests spasms, especially of smooth muscle.

spasmophilia (ˌspazmə'fili·ə) abnormal tendency to convulsions; abnormal sensitivity of motor nerves to stimulation with a resultant tendency to spasm.

spasmus ('spazməs) [L.] *spasm*.

s. nutans nodding spasm.

spastic ('spastik) characterized by spasms, or tightening of the muscles, causing stiff and awkward movements and in some cases a scissor-like gait. The term is often used to describe a person suffering from CEREBRAL PALSY.

spasticity (spa'stisitee) continuous resistance to stretching by a muscle due to abnormally increased tension, with heightened deep tendon reflexes.

spatial ('spayshəl) pertaining to space.

spatium ('spayshi·əm) pl. *spatia* [L.] space.

spatula ('spatyuhlə) a wide, flat, blunt, usually flexible instrument of little thickness, commonly used for spreading material on a smooth surface or mixing.

spatulate ('spatyuhlət) 1. having a flat blunt end. 2. to mix or manipulate with a spatula.

spatulation (ˌspatyuh'layshən) the combining of materials into a homogeneous mixture by continuously heaping them together and smoothing the mass out on a smooth surface with a spatula.

spay (spay) to remove the ovaries.

specialist ('speshəlist) a doctor whose practice is limited to a particular branch of medicine or surgery, especially one who, by virtue of advanced training, is recognized to be qualified to so limit his practice. See also clinical NURSE SPECIALIST.

speciality (ˌspeshi'alətee) the field of practice of a specialist. Sometimes spelled *specialty*.

species ('speesheez) a taxonomic category subordinate to a genus (or subgenus) and superior to a subspecies or variety; composed of individuals similar in certain morphological and physiological characteristics.

type s. the original species from which the description of the genus is formulated.

species-specific (ˌspeesheez·spə'sifik) characteristic of a particular species; having a characteristic effect on, or interaction with, cells or tissues of members of a particular species; said of an antigen, drug, or infective agent.

specific (spə'sifik) pertaining to a species. 1. produced by a single kind of microorganism. 2. restricted in application, effect, etc., to a particular structure, function, etc. 3. a remedy specially indicated for any particular disease. 4. in immunology, pertaining to the special affinity of antigen for the corresponding antibody.

s. gravity the weight of a substance compared with the weight of an equal amount of some other substance taken as a standard. For liquids the usual standard is water. The specific gravity of water is 1; if a sample of urine shows a specific gravity of 1.025, this means that the urine is 1.025 times heavier than water. Specific gravity is measured by means of a hydrometer.

specificity (ˌspesi'fisitee) the quality of having a certain action, as of affecting only certain organisms or tissues, or reacting only with certain substances, as antibodies with certain antigens (antigen specificity).

host s. the natural adaptability of a particular parasite to a certain species or group of hosts.

specimen ('spesimən) a small sample or part taken to show the nature of the whole, as a small quantity of urine for urinalysis, or a small fragment of tissue for microscopic study.

spectacles ('spektək'lz) a pair of LENSES in a frame which is worn to assist vision (see also GLASSES).

spectinomycin (ˌspektinoh'miesin) an antibiotic derived from *Streptomyces spectabilis*, used in treatment of gonorrhoea.

spectra ('spektrə) plural of *spectrum*.

spectrin ('spektrin) a contractile protein attached to glycophorin at the cytoplasmic surface of the cell membrane of erythrocytes, considered to be important in the determination of red cell shape.

spectrometry (spek'tromətree) determination of the place of lines in a spectrum.

spectrophotometer (ˌspektrohfə'tomitə) 1. an apparatus for measuring light sense by means of a spectrum. 2. an apparatus for determining the quantity of colouring matter in a solution by measurement of transmitted light.

spectrophotometry (ˌspektrohfə'tomətree) the use of the spectrophotometer.

spectroscope ('spektrəˌskohp) an instrument for developing and analysing the spectrum of a substance.

spectroscopy (spek'troskəpee) examination by means of a spectroscope.

spectrum ('spektrəm) pl. *spectra,spectrums* [L.] 1. the series of images resulting from the refraction of electromagnetic radiation (e.g., light, x-rays) and their arrangement according to frequency or wavelength. 2. range of activity, as of an antibiotic, or of manifestations, as of a disease. adj. **spectral**.

absorption s. one obtained by passing radiation with a continuous spectrum through a selectively absorbing medium.

broad-s. effective against a wide range of microorganisms.

visible s. that portion of the range of wavelengths of electromagnetic vibrations (from 770 to 390 nanometers) which is capable of stimulating specialized sense organs and is perceptible as light.

speculum ('spekyuhləm) an instrument for opening or expanding an orifice or cavity to permit visual inspection and operative manoeuvre.

speech (speech) the utterance of vocal sounds conveying ideas; the faculty of conveying thoughts and ideas by vocal sounds. The process is controlled through a speech centre located in the frontal lobe of the human brain.

THE MECHANICS OF SPEECH. The voice originates in the larynx, which is in the upper end of the air passage to the lungs and is located behind the thyroid cartilage. The larynx, in cooperation with the mouth, tongue, throat, trachea, and lungs, works on the same principle as an organ or an oboe, in which air is forced over a thin reed to produce sound. The vocal cords, two reedlike bands, are attached in front to the wall of the larynx behind the Adam's apple; posteriorly they are attached to movable cartilages. When the voice is not being used, muscles move these cartilages outward and hold the vocal cords open so that breathing is not obstructed. When one starts to speak, sing, grunt, or shout, the ends of the vocal cords connected to the cartilages are brought together. As air is forced through, the cords vibrate, producing sound waves, the voice.

In speaking, the size and shape of the mouth and pharynx are varied as the sound goes through, by means of muscles of the mouth, throat, and tongue. Vowel sounds are initiated in the throat and are given their distinctive 'shapes' by movements of the mouth and tongue. Consonants are formed by controlled interruptions of exhaled air.

VOLUME, PITCH AND QUALITY. The voice itself has three characteristics—volume, pitch, and quality. Volume depends on the effort made in forcing air through the vocal cords.

Pitch of the voice depends on the amount of tension in the vocal cords, and on their length and thickness. Children's and women's vocal cords are short, giving them higher-pitched voices. A man's are longer and thicker and his voice is deeper.

Quality is affected by the size and shape of the individual's various resonating chambers—mouth, pharynx, and chest. Singers can be trained to perfect the control of the voice mechanism, the mouth, and the chest cavities.

SPEECH DEFECTS. Over 100 muscles are involved in the utterance of a simple word, and the construction of a simple sentence is a feat so complicated that it is far beyond the capacity of any living thing except man.

A baby learns to make sounds by babbling and cooing. Gradually he becomes able to put these sounds together to form intelligible speech in imitation of his parents and other speakers. This complicated process is sometimes disturbed if the child is handicapped by congenital physical defects, deafness, illness, or psychological difficulties. As a result, speech disorders may occur.

Congenital Causes. Prominent among the congenital defects that may cause speech problems are CLEFT LIP and CLEFT PALATE. These abnormalities are evident at birth and are corrected by surgery at an early age.

Congenital deafness may prevent a child from learning to speak in the usual way. It is essential that this is detected early and that the child is fitted with a hearing aid if appropriate and given speech therapy.

Malformations of the nasal passages, larynx, or other parts of the vocal tract may cause problems with the voice. Such defects can sometimes be corrected by minor surgery.

Other Causes. By the age of 5 or 6 years, most children have mastered the basic art of talking. Serious difficulties that persist or appear for the first time after this age, and that are not due to congenital defects, are likely to arise from illness, injury, or a psychological disturbance. Damage to speech centres of the brain by multiple sclerosis, syphilis, or Parkinson's disease, for example, may cause speech to be singsong, explosive, mechanical, or slurred.

Poor alignment of the front teeth also may interfere somewhat with clear speech.

Stuttering (or Stammering). Stuttering is characterized by blocking or involuntary pauses in speech. There is often the spasmodic repetition of one sound with the apparent inability to pass on to the next one.

The cause of stuttering is unknown, but it commonly starts in childhood, about the age of 4 or 5 years.

Parents and other adults in a household can help to encourage clear speech and to prevent the onset of stuttering by listening to what the child says. It is best to avoid criticism of the child's pronunciation and other speech habits—especially criticism in the form of nagging interruptions—that is likely to make him self-conscious, uncertain, and awkward.

Stuttering often occurs when a child is addressing an angry or impatient parent or someone else who represents authority. The child's speech may become disorganized by fear of punishment or disapproval. He is often anxious to get his words out before his listener interrupts or turns away. Patience and calm will alleviate a child's anxiety and encourage clear speech. Counselling of the parents is helpful when the problem is present in a young child. Some therapists use a programmed and structured regimen that teaches the stutterer a new way to talk; others emphasize activities designed to change the client's attitudes, help him overcome his anxiety, and develop a healthier self-concept.

An organization that was formed to link individual stammerers with self-help groups is the Association for Stammerers, c/o The Finsbury Health Centre, Pine Street, London EC1R 0JH.

oesophageal s. speech produced by injecting air into the top part of the oesophagus then bringing it back, thereby vibrating the pharyngoesophageal segment, which serves as a substitute voice source; used after LARYNGECTOMY.

s. reading see LIP READING.

speech therapist a professional trained to identify, assess, and rehabilitate persons with speech or language disorders such as articulation problems, language problems (e.g., aphasia, delayed language development), stuttering, voice problems, and feeding difficulties.

Spencer Wells forceps (ˌspensə 'welz) artery forceps (see FORCEPS).

sperm (spərm) the male germ cell, which unites with an ovum in sexual reproduction to produce a new individual (see also SPERMATOZOON).

sperm(o)- word element. [Gr.] *seed;* specifically used to refer to the male germinal element.

spermatic (spər'matik) pertaining to the spermatozoa or to semen.

s. cord the structure extending from the abdominal inguinal ring to the testis, comprising the pampiniform plexus, nerves, ductus deferens, testicular artery, and other vessels.

spermatid ('spərmətid) a cell produced by meiotic division of a secondary spermatocyte; it develops into the spermatozoon.

spermatitis (ˌspərmə'tietis) inflammation of a vas deferens; deferentitis.

spermato- word element. [Gr.] *seed;* specifically used to refer to the male germinal element.

spermatoblast ('spərmətoh,blast) spermatid.

spermatocele ('spərmətoh,seel) a cyst of epididymis or rete testis.

spermatocelectomy (ˌspərmətohsi'lektəmee) excision of a spermatocele.

spermatocidal (ˌspərmətoh'sied'l) destructive to spermatozoa.

spermatocyst ('spərmətoh,sist) 1. a seminal vesicle. 2. spermatocele.

spermatocystectomy (ˌspərmətohsi'stektəmee) excision of a seminal vesicle.

spermatocystitis (ˌspərmətohsi'stietis) inflammation of a seminal vesicle.

spermatocystotomy (ˌspərmətohsi'stotəmee) incision of a seminal vesicle, for the purpose of drainage.

spermatocyte ('spərmətoh,siet) the mother cell of a spermatid.

primary s. the original large cell into which a spermatogonium develops before the first meiotic division.

secondary s. a cell produced by meiotic division of the primary spermatocyte, and which gives rise to the spermatid.

spermatocytogenesis (ˌspərmətoh,sietoh'jenəsis) the first stage of formation of spermatozoa, in which the spermatogonia develop into spermatocytes and then into spermatids.

spermatogenesis (ˌspərmətoh'jenəsis) the development of mature spermatozoa from spermatogonia; it includes spermatocytogenesis and spermiogenesis..

spermatogenic (ˌspərmətoh'jenik) giving rise to sperm.

spermatogonium (ˌspərmətoh'gohni·əm) pl. *spermatogonia* [Gr.] an undifferentiated male germ cell, originating in a seminal tubule and dividing into two spermatocytes.

spermatoid ('spərmə,toyd) resembling semen.

spermatolysin (ˌspərmə'tolisin) a lysin destructive to spermatozoa.

spermatolysis (ˌspərmə'tolisis) dissolution of spermatozoa. adj. **spermatolytic.**

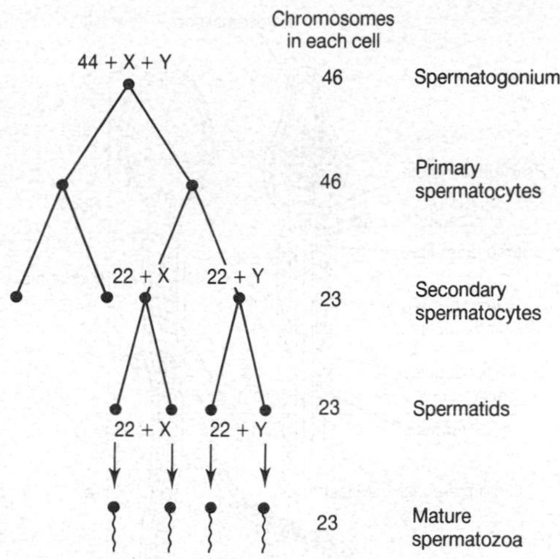

Summary of spermatogenesis demonstrating how each spermatogonium yields 8 mature spermatozoa

spermatopathia (ˌspərmətoh'pathi·ə) abnormality of the semen.

spermatorrhoea (ˌspərmətə'reeə) involuntary escape of semen, without orgasm.

spermatoschesis (ˌspərmə'toskisis) suppression of the semen.

spermatoxin (ˌspərmə'toksin) a toxin that destroys spermatozoa.

spermatozoicide (ˌspərmətoh'zoh·i,sied) an agent that destroys spermatozoa; spermicide.

spermatozoon (ˌspərmətoh'zoh·on) pl. *spermatozoa* [Gr.] a mature male germ cell, the specific output of the testes, which impregnates the ovum in sexual reproduction. adj. adj. **spermatozoal.** The mature sperm cell is microscopic in size. It looks like a translucent tadpole, and has a flat, elliptical head containing a spherical centre section, and a long tail by which it propels itself with a vigorous lashing movement. See accompanying illustration.

Spermatozoa are produced in the seminiferous tubules of the testes. The developmental stages are spermatogonia, spermatocytes, spermatids, and spermatozoa. When mature, the sperm are carried in the semen. At the climax of coitus, the semen is discharged into the vagina of the female. A single discharge (about a teaspoonful of semen on the average) may contain more than 250 million spermatozoa. Only a few of these will travel as far as the uterine tubes; if an ovum is present there, and if the head of a single sperm penetrates the ovum, fertilization takes place. See also REPRODUCTION.

spermaturia (ˌspərmə'tyooə·ri·ə) semen in the urine.

spermectomy (spər'mektəmee) excision of part of the spermatic cord.

spermicide ('spərmi,sied) an agent destructive to spermatozoa. adj. **spermicidal.**

spermidine ('spərmi,deen) a polyamine first found in human semen but now known to occur in almost all tissues, in association with nucleic acids.

spermiduct ('spərmi,dukt) the ejaculatory duct and vas

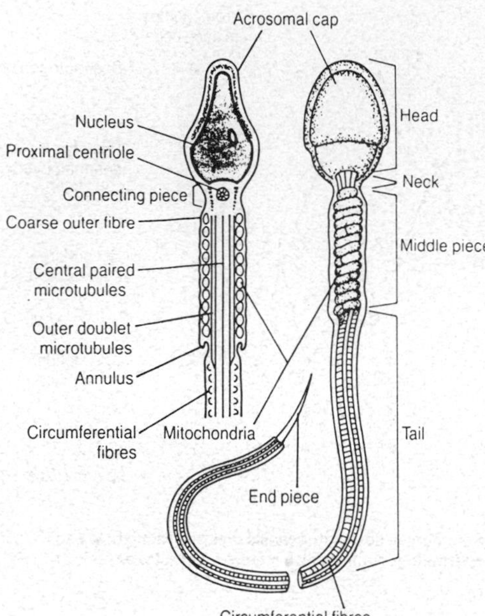

Human spermatozoon: side view (in cross-section) and flat view

deferens together.

spermine ('spərmeen) a polyamine first found in human semen but now known to occur in almost all tissues, in association with nucleic acids.

spermiogenesis (ˌspərmioh'jenəsis) the second stage in the formation of spermatozoa, in which the spermatids transform into spermatozoa.

spermioteleosis (ˌspərmiohˌteeli'ohsis) progressive development of the spermatogonium through various stages to the mature spermatozoon.

spermolith ('spərmohˌlith) a calculus in the vas deferens.

spermoneuralgia (ˌspərmohnyuh'raljə, -ji·ə) neuralgic pain in the spermatic cord.

spermophlebectasia (ˌspərmohˌflebek'tayzi·ə) varicose state of the spermatic veins.

spermotoxin (ˌspərmoh'toksin) a toxin lethal to spermatozoa; especially an antibody produced by injection of an animal with spermatozoa.

sphacelate ('sfasəˌlayt) to become gangrenous.

sphacelation (ˌsfasə'layshən) the formation of sphacelus; mortification.

sphacelism ('sfasəˌlizəm) sphacelation or necrosis; sloughing.

sphaceloderma (ˌsfasəloh'dərmə) gangrene of the skin.

sphacelous ('sfasələs) gangrenous; sloughing.

sphacelus ('sfasələs) a slough; a mass of gangrenous tissue.

sphenion ('sfeeni·ən) the point at the sphenoid angle of the parietal bone.

spheno- word element. [Gr.] *wedge-shaped*, *sphenoid bone*.

sphenoid ('sfeenoyd) wedge-shaped; designating especially a very irregular wedge-shaped bone at the base of the skull.

sphenoidal (sfee'noyd'l) pertaining to the sphenoid bone.

sphenoiditis (ˌsfeenoy'dietis) inflammation of the sphenoid sinus.

sphenoidotomy (ˌsfeenoy'dotəmee) incision of a sphenoid sinus.

sphenomaxillary (ˌsfeenohmak'silə·ree) pertaining to the sphenoid bone and the maxilla.

sphenopalatine (ˌsfeenoh'paləˌtien) pertaining to the sphenoid and palatine bones.

sphenotresia (ˌsfeenoh'treezi·ə) perforation of the base of the fetal skull in craniotomy.

sphenotribe ('sfeenohˌtrieb) an instrument used for crushing the base of the fetal skull.

sphere (sfiə) a ball or globe. adj. **spherical.**

attraction s. centrosome.

segmentation s. 1. the morula. 2. a blastomere.

sphero- word element. [Gr.] *round*, *a sphere*.

spherocyte ('sfiə·rohˌsiet) a small, globular, completely haemoglobinated erythrocyte without the usual central pallor; characteristically found in hereditary spherocytosis but also in acquired haemolytic anaemia. adj. **spherocytic.**

spherocytosis (ˌsfiə·rohsie'tohsis) the presence of spherocytes in the blood.

hereditary s. a congenital hereditary form of haemolytic anaemia characterized by spherocytosis, abnormal fragility of erythrocytes, jaundice, and splenomegaly.

spheroid ('sfiə·royd) a spherelike body.

spheroidal (sfiə'royd'l) resembling a sphere.

spheroma (sfiə'rohmə) a globular tumour.

sphincter ('sfingktə) a circular muscle that constricts a passage or closes a natural orifice. When relaxed, a sphincter allows materials to pass through the opening. When contracted, it closes the opening.

There are four main sphincter muscles along the alimentary canal that aid in digestion. The *cardiac sphincter*, between the oesophagus and the stomach, opens at the approach of food, which is then swept into the stomach by rhythmic peristaltic waves. The *pyloric sphincter* controls the opening from the stomach into the duodenum. It is usually closed, opening only for a moment when a peristaltic wave passes over it. Two *anal sphincters*, internal and external, control the anus, allowing the evacuation of faeces.

In addition, there are sphincters in the iris of the eye, the bile duct (sphincter of Oddi), the urinary tract, and elsewhere in the body.

sphincteralgia (ˌsfingktə'ralji·ə) pain in a sphincter muscle.

sphincterectomy (ˌsfingktə'rektəmee) excision of a sphincter.

sphincterismus (ˌsfingktə'rizməs) spasm of a sphincter.

sphincteritis (ˌsfingktə'rietis) inflammation of a sphincter, particularly the sphincter of Oddi.

sphincterolysis (ˌsfingktə'rolisis) surgical separation of the iris from the cornea in anterior synechia.

sphincteroplasty ('sfingktə·rohˌplastee) plastic reconstruction of a sphincter.

sphincterotomy (ˌsfingktə'rotəmee) incision of a sphincter.

sphingolipid (ˌsfing·goh'lipid) a phospholipid containing sphingosine (e.g., ceramides, sphingomyelins, gangliosides, and cerebrosides), occurring in high concentrations in the brain and other nerve tissue.

sphingolipidosis (ˌsfing·gohˌlipi'dohsis) pl. *sphingolipidoses* [Gr.] a general designation applied to diseases characterized by abnormal storage of sphingolipids, such as Gaucher's disease, Niemann–Pick disease, Hurler's syndrome, and Tay–Sachs disease. All are associated with mental handicap and premature death.

sphingolipodystrophy (ˌsfing·gohˌlipoh'distrəfee) any

of a group of disorders of sphingolipid metabolism. See SPHINGOLIPIDOSIS.

sphingomyelin (ˌsfing·goh'mieəlin) a group of phospholipids that on hydrolysis yield phosphoric acid, choline, sphingosine, and a fatty acid.

sphingosine ('sfing·goh,seen) a basic amino alcohol present in sphingomyelin.

sphygmic ('sfigmik) pertaining to the pulse.

s. period the second phase of ventricular systole (0.21–0.30 s), between the opening and closing of the semilunar valves, while the blood is discharged into the aorta and pulmonary artery.

sphygmo- word element. [Gr.] *the pulse.*

sphygmobolometer (ˌsfigmohboh'lomitə) an instrument for recording the energy of the pulse wave, and so, indirectly, the strength of the systole.

sphygmocardiograph (ˌsfigmoh'kahdioh,grahf, -ˌgraf) an instrument that records both the pulse waves and heartbeat.

sphygmochronograph (ˌsfigmoh'kronə,grahf, -ˌgraf, -'krohnə-) a self-registering sphygmograph.

sphygmodynamometer (ˌsfigmoh,dienə'momitə) an instrument for measuring the force of the pulse.

sphygmogram ('sfigmoh,gram) the record or tracing made by a sphygmograph; called also pulse tracing..

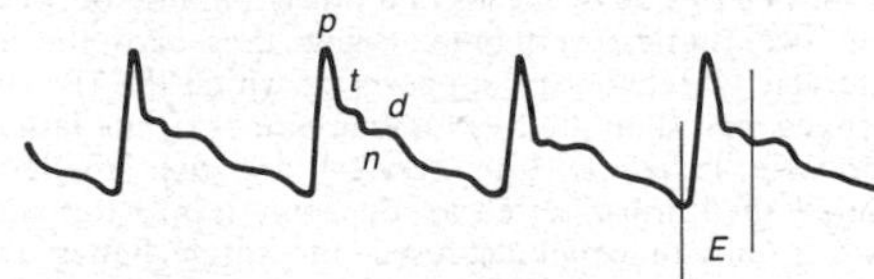

Radial sphygmogram from a healthy person. *p*, The percussion wave; *t*, tidal or predicrotic wave; *n*, dicrotic or aortic notch; *d*, dicrotic wave; *E*, the sphygmic period during which the semilunar valves are open

sphygmograph ('sfigmoh,grahf, -ˌgraf) an apparatus for registering the movements of the arterial pulse. adj. **sphygmographic.**

sphygmoid ('sfigmoyd) resembling the pulse.

sphygmomanometer (ˌsfigmohmə'nomitə) an instrument for measuring arterial blood pressure.

sphygmometer (sfig'momitə) an instrument for measuring the force and frequency of the pulse.

sphygmoscope ('sfigmə,skohp) a device for rendering the pulse beat visible.

sphygmotonometer (ˌsfigmohtə'nomitə) an instrument for measuring the elasticity of arterial walls.

sphyrectomy (sfie'rektəmee) excision of the malleus, or hammer, of the ear.

sphyrotomy (sfie'rotəmee) division of the malleus.

spica ('spiekə) a figure-of-8 bandage, with turns crossing and overlapping each other.

spicule ('spikyool) a sharp, needle-like body or spike.

spider ('spiedə) 1. an arthropod of the class Arachnida. 2. a spider-like naevus; a vascular spider.

vascular s. a telangiectasis composed of small vessels radiating from a central arteriole, the whole resembling spider legs, occurring most often on the upper arms and chest, usually in children and pregnant women, but also in persons with liver disease. Called also *naevus arachnoideus* and *spider naevus*.

Spielmeyer–Vogt disease (ˌshpeelmieə'fohkt) the juvenile form of AMAUROTIC FAMILIAL IDIOCY occurring between 5 and 10 years of age, and marked by 'salt and pepper' pigmentation of the retinas. It differs from the infantile form (TAY-SACHS DISEASE) in that it shows no racial predilection.

Spigelius lobe (spi'gayliəs) the small lobe on the under surface of the liver.

spigot ('spigət) a small peg used to close the opening of a tube.

spike (spiek) a sharp upward deflection in a curve or tracing, as on the encephalogram.

spina ('spienə) pl. *spinae* [L.] spine; used in anatomical nomenclature to designate a slender, thornlike process such as occurs on many bones.

s. bifida a developmental anomaly characterized by defective closure of the bony encasement of the spinal cord through which the spinal cord and meninges may or may not protrude.

Developmental defects of the neural tube tend to run in families. The genetic predisposition is inheritable, and the family history is significant in predicting the risk of recurrence. For example, a couple who has had one child with such a defect has a one in 20 (5%) risk of having a second child so affected. The risk is doubled to one in ten (10%) if two of their children have the disorder. Siblings of an affected child are at greater than average risk of producing a child with a similar problem.

Surgical correction may be required to relieve pressure on the spinal cord and prevent progressive neurological involvement with paralysis, musculoskeletal deformities, and bowel and bladder dysfunction. If HYDROCEPHALUS develops, the treatment of choice is a ventriculoperitoneal shunt or some other procedure to decompress the fluid-filled ventricles.

Other modes of therapy are dictated by the degree of neurological involvement and the special problems encountered by the affected child and his family. The familial tendency toward neural tube defects demands that genetic counselling be available to the family and that they receive psychological and emotional support to help them cope with their problems.

s. bifida anterior a defect of closure on the anterior surface of the bony spinal canal, often associated with defective development of the abdominal and thoracic viscera.

s. bifida cystica spina bifida in which there is protrusion through the defect of a cystic swelling involving the meninges (meningocele), spinal cord (myelocele), or both (meningomyelocele).

s. bifida occulta spina bifida in which there is a defect of the bony spinal canal without protrusion of the cord or meninges.

s. ventosa dactylitis of the bones of the hands or feet, occurring mostly in infants and children, with enlargement of digits, caseation, sequestration, and sinus formation.

spinal ('spien'l) pertaining to a spine or to the vertebral column.

s. canal the canal formed by the series of vertebral foramina together, enclosing the spinal cord and meninges; called also vertebral canal.

s. column the spine, or vertebral column.

s. cord that part of the central nervous system lodged in the spinal canal, extending from the foramen magnum to the upper part of the lumbar region.

s. fusion surgical creation of ankylosis of contiguous vertebrae; used in treatment of spondylosis and prolapsed intervertebral (slipped) disc.

s. nerve any of the 31 pairs of nerves arising from the spinal cord and passing out between the vertebrae, including eight cervical, twelve thoracic, five lumbar, five sacral, and one coccygeal.

s. puncture introduction of a hollow needle into the subarachnoid space of the spinal canal, usually between the fourth and fifth lumbar vertebrae; called also LUMBAR PUNCTURE or RACHICENTESIS. In some cases the doctor may choose to perform a CISTERNAL PUNCTURE, in which the needle is inserted immediately below the occipital bone into the cisterna cerebellomedullaris.

A spinal puncture may be done for diagnostic purposes to determine the pressure within the cerebrospinal cavities, to determine the presence of an obstruction to the flow of CEREBROSPINAL FLUID, to remove a specimen of cerebrospinal fluid for laboratory examination, or to inject air or other contrast medium into the spinal canal for the purpose of obtaining x-ray film of the cerebrospinal system.

PATIENT CARE. Before the procedure is begun the patient should be given an explanation of the nature and purpose of the test. He should be told that there is no danger of damage to the spinal cord during a lumbar puncture because the spinal cord does not extend below the second lumbar vertebra. For a cisternal puncture, the back of the neck may be shaved. The doctor should satisfy himself that the patient does not have raised intracranial pressure. The insertion of a needle at the lumbar region will act as a release valve and encourage further herniation, leading in some rare cases to death.

The patient is positioned so that his knees and head are flexed as much as possible, and he is assisted in maintaining this position during the entire procedure. A local anaesthetic such as 1 per cent procaine is injected subcutaneously to anaesthetize the skin and underlying tissues. The patient should be warned not to move suddenly and should be told that he will experience slight pressure when the puncture needle is inserted.

Strict adherence to the rules of aseptic technique is necessary to avoid the possibility of introducing microorganisms into the spinal canal. The attendant may be asked to assist in the Queckenstedt test during the spinal puncture. This test involves compression of the veins of the neck, first on one side, then on the other and finally on both sides at once. The cerebrospinal fluid pressure is measured each time the veins are compressed. This test determines whether there is an obstruction in the spinal canal. Care must be taken that the trachea is not constricted while the neck veins are being compressed.

Specimens of cerebrospinal fluid are collected into sterile containers and sent for examination for organisms and culture, and a sugar and protein count. Other investigations include virology studies or searching for cancerous cells. After the procedure the patient is observed for changes in the level of consciousness and vital signs, including the respiratory pattern. These rarely occur, but headache is common. Mild analgesia, and rest after the procedure, may help to relieve any discomfort.

spinalgia (spie'nalji·ə) pain in the spinal region.

spinate ('spienayt) thorn-shaped; having thorns.

spindle ('spind'l) 1. mitotic spindle; the fusiform figure occurring during metaphase of cell division, composed of microtubules radiating from the centrioles and attached to the chromosomes at their centromeres. 2. muscle spindle.

muscle s. a mechanoreceptor found between the skeletal muscle fibres; the muscle spindles are arranged in parallel with muscle fibres, and respond to passive stretch of the muscle but cease to discharge if the muscle contracts isotonically, thus signalling muscle length. The muscle spindle is the receptor responsible for the stretch or myotatic reflex.

sleep s. a particular wave form in the electroencephalogram during sleep.

spine (spien) 1. a thornlike process or projection; called also spina. 2. the backbone, or vertebral column. The spine is the axis of the skeleton; the skull and limbs are in a sense appendages. An intricate structure, the spine is composed of the vertebrae. These bones can move to a certain extent and so give flexibility to the spine, allowing it to bend forward, sideways and, to a lesser extent, backward. In the areas of the neck and lower back, the spine also can pivot, which permits the turning of the head and torso.

STRUCTURE OF THE SPINE. Each vertebra consists of two main parts: the body and, behind it, the vertebral arch. The body is a cylinder of bone, separated from the cylinders of neighbouring vertebrae by intervertebral discs, layers of cartilage that act as cushions and allow some movement. Projecting backward from each body are two short, thick bony processes (projections) called pedicles. From the ends of these pedicles project two bony plates (laminae), which join together to form the hollow vertebral arch. Through this arch, and protected by it, passes the spinal cord, which is further protected by the meninges and bathed by the cerebrospinal fluid, which serves as a shock absorber.

There are usually 24 movable vertebrae and nine that are fused together. The topmost are the seven cervical vertebrae, which form the back of the neck, supporting the skull and allowing the head to turn from side to side by means of a pivotal motion between the two highest vertebrae. Below these are the 12 thoracic vertebrae, the supports on which the ribs are hinged, and then the five lumbar vertebrae, the largest movable vertebrae (the cervical are the smallest). Below the lumbar vertebrae, the spine terminates with two groups of vertebrae fused into single bones: the sacrum, composed of five vertebrae, and the coccyx, composed of four vertebrae.

Viewed from the side of the body, the spine as a whole has the shape of a gentle double S curve.

SPINAL INJURIES. Fracture, the most serious injury the spine can suffer, has become increasingly common as the number of road traffic accidents has increased. When the spine is fractured, the greatest danger comes from the possibility that the spinal cord may be injured by movement of the fractured vertebrae. Injury to the cord can cause paralysis of all muscles lying below the point of injury. Therefore it is important not to lift or move a person who may have suffered fracture of the spine. If he must be moved before experienced first aid help arrives, he should be drawn carefully backwards or ahead, pulled by both legs or both armpits; any sideways motion must be avoided. See also PARAPLEGIA and QUADRIPLEGIA.

In a prolapsed intervertebral DISC the pulpy centre of the disc, the nucleus pulposus, herniates through a weakened annulus fibrosum (peripheral part of the disc). The nucleus pulposus may press on the spinal cord or one of the spinal nerves and cause pain, sometimes extremely severe. The disc may slip back into place after a period of bed rest, though sometimes the condition must be corrected surgically.

MALFORMATIONS OF THE SPINE. Of the various types of spinal malformations, some are congenital and others the result of postural defects or injuries. Spina bifida is congenital. KYPHOSIS (hunchback) may occasionally be congenital, but more often it is caused by one of the diseases that attack the structure of the bones. The most common of these is POTT'S DISEASE, or tuberculosis affecting the vertebrae and soft tissues of the spine. Another is osteitis deformans, a type of bone inflammation in which parts of the bone are replaced by softer tissue.

Less serious malformations include round shoulders,

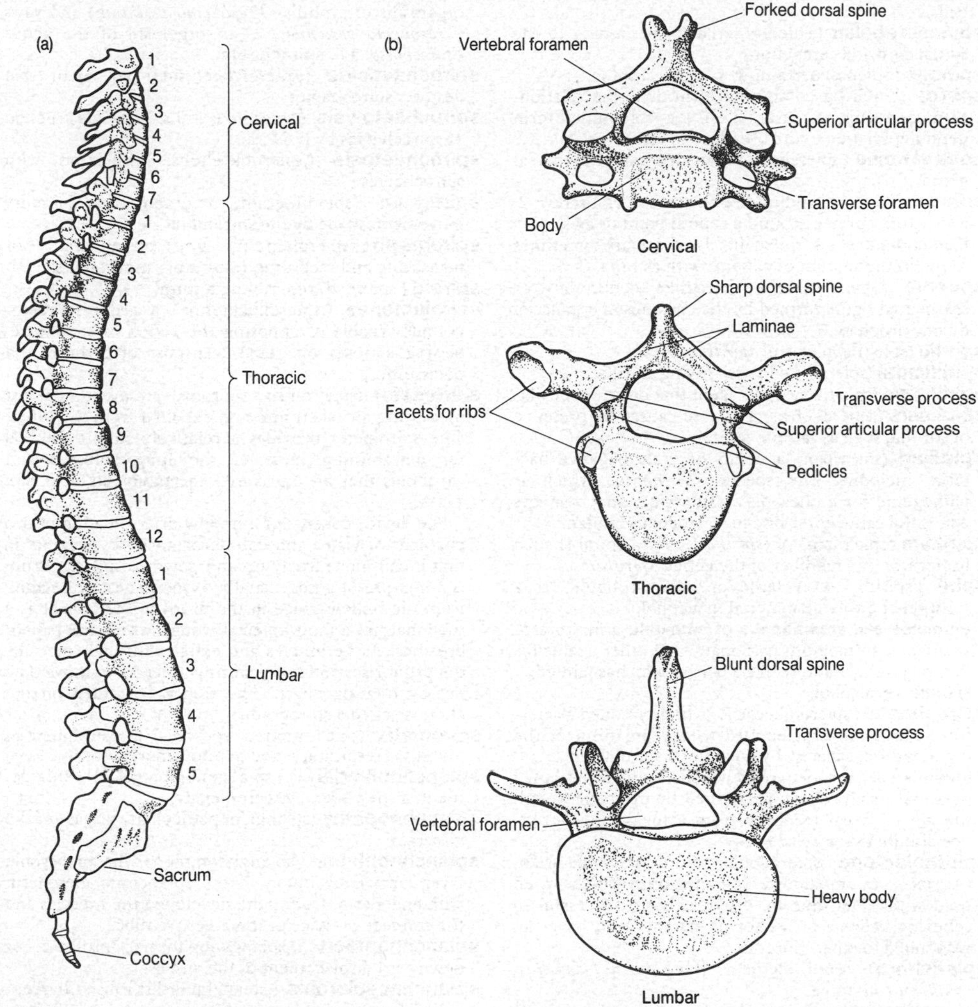

Spine. (a) The spinal column. (b) Typical vertebrae as viewed from above

which may sometimes result from poor posture; the condition warrants corrective treatment for it may cause a strain on the heart. A curvature of the spine toward one side (scoliosis) sometimes is caused by a difference in the length of the legs and can be corrected with the use of a built-up shoe. Occasionally the spine is bent backward, perhaps in an effort to correct a heavy abdomen or for the sake of fashion.

Spinal curvature can also result from certain diseases; it can be the cause or symptoms of serious disorders.

Other Spinal Disorders. Many of the various forms of arthritis may attack the spine. Among these is rheumatoid spondylitis, or Marie–Strümpell disease, which causes inflammation of cartilage between the vertebrae and eventually can cause the neighbouring vertebrae to fuse together, preventing movement. Occasionally the whole spine becomes stiffened, a condition sometimes called poker spine. Loss of spinal flexibility may also be caused by osteoarthritis, the relatively mild arthritic condition that may develop in the later years. Spinal meningitis is an inflammation of the meninges, the membranes that cover the spinal cord..

spinifugal (spie'nifyuhg'l) conducting or moving away from the spinal cord.

spinipetal (spie'nipit'l) conducting or moving toward the spinal cord.

spinnbarkeit ('spinbah,kiet) [Ger.] the formation of a thread by mucus from the cervix uteri when spread onto a glass slide and drawn out by a coverglass; the time at which it can be drawn to the maximum length usually precedes or coincides with the time of ovulation.

spinobulbar (,spienoh'bulbə) pertaining to the spinal cord and medulla oblongata.

spinocellular (ˌspienoh'selyuhlə) pertaining to prickle cells.

spinocerebellar (ˌspienohˌseri'belə) pertaining to the spinal cord and cerebellum.

spinous ('spienəs) pertaining to or like a spine.

spir(o)- 1. [Gr.] a combining form denoting relationship to a coil or spiral. 2. [L.] a combining form denoting relation to the breath or to breathing.

spiradenoma (ˌspieradə'nohmə) adenoma of the sweat glands.

spiral ('spierəl) 1. winding like the thread of a screw. 2. a structure curving around a central point or axis.
Curschmann's s's coiled fibrils of mucin sometimes found in the sputum of patients with asthma.

spireme ('spiereem) the threadlike continuous or segmented figure formed by the chromosome material during prophase.

spirilla (spie'rilə) plural of *spirillum.*

spirillicidal (spieˌrili'sied'l) destroying spirilla.

spirillicide (spie'riliˌsied) an agent that destroys spirilla.

spirillosis (ˌspierili'ohsis) a disease caused by presence of spirilla, such as rat-bite fever.

Spirillum (spie'riləm) a genus of gram-negative bacteria, including one species, *S. minus*, which is pathogenic for guinea pigs, rats, mice, and monkeys and is the cause of rat-bite fever (sodoku) in man.

spirillum (spie'riləm) pl. *spirilla* [L] 1. a spiral-shaped bacterium. 2. a member of the genus *Spirillum.*

spirit ('spirit) 1. a volatile or distilled liquid. 2. a solution of a volatile material in alcohol.
ammonia s's, aromatic s's of ammonia a mixture of ammonia, ammonium carbonate, and other agents for use as an inhalant to revive a person who has fainted.
rectified s. alcohol.

spirochaete ('spierohˌkeet) 1. a highly coiled bacterium; a general term applied to any organism of the order Spirochaetales, which includes the causative organisms of syphilis (*Treponema pallidum*) and yaws (*Treponema pertenue*). 2. an organism of the genus *Spirochaeta*. adj. **spirochaetal.**

spirochaeticide (ˌspieroh'keetiˌsied) an agent that destroys spirochaetes.

spirochaetolysis (ˌspierohkee'tolisis) the destruction of spirochaetes by lysis.

spirochaetosis (ˌspierohkee'tohsis) infection with spirochaetes.

spirogram ('spierohˌgram) a graph of respiratory movements made by the spirometer.

spirograph ('spierohˌgrahf, -ˌgraf) an apparatus for measuring and recording respiratory movements.

spiroid ('spieroyd) resembling a spiral.

spirolactones (ˌspieroh'laktohnz) a group of compounds capable of opposing the action of sodium-retaining steroids on renal transport of sodium and potassium.

spirometer (spie'romitə, spi'rom-) an instrument for measuring air taken into and expelled from the lungs. The spirometer provides a relatively simple method for determining most of the lung volumes and capacities that are measured in PULMONARY FUNCTION TESTS.

The device consists of a hollow drum floating over a chamber of water and counterbalanced by weights so that it can move freely up and down. Inside the drum is a mixture of gases, usually oxygen and air. Leading from the hollow space in the drum to the outside is a tube that has a mouthpiece through which the patient breathes. As he inhales and exhales through the tube the drum rises and falls, causing a needle to move on a nearby rotating chart. The tracing recorded on the chart is called a spirogram.

spirometry (spie'romətree, spi'rom-) measurement of digestive, respiratory, and genitourinary systems. the breathing capacity by means of a spirometer.
incentive s. a manoeuvre in which voluntary sustained maximal inspiration is performed by the patient with the aid of visual feedback from a measuring device. See also INCENTIVE SPIROMETRY.

spironolactone (ˌspierənoh'laktohn) one of the SPIROLACTONES, an oral aldosterone antagonist which, when used with other diuretic drugs, is often successful in relieving oedema or ascites in patients who have not responded to other diuretics.

splanchn(o)- word element. [Gr.] *viscus (viscera), splanchnic nerve.*

splanchnaesthesia (ˌsplangknis'theezi·ə) visceral sensation. adj. **splanchnaesthetic.**

splanchnapophysis (ˌsplangknə'pofisis) a skeletal element, such as the lower jaw, connected with the alimentary canal.

splanchnectopia (ˌsplangknek'tohpi·ə) displacement of a viscus or of the viscera.

splanchnic ('splangknik) pertaining to the viscera.
s. nerves a group of nerves serving the blood vessels and viscera. See splanchnic NERVES.

splanchnicectomy (ˌsplangkni'sektəmee) excision of part of the greater splanchnic nerve.

splanchnicotomy (ˌsplangkni'kotəmee) transection of a splanchnic nerve.

splanchnocele ('splangknohˌseel) hernial protrusion of a viscus.

splanchnocoele ('splangknohˌseel) the portion of the embryonic body cavity from which the abdominal, pericardial, and pleural cavities are formed.

splanchnodiastasis (ˌsplangknohdie'astəsis) displacement of a viscus or viscera.

splanchnolith ('splangknohˌlith) intestinal calculus.

splanchnology (splangk'noləjee) scientific study or description of the organs of the body, as of the

splanchnomegaly (ˌsplangknoh'megəlee) enlargement of the viscera; visceromegaly.

splanchnopathy (splangk'nopəthee) any disease of the viscera.

splanchnopleure ('splangknohˌplooə) the embryonic layer formed by union of the splanchnic mesoderm with endoderm; from it are developed the muscles and the connective tissue of the digestive tube.

splanchnoptosis (ˌsplangknop'tohsis) prolapse or downward displacement of the viscera.

splanchnosclerosis (ˌsplangknohsklə'rohsis) hardening of the viscera.

splanchnoskeleton (ˌsplangknoh'skelitən) skeletal structures connected with viscera.

splanchnotomy (splangk'notəmee) anatomy or dissection of the viscera.

splanchnotribe ('splangknohˌtrieb) an instrument for occluding the intestinal lumen and crushing its wall in preparation for resection and anastomosis.

splayfoot ('splayˌfuht) flatfoot; talipes valgus.

spleen (spleen) a large glandlike but ductless organ situated in the upper part of the abdominal cavity on the left side and lateral to the cardiac end of the stomach. adj. **splenic.** Called also *lien*.

The spleen is the largest collection of reticuloendothelial cells in the body. It is composed of a spongelike tissue, and is distinguished by two types of tissue: *red pulp*, which is the dark reddish brown substance that fills the interspaces of the sinuses of the spleen, and *white pulp*, which consist of sheaths of lymphatic tissue surrounding the arteries of the spleen. It is enclosed in a dense capsule. In a normal adult the spleen is about 125 mm (5 inches) long and weighs from approximately 140 to 200 grams.

In the unborn child the spleen, with the liver,

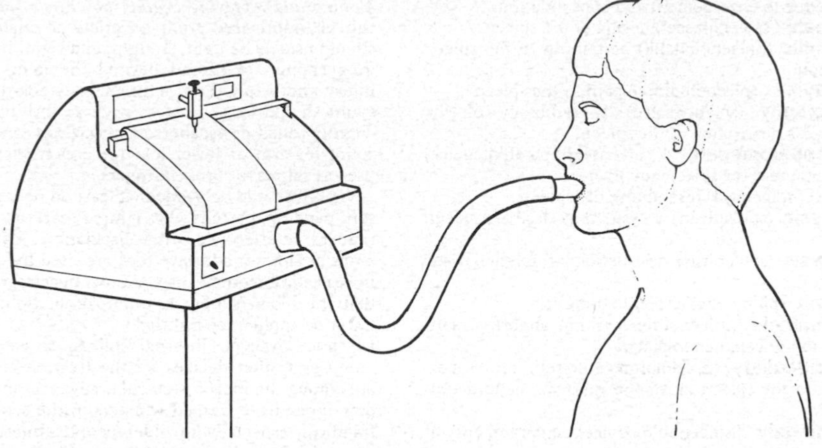

Spirometer

produces erythrocytes. After birth, this function is taken over by the bone marrow. However, if there is bone marrow failure, the spleen may again produce red blood cells. In the normal adult the spleen is a reservoir for blood, and contains a high concentration of erythrocytes. In times of exertion, emotional stress, pregnancy, severe bleeding, carbon monoxide poisoning, or other occasions when the oxygen content of the blood must be increased, the spleen contracts rhythmically to release its store of red cells into the bloodstream.

The spleen also acts to help keep the blood free from unwanted substances, including wastes and infecting organisms. The blood is delivered to the spleen by the splenic artery, and passes through smaller branch arteries into a network of channels lined with leukocytes known as phagocytes (see RETICULOENDOTHELIAL SYSTEM). These clear the blood of old erythrocytes, damaged cells, parasites, and other toxic or foreign substances. Haemoglobin from the removed red cells is temporarily stored.

DISORDERS OF THE SPLEEN. Because of its functions of blood formation, storage, and filtration, the spleen is subject to a host of disorders that are secondary to disease elsewhere in the body or in the blood stream. Both acute infections, such as typhoid fever, subacute bacterial endocarditis, and measles, and chronic infections, such as malaria, syphilis, and tuberculosis, can involve the spleen. Overactivity of the spleen (*hypersplenism)* results in faulty regulation of the number of blood cells in circulation. The cause of this hyperactivity of the spleen is not known. Splenomegaly is characteristically present in other disorders, such as Felty's syndrome (a form of rheumatoid arthritis), Banti's disease, and cirrhosis of the liver. Though they are rare, both benign and malignant tumours can develop in the spleen. A more common indication for splenectomy is traumatic injury from a physical blow.

s. atrophy wasting of the spleen. Splenic atrophy and consequent decreased splenic function (hyposplenism) can occur in patients with coeliac disease, and sickle cell disease. In young children this may lead to an increased susceptibility to infection.

accessory s. a small mass of tissue elsewhere in the body, histologically and functionally identical with that composing the normal spleen.

splen(o)- word element. [Gr.] *spleen.*

splenadenoma (ˌsplenadəˈnohmə) hyperplasia of the spleen pulp.

splenalgia (spliˈnalji·ə) pain in the spleen.

splenectasis (spliˈnektəsis) splenomegaly.

splenectomy (spliˈnektəmee) excision of the SPLEEN. Indications for this procedure include severe trauma to or rupture of the spleen, enlargement (splenomegaly) when the destructive properties of the organ are greatly accelerated, and such blood disorders as idiopathic thrombocytopenic purpura and hereditary spherocytosis. The latter two conditions respond well to splenectomy. In blood dyscrasias in which parts of the reticuloendothelial system other than the spleen are involved, splenectomy may be of little value.

Other indications for splenectomy include lymphoma, transplant rejection, sickle cell disease, abscesses, a clot in a major blood vessel serving the spleen, and hepatic cirrhosis. In recognition that the spleen has important immunological functions, current therapy is directed toward salvage of the injured spleen, if possible.

Other reticuloendothelial cells scattered throughout the body take over once the spleen is removed. However, those persons who no longer have a functioning spleen, either as a result of splenectomy or because of a destructive disease process, are at high risk from life-threatening infections, especially those caused by pneumococci. They should receive the vaccine against 14 strains of pneumococcal bacteria, and be sure to consult a doctor and take preventive antibiotics as prescribed even though they may seem to have a trivial infection or a mild case of the 'flu'.

splenectopia, splenectopy (ˌsplenekˈtohpi·ə; spliˈnektəpee) displacement of the spleen.

spleneolus (spliˈneeələs) an accessory spleen.

splenic (ˈsplenik) pertaining to the spleen.

splenitis (spliˈnietis) inflammation of the spleen, a condition that is attended by enlargement of the organ and severe local pain.

splenium (ˈspleeni·əm) a compress or bandage; a bandlike structure.

s. corporis callosi the posterior, rounded end of the corpus callosum.

splenization (ˌsplenieˈzayshən) the conversion of a tissue, as of the lung, into tissue resembling that of the spleen, due to engorgement and consolidation.

splenocele ('spleenoh,seel) hernia of the spleen.

splenocolic (,spleenoh'kolik) pertaining to the spleen and colon.

splenodynia (,spleenoh'dini·ə) pain in the spleen.

splenography (spli'nogrəfee) 1. radiology of the spleen. 2. a description of the spleen.

splenohepatomegaly (,spleenoh,hepətoh'megəlee) enlargement of the spleen and liver.

splenoid ('spleenoyd) resembling the spleen.

splenolysin (spli'nolisin) a lysin that destroys spleen tissue.

splenolysis (spli'nolisis) destruction of splenic tissue by a lysin.

splenoma (spli'nohmə) a splenic tumour.

splenomalacia (,spleenohmə'layshi·ə) abnormal softness of the spleen; lienomalacia.

splenomedullary (,spleenohmə'dulə·ree) of or pertaining to the spleen and bone marrow; lienomedullary.

splenomegaly (,spleenoh'megəlee) enlargement of the spleen.

congestive s. splenomegaly secondary to portal hypertension, with ascites, anaemia, thrombocytopenia, leukopenia, and episodic haemorrhage from the intestinal tract.

haemolytic s. that associated with haemolytic anaemia.

siderotic s. splenomegaly with deposit of iron and calcium.

splenometry (spli'nomətree) determination of the size of the spleen.

splenomyelogenous (,spleenoh,mieə'lojənəs) formed in the spleen and bone marrow; lienomyelogenous.

splenoncus (spli'nongkəs) splenoma.

splenopancreatic (,spleenoh,pangkri'atik) pertaining to the spleen and pancreas.

splenopathy (spli'nopəthee) any disease of the spleen.

splenopexy ('spleenoh,peksee) surgical fixation of the spleen.

splenopneumonia (,splenohnyoo'mohni·ə) pneumonia attended with splenization of the lung.

splenoportography (,splenohpaw'togrəfee) radiology of the portal venous circulation by direct injection of contrast medium through a needle inserted percutaneously into the spleen. See also SELDINGER TECHNIQUE.

splenoptosis (,spleenop'tohsis) downward displacement of the spleen.

splenorenal (,spleenoh'reen'l) pertaining to the spleen and kidney, or to splenic and renal veins.

splenorrhagia (,spleenə'rayji·ə) haemorrhage from the spleen.

splenorrhaphy (spli'no·rəfee) suture of the spleen.

splenotomy (spli'notəmee) incision of the spleen.

splenotoxin (,spleenoh'toksin) a toxin produced by or acting on the spleen; lienotoxin.

splenunculus (sple'nunkyuhləs) a tiny spleen closely related to the larger organ—either in the hilum or in one of the suspensory ligaments of the spleen.

splint (splint) a rigid or semirigid appliance, its common purpose being to prevent movement at the site of fracture, dislocation or soft tissue injury. It is used less commonly for the correction of deformity. Splints can be external or internal. See accompanying illustration.

EXTERNAL SPLINTS. The usual method of external splintage of fractures is by plaster-of-Paris cast. In a pelvic or spinal fracture, splinting is achieved by placing the patient on a stretcher or board. Breaks of the ribs and of face and skull bones usually do not require splints, since these parts remain fixed by adjacent bone and tissue.

Making and Applying Splints For First Aid. A splint can be improvised from a variety of materials, but should usually be light, straight, and rigid. It should be long enough to extend beyond the joint above the injury and below the fracture site. A board used as a splint should be at least as wide as the injured part. Tightly rolled newspapers or magazines can serve as a splint for arm or lower leg. Ice cream sticks may be used as splints for broken fingers.

A splint should be padded, at least on one side. Thick soft padding permits the injured part to swell and reduces interference with circulation. Bandages or strips of cloth or adhesive tape are used to hold splints in place. Subsequent inspection is necessary to ensure that the blood supply is unimpaired. Splints should never be applied too tightly.

INTERNAL SPLINTS. Internal splints, as well as pins, wires, and other devices for the fixation of fractures, are among the more spectacular advances in orthopaedics. They have worked wonders in the setting of hip fractures, especially in older people. Internal splints are available for almost every type of fracture. Stainless steel and Vitallium are the most commonly used materials. Splints and devices of this type require surgery for insertion, but are less cumbersome than external splints and permit earlier use of the fractured bone.

airplane s. one that holds the splinted arm in abduction.

Balkan s. Balkan Beam.

coaptation s's small splints adjusted about a fractured limb to produce coaptation of fragments.

cap s. metal cap splints which are cemented onto the teeth are a common form of immobilization of fractures of the jaw.

Gunning s. one in which modified upper and lower dentures are wired into place. It may be used to immobilize fractured jaws in edentulous patients.

spodo- word element. [Gr.] *waste material.*

spodogenous (spoh'dojənəs) caused by accumulation of waste material in an organ.

spondyl(o)- word element. [Gr.] *vertebra, vertebral column.*

spondylalgia (,spondi'lalji·ə) pain in the vertebrae.

spondylarthritis (,spondilah'thrietis) arthritis of the spine and joints as seen in the seronegative arthritides ankylosing spondylitis, psoriatic arthritis, Reiter's syndrome, and Crohn's and colitic arthritis.

spondylitic (,spondi'litik) pertaining to or marked by spondylitis.

spondylitis (,spondi'lietis) inflammation of the vertebrae. Almost always a serious chronic disorder, spondylitis may be associated with tuberculosis of the bones, in which case it is called POTT'S DISEASE. The vertebrae become eroded and collapse, causing KYPHOSIS (hunchback).

Spondylitis may also be associated with other infectious diseases, such as brucellosis, or undulant fever. The intervertebral discs and the vertebrae are affected and sometimes destroyed, and permanent stiffening, or ankylosis, of the back results.

Rheumatoid spondylitis, called also *Marie–Strümpell disease* or *ankylosing spondylitis*, is a of rheumatoid arthritis that affects the spine, and is characterized by inflammation of the cartilage in the joints between vertebrae, and inflammation of the gliding joints between the vertebral arches. It affects males almost exclusively. There is stiffening of the spinal joints and ligaments, so that movement becomes increasingly painful and difficult. When it runs its full course, it results in bony ankylosis of the vertebral joints. The stiffening may extend to the ribs and limit the flexibility of the rib cage, so that breathing is impaired.

Kümmel's spondylitis or post-traumatic spondylitis, is compression fracture of a vertebra, with symptoms occurring a few weeks after injury (see also KÜMMEL'S DISEASE).

spondylizema (ˌspondilie'zeemə) downward displacement of a vertebra because of destruction or softening of the one below it.

spondyloarthropathy (ˌspondiloh·ah'thropəthee) disease affecting the joints of the spine as well as peripheral joints. See also ANKYLOSING SPONDYLITIS, PSORIATIC ARTHRITIS, REITER'S SYNDROME and COLITIC ARTHRITIS.

spondylocace (ˌspondi'lokəsee) tuberculosis of the vertebrae.

spondylodymus (ˌspondi'lodiməs) twin fetuses united by the vertebrae.

spondylodynia (ˌspondiloh'dini·ə) pain in a vertebra.

spondylolisthesis (ˌspondilohlis'theesis) forward displacement of a vertebra over a lower segment due to a congenital defect or fracture in the pars interarticularis, usually of the fifth lumbar over the sacrum, or of the fourth lumbar over the fifth. adj. **spondylolisthetic**.

spondylolysis (ˌspondi'lolisis) the breaking down of a vertebra. adj. **spondylolytic**.

spondylopathy (ˌspondi'lopəthee) any disease of the vertebrae.

spondylopyosis (ˌspondilohpie'ohsis) suppuration of a vertebra.

spondyloschisis (ˌspondi'loskisis) congenital fissure of a vertebral arch; spina bifida.

spondylosis (ˌspondi'lohsis) ankylosis of a vertebral joint; also, a general term for degenerative changes in the spine.

rhizomelic s. rheumatoid spondylitis.

spondylosyndesis (ˌspondiloh'sindisis) surgical creation of ankylosis between contiguous vertebrae; spinal fusion.

sponge (spunj) 1. a porous, absorbent mass, as a pad of gauze or cotton surrounded by gauze. 2. the elastic fibrous skeleton of certain species of marine animals.

gelatin s., absorbable a sterile, absorbable, water-insoluble, gelatin-base material used in the control of bleeding.

spongi(o)- word element. [L., Gr.] *sponge, spongelike.*

spongiform ('spunjiˌfawm) resembling a sponge.

sponging ('spunjing) a method of reducing a high temperature by encouraging evaporation of water from the skin. The temperatures suggested for the sponge water are approximate, but suitable ones are: *cold s.* 20 °C, *tepid s.* 30 °C, *hot s.* 40 °C.

spongioblast ('spunjiohˌblast) 1. any of the embryonic epithelial cells developed about the neural tube, which become transformed, some into neuroglial and some into ependymal cells. 2. amacrine.

spongioblastoma (ˌspunjiohbla'stohmə) a tumour containing spongioblasts; gliosarcoma or glioblastoma.

spongiocyte ('spunjiohˌsiet) 1. a neuroglia cell. 2. one of the cells with spongy vacuolated protoplasm in the adrenal cortex.

spongioid ('spunjiˌoyd) resembling a sponge.

spongioplasm ('spunjiohˌplazəm) 1. a substance forming the network of fibrils pervading the cell substance and forming the reticulum of the fixed cell. 2. the granular material of an axon.

spongiosa (ˌspunji'ohsə) spongy; sometimes used alone to mean the spongy substance of bone (substantia spongiosa ossium).

spongiosaplasty (ˌspunji'ohsəˌplastee) autoplasty of the spongy substance of bone (substantia spongiosa ossium) to potentiate formation of new bone or to cover bone defects.

spongiosis (ˌspunji'ohsis) intercellular oedema within the epidermis.

spongiositis (ˌspunjioh'sietis) inflammation of the corpus spongiosum of the penis.

spongy ('spunjee) of spongelike appearance or texture.

s. degeneration of central nervous system, s. degeneration of white matter see spongy DEGENERATION of central nervous system.

spontaneous (spon'tayni·əs) 1. occurring without apparent cause. 2. occurring naturally, not induced. 3. unpremeditated, not deliberate.

s. abortion see spontaneous ABORTION.

s. fracture see spontaneous FRACTURE.

s. labour see spontaneous LABOUR.

sporadic (spə'radik) occurring singly; widely scattered; not epidemic or endemic.

spore (spor) 1. a refractile, oval body formed within bacteria, especially *Bacillus* and *Clostridium*, which is regarded as a resting stage during the life history of the cell, and is characterized by its resistance to environmental changes. 2. the reproductive element, produced sexually or asexually, of one of the lower organisms, such as protozoa, fungi, or algae.

sporicide ('spor·riˌsied) an agent that kills spores. adj. **sporicidal**.

sporocyst ('spor·rohˌsist) 1. any cyst or sac containing spores or reproductive cells; the oocyst of certain protozoa in which sporozoites develop. 2. the larval stages of flukes in snails.

sporogenic (ˌspor·roh'jenik) producing spores.

sporogony (spor'rogənee, -'roj-, spo-) the sexual stage in the life cycle of a sporozoan parasite, with development of the zygote into one or several haploid spores, each containing a distinctive number of sporozoites. adj. **sporogonic**.

sporont ('spor·ront) a mature protozoon in its sexual cycle.

sporoplasm ('spor·rohˌplazəm) the protoplasm of a spore.

Sporothrix ('spor·rohˌthriks) a genus of fungi, including *S. schenckii*, which causes sporotrichosis, and *S. carnis*, which causes formation of white mould on meat in cold storage.

sporotrichosis (ˌspor·rohtri'kohsis) a chronic fungal infection caused by *Sporothrix schenckii*, occurring in three forms. The *cutaneous lymphatic form* is characterized by a single pustule, papule, or nodule at the site of invasion, followed by lymphatic spread and the development of multiple, painless, subcutaneous granulomas, which tend to break down and form indolent ulcers or cold abscesses. The *disseminated form* is marked by multiple, painless, cutaneous or subcutaneous nodules, which may form cold abscesses, ulcers, or fistulas; this form may involve the muscles, joints, bones, eyes, gastrointestinal system, mucous membranes, and nervous system. The *pulmonary form* results from the inhalation of spores and causes acute disease or chronic granulomas similar to those seen in other mycoses.

Sporozoa (ˌspor·rə'zoh·ə) a subphylum of endoparasitic protozoa, marked by the lack of locomotor organs in adult stages and a complex life cycle usually involving an alternation of a sexual with an asexual cycle.

sporozoa (ˌspor·rə'zoh·ə) plural of *sporozoon.*

sporozoan (ˌspor·rə'zoh·ən) 1. pertaining to the Sporozoa. 2. an individual of the Sporozoa.

sporozoite (ˌspor·rə'zoh·iet) a spore formed after fertilization; any one of the sickle-shaped nucleated germs formed by division of the protoplasm of a spore of a sporozoan organism. In malaria, the sporozoites are the forms of the plasmodium that are liberated from the oocysts in the mosquito, that accumulate in the salivary glands and that are transferred to man in the act of feeding.

sporozoon (ˌspor·rə'zoh·on) pl. *sporozoa* [Gr.] an individual organism of the Sporozoa.

sports injuries (spawts 'injə·riz) see REPETITIVE STRAIN INJURY.

sporulation (ˌspo·ryuh'layshən) formation of spores.

spot map (spot) one used to plot epidemic disease by placing a spot on the map to represent each case or group of cases.

spotted fever ('spotid) a febrile disease characterized by a skin eruption, such as Rocky Mountain spotted fever, boutonneuse fever, and other infections due to tickborne rickettsiae.

sprain (sprayn) wrenching or twisting of a joint, with partial rupture of its ligaments. There may also be damage to the associated blood vessels, muscles, tendons, and nerves.

A sprain is more serious than a strain, which is simply the overstretching of a muscle, without swelling. Severe sprains are so painful that the joint cannot be used. There is much swelling, with reddish to blue discoloration owing to haemorrhage from ruptured blood vessels.

First aid for a sprain includes immediate rest with no weight bearing in order to prevent further damage. The injured part should be elevated to decrease swelling. Applications of ice or cold compresses (not heat) to the injured part during the first 12 hours also will relieve pain and help prevent swelling. If there is severe tearing or rupture of a ligament or tendon the condition will require immobilization in a cast or surgical repair or both.

Sprengel's deformity (shoulder) ('sprengəlz) a congenital deformity in which one scapula is higher than the other, causing some limitation in abduction of the shoulder.

sprue (sproo) a chronic form of malabsorption syndrome occurring in both tropical and nontropical forms; called also *pigmentosa*.

nontropical s. a malabsorption syndrome affecting both children and adults, precipitated by ingestion of gluten-containing foods (see also COELIAC DISEASE).

tropical s. a chronic disease, affecting the digestive system, that is marked by imperfect absorption of food elements, especially fats but also certain vitamins, from the small intestine. The condition is closely related to COELIAC DISEASE and may be identical with it.

The name sprue derives from a Dutch word describing inflammation of the mouth, which is a frequent symptom. The disease has been recognized for more than 2000 years. It occurs mostly, but not exclusively, in the tropics.

SYMPTOMS AND TREATMENT. Symptoms are loss of appetite, flatulence, anaemia, diarrhoea, stomach cramps, and extreme loss of weight. Stools are usually pale, greasy, unformed, and foul-smelling, but at times become watery. If a deficiency of vitamin B complex is also present, cracks develop at the corners of the mouth and the tongue becomes smooth, glossy, and bright red.

Treatment consists of a special diet of foods that are low in fat, high in protein, and fairly bland. Diets free of gluten, a viscid grain protein, may be prescribed. Liver preparations, folic acid, calcium lactate tablets, vitamin B_{12}, and iron supplements to provide food elements that are not absorbed, as well as skimmed milk and ripe bananas, have produced favourable results. Antibiotics and cortisone have proved temporarily successful, but their prolonged use is not recommended. In critical cases, repeated small blood transfusions have been beneficial.

Cases of sprue that are recognized early respond better to treatment than do cases of long standing. Appetite and weight return rapidly. The time required for complete recovery is prolonged, however, especially in extreme cases.

spud (spud) a flat, blunt blade used for removing foreign bodies from the eye.

spur (spər) a projecting body, as from a bone.

spurious ('spyooə·ri·əs) simulated; not genuine; false.

sputum ('spyootəm) mucous secretion from the lungs, bronchi, and trachea which is ejected through the mouth, in contrast to saliva which is the secretion of the salivary glands.

s. specimen a sample of mucous secretion from the bronchi and lungs. The specimen may be examined microscopically for the presence of malignant cells *(cytological examination)* or tested to identify pathogenic bacteria *(bacteriological examination)*.

It is essential that the specimen obtained be mucus from the lungs and bronchi and not saliva. For those who are unable to produce sputum for examination, an AEROSOL may be used to increase the flow of secretions and stimulate coughing. The optimum time for collection of a sputum specimen is in the morning before breakfast. At this time secretions accumulated in the bronchi through the night are more readily available, and, should the coughing produce gagging, the patient is less likely to vomit if his stomach is empty. Specimens collected for bacteriological culture must be placed in a sterile container and handled with care to avoid contamination from sources other than the sputum.

squalene ('skwayleen) an unsaturated terpene, which is an intermediate in cholesterol synthesis, and occurs normally at low levels in blood plasma and at elevated levels in viral influenza; used as a vehicle for pharmaceuticals.

squama ('skwaymə) pl. *squamae* [L.] a scale, or thin, platelike structure.

squame (skwaym) a scale or scalelike mass.

squamoparietal, squamosoparietal (ˌskwaymohpə'rieət'l; skwayˌmohsohpə'rieat'l) pertaining to the pars squamosa, or squamous portion of the temporal bone, and the parietal bone.

squamous ('skwayməs) scaly or platelike.

s. bone the pars squamosa, or squamous portion of the temporal bone.

s. epithelium epithelium composed of flat, scale-like cells.

s. cell carcinoma a malignancy of the squamous epithelial cells of the bronchus.

squatting ('skwoting) a position with the hips and knees flexed, the buttocks resting on the heels; sometimes adopted by the parturient at delivery or by children with certain types of cardiac defects.

squill (skwil) the fleshy inner scales of the bulb of the white variety of *Urginea maritima;* it contains several cardioactive glycosides. The red variety is used as a rat poison.

squint (skwint) strabismus.

SR sedimentation rate.

Sr chemical symbol, *strontium*.

SRH somatotrophin releasing hormone (growth hormone releasing hormone).

SRN State Registered Nurse.

SRS, SRS-A slow-reacting substance (of anaphylaxis).

ss. *semis* (one half).

SSStJ Serving Sister of the Order of St John of Jerusalem.

StAAA St Andrew's Ambulance Association.

stability (stə'bilitee) the quality of maintaining a

constant character despite forces that threaten to disturb it.

stabilization (ˌstaybilie'zayshən) the process of making firm and steady.

Stabillin V-K (ˌstaybilin vee'kay) trademark for a preparation of penicillin V.

stable ('stayb'l) not readily subject to change.

stactometer (stak'tomitə) a device for measuring drops.

stadium ('staydi·əm) the stage of a disease.

s. decrementi the period of decline in severity; defervescence.

s. incrementi the stage when symptoms are developing.

s. incubationis the incubation period.

s. invasionis the incubation period.

staff (stahf) 1. a wooden rod or rodlike structure. 2. a grooved director used as a guide for the knife in lithotomy. 3. the personnel employed by a health authority or other organisation.

s. of Æsculapius see ÆSCULAPIUS.

stage (stayj) 1. a definite period or distinct phase, as of development of a disease or of an organism. 2. the platform of a microscope on which the slide containing the object to be studied is placed.

staging ('stayjing) 1. the determination of distinct phases or periods in the course of a disease, the life history of an organism, or any biological process. 2. the classification of neoplasms according to the extent of the tumour.

TNM s. staging of tumours according to three basic components: primary tumour (T), regional nodes (N), and metastasis (M). Subscripts are used to denote size and degree of involvement; for example, 0 indicates undetectable, and 1, 2, 3, and 4 a progressive increase in size or involvement. Thus, a tumour may be described as $T_1N_2M_0$. See also CANCER.

stain (stayn) 1. a substance used to impart colour to tissues or cells, to facilitate microscopic study and identification. 2. an area of discoloration of the skin.

differential s. one which facilitates differentiation of various elements in a specimen.

Giemsa s. a solution containing azure II-eosin, azure II, glycerin, and methanol; used for staining protozoan parasites, such as trypanosomes, *Leishmania*; etc., and *Leptospira*, *Borrelia*, viral inclusion bodies, and *Rickettsia*.

Gram's s. a staining procedure in which bacteria are stained with crystal violet, treated with strong iodine solution, decolorized with ethanol or ethanol-acetone, and counterstained with a contrasting dye; those retaining the stain are gram-positive, and those losing the stain but staining with the counterstain are gram-negative.

haematoxylin and eosin s. a mixture of haematoxylin in distilled water and aqueous eosin solution, employed universally for routine examination of tissues.

metachromatic s. one that produces in certain elements colour different from that of the stain itself.

nuclear s. one that selectively stains cell nuclei, generally a basic stain.

port-wine s. naevus flammeus.

supravital s. a dye with an ability to stain living tissue or viable cells after their removal from the body.

tumour s. an area of increased density in a radiograph, due to collection of contrast material in distorted and abnormal vessels, prominent in the capillary and venous phases of arteriography, and presumed to indicate neoplasm.

vital s. a stain introduced into the living organism, and taken up selectively by various tissue or cellular elements.

Wright's s. a mixture of eosin and methylene blue, used for demonstrating blood cells and malarial parasites.

staining ('stayning) artificial coloration of a substance to facilitate examination of tissues, microorganisms, or other cells under the microscope. For various techniques, see under STAIN.

stalagmometer (ˌstaləg'momitə) an instrument for measuring surface tension by determining the exact number of drops in a given quantity of a liquid.

stammering ('stamə·ring) a speech problem characterized by involuntary pauses in speaking, often with repetition of sounds. See also SPEECH.

standard ('standəd) something established as a measure or model to which other similar things should conform.

standard deviation a measure of the dispersion of a random variable: the square root of the average squared deviation from the mean. For data that have a normal distribution about 68 per cent of the data points fall within one standard deviation from the mean and about 95 per cent fall within two standard deviations. Symbol σ.

standardization (ˌstandədie'zayshən) a statistical technique to enable comparison of morbidity and mortality rates in populations of different age and sex structures. The standardized rates take into account these differences.

standstill ('standˌstil) cessation of motion, as of the heart (cardiac standstill) or chest (respiratory standstill).

stannous ('stanəs) containing tin as a bivalent element.

stannum ('stanəm) [L.] *tin* (symbol Sn).

stanozolol (stan'ohzohˌlol) an androgenic anabolic steroid to increase haemoglobin levels in some patients with aplastic anaemia.

Stanton's disease ('stantənz) melioidosis.

stapedectomy (ˌstaypi'dektəmee) surgical removal of the stapes (stirrup of the middle ear), which is then replaced with a prosthetic device composed of stainless steel, Teflon, or a similar substance. The surgical procedure is performed for the relief of deafness produced by OTOSCLEROSIS, or fixation of the minute bones of the middle ear. Replacement of the fixed stapes with a device capable of vibrating permits the transmission of sound waves from the outer ear to the inner ear, and hearing is thus restored.

Because the stapes is one of the smallest bones in the body, this procedure is very delicate and must be performed under an operating microscope. Very fine instruments, designed specifically for this procedure, are used.

The procedure is done under local anaesthesia and the patient is allowed out of bed within 48 hours after surgery and usually can go home on the third postoperative day. Vertigo (dizziness) is common following stapedectomy but it is only temporary. The patient must be protected from falls and self-injury until he regains his sense of balance. Care must also be taken to prevent infection and the patient must be cautioned against blowing his nose and getting water in his ear while bathing until the operative site is completely healed.

stapedial (stə'peedi·əl) pertaining to the stapes.

stapediolysis (stəˌpeedi'olisis) an operation in which the footpiece of the stapes is mobilized to aid conduction in deafness from otosclerosis.

stapediotenotomy (stəˌpeediohtə'notəmee) cutting of the tendon of the stapedius muscle.

stapediovestibular (stəˌpeediohve'stibyuhlə) pertaining to the stapes and vestibule.

stapes ('staypeez) the innermost of the three ossicles of the ear; called also stirrup.

staphyl(o)- word element. [Gr.] *uvula, resembling a bunch of grapes, staphylococci.*

staphylectomy (ˌstafiˈlektəmee) uvulectomy.

staphyline (ˈstafiˌlien) 1. pertaining to the uvula. 2. shaped like a bunch of grapes.

staphylitis (ˌstafiˈlietis) inflammation of the uvula.

staphylococcaemia (ˌstafilohkokˈseemi·ə) staphylococci in the blood.

Staphylococcus (ˌstafilohˈkokəs) a genus of gram-positive bacteria made up of spherical microorganisms, tending to occur in grapelike clusters; they are constantly present on the skin and in the upper respiratory tract and are the most common cause of localized suppurating infections. There are several species, some of which are pathogenic, including *S. albus* (*S. epidermidis*).

staphylococcus (ˌstafilohˈkokəs) pl. *staphylococci* [Gr.] any organism of the genus *Staphylococcus.* adj. **staphylococcal.**

staphyloderma (ˌstafilohˈdərmə) pyogenic skin infection by staphylococci.

staphylodialysis (ˌstafilohdieˈaləsis) elongation of the uvula.

staphyloedema (ˌstafiliˈdeemə) oedema of the uvula.

staphylokinase (ˌstafilohˈkienəyz) a bacterial kinase produced by certain strains of staphylococci; it induces fibrinolysis by converting plasminogen to plasmin.

staphylolysin (ˌstafiˈlolisin) a substance produced by staphylococci that causes haemolysis.

staphyloma (ˌstafiˈlohmə) protrusion of the sclera or cornea, usually lined with uveal tissue, due to inflammation.

anterior s. staphyloma in the anterior part of the eye.

corneal s. 1. bulging of the cornea with adherent uveal tissue. 2. one formed by protrusion of the iris through a corneal wound.

posterior s. backward bulging of sclera at posterior pole of eye.

scleral s. protrusion of the contents of the eyeball where the sclera has become thinned.

staphyloncus (ˌstafiˈlongkəs) a tumour or swelling of the uvula.

staphyloplasty (ˈstafilohˌplastee) plastic repair of the soft palate and uvula.

staphyloptosis (ˌstafilopˈtohsis) elongation of the uvula.

staphylorrhaphy (ˌstafiˈlo·rəfee) surgical correction of a midline cleft in the uvula and soft palate.

staphyloschisis (ˌstafiˈloskisis) fissure of the uvula and soft palate.

staphylotomy (ˌstafiˈlotəmee) 1. incision of the uvula. 2. excision of a staphyloma.

starch (stahch) 1. any of a group of polysaccharides of the general formula, $(C_6H_{10}O_5)_n$; it is the chief storage form of CARBOHYDRATES in plants. 2. granular material separated from mature grain of *Zea mays* (Indian corn, or maize); used as a dusting powder and tablet disintegrant in pharmaceuticals.

starvation (stahˈvayshən) long-continued deprival of food and its morbid effects.

stasis (ˈstaysis) a stoppage or diminution of flow, as of blood or other body fluid, or of intestinal contents.

-stasis word element. [Gr.] *maintenance of (or maintaining) a constant level, preventing increase or multiplication.* adj. **-static.**

stat. [L.] *statim* (at once).

state (stayt) condition or situation.

alpha s. the state of relaxation and peaceful awakefulness associated with prominent alpha brain wave activity.

dream s. a state of defective consciousness in which the environment is imperfectly perceived.

excited s. the condition of a nucleus, atom, or molecule produced by the addition of energy to the system as the result of absorption of photons or of inelastic collisions with other particles or systems.

ground s. the condition of lowest energy of a nucleus, atom or molecule.

refractory s. a condition of subnormal excitability of muscle and nerve following excitation.

resting s. the physiological condition achieved by complete bed rest for at least 1 hour.

steady s. dynamic equilibrium.

static (ˈstatik) stationary; at rest.

s. electricity The build-up of an electrical charge in a nonconductor, which may cause a spark, and an explosion of oxygen or an explosive anaesthetic gas if such are present.

statim (ˈstaytim) [L.] *at once;* abbreviated stat.

station (ˈstayshən) 1. the position assumed in standing; the manner of standing; in ataxic conditions it is sometimes pathognomonic. 2. the location of the presenting part of the fetus in the birth canal, designated as −5 to −1 according to the number of centimetres the part is above an imaginary plane passing through the ischial spines, 0 when at the plane, and +1 to +5 according to the number of centimetres the part is below the plane.

statistics (stəˈtistiks) 1. numerical facts pertaining to a particular subject or body of objects. 2. the science dealing with the collection, tabulation, and analysis of numerical facts.

statoacoustic (ˌstatoh·əˈkoostik) pertaining to balance and hearing.

statoconia (ˌstatəˈkohni·ə) plural of *statoconium.* [Gr.] minute calcareous particles in the gelatinous membrane surmounting the macula in the inner ear. Called also *otoconia.*

statolith (ˈstatohˌlith) 1. a granule of the statoconia. 2. a solid or semisolid body occurring in the labyrinth of animals.

stature (ˈstachə) the height or tallness of a person standing.

status (ˈstaytəs) [L.] *condition, state.*

s. asthmaticus asthmatic crisis; a sudden intense and continuous asthmatic attack, with dyspnoea to the point of exhaustion and no response to the usual therapy.

s. epilepticus rapid succession of epileptic spasms without intervals of consciousness; brain damage may result.

s. lymphaticus lymphatism.

s. thymicolymphaticus a condition resembling lymphatism, with enlargement of lymphadenoid tissue and of the thymus as the special influencing factor; formerly thought to be the cause of sudden death in children.

s. verrucosus a wartlike appearance of the cerebral cortex, produced by disorderly arrangement of the neuroblasts, so that the formation of fissures and sulci is irregular and unpredictable.

staxis (ˈstaksis) haemorrhage.

steapsin (stiˈapsin) the fat-splitting enzyme (lipase) of the pancreatic juice.

stear(o)- word element. [Gr.] *fat.*

stearate (ˈsteeə·rayt) any compound of stearic acid.

stearic acid (stiˈarik) a saturated fatty acid from animal and vegetable fats.

steat(o)- word element. [Gr.] *fat, oil.*

steatitis (stiəˈtietis) inflammation of fatty tissue.

steatocystoma (ˌstiətohsiˈstohmə) an epithelial cyst.

s. multiplex steatomatosis, a rare hereditary condition in which multiple cutaneous epithelial cysts contain-

ing oily liquid, abortive hair follicles, and sebaceous glands occur on the trunk and limbs.
steatogenous (stiə'tojənəs) producing fat; lipogenic.
steatolysis (stiə'tolisis) the emulsification of fats preparatory to absorption. adj. **steatolytic.**
steatoma (stiə'tohmə) pl. *steatomata, steatomas.* 1. lipoma. 2. a fatty mass retained within a sebaceous gland.
steatomatosis (ˌstiətohmə'tohsis) the presence of numerous sebaceous cysts; steatocystoma multiplex.
steatonecrosis (ˌstiətohnə'krohsis) fat necrosis.
steatopathy (stiə'topəthee) disease of the sebaceous glands.
steatopygia (ˌstiətoh'piji·ə) excessive fatness of the buttocks. adj. **steatopygous.**
steatorrhoea (ˌstiətə'reeə) excess fat in the faeces due to a malabsorption syndrome caused by disease of the intestinal mucosa (e.g., sprue) or pancreatic enzyme deficiency.
steatosis (stiə'tohsis) fatty degeneration.
Steele–Richardson–Olszewski syndrome (ˌsteel-ˌrichədsənol'zooskee) a progressive neurological disorder, having an onset during the sixth decade, characterized by supranuclear ophthalmoplegia, especially paralysis of the downward gaze, pseudobulbar palsy, dysarthria, dystonic rigidity of the neck and trunk, and dementia.
stegnosis (steg'nohsis) constriction; stenosis.
Stein–Leventhal syndrome (ˌstien'levənthal) oligomenorrhoea or amenorrhoea, anovulation, and hirsutism associated with bilateral polycystic ovaries, but normal excretion of follicle-stimulating hormone and 17-ketosteroids.
Steinert's disease ('stienərts) myotonia dystrophica.
Steinmann extension ('stienmən) extension exerted on a limb, e.g. in a fractured limb by means of a nail or pin (Steinmann pin) driven into the bone distal to the fractured bone. Called also *nail extension.*
Steinmann pin ('stienmən) a pin to which a weight can be attached by way of a stirrup for extension of a bone. See also STEINMANN EXTENSION.
Stelazine ('steləˌzeen) trademark for preparations of trifluoperazine hydrochloride, a neuroleptic.
stella ('stelə) pl. *stellae* [L.] star.
stellate ('stelayt) star-shaped; arranged in rosettes.
s. ganglion cervicothoracic ganglion.
stellectomy (ste'lektəmee) excision of a portion of the stellate (cervicothoracic) ganglion.
Stellwag's sign ('stelvahgz) a 'widening' of the eyes with infrequent blinking, as may occur in exophthalmos.
stem (stem) stalk; a stalklike supporting structure.
brain s. the stemlike portion of the brain connecting the cerebral hemispheres with the spinal cord, and comprising the pons, medulla oblongata, and midbrain; considered by some to include the diencephalon. See also under BRAIN.
s. cells see under CELL.
Stemetil ('stemətil) trademark for preparations of prochlorperazine, a major tranquillizer and antiemetic.
steno- word element. [Gr.] *narrow, contracted, constriction.*
stenocardia (ˌstenoh'kahdi·ə) angina pectoris.
stenocephaly (ˌstenoh'kefəlee, -'sef-) narrowness of the head or cranium. adj. **stenocephalous.**
stenochoria (ˌstenoh'kor·ri·ə) stenosis.
stenocoriasis (ˌstenohkə'rieəsis) contraction of the pupil.
stenopeic (ˌstenoh'pee·ik) having a narrow opening or slit.
stenosed (stə'nohzd) narrowed; constricted.
stenosis (stə'nohsis) narrowing or contraction of a body passage or opening.
aortic s. obstruction to the outflow of blood from the left ventricle into the aorta.
idiopathic hypertrophic subaortic s. a cardiomyopathy of unknown cause, in which the left ventricle is hypertrophied and the cavity is small; it is marked by obstruction to left ventricular outflow.
mitral s. a narrowing of the left atrioventricular orifice. See also mitral COMMISSUROTOMY.
pulmonary s. narrowing of the opening between the pulmonary artery and the right ventricle.
pyloric s. obstruction of the pyloric orifice of the stomach (see also PYLORIC STENOSIS).
tricuspid s. narrowing or stricture of the tricuspid orifice of the heart.
stenostomia (ˌstenoh'stohmi·ə) narrowing of the mouth.
stenothermal, stenothermic (ˌstenoh'thərməl; ˌstenoh'thərmik) pertaining to or characterized by tolerance of only a narrow range of temperature.
stenothorax (ˌstenoh'thor·raks) abnormal narrowness of the chest.
stenotic (stə'notik) marked by abnormal narrowing or constriction.
Stensen's duct ('stensənz) the duct of the parotid gland, opening into the mouth opposite the second upper molar.
stent (stent) a mould used in dentistry and for keeping a skin graft in place.
sterco- word element. [L.] *faeces.*
stercobilin (ˌstərkoh'bielin) a bile pigment derivative formed by air oxidation of stercobilinogen; it is a brown–orange–red pigmentation contributing to the colour of faeces and urine.
stercobilinogen (ˌstərkohbie'linəjən) a bilirubin metabolite and precursor of stercobilin, formed by reduction of urobilinogen.
stercolith ('stərkohˌlith) a hard mass of faeces in the bowel. Called also a *faecalith.*
stercoraceous (ˌstərkə'rayshəs) faecal, or containing faeces.
s. vomit vomit containing faeces; caused by an overflow of faeces into the stomach due to intestinal obstruction.
stercorolith ('stərkə·rohˌlith) faecalith; an intestinal concretion formed around a centre of faecal matter.
stercoroma (ˌstərkə'rohmə) a tumour-like mass of faecal matter in the rectum; faecaloma.
sterculia gum (stər'kyooli·ə) karaya gum.
stercus ('stərkəs) [L.] *dung, faeces.* adj. **stercoral, stercorous.**
stereo- word element. [Gr.] *solid, firm, three dimensional.*
stereoarthrolysis (ˌsterioh·ah'throlisis, ˌstiə-) surgical formation of a movable new joint in cases of bony ankylosis.
stereoauscultation (ˌsteriohˌawskəl'tayshən, ˌstiə-) auscultation with two stethoscopes, on different parts of the chest.
stereocampimeter (ˌsteriohkam'pimitə, ˌstiə-) an instrument for studying unilateral central scotomas and central retinal defects.
stereochemistry (ˌsterioh'kemistree, ˌstiə-) the branch of chemistry treating of the space relations of atoms in molecules. adj. **stereochemical.**
stereocinefluorography (ˌsteriohˌsiniˌflooə'rogrəfee, ˌstiə-) recording by motion picture camera of images observed by steroscopic fluoroscopy, affording three-dimensional visualization.
stereoencephalotomy (ˌsterioh·enˌkefə'lotəmee, ˌstiə-, -ˌsef-) stereotaxic surgery.

stereognosis (ˌsteriog'nohsis, ˌstiə-) the sense by which the form of objects is perceived. adj. **stereognostic**.

stereoisomer (ˌsterioh'iesəmə, ˌstiə-) a compound showing stereoisomerism.

stereoisomerism (ˌsterioh·ie'somaˌrizəm, ˌstiə-) isomerism in which the compounds have the same structural formulae, but the atoms are distributed differently in space. adj. **stereoisomeric**.

stereoradiography (ˌsterioh'raydi'ografee, ˌstiə-) the making of a stereoscopic radiograph.

stereoscope ('sterioh,skohp, ˌstiə-) an instrument for producing the appearance of solidity and relief by combining the images of two similar pictures of an object.

stereoscopic (ˌsterioh'skopik, ˌstiə-) three-dimensional; having depth, as well as height and width.

stereospecific (ˌsteriohspə'sifik, ˌstiə-) pertaining to enzymes that interact only with substrates of very specific structure.

stereotactic, stereotaxic (ˌsterioh'taktik, ˌstiə-; ˌsterioh'taksik, stiə-) pertaining to or characterized by precise positioning in space; said especially of discrete areas of the brain that control specific functions.

s. surgery the production of sharply localized lesions in the brain after precise localization of the target tissue by use of three-dimensional coordinates.

stereotaxis, stereotropism (ˌsterioh'taksis, ˌstiə-; ˌsterioh'tropizəm, ˌstiə-) 1. movement or growth in response to contact with a solid or rigid surface. 2. a technique for locating structures in the brain.

stereotypy ('sterioh,tiepee, 'stiə-) persistent repetition of senseless acts or words. It may be a persistent maintaining of a bodily attitude (stereotypy of attitude), repetition of senseless movements (stereotypy of movement), or constant repetition of certain words or phrases (stereotypy of speech).

sterilant ('sterilənt) a sterilizing agent, i.e., an agent that destroys microorganisms.

sterile ('steriel) 1. not fertile; barren; not producing young. See also FERTILITY. 2. aseptic; not producing microorganisms; free from living microorganisms.

sterility (stə'rilətee) the state of being sterile.

sterilization (ˌsterilie'zayshən) 1. the process of rendering an individual incapable of reproduction, by castration, vasectomy, salpingectomy, or other procedure (see below). 2. the process of destroying or removing all living microorganisms. This is accomplished by heat (wet steam under pressure or dry heat) or by bactericidal chemical compounds. See Appendix 9 for further details. In sterilizing objects or substances, the high resistance of bacterial spore cells must be taken into account. Most dangerous bacteria are destroyed at a temperature of 50 to 60 °C (122 to 140 °F). Therefore, pasteurization of a fluid, which is the application of heat at about 60 °C, destroys most disease-causing bacteria. However, temperatures almost twice as high are usually required to destroy the spore cells. The discovery that heat, in the form of flame, steam, or hot water, kills bacteria made possible the advances of modern surgery, which is based on freedom from microorganisms, or asepsis, and prevention of contamination. Sterilization of all equipment used during an operation, and of anything that in any way may touch the operative area, is carried out scrupulously in hospitals. Doctors and nurses wear sterile clothing. Instruments are sterilized by autoclaving or by chemical antiseptics.

culdoscopic s. use of an endoscope to visualize the uterine tubes for the purpose of preventing conception. The endoscope is inserted through an incision in the vaginal wall behind the cervix. After the uterine tubes are located each tube is drawn out through the vaginal incision and severed. The major advantage of this procedure is that it can be done on an outpatient basis. A disadvantage is the complication of infection, a very real possibility owing to the unsterile nature of the vagina.

hysteroscopic s. use of an endoscopic instrument to visualize the interior of the uterus and uterine tubes for the purpose of preventing conception. The hysteroscope is inserted through the dilated cervix and on through the uterine cavity to the point at which each tube joins the uterus. A cautery is then used to electrocoagulate each tube. Occlusion of the tubes is accomplished by scar tissue that forms at the sites of cauterization.

laparoscopic s. that which employs an endoscope to visualize the uterine tubes and surrounding structures for the purpose of occluding the tubes. The instrument is guided into the abdominal cavity through a small puncture made by a trochar inserted immediately below the umbilicus. A second small puncture is made in the lower abdomen through which cautery forceps are inserted. The forceps are applied approximately 2 cm from the point at which each of the tubes joins the uterus. In this way each tube is electrocoagulated and severed. An alternative to cauterization and severance of the tubes is the application of clips. However, there is the possibility that the clips may not completely occlude the tubes, allowing passage of the ovum and impregnation.

sterilize ('steri,liez) to subject to sterilization.

sterilizer ('steri,liezə) an apparatus used in ridding instruments, dressings, etc., of all living microorganisms. See also AUTOCLAVE.

Sterispon ('sterispon) trademark for preparations of absorbable gelatin sponge, used as a local haemostatic.

stern(o)- word element. [L., Gr.] *sternum*.

sternal ('stərnəl) pertaining to the sternum.

s. puncture insertion of a hollow needle into the manubrium of the sternum for the purpose of obtaining a sample of bone marrow. The sternum is chosen because of its accessibility and because it is a thin, flat bone. The procedure must be done under surgical asepsis. The doctor anaesthetizes the skin and periosteum with 1 per cent procaine hydrochloride before introducing the sternal needle. The needle is designed with a special guard to prevent penetration beyond the desired depth. When the cells are being aspirated into the syringe the patient may experience a sharp pain.

The bone marrow samplings are examined for the presence of abnormal cells for the proportion of cells in their various stages of development and for the characteristics of the blood cells that predominate. This information is used in conjunction with clinical findings and other tests in the diagnosis of blood disorders such as the leukaemias and anaemia.

sternalgia (stər'nalji·ə) pain in the sternum.

Sternberg's giant cells ('stərnbərgz) Sternberg–Reed cells.

Sternberg–Reed cells (ˌstərnbərg'reed) enlarged, atypical histiocytes with multiple or hyperlobulated nucleoli; a characteristic feature of Hodgkin's disease.

sterno- word element. [L., Gr.] *sternum*.

sternoclavicular (ˌstərnohklə'vikyuhlə) pertaining to the sternum and clavicle.

sternocleidomastoid (ˌstərnoh,kliedoh'mastoyd) pertaining to the sternum, clavicle, and mastoid process.

sternocostal (ˌstərnoh'kost'l) pertaining to the sternum and ribs.

sternodymia (ˌstərnoh'dimi·ə) union of two fetuses by the anterior chest wall.

sternodymus (stər'nodiməs) conjoined twins united at the anterior chest wall.
sternohyoid (ˌstərnoh'hieoyd) pertaining to the sternum and hyoid bone.
sternoid ('stərnoyd) resembling the sternum.
sternomastoid (ˌstərnoh'mastoyd) pertaining to the sternum and the mastoid process of the temporal bone.
sternopericardial (ˌstərnohˌperi'kahdi·əl) pertaining to the sternum and pericardium.
sternoschisis (stər'noskisis) congenital fissure of the sternum.
sternothyroid (ˌstərnoh'thieroyd) pertaining to the sternum and thyroid cartilage or gland.
sternotomy (stər'notəmee) incision of the sternum.
sternum ('stərnəm) a plate of bone forming the middle of the anterior wall of the thorax and articulating with the clavicles and the cartilages of the first seven ribs. It consists of three parts, the manubrium, the body, and the xiphoid process.
sternutator ('stərnyuhˌtaytə) a substance which causes wheezing.
sternutatory (ˌstərnyuh'taytə·ree) 1. causing sneezing. 2. an agent that causes sneezing.
steroid ('steroyd, 'stiə-) a complex molecule containing carbon atoms in four interlocking rings forming a hydrogenated cyclopentophenanthrene-ring system; three of the rings contain six carbon atoms each and the fourth contains five. See accompanying illustration.

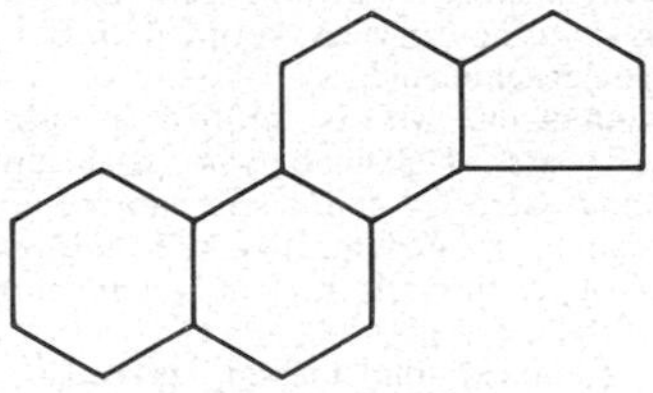

Cyclopentophenanthrene ring

Steroids are important in body chemistry. Among them are the male and female sex hormones, such as testosterone and oestrogen, and the hormones of the cortices of the adrenal glands, including cortisone. Vitamins of the D group are steroids involved in calcium metabolism. The cardiac glycosides, a group of compounds derived from certain plants, are partly steroids. Sterols, including cholesterol, are steroids. Cholesterol is the main building block of steroid hormones in the body; it is also converted into bile salts by the liver.

anabolic s. any of a group of synthetic derivatives of testosterone, having pronounced anabolic properties and relatively weak androgenic properties, which are used clinically mainly to promote growth and repair of body tissues in senility, debilitating illness, and convalescence.

s. purpura subcutaneous, blotchy, haemorrhagic staining of the back of the hands, forearms or shins caused by thinning and weakening of dermal and vascular connective tissue by longterm treatment with adrenocortical steroid hormones.

steroidogenesis (steˌroydoh'jenəsis) production of steroids, as by the adrenal glands.
sterol ('sterol, 'stiə·rol) any steroid, e.g., cholesterol and ergosterol, having long (8 to 10 carbons) aliphatic side-chains at position 17 and at least one alcoholic hydroxyl group; the sterols have lipid-like solubility.
stertor ('stərtə) snoring; sonorous respiration, usually due to partial obstruction of the upper airway. adj. **stertorous.**
steth(o)- word element. [Gr.] *chest.*
stethalgia (ste'thalji·ə) pain in the chest or chest wall.
stethogoniometer (ˌstethohˌgohni'omitə) an apparatus for measuring the curvature of the chest.
stethometer (ste'thomitə) an instrument for measuring the expansion of the chest.
stethoscope ('stethəˌskohp) an instrument used to hear and amplify the sounds produced by the heart, lungs and other internal organs. adj. **stethoscopic.** As first introduced by the 19th century French physician, René Laënnec, the stethoscope was a simple wooden tube with a bell-shaped opening at one end. The modern stethoscope is binaural, with two earpieces and flexible tubing leading to them from the two-branched opening of the bell or cone. In this way, sound travels simultaneously through both of the branches to the earpieces.

Pinard's s. a specially designed stethoscope for listening to the fetal heartbeat, called also *fetal* or *monoaural s.*

stethospasm ('stethohˌspazəm) spasm of the chest muscles.
Stevens–Johnson syndrome (ˌsteevənz'jonsən) a severe form of erythema multiforme in which the lesions may involve the oral and anogenital mucosa, eyes, and viscera, associated with such constitutional symptoms as malaise, headache, fever, arthralgia, and conjunctivitis.
STH somatotrophic (growth) hormone.
sthenia ('stheeni·ə) a condition of abnormally great strength and activity.
sthenic ('sthenik) active; strong.
stibialism ('stibi·əˌlizəm) antimony poisoning.
stibium ('stibi·əm) [L.] *antimony;* (symbol Sb).
stibogluconate (stiboh'glookəˌnayt) an antimony compound used in the treatment of leishmaniasis.
stibophen ('stibohˌfen) a sodium salt of antimony formerly given intramuscularly in the treatment of schistosomiasis.
stichochrome ('stikohˌkrohm) any neuron having the stainable substance arranged in more or less regular layers.
Stieda's fracture ('steedəz) fracture of the internal condyle of the femur.
stiff-man syndrome ('stifman) a condition of unknown aetiology marked by progressive fluctuating rigidity of axial and limb muscles in the absence of signs of cerebral and spinal cord disease but with continuous electromyographic activity.
stigma ('stigmə) pl. *stigmas,stigmata* [Gr.] 1. any mental or physical mark or peculiarity that aids in identification or diagnosis of a condition. 2. *stigmata,* purpuric or haemorrhagic lesions of the hands and/or feet, that resembles crucifixion wounds. adj. **stigmatic.**
stigmatization (ˌstigmətie'zayshən) the formation of stigmas.
stilboestrol (stil'beestrol) a synthetic oestrogen preparation used in the treatment of cancer of the prostate and sometimes of postmenopausal breast cancer.
Still's disease (stilz) See juvenile chronic ARTHRITIS.
Still's murmur a functional cardiac murmur of childhood, heard in midsystole.
stillbirth ('stilˌbərth) a baby delivered after the 28th week of pregnancy which did not, at any time after being completely expelled fron its mother, breathe or show any sign of life. adj. **stillborn.**
stimulant ('stimyuhlənt) 1. producing stimulation. 2. an agent that stimulates.

stimulate ('stimyuh,layt) to excite functional activity in a part.

stimulation (,stimyuh'layshən) the act or process of stimulating; the condition of being stimulated.

stimulus ('stimyuhləs) pl. *stimuli* [L.] any agent, act, or influence that produces functional or trophic reaction in a receptor or an irritable tissue.

conditioned s. a neutral object or event that is psychologically related to a naturally stimulating object or event and which causes a CONDITIONED RESPONSE (see also CONDITIONING).

discriminative s. a stimulus associated with reinforcement, which exerts control over a particular form of behaviour; the subject discriminates between closely related stimuli and responds positively only in the presence of that stimulus.

eliciting s. any stimulus, conditioned or unconditioned, which elicits a response.

structured s. a well-organized and unambiguous stimulus, the perception of which is influenced to a greater extent by the characteristics of the stimulus than by those of the perceiver.

threshold s. a stimulus that is just strong enough to elicit a response.

unconditioned s. any stimulus that is capable of eliciting an unconditioned response (see also CONDITIONING).

unstructured s. an unclear or ambiguous stimulus, the perception of which is influenced to a greater extent by the characteristics of the perceiver than by those of the stimulus.

sting (sting) 1. injury caused by a poisonous substance produced by an animal or plant (biotoxin) introduced into an individual or with which he comes in contact, together with mechanical trauma incident to its introduction. See also INSECT BITES AND STINGS. 2. the organ used to inflict such injury.

stippling ('stipling) a spotted condition or appearance, such as an appearance of the retina as if dotted with light and dark points, or the spotted appearance of the erythrocytes in basophilia.

stirrup ('stirəp) the stapes, the innermost of the three ossicles of the ear.

stitch (stich) 1. a sudden transient cutting pain, generally in the flank. 2. a loop made in sewing or suturing.

StJAA St. John Ambulance Association.

StJAB St. John Ambulance Brigade.

stochastic (sto'kastik) arrived at by skilful conjecturing.

stoichiology (,stoyki'oləjee) the science of elements, especially the physiology of the cellular elements of tissues. adj. **stoichiological**.

stoichiometry (,stoyki'omətree) the determination of the relative proportions of the compounds involved in a chemical reaction. adj. **stoichiometric**.

stoke (stohk) a unit of kinematic viscosity, that of a fluid with a dynamic viscosity of 1 poise and a density of 1 gram per cubic centimetre. Abbreviated St.

Stokes–Adams disease (,stohks'adəmz) a condition due to heart block and marked by sudden attacks of unconsciousness, with or without convulsions; called also Adams–Stokes disease or syndrome.

Stokes' disease (stohks) Graves' disease.

stoma ('stohmə) pl. *stomas,stomata* [Gr.] an artificial orifice, either temporary or permanent, from the gastrointestinal, urinary or upper respiratory tracts. adj. **stomal**.

PATIENT CARE. Care of the patient with a stoma, for whatever reason it may have been created, is primarily concerned with developing in the patient an attitude of independence and freedom from restrictions on his physical, social, and recreational activities once he has been discharged from the hospital.

He will need instruction in obtaining and caring for the special appliance that is worn for the collection of body waste, faecal or urinary. Protection of the skin around the stoma is of particular concern, as is the control of odour and regulation of the flow of faeces and urine. He must be aware of the complications that may develop and the signs and symptoms that should be reported to his doctor.

In recent years there has been a new health care speciality developing to meet the particular needs of patients with stomas. Ostomy clubs composed of stoma patients and often conducted under the guidance of stoma care nurses (see below) have been formed in many communities. At regularly held meetings the members find assistance in resolving their physical problems, and gain psychological support from one another in adjusting to their new body image. Those members of the club who have been able to adjust to their stomas are frequently available for visits to patients who are in the hospital or have just returned home after surgery.

Information about local resources available to the stoma patient can be obtained from the Colostomy Welfare Group, 38–39 Ecclestone Square, London SW1V 1PB; also from the Colostomy/Ileostomy Advisory Service, Saltair House, Lord Street, Nechells, Birmingham B7 4DS, which has a number of branches in the UK; and from other agencies concerned with meeting the needs of patients with stomas, providing visiting services, printed material, and audio-visual teaching aids.

s. care nurse one who is certified to assist in the specialized care of patients who have undergone enterostomy. Certified stoma care nurses in a community can be located through the addresses mentioned above, or through the family general practitioner.

stomach ('stumək) the curved, muscular, saclike structure that is an enlargement of the alimentary canal between the oesophagus and the small intestine; called also *gaster*.

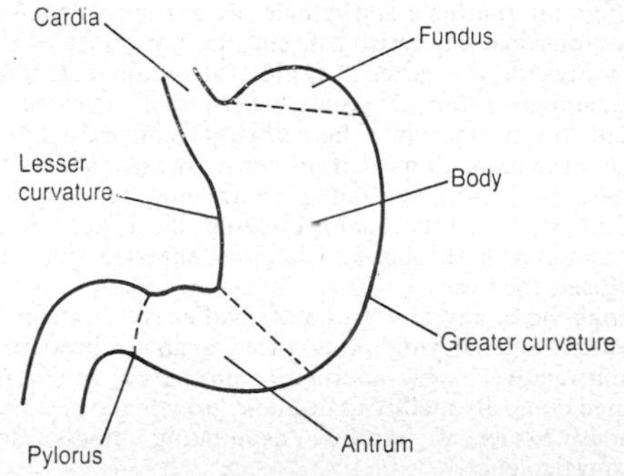

Parts of the stomach

The wall of the stomach consists of four coats: an outer serous coat; a muscular coat, made up of longitudinal, circular, and oblique muscle fibres; a submucous coat; and a mucous coat or membrane forming the inner lining. The muscles account for the stomach's ability to expand when food enters it. The muscle fibres slide over one another, reducing the thickness of the stomach wall while increasing its area. When empty, the stomach has practically no cavity at all, since its walls are pressed tightly together. When full, the average stomach holds about 1.7 litres.

The stomach muscles perform another function. When food enters the stomach, the muscles contract in rhythm. Their combined action sends a series of wavelike contractions from the upper end of the stomach to the lower end. These contractions, known as peristalsis, mix the partially digested food with the stomach secretions and ingested liquid until it has the consistency of a thick soup called *chyme;* the contractions then push it into the small intestine.

The stomach is emptied of its digested contents in 1 to 4 hours, or longer, depending upon the amount and type of food eaten. Foods rich in carbohydrates leave the stomach more rapidly than proteins, and proteins more rapidly than fats.

The stomach may continue to contract after it is empty. The contraction of the empty stomach stimulates nerves in its wall and may cause hunger pangs.

The mucous membrane lining the stomach contains innumerable gastric glands; their secretion, known as gastric juice, contains enzymes, mucin, and hydrochloric acid. Enzymes help to split the food molecules into smaller parts during digestion. Mucin acts on certain sugars and also protects the mucous lining of the stomach from coarse particles and from the corrosive hydrochloric acid. Hydrochloric acid aids in dissolving the food before the enzymes begin working on it. See also DIGESTIVE SYSTEM.

DISORDERS OF THE STOMACH. Disturbances in the functioning of the stomach include indigestion and nausea; organic diseases include peptic ULCER and cancer.

Care given to establishing good eating habits will help to prevent stomach distress. Food should be wholesome, well prepared, and properly cooked. Heavy, fried and fatty foods, highly spiced food, too much roughage, and foods to which one has shown a sensitivity should be avoided. When nervous tension and anxiety are the underlying cause of a stomach disorder, an effort should be made to resolve the basic problems causing emotional distress.

The diagnosis and treatment of stomach disorders has changed considerably with the development of endoscopy. This procedure permits direct examination and biopsy of the stomach, thereby increasing the accuracy of diagnosis and treatment. Surgery of the stomach has become increasingly conservative with a greater understanding of the organ's physiology. Such procedures as VAGOTOMY which reduces acid secretion, and the introduction of new medications that also reduce gastric acid secretion and increase gastric motility, have overall decreased the need for surgery for peptic ulcer disease.

Two common forms of gastric discomfort are belching (eructation) and heartburn. Usually belching results from swallowing air while eating, and heartburn, a burning sensation below the sternum, is thought to be caused by distention of the lower part of the oesophagus, possibly from gulping food or from other faulty eating habits. Both may be associated with peptic ulcer or hiatus hernia.

GASTRITIS, inflammation of the lining of the stomach, is a common disorder. It may be acute, chronic, or toxic.

SURGERY OF THE STOMACH. Surgical procedures of the stomach are most often done as treatment for malignant disease or for chronic ulcers that are complicated by haemorrhage or perforation. Surgical removal of the whole stomach is called total gastrectomy; excision of a portion of it is called subtotal or partial gastrectomy. When partial gastrectomy is done, the remaining portion of the stomach is anastomosed to a loop of intestine (gastroenterostomy), usually of the jejunum (gastrojejunostomy). This is done to maintain continuity of the digestive tract. When total gastrectomy is performed, continuity is restored by an anastomosis between the end of the oesophagus and the jejunum.

Another surgical procedure involving the stomach is GASTROSTOMY. This is a surgical incision into the stomach with the creation of a permanent opening to the surface of the body. Its purpose is the administration of feedings and fluids when strictures or obstruction of the oesophagus makes swallowing impossible.

PATIENT CARE. Unless there is an emergency situation such as haemorrhage, the patient who is to undergo gastric surgery will have several diagnostic tests before the operation, including GASTRIC ANALYSIS, a gastrointestinal series of x-rays (see BARIUM TEST), and GASTROSCOPY.

Before the operation a Ryles tube may be inserted and aspiration is used to remove gastric secretions and prevent distention. For other routine preoperative procedures, see PREOPERATIVE CARE.

Routine POSTOPERATIVE CARE, including observations of the patient and prevention of complications, is discussed under that heading. Immediately after surgery the patient who has undergone gastric surgery should be checked for tubes and drains that may have been inserted. In most instances the Ryles tube will be left in place and aspiration resumed after surgery. Drainage from this tube will be dark brown at first and may be streaked with bright red blood. The colour should gradually become lighter until it is a greenish yellow and the appearance of flecks or streaks of blood should diminish. If there is continued evidence of fresh bleeding the surgeon should be notified at once.

Fluids by mouth are restricted until peristalsis resumes and the nasogastric tube is removed. Irrigation of the tube may be done as ordered to assure proper drainage. The irrigations should be done gently and only as frequently as ordered because continuous washing can lead to excessive removal of electrolytes from the stomach. Mouth care and care of the nostrils are necessary as long as the tube is in place. Fluids are given intravenously until the patient is able to retain liquids and food by mouth.

After the tube is removed the surgeon will give instructions regarding liquids and foods permitted. Usually a very small amount of water is given at hourly intervals and the amount increased according to the patient's tolerance. Later, bland liquids and foods are added until the patient has progressed to a full diet. The hospital dietitian usually works closely with the patient in planning his diet so that when he returns home he will have well balanced meals that can be tolerated without difficulty.

Before the patient is discharged from the hospital he may be scheduled for another series of x-rays of the upper intestinal tract. This is done to observe the continuity of the digestive tract and to be sure it is functioning satisfactorily. A group of symptoms known as the 'dumping syndrome' sometimes develops after gastrectomy. They are the result of rapid emptying of gastric contents into the small intestine. These symptoms usually are mild and include palpitation, a feeling of weakness or fainting, and sweating; they may last for a few minutes or for as long as an hour. It is believed that meals high in carbohydrates and salt trigger the dumping syndrome because these substances must be diluted in the small intestine before they can be absorbed. To provide for this dilution, the jejunal loop becomes distended and fills with fluids that have shifted from the circulating blood. The symptoms produced by this condition can be relieved somewhat by limiting the intake of salt and carbohydrates and by restricting the amount of liquids taken with each meal.

When the stomach has been removed, the production of intrinsic factor, necessary for the absorption of vitamin B_{12} from the intestinal tract, is brought to a halt. Following the depletion of the reserve of B_{12}, which is stored in the liver, this condition must be corrected by monthly injections of vitamin B_{12} for the rest of the patient's life.

cascade s. an atypical form of hourglass stomach, characterized on x-ray by a drawing up of the posterior wall; an opaque medium first fills the upper sac and then cascades into the lower sac.

hourglass s. one shaped somewhat like an hourglass.

leather bottle s. linitis plastica.

s. pump an apparatus used to remove material from the stomach. It consists of a rubber stomach tube to which a bulb syringe is attached. The tube is inserted into the mouth or nose and passed down the oesophagus into the stomach. Suction from the syringe brings the contents of the stomach up through the tube.

A stomach pump can be used either to remove material from the stomach in case of emergency—for example, when a person has swallowed poison—or to obtain a specimen for chemical analysis, as in diagnosis of peptic ulcer or other stomach disorders.

s. tube a flexible tube used for introducing food, medication, or other material directly into the stomach. It can be passed into the stomach by way of either the nose or the mouth. See also TUBE FEEDING.

A stomach tube may be employed in emergency feeding, during coma, or when patients refuse food. It is also used to dilute the contents of the stomach when a person has swallowed poison or to lavage the stomach before the contents are pumped out. Stomach tubes are also inserted to decompress the stomach when it becomes abnormally distended after certain abdominal operations.

water-trap s. a stomach with an extremely high pylorus, so that it does not readily empty itself.

stomachal ('stuməkəl) pertaining to the stomach; stomachic.

stomachalgia (,stumə'kalji·ə) pain in the stomach.

stomachic (stə'məkik) 1. pertaining to the stomach. 2. a stimulant of gastric activity.

stomat(o)- word element. [Gr.] *mouth*.

stomatalgia (,stohmə'talji·ə) pain in the mouth.

stomatitis (,stohmə'tietis) inflammation of the mucosa of the mouth. It may be caused by one of many diseases of the mouth or it may accompany another disease. Both gingivitis (inflammation of the gums) and glossitis (inflammation of the tongue) are forms of stomatitis.

CAUSES. The causes of stomatitis vary widely, from a mild local irritant to a vitamin deficiency or infection by possibly dangerous disease-producing organisms.

Inflammation may arise from actual injury to the inside of the mouth, as from cheek-biting, jagged teeth, tartar accumulations, and badly fitting dentures. Irritating substances, including alcohol, tobacco, and excessively hot or spicy food, may also cause stomatitis.

Other causes may be infectious bacteria, such as streptococci and gonococci or those causing TRENCH MOUTH, diphtheria, and tuberculosis; the fungus causing THRUSH; or the viruses causing herpes simplex and measles. Extreme vitamin deficiencies can result in mouth inflammation, as can certain blood disorders. Poisoning with heavy metals, such as lead or mercury, can cause stomatitis.

SYMPTOMS. There is generally swelling and redness of the tissues of the mouth, which may become quite sore, particularly during eating. The mouth may have an unpleasant odour. In some types of stomatitis the mouth becomes dry, but in others there is excessive salivation. Ulcerations may appear, and, in extreme cases, gangrene (gangrenous stomatitis).

Other forms of stomatitis may occasionally cause more severe symptoms, including chills, fever, and headache. Sometimes bleeding or white patches in the mouth can be seen. In thrush, the symptoms themselves may be slight (white spots in the mouth resembling milk clots) but the disease may give rise to serious infections elsewhere in the body. In some cases, stomatitis causes inflammation of the parotid glands.

Stomatitis resulting from certain diseases presents special identifying symptoms. Syphilitic stomatitis produces patches in the mouth; in scarlet fever the tongue first has a strawberry colour, which then deepens to a raspberry hue; in measles, Koplik's spots appear.

TREATMENT AND PREVENTION. The treatment varies according to the cause. When the inflammation is caused by anaemia, vitamin deficiency, or any infection of the body, both the underlying disease and the stomatitis are treated.

Appropriate antibiotics often are effective against the inflammation and prevent its spreading to the parotid glands. Mouthwashes may be used under a doctor's direction after he has determined the cause of the stomatitis. Gentian violet solution may be applied to the lesions of thrush; other forms of stomatitis may be swabbed with sodium bicarbonate, sodium perborate solution, or hydrogen peroxide.

With proper care, many cases of stomatitis can be prevented. Cleanliness is essential, especially of the mouth, teeth, dentures, and feeding utensils. Infants may acquire mouth infection from dirty bottles or from the mother's nipples. In the case of a prolonged fever or of any severe general illness, dryness of the mouth should be avoided by ingestion of increased amounts of fluids, particularly fruit juices.

angular s. superficial erosions and fissuring at the angles of the mouth; it may occur in riboflavin deficiency and in pellagra or result from overclosure of the jaws in denture wearers. Called also *perlèche*.

aphthous s. an acute infection of the oral mucosa caused by the virus of herpes simplex, with vesicle formation; called also canker sore.

gangrenous s. see NOMA.

herpetic s. an acute infection of the oral mucosa with vesicle formation, due to the herpes simplex virus.

necrotizing ulcerative s. necrotizing ulcerative gingivostomatitis.

stomatodynia (,stohmətoh'dini·ə) pain in the mouth.

stomatogastric (,stohmətoh'gastrik) pertaining to the stomach and mouth.

stomatognathic (,stomətoh'nathik) denoting the mouth and jaws collectively.

stomatology (,stohmə'toləjee) that branch of medicine which treats of the mouth and its diseases. adj. **stomatological**.

stomatomalacia (,stohmətohmə'layshiə) softening of the structures of the mouth.

stomatomenia (,stohmətoh'meeni·ə) the phenomenon of bleeding from the mucous membrance of the mouth when menstruation occurs.

stomatomycosis (,stohmətohmie'kohsis) any fungal

disease of the mouth.

stomatonecrosis, stomatonoma, stomatitis gangrenosa (ˌstohmətohnəˈkrohsis; ˌstohmətəˈnohmə) gangrene of the mouth; see NOMA.

stomatopathy (ˌstohməˈtopəthee) any disorder of the mouth.

stomatoplasty (ˈstomətohˌplastee) plastic reconstruction of the mouth. adj. **stomatoplastic.**

stomatorrhagia (ˌstohmətəˈrayji·ə) haemorrhage from the mouth.

stomocephalus (ˌstohmohˈkefələs, -ˈsef-) a fetus with rudimentary jaws and mouth.

stomodeum (ˌstohməˈdeeəm, ˈstom-) the ectodermal depression at the head end of the embryo, which becomes the front part of the mouth.

-stomy word element. [Gr.] *creation of an opening into;* or *a communication between.*

stone (stohn) 1. a calculus. 2. a unit of weight, equivalent to 14 lb (6.35 kg).

stool (stool) the faecal discharge from the bowels (see also FAECES).

lienteric s. faeces containing much undigested food.

rice water s. the watery stool flecked with fragments of necrotic mucosal epithelium, characteristic of cholera.

silver s. stools having the colour of aluminium or silver paint, due to a mixture of melaena and white fatty stools; it occurs in tropical sprue and carcinoma of the ampulla of Vater, and in children with diarrhoea taking sulphonamides.

stopcock (ˈstopˌkok) a valve that regulates the flow of fluid through a tube.

storage disease (ˈstor·rij) any metabolic disorder in which some substance (e.g., fats, proteins, or carbohydrates) accumulates in certain cells in abnormal amounts; called also *thesaurismosis.*

storage pool disease a blood coagulation disorder due to failure of the platelets to release ADP in response to aggregating agents (collagen, adrenaline, exogenous ADP, thrombin, etc.); characterized by mild bleeding episodes, prolonged bleeding time, and reduced aggregation response to collagen or thrombin.

storiform (ˈstor·riˌfawm) denoting a matted, irregularly whorled pattern, somewhat resembling that of a straw mat; said of a microscopic appearance in malignant fibrous histiocytomas.

stosstherapy (ˈstosˌtherəpee) treatment of a disease by a single massive dose of therapeutic agent or short-term administration of unphysiologically large doses.

STPD standard temperature and pressure, dry; denoting a volume of dry gas at 0 °C and a pressure of 760 mmHg.

strabismus (strəˈbizməs) deviation of the eye that the patient cannot overcome; the visual axes assume a position relative to each other different from that required by the physiological conditions; called also *squint* and HETEROTROPIA. adj. **strabismic.**

The various forms of strabismus may be referred to as tropias, their direction being indicated by the appropriate prefix, as *cyclo*tropia, *eso*tropia, *exo*tropia, *hyper*tropia, and *hypo*tropia.

For further information on the functioning of the eyes, see EYE.

concomitant s. that in which the angle of deviation of the visual axis of the squinting eye is always the same in relation to the other eye, no matter what the direction of the gaze; due to faulty insertion of the eye muscles.

convergent s. that in which the visual axes converge; esotropia.

divergent s. that in which the visual axes diverge; called also *exotropia.*

horizontal s. that in which the visual axis of the squinting eye deviates in the horizontal plane (esotropia or exotropia).

inconcomitant s. that in which the amount of deviation of the squinting eye varies according to the direction in which the eyes are turned.

vertical s. that in which the visual axis of the squinting eye deviates in the vertical plane (hypertropia or hypotropia).

strain (strayn) 1. to overexercise. 2. to filter. 3. an overstretching or overexertion of some part of the musculature. 4. excessive effort. 5. a group of organisms within a species or variety, characterized by some particular quality, as rough or smooth strains of bacteria.

strait (strayt) a narrow passage.

s's of the pelvis the pelvic inlet (*superior pelvic strait*) and pelvic outlet (*inferior pelvic strait*).

stramonium (strəˈmohni·əm) a vegetable drug containing the alkaloid hyoscyamine, which in its action resembles belladonna.

strangulated (ˈstrang·gyuhˌlaytid) congested by reason of constriction or hernial restriction, as strangulated HERNIA.

strangulation (ˌstrang·gyuhˈlayshən) 1. arrest of respiration by occlusion of the air passages. 2. impairment of the blood supply to a part by mechanical constriction of the vessels.

strangury (ˈstrang·gyuhree) slow and painful discharge of urine due to spasm of the urethra and bladder.

strap (strap) 1. a band or slip, as of adhesive plaster, used in attaching parts to each other. 2. to bind down tightly.

stratification (ˌstratifiˈkayshən) arrangement in layers.

stratiform (ˈstratiˌfawm) occurring in layers.

stratigraphy (strəˈtigrəfee) a method of body-section radiology.

stratum (ˈstrahtəm, ˈstray-) pl. *strata* [L.] a sheetlike mass of tissue of fairly uniform thickness; used in anatomical nomenclature to designate distinct layers making up various tissues or organs, as of the skin, brain, retina.

s. corneum the outer horny layer of the epidermis, consisting of cells that are dead and desquamating.

s. germinativum 1. the basal layer and the prickle-cell layer of the skin considered together; called also malpighian layer. 2. the lower layer of the nail, from which the nail grows. Called also *germinative layer.*

s. granulosum 1. the layer of cells between the stratum lucidum and the stratum spinosum of the skin. 2. the deep layer of the cortex of the cerebellum. 3. the layer of follicle cells lining the theca of the vesicular ovarian follicle. Called also *granular layer.*

s. lucidum the clear translucent layer of the skin, just beneath the stratum corneum.

s. spinosum the layer of the epidermis between the stratum granulosum and the stratum basalis, marked by the presence of prickle cells; called also *spinous layer* and *prickle-cell layer.*

strawberry mark (ˈstrawbree, -bəree) congenital haemangioma.

streak (streek) a line or stripe.

angioid s's red to black irregular bands in the ocular fundus running outward from the optic disc. So named because of the appearance resembling blood vessels.

primitive s. a faint white trace at the caudal end of the embryonic disc, formed by movement of cells at the onset of mesoderm formation, providing the first evidence of the embryonic axis.

strephosymbolia (ˌstrefohsimˈbohli·ə) 1. a reading difficulty inconsistent with a child's general intelligence with confusion between similar but oppositely oriented letters (b–d, p–q), and a tendency to read backward. 2. a perceptual disorder in which objects are perceived as mirror images.

strepto- word element. [Gr.] *twisted.*

Streptobacillus (ˌstreptohbəˈsiləs) a genus of gram-negative bacteria.

s. moniliformis an organism that causes Haverhill fever, a form of RATBITE FEVER.

streptobacillus (ˌstreptohbəˈsiləs) pl. *streptobacilli.* 1. a group of rod-shaped bacteria that remain loosely attached end-to-end in long chains as a result of failure of daughter cells to separate after cell division. 2. an organism of the genus *Streptobacillus.*

streptocerciasis (ˌstreptohsərˈkieəsis) infection with *Dipetalonema streptocerca,* whose microfilariae may produce a pruritic rash resembling that in onchocerciasis; transmitted by midges of the genus *Culicoides*, it occurs in West and Central Africa.

Streptococcaceae (ˌstreptohkoˈkaysi·ee) a family of gram-positive, usually nonmotile, facultative anaerobic cocci, occurring in pairs, chains, or tetrads.

streptococcaemia (ˌstreptohkokˈseemi·ə) the presence of streptococci in the blood.

streptococcal (ˌstreptohˈkokəl) pertaining to or due to a streptococcus.

s. sore throat, 'strep throat' a sore throat caused by a streptococcus. (See also SCARLET FEVER.) The symptoms are more severe than in ordinary sore throat. There may be high fever, swelling of the glands of the neck and a rash. Treatment is usually with penicillin or other antibiotics. See also RHEUMATIC FEVER.

Streptococcus (ˌstreptohˈkokəs) a genus of gram-positive, facultatively aerobic cocci (family Streptococcaceae) occurring in pairs or chains. It is separable into the pyogenic group, the viridans group, the enterococcus group, and the lactic group. The first group includes the beta-haemolytic human and animal pathogens; the second and third include alpha-haemolytic parasitic forms occurring as normal flora in the upper respiratory tract and the intestinal tract, respectively; and the fourth is made up of saprophytic forms.

S. mutans a species implicated in dental caries.

S. pneumoniae pneumococcus, the most common cause of lobar pneumonia; it also causes serious forms of meningitis, septicaemia, empyema, and peritonitis. There are some 80 serotypes distinguished by the polysaccharide hapten of the capsular substance. Called also *Diplococcus pneumoniae.*

S. pyogenes beta-haemolytic, toxigenic pyogenic streptococci causing septic sore throat, scarlet fever, rheumatic fever, puerperal fever, acute glomerulonephritis, and other conditions in man.

streptococcus (ˌstreptohˈkokəs) pl. *streptococci* [Gr.] an organism of the genus *Streptococcus.* adj. **streptococcal.**

haemolytic s. any streptococcus capable of haemolysing erythrocytes, classified as *α-haemolytic* or *viridans type*, producing a zone of greenish discoloration much smaller than the clear zone produced by the β type about the colony on blood agar; and the *β-haemolytic type*, producing a clear zone of haemolysis immediately around the colony on blood agar. The most virulent streptococci belong to the latter group. The β-haemolytic streptococci are divided into serotype groups designated by letters (e.g., Group A).

streptodornase (ˌstreptohˈdornayz) an enzyme produced by haemolytic streptococci that catalyses the depolymerization of deoxyribonucleic acid (DNA).

streptokinase (ˌstreptohˈkienayz) an enzyme produced by streptococci that catalyses the conversion of plasminogen to plasmin. Streptokinase, when administered as a thrombolytic, requires careful usage to avoid haemorrhage. It also is capable of producing severe antigenic reactions upon readministration. See also ANTICOAGULANT.

s.-streptodornase a mixture of enzymes elaborated by haemolytic streptococci; used as a proteolytic and fibrinolytic agent.

streptolysin (strepˈtolisin) the haemolysin of haemolytic streptococci.

Streptomyces (ˌstreptohˈmieseez) a genus of bacteria, usually soil forms, but occasionally parasitic on plants and animals, and notable as the source of various antibiotics, e.g., the tetracyclines.

streptomycin (ˌstreptohˈmiesin) an antibiotic substance produced by *Streptomyces griseus*, used chiefly in the treatment of tuberculosis.

streptosepticaemia (ˌstreptohˌseptiˈseemi·ə) septicaemia due to streptococci.

streptozocin (ˌstreptohˈzohsin) an antineoplastic antibiotic derived from *Streptomyces achromogenes*; used principally in the treatment of islet-cell tumours of the pancreas.

stress (stres) 1. forcibly exerted influence; pressure. 2. in dentistry, the pressure of the upper teeth against the lower. 3. the sum of the biological reactions to any adverse stimulus, physical, mental, or emotional, internal or external, that tends to disturb the homeostasis of an organism. Should these reactions be inappropriate, they may lead to disease states. The term is also used to refer to the stimuli that elicit the reactions. Just as a bridge is structurally capable of adjusting to certain physical stresses, the human body and mind are normally able to adapt to the stresses of new situations. However, this ability has definite limits beyond which continued stress may cause a breakdown, although this limit varies from person to person.

PHYSICAL STRESS. There are many kinds of physical stress, but they can be divided into two principal types, to which the body reacts in different ways. There is emergency stress, a situation that poses an immediate threat, such as a near accident in an automobile, a wound, or an injury. There is also continuing stress, such as that caused by changes in the body during puberty, pregnancy, menopause, acute and chronic diseases, and continuing exposure to excessive noise, vibration, fumes, chemicals, or other agents.

The body's reaction to emergency stress is set off by the adrenal medulla. The medulla of each adrenal gland is directly connected to the nervous system. When an emergency arises, it pours the hormone adrenaline into the bloodstream. This has the effect of speeding up the heart and raising the blood pressure, emptying sugar supplies swiftly into the blood, and dilating the blood vessels in the muscles to give them immediate use of this energy. At the same time, the pupils of the eyes dilate. See also ALARM REACTION.

The reaction of the body to continuing stress is even more complex. Again the principal organs are the adrenal glands, but after the first phase of alarm, the glands continue to produce a steady supply of hormones that apparently increase the body's resistance. This is in addition to specific defences such as the production of antibodies to fight infection. If the stress is overwhelming, as in the case of an extensive third-degree burn or an uncontrollable infectious disease, the third phase, exhaustion of the adrenal glands, sets in, sometimes with fatal results.

PSYCHOLOGICAL STRESS. The emergency response of the body comes into play when a person merely foresees or imagines danger, as well as in real emergency situations. The thought of danger, or the vicarious experience of danger in a thrilling story, play, or film, may be enough to cause the muscles to tense and start the heart pounding. Psychological situations can have the same effect. One of the best-known examples of this is 'stage fright', often characterized by tensed muscles and an increased heart rate. At times the person may not even be aware of the unconscious thought that produces this dramatic reaction.

STRESS AND DISEASE. In recent years, there have been numerous attempts to find a direct correlation between certain diseases and a stressful environment or a personality type that responds to the environment in a certain way. However, while inappropriate activity and a 'hectic' lifestyle can cause illness in some persons, a busy and productive person can actually be subject to less stress than one who feels trapped in a limited position with no hope for release or a sense of accomplishment.

The diseases most often associated with a stressful environment are, according to some scientists, coronary artery disease and 'heart attack', high blood pressure, and cancer. Studies of laboratory animals have demonstrated a connection between isolated and specific stimuli such as electric shock and separation from mates and the development of heart disease in these animals. The stressful variables in the human environment are, however, much more complex, and a stressful environment can be related to heart disease only as a risk factor (see TYPE A BEHAVIOUR).

The postulated relationship between stress and the development of a malignancy is based on the theory that destructive emotions affect and in some way weaken the body's surveillance system, causing its immune response to fail to recognize and destroy malignant cells.

Although relaxation techniques can reduce blood pressure in persons with mild hypertension, there is no evidence that tension and stress cause the blood pressure to rise and stay at levels above normal.

Other diseases considered by some to be related to stress include asthma, allergies, colitis, migraine headaches, and peptic ulcers. Even though the relationship is not clear and there is currently no hard evidence to support such a claim, most health care providers are convinced that stress contributes to the worsening of symptoms and influences the impact a disease will have on the life of some patients while other patients adapt to stress and seem to have no long-term deleterious reaction to it.

COPING MECHANISMS. Unhealthy ways to cope with psychological stress include alcohol and drug abuse, smoking, abusive and violent behaviour, and working harder to accomplish unrealistic or poorly defined goals. In order to deal with stress in an effective and healthy way, one must first identify sources of stress, either within oneself or in one's environment.

Job stressors are frequently related to disorganisation in the work place, poor time management, and unrealistic or uncommunicated expectations of the employer. Another source of stress for the working person may be the lack of time for family and recreation because of job demands. Once job stressors are identified, some options are to change the stressful situation, modify the way one responds to stressors, or seek another job that is less stressful. In some instances learning to be more assertive and better able to communicate with supervisors and co-workers can reduce job-related stress.

Stressors in the home environment include negative self-concept; inadequate physical, cognitive, or behavioural resources; poor problem-solving skills; marital discord; ineffective parenting or lack of parenting skills; and lack of family support. Effective coping may require strategies to improve self-concept and build self-esteem, develop problem-solving skills, learn effective parenting, and establish a network of people who can give support. Exercise, improving one's nutritional status, making time for recreational activities, and utilising relaxation techniques to relieve tension can also be healthy ways to cope with stress.

s. polycythaemia elevated haemoglobin or packed cell volume resulting from contraction of plasma volume without an absolute increase in red cell mass. Also known as apparent, spurious, pseudo or benign polycythaemia and as Gaisbock's disease. Often found in elderly male smokers.

stress testing a technique for evaluating circulatory response to physical stress produced by exercise (see also EXERCISE TESTING).

stressor ('stresor) any factor that disturbs homeostasis producing stress.

stretcher ('strechə) a contrivance for carrying the sick or wounded.

stria ('strieə) pl. *striae* [L.] 1. a streak or line. 2. a narrow, bandlike structure; used in anatomic nomenclature to designate longitudinal collections of nerve fibres in the brain.

atrophic striae, striae atrophicae atrophic, pinkish or purplish, scarlike lesions, later becoming white (lineae albicantes), on the breasts, thighs, abdomen, and buttocks, due to weakening of elastic tissues, associated with pregnancy (striae gravidarum), overweight, rapid growth during puberty and adolescence, Cushing's syndrome, and topical or prolonged treatment with corticosteroids.

striae gravidarum striae atrophicae occurring in pregnancy.

striae medullares bundles of white fibres across the floor of the fourth ventricle.

striate, striated ('strie·ayt; strie'aytid) having streaks or striae.

striation (strie'ayshən) 1. the quality of being streaked. 2. a streak or scratch, or a series of streaks.

striatonigral (ˌstrieətoh'niegrəl) projecting from the corpus striatum to the substantia nigra.

stricture ('strikchə) an abnormal narrowing of a duct or passage.

stricturization (ˌstrikchə·rie'zayshən) the process of decreasing in calibre or of becoming narrowed or constricted.

stridor ('striedor) a shrill, harsh sound, especially the respiratory sound heard during inspiration in laryngeal obstruction. adj. **stridulous**.

laryngeal s. that due to laryngeal obstruction. A *congenital* form, marked by stridor and dyspnoea, is due to an infolding of a congenitally flabby epiglottis and aryepiglottic folds during inspiration; it is usually outgrown by two years of age.

stridulous ('stridyuhləs) relating to stridor. See LARYNGISMUS.

striocerebellar (ˌstrieohˌseri'belə) pertaining to the corpus striatum and cerebellum.

strip (strip) 1. to divest, to make bare; to dissect with blunt instruments. 2. to excise lengths of varicose veins and incompetent tributaries by the use of a stripper. 3. to remove tooth structure or restorative material from the mesial or distal surfaces of teeth, utilizing abrasive strips.

strobila (stroh'bielə) pl. *strobilae* [L., Gr.] the chain of proglottids constituting the bulk of the body of adult tapeworms; considered by some to comprise the entire body, including the head, neck, and proglottids.

stroke (strohk) a disorder of the blood vessels serving the cerebrum, resulting from an impaired blood supply to parts of the brain. Formerly called a cerebrovascular accident (CVA).

Strokes are more common than is generally realized. It is estimated that by the age of 30, one out of four persons has sufficient change in the cerebral arteries to provide a setting for a stroke at any time. Autopsy studies show that nearly half of those who die from other causes have had minor strokes without ever having been aware of them.

Attacks that are sometimes called 'little strokes' may last from a few minutes to almost 24 hours. These attacks have been termed TRANSIENT ISCHAEMIC ATTACKS (TIA). The term arises from the nature of the attack, which is only temporary and leaves no noticeable residual effects, and from the ischaemia or deficiency of blood supply to the cerebral tissues. These attacks are considered as warnings that a more severe attack will probably occur unless steps are taken to improve blood flow through the arteries. Those vessels most commonly affected are the extracranial arteries, particularly the carotid and vertebral arteries in the neck.

A second type of attack lasts for several days and then subsides with some minor residual effects. This type is termed TIA-IR (incomplete recovery). An attack of cerebral ischaemia that presents the more severe symptoms usually associated with stroke is diagnosed as (CS) completed stroke.

CAUSES. There are three main causes of stroke, all of which are related to a pathological condition of the arteries and associated with cerebral infarction, i.e., a necrotic area in the brain tissue. They are cerebral embolism, cerebral thrombosis, and cerebral haemorrhage. Other causes include compression of cerebral vessels, as from tumour or oedema, and arterial spasm.

Cerebral Embolism. An embolus is a small mass of material circulating in the blood vessels. It can consist of air, fat, or other material introduced into the circulatory system; or, as is most often the case, it is a detached portion of a thrombus that settles in a cerebral vessel. Damage from cerebral embolism is often less extensive and recovery more rapid than in strokes from thrombosis and cerebral haemorrhage.

Cerebral Thrombosis. A thrombus, or clot, in a blood vessel of the brain is by far the most common cause of stroke. Most often the thrombosis occurs where there is narrowing of the lumen of a vessel, usually caused by ATHEROSCLEROSIS. The thrombosis produces ischaemia, oedema, and congestion of the brain tissues surrounding the area. Symptoms appear more gradually in this type of stroke.

Cerebral Haemorrhage. A rupturing of a blood vessel, usually an artery, within the brain. The haemorrhage is frequently associated with preexisting HYPERTENSION. There often is weakening of the vessel wall as well. Healthy arteries can withstand considerable pressure because of their elasticity, but in persons with ARTERIOSCLEROSIS this elasticity is lost and the blood vessel may rupture from the increased pressure within it. In other situations the cerebral vessel wall may be weakened by an ANEURYSM, and thus is susceptible to rupture and haemorrhage into the brain tissues.

Stroke from cerebral haemorrhage is most common after the age of 50 and usually produces more extensive neurological defects with slower recovery than does stroke from other causes.

SYMPTOMS. The symptoms of stroke vary widely, depending on its cause, location of ischaemia, and extent of damage to brain cells. The onset is sudden in cerebral haemorrhage and cerebral embolism because the interruption of blood flow happens quickly. Its effects are noticed almost immediately. Strokes from cerebral haemorrhage occur most often in the daytime while the person is active. In cerebral thrombosis the clot gradually occludes the blood vessels, therefore the onset is gradual. A stroke caused by thrombosis tends to occur while the patient is sleeping or within an hour after arising.

There may be preliminary symptoms, particularly with thrombosis. The patient may experience dizziness, headache, mental confusion, and poor coordination. More often there is a sudden and dramatic onset with loss of consciousness; convulsions may occur. The unconsciousness may last for a few minutes or continue for weeks; it can terminate in a slow recovery or death. Sudden death rarely occurs as a result of stroke.

There are usually neurological symptoms related to the site of ischaemia; for example, hemiplegia, loss of sensation, and reflex changes. The area of paralysis is directly related to the area of cerebral ischaemia. If the left side of the brain is affected, the paralysis of the face, arm, and leg will be present on the opposite or right side. Speech disturbances also are related to the area of brain cell damage; if the left side of the brain, which is the location of the speech centre in right-handed persons, is affected, then aphasia as well as hemiplegia will be present.

Involvement of the region of the thalamus produces a sensation of pain in the hemiplegic area, especially the hand. The discomfort begins several weeks after the stroke.

Emotional disturbances also accompany thalamic involvement. The patient has difficulty controlling his emotions; he may laugh or cry with little or no provocation.

The symptoms of stroke are almost unlimited in type, severity, and permanency. Some may eventually subside, while others are never completely eliminated. Anyone concerned with the care of the stroke victim should be alert to all signs and symptoms that occur. These observations can be extremely helpful in establishing a definite diagnosis and planning a regimen of patient care.

PREVENTION AND TREATMENT. The overall goal in the prevention of stroke of any type is prevention or removal of the established primary cause; i.e., atherosclerosis, arteriosclerosis, aneurysm, and hypertension. Specific techniques in the prevention of stroke are related to the improvement of blood supply to the brain tissue within the limitations imposed by the particular pathological condition producing either impaired blood flow or intracranial bleeding, the surgical techniques and medical care available, and the general condition of the patient and his potential for survival.

Surgical procedures sometimes employed to prevent stroke, or lessen the severity of its effects once it has occurred, include: (1) endarterectomy to remove thickened areas from the inner lining of the carotid or vertebral arteries in the neck (to prevent TIA), (2) patching with a graft a section of artery in which there is an aneurysm, or removal of a section of artery so affected, and (3) evacuation of haematoma after intercerebral haemorrhage.

Surgery for stroke remains controversial and should only be undertaken in specialist units.

The choice of medical prevention and treatment is governed by the conditions which predispose the patient to stroke,and, in the event that a stroke has already occurred, the potential of the individual patient to benefit from the treatment. ANTICOAGULANT drugs are employed only when haemorrhage has been ruled out as a possibility and clot formation has been found to be either the potential or actual cause of decreased blood flow. Antihypertensive drugs are used to reduce pressure within the blood vessel and thereby avoid rupture.

EMERGENCY AND ACUTE CARE. Emergency care consists of loosening all constricting clothing, especially around the neck, to improve respiration and circulation to the head. The patient's head should be turned to the affected side to prevent aspiration of saliva and mucus. He is kept calm and quiet and reassured that he is being cared for. If he is conscious he may sit up or his head may be elevated to reduce blood pressure within the head.

After admission and during the acute stage of stroke, it is extremely important to assess the patient's condition frequently to determine the neurological effects of the stroke and to ascertain whether there is evidence of recurrent strokes. Observations of the patient are valuable in determining the cause of the stroke and the choice of treatment.

Maintenance of a patent AIRWAY and adequate oxygenation are critical. SUCTIONING may be necessary if paralysis prevents normal swallowing of saliva. An artificial airway is inserted if the patient cannot maintain an adequate airway on his own.

The vital signs are taken and recorded at frequent intervals during the 24 hours of the day. An elevated temperature, with decrease in the pulse and respiratory rates, indicates a poor prognosis.

GENERAL CARE. To avoid complications that can develop very quickly in a stroke victim, it is necessary to attend to proper positioning, good body alignment, and frequent turning. (See accompanying illustration.) The patient is turned at least every two to three hours. Because of poor circulation to the affected area, he should not be left to lie on his affected side for more than 20 minutes, four times a day.

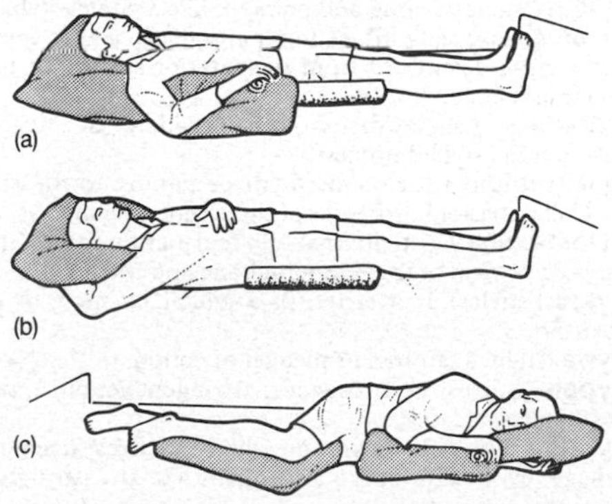

Positioning in stroke. (a) A pillow is placed next to the body on the weak side. The weak arm is placed on the pillow. Make sure that the elbow points away from the body and that the lower arm and hand are placed alongside the body and about 12 inches away from it. A rolled napkin or small towel is placed under the weak hand to keep the fingers open. Note trochanter roll along affected side to keep hip from rotating. (b) The affected arm is tucked under the pillow with the hand flattened to prevent curling of the fingers. (c) In this side-lying position, a pillow is used to support the weak arm. Another pillow is used to support the weak leg.

The amount of activity allowed the patient will depend on the cause of the stroke and the stage of illness. Those who have increased intracranial pressure from haemorrhage and oedema will be placed on complete bed rest. Others who are comatose will require continuous care to avoid complications arising from inactivity (see also COMA).

Complications to be avoided in the patient who has suffered a stroke include PRESSURE SORES, hypostatic PNEUMONIA, THROMBOSIS and other conditions resulting from circulatory stasis, kidney stones and urinary infections, and such orthopaedic deformities as foot and wrist drop and CONTRACTURES. Unless contraindicated, the joints are put through their full range of motion at least once a day (see also therapeutic EXERCISE). A programme of PHYSICAL THERAPY is planned and started as soon as possible to assure maximum rehabilitation.

Nutrition is maintained by whatever means necessary, depending on the patient's ability to chew, handle food in his mouth, and swallow. In some cases NASOGASTRIC TUBE feeding may be the only method by which food is administered. If the patient is able to swallow, but has difficulty moving the food about in his mouth, he should be turned to the affected side while he is being fed. Rinsing the mouth after meals and frequent mouth care help eliminate accumulation of food in the mouth and halitosis. The lips should be kept lubricated with cold cream or mineral oil to keep them from drying and cracking.

INCONTINENCE of urine and faeces sometimes accompanies a stroke. A regular schedule of offering the bedpan, especially after each meal, may help establish a routine of elimination. It is also helpful to get the patient up to the bathroom or to a bedside commode whenever this is possible. In any event the patient must be kept clean and dry and skin care must be given frequently to avoid pressure sores. Faecal impaction and urinary retention may occur and can be avoided by intelligent observation and recording of bowel movements and urinary output. The doctor may order an enema to be given periodically if constipation becomes a problem. See also BLADDER TRAINING and BOWEL TRAINING.

Rehabilitation of the patient begins the moment he enters the hospital. This means that all measures taken to maintain bodily functions and to avoid complications are aimed at the ultimate goal of getting the patient back to a state as near normal as possible. His reaction to his illness, his family's attitude, the quality of care he receives, and the attitude of those caring for him will greatly affect the eventual outcome of his illness. There may be a tendency on the part of the hospital staff and the patient's family to do everything for the patient when he seems so helpless and handicapped. Certainly he should be helped with the things he cannot do for himself, but total dependence on others can become very demoralizing and for the patient's sake he must be encouraged to help himself. This may be a slow and demanding process, requiring much patience and optimism. One can begin by providing the means by which the patient can gradually begin to bathe, feed, and dress himself.

Special equipment, such as an overbed table made of cardboard or plywood, can be used so that the patient can reach the bath water, toilet articles, and other things he needs. His food should be prepared and arranged on his tray so that he can handle it without great difficulty. If his first movements are awkward and messy, no mention should be made of this and he must never be made to feel that he has caused an inconvenience to anyone through his efforts to help himself.

There has been much interest in the rehabilitation of stroke patients in recent years and there is a wealth of information and help available for the stroke victim and his family. Pamphlets dealing with the special problems of this illness are readily available from the Chest, Heart and Stroke Association, Tavistock House

North, Tavistock Square, London WC1H 9JE. A volunteer stroke scheme exists to aid rehabilitation and volunteers will pay home visits to aid those patients with speech difficulties. In some areas stroke clubs are organized and patients can attend on a regular basis. The Association also offers a welfare and counselling service.

heat s. a condition caused by exposure to excessive heat; see also SUNSTROKE.

stroma ('strohmə) pl. *stromata* [Gr.] the tissue forming the ground substance, framework, or matrix of an organ, as opposed to the functioning part or parenchyma. adj. **stromal, stromatic.**

Stromba ('strombə) trademark for a preparation of stanozolol, an anabolic steroid.

stromuhr ('strohm·ooə) an instrument for measuring the velocity of the blood flow.

Strongyloides (ˌstronji'loydeez) a genus of nematode parasites.

S. stercoralis a species found in the intestine of man and other mammals, primarily in the tropics and subtropics, usually causing diarrhoea and intestinal ulceration, although a wide range of other symptoms may result.

strongyloidiasis, strongyloidosis (ˌstronjiloy'dieəsis; ˌstronjiloy'dohsis) infection with organisms of the genus *Strongyloides.*

strontium ('stronti·əm) a chemical element, atomic number 38, atomic weight 87.62, symbol Sr. See table of elements in Appendix 2.

strophulus ('strofyuhləs) a papular urticaria occurring in infants.

struma ('stroomə) enlargement of the thyroid gland; goitre.

Hashimoto's s., s. lymphomatosa a progressive disease of the thyroid gland with degeneration of its epithelial elements and replacement by lymphoid and fibrous tissue.

s. maligna carcinoma of the thyroid gland.

s. ovarii a teratoid ovarian tumour composed of thyroid tissue.

Riedel's s. a chronic, fibrosing, inflammatory process involving usually one but sometimes both lobes of the thyroid gland, as well as the trachea and other adjacent structures.

strumectomy (stroo'mektəmee) excision of a goitre.

strumitis (stroo'mietis) thyroiditis.

Strümpell's disease ('stroompelz) 1. hereditary lateral sclerosis with the spasticity mainly limited to the legs. 2. polioencephalomyelitis.

Strümpell–Leichtenstern disease (ˌstroompel'liekhtənˌstərn) haemorrhagic encephalitis.

Strümpell–Marie disease (ˌstroompelmə'ree) rheumatoid spondylitis.

strychnine ('strikneen) a very poisonous alkaloid from seeds of *Strychnos nux-vomica* and other species of *Strychnos.*

Stryker frame ('striekə) an apparatus specially designed for care of patients with injuries of the spinal cord or paralysis. It is constructed of pipe and canvas and is designed so that one nurse can turn the patient without difficulty. The frame on which the patient lies while in the supine position is called the posterior frame; the anterior frame is used when the patient is turned on his abdomen. There are perineal openings in both frames for use of a bedpan.

Stuart factor ('styooət) clotting factor X.

Stugeron ('stərgə·ron) trademark for a preparation of cinnarizine, an antiemetic.

stump (stump) the proximal end remaining after amputation.

stupe (styoop) a hot, wet cloth or sponge, charged with a medication for external application.

stupefacient (ˌstyoopi'fayshənt) 1. inducing stupor. 2. an agent that induces stupor.

stupefactive (ˌstyoopi'faktiv) producing narcosis or stupor.

stupor ('styoopə) partial or nearly complete unconsciousness; a state of lethargy and immobility with diminished responsiveness to stimulation. adj. **stuporous.**

Sturge–Weber syndrome (disease) (ˌstərj'webə) a condition in which distended and overgrown blood vessels on the surface of a brain compress the underlying cerebral tissues, eventually leading to areas of cerebral calcification. The syndrome is often associated with a naevus on the face, and common symptoms are epilepsy, hemiplegia, and mental handicap.

stuttering ('stutə·ring) a speech problem involving three definitive factors: (1) speech disfluency, most significantly the repetition of parts of words or whole words, prolongation of sounds or words and unduly prolonged pauses; (2) unfavourable reactions of listeners to the speaker's speech defect; and (3) the reactions of the speaker to the listeners' reactions, as well as to his own speech problems and to his conception of himself as a stutterer. See also SPEECH.

sty, stye (stie) inflammation of one or more of the sebaceous (meibomian or zeisian) glands of the eyelid. Called also *hordeolum.*

styl(o)- word element. [L., Gr.] *stake, pole, styloid process of the temporal bone.*

stylet ('stielit) 1. a wire run through a catheter or cannula to render it stiff or to remove debris from its lumen. 2. a slender probe.

stylohyoid (ˌstieloh'hieoyd) pertaining to the styloid process and hyloid bone.

styloid ('stieloyd) long and pointed, like a pen or stylus.

s. process a bony projection, particularly a long spine projecting downward from the inferior surface of the temporal bone.

styloiditis (ˌstieloy'dietis) inflammation of tissues around the styloid process.

stylomastoid (ˌstieloh'mastoyd) pertaining to the styloid and mastoid processes of the temporal bone.

stylomaxillary (ˌstielohmak'silə·ree) pertaining to the styloid process of the temporal bone and the maxilla.

stylus ('stieləs) 1. a stylet. 2. a pencil or stick, as of caustic.

stype (stiep) a tampon or pledget of cotton.

stypsis ('stipsis) 1. astringency; astringent action. 2. use of styptics.

styptic ('stiptik) 1. having the ability to arrest haemorrhage by means of an astringent. 2. an astringent remedy.

sub (sub) preposition. [L.] *under.*

sub- word element. [L.] *under, less than.*

subabdominal (ˌsubab'domin'l) below the abdomen.

subacromial (ˌsubə'krohmi·əl) below the acromion.

subacute (ˌsubə'kyoot) somewhat acute; between acute and chronic.

subalimentation (ˌsubalimen'tayshən) insufficient nourishment.

subaponeurotic (ˌsubəˌponyuh'rotik) below an aponeurosis.

subarachnoid (ˌsubə'raknoyd) between the arachnoid and the pia mater.

subareolar (ˌsubaree'ohlə) beneath the areola of the nipple.

subastragalar (ˌsubə'stragələ) below the astragalus (talus).

subaural (sub'or·rəl) below the ear.

subcapsular (sub'kapsyuhlə) below a capsule, especially the capsule of the brain.

subcartilaginous (ˌsubkahti'lajinəs) 1. below a cartilage. 2. partly cartilaginous.

subclass ('subˌklahs) a taxonomic category subordinate to a class and superior to an order.

subclavian, subclavicular (sub'klayvi·ən; ˌsubklə'vikyuhlə) below the clavicle.

subclavian steal syndrome (sub'klayvi·ən steel) cerebral or brain stem ischaemia resulting from diversion of blood flow from the basilar artery to the subclavian artery, in the presence of occlusive disease of the proximal portion of the subclavian artery.

subclinical (sub'klinik'l) without clinical manifestations; said of the early stages or a very mild form of a disease.

subconjunctival (ˌsubkonjunk'tiev'l) beneath the conjunctiva.

subconscious (sub'konshəs) 1. imperfectly or partially conscious, yet capable of being made conscious by an effort of memory or by association of ideas; called also preconscious. 2. the area of mental activity below the level of conscious perception.

subconsciousness (sub'konshəsnəs) 1. partial unconsciousness. 2. the area of mental activity below the level of conscious perception.

subcoracoid (sub'ko·rəˌkoyd) situated under the coracoid process.

subcortex (sub'kawteks) the brain substance underlying the cortex. adj. **subcortical**.

subcostal (sub'kost'l) below a rib or ribs.

subcranial (sub'krayni·əl) below the cranium.

subcrepitant (ˌsub'krepitənt) somewhat crepitant in nature; said of a rale.

subculture ('subˌkulchə) a culture of bacteria derived from another culture.

subcutaneous (ˌsubkyoo'tayni·əs) beneath the layers of the skin.

s. infusion infusion of fluids directly into the subcutaneous tissues.

s. injection an injection made into the subcutaneous tissues (see also subcutaneous INJECTION).

subcuticular (ˌsubkyoo'tikyuhlə) below the epidermis.

subdiaphragmatic (ˌsubdieəfrag'matik) below the diaphragm.

subduct (sub'dukt) to draw down.

subdural (sub'dyooə·rəl) between the dura mater and the arachnoid.

subendocardial (ˌsubendoh'kahdi·əl) beneath the endocardium.

subendothelial (ˌsubendoh'theeli·əl) beneath an endothelial layer.

subepidermal (ˌsubepi'dərməl) beneath the epidermis.

subepithelial (ˌsubepi'theeli·əl) beneath the epithelium.

subfamily (sub'familee) a taxonomic division sometimes established, subordinate to a family and superior to a tribe.

subfascial (sub'fashi·əl) beneath a fascia.

subfebrile (sub'feebriel, -'feb-) somewhat febrile.

subgenus (sub'jeenəs) a taxonomic category sometimes established, subordinate to a genus and superior to a species.

subglenoid (sub'gleenoyd) beneath the glenoid (mandibular) fossa.

subglossal (sub'glos'l) below the tongue.

subgrondation (ˌsubgron'dayshən) depression of one fragment of bone beneath another.

subhepatic (ˌsubhi'patik) below the liver.

subhyoid (sub'hieoyd) below the hyoid bone.

subiculum (syuh'bikyuhləm) an underlying or supporting structure.

subiliac (sub'iliˌak) below the ilium.

subilium (sub'ili·əm) the lowest portion of the ilium.

subinvolution (ˌsubinvə'looshən) incomplete involution; failure of a part to return to its normal size and condition after enlargement from functional activity.

subjacent (sub'jays'nt) located below.

subject ('subjikt) a person or animal subjected to treatment, observation, or experiment.

subjective (səb'jektiv) perceived only by the affected individual and not by the examiner.

subjugal (sub'joog'l) below the zygomatic bone.

sublatio retinae (subˌlayshioh 'retinie) detachment of the retina of the eye (see DETACHMENT OF RETINA).

sublesional (sub'leezhən'l) performed or situated beneath a lesion.

sublethal (sub'leethəl) insufficient to cause death.

sublimate ('subliˌmayt) 1. a substance obtained by sublimation (1). 2. to accomplish sublimation.

sublimation (ˌsubli'mayshən) 1. the conversion of a solid directly into the gaseous state. 2. a defence mechanism in which an individual diverts socially unacceptable instinctive drives into personally approved and socially acceptable channels. Mental conflicts may be resolved by this means although the person achieves only partial satisfaction of his impulses.

Sublimaze ('sublimayz) trademark for a preparation of fentanyl, an opiate used in anaesthesia.

subliminal (sub'limin'l) below the threshold of sensation or conscious awareness.

sublingual (sub'ling·gwəl) beneath the tongue.

s. gland a salivary gland on either side under the tongue.

sublinguitis (ˌsubling'gwietis) inflammation of the sublingual gland.

subluxate (sub'luksayt) to partially dislocate.

subluxation (ˌsubluk'sayshən) incomplete or partial DISLOCATION.

submammary (sub'mamə·ree) below the mammary gland.

submandibular (ˌsubman'dibyuhlə) below the mandible.

submaxilla (ˌsubmak'silə) the mandible.

submaxillaritis (subˌmaksilə'rietis) inflammation of the submaxillary gland.

submaxillary (ˌsubmak'silə·ree) below the maxilla.

s. gland a salivary gland on the inner side of each ramus of the lower jaw.

submental (sub'ment'l) below the chin.

submersion (sub'mərshən) the act of placing or the condition of being under the surface of a liquid.

submetacentric (ˌsubmetə'sentrik) having the centromere almost, but not quite, at the metacentric position.

submicroscopic (ˌsubmiekrə'skopik) too small to be visible with the microscope.

submucosa (ˌsubmyoo'kohsə) areolar tissue situated beneath a mucous membrane.

submucous (sub'myookəs) beneath a mucous membrane.

subnarcotic (ˌsubnah'kotik) moderately narcotic.

subneural (sub'nyooə·rəl) beneath a nerve.

subnormal (sub'nawm'l) below or less than normal.

subnormality (ˌsubnaw'malitee) a state less than normal or that usually encountered, as mental subnormality, generally considered characterized by an intelligence quotient under 69.

suboccipital (ˌsubok'sipit'l) below the occiput.

suborbital (sub'awbit'l) beneath the orbit.

suborder (sub'awdə) a taxonomic category sometimes established, subordinate to an order and superior to a family.

subpapular (sub'papyuhlə) indistinctly papular.

subpatellar (ˌsubpə'telə) below the patella.
subpericardial (ˌsubperi'kahdi·əl) beneath the pericardium.
subperiosteal (ˌsubperi'osti·əl) beneath the periosteum.
subperitoneal (ˌsubperitə'neeəl) beneath the peritoneum.
subpharyngeal (ˌsubfə'rinji·əl, subˌfarin'jeeəl) beneath the pharynx.
subphrenic (sub'frenik) beneath the diaphragm.
subphylum (sub'fieləm) pl. *subphyla* [L., Gr.] a taxonomic category sometimes established, subordinate to a phylum and superior to a class.
subplacenta (ˌsubplə'sentə) the decidua basalis.
subpleural (sub'plooə·rəl) beneath the pleura.
subpreputial (ˌsubpree'pyooshəl) beneath the prepuce.
subpubic (sub'pyoobik) beneath the pubic bone.
subpulmonary (sub'pulmənə·ree, -'puhl-) beneath the lung.
subretinal (sub'retinəl) beneath the retina.
subscapular (sub'skapyuhlə) below the scapula.
subserous (sub'siə·rəs) beneath a serous membrane.
subspecies (sub'speesheez) a subdivision of a species; a variety or race.
substage ('subˌstayj) the part of the microscope underneath the stage.
substance ('substəns) the material constituting an organ or body.
black s. substantia nigra.
depressor s. a substance that tends to decrease activity or blood pressure.
ground s. the gel-like material in which connective tissue cells and fibres are embedded.
medullary s. 1. the white matter of the central nervous system, consisting of axons and their myelin sheaths. 2. the soft, marrow-like substance of the interior of such structures as bone, kidney, and adrenal gland.
s. P a peptide of 11 amino acids present in the intestine, where it induces contraction of the intestine and dilation of blood vessels; it is also present in a number of neuronal pathways in the brain and in primary sensory fibres of peripheral nerves, and may be a neurotransmitter associated with transmission of pain impulses.
perforated s. 1. *anterior perforated substance*, an area anterolateral to each optic tract, pierced by branches of the anterior and middle cerebral arteries. 2. *posterior perforated substance*, an area between the cerebral peduncles, pierced by branches of the posterior cerebral arteries.
pressor s. a substance that raises blood pressure.
reticular s. the netlike mass of threads seen in erythrocytes after vital staining.
slow-reacting s. a substance released in the anaphylactic reaction that induces slow, prolonged contraction of certain smooth muscles. Symbol SRS or SRS-A.
threshold s's those substances (e.g., glucose) excreted into the urine only when their concentration in plasma exceeds a certain value.
transmitter s. a chemical substance mediator that induces activity in an excitable tissue.
substantia (sub'stanshi·ə) pl. *substantiae* [L.] substance; used in anatomical nomenclature in naming various components of various tissues and structures of the body.
s. gelatinosa the substance sheathing the posterior horn of the spinal cord and lining its central canal.
s. nigra the layer of grey substance separating the tegmentum of the midbrain from the crus cerebri.
substernal (sub'stərnəl) below the sternum.
substituent (sub'stityooənt) 1. a substitute; especially an atom, radical, or group substituted for another in a compound. 2. of or pertaining to such an atom, radical, or group.
substitution (ˌsubsti'tyooshən) 1. the act of putting one thing in the place of another, especially the chemical replacement of one atom or substituent group by another. 2. a defence mechanism in which an individual replaces an unattainable or unacceptable goal, emotion, or motive with one that is attainable or acceptable.
substrate ('substrayt) any substance upon which an enzyme acts.
substructure ('subˌstrukchə) the underlying or supporting portion of an organ or appliance.
subsylvian (sub'silvi·ən) situated deep in the lateral sulcus (sylvian fissure).
subtarsal (sub'tahs'l) below the tarsus.
subtentorial (ˌsubten'tor·ri·əl) beneath the tentorium of the cerebellum.
subtertian (sub'tərshən) pertaining to a form of malaria in which there is continuous or remittent fever, caused by infection by *Plasmodium falciparum*.
subthalamus (sub'thaləməs) the ventral thalamus or subthalamic tegmental region: a transitional region of the diencephalon interposed between the (dorsal) thalamus, the hypothalamus, and the tegmentum of the mesencephalon (midbrain); it includes the subthalamic nucleus, Forel's fields, and the zona incerta. adj. **subthalamic.**
subtle ('sut'l) 1. very fine, as a subtle powder. 2. very acute, as a subtle pain.
subtotal (sub'toht'l) incomplete.
subtraction (səb'trakshən) in diagnostic radiology a technique which subtracts unwanted information from a radiograph, usually the subtraction of bone densities from radiographs of contrast media in vessels to leave only the image of the contrast medium. The method of subtraction may be photographic or computerized. Called also *digital vascular imaging (DVI)* or *digital vascular subtraction (DVS)*.
subtribe ('subˌtrieb) a taxonomic category sometimes established, subordinate to a tribe and superior to a genus.
subtrochanteric (ˌsubtrohkan'terik) below the trochanter.
subtympanic (ˌsubtim'panik) somewhat tympanic in quality.
subungual (sub'ung·gwəl) beneath a nail.
suburethral (ˌsubyuh'reethrəl) beneath the urethra.
subvaginal (ˌsubvə'jien'l, sub'vajin'l) under a sheath, or below the vagina.
subvertebral (sub'vərtibrəl) on the ventral side of the vertebrae.
subvirile (sub'viriel) having deficient virility.
subvolution (ˌsubvə'looshən) turning a flap under, usually in reference to ophthalmic operations.
succenturiate (ˌsuksən'tyooə·ri·ət) accessory; serving as a substitute.
succinate ('suksiˌnayt) any salt of succinic acid.
succinic acid (suk'sinik) an intermediate in the tricarboxylic acid cycle.
succinylcholine chloride (ˌsuksiniel'kohleen) see SUXAMETHONIUM CHLORIDE.
succinylsulphathiazole (ˌsuksinilˌsulfə'thieəˌzohl) a sulphonamide preparation used for intestinal infections. It is not absorbed from the alimentary tract.
succorrhoea (ˌsukə'reeə) excessive flow of a natural secretion.
succus ('sukəs) pl. *succi* [L.] any fluid derived from living tissue; bodily secretion; juice.
succussion (su'kushən) a splashing sound elicited when a patient is shaken, indicative of fluid and air in

a body cavity.

sucralfate (soo'kralfayt) a complex of aluminium hydroxide and sulphated sucrose used for short-term treatment of peptic ulcer; it forms a complex with proteins that resists digestion by acid and pepsin thereby making a protective coating for the ulcer.

sucrose ('sookrohz, -ohs) a sugar obtained from sugar cane, sugar beet, or other sources; used as a food and sweetening agent.

suction, suctioning ('sukshən; 'sukshəning) removal of material by aspiration, as from an operative wound.

Suctioning of the nose and mouth is a relatively simple procedure requiring only cleanliness and sensible care in the removal of liquids that are obstructing the nasal and oral passages. Suctioning of the deeper respiratory structures ('deep' and 'endotracheal' suctioning), an aseptic technique, demands special skill and meticulous care to avoid traumatizing the delicate mucous membranes and introducing infection into the respiratory tree. See also ASEPTIC TECHNIQUE.

Another complication arising from improper tracheal suctioning is HYPOXIA, which occurs when prolonged suctioning removes the oxygen from the patient's airway and thus adds to his respiratory distress. The use of a catheter too large in diameter can cause obstruction of the bronchus and subsequent collapse of a lobe of the lung.

Because of the potential hazards inherent in the procedure, tracheal suctioning should be reserved only for those patients too weak and debilitated to cough up thick and tenacious sputum. When deep suctioning is necessary, it should be done only by those persons who are skilful in the technique and knowledgeable about the complications that can result from improper use of the suctioning equipment.

post-tussive s. a sucking sound heard over a lung cavity just after a cough.

suctorial (suk'tor·ri·əl) adapted for sucking.

Sudafed ('soodə,fed) trademark for preparations of pseudoephedrine, a nasal decongestant.

sudamen (soo'daymen) pl. *sudamina* [L.] a small whitish vesicle caused by retention of sweat in the layers of the epidermis.

Sudan (soo'dan) a group of azo compounds used as biological stains for fats.

sudanophilia (,soodanə'fili·ə) 1. affinity for a Sudan stain. 2. a condition in which the leukocytes contain particles staining readily with Sudan red III.

sudation (syoo'dayshən) the process of sweating.

sudatorium (syoodə'tor·ri·əm) pl. *sudatoria* [L.] a hot air bath or sweat bath.

sudden infant death syndrome (sud'n) the sudden and unexpected death of an apparently healthy infant, typically occurring between the ages of three weeks and five months, and not explained by careful postmortem studies. Abbreviated SIDS. Called also *crib* or *cot death* because the infant often is found dead in the cot.

Sudeck's disease ('syoodeks) post-traumatic osteoporosis.

sudomotor (,syoodoh'mohtə) stimulating the sweat glands.

sudor ('syoodor) sweat; perspiration.

sudoral ('syoodə·rəl) characterized by profuse sweating.

sudoresis (,syoodə'reesis) profuse sweating.

sudoriferous (,syoodə'rifə·rəs) 1. conveying sweat. 2. sudoriparous.

sudorific (,syoodə'rifik) 1. promoting sweating; diaphoretic. 2. an agent that causes sweating.

sudoriparous (,syoodə'ripə·rəs) secreting or producing sweat.

suffocation (,sufə'kayshən) the stoppage of breathing, or the asphyxia that results from it. If suffocation is complete—that is, no air at all reaches the lungs—the lack of oxygen and excess of carbon dioxide in the blood will cause almost immediate loss of consciousness. Though the heart continues to beat briefly, death will follow in a matter of minutes unless emergency measures are taken to get breathing started again.

Suffocation can be caused by drowning, electric shock, gas or smoke poisoning, strangulation, or choking on a foreign body in the trachea. Once the cause of suffocation has been removed, the most important first-aid measure is ARTIFICIAL RESPIRATION, preferably the mouth-to-mouth technique.

FIRST AID IN CASES OF SUFFOCATION. In any emergency when breathing has stopped, have someone get help from the emergency services. Meanwhile, give first aid as directed below. Artificial respiration, when called for, should be given preferably by the mouth-to-mouth method.

Drowning:
(1) Clear sand and other material from the mouth.
(2) Give artificial respiration.

Gas Poisoning:
(1) Drag victim into open air.
(2) Give artificial respiration.

Electric Shock:
(1) If victim is in contact with live wire or other electrical source, turn off electric current; if this is impossible, break contact by using a dry board or other nonconductor of electricity.
(2) Give artificial respiration.

Strangulation:
(1) Remove whatever is causing strangulation if it is still present.
(2) Give artificial respiration.

Choking on Foreign Body:
(1) Perform HEIMLICH MANOEUVRE.
(2) Try to remove object with fingers or forceps.

suffusion (sə'fyoozhən) 1. the process of overspreading, or diffusion. 2. the condition of being moistened or permeated through.

sugar ('shuhgə) a sweet carbohydrate of both animal and vegetable origin, the two principal groups of which are the disaccharides and the monosaccharides.

suggestibility (sə,jestə'bilətee) inclination to act on suggestions of others.

suggestible (sə'jestəb'l) inclined to act on the suggestion of another.

suggestion (sə'jeschən) 1. impartation of an idea to a subject from without. 2. an idea introduced from without.

hypnotic s. one imparted to a person in the hypnotic state.

posthypnotic s. implantation in the mind of a subject during hypnosis of a suggestion to be acted upon after recovery from the hypnotic state.

suggillation (,suji'layshən) an ecchymosis.

suicide ('sooi,sied) the taking of one's own life; also any person who voluntarily and intentionally takes his own life. Legally, a death suspected of being due to violence that is self-inflicted is not termed a suicide unless there is positive evidence of the victim's intent to destroy himself, or the method of death is such that a verdict of suicide is inevitable. This means that many deaths that would be termed suicide according to medicopsychological criteria are reported as accidental or from undetermined cause.

The difficulty of positively identifying a death as suicide is further complicated by the complexities of determining true intent and the psychological motivation a person may have had for ending his own life.

INCIDENCE. Statistical evidence of the actual suicide rate for a specific population is difficult to compile because of the ambiguity of the term, a lack of criteria by which a death may be judged suicidal, and a lack of agreement among those reporting deaths as to what does, indeed, constitute a suicide. In spite of these difficulties, some inferences can be drawn from the data at hand.

More males than females commit suicide, but more females than males commit acts of deliberate self-harm (parasuicide). The actual suicide rate is higher among elderly males, whereas the parasuicide rate is higher in young females, though, as a general rule, suicide rates increase with age. In recent years there has been an alarming increase in the incidence of suicide among university students throughout the world.

Other high-risk groups include the elderly, the sick, and the mentally ill. There is a tendency of suicides to occur in families, but there is no evidence of a genetically determined suicidal behaviour pattern. There are also seasonal fluctuations in the suicidal rates, with the highest number occurring in the spring and autumn.

Approximately one-third of all suicides have occurred in persons who have received psychiatric treatment. Depression is present in 95 per cent of all suicidal cases, but these persons are most suicidal when they are just entering into or recovering from an attack of depression.

SUICIDAL TENDENCIES. All deeply depressed people are potential suicides. Their depression may be set off by illness or an external event, such as the death of a friend or relative, or there may be no apparent cause. However, depressed people do not always admit their suicidal thoughts; in fact, they often deny them. The suicidal impulse appears to arise in many cases from a combination of hate, rage, revenge, a sense of guilt, and a feeling of unbearable frustration. Suicide often appears to be an act of spite in which the person who takes his own life expresses toward himself the resentment he feels toward other people or the world in general. Simultaneously, he dramatically punishes himself for his own shortcomings.

Early signs of suicidal tendencies include low moods, with expressions of guilt, tension, and agitation; insomnia, early morning awakenings, requests for more sleeping pills; neglected personal appearance in one who is normally tidy; loss of weight and appetite; inability to concentrate; preoccupation with death; crumpled copies of tentative suicide notes, left in wastebaskets or on desks; and heavier drinking, to give the person the courage to act.

TREATMENT AND PREVENTION. The suicidal person requires psychiatric care to relieve the depression, hostility, aggression, and other extremes of mood that cause him to contemplate taking his own life. Early recognition and treatment of mental illness, particularly depression, can do much to prevent many suicides.

The World Health Organization offers the following suggestions for prevention of suicide: (1) availability of emergency medical services and poison control centres to prevent the fatal outcome of suicidal acts; (2) recognition of the early signs of suicidal tendencies and prompt treatment. Any suicide threat must be taken seriously. The widespread belief that no one who talks about suicide is likely to attempt it is false. Of those who commit suicide, at least 80 per cent have discussed it with someone else; (3) special medical and social attention to high-risk groups. Measures should be taken against social isolation and neglect of those who are already suffering from a feeling of worthlessness and despair. These persons need satisfying social relations within the family and in the larger community so that they can receive continued support from others and experience a sense of self-worth and dignity.

Samaritans Inc., 17 Uxbridge Road, Slough, Berkshire SL1 1SN, was founded in 1953 to help the suicidal and the despairing, and to offer a 24-hour 'befriending' service based on initial telephone contacts. There are 180 Samaritan branches in the UK and Irish Republic, and Samaritans are all volunteers who choose to devote part of their spare time to helping the distressed. Many Samaritans are ex-clients of the organization.

sulcate ('sulkayt) furrowed; marked with sulci.

sulcus ('sulkəs) pl. *sulci* [L.] a groove or furrow; used in anatomical nomenclature to designate a linear depression, especially one separating the gyri of the brain.

calcarine s. a sulcus of the medial surface of the occipital lobe, separating the cuneus from the lingual gyrus.

central s. fissure of Rolando.

collateral s. collateral fissure.

sulci cutis fine depressions of the skin between the ridges of the skin.

gingival s. the groove between the surface of the tooth and the epithelium lining the free gingiva.

hippocampal s. hippocampal fissure.

sulf- for words beginning thus, see those beginning *sulph-*.

sulindac (sə'lindak) an anti-inflammatory, analgesic, and antipyretic used in the treatment of rheumatic disorders.

sulpha drugs ('sulfə) a group of chemical compounds used as antibacterial agents; called also *sulphonamides.*

sulphacetamide (,sulfə'setə,mied) an antibacterial sulphonamide used in infections of the eye.

sulphadiazine (,sulfə'dieə,zeen) a rapidly absorbed and readily excreted antibacterial agent.

silver s. the silver derivative of sulphadiazine; used in the form of a cream in the treatment of burns.

sodium s. an antibacterial compound used intravenously.

sulphadimidine (,sulfə'diemi,deen) a sulphonamide of which a high blood level can be obtained but toxic effects are rare. Used in the treatment of urinary tract infections.

sulphaemoglobin (,sulfheemə'glohbin) the substance produced in the blood by an excess of sulphur, which gives rise to sulphaemoglobinaemia. Called also *sulphmethaemoglobin.*

sulphaemoglobinaemia (,sulfheemə,glohbi'neemi·ə) sulphaemoglobin in the blood.

sulphafurazole (,sulfə'fyooə·rəzohl) an antibacterial compound used orally, topically, and parenterally, in infections of the urinary and respiratory tracts and of soft tissues.

s. acetyl the acetic acid amide of sulphafurazole, used as an antibacterial.

sulphaguanidine (,sulfə'gwahni,deen) a poorly absorbed sulphonamide formerly used in the treatment of bacillary dysentery.

sulphamethizole (,sulfə'methi,zohl) an antibacterial compound used mainly in urinary tract infections.

sulphamethoxazole (,sulfəmə'thoksə,zohl) an antibacterial sulphonamide, especially useful in acute urinary tract infections and pyodermata and in infections of wounds and soft tissues.

sulphanilamide (,sulfə'nilə,mied) a potent antibacterial compound, the first of the sulphonamides discovered.

sulphasalazine (ˌsulfə'saləˌzeen) a combination of sulphapyridine and salicylic acid, used in the treatment and prophylaxis of ulcerative colitis.
sulphatase ('sulfəˌtayz) an enzyme that catalyses the hydrolysis of sulphate esters.
sulphate ('sulfayt) a salt of sulphuric acid.
sulphathiazole (ˌsulfə'thieəˌzohl) a sulphonamide used as an antibacterial agent.
sulphatide ('sulfəˌtied) any of a class of cerebroside sulphuric esters.
sulphhydryl (sulf'hiedril) the univalent radical, –SH.
sulphide ('sulfied) any binary compound of sulphur; a compound of sulphur with another element or base.
sulphinpyrazone (ˌsulfin'pierəˌzohn) a uricosuric compound used in gout to promote excretion of uric acid.
sulphmethaemoglobin (ˌsulfmetˌheemə'globin) see SULPHAEMOGLOBIN.
sulphobromophthalein sodium (ˌsulfohˌbrohmoh-'thalee·in) see BSP.
sulphonamide (sul'fonəˌmied) 1. any compound containing the $-SO_2NH_2$ group. 2. any of a group of drugs that are derivatives of sulphanilamide, which competitively inhibit folic acid synthesis in microorganisms, and are bacteriostatic against gram-positive cocci (streptococci and pneumococci), gram-negative cocci (meningococci and gonococci), gram-negative bacilli (*Escherichia coli* and shigellae), and a wide variety of other bacteria. Sulphonamides have been supplanted by more effective and less toxic antibiotics in most uses. Called also *sulpha drug*.
sulphone ('sulfohn) a compound containing two hydrocarbon radicals attached to the $-SO_2-$ group, especially dapsone (4,4-sulfonylbisbenzenamine) and its derivatives, which are potent antibacterials effective against many gram-positive and gram-negative organisms, and are widely used as leprostatics.
sulphonylurea (ˌsulfoni'lyooə·ri·ə) a class of chemical compounds that includes the oral HYPOGLYCAEMIC AGENTS acetohexamide, chlorpropamide, tolazamide, and tolbutamide.
sulphoxide (sul'foksied) 1. the divalent radical =SO. 2. an organic compound intermediate between a sulphide and a sulphone.
sulphur ('sulfə) a chemical element, atomic number 16, atomic weight 32.064, symbol S. See table of elements in Appendix 2.
precipitated s. a fine, pale yellow powder; used as a scabicide, antiparasitic, antifungal, and keratolytic.
s. sublimatum, sublimed s. a fine yellow crystalline powder; used as a parasiticide and scabicide.
sulphurated ('sulfyuhˌraytid) combined with sulphur.
sulphuric acid (sul'fyooə·rik) an oily, highly caustic, poisonous compound, H_2SO_4.
sulthiame (sul'thieˌaym) an anticonvulsant drug used in the treatment of epilepsy.
Sultrin ('sultrin) trademark for a fixed combination preparation of sulphathiazole, sulphacetamide, and sulphabenzamide; an antibiotic for vaginitis and cervicitis.
sunburn ('sunˌbərn) inflammation—an actual burn—of the skin caused by exposure to ultraviolet rays of the sun. Depending on how severe the burn is, the skin may simply redden or it may become blistered and sore—a second-degree burn. In extreme cases there may be fever.
sunstroke ('sunˌstrohk) a profound disturbance of the body's heat-regulating mechanism caused by prolonged exposure to excessive heat from the sun, particularly when there is little or no circulation of air. Persons over 40 and those in poor health are most susceptible to it.

The condition is called also heat stroke, a somewhat broader term that covers disorders caused by other forms of intense heat as well as those caused by the sun.

RECOGNITION. Sunstroke is not the same as HEAT EXHAUSTION, a less serious disorder in which the amount of salt and fluid in the body falls below normal. In sunstroke there is a disturbance in the mechanism that controls perspiration. Since sunstroke is much more dangerous than heat exhaustion and is treated differently, it is of the utmost importance to distinguish between the two. The first symptoms of both disorders may be similar: headache, dizziness, and weakness. But later symptoms differ sharply. In heat exhaustion, there is perspiration and a normal or below normal temperature, whereas in sunstroke there is extremely high fever and absence of sweating. Sunstroke also may cause convulsions and sudden loss of consciousness. In extreme cases it may be fatal.

TREATMENT. In treatment of sunstroke, immediate steps must be taken to lower the body temperature, which may rise as high as 42 to 45 °C (108 to 112 °F). The patient should be placed in a shady, cool place and most of his clothing should be removed. Cold water is sprinkled on the patient or he is sprayed gently with a garden hose. The arms and legs should be massaged to maintain circulation.

Further treatment consists of measures to lower the body temperature, including ice packs, cold water enemas, and iced drinks by mouth. After the temperature has returned to normal, it is best for the patient to rest in bed for several days in a cool, well ventilated room.

super- word element. [L.] *above, excessive*.
superalimentation (ˌsoopəˌralimen'tayshən) excessive feeding; sometimes used in the treatment of wasting diseases.
superalkalinity (ˌsoopəˌralkə'linitee) excessive alkalinity.
supercilium (ˌsoopə'sili·əm) pl. *supercilia* [L.] 1. *supercilium*, eyebrow; the transverse elevation at the junction of the forehead and upper eyelid. 2. *supercilia*, eyebrows; the hairs on the arching protrusion over the eyes.
superclass ('soopəˌklahs) a taxonomic category sometimes established, subordinate to a phylum and superior to a class.
superego (ˌsoopə'reegoh, -'regoh) a part of the psyche derived from both the ID and the EGO, which acts, largely unconsciously, as a monitor over the ego. It is that part of the personality concerned with social standards, ethics, and conscience. Early in life the superego is formed by the infant's identification with his parents and other significant and esteemed persons in his life. The real or supposed expectations of these persons gradually are accepted as general rules of society and help form the 'conscience'. The superego tends to be self-critical and in psychotic and neurotic persons strong feelings of guilt and unworthiness can lead to self-punitive measures in an effort to resolve conflicts between the id, ego, and superego. See also NEUROSIS and PSYCHOSIS.
superexcitation (ˌsoopəˌreksie'tayshən) excessive excitation.
superfamily ('soopəˌfamilee) a taxonomic category sometimes established, subordinate to an order and superior to a family.
superfecundation (ˌsoopəˌfekən'dayshən, -ˌfee-) fertilization of two or more ova during the same ovulatory cycle, by separate coital acts.
superfetation (ˌsoopəfee'tayshən) the fertilization and subsequent development of an ovum when a fetus is

already present in the uterus, a result of fertilization of ova during different ovulatory cycles and yielding fetuses of different ages.

superficial (,soopə'fishəl) situated on or near the surface.

superficialis (,soopə,fishi'aylis) superficial.

superficies (,soopə'fisheez) an outer surface.

superinduce (,soopə·rin'dyoos) to bring on in addition to an already existing condition.

superinfection (,soopə·rin'fekshən) a new infection complicating the course of antibiotic therapy of an existing infection, due to invasion by bacteria or fungi resistant to the drug(s) in use.

superinvolution (,soopə,rinvə'looshən) prolonged involution of the uterus after delivery, to a size much smaller than the normal, occurring in breast feeding mothers.

superior (soo'piə·ri·ə) situated above, or directed upward; in official anatomical nomenclature, used in reference to the upper surface of an organ or other structure, or to a structure occupying a higher position.

superjacent (,soopə'jays'nt) located just above.

superlactation (,soopəlak'tayshən) oversecretion of milk; hyperlactation.

superlethal (,soopə'leethəl) more than sufficient to cause death.

supermotility (,soopəmoh'tilitee) excessive motility.

supernatant (,soopə'naytənt) the liquid lying above a layer of precipitated insoluble material.

supernumerary (,soopə'nyoomə·rə·ree) in excess of the regular number.

supernutrition (,soopənyoo'trishən) excessive nutrition.

superolateral (,soopə·roh'latə·rəl) above and to the side.

superoxide (,soopə'roksied) any compound containing the highly reactive superoxide ion O_2^-, a common intermediate in numerous biological oxidations.

supersaturate (,soopə'sachə,rayt) to add more of an ingredient than can be held in solution permanently.

supertension (,soopə'tenshən) extreme tension.

supervascularization (,soopə,vaskyuhlə·rie'zayshən) in radiotherapy, the relative increase in vascularity that occurs when tumour cells are destroyed so that the remaining tumour cells are better supplied by the (uninjured) capillary stroma.

supervoltage ('soopə,vohltij) in radiotherapy, pertaining to x-rays produced by a tube voltage in the range of 500–1000 kilovolts.

supinate ('soopi,nayt) the act of turning the palm foward or upward, or of raising the medial margin of the foot.

supination (,soopi'nayshən) the act of assuming the supine position; placing or lying on the back. Applied to the hand, the act of turning the palm upward.

supine ('soopien) lying with the face upward, or on the dorsal surface.

suppository (sə'pozitə·ree) an easily fusible medicated mass for introduction into the rectum, urethra, or vagina.

suppressant (sə'presənt) 1. inducing suppression. 2. an agent that stops secretion, excretion, or normal discharge.

suppression (sə'preshən) 1. sudden stoppage of a secretion, excretion, or normal discharge. 2. conscious inhibition as contrasted with repression, which is unconscious. 3. in genetics, restoration of a lost function by a second mutation either in a gene other than that involved in the primary mutation, or within the same gene.

suppurant ('supyuhrənt) 1. promoting suppuration. 2. an agent causing suppuration.

suppuration (,supyuh'rayshən) formation or discharge of pus. adj. **suppurative.**

supra- word element. [L.] *above.*

supra-acromial (,sooprə·ə'krohmi·əl) above the acromion.

supra-auricular (,sooprə·or'rikyuhlə) above the auricle of the ear.

suprachoroid (,sooprə'ko·royd) above or upon the choroid.

suprachoroidea (,sooprəko'roydi·ə) the outermost layer of the choroid.

supraclavicular (,sooprəklə'vikyuhlə) above the clavicle.

supracondylar (,sooprə'kondilə) above a condyle.

supracostal (,sooprə'kost'l) above or outside the ribs.

supracotyloid (,sooprə'koti,loyd) above the acetabulum.

supradiaphragmatic (,sooprə,dieəfrag'matik) above the diaphragm.

supraduction, sursumduction (,sooprə'dukshən; ,sərsəm'dukshən) the turning upward of a part, especially the eyes.

supraepicondylar (,sooprə,epi'kondilə) above the epicondyle.

suprahyoid (,sooprə'hieoyd) above the hyoid bone.

supraliminal (,sooprə'limin'l) above the threshold of sensation.

supralumbar (,sooprə'lumbə) above the loin.

supramaxillary (,sooprəmak'silə·ree) pertaining to the upper jaw.

supraorbital (,sooprə'awbit'l) above the orbit.

suprapelvic (,sooprə'pelvik) above the pelvis.

suprapharmacological (,sooprə,fahməkə'lojik'l) much greater than the usual therapeutic dose or pharmacological concentration of a drug.

suprapontine (,sooprə'pontien) above or in the upper part of the pons.

suprapubic (,sooprə'pyoobik) above the pubes.

suprarenal (,sooprə'reen'l) above a kidney; adrenal.
s. gland adrenal gland.

suprarenalectomy (,sooprə,reenə'lektəmee) adrenalectomy; excision of one or both adrenal glands.

suprascapular (,sooprə'skapyuhlə) above the scapula.

suprascleral (,sooprə'skliə·rəl) on the outer surface of the sclera.

suprasellar (,sooprə'selə) above the sella turcica.

supraspinal (,sooprə'spien'l) above the spine.

suprasternal (,sooprə'stərnəl) above the sternum.

supratrochlear (,sooprə'trokli·ə) above the trochlea.

supravaginal (,sooprəvə'jien'l, -'vajin'l) outside or above a sheath, specifically, above the vagina.

supraventricular (,sooprəven'trikyuhlə) situated or occurring above the ventricles, especially in an atrium or atrioventricular node.

supravergence, sursumvergence (,sooprə'vərjəns; ,sərsəm'vərjəns) an upward movement, especially of an eye, the other eye not moving.

supraversion (,sooprə'vərshən) 1. abnormal elongation of a tooth from its socket. 2. an act of turning or directing upward, especially the simultaneous and equal upward turning of the eyes; sursumversion.

sura ('syooə·rə) [L.] calf of the leg. adj. **sural.**

surditas ('sərdi,tas) deafness.

surface ('sərfis) the outer part or external aspect of a solid body.
s.-active agent any substance capable of altering the physicochemical nature of surfaces and interfaces; an example is a detergent. Called also *surfactant.*
s. immunoglobulin see surface IMMUNOGLOBULIN.

surfactant (sər'faktənt) a surface-active agent, such as soap or a synthetic detergent. In pulmonary physiology, a mixture of phospholipids (chiefly lecithin and sphingomyelin) secreted by the great alveolar (type II) cells into the alveoli and respiratory air passages, which reduces the surface tension of pulmonary fluids and thus contributes to the elastic properties of pulmonary tissue. See also HYALINE MEMBRANE DISEASE.

Surgam ('sərgam) trademark for preparations of tiaprofenic acid.

surgeon ('sərjən) a medical practictioner who specializes in surgery.

surgery ('sərjə·ree) 1. that branch of medicine which treats diseases, injuries, and deformities by manual or operative methods. 2. a room or office where a doctor sees and treats patients. adj. **surgical.**

Surmontil (sər'montil) trademark for preparations of trimipramine, a tricyclic antidepressant.

surrogate ('surəgət) a substitute; a thing or person that takes the place of something or someone else, as a drug used in place of another, or, in psychiatry, a person who takes the place of another in the subconscious or in dreams.

s. mother a woman who carries a child for another (the commissioning mother) with the intention that the child be handed over after birth. The pregnancy is usually established using artificial insemination or in vitro fertilization. The genetic parents of the child can vary; the commonest situation is the artificial insemination of the surrogate mother (who therefore provides the ovum) with sperm from the commissioning mother's partner.

sursumversion (,sərsəm'vərshən) see SUPRAVERSION (2).

surveillance (sər'vayləns) close supervision or observation.

individual s. monitoring the health of an individual exposed to infection.

population or epidemiological s. continuous watchfulness over infection in a population.

survey ('sərvay) the systematic collection of information, not forming part of a scientific epidemiological study.

survival rate (sər'vievəl) see RATE.

susceptibility (sə,septə'bilitee) the state of being susceptible.

susceptible (sə'septəb'l) readily affected or acted upon; lacking immunity or resistance.

suscitate ('susi,tayt) to arouse to great activity.

suscitation (,susi'tayshən) arousal to greater activity.

suspension (sə'spenshən) 1. temporary cessation, as of pain or a vital process. 2. a supporting from above, as in treatment of spinal disorders. 3. a preparation of a finely divided, undissolved substance dispersed in a liquid vehicle.

colloid s. one in which the suspended particles are very small.

suspensoid (sə'spensoyd) a colloid system in which the disperse phase consists of particles of any insoluble substance, as a metal, and the dispersion medium may be gaseous, liquid, or solid.

suspensory (sə'spensə·ree) 1. serving to hold up a part. 2. a ligament, bone, muscle, bandage, or sling for supporting a part.

Sustac ('sustak) trademark for a preparation of glyceryl trinitrate.

Sustanon ('sustənon) trademark for a sustained-action preparation of testosterone.

sustentacular (,susten'takyuhlə) supporting; sustaining.

sustentaculum (,susten'takyuhləm) pl. *sustentaculi* [L.] a support.

susurrus (syoo'surəs) [L.] *murmur.*

Sutton's disease ('sutənz) 1. halo naevus. 2. periadenitis mucosa necrotica recurrens. 3. granuloma fissuratum.

Sutton's naevus ('sutənz) halo naevus.

sutura (soo'tyooə·rə) pl. *suturae* [L.] suture; used in anatomical nomenclature to designate a type of joint in which the apposed bony surfaces are united by fibrous tissue, permitting no movement; found only between bones of the skull.

suture ('soochə) 1. sutura, the line of union of adjoining bones of the skull. 2. a stitch or series of stitches made to secure apposition of the edges of a surgical or traumatic wound; used also as a verb to indicate application of such stitches. 3. material used in closing a wound with stitches.

absorbable s. a strand of material used for closing wounds, which becomes dissolved in the body fluids and disappears, such as catgut and tendon.

catgut s. an absorbable suture, prepared from submucous connective tissue of the small intestine of healthy sheep.

coronal s. the line of union between the frontal bone and the parietal bones.

cranial s. the lines of junction between the bones of the skull.

Czerny's s. 1. an intestinal suture in which the thread is passed through the mucous membrane only. 2. union of a ruptured tendon by splitting one of the ends and suturing the other end into the slit.

interrupted s. one in which each stitch is made with a separate piece of material.

lambdoid s. the line of union between the upper borders of the occipital and parietal bones, shaped like the Greek letter lambda (λ).

Lembert's s. see LEMBERT'S SUTURE.

lock-stitch s. a continuous haemostatic suture in which the needle is passed through the loop of the preceding stitch.

mattress s. the stitches parallel with (*horizontal mattress suture*) or at right angles to (*vertical mattress suture*) the wound edges.

purse-string s. a continuous running suture being placed about the opening, and then drawn tight in order to invaginate.

relaxation s. any suture so formed that it may be loosened to relieve tension as necessary.

sagittal s. the line of union of the two parietal bones.

squamous s. the suture between the pars squamosa of the temporal bone and parietal bone.

subcuticular s. a continuous suture placed in the subcuticular tissues parallel with the line of the wound.

tension s. a suture taking a wide bite through all layers of a wound and tied on the surface in order to take tension off the wound as it heals.

suxamethonium chloride (,suksəmee'thohni·əm) a short-acting depolarizing muscle-relaxant that may be used to get good muscle relaxation during surgery performed under general anaesthesia and during electroconvulsive therapy. The main use of suxamethonium chloride is to provide rapid intense muscle relaxation to facilitate endotracheal intubation, less commonly to provide relaxation during surgery, and to prevent injury during electroconvulsive therapy.

svedberg ('sfedbərg) a unit equal to 10^{-13} second, used to express sedimentation coefficients. Symbol S.

swab (swob) 1. a pad of cotton, gauze or other sterilized material to mop up and cleanse wounds, surgical and traumatic. 2. to mop up moisture generally. 3. a small pledget of cotton wool wrapped around a slender shaft of wood or other flexible material, used for applying medications or for obtaining specimens of secretions etc. from body surfaces or orifices.

swage (swayj) 1. to shape metal by hammering or by

adapting it to a die. 2. to fuse, as suture material to the end of a suture needle.

swallowing ('swoloh·ing) the taking in of a substance through the mouth and pharynx and into the oesophagus. It is a combination of a voluntary act and a series of reflex actions. Once begun, the process operates automatically. Called also *deglutition*.

THE THREE STAGES OF SWALLOWING. In the first, voluntary, stage of swallowing, the cheeks are sucked in slightly and the tongue is arched against the hard palate, so that the bolus, or ball of chewed food, is moved to the pharynx.

Normally, air is free to pass from the nose or mouth to the lungs and back again. But the moment the bolus approaches the fauces, the passage from the mouth to the pharynx, nerve centres are triggered that control a series of reflex actions. After one quick inhalation, breathing is halted for the brief instant of the next stage.

In this second, involuntary, stage of swallowing, the rear edge of the soft palate, which hangs down from the roof of the mouth, swings up against the back of the pharynx and blocks the passages to the nose. The back of the tongue fits tightly into the space between two muscular pillars at each side of the fauces, sealing the way back to the mouth. Simultaneously, the larynx moves upward against the epiglottis, effectively closing the entrance to the trachea.

Sometimes the larynx does not move up quickly enough and food gets into the air passage, stimulating a coughing reaction. With the one-way route to the stomach firmly established, however, the muscular coat of the pharynx contracts, squeezing the ball of food and forcing its passage into the oesophagus.

In the third stage, the rhythmic contraction (peristalsis) of the muscles of the oesophagus moves the food on to the stomach. The cardiac sphincter keeps the stomach entrance closed until food is swallowed. As the food approaches, moved by the wavelike contractions of the oesophagus, the advancing portion of the wave causes the sphincter to relax and open, while the rear and contracting portion forces the ball of food through the entrance.

DISORDERS OF SWALLOWING. Difficulty in swallowing, dysphagia, is a symptom of most diseases of the oesophagus. ACHALASIA is failure of the smooth muscles to relax sufficiently during swallowing. This disorder, found mostly in the elderly, may result in complete or partial oesophageal obstruction. Acute and chronic oesophagitis can produce difficulty in swallowing as can oesophageal stricture. Although benign tumours of the oesophagus may occur, most of them are malignant and are accompanied by progressive difficulty in swallowing.

The feeling that there is a lump in the throat or that food sticks there may also be caused by hysteria, in which case it is known as globus hystericus. It is rare and occurs most often in young girls.

The swallowing process can also be impeded by illnesses such as cerebral palsy, stroke, and paralysis.

In diagnosing disorders of swallowing, x-rays and OESOPHAGOSCOPY are used. Treatment may consist of a special diet, dilation of the oesophagus, or surgery. With proper care most cases can be cured; early treatment is important.

Swan-Ganz catheter (ˌswon'gants) see PULMONARY ARTERY FLOTATION CATHETER.

sweat (swet) the excretion of the sweat (sudoriparous) glands of the skin; PERSPIRATION. Sweating produces an evaporative cooling of the body and also serves an excretory function. Substances eliminated in sweat include water, sodium chloride, and small amounts of urea, lactic acid, and potassium ions. During maximal sweating, as in extremely hot weather, the amount of water eliminated can account for a loss of as much as 3.5 kg of body weight per day.

Excessive sweating is called diaphoresis.

s. glands the glands that secrete sweat, situated in the dermis or subcutaneous tissue, and opening by a duct on the surface of the body. They are of two types. The ordinary or eccrine sweat glands are unbranched, coiled, tubular glands that are distributed over almost all of the body surface, and promote cooling by evaporation of their secretion. The apocrine sweat glands are large, branched, specialized glands that empty into the upper portion of a hair follicle instead of directly onto the skin surface, and are found only on certain areas of the body, such as around the anus and in the axilla. Called also sudoriferous, or sudoriparous, glands.

The sweat glands are innervated by cholinergic nerve fibres of the parasympathetic nervous system. They also can be stimulated by the hormones adrenaline and noradrenaline circulating in the blood.

sweetbread ('sweetˌbred) the pancreas or thymus of a food animal.

swelling ('sweling) 1. transient abnormal enlargement of a body part or area not due to cell proliferation. 2. an eminence, or elevation.

cloudy s. an early stage of toxic degenerative changes, especially in protein constituents of organs in infectious diseases, in which the tissues appear swollen, parboiled, and opaque but revert to normal when the cause is removed. Called also albuminoid, or albuminous, degeneration.

Swift's disease (swifts) acrodynia.

sycosiform (sie'kohsiˌfawm) resembling sycosis.

sycosis (sie'kohsis) a papulopustular inflammation of the hair follicles, usually of the beard.

s. barbae a staphylococcal infection and irritation of the hair follicles in the beard region. It may be associated with other superficial bacterial infections, such as impetigo or furunculosis.

The symptoms include burning, itching, and pain, with the formation of small papules and pustules that drain and form crusts. The pustules leave scars when they heal.

The condition is treated with bland hot compresses, antibiotics applied locally and administered parenterally, and manual epilation of the infected hairs. Scrupulous cleanliness and personal hygiene are necessary to prevent reinfection. Called also barber's itch, folliculitis barbae, and sycosis vulgaris.

lupoid s. a chronic, scarring form of deep sycosis barbae.

s. vulgaris sycosis barbae.

Sydenham's chorea ('sid'n'mz) a disorder of the central nervous system closely linked with rheumatic fever; called also Saint Vitus' dance.

The condition, usually self-limited, is characterized by purposeless, irregular movements of the voluntary muscles that cannot be controlled by the patient. The spasmodic jerking movements may be mild or severe and frequently begin as awkwardness and facial grimaces which can cause the child considerable embarassment since he has no control over them. Emotional instability and extreme nervousness usually accompany the physical symptoms.

Treatment and nursing care are based on relief of symptoms. Complete mental and physical rest are prescribed and mild sedatives such as phenobarbitone or one of the tranquillizers may be given to promote relaxation. The prognosis for Sydenham's chorea is good and complete recovery is the rule.

sylvian fissure ('silvi·ən) a fissure extending laterally between the temporal and frontal lobes, and turning posteriorly between the temporal and parietal lobes. Called also fissure of Sylvius.

symballophone (sim'balə,fohn) a stethoscope with two chest pieces, making possible the comparison and localization of sounds.

symbiont ('simbieont, -biont) an organism or species living in a state of symbiosis.

symbiosis (,simbie'ohsis) 1. in parasitology, the biological association of two individuals or populations of different species, classified as mutualism, commensalism, parasitism, amensalism, or synnecrosis, depending on the advantage or disadvantage derived from the relationship. 2. in pyschiatry, a mutually reinforcing relationship between persons who are dependent on each other; a normal characteristic of the relationship between a mother and infant. adj. **symbiotic**.

symbiote ('simbieoht, -bioht) symbiont.

symblepharon (sim'blefə·ron) adhesion of the tarsal to the bulbar conjunctiva, resulting in obliteration of the fornices.

symblepharopterygium (sim,blefə·rohtə'riji·əm) symblepharon in which the adhesion is a cicatricial band resembling a pterygium.

symbolism ('simbə,lizəm) 1. an abnormal mental state in which every occurrence is conceived of as a symbol of the patient's own thoughts. 2. in psychoanalysis, a mechanism of unconscious thinking, usually of a sexual nature, whereby the real meaning becomes transformed so as not to be recognized as sexual by the superego.

symbolization (,simbəlie'zayshən) a mental mechanism of the subconscious which consists in the representation of one object, idea, or quality by another.

Syme's amputation (siemz) amputation of the foot above the ankle-joint.

symmelus ('siməlǝs) a fetus with fused legs.

Symmetrel ('simǝtrel) tradename for amantadine, an antiviral and antiparkinsonism drug.

symmetry ('simitree) correspondence in size, form, and arrangement of parts on opposite sides of a plane, or around an axis. adj. **symmetrical**.

bilateral s. the configuration of an irregularly shaped body (such as the human body or that of higher animals) that can be divided by a longitudinal plane into halves that are mirror images of each other.

radial s. that in which the body parts are arranged regularly around a central axis.

sympathectomize (,simpə'thektə,miez) to deprive of sympathetic innervation.

sympathectomy (,simpə'thektəmee) excision or interruption of some portion of the sympathetic nervous pathway.

chemical s. the interruption of the transmission of impulses through a sympathetic nerve by chemical agents.

periarterial s. surgical removal of the sheath of an artery containing the sympathetic nerve fibres.

sympathetic (,simpə'thetik) 1. pertaining to or caused by sympathy. 2. pertaining to the sympathetic nervous system.

s. blockade block of nerve impulse transmission between a preganglionic sympathetic fibre and the ganglion cell.

s. nerves 1. see SYMPATHETIC TRUNK. 2. any nerve of the sympathetic nervous system.

s. nervous system the thoracolumbar part of the autonomic NERVOUS SYSTEM, the preganglionic fibres of which arise from cell bodies in the thoracic and first three lumbar segments of the spinal cord; postganglionic fibres are distributed to the heart, smooth muscle, and glands of the entire body.

s. trunk two long ganglionated nerve strands, one on each side of the vertebral column, extending from the base of the skull to the coccyx.

sympathicoblast (sim'pathikoh,blast) an embryonic cell that develops into sympathetic nerve cell.

sympathicoblastoma (sim,pathikohbla'stohmə) a malignant tumour containing sympathicoblasts.

sympathicolytic (sim,pathikoh'litik) sympatholytic.

sympathicomimetic (sim,pathikohmi'metik) sympathomimetic.

sympathicotonia (sim,pathikə'tohni·ə) a stimulated condition of the sympathetic nervous system marked by vascular spasm, heightened blood pressure, and the dominance of other sympathetic functions. adj. **sympathicotonic**.

sympathicotripsy (sim,pathikoh'tripsee) surgical crushing of a nerve, ganglion, or plexus of the sympathetic nervous system.

sympathicotropic (sim,pathikoh'tropik) 1. having affinity for or exerting its principal effect on the sympathetic nervous system. 2. an agent with such properties.

sympathicus (sim'pathikəs) the sympathetic nervous system.

sympathin ('simpəthin) a neurohormonal mediator of nerve impulses at sympathetic nerve synapses; the term is used only when the nature of the mediator is unknown.

sympathism ('simpə,thizəm) suggestibility.

sympathoadrenal (,simpəthoh·ə'dreen'l) 1. pertaining to the sympathetic nervous system and the adrenal medulla. 2. involving the sympathetic nervous system and the adrenal glands, especially increased sympathetic activity that causes increased secretion of adrenaline by the adrenal medulla and noradrenaline by the postganglionic sympathetic nerve endings.

sympathoblast (sim'pathoh,blast) sympathicoblast.

sympathoblastoma (,simpəthohbla'stohmə) sympathicoblastoma.

sympathogonia (,simpəthoh'gohni·ə) plural of *sympathogonium*. [Gr.] undifferentiated embryonic cells which develop into sympathetic cells.

sympathogonioma (,simpəthoh,goni'ohmə) a tumour composed of sympathogonia.

sympathogonium (,simpəthoh'gohni·əm) pl. *sympathogonia* [Gr.] an undifferentiated embryonic cell that develops into a sympathetic cell.

sympatholytic (,simpəthoh'litik) antiadrenergic: blocking transmission of impulses from the adrenergic (sympathetic) postganglionic fibres to effector organs or tissues, inhibiting such sympathetic functions as smooth muscle contraction and glandular secretion. Also, an agent that produces such an effect.

sympathomimetic (,simpəthohmi'metik) adrenergic: producing effects resembling those of impulses transmitted by the postganglionic fibres of the sympathetic nervous system. Also, an agent that produces such an effect.

sympathy ('simpəthee) 1. an influence produced in any organ by disease or disorder in another part. 2. compassion for another's grief or loss. 3. the influence exerted by one individual upon another, or received by one from another, and the effects thus produced, as in hypnotism or in yawning.

symphalangism (,simfə'lanjizəm) congenital ankylosis of the proximal phalangeal joints.

symphyseal, symphysial (sim'fizi·əl) pertaining to a symphysis.

symphysiectomy (,simfizi'ektəmee) surgical removal of a part of the symphysis pubis to facilitate a subsequent delivery; now rarely undertaken.

symphysiorrhaphy, symphyseorrhaphy (sim,fizi'o·rəfee) suture of a divided symphysis.

symphysiotomy (sim,fizi'otəmee) division of the symphysis pubis to facilitate delivery.

symphysis ('simfisis) pl. *symphyses* [Gr.] a site or line of union; a type of joint in which the apposed bony surfaces are firmly united by a plate of fibrocartilage.

pubic s., s. pubis the line of union of the bodies of the pubic bones in the median plane.

sympodia (sim'pohdi·ə) fusion of the lower extremities.

symport ('simpawt) a structure that transports two compounds simultaneously across a cell membrane in the same direction, one compound being transported down a concentration gradient, the other against a gradient.

symptom ('simptəm) any indication of disease perceived by the patient.

cardinal s's 1. symptoms of greatest significance to the doctor, establishing the identity of the illness. 2. the symptoms shown in the temperature, pulse, and respiration.

dissociation s. anaesthesia to pain and to heat and cold, without impairment of tactile sensibility.

objective s. one perceptible to others than the patient, as pallor, rapid pulse or respiration, restlessness, and the like.

presenting s. the symptom or group of symptoms about which the patient complains or from which he seeks relief.

signal s. a sensation, aura, or other subjective experience indicative of an impending epileptic or other seizure.

subjective s. one perceptible only to the patient, as pain, pruritus, vertigo, and the like.

withdrawal s's symptoms which follow sudden abstinence from a drug on which a person is dependent (see also WITHDRAWAL SYMPTOMS).

symptomatic (,simptə'matik) 1. pertaining to or of the nature of a symptom. 2. indicative (of a particular disease or disorder). 3. exhibiting the symptoms of a particular disease but having a different cause. 4. directed at the allaying of symptoms, as symptomatic TREATMENT.

symptomatology (,simptəmə'toləjee) 1. the branch of medicine dealing with symptoms. 2. the combined symptoms of a disease. Called also *semeiology*.

symptomatolytic (,simptə,matə'litik) causing the disappearance of symptoms.

sympus ('simpəs) a fetus with feet and legs fused.

syn- word element. [Gr.] *union, association*.

synaesthesia (,sinis'theezi·ə) a secondary sensation accompanying an actual perception; the experiencing of a sensation in one place, due to stimulation applied to another place; also, the condition in which a stimulus of one sense is perceived as sensation of a different sense, as when a sound produces a sensation of colour.

synaesthesialgia (,sinis,theezi'alji·ə) a condition in which a stimulus produces pain on the affected side but no sensation on the normal side of the body.

Synalar ('sinə,lah) trademark for preparations of fluocinolone acetonide, a glucocorticoid used topically.

synalgia (si'nalji·ə) pain felt in one part of the body but caused by inflammation of or injury to another part. Referred pain.

synapse ('sienaps) the junction between the processes of two neurons or between a neuron and an effector organ, where neural impulses are transmitted by chemical means. The impulse causes the release of a neurotransmitter (e.g., acetylcholine or noradrenaline) from the presynaptic membrane of the axon terminal. The neurotransmitter molecules diffuse across the synaptic cleft, bind with specific receptors on the postsynaptic membrane, causing depolarization or hyperpolarization of the postsynaptic cell. See also NEURON.

axoaxonic s. one between the axon of one neuron and the axon of another neuron.

axodendritic s. one between the axon of one neuron and the dendrites of another.

axodendrosomatic s. one between the axon of one neuron and the dendrites and body of another.

axosomatic s. one between the axon of one neuron and the body of another.

dendrodendritic s. one from a dendrite of one cell to a dendrite of another.

synapsis (si'napsis) the pairing off and union of homologous chromosomes from male and female pronuclei at the start of meiosis.

synaptic (si'naptik) pertaining to a synapse or to a synapsis.

synarthrodia (,sinah'throhdi·ə) synarthrosis. adj. **synarthrodial**.

synarthrophysis (sin,ahthrə'fiesis) any ankylosing process.

synarthrosis (,sinah'throhsis) pl. *synarthroses* [Gr.] a form of joint in which the bony elements are united by continuous intervening fibrous tissue; called also fibrous joint.

syncanthus (sin'kanthəs) adhesion of the eyeball to the orbital structures.

syncephalus (sin'kefələs, -'sef-) a twin fetus with heads fused into one, there being a single face, with four ears.

synchilia (sin'kieli·ə) cogenital adhesion of the lips.

synchiria (sin'kieri·ə) reference of sensation to the opposite side on application of a stimulus.

synchondrosis (,sinkon'drohsis) pl. *synchondroses* [Gr.] a type of cartilaginous joint in which the cartilage is usually converted into bone before adult life.

synchondrotomy (,sinkon'drotəmee) division of a synchondrosis.

synchronism ('singkrə,nizəm) occurrence at the same time.

synchronous ('singkrənəs) occurring at the same time.

synchysis ('singkisis) a softening or fluid condition of the vitreous body of the eye.

s. scintillans floating cholesterol crystals in the vitreous, developing as a degenerative change. Of no practical consequence.

synclitism ('singkli,tizəm) parallelism between the planes of the fetal head and those of the maternal pelvis. adj. **synclitic**.

synclonus ('singklohnəs) muscular tremor or successive clonic contraction of various muscles together.

syncope ('singkəpee) a temporary suspension of consciousness due to cerebral anaemia; fainting. adj. **syncopal, syncopic**.

cardiac s. sudden loss of consciousness, with momentary premonitory symptoms or without warning, due to cerebral anaemia caused by ventricular asystole, extreme bradycardia, or ventricular fibrillation.

laryngeal s. tussive syncope.

stretching s. syncope associated with stretching the arms upward with the spine extended.

swallow s. syncope associated with swallowing, a disorder of atrioventricular conduction mediated by the vagus nerve.

tussive s. brief loss of consciousness associated with paroxysms of coughing.

vasovagal s. vasovagal attack.

syncytioma (sin,siti'ohmə) syncytial endometritis.

s. malignum choriocarcinoma.

syncytiotrophoblast (sin,sitioh'trofə,blast, -'troh-) the outer syncytial layer of the trophoblast.
syncytium (sin'siti·əm) a multinucleate mass of protoplasm produced by the merging of cells. adj. **syncytial**.
syndactyly (sin'daktilee) the most common congenital anomaly of the hand, marked by the persistence of the webbing between adjacent digits, so they are more or less completely attached; generally considered an inherited condition, the anomaly may also occur in the foot.
syndesis ('sindisis, sin'deesis) 1. arthrodesis. 2. synapsis.
syndesm(o)- word element. [Gr.] *connective tissue, ligament*.
syndesmectomy (,sindes'mektəmee) excision of a portion of ligament.
syndesmitis (,sindes'mietis) inflammation of a ligament.
syndesmography (,sindes'mogrəfee) a description of the ligaments.
syndesmology (,sindes'moləjee) scientific study of the ligaments and joints.
syndesmoma (,sindes'mohmə) a tumour of connective tissue.
syndesmoplasty (sin'desmoh,plastee) plastic repair of a ligament.
syndesmosis (,sindes'mohsis) pl. *syndesmoses* [Gr.] a joint in which the bones are united by fibrous connective tissue forming an interosseous membrane or ligament.
syndesmotomy (,sindes'motəmee) incision of a ligament.
syndrome ('sindrohm) a combination of symptoms resulting from a single cause or so commonly occurring together as to constitute a distinct clinical picture. For specific syndromes, see under the specific name, as ADRENOGENITAL SYNDROME.
syndrome of inappropriate secretion of antidiuretic hormone a syndrome in which the secretion of antidiuretic hormone (ADH) is not inhibited by hypotonicity of extracellular fluid and hyponatraemia is produced. Abbreviated SIADH. It occurs in conjunction with oat cell carcinoma of the lung and certain other malignant tumours and is caused by production of ADH by the tumour (see also ECTOPIC HORMONES).
syndromic (sin'drohmik, -'drom-) occurring as a syndrome.
syndromology (,sindrə'moləjee) the field concerned with the taxonomy, aetiology, and patterns of congenital malformations.
synechia (si'neeki·ə) pl. *synechiae* [Gr.] adhesion, as of the iris to the cornea or the lens.
annular s. adhesion of the whole rim of the iris to the lens.
anterior s. adhesion of the iris to the cornea.
posterior s. adhesion of the iris to the capsule of the lens or to the surface of the vitreous body.
total s. adhesion of the whole surface of the iris to the lens.
s. vulvae a congenital condition in which the labia minora are sealed in the midline, with only a small opening below the clitoris through which urination and menstruation may occur.
synencephalocele (,sinen'kefəloh,seel, -'sef-) encephalocele with adhesions to adjoining parts.
syneresis (si'nerisis) a drawing together of the particles of the disperse phase of a gel, with separation of some of the disperse medium and shrinkage of the gel, such as occurs in the clotting of blood.
synergism ('sinə,jizəm, si'nər-) the joint action of agents so that their combined effect is greater than the algebraic sum of their individual parts. adj. **synergistic**.
synergist ('sinə,jist, si'nər-) an agent that acts with or enhances the action of another.
synergy ('sinəjee) correlated action or cooperation by two or more structures or drugs.
syngamy ('sing·gəmee) a method of reproduction in which two individuals (gametes) unite permanently and their nuclei fuse; sexual reproduction.
syngeneic (,sinjə'nee·ik, -'nayik) in transplantation biology, denoting individuals or tissues having identical genotypes, i.e., identical twins or animals of the same inbred strain, or their tissues. Called also isogeneic.
syngenesis (sin'jenəsis) 1. the origin of an individual from a germ derived from both parents and not from either one alone. 2. the state of having descended from a common ancestor.
synkaryon (sin'karion) a nucleus formed by fusion of two pronuclei, the fertilization nucleus.
synkinesis (,sinki'neesis) an associated movement; an unintentional movement accompanying a volitional movement. adj. **synkinetic**.
synnecrosis (,sin·nə'krohsis) symbiosis in which the relationship between populations (or individuals) is mutually detrimental.
synorchidism (si'nawki,dizəm) synorchism.
synorchism (si'nawkizəm) congenital fusion of the testes into one mass.
synoscheos (si'noskios) adhesion between the penis and scrotum.
synosteotomy (,sinosti'otəmee) dissection of the joints.
synostosis (,sino'stohsis) pl. *synostoses* [Gr.] normal or abnormal union of two bones by osseous material. adj. **synostotic**.
synotia (si'nohshi·ə) a developmental anomaly with fusion of the ears, or their location near the midventral line in the upper part of the neck.
synotus (si'nohtəs) a fetus exhibiting synotia.
synovectomy (,sienoh'vektəmee, ,si-) excision of a synovial membrane, as of that lining the capsule of the knee joint.
synovia (sie'nohvi·ə, si-) synovial fluid; the transparent viscid fluid secreted by the synovial membrane and found in joint cavities, bursae, and tendon sheaths.
synovial (sie'nohvi·əl, si-) of, pertaining to, or secreting synovia.
s. fluid synovia.
s. joint a specialized form of articulation permitting more or less free movement, the union of the bony elements being surrounded by an articular capsule enclosing a cavity lined by synovial membrane; called also diarthrosis.
s. membrane the inner of the two layers of the articular capsule of a synovial joint; composed of loose connective tissue and having a free smooth surface that lines the joint cavity; it secretes the synovia.
s. villi slender projections from the surface of the synovial membrane into the cavity of a joint.
synovialis (sie,nohvi'aylis) synovial.
synovialoma, synovioma (sie,nohvi·ə'lohmə; sie-,nohvi'ohmə) a tumour of synovial membrane origin.
synoviorthese (si'nohviaw,theez) irradiation of the synovium by intra-articular injection of radiocolloids to destroy inflamed synovial tissue.
synovitis (,sienoh'vietis) inflammation of a synovial membrane, usually painful, particularly on motion, and characterized by fluctuating swelling, due to effusion in a synovial sac. It may be caused by rheumatic fever, rheumatoid arthritis, tuberculosis, trauma, gout, etc.

dry s. synovitis with little effusion.
purulent s. synovitis with effusion of pus in a synovial sac.
serous s. synovitis with copious nonpurulent effusion.
s. sicca dry synovitis.
simple s. synovitis with clear or slightly turbid effusion.
tendinous s. inflammation of a tendon sheath.
villonodular s. proliferation of synovial tissue, especially of the knee joint, composed of synovial villi and fibrous nodules infiltrated by giant cells and macrophages.

synovium (sie'nohvi·əm) a synovial membrane.

Syntaris (sin'tahris) trademark for a preparation of flunisolide, an anti-inflammatory steroid used for seasonal and perennial rhinitis.

synteny ('sintənee) the presence together on the same chromosome of two or more gene loci whether or not in such proximity that they may be subject to linkage. adj. **syntenic.**

synthase ('sinthayz) any enzyme, especially a lyase, which catalyses a synthesis that does not involve the breakdown of a pyrophosphate bond, as opposed to *ligase.*

synthesis ('sinthəsis) 1. creation of a compound by union of elements composing it, done artificially or as a result of natural processes. 2. the process of bringing back into consciousness activities or experiences that have become split off or disassociated. adj. **synthetic.**

synthesize ('sinthə,siez) to produce by synthesis.

synthetase ('sinthə,tayz) ligase; any of a class of enzymes that catalyse the joining together of two molecules coupled with the breakdown of a pyrophosphate bond in ATP or a similar triphosphate.

syntonic (sin'tonik) pertaining to a stable, integrated personality.

syntrophoblast (sin'trohfoh,blast) syncytiotrophoblast.

syntropic (sin'tropik) 1. turning or pointing in the same direction. 2. denoting correlation of several factors, as the relation of one disease to the development or incidence of another. 3. pertaining to a well-balanced personality.

syntropy ('sintrəpee) the state of being syntropic.

syphilid ('sifilid) any cutaneous lesion of syphilitic origin. It may be macular, papular, pustular, or, in tertiary syphilis, a gumma.

syphilis ('sifilis) an infectious venereal disease leading to many structural and cutaneous lesions; called also *lues.*

Syphilis is caused by a spiral-shaped bacterium (spirochete), *Treponema pallidum.* It is a SEXUALLY TRANSMITTED DISEASE (STD) with the exception of congenital syphilis acquired by an infant from the mother in utero.

DIAGNOSIS. The major kinds of tests used for the detection of syphilis are: (1) complement fixation tests, which rely on an antigen–antibody reaction and haemolysis to detect the presence of antibodies to *Treponema pallidum* in the blood, e.g. the Reiter test; (2) flocculation tests, e.g. the Venereal Disease Research Laboratory test (VDRL), which has now replaced the Wasserman Reaction (WR) and the rapid plasma reagin (RPR) test; (3) the fluorescent antibody test (FTA-ABS); and (4) haemagglutination tests, e.g., the TPHA test.

The VDRL and RPR tests are themselves tests for (serum) antibody; they detect antibody to cardiolipin. Tests such as the TPHA and FTA are more specific, i.e. the antibody they detect is antibody to *Treponema pallidum.*

CONGENITAL SYPHILIS. Congenital syphilis is transmitted from a diseased mother to her unborn child through the placenta. Often this results in spontaneous abortion or stillbirth.

If the infant is born alive, he may have snuffles, caused by inflammation of the nose, and may be generally weak and sickly. Syphilitic rashes, especially in the genital area, may occur when the baby is 3 to 8 weeks old. Children with congenital syphilis are often born deformed, and may become blind, deaf, paralysed, or insane. See also HUTCHINSON'S INCISORS/MULBERRY MOLARS.

To prevent congenital syphilis all pregnant women should have a blood test for syphilis during the early months of pregnancy. Treatment before the fifth month will always prevent infection of the unborn child. A syphilitic mother who is not treated early has only one chance in six of having a healthy child. If a child is born with syphilis, immediate treatment may be effective if the disease has not progressed too far.

PREVENTION. Syphilis can be prevented and controlled through education. Educational campaigns have been effective in reducing the number of cases of syphilis, but the disease is still widespread, particularly in the 20–24-year-old age group.

nonvenereal s. a chronic treponemal infection mainly seen in children, occurring in many areas of the world, caused by an organism indistinguishable from *Treponema pallidum*, and transmitted by direct nonsexual contact and indirectly by common use of table and drinking utensils. The first lesions are usually oral mucous patches; subsequent lesions are concentrated in the axillae, inguinal region, and rectum. Then, after a latent period, there develop destructive lesions of the skin and bones. Some authorities believe that venereal and nonvenereal syphilis are the same disease.

syphilitic (,sifi'litik) affected with, caused by, or pertaining to syphilis.

syphiloderm ('sifiloh,dərm) syphilid.

syphilogenesis (,sifiloh'jenəsis) the development of syphilis.

syphiloid ('sifi,loyd) 1. resembling syphilis. 2. a disease like syphilis.

syphilologist (,sifi'loləjist) a specialist in syphilology.

syphilology (,sifi'loləjee) the sum of knowledge about syphilis, its pathology and treatment.

syphiloma (,sifi'lohmə) a tumour of syphilitic origin; a gumma.

syphilophyma (,sifiloh'fiemə) any syphilitic growth or excrescence.

syring(o)- word element. [Gr.] *tube, fistula.*

syringe (si'rinj) an instrument for introducing fluids into or withdrawing them from the body.
hypodermic s. one for introduction of liquids through a hollow needle into subcutaneous tissues.

syringectomy (,sirin'jektəmee) excision of a fistula.

syringitis (,sirin'jietis) inflammation of the pharyngotympanic tube.

syringoadenoma (si,ring·goh,adə'nohmə) syringocystadenoma.

syringobulbia (si,ring·goh'bulbə) the presence of fluid-filled cavities in the medulla oblongata and pons.

syringocarcinoma (si,ring·goh,kahsi'nohmə) cancer of a sweat gland.

syringocele (si'ring·goh,seel) a cavity-containing herniation of the spinal cord through the bony defect in spina bifida.

syringocoele (si,ring·goh,seel) the central canal of the spinal cord.

syringocystadenoma (si,ring·goh,sistadə'nohmə) adenoma of the sweat glands; called also hidradenoma.

syringocystoma (si,ring·gohsi'stohmə) a cystic tumour of a sweat gland.

syringoma (ˌsiring'gohmə) syringocystadenoma.
syringomeningocele (siˌring·gohmə'ning·gohˌseel) meningocele resembling syringomyelocele.
syringomyelia (siˌring·gohmie'eeli·ə) the presence of fluid-filled cavities in the substance of the spinal cord, with destruction of nerve tissue.
syringomyelitis (siˌring·gohˌmieə'lietis) inflammation of the spinal cord with the formation of cavities.
syringomyelocele (siˌring·goh'mieəlohˌseel) hernial protrusion of the spinal cord through the bony defect in spina bifida, the mass containing a cavity connected with the central canal of the spinal cord.
syringotomy (ˌsiring'gotəmee) incision of a fistula.
syrinx ('siringks) a tube or pipe; a fistula.
syrup ('sirəp) a viscous concentrated solution of a sugar, such as sucrose, in water or other aqueous liquid; combined with other ingredients, such a solution is used as a flavoured vehicle for medications.
systaltic (si'staltik) alternately contracting and dilating; pulsating.
system ('sistəm) 1. a set or series of interconnected or interdependent parts or entities (objects, organs, or organisms) that act together in a common purpose or produce results impossible by action of one alone. 2. an organized set of principles or ideas. adj. **systematic, systemic.**

The parts of a system can be referred to as its elements or components; the environment of the system is defined as all of the factors that affect the system and are affected by it. A living system is capable of taking in matter, energy, and information from its environment (input), processing them in some way, and returning matter, energy, and information to its environment as output.

An *open* system is one in which there is an exchange of matter, energy, and information with the environment; in a *closed* system there is no such exchange. A living system cannot survive without this exchange, but in order to survive it must maintain pattern and organization in the midst of constant change. Control of self-regulation of an open system is achieved by dynamic interactions among its elements or components. The result of self-regulation is referred to as the steady state; that is, a state of equilibrium. HOMEOSTASIS is an assemblage of organic regulations that act to maintain steady states of a living organism.

A system can be divided hierarchically into sub-systems, which can be further subdivided into sub-sub-systems and components. A system and its environment could be considered as a unified whole for purposes of study, or a sub-system could be studied as a system. For example, the collection of glands in the endocrine system can be thought of as a system, each endocrine gland could be viewed as a system, or even specific cells of a single gland could be studied as a system. It is also possible to think of the human body as a living system and the endocrine system as a sub-system. The division of a system into a sub-system and its environment is dependent on the perspective chosen by the person studying a particular phenomenon.

alimentary s. digestive system.
autonomic nervous s. the portion of the NERVOUS SYSTEM concerned with regulation of activity of cardiac muscle, smooth muscle, and glands.
cardiovascular s. the heart and blood vessels, by which blood is pumped and circulated through the body (see also CIRCULATORY SYSTEM).
central nervous s. the portion of the NERVOUS SYSTEM consisting of the brain and spinal cord.
centrencephalic s. the neurons in the central core of the brain stem from the thalamus down to the medulla oblongata, connecting the two hemispheres of the brain.
circulatory s. the channels through which nutrient fluids of the body flow (see also CIRCULATORY SYSTEM).
conduction s., conductive s. (of heart) the system comprising the sinoatrial and atrioventricular nodes, atrioventricular bundle, and Purkinje fibres.
digestive s. the organs concerned with the ingestion and digestion of food (see also DIGESTIVE SYSTEM).
endocrine s. the system of glands and other structures that elaborate internal secretions (hormones) which are released directly into the circulatory system, influencing metabolism and other body processes; included are the pituitary, thyroid, parathyroid, and adrenal glands, gonads, pancreas, and paraganglia.
extrapyramidal s. a functional, rather than an anatomical, unit comprising the nuclei and fibres (excluding those of the pyramidal tract) involved in motor activities (see also EXTRAPYRAMIDAL SYSTEM).
general s's theory a theory of organization proposed by Ludwig von Bertalanffy in the 1950s as a means by which various disciplines could communicate with one another and duplication of efforts among scientists could be avoided. The theory sought universally applicable principles and laws that would hold true regardless of the kind of system under study, the nature of its components, or the interrelationships among its components. Since the introduction of the general systems theory, theoretical models, principles, and laws have been developed that are of great value to scientists in all fields, including those of medicine, nursing, and other health-related professions.
genitourinary s. urogenital system; the organs concerned with production and excretion of urine, together with the REPRODUCTIVE ORGANS.
haversian s. a haversian canal and its concentrically arranged lamellae, constituting the basic unit of structure in compact bone (osteon).
haematopoietic s. the tissues concerned in the production of blood, including bone marrow and lymph nodes. **heterogeneous s.** a system or structure made up of mechanically separable parts, as an emulsion or suspension.
homogeneous s. a system or structure made up of parts that cannot be mechanically separated, as a solution.
hypophyseoportal s. the venules connecting the capillaries (gomitoli) in the median eminence of the hypothalamus with the sinusoidal capillaries of the anterior pituitary.
limbic s. a system of brain structures common to the brains of all mammals, comprising the phylogenetically old cortex (archipallium and paleopallium) and its primarily related nuclei. It is associated with olfaction, autonomic functions, and certain aspects of emotion and behaviour.
lymphatic s. the lymphatic vessels and lymphoid tissue, considered collectively (see also CIRCULATORY SYSTEMS and LYMPHATIC SYSTEM).
lymphoid s. the lymphoid tissue of the body, collectively; it consists of the bone marrow, thymus, lymph nodes, spleen, and gut-associated lymphoid tissue (tonsils, Peyer's patches).
metric s. a system of weights and measures based on the metre and having all units based on some power of 10.
mononuclear phagocyte s. the group of highly phagocytic cells that have a common origin from stem cells of the bone marrow and develop circulating monocytes and tissue macrophages, which develop from monocytes that have migrated to connective tissue of the liver (Kupffer's cells), lung, spleen, and

lymph nodes. The term has been proposed to replace *reticuloendothelial system*, which includes some cells of different origin.

nervous s. the organ system that along with the endocrine system, correlates the adjustments and reactions of an organism to internal and environmental conditions, comprising the central and peripheral nervous systems (see also NERVOUS SYSTEM).

parasympathetic nervous s. the craniosacral portion of the autonomic NERVOUS SYSTEM. Its preganglionic fibres leave the central nervous system with cranial nerves III, VII, IX and X and with the second to fourth sacral ventral roots; postganglionic fibres innervate the heart, smooth muscles, and glands of the head and neck, and thoracic, abdominal, and pelvic viscera.

peripheral nervous s. the portion of the NERVOUS SYSTEM consisting of the nerves and ganglia outside the brain and spinal cord.

portal s. an arrangement by which blood collected from one set of capillaries passes through a large vessel or vessels and another set of capillaries before returning to the systemic circulation, as in the pituitary gland and liver.

respiratory s. the tubular and cavernous organs that allow atmospheric air to reach the membranes across which gases are exchanged with the blood (see also RESPIRATORY SYSTEM).

reticuloendothelial s. a network of cells and tissues found throughout the body that is concerned in blood cell formation and destruction, storage of fatty materials and the metabolism of iron and pigment, and plays a defensive role in inflammation and immunity (see also RETICULOENDOTHELIAL SYSTEM).

skeletal s. the body's framework of bones; the skeleton (see also SKELETAL SYSTEM).

sympathetic nervous s. the thoracolumbar part of the autonomic NERVOUS SYSTEM, the preganglionic fibres of which arise from cell bodies in the thoracic and first three lumbar segments of the spinal cord; postganglionic fibres are distributed to the heart, smooth muscle, and glands of the entire body.

urinary s. the system formed in the body by the KIDNEYS, the urinary BLADDER, the URETERS, and the URETHRA, the organs concerned in the production and excretion of urine.

urogenital s. genitourinary system.

vascular s. the vessels of the body, especially the blood vessels.

vasomotor s. the part of the nervous system that controls the calibre of the blood vessels.

systema (si'steemə) [Gr.] *system.*

systemic (si'stemik) pertaining to or affecting the body as a whole.

s. circulation the flow of oxygenated blood from the left ventricle through the aorta, carrying oxygen and nutrient material to all the tissues of the body, and returning the venous blood through the superior and inferior venae cavae to the right atrium. See also CIRCULATORY SYSTEM.

s. lupus erythematosus (SLE) see systemic LUPUS erythematosus.

s. sclerosis see SCLEROSIS.

systole ('sistəlee) the contraction, or period of contraction, of the heart, especially of the ventricles, during which blood is forced into the aorta and pulmonary artery. adj. **systolic**.

atrial s. contraction of the atria by which blood is forced into the ventricles; it precedes the true or ventricular systole.

extra s. extrasystole; an atrial or ventricular contraction occurring prematurely, while the basic rhythm of the heart is maintained.

ventricular s. contraction of the ventricles, forcing blood into the aorta and pulmonary artery.

systremma (si'stremə) a cramp in the muscles of the calf of the leg.

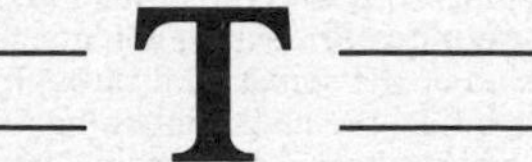

T symbol, *tesla; tera-;* (absolute) temperature.

2,4,5-T a toxic chlorphenoxy herbicide (2,4,5-trichlorophenoxyacetic acid), a component of Agent Orange.

T_3 symbol for triiodothyronine.

T_4 symbol for thyroxine.

T_m tubular maximum (of the kidneys); used in reporting kidney function studies, with inferior letters representing the substance used in the test, as T_{mPAH} (tubular maximum for *p*-aminohippuric acid).

t in genetics, symbol for translocation.

T cell ('tee ˌsel) a lymphocyte which is derived from the thymus and is responsible for cell-mediated immunity.

T group ('teegroop) training group; see under GROUP.

TA toxin–antitoxin.

Ta chemical symbol, *tantalum.*

TAB a vaccine prepared from killed typhoid, paratyphoid A and paratyphoid B bacilli.

tabacosis (ˌtabə'kohsis) poisoning by tobacco, chiefly by inhaling tobacco dust; a form of PNEUMOCONIOSIS attributed to tobacco dust.

tabanid ('tabənid) any gadfly of the family Tabanidae, including the horseflies and deerflies.

Tabanus (tə'baynəs) a genus of bloodsucking biting flies (horseflies or gadflies) which transmit trypanosomes and anthrax to various animals.

tabardillo (ˌtabah'deeyoh) murine typhus, an infectious disease of Mexico resembling typhoid fever.

tabes ('taybeez) 1. any wasting of the body; progressive atrophy of the body or a part of it. 2. tabes dorsalis. adj. **tabetic**.

t. dorsalis a slowly progressive nervous disorder, from degeneration of the dorsal columns of the spinal cord and sensory nerve trunks, resulting in disturbances of sensation and interference with reflexes and consequently with movements; called also locomotor ataxia. It is caused by SYPHILIS and may appear 5 to 20 years after initial infection. The first symptoms are pain (often in the legs, although it may occur in the arms or trunk) and loss of position sense. The pupils are uneven and do not react to light (Argyll Robertson pupils). Unless the patient looks down at his legs he does not know where they are and must depend on his vision for each step. The typical gait of a tabetic patient is jerky and wide-based. Its course is slow but progressive; it can often be arrested, but complete cure is rare.

t. mesenterica tuberculosis of the mesenteric glands in children.

tabescent (tə'bes'nt) growing emaciated; wasting away.

tabetiform (tə'betiˌfawm) resembling tabes.

tablature ('tablәchә) separation of the chief cranial bones into inner and outer tables, separated by a diploë.

table ('tayb'l) a flat layer or surface.

inner t. the inner compact layer of the bones covering the brain.

outer t. the outer compact layer of the bones covering the brain.

vitreous t. inner table.

tablespoon ('tayb'lˌspoon) a household unit of volume

or capacity, equivalent to three teaspoons or approximately 15 millilitres.

tablet ('tablit) a solid dosage form containing a medicinal substance with or without a suitable diluent.

buccal t. one which dissolves when it is held between the cheek and gum, permitting direct absorption of the active ingredient through the oral mucosa.

enteric-coated t. one coated with material that delays release of the medication until after it leaves the stomach.

sublingual t. one that dissolves when held beneath the tongue, permitting direct absorption of the active ingredient by the oral mucosa.

taboo (tə'boo) any of the negative traditions and behaviours generally regarded as harmful to social welfare.

taboparesis (ˌtaybohpə'reesis) tabes with general paresis.

tabular ('tabyuhlə) resembling a table.

tache (tash, tahsh) [Fr.] *a spot or blemish.*

t. blanche ('white spot'), a white spot on the liver in certain infectious diseases.

t's bleuâtres ('bluish spots'), maculae caeruleae.

t. cérébrale ('cerebral spot'), a congested streak produced by drawing the nail across the skin; a concomitant of various nervous or cerebral diseases.

t. motrice ('motor spot'), a motor nerve ending in which the nerve fibril passes to a muscle cell, where it ends in a slight enlargement.

t. noire ('black spot'), an ulcer covered with a black crust, a characteristic local reaction at the presumed site of the infective bite in certain tickborne rickettsioses.

tachogram ('takəˌgram) the graphic record produced by tachography.

tachography (ta'kogrəfee) the recording of the movement and speed of the blood current.

tachy- word element. [Gr.] *rapid, swift.*

tachyarrhythmia (ˌtaki·ə'ridhmi·ə) tachycardia associated with an irregularity in the normal heart rhythm.

tachycardia (ˌtaki'kahdi·ə) abnormally rapid heart rate, usually taken to be over 100 beats per minute. adj. **tachycardiac.**

atrial t. a rapid cardiac rate, usually 160–190 beats per minute, originating from an atrial locus.

ectopic t. rapid heart action in response to impulses arising outside the sinoatrial node.

junctional t. that arising in response to impulses originating in the atrioventricular junction, i.e., the atrioventricular node.

orthostatic t. disproportionate rapidity of the heart rate on arising from a reclining to a standing position.

paroxysmal t. rapid heart action that starts and stops abruptly.

supraventricular t. a combination of junctional tachycardia and atrial tachycardia.

ventricular t. an abnormally rapid ventricular rhythm with aberrant ventricular excitation, usually above 150 beats per minute, generated within the ventricle, and most often associated with atrioventricular dissociation.

tachylalia (ˌtaki'layli·ə) rapidity of speech.

tachymeter (ta'kimitə) an instrument for measuring rapidity of motion.

tachyphagia (ˌtaki'fayji·ə) rapid eating.

tachyphasia, tachyphrasia (ˌtaki'fayzi·ə; ˌtaki'frayzi·ə) extreme volubility of speech.

tachyphrenia (ˌtaki'freeni·ə) mental hyperactivity.

tachyphylaxis (ˌtakifi'laksis) 1. rapid immunization against the effect of toxic doses of an extract by previous injection of small doses of it. 2. rapidly decreasing response to a drug or physiologically active agent after administration of a few doses. adj. **tachyphylactic.**

tachypnoea (ˌtakip'neeə) very rapid respirations. These are seen in high fever when the body attempts to rid itself of excess heat. Other causes include pneumonia, compensatory respiratory alkalosis as the body tries to 'blow off' excess carbon dioxide, respiratory insufficiency, lesions in the respiratory control centre of the brain, and salicylate poisoning.

tachyrhythmia (ˌtaki'ridhmi·ə) tachycardia.

tachysterol (taki'stiə·rol) an isomer of ergosterol, an antirachitic substance, produced by irradiaton of ergosterol.

tactile ('taktiel) pertaining to touch.

tactometer (tak'tomitə) an instrument for measuring tactile sensibility; aesthesiometer.

tactus ('taktəs) [L.] *touch.* adj. **tactual.**

t. eruditus delicacy of touch acquired by practice.

Taenia ('teeni·ə) a genus of TAPEWORMS.

T. saginata a species 3.5–7.5 m long, found in the adult form in the human intestine and in the larval state in muscles and other tissues of cattle and other ruminants; human infection usually results from eating inadequately cooked beef.

T. solium a species 2–3.5 m long, found in the adult intestine; the larval form most often is found in muscle and other tissues of the pig; human infection results from eating inadequately cooked pork. See also CYSTICERCOSIS.

taenia ('teeni·ə) pl. *taeniae* [L] 1. a flat band or strip of soft tissue; used in anatomical nomenclature to designate various structures. 2. a TAPEWORM of the genus *Taenia.*

taeniae coli the three thickened bands (taenia libera, taenia mesocolica, and taenia omentalis) formed by longitudinal fibres in the tunica muscularis of the large intestine, extending from the root of the vermiform appendix to the rectum.

taeniacide ('teeni·əˌsied) 1. lethal to tapeworms. 2. an agent lethal to tapeworms.

taeniafuge ('teeni·əˌfyooj) a medicine for expelling tapeworms.

taeniamyotomy (ˌteeni·əmie'otəmee) an incision or a series of incisions into the taeniae coli; done in diverticular disease.

taeniasis (tee'nieəsis) infection with tapeworms of the genus *Taenia.*

TAF toxoid-antitoxin floccules. A vaccine used for diphtheria immunization. See also TOXOID.

tag (tag) 1. a small appendage, flap, or polyp. 2. label.

radioactive t. a radioisotope that has been incorporated in a chemical compound.

Tagamet ('tagəmet) trademark for preparations of cimetidine; an H_2-receptor blocker used for treatment of peptic ulcer.

Takayasu's arteritis (disease) (ˌtaka'yasooz) pulseless disease.

talc (talk) a native hydrous magnesium silicate, sometimes with a small amount of aluminium silicate; used as a dusting powder.

talcosis (tal'kohsis) a condition due to inhalation or implantation in the body of talc.

talcum ('talkəm) talc.

talipes ('talipeez) CLUBFOOT; a congenital deformity of the foot, which is twisted out of shape or position; the foot may have an abnormally high longitudinal arch (talipes cavus) or it may be in dorsiflexion (talipes calcaneus) or plantar flexion (talipes equinus), abducted, everted (talipes valgus), abducted, inverted (talipes varus), or various combinations of these (talipes calcaneovalgus, talipes calcaneovarus, talipes equinovalgus or talipes equinovarus)..

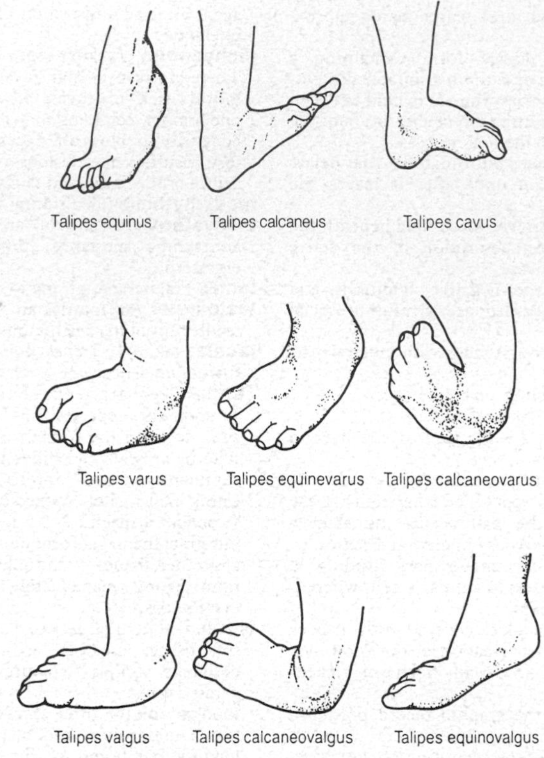

Talipes

talipomanus (ˌtalipoh'manəs) clubhand.

talocalcanean (ˌtaylohkal'kayni·ən) pertaining to the talus and calcaneus.

talocrural (ˌtayloh'krooə·rəl) pertaining to the talus and the leg bones.

talofibular (ˌtayloh'fibyuhlə) pertaining to the talus and fibula.

talonavicular (ˌtaylohnə'vikyuhlə) pertaining to the talus and navicular bone.

talus ('tayləs) ankle bone; the highest of the tarsal bones.

Tamofen ('tamohfen) trademark for a preparation of tamoxifen.

tamoxifen (tə'moksifen) a nonsteroidal oral antioestrogen used in the palliative treatment of breast cancer in postmenopausal women and to stimulate ovulation in infertility.

tampon ('tampon) a pack, pad, or plug made of cotton, sponge, or other material, variously used in surgery to control haemorrhage by pressure or to absorb secretions.

tamponade ('tampəˌnayd) 1. surgical use of a tampon. 2. pathological compression of a part.

cardiac t. compression of the heart due to collection of fluid or blood in the pericardium.

Tangier disease (tan'jiə) a familial disease characterized by a deficiency of high-density lipoproteins in the blood serum, with storage of cholesterol esters in the tonsils and other tissues.

tank (tangk) an artificial receptacle for liquids.

Hubbard t. a tank in which exercises may be performed under water.

tannate ('tanayt) any of the salts of tannic acid, all of which are astringent.

tannic acid ('tanik) a substance obtained from bark and fruit of many plants, used as an astringent.

tannin ('tanin) tannic acid.

tantalum ('tantələm) a chemical element, atomic number 73, atomic weight 180.948, symbol Ta. (See table of elements in Appendix 2.) It is a noncorrosive and malleable metal which is inert and can be implanted.

tantrum ('tantrəm) a violent display of temper.

tap (tap) 1. a quick, light blow. 2. to drain off fluid by PARACENTESIS.

spinal t. lumbar puncture.

tape ('tayp) a long, narrow strip of fabric or other flexible material.

adhesive t. a strip of fabric or other material evenly coated on one side with a pressure-sensitive adhesive material.

tapeinocephaly (ˌtapinoh'kefəlee, -'sef-) flattening or depression of the skull. adj. **tapeinocephalic.**

tapetum (tə'peetəm) pl. *tapeta* [L.] 1. a covering structure or layer of cells. 2. a stratum in the human brain composed of fibres from the body and splenium of the corpus callosum sweeping around the lateral ventricle.

t. lucidum the iridescent epithelium of the choroid of animals that gives their eyes the property of shining in the dark.

tapeworm ('taypwərm) a parasitic cestode worm having

a flattened bandlike form, which lodges in the intestines of animals and human beings. They are transmitted to man in larval form, embedded in cysts, in meat or fish that is not properly cooked. In the human they develop to maturity and attach themselves to the wall of the intestine, where they grow and release eggs.

Although a large number of adult tapeworms are considered human parasites, only a few infect man to any great degree. *Taenia saginata*, the beef tapeworm, and *T. solium*, the pork tapeworm, are widespread and quite common in some parts of the world. Beef tapeworms grow to a length of 3.5 to 7.5 m, and adult pork tapeworms average 2 to 3.5 m in length. Both species release white, egg-containing proglottids, or segments of the body, which make their way to the anus and may be found in clothes or bedding. *Diphyllobothrium latum* is the fish tapeworm, and is found predominantly in North America, northern Europe, and Japan. It may grow as long as 18 m. *Hymenolepis nana* and *H. diminuta* are dwarf tapeworms that are common in the tropics and subtropics.

The diagnosis of a tapeworm infection is made when segments of the worm are found in clothing or bedding or when characteristic eggs or segments are found in the stool. Occasionally diarrhoea, vague abdominal cramps, flatulence, distention, and nausea occur. Mental deterioration and seizures are rare and occur only when larval forms of *T. solium* invade brain tissue (CYSTICERCOSIS).

Tapeworm infection can be prevented by cooking pork, beef, and fish properly. Although most meats and fish are inspected under government supervision, eggs and larvae are not always detectable; the only certain protection is proper cooking.

Once it is inside the body, the tapeworm can be eliminated by specific anthelmintic drugs. The drug of choice is niclosamide. Mepacrine hydrochloride is now seldom used. The drug should be given in a single dose large enough to cause the worm to release its hold and allow for its passage through the intestinal tract. If the head is not found in the evacuated faeces, there is the possibility that the worm will regenerate in two to three months, and segments will reappear in the stools. If the head is found, no further treatment is necessary. Dichlorophen and its derivatives are also active taeniacides. They have the disadvantage of disintegrating the worm so that the head cannot be identified and thus there is no proof of cure. A follow-up after at least three months is recommended when these drugs are used.

Echinococcus granulosus and *E. multilocularis* differ from other tapeworms in that the adults infect animal hosts and the larval forms are found in man. The larvae develop in the human intestine, penetrate its wall and are carried by the lymphatics to various organs of the body where they form slowly growing cysts (hydatid cysts). The liver is the organ most commonly involved. Treatment is by surgical removal of the cyst. Echinococcosis (HYDATID DISEASE) is found where herding dogs are used and have close contact with man.

armed t. *Taenia solium.*

beef t. *Taenia saginata.*

broad t. *Diphyllobothrium latum.*

dog t. *Dipylidium caninum.*

fish t. *Diphyllobothrium latum.*

hydatid t. *Echinococcus granulosus.*

pork t. *Taenia solium.*

unarmed t. *Taenia saginata.*

taphophilia (ˌtafoh'fili·ə) morbid interest in graves and cemeteries.

tapotement (ˌtapoht'monh) [Fr.] a tapping manipulation in massage.

tapping ('taping) see PARACENTESIS.

tar (tah) a dark-brown or black, viscid liquid obtained from various species of pine or from bituminous coal.

coal t. a by-product obtained in destructive distillation of bituminous coal; used in ointment or solution in treatment of eczema and psoriasis.

juniper t. a volatile oil obtained from wood of *Juniperus oxycedrus*; used topically in the treatment of eczema.

pine t. a product of destructive distillation of the wood of various pine trees; used as a local antieczematic and rubefacient.

tarantula (tə'rantyuhlə) a venomous spider.

tardive ('tahdiv) late; applied to a disease in which the characteristic lesion is late in appearing.

tare (tair) 1. the weight of the vessel in which a substance is weighed. 2. to weigh a vessel which is to contain a substance in order to allow for it when the vessel and substance are weighed together.

target ('tahgit) 1. an object or area toward which something is directed. 2. the area of the anode of an x-ray tube where the electron beam collides causing the emission of x-rays. 3. a cell or organ that is affected by a particular agent, e.g., a hormone or drug.

t. cell see LEPTOCYTE.

tarichatoxin (ˌtarikə'toksin) a neurotoxin from the newt (*Taricha)*, identical with tetrodotoxin.

tars(o)- word element. [Gr.] *edge of eyelid*, *tarsus of foot*, *instep.*

tarsal ('tahs'l) pertaining to the tarsus of an eyelid or of the foot.

t. tunnel the osseofibrous passage for the posterior tibial vessels, tibial nerve, and flexor tendons, formed by the flexor retinaculum and the tarsal bones.

t. tunnel syndrome a complex of symptoms resulting from compression of the posterior tibial nerve or of the plantar nerves in the tarsal tunnel, with pain, numbness, and tingling paraesthesia of the sole of the foot.

tarsalgia (tah'salji·ə) pain in a tarsus.

tarsalia (tah'sayli·ə) the bones of the tarsus.

tarsalis (tah'saylis) [L.] *tarsal.*

tarsectomy (tah'sektəmee) 1. excision of one or more bones of the tarsus. 2. excision of the cartilage of the eyelid.

tarsoclasis (ˌtahsoh'klaysis) surgical fracture of the tarsus of the foot.

tarsomalacia (ˌtahsohmə'layshi·ə) softening of the tarsal cartilage of an eyelid.

tarsometatarsal (ˌtahsohˌmetə'tahs'l) pertaining to the tarsus and metatarsus.

tarsophyma (ˌtahsoh'fiemə) 1. any tumour of the tarsus. 2. a growth on the tarsus of the eyelid.

tarsoplasty ('tahsohˌplastee) plastic repair of the tarsus of the eyelid.

tarsoptosis (ˌtahsop'tohsis) falling of the tarsus; flatfoot.

tarsorrhaphy (tah'so·rəfee) suture of a portion of or the entire upper and lower eyelids for the purpose of reducing or closing the palpebral fissure.

tarsotomy (tah'sotəmee) surgical incision of a tarsus, or an eyelid.

tarsus ('tahsəs) 1. the seven bones—talus, calcaneus, navicular, medial, intermediate and lateral cuneiform, and cuboid—composing the articulation between the foot and leg; the ankle or instep. 2. the cartilaginous plate forming the framework of either (upper or lower) eyelid.

tartar ('tahtə) 1. the recrystallized sediment of wine casks; crude potassium bitartrate. 2. a yellowish film formed of calcium phosphate and carbonate, food particles, and other organic matter, deposited on the teeth by the saliva; called also dental calculus. Tartar should be removed regularly by a dentist. If neglected, it can cause bacterial plaque to lodge between the gums and the teeth, causing gum infection, dental caries, loosening of the teeth, and other disorders.

tartaric acid (tah'tarik) a compound used in preparing refrigerant drinks and effervescent powders.

tartrate ('tahtrayt) a salt of tartaric acid.

tastant ('taystənt) any substance, e.g., salt, capable of eliciting gustatory excitation, i.e., stimulating the sense of taste.

taste (tayst) the peculiar sensation caused by the contact of soluble substances with the tongue; the sense effected by the tongue, the gustatory and other nerves, and the gustatory centre.

The organs of taste are the taste buds, bundles of slender cells with hairlike branches that are packed together in groups that form the projections called papillae at various places on the tongue. When a substance is introduced into the mouth, its molecules enter the pores of the papillae and stimulate the taste buds directly. In order to do this, the substance has to be dissolved in liquid. If it is not liquid when it enters the mouth, then it melts or is chewed and becomes mixed with saliva.

There are four basic tastes: sweet, salt, sour, and bitter. Sometimes alkaline and metallic are also included as basic tastes. All other tastes are combinations of these. The taste buds are specialized, and each responds only to the kind of basic taste that is its speciality. The sweet and salt taste buds are most numerous on the tip and front part of the tongue, sour taste buds are mainly along the edges, and bitterness is tasted at the back of the tongue. Bitter–sweet substances are tasted in two stages, first sweet, then bitter. The solid centre of the tongue's surface has very few taste buds.

Other senses, including smell and touch, also play an important role in tasting.

taster ('taystə) an individual capable of tasting a particular substance, such as phenylthiocarbamide, used in certain genetic studies.

TAT thematic apperception test.

tattooing (ta'tooing) the introduction, by punctures, of permanent colours into the skin.

t. of cornea permanent colouring of the cornea, chiefly to conceal leukomatous spots.

taurine ('tor·reen) a crystallized acid from the bile; found also in small quantities in lung and muscle tissues.

taurocholate (ˌtor·roh'kohlayt) a salt of taurocholic acid, one of the bile acids.

taurocholic acid (ˌtor·roh'kohlik) a bile acid; when hydrolysed it splits into taurine and cholic acid.

Taussig–Bing syndrome (ˌtawsig'bing) transposition of the great vessels of the heart and a ventricular septal defect straddled by a large pulmonary artery.

Taussig's operation ('tawsigz) block dissection of the pelvic lymphatic glands.

tautomer ('tawtəmə) a chemical compound exhibiting, or capable of exhibiting, tautomerism.

tautomeral (taw'tomə·rəl) pertaining to the same part; said especially of neurons and neuroblasts sending processes to aid in formation of the white matter in the same side of the spinal cord.

tautomerase (taw'tomə,rayz) an enzyme that catalyses tautomeric reactions.

tautomeric (ˌtawtə'merik) exhibiting, or capable of exhibiting, tautomerism.

tautomerism (taw'tomə,rizəm) stereoisomerism in which the compounds are mutually interconvertible, under normal conditons, forming a mixture that is in dynamic equilibration.

Tawara's node (tə'wahrə) the atrioventricular node. See NODE.

taxis ('taksis) 1. an orientation movement of a motile organism in response to a stimulus; it may be either toward (positive) or away from (negative) the source of the stimulus; used also as a word ending, affixed to a stem denoting the nature of the stimulus. 2. manual replacement of a displaced organ or part, or reduction of a hernia.

taxon ('takson) pl. *taxa* [Gr.] 1. a particular taxonomic grouping, e.g., a particular species, genus, family, order, class, phylum, or kingdom. 2. the name applied to a taxonomic grouping.

taxonomy (tak'sonəmee) the orderly classification of organisms into appropriate categories (taxa), with application of suitable and correct names. adj. **taxonomic.**

numerical t. a method of classifying organisms solely on the basis of the number of shared phenotypic characters, each character usually being given equal weight; used primarily in bacteriology.

Tay–Sachs disease (ˌtay'saks) the infantile form of amaurotic familial idiocy, inherited as an autosomal recessive trait and affecting chiefly Ashkenazic Jews. It is a progressive disorder marked by degeneration of brain tissue and the maculas (with the formation of a cherry-red spot on both retinas) and by dementia, blindness, and death. Tay–Sachs disease is a sphingolipidosis in which the inborn error of metabolism is a deficiency of the enzyme hexosaminidase A that results in accumulation of GM_2 ganglioside in the brain.

It is possible to test for this disease in the unborn fetus at 14 weeks of pregnancy. An absence of the enzyme hexosaminidase A indicates conclusively that the fetus has Tay–Sachs disease. Carriers of the trait have lowered levels of the enzyme in their blood, thus permitting screening of populations most susceptible to transmission of the trait to their offspring and genetic counselling of known carriers.

Tay's spot ('tayz) the choroid appearing as a red circular area surrounded by grey-white retina, as viewed through the fovea centralis in Tay–Sachs disease. Called also *cherry-red spot.*

Taylor splint ('taylə) a horizontal pelvic band and long lateral posterior bars; used to apply traction to the lower extremity. Called also *Taylor brace.*

Tb chemical symbol, *terbium.*

tb tuberculosis; tubercle bacillus.

Tc chemical symbol, *technetium.*

TCID tissue culture infective dose; that amount of a pathogenic agent that will produce pathological change when inoculated on tissue cultures.

$TCID_{50}$ median tissue culture infective dose; that amount of a pathogenic agent that will produce pathological change in 50 per cent of cell cultures inoculated.

TdT terminal deoxynucleotidyl transferase.

Te chemical symbol, *tellurium.*

tea (tee) 1. the dried leaves of *Thea chinensis*, containing caffeine and tannic acid, or a decoction thereof. 2. any decoction or infusion.

pectoral t. an aqueous infusion of expectorant and demulcent herbs and aromatics.

tears (tiəz) the watery, slightly alkaline and saline secretion of the lacrimal glands that moistens the conjunctiva. See also LACRIMAL APPARATUS.

syndrome of crocodile t. spontaneous lacrimation occurring parallel with the normal salivation of eating. It follows facial paralysis and seems to be due to straying of the regenerating nerve fibres, some of those destined for the salivary glands going to the lacrimal glands.

tease (teez) to pull apart gently with fine needles to permit microscopic examination.

teaspoon ('tee,spoon) a household unit of volume or capacity approximately equal to 5 millilitres.

teat (teet) 1. the nipple of the mammary gland. 2. a man-made nipple used on infants' feeding bottles.

technetium (tek'neeshi·əm) a chemical element, atomic number 43, atomic weight 99, symbol Tc. See table of elements in Appendix 2.

t.-99m the most frequently used radioisotope in nuclear medicine, a gamma emitter having a half-life of 6.04 hours and a primary photon energy of 140 keV. It can be used as simple sodium pertechnetate or tagged to various chemicals so that specific organs can be imaged, e.g., ^{99}Tc^{m}-sulphur colloid for liver and spleen scanning, ^{99}Tc^{m}-dimethyl sulphonic acid (DMSA) for renal scanning, ^{99}Tc^{m}-methylene diphosphate (MDP) for bone scanning, and ^{99}Tc^{m}-pyrophosphate for imaging myocardial infarctions.

technician (,tek'nishən) a person skilled in the performance of the technical or procedural aspects of a health care profession.

technique (tek'neek) the method of procedure and details of a mechanical process or surgical operation.

technologist (tek'noləjist) a person skilled in the theory and practice of a technical profession.

tectorial (tek'tor·ri·əl) of the nature of a roof or covering.

tectorium (tek'tor·ri·əm) Corti's membrane.

tectospinal (,tektoh'spien'l) extending from the tectum of the midbrain to the spinal cord.

tectum ('tektəm) a rooflike structure.

t. of mesencephalon, t. of midbrain the dorsal portion of the midbrain.

TED threshold erythema dose.

teeth (teeth) plural of *tooth*.

teething ('teedhing) eruption of the teeth through the gums. The average infant cuts his first tooth between the sixth and ninth months. The full set of 20 baby teeth erupt gradually over a period up to about 30 months, the customary pattern being the arrival of two teeth, one on each side of the jaw, at a time.

Evidence of teething includes drooling, a compulsion to put objects into the mouth, and general fretfulness. Some babies seem to be more bothered by teething than others, and different teeth affect the same baby in different ways.

It was long fashionable to ascribe any baby ailment to teething, despite the considerable harm such a hasty diagnosis often did by delaying recognition of the real trouble. Although teething sometimes may cause a slight fever, any such symptom should be watched carefully for further developments.

Teflon ('teflon) trademark for tetrafluoroethylene fluorocarbon polymers; used as a surgical implant material.

tegmen ('tegmen) pl. *tegmina* [L.] a covering structure or roof.

t. tympani 1. the thin layer of bone separating the tympanic antrum from the cranial cavity. 2. the roof of the tympanic cavity, related to part of the petrous portion of the temporal bone.

tegmentum (teg'mentəm) pl. *tegmenta* [L.] 1. a covering. 2. the part of the cerebral peduncle dorsal to the substantia nigra. adj. **tegmental.**

Tegretol ('tegri,tol) trademark for a preparation of carbamazepine, an anticonvulsant.

tegument ('tegyuhmənt) the skin.

teichoic acids (tie'koh·ik) antigenic polymers of glycerol or ribitol phosphates found attached to the cell walls or in intracellular association with membranes of gram-positive bacteria; they determine group specificity of some species, e.g., the staphylococci.

teichopsia (tie'kopsi·ə) scintillating scotoma; the sensation of a luminous appearance before the eyes, with a zigzag, wall-like outline.

tela ('teelə) pl. *telae* [L.] a thin, weblike structure or tissue; used in naming various anatomic structures.

t. conjunctiva connective tissue.

t. elastica elastic tissue.

t. subcutanea the subcutaneous connective tissue or superficial fascia.

telaesthesia (,telis'theezi·ə) telepathy; perception at a distance.

telalgia (tə'lalji·ə) referred pain; pain occurring in a part distant from the lesion.

telangiectasia (tə,lanjiek'tayzi·ə) a vascular lesion formed by dilation of a group of small blood vessels. adj. **telangiectatic. hereditary haemorrhagic t.** a hereditary condition marked by multiple small angiomas of the skin and mucous membranes, often with nosebleed or gastrointestinal bleeding and sometimes with arteriovenous fistula of the lung or liver.

telangiectasis (tə,lanji'ektəsis) pl. *telangiectases;* telangiectasia.

spider t. vascular spider.

telangioma (tə,lanji'ohmə) a tumour of the blood capillaries.

telangiosis (tə,lanji'ohsis) any disease of the capillaries.

tele- word element. [Gr.] *far away*, *operating at a distance*, *an end*.

telecanthus (,teli'kanthəs) abnormally increased distance between the medial canthi of the eyelids.

telecardiography (,teli,kahdi'ografee) the recording of an electrocardiogram by transmission of impulses to a site at a distance from the patient.

telecardiophone (,teli'kahdioh,fohn) an apparatus for making heart sounds audible at a distance from the patient.

teleceptor ('teli,septə) telereceptor.

telecinesia (,telisi'neezi·ə) telekinesis.

telediagnosis (,teli,dieəg'nohsis) determination of the nature of a disease at a site remote from the patient on the basis of transmitted telemonitoring data or closed-circuit television consultation.

telefluoroscopy (,teli,flooə'roskəpee) television transmission of fluoroscopic images for study at a distant location.

telekinesis (,teliki'neesis) 1. movement of an object produced without contact. 2. the ability to produce such movement. adj. **telekinetic.**

telemedicine (,teli'medisin, -'medsin) the provision of consultant services by off-site specialists to health care professionals on the scene, as by means of closed-circuit television.

telemetry (tə'lemətree) the making of measurements at a distance from the subject, the measurable evidence of phenomena under investigation usually being transmitted by radio signals.

telencephalon (,telen'kefəlon, -'sef-) endbrain. 1. the paired brain vesicles, which are the anterolateral outpouchings of the forebrain, together with the median, unpaired portion, the terminal lamina of the hypothalamus; from it the cerebral hemispheres are derived. 2. the anterior of the two vesicles formed by specialization of the forebrain in embryonic development. adj. **telencephalic.**

teleneurite (,teli'nyooə·riet) an end expansion of an axon.

teleneuron (,teli'nyooə·ron) a nerve ending.

teleological (,teli·ə'lojik'l) serving an ultimate purpose in development.

teleology (ˌteli'oləjee) the doctrine that the explanation of phenomena is to be found in terms of their purpose.

teleomitosis (ˌteliohmie'tohsis) completed mitosis.

teleopsia (ˌteli'opsi·ə) a visual disturbance in which objects appear to be farther away than they actually are.

teleorganic (ˌteli·aw'ganik) necessary to life.

Telepaque ('teliˌpayk) trademark for a preparation of iopanoic acid, a radiopaque medium used in oral cholecystography.

telepathy (tə'lepəthee) the communication of thought through extrasensory perception.

teleradiography (ˌteliˌraydi'ogrəfee) radiography with the x-ray tube about 2 m away from the plate in order to more nearly secure parallelism of the rays.

teleradiotherapy (ˌteliˌraydi'therəpee) treatment with ionizing radiations from an x-ray source located at a distance from the body.

telereceptor (ˌteliri'septə) a sensory nerve ending which can respond to distant stimuli. Those of the eyes, ears and nose are examples. Called also *teleceptor*.

telergy ('teləjee) 1. automatism. 2. a hypothetical action of one brain on another at a distance.

telescope ('teliˌskohp) a cylinder or set of cylinders sliding into each other, with a mirror, lens or both for focusing light from a distant object and magnifying its image.

telescopic (ˌteli'skopik) expanding and contracting like a telescope.

teletherapy (ˌteli'therəpee) treatment in which the source of the therapeutic agent, e.g., radiation, is at a distance from the body.

telluric (te'lyooə·rik) 1. pertaining to tellurium. 2. pertaining to or originating from the earth.

tellurium (te'lyooə·ri·əm) a chemical element, atomic number 52, atomic weight 127.60, symbol Te. See table of elements in Appendix 2.

telo- word element. [Gr.] *end*.

telocentric (ˌteloh'sentrik) having the centromere at one end of the chromosome so that the chromosome has only one arm.

telodendron (ˌteloh'dendron) any of the fine terminal branches of an axon.

telogen ('teləjən) the quiescent or resting phase of the hair cycle, following catagen, the hair having become a club hair and not growing further.

telognosis (ˌtelog'nohsis) diagnosis based on interpretation of radiographs transmitted by radio or telephonic communication.

telolemma (ˌteloh'lemə) the covering of a motor end-plate, made up of sarcolemma and an extension of Henle's sheath.

telomere ('telohˌmiə) an extremity of a chromosome, which has specific properties, one of which is a polarity that prevents reunion with any fragment after a chromosome has been broken.

telophase ('telohˌfayz) the last of the four stages of mitosis and of the two divisions of meiosis.

temazepam (te'maziˌpam) a benzodiazepine tranquillizer used as a hypnotic.

Temgesic (tem'jeezik) trademark for preparations of buprenorphine, an analgesic.

temperament ('temprəmənt) the peculiar physical character and mental cast of an individual.

temperature ('temprəchə) the degree of sensible heat or cold, expressed in terms of a specific scale.

Body temperature is measured by a clinical thermometer and represents a balance between the heat produced by the body and the heat it loses. Though heat production and heat loss vary with circumstances, the body regulates them, keeping a remarkably constant temperature. An abnormal rise in body temperature is called FEVER.

See also table of comparative temperatures in Appendix 2.

NORMAL BODY TEMPERATURE. Body temperature is usually measured by a thermometer placed in the mouth or in the rectum. The normal oral temperature is 37 °C (98.6 °F); rectally, it is 37.3 °C (99.2 °F). These values are based on a statistical average. Normal temperature varies somewhat from person to person and at different times in each person.

Body temperature is usually slightly higher in the evening than in the morning. It is also higher during and immediately after eating, exercise, or emotional excitement. Temperature in infants and young children tends to vary more than in adults.

TEMPERATURE REGULATION. To maintain a constant temperature, the body must be able to respond to changes in the temperature of its surroundings. When the outside temperature drops, nerve endings near the skin surface sense the change and communicate it to the hypothalamus. Certain cells of the hypothalamus then signal for an increase in the body's heat production. This heat is conducted to the blood and distributed throughout the body. At the same time, the body acts to conserve its heat. The arterioles constrict so that less blood will flow near the body's surface. The skin becomes pale and cold. Sometimes it takes on a bluish colour, the result of a colour change in the blood, which occurs when the blood, flowing slowly, gives off more of its oxygen than usual. Another signal from the brain stimulates muscular activity, which releases heat. Shivering is a form of this activity.

When the outside temperature goes up, the body's cooling system is ordered into action. Sweat is released from sweat glands beneath the skin, and as it evaporates, the skin is cooled. Heat is also eliminated by the evaporation of moisture in the lungs. This process is accelerated by panting.

An important regulator of body heat is the peripheral capillary system. The vessels of this system form a network just under the skin. When these vessels dilate, they allow more warm blood from the interior of the body to flow through them, where it is cooled by the surrounding air.

ABNORMAL BODY TEMPERATURE. Abnormal temperatures occur when the body's temperature-regulating system is upset by disease or other physical disturbances. FEVER usually accompanies infection and many other disease processes. In most cases when the oral temperature is 37.8 °C (100 °F) or over, fever is present. Temperatures of 40 °C (104 °F) or over are common in serious illnesses, although occasionally very high fever accompanies an illness that causes little concern. Temperatures as high as 41.7 °C (107 °F) or higher sometimes accompany diseases in critical stages.

Subnormal temperatures, below 35.6 °C (96 °F) occur in cases of collapse (see also symptomatic HYPOTHERMIA).

absolute t. that reckoned from absolute zero (-273.15 °C or -459.67 °F).

critical t. that below which a gas may be converted to a liquid by pressure.

normal t. that usually registered by a healthy person (37 °C or 98.6 °F).

template ('templayt) a pattern or mould. In dentistry, a curved or flat plate used as an aid in setting teeth for a denture. In theoretical immunology, an antigen that determines the configuration of combining (antigen-binding) sites of antibody molecules. In genetics, a strand of DNA which specifies the synthesis of a complementary strand of RNA (messenger RNA, ribosomal RNA, or transfer RNA); mRNA in turn serves as a template for the synthesis of nucleic acids or proteins.

temple ('temp'l) the lateral region on either side of the head, above the zygomatic arch.

tempolabile (,tempoh'laybiel) subject to change with the passage of time.

tempora ('tempora) [L.] *the temples.*

temporal ('tempə·rəl) 1. pertaining to the temple. 2. pertaining to time; limited as to time; temporary.

t. bone one of the two irregular bones forming part of the lateral surfaces and base of the skull, and containing the organs of hearing.

t. lobe a long, tongue-shaped process constituting the lower lateral portion of the cerebral hemisphere.

temporomandibular (,tempə·rohman'dibyuhlə) pertaining to the temporal bone and mandible.

t. joint (TMJ) syndrome dysfunction of the temporomandibular joint, marked by a clicking or grinding sensation in the joint and often by pain in or about the ears, tiredness and slight soreness of the jaw muscles upon waking, and stiffness of the jaw or actual trismus; it results from mandibular overclosure, condylar displacement, or stress associated with bruxism, with deforming arthritis an occasional factor.

Treatment may include medical or dental therapy or a combination of these. Dental treatment usually involves insertion of a bite plane which prevents the teeth from meeting and grinding against one another. The bite plane relieves pain and promotes normal positioning of the mandible, which allows the inflamed joint to rest and heal. Once the inflammation has subsided and normal neuromuscular function returns, the dentist may attempt to correct malocclusion.

Medical therapy may include local heat applications to improve circulation and promote relaxation, corticosteroid injections into the joint, jaw exercises, and analgesics and anti-inflammatory agents.

temporomaxillary (,tempə·rohmak'silə·ree) pertaining to the temporal bone and maxilla.

temporo-occipital (,tempə·roh·ok'sipit'l) pertaining to the temporal and occipital bones.

temporosphenoid (,tempə·roh'sfeenoyd) pertaining to the temporal and sphenoid bones.

tempostabile (,tempoh'staybiel) not subject to change with time.

tenacious (tə'nayshəs) viscid; adhesive.

tenaculum (tə'nakyuhləm) a fine hook used for grasping and holding tissue during an operation.

tenalgia (te'nalji·ə) pain in a tendon.

tenderness ('tendənəs) a state of unusual sensitivity to touch or pressure.

rebound t. a state in which pain is felt on the release of pressure over a part.

tendinitis (,tendi'nietis) inflammation of tendons and of tendon–muscle attachments. It is one of the commonest causes of acute pain in the shoulder. Tendinitis is frequently associated with a calcium deposit (calcific tendinitis), which may also involve the bursa around the tendon or near the joint, causing bursitis.

Shoulder pain associated with calcific tendinitis is most pronounced when the affected arm is abducted between 50 and 130 degrees—the so-called painful arc. Short-term therapy is aimed at relieving pain and decreasing inflammation so that exercise is possible and permanent immobility of the shoulder is avoided.

Among the drugs that may be given are long-acting corticosteroids, which are given by injection directly into the painful area, short-term analgesics such as codeine and paracetamol with codeine, and oral anti-inflammatory agents. Applications of ice are more helpful in relieving pain than heat, which usually aggravates the pain of calcific tendinitis.

Once the patient is free of pain, exercise is begun to preserve motion. If the joint becomes fixed, surgical intervention may be necessary to break up adhesions and restore full mobility to the joint.

tendinoplasty ('tendinoh,plastee) tenoplasty.

tendinosuture (,tendinoh'soochə) tenorrhaphy.

tendinous ('tendinəs) pertaining to, resembling, or of the nature of a tendon.

tendo ('tendoh) pl. *tendines* [L.] tendon; used in anatomical nomenclature.

t. Achillis, t. calcaneus Achilles tendon.

tendolysis (ten'dolisis) tenolysis; the freeing of a tendon from adhesions.

tendon ('tendən) a cord or band of strong white fibrous tissue that connects a muscle to a bone. When the muscle contracts, or shortens, it pulls on the tendon, which moves the bone. Tendons are so tough they are seldom torn, even when an injury is severe enough to break a bone or tear a muscle. One of the most prominent tendons is the Achilles tendon, which can be felt at the back of the ankle just above the heel; it attaches the triceps surae muscle to the calcaneus.

tendonitis (,tendə'nietis) tendinitis.

tendovaginal (,tendohvə'jien'l, -'vajin'l) pertaining to a tendon and its sheath.

tenectomy (tə'nektəmee) excision of a lesion of a tendon or of a tendon sheath.

tenesmus (tə'nezməs) ineffectual and painful straining at stool or in urinating. adj. **tenesmic**.

tennis elbow ('tenis) a painful condition localized to the outer aspect of the elbow, due to inflammation of the extensor tendon attachment to the lateral humeral condyle.

teno- word element. [Gr.] *tendon.*

tenodesis (tə'nodisis) suture of the end of a tendon to a bone.

tenodynia (,tenoh'dini·ə) tenalgia.

tenolysis (tə'nolisis) the operation of freeing a tendon from adhesions.

tenomyoplasty (,tenoh'mieoh,plastee) plastic repair of a tendon and muscle, applied especially to an operation for inguinal hernia.

tenomyotomy (,tenohmie'otəmee) excision of a portion of a tendon and muscle.

Tenon's capsule (tə'nonhz) the connective tissue enveloping the posterior eyeball.

tenonectomy (,tenə'nektəmee) excision of part of a tendon to shorten it.

tenonitis (,tenə'nietis) 1. tendinitis. 2. inflammation of Tenon's capsule, the connective tissue enclosing the eyeball.

tenontitis (,tenən'tietis) tendinitis.

tenonto- word element. [Gr.] *tendon.*

tenontodynia (tə,nontoh'dini·ə) tenalgia.

tenontography (,tenən'togrəfee) a written description or delineation of the tendons.

tenontology (,tenən'toləjee) the sum of what is known about the tendons.

tenontothecitis (tə,nontoh·thee'sietis) tenosynovitis.

tenophyte ('tenoh,fiet) a growth or concretion in a tendon.

tenoplasty ('tenoh,plastee) plastic repair of a tendon. adj. **tenoplastic**.

tenoreceptor (,tenohri'septə) a nerve receptor in a tendon.

Tenormin ('tenormin) trademark for a preparation of atenolol, an antihypertensive (beta-blocker).

tenorrhaphy (te'no·rəfee) suture of a tendon.

tenositis (ˌtenohˈsietis) tendinitis.
tenostosis (ˌtenoˈstohsis) conversion of a tendon into bone.
tenosuspension (ˌtenohsəˈspenshən) an operation for stabilizing a joint, using a tendon as an artificial ligament, e.g., attachment of the head of the humerus to the acromion by a strip of tendon; it is done for habitual dislocation of the shoulder.
tenosuture (ˌtenohˈsoochə) tenorrhaphy.
tenosynovectomy (ˌtenohˌsienohˈvektəmee) excision or resection of a tendon sheath.
tenosynovitis (ˌtenohˌsienohˈvietis) inflammation of a tendon and its sheath, the lubricating layer of tissue in which the tendon is housed and through which it moves. Tenosynovitis resulting from intense and continued use occurs most frequently in the hands and wrists or feet and ankles. It is painful, and may temporarily disable the affected part.

Rheumatoid and other types of arthritis frequently involve tendon sheaths. Infective and suppurative tenosynovitis is now uncommon; it can be the result of tuberculous or gonorrhoeal infection.

Treatment is by immobilization of the limb or surgical release of the tendon from its constricting sheath. Infective cases are treated by antibiotics. If suppuration is suspected, incision of the sheath is required for drainage.

villonodular t. a condition marked by exaggerated proliferation of synovial membrane cells, producing a solid tumour-like mass, commonly occurring in periarticular soft tissues and less frequently in joints.

tenotomy (təˈnotəmee) transection of a tendon.

graduated t. partial transection of a tendon.

tenovaginitis (ˌtenohˌvajiˈnietis) tenosynovitis.
TENS transcutaneous electrical neural stimulation. It is used for pain relief in accordance with the *'Gate Control'* theory. See also PAIN.
tension (ˈtenshən) 1. the act of stretching or the condition of being stretched or strained. 2. the partial pressure of a component of a gas mixture or of a gas dissolved in a fluid, e.g., of oxygen in blood. 3. voltage.

arterial t. blood pressure within an artery.

intraocular t. intraocular pressure.

t. pneumothorax accumulation of air or gas within the pleural cavity which, if not relieved, can lead to lung collapse and MEDIASTINAL SHIFT. See also PNEUMOTHORAX.

premenstrual t. a complex of symptoms, including emotional instability and irritability, sometimes occurring in the 10 days before menstruation; other symptoms include pain in the breasts, headache, nausea, anorexia, constipation, and pelvic discomfort. See also PREMENSTRUAL TENSION.

surface t. tension or resistance that acts to preserve the integrity of a surface.

tissue t. a state of equilibrium between tissues and cells that prevents overaction of any part.

tensor (ˈtensə, -sor) any muscle that stretches or makes tense.
tent (tent) 1. a covering designed to enclose an open space, especially such a covering over a patient's bed for administering oxygen or vaporized medication by inhalation. 2. a conical or cylindrical expansible plug of soft material for dilating an orifice or for keeping a it open.

Laminaria t. a conical plug made from the dried stems of *Laminaria digitata*, a genus of kelp seaweed which expands when moist. Used to dilate the cervical os and thereby induce abortion.

sponge t. a conical plug made of compressed sponge used to dilate the cervical os.

tentacle (ˈtentək'l) a slender, whiplike appendage in animals that may function in prehension and feeding or as a sense organ.
tentorium (tenˈtor·ri·əm) pl. *tentoria* [L.] an anatomical part resembling a tent or covering. adj. **tentorial.**

t. cerebelli the process of the dura mater supporting the occipital lobes and covering the cerebellum.

Tenuate Dospan (ˌtenyooˌayt ˈdospan) trademark for preparations of diethylpropion hydrochloride; an anorexic.
tephromyelitis (ˌtefrohˌmieəˈlietis) inflammation of the grey matter of the spinal cord.
tephrosis (teˈfrohsis) incineration or cremation.
tepor (ˈteepor) [L.] *gentle heat.*
ter- word element. [L.] *three, three-fold.*
ter in die (ˌtər in ˈdeeay) [L.] *three times a day.*
tera- word element. [Gr.] *monster;* used in naming units of measurement to designate an amount 10^{12} (a billion, or million million) times the unit specified by the root to which it is joined; symbol T.
teras (ˈterəs) pl. *terata* [L., Gr.] a malformed fetus or infant. adj. **teratic.**
teratism (ˈterəˌtizəm) an anomaly of formation or development.
terato- word element. [Gr.] *monster, monstrosity.*
teratoblastoma (ˌterətohblaˈstohmə) a neoplasm containing embryonic elements, differing from a teratoma in that its tissue does not represent all germinal layers.
teratocarcinoma (ˌterətohˌkahsiˈnohmə) a malignant neoplasm consisting of elements of teratoma with those of embryonal carcinoma or choriocarcinoma, or both; occurring most often in the testis.
teratogen (ˈterətohˌjen) an agent or influence that causes physical defects in the developing embryo. adj. **teratogenic.**
teratogenesis (ˌterətohˈjenəsis) the production of deformity in the developing embryo. adj. **teratogenetic.**
teratogenous (ˌterəˈtojənəs) developed from fetal remains.
teratogeny (ˌterəˈtojənee) teratogenesis.
teratoid (ˈterəˌtoyd) resembling a monster.
teratology (ˌterəˈtoləjee) that division of embryology and pathology dealing with abnormal development and congenital deformations. adj. **teratological.**
teratoma (ˌterəˈtohmə) a true neoplasm made up of a number of different types of tissue, none of which is native to the area in which it occurs; usually found in the ovary or testis.

malignant t. a solid, malignant tumour composed of immature embryonal or extraembryonal elements derived from all three germ layers.

teratomatous (ˌterəˈtohmətəs) pertaining to or of the nature of teratoma.
terbium (ˈtərbi·əm) a chemical element, atomic number 65, atomic weight 158.924, symbol Tb. See table of elements in Appendix 2.
terbutaline (tərˈbyootəˌleen) a β-adrenergic receptor antagonist used as a bronchodilator.
terebration (ˌteriˈbrayshən) the act of boring or trephining; also, a boring pain.
teres (ˈtiə·reez) [L.] *long and round.*
term (tərm) a definite period, especially the period of gestation, or pregnancy.
terminal (ˈtərmin'l) 1. forming or pertaining to an end. 2. a termination, end or extremity, especially a nerve ending.
terminal deoxynucleotidyl transferase an enzyme present in stem cells of both B- and T-cell lineage; abbreviated TdT. A useful marker in the diagnosis of the leukaemias (acute lymphoblastic leukaemia is usually TdT positive; acute myeloid leukaemia rarely so) and lymphomas.

terminatio (ˌtərmi'nayshioh) pl. *terminationes* [L.] an ending; used in anatomical nomenclature to designate the site of discontinuation of a structure, as the free nerve endings (terminationes nervorum liberae), in which the peripheral fibre divides into fine branches that terminate freely in connective tissue or epithelium.

terminology (ˌtərmi'noləjee) 1. the vocabulary of an art or science. 2. the science that deals with the investigation, arrangement, and construction of terms.

terminus ('tərminəs) pl. *termini* [L.] an ending.

ternary ('tərnə·ree) 1. third in order. 2. made up of three elements or radicals.

terpene ('tərpeen) any hydrocarbon of the formula $C_{10}H_{16}$.

terpin ('tərpin) a product obtained by the action of nitric acid on oil of turpentine and alcohol, used as an expectorant in the form of the hydrate.

Terramycin (ˌterə'miesin) trademark for preparations of oxytetracycline, an antibiotic.

terror ('terə) an attack of extreme fear or dread.

night t. an extreme fear reaction in a child during sleep or at night.

tertian ('tərshən) recurring in 3-day cycles (every second day); applied to the type of fever caused by certain forms of malarial parasites (see also MALARIA).

tertiary ('tərshə·ree) third in order.

Tertroxin (tər'troksin) trademark for a preparation of liothyronine sodium, a thyroid hormone preparation.

tesla ('teslə) the SI unit of magnetic flux density, equal to one weber per square metre. Symbol T.

tessellated ('tesəˌlaytid) divided into squares, like a draughtboard.

test (test) 1. an examination or trial. 2. a significant chemical reaction. 3. a reagent. See also specific names of tests, as SCHILLING TEST.

acid elution t. air-dried blood smears are fixed in 80 per cent methanol and immersed in a pH 3.3 buffer; all haemoglobins are eluted except fetal haemoglobin (HbF), which is seen in red cells after staining. The test is for the presence of HbF.

agglutination t. one whose results depend on agglutination of bacteria or other cells; used in diagnosing certain infectious diseases and rheumatoid arthritis, and the cross-matching of blood.

alkali-denaturation t. a spectrophotometric method for measuring the concentration of fetal haemoglobin (HbF).

aptitude t. one designed to measure the capacity for developing general or specific skills.

association t. one based on associative reaction, usually by mentioning words to a patient and noting what other words the patient will give as the ones called up in his mind.

autohaemolysis t. determination of spontaneous haemolysis in a blood specimen maintained under certain conditions, to detect the presence of certain haemolytic states.

biuret t. see BIURET.

cis–trans t. a test in microbial genetics to determine whether two mutations that have the phenotypic effect, in a haploid cell or a cell with single phage infection, are located in the same gene or in different genes; the test depends on the independent behaviour of two alleles of a gene in a diploid cell or in a cell infected with two phages carrying different alleles.

complement-fixation t's tests that utilize antigen–antibody reaction and result in haemolysis to determine the presence of various organisms in the blood (see also COMPLEMENT FIXATION).

concentration t. a test of renal function based on the patient's ability to concentrate urine.

conjunctival t. itching and conjunctival congestion after instillation into the conjunctiva of a pollen or pollen extract to which the person is sensitive.

creatinine clearance t. a test for renal function based on the rate at which ingested creatinine is filtered through the renal glomeruli.

double-blind t. a study of the effects of a specific agent in which neither the investigator nor the recipient, at the time of administration, knows whether the active or an inert substance is being used.

early pregnancy t. a do-it-yourself immunological test for pregnancy, performed as early as 9 days after menstruation (missed period) was expected.

exercise stress t's tests for detecting previously undetected coronary artery disease; they are graded tests of coronary fitness in which the subject performs exercise, as by walking a treadmill or pedalling a stationary bicycle, while under continuous electrocardiographic monitoring, before, during, and after the exercise.

finger–nose t. a test for coordinated movements of the extremities; the patient is directed to close his eyes, and, with arm extended to one side, slowly endeavour to touch the end of his nose with the tip of his index finger.

galactose tolerance t. a test of carbohydrate tolerance of the liver by measuring the amount of galactose eliminated in the urine after oral or intravenous administration of galactose.

glucagon stimulation t. a provocative test of growth hormone (GH) function in which the fasting serum level of GH is measured after administration of glucagon.

glucose tolerance t. a metabolic test of carbohydrate tolerance. See GLUCOSE TOLERANCE TEST.

glycosylated haemoglobin t. measurement of the percentage of haemoglobin A molecules that form a stable ketoamine linkage between the amino terminal valine residue of the beta chain and a glucose moiety; used to assess diabetic control. In normal persons, this amounts to about 7 per cent of the total, in uncontrolled DIABETES MELLITUS about 14.5 per cent. See also HAEMOGLOBIN A_{1c}.

guaiac t. one for occult blood; glacial acetic acid and guaiac are mixed with the specimen; on addition of hydrogen peroxide, the presence of blood is indicated by a blue tint.

histamine t. 1. subcutaneous injection of 0.1 per cent solution of histamine to stimulate gastric secretion in order to measure maximal acid output. 2. after rapid intravenous injection of histamine phosphate, normal persons experience a brief fall in blood pressure, but in those with phaeochromocytoma, after the fall, there is a marked rise in blood pressure.

human erythrocyte agglutination t. one for rheumatoid arthritis, depending on agglutination by the patient's serum of human Rh-positive cells sensitized with incomplete anti-Rh antibody.

intracutaneous t. one that involves introduction of an antigen between the layers of the skin and evaluation of the reaction elicited by it.

latex-agglutination t., latex-fixation t. a serological test for rheumatoid factor, helpful in the diagnosis of rheumatoid arthritis.

LE t. serum from patients with systemic lupus erythematosus is combined with normal leukocytes; following incubation at 37 °C., polymorphonuclear leukocytes engulf nuclei or nuclear fragments of cells to form LE cells.

migration inhibition t. an in vitro test for detection of cell-mediated immunity (or delayed hypersensitivity) in which peritoneal exudate cells (lymphocytes and macrophages) are packed in capillary tubes; if the medium contains an antigen to which the lymphocytes are primed, macrophage migration from the tubes is inhibited by lymphokines (macrophage inhibiting factor) released by the lymphocytes.

monospot t. see PAUL–BUNNEL TEST.

multiple-puncture t. an intracutaneous test in which the material used (e.g., tuberculin) is introduced into the skin by pressure of several needles or pointed tines or prongs.

neutralization t. one for the bacterial neutralization power of a substance by testing its action on the pathogenic properties of the organism concerned.

patch t. a test for hypersensitivity, performed by observing the reaction to application to the skin of filter paper or gauze saturated with the substance in question (see also SKIN TEST).

precipitation t., precipitin t. any test in which the positive reaction consists in the formation and deposit of a precipitate in the fluid being tested.

pregnancy t's laboratory procedures for early determination of pregnancy (see also PREGNANCY tests).

prothrombin consumption t. a test to measure the formation of intrinsic thromboplastin by determining the residual serum prothrombin after blood coagulation is complete.

psychological t., psychometric t. any test to measure such factors as one's development, achievement, personality, intelligence, and thought processes.

pulmonary function t's see under PULMONARY.

radioallergosorbent t. (RAST) a radioimmunoassay for the measurement of extremely small amounts of specific IgE antibody to a variety of allergens, using antigen fixed in a solid-phase matrix and radiolabelled anti-gamma globulin.

radioimmunosorbent t. (RIST) a radioimmunoassay technique for measuring IgE immunoglobulins in serum, using radiolabelled IgE and anti-human IgE bound to an insoluble matrix.

rapid plasma reagin (RPR) t. a group of screening flocculation tests for syphilis, using a modified VDRL antigen.

renal clearance t's laboratory tests that determine the ability of the kidney to remove certain substances from the blood. The most commonly used is the clearance of endogenous creatinine, which is a measure of the glomerular filtration rate.

scratch t. a test for hypersensitivity in which a minute amount of the substance in question is inserted in small scratches made in the skin. A positive reaction is swelling or redness at the site within 30 minutes. Used in ALLERGY testing and in testing for tuberculosis (Pirquet's reaction). See also SKIN TEST.

serological t. one involving examination of blood serum.

sickling t. a method to demonstrate haemoglobin S and the sickling phenomenon in erythrocytes, performed by reducing the oxygen concentration to which the red cells are exposed.

significance t. a statistical test to estimate the probability of the association between two independent variables being due to chance. The probability is designated by *P*.

single-blind t. a study of the effects of a specific agent in which the investigator, but not the recipient, knows whether the active or an inert substance is being used.

thematic apperception t. (TAT) a projective test in which the subject tells a story based on each of a series of standard ambiguous pictures, so that his responses reflect a projection of some aspect of his personality and his current psychological preoccupations and conflicts.

tine t. a tuberculin skin test employing a multiple-puncture, disposable device (see also TINE TEST).

tolerance t. 1. an exercise test to determine the efficiency of the circulation. 2. a test to determine the body's ability to metabolize a substance or to endure administration of a drug.

tourniquet t. one involving the application of a tourniquet to an extremity, as in determination of capillary fragility (denoted by the appearance of petechiae) or of the status of the collateral circulation.

Treponema pallidum haemagglutination (TPHA) t., Treponema pallidum immobilization (TPI) t. serological tests related directly to the causative organism, used in the diagnosis of syphilis.

tuberculin t. a test for the presence of active or inactive TUBERCULOSIS, consisting in the subcutaneous injection of 5 mg of tuberculin; a positive test is denoted by redness and induration at the injection site (see also MANTOUX TEST).

VDRL t. a slide flocculation test for syphilis designed by the Venereal Disease Research Laboratory, United States. It has now superseded other tests in the United Kingdom, e.g., the Wassermann and the Kahn tests.

test meal a portion of food or foods given for the purpose of determining the functioning of the digestive tract.

test tube a tube of thin glass, closed at one end; used in chemical tests and other laboratory procedures.

test type printed letters of varying size, used in the testing of visual acuity.

testalgia (te'stalji·ə) testicular pain.

testectomy (te'stektəmee) ORCHIECTOMY, the removal of a testis.

testes ('testeez) [L.] plural of *testis.*

testicle ('testik'l) testis.

testicular (te'stikyuhlə) pertaining to the testis.

t. feminization syndrome an extreme form of male pseudohermaphroditism, with female external development, including secondary sexual characteristics, but with the presence of testes and absence of uterus and tubes; it is due to end-organ resistance to the action of testosterone.

testis ('testis) pl. *testes* [L.] the male gonad; either of the paired, egg-shaped glands normally situated in the scrotum; called also *testicle.* The testes produce the spermatozoa, the male reproductive cells, which are ejaculated into the female vagina during coitus, and the male sex hormone, testosterone, which is responsible for the secondary sexual characteristics of the male.

If the testes are removed (castration, bilateral ORCHIECTOMY) before puberty, the male is sterile and will never develop all the adult masculine characteristics. If the testes are removed after puberty, the male becomes sterile and his masculine characteristics will diminish unless he receives injections of male hormones. With ageing, there is a gradual decrease in the production of testosterone.

In the unborn child, the testes lie close to the kidneys. During approximately the seventh month of fetal life, the testes begin to descend through the abdominal wall at the groin and enter the scrotum. As they descend they are accompanied by blood vessels, nerves, and ducts, all contained within the spermatic cord. The passageway through which the testes and spermatic cord descend is called the inguinal canal. Failure of a testis to descend into the scrotum is called CRYPTORCHIDISM.

The testis is divided internally into about 250 compartments or lobules, each of which contains one to three extremely small and convoluted tubules, within which spermatozoa are produced. When mature, the spermatozoa leave the tubules and enter the epididymis situated on top of and behind each testis. The spermatozoa are stored in the epididymis until such time as they are mixed in the semen and ejaculated during coitus. See also REPRODUCTION and male REPRODUCTIVE ORGANS.

Testicular tumours are the most common form of cancer to afflict men between the ages of 20 and 35 years, but they account for less than 1 per cent of all cancers in males. An estimated 900 cases of testicular cancer are diagnosed each year in the United Kingdom. It is, however, one of the most curable forms of cancer when detected early and treated promptly.

In order to ensure early detection of cancer of the testis, men should be urged to conduct a monthly self-examination of the testes. The self-examination involves the use of both hands to examine each of the testes. The index and middle fingers are placed below the testis and the thumbs on top. With a gentle motion each testis is rolled between the thumbs and fingers to discover any lump (usually about the size of a pea), thickening, or change in the consistency of the tissues. It is important that the man become familiar with the feel of the epididymis so that he doesn't confuse this normal structure with an abnormal lump. Should a lump or any other abnormality be found, a doctor should be consulted immediately. An increasing awareness of testicular cancer has resulted in some educational material on testicular self-examination (TSE).

The surgical treatment of testicular cancer may or may not render the patient impotent and sterile. If there is no metastasis, only the affected testis need be removed. The remaining testis will retain its normal function and the patient should be able to have normal sexual intercourse and be fertile. However, if more radical surgery is called for and both testes and the lymph nodes are dissected, and if there has been no damage to nerves during surgery, the patient may be able to have sexual intercourse but no seminal fluid will be emitted. A young man who is looking forward to having children may consider banking his sperm prior to surgery so that he might father children by artificial insemination.

testitis (te'stietis) inflammation of a testis; called also ORCHITIS.

testoid ('testoyd) a term applied to testicular hormones and other natural or synthetic compounds having a similar effect.

testosterone (tes'tostə,rohn) the most important of the male sex hormones, or ANDROGENS, that are produced by the Leydig cells of the testes in response to luteinizing hormone (LH) secreted by the pituitary. Its chief function is to stimulate the development of the male reproductive organs, including the prostate, and the secondary sexual characteristics, such as the beard. It encourages growth of bone and muscle, and helps maintain muscle strength.

Testosterone is obtained for therapeutic purposes by extraction from animal testes or by synthesis from cholesterol. It is used generally in all cases of hypogonadism, i.e. underfunctioning of the testes. It is also used to relieve some forms of breast cancer. Women normally secrete a certain amount of male hormones; however, if the hormone balance is disturbed and there is overproduction of male hormones in a woman, signs of masculinity may develop.

tetanic (te'tanik) pertaining to tetanus.

tetaniform (te'tani,fawm) resembling tetanus.

tetanigenous (,tetə'nijənəs) producing tetanic spasms.

tetanism ('tetə,nizəm) persistent muscular hypertonicity, as in the newborn.

tetanization (,tetənie'zayshən) the induction of tetanic convulsions or symptoms.

tetanize ('tetə,niez) to induce tetanic convulsions or symptoms.

tetanode ('tetə,nohd) the unexcited stage of tetany.

tetanoid ('tetə,noyd) resembling tetanus.

tetanolysin (,tetə'nolisin) the haemolytic fraction of the exotoxin formed by *Clostridium tetani*, the causative organism of tetanus.

tetanospasmin (,tetənoh'spazmin) the neurotoxic component of the tetanus toxin, which causes the muscle spasms of tetanus.

tetanus ('tetənəs) an acute, often fatal, especially if untreated, disease caused by the tetanus bacillus (*Clostridium tetani*) and characterized by muscle spasm and convulsions. Because stiffness of the jaw is often the first symptom, it is known also as lockjaw. adj. **tetanic.**

Tetanus is a serious illness, but because of widespread immunization in childhood, it is now uncommon in the United Kingdom. It is a notifiable disease.

Tetanus bacilli, which grow in the intestines of animals and man, are prevalent in rural areas. They are found in soil and dust, and are spread by animal and human faeces. The organisms enter the body through a break in the skin, particularly in puncture wounds, but also through lacerations and burns. Occasionally, the original wound appears trivial and heals quickly; more often, there is obvious infection.

SYMPTOMS. Stiffness of the jaw is usually the first definite indication of tetanus. Difficulty in swallowing, stiffness of the neck, restlessness, irritability, headache, chills, fever, and convulsions are also among the early symptoms.

Muscles in the abdomen, back, neck, and face may go into spasm. If the infection is severe, convulsions are set off by slight disturbances, such as noises and draughts. During convulsions, there is difficulty in breathing and the possibility of asphyxiation.

TREATMENT. If there is any suspicion of contamination by tetanus bacilli, medical treatment should be obtained. This may include a booster injection of tetanus toxoid (see below) plus, where appropriate, an adequate dose of tetanus immune globulin to counteract any possible tetanus infection. In any case, the wound area must be carefully cleaned, and all dead tissue and foreign substances removed.

During a tetanus attack, sedatives are given to reduce the frequency of convulsions. Antibiotics are also advised, e.g. penicillin. More recently, hyperbaric oxygenation, providing oxygen under high pressure, has been used in treatment of tetanus.

PATIENT CARE. Because the toxin from *Clostridium tetani* attacks the central nervous system it is extremely important to provide a nonstimulating environment for patients with tetanus. The room must be kept dark and quiet, and draughts of cold air, noises, and other external stimuli must be avoided because they may precipitate convulsive muscle spasms. As for any patient subject to convulsions, padded side rails are applied to the bed to prevent injury to the patient during a seizure. The head board is also padded with a cotton blanket or pillow. Prevention of injury to and assessment of a patient with convulsive seizures are discussed under CONVULSION.

Fluids and nourishment usually are given intravenously during the acute stage of the disease. The patient's intake and output are carefully measured and recorded. Sedatives and antibiotic drugs are administered as ordered to reduce irritability and to combat secondary bacterial infections.

As long as the patient is acutely ill and likely to suffer

from convulsive seizures, someone should be in constant attendance. Signs of respiratory difficulty, changes in pulse and blood pressure, and frequent and prolonged muscle spasms should be reported immediately to the doctor in charge. A tracheostomy set should be readily available in the event severe dyspnoea should develop.

PREVENTION. The most important weapon against tetanus is adequate IMMUNIZATION. Tetanus toxoid in combination with diphtheria toxoid and pertussis vaccine (DTPer/Vac/Ads) is given at three months of age and repeated at approximately five months and nine months: a further booster, together with diphtheria toxoid (DT/Vac/Ads), is given between four and six years of age, and, finally, as a single vaccine, at school leaving age.

Routine tetanus immunization began in the UK in 1961, thus individuals born before that year will not have been immunized in infancy. A full course of immunization may be required unless it has been given previously as for instance in the armed services.

At the time of injury tetanus toxoid is given, either as an initial immunizing dose, the course being completed subsequently, or as a booster for previous immunization, unless the patient has received a booster or completed his initial immunization within the past five years. Patients who have not been previously immunized may require passive immunity with human tetanus immunoglobulin as well as active immunization, especially if the wound is severe, neglected, or over 6 hours old.

infantile t., t. neonatorum tetanus of very young infants, usually due to infection of the umbilicus; it is an important cause of death in many countries of Asia, Africa and South America. World-wide elimination of neonatal tetanus by the year 2000 is one of WHO targets.

tetany ('tetənee) 1. continuous tonic spasm of a muscle; steady contraction of a muscle without distinct twitching (also called *tetanic* CONVULSION). 2. a syndrome manifested by sharp flexion of the wrist and ankle joints (carpopedal spasm), muscle twitchings, cramps, and convulsions, sometimes with attacks of stridor. It is due to abnormal calcium metabolism, and occurs in parathyroid hypofunction, vitamin D deficiency, and alkalosis, and also as a result of ingestion of alkaline salts.

TREATMENT. Treatment for tetany varies according to the cause and is usually successful. It may include the administration of vitamin D, calcium, parathyroid hormone, or other remedies. In chronic cases, as in the loss of the parathyroid glands, treatment may have to be continued indefinitely.

duration t. a continuous tetanic contraction in response to a strong continuous current, occurring especially in degenerated muscles.

gastric t. a severe form due to disease of the stomach, attended by difficult respiration and painful tonic spasms of the extremities.

hyperventilation t. tetany produced by forced inspiration and expiration continued for a considerable time.

latent t. tetany elicited by the application of electrical and mechanical stimulation.

parathyroid t., parathyroprival t. tetany due to removal or hypofunctioning of the parathyroid glands.

tetartanopia, tetartanopsia (ˌtetahtə'nohpi·ə; ˌtetahtə'nopsi·ə) 1. quadrantanopia; loss of vision in one-fourth of the visual field. 2. a type of defective colour vision in which there is perception of red and green only, with blue and yellow perceived as an achromatic (grey) band.

tetra- word element. [Gr.] *four.*

tetrabrachius (ˌtetrə'brayki·əs) a double fetus having four arms.

tetrachloroethylene (ˌtetrəˌklor·roh'ethiˌleen) a clear, colourless liquid used as an anthelmintic.

tetracosactrin (ˌtetrəkoh'saktrin, -zak-) a synthetic corticotropin used in the screening of adrenal insufficiency on the basis of plasma cortisol response after intramuscular or intravenous injection.

tetracrotic (ˌtetrə'krotik) having four sphygmographic waves or elevations to one beat of the pulse.

tetracycline (ˌtetrə'siekleen) an antibiotic substance that is effective against many different microorganisms, including rickettsiae, certain viruses, and both gram-negative and gram-positive microorganisms. Preparations include chlortetracycline hydrochloride, tetracycline hydrochloride, and demeclocycline hydrochloride.

tetrad ('tetrad) a group of four similar or related entities, as (1) any element or radical having a valency, or combining power, of four; (2) a group of four chromosomal elements formed in the pachytene stage of the first meiotic prophase; (3) a square of cells produced by division into two planes of certain cocci (*Sarcina*).

tetradactyly (ˌtetrə'daktilee) the presence of four digits on the hand or foot.

tetragonum (ˌtetrə'gohnəm) [L.] *a four-sided figure.*

t. lumbale the quadrangle bounded by the four lumbar muscles.

tetrahydrocannabinol (ˌtetrəˌhiedrohkə'nabinol) the active principle of cannabis, occurring in two isomeric forms, both considered psychomimetically active. Abbreviated THC.

tetraiodothyronine (ˌtetrəˌieədoh'thierəˌneen) thyroxine.

tetralogy (te'traləjee) a group or series of four.

t. of Fallot a congenital defect of the heart that combines four structural anomalies: pulmonary stenosis (narrowing of the pulmonary artery); ventricular septal defect, or abnormal opening between the right and left ventricles; dextroposition of the aorta, in which the aortic opening overrides the septum and receives blood from both the right and left ventricles; and right ventricular hypertrophy, or increase of volume of the myocardium of the right ventricle.

Infants with this condition are sometimes referred to as blue babies because of the presence of cyanosis, an outstanding symptom of tetralogy of Fallot. The cyanosis is due to mixing of poorly oxygenated blood from the systemic circulation with oxygenated blood from the lungs, because of the position of the aorta. Other symptoms include clubbing of the ends of the fingers, haemoptysis, dyspnoea on exertion, and a slight delay in growth and development.

Treatment of tetralogy of Fallot involves surgical correction whenever possible. Without corrective surgery the prognosis is extremely poor for children who are deeply cyanotic and have dyspnoea on slight exertion.

Surgical procedures for correction of the defects in the heart and great vessels vary according to the severity of symptoms and the age of the patient. In some cases an anastomosis of the arteries may be done as a temporary measure until more extensive surgery is feasible. In most cases open heart surgery is most successful in relieving symptoms and produces the most lasting benefits.

tetramastigote (ˌtetrə'mastiˌgoht) 1. having four flagella. 2. an organism having four flagella.

tetrameric (ˌtetrə'merik) having four parts.

tetranopsia (ˌtetrə'nopsi·ə) obliteration of one quadrant of the visual field.

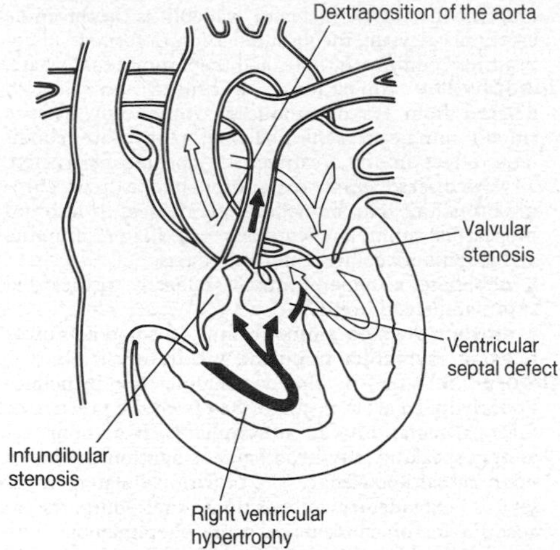

Tetralogy of Fallot.

tetraparesis (ˌtetrəpə'reesis) muscular weakness affecting all four extremities.

tetrapeptide (ˌtetrə'peptied) a peptide which, on hydrolysis, yields four amino acids.

tetraplegia (ˌtetrə'pleeji·ə) paralysis of all four extremities; QUADRIPLEGIA.

tetraploid ('tetrəˌployd) 1. characterized by tetraploidy. 2. an individual or cell having four sets of chromosomes.

tetraploidy ('tetrəˌploydee) the state of having four sets of chromosomes (4n).

tetrapus ('tetrəˌpəs) a fetus or infant with four feet.

tetrascelus (te'trasələs) a fetus or infant with four legs.

tetrasomy ('tetrəˌsohmee) the presence of two extra chromosomes of one type in an otherwise diploid cell. adj. **tetrasomic.**

tetraster (te'trastə) a figure in mitosis produced by quadruple division of the nucleus.

tetravalent (ˌtetrə'vaylənt) having a valency of four.

tetrodotoxin (teˌtrohdoh'toksin) a highly lethal neurotoxin present in numerous species of puffer fish (suborder Tetraodontoidea) and in newts of the genus *Taricha* (tarichatoxin); ingestion results, within minutes, in malaise, dizziness, and tingling about the mouth, which may be followed by ataxia, convulsions, respiratory paralysis, and death.

Tet/Vac/Ads tetanus vaccine, adsorbed.

textiform ('tekstiˌfawm) formed like a network.

textoblastic (ˌtektoh'blastik) forming adult tissue; regenerative; said of cells.

texture ('tekschə) the structure or constitution of tissues. adj. **textural.**

Th chemical symbol, *thorium.*

thalamencephalon (ˌthalәmen'kefəlon, -'sef-) that part of the diencephalon including the thalamus, metathalamus, and epithalamus.

thalamocoele ('thaləmohˌseel) the third ventricle of the brain.

thalamocortical (ˌthaləmoh'kawtik'l) pertaining to the thalamus and cerebral cortex.

thalamolenticular (ˌthaləmohlen'tikyuhlə) pertaining to the thalamus and lenticular nucleus.

thalamotomy (ˌthalə'motəmee) destruction of specific groups of cells within the thalamus, as for the relief of pain or for relief of tremor and rigidity in Parkinson's disease.

thalamus ('thaləməs) pl. *thalami* [L.] either of two large ovoid structures composed of grey matter and situated at the base of the cerebrum. See also BRAIN. adj. **thalamic.** The thalamus functions as a relay station in which sensory pathways of the spinal cord and brain stem form synapses on their way to the cerebral cortex. Specific locations in the thalamus are related to specific areas on the body surface and in the cerebral cortex. A sensory impulse from the body surface travels upward to the thalamus, where it is received as a primitive sensation and then is sent on to the cerebral cortex for interpretation as to location, character, and duration.

The thalamus has numerous connections to other areas of the brain as well, and these are thought to be important in the integration of cerebral, cerebellar, and brain stem activity.

thalassaemia (ˌthalə'seemi·ə) a heterogeneous group of hereditary haemolytic anaemias marked by a decreased rate of synthesis of one or more haemoglobin polypeptide chains, classified according to the chain involved (α, β, δ); the two major categories are α- and β-thalassaemia.

α-t., alpha-t. that caused by diminished synthesis of alpha chains of haemoglobin. The *homozygous* form is incompatible with life, the stillborn infant displaying severe hydrops fetalis. The *heterozygous* form may be asymptomatic or marked by mild anaemia.

β-t., beta-t. that caused by diminished synthesis of beta chains of haemoglobin. The *homozygous* form (Cooley's, Mediterranean, or erythroblastic anaemia; thalassaemia major), in which haemoglobin A is completely absent, appears in the newborn period and is marked by haemolytic, hypochromic, microcytic anaemia, hepatosplenomegaly, skeletal deformation, mongoloid facies, and cardiac enlargement. The *heterozygous* form (thalassaemia minor) is usually asymptomatic, but there is mild anaemia. **t. major** see beta-thalassaemia (above).

t. minor see beta-thalassaemia (above).

sickle cell-t. a hereditary anaemia involving simultaneous heterozygosity for haemoglobin S and thalassaemia.

thalassoposia (thəˌlasoh'pohzi·ə) the drinking of sea water.

thalassotherapy (thəˌlasoh'therəpee) treatment involving sea bathing or a sea voyage.

thalidomide (thə'lidəˌmied) a sedative and hypnotic compound whose use during early pregnancy was frequently followed by the birth of infants showing serious developmental deformities, notably malformation of a limb or limbs.

thallium ('thali·əm) a chemical element, atomic number 81, atomic weight 204.37, symbol Tl. (See table of elements in Appendix 2.) Its salts are active poisons.

t.-201 a radioactive isotope of thallium having a half-life of 73.5 hours; the principal emission is 71 keV x-rays.

thallium scan a scintillation scan involving the use of thallium-201. The radioisotope is administered intravenously and localizes, like potassium, in the myocardium. A scintillation camera produces an image of the distribution of the radioisotope. Areas of inadequate perfusion appear as 'cold spots', thus pinpointing the site of occlusions of the coronary arteries.

The thallium scan offers many advantages. It is noninvasive except for the administration of the radioisotope, which involves a radiation dose slightly larger than that received during a chest radiograph, and is extremely accurate.

The thallium-201 may be administered while the patient is exercising on a treadmill and being monitored by electrocardiogram. Subsequent scintigrams show areas of inadequate perfusion. This test is less likely than conventional exercise or stress testing to indicate disease when none is present and is more likely to detect disease when it is present.

thallous chloride Tl 201 ('thaləs) the form in which thallium-201 is injected intravenously for myocardial perfusion imaging.

thallus ('thaləs) 1. a simple plant body not differentiated into root, stem, and leaf, characteristic of mycelial fungi and some algae. 2. the actively growing vegetative organism as distinguished from reproductive or resting portions, as in fungi.

thanato- word element. [Gr.] *death.*

thanatobiological (ˌthanətohbieə'lojik'l) pertaining to life and death.

thanatognomonic (ˌthanətohnə'monik) indicating the approach of death.

thanatoid ('thanəˌtoyd) resembling death.

thanatology (ˌthanə'toləjee) the medicolegal study of death and conditions affecting dead bodies.

thanatophobia (ˌthanətoh'fohbi·ə) unfounded apprehension of imminent death.

THC tetrahydrocannabinol.

thebaine (thi'bayeen) a crystalline, poisonous, and anodyne alkaloid from opium, having properties similar to those of strychnine.

thebesian foramina (thi'beezi·ən) minute openings in the walls of the right atrium through which the smallest cardiac veins empty into the heart.

thebesian valve coronary vein.

thebesian veins smallest cardiac veins: numerous small veins arising in the muscular walls and draining independently into the cavities of the heart, and most readily seen in the atria.

theca ('theekə) pl. *thecae* [L.] a case or sheath. adj. **thecal.**

t. cordis pericardium.

t. folliculi an envelope of condensed connective tissue surrounding a vesicular ovarian follicle, comprising an internal vascular layer (*theca interna*) and an external fibrous layer (*theca externa*).

thecitis (thee'sietis) tenosynovitis.

thecoma (thee'kohmə) theca cell tumour.

thecostegnosis (ˌtheekohsteg'nohsis) contraction of a tendon sheath.

theism ('thee·izəm) chronic poisoning resulting from excessive tea drinking. Called also *theinism.*

thelalgia (thi'lalji·ə) pain in the nipples.

thelarche (thi'lahkee) beginning of development of the breast at puberty.

theleplasty ('theeliˌplastee) a plastic operation on the nipple.

thelerethism (thi'leriˌthizəm) erection of the nipple.

thelitis (thee'lietis) inflammation of a nipple.

thelium ('theeli·əm) 1. a papilla. 2. a nipple.

thelorrhagia (ˌtheelə'rayji·ə) haemorrhage from the nipple.

thelygenic (ˌtheli'jenik) producing only female offspring.

thenad ('theenad) toward the thenar or toward the palm.

thenar ('theenah) 1. the fleshy part of the hand at the base of the thumb. 2. pertaining to the palm.

Theo-Dur ('theeohˌdər) trademark for preparations of theophylline, a bronchodilator.

theobromine (ˌtheeoh'brohmeen) an alkaloid prepared from dried ripe seed of the tropical American tree *Theobroma cacao*; or made synthetically from xanthine; used as a diuretic, myocardial stimulant, vasodilator, and smooth muscle relaxant; available as theobromine calcium salicylate, theobromine sodium formate, theobromine sodium salicylate, and theobromine salicylate.

theophylline (thi'ofiˌleen, ˌthi·ə'fileen) an alkaloid derived from tea or produced synthetically; it is a smooth muscle relaxant used chiefly for its bronchodilator effect in the treatment of chronic obstructive airways disease, emphysema, bronchial asthma, chronic bronchitis, and bronchospastic distress. It also has myocardial stimulant, coronary vasodilator, diuretic, and respiratory centre stimulant effects.

t. cholinate a smooth muscle relaxant, myocardial stimulant, and diuretic.

t. ethylenediamine aminophylline, a smooth muscle relaxant, myocardial stimulant, and diuretic.

theory ('thi·ə·ree) 1. the doctrine or the principles underlying an art as distinguished from the practice of that particular art. 2. a formulated hypothesis or, loosely speaking, any hypothesis or opinion not based upon actual knowledge. 3. a provisional statement or set of explanatory propositions that purports to account for or characterize some phenomenon. The concepts and provisions set forth in a theory are more specific and concrete than those of a conceptual model. Hence a theory is derived from a conceptual model to fully describe, explain and predict phenomena within the domain of the model.

cell t. all organic matter consists of cells, and cell activity is the essential process of life.

clonal-selection t. of immunity immunological specificity is preformed during embryonic life and mediated through cell clones.

germ t. 1. all organisms are developed from a cell. 2. infectious diseases are of microbial origin.

information t. a mathematical theory dealing with messages or signals, the distortion produced by statistical noise, and methods of coding that reduce distortion to the irreducible minimum.

quantum t. radiation and absorption of energy occur in quantities (quanta) which vary in size with the frequency of the radiation.

recapitulation t. ontogeny recapitulates phylogeny (see also RECAPITULATION THEORY).

theque (tek) [Fr.] a round or oval collection, or nest, of melanin-containing naevus cells occurring at the dermoepidermal junction of the skin or in the dermis proper.

therapeutic (ˌtherə'pyootik) pertaining to therapeutics, or treatment of disease; curative.

t. community any treatment setting (usually psychiatric) which provides a living-learning situation through group processes emphasizing social, environmental and personal interactions and which encourages the individual to learn socially from these processes. Self-determination, trust, respect, and group consensus contrast with the usual hierarchical and authoritarian organization of therapeutic services. Feed-back from the peer group increases self-awareness and group support increases the motivation to revise self-damaging or negative behaviours and attitudes.

t. environment see therapeutic community (above), (an environmental milieu in which the client can experience 'experiments in living', i.e. can try alternative approaches to life difficulties and can benefit from support and feedback from his/her peers. Traditional hierarchial roles and authority structures are minimized and the emphasis is on democracy and communalism).

t. touch alleged by the transfer of energy from healer to client.

t. use of self the ability of the psychiatric nurse to use therapy and experimental knowledge along with self-awareness and the ability to explore, and use, one's personal impact on others.

therapeutics (,therə'pyootiks) 1. the science and art of healing. 2. a scientific account of the treatment of disease.

therapeutist (,therə'pyootist) therapist.

therapist ('therəpist) a person skilled in the corrective treatment of disease or other disorders. The therapist has both a theoretical and practical training and plans and implements programmes of therapy appropriate for each patient.

occupational t. a person skilled in the provision of services to patients with performance deficits that reduce their abilities to cope with the tasks of everyday living (see also OCCUPATIONAL THERAPIST).

physical t. a person skilled in the techniques of physiotherapy; term used in the USA (see also PHYSIOTHERAPIST).

remedial t. no longer exists as a profession in the United Kingdom. Remedial therapists have now amalgamated with physiotherapists, and are required to undertake an educational course to enable them to treat patients in all the fields that physiotherapists specialize in.

therapy ('therəpee) the treatment of disease; therapeutics. See also TREATMENT.

anticoagulant t. the use of drugs to render the blood sufficiently incoagulable to discourage thrombosis.

aversion t. therapy directed at associating an undesirable behaviour pattern with unpleasant stimulation and thus conditioning an aversion to the undesirable behaviour.

behaviour t. a form of psychotherapy focused primarily on the patient's observable behaviour (see also BEHAVIOUR THERAPY).

collapse t. collapse and immobilization of the lung in treatment of pulmonary disease. Very rarely used now.

electroconvulsive t. (ECT), electroshock t. (EST) a form of shock therapy used primarily in the treatment of depression, in which a general tonic-clonic seizure is produced by the application of an electric current through the brain (see also ELECTROCONVULSIVE THERAPY).

group t. psychotherapy carried out with a group of patients under the guidance of a single therapist.

immunosuppressive t. treatment with agents, such as x-rays, corticosteroids, and cytotoxic chemicals, which suppress the immune response to antigen(s); used in organ transplantation, autoimmune disease, allergy, multiple myeloma, etc.

inhalation t. breathing in of a gas, vapour or aerosol for the treatment of conditions affecting the respiratory tract.

milieu t. daily participation in group psychiatric therapy at a hospital, providing for observation and utilization of the patients' interpersonal relationships in a social setting, as well as occupational, physical, and individual psychotherapy.

occupational t. the teaching of useful skills or hobbies to sick or handicapped persons in order to promote their rehabilitation and recovery or to facilitate their ability to make a living (see also OCCUPATIONAL THERAPY, occupational THERAPIST).

oxygen t. the administration of supplementary oxygen to relieve hypoxaemia and prevent damage to the tissue cells as a result of oxygen lack (hypoxia) (see also OXYGEN THERAPY).

physical t. see PHYSIOTHERAPY.

play t. a method used in child psychotherapy in which play is used to reveal unconscious material (see also PLAY THERAPY).

radiotherapy treatment of disease by means of penetrating radiation or implantation of radioactive material within the body.

replacement t. treatment to replace deficient formation or loss of body products by administration of the natural body products or synthetic substitutes.

serum t. serotherapy; treatment of disease by injection of serum from immune individuals.

shock t. any somatic therapy for the treatment of mental illness in which some type of shock is delivered to the central nervous system producing coma or convulsions, e.g., electroconvulsive therapy or insulin shock therapy.

speech t. the use of special techniques for correction of speech and language disorders (see also SPEECH THERAPIST).

substitution t. the administration of a hormone to compensate for glandular deficiency.

therm(o)- word element. [Gr.] *heat.*

thermaesthesia (,thərmis'theezi·ə) perception of heat or cold.

thermaesthesiometer (,thərmis,theezi'omitə) an instrument for measuring sensibility to heat.

thermal ('thərməl) pertaining to heat.

thermalgesia (,thərmal'jeezi·ə) painful sensation produced by heat.

thermalgia (thər'malji·ə) causalgia.

thermanaesthesia (,thərmanəs'theezi·ə) inability to recognize heat and cold.

thermanalgesia (,thərman'l'jeezi·ə) absence of sensibility to heat.

thermelometer (,thərmə'lomitə) an electric thermometer for measuring small temperature changes.

thermhypaesthesia (,thərmhiepis'theezi·ə) decreased sensibility to high temperatures.

thermhyperaesthesia (,thərmhiepə·ris'theezi·ə) increased sensibility to high temperatures.

thermic ('thərmik) pertaining to heat.

thermistor ('thərmistə, thər'mistə) a thermometer whose electrical impedance varies with ambient temperature and so is able to measure extremely small temperature changes.

thermocautery (,thərmoh'kawtə·ree) cauterization by a heated wire or point.

thermochemistry (,thərmoh'kemistree) the aspect of physical chemistry dealing with temperature changes that accompany chemical reactions.

thermocoagulation (,thərmohkoh,agyuh'layshən) coagulation of tissue with high-frequency currents.

thermocouple ('thərmoh,kup'l) a pair of dissimilar electric conductors so joined that with the application of heat an electromotive force is established; used for measuring small temperature differences.

thermodiffusion (,thərmohdi'fyoozhən) diffusion influenced by a temperature gradient.

thermoduric (,thermoh'dyooə·rik) able to endure high temperatures.

thermodynamics (,thərmohdie'namiks) the branch of science dealing with heat and energy, their interconversion, and problems related thereto.

thermoexcitory (,thərmoh·ek'sietə·ree) stimulating production of bodily heat.

thermogenesis (,thərmoh'jenəsis) the production of heat, especially within the animal body. adj. **thermogenetic, thermogenic.**

thermogram ('thərmoh,gram) 1. a graphic record of temperature variations. 2. the visual record obtained by thermography.

thermograph ('thərmoh,grahf, -,graf) 1. an instrument for recording temperature variations. 2. thermogram (2). 3. the apparatus used in thermography.

thermography (,thər'mogrəfee) a technique wherein

an infrared camera photographically portrays the body's surface temperature, based on self-emanating infrared radiations; used as a diagnostic aid in the detection of breast tumours and the assessment of rheumatic joints; also used in the study of pain.

thermohyperaesthesia (ˌthərmohˌhiepə·ris'theezi·ə) extreme sensitiveness to heat.

thermohyperalgesia (ˌthərmohˌhiepə·ral'jeezi·ə) extreme thermalgesia.

thermoinhibitory (ˌthərmoh·in'hibitə·ree) retarding generation of bodily heat.

thermolabile (ˌthərmoh'laybiel) easily affected by heat.

thermolysis (thər'molisis) 1. chemical dissociation by means of heat. 2. dissipation of bodily heat by radiation, evaporation, etc. adj. **thermolytic**.

thermomassage (ˌthərmoh'masahzh, -sahj) massage with heat.

thermometer (thə'momitə) an instrument for determining temperatures, in principle making use of a substance (such as alcohol or mercury) with a physical property that varies with temperature and is susceptible of measurement on some defined scale.

Celsius t. one employing the Celsius scale, that is, with the ice point at 0 and the normal boiling point of water at 100 degrees (100 °C). For equivalents of Celsius and Fahrenheit temperatures, see Appendix 2.

centigrade t. one having the interval between two established reference points divided into 100 equal units, as the Celsius thermometer.

clinical t. one used to determine the temperature of the human body.

electronic t. a clinical thermometer using a sensor based on thermistors, solid-state electronic devices whose electrical characteristics change with temperature. The reading is recorded within seconds, some having a red light or other device to indicate when maximum temperature is reached. Available models include hand-held, desk-top, and wall-mounted units, all having probes that are inserted orally or rectally. It is expected that in the future an electronic thermometer to be worn on the wrist will be available.

Fahrenheit t. one employing the Fahrenheit scale, that is, with the ice point at 32 and the normal boiling point of water at 212 degrees (212 °F). For equivalents of Fahrenheit and Celsius temperatures, see Appendix 2.

Kelvin t. one employing the KELVIN SCALE. **oral t.** a clinical thermometer whose mercury containing bulb is placed under the tongue.

recording t. a temperature-sensitive instrument by which the temperature to which it is exposed is continuously recorded.

rectal t. a clinical thermometer that is inserted in the rectum for determining body temperature.

resistance t. one that uses the electric resistance of metals for determining temperature (thermocouple).

self-registering t. recording thermometer, usually indicating the maximum temperature during a given period.

thermometry (thə'momətree) measurement of temperature.

thermophile ('thərmohˌfiel) a microorganism that grows best at elevated temperatures. adj. **thermophilic**.

thermophore ('thərmohˌfor) 1. a device or apparatus for retaining heat. 2. an instrument for estimating heat sensibility.

thermopile ('thərmohˌpiel) a number of thermocouples in series, used to increase sensitivity to change in temperature or for direct conversion of heat into electric energy.

thermoplacentography (ˌthərmohˌplasen'togrəfee) use of thermography for determination of the site of placental attachment.

thermoplegia (ˌthərmoh'pleeji·ə) heat stroke or sunstroke.

thermopolypnoea (ˌthərmohˌpolip'neeə) quickened breathing due to great heat.

thermoreceptor (ˌthərmohri'septə) a nerve ending sensitive to stimulation by heat.

thermoregulation (ˌthərmohˌregyuh'layshən) heat regulation.

thermostabile (ˌthərmoh'staybiel) not affected by heat.

thermostasis (ˌthərmoh'staysis) maintenance of temperature, as in warm-blooded animals.

thermostat ('thərməˌstat) a device interposed in a heating system by which temperature is automatically maintained between certain levels.

thermosteresis (ˌthərmohstə'reesis) deprivation of heat.

thermosystaltic (ˌthərmohsi'staltik) contracting under the stimulus of heat.

thermotaxis (ˌthərmoh'taksis) 1. normal adjustment of bodily temperature. 2. movement of an organism in response to the stimulation of a temperature gradient. adj. **thermotactic, thermotaxic**.

thermotherapy (ˌthərmoh'therəpee) therapeutic use of heat.

thermotonometer (ˌthərmohtə'nomitə) an instrument for measuring the amount of muscular contraction produced by heat.

thermotropism (thər'motrəˌpizəm) the orientation of a living cell in response to a heat stimulus. adj. **thermotropic**.

thesaurismosis (theeˌsawriz'mohsis) a metabolic disorder in which a substance accumulates in certain cells in abnormal amounts. The stored substances may be fats, proteins, carbohydrates, or other substances.

thesaurosis (ˌtheesaw'rohsis) a condition due to the storing up in the body of unusual amounts of normal or foreign substance.

thi(o)- word element. [Gr.] *sulphur*.

thiabendazole (ˌthieə'bendəˌzohl) a broad-spectrum anthelmintic found useful in ancylostomiasis and strongyloidiasis.

thiaemia (thie'eemi·ə) sulphur in the blood.

thiamin ('thieəmin) thiamine.

thiaminase (thie'amiˌnayz) an enzyme that catalyses the splitting of thiamine into a pyrimidine and a thiazole derivative.

thiamine ('thieəˌmeen) vitamin B_1; a component of the B complex group of vitamins, found in various foodstuffs and present in the free state in blood plasma and cerebrospinal fluid. Deficiency results in neurological symptoms, cardiovascular dysfunction, oedema, and reduced intestinal motility. See also VITAMIN.

thiazide ('thieəˌzied) any of a group of benzothiadiazinesulphonamide derivatives, typified by chlorothiazide, that act as diuretics by inhibiting the reabsorption of sodium in the proximal renal tubule and stimulating chloride excretion, with resultant increase in excretion of water.

Thiersch graft ('teeəsh) a thin split-skin graft (Called also OLLIER–THIERSCH GRAFT).

thiethylperazine (thieˌethil'perəˌzeen) a phenothiazine derivative useful as an antiemetic and antinauseant.

thigh (thie) the portion of the leg above the knee; the femur.

t. bone femur.

thigmaesthesia (ˌthigmis'theezi·ə) tactile sensibility.

thigmotaxis (ˌthigmoh'taksis) movement of an organism in response to contact. adj. **thigmotactic, thigmotaxic**.

thigmotropism (ˌthigmoh'trohpizəm) the orientation

of an organism in response to the stimulus of contact. adj. **thigmotropic**.

thinking ('thingking) the formulation of images or concepts in one's mind.

thiocyanate (ˌthieoh'sieəˌnayt) a salt analogous in composition to a cyanate, but containing sulphur instead of oxygen.

thioguanine (ˌthieoh'gwahneen) an antineoplastic (2-aminopurine-6-thiol) used in leukaemia.

thionine ('thieohˌneen) a dark-green powder, purple in solution, used as a metachromatic stain in microscopy.

thiopentone (ˌthieoh'pentohn) a widely used ultrashort-acting barbiturate given intravenously to induce general anaesthesia. Also used as an anticonvulsant in the treatment of status epilepticus or fits due to local anaesthetic overdose.

thioridazine (ˌthieə'ridəˌzeen) a phenothiazine compound used in the form of the hydrochloride salt as a tranquillizer.

thiosulphate (ˌthieoh'sulfayt) any salt of thiosulphuric acid.

thiotepa (ˌthieoh'teepə) a cytotoxic alkylating agent used as an antineoplastic agent.

thiothixene (ˌthieoh'thikseen) a thioxanthine neuroleptic.

thioxanthene (ˌthieoh'zantheen) a class of structurally related neuroleptic drugs, including chlorprothixene and thiothixene.

thirst (thərst) a sensation, often referred to the mouth and throat, associated with a craving for drink; ordinarily interpreted as a desire for water.

thixotropism, thixotropy (thik'sotrəˌpizəm; thik'sotrəpee) the property of certain gels of becoming fluid when shaken and then becoming solid again.

thlipsencephalus (ˌthlipsen'kefələs, -'sef-) a fetus or infant with a defective skull.

Thomas splint ('tomәs) two round iron rods joined at the upper end by a padded oval iron ring, or half-ring, and bent at the lower end to form the letter W; used to give support to the lower extremity and to remove the weight of the body from the knee joint by transferring it to the pelvis.

Thomsen's disease ('tomsənz) myotonia congenita.

thorac(o)- word element. [Gr.] *chest*.

thoracalgia (ˌthor·rə'kalji·ə) pain in the chest wall.

thoracectomy (ˌthor·rə'sektəmee) thoracotomy with resection of part of a rib.

thoracentesis (ˌthor·rəsen'teesis) surgical puncture and aspiration or drainage of the thoracic cavity. This procedure is used as a therapeutic measure to remove accumulations of fluid from the thoracic cavity or may be performed as an aid to the diagnosis of inflammatory or neoplastic diseases of the lung or pleura.

The patient sits up for this procedure, his arms and head resting on the overbed table or over the back of a chair he is straddling. If the patient is unable to sit up he is turned onto his unaffected side. The skin at the site of insertion of the needle is cleansed with an antiseptic, and a local anaesthetic is injected. The site most often used is the seventh intercostal space, just below the angle of the scapula.

Equipment needed includes a 50 ml syringe and an aspirating needle, a stopcock and rubber tubing, a haemostat, sterile gauze dressings, sterile towels, and a sterile specimen tube.

After the procedure is completed the wound usually is sealed and covered with a sterile dressing. The site is checked frequently for signs of leakage, which should be reported to the doctor.

The total amount and character of the fluid obtained is noted on the patient's chart. Samples of fluid are sent to the laboratory for evaluation if requested.

Immediately following the thoracocentesis the patient is positioned on his unaffected side to rest the site of insertion of the trochar and allow it to seal itself. The patient is observed for signs of dizziness, changes in skin colour, and respiratory and heart rate changes. Other signs of complications following thoracocentesis include excessive coughing, blood-tinged sputum, and tightness of the chest.

Possible after-effects of the procedure include PNEUMOTHORAX, subcutaneous emphysema and bacterial infection. MEDIASTINAL SHIFT resulting from removal of large amounts of fluid from the thoracic cavity may produce cardiac distress and pulmonary oedema.

thoracic (thor'rasik) pertaining to the chest.

t. cage the bony structure forming the walls of the thorax, consisting of the ribs, vertebral column, and sternum.

t. duct a lymphatic duct beginning in the cisterna chyli and emptying into the venous system at the junction of the left subclavian and left internal jugular veins. It acts as a channel for the collection of the lymph from the body below the diaphragm and from the left side of the body above the diaphragm.

t. outlet syndrome compression of the brachial plexus nerve trunks, with pain in the arms, paraesthesia of fingers, vasomotor symptoms, and weakness and wasting of the small muscles of the hand; it may be caused by a drooping shoulder girdle, a cervical rib or fibrous band, an abnormal first rib, continual hyperabduction of the arm (as during sleep), or compression between the edge of scalenus anterior muscle and the first rib.

t. surgery surgical procedures involving entrance into the chest cavity. Until techniques for endotracheal anaesthesia were perfected, this type of surgery was extremely dangerous because of the possibility of lung collapse. By administering anaesthesia under pressure through an endotracheal tube it is now possible to keep one or both lungs expanded, even when they are subjected to atmospheric pressure.

Surgical procedures involving the lungs, heart, and great vessels are included under thoracic surgery as are tracheal resection, oesophagogastrectomy, and repair of hiatal hernia. In order to give intelligent care to the patient before and after surgery, one must have adequate knowledge of the anatomy and physiology of the chest and thoracic cavity. It is especially important to know the differences in pressures within and outside the thoracic cavity. See also LUNG, Mechanism of Inflation and Deflation.

PATIENT CARE. Prior to surgery the care of the patient will depend on the specific operation to be done and the particular disorder requiring surgery. (See also surgery of the LUNG, and HEART surgery.) In general, the patient should be given an explanation of the operative procedure anticipated and the type of equipment that will be used in the postoperative period. He will be taught the proper method of coughing to remove secretions accumulated in the lungs.

The development of intensive care units has sharply improved the care of the post-thoracotomy patient. The availability of monitors, ventilators and special assistance devices has increased not only the safety of the operation but also the comfort of the patient. Most patients return from the operating room with endotracheal tubes still in place, ventilated by machines, and monitored with such specialised equipment as Swan–Ganz catheters for observation of cardiac output, oxygenation and level of hydration.

During the postoperative period, alteration in respiratory status is a major potential problem for patients having thoracic surgery. Impaired gas exchange can result from atelectasis, pneumothorax, mediastinal shift, bronchopulmonary fistula, pneumonia, pleural effusion, pulmonary oedema, narcotics, or abdominal distention. To identify any change in respiratory status, the patient's arterial blood gases are serially monitored, breath sounds are auscultated, and the rate and character of respirations are assessed.

Although coughing may be painful in the immediate postoperative period and may require analgesic medication to relieve the discomfort, if the patient understands the need for coughing up the secretions he will be more cooperative. He may be given special exercises to preserve muscular action of the shoulder on the affected side and to maintain proper alignment of the upper portion of his body and arm. Usually the physiotherapist supervises these exercises, but the nursing staff must cooperate in seeing that they are done.

Narcotics are always used with caution before thoracic surgery because they can depress respiration. Usually the preoperative medication is atropine in combination with a barbiturate.

Postoperative care includes care of CHEST drains, positioned as specified by the surgeon, and suction as needed. When a patient cannot force out accumulated secretions by coughing, a chest suction machine may be used. These machines incorporate the principle of closed drainage and also provide negative pressure. Whatever the type of equipment used, the nurse should become familiar with its purpose and check frequently to be sure it is in good working order.

The nursing staff are usually responsible for measuring and recording the amount of drainage from the chest drains at regular intervals. This requires strict attention to proper clamping and reconnecting of the tubes before and after the bottles are removed.

Analgesics are administered postoperatively with caution to avoid depression of the respiratory centre or sedation to the point that the patient cannot cough or perform deep breathing exercises effectively. Fluid intake and output are carefully monitored. A pulmonectomy patient can become overloaded with fluids very quickly and, therefore, must be watched closely for signs such as high central venous pressure, rales, and distention of the jugular vein.

As the operative site heals and the lung expands, the chest drains can be safely removed. After their removal an airtight bandage is applied to the area. As a further precaution against leakage of air into the chest cavity, a purse-string suture is often put around the tube at the time of insertion and tied off as the tube is withdrawn.

t. vertebrae the 12 vertebrae between the cervical and lumbar vertebrae, giving attachment to the ribs and forming part of the posterior wall of the thorax.

thoracoacromial (ˌthor·rəkoh·ə'krohmi·əl) pertaining to the chest and acromion.

thoracoceloschisis (ˌthor·rəkohsi'loskisis) congenital fissure of the thorax and abdomen.

thoracocentesis (ˌthor·rəkohsen'teesis) thoracentesis.

thoracocyllosis (ˌthor·rəkohsi'lohsis) deformity of the thorax.

thoracocyrtosis (ˌthor·rəkohsər'tohsis) abnormal curvature of the chest wall.

thoracodelphus (ˌthor·rəkoh'delfəs) a double fetus with one head, two arms, and four legs, the bodies being joined above the navel.

thoracodidymus (ˌthor·rəkoh'didiməs) thoracopagus.

thoracodynia (ˌthor·rəkoh'dini·ə) pain in the thorax.

thoracogastroschisis (ˌthor·rəkohga'stroskisis) a developmental anomaly resulting from faulty closure of the body wall along the midventral line, involving both thorax and abdomen, i.e., fissure of the thorax and abdomen.

thoracolumbar (ˌthor·rəkoh'lumbə) pertaining to the thoracic and lumbar vertebrae.

thoracolysis (ˌthor·rə'kolisis) the freeing of adhesions of the chest wall.

thoracomelus (ˌthor·rə'koməlus) a fetus or infant with a supernumerary limb attached to the thorax.

thoracometer (ˌthor·rə'komitə) stethometer.

thoracomyodynia (ˌthor·rəkohˌmieoh'dini·ə) pain in the muscles of the chest.

thoracopagus (ˌthor·rə'kopəgəs) conjoined twins united at the thorax.

thoracopathy (ˌthor·rə'kopəthee) any disease of the thoracic organs or tissues.

thoracoplasty ('thor·rəkohˌplastee) surgical removal of ribs to achieve permanent collapse of a lung infected with tuberculosis or harbouring a lung abscess. Now obsolete.

thoracoschisis (ˌthor·rə'koskisis) congenital fissure of the chest wall.

thoracoscope (thor'rakohˌskohp) an endoscope for examining the pleural cavity through an intercostal space.

thoracoscopy (ˌthor·rə'koskəpee) examination of the pleural space with a thoracoscope.

thoracostenosis (ˌthorəkohstə'nohsis) abnormal contraction of the thorax.

thoracostomy (ˌthor·rə'kostəmee) incision through the chest wall, with maintenance of an opening for drainage.

thoracotomy (ˌthor·rə'kotəmee) incision through the chest wall.

thorax ('thor·raks) the part of the body between the neck and abdomen; the chest. It is separated from the abdomen by the diaphragm. The walls of the thorax are formed by the 12 pairs of ribs, attached to the sides of the spine and curving toward the front. The upper seven ribs are attached to the sternum, the next three connect with cartilage below and the last two (the floating ribs) are unattached in the front. The principal organs in the thoracic cavity are the heart with its major blood vessels, and the lungs with the bronchi, which bring in the body's air supply. The trachea enters the thorax to connect with the lungs, and the oesophagus travels through it to connect with the stomach below the diaphragm. See also THORACIC SURGERY.

Thorel's bundle ('torelz) a bundle of muscle fibres in the human heart connecting the sinoatrial and atrioventricular nodes.

thorium ('thor·ri·əm) a chemical element, atomic number 90, atomic weight 232.038, symbol Th. (See table of elements in Appendix 2.) Formerly used as a radiographic contrast medium.

Thorotrast ('thorohtrahst) a radiological contrast medium containing thorium used for angiography in the 1930s. It is not excreted from the body but stored in the reticuloendothelial system and because it emits alpha particles and has a half-life of 10^{10} years its use was complicated by the late development of malignancies.

threadworm ('thredˌwərm) any nematode worm, e.g., *Enterobius vermicularis* (see also WORM).

threonine ('threeəˌneen) a naturally occurring amino acid, one of those essential for human metabolism.

threpsology (threp'soləjee) the scientific study of nutrition.

threshold ('thresh·hohld) the level that must be reached for an effect to be produced, as the degree of intensity of stimulus which just produces a sensation.

auditory t. the slightest perceptible sound.
renal t. that concentration of a substance in plasma at which it begins to be excreted in the urine.
t. of consciousness the lowest limit of sensibility; the point of consciousness at which a stimulus is barely perceived.

thrill ('thril) a vibration felt by the examiner on palpation.
diastolic t. one felt over the precordium during diastole in advanced aortic insufficiency.
hydatid t. one felt on percussing over a hydatid cyst.
presystolic t. one felt just before systole over the apex of the heart.
systolic t. one felt over the precordium during systole in aortic stenosis, pulmonary stenosis, and ventricular septal defect.

thrix (thriks) [Gr.] *hair*.
t. annulata a condition in which a hair appears to be marked by alternating bands of white; called also *ringed hair*.

-thrix (thriks) word element. [Gr.] *hair*.

throat (throht) 1. the area that includes the LARYNX and PHARYNX, passageways that link the nose and mouth with the respiratory and digestive systems of the body. 2. the fauces. 3. the anterior part of the neck.

throb (throb) a pulsating movement or sensation.

thromb(o)- word element. [Gr.] *clot*, *thrombus*.

thrombapheresis (ˌthrombafə'reesis) thrombocytapheresis.

thrombasthenia (ˌthrombəs'theeni·ə) a platelet abnormality characterized by defective clot retraction and impaired ADP-induced platelet aggregation; it is manifested clinically as Glanzmann's disease, with epistaxis, inappropriate bruising, and excessive post-traumatic bleeding.
Glanzmann's t. thrombasthenia.

thrombectomy (throm'bektəmee) surgical removal of a clot from a blood vessel.
medical t. enzymatic dissolution of a blood clot in situ.

thrombin ('thrombin) an enzyme resulting from activation of prothrombin, which catalyses the conversion of fibrinogen to fibrin; a preparation from prothrombin of bovine origin is used as a topical haemostatic.
t. time a laboratory test used to measure fibrinogen concentration and function; used also to monitor heparin therapy.

thromboangiitis (ˌthrombohˌanji'ietis) inflammation of a blood vessel, with thrombosis.
t. obliterans thromboangiitis with contraction of the vessel about the clot, leading to diminution of blood flow distal to the site; most frequently the lower extremities are affected. Shows a strong relationship to heavy cigarette smoking. Called also BUERGER'S DISEASE.

thromboarteritis (ˌthrombohˌahtə'reitis) thrombosis associated with arteritis.

thromboasthenia (ˌthromboh·əs'theeni·ə) thrombasthenia.

thromboclasis (ˌthromboh'klaysis) the dissolution of a thrombus. adj. **thromboclastic**.

thrombocyst, thrombocystis ('thrombohˌsist; ˌthromboh'sistis) a sac formed around a clot or thrombus.

thrombocytapheresis (ˌthrombohsieˌtafə'reesis) the selective separation and removal of thrombocytes (platelets) from withdrawn blood, the remainder of the blood then being retransfused into the donor. Called also *plateletpheresis* and *thrombapheresis*.

thrombocyte ('thrombohˌsiet) a blood platelet (see also PLATELET). adj. **thrombocytic**.

thrombocythaemia (ˌthrombohsie'theemi·ə) an increase in the number of circulating blood platelets.
essential t., haemorrhagic t. a clinical syndrome with repeated spontaneous haemorrhages, either external or into the tissues, and greatly increased number of circulating platelets.

thrombocytocrit (ˌthromboh'sietohˌkrit) the volume of packed blood platelets in a given quantity of blood; also, the instrument used to measure platelet volume.

thrombocytolysis (ˌthrombohsie'tolisis) destruction of blood platelets (thrombocytes).

thrombocytopathy (ˌthrombohsie'topəthee) any qualitative disorder of blood platelets.

thrombocytopenia (ˌthrombohˌsietoh'peeni·ə) decrease in number of platelets in circulating blood. adj. **thrombocytopenic**. The condition can result from decreased or defective platelet production or from accelerated platelet destruction. Conditions related to defective production include hypoplastic and aplastic anaemia, infiltration of bone marrow by malignant cells or myelofibrosis, viral infections, nutritional deficiency and thrombocytopenic purpura. Increased destruction of platlets can be caused by infections, certain drugs, transfusion related purpuras, idiopathic thrombocytopenic purpura, and disseminated intravascular coagulation.

thrombocytopoiesis (ˌthrombohˌsietohpoy'eesis) the production of blood platelets (thrombocytes). adj. **thrombocytopoietic**.

thrombocytosis (ˌthrombohsie'tohsis) increase in the number of platelets in the circulating blood.

thromboembolism (ˌthromboh'embəˌlizəm) obstruction of a blood vessel with thrombotic material carried by the blood from the site of origin to plug another vessel.

thromboendarterectomy (ˌthrombohˌendahtə'rektəmee) removal of an obstructing thrombus together with a portion of the inner lining of the obstructed artery.

thromboendarteritis (ˌthrombohˌendahtə'rietis) inflammation of the innermost coat of an artery, with thrombus formation.

thromboendocarditis (ˌthrombohˌendohkah'dietis) formation of a thrombus on a heart valve which has previously been eroded.

thrombogenesis (ˌthromboh'jenəsis) clot formation. adj. **thrombogenic**.

thromboid ('thromboyd) resembling a thrombus.

thrombokinase (ˌthromboh'kienayz) activated clotting factor X.

thrombokinetics (ˌthrombohki'netiks) the dynamics of blood coagulation.

thrombolymphangitis (ˌthrombohˌlimfan'jietis) inflammation of a lymph vessel due to a thrombus.

thrombolysis (throm'bolisis) dissolution of a thrombus.

thrombolytic (ˌthromboh'litik) 1. dissolving or splitting up a thrombus. 2. an agent that dissolves or splits up a thrombus.

thrombopathy (throm'bopəthee) thrombocytopathy.

thrombopenia (ˌthromboh'peeni·ə) thrombocytopenia.

thrombophilia (ˌthromboh'fili·ə) a tendency to the occurrence of thrombosis.

thrombophlebitis (ˌthrombohfli'bietis) inflammation of a vein associated with thrombus formation. See also venous THROMBOSIS.
t. migrans a recurrent condition involving different vessels simultaneously or at intervals; frequently a manifestation of an occult carcinoma.
postpartum iliofemoral t. thrombophlebitis of the iliofemoral vein following childbirth.

thromboplastic (ˌthromboh'plastik) causing or accelerating clot formation in the blood.

thromboplastin (ˌthromboh'plastin) a substance in blood and tissues which, in the presence of ionized calcium, aids in the conversion of prothrombin to thrombin. Extrinsic and intrinsic thromboplastin are formed as the result of the interaction of different clotting factors; the factors that combine to form extrinsic thromboplastin are not all derived from intravascular sources, whereas those that form intrinsic thromboplastin are.

tissue t. Factor III, a material derived from several sources in the body (e.g., brain, lung). It is important in the formation of extrinsic prothrombin converting principle in the extrinsic pathway of blood coagulation. Called also *tissue factor*.

thrombopoiesis (ˌthrombohpoy'eesis) 1. thrombogenesis. 2. thrombocytopoiesis. adj. **thrombopoietic.**

thrombosis (throm'bohsis) formation, development, or presence of a thrombus. adj. **thrombotic.**

A thrombus may form whenever the flow of blood in the arteries or the veins is impeded. Many factors can interfere with the normal flow of the blood. Sometimes heart failure or physical inactivity retards circulation generally, or a change in the shape or inner surface of a vessel wall impedes the flow of blood, as in atherosclerosis. Any mass that has grown inside the body can exert pressure on a vessel, or the vessel wall can be injured and roughened by an accident, surgery, a burn, cold, inflammation, or infection.

If the thrombus detaches itself from the wall and is carried along by the bloodstream, the clot is called an embolus. The condition is known as EMBOLISM.

A thrombus may form in the heart chambers. This sometimes occurs after coronary thrombosis (see below) at the place where the wall of the heart is weakened or in the dilated atria in some cases of cardiac failure.

Because blood normally flows more slowly through the veins than through the arteries, thrombosis is more common in the veins than in the arteries.

VENOUS THROMBOSIS. Venous thrombosis occurs most often in the legs or pelvis. It may be a complication of phlebitis or may result from injury to a vein or from prolonged bed rest. The symptoms of venous thrombosis—a feeling of heaviness, pain, warmth, or swelling in the affected part, and possibly chills and fever—do not necessarily indicate its severity. Immediate medical attention is necessary in any case. Under *no* circumstances should the affected limb be massaged.

In a thrombosis of the superficial veins, bed rest with the legs elevated and application of heat to the affected area may be all that is necessary. In a thrombosis of the deep veins, the affected part must be immobilized to prevent the clot from spreading or turning into an embolus, and anticoagulant drugs may be given. With proper treatment, recovery occurs within a short time unless an embolism develops. Occasionally an operation is performed and the veins in which the thrombi have formed are tied off. Ordinarily, other veins take over their task and the circulation returns to normal.

PREVENTION. Immobility is a prime factor in the development of thrombosis; hence, all patients should be mobilized as soon as possible after surgery or an illness that requires bed rest or produces paralysis. Patients who cannot get out of bed should follow an exercise routine involving either active or passive motion of the extremities. For those who can perform active exercises, a footboard, rolled blanket, or pillow placed at the patient's feet can be used to encourage walking motions of the legs and stretching of the muscles. The bed clothes should be loose enough to permit free movement of the legs and feet.

ARTERIAL THROMBOSIS. The main types of arterial thrombosis are related to atherosclerosis, although thrombosis can result from infection or from injury to an artery. The pathogenesis of atherosclerosis is controversial. It may be related to diet although it is possible that diet only influences the complications such as thrombosis. It is associated with hypertension, with diabetes mellitus, and with some hereditary disorders of lipid metabolism. Coronary thrombosis is a complication of coronary artery ATHEROSCLEROSIS and will block off part of the blood supply to a region of heart muscle causing infarction (heart attack). (See also MYOCARDIAL INFARCTION.) This constitutes a medical emergency.

In cerebral thrombosis, the thrombus obstructs the supply of blood to the brain and is one of the causes of STROKE.

In advanced cases of atherosclerosis, thrombus may occlude the arteries of the legs. The onset, which is often sudden, is characterized by either a tingling feeling or numbness and coldness in the limb. Pain is not always present. Immediate treatment with anticoagulants to discourage clotting is necessary. If this is not effective, surgery may be required. This condition is most common in the elderly and in diabetics. Modern methods of treatment can often save the limb.

In addition to the surgical removal of a thrombus or an embolus, in some cases surgery of the blood vessels also involves the removal of old, narrowed, or deteriorated vessels and their replacement with grafts.

thrombostasis (ˌthromboh'staysis) stasis of blood in a part with formation of thrombus.

thromboxane (throm'boksayn) an intermediate in the metabolic pathway of arachidonic acid, formed from prostaglandin endoperoxides, and released from suitably stimulated platelets; the unstable form, thromboxane A_2, is a potent inducer of platelet aggregation and constrictor of arterial smooth muscle.

thrombus ('thrombəs) a solid aggregation of blood—primarily platelets and fibrin with entrapment of cellular elements, frequently causing vascular obstruction at the point of its formation. The sequence is usually initiated by platelet aggregation. As the platelets aggregate and degranulate they activate the clotting cascade with the formation of the fibrin mesh. Thrombus forms in situ in the vascular compartment and should be distinguished from clotting, which occurs to blood in the extravasular compartments, when taken for laboratory investigations and as a postmortem change.

mural t. one attached to the wall of the endocardium in a diseased area.

occluding t. one that occupies the entire lumen of a vessel and obstructs blood flow.

parietal t. one attached to a vessel or heart wall.

thrush (thrush) infection of the oral mucous membrane by the fungus *Candida albicans*. It is characterized by white patches on a red, moist inflamed surface, occurring anywhere in the mouth, including the tongue, but usually on the inner cheeks. These patches are occasionally accompanied by pain and fever. In babies they are distinguished from milk curds by the red, raw area which appears when they are wiped away.

Approximately 20 to 30 per cent of the population harbours *Candida albicans*, but the disease develops in only a very small number of this group. Those who are most susceptible are artificially fed infants and adults who are in a weakened condition from infection, dietary deficiency (malnutrition), or uncontrolled diabetes mellitus, or who have been treated with antibiotics for a long time.

Any baby who has a sore throat and shows discomfort while feeding may have oral or anal thrush. If the white patches that appear remain untreated, they will become larger and will tend to grow together and also spread to other parts of the gastrointestinal tract. An erythmatous napkin rash with small, white-headed pustules is usually due to *Candida albicans*.

Thrush is likely to occur in pregnancy due to altered vaginal pH (see DÖDERLEIN'S BACILLUS) and should be treated before delivery to prevent cross-infection of the child.

Thrush itself is treated with antibiotics and fungicidal drugs. The best preventive measures are good general health, a well-balanced diet, and good mouth hygiene.

thrypsis ('thripsis) a comminuted fracture.

thulium ('thyooli·əm) a chemical element, atomic number 69, atomic weight 168.934, symbol Tm. See table of elements in Appendix 2.

thumb (thum) the radial or first digit of the hand; it has only two phalanges and is apposable to the four fingers of the hand.

tennis t. tendinitis of the tendon of the long flexor muscle of the thumb, with calcification.

thumbprinting ('thum,printing) a radiographic sign appearing as smooth indentations on the barium-filled colon, as though made by depression with the thumb; seen in various disorders of the colon, especially ischaemic colitis.

thym(o)- word element. [Gr.] *thymus; mind, soul* or *emotions*.

thymectomy (thie'mektəmee) excision of the thymus.

thymelcosis (,thiemel'kohsis) ulceration of the thymus.

thymergasia (,thiemə'gayzi·ə) an affective or reaction-type psychosis, such as manic-depressive psychosis. adj. **thymergasic, thymergastic.**

-thymia ('thiemi·ə) word element. [Gr.] *condition of mind*. adj. **-thymic.**

thymic ('thiemik) pertaining to the thymus.

thymicolymphatic (,thiemikohlim'fatik) pertaining to the thymus and lymphatic nodes.

thymidine ('thiemi,deen) a nucleoside of DNA.

thymin ('thiemin) former name for thymopoietin.

thymine ('thiemeen) a pyrimidine base in DNA.

thymitis (thie'mietis) inflammation of the thymus.

thymocyte ('thiemoh,siet) a lymphocyte arising in the thymus.

thymogenic (,thiemoh'jenik) of affective or hysterical origin.

thymokesis (,thiemoh'keesis) persistence of the thymus gland in an adult.

thymokinetic (,thiemohki'netik) tending to stimulate the thymus.

thymol ('thiemol) a phenol obtained from thyme oil and other volatile oils or produced synthetically; used as a topical antifungal and antibacterial, and as an antibiotic agent in trichloroethylene.

t. iodide a mixture of iodine derivatives of thymol, containing not less than 43 per cent of iodine; mild antiseptic.

thymoleptic (,thiemoh'leptik) any drug that favourably modifies mood in serious affective disorders such as depression or mania; the main categories of thymoleptics include the tricyclic antidepressants, monoamine oxidase inhibitors, and lithium compounds. Called also *antidepressant*.

thymoma (thie'mohmə) a tumour derived from the epithelial or lymphoid elements of the thymus.

thymopathy (thie'mopəthee) any disease of the thymus.

thymopoietin (,thiemohpoy'eetin) a polypeptide hormone secreted by the thymus, which induces the proliferation of lymphocyte precursors and their differentiation into T-lymphocytes.

thymoprivic, thymoprivous (,thiemoh'prievik; ,thiemoh'prievəs) pertaining to or resulting from removal or atrophy of the thymus.

thymosin ('thiemoh,sin) a humoural factor secreted by the thymus, which promotes the maturation of T-lymphocytes. See also THYMUS.

thymus ('thieməs) a ductless glandlike body lying in the upper mediastinum beneath the sternum, which reaches its maximum development during puberty and continues to play an immunological role throughout life, even though its function declines with age.

During the last stages of fetal life and the early neonatal period, the reticular structure of the thymus entraps immature 'stem' cells arising from the bone marrow and circulating in the blood. The thymus preprocesses these cells, causing them to become sensitized and therefore capable of maturing into a type of lymphocyte that is essential to the development of cell-mediated IMMUNITY. After sensitization by the thymus, these lymphocytes reenter the blood and are transported to developing lymphoid tissue, where they seed the cells that eventually become thymus-dependent or T-lymphocytes. If the thymus is removed or becomes nonfunctional during fetal life, the lymphoid tissue fails to become seeded with the sensitized lymphocytes and the body's cell-mediated arm of immunity fails to develop. It is this arm of immunity that is mainly responsible for rejection of organ transplants and resistance to intracellular microbial infection, and perhaps plays a role in natural resistance to cancer.

In the 1960s Dr. Allan L. Goldstein discovered and isolated a humoral factor, believed to be a hormone from the thymus, which they named *thymosin*. It is hoped that eventually this hormone will prove to be of value in restoring immunological capability to immune-deficient patients. Another possibility is the development of an antithymosin serum, which could be effectively employed in the selective suppression of the immune systems of persons suffering from transplant rejection. It is proposed that the serum would suppress only the T-cell immune system, leaving the remaining humoral system intact and capable of producing antibodies against bacterial invasion. In addition to thymosin the thymus also secretes *thymopoietin* (formerly called thymin), which induces the proliferation of lymphocyte precursors and their differentiation into T-lymphocytes.

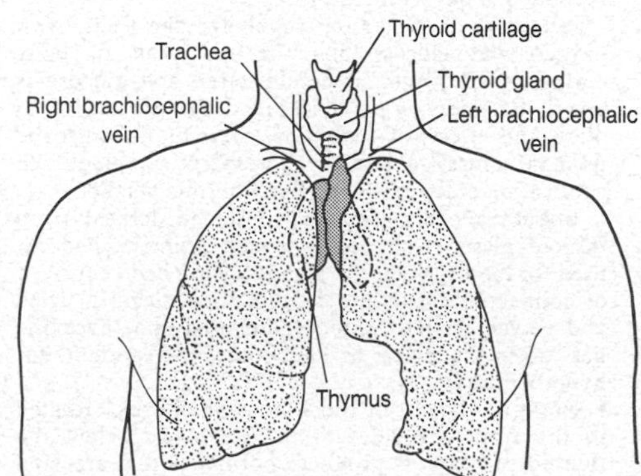

Thymus

thyro- word element. [Gr.] *thyroid.*
thyroadenitis (ˌthierohˌadəˈnietis) thyroiditis.
thyroaplasia (ˌthieroh·əˈplayzi·ə) defective development of the thyroid with deficient activity of its secretion.
thyroarytenoid (ˌthierohˌariˈteenoyd) pertaining to the thyroid and arytenoid cartilages.
thyrocalcitonin (ˌthierohˌkalsiˈtohnin) calcitonin.
thyrocardiac (ˌthierohˈkahdiˌak) pertaining to the thyroid and heart.
t. disease thyrotoxic heart disease.
thyrocele (ˈthierohˌseel) tumour of the thyroid gland; goitre.
thyrochondrotomy (ˌthierohkonˈdrotəmee) surgical incision of the thyroid cartilage.
thyrocricotomy (ˌthierohkrieˈkotəmee) incision of the cricothyroid membrane to achieve TRACHEOSTOMY.
thyroepiglottic (ˌthierohˌepiˈglotik) pertaining to the thyroid and epiglottis.
thyrogenic, thyrogenous (ˌthierohˈjenik; thieˈrojənəs) originating in the thyroid.
thyroglobulin (ˌthierohˈglobyuhlin) an iodine-containing glycoprotein of high molecular weight, occurring in the colloid of the follicles of the thyroid gland; the iodinated tyrosine moieties of thyroglobulin form the active hormones thyroxine and triiodothyronine.
thyroglossal (ˌthierohˈglosˈl) pertaining to the thyroid and tongue.
thyrohyal (ˌthierohˈhieəl) pertaining to the thyroid cartilage and the hyoid bone.
thyrohyoid (ˌthierohˈhieoyd) pertaining to the thyroid gland or cartilage and the hyoid bone.
thyroid (ˈthieroyd) 1. resembling a shield. 2. the thyroid gland. 3. a pharmaceutical preparation of cleaned, dried, powdered thyroid gland, obtained from those domesticated animals used for food by man.
t. cartilage the shield-shaped cartilage of the larynx; the prominence it produces on the neck is the Adam's apple.
t. crisis a sudden and dangerous increase of the symptoms of thyrotoxicosis; called also *thyroid storm.* The condition may occur in patients with severe HYPERTHYROIDISM and in the immediate postoperative period following THYROIDECTOMY. It is a serious event that can be fatal if not brought under control.

In thyroid crisis all of the body processes are accelerated to dangerously high levels. The pulse may rise to 200 beats per minute, and there is concurrent rise in the respiratory rate. The temperature control centre loses control, bringing about a rapid and steady increase in body temperature.

Treatment is aimed at supplying the cells with oxygen and glucose and the reduction of body temperature. Oxygen is administered and glucose is given. Beta-adrenergic blocking drugs are useful to offset the effects of thyroxine. Steroids may also be used. Measures to reduce hyperthermia include the application of ice packs or a hypothermia blanket.

t. extract a pharmaceutical substance derived from thyroid glands from domesticated animals that are used for food by man, the glands having been deprived of connective tissue and fat and then cleaned, dried and powdered. It is now seldom used and thyroxine has taken its place as the specific treatment for hypothyroidism.
t. gland the largest of the ENDOCRINE GLANDS, situated in the front and sides of the neck just below the thyroid cartilage. It produces hormones that are vital in maintaining normal growth and metabolism. It also contains most of the body's iodine content organically bound as thyroid hormone or in thyroglobulin.

Excessive thyroid activity increases metabolism, causing nervousness, heart palpitations, restlessness, and insomnia (see also HYPERTHYROIDISM). Deficient thyroid activity produces fatigue, and lethargy (see also HYPOTHYROIDISM); marked deficiency causes weight gain, coarsened features and thick, scaly skin (MYXOEDEMA). Enlargement of the thyroid gland is called GOITRE, and it often accompanies hyperthyroidism.

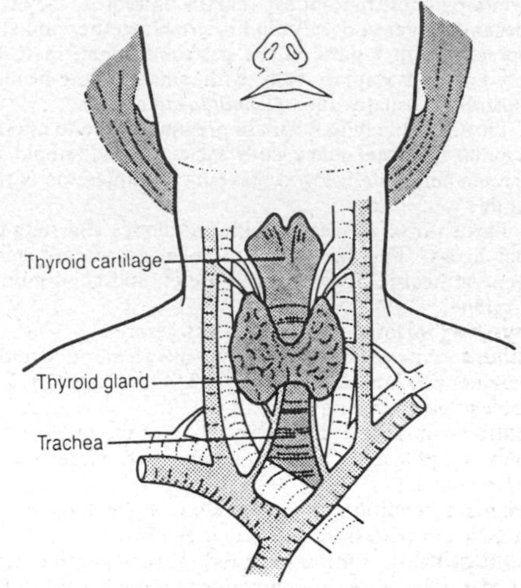

Thyroid gland

Diagnostic tests for thyroid disorders include radioimmunoassay for T_3, T_4, and thyroid-stimulating hormone (TSH), free thyroxine serum concentration, and free thyroxine index (FTI). These and other thyroid function tests can be distorted by preparations and foods containing iodine, and by oral contraceptives, phenytoin and several other drugs. The *thyroid scan* is useful in detecting nodules and active thyroid tissue and, combined with radioactive iodine uptake, measures the ability of the thyroid gland to take in ingested iodine. Ultrasound scans will determine if nodules in the thyroid gland are solid or cystic.

Persons who received radiation to the head and neck as children are at higher than normal risk for development of thyroid abnormalities. Of these disorders about one-third are carcinomas of the thyroid. Other problems related to radiation early in life include adenomas and other malignant and benign tumours, hypo- and hyperthyroidism, and thyroiditis.

t. hormones iodothyronines secreted by the thyroid gland, principally thyroxine (tetraiodothyronine, T_4) and triiodothyronine (T_3). The serum level of T_4 is normally 45 to 50 times the level of T_3. However, T_3 is several times more active than T_4, and most T_3 is produced by metabolism of T_4 in peripheral tissues. The pharmaceutical names for T_4 and T_3 are thyroxine and liothyronine, respectively. Thyroid hormones influence many metabolic processes. They stimulate the cellular production of heat, stimulate protein synthesis, regulate many aspects of carbohydrate metabolism, stimulate lipid synthesis, mobilization, and degradation, stimulate the synthesis of coenzymes from vitamins, and may affect the response of tissues to adrenaline and noradrenaline.

Elaboration of thyroid hormones is regulated by the hypothalamus–pituitary–thyroid control system. Internal environmental conditions, such as low thyroid hormone and noradrenaline serum levels, or external factors, such as cold and stress, activate the hypothalamus, which secretes thyrotrophin-releasing hormone (TRH). This hormone acts on the pituitary gland and brings about the release of thyroid-stimulating hormone (TSH). The TSH then stimulates the release of thyroid hormones T_3 and T_4 from the thyroid gland. When sufficient levels of serum thyroxine have been reached, there is negative feedback to the hypothalamus and TRH is no longer secreted.

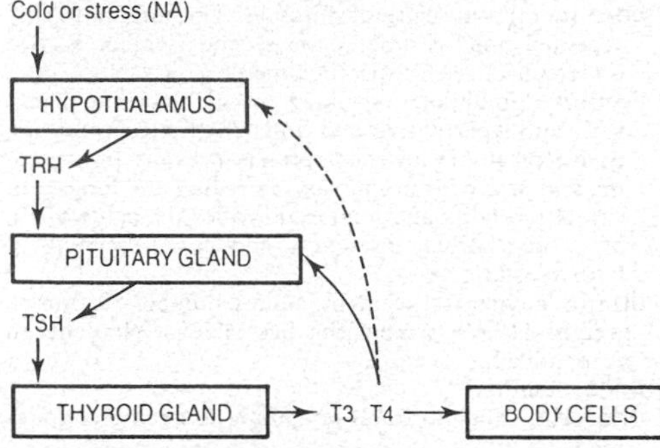

Hypothalamus – pituitary – thyroid axis. The cycle for regulation of thyroid hormone (triiodothyronine, T_3: thyroxine, T_4) involves either cold or noradrenaline (NA), which stimulates thyrotrophin-releasing hormone (TRH). This hormone, in turn, triggers the release of thyroid-stimulating hormone (TSH), which then stimulates the release of T_3 and T_4. Feedback from T_3 and T_4 reaches the pituitary gland and, probably, the hypothalamus

thyroidectomy (ˌthieroy'dektəmee) partial or total excision of the thyroid gland.

Total thyroidectomy may be performed in cases of cancer of the thyroid. Hemithyroidectomy may be performed for single solid adenomas. Subtotal thyroidectomy, in which more than two-thirds of the gland is removed, is performed in patients suffering from intractable HYPERTHYROIDISM. The remaining portion of the gland continues to function and produce the necessary hormones. Partial thyroidectomy, the commonest operation, is undertaken for benign goitrous enlargement of the gland which is unsightly or a cause of respiratory embarrassment due to impingement at the thoracic inlet.

thyroidism ('thieroyˌdizəm) hyperthyroidism; also, a morbid condition due to excess doses of thyroid.

thyroiditis (ˌthieroy'dietis) inflammation of the thyroid. Acute thyroiditis, usually due to a virus infection, is characterized by sore throat, fever, and painful enlargement of the gland.

Hashimoto's t. struma lymphomatosa, a progressive autoimmune disease of the thyroid gland with degeneration of its epithelial elements and replacement by lymphoid and fibrous tissue.

thyroidotomy (ˌthieroy'dotəmee) incision of the thyroid.

thyromegaly (ˌthieroh'megəlee) goitre.

thyromimetic (ˌthierohmi'metik) producing effects similar to those of thyroid hormones or the thyroid gland.

thyroparathyroidectomy (ˌthierohˌparəˌthieroy'dektəmee) excision of the thyroid and parathyroids.

thyroprival, thyroprivic (ˌthieroh'prievəl; ˌthieroh'prievik) pertaining to, marked by, or due to deprivation or loss of thyroid function.

thyroptosis (ˌthierop'tohsis) downward displacement of a goitrous thyroid.

thyrosis (thie'rohsis) any disease based on disordered thyroid action.

thyrotherapy (ˌthieroh'therəpee) treatment with preparations of thyroid.

thyrotomy (thie'rotəmee) 1. surgical division of the thyroid cartilage. 2. incision of the thyroid gland.

thyrotoxic (ˌthieroh'toksik) marked by toxic (excessive) activity of the thyroid.

t. crisis a fulminating increase in all the symptoms of thyrotoxicosis.

t. heart disease heart disease associated with hyperthyroidism, marked by atrial fibrillation, cardiac enlargement, and congestive heart failure. Called also *thyrocardiac disease.*

t. storm thyrotoxic crisis.

thyrotoxicosis (ˌthierohˌtoksi'kohsis) a morbid condition due to overactivity of the thyroid gland.

thyrotrope ('thierohˌtrohp) one of the basophils (beta cells) of the adenohypophysis, the granules of which secrete thyrotrophin.

thyrotroph ('thierohˌtrohf) thyrotrope.

thyrotrophic (ˌthieroh'trohfik) having an influence on the thyroid gland.

thyrotrophin (ˌthieroh'trohfin) a hormone secreted by the anterior lobe of the pituitary gland that has an affinity for and specifically stimulates the thyroid gland. Called also *thyroid-stimulating hormone (TSH).*

thyrotropic (ˌthieroh'tropik) thyrotrophic.

thyrotropin (ˌthieroh'trohpin) thyrotrophin.

thyrotropism (ˌthieroh'trohpizəm) affinity for the thyroid gland. adj. **thyrotropic.**

thyroxine (thie'rokseen) a hormone of the THYROID GLAND that contains iodine and is a derivative of the amino acid tyrosine. The chemical name for thyroxine is tetraiodothyronine (symbol, T_4); it is formed and stored in the thyroid follicles as thyroglobulin, the storage form. Thyroxine is released from the gland by the action of a proteolytic enzyme. T_4 is deiodinated in peripheral tissues to form triiodothyronine (T_3), which has a greater biological activity.

Thyroxine acts as a catalyst in the body and influences a great variety of effects, including metabolic rate (oxygen consumption); growth and development; metabolism of carbohydrates, fats, proteins, electrolytes, and water; vitamin requirements; reproduction; and resistance to infection.

Thyroxine can be extracted from animals or made synthetically; it is prescribed for hypothyroidism and for some types of goitre.

Ti chemical symbol, *titanium.*

TIA transient cerebral ischaemic attacks (see TRANSIENT ISCHAEMIC ATTACKS and STROKE).

tiaprofenic acid (ˌtiəproh'fenik) a nonsteroidal anti-inflammatory drug used in rheumatic conditions.

tibia ('tibi·ə) the inner and larger bone of the leg below the knee; it articulates with the femur and head of the fibula above and with the talus below. adj. **tibial.**

t. valga a bowing of the leg in which the angulation is away from the midline of the body.

t. vara a bowing of the leg in which the angulation is toward the midline of the body; bowleg.

tibialis (ˌtibi'aylis) [L.] *tibial.*

tibiofemoral (ˌtibioh'femə·rəl) pertaining to the tibia and femur.

tibiofibular (ˌtibioh'fibyuhlə) pertaining to the tibia and fibula.

tibiotarsal (ˌtibioh'tahs'l) pertaining to the tibia and tarsus.

tic (tik) a spasmodic twitching movement made involuntarily by muscles that are ordinarily under voluntary control. Twitching of the eyelid, of muscles of the face, and of the diaphragm (hiccupping) are examples. In general, tics are of psychological origin; they tend to develop in young persons of nervous temperament and occasionally persist into adulthood.

t. douloureux trigeminal neuralgia, a painful disorder of the trigeminal nerve (the fifth cranial nerve). The disorder is characterized by severe pain in the face and forehead on the affected side. The pain extends to the midline of the face and head and may be triggered by cold draughts, chewing, drinking cold liquids, brushing the hair, or washing the face.

TREATMENT. Drug therapy comprises the use of carbamazepine, although for some patients the level of medication needed to control the facial pain produces intolerable side-effects, including drowsiness. If drug therapy fails, trigeminal thermocoagulation may be considered. A cryoprobe is applied to the trigeminal nerve under intermittent general anaesthesia. With previous, cruder, surgical techniques the patient's cornea was often left unprotected; however, this is not now such a common problem. When it does occur the patient will need to be taught how to care for and protect the vulnerable eye.

facial t. spasm of the facial muscles.

Ticar ('tiekah) trademark for a preparation of ticarcillin disodium, a penicillin antibiotic.

ticarcillin (tie'kahsilin) a semisynthetic penicillin that is bactericidal against both gram-negative and gram-positive organisms.

tick (tik) a blood-sucking arachnid parasite. There are two types, hard and soft. Hard ticks have a smooth, hard cover that shields the entire back of the male but only the anterior portion of the back in the female. Soft ticks lack this shield.

Ticks are visible to the human eye. A hard tick can be seen on the skin, where it burrows into the outer layer with its knifelike tongue; it must be removed from the skin with care. Soft ticks do not bore into the skin. The two varieties carry different diseases but both thrive in the spring and early summer and inhabit wooded areas, brush, or grass.

Ticks serve as vectors for viruses causing Colorado and other tick fevers and some forms of encephalitis and for rickettsiae that cause such diseases as ROCKY MOUNTAIN SPOTTED FEVER (also called *tick fever* and *tick typhus*) and boutonneuse fever. A progressive ascending flaccid paralysis (tick paralysis) may follow the bite of certain ticks, usually *Dermacentor andersoni*.

REMOVAL OF HARD TICKS. If hard ticks are extracted from the skin immediately, before they begin to suck blood, the chances of their transmitting disease are lessened; probably the only damage done will be an irritating itch at the site.

Ticks should be extracted whole; if they are carelessly pulled off the body, all or part of the mouth may be left in the skin. To loosen the tick's grasp, heavy oil, petroleum, or turpentine is applied to the area and left for half an hour. Once the tick has relinquished its hold, it should be carefully removed with tweezers. The tick should be destroyed, but not with the bare hands. The site should be washed with soap and water and an antiseptic should be applied to prevent infection.

t.i.d. [L.] *ter in die* (three times a day).

tidal volume ('tied'l) the amount of gas passing into and out of the lungs in each respiratory cycle.

tide (tied) a physiological variation or increase of a certain constituent in body fluids.

acid t. a temporary increase in the acidity of the urine that sometimes follows fasting.

alkaline t. a temporary increase in the alkalinity of the urine during gastric digestion.

fat t. the increase of a fat in the lymph and blood following a meal.

Tigason ('tigəson) trademark for a preparation of etretinate.

Tildiem (til'dee·em) trademark for a preparation of diltiazem, a calcium antagonist.

tilt-table ('tilt·tayb'l) a device resembling a stretcher, the top of which can be tilted gradually from a horizontal to a vertical position; it enables a paralysed person to assume an erect standing position.

timbre ('tambə) the musical quality of a tone or sound.

time (tiem) a measure of duration. The internationally accepted unit of time is the second (symbol s). See under adjectives for specific times, e.g., BLEEDING TIME.

timolol ('timoh,lol) a beta-adrenergic blocking agent with antihypertensive and antiarrhythmic properties; used topically to lower intraocular pressure in glaucoma and orally for prophylaxis to reduce the long-term risk of mortality and reinfarction after the acute phase of a myocardial infarction and for treatment of hypertension.

tin (tin) a chemical element, atomic number 50, atomic weight 118.69, symbol Sn. See table of elements in Appendix 2.

tinct. tincture.

tinctorial (tingk'tor·ri·əl) pertaining to dyeing or staining.

tincture ('tingkchə) an alcoholic or hydroalcoholic solution prepared from an animal or vegetable drug or a chemical substance.

benzoin t., compound a mixture of benzoin, aloes, storax, and tolu balsam in alcohol; used as a topical protectant.

iodine t. a mixture of iodine and sodium iodide in a menstruum of alcohol and water; used as an anti-infective for the skin.

tine test (tien) a tuberculin skin test employing a multiple-puncture, disposable device. It is especially useful in mass screening of children, but is less accurate than the Mantoux test. Any doubtful reaction to the tine test should be rechecked by a Mantoux test before a follow-up chest radiograph is recommended. The test is read 48 to 72 hours after injection.

tinea ('tini·ə) RINGWORM; a name applied to many different kinds of fungal infection of the skin, the specific type (depending on characteristic appearance, aetiologic agent and site) usually being designated by a modifying term.

t. barbae infection of the bearded parts of the face and neck caused by *Trichophyton*; called also *ringworm of the beard*.

t. capitis fungal infection of the scalp caused by various species of *Microsporum* and *Trichophyton*. Generally it is characterized by one or more small, round, elevated patches, scaling of the scalp, and dry and brittle hair. Called also *ringworm of the scalp*.

t. corporis fungal infection of the glabrous skin, usually due to species of *Tricophyton* or *Microsporum*.

t. cruris a fungal infection common in males, starting in the perineal folds and extending onto the inner surface of the thighs, caused by *Epidermophyton floccosum* or species of *Trichophyton*; called also *eczema marginatum, epidermophytosis cruris,* and *jock itch*.

t. imbricata a distinctive type of tinea corporis occurring in tropical countries and caused by *Trichophyton concentricum*; the early lesion is annular, with a circle of scales at the periphery, characteristically attached along one edge. New and larger scaling rings form, sometimes reaching as many as 10 per lesion. Called also *Malabar itch* and *Burmese ringworm*.

t. kerion a highly inflammatory and suppurative

fungal infection of the scalp or beard region.
t. pedis a chronic superficial fungal infection of the skin of the foot, especially of that between the toes and on the soles, characterized by maceration, scaling, and itching, and caused by species of *Trichophyton* or by *Epidermophyton floccosum* (see also ATHLETE'S FOOT).
t. profunda trichophytic granuloma.
t. sycosis an inflammatory, deep type of tinea barbae, due to *Trichophyton violaceum* or *T. rubrum*.
t. unguium onychomycosis; fungal infection of the nails.
t. versicolor a chronic, noninflammatory, usually asymptomatic disorder due to *Pityrosporon orbiculare*, marked only by multiple macular patches. Called also *pityriasis versicolor*.

Tinel's sign (ti'nelz) a tingling sensation in the distal end of a limb when percussion is made over the site of a divided nerve; it indicates a partial lesion or the beginning regeneration of the nerve.

tingible ('tinjib'l) stainable.

tinnitus (ti'nietəs) a noise in the ears, as ringing, buzzing, or roaring, which may at times be heard by others than the patient.
t. aurium a subjective sensation of noise in the ears.

tintometer (tin'tomitə) an instrument by which changes in colour of a fluid can be measured.

tissue ('tisyoo, 'tishoo) a group or layer of similarly specialized cells that together perform certain special functions.
adenoid t. lymphoid tissue.
adipose t. connective tissue made of fat cells in a meshwork of areolar tissue. **areolar t.** connective tissue made up largely of interlacing fibres.
bony t. bone.
brown adipose t., brown fat t. a thermogenic type of adipose tissue containing a dark pigment, and arising during embryonic life in certain specific areas in many mammals, including man; it is prominent in the newborn.
bursal equivalent t. an unidentified component of the lymphoid system, analogous to the bursa of Fabricius in birds, which is considered to be the primary site of the origin of B-lymphocytes.
cancellous t. the spongy tissue of bone.
cartilaginous t. the substance of cartilage.
chordal t. the tissue of the notochord.
chromaffin t. a tissue composed largely of chromaffin cells, well supplied with nerves and vessels; it occurs in the adrenal medulla and also forms the paraganglia of the body.
cicatricial t. the dense fibrous tissue forming a cicatrix, derived directly from granulation tissue.
connective t. the tissue that binds together and is the support of the various structures of the body; it consists mainly of fibroblasts and collagen and elastic fibrils. See also CONNECTIVE TISSUE.
elastic t. connective tissue made up of yellow elastic fibres, frequently massed into sheets.
endothelial t. cells lining vascular and lymph spaces.
epithelial t. a general name for tissues not derived from the mesoderm.
erectile t. spongy tissue that expands and becomes hard when filled with blood.
fatty t. connective tissue made of fat cells in a meshwork of areolar tissue.
fibrous t. the common connective tissue of the body, composed of yellow or white interlacing elastic and collagen fibres.
t. fluid the extracellular fluid that constitutes the environment of the body cells. It is low in protein, is formed by filtration through the capillaries, and drains away as lymph.
gelatinous t. mucous tissue.
granulation t. material formed in repair of wounds of soft tissue, consisting of connective tissue cells and ingrowing young capillaries; it ultimately forms cicatrix.
gut-associated lymphoid t. (GALT) lymphoid tissue associated with the gut, including the tonsils, Peyer's patches, lamina propria of the gastrointestinal tract, and appendix.
indifferent t. undifferentiated embryonic tissue.
interstitial t. connective tissue between the cellular elements of a structure.
lymphadenoid t. tissue resembling that of lymph nodes, spleen, bone marrow, tonsils, and lymph vessels.
lymphoid t. a lattice work of reticular tissue, the interspaces of which contain lymphocytes.
mesenchymal t. embryonic connective tissue composed of stellate cells and a ground substance of mucins and proteoglycans.
muscular t. the substance of muscle.
myeloid t. red bone marrow.
nerve t., nervous t. the specialized tissue forming the elements of the nervous system.
osseous t. the specialized tissue forming the bones.
reticular t., reticulated t. connective tissue composed predominantly of spindle and stellate cells with interlacing reticular fibres.
scar t. cicatricial tissue.
sclerous t's the cartilaginous, fibrous, and osseous tissues.
skeletal t. the bony, ligamentous, fibrous, and cartilaginous tissue forming the skeleton and its attachments.
splenic t. red pulp.
subcutaneous t. the layer of loose connective tissue directly under the skin.
t. typing identification of tissue types for purposes of predicting acceptance or rejection of grafts and organ transplants or for disease association. The process and purposes of tissue typing are essentially the same as for blood typing. The major difference lies in the kinds of antigens being evaluated. The acceptance of allografts depends on the HLA antigens. If the donor and recipient are not HLA identical, the allograft is rejected.

The HLA genes are located in the major histocompatibility complex (MHC), a region on the short arm of chromosome 6. The HLA antigens are involved in cell–cell interaction, immune response, organ transplantation, development of cancer, and susceptibility to disease. There are five genetic loci, designated HLA-A, HLA-B, HLA-C, HLA-D, and HLA-DR. At each locus, there can be any of several different alleles.

Each person inherits one chromosome 6 from the mother and one from the father; that is, each parent transmits to the child one allele for each kind of antigen (A, B, C, D, and DR). If the parents are different at both alleles of a locus, the statistical chance of one sibling being identical to another is one in four (25 per cent), the chance of being identical at one allele only (haplo-identical) is 50 per cent, and the chance of a total mismatch is 25 per cent.

TECHNIQUES FOR TISSUE TYPING. Histocompatibility testing involves two basic methods of assay for HLA differences. *Serological methods* are used to detect serologically defined (SD) antigens on the surfaces of cells. In general, HLA-A, -B, and -C determinants are primarily measured by serological techniques. The second method involves lymphocyte reactivity in a mixed lymphocyte culture (MLC). HLA-D or lymphocyte-defined antigens are determined by this method.

Essentially, the *serological method* is performed by incubating target lymphocytes (isolated from fresh peripheral blood) with antisera that recognize all known HLA antigens. The cells are spread in a tray with microscopic wells containing various kinds of antisera. The cells are incubated for 30 minutes, followed by an additional 60-minute complement incubation. If the lymphocytes have on their surfaces antigens recognized by the antibodies in the antiserum, the lymphocytes are lysed. A dye is added to show changes in the permeability of the cell membrane and cellular death. The proportion of cells destroyed by lysis indicates the degree of histological incompatibility. If, for example, the lymphocytes from a person being tested for HLA-A3 are destroyed in a well containing antisera for HLA-A3, the test is positive for this antigen group.

Mixed lymphocyte culture is based on the fact that when two allogenic lymphocyte populations (one from the recipient, the other from the donor) are cultured together, the lymphocytes synthesize DNA and divide. Radioactive thymidine is incorporated into the DNA and can be used to measure the lymphocyte reactivity. Following treatment by radiation, the ability of a lymphocyte to respond can be eliminated; hence, one-directional MLC is possible; that is, only the peripheral blood lymphocytes of a potential recipient will divide in response to the presence of foreign antigens on the irradiated stimulating cells of the potential donor. The primary use for MLC has been to measure the capability of the recipient to respond to antigens of the donor, as in organ and bone marrow transplantation.

white adipose t., yellow adipose t. the adipose tissue composing the bulk of the body fat.

titanium (ti'tayni·əm, tie-) a chemical element, atomic number 22, atomic weight 47.90, symbol Ti. See table of elements in Appendix 2.

t. dioxide a white powder used in ointment or lotion to protect the skin from the rays of the sun.

titrate ('tietrayt) to analyse by titration.

titration (tie'trayshən) determination of a given component in solution by addition of a liquid reagent of known strength until a given end point, e.g., change in colour, is reached indicating that the component has been consumed by reaction with the reagent.

Dean and Webb t. a test for measuring antibody in which varying dilutions of antibody are mixed with a constant quantity of antiserum; antibody activity is determined by the dilution in which flocculation occurs most rapidly, i.e., the end point.

titre ('tietə, 'tee-) the quantity of a substance required to react with or to correspond to a given amount of another substance.

agglutination t. the highest dilution of a serum which causes clumping of microorganisms or other particulate antigens.

titrimetry (tie'trimətree) analysis by titration. adj. **titrimetric**.

titubation (ˌtityuh'bayshən) the act of staggering or reeling; a staggering gait with shaking of the trunk and head, commonly seen in cerebellar disease.

Tl chemical symbol, *thallium*.

TLC tender loving care; thin layer chromatography; total lung capacity.

Tm 1. chemical symbol, *thulium*. 2. tubular maximum (in renal excretion).

TMJ syndrome temporomandibular joint syndrome.

TNM a system of CANCER staging.

TNT trinitrotoluene.

tobacco (tə'bakoh) the dried prepared leaves of *Nicotiana tabacum*, an annual plant widely cultivated in North and South America, the USSR, India, and Turkey, the source of various alkaloids, the principal one being nicotine (see also SMOKING).

tobramycin (ˌtohbrə'miesin) an aminoglycoside antibiotic produced by *Streptomyces tenebrarius*.

toco-, toko- word element. [Gr.] *childbirth, labour*.

tocograph, tokograph ('tokohgraf, -grahf) see CARDIOTOCOGRAPH.

tocography, tokography (to'kogrəfee) see CARDIOTOCOGRAPHY.

tocology, tokology (to'koləjee) the science of reproduction and the art of obstetrics.

tocometer, tokometer (toh'komitə) an instrument for measuring and recording the expulsive force of uterine contractions. Called also *tokodynamometer*. See also CARDIOTOCOMETER.

tocopherol (to'kofə·rol) an alcohol isolated from wheat germ oil or produced synthetically; it has the properties of vitamin E. In animals it is needed in the diet to insure reproduction, but its role in humans is unclear.

alpha t. vitamin E.

toe (toh) a digit of the foot.

hammer t. a flexion deformity of the proximal interphalangeal joint with compensatory hyperextension of the metatarsophalangeal and distal interphalangeal joints. It most often affects the second toe.

Morton's t. a painful condition of the third and fourth toes due to a neuroma of the interdigital nerve supplying them. It is caused by pressure on the nerve at the metatarsophalangeal joint. Called also *Morton's plantar neuralgia* and *Morton's disease*.

pigeon t. a permanent toeing-in position of the feet. Called also *pes adductus*.

webbed t's toes abnormally joined by strands of tissue at their base.

toenail ('tohˌnayl) the nail on any of the digits of the foot.

ingrowing t. aberrant growth of a toenail, with one (usually the outer) margin growing deeply into the nail groove and surrounding tissues.

Tofranil (toh'fraynil) trademark for preparations of imipramine, an antidepressant.

togavirus ('tohgəˌvierəs) a subgroup of arboviruses, including mosquito- and tickborne viruses that cause haemorrhagic fever; they are RNA viruses with envelopes (or 'togas').

toilet ('toylit) the cleansing and dressing of a wound.

token economy programme ('tohkən i'konəmee) a behavioural approach to modifying troublesome behaviours and restoring lost self-help behaviours by the systematic rewarding of desired behaviour by giving tokens which may be exchanged for goods or privileges. Abbreviated TEP. There is a clearly defined range of behaviours (target behaviours), each of which is assigned a value in tokens by the staff. This approach has proved to be of value with the chronically socially disabled and the mentally handicapped.

toko- for words beginning thus, see those beginning *toco-*.

Tolanase ('toliˌnayz) trademark for tolazamide, an oral hypoglycaemic agent.

tolazamide (to'lazəˌmied) a hypoglycaemic agent.

tolazoline (to'lazohˌleen) a smooth muscle relaxant and peripheral vasodilator; used as the hydrochloride salt.

tolbutamide (tol'byootəˌmied) an oral hypoglycaemic agent.

Tolectin ('tolektin) trademark for a preparation of tolmetin sodium; a nonsteroidal anti-inflammatory agent.

tolerance ('tolə·rəns) the ability to endure without effect or injury. adj. **tolerant**.

drug t. decrease of susceptibility to the effects of a drug due to its continued administration.

immunological t. specific nonreactivity of lymphoid tissues to a particular antigen capable under other conditions of inducing immunity.

tolerogen ('tolə·rə,jen) an antigen that induces a state of specific immunological unresponsiveness to subsequent challenging doses of the antigen.

tolerogenesis (,tolə·roh'jenəsis) induction of immunological tolerance.

tolmetin ('tolmetin) an anti-inflammatory, analgesic, and antipyretic used in the treatment of certain cases of rheumatoid arthritis.

tolnaftate (tol'naftayt) a topical antifungal.

toluene ('tolyoo,een) the aromatic hydrocarbon $C_6H_5CH_3$.

-tome word element. [Gr.] *an instrument for cutting, a segment.*

tomo- word element. [Gr.] *a section, a cutting.*

tomogram ('tohmə,gram) an image of a tissue plane or slice produced by tomography.

tomograph ('tohmə,grahf, -,graf) an apparatus in which the x-ray tube and film are moved in opposite directions during an exposure so that only a single plane of tissue remains in focus during the exposure. Other planes above and below are blurred by the motion.

tomography (tə'mogrəfee) any method that produces images of single tissue planes. In conventional radiology, tomographic images (body section radiographs) are produced by motion of the x-ray tube and film or by motion of the patient that blurs the image except in a single plane. In reconstruction tomography (CT and PET) the image is produced by a computer program.

computed t. (CT) a radiological imaging modality that uses computer processing of x-ray photons detected by a detector bank after passing through the patient. The image generated is a representation of tissue densities within a 'slice', 1 to 10 mm thick, through the patient's body. Called also *computerized axial tomography* (*CAT*).

Since its introduction in 1972, the use of CT has grown rapidly. Because CT is noninvasive and has high contrast resolution, it has replaced some radiographic procedures using contrast media. CT also has a better spatial resolution than scintillation imaging (about 1 mm for CT compared with 15 mm for a scintillation camera).

A CT scan is divided into a square matrix of *pixels* (picture elements). The newer CT scanners use a high resolution matrix with 512 × 512 pixels. The region of the tissue slice corresponding to a pixel has a cross-sectional area of 1 × 1 mm to 2 × 2 mm; because of the thickness of the slice, it has a finite height and is therefore referred to as a *voxel* (volume element).

The actual measurements made by the scanner are the x-ray attenuations along thousands of rays traversing the slice at all angles. The attenuation value for a ray is the sum of the values for all of the voxels it passes through. A computer program called a *reconstruction algorithm* can solve the problem of assigning attenuation values for all the pixels that add up to the measured values along each ray.

The attenuation values are converted to CT numbers by subtracting the attenuation value of water and multiplying by an arbitrary coefficient to produce values ranging from -1000 for air to +1000 for compact bone with water as 0. CT numbers are sometimes said to be expressed in 'Hounsfield units', named after the inventor of the CT scanner Godfrey Hounsfield, who was a co-winner, with Allan Cormack, of the 1979 Nobel Prize in physiology or medicine for the development of computed tomography.

The design of CT scanners is changing rapidly. The first scanners had only one detector which moved with the x-ray tube around the patient in a complicated pattern of rotations and translations, and a scan of three to five minutes. The newest scanners (third and fourth generation) use multiple detectors and are much faster. Scans can now be performed in less than a second, although 3 to 10 seconds is routine. At this speed useful CT images can now be made of the heart and viscera.

positron emission t. (PET) a combination of computed tomography and scintillation scanning. Natural biochemical substances or drugs tagged with a positron-emitting radioisotope are administered to the subject. After injection, the tagged substance (tracer) is localized in specific tissues like its natural analogue. When the isotope decays, it emits a positron, which then annihilates with an electron of a nearby atom, producing two 511 keV gamma rays travelling in opposite directions 180 degrees apart. When the gamma rays trigger a ring of detectors around the subject, the line between the detectors on which the decay occurred is stored in the computer. A computer program (reconstruction algorithm), like those used in computed tomography, produces an image of the distribution of the tracer in the plane of the detector ring.

Most of the isotopes used in PET scanning have a half-life of only 2 to 10 minutes. Therefore, they must be produced by an on-site cyclotron and attached chemically to the tracer and used within minutes. Because of the expense of the scanner and cyclotron, PET is used only in research centres. However, PET is important because it provides information that cannot be obtained by other means. By labelling the blood with ^{11}C-carbon monoxide, which binds to haemoglobin, images can be obtained showing the regional perfusion of an organ in multiple planes. By using labelled metabolites, images can be obtained showing metabolic activity of an organ. ^{15}O-oxygen and ^{11}C-glucose have been used for brain imaging and ^{11}C-palmitate for heart imaging. ^{81}Rb, which is distributed like potassium, is also used for heart imaging. By using labelled neurotransmitters, hormones, and drugs the distribution of receptors for these substances in the brain and other organs can be mapped.

ultrasonic t. the ultrasonographic visualization of a cross-section of a predetermined plane of the body; see B-mode ULTRASONOGRAPHY.

-tomy word element. [Gr.] *incision, cutting.*

tone (tohn) 1. normal degree of vigour and tension; in muscle, the resistance to passive elongation or stretch. 2. a healthy state of a part; tonus. 3. a particular quality of sound or voice.

tongue (tung) a muscular organ on the floor of the mouth; it aids in chewing, swallowing, and speech, and is the location of organs of TASTE. The taste buds are located in the papillae, which are projections on the upper surface of the tongue.

The condition of the tongue can sometimes be a guide to the general condition of the body. Inflammation of the tongue, or glossitis, can accompany anaemia, scarlet fever, nutritional deficiencies, and most general infections. Sometimes it is part of an adverse reaction to medication. One form of glossitis causes a smooth tongue, with a red, glazed appearance. A coated or furry tongue may be present in a variety of illnesses, but does not necessarily indicate illness. A dry tongue sometimes indicates insufficiency of fluids in the body, or it may result from fever. When the tongue is extremely dry and has a leathery appearance, the cause may be uraemia.

bifid t. a tongue with a lengthwise cleft.

black t. blackening and elongation of the papillae of the tongue.

cleft t. bifid tongue.

coated t. one covered with a whitish or yellowish layer consisting of desquamated epithelium, debris, bacteria, fungi, etc.

fissured t., furrowed t. a tongue with numerous furrows or grooves on the dorsal surface, often radiating from a groove on the midline.

geographic t. a tongue with denuded patches, surrounded by thickened epithelium. Called also *erythema migrans*.

hairy t. one with the papillae elongated and hairlike.

raspberry t. a diffusely reddened and swollen, uncoated tongue, as seen several days after the onset of the rash in scarlet fever.

scrotal t. fissured tongue.

strawberry t. a coated tongue with enlarged red fungiform papillae, seen 24 hours after onset of the rash in scarlet fever.

trombone t. involuntary movement of the tongue, consisting of vigorous alternating protrusion and retraction.

tongue-tie ('tung,tie) abnormal shortness of the frenulum of the tongue, resulting in limitation of its motion; called also *ankyloglossia*.

tonic ('tonik) 1. producing and restoring normal tone. 2. characterized by continuous tension. 3. an agent that tends to restore normal tone.

tonicity (toh'nisitee) the state of tissue tone or tension; in body fluid physiology, the effective osmotic pressure equivalent.

tono- word element. [Gr.] *tone, tension*.

tonoclonic (,tohnoh'klonik) both tonic and clonic; said of muscular spasms.

tonofibril (,tohnoh'fiebril) one of the fine fibrils in epithelial cells, thought to give a supporting framework to the cell.

tonogram ('tohnoh,gram) the record produced by tonography.

tonograph ('tohnoh,grahf, -,graf) a recording tonometer.

tonography (toh'nogrəfee) the recording of changes in intraocular pressure due to sustained pressure on the eyeball.

carotid compression t. a test for occlusion of the carotid artery by measuring ocular pressure and pulse before, during, and after the proximal portion of the carotid artery is compressed by the fingers.

tonometer (toh'nomitə) an instrument for measuring tension or pressure, especially intraocular pressure.

tonometry (toh'nomətree) measurement of tension or pressure, e.g., intraocular pressure.

digital t. estimation of the degree of intraocular pressure by pressure exerted on the eyeball by the finger of the examiner.

tonoplast ('tohnoh,plast) the limiting membrane of an intracellular vacuole, the vacuole membrane.

tonoscope ('tohnoh,skohp) 1. an apparatus for rendering sound visible by registering the vibrations on a screen. 2. a device for examining the head or brain by means of sound. 3. tonometer.

tonsil ('tonsil) a small, rounded mass of tissue, especially of lymphoid tissue; generally used alone to designate the palatine tonsil. adj. **tonsillar**.

There are three different kinds of tonsils. The structures usually referred to as the tonsils are the palatine tonsils, a pair of oval-shaped structures, about the size of almonds, partially embedded in the mucous membrane, one on each side of the back of the throat. Below them, at the base of the tongue, are the lingual tonsils. On the upper rear wall of the mouth cavity are the pharyngeal tonsils, or adenoids, which are of fair size in childhood but usually shrink after puberty.

These tissues are part of the lymphatic system and help to filter the circulating lymph of bacteria and any other foreign material that may enter the body, especially through the mouth and nose. In the process of fighting infection the palatine tonsils and the adenoids sometimes become enlarged and inflamed (see also TONSILLITIS).

t. of cerebellum a rounded mass forming part of the cerebellum on its inferior surface.

tonsillectomy (,tonsi'lektəmee) excision of tonsils. The procedure is performed in treatment of chronic infection of the tonsils.

PATIENT CARE. Since most patients undergoing tonsillectomy are children, it is important that the preoperative period include adequate emotional preparation of the patient and his family. The child should be told in advance of the admission to the hospital and given some idea of what he can expect. He should not be deceived about the possibility of discomfort, but it is best to stress the positive aspects of surgery, such as the fact that he will not suffer as many colds and attacks of sore throat once the surgery is performed and his throat has healed.

Although tonsillectomy may be considered minor surgery, there is always the possibility of serious haemorrhage after surgery. The child should be placed on his abdomen with head on one side on returning to the ward after surgery, to allow for adequate drainage of blood and mucus from the throat and mouth and avoid aspiration. Signs of excessive bleeding from the operative site include bright red blood from the mouth or nose, frequent swallowing, and extreme restlessness.

During the immediate postoperative period the diet is restricted to liquids and soft solids. As the throat heals and oedema subsides, more solid food is gradually added to the diet.

tonsillitis (,tonsi'lietis) inflammation and enlargement of a tonsil, especially the palatine tonsils.

Enlarged tonsils need not be a cause for concern unless they become a source of chronic infection or interfere with swallowing or breathing. They may become enlarged in the process of filtering out frequent, mild infections.

Tonsils are part of the lymphatic system, which aids the body in fighting off infections and 'invasions' of foreign matter. Although the exact purpose of the tonsils is unknown, they are believed to act as filters and fighters of bacteria, guarding the entrances to the throat and nasal passages. Sometimes, however, they are overcome by the invading bacteria and become infected. One form of infection sometimes causing tonsillitis is streptococcal infection of the throat.

SYMPTOMS AND TREATMENT. A mild case of tonsillitis may appear to be only a slight sore throat. Symptoms of acute tonsillitis are inflamed, swollen tonsils and a very sore throat, with high fever, rapid pulse and general weakness. Swallowing is difficult and the lymph nodes in the neck may become swollen and painful.

Occasionally in an attack of severe tonsillitis an abscess may form around the tonsil, a condition called quinsy.

Treatment of tonsillitis usually consists of administration of antibiotics, gargles, and bed rest. When tonsillitis is recurrent and troublesome, however, it may be necessary to remove the tonsils surgically (see also TONSILLECTOMY).

follicular t. tonsillitis especially affecting the crypts.

parenchymatous t., acute that affecting the whole substance of the tonsil.

pustular t. a variety characterized by formation of pustules.

tonsilloadenoidectomy (ˌtonsilohˌadənoy'dektəmee) excision of lymphoid tissue from the throat and nasopharynx (tonsils and adenoids).

tonsillolith (ton'silohˌlith) a calculus in a tonsil.

tonsillotomy (ˌtonsi'lotəmee) incision of a tonsil.

tonus ('tohnəs) tone or tonicity; the slight, continuous contraction of a muscle, which in skeletal muscles aids in the maintenance of posture and in the return of blood to the heart.

tooth (tooth) pl. *teeth;* one of the small, bonelike structures of the jaws for the biting and mastication of food; the teeth also assist in shaping sounds and forming words in speech.

STRUCTURE. The portion of a tooth that rises above the gum is the crown; the portion below is the root. The crown is covered by enamel, which is related to the epithelial tissue of the skin and is the hardest substance in the human body. The surface of the root is composed of a bonelike tissue called cementum. Underneath the surface enamel and cementum is a substance called dentine, which makes up the main body of the tooth. Within the dentine, in a space in the centre of the tooth, is the dental pulp, a soft, sensitive tissue that contains nerves and blood and lymph vessels. The cementum, dentine, and pulp are formed from connective tissue.

Covering the root of the tooth and holding it in place in its socket, or alveolus, in the jaw is a fibrous connective tissue called the periodontium. Its many strong fibres are embedded in the cementum and also the wall of the tooth socket. The periodontium not only helps hold the tooth in place but also acts to cushion it against the pressure caused by biting and chewing.

There are 20 deciduous teeth, called also baby teeth or milk teeth, which are eventually replaced by 32 permanent teeth, evenly divided between upper and lower jaw.

Teeth have different shapes because they have different functions. The incisors, in the front of the mouth, are shaped like a cone with a sharp flattened end. They cut the food. There are eight deciduous and permanent incisors, four upper and four lower. The cuspids, at the corners of the mouth, shaped like simple cones, tear and shred food. There are four permanent cuspids; they are called also canines, and the two in the upper jaw are called eyeteeth. The premolars, or bicuspids, flanking the cuspids, consist of two cones, or cusps, fused together. They tear, crush, and grind the food. There are eight permanent premolars. The molars are in the back of the mouth. They have between three and five cusps each, and their function is to crush and grind food. There are 12 permanent molars in all, three on each side of both the upper and lower jaw. The hindmost molar in each of these groups, and the last one to emerge, is often called a wisdom tooth.

DEVELOPMENT AND ERUPTION. Both the deciduous teeth and the permanent teeth begin to develop before birth. Because of this, it is vitally important that expectant mothers receive foods that will supply the calcium, phosphorus, and vitamins necessary for healthy teeth.

The deciduous teeth begin to form about the sixth week of prenatal life, with calcification beginning about the sixteenth week. A considerable part of the crowns of these teeth is formed by the time the child is born.

Eruption, or cutting of teeth is slower in some children than others, but the deciduous teeth generally begin to appear when the infant is between 6 and 9 months of age, and the process is completed by the time a child is 2 to 2½ years old.

When the child is about 6, the first permanent molar comes in just behind the second molar of the deciduous teeth. About the same time, shedding of the baby teeth begins. The permanent teeth form in the jaw even before the baby teeth have erupted, with the incisors and the cuspids beginning to calcify during the first 6 months of life. Calcification of the others takes place shortly after. As the adult teeth calcify, the roots of the baby teeth gradually disappear, or resorb, and are completely gone by the time the permanent teeth are ready to appear. Occasionally a baby tooth root does not resorb, and as a result the permanent tooth comes in outside its proper position. When resorption does not occur, it is necessary to remove the baby tooth and root.

The first teeth to be shed, about the sixth year, are the central incisors. The permanent incisors erupt shortly afterward. The lateral incisors are lost and replaced during the seventh to ninth years, and the cuspids in the ninth to twelfth years. The first premolars generally appear between the ages of 10 and 12, the second molars between 11 and 13 and the third molars, or wisdom teeth, between 17 and 22. It is not uncommon for the third molars to fail to erupt.

Occasionally there is a partial or total lack of either the deciduous or permanent teeth. In some cases this anodontia is hereditary, or it may be related to endocrine gland disturbances. TOOTH DECAY AND ITS PREVENTION. Dental caries begins on the outside of the teeth in the enamel. Bacteria and food adhere to the tooth surface to form plaque. The action of the bacteria on starchy and sugary foods produces acid, which is believed to dissolve the enamel. Once there is a breakthrough in the enamel, the decaying process moves on into the dentine and then to the pulp, attacking the nerves and causing toothache.

Flossing and Brushing the Teeth. Cleanliness is the best weapon against caries and PERIODONTITIS. Bacteria and food particles must be removed before the enamel is penetrated. This means thorough brushing regularly each day, preferably after every meal. If it is impossible to brush after every meal, it is helpful to rinse the mouth by swishing water vigorously back and forth between and around the teeth. When the teeth are brushed, food particles that lodge between the teeth should also be removed with dental floss.

The dental floss should be strung tightly between the two index fingers or between the bows of a floss holder. Flossing and brushing should be done in an orderly sequence so that no area is neglected. The usual pattern is beginning at the upper right, progressing to the upper left, and then from the lower left to the lower right. The floss is gently inserted between the teeth and pulled against the surface of one tooth to a point slightly under the tissue of the gum. It is then moved up and down for several strokes. The adjacent tooth is cleaned in the same manner.

The 'sulcular' technique for brushing the teeth is so called because the bristles of the brush are worked beneath the free gingival margin and into the space between the tooth and the gum (the *sulcus).* To accomplish this the bristles are placed at a 45 degree angle to the gum line. Pressure is then used to move the brush back and forth horizontally. The brushing is continued around the mouth in the same pattern as the flossing.

A disclosing dye may be used to determine the presence of plaque on the teeth. Flavoured mouthwash does not reduce plaque formation and is useful only to moisturize the tissues and improve mouth taste.

Proper Diet. In order to help maintain healthy teeth, the diet should include all the essential elements of good NUTRITION. Tooth decay can be reduced by limiting the intake of certain forms of sugar, especially the rich or highly concentrated ones such as sweets or rich desserts.

Fluoridation. Another important means of preventing caries is through the use of fluoride. Some authorities whose water is lacking in an adequate natural supply of fluoride add the chemical to their water supply. FLUORIDATION is effective for children and adolescents, but less so for adults, and children raised on fluoridated water retain resistance to tooth decay when they become adults. In areas that do not have fluoridation, dentists often suggest the use of fluoride drops or tablets to achieve an optimum fluoride intake of one part per million.

Correction of Malocclusion. Another factor leading to tooth decay is poor position of the teeth, resulting in faulty closure of the jaws and uneven meeting of the teeth. This condition is called malocclusion. It should be corrected early because it also can lead to inadequate nutrition because of difficulty in chewing, and if it is severe enough to distort the face, it may have psychological effects.

accessional teeth the permanent molars, so called because they have no deciduous predecessors in the dental arch.

impacted t. one so placed in the jaw that it is unable to erupt or to attain its normal position in occlusion.

toothpaste ('toothpayst) a preparation for cleansing and polishing the teeth. Those containing fluoride inhibit the formation of dental caries.

top(o)- word element. [Gr.] *particular place or area.*

topaesthesia (ˌtohpis'theezi·ə) ability to recognize the location of a tactile stimulus.

topagnosia (ˌtopag'nohzi·ə) 1. loss of touch localization. 2. loss of ability to recognize familiar surroundings.

topalgia (toh'palji·ə) fixed or localized pain.

topectomy (toh'pektəmee) ablation of a small and specific area of the frontal cortex in the treatment of mental illness.

tophaceous (toh'fayshəs) gritty or sandy; pertaining to tophi.

tophus ('tohfəs) pl. *tophi* [L.] a chalky deposit of sodium urate occurring in GOUT; tophi form most often around the joints in cartilage, bone, bursae, and subcutaneous tissue and in the external ear, producing a chronic, foreign-body inflammatory response.

t. syphiliticus a syphilitic node.

topical ('topik'l) pertaining to a particular area, as a topical anti-infective applied to a certain area of the skin and affecting only the area to which it is applied.

topoanaesthesia (ˌtohpohˌanəs'theezi·ə) inability to recognize the location of a tactile stimulus.

topographic (ˌtopə'grafik, ˌtoh-) describing or pertaining to special regions.

topography (tə'pogrəfee, toh-) 1. a special description of an anatomical region or a special part. 2. electrohysterography.

torcular Herophili (ˌtawkyuhlah he'rofiˌlie) a depression in the occipital bone at the confluence of a number of cerebral venous sinuses.

Torecan ('tawrəkan) trademark for preparations of thiethylperazine, an antiemetic.

torpid ('tawpid) not acting with normal vigour and facility.

torque ('tawk) a rotatory force.

torsion ('tawshən) the act of twisting; the state of being twisted. adj. **torsive**.

torsiversion (ˌtawsi'vərshən, -zhən) turning of a tooth

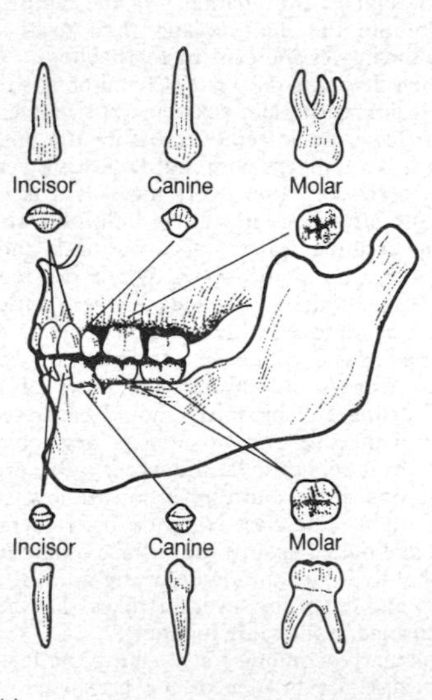

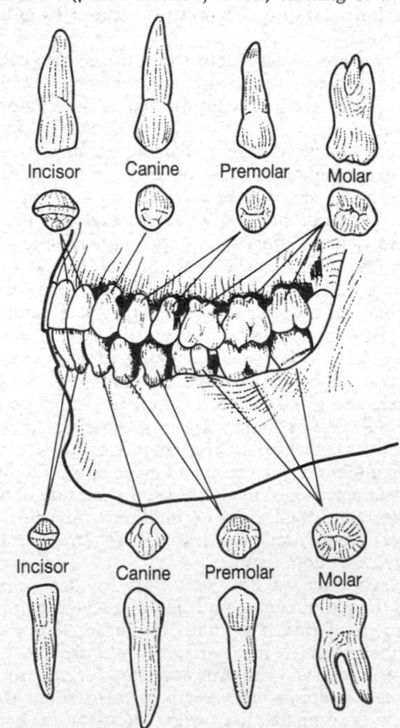

Teeth. (a) Typical deciduous teeth. (b) Typical permanent teeth

on its long axis out of normal position.

torso ('tawsoh) the body, exclusive of the head and limbs.

torticollis (ˌtawti'kolis) wryneck, a contracted state of the cervical muscles, producing torsion of the neck. The deformity may be congenital, hysterical, or secondary to pressure on the accessory nerve, to inflammation of glands in the neck, or to muscle spasm.

tortipelvis (ˌtawti'pelvis) distortions of the spine and hip produced by a disorder marked by irregular muscular contractions of the trunk and extremities.

tortuous ('tawtyoo·əs) twisted; full of turns and twists.

toruloid ('to·ryuhˌloyd, 'tor·rə-) knotted or beaded, like a yeast cell.

torulus ('to·ryuhləs, 'tor·rə-) [L.] *a small elevation*.

t. tactilis a tactile elevation in the skin of the palms and soles.

torus ('tor·rəs) pl. *tori* [L.] a *swelling* or *bulging projection*.

totipotential (ˌtohtipə'tenshəl) exhibiting totipotency; characterized by the ability to develop in any direction; said of cells that can give rise to cells of all types. adj. **totipotent**.

touch (tuch) 1. the sense by which contact of an object with the skin is recognized. 2. palpation with the finger.

Touch is actually not a single sense, but several. There are separate nerves in the skin to register heat, cold, pressure, pain, and touch. These thousands of nerves are distributed unevenly over the body, so that some areas are more responsive to cold, others to pain, and others to heat or pressure.

Each of these types of nerves has a different structure at the receiving end. A touch nerve has an elongated bulb-shaped end, and a nerve responsive to cold a squat bulb; the nerve that registers warmth has what looks like twisted threads, and the nerve for deep pressure has an egg-shaped end. Pain receptors have no protective sheath.

If the sensory nerves were evenly distributed over the whole body, each square centimetre of skin would have about 8 heat receptors, 1 for cold, 16 for touch and 125 for pain. The sensitivity of a given spot depends in part on how thickly receptors of a particular kind are clustered in that spot, and localization of particular sensation depends on the concentration of the particular nerve endings in an area. Touch, pressure, and pain are sensations that can be localized quite accurately, but sensations of cold and heat are more diffuse.

The thickness of the skin in a given area and its supply of hairs also contribute to its touch sensitivity. A touch as light as 0.4 grams on the thin skin of the forehead can be felt, whereas a touch must be two and a half times as heavy to be felt on a fingertip. Hairs grow almost everywhere on the skin except the palms of the hands and the soles of the feet. They grow at a slant, and touch spots cluster in the skin near each of them. Even a light touch on the tip of a hair bends it back, and like a tiny lever it communicates the touch to the nerve endings.

The tactile sense develops with learning and experience. A simple test is to hold a pea between the first and second fingers. With the eyes closed, it is easy to tell that it is one object. However, if the fingers are crossed first, it will seem that there are two peas, because ordinarily it takes two objects to stimulate the touch receptors on the opposite sides of the fingers.

tourniquet ('tooəniˌkay, 'tawni-) a device for compression of an artery or vein. It is used to stop excessive bleeding, and to facilitate obtaining blood samples or giving intravenous injections, and to prevent the spread of snake venom.

For haemorrhage, a tourniquet should be used only as a last resort, when the bleeding is so severe that it obviously threatens the life of the injured person and cannot be stopped by direct pressure.

A loosely applied tourniquet inhibits blood flow in the superficial veins, making them more prominent; this is helpful when a vein is being sought for an intravenous injection or for drawing blood.

In the case of snakebite, the use of tourniquets to impede the spread of venom remains controversial. However, a moderately tight tourniquet that impedes the spread of venom but does not stop arterial blood flow may be applied in some cases.

Applying a Tourniquet. There are two places on the body where a tourniquet is effective in stopping profuse bleeding from an artery. If blood comes from a wound on the arm, the tourniquet is applied a hand's width below the armpit. If the bleeding is from a leg wound, the tourniquet should be placed a hand's width below the groin.

Any wide, flat piece of cloth long enough to circle the arm or leg twice may be used for a tourniquet. A necktie, scarf, or strip of heavy material is suitable. The cloth strip should be placed over a thick pad made of gauze or cloth, then wrapped around the limb and tied with a half knot. A small stick is placed over the half knot, and a square knot is tied over the stick. The tourniquet is tightened by slowly twisting the stick; bleeding will stop suddenly when the tourniquet is twisted tight enough.

Ten minutes after the tourniquet is applied, it should be loosened for exactly 1 minute to permit circulation of the blood in the arm or leg. During this period, a hand should be pressed against the wound. If severe bleeding does not recur during the time the tourniquet is loose, it need not be retightened but should be left in position in case bleeding becomes heavy again.

Tourniquets should never be covered by bandages, clothing, or blankets. If it is not possible to leave the tourniquet exposed, the letters T K, with location of the tourniquet, should be written on the patient's forehead.

tox(o)- word element. [Gr., L.] *toxin, poison*.

toxaemia (tok'seemi·ə) 1. the condition resulting from the spread of bacterial products (toxins) by the bloodstream. 2. a condition resulting from metabolic disturbances, e.g., toxaemia of pregnancy. adj. **toxaemic**.

alimentary t. toxaemia due to absorption from the alimentary canal of chemical poisons generated therein; a form of autointoxication.

t. of pregnancy a group of pathological conditions, essentially metabolic disturbances, occurring in pregnant women, manifested by preeclampsia and fully developed ECLAMPSIA.

toxic ('toksik) poisonous; pertaining to poisoning.

toxic(o)- word element. [Gr.] *poison, poisonous*.

toxic shock syndrome ('toksik shok) a severe illness characterized by high fever of sudden onset, vomiting, diarrhoea, and myalgia, followed by hypotension and, in severe cases, shock and death. A sunburn-like rash with peeling of the skin, especially of the palms and soles, occurs during the late phase. The syndrome affects almost exclusively menstruating women using tampons, although a few women who do not use tampons and a few males have been affected. It is thought to be caused by infection with *Staphylococcus aureus*.

toxicant ('toksikənt) 1. poisonous. 2. a poison.

toxicity (tok'sisitee) the quality of being poisonous,

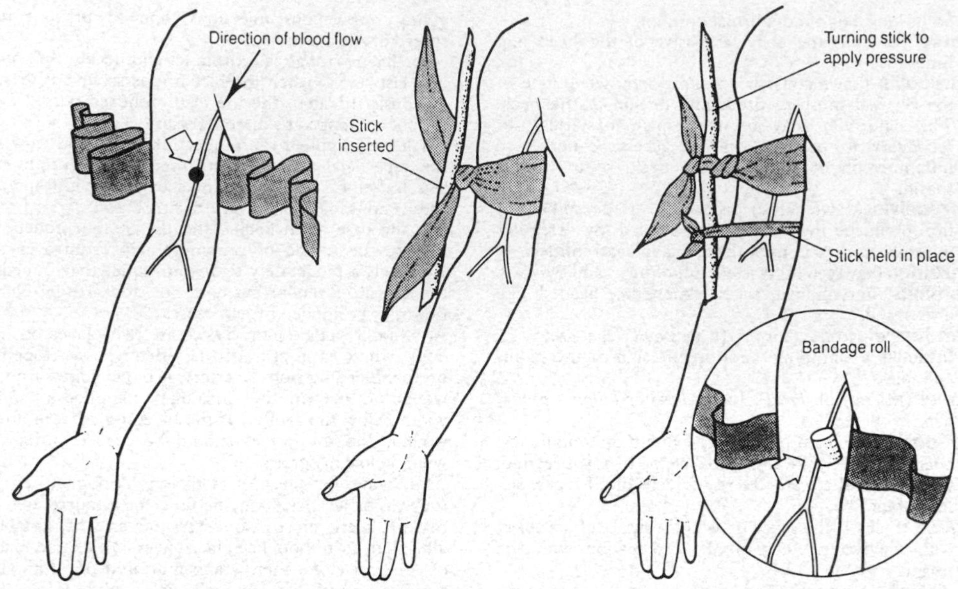

To apply a tourniquet for first aid control of arterial bleeding from the arm, wrap a gauze pad twice with a strip of cloth just below the armpit and tie with a half knot. Tie a stick at the knot with a square knot. Slowly twist stick to tighten

especially the degree of virulence of a toxic microbe or of a poison.

Toxicodendron (ˌtoksikoh'dendron) *Rhus.*

toxicogenic (ˌtoksikoh'jenik) producing or elaborating toxins.

toxicoid ('toksiˌkoyd) resembling a poison.

toxicologist (ˌtoksi'koləjist) a specialist in toxicology.

toxicology (ˌtoksi'koləjee) the science or study of poisons. adj. **toxicological**.

toxicomania (ˌtoksikoh'mayni·ə) intense desire for poisons or intoxicants.

toxicopathy (ˌtoksi'kopəthee) toxicosis. adj. **toxicopathic**.

toxicopexy ('toksikohˌpeksee) the fixation or neutralization of a poison in the body. adj. **toxicopectic, toxicopexic**.

toxicophidia (ˌtoksikoh'fidi·ə) venomous serpents collectively.

toxicophobia (ˌtoksikoh'fohbi·ə) morbid dread of poisons.

toxicophylaxin (ˌtoksikohfi'laksin) a phylaxin that destroys the poisons produced by microorganisms.

toxicosis (ˌtoksi'kohsis) any diseased condition due to poisoning.

toxiferous (tok'sifə·rəs) conveying or producing a poison.

toxigenic (ˌtoksi'jenik) caused by or producing toxins.

toxigenicity (ˌtoksijə'nisitee) the property of producing toxins.

toxin ('toksin) a poison, especially a protein or conjugated protein produced by certain animals, some higher plants, and pathogenic bacteria.

It is characteristic of bacterial toxins that they do not cause symptoms until after a variable period of incubation while the microbes multiply, or, as is the case in botulism, the preformed toxin reaches and affects the tissue. Usually only a few toxin-producing agents are introduced into the body, and it is not until there are enough of them to overwhelm the leukocytes and other types of antibodies that symptoms occur. In some cases of food poisoning, symptoms are almost immediate because the toxin is taken directly with the food.

Toxins cause antitoxins to form in the body, thus providing a means for establishing IMMUNITY to certain diseases. **bacterial t's** toxins produced by bacteria, including exotoxins, endotoxins, and toxic enzymes.

botulinus t. one of at least six type-specific, immunologically differentiable exotoxins (types A to F) produced by *Clostridium botulinum*.

dermonecrotic t. an exotoxin produced by certain bacteria that causes extensive local necrosis on intradermal inoculation.

Dick t. erythrogenic toxin.

diphtheria t. a protein exotoxin produced by *Corynebacterium diphtheriae* that is primarily responsible for the pathogenesis of diphtheritic infection; it is an enzyme that activates transferase II of the mammalian protein synthesizing system.

diphtheria t. for Schick test a sterile solution of the diluted, standardized toxic products of *Corynebacterium diphtheriae*; used as a dermal reactivity indicator.

dysentery t. one produced by organisms of various species of *Shigella*.

erythrogenic t. a bacterial toxin from certain strains of *Streptococcus pyogenes* that produces an erythematous reaction when injected intradermally and is responsible for the rash in scarlet fever.

extracellular t. exotoxin.

intracellular t. endotoxin.

tetanus t. the potent exotoxin produced by *Clostridium tetani*, consisting of two components, one a neurotoxin (*tetanospasmin)* and the other a haemolysin (*tetanolysin)*.

toxinology (ˌtoksi'noləjee) the science dealing with the toxins produced by certain higher plants and animals and by pathogenic bacteria.

toxipathic (ˌtoksi'pathik) pertaining to or caused by the pathogenic action of toxins, of whatever origin.

toxipathy (tok'sipəthee) toxicosis.

Toxocara (ˌtoksoh'kair·rə) a genus of nematode parasites found in the dog (*T. canis*) and cat (*T. cati*); the larvae are sometimes found in man, especially in children.

toxocariasis (ˌtoksohkə'rieəsis) infection by worms of the genus *Toxocara.*

toxoid ('toksoyd) a toxin treated by heat or chemical agent to destroy its deleterious properties without destroying its ability to combine with or stimulate the formation of antitoxin.

diphtheria t. a sterile preparation of formaldehyde-treated products of the growth of *Corynebacterium diphtheriae*, used as an active immunizing agent.

tetanus t. a sterile preparation of formaldehyde-treated products of the growth of *Clostridium tetani*, used as an active immunizing agent.

toxophilic (ˌtoksoh'filik) easily susceptible to poison; having affinity for toxins.

toxophore ('toksohˌfor) the group of atoms in a toxin molecule that produces the toxic effect.

toxophorous (tok'sofə·rəs) bearing poison; producing the toxic effect.

Toxoplasma (ˌtoksoh'plazmə) a genus of sporozoan parasites in man, other mammals and some birds; it includes one species, *T. gondii*, which is frequently transmitted from an infected mother to an infant in utero or at birth. The infection may be asymptomatic or may produce encephalomyelitis with cerebral calcification and choriodoretinitis (see TOXOPLASMOSIS).

toxoplasmin (ˌtoksoh'plazmin) an antigen prepared from mouse peritoneal fluids rich with *Toxoplasma gondii*; injected intracutaneously as a test for toxoplasmosis.

toxoplasmosis (ˌtoksohplaz'mohsis) a disease due to *Toxoplasma gondii.* The *congenital* form is marked by central nervous system lesions, which may lead to blindness, brain defects, and death. The acquired infection is often asymptomatic, and the clinical disease occurs in two forms: *lymphadenopathic toxoplasmosis*, closely resembling infectious mononucleosis, and, much more rarely, *disseminated toxoplasmosis*, with lesions involving the lungs, liver, heart, skin, muscle, brain, and meninges. Choroidoretinitis is very common in the congenital form, and may occur, in the chronic form, after many years of delay.

The only effective treatment of toxoplasmosis is the combination of pyrimethamine and sulphadiazine or triple sulphonamides given for a total of 30 days. Treatment is not usually necessary and is reserved for those with serious complications or who are not immunologically competent. Treatment during pregnancy will not eliminate congenital toxoplasmosis but it can minimize its effects.

Prevention of infection with the protozoan parasite is aimed at avoiding ingestion of infective cysts in raw meat and eliminating contact with cat faeces. Mutton, pork, and goat meat are more likely to be contaminated than beef; however, all meats should be thoroughly cooked, cured, or smoked before ingestion. Careful handling and disposal of cat litter can reduce the possibility of contamination from the faeces of a pet cat, but it is difficult to determine when the cat has become infected.

TPA total parenteral alimentation; see parenteral NUTRITION.

TPN total parenteral nutrition; see parenteral NUTRITION.

TPR temperature, pulse, respiration.

tr. tincture.

trabecula (trə'bekyuhlə) pl. *trabeculae* [L.] a small beam or supporting structure; used in anatomical nomenclature to designate various fibromuscular bands or cords providing support in various organs, as heart, penis, and spleen. adj. **trabecular.**

trabeculae of bone anastomosing bony spicules in cancellous bone which form a meshwork of intercommunicating spaces that are filled with bone marrow.

trabeculate (trə'bekyuhlət) marked with crossbars or trabeculae.

trabeculation (trəˌbekyuh'layshən) the formation of trabeculae in a part.

trabeculectomy (trəˌbekyuh'lektəmee) an operation to lower the intraocular pressure in glaucoma.

trabeculotomy (trəˌbekyuh'lotəmee) an operation for glaucoma, usually performed using a laser.

tracer ('traysə) a means by which something may be followed, as (1) a mechanical device by which the outline or movements of an object can be graphically recorded, or (2) a material by which the progress of a compound through the body may be observed.

radioactive t. a radioactive isotope replacing a stable chemical element in a compound introduced into the body, enabling its metabolism, distribution and elimination to be followed.

trachea (trə'keeə, 'traki·ə) the air passage extending from the throat and larynx to the main bronchi; called also the windpipe. adj. **tracheal.** This tube, about 12 millimetres wide and 10 centimetres long, is reinforced at the front and sides by a series of C-shaped rings of cartilage that keep the passage uniformly open. The gaps between the rings are bridged by strong fibroelastic membranes.

The trachea is lined with mucous membrane covered with small hairlike processes called cilia. These continously sweep foreign material out of the breathing passages toward the mouth. The process is retarded by cold but speeded by heat.

Although the trachea is closed off during swallowing by the epiglottis, a sort of lid, a foreign body, such as a piece of meat, occasionally becomes lodged in it and causes choking. Surgical incision of the trachea, called tracheotomy, may be necessary for removal of the foreign body. See also HEIMLICH MANOEUVRE.

TRACHEOSTOMY, incision of the trachea with insertion of a tube for passage of air, may be necessary if the trachea is obstructed by swelling due to infection or allergic reaction, by accumulation of tracheobronchial secretions or by a growth such as a polyp or tumour. It is also performed when a patient requires long-term mechanical ventilation.

trachealgia (ˌtraki'alji·ə) pain in the trachea.

tracheitis (ˌtraki'ietis) inflammation of the trachea.

trachel(o)- word element. [Gr.] *neck, necklike structure,* especially the uterine cervix.

trachelagra (ˌtrakə'lagrə) gout in the neck.

trachelectomy (ˌtrakə'lektəmee) excision of the uterine cervix.

trachelhaematoma, trachelematoma (ˌtrakəlˌheemə'tohmə; ˌtrakəˌlemə'tohmə) a haematoma on the sternocleidomastoid muscle.

trachelism, trachelismus ('trakəˌlizəm; ˌtrakə'lizməs) spasm of the neck muscles; spasmodic reaction of the head in epilepsy.

trachelitis (ˌtrakə'lietis) cervicitis; inflammation of the uterine cervix.

trachelocystitis (ˌtrakəlohsi'stietis) inflammation of the neck of the bladder.

trachelodynia (ˌtrakəloh'dini·ə) pain in the neck.

trachelomyitis (ˌtrakəlohmie'ietis) inflammation of the muscles of the neck.

trachelopexy ('trakəlohˌpeksee) fixation of the uterine cervix.

tracheloplasty ('trakəlohˌplastee) plastic repair of the uterine cervix.

trachelorrhaphy (ˌtrakə'lo·rəfee) suture of the uterine cervix.

trachelotomy (ˌtrakə'lotəmee) incision of the uterine cervix.

tracheo- ('trakioh) word element. [Gr.] *trachea.*

tracheoaerocele (ˌtrakioh'air·rohˌseel) tracheal hernia containing air.

tracheobronchial (ˌtrakioh'brongki·əl) pertaining to the trachea and bronchi.

tracheobronchitis (ˌtrakiohbrong'kietis) inflammation of the trachea and bronchi.

tracheobronchoscopy (ˌtrakiohbrong'koskəpee) inspection of the interior of the trachea and bronchus.

tracheocele ('trakiohˌseel) hernial protrusion of the tracheal mucous membrane.

tracheolaryngeal (ˌtrakiohlə'rinji·əl, -ˌlarin'jeeəl) pertaining to the trachea and larynx.

tracheolaryngotomy (ˌtrakiohˌlaring'gotəmee) incision of the larynx and trachea.

tracheomalacia (ˌtrakiohmə'layshi·ə) softening of the tracheal cartilages.

tracheo-oesophageal (ˌtrakioh·iˌsofə'jeeəl) pertaining to the trachea and oesophagus.

tracheopathy (ˌtraki'opəthee) disease of the trachea.

tracheopharyngeal (ˌtrakiohfə'rinji·əl, -ˌfarin'jeeəl) pertaining to the trachea and pharynx.

tracheophony (ˌtraki'ofənee) a sound heard in auscultation over the trachea.

tracheoplasty ('trakiohˌplastee) plastic repair of the trachea.

tracheopyosis (ˌtrakiohpie'ohsis) purulent tracheitis.

tracheorrhagia (ˌtraki·ə'rayji·ə) haemorrhage from the trachea.

tracheoschisis (ˌtraki'oskisis) fissure of the trachea.

tracheoscopy (ˌtraki'oskəpee) inspection of the interior of the trachea. adj. **tracheoscopic.**

tracheostenosis (ˌtrakiohstə'nohsis) constriction of the trachea.

tracheostomy, tracheotomy (ˌtraki'ostəmee; ˌtraki'otəmee) creation of an opening into the trachea through the neck, with insertion of an indwelling tube, undertaken in an emergency to restore the airway in acute obstruction, electively to improve the airway and aspirate secretions in chronic respiratory disease, or as part of an operation on the head or neck.

During the operation the patient is placed on his back with a pillow or roll of fabric under his shoulders so that the neck is extended and the trachea is prominent.

Tracheostomy Tubes. There are many types of tracheostomy tubes available, but the basic structure is the same. All are curved to accommodate the anatomy of the trachea and most consist of an outer cannula to maintain the patency of the airway and an inner cannula that fits snugly inside the outer cannula and can be removed for cleaning and removal of accumulated secretions without disturbing the operative site. An accessory to the tracheostomy tubes is the obturator (pilot), which is an olive-tipped curved rod that is used to guide the outer cannula and prevent scraping of the tracheal walls while the tube is being inserted.

Tracheostomy tubes are usually made of plastic and often have an inflatable cuff attached.

Patient Care. The primary concerns of tracheostomy care are maintenance of an adequate airway by keeping the tube free of secretions and prevention of infection. During the first 24 hours after the operation the patient should have someone in constant attendance. Because he cannot call for help and will not be able to cough up and expectorate accumulations of secretions in the trachea, the patient may easily panic and feel that he is suffocating.

The patient is observed closely for signs of respiratory difficulty. If there is a change in the respiratory rate or a wheezing or crowing sound on inspiration the tube may be obstructed. If suction does not relieve the situation a doctor should be called immediately. Restlessness, pallor, or the development of cyanosis is an indication of inadequate ventilation of the lungs resulting from obstruction of the airway.

Accidental expulsion of the outer cannula due to violent coughing or improperly tied tapes rarely occurs; should it happen, however, a dilator or haemostat must be used to hold open the incision while another tube is inserted.

The mucus will be slightly blood-tinged immediately after the tracheostomy is performed, but it should gradually assume a normal colour. If there is evidence of persistent bleeding, this should be reported, as it may indicate internal haemorrhage. The mucus is removed by suction as necessary. The size of the catheter to be used for suction will depend on the size of the tracheostomy tube. The catheter should be small enough to move freely into and out of the tube and large enough to aspirate secretions effectively.

It is recommended that aspiration of the tracheostomy tube be done under aseptic technique. Under no circumstances except dire emergency should the catheter used for suction of the tracheostomy tube be the same as that used for oral and nasal suction, unless it is used first for the tracheostomy tube and then discarded after suction of the nose and mouth. Suction should be done only as necessary and for no more than 20 seconds at a time. The patient should be reoxygenated for at least five deep breaths before suction is repeated. It is an irritating procedure that carries with it the hazards of infection and depletion of inhaled oxygen supply. See also suction.

A sterile dressing, slit so that it fits around the tube, is applied at the time of the tracheostomy and is changed as often as necessary. Sterile gloves should be worn for all handling of the site, and the area should be cleaned with an antibiotic solution at least every 8 to 12 hours. Gauze used as dressings around the site should never be cut, because strings from the dressing could be aspirated; instead, a gauze square is folded to fit.

The tracheostomy tube is usually changed 4 to 5 days after surgery and every 2 to 4 days thereafter. If the tracheostomy is permanent and the trachea has been sutured to the opening in the skin, there is less danger in removing the outer cannula because there are no loose flaps of skin to cover the opening while the tube is out of place.

The patient with a permanent tracheostomy must be taught self-care before he leaves the hospital. As he becomes accustomed to breathing through the tube, applying suction as necessary and replacing the dressings, he will become less apprehensive. He must be cautioned against swimming, and should be warned to use care when taking a shower or bath that water is not aspirated through the tracheostomy.

tracheotome ('trakiohˌtohm) an instrument for incising the trachea.

tracheotomy (ˌtraki'otəmee) tracheostomy.

trachoma (trə'kohmə) a chronic infectious disease of the conjunctiva and cornea, producing photophobia, pain, and lacrimation, caused by an organism once thought to be a virus but now classified as a strain of the bacteria *Chlamydia trachomatis*.

Trachoma is more prevalent in Africa and Asia than in other parts of the world; in North Africa few persons reach adulthood without having contracted the infection.

A condition closely related to trachoma in cause, manifestations, and epidemiological pattern is inclusive conjunctivitis. This is fundamentally a disease of the adult genital tract, transmitted as a venereal disease. The agents of trachoma and inclusive conjunctivitis are called TRIC agents.

SYMPTOMS. Clinically, trachoma in children and adults begins with a conjunctivitis that is marked by tiny follicles on the upper eyelids and tarsal plate. The follicles become increasingly larger and there is granulation of the cornea and impairment of vision. Eventually there is severe scarring which results in blindness.

TREATMENT AND PREVENTION. The drugs of choice in the treatment of trachoma are the tetracyclines and sulphonamides administered topically in the form of suspensions or ointments that adhere to the conjunctiva for prolonged effect.

Prevention of trachoma begins with an adequate water supply for washing the hands and bathing, control of flies, and education of the local population about the cause and spread of the disease. Early treatment of young children reduces the source of infection and avoids the complication of blindness. Repeated treatment programmes for adults aid in controlling the spread of infection.

t. bodies inclusion bodies found in clusters in the cytoplasm of the epithelial cells of the conjunctiva in trachoma.

trachomatous (trə'kohmətəs) pertaining to or of the nature of trachoma.

trachyphonia (ˌtrayki'fohni·ə) roughness of the voice.

tracing ('traysing) a graphic record produced by copying another, or scribed by an instrument capable of making a visual record of movements.

tract (trakt) a longitudinal assemblage of tissues or organs, especially a bundle of nerve fibres having a common origin, function, and termination, or a number of anatomical structures arranged in series and serving a common function.

alimentary t. alimentary canal.

biliary t. the organs, ducts, etc., participating in secretion (the liver), storage (the gallbladder), and delivery (hepatic and bile ducts) of bile into the duodenum.

digestive t. alimentary canal (see also DIGESTIVE SYSTEM).

dorsolateral t. a group of nerve fibres in the lateral funiculus of the spinal cord dorsal to the posterior column.

extrapyramidal t. see EXTRAPYRAMIDAL SYSTEM.

gastrointestinal t. the stomach and intestine in continuity (see also DIGESTIVE SYSTEM).

iliotibial t. a thickened longitudinal band of fascia lata extending from the tensor muscle downward to the lateral condyle of the tibia.

intestinal t. the small and large intestines in continuity (see also INTESTINAL TRACT).

optic t. the nerve tract proceeding backward from the optic chiasm, around the cerebral peduncle, and dividing into a lateral and medial root, which end in the superior colliculus and lateral geniculate body, respectively.

pyramidal t's collections of motor nerve fibres arising in the brain and passing down through the spinal cord to motor cells in the anterior horns.

respiratory t. the organs that allow entrance of air into the lungs and exchange of gases with the blood, from the air passages in the nose to the pulmonary alveoli.

urinary t. the organs concerned in the production and excretion of urine: the KIDNEYS, the urinary BLADDER, the URETERS, and the URETHRA.

uveal t. the vascular tunic of the eye, comprising the choroid, ciliary body, and iris.

traction ('trakshən) the exertion of a pulling force, as that applied to a fractured bone or dislocated joint to maintain proper position and facilitate healing, or, in obstetrics, that along the axis of the pelvis to assist in delivery of a fetal part, or the placenta and membranes.

Traction also may be used to overcome muscle spasms in musculoskeletal disorders, such as 'slipped disc', to lessen or prevent contractures and to correct or prevent a deformity.

Traction may be applied by means of a weight connected to a pulley mechanism over the patient's bed; this is known as weight traction. In skeletal traction, force is applied directly upon a bone by means of surgically installed pins and wires or tongs. Splints and reinforced garments, such as surgical corsets and collars, also may be employed to provide forms of traction. In skin traction foam-backed or adhesive extensions are applied to the affected limb, and bandaged in place. Traction is applied to the extensions by the use of weights.

PATIENT CARE. The patient in constant traction must receive special skin care frequently to prevent breakdown of the skin. Since he often cannot move certain parts of his body without help, a regular schedule of changing and alternating positions should be instituted. Bony prominences are checked frequently for signs of pressure and irritation.

The installation of a trapeze bar over the bed can give the patient greater freedom in moving himself about in bed and make him feel less dependent on the nursing staff. The patient should be instructed to lift himself straight up so as not to alter the position of the affected limb in traction.

The apparatus used for traction must be checked frequently to be sure the weights are hanging free and exerting the required amount of pull. The patient's body weight should counteract the pull of the weights; i.e., his feet should not be resting against the footboard nor should his body position interfere in any way with the tension on the ropes of the traction apparatus.

When traction is applied to the neck with a head halter or other apparatus, it may be best to have the patient's head at the foot of the bed. This facilitates observation of the patient, changing of dressings and other treatments.

To disturb the patient as little as possible during the changing of the bottom linen, it is best to start the linen change on the unaffected side, or from the top of the bed to the bottom, as this will not cause rotation of the limb. If the limb in traction feels cold to the touch or the patient complains of chilling, a small blanket may be used to cover the limb. Care must be taken that other top covers on the bed do not interfere with the traction apparatus.

tractotomy (trak'totəmee) transection of a nerve tract in the central nervous system, usually for the relief of intractable pain.

tractus ('traktəs) pl. *tractus* [L.] tract; used in anatomical nomenclature to designate certain collections of nerve fibres in the central nervous system.

tragacanth ('tragə,kanth) the dried gummy exudation from *Astragalus gummifer* or other species of *Astragalus;* used as a suspending agent for drugs.

tragomaschalia (,tragohma'skali·ə) odorous perspiration from the axilla.

tragus ('traygəs) pl. *tragi* [L.] a cartilaginous projection anterior to the external opening of the ear; used also in the plural to designate hairs growing on the pinna of the external ear, especially on the anterior cartilaginous projection. adj. **tragal.**

trainable ('traynəb'l) capable of being trained; the term is used with special reference to persons with moderate mental handicap (IQ approximately 36–51), who are capable of achieving self-care, social adjustment at home, and economic usefulness under close supervision.

trait (trayt) 1. any genetically determined condition; also, the condition prevailing in the heterozygous state of a recessive disorder, as the sickle cell trait. 2. a distinctive behaviour pattern.

trance (trahns) profound or abnormal sleep from which the patient cannot be aroused easily, and not due to organic disease. It is usually due to hysteria or other psychiatric disturbance and may be induced by hypnotism.

Trandate ('trandayt) trademark for preparations of labetolol, an antihypertensive.

tranquillizer ('trangkwi,liezə) any of a group of compounds that calm or quiet an anxious patient. There are two types: the *major tranquillizers* (also called NEUROLEPTICS or antipsychotic agents), such as chlorpromazine, and the *minor tranquillizers* (also called anxiolytics or antianxiety agents), such as diazepam, chlordiazepoxide, and meprobamate.

trans (tranz) 1. in organic chemistry, having certain atoms or radicals on opposite sides of a nonrotatable parent structure. 2. in genetics, having unlike members of a pseudoallelic, or closely linked, gene pair on the same member of a pair of homologous chromosomes. cf. *cis.*

trans- word element. [L.] *through, across, beyond.*

transabdominal (,tranzab'domin'l, ,trahnz-) across the abdominal wall or through the abdominal cavity.

transactional analysis (tran'zakshən'l, trahn-) a theory of personality structure and a psychotherapeutic method originated by Dr. Eric Berne. According to this theory the human personality is viewed as consisting of three ego states: the Parent, the Adult, and the Child. These ego states are described by Dr. Berne as being 'coherent systems of thought and feeling manifested by corresponding patterns of behaviour'.

The word *transaction* in this term is in reference to the communication that takes place between two people, or, more precisely, what occurs when a stimulus from the ego state of one person elicits a response from the ego state of another individual. *Analysis* refers to an investigation into the feelings and behaviour patterns that are demonstrated during the transaction. In a successful or complementary transaction, the stimulus and response are between the same ego states; for example, Parent–Parent and Adult–Adult. In unsuccessful transactions one individual is speaking from one ego state, but gets a response from a different ego state. The interaction between the two is then either terminated or switched to another focus.

The therapeutic effect of transactional analysis is believed to be derived from an understanding of the origin of each of the three ego states, recognition of their influence on behaviour, and an awareness of the options one has for dealing with reality in an effective and satisfying manner so that he can take care of his own needs and feel good about himself and other people.

transamidase (tran'zami,dayz) an enzyme that catalyses the transfer of an amide group from one molecule to another.

transaminase (tran'zami,nayz) an enzyme that catalyses the transfer of an amino group from one molecule to another. See also TRANSFERASE.

glutamic-oxaloacetic t. (GOT) see ASPARTATE AMINOTRANSFERASE.

glutamic-pyruvic t. (GPT) see ALANINE AMINOTRANSFERASE.

transamination (,tranzami'nayshən) the reversible exchange of amino groups between different amino acids.

transanimation (,tranzani'mayshən, ,trahnz-) resuscitation of an asphyxiated person by mouth-to-mouth breathing (see also ARTIFICIAL RESPIRATION).

transaortic (,tranzay'awtik, ,trahnz-) performed through the aorta.

transatrial (tran'zaytri·əl, trahn-) performed through the atrium.

transaudient (tran'zawdi·ənt, trahn-) penetrable by sound waves.

transaxial (tran'zaksi·əl, trahn-) directed at right angles to the long axis of the body or a part.

transbasal (tranz'bays'l, trahnz-) through the base, as a surgical approach through the base of the skull.

transcalent (tran'skaylənt, trahn-) penetrable by heat rays.

transcalvarial (,tranzkal'vair·ri·əl, ,trahnz-) through or across the calvaria.

transcendental meditation ('transen,dent'l ,medi'tayshən, 'trahn-) a technique for attaining a state of physical relaxation and psychological calm by the regular practice of a relaxation procedure which entails the repetition of a mantra.

transcervical (tranz'sərvik'l, -sə'viek'l, trahnz-) 1. performed through the cervical opening of the uterus. 2. across or through the neck of a structure.

transcobalamin (,tranzkoh'baləmin, ,trahnz-) a group of proteins (of intestinal cells) that bind to cyanocobalamin (vitamin B_{12}) and transport it to other tissues.

transcortical (,tranz'kawtik'l, ,trahnz-) connecting two parts of the cerebral cortex.

transcortin (,tran'skawtin) an α-globulin that binds and transports biologically active, unconjugated cortisol in plasma.

transcriptase (tran'skriptayz, trahn-) RNA polymerase; an enzyme that catalyses the synthesis (polymerization) of RNA from ribonucleoside triphosphates, with DNA serving as a template.

reverse t. RNA-directed DNA polymerase; an enzyme of RNA viruses that catalyses the transcription of RNA to DNA, which is then incorporated into the genome of the host cell.

transcription (tran'skripshən, trahn-) the synthesis of RNA using a DNA template catalysed by an RNA polymerase; the base sequences of the RNA and the DNA template are complementary.

transcutaneous electrical nerve stimulation (,transkyoo'tayni·əs, ,trahns-) a procedure in which mild electrical stimulation is applied by electrodes in contact with the skin over a painful area. Abbreviated TENS.

TENS stimulates the large myelinated nerve fibres and relieves pain in line with the gate control theory. It also causes the release of endogenous opiates or endorphins in the cerebrospinal fluid, thereby weakening the operator's perception of pain.

The primary use of TENS is for analgesia for

mothers in labour. The unit has four electrodes which should be placed parallel with and close to the spine between T10 and L1 and in the sacral area between S2–4. Pain relief is controlled by the mother who is able to increase the degree of stimulation during a contraction, and is able to be mobile while it is operating. As a non-invasive technique it is preferred by mothers who wish to avoid drugs or epidural analgesia. It has proved effective in early labour but most mothers require additional pain relief in the later stages.

It may interfere with CARDIOTOCOGRAPH recordings if the mother requires continuous FETAL MONITORING. The UKCC has recently accepted that at present this form of pain relief should not be used by midwives on their own responsibility, although this does not prevent it being used under medical supervision by mothers in their care.

transducer (tranz'dyoosə, trahnz-) a device that translates one physical quantity to another, e.g., pressure or temperature to an electrical signal.

neuroendocrine t. a neuron, such as a neurohypophyseal neuron, that on stimulation secretes a hormone, thereby translating neural information into hormonal information.

transduction (tranz'dukshən, trahnz-) the transfer of a genetic fragment from one microorganism to another by bacteriophage.

transdural (tranz'dyooə·rəl, trahnz-) through or across the dura mater.

transection (tran'sekshən, trahn-) a cross section; division by cutting transversely.

transepithelial (ˌtranzepi'theeli·əl, ˌtrahnz-) occurring through or across an epithelium.

transfer factor ('transfər, 'trahns-) a factor occurring in sensitized lymphocytes that has the capacity to transfer delayed hypersensitivity to a normal (nonreactive) individual. Abbreviated TF. Originally described by H.S. Lawrence, it confers cell-mediated IMMUNITY and therefore has been found to be useful in treating conditions in which there is a disorder of IMMUNE RESPONSE. As an adjunct to antibiotic therapy it is useful in the treatment of such antibiotic-resistant diseases as candidiasis, coccidioidomycosis, and leprosy.

transferase ('transfəˌrayz, 'trahns-) an enzyme that catalyses the transfer, from one molecule to another, of a chemical group that does not exist in free state during the transfer. See also TRANSAMINASE.

alanine aminotransferase (ALT) see ALANINE AMINOTRANSFERASE.

aspartate aminotransferase (AST) see ASPARTATE AMINOTRANSFERASE.

transference ('transfə·rəns, trans'fər·rəns, 'trahns-) 1. the passage of a symptom or affection from one part to another. 2. in psychiatry, the shifting of an affect from one person to another or from one idea to another; especially the transfer by the patient to the analyst of emotional tones, of either affection or hostility, based on unconscious identification.

transferrin (trans'ferin) a serum globulin that binds and transports iron.

transfix (trans'fiks, trahns-) to pierce through or impale.

transfixion (trans'fikshən, trahns-) a cutting through from within outward, as in amputation.

transforation (ˌtransfo'rayshən, ˌtrahns-) perforation of the fetal skull.

transformation (ˌtransfə'mayshən, ˌtrahns-) change of form or structure; conversion from one form to another. In oncology, the change that a normal cell undergoes as it becomes malignant.

bacterial t. the process of intercellular transfer of genetic information in which a small portion of the total DNA of a lysed bacterium enters a related bacterium and is incorporated into its genetic constitution.

transformer (trans'fawmə, trahns-) an induction apparatus for changing electrical energy at one voltage and current to electrical energy at another voltage and current, through the medium of magnetic energy, without mechanical motion.

step-down t. one for lowering the voltage of the original current.

step-up t. one for raising the voltage of the original current.

transfusion (trans'fyoozhən, trahns-) the introduction of whole blood or blood components directly into the bloodstream. Among the elements transfused are packed red blood cells, plasma, platelets, granulocytes, and cryoprecipitate, a plasma protein rich in antihaemophilic factor VIII. The current trend is to transfuse blood components rather than whole blood because by so doing the utility of each unit of blood can be extended and the treatment provided more nearly meets the specific needs of the patient.

Transfusion is most often indicated to maintain or replace blood volume, to provide deficient blood elements and improve coagulation, to maintain or improve transport of oxygen, and in exchange for blood that has been removed in the treatment of Rh incompatibility in the newborn, liver failure in which toxins accumulate in the blood, or in some other types of toxaemia.

TRANSFUSION METHODS. There are several different methods of transfusion. Direct transfusion, in which blood from one person is directly transferred to another person, is now rarely used. The usual method is indirect transfusion, in which blood is drawn from a donor, stored in a sterile container and later given to a recipient. Exchange transfusion, in which blood is removed from a person and simultaneously replaced by donor blood, is used mainly in treating HAEMOLYTIC DISEASE OF THE NEWBORN.

Intrauterine Transfusion. Intrauterine transfusion involves direct transfusion of Rh-negative packed blood cells into the fetal peritoneal cavity. It is done to prevent death as a result of maternal-fetal blood incompatibility in which the fetal blood cells are destroyed (HAEMOLYTIC DISEASE OF THE NEWBORN).

The first step in a fetal transfusion is injection of a radiopaque dye into the amniotic fluid. After the fetus ingests the dye, his intestinal tract can be visualized by radiography and serves as a guide for location of the abdominal cavity. A long pudendal needle is then inserted through the mother's abdomen and guided through the uterine wall, through the fetal abdomen, and into the peritoneal cavity. Another radiograph is taken to confirm correct placement of the needle and then the erythrocytes are transfused.

This procedure is obviously not without hazard and is done only if the fetus cannot be expected to survive without it. The treatment may need to be repeated several times before birth.

BLOOD TYPING AND CROSSMATCHING. Transfusions were not practicable until the four main hereditary blood types, A, B, AB, and O, were discovered at the beginning of this century. Until these blood types were identified, antigen–antibody reactions could not be predicted and transfusion reactions (often fatal) were a matter of chance. There are certain antigens on the surface of red blood cells which can precipitate a transfusion reaction when incompatible blood types are mixed. In the ABO system the types are dictated by

A antigen and B antigen. They stimulate the production of anti-A and anti-B antibodies, respectively. A person who is type A has only A antigen on red cells; one who is type B has only B antigen; one who is type AB has both A and B antigens; and one who is type O has neither. Usually, a person has antibodies against foreign antigens: type A has anti-B; type B has anti-A; type O has both; and type AB has neither.

In the Rh blood group the D antigen is clinically the most important. Rh negative individuals lack D antigen on red cells. They do not produce anti-D antibodies unless they are directly exposed to Rh positive blood, as may occur from a fetal–maternal haemorrhage or from transfusion of platelet or granulocyte concentrate containing Rh positive red cells.

Another system of blood typing is sometimes considered prior to transfusion of granulocytes or for long-term platelet administration. The typing identifies the HLA antigens that occur on leukocytes and platelets. See also HLA and TISSUE TYPING.

Crossmatching is the standard way in which blood is tested for compatibility prior to transfusion. It involves placing the cells of the donor in a sample of the recipient's serum, and cells of the recipient in a sample of the donor's serum. Absence of agglutination, haemolysis, and cytotoxicity indicates that the two blood specimens are compatible.

ADVERSE REACTIONS. Among the most severe transfusion reactions are antigen–antibody reactions resulting from blood type incompatibility. When blood groups are incompatible there is agglutination (clumping) of cells, haemolysis, and release of cellular elements into the serum. Signs and symptoms indicating such a reaction include burning sensation along the vein where the transfusion is given, facial flushing, chills and fever, headache, low back pain, rash, red urine, and shock. Other reactions include febrile reaction, allergic reaction with hives, wheezing, and anaphylaxis, and response to bacterial contamination.

Every hospital in which transfusions are administered should have a written policy regarding the correct steps to take in the event a patient begins to show signs of a reaction. In general, should such signs occur, the transfusion is stopped immediately, the venous line is kept open with normal saline, and the doctor is notified.

High levels of potassium in donor blood can occur when the bank blood is several days old and rarely may cause problems due to HYPERKALAEMIA in patients with cardiac or renal disease when large quantities of blood are transfused.

Another possible complication is hypocalcaemia, which can occur when large amounts of blood containing the additive acid citrate dextrose (ACD) are given rapidly. The ACD anticoagulant binds with calcium ions in the recipient's blood, removing them from circulation and thereby reducing the calcium level below that essential for normal coagulation.

Circulatory overload is a possibility any time blood is administered rapidly in large amounts. Patients who are particularly susceptible to this eventuality are the very young, the very old, and those suffering from a pre-existing cardiopulmonary or renal problem. Another difficulty that may be encountered when blood is administered rapidly under pressure is that of air embolism.

PATIENT CARE. Every patient receiving a blood transfusion should be monitored closely for early signs of transfusion reactions and complications. Although transfusion of whole blood is a relatively common procedure, it is a highly complex one and not without danger to the patient. Should early signs of a reaction develop, the transfusion should be discontinued and the doctor notified immediately.

Each unit of blood must be labelled carefully and accurately with the patient's name, hospital number, and blood group. The label is read carefully immediately before administration to assure that the patient is receiving compatible blood. Although many complications and reactions cannot be anticipated and prevented, carelessness in the handling and administration of blood can result in unnecessary discomfort and danger to the patient.

transglutaminase (transgloo'tami,nayz) the activated form of protransglutaminase, which forms stabilizing covalent bonds within fibrin strands; called also *coagulation factor XIIIa.*

transient ischaemic attack ('tranziənt) a sudden episode of temporary or passing symptoms typically due to diminished blood flow through the carotid blood vessels, but sometimes related to impaired blood flow through the vertebrobasilar vessels. Abbreviated TIA. The symptoms may be warning signals of impending stroke; approximately one in three persons experiencing a TIA will have a STROKE within five years.

The symptoms of TIA can range from obvious loss of sensation or motor function to more subtle changes in speech or mental acuity. During the attack the person may feel numbness or weakness or both on one side of the body, slurring of speech or inability to talk, or difficulty in thinking. Disturbance in the vision of one eye and double vision also are typical of TIA.

Because these signs are short lived, many persons may be inclined to ignore them unless they are informed of their importance and of the need to consult medical help before a catastrophic stroke occurs. Carotid artery occlusions usually can be corrected by surgery.

transiliac (tran'zili,ak, trahn-) across the two ilia.

transillumination (,tranzi,loomi'nayshən, ,trahnz-) the passage of strong light through a body structure, to permit inspection by an observer on the opposite side.

translation (trans'layshən, ,trahns-) the synthesis of a polypeptide using messenger RNA as a template, a complex process involving ribosomes and transfer RNAs; every three bases (a codon) along the mRNA beginning with the start codon specifies one amino acid in the polypeptide chain.

translocation (,tranzloh'kayshən, ,trahnz-) the attachment of a fragment of one chromosome to a nonhomologous chromosome.

reciprocal t. the mutual exchange of fragments between two broken chromosomes, one part of one uniting with part of the other.

robertsonian t. that in which the breaks occur at the centromeres and entire chromosome arms are exchanged, usually involving two acrocentric chromosomes.

translucent (tranz'loos'nt, trahnz-) slightly penetrable by light rays.

transmethylase (tranz'methi,layz) an enzyme that catalyses transmethylation.

transmethylation (,tranzmethi'layshən) the transfer of a methyl group (CH_3–) from the molecules of one compound to those of another.

transmigration (,tranzmie'grayshən, ,trahnz-) 1. diapedesis. 2. change of place from one side of the body to the other.

transmission (tranz'mishən, trahnz-) 1. transfer, as of a disease from one person to another. 2. heredity.

transmural (tranz'myooə·rəl, trahnz-) through the wall of an organ; extending through or affecting the entire thickness of the wall of an organ or cavity.

transmutation (ˌtranzmyoo'tayshən, ˌtrahnz-) 1. evolutionary change of one species into another. 2. the change of one chemical element into another.

transorbital (tran'zawbit'l, trahn-) performed through the bony socket of the eye.

transparent (tran'sparənt, trahn-) permitting the passage of rays of light so that objects may be seen through the substance.

transpeptidase (tranz'peptiˌdayz) an enzyme that catalyses the transfer of an amino or peptide group from one molecule to another.

transphosphorylase (ˌtranzfos'fo·riˌlayz) an enzyme that catalyses the transfer of a phosphate group from one molecule to another.

transphosphorylation (ˌtranzfosˌfo·ri'layshən) the exchange of phosphate groups between organic phosphates, without their going through the stage of inorganic phosphates.

transpiration (ˌtranspi'rayshən, ˌtrahns-) discharge of air, vapour, or sweat through the skin.

transplacental (ˌtranspla'sent'l, ˌtrahns-) through the placenta.

transplant ('transplahnt, 'trahns-) 1. an organ or tissue taken from the body and grafted into another area of the same individual or another individual. 2. to transfer tissue from one part to another or from one individual to another.

transplantation (ˌtransplahn'tayshən, ˌtrahns-) the transfer of living organs from one part of the body to another (autotransplant) or from one individual to another (allograft). Transplantation is often called grafting, though the term grafting is more commonly used to refer to the transfer of skin (see GRAFTING).

In dentistry, transplantation refers to the insertion into a prepared dental alveolus of an autogenous or homologous tooth; it may be a developing tooth germ from the same mouth, or a frozen homologous transplant.

In 1954 surgeons in Boston, USA successfully transplanted a kidney from one identical twin into the other to replace his diseased kidneys. Kidneys are the most commonly transplanted organ partly because they are a paired organ but also because the recipient may live a healthy life on dialysis whilst awaiting transplant. Most transplants are performed from cadaver donors who are certified brain dead before removal of organs. Survival of patients and graft for one year is 80 to 90 per cent. Live-related donation may occur by elective nephrectomy from a healthy person who donates his kidney for transplantation into a closely blood related recipient. One year survival is slightly improved and is over 90 per cent. Screening of donor and careful psychosocial counselling of donor and recipient must be performed prior to donation.

In 1967 the South African surgeon Christiaan N. Barnard transplanted a human heart and more recently liver and pancreas transplants have been performed. Multiorgan transplantation is becoming increasingly common. Ethical and legal discussion still occurs concerning cadaver donation and brain death criteria.

Nursing care starts when the patient is first considered for transplantation. Patients' emotions differ greatly, ranging from intense fear to desperate desire for a transplant. It is important that the positive aspects of a successful graft are emphasized, with a mention of the small chance that a kidney might fail or a suitable one not be found for many years. Some patients imagine that a transplant will solve not only their renal failure but also their marital, financial and employment problems and are bitterly disappointed when it does not.

Immediately after renal transplantation it is essential to maintain correct fluid balance and a good circulating volume so that the kidney is adequately perfused. All transplant patients need administration of immunosuppressive drugs and vigilance for signs of rejection or infection. The first few months are the most crucial for infection and rejection, as immunosuppression is adjusted to suit the patient. Too little may cause rejection, while too much may allow fatal infection to occur. The patient and his family must be kept well informed of progress and plans. The uncomplicated graft will be a joy to manage, but the patient with complications will need greater support to accept the temporary loss of security and independence from dialysis until the certainty of his transplant is established.

Rejection is a major problem in transplantation. Organs such as the cornea, skin, and bone can be transplanted successfully because, in the case of the cornea, the vascular supply is not involved, or, in skin and bone, the transplant serves as a structural foundation into which the new tissue grows. In the case of intact organs such as the kidney, heart, lung, liver, and pancreas, a generous blood supply is essential to their survival in the recipient's body. Specific cells in the recipient's blood recognize the transplanted organ as foreign and set up an IMMUNE RESPONSE by producing antibodies to the antigens of the donor. These antibodies are capable of inhibiting metabolism of the cells within the transplanted organ and eventually actively cause their destruction. This may occur initially or many weeks later. In order to achieve the greatest chance of graft survival, cross-matching is done between donor and recipient. ABO blood type compatibility is essential. TISSUE TYPING is done to identify the protein antigens that are specific to each individual. These antigens are the human leukocyte antigens (HLA), so called because they are easily identifiable on leukocytes. The significance of HLA matching is not proven, but a specific HLA antigen will not be given to a recipient who has a corresponding antibody. A third test is *cross-matching*, which involves mixing the intended recipient's serum with lymphocytes from the potential donor. A positive reaction would show destruction of the donor's cells by antibodies in the recipient's serum, thus eliminating the possibility of using an organ from that particular donor.

Control of the immune response in the recipient is attempted by the use of immunosuppressive agents. Corticosteroids are used in all transplant centres. Doses normally range from 1 mg/kg to 0.2 mg/kg body weight depending on the centre, reducing over the first year. Higher dose oral steroids have been clearly associated with sepsis and increased peptic ulceration and bleeding. Rejection crises are treated with methylprednisolone intravenously. One or a combination of the drugs azathioprine cyclophosphamide and cyclosporin A may be used in conjunction with steroids to prevent rejection. Cyclosporin A, though expensive, is the most popular, though accurate monitoring of blood levels is needed to prevent profound nephrotoxicity. Antilymphocyte or antithymocyte globulin may be given intravenously to treat an acute rejection episode.

transport ('transpawt, 'trahn-) movement of materials in biological systems, particularly into and out of cells and across epithelial layers.

active t. movement of materials across cell membranes and epithelial layers resulting directly from expenditure of metabolic energy.

transposition (ˌtranzpəˈzishən, ˌtrahnz-) displacement to the opposite side; in genetics, the nonreciprocal insertion of material deleted from one chromosome into another, nonhomologous chromosome.

t. of great vessels a CONGENITAL HEART DEFECT, in which the position of the chief blood vessels of the heart is reversed.

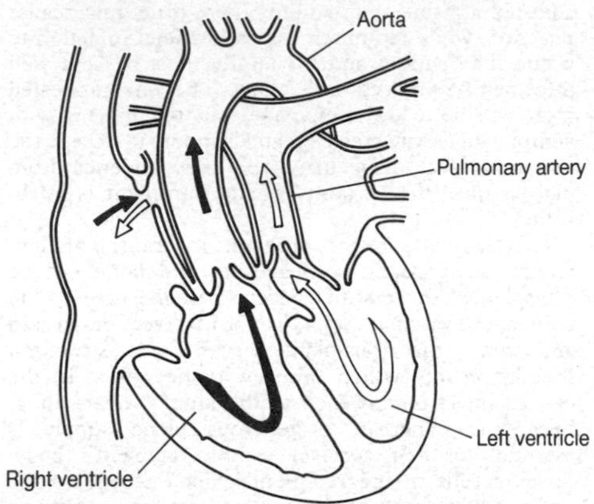

Transposition of the great vessels. Life cannot be sustained unless there is some communication between the systemic and pulmonary circulations, such as a persistent foramen ovale, an atrial septal defect, a ventricular septal defect, or a persistent ductus arteriosus

transposon (tranzˈpohzon) any discrete and characteristic genetic unit (DNA sequence) that may be transferred from one cell to another and be inserted into any of multiple sites in the recipient cell's plasmid- or chromosomal-DNA.

transpubic (tranzˈpyoobik, trahnz-) performed through the pubic bone after removal of a segment of the bone.

transsegmental (ˌtranz·segˈmentˈl, ˌtrahnz-) extending across segments.

transseptal (tranzˈseptˈl, trahnz-) extending or performed through or across a septum.

transsexual (tranzˈseksyooəl, trahnz-) 1. a person affected by transsexualism. 2. a person whose external anatomy has been changed to resemble that of the opposite sex.

transsexualism (tranzˈseksyooəˌlizəm, trahnz-) a disturbance of gender identity in which the affected person has an overwhelming desire to change anatomical sex, stemming from the fixed conviction that he or she is a member of the opposite sex; such persons often seek hormonal and surgical treatment to bring their anatomy into conformity with their belief.

transthalamic (ˌtranzthəˈlamik, ˌtrahnz-) across the thalamus.

transthoracic (ˌtranzthorˈrasik, ˌtrahnz-) through the thoracic cavity or across the chest wall.

transtympanic (ˌtranztimˈpanik, ˌtrahnz-) across the tympanic membrane or the cavity of the middle ear.

transudate (ˈtransyuhˌdayt, ˈtrahn-) a fluid substance that has passed through a membrane or has been extruded from a tissue; in contrast to an exudate, a transudate is characterized by high fluidity and a low content of protein, cells, or solid matter derived from cells.

transudation (ˌtransyuhˈdayshən, ˌtrahn-) 1. passage of serum or other body fluid through a membrane or tissue surface. 2. transudate.

transurethral (ˌtranzyuhˈreethrəl, ˌtrahn-) performed through the urethra.

transvaginal (ˌtranzvəˈjienˈl, -ˈvajinˈl, ˌtrahnz-) through the vagina.

transversalis (ˌtranzvərˈsaylis, ˌtrahnz-) [L.] transverse.

transverse (tranzˈvərs, trahnz-) extending from side to side; situated at right angles to the long axis.

transversectomy (ˌtranzvərˈsektəmee, ˌtrahnz-) excision of a transverse process of a vertebra.

transversus (tranzˈvərsəs) [L.] transverse.

transvesical (tranzˈvesikˈl, trahnz-) through the bladder.

transvestism (tranzˈvestizəm, trahnz-) the condition of being a transvestite.

transvestite (tranzˈvestiet, trahnz-) a person who experiences a habitual and strongly persistent desire to dress as a member of the opposite sex ('cross dressing'). The majority are male and have no desire to physically change sex (by surgery). Usually regarded as a relatively harmless disorder of gender identity.

Trantas' dots (ˈtrantəs) small, white calcareous-looking dots in the limbus of the conjunctiva in vernal conjunctivitis.

Tranxene (ˈtranzeen) trademark for a preparation of clorazepate dipotassium; an anxiolytic and anticonvulsant.

tranylcypromine (ˌtranilˈsieprohmeen) a monoamine oxidase inhibitor used as an antidepressant.

trapezium (trəˈpeezi·əm) an irregular, four-sided figure with two of its sides parallel.

trapezius (trəˈpeezi·əs) one of two large muscles situated between the shoulders and at the back of the neck. It controls some of the movements of the scapula and draws the head backward and to the side.

Trasicor (ˈtrazikor) trademark for preparations of oxprenolol, an antihypertensive.

Trasiderm-Nitro (ˌtrazidərmˈnietroh) trademark for a preparation of glyceryl trinitrate transdermal infusion, a coronary vasodilator.

trauma (ˈtrawmə) injury.

birth t. an injury to the infant during the process of being born. In some psychiatric theories, the psychological shock produced in an infant by the experience of being born.

psychological t. an emotional shock that makes a lasting impression.

traumat(o)- word element. [Gr.] *trauma.*

traumatic (trawˈmatik) pertaining to, resulting from, or causing trauma.

traumatism (ˈtrawməˌtizəm) 1. the physical or psychological state resulting from an injury or wound. 2. a wound.

traumatology (ˌtrawməˈtoləjee) the branch of surgery dealing with wounds and disability from injuries.

traumatopnoea (ˌtrawmətopˈneeə) passage of air through a wound in the chest wall or the apnoea that results.

travail (ˈtravayl, trəˈvayl) labour; childbirth.

travel sickness (ˈtravəl) see MOTION SICKNESS.

tray (tray) a flat-surfaced utensil for the conveyance of various objects or material.

Treacher Collins syndrome (ˌtreechə ˈkolinz) see mandibulofacial DYSOSTOSIS.

treatment (ˈtreetmənt) management and care of a patient or the combating of disease or disorder.

active t. treatment directed immediately to the cure of the disease or injury.

Banting t. treatment of obesity by a low carbohydrate diet rich in nitrogenous matter.

causal t. treatment directed against the cause of a disease.

conservative t. treatment designed to avoid radical

medical therapeutic measures or operative procedures.
empirical t. treatment by means that experience has proved to be beneficial.
expectant t. treatment directed toward relief of untoward symptoms, leaving the cure of the disease to natural forces.
Kenny's t. treatment of poliomyelitis by wrapping the patient in woollen cloths wrung out of hot water and re-educating muscles by passive exercise after pain has subsided.
palliative t. treatment that is designed to relieve pain and distress, but does not attempt a cure.
preventive t., prophylactic t. that in which the aim is to prevent the occurrence of the disease.
rational t. that based upon knowledge of disease and the action of the remedies given.
specific t. treatment particularly adapted to the special disease being treated.
supporting t. that which is mainly directed to sustaining the strength of the patient.
symptomatic t. treatment of symptoms per se where cure is not possible or practical (e.g., functional disorders, terminal cancer) or where self resolution is expected (e.g., virus infections).

tree (tree) an anatomical structure with branches resembling a tree.
bronchial t. the bronchi and their branching structures.
tracheobronchial t. the trachea, bronchi, and their branching structures.

Trematoda (ˌtreməˈtohdə, ˌtree-) a class of the phylum Platyhelminthes that includes the flukes. The trematodes or flukes are parasitic in man and animals, infection by most species resulting from the ingestion of insufficiently cooked fish, crustaceans, or vegetation which contain larvae. The important trematodes which infect man belong to the genera *Schistosoma*, *Echinostoma*, *Fasciolopsis*, *Gastrodiscoides*, *Heterophyes*, *Metagonimus*, *Clonorchis*, *Fasciola*, *Dicrocoelium*, *Opisthorchis*, and *Paragonimus*. See also WORM.

trematode (ˈtreməˌtohd, ˈtree-) an individual of the class Trematoda.

tremor (ˈtremə) an involuntary trembling of the body or limbs. It may have either a physical or a psychological cause.

Often tremors are associated with Parkinson's disease, in which nerve centres in the brain that control the muscles are affected. Early symptoms include trembling of the hands and nodding of the head. Tremors occur also in cerebral palsy and hyperthyroidism, and in narcotic addicts and alcoholics during withdrawal. They tend to develop as one of the results of ageing.

Tremors are sometimes symptoms of temporary abnormal conditions, as, for example, insulin shock, or of poisoning, especially metallic poisoning. They sometimes appear with a high fever resulting from an infection.

Tremors of psychological origin take many forms, some minor and some serious. If there is no physiological cause, they may be a sign of general tension, as when a person holding a full cup of coffee seems compelled to shake and spill it. Violent, uncontrollable trembling is often seen in certain phases of severe mental disorder.
action t. rhythmic, oscillatory, involuntary movements of the outstretched upper limb, as when writing or lifting a cup; it may also affect the voice and other parts.
coarse t. that involving large groups of muscle fibres contracting slowly.
fibrillary t. rapidly alternating contraction of small bundles of muscle fibres.
fine t. one in which the vibrations are rapid.
flapping t. asterixis.
Hunt's t. tremor associated with every voluntary movement; characteristic of cerebellar lesions.
intention t. one occurring when the patient attempts voluntary movement.
rest t. tremor occurring in a relaxed and supported limb, as in parkinsonism.
senile t. tremor due to the infirmities of old age.
volitional t. trembling of the entire body during voluntary effort; seen in multiple sclerosis.

tremulous (ˈtremyuhləs) shaking, trembling, or quivering.

trench fever (trench) a louseborne rickettsial disease due to *Rickettsia quintana*, with febrile paroxysms, leg pains, chills, sweating, rash, splenomegaly, and a tendency to relapse.

trench foot a condition of the feet resembling frostbite, due to the prolonged action of water on the skin combined with circulatory disturbance due to cold and inaction.

trench mouth an acute or chronic gingival infection; called also *necrotizing ulcerative gingivitis*. The name trench mouth was given to the disease during World War I, when it was common among soldiers in the trenches. It is relatively uncommon now and responds readily to antibiotic therapy.

When the condition extends to other parts of the oral mucosa, with lesions involving the palate or pharynx, it is termed Vincent's ANGINA or necrotizing ulcerative gingivostomatitis.

Trendelenburg's position (trenˈdelənˌbərgz) the patient is placed head downwards and supine on a surface inclined at 45 degrees or more, with his legs flexed over the upper end.

Trendelenburg's sign abnormality of the pelvis seen in cases of instability of the hip from dislocation, fracture of the femoral neck or paralysis of the gluteus medius muscle. When standing on the affected leg and flexing the opposite knee and hip, the pelvis drops downwards on the unsupported side rather than rising.

trendscriber (ˈtrendskriebə) the apparatus used in trendscription.

trendscription (trendˈskripshən) a programmed method of continuous electrocardiographic monitoring, wherein the tracing is condensed on a rotating drum recorder and the programme permits selective sampling of rhythm data.

trepanation, trephination (ˌtrepəˈnayshən; ˌtrefiˈnayshən) use of the trephine for creating an opening in the skull or in the sclera.

trephine (triˈfien, -ˈfeen) 1. a crown saw for removing a circular disc of bone, chiefly from the skull. 2. an instrument for removing a circular area of cornea. 3. to remove with a trephine.

trepidation (ˌtrepiˈdayshən) 1. a trembling or oscillatory movement. 2. nervous anxiety and fear. adj. **trepidant.**

Treponema (ˌtrepəˈneemə) a genus of spirochetes (family Treponemataceae), some of them being pathogenic and parasitic for man and other animals, including the aetiological agents of pinta (*T. carateum*), syphilis (*T. pallidum*), and yaws (*T. pertenue*).

treponema (ˌtrepəˈneemə) an organism of the genus *Treponema*. adj. **treponemal.**

Treponemataceae (ˌtrepəˌneeməˈtaysi·ee) a family of bacteria that commonly occur as parasites in vertebrates, some of them causing disease. They are coarse or slender spiral forms, and are sometimes visible only with a darkfield microscope.

treponematosis (ˌtrepəˌneeməˈtohsis) infection with

organisms of the genus *Treponema.*
treponemicidal (ˌtrepə·neemi'sied'l) destroying treponemas.
trepopnoea (trə'popni·ə) a condition in which respiration is more comfortable with the patient turned in a definite recumbent position.
treppe ('trepə) [Ger.] the gradual increase in muscular contraction following rapidly repeated stimulation.
tresis ('treesis) perforation.
tretinoin (ˌtreti'noh·in) the all-trans stereoisomer of retinoic acid, used as a topical keratolytic, especially in the treatment of certain cases of acne vulgaris.
TRH thyrotrophin (TSH) releasing hormone.
tri- word element. [Gr., L.] *three.*
triacylglycerol (trieˌasil'glisəˌrol) the systematic chemical name for triglyceride.
triad ('triead) 1. an element with a valency of three. 2. a group of three similar bodies, or a complex composed of three items or units.
triage (tree'ahzh) [Fr.] the assessment and classification of casualties according to the type and severity of their injuries in order to assign them for treatment.
triamcinolone (ˌtrieam'sinəˌlohn) a prednisolone derivative used as an anti-inflammatory glucocorticoid in the form of the acetonide derivative and the diacetate ester.
triamterene (trie'amtəˌreen) a diuretic which increases sodium and chloride excretion, but not potassium excretion.
triangle ('trieˌang·g'l) a three-cornered object, figure, or area, as such an area on the surface of the body capable of fairly precise definition.

carotid t., inferior that between the median line of the neck in front, the sternocleidomastoid muscle, and the anterior belly of the omohyoid muscle.

carotid t., superior that between the anterior belly of the omohyoid muscle in front, the posterior belly of the digastric muscle above, and the sternocleidomastoid muscle behind.

cephalic t. one on the anteroposterior plane of the skull, between lines from the occiput to the forehead and to the chin, and from the chin to the forehead.

digastric t. submandibular triangle.

t. of elbow a triangular area on the front of the elbow, bounded by the brachioradial muscle on the outside and the round pronator muscle inside, with the base toward the humerus.

t. of election superior carotid triangle.

facial t. a triangular area whose points are the basion and the alveolar and nasal points.

femoral t. the area formed superiorly by the inguinal ligament, laterally by the sartorius muscle, and medially by the adductor longus muscle; called also *Scarpa's triangle.*

infraclavicular t. that formed by the clavicle above, the upper border of the greater pectoral muscle on the inside, and the anterior border of the deltoid muscle on the outside.

inguinal t. the triangular area bounded by the inner edge of the sartorius muscle, the inguinal ligament, and the outer edge of the long adductor muscle.

lumbocostoabdominal t. that lying between the external oblique muscle of the abdomen, the posterior inferior serratus muscle, the erector muscle of the spine, and the internal oblique muscle of the abdomen.

t. of necessity inferior carotid triangle. **occipital t.** the area bounded by the sternocleidomastoid muscle in front, the trapezius muscle behind, and the omohyoid muscle below.

Scarpa's t. femoral triangle.

subclavian t. a triangular area bounded by the clavicle, the sternocleidomastoid muscle, and the omohyoid muscle.

submaxillary t. that bounded by the lower jaw bone above, the posterior belly of the digastric muscle and the stylohyoid muscle below and the median line of the neck in front.

suboccipital t. that lying between the posterior greater rectus muscle of the head and the superior and inferior oblique muscles of the head.

triangular (trie'ang·gyuhlə) having three angles or corners.
triangularis (trieˌang·gyuh'lair·ris) [L.] *triangular.*
Triatoma (trie'atəmə) a genus of bugs (order Hemiptera), the cone-nosed bugs, important in medicine as vectors of *Trypanosoma cruzi.*
triazolam (trie'ayzohlam) a benzodiazepine derivative with hypnotic properties.
tribe (trieb) a taxonomic category subordinate to a family (or subfamily) and superior to a genus (or subtribe).
triboluminescence (ˌtriebohˌloomi'nes'ns) luminescence produced by mechanical energy, as by the grinding, rubbing, or breaking of certain crystals.
tribrachius (trie'brayki·əs) a fetus or infant with three arms.
TRIC agents (trik 'ayjəns) those causing TRACHOMA and inclusive conjunctivitis.
tricarboxylic acid cycle (ˌtriekahbok'silik) the cyclic metabolic mechanism by which the complete oxidation of the acetyl moiety of acetyl-coenzyme A is effected; it is the chief source of mammalian energy, during which carbon chains of sugars, fatty acids, and amino acid are metabolized to yield carbon dioxide, water, and high-energy phosphate bonds. Called also *Krebs cycle* and *citric acid cycle.*
tricephalus (trie'kefələs, -'sef-) a fetus or infant with three heads.
triceps ('trieseps) a muscle having three heads; the triceps muscle of the arm extends the forearm.
trich(o)- word element. [Gr.] *hair.*
trichiasis (tri'kieəsis) 1. a condition of ingrowing hairs about an orifice, or ingrowing eyelashes. 2. the appearance of hairlike filaments in the urine.
trichilemmal (ˌtriki'leməl) pertaining to the outer root sheath of a hair.
trichilemmoma (ˌtrikilə'mohmə) a benign neoplasm of the lower outer root sheath of the hair.
Trichinella (ˌtriki'nelə) a genus of nematode parasites.

T. spiralis a species found in the striated muscle of various animals, a common cause of infection in man as a result of ingestion of poorly cooked pork. See TRICHINIASIS.

trichiniasis (triki'nieəsis) a disease caused by a roundworm, *Trichinella spiralis*, whose larvae, when ingested in pork or wild animal meat, migrate to and become encapsulated in the muscles. Very heavy infections can be fatal. Now rare in the United Kingdom. Called also *trichinosis, trichinelliasis.*

TREATMENT AND PREVENTION. With its varying symptoms, trichiniasis is sometimes difficult to diagnose, but serological tests have been developed that make identification of the disease easier. Chest radiographs and microscopic examination of muscle tissue also can be useful in diagnosis.

The anthelmintic mebendazole has been recommended for both the intestinal and muscle invasion stages, otherwise recovery is a matter of bed rest and time, which allow the body's natural defences to overcome the parasites. Corticosteroids may be prescribed to relieve muscular pain and other symtoms.

The only certain safeguard against trichiniasis is the thorough cooking of all meat products to ensure destruction of any encysted *Trichinella* larvae. Pork should be cooked until the meat is grey in colour; if it is pink it is underdone. Cooking in this manner ensures that all parts of the roast will be heated well above 68 °C (154 °F), the thermal death point of the larvae.

trichinous ('trikinəs) affected with or containing *trichinella.*

trichloroacetic acid (trie,klor·roh·ə'seetik) an extremely caustic acid, CCl_3COOH, used in medicine as a topical caustic for local destruction of lesions and in clinical chemistry as a protein precipitating agent.

trichloroethylene (trie,klor·roh'ethi,leen) a clear, mobile liquid still occasionally used as an inhalation analgesic and anaesthetic for short operative procedures. It is a widely used industrial solvent; exposure to high vapour concentrations can cause fatal poisoning.

trichoaesthesia (,trikoh·is'theezi·ə) sensibility of the hair to touch.

trichoanaesthesia (,trikoh,anəs'theezi·ə) loss of hair sensibility.

trichobezoar (,trikoh'beezor) a bezoar composed of hair; hairball.

trichocardia (,trikoh'kahdi·ə) a hairy appearance of the heart due to exudative pericarditis.

trichoclasia (,trikoh'klayzi·ə) brittleness of the hair.

trichoepithelioma (,trikoh,epi,theeli'ohmə) a benign skin tumour originating in the follicles of the lanugo; it may occur as an inherited condition marked by multiple tumours (trichoepithelioma papillosum multiplex). Called also *epithelioma adenoides cysticum.*

trichoglossia (,trikoh'glosi·ə) hairy tongue, due to thickening of the papillae.

trichoid ('trikoyd) resembling hair.

trichologia (,trikə'lohji·ə) the pulling out of the hair by delirious or insane patients.

trichology (tri'koləjee) the sum of knowledge about the hair.

trichomadesis (,trikohmə'deesis) abnormally rapid or premature loss of the scalp hair.

trichome ('triekohm, 'tri-) a filamentous or hairlike structure.

trichomonacide (,trikoh'mohnə,sied) an agent destructive to trichomonads.

trichomonad (,trikoh'mohnad) a parasite of the genus *Trichomonas.*

Trichomonas (,trikoh'mohnas) a genus of flagellate protozoa parasitic in animals and birds and in man.

T. hominis a nonpathogenic species found in the human mouth and intestines. **T. tenax** a nonpathogenic species found in the human mouth.

T. vaginalis a species causing trichomoniasis.

trichomoniasis (,trikohmə'nieəsis) a SEXUALLY TRANSMITTED DISEASE caused by *Trichomonas vaginalis.* In females, vaginal or urethral infections may be asymptomatic or may produce itching or burning, dysuria, and vaginal or urethral discharge. Infected males are usually asymptomatic carriers. Trichomonacides such as metronidazole are used in treatment. Both symptomatic patients and their sexual partners must be treated to avoid reinfection.

trichomycosis (,trikohmie'kohsis) any disease of the hair caused by fungi.

t. axillaris infection of the axillary and sometimes of the pubic hair, due to *Corynebacterium tenuis* and not a fungus, with development of clumps of bacteria on the hairs, appearing as red, yellow, or black nodules. Called also *lepothrix.*

trichonodosis (,trikohnoh'dohsis) a condition characterized by apparent or actual knotting of the hair.

trichopathy (tri'kopəthee) disease of the hair.

trichophytid (,trikoh'fietid) a secondary skin eruption that is the expression of an allergic reaction to a trichophyton infection and that occurs in an area remote from the site of infection.

trichophytin (,trikoh'fietin) a filtrate from cultures of *Trichophyton;* used in testing for trichophytosis.

trichophytobezoar (,trikoh,fietoh'beezor) a bezoar composed of animal hair and vegetable fibre.

Trichophyton (,trikoh'fieton) a genus of fungi that may cause various infections of the skin, hair, and nails.

trichophytosis (,trikohfie'tohsis) infection with fungi of the genus *Trichophyton.* adj. **trichophytic.**

trichoptilosis (,trikopti'lohsis) splitting of hairs at the end.

trichorrhexis (,trikə'reksis) the condition in which the hairs are split and feather-like.

t. nodosa bamboo hair; a condition marked by fracture and splitting of the cortex of a hair into strands, giving the appearance of white nodes at which the hair is easily broken.

trichoschisis (tri'koskisis) trichoptilosis.

trichoscopy (tri'koskəpee) examination of the hair.

trichosis (tri'kohsis) any disease or abnormal growth of the hair.

Trichosporon (trikoh'spor·ron) a genus of fungi that are normal flora of the respiratory and digestive tracts of man and animals, and may infect the hair.

trichosporosis (,trikohspə'rohsis) infection with *Trichosporon.*

trichostasis spinulosa (tri,kostəsis ,spinyuh'lohsə) obstruction of the hair follicles with a spinulous dark plug, consisting of many lanugo hairs in a horny mass, affecting the skin of the alae nasi and other facial areas, or of the arms, chest, abdomen, or interscapular area.

trichostrongyliasis, trichostrongylosis (,trikoh-,stronji'lieəsis; ,trikoh,stronji'lohsis) infection by nematodes of the genus *Trichostrongylus.*

Trichostrongylus (,trikoh'stronjiləs) a genus of nematode parasites infecting animals and man.

trichotillomania (,trikoh,tilə'mayni·ə) compulsion to pull out one's hair.

trichotomous (trie'kotəməs) divided into three parts.

trichroism ('triekroh,izəm, trie'kroh·izəm) the condition or quality of exhibiting three different colours when viewed from three different aspects. adj. **trichroic.**

trichromatopsia (,triekrohmə'topsi·ə) normal colour vision for all three primary colours, red, green, and blue.

trichrome ('triekrohm) a combination of dyes used to identify parenchyma, connective tissue, red blood cells, and fibrin by their distinctive coloration. The different trichromes, e.g., Masson, Goldner, Mallory, Picro-Mallory V, or MSB, produce particular combinations of colours in tissues.

trichromic (trie'krohmik) 1. pertaining to or exhibiting three colours. 2. able to distinguish only three of the seven colours of the spectrum.

trichuriasis (,trikyuh'rieəsis) infection with *Trichuris.*

Trichuris (tri'kyoo·ris) a genus of nematodes parasitic in the intestinal tract, including *T. trichiura,* the whipworm, found in man, which in heavy infections may cause diarrhoea, and, in children, rectal prolapse, but often produces no symptoms.

tricipital (trie'sipit'l) 1. three-headed. 2. relating to the triceps muscle.

triclofos ('triekloh,fos) a hypnotic and sedative.

tricornute (trie'kawnyoot) having three horns, cornua, or processes.

tricrotism ('triekro,tizəm) the quality of having three

sphygmographic waves or elevations to one beat of the pulse. adj. **tricrotic**.

tricuspid (trie'kuspid) having three points or cusps, as a valve of the heart.

t. valve the valve that guards the opening between the right atrium and right ventricle.

tricyclic (trie'sieklik) containing three fused rings in the molecular structure; see also ANTIDEPRESSANT.

tridactylism (trie'dakti,lizəm) the presence of only three digits on the hand or foot.

tridentate (trie'dentayt) having three prongs.

tridermic (trie'dərmik) derived from the ectoderm, entoderm, and mesoderm.

Tridil ('triedil) trademark for a preparation of glyceryl trinitrate.

triethanolamine (,trie·ethə'nolə,meen) trolamine.

trifid ('trifid) split into three parts.

trifluoperazine (,triefloo·oh'perə,zeen) a phenothiazine derivative; its hydrochloride salt is used as a major tranquillizer.

trifocal (trie'fohk'l) pertaining to a spectacle lens which has three foci, one for distant, one for intermediate and one for near vision.

trifurcation (,triefər'kayshən) division or the site of separation into three branches.

trigeminal (trie'jemin'l) 1. triple. 2. pertaining to the fifth cranial (trigeminal) nerve.

t. nerve the fifth cranial nerve; it arises in the pons, is composed of sensory and motor fibres, and has three divisions: ophthalmic, maxillary, and mandibular. The ophthalmic division supplies sensory fibres to the skin of the upper eyelid, side of the nose, forehead, and anterior half of the scalp. The maxillary division carries sensory impulses from the mucous membranes of the nose, the skin of the cheek and side of the forehead, and the upper lip and upper teeth. The mandibular division carries sensory impulses from the side of the head, chin, mucous membrane of the mouth, lower teeth, and anterior two-thirds of the tongue. (One can readily see why this nerve is sometimes called the great sensory nerve of the head.) The motor fibres are part of the mandibular branch and supply several of the muscles of chewing.

t. neuralgia pain arising from irritation of the fifth cranial (trigeminal) nerve. The disorder is characterized by brief attacks of severe pain in the face and forehead of the affected side. The cause is unknown. Many patients describe sensitive areas about the nose and mouth which, when touched, excite an attack. Attacks also may be brought on by exposure to cold, eating and drinking, and washing the face. Treatment may be palliative or surgical. Called also TIC DOULOUREUX.

trigeminy (trie'jeminee) the condition of occurring in threes, especially the occurrence of three pulse beats in rapid succession.

trigger finger ('trigə ,fing·gə) the temporary fixation of the finger in flexion, caused by stenosis of the flexor tendon sheath and secondary thickening of the tendon. A force from the opposite hand may be required to straighten the finger. A distinct snap is heard as the extended position is reached.

triglyceride (trie'glisə,ried) a compound consisting of three molecules of fatty acids bound with one molecule of glycerol; a neutral fat that is the usual storage form of lipids in animals.

Elevated serum triglycerides are now considered as important as high cholesterol levels in the development of ischaemic heart disease. The normal range for serum triglycerides is 0.4 to 1.5 g/l.

trigonal ('trigən'l) 1. triangular. 2. pertaining to a trigone.

trigone ('triegohn) 1. a triangular area. 2. the first three cusps of an upper molar tooth.

t. of bladder vesical trigone.

carotid t. the triangular area bounded by the posterior belly of the digastric muscle, the sternocleidomastoid muscle, and the anterior midline of the neck.

olfactory t. the triangular area of grey matter between the roots of the olfactory tract.

vesical t. a triangular region of the wall of the urinary bladder, the three angles corresponding with the orifices of the ureters and urethra; it is an area in which the muscle fibres are closely adherent to the mucosa and is more highly innervated than the rest of the bladder due to its embryonic origination. Faulty positioning of a self-retaining urinary catheter pressing on this area may cause severe pain. See also CATHETERIZATION.

trigonectomy (,triegoh'nektəmee) excision of the vesical trigone.

trigonitis (,triegoh'nietis) inflammation or localized hyperaemia of the vesical trigone.

trigonocephalus (,trigənoh'kefələs, -'sef-) an individual exhibiting trigonocephaly.

trigonocephaly (,trigənoh'kefəlee, -'sef-) triangular shape of the head due to sharp forward angulation at the midline of the frontal bone. adj. **trigonocephalic**.

trigonum (trie'gohnəm) pl. *trigona* [L.] trigone, or triangle; used in anatomical nomenclature to designate various regions or structures.

triiodothyronine (trie,ieədoh'thierə,neen) one of the thyroid hormones; an organic iodine-containing compound liberated from thyroglobulin by hydrolysis. It has several times the biological activity of thyroxine.

trilabe ('trielayb) a three-pronged lithotrite.

trilaminar (trie'laminə) three-layered.

trilobate (trie'lohbayt, 'trielə,bayt) having three lobes.

trilocular (trie'lokyuhlə) having three loculi or cells.

trilogy ('triləjee) a group or series of three.

t. of Fallot a term sometimes applied to concurrent pulmonary stenosis, atrial septal defect, and right ventricular hypertrophy.

trimanual (trie'manyooəl) accomplished by the use of three hands.

trimensual (trie'mensyooəl) occurring every 3 months.

trimeprazine (trie'meprə,zeen) a drug with mild central nervous depressant, moderate antiemetic and anticonvulsant, and powerful antihistaminic action; used as an antipruritic in the form of the tartrate salt.

trimester (trie'mestə) a period of 3 months.

trimethaphan (trie'methəfan) a compound used in ganglionic blockade and as an antihypertensive.

trimethoprim (trie'methohprim) an antibacterial closely related to pyrimethamine; sometimes administered in combination with a sulphonamide because these drugs blockade two consecutive steps in the synthesis of tetrahydrofolate by microorganisms; used primarily for the treatment of urinary tract infections.

trimipramine (trie'miprə,meen) a tricyclic antidepressant used for treatment of major depression.

trimorphous (trie'mawfəs) existing in three different forms.

trinitrophenol (trie,nietroh'feenol) a substance used as dye, tissue fixative, antiseptic, astringent, and stimulant of epithelialization; it can be detonated on percussion or by heating above 300 °C. Called also *picric acid*.

trinitrotoluene (trie,nietroh'tolyoo,een) a high explosive derived from toluene; abbreviated TNT. It sometimes causes poisoning in those who work with it, marked by dermatitis, gastritis, abdominal pain, vomiting, constipation, and flatulence.

Trinordil (trie'nordil) trademark for a combination

preparation of ethinyloestradiol and levonorgestrel, an oral contraceptive.

triocephalus (ˌtrieoh'kefələs, -'sef-) a fetus or infant with no organs of sight, hearing, or smell, the head being a nearly shapeless mass.

triol ('trieol) an organic compound containing three hydroxy groups, a trihydric alcohol, e.g., glycerol.

triolism ('trieohˌlizəm) sexual interests or practices involving three persons of both sexes.

triorchidism (trie'awkiˌdizəm) the presence of three testes.

triose ('trieohz) a monosaccharide containing three carbon atoms in a molecule.

tripelennamine (ˌtriepə'lenəˌmeen) an antihistaminic used orally, parenterally, and topically in the symptomatic treatment of various allergic disorders.

tripeptide (trie'peptied) a peptide formed from three amino acids.

triphalangism (ˌtriefə'lanˌjizəm) three phalanges in a digit normally having only two.

triphasic (trie'fayzik) having three phases.

triphenylmethane (triˌfeenil'meethayn) a substance from coal tar, the basis of various dyes and stains, including aurin, rosaniline, basic fuchsin, and gentian violet.

triplegia (trie'pleeji·ə) paralysis of three extremities.

triplet ('triplit) 1. one of three offspring produced at one birth. 2. a combination of three objects or entities acting together, as three lenses or three nucleotides.

triplex ('tripleks) triple or threefold.

triploid ('triployd) having triple the haploid number of chromosomes (3n).

triplokoria (ˌtriploh'kor·ri·ə) the presence of three pupils in an eye.

triplopia (tri'plohpi·ə) defective vision, objects being seen as threefold; usually a hysterical symptom.

triprolidine (trie'prohliˌdeen) a compound used as an antihistamine.

-tripsy word element. [Gr.] *crushing;* used to designate a surgical procedure in which a structure is intentionally crushed.

Triptafen ('triptəfen) trademark for a fixed combination preparation of perphenazine and amitriptyline hydrochloride; a tranquillizer.

tripus ('triepəs) a conjoined twin fetus having three feet.

trisaccharide (trie'sakəˌried) a sugar, each molecule of which yields three molecules of monosaccharides on hydrolysis.

trismus ('trizməs) motor disturbance of the trigeminal nerve, especially spasm of the masticatory muscles, with difficulty in opening the mouth (lockjaw); a characteristic early symptom of tetanus.

trisomy ('triesəmee) the presence of an additional (third) CHROMOSOME of one type in an otherwise diploid cell (2n + 1). adj. **trisomic.**

t. 8 syndrome a syndrome associated with an extra chromosome 8, usually mosaic (trisomy 8/normal), characterized by mild to severe mental handicap, prominent forehead, deep-set eyes, thick lips, prominent ears, and camptodactyly.

t. 13 syndrome holoprosencephaly due to an extra chromosome 13, in which central nervous system defects are associated with mental handicap, along with cleft lip and palate, polydactyly, and dermal pattern anomalies, and abnormalities of the heart, viscera, and genitalia. *Called also Patau's syndrome.*

t. 18 syndrome a condition due to the presence of an extra chromosome 18, characterized by neonatal hepatitis, mental handicap, scaphocephaly or other skull abnormality, micrognathia, blepharoptosis, low-set ears, corneal opacities, deafness, webbed neck, short digits, ventricular septal defects, Meckel's diverticulum, and other deformities. Called also *Edwards' syndrome.*

t. 21 syndrome Down's syndrome.

t. 22 syndrome a syndrome due to an extra chromosome 22, characterized typically by mental handicap and growth retardation, microcephaly, low-set or malformed ears, micrognathia, long philtrum, preauricular skin tag or sinus, and congenital heart disease. In males, there is small penis or undescended testes.

trisplanchnic (trie'splangknik) pertaining to the three great visceral cavities, the skull, thorax, and abdomen.

tristichia (trie'stiki·ə) the presence of three rows of eyelashes.

trisulcate (trie'sulkayt) having three furrows.

trisulphide (trie'sulfied) a sulphur compound containing three atoms of sulphur.

tritanomalopia (ˌtritəˌnomə'lohpi·ə) a rare form of defective colour vision, similar to but milder than tritanopia, in which there is decreased sensitivity to, rather than absence of, blue-sensitive visual pigment. adj. **tritanomalous.**

tritanomaly (tritə'nomələe) tritanomalopia.

tritanope ('tritəˌnohp) a person exhibiting tritanopia.

tritanopia (ˌtritə'nohpi·ə) defective colour vision in which the blue-sensitive pigment of the retinal cones is absent. adj. **tritanopic.**

tritium ('triti·əm) the mass 3 isotope of hydrogen, symbol ^{3}H or T, obtained by bombardment of beryllium in the cyclotron with deuterium ions. It has a half-life of about 31 years, and is used as an indicator or tracer in metabolic studies.

triturable ('trityuhrəb'l) susceptible of being triturated.

triturate ('trityuhˌrayt) 1. to reduce to powder by rubbing. 2. a substance powdered fine by rubbing.

trituration (ˌtrityuh'rayshən) 1. reduction to powder by friction or grinding. 2. a finely powdered substance.

triturator ('trityuhˌraytə) an apparatus in which substances can be continuously rubbed.

trivalent (trie'vaylənt) having a valency of three.

tRNA transfer RNA (ribonucleic acid).

trocar ('trohkah) a sharp-pointed instrument equipped with a cannula; used to puncture the wall of a body cavity or a cyst and withdraw fluid.

Duchenne's t. a trocar for obtaining specimens of deep-seated tissues.

trochanter (troh'kantə) a broad, flat process on the femur, at the upper end of its lateral surface (greater trochanter), or a short conical process on the posterior border of the base of its neck (lesser trochanter). adj. **trochanteric, trochanterian.**

troche ('trohkee) a medicinal preparation for solution in the mouth, consisting of an active ingredient incorporated in a mass made of sugar and mucilage or fruit base.

trochlea ('trokli·ə) pl. *trochleae* [L.] a pulley-shaped part or structure; used in anatomical nomenclature to designate various bony or fibrous structures through or over which tendons pass or with which other structures articulate.

trochlear ('trokli·ə) 1. pertaining to a trochlea. 2. pertaining to the fourth cranial (trochlear) nerve.

t. nerve the fourth cranial nerve; it supplies muscle sense and the impulse for movement to the superior oblique muscle of the eyeball.

trochocephaly (ˌtrokoh'kefəlee, -'sef-) a rounded appearance of the head due to synostosis of the frontal and parietal bones.

trochoid ('trohkoyd) pivot-like, or pulley-shaped.

trochoides (troh'koydeez) a pivot joint.

Troisier's node ('twahziˌayz) an enlarged supraclavicular lymph node, often the first sign of a malignant abdominal tumour. Called also *sentinel node* or *signal* *node.*

Trombicula (trom'bikyuhlə) a genus of mites (family Trombiculidae), including *T. akamushi*, and *T. deliensis*, whose larvae (CHIGGERS) are vectors of *Rickettsia tsutsugamushi*, the cause of scrub typhus.

trombiculiasis (trom,bikyuh'lieəsis) infestation with mites of the genus *Trombicula.*

Trombiculidae (,trombikyuh'liedee) a family of mites cosmopolitan in distribution, whose parasitic larvae (CHIGGERS) infest vertebrates.

troph(o)- word element. [Gr.] *food, nourishment.*

trophectoderm (tro'fektoh,dərm) the earliest trophoblast.

trophesy ('trofəsee) defective nutrition due to disorder of the trophic nerves.

trophic ('trofik) pertaining to nutrition.

-trophic, -trophin word element. [Gr.] *nourishing, stimulating.*

trophoblast ('trofoh,blast) the peripheral cells of the blastocyst, which attach the fertilized ovum to the uterine wall and become the placenta and the membranes that nourish and protect the developing organism. The inner cellular layer is the cytotrophoblast and the outer layer is the syntrophoblast.

trophoblastoma (,trofohbla'stohmə) choriocarcinoma.

trophodermatoneurosis (,trofoh,dərmətohnyuh'rohsis) acrodynia.

trophoedema (,trofi'deemə) a chronic disease with permanent oedema of the feet or legs.

trophology (tro'foləjee) the science of nutrition of the body.

trophoneurosis (,trofohnyuh'rohsis) any functional nervous disease due to failure of nutrition from defective nerve influence. adj. **trophoneurotic.**

trophonosis (,trofə'nohsis) any disease due to nutritional causes.

trophonucleus (,trofoh'nyookli·əs) macronucleus.

trophopathy (tro'fopəthee) any derangement of nutrition.

trophoplast ('trofoh,plast) a granular protoplasmic body.

trophotaxis (,trofoh'taksis) taxis in relation to nutritive materials.

trophotherapy (,trofoh'therəpee) treatment of disease by dietary measures.

trophozoite (,trofoh'zoh·iet) the active, motile feeding stage of a sporozoan parasite.

tropia ('trohpi·ə) a manifest deviation of an eye from the normal position when both eyes are open and uncovered. See also STRABISMUS.

-tropic word element. [Gr.] *turning toward, changing, tending to turn or change.*

tropical ('tropik'l) pertaining to the tropics, the regions of the earth lying between the tropic of Cancer north of the Equator and the tropic of Capricorn south of it.

t. anhidrotic asthenia a condition due to inhibition of sweating after prolonged exposure to high temperatures.

tropine ('trohpeen) a crystalline alkaloid from atropine and various plants.

tropism ('trohpizəm) a growth response in a nonmotile organism elicited by an external stimulus, and either toward (positive tropism) or away from (negative tropism) the stimulus; used as a word element combined with a stem indicating nature of the stimulus (e.g., phototropism) or material or entity for which an organism (or substance) shows a special affinity (e.g., neurotropism).

tropocollagen (,trohpoh'koləjən) the molecular unit of all forms of collagen; it is a helical structure of three polypeptides.

tropomyosin (,trohpoh'mieəsin) a muscle protein of the I band that inhibits contraction by blocking the interaction of actin and myosin, except when influenced by troponin.

troponin ('trohpənin) a complex of muscle proteins which, when combined with Ca^{2+}, influence tropomyosin to initiate contraction.

Trousseau's sign ('troosohz) 1. spontaneous peripheral venous thrombosis, suggestive of visceral carcinoma, especially carcinoma of the pancreas. 2. a sign for tetany in which carpal spasm can be elicited by compressing the upper arm and causing ischaemia to the nerves distally.

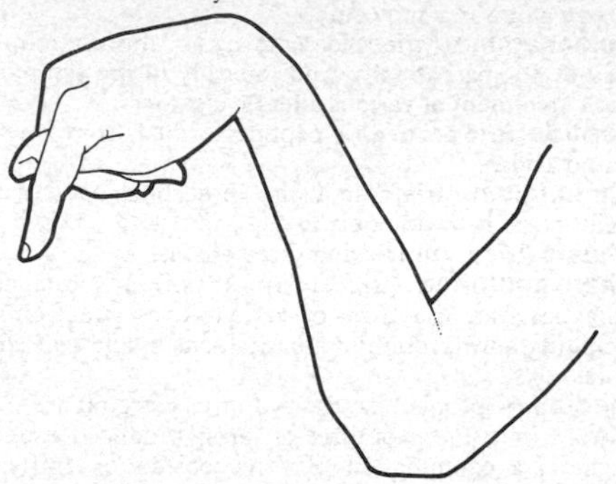

Trousseau's sign (carpopedal spasm) with hypocalcaemia.

Trousseau's syndrome spontaneous venous thrombosis of the upper and lower extremities occurring in association with visceral carcinoma.

truancy ('trooənsee) absence of a child from school without leave. A disorder of conduct which may result from emotional insecurity or a feeling of unfairness.

truncate (trung'kayt, 'trungkayt) 1. to amputate; to deprive of limbs. 2. having the end cut squarely off.

truncus ('trungkəs) pl. *trunci* [L.] trunk; used in anatomical nomenclature.

t. arteriosus an artery connected with the fetal heart, developing into the aortic and pulmonary arches.

t. brachiocephalicus a vessel arising from the arch of the aorta and giving origin to the right common carotid and right subclavian arteries.

t. coeliacus coeliac trunk.

t. pulmonalis pulmonary trunk.

trunk (trungk) the main part, as the part of the body to which the head and limbs are attached, or a larger structure (e.g., vessel or nerve) from which smaller divisions or branches arise, or which is created by their union. adj. **truncal.**

coeliac t. the arterial trunk arising from the abdominal aorta and giving origin to the left gastric, common hepatic, and splenic arteries.

lumbosacral t. a trunk formed by union of the lower part of ventral branch of the fourth lumbar nerve with the ventral branch of the fifth lumbar nerve.

pulmonary t. a vessel arising from the conus arteriosus of the right ventricle and bifurcating into the right and left pulmonary arteries.

sympathetic t. two long ganglionated nerve strands, one on each side of the vertebral column, extending from the base of the skull to the coccyx.

truss (trus) an elastic, canvas, or metallic device for retaining a reduced hernia within the abdominal cavity.

trypanocidal (,tripənoh'sied'l) destructive to trypanosomes.

trypanolysis (,tripə'nolisis) the destruction of trypanosomes. adj. **trypanolytic.**

Trypanosoma (,tripənoh'sohmə) a multispecies genus

of protozoa parasitic in the blood and lymph of invertebrates and vertebrates, including man; most species live part of their life cycle in the intestines of insects and other invertebrates, the typical adult stage being found only in the vertebrate host. Trypanosomal infections of man include Gambian and Rhodesian forms of African trypanosomiasis (caused by *T. gambiense* and *T. rhodesiense*, respectively) and South American trypanosomiasis (caused by *T. cruzi*). Other species cause serious diseases of domestic animals, including *T. brucei*, *T. congolense*, *T. evansi*, etc.

trypanosome ('tripənoh,sohm) an individual of the genus *Trypanosoma*. adj. **trypanosomal, trypanosomic.**

trypanosomiasis (,tripənohsə'mieəsis) infection with trypanosomes, parasitic protozoa found in the blood and lymph of infected animals and humans.

African t. a fatal disease of Africa caused by *Trypanosoma gambiense* or *T. rhodesiense* and involving the central nervous system. The parasites are transmitted to man from man (*T. gambiense*) or from man, cattle or other animals by the bite of the tsetse fly (*T. rhodesiense*). Usually the first symptom is inflammation at the site of the bite, appearing within 48 hours. Within several weeks the parasites invade the blood and lymph; eventually they attack the central nervous system. Characteristic symptoms include intermittent fever, rapid heartbeat, and enlargement of the lymph nodes and spleen. In the advanced stage of the disease there are personality changes, apathy, sleepiness, disturbances of speech and gait, and severe emaciation. Known also as SLEEPING SICKNESS.

Suramin, pentamidine isethionate, and melarsoprol are used in the treatment of African trypanosomiasis. Prevention includes injections of pentamidine isethionate or suramin to remove the parasites from the blood or lymph nodes, but the most effective measure would be eradication of the tsetse fly. See also GLOSSINA.

South American t. a form found in Mexico and Central and South America, caused by *Trypanosoma cruzi*; called also *Chagas' disease*. It is transmitted from wild animals by means of the faeces of a blood-sucking bug. The parasites multiply around the points of entry before entering the blood and eventually attacking the heart, brain, and other tissues.

The acute form usually attacks children. Early symptoms include swelling of the eyelids and the development of a hard, red, painful nodule on the skin. Enlargement of the lymph nodes, liver, and spleen occurs, along with inflammation of the heart muscle, psychological changes, and general debility. In adults the chronic form often resembles heart disease.

Preventive measures, such as the improvement of housing conditions, the wearing of protective clothing, and the use of insecticides, are of primary importance since there are no effective drugs for treatment.

trypanosomicide (,tripənoh'sohmi,sied) 1. lethal to trypanosomes. 2. an agent lethal to trypanosomes.

trypanosomid (,tripənoh'sohmid) a skin eruption occurring in trypanosomiasis.

trypsin ('tripsin) a proteolytic enzyme formed in the intestine by the cleavage of trypsinogen by enterokinase. It is an endopeptidase that hydrolyses peptides of arginine or lysine.

trypsinogen (trip'sinəjən) the inactive precursor of trypsin, secreted by the pancreas and activated to trypsin by contact with enterokinase.

tryptic ('triptik) relating to or resulting from digestion by trypsin.

Tryptizol ('triptizol) trademark for preparations of amitriptyline hydrochloride, an antidepressant.

tryptophan ('triptə,fan) a naturally occurring amino acid, existing in proteins and essential for human metabolism.

tryptophanase (,triptə'fanayz) an enzyme that catalyses the cleavage of tryptophan into indole, pyruvic acid, and ammonia.

tryptophanuria (,triptohfə'nyooə·ri·ə) excessive urinary excretion of tryptophan.

TSE testicular self-examination.

tsetse ('tetsee, 'tse-) an African fly of the genus *Glossina*, which transmits trypanosomiasis.

TSH thyroid-stimulating hormone (thyrotrophin, thyrotrophic hormone).

tsutsugamushi fever (disease) (,tsootsoogə'mooshee) scrub typhus.

TU tuberculin unit.

tuba ('tyoobə) pl. *tubae* [L.] tube.

tubal ('tyoob'l) relating to a tube.

t. pregnancy extrauterine pregnancy where the embryo develops in the uterine tube; an example of ectopic pregnancy.

tube (tyoob) a hollow cylindrical organ or instrument. adj. **tubal.**

auditory t. the narrow channel connecting the middle ear and nasopharynx (see also PHARYNGOTYMPANIC TUBE).

chest t. one or more tubes inserted into the pleural space to provide relief from either PNEUMOTHORAX or accumulations of fluid within the thoracic cavity and to allow for re-expansion of the lung (see also CHEST drain).

drainage t. a tube used in surgery to facilitate escape of fluids.

endobronchial t. a double-lumen tube inserted into the bronchus of one lung, permitting complete deflation of the other lung; used in anaesthesia for thoracic surgery.

endotracheal t. a tube inserted into the trachea either via the nose or mouth. It may have an inflatable cuff. See also ENDOTRACHEAL TUBE.

eustachian t. the narrow channel connecting the middle ear and the nasopharynx (see also PHARYNGOTYMPANIC TUBE).

fallopian t. uterine tube.

feeding t. one for introducing nutritious fluids into the stomach. A fine-bore feeding tube, which is made of a soft, flexible material such as polyurethane and has an internal diameter of approximately 1 mm, is introduced into the stomach via the nose, using a flexible guide-wire inside the tube. The guide-wire is removed when the tube is in position.

fermentation t. a U-shaped tube with one end closed, for determining gas production by bacteria.

grommet drain t. a double-cuffed tube that is inserted in the eardrum (tympanic membrane) to allow drainage of fluid from the middle ear in secretory otitis media.

intubation t. a breathing tube introduced through the vocal cords into the trachea.

nasogastric t. a tube of soft rubber or plastic inserted through a nostril and into the stomach, for instilling liquid foods or other substances, or for withdrawing gastric contents. See also TUBE FEEDING.

neural t. the epithelial tube produced by folding of the neural plate in the early embryo.

otopharyngeal t. auditory tube.

photomultiplier t. a vacuum tube that produces an electric current proportional to the intensity of light falling on its photocathode; it is sensitive enough to detect single photons.

Ryle's t. a trademark for a nasogastric tube (see also NASOGASTRIC TUBE).

Sengstaken–Blakemore t. an instrument used for tamponade of bleeding oesophageal varices (see also SENGSTAKEN–BLAKEMORE TUBE).

stomach t. one that is passed through the oesophagus to the stomachfor gastric analysis or lavage (see also STOMACH TUBE).

test t. a tube of thin glass, closed at one end; used in chemical tests and other laboratory procedures.

thoracostomy t. one inserted through an opening in the chest wall for drainage of the pleural cavity or to facilitate reexpansion of the lung in spontaneous pneumothorax (see also CHEST drain).

tracheostomy t. a curved tube that is inserted into the trachea through the opening made in the neck at TRACHEOSTOMY.

uterine t. a slender tube extending laterally from the uterus toward the ovary on the same side, conveying ova to the cavity of the uterus and permitting passage of spermatozoa in the opposite direction; called also *fallopian tube* (see also UTERINE TUBE).

tube feeding administration of liquid and semisolid foods through a nasogastric, gastrostomy, or enterostomy tube. Nasogastric tube feedings are administered to patients who are unable to take foods by mouth. These would include psychiatric patients who refuse to eat, debilitated and elderly patients who cannot swallow, and the newborn preterm infant who has immature swallowing and gag reflexes. Gastrostomy tube feedings are administered directly into the stomach via a gastrostomy tube. Enterostomy tube feedings are administered into the small intestine to patients who are unable to take food into the stomach.

PATIENT CARE. The major goal of care of a patient being fed by tube is prevention of dehydration, starvation, and subsequent fluid and electrolyte disturbances. This is particularly true in cases of prolonged tube feeding, in which there is always the possibility that fluid and electrolyte imbalances may become serious enough to present neurological symptoms and even death. Early detection and correction of dehydration depend on careful monitoring of the patient and periodic evaluation of electrolyte status through laboratory tests. Patients receiving tube feedings are not always aware of thirst or are unable to communicate their desire for water.

The social aspect of meal times should not be ignored and, where possible, the nurse should aim to sit down and converse with the patient during the tube feedings.

All tube-fed patients require good mouth care. If the feeding is through a nasogastric tube, the patient will be forced to breathe through his mouth which contributes to dryness of the oral mucosa. Adequate mouth care can help in differentiating between thirst due to dryness of the mouth and thirst resulting from systemic dehydration.

tubectomy (tyoo'bektəmee) excision of a portion of the uterine tube.

tuber ('tyoobə) a swelling or protuberance.

t. cinereum an area of the undersurface of the forebrain to which the stalk of the pituitary gland is attached.

tubercle ('tyoobək'l) 1. a small, rounded nodule produced by the bacillus of tuberculosis (*Mycobacterium tuberculosis*). It is made up of small spherical cells that contain giant cells and are surrounded by spindle-shaped epithelioid cells. 2. a nodule or small eminence, especially one on a bone, for attachment of a tendon. adj. **tubercular.**

fibrous t. a tubercle of bacillary origin that contains connective tissue elements.

mental t. a prominence on the inner border of either side of the mental protuberance of the mandible.

miliary t. one of the many minute tubercles formed in many organs in acute miliary tuberculosis.

pubic t. a prominent tubercle at the lateral end of the pubic crest.

supraglenoid t. one on the scapula for attachment of the long head of the biceps muscle.

tubercular (tyuh'bərkyuhlə) pertaining to tubercles.

tuberculate, tuberculated (tyuh'bərkyuhlət; tyuh'bərkyuh,laytid) covered or affected with tubercles.

tuberculid (tyuh'bərkyuhlid) a papular skin eruption usually attributed to allergy to tuberculosis.

papulonecrotic t. an eruption of crops of deep-seated papules or nodules, with central necrosis or ulceration.

tuberculigenous (tyuh,bərkyuh'lijənəs) causing tuberculosis.

tuberculin (tyuh'bərkyuhlin) a sterile liquid containing the growth products of, or specific substances extracted from, the tubercle bacillus; used in various forms in the diagnosis of tuberculosis.

New T. a suspension of the fragments of tubercle bacilli, freed from all soluble materials and with glycerin added.

Old T. a sterile solution of concentrated, soluble products of the growth of the tubercle bacillus, adjusted to standard potency by addition of glycerin and isotonic sodium chloride solution, the final glycerin content being about 50 per cent.

purified protein derivative (PPD) of t. a sterile, soluble, partially purified product of the growth of the tubercle bacillus in a special liquid medium free from protein.

tuberculitis (tyuh,bərkyuh'lietis) inflammation of or near a tubercle.

tuberculocele (tyuh'bərkyuhloh,seel) tuberculous disease of a testis.

tuberculofibroid (tyuh,bərkyuhloh'fiebroyd) characterized by a tubercle that has undergone fibroid degeneration.

tuberculoid (tyuh'bərkyuh,loyd) resembling a tubercle or tuberculosis.

tuberculoma (tyuh,bərkyuh'lohmə) a tumour-like mass resulting from enlargement of a caseated tuberculous granuloma.

tuberculosilicosis (tyuh,bərkyuhloh,sili'kohsis) silicosis complicated by pulmonary tuberculosis.

tuberculosis (tyuh,bərkyuh'lohsis) an infectious, inflammatory, notifiable disease that is chronic in nature and commonly affects the lungs (pulmonary tuberculosis), although it may occur in almost any part of the body.

The causative agent is the tubercle bacillus (*Mycobacterium tuberculosis*). Until recently, the only other mycobacteria thought to be pathogenic to humans were *M. bovis* and *M. avium.* It is now known that other 'atypical' mycobacteria can produce diseases similar to true tuberculosis.

The most common mode of transmission of tuberculosis in the United Kingdom is inhalation of infected droplet nuclei. In some other parts of the world bovine tuberculosis, which is carried by milk and other dairy products from tuberculous cattle, is more prevalent. A rare mode of transmission is by infected urine, especially for young children using the same toilet facilities.

The tubercle bacillus is capable of surviving for months in dried sputum that is not exposed to sunlight. Within the body it can lie dormant for decades and then become reactivated years after an initial infection. This secondary tuberculosis infection (endogenous reinfection) can occur at any time the patient's resistance is lowered. For this reason, periodic evaluation for evidence of the disease is extremely important for anyone who has had a primary tuberculosis infection.

The tubercle bacillus is destroyed by boiling for 5 minutes, by autoclaving, by contact with coal tar preparations, e.g., phenol, and by ultraviolet radiation.

Primary and Secondary Tuberculosis. The first or primary infection with tuberculosis bacilli usually presents no symptoms. In about 99 per cent of those who are infected, the disease remains quiescent after the development of a hypersensitivity to the tuberculin microorganism and is no longer clinically significant.

The primary infection usually involves the middle or upper lung area. (See also GHON FOCUS.) The primary lesion consists of a small area of exudation in the lung parenchyma which quickly becomes caseous (cheese-like) and spreads to the bronchopulmonary lymph nodes, where it gains access to the blood stream. Thus the stage is set for the development of a chronic pulmonary and extrapulmonary tuberculosis at a later time. In most instances, however, a secondary reinfection from inside the body (endogenous) or outside the body (exogenous) does not occur because of the subsequent development of tuberculin hypersensitivity and cellular immunity. The presence of antigen concentrations at the initial site of infection brings about necrosis and eventually fibrosis and calcification of the tissues, which arrests the infection and renders the disease inactive. If, however, the infection is not controlled, the patient develops the symptoms of progressive primary tuberculosis.

Secondary tuberculosis develops as a result of either endogenous or exogenous reinfection by the tubercle bacillus. This is the most common form of clinical tuberculosis. In the United Kingdom development of secondary tuberculosis is almost always the result of an endogenous reinfection, which occurs when the primary lesion becomes active. This most frequently happens in debilitated persons who have lowered resistance to disease.

Resistance to tuberculosis depends on the general health and living conditions of the individual. Poor health, crowded and unsanitary housing, malnutrition, and other illnesses can lower the body's defences. A second factor that can lead to activation of the disease is frequent exposure to the bacilli or exposure to such numbers that even a healthy person cannot escape infection.

Tuberculin Testing. Within 3 to 10 days after the initial entry of the tubercle bacillus into the body, a sensitivity to the bacillus is present in all of the body cells. This sensitivity is the basis of tuberculin testing.

The most commonly used test is the MANTOUX TEST, which consists of an intradermal injection of a purified protein derivative of tuberculin. An indurated area (wheal) of 8 to 10 mm in diameter 48 to 72 hours after injection is considered positive. Induration must be present; a reddened area is not indicative of a positive reaction. If the test is positive for tuberculin sensitivity, further studies, including radiographs, are indicated before a definite diagnosis of tuberculosis is established. False negative results can occur with acute viral infections and some neoplastic diseases, e.g., Hodgkin's disease. See also IMMUNIZATION for the recommended tuberculin testing of children.

Symptoms. A child or young person with active tuberculosis usually suffers from one or more of the following symptoms: loss of energy, poor appetite, loss of weight, and fever. Even though these symptoms may have causes other than tuberculosis, they must be regarded as warning signals.

In adults, listlessness and vague pains in the chest may go unnoticed, since they are often not severe enough to attract attention. Unfortunately, the symptoms that most people associate with tuberculosis—cough, expectoration of purulent sputum, fever, night sweats, and haemorrhage from the lungs—do not appear in the early, most easily curable stage of the disease; often their appearance is delayed until a year or more after the initial exposure to the bacilli.

Chronic pulmonary tuberculosis is often accompanied by pleurisy. Pleurisy with effusion often is the first symptom of tuberculosis. In certain cases, complications are possible and each has its characteristic symptoms. At a fairly late stage, the tuberculosis bacillus may cause ulcers or inflammation around the larynx (tuberculous laryngitis). Less often, tuberculous ulcers form on the tongue or tonsils. Sometimes intestinal infections develop; they are probably caused by swallowed bacteria-contaminated sputum. A most serious complication is the sudden collapse of a lung, the indication that a deep tuberculous cavity in the lung has perforated, or opened into the pleural cavity, allowing air and infected material to flow into it.

When a fairly large and previously walled-off lesion, or infected area, suddenly discharges its contents into the bronchial tree, the result is the infection of a large part of the lung, an acute and dangerous complication which causes tuberculous pneumonia.

Tuberculosis bacilli can spread to other parts of the body by way of the blood, producing the condition called miliary tuberculosis. When a large number of bacilli suddenly enter the circulatory system, they are carried to all areas of the body and may lodge in any organ. Minute tubercles form in the tissues of the organs affected; these lesions are about the size of a pinhead or millet seed (hence the name 'miliary'). Unless promptly treated, and occasionally even then, the tiny lesions spread, join, and produce larger areas of infection.

Tuberculous pneumonia can begin in this way, as can tuberculosis of any other organ. Miliary infections involving the meninges produce a particularly serious disease; indeed, until the development of antibiotics and similar medicines, this condition nearly always proved fatal.

Practically all parts and organs of the body can be secondarily invaded by tubercle bacilli, a common type being involvement of the kidneys, which often spreads to the bladder and genitalia. Bone involvement, particularly of the spine (POTT'S DISEASE), was once common, especially among children.

Lupus, or lupus vulgaris, tuberculosis of the skin, is characterized by brown nodules on the dermis; another form of tuberculosis of the skin is tuberculosis indurativa, a chronic disease in which indurated nodules form on the skin. When the adrenal glands are affected by tuberculosis, a rare occurrence, the condition can cause ADDISON'S DISEASE.

Treatment and Care. Most tuberculous patients are cared for at home under supervision. Hospitalization may be required for those patients who experience complications or who are beginning chemotherapy. The length of stay varies, but the advent of effective drug therapy has all but eradicated lengthy stays at special sanitoria and hospitals.

During hospitalization the patient should be taught how the disease is transmitted and how he can avoid spreading the infection to others. Patient education also should include information on the importance of a well-balanced diet and good health habits in the control of his disease.

It should be remembered that tuberculosis is an airborne infection. The patient's room should be adequately ventilated, but with the door to the hall kept closed. Ultraviolet radiation is most effective in decontamination. Masks may be necessary for those having intimate contact with a patient who is just beginning chemotherapy, and in caring for patients who cannot or will not take precautions against spreading the infection. Handwashing is essential to prevention of cross-infection. Fomites are not considered important in the transmission of tuberculosis and so no special precautions are required for eating utensils and other inanimate articles in the patient's room.

Drugs. Combination therapy with 3 or 4 drugs is now routine. Isoniazid, rifampicin and ethambutol are the mainstays of treatment, with pyrazinamide added as the fourth drug in some regimens. Streptomycin is still an important drug but tends to be reserved for infections which are resistant to any of the above agents, or when side-effects prevent their use. Treatment is usually continued for 9 months, with careful observation and follow up.

Surgical Procedures. In the past, the isolation hospital rest cure was frequently augmented by one of the surgical procedures which aid healing by resting an infected lung for a period of time.

The best-known of these operations, artificial pneumothorax, involved collapsing the lung by injecting air into the pleural cavity. A lung could also be rested by inactivating the phrenic nerve, which carries impulses to the diaphragm from the brain and so helps to control breathing; if the left or right phrenic nerve is inactivated, the diaphragm and lung on the same side will not move.

With the successful treatment of tuberculosis by the new drugs, these operations have become obsolete.

PREVENTION. Tuberculosis is one of the most easily avoided of all the serious diseases. The best precautions are (1) maintenance of good health, (2) avoidance of unnecessary exposure to tuberculosis organisms, and (3) detection of the disease in its earliest stages.

BCG Vaccine. Some success in preventing tuberculosis has been attained by vaccination with BCG (bacille Calmette-Guérin)—a vaccine evolved from strains of *Mycobacterium tuberculosis* taken from cattle. It provides at least partial immunity in most people, although it takes about 2 months to do so. BCG is recommended for those repeatedly exposed to tuberculosis, such as health professionals, travellers to high-prevalence areas, contacts, people living in communities where there is a high incidence of infection, and, at the current time, school-children aged 11 to 13 years, although this is being carefully reviewed with a view to dicontinuation once infection rates are reduced to an acceptable level. After vaccination with BCG, the patient will have a positive response to the tuberculin test. See also BCG VACCINE.

avian t. a form affecting various birds, due to *Mycobacterium avium*, which may be communicated to man and other animals.

bovine t. an infection of cattle caused by *Mycobacterium bovis*, transmissible to man and other animals.

endogenous t. that arising from within the body and transmitted by blood to another organ.

exogenous t. that arising from a source outside the body.

haematogenous t. that carried through the bloodstream to other organs from the primary site of infection.

open t. 1. that in which there are lesions from which tubercle bacilli are being discharged out of the body. 2. tuberculosis of the lungs with cavitation. **t. verrucosa, warty t.** a condition usually resulting from external inoculation of the tubercle bacilli into the skin, with wartlike papules coalescing to form distinctly verrucous patches with an inflammatory, erythematous border.

tuberculostatic (tyuh,bərkyuhloh'statik) 1. inhibiting the growth of *Mycobacterium tuberculosis.* 2. a tuberculostatic agent.

tuberculotic (tyuh,bərkyuh'lotik) pertaining to or affected with tuberculosis.

tuberculous (tyuh'bərkyuhləs) pertaining to or affected with tuberculosis; caused by *Mycobacterium tuberculosis.*

tuberculum (tyuh'bərkyuhləm) pl. *tubercula* [L.] a tubercle, nodule, or small eminence; used in anatomical nomenclature to designate principally a small eminence on a bone.

tuberosis (,tyoobə'rohsis) a condition characterized by the presence of nodules.

tuberositas (,tyoobə'rositas) pl. *tuberositates* [L.] tuberosity; used in anatomical nomenclature to designate elevations on bones to which muscles are attached.

tuberosity (,tyoobə'rositee) an elevation or protuberance.

tuberous ('tyoobə·rəs) covered with tubers; knobby.

t. sclerosis a familial disease with tumours on the surfaces of the lateral ventricles of the brain and sclerotic patches on its surface, and marked by mental deterioration and epileptic attacks.

tubo- word element. [L.] *tube.*

tubocurarine (,tyoobohkyoo'rahreen) an alkaloid from the bark and stems of *Chondrodendron tomentosum*, used as a skeletal muscle relaxant.

tuboligamentous (,tyooboh,ligə'mentəs) pertaining to the uterine tube and broad ligament.

tubo-ovarian (,tyooboh·oh'vair·ri·ən) pertaining to the uterine tube and ovary.

tuboperitoneal (,tyooboh,peritə'neeəl) pertaining to the uterine tube and the peritoneum.

tuboplasty ('tyooboh,plastee) 1. salpingoplasty. 2. plastic repair of a tube, such as the pharyngotympanic tube.

tubouterine (,tyooboh'yootə,rien) pertaining to the uterine tube and uterus.

tubule ('tyoobyool) a small tube. adj. **tubular.**

collecting t's the terminal channels of the nephrons which open on the summits of the renal pyramids in the renal papillae.

convoluted t's channels that follow a tortuous course; there are convoluted renal tubules and convoluted seminiferous tubules.

dentinal t's the tubular structures of the teeth.

galactophorous t's small channels for the passage of milk from the secreting cells in the mammary gland.

Henle's t's the straight ascending and descending portions of a renal tubule forming Henle's loop.

lactiferous t's galactophorous tubules. **mesonephric t's** the tubules comprising the mesonephros, or temporary kidney, of amniotes.

metanephric t's the tubules comprising the permanent kidney of amniotes.

renal t's the minute canals made up of basement membrane and lined with epithelium, composing the substance of the kidney and secreting, collecting and conducting the glomerular filtrate and urine.

seminiferous t's the tubules of the testis, in which spermatozoa develop and through which they leave the gland.

uriniferous t's renal tubules; channels for the passage of glomerular filtrate and urine.

tubulin ('tyoobyuhlin) the constituent protein of microtubules; thought to be involved in phagocyte motility.

tubulorrhexis (ˌtyoobyuhlə'reksis) rupture of the tubules of the kidney.

tubulus ('tyoobyuhləs) pl. *tubuli* [L.] tubule; a minute canal found in various structures or organs of the body.

tuft (tuft) a small clump or cluster; a coil.

malpighian t. renal glomerulus.

tuftsin ('tuftsin) a basic tetrapeptide produced in the spleen that stimulates phagocytosis in polymorphonuclear leukocytes and in macrophages.

tugging ('tuging) a pulling sensation, as a pulling sensation in the trachea (tracheal tugging), due to aneurysm of the arch of the aorta.

Tuinal ('tyooinal) trademark for a preparation of amylobarbitone, a hypnotic.

tularaemia (ˌtoolə'reemi·ə) a plaguelike disease of rodents, caused by *Francisella (Pasteurella) tularensis*, which is transmissible to man.

The illness can be contracted by handling diseased animals or their hides, eating infected wild game or being bitten by insects, such as horseflies and deer flies, that have fed on infected animals.

SYMPTOMS AND TREATMENT. Tularaemia begins with a sudden onset of chills and fever, accompanied by headache, nausea, vomiting, and severe weakness. A day or so later, a small sore usually develops at the site of the infection, and it becomes ulcerated. There may also be enlargement and ulceration of the lymph nodes and a generalized red rash. In untreated cases, the fever may last for weeks or months. Treatment is with antibiotics, such as tetracycline, streptomycin, and chloramphenicol.

PREVENTION. Tularaemia is usually thought of as an occupational disease. Those who may be exposed to it, such as game wardens and hunters, should take certain precautions, such as wearing gloves when handling wild animals, particularly rabbits and squirrels, and wearing adequate clothing in the woods to prevent bites by insect vectors of the disease. Wild game must be especially well cooked, in order to kill the tularaemia organism.

tulle gras (ˌtyool 'grah) a preparation of gauze impregnated with petroleum jelly. Other drugs may be added. Most useful on a granulating surface to stop a dressing adhering.

tumefacient (ˌtyoomi'fayshənt) producing tumefaction.

tumefaction (ˌtyoomi'fakshən) a swelling; the state of being swollen, or the act of swelling; puffiness; oedema.

tumescence (tyoo'mes'ns) 1. the condition of being swollen. 2. a swelling.

tumid ('tyoomid) swollen; oedematous.

tumor ('tyoomaw) swelling, one of the cardinal signs of inflammation.

tumoricidal (ˌtyoomo·ri'sied'l) destructive to cancer cells.

tumorigenesis (ˌtyoomo·ri'jenəsis) the production of tumours. adj. **tumorigenic**.

tumour ('tyoomə) neoplasm; a new growth of tissue in which cell multiplication is uncontrolled and progressive. adj. **tumorous.**

Neoplasms, being composed of new and actively growing tissue, have a faster growth rate than that of normal tissue, continuing after cessation of the stimuli that evoked the growth, and serving no useful physiological purpose. Tumours are classified in a number of ways, one of the simplest being according to their origin and whether they are malignant or benign. Tumours of mesenchymal origin include fibroelastic tumours and those of bone, fat, blood vessels, and lymphoid tissue. They may be benign or malignant (sarcoma). Tumours of epithelial origin may be benign or malignant (carcinoma); they are found in glandular tissue and such organs as the breast, stomach, uterus, or skin. Mixed tumours contain different types of cells derived from the same primary germ layer, and teratomas contain cells derived from more than one germ layer; both kinds may be benign or malignant.

BENIGN TUMOURS. Benign tumours do not endanger life unless they interfere with normal functions of other organs or affect a vital organ. They grow slowly, pushing aside normal tissue but not invading it. They are usually encapsulated, well demarcated growths. They are not metastatic; that is, they do not spread to form secondary tumours in other organs. Benign tumours usually respond favourably to surgical treatment and some forms of RADIATION THERAPY.

MALIGNANT TUMOURS. These tumours are composed of embryonic, primitive, or poorly differentiated cells. They grow in a disorganized manner and so rapidly that nutrition of the cells becomes a problem. For this reason necrosis and ulceration are characteristic of malignant tumours. They also invade surrounding tissues and are metastatic, initiating the growth of similar tumours in distant organs. See also CANCER.

Brenner t. an ovarian tumour of epithelial cells with much stromal overgrowth. The epithelial cells are thought to be derived from the germinal surface epithelium of the ovary. The tumour is benign, though very rare malignant variants have been described.

brown t. a giant-cell granuloma produced in and replacing bone, occurring in osteitis fibrosa cystica and due to hyperparathyroidism.

carotid body t. a firm, round mass at the bifurcation of the common carotid artery.

connective tissue t. any tumour arising from a connective tissue structure, e.g., a fibroma or sarcoma.

desmoid t. desmoid (1).

erectile t. cavernous haemangioma.

Ewing's t. See Ewing's SARCOMA.

false t. structural enlargement due to extravasation, exudation, echinococcus, or retained sebaceous matter.

fibroid t. a common benign tumour of the uterus, properly designated as LEIOMYOMA UTERI; a fibroma.

giant cell t. 1. a bone tumour, ranging from benign to frankly malignant, composed of cellular spindle cell stroma containing multinucleated giant cells resembling osteoclasts. 2. a benign, small, yellow, tumour-like nodule of tendon sheath origin, most often of the wrist and fingers or ankle and toes, laden with lipophages and containing multinucleated giant cells. Despite its name, this tumour is more analagous to villonodular synovitis of large joints than the giant cell tumour of bone.

granulosa t., granulosa cell t. an ovarian tumour originating in the cells of the cumulus oophorus of the follicle (see also GRANULOSA CELL TUMOUR).

granulosa–theca cell t. an ovarian tumour composed of granulosa (follicular) cells and theca cells; either form may predominate (see also GRANULOSA–THECA CELL TUMOUR).

heterologous t. one made up of tissue differing from that in which it grows.

homoiotypic t., homologous t. one made up of tissue resembling that in which it grows.

Hürthle cell t. a new growth of the thyroid gland composed wholly or predominantly of Hürthle cells (see also HÜRTHLE CELL TUMOUR).

islet cell t. a tumour of the islets of Langerhans, which may produce the hormone(s) normally found in the cell of origin. Most commonly this is insulin, but production of other hormones, including glucagon and gastrin, has been well described. Symptoms may be produced by the autonomous tumorous overproduction of the hormone.

Krukenberg's t. a metastatic carcinoma of the ovary, usually metastatic from gastrointestinal cancer, marked by areas of mucoid degeneration and by the presence of signet-ring-like cells (see also KRUKENBERG'S TUMOUR).

lipoid cell t. of ovary a usually benign ovarian tumour composed of eosinophilic cells or cells with lipoid vacuoles; it causes masculinization.

mast cell t. a benign, local aggregation of mast cells forming a nodulous tumour.

melanotic neuroectodermal t. a benign, rapidly growing, dark tumour of the jaw and occasionally of other sites; almost always seen in infants.

mixed t. one composed of more than one type of neoplastic tissue.

organoid t. teratoma.

phantom t. abdominal or other swelling not due to structural change.

sand t. psammoma.

theca cell t. fibroid-like tumour of the ovary containing yellow areas rich in lipid-laden theca cells.

true t. a neoplasm.

turban t's multiple CYLINDROMAS of the scalp grouped together so as to cover the entire scalp.

Wilms' t. a rapidly developing malignant tumour of the kidneys, made up of embryonal elements, and occurring chiefly in children before the fifth year; called also *embryonal carcinosarcoma* and *nephroblastoma*.

tumultus (tyoo'multəs) excessive organic action or motility.

Tunga ('tuhngə) a genus of fleas native to tropical and subtropical America and Africa.

T. penetrans the chigoe flea, the female of which buries herself almost completely under the skin of human beings and pigs in particular, but also of other animals, and causes intense skin irritation (see also CHIGOE).

tungsten ('tungstən) a chemical element, atomic number 74, atomic weight 183.85, symbol W. See table of elements in Appendix 2.

tunic ('tyoonik) a covering or coat.

Bichat's t. tunica intima.

tunica ('tyoonikə) pl. *tunicae* [L.] a covering or coat; used in anatomical nomenclature to designate a membranous covering of an organ or a distinct layer of the wall of a hollow structure, as a blood vessel.

t. adventitia the outer coat of various tubular structures.

t. albuginea a dense, white, fibrous sheath enclosing a part or organ.

t. conjunctiva the conjunctiva.

t. dartos dartos.

t. externa an outer coat, especially the fibroelastic coat of a blood vessel.

t. intima the innermost coat of blood vessels; called also *Bichat's tunic*.

t. media the middle coat of blood vessels.

t. mucosa the mucous membrane lining of various tubular structures.

t. muscularis the muscular coat or layer surrounding the tela submucosa in most portions of the digestive, respiratory, urinary, and genital tracts.

t. propria the proper coat or layer of a part, as distinguished from an investing membrane.

t. serosa the membrane lining the external walls of the body cavities and reflected over the surfaces of protruding organs; it secretes a watery exudate.

t. vaginalis the serous membrane covering the front and sides of the testis and epididymis.

t. vasculosa a vascular coat, or a layer well supplied with blood vessels.

tuning fork ('tyooning) a two-pronged forklike instrument of steel, the prongs of which give off a musical note when struck; used in detection of DEAFNESS.

tunnel ('tun'l) a passageway of varying length through a solid body, completely enclosed except for the open ends, permitting entrance and exit.

carpal t. the osseofibrous passage for the median nerve and the flexor tendons, formed by the flexor retinaculum and the carpal bones (see also CARPAL TUNNEL SYNDROME).

flexor t. carpal tunnel.

tarsal t. the osseofibrous passage for the posterior tibial vessels, tibial nerve, and flexor tendons, formed by the flexor retinaculum and the tarsal bones.

t. vision a condition of concentric reduction in the visual field, as though the subject were looking through a long tunnel or tube.

turbid ('tərbid) cloudy.

turbidimeter (ˌtərbi'dimitə) an apparatus for measuring turbidity of a solution.

turbidimetry (ˌtərbi'dimətree) the measurement of the turbidity of a liquid.

turbidity (tər'biditee) cloudiness; disturbance of solids (sediment) in a solution, so that it is not clear. adj. **turbid.**

turbinal, turbinate ('tərbin'l; 'tərbinət, -ˌnayt) 1. shaped like a top. 2. turbinate bone (concha nasalis ossea).

turbinectomy (ˌtərbi'nektəmee) excision of a turbinate bone (nasal concha).

turbinotomy (ˌtərbi'notəmee) incision of a turbinate bone.

Turcot's syndrome ('tərkohz) familial polyposis of the colon associated with malignant tumours of the central nervous system.

turgescence (tər'jes'ns) distention or swelling of a part.

turgescent (tər'jes'nt) becoming swollen.

turgid ('tərjid) swollen and congested.

turgor ('tərgə) the condition of being turgid; normal or other fullness.

turmschädel ('tooəmshayd'l) a developmental anomaly in which the head is high and rounded, due to early synostosis of the three major sutures of the skull.

Turner's syndrome ('tərnəz) a chromosomal defect in females, causing short stature and gonadal dysgenesis. Classically, an absence of one X chromosome (karotype 45X) but variants have an abnormality of the X chromosome or mosaicism. Affects one in 3000 live female births. The majority have streak ovaries leading to an absence of puberty and infertility and therefore require oestrogen therapy. Other features may include webbing of the neck, cubitus valgus, nail abnormalities and coarctation of the aorta. Intelligence is usually normal.

Turner tooth ('tərnə) enamel hypoplasia affecting a single tooth only. The defect may range from mild discoloration to severe irregularities in tooth shape.

turricephaly (ˌturi'kefəlee, -'sef-) oxycephaly.

tussigenic (ˌtusi'jenik) causing cough.

tussis ('tusis) [L.] *cough*.

tussive ('tusiv) pertaining to or due to a cough.

tutamen ('tyootaymən) pl. *tutamina* [L.] a protective covering or structure.

tutamina oculi the protecting appendages of the eye, as the eyelids, eyelashes, etc.

Tween (tween) trademark for preparations of polysorbates; used with a numerical suffix, e.g., Tween 80 is a trademark for polysorbate 80.

twin (twin) one of two offspring produced in the same pregnancy. Twins occur approximately once in every 89 births. See also HELLIN'S LAW.

Dizygotic, or fraternal, twins develop from two separate ova fertilized at the same time. They may be of the same sex or of opposite sexes, and are no more similar than any other two children of the same parents. Called also *binovular*, *dichorial*, *dissimilar*, and *unlike twins*.

Monozygotic, or identical, twins develop from a single ovum that divides after fertilization. Because they share the same set of chromosomes, they are always of the same sex, and are remarkably similar in hair colour, finger and palm prints, teeth, and other respects. Monozygotic twins have exactly the same blood type and can accept tissue or organ transplants from each other. Called also *uniovular, enzygotic, monochorial*, *mono-ovular*, *similar*, or *true twins*.

Approximately one-third of all twins are identical; the rest are fraternal. It is not clearly understood exactly what causes a single ovum to divide shortly after conception and thereby produce identical twins, although it seems to be a chance occurrence. The reasons for the production and fertilization of two separate ova that result in fraternal twins are not well understood either, but it is thought that a tendency toward fraternal twins runs in families and is transmitted through the genes of the mother. Women are more likely to have fraternal twins in their later childbearing years, between the ages of 30 and 38 years, than earlier. Older age in the father also seems to be a factor with fraternal twins. Diagnosis of monozygotic and dizygotic twins may be obtained from examination of the placenta and membranes. Uniovular twins may have one chorion and two amnia.

conjoined t's monozygotic twins whose bodies are joined (see also SIAMESE TWINS). **impacted t's** twins so situated during delivery that pressure of one against the other prevents complete engagement of either. Management usually requires decapitation of one twin. The condition may be fatal to both infants. Called also *locked twins*.

locked t's impacted twins.

Siamese t's conjoined twins.

unequal t's twins of which one is incompletely developed.

twinning ('twining) 1. the production of symmetrical structures or parts by division. 2. the simultaneous intrauterine production of two or more embryos.

twitch (twich) a brief, contractile response of a skeletal muscle elicited by a single maximal volley of impulses in the neurons supplying it.

twitching ('twiching) the occurrence of a single contraction or a series of contractions of a muscle.

tychastics (tie'kastiks) the study of industrial accidents.

tyloma (tie'lohmə) a callus or callosity.

tylosis (tie'lohsis) formation of callosities. adj. **tylotic**.

tympanal ('timpən'l) pertaining to the tympanum or to the tympanic membrane.

tympanectomy (ˌtimpə'nektəmee) excision of the tympanic membrane.

tympanic (tim'panik) 1. of or pertaining to the tympanum. 2. bell-like; resonant.

t. membrane a thin, semitransparent membrane, nearly oval in shape, that stretches across the ear canal separating the tympanum (middle ear) from the external acoustic meatus (outer ear); called also the *eardrum*. It is composed of fibrous tissue, covered with skin on the outside and mucous membrane on the inside. It is constructed so that it can vibrate freely with audible sound waves that travel inward from outside. The handle of the malleus (hammer) of the middle ear is attached to the centre of the tympanic membrane and receives the vibrations collected by the membrane, transmitting them to other bones of the middle ear (the incus and stapes) and eventually to the fluid of the inner ear.

Perforation of the tympanic membrane can cause some loss of hearing, the degree of loss depending on the size and location of the perforation. Since vibrations can still be transmitted to the inner ear by way of the bones of the skull, even nearly total destruction of the tympanic membrane does not produce total deafness. Surgical incision of the eardrum (myringotomy) may be done to relieve pressure and provide for drainage in an infection of the middle ear (see also OTITIS MEDIA).

t. membrane, secondary the membrane enclosing the fenestra cochlearis; called also *Scarpa's membrane*.

t. notch Rivinus' incisure.

t. plexus a network of nerve fibres supplying the mucous lining of the tympanic tube.

tympanism, tympanites ('timpəˌnizəm; ˌtimpə'nieteez) drumlike distention of the abdomen due to air or gas in the intestine or peritoneal cavity. adj. **tympanitic**.

tympanitic (ˌtimpə'nitik) 1. pertaining to or affected with tympanism. 2. bell-like; tympanic.

tympanitis (ˌtimpə'nietis) otitis media.

tympanocentesis (ˌtimpənohsen'teesis) surgical puncture of the tympanic membrane or tympanum.

tympanogenic (ˌtimpənoh'jenik) arising from the tympanum or middle ear.

tympanogram ('timpənohˌgram) a graphic representation of the relative compliance and impedance of the tympanic membrane and ossicles of the middle ear obtained by tympanometry.

tympanomastoiditis (ˌtimpənohˌmastoy'dietis) inflammation of the middle ear and the pneumatic cells of the mastoid process.

tympanometry (ˌtimpə'nomətree) indirect measurement of the compliance (mobility) and impedance of the tympanic membrane and ossicles of the middle ear; it is done by subjecting the external acoustic meatus to positive, normal, and negative air pressure and monitoring the resultant sound energy flow.

tympanoplasty ('timpənohˌplastee) plastic reconstruction of the bones of the middle ear, with establishment of ossicular continuity from the tympanic membrane to the oval window. This surgical procedure is performed when chronic infection or tumour has led to destruction of the ossicles, of the pars petrosa of the temporal bone, or both. Because the ossicles are so small, the surgery must be done under magnification with an operating microscope. Tympanoplasty requires great surgical skill and the use of specially designed instruments. It is often done in preference to radical MASTOIDECTOMY and offers the advantage of greater preservation of hearing. For patient care after tympanoplasty, see surgery of the EAR. adj. **tympanoplastic.**

tympanosclerosis (ˌtimpənohsklə'rohsis) a condition characterized by the presence of masses of hard, dense connective tissue around the auditory ossicles in the middle ear.

tympanotomy (ˌtimpə'notəmee) myringotomy.

tympanous ('timpənəs) distended with gas.

tympanum ('timpənəm) the part of the cavity of the middle ear, in the temporal bone, just medial to the tympanic membrane.

tympany ('timpənee) 1. tympanitis. 2. a tympanic, or

bell-like, percussion note.

type (tiep) the general or prevailing character of any particular case of disease, person, substance, etc.

asthenic t. a type of physical constitution, with long limbs, small trunk, flat chest, and weak muscles.

athletic t. a type of physical constitution with broad shoulders, deep chest, flat abdomen, thick neck, and good muscular development.

blood t's see BLOOD GROUP.

phage t. a subgroup of a bacterial species susceptible to a particular bacteriophage and demonstrated by phage TYPING. Called also *lysotype* and *phagotype*.

pyknic t. a type of physical constitution marked by rounded body, large chest, thick shoulders, broad head, and short neck.

type A behaviour (tiep 'ay) a behaviour pattern associated with the development of coronary heart disease, characterized by excessive competitiveness and aggression and a fast-paced life style. Persons exhibiting type A behaviour are constantly struggling to accomplish ill-defined goals in the shortest possible time. In several studies this type of behaviour has been shown to be as significant as other risk factors, such as smoking and hypertension, in the development of coronary artery disease and myocardial infarction. The opposite type of behaviour exhibited by individuals who are relaxed, unhurried, and less aggressive is called type B.

typhl(o)- word element. [Gr.] *caecum, blindness.*

typhlectasis (ti'flektəsis) distention of the caecum.

typhlitis (ti'flietis) inflammation of the caecum.

typhlodicliditis (,tifloh,dikli'dietis) inflammation of the ileocaecal valve.

typhlolexia (,tifloh'leksi·ə) visual aphasia; loss of ability to comprehend written language.

typhlolithiasis (,tiflohli'thieəsis) the presence of calculi in the caecum.

typhlon ('tiflon) the caecum.

typhlotomy (tif'lotəmee) incision into the caecum.

typhoid ('tiefoyd) 1. resembling typhus. 2. typhoid fever.

t. fever a notifiable bacterial infection transmitted by contaminated water, milk or other foods, especially shellfish. The causative organism is *Salmonella typhi*, found in the excreta of human carriers.

Entering the body through the intestinal tract, the typhoid bacillus starts multiplying in the bloodstream, causing fever, headache, and malaise. The usual incubation period is 7 to 14 days. Later the bacilli localize in the intestinal tract, the gallbladder, or, less often, the kidneys.

SYMPTOMS. The first symptoms of typhoid are headache, perhaps sore throat and a fever that may reach 40.5 °C (105 °F). The pulse is relatively slow. The temperature rises daily, reaching a peak in 7 to 10 days, maintaining this level for about another week, and then subsiding by the end of the fourth week. Periods of chills and sweating may occur, with loss of appetite. A watery, greyish or greenish diarrhoea may occur, but constipation is commoner in the first week of illness. After 2 weeks, red spots may be seen on the chest and abdomen. If the case is severe, the patient may lapse into states of delirious muttering and staring into space. About the third to fourth week an improvement is noticeable, and steady recovery then follows in most cases. The disease is a serious one, however, and may, if untreated, be fatal.

TRANSMISSION. A person who has had typhoid fever gains immunity from it but may become a carrier. Although perfectly well, he harbours the bacteria and passes them out in his faeces or urine. The typhoid bacillus often lodges in the gallbladder of carriers. In cities, food handled by carriers is the principal source of infection. In rural areas carriers may infect food–fruit and fresh vegetables, for example–that they raise. When sewage and sanitation systems are poor, the organisms may enter the water supply and outbreaks may then occur. They can also be spread to food and water by flies that have been in contact with body eliminations. Contamination is more likely if human faeces are used to fertilize the crops, as they are in some parts of the world.

PREVENTION AND TREATMENT. Once a widespread disease, typhoid fever has now been greatly reduced in countries with advanced sanitation. Proper sanitation involves (1) good sewage systems to dispose of human wastes and (2) proper measures for keeping foods uncontaminated. Food should be carefully protected from flies and food handlers must maintain a good standard of hygiene. Effective medicines, such as the antibiotic chloramphenicol, are available for the treatment of the disease.

Another disease whose symptoms resemble those of typhoid fever, although it tends to be less severe, is paratyphoid fever, also transmitted by contaminated food or liquids.

PATIENT CARE. Patients with typhoid and paratyphoid fevers are placed under enteric precautions until the urine and faeces are clear of the bacilli. (See ISOLATION TECHNIQUE.) If sewage treatment for the community is adequate, the stools and urine need not be disinfected, but if there is danger of incomplete destruction of the bacilli by sewage treatment methods, the urine and faeces should be disinfected by chlorinated lime or a 4 per cent Lysol solution before disposal. Other precautionary measures to prevent the spread of the disease include adequate screening of windows and doors so that flies may not come in contact with excreta.

Many patients with typhoid fever require measures to lower the body temperature when fever is extreme. These include cool sponge baths, application of ice bags, and administration of antipyretic drugs as ordered. Plenty of fluids should be given to prevent dehydration. The diet should consist of soft, bland, easily digested, and nourishing foods.

Observations of the patient include watching for sudden temperature changes, signs of intestinal bleeding, and symptoms of intestinal perforation.

Kaolin or a similar antidiarrhoeal agent may be needed to help control diarrhoea. If constipation becomes a problem, a low saline enema should be given if absolutely necessary. Cathartics are contraindicated because of the danger of intestinal perforation.

Good oral hygiene and care of the lips and mouth are essential, as for any patient with a prolonged febrile condition. In addition, the patient must be kept clean and dry and turned frequently to avoid the development of PRESSURE SORES. During the convalescent period the patient will need adequate rest and a well-balanced diet to help him recover from this debilitating illness.

typhoidal (tie'foyd'l) resembling typhoid fever.

typhopneumonia (,tiefohnyoo'mohni·ə) pneumonia with typhoid fever.

typhus ('tiefəs) an acute, notifiable, infectious disease caused by species of the parasitic microorganism *Rickettsia*. The organisms are usually transmitted from infected rats and other rodents to man by lice, fleas, ticks and mites.

Rickettsiae enter the human body through cuts or breaks in the skin made by the bites of the lice or other pests.

TYPES AND TREATMENT. The principal types of the diseases are louse-borne typhus (epidemic or classic typhus) caused by *Rickettsia prowazekii*, murine (flea-borne) typhus caused by *R. typhi*, scrub typhus caused by *R. tsutsugamushi*, and recrudescent typhus.

Louse-Borne Typhus. Louse-borne typhus (epidemic or classic typhus) occurs after faeces of an infected louse are rubbed into a break in the skin. After an incubation period of 6 to 15 days, the symptoms begin to appear—headache, runny nose, cough, nausea, and chest pain. These are followed in a few days by high fever and chills, vomiting, constipation or diarrhoea, muscular aching, and perhaps delirium or stupor. A red rash, which may bleed, appears on the trunk and spreads to the arms and legs.

After about 2 weeks the symptoms usually subside. Ordinarily louse typhus is not fatal, but it can be, particularly if pneumonia develops or if the afflicted person has heart disease.

Louse typhus is called epidemic typhus because of the devastation it has caused throughout history. It tends to appear where people are crowded together and are weakened by cold, disease, and starvation. It has many colloquial names, such as war fever, camp fever, or gaol fever.

Murine Typhus. Murine typhus is a less common variety. It is called also endemic, rat, or flea typhus. As the name 'murine' indicates, it is transmitted by the bites of rat or mouse fleas. The symptoms are like those of louse typhus but are less severe, and recovery occurs sooner. Antibiotics are used in treatment.

Scrub Typhus. Scrub typhus, called also *Japanese river fever* and *tsutsugamushi fever*, is prevalent in eastern Asia and has been carried to other areas by infected persons. It is transmitted by mites and hence is often called mite fever. The rodent responsible for this illness is the field mouse. The rickettsiae are transferred to humans by the bite of the larval form of the mite, usually in the groin or neck. The fever of scrub typhus and its other symptoms are very similar to those of other forms of typhus. It is treated with chloramphenicol and the tetracyclines.

Recrudescent Typhus. Recrudescent typhus, or Brill-Zinsser disease, is caused by *Rickettsia prowazekii*, the aetiological agent of louse-borne typhus. The rickettsiae, however, remain in the body after a first attack of typhus and can cause a recurrence (a recrudescence) as long as years after the first attack. The recrudescence is milder than the initial infection, however. Treatment is similar to that for epidemic typhus.

Closely related to these forms of typhus are tick-borne rickettsial diseases, such as ROCKY MOUNTAIN SPOTTED FEVER.

PREVENTION. Immunizing vaccines are available if an outbreak of typhus occurs or threatens. They greatly reduce the chance of infection, or modify the effects of the disease. Travellers should be vaccinated before visiting countries where the disease is prevalent. Some countries require proof of such protection before admitting a visitor.

Insect and rodent control are of great importance in the prevention and control of typhus. Adult lice can be destroyed by spraying garments with DDT. Frequent bathing and changes of underclothes are vital. Outer garments should be sterilized by steam to kill the louse eggs.

Fleas and mites are more difficult to control than lice. The best method is to destroy the rodents on which they live.

PATIENT CARE. The patient with typhus is initially isolated until he is free of body lice or mites. He is not capable of transmitting the disease without the aid of these vectors. To accomplish removal of lice or mites the patient should be washed with a 1 per cent solution of Lysol upon admission and his clothing must be disinfected or destroyed. Several shampoos may be necessary to eliminate parasites from the hair. Gentle, thorough cleaning is necessary and every effort must be made to avoid damage to the skin.

The patient is given a soft diet and ample fluids, to prevent dehydration. Efforts are made to conserve the patient's strength and to protect him during periods of delirium, which are common.

Typhus is a very debilitating disease and requires a long period of convalescence in which the patient's general health must be improved. Nervous and mental symptoms may persist long after the acute phase of the disease subsides.

typing ('tieping) in transplantation immunology, a method of measuring the degree of organ, solid tissue, or blood compatibility between two individuals, in which specific histocompatibility antigens (e.g., those present on leukocytes or erythrocytes) are detected by means of suitable isoimmune antisera.

t. of blood determining the character of the blood on the basis of agglutinogens in the erythrocytes. See also BLOOD GROUP. **phage t.** characterization of bacteria, extending to strain differences, by demonstration of susceptibility to one or more (a spectrum) races of bacteriophage; widely applied to staphylococci, typhoid bacilli, etc., for epidemiological purposes.

tissue t. the identification of the HLA antigens of the donor and recipient of a transplant or transfusion (see also TISSUE TYPING).

typology (tie'poləjee) the study of types; the science of classifying, as bacteria according to type.

tyramine ('tierə,meen, 'ti-) a decarboxylation product of tyrosine, which may be converted to cresol and phenol, found in decayed animal tissue, ripe cheese, and ergot. Closely related structurally to adrenaline and noradrenaline, it has a similar but weaker action.

tyrogenous (tie'rojənəs, ti-) originating in cheese.

tyroid ('tieroyd, 'ti-) of cheesy consistency; caseous.

tyroma (tie'rohmə, ti-) a caseous tumour.

tyromatosis (,tierohmə'tohsis, ,ti-) a condition characterized by caseous degeneration.

tyrosine ('tieroh,seen, 'ti-) a naturally occurring amino acid present in most proteins; it is a product of phenylalanine metabolism and a precursor of melanin, catecholamines, and thyroid hormones.

tyrosinosis (,tierohsi'nohsis, ,ti-) a condition characterized by a faulty metabolism of tyrosine in which an intermediate product, parahydroxyphenyl pyruvic acid, appears in the urine and gives it an abnormal reducing power.

tyrosinuria (,tierohsi'nyooə·ri·ə, ,ti-) the presence of tyrosine in the urine.

tyrosis (tie'rohsis, ti-) caseation (2).

tyrosyluria (,tierohsi'lyooə·ri·ə, ,ti-) increased urinary secretion of para-hydroxyphenyl compounds derived from tyrosine, as in tyrosinuria.

tyrotoxism (,tieroh'toksizəm, ,ti-) poisoning from a toxin present in milk or cheese.

Tyson's glands ('tiesənz) sebaceous glands of the corona of the penis and inner surface of the prepuce-they secrete smegma; called also *preputial glands*.

tysonitis (,tiesə'nietis) inflammation of Tyson's glands (preputial glands).

tyvelose ('tievə,lohs) an unusual sugar that is a polysaccharide somatic antigen of *Salmonella* species.

Tzanck's test (tsangks) cytological examination of scrapings from the base of herpetic lesions, useful in the diagnosis of HERPES SIMPLEX and HERPES GENITALIS. The scrapings are fixed on a slide with absolute or methyl alcohol for 10 minutes and stained with Giesma stain. The findings of multinucleated giant cells or of typical eosinophilic intranuclear inclusions is diagnostic of herpesvirus infection.

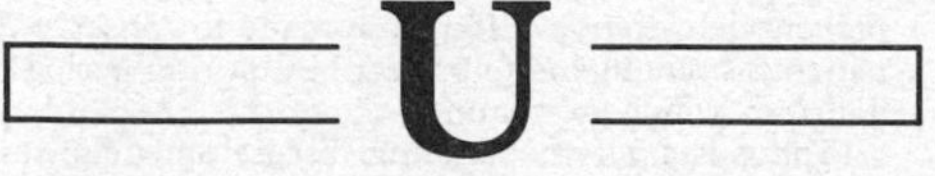

U chemical symbol, *uranium;* unit.

ubiquinol (yoo'bikwi,nol) the form of ubiquinone when reduced by two electrons.

ubiquinone (yoo'bikwi,nohn) coenzyme Q.

Ubretid (yoo'bretid) tradename for distigmine, a cholinesterase inhibitor used in the treatment of a neurogenic bladder.

UDP uridine diphosphate.

UICC International Union Against Cancer (see CANCER).

UKCC (,yookatsee'see) United Kingdom Central Council (for Nursing, Midwifery and Health Visiting). See under UNITED KINGDOM.

ulcer ('ulsə) an area of loss of epithelium from skin or mucosa resulting from a wide variety of causes—direct, physical and chemical trauma; infection; neoplasia; allergy.

chronic leg u. ulceration of the lower leg caused by peripheral vascular disease involving either the arteries and arterioles or the veins and venules of the affected extremity. Chronic leg ulcers result in social and industrial incapacity. Approximately 0.5 per cent of the population of the United Kingdom are affected. Arterial and venous ulcers are quite different and require different modes of treatment.

Arterial ulcer disease usually is caused by occlusion of small arteries or arterioles at the extremity. Ulceration is likely to occur in diabetics and in patients with atherosclerosis. The extremity is cold and pale with loss of hair and atrophy of the skin. If ulceration develops, it is treated by keeping the ulcer clean and dry and free from pressure. The patient must be taught to care for his feet and to avoid trauma from pressure and from physical injury. *Venous* ulceration occurs as a result of chronic venous stasis either from varicose veins or one or more episodes of thrombophlebitis. The ulcers almost always occur in the lower third of the leg. Treatment consists of elevating the leg, the feet being higher than the hips, to promote venous and tissue fluid return. Prolonged bed rest is contraindicated except in cases of gross oedema and severe infection. Physiotherapy should be instituted to correct any deformity and maintain mobility. The patient is taught a correct gait to allow efficient emptying of the deep veins. Elastic bandages or stockings are worn to give support to the superficial veins and reduce oedema. Local pressure may be applied directly over the granulating tissue of the ulcer by using 4 × 4 non-adhesive gauze squares cut to exact size and changed as necessary. As the ulcer heals, the gauze is cut smaller. An elastic bandage is then wrapped from the toes up to the groin. The purpose of this treatment is to collapse perforating venules and prevent the transmission of hydrostatic pressure to the tissues under the ulcer.

A clean ulcer should be disturbed as little as possible. Débridement may be necessary for necrotic ulcers. Cleansing agents can be used to remove areas of slough (eusol, aqueous silver nitrate, and acetic acid lotion), but should only be used for a week at a time to prevent colonization of bacteria.

Analgesia is required at four- to six-hourly periods since persistent pain will limit mobility. Medications in the form of topical antibiotics, steroids, and creams are not recommended because of the potential problem of contact dermatitis. Systematic antibiotics are given when the ulcer is infected, according to the sensitivity of the infecting organism. Clean, non-infective ulcers may be treated surgically with pinch grafts.

Chronic leg ulcers are slow to heal and may reoccur. Patients should be advised to: (1) avoid prolonged standing, (2) continue leg and feet exercises, (3) avoid constrictive garters or corsets, (4) avoid obesity, (5) rest with elevated legs, (6) keep legs warm, and (7) wear well-fitting, supportive shoes with low heels.

Curling's u. acute ulceration of the duodenum seen after a severe burn.

decubitus u. pressure sore, bedsore; ulceration caused by pressure on a body area in a recumbent patient. See PRESSURE SORE.

Hunner's u. a persistent and painful ulcer of the bladder wall, occurring in chronic interstitial cystitis.

marginal u. a descriptive term of no nosological significance. In ophthalmology used to indicate corneal ulceration adjacent to the limbus. In gastroenterology it often refers to anastomotic ulceration.

peptic u. a focal loss of tissues lining any part of the lower oesophagus, the stomach, and the duodenum. Acute lesions that do not extend through the muscularis mucosae are called erosions. Chronic lesions, which are almost always called ulcers, involve the muscular coat, destroying the musculature and replacing it with permanent scar tissue at the site of healing.

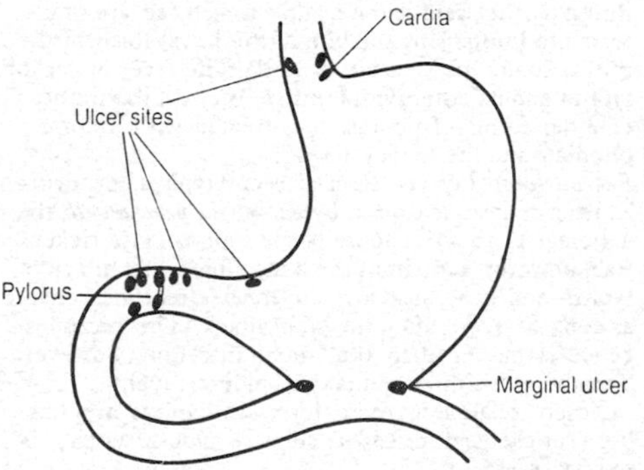

Common sites of peptic ulcer. Marginal ulcers occur where an abnormal opening is made between the stomach and some portion of the small intestine

CAUSE. While gastric acid and pepsin may be responsible for ulcer formation, it is not known why mucosal resistance to them should become impaired. Duodenal ulcers and some prepyloric gastric ulcers are associated with hyperacidity of the gastric juice. Gastric ulcers, on the other hand, are not usually associated with abnormal acid levels.

Theories about genetic and environmental causes of peptic ulcer abound. Both gastric and duodenal ulcers tend to occur in families; gastric ulcer is three times more common in relatives of persons with gastric ulcers than in the population generally. The same is true of duodenal ulcers. There is evidence that the increased familial incidence of both gastric and duodenal ulcers is not just due to a shared environment. There is as yet no direct evidence that either diets or particular elements of diets, such as hot spices, cause ulcers. However, gastric ulcer is more likely to occur in those who are poorly nourished and is primarily a disease of the lower socioeconomic levels of society. Despite the stereotype of the hard-driving executive who suffers from an ulcer, there is actually little difference in the incidence of ulcer in various occupations.

Psychosomatic factors do play some role in the development of peptic ulcers. Stress can and does alter gastric function. Prolonged psychological or physiological stress produces what is known as a *stress ulcer*, believed to be the result of persistent vagal stimulation. A stress ulcer differs from a chronic peptic ulcer: it is more acute and more likely to produce haemorrhage, perforation occurs occasionally and pain is rare.

Conditions that are often associated with stress ulcers include severe trauma, surgery, advanced malignancy, extensive burns (Curling's ulcer), and brain injury.

Drug-induced ulcers are most commonly caused by the ingestion of aspirin, other nonsteroidal anti-inflammatory drugs (NSAIDs) or alcohol. Corticosteroids, especially glucocorticoids, are also probably ulcerogenic.

SYMPTOMS. The cardinal symptom of peptic ulcer is intermittant epigastric pain described as burning, gnawing, cramping, or aching. The pattern of pain can reflect the site of the ulcer. Preprandial and night pain relieved by taking food may be indicative of duodenal or prepyloric ulcer, pain occuring with food or postcibally is typical of gastric ulcer. Pain of duodenal ulcer tends to occur in episodes of three or four days or weeks and then subsides to reappear weeks or months later. Conversion to continuous pain occurs as ulceration penetrates and inflammation begins to involve the posterior abdominal wall, when it may also radiate to the back.

COMPLICATIONS. The three major complications of ulcer are haemorrhage, perforation, and obstruction. Bleeding results from ulceration of an arteriole or artery and may present with haematemesis or melaena or evidence of sudden occult bleeding such as faintness, shock and pallor. More commonly bleeding loss is slow but continuous, leading imperceptibly to anaemia.

Perforation is a surgical emergency requiring urgent operation.

Obstruction due to persistent scarring presents as pyloric stenosis, uncommonly as an hour glass stomach. It is manifested by cumulative vomiting, a forceful emesis of large volume occuring once towards the end of the day with items of food undigested and recognisable in the vomit. At this stage ALKALOSIS develops, through loss of hydrogen ions. The condition is usually corrected surgically, although endoscopic balloon dilation can now be employed, and the condition may improve following medical treatment of an active duodenal ulcer by, for example, H_2 antagonists.

Gastric ulcers have the potential to become malignant, and histology should always be obtained as gastric cancer has a very poor survival rate if not detected early.

DIAGNOSIS is made directly by endoscopy or indirectly by radiology. In haematemesis, GASTROSCOPY can indicate whether the source of bleeding lies in the duodenum, stomach or oesophagus, and allows therapeutic measures such as thermocoagulation by laser or heater probe. Endoscopy is also important in obtaining a tissue diagnosis in the case of gastric ulcer where malignancy must always be suspected.

TREATMENT. The primary goals of medical treatment of peptic ulcers are: (1) relief of symptoms, (2) promotion of healing, (3) prevention of complications, and (4) prevention of recurrences.

In general the treatment of ulcer disease now lies in the administration of H_2-receptor antagonists that reduce gastric acid secretion in response to all stimuli, and they relieve pain.

It is becoming increasingly recognized that nocturnal acid secretion is most responsible for ulcer development, and by giving a single night time dose of an H_2 antagonist, ulcer healing occurs usually within 2–4 weeks. This allows normal acid levels during the day to help with digestion and prevents bacterial colonization of the stomach. This regimen is effective in gastric ulcer as well as duodenal ulcer.

Alternative forms of therapy include high dose antacids, carbenoxolone, sucralfate and liquorice preparations. Bismuth is being increasingly used and seems to reduce the incidence of relapse in duodenal ulcer more than other forms of therapy.

There is no doubt that smoking delays ulcer healing and increases the likelihood of relapse, and patients should be strongly urged to stop.

Operation may be necessary when medical treatment fails and for complications described above. Selective vagotomy is the operation of choice for duodenal and prepyloric ulcers, gastrectomy being reserved for the complications and gastric ulcer.

perforating u. one that involves the entire thickness of an organ, either creating an opening on both surfaces or penetrating adjacent structures.

phagedenic u. a necrotizing lesion in which tissue destruction is prominent.

rodent u. a slow growing malignant tumour of the face, edge of the eyelids, lips or nostril. Rodent ulcers usually occur in middle age or later. If untreated they will quickly destroy skin, muscle, and bone, but they do not spread to other parts of the body.

stress u. peptic ulcer, usually gastric, resulting from stress; possible predisposing factors include changes in the microcirculation of the gastric mucosa, and increased permeability of the gastric mucosa barrier to H^+.

trophic u. a chronic and intractable ulcer developing in an area with loss of sensation, usually at site of pressure within such an area as the ball or heel of the foot.

tropical u. a chronic, sloughing ulcer usually on the lower extremities, occurring in certain tropical countries.

varicose u. an ulcer in the leg situated above the medial malleolus due to varicose veins, often within an area of varicose eczema. See VARICOSE veins.

venereal u. a chancre or chancroid.

ulcerate ('ulsə,rayt) to undergo ulceration.

ulceration (,ulsə'rayshən) 1. formation or development of an ulcer. 2. an ulcer.

ulcerative ('ulsə,raytiv) pertaining to or characterized by ulceration.

u. colitis a recurrent acute and chronic disorder characterized by extensive inflammatory ulceration in the colon, chiefly of the mucosa and submucosa. The aetiology is unknown; hence, the term *idiopathic* is used in reference to ulcerative colitis. The disorder is not always limited to pathological changes in the colon, but may become systemic, involving the joints and causing migratory arthritis, sacroileitis, and ankylosing spondylitis. Other organs that can become involved are the liver and the skin.

Ulcerative colitis shares many of the same characteristics with regional ileitis or CROHN'S DISEASE; the two are often included in the broader diagnostic entity called *inflammatory bowel disease* (IBD). There are some who believe that both disorders are immunological responses to the same as yet unknown aetiological agent.

Genetic predisposition to IBD is a possibility because there is a higher incidence of ulcerative colitis and Crohn's disease among close relatives. Ulcerative colitis is slightly more prevalent in females than in males and most often appears between the ages of 30 and 60 years. Crohn's disease follows a similar pattern of incidence.

CLINICAL MANIFESTATIONS AND COMPLICATIONS. The patient with ulcerative colitis suffers from attacks of bloody, mucoid diarrhoea that are usually precipitated by physical or emotional stress. These acute attacks can last for days, weeks, or even months and are followed by periods of remission that can extend from a few weeks to several decades. Some patients experience relatively few attacks throughout their lifetime, while others have frequent, prolonged, and potentially serious attacks that predispose the colon to malignant changes. Both acute and chronic diarrhoéa can upset the fluid and electrolyte balance, interefere with normal nutrition, and produce fever, abdominal cramps, and weight loss.

A sudden and severe attack of the disease can lead to cessation of bowel function and *toxic megacolon* or dilation of the colon by accumulating faeces, fluid, and toxic substances. Other complications include severe blood loss and anaemia, systemic toxicity, and metabolic disturbances. These conditions contribute to the 20 per cent mortality rate during the first ten years of the disease. A serious sequela of long-term chronic and continuous ulcerative colitis is carcinoma of the colon. The risk for this complication is lower for those persons who have infrequent relapses than for those who are symptomatic for years.

PATIENT CARE. During acute attacks of the disease the patient will most likely present problems related to fluid volume deficit, alteration in nutrition, loss of electrolytes, potential for skin breakdown in the anal region, disturbance of sleep and rest, and discomfort from abdominal cramps. Long-term problems are likely to be related to anxiety, alterations in self-concept, social isolation, and fear of malignancy.

The plan of care should include observation of the number and character of stools, periodic auscultation of bowel sounds, measurement of fluid intake and output, daily weight, checking for signs of bleeding and anaemia, and monitoring of blood gases, electrolytes, and pH for evidence of acid-base imbalance or abnormal electrolyte values. It also is important to be alert for signs of inflammatory changes in the joints or lesions on the skin.

When diagnostic procedures such as sigmoidoscopy, barium enema, and stool analyses are necessary, the patient should have a satisfactory explanation of the purpose of these tests and what is expected of him before, during, and after each procedure.

Long-term goals of care should help the patient comply with the prescribed medical regimen, which usually consists of antidiarrhoeic agents, anticholinergic drugs to relieve abdominal cramps, mild sedatives, and dietary advice according to the patient's needs. Antibiotics are sometimes needed to control infections of the bowel.

Surgical intervention may be the only alternative when more conservative treatments fail. The surgery usually involves creation of a permanent ILEOSTOMY, which predisposes to a new set of problems.

There is no cure for ulcerative colitis, and it is a debilitating disorder that can create many physiological, psychological, and social problems for the patient. The frequent bouts of severe diarrhoea and discomfort can be embarrassing and depressing. Emotional support, empathetic listening, and cooperative problem solving are essential components of patient care.

ulcerogangrenous (ˌulsə·roh'gang·grinəs) characterized by both ulceration and gangrene.

ulcerogenic (ˌulsə·roh'jenik) causing ulceration; leading to the production of ulcers.

ulceromembranous (ˌulsə·roh'membrənəs) characterized by ulceration and a membranous exudation.

ulcerous ('ulsə·rəs) 1. of the nature of an ulcer. 2. affected with ulceration.

ulcus ('ulkəs) pl. *ulcera* [L.] ulcer.

ulectomy (yoo'lektəmee) 1. excision of scar tissue. 2. excision of the gums; gingivectomy.

ulerythema (ˌyooleri'theemə) an erythematous disease of the skin with formation of cicatrices and atrophy.

u. ophryogenes a hereditary form in which keratosis pilaris involves the follicles of the eyebrow hairs.

ulna ('ulnə) pl. *ulnae* [L.] the inner and larger bone of the forearm, on the side opposite the thumb. It articulates with the humerus and with the head of the radius at its proximal end; with the radius and bones of the carpus at the distal end.

ulnad ('ulnad) toward the ulna.

ulnar ('ulnə) pertaining to the ulna or to the ulnar (medial) aspect of the arm as compared to the radial (lateral) aspect.

ulnaris (ul'nair·ris) [L.] *ulnar.*

ulnocarpal (ˌulnoh'kahp'l) pertaining to the ulna and carpus.

ulnoradial (ˌulnoh'raydi·əl) pertaining to the ulna and radius.

uloid ('yooloyd) scar-like lesion in the dermis due to degeneration. Characteristic of syphilis.

ulotomy (yoo'lotəmee) 1. incision of scar tissue. 2. incision of the gums.

ultra- word element. [L.] *beyond, excess.*

ultrabrachycephalic (ˌultrəˌbrakikə'falik, -sə'falik) having a cephalic index of more than 90.

ultracentrifugation (ˌultrəˌsentrifyuh'gayshən) subjection of material to an exceedingly high centrifugal force, which will separate and sediment the molecules of a substance.

ultracentrifuge (ˌultrə'sentriˌfyooj) the centrifuge used in ultracentrifugation.

ultradian (ul'traydi·ən) pertaining to a period of less than 24 hours; applied to the rhythmic repetition of certain phenomena in living organisms occurring in cycles of less than a day (ultradian rhythm).

ultrafilter (ˌultrə'filtə) the filter used in ultrafiltration.

ultrafiltration (ˌultrəfil'trayshən) filtration through a filter capable of removing colloidal particles from a dispersion medium, as in the filtration of plasma at the capillary membrane.

ultramicroscopic (ˌultrəˌmiekrə'skopik) too small to be seen with the ordinary light microscope.

ultrasonic (ˌultrə'sonik) beyond the audible range; relating to sound waves having a frequency of more than 20,000 cycles per second.

ultrasonics (ˌultrə'soniks) that part of the science of acoustics dealing with the frequency range beyond the upper limit of perception by the human ear (above 20,000 cycles per second), but usually restricted to frequencies above 50,000 hertz. Ultrasonic radiation is injurious to tissues because of its thermal and mechanical effects when passing through living matter, but in controlled amounts it is used therapeutically to selectively break down pathological tissues, as in treatment of arthritis, gallstones, and lesions of the nervous system, and also as a diagnostic aid by visually displaying echoes received from insonated tissues, as in ECHOCARDIOGRAPHY and echoencephalography. See also ULTRASONOGRAPHY.

ultrasonogram (,ultrə'sonə,gram) the record obtained by ultrasonography.

ultrasonography (,ultrəsə'nogrəfee) a radiological technique in which deep structures of the body are visualized by recording the reflections (echoes) of ultrasonic waves directed into the tissues. adj. **ultrasonographic.** Frequencies in the range of 2.5 million to 10 million hertz are used in diagnostic ultrasonography. The lower frequencies provide a greater depth of penetration and are used to examine abdominal organs; those in the upper range provide less penetration but better resolution and are used predominantly to examine more superficial structures such as the eye.

The basic principle of ultrasonography is the same as that of depth-sounding in oceanographic studies of the ocean floor. The ultrasonic waves are confined to a narrow beam that may be transmitted through, refracted, absorbed, or reflected by the medium toward which they are directed, depending on the nature of the surface they strike.

In diagnostic ultrasonography the ultrasonic waves are produced by electrically stimulating a crystal called a *transducer.* As the beam strikes an interface or boundary between tissues of varying density (e.g., muscle and blood) some of the sound waves are reflected back to the transducer as echoes. The echoes are then converted into electrical impulses that are displayed as a television immage, presenting a 'picture' of the tissues under examination.

Ultrasonography can be utilized in examination of the heart (echocardiography), in location of aneurysms of the aorta and other abnormalities of the major blood vessels, and in identifying size and structural changes in organs in the abdominopelvic cavity. It is of supreme value in distinguishing solid from cystic masses. The technique also may be used to evaluate tumours and foreign bodies of the eye, and to demonstrate retinal detachment. It is also a valuable tool in imaging the infant brain. Ultrasonography is not, however, of much value in examination of the lungs because ultrasound waves do not pass through structures that contain air; the presence of bowel gas may also limit the visualization of abdominal organs.

A particularly important use of ultrasonography is in the field of obstetrics and paediatrics, where ionizing radiation is to be avoided whenever possible. The technique can evaluate fetal size and maturity and fetal and placental position. It is a fast, relatively safe, and reliable technique for diagnosing multiple pregnancies. Fetal abnormalities may be detected, making it possible to offer a termination of pregnancy at an early stage. Uterine tumours and other pelvic masses, including abscesses, can be identified by ultrasonography by the demonstration of mid-line shift.

A-mode u. that in which on the cathode-ray tube (CRT) display one axis represents the time required for the return of the echo and the other corresponds to the strength of the echo, as in echoencephalography.

B-mode u. that in which the position of a spot on the CRT display corresponds to the time elapsed (and thus to the position of the echogenic surface) and the brightness of the spot to the strength of the echo; movement of the transducer produces a sweep of the ultrasound beam and a tomographic scan of a cross section of the body (a compound B-scan).

Modern B-mode ultrasonography translates the brightness of the echoes into shades of grey. Called also GREY-SCALE ULTRASONOGRAPHY.

Doppler u. that in which measurement and a visual record are made of the shift in frequency of a continuous or pulsed ultrasonic wave proportional to the blood-flow velocity in underlying vessels; used in diagnosis of occlusive vascular disease. It is also used in detection of the fetal heart beat and the velocity of blood across a stenotic heart valve, which can then be used to estimate the pressure gradient across it.

grey-scale u. B-mode ultrasonography.

M-mode u. that in which the B-mode display is moved across the monitor screen by a time-base generator. In this way a recording of the movement of structures is made. This method is particularly applicable to study of cardiac structures.

real-time u. B-mode ultrasonography using an array of detectors so that scans can be made electronically at a rate of 30 frames a second and viewed as a moving image.

ultrasound ('ultrə,sownd) sound at frequencies above the upper limit of normal hearing, i.e., greater than about 20,000 Hz (cycles per second); used in medicine in the technique of ULTRASONOGRAPHY.

ultrastructure ('ultrə,strukchə) the structure visible only under the electron microscope.

ultraviolet (,ultrə'vieələt) denoting electromagnetic radiation of wavelength shorter than that of the violet end of the spectrum, having wavelengths of 4–400 nanometers.

u. rays electromagnetic radiation beyond the violet end of the visible spectrum and therefore not visible to man. They are produced by the sun but are absorbed to a large extent by ozone and particles of dust and smoke in the earth's atmosphere. They are also produced by the so-called sun lamps.

Ultraviolet rays can produce sun-burning and affect skin pigmentation, causing tanning. When they strike the skin surface, these rays transform provitamin D, secreted by the glands of the skin, into vitamin D, which is then absorbed into the body.

Because ultraviolet rays are capable of killing bacteria and other microorganisms, they are sometimes utilized in specially designed cabinets to sterilize objects, and may also be used to sterilize the air in operating rooms and other areas where destruction of bacteria is necessary.

u. therapy the employment of ultraviolet radiation in the treatment of various diseases, particularly those affecting the skin. Among those diseases which respond to this form of therapy are ACNE VULGARIS, PSORIASIS, and ulcerations, as in DECUBITIS ULCERS.

DOSAGE. The dosage unit of ultraviolet radiation is expressed as minimal erythema dose (MED). Because of varying degrees of skin thickness and pigmentation, human skin varies widely in its sensitivity to ultraviolet radiation. The MED refers to the amount of radiation that will produce, within a few hours, minimal *erythema* (redness caused by engorgement of capillaries) in the average Caucasian skin. Dosage for individual patients is prescribed according to probable sensitivity as determined by that individual's skin type as compared to average sensitivity.

DEGREES OF ERYTHEMA. Minimal erythema is a *first degree* erythema. It usually is produced after about 15 seconds of exposure to a high-pressure mercury arc in a quartz burner that is placed at a distance of 75 centimetres from the skin. A *second degree* erythema results from a dose of about 2.5 MED Its effects become apparent about four to six hours after application and is followed by slight peeling of the skin. A *third degree* erythema is produced by about 5 MED. It may become apparent within two hours after application and is accompanied by oedema followed by marked desquamation. A *fourth degree* erythema is produced by about 10 MED and is characterized by blistering.

PRECAUTIONS. It is apparent that ultraviolet therapy is safe only in the hands of a skilled and knowledgeable therapist. Areas of 'thin skin' that may be burned more readily than that receiving treatment must be protected by wet towels or dressings. The eye is highly sensitive to ultraviolet radiation; therefore some form of protection, such as goggles, compresses, or cotton balls, should be provided for the patient and the therapist to avoid damage to the conjunctiva and cornea.

Certain drugs, for example the sulphonamides, greatly increase sensitivity to ultraviolet radiation. All patients scheduled for this form of therapy should be questioned in regard to the medication they are taking so the dosage can be adjusted accordingly or the treatment deferred.

ululation (ˌyoolyuh'layshən, ˌulyuh-) loud crying or wailing.

umbilical (um'bilik'l, ˌumbi'liek'l) pertaining to the umbilicus.

u. cord the structure that connects the fetus and placenta. This cord is the lifeline of the fetus in the uterus throughout pregnancy.

Nourishment and oxygen pass along the umbilical vein from the placenta to the fetus, and waste products pass from the fetus to the placenta via two umbilical arteries. These vessels are surrounded and protected by Wharton's jelly.

Soon after birth, the umbilical cord is clamped and then cut. The length of cord that is attached to the placenta, still in the uterus, is expelled with the placenta. The stump that remains attached to the baby's abdomen is about 5 centimetres long. After a few days it separates naturally by a process of dry, aseptic NECROSIS.

u. hernia protrusion of abdominal contents through the abdominal wall at the umbilicus, the defect in the abdominal wall and protruding intestine being covered with skin and subcutaneous tissue.

During the growth of the fetus, the intestines grow more rapidly than the abdominal cavity. For a period, a portion of the intestines of the unborn child usually lies outside his abdomen in a sac within the umbilical cord. Normally, the intestines return to the abdomen, and the defect is closed by the time of birth. Occasionally the abdominal wall does not close solidly, and umbilical hernia results. This defect is more likely to be seen in preterm infants and in girls rather than boys.

The defect in the abdominal wall usually closes by itself. Coughing, crying, and straining temporarily cause the sac to enlarge, but the hernia never bursts and digestion is not affected. The hernia may be strapped with adhesive or elastic tape or a truss may be used, but the effectiveness of these methods is doubtful. If the defect in the abdominal wall has not repaired itself by the time the child is 2 years old, surgery to correct the condition (HERNIORRHAPHY) can then be performed.

Umbilical hernia should be distinguished from exomphalos, in which the intestines protrude directly into the umbilical cord and are covered only by a thin membrane. Exomphalos is a surgical emergency that must be treated immediately after birth. See also *umbilical* RING.

umbilicated (um'biliˌkaytid) marked by depressed spots resembling the umbilicus.

umbilication (umˌbili'kayshən) a depression resembling the umbilicus.

umbilicus (um'bilikəs, ˌumbi'liekəs) the (usually) depressed scar marking the site of entry of the umbilical cord in the fetus; called also *navel*.

umbo ('umboh) pl. *umbones* [L.] 1. a rounded elevation. 2. the slight projection at the centre of the outer surface of the tympanic membrane.

unciform ('unsiˌfawm) hooked or shaped like a hook.

uncinate ('unsiˌnayt) 1. unciform. 2. relating to or affecting the uncinate gyrus.

uncipressure ('unsiˌpreshə) pressure with a hook to stop haemorrhage.

unconscious (un'konshəs) 1. insensible; incapable of responding to sensory stimuli and of having subjective experiences. 2. that part of the mental activity which includes primitive or repressed wishes, concealed from consciousness by the psychological censor.

collective u. in jungian psychology, the portion of the unconscious which is theoretically common to mankind.

unconsciousness (un'konshəsnəs) an abnormal state of lack of response to sensory stimuli, resulting from injury, illness, shock or some other bodily disorder. A brief loss of unconsciousness from which the person recovers spontaneously or with slight aid is called fainting. Deep, prolonged unconsciousness is known as COMA (see also levels of CONSCIOUSNESS).

unction ('ungkshən) 1. an ointment. 2. application of an ointment or salve; inunction.

unctuous ('ungktyooəs) greasy or oily.

uncus ('ungkəs) the medially curved anterior part of the hippocampal gyrus. adj. **uncal**.

undecenoic acid ('undekəˌnoh·ik) an antifungal agent used in the treatment of such infections as athlete's foot. May be used in powder, ointment, lotion, or spray form.

undifferentiated (ˌundifə'renshiˌaytid) not differentiated; primitive.

undine ('undeen) a small glass flask for irrigating the eye.

UNDP United Nations Development Programme.

undulant fever ('undyuhlənt) brucellosis.

undulation (ˌundyuh'layshən) a wavelike motion in any medium; a vibration.

ung. *unguentum* (ointment).

ungual ('ung·gwəl) pertaining to the nails.

unguent ('ung·gwənt) an ointment.

unguentum (ung'gwentəm) pl. *unguenta* [L.] ointment.

unguiculate (ung'gwikyuhlət) having claws; clawlike.

unguinal ('ung·gwin'l) pertaining to a nail.

unguis ('ung·gwis) pl. *ungues* [L.] the horny cutaneous plate on the surface of the distal end of finger or toe; a fingernail or toenail. See also NAIL.

Unh chemical symbol, *unnilhexium*.

uni- word element. [L.] *one*.

uniaxial (ˌyooni'aksi·əl) 1. having only one axis. 2. developed in an axial direction only.

unicameral (ˌyooni'kamə·rəl) having only one cavity or compartment.

UNICEF ('yoonisef) United Nations International Children's Emergency Fund.

unicellular (ˌyooni'selyuhlə) made up of a single cell, as the bacteria.

uniglandular (ˌyooni'glandyuhlə) affecting only one gland.

unilateral (ˌyooni'latə·rəl) affecting only one side.

unilocular (ˌyooni'lokyuhlə) having only one loculus or compartment; monolocular.

uninucleated (ˌyooni'nyookliˌaytid) mononuclear.

uniocular (ˌyooni'okyuhlə) monocular.

union ('yooni·ən) the growing together of tissues separated by injury, as of the ends of a fractured bone, or of the edges of a wound.

uniovular (ˌyooniˈohvyuhlə, -ˈov-) monovular, monozygotic.

uniparous (yooˈnipə·rəs) 1. producing only one ovum or offspring at a time. 2. primiparous.

unipolar (ˌyooniˈpohlə) having a single pole or process, as a nerve cell.

unipotent, unipotential (yooˈnipətənt; ˌyoonipəˈtenshəl) having only one power, as giving rise to cells of one order only.

unit (ˈyoonit) 1. a single thing; one segment of a whole that is made up of identical or similar segments. 2. a specifically defined amount of anything subject to measurement, as of activity, dimension, velocity, volume, or the like. **Angström u.** angström.

atomic mass u. the unit of mass equal to one-twelfth the mass of the nuclide of carbon-12. Called also *dalton*.

electrostatic u's that system of units which is based on the fundamental definition of a unit charge as one that will repel a similar charge with a force of 1 dyne when the two charges are 1 cm apart in a vacuum.

International u. 1. a unit of enzyme activity equal to the amount of enzyme that catalyses the conversion of one micromole of substrate or coenzyme per minute under specified conditions (temperature, pH, and substrate concentration) of the assay method. Abbreviated U. 2. any of several arbitrary units that have been adopted by international bodies to express the quantities of certain vitamins (A, C, D, and thiamine hydrochloride), hormones (androgen, chorionic gonadotropin, oestradiol benzoate, oestrone, insulin, progesterone, and prolactin), and drugs (digitalis and penicillin).

Kienböck's u. a unit of x-ray exposure equal to 0.1 erythema dose; symbol X.

motor u. the unit of motor activity formed by a motor nerve cell and its many innervated muscle fibres.

SI u. any unit of the International System of units (the metric system). See SI UNITS.

Svedberg u. svedberg.

unitary (ˈyoonitə·ree) pertaining to a single object or individual.

United Kingdom Central Council (UKCC), United Kingdom Central Council for Nursing, Midwifery and Health Visiting (yooˌnietid ˈkingdəm) set up as a result of the 1979 Nurses, Midwives, and Health Visitors' Act; abbreviated UKCC. Its functions are to:

(1) Establish and improve standards of training and professional conduct for nurses, midwives, and health visitors.

(2) Ensure that standards of training meet any community obligations of the United Kingdom.

(3) Determine by means of rules the conditions of a person being admitted to training and the kind and standards of training to be undertaken, with a view to registration.

(4) Make provision within the rules for the kind and standards of further training available to persons who are already registered.

(5) Provide in such manner as it thinks fit advice for nurses, midwives, and health visitors on standards of professional conduct.

(6) Have proper regard for the interests of all groups within the professions, including those with minority representation.

UKCC code of professional conduct for the nurse, midwife and health visitor revised periodically, this code is intended to provide definite standards of practice and conduct that are essential to the ethical discharge of the nurse's responsibility.

The code is reproduced at the end of Appendix 1. Further information on the code, interpretative statements that clarify it, and guidance in implementing it in specific situations can be obtained from the UKCC (PC Division), 23 Portland Place, London W1N 3AF.

United States Pharmacopeia (yooˌnietid ˈstayts) see USP.

univalent (ˌyooniˈvaylənt) having a valency of one.

unmyelinated (unˈmieəliˌnaytid) not having a myelin sheath.

Unna's paste boot (ˈuhnəz) a dressing for varicose ulcers that consists of a gelatin, zinc oxide, and glycerin paste and spiral bandages applied in alternate layers on the entire leg to make a rigid boot.

unnilhexium (unilˈheksi·əm) a chemical element, atomic number 106, atomic weight 263, symbol Unh. See table of elements in Appendix 2.

unnilpentium (unilˈpenti·əm) a chemical element, atomic number 105, atomic weight 262, symbol Unp. See table of elements in Appendix 2.

unnilquadrium (unilˈkwodri·əm) a chemical element, atomic number 104, atomic weight 261, symbol Unq. See table of elements in Appendix 2.

unnilseptium (unilˈsepti·əm) a chemical element, atomic number 107, atomic weight 264, symbol Uns. See table of elements in Appendix 2.

Unp chemical symbol, *unnilpentium*.

unphysiological (ˌunfizi·əˈlojikˈl) not in harmony with the laws of physiology.

Unq chemical symbol, *unnilquadrium*.

UNRAA United Nations Relief and Rehabilitation Administration.

Uns chemical symbol, *unnilseptium*.

unsaturated (unˈsachəˌraytid) 1. not having all affinities of its elements satisfied (unsaturated compound). 2. not holding all of a solute which can be held in solution by the solvent (unsaturated solution). 3. denoting compounds in which two or more atoms are united by double or triple bonds.

unsealed radiation sources (unˈseeld) see RADIATION THERAPY.

unsex (unˈseks) to deprive of the gonads.

unstriated (unˈstrieaytid) having no striations, as smooth muscle.

Unverricht's disease (syndrome) (ˈuhnferikhts) myoclonus epilepsy.

ur-defence (ˈərdiˌfens) a belief essential to the psychological integrity of the individual. Such beliefs include faith in personal survival, in religious, philosophical, or scientific systems, and in human succorance.

urachus (ˈyooə·rəkəs) a fetal canal connecting the bladder with the allantois, persisting throughout life as a cord (median umbilical ligament). adj. **urachal.**

uracil (ˈyooə·rəsil) a pyrimidine base obtained from nucleic acid.

uracrasia (ˌyooə·rəˈkrayzi·ə) disordered state of the urine.

uraemia (yuhˈreemi·ə) 1. an excess in the blood of urea, creatinine, and other nitrogenous end products of protein and amino acid metabolism; sometimes referred to as *azotaemia*. 2. in current usage, the entire complex of signs and symptoms of chronic RENAL FAILURE. As the glomerular filtration rate falls in either acute tubular necrosis or chronic renal failure, serum urea and creatinine rise to very high levels. However, urea and creatinine measurements are only roughly correlated with uraemic symptoms. Other nitrogenous compounds present in small amounts may produce most of the toxic effects. Some uraemic symptoms are due to losses of kidney function that do not involve uraemia. adj. **uraemic.**

SYMPTOMS. The signs and symptoms of uraemia are those of end-stage renal disease. In this phase,

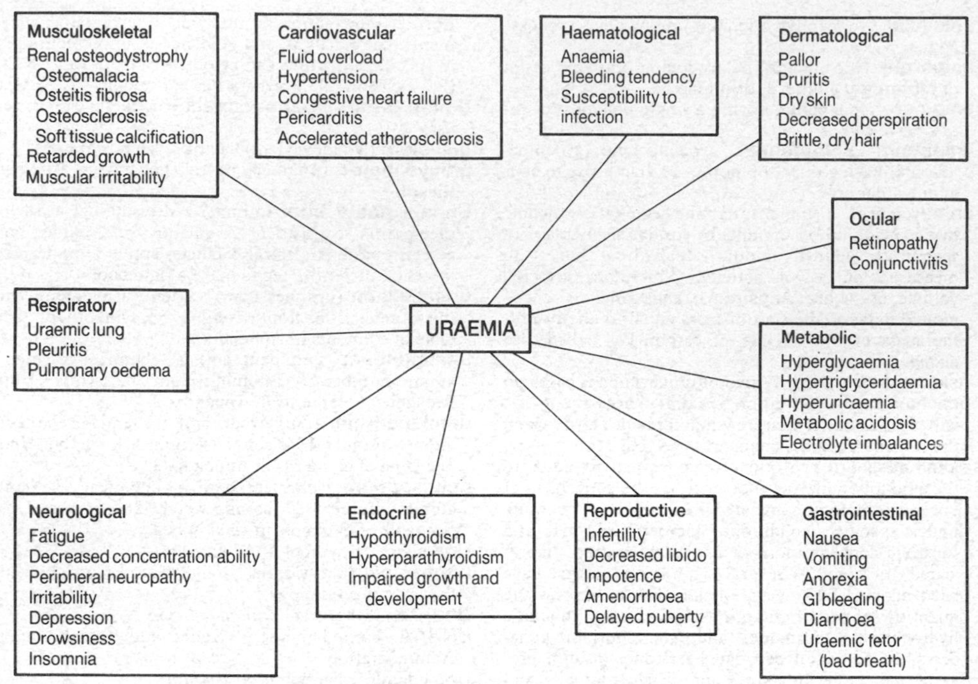

Systemic effects of uraemia

pathophysiological changes are evident in all of the body systems. A major threat is hyperkalaemia, which leads to cardiac abnormalities and can produce cardiac arrest. Warning signs that the heart muscle is failing can be seen on electrocardiographic tracings that show a flattened P wave, widened QRS complex, and peaked T wave.

HYPERTENSION is another threat to survival, second only to primary renal failure as a cause of death. Some patients develop an accelerated or malignant hypertension that is particularly resistant to drug therapy.

Susceptibility to infection is usually considered characteristic of uraemia, but the exact reason for this is not known. Superinfection with *Candida albicans* and *Herpes simplex* is common in patients receiving haemodialysis.

Gastrointestinal problems include stomatitis, duodenal ulcer, and ulcerations of the gut which produce diarrhoea; however, most uraemic patients complain of constipation. Anorexia is common and progresses to nausea, vomiting, and eventually continuous dry retching. An exceedingly dry mouth, metallic taste, and 'uraemic breath' contribute to the anorexia and nausea.

There is some tendency toward anaemia in uraemic patients because of decreased production of erythropoietin by the kidney and attendant decrease in the production of red blood cells. Bleeding tendencies also are present because of increased capillary fragility and a reduction in the adhesive properties of the platelets. The bleeding is rarely life-threatening, but it does contribute to the general weakness and discomfort of the patient.

Neurological changes predispose the uraemic patient to restlessness of the limbs, persistent hiccups, alterations in level of consciousness, and in uncontrolled uraemia to convulsive seizures that are usually of the grand mal type and often occur in rapid succession.

The skin of the patient with uraemia is a sallow, greyish-yellow colour due to anaemia and accumulations of the urinary pigment that gives urine its yellow colour. The sebaceous glands decrease production and the skin becomes dry and flaky. Pruritus, which is common in the uraemic patient, is due to the dryness and to deposits of urea crystals on the skin (uraemic frost).

Fluid and electrolyte imbalance can lead to either dehydration due to sodium and water loss or oedema due to sodium and water retention. Dehydration is most likely to occur in the early phase of renal failure. Later, the renin–angiotensin–aldosterone system, activated by ischaemic kidney cells, further compounds the retention of sodium and water and causes a generalized oedema.

ACIDOSIS is an expected outcome of a severely damaged kidney. Probably the major reason for the acidosis is reduced capacity to excrete hydrogen ions and retain bicarbonate. Compensatory hyperventilation occurs in response to the systemic acidosis.

TREATMENT. The treatment of acute renal failure and uraemia is primarily concerned with the institution of early and frequent dialysis; either peritoneal dialysis or haemodialysis may be employed. If the patient is not dialysed, he is placed on fluid and sodium restriction and a low-protein diet. The prevention of progressive hyperkalaemia is extremely important and is accomplished by administration of a potassium-binding resin. Acidosis is controlled by the intravenous administration of sodium bicarbonate. Antibiotics, diuretics, and digitalis may be prescribed as indicated to manage complications. Once the immediate problem of acute renal failure is resolved and extrarenal complications are avoided, the patient's prognosis for long-term survival is good. If the renal damage is irreversible, the patient becomes a candidate for renal replacement therapy.

Patients with uraemia resulting from chronic renal failure also are candidates for haemodialysis, peritoneal dialysis and transplantation.

uraemigenic (yuh,reemi'jenik) 1. caused by uraemia. 2. causing uraemia.

uragogue ('yooə·rə,gog) diuretic.

uran(o)- word element. [Gr.] *palate.*

uraniscoplasty (yooə·rə'niskohplastee) an operation for repair of a cleft palate.

uraniscorrhaphy (,yooə·rənis'ko·rəfee) suture of a cleft palate; staphylorrhaphy.

uraniscus (,yooə·rə'niskəs) the palate.

uranium (yuh'rayni·əm) a chemical element, atomic number 92, atomic weight 238.03, symbol U. See table of elements in Appendix 2.

uranoplasty ('yooə·rənoh,plastee) plastic repair of the palate; palatoplasty. adj. **uranoplastic.**

uranorrhaphy (,yooə·rə'no·rəfee) suture of the palate; staphylorrhaphy.

uranoschisis (,yooə·rə'noskisis) cleft palate.

uranostaphyloschisis (,yooə·rənoh,stafi'loskisis) fissure of the soft and hard palates.

uranyl ('yooə·rənil) the UO_2^{2+} ion, as in uranyl sulphate.

urarthritis (,yooə·rah'thrietis) gouty arthritis.

urataemia (,yooə·rə'teemi·ə) urates in the blood.

urate ('yooə·rayt) a salt of uric acid.

uratic (yuh'ratik) pertaining to urates or to gout.

uratoma (,yooə·rə'tohmə) a concretion made up of urates; tophus.

uratosis (,yooə·rə'tohsis) the deposit of urates in the tissues.

uraturia (,yooə·rə'tyooə·ri·ə) urates in the urine.

urceiform (ər'see·i,fawm) pitcher-shaped.

urea (yuh'reeə, 'yooə·ri·ə) 1. the diamide of carbonic acid found in urine, blood, and lymph, the chief nitrogenous constituent of urine, and the chief nitrogenous end-product of protein metabolism; it is formed in the liver from amino acids and from ammonia compounds. 2. a pharmaceutical preparation of urea occasionally used to lower intracranial pressure. adj. **ureal.**

The amount of urea in the urine increases with the quantity of protein in the diet. This is because urea is an endogenous and exogenous waste product: endogenous because some of it is derived from the breakdown of body protein as the tissues undergo disintegration and repair, and exogenous because some of it is derived from the deamination of amino acids absorbed from the intestinal tract but not utilized by the body.

In severe nephritis or other disorders leading to renal failure, the concentration of urea in the blood may be greatly increased, as revealed by measurement of the blood urea nitrogen (BUN).

u. cycle a cyclic series of reactions that produce urea, a major route for removal of the ammonia produced in the metabolism of amino acids in the liver and kidney.

u. nitrogen the urea concentration of serum or plasma, conventionally specified in terms of nitrogen content and called *blood urea nitrogen* (BUN), an important indicator of renal function.

Ureaplasma urealyticum (,yooə·ri·ə'plazmə ,yooə·reeə'litikəm) a species of nonmotile pleomorphic, gram-negative bacteria, lacking a cell wall and forming very small granular colonies, 15–25 μm in diameter; they are associated with nonspecific urethritis in males and genital tract infections in females.

ureapoiesis (yuh,reeəpoy'eesis) formation of urea. adj. **ureapoietic.**

urease ('yooə·ri,ayz) an enzyme that catalyses the decomposition of urea to ammonia and carbon dioxide.

urecchysis (yuh'rekisis) an effusion of urine into cellular tissue.

urelcosis (,yooə·rel'kohsis) ulceration in the urinary tract.

ureotelic (,yooə·rioh'telik) having urea as the chief excretory product of nitrogen metabolism.

uresiaesthesis (yuh,reesee·is'theesis) the normal impulse to pass the urine.

uresis (yuh'reesis) the passage of urine; urination.

-uresis word element. [Gr.] *urinary excretion of.* adj. **-uretic.**

ureter (yuh'reetə, 'yooə·ritə) the fibromuscular tube, 25–30 centimetres long, through which the urine passes from the kidney to the bladder. adj. **ureteral, ureteric.** As urine is produced by each kidney, it passes into the ureter, which, by contracting rhythmically, forces the urine along and empties it in spurts into the bladder. After being stored temporarily in the bladder, the urine passes out of the body by way of the urethra.

Rarely, a small calculus, or stone, formed in a kidney, passes into a ureter and obstructs it. The result is the sudden severe pain known as renal or ureteric colic. In such cases the aim of medical treatment is to relieve the pain and obstruction and to eliminate the condition that causes the stone.

ureter(o)- word element. [Gr.] *ureter.*

ureteralgia (yuh,reetə'ralji·ə) pain in the ureter.

ureterectasis (yuh,reetə'rektəsis) distention of the ureter.

ureterectomy (yuh,reetə'rektəmee) excision of a ureter.

ureteritis (yuh,reetə'rietis) inflammation of a ureter.

ureterocele (yuh'reetə·roh,seel) ballooning of the lower end of the ureter into the bladder.

ureterocelectomy (yuh,reetə·rohsi'lektəmee) excision of a ureterocele.

ureterocolostomy (yuh,reetə·rohkə'lostəmee) anastomosis of a ureter to the colon.

ureterocystoscope (yuh,reetə·roh'sistə,skohp) a cystoscope with a catheter for insertion into the ureter.

ureterocystostomy (yuh,reetə·rohsi'stostəmee) ureteroneocystostomy.

ureterodialysis (yuh,reetə·rohdie'aləsis) rupture of a ureter; ureterolysis.

ureteroenterostomy (yuh,reetə·roh,entə'rostəmee) anastomosis of one or both ureters to the wall of the intestine.

ureterography (yuh,reetə'rografee) radiography of the ureter, after injection of a contrast medium.

ureteroheminephrectomy (yuh,reetə·roh,heminə'frektəmee) excision of the diseased portion of a reduplicated kidney and its ureter.

ureteroileostomy (yuh,reetə·roh,ili'ostəmee) anastomosis of the ureters to an isolated loop of the ileum to form a urinary conduit.

ureterolith (yuh'reetə·roh,lith) a calculus in the ureter.

ureterolithiasis (yuh,reetə·rohli'thieəsis) formation of a calculus in the ureter.

ureterolithotomy (yuh,reetə·rohli'thotəmee) incision

of a ureter for removal of calculus.

ureterolysis (yuh,reetə'rolisis) 1. rupture of the ureter; ureterodialysis. 2. paralysis of the ureter. 3. the operation of freeing the ureter from adhesions.

ureteroneocystostomy (yuh,reetə·roh,neeohsi'stostəmee) surgical transplantation of a ureter to a different site in the bladder; ureterocystostomy.

ureteronephrectomy (yuh,reetə·rohnə'frektəmee) excision of a kidney and ureter.

ureteropathy (yuh,reetə'ropəthee) any disease of the ureter.

ureteropelvioplasty (yuh,reetə·roh'pelvioh,plastee) surgical reconstruction of the junction of the ureter and renal pelvis. Called aslo *ureteroneopyelostomy, ureteropyelostomy, ureteropyeloplasty.*

ureteropexy (yuh'reetə·rohpeksee) fixation of the ureter.

ureteroplasty (yuh'reetə·roh,plastee) plastic repair of a ureter.

ureteropyelitis (yuh,reetə·roh,pieə'lietis) inflammation of a ureter and renal pelvis.

ureteropyelography (yuh,reetə·rohpieə'logrəfee) radiography of the ureter and renal pelvis.

ureteropyelonephritis (yuh,reetə·roh,pieəlohnə'frietis) inflammation of the ureter, renal pelvis, and kidney.

ureteropyosis (yuh,reetə·rohpie'ohsis) suppurative inflammation of the ureter.

ureterorenoscope (yuh,reetə·roh'reenoh,skohp) a fibreoptic endoscope used in uterorenoscopy.

ureterorenoscopy (yuh,reetə·rohree'noskəpee) visual inspection of the interior of the ureter and kidney by means of a fibreoptic endoscope for such purposes as biopsy, removal or crushing of stones, or other procedures.

ureterorrhagia (yuh,reetə·roh'rayji·ə) discharge of blood from the ureter.

ureterorrhaphy (yuh,reetə'ro·rəfee) suture of the ureter.

ureterosigmoidostomy (yuh,reetə·roh,sigmoy'dostəmee) anastomosis of one or both ureters to the sigmoid colon, now seldom performed.

ureterostomy (yuh,reetə'rostəmee) creation of a new outlet for a ureter.

cutaneous u. a type of urinary diversion in which one or both ureters are detached from the bladder and brought to the skin. A collecting pouch fitted with a belt is then worn snugly against the abdomen and over the 'ureteral buds' or stomas.

Indications for ureterostomy include malignancy or any cause necessitating removal of the bladder, when an ileal conduit is contraindicated.

Patient care is similar to that for any patient with a diversion of urinary flow and is primarily concerned with teaching the patient how to care for his own appliance, and avoidance of complications arising from the creation of the stoma. See also STOMA and ILEAL CONDUIT.

ureterotomy (yuh,reetə'rotəmee) incision into a ureter.

ureteroureterostomy (yuh,reetə·roh·yuh,reetə'rostəmee) end-to-end anastomosis of the two portions of a transected ureter.

ureterovaginal (yuh,reetə·rohvə'jien'l, -'vajin'l) pertaining to or communicating with a ureter and the vagina.

ureterovesical (yuh,reetə·roh'vesik'l) pertaining to a ureter and the bladder.

urethr(o)- word element. [Gr.] *urethra.*

urethra (yuh'reethrə) the tubular passage through which urine is discharged from the bladder to the exterior of the body. adj. **urethral.**

The external urinary opening is called the urinary meatus. In men the urethra conveys both urine and the secretions of the reproductive organs.

The female urethra is about 3.5 centimetres long. The opening is situated between the clitoris and the opening of the vagina.

The male urethra is about 18 centimetres long and is narrower than that of the female. It has three sections—prostatic, membranous, and penile. It extends downward from the bladder through the prostate, which secretes into it a thin fluid. The membranous portion of the urethra receives the secretion of the bulbourethral glands. The urethra then extends down through the main body of the penis to the opening, or meatus, at the tip. Along the entire length of the passage are mucous glands.

DISORDERS OF THE URETHRA. Urethritis, inflammation of the urethra, occurs mainly in gonorrhoea. Urethral strictures in men, caused by bands of fibrous tissue which obstruct the passage of urine, are also most often caused by neglected gonorrhoea but may sometimes be caused by any infection, or by injury. They may be treated surgically or by dilation. Kidney stones, or calculi, may rarely lodge in the urethra. They usually pass spontaneously but if not, may be removed with forceps or crushed.

In women, urethral caruncles, small, fleshy, red masses, sometimes form near the opening of the urethra, usually at the time of menopause. Caruncles are not dangerous unless they cause bleeding and painful urination; then surgical removal is required.

urethralgia (,yooə·ri'thralji·ə) pain in a urethra; urethrodynia.

urethratresia (yuh,reethrə'treezi·ə) imperforation of the urethra.

urethrectomy (,yooə·ri'threktəmee) excision of the urethra.

urethremphraxis (yuh,reethrem'fraksis) obstruction of the urethra.

urethrism (yuh'reethrizəm) irritability or chronic spasm of the urethra.

urethritis (,yooə·ri'thrietis) inflammation of the urethra. The condition is frequently a symptom of gonorrhoea but may be caused by other infectious organisms.

In urethritis the urethra swells and narrows, and the flow of urine is impeded. Both urination and the urgency to urinate increase. Urination is accompanied by burning pain. There may be a purulent discharge.

Urethritis usually responds to treatment with antibiotics or sulphonamides.

nonspecific u. (NSU) a sexually transmitted inflammation of the urethra caused by a variety of organisms other than gonococci, e.g. *Chlamydia trachomatis, Ureaplasma urealyticum* and *Trichomonas vaginalis.* It is believed to be the most common sexually transmitted urethritis in males in the United Kingdom. NSU usually responds to treatment with antibiotics.

urethrobulbar (yuh,reethroh'bulbə) pertaining to the urethra and the bulb of the penis.

urethrocele (yuh'reethroh,seel) prolapse of the female urethra through the urinary meatus.

urethrocystitis (yuh,reethrohsi'stietis) inflammation of the urethra and bladder.

urethrodynia (yuh,reethroh'dini·ə) urethralgia.

urethrography (,yooə·ri'throgrəfee) radiography of the urethra.

urethrometry (,yooə·ri'thromətree) 1. determination of the resistance of various segments of the urethra to retrograde flow of fluid. 2. measurement of the urethra.

urethropenile (yuh,reethroh'peeniel) pertaining to the urethra and penis.

urethroperineal (yuh,reethroh,peri'neeəl) pertaining to the urethra and perineum.
urethroperineoscrotal (yuh,reethroh,peri,neeoh-'skroht'l) pertaining to the urethra, perineum, and scrotum.
urethrophraxis (yuh,reethroh'fraksis) obstruction of the urethra.
urethrophyma (yuh,reethroh'fiemə) a tumour or growth in the urethra.
urethroplasty (yuh'reethroh,plastee) plastic repair of the urethra.
urethroprostatic (yuh,reethrohpro'statik) pertaining to the urethra and prostate.
urethrorectal (yuh,reethroh'rekt'l) pertaining to the urethra and rectum.
urethrorrhagia (yuh,reethrə'rayji·ə) a flow of blood from the urethra.
urethrorrhaphy (,yooə·ri'thro·rəfee) suture of a urethra in the case of urethral fistula or injury.
urethrorrhoea (yuh,reethrə'reeə) abnormal discharge from the urethra.
urethroscope (yuh'reethrə,skohp) an instrument for viewing the interior of the urethra.
urethroscopy (,yooə·ri'throskəpee) visual inspection of the urethra. adj. **urethroscopic**.
urethrospasm (yuh'reethroh,spazəm) spasm of the urethral muscular tissue.
urethrostaxis (yuh,reethroh'staksis) oozing of blood from the urethra.
urethrostenosis (yuh,reethrohstə'nohsis) constriction of the urethra.
urethrostomy (,yooə·ri'throstəmee) creation of a permanent opening for the urethra in the perineum.
urethrotome (yuh'reethrə,tohm) an instrument for cutting a urethral stricture.
urethrotomy (,yooə·ri'throtəmee) incision into the urethra.
urethrotrigonitis (yuh,reethroh,triegoh'nietis) inflammation of the urethra and trigone of the bladder (vesical trigone).
urethrovaginal (yuh,reethrohvə'jien'l, -'vajin'l) pertaining to the urethra and vagina.
urethrovesical (yuh,reethroh'vesik'l) pertaining to the urethra and bladder.
urgency ('ərjənsee) the sudden compelling desire to urinate.
urhidrosis (,yooəhi'drohsis) the presence in the sweat of urinous materials, chiefly uric acid and urea.
-uria word element. [Gr.] *condition of the urine*. adj. **-uric**.
uriaesthesis (,yooə·ri·is'theesis) uresiaesthesis.
uric ('yooə·rik) pertaining to the urine.

u. acid the end product of purine metabolism or oxidation in the body. It is present in blood in a concentration of about 0.13–0.42 mmol/l and is excreted in the urine in amounts of a little less than 1 g per day. In GOUT there is an excess of uric acid in the blood, and salts of uric acid (urates) form insoluble stones in the urinary tract, or they may crystallize and form deposits (tophi) in the joints and tissues.

The presence of high concentrations of uric acid in the urine is significant in the diagnosis of gout, but is of little significance in urinary disorders.

uricacidaemia (,yooə·rik,asi'deemi·ə) uric acid in the blood.
uricaciduria (,yooə·rik,asi'dyooə·ri·ə) excess of uric acid in the urine.
uricaemia (,yooə·ri'seemi·ə) uricacidaemia.
uricase ('yooə·ri,kayz) an enzyme that catalyses the conversion of uric acid to allantoin.
uricolysis (,yooə·ri'kolisis) the cleavage of uric acid or urates. adj. **uricolytic**.
uricosuria (,yooə·rikoh'syooə·ri·ə) excretion of uric acid in the urine.
uricosuric (,yooə·rikoh'syooə·rik) 1. pertaining to, characterized by, or promoting uricosuria. 2. an agent that promotes uricosuria.
uricotelic (,yooə·rikoh'telik) having uric acid as the chief excretory product of nitrogen metabolism.
uridine ('yooə·ri,deen) a ribonucleoside containing uracil.

u. diphosphate (UDP) a nucleotide that participates in glycogen metabolism and in some processes of nucleic acid synthesis.

uridrosis (,yooə·ri'drohsis) urhidrosis.
urin(o)- word element. [Gr., L.] *urine*.
urina (yuh'rienə) [L.] *urine*.
urinaemia (,yooə·ri'neemi·ə) uraemia.
urinal (yuh'rien'l, 'yooə·rin'l) a receptacle for urine.
urinalysis (yooə·ri'nalisis) analysis of the urine as an aid in the diagnosis of disease. Many types of tests are used in analysing the urine in order to determine whether it contains abnormal substances indicative of disease. The most significant substances normally absent from urine and detected by urinalysis are protein, glucose, ketones, blood, pus, and casts.
urinary ('yooə·rinə·ree) pertaining to the urine; containing or secreting urine.

u. bladder the musculomembranous sac in the anterior part of the pelvic cavity that serves as a reservoir for urine (see also BLADDER).

u. system, u. tract the system formed in the body by the KIDNEYS, the urinary BLADDER, the URETERS, and the URETHRA, the organs concerned in the production and excretion of urine.

urinate ('yooə·ri,nayt) to void urine.
urination (,yooə·ri'nayshən) the discharge of urine from the bladder; called also *voiding the urine* and *micturition*. Urine from the kidneys is passed in spurts every few seconds along the ureters to the bladder, where it collects until voided. During the act of urination the urine passes from the bladder to the outside via the urethra.

THE URINARY PROCESS. Urination is a complex process controlled by several sets of muscles, including the internal and external sphincters, which are circular muscles surrounding the urethra; they have the power to contract and prevent flow through it. The internal sphincter is at the outlet of the bladder and works automatically. The external sphincter, situated along the urethra below the prostate in males and at an equivalent position in females, is controlled voluntarily.

As the bladder fills, the bladder muscle tends to contract automatically. The urge to urinate enters consciousness, but voiding may be controlled consciously to some extent. When the person decides to urinate, the bladder muscle contracts and both sphincters relax.

BED-WETTING AND INCONTINENCE. Control of the sphincters is late in developing. For the first year of life there is no control at all. Conscious control of the external sphincter develops in the second year, but complete control during sleep does not develop until the sphincters can deal automatically with the total amount of urine excreted during the night. This is why bed-wetting can continue until comparatively late in young children.

Extreme fear in emergency situations may cause automatic relaxation of the sphincters with loss of control of urination, or INCONTINENCE. Incontinence also may occur in epileptic seizures, strokes, or other neurological illness. In elderly men it may be due to hypertrophy of the prostate. Infection of the bladder or urethra in both men and women may impair control of urination.

Normally 1.1 to 1.7 litres of urine is passed each day, but the amount is increased by a large intake of liquid or by cold weather. It is decreased in hot weather, when more fluid is eliminated through the skin by perspiration. Urination is usually necessary three or four times a day.

DISORDERS OF URINATION. Excessive secretion of urine (polyuria) may indicate diabetes mellitus, and diminution of urinary secretion (oliguria) may occur in nephritis. Frequent urination is a symptom of cystitis. Painful urination (dysuria) is characteristic of some bladder diseases, inflammation of the prostate, and certain infections, including gonorrhoea. Nocturia, or excessive urination at night, is a symptom of some urinary system diseases. It often occurs in acute prostatitis.

Urinary suppression is failure of the kidneys to produce urine and results in uraemia if not corrected. This condition is brought about by severe disease or injury to the renal cells. Urinary retention is the accumulation of urine within the bladder because of inability to urinate.

urine ('yooə·rin) the fluid containing water and waste products that is secreted by the KIDNEYS, stored in the bladder and discharged by way of the urethra.

CONTENTS OF THE URINE. Several different types of waste products are eliminated in urine—for example, urea, uric acid, ammonia, and creatinine—none of which is useful in the blood. The largest component of urine by weight (apart from water) is urea, which is derived from the breakdown of proteins and amino acids in the diet and in the body itself. Its amount varies greatly from person to person, however, depending on the amount of protein in the diet. Besides waste materials, urine also contains surpluses of products that are necessary for bodily functioning. The kidneys remove not only excess water but also excess sodium chloride and other chemicals. Thus in a typical specimen of urine there will be sodium, potassium, calcium, magnesium, chloride, phosphate, and sulphate ions.

The colour of urine is due to the presence of the yellow pigment urochrome. Individual ingredients of urine are not usually visible, but when the urine is alkaline some of the ingredients may form sediments of phosphates and urates. It may also become cloudy from the presence of mucus. Persistent cloudiness may indicate the presence of pus or blood.

CHANGES IN THE URINE AS A SIGN OF ILLNESS. Changes in the urine can be an important warning of illness. The presence of glucose may signify the development of diabetes mellitus. If the urine is red or brown, this may indicate kidney disease, since the colour may be due to blood in the urine (haematuria). A pink hue is not always caused by blood but may be due to certain foods such as beets and rhubarb, and cathartics containing senna, phenolphthalein, or cascara. A smoky colour may indicate old blood in the urine. With jaundice the urine may become dark or brown-coloured.

u. osmolality a measure of the number of dissolved particles per unit of water in urine (see also urine OSMOLALITY).

residual u. urine remaining in the bladder after urination; seen in bladder outlet obstruction (as by prostatic hypertrophy) and disorders affecting nerves controlling bladder function.

uriniferous (ˌyooə·ri'nifə·rəs) transporting or conveying urine.

uriniparous (ˌyooə·ri'nipə·rəs) excreting urine.

urinogenital (ˌyooə·rinoh'jenit'l) urogenital.

urinogenous (ˌyooə·ri'nojənəs) of urinary origin.

urinology (ˌyooə·ri'noləjee) urology.

urinoma (ˌyooə·ri'nohmə) a cyst containing urine.

urinometer (ˌyooə·ri'nomitə) an instrument for determining the specific gravity of urine.

urinous ('yooə·rinəs) pertaining to or of the nature of urine.

uriposia (ˌyooə·ri'pohzi·ə) the drinking of urine.

Urispas ('yooə·riˌspaz) trademark for a preparation of flavoxate, a smooth muscle relaxant.

uro- word element. [Gr.] *urine* (urinary tract, urination).

urobilin (ˌyooə·roh'bielin) a brownish pigment formed by oxidation of urobilinogen; found in the faeces and sometimes in the urine after standing in the air.

urobilinaemia (ˌyooə·rohˌbieli'neemi·ə) urobilin in the blood.

urobilinogen (ˌyooə·rohbie'linəjən) a colourless compound formed in the intestines by the reduction of BILIRUBIN. Normally about 1 per cent of the bilirubin produced in the body by the breakdown of haemoglobin is excreted in the urine as urobilinogen. Increased amounts of urobilinogen in the urine indicate an excessive amount of bilirubin in the blood. Determination of the amount of urobilinogen excreted in a given period makes it possible to evaluate certain types of haemolytic anaemia and also is of help in diagnosing liver dysfunction.

Laboratory tests for urobilinogen require collection of urine for a 24-hour period or for a 2-hour period. The specimen should be taken to the laboratory immediately since bacteria which may be present in the urine can oxidize urobilinogen and change it to urobilin.

urocele ('yooə·rohˌseel) distention of the scrotum with extravasated urine.

urochezia (ˌyooə·roh'keezi·ə) discharge of urine in the faeces.

urochrome ('yooə·rohˌkrohm) a breakdown product of haemoglobin related to the bile pigments, found in the urine and responsible for its yellow colour.

uroclepsia (ˌyooə·roh'klepsi·ə) the involuntary escape of urine.

urocrisia (ˌyooə·roh'krisi·ə) diagnosis by examining the urine.

urocyst ('yooə·rohˌsist) the urinary bladder. adj. **urocystic.**

urocystitis (ˌyooə·rohsi'stietis) inflammation of the urinary bladder.

urodynamics (ˌyooə·rohdie'namiks) the dynamics of the propulsion and flow of urine in the urinary tract. adj. **urodynamic.**

urodynia (ˌyooə·roh'dini·ə) pain accompanying urination.

uroedema (ˌyooə·ri'deemə) swelling from extravasated urine.

urogastrone (ˌyooə·roh'gastrohn) a polypeptide secreted by the salivary glands and by Brunner's glands, which is a potent inhibitor of gastric acid secretion.

urogenital (ˌyooə·roh'jenit'l) pertaining to the urinary system and genitalia; urinogenital; genitourinary.

u. system genitourinary system.

urogenous (yuh'rojənəs) 1. producing urine. 2. produced from or in the urine.

Urografin (ˌyooə·roh'grafin) trademark for a contrast medium series containing diatrizoate as the anion.

urogram ('yooə·rohˌgram) a film obtained by urography.

urography (yuh'rografee) radiography of the urinary tract after the injection of a radiopaque, water-soluble, iodine-containing medium.

excretion u., intravenous u. the contrast medium is

injected as a rapid bolus and radiographs are exposed at predetermined intervals, thus recording its excretion by the kidney, opacification of the calyces and pelvis, and filling of the ureters and bladder. It is common practice to give the patient nothing by mouth for five hours prior to the injection, but dehydration is contraindicated in the presence of renal failure and myeloma and in young infants because of the increased likelihood of CONTRAST MEDIUM REACTIONS. Preparation of the patient may also include the prescribing of a laxative so that bowel contents will not obscure visualization of the urinary tract.

urokinase (ˌyooə·roh'kienayz) an enzyme found in the urine of man and other mammals which is secreted by kidney parenchymal cells and converts plasminogen to plasmin and activates the fibrinolytic system; used as a fibrinolytic agent.

urolith ('yooə·rohˌlith) a calculus in the urine or the urinary tract. adj. **urolithic**.

urolithiasis (ˌyooə·rohli'thieəsis) formation of urinary calculi, or the condition associated with urinary calculi.

urologist (yuh'roləjist) a specialist in urology.

urology (yuh'roləjee) the branch of medicine dealing with the urinary system in the female and genitourinary system in the male. adj. **urological**.

uromelus (yuh'romələs) a fetus or infant with fused legs and a single foot.

urometry (yuh'romətree) the measurement and recording of pressure changes caused by contraction of the ureter during ureteral peristalsis. adj. **urometric**.

Uromiro (ˌyuhroh'mieroh) trademark for a contrast medium series containing iodamide as the anion.

uroncus (yuh'rongkəs) a swelling caused by retention or extravasation of urine.

uronephrosis (ˌyooə·rohnə'frohsis) distention of the renal pelvis and tubules with urine.

uropathy (yuh'ropəthee) any disease in the urinary tract.

urophanic (ˌyooə·roh'fanik) appearing in the urine.

uroplania (ˌyooə·roh'playni·ə) the presence of urine in, or its discharge from, organs not of the genitourinary system.

uropoiesis (ˌyooə·rohpoy'eesis) the formation of urine. adj. **uropoietic**.

uroporphyria (ˌyooə·rohpaw'firi·ə) porphyria with excessive excretion of uroporphyrin.

uroporphyrin (ˌyooə·roh'pawfirin) one of a group of porphyrins produced during biosynthesis of natural porphyrins and excreted in urine.

uroporphyrinogen (ˌyooə·rohˌpawfi'rinəjən) a precursor of uroporphyrin and coproporphyrinogen.

uropsammus (ˌyooə·roh'saməs) urinary gravel.

uroradiology (ˌyooə·rohˌraydi'oləjee) radiology of the urinary tract.

urorrhagia (ˌyooə·rə'rayji·ə) excessive secretion of urine.

urorrhoea (ˌyooə·rə'reeə) involuntary flow of urine.

uroscheocele (yuh'roskiohˌseel) urocele.

uroschesis (yuh'roskisis) retention or suppression of the urine.

uroscopy (yuh'roskəpee) diagnostic examination of the urine. adj. **uroscopic**.

urosepsis (ˌyooə·roh'sepsis) septic poisoning from retained and absorbed urinary substances. adj. **uroseptic**.

urostealith (ˌyooə·roh'stiəlith) a urinary calculus having fatty constituents.

urostomy (yuh'rostəmee) an artificial urinary conduit to deflect urine from the ureters to the abdominal wall; usually constructed from a transposed section of ileum taken out of intestinal circuit, the external portion being everted as for ileostomy the ureters being inserted into the closed inner end. It serves the purpose of permanent urinary diversion from the bladder and beyond, and is a necessary preliminary to total cystectomy; it is controlled by an appliance made to adhere to the peristomal skin.

urotoxia (ˌyooə·roh'toksi·ə) 1. the toxicity of the urine. 2. the toxic substances of the urine. 3. the unit of toxicity of the urine or a quantity sufficient to kill 1 kg of living substance. adj. **urotoxic**.

uroureter (ˌyooə·roh·yuh'reetə, -'yooə·ritə) distention of the ureter with urine.

urticant ('ərtikənt) producing urticaria.

urticaria (ˌərti'kair·ri·ə) a vascular reaction of the skin marked by transient appearance of slightly elevated patches (wheals) which are redder or paler than the surrounding skin and often attended by severe itching; called also *nettle rash*. The cause may be certain foods, infection, or emotional stress. adj. **urticarial**. Called also *hives*.

giant u., u. gigantea angioneurotic oedema.

u. haemorrhagica purpura with urticaria. **u. medicamentosa** that due to use of a drug.

papular u., u. papulosa an allergic reaction to the bite of various insects, with appearance of lesions that evolve into inflammatory, increasingly hard, red or brownish, persistent papules.

u. pigmentosa mastocytosis manifested as persistent pink to brown macules or soft plaques of various size; pruritus and urtication occur on stroking the lesions.

u. pigmentosa, juvenile urticaria pigmentosa present at birth or in the first few weeks of life, usually disappearing before puberty, taking the form of a single nodule or tumour or of a disseminated eruption of yellowish brown to yellowish red macules, plaques, or bullae.

solar u. a rare form produced by exposure to sunlight.

urtication (ˌərti'kayshən) 1. the development or formation of urticaria. 2. a burning sensation, as of the sting of nettles.

urushiol (ə'rooshiol) the toxic irritant principle of poison ivy and various related plants.

US ultrasonic; ultrasound.

USP United States Pharmacopeia, a legally recognized compendium of standards for drugs, published by the United States Pharmacopeial Convention, Inc., and revised periodically; it also includes assays and tests for determination of strength, quality, and purity.

USS ultrasound scan.

ustilaginism (ˌusti'lajiˌnizəm) a condition resembling ergotism due to ingestion of maize containing *Ustilago maydis*.

uter(o)- word element. [L.] *uterus*.

uteralgia (ˌyootə'ralji·ə) pain in the uterus.

uterine ('yootəˌrien) pertaining to the uterus.

u. tube a slender tube arising from the cornu of the uterus, extending laterally to the ovary on the same side. The other ovary is similarly connected to the uterus. The tubes permit the passage of spermatozoa and convey the fertilized ovum to the uterus in the opposite direction. Following ovulation, oestrogen causes the fimbria ovarica to curve toward the ovum in order to sweep it into the fimbriated end of the tube. The ampulla is the usual site of fertilization, following which the ovum is propelled by peristalsis and the action of cilia lining the tube toward the uterus. The journey takes 4–5 days during which time the ovum is nourished by mucus secreted by the goblet cells lining the tube. Called also *oviduct* or *fallopian tube*.

Obstruction of the tube is a likely complication because of its highly convoluted lining and narrow lumen, and may follow salpingitis or gonorrhoea, possibly resulting in a fertilzed ovum implanting within the tube to cause ectopic, or tubal, PREGNANCY.

uteroabdominal (ˌyootə·roh·ab'domin'l) pertaining to the uterus and abdomen.

uterocele ('yootə·roh,seel) a hernia of the uterus. A hysterocele.

uterocervical (ˌyootə·roh'sərvik'l, -sə'viek'l) pertaining to the uterus and uterine cervix.

uterofixation (ˌyootə·rohfik'sayshən) hysteropexy; surgical fixation of the uterus.

uterogenic (ˌyootə·roh'jenik) formed in the uterus.

uterogestation (ˌyootə·rohje'stayshən) uterine gestation; normal pregnancy.

uterography (ˌyootə'rogrəfee) radiographic examination of the uterus; hysterography.

uterolith ('yootə·roh,lith) a uterine calculus; hysterolith.

uterometer (ˌyootə'romitə) an instrument for measuring the uterus; hysterometer.

utero-ovarian (ˌyootə·roh·oh'vair·ri·ən) pertaining to the uterus and ovary.

uteropexy ('yootə·roh,peksee) hysteropexy.

uteroplacental (ˌyootə·rohplə'sent'l) pertaining to the placenta and uterus.

uteroplasty ('yootə·roh,plastee) plastic repair of the uterus.

uterorectal (ˌyootə·roh'rekt'l) pertaining to or communicating with the uterus and rectum.

uterosacral (ˌyootə·roh'saykrəl) pertaining to the uterus and sacrum.

uterosalpingography (ˌyootə·roh,salping'gogrəfee) radiography of the uterus and uterine tubes; hysterosalpingography.

uteroscope ('yootə·roh,skohp) an instrument for viewing the interior of the uterus; hysteroscope.

uterotomy (ˌyootə'rotəmee) hysterotomy; incision of the uterus.

uterotonic (ˌyootə·roh'tonik) 1. increasing the tone of uterine muscle. 2. a uterotonic agent.

uterotubal (ˌyootə·roh'tyoob'l) pertaining to the uterus and uterine tubes.

uterovaginal (ˌyootə·rohvə'jien'l, -'vajin'l) pertaining to the uterus and vagina.

uterovesical (ˌyootə·roh'vesik'l) pertaining to the uterus and bladder.

uterus ('yootə·rəs) the hollow muscular organ in female mammals in which the fertilized ovum normally becomes embedded and in which the developing embryo and fetus is nourished. The human uterus, or womb, is normally about the size and shape of a pear. The upper part, or fundus, is broad and flattened; the middle portion is the body, or corpus; the lower part, or cervix, is narrow and tubular. The cervix opens downward into the VAGINA. Two UTERINE TUBES enter the uterus at the upper end, one on each side.

The walls of the uterus are composed of muscle, the myometrium; its lining is endometrium. Between puberty and menopause, the lining goes through a monthly cycle of growth and discharge, known as the MENSTRUAL CYCLE. Menstruation occurs when the tissue prepared by the uterus for a possible embryo or fertilized egg, is unused and is reabsorbed.

The menstrual cycle is interrupted by pregnancy when a mature ovum is fertilized by a spermatozoon. Fertilization usually takes place in the uterine tube; the fertilized ovum continues moving along the tube and comes to rest in the uterus, where it implants in the endometrium. The endometrium then serves to anchor the placenta, which filters nutrients from the mother's blood into the blood of the growing fetus. See also REPRODUCTION and female REPRODUCTIVE ORGANS.

DISORDERS OF THE UTERUS. The main organs of the female reproductive system—uterus, uterine tubes, and ovaries—are connected to each other by ligaments that normally hold each in its proper place. Occasionally childbirth starts a chronic displacement of the uterus. The ligaments may stretch and weaken enough to allow the uterus to bulge into the vagina. This is called a prolapsed uterus. Uterine displacement may give rise to difficulties in urination and at times in conception. Internal supportive pessaries are sometimes prescribed for these conditions. Some can be corrected surgically.

The uterus is a frequent site of cancer, both of the cervix and of the corpus of the uterus. Regular medical examinations help to detect such growths promptly, and early diagnosis makes for successful treatment. Any irregular vaginal bleeding or discharge may be a symptom of such a growth and should have prompt attention.

Benign growths in the uterine walls, LEIOMYOMAS (called myomas, fibroid tumours, or fibroids) are common, and are not removed unless they produce symptoms or threaten to interfere with a desired pregnancy. They may occur in any part of the uterus. Leiomyomas are often numerous, although a single tumour may occur. They are usually small but sometimes grow quite large and may fill the whole uterus. After menopause, their growth usually ceases. Large tumours may cause pressure on neighbouring organs, such as the bladder. Symptoms vary according to the location and size of the tumours. As they grow, they may cause painful menstruation, profuse and irregular menstrual bleeding, vaginal discharge, or frequent urination, as well as irregular enlargement of the uterus. If the tumour becomes twisted, there may be severe pelvic pain. They may also be the cause of infertility.

In pregnancy, the tumours can interfere with the natural enlargement of the uterus with the growing fetus. They may also cause spontaneous abortion and death of the fetus. Those in the lower part of the uterus may block the birth canal, in which case caesarean section may be necessary. Most commonly, however, they have no effect on a pregnancy; a woman with fibroids should seek medical care early in pregnancy, but will probably proceed normally.

Medical examination is wise if one or more of the symptoms mentioned occur. Small leiomyomas are usually left and are checked at frequent intervals. Larger tumours may be removed surgically. In some instances, hysterectomy is performed. It is reassuring that only a very small percentage of such tumours ever become malignant, usually in later life.

Other frequent disorders associated with the uterus are menstrual problems, including painful menstruation (DYSMENORRHOEA) and excess blood flow (MENORRHAGIA). These disorders are among the most common causes of temporary female disability and are often difficult to correct, but they may also be symptoms of serious conditions. Excessive menstruation may cause anaemia.

SURGERY OF THE UTERUS. Surgical procedures involving the uterus include various operations for shortening the ligaments supporting the uterus, for the purpose of correcting uterine displacement, and hysterectomy, or surgical removal of the uterus.

Subtotal hysterectomy involves removal of all of the uterus except the cervix. This operation is most commonly performed in the case of a large leiomyoma. After the operation pregnancy is no longer possible and menstruation ceases, but glandular functions continue. MENOPAUSE does not occur prematurely, since the ovaries still produce oestrogen and progesterone.

If the cervix as well as the corpus of the uterus is removed, the operation is called total hysterectomy. Sometimes one or both of the uterine tubes and the ovaries are removed as well. The operation is sometimes necessary in conditions such as cysts and large leiomyomas, and is usual in malignant conditions.

As long as one ovary remains, menopause is not brought on by the operation. If both ovaries are removed, artificial menopause occurs; hormones or other medications may be given to facilitate this period of hormonal adjustment. Sexual activity is usually not affected.

Radical hysterectomy is one in which an upper portion of the vagina, the surrounding lymph nodes and the supporting ligaments of the pelvic organs are removed, in additon to the entire uterus. This operation may be performed in some cases of cancer of the cervix, although radiotherapy is usually preferred.

Usually in a hysterectomy the incision is made in the abdominal wall (abdominal hysterectomy), but in some instances the operation is performed by way of the vagina. A vaginal hysterectomy avoids the discomfort of an abdominal incision. This method may be used in certain benign conditions when other factors are favourable. When the cervix is not removed with the uterus, the procedure usually cannot be performed vaginally.

Patient Care. Preoperative procedures may include complete shaving of the lower abdomen and perineum, administration of a cleansing enema and a vaginal douche the evening before surgery and restriction of food and fluids as for any other type of abdominal surgery.

Postoperatively, the patient is observed frequently for signs of haemorrhage. Although some serosanguineous discharge is to be expected, bleeding that exceeds a normal menstrual flow should be reported. The number of perineal pads soiled during an 8-hour period should be noted. Intra-abdominal bleeding may be recognized by such changes as restlessness, falling blood pressure, pallor, tachycardia, thirst, and excessive perspiration.

Complications include thrombophlebitis, abdominal distention, and urinary retention. To avoid the development of a thrombus in the legs or pelvis the patient is encouraged to exercise her legs and to breathe deeply to improve pelvic circulation. Fowler's position and pillows beneath the knees are not allowed. Any complaint of pain, tenderness, or redness in the calf of the leg should be reported immediately. Early ambulation is the best preventive for most complications arising from a hysterectomy.

Abdominal distention is often avoided by insertion of a nasogastric tube prior to surgery. Urinary retention usually is prevented by insertion of a catheter while the patient is anaesthetized; this is left in place until the third or fourth postoperative day.

Postoperative infection is relatively rare, but when it does occur the first symptoms develop about the third or fourth postoperative day. Elevation of temperature, malaise, and foul vaginal discharge are indicative of this complication.

Emotional aspects of care must not be forgotten. The patient and her partner should fully understand the implications of hysterectomy prior to surgery. In the post-operative period the patient may require encouragement to discuss her self-concept. It is not uncommon for these patients to regard the operation as having removed their womanhood and a great deal of tact and understanding are required to help such patients accept themselves again.

utricle ('yootrik'l) 1. any small sac. 2. the larger of the two divisions of the membranous labyrinth of the inner ear.

prostatic u., urethral u. a small blind pouch in the substance of the prostate.

utricular (yoo'trikyuhlə) 1. bladder-like. 2. pertaining to the utricle.

utriculitis (yoo,trikyuh'lietis) inflammation of the prostatic utricle or of the utricle of the ear.

utriculosaccular (yoo,trikyuhloh'sakyuhlə) pertaining to the utricle and saccule of the membranous labyrinth of the inner ear.

uve(o)- word element. [L.] *uvea.*

uvea ('yoovi·ə) [L.] the iris, ciliary body, and choroid together. adj. **uveal.**

uveitis (,yoovi'ietis) inflammation of the uvea. adj. **uveitic.**

heterochromic u. heterochromic iridocyclitis.

sympathetic u. sympathetic ophthalmia.

uveoparotid fever (,yooviohpə'rotid) a manifestation of sarcoidosis, marked by chronic inflammation of the parotid gland and uvea, with chronic iridocyclitis, unilateral facial paralysis, lassitude, and a subfebrile temperature.

uveoparotitis (,yoovioh,parə'tietis) uveoparotid fever.

uveoscleritis (,yooviohsklə'rietis) scleritis due to extension of uveitis.

uviform ('yoovi,fawm) shaped like a grape.

uvula ('yoovyuhlə) pl. *uvulae* [L.] a pendant, fleshy mass, specifically the palatine uvula. adj. **uvular.**

u. of bladder a rounded elevation at the neck of the bladder, formed by convergence of muscle fibres terminating in the urethra. Called also *uvula vesicae.*

u. cerebelli a lobule that is the posterior limit of the fourth ventricle of the brain. Called also *uvula vermis.*

u. palatina, palatine u. the small, fleshy mass hanging from the soft palate above the root of the tongue.

u. vermis the part of the vermis of the cerebellum between the pyramid and nodule.

u. vesicae uvula of bladder.

uvulectomy (,yoovyuh'lektəmee) excision of the uvula; cionectomy.

uvulitis (,yoovyuh'lietis) inflammation of the uvula.

uvuloptosis (,yoovyuhlop'tohsis) a relaxed, pendulous state of the uvula.

uvulotomy (,yoovyuh'lotəmee) the cutting off of the uvula or a part of it.

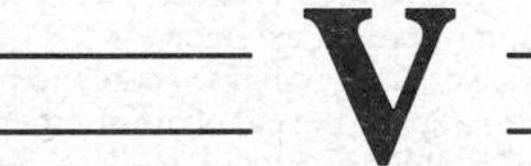

V

V chemical symbol, *vanadium;* symbol for *volt.* V stands for precordial lead, see precordial LEAD.

V_T tidal volume.

v. [L.] *vena* (vein).

vaccigenous (vak'sijənəs) producing vaccine.

vaccina (vak'sienə) vaccinia.

vaccinable (vak'sinəb'l) susceptible of being successfully vaccinated.

vaccinal ('vaksinəl) 1. pertaining to vaccinia, to vaccine, or to vaccination. 2. having protective qualities when used by way of inoculation.

vaccinate ('vaksi,nayt) to inoculate with vaccine to produce immunity.

vaccination (,vaksi'nayshən) the introduction of vaccine into the body to produce immunity to a specific disease. The term vaccination comes from the Latin *vacca,* cow, and was coined when the first inoculations were given with organisms that caused the mild disease cowpox to produce immunity against smallpox. See also INOCULATION and IMMUNIZATION.

vaccine ('vakseen) a suspension of attenuated or killed microorganisms (viruses, bacteria, or rickettsiae), administered for prevention, amelioration, or treatment of infectious diseases.

attenuated v. a vaccine prepared from live microorganisms or viruses cultured under adverse conditions, leading to loss of their virulence but retention of their ability to induce protective immunity.

autogenous v. a bacterial vaccine prepared from cultures of material derived from a lesion of the patient to be treated.

bacterial v. a preparation of attenuated or killed bacteria, used to increase immunity to the organisms injected, or sometimes for pyrogenetic effects in treatment of certain noninfectious diseases.

BCG v. a preparation used as an active immunizing agent against tuberculosis, consisting of a dried, living, avirulent culture of the Calmette–Guérin strain of *Mycobacterium bovis* (see also BCG VACCINE).

caprinized v. a vaccine prepared from microorganisms that have been attenuated by passage in goats.

live v. a vaccine prepared from live microorganisms or viruses that have been attenuated but that retain their immunogenic properties.

v. lymph material containing vaccinia virus collected from vaccinial vesicles of calves; used for active immunization against smallpox.

polyvalent v. one prepared from more than one strain or species of microorganisms.

vaccinia (vak'sini·ə) a viral disease of cattle; called also *cowpox*.

vaccinial (vak'sini·əl) pertaining to or characteristic of vaccinia (cowpox).

vacciniform (vak'sini,fawm) resembling vaccinia.

vacciniola (,vaksini'ohlə) generalized vaccinia.

vaccinotherapy (,vaksinoh'therəpee) therapeutic use of vaccines.

vacuolar ('vakyooələ, ,vakyoo'ohlə) containing, or of the nature of, vacuoles.

vacuolated ('vakyooə,laytid) containing vacuoles.

vacuolation (,vakyooə'layshən) the process of forming vacuoles; the condition of being vacuolated.

vacuole ('vakyoo,ohl) a space or cavity in the protoplasm of a cell.

contractile v. a small fluid-filled cavity in the protoplasm of certain unicellular organisms; it gradually increases in size and then collapses, its function is thought to be respiratory and excretory.

vacuolization (,vakyooəlie'zayshən) vacuolation.

vacuum ('vakyoom) a space devoid of air or other gas.

VAD Voluntary Aid Detachment.

vagabond's disease ('vagəbondz) discoloration of the skin in persons subjected to louse bites over long periods.

vagal ('vayg'l) pertaining to the vagus nerve.

v. attack vasovagal attack.

vagectomy (vag'ektəmee) surgical excision of a segment of the vagal nerve.

vagina (və'jienə) 1. any sheath or sheathlike structure. 2. the canal in the female, from the external genitalia (vulva) to the uterine cervix. The adult vagina is normally about 10 cm in length, measured along the posterior wall, and 7.5 cm anteriorly, and slopes upward and backward. Internally, the bladder is in front of the vagina and the rectum behind.

The vagina receives the erect penis in coitus. The spermatozoa are discharged into the vagina, swim through the cervical canal, and enter the uterus. The vagina is also the passage for menstrual discharge and functions as part of the birth canal.

The interior lining of the vagina is squamous epithelium. Muscles and fibrous tissue form the vaginal walls. In pregnancy, changes occur in these tissues, enabling the vagina to stretch to many times its usual size during delivery of the infant.

In a virgin, the opening of the vagina is usually, but not necessarily, partially closed by a membrane, the hymen. Usually the hymen breaks at first intercourse; occasionally it ruptures during physical exercise. Shreds of ruptured hymen may be seen in multigravidas, and are called CURUNCULATE MYRTIFORMES.

In a normal state, DÖDERLEIN'S BACILLUS acts on the glycogen within the epithelium of the vaginal walls to produce lactic acid. This acidity probably helps to protect the vagina from invasion by other organisms. Douching as a regular practice should not be employed except when recommended by a doctor.

VAGINAL EXAMINATION WHEN THE PATIENT IS NOT PREGNANT OR DURING EARLY PREGNANCY. Since cancer of the female reproductive organs is a relatively common occurrence and is curable if detected early, gynaecologists recommend that women of reproductive age and beyond have a regular vaginal or pelvic examination. This is a simple procedure that is only mildly uncomfortable if the woman relaxes and appreciates its purpose.

The patient lies on her back on an examination couch or bed with her knees flexed and apart and her heels together. The gynaecologist/obstetrician inserts a speculum to spread the vagina open. He is able to observe the cervix and the lining of the vagina directly, and may take smears for microscopic examination to detect infection or cancer. See also PAPANICOLAOU TEST.

After removing the speculum the examiner inserts rubber-gloved fingers into the vagina and places the other hand on the abdomen. In this way he is able to palpate the female reproductive organs, including the uterus and ovaries, between his hands. These organs are otherwise difficult or impossible to examine.

Patient Care. Ideally, a vaginal examination should be done between menstrual periods; however, vaginal bleeding is not a contraindication to this procedure, except for the six week post-natal examination.

VAGINAL EXAMINATION DURING LABOUR. The examination is a sterile procedure and may be undertaken by either a doctor or a midwife. The purpose is always to obtain the maximum amount of information possible, whatever the specific reason for performing the examination. In modern obstetric practice vaginal examinations may be performed as often as two-hourly on a routine basis. In natural childbirth vaginal examination may be performed only to exclude prolapse of the cord when the fetal membranes rupture and to confirm full dilation of the cervix before allowing the mother to push in the second stage. Vaginal examination for this purpose is also essential in all cases of premature labour and breech presentation. Vaginal examination may sometimes be made to confirm the presenting part, or prior to giving analgesia in labour.

The information that may be obtained during vaginal examination is: (1) the condition of the perineum and external genitalia, particularly noting the presence of any scars, evidence of infection, or varicose veins; (2) the tone of the vagina; (3) the length and degree of effacement of the cervix, and whether it is thick or thin, around the external os; (4) the dilation of the external os measured in centimetres; (5) whether the fetal membranes are present or have been ruptured; (6) the colour of any liquor which is draining; (7) the level of the presenting part of the fetus in relation to the ischial spines of the maternal pelvis; (8) the landmarks of the presenting part in order to confirm the lie, presentation, position, and attitude of the fetus; (9) the contors of the pelvic outlet, in particular the prominence of the ischial spines and the angle of the subpubic arch.

An abdominal examination should always precede a vaginal examination and the fetal heart rate listened to before and after the procedure. The findings are recorded on the mother's partogram.

vaginal (və'jien'l, 'vajin'l) pertaining to the vagina, the tunica vaginalis testis, or to any sheath.

v. discharge excessive discharge may indicate an abnormal condition. Yellowish or creamy white discharge, especially if it is thick, often contains pus and provides evidence of infection. Thinner discharge, and the kinds that seem to be clear mucus, especially if irritating or offensive, indicate that the disorder is chronic, but of less significance.

CAUSES. A frequent cause of vaginal discharge is trichomoniasis. The discharge is usually yellowish, profuse, has an unpleasant odour and may be accompanied by itching.

Another cause of vaginal discharge is infection of the cervix during pregnancy. This infection irritates the mucous glands of the cervix, causing them to secrete an excessive amount of mucus. Sexually transmitted disease, especially gonorrhoea, is also a common cause of abnormal vaginal discharge. When there is a burning sensation during urination, gonorrhoea should be suspected.

Other bacteria and fungi may be causes of vaginal discharge. Infections of the genital tract that cause abnormal discharge may originate from foreign bodies, such as tampons, diaphragms, and pessaries, left in the vagina over too long a period.

Discharge sometimes is an early indication of cervical cancer, or of benign conditions, such as polyps or leiomyoma (myoma) of the uterus. It may also be caused by pelvic congestion associated with heart disease, by malnutrition, or by inflammation of the uterine (fallopian) tubes as a result of tuberculosis. In later years, the disorder may be caused by debility.

TREATMENT. Vaginal discharge caused by an infection of the reproductive organs is usually treated by an appropriate antibiotic or antimycotic.

vaginalectomy (və,jienə'lektəmee, ,vaji-) vaginectomy.

vaginalitis (və,jienə'lietis, ,vaji-) inflammation of the tunica vaginalis testis; periorchitis.

vaginate ('vajinət) enclosed in a sheath.

vaginectomy (,vaji'nektəmee) 1. resection of the tunica vaginalis testis. 2. excision of the vagina.

vaginismus (,vaji'nizməs) painful spasms of the muscles of the vagina.

vaginitis (,vaji'nietis) 1. inflammation of the vagina; colpitis. 2. inflammation of a sheath.

adhesive v. that in which ulceration and exfoliation of the mucosa result in adhesions of the membranes. See atrophic VAGINITIS.

atrophic v. vaginitis occurring in postmenopausal women and associated with oestrogen deficiency. The common types are: *senile vulvovaginitis*, in which there is intense itching around the vagina, almost complete lack of vaginal secretions, and evidence of tissue atrophy; and *senile vaginitis* or *adhesive vaginitis*, marked by the formation of superficial erosions, which often adhere to opposed surfaces, sometimes causing obliteration of the vaginal canal.

desquamative inflammatory v. a form resembling atrophic vaginitis but affecting women with normal oestrogen levels.

emphysematous v. inflammation of the vagina and adjacent cervix, characterized by numerous, asymptomatic, gas-filled cystlike lesions.

senile v. atrophic vaginitis.

vaginoabdominal (və,jienoh·ab'domin'l, ,vaji-) pertaining to the vagina and abdomen.

vaginocele ('vajinoh,seel) colpocele; vaginal hernia.

vaginodynia (,vajinoh'dini·ə) pain in the vagina.

vaginofixation (,vajinohfik'sayshən) vaginopexy; colpopexy.

vaginolabial (və,jienoh'laybi·əl, ,vaji-) pertaining to the vagina and labia.

vaginomycosis (və,jienohmie'kohsis, ,vaji-) any fungal disease of the vagina.

vaginopathy (,vaji'nopəthee) any disease of the vagina.

vaginoperineal (və,jienoh,peri'neeəl, ,vaji-) pertaining to the vagina and perineum.

vaginoperineorrhaphy (və,jienoh,perini'o·rəfee) suture of the vagina and perineum; colpoperineorrhaphy.

vaginoperineotomy (və,jienoh,perini'otəmee, ,vaji-) incision of the vagina and perineum.

vaginoperitoneal (və,jienoh,peritə'neeəl, ,vaji-) pertaining to the vagina and peritoneum.

vaginopexy (və'jienoh,peksee, 'vaji-) colpopexy; vaginofixation; suturing of the vagina to the abdominal wall.

vaginoplasty (və'jienoh,plastee, 'vaji-) colpoplasty; plastic repair of the vagina.

vaginotomy (,vaji'notəmee) colpotomy; incision of the vagina.

vaginovesical (və,jienoh'vesik'l, ,vaji-) pertaining to the vagina and bladder.

vagitus (və'jietəs) the cry of an infant.

v. uterinus the cry of an infant in the uterus.

vagolytic (,vaygoh'litik) having an effect resembling that produced by interruption of impulses transmitted by the vagus nerve; parasympatholytic.

vagomimetic (,vaygohmi'metik) having an effect resembling that produced by stimulation of the vagus nerve.

vagotomy (vay'gotəmee) division of the vagus nerves to reduce gastric acidity as treatment for gastric or duodenal ULCER.

highly selective v. division of only those vagal fibres supplying the acid-secreting glands of the stomach, with preservation of those supplying the antrum as well as the hepatic and coeliac branches.

medical v. interruption of impulses carried by the vagus nerve by administration of suitable drugs.

parietal cell v. selective severing of the vagus nerve fibres supplying the proximal two-thirds (parietal area) of the stomach.

selective v. division of the vagal fibres to the stomach with preservation of the hepatic and coeliac branches.

vagotonia (,vaygoh'tohni·ə) irritability of the vagus nerve, characterized by vasomotor instability, sweating, disordered peristalsis, and muscle spasms. adj. **vagotonic.**

vagotonin (,vaygoh'tohnin) a preparation of hormone from the pancreas that increases vagal tone, slows the heart, and increases the store of glycogen in the liver.

vagotropic (,vaygoh'trohpik) having an effect on the vagus nerve.

vagovagal (,vaygoh'vayg'l) arising as a result of afferent and efferent impulses mediated through the vagus nerve.

vagus nerve ('vaygəs) the tenth cranial nerve; it has the most extensive distribution of the cranial nerves, serving structures of the chest and abdomen as well as the head and neck.

Afferent fibres of the vagus nerve serve the mucous

membrane of the larynx, trachea, and bronchi, lungs, arch of the aorta, oesophagus, and stomach. Some of the functions affected by this nerve are coughing, sneezing, reflex inhibitions of the heart rate, and the sensation of hunger.

Motor fibres of the vagus nerve are concerned with swallowing, speech, peristalsis, and secretions from the glands of the stomach and the pancreas and contractions of the trachea, bronchi, and bronchioles.

valency ('vaylənsee) the numerical measure of the capacity to combine; in chemistry, an expression of the number of atoms of hydrogen (or its equivalent) that one atom of a chemical element can hold in combination, if negative, or displace in a reaction, if positive; in immunology, an expression of the number of antigenic determinants with which one molecule of a given antibody can combine or of the number of different organisms or antigens attacked by a vaccine or antiserum. Called also *valence*.

valgus ('valgəs) [L.] *bent outward*, *twisted;* denoting a deformity in which the angulation is away from the midline of the body, as in talipes valgus.

valinaemia (ˌvali'neemi·ə) hypervalinaemia; elevated levels of valine in the blood and urine.

valine ('valeen) a naturally occurring amino acid, one of those essential for human metabolism.

Valium ('vali·əm) trademark for a preparation of diazepam, an anxiolytic and skeletal muscle relaxant.

vallate ('valayt) having a wall or rim; rim-shaped.

vallecula (və'lekyuhlə) pl. *valleculae* [L.] a depression or furrow.

v. cerebelli a longitudinal fissure on the inferior cerebellum, in which the medulla oblongata rests.

v. sylvii a depression made by the fissure of Sylvius at the base of the brain.

v. unguis the sulcus of the matrix of the nail.

Valleix's points ('valeksiz) tender points along the course of certain nerves in neuralgia; called also *puncta dolorosa*.

Vallergan ('valəgən) trademark for preparations of trimeprazine, a systemic antipruritic.

Valley fever ('valee) coccidioidomycosis.

valproic acid (val'proh·ik) an anticonvulsant used for the control of absence seizures.

Valsalva's manoeuvre (val'salvəz) 1. increase of intrathoracic pressure by forcible exhalation against the closed glottis. The manoeuvre causes a trapping of blood in the great veins, preventing it from entering the chest and right atrium. When the breath is released, the intrathoracic pressure drops and the trapped blood is quickly propelled through the heart, producing an increase in the heart rate (tachycardia) and the blood pressure. Immediately after this event a reflex bradycardia ensues. Valsalva's manoeuvre occurs when a person strains to defecate or urinate, uses his arm and upper trunk muscles to move up in bed, or strains during coughing, gagging, or vomiting. The increased pressure, immediate tachycardia, and reflex bradycardia can bring about cardiac arrest in vulnerable heart patients. 2. increase in the pressure in the pharyngotympanic tube and middle ear by forcible exhalation against closed nostrils and mouth.

value ('valyoo) a measure of worth or efficiency; a quantitative measurement of the activity, concentration, etc., of specific substances.

normal v's the range in concentration of specific substances found in normal healthy tissues, secretions, etc.

valva ('valvə) pl. *valvae* [L.] a valve.

valve (valv) a membranous fold in a canal or passage that prevents backward flow of material passing through it.

aortic v. that guarding the entrance to the aorta from the left ventricle.

atrioventricular v's the valves between the right atrium and right ventricle (tricuspid valve) and the left atrium and left ventricle (mitral valve).

bicuspid v. mitral valve.

cardiac v's valves that control flow of blood through and from the heart.

coronary v. a valve at entrance of the coronary sinus into right atrium.

flair v. a cardiac valve having a cusp that has lost its normal support (as in ruptured chordae tendineae) and flutters in the blood stream.

ileocaecal v., ileocolic v. that guarding the opening between the ileum and caecum.

mitral v. that between the left atrium and left ventricle, usually having two cusps (anterior and posterior).

pulmonary v. that at the entrance of the pulmonary trunk from the right ventricle.

pyloric v. a prominent fold of mucous membrane at the pyloric orifice of the stomach.

semilunar v's valves made up of semilunar segments or cusps (valvulae semilunares), guarding the entrances into the aorta and pulmonary trunk from the cardiac ventricles.

thebesian v. coronary valve.

tricuspid v. that guarding the opening between the right atrium and right ventricle.

valvotomy (val'votəmee) incision of a valve.

valvula ('valvyuhlə) pl. *valvulae* [L.] a small valve.

valvular ('valvyuhlə) pertaining to, affecting or of the nature of a valve.

valvulitis (ˌvalvyuh'lietis) inflammation of a valve, especially of a valve of the heart.

valvuloplasty ('valvyuhloh,plastee) plastic repair of a valve, especially a valve of the heart.

valvulotome ('valvyuhloh,tohm) an instrument for cutting a valve.

valvulotomy (ˌvalvyuh'lotəmee) valvotomy.

van den Bergh's test ('van dən ˌbərgz) a chemical test of bilirubin in serum to aid the diagnosis of jaundice.

van der Hoeve's syndrome (ˌvan dər 'hohvz) see OSTEOGENESIS IMPERFECTA.

Van der Waals forces (ˌvan dər 'wahlz) the relatively weak, short-range forces of attraction existing between atoms and molecules, which results in the attraction of nonpolar organic compounds to each other (hydrophobic bonding).

van't Hoff's rule (law) (ˌvant 'hofs) the velocity of chemical reactions is increased twofold or more for each rise of 10 °C in temperature.

vanadium (və'naydi·əm) a chemical element, atomic number 23, atomic weight 50.942, symbol V. (See table of elements in Appendix 2.) Its salts have been used in treating various diseases. Absorption of its compounds, usually via the lungs, causes chronic intoxication, the symptoms of which include respiratory tract irritation, pneumonitis, conjunctivitis, and anaemia.

vancomycin (ˌvankoh'miesin) an antibiotic produced by *Streptomyces orientalis*, highly effective against gram-positive bacteria, especially against staphylococci; it is used as the hydrochloride salt. The toxic effects are quite severe and include damage to the eighth cranial (vestibulocochlear) nerve and renal disorders.

vanillism (və'nilizəm) dermatitis, coryza, and malaise seen in handlers of raw vanilla, due to the mite *Acarus siro*.

vanillylmandelic acid (vəˌnililman'delik) an excretory product of the catecholamines, used as a test for adrenaline metabolism.

vaporization (ˌvaypə·rie'zayshən) 1. the conversion of a

solid or liquid into a vapour without chemical change; distillation. 2. treatment by vapours; vapotherapy.
vaporize ('vaypə,riez) to convert into vapour or to be transformed into vapour.
vapour ('vaypə) steam, gas, or exhalation.
Vaquez's disease ('vakeziz) polycythaemia vera.
variability (,vair·ri·ə'bilitee) the state of being variable.
variable ('vair·ri·əb'l) in epidemiology any measurement that can have different values.
confounding v. a term used in epidemiological studies to mean a factor which distorts the time association between two variables.
dependent v. a variable which is dependent on the effect of other variables in an epidemiological study.
independent v. a variable not influenced by other variables in an epidemiological study but which may be the cause of alterations in these variables.
variance ('vair·ri·əns) a measure of the variation seen in a set of data.
varicectomy (,vari'sektəmee) excision of a varicose vein.
varicella (,vari'selə) chickenpox.
varicelliform (,vari'seli,fawm) resembling chickenpox.
varices ('vari,seez) [L.] plural of *varix*.
variciform (və'risi,fawm) resembling a varix; varicose.
varicoblepharon (,varikoh'blefə·ron) a varicose swelling of the eyelid.
varicocele ('varikoh,seel) varicosity of the pampiniform plexus of the spermatic cord, forming a scrotal swelling that feels like a 'bag of worms'.
varicocelectomy (,varikohsi'lektəmee) excision of a varicocele.
varicography (,vari'kogrəfee) radiographic visualization of varicose veins.
varicomphalos (,vari'komfəlos) a varicose tumour of the umbilicus.
varicophlebitis (,varikohfli'bietis) varicose veins with inflammation.
varicose ('vari,kohs) of the nature of or pertaining to a varix; unnaturally and permanently distended (said of a vein); variciform.
v. eczema pigmented discoloration with thickening of the skin of the leg resulting from chronic venous stasis due to varicose veins.
v. ulcer chronic ulceration developing on the inner leg, just above the medial malleolus, sometimes persistent. It may respond to supportive bandages to the leg, or prolonged bed rest, but is likely to recur until the varicose condition is corrected by operation.
v. veins swollen, distended, and tortuous veins, usually in the subcutaneous tissues of the leg. Usually the result of incompetence of the valves in the long saphenous vein, sometimes of the short saphenous vein, occasionally both.

The tendency to develop varicose veins may be inherited. Pregnancy sometimes precipitates the development of the condition through pressure of the gravid uterus on the iliac veins, sometimes following deep vein thrombosis.

Many cases of varicose veins require no treatment. The occasional superficial varicosity if unsightly, may be obliterated by a sclerosing agent. When operation has to be undertaken, either for unsightliness, aching and general discomfort, or varicose ulceration, it almost always includes long saphenous ligation in the groin in association with such manoeuvres as multiple distal ligatures, repeated sclerosing injections postoperatively or selective removal of varicosities. In the rarer event of incompetence of the short saphenous system, that vein is ligated behind the knee.
varicosity (,vari'kositee) 1. a varicose condition; the quality or fact of being varicose. 2. a varix, or varicose vein.

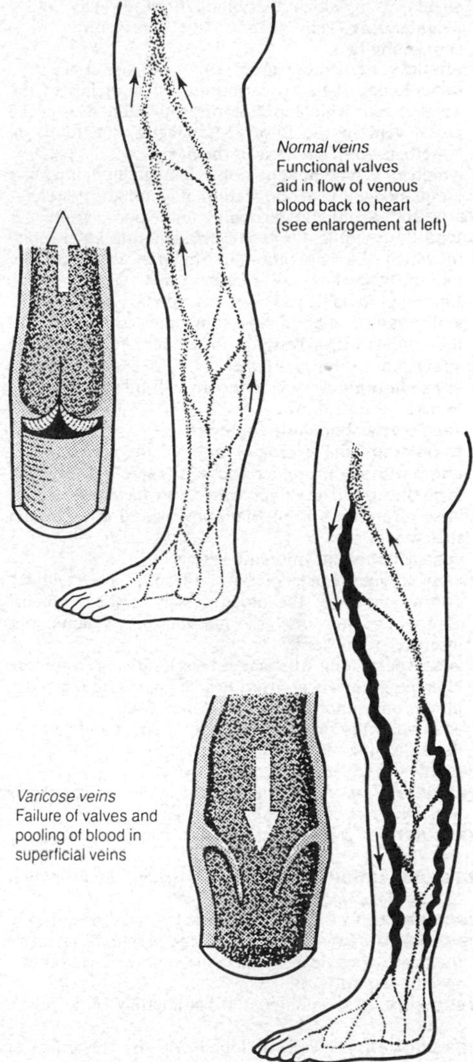

Comparison of normal veins and varicose veins in the leg

varicotomy (,vari'kotəmee) treatment of a varix or of a varicose vein by incision.
varicula (və'rikyuhlə) a varix of the conjunctiva.
variety (və'rieətee) a taxonomic subcategory of a species.
variola (və'rieələ) smallpox. adj. **variolar, variolous.**
v. minor a mild form of smallpox having a low fatality rate.
variolate ('vair·ri·ə,layt) 1. having the nature of appearance of smallpox. 2. to inoculate with smallpox virus.
varioliform (,vair·ri'ohli,fawm) resembling smallpox.
varix ('vair·riks) pl. *varices* [L.] an enlarged, tortuous vein, artery, or lymphatic vessel.
aneurysmal v. a markedly dilated tortuous vessel; sometimes used to denote a form of arteriovenous

aneurysm in which the blood flows directly into a neighbouring vein without the intervention of a connecting sac.

arterial v. a racemose aneurysm or varicose artery.

oesophageal varices varicosities of branches of the azygous vein which anastomose with tributaries of the portal vein in the lower oesophagus, due to portal hypertension in cirrhosis of the liver.

lymph v., v. lymphaticus a soft, lobulated swelling of a lymph node, due to obstruction of lymphatic vessels.

varolian (və'rohli·ən) pertaining to the pons varolii.

varus ('vair·rəs) [L.] *bent inward;* denoting a deformity in which the angulation of the part is toward the midline of the body, as in talipes varus.

vas (vas) pl. *vasa* [L.] a vessel. adj. **vasal**.

v. aberrans 1. a blind tube sometimes connected with the epididymis; a vestigial mesonephric tube. 2. any anomalous or unusual vessel.

vasa afferentia vessels that convey fluid to a structure or part.

vasa brevia short gastric arteries.

v. deferens the excretory duct of the testis, which unites with the excretory duct of the seminal vesicle to form the ejaculatory duct; called also *ductus deferens.*

vasa efferentia vessels that convey fluid away from a structure or part.

vasa lymphatica lymphatic vessels.

vasa previa the presentation, in front of the fetal head during labour, of the blood vessels of the umbilical cord where they enter the placenta in a velamentous insertion of the cord.

vasa recta long U-shaped vessels arising from the efferent glomerular arterioles of juxtamedullary nephrons and supplying the renal medulla.

vasa vasorum the small nutrient arteries and veins in the walls of the larger blood vessels.

vas(o)- word element. [L.] *vessel, duct.*

vascular ('vaskyuhlə) pertaining to blood vessels or indicative of a copious blood supply.

vascularity (ˌvaskyuh'laritee) the condition of being vascular.

vascularization (ˌvaskyuhlə·rie'zayshən) the formation of new blood vessels in tissues.

vascularize ('vaskyuhlə,riez) to supply with vessels.

vasculature ('vaskyuhləchə) 1. the vascular system of the body, or any part of it. 2. the supply of vessels to a specific region.

vasculitis (ˌvaskyuh'lietis) inflammation of a vessel; angiitis.

vasculopathy (ˌvaskyuh'lopəthee) any disorder of blood vessels.

vasectomy (və'sektəmee) resection of the vas (ductus) deferens with ligation.

vasifactive (ˌvasi'faktiv) vasoformative.

vasiform ('vasi,fawm) resembling a vessel.

vasitis (və'sietis) inflammation of the vas (ductus) deferens.

vasoactive (ˌvayzoh'aktiv) exerting an effect on the calibre of blood vessels.

vasoactive intestinal peptide a peptide hormone that, in addition to its vasoactive properties, stimulates intestinal secretion of water and electrolytes, inhibits gastric secretion, promotes glycogenesis, causes hyperglycaemia, and stimulates production of pancreatic juice. Abbreviated VIP.

vasoconstriction (ˌvayzohkən'strikshən) decrease in the calibre of blood vessels. adj. **vasoconstrictive**.

vasoconstrictor (ˌvayzohkən'striktə) 1. causing constriction of the blood vessels. 2. a vasoconstrictive agent.

vasodepression (ˌvayzohdi'preshən) decrease in vascular resistance with hypotension.

vasodepressor (ˌvayzohdi'presə) 1. having the effect of lowering the blood pressure through reduction in peripheral resistance. 2. an agent that causes vasodepression.

vasodilation, vasodilatation (ˌvayzoh,die'layshən; ˌvayzoh,dielə'tayshən) a state of increased calibre of blood vessels. adj. **vasodilative**.

vasodilator (ˌvayzohdie'laytə) 1. causing dilation of blood vessels. 2. a nerve or agent that causes dilation of blood vessels.

vasoepididymography (ˌvasoh,epididi'mogrəfee) radiography of the vas deferens and epididymis after injection of a contrast medium.

vasoepididymostomy (ˌvasoh,epididi'mostəmee) anastomosis of the vas (ductus) deferens and the epididymis.

vasoformative (ˌvayzoh'fawmətiv) pertaining to or promoting the formation of blood vessels.

vasoganglion (ˌvayzoh'gang·gli·ən) a vascular ganglion or rete.

vasohypertonic (ˌvayzoh,hiepə'tonik) vasoconstrictor.

vasohypotonic (ˌvayzoh,hiepoh'tonik) vasodilator.

vasoinhibitor (ˌvayzoh·in'hibitə) an agent that inhibits vasomotor nerves. adj. **vasoinhibitory**.

vasoligation (ˌvasohlie'gayshən) ligation of the vas (ductus) deferens.

vasomotion (ˌvayzoh'mohshən) change in calibre of blood vessels.

vasomotor (ˌvayzoh'mohtə) 1. having an effect on the calibre of blood vessels. 2. a vasomotor agent or nerve.

vasoneuropathy (ˌvayzohnyuh'ropəthee) a condition caused by combined vascular and neurological defect, resulting from simultaneous action or interaction of the vascular and nervous systems.

vasoneurosis (ˌvayzohnyuh'rohsis) angioneurosis.

vaso-orchidostomy (ˌvasoh,awki'dostəmee) anastomosis of the epididymis to the severed end of the vas (ductus) deferens.

vasoparesis (ˌvayzohpə'reesis) paralysis of vasomotor nerves.

vasopermeability (ˌvayzoh,pərmi·ə'bilitee) the permeability of a blood vessel; the extent to which a blood vessel is permeable.

vasopressin (ˌvayzoh'presin) a pressor agent produced in the pituitary gland. Also known as antidiuretic hormone. Used in the treatment of diabetes insipidus and bleeding from oesophageal varices.

vasopressor (ˌvayzoh'presə) 1. stimulating contraction of the muscular tissue of the capillaries and arteries. 2. a vasopressor agent.

vasopuncture ('vasoh,pungkchə) surgical puncture of the vas (ductus) deferens.

vasoreflex (ˌvayzoh'reefleks) a reflex of blood vessels.

vasorelaxation (ˌvayzoh,reelak'sayshən) decrease of vascular pressure.

vasorrhaphy (və'so·rəfee) suture of the vas (ductus) deferens.

vasosection (ˌvasoh'sekshən) the severing of a vessel or vessels, sometimes referring to the vas deferens (ductus deferentes).

vasosensory (ˌvayzoh'sensə·ree) supplying sensory filaments to the vessels.

vasospasm ('vayzoh,spazəm) spasm of blood vessels, decreasing their calibre. adj. **vasospastic**.

vasostimulant (ˌvayzoh'stimyuhlənt) stimulating vasomotor action.

vasostomy (və'sostəmee) surgical formation of an opening into the vas (ductus) deferens.

vasotomy (və'sotəmee) incision of the vas (ductus) deferens.

vasotonia (ˌvayzoh'tohni·ə) tone or tension of the vessels.

vasotonic (ˌvayzoh'tonik) pertaining to, characterized by, or increasing vasotonia.
vasotrophic (ˌvayzoh'trohfik) affecting nutrition through alterations of the calibre of the blood vessels.
vasotropic (ˌvayzoh'tropik) exerting an influence on the blood vessels, causing either constriction or dilation.
vasovagal (ˌvayzoh'vayg'l) vascular and vagal.
v. attack, v. syncope a transient vascular and neurogenic reaction marked by pallor, nausea, sweating, bradycardia, and rapid fall in arterial blood pressure which, when below a critical level, results in loss of consciousness and characteristic electroencephalographic changes. It is most often evoked by emotional stress associated with fear or pain. Called also *vagal attack*.
vasovasostomy (ˌvasohvə'sostəmee) anastomosis of the ends of the severed vas (ductus) deferens.
vasovesiculectomy (ˌvasohvəˌsikyuh'lektəmee) excision of the vas (ductus) deferens and seminal vesicle.
vasovesiculitis (ˌvasohveˌsikyuh'lietis) inflammation of the vas (ductus) deferens and seminal vesicles.
vastus ('vastəs) [L.] *great*.
Vater's papilla ('vahtəz) major duodenal papilla.
Vc vital capacity.
VCG vector cardiogram.
V-Cil-K trademark for preparations of penicillin V.
VD venereal disease.
VDRL Venereal Disease Research Laboratory. See also VDRL TEST.
vection ('vekshən) the carrying of disease germs from an infected person to a well person.
vectis ('vektis) a curved lever for making traction on the fetal head in labour.
vector ('vektə) 1. a carrier, especially the animal (usually an arthropod) which transfers an infective agent from one host to another. The mosquito, which carries the malaria parasite, *Plasmodium*, from man to man, and the tsetse fly, which carries trypanosomes from beast to man, are vectors, as are dogs, bats, and other animals that transmit the rabies virus to man. 2. a quantity possessing magnitude, direction, and sense (positivity or negativity). adj. **vectorial**.
biological v. an arthropod vector in whose body the infecting organism develops or multiplies before becoming infective to the recipient individual.
mechanical v. an arthropod vector that transmits the infective organisms from one host to another but is not essential to the life cycle of the parasite.
vectorcardiogram (ˌvektə'kahdiohˌgram) the record, usually a photograph, of the loop formed on the oscilloscope in vectorcardiography.
vectorcardiography (ˌvektəˌkahdi'ogrəfee) the registration, usually by formation of a loop on an oscilloscope, of the direction and magnitude (vector) of the moment-to-moment electromotive forces of the heart during one complete cycle. adj. **vectorcardiographic**.
vecuronium (ˌvekyuh'rohni·əm) a newly introduced neuromuscular blocking agent of a non-depolarizing type closely related to pancuronium but having a much shorter duration of action and no adverse effects on the cardiovascular system. Unlike most other muscle relaxants of this type, it does not release histamine.
vegan ('veegən) a vegetarian who excludes from his diet all foods of animal origin.
veganism ('veegəˌnizəm) strict adherence to a vegetable diet, with exclusion of all foods of animal origin.
vegetable ('vejtəb'l) 1. pertaining to or derived from plants. 2. any plant or species of plant, especially one cultivated as a source of food.
vegetal ('vejit'l) 1. pertaining to plants or a plant. 2. vegetative.
vegetarian (ˌveji'tair·ri·ən) one who eats only foods of vegetable origin.
v. diet one in which no meat is eaten. The strictly vegetarian diet (called also the *vegan* diet) allows no foods of animal origin. Maintenance of this diet requires a firm commitment to restriction of dietary intake, an extensive knowledge of dietary principles, and detailed planning to ensure nutritional adequacy. Deficiencies most likely to occur in a person who faithfully adheres to a vegetarian diet are those of protein, vitamin B_{12}, riboflavin, vitamin D, and calcium.
There are several variations of the so-called vegetarian diet; some are not strictly vegetarian inasmuch as animal products such as eggs and cheese are allowed. A *lacto-vegetarian* diet prohibits the intake of meat, poultry, fish, and eggs. It does, however, permit milk and dairy products. An *ovo-lacto-vegetarian* diet allows all foods from plants plus eggs, milk, and other dairy products. An *ovo-vegetarian* diet allows eggs and foods of plant origin but prohibits all animal and dairy products.
vegetarianism (ˌveji'tair·ri·əˌnizəm) the restriction of one's food to substances of vegetable origin.
vegetation (ˌveji'tayshən) any plantlike fungoid neoplasm or growth; a luxuriant fungus-like growth of pathological tissue composed of a mixture of fibrin, blood clot, macrophages and frequently, though not invariably, microorganisms.
vegetative ('vejitətiv) 1. concerned with growth and nutrition. 2. functioning involuntarily or unconsciously. 3. resting; denoting the portion of a cell cycle during which the cell is not replicating. 4. pertaining to plants. 5. pertaining to asexual reproduction.
vehicle ('veeək'l) 1. a transporting agent, especially the component of a medication (prescription) serving as a solvent or to increase the bulk or decrease the concentration of the mixture. 2. any medium through which an impulse is propagated.
veil (vayl) 1. a covering structure. 2. a caul or piece of amniotic sac occasionally covering the face of a newborn child. 3. slight huskiness of the voice.
vein (vayn) a vessel through which blood passes from various organs or parts back to the heart, in the systemic circulation carrying blood that has given up most of its oxygen. Veins, like arteries, have three coats, an inner, middle, and outer, but the coats are not so thick and they collapse when the vessel is cut. Many veins, especially the superficial, have valves formed of reduplication of their lining membrane.
afferent v's veins that carry blood to an organ.
allantoic v's paired vessels that accompany the allantois, growing out from the primitive hindgut and entering the body stalk of the early embryo.
cardinal v's embryonic vessels that include the pre- and postcardinal veins and the ducts of Cuvier (common cardinal veins).
emissary v. one passing through a foramen of the skull and draining blood from a cerebral sinus into a vessel outside the skull.
postcardinal v's paired vessels in the early embryo that return blood from regions caudal to the heart.
precardinal v's paired venous trunks in the embryo cranial to the heart.
pulp v's vessels draining the venous sinuses of the spleen.
subcardinal v's paired vessels in the embryo, replacing the postcardinal veins and persisting to some degree as definitve vessels.
sublobular v's tributaries of the hepatic veins that

receive the central veins of hepatic lobules.

supracardinal v's paired vessels in the embryo developing later than the subcardinal veins and persisting chiefly as the lower segment of the inferior vena cava.

thebesian v's smallest cardiac veins: numerous small veins arising in the muscular walls and draining independently into the cavities of the heart, and most readily seen in the atria. **trabecular v's** vessels coursing in splenic trabeculae, formed by tributary pulp veins.

varicose v's permanently dilated, tortuous veins, usually in the subcutaneous tissues of the leg; incompetency of the venous valve is associated (see also VARICOSE veins).

vitelline v's veins that return the blood from the yolk sac to the primitive heart of the early embryo.

velamen (və'laymen) pl. *velamina* [L.] a membrane, meninx, or velum.

velamentous (,velə'mentəs) membranous and pendent; like a veil.

v. insertion of the umbilical cord a placenta in which the umbilical cord vessels divide before reaching the placenta. See also vasa previa under VAS.

vellus ('veləs) the coat of fine hairs that appears after the lanugo hairs are cast off and persists until puberty.

velopharyngeal (,velohfə'rinji·əl, -,farin'jeeəl) pertaining to the velum palatinum (soft palate) and pharynx.

Velosef ('veloh,sef) trademark for preparations of cephradine, a cephalosporin antibiotic.

velum ('veləm) pl. *vela* [L.] a covering structure or veil. adj. **velar.**

v. interpositum the membranous roof of the third ventricle of the brain.

medullary v. one of the two portions (superior medullary velum and inferior medullary velum) of the white matter of the hindbrain that form the roof of the fourth ventricle.

palatine v., v. palatinum soft palate.

ven-, vene-, veni-, veno- word element. [L.] *vein.*

vena ('veenə) pl. *venae* [L.] vein.

venectasia (,veenək'tayzi·ə) phlebectasia.

venectomy (və'nektəmee) excision of a vein.

venenation (,venə'nayshən) poisoning; a poisoned condition.

venenous ('venənəs) venomous.

venepuncture ('veni,pungkchə) the insertion of a needle into a vein, usually to obtain a blood specimen.

venereal (və'niə·ri·əl) due to or propagated by sexual intercourse.

v. disease a disease transmitted by sexual intercourse or other genital contact. In the UK, GONORRHOEA, SYPHILIS, and CHANCROID are defined in law as venereal diseases. The term venereal disease (VD) is being replaced by the term SEXUALLY TRANSMITTED DISEASE (STD) or the specialty of GENITOURINARY MEDICINE. The diseases included in this classification are those that are *usually* transmitted by means of either heterosexual or homosexual intercourse, or by intimate contact with the genitals, mouth, and rectum.

venereologist (və,niə·ri'oləjist) a specialist in venereology.

venereology (və,niə·ri'oləjee) a branch of medicine which deals with venereal disease; see VENEREAL DISEASE and GENITOURINARY MEDICINE.

venery ('venə·ree, 'vee-) coitus.

venesection ('veni,sekshən) cuting into or division of a vein.

venipuncture ('veni,pungkchə) venepuncture.

venisuture ('veni,soochə) repair of a vein.

venoclysis (vee'noklisis) injection of fluid into a vein; phleboclysis (see also INTRAVENOUS INFUSION).

venogram ('veenə,gram) 1. phlebogram. 2. venous-pulse tracing.

venography (vee'nogrəfee) phlebography.

venom ('venəm) poison, especially a toxic substance normally secreted by a snake, insect, or other animal.

Russell's viper v. the venom of the Russell viper (*Vipera russelli)*, which acts in vitro as an intrinsic thromboplastin and is useful in defining deficiencies of clotting factor X.

venomotor (,veenoh'mohtə) controlling dilation or constriction of the veins.

venomous ('venəməs) secreting poison; poisonous.

veno-occlusive (,veenoh·ə'kloosiv) pertaining to or characterized by obstruction of the veins.

v. disease of liver acute or chronic, partial or complete, occlusion of the branches of the hepatic veins by endophlebitis and thrombosis, leading to centrilobular necrosis, fibrosis, and ascites; most often seen in children.

venoperitoneostomy (,veenoh,peritəni'ostəmee) anastomosis of the saphenous vein with the peritoneum for drainage of ascites.

venosclerosis (,veenohsklə'rohsis) sclerosis of veins; phlebosclerosis.

venosity (vi'nositee) 1. excess of venous blood in a part. 2. a plentiful supply of blood vessels or of venous blood.

venostasis (,veenoh'staysis) retardation of the venous outflow in a part, as from the leg on standing when venous valves are incompetent (see also PHLEBOSTASIS).

venotomy (vi'notəmee) phlebotomy.

venous ('veenəs) pertaining to the veins.

v. return the flow of blood into the heart from the peripheral vessels.

v. thrombosis the presence of a thrombus in a vein (see also venous THROMBOSIS).

venovenostomy (,veenohvi'nostəmee) anastomasis between two veins.

vent (vent) an opening or outlet, such as an opening that discharges pus, or the anus.

venter ('ventə) pl. *ventres* [L.] 1. any belly-shaped part; a fleshy contractible part of a muscle. 2. the abdomen or stomach. 3. a hollowed part or cavity.

ventilation (,venti'layshən) 1. the process or act of supplying a house or room continuously with fresh air. 2. in respiratory physiology, the process of exchange of air between the lungs and the ambient air. *Pulmonary ventilation* (usually measured in litres per minute) refers to the total exchange, whereas *alveolar ventilation* refers to the effective ventilation of the alveoli, where gas exchange with the blood takes place. 3. in psychiatry, the free discussion of one's problems or grievances.

alveolar v. the amount of gas expelled from the alveoli to the outside of the body per minute.

intermittent mandatory v. (IMV) a type of mechanical ventilation in which the VENTILATOR is set to deliver a prescribed tidal volume at specified intervals and a high-flow gas system permits the patient to breathe spontaneously between cycles. The ventilator rate is set to maintain the patient's $P_{a}CO_2$ at normal levels and is reduced gradually to zero as the patient's condition improves.

intermittent positive-pressure v. (IPPV) the provision of mechanical ventilation by a machine designed to deliver breathing gas until equilibrium is established between the patient's lungs and the VENTILATOR. IPPV machines are positive-pressure, pressure-cycled, assistor-controller (pneumatic) devices.

Because of their compact size and capability of operating independently of an electrical current, the IPPV machines have the most widespread applicability in the employment of a form of treatment called INTERMITTENT POSITIVE-PRESSURE BREATHING. Examples of the ventilators utilized in IPPV include the Bird respirator and the Bennett 7200a model. Several newer machines employed specifically for IPPV and relatively simple in design are now available.

maximal voluntary v. (MVV) the maximal volume that can be exhaled per minute by the patient breathing as rapidly and deeply as possible.

mechanical v. that accomplished by extrinsic means.

minute v. the total amount of gas (in litres) expelled from the lungs per minute.

ventilator ('venti,laytə) an apparatus designed to qualify the air that is breathed through it or to either intermittently or continuously control pulmonary ventilation; called also *respirator*. Use of a mechanical ventilator is indicated as a supportive measure in patients suffering from respiratory paralysis and in those with ventilatory failure manifested by either alveolar hypoventilation or ventilation/perfusion inequality (distributive HYPOXIA), or both.

In alveolar hypoventilation gas exchange with the blood is inadequate for the removal of carbon dioxide, and hypercapnia results. When breathing air, as there is an inverse relationship between carbon dioxide and oxygen in the alveoli, any increase in carbon dioxide is accompanied by a fall in oxygen, and hypoxia occurs. The hypercapnia causes respiratory ACIDOSIS. Thus the patient shows hypoxia, hypercapnia, and respiratory acidosis.

In an ideal lung each alveolus would receive its fair share of respiratory gases and its fair share of pulmonary blood flow in relation to its ventilation. In other words, ventilation and perfusion would be perfectly matched. However, in a real lung, even in a healthy man, neither alveolar ventilation nor pulmonary blood flow is distributed perfectly, and in patients with cardiorespiratory problems the uneven matching of ventilation to perfusion is the most common cause of hypoxaemia. In those areas of the lung where alveoli are ventilated but not perfused, or where ventilation is greater than perfusion, some or all of this ventilation is wasted and adds to what is known as 'dead-space'. Increased dead-space leads to carbon dioxide retention. Whether this leads to hypercapnia depends on whether the patient can respond by increasing his ventilation. Where alveoli are perfused but not ventilated, or where perfusion is greater than ventilation, some or all of the perfused blood is not being oxygenated and adds to what is known as 'shunt'. Increased shunt leads to hypoxaemia. If the patient can respond to this hypoxaemia by increasing his ventilation then the carbon dioxide level in the blood will fall (hypocapnia). This hypocapnia is the cause of respiratory ALKALOSIS.

In either case, the ventilator is used to improve alveolar ventilation, re-establish a normal ACID–BASE BALANCE, and correct the associated hypoxia. It is important, however, that the primary cause of a patient's ventilatory failure be known and that his blood gases be evaluated frequently during controlled ventilation so that the mechanical ventilator can be used to its best advantage and greatest benefit to the individual patient.

TYPES OF VENTILATORS. There are two major groups of ventilators:

Negative-pressure ventilators generate negative pressure on the exterior surface of the chest. Among the ventilators of this type are the body tank (IRON LUNG, or Drinker respirator) and the chest and chest-abdomen respirators such as the Emerson cuirass. These machines exert negative (subatmospheric) pressure on the exterior chest wall which is transmitted to the interior of the thorax, creating a suction effect and causing air to flow into the lungs. The lungs are allowed to exhale passively before the next inspiratory cycle. Full-body and chest ventilators are not effective in relief of ventilatory failure resulting from increased airway resistance due to intrapulmonary diseases, such as CHRONIC OBSTRUCTIVE AIRWAYS DISEASE (COAD). They are, therefore, limited to the treatment of patients whose ventilatory problems are caused by respiratory paralysis rather than obstructive lung disease and whose condition limits the employment of intubation.

Positive-pressure ventilators force air directly into the lungs under positive pressure, causing the lungs and chest to expand. Ventilators of this type are indicated in a wide variety of conditions that produce either acute respiratory distress or chronic respiratory insufficiency, or both.

There is at the present time no mechanical ventilator that exactly duplicates all of the physiological mechanisms involved in the spontaneous breathing patterns of a healthy person during various stages of rest and activity. Each model is designed to utilize one or more physiological and mechanical principles to assist the patient in respiratory failure; selection of the type of ventilator for the individual patient is based on that patient's particular needs.

All mechanical ventilators can be used for controlled ventilation, that is the machine can ventilate automatically the lungs of a patient who cannot breathe on his own or whose breathing is erratic. In addition, other features may be incorporated, such as negative end-expiratory pressure, positive end-expiratory pressure, the assist mode, where the patient's own inspiration triggers the machine, and various other modes that help wean the patient from the machine.

Ventilators may be regarded as producing inspiration by exerting either a predetermined flow of gas (flow generators) or a predetermined pressure (pressure generators). Pressure generators generally exert a constant pressure and, as the pressure in the airway is zero at the start of inspiration, gas flow is rapid initially, but then falls off as the pressure gradient between machine and airway decreases. Pressure generators compensate for small leaks in the circuit, but if there is increased resistance to flow in the machine, the ventilator tubing, or the patient, the volume of gas delivered to the patient will fall. Flow generators may or may not produce a constant flow, but they are able to compensate for changes in resistance, though not for leaks. Pressure generators include the Blease and the East Radcliffe, whilst flow generators include the Cape and the Bird.

There are three main ways in which the change-over from inspiration to expiration is controlled (cycling):

Pressure-cycled ventilators (e.g., Bird) are those in which inspiration stops when a certain pressure is reached in the patient's airway. Tidal volume can therefore be altered by manipulating the pressure control. In the presence of increased airway resistance or increased stiffness of the patient's lungs, the cycling pressure is reached earlier and tidal volume decreases. These ventilators are often fitted with a triggering device whereby the inspiratory effort of the patient triggers the ventilator. The amount of inspiratory effort required by the patient to do this can be altered using the sensitivity control.

Volume-cycled ventilators (e.g., Manley and Cape) rely upon a predetermined volume as the cycling monitor. Increases in airway resistance or stiffness in the lungs of the patient do not diminish the volume delivered, though the pressure required to do so rises.

In order to avoid damage to the lungs there is an upper limit to the pressure allowed. Volume-cycled ventilators are particularly useful in patients with asthma and chronic obstructive airways disease (COAD).

In *time-cycled ventilators* (e.g., Nuffield and Servo) the cycling pattern is determined by controls that set the length of a breath, and thus the number of breaths per minute. The length of the inspiratory and expiratory phases may be adjustable separately, or the ratio between the two may be alterable. The flow rate is adjusted so that the tidal volume required can be delivered in the time allotted for inspiration. Although pressure plays no direct role in governing the cycling pattern, the variables of time and flow do, of course, affect the pressure.

Some machines can be used in different cycling modes, e.g., the Bennett. Ventilators are powered either by electricity (e.g., Cape), compressed gases (e.g., Nuffield), by gases supplied from an anaesthetic machine (e.g., Manley), or a combination of electricity and compressed gases (e.g., Servo).

The expiratory phase is usually passive, that is the expiratory limb is connected to the atmosphere and the pressure in the airways falls to zero. Some machines can add a subatmospheric (negative) pressure during expiration, but this is seldom, if ever, used. More useful is the facility to keep the pressure positive during expiration, a manoeuvre known as adding positive end-expiratory pressure (PEEP). This has the effect of holding the smaller air passages open, increasing the functional residual capacity of the lung and preventing atelectasis. This usually improves the oxygenation of the patient without the need to increase the inspiratory oxygen concentration and thereby run the risk of oxygen toxicity. Whereas PEEP is applied to patients who are intubated and ventilated, positive pressure can be applied to patients who are breathing spontaneously, a manoeuvre known as continuous positive airway pressure (CPAP). PEEP, the level of which is commonly between 5 and 15 mmH_20, is, however, associated with an increased risk of problems due to increased pressure within the airways, such as pneumothorax. CPAP has similar advantages to PEEP but is not accompanied by as many problems related to increased airway pressure.

Other variations of controlled ventilation which are often used when trying to wean a patient from the machine include *intermittent mandatory ventilation* (IMV) and *synchronized intermittent mandatory ventilation* (SIMV). IMV allows the patient to take spontaneous breaths between the controlled number of breaths for which the machine has been set. The number of programmed breaths can be gradually reduced as the patient becomes better able to breathe effectively on his own. SIMV is similar to IMV except that delivery of positive pressure is synchronized with the patient's breathing pattern. In theory this eliminates the possibility of the machine delivering positive pressure at the peak of the patient's spontaneous respiration, which could overdistend the lungs. In practice this does not seem to occur, so SIMV has no advantage over IMV.

High frequency ventilation is a technique of ventilating the lungs with small tidal volumes but at far greater frequency than normal. In *high frequency positive pressure ventilation* (HFPPV) frequencies of 60–100 breaths per minute at tidal volumes about half that of normal are used to maintain adequate gaseous exchange. Some conventional ventilators can, or can be adapted to, deliver this sort of ventilation. In *high frequency jet ventilation* (HJV) small pulses of high pressure gas are delivered to the airway by some form of injector. Frequencies of 80–600 breaths per minute are achieved by interrupting at rapid frequency a high pressure flow of gas. Purpose-designed ventilators are required. In *high frequency oscillation* (HFO) frequencies of 300–2400 breaths per minute are achieved using a loudspeaker cone or piston pump.

The advantage of high frequency ventilation is that adequate gas exchange can be achieved with lower airway pressures and therefore less risk of damage to lungs, less adverse effect on the cardiovascular system, improved patient tolerance, and therefore less need for sedation, and the allowance of adequate ventilation in the presence of disrupted airways, e.g., bronchopleural fistulas. The disadvantages include the need for specialized equipment, difficulty in humidification and difficulty in monitoring what is actually occurring. Its role in the management of respiratory failure awaits clarification, but it does have a part to play in certain specific situations, e.g., laryngeal surgery.

PATIENT CARE. Regardless of the model and capabilities of the mechanical ventilator being used in the treatment of a patient with inadequate ventilation, there are certain general principles that are basic to the competent care of that patient. It is essential that those responsible for the care of the patient be fully aware of the physiological effects of mechanical ventilation. A major contribution of mechanical ventilation should be the normalization of blood gases and avoidance of the extremes of respiratory ACIDOSIS and respiratory ALKALOSIS. Thus careful monitoring of the blood gases and the pH is an essential part of patient care during mechanical ventilation.

A second consideration is the influence of mechanical ventilation on circulation. The intrathoracic pressure that accompanies positive pressure ventilation will impede venous return to the heart and lead to a fall in cardiac output and a drop in blood pressure. This effect is exaggerated if the patient already has a reduced intravascular volume or if PEEP is added. Normally, the body compensates for this fall in venous return and the application of intermittent positive pressure ventilation does not lead to adverse cardiovascular changes. Frequent determinations of pulse and blood pressure are necessary, especially when the patient is first put on the ventilator, and any fall in blood pressure probably requires volume replacement. It should be noted that the interference with the venous return to the right side of the heart can bring about a therapeutic effect in patients with pulmonary oedema. Thus, a potentially hazardous side-effect of an increase in intrathoracic pressure can be of benefit to the patient when used judiciously by a doctor who is knowledgeable about all aspects of ventilatory therapy.

A third consideration is that of the effects of mechanical ventilation on fluid balance. Retention of water and sodium occurs when patients are put on ventilators, an effect due partly to a rise in the level of antiduiretic hormone in the blood and partly to the cardiovascular changes. The situation can lead to pulmonary oedema and further interference with the patient's ventilation. Accurate records of fluid intake and output are necessary and the patient is kept on the 'dry side', that is, given less fluid than if he was not on a ventilator.

A thorough knowledge of the apparatus being used for mechanical ventilation is vital to competent care of the patient. No one should attempt to give patient care without prior instruction in the purpose of the machine and the physiological and physical principles upon which it operates. Furthermore, a means of ventilating the patient, e.g., bag and mask, must be available should the machine develop a fault.

TRACHEOSTOMY care is of vital importance when the patient is being maintained on a respirator with controlled ventilation and positive pressure is being delivered via a tracheostomy tube. Suction is applied as necessary. Whether the patient has a tracheostomy or not, the air passages must be kept moist whenever a respirator is used for a prolonged period. See also TRACHEOSTOMY.

If AEROSOL medications are administered by use of a respirator, it is important to know the type of medication being used, its desired effects and the signs and symptoms of overdosage or toxic side-effects. When such symptoms appear the rate of nebulization requires adjustment.

The psychological implications of the use of a respirator are manifold. If he is conscious or semiconscious, the patient is aware that the machine is concerned with maintaining his very 'breath of life' and he is understandably apprehensive about its use and effects on his breathing. When a respirator is used for a brief period as a means of therapy, the patient can be told that he can control the cycle by the slightest effort on his part. Once he understands the way the machine works and his questions are answered to his satisfaction his fears can be allayed. The patient who is partially or totally dependent on a respirator will need more reassurance. He should be assured that someone will be near at all times in case the apparatus needs adjusting. Much of his panic and fear can be relieved if the nursing staff exercises patience and maintains a calm attitude when helping him adjust to the respirator.

WEANING FROM THE VENTILATOR. Gradual withdrawal of the support of the ventilator ('weaning') begins as soon as the patient's blood gases, spontaneous breathing capabilities, and clinical status indicate that he may be able to start breathing on his own. Some patients view with alarm the prospect of trying to breathe without the aid of the ventilator while others may be overenthusiastic and wish to end their dependence on the machine before they are ready to do so. Difficulties are more likely to develop in those who have had prolonged controlled ventilation than in those who have had assisted ventilation. Classical weaning involves taking the patient off the machine for gradually increasing periods until he can manage on his own. Alternatively, the patient is transferred from controlled to intermittent mandatory ventilation with a decreasing number of breaths being contributed by the machine.

Prior to the actual removal of ventilatory assistance the patient should be taught abdominal breathing and informed that a deep controlled breathing pattern will be more advantageous than rapid shallow breaths. He will need calm assurance that he will not be expected to endure any distress beyond his capability to cope, and that a person in whom he has confidence will remain with him while he is off the respirator.

It is recommended that weaning be initiated during the morning hours when the patient is most rested and relaxed. During the time the patient is off the ventilator he is given warmed, humidified, oxygenated air via the endotracheal tube or tracheostomy. Such measures will enhance the patient's tolerance to the weaning process. Once he is able to breathe adequately independently of the ventilating machine, a simple ventilator may be kept close at hand in the event the patient should express or exhibit a need for it. During this time he is observed regularly to make certain he is able to breathe adequately on his own.

Ventolin ('ventohlin) trademark for a salbutamol metered-dose inhaler; a bronchodilator.

ventr(i)-, ventr(o)- word element. [L.] *belly, front (anterior) aspect of the body, ventral aspect.*

ventrad ('ventrad) toward a belly, venter, or ventral aspect.

ventral ('ventrəl) 1. pertaining to the abdomen or to any venter. 2. directed toward or situated on the belly surface; opposite of dorsal.

ventralis (ven'traylis) [L.] *ventral.*

ventricle ('ventrik'l) a small cavity or chamber, as in the brain or heart.

v. of Arantius 1. the rhomboid fossa, especially its lower end. 2. fifth ventricle.

fifth v. the median cleft between the two laminae of the septum lucidum.

fourth v. a median cavity in the hindbrain, containing cerebrospinal fluid.

v. of larynx the space between the true and false vocal cords.

lateral v. the cavity in each cerebral hemisphere, derived from the cavity of the embryonic tube, containing cerebrospinal fluid.

left v. the lower chamber of the left side of the heart, which pumps oxygenated blood out through the aorta to all the tissues of the body.

Morgagni's v. ventricle of larynx.

pineal v. an extension of the third ventricle into the stalk of the pineal body.

right v. the lower chamber of the right side of the heart, which pumps venous blood through the pulmonary trunk and arteries to the capillaries of the lung.

third v. a narrow cleft below the corpus callosum, within the diencephalon between the two thalami.

ventricornu (ˌventri'kawnyoo) the anterior horn of grey matter in the spinal cord. adj. **ventricornual.**

ventricular (ven'trikyuhlə) pertaining to a ventricle.

v. septal defect a CONGENITAL HEART DEFECT in which there is persistent patency of the ventricular septum in either the muscular or fibrous portion most often due to failure of the bulbar septum to completely close the interventricular foramen. The defect permits flow of blood directly from one ventricle to the other, resulting in bypassing of the pulmonary circulation and producing varying degrees of cyanosis because of oxygen deficiency.

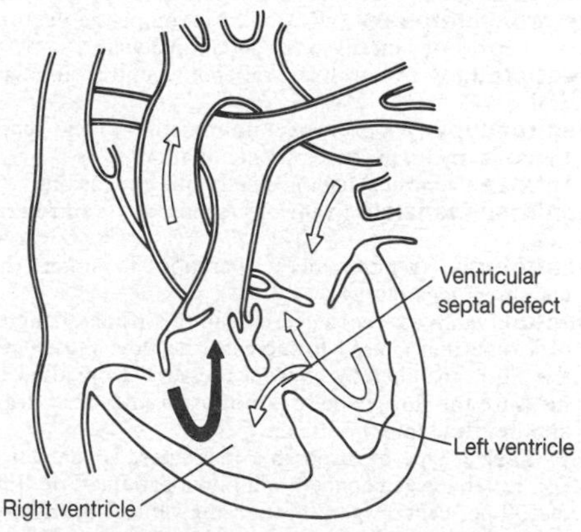

Ventricular septal defect.

ventriculitis (venˌtrikyuh'lietis) inflammation of a ventricle, especially a cerebral ventricle.

ventriculoatriostomy (venˌtrikyuhlohˌaytri'ostəmee) introduction of a catheter with a one-way valve to drain cerebrospinal fluid from a cerebral ventricle to the right atrium via the jugular vein, for relief of hydrocephalus.

ventriculocisternostomy (ven,trikyuhloh,sistər'nostəmee) surgical creation of a communication between the third ventricle and the interpeduncular cistern, for drainage of cerebrospinal fluid.

ventriculocordectomy (ven,trikyuhlohkaw'dektəmee) punch resection of the vocal cords.

ventriculogram (ven'trikyuhloh,gram) radiograph of the cerebral ventricles.

ventriculography (ven,trikyuh'logrəfee) 1. radiography of the cerebral ventricles after introduction of air or other contrast medium. 2. radiography of a ventricle of the heart after injection of a contrast medium.

ventriculometry (ven,trikyuh'lomətree) measurement of intracranial pressure.

ventriculonector (ven,trikyuhloh'nektor) the bundle of His.

ventriculopuncture (ven'trikyuhloh,pungkchə) surgical puncture of a lateral ventricle of the brain.

ventriculoscopy (ven,trikyuh'loskəpee) endoscopic examination of the cerebral ventricles.

ventriculostomy (ven,trikyuh'lostəmee) surgical creation of a free communication between the third ventricle and the interpeduncular cistern for relief of hydrocephalus.

ventriculosubarachnoid (ven,trikyuhloh,subə'raknoyd) pertaining to the cerebral ventricles and subarachnoid space.

ventriculotomy (ven,trikyuh'lotəmee) incision of a ventricle of the heart.

ventriculus (ven'trikyuhləs) pl. *ventriculi* [L.] 1. a ventricle. 2. the stomach.

ventricumbent (,ventri'kumbənt) prone; lying on the belly.

ventriduct ('ventri,dukt) to bring or carry ventrad.

ventriflexion (,ventri'flekshən) bending towards a belly or anterior surface.

ventrimeson (,ventri'meson, -'meez-) the median line on the ventral surface. adj. **ventrimesal**.

ventrofixation, ventrifixation (,ventrohfik'sayshən; ,ventrifik'sayshən) fixation of a viscus, e.g., the uterus, to the abdominal wall; ventrosuspension.

ventrohysteropexy (,ventroh'histə·roh,peksee) suture of a retroverted uterus to the abdominal wall.

ventrolateral (,ventroh'latə·rəl) both ventral and lateral.

ventroscopy (ven'troskəpee) illumination of the abdominal cavity for purposes of examination.

ventrose ('ventrohs) having a belly-like expansion.

ventrosuspension (,ventrohsə'spenshən) ventrofixation.

ventrotomy (ven'trotəmee) operation to enter the abdomen; laparotomy.

venturi (ven'tyooə·ree) a decrease in the inside diameter of a tube that is used to increase the flow velocity of the fluid and thereby cause a pressure drop; used to measure the flow velocity (a *venturi meter)* or to draw another fluid into the stream.

v. mask a type of disposable mask used to deliver a controlled oxygen concentration to a patient. The flow of 100 per cent oxygen through the venturi draws in a controlled amount of room air (21 per cent oxygen). Commonly available masks deliver 24, 28, 35, or 40 per cent oxygen. At concentrations above 24 per cent, humidification may be required. See also OXYGEN THERAPY.

v. nebulizer a type of nebulizer used in AEROSOL therapy. The pressure drop of gas flowing through the venturi draws liquid from a capillary tube. As the liquid enters the gas stream it breaks up into a spray of small droplets.

venula ('venyuhlə) pl. *venulae* [L.] venule.

venule ('venyool) any of the small vessels that collect blood from the capillary plexuses and join to form veins. adj. **venular**.

verapamil (ve'rapə,mil) a calcium channel blocking agent used as a coronary vasodilator in the treatment of angina pectoris.

verbigeration (,vərbijə'rayshən) abnormal repetition of meaningless words and phrases.

verge (vərj) a circumference or ring.

anal v. the opening of the anus on the surface of the body.

vergence ('vərj'ns) disjunctive movement of the eyes in opposite directions in adjusting to near or far vision; convergence or divergence.

vermicide ('vərmi,sied) an agent lethal to parasitic intestinal worms; an anthelmintic.

vermicular (vər'mikyuhlə) wormlike in shape or appearance.

vermiculation (vər,mikyuh'layshən) peristaltic motion; peristalsis.

vermiculous (vər'mikyuhləs) 1. wormlike. 2. infected with worms.

vermiform ('vərmi,fawm) worm-shaped.

v. appendix a small appendage near the juncture of the small intestine and the large intestine (ileocaecal valve); often called simply appendix. An apparently useless structure, it can be the source of a serious illness, APPENDICITIS.

vermifugal (,vərmi'fyoog'l, vər'mifyuhg'l) expelling parasitic worms from the intestine.

vermifuge ('vərmi,fyooj) any agent that expels parasitic intestinal worms; an anthelmintic.

vermilion border (və'mili·ən) the exposed red portion of the upper or lower lip.

vermilionectomy (və,mili·ə'nektəmee) excision of the vermilion border of the lip.

vermin ('vərmin) an external animal parasite; such parasites collectively.

vermination (,vərmi'nayshən) infestation with vermin or infection with worms.

verminous ('vərminəs) pertaining to, due to, or abounding in worms or in vermin.

vermis ('vərmis) [L.] 1. a worm, or wormlike structure. 2. vermis cerebelli.

v. cerebelli the median part of the cerebellum, between the two hemispheres.

nodule of v. the part of the vermis of the cerebellum, on the ventral surface, where the inferior medullary velum attaches.

vermix ('vərmiks) the vermiform appendix.

Vernet's syndrome ('vərnayz) paralysis of the glossopharyngeal, vagus, and spinal accessory nerves due to a lesion in the region of the jugular foramen.

vernix ('vərniks) [L.] *varnish*.

v. caseosa the unctuous substance composed of sebum and desquamated epithelial cells, covering the skin of the fetus between 30 and 37 weeks' gestation; designed to protect the fetal skin from the effects of the amniotic fluid.

verruca (və'rookə) pl. *verrucae* [L.] 1. a WART. 2. one of the wartlike elevations on the endocardium in various types of endocarditis. adj. **verrucose, verrucous. v. plana** a small, smooth, usually skin-coloured or light brown, slightly raised wart sometimes occurring in great numbers; seen most often in children.

v. plantaris a viral epidermal tumour on the sole of the foot (see also PLANTAR WART).

verruciform (və'roosi,fawm) wartlike.

verruga (və'roogə) wart.

v. peruana a haemangioma-like tumour or nodule occurring in Carrión's disease.

version ('vərshən, -zhən) the act of turning; especially the manual turning of the fetus in delivery.

bipolar v. turning effected by acting upon both poles of the fetus either by external or combined version.

cephalic v. turning of the fetus so that the head presents.

external v. that effected by outside manipulation.

external cephalic v. a procedure (not favoured by some obstetricians) where the fetus presenting by the breech may be turned into cephalic presentation by means of manipulation through the abdominal wall.

internal v. that effected by the hand or fingers inserted through the dilated cervix.

pelvic v. version by manipulation of the breech.

podalic v. conversion of a more unfavourable presentation into a footling presentation.

spontaneous v. one that occurs without aid from any extraneous force.

vertebr(o)- word element. [L.] *vertebra, spine.*

vertebra ('vərtibrə) pl. *vertebrae* [L.] any of the separate segments comprising the spine (vertebral column). See also SPINE.

The vertebrae support the body and provide the protective bony corridor through which the spinal cord passes. The 33 bones that make up the spine differ considerably in size and structure according to location. There are seven cervical (neck) vertebrae, 12 thoracic (high back), five lumbar (low back), five sacral (near the base of the spine), and four coccygeal (at the base). The five sacral vertebrae are fused to form the sacrum, and the four coccygeal vertebrae are fused to form the coccyx.

The weight-bearing portion of a typical vertebra is the vertebral body, the most forward portion. This is a cylindrical structure that is separated from the vertebral bodies above and below by discs of cartilage and fibrous tissue. These intervertebral discs act as cushions to absorb the mechanical shock of walking, running, and other activity. Rupture of an intervertebral disc is known popularly as slipped DISC. A semicircular arch of bone protrudes from the back of each vertebral body, surrounding the spinal cord. Directly in its midline a bony projection, the spinous process, grows backward from the arch. The spinuous process can be felt on the back as a hard knob. Three pairs of outgrowths project from the arch. One of these protrudes horizontally on each side and in the thorax connects with the ribs. The remaining two form joints with the vertebrae above and below. The joints permit the spine to bend flexibly. The vertebrae are held firmly in place by a series of strong ligaments.

cranial v. the segments of the skull and facial bones, regarded by some as modified vertebrae.

v. dentata the second cervical vertebra, or axis.

dorsal vertebrae thoracic vertebrae.

false vertebrae those vertebrae which normally fuse with adjoining segments: the sacral and coccygeal vertebrae.

v. magnum the sacrum.

odontoid v. the second cervical vertebra, or axis.

v. plana a condition of spondylitis in which the body of the vertebra is reduced to a sclerotic disc.

true vertebrae those segments of the vertebral column that normally remain unfused throughout life: the cervical, thoracic, and lumbar vertebrae.

vertebral ('vərtibrəl) of or pertaining to a vertebra.

v. canal the canal formed by the series of vertebral foramina together, containing the spinal cord and meninges. Called also *spinal canal.*

v. column the spine; the rigid structure in the midline of the back, composed of the vertebrae.

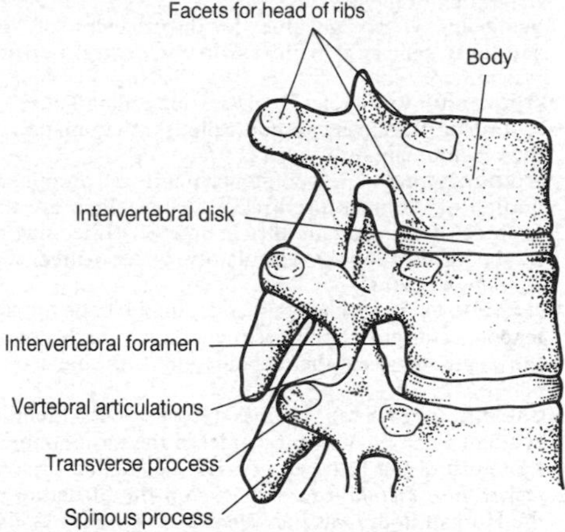

Structure of vertebral column

vertebrarium (ˌvərti'brair·ri·əm) the spine, or vertebral column.

Vertebrata (ˌvərti'brahtə) a subphylum of the Chordata, comprising all animals having a vertebral column, including mammals, birds, reptiles, amphibians, and fishes.

vertebrate ('vərtiˌbrət, -ˌbrayt) 1. having a vertebral column. 2. an animal with a vertebral column; any member of the Vertebrata.

vertebrectomy (ˌvərti'brektəmee) excision of a vertebra.

vertebrobasilar (ˌvərtibroh'basilə) pertaining to or affecting the vertebral and basilar arteries.

vertebrochondral (ˌvərtibroh'kondrəl) pertaining to a vertebra and a costal cartilage.

vertebrocostal (ˌvərtibroh'kost'l) pertaining to a vertebra and a rib.

vertebrogenic (ˌvərtibroh'jenik) arising in a vertebra or in the vertebral column.

vertebrosternal (ˌvərtibroh'stərnəl) pertaining to a vertebra and the sternum.

vertex ('vərteks) the summit or top, especially the top of the head (vertex cranii).

vertical ('vərtik'l) 1. perpendicular to the plane of the horizon. 2. relating to the vertex.

verticalis (ˌvərti'kaylis) [L.] *vertical.*

verticillate (vər'tisilət, ˌvərti'silayt) arranged in whorls.

vertigo ('vərtiˌgoh) a sensation of rotation or movement of one's self (subjective vertigo) or of one's surroundings (objective vertigo) in any plane. The term is sometimes used erroneously as a synonym for dizziness. Vertigo may result from diseases of the inner ear or may be due to disturbances of the vestibular centres or pathways in the central nervous system.

auditory v., aural v. Menière's disease. **benign paroxysmal positional (or postural) v.** recurrent vertigo and nystagmus occurring when the head is placed in certain positions, usually not associated with lesions of the central nervous system.

central v. that due to disorder of the central nervous system.

labyrinthine v. a form associated with disease of the labyrinth of the ear.

organic v. that caused by vestibular brain disease or to tabes dorsalis.

peripheral v. vestibular vertigo.

positional p., postural p. that associated with a specific position of the head in space or with changes in position of the head in space.

vestibular v. vertigo due to disturbances of the vestibular centres or pathways in the central nervous system.

vertigraphy (vər'tigrəfee) body-section radiography.

verumontanitis (ˌveryooˌmontə'nietis) inflammation of the verumontanum.

verumontanum (ˌveryoomon'taynəm) a prominent portion of the male urethral crest, on which are the opening of the prostatic utricle and, on either side of it, the orifices of the ejaculatory ducts; called also *seminal colliculus*.

vesalianum (vəˌsayli'aynəm) a sesamoid bone in the tendon of origin of the gastrocnemius muscle, or in the angle between the cuboid and fifth metatarsal bones.

Vesalius (ve'sayli·əs) Andreas (1514–1564). Flemish anatomist and physician, considered the most eminent anatomist of the 16th century. His *De humani corporis fabrica libri septum* (Seven Books on the Structure of the Human Body) was published in 1543. He was also a pioneer in ethnic craniology and experimental and comparative psychology.

vesic(o)- word element. [L.] *blister, bladder.*

vesica ('vesikə) pl. *vesicae* [L.] bladder. adj. **vesical.**

vesicant ('vesikənt) 1. producing blisters. 2. an agent that produces blisters.

vesication (ˌvesi'kayshən) 1. the process of blistering. 2. a blistered spot or surface.

vesicle ('vesik'l) 1. a small bladder or sac containing liquid. 2. a small circumscribed elevation of the epidermis containing a serous fluid; a small blister.

allantoic v. the internal hollow portion of the allantois.

auditory v. a detached ovoid sac formed by closure of the auditory pit in the early embryo, from which the percipient parts of the inner ear develop. **brain v's** the five divisions of the closed neural tube in the developing embryo, including the telencephalon, diencephalon, mesencephalon, metencephalon, and myelencephalon.

brain v's, primary the three earlier subdivisions of the embryonic neural tube, including the forebrain, midbrain, and hindbrain.

brain v's, secondary the four brain vesicles formed by specialization of the forebrain and of the hindbrain in later embryonic development.

chorionic v. the developing ovum at the time of its invasion of the endometrium of the uterus.

compound v. multilocular vesicle.

encephalic v's brain vesicles.

germinal v. the fluid-filled nucleus of an oocyte toward the end of prophase of its meiotic division.

lens v. a vesicle formed from the lens pit of the embryo, developing into the crystalline lens.

multilocular v. one with multiple chambers or compartments.

olfactory v. 1. the vesicle in the embryo which later develops into the olfactory bulb and tract. 2. a bulbous expansion at the distal end of an olfactory cell, from which the olfactory hairs project.

optic v. an evagination on either side of the forebrain of the early embryo, from which the percipient parts of the eye develop.

otic v. auditory vesicle.

seminal v. paired sacculated pouches attached to the posterior urinary bladder; the duct of each joins the ipsilateral vas (ductus) deferens to form the ejaculatory duct.

umbilical v. the pear-shaped expansion of the yolk sac growing out into the cavity of the chorion, joined to the midgut by the yolk stalk.

vesicocele ('vesikohˌseel) hernia of the bladder.

vesicocervical (ˌvesikoh'sərvik'l, -sə'viek'l) pertaining to the bladder and uterine cervix.

vesicoclysis (ˌvesi'koklisis) introduction of fluid into the bladder.

vesicoenteric, vesicointestinal (ˌvesikoh·en'terik; ˌvesikoh·in'testin'l) pertaining to or communicating with the urinary bladder and intestine.

vesicofixation (ˌvesikohfik'sayshən) 1. fixation of the urinary bladder (cystopexy). 2. fixation of the uterus to the bladder.

vesicoprostatic (ˌvesikohpro'statik) pertaining to the bladder and prostate.

vesicopubic (ˌvesikoh'pyoobik) pertaining to the bladder and pubes.

vesicosigmoidostomy (ˌvesikohˌsigmoy'dostəmee) the creation of a permanent communication between the urinary bladder and the sigmoid flexure.

vesicospinal (ˌvesikoh'spien'l) pertaining to the bladder and spine.

vesicostomy (ˌvesi'kostəmee) the formation of an opening into the bladder; cystostomy.

vesicoureteral, vesicoureteric (ˌvesikoh·yuh'reetə·rəl; ˌvesikoh·yoori'terik) pertaining to the bladder and ureter.

vesicouterine (ˌvesikoh'yootəˌrien) pertaining to the bladder and uterus.

vesicovaginal (ˌvesikohvə'jien'l, -'vajin'l) pertaining to the bladder and vagina.

vesicula (ve'sikyuhlə) pl. *vesiculae* [L.] vesicle.

vesicular (ve'sikyuhlə) 1. composed of or relating to small, saclike bodies. 2. pertaining to or made up of vesicles on the skin.

vesiculation (veˌsikyuh'layshən) formation of vesicles.

vesiculectomy (veˌsikyuh'lektəmee) excision of a vesicle, especially the seminal vesicle.

vesiculiform (ve'sikyuhliˌfawm) shaped like a vesicle.

vesiculitis (veˌsikyuh'lietis) inflammation of a vesicle, especially a seminal vesicle (seminal vesiculitis).

vesiculocavernous (veˌsikyuhloh'kavənəs, -kə'vərnəs) both vesicular and cavernous.

vesiculogram (ve'sikyuhlohˌgram) a radiograph of the seminal vesicles.

vesiculography (veˌsikyuh'logrəfee) radiography of the seminal vesicles.

vesiculopapular (veˌsikyuhloh'papyuhlə) marked by or having the characteristics of vesicles and papules.

vesiculopustular (veˌsikyuhloh'pustyuhlə) marked by or having the characteristics of vesicles and pustules.

vesiculotomy (veˌsikyuh'lotəmee) incision into a vesicle, especially the seminal vesicle.

vesiculotympanic (veˌsikyuhlohtim'panik) having both a vesicular and tympanic quality; said of percussion sounds.

vessel ('ves'l) any channel for carrying a fluid, such as blood or lymph (see also VAS).

absorbent v's lymphatic vessels.

blood v. any of the vessels conveying the blood; an artery, arteriole, vein, venule, or capillary.

collateral v's 1. a vessel that parallels another vessel, a nerve, or other structure. 2. a vessel important in establishing and maintaining a collateral circulation.

great v's the large vessels entering the heart, including the aorta, the pulmonary arteries and veins, and the venae cavae. **lacteal v's** those that take up chyle from the intestinal wall during digestion.

lymphatic v's the capillaries, collecting vessels, and trunks that collect lymph from the tissues and carry it to the blood stream.

nutrient v's vessels supplying nutritive elements to special tissues, as arteries entering the substance of bone or the walls of large blood vessels.

vestibular (ve'stibyuhlə) relating to a vestibule.

v. glands those in the vestibule of the vagina, including Bartholin's glands.

v. nerve a branch of the vestibulocochlear (eighth) nerve supplying the semicircular canals and concerned with balance and equilibrium.

vestibule ('vesti,byool) a space or cavity at the entrance to another structure. adj. **vestibular**.

v. of aorta a small space at the root of the aorta.

v. of ear an oval cavity in the middle of the bony labyrinth.

v. of mouth the portion of the oral cavity bounded on the one side by teeth and gingivae, or the residual alveolar ridges, and on the other by the lips (labial vestibule) and cheeks (buccal vestibule).

v. of nose the anterior part of the nasal cavity.

v. of pharynx 1. the fauces. 2. oropharynx.

v. of vagina the space between the labia minora into which the urethra and vagina open.

vestibulocochlear nerve (ve,stibyuhloh'kokli·ə) the eighth cranial nerve, which emerges from the brain between the pons and medulla oblongata, behind the facial nerve. The vestibular division serves the vestibule of the ear and the semicircular canals, carrying impulses for equilibrium. The cochlear division serves the cochlea and carries impulses for the sense of hearing. Called also *acoustic nerve* and *auditory nerve*.

vestibulogenic (ve,stibyuhloh'jenik) arising in a vestibule, as that of the ear.

vestibulo-ocular (ve,stibyuhloh'okyuhlə) pertaining to the vestibular and oculomotor nerves; or to the maintenance of visual stability during head movements.

vestibuloplasty (ve'stibyuhloh,plastee) surgical modification of gingiva-mucous membrane relationships in the vestibule of the mouth.

vestibulotomy (ve,stibyuh'lotəmee) incision into the vestibule of the ear.

vestibulourethral (ve,stibyuhloh·yuh'reethrəl) pertaining to vestibule of the vagina and the urethra.

vestibulum (ve'stibyuhləm) pl. *vestibula* [L.] vestibule.

vestige ('vestij) the remnant of a structure that functioned in a previous stage of species or individual development. adj. **vestigial**.

vestigium (ve'stiji·əm) pl. *vestigia* [L.] vestige.

veterinary ('vetrinree) pertaining to domestic animals and their diseases.

v. surgeon a person trained and authorized to practice veterinary medicine and surgery; a doctor of veterinary medicine. Called also *veterinarian*.

v.f. visual field.

via ('vieə) pl. *viae* [L.] way, channel.

viability (,vieə'bilitee) the state or quality of being viable.

viable ('vieəb'l) able to maintain an independent existence; able to live after birth.

vial ('vieəl) a small bottle.

vibex ('viebeks) pl. *vibices* [L.] a narrow linear mark or streak; a linear subcutaneous effusion of blood.

Vibramycin (,viebrə'miesin) trademark for preparations of doxycycline; a tetracycline antibiotic.

vibratile ('viebrə,tiel) swaying or moving to and fro; vibratory.

vibration (vie'brayshən) 1. a rapid movement to and fro; oscillation. 2. the shaking of the body tissues to have a stimulating effect. 3. a form of massage.

vibrator (vie'braytə) an apparatus used in vibratory treatment.

vibratory (vie'braytə·ree, 'viebrətə·ree) vibrating or causing vibration; vibratile.

Vibrio ('vibrioh) a genus of gram-negative bacteria (family Spirillaceae).

V. cholerae the aetiological agent of classic (Asiatic) cholera in man.

vibrio ('vibrioh) an organism of the genus *Vibrio*, or other spiral motile organism.

cholera v. *Vibrio cholerae*.

vibriocidal (,vibrioh'sied'l) destructive to organisms of the genus *Vibrio*, especially *V. cholerae*.

vibrissa (vie'brisə) pl. *vibrissae* [L.] one of the hairs growing in the vestibule of the nose in man or about the nose (muzzle) of an animal.

vibrocardiogram (,viebroh'kahdioh,gram) the record produced by vibrocardiography.

vibrocardiography (,viebroh,kahdi'ografee) graphic recording of vibrations of the chest wall of relatively high frequency that are produced by the action of the heart.

vibrotherapeutics (,viebroh,therə'pyootiks) the therapeutic use of vibrating appliances.

Vic d'Azyr's bundle (,veek də'zeeəz) a band of fibres extending from the mamillary body to the anterior nucleus of the thalamus.

vicarious (vi'kairi·əs, vie-) 1. substituted for another; used when one organ functions instead of another. 2. occurring in circumstances where not normally expected.

Vicia ('visi·ə) a genus of herbs.

V. faba (V. fava) the fava or broad bean, whose beans or pollen contain a component capable of causing favism in susceptible persons.

vidarabine (vie'darə,been) a purine analogue, adenine arabinoside (ara-A), that inhibits DNA synthesis; used as an antiviral agent to treat herpes simplex keratitis and encephalitis.

videognosis (,vidiog'nohsis) diagnosis based on the interpretation of radiographs transmitted by television techniques to a radiological centre.

vigilambulism (,viji'lambyuh,lizəm) a state resembling somnambulism, but not occurring in sleep.

Villaret's syndrome ('vilə,rayz) unilateral paralysis of the glossopharyngeal, vagus, spinal accessory, and hypoglossal nerves and sometimes the facial nerve, due to a lesion in the retroparotid space.

villi ('vilie) [L.] plural of *villus*.

villoma (vi'lohmə) a papilloma, chiefly of the rectum.

villositis (,viloh'sietis) a bacterial disease with alterations in the villi of the placenta.

villosity (vi'lositee) 1. condition of being covered with villi. 2. a villus.

villouse (vi'looz) shaggy with soft hairs; covered with villi.

villus ('viləs) pl. *villi* [L.] a small vascular process or protrusion, as from the free surface of a membrane.

arachnoid villi microscopic projections of the arachnoid into some of the venous sinuses through which cerebrospinal fluid is reabsorbed.

chorionic villi threadlike projections originally occurring uniformly over the external surface of the chorion.

intestinal villi multitudinous threadlike projections covering the surface of the mucous membrane lining the small intestine, serving as the sites of absorption of fluids and nutrients.

synovial villi slender projections from the surface of the synovial membrane into the cavity of a joint; called also *haversian glands*.

villusectomy (,vilə'sektəmee) synovectomy; excision of a synovial villus.

vinblastine (vin'blasteen) a vinca alkaloid used as an antineoplastic in the treatment of Hodgkin's disease and testicular germinal cell cancer, usually in combination with other antineoplastic agents.

vinca alkaloids ('vingkə) a group of alkaloids, including vinblastine and vincristine, extracted from the periwinkle plant (*Vinca rosea)*, which arrest cell division in metaphase by disrupting the microtubules that form the spindle apparatus; used as antineoplastic agents.

Vincent's angina ('vinsənts) see under ANGINA.

Vincent's disease (gingivitis) trench mouth.

vincristine (vin'kristeen) a vinca alkaloid used as an antineoplastic in the treatment of acute leukaemias, Hodgkin's disease and non-Hodgkin's lymphomas, lymphosarcoma, rhabdomyosarcoma, neuroblastoma, and Wilms' tumour, usually in combination with other antineoplastic agents.

vinculum ('vingkyuhləm) pl. *vincula* [L.] a band or bandlike structure.

vincula tendinum filaments that connect the phalanges with the flexor tendons.

vinyl ('vien'l) the univalent group, CH_2CH, from vinyl alcohol.

violet ('vieələt) the reddish blue colour produced by the shortest rays of the visible spectrum.

crystal v., gentian v., methyl v. a dye derived from triphenylmethane, used as a topical anti-infective, stain, and internal anthelmintic; called also *methylrosaniline chloride*.

viper ('viepə) any venomous snake, especially any member of the families Viperidae (true vipers) and Crotalidae (pit vipers).

viraemia (vie'reemi·ə) the presence of viruses in the blood.

viral ('vierəl) pertaining to or caused by a virus.

Virales (vie'rayleez) the taxonomic order comprising the viruses.

Virchow's node ('fiəkohz) an enlarged supraclavicular lymph node; often the first sign of a malignant abdominal tumour. Called also sentinel, or signal, node.

virgin ('vərjin) a female or male who has not had coitus.

virile ('viriel) 1. peculiar to men or the male sex. 2. possessing masculine traits, especially copulative power.

virilescence (,viri'les'ns) the development of male secondary sexual characteristics in the female.

virilism ('viri,lizəm) the presence of male characteristics in the female. See also VIRILIZATION.

virility (vi'rilitee) possession of normal primary sexual characteristics in a male.

virilization (,virilie'zayshən) induction or development of male secondary sexual characteristics, especially the appearance of such changes in the female. Called also *masculinization*.

virion ('vieə·ri,on) the complete viral particle, found extracellullarly and capable of surviving in crystalline form and infecting a living cell; it comprises the nucleoid (genetic material) and the capsid.

virolactia (,vieroh'lakshi·ə) secretion of viruses in the milk.

virologist (vie'roləjist) microbiologist specializing in virology.

virology (vie'roləjee) the study of viruses and viral diseases.

Virormone ('vierormohn) trademark for preparations of testosterone, a male sex hormone.

virucidal (,vierə'sied'l) capable of neutralizing or destroying a virus.

virucide ('vierə,sied) an agent that neutralizes or destroys a virus.

virulence ('virələns) the degree of pathogenicity of a microorganism as indicated by case fatality rates and/or its ability to invade the tissues of the host; the competence of any infectious agent to produce pathological effects. adj. **virulent**.

viruliferous (,viryuh'lifə·rəs) conveying or producing a virus or other noxious agent.

viruria (vie'roo·ri·ə) the presence of viruses in the urine.

virus ('vierəs) any member of a unique class of infectious agents, which were originally distinguished by their smallness (hence, they were described as 'filtrable' because of their ability to pass through bacteria-retaining filters) and their inability to replicate outside of a living host cell; because these properties are shared by certain other microorganisms (rickettsiae, chlamydiae), viruses are now characterized by their simple organization and their unique mode of replication. A virus consists of genetic material, which may be either DNA or RNA, and is surrounded by a protein coat and, in some viruses, by a membranous envelope.

Unlike cellular organisms, viruses do not contain the biochemical mechanisms for their own replication; viruses replicate by using the biochemical mechanisms of a host cell to synthesize and assemble their separate components. When a complete virus particle (virion) comes in contact with a host cell, only the viral nucleic acid and, in some viruses, a few enzymes are injected into the host cell.

Within the host cell the genetic material of a DNA virus is replicated and transcribed into messenger RNA by host cell enzymes, and proteins coded for by viral genes are synthesized by host cell ribosomes. These are the proteins that form the capsid (protein coat); there may also be a few enzymes or regulatory proteins involved in assembling the capsid around newly synthesized viral nucleic acid, in controlling the biochemical mechanisms of the host cell, and in lysing the host cell when new virions have been assembled.

Because host cells do not have the ability to replicate RNA, RNA viruses must contain enzymes to produce genetic material for new virions. For certain viruses the RNA is replicated by a viral enzyme (transcriptase) contained in the virion, or produced by the host cell using the viral RNA as a messenger. In other viruses a reverse transcriptase contained in the virion transcribes the genetic message on the viral RNA into DNA, which is then replicated by the host cell.

In viruses that have membranes, membrane-bound viral proteins are synthesized by the host cell and move, like host cell membrane proteins, to the cell surface. When these proteins assemble to form the capsid, part of the host cell membrane is pinched off to form the envelope of the virion.

Some viruses have only a few genes coding for capsid proteins. Other more complex viruses may have a few hundred genes. But no virus has the thousands of genes required by even the simplest cells.

Some viruses do not produce rapid lysis of host cells. They remain latent for long periods in an infected host before the appearance of clinical symptoms. This carrier state can arise by several mechanisms. Most of the host cells may be protected from infection by immune mechanisms involving antibodies to the viral particles or interferon. Some enveloped RNA viruses can be produced in infected cells that grow and divide without being killed by the virus. This probably involves some sort of intracellular regulation of viral growth. It is also possible for the DNA of some viruses to be incorporated into the host cell DNA, producing a carrier state.

Viruses cause many diseases, including smallpox (variola), chickenpox (varicella), herpes zoster (shingles), herpes infections, measles (rubeola), German measles (rubella), mumps, infectious mononucleosis, hepatitis A and B, yellow fever, the common cold, influenza, certain types of pneumonia and croup and other respiratory infections, poliomyelitis, and several types of encephalitis. There is evidence that certain viruses may be capable of causing cancer.

Viruses do not produce toxins, but they are highly antigenic. Mechanisms of pathological injury include cell lysis, induction of cell proliferation (as in viral wart and molluscum contagiosum), the formation of giant cells or intracellular inclusion bodies caused by the virus, and symptoms caused by the host's immune response, such as inflammation or the deposition of antigen–antibody complexes in tissues. Because viral reproduction is almost completely carried out by host cell mechanisms, there are few points in the process where stopping viral reproduction will not also kill host cells. For this reason there are no chemotherapeutic agents for most viral diseases, but advances are being made. A number of agents are now available for the treatment of herpesviruses, principally nucleoside analogues such as acyclovir and idoxuridine. Cytomegalovirus infections can now also be treated and various drugs are being assessed against the AIDS virus. Another promising approach involves INTERFERONS—antiviral proteins produced naturally by cells and some of which can now be made commercially by genetic engineering. Some viral infections are preventable by vaccination (active immunization) or treated by passive immunization with immune globulin.

arbor v. arbovirus (*ar*thropod-*bor*ne).

attenuated v. one whose pathogenicity has been reduced by serial animal passage or other means.

bacterial v. one that is capable of producing transmissible lysis of bacteria (see also BACTERIOPHAGE).

Coxsackie v. coxsackievirus.

defective v. one that cannot be completely replicated or cannot form a protein coat; in some cases replication can proceed if missing gene functions are supplied by other viruses (see helper VIRUS).

Ebola v. an RNA virus almost identical to the Marburg virus but serologically distinct; it causes a disease similar to that caused by the Marburg virus.

ECHO v. echovirus (*e*nteric *c*ytopathogenic *h*uman *o*rphan).

EB v. Epstein-Barr virus.

encephalomyocarditis v. an enterovirus that causes mild aseptic meningitis and encephalomyocarditis.

enteric v. enterovirus.

enteric orphan v's orphan viruses isolated from the intestinal tract of man and other animals.

Epstein–Barr v. (EB v.; EBV) a herpes-like virus that causes infectious mononucleosis and is associated with Burkitt's lymphoma and nasopharyngeal carcinoma (see also EPSTEIN–BARR VIRUS).

filterable v., filtrable v. a pathogenic agent capable of passing through fine filters of diatomite or unglazed porcelain; ultravirus.

v. fixé, fixed v. rabies virus whose virulence and incubation period have been stabilized by serial passage and have remained fixed during further transmission; used for inoculating animals from which rabies vaccine is prepared.

HB_sAg v. a serum market for hepatitis B; initially called the Australia antigen and thought to be the causative agent, subsequently shown to be excess viral coat particles.

helper v. one that aids in the development of a defective virus by supplying or restoring the activity of the viral gene or enabling it to form a protein coat.

hepatitis A v. (HAV) a virus, 27 nm in diameter, that causes hepatitis A (infectious hepatitis), which is usually transmitted by the faecal–oral route.

hepatitis B v. (HBV) a double-shelled DNA virus, 42 nm in diameter, that causes hepatitis B (serum hepatitis), which can be transmitted parenterally, vertically (mother to infant), and nonparenterally by the faecal–oral route.

hepatitis C v. the aetiological agent of non-A, non-B viral hepatitis, a frequent cause of post-transfusion hepatitis similar to hepatitis B.

herpes v herpesvirus.

influenza v. any of a group of myxoviruses that causes influenza, including at least three serotypes (A, B, and C). Serotype A viruses are subject to major antigenic changes (antigenic shifts) as well as minor gradual antigenic changes (antigenic drift) and cause widespread epidemics and pandemics. Serotypes B and C are chiefly associated with sporadic epidemics. See also INFLUENZA.

Lassa v. see LASSA FEVER.

latent v. one that ordinarily occurs in a noninfective state and is demonstrable by indirect methods that activate it.

lytic v. one that is replicated in the host cell and causes death and lysis of the cell.

Marburg v. an RNA virus occurring in Africa, transmitted by insect bites, and causing Marburg disease.

masked v. latent virus.

orphan v's viruses isolated in tissue culture, but not found specifically associated with any disease.

parainfluenza v. one of a group of viruses isolated from patients with upper respiratory tract disease of varying severity.

pox v. poxvirus.

rabies v. an RNA virus of the rhabdovirus group that causes rabies.

respiratory syncytial v. a virus isolated from children with bronchopneumonia and bronchitis, characteristically causing syncytium formation in tissue culture.

slow v. any virus that remains latent for long periods in the infected host before the appearance of clinical symptoms.

street v. rabies virus from a naturally infected animal, as opposed to a laboratory-adapted strain of the virus.

vis (vis) pl. *vires* [L.] force, energy.

viscer(o)- word element. [L.] *viscera.*

viscera ('visə·rə) [L.] plural of *viscus.*

viscerad ('visə,rad) toward the viscera.

visceral ('visə·rəl) pertaining to a viscus.

visceralgia (,visə'ralji·ə) pain in any viscera.

visceroinhibitory (,visə·roh·in'hibitə·ree) inhibiting the essential movements of any viscus.

visceromegaly (,visə·roh'megəlee) splanchnomegaly.

visceromotor (,visə·roh'mohtə) concerned in the essential movements of the viscera.

visceroparietal (,visə·rohpə'rieət'l) indicating the relationship of a viscus to the abdominal wall.

visceroperitoneal (,visə·roh,peritə'neeəl) pertaining to the viscera and peritoneum.

visceropleural (,visə·roh'plooə·rəl) pertaining to the viscera and the pleura.

visceroptosis (,visə·rop'tohsis) splanchnoptosis; prolapse or downward displacement of the viscera.

viscerosensory (,visə·roh'sensə·ree) pertaining to sensation in the viscera.

visceroskeletal (,visə·roh'skelit'l) pertaining to the visceral skeleton.

viscerosomatic (,visə·rohsoh'matik) pertaining to the viscera and the body.

viscerotropic (,visə·roh'tropik) acting primarily on the viscera; having a predilection for the abdominal or thoracic viscera.

viscid ('visid) glutinous or sticky.

viscidity (vi'siditee) the property of being viscid.
viscosimeter (viskoh'simitə) an apparatus used in measuring viscosity of a substance.
viscosity (vi'skositee) resistance to flow; a physical property of a substance that is dependent on the friction of its component molecules as they slide by one another.
viscous ('viskəs) sticky or gummy; having a high degree of viscosity.
viscus ('viskəs) pl. *viscera* [L.] any large interior organ in any of the great body cavities, especially those in the abdomen.
vision ('vizhən) the faculty of seeing; sight. adj. **visual.** The basic components of vision are the eye itself, the visual centre in the brain, and the optic nerve, which connects the two.

How the Eye Works. The eye works like a camera. Light rays enter it through the adjustable iris and are focused by the lens onto the retina, a thin light-sensitive layer which corresponds to the film of the camera. The retina converts the light rays into nerve impulses, which are relayed to the visual centre. There the brain interprets them as images.

Like a camera lens, the lens of the eye reverses images as it focuses them. The images on the retina are upside down and they are 'flipped over' in the visual centre. In a psychology experiment, a number of volunteers wore glasses that inverted everything. After 8 days, their visual centres adjusted to this new situation, and when they took off the glasses, the world looked upside down until their brain centres re-adjusted. The retina is made up of millions of tiny nerve cells that contain specialized chemicals that are sensitive to light. There are two varieties of these nerve cells, rods and cones. Between them they cover the full range of the eye's adaptation to light. The cones are sensitive in bright light, and the rods in dim light. At twilight, as the light fades, the cones stop operating and the rods go into action. The momentary blindness experienced on going from bright to dim light, or from dim to bright, is the pause needed for the other set of nerve cells to take over.

The rods are spread toward the edges of the retina, so that vision in dim light is general but not very sharp or clear. The cones are clustered thickly in the centre of the retina, in the fovea centralis. When the eyes are turned and focused on the object to be seen the image is brought to the central area of the retina. In very dim light, on the other hand, an object is seen more clearly if it is not looked at directly because then its image falls on an area where the rods are thicker.

Colour Vision. Colour vision is a function of the cones. The most widely accepted theory of colour vision is that there are three types of cones, each type containing chemicals that respond to one of the three primary colours–red, green, and violet. White light stimulates all three sets of cones; any other colour stimulates only one or two sets. The brain can then interpret the impulses from these cones as various colours. Man's colour vision is amazingly delicate; a trained expert can distinguish among as many as 300,000 different hues.

colour blindness is the result of a disorder of one or more sets of cones. The great majority of people with some degree of colour blindness lack either red or green cones, and cannot distinguish between the two colours. True colour blindness, in which none of the sets of colour cones works, is very rare. Most colour blindness is inherited, and mostly by male children through their mothers from a colour-blind grandfather.

Stereoscopic Vision. Stereoscopic vision, or vision in depth, is caused by the way the eyes are placed. Each eye has a slightly different field of vision. The two images are superimposed on one another, but because of the distance between the eyes, the image from each eye goes slightly around its side of the object. From the differences between the images and from other indicators such as the position of the eye muscles when the eyes are focused on the object, the brain can determine the distance of the object.

Stereoscopic vision works best on nearby objects. As the distance increases, the difference between the left-eyed and the right-eyed views becomes less, and the brain must depend on other factors to determine distance. Among these are the relative size of the object, its colour and clearness, and the receding lines of perspective. These factors may fool the eye; for example, in clear mountain air distant objects may seem to be very close. This is because their sharpness and colour are not dulled by the atmosphere as much as they would be in more familiar settings.

Disorders of Vision. Imperfect vision is most commonly caused by abnormal shape of the eyeball. In the normal eye, the lens focuses the image on the retina. This is 6/6 vision. The figures refer to the distance at which a standard object can be recognized. A person who is nearsighted, for example, may only be able to recognize at 6 m an object that a person with perfect vision can recognize at 60 m. In this case he is said to have 6/60 vision. For the sake of convenience, eye charts with letters of different sizes are used rather than objects placed at different distances.

Nearsightedness, or myopia, is the result of an eyeball that is longer than usual from front to back, so that the image falls in front of the retina. The lens can bring nearby objects into focus, but not those farther away. Longsightedness, or hypermetropia, is caused by an eyeball that is shorter than normal, in which the image focuses behind the retina. astigmatism is impaired vision caused by irregularities in the curvature of the cornea or lens. All of these conditions can usually be corrected with prescription lenses.

achromatic v. vision characterized by lack of colour vision.
binocular v. the use of both eyes together, without diplopia.
central v. that produced by stimulation of receptors in the fovea centralis.
day v. visual perception in the daylight or under conditions of bright illumination.
dichromatic v. that in which colour perception is restricted to a pair of primaries, either blue and yellow or (rarely) red and green.
double v. diplopia.
indirect v. peripheral vision.
low v. impairment of vision such that there is significant visual handicap but also significant usable residual vision; such impairment may involve visual acuity, visual fields, or ocular motility.
monocular v. vision with one eye.
multiple v. polyopia.
night v. visual perception in the darkness of night or under conditions of reduced illumination.
oscillating v. oscillopsia.
peripheral v. that produced by stimulation of receptors in the retina outside the macula lutea.
tunnel v. a condition of concentric reduction in the visual field, as though the subject were looking through a long tunnel or tube.
visual analogue scale ('vizhyooəl 'anəlog) a method of quantifying subjective feelings such as pain, sedation, etc. Consists of a line exactly 10 centimetres long with the extremes of the parameter being considered

at each end, for instance, absence of pain and the worst pain imaginable. The patient or volunteer marks a point along the line which represents the pain or other sensation he is feeling at that moment. The number of centimetres the marked point is from the left-hand end of the line represents a numerical assessment of the pain or other sensation.

visualization (ˌvizhyooəlie'zayshən) the act of viewing or of achieving a complete visual impression of an object.

visuoauditory (ˌvizhyoo·oh'awditə·ree) pertaining to sight and hearing.

visuognosis (ˌvizhyoo·og'nohsis) recognition and interpretation of visual impressions.

visuolexic (ˌvizhyoo·oh'leksik) pertaining to the visual aspects of language, as in perception of written language.

visuopsychic (ˌvizhyoo·oh'siekik) visual and psychic; applied to the area of the cerebral cortex concerned in judgement of visual sensation.

visuosensory (ˌvizhyoo·oh'sensə·ree) pertaining to perception of visual impressions.

visuospatial (ˌvizhyoo·oh'spayshəl) pertaining to visual perception of spatial relationships.

vita glass ('vietə ˌglahs) quartz glass which is capable of transmitting ultraviolet rays of light.

vital ('viet'l) pertaining to life; necessary to life.

v. capacity the greatest volume of gas that, following maximum inspiration, can be expelled during a complete, slow, unforced expiratory manoeuvre; equal to inspiratory capacity plus expiratory reserve volume.

Forced vital capacity (FVC) is the greatest volume of air that can be expelled when a person performs a rapid, forced expiratory manoeuvre. This usually takes a total of about five seconds. The greatest volume of air a person can exhale during one, two, three, or more seconds of forced expiration is called the forced expiratory volume (FEV). A subscript is added to the abbreviation FEV to indicate the time during which the particular amount or volume of air is exhaled. A volume exhaled during the first second is designated $FEV_{1.0}$, a volume exhaled during the first two seconds is designated as $FEV_{2.0}$, and so on. The rate at which a specified volume of air is exhaled during a forced expiratory movement is called forced expiratory flow (FEF). The rate at which air is exhaled from an FEV of 200 ml to an FEV of 1200 ml is designated $FEF_{200-1200}$ (formerly called maximal expiratory flow rate, MEFR); the rate from 25 to 75 per cent of the FVC is designated $FEF_{25-75\%}$ (formerly called maximal midexpiratory flow rate, MMFR).

Laboratory values for vital capacity, FVC, FEV, and FEF are usually reported both as absolute values and as statistically derived predicted values based on the age, sex, and height of a patient. The statistical value is reported as a percentage. See also PULMONARY FUNCTION TESTS.

v. signs the signs of life, namely pulse, respiration, and temperature.

v. statistics that branch of biometry dealing with the data and laws of human mortality, morbidity, births, marriages and divorce. Statistics are expressed as percentages, ratios and rates.

vitamer ('vietəmə) a substance or compound that has vitamin activity.

vitamin ('vitəmin) an organic substance found in foods and essential in small quantities for growth, health, and the preservation of life itself. The body needs vitamins just as it requires other food constituents such as proteins, fats, carbohydrates, minerals, and water. The absence of one or more vitamins from the diet, or poor absorption of vitamins, can cause deficiency diseases such as rickets, scurvy, and beriberi.

Vitamins serve as coenzymes or cofactors in enzymatic reactions. They are required only in trace quantities because they are not consumed in the reactions.

The major vitamins are designated by the letters A, C, D, E, and K, and the term B complex. The B vitamins and vitamin C are water-soluble. The rest are fat soluble and are not absorbed unless the body's digestion and absorption of fats is normal. Deficiencies of the fat-soluble vitamins can be produced by various malabsorption syndromes.

VITAMIN A. Vitamin A helps to maintain epithelial tissues which cover the body and line certain internal organs. This vitamin also is essential for the proper growth of skeletal and soft tissues, and for synthesizing rhodopsin, a light-sensitive pigment in the eye that makes night vision possible. The particular manifestation of vitamin A deficiency depends upon the age of the patient. Among the commonest symptoms of vitamin A deficiency is night blindness. The skin may also be affected, becoming dry and pimply like a toad's skin.

Vitamin A occurs in nature in two forms: retinol (vitamin A_1) and dehydroretinol (vitamin A_2). It is manufactured by animals and man from carotenes found in green leafy and yellow vegetables, including kale, broccoli, spinach, carrots, marrow, and sweet potatoes. It is obtained directly by eating animal products such as liver, eggs, whole milk, cream, and cheese.

A toxic syndrome (hypervitaminosis A) can result from excessive vitamin intake. It is marked by generalized pruritus, desquamation of the skin, loss of hair, and hyperostoses.

THE B COMPLEX. The original 'vitamin B' was found to be a group of vitamins, each differing chemically and each individually important in the body. For convenience, these vitamins are referred to as one group since they are often found together in foods. Deficiency in only one of these vitamins is rare, and the deficiency disease attributed to lack of one vitamin B usually is complicated by deficiencies of the others as well.

Vitamin B_1 (Thiamine). This vitamin is necessary to break down and release energy from carbohydrates. Lack of thiamine can cause loss of appetite, certain types of neuritis, and, in severe cases, BERIBERI, which affects the brain, heart, and nerves.

The best sources of thiamine are yeasts, ham, and certain pork cuts, liver, peanuts, whole and fortified cereals, and milk. The vitamin is easily destroyed by cooking and may also be lost by dissolving in the cooking water. Because the body does not store thiamine well, foods that are good sources of it should be included in each day's diet.

Vitamin B_2 (Riboflavin). This vitamin functions as a coenzyme concerned with oxidative processes. There is a widespread incidence of riboflavin deficiency (ariboflavinosis) which may occur for a long time but only cause relatively few problems. The symptoms include open sores at the corners of the mouth and on the lips, a purple-red, inflamed tongue, seborrhoeic dermatitis, and corneal and other eye changes.

The main food sources of riboflavin are milk, liver, kidney, heart, green vegetables, dried yeasts, and enriched cereals. It is not usually affected by cooking, but is destroyed by light.

Niacin (Nicotinic Acid). This vitamin B appears to act in enzyme systems to utilize carbohydrates, fats, and amino acids. Niacin deficiency causes PELLAGRA. Symptoms of pellagra involve the skin and digestive

Sources and characteristics of major vitamins

Vitamin	Major sources	Functions	Effect of deficiency	Chemical and physiological characteristics	Recommended daily adult allowance
Vitamin A (retinol)	Dairy fats, fish oil, egg yolk, liver	Formation of rhodopsin – required for visual acuity in poor light Essential for normal growth and reproduction	Night blindness; keratinization of mucous membranes	Insoluble in water; fat-soluble; stable in cooking	750 μg retinol equivalent
Carotene	Carrots, pumpkin, spinach, broccoli, apricots, yellow peaches	As vitamin A	As vitamin A	Water-soluble; converted to vitamin A in the body; stable in cooking	5000 IU
Thiamine (vitamin B_1)	Milk, meats, particularly organ meat, wholegrain products, green leafy vegetables	Coenzyme in carbohydrate metabolism	Beri-beri in severe cases; in moderate deficiency cases loss of appetite and weight, emotional and psychological symptoms	Water-soluble; destroyed by heat in alkaline medium, heat-stable in acid medium	1.3 mg (approx. 0.5 mg per 4200 kJ)
Riboflavin	Milk, meats, particularly organ meat, wholegrain cereals, green leafy vegetables	Essential for normal cell growth and development	Cheilosis (cracks at the corners of the mouth), burning eyes and affected vision	Slightly soluble in water, unstable in light	1.6 mg (approx. 0.6 mg per 4200 kJ)
Niacin	Wholegrain cereals, lean meat, poultry, fish and organ meats, green vegetables	Active compound of enzyme systems involved with energy production	Pellagra. Early symptoms: loss of appetite and weight, weakness	Slightly soluble in water; unaffected by external factors such as light, alkali, acid, etc.	18 mg nicotinic acid equivalent

Vitamin B_{12}	Liver and kidneys, meat, milk	Participates in production of nucleic acid, necessary for haemopoiesis	Pernicious anaemia; long-term deficiency results in subacute degeneration of the spinal cord	Absorption dependent on Castle's intrinsic factor. Heat-stable; adversely affected by light, alkalis and strongly acid media	3 μg
Folic acid	Dark green vegetables, liver and kidneys, yeast	As vitamin B_{12}	Megaloblastic anaemia	Fairly stable in water; unstable in light and strongly acid media	300 μg
Ascorbic acid (vitamin C)	Citrus fruits, tomatoes, potatoes, strawberries	Maintains intercellular substances; assists in iron absorption	Scurvy, evidenced by bleeding gums, subcutaneous bleeding, corkscrew hair follicles	Water-soluble; adversely affected by light, heat, air, alkalis; minimal reserves retained in body	30 mg
Vitamin D	Sunlight, fish-liver oil, fortified milk, margarine	Necessary for efficient calcium metabolism and deposition, thus essential for development of bones and teeth	Rickets: soft, fragile bones, skeletal deformities, retarded growth. Osteomalacia in adults; dental caries; tetany	Ultraviolet light synthesizes the vitamin in the skin; fat-soluble; stable in air and heat	0–10 μg 400 IU
Vitamin E (tocopherols)	Oils of vegetable origin (e.g. sunflower seed oil, nut oils), peas, beans, leafy vegetables, wheatgerm	Counteracts oxidation of certain essential components (e.g. vitamin A) in the body, needed for cell respiration	Not seen in humans under normal conditions	Fat-soluble; antioxidant of oil; protects red blood cells against haemolysis	15 IU
Vitamin K	Green leafy vegetables	Essential for blood clotting	Haemorrhagic disease of the newborn; increased tendency to bleed	Fat and water-soluble; can be synthesized in gut; heat-stable	Dietary deficiency unlikely

From Huskisson, J. (1985) *Applied Nutrition and Dietetics*, 2nd edn. Baillière Tindall, pp. 24–25.

and nervous systems. The vitamin also has vasodilating activity.

Food sources of niacin are various high-protein foods such as liver, yeast, bran, peanuts, lean meats, fish, and poultry.

Vitamin B_{12}. This vitamin contains a metal, cobalt. It is called also *cyanocobalamin* and *extrinsic factor*, and is needed for the efficient production of blood cells and for the health of the nervous system. Only small amounts of B_{12} are required by the body. The activity of this vitamin is associated with that of another B vitamin, folic acid.

Inability to absorb vitamin B_{12} occurs in PERNICIOUS ANAEMIA, in which a substance normally secreted by the stomach, called intrinsic factor, is missing. Intrinsic factor is needed to absorb vitamin B_{12} in the small intestine. Injections of vitamin B_{12} can control pernicious anaemia. Poor absorption of vitamin B_{12} also occurs in sprue.

Vitamin B_{12} is not found in plant foods. The main sources in the human diet are animal products such as milk, eggs, and liver. Probably the ultimate source of B_{12} is bacterial production in animal intestines. This production occurs in man, and in normal persons probably meets some or perhaps all of the body's requirements.

Other B Vitamins. These include vitamin B_6 (pyridoxine), biotin, folic acid, pantothenic acid, choline, inositol, and para-aminobenzoic acid. Vitamin B_6 deficiency can cause convulsions, lethargy, mental changes and handicap, inflammation of the skin, and anaemia.

These vitamins, like most other members of the B complex, are widely found in fruits, vegetables, meat, and whole-grain cereals.

VITAMIN C (ASCORBIC ACID). This vitamin is necessary for the health of supporting tissues such as bone, cartilage, and connective tissue (see also ASCORBIC ACID). Deficiency produces SCURVY.

Vitamin C is found in fresh fruits and vegetables, including citrus fruits, tomatoes, brussels sprouts, and to some extent whole potatoes. Cooking and storage destroys much of the vitamin C content of foods.

VITAMIN D. The action of sunlight on the skin changes certain substances in the body into vitamin D, a term for any of several active substances required for the utilization of calcium and phosphorus, essential for the growth and maintenance of bone, including cholecalciferol and ergocalciferol (know collectively as calciferol). Vitamin D deficiency causes RICKETS in children and OSTEOMALACIA and OSTEOPOROSIS in adults. Rickets is usually caused either by a diet deficient in vitamin D or by insufficient exposure to sunlight.

Few foods contain vitamin D. The only rich natural sources are fish liver oil and the livers of animals feeding on fish. For this reason vitamin D is added to margarines in the UK.

A toxic syndrome (hypervitaminosis D) can result from excessive vitamin intake. It results in hypercalcaemia with its typical symptoms of weakness, fatigue, loss of weight, and impairment of renal function.

VITAMIN E. The role of this vitamin in human nutrition is uncertain. It is necessary in the diet of many species for normal reproduction, normal muscular development, normal resistance of erythrocytes to haemolysis, and various other biochemical functions; chemically, it is α-tocopherol, found in wheat germ oil, cereals, egg yolk, and beef liver, or produced synthetically.

VITAMIN K. Any of a group of vitamins including vitamin K_1 (phytonadione) and vitamin K_2 (menaquinone) found in alfalfa, spinach, cabbage, putrefied fish meal, and hempseed.

Generally, the bacteria of the intestine produce vitamin K in quantities that are adequate (provided it can be absorbed), except in newborn infants, in whom the deficiency is most frequently found.

Vitamin K is needed for the γ-carboxylation of the inert precursor protein of prothrombin and the other vitamin-K-dependent coagulation factors, enabling them to bind calcium and promote clotting. Deficiency of vitamin K is seen in malabsorption, obstructive jaundice, and in newborn infants, and may lead to a haemorrhagic disorder.

VITAMIN SUPPLEMENTS. The exact vitamin requirements for good health often are not known with accuracy; they vary with age, weight, sex, and state of health. The need for certain vitamins increases with fever, some diseases, heavy exercise, pregnancy, and lactation.

If a person eats an adequate, varied diet of meats, fish, vegetables, and dairy products, he will receive enough vitamins to meet his usual requirements. Public health measures such as the addition of vitamin D to milk and the B vitamins to bread and other cereal products have helped to combat deficiency diseases.

The use of vitamin supplements is expensive and in general unnecessary. Specialists in nutrition advise against taking supplementary vitamins unless they are prescribed for a specific reason by a doctor. Vitamins should not be used as 'tonics'. There is a distinct possibility that the indiscriminate use of vitamin preparations may sometimes lead to overdosage, a problem that has arisen in recent years. For example, overdoses of vitamins D, A, or K may result in serious disease, the excess vitamins acting like poisons. Also, tests suggest that large doses of vitamin D taken by a woman during pregnancy may have undesirable effects on her unborn child. Though these tests are not conclusive, they confirm the need for caution in the use of vitamins.

Vitamins are commonly prescribed in infancy and childhood, during pregnancy and breast feeding, for elderly patients whose dietary habits are poor, and in clearly diagnosed deficiency states. These include not only the more familiar deficiency diseases already described but also alcoholism and chronic wasting diseases..

vitellin (vie'telin) the chief protein of egg yolk.

vitelline (vi'telien) resembling or pertaining to the yolk of an egg or ovum.

vitellus (vie'teləs) the yolk of an egg.

vitiligines (,viti'liji,neez) depigmented areas of the skin.

vitiligo (,viti'liegoh) a condition in which destruction of melanocytes in small or large circumscribed areas results in patches of depigmentation often having a hyperpigmented border, and often enlarging slowly. adj. **vitiliginous**.

vitrectomy (vi'trektəmee) surgical removal of a diseased vitreous of the eye. Vitreous is removed with a specially designed infusion cutter which delivers a physiological solution (e.g., Ringer's solution) to maintain intraocular pressure, and withdraws the diseased vitreous by suction and cutting.

Vitrectomies may be performed for the treatment of advanced diabetic RETINOPATHY in order to prevent blindness. The procedure also is indicated in the treatment of vitreous haemorrhage and retinal detachment due to other causes, such as penetrating injuries to the eye, central vein occlusion, and some forms of retinal detachments.

vitreodentine (,vitrioh'denteen) an unusually hard and glasslike form of dentine.

vitreous ('vitri·əs) 1. glasslike or hyaline. 2. the vitreous

body.
v. body the transparent gel filling the inner part of the eyeball between the lens and retina.
v. humour 1. vitreous body. 2. the watery substance contained within the interstices of the stroma in the vitreous body.
persistent hyperplastic v. a congenital anomaly, usually unilateral, due to persistence of embryonic remnants of the fibromuscular tunic of the eye and part of the hyaloid vascular system. Clinically, there is a white pupil, elongated ciliary processes, and often microphthalmia; the lens, although clear initially, may become completely opaque.
vitropression (,vitroh'preshən) exertion of pressure on the skin with a slip of glass, forcing blood from the area.
vitrum ('vitrəm) [L.] *glass.*
vivi- word element. [L.] *alive, life.*
vividialysis (,vividie'aləsis) dialysis through a living membrane (see also PERITONEAL DIALYSIS).
vividiffusion (,vividi'fyoozhən) circulation of the blood through a closed apparatus in which it is passed through a membrane for removal of substances ordinarily removed by the kidneys (see also HAEMODIALYSER).
vivification (,vivifi'kayshən) conversion of lifeless into living protein matter by assimilation.
viviparous (vi'vipə·rəs) giving birth to living young which develop within the maternal body.
vivisection (,vivi'sekshən) surgical procedures performed upon a living animal for purpose of physiological or pathological investigation.
vivisectionist (,vivi'sekshənist) one who practices or defends vivisection.
VLDL very low-density lipoproteins.
VMA vanillylmandelic acid.
vocal ('vohk'l) pertaining to the voice.
v. cords the folds of mucous membrane in the LARYNX, the superior pair being called the false, and the inferior pair the true, vocal cords. These thin, reedlike bands vibrate to make vocal sounds during speaking, and are capable of producing a vast range of sounds.

One end of each cord is attached to the front wall of the larynx. These ends are close together. The opposite ends are connected to two tiny cartilages near the back wall of the larynx. The cartilages can be rotated so as to swing the cords far apart or bring them together. When the cords are apart, the breath passes through silently, unobstructed. When they are closer together, the cords partly obstruct the air passage, and as the air is forced through them, the cords vibrate like the reeds of a pipe organ, producing sound waves. These waves are what we call the voice. See also SPEECH.

Various disorders may affect the larynx and vocal cords. LARYNGITIS may be acute or chronic and is usually caused by continual irritation of the vocal cords by overuse or by inhaled irritants such as tobacco smoke. The voice may be 'lost' and then regained after a few days of rest and medication, if the cause has been removed. Prolonged or repeated impairment of the voice requires medical diagnosis.

Partial or total removal of the larynx, usually is performed as treatment for cancer of the larynx. See also LARYNGECTOMY.
voice (voys) the sound produced by the SPEECH organs and uttered by the mouth.
void (voyd) to cast out as waste matter, especially the urine.
vol. volume.
vola ('vohlə) a concave or hollow surface.
v. manus the palm.
v. pedis the sole.
volar ('vohlə) pertaining to the sole or palm; indicating the flexor surface of the forearm, wrist, or hand.
volaris (voh'lair·ris) palmar.
volatile ('volə,tiel) evaporating rapidly.
volatilization (vo,latilie'zayshən) conversion into a vapour or gas without chemical change.
volition (ve'lishən) the act or power of willing. adj. **volitional.**
Volkmann's canals ('vohlkmənz) canals communicating with haversian canals, for passage of blood vessels through bone.
Volkmann's contracture contraction of the fingers and sometimes of the wrist or of analogous parts of the foot, with loss of power, after severe injury or improper use of a tourniquet or cast.
Volkmann's disease congenital deformity of the foot due to tibiotarsal dislocation.
Volkmann's paralysis ischaemic paralysis.
volley ('volee) a rhythmical succession of muscular twitches artificially induced; the aggregate of nerve impulses set up by a single stimulus.
volsella (vol'selə) a forceps with clawlike hooks at the end of each blade. Called also *vulsella, vulsellum.*
volt (vohlt) the unit of electromotive force; 1 ampere of current against 1 ohm of resistance.
electron v. (eV) a unit of energy equal to the energy acquired by an electron in being accelerated through a potential difference of 1 volt; equal to 1.602×10^{-19} joule.
voltage ('vohltij) electromotive force measured in volts.
Voltarol ('voltərol) trademark for preparations of diclofenac, a nonsteroidal anti-inflammatory drug used in arthritic conditions.
voltmeter ('vohlt,meetə) an instrument for measuring electromotive force in volts.
volume ('volyoom) the space occupied by a substance or a three-dimensional region; the capacity of such a region or of a container.
closing v. (CV) the volume of gas in the lungs in excess of the residual volume at the time when small airways in the dependent portions close during maximal exhalation (see also CLOSING VOLUME).
forced expiratory v. (FEV) the volume that can be exhaled from full inspiration exhaling as forcefully and rapidly as possible for a timed period. $FEV_{0.5}$, $FEV_{1.0}$, $FEV_{2.0}$, $FEV_{3.0}$, denote the FEV for 0.5, 1, 2, and 3 seconds.
expiratory reserve v. the maximal amount of gas that can be expired from the end-expiratory level.
inspiratory reserve v. the maximal amount of gas that can be inspired from the end-inspiratory position.
minute v. the volume of air expelled from the lungs per minute.
packed-cell v. the volume of packed red cells in millilitres per 100 ml of centrifuged blood; abbreviated PCV.
residual v. the amount of gas remaining in the lung at the end of a maximal expiration.
stroke v. the quantity of blood ejected from a ventricle at each beat of the heart.
tidal v. the amount of gas passing into and out of the lungs in each respiratory cycle.
volumetric (,volyuh'metrik) pertaining to or accompanied by measurement in volumes.
voluntary ('volantə·ree) accomplished in accordance with the will.
volute ('volyoot, və'lyoot) rolled up.
volvulosis (,volvyuh'lohsis) onchocerciasis due to *Onchocerca volvulus.*
volvulus ('volvyuhləs) [L.] torsion of a loop of intestine, causing obstruction with or without strangulation.

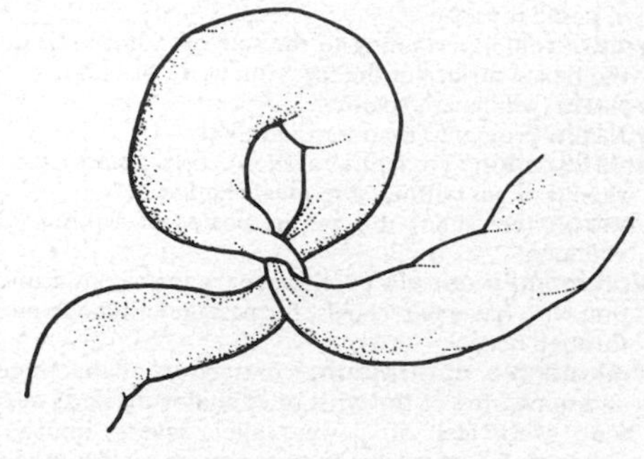

Volvulus

vomer ('vohmə) a bone forming part of the nasal septum. adj. **vomerine**.

vomica ('vomikə) pl. *vomicae* [L.] 1. the profuse and sudden expectoration of pus and putrescent matter. 2. an abnormal cavity in an organ, especially in the lung, caused by suppuration and the breaking down of tissue.

vomit ('vomit) 1. matter expelled from the stomach by the mouth. 2. to eject stomach contents through the mouth.

black v. vomit consisting of blood which has been acted upon by the gastric juice, seen in yellow fever and other conditions in which blood collects in the stomach.

coffee-ground v. dark granular material ejected from the stomach, produced by mixture of blood with gastric contents; it is a sign of bleeding in the upper alimentary canal.

vomiting ('vomiting) forcible ejection of contents of stomach through the mouth.

cyclic v. recurring attacks of vomiting. **dry v.** attempts at vomiting, with the ejection of nothing but gas.

pernicious v. vomiting in pregnancy so severe as to threaten life.

v. of pregnancy vomiting occurring in pregnancy, especially early morning vomiting (see also MORNING SICKNESS).

projectile v. vomiting with the material ejected with great force; seen commonly in congenital pyloric stenosis.

stercoraceous v. vomiting of faecal matter.

vomitory ('vomitə·ree) an emetic.

vomiturition (ˌvomityuh'rishən) repeated ineffectual attempts to vomit; retching.

vomitus ('vomitəs) 1. vomiting. 2. matter vomited.

von Gierke's disease (von 'giəkəz) glycogenosis (type I) (see also GIERKE'S DISEASE).

von Hippel's disease (von 'hip'lz) angiomatosis confined chiefly to the retina.

von Hippel–Lindau disease (von ˌhip'l'lindow) Lindau–von Hippel disease.

von Jaksch's disease (von 'yaksh) anaemia pseudoleukaemia infantum.

von Recklinghausen's disease (von 'rekling-ˌhowzənz) 1. neurofibromatosis. 2. see OSTEITIS FIBROSA CYSTICA.

von Willebrand's disease (von 'viliˌbrants) a congenital haemorrhagic diathesis, inherited as an autosomal dominant trait (rarely recessive), characterized by a prolonged bleeding time, deficiency of coagulation factor VIII, and often impairment of platelet adhesion, and associated with epistaxis and increased bleeding after trauma or surgery, menorrhagia, and postpartum bleeding. Called also *angiohaemophilla and pseudohaemophilia.*

vortex ('vawteks) pl. *vortices* [L.] a whorled or spiral arrangement or pattern, as of muscle fibres, or of the ridges or hairs of the skin.

vox (voks) [L.] *voice.*

v. cholerica the peculiar suppressed voice of true cholera.

voxel ('voksel) a volume element; the region in a tissue slice that corresponds to a *pixel* (picture element) in an image. See also computed TOMOGRAPHY.

voyeurism ('vwieəˌrizəm) a form of sexual aberration in which gratification is derived from looking at sexual objects or acts.

VR vocal resonance.

VS volumetric solution.

v.s. vibration seconds (the unit of measurement of sound waves).

vulgaris (vul'gair·ris) [L.] *ordinary, common.*

vulnerability (ˌvulnə·rə'bilitee) weakness; susceptibility to injury or infection.

vulnerary ('vulnə·rə·ree) 1. pertaining to wounds or the healing of wounds. 2. an agent that promotes the healing of wounds.

vulnus ('vulnəs) pl. *vulnera* [L.] a wound.

vulva ('vulvə) the external genital organs in the female. adj. **vulval, vulvar**.

Two pairs of skin folds protect the vaginal opening, one on each side. The larger outer folds are the labia majora, and the more delicate inner folds are the labia minora. In a virgin, a thin membrane, the hymen, usually partially covers the opening of the vagina. Normally, the hymen is well perforated, to permit the menstrual flow. Occasionally it is not, and a minor surgical procedure may be necessary.

The upper or forward ends of the labia minora join around the clitoris, a small projection that is composed of erectile tissue like the male penis and has erotic functions. The opening of the urethra, which empties urine from the bladder, lies between the clitoris and the vagina. See also female REPRODUCTIVE ORGANS.

vulvectomy (vul'vektəmee) excision of the vulva.

vulvismus (vul'vizməs) vaginismus.

vulvitis (vul'vietis) inflammation of the vulva.

vulvocrural (ˌvulvoh'krooə·rəl) pertaining to the vulva and thigh.

vulvouterine (ˌvulvoh'yootəˌrien) pertaining to the vulva and uterus.

vulvovaginal (ˌvulvohvə'jien'l, -'vajin'l) pertaining to the vulva and vagina.

vulvovaginitis (ˌvulvohˌvaji'nietis) inflammation of the vulva and vagina.

vv. [L.] *venae* (veins).

v/v volume (of solute) per volume (of solvent).

vyprinium an anthelmintic used for intestinal pinworms in the form of the embonate salt.

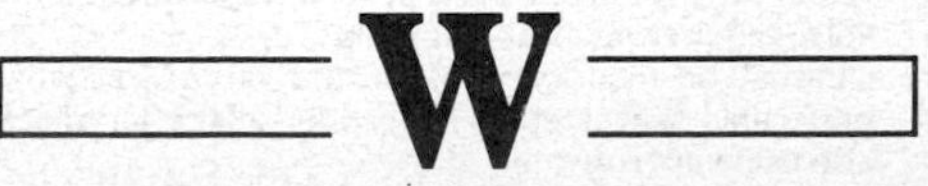

W

W chemical symbol, *tungsten* (Ger. *wolfram*); symbol for *watt*.

Waardenburg's syndrome ('vahdənbərgz) a hereditary disorder, transmitted as an autosomal dominant trait, characterized by wide bridge of the nose due to lateral displacement of the inner canthi and puncta;

pigmentary disturbances, including white forelock, heterochromia iridis, white eyelashes, and leukoderma; and sometimes cochlear deafness.

wafer ('wayfə) a thin double layer of flour paste sometimes used to enclose a dose of medicinal powder. A cachet.

waist (wayst) the portion of the body between the thorax and the hips.

Waldenström's disease ('valdən,strərmz) osteochondrosis of the capitular femoral epiphysis.

Waldenström's macroglobulinaemia a malignant lymphoma of B-cell lymphocytes with plasmacytoid features. There is always a monoclonal increase in IgM which can be marked, giving rise to the hyperviscosity syndrome. Hepatosplenomegaly and lymphadenopathy are often present; bone lesions are unusual. Treatment is of the underlying lymphoma: plasmapheresis may be necessary.

Waldeyer's glands ('valdieəz) glands in the attached edge of the eyelid.

Waldeyer's ring ('valdieəz) the circle of lymphoid tissue in the pharynx formed by the lingual, faucial, and pharyngeal tonsils.

wall (wawl) a structure bounding or limiting a space or a definitive mass of material.

cell w. a rigid structure that lies just outside of and is joined to the plasma membrane of plant cells and most prokaryotic cells, which protects the cell and maintains its shape.

wallerian degeneration (wə'liə·ri·ən) fatty degeneration of a nerve fibre that has been severed from its nutritive source.

Walthard's rests ('valtahts) microscopic inclusions of the ovarian germinal epithelium into the wall of the uterine tube or hilum of the ovary, which have been implicated in the development of Brenner tumours.

Walther's ganglion ('valtəz) glomus coccygeum.

Wangensteen tube ('wangen,steen) a small nasogastric tube connected with a special suction apparatus to maintain gastric and duodenal decompression.

warfarin ('wawfə·rin) an ANTICOAGULANT, usually used as the sodium salt.

wart (wawt) an epidermal tumour of viral origin; the term is also applied loosely to any of various benign, wartlike epidermal proliferations of nonviral origin. Called also verruca. Warts are generally more common among children and young adults than among older persons. Most warts are less than 5 mm in diameter; they may be flat or raised, dry or moist. Usually they have a rough and pitted surface, either flesh-coloured or darker than the surrounding skin.

Warts develop usually on the exposed parts of the fingers and hands, but also on the elbows, face, scalp, and other areas. When on especially vulnerable parts of the body, such as the knee or elbow, they are subject to irritation and may become quite tender. PLANTAR WARTS, which occur on the soles of the feet, become very sensitive because of pressure. Anal warts cause itching. Warts can also block a nostril or an external acoustic meatus.

A wart develops between 1 and 8 months after the virus becomes lodged in the skin. The virus is often spread by scratching, rubbing, and slight razor cuts. In more than half the cases, warts disappear without treatment, but some remain for years.

TREATMENT. Many popular 'cures' for warts have been suggested, but are generally useless. Furthermore, self-treatment by cutting, scraping, or using acids or patent medicines, may cause bacterial infection, scarring, and other harm—without eliminating the warts.

A troublesome wart should be removed only by a doctor or dermatologist, who may use acid podophyllin, curettage and cautery freezing liquid nitrogen, or carbon dioxide snow for the purpose. Warts are notoriously stubborn. Often the virus remains in the skin, and the wart grows again.

It is generally advised that warts on children be removed early. Otherwise they tend to be spread by the child's scratching and other activities. The tendency of warts to spread is less evident in adults.

genital w's sexually transmitted venereal papillomatous lesions caused by the human papillomavirus. The incubation period is one to three months. The growths are pinkish or flesh-coloured and occur around the cervix, vulva, perineum, anus and anal canal, urethra, and glans penis.

Genital warts (*condylomata acuminata*) are treated with weekly applications of podophyllin, 10 to 25 per cent in tincture of benzoin. Especially resistant and extensive involvement may require electrocautery and cryosurgery.

wash (wosh) a solution used for cleansing or bathing a part, as an eye or the mouth.

Wassermann test (reaction) ('vasəmən) a complement-fixation test used in the diagnosis of syphilis.

waste (wayst) 1. gradual loss, decay, or diminution of bulk. 2. useless and effete material, unfit for further use within the organism. 3. to pine away or dwindle.

water ('wawtə) 1. a clear, colourless, odourless, tasteless liquid, H_2O. 2. an aqueous solution of a medicinal substance.

distilled w. water that has been purified by distillation.

water brash ('wawtə ,brash) heartburn with regurgitation of sour fluid or almost tasteless saliva into the mouth.

Waterhouse–Friderichsen syndrome (,wawtəhows'freedriksən) the malignant or fulminating form of meningococcal MENINGITIS, which is marked by sudden onset and short course, fever, coma, collapse, cyanosis, haemorrhages from the skin and mucous membranes, and bilateral adrenal haemorrhage.

waters ('wawtəz) popular name for amniotic fluid.

Waterston's operation ('wawtəstənz) anastomosis of the right pulmonary artery to the ascending aorta to relieve tricuspid atresia in the young child.

Watson–Crick helix (,wotsən 'krik) double helix; a representation of the structure of DEOXYRIBONUCLEIC ACID (DNA), consisting of two coiled chains, each of which contains information completely specifying the other chain.

watt (wot) a unit of power, being the work done at the rate of 1 joule per second. Electrically, it is equivalent to 1 ampere under pressure of 1 volt. Abbreviated W.

wattage ('wotij) the output or consumption of an electric device expressed in watts.

wattmeter ('wot,meetə) an instrument for measuring wattage.

wave (wayv) a uniformly advancing disturbance in which the parts undergo a double oscillation, as a progressing disturbance on the surface of a liquid or the rhythmic variation occurring in the transmission of electromagnetic energy.

alpha w's electroencephalographic waves having a frequency of 8 to 13 per second, typical of a normal person awake in a quiet resting state. They occur primarily in the occipital region. See also ELECTROENCEPHALOGRAPHY.

beta w's waves in the electroencephalogram having a frequency of 18 to 30 per second, typical during periods of intense central nervous system activity. They occur primarily in the parietal and frontal regions.

brain w's changes in electric potential of different areas of the brain, as recorded by electroencephalography.

delta w's 1. electroencephalographic waves having a frequency below 3.5 per second, typical in deep sleep, in infancy, and in serious brain disorders. See also ELECTROENCEPHALOGRAPHY. 2. an early QRS vector in the electrocardium in Wolff–Parkinson–White syndrome.

electromagnetic w's the entire series of ethereal waves which are similar in character, and which move with the velocity of light, but which vary enormously in wavelength. The unbroken series is known from the hertzian waves used in radio transmission, which may be miles in length (one mile equals 1.6×10^5 cm), through heat and light, the ultraviolet, x-rays, and gamma rays of radium to the cosmic rays, the wavelength of which may be as short as 40 femtometers (4×10^{-14} nm.

light w's the electromagnetic waves that produce sensations on the retina. See also VISION.

P w. a deflection in the normal electrocardiogram produced by the wave of excitation passing over the atria.

pulse w. the elevation of the pulse felt by the finger or shown graphically in a recording of pulse pressure.

Q w. in the QRS complex, the initial electrocardiographic downward (negative) deflection, related to the initial phase of depolarization.

R w. the initial upward deflection of the QRS complex, following the Q wave in the normal electrocardiogram.

S w. a downward deflection of the QRS complex following the R wave in the normal electrocardiogram.

T w. the second major deflection of the normal electrocardiogram, reflecting the potential variations occurring with repolarization of the ventricles.

theta w's electroencephalographic waves having a frequency of 4 to 7 per second, occurring mainly in children but also in adults under emotional stress. See also ELECTROENCEPHALOGRAPHY.

wavelength ('wayv,length) the distance between a point on one wave and the point in the identical phase in the succeeding one in the advance of waves of radiant energy.

wax (waks) a plastic solid of plant or animal origin or produced synthetically. adj. **waxy**.

ear w. cerumen.

waxy flexibility (,waksi ,fleksi'bilitee) a cataleptic state in which a patient's limbs are held indefinitely in any position in which they have been placed. Called also FLEXIBILITAS CEREA. See also CATATONIA.

Wb weber.

WBC white blood cell (leukocyte); white blood (cell) count.

weal (weel) a raised stripe on the skin, as is caused by the lash of a whip. Typical of urticaria.

wean (ween) 1. to discontinue breast feeding and substitute other feeding habits. 2. in respiratory therapy, to gradually decrease dependence on assisted ventilation until the patient is able to breathe spontaneously. See also VENTILATOR.

weanling ('weenling) an animal newly changed from breast feeding to other forms of nourishment.

webbed (webd) connected by a membrane or strand of tissue.

weber ('webə, 'vaybə) the SI unit of magnetic flux which, linking a circuit of one turn, produces in it an electromotive force of one volt as it is reduced to zero at a uniform rate in one second. Abbreviated Wb.

Weber–Christian disease (,webə'krischən) nodular nonsuppurative panniculitis.

Weber's glands ('vaybəz) the tubular mucous glands of the tongue.

Weber test ('vaybə) a hearing test made by placing a vibrating tuning fork at some point on the midline of the head and noting whether it is perceived as heard in the midline (normal) or referred to either ear (middle ear disease). If it is heard best in the affected ear, there is conductive hearing impairment; if it is heard best in the normal ear, there is sensineural hearing impairment.

Wegener's granulomatosis ('vaygənəz) a progressive disease, with granulomatous lesions of the respiratory tract, focal necrotizing arteriolitis with mainly glomerular renal involvement and, finally, widespread inflammation of all organs of the body.

weight (wayt) heaviness; the degree to which a body is drawn toward the earth by gravity.

apothecaries' w. a system of weight used in compounding prescriptions based on the grain (equivalent 64.8 mg). Its units are the scruple (20 grains), dram (3 scruples), ounce (8 drams), and pound (12 ounces).

atomic w. the weight of an atom of a chemical element, compared with the weight of an atom of carbon-12, which is taken as 12.00000.

avoirdupois w. the system of weight commonly used for ordinary commodities in English-speaking countries. Its units are the dram (27.344 grains), ounce (16 drams), and pound (16 ounces).

equivalent w. the weight in grams of a substance that is equivalent in a chemical reaction to 1.008 g of hydrogen (see also chemical EQUIVALENT).

molecular w. the weight of a molecule of a chemical compound as compared with the weight of an atom of carbon-12; it is equal to the sum of the weights of its constituent atoms. Abbreviated mol. wt.

Weil's disease ('vielz) leptospiral jaundice.

Weil–Felix reaction (,viel'feeliks) an agglutination test of blood serum used in the diagnosis of typhus.

Weitbrecht's foramen ('vietbrekhts) a foramen in the capsule of the shoulder joint.

Weitbrecht's ligament a small ligamentous band extending from the ulnar tuberosity to the radius.

Welldorm ('weldawm) trademark for preparations of dichlophenazone, a hypnotic.

wellness ('welnəs) the development of a personal lifestyle which promotes feelings of well-being, achieves the highest level of health within one's capability, and minimizes one's chances of becoming ill. It is guided by a developing sense of self-awareness and self-responsibility encompassing emotional, mental, physical, social, spiritual, and environmental health and results in growth toward harmony and balance.

wen (wen) 1. a sebaceous or epidermal inclusion cyst. 2. pillar cyst.

Wenckebach period ('venkə,bahk) a phenomenon characterized by a progressive lengthening of the P–R interval until a ventricular (QRST) complex fails to follow an atrial (P wave) complex.

Wenckebach type A-V block type 1 second degree atrioventricular (A-V) block characterized by the Wenckebach period.

Werdnig–Hoffmann disease (,vərdnig'hofmən) disease characterized by progressive spinal muscular atrophy affecting the shoulder, neck, pelvis, and eventually the respiratory muscles of infants.

Werner's syndrome ('vərnəz) a hereditary condition characterized by cataracts, osteoporosis, stunted growth and premature greying of the hair.

Wernicke's encephalopathy (disease, syndrome) ('vərnikəz) an inflammatory haemorrhagic encephalopathy due to thiamine deficiency associated with chronic alcoholism, but also occurring as a complication of certain other diseases, with paralysis of the eye muscles, diplopia, nystagmus, ataxia, and mental changes ranging from deterioration and forgetfulness to delirium tremens and KORSAKOFF'S SYNDROME. See also WERNICKE–KORSAKOFF SYNDROME.

Wernicke–Korsakoff syndrome (ˌvərnikə'kawsəkof) a disorder of the central nervous system, usually associated with chronic alcoholism and nutritional deficiency. Sometimes called cerebral beriberi because of the severe depletion of vitamin B_1, or thiamine, which is typical of the disorder.

It is characterized by a combination of motor and sensory disturbances (WERNICKE'S ENCEPHALOPATHY or disease) and disordered memory function (KORSAKOFF'S SYNDROME or psychosis). The condition typically has an abrupt onset, manifested by ocular motility, ataxia, diplopia, and horizontal nystagmus. Many patients are unaware of their unsteady gait and decreased mental acuity and other signs of cognitive dysfunction.

There usually is an immediate improvement in ocular disturbances once vitamin therapy is begun. The ataxia and diminished perceptual function and concept formation show a much slower rate of improvement. Only about one-third of those with Korsakoff's psychosis can fully recover. The mortality rate for the syndrome may be as high as 17 per cent during the acute phase.

Wertheim's operation ('vərt·hiemz) see HYSTERECTOMY.

Westphal–Strümpell pseudosclerosis (disease) (ˌvestfahl'stroompel) hepatolenticular degeneration.

wet brain (wet brayn) brain oedema.

wet-nurse ('wetˌnərs) a woman who breast feeds infants other than her own.

Wetzel grid ('wetsel) a direct-reading chart for evaluating physical fitness in terms of body build, development level, and basal metabolism.

Wharton's duct ('wawtənz) the duct of the submandibular gland.

Wharton's jelly the soft, jelly-like intracellular substance of the umbilical cord.

wheal (weel) a localized area of oedema on the body surface, often attended with severe itching and usually evanescent. It is the typical lesion of urticaria.

wheat germ ('weet ˌjərm) the embryo of wheat, which contains tocopherol, thiamine, riboflavin, and other vitamins.

wheeze (weez) a whistling respiratory sound.

wheezing ('weezing) breathing with a rasp or whistling sound. It results from constriction or obstruction of the throat, pharynx, trachea, or bronchi.

Wheezing is commonly a symptom of ASTHMA. In an asthmatic attack, spasm of the bronchi occurs, and air can be forced only with difficulty into and from the lungs through the trachea.

Another cause of wheezing is congestive HEART FAILURE, in which there is difficulty in breathing, and frequently the lips have a bluish colour and the veins in the neck are distended.

When wheezing is persistent and is not asthmatic, the cause may be an obstruction, such as a foreign body or tumour, somewhere in the breathing passages.

whiplash ('wipˌlash) a nonspecific term applied to injury to the spinal cord and spine due to sudden extension of the neck, as in sudden stopping or propulsion of a vehicle.

whiplash shake syndrome ('wipˌlash shayk) a constellation of injuries to the brain and eye that may occur when a child less than 3 years old, usually less than 1 year old, is shaken vigorously while being held by the trunk or limbs with the head unsupported. This causes stretching and tearing of the cerebral vessels and brain substance, commonly leading to subdural haematomas and retinal haemorrhages, but may also be associated with cerebral contusion. It may result in paralysis, blindness and other visual disturbances, convulsions, and death.

Whipple's disease ('wip'lz) intestinal lipodystrophy.

Whipple's operation see PANCREATODUODENECTOMY.

whipworm ('wipˌwərm) *Trichuris trichiura.*

white cell, white blood cell (wiet) leukocyte.

white leg milk leg. See PHLEGMASIA.

white matter, white substance the white nervous tissue, constituting the conducting portion of the brain and spinal cord, composed mostly of myelinated nerve fibres. Grey matter or substance is the term used to describe the tissues composed of unmyelinated fibres.

Whitfield's ointment ('witfeeldz) compound ointment of benzoic acid used in the treatment of fungal diseases.

whitlow ('witloh) felon.

melanotic w. a malignant tumour of the nail bed characterized by formation of melanotic tissue.

Whitmore's disease ('witmorz) melioidosis.

WHO (hoo) World Health Organization.

whole blood coagulation time (hohl blud) a simple, rather crude test of the coagulation factors. It has been used to monitor heparin therapy.

whoop (hoop) the sonorous and convulsive inspiration of whooping cough.

whooping cough ('hooping ˌkof) a notifiable infectious disease characterized by catarrh of the respiratory tract and paroxysms of coughing, ending in a prolonged crowing or whooping respiration; called also pertussis. The causative organism is *Bordetella pertussis.* Whooping cough is a serious disease.Although it may attack at any age, most cases occur in children under 10 years, and half of these are in children under 5 years.

The organisms of whooping cough are spread by droplet infection and contact with discharges of the respiratory tract particularly during the early catarhal phase of the illness, although patients may be infectious for several weeks.The incubation period is usually about 7 days, although it may vary between 2 and 21 days.

PREVENTION. Immunization is the main method of prevention and is recommended in three doses beginning at age 3 months in combination with diphtheria and tetanus toxoids (DTPer/Vac/Ads). Side-effects include local reactions, transient fever, and possibly neurological reactions. Vaccinations should be postponed if the child is febrile, and should not be given if there is a history of a severe local or general reaction after a previous dose. In the management of an outbreak, vaccination has been recommended for close contacts under 5 years of age who are inadequately immunized. Health care professionals may develop whooping cough: they should not be immunized, but should be advised of the possibility of infection and removed from duty if catarrhal symptoms develop.

whorl (wərl) a spiral arrangement, as in the ridges on the finger that make up a fingerprint.

Widal test (vee'dahl) a test for the diagnosis of typhoid fever, based on agglutination of *Salmonella typhosa* by dilutions of the patient's serum.

Wilms' tumour (vilmz) a rapidly developing malignant mixed tumour of the kidneys, made up of embryonal elements, and occurring chiefly in children before the fifth year; called also embryonal carcinosarcoma and nephroblastoma.

Wilson's disease ('wilsənz) hepatolenticular degeneration.

Wilson–Mikity syndrome (ˌwilsən'mikitee) a rare form of pulmonary insufficiency in low-birth-weight infants, marked by hyperpnoea and cyanosis of insidious onset during the first month of life and often resulting in death. Radiographically, there are multiple cystlike foci of hyperaeration throughout the lung, with coarse thickening of the interstitial supporting structures. Called also pulmonary dysmaturity.

Winckel's disease ('vingkelz) a fatal disease of the newborn, with jaundice, haemoglobinuria, bloody urine, haemorrhage, cyanosis, collapse, and convulsions.

window ('windoh) a circumscribed opening in a plane surface.

aortic w. a transparent region below the aortic arch, formed by the bifurcation of the trachea, visible in the left anterior oblique radiograph of the heart and great vessels.

oval w. an oval opening in the inner wall of the middle ear, which is closed by the stapes; called also *fenestra vestibuli, fenestra ovalis*.

round w. a round opening in the middle ear covered by the secondary tympanic membrane; called also *fenestra cochleae, fenestra rotunda*.

ultrasound w. an access point for an ultrasound beam to image an organ.

windpipe ('windˌpiep) the trachea.

winking ('wingking) quick opening and closing of the eyelids.

jaw w. involuntary closing of the eyelids associated with jaw movements.

wintergreen oil ('wintəˌgreen) methyl salicylate.

wiring ('wieəring) the fixing together of a broken or split bone by the use of a wire. Commonly used for the jaw, the patella and the sternum. The most widely used form of fixation in fractures of the jaw is undoubtedly dental wiring. It is quick to apply, cheap, and effective. Stainless steel wire of 0.35 mm diameter is used.

circumferential w. a wire passing around the mandible, commonly used to retain a gunning splint.

transosseous w. the wiring of fractured bone ends together under direct vision. Immobilization of the jaws is still required for adequate stability.

interdental eyelet w. loops of wire fixed around individual teeth in opposing dental arches to provide fixation points to wire the jaws together.

wisdom teeth ('wizdəm ˌteeth) the back molar teeth, the appearance of which is often delayed until maturity.

Wiskott–Aldrich syndrome (ˌwiskot'awldrich) a condition characterized by chronic eczema, chronic suppurative otitis media, anaemia, and thrombocytopenic purpura; it is an immunodeficiency syndrome transmitted as an X-linked recessive trait, in which there is poor antibody response to polysaccharide antigens and dysfunction of cell-mediated immunity. Called also Aldrich's syndrome.

witch-hazel ('wich ˌhayz'l) hamamelis.

withdrawal (widh'dror'l) 1. a pathological retreat from reality. 2. abstention from drugs to which one is habituated or addicted; also denoting the symptoms occasioned by such withdrawal (see also DRUG ADDICTION).

w. symptoms a group of symptoms brought about by abrupt withdrawal of a narcotic or other drug to which a person has become addicted; called also *abstinence syndrome*. The usual reactions to alcohol withdrawal are anxiety, weakness, gastrointestinal symptoms, nausea and vomiting, tremor, fever, rapid heartbeat, convulsions, and delirium (see also DELIRIUM TREMENS). Similar effects are produced by withdrawal of barbiturates and in this case convulsions occur very frequently, often followed by psychosis with hallucinations.

Morphine withdrawal produces a standard pattern of reactions beginning with restlessness, which later becomes extreme. There may be slight fever, elevated blood pressure, and mild hyperglycaemia, with lack of appetite and vomiting. The symptoms begin to decline by the third day and usually disappear by about the fourteenth day. The various morphine-like drugs produce similar symptoms, in some instances more acute and in others milder.

Treatment consists of providing a substitute drug such as a mild sedative, along with treatment of the symptoms as needed. Parenteral fluids are often required.

witzelsucht ('vitsəlˌzuhkht) [Ger.] a mental condition marked by the making of poor jokes and puns and the telling of pointless stories at which the speaker is intensely amused; a condition characteristic of frontal lobe lesions.

wolffian body ('wuhlfi·ən, 'volfi·ən) mesonephros.

Wolff–Parkinson–White syndrome (ˌwuhlfˌpahkinsən'wiet) the association of paroxysmal tachycardia (or atrial fibrillation) and preexcitation, in which the electrocardiogram displays a short P–R interval and a wide QRS complex which characteristically shows an early QRS vector (delta wave). Called also anomalous atrioventricular excitation.

Wolf–Hirschhorn syndrome (ˌwuhlf'hiəsh·hawn) a syndrome associated with partial deletion of the short arm of chromosome 4, characterized by microcephaly, ocular hypertelorism, epicanthus, cleft palate, micrognathia, low-set ears simplified in form, cryptorchidism, and hypospadias.

wolfram ('wuhlfrəm) tungsten (symbol W).

Wolman's disease ('wolmənz) primary familial xanthomatosis in infants; associated with involvement and calcification of the adrenal glands, failure to thrive, vomiting, diarrhoea, hepatomegaly, splenomegaly, foam cells in the bone marrow and other tissues, and early death.

womb (woom) uterus.

Wood's filter (wuhdz) see WOOD'S LIGHT.

Wood's light ultraviolet radiation from a mercury vapour source, transmitted through a nickel-oxide filter (Wood's filter), which holds back all but a few violet rays and passes ultraviolet wavelengths of about 365 nm; used in diagnosis of fungal infections of the scalp and erythrasma, and to reveal the presence of porphyrins and fluorescent minerals.

wood alcohol (wuhd 'alkəˌhol) methyl alcohol.

woolsorter's disease ('wuhlsawtəz) pulmonary anthrax.

work-up ('wərkup) the procedures done to arrive at a diagnosis, including history taking, laboratory tests, radiograms and so on.

World Health Organization (wərld) the specialized agency of the United Nations that is concerned with health on an international level. Abbreviated WHO. The agency was founded in 1948 and in its constitution are listed the following objectives.

Health is a state of complete physical and social well-being, and not merely the absence of disease or infirmity. The enjoyment of the highest attainable standards of health is one of the fundamental rights of every human being without distinction of race, religion, political belief, economic or social condition. The health of all peoples is fundamental to the attainment of peace and security and is dependent upon the fullest cooperation of individuals and States. The achievement of any State in the promotion and protection of health is of value to all.

The major specific aims of the WHO are:

(1) To strengthen the health services of member nations, improving the teaching standards in medicine and allied professions, and advising and helping generally in the field of health.

(2) To promote better standards for nutrition, housing, recreation, sanitation, economic and working conditions.

(3) To improve maternal and child health and welfare.

(4) To advance progess in the field of mental health.

(5) To encourage and conduct research on problems of public health.

In carrying out these aims and objectives the WHO functions as a directing and coordinating authority on international health. It serves as a centre for all types of global and health information, promotes uniform quarantine standards and international sanitary regulations, provides advisory services through public health experts in control of disease and sets up international standards for the manufacture of all important drugs. Through its teams of doctors, nurses, and other health personnel it provides modern medical skills and knowledge to communities throughout the world. See also HEALTH.

worm (wərm) any of the soft-bodied, elongated, naked invertebrates of the phyla Annelida, Acanthocephala, Aschelminthes, and Platyhelminthes. Worms are often found as parasites in man and other animals. RINGWORM is not caused by a worm but is a form of fungal infection of the skin.

Most worm infections are transmitted from person to person via faeces that contaminate food and water. Serious worm infections may cause anaemia, listlessness, fatigue, irritability, abdominal pain, diarrhoea, and weight loss.

Parasitic worms usually live in relative balance with their human hosts, taking enough nutrients to survive without destroying the health of the host. However, they reduce the strength and energy of the bodies they inhabit and often produce very uncomfortable symptoms.

Suspected cases of worm infestation should be brought to the attention of a doctor, for self-treatment may be ineffective and even harmful. Effective medications against certain worms can be prescribed only by a doctor.

ROUNDWORMS (NEMATODA). Roundworms somewhat resemble common earthworms in appearance. The varieties most frequently infecting man include *Ascaris lumbricoides*, pinworms, hookworms, filaria, and *Trichinella spiralis*, the cause of TRICHINOSIS.

Ascaris lumbricoides. The largest of the roundworms that infect man, *Ascaris lumbricoides*, occurs worldwide, but is particularly common in moist tropical and sub-tropical areas. It is transmitted when infective eggs in soil, or in uncooked produce contaminated with the soil, are ingested. The *Ascaris* eggs leave the body in the faeces and develop in the soil and on growing plants on which the infected faeces have been deposited. When such soil is swallowed, as may happen with young children, or when vegetables from these areas are eaten without having been properly washed or thoroughly cooked, larvae hatch out from the eggs in the digestive system. Migrating from the intestines into the blood, then to the lungs and the oesophagus, the larvae finally return to the intestines, where they grow to maturity, reaching a length ranging from 15 to 35 cm.

Ascaris infection may go unsuspected until a worm is passed in the stool. But there may be colic or other abdominal symptoms, and occasionally the worms are vomited during their passage through the oesophagus. If heavily infected, children may be thin because the worms consume vital nutrients and inhibit the digestion of proteins. Intestinal obstruction, perforation and volvulus have been reported. Loss of appetite and angioneurotic oedema are common.

Accurate diagnosis of the presence and extent of *Ascaris* infection usually depends on the detection of eggs in a stool sample examined microscopically. Treatment involves the use of anthelmintics such as piperazine or mebendazole, and is completely successful in nearly every case.

Prevention of *Ascaris* infection depends primarily on the sanitary disposal of human faeces and discontinuing their use as fertilizer. Also important are the thorough washing of hands before eating and the careful cleaning and cooking of possibly infected foods.

Enterobius vermicularis. *Enterobius vermicularis*, called also *pinworm* or *threadworm*, is a spindle-shaped roundworm of worldwide distribution. It is less than 15 mm long and normally inhabits the upper part of the large intestine, more commonly in children than adults. Pinworms do not produce the abdominal symptoms, or the fatigue and loss of weight that may occur in *Ascaris* infection, but when the adult female worms migrate to the anal region, usually at night, and deposit eggs, irritation of the skin around the anus, leading to painful scratching and restless sleep, may result.

This irritation is the usual sign of pinworm infection, although there may also be vague intestinal discomfort. Adult worms may appear in the faeces, but the infection is transmitted by the eggs, which may be transferred to clothing, bedclothes, and toilet seats from the skin around the anus.

In scratching, the infected person is likely to collect the minute eggs on his hands and under his fingernails, and, until he washes thoroughly, he will shed the eggs on anything he touches.

The infection spreads to other persons when the eggs are carried to their mouths on contaminated food, or on hands, or even in contaminated house dust by inhalation. Widespread pinworm infection is explained by the fact that the eggs, which develop into mature worms only in a human body, can remain dormant but alive and infective for a considerable time in dust or air; they are not killed by most household disinfectants.

Enterobius vermicularis infection is treated by an anthelmintic such as mebendazole, or piperazine citrate. Where more than one member of the family is infected, it is probably best to treat the whole family simultaneously. Equally important, instructions for disinfecting bedclothes and other material that may harbour eggs must be followed carefully to avoid reinfection and spread of pinworms to other members of the family.

Prevention of pinworms is largely a matter of hygiene. Children should be taught to wash their hands well with soap and water before meals and after using the toilet. Care and cleanliness in the preparation of food is essential. If a case of pinworms develops in a family, extra precautions should be taken; toilet seats should be scrubbed daily with soap and water, and the bedding and nightclothes of the infected person should be disinfected by boiling at least twice a week.

Hookworm. Hookworms are small—about 15 mm long—and are particularly common in tropical and subtropical countries wherever disposal of human faeces is inadequate. Their larvae develop in soil contaminated by faeces from infected persons and they enter the body through the skin, usually through the sole of the foot. Children who go barefoot are especially susceptible. They travel by way of the blood to the lungs and then to the intestines, where the worms, by now full-grown, attach themselves to the intestinal wall and suck blood from it for nourishment. If the worm load is small, there may be no symptoms at all, but in heavier infections there may be severe blood loss and iron-deficiency anaemia, and eventually retardation of growth and mental development and even death if other infections intervene. Diagnosis is made by detection of eggs in the faeces. The infection is treated by administration of anthelmintic drugs such as mebendazole. It is prevented by improvement in sanitation facilities and wearing shoes out of doors. See also HOOKWORM.

Filaria. Another type of threadlike roundworm; it causes a tropical disease known as FILARIASIS, which affects lymphoid tissues.

FLATWORMS (PLATYHELMINTHES). Flatworms infecting man include tapeworms and flukes.

Tapeworm. Several species of tapeworms infect man; all depend on two hosts, one human and one animal, for development through their full life cycle (egg to larva to adult). Usually larvae are found in animal hosts and adult worms in man.

The tapeworms most commonly found in man (though the incidence of each species varies widely) enter human bodies in contaminated and insufficiently cooked pork (*Taenia solium*), beef (*T. saginata*), or fish (*Diphyllobothrium latum*). The larvae, embedded in cysts in the meat or fish, develop to maturity in the human intestine and attach themselves to the intestinal wall; from there they release eggs, or, in the case of *Taenia* species, egg-laden segments of the body called proglottids.

In mild or even moderate infections, tapeworms cause few or no symptoms. In heavy infections there may be diarrhoea, abdominal cramps (resembling hunger pains), flatulence, distention, and nausea. In most cases, before these symptoms have developed, the infected person discovers the tapeworm segments in his clothes or bedding.

Niclosamide is the drug of choice in the treatment of tapeworm infection. Three months freedom from recurrence of the passage of segments indicates cure. Prevention depends on thorough cooking of fish and meat.

Echinococcus granulosus. This tapeworm reverses the usual process of development in human and animal hosts. The adult *Echinococcus* is found in the intestine of dogs. The larva develops in the human intestine, penetrating the intestinal wall, and settling in various organs—most often the liver—where it forms a cyst (hydatid cyst) that grows slowly. Treatment is by surgical removal of the cyst. See also TAPEWORM.

Flukes (Trematoda). Flukes are a serious problem in many tropical, and subtropical countries. The Chinese liver fluke, *Clonorchis sinensis*, enters the body in raw or improperly cooked fish and may cause enlargement of the liver, jaundice, anaemia, and weakness. Another liver fluke, *Fasciola hepatica*, is occasionally found in man; it causes obstruction of the bile ducts and enlargement of the liver. Blood flukes such as *Schistosoma* penetrate the skin, make their way to the blood and travel to various parts of the body (see also SCHISTOSOMIASIS).

Treatment varies according to the type of fluke involved and requires careful medical supervision. Proper cooking of fish provides protection against *Clonorchis* infection. Since snails are carriers of flukes, their destruction, usually by poison, is an effective preventive measure in areas where fluke infection is a problem.

PATIENT CARE. The patient suffering from infection with worms may be malnourished and anaemic. Special attention should be given to the diet so that these conditions can be relieved. The patient may also need adequate rest and other general measures to improve his state of health.

Some types of worms or eggs are best destroyed before they can be flushed into the sewage system. This will depend on the community's sewage treatment plant and the type of worm involved. If there is any doubt that the worms will be destroyed it is best to disinfect the stool with chlorinated lime before disposal in the sewage system.

wound (woond) a bodily injury caused by physical means, with disruption of the normal continuity of structures.

contused w. one created by a blow without breaking the skin.

w. drain any device by which a channel or open area may be established for the exit of material from a wound or cavity. See also WOUND HEALING.

w. healing the restoration of integrity to injured tissues by replacement of dead tissue with viable tissue. The process starts immediately after an injury and may continue for months or years, and is essentially the same for all types of wounds. Variations in wound healing are the result of differences in location, severity of the wound, and the extent of injury to the tissues. Other factors affecting wound healing are the age, nutritional status, and general state of health of the patient and his body reserves and resources for the regeneration of tissue.

Healing may occur by regeneration or repair, most commonly by a combination of both. *Regeneration* is where structures are replaced by proliferation of similar cells, e.g., those of liver and squamous epithelium. *Repair* involves formation of new fibrous tissue with some degree of subsequent contraction. Since most wounds extend to more than one type of tissue, complete regeneration is unusual and scar formation is to be expected.

In *healing by first intention* (primary union), restoration of tissue continuity occurs directly, without granulation; in *healing by second intention* (secondary union), wound repair following tissue loss (as in ulceration) is accomplished by closure of the wound with granulation tissue. This tissue is formed by extensive capillary budding at the outer edges and base of the wound cavity followed by proliferation of fibroblasts and formation of new collagen and slowly extends from the base and sides of the wound toward its centre. If, however, the wound is very deep and extensive, granulation tissue cannot fill the defect and grafting may be needed to cover the space and avoid severe contracture due to scarring and loss of function. *Healing by third intention* (delayed primary closure) occurs when a wound is initially too contaminated to close and is closed surgically 4 or 5 days after the injury.

The insertion of drains can facilitate healing by providing an outlet for removing accumulations of serosanguineous fluid and purulent material, and obliterating dead space such as that created by surgical removal of an organ.

If the area of injury is not very large, the products of inflammation, small blood clots, and other debris from the wound can be absorbed into the blood stream and disposed of. Wounds that are filled with large amounts of dead cells, blood clots, and other debris must be

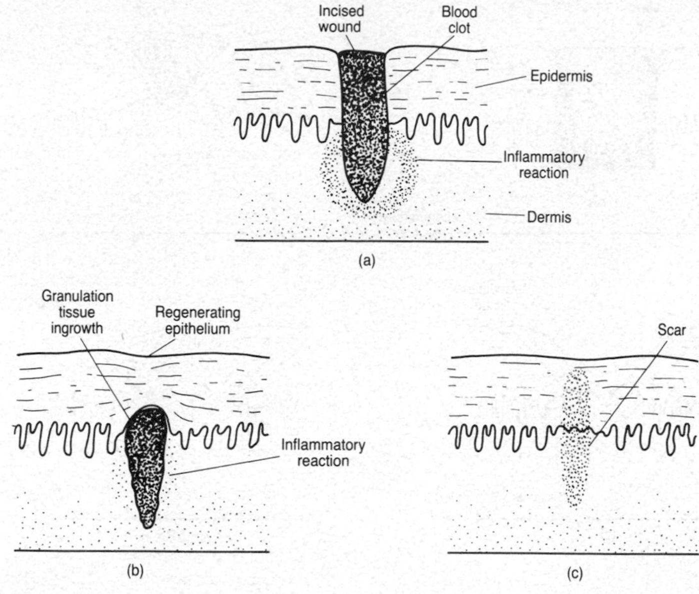

Wound healing by primary, or first, intention. In primary wound healing there is no tissue loss. (a) Incised wound is held together by a blood clot and possibly by sutures or surgical clamps. An inflammatory process begins in adjacent tissue at moment of injury. (b) After several days, granulation tissue forms as a result of migration of fibroblasts to the area of injury and formation of new capillaries. Epithelial cells at wound margin migrate to the clot and seal the wound. Regenerating epithelium covers the wound. (c) Scarring occurs as granulation tissue matures and injured tissue is replaced with connective tissue

cleansed in order to prevent bacterial growth and for healing to take place. This can be accomplished by surgical débridement or by irrigations. Enzymes such as streptokinase are sometimes used to remove the debris by enzymatic action. Since foreign bodies, such as sutures, slivers of glass, splinters, and the like, can delay healing, they too must be removed from the wound to facilitate healing.

Patient Care. Assessment of the progress of wound healing begins with frequent inspection of the site for signs of bleeding in or around the wound. Discoloration of the skin adjacent to a surgical or traumatic wound that has been sutured may indicate a pooling of blood in the tissue spaces and the beginning stages of a haematoma. Bleeding in a wound and clot formation can delay healing. Accumulations of serosanguineous fluid and purulent drainage also must be watched for, because they also retard the healing process. If a drain has been inserted to remove excess fluid, the colour, amount, odour, and other characteristics of the drainage must be noted and recorded. If there is more than one drain, the drainage from each should be noted separately.

Dressings also must be observed frequently, especially a pressure dressing, which can become dangerously restrictive if there is swelling. Any change in sensation, e.g., tingling and numbness, signs of impaired circulation, or complaint of discomfort, should be noted.

Other data important to the ongoing assessment of wound healing are the leukocyte count, coagulation tests, and electrolyte levels. An elevated body temperature can signal local or systemic infection. Another sign of infection is the presence of purulent drainage. The colour of the drainage is often indicative of the particular infecting organism. For example, a yellow colour may indicate the presence of *Staphylococcus aureus*, and a blue-green colour may indicate infection with *Pseudomonas aeruginosa*.

In a surgical wound, a discharge of serosanguineous fluid at any time during the first postoperative week may signal wound DEHISCENCE and, therefore, should be reported immediately to the surgeon.

During the scarring phase of healing, the wound is inspected for changes in size, colour, and shape. These changes can continue for months, even in superficial wounds. New scar tissue is usually raised, irregular, and purplish in colour. With time, the colour fades, the scar contracts and its surface and edges become less irregular. Sometimes the scar tissue grows to excess and extends beyond the normal limits of the wound. This is called a KELOID or hypertrophic scar and may require steroid injections or surgical removal.

In order to achieve adequate and uneventful healing of a wound the patient must be in a good state of nutrition. Nutrition plays an important role in the healing process; hence, a wide range of dietary nutrients must be supplied, either through oral feedings, supplementary vitamins and protein, or parenteral NUTRITION. Oxygen is also essential to the healing process and measures must be taken to ensure adequate circulation of blood to the wound, including exercise, ambulation when possible, and applications of warmth when prescribed. Positioning also is important to avoid prolonged pressure against blood vessels serving the wounded area. Adequate rest is needed to facilitate healing. The patient should understand the need for rest and the purpose of splints, casts, and other devices employed for immobilization of a wounded part.

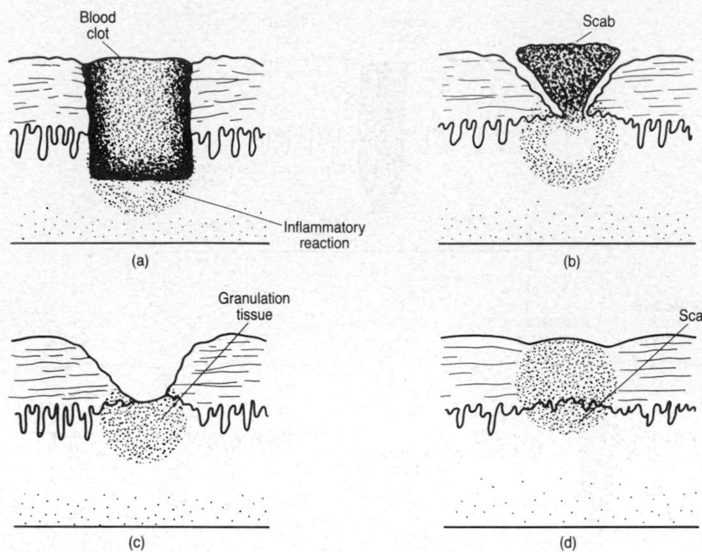

Wound healing by second intention. (b) Occurs when there is tissue loss, as in extensive burns and deep ulcers. The healing process is more prolonged than in healing by primary intention because large amounts of dead tissue must be removed and replaced with viable cells. (a) Open area is more extensive; inflammatory reaction is more widespread and tends to become chronic. (b) Healing may occur under a scab formed of dried exudate, or dried plasma proteins and dead cells [eschar]. (c) Fibroblasts and capillary buds migrate towards centre of wound to form granulation tissue, which becomes a translucent red colour as capillary network develops. Granulation tissue is fragile and bleeds easily. (d) As granulation tissue matures, marginal epithelial cells migrate and proliferate over connective tissue base to form a scar. Contraction of skin around scar is result of movement of epithelial cells towards centre of wound in an attempt to close defect. Surrounding skin moves towards centre of wound in an effort to close defect.

Mechanical injury to a wound can greatly impede healing by damaging the tissues involved in the healing process. The wound should be protected from friction and direct blows. The affected part must be handled gently, and great care must be used in applying and removing dressings and bandages.

Other factors that work against optimal healing are stress, old age, smoking, obesity, and diabetes mellitus. Poorly controlled diabetic patients have an abnormal function of the phagocytes, which predisposes wounds to infection. Radiotherapy, steroids, and antineoplastic drugs, and general debility of the patient compromise healing.

incised w. one caused by a sharp instrument.

lacerated w. one in which the tissues are torn or cut apart.

open w. one that communicates directly with the atmosphere.

penetrating w. one caused by a sharp, usually slender object, which passes through the skin into the underlying tissues.

perforating w. a penetrating wound which extends into a viscus or bodily cavity.

puncture w. penetrating wound with a small orifice.

sucking w. wound of the chest through which air is drawn in and out with respiratory movements.

WPHOA Women Public Health Officers' Association.

Wrisberg's ganglia ('risbərgz) cardiac ganglia.

wrist (rist) the region of the joint between the hand and the forearm; called also the carpus.

There are eight carpal bones in the wrist, arranged in two rows. The joint surfaces of these bones glide upon each other in four directions. The carpals join the bones of the forearm, the radius and ulna, and the bones of the hands, the metacarpals. The bones are bound together and protected by tough ligaments and capsules, the enveloping structures. The major arteries, nerves, veins, and tendons that serve the hand and fingers run across the wrist. Both tendons and the joint are lined with synovial membrane.

DISORDERS OF THE WRIST. The wrist is a strong but complicated joint and can suffer the same disorders as any other joint. The hands are constantly being used, and any sudden or strong movement or exertion may cause a structure to stretch, tear, or become dislocated.

A strained wrist, caused by overstretching or overexertion, is usually treated by rest and the application of heat and light massage. Injury of the joint ligaments is called a SPRAIN and is a common disorder. DISLOCATION, or displacement of the bones of the wrist from their normal relationship, and FRACTURE, which causes swelling and pain on movement, may also occur. Often a fracture is difficult to distinguish from a bad sprain, and radiographical examination may be necessary for diagnosis.

Severe pain, swelling, and reddish blue discoloration may be a symptom of any of these cases of wrist injury. An ice pack is often recommended for swelling.

Other disorders of the wrist include ARTHRITIS, infection, ganglion (a form of cystic tumour), and TENOSYNOVITIS..

wristdrop ('rist,drop) paralysis of the extensor muscles of the hand and fingers; it may be due to metallic poisoning.

WRVS Women's Royal Voluntary Service.

wryneck ('rie,nek) torticollis.

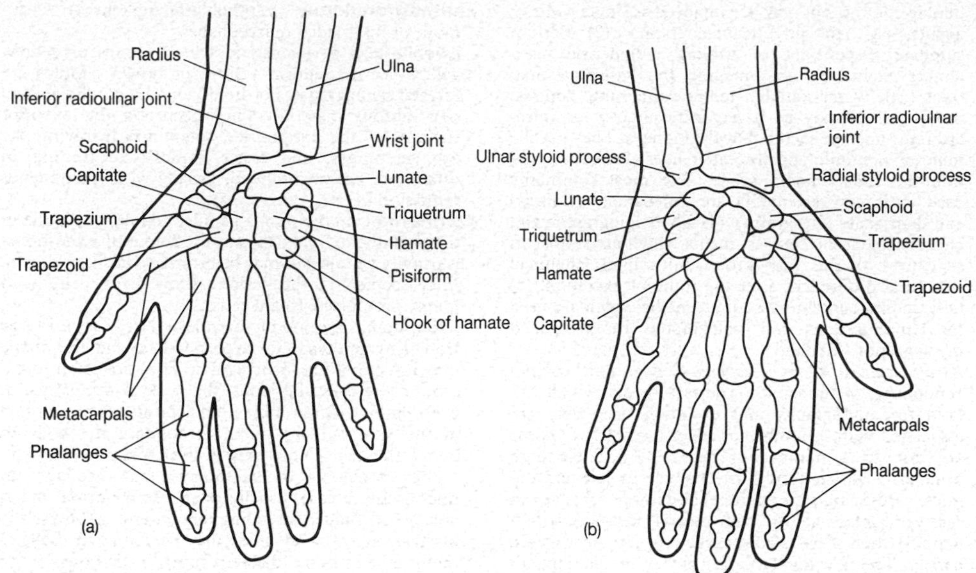

Bones of the wrist (carpal bones). (a) Anterior view, right arm. (b) Posterior view, right arm

wt. weight.

Wuchereria (ˌvookəˈriə·ri·ə) a genus of filarial nematodes indigenous to the warmer regions of the world.

W. bancrofti a species widely distributed in tropical and subtropical countries, causing ELEPHANTIASIS, lymphangitis, and chyluria by interfering with the lymphatic circulation (see also FILARIASIS).

w/v weight (of solute) per volume (of solvent).

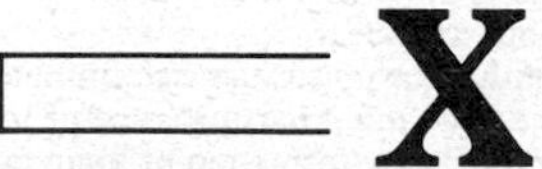

X symbol, *Kienböck's unit* (of x-ray exposure).

X-chromosome (ˈeksˌkrohməˌsohm) the female sex chromosome, being present in all female gametes and only half the male gametes. When union takes place two X-c's result in a female child (XX) but one of each results in a male child (XY). See Y-CHROMOSOME.

X-linked (ˈeksˌlinkt) transmitted by genes on the X chromosome; sex-linked.

x-rays (ˈeksˌrayz) high-energy electromagnetic radiation produced by the collision of a beam of electrons with a metal target in an x-ray tube. Called also *roentgen rays*. The penetrability and hardness of the x-rays increases with the voltage applied to the x-ray tube, which controls the speed with which the electrons strike the target. For diagnostic radiography, tube voltages in the range 60 to 120 kilovolts peak (kVp) are normally used. For radiotherapy, voltages in the 1 to 2 megavolt range are used for most treatment. Accelerating electrons to speeds high enough to produce megavoltage x-rays requires a linear accelerator (lineac).

The x-ray exposure is proportional to the tube current (milliamperage) and also to the exposure time. In diagnostic radiography, the tube voltage and current and exposure time are selected to produce a high-quality radiograph with the correct contrast and film density. In radiotherapy, these exposure factors are selected to deliver a precisely calculated radiation dose to the tumour. The total dose is usually fractionated so that tumour cells can be oxygenated as surrounding cells die; this increases the sensitivity of the cells to radiation.

Body tissues and other substances are classified according to the degree to which they allow the passage of x-rays (*radiolucency*) or absorb x-rays (*radiopacity*). Gases are very radiolucent; fatty tissue is moderately radiolucent. Compounds containing high-atomic-weight elements, such as barium and iodine, are very radiopaque; bone and deposits of calcium salts are moderately radiopaque. Water; muscle, skin, blood, and cartilage and other connective tissue; and cholesterol and uric acid stones have intermediate density. See also RADIATION and RADIOTHERAPY.

X-RAY CONTRAST MEDIA. Substances employed to increase or create a density difference in diagnostic radiology. X-ray contrast media may be denser than adjacent tissues (radiopaque) or less dense (radiolucent). When only one contrast medium is used the radiological technique may be described as single contrast and when two contrast media of differing densities are used the term double contrast is used. A good example of a double contrast technique is the double contrast barium meal in which the gastric mucosa is visualized by coating it with a radiopaque barium sulphate suspension and the lumen is distended with radiolucent carbon dioxide.

Contrast media fall into a number of types with differing uses: (1) Gases, which are either air or carbon dioxide. They are most frequently used to provide double contrast but may be employed as single contrast agents, e.g., in air encephalography. (2) Barium sulphate suspensions of varying radiodensity used almost exclusively for imaging the gastrointestinal tract. (3) Water-soluble, iodine-containing contrast media which may be given intravenously or intra-arterially and are excreted by the kidneys. They may be ionic or nonionic and the latter may also be injected into the subarachnoid space. The most commonly used ionic contrast media are iothalamate (Conray) and diatrizoate (Urografin). (4) Cholangiographic and cholecystographic contrast media which are similar in structure to the last group but slight chemical structural differences alter the route of excretion. (5) Oily, iodine-containing contrast media which are used for lymphography and sialography (Lipiodol) and myelography (Myodil).

X-ray Contrast Media Reactions. Conventional iodine-containing, water-soluble contrast media which are used for angiography and excretion urography are associated with a number of adverse reactions. These are due to a number of factors: (1) Their high osmolarity which results in changes in haemodynamics, cardiac output, endothelial damage, changes in red cell deformability and central nervous system toxicity when there is a breakdown in the blood-brain barrier. The new low-osmolar contrast media (iopamidol, iohexol, ioxaglate, and metrizamide) are associated with less of these adverse reactions. (2) The electric charge on the molecule. This is the probable cause of CNS toxicity when ionic contrast media are injected intrathecally. Nonionic contrast media (iopamidol, iohexol, and metrizamide) are safe in the subarachnoid space. (3) Chemotoxicity of the molecule itself. This may be reflected in the degree of inhibition of acetylcholinesterase and the symptoms (e.g., vomiting and flushing) so produced. (4) A direct hypersensitivity response to the molecule. Contrast media reactions are more common in allergic patients. Whenever contrast medium is given intravenously or intra-arterially drugs such as adrenaline and hydrocortisone and facilities for resuscitation should be on hand.

Xanax ('zanaks) trademark for a preparation of alprazolam, an anxiolytic.

xanth(o)- word element. [Gr.] *yellow*.

xanthaemia (zan'theemi·ə) the presence of yellow colouring matter in the blood; carotenaemia.

xanthelasma (ˌzanthə'lazmə) xanthoma affecting the eyelids and characterized by soft yellowish spots or plaques.

xanthic ('zanthik) 1. yellow. 2. pertaining to xanthine.

xanthine ('zantheen) a purine compound found in most bodily tissues and fluids; it is a precursor of uric acid.

dimethyl x. theobromine.

trimethyl x. caffeine.

xanthinuria (ˌzanthi'nyooə·ri·ə) excess of xanthine in the urine, due to a hereditary disorder of purine metabolism in which there is a deficiency of the enzyme xanthine oxidase.

xanthochromatic (ˌzanthohkrə'matik) yellow-coloured.

xanthochromia (ˌzanthoh'krohmi·ə) yellowish discoloration of the skin or spinal fluid. Xanthochromic spinal fluid usually indicates haemorrhage into the central nervous system and is due to the presence of xanthematin.

xanthochromic (ˌzanthoh'krohmik) yellow-coloured.

xanthocyanopsia (ˌzanthohˌsieə'nopsi·ə) inability to perceive red or green tints, vision being limited to yellow and blue.

xanthogranuloma (ˌzanthohˌgranyuh'lohmə) a tumour of lipid-laden macrophages.

juvenile x. a dermatosis in which groups of yellow, yellow-brown, reddish yellow, or brown papules are formed by aggregates of lipid-laden macrophages and new fibrous material. They occur on the extensor surfaces of the extremities, sometimes involving the eye, meninges, and testes, typically beginning in infancy or early childhood, usually with spontaneous remission in one to three years.

xanthoma (zan'thohmə) a papule, nodule, or plaque in the skin due to lipid deposits; the colour of a xanthoma is usually yellow, but may be brown, reddish, or cream. Microscopically, the lesions show light cells with foamy protoplasm (foam cells).

Xanthomas are usually harmless. They range in size from tiny pinheads to large nodules, and the shape may be round, flat, or irregular. They are often found around the eyes, the joints, the neck or the palms, or over tendons. Often these lipid deposits are not limited to the skin but are found throughout the body in bones, the heart, blood vessels, liver, and other organs.

The formation of xanthomas may indicate an underlying disease, usually related to abnormal metabolism of lipids, including cholesterol. Abnormally high levels of blood lipids may be found in diabetes mellitus (xanthoma diabeticorum), in diseases of the liver, kidney, and thyroid gland, and in several hereditary metabolic diseases. The excessive lipids carried in the blood may then be deposited as xanthomas.

Another group of diseases producing xanthomas affect the reticuloendothelial system, a widespread system of cells that have several functions, including an influence in the storage of fatty materials. These diseases are thought to have a similar basic mechanism but they have many different manifestations, which may include the formation of xanthomas. The xanthomas are usually found in the reticuloendothelial disorder called Hand-Schüller-Christian disease.

Treatment of xanthomas includes surgery, application of acids directly to the lipid deposits and management of the disease that causes them, as in diabetes mellitus.

diabetic x. an eruptive xanthoma associated with diabetes mellitus; when the diabetes is brought under control, the skin lesions disappear.

xanthomatosis (ˌzanthohmə'tohsis) an accumulation of excess lipids in the body due to disturbance of lipid metabolism and marked by the formation of foam cells in skin lesions. See XANTHOMA.

x. bulbi fatty degeneration of the cornea due to disorder of lipid metabolism, marked by the presence of xanthomas.

xanthomatous (zan'thohmətəs) pertaining to xanthoma.

xanthophose ('zanthohˌfohz) a yellow phose.

xanthopsia (zan'thopsi·ə) chromatopsia in which objects are seen as yellow.

xanthosine ('zanthohˌseen) a nucleoside composed of xanthine and ribose.

xanthosis (zan'thohsis) yellowish discoloration; degeneration with yellowish pigmentation.

xanthurenic acid (ˌzanthyuh'renik) a metabolite of L-tryptophan, present in normal urine and in increased amounts in vitamin B_6 deficiency.

Xe chemical symbol, *xenon*.

xenodiagnosis (ˌzenohˌdieəg'nohsis) diagnosis of a communicable disease by finding the causal organism in (1) a vector fed on the patient (e.g., Chagas' disease) or (2) a suitable animal host fed on suspect food (e.g., trichinosis). adj. **xenodiagnostic**.

xenogeneic (ˌzenohjə'nee·ik, -'nayik) in transplantation biology, denoting individuals or tissues from individuals of different species and hence of disparate cell type.
xenogenesis (ˌzenoh'jenəsis) 1. heterogenesis (1). 2. production of offspring unlike either parent.
xenogenous (zə'nojənəs) caused by a foreign body, or originating outside the organism.
xenograft ('zenohˌgrahft) a graft of tissue transplanted between animals of different species; a heterograft.
xenomenia (ˌzenoh'meeni·ə) vicarious menstruation. See also MENSTRUATION.
xenon ('zeenon, 'zen-) a chemical element, atomic number 54, atomic weight 131.30, symbol Xe. See table of elements in Appendix 2.
x.-133 a radioisotope of xenon having a half-life of 5.3 days and a principal gamma ray photon energy of 81 keV; used for pulmonary ventilation imaging. Symbol ^{133}Xe.
xenoparasite (ˌzenoh'parəˌsiet) an organism not usually parasitic on a particular species, but becomes so because of a weakened condition of the host.
xenophobia (ˌzenoh'fohbi·ə) morbid dread of strangers.
xenophonia (ˌzenoh'fohni·ə) alteration in the quality of the voice.
xenophthalmia (ˌzenof'thalmi·ə) inflammation caused by a foreign body in the eye; called also ophthalmoxerosis.
Xenopsylla (ˌzenop'silə) a genus of fleas, including more than 30 species, many of which transmit disease-producing microorganisms.
X. cheopis the rat flea, which transmits *Pasteurella pestis*, the causative organism of plague and *Rickettsia typhi*, the causative organism of murine typhus.
xer(o)- word element. [Gr.] *dry, dryness*.
xerocheilia (ˌziə·roh'kieli·ə) dryness of the lips.
xeroderma (ˌziə·roh'dərmə) a mild form of ichthyosis; excessive dryness of the skin.
x. pigmentosum a rare and frequently fatal pigmentary and atrophic disease in which the skin and eyes are extremely sensitive to light. It begins in childhood and progresses to early development of telangiectases, carcinoma, and melanoma. Ocular symptoms include photophobia, opacities, and tumours. It is inherited as an autosomal recessive trait involving a defect in the enzymes active in the repair of DNA damaged by ultraviolet irradiation. Total protection from sunlight prevents the development of lesions.
xerography (zi'rogrəfee) xeroradiography.
xeroma (zi'rohmə) abnormal dryness of the conjunctiva; xerophthalmia.
xeromammography (ˌziə·rohmə'mogrəfee) xeroradiography of the breast.
xeromenia (ˌziə·roh'meeni·ə) the appearance of constitutional symptoms at the menstrual period without any flow of blood.
xerophagia (ˌziə·roh'fayji·ə) the eating of dry food.
xerophthalmia (ˌziə·rof'thalmi·ə) abnormal dryness and thickening of the surface of the conjunctiva and cornea due to a deficiency of vitamin A or to local disease.
xeroradiography (ˌziə·rohˌraydi'ogrəfee) the making of radiographs by a dry, totally photoelectric process, using metal plates coated with a semiconductor, such as selenium.

The image produced by this process differs from conventional radiographs in that margins between tissues of varying densities are more clearly defined. Hence, edge enhancement is especially beneficial in the diagnosis of soft tissue abnormalities, especially breast disease. It does, however, require higher doses of radiation. Called also *xerography*.
xerosialography (ˌziə·rohˌsieə'logrəfee) sialography in which the images are recorded by xerography.
xerosis (zi'rohsis) abnormal dryness, as of the eye (xerophthalmia), skin (xeroderma), or mouth (xerostomia).
xerostomia (ˌziə·roh'stohmi·ə) dryness of the mouth from lack of the normal secretion.
xerotomography (ˌziə·rohtə'mogrəfee) tomography in which the images are recorded by xeroradiography.
xiph(o)- word element. [Gr.] *xiphoid process*.
xiphisternum (ˌzifi'stərnəm) xiphoid process. adj. **xiphisternal**.
xiphocostal (ˌzifi'kost'l) pertaining to the xiphoid process and ribs.
xiphoid ('zifoyd) 1. sword-shaped; ensiform. 2. xiphoid process.
x. process the pointed process of cartilage, supported by a core of bone, connected with the lower end of the body of the sternum.
xiphoiditis (ˌzifoy'dietis) inflammation of the xiphoid process.
xiphopagus (zi'fopəgəs) symmetrical conjoined twins united in the region of the xiphoid process.
XO symbol for the karyotype observed in most cases of Turner's syndrome, in which there is only one sex chromosome, an X chromosome.
xylene ('zieleen) xylol, dimethylbenzene. A clear inflammable liquid resembling benzene. Used as a solvent for rubber and in the preparation of tissues and sections for microscopy.
Xylocaine ('ziehlohˌkayn) trademark for preparations of lignocaine, a topical anaesthetic.
xylometazoline (ˌzielohme'tazəˌleen) an adrenergic used as a topical nasal decongestant in the form of the hydrochloride salt.
xylose ('zielohz) a pentose occurring in mucopolysaccharides of connective tissue and sometimes in the urine; also obtained from vegetable gum. D-Xylose is used in a diagnostic test of intestinal absorption.
xylulose ('zielyuhlohz) a pentose sugar occurring as D-xylulose and as L-xylulose, one of the few L sugars found in nature; it is sometimes excreted in the urine (see PENTOSURIA).
xysma ('zismə) material resembling bits of membrane in stools of diarrhoea.
xyster ('zistə) a filelike instrument used in surgery; raspatory.
XYY syndrome (ˌeksˌwie'wie) an extremely rare condition in males in which there is an extra Y chromosome, making a total of 47 in each body cell. Often the affected individuals are very tall and liable to exhibit aggressive and antisocial behavioural patterns.

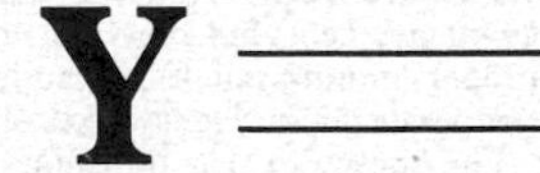

Y chemical symbol, *yttrium*.
Y-chromosome ('wieˌkrohməˌsohm) the male sex chromosome, being present in half the male gametes and none of the female. It carries few major genes. See X-CHROMOSOME.
yard (yahd) a unit of linear measure, 3 feet, or 36 inches, equivalent to 86.44 cm.
yaw (yor) a lesion of YAWS.
mother y. the initial cutaneous lesion of YAWS; called also framboesioma.

yawning ('yawning) a deep, involuntary inspiration with the mouth open, often accompanied by the act of stretching.

yaws (yorz) a highly infectious disease caused by the spirochete *Treponema pertenue*; called also framboesia.

Yaws is common among people, especially children, who live under primitive conditions in equatorial Africa, South America, and the East and West Indies. Mass control measures lower the incidence dramatically, but surveillance must continue in order to maintain a low incidence.

TRANSMISSION AND SYMPTOMS. Yaws is transmitted by direct contact. The first symptom, appearing usually about a month after exposure, is a single granulomatous lesion, an inflammatory but painless elevation of the skin. Called the 'mother yaw', this soon ulcerates. Open, oozing sores appear a few weeks later on the hands, feet, face, scalp, and trunk. Eventually, after several years, the disease causes tissue destruction, bone changes, and shortening of the fingers or toes.

The causative organism of yaws is closely related to that of syphilis, and both diseases give a positive result in the Wassermann test. Yaws is classified as a nonvenereal disease and is not primarily communicated by coitus. TREATMENT AND PREVENTION. Effective treatment is afforded by antibiotics, particularly penicillin.

Unsanitary living conditions unquestionably encourage the spread of the disease. Ideally, all clothing that has come in contact with yaws lesions should be sterilized and the sores cleaned with antiseptic and covered with clean dressings.

There is as yet no immunizing vaccine for yaws.

Yb chemical symbol, *ytterbium.*

yeast (yeest) a general term including unicellular, nucleated, usually rounded fungi that reproduce by budding; some are fermenters of carbohydrates, and a few are pathogenic for man.

brewer's y. *Saccharomyces cerevisiae*, used in brewing beer, making alcoholic liquors, and baking bread.

dried y. dried cells of any suitable strain of *Saccharomyces cerevisiae*, usually a byproduct of the brewing industry; used as a natural source of protein and B-complex vitamins.

yellow ('yeloh) 1. the colour produced by stimulation by light waves of wavelength of 571.5 to 578.5 nm. 2. a dye or stain that produces a yellow colour.

y. fever an acute, notifiable, infectious viral disease, transmitted by the female of certain types of mosquitoes, and characterized by fever, jaundice due to necrosis of the liver, and albuminuria.

Yellow fever is less rampant today largely because of vaccination and better control of the mosquitoes, but it is still a potential danger in tropical America and Africa. Among native inhabitants who contract the disease there is a mortality rate of about 5 per cent. In visitors from other climates, fatalities once ran as high as 40 per cent, but they are now much lower. With proper immunization precautions, a visitor from a temperate country today takes only a minimal risk.

The mosquito that transmits classic 'urban' yellow fever is *Aedes aegypti.* In the jungles of Brazil and in parts of Africa, in the absence of *Aedes aegypti*, the disease may be carried by a different type of mosquito, which lives in treetops. These forest mosquitoes can communicate the disease to forest workers and also to certain animals, such as monkeys and marmosets, which then serve as virus reservoirs and as sources of reinfection for man. This form of the disease is called jungle or sylvan yellow fever, and is difficult to control because of the virtual impossibility of eradicating the tropical tree-inhabiting mosquitoes.

SYMPTOMS AND TREATMENT. Yellow fever has an incubation period of 3 to 6 days. It then manifests itself suddenly and intensely with fever, headache, muscular aches, abdominal pain, vomiting, and prostration. A few days later, jaundice, usually mild, appears and the temperature suddenly falls. In the more serious cases, after up to 2 days of remission, the fever returns and the general symptoms having abated, worsen.

The disease runs its course in a little more than a week. Those who survive (and the great majority do) suffer no permanent damage. The jaundice completely disappears. Furthermore, these persons are immune from a second attack. In fatal cases, death is usually due to kidney, vascular, or, less often, liver failure.

There is no specific drug for the cure of yellow fever. The effects of the disease can be mitigated by analgesics, sedatives, strict bed rest, and a high-calorie, high-carbohydrate diet.

PATIENT CARE. The patient's fever is controlled with cold or tepid sponges and other measures to lower body temperature. (See also FEVER.) The diet consists of liquids and easily digested foods until the vomiting stops, and then is gradually increased. Intravenous infusions may be required if there is much vomiting and/or dehydration. The patient's bed and room should be well screened to prevent transmission of the fever to others via mosquitoes.

PREVENTION. Urban yellow fever can be controlled by eradication of *Aedes aegypti.* Travellers to endemic areas should be vaccinated. This gives protection for at least 10 years.

visual y. all-*trans* retinal (see RETINAL [2]).

Yersinia (yər'sini·ə) a genus of nonmotile, ovoid or rod-shaped, nonencapsulated, gram-negative bacteria (family Enterobacteriaceae); *Y. pestis* causes plague in man and rodents, transmitted from rat to rat and from rat to man by the rat flea, and from man to man by the human body louse; *Y. pseudotuberculosis* causes pseudotuberculosis in rodents and mesenteric lymphadenitis in man.

yoghurt ('yogət) a form of curdled milk produced by fermentation with organisms of the genus *Lactobacillus.*

yoke (yohk) a connecting structure; a depression or ridge connecting two structures.

yolk (yohk) the stored nutrient of the ovum.

Young–Helmholtz theory (,yung'helmhohlts) the theory that colour vision depends on three sets of retinal receptors, corresponding to the colours red, green, and violet.

Young's rule (yungz) the dose of a drug for a child is obtained by multiplying the adult dose by the child's age in years and dividing the result by the sum of the child's age plus 12.

ytterbium (i'tərbi·əm) a chemical element, atomic number 70, atomic weight 173.04, symbol Yb. See table of elements in Appendix 2.

yttrium ('itri·əm) a chemical element, atomic number 39, atomic weight 88.905, symbol Y. See table of elements in Appendix 2.

Z

Z symbol, *atomic number.*

Z-plasty ('zed,plastee) a method of excising a scar (or skin defect) and resuturing it in a plane at right angles to its original direction, thus overcoming a contracture; achieved by means of relieving incisions placed one at each end of the scar but on opposing sides and transposing the triangular flaps thus created.

Zantac ('zantak) trademark for preparations of ranitidine, an ulcer-healing drug.

Zarontin (zə'rontin) trademark for a preparation of ethosuximide, an anticonvulsant.

zein ('zee·in) maize protein.

Zen (Zen Buddhism) (zen) eastern teaching that a form of meditation which consists of contemplating one's essential nature, to the exclusion of all else, thus achieving a 'stilling of the mind', provides the way to enlightenment. This state of enlightenment enables one to appreciate the true, mystical, unanalysed nature of things beyond the normal, rational, conscious manner of ordinary knowing. Zen has influenced many humanistic approaches to psychotherapy.

Zenker's necrosis (degeneration) ('zengkəz) hyaline degeneration and necrosis of striated muscle.

zero ('ziə·roh) the point on a thermometer scale from which the graduations begin. The zero of the Celsius (centigrade) scale is the ice point; on the Fahrenheit scale it is 32 degrees below the ice point.

absolute z. the lowest possible temperature, designated 0 on the Kelvin or Rankine scale, the equivalent of –273.15 °C or –459.67 °F.

Ziehl–Neelsens's method (,ziel'neelsənz) a method of staining tubercle bacilli for microscopic study.

Zieve's syndrome (zeevz) an acute self-limiting haemolytic anaemia, associated with hyperlipaemia and usually following alcoholic intoxication.

zimmer ('zimə) the tradename of a metal, light-weight walking aid, and commonly applied to other products of similar design and weight. Predominately used by the elderly to assist in rehabilitation.

Zinacef ('zinəsef) trademark for preparations of cefuroxime, an antibiotic.

zinc (zingk) a chemical element, atomic number 30, atomic weight 65.37, symbol Zn. See table of elements in Appendix 2. Zinc is a trace element that is a component of several enzymes, including DNA and RNA polymerases, and carbonic anhydrase. It is abundant in red meat, shellfish, liver, peas, lentils, beans, and rice. A well-balanced diet assures adequate intake of zinc. Those who may suffer from zinc deficiency include persons on a strictly vegetarian diet and those who are on a high-fibre diet. In the latter case, the zinc is bound to the fibre and is eliminated in the faeces without having been absorbed through the intestinal wall. Poor absorption of zinc also can occur in persons with chronic and severe bowel disease.

The recommended daily intake of zinc is 15 mg for an adult. A severe deficiency of zinc can retard growth in children, cause a low sperm count in adult males, and retard wound healing. Signs of a deficiency include anorexia and a diminished sense of taste. An excessive intake of zinc can interfere with the body's utilization of copper and other trace elements, and produce diarrhoea, nausea, vomiting, and other signs of intestinal irritation.

z. acetate a salt used as an astringent and styptic.

z. chloride a salt used topically as an astringent desensitizer for dentine, caustic antiseptic, and deodorant.

z. gelatin a mixture of zinc oxide, gelatin, glycerin and purified water; used topically as a protectant.

z. ointment a preparation of zinc oxide and mineral oil in white ointment; used topically as an astringent and protectant.

z. oxide a compound used as a topical astringent and protectant.

z. stearate a compound of zinc with stearic and palmitic acids; used as a water-repellent protective powder in dermatoses.

z. sulphate a compound used as an ophthalmic astringent.

z. undecylenate a compound used topically in 20 per cent ointment as an antifungal agent.

zirconium (zər'kohni·əm) a chemical element, atomic number 40, atomic weight 91.22, symbol Zr. See table of elements in Appendix 2.

Zn chemical symbol, *zinc.*

zo(o)- word element. [Gr.] *animal.*

zoacanthosis (,zoh·akən'thohsis) a dermatitis caused by penetration into the skin, of bristles, hairs, etc., of lower animals.

zoanthropy (zoh'anthrəpee) the delusion that one has become a beast adj. adj. **zoanthropic.**

zoetic (zoh'etik) pertaining to life.

Zollinger–Ellison syndrome (,zolinjə'elisən) a triad comprising intractable, sometimes fulminating, atypical peptic ulcers; extreme gastric hyperacidity; and nonbeta-cell, gastrin-secreting islet cell tumours (gastrinomas) of the pancreas, which might be single or multiple, small or large, benign or malignant.

zona ('zohnə) pl. *zonae* [L.] 1. zone. 2. herpes zoster.

z. fasciculata the thick middle layer of the adrenal gland.

z. glomerulosa the outermost layer of the adrenal cortex.

z. ophthalmica herpetic infection of the cornea.

z. pellucida 1. the transparent, noncellular, secreted layer surrounding an ovum. 2. area pellucida.

z. radiata a zona pellucida exhibiting conspicuous radial striations.

z. reticularis the innermost layer of the adrenal cortex.

z. striata a zona pellucida exhibiting conspicuous striations.

zone (zohn) an encircling region or area; by extension, any area with specific characteristics or boundary.

ciliary z. the outer of the two regions into which the anterior surface of the iris is divided by the angular line.

comfort z. an environmental temperature between 13 and 21 °C (55 and 70 °F) with a humidity of 30 to 55 per cent.

epileptogenic z. an area, stimulation of which may provoke an epileptic seizure.

erogenous z's, erotogenic z's areas of the body whose stimulation produces erotic desire, e.g., the oral, anal, and genital orifices, and the nipples.

hypnogenic z., hypnogenous z. an area of the body pressure on which will characteristically induce sleep.

transitional z. the circle in the equator of the lens of the eye in which epithelial fibres are developed into lens fibres.

zonethesia (,zohnis'theezi·ə) a sensation of constriction, as by a girdle.

zonifugal (zoh'nifyuhg'l) passing outward from a zone or region.

zonipetal (zoh'nipit'l) passing toward a zone or region.

zonography (zə'nogrəfee) thick-slice tomography.

zonula ('zohnyuhlə) pl. *zonulae* [L.] zonule.

zonular ('zonyuhlə) pertaining to a zonule.

z. fibres the suspensory ligaments that support the lens.

zonule ('zohnyool, 'zo-) a small zone.

ciliary z., z. of Zinn a series of fibres connecting the ciliary body and lens of the eye, holding the lens in place.

zonulitis (,zohnyuh'lietis) inflammation of the ciliary

zonule.

zonulolysis (ˌzonyuh'lolisis) dissolution of the ciliary zonule by use of enzymes, to permit surgical removal of the lens.

zonulotomy (ˌzonyuh'lotəmee) incision of the ciliary zonule.

zonulysin (ˌzonyuh'liesin) a proteolytic enzyme that may be used in eye surgery to dissolve the suspensory ligament.

zoo- word element. [Gr.] *animal.*

zoodermic (ˌzoh·ə'dərmik) performed with the skin of an animal, especially in reference to skin grafts.

zoogenous (zoh'ojənəs) 1. acquired from animals. 2. viviparous.

zoogeny (zoh'ojənee) the development and evolution of animals.

zoogony (zoh'ogənee) the production of living young from within the body. adj. **zoogonous.**

zoografting ('zoh·ohˌgrahfting) heterogenous grafting of animal tissue or organs to man.

zooid ('zoh·oyd) 1. animal-like. 2. an animal-like object or form. 3. an individual in a united colony of animals.

zoolagnia (ˌzoh·ə'lagni·ə) sexual attraction toward animals. Called also *bestiality.*

zoology (zoh'oləjee, zoo-) the biology of animals.

Zoomastigophora (ˌzoh·ohˌmasti'gofə·rə) a class of protozoa (subphylum Mastigophora), including all the flagellates that parasitize higher animals.

zoonosis (ˌzoh·ə'nohsis, ˌzooə'nohsis) pl. *zoonoses;* disease of animals transmissible to man. adj. **zoonotic.**

zooparasite (ˌzoh·oh'parəˌsiet) any parasitic animal organism or species. adj. **zooparasitic.**

zoopathology (ˌzoh·ohpə'tholəjee) the science of the diseases of animals.

zoophagous (zoh'ofəgəs) carnivorous.

zoophilia (ˌzoh·ə'fili·ə) abnormal fondness for animals.

zoophobia (ˌzoh·ə'fohbi·ə) abnormal fear of animals.

zooplasty ('zoh·əˌplastee) zoografting.

zoopsia (zoh'opsi·ə) a hallucination with vision of animals.

zoospore ('zoh·ohˌspor) a motile mitospore; a motile, flagellated, asexual spore, as produced by certain algae and fungi.

zootoxin (ˌzoh·oh'toksin) a toxic substance of animal origin, e.g., venom of snakes, spiders, and scorpions.

zoster ('zostə) herpes zoster.

zosteriform, zosteroid (zo'steriˌfawm; 'zostəˌroyd) resembling herpes zoster.

Zovirax ('zohviraks) trademark for preparations of acyclovir, an antiviral.

Zr chemical symbol, *zirconium.*

zwitterion ('tsvitə·rieən) an ion that has both positive and negative regions of charge. Called also dipolar ion.

zyg(o)- word element. [Gr.] *yoked, joined, a junction.*

zygal ('zieg'l) shaped like a yoke.

zygapophysis (ˌziegə'pofisis) the articular process of a vertebra.

zygion ('ziji·ən) the most lateral point on the zygomatic arch.

zygodactyly (ˌziegoh'daktilee, ˌzi-) union of digits by soft tissues (skin), without bony fusion of the phalanges involved.

zygoma (zie'gohmə, zi-) 1. the zygomatic process of the temporal bone. 2. zygomatic arch. 3. a term sometimes applied to the zygomatic bone.

zygomatic (ˌziegoh'matik, ˌzi-) pertaining to zygomatic bone.

z. arch the arch formed by the processes of the zygomatic and temporal bones.

z. bone the bone forming the hard part of the cheek and the lower, lateral portion of the rim of the orbit.

z. process a projection from the frontal or temporal bone, or from the maxilla, by which they articulate with the zygomatic bone.

zygomaticofacial (ˌziegohˌmatikoh'fayshəl, ˌzi-) pertaining to the zygoma and face.

zygomaticotemporal (ˌziegohˌmatikoh'tempə·rəl, ˌzi-) pertaining to the zygoma and temporal bone.

zygon ('ziegon, 'zi-) the stem connecting the two branches of a zygal fissure.

zygosity (zie'gositee, zi-) the condition relating to conjugation, or to the zygote, as *(a)* the state of a cell or individual in regard to the alleles determining a specific character, whether identical (homozygosity) or different (heterozygosity); or *(b)* in the case of twins, whether developing from one zygote (monozygosity) or two (dizygosity).

zygote ('ziegoht, 'zi-) the cell resulting from union of a male and a female gamete; the fertilized ovum. More precisely, the cell after synapsis at the completion of fertilization until first clevage. adj. **zygotic.** See also REPRODUCTION.

zygotene ('ziegohˌteen, 'zi-) the synaptic phase of the first meiotic prophase in which the two leptotene chromosomes undergo pairing by the formation of synaptonemal complexes to form a bivalent.

Zyloric trademark for preparations of allopurinol, an inhibitor of uric acid production in the body; used in prevention of acute attacks of gout.

zym(o)- word element. [Gr] *enzyme, fermentation.*

zymase ('ziemayz) enzyme.

zymic ('ziemik) pertaining to enzymes or fermentation.

zymogen ('ziemohˌjen) an inactive precursor that is converted into an active enzyme by action of an acid or another enzyme or by other means; a proenzyme. adj. **zymogenic.**

zymosis (zie'mohsis) 1. fermentation. 2. the development of an infectious disease.

Appendices

1. Degrees, Organizations and Abbreviations
2. Units of measurement and Table of Chemical Elements
3. Useful Addresses

Appendix 1

Degrees, Organizations and Abbreviations

Degrees

ADM Advanced Diploma in Midwifery
BA Bachelor of Arts
BAO Bachelor of the Art of Obstetrics
BC, BCh, BChir Bachelor of Surgery
BChD, BDS Bachelor of Dental Surgery
BHyg Bachelor of Hygiene
BM Bachelor of Medicine
BS, ChB Bachelor of Surgery
CM, ChM Master of Surgery
CNN Certificated Nursery Nurse
CPH Certificate of Public Health
CSP Chartered Society of Physiotherapists
DA Diploma in Anaesthetics
DCH Diploma in Child Health
DCh Doctor of Surgery
DChO Doctor of Opthalmic Surgery
DCMT Doctor of Clinical Medicine of the Tropics
DCP Diploma in Clinical Pathology
DDH Diploma in Dental Health
DDO Diploma in Dental Orthopaedics
DDPH Diploma in Dental Public Health
DDS Doctor of Dental Surgery
DGO Diploma in Gynaecology and Obstetrics
DHyg Doctor of Hygiene
DIH Diploma in Industrial Health
DLO Diploma in Laryngology and Otology
DM Doctor of Medicine
DMD Doctor of Dental Medicine
DMR Diploma in Medical Radiology
DMRE Diploma in Medical Radiology and Electrology
DN Diploma in Nursing, Doctor of nursing
DNE Diploma in Nursing Education
DO Diploma in Opthalmology
DObstRCOG Diploma in Obstetrics of the Royal College of Obstetricians and Gynaecologists
DOMS Diploma in Ophthalmological Medicine and Surgery
DOrth Diploma in Orthodontics
DPA Diploma in Public Administration
DPD Diploma in Public Dentistry
DPhysMed Diploma in Physical Medicine
DPH Diploma in Public Health
DPhil Doctor of Philosophy
DPM Diploma in Psychological Medicine
DR Diploma in Radiology
DRCPath Diploma of the Royal College of Pathologists
DSc Doctor of Science

DSSc Diploma in Sanitary Science
DTH Diploma in Tropical Hygiene
DTM Diploma in Tropical Medicine
EN(G) Enrolled Nurse (General)
EN(M) Enrolled Nurse (Mental)
EN(MH) Enrolled Nurse (Mental Handicap)
FACP Fellow of American College of Physicians
FACS Fellow of American College of Surgeons
FBPsS Fellow of British Psychological Society
FCSP Fellow of the Chartered Society of Physiotherapists
FETC Further Education Teaching Certificate
FDS Fellow of Dental Surgery
FFA Fellow of Faculty of Anaesthetists
FFARCS Fellow of the Faculty of Anaesthetists, Royal College of Surgeons
FFHom Fellow of Faculty of Homeopathy
FFR Fellow of Faculty of Radiologists
FLS Fellow of Linnean Society
FPS Fellow of the Pharmaceutical Society
FRACP Fellow of Royal Australian College of Physicians
FRACS Fellow of Royal Australian College of Surgeons
FRCGP Fellow of Royal College of General Practitioners
FRCOG Fellow of Royal College of Obstetricians and Gynaecologists
FRcn Fellow of the Royal College of Nursing
FRCP Fellow of Royal College of Physicians of London
FRCPE* Fellow of Royal College of Physicians of Edinburgh
FRCPI Fellow of the Royal College of Physicians of Ireland
FRCPath Fellow of Royal College of Pathologists
FRCPsych Fellow of the Royal College of Psychiatrists
FRCS Fellow of Royal College of Surgeons of England
FRCSE Fellow of Royal College of Surgeons of Edinburgh
FRCSI Fellow of the Royal College of Surgeons of Ireland
FRES Fellow of Royal Entomological Society
FRFPS Fellow of the Royal Faculty of Physicians and Surgeons
FRIPHH Fellow of Royal Institute of Public Health and Hygiene
FRS Fellow of Royal Society
FRSE Fellow of the Royal Society of Edinburgh
FRSH Fellow of the Royal Society of Health
FRSM Fellow of the Royal Society of Medicine
FRSanI Fellow of Royal Sanitary Institute
FSR(R) Fellow of the Society of Radiographers (Radiography)
FSS Fellow of Royal Statistical Society
HVCert Health Visitors Certificate
LAH Licentiate of Apothecaries Hall, Dublin
LDS Licentiate in Dental Surgery
LDSc Licentiate in Dental Science
LM Licentiate in Midwifery
LMS Licentiate in Medicine and Surgery
LMSSA Licentiate in Medicine and Surgery, Society of Apothecaries
LRCP Licentiate of Royal College of Physicians
LRCPE Licentiate of Royal College of Physicians (Edinburgh)
LRFPS Licentiate of Royal Faculty of Physicians and Surgeons
LSA Licentiate of Society of Apothecaries
LSSc Licentiate of Sanitary Science
MA Master of Arts
MAO Master of the Art of Obstetrics
MAOT Member of the Association of Occupational Therapists
MB Bachelor of Medicine
M-C Medico-Chirurgical
MC, MCh, MChir Master of Surgery

MChD Master of Dental Surgery
MChOrth Master of Orthopaedic Surgery
MChS Member of the Society of Chiropodists
MCPath Member of College of Pathology
MCPS Member of College of Physicians and Surgeons
MCSP Member of the Chartered Society of Physiotherapists
MD Doctor of Medicine
MDentSc Master of Dental Science
MDS Master of Dental Surgery
MFCP Member of the Faculty of Community Physicians
MFHom Member of the Faculty of Homeopathy
MHyg Master of Hygiene
MMSA Master of Midwifery of Society of Apothecaries
MPH Master of Public Health
MPS Member of the Pharmaceutical Society
MRCGP Member of Royal College of General Practitioners
MRCOG Member of Royal College of Obstetricians and Gynaecologists
MRCP Member of Royal College of Physicians of London
MRCPath Member of Royal College of Pathologists
MRCPsych Member of the Royal College of Psychiatrists
MRCS Member of Royal College of Surgeons of England
MS Master of Surgery
MRSH Member of the Royal Society for the Promotion of Health
MSA Member of the Society of Apothecaries
MSRG Member of the Society of Remedial Gymnasts
MSR(R) Member of the Society of Radiographers (Radiography)
MSR(T) Member of the Society of Radiographers (Radiotherapy)
MSc Master of Science
MTD Midwife Teachers' Diploma
OHNC Occupational Health Nursing Certificate
ONC Orthopaedic Nursing Certificate
OND Ophthalmic Nursing Diploma
PhD Doctor of Philosophy
RCNT Registered Clinical Nurse Teacher
RFN Registered Fever Nurse
RGN Registered General Nurse
RHV Registered Health Visitor
RM Registered Midwife
RMN Registered Mental Nurse
RN Registered Nurse (USA and other overseas countries)
RNMD Registered Nurse for Mental Defectives
RNMH Registered Nurse for the Mentally Handicapped
RNMS Registered Nurse for the Mentally Subnormal
RNT Registered Nurse Tutor
RSCN Registered Sick Children's Nurse
ScD Doctor of Science
SCM State Certified Midwife
SEN State Enrolled Nurse
SRN State Registered Nurse
TDD Tuberculous Diseases Diploma

*This may be written as FRCPEd, FRCP(Ed), FRCP(Edin), or FRCPE. It is correct to add the College after the MRCP or FRCS of the Scottish Royal Colleges.

Organizations

ABPN Association of British Paediatric Nurses
ASTMS Association of Scientific Technical and Managerial Staffs
BDA British Dental Association

BMA British Medical Association
BP British Pharmacopoeia
BRCS British Red Cross Society
CCD Central Council for the Disabled
CCHE Central Council for Health Education
CMB Central Midwives' Board
CoHSE Confederation of Health Service Employees
CSP Chartered Society of Physiotherapists
CU Casualties Union
DDA Dangerous Drugs Act
DNA District Nursing Association
FNIF Florence Nightingale International Foundation
GMC General Medical Council
HSA Hospital Savings Association
ICN International Council of Nurses
ICW International Council of Women
IHF International Hospitals Federation
MIND National Association for Mental Health
NALGO National Association of Local Government Officers
NAMCW National Association for Maternal and Child Welfare
NAMH National Association for Mental Health
NAWCH National Association for the Welfare of Children in Hospital
NHS National Health Service
NHSR National Hospital Service Reserve
NNEB National Nursery Exmination Board
NUPE National Union of Public Employees
PMRAFNS Princess Mary's Royal Air Force Nursing Service
QARANC Queen Alexandra's Royal Army Nursing Corps
QARNNS Queen Alexandra's Royal Naval Nursing Service
QHP Queen's Honorary Physician
QHNS Queen's Honorary Nursing Sister
QHS Queen's Honorary Surgeon
QIDN Queen's Institute of District Nursing
RADC Royal Army Dental Corps
RAMC Royal Army Medical Corps
RCM Royal College of Midwives
Rcn Royal College of Nursing and National Council of Nurses of the United Kingdom
RHA Regional Health Authority
RMO Resident Medical Officer
RRC Royal Red Cross
StAAA St Andrew's Ambulance Association
StJAA St John Ambulance Association
StJAB St John Ambulance Brigade
VAD Voluntary Aid Detachment
WHO World Health Organization
WPHOA Women Public Health Officers' Association
WRVS Women's Royal Voluntary Service

Appendix 1

Medical Abbrevations

The use of abbreviations is a practice forced upon health professionals by the necessity to be brief and quick when writing notes or instructions. Abbreviations are so easy to misinterpret that great care should be exercised in their use. The problem is that there is only a little standardization and therefore the list contains only those that are generally and widely used and are not peculiar to one hospital or one department. Many medical abbreviations have a Latin origin and when this is the case the Latin words are given in brackets after the abbreviation.

aa (ana) of each
a.c. (ante cibum) before meals
ad to; up to
ad lib. (ad libitum) as much as needed
aet. (aetas) aged
A/G *ratio* albumin/globulin ratio
AHA Area Health Authority
alb. albumin
alt. dieb. (alternis diebus) every other day
alt. hor. (alternis horis) every other hour
alt. noct. (alternis noctibus) every other night
AN antenatal
ante *(ante)* before
AP anteroposterior
APH antepartum haemorrhage
APT alum-precipitated toxoid
aq. (aqua) water
aq.-dist. (aqua distillata) distilled water
ARM artificial rupture of membranes
Ba.E barium enema
Ba.M barium meal
BBA born before arrival
BCG Bacille Calmette-Guérin
b.d. or ***b.i.d. (bis in die)*** twice daily
BI bone injury
bib. (bibe) drink
BID brought in dead
BMR basal metabolic rate
BNF British National Formulary (with date)
BO bowels opened
BP blood pressure or British Pharmacopoeia (with date)
BPC British Pharmaceutical Codex (with date)
BS breath sounds
C *(centum gradus)* centigrade
c. (circa) about
c. (cum) with
Ca. carcinoma
caps (capsula) capsule
CCF congestive cardiac failure
cf. compare
circ. circumcision
CF cystic fibrosis
cm centimetre
CNS central nervous system
c.o. complains of
Crem (cremor) cream
CSF cerebrospinal fluid
CSOM chronic suppurative otitis media
CSU catheter specimen of urine
CVS cardiovascular system
Cx cervix
D&C dilatation and curettage
DDA Dangerous Drugs Act
dil. (dilutus) dilute
DMC District Medical Committee
DMT District Management Team
DNA did not attend
DT delirium tremens
D and V diarrhoea and vomiting
DU duodenal ulcer
DXR deep X-ray
ECG electrocardiogram
ECT electroconvulsive therapy
EDC expected date of confinement
EDD expected date of delivery
EEG electroencephalogram
ENT ear, nose and throat
e.s. (enema saponis) soap enema
ESN educationally subnormal
ESR erythrocyte sedimentation rate
EUA examination under anaesthesia
ext. (extractum) extract
F Fahrenheit
FB foreign body
FH fetal heart or family history
FHH fetal heart heard
FHNH fetal heart not heard
Fib. fibula
fl. (fluidum) fluid
FMF fetal movements felt
FPC Family Practitioner Committee
ft. (fiat) let there be made
FTM fractional test meal
g gram
GA general anaesthetic
G and O gas and oxygen
GB gall-bladder
GC gonorrhoea
GCFT gonorrhoea complement fixation test
GI gastrointestinal
GP general practitioner
GPI general paralysis of insane
GTT glucose tolerance test
GU gastric ulcer

***gt.* (*gutta*)** drop (eye-drops)
Gyn. gynaecology
h.* (*hora*) *hour
Hb haemoglobin
HMC Hospital Management Committee
HP house physician
HS house surgeon
***h.s.* (*hora somni*)** at bedtime
HV health visitor
***id.* (*idem*)** the same
***i.e.* (*id est*)** that is
***in d.* (*in dies*)** daily
IP inpatient
IQ intelligence quotient
***ISQ* (*in statu quo*)** without change
IV intravenous
IVP intravenous pyelogram
IZS insulin zinc suspension
KJ knee jerk
KP keratitis punctata
l litre (should be written in full)
LA local anaesthetic or local authority
Lab. laboratory
LE cells lupus erythematosus cells
LHA Local Health Authority
LIF left iliac fossa
LIH left inguinal hernia
***liq.* (*liquor*)** a solution in water
LMC Local Medical Committee
LMP last menstrual period
LOA left occipitoanterior
LOP left occipitoposterior
LSCS lower segment caesarean section
LV left ventricle
***M.* (*misce*)** mix
m. minim
mCi millicurie
MCD mean corpuscular diameter
MCH mean corpuscular haemoglobin
MCHC mean corpuscular haemoglobin concentration
MCV mean corpuscular volume
mEq milliequivalent
***mist.* (*mistura*)** mixture
mm millimetre
mmHg millimetres of mercury
MMR mass miniature radiography
MO Medical Officer
MOH Medical Officer of Health
MRC Medical Research Council
MS multiple sclerosis
MSU midstream urine
MSW medical social worker (almoner)
NAD no abnormality detected
NBI no bone injury
neg. negative
NG new growth
***no.* (*numero*)** number
***noct.* (*nocte*)** at night
NOTB National Ophthalmic Treatment Board
***n.p.* (*nomen proprium*)** give proper name
NPU not passed urine
OA osteo-arthritis
Ob. obstetrics
OE on examination
***Omn. hor.* (*omni hora*)** every hour
***Omn. noct.* (*omni nocte*)** every night
Op. operation
OP outpatient
PA pernicious anaemia
Path. pathology
PBI protein bound iodine
***p.c.* (*post cibum*)** after meals
PCO patient complains of
PID prolapsed intervertebral disc
PMH previous medical history
PN post-natal
POP plaster of Paris
PP private patients
PPH post-partum haemorrhage
***p.r.* (*per rectum*)** rectal examination or by the rectum
***p.r.n.* (*pro re nata*)** whenever necessary
PSW psychiatric social worker
PY physiotherapy
PU passed urine
PUO pyrexia of unknown origin
***p.v.* (*per vaginam*)** vaginal examination or by the vagina
PZI protamine zinc insulin
***q.* (*quaque*)** every
***q.h.* (*quaque hora*)** every hour
***q.i.d.* (*quater in die*)** four times a day
***quotid.* (*quotidie*)** daily
***q.s.* (*quantum sufficiat*)** sufficient quantity
Rx (*recipe*) take
RA rheumatoid arthritis
RBC red blood corpuscle
Rh. rhesus factor
RHA Regional Health Authority
RIF right iliac fossa
RIH right inguinal hernia
RLL right lower lobe
RMO Resident Medical Officer
ROA right occipitoanterior
ROL right occipitolateral
ROP right occipitoposterior
RS respiratory system
RSO Resident Surgical Officer
***s.* (*sine*)** without
SB stillborn
SG specific gravity
***sig.* (*signetur*)** let it be labelled
SMR submucous resection
***sol.* (*solutis*)** solution

***s.o.s.* (*si opus sit*)** if necessary
sp. gr. specific gravity
***ss.* (*semis*)** half
***stat.* (*statim*)** at once
SWD short wave diathermy
***syr.* (*syrupus*)** syrup
T and A tonsils and adenoids
TAB typhoid and paratyphoid A and B
TB tuberculosis
TCA to come again
TCI to come in
***t.i.d.* (*ter in die*)** three times a day
TPR temperature, pulse and respiration
***tr.* (*tinctura*)** tincture
***Ung.* (*unguentum*)** ointment
VD venereal disease
***vi* (*virgo intacta*)** virgin
***Vin.* (*vinum*)** wine
VV varicose vein
Vx vertex
WBC white blood corpuscle
WR Wassermann reaction
wt weight
XR X-ray
YOB year of birth

Appendix 2
Units of Measurement and
Table of Chemical Elements

SI Units (Système Internationale d'Unités)

Base units

Physical quantity	Name of unit	Symbol
mass	kilogram	kg
length	metre	m
time	second	s
electric current	ampere	A
temperature	kelvin	K
luminous intensity	candela	cd
amount of substance	mole	mol

Derived units

Derived units to measure other quantities are obtained by multiplying or dividing any two or more of the seven base units. Some of these have their own names and symbols. For example:

Physical quantity	Name of unit	Symbol	Base units
force	newton	N	kg m/s^2 ($kg{\cdot}m{\cdot}s^{-2}$)
pressure	pascal	Pa	N/m^2 ($N{\cdot}m^{-2}$)
energy, work, heat	joule	J	N m ($N{\cdot}m$)
power	watt	W	J/s ($J{\cdot}s^{-1}$)

Prefixes used for multiples

Figure	Prefix	Sign
10^{-12}	pico-	p
10^{-9}	nano-	n
10^{-6}	micro-	μ
10^{-3}	milli-	m
10^{-2}	centi-	c
10^{-1}	deci-	d
10	deca-	da
10^2	hecto-	h
10^3	kilo-	k
10^6	mega-	M
10^9	giga-	G
10^{12}	tera-	T

Appendix 2

Capacity

The SI unit of *volume* is the cubic metre (m^3), but the litre (l) is more commonly and acceptedly used (it is equivalent to 1 dm^3).

1000 microlitres (μl)	=	1 millilitre (ml)		
10 millilitres	=	1 centilitre (cl)		
100 millilitres	=	10 centilitres	=	1 decilitre (dl)
1000 millilitres	=	100 centilitres	=	10 decilitres = 1 litre (l)

1 cubic centimetre (cm^3 *or* cc) = 1 millilitre
1 cubic decimetre (dm^3) = 1 litre

Domestic equivalents (approximate)

1 teaspoon	=	5 ml
1 dessertspoon	=	10 ml
1 tablespoon	=	20 ml
1 sherryglass	=	60 ml
1 teacup	=	142 ml
1 breakfastcup	=	230 ml
1 tumbler	=	285 ml

Weights

1000 micrograms (μg) = 1 milligram
1000 milligrams (mg) = 1 gram
1000 grams (g) = 1 kilogram
1000 kilograms (kg) = 1 metric tonne

Energy

A dietetic Calorie is the amount of heat required to raise the temperature of 1 litre of water 1 °C and is equal to 4.184 kilojoules.

1 gram of fat will produce 38 kilojoules or 9 Calories.
1 gram of protein will produce 17 kilojoules or 4 Calories.
1 gram of carbohydrate will produce 17 kilojoules or 4 Calories.

Comparative Temperatures

Celsius (°C)		Fahrenheit (°F)	Celsius (°C)	Fahrenheit (°F)
100	Boiling point	212	55	131
			50	122
95		203	45	113
90		194	44	112.2
85		185	43	109.4
80		176	42	107.6
75		167	41	105.8
70		158	40	104
65		149	39.5	103.1
60		140	39	102.2

Comparative Temperatures

Celsius (°C)	Fahrenheit (°F)	Celsius (°C)		Fahrenheit (°F)
38.5	101.3	32		89.6
38	100.4	31		87.8
37.5	99.5	30		86
37	98.6	25		77
36.5	97.7	20		68
36	96.8	15		59
35.5	95.9	10		50
35	95	5		41
34	93.2	0	Freezing point	32
33	91.4			

To convert readings of the Fahrenheit scale into Celsius degrees subtract 32, multiply by 5, and divide by 9, as follows:

$$98 - 32 = 66 \times 5 = 330 \div 9 = 36.6. \text{ Therefore } 98\ °F = 36.6\ °C.$$

To convert readings of the Celsius scale into Fahrenheit degrees multiply by 9, divide by 5, and add 32, as follows:

$$36.6 \times 9 = 330 \div 5 = 66 + 32 = 98. \text{ Therefore } 36.6\ °C = 98\ °F.$$

The term 'Celsius' (from the name of the Swede who invented the scale in 1742) is now being internationally used instead of 'centigrade', which term is employed in some countries to denote fractions of an angle.

Table of Chemical Elements

Element (date of discovery)	Symbol	Description
actinium (1899)	Ac	radioactive element associated with uranium
aluminium (1827)	Al	silvery-white metal, abundant in earth's crust, but not in free form
americium (1944)	Am	fourth transuranium element discovered
antimony (prehistoric)	Sb	exists in 4 allotropic forms
argon (1894)	Ar	colourless, odourless gas
arsenic (1250)	As	grey, black or yellow semimetallic solid
astatine (1940)	At	radioactive halogen
barium (1808)	Ba	silvery-white, alkaline earth metal
berkelium (1949)	Bk	fifth transuranium element discovered
beryllium (1798)	Be	light, steel-grey metal
bismuth (1753)	Bi	pinkish-white, crystalline, brittle metal
boron (1808)	B	crystalline or amorphous element, not occurring free in nature
bromine (1826)	Br	mobile, reddish-brown liquid, volatilizing readily to red vapour with disagreeable odour
cadmium (1817)	Cd	soft, bluish-white metal
caesium (1869)	Cs	silvery-white, soft, alkaline metal
calcium (1808)	Ca	metallic element, forming more than 3 per cent of earth's crust

Contd.

Appendix 2

Table of Chemical Elements

Element (date of discovery)	Symbol	Description
californium (1950)	Cf	sixth transuranium element discovered
carbon (prehistoric)	C	element widely distributed in nature
cerium (1803)	Ce	most abundant rare earth metal
chlorine (1774)	Cl	greenish-yellow, gas of the halogen group
chromium (1797)	Cr	steel-grey, lustrous, hard metal
cobalt (1735)	Co	brittle, hard metal
copper (prehistoric)	Cu	reddish, lustrous, malleable metal
curium (1944)	Cm	third transuranium element discovered
dysprosium (1886)	Dy	rare earth metal with metallic bright silver lustre
einsteinium (1952)	Es	seventh transuranium element discovered
element 108		no name yet proposed
element 109		no name yet proposed
erbium (1843)	Er	soft, malleable rare earth metal
europium (1896)	Eu	lustrous, silvery-white rare earth metal
fermium (1953)	Fm	eighth transuranium element discovered
fluorine (1771)	F	pale yellow, corrosive gas of the halogen group
francium (1939)	Fr	product of alpha disintegration of actinium
gadolinium (1880)	Gd	lustrous silvery-white rare earth metal
gallium (1875)	Ga	beautiful, silvery-appearing metal
germanium (1886)	Ge	greyish-white, brittle metal
gold (prehistoric)	Au	malleable yellow metal
hafnium (1923)	Hf	grey metal associated with zirconium
helium (1895)	He	inert gas
holmium (1879)	Ho	relatively soft and malleable rare earth metal
hydrogen (1766)	H	most abundant element in the universe
indium (1863)	In	soft, silvery-white metal
iodine (1811)	I	greyish-black, lustrous solid or violet-blue gas
iridium (1803)	Ir	white, brittle metal of platinum family
iron (prehistoric)	Fe	fourth most abundant element in earth's crust
krypton (1898)	Kr	inert gas
lanthanum (1839)	La	silvery-white, ductile, rare earth metal
lawrencium (1961)	Lr	tenth transuranium element discovered
lead (prehistoric)	Pb	bluish-white, lustrous, malleable metal
lithium (1817)	Li	lightest of all metals
lutetium (1907)	Lu	rare earth metal
magnesium (1808)	Mg	silvery-white metallic element, eighth in abundance in earth's crust
manganese (1774)	Mn	exists in 4 allotropic forms
mendelevium (1955)	Md	ninth transuranium element discovered
mercury (prehistoric)	Hg	heavy, silvery-white metal, liquid at ordinary temperatures
molybdenum (1782)	Mo	silvery-white, very hard metal
neodymium (1885)	Nd	exists in 2 allotropic forms
neon (1898)	Ne	inert gas
neptunium (1940)	Np	first transuranium element discovered
nickel (1751)	Ni	silvery-white, malleable metal
niobium (1801)	Nb	shiny white, soft ductile metal
nitrogen (1772)	N	colourless, odourless, inert element, making up 78 per cent of the air
nobelium (1958)	No	acceptance of this element considered premature
osmium (1803)	Os	bluish-white, hard metal of platinum family

Contd.

Appendix 2

Table of Chemical Elements

Element (date of discovery)	Symbol	Description
oxygen (1774)	O	colourless, odourless gas, third most abundant element in the universe
palladium (1803)	Pd	steel-white metal of the platinum family
phosphorus (1669)	P	white, red or black waxy solid, transparent when pure
platinum (1735)	Pt	silvery-white, malleable metal
plutonium (1940)	Pu	second transuranium element discovered
polonium (1898)	Po	very rare natural element
potassium (1807)	K	soft, silvery, alkali metal, seventh in abundance in earth's crust
praseodymium (1885)	Pr	soft, silvery rare earth metal
promethium (1941)	Pm	produced by irradiation of neodymium and praseodymium; identity established in 1945
protactinium (1917)	Pa	bright lustrous metal
radium (1898)	Ra	brilliant white, radioactive metal
radon (1900)	Rn	heaviest known gas
rhenium (1925)	Re	silvery-white lustrous metal
rhodium (1803)	Rh	silvery-white metal of platinum family
rubidium (1861)	Rb	soft, silvery-white, alkali metal
ruthenium (1844)	Ru	hard white metal of platinum family
samarium (1879)	Sm	bright silver lustrous metal
scandium (1879)	Sc	soft, silvery-white metal
selenium (1817)	Se	exists in several allotropic forms
silicon (1823)	Si	a relatively inert element, second in abundance in earth's crust
silver (prehistoric)	Ag	malleable, ductile metal with brilliant white lustre
sodium (1807)	Na	most abundant of alkali metals, sixth in abundance in earth's crust
strontium (1808)	Sr	exists in 3 allotropic forms
sulphur (prehistoric)	S	exists in several isotopic and many allotropic forms
tantalum (1802)	Ta	grey, heavy, very hard metal
technetium (1937)	Tc	first element produced artificially
tellurium (1782)	Te	silvery-white, lustrous element
terbium (1843)	Tb	silvery-grey, malleable, ductile rare earth metal
thallium (1861)	Tl	very soft, malleable metal
thorium (1828)	Th	silvery-white, lustrous metal
thulium (1879)	Tm	least abundant rare earth metal
tin (prehistoric)	Sn	malleable metal existing in 2 or 3 allotropic forms, changing from white to grey on cooling and back to white on warming
titanium (1791)	Tl	lustrous white metal
tungsten (1783)	W	steel-grey to tin-white metal
unnilhexium (1974)	Unh	thirteenth transuranium element discovered
unnilpentium (1970)	Unp	twelfth transuranium element discovered
unnilquadium (1969)	Unq	eleventh transuranium element discovered
unnilseptium (1981)	Uns	fourteenth transuranium element discovered
uranium (1789)	U	heavy, silvery-white metal
vanadium (1801)	V	bright, white metal
xenon (1898)	Xe	one of the so-called rare or inert gases
ytterbium (1878)	Yb	exists in 2 allotropic forms
yttrium (1794)	Y	rare earth metal with silvery metallic lustre
zinc (1746)	Zn	bluish-white, lustrous metal, malleable at 100–150°C
zirconium (1789)	Zr	greyish-white, lustrous metal

Appendix 2

Normal values

These normal values were compiled by Ruth Halliday SRN, St Bartholomew's Hospital, London.

Haematology

Basophil granulocytes	0.01–0.1 × 10^9/l
Eosinophil granulocytes	0.04–0.4 × 10^9/l
Erythrocyte sedimentation rate (ESR)	< 20 mm in 1 h
Haemoglobin	
male	14.0–17.7 g·dl^{-1}
female	12.2–15.2 g·dl^{-1}
Leukocytes	4.3–10.8 × 10^9/l
Mean corpuscular haemoglobin (MCH)	27–33 pg
Mean corpuscular haemoglobin concentration (MCHC)	32–35 g·dl^{-1}
Mean corpuscular volume (MCV)	80–96 fl
Monocytes	0.2–0.8 × 10^9/l
Neutrophil granulocytes	3.5–7.5 × 10^9/l
Packed cell volume (PCV)	
male	0.42–0.53 l·l^{-1}
female	0.36-0.45 l·l^{-1}
Plasma volume	45 ± 5 ml·kg^{-1}
Platelet count	150–400 × 10^9/l
Red cell folate	> 160 μg·l^{-1}
Red cell mass	
male	30 ± 5 ml·kg^{-1}
female	25 ± 5 ml·kg^{-1}
Reticulocyte count	0.5–2.5% of red cells
Serum B_{12}	150–675 pmol·l^{-1} (160–925 ng·l^{-1})
Serum folate	5–63 nmol·l^{-1} (3–20 μg·l^{-1})
Total blood volume	
male	75 ± 10 ml·kg^{-1}
female	70 ± ml·kg^{-1}
Coagulation	
Bleeding time (Ivy method)	3–8 min
Partial thromboplastin time (PTTK)	30–40 s
Prothrombin time	10–14 s

Biochemistry

Acid phosphatase	1–5 U·l^{-1}
Alanine aminotransferase (ALT)	5–30 U·l^{-1}
Albumin	34–48 g·l^{-1}
Alkaline phosphatase	25–115 U·l^{-1}
Alpha-l-antitrypsin	2–4 g·l^{-1}
Alpha-fetoprotein	< 10 kU·l^{-1}
Amylase	70–300 U·l^{-1}
Angiotensin-converting enzyme	204–360 U·l^{-1}
Aspartate aminotransferase (AST)	10–40 U·l^{-1}
Bicarbonate	22–30 mmol·l^{-1} (22–30 mEq·l^{-1})
Bilirubin	< 17 μmol·l^{-1} (0.3–1.5 mg·dl^{-1})
Calcium	2.2–2.67 mmol·l^{-1} (8.5–10.5 ng·dl^{-1})
Chloride	100–106 mmol·l^{-1} (100–106 mEq·l^{-1})

Appendix 2

Biochemistry

Cholinesterase	2.25–7.0 $U \cdot l^{-1}$
Copper	12–25 $\mu mol \cdot l^{-1}$ (100–200 $mg \cdot dl^{-1}$)
Complement—total haemolytic	150–250 $U \cdot mol^{-1}$
Creatinine	0.06–0.12 $mmol \cdot l^{-1}$ (0.6–1.5 $mg \cdot dl^{-1}$)
Creatinine kinase (CPK)	24–195 $U \cdot l^{-1}$
Ferritin	5.8–120 $nmol \cdot l^{-1}$ (15–250 $\mu g \cdot l^{-1}$)
Gamma glutamyl transferase (γ-GT)	10–40 $iu \cdot l^{-1}$
Glucose	4.5–5.6 $mmol \cdot l^{-1}$ (70–110 $mg \cdot dl^{-1}$)
Glycosylated haemoglobin (Hb_1Ac)	3.8–6.4%
Hydroxybutyric dehydrogenase (HBD)	40–125 $U \cdot l^{-1}$
Iron	13–32 $\mu mol \cdot l^{-1}$ (509–150 $\mu g \cdot dl^{-1}$)
Iron binding capacity (total)	42–80 $\mu mol \cdot l^{-1}$ (250–410 $\mu g \cdot dl^{-1}$)
Lactate dehydrogenase	240–525 $U \cdot l^{-1}$
Lead	1.8 $\mu mol \cdot l^{-1}$
Magnesium	0.7–1.1 $mmol \cdot l^{-1}$
Osmolality	280–296 $mmol \cdot kg^{-1}$ (280–296 $mosmol \cdot kg^{-1}$)
Phosphate	0.8–1.4 $mmol \cdot l^{-1}$
Potassium	3.5–5.0 $mmol \cdot l^{-1}$ (3.5–5.0 $mEq \cdot l^{-1}$)
Protein (total)	62–80 $g \cdot l^{-1}$ (6.2–8.0 $g \cdot dl^{-1}$)
Sodium	135–146 $mmol \cdot l^{-1}$ (135–146 $mEq \cdot l^{-1}$)
Urate	0.18–0.42 $mmol \cdot l^{-1}$ (3.0–7.0 $mg \cdot dl^{-1}$)
Urea	2.5–6.7 $mmol \cdot l^{-1}$ (8–25 $mg \cdot dl^{-1}$)
Vitamin A	0.5–2.1 $\mu mol \cdot l^{-1}$ (0.15–0.6 $\mu g \cdot ml^{-1}$)
Vitamin D	
—25-hydroxy	19.4–137 $nmol \cdot l^{-1}$ (8–55 $ng \cdot l^{-1}$)
—1,25-dihydroxy	62–155 $pmol \cdot l^{-1}$ (26–65 $pg \cdot l^{-1}$)
Zinc	7–18 $\mu mol \cdot l^{-1}$
Lipids and lipoproteins	
Cholesterol	3.9–7.8 $nmol \cdot l^{-1}$
Triglyceride	0.5–2.1 $nmol \cdot l^{-1}$
Phospholipid	2.9–5.2 $nmol \cdot l^{-1}$
Non-esterified fatty acids	
—male	0.19–0.78 $nmol \cdot l^{-1}$
—female	0.06–0.9 $nmol \cdot l^{-1}$
Lipoproteins	
—VLDL	0.128–0.645 $nmol \cdot l^{-1}$
—LDL	1.55–4.4 $nmol \cdot l^{-1}$
—HDL—male	0.7–2.0 $nmol \cdot l^{-1}$
—female	0.95–2.15 $nmol \cdot l^{-1}$
Lipids (total)	4.0–10 $g \cdot l^{-1}$ (400–1000 $mg \cdot dl^{-1}$)
Blood gases	
Arterial $P\text{CO}_2$	4.8–6.1 kPa (36–46 mmHg)
Arterial $P\text{O}_2$	10–13.3 kPa (75–100 mmHg); for every year over 60 *add* 0.13 kPa
Arterial $[H^+]$	35–45 $nmol \cdot l^{-1}$
Arterial pH	7.35–7.45
Urine values	
Calcium	7.5 mmol daily or less (300 mg daily or less)
Copper	0–1.6 μmol daily (0–100 μg daily)

Contd.

Appendix 2

Biochemistry

Creatinine	0.13–0.22 mmol·kg^{-1} body weight daily (15–25 mg·kg^{-1} body weight daily)
5-Hydroxyindole acetic acid	10–45 μmol daily (2–9 mg daily); amounts lower in females than males
Lead	0.39 μmol·l^{-1} or less (0.08 μg·ml^{-1} or 120 μg daily or less)
Protein (quantitative)	< 0.15 g per 24 h (< 150 mg per 24 h)

Thyroid Function Tests

Total serum thyroxine (T_4)	60–160 nmol·l^{-1}
Total serum triiodothyronine (T_3)	1.2–3.1 nmol·l^{-1}
Free serum thyroxine (T_4)	13–30 pmol·l^{-1}
Thyroid-stimulating hormone (TSH)	0.5–5.0 mu·l^{-1} (lower limit not definable on older assays)

Acceptable Weights

Acceptable weights as recommended by the Fogarty Conference (USA 1979) and the Royal College of Physicians (1983).

Height without shoes (m)	MEN Weight without clothes (kg)			WOMEN Weight without clothes (kg)		
	Acceptable average	Acceptable weight range	Obese	Acceptable average	Acceptable weight range	Obese
1.45				46.0	42–53	64
1.48				46.5	42–54	65
1.50				47.0	43–55	66
1.52				48.5	44–57	68
1.54				49.5	44–58	70
1.56				50.4	45–58	70
1.58	55.8	51–64	77	51.3	46–59	71
1.60	57.6	52–65	78	52.6	48–61	73
1.62	58.6	53–66	79	54.0	49–62	74
1.64	59.6	54–67	80	55.4	50–64	77
1.66	60.6	55–69	83	56.8	51–65	78
1.68	61.7	56–71	85	58.1	52–66	79
1.70	63.5	58–73	88	60.0	53–67	80
1.72	65.0	59–74	89	61.3	55–69	83
1.74	66.5	60–75	90	62.6	56–70	84

Acceptable Weights (cont.)

Acceptable weights as recommended by the Fogarty Conference (USA 1979) and the Royal College of Physicians (1983).

Height without shoes (m)	MEN Weight without clothes (kg)			WOMEN Weight without clothes (kg)		
	Acceptable average	Acceptable weight range	Obese	Acceptable average	Acceptable weight range	Obese
1.76	68.0	62–77	92	64.0	58–72	86
1.78	69.4	64–79	95	65.3	59–74	89
1.80	71.0	65–80	96			
1.82	72.6	66–82	98			
1.84	74.2	67–84	101			
1.86	75.8	69–86	103			
1.88	77.6	71–88	106			
1.90	79.3	73–90	108			
1.92	81.0	75–93	112			
BMI[1]	22.0	20.1–25.0	30.0	20.8	18.7–23.8	28.6

[1] *Body mass index* = weight/height^2 (kg/m^2).

From Bray, G. A. (ed.) (1979) *Obesity in America*, Proceedings of the Second Fogarty International Center Conference on Obesity, No. 79, Washington, US, DHEW.

Appendix 3
Useful Addresses

Accept Services UK (ACCEPT)
Accept Clinic
200 Seagrave Road
London SW6 1RQ

Action Health 2000/International Voluntary Health Association
35 Bird Farm Road
Fulbourn
Cambridge CB1 5DP

Action for Research into Multiple Sclerosis
4a Chapel Hill
Stansted
Essex CM24 8AG

Action on Smoking and Health (ASH)
Margaret Pyke House
5–11 Mortimer Street
London W1N 7RH

Age Concern England (National Old Peoples' Welfare Council)
60 Pitcairn Road
Mitcham
Surrey CR4 3LL

Al-Anon Family Groups UK and Eire
61 Great Dover Street
London SE1 4YF

Alcohol Concern (The National Agency of Alcohol Misuse)
305 Grays Inn Road
London WC1X 8QF

Alcoholics Anonymous
PO Box 514
11 Redcliffe Gardens
London SW10 9BQ

Alzheimer's Disease Society
3rd Floor
Bank Building
Fulham Broadway
London SW6 1EP

Anorexic Aid
The Priory Centre
11 Priory Road
High Wycombe
Bucks HP13 6SL

Anorexic Family Aid and National Information Centre
Sackville Place
44–48 Magdalen Street
Norwich
Norfolk NR3 1JE

Arthritis Care (formerly British Rheumatism and Arthritis Association)
6 Grosvenor Crescent
London SW1X 7ER

Arthritis and Rheumatism Council (ARC)
41 Eagle Street
London WC1R 4AR

Association for All Speech Impaired Children (AFASIC)
347 Central Markets
Smithfield
London EC1A 9NH

Association for Improvements in the Maternity Services (AIMS)
163 Liverpool Road
London N1 0RF

Association for Post-Natal Illness
7 Gowan Avenue
London SW6

Association for the Prevention of Addiction (APA)
56 New Oxford Street
London WC1A 1ES

Association for Research into Restricted Growth (ARRG)
7 Plover Road
Milborne Port
Dorset DT9 5DA

Association for Spina Bifida and Hydrocephalus (ASBAH)
22 Woburn Place
London WC1H 0EP

Association of Breast Feeding Mothers
131 Mayrow Road
London SE26

Association of British Paediatric Nurses (ABPN)
c/o Central Nursing Office
The Hospital for Sick Children
Great Ormond Street
London WC1

Association of Carers
First Floor
21–23 New Road
Chatham
Kent ME4 4JQ

Association of Community Health Councils for England and Wales
Mark Lemon Suite
Barclays Bank Chambers
254 Seven Sisters Road
London N4 2HZ

Association of Medical Secretaries
Tavistock House South
Tavistock Square
London WC1

Association of Nurse Administrators
13 Grosvenor Place
London SW1X 7EN

Association of Parents of Vaccine-Damaged Children
2 Church Street
Shipston-on-Stour
Warwickshire CV36 4AP

Association of Professions for Mentally Handicapped People (APMH)
Greytree Lodge
Second Avenue
Ross-on-Wye
Herefordshire HR9 7EG

Association of Radical Midwives
c/o Haringey Women's Centre
40 Turnpike Lane
London N8

Asthma Society
300 Upper Street
London N1 2XX

Baby Life Support Systems (BLISS)
44–45 Museum Street
London WC1A 1LY

Back Pain Association
31–33 Park Road
Teddington
Middx TW11 0AB

Birth Centre
101 Tufnell Park Road
London N7

British Agencies for Adoption and Fostering
11 Southwark Street
London SE1 1RQ

British Association for Cancer United Patients (BACUP)
121 Charterhouse Street
London EC1

British Association for Counselling
37a Sheep Street
Rugby
Warwickshire CV21 3BX

British Council for the Rehabilitation of the Disabled
25 Mortimer Street
London W1

British Deaf Association
38 Victoria Place
Carlisle
Cumbria CA1 1HU

British Diabetic Association
10 Queen Anne Street
London W1M 0BD

British Epilepsy Association
Anstey House
40 Hanover Square
Leeds LS3 1BE

British Geriatrics Society (BGS)
1 St. Andrew's Place
London NW1 4LB

British Guild for Sudden Infant Death Study
Pathology Department
Royal Infirmary
Cardiff CF2 1SZ

British Heart Foundation
102 Gloucester Place
London W1H 4DH

British Medical Association
BMA House
Tavistock Square
London WC1H 9JP

British Paediatric Association (BPA)
5 St. Andrew's Place
Regents Park
London NW1 4LB

British Pregnancy Advisory Service
Austry Manor
Wootton Wawen
Solihull
West Midlands B95 6DA

British Red Cross Society (BRCS)
9 Grosvenor Crescent
London SW1X 7EJ

British United Provident Association (BUPA)
24/27 Essex Street
London WC2

Brittle Bone Society
112 City Road
Dundee DD2 2PW

Appendix 3

Brook Advisory Centres
153a East Street
London SE17 2SD

Catholic Nurses' Guild of Great Britain
Bevendean Hospital
Brighton
East Sussex

Central Midwives Board
39 Harrington Gardens
London SW7 5JY

Central Midwives Board for Scotland
24 Dublin Street
Edinburgh EH1 3PU

Chest, Heart and Stroke Association
Tavistock House North
Tavistock Square
London WC1H 9JE

Children's Chest Circle
Tavistock House North
Tavistock Square
London WC1H 9JE

Cleft Lip and Palate Association
1 Eastwood Gardens
Kenton
Newcastle-upon-Tyne
NE3 3DQ

Coeliac Society
PO Box 220
High Wycombe
Bucks HP11 2HY

Colostomy Welfare Group
38–39 Eccleston Square
London SW1V 1PB

Committee on Safety of Drugs
Finsbury Square House
33/37a Finsbury Square
London EC2

Compassionate Friends
5 Lower Clifton Hill
Clifton
Bristol BS8

Council for the Education and Training of Health Visitors
Clifton House
Euston Road
London NW1 2RS

Cruse (National Organization for the Widowed and their Children)
Cruse House
126 Sheen Road
Richmond
Surrey TW9 1UR

Cystic Fibrosis Research Trust
Alexandra House
5 Blyth Road
Bromley
Kent BR1 3RS

Department of Health and Social Security (DHSS)
Alexander Fleming House
Elephant and Castle
London SE1 6BY

Depressives Associated
PO Box 5
Castle Town
Portland
Dorset DT5 1BQ

Down's Syndrome Association
12–13 Clapham Common Southside
London SW4 7AA

Drink Watchers
200 Seagrave Road
London SW6 1RQ

Emergency Bed Service
28 London Bridge Street
London SE1

English National Board for Nursing, Midwifery and Health Visiting (ENB)
Victory House
170 Tottenham Court Road
London W1P 0HA

Families Anonymous (FA)
88 Caledonian Road
London N1 9DN

Family Planning Association (FPA)
Margaret Pyke House
27–35 Mortimer Street
London W1N 7RJ

Family Welfare Association
501–505 Kingsland Road
Dalston
London E8 4AU

Federated Superannuation Scheme for Nurses and Hospital Officers
Rosehill
Park Road
Banstead
Surrey

Foresight – the Association for the Promotion of Preconceptual Care
The Old Vicarage
Church Lane
Witley
Godalming
Surrey GU8 5PN

Foundaton for the Study of Infant Deaths (Cot Death Research and Support)
15 Belgrave Square
London SW1X 8PS

Gamblers Anonymous and Gam-Anon
17–23 Blantyre Street
Cheyne Walk
London SW10 0DT

General Medical Council (GMC)
44 Hallam Street
London W1

General Nursing Council for England and Wales
23 Portland Place
London W1A 1BA

General Nursing Council for Scotland
5 Dunaway Street
Edinburgh EH3 6DP

General Register Office
Somerset House
Strand
London WC2

Gingerbread
Minerva Chambers
35 Wellington Street
London WC2E 7BN

Guild of St. Barnabas for Nurses
St. Helena's Retreat House
Drayton Green
London W13

Haemophilia Society
123 Westminster Bridge Road
London SE1 7HR

Health Education Council (HEC)
78 New Oxford Street
London WC1A 1AH

Health Services Superannuation Division
Hesketh House
200–220 Broadway
Fleetwood
Lancs FL7 8LG

Health Visitors' Association (HVA)
36 Eccleston Square
London SW1V 1PF

Help the Aged
16–18 St. James's Walk
London EC1R 0BE

Her Majesty's Prisons and Borstal Institutions Nursing Service
Her Majesty's Prison
Holloway
London N5 1PL

Hospital Administrative Staff College
2 Palace Court
London W2 4HS

Hospital Savings Association
30 Lancaster Gate
London W2 3LT

Hysterectomy Support Group (HSG)
11 Henryson Road
London SE4 1HL

Ileostomy Association of Great Britain and Ireland
Amblehurst House
Chobham
Woking
Surrey GU24 8PZ

Imperial Cancer Research Fund (ICRF)
PO Box 123
Lincoln's Inn Fields
London WC2A 3PX

Institute for the Study of Drug Dependence
1–4 Hatton Place
Hatton Garden
London EC1N 8ND

Institution of Environmental Health Officers
Chadwick House
48 Rushworth Street
London SE1 0QT

International Confederation of Midwives (ICM)
57 Lower Belgrave Street
London SW1W 0LR

International Council of Nurses
37 rue Vermont
1202 Geneva
Switzerland

International Voluntary Service (IVS)
(UK Branch of Service Civil International)
53 Regent Road
Leicester LE1 6YL

Invalid Children's Aid Association (ICAA)
126 Buckingham Palace Road
London SW1W 9SB

Invalids at Home
23 Farm Avenue
London NW2 2BJ

Joint Board of Clinical Nursing Studies
178–202 Great Portland Street
London W1N 6TB

King Edward's Hospital Fund for London
2 Palace Court
London W2 4HT

King's Fund Centre (KFC)
126 Albert Street
London NW1 7NF

Lady Hoare Trust for Physically Disabled Children (Associated with Arthritis Care)
7 North Street
Midhurst
West Sussex GU29 9DJ

Let Live Association
56a Kyverdale Road
London N16

Leukaemia Research Fund
43 Great Ormond Street
London WC1N 3JJ

Leukaemia Society
28 Eastern Road
London N2

Marie Curie Memorial Foundation
28 Belgrave Square
London SW1X 8QG

Marie Stopes Clinic
Well Woman Centre
108 Whitfield Street
London W1P 6BE

Mastectomy Association of Great Britain
26 Harrison Street
London WC1H 8JG

Maternity Alliance
59–61 Camden High Street
London NW1 7JL

Medical Council on Alcoholism
31 Bedford Square
London WC1

Medical Defence Union Ltd
3 Devonshire Place
London W1

Medic-Alert Foundation
11–13 Alfton Terrace
London N4 3JP

Medical Protection Society Ltd
50 Hallam Street
London W1

Medical Research Council (MRC)
20 Park Crescent
London W1N 4AL

Mental After Care Association
Eagle House
110 Jermyn Street
London SW1Y 6HB

Midwife Teachers Training College
High Coombe
Warren Road
Kingston Hill
Surrey

Midwives Information and Resource Service (MIDIRS)
National Temperance Hospital
12 Hampstead Road
London NW1 2LT

MIND (National Association for Mental Health)
22 Harley Street
London W1N 2ED

Miscarriage Association (MA)
18 Stonybrook Close
West Bretton
Wakefield
West Yorkshire WF4 4TP

Motor Neurone Disease Association
61 Derngate
Northampton NN1 1UE

Multiple Sclerosis Society of Great Britain and Northern Ireland
25 Effie Road
Fulham
London SW6 1EE

Muscular Dystrophy Group of Great Britain and Northern Ireland
Nattrass House
35 Macaulay Road
London SW4 0QP

Narcotics Anonymous
PO Box 246
London SW1

National Advisory Centre on the Battered Child
Denver House
The Drive
Bounds Green Road
London N11

National Ankylosing Spondylitis Society
6 Grosvenor Crescent
London SW1X 7ER

National Association for Colitis and Crohn's Disease (NACC)
98a London Road
St Albans
Herts AL1 7NX

National Association for Deaf–Blind and Rubella Handicapped (SENSE)
311 Grays Inn Road
London WC1X 8PT

National Association for Gifted Children
1 South Audley Street
London W1Y 5DQ

National Association of Laryngectomee Clubs
4th Floor
39 Eccleston Square
London SW1V 1PB

National Association for Maternal and Child Welfare (NAMCW)
1 South Audley Street
London W1Y 6JS

National Association of State Enrolled Nurses
1 Vere Street
London W1

National Association for the Education of the Partially Sighted
Joseph Clark School
Vincent Road
Higham Park
London E4

National Association for the Relief of Paget's Disease
413 Middleton Road
Middleton
Manchester M24 4QZ

National Association for the Welfare of Children in Hospital (NAWCH)
Argyle House
29–31 Euston Road
London NW1 2SD

National Autistic Society
276 Willesden Lane
London NW2 5RB

National Blood Transfusion Service
Moor House
London Wall
London EC2

National Board for Nursing, Midwifery and Health Visiting for Northern Ireland
123/137 York Street
Belfast BT15 1JB

National Board for Nursing, Midwifery and Health Visiting for Scotland
Trinity Park House
South Trinity Road
Edinburgh EH5 3SF

National Campaign Against Solvent Abuse
Box 513
245a Coldharbour Lane
London SW9 8RR

National Childbirth Trust (NCT)
9 Queensborough Terrace
London W2 3TB

National Council for One Parent Families
255 Kentish Town Road
London NW5 2LX

National Council for Special Education (NCSE)
1 Wood Street
Stratford-on-Avon
Warwickshire CV37 6JE

National Deaf Children's Society
45 Hereford Road
London W2 5AH

National Diabetes Foundation
177a Tennison Road
London SE25 5NF

National Eczema Society
Tavistock House North
Tavistock Square
London WC1H 9SR

National Federation of Kidney Patients' Associations
Acorn Lodge
Woodsets
Nr Worksop
Notts S81 8AT

National Fund for Nurses
1 Henrietta Place
Cavendish Square
London W1M 0AB

National Health Service Retirement Fellowship
St Mary Abbots Hospital
Marloes Road
London W8 4LG

National Marriage Guidance Council
Herbert Gray College
Little Church Street
Rugby
Warwickshire CV21 3AP

National Rubella Campaign
105 Gower Street
London WC1E 6AH

National Schizophrenia Fellowship
79 Victoria Road
Surbiton
Surrey KT6 4NS

National Society for Autistic Children
1a Golders Green Road
London NW11

National Society for Cancer Relief (NSCR)
Anchor House
15–19 Britten Street
London SW3 3TY

National Society for Epilepsy
Chalfont Centre for Epilepsy
Chalfont St. Peter
Gerrards Cross
Bucks SL9 0RJ

National Society of Phenylketonuria and Allied Disorders
6 Rawdon Close
Palace Fields
Runcorn
Cheshire

National Society for the Prevention of Cruelty to Children (NSPCC)
67 Saffron Hill
London EC1N 8RS

New Life Foundation Trust
The Red House
Kelham
Newark
Notts NG23 5QP

Northern Ireland Council for Nurses and Midwives
216 Belmont Road
Belfast BT4 2AT

Northern Ireland Council on Alcoholism
36/40 Victoria Street
Belfast

Nuffield Foundation
Nuffield Lodge
Regent's Park
London NW1 4RS

Nuffield Provincial Hospitals Trust
3 Prince Albert's Road
London NW1

Nursing and Hospital Careers Information Centre
121 Edgware Road
London W2 2HX

Nursing Education Research Unit (NERU)
Chelsea College Road
London SW3 6LX

Nursing Practice Research Unit
Northwick Park Hospital
Watford Road
Harrow
Middlesex HA1 3UJ

Office of Population Censuses and Surveys (OPCS)
St. Catherine's House
10 Kingsway
London WC2B 6TP

Open Door Association
447 Pensby Road
Heswall
Wirral
Merseyside

Open University
Milton Keynes
Bucks MK7 6AA

Parkinson's Disease Society
36 Portland Place
London W1N 3DG

Partially Sighted Society
40 Wordsworth Street
Hove
East Sussex BN3 5BH

Phobias Confidential
1 Clovelly Road
Ealing
London W5 5HF

Play Board (formerly Toy Libraries Association)
68 Churchway
London NW1 1LT

Poisons Unit
New Cross Hospital
Avonley Road
London SE14

Pregnancy Advisory Service
13 Charlotte Street
London W1P 1HD

Princess Mary's Royal Air Force Nursing Service (PMRAFNS)
Ministry of Defence
First Avenue House
High Holborn
London WC1V 6HD

Psoriasis Association
7 Milton Street
Northampton NN2 7JG

Psychiatric Rehabilitation Association
21a Kingsland High Street
London E8 2JS

Queen Alexandra's Royal Army Nursing Corps (QARANC)
Ministry of Defence
First Avenue House
High Holborn
London WC1V 6HD

Queen Alexandra's Royal Naval Nursing Service (QARNNS)
Ministry of Defence
First Avenue House
High Holborn
London WC1V 6HD

Queen's Nursing Institute (QNI)
57 Lower Belgrave Street
London SW1W 0LR

Raynaud's Association Trust
40 Bladon Crescent
Alsager
Cheshire ST7 2BG

Release
169 Commercial Street
London E1 6BW

Renal Society
64 South Hill Park
London NW3 2SJ

Re-Solv- The Society for the Prevention of Solvent and Volatile Substance Abuse
St Mary's Chambers
19 Station Road
Stone
Staffs ST15 8JP

Royal Association in Aid of the Deaf and Dumb
27 Old Oak Road
London W3 7SL

Royal British Nurses Association Club
194 Queen's Gate
London SW7 3DL

Royal College of General Practitioners (RCGP)
14 Prince's Gate
Hyde Park
London SW7

Royal College of Midwives (RCM)
15 Mansfield Street
London W1M 0BE

Royal College of Nursing and National Council of Nurses of the United Kingdom (RCN)
20 Cavendish Square
London W1M 0AB

Royal College of Nursing and National Council of Nurses of the UK (RCN) Scotland
44 Heriot Row
Edinburgh EH3 6EY

Royal College of Nursing and National Council of Nurses of the UK (RCN) Welsh Board
Ty Maeth
King George V Drive
East Cardiff CF4 4XZ

Royal College of Obstetricians and Gynaecologists
27 Sussex Place
Regent's Park
London NW1

Royal College of Pathologists
2 Carlton House Terrace
London SW1

Royal College of Physicians
11 St. Andrew's Place
London NW1

Royal College of Physicians of Edinburgh
9 Queen Street
Edinburgh EH2

Royal College of Physicians and Surgeons of Glasgow
242 St. Vincent Street
Glasgow G2

Royal College of Psychiatrists
17 Belgrave Square
London SW1

Royal College of Surgeons
Nicholson Street
Edinburgh EH8

Royal College of Surgeons of England
35 Lincoln's Inn Fields
London WC2

Royal Commonwealth Society for the Blind
Heath Road
Haywards Heath
West Sussex RH16 3AZ

Royal Institute of Public Health and Hygiene
28 Portland Place
London W1N 4DE

Royal National Institute for the Blind (RNIB)
224 Great Portland Street
London W1N 6AA

Royal National Institute for the Deaf (RNID)
105 Gower Street
London WC1E 6AH

Royal National Pension Fund for Nurses
Burdett House
15 Buckingham Street
Strand
London WC2N 6ED

Royal Society of Health
13 Grosvenor Place
London SW1X 7EN

Royal Society of Medicine
1 Wimpole Street
London W1M 8AE

Royal Society for the Prevention of Accidents (RoSPA)
Cannon House
The Priory Queensway
Birmingham B4 6BS

St. Andrew's Scottish Ambulance Association (StAAA)
Milton Street
Glasgow G4

St John Ambulance Association (StJAA)
1 Grosvenor Crescent
London SW1X 7EF

Samaritans Incorporated
17 Uxbridge Road
Slough
Berkshire SL1 1SN

SANITY – Mental Illness and Biochemical and Nutritional Research Society
'Robina'
The Chase
Hurn Lane
Ashley
Nr. Ringwood
Dorset BN24 2AN

Schizophrenia Association of Great Britain (SAGB)
International Schizophrenia Centre
Bryn Hyfryd, The Crescent
Bangor
Gwynedd LL57 2AG

Scoliosis Association (UK)
380–384 Harrow Road
London W9 2HU

Scottish Association for Counselling
14 Caiystane Hill
Edinburgh EH10 6SL

Scottish Association for Mental Health
40 Shandwick Place
Edinburgh EH2 4RT

Scottish Association for the Deaf
158 West Regent Street
Glasgow G2

Scottish Board
22 Queen Street
Edinburgh EH2 1JX

Scottish Council for Health Education
21 Landsdowne Crescent
Edinburgh EH12

Scottish Council for the Care of Spastics
Rhuemore
Corstorphine Road
Edinburgh EH12

Scottish Council for the Unmarried Mother and her Child
44 Albany Street
Edinburgh EH1

Scottish Council on Alcoholism
147 Blythswood Street
Glasgow G2 4EN

Scottish Epilepsy Association
48 Govan Road
Glasgow G51

Scottish Home and Health Department (SHHD)
St. Andrew's House
Edinburgh EH1

Scottish National Federation for the Welfare of the Blind
39 St. Andrew's Street
Dundee

Scottish Society for the Mentally Handicapped
69 West Regent Street
Glasgow G2 2AN

Scottish Spina Bifida Association
190 Queensferry Road
Edinburgh EH4 2DW

Sickle Cell Society (SCS)
Green Lodge
Barretts Green Road
London NW10 7AP

Society for Advancement of Research into Anorexia
Stanthorpe
New Pound
Wisborough Green
West Sussex RH14 0EJ

Society for Registered Male Nurses
38 Marland Avenue
Oldham
Lancs

Society of Apothecaries
Blackfriars Lane
Queen Victoria Street
London EC4

Spastics Society
12 Park Crescent
London W1N 4EQ

Spinal Injuries Association
Yeoman House
76 St James's Lane
London N10

SPOD (Association to Aid the Sexual and Personal Relationships of People with a Disability)
286 Camden Road
London N7 OBJ

Standing Committee on Sexually-Abused Children (SCOSAC)
4th Floor
Crown House
London Road
Morden
Surrey
SM4 5DX

Standing Conference on Drug Abuse
1–4 Hatton Place
Hatton Garden
London EC1N 8ND

Stillbirth and Neonatal Death Society (SANDS)
Argyle House
29–31 Euston Road
London NW1 2SD

Stillbirth and Perinatal Death Association
37 Christchurch Hill
London NW3

Stress Syndrome Foundation
Cedar House
Yalding
Kent ME18 6JD

Student Nurses Association
Royal College of Nursing
1 Henrietta Place
Cavendish Square
London W1M 0AB

Tavistock Institute of Human Relations
Tavistock Centre
Belsize Lane
London NW3 5BA

Tay–Sachs and Allied Diseases Association
17 Sydney Road
Barkingside
Ilford
Essex IG6 2ED

Tenovus-Cancer Research Appeal
11 Whitchurch Road
Cardiff CF4 3JN

Terrence Higgins Trust
BM AIDS
London WC1N 3XX

Tranquilizer Withdrawal Support
160 Tosson Terrace
Heaton
Newcastle NE6 5EA

Tranx Release
106 Welstead Avenue
Aspley
Nottingham

TRANX UK Ltd – National Tranquilliser Advisory Council
17 Peel Road
Harrow
Middlesex HA3 7QX

Tuberous Sclerosis Association of Great Britain
Martell Mount
Holywell Road
Malvern Wells
Worcs WR14 4LF

Twins and Multiple Births Association
54 Broad Lane
Hampton
Middlesex TW12 3BG

United Kingdom Central Council for Nursing, Midwifery and Health Visiting (UKCC)
23 Portland Place
London W1N 3AF

United Nursing Services Club
40 South Street
London W1

Urostomy Association
8 Coniston Close
Dane Bank
Denton
Manchester M34 2EW

VAD Ladies Club
44 Great Cumberland Place
London W1H 8BS

Welsh Board of Health
Cathays Park
Cardiff

Welsh National Board for Nursing, Midwifery and Health Visiting
13th Floor, Pearl Assurance House
Greyfriars Road
Cardiff CF1 3AG

Women's Health Concern (WHC)
Ground Floor
17 Earls Terrace
London W8 6LP

Women's National Cancer Control Campaign
1 South Audley Street
London W1Y 5DQ

Women's Reproductive Rights Information Centre (WRRIC)
52–54 Featherstone Street
London EC1Y 8RT

Women's Royal Voluntary Service (WRVS)
17 Old Park Lane
London W1Y 4AJ

Women's Therapy Centre
6 Manor Gardens
London N7 6LA

World Health Organization
Geneva
Switzerland

Acknowledgements

The publishers would like to thank the following for permission to reproduce material in this dictionary.

W.B. Saunders for figures in abscess, acid–base balance, adenoid, adrenal, Æsculapius, airway, ankle, appendix, atrial, auricle, blood pressure, brain, breast, caduceus, cast, cell, circulation, clotting, coarctation, coronary, deoxyribonucleic acid, digestion, disc, dislocation, diverticulum, elbow, electromyogram, embolus, eye, fluid, goniometer, goniometry, graafian follicle, hair, heart, heat, hepatitis, hip, hormone, hyperbaric, hypothalmus, immunity, immunoglobulin, injection, intussusception, joint, kidney, knee, kyphosis, leukocyte, liver, lordosis, lymphatic, malaria, malocclusion, meiosis, menstrual, mitosis, muscle, need, nervous, nose, osmosis, ovulation, ovum, pancreas, patent, pelvic, peritoneal, pinocytosis, posture, pregnancy, pressure, prostate, pulmonary, pulse, radiation, reflex, regions, reproduction, scoliosis, shoulder, skin, skull, spermatozoon, sphygmogram, spine, spirometer, steroid, talipes, tetralogy, thymus, thyroid, tooth, tourniquet, transposition, Trousseau's sign, ulcer, varicose, ventricular, vertebral, volvulus, wound, wrist.

Tables in antibiotic, blood group, cancer, cranial, electrolyte, fracture, hepatitis, hormone, hypothalmus, parasite, position, secretin, somatostatin.

American College of Surgeons, figure in Lund and Browder chart.
Croom-Helm, figure in burn.
Harper & Row Ltd. Publishers, figures in gait.
Health Education Authority, figure in breast.
Laerdal Medical, figure in intubation.
Mark Allen Publishing, figure in fracture, table in insulin.
McGraw-Hill, Inc, figures in injection, oocyte, spermatogenesis.
Merck & Co Inc. figure in EEG's.
C V Mosby Co., figure in postural.
Oxford University Press, New York, figure in oedema.
Scutari Press, table in disinfectants.
Springer Verlag, table in cancer.
University of Washington, dept. of prosthetics, figure in amputation.
U.S. Government Printing Office, figure in stroke.
Werth Publishers, New York, figure in adenosine.
Year Book Medical Publishers, table in blood gas analysis.

Every effort has been made to contact copyright holders of material reproduced in this dictionary. In the few instances where this has not been possible the publishers invite such copyright holders to contact them.